How to Use MOSBY'S MANUAL OF CLINICAL NURSING to Develop or Individualize a Care Plan

Use PART ONE if

Your patient has a medical diagnosis

↓

Look up the medical diagnosis in the index

↓

Turn to appropriate medical diagnosis in Part One

↓

OPTIONAL

For the specific disease:
- Review definition
- Review pathophysiology
- Review list of diagnostic studies
- Review medical plan

For the related body system:
- Review A & P, normal findings, and normal lab data

↓

1. Prepare assessment checklist
2. Identify patient-specific nursing diagnoses
3. Identify patient-specific nursing interventions
4. Identify relevant patient teaching interventions
5. Identify relevant patient outcomes
6. Identify relevant data indicating that outcomes are reached

Use PART TWO if

Your patient is admitted for tests

↓

Look up the diagnostic test in the index

↓

Turn to appropriate diagnostic test in Part Two

↓

OPTIONAL

Consult index at beginning of Part Two to review other tests related to the body system

↓

1. Review nursing care section for patient-specific interventions

Use PART THREE if

Your patient has a nursing diagnosis

↓

Look up the nursing diagnosis in the index

↓

Turn to appropriate nursing diagnosis in Part Three

↓

OPTIONAL

- Review definition
- Read discussion
- Review defining characteristics
- Review related factors/risk factors

↓

1. Identify patient goals
2. Identify patient-specific nursing interventions
3. Identify relevant patient outcomes
4. Identify relevant data indicating that outcomes are reached

↓

WRITE THE CARE PLAN FOR YOUR PATIENT

Mosby's Manual of

Clinical Nursing

Mosby's Manual of Clinical Nursing

Second Edition

June M. Thompson, RN, MS
Assistant Professor, School of Nursing
University of Texas Health Science Center
Houston, Texas

Gertrude K. McFarland, RN, DNSc, FAAN
Health Scientist Administrator
Nursing Research Study Section, Division of Research Grants
U.S. Department of Health and Human Services
National Institutes of Health, USPHS
Bethesda, Maryland

Jane E. Hirsch, RN, MS
Associate Director of Nursing
University of California—San Francisco
San Francisco, California

Susan M. Tucker, RN, BSN
Director of Nursing
Parent Child Health and Skilled Nursing Facility
Kaiser Permanente Medical Center
East San Fernando Valley
Panorama City, California

Arden C. Bowers, RN, MS
Associate Professor Emeritus
Department of Nursing, College of Santa Fe
Santa Fe, New Mexico

Original illustrations by **George Wassilchenko**

The C.V. Mosby Company
ST. LOUIS • BALTIMORE • PHILADELPHIA • TORONTO 1989

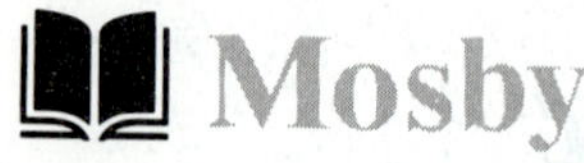

Editor: William Grayson Brottmiller
Senior Developmental Editor: Sally Adkisson
Project Manager: Patricia Tannian
Design: Liz Fett

The authors and publisher have made a conscientious effort to ensure that the drug information and recommended dosages in this book are accurate and in accord with accepted standards at the time of publication. However, pharmacology is a rapidly changing science, so readers are advised to check the package insert provided by the manufacturer before administering any drug.

Second Edition

Printed in the United States of America
The C.V. Mosby Company
11830 Westline Industrial Drive, St. Louis, Missouri 63146

Library of Congress Cataloging-in-Publication Data

Mosby's manual of clinical nursing.

Rev. ed. of: Clinical nursing. 1986.
Includes bibliographies and index.
1. Nursing. I. Thompson, June M., 1946-
II. Clinical nursing. [DNLM: 1. Nursing Care.
RT41.C65 1989 610.73 88-33042
ISBN 0-8016-5157-3

GW/D/D 9 8 7 6 5 4 3 2 1

Contributors

Mary A. Allen, RN, MS*
Clinical Nurse Specialist
National Institutes of Health
Clinical Center, Nursing Department
Bethesda, Maryland

Cynthia Reno Balkstra, RN, C, BSN
Clinical Nurse III
Medicine/Cardiology
The Medical Center at UCSF
San Francisco, California

Anne Elizabeth Belcher, RN, PhD
Associate Professor
Maryland Division, American Cancer Society;
Professor of Oncology Nursing
University of Maryland School of Nursing
Baltimore, Maryland

Arden C. Bowers, RN, MS
Associate Professor Emeritus
Department of Nursing
College of Santa Fe
Santa Fe, New Mexico

Priscilla C. Boykin, RN, MSN*
Clinical Nurse Educator
National Institutes of Health
Warren Grant Magnuson Clinical Center
Department of Nursing
Bethesda, Maryland

Debra C. Broadwell, RN, ET, PhD
Associate Professor
Emory University
Nell Hodgson Woodruff School of Nursing
Atlanta, Georgia

Dorothy Brundage, RN, PhD, FAAN
Associate Professor
Duke University School of Nursing
Durham, North Carolina

Ann W. Burgess, RN, CS, DNSc, FAAN
van Ameringen Professor of Psychiatric Mental Health Nursing
University of Pennsylvania
School of Nursing
Philadelphia, Pennsylvania

Victor G. Campbell, RN, PhD
Assistant Vice President, Nursing
Doctors Hospital West
Columbus, Ohio

Mary M. Canobbio, RN, MN
Cardiovascular Clinical Specialist;
Assistant Clinical Professor
UCLA School of Nursing
Los Angeles, California

MaryAnn Colletti, RN, MS
AIDS Clinical Nurse Specialist
Rush–Presbyterian–St. Luke's Medical Center
Chicago, Illinois

Joyce E. Dains, DrPH, RN
Assistant Professor
University of Texas Health Science Center at Houston
School of Nursing
Houston, Texas

Jacqueline Dienemann, RN, PhD
Assistant Professor;
Coordinator, Nursing Administration
George Mason University
School of Nursing
Fairfax, Virginia

Kathleen A. Dobkin, RN, BSN, CETN
Enterostomal Therapy Nursing Coordinator
Emory Clinic/Egelston Hospital
Atlanta, Georgia

Janice A. Drass, RN, BSN, CDE*
Clinical Nurse
National Institutes of Health
Clinical Center, Nursing Department
Bethesda, Maryland

Richard J. Fehring, BS, DNSc
Associate Professor
Marquette University
College of Nursing
Milwaukee, Wisconsin

Kay Fischer, RN, MN
Clinical Nurse Specialist in Private Practice
Children's Health Care, Inc.
Delafield, Wisconsin

Elizabeth K. Gerety, RN, MS, CS*
Clinical Nurse Specialist, Psychiatry
Psychiatry Consultation Service
Veterans Administration Medical Center
Portland, Oregon

Maggie German, RN, MSN
Department of Medical Nursing
Rush–Presbyterian–St. Luke's Medical Center
Chicago, Illinois

Anne Scott Grasberger, RN, BSN*
Head Nurse
National Institutes of Health
Bethesda, Maryland

Mikel Gray, PhD Candidate, CURN
Clinical Urodynamics
Henrietta Egelston Hospital for Children, Scottish Rite Children's Hospital, Shepherd Spinal Center
Atlanta, Georgia

*The opinions expressed herein are those of the authors and do not necessarily reflect those of the National Institutes of Health, USPHS, U.S. Department of Health and Human Services, or Veterans Administration.

Deanna Grimes, DrPH, RN
Assistant Professor
University of Texas Health Science Center at Houston
School of Nursing
Houston, Texas

Kathleen E. Gunta, RN, MSN, ONC
Clinical Nurse Specialist
Sinai Samaritan Medical Center
Milwaukee, Wisconsin

Janice C. Hallal, RN, DNSc
Assistant Professor
The Catholic University of America
School of Nursing
Washington, D.C.

Carol R. Hartman, RN, CS, DNSc
Professor Psych/Mental Health Nursing
Boston College
Chestnut Hill, Massachusetts

Karen D. Hench, RN, MS*
Associate Investigator, NICHHD
National Institutes of Health
Bethesda, Maryland

Jane E. Hirsch, RN, MS
Associate Director of Nursing
University of California—San Francisco
San Francisco, California

Lois Hoskins, RN, PhD
Dean and Associate Professor
The Catholic University of America
School of Nursing
Washington, D.C.

Jacqueline L. Kartman, RN, MS, CCRN
Cardiopulmonary Critical Care, Clinical Nurse Specialist
Lutheran Hospital—La Crosse
La Crosse, Wisconsin

Candice S. Korb, RN, MS
Formerly Pediatric Home Health Nurse
Jewish Social Service Agency
Rockville, Maryland

Carol Kupperberg, RN, MSN
Nursing Consultant
Home Care Program
Children's Hospital National Medical Center
Washington, D.C.

Rae Langford, RN, MS, EdD
Associate Professor
Prairie View A & M University
Houston, Texas

Estelle Codier Lincoln, RN, MSN, CNA*
National Institutes of Health
Bethesda, Maryland

Sylvia B. Lloyd, RN, MSN
Assistant Professor
Samuel Merritt College of Nursing
Oakland, California

Teresa Choate Loriaux, RN, MSN, CDE*
Clinical Nurse, Warren G. Magnuson Clinical Center
National Institutes of Health
Bethesda, Maryland

James C. McCann, RN, DNSc
Psychiatric Nurse Consultant
Office of Survey and Certification
Health Care Financing Administration
Baltimore, Maryland

Gertrude K. McFarland, RN, DNSc, FAAN*
Health Scientist Administrator
Nursing Research Study Section
Division of Research Grants
U.S. Department of Health and Human Services
National Institutes of Health, USPHS
Bethesda, Maryland

Elizabeth McFarlane, RN, DNSc
Associate Professor and Dean for Academic Affairs
The Catholic University of America
School of Nursing
Washington, D.C.

Audrey M. McLane, RN, PhD
Professor Emerita
College of Nursing
Marquette University
Milwaukee, Wisconsin

Ruth E. McShane, RN, PhD
Robert Wood Johnson Clinical Nurse Scholar
University of Rochester, School of Nursing
Rochester, New York

Victoria L. Mock, RN, DNSc
Assistant Professor
School of Nursing
Boston College
Boston, Massachusetts

Viola Morofka, RN, CS, PhD
Associate Professor of Nursing
Graduate Program
Psychiatric Mental Health Nursing
School of Nursing
Kent State University
Kent, Ohio

Martha M. Morris, RN, EdD
Director of Nursing
St. Louis State Hospital
St. Louis, Missouri

Leona Mourad, RN, MS
Associate Professor, Emeritus
The Ohio State University College of Nursing
Columbus, Ohio

Charlotte Naschinski, RN, MS
Acting Director for Nursing Education
District of Columbia Commission on Mental Health Services
Office of Training and Standards
Washington, D.C.

Barbara K. Redman, RN, PhD, FAAN
Executive Director
American Association of Colleges of Nursing
Washington, D.C.;
Adjunct Professor
University of Maryland
School of Nursing
Baltimore, Maryland

Patrice A. McCurley Robins, RN, BSN, C*
Nursing Systems Coordinator
Clinical Center, NIH
Bethesda, Maryland

M. Gaie Rubenfeld, RN, MS
Assistant Professor
Department of Nursing Education
Eastern Michigan University
Ypsilanti, Michigan

Polly Ryan, RN, MSN
Doctoral Student
University of Wisconsin—Milwaukee
Milwaukee, Wisconsin

Pamela M. Schroeder, RN, MSN
Staff Nurse, Mercy Health Center;
M.Div. Student, Wartburg Theological Seminary
Dubuque, Iowa

Marlene Schwartz, RN, MSN
Nurse Psychotherapist
Private Practice
Milwaukee, Wisconsin

Sylvia Rae Stevens, RN, MS, CS
Assistant Professor of Nursing
Graduate Department of Psychiatric-Mental Health Nursing,
The Catholic University of America
Washington, D.C.;
Private Practice of Psychotherapy
Washington, D.C.

June M. Thompson, RN, MS
Assistant Professor
School of Nursing
University of Texas Health Science Center at Houston
Houston, Texas

Jean O. Trotter, RN, C, MS
Assistant Professor
University of Maryland
School of Nursing
Baltimore, Maryland

Susan M. Tucker, RN, BSN
Director of Nursing
Parent Child Health and Skilled Nursing Facility
Kaiser Permanente Medical Center
East San Fernando Valley
Panorama City, California

Karin von Schilling, RN, MScN
Professor Emeritus
School of Nursing
Faculty of Health Sciences
McMaster University
Hamilton, Ontario, Canada

Evelyn L. Wasli, RN, DNSc
Clinical Specialist/Quality Assurance Coordinator
Emergency Psychiatric Response Division
District of Columbia Government
Washington, D.C.

Mary Wells, RN*
Clinical Nurse
National Institutes of Health
Warren Grant Magnuson Clinical Center
Department of Nursing
Bethesda, Maryland

Susan Fickertt Wilson, RN, PhD
Associate Professor
Texas Christian University
Harris College of Nursing
Ft. Worth, Texas

Janice M. Zeller, RN, PhD
Department of Medical Nursing
Rush–Presbyterian–St. Luke's Medical Center
Chicago, Illinois

Consultants

Susan Barbour, RN, MS
Clinical Nurse Specialist
General Surgery/Enterostomal Therapy
The Medical Center at UCSF
San Francisco, California

Sally Pomeranz Duchin, RN, PhD
Assistant Professor
Critical Care Nursing
Graduate Program
University of Texas Health Science Center at Houston
Houston, Texas

Eleanor C. Louie, RN, MS
Head Nurse
Gynecology, Urology, and Otolaryngology
The Medical Center at UCSF
San Francisco, California

Christine L. Mudge-Grout, RN, MS
Clinical Nurse Specialist
Nephrology/Transplant
The Medical Center at UCSF;
Assistant Clinical Professor
UCSF School of Nursing
San Francisco, California

Catherine H. Rickard, RN, MN
Clinical Nurse Specialist
Orthopaedics and Microvascular Surgery
The Medical Center at UCSF
San Francisco, California

Carol S. Viele, RN, MS
Clinical Nurse Specialist
Oncology, Hematology, Bone Marrow Transplant
The Medical Center at UCSF
San Francisco, California

Preface
to the second edition

We are extraordinarily grateful to the tens of thousands of nurses who made the first edition of this book so successful. Authors could scarcely hope for higher praise. Yet it is you, the user of this book, who deserves to be congratulated. As we noted in the preface to the first edition, you invented this book. It has succeeded only to the extent that it reflects the way you learn, create, and practice nursing.

Nurses and students familiar with the first edition of *Clinical Nursing* will notice that the title of the book has been expanded to *Mosby's Manual of Clinical Nursing*. We have done this because a book of this scope would not be possible without the resources of the world's largest publisher of texts and reference books for nurses. As authors, we take sole responsibility for the accuracy of the content. The publisher's contributions, however, are enormous. They developed the format, maintained the consistency, ensured the book's inclusiveness, and most of all, insisted that the book be made responsive to the needs of the profession. Manuals of nursing practice bearing the names of their publishers are not without precedent. None, however, has benefited from such a massive influx of resources and commitment to contemporary practice as this one.

As a comprehensive reference on nursing care, this book provides broad, practical, and detailed information on human responses to health states. Whether well or ill; whether at home, in a hospital, or in an intermediate care setting; whether under a physician's care, undergoing tests, or independently seeking the services of a professional nurse, consumers of nursing care are depicted in these pages not as types or groups, but as individuals with unique needs. The information in the manual includes virtually everything nurses need to provide personalized care for every single person who seeks or needs their services. In revising this book, we have again tried to mirror the advancing state of the art in the practice of nursing.

For ease of access, Part One continues to be organized by medical diagnoses, system by system, covering virtually every disease, disorder, or condition nurses are likely to encounter in their practice. Beyond the convenience of this organizational scheme, however, the emphasis lies squarely on nursing care, presented according to the nursing process. Nursing diagnoses, including those accepted in 1988 at the Eighth NANDA Conference, are integrated into each disease. Thousands of nursing interventions have been provided with rationales, printed in italics, because the practice of nursing advances when students and practitioners understand *why* they do *what* they do. Patient teaching guidelines, in colored boxes for emphasis in every discussion of nursing care, highlight the importance of the nurse's role as a teacher. The nursing care associated with every disease has been carefully evaluated and updated by nurse specialists, researchers, and educators. Even the nursing care associated with major medical interventions reflects current practice.

Added to all this is an in-depth review of anatomy and physiology for each system and a summary of the medical plan for each disease. In response to users' requests, the pathophysiology of every disease has been thoroughly evaluated, updated, and in many cases expanded, including the latest research on such pressing disorders as AIDS, Alzheimer's disease, and hemophilia, to name a few. Much of this information was previously available to nurses only in reference works and journal articles written by and for physicians. Here it is presented from a nursing point of view to facilitate the decision making expected of professional nurses.

Part Two, on diagnostic tests, is new to this edition. For the patient undergoing tests, whose health problems are as yet undefined, the nurse is provided with care-related information, test by test.

Part Three includes nursing care information for every nursing diagnosis currently accepted by NANDA. This part not only explains the nursing diagnoses themselves but also facilitates the care of patients who may or may not have a medical diagnosis, or may or may not even be ill.

The result is an authoritative source for developing detailed, informed, and highly individualized care plans.

Perhaps the hallmark of this edition is the accessibility of the information provided. Even though the content is comprehensive, it is simple to retrieve. A new design, making use of tabbed pages, prominent headings, and an extremely functional use of color, guides the user directly to whatever information is being sought. The organization has been made as obvious as possible, without complex numbering, coding, or cross-referencing schemes. Every effort was made to develop an index that won't fail, and specialized indexes have been added to the front matter to speed access, even though they duplicate citations included in the general index in the back of the book. We believe that users will be able to locate the precise information being sought in 15 or 20 seconds, every time.

Mosby's Manual of Clinical Nursing is the product of extensive formal market research, hundreds of comments from users and reviewers, numerous focus groups, and many personal conversations with nurses initiated by the authors and the publisher. It is written for students as well as practitioners. It reviews concepts, answers questions, and expands the scope of nursing knowledge. It is, we believe, the most efficient tool for creating high-caliber, individualized care plans ever developed. It attempts to be the definitive manual of clinical nursing, written by nurses for nurses, who developed the practice it reflects. We are honored that the first edition was named in an *American Journal of Nursing* poll as "Nursing's most indispensable reference." As one reviewer of the second edition put it, this is the manual for the 1990s and beyond.

But you can use it right now.

June M. Thompson
Gertrude K. McFarland
Jane E. Hirsch
Susan M. Tucker
Arden C. Bowers

Preface

to the first edition

We have developed what we believe to be the definitive reference source for the clinical nursing practice. No longer will you need to rely on the six or seven reference texts that you currently use. It's all here at last, a single text. A text that stands alone.

The Publisher

We didn't invent this text, you did. This text has evolved as a result of the demand by professional nurses from across the United States and Canada and in many parts of the world. Nurses said there was a need to clarify nursing practice—to "put it all together" in one book. They said, "Put together the nursing theories, nursing process including nursing diagnoses, and physiology and pathophysiology. Use those theory bases and an interdisciplinary health care approach to develop a contemporary and comprehensive text that reflects the potential scope and responsibilities of professional nursing practice."

So, here it is. We have written what we believe to be a succinct reference and text that is broad in scope and intensive in content. This text will permit nurses to easily relate nursing diagnosis to medical diagnosis and medical treatment to nursing process. *Clinical Nursing* is more than just "clinical nursing." It provides a strong foundation in nursing science, integrating the nursing process with nursing diagnoses throughout the text while at the same time providing thorough coverage in anatomy, physiology, pathophysiology, and the social sciences. The intent is to provide a single practical text that is also high level, theory based, interdisciplinary, contemporary, and comprehensive.

The framework for the text is *Nursing: A Social Policy Statement,* which was published by the American Nurses' Association Congress for Nursing Practice in 1980. This document defines nursing as "the diagnosis and treatment of human responses to actual or potential health problems."* According to definition, practice is built upon phenomena (observable manifestations), theory application, nursing actions, and evaluation of effects of action in relation to the phenomena. Therefore these are the underlying principles of the text.

*American Nurses' Association: Nursing: a social policy statement, Kansas City, 1980, p. 9.

Clinical Nursing is designed for convenient use by both students and practitioners. Theoretical content provides the solid background required for the implementation of sound clinical practice, and the ready-reference format permits easy access to the detailed information needed to assess and provide care for individuals with actual or potential health care problems. The systematic design, layout, and two-color format make it easy to find information or extract specific data. Whether the reader wants to develop a nursing care plan, look up the details of a particular chemotherapeutic agent, read about the pathophysiology of a disease, or review the theory base and clinical application of a specific nursing diagnosis, the information is readily accessible and richly detailed.

Many steps were taken throughout the development of this text to ensure its quality. Authors and contributors were selected because of their clinical, educational, and research expertise. Thus they represent both theory and practice. Each chapter was carefully reviewed by clinical and educational experts in nursing, medicine, physiology, pharmacology, and related fields. We also consulted many others in nursing regarding the content and design of the text. Ideas and prototypes were circulated among practicing nurses, students, and nursing educators to verify that this was the book they wanted. Laboratory and chemotherapeutic data were standardized where appropriate.*

This text is based on the complex foundation of nursing theory and nursing science. We believe that it is unique, in-depth, comprehensive, precise, contemporary, and interdisciplinary.

June M. Thompson
Gertrude K. McFarland
Jane E. Hirsch
Susan M. Tucker
Arden C. Bowers

*Laboratory values were taken from Jacobs, D., et al.: Laboratory test handbook, St. Louis, 1984, The C.V. Mosby Co. Chemotherapeutic data were taken from U.S. and Canadian sources: McEvoy, T.K., editor: American hospital formulary system: drug information 1985, Bethesda, Md., 1985, American Society of Hospital Pharmacists; and Canadian Pharmaceutical Association: Compendium of pharmaceuticals and specialties, ed. 20, Ottawa, Canada, 1985.

Contents

Detailed Contents

PART ONE Clinical Nursing Practice

CHAPTER 3 Neurologic System, 239

CHAPTER 4 Musculoskeletal System, 375

CHAPTER 5 Integumentary System, 476

PART TWO Diagnostic Procedures

PART THREE Nursing Diagnoses

Overview of Text

Mosby's Manual of Clinical Nursing was designed to blend the traditional body system–disease approach with contemporary theory-based nursing practice. The text is divided into three major parts. Part One, "Clinical Nursing Practice," is organized by body system and consists of 17 chapters. Part Two, "Diagnostic Procedures," includes common and not-so-common diagnostic studies. Part Three, "Nursing Diagnoses," includes 11 functional patterns subsuming all of the currently accepted nursing diagnoses.

Part One: Clinical Nursing Practice

Part One is organized by body system for easy reference. The description of each body system is divided into three sections:

Overview. The overview presents the system in terms of its importance and functioning. Presented in detail are:

- Normal anatomy and physiology of the system
- Normal clinical assessment findings for the system
- Normal laboratory values

Conditions, diseases, and disorders. Health problems related to the specific body system are presented using a systematic format:

- Definition of the condition, disease, or disorder
- Pathophysiology of the problem
- Diagnostic studies with anticipated findings
- Medical plan, including general management, medications, and surgery
- Assessment criteria
- Nursing diagnoses
- Nursing interventions and selected rationales
- Patient education
- Evaluation based on patient outcome criteria

Medical interventions and related nursing care. Major therapeutic interventions are presented and discussed thoroughly:

- Overview of intervention including description and rationale
- Contraindications and cautions
- Preprocedural nursing care
- Medical plan
- Assessment criteria
- Nursing diagnoses
- Nursing interventions and selected rationales
- Patient education
- Evaluation

Part Two: Diagnostic Procedures

Part Two presents more than 156 diagnostic tests within 15 categories for easy reference. The description, contraindications, complications, and nursing care are presented for each diagnostic test.

Part Three: Nursing Diagnoses

Part Three is organized into the 11 functional health patterns. It contains all of the nursing diagnoses accepted by the North American Nursing Diagnoses Association (NANDA). Each diagnosis includes the following information:

- Definition and brief description of the nursing diagnosis
- Related/risk factors and defining characteristics, including those accepted by NANDA and other research-based factors and characteristics determined by the authors
- Patient goals
- Nursing interventions
- Principles and rationale for nursing interventions
- Evaluation based on patient outcome criteria

In addition to the three major parts of the text, an appendix provides supplemental content on conversion factors to International System of Units (SI units). In May 1977, the Thirtieth World Health Assembly recommended that SI units be used in medicine. Although health care agencies in the United States continue to use the metric system, many health care systems throughout the world have adopted SI units.

Parts One, Two, and Three can be used independently or interdependently. The nurse can look up a particular disease in Part One and find virtually all the information needed to provide optimal care for the patient. The nurse can consult Part Two for additional information related to tests the patient may be undergoing. Part Two will be especially helpful in planning care for patients whose disease has not yet been diagnosed by a physician. The nurse can consult Part Three for a specific nursing diagnosis and can use the related or risk factors, defining characteristics, nursing interventions, and evaluation sections presented to implement a plan of care. Part Three will be an especially good resource in planning nursing care for people when a medical diagnosis is inappropriate, such as for well patients.

Although the nurse is concerned with medical diagnoses and nursing diagnoses as separate entities, the two should be integrated to deliver high-quality nursing care. Parts One and Three of this book facilitate this integration. The nurse can look up a particular disorder in Part One. Within that discussion, in the section "Nursing Dx & Intervention," are the details the nurse needs to provide nursing care for a patient with the disorder. In addition, many times cross-references are provided to specific nursing diagnoses discussed in Part Three. The expanded discussion in Parts Two and Three will help the nurse consider additional strategies of care.

The interrelationship of the three parts of the text provides the nurse with complete information that can be used to develop an effective plan of care for patients. This book offers all the information the nurse needs to determine, implement, and evaluate an individualized plan of nursing care.

INDEX TO

Conditions, Diseases, and Disorders

I

J

K

L

M

INDEX TO

Medical Interventions

INDEX TO

Diagnostic Procedures

INDEX TO

Nursing Diagnoses

Mosby's Manual of

Clinical Nursing

PART ONE

Clinical Nursing Practice

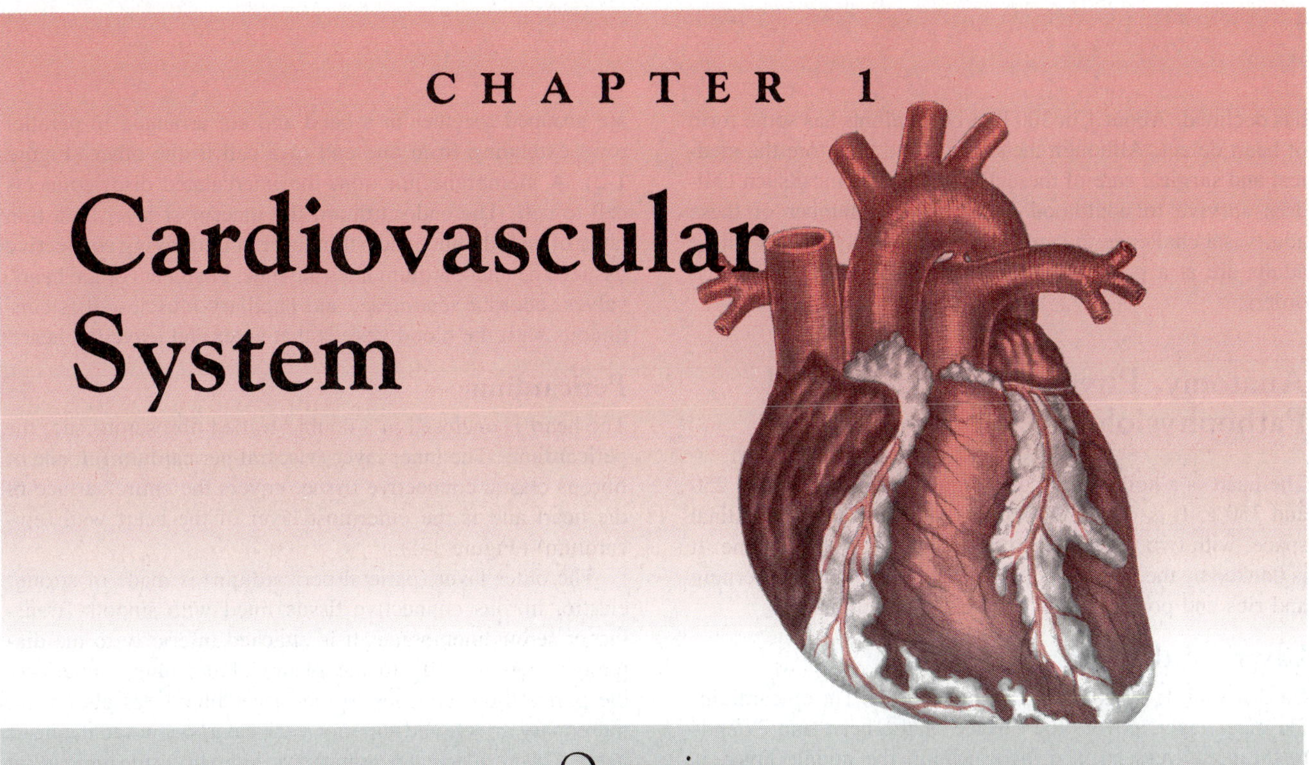

CHAPTER 1

Cardiovascular System

Overview

Despite recent advances in both medicine and surgery, cardiovascular disorders continue to be a principal cause of morbidity and mortality in the United States. In the day-to-day care of patients, nurses deal with cardiovascular disorders in terms of their physical signs and symptoms and appropriate therapeutic interventions. But they must also consider the socioeconomic and emotional impact of these disorders on the patient and family.

During the past 30 years, progress has been made in prevention, diagnosis, treatment, and rehabilitation. Yet, despite a demonstrated decrease in cardiac mortality, more people die from cardiovascular disease than from all other causes of death combined. Over 40 million Americans have some form of cardiovascular disease. This costs about 72 billion dollars per year.[4] Additional costs incurred through job-related losses are difficult to determine.

Cardiac diseases can be divided into those that are acquired during life and congenital defects.

Major acquired cardiovascular disorders, which cause approximately 1 million deaths per year, include hypertension (high blood pressure), myocardial infarction (heart attacks), congestive heart failure, cerebrovascular accident (stroke), and rheumatic heart disease.

High blood pressure, known as the silent killer, is a major factor contributing to heart attacks and strokes. Studies have estimated that one in four adults has high blood pressure.[74] Among black Americans the prevalence is 30% or greater. Research is now focusing on early detection because studies have identified high blood pressure in children as young as 4 years of age.[4]

Heart attacks are the number one cause of death in the United States.[4] About 4 million Americans are treated for heart attacks or angina pectoris each year. Major research has been undertaken to identify factors, such as occupation, sex, age, dietary habits, serum lipoprotein levels, and activity levels, that may be linked to many underlying diseases that contribute to death by heart attack.[49] In recent years health professionals and community organizations have made major efforts to inform the public about risk factors and early warning signals of heart attacks and strokes. Because fewer than half of cardiac deaths occur in hospitals, organizations such as the American Heart Association and the American Red Cross have initiated programs to teach the public the basic techniques of cardiopulmonary resuscitation.

Congestive heart failure is a consequence of a myocardial dysfunction. Although often controllable with drugs, it remains the major form of chronic cardiac disability. It is also one of the most expensive in terms of medical and nursing services, repeated hospital and nursing home services, drug costs, and job disability.

A stroke is most commonly the result of high blood pressure. About 2 million Americans have had strokes even though they can usually be prevented.[4]

Rheumatic heart disease occurs in both children and adults. It is the result of rheumatic fever, a preventable disease. Although the incidence of rheumatic fever has declined, it is still a problem in urban populations where preventive measures are inadequate. About 0.7% of deaths in the United States are associated with rheumatic heart disease.[4]

Congenital cardiovascular malformations are the major cause of death of children 5 years and younger. Since the advent of heart surgery, death from congenital heart disease has declined. About 1 in 300 live-born infants has some form of heart defect. Although the severity and therefore the medical and surgical care of these disorders vary, most such children survive to adulthood. The growing number of these adults is a challenge to caregivers, particularly because these adults are at a greater risk of acquiring cardiovascular disorders.

Anatomy, Physiology, and Related Pathophysiology

The heart is a hollow muscular organ weighing between 250 and 350 g. It is within the thoracic cavity in the mediastinal space, with two thirds extending to the left of the midline. It is flanked by the lungs and protected anteriorly by the sternum and ribs and posteriorly by the vertebral column.

Layers of the Heart

Cardiac muscle has three layers (Figure 1-1). The epicardium, the outer layer, covers the surface of the heart and extends to the great vessels. The myocardium, the middle layer, is responsible for the major pumping action of the ventricles. Cardiac muscle cells are made of striated muscle fibrils consisting of contractile elements known as myofibrils. The fibrils are grouped together in a band and are arranged in parallel rows extending from one end of a cell to the other (Figure 1-2). A membrane junction, the intercalated disc, connects cell to cell. The endocardium, the innermost layer, is a thin layer of endothelium and a thin layer of underlying connective tissue. The endocardium lines the inner chambers of the heart, valves, chordae tendineae, and papillary muscles. It is continuous with the blood vessels that enter and leave the heart.

Pericardium

The heart is enclosed in a double-walled fibroserous sac, the pericardium. The inner layer (visceral pericardium), made of fibrous elastic connective tissue, covers the entire surface of the heart and is the outermost layer of the heart wall (epicardium) (Figure 1-1).

The outer layer (parietal pericardium) is made of strong, elastic, fibrous connective tissue lined with smooth, translucent serous membrane. It is attached inferiorly to the diaphragm and laterally to the pleura of the lung. Superiorly the pericardium attaches to the larger blood vessels (aorta, pulmonary artery, and superior vena cava) but not to the heart itself. This results in a potential space known as the pericardial cavity.

The space between the visceral and parietal layers contains

Figure 1-1 Cross section of cardiac muscle showing its three layers (endocardium, myocardium, and epicardium) and pericardium.

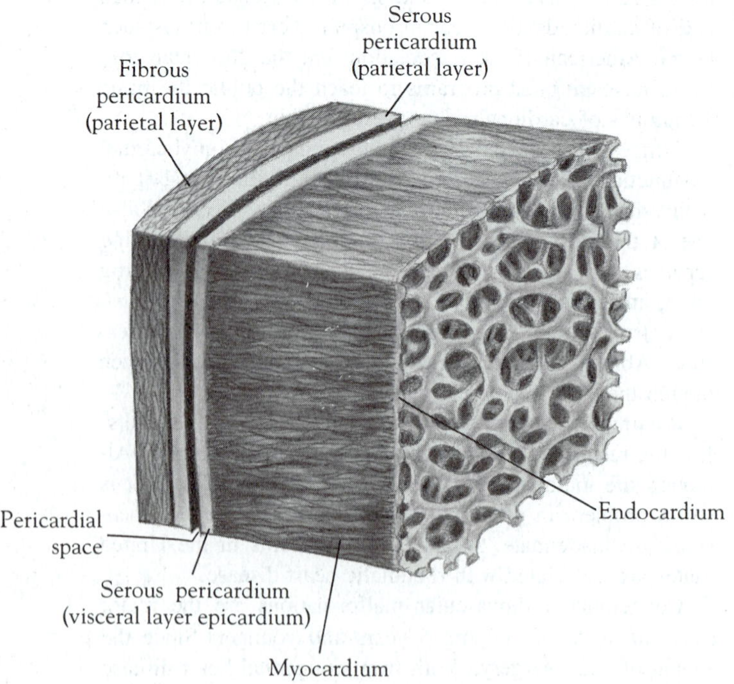

Figure 1-2 Histologic representation of myocardial tissue showing arrangement of myofibrils in relaxed state.

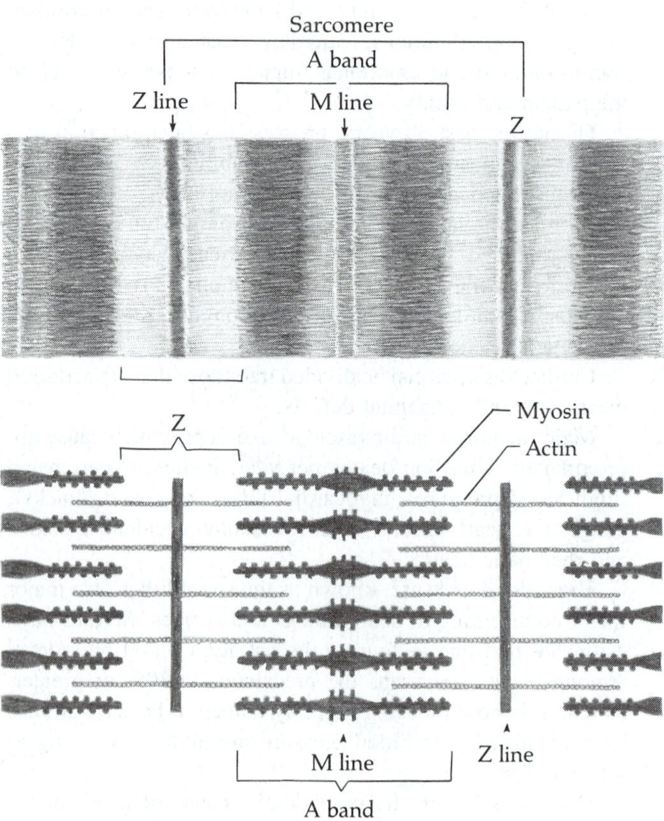

10 to 30 ml of clear, lymphlike fluid that helps the smooth, easy motion of the heart during contraction and expansion. The pericardial cavity can hold 300 ml of fluid without interference in cardiac function. It can hold up to 1 L in some chronic disease states. The degree to which pericardial fluid compromises cardiac function depends more on the rate of rise in intrapericardial volume than on the amount. During rapid filling, as little as 100 ml may cause acute tamponade,[11] but patients who have slowly developing pericardial effusions can hold up to 1 L of fluid without hampering heart function. The rate of filling is also more important than the amount in the relationship between intrapericardial fluid volume and intrapericardial pressure. Normal pressure is −2 to −5 mm Hg. A sudden increase in pressure may occur with rapid filling of fluid in the pericardial space, regardless of the amount of fluid.

The pericardium shields against infection and trauma and aids cardiac function by helping with the free pumping motion of the heart.

Chambers of the Heart

The heart is a four-chambered organ but functions as a two-sided pump (Figure 1-3). The right side is a low-pressure system pumping venous or deoxygenated blood to the lung. The left side is a higher-pressure system pumping arterial or oxygenated blood to the systemic circulation.

Right atrium. The right atrium (RA) is a thin-walled muscle that is a receiving chamber. It receives systemic venous blood from the superior vena cava (SVC), which drains the upper part of the body, and from the inferior vena cava (IVC), which drains blood from the lower extremities.

Figure 1-3 Frontal schematic view of heart.

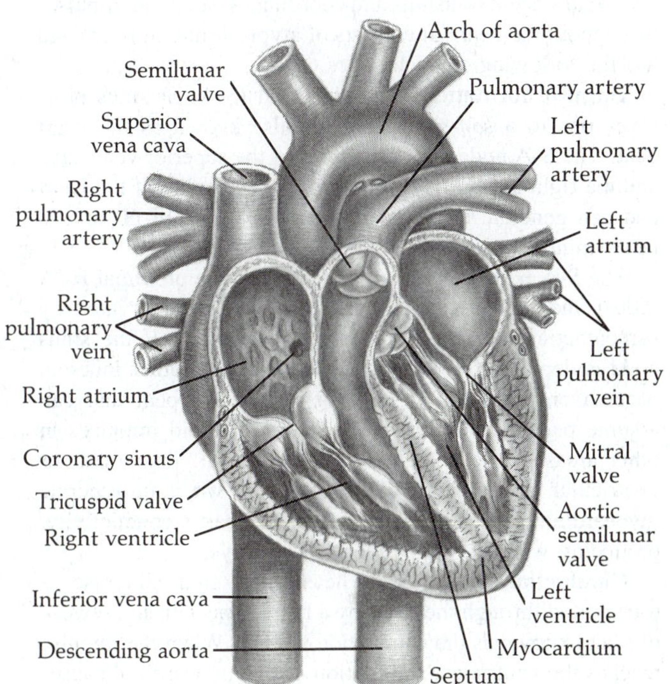

The coronary sinus, which drains venous blood from myocardial circulation, also empties into the RA just above the tricuspid valve. The pressure exerted during normal filling of the RA is 0 to 7 mm Hg and varies with respiration. During inspiration, RA pressure drops below the pressure in veins outside the chest cavity. Because blood flows from an area of high pressure to an area of lower pressure, blood flow to the RA occurs mainly during inspiration.

Oxygen saturation varies depending on the place of entry (IVC, 80%; SVC, 70%; coronary sinus, 30%), but the combined oxygen saturation of RA mixed venous blood is about 75% or 40 mm Hg.

Right ventricle. The right ventricle (RV) is normally the most anterior chamber of the heart, lying directly beneath the sternum. The RV functions as both an inflow and an outflow tract. The inflow tract includes the tricuspid area and the crisscross muscular bands (trabeculations) that make up the inner surface of the ventricle. The outflow tract is commonly referred to as the infundibulum.

During diastole blood enters the RV through the tricuspid valve and is ejected into the pulmonary circulation through the pulmonic valve. Because of low pulmonary resistance, systolic or ejection pressures of the RV are also low. RV pressures are 20 to 25/0 to 5 mm Hg. RV oxygen saturation is similar to that in the RA.

Left atrium. The left atrium (LA), the most posterior cardiac structure, receives oxygenated blood from the lungs via the right and left pulmonary veins. The wall of the LA is slightly thicker than that of the RA and exerts a filling pressure of 5 to 10 mm Hg with little breathing variation. The arterial oxygen saturation is 98% (95 mm Hg).

Left ventricle. The left ventricle (LV) lies posterior to and to the left of the RV. It is ellipsoid, with a wall made of thick muscular tissue measuring 8 to 16 mm, two to three times thicker than that of the RV. This increased muscle mass is necessary to generate enough pressure to move blood into the circulation. LV pressure is normally 100 to 120/0 to 10 mm Hg with oxygen saturation of 95%. The inflow tract is funnel shaped, formed by the mitral anulus, the two mitral leaflets, and the chordae tendineae. The outflow tract is surrounded by the anterior mitral leaflet, the interventricular septum, and the left ventricular free wall. During systole, blood is propelled above and to the right across the aortic valve.

Cardiac Valves

The heart's efficiency as a pump depends on the integrity of the cardiac valves (Figure 1-4). Their sole purpose is to ensure one-way forward blood flow.

Atrioventricular valves. The two atrioventricular (A-V) valves are similar in function but differ in several anatomic details. They are positioned along the atrioventricular groove, which separates the atria from the ventricles.

The tricuspid (right side) and mitral (left side) apparatus is composed of the anulus fibrosus, the valvular tissue (leaf-

Figure 1-4 Anatomic position of cardiac valves.

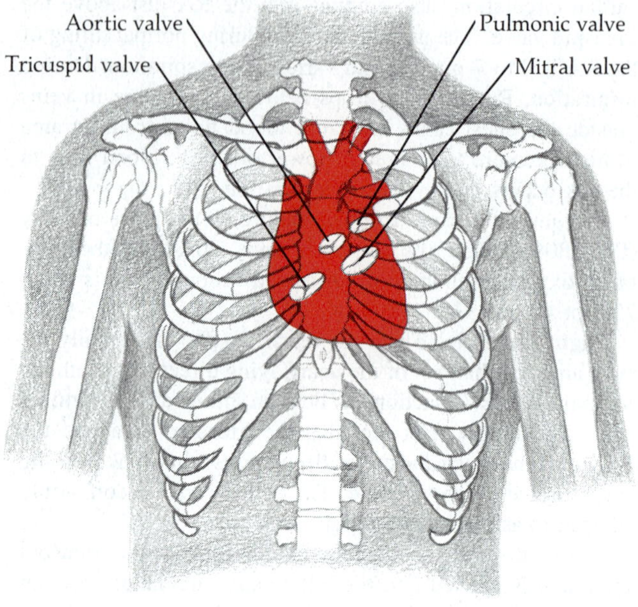

lets) to which the chordae tendineae are attached, and the papillary muscles connecting the chordae to the floor of the ventricular wall. This arrangement allows the leaflets to balloon upward during ventricular systole, but it prevents eversion of the cusps into the atria. These components are considered as a single unit, since disruption of any one element can result in serious hemodynamic dysfunction.

The tricuspid valve is larger and thinner than the mitral and has three separate leaflets: anterior, posterior, and septal. Competence of the anterior and posterior leaflets depends on RV lateral wall function. The septal leaflet attaches to portions of the interventricular septum and sits in close proximity to the A-V node.

The mitral valve is composed of two cusps: anterior and posterior. The anterior leaflet has a wide range of motion. It descends deep into the LV during diastole and rises quickly in systole to meet the posterior leaflet. The posterior leaflet is smaller and more restricted in its motion. The orifice is normally 4 to 6 cm^2 in adults.

Semilunar valves. The two semilunar valves are the aortic and pulmonic. They are smaller than the A-V valves and are similar to each other except that the aortic cusps tend to be thicker. The semilunar valves sit above the outflow tracts of their respective ventricles. Each is composed of a fibrous supporting ring called the anulus and three fibrous valve leaflet cusps. The normal valve orifice is 2.6 to 3.5 cm^2.

Coronary Circulation

The right and left coronary arteries, which arise from the aorta just above and behind the aortic valve, supply blood to the myocardium.

Right coronary artery. The right coronary artery (RCA) arises from the right aortic sinus of Valsalva and branches out along the atrioventricular groove to supply the anterior portion of the right ventricle. In 90% of persons the RCA curves posteriorly within the interventricular groove and supplies the posterior septum, the posterior left papillary muscle, and the sinus and A-V nodes.

Left coronary artery. The left coronary artery (LCA) arises from the left aortic sinus of Valsalva. It begins as a common artery referred to as the left main and then divides into the left anterior descending (LAD) artery and the circumflex artery. The LAD descends along the anterior intraventricular groove to nourish a large portion of the anterior left ventricular wall, including the anterior septum, the anterior papillary muscle, and the apical portion of the myocardium.

The circumflex artery extends from the left main coronary artery along a groove between the LA and LV. In some persons the circumflex artery supplies the inferior and posterior portions of the LV. This is known as left coronary dominance.

Cardiac veins. Three main divisions of cardiac veins comprise the venous circulation and closely parallel the coronary arteries. These include the thebesian veins, most of which empty into the atria; the anterior cardiac veins, which empty into the RA; and the coronary sinus, a short vein lying on the posterior side of the heart. Most venous circulation drains into the coronary sinus, which receives blood from the deeper myocardium and empties into the RA at the coronary sinus ostium between the tricuspid valve and the opening of the interior vena cava.

Conduction

A special system transmits and coordinates electrical impulses throughout the heart. It consists of atypical muscle fibers and has the following characteristics.

Impulse formation. The sinoatrial (S-A) or sinus node gives rise to a self-generating impulse known as the heart beat. The S-A node is at the border of the superior vena cava and the right atrium. It is the primary pacemaker of the heart and can generate electrical impulses at a rate of 60 to 100 beats/minute (Figure 1-5, *A*).

The S-A node is supplied primarily by the proximal RCA (60%) and the left circumflex artery and is innervated by sympathetic and parasympathetic nerve fibers. If the sinus node is depressed, escape ectopic beats from other inherent pacemakers in the A-V node or ventricle appear and can assume pacemaker function. In addition, rapid impulses in other areas of the heart may produce atrial, junctional, or ventricular tachycardias. These can occur when an ischemic myocardium causes an alteration in the heart's conductivity, producing what are called reentry pathways.

Conduction pathways. The normal sinus impulse is transmitted through the heart by a highly specialized network of fibers known as the conduction system. When the impulse reaches the ventricles, stimulation of the myocardium causes

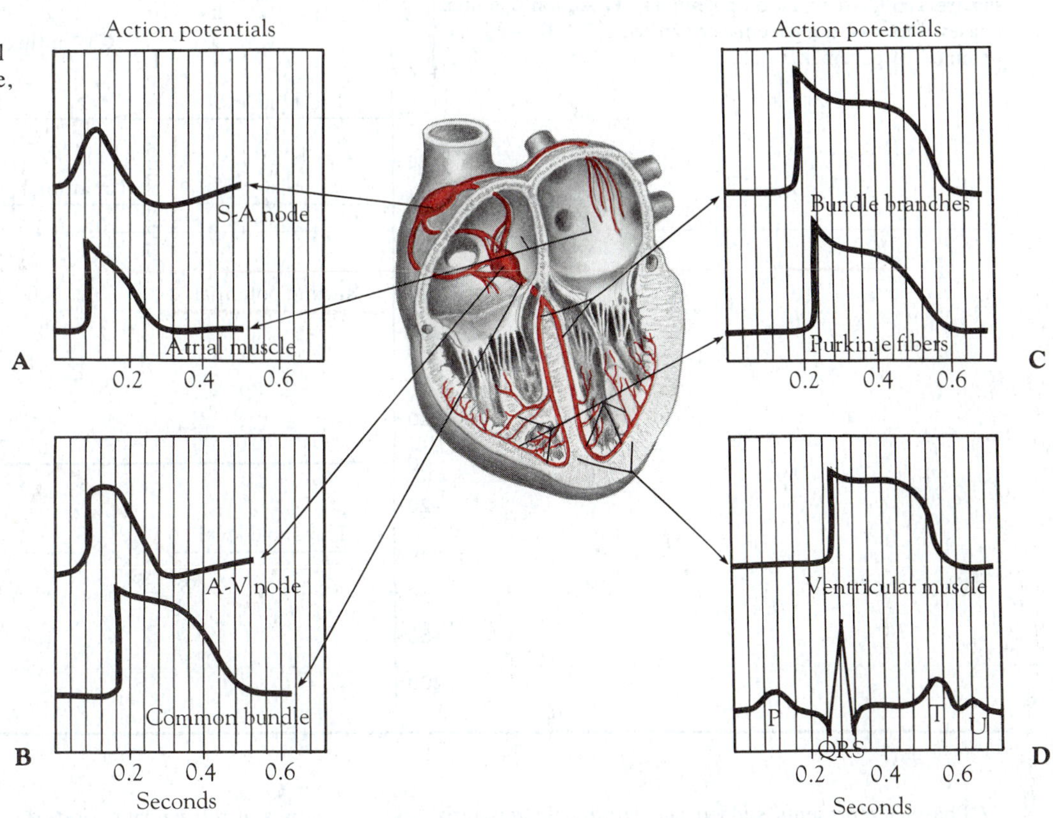

Figure 1-5 Heart with normal conduction pathways and transmembrane action potential of, **A,** S-A node, **B,** A-V node, **C,** bundle branches, and **D,** ventricular muscle.

depolarization of the cells, and contraction occurs.

The conduction system is made up of the A-V node, bundle of His, and right and left bundle branches. The A-V node filters atrial impulses as they pass through to the ventricles. It can initiate its own impulse, but usually at lower rates (40 to 60 beats/minute). It is generally supplied by the RCA and is also innervated by the autonomic nervous system (Figure 1-5, *B*).

The bundle of His provides infranodal conduction traversing the two sides of the intraventricular system, where it divides into the right and left bundle branches. The bundle branches end in a fine network of conductive tissue called the Purkinje fibers. These fibers extend to the papillary muscles and lateral walls of the ventricles. The His bundle and its branches are supplied by the proximal branches of the LAD coronary artery (Figure 1-5, *C*).

Electrophysiology. Transmission of the electrical impulse or action potential of the myocardium is preceded by a series of sequential ionic changes across the cardiac cell membrane, which results in depolarization and subsequent contraction of the myocardium. These events correspond in time to the mechanical events described on p. 8. After depolarization the cells return for recovery to a resting state called repolarization, diastole, or relaxation.

A resting (polarized) cell has a net charge of −90 mV. Potassium is the predominant intracellular cation, and sodium the predominant extracellular cation. The difference in concentrations of these ions results in a resting state of electrical potential commonly referred to as the resting membrane potential (RMP).

On initiation of an electrical stimulus, sodium ions move across the cell membrane, converting the net electrical force within the cell to a positive charge. The cell is then depolarized, resulting in shortening of the cell.

The electrical potential created by this ionic movement progresses through adjacent regions of the cell membrane and is referred to as the action potential. Figure 1-6 illustrates the five phases of the cardiac action potential and its relationship to the electrocardiogram.

Phase 0 represents the depolarization of the cell with the rapid influx of sodium causing a reversal of ionic changes (the inner surface of the cell becomes positive). This is depicted by the upstroke of the action potential curve (Figure 1-6, *A*).

Phase 1 is the brief rapid change toward the repolarization process, during which the membrane potential returns to 0 mV.

Phase 2 is a plateau or stabilization period caused by the slow influx of sodium and the slow exit of potassium. During this period, calcium ions enter the cell through slow calcium channels, triggering the release of large quantities of calcium. Calcium functions in the process of cellular contraction.

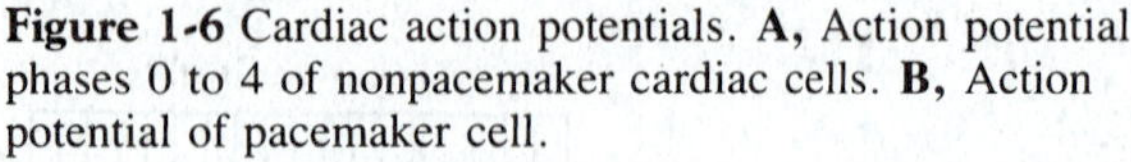

Figure 1-6 Cardiac action potentials. **A,** Action potential phases 0 to 4 of nonpacemaker cardiac cells. **B,** Action potential of pacemaker cell.

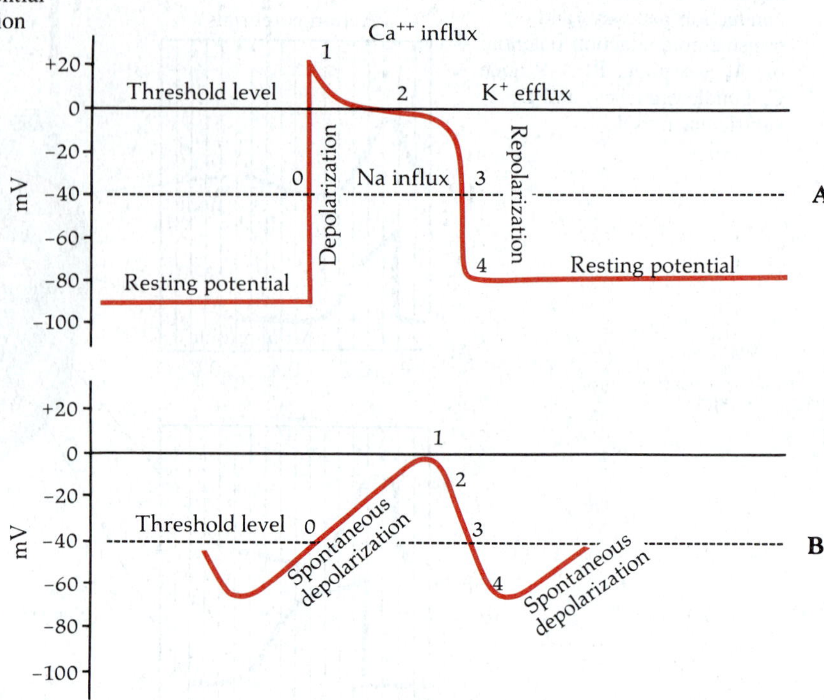

Phase 3 represents sudden acceleration in repolarization as potassium leaves rapidly, causing the inside of the cell to move toward a more negative state.

Phase 4 represents the return to the resting phase during which the intracellular charge is once again electronegative, leading to the initiation of the action potential (phase 0). Any excess sodium is eliminated from the cell in exchange for potassium that left the cell during phases 2 and 3.

Throughout these phases the cardiac cell goes through a series of refractory periods during which the cell is incapable of accepting another stimulus and responding with a full action potential. An *absolute refractory period* occurs during depolarization and at the beginning of repolarization (phases 0, 1, and 2). During this period, excitation of the cardiac cell will not result in another impulse no matter how strong the stimulus. The *relative refractory period* represents the time when the cell is once again electronegative. A stronger than threshold stimulus can initiate another impulse. A *vulnerable* or *supernormal period* occurs as phase 4 begins and the cell is returning to its resting potential. During this time a weaker than threshold stimulus can initiate an action potential.

Figure 1-7 Normal electrocardiographic waveform.
From Tucker.[104]

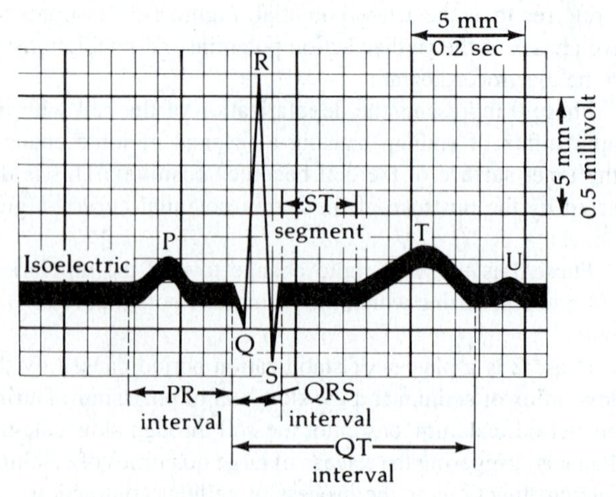

Electrocardiogram. The electromechanical events of the heart can be recorded and interpreted on the electrocardiogram (ECG). The various waveforms in Figure 1-7 have been correlated with the normal conduction sequence. Any deviation from normal indicates arrhythmia.

The cardiac cycle includes the following waveforms and time intervals:

P wave—the electrical activity associated with the sinus node impulse and its depolarization of the atria

PR interval—the time the impulse takes to travel through the atria to the A-V node, the bundle of His and bundle branches, and the ventricles; normal duration is 0.12 to 0.20 second

QRS complex—electrical depolarization and contraction of the ventricles

ST segment—the period between the completion of depolarization and the repolarization of the ventricles

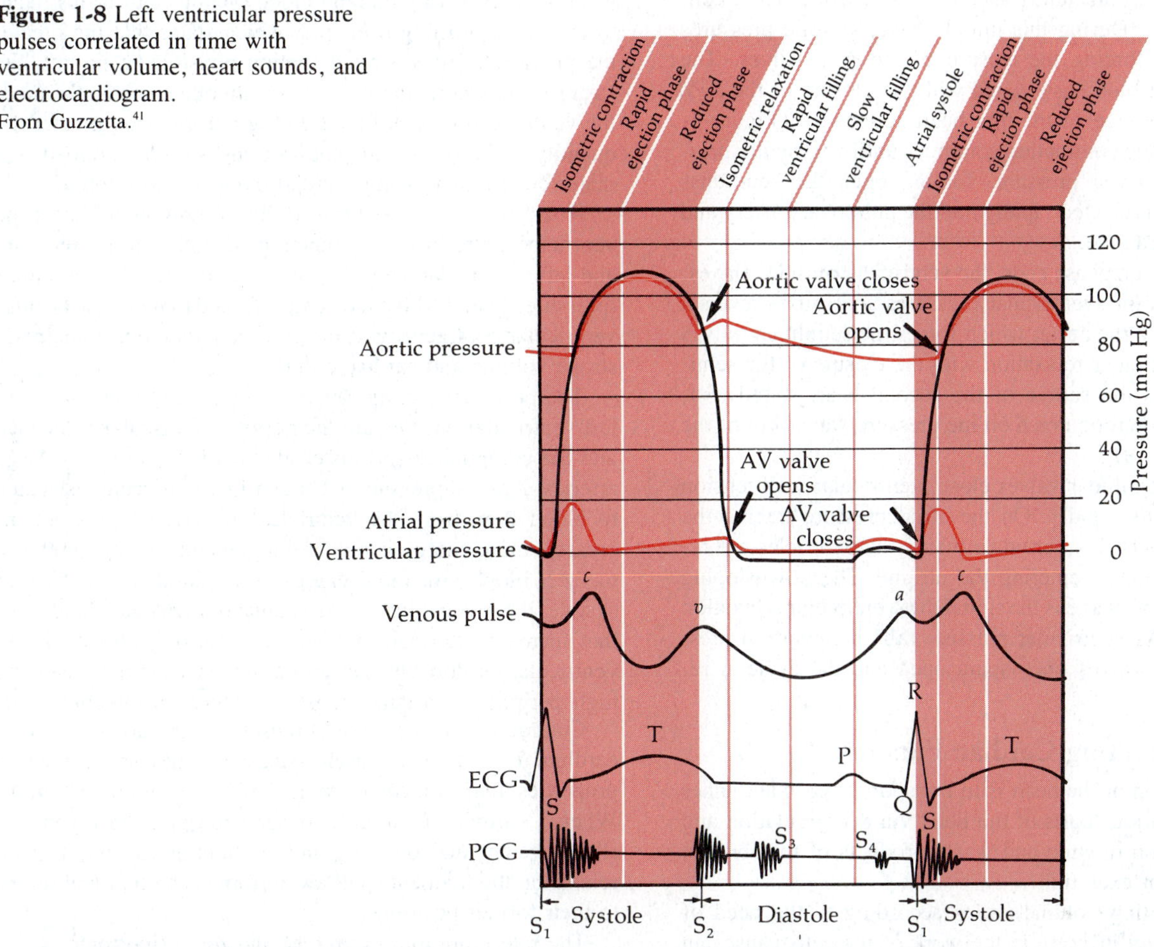

Figure 1-8 Left ventricular pressure pulses correlated in time with ventricular volume, heart sounds, and electrocardiogram.
From Guzzetta.[41]

T wave—the recovery or repolarization phase of the ventricles

Intervals between these waveforms reflect the time an impulse takes to travel through the heart.

Identification of rhythms, normal or otherwise, requires a careful systematic approach to interpretation. One method is described in the box at right.

Cardiac Cycle

The cardiac cycle is divided into two phases, systole and diastole. Systole is the time interval during which blood is ejected from the ventricles. Diastole is the time interval during which the ventricles are relaxed and filling with blood from the atria. Diastole is discussed first because filling pressures often predict the effectiveness of systolic ejection.

As described previously, the atria are reservoirs for blood entering the heart. During diastole the semilunar valves are closed, the ventricles are at rest, and the A-V valves are forced opened, allowing blood to flow from the atria into the ventricles. During the initial phase of diastole, approximately 70% of the blood flows rapidly into the ventricles. In the second half of diastole, blood flow slows until atrial contraction is accelerated, forcing the remainder of the blood into the ventricles. This added atrial thrust completes diastolic filling of the ventricle and is reflected as the "a" wave on the atrial pressure tracing (Figure 1-8). The blood present in the ventricles at the end of diastole is the end-diastolic volume.

Systematic Approach to ECG Interpretation

1. Calculate the heart rate. Calculate atrial (P waves) rate. Calculate ventricular (QRS complexes) rate.
2. Determine rhythm regularity.
3. Determine whether P waves are present. Determine the position of P waves with relation to the QRS complex.
4. Measure the PR interval.
5. Measure the QRS interval.
6. Identify and examine the ST segment and T wave.
7. Determine the origin of the rhythm. Is it of sinus, atrial, junctional, or ventricular origin?

With filling of the ventricles complete, isovolumetric contraction begins. During this initial phase, systolic pressures begin to rise, forcing the closure of the A-V valves. The deceleration of blood associated with the closure of the A-V valves is the source of the first heart sound (S_1) (Figure 1-8). Isovolumetric contraction continues until ventricular pressure exceeds aortic pressure, forcing open the semilunar valves. Blood is ejected rapidly into the pulmonary artery and aorta on the left side.

As the ejection phase ends, the ventricular muscle relaxes. This decreases intraventricular pressures and causes reversal of blood flow in the aorta, which forces the semilunar valves to close. Ventricular relaxation with the closure of the semilunar valves is the source of the second heart sound (S_2), reflected by a dicrotic notch on the pressure waveform of the aorta (Figure 1-8).

After the semilunar valves close, ventricular wall tension or pressure falls rapidly. On the atrial pressure tracing the "v" wave reflects this period in which the ventricles are relaxing and blood is entering the atrium. The downsloping following the "v" wave is the signal that ventricular relaxation is complete. As ventricular pressure falls below atrial pressure, the A-V valves once again open and the cycle is repeated.

Factors Affecting Cardiac Function

A basic function of the heart is to transport oxygen and other nutrients to various parts of the body via the circulation and to return carbon dioxide and waste products of metabolism to the lungs for excretion.

The circulating volume varies according to the need of tissue cells. Any increase in the work of the cells causes an increase in blood flow and thus increases the work of the heart and myocardial oxygen consumption (MVO_2).

The heart's function is governed by the closely integrated working of three major factors: intrinsic properties of the heart; extrinsic factors including nervous system, blood volume, and venous return; and peripheral circulation.

Cardiac function is based on the adequacy of the cardiac output (CO), which is the amount of blood pumped from the left ventricle per minute. CO is calculated by multiplying the amount of blood ejected from one ventricle with one heart beat (stroke volume, or SV) by the heart rate (HR): $CO = SV \times HR$. In a normal 70 kg (150-pound) adult at rest, the CO is 5 L/minute. The main factors affecting CO are preload (filling of the heart during diastole), afterload (the resistance against which the heart must pump), contractility of the heart muscle, and heart rate.

Preload is the degree of fiber stretch that occurs as a result of load or tension placed on the muscle before contraction. The term "load" refers to the quantity of blood and the term "tension" to the pressure it exerts in the left ventricle at the end of diastole (filling) just before systole (ejection). This is commonly referred to as left ventricular end-diastolic pressure (LVEDP).

The ability of the muscle fibers to stretch in response to increasing loads of incoming blood (venous return) is related to the Frank-Starling principle, which states that the greater the presystolic fiber stretch (within physiologic limits), the stronger the ventricular contraction. In other words, the more the ventricle fills with blood during diastole, the greater the quantity of blood it will pump during systole. Preload is a major determinant of myocardial oxygen consumption.

Afterload is the resistance to blood flow as it leaves the ventricles. Afterload is a function of both arterial pressure and left ventricular size. Any increase in vascular resistance (pressure against which the heart is forced to pump) will cause ventricular contractility to increase in an attempt to maintain stroke volume and cardiac output.

The principal factors causing impedance or resistance to left ventricular outflow are the peripheral vascular resistance and the compliance and distensibility of the aorta and large arteries. Arterial pressure is a major factor offering resistance to blood flow from the ventricles. As arterial pressure increases, more energy is required to generate enough pressure to eject blood. As more energy is required for ventricular systole, the myocardial oxygen demand increases. Conditions that increase afterload include those causing obstruction to ventricular outflow (such as aortic stenosis) and those causing high peripheral vascular resistance (such as hypertension).

Contractility is the force of muscle contraction. The myocardium is a unique muscle because it has some specific properties that contribute to its effective pumping action. When a stimulus is applied to heart muscle, the myofibrils slide together and overlap, and contraction occurs. During relaxation the filaments pull away from each other and return to their former positions.

The rate (chronotropic force) and force (inotropic force) of contraction can be increased by sympathetic nerve stimulation or administration of drugs with inotropic properties, such as isoproterenol, epinephrine, and dopamine. Depressed contractility is generally due to loss of contractile muscle mass through injury, disease, arrhythmias, or drugs.

The normal heart rate is 60 to 100 beats/minute. It is initiated by the S-A node within the heart, but other factors such as stimulation of the autonomic nervous system can greatly influence heart rate and rhythm.

Cardiac output can be depressed or increased, directly changing the heart rate. With a heart rate of less than 40 beats/minute, the cardiac output often falls, impairing cardiac performance. With low rates the tendency for arrhythmias increases because of the uncoordinated myocardial contraction, which further depresses contractility. With rapid pulse rates the length of time that the heart is in diastole is reduced. As a result, left ventricular filling is decreased as is coronary blood flow to the myocardium, which occurs primarily during diastole.

Peripheral Vascular System

The vascular system is composed of the arteries, capillaries, and veins; its main function is to distribute blood to body organs and tissues.

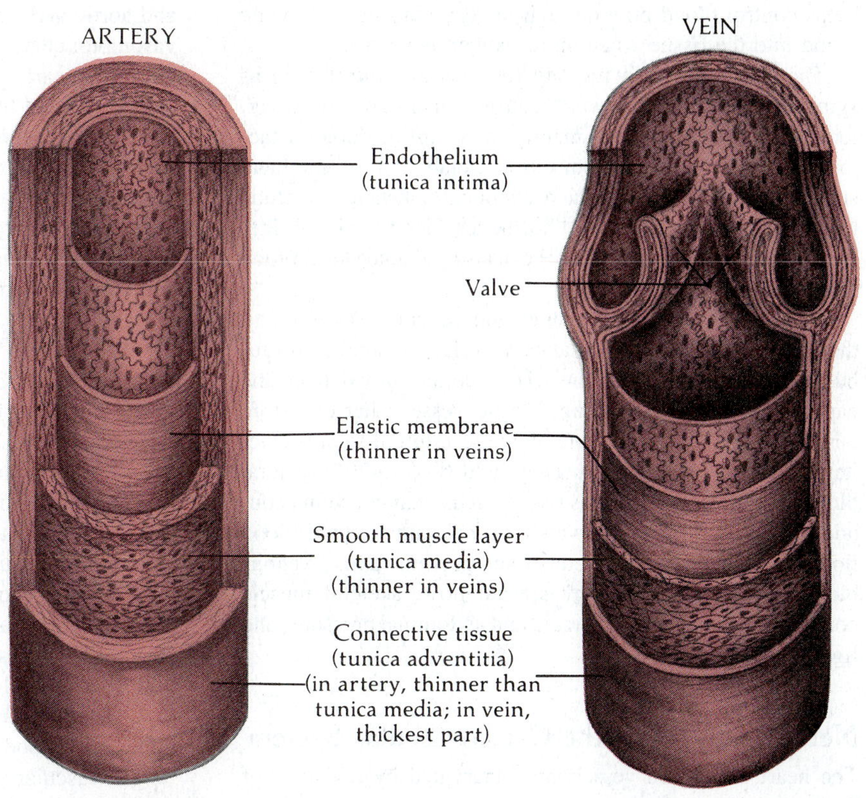

Figure 1-9 Cross section of artery and vein showing the three layers: tunica intima, tunica media, and tunica adventitia. Note difference in wall thickness between artery and vein.

The arterial tree, which carries oxygenated blood to all body tissues, is made up of arteries, arterioles, and capillaries. Arteries are easily distended, high-pressure conduits (Figure 1-9). Known as resistance vessels, they have a high elastic fiber content that can support high pressure and hold large volumes of blood. About 20% of the total circulating blood is contained within the arteries. Arterioles are smaller branches whose walls contain less elastic tissue and more smooth muscle. Constriction or dilation of the lumens of the arterioles is the major control of pressure and blood flow. By changing the diameter of the blood vessels, the volume of blood supplied to the tissues may be increased or decreased.

Arteries and arterioles respond to the autonomic nervous system and to chemical stimulation. Nerve impulses from reflex centers in the brain may constrict or dilate the vessels. Chemical substances may alter the size of a blood vessel by acting directly on the vessel or by stimulating sensory receptors, thus beginning reflex control. Temperature can also alter the size of the blood vessels.

Capillaries are microscopic (1 mm), inelastic endothelial vessels. The large capillary bed is permeable to the molecules that are exchanged between blood cells and tissue cells (Figure 1-10). The vital exchange of oxygen, nutrients, and metabolic waste products between blood and interstitial fluid occurs here. Blood flow through the capillaries is regulated by

Figure 1-10 Microcirculation involving blood, interstitial fluid, oxygen, and nutrients.

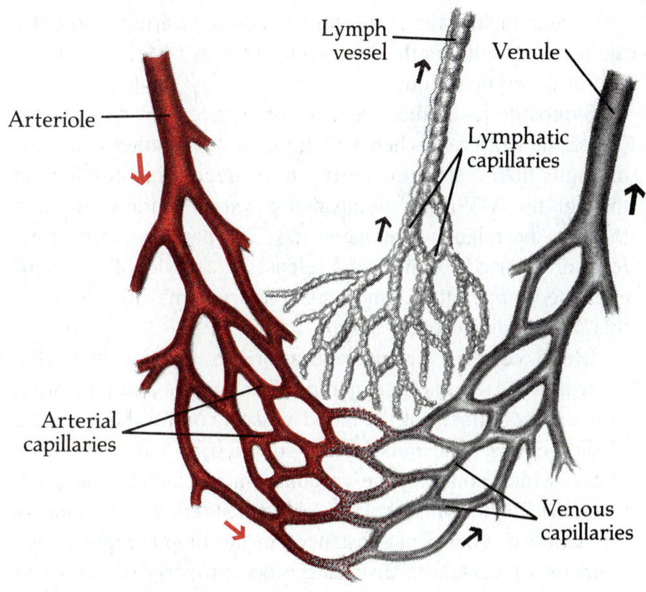

the demand for oxygen by cells. The precapillary sphincter helps control blood flow through the capillary bed, allowing blood into the tissue when more oxygen is needed.

The capillaries also respond to nervous control such as sympathetic stimulation, which causes constriction. However, local capillary response is mainly the result of humoral factors, that is, chemicals from tissue metabolism or chemical substances in the blood. Such chemical substances include histamine, which dilates, and hormones such as epinephrine, which constrict. Oxygen and pH can also influence local blood flow.

The venous system of venules and veins returns blood to the heart. Venules, the exchange vessels, are small, thin tubules that join to form veins. They collect blood from the capillary bed. Veins are thin, elastic vessels that can store large amounts of blood. Thus they are referred to as capacitance vessels (Figure 1-9). They hold 60% to 70% of total blood volume and change as tissue needs change. Veins contain valves at varying intervals that maintain forward blood flow to the heart (venous return) and prevent reflux. Venous blood flow is influenced by arterial flow, skeletal muscle contractions, changes in thoracic and abdominal pressure, and right atrial pressure.

Neural Control of the Cardiovascular System

The heart and blood vessels are innervated by divisions of the autonomic nervous system.

Heart. The heart can begin its own impulse through the S-A node. This is known as automaticity. It is influenced by both divisions of the autonomic nervous system. Sympathetic fibers innervate the heart through nerves arising from the cervical and upper thoracic ganglia of the sympathetic trunks and by the parasympathetic fibers arising in the vagal branches. Combined, they form the cardiac plexuses located close to the arch of the aorta.[6] From these plexuses, nerve fibers accompany the right and left coronary arteries to enter the heart. The fibers then extend to the S-A node, A-V node, and atrial myocardium.

Sympathetic cardiac nerves, or accelerator nerves, increase the heart rate when activated. Parasympathetic nerves, or vagus fibers, slow the heart rate by decreasing conduction through the A-V node. Sympathetic system action is effected through the release of epinephrine. The parasympathetic effects are caused by the vagal release of acetylcholine. Pain, exercise, temperature, emotions, and drugs may also activate this autonomic receptor system.

Blood vessels. Arteries and arterioles are also under the control of the sympathetic nerves. Contraction and relaxation of the muscle fibers of the blood vessels control the diameter of the vessels. The muscles are supplied by vasoconstrictor fibers, which constrict the vascular smooth muscle, and vasodilator fibers, which relax it. Vascular reflexes, helped by the action of chemical substances in the blood, regulate the diameter of vessels to distribute blood properly to tissues in response to their needs.

Baroreceptors. Baroreceptor cells are in the carotid sinus and aortic arch. Stimulation by stretch or pressure slows the vasomotor center, resulting in vasodilation. As more impulses go to the heart, stimulating parasympathetic fibers, the heart beat slows and the arterioles and venules dilate.

Chemoreceptors. Vasomotor chemoreceptors are in the aortic arch and carotid bodies. They are very sensitive to lowered Pao_2, raised Pco_2, and lowered pH. When stimulated, the chemoreceptors send impulses to the vasoconstrictor centers in the medulla, causing vasoconstriction of arterioles and the venous reservoir.

Arterial Blood Pressure

Arterial blood pressure is a measure of the pressure blood exerts within the blood vessels. This pressure depends largely on work of the heart (cardiac output), blood volume, and peripheral resistance, including the elasticity of arterial walls.

Peripheral resistance is the resistance to blood flow caused by the force created by the aorta, arteries, and arterioles. The amount of pressure on the blood is highest in the aorta (120 mm Hg) and becomes lower in arteries (80 mm Hg), arterioles (55 mm Hg), capillaries (30 mm Hg), and veins (20 mm Hg).[40] This pressure difference (gradient) determines blood flow, because blood flows naturally from high pressure to low. Other factors include the size and patency of the vessel lumen and blood viscosity.

The vascular tone of the arteries and arterioles allows them to constrict or dilate, influencing the resistance to flow. For example, the greater the resistance in the arteriole, the less the blood flow to capillaries. Therefore more blood remains in the arteries, creating a higher arterial pressure.

Blood viscosity depends on red blood cells and protein molecules in the blood. Greater pressure is needed to propel viscous, or thick, fluid. Altered blood protein levels or reduced red cell levels, as in anemia or hemorrhage, reduce peripheral resistance and arterial pressure.

Measurement of arterial pressure. Arterial pressure may be measured directly or indirectly. Direct measurement is done by placing a catheter, attached to a recording monitor, into the artery. Indirect measurement is performed with a stethoscope and a blood pressure cuff.

Fetal Development

From the onset of gestation the developing embryo undergoes rapid cellular diffusion, forming tissues that will later become the heart. By the third week a primitive single tubular structure made up of two layers of germ cells is formed. The mesoderm contributes to the pericardial wall (epicardium) and myocardium, and within this layer a single longitudinal tube is formed that will eventually become the endocardium.

The tube's position permits it to accommodate rapid growth. During the first 28 days the primitive cardiac tube grows and bends to the side, twisting into a loop. At this stage the cardiac structures are developing and identifiable; the sinuatrium, which connects the atria with the primitive ventricle; the conus cordis, which will later become the out-

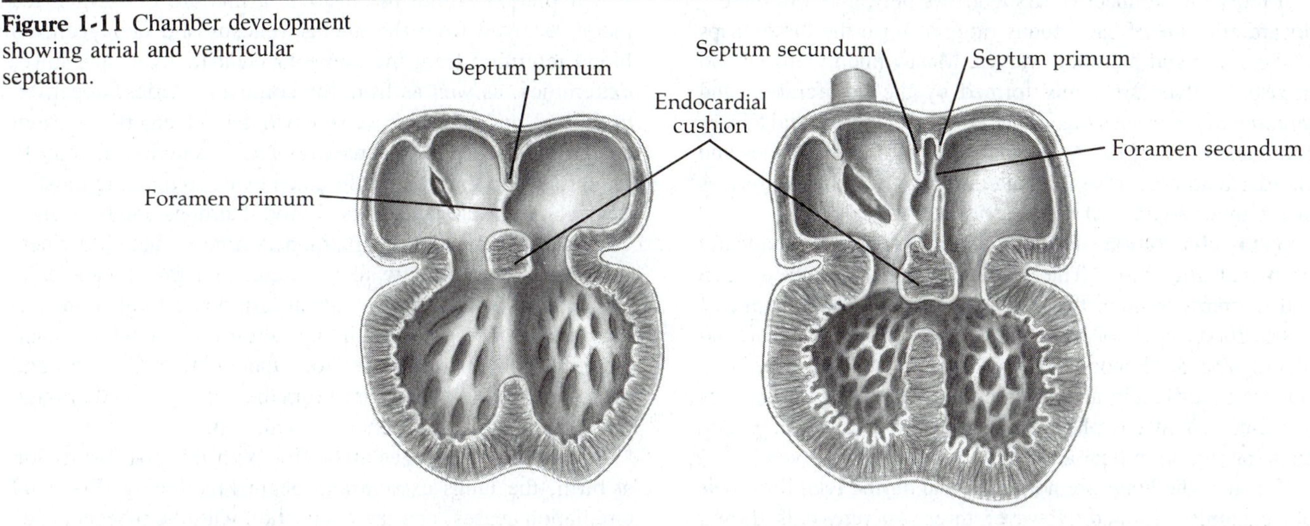

Figure 1-11 Chamber development showing atrial and ventricular septation.

flow tract for the ventricles; and the truncus arteriosus, which later divides into the aorta and pulmonary artery.

From the fourth through the eighth weeks, transition to a four-chambered heart occurs. A midline groove forms at the apex of the ventricular loop, beginning the division between the right and left sides. Blood flow remains undivided and continuously enters the atria and sinus venosus and leaves via the truncus arteriosus.

Atria. Atrial development begins from the common atrioventricular (A-V) canal. Two tissue bundles, the endocardial cushions, arise from the A-V canal, forming a dorsal (back) and ventral side. By the sixth week these tissues merge in the center of the heart, dividing the A-V canal into left and right channels and developing what will later be the tricuspid and mitral valves.

Atrial septation develops from the septum primum, which grows toward the A-V canal and endocardial cushions. An intercommunication between the left and right atria called the foramen primum remains (Figure 1-11, *A*). As atrial division continues, a second atrial septum (septum secundum) is established in the center and to the right of the septum primum. The septum primum continues to fuse with the endocardial cushions, obliterating the foramen primum. However, the lower portion remains as a flap valve that prevents blood flow from reversing to left to right. Throughout fetal life, blood flow is directed right to left through the foramen ovale, supplying oxygen to the left side of the heart and fetal structures (Figure 1-12). The foramen ovale closes shortly after birth.

Ventricles. Septation of the ventricles takes place during the second month of fetal development. Rapid growth occurs from the apex of the common ventricle upward toward the expanding endocardial cushions and A-V canal. This upward-growing muscular tissue does not merge with the cushions. Thus an interventricular communication is created that exists until the tissues from the endocardial cushion and conus ridges of the truncus arteriosus grow downward and eventually obliterate it. The upper portion of the septum thins out into a fibrous sheet referred to as the membranous portion of the septum, while the lower portion remains muscular.

Great vessels and cardiac valves. The truncus arteriosus, which is initially a single undivided tubular structure, undergoes its own partitioning process. The conus ridges in the ventricular septum fuse and divide the truncus into a left and a right side, forming the aorta and pulmonary artery. These vessels continue to develop in a spiral fashion, so the aorta receives blood from the left ventricle and the pulmonary artery receives blood from the right ventricle.

Figure 1-12 Blood flow being directed through foramen ovale.

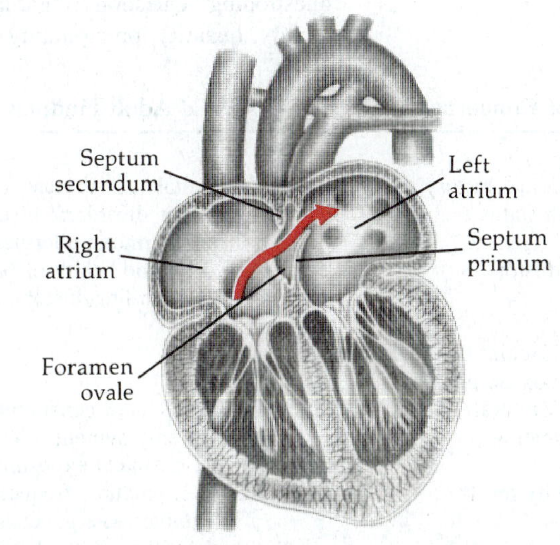

Embryonic connective tissue grows outward from the endocardial tissue of each conus ridge to form the three cusps of the aortic and pulmonic valves. Meanwhile the mitral and tricuspid valves are being formed by the proliferation and thinning of the tissues that project from the endocardial tissues and outer walls of the A-V canal. The papillary muscles and chordae tendineae arise from alteration of the muscular tissues of the inner sources of the ventricles.

Fetal circulation. Fetal circulation differs dramatically from that after birth. The developing fetus secures oxygen and nutrients through the placenta, where an interchange of gases, foods, and wastes occurs between fetal and maternal blood. The fetal blood receives oxygen and nutritive substances by diffusion and gives up waste products. The fetus is connected to the placenta by the umbilical cord, which contains two umbilical arteries and one umbilical vein.

Because the lungs are nonfunctional during fetal life, their blood supply is limited. However, three structures exist during the fetal life to ensure circulation within the heart. These are the foramen ovale in the interatrial septum, which allows the blood in the right atrium to pass directly into the left atrium; the ductus arteriosus, which connects the pulmonary artery directly with the aorta; and the ductus venosus, which allows blood to pass directly to the inferior vena cava.

The heart begins to beat in about the fourth week of fetal life. Fetal circulation of blood is similar to that in adults with the exception of the heart, lungs, and placenta. Blood reaches the placenta via the umbilical arteries. Within the placenta, blood passes through the capillaries of the villi and then returns to the fetus by way of the umbilical vein to the liver. Most of the blood is shunted directly to the inferior vena cava by way of the ductus venosus; the remainder is directed into the liver.

Circulation within the heart is a mixture of oxygenated blood received from the ductus venosus and deoxygenated blood returning from the alimentary canal, liver, and lower extremities, as well as from the coronary arteries, upper extremities, and superior vena cava. Blood enters the right atrium via the inferior vena cava and is shunted directly to the left atrium through the foramen ovale, bypassing most of the right ventricle and lungs. Blood that does enter the right ventricle is pumped to the pulmonary artery where it divides. A portion goes directly to the lung, and the remainder is shunted through the narrow ductus arteriosus to the descending aorta. Blood entering the left atrium mixes with a small amount of blood received from the pulmonary veins and passes into the left ventricle. From there it is pumped through the aorta and into the general circulation.

Circulatory changes at birth. With the first inspiration at birth, the lungs expand and begin functioning. Placental circulation ceases, and the connection with the placenta ends with the cutting of the umbilical cord, causing several major changes. During fetal life the lungs have a high vascular resistance. As a result, the blood ejected from the right ventricle into the pulmonary artery is shunted via the ductus arteriosus into the descending aorta. With the first breath the alveoli expand, the pulmonary vascular resistance drops rapidly, and pulmonary blood flow increases. Simultaneously, the loss of placental blood flow causes the right atrial pressure to drop. The combination of decreased pulmonary vascular resistance, increased pulmonary blood flow, and decreased right atrial pressure causes the left atrial pressure to rise above right atrial pressure. The foramen ovale then closes, and the increase in oxygen saturation following the changes in pulmonary vascular resistance stimulates constriction and eventual closure of the ductus arteriosus.

Normal Findings

The assessment of any patient begins with careful attention to the patient's chief complaint. The problem, whether chest pain, palpitations, or shortness of breath, should guide the direction of questioning. Questions regarding the problem may be organized into seven categories: location, quality, quantity, precipitating or aggravating factors, duration, and associated symptoms.

Area of Concern	Normal Adult Findings
History	
Past medical history and general health status	Congenital heart disease; childhood disease (rheumatic fever, scarlet fever); coronary artery disease; vascular disorders; bleeding disorders; hypertension; kidney disease; diabetes; hyperlipidemia; heart murmurs; allergies; genetic disorders, e.g., Marfan's syndrome
Family history	Age, sex, and health of parents, siblings, and children and cause of death for deceased members; data regarding history of hypertension, heart disease, diabetes, elevated lipid levels, sudden deaths
Cardiovascular risk factor profile (see box on p. 29)	
Sociocultural	Culture; alcohol consumption; economic situation
Occupation	Type of employment; physical and emotional demands; environmental hazards (actual, potential), e.g., chemical exposures, dust
Activity level	Exercise: amount, frequency, intensity; sexual: frequency, recent changes, problems or presence of symptoms, e.g., chest pain, shortness of breath during or after intercourse; sports: type, e.g., competitive versus leisure, contact, e.g., football, soccer

Area of Concern	Normal Adult Findings
Sleep	Number of pillows used; presence of paroxysmal nocturnal dyspnea; number of times up to urinate
Nutrition	Fluid and dietary restriction; any recent weight increases or decreases
Dental history	Major problems; last dental visit; knowledge regarding antibiotic prophylaxis if pertinent
Medications	Prescription and nonprescription drugs; contraceptives; regular use of street drugs, e.g., cocaine, crack
Smoking history	Type: cigarettes, cigars, pipe, chewing tobacco, snuff; duration; frequency
Female history	Birth control measures: intrauterine devices, diaphragm, sponge/foam, male contraception; hormone therapy: type and years used; pregnancies: para, gravida, any related complications
Psychosocial	Perception of illness; response to health problems; patterns of coping or adaptation; understanding of current and past health problems
Support system	Marital status; primary support system
General appearance	Level of consciousness (alert, oriented); respiratory rate and pattern (passive breathing 12-20/minute, respiratory/pulse rate ratio 1:4, no shortness of breath or dyspnea); nutritional state (well nourished); weight and height normal
Blood pressure	Systolic 100-140 mm Hg (tends to be 5-15 mm Hg higher in right arm); diastolic 60-90 mm Hg; pulse pressure 30-40 mm Hg *Older adult:* Maximum systolic pressure 160 mm Hg; with standing, there may be systolic drop of 10-15 mm Hg and diastolic drop of 5 mm Hg
Arterial pulse (heart rate)	60-90 beats/minute *Older adult:* Slows with age due to increase in vagal tone; wide range (40-100 beats/minute), occasional ectopic beats may be felt Rhythm (regular); amplitude and contour (upstroke full, strong, rounded, brisk); symmetric response (equal on right and left); timing (equal for all arterial pulsations, e.g., brachial, femoral); auscultation (no murmurs or bruits); amplitude: 4+ = strong, bounding (normal) 3+ = easily palpable 2+ = difficult to palpate 1+ = diminished, weak, thready 0 = absent *Older adult:* Amplitude and contour (upstroke more rapid, smooth)
Jugular venous pressure (JVP) (Figure 1-13)	Should not exceed 3 cm (1 inch) above level of sternal angle (Figure 1-13) with head of client elevated to 30-45 degrees

Figure 1-13 Inspection of external jugular venous pressure.

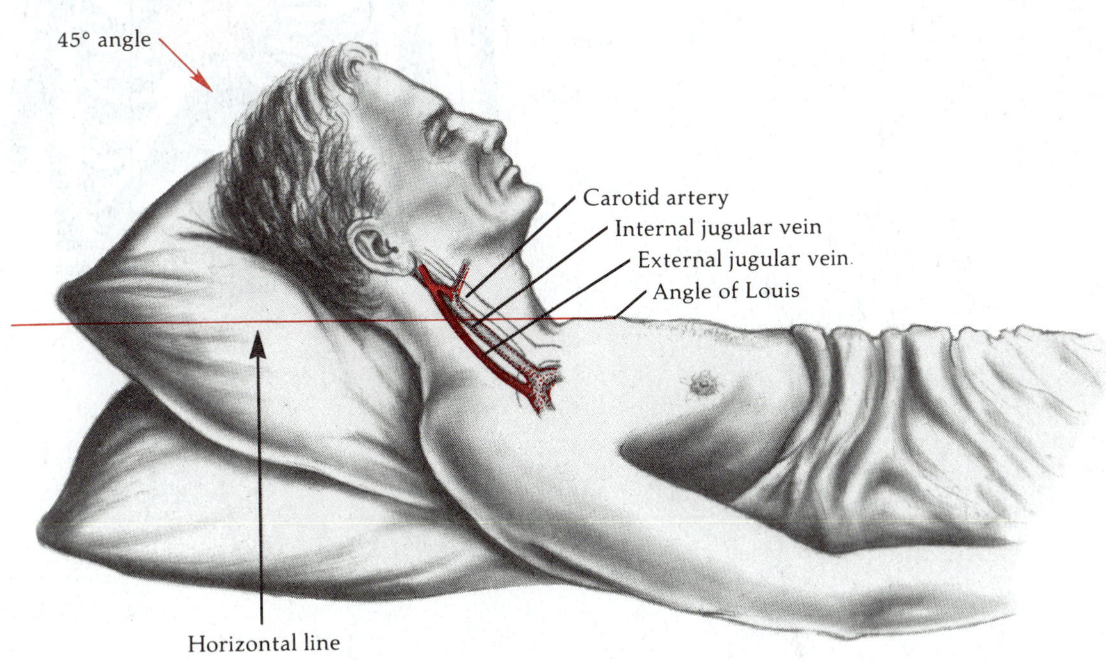

Area of Concern	Normal Adult Findings
Jugular pulsations	Undulations; movement with inspiration; increase or decrease with change in body position
Wave pulsations	
a wave	First positive wave visualized; coincides with S_1; represents right atrial contraction and retrograde transmission of pressure pulse to jugular veins
X descent	First negative "trough" undulation; occurs between S_1 and S_2; results from right atrial diastole, plus the effects of the tricuspid valve being pulled down during ventricular systole
v wave	Third positive wave; coincides with S_2; continued atrial filling
y descent	Represents fall in right atrial pressure from peak of v wave following tricuspid valve opening and occurs during period of rapid atrial emptying in early diastole
Precordium (Figure 1-14)	Point of maximum impulse (PMI) 5-7 cm left of midsternal border at fifth intercostal space (ICS) and 1-2 cm (⅓-½ inch) in diameter; palpable areas: aortic area—at second ICS to right of sternal border, pulmonic area—at second ICS to left of sternal border, apex—at fifth ICS 5-7 cm to left of sternal border; precordial motion symmetric, even with respiration
Heart sounds (Figure 1-8)	First heart sound (S_1) closing of A-V valves; components are tricuspid (T_1), located at fifth intercostal space (ICS) and left lower sternal border (LLSB), and mitral (M_1), located in apical area at fifth ICS and 5-7 cm left of sternal border; loudest at apical area; normal splitting heard LLSB at fifth ICS
	Second heart sound (S_2) closure of semilunar valves; components are aortic (A_2), located at second ICS to right of sternal border, and pulmonic (P_2), located at second ICS to left of sternal border; loudest at base; normal splitting heard at P_2

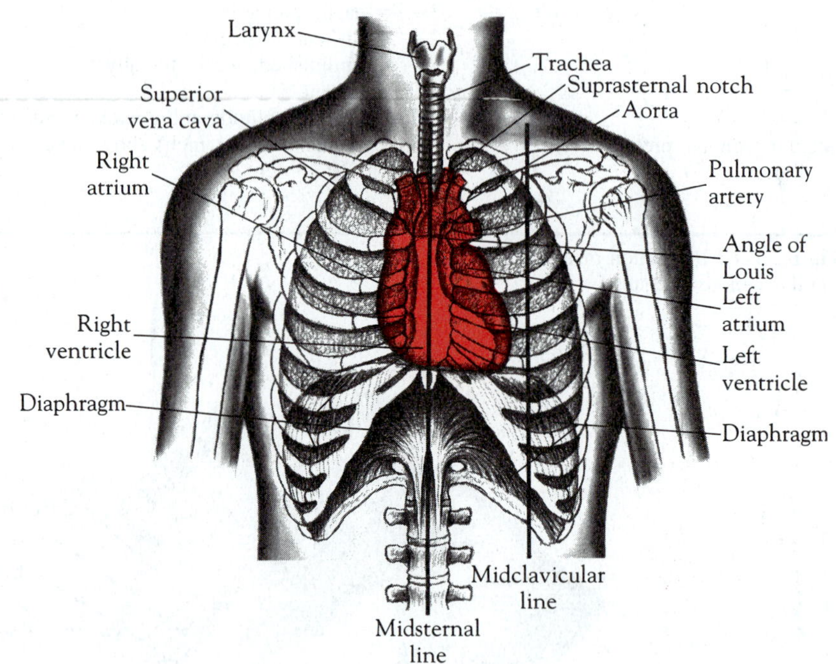

Figure 1-14 Chest wall landmarks for inspection, percussion, and palpation.

Normal Laboratory Data

Laboratory Test	Values
Complete blood count (CBC)	
Glycosylated hemoglobin	5.7%-8.8%
Plasma hemoglobin	1-5 mg/dl
Whole-blood hemoglobin	
Men	15.5 ± 1.1 g/dl
Women	13.7 ± 1.0 g/dl
Hematocrit	
Men	42%-52%
Women	35%-47%
Cardiac enzymes	
Creatine phosphokinase (CPK)	
Males	55-70 U/L
Females	15-57 U/L
CPK-MB (isoenzyme)	0-7 IU/L
SGOT	8-42 U/ML
Lactate dehydrogenase (LDH) isoenzymes (method dependent)	
LDH_1	22%-36%
LDH_2	35%-46%
LDH_3	13%-26%
LDH_4	3%-10%
LDH_5	2%-9%
LDH (specific for heart, kidney, blood cells)	0.17-0.27 of total LDH

Laboratory Test	Values
Lipid profile	
Total	400-800 mg/dl
Cholesterol	100-210 mg/dl
Triglycerides (at 95th percentile)	
White men	
25-29 yr	Up to 250 mg/dl
35-54 yr	Up to 320 mg/dl
55-64 yr	Up to 290 mg/dl
65 and older	Up to 260 mg/dl
White women	
35-39 yr	Up to 195 mg/dl
55-64 yr	Up to 250 mg/dl
Lipoproteins	
High density (HDL)	
Men 15-34 yr	30-65 mg/dl
Women	35-80 mg/dl
Low density (LDL)	
White men 35-39 yr	Up to 190 mg/dl
Phospholipids	150-380 mg/dl
Fatty acids	9-15 mmol/L
Drug levels	
Digoxin	
Therapeutic	1-2 ng/ml
Toxic	3 ng/ml
Underdigitalization	<0.5 ng/ml
Digitoxin	
Therapeutic	10-30 ng/ml
Toxic	>35 ng/ml

Conditions, Diseases, and Disorders

CARDIAC DISEASES

Cardiac arrhythmias

An arrhythmia is a disorder of the heart rate and rhythm caused by a conduction system disturbance.

Cardiac arrhythmias can cause sudden death resulting from electromechanical failure (as in ventricular fibrillation) or from impaired cardiac function.

Early recognition and treatment are needed because arrhythmias such as premature ventricular ectopic beats may spontaneously become frequent or multifocal. For example, in a patient with myocardial ischemia the ectopic beat may convert to ventricular tachycardia or ventricular fibrillation without warning. About 40% to 70% of deaths from acute myocardial infarction occur within the first hour, generally before the victim can reach a hospital.

Careful continuous ECG monitoring now enables early detection and prompt treatment of potentially serious arrhythmias. However, proper treatment involves diagnosis and a thorough understanding of the underlying etiologic factors.

Pathophysiology

Cardiac arrhythmias may be classified into abnormalities of impulse formation (sinus, atrial, ventricular) or impulse conduction or a combination.[44] Arrhythmias may also be described on the basis of rate (bradyarrhythmia, tachyarrhythmia) or seriousness (minor, life threatening). Arrhythmias may occur as a result of a primary cardiac disorder, as a secondary response to a systemic problem, or as a complication of drug toxicity or electrolyte imbalance.

Each of the major arrhythmias is described in the section on nursing assessment.

Diagnostic Studies and Findings

Electrocardiogram (ECG)

See "Nursing Assessment" for ECG characteristics and findings for specific arrhythmias

24-Hour Ambulatory Electrocardiogram

Electrophysiologic Studies

Medical Plan

Surgery

Surgical ablation or resection—specialized procedure performed in catheterization laboratory or by direct visualization in operating room; performed only on patients with highly refractory tachyarrhythmias and to identify accessory A-V bundles in patients with Wolff-Parkinson-White syndrome, since tracts can be excised surgically once irritable focus is located; can also be performed on patients with recurrent ventricular tachycardia through use of programmed stimulation, which allows cardiologist or surgeon to induce ventricular tachycardia, identify arrhythmogenic site, and excise ectopic focus

Medications

Antiarrhythmic drugs: group I—potent local anesthetic drugs that affect nerves as well as myocardial fibers; decrease conduction velocity by retarding influx of sodium and reduce maximum rate of depolarizing action potential

- Quinidine
  - Indications: Suppresses atrial, junctional, or ventricular ectopy, ventricular tachycardia, and paroxysmal atrial tachycardia; may be used to convert atrial fibrillation or flutter to sinus rhythm or to maintain sinus rhythm after cardioversion
  - Usual dosage: 200-400 mg po q4-6h
  - Onset of action: 15 min with peak activity in 2-4 h
  - Therapeutic blood levels: 2-6 mg/ml
  - Toxic signs: Widened QRS, prolonged QT bundle branch block, complete heart block, ventricular tachycardia, asystole
  - Sustained-release preparations: Quinidex, 300 mg q8-12h; Quinaglute, 324 mg q8-12h; Cardioquin, 275 mg q6h
- Procainamide (Pronestyl)
  - Indications: Similar to quinidine; suppresses ventricular ectopy; may be less effective in controlling atrial arrhythmias
  - Usual dosage: 250-750 mg po q4-6h; 100 mg q5-15 min for total of 1 g IV
  - Peak action: Within 30 min
  - Therapeutic blood levels: 4-8 mg/ml
  - Sustained-release preparations: Procan SR, 500-1000 mg q6h
- Disopyramide phosphate (Norpace)
  - Indications: Suppresses or prevents ventricular arrhythmias; not particularly effective in treating atrial arrhythmias
  - Usual dosage: 400-800 mg/day po in four doses with loading dose of 200 mg
  - Peak action: 2-4 h
  - Therapeutic blood levels: 2-4 mg/ml
- Lidocaine (Xylocaine)
  - Indications and actions: Controls ventricular arrhythmias by depressing automaticity in Purkinje network and increasing excitability threshold of ventricles
  - Usual dosage: 50-100 mg (1-2 mg/kg) by IV bolus followed by 1.5-4 mg/min
  - Onset of action: 45-90 sec
  - Duration of action: 20 min
  - Therapeutic blood levels: 1.5-5 mg/ml
- Phenytoin (Dilantin)
  - Indications and actions: Depresses automaticity
  - Usual dosage: 100 mg q6h po with loading dose of 200 mg or 50-100 mg IV over 5-10 min up to 1 g
  - Onset of action: Slow and variable
  - Therapeutic blood levels: 10-15 mg/ml
- Mexiletine
  - Indications: Investigational local anesthetic whose electrophysiologic properties closely resemble those of lidocaine; used in management of ventricular arrhythmias
  - Usual dosage: IV loading 10-15 mg/min (200-300 mg over 30 min), maintenance 250-500 mg/12 h; po loading 100-400 mg, maintenance 200-300 mg q8h
  - Onset of action: IV <5 min; po 1-2 h
  - Therapeutic blood levels: 0.5-2 μg/ml
- Tocainide (Tonocard)
  - Indications and actions: Class I antiarrhythmic similar to lidocaine given for control of ventricular arrhythmias; decreases excitability of myocardial cells
  - Usual dosage: Loading 400-600 mg po q8h, maintenance 1200-1800 mg, in divided doses over 8 h
  - Onset of action: 1½ h
  - Therapeutic blood levels: 6-12 μg/ml
- Aprindine
  - Indications: Used in control of supraventricular and ventricular arrhythmias resistant to traditional agents
  - Usual dosage: Loading 200-300 mg po, maintenance 100-150 mg/d
  - Onset of action: 2 h
  - Therapeutic blood levels: 1-2 μg/ml

Antiarrhythmic drugs: group II—control arrhythmias by blocking sympathetic stimulation, which shortens phase 4 depolarization of action potential

- Propranolol (Inderal)
  - Indications and actions: Controls supraventricular tachycardia resulting from reentry mechanism; used to control ventricular response to atrial fibrillation and flutter by depressing A-V nodal conduction
  - Usual dosage: 10-80 mg po qid; 0.5-1 mg IV push slowly to control heart rate
  - Onset of action: 1-1½ h (po)
  - Therapeutic blood levels: Not determined

Atenolol
Usual dosage: 50-100 mg/d
Pindolol
Usual dosage: 10-60 mg bid

Antiarrhythmic drugs: group III—act directly on myocardium, prolonging action potential
Bretylium tosylate (Bretylol)
Indications: Life-threatening ventricular arrhythmias; not recommended to treat asymptomatic ventricular ectopic beats
Usual dosage: 5-10 mg/kg IV push up to total of 30 mg/kg; may repeat in 15-30 min; slow continuous infusion 5-10 mg/kg q6-8h
Amiodarone
Indications: Effective in treatment and prevention of wide variety of atrial and ventricular arrhythmias
Usual dosage: 200-800 mg/d; loading dose 800-1200 mg/d for 1 wk
Onset of action: 4-8 h

Antiarrhythmic drugs: group IV—inhibit calcium transport into cells, depress activity of the S-A and A-V nodes, prolong conduction in A-V node, and increase A-V node refractoriness
Verapamil (Calan, Isoptin)
Indications: Reentrant paroxysmal supraventricular tachyarrhythmias; suppresses A-V junctional tachycardia and controls ventricular response to atrial fibrillation and flutter
Usual dosage: 5-10 mg (0.1 mg/kg) IV or 40-80 mg po q6-8h
Peak action: IV 3-5 min; po 3-4 h

General Management

Cardiac monitoring—continuous electrocardiographic monitoring provides most efficient and reliable method of detection of arrhythmias

Electrical countershock—often treatment of choice for tachyarrhythmias that are life threatening or producing a decrease in cardiac output and are resistant to pharmacologic interventions (see p. 98 for further discussion and nursing care)
Cardioversion—synchronized discharge of electrical impulse used to convert atrial fibrillation, atrial flutter, or supraventricular tachycardia to sinus rhythm
Defibrillation—emergency procedure that is unsynchronized; used in treatment of ventricular defibrillation

Cardiac pacemakers—battery-operated electrical devices used to initiate and control heart rate; system is composed of battery pack and electrodes through which electrical stimulation is delivered to myocardium; may be used as temporary assistive devices or implanted permanently; have variety of modalities that are selected on basis of rhythm disturbance; most common indication for pacemaker implantation is bradyarrhythmias, but recent advances in technology have broadened their use to treatment of suppressing supraventricular arrhythmias otherwise resistant to drug therapy (see p. 107 for further discussion)

Automatic implantable defibrillator—device capable of detecting the presence of ventricular tachyarrhythmias, and then deliver electrical countershock via cardioversion or defibrillation within 15 to 20 seconds (see p. 88 for further discussion)

Diet—restrictions usually directed to underlying disease process; patients with diagnosed supraventricular tachyarrhythmias instructed to avoid using stimulants such as caffeine, which is found in coffee, certain teas, soft drinks, and chocolate

Smoking—use of nicotine contraindicated because of its effect on ventricular threshold, which may be basis for dysrhythmias that could precipitate fatal rhythms

NURSING CARE

Nursing Assessment

Rhythm	Characteristics	Etiology	Clinical Significance	Management
Sinus origin Sinus tachycardia (Figure 1-15)	Regular rhythm; rate 100-180 beats/minute (higher in infants); normal P wave; normal QRS complex	Rate increase may be normal response to exercise, emotion, or abnormal stressors such as pain, fever, pump failure, hyperthyroidism, and certain pharmacologic agents, including caffeine, nitrates, atropine, epinephrine, isoproterenol, and nicotine	May have hemodynamic consequence in patient with damaged heart that is unable to sustain increased workloads brought on by persistent increases in heart rate	Correcting underlying factors; discontinuing offending drugs

Figure 1-15
From Andreoli.[5]

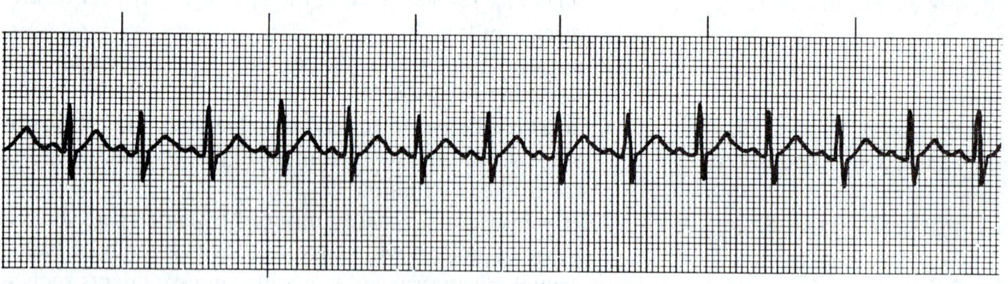

Rhythm	Characteristics	Etiology	Clinical Significance	Management
Sinus bradycardia (Figure 1-16)	Regular rhythm; rate less than 60 beats/minute; normal P wave; normal PR interval; normal QRS complex	Rate decrease may be normal response to sleep or in well-conditioned athlete; abnormal drops in rate may be caused by diminished blood flow to S-A node, vagal stimulation, hypothyroidism, increased intracranial pressure, or pharmacologic agents such as digoxin, propranolol, quinidine, or procainamide	None unless associated with signs of impaired cardiac output; symptoms: dizziness, syncope, chest pain	Correcting underlying cause; atropine 0.5-1 mg IV; transvenous pacemaker

Figure 1-16
From Andreoli.[5]

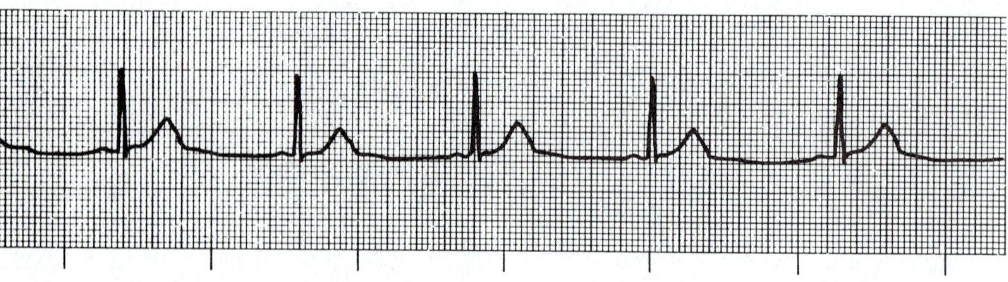

Rhythm	Characteristics	Etiology	Clinical Significance	Management
Sinus arrhythmia (Figure 1-17)	Irregular rhythm; may be phasic with respiration, slowing during inspiration and increasing with expiration; rate 60-100 beats/minute; normal PR interval; normal QRS complex	Sinus rhythm with cyclic variation caused by vagal impulses that influence rhythm during respiration; occurs commonly in children, young adults, and the elderly; usually disappears as heart rate increases	None unless heart rate decreases; symptoms: dizziness with decreased rate	None indicated unless heart rate decreases and symptoms occur

Figure 1-17
From Conover.[19]

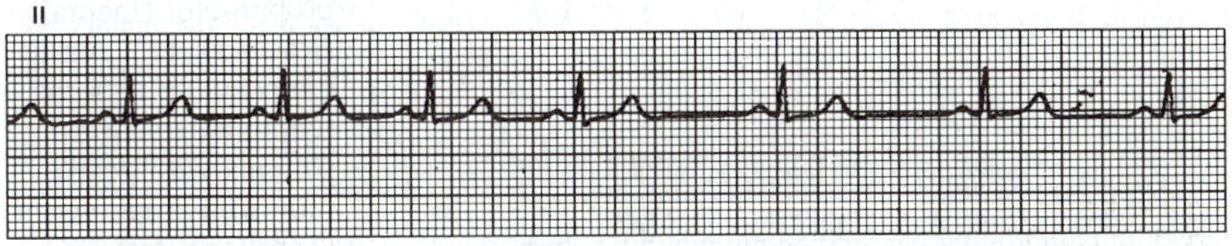

Rhythm	Characteristics	Etiology	Clinical Significance	Management
Atrial origin Atrial premature contractions (APCs, PACs) (Figure 1-18)	Irregular rhythm owing to ectopic beats followed by incomplete compensatory pause; rate normal or increased depending on number of ectopic beats; P wave present but different from normal underlying sinus beat; PR interval may be shorter or longer than normal sinus beat; normal QRS complex	May be precipitated in healthy persons by anxiety, fatigue, caffeine, smoking, and alcohol; observed in patients with ischemia or organic heart disease and those receiving digoxin	May indicate atrial strain or hypoxia; frequent PACs (more than 6/minute) reflect atrial irritability and often mark onset of atrial fibrillation	Correcting underlying cause; for frequent PACs, quinidine or pronestyl

Figure 1-18
From Conover.[21]

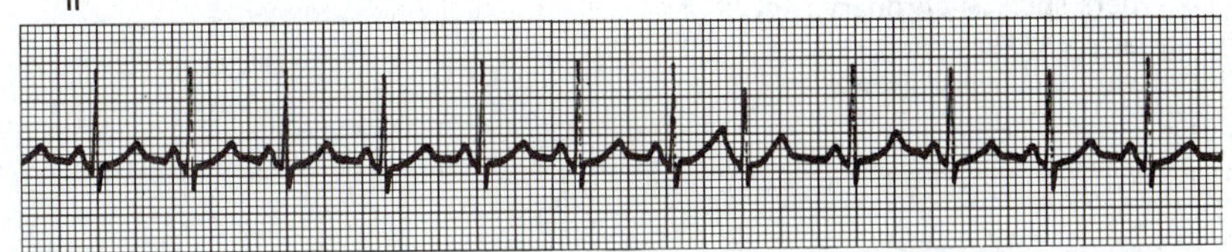

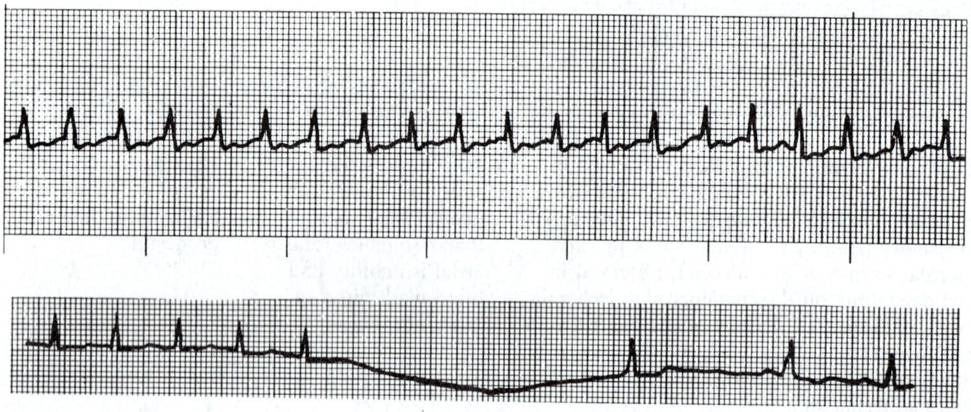

Rhythm	Characteristics	Etiology	Clinical Significance	Management
Paroxysmal supraventricular tachycardia (PSVT) (Figure 1-19)	Sudden, rapid onset of tachycardia with stimulus originating above A-V node; regular rhythm; rate 150-250 beats/minute; P wave uniform, may or may not be buried in preceding T wave; PR interval may vary, often difficult to measure; normal QRS complex	May begin and end spontaneously or be precipitated by excitement, fatigue, caffeine, smoking, or alcohol	Usually no significant impairment; patient complains of palpitations and shortness of breath; if persistent or occurring in patient with preexisting organic heart disease, may cause decrease in cardiac output and/or blood pressure resulting in pump failure or shock	Performing vagal stimulation with carotid sinus massage; using Valsalva maneuver to stimulate baroreceptors (may be used in conjunction with carotid sinus massage); decreasing ventricular response with medication to block A-V conduction; sedation to reduce sympathetic stimulation; verapamil 5-10 mg IV push; propranolol (Inderal) slowly IV in 1 mg increments up to 4 mg (contraindicated in patients with heart failure); edrophonium (Tensilon), test dose 1 mg followed by 10 mg IV; cardioversion if resistant to preceding
Atrial flutter (Figure 1-20)	Rhythm may be regular or irregular; rate: atrial 250-350 beats/minute, characterized by sawtooth flutter waves; ventricular depends on A-V conduction, may occur at 2:1, 3:1, or 4:1 ratio; PR interval not measurable; normal QRS complex	Results from rapidly firing ectopic atrial focus; most likely underlying mechanism is localized atrial reentry phenomenon; seen in patients with organic heart disorders such as coronary artery disease and valvular heart disease	Patient complains of palpitations, which may be associated with heart failure, and chest pain, particularly in presence of rapid ventricular rates	Cardioversion; digoxin if cardioversion is not used or is unsuccessful; quinidine or procainamide

Figure 1-19
From Andreoli.[5]

Figure 1-20
From Conover.[21]

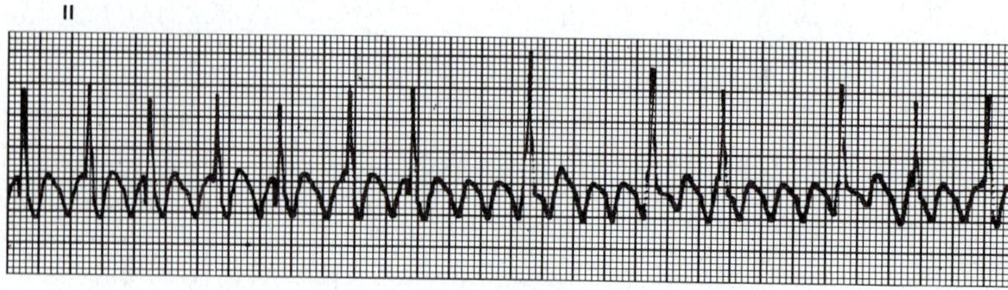

Rhythm	Characteristics	Etiology	Clinical Significance	Management
Atrial fibrillation (Figure 1-21)	Rhythm irregular; rate: atrial more than 350 beats/minute; absence of uniform atrial depolarization produces undulations (f waves); ventricular varies according to A-V conduction but may range between 50 and 150 beats/minute	Results from multiple atrial foci discharging almost simultaneously; atria never uniformly depolarize; reflects organic heart disease; may also occur with digitalis toxicity	With rapid ventricular rates, cardiac output may be impaired, resulting in heart failure, angina, and shock	Determination of underlying cause and whether acute or chronic; cardioversion for rapid ventricular response; digoxin if cardioversion is not used; quinidine; procainamide; verapamil

Figure 1-21
From Conover.[21]

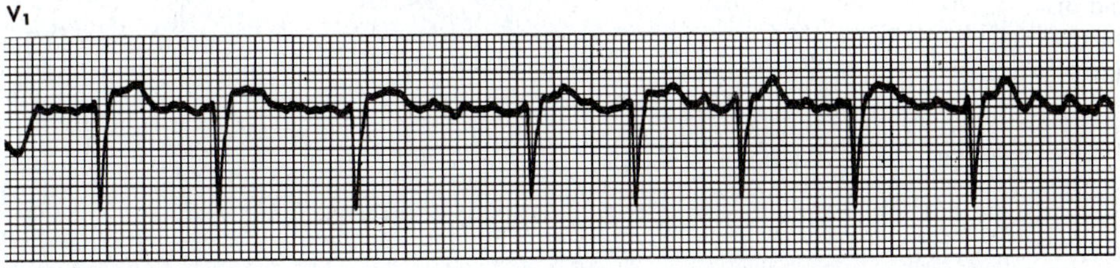

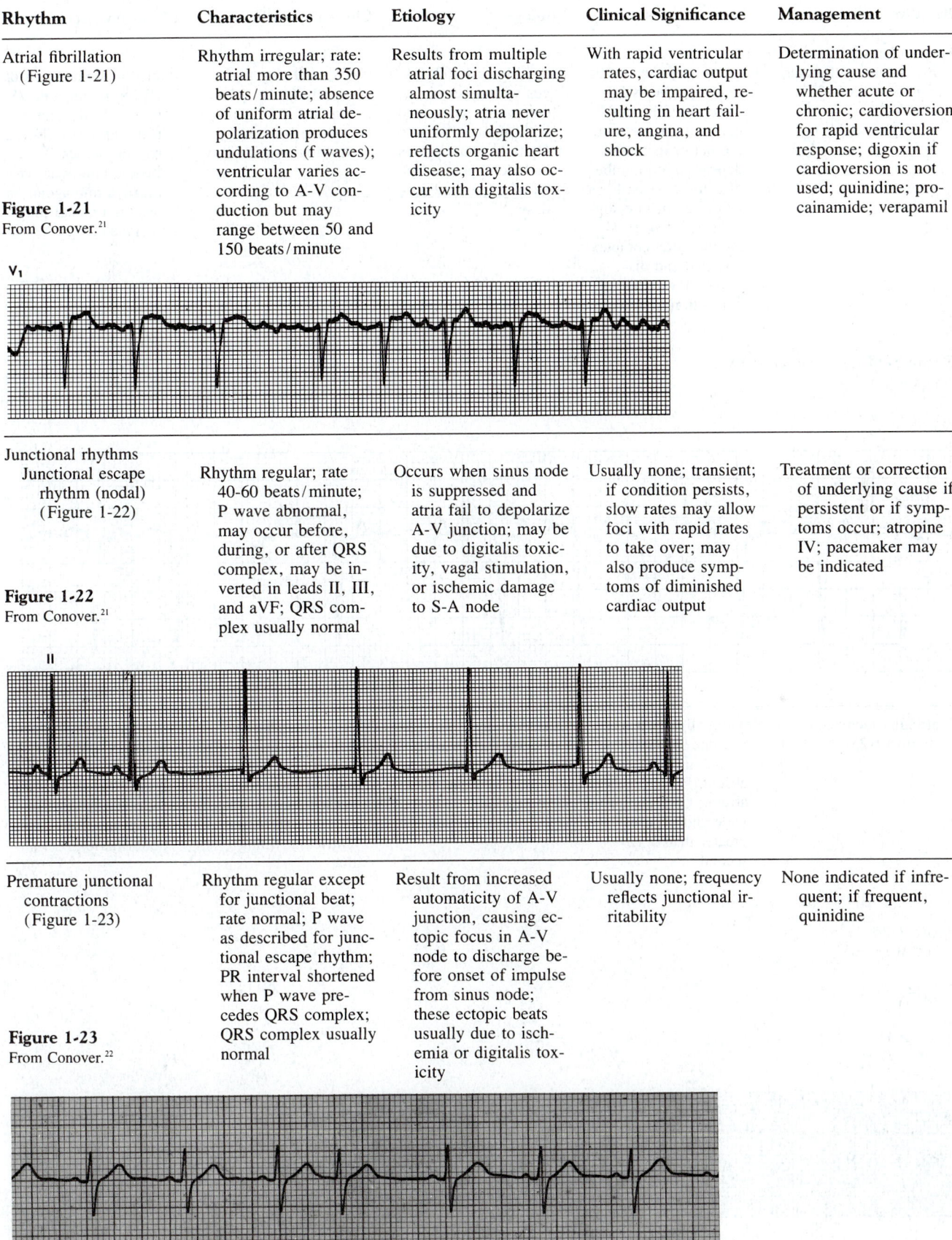

V1

Rhythm	Characteristics	Etiology	Clinical Significance	Management
Junctional rhythms Junctional escape rhythm (nodal) (Figure 1-22)	Rhythm regular; rate 40-60 beats/minute; P wave abnormal, may occur before, during, or after QRS complex, may be inverted in leads II, III, and aVF; QRS complex usually normal	Occurs when sinus node is suppressed and atria fail to depolarize A-V junction; may be due to digitalis toxicity, vagal stimulation, or ischemic damage to S-A node	Usually none; transient; if condition persists, slow rates may allow foci with rapid rates to take over; may also produce symptoms of diminished cardiac output	Treatment or correction of underlying cause if persistent or if symptoms occur; atropine IV; pacemaker may be indicated

Figure 1-22
From Conover.[21]

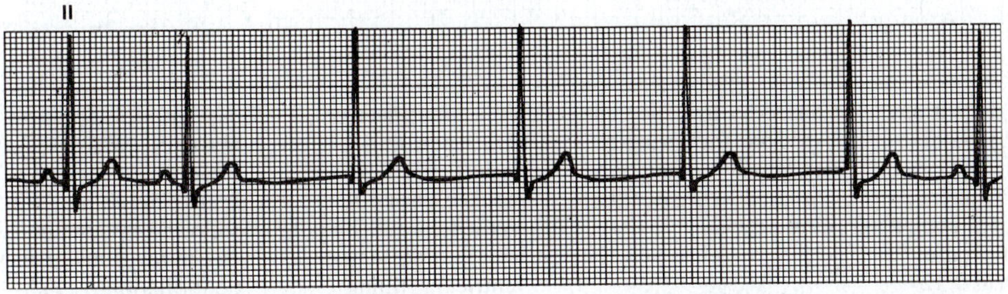

II

Rhythm	Characteristics	Etiology	Clinical Significance	Management
Premature junctional contractions (Figure 1-23)	Rhythm regular except for junctional beat; rate normal; P wave as described for junctional escape rhythm; PR interval shortened when P wave precedes QRS complex; QRS complex usually normal	Result from increased automaticity of A-V junction, causing ectopic focus in A-V node to discharge before onset of impulse from sinus node; these ectopic beats usually due to ischemia or digitalis toxicity	Usually none; frequency reflects junctional irritability	None indicated if infrequent; if frequent, quinidine

Figure 1-23
From Conover.[22]

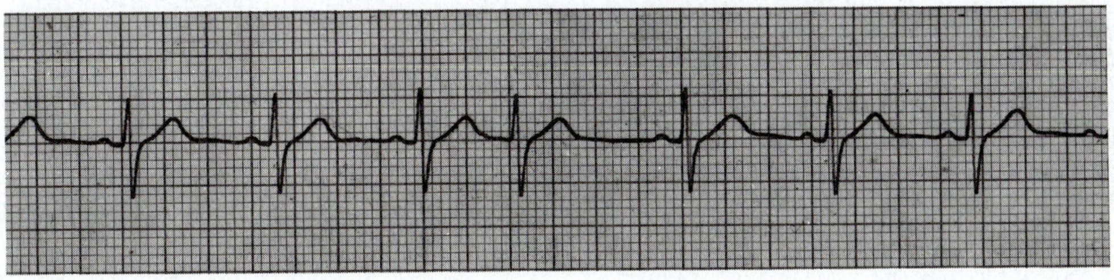

Rhythm	Characteristics	Etiology	Clinical Significance	Management
Ventricular arrhythmias				
Premature ventricular contractions (PVCs) (Figure 1-24)	Rhythm irregular owing to ectopic beats followed by full compensatory pause; rate normal or increased depending on number of ectopic beats; P wave absent in ectopic beat; PR interval absent; QRS complex widened and distorted; T wave is in opposition to R wave	Caused by irritable focus within ventricle, commonly associated with myocardial infarction; other causes include hypoxia, hypocalcemia, and acidosis	PVCs occurring frequently (more than 6/minute) or in pairs indicate increased ventricular irritability	Aimed at suppression of PVCs; if frequent, IV bolus of lidocaine (50-100 mg) followed by continuous IV infusion; additional antiarrhythmic agents in classes I and II may be given

Figure 1-24 Left ventricular PVC.
From Conover.[21]

V_1

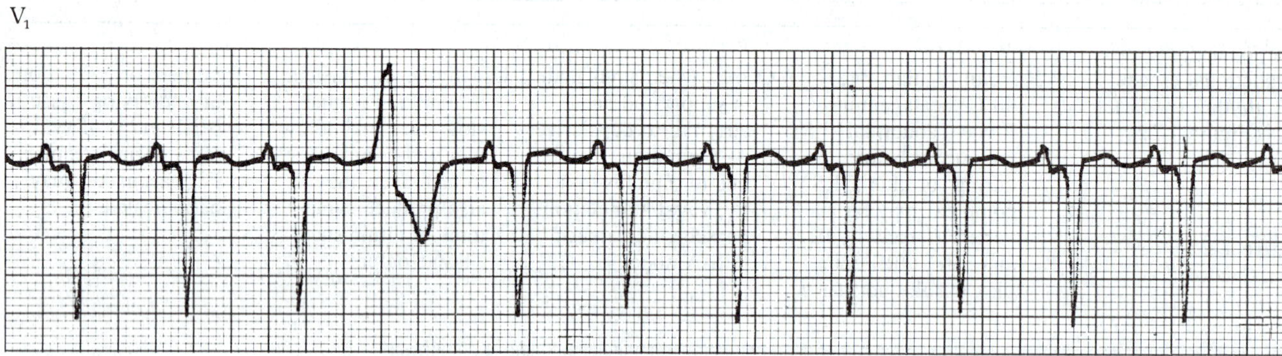

Rhythm	Characteristics	Etiology	Clinical Significance	Management
Ventricular tachycardia (Figure 1-25)	Rhythm slightly irregular; rate 100-200 beats/minute; P wave absent; PR interval absent; QRS complex wide and bizarre, greater than 0.12 second	Caused by irritable ventricular foci firing repetitively; commonly caused by myocardial infarction	Often a forerunner of ventricular fibrillation; if persistent and rapid, causes decreased cardiac output owing to decreased ventricular filling time	Most episodes terminate abruptly without treatment; lidocaine bolus 75-100 mg IV followed by continuous intravenous drip; defibrillation

Figure 1-25
From Conover.[22]

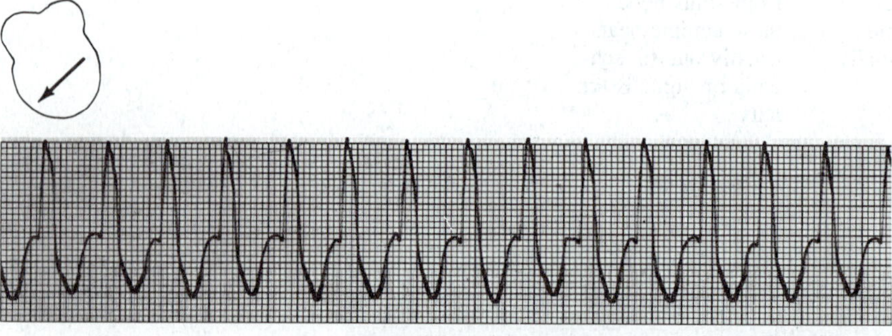

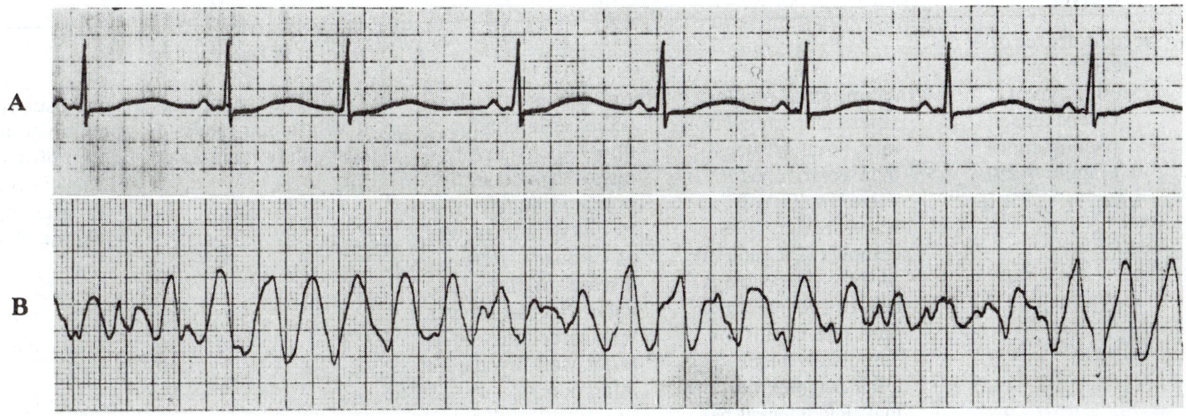

Rhythm	Characteristics	Etiology	Clinical Significance	Management
Torsades de pointes (polymorphous ventricular tachycardia) (Figure 1-26)	Atypical ventricular tachycardia occurring in setting of delayed repolarization (prolonged QT interval); rhythm regular or irregular; ventricular rate, 150-300 beats/minute; PR interval not measurable; QRS complex wide and bizarre in configuration lasting >0.12 second; amplitude and direction of QRS complex vary; QT interval during baseline rhythm >0.46 second or >33% of baseline; T wave during baseline rhythm very broad and flat	Drug toxicity (e.g., quinidine, procainamide, amiodarone); electrolyte imbalance (e.g., hypokalemia, hypomagnesemia)	Palpitations, which may lead to faintness, syncope; often forerunner of ventricular fibrillation and sudden death	Treatment initiated only if QT prolonged; if present, temporary overdrive ventricular or atrial pacing; IV magnesium sulfate: IV push 2 g over 1-2 min, IV infusion 1-2 g for 4-6 h
Ventricular fibrillation (Figure 1-27)	Rhythm irregular; rate: rapid repetitive waves or undulations that have no uniformity and are coarse or fine; P wave, QRS complex, and T wave cannot be identified	Lethal arrhythmia resulting from electrical stimulation of ventricular muscle, which leads to abrupt cessation of effective blood flow; occurs in severely damaged hearts as with ischemia, drug toxicity, trauma, or contact with high-voltage electricity	Loss of consciousness; decreases in blood pressure and peripheral pulse owing to loss of cardiac output	Cardiopulmonary resuscitation; defibrillation

Figure 1-26 Torsade de pointes. **A,** Sinus rhythm. T waves are flat, and QT interval is prolonged. Patient's serum potassium level was 3.1 mEq/L. **B,** Taken next day, characteristic torsade.
Courtesy Dr. Daniel H. Schwartz, South Fallsburg, N.Y. From Goldberger.[34]

Figure 1-27
From Conover.[22]

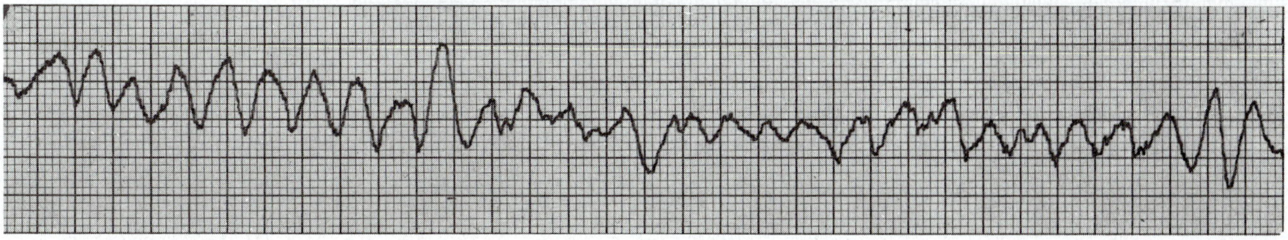

Rhythm	Characteristics	Etiology	Clinical Significance	Management
Conduction disturbances				
First-degree A-V heart block (Figure 1-28)	Rhythm regular; rate normal; P wave normal; PR interval prolonged to greater than 0.2 second; QRS complex normal	Represents delay in impulse conduction through A-V node; occurs as result of increased vagal tone, digoxin administration, or congenital anomalies	No associated symptoms	None indicated; digitalis discontinued if causative factor; observation for development of further A-V block

Figure 1-28
From Conover.[22]

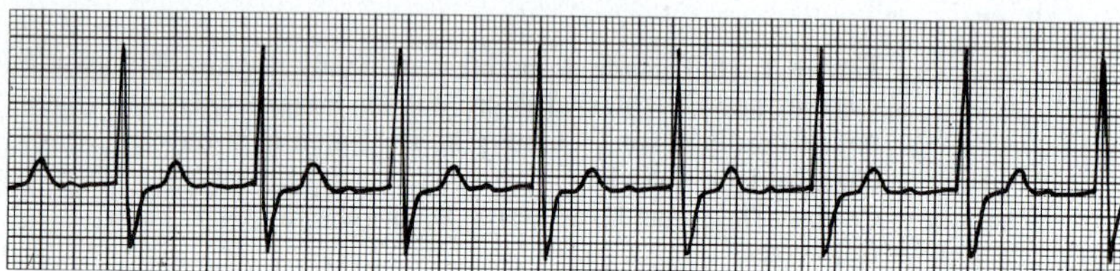

Rhythm	Characteristics	Etiology	Clinical Significance	Management
Second-degree A-V heart block Mobitz type I (Wenckebach phenomenon) (Figure 1-29)	Rhythm: atrial regular, ventricular irregular; rate: atrial greater than ventricular; P wave: multiple P waves before QRS complex; PR interval: progressive prolongation of PR interval until one impulse is completely blocked; QRS complex normal; RR interval becomes progressively shortened until one QRS complex is dropped	Represents progressive decrease in conduction velocity involving A-V node and proximal bundle of His; occurs as result of coronary artery disease, digitalis toxicity, rheumatic fever, viral infections, or inferior wall myocardial infarction	No associated symptoms if ventricular rate is adequately maintained	None usually indicated; elimination or correction of underlying cause; observation for progression to higher degree of block

Figure 1-29
From Conover.[20]

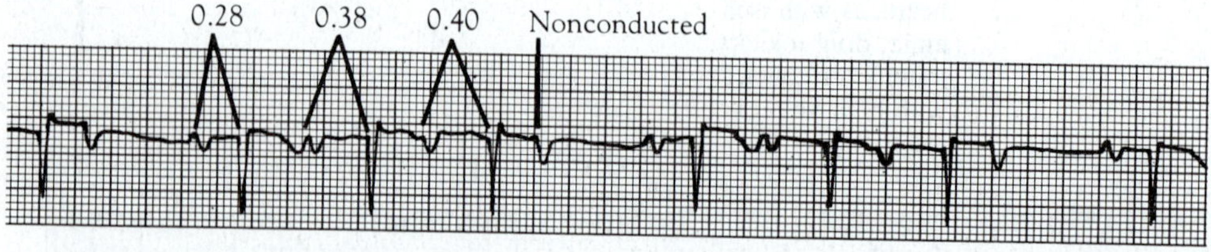

Rhythm	Characteristics	Etiology	Clinical Significance	Management
Mobitz type II (Figure 1-30)	Rhythm: atrial regular, ventricular varies; rate: atrial slow to normal, ventricular may be slow, usually half or one-third atrial rate; P wave normal, occurring in multiples before QRS complex; PR interval normal or slightly prolonged, always constant; QRS complex normal or slightly prolonged	Represents block of impulse below level of A-V node and within His-Purkinje system; occurs as result of ischemia, digitalis or quinidine toxicity, anterior wall myocardial infarction	No associated symptoms if ventricular rate is adequately maintained; if rate is slow, cardiac output may be impaired, causing dizziness and weakness	Correction or elimination of underlying cause; tends to be recurrent, may progress to complete heart block; transvenous demand pacing may be required

Figure 1-30
From Conover.[21]

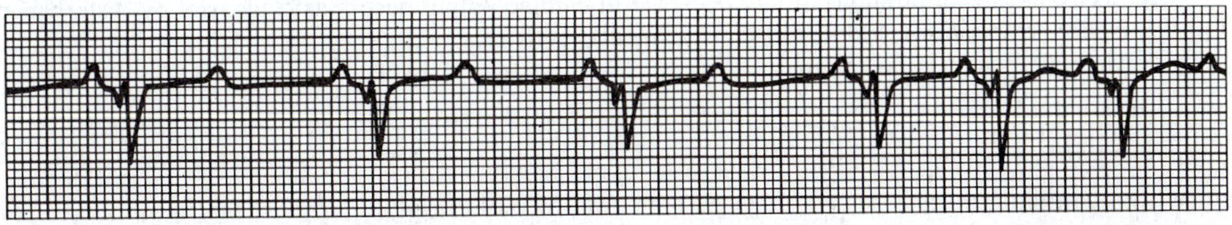

Rhythm	Characteristics	Etiology	Clinical Significance	Management
Third-degree A-V block (complete heart block) (Figure 1-31)	Rhythm: atrial and ventricular regular but act independent of each other; rate: atrial 60-90 beats/minute, ventricular 30-40 beats/minute; P wave normal but occurs in greater frequency than QRS complex; PR interval: no relationship with QRS complex, therefore never constant; QRS complex normal if ventricular depolarization initiated by junctional escape pacemaker, widened if depolarization initiated by ventricular pacemaker low in conduction system	Represents failure of A-V node to conduct impulse to ventricles; block may occur at any point in conduction system at or below level of A-V node; occurs as result of coronary artery disease, degenerative fibrosis of conduction system, congenital anomalies, myocarditis, drug toxicity (digitalis, quinidine, procainamide, verapamil), trauma	Symptoms associated with low cardiac output owing to slow ventricular rates; include syncope and signs of ventricular failure	Transvenous demand pacing; while awaiting pacemaker insertion, isoproterenol infusion to accelerate ventricular rate

Figure 1-31
From Andreoli.[5]

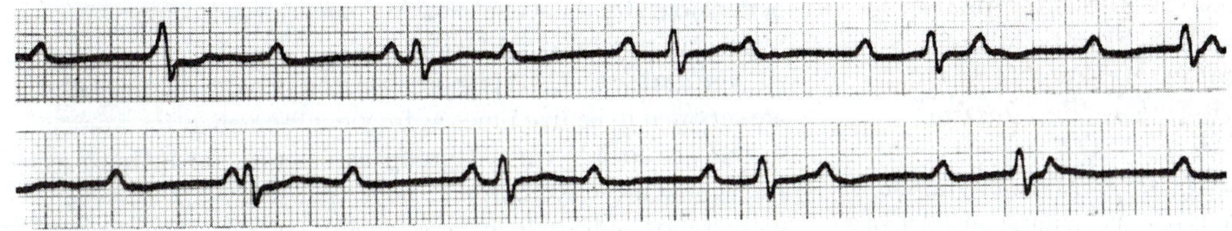

Nursing Dx & Intervention

Nursing Diagnosis	Nursing Intervention/Rationale
Anxiety related to altered heart action in response to perceived or actual threat to biologic integrity	• Assess degree of anxiety, level of understanding, and fears associated with arrhythmias and treatment. • Provide continual explanations for the various monitoring devices in use. • Promote physical rest *to reduce cardiac workload by maintaining bed rest, scheduled naptimes, and assistance with activities of daily living.* • Administer oxygen therapy *to increase cardiac oxygenation.* • Offer reassurance. • Administer sedation as ordered *to reduce anxiety and to promote rest.*
Decreased cardiac output	• Assess and monitor patient continuously *to determine cardiac rate, rhythm, and level of consciousness.* • Monitor vital signs frequently, according to policy and patient's condition. • Initiate prompt treatment of life-threatening arrhythmias per protocol: cardiopulmonary resuscitation (CPR), appropriate drug therapy, and preparation for pacemaker insertion. • Continue to monitor and record changes in ECG tracings. • Notify physician promptly if any decrease in cardiac output occurs as evidenced by disturbance in rate, respirations, blood pressure, or mental activity. • Maintain patent IV as ordered.

Patient Education

Instruction for a patient with a cardiac arrhythmia begins with the initial phase of care, whether in a coronary care unit or in an outpatient setting. The following points should be included:

1. Brief description of the disease etiology, rhythm disturbances, and associated symptoms
2. Explanation of any diagnostic or therapeutic procedures that are planned
3. Explanation of monitoring equipment that may be used
4. Dietary restrictions that may be prescribed; need to avoid caffeine and nicotine
5. Instructions regarding drug therapy, its purpose, desired effects, dosage, and side effects to report to the physician
6. Explanation and method of taking pulse

Evaluation

Patient Outcome	Data Indicating That Outcome is Reached
Heart returns to baseline rhythm.	ECG tracing reflects baseline rhythm. Blood pressure and heart rate are within normal limits. There is no ectopy.
Cardiac output is adequate to maintain cerebral perfusion.	Patient is alert and has no dizziness, syncopal episodes, or chest pains. Vital signs are stable. Peripheral perfusion is good.
Anxiety level is reduced.	Patient demonstrates decreased anxiety. Patient appears relaxed, with decreased tension. Patient verbalizes fears and asks questions.

Coronary artery disease

Coronary artery disease (CAD) is a disorder of the coronary arteries that disrupts blood supply to the myocardium. Permanent disruption of blood flow causes myocardial dysfunction, including sudden death.

The rate and severity of CAD vary considerably among world populations. Serious study of the natural history of CAD began in 1950 with the Framingham study and other projects.[49] The data collected in these early studies established certain factors related to the incidence and progression of coronary atherosclerotic disease. These include age, sex, hypertension, lipid levels, obesity, smoking, sedentary life-style, and psychosocial factors.

Age and sex. CAD is more common in older men. Deaths are reported to be five times as frequent for men as for women in the 35- to 40-year-old group and two to three times as frequent in those 60 years and older. In recent years, however, these ratios appear to have changed, probably because of changes in women's life-styles and an increase in smoking and the use of contraceptives. CAD in persons less than 30

Cardiovascular Risk Factor Profile

Family history of heart disease	Elevated serum level of lipids and fats
Sex	Diabetes mellitus
Males (35-55 years)	Physical inactivity; sedentary life-style
Females (>50 years or after menopause)	Stress
Hypertension	For women <50 years: use of estrogen (i.e., birth control pills) and smoking
Smoking	
Overweight/obesity	

From Tucker.[104]

years of age is usually linked to hyperlipidemia, hypertension, and smoking.

Hypertension. Although systolic hypertension is closely linked to cardiovascular disease, elevated systolic and diastolic pressures are associated with ischemic heart disease. Systolic pressures greater than 160 mm Hg or diastolic pressures greater than 95 mm Hg are considered a high risk factor for heart attacks, particularly in younger persons.[74]

Lipid levels. Of the various types of circulating lipoproteins, cholesterol and triglycerides are most commonly linked to CAD. Hyperlipidemia may be a primary disorder or may occur as a result of diabetes, myxedema, or alcoholism. Lipoproteins can now be broken down and measured separately to determine levels of those that are atherogenic. Low-density lipids (LDLs) carry a high percentage of cholesterol in plasma and in high levels help produce atheromas. High-density lipids (HDLs), however, are mostly protein and carry a smaller percentage of cholesterol, thereby helping to remove lipids from the cell through liver metabolism. Recent studies show that the ratio of HDLs to LDLs is lower in patients with CAD and that a high ratio of HDLs helps reduce vascular disease. HDLs are formed through exercise, fat-controlled diets, and estrogens.[11]

Obesity. Studies have shown that an increased food intake can elevate LDLs. Obese people tend to have hypertension and glucose intolerance.

Smoking. Cigarette smoking is now clearly linked to heart disease. Primarily through adrenergic stimulation, nicotine contributes to increases in heart rate, stroke volume, cardiac output, and blood pressure. Nicotine also causes peripheral vasoconstriction and in persons with decreased blood flow enhances ischemic changes. Smoking decreases the threshold for ventricular fibrillation because it interferes with oxygen binding with hemoglobin, thus slowing the diffusion of oxygen into mitochondria.

Sedentary life-style. Although the positive effects of exercise on the risk of CAD are difficult to assess, studies show that people who exercise heavily are at a decreased risk of having CAD. Inactivity is associated with decreases in HDLs.

Psychosocial factors. A person with a type A personality is at great risk of having CAD. This type of person is usually aggressive, competitive, and rushed. When the type A personality is combined with other risk factors such as age, high lipid levels, and smoking, the risk of heart disease may increase.

Other risk factors. Other factors have also been linked to heart disease, including diabetes, genetic factors, and oral contraceptives.

For reasons not understood, patients with diabetes have a high risk of CAD. The role of heredity is also unclear. Apparently a tendency toward hypertension, hyperlipidemia, and diabetes exists in some families. Whether the tendency is inherited or simply the result of life-style patterns is unknown. Oral contraceptives have been linked to CAD when taken by women 45 years or younger. This finding results from studies that show high serum cholesterol and triglyceride levels in women taking oral contraceptives.[4]

Pathophysiology

Atherosclerosis, the basic underlying disease affecting coronary lumen size, is marked by changes in the intimal lining of the arteries. It begins as an irregular thickening process producing fatty streaks. This becomes a more severe form combining large amounts of lipids with collagen to produce fibroblasts that lead to fibrous atherosclerotic plaques.

The severity of the disease is measured by the degree of obstruction within each artery, as well as the number of vessels involved. Obstructions of more than 75% of the lumen of one or more of the three coronary arteries increase the risk of death. The annual death rate of persons with one-vessel disease is 1% to 3%. Three-vessel disease increases the risk to 10% to 15%. Among people with 75% obstruction of the left main artery, however, the annual death rate is 30% to 40%.

Myocardial Perfusion

The basic physiologic changes resulting from the atherosclerotic process are problems of myocardial oxygen supply and demand. When myocardial oxygen demand exceeds the supply provided by the coronary arteries, ischemia results. Myocardial metabolism is oxygen dependent (aerobic), extracting up to 80% of the oxygen from the coronary blood supply. Blood flow to the myocardium occurs mainly during diastole. Factors influencing supply include cardiac output, intramyocardial tension, aortic pressure, and coronary artery resistance. Coronary blood flow can be increased by raising the cardiac output and aortic pressure and lowering coronary artery resistance and intramyocardial tension.

Factors determining myocardial oxygen demand are heart rate, myocardial wall tension, and contractile state of the myocardium. As the heart rate increases, so does the demand for oxygen to the myocardial cells. Myocardial wall tension occurs during contraction and is influenced by ventricular and systolic (arterial) pressure. Myocardial contractility is stimulated by the release of catecholamines or sympathetic stimulation. These increase wall tension and thus energy or oxygen demands.

Myocardial ischemia is the result of impaired myocardial perfusion. Coronary atherosclerotic heart disease is the cause of myocardial ischemia. Obstruction varies in degree and may be well tolerated as long as myocardial oxygen demand is low. As the demand increases and the obstruction persists or advances, ischemic changes result. Coronary blood vessel distribution is also important in providing oxygen to the myocardium. The coronary arteries sit on the epicardial surface of the heart. Blood travels in toward the endocardium. The inner subendocardial layers of the myocardium therefore are particularly at risk for ischemia. Increases in heart rate and wall tension can reduce flow to the endocardium.

The coronary arteries also supply major conduction structures within the myocardium. The right coronary artery (RCA) supplies the sinus node in 55% to 60% of persons. In the remainder it is supplied by a branch of the circumflex artery. The RCA also supplies the A-V node in 85% of persons. The remaining 15% is supplied by the left coronary artery (LCA). The septum is supplied mainly by the left anterior descending (LAD) artery, although part of the posterior wall is supplied by the RCA. An obstruction of any of the major arteries or their branches results in ischemia to the portion of myocardium supplied by that vessel. Obstruction of the LAD results in ischemic changes of the anterior wall of the ventricle. RCA obstruction results in infarction and ischemia of the right ventricle. The degree of obstruction and number of coronary arteries involved influence how serious the disease will be. CAD is described as single-, double-, or triple-vessel disease. When a major obstruction occurs in the first branch of the LCA or the left main artery before bifurcation, the risk for a major infarction and death rises. This is called left main disease.

The major signs of ischemia are chest pain and ECG changes. Other symptoms result from compromised cardiac function.

Angina Pectoris

The term "angina pectoris," which means chest pain, is used to describe pain as a symptom of myocardial ischemia. Myocardial ischemia is the result of an imbalance between myocardial oxygen supply and demand. It occurs most often with coronary atherosclerosis but can also occur in patients with normal coronary arteries. For example, patients with aortic stenosis, hypertension, and hypertrophic cardiomyopathy may have symptoms of angina pectoris. In these patients myocardial work is increased, but perfusion of the hypertrophied muscle is inadequate. This results in myocardial ischemia despite normal coronary arteries.

Various terms have been used to describe the many syndromes linked to myocardial ischemia. The following describe chest pain that is transient and linked to myocardial ischemia.

Stable angina pectoris is marked by chest discomfort caused by effort, with or without radiation, that lasts from a few seconds to 15 minutes. It is generally relieved by rest and the removal of provoking factors or by sublingual vasodilators.

Unstable angina pectoris is marked by pain that lasts longer, occurs more often, and may be caused by factors other than effort. Various names used to describe this syndrome include crescendo angina, preinfarction angina, angina decubitus, and noctural angina.

Variant (Prinzmetal's) angina is marked by chest pain that occurs at rest and is often linked to ST elevations on the ECG. The underlying cause is thought to be coronary artery spasm. Unlike angina pectoris, variant angina is caused by a sudden reduction in coronary blood flow brought on by the spasm and not by an increase in myocardial oxygen demand. The decrease in oxygen consumption occurring during sleep or rest may lead to coronary artery vasoconstriction and may be the cause of the spasm.[114]

Some have suggested a link between the spasm and stimulation of α (vasoconstriction) and β (vasodilation) adrenergic receptors.[114] Others have suggested various mechanisms involved in the cause of spasm, including parasympathetic nervous system activity[114] and possibly local abnormalities of vascular smooth muscle.[12]

Myocardial Infarction

Myocardial infarction is the development of ischemia and necrosis of myocardial tissue. It results from a sudden decrease in coronary perfusion or an increase in myocardial oxygen demand without adequate coronary perfusion.

Two types of infarction have been described. Subendocardial infarction is generally confined to small areas of myocardium. It is usually within the subendocardial wall of the left ventricle, the ventricular septum, and papillary muscles. Transmural, or full-thickness, infarction is widespread myocardial necrosis, extending from the endocardium to the epicardium.

Myocardial tissue death is usually preceded by sudden occlusion of a major coronary artery. Coronary thrombosis is the most common cause of infarction, but other factors may be responsible. These include coronary artery spasm, platelet aggregation and embolism from a mural thrombus, a thrombus on a prosthetic mitral or aortic valve, or a dislodged calcium plaque from a calcified aortic or mitral valve.

Persistent cellular ischemia interferes with myocardial tissue metabolism, causing a rapid development of permanent cell damage. At first there are three zones of tissue damage. The first is a central area of necrotic myocardial cells, capillaries, and connective tissue. Surrounding this tissue is a second zone of "injured" cells that are potentially viable if enough circulation is quickly restored. The third zone, characterized by ischemia, is also viable and can be expected to recover unless the ischemia persists or worsens. The severity or extension of a myocardial infarction often depends on the fate of the injured and ischemic zones. Ischemia may progress to necrosis if untreated. Because the infarction process may take up to 6 hours to complete, restoration of adequate myocardial perfusion is important to limit necrosis.

Diagnostic Studies and Findings

Study	Stable Angina Pectoris	Variant (Prinzmetal's) Angina	Unstable Angina Pectoris	Myocardial Infarction
Electrocardiogram (ECG)	Changes usually seen during anginal episodes; 50%-70% of patients have normal ECG during pain-free episodes; ischemia determined by horizontal ST segment or down-sloping with depression of 1 mm; T wave inversion represents impaired repolarization caused by ischemia	Ischemia appears as ST elevation during anginal attack but regresses as pain subsides; ECG changes may be seen before patient complains of chest pain or may be recorded in absence of pain; A-V conduction defects may occur, particularly when right coronary artery is involved, and include Mobitz type II and complete A-V block; ventricular irritability such as premature ventricular contractions, ventricular tachycardia, or fibrillation can occur, particularly during ischemic attack	Ischemia determined by horizontal ST segment or downsloping with depression of 1 mm; T wave inversion represents impaired repolarization caused by ischemia; ventricular irritability such as premature ventricular contractions, ventricular tachycardia, or fibrillation	Changes are evolutionary and indicate progression of infarction; in acute stage, ST elevations with subsequent T wave inversion and Q wave formation; Q waves indicate necrosis and are considered pathologic if they are 0.04 second or greater in duration, 0.4 mm or greater in depth, or present in leads that do not normally have Q waves; ST elevations reflect myocardial injury that interferes with polarization of cells, are seen in leads facing injured area, and return to normal (isoelectric) within days; ST elevations beyond 4-6 weeks should raise suspicion of ventricular aneurysm; infarction location determined by identifying leads that demonstrate characteristic ECG changes; such leads are those with positive terminals that face injured site of heart; reciprocal changes, seen in leads that face *opposite* surface of damaged heart, are absence of Q wave, increase in R wave amplitude, depressed ST segment, upright tall T wave
Laboratory tests Enzymes	No elevation; checked to rule out myocardial infarction	No elevation; checked to rule out myocardial infarction	No elevation; checked to rule out myocardial infarction	*Onset* / *Peak* / *Return to normal* SGOT: 6-12 hours / 36 hours / 5-7 days CPK-MB: 4-12 hours / 24 hours / 3-4 days LDH (isoenzyme): 24-48 hours / 3-6 days / 8-14 days
Complete blood count (CBC)	No elevation; checked to rule out anemia-induced angina	No elevation; checked to rule out anemia-induced angina	No elevation; checked to rule out anemia-induced angina	Elevated white count (WBC) and erythrocyte sedimentation rate (ESR) reflect myocardial damage

Continued.

Diagnostic Studies and Findings—cont'd

Study	Stable Angina Pectoris	Variant (Prinzmetal's) Angina	Unstable Angina Pectoris	Myocardial Infarction
Glucose	No elevation	No elevation	No elevation	Transiently elevated owing to adrenergic response
Lipid levels (triglycerides, cholesterol, high- and low-density lipids)	Checked to determine any lipoprotein abnormalities	Checked to rule out presence of atherosclerotic process	Checked to determine any lipoprotein abnormalities	Checked to determine any lipoprotein abnormalities
Exercise stress test (EST)	Chest pain; horizontal ST segment or downsloping of 1 mm or more; failure of systolic blood pressure to rise or drop; ST elevations	Normal stress test done to differentiate between variant and classic angina; ST elevation with or without associated chest pain occasionally develops	As in stable angina pectoris; should not be done until patient has been stable and pain free for 24 hours	Not done in presence of documented myocardial infarction; low-level test may be performed before discharge from hospital
Thallium-201 scintigraphy	Ischemic areas appear as "cold" areas, reflecting reduced thallium uptake; when ischemia relieved, "cold" areas show normal thallium uptake		Similar to stable angina pectoris	Similar to stable angina pectoris; used to confirm diagnosis; with decreased blood flow an area of decreased activity is visualized
Radionuclide blood pool imaging with technetium-99 m				Confirms myocardial damage by localizing and permitting estimation of size of transmural infarction; must be done within 2-6 days after acute infarction; determines wall motion abnormalities; permits estimation of ventricular function by determining ejection fractions
Cardiac catheterization and coronary angiography	Determines number and location of obstructive lesions, "graftability" of artery distal to obstructive lesion, and ventricular function	Distinguishes spasm in normal coronary arteries from those with severe obstructive lesions; intravenous injection of ergonovine maleate provokes coronary artery spasm in patients with variant angina	As in stable angina pectoris	Generally not performed as diagnostic procedure during acute period; procedures used in the administration of thrombolysis or percutaneous angioplasty

Medical Plan

Surgery

Coronary artery bypass grafting (CABG)—only direct method of increasing myocardial coronary blood flow; provides symptomatic relief in 80% of patients with significant angina and has low operative mortality
 Indications: Disabling angina that is refractory to medical therapy, significantly abnormal ECG response to exercise, 50% or greater obstruction of left main coronary artery, and significant obstructive lesions in all three coronary arteries (see p. 90 for care of patients undergoing open-heart surgery)

Percutaneous transluminal coronary angioplasty (PTCA)—alternative approach to coronary artery bypass surgery in selected patients; attempts to restore luminal patency by compressing atheromatous plaques
 Indications: Single-vessel disease in which there are high degree of stenosis, good left ventricular function, and recent onset of angina refractory to medical therapy

Thrombolytic therapy (intracoronary thrombolysis)—nonsurgical reperfusion procedure used in treatment of acute transmural myocardial infarction; purpose is to interrupt evolution of myocardial ischemia to necrosis and to limit infarction size; improvement of ischemic area can be achieved if therapy is initiated within 4 to 6 hours from onset of infarction (see p. 115 for care of patients undergoing thrombolytic therapy)
 Indications: Chest pain not relieved by nitroglycerin, 4 hours from onset of chest pain, and ST elevations with reciprocal ECG changes

Medications

Vasodilators
 Nitrates
  Short-acting nitrates: Sublingual nitroglycerin (0.4-0.6 mg); isosorbide dinitrate (5 mg)
   Duration of action: ½-2 h
  Long-acting oral nitrates: Isosorbide dinitrate (10-20 mg qid)
  Topical 2% nitroglycerin ointment (1-2 inches q4-6h)
   Duration of action: Up to 6 h or longer

β-Adrenergic blocking agents
 Propranolol (Inderal)
  Usual dosage: 10-20 mg po tid or qid; IV 1 mg/min not exceeding 3-5 mg
 Nadolol (Corgard)
  Indications: Treatment of angina and hypertension
  Usual dosage: 40-80 mg po up to 240 mg/d as necessary
  Duration of action: About 20-24 h
 Timolol (Blocadren)
  Indications: Reduction of mortality and reinfarction after myocardial infarctions; hypertension
  Usual dosage: 20-60 mg bid
 Atenolol (Tenormin)
  Indications: Approved for use of hypertension but may have potential use in treating angina and reducing infarct size
  Usual dosage: 50-100 mg/d

Calcium antagonists
 Nifedipine (Procardia)
  Indications: Angina pectoris caused by coronary artery spasm, chronic stable angina pectoris
  Usual dosage: 10 mg po; sublingual 10-40 mg q8h (not to exceed 180 mg); IV 5-15 mg/kg
 Verapamil (Calan, Isoptin)
  Usual dosage: 80-160 mg q8h (not to exceed 480 mg/d); IV 0.075-0.15 mg/kg (not to exceed 15 mg/30 min)
  Indications: Treatment of angina pectoris and coronary artery spasm
 Diltiazem (Cardizem)
  Indications: Treatment of variant angina
  Usual dosage: Initially 30 mg po qid, increasing gradually to 80 mg tid (total 240 mg/d)

Antihyperlipidemic agents—interfere with reabsorption of cholesterol and lower triglyceride levels
 Lovastatin (Mevacor)
  Usual dosage: 20 mg po bid
 Cholestyramine (Questran)
  Usual dosage: 8-12 g bid
 Neomycin sulfate
  Usual dosage: 0.5-2 g/d
 Clofibrate (Atromid-S)
  Usual dosage: 0.5 g tid
 Gemfibrozil (Lopid)
  Usual dosage: 0.6 g bid
 Niacin (nicotinic acid)
  Usual dosage: 0.5-1 g tid

Streptokinase
 Indications: Used in early myocardial infarction (within 4-6 h of onset) to restore myocardial oxygen supply, thereby preserving myocardium and limiting infarct size
 Usual dosage: 500,000-1.7 million U over 30-60 min

Antiplatelet agents
 Aspirin (acetylsalicylic acid, ASA)
  Indications: Used in setting of coronary artery thrombosis and in the prevention of further atherogenesis; because of possible beneficial effects, may be used in patients with unstable angina syndrome and myocardial infarction
  Usual dosage: 325-1300 mg/d

Dipyridamole (Persantine, Persantin)
 Indications: Used in combination with aspirin to maintain patency of saphenous vein coronary artery bypass grafts
 Usual dosage: 100 mg tid 1 h before meal (with ASA, 325 mg tid after meals)

General Management

Cardiovascular monitoring—used to assess and monitor for signs of life-threatening complications associated with severe myocardial ischemia and necrosis, including arrhythmias, heart failure, extension of myocardial infarction (MI), cardiogenic shock, ventricular or papillary muscle rupture, and ventricular aneurysm; complications occur within first 5 days in half of patients with acute MI; early detection depends on careful and frequent continuous monitoring of various hemodynamic parameters and clinical status that reflect left ventricular function: arterial pressure, pulmonary artery pressure (PAP), pulmonary capillary wedge pressure (PCWP)

Electrocardiogram (ECG)—used to detect changes in heart rhythms and to determine serial changes reflective of myocardial ischemia, injury, or extension of MI

Intra-aortic balloon counterpulsation (IABP)—used mainly in patients with acute myocardial infarction to protect ischemic myocardium by decreasing preload, afterload, and myocardial oxygen demand; diastolic pressure is supported, thus improving coronary perfusion and cardiac output; most successful in patients who are treated less than 6 hours after infarction, are undergoing their first MI, and have no aortic insufficiency (see p. 106 for specific care)

Admission to coronary care unit (CCU) or coronary observation unit—indicated for patients with acute chest pain for evaluation, surveillance, and management

Diet

Admission diet—depends on clinical status; during acute phase, patient may be permitted nothing by mouth (NPO) or receive clear liquids progressing to 1500-calorie, soft, low-fat, no-added-salt diet; iced beverages limited to 600 to 800 ml[57]; caffeine, a cardiac stimulant, restricted because it lowers threshold for certain arrhythmias[43,89]

Discharge diet—dependent on several factors including cholesterol and triglyceride levels, total body weight, and clinical status; American Heart Association suggests diet of reduced saturated fats, cholesterol, restriction of sodium, and limiting total caloric consumption to maintain ideal body weight[4]

Oxygenation—patients evaluated early for hypoxemia, which may result from ventilation-perfusion abnormalities; providing additional inspired oxygen to patient in absence of hypoxemia does not ensure increased oxygen delivery to myocardium and may rarely increase systemic vascular resistance and arterial pressure, with subsequent decrease in cardiac output and oxygen delivery to tissues; arterial oxygen tension (PaO_2) should be measured on admission to coronary care unit; if normal, oxygen therapy may be omitted; hypoxemic patients should receive oxygen therapy as required; serial arterial blood gas determinations to monitor effectiveness of therapy.

NURSING CARE

Nursing Assessment

Area of Concern	Stable Angina Pectoris	Variant (Prinzmetal's) Angina	Unstable Angina Pectoris	Myocardial Infarction
Chest pain				
Quality	Aching, sharp, tingling, or burning sensation or pressure	Similar to stable angina pectoris	Similar to stable angina pectoris but may be more severe	Crushing, squeezing, stabbing, oppressive sensation or as if heavy object is sitting on chest
Location and radiation	Substernal with radiation to left shoulder, down inner aspect of left arm or both arms; neck, jaw, and scapula may be additional sites of radiation	Similar to stable angina pectoris	Similar to stable angina pectoris	Retrosternal and left precordial radiating down left arm and to neck, jaws, teeth, epigastric area, and back
Precipitating factors	Onset classically associated with exercise or activities that increase myocardial oxygen demand, e.g., physical exercise, heavy lifting, emotional stress, cold temperatures	Onset at rest; pain is cyclic, often occurring during sleep	Pain may be brought on with less than usual exertion; may occur at rest	May occur at rest or during exertion

Area of Concern	Stable Angina Pectoris	Variant (Prinzmetal's) Angina	Unstable Angina Pectoris	Myocardial Infarction
Duration and alleviating factors	3-15 minutes; relieved by rest, stopping pain-inducing activities, taking sublingual nitroglycerin (NTG) tablet	Characteristically, pain intensifies quickly, tends to last longer than angina, and subsides with exercise	Prolonged and not usually as quickly relieved by rest or taking NTG	Described as continuous, lasting more than 30 minutes, unrelieved by rest, position change, or taking NTG tablets
Associated signs and symptoms	During anginal attack, dyspnea, anxiety, diaphoresis, cool clammy skin	Similar to stable angina pectoris	Similar to stable angina pectoris but symptoms may be more prominent and may persist; may be associated with nausea	Anxiety, restlessness, weakness, associated profuse diaphoresis, dyspnea, dizziness; signs of vasomotor response including nausea, vomiting, faintness, and cold clammy skin; hiccough and other gastrointestinal distress may be present; low-grade temperature elevations common for first 24-48 hours but may last several days (this is inflammatory response to myocardial tissue damage)
Physical examination	Normal during asymptomatic periods; during anginal attacks, increased heart rate, pulsus alternans, and transient abnormal findings including precordial bulge and atrial and ventricular gallops (S_3, S_4)	Similar to stable angina pectoris	Similar to stable angina pectoris; may also demonstrate irregular pulse, hypotension, or signs of left ventricular dysfunction	May be unremarkable unless signs of ventricular failure or cardiogenic shock are present; blood pressure normal, elevated, or decreased—initially elevated when pain is present but usually decreases for first few days; respirations: Cheyne-Stokes respiration owing to central nervous system hypoperfusion or opiate therapy; initial tachypnea returns to normal once pain subsides; heart sounds: S_3, S_4 gallops indicative of ventricular dysfunction; systolic murmurs reflecting papillary muscle dysfunction; diminished heart sounds and pericardial friction rub may occur; with left ventricular dysfunction: pulmonary rales, decreased urine output, increased amplitude of "a" wave in jugular vein; with right ventricular dysfunction: increased jugular venous distention, peripheral edema, liver tenderness; pulse often within normal limits; bradycardia present with inferior wall myocardial infarction; tachycardia with rates greater than 100 beats/minute may reflect compromised ventricle

Nursing Dx & Intervention

Nursing Diagnosis	Nursing Intervention/Rationale
Pain	*Acute care:* • Assess and record description of pain and activity that occurred before onset of pain *to determine etiology.* • Stop angina-inducing activity. • Maintain bed rest *to reduce myocardial oxygen demand.* • Administer drug therapy as ordered *to relieve pain;* assess and record response. • Administer oxygen therapy as ordered *to increase oxygen supply to myocardium.* • Obtain 12-lead ECG *to document ischemia during chest pain episode.* • Monitor vital signs frequently throughout episode of chest pain. *Convalescent care:* • Administer long-acting nitrates as ordered. • Encourage limitation of activities as needed to prevent pain.
Decreased cardiac output (potential) related to loss of myocardial contractility	*Acute care:* • Assess and report signs of decreased cardiac output: decreased blood pressure, increased heart rate, decreased urine output, fatigue, and cool clammy skin. • Monitor vital signs every 5 to 15 minutes. • Maintain bed rest *to reduce myocardial oxygen demand.* • Monitor ECG for dysrhythmias and alterations. • Maintain IV as ordered with 5% glucose in water for drug administration. • Auscultate breath sounds and heart tones every 1 to 4 hours. • Administer drug therapy as ordered. • Monitor hemodynamic parameters as indicated: arterial pressure, PA, pulmonary capillary wedge pressure (PCWP), and central venous pressure (CVP). *Convalescent care:* • Monitor for early complications: hypotension, arrhythmias, heart failure, and heart rupture. • Begin progressive ambulation as patient's condition stabilizes.
Impaired gas exchange	*Acute care:* • Assess and monitor for signs and symptoms of impaired gas exchange: restlessness, confusion, somnolence, dusky or cyanotic coloring, decreased breath sounds, tachypnea, and dyspnea. • Administer oxygen therapy as ordered. • Monitor arterial blood gases and report abnormal results. • Enforce safety precautions such as low oxygen concentrations for patients with chronic respiratory disease. • Prepare for possible intubation and assisted ventilation rehabilitation as ordered. • Begin respiratory exercises, especially for patients with chronic respiratory disease.
Altered nutrition	• Promote proper nutrition with liquid or soft diet as ordered. • Limit offerings of hot or cold beverages. Avoid offering caffeine beverage such as coffee, tea, or colas. • Restrict sodium intake as ordered. • Monitor intake and output closely *to detect or prevent circulatory overload.* • Provide IV fluids as ordered if patient is unable to eat because of nausea or vomiting.
Anxiety related to perceived or actual threat to biologic integrity	• Assess for signs and symptoms of fear and anxiety: verbalizations, restlessness, irritability, facial expressions, and noncompliance. • Offer reassurance during episodes of pain. • Initiate comfort measures such as quiet, restful environment and relaxation techniques. • Administer sedation as ordered. • Stay with patient as much as possible. Use calm, reassuring voice. • Allow family members to assist patient if possible. • Explain all procedures and routine care as they occur. • Encourage expressions of feelings. Permit crying.
Constipation	• Administer stool softeners as ordered. • Caution patient not to strain with bowel movements and to avoid Valsalva maneuvers. • Monitor output *to ensure normal bowel movements.*
Activity intolerance	*Acute care:* • Maintain bed rest *to reduce myocardial workload and increase oxygenation.* • Increase activities as ordered, using ECG changes, heart rate, blood pressure, and patient's clinical status (e.g., complicated versus uncomplicated myocardial infarction) as guidelines. Bed or tub

Nursing Diagnosis	Nursing Intervention/Rationale
	bath causes *fewer hemodynamic and postural changes than shower.*[57] Allow patient out of bed for toileting, since this does not seem to have adverse effects.[110] Backrubs may have a soothing effect.[57] • Perform passive range of motion (ROM) exercises to prevent thromboembolism, progressing to active ROM exercises (see box below). *Convalescent care:* • Begin phase I rehabilitation (see box below). • Teach necessity to increase activity gradually at home while continuing periods of rest.

Patient Education

1. Explain the disease process risk factors involved, methods of modification, associated symptoms, and actions to take when the symptoms occur. Associated complications are irregular heartbeats, chest pain, and shortness of breath.
2. Explain the name, purpose, side effects, and method of administration of all drugs.
3. Explain activity allowances and limitations, including the patient's return to work, resumption of sexual activity, and need to avoid or modify activity following heavy meals and alcohol consumption and in periods of emotional stress or extremes of temperatures.
4. Refer the patient to a rehabilitation program to assist with progressive increase in activity levels.
5. Teach the patient to avoid foods high in sodium, saturated fats, and triglycerides. Teach good nutritional habits and alternative ways of seasoning food to avoid cooking with salt and salt products.
6. Explain importance of controlling any coexisting condition that may aggravate recovery, such as hypertension, obesity, and diabetes.

Evaluation

Patient Outcome	Data Indicating That Outcome is Reached
Cardiac output is improved or maintained.	ECG, vital signs, and urine output are within normal limits.
Gas exchange is improved or maintained.	Po_2 and Pco_2 are within normal limits. Patient has no complaints about shortness of breath.
Patient is free from chest pain.	Patient verbalizes absence of pain. Blood pressure and heart rate are within normal limits. Patient engages in hospital routines and activities without pain. Patient appears relaxed and expresses a sense of calm.
Anxiety level is reduced.	Patient appears relaxed.

Phases of Cardiac Rehabilitation

Phase I: Inpatient activities; anywhere from 4 to 16 stages; patient should be at 3 to 5 metabolic equivalents of tasks (METs) at discharge

Phase II: Begins with discharge and continues until healing has been completed; patient is evaluated with a stress test that is symptom limited

Phase III: Begins 4 to 6 weeks after myocardial infarction or surgery; training phase; patient exercises two to five times a week under supervision for usually 12 weeks; patient should be able to perform at 10 METs or greater at the end of this phase

Phase IV: Begins at the end of the training phase and continues for another 3 to 6 months (some believe it continues for the patient's lifetime); patient maintains level of training by exercising two or three times a week; stress tests usually done at yearly intervals to measure effectiveness and amend exercise prescription

Modified from Guzzetta.[41]

Congestive heart failure

Congestive heart failure (CHF) is a complex clinical syndrome that results from the heart's inability to increase cardiac output sufficiently to meet the body's metabolic demands.

Pathophysiology

The underlying causes of CHF vary, but it ultimately results in the heart's inability to act as an effective pump.

Decreased myocardial contractility may result from a primary disorder or an excessive workload placed on the heart such as systemic hypertension or a valvular disorder. Causes of primary myocardial disorders and disorders that increase the heart's workload are summarized as follows:

- Causes of decreased myocardial contractility
  - Coronary artery disease
  - Myocarditis
  - Cardiomyopathies
    - Congestive
    - Restrictive
    - Hypertrophic
  - Infiltrative diseases
    - Amyloidosis
    - Tumors
    - Sarcoidosis
  - Collagen-vascular diseases
    - Systemic lupus erythematosus
    - Scleroderma
  - Iatrogenic factors
    - Drugs such as β-blockers; calcium antagonists
- Causes of increased myocardial workload
  - Hypertension
  - Pulmonary hypertension
  - Valvular heart disease
    - Aortic or pulmonic stenosis
    - Mitral, tricuspid, or aortic insufficiency
  - Hypertrophic cardiomyopathy
  - Intracardiac shunting
  - High-output states
    - Anemia
    - Hyperthyroidism
    - Beri-beri
    - Arteriovenous fistula

Disorders that interfere with the normal stretch of the ventricle, thereby decreasing ventricular filling, cause a drop in cardiac output. Pericardial tamponade and constrictive pericarditis are examples.

Persistent tachyarrhythmias reduce ventricular filling time, and marked bradyarrhythmias greatly reduce cardiac output because the ventricles cannot augment the stroke volume.

Loss of coordinated atrial contraction, as occurs in atrial fibrillation, can decrease cardiac output, probably because of loss of the atrial "booster pump" that contributes to normal ventricular filling.

The primary dysfunction in CHF is decreased myocardial contractility. However, secondary changes in preload and afterload also contribute to the heart failure.

Heart failure can be divided into left- and right-sided failure; they can occur independently or together.

Left-Sided Heart Failure

Any sustained elevation in left ventricular end-diastolic pressure (LVEDP) increases left atrial pressure. This is transmitted to the pulmonary vascular bed and is manifest as an increase in pulmonary capillary wedge pressure (PCWP). If the PCWP exceeds the colloid osmotic pressure of the pulmonary capillaries, transudation of fluid into the interstitial spaces and eventually into alveolar spaces will occur. This leads to hypoxia (resulting from poor oxygen exchange) and clinically to dyspnea, cough orthopnea, and paroxysmal nocturnal dyspnea.

Right-Sided Heart Failure

Persistent elevation of LVEDP eventually leads to right-sided failure marked by venous congestion in the systemic circulation. Right-sided heart failure may also occur as a primary disorder of the right ventricle as in tricuspid regurgitation, in right ventricular infarction, or as a result of cor pulmonale. Distended neck veins, hepatomegaly, and dependent edema occur.

Diagnostic Studies and Findings

Laboratory Tests

- Electrolytes
  - Hyponatremia owing to water retention; urinary sodium loss in response to diuretics; hypokalemia from excessive use of diuretics or as secondary manifestation of aldosteronism; hypochloremia as result of diuretic therapy; metabolic acidosis or alkalosis
- Blood chemistry
  - BUN, creatinine rise with decreased glomerular filtration; liver function values (SGOT, bilirubin, alkaline phosphatase) mildly increased; prothrombin time prolonged; glucose level elevated
- Arterial blood gases
  - Hypoxemia; decreased oxygen saturation; (early) mild respiratory alkalosis; (late) hypercarbia, hypoxia
- Urine studies
  - Urine output decreased; metabolic acidosis or alkalosis; specific gravity >1.010: excessive fluid intake, <1.035: decreased fluid intake; proteinuria; glucosuria
- Pulmonary function tests
  - Reduced vital capacity; reduced total lung capacity; increased residual volume

Chest Roentgenogram (Figures 1-32 and 1-33)

- Increased pulmonary congestion: redistribution of pulmonary blood flow, interstitial edema (intraseptal

Figure 1-32 Pulmonary congestion. Upper lobe distention *(arrows)*. Enlarged cardiac silhouette.
Courtesy P. Batra, M.D., Department of Radiology, UCLA School of Medicine, Los Angeles. From Michaelson.[68]

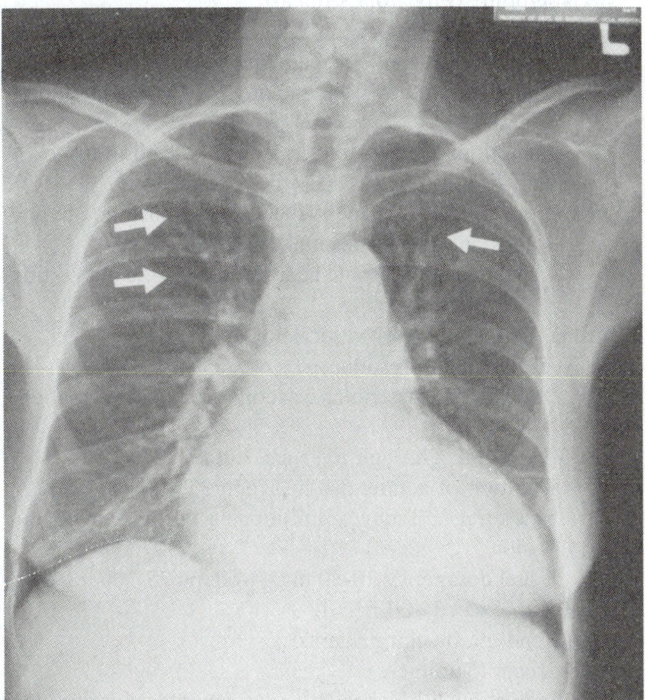

Figure 1-33 Interstitial edema. Hilar areas are blurred and hazy. Cardiac silhouette is enlarged. Fluid collected within intralobular septa of lungs is visible as Kerley-B lines *(arrow)*.
Courtesy P. Batra, M.D., Department of Radiology, UCLA School of Medicine, Los Angeles. From Michaelson.[68]

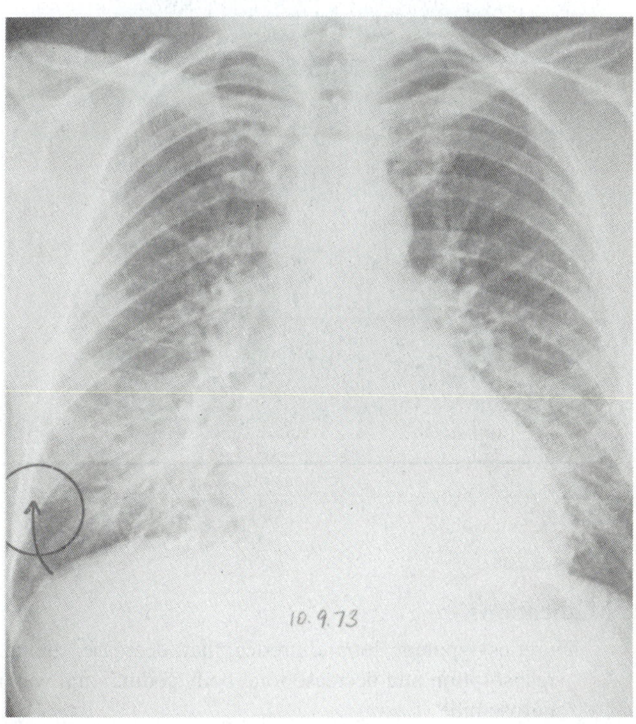

edema—Kerley-B lines; perivascular edema), alveolar edema, pleural effusion; (early) little or no change in size or contour of cardiac silhouette; (late) increased cardiothoracic ratio

Electrocardiogram (ECG)

Changes reflect primary disorders as well as chronic secondary effects of heart failure: left ventricular hypertrophy (LVH), right ventricular hypertrophy (RVH), atrial hypertrophy, tachycardia, arrhythmias

Radionuclide Angiography (Scintigraphy)

Detects presence and severity of ventricular dysfunction; used to predict prognosis based on etiology and/or determine response to therapeutic interventions, e.g., LV ejection pressures are found to be depressed in more than 90% of patients following an anterior MI[68] and in 50% of patients following an inferior MI; in general, LV ejection pressure of <0.30 mm is prognostic of high mortality

Echocardiogram (Figure 1-34)

Increased or decreased ventricular chambers or structures reflect primary disorder; left ventricular failure: increased LVEDP (>5.6 cm), decreased wall motion

Hemodynamic Monitoring (Right Heart Catheterization)

Left ventricular failure: elevated pulmonary capillary wedge pressure (PCWP) and pulmonary artery diastolic pressure (PADP), decreased cardiac output (CO), decreased ejection fractions; right ventricular failure: elevated pulmonary artery pressure (PAP), right ventricular pressure, and right atrial pressure (RAP)

Medical Plan

Surgery

Directed by underlying condition; mortality is greater among patients with left ventricular dysfunction

Figure 1-34 Patient with dilated left ventricle (6.7 cm) and normal intraventricular septum (1 cm).
Courtesy Non Invasive Labs, Division of Cardiology, UCLA School of Medicine, Los Angeles. From Michaelson.[68]

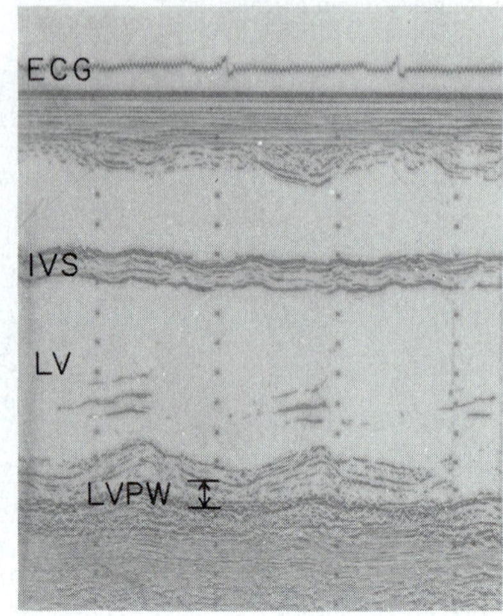

Medications

Diuretics—potent loop diuretics that decrease tubular reabsorption and decrease total body sodium and water
- Furosemide (Lasix)
  - Usual dosage: 20-300 mg/d
- Ethacrynic acid (Edecrin)
  - Usual dosage: 25-200 mg/d
- Thiazides
  - Indications: Oral agents used in management of chronic CHF

Vasodilators—used therapeutically to dilate arterioles and veins, thereby achieving the following hemodynamic effects: (1) improving ejection fraction, which decreases LVEDP (preload) and pulmonary congestion; (2) reducing wall tension, which reduces myocardial oxygen demand; (3) decreasing pressure work of a failing ventricle
- Nitrates—act directly on smooth muscle, causing dilation of arterial and venous beds; used to decrease preload in acute left ventricular failure and to decrease pulmonary and venous pressure
- Nitroprusside sodium (Nipride)
  - Indications: Decreases preload and afterload
  - Precautions: Excreted by kidney; requires careful monitoring of kidney function
  - Half-life: 2-5 min; light sensitive
  - Side effects: Hypotension, tachycardia, palpitations, dizziness, headache, nausea, and vomiting
  - Usual dosage: 3 μg/kg/min IV; average dose 200 μg/min; should not exceed 800 μg/min
- Isosorbide dinitrate (Isordil)
  - Indications: Relaxes vascular smooth muscle
  - Excretion: By liver
  - Onset of action: Sublingual 2-3 min; po 20-40 min; chewable 3-4 min
  - Side effects: Headache, flushing, dizziness
  - Usual dosage: 10-30 mg sublingually; 20-80 mg po; 10-30 mg chewable
- Nifedipine (Procardia, Adalat)
  - Indications: Potent vasodilator used as afterloading reducing agent in treatment of acute and chronic CHF caused by ischemic or hypertensive heart disease
  - Excretion: Metabolized in liver; excreted in urine
  - Half-life: 4-6 h
  - Side effects: Dizziness, headaches, flushing, hypotension, gastrointestinal upset
  - Usual dosage: Chronic heart failure, 10-20 mg po tid, maximum of 60 mg

Antihypertensives (for vasodilator effect)
- Hydralazine (Apresoline)
  - Indications: Arteriolar vasodilator, decreases afterload
  - Excretion: Through liver and kidney
  - Duration of action: 2-8 h (average 3 h)
  - Side effects: Tachycardia, lupus syndrome, hypotension
  - Usual dosage: IV 10-20 mg q4-6h; po 25-100 mg (not to exceed 400 mg/d)

α-Adrenergic blocking agents
- Prazosin (Minipress)
  - Indications: Relaxes vascular smooth muscle, decreases peripheral vascular resistance and venous return
  - Excretion: Through liver
  - Half-life: 3 h
  - Side effects: Syncope, dizziness, headache, drowsiness, nausea, orthostatic hypotension
  - Usual dosage: Initially 1-2 mg, increasing slowly to total of 20 mg bid or tid
- Phentolamine (Regitine)
  - Indications: Acts directly on vascular smooth muscle
  - Excretion: Unknown
  - Duration of action: IV 5-15 min; po 2-4 h
  - Side effects: Hypotension
  - Usual dosage: IV 0.2-2 mg/min; po 50-100 mg in four to six doses/d

Angiotensin-converting enzyme inhibitors
- Antihypertensive: Captopril (Capoten)
  - Indications: Patients who have failed to respond to conventional drug therapy; inhibit formation of angiotensin II, one of the most potent vasoconstrictors; decrease aldosterone secretion and renal-mediated vasoconstriction
  - Excretion: By kidney
  - Duration of action: 4-8 h
  - Side effects: Hypotension; metallic taste in mouth
  - Usual dosage: Initially 25 mg po tid, increasing to maximum dose of 150 mg

Morphine sulfate
  Indications: Venous dilation rapidly decreases preload; sedative effect relieves anxiety; decreases hyperventilation by depressing respiratory center
  Usual dosage: Slow IV push, 3-5 mg
Inotropic agents—increase contractile state of ventricle, thereby improving ejection fraction
  Cardiac glycosides: Digitalis
    Commonly used, but use is limited because toxic effects occur when blood levels exceed 2 ng/ml
    Excretion: By kidney; therefore daily dose should be reduced if renal function is impaired
    Half-life: 30 h
    Usual dosage: 0.25 mg/d
    Precautions: May have toxic effects when blood levels exceed 2 ng/ml; toxicity more likely to occur in patients who are small or elderly or have chronic obstructive pulmonary disease; hypokalemia and digitalis in combination with quinidine can also cause toxicity; common symptoms are arrhythmias, nausea, anorexia
  Adrenergic drugs: Dopamine (Intropin)
    Indications: Directly stimulates myocardial contractility through β-receptors; produces positive inotropic effects through release of norepinephrine; like other inotropic agents, increases force of contraction, resulting in improved ejection fraction
    Usual dosage: 5-20 μg/kg/min IV
    Side effects: Tachycardia, headache, nausea, vomiting
  Dobutamine (Dobutrex)
    Indications: Synthetic cardioactive derivative of dopamine that stimulates α- and β_1-adrenergic receptors; increases contractility and possesses slight chronotropic effects
    Usual dosage: 2.5-10 μg/kg/min
    Side effects: Tachycardia, palpitations, nausea, headache
  Milrinone (Amrinone)
    Indications: Positive inotropic agent that decreases systemic vascular resistance; used in patients with refractory heart failure
    Excretion: Renal
    Side effects: Nausea, anorexia
    Usual dosage: 5 mg q6h po; average dose 30 mg/d

General Management

Intra-aortic balloon pump (IABP)—counterpulsation device that assists failing heart by decreasing afterload and increasing coronary artery perfusion (see p. 105 for further discussion)
Hemodynamic monitoring—initiated as direct means of assessing hemodynamic status of heart and effectiveness of treatment; also assists in direction of therapy
Electrocardiogram—used to assess for drug-induced arrhythmias and for arrhythmias induced by an underlying disorder
Bed rest—head of bed elevated to 45 degrees to reduce myocardial oxygen demand and decrease circulating volume returning to heart
Restriction of sodium and water; weighing daily to monitor fluid retention
Oxygen therapy—initiated if patient is hypoxic
Rotating tourniquets—used for rapid reduction of circulating blood volume; however, effectiveness is questionable
Sodium-restricted diet—4 g is "no added salt," 2 g is all salt eliminated from cooking

NURSING CARE

Nursing Assessment

General Complaints

Dyspnea owing to increased pulmonary venous and interstitial pressures; variations: dyspnea on exertion (DOE), orthopnea, paroxysmal nocturnal dyspnea (PND)
Fatigue moderate to severe owing to diminished cardiac output
Gastrointestinal symptoms as result of splanchnic congestion: anorexia, nausea, vomiting, abdominal distention, right upper quadrant pain

Physical Examination

Decreased cardiac output: tachycardia, pulsus alternans, weak thready pulse, hypotension, narrowed pulse pressure, pallor, diaphoresis, cool skin, altered mental status, dizziness, syncope, decreased urine output
Increased pulmonary capillary pressure: rapid labored respiration, cough, frothy or blood-tinged sputum, moist rales on pulmonary auscultation, left ventricular S_3 and systolic murmur at apex on cardiac auscultation, precordial movement—displaced apical impulse and palpable thrills
Increased right atrial pressure: weight gain, elevated jugular venous pressure (rise in a and v waves), hepatojugular reflex, precordial movement (right ventricular impulse along lower left sternal border or subxiphoid), on auscultation right ventricular S_3 heard best at lower left sternal border; presence of systolic murmur, hepatomegaly, splenomegaly, peripheral edema, dilation of peripheral veins

Nursing Dx & Intervention

Nursing Diagnosis	Nursing Intervention/Rationale
Decreased cardiac output related to mechanical factors (preload, afterload, contractility)	• Assess and monitor for signs and symptoms indicative of decreased cardiac output: fatigue; skin pallor, diaphoresis, or cyanosis; oliguria; anuria; decreased peripheral pulses; cold, clammy skin; dyspnea; hypotension; and tachycardia. • Maintain bed rest *to conserve energy and decrease oxygen demand.* Elevate head of bed 30 to 60 degrees. Lean patient forward on padded over-bed table *to facilitate ventilation and decrease workload of breathing.* • Monitor hemodynamic parameters as ordered *to evaluate patient's clinical status and response to therapy.* Blood pressure and arterial pressures reflect tissue perfusion. Pulmonary artery pressure (PAP), pulmonary capillary wedge pressure (PCWP), and cardiac output (CO) reflect LVEDP and myocardial contractility. • Administer drug therapy as ordered. Monitor for signs of drug toxicity. • Monitor ECG rate and rhythms *to detect early arrhythmias.* • Limit IV fluids as ordered *to prevent circulatory overload.* • Restrict activities as indicated. Plan care to prevent fatigue, which increases oxygen demand. Provide rest periods between procedures.
Impaired gas exchange related to elevated pulmonary capillary pressure	• Assess for signs of impaired ventilation or perfusion: restlessness, confusion, somnolence, hypoxia, and hypercapnia. • Monitor arterial blood gas frequently. • Administer oxygen therapy as ordered, via nasal prongs, mask, or positive-pressure device. • Administer morphine sulfate IV per protocol *to reduce hyperventilation.* • Elevate head of bed. • Auscultate breath sounds every hour *to detect increases in congestion and determine adequacy of ventilatory effort.* • Prepare for intubation and assisted ventilation if required. • Explain all procedures and modalities briefly to patient *to prevent hyperventilation resulting from fear or anxiety.*
Fluid volume excess related to increased systemic venous congestion or right ventricular failure	• Inspect for increased or decreased jugular venous distention. • Auscultate heart sounds and breath sounds every 1 to 2 hours *to detect increased congestion and response to treatment.* • Maintain patent IV for drug administration. • Administer rapid-acting diuretics as ordered *to decrease circulating volume.* • Restrict sodium and fluid intake. • Weigh patient daily (same time of day, same amount of clothing) *to determine fluid loss or retention.* • Monitor intake and output; report output of less than 30 ml/hour. • Monitor serum electrolytes, especially sodium and potassium.
Altered nutrition: less than body requirements related to impaired absorption of nutrients, secondary to low cardiac output	• Observe daily for signs of malnutrition: dry body weight less than 20% of ideal weight for age, height, and body size; decreased triceps skinfold measurements; stomatitis; anorexia; increasing fatigue and weakness; decreased serum albumin, transferrin, and BUN levels. • Weigh patient daily: upon rising, after voiding, with same clothing *to obtain consistent and accurate body weight.* • Maintain diet as ordered. Do not force patient to eat, but offer small frequent meals, tempt appetite with food preferences compatible with diet restrictions and cultural values, and supplement with high-caloric feedings as indicated *to maintain minimum required caloric intake.* • Administer antiemetics and analgesics before meals *to ensure patient's comfort and improve appetite.* • Initiate caloric count if patient's nutritional status fails to improve. Obtain dietary consultation *to evaluate nutritional status and assist patient in selection of foods.*
Impaired skin integrity related to altered circulation and metabolic state	• Assess skin integrity, noting color, texture, temperature, and signs of redness, scaling, breaks, or ulcerations. • Turn and reposition every 2 to 4 hours *to relieve pressure areas and improve circulation, muscle tone, and joint mobility.* • Administer skin care daily. Massage bony pressure areas *to increase tissue perfusion to affected areas. To avoid causing skin excoriations,* do not massage reddened areas. • Anticipate and initiate preventive measures for a patient considered at high risk for skin breakdown: a cachectic, debilitated, or edematous patient who is immobile. • Use alternative preventive measures *to ensure skin integrity as indicated:* air pressure beds, alternating pressure mattress, sheepskin.

Nursing Diagnosis	Nursing Intervention/Rationale
	• Prevent and eliminate pressure and friction. Position pillows or other supports between pressure areas *to prevent friction, abrasions, and rubbing of two skin areas.* • Keep skin dry when diaphoretic, *since moisture contributes to skin breakdown and infection.* • Initiate aggressive decubitus care at first sign of reddened areas, tissue breakdown, or ulceration, *since decubiti can develop in a matter of hours.*

Patient Education

Instruction is directed toward long-term maintenance of the therapeutic program.

1. Describe the disease process, the underlying cause, and any precipitating factors.
2. Instruct the patient to report symptoms of increased failure to physician: weight gain of more than 2 pounds in 24 hours, dyspnea on exertion, paroxysmal nocturnal dyspnea, and decreased exercise tolerance.
3. Instruct the patient to limit physical activity and avoid fatigue.
4. Instruct the patient to limit the intake of salt in the diet and avoid foods that have a high sodium content; instruct the patient in label reading. Provide information about alternative ways to season food.
5. Teach the patient to weigh daily in the morning before the first meal with the same scale and wearing the same clothing.
6. Teach the patient the name and method of administration of drugs and their potential side effects.

Evaluation

Patient Outcome	Data Indicating That Outcome is Reached
Ventricular function is improved.	Heart rate and pulmonary capillary wedge pressure (PCWP) are decreased. Cardiac output is increased. Mental status is improved. Urine output is increased.
Fluid overload is decreased.	Patient loses weight. Jugular venous distention is decreased. Breath sounds are improved. Peripheral edema is decreased.
Gas exchange is improved.	Lung sounds are clear. Anxiety level is diminished. Orthopnea and dyspnea are reduced. Hypoxemia and hypercarbia are absent. Respirations are improved.
Knowledge level is increased.	Patient verbalizes knowledge regarding importance of daily weight, taking prescribed medication, activity allowances and limitation, and dietary restriction.
Anxiety level is decreased.	Patient appears relaxed. Patient demonstrates ability to rest and sleep without complaints. Patient verbalizes fears regarding disease process, asking appropriate questions.

Shock

(Hypovolemic, vasogenic, cardiogenic, neurogenic)

Shock is an abnormal physical state that is the first phase of the body's alarm reaction to stress.

Most commonly shock occurs as an extreme syndrome linked to abnormal cellular metabolism, which in most cases is caused by inadequate tissue perfusion. If shock is untreated, circulatory collapse and impaired cellular metabolism develop, leading eventually to death.

Pathophysiology

Various methods of classifying shock have been used. The following four categories based on causes are commonly used in the clinical setting:

- Hypovolemic
  - Loss of blood volume (hemorrhage)
  - Loss of plasma volume (dehydration)
- Vasogenic
  - Sepsis
  - Immune mediated (anaphylaxis)
  - Deep anesthesia effects
- Cardiogenic
  - Acute myocardial infarction
  - Other causes (pulmonary emboli, cardiac surgery, tamponade)
- Neurogenic
  - Spinal anesthesia
  - Damage or disease of upper spinal cord

Hypovolemic Shock

Hypovolemic or "cold" shock results from a decrease in intravascular volume and generally occurs when there is also a deficit involving at least 15% of the total blood volume. Hypovolemia is the most common cause of hypotension in critically ill patients, particularly in the postoperative phase.

Hypovolemic shock may be caused by excessive loss of plasma volume as occurs in burns or pancreatitis when extracellular fluid is sequestered in injured or inflamed tissue cells. Severe dehydration and hypovolemia may also be caused by diabetic ketoacidosis, extreme vomiting, or diarrhea. The most common cause of hypovolemic shock, however, is excessive blood loss through damage to a major blood vessel or organ such as the kidney, spleen, or liver; through injury or disease of the gastrointestinal system such as rupture of esophageal varices; or through ruptured aneurysms.

The severity of hypovolemic shock is related to the amount and rate of volume loss. If volume is replaced quickly, the shock state can be easily reversed. If low aortic pressures last longer than 60 minutes, the process may be irreversible.

The major hemodynamic changes linked to fluid loss are low cardiac output, increased systemic vascular resistance, and decreased central venous pressure. The patient usually has cool clammy skin, increased heart and respiratory rates, and decreased urine output, owing to compensatory vasoconstriction. The blood pressure may be normal or low, particularly in the early phase of "cold shock."

Vasogenic Shock

Unlike hypovolemic shock, which leads to vasoconstriction, vasogenic shock results in massive vasodilation from an increase in total vascular capacity. Circulating volume is lost because of venous pooling, increased capillary permeability, and third spacing of fluid. If intravascular volume is not replaced, hypovolemia occurs. Whereas a patient with hypovolemia has cold extremities as a result of vasoconstriction, a patient with vasogenic shock has warm extremities, giving rise to the term "warm shock." Warm shock is present in 30% to 50% of patients in the early phase of septic shock.

Sepsis is the most common form of vasogenic shock, but it may also occur as a result of other factors, including food allergies and anaphylactic reactions from drugs and insect stings.

Septic shock is commonly related to the release of bacterial endotoxins following a gram-negative bacterial infection. The organisms most often found in septic shock are the gram-negative bacteria *Escherichia coli, Klebsiella, Enterobacter, Pseudomonas, Serratia, Proteus,* and *Bacteroides fragilis;* the gram-positive bacteria *Staphylococcus, Pneumococcus,* and α- or β-*Streptococcus;* and the fungus *Candida.* Many are a part of the natural body flora or are commonly present in hospitals. The microbes linked to the highest death rate are *Proteus, Pseudomonas, Candida,* and *B. fragilis.* Although patients in critical care units are the most likely to acquire infections in the hospital, patients in general hospital units are also vulnerable. Patients particularly susceptible to septic shock are the elderly, immunosuppressed patients, patients who have indwelling catheters (urinary, intravenous, or intracardiac) or urinary tract infection, patients who have had surgery of the digestive tract or urinary tract, and patients who have undergone manipulative instrumentation.

Although deaths from septic shock have decreased since the 1960s, the death rate continues to be as high as 50%. This is the result of several factors, the most striking of which are the changing pattern of microbial resistance to antimicrobial agents[13,39] and the rapidly changing nature of microbes.

Certain hemodynamic changes have been recognized as probable causes of septic shock. In early phases a hyperdynamic state exists in which the cardiac output, stroke volume, and heart rate are increased and the systemic vascular resistance and central venous pressure are decreased. The patient appears warm, dry, and flushed because of generalized vasodilation and venous pooling. This state is probably caused by the effects of various substances released by exotoxins or from the injured or infected tissue.

The circulatory changes combined with the decreased systemic vascular resistance may stimulate a sympathetic response. This causes the increased heart rate and maintenance of normal blood pressure that occur during this "warm shock" phase.

If hyperdynamic shock continues, the continued increase in capillary leaking increases hypovolemia to the point that the process converts to a hypodynamic phase known as the "cold" phase of septic shock. In this state the systemic vascular resistance increases, cardiac output drops, and the patient appears cold, pale, and clammy. The cause of this change is related to ineffective circulating blood volume, sympathetic vasoconstriction, and pump failure.[60]

In *anaphylactic reactions* from drugs, insect stings, or food allergies, the mechanism involved is an antibody-antigen interaction that provokes the release of chemicals such as histamine. These mediators act mainly on the vascular membranes and smooth muscles. Histamine release causes veins and arterioles to dilate, decreasing cardiac output and arterial pressure. Histamine also increases capillary permeability, causing fluid to escape from the intravascular compartment into the interstitial space. The result is volume depletion; however, while plasma water is removed from the capillaries, the red cells remain and the hemoglobin levels and hematocrit values rise. The immediate reactions in anaphylaxis are pharyngeal and laryngeal edema, probably because of the effects of histamines, and bronchoconstriction with the immediate threat of death from asphyxiation.

Deep anesthesia can cause severe depression of the vasomotor centers of the brain, which may result in vasomotor collapse and venous pooling. These decrease venous return to the heart and diminish cardiac output.

Cardiogenic Shock

Cardiogenic shock occurs when the heart cannot maintain enough output to meet the body's demands.

Myocardial infarction is the most common cause of cardiogenic shock, but it may be the result of a variety of cardiac disorders: acute myocardial infarction, end-stage cardiomyopathy (congestive, hypertrophic, or restrictive), valvular heart disease, cardiopulmonary bypass, and cardiac tamponade. The major feature of cardiogenic shock is inadequate tissue perfusion and oxygen delivery resulting from a severely impaired ventricle.

The incidence of cardiogenic shock resulting from myocardial infarction is 10% to 15%, with a death rate greater than 60%. Current therapies focus on early intervention to reduce ischemia and limit permanent myocardial damage.

In patients with myocardial infarction, shock develops as a result of abnormal reflexes arising from the ischemic myocardium. The inability to increase systemic vascular resistance makes it difficult to maintain an adequate arterial pressure. This leads to hypoperfusion to an already ischemic myocardium, causing further insufficiency of the pumping action of the left ventricle. Failure of the left ventricle to generate enough energy to pump blood into the systemic circulation further decreases perfusion and myocardial oxygen supply.

Cardiogenic shock has been linked to the destruction of 40% or more of left ventricular muscle. The mechanism of cardiogenic shock is complex, with a vicious cycle of changes that lead rapidly to further deterioration of cardiac function. If left untreated, the reduction in tissue blood flow and oxygen delivery to the myocardium results in circulatory collapse, impaired cellular metabolism, and eventual death.

The basic pathophysiologic defect linked to severe myocardial ischemia or necrosis is drastically decreased function of the ventricle, which results in reduced cardiac output and inadequate tissue perfusion. The degree of reduced function of the ventricle is related to total myocardial damage and the balance between oxygen supply and demand.

Neurogenic Shock

Neurogenic shock is caused by damage to or blockage of the sympathetic nervous system, resulting in vasodilation. This leads to a relative hypovolemia brought on by a decrease in systemic vascular resistance with peripheral pooling and decrease in venous return. The result is a drop in cardiac output leading to tissue hypoperfusion.

Neurogenic shock is relatively rare and most commonly results from spinal anesthesia or damage or disease of the upper spinal cord. Brain trauma or injury rarely if ever causes shock.

Compensatory Mechanisms of Shock

A number of compensatory mechanisms are activated when arterial pressure and tissue perfusion are reduced. These mechanisms are controlled by the sympathetic nervous system and the release of endogenous vasoconstrictors and hormonal substances.[26]

Baroreceptors. A reduction in mean arterial pressure and pulse pressure is sensed by baroreceptors in the carotid sinus and aortic arch. By secreting epinephrine and norepinephrine, they produce a generalized sympathetic stimulation, resulting in increased peripheral vascular resistance, arterial pressure, and myocardial contractility.

Fluid shifts. The major endogenous vasoactive substances released during shock are catecholamines and vasopressin, which augment sympathetic activity when activated further. The release of these substances also reduces vascular capacity, which eases the osmotic movement of interstitial fluid into the vascular compartments to restore blood volume.

Renin-angiotensin-aldosterone system. When renal ischemia occurs, the renin-angiotensin-aldosterone system is activated to help maintain blood pressure and intravascular volume. Reducing renal perfusion pressure results in the release of renin, which in time is converted to angiotensin II, a powerful vasoconstrictor. Angiotensin II stimulates the release of aldosterone, which enhances sodium and water reabsorption by the renal tubules to help maintain intravascular volume.

Antidiuretic hormone. The release of antidiuretic hormone (ADH) from the posterior pituitary gland in response to hypotension plays a role in volume regulation during circulatory shock. ADH enhances reabsorption of sodium and water by increasing permeability of the renal tubules.

Progressive Shock

If the compensatory mechanisms cannot restore effective perfusion to vital organs, circulatory function deteriorates further, leading to a cycle of changes that decrease cardiac output. Figure 1-35 illustrates some of the changes that contribute to decreased cardiac output and circulatory collapse.

Cell deterioration. As shock becomes severe, local changes in cellular metabolism occur. Prolonged tissue ischemia results in incomplete oxidation at the cellular level, diminishing mitochondrial activity. Adenosine triphosphate (ATP) stores then begin to be used, and the cells resort to anaerobic metabolism of glucose to provide energy. This process of glycolysis produces lactic acid, which builds up in the blood. The effects of an acidic pH include depressed myocardial function and a decreased vascular response to epinephrine and norepinephrine, leading to vasomotor collapse late in shock.[3]

Another significant cellular change resulting from continued ischemia is the release of vasoactive metabolites into the circulation. Substances such as bradykinin, histamine, serotonin, and prostaglandins, along with decreased vascular tone, lead to increases in venous pooling and capillary permeability. Excessive vasodilation then decreases venous return and cardiac filling. The increased permeability of the capillaries allows large quantities of fluid to escape into the interstitial spaces.

Organ and Tissue Changes

As the shock syndrome becomes severe, generalized organ deterioration begins.

Renal function. Although reduced renal perfusion activates certain compensatory mechanisms, in the early phases of shock prolonged decreased renal blood flow leads to ischemia and acute tubular necrosis. This is marked by fluid, electrolyte, and metabolic disturbances.

Pulmonary function. Ischemia to the pulmonary circulation in the early phases of shock can damage pulmonary

Figure 1-35 Different types of feedback that can lead to progression of shock.
Modified from Guyton.[40]

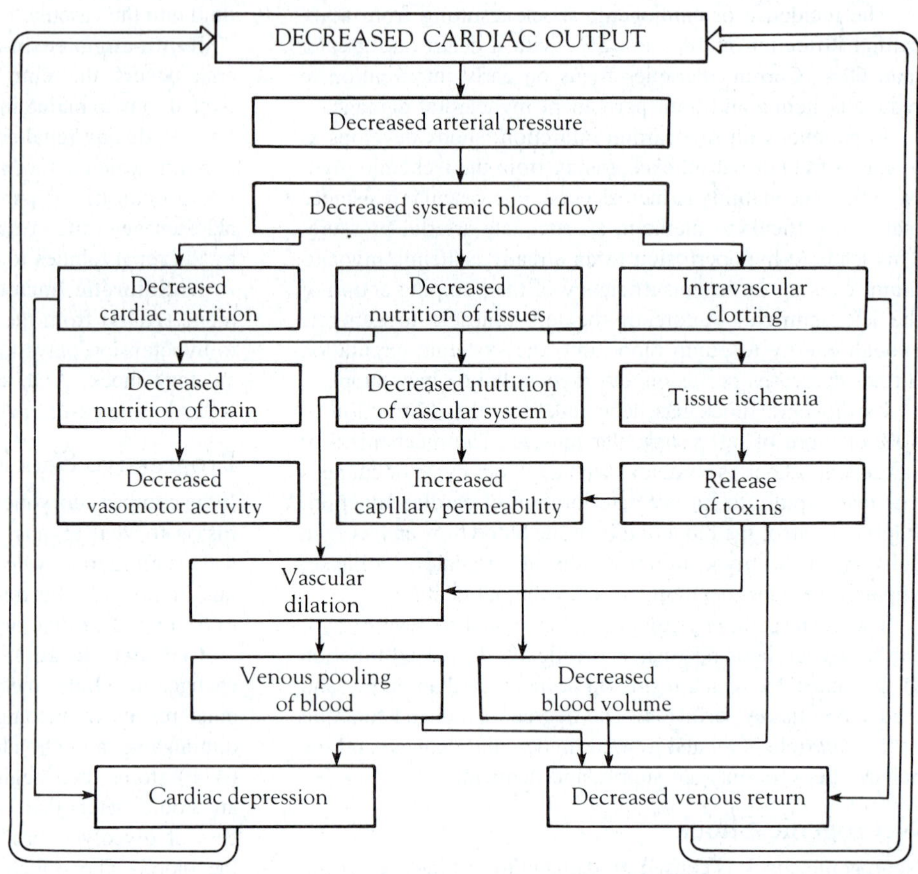

function to cause adult respiratory distress syndrome. Damage to the pulmonary capillary endothelial cells increases capillary permeability. This leads to interstitial and alveolar edema that impairs gas exchange. The resulting hypoxemia and respiratory acidosis further reduce tissue oxygen delivery and organ function.

Gastrointestinal function. Ischemic damage to the digestive tract causes a loss of the protective mucosal covering in the intestine. This can lead to intestinal damage and necrosis by digestive enzymes. It may also account for the release of bacteria and toxins into the bloodstream, causing sepsis and further circulatory problems.

The reticuloendothelial system may also be damaged during shock, impairing the patient's ability to withstand infection.

Intravascular clotting. As the products of cell deterioration begin to accumulate in the capillaries and vasodilation occurs, blood flow becomes sluggish. The stagnation, along with local chemical changes in the capillaries, leads to blood aggregation and intravascular clotting. The formation of microemboli enhances tissue ischemia by further decreasing blood flow through the capillaries. This hypercoagulability response may occur as an early compensatory mechanism, particularly with hemorrhage. In the late stages of shock, however, a reversal in clotting occurs, leading to a hypocoagulability state. This results from loss in clotting factors through bleeding or decreased production caused by poor tissue perfusion. It may also be the result of a consumption of clotting factors that occurs in disseminated intravascular coagulation.

Myocardial depression. Except with cardiogenic shock, the major cardiac effects of shock occur in the late stage and are by far the most important factor in the deterioration caused by shock. As arterial pressure continues to drop, so does coronary blood flow. This leads to depressed myocardial function and a further reduction in cardiac output. Myocardial contractility is depressed further by the combined effects of toxins, acidosis, and tissue hypoxia that result from cell deterioration. Thus circulatory failure is a syndrome that involves all systems, and it is usually the deterioration of heart function that makes shock irreversible.[3]

Diagnostic Studies and Findings

Laboratory Tests

Hematocrit
  Increased in volume deficits
Hemoglobin
  Decreased in hemorrhage
White blood cell count with differential
  Increased; leukopenia in gram-negative sepsis; leukocytosis with increased neutrophils in all forms of shock
Erythrocyte sedimentation rate
  Increased in response to tissue injury
Cultures (blood [obtain two to four cultures before initiation of antibiotic therapy], urine, sputum)
  Positive growth of an organism
Serum electrolytes
  Sodium
    Increased during diuretic phase of acute tubular necrosis; decreased with administration of hypotonic fluid following fluid loss
  Potassium
    Increased with cellular death during oliguric phase, in acidosis, and after transfusion reactions
Serum chemistry
  BUN, creatinine
    Increased, reflecting impaired renal function
  Lactate levels
    Increased
  Glucose levels
    Increased in early shock, reflecting release of liver glycogen stores in response to catecholamines
Prothrombin time
  Increased
Arterial blood gases
  Respiratory alkalosis; metabolic acidosis
Urine studies
  Specific gravity
    Increased in response to action of ADH and during oliguric phase
  Osmolality
    High during oliguric phase

Electrocardiogram (ECG) (12-Lead Continuous Monitoring)

To determine changes in heart rate and rhythm and ischemic changes

Chest Roentgenogram

To determine pulmonary status and rule out other causes of shock state

Hemodynamic Monitoring (Pulmonary Artery Pressure, Pulmonary Capillary Wedge Pressure, Cardiac Output)

To provide information regarding serial changes in left ventricular function in response to specific treatments, such as fluid replacement

Medical Plan

Medications

Fluid-volume regulation. Except with patients in cardiogenic shock, restoration of intravascular volume is the most significant therapeutic intervention, particularly in the early phases of therapy.

Volume replacement should be initiated rapidly with 3 to 5 L of saline or other volume expanders over a 30- to 60-minute period. Ringer's lactate provides effective intravascular expansion and is the usual fluid of choice; however, a buffered solution with lactate may be used for severe shock.

Regulation of fluids should be based on hemodynamic response to the rapid fluid infusion. Careful monitoring of mean arterial pressure, pulmonary capillary wedge pressure (PCWP) or central venous pressure (CVP), and urine output is used to guide fluid replacement.

Blood plasma expanders should be given after the initial volume deficit is corrected. In cases of massive hemorrhage, replacement should be with whole blood if the hematocrit value is less than 30%. If the hematocrit value is greater than 30%, plasma expanders may be given. Packed cells are used if the right atrial pressure or PCWP is elevated and in cases such as cardiogenic shock in which myocardial dysfunction limits the amount and speed of fluid replacement.

In a patient in shock after acute myocardial infarction, volume deficits may occur and fluid replacement may be necessary to restore a depressed cardiac output to normal. Continuous monitoring of the PCWP is the most precise method of determining volume deficits. If the PCWP is below the desired level of 15 to 18 mm Hg, fluid replacement may be given to increase cardiac output (Starling's law). The PCWP should be kept below 18 mm Hg to prevent pulmonary congestion.

If the PCWP of a patient in shock is elevated, fluid replacement is contraindicated and diuretics may be necessary to return the PCWP to therapeutic range. Diuretics are generally given only to patients in cardiogenic shock with an elevated PCWP. They reduce preload through their effect on venous capacitance and decrease total circulating fluid.

Maintenance of adequate hemodynamic state. In shock, myocardial dysfunction develops as a result of workload, limited coronary blood flow, and decreased myocardial oxygenation. Sympathomimetic agents are used to maintain an adequate hemodynamic state. The effects of these agents are mediated through the action of α- and β-adrenergic receptors. α-Receptors in the smooth muscle of the vascular bed cause vasoconstriction, thereby increasing peripheral resistance and venous return. By contrast, β_1-receptors are located in the myocardium, arteries, and lungs. Myocardial β_1-receptors act to increase heart rate and contractility, whereas activation of β_2-receptors causes vasodilation.

The various adrenergic drugs differ with respect to their relative α (peripheral) and β (peripheral, myocardial) effects. The rationale for selecting any drug depends on the specific vascular bed on which the drug acts and the desired cardiovascular effect. In cardiogenic shock, for example, drugs with positive inotropic and vasoconstrictor properties are used to increase cardiac output by augmenting myocardial contractility and to improve blood flow to vital organs by increasing total vascular resistance. Dopamine, norepinephrine, and epinephrine, which have both constrictor and inotropic properties, are commonly used in treatment of cardiogenic shock.

The following agents are most commonly used in the treatment of patients with shock.

Adrenergic drugs. Dopamine (Intropin) is one of the most widely used drugs in the treatment of shock. Its effects depend on the dose used. In low doses (2 to 5 μg/kg/min) it produces dilation of renal, mesenteric, coronary, and cerebral blood vessels. In higher doses (6 to 15 μg/kg/min) it improves cardiac output by increasing contractility (β effect) but has no effect on blood pressure. At therapeutic levels (10 to 15 μg/kg/min) dopamine increases cardiac output and blood pressure with little change or reduction in pulmonary vascular resistance. The increase in blood pressure is due primarily to an enhanced cardiac output. In addition, the vasodilator effect on renal blood vessels increases renal blood flow, which improves urine output. In very high doses (>20 μg/kg/min) dopamine causes generalized vasoconstriction (α effect), which opposes the desired vasodilator effect obtained with lower doses. Infusions should be started with low doses (3 to 5 μg/kg/min), increasing slowly until optimum arterial pressure is achieved.

Dobutamine (Dobutrex) is used primarily for its inotropic effect. It stimulates β_1-receptors to increase myocardial contractility and stroke volume, resulting in improved cardiac output. Since dobutamine has minimal β_2 and α effects, it produces little change in blood pressure and heart rate; however, systolic blood pressure may be increased because of increased cardiac output. Coronary blood flow and myocardial oxygen consumption (MVO_2) are also increased because of increased myocardial contractility. Infusions begin at 2 to 4 μg/kg/min, with therapeutic doses between 2.5 and 10 μg/kg/min.

Epinephrine is a potent β- and α-catecholamine causing vasoconstriction of the splanchnic and renal beds. Although it does increase cardiac output, its effects on peripheral resistance do not favor redistribution of blood flow to vital organs. It is also considered less advantageous than other adrenergic drugs because it increases automaticity, which can initiate serious arrhythmias.

Norepinephrine has both α and β actions. It increases myocardial contractility by stimulating β_1-receptors and causes arteriovenous constriction by stimulating α-receptors. Thus norepinephrine increases systemic arterial pressure by increasing the cardiac output and peripheral vascular resistance. Once again the actual hemodynamic effects depend on the dose employed. With small doses a β effect predominates, causing slight increases in blood pressure and cardiac output. With very high doses norepinephrine produces significant vasoconstriction, causing an increased systemic resistance and blood pressure. However, the cardiac output may fall despite the positive inotropic effect. The usual starting dose is 2 to 8 μg/minute. Norepinephrine should be administered through an indwelling catheter placed in a large vein, since it is known to cause tissue necrosis with extravasation. The disadvantage of this drug is its vasoconstricting effect on the kidneys, which can result in impaired renal perfusion and oliguria.

Isoproterenol (Isuprel) acts as a peripheral dilator through β_2 stimulation. More important is the β_1 effect, which augments myocardial contractility and heart rate, thereby improving cardiac output. However, it may cause a substantial increase in myocardial oxygen demand, which can exacerbate myocardial ischemia in a patient with cardiogenic shock.

Cardiac glycosides. The role of digitalis in the treatment of shock is being questioned. It has been noted that inotropic drugs such as digoxin become less effective as the degree of left ventricular failure increases. As an inotropic agent for treatment of severe or cardiogenic shock, digitalis is relatively weak when compared with the sympathomimetic drugs. In addition, it could be hemodynamically detrimental because of the increased MVO_2 produced by the increased contractility, as well as by the decrease in afterload associated with it. Furthermore, because of the impaired renal function, acidosis, and hypoxia occurring in shock states, the patient is predisposed to digitalis-induced arrhythmias.[26,28]

Vasodilators. Vasodilator therapy is generally limited to patients with failing ventricular function and is still debated in the routine treatment of cardiogenic shock. However, it may be of use in patients with severe hypotension whose severe vasoconstriction continues despite volume replacement. Excessive vasoconstriction, which occurs initially as a compensatory response to hypoperfusion, can reduce blood flow and oxygen delivery, as well as cause such a loss of intravascular volume that it leads to further reduction of cardiac output. The rationale for using vasodilator therapy in shock is to break this progressive positive-feedback cycle.

Vasodilator agents improve left ventricular function by decreasing myocardial oxygen demand through the reduction of preload and afterload. These drugs have no direct inotropic action on the heart. The increased cardiac output produced by vasodilators is caused by the changes in preload and afterload.

Arterial vasodilators are used to decrease peripheral vascular resistance, which then decreases resistance to left ventricular ejection and therefore afterload. Venodilators are used to increase venous capacitance, causing a decrease in venous return that decreases PCWP and preload.

The potential role of vasodilator therapy in cardiogenic shock merits further study. Although inappropriate as a single form of therapy, the use of vasodilators combined with external counterpulsation and other inotropic agents appears to be effective in providing efficient ventricular function. Nitroprusside and phentolamine are the vasodilator agents most commonly used in the treatment of cardiogenic shock.

Antihypertensive agents. Nitroprusside (Nipride, Nitropress) causes both arterial and venous dilation, thereby decreasing venous return and left ventricular filling (decreased preload), as well as resistance to left ventricular ejection (decreased afterload). The drug is administered intravenously with an initial dose of 0.5 to 10 μg/kg/min, which is increased in increments of 5 to 10 μg/kg/min every 5 minutes or until an improvement in hemodynamics is observed. Fluid replacement may be required if filling pressures drop excessively. Fluid volumes should be determined before administration of these agents. In hypovolemic patients, massive vasodilation only worsens the clinical picture by further decreasing venous return.

α-Adrenergic blocking agents. Phentolamine mesylate (Regitine) inhibits vasoconstriction by blocking α-adrenergic receptors. It lowers arterial pressure, thereby decreasing afterload. The drug is given intravenously at a dosage of 0.1 to 2 mg/minute.

General Management

Intra-aortic counterpulsation. Counterpulsation is the most frequently used method of mechanically assisting circulation to profound cardiovascular collapse. Counterpulsation augments aortic pressure during diastole with subsequent reduction of afterload, thus effectively reducing the work of the myocardium and improving coronary blood flow (see p. 105).

The intra-aortic balloon pump (IABP) is the most widely used counterpulsation technique. A catheter with a 10 to 50 cc balloon is inserted into the femoral artery and positioned in the thoracic aorta just distal to the left subclavian artery. With the ECG used for synchronization, the balloon is inflated during diastole and deflated during systole.

Oxygenation. Ventilation/perfusion ratios should be determined early to ensure adequate ventilation. Oxygen exchange may be impaired in patients with shock, especially if cardiac output is decreased. Oxygen therapy should be given from the onset of treatment to maintain an arterial Po_2 of at least 80 mm Hg. Intubation may be indicated if arterial blood gases show worsening hypoxemia despite high oxygen concentrations. The indications for mechanical ventilation are a Pao_2 of less than 50 mm Hg while the patient is receiving oxygen concentrations of 50%, a vital capacity of less than 15 ml/kg body weight, a Pco_2 of greater than 45 mm Hg, and an arterial pH of less than 7.25.

Hemodynamic monitoring. For diagnostic information and evaluation of ongoing therapy, arterial pressures, pulmonary artery pressure (PAP), and PCWP should be monitored initially every 5 to 10 minutes. A cardiac index of less than 2 L/minute is reflective of a shock state.

Nutrition. Patients in shock should receive nothing by mouth, but care must be taken to provide nutrition, preferably with hyperalimentation.

Acid-base balance. Frequent monitoring of acid-base balance is necessary to avert profound acidosis. Intravenous administration of sodium bicarbonate may be necessary to maintain or correct the pH to 7.35.

Renal function. Hourly urine output measurements with frequent checks are necessary to determine adequate kidney perfusion. Urine output of less than 30 ml/hour reflects inadequate renal perfusion. Elevated serum BUN and creatinine levels reflect renal dysfunction.

Activity. Efforts should be made to minimize energy expenditure. The patient should be maintained on complete bed rest in a supine position, with legs elevated to 45 degrees.

NURSING CARE

Nursing Assessment

Area of Concern	Hypovolemic Shock	Cardiogenic Shock	Vasogenic Shock	Neurogenic Shock
General appearance	Anxiety, restlessness	Anxiety, restlessness	Anxiety, vertigo, restlessness	Anxiety, restlessness
Level of consciousness	Lethargy, stupor, or coma	Lethargy, stupor, or coma	Lethargy, stupor, or coma	Lethargy, stupor, or coma
Temperature	Increased or decreased	Increased	Increased or decreased	Increased or decreased
Heart rate	Increased, pulse thready	Increased, pulse thready	Increased, pulse thready	Normal or slow
Auscultation		S_3, S_4; murmurs		
Blood pressure				
Early	Pulse pressure decreased; diastolic pressure increased	Pulse pressure decreased; diastolic pressure increased	Normal; pulse pressure decreased	Normal; pulse pressure decreased
Late	Systolic pressure decreased	Systolic pressure decreased	Systolic pressure decreased	Systolic pressure decreased

Area of Concern	Hypovolemic Shock	Cardiogenic Shock	Vasogenic Shock	Neurogenic Shock
Skin temperature and texture	Cool, moist, clammy, pale	Cool, moist, clammy, pale, cyanosis	Early: warm, dry; late: cool, moist, clammy; color: pale, cyanosis (late)	Early: warm, dry; late: cyanosis
Capillary refill time	Decreased	Decreased	Decreased	Decreased
Peripheral pulses	Absent or diminished	Absent or diminished	Absent or diminished (late)	Absent or diminished
Jugular venous distention	Absent or flat	Elevated		
Hemodynamic findings				
Central venous pressure	Decreased	Increased	Decreased	Decreased
Pulmonary capillary wedge pressure	Decreased	Increased	Decreased	Decreased
Cardiac output	Decreased	Decreased	Increased or decreased	Decreased
Peripheral vascular resistance	Decreased	Increased	Decreased or normal; late: increased	Decreased
Pulmonary function				
Respiratory rate	Increased; shallow or Cheyne-Stokes respirations	Increased; late: Cheyne-Stokes respirations, apnea	Increased; late: Cheyne-Stokes respirations	Varies
Auscultation	Early: clear; late: rales	Rales	Early: clear; late: rales	Early: clear; late: rales
Acid-base changes				
Early	Respiratory alkalosis	Respiratory alkalosis	Respiratory alkalosis	Respiratory alkalosis
Late	Metabolic (lactic) acidosis	Metabolic (lactic) acidosis	Metabolic (lactic) acidosis	Metabolic (lactic) acidosis
Urine output				
Early	Decreased (<20 ml/mm)	Decreased (<20 ml/mm)	Decreased (<20 ml/mm)	Decreased (<20 ml/mm)
Late	Anuria	Anuria	Anuria	Anuria
Urine sodium concentration	Decreased	Decreased	Decreased	Decreased
Urine osmolality	Increased	Increased	Increased	Increased

Nursing Dx & Intervention

Nursing Diagnosis	Nursing Intervention/Rationale
Altered renal, cerebral, cardiopulmonary, and peripheral tissue perfusion	• Assess for signs and symptoms indicative of altered tissue perfusion: cool skin temperature, pale or cyanotic color, decreased arterial pulsations, altered mental status, decreased blood pressure, tachycardia, decreased urine output, thirst. • Maintain complete bed rest *to minimize metabolic needs.* Maintain flat position or position that *facilitates or improves circulation.* • Keep patient warm *to minimize metabolic needs.* • Measure all body fluid loss. Estimate loss in dressings or perineal pads. • Measure intake and output every 1 to 2 hours or as indicated. • Administer parenteral therapy as ordered: whole blood, plasmanate, and volume expanders. • Permit nothing by mouth or give clear liquid diet. • Check blood pressure and peripheral pulses every 1 to 2 hours as ordered *to assess tissue perfusion.* • Apply support measures to control bleeding as indicated: pressure dressings, shock trousers.

Nursing Diagnosis	Nursing Intervention/Rationale
Decreased cardiac output related to mechanical factors (preload, afterload, contractility)	• Assess and monitor for signs and symptoms indicative of decreased cardiac output: fatigue, skin pallor, diaphoresis, oliguria, anuria, hypotension, tachycardia. • Maintain bed rest *to conserve energy and decrease oxygen demand.* • Monitor hemodynamic parameters as ordered *to evaluate patient's clinical status and response to therapy:* blood pressure, arterial pressure, pulmonary artery pressure (PAP), pulmonary capillary wedge pressure (PCWP), and cardiac output (CO) reflect LVEDP and myocardial contractility. • Calculate systemic vascular resistance as ordered. • Frequently assess cardiovascular response to drug therapy. Adjust flow and dosage according to blood pressure and heart rate response. • Administer sympathomimetic and vasodilator drugs as ordered *to increase myocardial contractility and reduce peripheral vascular resistance (PVR).* • Administer plasma volume expanders as ordered. Adjust flow rate according to PAP and PCWP readings. • Restrict activities as indicated. Plan care to prevent fatigue, which increases oxygen demand. Provide rest between procedures. • Initiate intra-aortic balloon pumping as indicated *to decrease cardiac workload and increase coronary perfusion.* • Measure intake and output every 1 to 2 hours. Monitor indices of renal function: BUN and creatinine levels.
Fluid volume deficit	• Assess for signs and symptoms of fluid volume deficit: hypotension and decreased venous filling, pulse volume, and pressure. • Assess skin for increased temperature, color, and turgor. • Administer fluids as ordered. • Monitor hemodynamic parameters, including pulmonary capillary wedge pressure, heart rate, urine output, and central venous pressure. • Maintain patient's core temperature by covering patient with blankets as needed. • Maintain accurate intake and output record. • Monitor electrolytes. • Measure fluid loss.
Impaired gas exchange	• Monitor arterial blood gas levels. • Administer oxygen as ordered, via mask or through endotracheal tube. • Auscultate breath sounds every hour *for increasing pulmonary congestion and atelectasis.* • Prepare for intubation and assisted ventilation as indicated. • Obtain chest roentgenograms as ordered. Assess for signs of increased congestion. • Monitor for signs of impairment in respiratory pattern by assessing skin color, respiratory rate, and breathing pattern.
Potential for trauma	• Implement safety precautions, including use of soft restraints and side rails, for patients who are restless or confused.
Potential impaired skin integrity	• Perform skin care every 1 to 2 hours, carefully observing bony prominences for pressure points and evidence of breakdown. • Provide egg-crate mattress, sheepskin mattress, or air-pressure mattress as ordered. • Turn patient every 1 to 2 hours as condition permits. • Begin passive range of motion exercises as condition permits.
Altered nutrition: less than body requirements	• Weigh daily. • Begin tube feedings, intralipids, and hyperalimentation as ordered.
Anxiety	• Explain all procedures and treatments. • Remain with patient to offer reassurance. • Maintain as quiet and calm an atmosphere as possible. • Allow family to be with patient as condition permits. • Provide alternative means of communication if patient is intubated or unable to verbalize fears and needs. • Administer medications as ordered for persistent chest pain or discomfort. • Maintain calm and reassuring manner.
Potential for infection	• Maintain strict asepsis of all invasive lines. • Administer antibiotics as ordered. • Turn patient every 1 to 2 hours as condition permits.

Patient Education

1. Explain all procedures and treatments as they occur. Refer to primary disorder for specific teaching protocol.

Evaluation

Patient Outcome	Data Indicating That Outcome is Reached
Cardiac output is improved.	Patient is normotensive. Cardiac output is 4 to 5 L/minute. Pulmonary capillary wedge pressure (PCWP) is 10 to 15 mm Hg. Skin is warm and dry. Patient is resting quietly.
Fluid volume is restored.	Patient is normotensive. PCWP is 10 to 15 mm Hg. Urine output is increased.
Gas exchange is improved.	Pa_{O_2} is 80 to 100 mm Hg. Pco_2 is 35 to 45 mm Hg. Lungs are clear. Patient verbalizes that breathing is easier.
Acid-base balance is normal.	CO_2 is 35 to 45 mm Hg. pH is 7.35 to 7.45.
Anxiety is decreased.	Patient verbalizes fears and asks questions. Patient appears relaxed and is resting quietly.

Cardiomyopathy

The term "cardiomyopathy" is applied to diseases that affect the myocardium, resulting in enlargement or ventricular dysfunction.

In the past three decades, great advances in the understanding of this complex disorder have been made. In an attempt to distinguish the various forms and causes of the myopathies, several classifications have been proposed. In *classifications according to cause,* terms such as "idiopathic cardiomyopathy" and "myocardiomyopathy" have been used to describe disease not caused by coronary artery, valvular, or congenital heart disease. Types of idiopathic cardiomyopathy include the following:

- Endocardial fibroelastosis
- Hypertrophic obstructive cardiomyopathy
- Primary myocardial disease
- Familial cardiomyopathies
  - Metabolic storage diseases
    - Pompe's disease (glycogen)
    - Fabry's disease (glycolipid)
  - Muscular dystrophies
  - Friedreich's ataxia
  - Sickle cell anemia

Secondary cardiomyopathies occur as a result of a disease process that affects other parts of the body before or after the myocardium is involved. The following are examples of such conditions:

- Inflammatory
  - Infectious
    - Viral (such as coxsackievirus, rubella)
    - Rickettsial (typhus, Q fever)
    - Bacterial (streptococcal)
    - Spirochetal (leptospirosis, syphilis)
    - Fungal (histoplasmosis, coccidioidomycosis)
    - Parasitic (Chagas' disease, schistosomiasis)
- Noninfectious (collagen)
  - Rheumatic heart disease
  - Scleroderma
  - Systemic lupus erythematosus
  - Polyarteritis
  - Löffler's disease
  - Dermatomyositis
- Infiltrative
  - Sarcoidosis
  - Amyloidosis
  - Neoplastic disease
- Metabolic
  - Endocrine disorders
    - Thyrotoxicosis
    - Myxedema
  - Nutritional
    - Starvation, malnutrition
    - Beri-beri
- Toxic
  - Alcohol
  - Carbon monoxide
  - Arsenic
  - Immunosuppressive drugs (doxorubicin)
  - Emetine
- Miscellaneous
  - Postpartum
  - Radiation

In *functional classifications* three types exist: hypertrophic, dilated, and restricted.

Pathophysiology

Hypertrophic Cardiomyopathy

Hypertrophic cardiomyopathy is the form of myocardial disease whose pathophysiologic, etiologic, and clinical features continue to receive the widest attention. As a result it has acquired an extensive list of identifying terms that generally describe features of the disease not present in all cases. These include idiopathic hypertrophic subaortic stenosis (IHSS), asymmetric septal hypertrophy (ASH), and hypertrophic obstructive cardiomyopathy (HOCM).

Hypertrophic cardiomyopathy is marked by a distinctive pattern of hypertrophy, with thickening of the interventricular septum when compared with the free wall of the left ventricle (Figure 1-36). The overgrowth of muscle mass makes the ventricular walls rigid, increasing resistance as blood enters from the left atrium. Obstruction of left ventricular outflow is another characteristic. Consequently, left ventricular ejection is impeded throughout systole. Contributing to outflow obstruction is the obstruction caused by opposition of the anterior mitral leaflet against the hypertrophied septum during midsystole. Systolic motion of the anterior mitral leaflet has been used to determine the severity of outflow obstruction.[34] Elevated systolic pressure gradients occur in the range of 70% to 90% of left ventricular volumes.[50] Failure occurs as resistance to diastolic filling increases as the result of a stiff, noncompliant left ventricle.

These hearts show massive overgrowth of myocardial tissue with small ventricular cavities. The atria are also hypertrophied and dilated, reflecting the high resistance to ventricular filling.

Histologically the heart muscle may show myocardial fiber disarray. First described in 1958 by Donald Teare, this form of hypertrophic cardiomyopathy is thought to reflect a genetic defect that results in abnormal heart structure. This feature is not limited to hypertrophic cardiomyopathy; similar disorganization has been seen in some cases of acquired or congenital heart disease.

Figure 1-36 Heart with hypertrophic cardiomyopathy. Interventricular septum, *IVS*, is thicker than posterior wall, *PW*. Histologic section *(lower illustration)* shows marked disorganization of myocardium that is especially prominent in septum. (Hematoxylin and eosin, ×50.)
From Bulkley, B.H.: Advances in cardiac pathology. In The heart, update I, by J. Willis Hurst, editor. Copyright © 1979, McGraw-Hill Book Co. Used with the permission of McGraw-Hill Book Co.

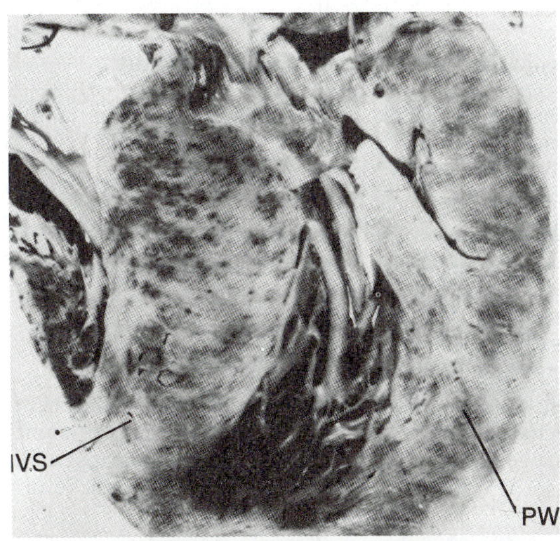

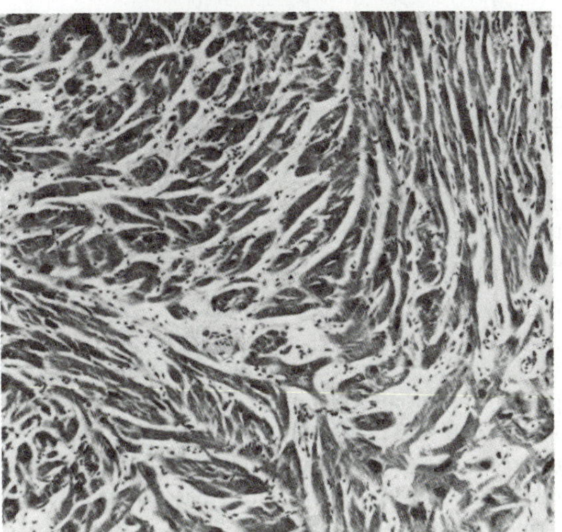

Figure 1-37 Heart with idiopathic dilated congestive cardiomyopathy. Opened left ventricle, *LV*, has dilated and globular configuration. Aortic valves, *AV*, and mitral valves, *MV*, are normal.
From Kaye.[50]

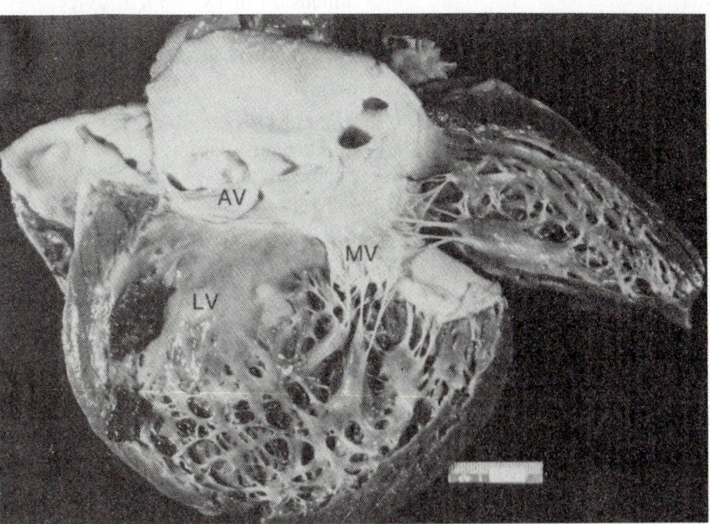

Dilated Cardiomyopathy

The second and most common form of cardiomyopathy is marked by gross dilation of the heart, interference with systolic function, and damage to myofibrils. Dilated cardiomyopathy is marked by impaired systolic ejection function and increased end-diastolic and end-systolic volumes.

The heart has a globular shape with enlargement and dilation of all four chambers (Figure 1-37). Although the heart may weigh up to 700 g (normal 350 g), the wall thickness may be normal or decreased. Left ventricular filling pressures are generally higher as a result of poor contractile function. The cardiac valves are basically normal, as are the coronary arteries. Endocardial thrombi are common, particularly in the ventricular apex.

Histologic examination reveals nonspecific changes including cell hypertrophy and extensive interstitial and perivascular fibrosis.

The cause of this disorder is not clear, but it has been linked to various factors that predispose to the development of cardiomyopathy, including alcohol, pregnancy, infections, and toxic agents.

Restrictive Cardiomyopathy

A less common form of cardiomyopathy, restrictive cardiomyopathy is marked by abnormal diastolic (filling) function and excessively rigid ventricular walls. Contractility is relatively unimpaired with normal systolic emptying of the ventricles. Hemodynamically, this group of cardiomyopathies resembles constrictive pericarditis.

The abnormal diastolic filling occurs as a result of infiltration of the endocardium or myocardium with fibroelastic tissue similar to that seen in Löffler's endocarditis, endomyocardial fibrosis, and amyloidosis.

Diagnostic Studies and Findings

Study	Hypertrophic Cardiomyopathy	Dilated Cardiomyopathy	Restrictive Cardiomyopathy
Chest roentgenogram	Enlarged cardiac silhouette (mild to moderate)	Enlarged cardiac silhouette; prominence of left ventricle (LV) (moderate to marked)	Cardiac enlargement (mild)
Electrocardiogram (ECG) (24-hour ambulatory monitor)	LV hypertrophy; ST segment and T wave changes; Q waves may be seen in precordial leads; atrial arrhythmias	LV hypertrophy; sinus tachycardia; atrial and ventricular arrhythmias; ST segment and T wave changes; conduction disturbances	Low-voltage; conduction disturbances
Echocardiogram	Asymmetric septal hypertrophy (ASH); narrow LV outflow tract; systolic anterior motion of mitral valve; decreased internal dimension of LV	LV dilation; abnormal diastolic mitral valve motion; enlarged atria	Increased LV wall thickness and mass; small or normal LV cavity; normal systolic function; pericardial effusion
Radionuclide studies	ASH; hyperdynamic systolic function; LV size small or normal	LV dilation and dysfunction	Myocardial infiltration; small or normal LV cavity; normal systolic function
Cardiac catheterization	Decreased LV compliance; mitral regurgitation; hyperdynamic systolic function; LV outflow obstruction	LV enlargement and dysfunction; mitral and tricuspid regurgitation; elevated diastolic filling pressures; decreased cardiac output	Decreased LV compliance; normal systolic function; elevated diastolic filling process

Medical Plan

Surgery

Myotomy-myectomy—for patient with hypertrophic cardiomyopathy who has intractable symptoms and severe obstruction; hypertrophied septum is excised, which diminishes left ventricular gradient and mitral regurgitation; procedure improves symptoms but has not been reported to prolong life

Excision of fibrotic endocardium—successful in limited number of cases of restrictive cardiomyopathy; procedure apparently decreases ventricular filling pressures and increases cardiac output

Cardiac transplantation—an alternative for certain patients

but requires careful evaluation of patient and family (see p. 94 for care of patient following transplantation)

Other surgical interventions—essentially nonexistent; valve replacement considered in individual cases but generally not favored

Medications

Hypertrophic cardiomyopathy—goals of drug therapy are to decrease ventricular contractility and increase ventricular volume and left ventricular outflow

Cardiac glycosides: digitalis

Indications: Not favored in management of hypertrophic cardiomyopathy because it increases contractility and therefore degree of obstruction; used in presence of atrial fibrillation with rapid ventricular rates or left ventricular dysfunction without obstruction

β-Adrenergic blocking agents: propranolol (Inderal)

Indications: Principal mode of therapy; has negative inotropic effects on myocardial contractility and thus is believed to prevent increase in outflow obstruction, decrease myocardial oxygen consumption, and exert antiarrhythmic actions

Antiarrhythmic drugs: verapamil (Calan)

Indications: Calcium channel blocking agent that has given best results in management of these patients; has been shown to decrease left ventricular outflow obstruction and increase exercise tolerance[14]

Usual dosage: 80-160 mg q8h (not to exceed 480 mg/d)

Dilated cardiomyopathy—cannot be halted or reversed by any pharmacologic agent; pharmacologic interventions directed largely by symptoms; as with any patient in congestive heart failure, digitalis, diuretic, and vasodilator therapy used (see p. 40); antiarrhythmics such as quinidine and procainamide used to treat arrhythmias

Restrictive cardiomyopathy—pharmacologic agents directed by underlying disorder; digitalis and diuretics often employed to treat arrhythmias and signs of failure, but their effectiveness is limited

General Management

Hemodynamic monitoring—initiated as means of assessing left ventricular function and cardiac output

Intra-aortic balloon counterpulsation—used to sustain severely depressed ventricular function

Cardiac monitoring—used to determine presence of atrial or ventricular arrhythmias or conduction defects and to assess effectiveness of antiarrhythmic agents

Cardioversion—used in treatment of atrial fibrillation with rapid ventricular response

Restriction of sodium and fluid intake

Oxygen therapy

NURSING CARE

Nursing Assessment

Area of Concern	Hypertrophic Cardiomyopathy	Dilated Cardiomyopathy	Restrictive Cardiomyopathy
General complaints	Dyspnea; shortness of breath; angina pectoris; fatigue; palpitations; syncope (may be exertional)	Dyspnea; fatigue; complaints associated with biventricular failure	Dyspnea; fatigue; complaints associated with right ventricular failure
Arterial pressure		Normal or low systolic; narrowed pulse pressure	
Arterial pulse	Brisk carotid upstroke	Low amplitude and volume; pulsus alternans	
Jugular venous pressure		Distended; prominent a and v waves	Distended
Palpation	Apical systolic thrill and heave	Apical impulse displaced laterally; parasternal impulses and heaves; pulsatile liver	Apical impulse difficult to palpate
Auscultation	Systolic murmur at lower left sternal border increasing in intensity with Valsalva maneuver; S_4 gallop	Murmurs of mitral and tricuspid regurgitation; S_3 and S_4 gallops; pulmonary rales	Murmurs of mitral regurgitation; S_3 and S_4 gallops; heart sounds distant

Nursing Dx & Intervention

Nursing Diagnosis	Nursing Intervention/Rationale
Decreased cardiac output	• Observe for signs and symptoms of decreased left ventricular functioning: chest pain, syncope, peripheral constriction, and cyanosis. • Encourage bed rest. Limit self-care activities *to conserve energy and decrease oxygen demand.* • Monitor arterial pressure, pulmonary capillary wedge pressure, cardiac output, and ECG as indicated. • Administer drugs as ordered. • Limit and monitor IV fluids as ordered. *Convalescent care:* • Progressively increase activity level as indicated by improvement in patient status. • Monitor vital signs and report any changes in heart rate or blood pressure. • Teach patient and family the importance of monitoring vital signs and how to check blood pressure and pulse accurately.
Ineffective individual coping	• Determine baseline knowledge of disease. • Answer all questions about disease and future health. • Encourage discussion of feelings of hopelessness and fears. • Assist patient to participate in decision-making process with regard to any adjustments in life-style. • Provide patient education. • Include family or significant other in care. • Encourage family to learn cardiopulmonary resuscitation.
Impaired gas exchange related to elevated pulmonary capillary pressure	• Assess for signs of impaired ventilation and perfusion; restlessness, somnolence, hypercapnia, hypoxia. • Monitor arterial blood gases frequently. • Administer oxygen therapy as ordered, via nasal prongs, mask, or positive-pressure device. • Administer IV morphine sulfate per protocol *to reduce hyperventilation.* • Elevate head of bed *to improve ventilation and decrease workload of breathing.* • Auscultate breath sounds every hour *to determine increases in congestion and adequacy of ventilatory effort.* • Prepare for intubation and assisted ventilation if required. • Explain all procedures and modalities briefly to patient *to prevent hyperventilation resulting from fear or anxiety.*
Fluid volume excess	• Observe for signs of decreased ventricular function and fluid retention: increased adventitious lung sounds, presence of S_3, shortness of breath, cough, peripheral edema, increased venous filling. • Maintain patent IV line for drug administration. • Administer diuretics as ordered *to decrease circulating volume.* • Restrict sodium and fluid intake. • Weigh patient daily (same time of day, same amount of clothing) *to determine fluid loss or retention.* • Monitor intake and output. • Monitor serum electrolytes, especially sodium and potassium. • Inspect for increased or decreased jugular venous distention. • Auscultate heart tones and breath sounds every 1 to 2 hours for increased congestion.
Altered nutrition: less than body requirements related to impaired absorption of nutrients	• Observe daily for signs of malnutrition: loss of dry body weight greater than 20% of ideal weight, anorexia, stomatitis, decreased skinfold measurements. • Weigh daily. • Maintain diet as ordered. Do not force patient to eat. Offer frequent small meals. Supplement meal with high-caloric feedings as ordered *to maintain nutrient intake.*
Pain	• Administer morphine sulfate as ordered. • Stay with patient as much as possible. • Explain all procedures and routines to patient. • Provide over-bed table and pillows as needed *to maintain position of comfort.* • Allow family to stay with patient and assist with patient care.

Patient Education

1. Describe the nature and type of cardiomyopathy.
2. Explain the limitations of the disease on life-style and the prognosis.
3. Explain the signs and symptoms to report to the physician.
4. Describe activity allowances and limitations; explain the importance of avoiding isometric exercises.
5. Explain dietary and fluid restrictions.
6. Explain the name, purpose, dosage, and side effects of prescribed medications; warn against the effects of abruptly stopping propranolol.
7. Explain the need for daily weighing when ordered.

Evaluation

Patient Outcome	Data Indicating That Outcome is Reached
Ventricular volume is increased; outflow obstruction is decreased.	Cardiac output and left ventricular end-diastolic pressure (LVEDP) are increased. Fatigue, dyspnea, and angina are relieved.
LV diastolic volume is decreased; ventricular contractility is improved.	LVEDP is decreased. Stroke volume is improved. Patient loses weight. Dyspnea and shortness of breath are relieved.
Patient copes effectively with diagnosis.	Patient follows up with medical therapy. Patient reports taking medications. Patient verbalizes feeling less anxious and fearful.

Valvular heart disease

Valvular heart disease (VHD) is an acquired or congenital disorder of a cardiac valve, marked by stenosis and obstructed blood flow or by valvular breakdown and regurgitation of blood.

With the introduction of antibiotic therapy and with improved diagnostic procedures, the incidence of VHD has declined over the past three decades. It is most commonly a chronic illness, and symptoms requiring therapy may take years to develop. VHD may also occur as an acute illness following trauma or myocardial infarction.

Pathophysiology

The etiology of VHD can be classified into congenital and acquired disorders.

Congenital disorders include bicuspid valve and pulmonary stenosis. Although not usually classified as VHD, tricuspid and pulmonary atresia, mitral valve prolapse, and Ebstein's anomaly are all defects involving valve function.

Rheumatic fever and endocarditis account for the greatest number of cases of acquired VHD.[3,11] Other disorders such as Marfan's syndrome, cardiomyopathy, myocardial infarction, myxomatous degeneration of the mitral valve, and trauma can also lead to valve dysfunction.

Cardiac valves are unidirectional, ensuring efficient flow of blood throughout the heart and the pulmonary and systemic circulation. Valve disorders occur when the integrity of the valve leaflets or the surrounding structures are disrupted.

Two basic valve abnormalities exist: stenosis and regurgitation. In stenosis the valve opening narrows as a result of thickening and rigidity of the valve leaflets. Stenosis blocks the flow of blood across the valve, increasing the pressure gradient. In regurgitation (insufficiency, incompetency), calcification, scarring, and retraction of the leaflets or adjacent structures lead to an incomplete valve closure that results in reversed blood flow.

Mixed lesions producing both stenosis and regurgitation can occur. In addition, more than one valve may be affected.

Mitral Stenosis

The most common cause of mitral stenosis is rheumatic valvulitis that leads to fibrotic thickening and fusion of the valve commissures. Scarring of the free margins of the leaflets occurs with shortening and thickening of the chordae tendineae, which may lead to regurgitation often seen with mitral stenosis.

The normal mitral valve opening is 4 to 6 cm^2. When this opening is reduced, flow across the valve is blocked, increasing the pressure gradient needed to eject blood from the left atrium to the left ventricle. The pressure gradient rises to maintain cardiac output. When the mitral orifice is decreased to 1.5 cm^2, cardiac output drops and symptoms appear with exertion. As the disease progresses, the mean left atrial pressure rises, causing the left atrial chamber to enlarge. The increased left atrial pressure is reflected in the pulmonary capillaries and pulmonary artery. As pulmonary capillary pressure rises, fluid flows back across the alveolar membrane, eventually exceeding oncotic pressure of the plasma proteins in the blood and forcing fluid out of the capillaries into the lung. If this fluid cannot be removed by drainage, pulmonary edema develops.

Mitral Regurgitation

Rheumatic fever, the usual cause of mitral regurgitation, causes thickening, scarring, rigidity, and calcification of the valve leaflets. The commissures become fused with the chordae tendineae, causing the leaflets to shorten and retract, which prevents them from complete closure during systole. A nonrheumatic cause of mitral regurgitation is myocardial infarction, which causes dilation of the left ventricle and displacement of the papillary muscles. Papillary muscle dysfunction may also occur as a result of rupture or fibrosis caused by ischemia, infarction, and ventricular aneurysm at the base of a papillary muscle. In addition, annular dilation may lead to an incompetent mitral apparatus. The most common cause is left ventricular dilation resulting from coronary artery disease or congestive cardiomyopathy.

As the mitral valve disorder progresses, the reverse flow to the left atrium causes left atrial pressure to rise. This pressure is reflected in the pulmonary veins, leading to leakage of fluid into the lungs.

The increase in backward flow causes atrial dilation and enlargement. The left ventricle becomes hypertrophied, because it must deal with the larger volume of blood that is lost to the left atrium during systole.

Aortic Stenosis

The most common cause of aortic stenosis is congenital bicuspid valve. This defect occurs in 1% of the population, more often in males (3:1).

The normal aortic valve opening measures 2.6 to 3.5 cm^2. Valve narrowing results from calcification of the leaflets. Calcification may extend into the aortic wall or onto the anterior leaflet of the mitral valve, which accounts for the mitral disease commonly occurring with aortic stenosis. Calcification may also extend into the conduction system, leading to conduction defects. As the disease progresses, calcification makes the valve inflexible, reducing the opening to a small slit.

As the aortic valve opening decreases, left ventricular pressure rises to create enough pressure to eject a normal stroke volume and propel flow across the valve into the aorta. This obstruction to left ventricular outflow leads to a pressure gradient between the aorta and left ventricle during systole. To maintain flow across the narrowed opening, wall thickness gradually increases in the pressure-overloaded left ventricle, leading to hypertrophy. In time the flow across the valve becomes fixed and cardiac output does not increase in response to demand. During exercise the increased flow to extremities with fixed cardiac output causes a decreased cerebral blood flow, resulting in dizziness or syncope.

Left atrial hypertrophy occurs in an attempt to increase cardiac output. To produce a forceful atrial contraction, left ventricular end-diastolic pressure (LVEDP) rises, which in turn increases the myocardial fiber stretch and leads to increased contraction and improved stroke volume.

The course of aortic stenosis depends on the size of the valve opening and the left ventricle. When myocardial contractility falls, the left ventricle dilates, causing diastolic and left atrial pressures to increase further.

The onset of symptoms of heart failure indicates moderate to severe disease, and death often occurs less than 5 years after symptoms appear. Sudden death is linked to severe aortic stenosis (0.5 to 0.7 cm^2).

Aortic Regurgitation

Rheumatic fever, syphilis, connective tissue disorder, and infective endocarditis are common causes of aortic valve disorders.

The basic hemodynamic problem in aortic regurgitation is a volume-overloaded left ventricle. Blood ejected during normal systole reenters the left ventricle in diastole. To compensate for this volume, the left ventricle must produce a higher stroke volume by increasing the systolic pressure, resulting in eventual hypertrophy of the left ventricle.

With time, LVEDP and left atrial pressure increase. As myocardial contractility diminishes and failure takes place, mitral regurgitation may occur as a result of the malpositioning of papillary muscles.

Diagnostic Studies and Findings

Study	Mitral Stenosis	Mitral Regurgitation	Aortic Stenosis	Aortic Regurgitation
Radionuclide studies	To determine resting and exercise ejection fraction	To determine resting and exercise ejection fraction	To determine resting and exercise ejection fraction	To determine resting and exercise ejection fraction
Cardiac catheterization	Pressure across mitral valve increased; left atrial (LA) pressure increased; PCWP increased; low cardiac output	Left ventricular end-diastolic pressure (LVEDP) increased; left atrial pressure (LAP) increased; angiography with contrast media performed to quantify regurgitation	Pressure gradient in systole across aortic valve; LVEDP increased	Pulse pressure increased; LVEDP increased; LAP increased; angiography with contrast media performed to quantify regurgitation
Electrocardiogram (ECG)	LA enlargement; notched P wave (P mitrale); right ventricular (RV) hypertrophy	LA enlargement; LV hypertrophy; atrial fibrillation	LV hypertrophy; conduction defects: first-degree A-V block, left bundle-branch block	LV hypertrophy
Chest roentgenogram	LA and RV enlargement; pulmonary venous congestion; interstitial pulmonary edema	LA and LV enlargement; pulmonary vascular congestion	Poststenotic aortic dilation; aortic valve calcification	Aortic valve calcification; LV enlargement; dilation of ascending aorta
Echocardiogram	Decreased excursion of leaflets; diminished E to F slope	LA enlargement; hyperdynamic LV	Nonrestricted movement of aortic valve; thickening of LV wall	LV dilation; diastolic fluttering of anterior leaflet

Medical Plan

Surgery

Indicated when medical therapy no longer alleviates clinical symptoms or when there is diagnostic evidence of progressive myocardial failure (such as progressive enlargement of heart)

Open mitral commissurotomy (valvulotomy)—surgical splitting of fused mitral valve leaflet with guidance and separating fused commissures; a palliative procedure performed only for pure mitral stenosis that involves leaflets and not chordae; contraindicated in patients with history of emboli

Valvular annuloplasty—reparative procedure of valve ring, chordae, or papillary muscle performed primarily for mitral and tricuspid regurgitation

Valve replacement—replacement of stenotic or incompetent valve with bioprosthetic or mechanical valve; commonly used valves include pynolite tilting disks, porcine heterografts, homografts, pericardial valves, and ball-in-cage valves

Medications

Guided by patient's clinical signs and symptoms

Digitalis and diuretics for heart failure (see pp. 40 and 41)

Quinidine, procainamide, propranolol for arrhythmias (see p. 18)

Anticoagulants for patients in atrial fibrillation who are at risk for systemic or pulmonary embolization; warfarin sodium (Coumadin) in doses titrated to maintain prothrombin time at two times control

Antibiotic prophylaxis before any procedure that increases risk of endocarditis (Table 1-3)

General Management

Cardioversion—indicated for patients with mitral stenosis in atrial fibrillation to decrease risk of emboli

Dictated by severity of valvular disorder (see pp. 28 and 42 for supportive care of patients in heart failure or with arrhythmias)

Diet therapy—sodium restriction for patients with mild to moderate signs of pulmonary congestion

NURSING CARE

Nursing Assessment

Area of Concern	Mitral Stenosis	Mitral Regurgitation	Aortic Stenosis	Aortic Regurgitation
General complaints	Fatigue; dyspnea on exertion; palpitations; hemoptysis; hoarseness; orthopnea; paroxysmal nocturnal dyspnea	Dyspnea; fatigue; exercise intolerance; orthopnea; palpitations	Fatigue; dyspnea; orthopnea; angina pectoris; dizziness; syncope	Dyspnea on exertion; palpitations; orthopnea; exertional chest pain
Physical examination	Resting tachycardia; irregular pulse; jugular venous distention increased in presence of right ventricular (RV) failure; prominent a wave in presence of pulmonary hypertension (absent in atrial fibrillation)	Irregular pulse; sharp upstroke of arterial pulse; jugular venous distention increased in presence of RV failure; prominent "a" wave in presence of increased RV pressure	Early: normal blood pressure; late: systolic pressure decreased; narrow pulse pressure; carotid pulse slow with small pulse volume	Arterial pulsations: bounding pulse with rapid rise and fall (water-hammer pulse); widened pulse pressure; head bobbing (Musset's sign); skin warm, damp, and flushed
Palpation	Diastolic thrill at apex	Apical impulse forceful and displaced downward and to left	Systolic thrill palpable at base of heart; apical pulse strong and sustained throughout systole	Diastolic thrill along left sternal border; laterally displaced apical impulse; systolic thrill in jugular notch and along carotid arteries
Auscultation (Figure 1-38)	Loud S_1; opening snap; low snap; low-pitched, rumbling diastolic murmur	Diminished or absent S_1; wide splitting of S_2; S_3, S_4 heard in severe regurgitation; holosystolic murmur heard best at apex	Diminished or absent A_2; crescendo-decrescendo harsh systolic murmur heard best at base (second intercostal space to right of sternum); aortic ejection sound	Decrescendo diastolic murmur (blowing), high pitched and heard best at base (second intercostal space to right of sternum); systolic ejection murmur heard best at base

Figure 1-38 Auscultation of valvular heart disease murmurs. **A,** Mitral stenosis. **B,** Mitral regurgitation. **C,** Aortic stenosis. **D,** Aortic regurgitation.
From Guzzetta.[41]

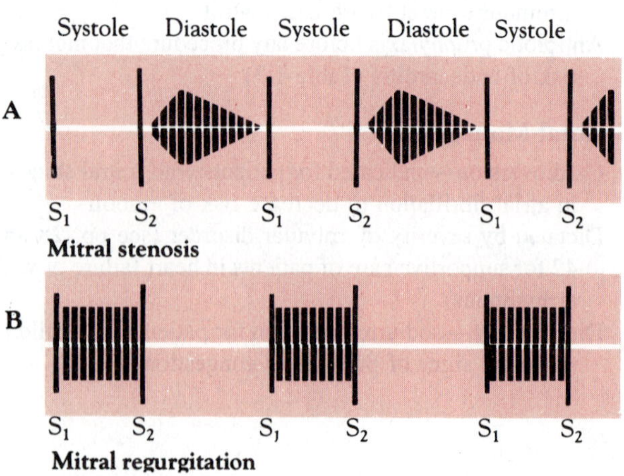

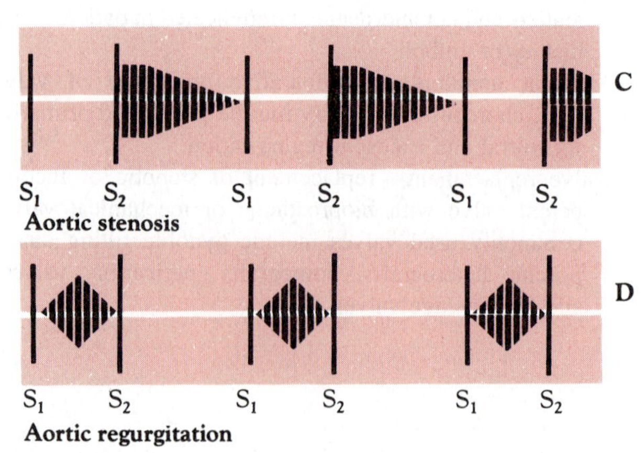

Nursing Dx & Intervention

Nursing Diagnosis	Nursing Intervention/Rationale
Decreased cardiac output (potential) related to valvular insufficiency (preload)	• Establish baseline assessment of cardiovascular status *to evaluate response to therapy.* • Monitor vital signs every 2 to 4 hours. • Administer medications as ordered *to maintain blood pressure.* • Maintain activities as tolerated; maintain planned rest periods.
Fluid volume excess (potential) related to cardiac decompensation	• Assess for signs and symptoms of fluid volume excess: weight gain, increased jugular venous pressure, lung congestion. • Administer diuretic and vasodilator therapy as ordered. • Auscultate lung sounds every 8 hours. • Monitor nutrition with dietary sodium and fluid restrictions. • Weigh patient daily (same time of day, same amount of clothing) *to detect fluid retention.* • Monitor intake and output *to determine response to therapy.* • Monitor electrolyte levels, blood chemistry findings, hemoglobin level, and hematocrit.

Patient Education

1. Assess the patient's level of knowledge and teach the patient about the disease, including etiology, medications, diet restrictions, exercise levels, and possible complications.
2. Assist the patient during diagnostic workup and assist with the decision for medical or surgical treatment.
3. Include the patient's family in the teaching and decision-making process.
4. Instruct the patient in the name, dosage, and purpose of medications.
5. Instruct the patient in the disease process and associated symptoms to report to the physician.
6. Explain activity allowances and limitations.
7. Explain diet and fluid restrictions.
8. Instruct the patient about antibiotic prophylaxis to prevent infectious endocarditis (Table 1-3).
9. Explain the importance of notifying the dentist, urologist, and gynecologist of valvular heart disease.
10. Provide a female patient with instruction regarding contraception and pregnancy.
11. Instruct the patient about maintaining good oral hygiene, daily care, and regular visits to dentist.

Evaluation

Patient Outcome	Data Indicating That Outcome is Reached
Cardiac output is maintained.	Lungs are clear. Patient reports improvement of symptoms. Heart rate is within acceptable limits.
Fluid balance is regained.	Baseline weight is achieved. There is no peripheral edema or sign of fluid overload.

Pericarditis

Pericarditis is an inflammatory process involving the parietal and visceral layers of the pericardium and outer myocardium.

Pericarditis may occur by itself or as a complication of another disease. Acute pericarditis, which can occur within 2 weeks of the offending condition, lasts up to 6 weeks. There may be effusion or tamponade. Chronic pericarditis may follow acute pericarditis and may last up to 6 months.

Pathophysiology

Because of the closeness of the pericardium to the pleura, lung, sternum, diaphragm, and myocardium, pericarditis may be the result of a number of disease states. The most common cause is probably viral; this generally has a good prognosis. The causes of pericarditis can be summarized as follows:

- Viral (idiopathic)—organism may never be isolated
- Infectious
  - Bacterial
  - Tuberculous
  - Fungal

Table 1-1
Characteristics of Pericardial Fluid

Characteristic	Normal Fluid	Exudate Effusion
Appearance	Clear	Clear or turbid with fibrin sheds; straw or amber color; may appear hemorrhagic because of RBCs; may be purulent
Volume	50 ml	>100 ml (up to 3 L)
Specific gravity	<1.015	>1.015 (usually >1.017)
Total protein	<2 g/dl	>3 g/dl
Seromucin clot	Negative	Positive
Coagulation	Uncommon	Usual
Cells	Few	Few
Glucose	Nearly equal to plasma glucose	Nearly equal to plasma glucose
Culture	Negative	Negative

Figure 1-39 In acute pericarditis, ST segment elevation is typically upward and concave in leads I, II, aV_f, and V_4 to V_6. From Guzzetta.[41]

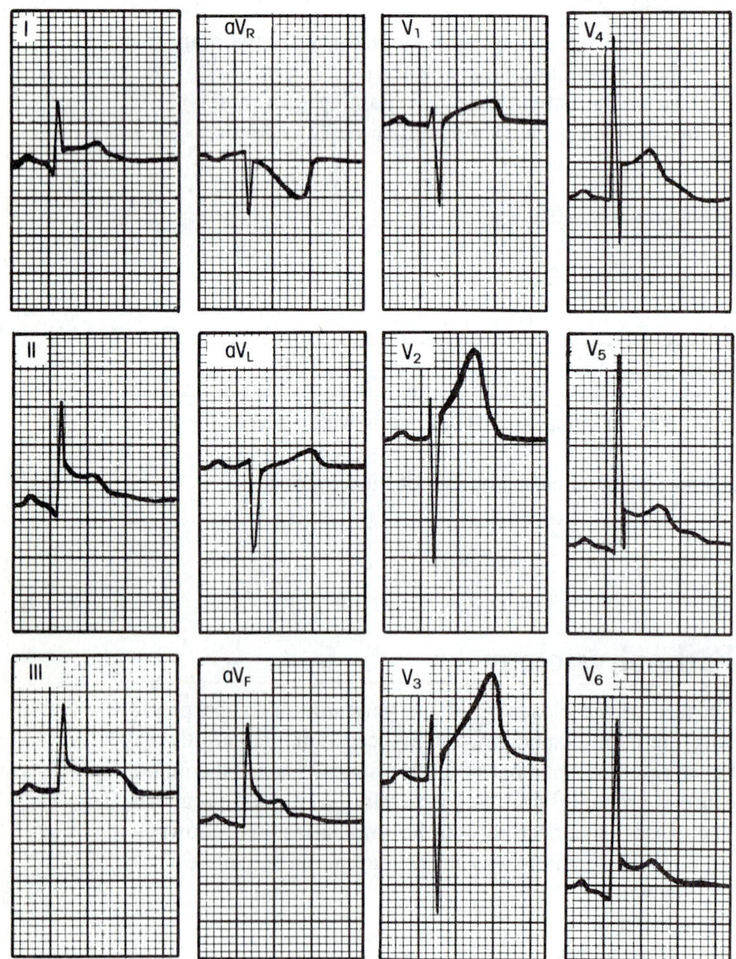

Following myocardial infarction
- Dressler's syndrome
- Postmyocardial infarction syndrome

Following cardiac surgery (postpericardiotomy syndrome)
Neoplastic diseases
Chemotherapy
Radiotherapy
Uremia
Trauma, blunt or penetrating
Connective tissue diseases
- Systemic lupus erythematosus
- Rheumatoid arthritis
- Scleroderma
- Dermatomyositis

Inflammation may occur by direct extension or by irritation. Under normal conditions the pericardial sac contains up to 50 ml of clear, serouslike fluid. When an injury occurs, an exudate of fibrin, white blood cells, and endothelial cells is released, covering the parietal and visceral layers of pericardium. Friction between the layers causes irritation and inflammation of the surrounding pleura and tissues. This may remain in one region of the heart or be widespread. Acute pericarditis may be "dry" and fibrinous or obstruct the heart's venous and lymphatic drainage, causing seepage into the pericardial sac, which creates pericardial effusion.[100]

Serofibrinous exudates occur in varying amounts from 100 ml to 3 L and may appear straw colored or turbid with fibrin strands. The exudate of pyrogenic pericarditis is purulent. The characteristics of pericardial exudate fluid are summarized in Table 1-1.

A slowly developing effusion of moderate amount (350 to 500 ml) may not alter the cardiovascular dynamics. However, a rapidly accumulating effusion, regardless of amount, can interfere with diastolic filling and lead to cardiac tamponade.

Chronic pericarditis can occur in a variety of forms, including chronic pericardial effusion and constrictive or adhesive pericarditis. Chronic effusion may lead to constrictive effusion.

Constrictive pericarditis is marked by pericardial thickening and scarring of the parietal or visceral pericardium. The layers adhere to each other, blocking out the pericardial space. This eventually involves the surface of the myocardium, causing the pericardium to become useless. In some cases the pericardium calcifies.

As the pericardium becomes scarred and rigid, normal diastolic filling of the heart is impeded. In severe cases, left ventricular end-diastolic volume may be less than stroke volume. This causes the stroke volume to be reduced with a subsequent drop in cardiac output. The normal tachycardia is unable to improve the cardiac output because of the constriction of the myocardium.

Constrictive pericarditis usually occurs in all four chambers but may be limited to certain areas such as the right ventricle, pulmonary artery, or aortic root. When all chambers are involved, left and right ventricular diastolic pressure and atrial pressures become equal. As stroke volume diminishes, left and right filling pressures rise. When this is combined with reduced cardiac output, systemic and pulmonary congestion results.

Diagnostic Studies and Findings

Laboratory Tests

- Complete blood count and differential
  - To determine infectious processes and inflammatory response
- Sedimentation rate
  - Usually elevated
- Viral serology studies
  - Performed during acute and convalescent periods
- Blood and urine cultures
  - Identification of organism in infectious process

Electrocardiogram (ECG)

- Acute pericarditis
  - Stage I (Figure 1-39)
    - ST-T segment elevation in left ventricular leads V_5, V_6, I, II, aV_L, and aV_F during first few days; PR interval depression
  - Stage II
    - Return of ST segment to baseline; PR interval depression may persist
  - Stage III
    - T wave inversions
  - Stage IV
    - Normalization of T waves
  - Low-voltage QRS complexes in presence of pericardial effusion
  - Atrial arrhythmias
- Constrictive pericarditis
  - Wide P wave in leads I, II, and V_6; Q waves deep and wide; T waves flattened or inverted; low QRS voltage

Figure 1-40 A, Normal chest roentgenogram. **B,** With pericardial effusion, cardiac silhouette is enlarged and has globular shape *(arrows)*.
From Guzzetta.[41]

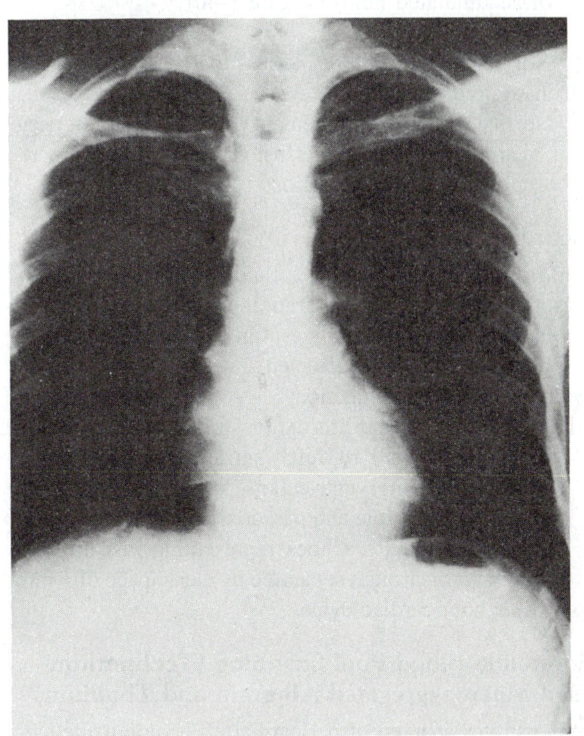

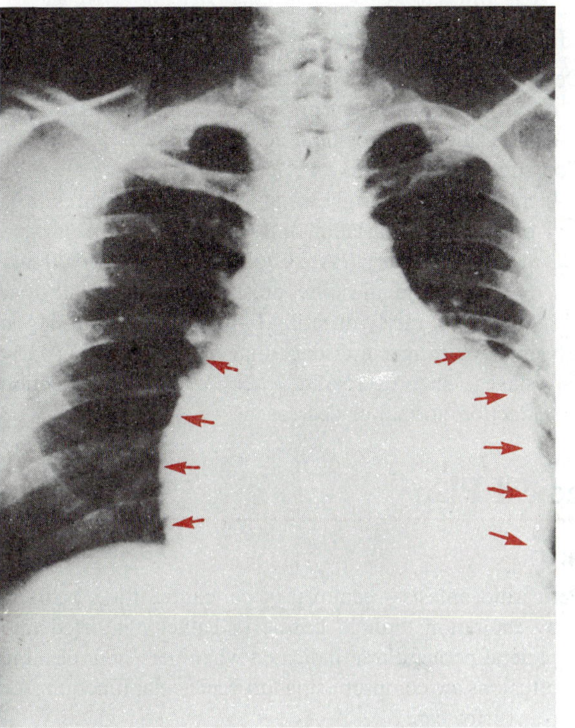

Chest Roentgenogram

Cardiac silhouette

Enlargement depends on underlying disease or amount of pericardial effusion (enlarges with 250 ml or more of accumulated fluid) (Figure 1-40)

Acute pericarditis

Normal if pericardial fluid less than 250 ml

Constrictive pericarditis

Normal or small; enlargement occurs as result of pericardial thickening or effusion; calcification of pericardium; pleural effusion

Echocardiogram

Confirms accumulation of free fluid in pericardial sac

As fluid accumulates, separation of pericardial and epicardial echoes occurs, resulting in echo-free space; minimum of 20 ml detected

Evaluates ventricular function

In constrictive pericarditis demonstrates reduced motion of posterior wall of left ventricle (LV); abnormal movement of interventricular septum characterized by flattening in systole and paradoxic movement in diastole; two separate echoes representing visceral and parietal pericardium separated by clear space of 1 mm throughout cardiac cycle

Radionuclide Blood Pool Scanning (Technetium-Labeled Macroaggregated Albumin and Thallium)

Demonstrates shadow of pericardial effusion outside cardiac chambers; seen as abnormal space between heart and liver or heart and lungs

Cardiac Catheterization

Demonstrates characteristic pericardial shadow outside opacified cardiac chambers, which are increased by pericardial thickening or fluid accumulation

Constrictive pericarditis

Increased left and right atrial (LA, RA) pressures; loss of respiratory variation of RA pressure curve; elevated pulmonary artery (PA) systolic pressure (35 to 40 mm Hg); elevated diastolic pressures equal in all four chambers, rarely differing by more than 5 mm Hg at rest or during exercise; cardiac output normal in early stages, later decreased (<2.3 L/min/m^2); ejection fraction normal or decreased

Medical Plan

Surgery

Pericardiocentesis—removal of pericardial fluid or blood by aspiration through needle or catheter inserted into parietal pericardium; indicated when persistent or large effusions are compromising left ventricular function (see p. 114 for care)

Pericardial window—open pericardial drainage implemented for acute suppurative and chronic effusions: has certain advantages over pericardiocentesis: multiple aspirations can be avoided, pericardial tissue can be obtained for culture, pericardium can be visualized, and clots and fibrin deposits can be removed

Pericardiectomy—surgical removal of visceral and parietal pericardium; has excellent long-term benefits; operative mortality of about 10%; best results when myocardial fibrosis and ventricular atrophy are not far advanced and when total or near-total pericardiectomy is performed; if hemodynamic improvement not seen immediately, elevated pressures and abnormal waveforms continue for several weeks owing to atrophy of ventricles that have been immobilized for long periods—thus early pericardiectomy is encouraged before dense fibrosis and myocardial atrophy occur; postoperative care similar to that of any cardiac surgical patient (see p. 91)

Medications

Acute pericarditis

Anti-inflammatory agents for symptomatic relief of chest pain, fever, and malaise in absence of clinical signs of cardiac tamponade

Analgesic-antipyretics: aspirin

Usual dosage: 600-900 mg to qid

Nonsteroidal anti-inflammatory agents: indomethacin (Indocin)

Usual dosage: Divided doses beginning with 25 mg qid, to maximum of 200 mg/d

Precautions: Patients should be instructed to take medicine on a full stomach

Corticosteroids

Indications: Less effective; given only in persistent recurring pericarditis and effusion

Constrictive pericarditis

Chemotherapeutic agents aimed at specific cause; for example, patients with known or suspected tuberculosis should receive antituberculous therapy before and after pericardiectomy

General Management

Electrocardiography—performed to rule out myocardial infarction, when cardiac tamponade is suspected, and if patient demonstrates signs of cardiac decompensation

Hemodynamic monitoring—indicated if cardiac tamponade is evident (see p. 66); for patients with constrictive pericarditis, closer monitoring of right atrial and pulmonary arterial pressures and cardiac output; after pericardiectomy, elevated pressures may continue for several weeks or months

Acute pericarditis

Bed rest with bathroom privileges during period of fever and pain; activity limited during acute period, with modification of all activities for 2 weeks to allow inflammatory reaction of the pericardium to resolve; regular diet; encourage fluids during febrile period

Constrictive pericarditis

Bed rest with activity limitations before pericardiectomy; extent of limitation dictated by degree of hemodynamic compromise and symptoms

NURSING CARE

Nursing Assessment

Area of Concern	Acute Pericarditis	Constrictive Pericarditis
General complaints	Chest pain: location retrosternal or precordial radiating to neck and back, sudden pleuritic-like pain that worsens with deep inspiration, movement, or lying down and is relieved by sitting up or leaning forward; sharp, deep, persistent ache; tachypnea; shallow breathing; dyspnea in presence of pleural effusion or owing to impaired cardiac filling from compression of heart; restlessness; anxiety; malaise; dysphagia	Exertional dyspnea; fatigue; orthopnea; palpitations; paroxysmal nocturnal dyspnea; cough; peripheral edema
Physical examination	Low-grade temperature (39° C [102° F]); may be associated with diaphoresis and chills; auscultation: pericardial friction rub—best heard with patient leaning forward, heard in second, third, or fourth intercostal space to left of sternal border or at apex, loudest during inspiration, varies in intensity (grade 4 to 5), may be transient, triphasic consisting of presystolic, systolic, and diastolic components, scratchy, grating	Afebrile; elevated jugular venous pressure with presence of Kussmaul's sign (increased distention during inspiration); arterial pressure normal or slightly reduced; diffuse precordial movement; decreased amplitude; absence of localized apical impulse; paradoxic pulse (rarely exceeds 15 mm Hg); auscultation: quiet, distant heart sounds, pericardial knock—early diastolic sound, accentuated with inspiration and heard best along lower left sternal border; clinical signs of elevated venous pressure: peripheral edema, hepatomegaly, ascites

Nursing Dx & Intervention

Nursing Diagnosis	Nursing Intervention/Rationale
Anxiety related to actual or perceived threat to biologic integrity	• Assess for signs of fear and anxiety: restlessness, facial expressions. • Provide supportive care. • Explain disease process and procedures as they are implemented. • Ensure quiet environment. Reduce external stimuli as much as possible. • Maintain family contact.
Pain related to pericardial friction rub	• Assess quality of chest pain. • Administer pain medication as ordered *to relieve pericardial chest pain.* • Encourage bed rest with head of bed elevated or in position of comfort. Instruct patient to lean forward on over-bed table *to reduce pain.*
Decreased cardiac output related to alteration in preload	• Assess for signs of cardiac tamponade (see p. 66): narrowing pulse pressure, pulsus paradoxus. • Monitor vital signs *to detect signs of ventricular decompensation.* • Prepare for pericardiocentesis or pericardiectomy as indicated by clinical status.
Fluid volume excess	• Auscultate heart and breath sounds every 1 to 2 hours during inflammatory period. • Observe for increase in jugular venous pressure. • Maintain accurate intake and output record. • Maintain patent IV.

Patient Education

1. Explain the underlying cause and disease process.
2. Instruct the patient in signs and symptoms of recurring inflammation and tell the patient to notify the physician if they occur.
3. Explain the purpose, method of administration, and side effects of medications.

Evaluation

Patient Outcome	Data Indicating That Outcome is Reached
Patient demonstrates decreased anxiety.	Patient verbalizes relief of pain. Patient demonstrates ability to rest and sleep without complaint. Patient appears relaxed. Patient tolerates routine activities and procedures without complaining of pain or shortness of breath.
There is no pericardial irritation.	ECG is normal. There is no friction rub or chest pain. White blood cell count and sedimentation rate are normal.
Patient shows an increased level of understanding.	Patient identifies signs and symptoms to report to physician. Patient verbalizes knowledge regarding disease, activity allowances and limitations, and medications.

Cardiac tamponade

Cardiac tamponade is acute cardiac compression caused when fluid accumulates within the pericardial sac and exerts increased pressure around the heart. The result is restricted blood flow in and out of the ventricles.

Pathophysiology

Tamponade is most commonly caused by acute pericarditis but is quite common in patients with malignant and uremic pericardial effusions. A hemopericardium, bleeding into the pericardial spaces, may occur as a result of chest trauma, cardiac surgery, myocardial rupture, aortic dissection, or anticoagulant therapy.

The pericardial sac normally holds 30 to 50 ml of fluid, creating pressures of approximately −1 to −3 mm Hg during expiration and −5 mm Hg with inspiration. An increase in pericardial fluid can cause a rise in intrapericardial pressure, first to 0 mm Hg and eventually to a positive value. However, it is the rate of accumulation, not the volume, that determines the degree to which filling becomes restricted and whether cardiac tamponade will ensue.

When pericardial fluid accumulates slowly, large volumes (1 to 2 L) can be readily accommodated because of the stretching of pericardial fibers. During rapid filling, however, the pericardium fails to stretch. This causes intrapericardial pressure to rise to a level exceeding normal filling pressure of the ventricles. When this occurs, filling is restricted, stroke volume decreases, and cardiac output falls. These alterations are followed by hypotension and shock. Pulsus paradoxus, an important hemodynamic feature of tamponade, is an abnormally large inspiratory fall in arterial pressure. When left ventricular filling and stroke volume are decreased, blood pools in the lung and right side of the heart during inspiration, increasing intrapericardial pressure. Therefore during inspiration a greater negative intrathoracic pressure occurs, resulting in a dramatic fall in systolic blood pressure and pulse volume. The arterial blood pressure may normally fall to 4 to 5 mm Hg during inspiration, but a decrease of 10 mm Hg or more is considered abnormal.

Diagnostic Studies and Findings

Chest Roentgenogram

Enlarged cardiac silhouette (globular configuration depending on degree of effusion); lung fields clear

Electrocardiogram (ECG)

Nonspecific ST and T wave changes; diminished voltage with specific alteration (electrical alternans) in QRS complex; peaked T waves in precordial leads associated with hemopericardium; changes associated with acute pericarditis (see p. 63)

Echocardiogram

Increased pericardial fluid; paradoxic septal motion; septum moves toward left ventricle during inspiration as right ventricle fills; may be possible to estimate fluid volume

Radionuclear Scan

May be possible to identify presence of pericardial fluid by demonstrating increased space between inferior border of the heart and liver

Cardiac Catheterization

Documents hemodynamic parameters associated with tamponade: decreased ventricular filling pressures, elevated right atrial pressure, alteration (equalization) of pressures during inspiration

Medical Plan

Surgery

Pericardiocentesis (see p. 113) or pericardial window (subxiphoid incision and placement of tube for continuous drainage) to remove pericardial fluid and relieve cardiac compression

Medications

Temporary supportive therapy—volume expansion with normal saline and infusion of inotropic agents to increase cardiac output and blood pressure

General Management

Careful, continuous monitoring of clinical signs and symptoms, as well as changes in hemodynamic parameters, to support patient until definitive treatment is initiated; arterial pressure monitored for pulsus paradoxus and hypotension; observe for decreased cardiac output, lowered left atrial pressure, elevated central venous pressure.

Bed rest with head of bed elevated to position of comfort; nothing by mouth (NPO) in anticipation of pericardiocentesis; parenteral therapy as ordered to maintain adequate blood pressure.

NURSING CARE

Nursing Assessment

General Complaints

Clinical presentation may vary from asymptomatic to dramatic and severe and is often nonspecific; anxiety; tachypnea; mild dyspnea to marked respiratory distress; lightheadedness; fatigue; chest discomfort (fullness, heaviness).

Physical Examination

Tachycardia; peripheral pallor and/or cyanosis

Peripheral pulses weak or absent

Arterial pressure

Decreased systolic blood pressure; narrowing pulse pressure; pulsus paradoxus greater than 10 mm Hg; soft or absent pulse during inspiration

Venous pressure

Elevated venous pressure; distended neck veins on inspiration (positive Kussmaul's sign)

Auscultation

Distant, often inaudible heart sounds; pericardial rubs may be heard, particularly in patients with uremia

Nursing Dx & Intervention

Nursing Diagnosis	Nursing Intervention/Rationale
Decreased cardiac output related to restricted ventricular filling pressure	• Assess jugular venous distention and determine degree of pulsus paradoxus. • Maintain bed rest. Elevate head of bed 45 degrees. • Monitor arterial pressure, pulse pressure, pulse volume, ECG voltage, and level of consciousness every 5 to 15 minutes. • Assist with pericardiocentesis or prepare patient for emergency surgery (pericardiectomy or pericardial window) as ordered. • Administer inotropic medications as ordered. Administer fluids as ordered. • Limit self-care activities.
Pain	• Assess quality and characteristics of chest pain. • Provide bed rest in position of comfort. • Provide medication as ordered *to alleviate chest pain.* • Provide emotional support. • Remain with patient as needed.

Patient Education

1. Provide an explanation of the condition.
2. Explain the need for and procedures regarding pericardiocentesis (see p. 113 for further detail) or for pericardiectomy as ordered.

Evaluation

Patient Outcome	Data Indicating That Outcome is Reached
Improved ventricular compliance is shown by absence of tamponade.	Pulsus paradoxus decreases. Jugular venous distention decreases. Ventilation is improved. Pulse pressure and arterial pressure are normalized. Kussmaul's sign is absent.
Patient comfort level is achieved.	Patient verbalizes relief of pain and dyspnea. Patient demonstrates ability to rest and sleep without complaint. Patient tolerates routine activities and procedures without complaint.

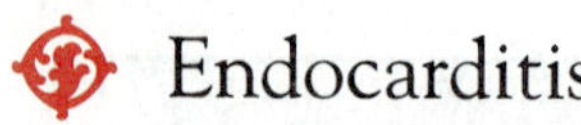

Endocarditis

Endocarditis is an inflammatory process involving the endothelial layer of the heart, including the cardiac valves and septal defects (if present).

The designation of acute or subacute endocarditis describes the virulence of the infecting organism and the rapidity of destruction. Acute bacterial endocarditis (ABE) is considered fulminant, whereas subacute bacterial endocarditis (SBE) may be indolent for up to 8 weeks.

The incidence of endocarditis is not known. In one report the frequency was about 0.16 to 5.4 cases per 1000 hospital admissions.[11] Endocarditis primarily involves older adults, with a mean age of 55 years. Men are affected more often by a ratio of 2:1 to 5:1 in several series.[11,36]

Persons at risk for endocarditis include patients who have a history of rheumatic heart disease, valvular heart disease, or congenital heart defects or who have prosthetic heart valves, arteriovenous shunts for dialysis, or pacemaker wires. Immunosuppressed patients are susceptible to transient bacteremia. The fatality rate remains at 30% to 90%. Congestive heart failure is the major cause of death.[83]

Pathophysiology

Endocarditis can be linked to a number of organisms. Diagnosis and treatment depend on isolating the organism.

Streptococcal strains account for 40% to 80% of all SBE cases. These low-virulence bacteria generally affect already damaged valves. *S. viridans*, the most commonly implicated α-hemolytic organism, is found in the mouth and upper respiratory tract.

Staphylococcus aureus, which affects normal valves, is responsible for 50% of cases of ABE. It is associated with a mortality ranging from 45% to 73%.[83] Less common enterococcal strains *(S. faecalis)* have increasingly been seen in both ABE and SBE. *Enterococcus* is found in the gastrointestinal and genitourinary tracts and the oral cavity. It occurs often in elderly patients, particularly men undergoing urologic procedures, and has been reported in women of childbearing age. *S. epidermidis* is commonly seen in endocarditis following prosthetic valve replacement.

Other known pathogens linked to endocarditis include gram-negative organisms, fungi, and yeast. Endocarditis caused by gram-negative cocci and bacilli *(Serratia marcescens, Klebsiella, Pseudomonas)* occurs in the elderly and mainline drug abusers. The increase in incidence of endocarditis caused by fungi *(Candida, Aspergillus)* may be linked to the increase in IV drug abuse and the widespread use of antimicrobial and corticosteroid therapies. Fungal vegetations tend to be large and to embolize in major blood vessels, particularly in the legs.

Endocarditis generally begins as a transient bacteremia (or fungemia) introduced into the circulation through several portals of entry (Table 1-2). Bacteria more commonly settle on cardiac structures that have already been damaged. The valves are especially susceptible. Ventricular septal defects, coarctation of aorta, patent ductus arteriosus, and unrepaired tetralogy of Fallot are also susceptible. Infected structures are often those in which turbulent blood flow is forced across an area of high pressure to low pressure. Trauma to the endothelial surface of the low-pressure side of the damaged site causes local clotting. As a result, an aggregation of platelets and fibrin thrombi forms on the injured structure. During the

Table 1-2
Possible Ports of Entry and Factors Predisposing to Bacteremia

Port of Entry	Infecting Organism
Oral cavity Extractions, teeth cleaning, periodontal disease (abscesses), periodontal operations, use of unwaxed dental floss, oral irrigation, bridgework	*Streptococcus, Staphylococcus epidermidis*
Upper respiratory tract Tonsilloadenoidectomy, orotracheal intubation, bronchoscopy (rigid tubes), pneumonia	*Staphylococcus aureus, Streptococcus, Haemophilus* species, *Streptococcus pneumoniae, S. epidermidis*
Gastrointestinal tract Barium enema, sigmoidoscopy, colonoscopy, percutaneous biopsy of liver	Gram-negative rods, *Enterobacter, Escherichia coli, Klebsiella*
Genitourinary system Catheterization, urethrotomy, transurethral prostatectomy, retropubic prostatectomy, cystoscopy	*E. coli*, gram-negative bacilli, *Enterococcus*
Female reproductive system Delivery, abortion (therapeutic, illegal), intrauterine devices	*E. coli*
Skin Furuncles, acne (infected, squeezed)	*S. aureus, S. epidermidis*
Other sources of infection Pacemaker (transvenous), prolonged use of polyethylene catheter (arterial), hemodialysis (arteriovenous cannulas), infection (hematogenous osteomyelitis, Q fever, meningococcemia)	

active phase of the infection these thrombi can foster the growth of microorganisms.

The pathogenesis of endocarditis is related to the adherence of infected thrombi to cardiac structures, which in the case of the valves can lead to scarring and retraction of the leaflets. The destruction may be sufficient to cause erosion of the leaflets and perforation leading to valvular insufficiency. The infectious process may also spread to the anulus, creating abscesses, or rupture the chordae tendineae. Mycotic aneurysms may result from septic embolization, which develops in the aorta, cerebral arteries, sinus of Valsalva, ligated ductus arteriosus, and smaller arterial vessels (of the lung, kidney, or spleen).

Diagnostic Studies and Findings

Laboratory Tests

- Complete blood count (CBC)
  - Anemia; elevated sedimentation rate; leukocytosis
- Blood cultures (four to six cultures from different venipuncture sites within 6 to 72 hours before therapy started)
  - Identification of causative organism
- Urine
  - Proteinuria; red cell or leukocyte casts; microhematuria
- Rheumatoid factor
  - Positive in 50% of patients with infection of 6 weeks' duration
- Blood chemistry
  - Elevated BUN and creatinine values in patients with renal complications

Echocardiogram

Presence of vegetations or abscesses; involvement or damage of cardiac valves; ventricular function; hemodynamic changes such as regurgitation

Electrocardiogram (ECG)

Conduction defects; atrial fibrillation, flutter

Medical Plan

Surgery

Surgical removal of vegetations and thrombi—not indicated unless uncontrollable sepsis occurs, and then combined with long-term antimicrobial therapy; if infectious process is fulminant and resistant to antimicrobial therapy, excision of vegetations, unroofing of abscesses, and valve replacement recommended; presence of congestive heart failure is a major indication for surgery, reducing the high mortality to 9% to 14%[80]

Medications

- Antibiotics—long-term IV antibiotic therapy inhibits bacterial growth; since appropriate therapy depends on isolation of infecting organism, serial blood cultures required *before* initiation of therapy; initiation of antibiotic therapy is guided by patient's clinical state: for subacute infection, delaying therapy until culture results are available will not endanger patient, but treatment for acutely ill patient should begin immediately; therapy usually continues 4-6 wk with parenteral administration as recommended route; in approximately 10%-20% of cases, primarily subacute bacterial endocarditis, culture findings are negative and therapy is directed at enterococcal infections, using combination of penicillin and streptomycin; blood cultures are obtained periodically to determine adequacy of regimen and sensitivity to antibiotics
- Analgesic-antipyretics (salicylates) given for elevated temperature
- Anticoagulants given prophylactically if large thrombus is visualized on echocardiogram or if atrial fibrillation develops
- Other agents dictated by presence of complications
  - Cardiac
    - Abscesses
    - Valvular dysfunction (see p. 57)
    - Heart failure (see p. 38)
    - Myocarditis
  - Embolization
    - Cerebral
    - Renal
    - Splenic
    - Coronary
  - Mycotic aneurysms

General Management

- Rest—encouraged during acute phase; patient often requires prolonged hospitalization (2 to 6 weeks)
- Vital signs—checked every 4 to 8 hours, decreasing frequency as indicated by improved clinical condition
- Diet—regular; patient may require high-caloric supplemental feedings; force fluids during periods of elevated temperature provided there is no ventricular failure
- Monitor parenteral therapy for rate and amount of infusion; check regularly for localized signs of inflammation, phlebitis

NURSING CARE

Nursing Assessment

General Complaints

- Acute: high-grade fever (39° to 40° C [102° to 104° F])
- Subacute: low-grade fever (less than 39.4° C [103° F]), weakness, malaise, weight loss, anorexia, arthralgia, sweats, headache, dyspnea

Signs of Embolization (Peripheral, Cerebral, Systemic)

Petechiae in conjunctivae, palate, buccal mucosa, and extremities; splinter hemorrhages (linear, dark-red streaks on nail beds); Osler's nodes (small, tender, raised nodules frequently found on finger and toe pads); Janeway lesions (nontender, flat, erythematous macules on palms and soles); splenomegaly; Roth's spots (retinal hemorrhages with white centers); neurologic changes (behavioral changes, aphasia, paralysis)

Auscultation

Murmurs not usually present in early phase of infection but become apparent if valvular damage occurs (see discussion of valvular heart disease, p. 57); ventricular gallop (S_3) occurs in setting of ventricular failure (see p. 39)

Splenomegaly

Present in only 44% of patients with subacute bacterial endocarditis and in 23% with acute endocarditis

Nursing Dx & Intervention

Nursing Diagnosis	Nursing Intervention/Rationale
Altered nutrition: less than body requirements related to anorexia or diminished energy reserve	• Assess patient for signs of malnutrition: dry weight below normal for age and height, fatigue, decreased triceps skinfold measurements. • Weigh patient daily. Decrease frequency as weight stabilizes. • Monitor daily caloric intake as indicated by patient's appetite and food intake. • Offer high-caloric, high-protein supplemental feedings *to ensure adequate intake of daily nutrients during anorexic periods.* • Ensure patient comfort during mealtime. Encourage patient participation in food selections.
Diversional activity deficit related to prolonged hospitalization (4 to 6 weeks)	• Assess level and type of diversional interest *to explore possible activities.* • Provide diversional activities such as occupational therapy, reading, television, radio, and out-of-hospital passes. • Encourage a daily structured exercise program unless contraindicated by clinical status.
Altered thought processes (potential) related to cerebral embolization	• Assess for signs of embolization each shift and as needed. Report any changes to physician immediately. • Administer anticoagulant therapy as ordered. Instruct patient about need to continue with anticoagulants, if ordered, *to prevent future embolic episodes.*
Fluid volume excess (potential)	• Assess for signs of increasing pulmonary congestion or the presence of new murmurs that may indicate a regurgitant or stenotic heart valve. • Monitor vital signs every 4 to 6 hours *to detect changes in heart rate, rhythm, temperature, and blood pressure.* • Assess peripheral extremities *for evidence of dependent edema.* • Weigh daily *to detect steady weight gain indicative of fluid retention.* • Monitor for jugular venous distention that may *indicate regurgitation of tricuspid valve or increased pulmonary congestion.*
Decreased cardiac output (potential)	• Assess for signs and symptoms of impending heart failure, and initiate nursing care if they are present.

Patient Education

1. Provide instruction regarding the disease process, purpose, and method of treatment.
2. Explain precipitating factors that can lead to bacteremia and reinfection: poor oral hygiene, dental work (gum cleaning or treatment, extractions), gastrointestinal or genitourinary procedures, vaginal deliveries, furuncles, staphylococcal infections, surgical procedures.
3. Encourage regular follow-up care with a medical physician.
4. Instruct the patient on the need for good oral hygiene and regular dental care.
5. Explain and reinforce the need for antibiotic prophylaxis before procedures that predispose to bacteremia (refer to Table 1-3 for specific recommendations).

Table 1-3
Recommended Antibiotic Coverage for Endocarditis Prophylaxis

Drug	Dosage
Penicillin For most patients: oral	Adults: 2 g of penicillin V 1 h before procedure and then 1 g 6 h after initial dose
Erythromycin For those allergic to penicillin; may also be selected for those receiving oral penicillin as continuous rheumatic fever prophylaxis	Adults: erythromycin 1 g po 1 h before procedure and then 500 mg 6 h after initial dose
Ampicillin plus gentamicin For patients at higher risk of infective endocarditis (especially those with prosthetic heart valves) who are not allergic to penicillin	Adults: ampicillin 1-2 g plus gentamicin 1.5 mg/kg IM or IV, both given 30 min before procedure; then penicillin V 1 g po 6 h after initial dose
Vancomycin intravenously and erythromycin orally For higher-risk patients (especially those with prosthetic heart valves) who are allergic to penicillin	Adults: vancomycin 1 g IV over 60 min, begun 60 min before procedure; no repeat dose is necessary

Modified from American Heart Association.[2]

Evaluation

Patient Outcome	Data Indicating That Outcome is Reached
There is absence of inflammatory processes.	Temperature, blood cultures, white cell count, and other laboratory findings are normal. Patient's sense of well-being is improved. Patient reports feeling less fatigued, improved appetite, weight gain, and absence of sweats and headache.
Nutritional status is improved and maintained.	Baseline or normal body weight is regained. Patient demonstrates improved appetite.

Congenital heart disease

A congenital heart disorder is any structural or functional abnormality or defect of the heart or great vessels existing from birth.

Congenital heart disease is a specialty of pediatrics. However, persons with congenital defects are now living longer and are being treated as adults. Although the incidence of congenital heart disease has decreased over the decades, it continues to occur at a rate of 5 to 8 per 1000 live births.[4]

Pathophysiology

In most cases the cause for the congenital defect cannot be determined. However, various factors are believed to contribute to these malformations.

Genetics. Several studies have demonstrated prevalence rates among siblings and blood relatives to be 1.5% to 5%,[73] suggesting a genetic link in the etiology of cardiac malformations. Also, certain chromosomal abnormalities, including Turner's syndrome and Down's syndrome, have been linked to heart defects.

Environmental factors. Although difficult to prove as isolated causes, environmental factors along with genetic factors have been linked to heart defects. Factors include pollution and smoking and alcohol use by the mother.

Teratogens. Use of certain drugs such as warfarin and exposure to viruses such as rubella during fetal development have been shown to cause not only heart defects but also widespread injury to the embryo.

Altitude. Altitude may cause the ductus arteriosus to fail to close after birth.

Common Defects in Which Prolonged Survival Occurs

Patent ductus arteriosus (Figure 1-41). The ductus arteriosus is a vascular connection that during fetal life directs blood flow from the pulmonary artery to the aorta, bypassing the lungs. Functional closure of the ductus occurs after birth. In some cases it takes 6 months to several years before complete closure. If the ductus remains patent, the direction of blood flow is reversed to left to right because of high systemic pressure in the aorta. Blood is shunted through the ductus to the pulmonary artery during both systole and diastole. This

Figure 1-41 Patent ductus arteriosus.
From Whaley.[109]

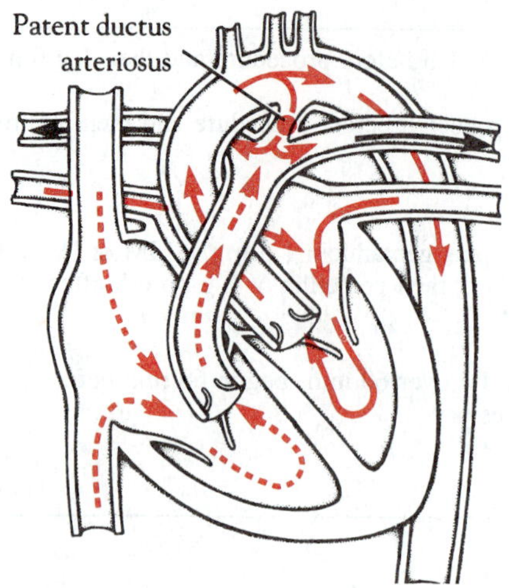

Figure 1-42 Atrial septal defect.
From Whaley.[109]

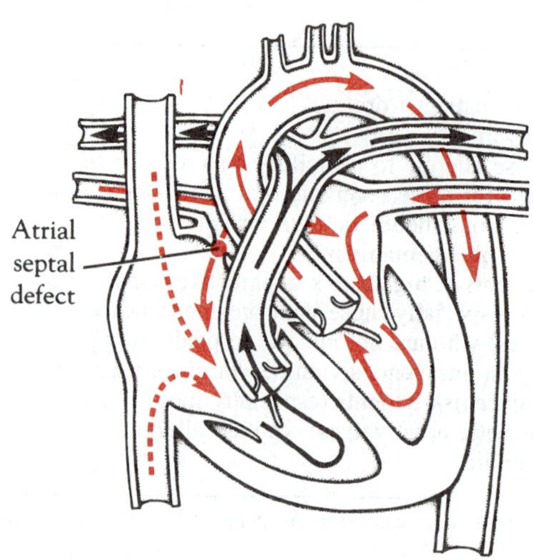

raises pressure in the pulmonary circulation and increases the pressure against which the right ventricle must work.

Survival into adulthood is possible. Patent ductus arteriosus occurs more often in girls and can be linked to other defects such as ventricular septal defect and coarctation of the aorta.

Atrial septal defect (Figure 1-42). An atrial septal defect is an abnormal opening between the right and left atria causing blood to be shunted from left to right. There are two common forms. In ostium secundum, the more common, the defect is in the middle of the septal wall near the fossa ovalis. Ostium primum results from failure of fusion of the left portions of the endocardial cushions occurring low in the atrial septum. An associated cleft (separation) is present in the anterior mitral valve leaflet, which can lead to mitral regurgitation.

Ventricular septal defect (Figure 1-43). A ventricular septal defect is an abnormal opening between the right and left ventricles. It varies in size (7 mm to 3 cm in diameter) and occurs in either the upper or lower portion of the ventricular septum. The size of the defect determines the extent

Figure 1-43 Ventricular septal defect.
From Whaley.[109]

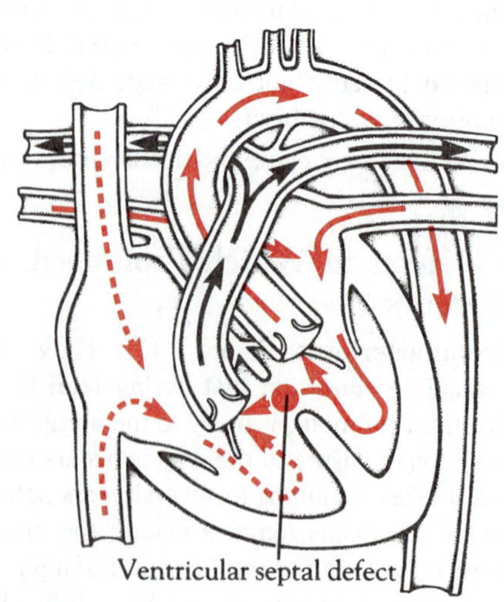

Figure 1-44 Tetralogy of Fallot.
From Whaley.[109]

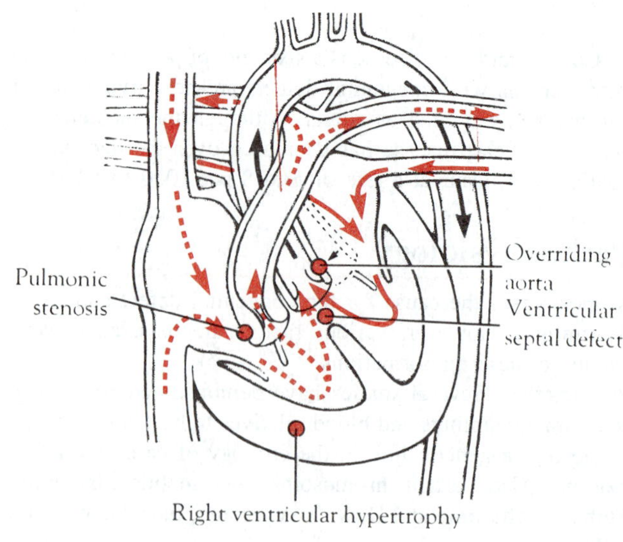

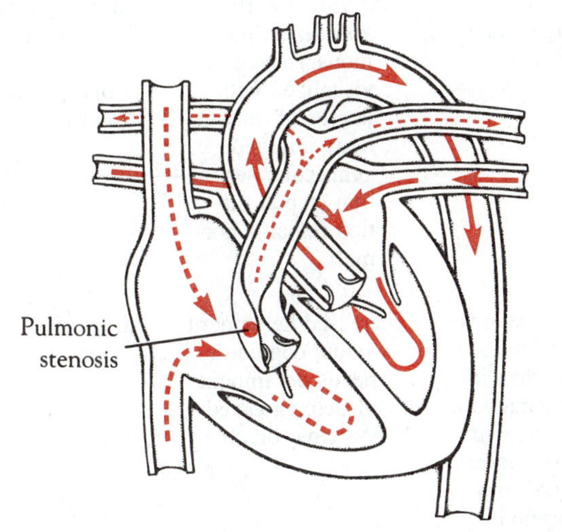

Figure 1-45 Pulmonic stenosis.
From Whaley.[109]

of the shunt from left to right ventricle. The larger the shunt, the greater the volume of blood ejected into the right ventricle and lungs. Therefore large defects cause a volume overload for both ventricles. Large defects can also lead to an increase in pulmonary vascular resistance, producing pulmonary hypertension. If this occurs, the shunt may be reversed to right to left, causing systemic cyanosis and Eisenmenger syndrome, which renders the patient inoperable.

Tetralogy of Fallot (Figure 1-44). Tetralogy of Fallot is an anomaly marked by four defects: ventricular septal defect, right ventricular outflow obstruction (pulmonic stenosis), deviation (dextroposition) of the aorta so it overrides the ventricular septum, and right ventricular hypertrophy. It is the most common cyanotic lesion in which survival to adulthood is expected. The severity of symptoms depends on the size of the ventricular septal defect, degree of pulmonic stenosis, and position of the aorta. Right ventricular outflow is obstructed, resulting in hypertrophy of the right ventricle and a right-to-left shunt. This produces a decrease in systemic arterial oxygen saturation, cyanosis, reduced pulmonary blood flow, and in some cases a hypoplastic pulmonary artery.

Pulmonic valvular stenosis (Figure 1-45). Congenital pulmonic valvular stenosis may occur by itself, with other defects such as atrial or ventricular septal defect, or as part of tetralogy of Fallot. If it occurs by itself, the chance of survival to adulthood is good. Pulmonic stenosis may occur as one of three types: valvular, subvalvular (infundibular), or supravalvular. The degree of right ventricular hypertrophy varies with the degree of obstruction.

Diagnostic Studies and Findings

Study	Patent Ductus Arteriosus	Atrial Septal Defect	Ventricular Septal Defect	Tetralogy of Fallot	Pulmonic Stenosis
Electrocardiogram (ECG)	Normal (small ductus); left ventricular hypertrophy (LVH); PR interval may be prolonged; atrial fibrillation in adults	Normal; right ventricular hypertrophy (RVH); right bundle-branch block; PR interval may be prolonged; left axis deviation (ostium primum); normal or right axis (ostium secundum)	Normal if defect is small; if moderate to large, LVH; LVH/RVH in presence of pulmonary hypertension	RVH	Normal if stenosis is mild; if moderate to severe, RVH and right axis deviation; if severe, right atrial hypertrophy (RAH)
Chest roentgenogram	Normal; with moderate to large shunt, enlarged cardiac silhouette with enlarged LA, LV, and pulmonary artery (PA); enlarged aorta; enlarged pulmonary trunk and increased pulmonary flow	Enlarged RA, RV, PA; increased pulmonary vascular markings; LA, LV, and aortic knob may be small	Mild LVH with small shunt; with large shunt, increased LV, dilation of PA, increased pulmonary vascular markings, enlarged LA	Small cardiac silhouette; small PA; prominent aorta (may arch to right in 25% of cases)	Enlarged RV and PA; if severe, decreased peripheral pulmonary vascular markings

Study	Patent Ductus Arteriosus	Atrial Septal Defect	Ventricular Septal Defect	Tetralogy of Fallot	Pulmonic Stenosis
Echocardiogram	Ductus not visualized; enlarged LA and LV owing to left-to-right shunt	With ostium secundum, enlarged RV, paradoxic movement of septum during systole; with ostium primum, mitral valve displaced inferiorly and anteriorly	Defect not visualized; large shunt; enlarged LA	Overriding aorta visualized; pulmonary stenosis visualized with degree of obstruction; enlarged ventricular septum (septal motion remains normal)	Normal if stenosis is mild; if moderate to severe, enlarged RA and RV
Laboratory tests	No specific findings	No specific findings	No specific findings unless patient is cyanotic, then increased hematocrit value, decreased hemoglobin level and arterial oxygen saturation	Increased hematocrit value; degree depends on amount of deoxygenated systemic blood	No specific findings
Cardiac catheterization	Increased pulmonary blood flow; increased oxygen saturation in PA; intracardiac pressures normal; RV and PA pressures may be slightly elevated	Left-to-right shunt at atrial level; increased oxygen saturation in RA; RA pressure usually normal; mitral regurgitation	Left-to-right shunt (LV to RV); study determines degree of shunt; increased pulmonary blood flow, oxygen saturation in RV, and systolic pressure in RV and PA	RV outflow obstruction; increased RV pressure; RV to LV shunt; decreased PA pressure as catheter crosses obstruction	Increased RA pressure, which determines systolic pressure gradient between RV and PA

Medical Plan

Surgery

Patent ductus arteriosus
- Ligation of ductus

Atrial septal defect
- Direct closure by suturing or placement of Dacron patch across defect
- Correction of mitral regurgitation by valvuloplasty or replacement (depends on degree of regurgitation)

Ventricular septal defect
- Direct closure by suturing or with placement of Dacron patch across defect

Tetralogy of Fallot
- Palliative procedures performed on infants to enhance blood flow to lungs, thereby reducing hypoxia
  - Blalock-Taussig procedure—anastomosis between subclavian artery and pulmonary artery
  - Potts' anastomosis—side-to-side anastomosis of left pulmonary artery to descending aorta
  - Waterston-Cooley procedure—anastomosis of right pulmonary artery to ascending aorta

Pulmonic stenosis
- Valvotomy; resection of excess infundibular muscle; valve replacement

Corrective surgery—intracardiac repair of ventricular septal defect and pulmonic stenosis; contraindicated if pulmonary artery is hypoplastic

Medications

Dictated by patient's clinical picture and presence of ventricular failure and arrhythmias

General Management

None specific unless indicated by complications such as heart failure, arrhythmias, or effects of polycythemia in cyanotic patient

NURSING CARE

Nursing Assessment

Area of Concern	Patent Ductus Arteriosus	Atrial Septal Defect	Ventricular Septal Defect	Tetralogy of Fallot	Pulmonic Stenosis
Physical examination	Small shunt: asymptomatic, increased respiratory infections, small for age; large shunt: exertional dyspnea, decreased exercise tolerance	Small shunt: asymptomatic; moderate to large shunt: exertional dyspnea, decreased exercise tolerance, palpitations	Small to moderate shunt: asymptomatic, exertional dyspnea; large shunt: failure in infancy, growth failure, feeding difficulties	In infancy: paroxysmal attacks of dyspnea with loss of consciousness ("blue" spells), small for age; in later childhood: cyanosis with clubbing of fingers and toes; in adulthood (following palliation): exertional dyspnea, cyanosis with clubbing	Asymptomatic during childhood; exertional dyspnea; decreased exercise tolerance
Palpation	Neck vessels dilated and pulsating	Left parasternal lift	Large shunt: left parasternal lift	Precordial prominence; parasternal heave	Left parasternal heave; subxiphoid pulsation
Auscultation	Systolic pressure normal; diastolic pressure low; wide pulse pressure; harsh, loud, continuous murmur in first, second, and third intercostal spaces (ICS) at lower sternal border (LSB); machinery-like murmur best heard when patient is lying down, becoming fainter when patient is standing	Soft blowing systolic murmur at second ICS at LSB	Small shunt: holosystolic at third, fourth, and fifth ICS, systolic thrill; large shunt: holosystolic murmur at third, fourth, and fifth ICS, splitting of S_2 during expiration, widening during inspiration, systolic ejection sound at second ICS at LSB	Single S_2; systolic ejection murmur at third ICS, may radiate upward to left side of neck	S_1 normal; early systolic ejection click heard at base; midsystolic murmur at second and third ICS at LSB, radiates to suprasternal notch and to left side of neck; S_2 widely split

Nursing Dx & Intervention

Nursing Diagnosis	Nursing Intervention/Rationale
Knowledge deficit	• Instruct parents on type of defect and how to manage at home, and provide referral services for assistance with home care. • For adult patients, provide detailed explanation of defect and surgical interventions and treatments as dictated by defect.
Anxiety related to actual or perceived threat to biologic integrity	• Assess level of anxiety: determine primary cause to identify any misconceptions, fears, and concerns. • Encourage verbalization of feelings. • Elicit questions and concerns of patient. • Assess usual coping mechanisms for dealing with stress to determine if they are adequate to control anxiety. • Assist the patient to deal realistically with anxiety, providing alternative methods for dealing with anxiety. • Refer the patient to long-term counseling if necessary.

Patient Education

1. Instruct the patient and family about the primary defect and any surgical procedures that have occurred. Explain the associated signs and symptoms and describe what is normal and abnormal.
2. Explain activity allowances and limitations, including schooling, sports, and occupation.
3. For adolescents and adults provide counseling on issues concerning genetics, marriage, contraception, and childbearing.
4. Explain dietary restrictions as indicated.
5. Explain the need to prevent endocarditis (see p. 68).

Evaluation

Patient Outcome	Data Indicating That Outcome is Reached
Level of knowledge is increased.	Patient and family verbalize knowledge regarding defect, prescribed care, medication, need for return visits, and endocarditis prophylaxis.
Anxiety is decreased.	Patient and family verbalize reeducation in anxiety level and demonstrate appropriate behavior in self-care management.

VASCULAR DISEASES

Systemic hypertension

An intermittent or sustained elevation in systolic or diastolic blood pressure, hypertension is a major cause of cerebrovascular accident (stroke), cardiac disease, and renal failure.

Nearly one sixth of all Americans (35 million persons) have hypertension, and an additional 25 million have borderline hypertension. Half of those affected are unaware of it.

Hypertension may be defined as a blood pressure greater than 160/95 mm Hg. Persons with blood pressures less than 140/90 mm Hg are normotensive; those with blood pressure between 140/90 and 160/95 mm Hg are considered borderline hypertensive.[91]

Although there is no way of predicting in whom high blood pressure will develop, hypertension can be detected easily. Therefore the major emphasis in the control of hypertension should be on early detection and effective treatment.

Pathophysiology

Primary (essential) hypertension is the most common form, accounting for 90% of all cases. It is an abnormal state in which excessive neurohumoral stimulation results in increased arterial tone. The cause is unknown, but certain risk factors have been identified. These include family history, age group, race, obesity, stress, cigarette smoking, and a diet high in salt and saturated fats.

Secondary hypertension occurs as a result of many factors:

- Renal parenchymal disorders
  - Pyelonephritis
  - Glomerulonephritis
  - Hydronephrosis
  - Polycystic kidney
  - Juxtaglomerular (renin-producing) tumors
  - Following kidney transplant
- Renal artery disease
  - Atherosclerosis
  - Arthritis
  - Embolism
  - Aneurysm
  - Diabetic nephrosclerosis
- Endocrine and metabolic disorders
  - Pheochromocytoma
  - Cushing's syndrome
  - Aldosteronism (primary)
  - Hypercalcemia
  - Acromegaly
  - Myxedema
  - Oral contraceptives
  - Chronic licorice use
- Central nervous system disorders
  - Increased intracranial pressure
  - Brain tumor
  - Neurogenic; psychogenic
  - Polyneuritis (porphyria)
- Coarctation of aorta

Accelerated (malignant) hypertension is a state in which the blood pressure is extremely high (diastolic pressure greater than 120 mm Hg). It is accompanied by acute hypertensive retinopathy, nephrosclerosis, and encephalopathy.

The pathogenesis of hypertension is complex because various homeostatic mechanisms contribute to the maintenance of normal arterial pressure.

Cardiac output (stroke volume times heart rate) and peripheral vascular resistance determine arterial pressure. Increases in blood volume (high-output states), heart rate, or arterial vasoconstriction that cause an increase in peripheral resistance can lead to hypertension.

Figure 1-46 Complex relationship between extracellular fluid volume and pressure as mediated by renal hormonal mechanisms. These involve production of renin and angiotensin. Latter is potent vasoconstrictor that stimulates aldosterone synthesis, resulting in sodium retention and increased volume.
From Kaye.[50]

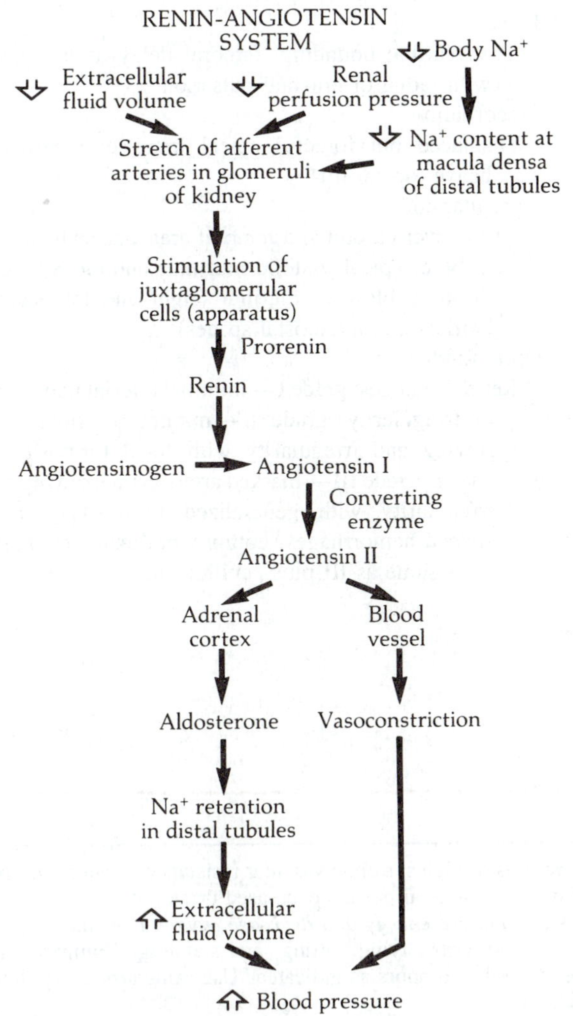

Stimulation of stretch receptors (baroreceptors) in the wall of the carotid sinus and the aortic arch increases vagal activity (parasympathetic component) and decreases sympathetic activity. The result is decreased peripheral resistance and reduced blood pressure. Researchers currently believe that increased sympathetic activity with reduced vagal activity causes an autonomic dysregulation in persons with primary hypertension.[91]

Stimulation and production of high plasma levels of renin (a proteolytic enzyme produced by juxtaglomerular cells) contribute to a complex relationship between extracellular fluid and pressure, leading to sympathetic activation and elevated arterial pressure. Figure 1-46 outlines the conversion of renin to angiotensin I and II.

Diagnostic Studies and Findings

Laboratory Tests

Urine studies including microscopic examination
- Proteinuria, hematuria

Blood chemistry
- BUN >20 mg/dl
- Creatinine >1.5 mg/dl
- Potassium >5 mEq/L in renal failure; <3.5 mEq/L in primary aldosteronism and with diuretic administration
- Cholesterol and lipid levels elevated in hyperlipidemia
- Uric acid level may increase with diuretic therapy
- Calcium level may increase with diuretic therapy

Electrocardiogram (ECG)

Evaluates presence of left ventricular hypertrophy and myocardial ischemia

Chest Roentgenogram

Cardiomegaly; aortic atherosclerosis

Medical Plan

Surgery

None for primary hypertension (see Chapter 11 for surgical interventions for renal disorders)

Medications

Diuretics
- Thiazides
  - Chlorothiazide (Diuril) (0.5-1 g/d)
  - Hydrochlorothiazide (Esidrix, Hydrodiuril) (50-100 mg/d)
  - Bendroflumethiazide (Naturetin) (2.5-10 mg/d)
- Loop diuretics
  - Furosemide (Lasix) (40-80 mg bid or qid)
  - Ethacrynic acid (Edecrin) (initial dose 25-50 mg)
- Potassium-sparing diuretics

Spironolactone (Aldactone) (100-400 mg bid or tid)
Triamterene (Dyrenium) (100-300 mg bid)
Amiloride (Midamor) (5-20 mg/d or bid)

β-Adrenergic blocking agents
Propranolol (Inderal) (10-80 mg po bid or qid)
Metoprolol tartrate (Lopressor) (50-200 mg po qd or bid)
Pindolol (Visken) (15-60 mg/d)
Atenolol (Tenormin) (50-100 mg/d)
Timolol maleate (Blocadren) (20-40 mg/d)
Nadolol (Corgard) (80-320 mg/d)

Antihypertensive agents
Methyldopa (Aldomet) (up to 2 g/d po bid, tid, or qid)
Guanethidine (Ismelin) (5-200 mg/d po)
Clonidine (Catapres) (0.1-1.2 mg bid po)
Captopril (Capoten) (24-150 mg tid)
Hydrazaline (Apresoline) (10-50 mg po qid)
Sodium nitroprusside (Nipride) (0.5-10 μg/kg/min IV)
Diazoxide (Hyperstat) (300 mg by rapid IV bolus)

α-Adrenergic blocking agents
Phentolamine (Regitine) (1-5 mg IV intermittently)
Prazosin (Minipress) (initial dose 1 mg po, slowly increased to 10-15 mg/d)

General Management

Cardiac monitoring for hypertensive crisis
Arterial pressure monitoring for hypertensive crisis
Dietary management
Sodium restriction—may range from mild to rigid restriction depending on degree of hypertension; recommended dietary restriction 2 to 6 g/day
Alcohol—limit intake to less than 3 drinks/day
Caffeine—restrict intake
Cholesterol, lipids, saturated fats—reduce intake
Weight control—recommend weight loss of 5% or more in obese patient
Exercise
Aerobic exercise appropriate for age and health status
Refer to cardiac rehabilitation for prescribed exercise program
Avoid isometric exercises
Stress reduction and management
Monitoring of blood pressure on regular basis; frequency determined by blood pressure elevations

NURSING CARE

Nursing Assessment

Symptoms

Mild to moderate hypertension
Asymptomatic
Moderate to severe hypertension
Headaches, dizziness, fatigue, vertigo, palpitations
Severe hypertension
Throbbing suboccipital headache (may be present when patient awakens in morning, disappearing spontaneously after several hours); epistaxis

Physical Examination

Mild to moderate hypertension
Normal with exception of blood pressure
Moderate hypertension
Blood pressure (in both arms; sitting, standing, and supine; determined over at least two visits)
160/90 mm Hg or higher
Pulse
Tachycardia; bounding; femoral delay as compared with radial or brachial pulsation
Precordium
Displaced but forceful apical impulse; ventricular heave (apical lift)
Auscultation
Bruits over carotid and femoral areas; accentuated S_2 at base; apical systolic murmur; audible S_4; early diastolic blowing murmur (right and left sternal borders and intercostal spaces)
Optic fundi
Retinal changes: grade I—minimal arterial narrowing or irregularity; grade II—marked arteriolar narrowing and irregularity with focal tortuosity or spasm; grade III—marked arteriolar narrowing and irregularity with generalized tortuosity, flame-shaped hemorrhages, cotton-wool exudates; grade IV—same as III plus papilledema

Nursing Dx & Intervention

Nursing Diagnosis	Nursing Intervention/Rationale
Decreased cardiac output (potential) related to mechanical factors (afterload)	• Assess and monitor for signs and symptoms of high systemic vascular resistance: elevated arterial pressure, increased pulse rate, diminished peripheral pulses, decreased urine output. • Maintain bed rest and limit activities *to conserve energy and decrease oxygen demand.* • Check blood pressure on admission in both arms, lying, sitting, and standing. Compare with arterial pressure monitor if available every 4 to 6 hours as indicated. Use same arm every time. • Maintain parenteral fluids as ordered. • Administer antihypertensive medications as ordered. Observe for side effects or toxic effects of

Nursing Diagnosis	Nursing Intervention/Rationale
	each medication. Monitor IV medications carefully, titrating according to prescribed blood pressure parameters ordered. • Attach patient to cardiac monitor as indicated for arrhythmias, sudden hypotensive response, or hypertensive crisis. • Measure intake and output. Report output of less than 30 ml/hour. • Monitor electrolytes, BUN, and creatinine levels. Check specific gravity as ordered. • Permit nothing by mouth (NPO) if nausea and vomiting are present. • Maintain a low-sodium, low-fat diet. Restrict fluids as ordered.
Pain (headache) related to increased cerebrovascular pressure	• Assess quality of pain and presence of associated symptoms such as nausea, vomiting, and epistaxis. • Initiate measures *to relieve pain and reduce external stimuli:* Maintain a quiet environment with reduced lighting. Limit activities. Avoid sudden jarring motion. Limit visitors. Use additional comfort measures such as cold packs and position changes. • Administer pain-relieving medications and antiemetics as ordered. • Assist with ambulation *because patient may experience dizziness.*
Potential for injury (cerebral) related to severe, accelerated, or malignant hypertension	• Assess and monitor level of consciousness. Check neurologic signs every hour during hypertensive crisis. Notify physician of any sudden changes in mentation, pupillary response, or movement of extremities. • Maintain seizure precautions as indicated.
Noncompliance (potential)	• Assess factors that will influence the patient's ability to adhere to the therapeutic plan: financial status, age, culture, health status, occupation. • Identify and clarify any misconceptions the patient has regarding disease state. • Design a program that is compatible with the patient's habits, life-style, and personality. Include the patient in program design. • Provide opportunities to discuss feelings toward recommended life-style changes.
Powerlessness (potential)	• Assess the patient's attitudes and feelings toward the health care regimen. • Identify any misconceptions and fears the patient has regarding this chronic illness, such as forced dependence on the health care system. • Encourage the patient to participate in determining the therapeutic plan. • Teach the patient and family members to monitor blood pressure at home and interpret results.

Patient Education

1. Instruct the patient and family in blood pressure monitoring, procedure for taking blood pressure at home, frequency of monitoring, influencing factors, interpretation of results, and actions to take if significant change occurs.
2. Explain diet therapy, including sodium, calorie, and lipid restrictions as ordered; include the rationale in explanation.
3. Explain the role of exercise in blood pressure regulation and weight control.
4. Explain the relationship between stress and hypertension, factors that produce stress, and methods to modify stress.
5. Explain antihypertensive therapy, including name, rationale, dosage, and side effects of all medications.

Evaluation

Patient Outcome	Data Indicating That Outcome is Reached
Blood pressure is within acceptable limits.	Blood pressure is 140/90 mm Hg or less. Patient has no complaints of headache or dizziness. Laboratory values are within normal limits.
Patient complies with therapeutic plan.	Patient is normotensive, reports taking medication, loses weight, and has no symptoms.

Acute arterial insufficiency

Arterial insufficiency is a sudden decrease in the arterial supply to an extremity.

Classified as an acute disorder, obstruction of any major artery produces symptoms.

Pathophysiology

The most common causes of acute arterial insufficiency are embolism, thrombosis, and trauma. Cardiac disorders are the main source of thrombi on the left side of the heart. Once dislodged, an embolus may travel throughout the systemic circulation, lodging in an arterial branch and stagnating blood flow in the distal circulation. This sets up a condition of distal clotting or the formation of another thrombus. When the collateral circulation is inadequate, acute arterial insufficiency occurs.

The legs are most commonly involved. The femoral artery is most often affected (46%), followed by the popliteal tibial tree (11%) and the iliac arteries (8%).[69]

Acute arterial obstruction may also occur as a result of injury produced by compression, shearing, or laceration of a vessel. Furthermore, severe hypothermia may produce sudden severe vasoconstriction.

Diagnostic Studies and Findings

Doppler Ultrasonography

Abnormal blood flow pattern proximal to occlusion; "pistol shot" sound characterizes absence of diastolic flow component; ankle/brachial index <0.25 reflects severe ischemia and impending gangrene

Arteriography

Determines location of obstruction and character of arterial circulation proximal and distal to obstruction

Medical Plan

Surgery

Embolectomy—embolus can be removed directly via femoral arteriotomy using soft balloon-tipped catheter known as Fogarty catheter; catheter is passed distal to occlusion, carefully inflated, and withdrawn

Medications

Anticoagulants
- Heparin sodium (Lipo-Hepin and others)
  - Indications: Initiated once diagnosis of embolization is made and before operative treatment is performed
  - Usual dosage: Loading, 5000-10,000 U IV; maintenance, dose given to keep partial thromboplastin time to two times normal

Fibrinolytic agents
- Streptokinase (Streptase), urokinase (Abbokinase)
  - Indications: Thrombolytic agents instilled by intra-arterial infusion into site of occlusion; method of action is fibrinolysis causing fibrin dissolution

General Management

Percutaneous transluminal angioplasty—nonsurgical procedure involving mechanical dilation of occluded artery performed under local anesthesia with fluoroscopy; lesions considered suitable are stenotic vessels with intraluminal diameter of 2.5 mm and length of not more than 10 cm

NURSING CARE

Nursing Assessment

Peripheral Extremity

Pain, sudden in onset; numbness; "embolic syndrome" characterized by five Ps: pain, pallor, paresthesia, pulselessness, and paralysis

Nursing Dx & Intervention

Nursing Diagnosis	Nursing Intervention/Rationale
Altered tissue perfusion related to interruption of arterial flow	• Assess arterial pulses distal to occlusion every 1 to 2 hours *to determine arterial blood flow patterns*. Evaluate signs of further ischemia by checking the color and temperature of the extremity, the presence or absence of sensation, and the level of motor deficit. • Provide bed rest during acute periods. • Administer anticoagulants as ordered *to prevent enlargement of thrombus and further embolization.* • Keep extremities below level of heart *to maintain optimum gravitational flow.*
Pain related to peripheral ischemia	• Provide for position of most comfort. • Do not raise knee gatch, elevate extremity, or allow hips to be maintained in prolonged flexion, *since these procedures can interfere with arterial circulation.* • Administer analgesics as ordered. • Protect affected extremity by using a bed cradle, cotton blankets, or sheepskin. • Provide regular active and passive range of motion exercises unless contraindicated.

Nursing Diagnosis	Nursing Intervention/Rationale
Anxiety	• Assess level of anxiety. • Offer a brief, accurate explanation of disease and therapeutic modalities. • Correct any misconception about diagnosis and outcomes. • Encourage verbalization, since the patient may fear loss of the extremity.

Patient Education

1. Instruct the patient and family about the disease process, possible causes, and therapeutic modalities.
2. At discharge explain anticoagulant therapy and the need for follow-up monitoring with clotting studies.
3. Instruct the patient and family to avoid situations that cause blood pooling or interruption of blood flow: crossing legs, smoking, sitting or standing for extended periods of time.

Evaluation

Patient Outcome	Data Indicating That Outcome is Reached
Peripheral perfusion is improved.	Pain is relieved. Distal and proximal pulses are present. Extremity has normal color. Normal motor function returns in affected extremity.

Chronic arterial insufficiency

Chronic arterial insufficiency is inadequate blood flow in arteries. It is caused by occlusive atherosclerotic plaques or emboli, damaged or diseased vessels, aneurysms, hypercoagulability states, or heavy use of tobacco.

Arteriosclerosis obliterans is the primary cause of chronic arterial insufficiency. Other causes, although rare, may lead to arterial insufficiency of the legs. These include thromboangiitis obliterans (Buerger's disease), cystic degeneration of the popliteal artery, popliteal entrapment, and some connective tissue disorders.

Arteriosclerosis obliterans, a progressive ischemic syndrome, is more common in men, and the incidence rises with age. It is a diffuse process but is generally confined to short segments of arteries near bifurcations and origins. The aortoiliac and femoropopliteal areas are common sites.

Pathophysiology

Progressive narrowing of the arterial tree by atherosclerotic plaques gives rise to collateral vessels that tend to ensure adequate blood supply and prevent peripheral ischemia. However, the effectiveness of these collateral pathways is limited by their small size and high resistance, as well as by the extent of occlusive disease. Progressive occlusion leads to hypoperfusion and ischemia. These are related directly to the number of occlusions and the adequacy of collateral vessels. The arms and legs are the most vulnerable to ischemia.

Diagnostic Studies and Findings

Doppler Ultrasonography

Quantitates degree of ischemia; ankle/brachial index: arterial pressure less than pressure in brachial artery

Plethysmography

Determines degree to which peripheral circulation is decreased

Angiography

Provides visualization of arterial tree with exact localization of obstruction

Medical Plan

Surgery

Arterial revascularization, reconstruction—performed to restore unimpeded pulsatile blood flow, usually beginning with proximal segments (aortoiliac-femoral)
- Endarterectomy—removal of atheromatous intima from artery
- Bypass graft surgery—use of Dacron conduit to deliver blood from aorta to femoral vessels, bypassing diseased segments (Figure 1-47)
- Femoropopliteal reconstruction
  - Femoropopliteal bypass
  - Profundoplasty—local endarterectomy of proximal profunda femoris artery

Figure 1-47 A, Arteriogram depicting complete occlusion of distal abdominal aorta *(arrows)*.
B, Aortobifemoral bypass graft using synthetic conduit.
From Guzzetta.[41]

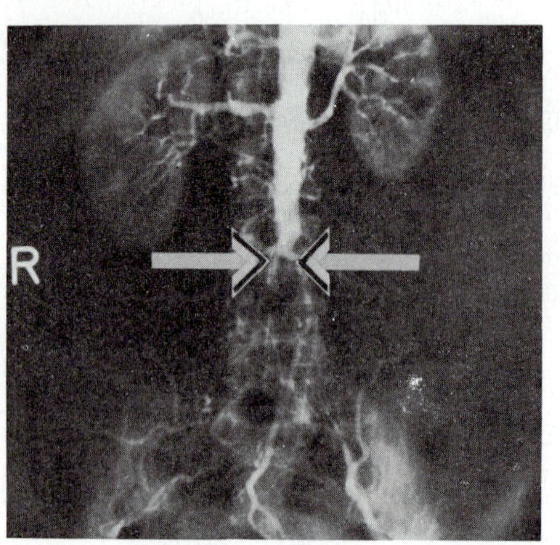

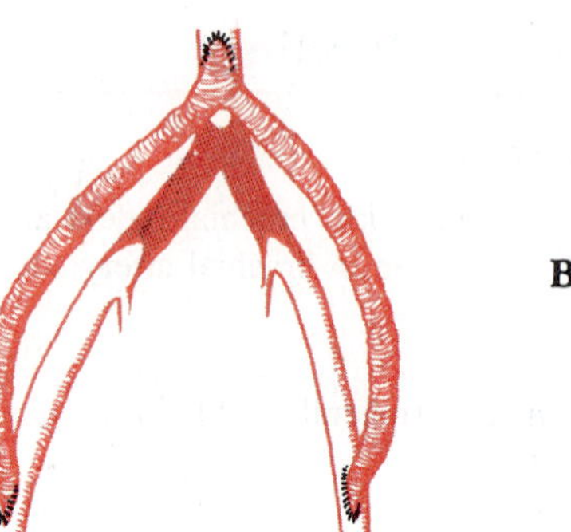

Lumbar sympathectomy—removal of second and third lumbar ganglia; performed to improve blood flow to skin

Amputation of limb—for severe, irreversible ischemia (gangrene)

Medications

Several drugs such as anticoagulants, vasodilators, and antiplatelets have been used but tend to be unhelpful or only palliative

General Management

Peripheral angioplasty (percutaneous transluminal angioplasty, PTA)—with inflatable balloon-tipped catheter, atheromatous plaque is mechanically compressed to increase lumen patency; vessels of iliac or femoral arteries are reported to respond best to PTA, but success has been reported for vessels of aorta, popliteal, superior mesenteric, subclavian, and brachial systems, as well as stenoses in peripheral arterial grafts[29]

Laser thermal angioplasty (LTA)—a new, experimental method of obliterating the atheromatous plaque by heat vaporization; with a fiberoptic catheter, energy from laser source is applied to occlusive lesion; often performed in conjunction with PTA

Risk reduction program aimed at weight reduction for the obese patient, smoking cessation, and a low-cholesterol, low–saturated fat diet; evaluation and control of diabetes and hyperlipidemia should be carried out to slow progression of atherosclerotic process

Daily foot care—inspection; cleaning; use of cotton socks; attention to nails, corns, calluses

Regular walking program to point of claudication several times a day may improve patient's walking distance; improvement may be due to development of increased collateral arterial flow, progressive adaptation to discomfort or gait modification, metabolic changes in the muscles, or redistribution of blood flow to the muscles[69]

NURSING CARE

Nursing Assessment

Peripheral Tissue Perfusion

Intermittent claudication
- Calf pain, fatigue induced by walking and relieved by rest, pain in thigh and buttocks (foot rarely involved)

Ischemic rest pain
- Continuous burning pain confined to toes, aggravated by elevation and improved by dependence; occurs at rest and improved with walking; may occur at night, interfering with sleep

Arterial Pulses

Palpation
- Ranges from slightly reduced to absent

Auscultation
- Presence of bruits at rest and after exercise; sites are abdominal aorta and iliac and femoral arteries

Skin, Nails, Hair

Ulcerations; glossy, cold, smooth skin; pallor—increasing with elevation of extremity; atrophic nails; hair loss

Nursing Dx & Intervention

Nursing Diagnosis	Nursing Intervention/Rationale
Altered peripheral tissue perfusion related to interruption of arterial flow	• Assess arterial pulses, determining pulse volume; auscultate for bruits before and after exercise. • Observe skin color changes (pallor) and venous filling with elevation and dependency procedures *to estimate the degree of ischemia.* • Avoid procedures or bed positions that *interfere with gravitational blood flow* (arterial flow is downward), such as elevating affected extremity or using knee gatch. • Protect the affected extremity: place bed cradle over affected areas, avoid use of heating devices on lower extremities. • Instruct the patient to avoid nicotine, *since it causes both small and larger vessels to constrict and damage intimal cells.*
Pain related to peripheral ischemia	• Assess quality and degree of pain; assist the patient to identify activities that precipitate or aggravate pain *to define a baseline for activity intolerance.* • Provide position of most comfort. Frequent, small position changes may be helpful during periods of restlessness brought on by pain. • Instruct the patient to stand or dangle at bedside *to obtain relief from ischemic pain.* • Begin a slow, progressive exercise program.
Impaired skin integrity (actual and potential) related to impaired circulation	• Assess skin color, temperature, and integrity *to observe for signs of necrosis.* • *Provide daily skin care to prevent fissures and infection.* Ensure that skin is thoroughly dried. • Treat ulcerations as they occur. Administer soaks, medications, and dressings as ordered. • Avoid using adhesive tape directly on skin. • Avoid use of tight constricting socks or hose; use cotton socks.

Patient Education

1. Provide information regarding the disease process and precipitating risk factors (see risk factor profile on p. 29).
2. Explain the importance of daily skin care. Tell the patient to wash with mild soap, dry well, and apply lanolin-based lotions.
3. Clean small cuts or abrasions with soap and water; report cuts or skin breaks that do not begin to heal in 2 to 3 days.
4. Nails, corns, and calluses should be managed professionally. Encourage the patient to wear well-fitted, hard-soled shoes.
5. Instruct the patient in a daily progressive walking program: walk until pain increases, stop and stand still to decrease pain, then continue walking.
6. Explain the need to avoid the use of nicotine.
7. Provide weight counseling for obese patients.
8. Explain the need for a low-cholesterol, low-fat diet.
9. Instruct the patient to avoid crossing legs and long periods of sitting and standing.

Evaluation

Patient Outcome	Data Indicating That Outcome is Reached
Peripheral perfusion is improved.	Patient reports relief of pain (claudication). Pulses are present, equal, and bilateral. Skin color is normal; skin is warm to touch.
Skin integrity is maintained.	Skin shows no signs of ulcerations. Skin color and temperature are normal.
Comfort level is achieved.	Patient verbalizes absence or control of pain. Patient demonstrates use of variety of strategies to reduce pain level.

Raynaud's disease

Raynaud's disease is a disorder of small cutaneous arteries, most frequently involving the fingers; it is marked by episodic vasospasm.

Raynaud's disease may occur by itself or may follow other disorders. By itself it occurs more commonly in young women, is often triggered by emotional stress and cold, and involves both hands.

Pathophysiology

Raynaud's disease involves three phases. First, severe constriction of cutaneous vessels results in blanching of the fingers. The vessels then dilate, slowing blood flow. This allows hemoglobin to release more oxygen into the tissues. During this ischemic phase the fingers are first white and then cyanotic, numb, and cold. This phase is followed by a reactive hyperemic phase during which the fingers become red and the patient has throbbing pain. Because attacks are often triggered by stress and cold, the disease may be related to vasoconstriction caused by the release of catecholamines. The attacks may last a few minutes or, in severe cases, several hours.

In severe cases, progressive ischemia with trophic skin changes may lead to recurring infection and gangrene. However, Raynaud's disease is rare and is most often seen in mild form.

Diagnostic Studies and Findings

Digital Plethysmography

Abnormal perfusion pressure and pulsatile contour

Peripheral Arteriography

Visualization of distal arteries of hands

Medical Plan

Surgery

- Sympathectomy
  - Lumbar ganglionectomy for relief of symptoms involving feet
  - Ganglionectomy for relief of symptoms involving hands
- Amputation of terminal phalanges (very rare)

Medications

- Antihypertensive agents
  - Reserpine (Serpasil, others)
    - Indications: Rauwolfia alkaloids that decrease vasoconstriction
    - Usual dosage: 0.25-0.5 mg/d po
- α-Adrenergic blocking agents
  - Phenoxybenzamine (Dibenzyline)
    - Dosage is variable
  - Tolazoline (Priscoline)
    - Usual dosage: 25-50 mg po tid; 10-50 mg parenterally qid
- Vasodilators
  - Nicotinyl alcohol (Roniacol)
    - Usual dosage: 50-100 mg po tid or 150 mg bid

General Management

Avoidance of exposure to irritants such as cold, mechanical or chemical injury, and stressful situations

NURSING CARE

Nursing Assessment

Hands and Fingers

Initially blanched and numb after exposure to cold or stress; then fingers become cyanotic; this is followed by change in color to red; trophic changes (ulcerations, chronic paronychia) may occur in long-standing disease

Nursing Dx & Intervention

Nursing Diagnosis	Nursing Intervention/Rationale
Pain related to ischemia	• Assess for aggravating factors leading to vasospasm. • Remove aggravating factors when possible; for example, provide warmth to fingers, have the patient stop smoking. • Assist the patient to modify stressful periods that may *aggravate vasospasm*. • Instruct the patient as to cause of pain.
Potential impaired skin integrity	• Perform daily assessment for color changes and ulcerations. • Treat ulcerations if they occur. • Avoid exposure to cold, mechanical and chemical irritants, or other stressful factors.

Patient Education

1. Instruct the patient to avoid exposure to cold temperatures and to wear gloves or mittens when handling cold items and in cold weather.
2. Instruct the patient to avoid smoking.
3. Explain the need to avoid stressful situations. Teach ways to deal with stress, such as relaxation techniques.
4. Explain the purpose, side effects, and dosage of medications.

Evaluation

Patient Outcome	Data Indicating That Outcome is Reached
Circulation in hands and fingers is improved.	There is no pain. Color is normal and skin is warm. Skin integrity is maintained.

Venous thrombosis

Venous thrombosis is an abnormal vascular condition in which a thrombus develops within a blood vessel.

Venous thrombosis is the most common venous disorder. The greatest incidence is in those having surgery (30% to 60%) and in patients receiving intravenous therapy, because of the embolization of a thrombus to the lungs. The incidence of pulmonary embolism in surgical patients has been estimated to be 7.3% to 54%, with the estimated number of deaths 200,000 per year.[69] The following terms are commonly used to describe venous disorders that reflect thrombus formation or inflammation:

phlebitis inflammation of vein.

phlebothrombosis (venous thrombosis) intraluminal thrombus with minimal or no inflammation, these have greater tendency to embolize.

thromboembolism the thrombus dislodgment and migration.

thrombophlebitis an acute condition marked by thrombus and inflammation in deep or superficial veins.

Pathophysiology

The triad of stasis, intimal damage, and hypercoagulability is responsible for most venous thrombosis.

Venous stasis occurs in persons who are inactive for a time because of bed rest or immobilization of the lower extremities. Thrombus formation results from a reduction of flow-induced dilution and a decrease in natural circulating anticoagulants (antithrombin III, platelet factor IV, and some prostaglandins).[69] Stasis caused by reduced flow increases the contact between platelets and coagulation factors that enhance platelet aggregation.

Intimal damage may occur as a result of internal or external trauma, usually involving IV therapy. Endothelial damage leads to exposure of the subintimal collagen membrane, which promotes platelet adherence, and activation of intrinsic coagulation factors, which contribute to thrombus formation.

Hypercoagulability reflects an alteration in coagulability. This occurs in some patients with disorders such as polycythemias and anemias, excessive estrogen or steroid use, or malignancies.

Once formed, the thrombus begins an inflammatory process leading to fibrosis. The enlarging thrombus eventually occludes the lumen of the vein or detaches and migrates to the systemic circulation.

Frequent sites for venous thrombus formation are the soleal and gastrocnemius venous sinus and the larger veins. Thrombosis of these veins is linked to increased risk of clotting. Thrombosis in subcutaneous veins rarely leads to pulmonary embolism.

Diagnostic Studies and Findings

Plethysmography

Shows decreased circulation distal to affected area

Doppler Ultrasonography

Identifies reduced blood flow to specific area; shows obstruction to venous flow

Phlebography

Confirms diagnosis; shows filling defects

^{125}I Fibrinogen Scan

Defines location of clot and any emboli that may have dislodged

Medical Plan

Surgery

Rarely indicated

Techniques used for deep vein thrombophlebitis necessitating venous interruption—ligation, vein plication, or clipping

Iliofemoral thrombectomy—may be considered for patients with acute iliofemoral thrombosis and compromised arterial perfusion that fail to respond to conventional therapy

Procedures to prevent distal embolization

- Extravascular vena cava interruption—application of a partitioning clip around the vein; used prophylactically for patients who are considered at high risk for embolization and are undergoing abdominal surgery for another reason
- Intracaval filters (Mobin-Uidden umbrella, Kimray-Greenfield filter)—interruption devices inserted into right internal jugular vein and advanced to vena cava via catheter; once in place, devices permit continuous venous flow while filtering clots, thus preventing further embolization

Medications

Anticoagulants

- Heparin sodium
  - Indications: Initially administered IV to augment fibrinolytic activity and aid in thrombolysis
  - Usual dosage: 300-500 U/kg followed by infusion of 1000 U/h
- Warfarin
  - Indications: Given later to maintain prothrombin time to twice control level; usually for 3 mo

Fibrinolytic agents

- Streptokinase (Streptase)
  - Indications: Produces total clot lysis and restores normal venous valve function
  - Usual dosage: IV initially 250,000 IU/30 min; maintenance 100,000 IU/h for 24-72 h

Antiplatelet agents (used in prevention of thrombus)

- Dipyridamole (Persantine)
  - Usual dosage: 800 mg/d; 400 mg/d if used with anticoagulants

General Management

Bed rest with elevation of affected extremity above level of right atrium

Warm, moist heat

Custom-fitted elastic stockings when ambulatory

Monitoring of partial thromboplastin time and/or prothrombin time while patient is receiving anticoagulant therapy

NURSING CARE

Nursing Assessment

Lower Extremity (Deep Veins)

Calf pain and tenderness; Homans' sign (calf pain on dorsiflexion of foot); dilated superficial veins; edema of involved extremity (30% to 50% of deep vein thromboses may be clinically silent); pain and tenderness over involved vein (for example, groin); increased size compared to unaffected side

Upper Extremity (Superficial Veins)

Redness, warmth, and tenderness over affected vein; veins visible and palpable

Nursing Dx & Intervention

Nursing Diagnosis	Nursing Intervention/Rationale
Impaired skin integrity related to venous stasis and fragility of small blood vessels	• Assess skin integrity daily; observe for signs of redness, breakdown, or ulcerations *reflective of venous stasis.* • Raise affected extremity above heart *to eliminate venous hypertension.* • Use elastic compression gradient stockings *to minimize peripheral edema.* • Administer daily hygiene measures. Use mild soap, rinse well, and dry gently but thoroughly. Avoid vigorous rubbing or massaging that may *lead to dislodgment of clot.*
Altered tissue perfusion related to interruption of venous flow	• Assess circulation of affected extremity and check pulses in all extremities. Use Doppler sensor if pulses seem absent. • Measure and record size of affected limb every day. • Maintain bed rest during acute phase; elevate affected extremity *to facilitate venous circulation toward the heart.* • Instruct patient to avoid positions that restrict venous blood flow such as use of knee gatch or crossing legs. • Administer anticoagulant and fibrolytic therapy as ordered. • Instruct patient to avoid use of nicotine *to prevent further constriction and damage to intimal cells.*

Nursing Diagnosis	Nursing Intervention/Rationale
	• Initiate a progressive exercise program as ordered: Never permit patient to dangle legs. Instruct patient to apply support stockings before ambulating, avoid standing for long periods, and alternate position by standing on toes, then on heels.
Pain related to inflammatory process	• Assess quality and location of pain. • Provide bed rest; limit self-care activities. • Elevate affected limb above level of right atrium. • Do not use knee gatch. • Administer analgesics as ordered. • Apply warm, moist compresses as ordered. • Measure calf or thigh or both daily and record. • Use elastic stockings as ordered.
Impaired gas exchange (potential) related to embolization of thrombus	• Observe for signs of pulmonary embolism: chest pain, dyspnea, tachypnea. • Monitor vital signs every 4 to 8 hours. • Maintain bed rest during acute period. Avoid exercising and massage affected extremity during acute phase. • Administer anticoagulant therapy as ordered. • Use elastic stockings during periods of ambulation.
Patient problem: hemorrhage	• Monitor anticoagulant therapy, including dosage, sites of administration, and bleeding (epistaxis, bleeding gums, petechiae). • Obtain daily coagulation laboratory values before administering medication. • Teach the patient and family the need for and proper administration of medication and the need for frequent laboratory evaluation.

Patient Education

1. Instruct the patient and family about the nature of the disorder and methods of preventing recurrence.
2. Instruct the patient to avoid constrictive clothing and crossing legs when sitting.
3. Instruct the patient and family in skin care.
4. Explain the value of rest periods with legs raised.
5. Explain the need to lose weight if the patient is obese.
6. Instruct the patient to avoid use of nicotine and oral contraceptives.
7. Explain the need for a regular or moderate exercise program.
8. Explain anticoagulant therapy and precautions.

Evaluation

Patient Outcome	Data Indicating That Outcome is Reached
Inflammation is decreased, and venous blood flow is improved.	Patient has relief of pain, swelling, and redness.
Skin integrity is maintained or improved.	Patient exhibits no ulcerations. Skin is free of infections.

Medical Interventions and Related Nursing Care

Automatic Implantable Cardioverter-Defibrillator

Description and Rationale

The automatic implantable cardioverter-defibrillator (AICD) is a self-contained system capable of identifying and treating life-threatening ventricular arrhythmias. Originally designed to correct ventricular fibrillation, AICD units now also have the capability to identify and treat ventricular tachycardia.[70,81]

The surgically implanted device continuously monitors and analyzes the patient's heart rate and waveform configuration. In the presence of ventricular tachycardia and ventricular fibrillation, electrical countershock is delivered directly to the heart via two transcardiac electrodes. One catheter electrode is positioned in the superior vena cava; the second may be a ventricular patch lead made of titanium mesh that is placed on the pericardium or myocardium during surgery.[16]

Patients for whom the AICD device is indicated include those who have survived sudden cardiac death not associated with acute MI and whose arrhythmias are not controlled with antiarrhythmic therapy, those who have had more than one cardiac arrest but whose arrhythmia cannot be induced during electrophysiologic testing, and those with sustained ventricular tachycardia not controlled with conventional antiarrhythmic agents.

Cautions

Safety from strong magnetic fields should be ensured, since they can activate or deactivate the AICD device.

Preprocedural Care

1. Initiate preoperative instruction for the patient and family, including information about the AICD device, its benefits and risks, the implantation procedure, and postoperative care. Include discussion regarding surgical approaches that may be used (thoracotomy, median sternotomy, or subxiphoid and subcostal approaches) and routine postoperative procedures and equipment of the intensive care unit where patients receiving implants stay for the first 24 to 48 hours postoperatively.
2. Obtain written informed consent.
3. Obtain baseline data as ordered: ECG (baseline rhythm), vital signs, and laboratory work (CBC, blood type and cross-match, electrolytes).
4. Perform skin preparation of chest and abdomen.
5. Permit nothing by mouth (NPO).
6. Deal with preoperative anxiety and fears of discomfort associated with shocks and possible malfunction of the device.

Medical Plan

Surgery

Approach for implantation determined by various clinical circumstances such as whether the patient has had previous chest surgery or will also undergo corrective cardiac surgery; surgical approaches used for AICD implantation include:
- Thoracotomy—for patient who previously underwent cardiac surgery and may have scar tissue around the heart
- Median sternotomy—used for patients undergoing concomitant cardiac surgery such as antiarrhythmic surgery or coronary artery bypass graft (CABG) surgery
- Subxiphoid—incision is made below the xiphoid process entering the pericardial space anteriorly
- Subcostal—similar to thoracotomy but requires a smaller incision and shorter recovery time

General Management

Continuous ECG monitoring during and after implantation, observing for inappropriate shocks during sinus rhythm or patient's preestablished rhythm
Diet as ordered
Intravenous therapy as ordered
Activity level determined by clinical status

NURSING CARE

Nursing Assessment

Malfunction of AICD Device

Sudden death

ECG Rhythm

Spontaneous uninterrupted appearance of malignant arrhythmias
False positive discharges of shocks in the presence of normal sinus rhythm; spurious shocks may be due to fractured leads or to miscounting of the heart rate because of oversensing
Using a low-level current, the malignant arrhythmias are induced to test the automatic functions of the device

Infection of the Pulse Generator Pocket Site

Redness, swelling, heat, fluid collection or drainage, skin irritation or breakdown

Nursing Dx & Intervention

Nursing Diagnosis	Nursing Intervention/Rationale
Fear related to anticipated shock, possible battery failure, or perceived loss of control	• Assess level of understanding, encouraging the patient to verbalize subjective feelings and perceptions. • Provide information to correct distorted perception. Assist the patient to identify sources of fear. • Assist the patient to cope with fears. Review strategies to cope with unpredictability of the arrhythmias and discomfort from the shocks. • Offer a brief description of the shock, including symptoms that may accompany it. • Review the signs and symptoms of battery failure or device malfunction and interventions to take if suspected.
Activity intolerance (actual and potential) related to functional limitations	• Assess the patient's tolerance or intolerance to activities of daily living. Determine whether intolerance is related to progressive heart disease or to perceived fear of the AICD device. • Discuss activity allowances and limitations. • Encourage the patient to engage in exercise activities as tolerated. Participation in a monitored exercise program may give the patient a sense of security when engaging in routine activities.

Patient Education

1. Instruct the patient and family about the purpose and basic function of the AICD device. Discuss benefits and limitations.
2. Describe the AICD device, discussing the signs and symptoms of defibrillation discharge.
3. Describe the signs and symptoms of AICD malfunction, such as inappropriate shocks or loss of consciousness, and the need to notify physician if suspected.
4. Explain the need for regular follow-up magnet testing to predict the end of generator life. Describe the use of the transtelephonic system if available.
5. Explain the signs and symptoms of wound or pocket infection, and instruct the patient or family to report any fever or drainage to the physician.
6. Instruct the patient in the need to protect the implantation site and to avoid constricting clothing such as belts and girdles.
7. Describe activity allowances and limitations. Explain that most former activities may be resumed, that driving is permitted unless the patient is bothered by neurologic symptoms or continues to have syncope after AICD implantation, and that sexual activity can be resumed without danger to patient or partner.
8. Discuss the need to avoid strong magnetic fields that may activate or deactivate the AICD unit, such as areas around radio or television transmitting towers and use of diathermy motors. Instruct the patient not to touch spark plugs of a running motor, as on a lawn mower or car.
9. Assure the patient that normal household appliances such as microwave ovens and hair dryers will not interfere with the AICD unit.
10. Assure the patient that routine contact with another person will not activate the unit; if the unit discharges during physical contact, the other person may feel a slight muscular contraction but will not be harmed.

Evaluation

Patient Outcome	Data Indicating That Outcome is Reached
AICD unit functions properly.	Patient demonstrates no further episode of syncope or cardiac arrest. AICD unit shows appropriate discharge response during magnet testing.
Fear level is reduced.	Patient is able to verbalize specific fears and concerns regarding AICD unit. Patient verbalizes comfort with AICD unit and asks appropriate questions regarding home maintenance hemodynamic monitoring.
Activity level returns to normal for patient.	Patient is able to return to activities of daily living and participates in exercise as allowed.

Cardiac Surgery

(Coronary artery bypass graft, valve surgeries, repair of septal defects, ventricular aneurysm resection, mapping, congenital defect repairs)

Description and Rationale

Surgical interventions for cardiac disorders may be employed as a corrective measure in congenital heart disease or as an alternative treatment modality when a patient's clinical course becomes refractory to medical management.

Cardiac surgery may be broadly classified as an open or a closed procedure. Open-heart techniques were made possible with the development of the cardiopulmonary bypass machine (extracorporeal circulation) in the early 1950s. Since that time, advances in myocardial preservation, in preoperative and postoperative support devices, and in pharmacology have contributed to improved mortality and morbidity and to a greater number of operative procedures for cardiac disorders.

Procedures for acquired disorders include the following:

- Coronary artery bypass graft (CABG) surgery—myocardial revascularization for coronary artery disease; aimed at relief of unstable angina pectoris
- Valve surgery—valvulotomy (commissurotomy), valvuloplasty (repair of valve), and replacement with prosthetic valve
- Resection of ventricular aneurysm—resection of nonviable myocardium
- Septal defects—closure of atrial or ventricular septal defect by direct suturing or placement of Dacron patch across defect
- Antiarrhythmia surgery—mapped (directed endocardial resection), and aneurysectomy

Procedures for congenital defects include these:

- Closure of patent ductus arteriosus
- Closure of atrial or ventricular septal defect
- Repair of coarctation of aorta
- Repair of tetralogy of Fallot
- Fontan or modified Fontan procedure for tricuspid atresia and single ventricle
- Mustard procedure for transposition of great vessels

Contraindications

Contraindications to cardiac surgery include bleeding disorders and acute (recent) cerebrovascular accident (stroke).

Cautions

Streptokinase should be administered within 24 hours before a cardiac surgical procedure. Cardiac surgery may be performed without added risk in the presence of pulmonary hypertension, in patients with an active infectious process, or in refractory ventricular failure.

Preprocedural Care

1. Determine the type of lesion and associated risks.
2. Initiate preoperative instruction for the patient and family, including information about the operative procedure and postoperative care: routine procedures of the intensive care unit (suctioning, coughing, turning, monitoring of vital signs); various tubes (endotracheal, chest, gastrointestinal, urinary catheter, intravenous); equipment (respirators, monitors); pain management; level of consciousness and emotional response; and visitor policies.
3. Obtain written informed consent.
4. Obtain baseline data: chest roentgenogram; ECG; laboratory work: complete blood count, blood type and crossmatch, electrolytes, serum chemistries, and urinalysis; weight; height; and vital signs.
5. Perform skin preparation: chest; legs for vein harvesting.
6. Hold or modify preoperative medications:
   - Digoxin—discontinued 24 to 36 hours before surgery
   - Antiplatelets—instruct patient not to take these up to 1 week before surgery
   - Anticoagulants—discontinue warfarin; initiate heparin therapy
   - Antiarrhythmics, antihypertensives—in most cases continue until hours before surgery
7. Initiate pulmonary preparation by instructing the patient to stop smoking, teaching the patient methods for coughing and deep breathing, and using an incentive spirometer.
8. Deal with preoperative anxiety, offering reassurance and support.
9. Assist with insertion of balloon flotation catheter, if ordered, before surgery.
10. Administer preoperative sedation.
11. Permit nothing by mouth for 24 hours before procedure.

Medical Plan

Surgery

Cardiopulmonary bypass machine (extracorporeal circulation; heart-lung machine)—assumes function of heart and lungs, providing quite bloodless operative field; procedure involves cannulation of great vessels, allowing drainage of unoxygenated blood that is emptied into venous reservoir; blood is then passed to oxygenator where it is fully saturated; to reduce tissue oxygen requirements, temperature of blood circulating in extracorporeal unit is lowered; cold blood is returned to patient, reducing total body temperature and slowing metabolic processes; myocardial preservation is required while the heart is arrested and includes coronary perfusion, topical cooling (profound hypothermia), and cold cardioplegia arrest

Medications

Preoperative management
- Cardiac glycosides
  - Digoxin (Lanoxin)
    - Indications: Atrial fibrillation and flutter
    - Usual dosage: 0.25 mg or 0.5 mg (to control rate)
- Antiarrhythmics
  - Lidocaine (Xylocaine)
    - Indications: Ventricular ectopy, tachycardia
    - Usual dosage: IV bolus 50-100 mg followed by continuous IV drip
  - Quinidine sulfate (Quinora, others)
    - Indications: Ventricular ectopy, tachycardia
    - Dosage varies
  - Procainamide (Pronestyl)
    - Indications: Ventricular ectopy, tachycardia
    - Usual dosage: 0.5-1 g IM; 0.2-1g IV
- Potassium replacement
  - Usual dosage: IV or po to maintain serum levels at 4-5 mEq/L

Postoperative management (based on clinical symptoms, complications, and progress of patient)
- Parenteral fluids
  - Usual dosage: Calculated on basis of procedure performed and patient's body surface area: CABG, 50 ml/h; valve replacement, 1000-1500 ml/24 h; pediatric dosage, 60 ml/kg for first 10 kg body weight, 30 ml/kg for next 10 kg, 15 ml/kg for remainder of weight
- Drugs to correct coagulopathy
  - Protamine sulfate
  - 6-Aminocaproic acid (Amicar)
  - Epsilon-aminocaproic acid (EACA)
  - Vitamin K

General Management

Intra-aortic balloon pump—used when severe ventricular dysfunction occurs as patient is removed from bypass; provides circulatory support to failing myocardium

Hemodynamic monitoring—arterial, left atrial, pulmonary artery, and pulmonary capillary wedge pressures; cardiac output measurements may be required

ECG monitoring—continuous evaluation of heart rate, rhythm

Pacemakers

Immediate postoperative
- Assisted ventilation
- Suctioning
- Chest tubes

Diet therapy—sodium and fluid restrictions on basis of patient's clinical status

Pulmonary toilet—encourage coughing, deep breathing, and use of incentive spirometry

NURSING CARE

Nursing Assessment

Level of Consciousness

Early
- Arousable

Late
- Alert and oriented

Pupils

May be small, but reactive to light

Sensory-Motor Function

As patient awakens, moves all extremities

Respiratory Function

Early
- Atelectasis; diminished breath sounds at base

Late
- Clear with full aeration; arterial blood gases normal

Cardiovascular System

Low cardiac output
- Narrow pulse pressure; thready, rapid pulse; decreased urine output; labored respiration; disorientation; increased pulmonary capillary wedge pressure (PCWP) and left atrial pressure (LAP)

Arrhythmias
- Atrial fibrillation and flutter; junctional rhythms; heart block; ventricular rhythms: premature ventricular contractions, tachycardia, fibrillation

Cardiac tamponade
- Hypotension; narrowed pulse pressure (10 mm Hg); pulsus paradoxus; widened mediastinal shadow on chest roentgenogram; increased venous pressure

Bleeding
- Chest tube drainage at least 250 ml/hour; hypotension; disorientation; prolonged prothrombin time and partial thromboplastin time; decreased platelet levels

Infection
- Elevated temperature; purulent drainage from suture sites; chills; diaphoresis; malaise

Pericarditis; postpericardiotomy syndrome
- Pericardial friction rub; low-grade fever; chills; diaphoresis; malaise; chest pain

Nursing Dx & Intervention

Nursing Diagnosis	Nursing Intervention/Rationale
Decreased cardiac output (potential) related to mechanical problems (altered preload, afterload, contractility, heart rate)	• Assess and monitor for signs and symptoms of decreased cardiac output: skin pallor, diaphoresis, hypotension, decreased urine output, tachycardia, diminished peripheral pulse, dyspnea. • Monitor pulmonary artery pressure (PAP), pulmonary capillary wedge pressure (PCWP), and arterial pressures every 15 minutes during the immediate postoperative period, decreasing frequency as the clinical status stabilizes. Then monitor vital signs every 2 to 4 hours. • Calculate cardiac output and systemic vascular resistance (SVR) as ordered. • Measure urine output every hour; report output of less than 30 ml per hour in an adult patient. • Check peripheral perfusion: pulses, skin temperature, color. • Auscultate chest for heart sounds to detect gallops, murmurs, or rubs. • Administer fluids and medications as ordered.
Ineffective breathing pattern related to decreased lung expansion, pain, or anxiety	• Assess respirations, lung sounds, skin color, use of accessory muscles, and arterial blood gases to determine lung expansion and detect diminished sounds that may be due to increased fluid or atelectasis. • Auscultate chest for diminished breath sounds, initially every 1 to 2 hours and later every 4 to 6 hours. • Observe and maintain patency of chest tubes to ensure proper drainage and lung expansion. • Reposition the patient from one side to the other during the immediate postoperative period to encourage lung expansion. • Assist the patient to cough and deep breathe, and use incentive spirometry. • Obtain serial chest roentgenograms to check for progressive or resolving atelectasis and pleural effusions.
Impaired gas exchange related to hypoventilation, ventilation-perfusion abnormalities	• Assess respirations, observing rate and quality as the patient is weaned from the respirator. • Administer oxygen therapy with assisted ventilation; check FIO_2 tidal volume to yield Pao_2 of about 100 mm Hg. • Observe for signs of progressive atelectasis: diminished breath sounds over affected area, restlessness, rales. • Obtain and monitor arterial blood gases for signs of respiratory acidosis or alkalosis. • Auscultate the chest for diminished or adventitious breath sounds every 1 to 2 hours. • Suction every 1 to 2 hours to maintain a patent airway. Oxygenate before suctioning procedure per institutional policy. Monitor and record any arrhythmia during the procedure. *Convalescent care:* • Assist and teach the patient to turn, cough, and deep breathe. • Encourage use of the incentive spirometer. • Auscultate lung sounds every 4 to 8 hours.
Fluid volume deficit	• Monitor for signs of hypovolemia, including decreased blood pressure, increased heart rate, decreased central venous pressure, decreased PAP, and oliguria. • During rewarming, check right atrial pressure, left atrial pressure, and PAP every 5 minutes until stable, then every 30 to 60 minutes. • Titrate parenteral fluids according to hemodynamic parameters per protocol. • Measure output every hour. Check specific gravity as ordered. • Limit fluid intake as ordered. • Monitor electrolyte, hemoglobin, and hematocrit values. • Weigh daily as indicated by clinical picture.
Potential for infection	• Observe for signs of generalized sepsis: elevated temperature, chills, diaphoresis. • Observe suture sites for local redness, drainage, and swelling; clean incisions and change dressing daily. • Check temperature every 2 hours for 48 hours, then every 4 hours for 48 hours, then every 8 hours. • Change IV and pressure lines and dressing as ordered, maintaining aseptic technique *to prevent nosocomial infections and cross-contamination.* • Obtain blood cultures as ordered. • Obtain complete blood count with differential as ordered.
Patient problem: potential hemorrhage	• Observe for signs of hemorrhage: decreased blood pressure, disorientation, and falling hemoglobin level. • Observe for signs of coagulopathy: blood oozing from incisions, bloody secretions from endotracheal tube, increased chest tube drainage, and hematuria. • Observe and measure chest tube drainage every 30 to 60 minutes.

Nursing Diagnosis	Nursing Intervention/Rationale
	• Report output in excess of 150 ml/hour for an adult or 5 ml/kg/hour for a child. • Check hemoglobin, hematocrit, and clotting studies on the patient's arrival in the intensive care unit and every 2 to 4 hours as ordered. • Administer blood and blood products as ordered. • Administer drugs as ordered.
Anxiety related to actual or perceived threat to biologic integrity	*Preoperative:* • Provide adequate instruction, answering questions and offering reassurance. • Explain the method of communication to be used after the operation while the patient is intubated. *Postoperative:* • Orient the patient to time, situation, and location. • Inform the patient that the surgery is over. • Assist with communication. • Anticipate needs if possible. • Allow family support and participation. • Provide reassurance of daily progress. • Encourage verbalization of fears and questions regarding the operation, recovery, and discharge. • Begin postoperative instruction.

Patient Education

General:

1. Review the surgical procedure, emphasizing any precautions or complications that may be associated with it.
2. Clarify what action(s) should be taken if symptoms of infection, bleeding, ventricular failure, or arrhythmias develop.
3. Review diet and fluid restrictions.
4. Review discharge medication, including purpose, dosages, side effects, and need for specific follow-up laboratory studies as indicated.
5. Discuss activity allowances or limitations. Refer patient to cardiac rehabilitation for progressive ambulation.
6. Discuss the importance of avoiding fatigue and sitting for prolonged periods of time.
7. Discuss care of incisions and symptoms of wound infection to report to the physician.

After valve replacement:

1. Discuss the importance of anticoagulation therapy.
2. Discuss the importance of reporting signs of endocarditis (see p. 69).
3. Discuss the importance of prophylactic antibiotic therapy before procedures that predispose to bacteremia (see p. 68).

Evaluation

Patient Outcome	Data Indicating That Outcome is Reached
Hemodynamic and electromechanical stability is achieved. Cardiac output is adequate.	Blood pressure, pulmonary artery pressure, and cardiac output are within acceptable range. There is no arrhythmia. ECG findings are within acceptable limits.
Oxygenation, ventilation, and lung perfusion are adequate.	PaO_2 and PCO_2 are within normal limits. There is no dyspnea or tachypnea. Lungs are clear on auscultation and radiography.
There is no infection.	Patient is afebrile.
Hematologic hemostasis is achieved.	Hematocrit and hemoglobin level are within normal limits. A progressive decline in chest drainage occurs.
Anxiety is reduced.	There is no pain. Anxiety is absent or decreased. Patient demonstrates appropriate behavior patterns: asking questions and participating in self-care.
Patient has knowledge and understanding of primary cardiac disorder, surgical procedure performed, and discharge instructions.	Patient is able to describe specific action to take regarding diet, medications, and care of incision(s). Patient is able to describe activity allowances and limitations.

 Cardiac Transplantation

Description and Rationale

Cardiac transplantation has evolved rapidly during the past 20 years, yet it was first performed in 1905 when Carrel and Guthrie transplanted the heart of one dog to another. However, it was not until 1967, when Christian Barnard performed the first human cardiac transplantation, that serious interest was stimulated. Because early survival rates were poor, transplantations continued to be performed on a limited basis. Since the introduction of the immunosuppressant agent cyclosporine in 1980, the number of centers performing heart transplantations has grown steadily.

By 1987 the number of medical centers with active transplant programs had increased throughout the world to 105, 90 of which were located in the United States. One-year survival rates are reported to be 88%, and 5-year survival is 78%.

Infection and organ rejection continue to be the most common medical complications and the primary causes of death in long-term follow-up. However, as survival time increases, other medical problems are being identified, and these have contributed to the increased morbidity and mortality of patients over time.

Infection remains a major cause of morbidity and mortality for long-term, immunosuppressed transplant recipients, although the incidence and severity of infections decrease after the first year. The more common sites of infections in this population include the respiratory tract, urinary tract, mediastinum, and retinitis. The organisms commonly involved in infections include bacteria *(Escherichia coli, Pseudomonas)*, viruses (cytomegalovirus, herpes simplex, herpes zoster), and fungi *(Candida, Aspergillus, Cryptococcus)*.

Rejection of the transplanted heart remains the major lifelong threat to the recipient. Cardiac rejection can occur as an acute episode or a chronic condition. The risk of acute rejection is highest in the first days and weeks after transplantation while immunosuppressant therapy is being adjusted. Although rejection rates decrease with each year of survival, the recipient is always at risk if therapy is interrupted or stopped. Immunosuppression is the only safeguard against acute rejection.

Graft atherosclerosis, or chronic rejection, has been reported to occur in approximately 35% to 40% of patients who survive 5 years after transplantation. The incidence among patients who had coronary artery disease before receiving the transplant is similar to that among patients with pretransplant cardiomyopathy. Furthermore, because the donor heart has been denervated, patients who develop diffuse occlusive CAD do not present clinically with angina pectoris. Thus, if not monitored carefully, they can die suddenly or develop ventricular failure.

Malignancies, particularly lymphomas of the histiocytic type, have been reported.[46] Their occurrence is thought to be associated with immunosuppression therapy, particularly including antithymocyte globulin in addition to cyclosporine. Other reported malignancies include epithelial tumors of the skin and leukemia.

Other late complications associated with lifelong immunosuppression in long-term survivors include osteoporosis (18.2%), spinal disorders (8.8%) and visual problems (14.3%).[65]

The quality of life following cardiac transplantation has also been evaluated. Lough and associates[65] reported that an average of 3.7 years after surgery 89% of heart recipients perceived their quality of life as good to excellent, and 82% reported satisfaction with life as good to very satisfactory. Factors associated with negative life change were reported to be financial status, physical appearance, and sexual function. All recipients were bothered by the side effects associated with immunosuppression therapy, but these were found to have little impact on their evaluation of quality of life and life satisfaction.[65]

Immunosuppression. Increased understanding of immune suppression and the introduction of various immunosuppressive agents have made organ transplantation a viable treatment modality. Since the late 1960s, a variety of nonselective immunosuppressive agents had been used in transplantations, but these were associated with impairment of the immune system, leaving the host vulnerable to any number of infections. With the introduction of cyclosporine A, morbidity and mortality figures were significantly reduced.

The primary goal of immunosuppressive therapy is to prevent rejection of the foreign graft (heart), yet retain the host's natural immune system, which protects him from infections.

The immune system is a complex response mechanism. Its purpose is to destroy any tissue invasion or foreign material in order to maintain hemostasis. There are two primary types of immune response, humoral and cell-mediated. Both are derived from lymphocytes.

Medical Plan

Medications

While there are a variety of immunosuppressant agents available, maintenance immunosuppression protocols for cardiac transplant patients can include the following.

Cyclosporine (Sandimmune)—naturally occurring polypeptide antibiotic produced by fungi; inhibits T cell lymphocyte proliferation and activity, which is responsible for tissue graft rejection

- Usual dosage: 1-10 mg/kg/d po; daily dose adjusted to maintain therapeutic levels (NOTE: therapeutic level dependent on biologic fluid, assay method)
- Half-life: 18-40 h (average 27 h)
- Excretion: Metabolized by liver; excretion in bile and urine
- Side effects: Hirsutism, acne, fragile skin, gingival hyperplasia, fine hand tremor
- Adverse reaction: Nephrotoxicity, hypertension, hepatotoxicity, infection (viral, bacterial, and fungal), lymphoma

Azathioprine (Imuran)—antimetabolite that produces immunosuppression by inhibiting purine and DNA synthesis
- Usual dosage: 1.5-2 mg/kg/d po (NOTE: dosage adjusted by CBC)
- Half-life: Approximately 3 h
- Excretion: Metabolized by liver; excreted in urine
- Side effects: Rash, bruising, nausea, vomiting, stomatitis, muscle wasting, arthralgia, fatigue, decreased libido, impotence
- Adverse reaction: Leukopenia, thrombocytopenia, anemia, hepatotoxicity, pancreatitis, jaundice

Antithymocyte globulin (ATG)—reduces T lymphocytes; used to prevent rejection, or as an adjunct to immunosuppression therapy during rejection episodes
- Usual dosage: Rabbit ATG-2 mg/kg/d IM, adjusted according to circulating T lymphocytes (WBCs); equine ATG-10 mg/kg/d IV, adjusted according to circulating T lymphocytes (rosette count)
- Side effects: Localized pain and inflammation with IM injection; chills, fever, hypotension
- Adverse reactions: Anaphylaxis

Corticosteroids—anti-inflammatory agents used to suppress both T and B lymphocyte function and to reverse capillary permeability, vasodilation, and edema; may be used as part of maintenance program to prevent rejection or as adjunct therapy when there is evidence of rejection
- Prednisone (Meticorten, Deltasone)—used as part of maintenance therapy
  - Usual dosage: 0.1-0.2 mg/kg/d po (NOTE: may be increased with rejection)
- Methylprednisone (Medrol, Depo-Medrol, Solu-Medrol)—used when there is evidence of rejection
  - Usual dosage: 1 g/d for 3 d IV
  - Half-life: 3½ h
  - Side effects: Cushingoid appearance, mood changes, GI distress, fragile skin, bruising, delayed wound healing
  - Adverse reactions: Infection, diabetes, thrombocytopenia, pancreatitis

General Management

ECG changes—reflect lack of autonomic innervation of heart that occurs as result of denervation when donor heart is removed
- Heart rate—resting heart rate generally higher (90-100 beats/minute); response to metabolic demands such as fever or exercise in a denervated patient is one in which heart rate changes gradually; as result of these changes, response to drugs whose effect on the heart is mediated by autonomic nervous system is also altered
- Rhythm—normal sinus but without respiratory variation
- P wave—transplant procedure generally involves retaining posterior portion of recipient's atria, which includes SA node; therefore second P wave is visible

Endomyocardial biopsy—after first year, endomyocardial biopsies are performed on an interval basis depending on recipient's clinical status

Diet—low saturated fat and cholesterol; moderate decrease in sodium intake

Laboratory studies—regular monitoring to detect adverse reactions to immunosuppressive therapy: CBC, serum BUN and creatinine, liver function (SGOT, SGPT, LDH), glucose, urinalysis

NURSING CARE

Nursing Assessment

Acute Rejection

Mild or early rejection—generally no symptoms associated; to detect early rejection, diagnosis is done with EMB

Severe rejection
- Weakness, fatigue, malaise
- Anorexia
- Nausea, vomiting
- Decreased urine output
- Weight gain
- Peripheral edema
- Distended neck veins
- Increased jugular venous pulsations and decreased perfusion: cool pale skin, diminished pulses, diaphoresis, confusion, restlessness
- Pulmonary venous congestion: dyspnea on exertion, cough, tachypnea
- Development of S_3 and S_4

Electrocardiogram (ECG)

Using conventional immunosuppression; 20% decrease in QRS voltage; right axis shift; atrial arrhythmias, e.g., PAC, atrial fibrillation, atrial flutter (with cyclosporine these ECG changes may not be seen)

Chest Roentgenogram

Increased cardiothoracic ratio (cardiomegaly)

Echocardiogram

Thickening of left ventricle; decreased left ventricular function; decreased contractility

Endomyocardial Biopsy (EMB)

Changes in lymphocytes; finding varies according to degree of rejection
- Mild—occasional WBCs
- Severe—extensive perivascular infiltration of lymphocytes, interstitial edema, and myocyte necrosis
- Increased CPK-MB, SGOT, LDH

Infection

Usual signs and symptoms of infection often absent in immunosuppressed patient

Fever—low grade; baseline temperature may be lower than before transplant, so elevation to 37.2° C (99° F) may be significant

Malaise

Nursing Dx & Intervention

Nursing Diagnosis	Nursing Intervention/Rationale
Potential for injury: rejection related to noncompliance with prescribed medical regimen	• Assess and evaluate patient for understanding and cognitive appraisal of prescribed lifelong therapy *to identify misconceptions and cues that may indicate potential adherence problems.* • Encourage discussion regarding changes in life-style that have been positive or negative. • Anticipate and allow questions regarding prescribed therapy.
Potential for infection	• Assess and monitor for signs of infection (see above). • Take temperature every 4 hours. • Obtain cultures as indicated: sputum, throat, urine, any suspicious drainage sites in wounds. • Obtain and assess complete blood count and chest roentgenogram as indicated. NOTE: Laboratory values may be altered owing to steroids. • Minimize or avoid use of invasive procedures that increase risk of infection: IV, indwelling catheters. • Change IV tubings, bags, and dressings daily using aseptic technique. • Avoid placing patient in room with other patient who is at risk for infection *to avoid potential cross-contamination.* • Administer antibiotic therapy as ordered.
Decreased cardiac output related to acute rejection	• Assess and monitor for signs and symptoms of decreased cardiac output and signs of rejection (see p. 95). • Auscultate heart sounds *assessing for changes in rhythm* and presence of S_3 and S_4. • Auscultate chest for lung sounds, *assessing for signs of increased pulmonary congestion.* • Weigh daily. • Prepare patient for EMB. • Administer immunosuppressive therapy as ordered.

Patient Education

1. Discuss and review signs and symptoms of rejection. Emphasize the importance of keeping scheduled EMB appointments, since there are usually *no* signs of early rejection and appearance of symptoms is associated with moderate to severe rejection.
2. Discuss and review the need to take medications lifelong and the need to take them *exactly* as prescribed. Caution the patient *never to stop* taking medication. Notify the physician if a dose was skipped. Review medications, checking dosage, method of administration, and side effects.
3. Discuss signs and symptoms of infection to report: elevation of baseline temperature; early signs of sore throat, cold, or flu; and cuts and lesions that do not heal.
4. Discuss the need to reduce risk of infection by avoiding individuals with infections or contagious diseases, avoiding large crowds, and wearing a face mask when traveling in crowded areas.
5. Discuss the importance of lifelong follow-up: clinic visits, endomyocardial biopsy (EMB) appointments, and periodic stress tests, radionuclide studies, and cardiac catheterization.
6. Discuss activities allowances and limitations. Tell the patient to check with the physician before engaging in strenuous or competitive activities or sports.

Evaluation

Patient Outcome	Data Indicating That Outcome is Reached
There is no infection.	The patient maintains baseline temperature. There is no sign of infection: complete blood count, urinalysis, and cultures are within normal limits.
There are no signs of rejection on biopsy.	There are no new changes in endomyocardial biopsy (EMB) results. There are no clinical signs of rejection.

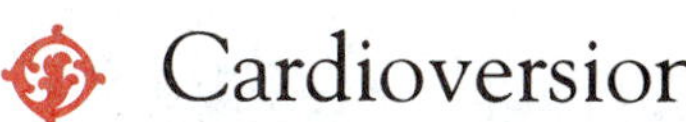

Cardioversion
(Synchronized cardioversion)

Description and Rationale

Synchronized cardioversion is the electrical conversion of a tachyarrhythmia, such as atrial fibrillation, atrial flutter, or supraventricular tachycardia, to a normal sinus rhythm. A synchronized electrical shock is released through the chest wall, depolarizing the myocardium and simultaneously making it refractory, thereby enabling the S-A node to resume its function as primary pacemaker.

Cautions

When cardioversion is performed, the electrical current must be timed so the discharge occurs at the apex of the R wave of the ECG pattern. Caution must be taken to avoid zones of vulnerability during which electrical current can produce ventricular fibrillation. The most vulnerable zone is the peak of the T wave on the ECG pattern. Grounding of equipment must be secure to avoid delivering current to the myocardium, which could lead to ventricular fibrillation.

Contraindications

Contraindications to cardioversion include atrial fibrillation of long standing or with slow ventricular rate, sick sinus syndrome with tachycardia, digitalis toxicity, and third-degree heart block.

Preprocedural Care

1. Explain the procedure to the patient and family, including rationale and associated risks.
2. Obtain written informed consent unless used in life-threatening situations.
3. Permit nothing by mouth for 6 to 8 hours before the procedure.
4. Withhold digitalis for 24 to 72 hours before the procedure.
5. Check digitalis and potassium levels.
6. Maintain an emergency cart at the bedside.
7. Obtain baseline ECG rhythm.
8. Insert an intravenous line.
9. Administer sedation as ordered (an anesthetist is usually in attendance).

Medical Plan

Medications

Antiarrhythmic drugs
- Quinidine sulfate (Quinora, others)
  - Indications: Atrial fibrillation or flutter
  - Usual dosage: 200-400 mg po q6h beginning 24-48 h before procedure
- Lidocaine (Xylocaine)
  - Indications: Ventricular tachycardia or fibrillation
  - Usual dosage: Bolus of 50-100 mg

Anesthesia during elective procedure—light intravenous anesthesia may be given by anesthetist

Tranquilizers
- Diazepam (Valium)
  - Usual dosage: IV in 5 mg increments

General Management

Cardiac monitoring—rhythm strip obtained before, during, and after procedure

Cardioverter electrical energy,[3] 50 to 100 joules (adults)
- Placement of paddles
  - Anterior-posterior—anterior paddle on left precordium, posterior paddle beneath patient
  - Standard—one paddle to right of upper sternum and below clavicle, second paddle to left of nipple with center of electrode in midaxillary line
- Saline-soaked gauze pads or electrode paste on electrode paddles

Oxygen therapy as ordered; intubation equipment on standby

Cardiopulmonary resuscitation in absence of breathing and pulse

Vital signs before, during, and after procedure

NURSING CARE

Nursing Assessment

After Procedure

Mental status
- Awake, alert

Vital signs
- Within normal limits

ECG
- Normal sinus rhythm

Precordial chest
- Observe skin for redness, irritation, excoriation

Complications

Ventricular fibrillation, cardiac arrest, pulmonary embolism, myocardial injury, hypotension, transient heart block

Nursing Dx & Intervention

Nursing Diagnosis	Nursing Intervention/Rationale
Impaired skin integrity	• Check area where electrode paddles were placed. • Wash area of electrode paddle placement with water and apply lanolin-based lotions as indicated.
Decreased cardiac output	• Assess level of consciousness and monitor blood pressure, apical and peripheral pulses, and respirations every 5 to 10 minutes after procedure to establish hemodynamic stability. • Monitor ECG every 2 to 4 hours as ordered after procedure to determine electromechanical stability. Compare with previous tracings. • Initiate hemodynamic monitoring as ordered.

Patient Education

1. Instruct the patient to notify the physician of recurrence of tachyarrhythmia symptoms such as dizziness or lightheadedness, sudden onset of palpitations, or rapid heart action.
2. Instruct the patient on pulse rate and rhythm checking.
3. Discuss care of skin burns: gently wash area where electrode paddles were placed with water, and apply lanolin-based lotions as required.

Evaluation

Patient Outcome	Data Indicating That Outcome is Reached
Sinus rhythm is reestablished.	ECG monitor shows normal sinus rhythm. Pulse rate is regular.

Defibrillation

(Unsynchronized countershock)

Description and Rationale

Defibrillation is the use of direct-current electrical countershock for treatment of malignant ventricular arrhythmias leading to asystole and cardiac arrest.

Considered an advanced life support measure, defibrillation is usually preceded by and performed in conjunction with cardiopulmonary resuscitation (CPR).

Current recommendations from the American Heart Association differentiate the management of patients with ventricular arrhythmias into hemodynamically stable (pulse present) and unstable (pulse absent).[3]

The recommendation sequence for treatment of a hemodynamically stable patient with ventricular tachycardia appears in Figure 1-48. For a hemodynamically unstable patient with ventricular tachycardia or ventricular fibrillation, emergency unsynchronized countershock is recommended. The management sequence is summarized in Figure 1-49.

Medical Plan

Medications

Epinephrine 1:10,000
- Indications: Administered during CPR following defibrillation to increase myocardial and central nervous system blood flow during chest compression and ventilation
- Usual dosage: 0.5-1 mg (5-10 ml of 1:10,000) IV q5 min during resuscitation

Lidocaine
- Indications: Recommended in ventricular tachycardia and ventricular fibrillation that is resistant to defibrillation
- Usual dosage: 1 mg/kg IV bolus

Bretylium
- Indiciations: Recommended for use only if lidocaine and defibrillation fail to convert ventricular fibrillation[4]
- Usual dosage: 5 mg/kg IV bolus

General Management

Energy requirements (adults)
- Ventricular fibrillation (and pulseless ventricular tachycardia)
  - Initial shock 200 joules
  - Second shock 200-300 joules
  - Third shock not to exceed 360 joules
- Ventricular tachycardia (pulse present)
  - Initial shock 50 joules
  - Second shock 100 joules
  - Third shock 200 up to 360 joules

Paddle electrode 10 cm in diameter

Oxygen therapy as ordered; intubation and assisted mechanical ventilation may be indicated

Cardiopulmonary resuscitation in absence of breathing and pulse

Figure 1-48 Sequence of treatment for ventricular tachycardia (VT).
From American Heart Association.[3]

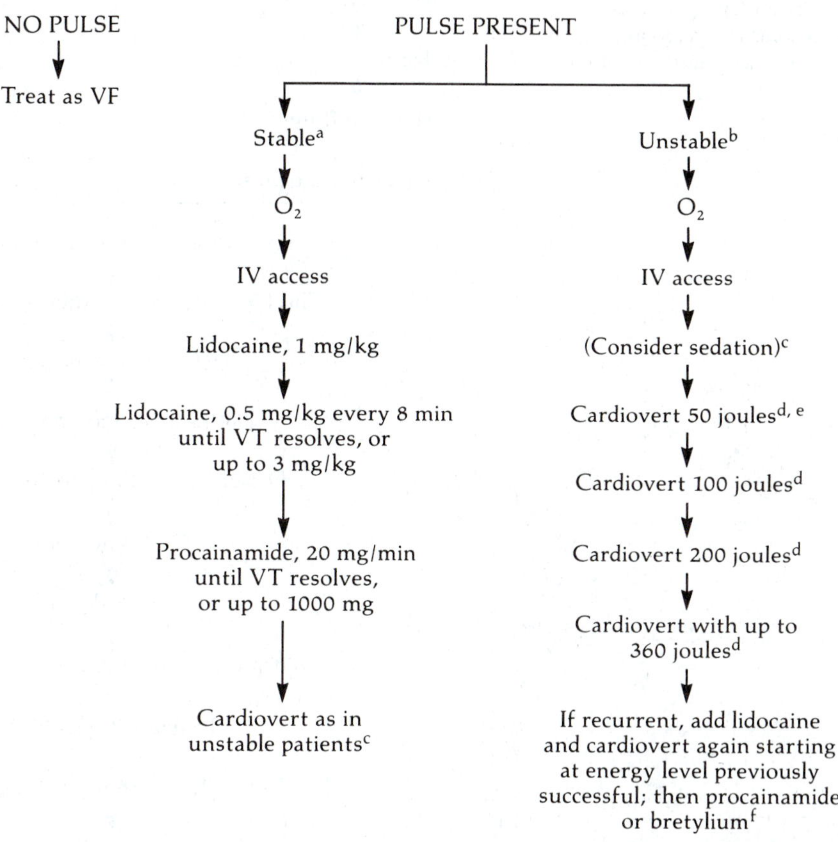

Sustained ventricular tachycardia (VT). Some patients may require care not specified herein. Flow of algorithm presumes that VT is continuing. VF indicates ventricular fibrillation.

[a]If patient becomes unstable (see footnote b for definition) at any time, move to "Unstable" arm of algorithm.

[b]Unstable indicates symptoms (eg, chest pain or dyspnea), hypotension (systolic blood pressure <90 mm Hg), congestive heart failure, ischemia, or infarction.

[c]Sedation should be considered for all patients, including those defined in footnote b as unstable, except those who are hemodynamically unstable (eg, hypotensive, in pulmonary edema, or unconscious).

[d]If hypotension, pulmonary edema, or unconsciousness is present, unsynchronized cardioversion should be done to avoid delay associated with synchronization.

[e]In the absence of hypotension, pulmonary edema, or unconsciousness, a precordial thump may be employed prior to cardioversion.

[f]Once VT has resolved, begin intravenous (IV) infusion of antiarrhythmic agent that has aided resolution of VT. If hypotension, pulmonary edema, or unconsciousness is present, use lidocaine if cardioversion alone is unsuccessful, followed by bretylium. In all other patients, recommended order of therapy is lidocaine, procainamide, and then bretylium.

NURSING CARE

Nursing Assessment

Preprocedure

Mental status: awake, unconscious
Pulse: present or absent
BP: present or absent
ECG: ventricular tachycardia, ventricular fibrillation, asystole

After Procedure

Mental status: awake, alert
Vital signs: within normal limits
ECG: normal sinus rhythm or return to baseline rhythm
Precordial chest examination: observe for signs of skin irritation or excoriation

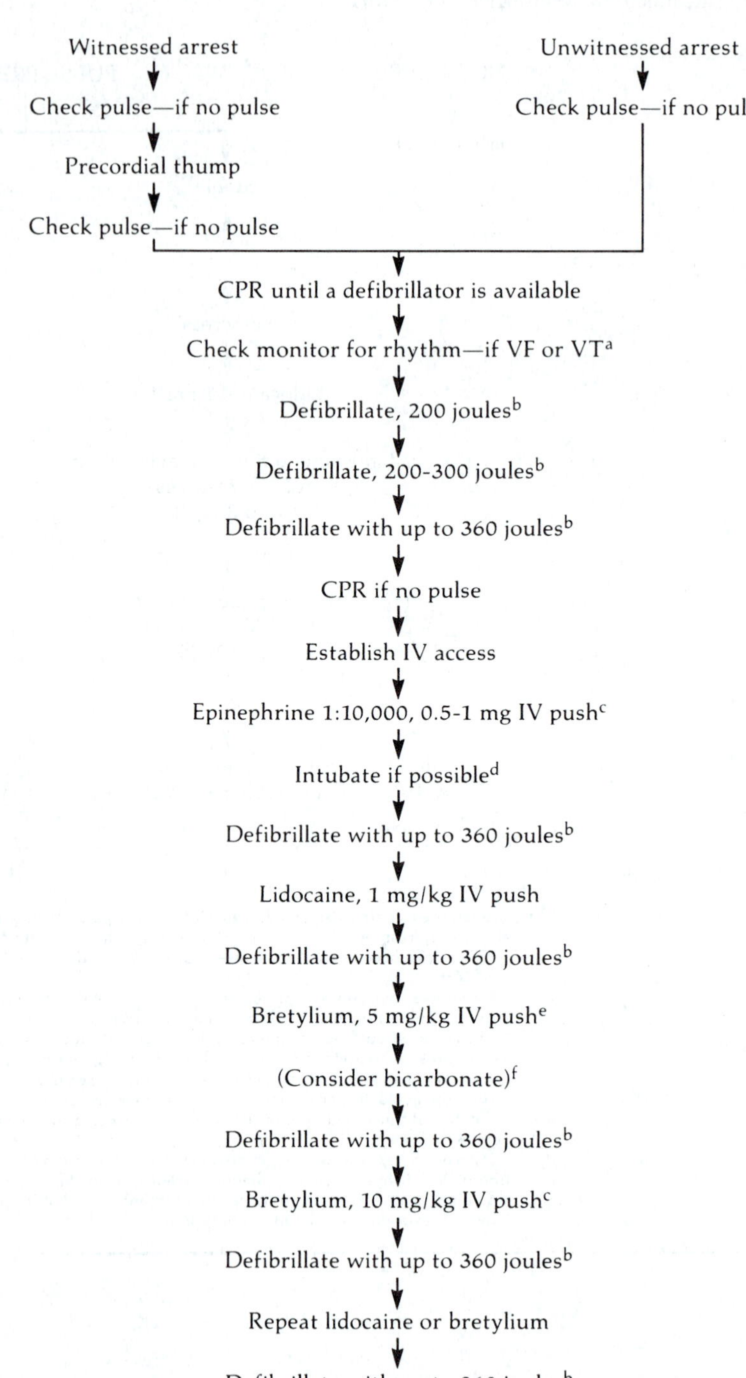

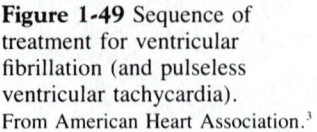

Figure 1-49 Sequence of treatment for ventricular fibrillation (and pulseless ventricular tachycardia). From American Heart Association.[3]

..—Ventricular fibrillation (and pulseless ventricular tachycardia). Some patients may require care not specified herein. Flow of algorithm presumes that VF is continuing. CPR indicates cardiopulmonary resuscitation.

[a]Pulseless VT should be treated identically to VF.

[b]Check pulse and rhythm after each shock. If VF recurs after transiently converting (rather than persists without ever converting), use whatever energy level has previously been successful for defibrillation.

[c]Epinephrine should be repeated every five minutes.

[d]Intubation is preferable. If it can be accomplished simultaneously with other techniques, then the earlier the better. However, defibrillation and epinephrine are more important initially if the patient can be ventilated without intubation.

[e]Some may prefer repeated doses of lidocaine, which may be given in 0.5-mg/kg boluses every eight minutes to a total dose of 3 mg/kg.

[f]Value of sodium bicarbonate is questionable during cardiac arrest and it is not recommended for routine cardiac arrest sequence. Consideration of its use in a dose of 1 mEq/kg is appropriate at this point. Half of original dose may be repeated every ten minutes if it is used.

Nursing Dx & Intervention

Nursing Diagnosis	Nursing Intervention/Rationale
Impaired skin integrity	• Inspect surface area where electrode paddles were placed, noting early signs of redness and burn. • Wash area of electrode paddle placement with water, and apply lanolin-based lotions as indicated.
Decreased cardiac output (actual and potential)	• Assess level of consciousness and monitor blood pressure, apical and peripheral pulses, and respirations every 5 to 10 minutes following procedure to establish hemodynamic stability. • Monitor ECG every 2 to 4 hours as ordered following procedure to determine electromechanical stability. Compare with previous tracings. • Initiate hemodynamic monitoring as ordered. Refer to p. 49 for management of patient in cardiogenic shock.

Evaluation

Patient Outcome	Data Indicating That Outcome is Reached
Sinus rhythm is reestablished.	ECG monitor shows normal sinus rhythm. Pulse rate is regular.

Hemodynamic Monitoring

Description and Rationale

Monitoring to assess a patient's circulatory status may be done by indirect (noninvasive) or direct (invasive) methods. Indirect methods include arterial pressure monitoring by sphygmomanometer and stethoscope, heart rate monitoring by chest electrode placement, and cardiac monitoring. Direct methods are indicated by the term "hemodynamic monitoring."

Hemodynamic monitoring is a technique that permits close examination of cardiac function in acutely ill patients. Used primarily in critical care units, hemodynamic monitoring permits rapid identification of complications of myocardial infarction, guides the diagnosis and management of patients with low cardiac output, and helps to differentiate pulmonary disease from left ventricular failure.[41]

With use of a balloon-tipped, flow-directed catheter to provide continuous monitoring of the pulmonary artery pressure and pulmonary capillary wedge pressure, myocardial function can be evaluated in terms of preload, afterload, and contractility. From these parameters the left ventricular end-diastolic pressure (LVEDP) can be estimated. Other possible measurements include cardiac output by the thermodilution method and sampling of arteriovenous oxygen differences. Hemodynamic monitoring also provides a direct means of assessing the patient's progress and response to fluid and drug management and permits careful titration of specific therapies.[101]

Pulmonary artery pressure and pulmonary capillary wedge pressure. Although the LVEDP is the major determinant of left ventricular function, it cannot be measured at the bedside. However, the LVEDP can be reflected by the pressure in the pulmonary capillaries and by the pulmonary artery pressure (PAP) at the end of diastole. The catheter, which is introduced via the subclavian vein or by cutdown, is passed through the right side of the heart into the pulmonary artery (Figure 1-50). There the balloon is inflated, occluding the artery. With the balloon inflated, the catheter is wedged in a distal branch of the capillaries (Figure 1-50). The pressure recorded reflects left atrial pressure, which corresponds to the LVEDP and is called the pulmonary capillary wedge pressure (PCWP).

Intra-arterial pressure (arterial line). Direct continuous monitoring of systemic arterial pressure is made possible by placement of an indwelling catheter, connected to a transducer and monitor, into a major artery. Central artery pressures, although more accurate, are used less frequently. The radial artery is the most common site for placement. The line also facilitates obtaining blood samples to measure arterial blood gases.

Cardiac output. The cardiac output, the volume of blood the heart pumps per minute, can be measured using a calibrated thermistor located near the tip of the pressure catheter. Based on the Fick principle, a thermodilution technique using blood temperature changes is used to produce cardiac output determinations. A known volume of solution is injected at a specific rate into the right atrium via the proximal port of a three- or four-lumen pulmonary pressure catheter. Although the standard practice has been to use an iced solution, studies now show that room temperature injectate produces the same results.[94] The temperature-sensitive thermistor records the temperature of the blood as it passes through the catheter. The difference in temperature between the iced injectate and the blood is calculated, and the cardiac output is then digitally displayed by a special computer.

Contraindications and Cautions

Patients with left bundle-branch block should be observed for development of right bundle-branch block during insertion and while the flotation catheter is in place. Insertion of the flotation catheter in a patient with right-sided endocarditis

Figure 1-50 Balloon-tipped flow-directed catheter.
A, Placement of flow-directed catheter via superior vena cava.
B, Balloon inflated and wedged in pulmonary artery.
From Tucker.[104]

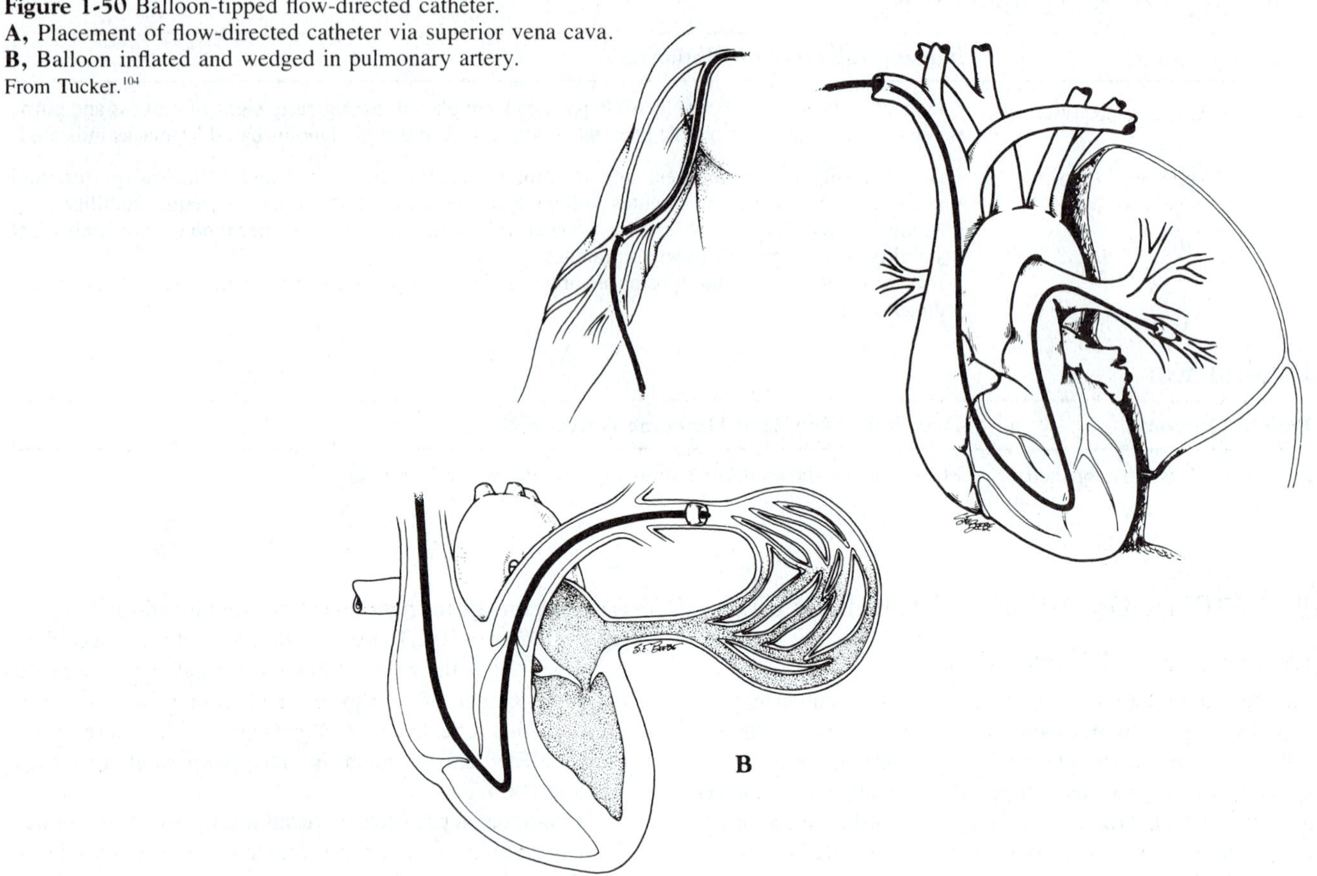

may cause dislodgment of septic emboli to the lung. Use of the radial artery for monitoring is contraindicated in the presence of inadequate circulation. Relative contraindications include severe bleeding disorders and severe immunosuppression.

Preprocedural Care

1. Pulmonary pressure catheters can be inserted at the bedside, or the patient may be transferred to a special procedure room for insertion under fluoroscopy. Intra-arterial lines are inserted at the bedside using sterile technique.
2. Explain the purpose, risks involved, and techniques of insertion.
3. Obtain written, informed consent.
4. Measure blood pressure, pulse, and respiration. If the cardiac output is to be measured, take the patient's temperature.
5. Connect the patient to a cardiac monitor, obtain a baseline rhythm strip.
6. Place the patient in a supine or slight Trendelenburg position.
7. Assemble the necessary equipment and supplies according to routine hospital policies:
   - Monitoring equipment
     - Pressure catheter with flush solution, related closed tubing, stopcocks, and a low-flush pressurized system
     - Transducer with oscilloscope
   - Insertion equipment
     - Local anesthetic
     - Skin preparation solution
     - Sterile gloves
     - Dressing supplies
8. Calibration of the pressure system is recommended to ensure accuracy of measurements, and to avoid spurious readings resulting from temperature changes, or changes in transducer level. Calibrate the pressure monitor according to the manufacturer's directions; for PAP readings, calibrate the transducer to the level of the right atrium.

Medical Plan

Surgery

Pulmonary pressure catheter (balloon flotation)—inserted via jugular, subclavian, brachial, or right femoral vein by cutdown or percutaneous puncture under local anesthesia

Arterial catheter—inserted via radial, brachial, or femoral artery by percutaneous method

Medications

Flushing system—continuous microdrip of heparinized solution (5% dextrose), kept in closed system under pressure greater than patient's systolic pressure (usually 300 mm Hg) by pressurized bag

General Management

Continuous ECG monitoring

Monitoring and recording of pressures every 1 to 2 hours or as ordered

Calibration of transducer and monitoring every 4 to 8 hours or as specified by manufacturer

Maintaining patency of catheters with continuous pressurized flushing device

Normal Ranges of Hemodynamic Parameters

Right atrial pressure	2-6 mm Hg (mean pressure)
Right ventricular pressure	Systolic: 20-30 mm Hg Diastolic: 0-5 mm Hg End-diastolic: 2-6 mm Hg
Pulmonary artery pressure (PAP)	Systolic: 20-30 mm Hg End-diastolic: 8-12 mm Hg Mean: 10-20 mm Hg
Pulmonary arterial wedge pressure (PAWP)	4-12 mm Hg (mean pressure)
Arterial pressure (intra-arterial)	Peak systolic: 100-140 mm Hg End-diastolic: 60-80 mm Hg Mean: 70-90 mm Hg
Cardiac output (CO)	4-8 L/min
Cardiac index (CO/body surface area)	2.5-4 L/min
Systemic vascular resistance (SVR)	800-1200 dynes/sec/cm^5
Pulmonary vascular resistance (PVR)	37-250 dynes/sec/cm^5

Table 1-4
Problems Observed in Pressure Waveforms

Observation	Etiologic Factors	Interventions
Loss of waveform on oscilloscope	Displacement of catheter	Reposition patient: notify physician
Loss of PAP; PCWP is displayed on monitor	Self-wedging	Instruct patient to cough Obtain x-ray examination
Loss of PWP	Displaced into PAP; balloon rupture	Use diastolic of PAP
Decreased amplitude of waveform (damped waveform)	Damping due to	
	Clot in catheter tip	Flush lines: *Do not force if resistance is met*
	Air bubbles	Check all connections for air leaks: flush air bubbles
	Kinking of catheter	Notify physician
	Occluded catheter	Reposition patient; have patient cough
	Tip against artery wall	
Loss of PCWP; no resistance with inflation	Rupture of balloon	Seal off balloon lumen: *Do not allow any injection of air*
Air bubbles in pressure lines Damping of waveform Inaccurate reading	Air leak in system	Check that all connections are secure
Artifacts and inadequate pressure readings	Respiratory interference from handling of pressure equipment during readings	Record pressure at end exhalation using printed waveform
	Inaccurate calibration of equipment	Check for possible interference with tubing during readings
	Faulty equipment	Check electrical system for grounding Check calibration of and level to RA of transducer Check all equipment for proper functioning

From Tucker.[104]

NURSING CARE

Nursing Assessment

Pulmonary Artery Pressure Catheters (Table 1-4)

Pneumothorax and arrhythmias during insertion; pulmonary and air embolism; pulmonary infarction; pulmonary perforation; sepsis or infection; thrombophlebitis at insertion site

Arterial Lines

Hemorrhage; clot formation; diminished or absent pulse distal to insertion site; hematoma at insertion site; infection

Nursing Dx & Intervention

Nursing Diagnosis	Nursing Intervention/Rationale
Impaired gas exchange (potential) related to embolization of thrombus from catheter migration or wedging	• Observe for signs of pneumothorax and pulmonary air embolism: chest pain, dyspnea, hemoptysis, tachypnea. • Observe for and prevent balloon rupture: Inflate balloon for few seconds only. Ensure balloon is deflated following wedge pressure measurement. Observe waveform for signs of self-wedge or damped tracing. Secure and label catheter and injection ports to avoid confusion of lines. • Obtain chest roentgenogram in first 12 hours or as ordered and check for catheter placement. • Auscultate chest sounds every 4 hours to assess for signs of diminished or adventitious sounds. • Monitor arterial blood gases as ordered to identify fall in arterial Po_2 or increase in Pco_2. • Administer oxygen therapy as ordered. • Check patency of lines, tubes, and connections. Never use force to flush or irrigate a line that is resistant.
Potential for infection related to contamination	• Observe for signs of local inflammation or infection. • Take measures to prevent infection: Maintain aseptic technique during insertion. Change flushing solution and tubing to catheter every day. Change dressing every day, cleaning insertion site with antiseptic agents. Observe for signs of local inflammation or infection.
Anxiety	• Provide continuous explanation of procedure. • Offer frequent reassurance, encouraging verbalization and questions regarding progress. • Allow family and significant others to visit patient when feasible.
Decreased cardiac output (potential) related to arrhythmias	• Observe and monitor ECG rhythm for ventricular arrhythmias (premature ventricular contractions, ventricular tachycardia) during and after insertion. • Keep lidocaine available at bedside during insertion. • Monitor vital signs every 30 to 60 minutes as ordered.

Patient Education

1. Instruct the patient and family in the purpose of the procedure, as cited in preprocedural care.
2. Instruct the patient not to move the insertion area.

Evaluation

Patient Outcome	Data Indicating That Outcome is Reached
Pressure lines are patent.	Waveform is normal.
There is no infection.	Patient is afebrile.
Anxiety is reduced.	Patient verbalizes absence of anxiety or decrease in anxiety level.
Lung aeration and perfusion are normal.	Lung sounds are clear to bases. There is bilateral aeration. Chest roentgenogram is normal.

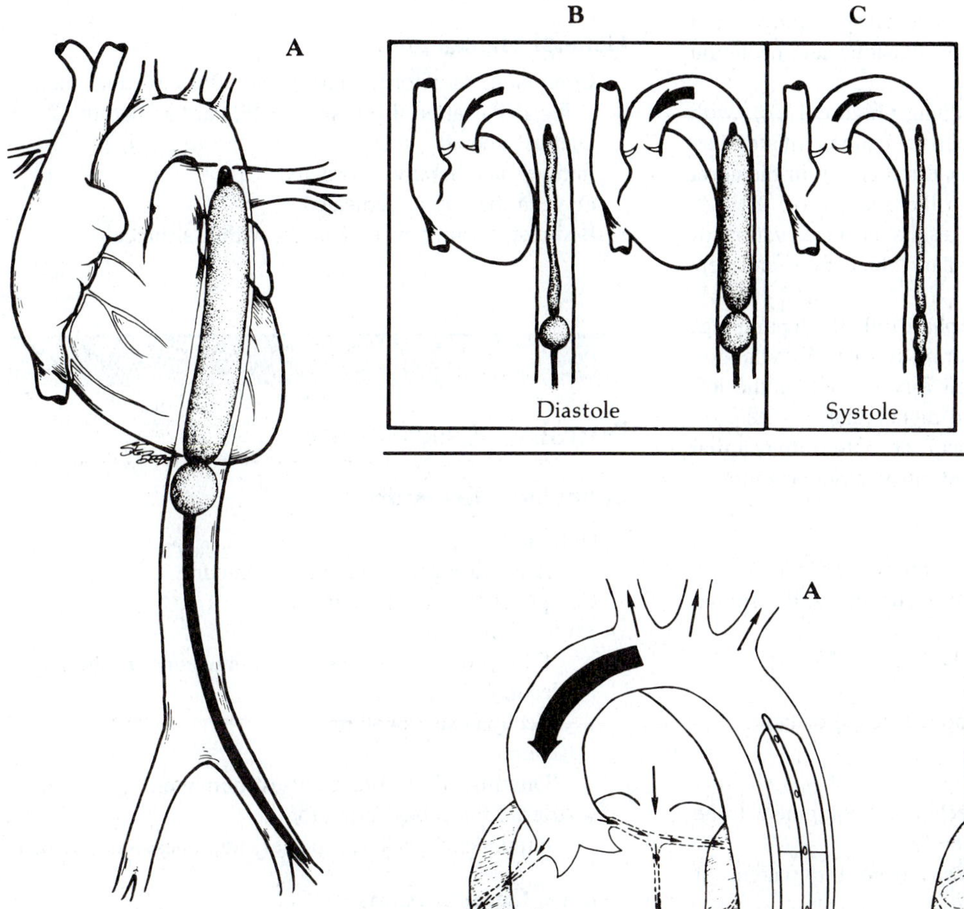

Figure 1-51 Intra-aortic balloon. **A,** Position of balloon catheter. **B,** During inflation (diastole). **C,** During deflation (systole).
From Tucker.[104]

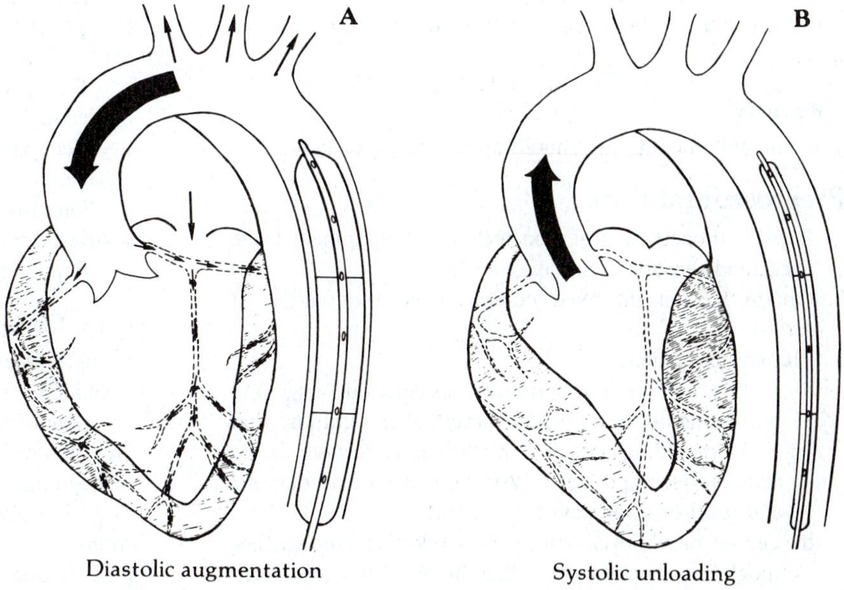

Figure 1-52 Two phases of balloon pumping. **A,** Balloon inflation occurs from closure of aortic valve to end of diastole. Inflation causes retrograde flow of blood in aorta, increasing coronary perfusion pressure without increasing myocardial work or oxygen demand. Inflation also causes antegrade flow, increasing mean arterial pressure, renal flow, and cerebral flow. **B,** Balloon deflation occurs from just before opening of aortic valve to closure of aortic valve. Deflation encourages antegrade flow, decreasing afterload or resistance to left ventricular ejection. Deflation also decreases oxygen required by left ventricle, shortens systolic ejection, and increases stroke volume.
From Michaelson.[68]

Intra-Aortic Balloon Pumping

Description and Rationale

An intra-aortic balloon pump (IABP) is a mechanical device that provides circulatory assistance to the failing myocardium. Using the principles of counterpulsation, the balloon inflates with diastole and inflates during systole.

A sausage-shaped balloon is inserted through the common femoral artery and passed upward into the aorta. It lies in the descending aorta just distal to the left subclavian artery (Figure 1-51). Externally the catheter is connected to a power console that has ECG input. Helium or carbon dioxide gas is used to inflate the balloon.

The IABP is used in the treatment of cardiogenic shock in low-cardiac output states, following cardiopulmonary bypass, in drug-resistant arrhythmias caused by ischemia, and in unstable angina. The effect of counterpulsation on left ventricular function is produced by diastolic augmentation and afterload reduction.

The first phase of balloon pumping (Figure 1-52), with diastolic augmentations, occurs when the balloon inflates during diastole. This displaces the blood remaining in the aorta after ventricular ejection back into the aortic root. The increased blood in the aortic root results in an elevation of diastolic pressure, increasing coronary blood flow and perfusion.

Afterload reduction, the second phase of balloon pumping, occurs when the balloon deflates during systole. With balloon deflation blood flow is encouraged forward out of the left ventricle. This produces decreased myocardial wall tension during diastole (decreased resistance), decreased myocardial oxygen consumption, and improved left ventricular output.

Contraindications

Contraindications to IABP include severe aortic regurgitation, aortic dissection, abdominal aortic aneurysm, and terminal illness.

Cautions

The cannulated extremity should not be flexed or bent.

Preprocedural Care

1. Explain procedure, insertion technique, equipment to be used, and sensations that may be felt.
2. Obtain written informed consent from the patient or family.
3. Prepare the patient:
   a. Assess and record peripheral circulation, checking pulses and noting color and warmth of extremities; vital signs, including heart and breath sounds; hemodynamic status (arterial pressure, PAP, PCWP, cardiac output); and level of awareness (mentation).
   b. Obtain baseline laboratory data (clotting studies, hemoglobin, hematocrit, white blood cell count, and platelets).
   c. Obtain baseline ECG rate and rhythm.
   d. Prepare groin area.

Medical Plan

Medications

Local anesthetic agents
Lidocaine (Xylocaine)

General Management

Continuous monitoring during and after insertion, including ECG, arterial pressure, PAP, cardiac output
Diet as ordered
Intravenous therapy as ordered
Oxygen therapy as indicated
Bed rest; turning every 2 hours with assistance

NURSING CARE

Nursing Assessment

Cannulated Extremity

- Normal
  - Decreased pulse volume and contour
- Complications at insertion site
  - Infection
    - Fever, local tenderness, swelling, purulent drainage
  - Bleeding, hematoma
    - Ecchymosis, swelling
  - Ischemia
    - Diminished or absent pulses, numbness, pallor, pain
  - Arterial thrombus formation
    - Diminished or absent pulses, numbness, pallor, pain

General Complications

- Aortic dissection, perforation
  - Sudden, severe, sharp pain in abdomen and back; hypotension; tachycardia; decreased hematocrit value
- Thrombocytopenia
  - Bleeding; decreased platelet count (fewer than 150,000/ml)
- Progressive myocardial failure
  - Decreased cardiac output, arterial pressure, and urine output; increased PCWP; rales, rhonchi
- Arrhythmias
  - Ventricular ectopy: pulmonary ventricular contractions and ventricular tachycardia; atrial fibrillation

Machine Console and Equipment

- Balloon synchronization
  - Inflation (augmentation) at dicrotic notch of aortic waveform; deflation at end of diastole
- Complications
  - Catheter kinking; malposition; balloon rupture

Nursing Dx & Intervention

Nursing Diagnosis	Nursing Intervention/Rationale
Altered peripheral tissue perfusion (potential)	• Assess skin color, temperature, and pulses, which are indicators of peripheral tissue perfusion. • Monitor peripheral extremities for decreased perfusion every 1 to 2 hours. • Provide protection to cannulated extremity with sheepskin, lamb's wool, or foot cradle. • Perform passive range of motion exercises every 4 hours. • Avoid bending extremity. • Check dressings every hour.
Decreased cardiac output (potential)	• Monitor arterial pressure, PAP, and PCWP every hour. • Assess cardiac output as ordered. • Monitor ECG rhythm every hour.
Altered cerebral, renal, and pulmonary tissue perfusion (potential)	• Assess level of consciousness. • Auscultate breath sounds. • Monitor arterial blood gases as ordered. • Maintain oxygen therapy as ordered. • Measure intake and output every hour. • Ensure that ordered chest roentgenogram is obtained.
Impaired skin integrity	• Assess for skin breakdown and decubitus formation. • Turn and position every 2 hours. • Provide skin care every 2 to 4 hours.
Anxiety	• Provide continued explanation of procedure and treatments. • Offer frequent reassurance, encouraging verbalization and questions regarding progress. • Allow family and significant others to visit patient when feasible.

Evaluation

Patient Outcome	Data Indicating That Outcome is Reached
Perfusion of cannulated extremity is adequate.	Extremity is warm. Capillary filling time is normal. Pulses are palpable. Color is normal. Mobility of extremity is normal.
Myocardial function is restored.	Arterial pressure, cardiac output, and PCWP are within normal limits. Urine output is restored to normal. Lungs are clear. S_3 and S_4 are absent.

Pacemakers

Description and Rationale

Pacemakers are battery-operated generators that initiate and control the heart rate by delivering an electrical impulse via an electrode to the myocardium. Implantation of myocardial electrodes is initiated when a patient has symptomatic atrioventricular block. However, since the development of pacemakers in 1960, their use has expanded to include treatment of symptomatic brachyarrhythmias from other causes and refractory tachyarrhythmias.

Pacemaker implantation may be performed for temporary or long-term pacing. Temporary cardiac pacing is most commonly used for hemodynamic or life support purposes. The therapeutic indications include prophylactic pacing for complete heart block, symptomatic bradyarrhythmias, particularly in the setting of acute myocardial infarction,[66] and as an emergency measure for malfunction of an implanted permanent pacemaker. In addition to control of heart rate, temporary pacing is often used in the electrophysiologic laboratory to evaluate cardiac arrhythmias and to interrupt tachycardias.

Permanent cardiac pacing is indicated in the presence of symptomatic bradyarrhythmias.

Based on a universal code, pacemakers are described using a three-letter designation for the mode of pacing and the chambers to be sensed and paced.[66] The first letter describes the chamber that will be paced: the atrium (A), ventricle (V), or both (dual) chambers (D). The second letter represents the chamber that will be sensed: atrium (A), ventricle (V), dual (D), or none (O). The third letter reflects the mode that will be used: triggered (T), inhibited (I), or both (D). For example:

VVI

V The pacemaker will pace the ventricle.

V The pacemaker will sense the ventricle.

I The pacemaker will inhibit pacing when the patient's own impulse is sensed.

There are three types of pacemakers:

Asynchronous or fixed rate, in which rate and rhythm of pacemaker beats are unaffected by spontaneous beats

Demand pacing or standby pacing, which discharges (fires) only when spontaneous beats drop below a preset minimum rate

Synchronous pacemakers, in which a sensing circuit is used to detect atrial and ventricular activity

Contraindications

Pacemaker implantation is contraindicated for patients with active infections. Potential contraindications include the presence of atrial fibrillation or any poorly controlled supraventricular tachycardia.

Cautions

Safety from electrical hazards should be ensured.

Preprocedural Care

1. Initiate preoperative instruction for the patient and family, including purpose and indications for pacemaker implantation, benefits and associated risks, information regarding method of insertion, type and mode of pacemaker to be used, and postoperative care including need for routine 24-hour ECG monitoring and need to restrict activities for 4 to 6 hours.
2. Obtain written informed consent.
3. Perform skin preparation.
4. Obtain baseline assessment data: underlying ECG rhythm, heart rate, pulse, respirations, blood pressure, and level of consciousness.
5. Permit nothing by mouth (NPO) 6 to 8 hours before procedure.
6. Initiate intravenous line.
7. Check functioning of external generator (for a temporary unit).

Medical Plan

Surgery

Method of implantation depends on whether pacing will be temporary or permanent

Temporary

Transvenous approach—most common technique for temporary pacing; catheter electrode is passed into right ventricle via peripheral vein (brachial, femoral, subclavian, or internal jugular); electrode is connected to external pulse generator that can be set manually for direct or demand pacing mode (Figure 1-53)

Transthoracic approach—used primarily after open heart surgery; catheter is passed directly into heart through chest wall

Permanent

Transvenous pacing—catheter electrode is passed into right ventricle and attached to small, sealed, battery-operated pulse generator that is planted subcutaneously in shoulder or upper left quadrant (Figure 1-54)

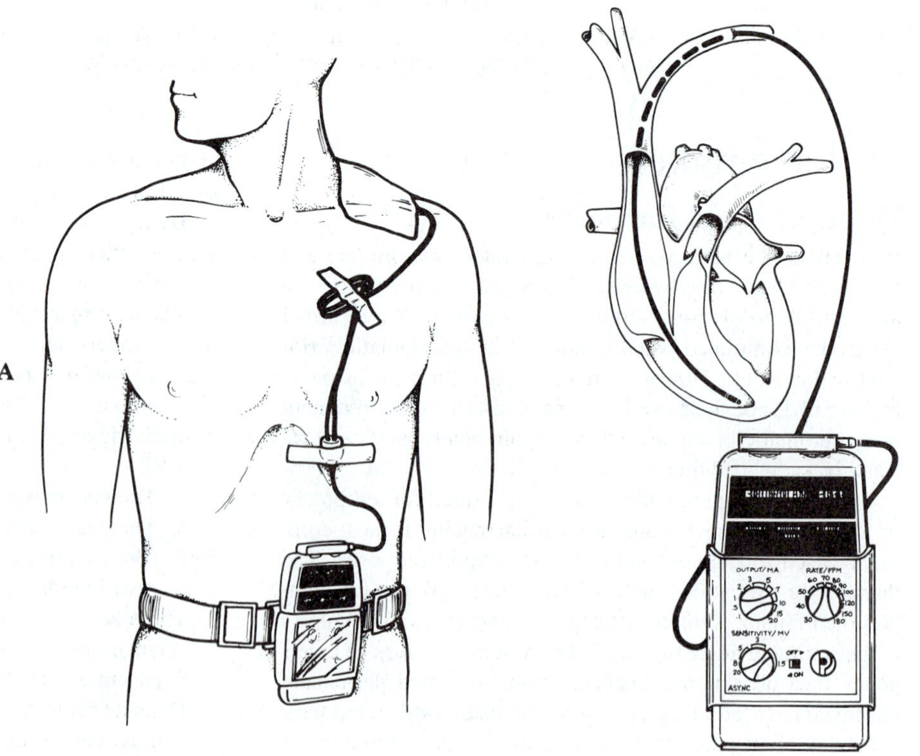

Figure 1-53 A, Temporary external pacemaker. **B,** Temporary pacemaker unit, transvenous approach.
From Tucker.[104]

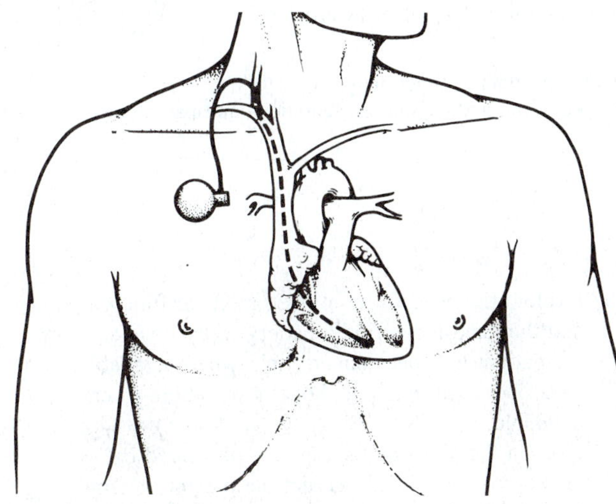

Figure 1-54 Permanent pacemaker.
From Tucker.[104]

Epicardial pacing—performed less frequently; electrode is sutured to epicardial surface of right ventricle; procedure requires a thoracotomy

Medications

Preoperative
- Mild sedation, tranquilizers

Intraoperative
- Local anesthesia, used for temporary and long-term transvenous pacing
- General anesthesia, used for transthoracic approach

General Management

Cardiac monitoring—ECG pattern observed for rate, pacemaker response, signs of pacemaker failure, and arrhythmias

Pacemaker unit
- Pulse generator—self-contained device consisting of electronic circuit and power source of lithium batteries; device is hermetically sealed for protection from biologic environment; lithium-powered pacemakers can last 5 to 8 years before battery change is required
- Pacing leads—pulse generators use either unipolar or bipolar leads, and most generators are programmable to both; with unipolar leads, electrode (negative terminal) is at distal tip of catheter touching endocardium or myocardium; with bipolar lead two electrodes are located at distal tip of catheter; current flows from pulse generator through distal electrodes into heart, where it stimulates myocardial contraction

Bed rest for 8 hours after implantation, keeping arm below level of shoulder

Range of motion exercises to affected extremity when ordered after third postoperative day

NURSING CARE

Nursing Assessment

Pacemaker Failure

Clinical symptoms
- Syncope, hypotension, bradycardia, pallor, shortness of breath, chest muscle spasm, hiccoughs

ECG rhythm
- Loss of pacemaker artifact, change in paced QRS complex, decreased amplitude of pacemaker artifact, competition between patient's underlying rhythm and paced beats, arrhythmias

Infection at Incision Site

Redness, swelling, heat, fluid collection and drainage, skin breakdown, soreness

Arrhythmias

Premature ventricular beats, ventricular tachycardia, patient complaints of palpitations

Nursing Dx & Intervention

Nursing Diagnosis	Nursing Intervention/Rationale
Anxiety related to perceived and/or actual change in health status, role functioning	• Assess level of anxiety, level of understanding, and fears associated with pacemaker implantation. • Provide explanation and rationale for pacemaker, gauging the patient's reactions. • Anticipate and allow the patient's questions regarding changes in life-style, cautions, and concerns over pacemaker management.
Decreased cardiac output (potential) related to electrical alterations in rate, rhythm, and conduction	• Assess the patient and pacemaker unit for signs of low cardiac output that is *reflective of pacemaker failure:* decreased blood pressure, pulse rate less than 60 beats per minute, lightheadedness, decreased amplitude of pulse, cool pale skin. • Monitor vital signs every 4 hours after insertion. • Monitor ECG rhythm strip every 4 hours for 24 hours after insertion. • Discourage use of nicotine, which causes vasoconstriction and reduces oxygen availability.

Nursing Diagnosis	Nursing Intervention/Rationale
Pain	• Assess quality and source of pain. • Administer pain medication as ordered. • Encourage range of motion exercises to affected shoulder as ordered.
Knowledge deficit	• Assess level of knowledge. • Correct any misconceptions regarding pacemaker function. • Initiate patient education program, providing audiovisual presentations and pamphlets. • Provide follow-up.

Patient Education

1. Instruct the patient and family about the purpose, rationale, and basic function of the permanent pacemaker.
2. Describe the type of pacemaker and the pacemaker's set rate. Instruct the patient on pulse rate and rhythm checking, emphasizing that pulse rate monitoring in lithium pacemakers needs to be done once a week or when symptoms occur.
3. Describe the signs and symptoms of pacemaker failure, including dizziness, weakness, lightheadedness, and drop in pacemaker's set rate. Discuss actions to take if pacemaker malfunction is suspected, including calling for a pacemaker check via transtelephonic monitoring and notifying the physician or pacemaker clinic.
4. Describe activity allowances and limitations. Tell the patient to avoid traveling and driving for first 4 weeks after insertion. Encourage the patient to resume normal daily activities and recreational interests, except competitive contact sports, which can increase the risk of lead dislodgment.
5. Discuss the need to avoid and protect against hazards from high-output electrical generators such as diathermy motors, welding equipment, and radar. Most household electrical devices (such as microwave ovens and blow dryers) are considered safe, but review symptoms that may reflect electromagnetic interference and the action to take if symptoms occur.
6. Explain the need for continued medical follow-up and the need for periodic battery replacements; refer the patient to a pacemaker clinic where available.
7. Describe the use of telephone transmitters where available.
8. Explain the signs and symptoms of wound or pocket infection, and instruct the patient or family to report to the physician if fever or drainage develops.
9. Instruct the patient in the need to protect the pacemaker site: avoid constricting clothing and direct contact or blows to the site; contact sports are usually contraindicated.
10. Explain the need to carry an identification card.
11. Reassure a female patient in her reproductive years that pregnancy is not contraindicated. Tell her to inform her physician of the desired pregnancy before conception so the pacemaker program can be checked and adapted to rate changes commonly associated with pregnancy.

Evaluation

Patient Outcome	Data Indicating That Outcome is Reached
Pacemaker functions properly.	Patient is normotensive and without dizziness, syncope, palpitations, chest pain, shortness of breath, or fatigue. Heart rate is acceptable. A temporary pacemaker fires at preset rate, sensing mechanism is visualized, and pacemaker artifact is visualized on ECG. A permanent pacemaker fires at preset rate, and pacemaker artifact is visualized on ECG.
Patient is free of infection and pain.	Patient is afebrile. Incisional site is clean with no swelling or redness. Patient verbalizes comfort.
Anxiety level is reduced.	Patient demonstrates reduced anxiety level and appears relaxed and less tense. Patient verbalizes feeling less fearful and asks appropriate questions.

Percutaneous Transluminal Coronary Angioplasty

Description and Rationale

Percutaneous transluminal coronary angioplasty (PTCA) is an invasive, nonsurgical, therapeutic procedure that restores arterial luminal patency, thereby relieving myocardial ischemia by compressing atheromatous plaques. PTCA has evolved over the past decade as an extension of peripheral balloon angioplasty. Intracoronary transluminal dilatation, first developed by Andreas Gruntzig in 1977, was at first used only on a highly selected population of patients with stable angina and discrete proximal noncalcified lesions of the coronary arteries. Since then, because of advances and modifications of the percutaneous catheter, the selection criteria of candidates for angioplasty has also widened. Current patient selection criteria focus on accessibility of the lesion, its compressibility, and whether there is single- or multi-vessel disease. The current recommendations from the National Heart, Lung, and Blood Institute PTCA registry[53] include the following guidelines:

Stable angina with symptoms refractory to medical therapy; single-vessel coronary stenosis

Objective evidence of myocardial ischemia by exercise treadmill, thallium scintigraphy with exercise, or gated blood pool studies

Lesions that are proximal, discrete, concentric, and noncalcified

The procedure, which is technically similar to a standard cardiac catheterization, involves passing a balloon-tipped catheter into a stenosed coronary artery where the balloon is then inflated and deflated using a hand-held syringe or pressure-controlled device. Successful dilatation is usually accompanied by reduction in the systolic gradient across the stenosis; however, the gradient may not be abolished and the inflation-deflation cycle may have to be repeated several times until the past-angioplasty arteriogram demonstrates improved luminal diameter. Successful PTCA is defined as an increase of at least 20% in lumen size. Currently, primary success rates are being achieved in 85% to 90% of patients undergoing PTCA. Symptomatic relief is being achieved in 80%, and long-term follow-up shows continued lumen patency and symptomatic improvement from 6 months to 2 years.[54]

The angioplasty procedure involves using a two-catheter system. First a guiding sheath is introduced percutaneously via the femoral or brachial artery cutdown. Once the guiding catheter is at the orifice of the stenosed coronary artery, a second double-lumen dilation catheter is inserted and advanced under fluoroscopy until the balloon straddles the lesion. Pressure is applied at 5 to 15 atmospheres for 4 to 5 seconds at a time. After angioplasty, the deflation catheter is removed, leaving the sheath in place.

Arteriograms are performed before and after the procedure, using the guiding catheter in the angiographic catheter. This allows evaluation of the results and decisions regarding the need for further dilation.

Contraindications

1. Left main coronary artery disease
2. Coronary artery spasm

Preprocedural Care

1. Initiate preprocedural instruction for patient and family.
2. Obtain written informed consent for PTCA. Be aware that consent must include consent for emergency CABG, which has been reported to occur in 2% of cases.[101] Operating room and cardiothoracic team must be on standby throughout procedure.
3. Obtain baseline data for PTCA and CABG: complete blood count; coagulation studies; electrolyte, BUN, and creatinine levels; blood type and cross-match; ECG; chest roentgenogram; vital signs.
4. Perform skin preparation of both right and left groin areas.
5. Permit nothing by mouth (NPO) for at least 8 hours before procedure.
6. Establish a patent intravenous line.
7. Administer medications as ordered.
8. Administer preoperative sedatives as ordered.

Medical Plan

Medications

- Before procedure
  - Antiplatelet agents: aspirin, 325 mg bid; dipyridamole 75 mg tid 48 h before procedure to decrease risk of platelet adhesion, which is thought to be cause of early restenosis after procedure[101]
  - Diphenhydramine to reduce risk of allergic reaction
  - Nitrates, calcium channel blockers to reduce risk of coronary artery spasm
  - Beta-blockers are held
- During procedure
  - Heparin infusion, 10,000 U by continuous drip
  - Intracoronary nitroglycerin (100-300 mg) and/or sublingual nifedipine (10 mg) to prevent coronary artery spasm as catheter is introduced
  - Thrombolytic agents as necessary (see p. 115)
- After procedure
  - Immediate
    - Heparin infusion (800-1200 U/h); tapered doses for 12-24 h to prevent coronary thrombosis from possible intimal tear
  - Long-term
    - Aspirin po for 6 mo; dosage will vary: 60 mg/d (baby aspirin); 325 mg po qd or bid
    - Nitrates and calcium channel blockers resumed while patient is in hospital and continued for 3-6 mo; dosage varies
    - Dipyridamole 75 mg po tid for 3 mo

General Management

Cardiac monitoring—ECG pattern observed for rate, dysrhythmias, signs of ischemia

Intra-arterial blood pressure—observed during and after procedure

Intra-aortic balloon pump—must be available on standby during procedure

Bed rest for first 6 hours after successful angioplasty following removal of catheters and until hemostasis has been reestablished

Laboratory studies: careful monitoring of partial thromboplastin time (PTT) and hemoglobin (Hgb), creatinine phosphokinase (CPK), potassium, and sodium levels

NURSING CARE

Nursing Assessment

Complications Related to Procedure

- Failure to dilate artery
- Development of acute thrombosis or occlusion
- Myocardial infarction
- Coronary artery rupture
- Clinical symptoms
  - Chest pain, ST depression or elevation, drop in blood pressure, tachycardia, dysrhythmias

Hemorrhage Related to Prolonged PTT; Drop in Hgb

Cannulated Extremity

- Complications at insertion site
  - Bleeding, hematoma
    - Ecchymosis, swelling
  - Ischemia
    - Diminished or absent pulses, numbness, pallor, pain
  - Arterial thrombosis formation
    - Diminished or absent pulses, numbness, pain, swelling, pale skin
    - See p. 1588 for other complications associated with catheterization

Nursing Dx & Intervention

Nursing Diagnosis	Nursing Intervention/Rationale
Anxiety (preoperative) related to perceived and actual threat to biologic integrity	• Assess level of anxiety and understanding associated with procedure *to determine source of fears and any misconceptions.* • Provide explanations and description of procedure, including sensations to be experienced. • Provide an opportunity for questions. Assist the patient to explore fears and discuss feelings. • Provide the patient with an opportunity to meet the catheterization staff and visit the laboratory and postangioplasty unit.
Decreased cardiac output (potential) related to mechanical or electrical problems associated with complications	• Assess for signs of diminished cardiac output. • Monitor blood pressure, heart rate, and respirations every 15 minutes immediately after the procedure, decreasing frequency as clinical status stabilizes. Then monitor vital signs every 4 hours for 24 hours. • Monitor ECG, observing for signs of ischemia or arrhythmias. Obtain 12-lead ECG without any episode of chest pain. • Monitor urine output hourly or for every voiding if the patient is not catheterized. Report outputs of less than 30 ml per hour or inability to void within first 4 hours. • Check peripheral perfusion: pulses, skin temperature, color. • Auscultate heart sounds, noting diminished or extra sounds. • Auscultate lung sounds for presence of adventitious sounds or diminished aeration. • Administer medications as ordered: IV nitroglycerin *to decrease incidence of coronary spasm* and antiplatelet agents *to reduce risk of restenosis.*
Altered peripheral tissue perfusion (potential) related to thrombus formation	• Inspect cannulated extremity for ecchymosis, swelling, pain, and warmth *reflective of hematoma formation or bleeding.* • Assess pulses distal to the site every 15 minutes for 1 hour, noting any decrease in amplitude. Decreasing frequency as ordered. Note skin color and temperature.

Nursing Diagnosis	Nursing Intervention/Rationale
	• Maintain bed rest in flat position until arterial sheaths are removed. Instruct the patient to keep the catheterized extremity immobile and extended *to decrease risk of bleeding*. After the catheter sheaths are removed, maintain pressure dressing with 5- to 10-pound sandbags over site. • Monitor coagulation studies, reporting prolonged partial thromboplastin time or abnormal results to the physician. • Administer antiplatelet agents as ordered *to reduce risk of restenosis*.

Patient Education

Preoperative:

1. Instruct the patient and family about purpose and indications for PTCA, its benefits, and associated risk.
2. Describe the procedure, explaining that it is similar to cardiac catheterization (see p. 1588) and that it may last 2 to 5 hours. Review sensations to be experienced, such as pressure during insertion of the catheter, but explain that there is no discomfort with actual balloon inflation.
3. Explain and review postprocedure routines: that 24-hour monitoring in the coronary care unit is needed, that the affected leg must be kept immobile immediately after the procedure, that patient will remain on bed rest for up to 8 hours, and that discharge home is usually within 48 hours.
4. Explain the need for consent for CABG surgery. Provide a brief review of differences in patient care after open-heart surgery.

After procedure:

1. Reinforce explanation of procedure and postprocedure results.
2. Describe activity allowances and limitations. Explain that, unless contraindicated by postprocedure status, the patient may resume work within a week after discharge.
3. Discuss the importance of avoiding nicotine, which is associated with an increased incidence of restenosis after PTCA.
4. Discuss the need to modify and/or continue to modify coronary risk factors.
5. Discuss the importance of continued follow-up. Explain that a postexercise ECG treadmill test will be required at 2 weeks and again at 3 months after PTCA.
6. Review medications, discussing dosage, method of administration, and side effects.
7. Discuss the need to modify or continue to modify coronary risk factors.

Evaluation

Patient Outcome	Data Indicating That Outcome is Reached
Anxiety level is reduced.	Patient demonstrates reduced anxiety level. Patient appears relaxed, with decreased tension. Patient verbalizes feeling less fearful and asks appropriate questions. Patient verbalizes understanding of procedures. Misconceptions are corrected.
Cardiac output is maintained.	Patient remains normotensive. Skin is warm and dry. Patient verbalizes no chest discomfort and rests quietly. Vital signs remain stable.
Tissue perfusion is maintained.	Pulses distal to cannulation site are palpable. Extremities are warm and dry. Coagulation studies are within normal limits.

Pericardiocentesis

Description and Rationale

Pericardiocentesis (Figure 1-55) is an invasive procedure performed by inserting a needle into the pericardial space (sac) to aspirate fluid. It may be done as a diagnostic procedure for analysis of pericardial fluid or as an emergency measure to relieve cardiac compression and drain the pericardial space.

Contraindications

The procedure is contraindicated in any patient who has been taking anticoagulants or who has a bleeding disorder or thrombocytopenia.

Cautions

All equipment must be secured and properly grounded to avoid delivering current to the myocardium, which would cause ventricular fibrillation.

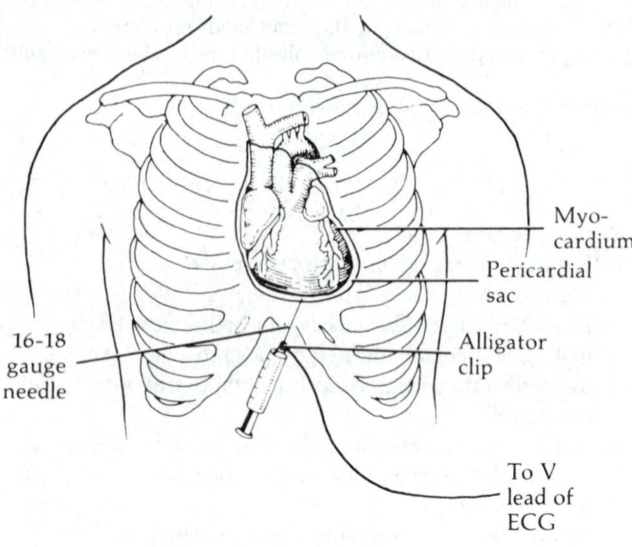

Figure 1-55 Pericardiocentesis.
From Sheehy.[93]

Complications

Complications include cardiac puncture with hemopericardium; air embolism; pneumothorax.

Preprocedural Care

1. Explain the procedure, its purpose, and associated risks to the patient and family.
2. Obtain written informed consent.
3. Initiate and maintain the intravenous line.
4. Have an emergency crash cart close by.
5. Assemble equipment:
   Pericardiocentesis tray with 50 ml syringe
   Local anesthetic agents (lidocaine) and equipment (needles, syringes)
   Percutaneous entry needle, guide wire, and catheter
   Sterile test tubes and drainage container
   Three-way stopcock
   Standard 12-lead ECG machine
   Kelly clamp
   Alligator clips
6. Perform skin preparation from the left costal margin to the xiphoid process.

Medical Plan

Surgery

Pericardial window if pericardiocentesis is unsuccessful

Medications

Tranquilizers
  Diazepam (Valium)
    Usual dosage: 5 mg IV

General Management

Cardiac monitoring during and after procedure
Oxygen therapy as ordered
Monitoring blood pressure, pulse, and respiration before and immediately after procedure

NURSING CARE

Nursing Assessment

ECG Changes

Ventricular irritation: premature ventricular contractions, ventricular tachycardia; ischemia: ST elevation

Cardiac Tamponade (Hemopericardium)

Distended neck veins; paradoxic pulse; narrowed pulse pressure; dyspnea; cyanosis; distant heart sounds

Other Complications

Air embolism; myocardial injury; shock; pneumothorax

Nursing Dx & Intervention

Nursing Diagnosis	Nursing Intervention/Rationale
Decreased cardiac output (potential)	• After procedure, monitor blood pressure, pulse, respirations, and heart sounds every 15 minutes until stable, then every 30 minutes for 2 hours, then every hour for 4 hours, then every 4 hours. • Assess for improvement of symptoms *to determine relief of cardiac compression.* • Check for pulsus paradoxus *to determine presence or absence of signs of cardiac tamponade.*
Potential for infection	• Ensure asepsis during procedure. • Check temperature every 4 hours after procedure.

Evaluation

Patient Outcome	Data Indicating That Outcome is Reached
Cardiac compression is relieved.	Pulse pressure is normal and pulsus paradoxus, if present, is less than 10 mm Hg. Symptoms of cardiac tamponade are relieved.

Thrombolytic Therapy for Acute Myocardial Infarction

(Fibrolytic therapy, acute myocardial infarction therapy)

Description and Rationale

It has long been recognized that long-term survival after myocardial infarction depends on maintaining ventricular function. However, only in the past decade have investigators actively sought interventions to retard myocardial necrosis. Thrombolytic therapy has emerged as a successful modality in the treatment of acute myocardial infarction (AMI); its use is based on studies that examined the role of coronary thrombosis as the precipitating factor of myocardial infarctions[27] and on studies that demonstrated how clot lysis and reperfusion of an infarct-related vessel can reduce infarct size and preserve myocardial function.[51,52] In the acute stage of myocardial infarction (first 6 hours), abrupt coronary occlusion in the setting of an already narrowed coronary artery is due to intracoronary thrombosis.[27] Total coronary occlusion from intraluminal thrombosis occurs in 80% to 90% of patients with transmural infarctions, and subtotal occlusion occurs in 15% to 20% of patients.[27,54]

Intracoronary infusion of thrombolytic agents, first reported by Rentrop,[84] achieves clot lysis, restores coronary blood flow, and limits myocardial ischemia. However, the extent to which thrombolytic therapy salvages myocardial function is time dependent. Kennedy and co-workers[52] found that the time from onset of clinical symptoms to initiation of intracoronary thrombolysis was the strongest predictor of achieving coronary reperfusion. It is now generally accepted that thrombolytic therapy initiated within the first 4 to 6 hours to patients with an evolving AMI can reduce in-hospital and 1-year mortality rates.

Because early intervention is critical in achieving clot lysis, intravenous administration of thrombolytic agents has more recently been advocated.[33] Its effectiveness is similar to that of intracoronary administration; each has certain advantages and disadvantages (Table 1-5).

Intracoronary thrombolysis is performed in the cardiac catheterization laboratory with selective angiography, whereas intravenous thrombolysis may be initiated in either the emergency department or the coronary care unit. In intravenous thrombolytic therapy, administration is via a peripheral vein.

Thrombolytic agents. Thrombogenesis, the result of a complex interplay of coagulation factors, begins with platelet

Table 1-5
Comparison of Intracoronary and Intravenous (Systemic) Thrombolytic Therapy of Acute Myocardial Infarction

Comparative Features	Intracoronary	Intravenous
Widespread availability	No	Yes
Delay in institution	1-2 hr frequent	None
Complexity	Yes	No
Risks of coronary catheterization	Yes	No
Risk of arterial puncture site complications	Yes	No
Risk of systemic bleeding complications	Probably less	Probably more
Cost	High	Low
Success in achieving prompt coronary thrombolysis*	75%-80%	50%-60% (75% with t-PA)
Risk of rethrombosis*	20%	20%
Time required for thrombolysis*	25-35 min	50-60 min
Doses of thrombolytic agent used*	Generally less; therefore early surgery possible	Larger—early surgery risks bleeding complications
Coronary anatomy	Known (initial and residual)	Not known or deferred to later study
Coronary angioplasty	May be first approach or may follow thrombolytic therapy	Not available
Documentation of success or failure	Yes	Not always possible

From Tilkian.[101]
*Applies to conventional agents (streptokinase, urokinase).

aggregation and adhesion. Prothrombin is then converted to thrombin, which contributes to the conversion of fibrinogen to fibrin. Fibrin stabilizes platelet aggregation, forming a hemostatic plug. The development of fibrin-specific thrombolytic agents has been the key to the dissolution of coronary thrombi. Lysis of thrombi results from two actions: invasion of the injury site by leukocytes and activation of the fibrinolytic system. Normally the fibrinolytic system, which involves plasminogen activators, converts plasminogen, a circulating proenzyme, to plasmin. Plasmin, the proteolytic enzyme responsible for clot lysis, degrades fibrin into soluble fragments that are removed in the microcirculation. This system is inadequate to dissolve the fibrin mass of a large thrombus. However, the introduction of exogenous plasminogen activators produces more plasmin, which depletes circulating fibrinogen and generates high titers of fibrinogen degradation products (FDPs), which promote lysis. Exogenous plasminogen activators also destroy coagulation factors V and VIII, causing a systemic lytic state that increases the risk of bleeding.[103,107]

Streptokinase. Streptokinase (SK, Streptase, Kabikinase), a synthetic protein, is derived from group C-hemolytic streptococci. It forms an activator complex with plasminogen to activate the fibrinolytic process.[103] In addition, SK depletes fibrinogen levels and other coagulation factors such as V and VIII, predisposing the patient to bleeding. Furthermore, since SK is a bacterial protein with antigenicity, it can lead to a variety of allergic reactions.

Urokinase. Urokinase (Abbokinase), a naturally occurring human proteolytic enzyme, is produced by the parenchymal cells of the kidney. It acts directly on circulating plasminogen to produce the fibrinolytic enzyme plasmin.

Tissue plasminogen activator. Tissue plasminogen activator (t-PA) is a naturally occurring human enzyme present in endothelium, circulating blood, and human tissue. Unlike SK and urokinase, which activate plasminogen systemically, t-PA is fibrin specific, activating plasminogen only after binding to the plasminogen bound to fibrin contained in the thrombus.[17] Thus t-PA is a clot-specific agent; since it produces relatively little circulating plasmin, it does not deplete other clotting factors, and therefore it reduces the risk of bleeding.[82,107]

Indications

1. Recent (within 30 minutes but not to exceed 4 to 6 hours) onset of chest pain unresponsive to conventional sublingual nitroglycerin therapy
2. ECG changes documenting acute myocardial injury: ST elevation greater than 0.1 mm with reciprocal changes
3. Less than 75 years of age

Contraindications

Absolute contraindications to thrombolytic therapy include bleeding disorders, acute or recent cerebrovascular events, uncontrolled hypertension (diastolic pressures at least 120 mm Hg), recent surgery or trauma, recent cardiopulmonary resuscitation (CPR), and pregnancy.[59,102] Relative contraindications include ongoing anticoagulation therapy, recent intraarterial procedures, and organ biopsies.

Preprocedural Care

1. Initiate preprocedural explanation of procedure to patient and family.
2. Obtain written informed consent for intravenous or intracoronary thrombolytic therapy. Be aware that the consent will include cardiac catheterization if intracoronary procedure is used. Consent may also include permission to perform angioplasty.
3. Obtain baseline laboratory data to determine hemostatic status and degree of myocardial injury: CBC with platelets, prothrombin time, fibrinogen and fibrin split product levels, creatine phosphokinase with isoenzyme levels; blood type and cross-match; electrolytes, BUN, creatinine; 12-lead ECG; chest roentgenogram; vital signs.
4. Prepare for cardiac catheterization as indicated for intracoronary thrombolysis.
5. Establish a patent intravenous line(s): one line for intracoronary procedure; two lines for intravenous procedure.
6. Administer medication as ordered; intravenous lidocaine may be given prophylactically.

Medical Plan

Medications

Streptokinase*

- Intracoronary—25,000-50,000 U bolus followed by continuous infusion of 2000-4000 U/min for 60 min (total dose 150,000-500,000 U); procedure is carried out in conjunction with angiography; infusions are continued for 30-60 min after antegrade flow has been established
- IV—10,000-20,000 U bolus followed by continuous infusion of 10,000-20,000 U administered over 30-60 min (total dose 750,000-1.5 million IU); infusion may be initiated in emergency room or coronary care unit
- Precede with diphenhydramine (Benadryl), 50 mg IV, to reduce allergic reaction (does not prevent anaphylactoid reaction)
- Half-life: α and β half-life during which serum levels can be detected is 18 min and enzymatic action persists 18 to 80 min; enzymatic action on coagulation system persists up to 24 h
- Side effects: Hypotension, which has been reported to occur in 15% of patients, may occur during rapid bolus infusions[103]; allergic reactions, which are reported to occur in 5% of patients, include fever, flushing, rash, periorbital swelling, and bronchospasms; anaphylaxis is rare

*Drug dosages are not standardized; bolus and maintenance dosages may have a wide range.

Urokinase*
- Intracoronary—10,000-30,000 U by bolus followed by continuous infusion of 2000-24,000 U/min; infusion procedure must be performed in conjunction with coronary angiography
- IV—10,000-20,000 U by bolus followed by continuous infusion of 10,000-20,000 U/min up to total of 2 or 3 million U
- Half-life: 10-20 min; prolonged action on coagulation persists up to 24 h
- Side effects: None specified; may be administered rapidly either by bolus or infusion without side effects

Tissue plasminogen activator
- Usual dosage: 0.5-0.75 mg/kg IV over 3 h with 60 mg given over the first h and 20 mg over the second and third h for total dose of 100 mg
- Half-life: 3-5 min
- Side effects: Bleeding

Heparin
- During streptokinase or urokinase infusion, 5000-10,000 U IV bolus followed by continuous infusion to maintain PTT, 1½ to 2 times control value; used to reduce risk of reocclusion immediately and after initial reperfusion
- After procedure, 600-700 U continuous IV once PTT levels have reached 2 times control value

General Management

Intra-arterial blood pressure—observe for changes in blood pressure during and following infusion; used for drawing of blood samping

Cardiac monitoring—ECG pattern observed for signs of reperfusion: resolution of preprocedure ECG changes; dysrhythmias

Hemodynamic monitoring—pulmonary artery and pulmonary capillary wedge pressures as indicated

PTCA—may be performed immediately after reperfusion or delayed 1 to 2 days

Coronary arteriograms—postprocedure arteriograms performed before discharge or as indicated by clinical signs

Bed rest—12 hours after intracoronary infusion; intravenous requires no bed rest restrictions

Diet—as ordered

Laboratory studies—careful monitoring during and after thrombolysis: serum fibrinogen levels (will be less 50 mg/dl after infusion of thrombolytic agent, returning to baseline within 24 hours of completion of thrombolytic infusion); partial thromboplastin time (PTT); hemoglobin; creatinine phosphokinase (CPK)

*Drug dosages are not standardized; bolus and maintenance dosages may have a wide range.

NURSING CARE

Nursing Assessment

Myocardial Ischemia

Preprocedure; 30 minutes of pain; chest discomfort of less than 4 to 6 hours' duration from onset of symptoms; ST elevation of 0.1 mm on ECG; hypotension; dysrhythmias

Reperfusion

Develops within 30 to 60 minutes of administration of thrombolytic therapy; abrupt cessation of chest discomfort; rapid fall in ST elevation; appearance of reperfusion arrhythmias may not be accurate indicator of reperfusion; sinus bradycardia and atrioventricular block with hypotension and asystole are more common with reperfusion of right coronary artery (inferior myocardial infarction); accelerated idioventricular rhythm; ventricular ectopy; peaking of CPK levels 3 to 4 hours after onset of symptoms

Bleeding and Hemorrhage

Related to intravascular fibrinogenolysis, which induces lytic state that is associated with bleeding[98]; bleeding at puncture sites; gastrointestinal or intracranial hemorrhage and hemopericardium

Recurrent Ischemia or Infarction

Related to reocclusion, which has been reported to occur in 20% to 40% of patients following successful recanalization[45]

Nursing Dx & Intervention

Nursing Diagnosis	Nursing Intervention/Rationale
Potential for injury: bleeding or hemorrhage related to thrombolysis-induced coagulopathy	• Assess for signs of bleeding: swelling, pain, or discoloration at puncture sites; petechiae; hematoma; flank pain indicating retroperitoneal bleeding; signs of internal bleeding or hemorrhage: tachycardia, tachypnea, hypotension, coolness of skin, pallor, thirst, restlessness, hematuria, occult blood in emesis or stool. • Monitor blood pressure, heart rate, and respiratory rate every 15 minutes during first hour, decreasing frequency thereafter. • Inspect puncture sites every 15 minutes. Apply manual pressure when removing catheters and after venipunctures *to control superficial bleeding*.

Nursing Diagnosis	Nursing Intervention/Rationale
	• Monitor coagulation values until hemostasis has been reestablished. • Avoid any interruption of vascular integrity following fibrinolytic therapy. • Avoid use of venous or arterial punctures. • Use heparin lock for blood sampling and IV access.
Decreased cardiac output (potential) related to reperfusion arrhythmias	• Assess and record changes in ECG tracing during and after thrombolytic therapy *to determine any changes in baseline cardiac rate or appearance of reperfusion arrhythmias.* • Monitor vital signs frequently according to protocol and the patient's condition. • Notify the physician promptly of any signs of decreased cardiac output as evidenced by changes in heart rate, blood pressure, and mental status. • Initiate prompt treatment for life-threatening arrhythmias per protocol: cardiopulmonary resuscitation (CPR), drug therapy, and preparation for pacemaker insertion.
Pain: chest (potential or actual), related to decreased myocardial oxygen supply	• Assess and record level of comfort including patient's verbal and nonverbal expressions. Compare with preprocedural chest pain complaints. • Record any activity that preceded onset of pain to determine etiology. • Maintain bed rest *to reduce myocardial oxygen demand.* • Obtain 12-lead ECG *to document recurrent ischemia.* • Administer drug therapy as ordered to relieve pain; assess and record response.
Altered cerebral, renal, or gastrointestinal tissue perfusion related to thrombolytic drug–induced coagulopathy	• Assess for changes in neurologic status, complaints of headache, or evidence of gastrointestinal bleeding such as occult blood in emesis or stool or hematuria for up to 24 hours after thrombolytic infusion. • Report any abrupt change from baseline *to determine need for change in or discontinuation of thrombolytic or anticoagulation therapy.*

Patient Education

Preoperative:

1. Instruct patient and family about purpose and indications for thrombolytic therapy, its benefits, and associated risks.
2. Describe the procedure: intracoronary—that it is similar to cardiac catheterization (see p. 1588), and may last 2 to 5 hours. Review sensations to be experienced, such as pressure during insertion of the catheter, but explain that there is no discomfort with infusion.
3. Explain and review procedures and routines associated with the procedure: monitoring in the coronary care unit for heart rhythm problems and bleeding, need for bed rest during and after administration of thrombolytic therapy, and need for frequent blood sampling to monitor clotting times.
4. Instruct the patient to inform a nurse if chest pain develops.

After procedure:

1. Review the explanation of the procedure and postprocedure results.
2. Instruct the patient to report any signs of bleeding: bruising, bleeding gums, hematuria, tarry stools.
3. Instruct the patient to report pain relief or new onset of pain.
4. Discuss activity allowances and limitations.
5. Discuss the need to modify and/or continue to modify coronary risk factors.
6. Discuss the importance of continued follow-up. Explain that coronary angiography may be necessary to evaluate the patency of coronary arteries.
7. Review medications, discussing dosage, method of administration, and side effects.

Evaluation

Patient Outcome	Data Indicating That Outcome is Reached
There is no evidence of bleeding.	Hemostasis is reestablished. Coagulation studies are within acceptable limits. There are no overt or covert signs of bleeding: no hematomas or petechiae. Vital signs are within normal limits. Patient is alert and oriented.
Comfort level is achieved.	Patient verbalizes absence of chest discomfort or pain. Patient is able to resume previous activity level without complaints of pain.

Patient Outcome	Data Indicating That Outcome is Reached
Cardiac output is maintained.	ECG remains stable. Arrhythmias are controlled. Vital signs are stable.
Tissue perfusion is maintained.	Patient is alert and oriented. Patient demonstrates no signs of intracranial bleeding. Urine output is within normal limits and clear.

References

1. Akhtar M: Practical considerations in the treatment of ventricular arrhythmias with Mexiletine, Am Heart J 107:1086, 1984.
2. American Heart Association: Recommendation for prophylaxis of infective endocarditis, Circulation 56:139A, 1985.
3. American Heart Association: Standards and guidelines for cardiopulmonary resuscitation and emergency cardiac care, JAMA 225:2841, 1986.
4. American Heart Association: Heart facts—1987, Dallas, 1987, National Center.
5. Andreoli K et al: Comprehensive cardiac care, ed 6, St Louis, 1987, The CV Mosby Co.
6. Anthony CP and Thibodeau GA: Textbook of anatomy and physiology, ed 11, St Louis, 1983, The CV Mosby Co.
7. Arnsdorf MF: Electrophysiologic properties of antiarrhythmic drugs as a rational basis for therapy, Med Clin North Am 60:213, 1976.
8. Barry J and Dieter WG: Endocarditis: an overview, Heart Lung 11:138, 1982.
9. Belloni FL: The local control of coronary blood flow, Cardiovasc Res 13:63, 1979.
10. Blake S: The clinical diagnosis of constrictive pericarditis, Am Heart J 106:432, 1983.
11. Braunwald E editor: Heart disease: a textbook of cardiovascular medicine, Philadelphia, 1980, WB Saunders Co.
12. Breu CS, Lindenmuth JE, and Tillisch JH: Treatment of patients with congestive cardiomyopathy during hospitalization: a case study, Heart Lung 11:229, 1982.
13. Brown WJ: A classification of microorganisms frequently causing sepsis, Heart Lung 5:397, 1976.
14. Bulkley BH, Weisfeldt ML, and Hutchins GM: Asymmetric septal hypertrophy and myocardial fiber disarray, Circulation 56:292, 1977.
15. Cain R, Ferguson RM, and Tillisch J: Variant angina: a nursing approach, Heart Lung 8:1122, 1979.
16. Cannom DS and Winkle RA: Implantation of the automatic implantable cardioverter defibrillator (AICD): practical aspects, Pace 9:723, 1987.
17. Collen D et al: Coronary thrombolysis with recombinant human tissue-type plasminogen activator: a prospective randomized, placebo controlled trial, Circulation 70:1012, 1984.
18. Conolly ME, Kersting F, and Dollery CT: The clinical pharmacology of beta-adrenoceptor-blocking drugs, Prog Cardiovasc Dis 19:203, 1976.
19. Conover MB: Cardiac arrhythmias: exercises in pattern interpretation, ed 2, St Louis, 1978, The CV Mosby Co.
20. Conover MB: Understanding electrocardiology: physiological and interpretive concepts, ed 3, St Louis, 1980, The CV Mosby Co.
21. Conover MB: Exercises in diagnosing ECG tracings, ed 3, St Louis, 1984, The CV Mosby Co.
22. Conover MB: Understanding electrocardiology: physiological and interpretive concepts, ed 4, St Louis, 1984, The CV Mosby Co.
23. Cooper DK et al: The impact of automatic implantable cardioverter defibrillator on quality of life, Clin Prog Electrophysiol Pacing 4:306, 1986.
24. Craven RF and Curry TD: When the diagnosis is Raynaud's, Am J Nurs 8:1007, 1981.
25. Dalen JE and Alpert JS: Natural history of pulmonary embolism, Prog Cardiovasc Dis 17:259, 1975.
26. da Luz PL, Weil MH, and Shubin H: Current concepts and mechanisms and treatment of cardiogenic shock, Am Heart J 92:103, 1976.
27. DeWood MA et al: Coronary arteriographic findings of acute transmural myocardial infarction, Circulation 58:139, 1983.
28. Dole WP and O'Rourke RA: Pathophysiology and management of cardiogenic shock, Curr Probl Cardiol 8:1, 1983.
29. Doyle JE: Treatment modalities in peripheral vascular disease, Nurs Clin North Am 58:139, 1983.
30. Fenster PE: Verapamil: new therapy for supraventricular arrhythmias, J Cardiovasc Med 7:410, 1982.
31. Gabriel Khan MI: Manual of cardiac drug therapy, London, 1984, Baulliere Tindall.
32. Ginzton LE and Laks MM: Acute pericarditis: recognition by ECG, Primary Cardiol 10:73, 1984.
33. GISSI trial: effectiveness of intravenous thrombolytic treatment in acute myocardial infarction, Lancet 1:397, 1986.
34. Goldberger E: Textbook of clinical cardiology, St Louis, 1982, The CV Mosby Co.
35. Goodwin JF: Hypertrophic cardiomyopathy: a disease in search of its own identity, Am J Cardiol 45:177, 1980.
36. Gregoratos G and Karliner JS: Infective endocarditis: diagnosis and management, Med Clin North Am 63:173, 1979.
37. Groër MW and Shekleton ME: Basic pathophysiology: a conceptual approach, St Louis, 1983, The CV Mosby Co.
38. Guazzi M et al: Repetitive myocardial ischemia of Prinzmetal type with angina pectoris, Am J Cardiol 37:923, 1976.
39. Guthrie MM, editor: Shock, New York, 1982, Churchill Livingstone, Inc.
40. Guyton AC: Textbook of medical physiology, ed 8, Philadelphia, 1980, WB Saunders Co.
41. Guzzetta CE and Dossey BM: Cardiovascular nursing: bodymind tapestry, St Louis, 1984, The CV Mosby Co.
42. Hardaway RM et al: The danger of hemolysis in shock, Ann Surg 189:373, 1979.
43. Harris L et al: The cardiovascular effects of caffeine post-myocardial infarction, Circulation 72(suppl III):116, 1985.
44. Hoffman BF and Cranefield PF: The physiological basis of cardiac arrhythmias, Am J Med 37:670, 1964.
45. Jaffe AJ and Sobel BE: Thrombolysis with tissue type plasminogen activator in acute myocardial infarction: potentials and pitfalls, JAMA 255:237, 1986.
46. Jamieson SW et al: Heart transplantation for end-stage ischemic heart disease: the Stanford experience, Heart Transplant 3:224, 1984.
47. Josephson M, Harken A, and Horowitz L: Endocardial excision: a new surgical technique for the treatment of recurrent ventricular tachycardia, Circulation 60:1430, 1979.
48. Josephson M and Horowitz L: Electrophysiologic approach to therapy of recurrent sustained ventricular tachycardia, Am J Cardiol 43:631, 1979.
49. Kannel WB, McGee D, and Gordon T: A general cardiovascular risk profile: the Framingham study, Am J Cardiol 38:46, 1976.
50. Kaye D and Rose LF: Fundamentals of internal medicine, St Louis, 1983, The CV Mosby Co.
51. Kennedy JW et al: Western Washington randomized trial of intracoronary streptokinase in acute myocardial infarction, N Engl J Med 309:1477, 1983.
52. Kennedy JW et al: Acute myocardial infarction treated with intracoronary streptokinase: a report of the society for cardiac angiography, Am J Cardiol 55:871, 1985.
53. Kent KM: Percutaneous transluminal angioplasty: report from the registry of National Heart Lung and Blood Institute, Am J Cardiol 49:2011, 1982.
54. Kent KM: Transluminal coronary angioplasty. In Rackey CE, editor: Advances in critical care cardiology, Cardiovasc Clin 16:53, 1986.
55. King SL: Patient care in vascular surgery, AORN J 33:843, 1981.

56. Kinney MR et al, editors: AACN's clinical reference for critical care nurses, New York, 1981, McGraw-Hill Book Co.
57. Kirchhoff KT: An examination of the physiologic basis for "coronary precautions," Heart Lung 15:874, 1981.
58. Kistner RL et al: Incidence of pulmonary embolism and thrombophlebitis of lower extremities, Am J Surg 124:169, 1972.
59. Laffel O and Brunwald E: Thrombolytic therapy: a new strategy for the treatment of acute myocardial infarction, Part I, N Engl J Med 311:710, 1984.
60. Lee NW: The diagnosis and treatment of endotoxin shock, Anesthesia 31:897, 1976.
61. Lees RS and Lees AM: Lipid lowering drugs: renewed enthusiasm, Drug Ther, 1984, p 57.
62. LeFrock JL et al: Transient bacteremia associated with sigmoidoscopy, N Engl J Med 289:469, 1973.
63. LeFrock JL et al: Transient bacteremia associated with nasotracheal suctioning, JAMA 236:1610, 1977.
64. Lewis SM and Collier IC: Medical surgical nursing: assessment and management of clinical problems, New York, 1983, McGraw-Hill Book Co.
65. Lough ME: Quality of life issues following heart transplantation, Prog Cardiovasc Nurs 1:17, 1986.
66. Ludmer P and Goldschlager N: Cardiac pacing in the 1980's, N Engl J Med 311:1671, 1984.
67. Massey JA: Diagnostic testing for peripheral vascular disease, Nurs Clin North Am 21:207, 1986.
68. Michaelson CR, editor: Congestive heart failure, St Louis, 1983, The CV Mosby Co.
69. Miller DC and Roon AJ: Diagnosis and management of peripheral vascular disease, Menlo Park, Calif, 1982, Addison-Wesley Publishing Co.
70. Mirowski N: The automatic implantable cardioverter-defibrillator: an overview, J Am Coll Cardiol 6:461, 1985.
71. Moore S: Pericarditis after acute myocardial infarction: manifestations and nursing implications, Heart Lung 8:551, 1979.
71a. Moore WS: What's new in peripheral vascular surgery, J Cardiovasc Surg 24:49, 1983.
72. Murdaugh C: Coronary artery disease in women, Prog Cardiovasc Nurs 1:2, 1986.
73. Neill CA: Etiology of congenital heart disease, Cardiovasc Clin 4:138, 1972.
74. The 1980 report of the Joint National Committee on Detection: evaluation and treatment of high blood pressure, Arch Intern Med 140:1280, 1980.
75. Noel DK et al: Challenging concerns for patients with automatic implantable cardioverter defibrillators, Focus Crit Care 13:50, 1986.
76. O'Rourke MF: Cardiogenic shock following myocardial infarction, Heart Lung 3:353, 1974.
77. Parsonnet V, Furman S, and Symth N: A revised code for pacemaker identification: pacemaker study group, Circulation 64:60A, 1981.
78. Perez MM and Pintos Diaz G: Arteriosclerosis obliterans of the lower limbs, Cardiovasc Rev 4:1357, 1983.
79. Perloff JK: Clinical recognition of congenital heart disease, Philadelphia, 1987, WB Saunders Co.
80. Rahimtoola S: Surgery for infective endocarditis, Crit Care Q 4:51, 1981.
81. Rahimtoola SH et al: Consensus statement of the conference on the state of the art of electrophysiologic testing in the diagnosis and treatments of patients with cardiac arrhythmias, Circulation 75(suppl III):3, 1987.
82. Rao AK and TIMI Investigators: Thrombolysis in myocardial infarction trial (phase I): effect of intravenous tissue plasminogen activator and streptokinase on plasma fibrinogen and the fibrinolytic system, Circulation 72(III):416, 1985.
83. Reid CL et al: Infective endocarditis: improved diagnosis and treatment, Curr Probl Cardiol 10:6, 1985.
84. Rentrop KP et al: Effects of intracoronary streptokinase and intracoronary nitroglycerin infusion on coronary angiographic patterns and mortality in patients with acute myocardial infarction, N Engl J Med 311:1457, 1984.
85. Roberts B: Balloon angioplasty in treatment of peripheral vascular disease, J Cardiovasc Surg 23:225, 1982.
86. Rosenbaum MB et al: Clinical efficacy of amiodarone as an antiarrhythmic agent, Am J Cardiol 38:934, 1976.
87. Sacksteder S, Gildea JH, and Dassy C: Common congenital cardiac defects, Am J Nurs 78:266, 1978.
88. Sawaya J, Muyais S, and Armenian H: Early diagnosis of pericarditis in acute myocardial infarction, Am Heart J 100:144, 1980.
89. Schneider JR: Effects of caffeine ingestion on heart rate, blood pressure, myocardial oxygen consumption, and cardiac rhythm in acute myocardial infarction patients, Heart Lung 16:167, 1987.
90. Schnittger I et al: Echocardiography: pericardial thickening and constrictive pericarditis, Am J Cardiol 42:388, 1978.
91. Schomerus M et al: Physiological disposition of verapamil in man, Cardiovasc Res 10:605, 1976.
92. Shabetai R: Cardiomyopathy: how far have we come in 25 years, how far yet to go? J Am Coll Cardiol 1:252, 1983.
93. Sheehy SB and Barber JM: Emergency nursing: principles and practice, ed 2, St Louis, 1985, The CV Mosby Co.
94. Shellock FG and Riedinger MS: Reproducibility and accuracy of using room temperature vs. ice temperature for thermodilution cardiac output determination, Heart Lung 12:175, 1983.
95. Shine, KI et al: Aspects of the management of shock, Ann Intern Med 93:723, 1980.
96. Silva J: Anaerobic infections, Heart Lung 5:406, 1976.
97. Singh BN, Collett JT, and Chew C: New perspectives in the pharmacologic therapy of cardiac arrhythmias, Prog Cardiovasc Dis 22:243, 1980.
98. Sobel BE: Fibrinolysis and activators of plasminogen, Heart Lung 16:776, 1987.
99. Spittell JA: Office and bedside diagnosis of occlusive arterial disease, Curr Probl Cardiol 7, May 1983.
100. Spodic DH: Acute pericardial disease, Heart Lung 14:599, 1985.
101. Tilkian AG and Daily EK: Cardiovascular procedures: diagnostic techniques and therapeutic procedures, St Louis, 1986, The CV Mosby Co.
102. TIMI Study Groups: The thrombolysis in myocardial infarction (TIMI) trial: phase 1 findings, N Engl J Med 312:932, 1985.
103. Topol EJ: Clinical use of streptokinase and urokinase therapy for acute myocardial infarction, Heart Lung 16:760, 1987.
104. Tucker SM et al: Patient care standards: nursing process, diagnosis, and outcome, ed 4, St Louis, 1988, The CV Mosby Co.
105. Tyndall A: A nursing perspective of the invasive electrophysiologic approach to treatment of ventricular arrhythmias, Heart Lung 12:620, 1983.
106. Urban N: Integrating hemodynamic parameters with clinical decision making, Crit Care Nurse 6:48, 1986.
107. Verstraete M et al: Randomized trial of intravenous streptokinase tissue-type plasminogen activator versus intravenous streptokinase in acute myocardial infarction, Lancet 1:842, 1985.
108. Watanakunakorn C: Changing epidemiology and newer aspects of infective endocarditis, Adv Intern Med 22:21, 1977.
109. Whaley LF and Wong DL: Nursing care of infants and children, ed 3, St. Louis, 1987, The CV Mosby Co.
110. Winslow EH: Cardiovascular consequences of bed rest, Heart Lung 14:236, 1985.
111. Winston TR, Henly WS, and Geis RC: Surgery for peripheral vascular disease, AORN J 33:849, 1981.
112. Wirsing P, Andriopoulous A, and Botticher R: Arterial embolectomies in the upper extremity after acute occlusion, J Cardiovasc Surg 24:40, 1983.
113. Wit AL and Rosen MR: Pathophysiologic mechanisms of cardiac arrhythmias, Am Heart J 106:798, 1983.
114. Yasue H et al: Prinzmetal's variant form of angina as a manifestation of alpha adrenergic receptor-mediated coronary artery spasm: documentation of coronary arteriography, Am Heart J 91:148, 1976.
115. Zipis DP and Troup PJ: New antiarrhythmic agents, Am J Cardiol 41:100, 1978.
116. Zsoter TT: Calcium antagonist, Am Heart J 99:805, 1980.

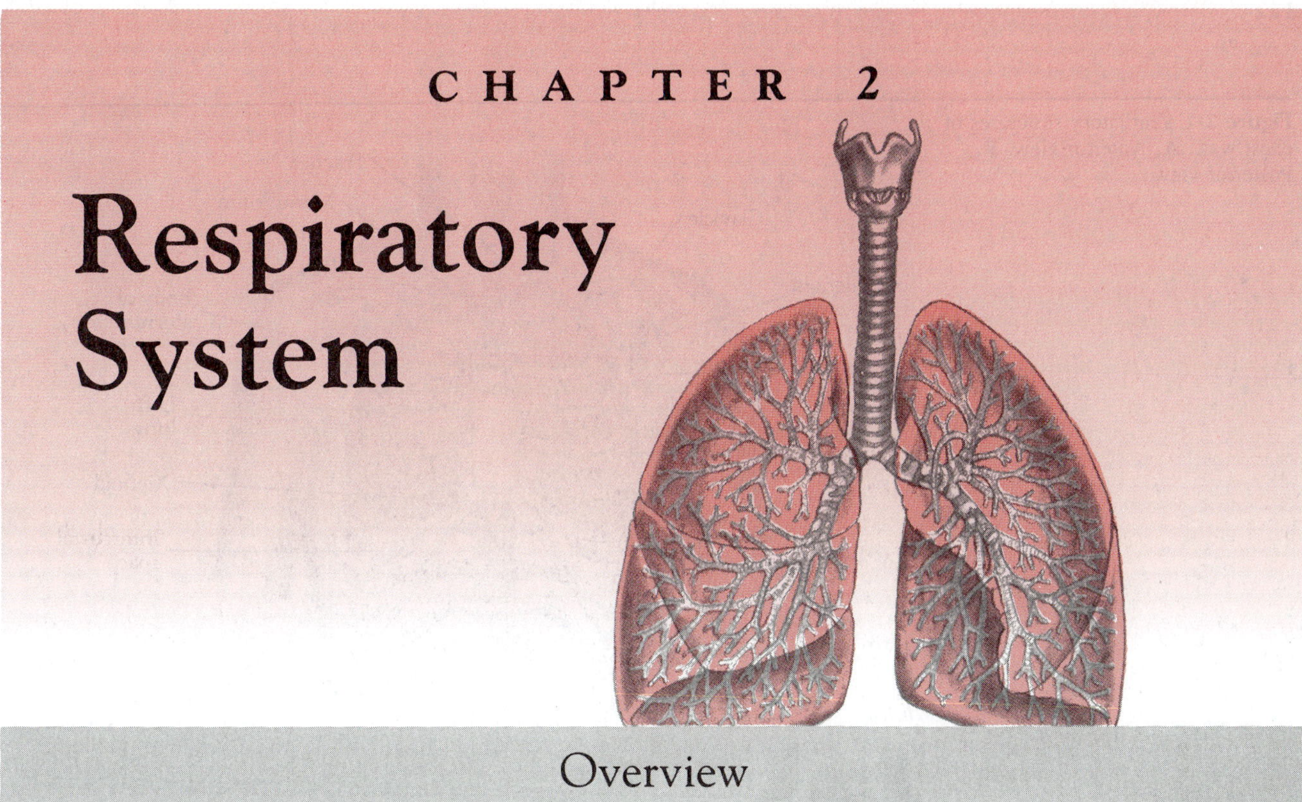

CHAPTER 2
Respiratory System

Overview

The main function of the respiratory system is to supply oxygen to the body cells and to remove carbon dioxide from the cells. Oxygen is used at the cellular level, where it combines with adenosine diphosphate (ADP) and simple sugar (CHO) to produce energy in the form of adenosine triphosphate (ATP). Carbon dioxide and water are by-products of this cellular function.

Smoking is the single most common cause of respiratory problems from an external source. It is considered to be the major cause of chronic bronchitis, emphysema, and lung cancer in the United States. Environmental factors have become more important over the past three decades as by-products of industrialization and urbanization have polluted the air. Small particles of air pollutants inhaled into the respiratory tract often cause disease states. Major air pollutants include sulfur dioxide and sulfur trioxide, nitrogen dioxide, carbon monoxide, chlorine, ammonia, hydrocarbons, silica, cobalt, asbestos, and coal dust.[82] These chemicals also cause smog and haze, which affects crop growth. Much of this pollution comes from motor vehicles and industrial plants.

Internal respiratory factors include ventilation, diffusion and perfusion, blood flow, and control of breathing. All these factors must function effectively for adequate breathing.

Anatomy, Physiology, and Related Pathophysiology

The anatomy of the respiratory system is discussed from a functional perspective within each of the following four levels:

1. Ventilation—the movement of air from outside to inside the body and its distribution within the tracheobronchial system to the gas exchange units of the lungs.
2. Diffusion and perfusion—the movement of oxygen and carbon dioxide across the alveolar-capillary membrane to the blood in the pulmonary capillaries.
3. Blood flow—the movement of respiratory gases through the pulmonary and arterial circulation, the distribution and exchange of oxygen and carbon dioxide at the peripheral tissues, and the return of respiratory gases to the lungs.
4. Control of breathing—the regulation of ventilation to maintain adequate gas exchange, usually in accord with changing metabolic demands or other special needs.

Ventilation

Ventilation is the process that moves air from outside the body to the gas exchange units of the lungs. The muscles of respiration must exert sufficient force to move the chest wall and expand the lungs. There must be enough force to overcome the resistance in the respiratory system so air will be drawn into the tracheobronchial tree. The volume of air that enters is determined by the mechanical properties of the lung parenchyma, airways, and chest wall.

Chest wall. The sternum, manubrium, and xiphoid process form the anterior border of the thorax. The posterior portion is formed by 12 thoracic vertebrae. The lateral boundaries are formed by 12 pairs of ribs, which have a posterior connection directly to the thoracic vertebrae. The first seven ribs also connect anteriorly to the sternum by the costal cartilages (Figure 2-1).

The major muscle groups used in the ventilatory process are the diaphragm and the intercostal muscles (Figure 2-2).

Figure 2-1 Ventilatory structures of chest wall. **A,** Anterior view. **B,** Posterior view.

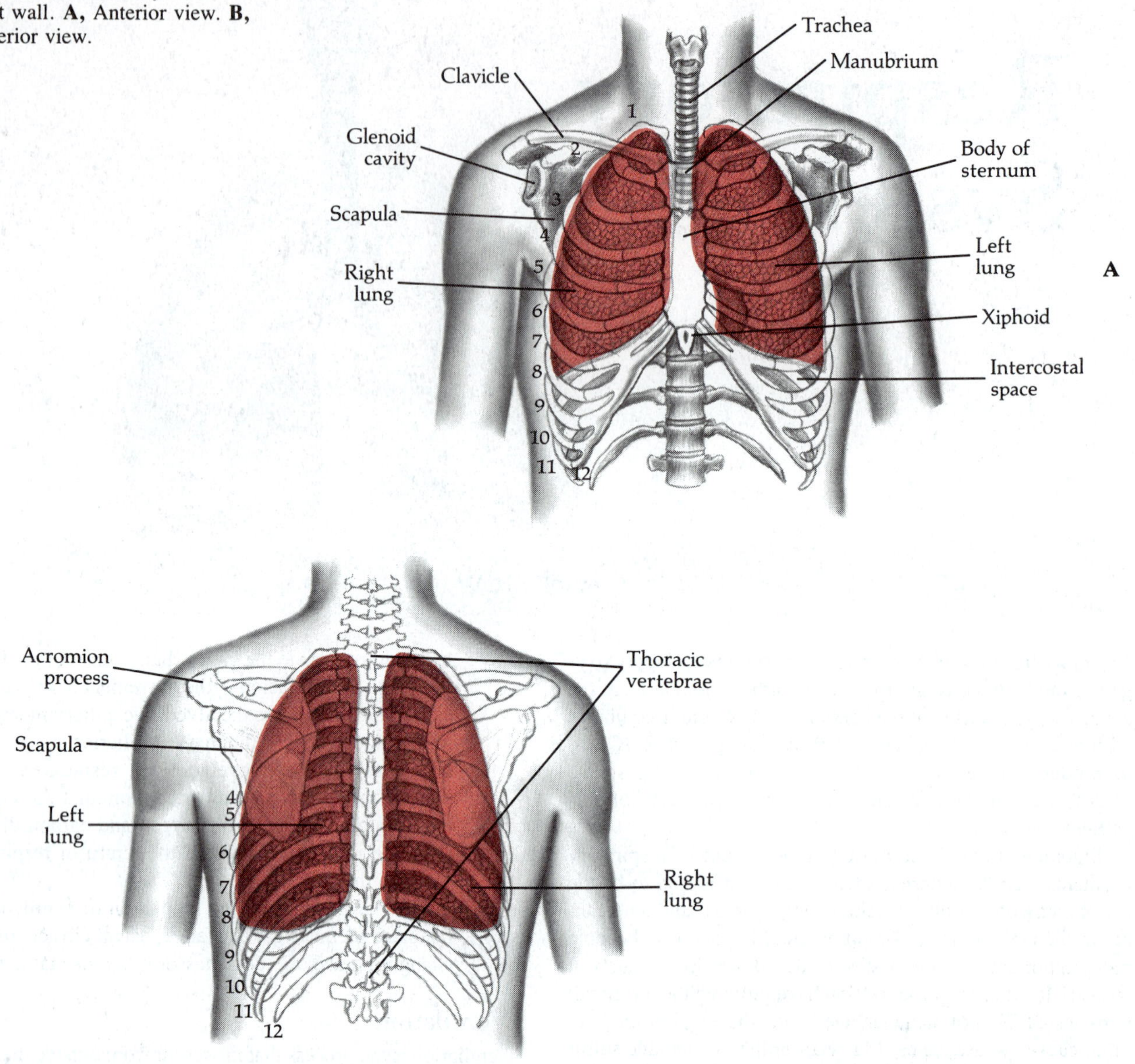

The diaphragm is the main muscle of inspiration. During deep inspiration the diaphragm contracts and moves downward. This contraction, which occurs because of stimulation by the phrenic nerve, forces two major movements to ease ventilation. The first raises the lower ribs upward and laterally, increasing the transverse and lateral intrathoracic space. The second action forces the abdominal contents downward.

The intercostal muscles are divided into the external and internal muscles. The external muscles contract to increase the anterior to posterior diameter of the thoracic cavity during inspiration. With deep breathing the internal muscles contract to decrease the transverse diameter during expiration.

Three muscles augment increased-effort breathing: the scalene, sternocleidomastoid, and abdominal muscles. During inspiration, the scalene muscles contract to raise the first two ribs and stabilize the upper chest wall. The sternocleidomastoid muscle contracts to raise the sternum. During expiration these muscles relax and the abdominal wall muscles contract. During quiet ventilation the abdominal wall muscles are not used. If expiration is forced, as during exercise, the abdominal muscles may depress the lower ribs of the chest wall to assist expiration.

Figure 2-2 Muscles of ventilation. **A,** Anterior view. **B,** Posterior view.

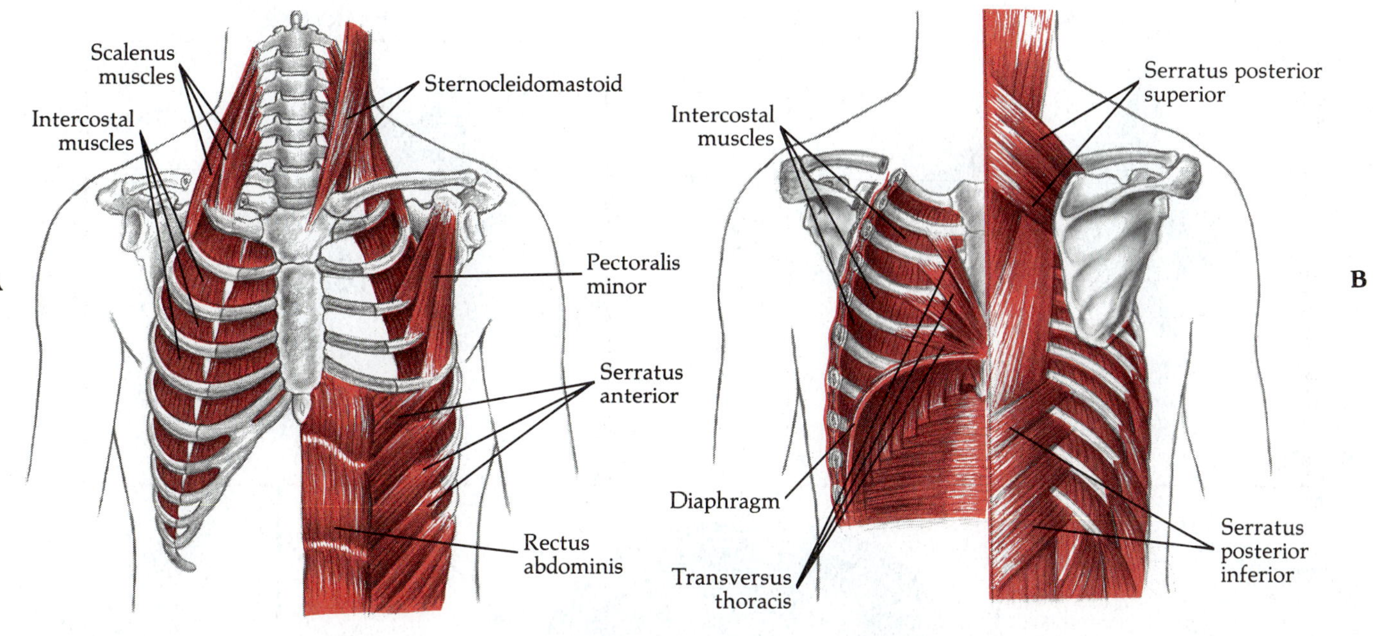

Figure 2-3 Chest cavity related structures. **A,** Anterior view. **B,** Cross section.

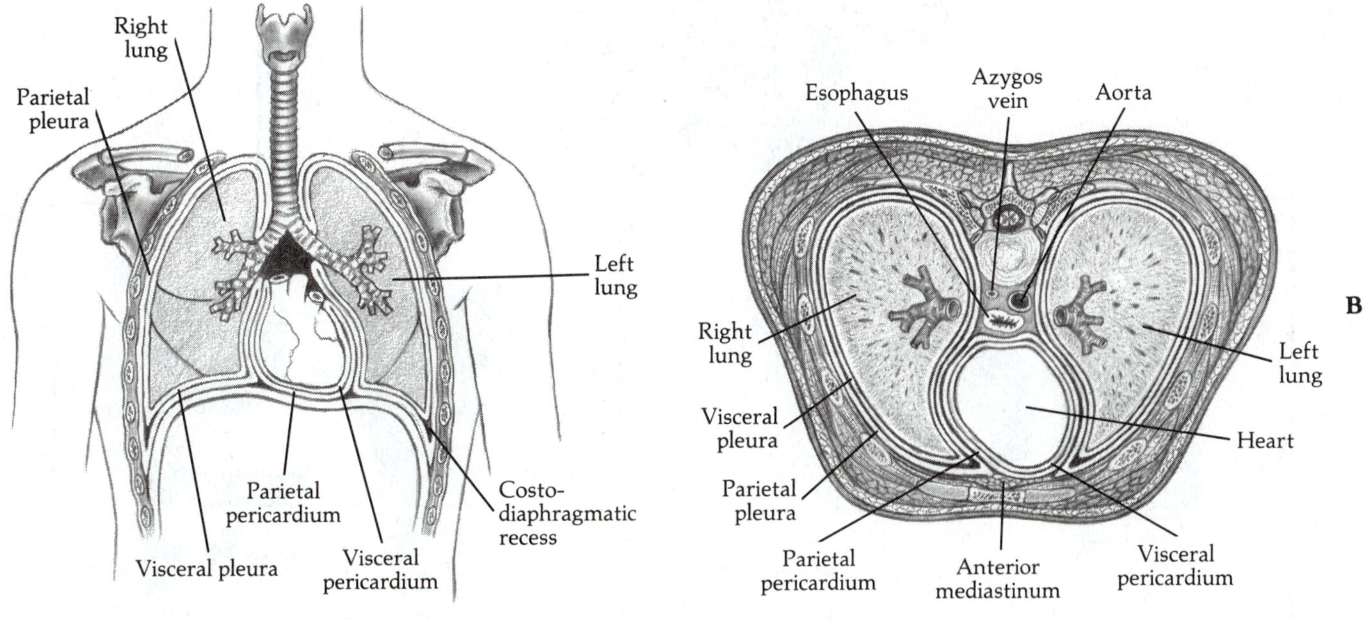

Figure 2-4 Structures of upper airway.

NASAL WALL

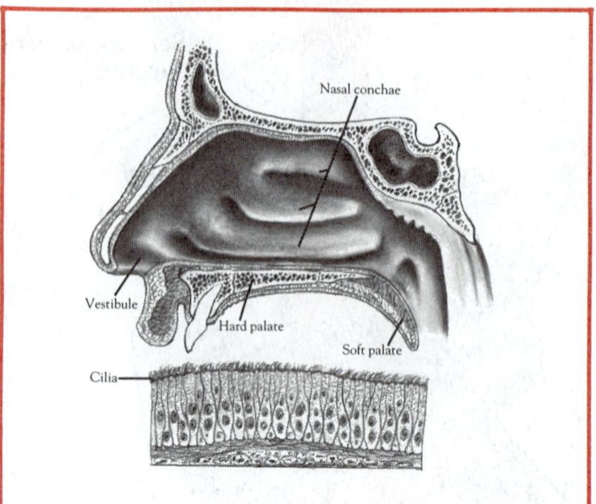

PHARYNX

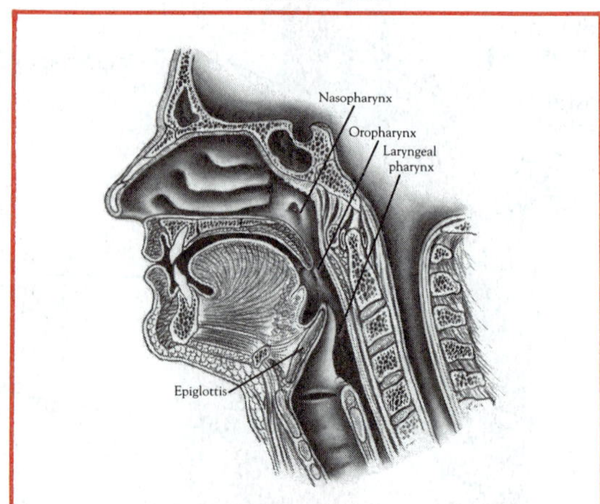

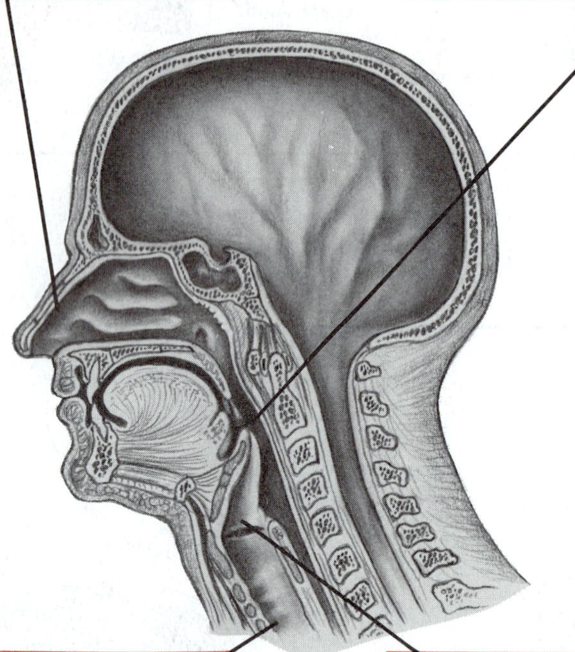

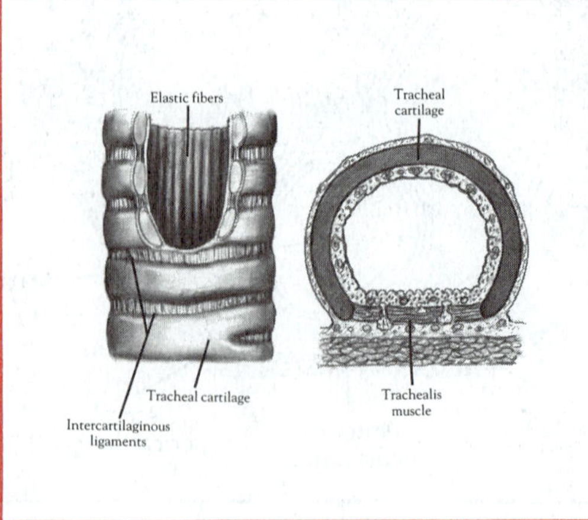

TRACHEA

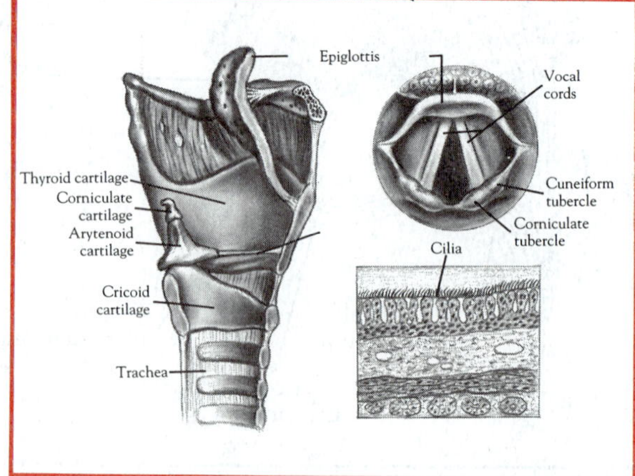

LARYNX

Thoracic cavity. The main structures of the thoracic cavity include the pleura, pleural space, mediastinum, and lungs. Figure 2-3 details this anatomy.

The pleura is a two-layered protective membrane. The first layer is the parietal pleura, which lines the thoracic cavity within the lung chambers. The second is the visceral or pulmonary pleura, which covers each lung. Although each is given a separate name, the pleurae are continuous with one another and form one closed sac. Between the two pleurae is a potential space, the pleural space, which contains a serous lubricant film that allows one pleura to slip over the other and thus helps the lungs move. The intrapleural space also maintains a subatmospheric pressure. At rest the pressure is 755 mm Hg; just before breathing this pressure drops to 751 mm Hg.

The mediastinum is the region between the right and left parietal pleurae. It is bordered by the sternum on the front and the thoracic vertebrae on the back. The heart, contained in its own pericardial sac, is in the middle of the mediastinum. Also in the mediastinum are the great vessels that enter and leave the heart, the bifurcation of the trachea, the large bronchi, part of the esophagus, the thymus gland, lymph nodes, and various nerves including the phrenic nerve, cardiac and splanchnic branches of the sympathetic system, and recurrent laryngeal and vagus branches of the parasympathetic system.

The hilum is at the center of the mediastinal surface. This area contains the root of the lung and is the place where the visceral and parietal pleurae join and form a sheath around the bronchi. It is also the place where blood vessels and nerves connect with the lungs.

The right lung contains three lobes, has 10 bronchopulmonary segments, and is responsible for 55% of all normal lung activity.

The left lung has eight bronchopulmonary segments and is responsible for 45% of all normal lung functioning. Blood is supplied to the tissue of both lungs by the bronchial arteries.

Upper airway. The upper airway, consisting of the nose, pharynx, larynx, and extrathoracic trachea (Figure 2-4), has three major functions:

1. To conduct air to the lower airway
2. To protect the lower airway from foreign matter
3. To warm, filter, and humidify inspired air

The nose warms, moistens, and filters inspired air. Temperature adjustment and proper humidification begin as soon as air hits the anterior nasal cavity. The structure of the nose, with its two nasal cavities, turbinates, and rich vasculature, provides maximum contact between inspired air and the nasal mucosa. By the time inspired air reaches the alveoli, it is 100% water vapor saturated.

Another function of the nose is to clear debris from the inspired air. The nasal cilia, hair, and moisture cluster small airborne particles. Sneezing is another means of clearing the inspired air. When a mechanical or chemical irritation occurs, sensory receptors in the nasal mucosa send impulses to the brain via the trigeminal and olfactory nerves, thus causing a sneeze.

Air passes from the nasal cavity into the three divisions of the pharynx: the nasopharynx, oropharynx, and laryngeal pharynx. The pharynx, which is covered with ciliated epithelium, filters and humidifies inspired air.

Figure 2-5 Structures of lower airway.
Modified from Weilbrel.[83]

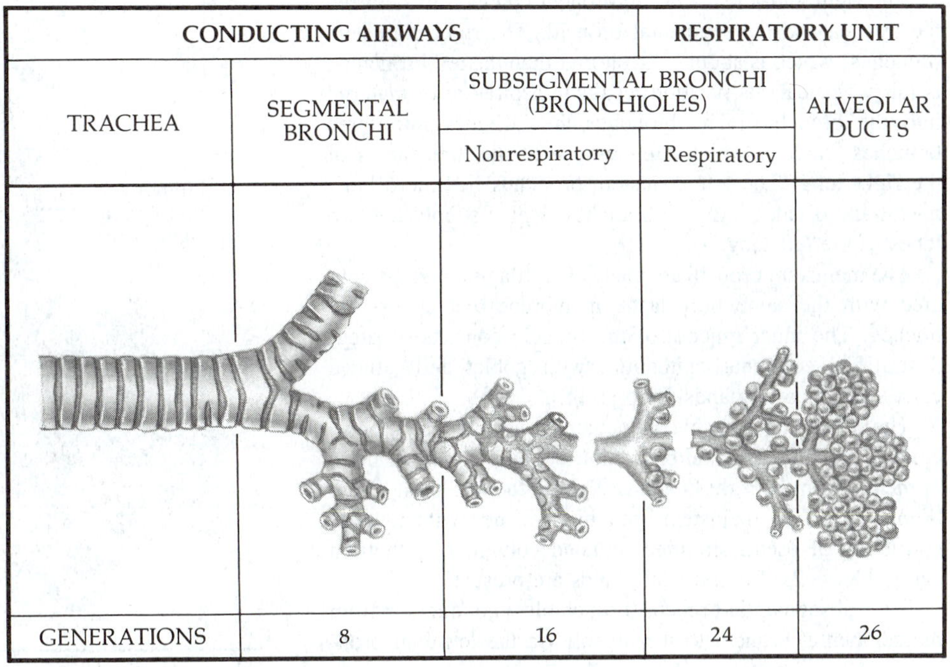

CONDUCTING AIRWAYS				RESPIRATORY UNIT
TRACHEA	SEGMENTAL BRONCHI	SUBSEGMENTAL BRONCHI (BRONCHIOLES)		ALVEOLAR DUCTS
		Nonrespiratory	Respiratory	
GENERATIONS	8	16	24	26

The larynx contains the vocal cords for phonation, prevents aspiration of food into the trachea, and helps to initiate coughing. It extends up to the level of the sixth cervical vertebra (C6) and is covered with the same pseudostratified ciliated columnar epithelium found in the nose and the pharynx.

The main cartilages of the larynx are the thyroid, arytenoid, and cricoid. Attached to the anterior surface of the thyroid cartilage is the epiglottis. The cricoid cartilage, beneath the thyroid cartilage, forms the narrowest part of the airway for infants and children. The larynx is innervated by two separate branches of the vagus nerve. The recurrent laryngeal nerve innervates the larynx, and the superior laryngeal nerve provides some motor and all sensory innervation. The sensory fibers are responsible for the cough reflex.

Lower airway. The lower airway, made up of the trachea, mainstem bronchi, segmental bronchi, subsegmental bronchioles, terminal bronchioles, and gas exchange units (Figure 2-5), has three main functions:

1. Air conduction to the alveolar level of the lungs
2. Mucociliary clearance
3. Pulmonary surfactant production by the type II cells of the alveoli

There is a range of 23 to 26 levels of branches of conducting airways and terminal respiratory units involved. These branch levels, called generations, are divided into two categories and five types (Figure 2-5).

The trachea, which is 4 to 5 cm wide and 11 to 12 cm long and which consists of C-shaped rings of cartilage, extends from the larynx and cricoid cartilage to the division of right and left mainstem bronchi at the level of the fifth thoracic vertebra (T5) in the chest.

The lining of the trachea consists of a pseudostratified, ciliated columnar epithelium mixed with mucus-producing goblet cells.

The right and left mainstem bronchi conduct air between the trachea and the segmental bronchi. The right mainstem bronchus, which is about 5 cm shorter than the left bronchus, is fairly vertical. Its position results in aspiration of material into the bronchus. The bronchus then divides into three branches, each of which supplies one of the three lobes of the right lung. The left mainstem bronchus lies more horizontal and divides into two branches, which supply the two lobes of the left lung.

The mainstem bronchi are made of cartilaginous rings covered with the same fibroelastic membrane that covers the trachea. The inner mucosa of the bronchi consists of pseudostratified columnar epithelium with goblet and ciliated cells. Submucosal glands are present.

The segmental bronchi conduct air between the main bronchi and the subsegmental bronchioles. There are 18 of these bronchi: 10 in the right lung and eight in the left lung. These bronchi, like the mainstem bronchi, are lined with mucosa consisting of pseudostratified, ciliated columnar epithelium and goblet cells. Submucosal glands are present.

The subsegmental bronchi (bronchioles) conduct air from the segmental bronchi to the alveoli via the terminal bronchioles. These airways have no cartilage, no goblet cells, and no submucosal glands. The bronchioles have a complete concentric ring of smooth muscle with two sets of smooth muscle fibers. When the muscle rings constrict as in asthma, the airways narrow.

The lower part of the bronchioles consists of units, called the terminal bronchi, that conduct air from the subsegmental bronchi to the alveolar ducts. There are about 35,000 of these small bronchioles throughout both lungs. They are clustered so that three to five of them form a pulmonary lobule. Their mucosal lining consists of cuboidal epithelium and Clara cells. They contain no goblet cells or submucosal glands.

The most distal section of the lower respiratory tract consists of the terminal respiratory units (acini), which include the respiratory bronchioles, the alveolar ducts, the alveolar sacs, and the terminal air sacs, called the alveoli. An acinus is the site of gas exchange. Figure 2-6 shows the cluster arrangement of these units.

The membrane surface of the terminal respiratory unit is a flattened, one-cell-thick epithelial surface. The type II cell of the alveolar epithelium secretes the lipoprotein substance called surfactant. Surfactant forms a thin layer between the surface of the alveoli and the air. Surfactant decreases the surface tension of the air-liquid interface in the alveoli. Without adequate surfactant, as occurs in hyaline membrane disease or respiratory distress syndrome, it is difficult for the

Figure 2-6 Terminal respiratory units.

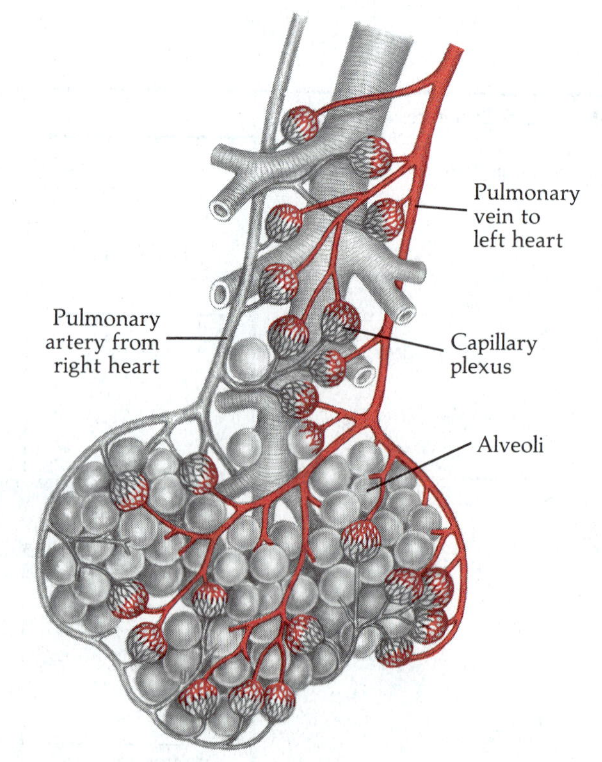

Figure 2-7 Alveolar wall and space.

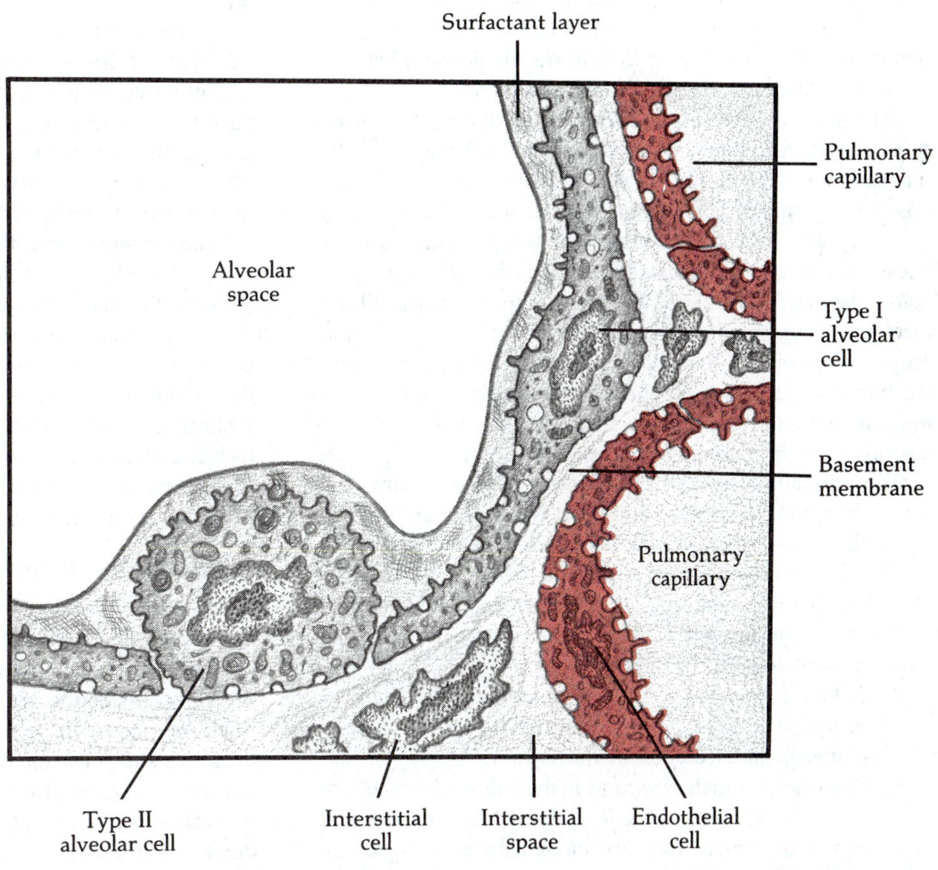

Figure 2-8 Structures of the ventilatory mucosa.

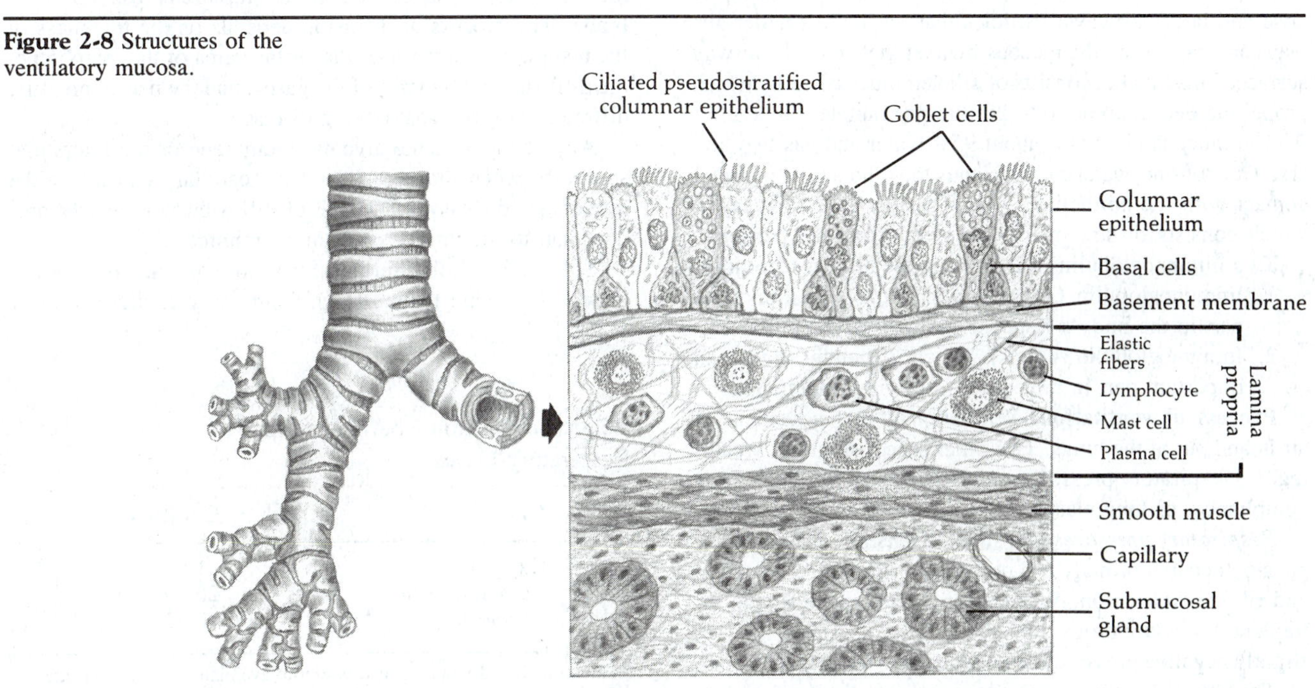

alveoli to inflate with inspiration because of the high pressure gradients needed to overcome the high surface tension.

The alveolar membrane is composed of five layers. This membrane, shown in Figure 2-7, forms the division between the alveolar space and the pulmonary capillary.

Histology of the respiratory tract. Mucosa lines most of the upper respiratory tract. As shown in Figure 2-8, this mucosa consists of an epithelial layer, a basement membrane, and lamina propria. The lamina propria, which has an elastic tissue layer boundary, contains lymphocytes, plasma cells, occasional polymorphonuclear leukocytes, and many mast cells. The mast cells release histamine in the antigen-antibody reactions occurring in asthma or allergic reactions. The lamina propria also contains lymphoid nodules at various sites along the tracheobronchial tree. These nodules participate in a variety of immune responses occurring in the lungs. They are also involved in making immunoglobulin A (IgA).

The epithelial layer of the mucosa contains many cell types. Following are three significant types of cells:

1. Ciliated, pseudostratified epithelial cells, which are found in the columnar epithelium of the larger airways and the cuboidal epithelium of the smaller airways. The main purpose of the cilia is to propel airway secretions toward the upper airway.
2. Goblet cells, which are found among the columnar epithelial cells of the larger airways. Their function is synthesis and secretion of mucus.
3. Clara cells, which are found in the cuboidal epithelium of the distal small airways. Although their exact function is unknown, they are thought to be at least one source of the fluid lining of the smallest airways.

The mucociliary system traps and transports airborne particles (between 2 and 10 μm in diameter) not filtered in the nose and larger airways. Particles that reach the smaller airways are trapped on the mucous blanket that coats the airway surface. This blanket consists of ciliated mucosal cells, which propel the debris up at 10 to 20 mm per minute.

The mucous blanket is about 95% water and has two layers. The bottom, watery layer cleans the cilia and is in direct contact with the epithelium. The top layer is the gel layer, which consists of streams of mucus that trap the particles.

Two immunoglobulins are found in the airway secretions:

1. Immunoglobulin G (IgG), which plays an important part in the body's response to bacterial infections
2. Immunoglobulin A (IgA), which is thought to play an important part in protection from viral infections

Process of ventilation. Ventilation is the movement of air in and out of the lungs. Two other processes affect breathing: (1) respiratory pressures and surface tension and (2) lung compliance, or lung elasticity.

Respiratory pressures and surface tension. Thoracic expansion occurs normally and quietly after muscle contraction and rib cage elevation. When the rib cage expands, the intrapleural pressure drops from about 755 to 751 mm Hg. This slightly negative pressure is enough to draw air into the lungs.

The alveoli's surface tension augments the normal tendency of the lungs to collapse and pull away from the chest wall.

A lipoprotein substance called surfactant, located where the alveolar lining interacts with the air in the alveoli, is important in decreasing the surface tension so the lungs inflate easily. Surfactant decreases the surface tension within the alveoli and assists even distribution of the gas over all the alveoli. When surfactant is absent or decreased, lung inflation becomes much more difficult.

Lung compliance. Compliance is a measure of the elasticity of the lungs and the thorax. It is determined by plethysmography. The inspired or expired gas volume (ΔV) and the intrapleural pressure (ΔP) are measured, and ΔV is divided by ΔP (see "Pulmonary Function Tests"). Generally, when the intrapleural pressure is increased by 1 cm H_2O, the lung volume increases 130 ml. Any condition that destroys lung tissue, causes it to become fibrotic or edematous, blocks the alveoli, or in any other way impedes lung expansion and contraction decreases lung compliance.

Diffusion and Perfusion

Once the air reaches the surface of the alveoli, the oxygen must cross the alveolar-capillary membrane and enter the pulmonary arterial system. Likewise the carbon dioxide in the unoxygenated venous blood must cross the alveolar-capillary membrane to be exhaled from the lungs. Diffusion of the gases and perfusion of the alveoli are the two components that must be considered.

Diffusion. Diffusion of gases depends on pressure gradients for exchange. The diffusing capacity of the alveolar-capillary membrane is determined by the volume of gas that diffuses through the membrane each minute, for each millimeter of mercury difference in the pressure across the membrane. The process of diffusion depends on the thickness of the respiratory membrane, the surface area of the membrane, the diffusion coefficients of the gases, and the partial pressure differences of the gases being diffused.

Any changes in the alveolar membrane or the interstitial spaces between the alveoli and the capillary can affect the rate of gas diffusion. The rate of diffusion is inversely proportional to the thickness of the membrane.

The total alveolar surface for a normal adult is approximately 80 square meters (M^2). Pulmonary capillaries cover

Table 2-1
Relative Diffusion Coefficients for Respiratory Gases

Gas	Coefficient
Oxygen	1.00*
Carbon dioxide	20.30
Nitrogen	0.53

*1 is an assigned value against which to evaluate the diffusion rate of the other gases.

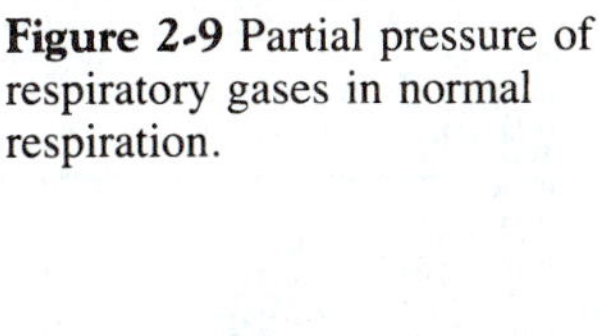

Figure 2-9 Partial pressure of respiratory gases in normal respiration.

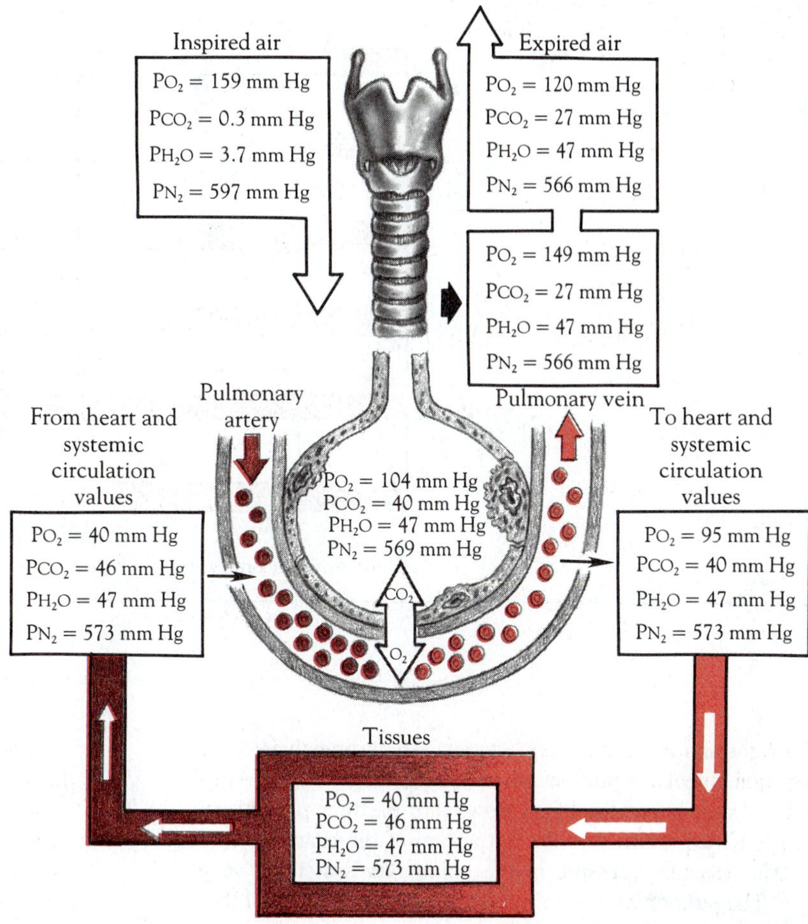

Figure 2-10 Alteration of gas diffusion by varying oxygen concentration.

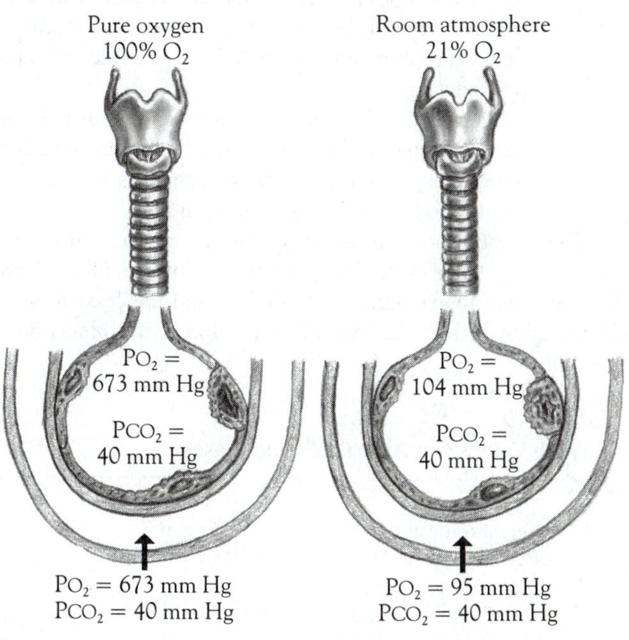

85% to 90% of this surface. Therefore the total surface for gas diffusion is about 70 M^2. Any alteration such as the removal of a lung or emphysema decreases the total surface area available for gas exchange. The pressure that gases exert against a surface is proportional to their concentrations. The diffusion coefficients are shown in Table 2-1.

The process of gas exchange between the air in the alveoli and the blood in the lung capillaries occurs because of a difference in the partial pressures of the gases. Figure 2-9 shows the partial pressures. Each gas diffuses from an area of high partial pressure to an area of low partial pressure.

When the concentration of oxygen is altered, as is done with oxygen therapy, the diffusion partial pressures of the gases are also altered (Figure 2-10).

Perfusion. The major purpose of the pulmonary circulation is to deliver blood in a thin film to the alveoli so oxygen can be taken in and carbon dioxide taken out. The pulmonary vascular system is a high volume–low pressure system. This means that a large amount of blood flows through the lungs and that the capillary resistance to that blood is very low.

Pulmonary circulation begins when carbon dioxide–saturated blood from the right ventricle of the heart drains into

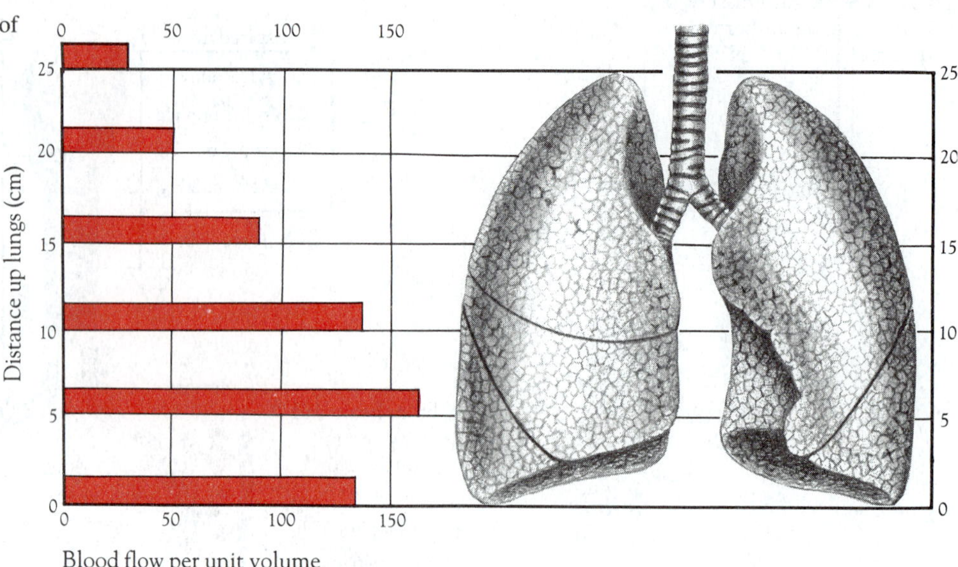

Figure 2-11 Measurements of distribution of blood flow in lungs of individual sitting in an upright position.
Modified from West.[86]

the right and left pulmonary arteries, which branch into the 6 billion alveolar capillaries where gas exchange occurs. After being oxygenated, the blood flows into the four pulmonary veins, which return it to the left atrium of the heart.

The vascular pressure in the pulmonary system is very low. The pulmonary arterial pressure is about one fifth of that within the systemic system. The mean pressure is about 15 mm Hg.

Under normal resting conditions only about 25% of the pulmonary capillaries are actively perfused. As cardiac output increases, the pulmonary arterial pressure remains fairly constant. This is possible because of two mechanisms:

1. Recruitment, which decreases pulmonary vascular resistance and thus permits increased blood flow through the vessels
2. Capillary dilation, which directly increases the capillary size

Both of these mechanisms can adjust to an increase in cardiac output. A malfunction of these mechanisms could lead to pulmonary hypertension. The Swan-Ganz catheter is commonly used to measure the pulmonary arterial pressure.

Common alterations in perfusion

1. Alveolar dead space. Alveolar dead space occurs when breathing is normal but the perfusion of a variable number of alveoli is reduced or absent. Either there is not enough blood, or the blood is blocked from reaching the alveoli. Among the many causes of this are gravitational shifts in pulmonary blood flow in a normal subject and impaired blood flow in an ill patient.[71]
2. Physiologic shunting. Physiologic shunting occurs when the pulmonary circulation is adequate but the air available in the alveoli is inadequate for normal diffusion. Thus part of the blood passing through the pulmonary system does not become oxygenated. Three types of shunting tend to occur:
   a. Anatomic shunting. This is the 2% to 5% of the cardiac output that normally bypasses the pulmonary arterial system. This blood is part of the bronchial, pleural, and coronary circulation.
   b. True shunt. The blood perfuses the alveoli, but for one reason or another the alveoli are totally unventilated. Thus little or no diffusion occurs. Mechanical ventilation may be needed to overcome this type of shunting.
   c. Shunt effect. This occurs when the alveoli are underventilated or the blood flows rapidly through the pulmonary system. Oxygen and perhaps mechanical ventilation help this type of shunting.

The distribution of blood flow throughout the pulmonary system is not uniform. The greatest amount of blood flow occurs in the lower parts of the lungs, and the least flow is in the apex. When the individual is supine, the blood flow

Table 2-2
Normal Values for Arterial Blood Gases

Po_2	90 ± 10 mm Hg
O_2 saturation	96% ± 1%
Pco_2	40 ± 3 mm Hg
pH	7.4 ± 0.03
Bicarbonate	22-26 mEq/L

distribution becomes more even. The distribution of pulmonary blood flow is easily measured by radioisotopes (Figure 2-11).

The arterial blood gases (Table 2-2) indicate the effectiveness of the ventilation, diffusion, and perfusion processes.

Blood Flow: Transportation of the Respiratory Gases

Following the diffusion of the gases at the alveolar level, they must be transported to the tissues for use. The following includes the analysis of oxygen and carbon dioxide movement and a discussion of blood gases that can be used to evaluate gas exchange.

Oxygen. Oxygen in the blood is carried two ways: dissolved in the liquid part of the blood plasma and in chemical combination with hemoglobin. Most oxygen is transported in the second manner.

The amount of dissolved oxygen carried in the plasma is directly proportional to the partial pressure of oxygen (Henry's law). There is 0.003 ml of oxygen dissolved in each 100 ml of blood for each 1 mm Hg partial pressure of oxygen. Thus at an ideal $Pa{O_2}$ of 100 mm Hg, only 0.3 ml of oxygen would be carried per 100 ml of plasma. The individual's normal resting cardiac output is about 5 L/minute.

Most oxygen in the body is transported to the cells in combination with hemoglobin. Oxygen combines loosely and reversibly with the heme portion of hemoglobin. When the $P{O_2}$ is high, as in the pulmonary capillaries, the oxygen readily combines with the hemoglobin. When the $P{O_2}$ is low, as in the tissue capillaries, the oxygen is released from the hemoglobin.

The amount of oxygen carried in the blood by hemoglobin is directly dependent on the concentration of hemoglobin. The average individual has about 15 g of hemoglobin in each 100 ml of blood. Each gram of hemoglobin has the maximum capability to combine with 1.34 ml of oxygen. Therefore a hemoglobin level of 15 g/100 ml would result in 20.1 ml of oxygen combined with hemoglobin and 100% saturation.

$$\frac{15 \text{ g Hb}}{100 \text{ ml blood}} \times \frac{1.34 \text{ ml } O_2}{1 \text{ g Hb}} = \frac{20.1 \text{ ml } O_2}{100 \text{ ml blood}}$$

Tisi[75] discusses three terms that must be differentiated:

1. Oxygen content is the total amount of oxygen carried in both a dissolved and combined state per 100 ml of blood.
2. Oxygen capacity is the maximum amount of oxygen that can be carried in both states per 100 ml of blood.
3. Percent saturation is the relationship between the amount of oxygen that is carried and the amount of oxygen that can be carried.

$$\text{Saturation} = \frac{\text{Content (amount dissolved)}}{\text{Capacity (amount dissolved)}} = \frac{\text{"Is"}}{\text{"Can"}}$$

The amount of oxygen combined with hemoglobin depends on the partial pressure of oxygen dissolved in the arterial blood ($Pa{O_2}$). The oxygen content at different partial pressures that combines with the hemoglobin is shown in the oxyhemoglobin dissociation curve (Figure 2-12). When the blood leaves the lungs, the $Pa{O_2}$ is about 100 mm Hg and the percent

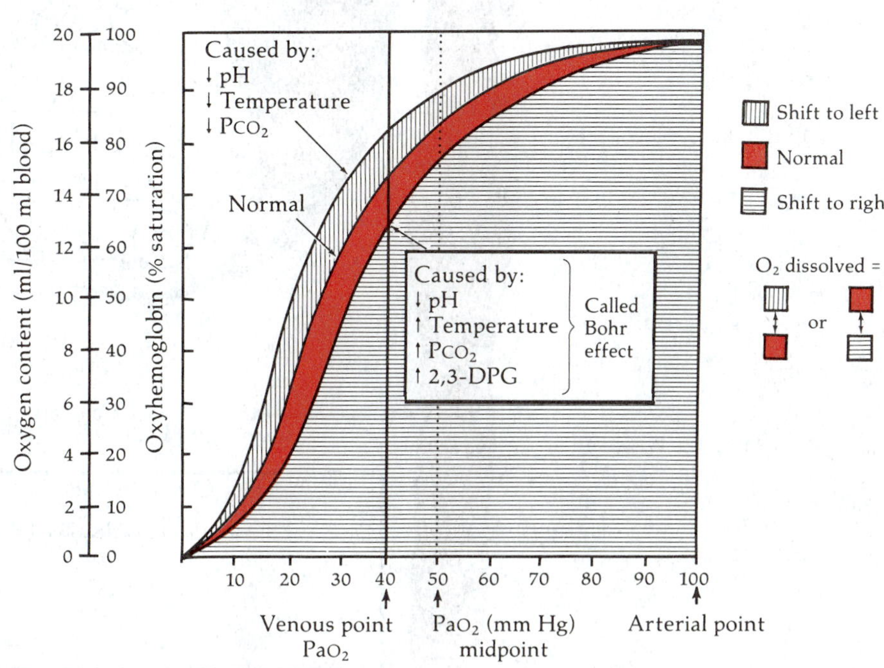

Figure 2-12 Oxyhemoglobin dissociation curve with pH 7.4 and temperature 98.6° F (37° C).
Modified from Guenter.[35]

saturation is 97.5. In normal mixed venous blood the $P\bar{v}O_2$ is about 40 mm Hg with a 75% saturation. Tisi points out three important areas along the curve: (1) at a $P\bar{v}O_2$ of 40 mm Hg the percent saturation is 75, (2) at a PaO_2 of 50 mm Hg the percent saturation is about 84, and (3) at a PaO_2 of 100 mm Hg the percent saturation is 97.5.[75] On the steep portion of the curve, between points 1 and 2, for every 10 mm Hg change in PO_2 there is a 10% saturation change. Note that between points 2 and 3 there is a 50 mm Hg change in the PO_2 but only a 13% change in saturation.

Various shifts in body functioning can also cause changes in the oxyhemoglobin dissociation curve (Figure 2-12). Shifts to the right are produced by a decrease in pH, a rise in $PaCO_2$, and an increase in body temperature. The curve can also be shifted to the right by an increase in 2,3-diphosphoglycerate (DPG) inside the red blood cells, which occurs as a result of prolonged hypoxia. A dissociation curve that shifts to the right means that something has weakened the hemoglobin's ability to hold on to oxygen and that higher gas pressure is needed for binding. Oxygen escapes hemoglobin more easily and is more available to the tissues.

Shifts to the left are produced by an increase in pH, a decrease in $PaCO_2$, and a decrease in body temperature. This shift may be important in explaining the difference between

Figure 2-13 Transport of carbon dioxide and other gases in the blood.

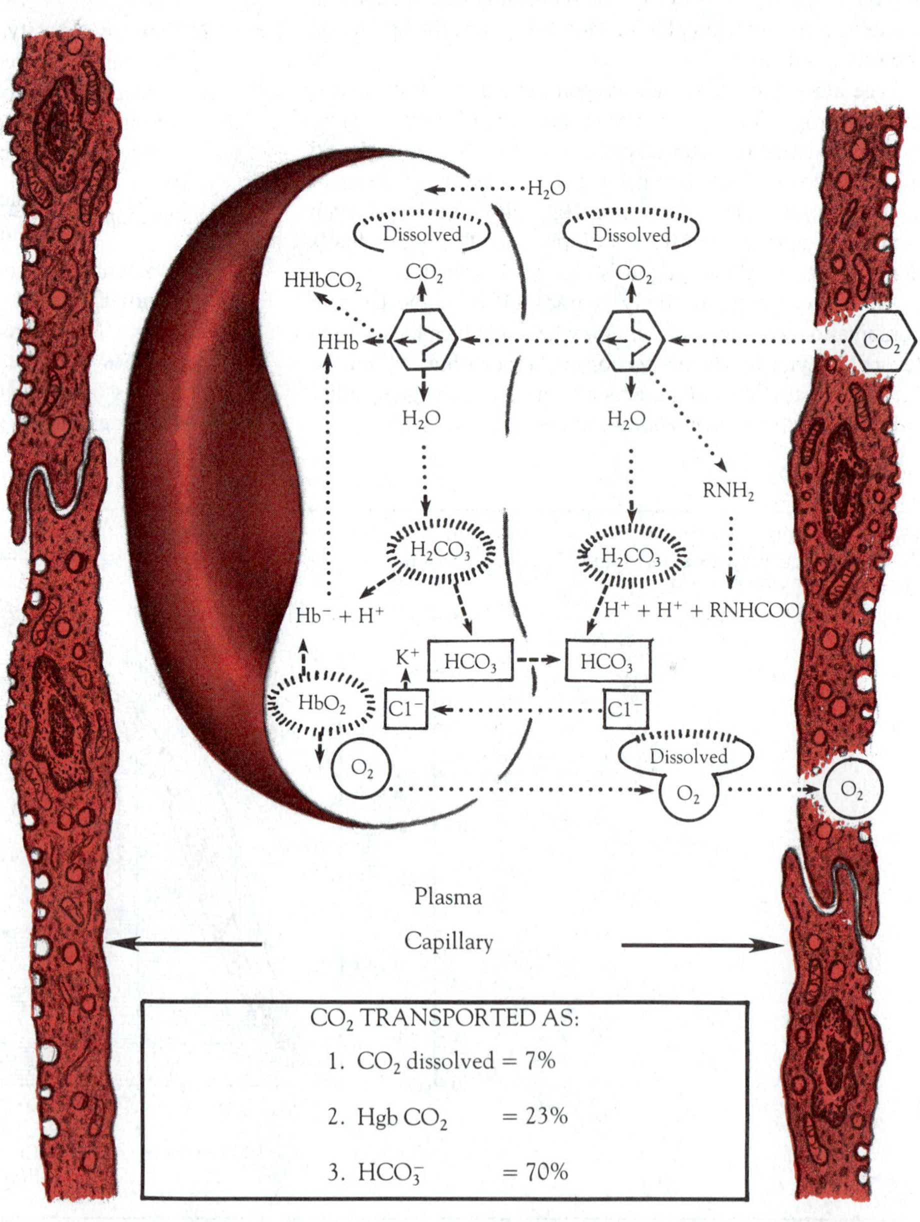

a patient's appearance and the arterial blood gas results. When there is a shift to the left, something has happened to increase the affinity of hemoglobin for oxygen. The hemoglobin holds the oxygen more firmly than normal, and although less pressure is needed to bind the two, it is more difficult to separate them at the cellular level.

Carbon dioxide. Carbon dioxide transport must be understood clearly because the amount of carbon dioxide in transit helps determine the acid-base balance of the body.[72] Most carbon dioxide is carried in three plasma and three erythrocyte compartments. In plasma it is bound to protein to form carbamino compounds, as a bicarbonate (HCO_3^-), and in physical solution dissolved in plasma. In erythrocytes it is dissolved in erythrocyte water, combined with the amino group of carbaminohemoglobin, and converts to carbonic acid (H_2CO_3). The carbonic acid further dissociates to form hydrogen and bicarbonate ions ([H^+] and [HCO_3^-]). Figure 2-13 summarizes the transport of carbon dioxide in the blood.

Just as the relationship between blood Pao_2 and oxygen saturation of hemoglobin was expressed by the oxygen saturation curve, so there is a relationship between blood $Paco_2$ and the whole blood content of carbon dioxide, which is calculated in volume percent. The carbon dioxide dissociation curve as seen in Figure 2-14 shows this relationship. The purpose of the curves is to show how carbon dioxide dissociates from, or leaves, the blood as its partial pressure drops. The curves also show that as the amount of carbon dioxide in the blood increases, so does the tension. When examining these curves note the influence of oxygen saturation (So_2) on the $Paco_2$ content ratio. This influence, referred to as the Haldane effect, demonstrates that So_2 determines the course of carbon dioxide dissociation.[72] Figure 2-14 shows some parts of the curves to include the range of $Paco_2$ from the arterial point, with a $Paco_2$ of 40 mm Hg, So_2 of 97.5%, and carbon dioxide content of 48 vol%, to the venous point, with a Pco_2 of 46 mm Hg, So_2 of 70%, and carbon dioxide content of 53 vol%.[72] Since oxygen saturation changes from arterial to venous blood, the true carbon dioxide dissociation curve must lie somewhere between these two curves.

Figure 2-14 Carbon dioxide dissociation curve.
Modified from Tisi.[75]

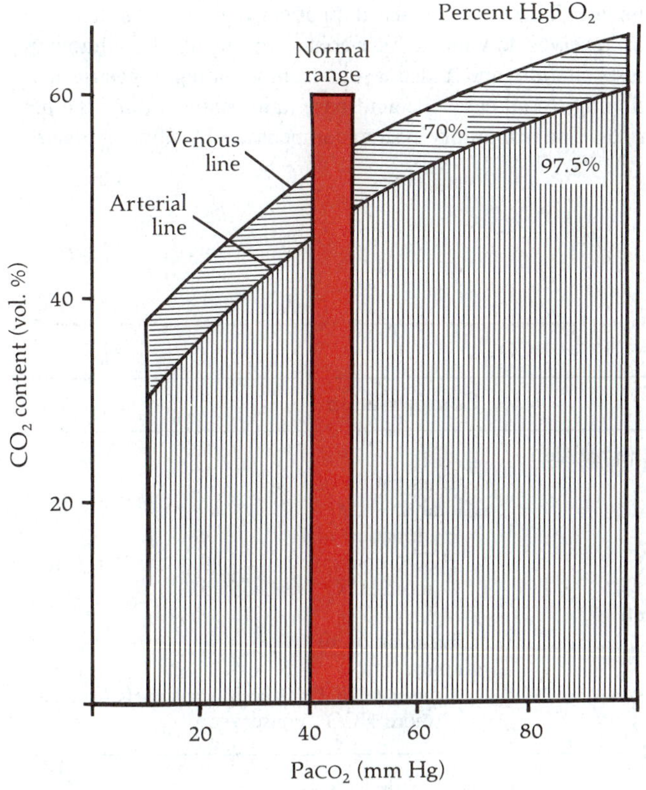

Acid-Base Balance and Blood Gases

The term *acid-base balance* refers to the ratio between carbonic acid and its salt, sodium bicarbonate. For body cells to function best, body fluids and blood must remain within a specific, narrow acid-base balance (pH). Deviations of body pH outside this narrow range interfere with cellular metabolism and can cause cell death. Interactions of substances in the body should produce a hydrogen ion concentration sufficient to maintain a blood pH of 7.35 to 7.45. This normal acid-base balance is maintained by respiration and kidney function. The respiratory system determines the carbon dioxide concentration, thereby regulating the hydrogen ion concentration. The renal system uses buffering mechanisms to regulate bicarbonate concentration. Following is the Henderson-Hasselbach equation for the calculation of blood pH:

$$pH = pK^* + \log \frac{\text{Base}}{\text{Acid}}$$

$$(1)\quad \frac{HCO_3^-}{H_2CO_3} = \frac{25.4 \text{ mEq/L}}{1.27 \text{ mEq/L}} = \frac{20}{1}$$

$$(2)\quad \text{Blood pK} = 6.1$$

$$pH = 6.1 + \log \frac{20}{1}$$

$$pH = 6.1 + 1.3 = 7.4$$

Blood pH depends on the ratio of bicarbonate to dissolved carbon dioxide. As long as that ratio is 20:1, the pH is 7.4. If the blood pH falls below the normal range, becoming less alkaline, acidemia occurs. If the pH is above normal, becoming more alkaline, alkalemia occurs.[1]

The body also has a buffer system that modifies large hydrogen ion concentrations to prevent wide swings in the pH. The buffering occurs mainly in the plasma and the eryth-

*The pK is the pH at which the substance is half dissociated and half undissociated.

rocytes. The carbonic acid–sodium bicarbonate buffer in the plasma is by far the most important of the buffers.[72]

Two types of disorders can cause an acid-base imbalance: respiratory disorders and metabolic disorders. An acid-base imbalance is referred to as acidosis or alkalosis. Acidosis caused by a respiratory disease is marked by an elevated arterial carbon dioxide tension. When acidosis has a metabolic cause, arterial bicarbonate concentration is lowered. Alkalosis is marked by lowered arterial carbon dioxide tension when it is the result of a respiratory disease and by an elevated arterial bicarbonate concentration when it is caused by a metabolic problem.

Disorders of the respiratory system upset the denominator of the acid-base ratio because ventilation disrupts the blood carbon dioxide concentration, and the body attempts to adjust the numerator. Metabolic disorders upset the numerator of the ratio because the bicarbonate is either raised or lowered, and compensation attempts to adjust the denominator.[72]

Acidosis states

Respiratory acidosis (↓ pH, ↑ Pa_{CO_2}). Respiratory acidosis is the result of alveolar hypoventilation. This may occur in response to cardiopulmonary, neuromuscular, skeletal, or obstructive lung disease, to acute infections, or to the actions of drugs such as narcotics or sedatives. The partial pressure of arterial carbon dioxide increases and pH drops.

The body attempts to compensate for the raised Pa_{CO_2} in two ways: by immediately trying to chemically buffer the excess hydrogen ions as they are produced, and by removing excess hydrogen ion in the urine in exchange for bicarbonate ions. The bicarbonate ions are concentrated in the blood plasma, where they help to restore the acid-base ratio and thus return the pH to normal. Through the process of compensation the patient may still have a raised Pa_{CO_2}, even though the pH may have returned to normal.[37]

Metabolic acidosis (↓ pH, ↓ HCO_3^-). Metabolic acidosis is caused in one of two ways: through the increase of fixed metabolic acids or through the loss of bicarbonate in the body fluids.

Examples of the first cause include salicylate poisoning, renal failure, diabetic ketoacidosis, and circulatory failure that produces a buildup of lactic acid. Persistent diarrhea, for example, causes bicarbonate loss. In all situations of acidosis the body responds to the increase in body acids by using bicarbonate ions as a buffer. As a result the bicarbonate levels are low. To compensate, the respiratory system increases ventilation and the kidneys retain bicarbonate. Table 2-3 summarizes this process.

Alkalosis states

Respiratory alkalosis (↑ pH, ↓ Pa_{CO_2}). Respiratory alkalosis occurs when excess amounts of carbon dioxide are exhaled. Alveolar hyperventilation removes carbon dioxide from the blood, decreasing the Pa_{CO_2} and elevating the pH. Hyperventilation from anxiety is perhaps the best example. Other causes of alkalosis include brain injury or brain tumors, gram-negative sepsis, and improper management of the patient attached to a ventilator.

The body attempts to compensate by increasing kidney excretion of bicarbonate, retaining chloride, and reducing the formation of ammonia and excretion of acid salts. These mechanisms lower the blood bicarbonate level and thus bring the acid-base ratio back into balance.[72]

Metabolic alkalosis (↑ pH, ↑ HCO_3^-). Metabolic alkalosis is caused by an increase in the body's level of bicarbonate. This occurs when the patient ingests too much base or receives too much bicarbonate during cardiopulmonary resuscitation, and it also results from vomiting or gastric suctioning. In all cases the acid-base ratio is altered, and the pH rises. The respiratory system compensates by slowing breath-

Table 2-3
Summary of the Acidosis Process

$$CO_2 + H_2O = H_2CO_3 = H^+ + HCO_3^-$$

	Initial Cause	Buffering	Compensation
Respiratory acidosis	↑ P_{CO_2}	Reaction moves to right to handle excess CO_2* ↑ HCO_3^-	Lungs Elimination of CO_2 Kidneys Elimination of H^+ HCO_3^- conserved (the higher the P_{CO_2}, the more HCO_3^- reabsorbed)
Metabolic acidosis	↓ Base ↑ Fixed acids	Reaction moves to the left to handle excess H^+ ↓ HCO_3^-	Lungs Elimination of CO_2 Kidneys Conserve HCO_3^- (the lower the HCO_3^-, the more HCO_3^- conserved)

From Harper.[37]
*Movement to the right refers to moving from the left side of the equation above to the right side, therefore decreasing CO_2 production.

Table 2-4
Summary of Alkalosis Process

$$CO_2 + H_2O = H_2CO_3 = H^+ + HCO_3^-$$

	Initial Cause	Buffering	Compensation
Respiratory alkalosis	↓ P_{CO_2}	Movement to left to form more CO_2* ↓ HCO_3^-	Kidneys Conservation of H^+ HCO_3^- excretion (the lower the P_{CO_2}, the less HCO_3^- reabsorbed)
Metabolic alkalosis	↑ Base ↓ Fixed acids	Movement to right to form more H^+ to offset increased base HCO_3^- ↑	Lungs ↓ Ventilation to ↑ P_{CO_2} Kidneys Conserve H^+ by excreting HCO_3^- (the higher the plasma HCO_3^-, the greater the HCO_3^- excretion)

From Harper.[37]
*Movement to the left refers to moving from the right side of the equation above to the left side, therefore increasing CO_2 production.

ing. This conserves carbon dioxide and raises the Pa_{CO_2}. The kidneys respond by increasing the removal of bicarbonate ions, thereby conserving hydrogen ions. As a result the pH decreases to normal levels. Table 2-4 summarizes these processes.

Control of Breathing

In the past, the control of ventilation was believed to be in a single respiratory center located in the medulla of the brain. However, recent studies more clearly indicate that the control mechanisms of breathing are complex and not entirely understood. The following discussion represents those factors generally accepted to be the prime determinants of ventilation.[72]

There are at least three respiratory centers: one in the medulla and two in the pons. In addition, there is a less well-located area in the medulla containing chemoreceptors. Similar chemoreceptors are found among the peripheral stimulators, along with reflexes from the lung and many other organs and tissues.

The medullary center is the final determinant of breathing patterns. It responds to the autonomic and voluntary stimuli of the higher centers of the cerebral cortex. The medullary center has two major functions: it coordinates data continuously received from sensory, gas exchange, and chemical units in the body, matching these needs and influences to determine the breathing pattern, and it sends nerve impulses to the two subcenters responsible for the muscles that control inspiration and expiration.

The chemoreceptors in the medulla as seen in Figure 2-15 are groups of specialized nerve cells that differentiate between concentrations of hydrogen ions and oxygen. The medulla chemoreceptors, also called central chemoreceptors, are the primary receptors. Other chemoreceptors, called peripheral chemoreceptors, are located at many body locations including the carotid arteries and the aortic arch. All chemoreceptors function basically the same way. They respond to the concentration of either oxygen or hydrogen ions crossing their membranes to send ventilatory stimulus impulses to the medullary center.

The two breathing centers in the pons are the apneustic center and the pneumotaxic center. The apneustic center, in the lower part of the pons, is also called the pontine center. Apneusis is a condition in which ventilation stops in the inspiratory position. The apneustic center is controlled by the pneumotaxic center and the inflation reflexes. Diseases of the pons may lead to abnormal stimulation of the apneustic center and apneustic breathing.

The pneumotaxic center controls the effect of the apneustic center and encourages rhythmic breathing. It is thought that the pneumotaxic center receives impulses from the medullary inspiratory subcenter and sends impulses to the medullary expiratory subcenter, thus limiting inspiration.

An inflation reflex, called the Hering-Breuer reflex, carries impulses from the lung to the brain through the vagus nerve. This stretch reflex, originating in the bronchiolar or alveolar walls, modifies the apneustic center's action by limiting inhalation and by helping the medullary center establish a smooth and easy combination of tidal volume and rate.

In addition to these major areas, there are many other reflexes that respond to pain, temperature, tissue pressure and stretch, and circulatory dynamics.

In summary, the greatest influences on the autonomic nervous system's ventilation control come from the blood's hydrogen ion concentration and oxygen content stimulation of the medullary center's chemoreceptors. These help correlate breathing with acid-base balance and with gas exchange needs. The whole breathing control system can be overridden by higher areas of the cerebral cortex.

Figure 2-15 Respiratory control system.

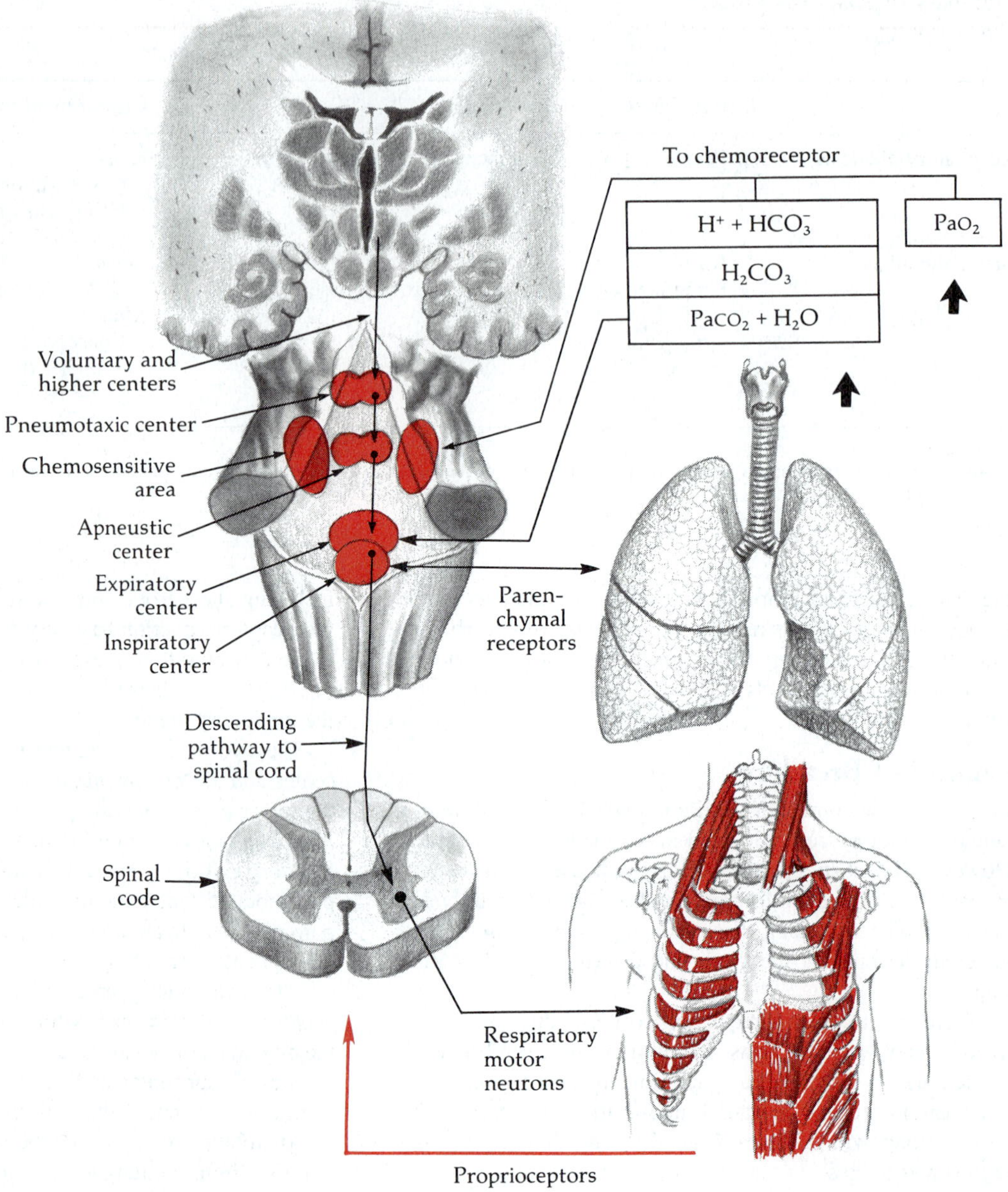

Normal Findings

Area of Concern	Normal Adult Findings
General appearance	Appears relaxed Breathing is quiet and easy without apparent effort Facial expressions and limb movements are relaxed
Breathing pattern	Diaphragmatic-thoracic pattern is smooth and regular May have occasional sighing respirations Breathing is quiet and passive *Older adult:* pattern is same as for adults, but calcification at rib articulation points may decrease chest expansion

Area of Concern	Normal Adult Findings
Respiratory rate	12-20 resp/min Ratio of pulse to respirations is 4:1
Skin	Appears well oxygenated; no cyanosis or pallor present Palpation of skin and chest wall reveals smooth skin and a stable chest wall; there are no crepitations, bulging, or painful spots
Nail bed, nail configuration	Minimum angulation between base of nail and finger No thickening of distal finger width
Chest wall configuration (Figure 2-16)	Symmetric, bilateral muscle development A:P to transverse ratio is 1:2 to 5:7; larger than these ratios is considered to be barrel chest Straight spinal processes Downward and equal slope of ribs; costal angle 90 degrees or less Deviation of chest wall configuration discussed in Chapter 4 (Figure 2-16) *Older adult:* kyphosis is a common finding in elderly persons; there is dorsal scoliosis with slight tracheal deviation; this may also cause a slight increase in A:P to transverse ratio
Tracheal position	Midline and straight directly above the suprasternal notch *Older adult:* may be slightly deviated if kyphosis is present
Vocal fremitus	Bilaterally equal mild sensation More intense vibratory feeling in upper posterior wall medial to scapula See box below
Respiratory excursion	Bilaterally equal expansion of ribs during deep inspiration *Older adult:* depth of breath may be less than in younger adult, but response should be the same
Percussion	Resonance heard throughout lung fields; see Figure 2-17 and Table 2-5 for percussion tone characteristics Percussion of diaphragmatic excursion should measure 4 to 6 cm; inhaled position is approximately at tenth posterior rib level
Auscultation	Quiet breathing heard throughout all lung fields; Figure 2-18 shows normal sounds heard in each lung field, and Table 2-6 describes the normal and abnormal breath and voice sounds *Older adult:* lung elasticity is diminished resulting in decreased pulmonary compliance; airway resistance increases

Overview of Vocal Fremitus

Vocal fremitus is the sensation of sound vibrations produced when the patient speaks.

The examiner may feel for these vibrations by placing the extended hand gently on the chest wall. The spoken voice produces low-frequency vibrations through the vocal cords, the airways, and the pleura. These vibrations are felt and compared bilaterally.

The examiner instructs the patient to say "one-two-three" or "how-now-brown-cow." As these words are spoken, the examiner feels for the vibrations.

Abnormal responses

Increased fremitus. An increase in the vibratory sensation is felt when there is consolidation of the lung caused by fluid-filled or solid structures, which would transmit the vibrations better than air-filled lungs. This occurs, for example, with pneumonia or a tumor of the lung.

Decreased fremitus. A decrease in the vibratory sensation is felt when more air than normal is blocked or trapped in the lungs or pleural space; vibrations of the spoken voice are decreased. This occurs, for example, with emphysema or a pneumothorax.

Table 2-5
Percussion Tones Heard over Chest

Type of Tone	Intensity	Pitch	Duration	Quality
Resonant	Loud	Low	Long	Hollow
Flat	Soft	High	Short	Extremely dull
Dull	Medium	Medium-high	Medium	Thudlike
Tympanic	Loud	High	Medium	Drumlike
Hyperresonant*	Very loud	Very low	Longer	Booming

*Hyperresonance is abnormal sound heard during percussion in adults. It represents air trapping such as occurs in obstructive lung diseases.

Figure 2-16 Landmarks and structures of chest wall. **A,** Anterior view. **B,** Posterior view.

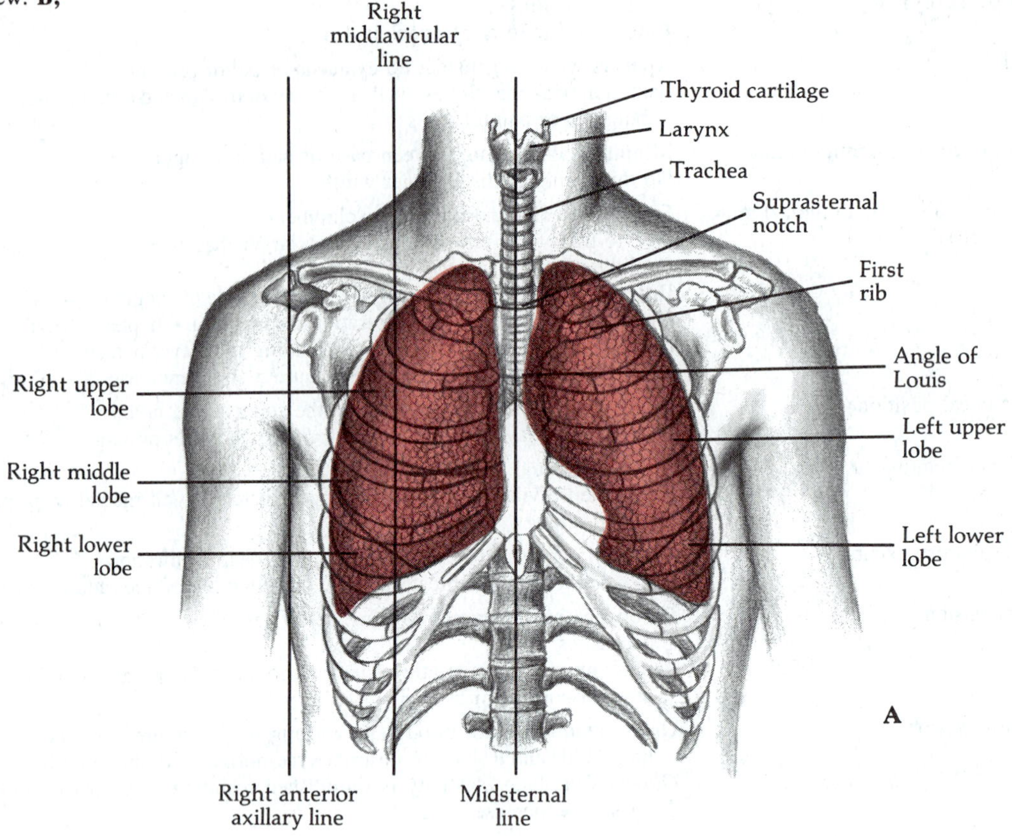

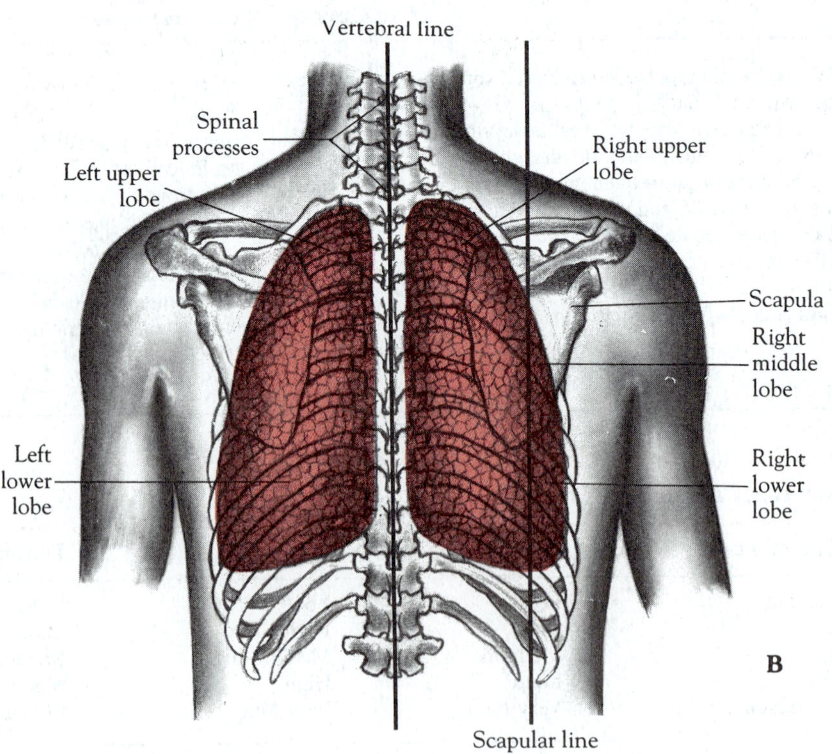

Figure 2-17 Percussion tones. **A,** Anterior view. **B,** Posterior view.

Resonance
Flat over heavy muscles and bones
Cardiac dullness
Liver dullness
Stomach tympany
Flat over spinous process
Flat over scapula and heavy muscles
B
Visceral flatness

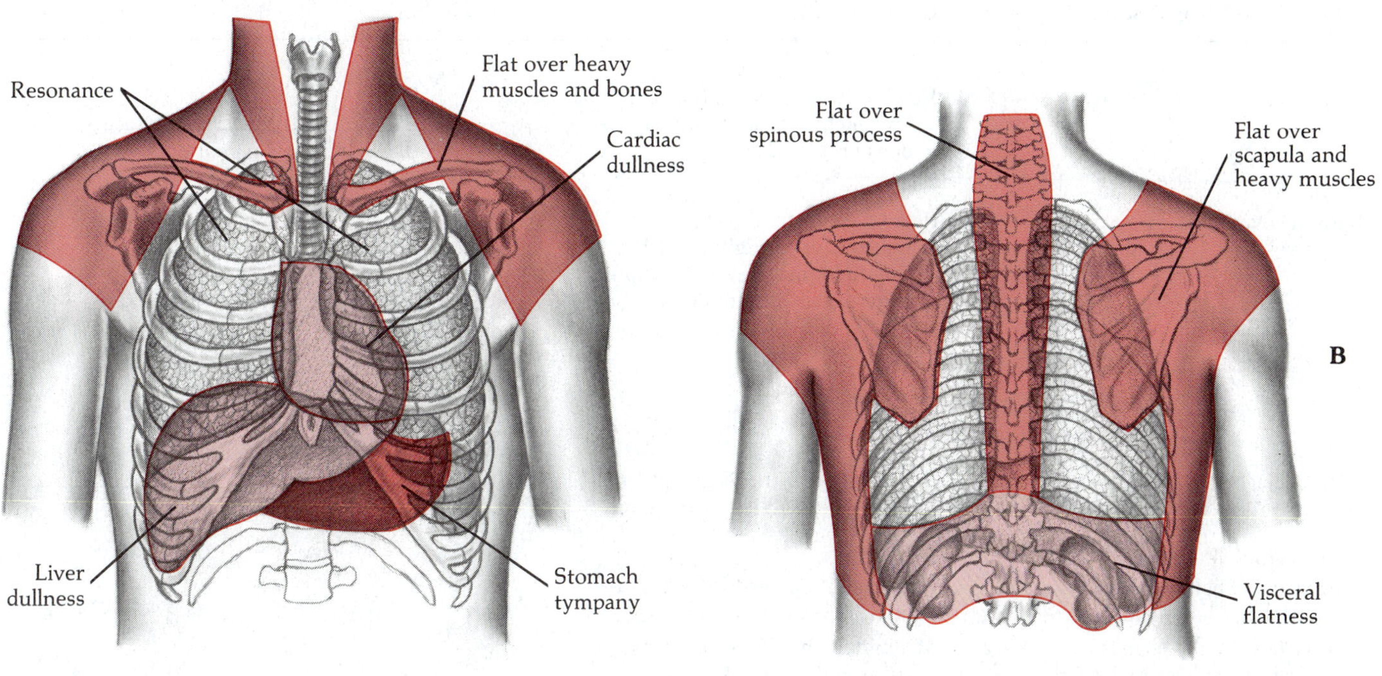

Figure 2-18 Normal auscultatory sounds. **A,** Anterior view. **B,** Posterior view.

KEY:
Bronchovesicular over main bronchi
Vesicular over lesser bronchi, bronchioles, and lobes
Bronchial over trachea
A
B

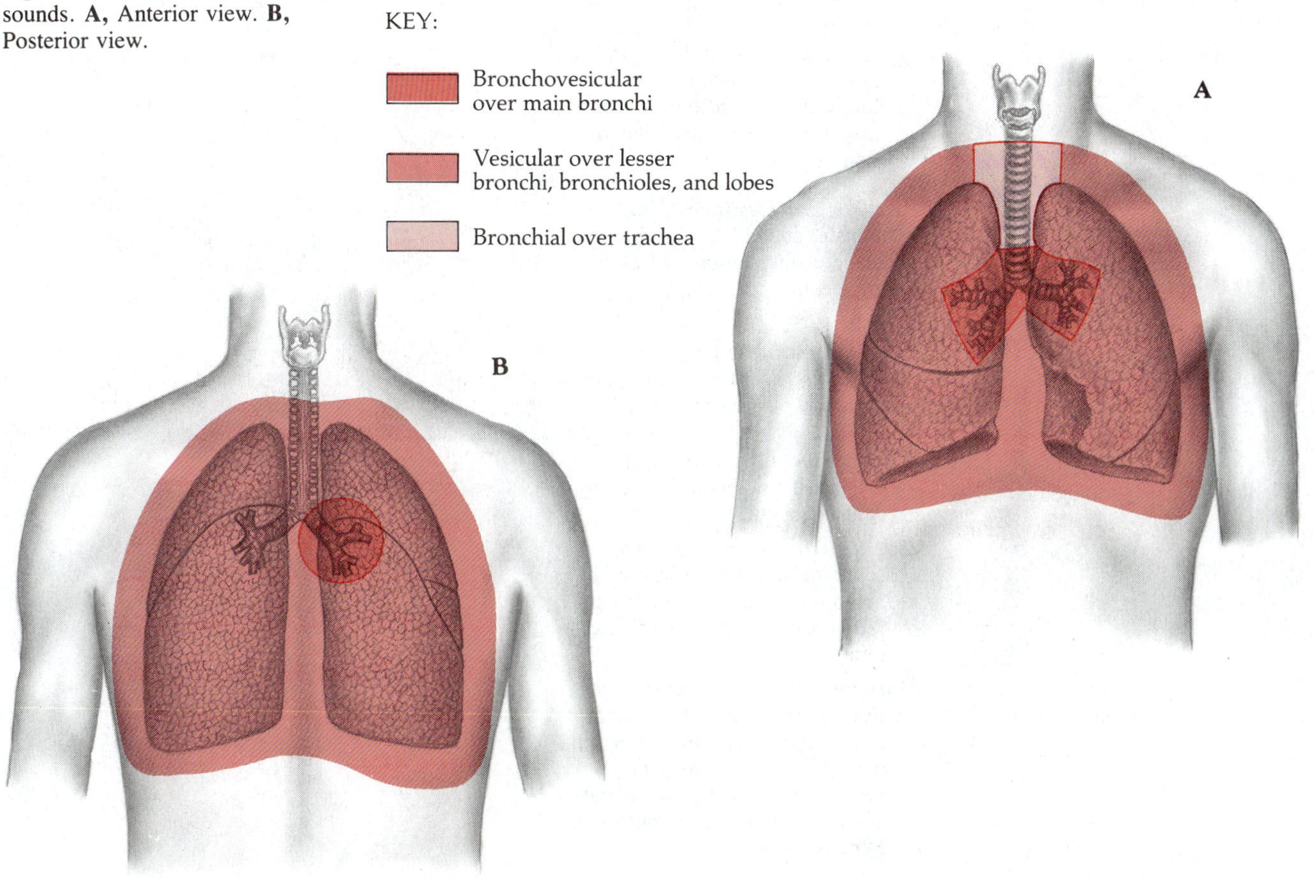

Table 2-6
Breath and Voice Sounds: Normal and Abnormal

Breath and Voice Sounds	Characteristics	Findings
Normal		
Vesicular	Heard over most of lung fields; low pitch; soft and short expirations (Figure 2-18)	Low pitch, soft expirations
Bronchovesicular	Heard over main bronchus area and over upper right posterior lung field; medium pitch; expiration equals inspiration	Medium pitch, medium expirations
Bronchial	Heard only over trachea; high pitch; loud and long expirations	High pitch, loud expirations
Abnormal		
Bronchial when heard over peripheral lung fields	High pitch; loud and long expirations	
Bronchovesicular sounds when heard over peripheral lung fields	Medium pitch with inspirations equal to expirations	
Adventitious	Crackles: discrete, noncontinuous sounds	
	Fine crackles (rales): high-pitched, discrete, noncontinuous crackling sounds heard during end of inspiration (indicates inflammation or congestion)	
	Medium crackles (rales): lower, moister sound heard during midstage of inspiration; not cleared by a cough	
	Coarse crackles (rales): loud, bubbly noise heard during inspiration; not cleared by a cough	
	Wheezes: continuous musical sounds; if low pitched, may be called rhonchi	
	Sibilant wheeze: musical noise sounding like a squeak; may be heard during inspiration or expiration; usually louder during expiration	
	Sonorous wheeze (rhonchi): loud, low, coarse sound like a snore heard at any point of inspiration or expiration; coughing may clear sound (usually means mucus accumulation in trachea or large bronchi)	

Table 2-6—cont'd
Breath and Voice Sounds: Normal and Abnormal

Breath and Voice Sounds	Characteristics	Findings
	Pleural friction rub: dry, rubbing, or grating sound, usually due to inflammation of pleural surfaces; heard during inspiration or expiration; loudest over lower lateral anterior surface	
Resonance of spoken voice	*Bronchophony:* using diaphragm of stethoscope, listen to posterior chest as patient says "ninety-nine"	Negative response: muffled "nin-nin" sound heard Positive response: clear, loud "ninety-nine" response heard because lung tissue is consolidated
	Whispered pectoriloquy: listen to posterior chest as patient whispers "one, two, three"	Negative response: muffled sounds heard Positive response: clear "one, two, three" is heard because of lung consolidation
	Egophony: listen to posterior chest as the patient says "e-e-e"	Negative response: muffled "e-e-e" sound heard Positive response: sound of "e" changes to "a-a-a" sound because of consolidation

Common Abnormal Findings

Cough. Cough is one of the important body reflexes. It is intended to maintain airway patency by eliminating materials accumulated or deposited on the mucosa of the respiratory tract, such as tracheobronchial secretions, blood, aspirated substances, and other foreign bodies. A nonproductive cough may be the result of acute inflammation of the respiratory mucosal membranes, the presence of a growth, or a reflex initiated in other areas.

The cough reflex is mediated through sensory interventions of cranial nerves X (vagus), IX (glossopharyngeal), and occasionally V (trigeminal), as well as motor nerves of the larynx and respiratory muscles. The cough reflex is in the medulla.

Although a common symptom, cough has limited diagnostic value. Only changes in the characteristics of the cough and expectoration are of concern. For smokers a change in the cough may be due to infection or a malignant neoplasm. Chronic cough among nonsmokers is more significant and diagnostically more helpful. It often suggests the presence of a serious underlying bronchopulmonary disease such as tuberculosis, bronchiectasis, or neoplasm. Cough of recent onset frequently is due to an acute infection of the larynx, trachea, bronchi, lung, or pleura.

The intensity of cough has no relationship to the severity or seriousness of underlying bronchopulmonary disease. It is not unusual for a patient with serious pulmonary disease to have minimal or no cough. On the other hand, a mild viral infection involving the trachea or the bronchi may cause a troublesome cough.[24]

Expectoration. Expectoration is the act of coughing up and spitting material raised from the lower respiratory tract. Sputum consists of secretions formed continuously by the mucous glands and the goblet cells of the tracheobronchial tree. The cilia along the mucosal lining of the bronchi propel the thin mucus secretions toward the upper airway.

In pathologic conditions, increased tracheobronchial secretions may be due to the stimulation of normal secretory cells or to an increase in the number of these cells. In acute situations, increased sputum production is the result of transient stimulation of mucous glands and goblet cells.

In addition to mucus, expectorated material may contain other fluids from various sites in the respiratory tract, including the alveoli. It may contain white blood cells accumulated for the purpose of fighting infection, necrotic material from tissue death, blood, aspirated vomitus, or other foreign material.

The gross appearance of sputum may suggest the underlying condition. Yellow sputum generally indicates the presence of large numbers of white blood cells, which are the major component of pus. Green discoloration signifies the production of an enzyme from stagnant pus cells. Red or brownish sputum is usually due to the presence of red blood cells.[24]

Dyspnea. Dyspnea is a shortness of breath or a difficulty in breathing. The awareness of breathing may range in intensity from mild discomfort to extreme distress. Dyspnea, like pain, is a subjective sign that is likely to be influenced by the patient's reaction, sensitivity, and emotional state. Dyspnea involves both a physiologic and a cognitive component.

Dyspnea as a result of increased work of breathing occurs under numerous clinical conditions. Some basic causes are increased airway resistance, as in upper airway obstruction, asthma, and other chronic obstructive pulmonary diseases; reduced pulmonary compliance as a result of pulmonary fibrosis, congestion, edema, and a variety of other parenchymal lung diseases; mechanical interference with the expansion of the lungs because of massive pleural effusion of pneumothorax; and abnormality of chest wall and respiratory muscles resulting in inefficient and wasteful respiratory efforts.

The circumstance in which the symptom occurs has diagnostic importance. Breathlessness may occur with certain body positions. Orthopnea refers to dyspnea upon lying down. Paroxysmal nocturnal dyspnea is the sudden onset of shortness of breath during the night. This occurs in cardiac patients. The cause is thought to be transient pulmonary congestion or edema.

A recent increase in dyspnea in a patient with chronic respiratory disease is indicative of an acute event. This may be due to increased airway resistance as with bronchospasm, secretions, and infection or to reduced pulmonary compliance as with pulmonary congestion or edema.[24]

Hemoptysis. Hemoptysis is the expectoration of blood originating from the respiratory tract below the pharynx. Blood-tinged or blood-streaked sputum is not usually called hemoptysis. Hemoptysis is the coughing up of a quantifiable amount of blood (as much as 600 ml within 24 hours), pure or mixed with sputum.

The causes of hemoptysis are many, and almost any pulmonary lesion may lead to it. The three major basic underlying pathologic conditions are infection, neoplasm, and cardiovascular disease. Common infectious causes of hemoptysis are pneumonia, tuberculosis, bronchiectasis, lung abscess, fungal infection, and parasitic lung diseases. Bronchogenic carcinoma is the neoplastic disease most commonly causing hemoptysis. Hemoptysis is a symptom of certain cardiovascular diseases, such as pulmonary embolism, congestive heart failure, and mitral stenosis.[24]

Chest pain. Chest pain of pulmonary origin can derive from the chest wall, parietal pleura, or visceral pleura. The thoracic wall is the most common source of chest pain; skin, muscles, nerves, and bones may be its cause in association with various clinical conditions. The lung parenchyma is insensitive to painful stimuli, and only the parietal layer of the pleura is very pain sensitive. Its direct or indirect involvement by various pathologic processes commonly causes a dull, constant ache or poorly localized chest pain. Pain with pneumonia and the other inflammatory diseases of the lung is usually due to pleural reaction. In lung cancer the chest pain is frequently indicative of pleural reaction or chest wall invasion.

Pulmonary arterial hypertension sometimes causes chest pain because of increased tension of arterial walls or strain of the right side of the heart muscle. The sudden and transient chest pain of pulmonary embolism results from a pleural reaction.

Pleuritic pain is a well-localized, constant ache or sharp chest pain that is produced or aggravated by deep breathing or other chest wall movement.[24]

Normal Laboratory Data

Laboratory Test	Normal Adult Values
Whole Blood	
pH	
Arterial range	7.35-7.45 (average 7.4)
Venous range	7.32-7.43
P_{CO_2}	
Arterial range	35-45 mm Hg (average 40 mm Hg)
Venous range	35-50 mm Hg
P_{O_2}	
Arterial range	80-95 mm Hg (average 95 mm Hg)
HCO_3^-	
Arterial range	21-28 mEq/L
Venous range	22-29 mEq/L
S_{O_2}	
Arterial range	95%-99% (average 97%)
Venous range	60%-85% (average 75%)
Pulmonary artery	75%-80%
O_2 content	
Arterial range	17-21 ml/100 ml or 17-21 vol%
Venous range	10-16 ml/100 ml or 10-16 vol%
CO_2 content	
Arterial range	22-29 mEq/L
Venous range	23-30 mEq/L
Plasma	
CO_2 content	
Arterial range	21-30 mEq/L
Venous range	24-34 mEq/L
Hemoglobin	
CO saturation (carboxyhemoglobin)	
Nonsmoker	0-2%
Smoker	3%-5%
Heavy smoker	9%-10%

Conditions, Diseases, and Disorders

Respiratory Insufficiency, Respiratory Failure

The precise definition of respiratory insufficiency leading to respiratory failure is a condition in which the arterial Pco_2 is above 50 mm Hg when the patient is at rest and breathing room air or in which the Pao_2 is less than 55 mm Hg.[34]

Respiratory insufficiency refers to the inability of the lungs to maintain adequate gas exchange. That is, not enough oxygen is taken up through ventilation to remove enough carbon dioxide to maintain normal partial pressures of these gases in the arterial blood. Respiratory insufficiency left untreated results in respiratory failure and thus physiologic decompensation.

Respiratory insufficiency and respiratory failure are not diseases but more correctly are disorders of ventilation that may be caused by many conditions either directly or indirectly.

Respiratory insufficiency and failure may be divided into three types.

Type I. Causes of severe hypoxemia with an abnormally low $Paco_2$ include the following:

1. Increased pulmonary capillary pressure resulting from such conditions as the following
   a. Left ventricular heart failure
   b. Pulmonary edema or fluid overload
2. Increased pulmonary capillary permeability from such conditions as the following
   a. Pneumonia
   b. Tuberculosis
   c. Fungal infections
   d. Near-drowning
   e. Chemical or smoke inhalation
   f. Liquid aspiration

In its most severe state, acute respiratory failure is referred to as adult respiratory distress syndrome (ARDS).

Type II. In type II respiratory failure the diseased lung is unable to remove carbon dioxide normally. Usually this occurs in some type of chronic breathing problem linked to such conditions as the following:

1. Chronic bronchitis
2. Emphysema
3. Massive obesity
4. Severe kyphoscoliosis
5. Asthma

Type III. The third type of respiratory failure is caused by the inability of the neuromuscular system to ventilate normal or nearly normal lungs. There are two basic causes for this:

1. Respiratory center depression caused by a malfunctioning central nervous system, which can result from the following
   a. Drug overdoses
   b. Central nervous system lesions or infections
2. Inability of a normally functioning central nervous system to generate respiratory muscle power; examples include the following
   a. Guillain-Barré syndrome
   b. Multiple sclerosis
   c. Spinal cord injury
   d. Myasthenia gravis
   e. Muscular dystrophies
   f. Poliomyelitis
   g. Tetanus

Pathophysiology

Each of the three types of respiratory insufficiency and respiratory failure has a specific pathophysiology.

Type I. The most important factor in type I respiratory failure is increased extravascular lung fluid. The cause may be increased pulmonary capillary pressure or increased pulmonary capillary permeability. Patients who have diffuse pulmonary edema and respiratory failure secondary to increased pulmonary-capillary permeability are said to have ARDS.

The process of hemodynamic pulmonary edema can be divided into three stages:

1. In the initial stage, pulmonary congestion and distended pulmonary vessels occur as the result of some specific condition. This leads to peripheral airway resistance and eventually to decreased lung compliance.
2. In the second stage, peripheral airway resistance increases as additional fluid collects in the interstitial spaces, compressing the peripheral airways.
3. In the third stage, the alveoli become filled with fluid and total lung capacity is decreased, causing intrapulmonary shunting and hypoxia. The edema also suppresses the formation and effectiveness of surfactant. The surfactant problem leads to microatelectasis and further reduction in functional residual capacity.

The severe hypoxemia that occurs in patients with ARDS and respiratory failure is primarily the result of the shunting of blood through fluid-filled alveoli and atelectatic alveoli. The small airways close and remain closed, leading to distal atelectasis and loss of lung volume. Because of reduced compliance, a greater than normal pressure is necessary to deliver the same tidal volume. As compliance decreases, overall lung volume also decreases.

Hypoxia is a major feature of type I respiratory failure and ARDS. Even though the alveoli receive enough blood, there is shunting in the lungs with little gas exchange. If shunting is uncorrected, acidosis results. Cardiac output and alveolar minute ventilation increase.

Diagnostic studies for type I respiratory failure include evaluating the $Paco_2$ (which is initially low when the body is still trying to compensate but then increases to greater than 50 mm Hg when compensation is no longer possible), pulmonary capillary wedge pressure (PCWP; significant below 12 mm Hg), and protein concentration of fluid aspirated from the lung.

Type II. The primary problem in type II respiratory failure is the inability to generate enough alveolar ventilation. This results in increased $Paco_2$ and decreased Pao_2.

The patient may have difficulty performing forced expiratory tests because of shortness of breath. In addition, because of the retention of carbon dioxide, the kidneys tend to retain bicarbonate, so the arterial pH remains above 7.3.

Type III. Type III respiratory failure can be subdivided into the two core divisions for the disorder.

Central nervous system depression. Respiratory failure from central nervous system (CNS) depression most commonly follows an overdose of opiates, alcohol, tricyclic antidepressants, barbiturates, or other sedative drugs. After the body takes in large quantities of any of these drugs, stimulation of the respiratory center is depressed and the rate of breathing is lowered with little change in tidal volume. The respiratory center does not appear to respond to the rising $Paco_2$.

Neuromuscular transmission difficulties. The main difficulty for patients with a neuromuscular disease is their inability to generate enough force for deep breathing or coughing. Exercise or a need for deep breathing may cause difficulty. Chronically poor breathing leads to secretion buildup and eventual airway obstruction. Because of the patient's inability to cough and thus clear the small airways, hypoventilation and an increase in $Paco_2$ occur.

• • •

The diagnostic evaluation and nursing care of the patient with respiratory insufficiency and respiratory failure are cause specific. The reader is referred to the specific causes for a detailed discussion.

Adult Respiratory Distress Syndrome

In adult respiratory distress syndrome (ARDS) capillary permeability is increased, creating a condition in which the lungs are wet and heavy, congested, hemorrhagic, stiff, and unable to diffuse oxygen.

ARDS left untreated leads to respiratory failure and death. The following are many of the disorders that may lead to ARDS:

- Trauma
  - Hypovolemic shock
  - Lung or cardiac contusion
  - Fat embolism
  - Head injury
- Inhaled toxins
  - Smoke
  - Chemicals
  - Oxygen toxicity
- Liquid aspiration
  - Gastric contents
  - Near-drowning
- Hematologic disorders
  - Disseminated intravascular coagulation (DIC)
  - Blood transfusions
- Infections
  - Gram-negative sepsis
  - Pneumonia
- Drug overdose
- Toxic metabolic disorders
  - Pancreatitis
  - Uremia
  - Eclampsia

This type of respiratory failure has been known for a long time. During World War I it was described as posttraumatic pulmonary insufficiency, during World War II it was called wet lung, and during the Vietnam War it was described as Da Nang lung. The following are among the many other synonyms for ARDS:

- Shock lung
- Pump lung
- Congestive atelectasis
- Acute pulmonary insufficiency
- Noncardiogenic pulmonary edema
- Stiff lung
- White lung
- Respirator lung
- Progressive pulmonary consolidation
- Adult hyaline membrane disease
- Acute ventilatory insufficiency

Because of the variability of its diagnosis, the incidence and survival rates of ARDS are difficult to state. Studies done since the early 1970s have shown survival rates to be between 30% and 50%.[50] Other authors suggest that with prompt treatment the survival rate may be increased to 60% to 70%. In all cases, early detection and aggressive interventions directly affect the patient's survival probability.

Pathophysiology

Regardless of the cause of ARDS, the tissue response of the lung and the response of the body do not vary. On biopsy examination the lung is congested and bleeding and looks like a liver. The amount of secretions in the large airways is insignificant, and there is no visible blockage of the major vessels.

There is always a time sequence in the development of ARDS. For example, it may be seen 12 to 24 hours after an injury resulting in hypovolemic shock or lung contusion, or it may appear 5 to 10 days following the development of sepsis. In either case the sequence of response and the symptoms remain the same. Figure 2-19 outlines the physiologic process.

As a result of this process the following major problems occur:

1. A reduction in the functional vital capacity
2. Bronchovascular edema, resulting in a decrease of the interstitial negative pressure, distal atelectasis, and decreased vital capacity
3. Decreased lung compliance caused by congestion, resulting in a decreased functional residual capacity (FRC)
4. Hypoxia caused by shunting in the lungs
5. Increased oxygen consumption, increased airway resistance, and increased venous blood return to the heart caused by the patient's attempt to increase minute breathing

Figure 2-19 Proposed pathogenesis for adult respiratory distress syndrome (ARDS).
From Martin.[52]

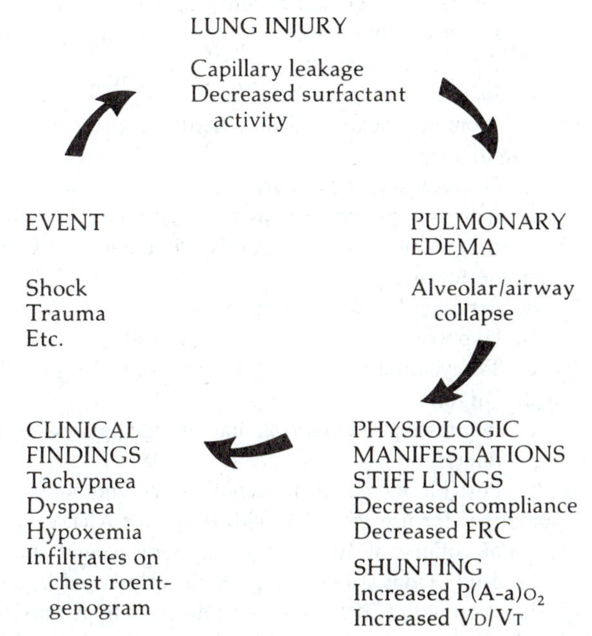

Diagnostic Studies and Findings

Pulmonary Function

Alveolar-arterial oxygen gradient $P(A\text{-}a)O_2$ (also A-a Do_2): 300-500 mm Hg; reflects the difficulty with which oxygen crosses the alveolar-capillary membrane

Shunt fraction (Qs-Qt): May be greater than 15%-20%; measures the degree of intrapulmonary shunting; normal value <6%

Functional residual capacity (FRC): Below normal

Compliance (C): Below normal

Pulmonary capillary wedge pressure (PCWP): Low to normal pressure seen in ARDS

Pulmonary capillary wedge pressure: 3-12 mm Hg

Arterial Blood Gases

Pao_2 <70 mm Hg

$Paco_2$ >35 mm Hg

HCO_3 <22 mEq/L

pH increased in beginning; as ARDS becomes worse, pH decreases

Lactic Acid Levels

Increased regardless of measurement technique

Normal values:

80-100 Wacker units

120-340 IU/I

150-450 Wroblewski units

Figure 2-20 Chest roentgenogram of patient with adult respiratory distress syndrome (ARDS). Heart is normal size; note diffuse infiltrates in upper and middle zones of lungs.
Courtesy R. Keith Wilson, M.D., Baylor College of Medicine, Houston, Texas.

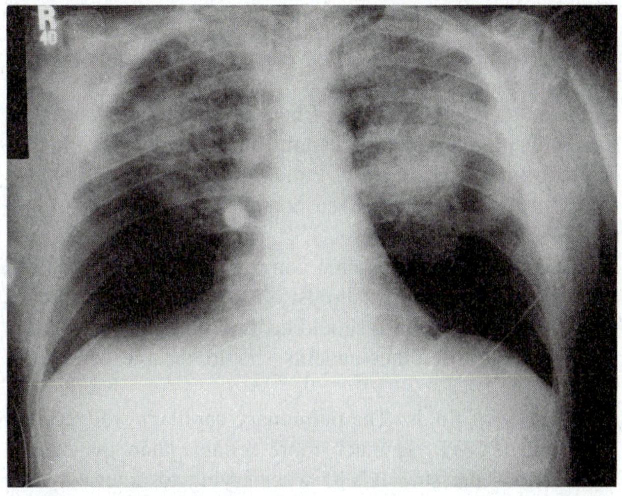

Chest Roentgenograms

There must be a large increase in lung fluid before abnormalities are observed on chest roentgenograms; early diagnostic radiographic changes include thickened or blurred margins of the bronchi or vessels; Figure 2-20 shows diffuse and hazy blurred appearance throughout the lung fields

Medical Plan

The major medical plan is focused in three areas:

1. Supportive, to provide adequate oxygenation and mechanical ventilation to reverse the hypoxemia and expand the distal gas exchange units so as to prevent further airway and alveolar collapse
2. Therapeutic, to treat the systemic responses caused by the alterations in pulmonary function
3. Curative, to locate and halt the causal insult

Medications

There are no specific drugs used to treat the syndrome. Drugs used are primarily supportive to other therapeutic measures such as mechanical ventilation.

Morphine (3 to 5 mg/h IV) may be given as sedation for mechanical ventilator patients who are restless and experiencing tachypnea.

Pancuronium bromide (Pavulon) may be used as a neuroblocking agent to completely paralyze the voluntary respirations of the patient. Dosage must be carefully and individually calculated for each patient. The initial intravenous dosage range for an adult is 0.04 to 0.1 mg/kg.

Corticosteroid use is controversial. Evidence remains speculative that they are helpful in reducing pulmonary edema and stabilizing pulmonary membranes.

Heparin has been advocated by some sources as a drug to combat microvascular emboli. Most authorities, however, question the real benefits of heparin and warn that its risks outweigh any potential benefit for these critically ill individuals.

General Management

Fluid and electrolyte therapy: Fluids are monitored carefully. Excessive intravascular fluid administration may result in cardiogenic pulmonary edema. Patients with capillary damage from ARDS are especially susceptible to fluid leakage into the alveolar spaces.

Fluid types: There is some controversy regarding the use of colloids and crystalloids. It is most generally believed that colloidal fluids should be used in hypoalbuminemic patients. All other patients should receive crystalloid fluids.[74]

Quantity of fluids: The pulmonary capillary wedge pressure (PCWP) is much more reliable than the central venous pressure (CVP) when trying to determine the quantity of fluids to be administered. In most situations, maintenance of the PCWP at 10 to 15 mm Hg provides adequate, but not excessive, intravascular volumes. Certainly clinical parameters such as pulse, urinary output, and peripheral vasoconstriction should also be considered as assessment variables.

Oxygenation: Oxygen support via mask may be used in the very early stages of ARDS but will not be sufficient as the syndrome becomes worse. The goal is to provide the lowest oxygen concentration to maintain the mixed venous oxygen at a level above 40 mm Hg (this may be measured by obtaining a blood sample from the distal lumen of the Swan-Ganz catheter). The $P\bar{v}O_2$ and PaO_2 must both be carefully monitored.

If oxygen concentrations of greater than 50% are required to maintain adequate blood gas oxygen levels, intubation and mechanical ventilation are indicated.

Mechanical ventilation: Early endotracheal intubation and mechanical ventilation should be considered as soon as subtle abnormalities in pulmonary function and laboratory and radiologic findings are observed. Unless the patient is to be maintained on the ventilator for longer than several weeks, tracheostomy is not usually required. See pp. 216 to 217 and 225 to 228 for discussion of endotracheal tubes and ventilatory maintenance.

The purpose of mechanical ventilation for ARDS is to produce a rapid inspiratory flow rate while also exerting a continuous positive end-expiratory pressure (PEEP). A pressure-cycled ventilator is therefore the ventilator of choice. For the acute stages of ARDS a continuous positive-pressure ventilator (CPPV) with PEEP is most commonly used. PEEP results in decreased shunt and an increase in PaO_2. The effects of PEEP in ARDS are[55]:

1. Pulmonary
   a. Increases mean airway pressure
   b. Increases functional residue capacity
   c. Increases compliance
   d. Decreases shunting
   e. Increases lung volumes
   f. Promotes clearing of lung fields
2. Circulatory
   a. Decreases venous return
   b. Increases pulmonary vascular resistance
3. Complications: may compromise circulation, resulting in the following
   a. Peripheral vasoconstriction
   b. Hypotension
   c. Tachycardia
   d. Oliguria
   e. Increased pulmonary capillary wedge pressure (>15 mm Hg)
   f. Possible increased incidence of pneumothorax[2]

Guidelines for use of CPPV with PEEP for ARDS:

1. Tidal volume of 10 to 20 ml/kg body weight should be used. Tidal volumes greater than this used in conjunction with CPPV may cause alveolar hypertension.
2. PEEP should be regulated between 5 and 10 cm H_2O.

Although a PEEP greater than 15 cm H_2O is generally contraindicated, many practitioners go much higher. The purpose of PEEP is to decrease the intrapulmonary shunting and to improve pulmonary compliance. Therefore PEEP should be considered for use when an inspired oxygen concentration of >50% is required to maintain an adequate Pa_{O_2} level. Optimal use of PEEP is to add it in small increments in an attempt to decrease the intrapulmonary shunt to the 15% to 20% range.

3. Physiologic respiratory rate should be between 10 and 20 per minute, although rates up to 30 per minute may be used.
4. The goal of mechanical ventilation is to keep the Pa_{CO_2} in the range of 35 to 40 mm Hg. A level below this will decrease cardiac output, increase airway resistance, and increase oxygen consumption.
5. If the patient fights the ventilator, sedation such as morphine or a neuroblocking agent such as pancuronium bromide may be necessary (see "Medications").
6. CPPV with PEEP should be used very cautiously in patients with low blood pressure. An increase in already high intrathoracic pressure may result. This in turn may compress thoracic vessels, leading to decreased venous return, decreased cardiac output, poor tissue perfusion, and a lactic acid buildup.

Other mechanical ventilation techniques used with ARDS:

Intermittent mandatory ventilation (IMV): This technique permits the patient to breathe spontaneously from a gas reservoir and still receive periodic mechanical hyperinflations. The patient's own spontaneous minute ventilation is thus augmented to a desired level by ventilator delivered breaths.

Continuous positive airway pressure (CPAP): For patients breathing on their own this technique provides a positive end-expiratory pressure to the end of each inhalation. It may be used in the patient who can maintain adequate Pa_{CO_2} levels without mechanical ventilation but who cannot maintain adequate arterial oxygen.

Cardiovascular monitoring: Invasive cardiovascular monitoring as with the Swan-Ganz catheter should be used whenever cardiovascular compromise is anticipated. Once the catheter is in place, the pulmonary capillary wedge pressure (PCWP) should be optimized to 13 to 17 mm Hg.

Electrocardiogram: Monitor cardiac response.

Alimentation: Alimentation should be undertaken from the onset. External alimentation with a small feeding tube is best, but intravenous hyperalimentation should be instituted if enteral alimentation is not possible. The use of antacids and H_2 blockers to maintain gastric pH above 4 is warranted for prophylaxis.[43]

Tracheobronchial suctioning: To remove mucus secretions and to ensure patent airway.

Monitoring of ventilatory sufficiency: The patient's vital capacity, minute volume, and intrapulmonary shunting ($\dot{Q}s/\dot{Q}t$) should be monitored.

Monitoring of blood gases and pressure response: The patient's blood gases, pulmonary-capillary wedge pressure, and alveolar-arterial oxygen gradient ($P[A\text{-}a]O_2$) should be monitored.

Monitoring of sputum and bronchial secretions: Frequent laboratory analysis of bronchial secretions should be made to watch for signs of pulmonary system infection.

Monitoring of chest roentgenograms: Frequent chest roentgenogram analysis is useful in monitoring the patient's response to the therapeutic treatment.

NURSING CARE

Nursing Assessment

One of the most important assessment rules in the care of the patient with ARDS or potential ARDS is to have good baseline data. Should the patient's condition deteriorate, subtle changes can be identified.

Respiratory Status

Respiratory distress: nasal flaring, chest wall retractions, tachypnea or bradypnea, decreased chest wall movement, labored breathing

Breath sounds: rales, rhonchi, wheeze, decreased, bilaterally unequal

Breathing pattern: labored, irregular

Increased sputum, persistent cough, wet-sounding breathing

Pulmonary function: decreased vital capacity, minute volume, and functional residual capacity; increased intrapulmonary shunting

Hypercapnia: headache, dizziness, confusion, unconsciousness, twitching, hypertension, sweating, flushed face

Hypoxia: restlessness, confusion, impaired motor function, hypotension, cyanosis, tachycardia

Laboratory Values

Blood gases: Pa_{CO_2}, Pa_{O_2}, $P\bar{v}_{O_2}$, $P_{A\text{-}a}O_2$, pH, HCO_3^-, lactic acid levels

Cardiovascular Status

Decreased cardiac output: restlessness, lethargy, tachycardia, hypotension, decreased urinary output

Pulmonary pressures: increased pulmonary wedge pressure (PWP), pulmonary artery pressure (PAP)

Fluid and Electrolytes

Intake and output, cardiovascular response, potassium, and sodium bicarbonate

Bronchopulmonary Infection

Temperature, sputum specimens for culture and sensitivity

Chest Roentgenograms

Serial chest roentgenograms to monitor the clearing of thickened or blurred margins of the bronchi or vessels

Psychosocial

Fear of suffocation, fear of being out of control if on ventilator, fear of unknown, family understanding, support, ability to communicate

Nursing Dx & Intervention

Nursing Diagnosis	Nursing Intervention/Rationale
Ineffective breathing pattern	• Assess ventilation to include evaluation of breathing rate, rhythm, and depth, chest expansion, presence of respiratory distress such as dyspnea, shortness of breath, nasal flaring, cyanosis, and changes in skin color including nail beds and mucous membranes. *Signs of respiratory distress may be present because of stiff lungs and shunting.* • Assess tidal volume, vital capacity and minute volume, and intrapulmonary shunting. • Identify contributing factors such as airway clearance or obstruction problem, pain, level of consciousness, or weakness. • Maintain patient position to facilitate ventilation (i.e., head of bed in semi-Fowler's position), cough, and deep breathing *to maximize breathing potential.* • Assess patient for tiring in relation to attempts to breathe; encourage pursed-lip breathing. • Initiate techniques of pulmonary toileting to liquefy secretions and minimize pulmonary congestion *to prevent secondary infections.* • Help to protect patient from known sources of secondary infection. • In collaboration with physician, prepare for and institute mechanical ventilation when breathing pattern cannot maintain adequate blood gas levels or when patient demonstrates tiring with breathing efforts. • When patient is receiving mechanical ventilation, provide care and monitoring consistent with the guidelines presented on pp. 225 to 228. • Assess patient to identify signs such as restlessness, confusion, and irritability, which may indicate the body's response to altered blood gas states.
Impaired gas exchange	• Monitor arterial blood gases; report increases or decreases of $Paco_2$ and Pao_2 of more than 10 to 15 mm Hg. • Assess pulmonary artery pressure and pulmonary capillary wedge pressure (PCWP). • Monitor alveolar-arterial oxygen gradient. • Be aware that *pathologic changes of this disease may impede gas diffusion. Alterations in the alveolar wall, focal atelectasis, congested capillaries, stiff lungs, and shunting may all cause decreased gas exchange.* • Prevent physiologic factors that promote restlessness or anxiety. *Altered blood gas states may alter patient's response.* • Monitor for signs of cor pulmonale: pulmonary hypertension, gradually increasing edema of the legs, increasing central venous pressure and pulmonary capillary wedge pressure, jugular venous distention, blood gas abnormalities, and hepatomegaly *related to stiff lungs and shunting.* • Monitor electrocardiogram and cardiac status for arrhythmias *secondary to alteration in blood gases.* • Monitor and record kidney functioning and urinary output, which may be affected *secondary to chronic tissue hypoxia and alterations in metabolism.* • In collaboration with the physician, administer oxygen *to maintain Pao_2 of at least 50 to 60 mm Hg; if blood gas levels cannot be maintained or if the concentration of oxygen exceeds 50%, mechanical ventilation must be considered.* • Monitor serum electrolytes; *these may change because of alterations in oxygenation and metabolism.* • Carefully monitor body temperature; *this may fluctuate because of alterations in metabolism or secondary infections.* • In collaboration with physician, administer respiratory-related medications and assess and document patient's response.
Fatigue	• Assess patterns of fatigue. • Assess factors related to fatigue and strategies for dealing with them. • Assess support systems and available resources. • Administer treatments or medications to relieve discomfort. • Enhance patient's ability to rest between specified activities.

Nursing Diagnosis	Nursing Intervention/Rationale
Ineffective airway clearance	• Assess patient to identify inability to move secretions; if inability is identified, assist with appropriate measures (coughing, positioning, suctioning, liquefying secretions, etc.) on a regular and scheduled basis every 30 minutes to every 2 hours. • Assist patient to maintain proper body positioning *to ensure patent airway.* • Carefully monitor fluid intake and the corresponding pulmonary capillary wedge pressure; *these may indicate fluid overload complicating pulmonary wetness.*
Potential for aspiration	• Avoid triggering gag mechanism when performing caretaking activities, including mouth care. • If swallowing reflex is diminished, elevate head of bed when performing mouth care. • Assess and document amount of secretions present, patient's level of consciousness, and patient's ability to swallow secretions effectively. • Administer suction when necessary to remove secretions and maintain patent airway. • If secretions are thick or inspissated, ensure adequate humidification to help liquefy secretions. • For patients with reduced level of consciousness, ensure that head of bed is elevated, unless contraindicated.
Altered nutrition: less than body requirements	• Assess for adequacy of fluid and caloric intake and ensure intake of required fluids and nutrients. • Maintain tube feedings or hyperalimentation in collaboration with physician. • Monitor for signs and symptoms of malnutrition.
Potential fluid volume deficit	• Assess for evidence of gastrointestinal bleeding *secondary to physiologic stress;* monitor serial hemoglobin and hematocrit; check all stools, emesis, and nasogastric aspirate *for presence of blood;* observe changes in vital signs or abdominal girth. • Initiate prevention measures: for example, minimize activities for uninterrupted periods of time, maintain calm and restful environment, encourage patient to participate in care as tolerated, explain all therapy before administering.
Impaired physical mobility	• See p. 1687 of text for associated care.
Potential impaired skin integrity	• See p. 1646 of text for associated care.
Impaired verbal communication (if patient is intubated or demonstrates significant dyspnea)	• Provide alternative method of communication appropriate to the patient's comprehension ability. • If patient is intubated, assure patient that speech will return as soon as endotracheal tube is removed. • Observe for signs of frustration or patient withdrawal secondary to the inability to speak. • Teach family members appropriate methods to communicate with patient.
Self-care deficit	• See p. 1692 of text for associated care.
Ineffective individual coping	• See p. 1804 of text for associated care.
Family coping: potential for growth	• See p. 1816 of text for associated care.

Patient Education

1. Teach the patient adaptive breathing techniques. Emphasize importance of periodic turning, coughing, and deep breathing.
2. Teach the importance of not fighting the ventilator and relaxing instead to permit maximum ventilation. Assure the patient that oxygen is being supplied.
3. Teach adaptive exercise and rest techniques.
4. Teach eating and food choice modifications.
5. Provide the patient and family with information regarding all medications the patient is taking.

Evaluation

Patient Outcome	Data Indicating That Outcome is Reached
Movement of air in and out of lungs is optimal. Airway is patent. Both lungs are fully aerated as visualized on roentgenograms.	Vital capacity measurements including tidal and minute volumes are optimal for patient's status. Pulmonary capillary wedge pressure is within normal limits. Blood gas values are within normal limits. Airways are clear and breathing occurs without obstruction.
Breathing pattern occurs without tiring patient. Breath sounds are clear in all areas.	Patient demonstrates modified breathing techniques that facilitate ventilatory capacity. Behavior is modified to conserve energy expenditure.
Physiologic function is stable.	Nutrition level is maintained. Kidney and bladder functioning is within normal limits. Gastrointestinal system is functioning adequately. Skin integrity is maintained. There are no secondary infections. Serum electrolytes are within normal limits.
Patient preserves pulmonary functioning by maintaining optimal activity level, preventing infection, and following prescribed treatments.	Patient demonstrates a variety of methods indicating ability to preserve and facilitate optimal respiratory functioning (e.g., breathing, exercises, modified activities or exercise, taking medications as prescribed).
Patient and family have sufficient information to comply with discharge regimen.	Patient and family are able at time of discharge to discuss medications (purpose, side effects, route, and schedule), dietary therapy regimen, activity progression regimen, signs of infection or respiratory deterioration, and plan for follow-up visits.

CHRONIC OBSTRUCTIVE PULMONARY DISEASE

Chronic obstructive pulmonary disease (COPD) is a group of diseases that includes asthma, bronchitis, emphysema, and bronchiectasis.[34] Recurrent obstruction of airflow is common to each of these diseases. At one end of the spectrum is periodic asthmatic attacks, and at the other end is pure emphysema.

COPD is a major cause of death and disability in the United States. About 15% of the older population have some degree of COPD. The estimated economic costs for treatment are greater than $1 billion per year.[26] The actual incidence of COPD is difficult to determine because of the lack of agreement regarding diagnosis and because two or more obstructive diseases may be present at the same time. In most patients with COPD two or more histopathologic elements aggravate the breathing process.[13]

Figure 2-21 illustrates the interrelatedness of these diseases and the many host and environmental factors that tend to affect them. The degree of involvement and the response to therapy are individual.

The most important task for the health professional is to determine and maintain maximum respiration for each patient. This means that the professional must be able to separate the reversible components of COPD from the irreversible components and to maximize each individual's potential.

Chronic bronchitis and emphysema

Obstructive airway disease refers to a continuum of pulmonary responses to various noxious stimuli. At one end of the spectrum is pure chronic bronchitis (e.g., congenital immune system dysfunction), and at the other end is pure emphysema (e.g., alpha-1-antitrypsin deficiency). Because of this complexity, these two pure disease states are discussed in combination. Where possible, their differences are pointed out.

Chronic bronchitis refers to excessive mucus secretion in the bronchial tree. This mucus causes chronic and recurrent productive coughing.

Emphysema refers to anatomic alterations of the air spaces distal to the conducting airways. There is an abnormal enlargement of the air spaces. This causes physiologic destruction of the alveolar walls, which in turn causes increased lung compliance, decreased diffusing capacity, and increased airway resistance.

Chronic bronchitis and emphysema represent a variety of respiratory disorders that all lead to a slowly progressive airway-obstructive disease. The airway obstruction is persistent and irreversible.

The development of chronic bronchitis or emphysema is determined by evaluating the interrelatedness of the individ-

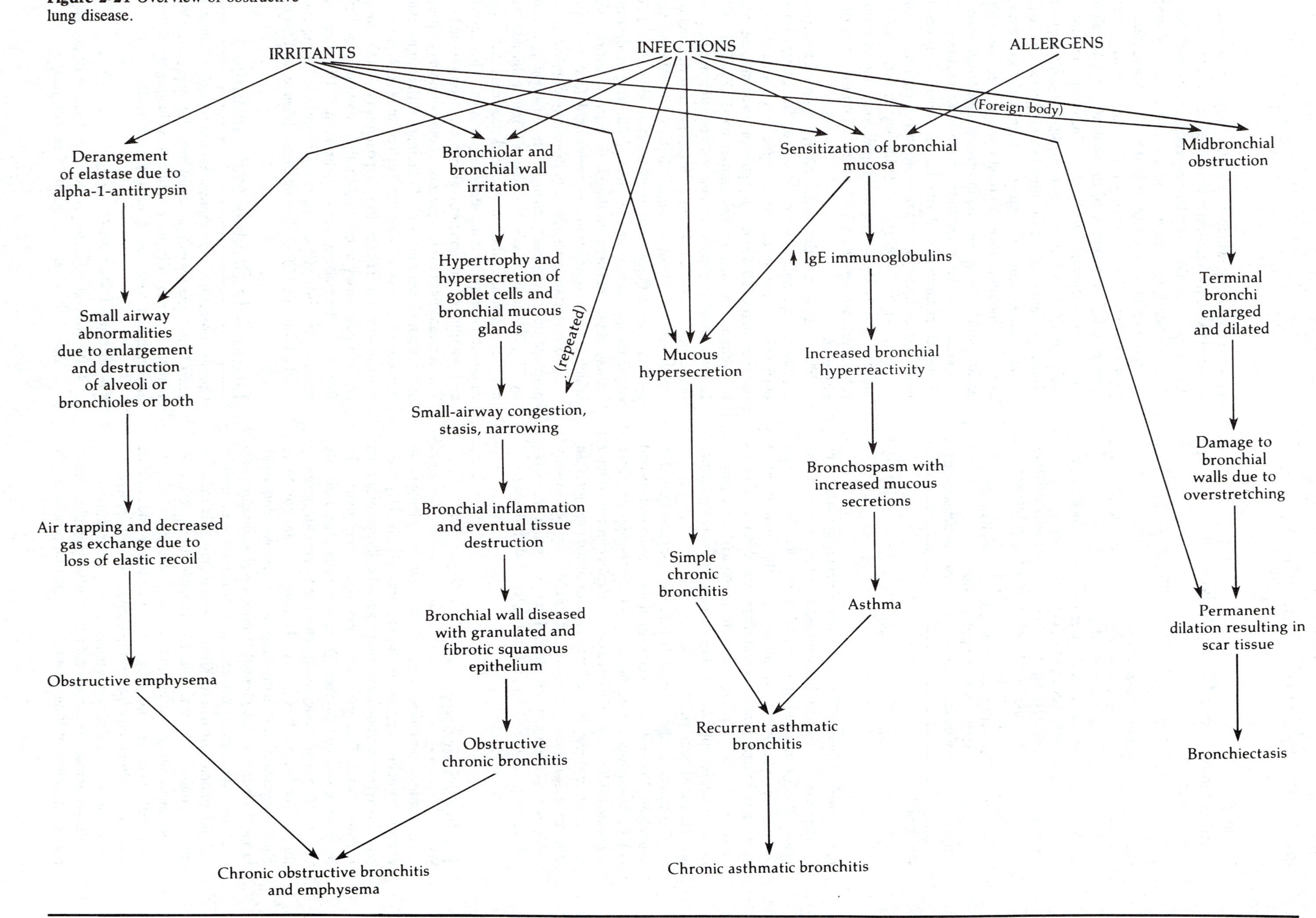

Figure 2-21 Overview of obstructive lung disease.

Table 2-7
Relationship between FEV_1 and Activities of Daily Living

FEV_1 (L)	Activity Response
3.7-4	Normal value for adult
2-1.5	Complaints of dyspnea on exertion such as carrying packages or climbing stairs
about 1	Breathlessness when trying to perform activities of daily living such as cooking, cleaning, bathing, dressing, walking
	Subject to complications of carbon dioxide retention and cor pulmonale
<0.75	Individual unable to work, usually housebound

Data from Fries.[29]

ual's genetic vulnerability and environmental factors.[34] The incidence of the diseases has increased dramatically in recent years. The American Lung Association attributes this increase to smoking and airborne irritants and to a better understanding of the physiologic processes and diagnostic criteria.[2] The incidence of chronic bronchitis and emphysema remains greater in men than in women, possibly because of smoking history and choice of occupation.

The course of the diseases before the symptoms develop is unclear. Probably the forced expiratory volume in 1 second (FEV_1) decreases before the signs of illness appear. Once signs are evident, the FEV_1 measurement (after bronchodilator administration) may be the best indicator of the prognosis. In addition to predicting outcome, the FEV_1 may be a useful guide for evaluating death rates. Table 2-7 summarizes the relationship between FEV_1 and activities of daily living.

Pathophysiology

Chronic bronchitis. One of the earliest changes in chronic bronchitis appears in the secretory glands. Hypertrophy and hypersecretion occur in the goblet cells and bronchial mucous glands. The goblet cells and the mucous gland cells increase in size and number. The goblet cells extend distally into the terminal bronchioles, where they are not normally found. The net result is increased amounts of sputum, bronchial congestion, and narrowing of bronchioles and small bronchi. With time the normally sterile lower respiratory tract becomes colonized by bacteria, and an increased number of polymorphonuclear neutrophil (PMN) leukocytes is found in the secretions.[34] These leukocytes probably stimulate further bronchial swelling and eventual tissue destruction.[70] As the bronchial wall becomes diseased, granulated and fibrotic squamous epithelium replaces the normal ciliated epithelium. This scarring leads to stenosis and airway obstruction.

Emphysema. The main defect underlying emphysema is the derangement of lung elastin by the neutral proteases, the most important of which is elastase. Elastase is made and released by PMN leukocytes and alveolar macrophages. Under normal conditions, proteases become fused with bacteria that find their way to the alveolar level. A fraction of the total protease produced is liberated in the lung in response to inhaling particles and following cell death. Normally there is a counterbalancing supply of the protease inhibitor alpha-1-antitrypsin. Recurrent infections, environmental irritants, and cigarette smoking, along with an alpha-1-antitrypsin deficiency, probably cause a situation in which elastin in the distal airways and alveoli is degraded.[34] There is also evidence that cigarette smoking alone depresses the activity of alpha-1-antitrypsin.[61] The imbalance in this elastase-antielastase system allows for the destruction of the basic elastin structure of the distal airways and alveoli. As septal walls are lost, blood vessel density is also reduced and emphysema results.[34]

NOTE: Alpha-1-antitrypsin deficiency is estimated to be present in only 0.06% of the population[23] and is probably responsible for less than 10% of the identified cases of emphysema.[34]

The lungs of a patient with emphysema appear large, overinflated, and pale. The walls of the bronchioles undergo destructive changes, and large bullae may form. If changes occur throughout the lobule and pulmonary acinus, the disease is referred to as panlobular emphysema (PLE). PLE, which is often found in elderly persons with no evidence of chronic bronchitis, shows a uniform enlargement and destruction of the alveoli throughout the acinus. Individuals with true alpha-1-antitrypsin deficiency are most likely to have PLE. In emphysema the normal architecture of the lung is destroyed. Lobule septal damage produces air sacs of various sizes, which leads to ventilation and perfusion defects.

Two important consequences of emphysema are air trapping and decreased gas exchange. The air trapping is caused by a loss of elastic recoil. Ventilation is regionally decreased, not only because of the elastic recoil problems, but also because of poor support of terminal airways. This increases collapsibility of the noncartilaginous peripheral bronchioles. The decreased gas exchange causes both pulmonary diffusion and perfusion abnormalities. Pulmonary diffusion is reduced because of a loss of alveolar surface area and pulmonary vasoconstriction. The resulting hypoxemia causes a more generalized pulmonary artery constriction, shunting blood away from even the normal areas of the lung.[45] The measurable result of these two processes is an increase in the functional residual capacity (FRC), increased compliance, and hypoxia.

Diagnostic Studies and Findings

Chronic bronchitis and emphysema are typically "silent" for years before the patient has even minimal symptoms. When symptoms appear, diagnostic studies evaluating the shortness of breath and cough are generally performed.

Pulmonary Function

FEV_1 (forced expiratory volume in 1 second): decreased, may fall as much as 50 to 75 ml per year

FVC (forced vital capacity): decreased
FEV_1/FVC ratio: decreased
TLC (total lung capacity): increased in emphysema because of decreased elastic recoil
RV (residual volume): increased in emphysema because of decreased elastic recoil and in chronic bronchitis because of air trapping
FRC (functional residual capacity): increased in emphysema because of decreased elastic recoil; may be normal in pure chronic bronchitis
C (compliance): increased in emphysema
R_{aw} (airway resistance): increased in both chronic bronchitis and emphysema
Ventilatory response: decreased with hypoxia and hypercapnia

Arterial Blood Gases

Alveolar-arterial (A-a) oxygen gradient: widened
Pao_2: decreased
$Paco_2$: increased; patients with pure chronic bronchitis are more prone to CO_2 retention than are those patients with emphysema of comparable severity

Chest Roentgenogram

May have flattened diaphragm and increased anterior-posterior (A-P) diameter
In emphysema, vascular markings may be decreased and intercostal spaces widened, and bullae may be present
Abnormalities such as hyperinflation and increased lung markings are usually due to concomitant emphysema or other complicating causes

Medical Plan

The medical plan for both of these diseases is to stop the progress of the disease and to maximize breathing by reducing airway secretions and inflammation and halting bronchospasms.

Medications

Acute exacerbation management
Ampicillin (Amcill, Omnipen, others), 250-500 mg po q6h for 10 d
Tetracycline (Achromycin, others), 250-500 mg po q6h for 10 d

Long-term management
Bronchodilators
Therapeutic theophylline levels should be maintained between 10 and 20 mEq/ml
Corticosteroids
If pulmonary function tests are improved after 3 to 4 weeks by corticosteroids, they may be continued at low doses; the goal is discontinuation of the medication
Influenza and pneumococcal vaccines
These vaccines are recommended for patients with chronic bronchitis and emphysema

General Management

Acute exacerbations

Oxygenation: Administered at rates sufficient to maintain a Pao_2 between 50 and 60 mm Hg, usually by nasal cannula at a flow rate of 1 to 3 L per minute. Because patients with chronic bronchitis and emphysema may have chronic hypercapnia, they are considered to be sensitive to increased alveolar oxygen. This means that their borderline or diminished ventilatory drive may be further suppressed by increasing the Pao_2. Care must be taken to closely monitor oxygen administration and to increase the flow slowly and carefully. Use of the Venturi mask allows more precise oxygen administration.

Mechanical ventilation: Intubation and mechanical ventilation may be necessary if supplemental oxygen cannot maintain the Pao_2 above 40 mm Hg with a pH greater than 7.25. If mechanical ventilation becomes necessary, the intermittent mandatory ventilation (IMV) technique becomes useful. The IMV allows the patient to breathe spontaneously with the exact amount of additional minute ventilation required to be delivered by the machine.

Long-term management

Oxygenation: Intermittent (at least 18 hours per day) oxygen therapy via nasal prongs may be indicated for patients who are unable to maintain a Pao_2 of at least 50 to 55 mm Hg while at rest and breathing room air. The flow rate should be adjusted to maintain a resting Pao_2 close to 60 mm Hg.

Chest physiotherapy: Percussion and postural drainage may be administered at regular intervals for patients with large amounts of sputum production. See pp. 221 to 225 for techniques.

Physical training program: Physical training programs are based on the premise that improved ventilatory and cardiac muscle function might compensate for nonreversible lung disease. Bicycle and treadmill training appears to lead to decreased oxygen consumption with exercise and increased work capacity. These physical training techniques are currently used as methods of rehabilitation.[55]

NURSING CARE

Nursing Assessment

History

Smoking history and history of known respiratory irritants including duration of exposure to each; history of previous respiratory diseases, infections, allergies, etc.; history of chronic cough and characteristics; family history of respiratory diseases; description of activity tolerance including fatigue and dyspnea precipitation

Current Medications

Careful and complete history of current respiratory-related medications, as well as use of over-the-counter medications and inhalers

Use of Oxygen

History of use of oxygen, intermittent positive-pressure breathing (IPPB), or other related respiratory assistive devices; history to include amount, frequency, duration, and therapeutic response

Respiratory Status

Respiratory distress as evidenced by dyspnea, cough, prolonged expiration; audible expiratory wheeze; diminished breath sounds over diseased area; anxiety; bronchospasm; sputum-producing cough; hyperresonance owing to overinflation of lungs; barrel chest; cyanosis of nail beds and mucous membranes; posturing and use of accessory muscles during breathing; respiratory failure signs (see discussion of respiratory failure at beginning of this chapter)

Hypoxia

Restlessness; tachycardia; confusion; hypotension; cyanosis; premature ventricular contractions and right bundle-branch block if hypoxia becomes severe; somnolence; loss of memory; pulsus paradoxus

Laboratory Values

Decreased chloride (from salt restriction and diuretics); decreased potassium (from diuretics)

ECG

May show atrial arrhythmias; tall, symmetric P waves in leads II, III, and aV_F; vertical QRS axis; and signs of right ventricular hypertrophy late in the disease

Pulmonary Function

FEV_1; residual volume; forced vital capacity; total lung capacity; functional residual capacity; compliance; R_{aw}

Infection Signs

Elevated temperature; purulent sputum; foul mouth odor or taste

GI Response

Malaise and anorexia owing to chronic hypoxic state; weight loss; constipation

Major Complications

Cor pulmonale and pneumothorax

Nursing Dx & Intervention

Nursing Diagnosis	Nursing Intervention/Rationale
Ineffective airway clearance	• Assess patient to identify inability to move secretions; if inability is identified, assist with appropriate measures (coughing, positioning, suctioning, liquefying secretions, etc.). • Administer bronchodilators, mucolytics, and expectorants as ordered; observe for therapeutic response; monitor theophylline level if appropriate. • Assist patient to maintain proper body positioning *to ensure maximum airway availability* (e.g., semi-Fowler's position or sitting upright and leaning on overbed table). • Provide hydration (up to 2000 ml/day) *to liquefy secretions and replace fluids*. • Administer vaporization therapy and perform postural drainage with percussion as ordered; at least 1 hour prior to meals; provide oral hygiene after treatment. • Carefully and frequently auscultate chest for quality of breath sounds and adventitious sounds; note cough and sputum characteristics.
Ineffective breathing pattern	• Assess ventilation to include evaluation of breathing rate, rhythm, and depth, chest expansion, presence of respiratory distress such as dyspnea, shortness of breath, nasal flaring, pursed-lip breathing or prolonged expiratory phase, use of accessory muscles. • Assist to assess total lung capacity (TLC), residual volume (RV), functional residual capacity (FRC), forced expiratory volume (FEV), and forced vital capacity (FVC) as ordered. • Identify contributing factors such as airway clearance, obstruction problem, or weakness. • Instruct patient in proper pulmonary routines such as coughing, deep breathing, pursed-lip breathing, and diaphragmatic breathing. • Suction as necessary to remove secretions. • Assess patient for tiring in relation to attempts to breathe. • Assist to protect patient from known sources of secondary infection or breathing irritation such as smoking. • Should mechanical ventilation become necessary, provide care and monitoring consistent with the guidelines given in medical intervention section of this chapter (pp. 225 to 228).
Impaired gas exchange	• Assess patient to identify signs such as restlessness, confusion, and irritability, which *may indicate the body's response to altered blood gas states*. • In collaboration with physician order, monitor arterial blood gases; report increases or decreases in $Paco_2$ and Pao_2 of more than 10 to 15 mm Hg. • Administer oxygen as ordered *to maintain Pao_2 of no less than 55 mm Hg;* this usually may be maintained by administration of oxygen by nasal cannula at a flow rate of 1 to 3 L/min;

Nursing Diagnosis	Nursing Intervention/Rationale
	if needed, a Venturi tube may be used; if blood gas levels cannot be maintained, mechanical ventilation must be considered. *Extreme caution must be exercised to maintain a low oxygen flow not to exceed 3 L/min.* • Monitor electrocardiogram and cardiac status for arrhythmias *secondary to alterations in blood gases.* • If patient is seriously ill, monitor for signs of cor pulmonale such as pulmonary hypertension, gradually increasing edema of the legs, increasing central venous pressure, jugular venous distention, blood gas abnormalities, and hepatomegaly. *These are all signs of respiratory compromise and malfunction.* • Monitor and record kidney function and urinary output, which *may be affected secondary to chronic tissue hypoxia and alterations in metabolism.* • Monitor serum electrolytes, which *may change because of alterations in oxygenation and metabolism.* • Carefully monitor body temperature, which *may fluctuate because of alterations in metabolism or secondary infections.*
Altered oral mucous membrane	• Assess oral mucosa for presence of mouth irritation; consult physician if noted. • Instruct patients using aerosolized corticosteroids to perform thorough mouth washing after each use *to prevent secondary infections of oral candidiasis.*
Altered nutrition: less than body requirements	• Assess for signs and symptoms of malnutrition. • Assist patient to choose foods that are easy to chew and swallow; assist by cutting and feeding if patient tires easily. *Medications, sputum, and shortness of breath may cause anorexia, nausea, and vomiting.* • Diet should consist of high-protein and high-carbohydrate foods and fluids. • Avoid gas-producing foods. • Encourage smaller, more frequent meals. • Encourage fluid intake of at least 2 L per day *to facilitate liquefying secretions and promote urinary output.* (If patient has compromised cardiac or renal condition, fluid intake must be determined in collaboration with physician.) • If indicated, and in consultation with physician, administer stool softeners *to relieve constipation.*
Fatigue	• Assess patterns of fatigue. • Assess factors related to fatigue and strategies for dealing with them. • Assess support systems and available resources. • Administer treatments or medications to relieve discomfort. • Enhance patient's ability to rest between specified activities.
Potential for infection	• Assess for signs and symptoms of infection, fever, dyspnea, and change in sputum color, amount, or odor. • Obtain sputum for culture and sensitivity. • Protect patients from known sources of secondary infection.
Knowledge deficit related to disease process	• Explain and reinforce explanation of the disease and medications. • Encourage patient and family to ask questions. • Explain and discuss different medications necessary for treating the disease.
Potential fluid volume deficit	• In the seriously ill patient, assess for evidence of gastrointestinal bleeding *secondary to physiologic stress;* monitor serial hemoglobin and hematocrit; check all stools, emesis, and nasogastric aspirate for presence of blood; observe changes in vital signs or abdominal girth.
Impaired physical mobility	• Encourage patient to use adaptive breathing techniques *to decrease the work of breathing.* • Assist patient to space activities *to provide periods of rest in between.* • Encourage gradual increase of activities as tolerated *to prevent "pulmonary crippling."* • Problem solve with patient to determine methods of conserving energy while still performing activities of daily living (e.g., using stool to sit while in the bathroom shaving). • Assess and document activities that cause patient to tire easily and become short of breath. • If patient is seriously ill and maintained on bed rest, encourage or provide active or passive range of motion exercises *to maintain adequate muscle tone.*
Fear	• Assess for signs of frustration or fear secondary to hypoxia.
Self-care deficit	• See p. 1692 for nursing care.
Altered health maintenance	• Assess with patient and family home and personally used irritants (smoking, fumes, vapors) that *may exacerbate the chronic respiratory condition.*

Nursing Diagnosis	Nursing Intervention/Rationale
	• Provide education regarding need to avoid irritants in home, work, and community environments. • Provide education regarding need to identify early signs of complications and need for medical consultation.
Ineffective individual coping	• Assess patient's ability to cooperate with health care providers regarding intervention strategies such as breathing techniques, exercise progression, and alterations in the activities of daily living. • Listen carefully to collect information significant to the current health care problem and the patient's perception of ability to deal with alterations it is causing. • Assist patient to develop appropriate coping strategies based on personal strengths and past experience.
Family coping: potential for growth	• See p. 1816 for associated nursing care.

Patient Education

1. Teach patient adaptive breathing techniques, and work with family to teach postural drainage techniques.
2. Teach importance of avoiding contact with persons who have upper respiratory infections and influenza.
3. Teach facts about and importance of prescribed medications such as bronchodilators and corticosteroids.
4. Provide patient and family with information regarding chronic lung diseases, how to assess individual capabilities and responses, and what to do during an acute episode of difficult breathing.
5. Teach change in health status that must be reported to the patient's health care providers; indicators of change may include change in sputum characteristics or color, decreased activity tolerance, increased use of IPPB or oxygen, decreased appetite, and fever.
6. Teach importance of consuming large quantities of fluid.
7. Teach importance of not smoking and of avoiding dust-producing articles (feathers, animal dander, cleaning equipment) and strong cooking odors, which may irritate the respiratory tract.
8. Teach eating and food choice modifications.
9. Provide patient and family with information regarding the care, cleaning, and maintenance of inhalation or oxygen equipment being used in the hospital or to be used at home, as well as signs of oxygen toxicity.
10. Provide patient and family with respiratory-related health information such as pollution indexes, secondary infection exposure, and community support groups.
11. Advise patient to avoid using powders and aerosol products, which may cause bronchospasm.

Evaluation

Patient Outcome	Data Indicating That Outcome is Reached
Air moves optimally in and out of lungs.	Vital capacity measurements including FEV_1, FVC, TLC, RV, and FRC are optimal for patient's status. Blood gas values are within acceptable limits for patient.
Airway is patent.	Airway clearance and breathing occur without obstruction and are optimal for patient.
Breathing pattern occurs without tiring patient.	Patient demonstrates modified breathing techniques that facilitate ventilatory capacity. Behavior is modified to conserve energy expenditure.
Physiologic function is stable.	Nutrition level is maintained. Kidney and bladder are functioning adequately. There are no secondary infections. Serum electrolytes are within normal limits.
Patient understands importance of daily pulmonary exercises.	Patient demonstrates pulmonary exercises and states rationale and importance of maintaining daily exercise routine.
Patient preserves pulmonary functioning by maintaining optimal activity level, preventing infection, and following prescribed treatments.	Patient demonstrates a variety of methods indicating ability to preserve and facilitate optimal respiratory functioning (e.g., breathing exercises, modified exercises, modified activities or exercise, taking medications as prescribed).
Patient and family have sufficient information to comply with discharge regimen.	Patient and family are able at time of discharge to discuss medications—purpose, side effects, route, and schedule; dietary therapy regimen; activity progression regimen; signs of infection or respiratory deterioration; and plan for follow-up visits.

Bronchial asthma

Asthma, a disease marked by increased responsiveness of the trachea and bronchi to various stimuli, results in widespread narrowing of the airways that improves either spontaneously or as a result of therapy.[4]

Status asthmaticus is an intense, unrelenting attack that does not respond to the usual modes of therapy.

Bronchial asthma is a broad clinical syndrome rather than a specific disease. There is bronchial hypersensitivity marked by reversible airway bronchospasm. The bronchospasm causes increased mucosal edema; constriction of the bronchial muscles; production of viscous mucus, which eventually leads to increased mucus plugs; bronchial airway obstruction; and overdistention of the lungs.

Asthma affects about 2% to 3% of the U.S. population and has a death rate of 1 per 100,000 persons.[73] In about 50% of patients the disease begins before 10 years of age, and in another 30% it occurs before age 40. During childhood there is a 2:1 male/female prevalence. This ratio equalizes during adolescence and thereafter.[29]

Asthma is the most common chronic disease for children and adults. It is responsible for about 150,000 hospital admissions and 1,275,000 hospital days a year. Asthma accounts for at least 85 million days of restricted work and 5 million days of work lost each year.[29]

Asthma may be divided into two types: extrinsic (atopic) asthma and intrinsic (nonatopic) asthma.

Extrinsic or *atopic asthma* is caused by external agents such as dust, lint, insecticides, mold spores, or foods. This type is best understood as a reaction to specific allergens. Exposure to an allergen can cause an attack.

Table 2-8
Intrinsic Versus Extrinsic Asthma

Characteristic	Extrinsic	Intrinsic
Allergens as precipitants	Yes	No
Immediate skin test	Positive	Negative
Elevated IgE	Common	Uncommon
Eosinophilia	Yes	Yes
Childhood onset	Common	Uncommon
Other allergies	Common	Uncommon
Family history of multiple allergies	Common	Uncommon
Hyposensitization therapy	Helpful	Equivocal
Typical attack	Acute and self-limiting	Often fulminant and severe
Relationship of attack to infection	May be present	Common
Aspirin sensitivity	Uncommon	Uncommon

Data from Miller[55] and Weiss.[84]

Intrinsic or *nonatopic asthma* indicates that the specific causes cannot be identified. It may be precipitated by many situations such as a common cold, upper respiratory infection, or even exercise. This type usually begins in persons over 35 years of age and develops into a lifelong condition, becoming worse and occurring more often.

In asthma there is increased reactivity to nonspecific factors such as cold air, dust, fumes, exercise, occupational exposure, emotions, and respiratory infections.

Status asthmaticus has been defined as a severe asthmatic attack that does not respond to pharmacologic treatment within a few hours. Status asthmaticus is an acute progressive and life-threatening event that leads to respiratory failure if not properly treated.

Table 2-8 shows the characteristics of intrinsic and extrinsic asthma.

Pathophysiology

Whereas the trigger mechanism and physiologic response for intrinsic and extrinsic asthma differ, the clinical response appears the same. Figure 2-22 summarizes the proposed pathogenesis for the two causes of an asthmatic response.

Diagnostic Studies and Findings

Arterial Blood Gases

$Pa{O_2}$: normal or slightly decreased secondary to decreased $\dot{V}/\dot{Q}$; has direct linear relationship with FEV_1 (as FEV_1 decreases, so does $Pa{O_2}$ [<60 mm Hg])

$Pa{CO_2}$: increases only when FEV_1 is decreased by at least 20% (≥40 mm Hg)

pH: normal or decreased

HCO_3^-: normal or decreased

Pulmonary Function

FEV_1 (young healthy adult individual):
- Asthma before treatment: abnormally low
- After treatment: at least 2 L

PEFR (peak flow) (young healthy adult individual):
- Asthma before treatment: as low as 100 L/min
- After treatment: at least 300 L/min

TLC: increases during acute episode because of air trapping

RV: increases during acute episode

VC: <1 L

Sputum Examination

Gross examination of sputum indicates sputum with increased viscosity and plugs

Complete Blood Count (CBC)

Eosinophilia usually seen, which indicates allergic response

Increased hematocrit (Hct)

Figure 2-22 Proposed pathogenesis of bronchial asthma.

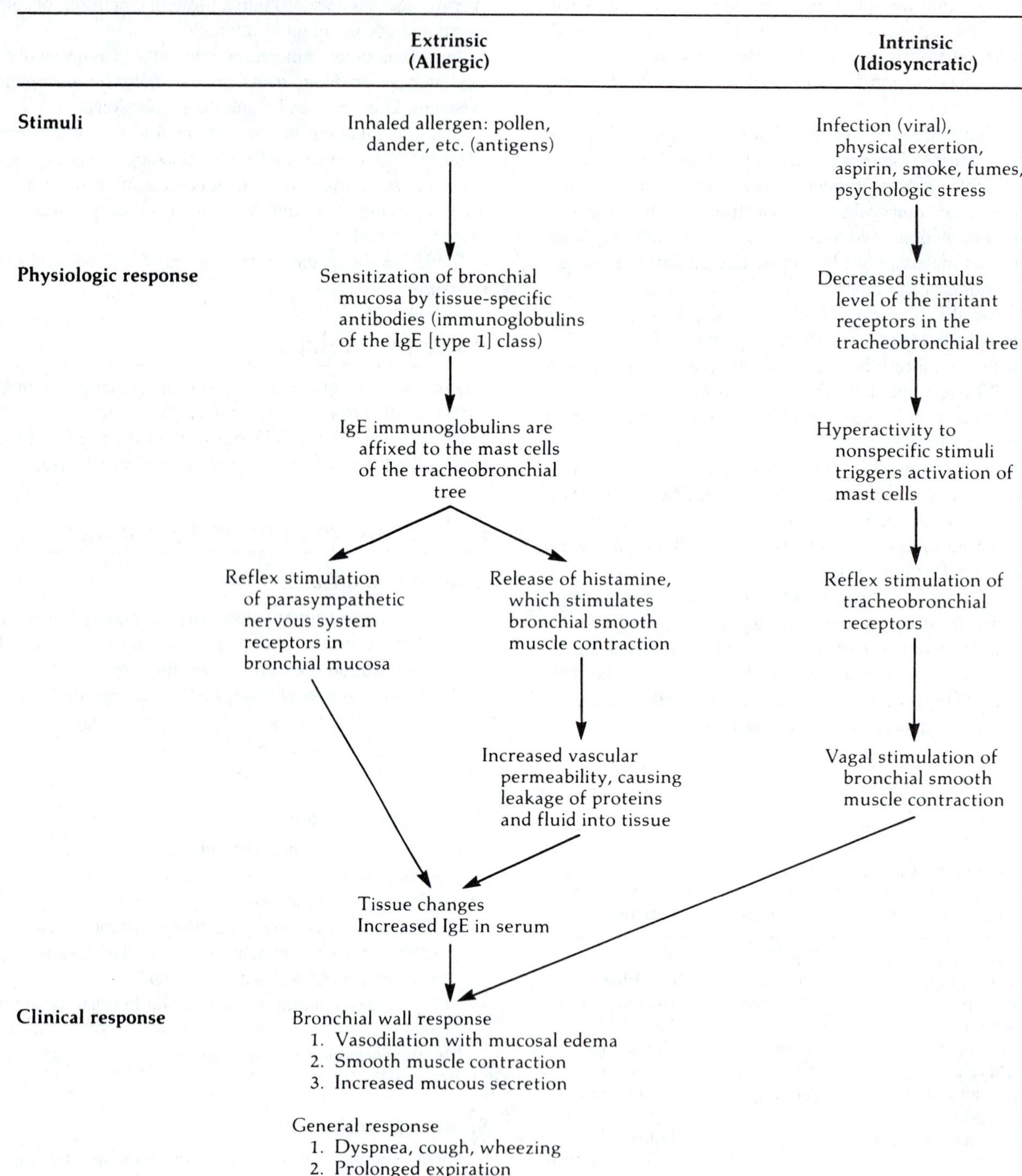

Chest Roentgenogram

Roentgenogram usually clear; hyperinflation secondary to air trapping may be seen in persistent and long-standing cases; transient migratory pulmonary infiltrations may also be seen

Electrocardiogram (ECG)

Sinus tachycardia may be seen in acute episodes; prominent P waves occur in chronic asthma

Theophylline Level

Any asthmatic patient taking theophylline should have baseline monitoring of theophylline levels; therapeutic level of theophylline in the blood is 10 to 20 μg/ml

Medical Plan

The intent of the immediate medical plan is to decrease the amount of bronchospasm and to increase pulmonary ventilation.

After the acute event is passed, the medical plan is to identify precipitating stimuli and to promote maximum health with this potentially degenerative chronic disease.

Surgery

Bronchoscopy: On the rare occasions when conventional therapy fails to produce an improvement, a bronchoscopy for aspiration and saline lavage of secretions may be performed.

Medications

Drug therapy for asthma can be divided into three categories: I, acute phase therapy; II, status asthmaticus therapy; and III, interim therapy. For each of these treatment categories, two types of pharmacologic agents are used. Bronchodilators are used to increase the airway diameter, and corticosteroids are used to reduce the inflammatory response.

Category I: acute phase

Bronchodilators

Parenteral

Epinephrine 1:1000, 0.3-0.8 ml subcutaneously q15-30 min

Theophylline (Quibron, Theo-Dur), loading dose 5-6 mg/kg in normal saline over 20 min; lower dose for patients over 40 years of age; obtain theophylline levels in 12-24 h and maintain level at 10-20 μg/ml

Terbutaline (Brethine, Bricanyl), 0.2-0.3 ml subcutaneously q30 min for 3 doses

Aminophylline, 250 mg in 20-30 ml normal saline IV (or 5.6-6 mg/kg in 100 ml normal saline); maximum rate 25 mg/min

Aerosols: 1 or 2 inhalations from hand nebulizer q3-4h or 0.5 ml in 2.5 or 3 ml normal saline by nebulization

Isoproterenol (Isuprel) 1:200

Isoetharine (Bronkosol) 1:200

Corticosteroids

Parenteral

Hydrocortisone sodium succinate (Solu-Cortef), 100-250 mg

Oral

Prednisone (Deltasone, others), 40-60 mg/d in divided doses; tapered rapidly over 3 wk if possible

Category II: status asthmaticus

Bronchodilators

Epinephrine: same as for category I

Aminophylline (loading dose): 5.6-6 mg/kg in 100 ml normal saline for 20-30 min; maximum rate 25 mg/min

Continued therapy dose

Young adult smokers: 1 mg/kg/h for 12 h, then reduce to 0.8 mg/kg/h

Healthy, nonsmoking adults: 0.7-0.9 mg/kg/h for 12 h; then reduce to 0.5 mg/kg/h

Older adults with cor pulmonale: 0.6 mg/kg/h for 12 h; then reduce to 0.3 mg/kg/h

Adults with congestive heart failure and liver failure: 0.5 mg/kg/h for 12 h; then reduce to 0.1-0.2 mg/kg/h

Subsequent doses should be determined by therapeutic serum level of aminophylline of 10-20 μg/ml

Corticosteroids

Parenteral

Hydrocortisone sodium succinate (Solu-Cortef), 4 mg/kg IV q4h

Methylprednisolone sodium succinate (Solu-Medrol), 2 mg/kg IV q4h

Oral: may also start on oral medications then reduce IV medications

Hydrocortisone sodium succinate (Solu-Cortef), 300 mg/d divided into 4 doses

Prednisone (Deltasone, others), 20 mg/d divided into 4 doses

Methylprednisolone (Medrol), 16 mg/d divided into 4 doses

Category III: interim phase

Bronchodilator: maintenance doses to keep serum level at 10-20 μg/ml

Oral

Theophylline (Aerolate, Elixophyllin, Quibron, Tedral, Theo-Dur, Theolair), 16 mg/kg/d in single dose or divided doses

Aminophylline (Aminodur, Aminophyl, Somophyllin), 3.5-5 mg/kg q6h

Aerosol

Albuterol (Proventil Inhaler, Ventolin Inhaler) 1-2 inhalations q4-6h

Corticosteroids

Aerosol

Beclomethasone dipropionate (Vanceril inhaler, others), 2 inhalations qid; long acting and not systematically absorbed

Fluid and electrolyte therapy: The purpose of fluid therapy is to liquefy secretions and to have a method by which to administer intravenous drugs. Providing that the patient has no cardiovascular dysfunction, fluid therapy should be aggressive. Dextrose 5% in water or 5% dextrose in 0.02 normal saline are adequate intravenous solutions. Electrolytes must be monitored frequently and replaced as indicated.

General Management

Oxygenation: Humidified oxygen should be administered by nasal cannula or mask to counteract clinical and laboratory signs of hypoxemia. Oxygen is administered to keep PaO_2 in range of 60 to 70 mm Hg to result in oxygen saturation greater than 90%.

Volume-cycled ventilator: Should the patient's condition continue to deteriorate despite aggressive therapy (1% to 3% of hospitalized asthma patients), endotracheal intubation and mechanical ventilation may become necessary.

The goal of ventilation by this method is to ensure adequate alveolar ventilation without hypercapnia or hypocapnia. To do this the practitioner should:

1. Decrease tidal volume as tolerated to allow lower cycling pressures
2. Decrease respiratory rate as tolerated to allow adequate duration of expiration
3. Supply heated, humidified oxygen to maintain PaO_2
4. Sedate patient as required and ordered
5. Continue to administer medications as listed under the drug section
6. Administer chest physiotherapy and continue to encourage coughing[55]

Chest physiotherapy: Postural drainage with chest percussion should be administered at least every 2 to 4 hours as long as the patient has congestion. See pp. 221 to 225 for techniques.

Environment: Provide an atmosphere void of known allergens.

NURSING CARE

Nursing Assessment

Asthma must be assessed not only in the areas of concern listed but also as to its overall severity on both a short- and long-term basis. Table 2-9 summarizes this assessment.

Table 2-9
Assessment of Severity of Asthma

	Mild	Moderate	Severe
Episode Severity Analysis*			
Acute phase	Mild dyspnea Diffuse wheezes Adequate air exchange	Respiratory distress at rest Hyperpnea Marked wheezes Air exchange normal or ↓	Marked respiratory distress Marked wheezes or absent breath sounds Pulsus paradoxus >10 mm Chest wall retractions
	FEV_1 = 80% normal pH = Normal or ↑ PaO_2 = Normal or ↓ $PaCO_2$ = Normal or ↓	FEV_1 = 50% normal pH = Generally ↑ PaO_2 = ↓ $PaCO_2$ = Generally ↓	FEV_1 = 25% normal pH = Normal or ↓ PaO_2 = ↓ $PaCO_2$ = Normal or ↑
Disease Severity Analysis†			
General assessment	Attacks no more than once per week Responds to bronchodilators in 24 hours No signs of asthma between episodes No sleep interruption due to asthma No hyperventilation Normal chest roentgenogram Minimal evidence of airway obstruction No to minimal degree of increase in lung volume	Cough and wheeze episodes more than once per week Cough and low-grade wheeze between acute episodes Exercise tolerance diminished May be up at night because of cough and wheeze Hyperinflation seen on chest roentgenogram Lung volumes increased	Daily wheezing Frequent severe episodes Hospitalization frequently required to break cycle Poor exercise tolerance Much sleep interruption Chest deformity due to chronic hyperinflation Airway obstruction not completely reversible by bronchodilators Lung volumes markedly increased

*Modified from Berkow.[7]
†From Ellis.[22]

History

Known family or personal history of allergy, infantile eczema, or previous episodes of asthma
Previous recent severe attack
Prolonged attack (greater than 24 to 36 hours)
Previous hospitalization for asthma

Current Medications

Careful and complete history of current respiratory-related medications, as well as most recent dose and time before hospital arrival

Respiratory Status

Airway obstruction: with severe airway obstruction, breath sounds diminished in certain lung regions
Respiratory distress: dyspnea, tachypnea, cough, prolonged expiration, use of accessory muscles during breathing, retractions
Breath sounds: inspiratory and expiratory wheeze, coarse rhonchi; in severe cases only coarse bronchial sounds heard; bilateral sounds heard throughout chest

Skin

Increased diaphoresis as respiratory distress increases

Hypoxia

Restlessness, tachycardia; respiratory rate greater than 30 per minute; pulse greater than 130 per minute; pulsus paradoxus greater than 15 per minute; confusion, hypotension, cyanosis, premature ventricular contractions, right bundle-branch block with severe hypoxia

Pulmonary Function

FEV_1 decreased, peak expiratory flow rate decreased, total lung capacity increased, residual volume increased

Laboratory Values

Blood gases: decreased Pao_2, increased $Paco_2$, decreased pH
CBC: eosinophilia, increased Hct

Chest Roentgenogram

Unilateral obstruction or infiltration

Hydration

Intake and output to monitor hydration

Psychosocial

Fear of suffocation

Nursing Dx & Intervention

Nursing Diagnosis	Nursing Intervention/Rationale
Ineffective breathing pattern	• Assess ventilation to include evaluation of breathing rate, rhythm, and depth; chest expansion; presence of respiratory distress such as dyspnea; shortness of breath; nasal flaring; pursed-lip breathing or prolonged expiratory phase; and use of accessory muscles *to evaluate respiratory status and effectiveness of treatment measures*. • Assess peak expiratory flow rate or forced expiratory volume as ordered. • Assess patient for tiring in relation to attempts to breathe. • Identify contributing factors such as allergens in immediate environment or other irritants that may exacerbate condition. • Maintain patient positioning *to facilitate ventilation* (i.e., sitting upright and leaning forward on overbed table). • Instruct patient in pulmonary hygiene routines *that facilitate breathing and minimize pulmonary congestion that could lead to secondary infections*. • Initiate preventive measures such as uninterrupted periods of quiet time; maintain calm and restful environment; encourage patient to participate in care as tolerated; explain all therapy before administering *to improve breathing pattern*. • Encourage patient to use adaptive breathing techniques *to decrease work of breathing*. • Assist patient to space activities *to provide periods of rest in between*. • Cover pillows with allergen-proof covers *to eliminate dust and other irritants*. • Problem solve with patient to determine methods of conserving energy while still performing activities of daily living *to prevent further depression of respiratory status*. • Assist to protect patient from known sources of secondary infection. • If mechanical ventilation is required, provide care and monitoring consistent with the guidelines presented on pp. 225 to 228.
Fatigue	• Assess patterns of fatigue. • Assess factors related to fatigue and strategies for dealing with them. • Assess support systems and available resources. • Administer treatments or medications to relieve discomfort. • Enhance patient's ability to rest between specified activities.

Nursing Diagnosis	Nursing Intervention/Rationale
Potential for infection	• Assess mouth and oral mucosa for presence of mouth irritation *to prevent possible mouth infection secondary to corticosteroids.* • Instruct patient using aerated corticosteroids to perform thorough mouth washing after each use *to prevent mouth irritation.* • Assess for secondary respiratory infection resulting from congested condition. • Monitor results of complete blood count and report abnormal leukocyte level. • Encourage optimum nutrition; encourage fluids up to 2600 ml/day unless otherwise contraindicated.
Impaired verbal communication	• Assess for signs of frustration or fear secondary to hypoxia that is causing fatigue when patient attempts to talk.
Self-care deficit	• Assess level of self-care deficit secondary to patient's current condition. • Provide assistive interventions for such activities of daily living as toileting, bathing, and feeding *to minimize patient's energy expenditures.*
Altered health maintenance	• Assess with patient or family home and environmental stimulants (allergens) that may exacerbate asthma episode. • Provide education regarding need to avoid contact with irritant allergens. • Assist with allergy testing and desensitization if indicated. • Assess for adverse systemic allergic response during allergy testing or desensitization process.
Ineffective individual coping	• Assess patient's response and perception related to present breathing difficulties. • Determine patient's ability to cooperate with health care providers regarding intervention strategies such as breathing techniques, exercise progression, and alterations in activities of daily living. • Listen carefully to collect information regarding significance of asthma and patient's perception of ability to deal with alterations it is causing.
Family coping: potential for growth	• Assess family's anxiety related to limited understanding of diagnostic procedures, disease process and prognosis, and therapies employed. • Provide information in areas needed *to assist family to become informed about asthma as a disease.* • Explain relationship of disease process and rationale for various therapeutic interventions at a level appropriate for comprehension and degree of anxiety. • Involve family in care as appropriate. • Encourage family to verbalize questions and concerns.

Patient Education

1. Teach facts about and importance of prescribed medications such as bronchodilators and corticosteroids.
2. Provide the patient and family with information about asthma as a disease, how to assess an asthmatic response, what to do during the process of care, criteria for requesting professional assistance, and acute emergency care.
3. Assist the patient and family to examine secondary factors that may precipitate asthmatic episodes such as emotional stress, fatigue, or environmental changes or specific allergen contacts such as dust, animal dander, feathers, and pollen.
4. Teach the patient adaptive breathing techniques and breathing exercises such as pursed-lip breathing and positioning.
5. Teach the importance of consuming large quantities of fluid to maintain secretion liquefaction.
6. Teach adaptive exercise and rest techniques.
7. Provide the patient and family with information regarding the care, cleaning, and maintenance of inhalation equipment being used in the hospital or to be used at home.
8. Provide the patient and family with respiratory-related health information such as pollution indexes, secondary infection exposure, and community support groups.

Evaluation

Patient Outcome	Data Indicating That Outcome is Reached
Air moves optimally in and out of lungs. Airway is patent. Lungs are fully aerated as visualized on chest roentgenogram.	Vital capacity measurements including FEV_1, TLC, and RV are optimum for patient's status. Serum level of IgE is normal for patient. WBC is within normal limits. Blood gas values are within normal limits. Airways are clear, breath sounds are clear, and breathing occurs without obstruction.
Breathing pattern occurs without tiring patient. Clear breath sounds are heard in all areas.	Patient demonstrates modified breathing techniques that facilitate ventilatory capacity. Behavior is modified to conserve energy expenditure.
Physiologic function is stable.	Hydration level is maintained within normal limits. Gastrointestinal system is functioning adequately. There are no secondary infections. Serum electrolytes are within normal limits.
Patient relates importance of pulmonary exercises.	Patient demonstrates pulmonary exercises and states rationale and importance of maintaining daily exercise routine.
Patient preserves pulmonary functioning by maintaining optimum activity level, preventing infection, and following prescribed treatments.	Patient demonstrates a variety of methods indicating ability to preserve and facilitate optimum respiratory functioning (e.g., breathing exercises, modified activities or exercise, taking medications as prescribed).
Patient and family have sufficient information to comply with discharge regimen.	Patient and family are able at time of discharge to discuss medications (purpose, side effects, route, and schedule), activity regimen, signs of infection or respiratory deterioration, and plan for long-term follow-up maintenance.
Patient and family have sufficient information to assist with preventing further asthma episodes or reduce severity of episodes.	Patient and family discuss pathophysiology of asthma, precipitating factors, and factor avoidance techniques, as well as treatment interventions should episode occur.

Bronchiectasis

Bronchiectasis is the chronic dilation of the medium-sized bronchi with eventual destruction of the bronchial elastic and muscular elements. Usually the result of repeated pulmonary infections or bronchial obstruction, this chronic dilation leads to the eventual malfunctioning of bronchial muscle tone and elasticity.

The incidence of this acquired disorder has decreased greatly since the development of antibiotics and aggressive management of pulmonary infections. Before the use of antibiotics, pulmonary infections sometimes lingered and a second pulmonary obstruction occurred below the buildup of sputum and bronchial secretions. The chronic obstruction and tissue stretching eventually progress to the destruction of bronchial elasticity and actual malfunctioning of bronchial muscle tone.

Children are at high risk for the development of bronchiectasis. This is because their bronchi are small and soft and easily damaged by prolonged overinflation caused by infection or bronchial foreign body obstruction. The prevalence of childhood bronchiectasis is decreasing because of the use of antibiotics, but it is still seen in children with cystic fibrosis and immune deficiency diseases.

Although disease onset, especially in children, may follow a single episode of pulmonary disease, most adults have a history of numerous pulmonary infections such as pneumonia and a chronic bronchitis type of cough. Delayed resolution of any type of pulmonary disease should raise suspicion of bronchiectasis.

Pathophysiology

Bronchiectasis is almost always caused by a failure of normal lung defenses to infection and a failure to clear bronchial secretions. This may be the result of primary or secondary ciliary dysfunction, aspiration of gastric acid or a foreign body, bronchial obstruction by a tumor, or abnormal mucus clearance of cystic fibrosis or allergic aspergillosis. Failure of the immune system may also predispose an individual to infection leading to bronchiectasis. These various factors often occur together and are more likely to cause severe, chronic airway and pulmonary injury in the developing bronchial tree of the child. The most important interrelationships are shown in Figure 2-23.[17]

The development of bronchiectasis usually occurs over a period of time where a recurrence of an inflammatory and infectious process slowly alters the structure of the bronchial

Figure 2-23 Pathogenesis of bronchiectasis.
From Cherniack.[17]

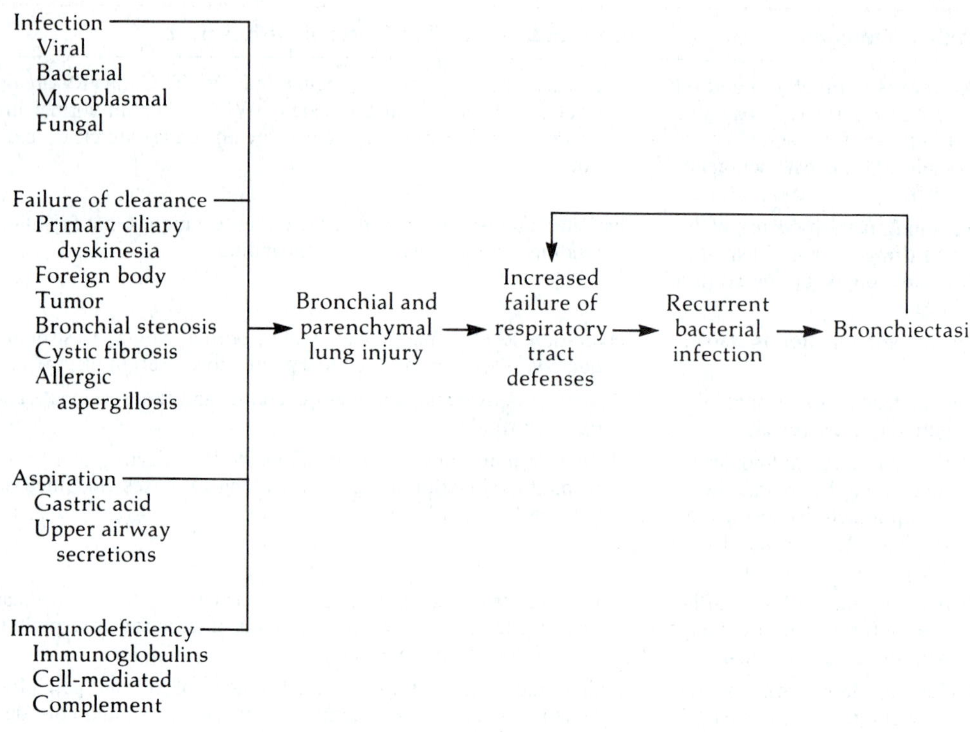

walls and their elastic and muscular response. Once the alterations have occurred, they are irreversible.

Diagnostic Studies and Findings

Clinical Examination

Severe and chronic, mucopurulent, sputum-producing cough; hemoptysis; moist rales and rhonchi heard over the lower lobes; dyspnea; fatigue; and general signs of pulmonary insufficiency

Bronchography

Definitive diagnostic procedure of bronchiectasis; bronchography outlines walls of bronchi and clearly shows bronchiectatic areas

Sputum Examination

Gross examination shows that the sputum has three layers (sediment, fluid, and foam); a sputum smear is done to rule out tuberculosis and identify secondary bacterial infections such as those caused by pneumococci, *Pseudomonas,* and *Enterobacter;* large numbers of white blood cells and bacteria that mostly include pharyngeal flora, including anaerobic organisms, are usually seen; the decision on choice of antibiotics in the treatment of the intercurrent infection depends on the result of culture and sensitivity studies of sputum

Complete Blood Count (CBC)

With severe hypoxia may show polycythemia secondary to pulmonary insufficiency

Pulmonary Function

Spirometry may reveal a decreased forced expiratory volume (FEV_1) and a decreased forced vital capacity (FVC); many patients with mild to moderate bronchiectasis will have no abnormality detectable by routine spirometry and arterial blood gas analysis

Chest Roentgenogram

Clear but may show patches of inflammation with increased pulmonary markings at the lung bases

Medical Plan

The goals of the medical plan are to maintain maximum ventilation by controlling infections and removing secretions.

Surgery

Bronchial resection—may rarely be performed on patients with isolated areas of bronchiectasis that do not respond to conservative treatment; for this disease must be localized enough to permit complete resection without inadvertently compromising pulmonary function

Medications

Mucolytic agents

Acetylcysteine (Mucomyst), nebulization q2-6h with 20% solution (1-10 ml) or 10% solution (2-20 ml)

Anti-infective agents

Antibiotic therapy should be specific to the organism identified in the sputum evaluation

Bronchodilators

Ipratropium bromide (Atrovent), 40-80 μg q6h

Theophylline used in rare cases, long acting, 200 mg q12h increased in a few days to 300 mg q12h

General Management

Warm or cool mist via vaporizer to assist in liquefying of secretions

Physiotherapy with postural drainage for at least 10 minutes 3 or 4 times a day (see p. 221 for technique)

Warm, dry climate void of smoke, fumes, and air pollution

Patient discouraged from smoking

Fluid increase to liquefy secretions and maintain hydration

Periodic sputum culture to identify presence of secondary infections

NURSING CARE

Nursing Assessment

Respiratory Status

Breath sounds: rales and rhonchi over lower lobes

Breathing patterns: may be labored with prolonged expiration; increased dyspnea

Cough: chronic with production of large quantities of purulent sputum (coughing and sputum production may become worse with changes in posture and activity)

Hemoptysis in 50% of cases

Chest wall may have retractions during breathing and decreased expiratory excursion

Respiratory failure will eventually develop

Chest Roentgenogram

Clear but may show some areas of inflammation with increased markings at the base

Mediastinal shift may be seen secondary to overinflation of specific lobes of the lung

Cardiovascular Response

In advanced cases, cyanosis and clubbing of fingers

Generalized Response

Weight loss, night sweats, fever, gradual emaciation may be indications of disease progression with possible secondary infections

Nursing Dx & Intervention

Nursing Diagnosis	Nursing Intervention/Rationale
Ineffective airway clearance	• Assess patient to identify inability to move secretions; promote aggressive techniques such as positioning, postural drainage, coughing, suctioning, and fluid promotion *to liquefy and drain excessive secretions*. (See pp. 221 to 225 for techniques of postural drainage.) • Assist patient to maintain proper body positioning and frequent alteration of body position *to ensure patent airway and secretion drainage*. • Suction if necessary *to remove secretions*. • In collaboration with physician administer mucolytic drugs and antibiotics; assess and document patient response. • Provide oral hygiene before and after respiratory therapy *because of medication taste and increased sputum production*.
Ineffective breathing pattern	• Assess ventilation to include evaluation of breathing rate, rhythm, and depth, chest expansion, presence of respiratory distress such as dyspnea, shortness of breath, nasal flaring, pursed-lip breathing or prolonged expiratory phase, use of abdominal muscles. • Periodically assess forced expiratory volume (FEV_1) and forced vital capacity (FVC) *to evaluate pulmonary function*. • Instruct patient in hygiene routines that facilitate easy and effective breathing. • Assess patient for tiring in relation to attempts to breathe.
Impaired gas exchange	• Assess patient to identify signs such as restlessness, confusion, and irritability, which *may indicate the body's response to altered blood gas states*. • Carefully monitor body temperature, sputum characteristics, and cough characteristics, which *may indicate the presence of secondary infection and which may lead to respiratory insufficiency if not properly treated*.

Nursing Diagnosis	Nursing Intervention/Rationale
	• Assist patient to avoid environmental irritants such as smoke, fumes, and air pollution; patient should also be instructed not to smoke. • Monitor and record kidney function and urinary output, which *may be affected secondary to chronic tissue hypoxia and alterations in metabolism.* • Monitor serum electrolytes, which *may change because of alterations in oxygenation and metabolism.*
Potential for infection	• Assess for signs and symptoms of infection, fever, dyspnea, and change in sputum color, amount, or odor. • Obtain sputum for culture and sensitivity. • Protect patient from known source of secondary infection, which may lead to respiratory insufficiency.
Altered nutrition: less than body requirements	• Assess for signs and symptoms of malnutrition. • Assist patient to choose foods that are easy to chew and swallow; assist by cutting and feeding if patient tires easily. • Encourage smaller, more frequent meals. • Encourage fluid intake of at least 2 L/day *to facilitate liquefying of secretions and promote urinary output.* (If patient has compromised cardiac or renal condition, fluid intake must be determined in collaboration with physician.)
Impaired physical mobility	• Encourage patient to use adaptive breathing techniques *to decrease the work of breathing.* • Assist patient to space activities *to provide periods of rest in between.* • Encourage gradual increase of activities as tolerated *to prevent "pulmonary crippling."* • Problem solve with patient to determine methods of conserving energy while still performing activities of daily living. • Assess and document activities that cause patient to tire easily and become short of breath. • If patient is seriously ill and maintained on bed rest, encourage or provide active or passive range of motion exercises *to maintain adequate muscle tone.*
Self-care deficit	• See p. 1692 for associated care.
Anxiety	• Assess patient's level of anxiety related to the present health state. • Assess patient's level of anxiety related to chronic cough and sputum production.
Ineffective individual coping	• Assess patient's ability to cooperate with health care providers regarding intervention strategies such as breathing techniques, exercise progression, and alterations in the activities of daily living. • See p. 1804 for additional strategies.
Family coping: potential for growth	• See p. 1816 for additional nursing care.

Patient Education

1. Teach patient adaptive breathing techniques such as pursed-lip and abdominal breathing.
2. Teach patient to prevent secondary infections by coughing and deep breathing, which will prevent the accumulation of secretion buildup in the lungs.
3. Teach importance of not smoking and avoiding fumes or smoke during active disease state.
4. Teach adaptive exercise and rest techniques.
5. Teach eating and food choice modifications.
6. Teach importance of getting immunizations to prevent illnesses.
7. Teach facts about and importance of prescribed medications.
8. Provide patient and family with respiratory-related health information such as pollution indexes, home humidification techniques, and climate changes.
9. Teach importance of avoidance of contact with other persons who may expose patient to a secondary infection.
10. Teach signs of secondary infection such as change in characteristics of sputum or prolonged fever.

Evaluation

Patient Outcome	Data Indicating That Outcome is Reached
Air moves optimally in and out of lungs.	Coughing if present is productive of sputum.
Airway is patent.	Airways are clear and breathing occurs without obstruction.
Chest roentgenogram is clear.	No evidence of overinflation or infiltration is seen.
Patient is free of secondary respiratory infection.	Sputum evaluation shows no evidence of a secondary respiratory infection.
Breathing pattern occurs without tiring patient.	Patient demonstrates modified breathing techniques that facilitate ventilatory capacity. Behavior is modified to conserve energy expenditure.
Physiologic function is stable.	Nutrition level is maintained.
Patient relates importance of daily pulmonary exercises.	Patient demonstrates pulmonary exercises and states rationale and importance of maintaining daily exercise routine.
Patient preserves pulmonary functioning by maintaining optimal activity level, preventing infection, and following prescribed treatments.	Patient demonstrates a variety of methods indicating ability to preserve and facilitate optimal respiratory functioning (e.g., breathing exercises, modified activities or exercise, taking medications as prescribed).
Patient and family have sufficient information to comply with discharge regimen.	Patient and family are able at time of discharge to discuss medications (purpose, side effects, route, and schedule), activity progression regimen, signs of infection or respiratory deterioration, and plan for follow-up visits.

Cystic Fibrosis

Cystic fibrosis (CF) is an autosomal recessive disorder of the exocrine glands that causes those glands to produce abnormally thick secretions of mucus. The glands most affected are the respiratory, pancreatic, and sweat glands.

In the United States, CF is the most common cause of life-threatening pulmonary disease of whites during childhood and adolescence. The disease incidence is 1 in 1500 to 2000 live births. CF is least prevalent in blacks, American Indians, and persons of Asian ancestry. Boys and girls are equally affected.

CF is the primary cause of pancreatic deficiency and chronic malabsorption in children. It is also responsible for many cases of intestinal obstruction in newborns. Although CF is a widespread multisystem disease, the progressive pulmonary infections are the most important clinical problem and are responsible for most of the morbidity and mortality.[82] Advances in the treatment of the respiratory components of the disease have been important in improving the prognosis, but maximum success cannot be achieved unless gastrointestinal, hepatic, and psychologic components and sweat abnormalities are also managed.

There is no known cure for CF, but much has been done to lengthen the survival of patients. Without knowledge of the underlying biochemical defect, treatment focuses on the effects of the disease. Despite marked improvement in prognosis since CF was first described in the 1930s, the disease remains uniformly fatal, the median age of death being approximately 22 years for females and 28 years for males.[17]

Therapy for patients with CF is aimed at improving the nutritional status and minimizing pulmonary involvement. Respiratory and cardiac complications (e.g., hemoptysis, pneumothorax, pulmonary insufficiency, cor pulmonale, and cardiac failure) are additive and tend to become more severe with increasing age. Death is most commonly caused by cardiac and respiratory insufficiency.

CF can be an extremely expensive disease. Average costs just for drugs, laboratory tests, and clinic visits are estimated to be at least $2000 annually. The costs are much higher for patients requiring hospitalization, home oxygenation, or home nursing care.[29]

Pathophysiology

CF (mucoviscidosis) is a pancreatic enzyme deficiency affecting the exocrine glands throughout the body, both mucus producing and other. Despite intensive research the exact defect in CF remains unknown.

The goblet cells of the mucus-producing (exocrine) glands of the body produce abnormal secretions. These secretions, instead of being thin and free flowing, are thick mucoproteins that coagulate to form eosinophilic concentrations in the glands or ducts. The glands and ducts clog and widen, causing pathologic changes and thus symptoms. The pathologic changes are thought to be caused by the obstruction, not the abnormal condition of the secretions. Abnormalities of the non-mucus-producing glands are seen in saliva and sweat.

CF has a significant and predictable impact throughout the body.

Pancreas. Thick secretions block the pancreatic ducts, causing cystic widenings of the small lobes of the acini. Degenerative and fibrotic changes in the pancreas result, and the essential pancreatic enzymes (trypsin, amylase, and lipase) are unable to participate in food absorption and digestion. Thus digestion of fats, proteins, and carbohydrates is disturbed, as evidenced by increased stool fat and protein. Generalized pancreatic dysfunction places patients with CF at higher risk for diabetes mellitus.

Pulmonary system. The thick mucus causes bronchial and bronchiolar obstruction. This leads at first to areas of atelectasis and hyperinflation. As lung involvement progresses, reduction of oxygen and retention of oxygen and carbon dioxide result in hypoxia, hypercapnia, and acidosis. The heavy mucous secretions also decrease ciliary activity and thus contribute to mucous obstruction. Mucous stasis encourages bacterial growth and resulting infection. With severe lung involvement, compression of pulmonary blood vessels and progressive lung dysfunction frequently lead to pulmonary hypertension and cor pulmonale.

Cardiac system. Cardiac changes such as right ventricular hypertrophy occur as a result of obstructive bronchial disease, cor pulmonale, and pulmonary hypertension.

Biliary system. Foci of biliary blockage and fibrosis are common and become progressively worse, resulting in a type of multilobular biliary cirrhosis. If liver involvement is extensive, portal hypertension and an enlarged spleen may also occur. Jaundice may be evidence of gallbladder obstruction.

Reproductive organs. In girls the cervical mucous glands may be dilated. Boys may have abnormal development and function of the epididymis, vas deferens, and seminal vesicles as a result of abnormal secretions during fetal development.

Non-mucus-producing glands. Sweat and salivary gland secretions have abnormally high levels of sodium and chloride. There are no histologic abnormalities.

Diagnostic Studies and Findings

Cystic fibrosis may occur at any age from infancy to adulthood. Diagnosis is based on clinical presentation (Table 2-10) and is confirmed by an elevated sweat chloride level, the most consistent diagnostic test available, although even this has a 2% false positive and false negative rate. A sweat chloride concentration greater than 60 mEq/L is considered diagnostic.[17]

Table 2-10
Clinical Presentation of Cystic Fibrosis

Age	Clinical Features
Infancy	Meconium ileus, protracted neonatal jaundice, hyponatremic dehydration
Childhood	Recurrent or chronic chest infection, malnutrition, intussusception, volvulus, meconium ileus equivalent, fat-soluble vitamin deficiency, pancreatitis, recurrent nasal polyps, chronic sinusitis
Adolescence	Recurrent or chronic chest infection, cor pulmonale, diabetes mellitus, male infertility

From Cherniack.[17]

Family History

History of siblings or other family members with cystic fibrosis

Sweat Electrolytes

Normal mean value approximately 18 mEq/L (varies with age); sweat chloride 40-60 mEq/L suggestive of CF; sweat chloride over 60 mEq/L diagnostic of CF

Pancreatic Enzymes

Examination of duodenal secretions or stool for presence of trypsin and chymotrypsin; absence of enzymes suggestive of potential CF

Stool Examination for Fat

Fat absorption tests conducted for 5 days to calculate ratio of fat in oral intake to fat in stool; impaired fat absorption in intestine, resulting in large volumes excreted in the stool (steatorrhea), suggestive of CF

Figure 2-24 Chest roentgenogram of patient with cystic fibrosis. Note bronchial thickening and ill-defined shadows.

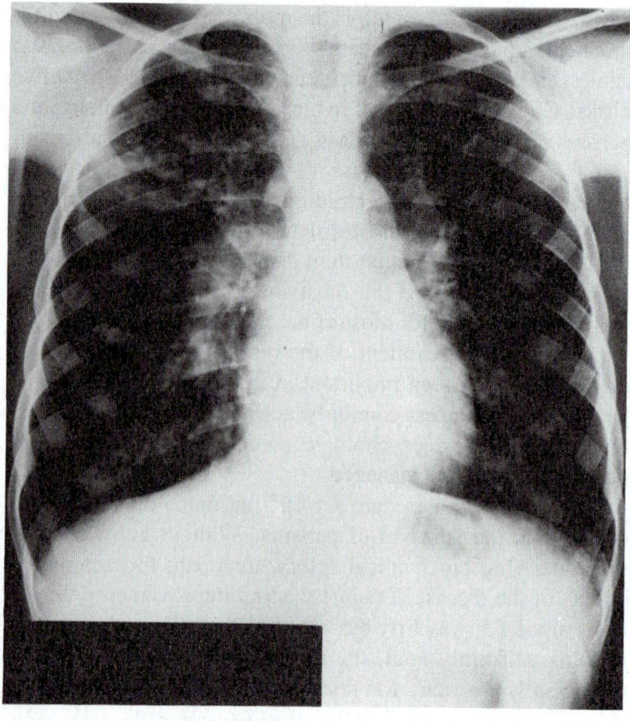

Chest Roentgenogram

Evidence of generalized obstructive emphysema suggestive of CF (Figure 2-24); in advanced disease patchy atelectasis and disseminated infiltration pattern may be seen

Medical Plan

Treatment is aimed at minimizing the bronchial plugging and attempting to inhibit the bacterial colonization.

Surgery

Pulmonary lavage or bronchial washing—may be used for seriously ill patients whose bronchial airways cannot be cleared by other means

Resection of blebs and pleural scars—may be attempted if pulmonary disease is localized; purpose is resection of blebs and pleural scars by pleural stripping

Tracheostomy or endotracheal intubation—may be carried out for seriously ill patients; permits mechanical ventilation and facilitates mechanical pulmonary toileting

Medications

Mucolytic agents

- Acetylcysteine (Mucomyst), nebulization q8-12h with 10% solution (2-3 ml)

Anti-infective agents

- May be prescribed only at time of illness and infection or prophylactically; if prescribed for infection, antibiotic of choice depends on organism

Expectorants

- Iodinated glycerol (Organidin), 60 mg q6h taken with liquid
- Potassium iodide (Ki-N, Pima), 300-600 mg q4-6h

Bronchodilators

- Salbutamol, metered aerosol 1-2 puffs q4-6h
  - Inhalation solution, inhalation 0.01-0.03 mg/kg/day
- Theophylline po or IV 18-24 mg/kg/day
- Fenoterol, metered aerosol, inhalation, 1-2 puffs q4-6h

Digestive agents

- Rationale: Provide enzymatic activity necessary to assist in digestion of carbohydrates, fats, and proteins
- Pancreatin (Elzyme, Viokase), 325-1000 mg with meals or snacks
- Pancrelipase (Cotazym, Ilozyme, Ku-Zyme HP, Pancrease), 1-3 tablets or capsules, 0.43-1.29 g powder, or 1-2 powder packets before or with meals or snacks; has 12 times the lipase and four times the amylase and protease activity of pancreatin
- Contraindication: Hypersensitivity to pork or beef
- Common side effects: Nausea, diarrhea, vomiting, anorexia

Immunizations

- Routine immunizations against diphtheria, tetanus, pertussis, poliomyelitis, measles, mumps, and influenza recommended as preventive measures

General Management

Oxygenation—may be indicated for persons unable to maintain adequate oxygen levels; oxygen concentrations should be as low as possible while maintaining adequate Pa_{O_2} level; oxygen concentration should not exceed 24% to 40%; therapy may be initiated during times of infection or disease exacerbation

Aerosol therapy—may be used intermittently in conjunction with physiotherapy

Diet—sufficient calories to promote normal growth (exceeding daily requirements by at least 25%); high protein (at least 1.5 to 2 g/lb/day for infants and 1.25 g/lb/day for adults); low fat (no more than 50% of normal); multivitamins with addition of vitamins A, D, and E; vitamin K if hypoprothrombinemia present; supplemental salt in hot weather

Physiotherapy—time-honored part of the treatment of CF; standard techniques of chest percussion and postural drainage are used to help patient expectorate mucus from various pulmonary segments; recommended treatment plan is physiotherapy for 20 minutes twice or three times daily, depending on amount of sputum produced; see pp. 221 to 225 for techniques

NURSING CARE

Nursing Assessment

Respiratory Status

Respiratory distress: cough; congestion; tachypnea; retractions; decreased chest wall movement; labored breathing; dyspnea

Examination: barrel chest; tympanic percussion tone over consolidation or areas of atelectasis; clubbing of fingers and toes

Breath sounds: moist rales and rhonchi; decreased or unequal breath sounds

Sputum: productive cough with thick sputum; hemoptysis

Pulmonary function: decreased vital capacity; decreased FEV_1; decreased tidal volume; increased airway resistance

Acute respiratory complications: lobar atelectasis; lung abscess; spontaneous pneumothorax; cor pulmonale; congestive heart failure

Hypercapnia

Headache; dizziness; confusion; unconsciousness; twitching; sweating

Hypoxia

Restlessness; confusion; impaired motor function; cyanosis; tachycardia

Laboratory Values

Blood gases: pH; $Paco_2$; Pao_2
Serum levels: bicarbonate; sodium; chloride; potassium
Hematology: hematocrit; hemoglobin level
Sweat test: chloride concentrations greater than 60 mEq/L
Stool: no presence of pancreatic enzymes trypsin and chymotrypsin; increased fat in stool

Nutritional Status

Appetite; percentages of carbohydrate, fat, and protein in diet; salt supplementation; evidence of malnutrition

Hepatic and Biliary Function

Jaundice; enlarged liver; ascites; abnormal liver function findings

Gastrointestinal Function

Insufficient digestion producing bulky, foul-smelling, pale, watery stools; evidence of intestinal obstruction, fecal impaction, or rectal prolapse; evidence of gastrointestinal bleeding: tarry stools, positive guaiac findings

Cardiovascular Status

Decreased cardiac output: restlessness; lethargy; tachycardia

Bronchopulmonary Infection

Temperature; sputum specimens for culture and sensitivity; chest roentgenogram

Psychosocial

Support systems; networking with cystic fibrosis resource groups; activities of daily living; self-esteem; interaction with peers; sexuality

Nursing Dx & Intervention

Nursing Diagnosis	Nursing Intervention/Rationale
Ineffective airway clearance	• Assess patient's ability to move secretions. If inability is identified, assist with appropriate measures (such as coughing, positioning, suctioning, and liquefying secretions). • Promptly administer mucolytics and expectorants as ordered. Observe for therapeutic response and side effects. • Assist patient to maintain body position that *ensures maximum airway availability* (semi-Fowler's position or sitting upright). • Provide hydration *to liquefy secretions and replace fluids.* • Administer aerosol and perform postural drainage with percussion at least 1 hour before meals; provide oral hygiene after treatment. • Carefully and frequently auscultate chest for quality of breath sounds and adventitious sounds. Note cough and sputum characteristics. • Perform chest physiotherapy including percussion and postural drainage *to clear mucus and open airways.*
Ineffective breathing pattern	• Assess ventilation to include evaluation of breathing rate, rhythm, and depth; chest expansion; presence of respiratory distress such as dyspnea, shortness of breath, nasal flaring, pursed-lip breathing, or prolonged expiratory phase; and use of accessory muscles. • Identify contributing factors such as airway clearance or obstruction problem or weakness. • Maintain patient positioning *to facilitate easy ventilation* (head of bed in semi-Fowler's position). • Instruct patient in pulmonary hygiene routines *that will promote easy and effective breathing, facilitate removal of secretions from the tracheobronchial tree, and minimize pulmonary congestion that could lead to secondary infections.* • Suction if necessary *to remove secretions.* • Assess patient for tiring in relation to attempts to breathe. • Encourage patient to use adaptive breathing techniques *to decrease work of breathing and to alternate activities with periods of rest.* • Protect patient from known sources of secondary infection or breathing irritation such as smoking. • If mechanical ventilation is necessary, provide care and monitoring consistent with guidelines provided on pp. 225 to 228.
Impaired gas exchange	• Assess patient to identify signs, such as restlessness, confusion, and irritability, *that may indicate body's response to altered blood gas states.* • If patient is very ill, monitor arterial blood gases. Report increases or decreases of more than 10 to 15 mm Hg in $Paco_2$ and Pao_2. • Administer oxygen as ordered and monitor *to maintain* Pao_2 *between 45 and 60 mm Hg.* This may usually be maintained by administering oxygen by nasal cannula at flow of 1 to 3 L/minute. Venturi mask may be used if needed. If adequate blood gas levels cannot be maintained, mechanical ventilation must be considered.

Nursing Diagnosis	Nursing Intervention/Rationale
	• If patient is very ill, monitor electrocardiogram and cardiac status *for arrhythmias resulting from alterations in blood gases.* • Monitor and record kidney functioning and urinary output, which may be affected by chronic tissue hypoxia and alterations in metabolism. • Monitor serum electrolytes, which *may change owing to alterations in oxygenation and metabolism.* • Carefully monitor body temperature, which *may fluctuate owing to alterations in metabolism or secondary infections.*
Fatigue	• Assess patterns of fatigue. • Assess factors related to fatigue and strategies for dealing with them. • Assess support systems and available resources. • Administer treatments or medications to relieve discomfort. • Enhance patient's ability to rest between specified activities.
Altered nutrition: less than body requirements	• Assess nutritional status by daily weighing, monitoring intake and output, and observing skin turgor and muscle tone. • Provide small, frequent feedings of high-calorie, high-protein, low-fat foods with supplemental vitamins. Assist by cutting food and feeding if patient tires easily. • Administer pancreatic enzyme medications at mealtime. • Monitor serum levels of sodium and chloride. Observe for lethargy and signs of dehydration. Consult physician to administer sodium chloride should deficits occur. • If indicated and in consultation with physician, administer stool softeners *to relieve constipation.* • Monitor for signs and symptoms of malnutrition.
Potential for infection	• Assess for signs and symptoms of infection, fever, dyspnea, and change in sputum color, amount, or odor. • Obtain sputum for culture and sensitivity. • Protect patient from known sources of secondary infection.
Potential fluid volume deficit	• If patient is seriously ill, assess for evidence of gastrointestinal bleeding *related to physiologic stress;* monitor serial hemoglobin levels and hematocrit; check all stools, emesis, and nasogastric secretions *for presence of blood;* and observe changes in vital signs or abdominal girth.
Impaired physical mobility	• Encourage patient to use adaptive breathing techniques *to decrease work of breathing.* • Assist patient to alternate activities with periods of rest. • See p. 1687 for additional strategies.
Impaired verbal communication	• Assess for signs of frustration or fear, fatigue, and tiring with attempts to communicate *as result of hypoxia.*
Self-care deficit	• Assist with activities of daily living such as toileting, bathing, and feeding *to minimize patient's energy expenditures.* • See p. 1692 for additional strategies.
Altered health maintenance	• With patient and family, assess home and personally used irritants (smoking, fumes, vapors) that may exacerbate chronic respiratory condition. • Provide education regarding need to avoid irritants in home, work, and community environments.
Constipation	• Assess stool; note odor, color, amount, frequency, and consistency. • Observe for signs of intestinal obstruction or prolapse of rectum. • Administer stool softener as ordered and report results. • Observe for presence of blood in stool.
Ineffective individual coping	• Assess patient's perception of present and chronic disease state. • Assess patient's level of frustration related to feeling of air hunger. • Determine patient's ability to cooperate with health care providers in interventions such as breathing techniques, exercise progression, and alterations in activities of daily living. • Listen carefully to collect information regarding significance of current health care problem and patient's perception of *ability to deal with alterations caused by CF.* • Assist patient to develop appropriate coping strategies based on personal strengths and past experience. • Explain all treatments and procedures in manner appropriate for patient's age and comprehension. • Assist patient to participate in care. • Encourage patient to maintain usual activities, especially school activities if patient is child. • Arrange for continued schooling and peer contacts when patient is in hospital.

Nursing Diagnosis	Nursing Intervention/Rationale
Family coping: potential for growth	• Assess family's understanding of diagnostic procedures, disease process and prognosis, and therapies employed. • Explain relationship of disease processes and rationale for various therapeutic interventions at level appropriate for family members' comprehension and emotional state. • Involve family in care as appropriate.

Patient Education

1. Teach the patient adaptive breathing techniques and work with the family to teach postural drainage techniques.
2. Teach the importance of avoiding contact with persons who have respiratory infections.
3. Teach the importance of obtaining appropriate immunizations and vaccinations to prevent as many childhood and communicable diseases as possible.
4. Teach the facts about and importance of prescribed medications and diet modifications.
5. Provide the patient and family with information regarding CF, assessment of individual capabilities and responses, and actions to take during an acute episode of difficult breathing.
6. Inform the patient and family that a change in health status must be reported to the patient's health care providers. Indicators of change include change in sputum characteristics or color, decreased activity tolerance, nutrition or gastrointestinal changes, weight loss, fever, or stress symptoms indicating an inability to tolerate the disease state.
7. Teach adaptive exercise and rest techniques.
8. Provide the patient and family with information regarding the care, cleaning, and maintenance of inhalation or oxygen equipment used in the hospital or at home, as well as signs of oxygen toxicity.
9. Provide the patient and family with information related to respiratory health, such as pollution indexes, secondary infection exposure, and community support groups.

Evaluation

Patient Outcome	Data Indicating That Outcome is Reached
Movement of air in and out of lungs is optimum.	Vital capacity measurements are optional for patient's health status.
Airway is patent.	Airways are clear and breathing is as optimum as possible for patient.
Breathing occurs without tiring patient. Breath sounds are clear in all areas.	Patient demonstrates modified breathing techniques that facilitate ventilatory capacity. Patient's behavior is modified to conserve energy expenditure.
Physiologic stability is achieved.	Nutrition level is maintained. Kidney and bladder functioning is within normal limits. Gastrointestinal system is functioning adequately. There are no secondary infections. Serum electrolyte levels are within normal limits. Stool enzymes are present in normal levels. Stool fat content is within normal concentration.
Patient understands importance of daily pulmonary exercises.	Patient demonstrates pulmonary exercises and states rationale and importance of maintaining daily exercise routine.
Patient preserves pulmonary functioning by maintaining optimum activity level, avoiding infection, and following prescribed treatments.	Patient demonstrates variety of methods indicating ability to preserve and facilitate respiratory functioning (breathing exercise, taking medications as prescribed).
Patient and family have sufficient information to comply with discharge regimen.	Patient and family at time of discharge are able to discuss medications (purpose, side effects, route, and schedule), dietary therapy regimen, activity progression regimen, signs of infection or respiratory deterioration, and plan for follow-up visits.
Patient and family understand disease process and complications.	Patient and family discuss CF as disease: its consequences, outcome, and support strategies.

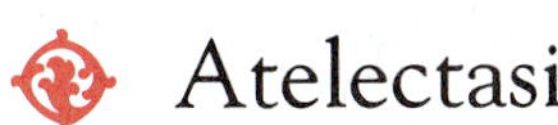

Atelectasis

Atelectasis is failure of the lung to expand.

Atelectasis is an acquired condition in which all or part of the normally aerated and expanded lung collapses. It may be prevented by comprehensive nursing care of postoperative patients and injured patients with pneumothorax or hemothorax.

Atelectasis is a common complication of thoracic or upper abdominal surgery. The problem is caused mostly by hypoventilation, which commonly leads to a bronchial obstruction with mucus. It may also be caused by compression of the lung tissue from hemothorax, pneumothorax, emphysema, oxygen therapy, or tumor.

Pathophysiology

Atelectasis may occur suddenly and be extensive, or it may occur slowly and cause minor pulmonary problems. Atelectasis may be defined as collapse of the lung from absence of air within the alveoli. The extent of the atelectasis depends on the site and rapidity of the blockage. If the mainstem bronchus to one lung is blocked, the entire lung becomes atelectatic and respiratory compromise is great. If only a small bronchiole becomes slowly blocked because of a buildup of secretions, symptoms may be minor and the respiratory system is able to compensate. In both cases, infection and lung tissue damage are possible.

The collapse of lung tissue results in hypoxia. Once blockage has occurred, the gas distal to the obstruction is absorbed into the circulation because the oxygen tension in the pulmonary arteries is lower than in the alveoli. The higher the concentration (FIO_2) of the inspired gas at the time of the blockage, the faster the alveolar collapse.

Surfactant levels may be an important factor in atelectasis because decreased surfactant levels are thought to be a cause of the collapse of alveoli. Decreased blood flow after surgery may cause decreased surfactant levels. The actual cause is yet to be determined.

Diagnostic Studies and Findings

Arterial Blood Gases

Pao_2 less than 80 mm Hg initially, often improving during first 24 hours; $Paco_2$ often normal or low owing to hyperventilation

Serial Chest Roentgenograms

Airless area over region of atelectasis; trachea, heart, and mediastinum deviated toward atelectatic area; diaphragm elevated on affected side; rib spaces narrowed

Clinical Examination

Rapid occlusion with massive collapse: hyperventilation, dyspnea, cyanosis, tachycardia, elevated temperature, diminished breath sounds over affected area, dull or flat percussion tones, restlessness, rales on auscultation

Slow occlusion with minor collapse; may be asymptomatic or have minor pulmonary symptoms

Bronchoscopy

May show bronchial obstruction

Medical Plan

The ultimate treatment plan for atelectasis is removal of the underlying cause.

Surgery

Surgical excision or insertion of drainage tube—performed to relieve atelectasis caused by compression component such as tumor, hemothorax, or pneumothorax

Bronchoscopy—may be performed when atelectasis is not relieved by suction, coughing and deep breathing, or postural drainage

Medications

Bronchodilators
- Isoetharine (Bronkosol), 2-4 ml of 0.125%-0.25% solution q4h
- Metaproterenol sulfate (Alupent), 2-3 inhalations q3-4h

Anti-infective agents (use is controversial)
- Broad-spectrum antibiotic (such as penicillin or ampicillin) given as soon as symptoms are noted; drug may be modified appropriately if specific pathogen is isolated from bronchial secretions

Mucolytic agents such as *N*-acetylcysteine can be given by intermittent positive-pressure breathing (IPPB) or nebulizer

General Management

High tidal volumes and/or positive end-expiratory pressure (PEEP)—used to maintain open alveoli if patient is intubated

Saline irrigation with suctioning—may help loosen secretions and enhance removal

IPPB—inspiratory volumes are increased by over 500 ml

Positioning—patient placed with uninvolved side in dependent position to promote drainage of affected area; patient repositioned at least every hour

Chest physiotherapy with coughing and deep breathing

Ambulation as quickly as possible

NURSING CARE

Nursing Assessment

Respiratory Status

Tachypnea; retractions; labored breathing; dyspnea; nasal flaring; rales; pleural friction rub; diminished breath sounds over area of consolidation; hypoventilation; labored or irregular breathing; breathing tiring for patient; percussion tone dull over area of consolidation

Hypoxia

Restlessness; confusion; hypertension early; hypotension late; cyanosis; tachycardia

Inspired air should be humidified to avoid inspissation of tracheobronchial secretions; supplemental oxygen may be given to maintain arterial $PO_2 \geq 80$ torr (must accept lower value in patients with severe chronic pulmonary diseases)

Laboratory Values

Blood gases: pH; Pa_{O_2}; Pa_{CO_2}

Serum electrolyte levels: bicarbonate; sodium; potassium; chloride

Hematology: hematocrit; hemoglobin level

Bronchopulmonary Infection

Temperature; characteristics of sputum; sputum specimens for culture and sensitivity

Chest Roentgenogram

Periodic evaluation to monitor atelectasis region

Psychosocial

Fear of air hunger; fear of complications such as atelectasis

Nursing Dx & Intervention

Nursing Diagnosis	Nursing Intervention/Rationale
Ineffective airway clearance (potential)	• Assess patient's respiratory status frequently after surgery. • Prevent buildup of respiratory secretions after surgery by encouraging deep breathing and coughing; repositioning patient every hour; ambulating patient as soon as possible; not administering large doses of sedatives, which depress cough reflex and respirations; liquefying secretions by administering aerosol or intermittent positive-pressure breathing (IPPB) treatments, humidifying inspired air, and maintaining body hydration; and using incentive spirometer *to encourage deep breathing*. • After surgery, position patient with pillow along incision site *to function as splint*. Administer analgesic medications before initiating deep breathing and coughing exercises.
Ineffective airway clearance	• Assess patient to identify inability to move secretions. If inability is identified, assist with appropriate measures (such as coughing, positioning, suctioning, and liquefying secretions). • Promptly administer bronchodilators, mucolytics, and expectorants per protocol *to dilate bronchioles and remove secretions*. Observe for therapeutic response and side effects. • *Assist patient to maintain body position that ensures maximum airway availability and draining of affected side* (uninvolved side is in dependent position). • Provide hydration *to liquefy secretions and replace fluids*. • Administer IPPB and perform postural drainage with percussion. • Carefully and frequently auscultate chest for quality of breath sounds and adventitious sounds. Note cough and sputum characteristics.
Ineffective breathing pattern	• Assess ventilation to include evaluation of breathing rate, rhythm, and depth; chest expansion; presence of respiratory distress such as dyspnea, shortness of breath, nasal flaring, pursed-lip breathing or prolonged expiratory phase; and use of accessory muscles. • If possible, maintain patient in position *that facilitates easy ventilation* (head of bed in semi-Fowler's position or patient sitting and leaning forward on overbed table). • Instruct patient in pulmonary hygiene routines *that will promote easy and effective breathing, facilitate removal of secretions from tracheobronchial tree, and minimize pulmonary congestion that may lead to secondary infections*. • Suction if necessary *to remove secretions*. • Assess patient for tiredness in relation to attempts to breathe. • Protect patient from known sources of secondary infection or breathing irritation such as smoking.
Impaired gas exchange	• Assess patient to identify signs, such as restlessness, confusion, and irritability, *that may indicate body's response to altered blood gas states*.

Nursing Diagnosis	Nursing Intervention/Rationale
	• In collaboration with physician's order, monitor arterial blood gases. Report increases or decreases of more than 10 to 15 mm Hg in $Paco_2$ and Pao_2. • Monitor electrocardiogram and cardiac status *for arrhythmias resulting from alterations in blood gases.* • Monitor serum electrolyte levels, *which may change owing to alterations in oxygenation and metabolism.* • Carefully monitor body temperature, *which may fluctuate owing to alterations in metabolism or secondary infections.*
Fatigue	• Assess patterns of fatigue. • Assess factors related to fatigue and strategies for dealing with them. • Assess support systems and available resources. • Administer treatments or medications to relieve discomfort. • Enhance patient's ability to rest between specified activities.
Impaired physical mobility	• Encourage ambulation of patient as quickly as possible *to encourage deeper breathing and lung expansion.* • Closely monitor amount of deep breathing and activity patient can tolerate before dyspnea occurs. • Encourage early mobilization and ambulation.
Fear	• Observe for signs of frustration or fear, fatigue, and tiring with attempts to communicate that result from hypoxia. • Assess patient's level of fear related to current health state. • Assess patient's level of fear related to feeling of air hunger.
Self-care deficit	• Assess level of self-care deficit resulting from patient's current condition. • Assist with activities of daily living, such as toileting, bathing, and feeding, *to minimize patient's energy expenditures.*
Ineffective individual coping	• Determine patient's ability to cooperate with health care providers regarding intervention strategies such as deep breathing and coughing techniques and exercise progression.

Patient Education

1. Teach the patient deep breathing and coughing techniques, as well as increased movement and splinting when coughing.
2. Teach the patient facts about and the importance of prescribed medications such as bronchodilators and antibiotics.
3. If the patient has undergone surgery and does not have atelectasis, provide the patient and family with information about techniques such as movement, deep breathing, and coughing and use of an incentive spirometer to facilitate aeration of the lungs.
4. Provide the patient and family with information regarding the care, cleaning, and maintenance of inhalation or oxygen equipment in the hospital or at home.

Evaluation

Patient Outcome	Data Indicating That Outcome is Reached
Movement of air in and out of lungs is optimum.	Chest roentgenogram shows bilaterally equal and aerated lung fields.
Airway is patent.	Blood gas findings are within normal range for patient. No signs of respiratory distress are noted. Airways are clear, and breathing occurs without obstruction. Breath sounds are clear throughout.

Pleural Effusion
(Pleurisy with effusion)

A pleural effusion develops when excess nonpurulent fluid accumulates in the pleural space between the visceral and parietal pleurae.

Pleural effusion is rarely a disease by itself. It generally occurs as a secondary problem when the physiologic processes of capillary fluids, lymphatic drainage, membrane hydrostatic pressures, and colloidal osmotic pressures of the pleurae are disturbed.

Pleural effusions may be divided into two categories, transudates and exudates. They are determined by the presence and amount of protein in the aspirated fluid. Following are the common causes of pleural effusions:

- Exudates
  - Viral infections
  - Tuberculosis
  - Bacterial infections
  - Chest trauma
  - Pancreatitis
  - Rheumatic fever
  - Collagen-vascular diseases
  - Metastatic diseases
  - Uremia
  - Subphrenic abscess
  - Pulmonary infarction
- Transudates
  - Peritoneal dialysis
  - Pericarditis
  - Cirrhosis
  - Congestive heart failure
  - Myxedema
  - Kidney disease
  - Sarcoidosis
  - Hypoproteinemia

Pathophysiology

The visceral and parietal pleurae form a continuous sac between the lung and the chest wall. Normally only a potential space containing less than 10 ml of fluid separates these surfaces. The fluid is continuously moving in and out of this space because of a balance between hydrostatic pressures, colloidal osmotic pressures, and the surface characteristics of capillaries and the pleurae. Any alteration in pressure gradients or surface characteristics can lead to the formation of an effusion.

The distinction between transudate and exudate is based on protein content. Transudates (hydrothorax) are produced when the flow of protein-free fluid into the pleural space is disturbed. Aspirated fluid is clear or pale yellow, has a specific gravity of 1.015 or less, and has a protein content that is either normal or less than 3 g/dl. Exudates result from a disease of the pleural surface or an obstruction in the lymphatic system that inhibits the drainage of proteins. The fluid is often dark yellow or amber and has a specific gravity greater than 1.016 and a protein content greater than 3 g/dl.

When fluid accumulates as the result of a disturbance in plasma oncotic pressure, it is a transudate. Increased capillary pressure in heart failure and reduced plasma oncotic pressure in certain kidney or liver diseases are the known causes of transudate fluid. This type of fluid has a low specific gravity, a low protein content, and usually a low cell count.

When increased fluid formation is the result of capillary permeability, as in inflammation, it is an exudate. The exudative fluid has a high specific gravity, higher protein content, and often an increased cell count. It may have a large number of white cells, to the point of gross purulent appearance.

The accumulation of pleural fluid in association with pneumonia is called pneumonic effusion. Pleural empyema refers to pus in the pleural cavity; however, pleural fluid with a large number of polymorphonuclear leukocytes in the presence of pyogenic organisms can be an empyema. The accumulation of blood in the pleural cavity is called hemothorax; the presence of chyle (a milky intestinal lymph) is known as chylothorax. Air and fluid together results in hydropneumothorax; if the fluid is pus or blood, it is a pyopneumothorax or hemopneumothorax.[24]

Diagnostic Studies and Findings

Clinical Examination

Dullness to percussion, which shifts with change in position; decreased or absent breath sounds over affected area; egophony above effusion site; dyspnea if effusion has occurred rapidly; if effusion is large, intercostal bulging or decreased chest wall movement during breathing

Chest Roentgenogram

Effusions typically located at base of pleural space; moderate amount of fluid (250 to 300 ml) must accumulate to be seen on upright posterior-anterior, decubitus, or lateral chest roentgenogram; effusion seen as dense opacity (Figure 2-25); large effusions may obliterate hemothorax, simulating lung collapse; distinction between effusion and collapse based on shift of mediastinum away from effusion but toward lung collapse[55]

Thoracentesis

For pleural fluid analysis; submit several hundred milliliters if possible (Table 2-11)

Stain, Culture, and Sensitivity of Pleural Fluid

Identification of causative agent (bacterial, fungal, or viral)

Cytologic Examination of Pleural Fluid

Evaluation of potential neoplastic involvement

Bloody effusion without history of chest trauma suggestive of malignancy or pulmonary embolism

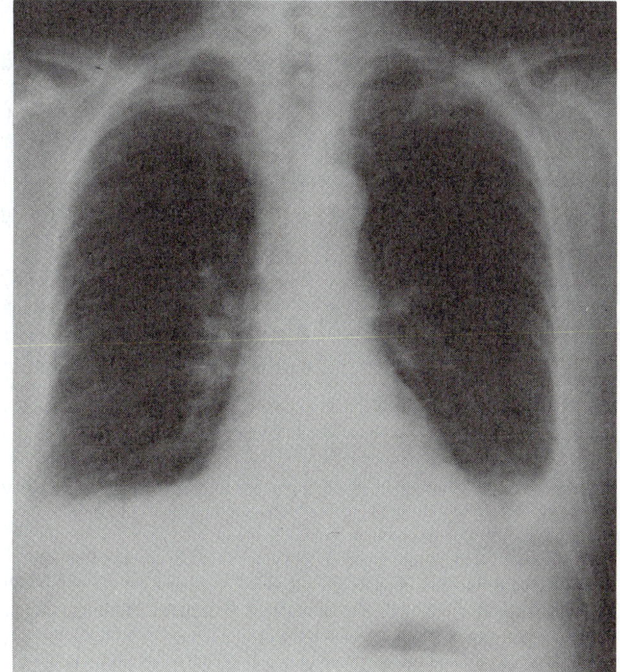

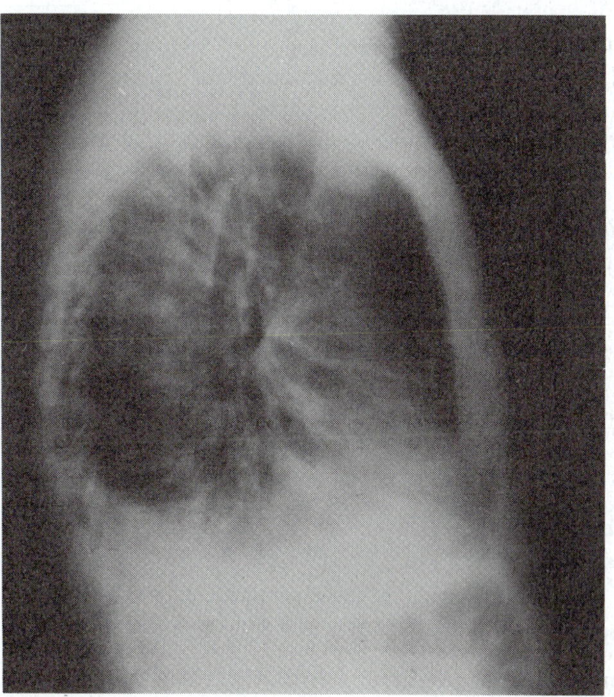

Figure 2-25 Chest roentgenogram of patient with pleural effusion. **A,** PA view: note obliteration of costophrenic angles bilaterally; pulmonary vasculature appears normal. **B,** Lateral view: note lack of costophrenic angles.
Courtesy R. Keith Wilson, M.D., Baylor College of Medicine, Houston, Texas.

Table 2-11
Pleural Fluid Analysis

Measurement	Transudate	Exudate
Color	Pale yellow	Dark amber, blood or pus
Red blood cells (RBCs)	May increase	>5000 RBCs/mm^3; may increase
Protein	<3 g/dl	>3 g/dl
Specific gravity	<1.016	>1.016
Lactic dehydrogenase (LDH)	<200 U/dl	>200 U/dl
Pleural LDH/serum LDH	<0.6	>0.6
White blood cells (WBCs)	Increase indicates empyema or infected effusion	
Amylase	Exceeds serum amylase level	
Glucose	Less than serum glucose level	
Triglyceride	May be increased	
pH	<7.3	>7.3

Modified from Miller.[55]

Pleural Biopsy with Tissue Analysis

Indicated when fluid analysis fails to establish cause

Medical Plan

The treatment of pleural effusion depends on the etiology and clinical consequences. The following discussion refers to the general treatment of effusion. The reader is referred to the section of the text dealing with the cause of the effusion.

Surgery

- Thoracentesis—to drain excess fluid from pleural space and relieve dyspnea or hypoxemia; because of potential cardiovascular response to rapid removal of pleural fluids, removal limited to 1200 to 1500 ml at any one time; another complication of thoracentesis is pneumothorax (see pp. 206-211)
- Insertion of small chest tube
  - Tube may be connected to underwater seal drainage system and left in place if accumulation of fluids is large and compromising respiratory function
  - If pleural effusion is caused by malignancy, tube may be inserted to drain fluid and left in place to provide insertion point for medications and therapeutic techniques

Medications

- Antibiotics
  - Antibiotics specific to cause administered if effusion is thought to be caused by infectious process

General Management

- Treatment of underlying disease or problem
- Deep breathing and coughing to encourage maximal ventilation; incentive spirometer may be used
- Bed rest, which causes most effusions to absorb spontaneously

NURSING CARE

Nursing Assessment

Respiratory Insufficiency Resulting from Fluid in Pleural Space

- Respiratory distress: nasal flaring; tachypnea; decreased chest wall movement; dyspnea; restlessness; tachycardia; decreased breath sounds; paradoxic breathing; dull percussion tone
- Pulmonary function studies: decreased vital capacity and minute volume

Reaccumulation of Fluid in Pleural Space after Drainage by Thoracentesis

- Assessment of potential respiratory distress as discussed above

Cardiovascular Response to Removal of Large Quantity of Pleural Fluid during Thoracentesis

- Hypotension; tachycardia; cardiac arrhythmias; syncopy; clammy skin; paleness

Bronchopulmonary Infection

- Temperature; sputum specimen for culture and sensitivity

Psychosocial

- Fear of dyspnea or not being able to get enough air; potential fear of unknown cause of pleural effusion

Nursing Dx & Intervention

Nursing Diagnosis	Nursing Intervention/Rationale
Fluid volume excess	• Assess for signs of respiratory distress *caused by fluid buildup in pleural space.* • Position patient so maximum ventilation can occur (semi-Fowler's or upright position). • Assist with thoracentesis procedure and *monitor patient's response after procedure.* • Assess for signs of secondary infection in pleural area or in lungs themselves. • If chest tube is in place, assess and provide care as indicated on pp. 222-225.
Impaired gas exchange	• Assess for signs of restlessness, confusion, change in respiratory pattern, or irritability *that may indicate altered blood gas levels resulting from compromised breathing.* • Monitor for signs of atelectasis resulting from decreased ventilation. • Turn patient frequently *to prevent pooling of secretions within lungs and pleural space.*

Patient Education

1. Teach the patient the importance of positioning to facilitate ventilatory effort.
2. Teach the patient the importance of deep breathing and coughing to keep the lungs aerated and to prevent complications.
3. If pleural effusion is a recurrent problem, ensure that the patient is able to identify signs of accumulating fluid so care can be sought early.
4. Prepare the patient for thoracentesis.

Evaluation

Patient Outcome	Data Indicating That Outcome is Reached
Minimal fluid remains in pleural space.	Chest roentgenogram shows no evidence of fluid accumulation.
Movement of air in and out of lungs is optimum.	Breath sounds are clear and bilaterally equal; percussion tone is resonant over all lung fields.
Cause of pleural effusion is identified and treated.	There is no recurrence of disease.

INFECTIOUS AND INFLAMMATORY DISEASES

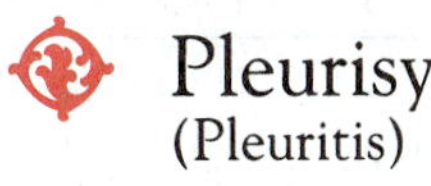

Pleurisy
(Pleuritis)

Pleurisy is an inflammation of the visceral and parietal pleura. It is also referred to as dry pleurisy or fibrinous pleurisy.

Pleurisy often occurs as a result of pulmonary bacterial infections such as pneumonia or pulmonary infarction, viral infections of the intercostal muscles, transport of an infectious agent or neoplastic cells directly to the pleura by the bloodstream or lymphatics, pleural trauma, asbestos-related pleural diseases, or early stages of tuberculosis or lung tumor. The size of the affected area varies greatly. The disease onset is usually sudden, and the diagnosis is easily made based on the characteristic pleuritic pain and pleural friction rub.

Pathophysiology

The visceral pleura attaches to the lung's surface, whereas the parietal pleura lines the costal, diaphragmatic, mediastinal, and cervical regions of the thoracic cavity. Under normal circumstances these membranes slide easily over each other to reduce friction during breathing. During the development of pleurisy the pleura becomes edematous and congested, an exudate collects on the pleural surface, and cell infiltration occurs. The exudate develops from plasma proteins leaking from damaged vessels. It may be reabsorbed into the fibrous tissue, causing pleural adhesions. The buildup of the fibrinous exudate causes the pleural surfaces to rub roughly together. This causes the audible pleural friction rub.

The pain felt in pleurisy is caused by stretching of the inflamed pleura. The pain is usually felt in the chest wall and occasionally the abdominal wall. If the pleuritic area is along the diaphragm border, pain is referred to the shoulder.

Diagnostic Studies and Findings

Clinical Examination

Auscultation during late inspiration and early expiration reveals dry rubbing sound (may not occur until 24 to 36 hours after onset of pain); history of pain with deep breath or coughing; with diaphragmatic pleurisy, pain referred to shoulder; respirations rapid and shallow; breath sounds diminished; if pleural effusion develops, pain subsides and fever and dry cough occur

Chest Roentgenogram

Limited value in diagnosing pleurisy; diagnostic if fluid accumulates as in pleural effusion

Medical Plan

Medications

Local anesthetics
- Paravertebral infiltration of anesthetic to block intercostal nerves

Narcotic analgesics
- Analgesics to relieve discomfort; narcotics such as me-

peridine (Demerol), 50-75 mg q4-6h IM or IV, or morphine, 15 mg q4-6h IM, to decrease pain while patient takes deep breaths and coughs

Analgesic-antipyretics

Acetaminophen (Tylenol), 600 mg q4-6h

General Management

Treatment of underlying disease or problem

Positioning patient on affected side to splint chest

Deep breathing and coughing to prevent atelectasis and pneumonia

Heat to affected area

NURSING CARE

Nursing Assessment

Respiratory Status

Pleural friction rub heard during late inspiration and early expiration

Pleural Effusion

Purulent sputum; fluid accumulation on chest roentgenogram; subsidence of pleural pain; dyspnea; dull percussion tone over chest

Pain

Relationship between patient's level of pain and ability to cough and deep breathe; ability of analgesic or narcotic to relieve patient's pain

Bronchopulmonary Infection

Presence of fever; altered hematologic findings; sputum characteristics that might indicate secondary infection

Nursing Dx & Intervention

Nursing Diagnosis	Nursing Intervention/Rationale
Pain	• Assess and document patient's degree of discomfort. • Position patient on affected side *to splint chest and minimize pain.* • In collaboration with physician, administer analgesic or narcotic medication as needed *to minimize discomfort.* • Splint chest with pillow or other object during deep breathing and coughing.
Impaired gas exchange	• Assess for signs of restlessness, confusion, and irritability, *which may indicate altered blood gas levels resulting from shallow breathing.* • Monitor for signs of atelectasis (see pp. 173-175). • Monitor for signs of pleural effusion (see pp. 176-179). • Protect patient from known sources of secondary infection. • Turn patient frequently *to prevent pooling of secretions and promote expansion of all lung lobes.* • Position patient *to facilitate maximum ventilation.*
Fatigue	• Assess patterns of fatigue. • Assess factors related to fatigue and strategies for dealing with them. • Assess support systems and available resources. • Administer treatments or medications to relieve discomfort. • Enhance patient's ability to rest between specified activities.

Patient Education

1. Teach the patient the importance of deep breathing and coughing to keep the lungs aerated.
2. Teach the patient splinting during deep breathing and coughing.

Evaluation

Patient Outcome	Data Indicating That Outcome is Reached
Movement of air in and out of the lungs is optimum.	Breath sounds are clear with no evidence of pleural friction rub during inspiration and expiration.
There is no pain with breathing.	Patient is able to take deep breaths and cough without discomfort.
Disease state is corrected without atelectasis or secondary infection.	Patient recovers without development of atelectasis or secondary infection such as pneumonia.

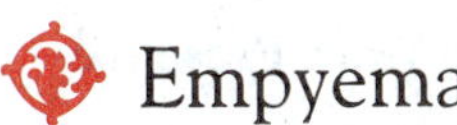

Empyema

Empyema is the accumulation of infected fluid or pus in the pleural space.

The accumulation of purulent exudate in the pleural cavity may occur in several ways. The most common cause is direct extension from adjacent structures as occurs in pneumonia, tuberculosis, pulmonary abscess, bronchiectasis, or esophageal rupture. Exudate accumulation may also occur from direct contamination such as that caused by penetrating chest wounds or chest surgery. Empyema is an uncommon but serious disorder that occurs most often in debilitated patients. If identified early and treated promptly with antibiotics, it can usually be controlled.

Pathophysiology

Both kinds of empyema, acute and chronic, may affect a small area of pleura or may involve the entire pleural cavity. In the acute stage the affected area appears inflamed and has a thin layer of exudate with a low leukocyte count. If untreated, the exudate thickens and pus may accumulate. The pleura may thicken, and adhesions may occur. Chronic empyema develops when there are recurrent infections or when treatment of a previous infection was incomplete. Treatment of chronic empyema is difficult because the pleura often becomes thickened and fibrous, and the lung may stick to the chest wall, decreasing ventilation. Pleural fibrosis with secondary limited ventilatory capacity may result. The multiloculated cavities within the pleural space fill with pus and are difficult to drain.

Diagnostic Studies and Findings

History

Recent thoracic or abdominal surgery; blunt or penetrating chest trauma; esophageal fistula; lung infections; aspiration; recent thoracentesis; persistent fever despite administration of antibiotics

Physical Examination

Foul-smelling sputum; pleural friction rub; localized chest pain; dullness to percussion; decreased breath sounds at lung bases; decreased vocal fremitus

Chest Roentgenogram

Pleural fluid, usually unilateral, with associated lung lesion

Thoracentesis

Evidence of pus in pleural exudate (because pus is difficult to aspirate, 18-gauge or larger needle must be used)

Laboratory Examination of Pleural Exudate

Odor and general appearance; specific gravity; cell count; Gram stains; aerobic and anaerobic cultures (NOTE: When materials are sent for culture, all air must be expressed from syringe and sample must be quickly transported to laboratory for anaerobic evaluation)

pH

Of special diagnostic value; fluid collected and analyzed in same manner as for arterial blood gases (using capped, 5 to 10 cc heparinized syringe); pH less than 7.21 suggestive of empyema that necessitates chest tube drainage

Medical Plan

Surgery

Thoracentesis—may be performed to drain purulent drainage if area is small and localized

Thoracic drainage—closed or open drainage system for large areas or quantities of collected pus; if intrapleural fluid and pus are thin and localized, large-diameter thoracotomy tube may be inserted and connected to closed system under water-seal drainage; open drainage possible only if there is no danger of lung collapse when atmospheric pressure enters pleural space; for open drainage, thoracotomy tube exits to room air and is covered with large, absorbent, sterile dressing (see pp. 222-225 for detailed discussion of thoracic drainage systems)

Intrapleural aspiration and instillation of medications—chest tube may be used to aspirate pleural drainage and as vehicle for instillation of antibiotics and fibrinolytic enzymes

Thoracotomy—may be necessary for patients not effectively treated by tube drainage system; area with empyema is resected and thickened membrane is stripped by process called decortication to permit reexpansion of lung

Medications

Anti-infective agents

Antibiotic therapy based initially on results of Gram stain; alterations made if necessary when culture results are available

Fibrinolytic agents

Controversial; recommended by several researchers as method to decrease viscosity of pus and dissolve fibrin clots

Trypsin (Granulex) as aerosol, 0.1 mg/0.82 ml with balsam of Peru and castor oil; spray bid to debride necrotic areas

Streptokinase (Kabikinase, Streptase), 100,000 U/h IV over 24-72 h for adults; converts plasminogen to proteolytic enzyme fibrinolysin, which breaks down fibrin clots

General Management

Oxygen support—may be necessary if signs of hypoxia are present

Irrigation of pleural cavity with sterile solution—periodically for patient with thoracotomy tube in place to flush out purulent and necrotic materials

Bed rest—while patient is febrile and has drainage mechanism in process

Deep breathing and coughing—to encourage maximum ventilation and decrease congestion resulting from pulmonary problem and bed rest; incentive spirometer may be used

NURSING CARE

Nursing Assessment

Respiratory Insufficiency Resulting from Presence of Pus in Pleural Space

Nasal flaring; tachypnea; decreased chest wall movement; dyspnea; restlessness; tachycardia; decreased breath sounds; paradoxic breathing; dull percussion tone; decreased vital capacity and minute volume; arterial blood gases must be assessed if signs of hypoxia are present

Characteristics and Amount of Purulent Drainage from Pleural Cavity and Physiologic Response to Accumulation

Amount, odor, and color of drainage; specimens sent periodically to laboratory for analysis and culture; response to purulent accumulation, including fever, respiratory distress, and pain

Bronchopulmonary Infection

Temperature; sputum specimen for culture and sensitivity

Common Complications (Pericarditis, Endocarditis, Meningitis, Brain Abscess)

Signs that patient is becoming more ill; for specific signs refer to appropriate sections in text

Nursing Dx & Intervention

Nursing Diagnosis	Nursing Intervention/Rationale
Ineffective breathing pattern	• Assess ventilation, including evaluation of breathing rate, rhythm, and depth; chest expansion; and presence of respiratory distress such as dyspnea, shortness of breath, nasal flaring, or prolonged expiratory phase. • Assess potential of purulent collection to interfere with ventilation and vital capacity. • Identify contributing factors such as airway clearance or obstruction, pain, level of consciousness, or weakness. • Maintain patient in position *that facilitates easy ventilation* (head of bed in semi-Fowler's position). • Encourage deep breathing, coughing, and use of incentive spirometer.
Impaired gas exchange	• Assess for signs of restlessness, confusion, and irritability, *which may indicate altered blood gas levels resulting from compromised breathing*. • Assess blood gases if hypoxia is anticipated. • Monitor for signs of atelectasis *resulting from decreased ventilation*. • Encourage deep breathing and coughing *to loosen secretions and facilitate expectoration*. Incentive spirometry may be used. • Turn patient frequently *to prevent pooling of secretions within lungs and pleural space*.
Self-care deficit	• Assess level of self-care deficit resulting from empyema and associated chest tubes (if used). • Assist with activities of daily living as needed. • Encourage progressive activity after fever and acute stage are over.

Nursing Diagnosis	Nursing Intervention/Rationale
Potential fluid volume deficit	• If patient is febrile because of empyema, monitor hydration and maintain at adequate level.
Potential for infection	• Carefully assess for signs that could indicate a secondary infection; report observations to physician. • Protect patient from known sources of secondary infection.

Patient Education

1. Teach the patient the importance of positioning to facilitate the ventilatory effort.
2. Teach the patient the importance of deep breathing and coughing to keep the lungs aerated and prevent complications.
3. If empyema is a recurrent problem, teach the patient to identify signs of the problem so care can be sought early.
4. Prepare the patient for thoracentesis or the insertion of chest tubes (see pp. 222 to 225).
5. If the patient is to go home with an open chest tube left in place for drainage, teach care techniques (such as aseptic dressing change).
6. Teach the patient and family about empyema; inform them that the healing process may be slow and that repeated treatments, drainage, irrigation, and chest roentgenograms may be necessary.

Evaluation

Patient Outcome	Data Indicating That Outcome is Reached
No purulent material remains in pleural space.	Chest roentgenogram shows no evidence of pus accumulation.
Movement of air in and out of lungs is optimum.	Breath sounds are clear and bilaterally equal; percussion tone is resonant over all lung fields.

Acute bronchitis

Acute bronchitis is an inflammation of the bronchi or trachea or both that results from irritation or infection.

Acute bronchitis usually heals by itself. It is most common in winter. Acute bronchitis may occur alone and also occurs with many chronic diseases such as bronchiectasis, emphysema, or tuberculosis. It may also be linked to systemic illnesses such as chickenpox, measles, and influenza. Once the disease is in process, exposure to air pollutants or physical disabilities such as malnutrition or fatigue may make it worse. If the patient already has a chronic disease such as pulmonary or cardiovascular disease, acute bronchitis may become serious. Pneumonia is perhaps the most common complication. If the patient already has impaired cough, lung, or bronchial functioning, acute bronchitis may lead to respiratory failure.

In most cases infective acute bronchitis is viral, but bacterial causes (e.g., *Streptococcus pneumoniae, Haemophilus influenzae*) are also common. Irritative bronchitis may be caused by dust or fumes, such as from strong acids, ammonia, chlorine, bromide, or smoke.

Pathophysiology

Congestion of the bronchial mucous membranes is the earliest physiologic change. This is followed by desquamation or shedding of the submucosa. The congestion and shedding process causes submucosal edema with leukocyte infiltration. This process interferes with the normal function of the ciliated bronchial epithelium and the phagocytes. The result is a sticky or mucopurulent exudate that stays in the bronchi until coughed out.

Because the normally sterile bronchial system is contaminated, bacteria may move in to cause secondary bacterial infection. At the beginning of the disease process the sputum of a patient with acute bronchitis is normally mucoid. If the sputum becomes mucopurulent or purulent, a superimposed bacterial infection can be suspected (Table 2-12).

Diagnostic Studies and Findings

Clinical Examination

Cough initially dry and nonproductive but may produce mucoid sputum within a few days; fever (38.3° to 38.9° C [101° to 102° F]); if cause is bacterial, midsternal chest pain, malaise, sore throat, diffuse rales and rhonchi throughout chest; if patient already has chronic lung disease, sputum may change from clear and thin to thick and tenacious or purulent

Chest Roentgenogram

Clear; no evidence of lung consolidation

Table 2-12
Agents Commonly Causing Acute Bronchitis and Pneumonitis

Product	Industry	Injury
Aldehydes (acrylaldehyde, formaldehyde, and acetaldehydes)	Plastic, rubber, textiles, resins, disinfectant	Bronchitis, asthma
Ammonia	Fertilizer, explosives, refrigeration	Tracheobronchitis, pulmonary edema
Chlorine and hydrochloric acid	Bleaches, disinfectants, plastics, refining, dye making, organic chemical synthesis	Tracheobronchitis, pulmonary edema
Nitrogen dioxide	Fertilizer, dyes, explosives, farming, rockets, arc welding	Tracheobronchitis, pulmonary edema, bronchiolitis obliterans
Ozone	Arc welding, sewage and water treatment	Tracheobronchitis
Phosgene	Chemical industry, dyes, insecticides	Tracheobronchitis, pulmonary edema
Sulfur dioxide	Bleaching, smelting, paper manufacture, refrigeration	Tracheobronchitis, pulmonary edema (rare)

From Cherniack.[17]

Sputum

Mucoid; may be thick; purulent sputum suggestive of superimposed infection

Medical Plan

The goals of the treatment plan are to provide supportive therapy during the course of the self-limited disease and to prevent secondary infections.

Medications

Antitussive agents
- Cough suppressants (use with extreme caution in patients with chronic lung disease)
  - Hydrocodone bitartrate (Codone, Dicodid, Hycodan), 5-10 mg tid or qid
  - Codeine phosphate (tablets and in mixture form in numerous syrups), 10-20 mg q4-6h

Nonnarcotic analgesic agents
- Many agents available; following is incomplete list
  - Dextromethorphan (Romilar, Benylin CM, Pertussin, Congespirin), 10-20 mg q4h or 30 mg q6-8h
  - Noscapine (Tusscapine, Narcotine), 15-30 mg tid or qid
  - Levopropoxyphene napsylate (Novrad), 50-100 mg q4-6h

Bronchodilators
- Terbutaline (Brethine, Bricanyl), 2.5-5 mg tid
- Theophylline (Aerolate, Theolair, Slo-Phyllin, Theo-Dur, Bronkodyl, Elixophyllin, others); *dosage highly individualized based on serum theophylline levels;* therapeutic level 10-20 µg/ml; 200-250 mg q6h or 1-2 timed-release preparations q8-12h (3.5-5 mg/kg)

Anti-infective agents
- Antibiotics when superimposed respiratory infection is suspected on basis of clinical evidence such as purulent sputum, high fever, and ill-appearing patient; antibiotics also indicated for patients with chronic obstructive lung disease
  - Doxycycline (Vibramycin), oxytetracycline (Terramycin), others, 250-500 mg po qid
- Ampicillin (Amcill, Omnipen, others), 250-500 mg po qid
- Antipyretic-analgesics
  - To reduce fever and relieve malaise

General Management

- Increase in fluid intake—up to 4000 ml/day to liquefy secretions and maintain hydration
- Steam or mist vaporizer to humidify air surrounding patient
- Rest to conserve energy
- Culture of sputum if sputum becomes purulent or patient's illness becomes progressively worse

NURSING CARE

Nursing Assessment

Because acute bronchitis is generally a self-limited disease, assessment is important to identify complications, superimposed infections, or adverse effects of therapy.

Respiratory Status

Sibilant and sonorous rhonchi; wet rales at base; labored or irregular breathing; dyspnea; substernal tightness with breathing; back pain; cough characteristics and duration

Chest Roentgenogram

No evidence of lung consolidation

Bronchopulmonary Infection

If bacterial, fever (38.3° to 38.9° C [101° to 102° F]) lasting several days; mucopurulent or purulent sputum; send sputum specimen for culture and sensitivity

Nursing Dx & Intervention

Nursing Diagnosis	Nursing Intervention/Rationale
Ineffective breathing pattern	• Assess ventilation to include evaluation of breathing rate, rhythm, and depth; chest expansion; presence of respiratory distress such as dyspnea, shortness of breath, nasal flaring, pursed-lip breathing, or prolonged expiratory phase; and use of accessory muscles. • Maintain patient in position *that facilitates easy ventilation* (patient sitting upright and leaning on overbed table). • See p. 1704 for additional strategies.
Impaired gas exchange	• Assess patient to identify signs, such as restlessness, confusion, and irritability, *that may indicate body's response to altered blood gas states.* • Assist patient to avoid smoking, fumes, smoke, or other inhaled irritants *that may aggravate current disease state.* • See p. 1706 for additional strategies.
Fatigue	• Assess patterns of fatigue. • Assess factors related to fatigue and strategies for dealing with them. • Assess support systems and available resources. • Administer treatments or medications to relieve discomfort. • Enhance patient's ability to rest between specified activities.
Ineffective airway clearance	• Assess patient to identify inability to move secretions. If inability is identified, assist with appropriate measures (coughing, positioning, suctioning, liquefying secretions, and so on). • Provide adequate hydration *to ensure liquefaction of secretions.* Avoid offering dairy products, which tend to increase viscosity of mucus.
Self-care deficit	• See p. 1692 for associated nursing care.
Family coping: potential for growth	• Assess family's level of understanding of diagnostic procedures, disease process and prognosis, and therapies employed. • See p. 1816 for associated nursing care.
Potential for infection	• Assess for signs and symptoms of infection, fever, dyspnea, and change in sputum color, amount, or odor. • Obtain sputum for culture and sensitivity. • Protect patient from known sources of secondary infection.

Patient Education

1. Teach the patient the importance of consuming large quantities of fluid.
2. Teach the patient the importance of not smoking and of avoiding fumes or smoke when the disease is active.
3. Teach the patient the importance of rest during the course of the disease.
4. Teach the patient facts about and the importance of prescribed medications.
5. Teach the patient how to use antipyretic-analgesics to reduce fever and relieve malaise.
6. Teach the patient the importance of avoiding contact with others, who may transmit infection.
7. Teach the patient signs of secondary infection such as a change in sputum characteristics or prolonged fever that may be suggestive of secondary infection.

Evaluation

Patient Outcome	Data Indicating That Outcome is Reached
Movement of air in and out of lungs is optimum.	Breath sounds are clear with no evidence of adventitious sounds.
Airways are patent.	Breathing occurs without cough or substernal tightness. Chest roentgenogram is clear.
Tracheobronchial tree returns to noninflamed, predisease state.	Cough is decreased. Sputum if present is mucoid.

Lung abscess

Lung abscess is an inflammatory lesion in the lung accompanied by necrosis. The abscess usually has well-defined borders and may be putrid (containing anaerobic bacteria) or nonputrid (containing aerobic bacteria).

The incidence of lung abscess has dropped significantly because of the availability of effective antibiotics and the increased willingness of individuals to seek medical care. Lung abscesses are generally caused by aspiration of infected material, which may occur during unconsciousness, general anesthesia, alcoholism, near-drowning, diabetic coma, or drug sedation. It can also occur as a result of poor oral hygiene, gum disease, infected tonsils, or aspiration of food. Bronchial carcinoma (squamous cell type) is also considered to be a common cause of lung abscess for male smokers over 55 years of age. Other, less common causes of lung abscess include septic pulmonary emboli and abscess transfers from the liver. The following are predisposing factors[17]:

- Massive inoculum
  - Aspiration*
    - Stupor, coma, seizure, intoxication
    - Anesthesia
    - Laryngeal dysfunction
  - Dental and gingival infection*
  - Hematogenous dissemination
    - Intravenous drug abuse
    - Right-sided endocarditis
    - Septic phlebitis
    - Osteomyelitis or other septic focus
- Local pathology
  - Obstructing neoplasm
  - Foreign body
  - Distortion by fibrosis
  - Bronchostenosis
  - Cysts, bullae
  - Sequestration
  - Contusion or trauma
  - Gastric acid
- Necrotizing vascular disorders
  - Embolic infarction
  - Vasculitis (Wegener's, rheumatoid arthritis, polyarteritis)
  - Necrosis within neoplasm
  - Necrotizing conglomerate pneumoconiosis
  - Chronic eosinophilic pneumonia
- Impaired host resistance
  - Alcoholism*
  - Diabetes
  - Chronic debilitating disease
  - Malnutrition*
  - Impaired humoral resistance
    - Leukopenia
    - Hypoglobulinemia
  - Impaired tissue-mediated immunity
    - Acquired immunodeficiency
    - Radiation exposure
    - Chemotherapy
    - Steroid therapy
    - Neoplasia; Hodgkin's disease, lymphomas

*Circumstances commonly associated with primary lung abscess.

Pathophysiology

The site of the abscess is determined by the body's position at the time of the inhalation. The aspirated material moves to the most dependent position in the lung. Once it has settled, a fibrous granulation tissue forms around it and it embeds itself in the parenchyma.

As the abscess develops, it fills with pus. Pressure develops, and the infected tissue ruptures into the bronchus. Drainage of foul-smelling, pus-filled, or bloody sputum results. The expectoration of purulent sputum may lead to partial healing and cavity formation. However, if the cavity does not drain adequately, small abscesses may form within the lung. The following is a partial list of etiologic organisms[17]:

- Pyogenic aerobic bacteria
  - *Staphylococcus aureus*
  - Gram-negative bacilli (*Klebsiella, Proteus,* and others)
  - *Streptococcus pneumoniae*
  - Group A streptococci
  - *Legionella*

Pyogenic anaerobes*
- *Fusobacterium nucleatum* and other species
- *Bacteroides melaninogenicus, B. fragilis,* and other species
- Peptostreptococci
- *Treponema macrodentium*

Nocardia

Mycobacteria—*M. tuberculosis, M. kansasii, M. intracellulare,* and other species

Fungi
- *Histoplasma*
- *Coccidioides*
- *Blastomyces*
- *Actinomyces*
- *Sporothrix*
- *Aspergillus*
- *Cryptococcus*
- *Phycomycetes*

Parasites
- *Entamoeba histolytica*
- *Paragonimus*
- *Echinococcus*

Diagnostic Studies and Findings

Clinical Examination

Initial signs resembling pneumonia; cough producing bloody, purulent, foul-smelling sputum; general malaise; sporadic fever; pleuritic pain; dyspnea if abscess is large; dull percussion tone; rales; decreased or absent breath sounds over abscess area; pleural friction rub; if abscess left untreated and becomes chronic, auscultation may detect only fine rales or rhonchi; may be weight loss, anemia, and hypertrophic pulmonary osteoarthropathy

Chest Roentgenogram

Initially, lobar consolidation, which becomes globular as disease progresses; rupture of consolidation causes fluid level, which indicates communication with bronchus; when fluid level is apparent, diagnosis can be narrowed to either empyema with a bronchopleural fistula or a lung abscess

Laboratory Examination of Pleural Exudate

Odor and general appearance; specific gravity; cell count; Gram stains; aerobic and anaerobic cultures to determine infective organisms; therapeutic intervention based on agent identification (NOTE: When material is sent for culture, all air must be expressed from syringe and sample must be quickly transported to laboratory for anaerobic evaluation)

White Blood Cell Count

Leukocytosis common

Bronchoscopy

Unnecessary if roentgenography shows rapid resolution of abscess but may be needed to verify presence of abscess or determine its severity if patient's condition does not improve

Medical Plan

The ability of the lung abscess to heal depends primarily on its ability to drain adequately through the bronchus. With free drainage, resolution occurs. Without free drainage, and without prompt antibiotic therapy, the abscess may become chronic.

Surgery

Bronchoscopy—occasionally necessary to remove thick, tenacious sputum

Pulmonary resection—necessary in rare cases if lung abscess does not respond to antibiotic therapy; single lesions removed by lobectomy and multiple lesions removed by pneumonectomy

Medications

Anti-infective agents

Antibiotic therapy directed at causative agent; should be monitored and perhaps changed depending on patient's clinical response; should begin as soon as initial sputum specimens have been collected; drug of choice while awaiting test results is penicillin G, 1.2 million U po qid, or 300,000-600,000 U IM q6-8h; if after 4-7 d patient is not improved and specific organism is still not identified, medication may be changed to tetracycline (Achromycin, others), 500 mg po qid; antibiotic therapy continued until all signs of abscess are resolved on serial chest roentgenograms

General Management

Postural drainage—extremely important to drain abscess (see pp. 221-222 for techniques)

Percussion—to loosen secretions and enhance their removal

Daily measurement of sputum volume output and assessment of sputum characteristics

*Primary lung abscess is caused by combinations of these anaerobes with *S. viridans, Neisseria* species, and other normal oral flora.

NURSING CARE

Nursing Assessment

Characteristics and Amount of Purulent Drainage from Pleural Cavity and Physiologic Response to Infection

Amount, odor, and color of drainage; periodic specimens to laboratory for analysis and culture; body response to infectious process, including fever, respiratory distress, pleuritic chest pain, chills, diaphoresis, and weight loss; evidence that abscess continues to drain freely

Respiratory Insufficiency Resulting from Presence of Abscess in Pleural Cavity

Dyspnea; restlessness; tachycardia; decreased breath sounds; evidence of pleural friction rub; rales; rhonchi; dull percussion tones

Chest Roentgenogram

Serial chest roentgenograms to monitor healing process of lung abscess

Response to Antibiotic Therapy

Monitoring of response to treatment process; if not improved, assessment for additional underlying cause of abscess such as tumor or foreign body

Psychosocial

Concern that there is infection that must be treated for extended period

Nursing Dx & Intervention

Nursing Diagnosis	Nursing Intervention/Rationale
Ineffective airway clearance	• Assess patient to identify inability to move secretions. If inability is identified, assist with appropriate measures (such as coughing, positioning, suctioning, and liquefying secretions). • Assist patient to maintain proper body positioning *to ensure maximum airway availability and to promote drainage position that will facilitate drainage of lobe*. • Provide hydration to liquefy secretions and replace fluids. • Perform postural drainage with percussion at least 1 hour before meals; provide oral hygiene after treatment. • Carefully and frequently auscultate chest for quality of breath sounds and adventitious sounds. • Assess potential of purulent collection to interfere with ventilation. • If necessary provide suctioning *to remove sputum drainage*. • Note color, odor, and amount of sputum daily. • Administer antibiotics as ordered.
Ineffective breathing pattern	• Assess ventilation, including evaluation of breathing rate, rhythm, and depth, chest expansion, breathing difficulty, or dyspnea. • Identify contributing factors such as airway clearance, obstruction problem, or weakness. • Assess patient for tiring in relation to attempts to breathe. • Protect patient from known sources of secondary infection or breathing irritation such as smoking.
Impaired gas exchange	• Assess for signs of restlessness, confusion, and irritability, which may indicate altered blood gas levels resulting from compromised breathing. • Assess blood gases if hypoxia is anticipated. • Monitor for signs of atelectasis resulting from decreased ventilation. • Encourage deep breathing and coughing *to loosen secretions and facilitate expectoration*. • Assist patient to turn frequently *to prevent pooling of secretions within lungs*. • Monitor white blood cells and electrolytes *to evaluate changes that may be due to alterations in oxygenation, metabolism, and infection*. • Carefully monitor body temperature, *which may fluctuate owing to alterations in metabolism or infectious process*.
Bathing/hygiene self-care deficit	• Provide mouth care and toothbrushing after postural drainage and chest physiotherapy, as well as every several hours as long as abscess is draining. • Encourage use of mouthwash *to remove tastes associated with drainage*.
Anxiety	• Assess patient's level of anxiety related to present health state. • See p. 1743 for additional strategies.

Nursing Diagnosis	Nursing Intervention/Rationale
Ineffective individual coping	• Assess patient's ability to cooperate with health care providers regarding intervention strategies, such as frequent postural drainage sessions and need to sleep in positions *that will facilitate abscess drainage*. • See p. 1804 for additional strategies.
Potential for infection	• Observe for signs or symptoms of infection; fever; dyspnea; change in sputum color, amount, or odor. • Obtain sputum for culture and sensitivity. • Protect patient from known sources of secondary infection.

Patient Education

1. Teach the patient the importance of positioning to facilitate abscess drainage.
2. Teach the patient the importance of deep breathing and coughing to keep the lung aerated and to prevent secondary complications.
3. Teach the patient facts about and the importance of prescribed medications such as antibiotics.
4. Provide the patient and family with information regarding lung abscess and the treatment protocol, which may last as long as 6 to 8 weeks.
5. Teach the patient the importance of good oral hygiene, especially as long as there is active lung drainage.
6. Teach the patient methods to reduce the chances of a lung abscess in the future, such as good oral hygiene, avoidance of aspiration, and prompt medical attention for potential bacterial infection of the mouth or respiratory tract.

Evaluation

Patient Outcome	Data Indicating That Outcome is Reached
No purulent material remains in lungs, and there is no evidence of lung abscess.	Serial chest roentgenograms show progressive improvement and healing. Temperature and laboratory values return to normal.
Movement of air in and out of lung is optimum.	Airways are clear and breathing occurs without obstruction. Breath sounds are clear and bilaterally equal; percussion tone is resonant over all lung fields.
Cause of lung abscess has been identified and treated.	Disease state does not recur.
Patient and family have sufficient information to comply with discharge regimen.	Patient and family at time of discharge are able to discuss medications (purpose, side effects, and route) and signs of additional infection or respiratory deterioration.

Pneumonia and pneumonitis

Pneumonia is an inflammatory process of the respiratory bronchioles and the alveolar spaces that is caused by infection. Pneumonitis is noninfectious bronchial and alveolar inflammation. Together, these terms are used to refer to inflammatory processes of the parenchyma of the lung.

Pneumonia is the most common cause of death from infectious disease in North America. It is also considered to be the major source of disease and death in critically ill patients.[45] Despite the use of antibiotics, pneumonia still accounts for 27.7 of every 100,000 deaths.[56]

Pneumonia may be caused by bacteria, viruses, *Mycoplasma,* fungi, and parasites. Currently about half of pneumonia cases are caused by bacteria and half by virus. Up to 96% of bacterial pneumonia is caused by three organisms. Since most of the organisms require specific therapy, it is important to identify the agent causing the disease.

Pneumonia occurs most often during the winter and early spring and in persons 60 years or older. The disease usually resolves within 2 to 3 weeks.

Bacterial Pneumonia

***Streptococcus pneumoniae* (pneumococcal) pneumonia.** *S. pneumoniae* (hemolytic streptococcus type A), a gram-positive diplococcus, is by far the most common and important cause of bacterial pneumonia, accounting for 90% of cases. The infection usually involves extensive consolidation of part or all of the parenchyma of the lobe. *S. pneumoniae* pneumonia is often seen in infants, the elderly, and patients with sickle cell disease, congestive heart failure, alcoholism, or diabetes mellitus. A vaccine is now available and is 80% to 90% effective against this type of pneumonia in adults.

***Staphylococcus aureus* pneumonia.** *S. aureus,* a gram-positive coccus, may cause pneumonia in infants and the elderly and commonly causes pneumonia as a complication of influenza or in hospitalized patients as a secondary infection after surgery, tracheostomy, coma, or immunosuppressive therapy. It accounts for 3% to 5% of bacterial pneumonia.

***Haemophilus influenzae* (type B) pneumonia.** *H. influenzae,* a gram-negative bacillus, causes lobar-type pneumonia, bronchopneumonia, or bronchiolitis in adults. It accounts for 1% of bacterial pneumonia.

Nonbacterial Pneumonia

Atypical pneumonia

Mycoplasma pneumoniae *pneumonia.* Infection with *M. pneumoniae,* which is most common in school-aged children and young adults, spreads among family members. Transmission is believed to be by infected respiratory secretions. *M. pneumoniae* pneumonia is a type of bronchopneumonia.

Legionnaires' disease. *Legionella pneumophila* is a weakly organized gram-negative organism that is identified with a special fluorescent antibody stain. Legionnaires' disease occurs most commonly in older adults and in persons who smoke or have chronic disease such as diabetes, renal disease, cancer, chronic bronchitis, or emphysema. It is three times more common in men than in women.

Pneumocystis carinii *pneumonia.* *P. carinii* pneumonia, caused by a protozoal organism, is discussed in Chapter 14.

Aspiration Pneumonia Syndrome

Aspiration pneumonia syndrome occurs most commonly as a result of aspiration when the patient is in an altered state of consciousness owing to a seizure, drugs, alcohol, anesthesia, acute infection, or shock. It may also occur when the anatomy is altered by esophageal stricture, tracheal fistula, a nasogastric tube, or a tracheotomy. Aspiration pneumonia may be acquired through foreign body aspiration. Nonbacterial aspiration pneumonia may follow aspiration of toxic materials such as toxic fluids and inert substances; bacterial aspiration pneumonia may occur as a secondary problem.

The causative agents of bacterial pneumonia include the gram-positive coccus *Staphylococcus aureus,* the gram-negative coccus *Escherichia coli,* and the gram-negative bacilli *Klebsiella pneumoniae, Pseudomonas aeruginosa, Proteus,* and *Enterobacter.*

All of these bacterial aspiration pneumonias have a poor prognosis even with antibiotic therapy. They may cause extensive lung damage resulting in lung abscess or empyema. Mortality is 70% with *P. aeruginosa,* 45% with *E. coli,* 25% to 50% with *K. pneumoniae,* and 15% to 50% with *S. aureus.*[59]

Pathophysiology

The pathophysiology depends on the etiologic agent. Bacterial pneumonia is marked by an intra-alveolar suppurative exudate with consolidation. Lobar pneumonia causes consolidation of the entire lobe (Figure 2-26). Bronchopneumonia causes a patchy distribution of infectious areas around and involving the bronchi. A chest roentgenogram of bronchopneumonia shows patchy segmental or subsegmental infiltration in one or more dependent lobes.

Mycoplasmal and viral pneumonias produce interstitial inflammation with accumulation of an infiltrate in the alveolar walls. There is no consolidation or exudate.

Fungal and mycobacterial pneumonias are marked by patchy distribution of granulomas that may undergo necrosis with the development of cavities.

The most extensively studied type of pneumonia is pneumococcal or streptococcal pneumonia. The bacteria are thought to reach the alveoli in mucus or saliva. In the alveoli they undergo four predictable phases[59]:

Engorgement (first 4 to 12 hours). Serous exudate pours into alveoli from the dilated, leaking blood vessels.

Figure 2-26 Chest roentgenogram of patient with pneumonia. Note infiltrate of right middle and lower zones with air bronchogram seen; right heart border not obliterated. Also note monitor electrodes, gown snaps, endotracheal tube, and ventilator tubing.
Courtesy R. Keith Wilson, M.D., Baylor College of Medicine, Houston, Texas.

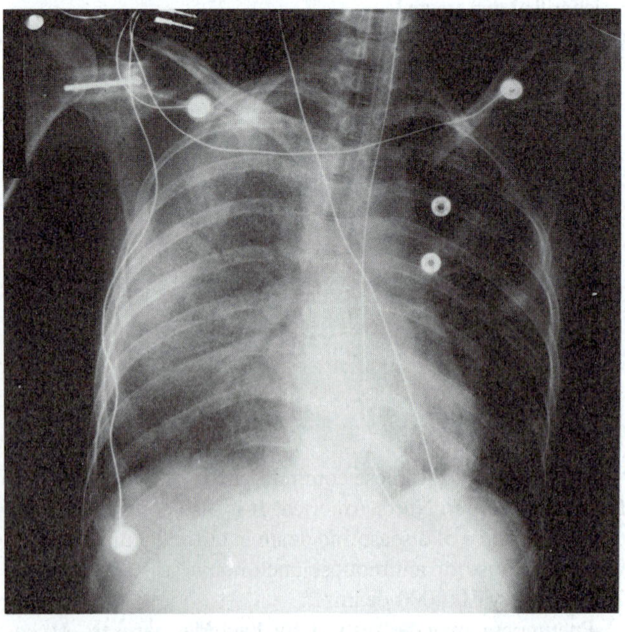

Red hepatization (next 48 hours). The lung assumes a red granular appearance as red blood cells, fibrin, and polymorphonuclear leukocytes fill the alveoli.

Gray hepatization (3 to 8 days). The lung assumes a grayish appearance as the leukocytes and fibrin consolidate in the involved alveoli.

Resolution (7 to 11 days). Exudate is lysed and resorbed by macrophages, restoring the tissue to its original structure.

These stages represent the course of untreated pneumococcal pneumonia. With the use of antibiotics the course should run 3 to 5 days.

Viral pneumonia affects the tissues differently. The inflammatory response in the bronchi damages the ciliated epithelium. The lungs are congested and in some cases hemorrhagic. The inflammatory response is composed of mononuclear cells, lymphocytes, and plasma cells in proportions that vary with the type of virus causing the disease. In severe types of viral pneumonia the alveoli contain hyaline membranes. Characteristic intracellular viral inclusions may be seen in adenovirus, cytomegalovirus, respiratory syncytial virus, or varicella virus infections.

Aspiration pneumonia presents a still different physiologic response, which is based on the pH of the aspirated substance. If the pH is 2.5 or above, little necrosis results. However, if the pH is below 2.5, atelectasis occurs, followed by pulmonary edema, hemorrhage, and type II cell necrosis. The alveolar-capillary "membrane" may be damaged, leading to exudation and in severe cases adult respiratory distress syndrome.[55]

Diagnostic Studies and Findings

Clinical Examination (Depends on Type of Pneumonia)

Streptococcal, pneumococcal

Sudden onset; chest pain; chills; fever; headache; cough; rust-colored sputum; rales and possibly friction rub; hypoxemia as blood is shunted away from area of consolidation; cyanosis; area of consolidation visible on chest roentgenogram; sputum culture needed to determine causative agent

Staphylococcal

Many of same signs as streptococcal; sputum copious and salmon colored

Klebsiella

Many of same signs as streptococcal; onset more gradual; more bronchopneumonia visible on chest roentgenogram; if treatment delayed beyond second day after onset, patient will become critically ill; mortality high

Haemophilus

Commonly follows upper respiratory infection; low-grade fever; croupy cough; malaise; arthralgias; yellow or green sputum

Mycoplasmal

Gradual onset; headache; fever; malaise; chills; cough severe and nonproductive; decreased breath sounds and rales; chest roentgenogram clear; white blood cell count normal

Viral

Symptoms generally mild; cold symptoms; headache; anorexia; fever; myalgia; irritating cough that produces mucopurulent or bloody sputum; bronchopneumonic type of infiltration on chest roentgenogram; white blood cell count usually normal; rise in antibody titers

Sputum Examination

Sputum from lower respiratory tract needed for assessment; if necessary, may be obtained by needle aspiration, transtracheal aspiration, fiberoptic bronchoscopy, or open lung biopsy; sputum *must* be examined before initiation of antibiotic therapy

Macroexamination for odor, consistency, amount, color (see above for anticipated color)

Microexamination including Gram stain for etiologic agent, neutrophilia, increased epithelial cells, presence of other organisms

Sputum culture for organism identification; although routinely performed, culture thought to be only 50% sensitive for pneumococcal disease and only 35% to 50% sensitive for pneumonia caused by *Haemophilus influenzae*[55]

Blood Cultures

May be transient bacteremia in pneumococcal pneumonia

Acid-Fast Stains and Cultures

To rule out tuberculosis

Serum Specimen for Cold Agglutinins

Test requires 10 ml of clotted blood; used for differential diagnosis of viral or mycoplasmal infections; cold agglutinins present in about 50% of diseases caused by these two agents

White Blood Cell Count

Leukocytosis (15,000 to 25,000/mm^3); neutrophilia (normal or low white blood cell count in mycoplasmal or viral infection)

Chest Roentgenogram

Presence of density changes involving primarily lower lobes (Figure 2-26)

Lung Function Studies

Volumes—congestion and collapse of alveoli; decreased lung volumes

Pressures—in increased airway resistance and decreased compliance

Gas exchange—shunting as a result of hypoxemia

Table 2-13
Antibiotic Therapy for Pneumonia

Organism	Agent of First Choice	Adult Daily Dose	Duration (Days)	Alternate Agents
Streptococcus pneumoniae				
Mild	Penicillin	Penicillin V, 500 mg po q6h	7-10	Erythromycin 500 mg q6h
Fulminant	Penicillin	Penicillin G, 2 × 10^6 U q4h	7	Cefazolin 1 g q8h Vancomycin 1 g q12h
Streptococcus pyogenes (group A)	Penicillin G	2 × 10^6 units q4h	14-21	Cefazolin[a]
Staphylococcus aureus				
Nonbacteremic	Nafcillin	1.5-2 g q4-6h	21	Cefazolin[a]
Bacteremic	Nafcillin	1.5-2 g q4-6h	28	Vancomycin[b]
Anaerobic mouth flora (peptostreptococci, *Bacteroides melaninogenicus*)	Penicillin	2 × 10^6 U q4h followed by penicillin V 0.5-1 g q6h	10-14 14-30	Clindamycin 600 mg q8h followed by 300 mg q6h
Mycoplasma pneumoniae	Erythromycin	250 mg q6h	21	Tetracycline 250 mg q6h
Legionella spp.	Erythromycin	1 g q6h IV followed by 250 mg q6h po	7-14 14-21	Rifampin 300 mg q8h po
Escherichia coli	Third-generation cephalosporin[c]	1-2 g q8h	14	Imipenem 500 mg q6h Aztreonam 1 g q8h
Providencia spp. or *Morganella*	Third-generation cephalosporin[c]	2 g q8h	14	TMP/SMX[d]
Chlamydia psittaci	Tetracycline	500 mg q6h	14	
Francisella tularensis	Streptomycin *plus* Tetracycline	1 g q12h IM 500 mg q6h	14	TMP/SMX[d]
Yersinia pestis	Streptomycin *plus* Tetracycline	1 g q12h	21	
Haemophilus influenzae	Cefuroxime	0.75 g q8h	14	Third-generation cephalosporin,[c] aztreonam TMP/SMX[d]
Klebsiella pneumoniae	Third-generation cephalosporin[c]	2 g q8h	21	TMP/SMX,[d] aztreonam *or* Aminoglycoside[e]
Pseudomonas aeruginosa	Antipseudomonas penicillin[f] *or* aztreonam *plus* aminoglycoside[g]	18 g IV 2 g q8h IV	21	Imipenem 500 mg q6h *plus* Aminoglycoside
Acinetobacter calcoaceticus	Ticarcillin *plus* Tobramycin[g]	3 g q4h 2 mg/kg q8h[g]	14-21	Imipenem 500 mg q6h
Serratia marcescens	TMP/SMX	15 mg/75 mg/kg/day in 3 doses	14-21	Third-generation cephalosporin[c] *plus* Aminoglycoside *or* Imipenem[h]
Enterobacter spp.	TMP/SMX	15 mg/75 mg/kg/day in 3 doses	14-21	Imipenem 500 mg q6h *plus* Aminoglycoside

From Rakel.[60]
[a]Cefazolin—1 g q8h; [b]Vancomycin—500 mg q6h or 1 g q12h; [c]Cefotaxime—2 g q2h, ceftizoxime 2 g q8h, ceftriaxone 2 g q12h, ceftazidime 1-2 g q8h; [d]TMP/SMX—15 mg/kg of trimethoprim, 75 mg/kg sulfamethoxazole per day given as three divided doses; [e]Gentamicin—2 mg/kg q8h, tobramycin 2 mg/kg q8h, amikacin 5 mg/kg q8h; [f]Anti-*Pseudomonas* penicillin—azlocillin, piperacillin, ticarcillin 3 g q4h; adjust dose of ticarcillin if creatinine clearance less than 30 ml/min. Aztreonam 2 g q8h; [g]Adjust dose depending on renal function status; [h]Imipenem 0.25 to 1 g q6h; adjust dose in presence of renal failure.

Medical Plan

Surgery

Thoracentesis with chest tube insertion—may be necessary if secondary problem such as empyema occurs

Medications

Anti-infection agents
See Table 2-13 for complete list of anti-infective agents

General Management

Humidification—humidifier or nebulizer if secretions are thick and copious
Oxygenation—if patient has $Pa{O_2}$ less than 60 mm Hg; Venturi mask or nasal prongs commonly used
Physiotherapy—role in hastening resolution of pneumonia uncertain; patient should be encouraged at least to cough and deep breathe to maximize ventilatory capabilities[55]
Hydration—monitoring of intake and output; supplemental fluids to maintain hydration and liquefy secretions

NURSING CARE

Nursing Assessment

Respiratory Status

Tachypnea; retractions; labored breathing; dyspnea; nasal flaring; rales; pleural friction rub; diminished breath sounds over area of consolidation; hypoventilation; labored or irregular breathing; breathing tiring for patient; percussion tone dull over area of consolidation

Hypoxia

Restlessness; confusion; tachycardia; cyanosis

Laboratory Values

If patient seriously ill, monitor for decreased pH and $Pa{O_2}$ and increased $Pa{CO_2}$; evidence of elevated leukocyte count

Temperature

Must be carefully monitored and controlled because of nature of infection

Cough and Sputum

Amount and productivity of coughing; color, consistency, odor, and amount of sputum; fatigue related to coughing; periodic laboratory evaluation of sputum needed to evaluate patient's response to treatment

Hydration State

Intake and output; tissue turgor; liquidity of sputum; electrolytes

Chest Roentgenogram

Periodic evaluation to monitor improvement

Potential Complications

Complications most common with pneumonia caused by gram-negative bacteria

Pleurisy
Pleuritic pain; fever; shallow, rapid breathing; dull percussion tones; occasional hemoptysis with coughing; pleural friction rub

Atelectasis
Pleuritic pain; tachypnea; dyspnea; absence of breath sounds over affected area; anxiety; cyanosis; flat percussion tone over area; mediastinal shift toward affected side

Empyema
Persistent fever despite antibiotics; foul-smelling sputum; pleural friction rub; localized chest pain; dullness to percussion; decreased breath sounds at bases of lung; decreased vocal fremitus

Lung abscess
Usually foul-smelling and purulent sputum (unless abscess is walled off); high fever; chest pain; persistent fever despite antibiotics

Pulmonary edema
Acute respiratory distress; frothy, red-tinged sputum; coarse rales or rhonchi; tachycardia and tachypnea; diaphoresis; moist, noisy breathing

Superinfection pericarditis
Sharp, sudden chest pain that radiates to neck, shoulders, and back; pericardial friction rub; tachycardia; fever; dyspnea; possible pulsus paradoxus; elevated ST segment on electrocardiogram; elevated white blood cell count; widened space between pericardial layers on echocardiogram; erythrocyte sedimentation rate elevated

Meningitis
Nuchal rigidity; altered neurologic signs; fever; papilledema; positive Kernig's sign; projectile vomiting

Nursing Dx & Intervention

Nursing Diagnosis	Nursing Intervention/Rationale
Ineffective airway clearance	• Assess patient to identify inability to move secretions. If inability is identified, assist with appropriate measures (such as coughing, positioning, suctioning, and liquefying secretions). • Promptly administer bronchodilators, mucolytics, and expectorants per protocol *to dilate bronchioles and remove secretions*. Observe for therapeutic response and side effects. • Assist patient to maintain body position *that ensures maximum airway availability* (semi-Fowler's position or sitting upright and leaning on overbed table). • Provide hydration *to liquefy secretions and replace fluids*. • Carefully and frequently auscultate chest for quality of breath sounds and adventitious sounds. Note cough and sputum characteristics.
Ineffective breathing pattern	• Assess ventilation to include evaluation of breathing rate, rhythm, and depth; chest expansion; presence of respiratory distress such as dyspnea, shortness of breath, nasal flaring, pursed-lip breathing, or prolonged expiratory phase; and use of accessory muscles. • Identify contributing factors such as airway clearance or obstruction problem or weakness. • Maintain patient in position *that facilitates ventilation* (head of bed in semi-Fowler's position or patient sitting and leaning forward on overbed table). • Instruct patient in proper pulmonary hygiene routines *that will promote easy and effective breathing, facilitate removal of secretions from tracheobronchial tree, and minimize pulmonary congestion,* which could lead to superinfections. • Assess patient for tiring in relation to attempts to breathe. • Protect patient from known sources of secondary infection.
Impaired gas exchange	• Assess patient to identify signs, such as restlessness, confusion, and irritability, *that may indicate body's response to altered blood gas states*. • If necessary and with physician consultation, administer oxygen by nasal cannula or Venturi mask *to maintain* Pa_{O_2} *above 60 mm Hg*. • Monitor serum electrolytes that may change *owing to alterations in oxygenation and metabolism*. • Carefully monitor body temperature, which may fluctuate *owing to alterations in metabolism or infection*.
Fatigue	• Assess patterns of fatigue. • Assess factors related to fatigue and strategies for dealing with them. • Assess support systems and available resources. • Administer treatments or medications to relieve discomfort. • Enhance patient's ability to rest between specified activities.
Altered health maintenance	• Provide strict isolation for patient with pneumonia caused by *Staphylococcus* (see Chapter 13 for techniques). • Adhere to strict handwashing *to prevent spread of disease*.
Altered nutrition: less than body requirements	• Help patient choose foods that are easy to chew and swallow. Assist by cutting and feeding if patient tires easily. • See p. 1630 for additional strategies.
Potential fluid volume deficit	• If patient is seriously ill, assess for evidence of dehydration resulting from fever and lack of fluid intake. • Carefully monitor intake and output. Encourage fluid intake if needed.
Impaired physical mobility	• Encourage patient to use adaptive breathing techniques *to decrease work of breathing*. • Assist patient to alternate activities with periods of rest. • Encourage gradual increase of activities as tolerated. • If patient is seriously ill and maintained on bed rest, encourage or provide active or passive range of motion *to maintain adequate muscle tone*.
Self-care deficit	• Assess level of self-care deficit resulting from patient's current condition.
Anxiety	• Assess patient's level of anxiety related to present health state.
Defensive coping	• Assess patient's emotional response to feeling of air hunger or pulmonary congestion. • Determine patient's ability to cooperate with health care providers in intervention strategies such as breathing techniques and coughing exercises. • See p. 1808 for additional strategies.

Nursing Diagnosis	Nursing Intervention/Rationale
Family coping: potential for growth	• Assess family's understanding of diagnostic procedures, disease process and prognosis, and therapies employed. • Involve family in care as appropriate. • Teach family about strict handwashing *to prevent spread of pneumonia*.
Potential for infection	• Observe for signs and symptoms of infection; fever; dyspnea; and change in sputum color, amount, or odor. • Obtain sputum for culture and sensitivity. • Protect patient from known sources of secondary infection.

Patient Education

1. Teach the patient deep breathing and coughing techniques.
2. Teach the family the importance of handwashing when working with the patient to prevent the spread of the disease.
3. Teach the patient and family facts about and the importance of prescribed medications such as antibiotics.
4. Provide the patient and family with information regarding the specific type of pneumonia the patient has, treatment, anticipated response, possible complications, and probable disease duration.
5. Inform the patient and family that a change in health status must be reported to the patient's health care providers. Indicators of change may include a change in sputum characteristics or color, decreased activity tolerance, fever despite the antibiotics, increasing chest pain, or a feeling that things are not getting better.
6. Teach the patient the importance of consuming large quantities of fluid.
7. Teach the patient adaptive exercise and rest techniques.

Evaluation

Patient Outcome	Data Indicating That Outcome is Reached
Movement of air in and out of lungs is optimum.	Airways are clear, and breathing occurs without obstruction.
Airway is patent.	There is no cough or pulmonary congestion and no sputum production.
Breath sounds are clear in all areas.	Bronchovesicular breath sounds are heard throughout lungs. There are no areas of decreased breath sounds or consolidation.
Physiologic stability is achieved after pneumonia.	Nutrition level is maintained. Kidney and bladder functioning is within normal limits. There is no secondary infection. Serum electrolytes are within normal limits.
Patient and family have sufficient information to comply with discharge regimen.	Patient and family at time of discharge are able to discuss medications (purpose, side effects, route, and schedule), dietary therapy regimen, activity progression regimen, and signs of secondary infection.

Cor Pulmonale and Pulmonary Hypertension

Cor pulmonale is a condition of hypertrophy and dilation of the right ventricle of the heart resulting from a disease process that affects the function or structure of the lung or its vasculature. This may occur with or without heart failure. Pulmonary hypertension is an increase in the main pulmonary artery pressure at rest or during exercise. This means that the systolic/diastolic pressure in the pulmonary artery exceeds 30/15 mm Hg at rest.

Cor pulmonale occurs as a secondary process following a primary pulmonary disease. The four most common disorders leading to cor pulmonale are obstructive lung diseases, vascular diseases, restrictive lung diseases, and chest wall disorders.

Obstructive lung diseases
- Chronic bronchitis
- Emphysema
- Asthma

Cystic fibrosis
Bronchiectasis
Vascular disease—thromboembolism
Restrictive lung diseases
Atelectasis
Pneumonia
Interstitial fibrosis
Sarcoidosis
Chest wall disorders—kyphoscoliosis

Chronic obstructive pulmonary disease accounts for about 75% of cases of cor pulmonale in the United States.

There are four primary factors in the development of cor pulmonale and right-sided failure: (1) reduction in the size of the pulmonary vascular bed as a result of destruction of pulmonary capillaries or loss of large amounts of lung tissue; (2) increased resistance in the pulmonary vascular bed; (3) shunting of nonaerated blood; and (4) the effect of reduced oxygen in causing pulmonary vasoconstriction and elevation of pressure in the pulmonary artery.[51] The most common direct cause of cor pulmonale is pulmonary hypertension. Right-sided heart failure is most frequently the terminal event in the disease process.

Figure 2-27 Etiology and pathogenesis of cor pulmonale. From Price.[59]

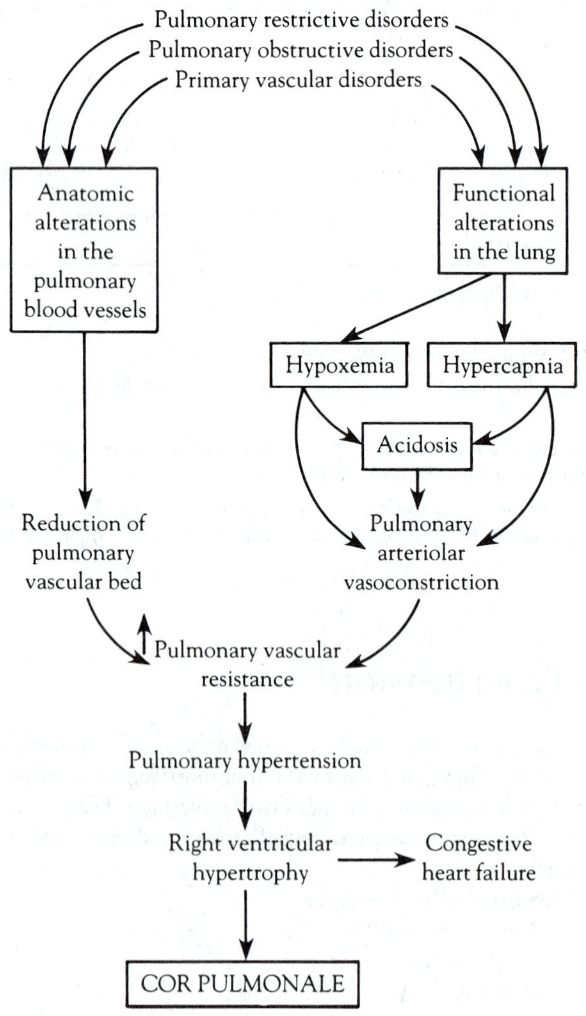

Pathophysiology

The pulmonary circulation is normally a low-pressure, low-resistance system that may increase output, without increasing pulmonary pressure, to increase cardiac output. As pulmonary vascular resistance of the small arterioles and arteries increases in some types of disease, pulmonary hypertension results. Pulmonary hypertension, in turn, increases the workload of the right side of the heart, causing it to hypertrophy and eventually fail.[59]

A second major process causing pulmonary hypertension is an alteration in pulmonary arteriolar vasoconstriction. Chronic vasoconstriction, resulting from hypoxemia, and acidosis may lead to pulmonary hypertension. Figure 2-27 shows the pathogenesis of cor pulmonale.

Diagnostic Studies and Findings

Clinical Examination

Evidence of other chronic lung diseases; dyspnea; cough; cyanosis; wheezing; distended neck veins; loud pulmonic secondary sound on cardiac auscultation; gallop rhythm and occasional murmur resulting from functional insufficiency of tricuspid and pulmonic valves

Chest Roentgenogram

Right ventricular hypertrophy

Echocardiogram

Right ventricular enlargement

Arterial Blood Gases

Decreased PaO_2 in range of 40 to 60 mm Hg; $PaCO_2$ in range of 40 to 70 mm Hg

Electrocardiogram

Arrhythmias resulting from hypoxia; right bundle-branch block; right axis deviation; right ventricular hypertrophy

Complete Blood Count

Elevated hemoglobin level and hematocrit value and polycythemia resulting from chronic hypoxia

Pulmonary Arterial Pressure

Systolic pressure above 30 mm Hg; diastolic pressure above 15 mm Hg; pulmonary function findings consistent with underlying pulmonary disease

Medical Plan

The underlying pulmonary and cardiac diseases must be treated first. (See Chapter 1 for cardiac disease guidelines.)

Medications

Diuretics
- Initial diuresis can lower pulmonary artery pressure by decreasing total blood volume; careful monitoring of serum electrolytes needed when administering diuretics
- Furosemide (Lasix), 20-80 mg/d to maximum of 600 mg/d

Bronchodilators
- Concomitant administration of theophylline and terbutaline recommended to improve airway obstruction and reduce afterload on right and left sides of heart, thereby improving cardiac output[34]
- Theophylline (Theo-Dur, Theolair, Elixophyllin, others), 16 mg/kg divided into 3 or 4 doses
- Terbutaline (Brethine, Bricanyl), 2.5-5 mg po tid

Anti-infective agents
- Antibiotics administered after Gram stain analysis of sputum specimens

General Management

Oxygenation—administered in concentrations ranging from 24% to 40% unless contraindicated by underlying pulmonary disease; 85% to 95% arterial oxygen saturation or arterial oxygen tension greater than 55 mm Hg[34]; ventilation and oxygenation cannot be overemphasized

Sodium-restricted diet

Bed rest during acute episodes to conserve energy and pulmonary effort

NURSING CARE

Nursing Assessment

Primary Disease State

See assessment for specific primary disease state

Pulmonary Artery Pressure

Carefully monitored

Arterial Blood Gases

Pa_{O_2}; Pa_{CO_2}; pH

Laboratory Values

Hemoglobin; hematocrit; serum electrolytes

Sputum Characteristics

Periodic laboratory analysis of sputum specimens

Fluid Retention

Careful monitoring of intake and output

Presence of Complications

Ankle edema; distended neck veins; abdominal pain; hepatomegaly; cardiac ventricular gallop (S_3); tachycardia; tachypnea

Nursing Dx & Intervention

The primary nursing diagnoses and nursing care should be directed toward the primary disease state. In addition, the following diagnoses and care strategies are specific for cor pulmonale.

Nursing Diagnosis	Nursing Intervention/Rationale
Impaired gas exchange	• Assess patient to identify signs, such as restlessness, confusion, and irritability, that may indicate body's response to altered blood gases. • In collaboration with physician, order and monitor arterial blood gas studies. • In collaboration with physician, administer oxygen *to maintain oxygen saturation between 85% and 95%*. If patient has chronic obstructive lung disease, adminster oxygen at low flow and with extreme caution. • Administer and monitor bronchodilators as ordered. Monitor patient response. • Monitor electrocardiogram and cardiac status for arrhythmias resulting from alterations in blood gases. • Monitor for signs of increasing cor pulmonale such as increased pulmonary artery pressure, increased edema in extremities, jugular venous distention, and hepatomegaly. • Monitor body temperature, which may fluctuate *owing to alterations in metabolism or secondary infection*.

Nursing Diagnosis	Nursing Intervention/Rationale
	• Evaluate for need to continue low-flow oxygen use at home *to maintain arterial blood gas level*. Indicators include continued reduced Pa_{O_2} (50 to 55 mm Hg while patient is at rest), continuing pulmonary artery hypertension, and clinically apparent right ventricular failure.[34]
Fluid volume excess	• Monitor and record weight daily. • Carefully monitor and record intake and output. • In collaboration with physician, administer diuretic medications. • Assist patient to maintain sodium-restricted diet. • Assist patient to limit fluid intake. • Monitor serum electrolytes, which may change owing to administration of diuretics or alterations in metabolism.
Potential for infection	• Assess for signs and symptoms of infection; fever; dyspnea; and change in sputum color, amount, or odor. • Obtain sputum for culture and sensitivity. • Protect patient from known sources of secondary infection.

Patient Education

The primary education is directed toward the patient's primary disease state; refer to patient education for specific primary disease.

1. Teach the patient the importance of restricting salt intake and limiting fluid intake.
2. Teach the patient to weigh self daily.
3. Provide the patient and family with information regarding chronic lung diseases, assessment of the patient's capabilities and responses, and actions to take during an acute episode.
4. Teach the patient the importance of avoiding environmental pollutants and not smoking.
5. Teach the patient facts about and importance of prescribed medications.
6. Provide the patient and family with information regarding the care, cleaning, and maintenance of inhalation or oxygen equipment being used in the hospital or to be used at home, as well as the signs of oxygen toxicity.

Evaluation

Also see the patient outcomes for the underlying disease state.

Patient Outcome	Data Indicating That Outcome is Reached
Breathing pattern occurs without tiring patient.	Modified breathing technique is maintained.
Optimum gas exchange occurs throughout lungs.	Blood gas values are within normal limits for patient's condition.
Fluid and electrolyte balance is restored.	There is no evidence of fluid retention; serum electrolytes are within normal limits.
Patient and family have sufficient information to comply with discharge regimen.	Patient and family at time of discharge are able to discuss medications, dietary therapy, activity progression, evidence of respiratory infection or compromise, and plan for follow-up visit.

Pulmonary Edema

Pulmonary edema is the accumulation of serous fluid in the interstitial tissue of the lung.

Pulmonary edema may result from many causes:

Heart failure owing to arteriosclerosis, mitral valve disease, or hypertension
Near-drowning
Pulmonary embolism
Overdose from heroin, barbiturates, or opiates
Overload or rapid infusion of intravenous fluids, plasma, or blood products
Renal disease
Pulmonary disease
Diffuse infections
Hemorrhagic pancreatitis

Pulmonary edema is acute and extensive and may lead to death unless treated rapidly. Pulmonary edema results from one of three conditions: damage to the capillary walls, a decrease in colloid osmotic pressure as occurs in nephritis, or an increase in hydrostatic pressure within the pulmonary capillary walls. Pulmonary edema has therefore been divided into cardiogenic and noncardiogenic types. The remainder of this section is devoted to the cardiogenic type. For discussion of the noncardiogenic type, see the discussion of adult respiratory distress syndrome (pp. 144-150). The most common cause of cardiogenic pulmonary edema is left ventricular failure resulting from heart disease.

Pathophysiology

Pulmonary edema occurs when left ventricular failure or fluid overload causes fluid to leave the vascular space and collect in the interstitial tissue of the lungs, increasing hydrostatic pressure and altering pulmonary capillary dynamics.

The formation of pulmonary edema has two stages: engorgement and fluid movement. In the first stage, interstitial edema causes engorgement of the perivascular and peribronchial spaces. The body has three safety mechanisms to protect against alveolar flooding.[34] First, lung lymph flow increases to help clear the edema fluid from the lung. Second, the concentration of protein in the interstitial space falls because of an increase of water and solutes entering the interstitial space around the alveolar vessels. This leads to an oncotic pressure difference between the plasma and the interstitial fluid, resulting in resorption of fluid into the circulation. The third safety factor is the capacity of the interstitial spaces in the lung, which can contain up to 500 ml of edema fluid in the bronchovascular cuffs before edema symptoms become severe.

Once engorgement reaches its limits and the safety factors are overwhelmed, alveolar edema occurs and fluid moves into the alveolar spaces. Blood plasma pours into the alveoli faster than coughing or the safety factors can clear it.[59] The result of this process is acute pulmonary edema, which causes interference with the diffusion of oxygen, tissue hypoxia, and asphyxia. Without emergency treatment, respiratory failure occurs.

Diagnostic Studies and Findings

Clinical Examination

Severe dyspnea; grunting and labored respirations; tachypnea; cyanosis; tachycardia; cough; rales; frothy, blood-tinged sputum; distended neck veins; restlessness; vague uneasiness; agitation or confusion resulting from hypoxia; diaphoresis

Chest Roentgenogram

Prominent interlobular septa (Kerley-B lines) (Figure 2-28)

Figure 2-28 Chest roentgenogram of patient with pulmonary edema. Note cardiomegaly, increased pulmonary vascularity, and obliteration of costophrenic angles indicating increase of pleural space fluid. Note infiltration of fluid indicating alveolar edema.
Courtesy R. Keith Wilson, M.D., Baylor College of Medicine, Houston, Texas.

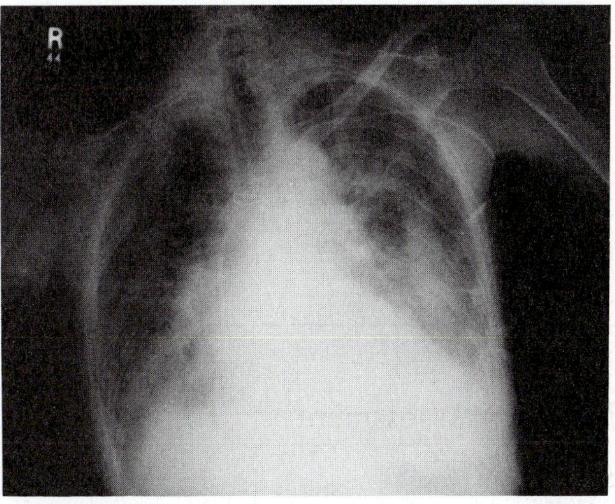

Pulmonary Capillary Wedge Pressure

Left atrial pressure increased: 14 to 20 mm Hg in mild cases, 25 to 30 mm Hg in severe cases[34]

Arterial Blood Gases

Pa_{O_2} and Pa_{CO_2} variable; respiratory alkalosis or acidosis may occur

Medical Plan

Medications

- D5W IV with microdrip tubing running at keep-open rate for medication infusion
- Narcotic analgesics
  - Morphine sulfate, 10-15 mg IV, to reduce anxiety, slow respirations, and reduce venous return
- Diuretics
  - Furosemide (Lasix), loading dose of 40 mg IV over 1-2 min, increasing to 80 mg IV after 1 h
  - Ethacrynic acid (Edecrin), loading dose of 50 mg slow IV push (may be repeated once if needed); monitor serum potassium level
- Bronchodilators
  - Aminophylline, 250-500 mg (diluted in 50 mg IV solution) IV over 15-20 min
- Other drugs to treat underlying cause of pulmonary edema, e.g., cardiac drugs for cardiac-related problem

General Management

Rotation of tourniquets (infrequently used)—manually or by machine; pressure applied to three limbs at a time; cuff inflation slightly above patient's diastolic blood pressure; cuff inflated for 45 minutes followed by 15 minutes free of compression

Oxygenation—high flow by Venturi mask at 50% concentration or intermittent positive-pressure breathing treatment; short-term intubation with mechanical ventilatory support if patient unable to maintain adequate arterial blood gas levels and adequate tidal volume

Foley catheter attached to closed-system drainage—for careful monitoring of intake and output

Cardiac monitoring

Pulmonary capillary wedge pressure monitoring

High Fowler's position or patient permitted to sit on edge of bed and dangle legs

NURSING CARE

Nursing Assessment

Respiratory Status

Nasal flaring; retractions; tachypnea; labored noisy breathing; diaphoresis; rales; wheezing; noisy, wet breathing; cough productive of sputum; frothy, blood-tinged sputum; persistent cough; decreased vital capacity; decreased minute volume; increased intrapulmonary shunting

Tourniquets

Careful monitoring and systematic rotation of tourniquets; patient's response; tissue oxygenation and pulses distal to tourniquets

Hypoxia

Restlessness; confusion; hypotension, anxiety; tachycardia

Laboratory Values

$Paco_2$; Pao_2; pH; HCO_3^-; alveolar-arterial oxygen gradient; potassium; sodium

Cardiovascular Status

Decreased cardiac output; restlessness; lethargy; tachycardia; hypotension

Intake and Output

Careful monitoring of intake and urinary output

Pulmonary Pressures

Pulmonary capillary wedge pressure; pulmonary artery pressure

Bronchopulmonary Infection

Temperature; sputum specimens for periodic culture and sensitivity

Chest Roentgenogram

Serial chest roentgenograms to monitor clearing of edema

Psychosocial

Fear of suffocation

Associated Complications or Indications That Condition is Worsening

Sudden weight gain; swollen feet or ankles; chest pain; decreased urinary output; persistent cough

Nursing Dx & Intervention

Nursing Diagnosis	Nursing Intervention/Rationale
Fluid volume excess	• Assess patient's volume status continuously. • In collaboration with physician apply and monitor tourniquets. Rotate tourniquets, with 45 minutes on and 15 minutes off. Keep pressure slightly above patient's diastolic pressure. Carefully observe color and temperature of limb distal to each tourniquet. To discontinue tourniquets, remove one at a time, waiting at least 15 minutes before removing another. Carefully monitor cardiovascular and respiratory system response. • Carefully monitor intake and output. • Monitor pulmonary capillary wedge pressure as ordered (may indicate fluid overload complicating pulmonary wetness). • Administer diuretics, and monitor and record patient response as ordered. • Monitor serum electrolytes as ordered (may change owing to diuretics and alterations in oxygenation and metabolism). • Weigh patient at same time each day.
Ineffective breathing pattern	• Assess ventilation to include evaluation of breathing rate, rhythm, and depth; chest expansion; presence of respiratory distress such as dyspnea, shortness of breath, nasal flaring, pursed-lip breathing, or prolonged expiratory phase; and use of accessory muscles.

Nursing Diagnosis	Nursing Intervention/Rationale
	• Assess tidal volume, vital capacity, minute volume, functional residual capacity, and intrapulmonary shunting. • Identify contributing factors such as airway clearance or obstruction problem or weakness. • Position patient in high Fowler's position or sitting and leaning forward on overbed table *to facilitate ventilation.* • Suction if necessary *to remove secretions.* • Assess patient for tiring in relation to attempts to breathe. • Collaborate with physician to prepare for and administer mechanical ventilation *when breathing pattern is unable to maintain adequate blood gas levels or when patient demonstrates tiring with breathing efforts.*
Ineffective airway clearance	• Assess patient to identify inability to move secretions. If inability is identified, assist with appropriate measures (such as coughing, positioning, suctioning, and liquefying secretions). • Promptly administer bronchodilators as ordered *to dilate bronchioles and remove secretions.* Monitor serum theophylline level. • Assist patient to maintain body position *that ensures maximum airway availability.* • Carefully and frequently auscultate chest for quality of breath sounds and adventitious sounds. Note cough and sputum characteristics.
Impaired gas exchange	• Assess patient to identify signs, such as restlessness, confusion, and irritability, *that may indicate body's response to altered blood gas states.* • In collaboration with physician, monitor arterial blood gases. Report increases or decreases of more than 10 to 15 mm Hg in $Paco_2$ and Pao_2. • In collaboration with physician, administer oxygen and intermittent positive-pressure breathing. • Monitor electrocardiogram and cardiac status for arrhythmias *resulting from alterations in blood gases.* • Monitor for signs of cor pulmonale such as pulmonary hypertension, gradual increasing edema of legs, increasing central venous pressure and pulmonary capillary wedge pressure, jugular venous distention, blood gas abnormalities, and hepatomegaly. • Carefully monitor body temperature, which may fluctuate *owing to alterations in metabolism or secondary infection.* • In collaboration with physician, administer respiratory and cardiac medications and assess and document patient response.
Fatigue	• Assess patterns of fatigue. • Assess factors related to fatigue and strategies for dealing with them. • Assess support systems and available resources. • Administer treatments or medications to relieve discomfort. • Enhance patient's ability to rest between specified activities.
Impaired physical mobility	• Encourage patient to use adaptive breathing techniques *to decrease work of breathing.* • Assist patient to alternate activities with periods of rest. • Provide active or passive range of motion exercises *to maintain adequate muscle tone.*
Potential impaired skin integrity	• Assess skin for hygiene and potential for skin breakdown, and provide meticulous skin care. • Reposition patient at least every 2 hours *to prevent extended periods of lying on known pressure points.*
Fear	• Observe for signs of frustration, fear, fatigue, and tiring with attempts to communicate *resulting from hypoxia.*
Self-care deficit	• Assess patient's level of fear related to present health state. • Assess patient's level of fear related to feeling of air hunger. • Assess level of self-care deficit resulting from patient's current condition. • Assist with activities of daily living such as toileting, bathing, and feeding *to minimize patient's energy expenditures.*
Ineffective individual coping	• Determine patient's ability to cooperate with health care providers in intervention strategies.
Family coping: potential for growth	• Assess family's understanding of diagnostic procedures, disease process and prognosis, and therapies employed. • Provide information in areas needed. • See p. 1816 for additional strategies.

Patient Education

1. Teach the patient adaptive breathing techniques.
2. Teach the patient the importance of avoiding contact with persons who have upper respiratory infections.
3. Teach the patient facts about and the importance of prescribed medications such as bronchodilators and diuretics.
4. Teach the patient the importance of maintaining a low-sodium diet.
5. Inform the patient that a change in health status must be reported to the patient's health care providers. Indicators of change may include change in sputum characteristics or color, decreased activity tolerance, increased cough or chest fullness, noisy wet breathing, or leg or ankle edema.
6. Teach the patient adaptive exercises and rest techniques.

Evaluation

Patient Outcome	Data Indicating That Outcome is Reached
Movement of air in and out of lungs is optimum. Airway is patent.	Vital capacity measurements including tidal and minute volumes are normal for patient.
Both lungs are fully aerated as visualized on chest roentgenogram.	Blood gas values are within normal limits. Airways are clear, and breathing occurs without obstruction.
Breathing pattern occurs without tiring patient.	Patient demonstrates modified breathing techniques that facilitate ventilator capacity. Behavior is modified to conserve energy expenditure.
Physiologic stability is achieved after respiratory insult.	Nutrition level is maintained. Kidney and bladder functioning is within normal limits. Gastrointestinal system functions adequately. There is no secondary infection. Serum electrolytes are within normal limits.
Patient understands importance of daily pulmonary exercises.	Patient demonstrates pulmonary exercises and states rationale and importance of maintaining daily exercise routine.
Patient preserves pulmonary functioning by maintaining optimum activity level, preventing infection, and following prescribed treatments.	Patient demonstrates variety of methods indicating ability to preserve and facilitate optimum respiration (e.g., breathing exercises, modified activities or exercise, taking medications as prescribed).
Patient and family have sufficient information to comply with discharge regimen.	Patient and family at time of discharge are able to discuss medications (purpose, side effects, route, and schedule), dietary therapy regimen, activity progression regimen, signs of infection or respiratory deterioration, and plan for follow-up visits.

Pulmonary Embolism and Pulmonary Infarction

Pulmonary embolism is the blockage of a pulmonary artery by foreign matter such as a thrombus that usually arises from a peripheral vein, fat, air, or tumor tissue. Subsequent to the blockage is obstruction of blood supply to the lung tissue.

Pulmonary infarction is an uncommon complication of pulmonary embolism resulting in a localized area of lung tissue ischemic necrosis distal to the area of embolus.

The formation of a pulmonary embolism usually occurs in patients with well-defined risk factors. Following are the most common predisposing factors:

- Thrombophlebitis
- Major surgery
- Use of estrogens
- Pregnancy
- Recent childbirth
- Leg trauma
- Myocardial infarction
- Elderly
- Chronic illness
- Congestive heart failure
- Obesity
- Venous insufficiency
- Immobilization from fracture
- Polycythemia vera

Common to all of these predisposing factors is immobilization. It has been suggested that up to 5% of hospital deaths may be caused by pulmonary embolism resulting partly from immobilization.[29]

Death from pulmonary embolism usually occurs within the

first 24 hours. After that time and with proper treatment the death rate drops significantly. Resolution of the embolus occurs within 7 to 10 days.

Pathophysiology

Three factors (Virchow's triad) are related to the development of a venous thrombus: venous stasis, injury to the vein wall, and increased blood coagulability.

The most common sites for thrombus formation are the deep veins of the legs (90%) and the pelvic veins. At some point the thrombus breaks loose and travels to and lodges in one of the pulmonary arteries.

A pulmonary embolism produces an area of the lung that is ventilated but underperfused. This results in an increase in physiologic dead space ventilation. Reflex bronchoconstriction occurs in the affected area and is thought to result from the release of histamine or serotonin from the clot.[45] If the embolism is large and sufficiently reduces the pulmonary perfusion, pulmonary hypertension may result.

If the embolism lodges in a large or medium-size artery, there may be insufficient collateral bronchial blood circulation. If this occurs, there may be significant tissue underperfusion, and pulmonary infarction may result.

Figure 2-29 Lung scan showing pulmonary embolism. Note decreased perfusion of right upper lobe indicative of pulmonary embolism.
Courtesy R. Keith Wilson, M.D., Baylor College of Medicine, Houston, Texas.

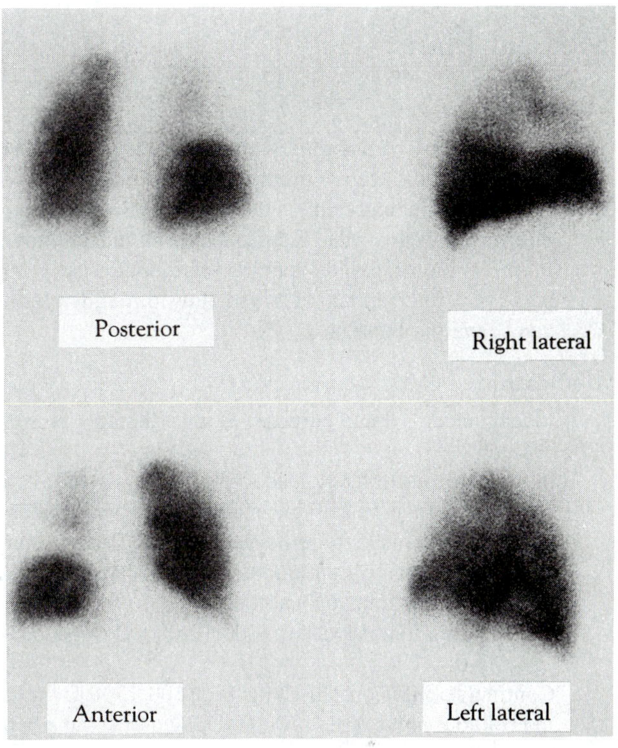

Diagnostic Studies and Findings

Clinical Examination

Dyspnea, pleuritic pain, apprehension, cough, unexplained hemoptysis, sweats, tachypnea, localized rales, pleural friction rub, tachycardia, cyanosis, low-grade fever, thrombophlebitis

Blood Gases

PaO_2 less than 60 mm Hg in association with hyperventilation leads to $PaCO_2$ less than 40 mm Hg; alveolar arterial oxygen tension gradient ($PA\text{-}aO_2$) increased

Electrocardiogram

The following classic signs help to differentiate pulmonary embolism from myocardial infarction: right axis deviation, incomplete or complete right bundle-branch block, tall peaked P waves, S wave in lead I, a Q wave in lead III, T wave insertion, ST and T wave changes in the right precordial leads

Chest Roentgenogram

Unilateral diaphragm elevation, enlarged main pulmonary artery associated with decreased vascular markings on one side, unilateral pulmonary effusion, occasional wedge-shaped area of consolidation

Lung Scans

Rapid, relatively safe and easy screening tests for establishing the diagnosis (Figure 2-29); if the patient has a chronic lung disease, asthma, or congestive heart failure, the lung scan is of little diagnostic value; two scans are commonly used sequentially: perfusion lung scan and ventilation lung scan; comparison of scans may be diagnostic of pulmonary embolism

Perfusion lung scan

This study involves the intravenous injection of serum albumin tagged with tracer amounts of a radioisotope; the radioactive particles pass through the right side of the heart and lodge in the pulmonary capillary bed; significant diagnostic findings reveal an area deficient in radioactivity

Ventilation lung scan

The patient initially breathes a radioactive gas through a carefully sealed system for several minutes; during this time the lungs are scanned by a gamma camera

Pulmonary Angiography

Although it is the most specific diagnostic procedure, pulmonary angiography also has the most risk; the two diagnostic criteria of this technique are intra-arterial filling defects and complete obstruction of a pulmonary artery branch

Laboratory Tests

Serum assays (looking for the triad of elevated lactate dehydrogenase [LDH] and bilirubin with a normal serum glutamic-oxaloacetic transaminase [SGOT] and white blood cell count [WBC] [less than 15,000], and elevated fibrin split products [FSP])

Medical Plan

Surgery

Surgical therapy of pulmonary embolism infrequently indicated; when there are multiple emboli, umbrella filter (Mobin-Uddin umbrella) may be surgically placed in inferior vena cava; other techniques are surgical removal of the embolus, which requires cardiopulmonary bypass, and interruption of blood flow through inferior vena cava via ligation

Medications

Anticoagulants—main purpose of this therapy is supportive

Heparin: does not directly lead to clot lysis; instead, heparin halts clot propagation, enabling endogenous fibrinolytic mechanisms to remove the clot.[55] Heparin may be administered by continuous intravenous infusion or by intermittent intravenous injections.

Initial bolus loading dose: 5000-10,000 U subcutaneously q8-12h

Continuous infusion: 20 U/kg/h or 800-1500 U/h

Intermittent bolus doses: 70-100 U/kg q4h using a heparin lock

The dose of heparin is best monitored and regulated by obtaining serial venous samples for partial thromboplastin time (PTT) coagulation studies. The dose should be adjusted to maintain clotting times in the range of 1.5 to 2.5 times the control values. The drug is generally continued for 7 to 14 days.

Should a severe bleeding event occur secondary to the use of heparin, protamine sulfate may be given intravenously. In such a case, 1 mg of protamine is given for every 100 U of heparin received in the dose prior to the bleeding episode. The drug should be administered slowly over 3 to 5 minutes in 20 ml saline. The total amount of protamine should not exceed 100 mg.

Long-term anticoagulation: necessary when the patient is predisposed to another pulmonary embolus.

Warfarin (Coumadin): should be started before the heparin is terminated.

Oral dose: 5-10 mg daily

Warfarin may be used for 6 months up to life in some cases. Clotting time should be monitored by the prothrombin time (PT).

Fibrinolytic enzymes: some authors believe fibrinolytic therapy to be superior to heparin therapy.[55] The two drugs of choice are:

Urokinase (Abbokinase, Breokinase): 4400 U/kg IV over 10 min, followed by 4400 U/kg/h for 12 h; thrombin time (TT) or PTT should be monitored after 2 h

Streptokinase (Kabikinase, Streptase): 250,000 U IV over 20-30 min followed by 100,000 U/h over 24-72 h; TT or PTT should be monitored after 2 h

The main side effects of these two drugs are bleeding and allergic reactions.

Dextran: Dextran is a carbohydrate polymer available in two preparations, dextran 40 and dextran 70. Dextran has antithrombotic effects, which are attributed to a decrease in platelet aggregability, alterations in factor VIII activity, and interference with fibrin formation. Dextran 70 has been shown to be as effective as low-dose heparin. Major side effects of dextran are anaphylaxis, volume overload, renal failure, and excessive bleeding. Dextran is a suitable alternative to low-dose heparin when the latter is contraindicated.

General Management

Oxygen therapy—administer oxygen by mask or cannula to maintain blood gas levels

Bed rest for first 2 or 3 days; following that, mobilization should be gradually increased

NURSING CARE

Nursing Assessment

Respiratory Status

Respiratory distress: tachypnea, labored breathing, dyspnea, coughing, shallow breathing

Breath sounds: rales or pleural friction rub

Hypoxia

Restlessness, confusion, tachycardia, cyanosis

Laboratory Values

Blood gases: monitor pH, Pa_{O_2}, Pa_{CO_2}

As long as patient is receiving anticoagulants, daily monitor clotting time, hematocrit, urinalysis, and stool for occult blood

Platelet count should be monitored at least twice weekly for thrombocytopenia

Cough, Sputum

Characteristics of cough and sputum should be monitored daily

Chest Roentgenogram

Should be monitored periodically for changes

Potential Complications

Cardiac arrhythmias, cor pulmonale, hypotension, severe hypoxemia, pulmonary hypertension, atelectasis, chest congestion

Psychosocial

Fear, air hunger, pain, confusion

Potential Risk for Pulmonary Embolism

Identification of persons at risk for development of pulmonary embolism

Preoperative teaching and postoperative care to maximize early ambulation of surgical patients

Leg exercises to maintain peripheral circulation and antiembolism stockings

Nursing Dx & Intervention

Nursing Diagnosis	Nursing Intervention/Rationale
Impaired gas exchange	• Assess patient to identify signs such as restlessness, confusion, and irritability, which may indicate the body's response to altered blood gas states. • In collaboration with physician order, monitor arterial blood gases; report increases or decreases in Pa_{CO_2} and Pa_{O_2} of more than 10 mm Hg. • In collaboration with physician, administer oxygen *to maintain adequate blood gas levels.* • Monitor electrocardiogram and cardiac status *for arrhythmias secondary to alterations in blood gases.* • If patient is seriously ill, monitor for signs of cor pulmonale such as pulmonary hypertension, cardiac compromise, jugular venous distention, blood gas abnormalities, and hepatomegaly. • Monitor and record kidney functioning and urinary output, which may be affected *secondary to tissue hypoxia and alterations in metabolism.* • Monitor serum electrolytes, which may change *because of alterations in oxygenation and metabolism.* • Carefully monitor body temperature, which may fluctuate *because of alterations in metabolism or secondary infections.* • As long as patient has an active pulmonary embolism, maintain bed rest; proceed with ambulation as quickly as possible.
Ineffective breathing pattern	• Assess ventilation to include evaluation of breathing rate, rhythm, and depth, chest expansion, presence of respiratory distress such as dyspnea, shortness of breath, tachypnea, shallow breathing, ineffective breathing, and use of accessory muscles. • Carefully and frequently auscultate chest for quality of breath sounds and adventitious sounds; *note cough and sputum characteristics.* • Help to assess total lung capacity (TLC), residual volume (RV), functional residual capacity (FRC), and forced vital capacity (FVC) as ordered. • Identify contributing factors such as airway clearance or obstruction problem, or weakness. • Maintain patient positioning *to facilitate easy ventilation* (i.e., head of bed in semi-Fowler's position). • Assess patient for tiring in relation to attempts to breathe. • Encourage patient to use adaptive breathing techniques *to decrease the work of breathing* and to space activities *so as to provide periods of rest in between.*
Fatigue	• Assess patterns of fatigue. • Assess factors related to fatigue and strategies for dealing with them. • Assess support systems and available resources. • Administer treatments or medications to relieve discomfort. • Enhance patient's ability to rest between specified activities.
Impaired physical mobility	• Encourage patient to use adaptive breathing techniques *to decrease the work of breathing.* • Provide range of motion exercises for legs as soon as ordered. • Provide antiembolism stockings. • See p. 1687 for additional strategies.
Anxiety	• Assess patient's level of anxiety related to feeling of air hunger.
Defensive coping	• Listen carefully to collect information regarding the significance of the current health care problem and the patient's perception of his ability to deal with alterations it is causing.
Family coping: potential for growth	• See p. 1816 for associated nursing care.

Patient Education

1. Teach the patient about medications (including side effects) that are currently being used to treat the pulmonary embolism.
2. Teach preventive measures to all high-risk patients preoperatively and initiate interventions postoperatively that will help to prevent pulmonary embolism.
3. Teach strategies for persons at high risk to prevent venous pooling, which may lead to thrombophlebitis.
4. Changes in the health status of a patient recovering from pulmonary embolism must be reported immediately to the patient's health care provider. Changes include chest pain, shortness of breath, tachypnea, blood-tinged sputum, and blood in the stool or urine.

Evaluation

Patient Outcome	Data Indicating That Outcome is Reached
Optimum movement of air in and out of lungs occurs.	Vital capacity measurements are optimum for patient's status.
Airway is patent.	Blood gas values are within normal limits for patient. Airways are clear, and breathing occurs without obstruction. Chest roentgenogram or lung scan shows no evidence of pulmonary embolism.
Breathing pattern is adequate.	There is no shortness of breath, dyspnea, tachypnea, or shallow breathing. Clear breath sounds are heard in all areas.
Physiologic stability occurs secondary to respiratory insult.	Nutrition level is maintained. Kidney and bladder functioning is within normal limits. Gastrointestinal system functioning is adequate. Secondary infections do not occur. Serum electrolytes are within normal limits.
Patient and family have sufficient information to comply with discharge regimen.	Patient and family are able at time of discharge to discuss medications—purpose, side effects, route, and schedule; dietary therapy regimen; activity progression regimen; signs of infection or respiratory deterioration; and plan for follow-up visits.

Pneumothorax and Hemothorax

The presence of air in the pleural space between the parietal and visceral pleurae is a pneumothorax. The presence of blood in the pleural space is a hemothorax. Many times, especially with trauma, victims have both pneumothorax and hemothorax. In these cases the term "hemopneumothorax" is used.

A pneumothorax may be caused by trauma or surgery or may occur spontaneously. A penetrating injury to the chest wall can permit air to enter the pleural space directly. An injury may also cause a broken rib, which tears the lung surface from the inside. In either case, air may gather in the pleural space, resulting in a pneumothorax.

A spontaneous pneumothorax occurs suddenly without injury and may or may not be the result of underlying pulmonary disease. Specifically, there is a rupture of the bronchus or alveolus. Pulmonary diseases such as emphysema, pneumonia, and neoplasms may result in weak tissue where a spontaneous pneumothorax may occur. It may occur in apparently healthy persons, usually between 20 and 40 years of age. For these persons there may be a rupture of a subpleural bleb after a hard cough or sneeze, allowing air to leak from the lungs into the pleural space.

A pneumothorax can occur after certain kinds of chest surgery, such as thoracotomy or a thoracentesis. A pneumothorax may also be classified by its type: open pneumothorax, closed pneumothorax, or tension pneumothorax.

An open pneumothorax is one that is communicating with the outside air (also called a sucking chest wound). The cause of this type of pneumothorax is almost always a penetrating injury.

Pathophysiology

The pleural space normally maintains a negative pressure between −10 and −12 mm Hg. This negative pressure facilitates lung expansion during ventilation. When there is penetration into the pleural space by an object external to the chest wall (such as a knife or needle) or when there is penetration into the pleural space by an internal mechanism (such as a broken rib or bleb rupture of the lung), air enters the pleural space and the negative pressure is decreased. Depending on the amount of air that enters initially and the amount that continues to enter, such as with a tension pneumothorax, the lung is no longer able to remain fully inflated.

As the pleural space pressure increases and the lung collapses, there is a mediastinal shift toward the unaffected side. This shift causes pressure on the great vessels returning to the heart and thus a decreased venous return. If pneumothorax is left untreated, cardiac output is compromised and a shutdown systemic response may occur.

Diagnostic Studies and Findings

The types of pneumothorax and hemothorax have both similarities and differences. The following diagnostic studies discuss the differences where they exist.

Spontaneous, Simple, or Noncommunicating Pneumothorax

History

Patient generally is male between the ages of 20 and 40 years and is in good health

Patient is older and has a chronic obstructive pulmonary disease, pneumonia, or a neoplasm

Patient usually awakens to note shortness of breath and chest pain

Clinical examination

Shortness of breath and chest pain in only 50% of all cases; patient may appear acutely ill with cyanosis and tachypnea or may appear to be healthy; the difference in the clinical signs is dependent on the size of the pneumothorax; breath sounds are generally diminished; percussion tones are hyperresonant over involved area; approximately 25% of patients have subcutaneous emphysema[81]; in addition the patient demonstrates syncope and Hamman's sign (a crunching sound with each heartbeat owing to mediastinal air accumulation)

Chest roentgenogram

The characteristic finding shows air in the pleural cavity without the lateral markings of the lungs; instead there is a sharp pleural margin seen medially, indicating that the lung has collapsed; if the lung is not entirely collapsed, this margin may not be as obvious; it is therefore desirable to take an expiratory film with the patient sitting upright; because intrapleural air first collects in the apex, partial pneumothorax identification may be made; Figure 2-30 shows a classic picture of a pneumothorax

Figure 2-30 Chest roentgenogram of patient with pneumothorax. Note narrowing of pleural edge at arrow point and lack of lung markings beyond pleural line.
Courtesy R. Keith Wilson, M.D., Baylor College of Medicine, Houston, Texas.

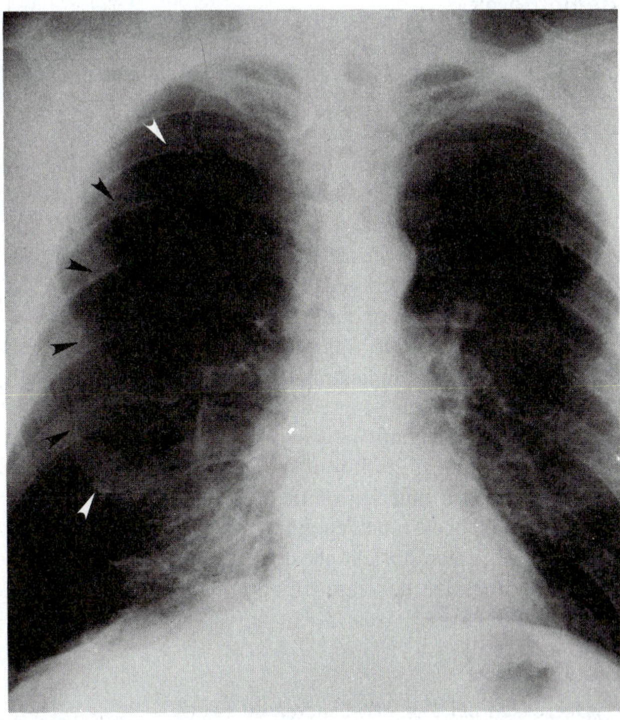

Open, Communicating, Penetrating-Trauma Pneumothorax

History

Some event that has caused a penetration of the chest wall

Clinical examination

Penetration of the chest wall, a sucking sound on inspiration as the chest wall rises, and varying signs of respiratory distress depending on the size of the pneumothorax

Chest roentgenogram

See "Spontaneous, Simple, or Noncommunicating Pneumothorax" above

Tension Pneumothorax

History

Blunt trauma to the chest that may have resulted in fractured ribs or penetrating injury to the chest that permits air to enter the chest wall but then seals off as the air tries to escape

Clinical examination

As the positive pressure on the affected side increases, the clinical signs will become more severe; these include neck vein enlargement owing to pressure on the superior vena cava, dyspnea, cardiogenic shock because of the lack of oxygenated blood, paradoxic movement of the chest, deviated trachea toward the unaffected side, cyanosis, distant heart sounds, absence of breath sounds on the affected side, and hyperresonance on percussion of the affected side

The chest roentgenogram of an individual with a tension pneumothorax shows complete lung collapse and a shift of mediastinal structures toward the unaffected side

Hemothorax

History

Same as for open pneumothorax or tension pneumothorax

Clinical examination

Same as above with the addition of tachycardia, hypotension, dullness on chest percussion, and signs of hypovolemic shock such as pallor and anxiety; the severity of the hemothorax may be determined by the amount of blood accumulation: less than 300 ml is considered minor and may not cause significant clinical signs; 300 to 1400 ml is moderate; and over 1400 ml is severe, indicating that most clinical signs will also be present

Chest roentgenogram

A minimum of 250 ml of intrapleural fluid is required to show a blunting of the costophrenic angle on an upright chest roentgenogram[47]; it is therefore desirable to obtain an upright chest roentgenogram if possible; findings are decreased lung expansion as in Figure 2-30

Blood Gases

Decreased pH and PaO_2; increased $PaCO_2$

Medical Plan

Surgery

Closed-tube thoracostomy (chest tube): this technique is used to treat most types of pneumothorax. The exception is a small, spontaneous pneumothorax in an otherwise healthy individual. The indications for closed-tube thoracostomy include the following[66]:

Traumatic causes
Pneumothorax with respiratory distress
Recurrent pneumothorax
Necessity for ventilatory support
Moderate to large pneumothorax
Pneumothorax that continues to grow despite treatment
Associated hemothorax
Tension pneumothorax

The chest tube should be inserted in the fifth or sixth intercostal space at the midaxillary line. If the tube is positioned posteriorly and toward the apex of the lung, it can effectively remove air and fluid. The lateral placement is preferred not only because it is most efficient but also because it does not produce a cosmetic defect, as does the anterior site of the second intercostal space at the midclavicular line.[81] See pp. 222 to 225 for discussion of chest tubes.

Tension pneumothorax requires immediate and specific medical intervention. The building pressure in the pleural space must be reversed. A mechanism must be provided to release the pressure. The most effective way to release the pressure is to insert a large-bore needle (16 to 18 gauge) either anteriorly at the midclavicle line between the second and third intercostal space or at the midlateral line between the fifth and sixth intercostal space. Once the needle is inserted, the patient's condition should improve remarkably.

Thoracotomy: A hemothorax may require a thoracotomy for correction. Indications for this procedure include initial thoracostomy tube drainage greater than 1500 ml of blood; persistent bleeding rate greater than 500 ml/h; increasing hemothorax seen on chest roentgenogram; patient in an unstable and hypotensive state despite adequate blood replacement.[66]

Medications

Hemothorax requires aggressive intravenous therapy to restore the circulating blood volume

Narcotic analgesics: Analgesics such as meperidine (Demerol) may be given for pain if respirations are adequate; drugs such as morphine and barbiturates are generally contraindicated because they may cause respiratory depression

Adrenergic agents: Antihypotensives such as dopamine may be indicated

Dopamine (Intropin)

Dilute 1 ampule (200 mg) in 250 ml D5W; use with microdrip administration set; usual dose is 2-5 mg/kg/min initially; then titrate to desired response

General Management

Airway maintenance—done by positioning, a simple airway, or endotracheal intubation, depending on patient's condition

Oxygenation—provide oxygen to maintain adequate blood gas levels

Mechanical ventilation with PEEP—if patient shows evidence of respiratory failure, may be initiated after chest tubes have been inserted and determined to be functioning adequately; see p. 225 for discussion of technique

If the patient has active and communicating pneumothorax, entrance wound into the chest wall should be immediately covered by petrolatum jelly gauze; three sides of the gauze pad should be taped; the fourth is left open to permit exhale ventilation; if gauze is placed on too tightly, tension pneumothorax may result

NURSING CARE

Nursing Assessment

Respiratory Status

Respiratory distress to include dyspnea, tachypnea, retractions, labored breathing, nasal flaring

Breath sounds distant, bilaterally unequal, diminished; vocal fremitus on the affected side; hyperresonance to percussion on affected side

Breathing pattern may show presence of splinting or hypoventilation that may lead to atelectasis; breathing seems inadequate, causing patient to tire but still be "air hungry"

Evaluate chest wall for stability and movement

Tracheal deviation noted with palpation

Evaluate for presence of crepitation

Cough, characteristics and amount; sputum, amount and characteristics

Hypoxia

Restlessness, confusion, tachycardia, cyanosis; note mucous membranes, nail beds

Cardiovascular Status

Blood pressure, heart rate, auscultation quality, tissue perfusion, urinary output

Laboratory Values

Blood gases; electrolytes; CBC

Chest Roentgenogram

For presence of pneumothorax and change since last chest roentgenogram

Chest Tube Drainage

Assess intact drainage system and amount and characteristics of drainage

Anxiety

Fear, air hunger, pain, confusion

Secondary Complications

Atelectasis, ARDS, chest congestion, infection, pulmonary edema, pulmonary embolus

Nursing Dx & Intervention

Nursing Diagnosis	Nursing Intervention/Rationale
Ineffective breathing pattern	• Assess ventilation to include evaluation of breathing rate, rhythm, and depth, chest expansion, presence of respiratory distress such as dyspnea, shortness of breath, nasal flaring, anxiety, retractions, prolonged expiratory phase, use of accessory muscles. • Assist to insert chest tubes as indicated. • Provide chest tube care consistent with the guidelines presented on pp. 222 to 225; carefully maintain *to avoid interruption in the airtight system via dislodgment of the tubing or breaking of the bottles.* • Identify contributing factors such as airway clearance or obstruction problem or weakness that may contribute to the patient's respiratory distress. • Maintain patient positioning *to facilitate easy ventilation* (i.e., head of bed in semi-Fowler's position). • Suction if necessary *to remove secretions.* • Assess patient for tiring in relation to attempts to breathe. • Encourage patient to breathe deeply but also to use adaptive breathing techniques *to decrease the work of breathing* and to space activities *so as to provide periods of rest in between.* • Assist to protect patient from known sources of secondary infection. • Should mechanical ventilation become necessary, provide care and monitoring consistent with the guidelines on pp. 225 to 228.
Inpaired gas exchange	• Assess patient to identify signs such as restlessness, confusion, and irritability, *which may indicate the body's response to altered blood gas states.* • In collaboration with physician, monitor arterial blood gases; report increases or decreases in $Paco_2$ and Pao_2 of more than 10 to 15 mm Hg. • Administer oxygen *to maintain the arterial blood gases as ordered.* • Monitor electrocardiogram and cardiac status *for arrhythmias secondary to alterations in blood gases.* • Monitor and record kidney functioning and urinary output, which may be affected *by chronic tissue hypoxia and alterations in metabolism.* • Monitor serum electrolytes, which may change *because of alterations in oxygenation and metabolism.* • Carefully monitor body temperature, which may fluctuate *because of alterations in metabolism or secondary infections.*

Nursing Diagnosis	Nursing Intervention/Rationale
Ineffective airway clearance	• Assess patient to identify inability to move secretions; if inability is identified, assist with appropriate measures (coughing, positioning, suctioning, liquefying secretions, etc.). • Assist patient to maintain proper body positioning *to ensure maximum airway availability* (e.g., semi-Fowler's position). • Carefully and frequently auscultate chest for quality of breath sounds and adventitious sounds; note cough and sputum characteristics.
Fatigue	• Assess patterns of fatigue. • Assess factors related to fatigue and strategies for dealing with them. • Assess support systems and available resources. • Administer treatments or medications to relieve discomfort. • Enhance patient's ability to rest between specified activities.
Altered nutrition: less than body requirements	• See p. 1630 for associated nursing care.
Potential fluid volume deficit	• In the seriously ill patient, assess for evidence of gastrointestinal bleeding secondary to physiologic stress; monitor serial hemoglobin and hematocrit; check all stools, emesis, and nasogastric aspirate for presence of blood; observe changes in vital signs or abdominal girth.
Impaired physical mobility	• Encourage patient to use adaptive breathing techniques *to decrease the work of breathing*. • See p. 1687 for additional strategies.
Fear	• Assess patient's level of fear related to the present health state. • Assess patient's level of fear related to feeling of air hunger.
Self-care deficit	• Assess the level of self-care deficit secondary to the patient's current condition. • See p. 1692 for additional strategies.
Defensive coping	• Listen carefully to collect information regarding the significance of the current health care problem and the patient's perception of ability to deal with alterations it is causing.
Family coping: potential for growth	• Assess family's understanding of diagnostic procedures, disease process and prognosis, and therapies employed. • See p. 1816 for additional strategies.

Patient Education

1. Teach the patient and family about the chest tubes, their purpose, function, and care that must be taken during their use.
2. Teach the patient adaptive breathing techniques to maximize lung reexpansion and prevent complications.
3. Teach importance of avoiding contact with persons who have upper respiratory infections and influenza.
4. Teach importance of regular medical reevaluations for an extended period following the pneumothorax.

Evaluation

Patient Outcome	Data Indicating That Outcome is Reached
Full expansion of lungs is achieved.	Chest roentgenograms show full lung expansion with no evidence of pneumothorax or hemothorax.
Optimum movement of air in and out of lungs occurs.	Vital capacity measurements are optimum for patient. Blood gas values are within normal limits. Airways are clear, and breathing occurs without obstruction. Clear breath sounds are heard in all areas. Behavior is modified to conserve energy expenditure.
Physiologic stability occurs secondary to respiratory insult.	Nutrition level is maintained. Kidney and bladder functioning is within normal limits. Gastrointestinal system functioning is adequate. Secondary infections do not occur. Serum electrolytes are within normal limits.

Patient Outcome	Data Indicating That Outcome is Reached
Patient understands importance of daily pulmonary exercises until pneumothorax is completely healed.	Patient demonstrates pulmonary exercises and states rationale and importance of maintaining daily exercise routine.
Patient and family have sufficient information to comply with discharge regimen.	Patient and family are able at time of discharge to discuss medications—purpose, side effects, route, and schedule; dietary therapy regimen; activity progression regimen; signs of infection or respiratory deterioration; and plan for follow-up visits.

Pneumoconioses

(Occupational lung disease)

Industrial and work-related lung diseases are caused by inhaling inorganic dusts or gaseous or particulate matters in the air. They are referred to as pneumoconioses (*pneuma,* lung; *konia,* dust; *osis,* condition).[24] The three major pneumoconioses are silicosis, asbestosis, and coal workers' pneumoconiosis.

Pathophysiology

Fine particles and gaseous agents entering the lung encounter little, if any, resistance. Once inhaled, particulate matters are deposited on various areas of the respiratory tract. Particles deposited on the mucous surfaces of the nose and upper airways are readily moved toward the pharynx, from which they are swallowed or coughed out.

The ciliated pseudostratified epithelium is covered by a mucous blanket. The rhythmic beating of the epithelium moves inhaled particles along. The speed of the mucus movement has been estimated to be between 10 and 20 mm/minute. Thus 90% of the deposited material is physically cleared in less than 1 hour.[24]

The irritating effects of certain particles and gases increase mucous production. With repeated exposures the mucous glands hypertrophy and secrete more mucus in response to a variety of inhaled irritants. This may result in a type of chronic bronchitis.

Bronchioles and alveoli have no epithelium, mucous glands, or goblet cells; therefore particles deposited in their lumen are not as easily removed. Alveolar clearance involves more complex pathways of cellular and fluid transport. Phagocytic cells in the alveoli play the major role in disposing of the particles reaching this part of the respiratory tract. In addition, alveolar surfactant and fluid produced from capillary transudation help in moving the particles to the lymph channels. Disposal of particles from the alveoli is a very slow process, and the respiratory membrane remains exposed to their harmful effects until they are removed. Coating of the particles by surfactant and certain chemical reactions, as well as some enzymatic actions, reduce their harmful effects.

Once phagocytized, the particles are processed by the metabolic and enzymatic apparatus of the alveolar macrophages. The phagocytic effectiveness of these cells is influenced by many exogenous and endogenous factors. Sometimes the offending agents impair the function of these cells.

When the primary disposing mechanisms fail to control the agents' harmful effects, the secondary cellular and humoral defense mechanisms are brought into action. These mechanisms result in inflammation, which consists of dilation and increased permeability of capillaries, exudation of fluid, and infiltration of white blood cells. The immunologic system plays a major part in this process. It therefore seems that the pathologic changes are at least partly the result of these secondary defense mechanisms.[24]

Silicosis

Silicosis is the most important of the pneumoconioses. It is a progressive pulmonary disease marked by nodular lesions, which often progress to fibrosis. This disease often shows no symptoms. It is caused by the inhalation and pulmonary deposition of crystalline silicon dioxide dust, mostly from quartz.

Industrial sources of silica in its pure form include the manufacture of ceramics (flint) and building materials (sandstone). It occurs in mixed form in the production of construction materials such as cement. Silica is found in powder form in paints, porcelain, scouring soaps, and wood fillers. It may also be found in the mining of gold, coal, lead, zinc, and iron. Sources of free silica dust include industries such as mining, quarrying, tunneling, stone cutting, abrasive industry, pottery, and tile manufacturing.

The development of silicosis depends on the size of the silica particle, its concentration in the air, length of exposure, and susceptibility of the individual. Very heavy exposure, as sometimes occurs in sandblasters, may result in a more acute form of silicosis after brief exposure.

Pathophysiology. The silica particles deposited in the alveoli are 1 to 3 μm in diameter. These are phagocytized by the macrophages. In the process, part of these cells containing the particles is damaged. Cellular enzymes dispersing in cytoplasm cause death of the macrophages and release of their contents, including the silica particles. More macrophages are attracted to the area and are also killed. The production of fibrosis, the major pathologic finding, has been attributed to the release of certain fibrogenic factors. The pathologic process continues even after the environmental exposure has ceased.

The characteristic pathologic changes are the silicotic nodules, which are fibrotic lesions. In simple silicosis the nodules may measure 2 to 3 mm in diameter and are unevenly scattered throughout the lungs. They are surrounded by distorted lung tissue, which may show emphysematous changes. As the disease state progresses, these changes are characteristic of progressive massive fibrosis (PMF) and indicate complicated silicosis. With progressive massive fibrosis, the upper lobes may show evidence of emphysema, sometimes with large bullous changes.[24]

Asbestosis

Asbestos, the name given to a number of fibrous silicates, is mined principally in Canada, South Africa, and Russia. Raw asbestos is first processed to release asbestos fibers from the parent rock and then transported for use in a variety of industries. In the United States most asbestos is used to fireproof and insulate buildings. Workers in these industries may be exposed to asbestos dust. Symptoms of asbestosis do not usually appear until the individual has been exposed to asbestos dust for at least 10 years.[86]

Pathophysiology. Asbestosis is caused by deposition of small asbestos particles on bronchioles or alveolar walls where they are ingested by cells. This swells the alveolar wall by a process that is not fully understood.

Fibrosis in asbestosis, unlike silicosis, is nonnodular, involves mostly the lower lungs, and often has pleural thickening. Pleural thickening, plaque formation, and pleural calcification are common with asbestos exposure. Pleural effusion, sometimes bloody, is a fairly common form of pleural reaction.

Bronchogenic carcinoma often occurs with asbestosis. However, the relationship is mostly because of the combined effect of asbestos and cigarette smoking. Heavy smokers who are also exposed to asbestos have 80 to 90 times the risk of nonsmokers for having bronchogenic carcinoma.[24]

Coal Workers' Pneumoconiosis (Black Lung)

Coal workers' pneumoconiosis (CWP) is a chronic pathologic condition resulting from prolonged exposure to coal dust. Although carbon is not a fibrogenic agent, with massive and prolonged exposure the clearance mechanisms of the lung are overwhelmed, and coal dust accumulates in terminal air spaces, resulting in pulmonary problems.

The incidence of pneumoconiosis in anthracite mining is much higher than in soft (bituminous) coal mining. An estimated 10 to 12 years of mining work is needed for the development of this disease.[24]

Pathophysiology. After the deposition of coal dust in the respiratory bronchioles and alveoli, the first reaction is phagocytosis of the particles by increasing numbers of macrophages, which move to the terminal bronchioles. An excessive dust load overwhelms the pulmonary clearing mechanism. Fibroblasts appear in this area, laying a thin network of reticulin fibers without significant collagen formation. The aggregations of macrophages and dust particles enmeshed in reticulin fibers are called coal macules because they appear as black dots on the lung sections. These spots are often linked with dilation of respiratory bronchioles, called focal centrilobular emphysema. These changes are often seen in simple CWP. The complicated form of the disease is marked by massive fibrosis, involving mostly the upper lobes.[24]

Diagnostic Studies and Findings

Clinical History

Occupational exposure to silica dust, asbestos, or coal dust

Clinical Examination

Patients with all three of these diseases are often asymptomatic. The main symptoms may be tachypnea and dyspnea with or without a dry cough. The cough is worse in the morning. The severity of dyspnea is usually progressive. The dyspnea is more evident in patients who also smoke. Patients may have 10 or more years of exposure before clinical symptoms are noticed.

As the disease progresses, respiratory failure may develop and clinical evidence of respiratory failure, pulmonary hypertension, or cor pulmonale may appear. Relatively few physical findings are apparent until the development of cor pulmonale. Rales, clubbing, and other findings associated with chronic lung disease may or may not be present.

Other clinical signs are decreased chest expansion, diminished breath sounds, and areas of hyporesonance and hyperresonance.

Patients with CWP have expectoration of black material.

Chest Roentgenogram

Silicosis

The initial manifestation of silicosis is the development of small nodules on the chest roentgenogram. At this point in the disease the patient is usually asymptomatic. Exposure to silica may have been going on for 10 to 20 years.

With the development of massive fibrosis, the upper lobes show evidence of volume loss. The lower lobes show emphysematous changes.

In complicated silicosis, massive densities may be seen in the fields. Progressive changes from simple nodular form to massive fibrosis may take place within 5 years.

Asbestosis

Asbestosis is manifest as interstitial markings with reticular density, predominantly involving the lower lung fields. Sometimes a marked honeycomb pattern is present. The lung volume is often diminished. Common pleural changes include thickening, plaques, calcification, and effusion.

Coal workers' pneumoconiosis

CWP usually does not appear until the worker has been exposed to coal dust for approximately 10 years. The roentgenogram shows the presence of small opacities or nodular densities through the lung fields. These lesions are usually confined to the upper lung fields. The nodular densities are often smaller and less defined than those of silicosis.[24]

Pulmonary Function Tests

These may be normal in early disease. As the diseases progress, abnormalities may be seen. These changes may indicate both obstructive and restrictive lung damage. Test findings may include decreases in FVC, FEV_1, reduced diffusing capacity of CO (DLco), reduced total lung capacity (TLC), and static lung compliance.

Blood Gas Studies

These are normal early in the diseases. As the diseases progress, decreased Po_2 and increased Pco_2 may occur. Hypoxemia may become severe.

Medical Plan

Surgery

Biopsy—may be necessary for diagnostic evaluation

Medications

None specific; treat complications of disease such as infection, pulmonary hypertension, and cor pulmonale

General Management

Prevention of secondary infections
Chest physical therapy
Steam inhalation
Oxygen by cannula, 1 to 2 L/minute
Increased fluids

NURSING CARE

Nursing Assessment

Respiratory Status

Dyspnea, respiratory distress
Breath sounds: decreased, bilaterally unequal, rales, rhonchi
Increased sputum, persistent cough, wet-sounding breathing
Pulmonary function: decreased vital capacity, minute volume, and functional residual capacity; increased intrapulmonary shunting
Hypoxia: restlessness, confusion, impaired motor function, hypotension, tachycardia

Laboratory Values

Monitor blood gas values

Secondary Infection

Resulting decreased ability to move secretions; increased risk of tuberculosis; monitor temperature, sputum amount, and characteristics

Cor Pulmonale and Pulmonary Hypertension

Monitor for presence (see p. 195)

Chest Roentgenogram

Monitor for disease progression

Nursing Dx & Intervention

Nursing Diagnosis	Nursing Intervention/Rationale
Knowledge deficit related to unfamiliarity with disease process	• Assess patient's and family's level of knowledge about these pneumoconioses. • Inform patient that prevention is the most important aspect of the management of the disease. The disease may not become apparent until after 20 years of exposure. Protective hoods and clothing should be used during times of exposure. • Instruct patient to maintain regular follow-up examinations and to report new symptoms or exposure to other respiratory diseases.
Potential for infection	• Instruct patient about increased risk for acquiring tuberculosis and other infectious diseases and about need for frequent medical evaluations. • Instruct patient to avoid persons with known respiratory infections. • Assess patient for weight loss, anorexia, and fever, which may be present in the presence of an infection.
Potential for injury	• Inform patient that exposure to these dusts will make the disease worse. Continued dust exposure should be avoided.
Impaired gas exchange	• Assess patient to identify signs, such as restlessness, confusion, and irritability, *that may indicate the body's response to altered blood gases.*

Nursing Diagnosis	Nursing Intervention/Rationale
	• Monitor for signs of increasing cor pulmonale such as increased pulmonary artery pressure, increased edema in extremities, jugular venous distention, and hepatomegaly. • Administer and monitor bronchodilators as ordered. • Schedule blood gases and pulmonary function testing on a periodic basis. • Ensure that patient is aware that the disease progresses even if the patient is removed from further dust exposure. The patient should be frequently monitored for condition deterioration.

Patient Education

Education should be directed to the predisease state. These diseases are preventable if precautions are taken on a regular basis.

1. Teach the patient that protective head hoods should be used at work when dust production is heavy. Exposure to crystalline silica, asbestos, or coal dust may occur during mining or quarrying for the material. In addition, individuals who work in foundries; who are involved in abrasive blasting, stone cutting, or other masonry work; or who work in areas where glass, pottery, or porcelain is manufactured may be at risk for silicosis.
2. Teach the patient and the family to watch for other pulmonary signs that may indicate infection or complications of the disease. Such signs may be dyspnea, cough, worsening expectoration, or hemoptysis.
3. Teach the patient the importance of avoiding environmental pollutants and not smoking.
4. Teach the patient adaptive breathing techniques if dyspnea and shortness of breath are present.

Evaluation

Patient Outcome	Data Indicating That Outcome is Reached
Further lung injury is prevented.	Patient uses protective headwear so further respiratory damage is prevented.
Air moves optimally in and out of the lungs.	Vital capacity measurements are optimum for the patient's status. Blood gases are within normal limits for the patient.
Breathing pattern occurs without tiring the patient.	Patient demonstrates modified breathing techniques that facilitate ventilatory capacity.
Physiologic function is stable.	Nutrition is maintained. There are no secondary infections. Serum electrolytes are within normal limits.
Patient preserves pulmonary functioning by maintaining optimum activity level, preventing infection, and following prescribed treatments.	Patient demonstrates a variety of methods indicating ability to preserve and facilitate optimum respiratory functioning (e.g., breathing exercises, modified exercises, modified activities or exercises, taking medications as prescribed).
Patient and family have sufficient information to comply with discharge regimen.	Patient and family are able to discuss medications, activity progression, signs of infection, breathing exercises, and plan for follow-up visits.

Medical Interventions and Related Nursing Care

Airway Maintenance

Airway maintenance may occur in many forms including the following:

Suctioning
Oropharyngeal airway
Nasopharyngeal airway
Endotracheal intubation
Tracheostomy (see Chapter 7 for procedures)

Regardless of technique, the purpose of maintaining a patent airway is so ventilation may occur. Certain airway maintenance methods such as endotracheal intubation are usually connected to oxygen sources or mechanical ventilators.

Preprocedural Care

Clinical assessment indicating airway obstruction

Restlessness
Wheezing
Noisy respirations
Difficulty breathing
Tachycardia
Rhonchi over large airways
Decreased breath sounds
Retractions: intercostal, suprasternal, supraclavicular, nasal flaring
Stridor
Mouth breathing
Low tidal volume

Preprocedural teaching. Because of the patient's situation requiring airway maintenance procedures, preprocedural teaching may seem inappropriate. The care provider is still required to anticipate teaching opportunities and to provide the following information as appropriate:

1. Explain procedure to patient and family members
2. Discuss with patient and family what procedure will be like for the patient
3. Demonstrate equipment and its purpose

Procedural Techniques and Associated Care[37,38,42,45,77]

Orotracheal or Nasotracheal Suctioning

Indications:

Signs of respiratory distress
Noisy, wet breathing

Contraindications:

Tight wheeze with bronchospasm or croup

Procedural guidelines:

1. If possible, position patient in semi-Fowler's position.
2. Use sterile, gloved technique.
3. Use smallest catheter size possible to remove secretions.
4. Hyperoxygenate patient before suctioning procedure if patient is attached to respiratory assistance ventilator.
5. Encourage patient to breathe slowly during procedure.
6. Lubricate catheter tip with sterile saline or water before procedure.
7. Insert vented catheter for suctioning.
8. Insert and advance catheter as patient breathes slowly.
9. Do not apply suction while catheter is fully inserted.
10. Once catheter is in place, apply suction for 5- to 10-second interval; rotate and slowly withdraw catheter during suctioning.
11. Allow at least 3 minutes between suctioning periods; during this time, administer oxygen.
12. Note and record amount and characteristics of sputum.
13. Note and record patient's response to suctioning procedure.
14. Discard catheter after each treatment.
15. Change vacuum container and tubing every day.

Complications:

Wheezing or crowing respiratory sounds after or during procedure indicating potential bronchospasm or laryngospasm (if noted, administer oxygen and contact physician)
Bloody drainage owing to trauma or respiratory secretions
Prolonged spasmodic coughing
Traumatic ulceration of the airways
Infection
Atelectasis if catheter greater than two thirds the size of bronchus is used
Hypoxemia
Cardiac rhythm and rate disturbance

Oropharyngeal or Nasopharyngeal Airways

Indications:

Potential or actual upper airway obstruction owing to altered levels of consciousness resulting in relaxation of the tongue against the hypopharynx
Trauma-induced upper airway obstruction

Procedural guidelines:

1. Determine type of airway according to individual patient needs:
   a. Oropharyngeal airway: length should be from teeth to the mandibular end of jaw.
   b. Nasopharyngeal airway: may be indicated if patient has associated mouth injury; the length

should be slightly narrower than the nares diameter

2. Insertion techniques:
   a. Oropharyngeal airway: insert airway upside down to prevent tongue from being pushed posteriorly; as the airway passes the uvula, rotate the airway 180 degrees; the flange of the airway should be securely positioned outside the lips.
   b. Nasopharyngeal airway: should be inserted in anatomic line with the nasal passage.
3. Position patient on side to facilitate drainage.
4. Remove and change airway at least every 6 to 8 hours; observe for ulcerations of mucous membranes.
5. Remove and change nasal airway at least every 72 hours; rotate to other nares; observe for ulcerations of mucous membranes.
6. Carefully observe position of airway at least every hour; suction if needed.
7. Provide mouth and nose care at least every 2 hours.
8. Airway removal: observe patient's level of consciousness and presence of gag and swallow reflexes; when patient is awake, instruct him to push airway out with tongue; carefully observe patient for adequate airway maintenance after removal.

Complications:

Will not prevent aspiration of secretions; suction must be available

May cause patient to gag

May become clogged

May become dislodged if not secured in place

Bleeding secondary to trauma of insertion

Potential infection secondary to airway

Ulceration of nares or pharynx secondary to prolonged insertion

Observe for mucus plugs or other signs of noisy breathing, restlessness, or malpositioning of airway, which indicate blockage of airway or malpositioning

Endotracheal Intubation

Indications:

Intubation:

Airway obstruction that occurs despite the use of an oral airway

To prevent possible aspiration in an unconscious patient

To remove secretions from the tracheobronchial tree

To provide controlled ventilation, which may or may not be accomplished by face masks

To provide high concentrations of oxygen

Extubation:

Should be attempted only in a planned and controlled environment

Procedural guidelines:

1. Assemble all equipment before attempting intubation procedure.
2. Check the cuff on endotracheal tubes for leakage.
3. Assist to position patient so the neck is flexed and the head is extended; this should bring the mouth, larynx, and trachea in line.
4. If patient is awake or combative, succinylcholine may be given to block voluntary ventilation; before administration of this drug, ventilatory assistance equipment must be available for immediate use.
5. Before intubation, explain the procedure and ensure that any false teeth or bridges have been removed.
6. Before intubation, hyperventilate patient using an Ambu bag with supplemental 100% oxygen.
7. If intubation is prolonged, interrupt the procedure and oxygenate the patient.
8. Once the endotracheal tube is in place, assist to determine proper endotracheal tube placement; this is done by considering the following:
   a. Correct placement: bilateral lung inflation, breath sounds heard equally throughout all lobes.
   b. Incorrect placement:

      Esophagus: absence of breath sounds, respiratory distress and cyanosis; if these are noted, the endotracheal tube should be removed and reinserted.

      Right mainstem bronchus or carina: the endotracheal tube has been inserted too far; clinical signs include unilateral breath sounds, lung inflation, and coughing; if this is noted and confirmed by x-ray examination, the endotracheal tube should be retracted slightly and resecured; reassessment should indicate proper placement.
9. Once the endotracheal tube is in correct position, tape it securely so movement of tube is impossible.
10. Monitor tube placement and patency at least every hour; this assessment should include:
    a. Tube position
    b. Tube patency
    c. Lung inflation
    d. Absence of respiratory distress
    e. Generalized respiratory response
    f. Monitoring of arterial blood gases
11. Provide ongoing care for patients with endotracheal tube in place:
    a. Provide mouth care every 2 hours.
    b. Clean nares and around endotracheal tube at least every 6 to 8 hours.
    c. Reposition and retape endotracheal tube at least every 6 to 8 hours.
    d. Take precaution not to dislodge tube position.
12. If tube has cuff, use minimal leak technique or deflate cuff every 4 to 5 hours for at least 20 minutes (prolonged cuff deflation will not work if patient is attached to ventilator); this should follow careful and thorough suctioning of oral secretions; the cuff should then be reinflated until no air leakage is noted; record the amount of air inserted to inflate the cuff.

13. Use bite block if the patient bites the endotracheal tube.
14. Remove any mucus plugs by instillation of 8 to 10 ml of saline into the endotracheal tube.
15. Perform chest physiotherapy at least every 4 hours.
16. Patient should receive humidified oxygen while intubated.
17. If patient is awake, provide writing materials for communication.
18. Extubation:
    a. Assess patient's ability to breathe on own before extubation.
    b. Determine that patient is able to maintain spontaneous respiratory rate sufficient to maintain stable blood gas values.
    c. Carefully suction endotracheal tube and mouth before extubation.
    d. Immediately after extubation, assess for signs of respiratory distress or laryngeal spasm such as dyspnea, noisy breathing, use of abdominal or accessory muscles, restlessness, irritability, tachycardia, tachypnea, decreased $Pa{O_2}$, increased $Pa{CO_2}$; if these are noted, consult physician immediately and prepare for reinsertion of endotracheal tube.

Complications:

Delay of oxygenation or ventilation during intubation procedure

Placement of endotracheal tube into right mainstem bronchus, resulting in unilateral and thus diminished lung aeration

Ulceration of trachea or tracheoesophageal fistula resulting from endotracheal tube cuff inflated for more than 8 hours

Mucus plugs or other blockage of endotracheal tube may lead to hypoxia and respiratory distress

Unplanned extubation by combative patient or secondary to poor securement of tube will require immediate airway and ventilatory assessment by the nurse as well as potential need for oral airway, patient positioning, and ventilation by Ambu bag with supplemental oxygen

Aspiration of secretions secondary to poorly inflated cuff, inadequate suctioning before cuff deflation, or too small noncuffed endotracheal tube used

Potential laryngospasm or edema following intubation

NURSING CARE

Nursing Assessment

Inability to Maintain Patent Airway

Despite the selected technique, patent airway is not obtained; patient continues to have same or different airway obstruction signs as noted during preprocedural assessment (see above)

Carefully observe patent condition of tubing; clean or reposition as necessary to maximize airway potential

For tracheostomy and endotracheal intubation, obtain a chest roentgenogram after insertion to ascertain exact positioning of tube

Positioning to Maximize Airway Potential

Carefully assess for patent airway, presence of bilaterally equal breath sounds, and bilateral expansion of chest wall

Bleeding or Trauma Caused by the Airway Maintenance Technique

Observe for presence of bleeding and for wet breath sounds; bleeding is usually self-limited unless the patient is receiving anticoagulants or has a bleeding disorder

Potential Dental Damage Secondary to Insertion

Observe condition of patient's teeth

Ulcerations of Nasal Tissue or Pharynx

Carefully observe tissue around the airway mechanism; when possible, change position of the mechanism or its taped location

Infection Secondary to Airway Maintenance Mechanism

Observe for signs of infection such as increased temperature, change in secretions, or foul odor

Nursing Dx & Intervention

Nursing Diagnosis	Nursing Intervention/Rationale
Ineffective airway clearance	• Assess patient for signs of hypoxia or airway blockage as indicated in the preprocedural assessment section. • Position patient *to maximize airway potential.* • Using sterile technique, suction as needed *to maintain airway.* • At least hourly, auscultate chest for presence and quality of bilateral breath sounds and adventitious sounds. • If patient has endotracheal tube in place, provide oropharyngeal airway or bite block *to prevent biting* on the endotracheal tube.

Nursing Diagnosis	Nursing Intervention/Rationale
Anxiety	• Assess for signs of anxiety secondary to airway blockage or hypoxia. • Observe for signs of anxiety secondary to the airway maintenance procedure.
Ineffective breathing pattern	• Assess breathing pattern that is secondary to airway maintenance procedure or remains ineffective despite the airway maintenance procedure; in collaboration with physician prepare *to administer supportive ventilation*.
Impaired gas exchange	• Assess arterial blood gases secondary to airway maintenance procedure; in collaboration with physician prepare to administer oxygen therapy secondary to airway maintenance procedure.
Potential for aspiration	• Avoid triggering gag mechanism when performing caretaking activities, including mouth care. • If swallowing reflex is diminished, elevate head of bed when performing mouth care. • Assess and document amount of secretions present, patient's level of consciousness, and patient's ability to swallow secretions effectively. • Administer suction when necessary to remove secretions and maintain patent airway. • If secretions are thick or inspissated, ensure adequate humidification to help liquefy secretions. • For patients with reduced level of consciousness, ensure head of bed is elevated, unless contraindicated.
Altered oral mucous membrane	• Assess integrity of oral mucous membranes frequently. • Provide mouth care at least every 2 hours for those patients with an airway maintenance device left in place.
Potential impaired skin integrity	• Assess skin around the airway maintenance device often for skin erosion or irritation. • Provide careful skin care around the airway maintenance device at least every 4 hours. • If taping is involved, rotate the taping site often.
Impaired verbal communication	• Provide patient with note paper and pencil or Magic Slate for easy communication. • Place call-light cord in easy reach.
Potential for injury	• Should patient demonstrate restlessness and confusion secondary to hypoxia or systemic condition, provide soft restraints for the patient's wrists so that airway does not become dislodged.

Evaluation

Patient Outcome	Data Indicating That Outcome is Reached
Airway is patent.	Breath sounds are clear and bilaterally equal. There are no adventitious sounds. Breathing occurs easily and seems to be adequate for patient's attempt.
Gas exchange is adequate.	Blood gas values are within normal limits.

Breathing Techniques

Following are some breathing techniques that may be taught to the patient that will facilitate effective ventilation:

Abdominal or diaphragmatic breathing
Pursed-lip breathing
Deep breathing: coughing and splinting
Incentive spirometer

These are useful and specific measures to increase the volume of air entering the lungs as well as being expelled from the lungs. These techniques are discussed according to indications and procedural techniques.

Abdominal or Diaphragmatic Breathing

Indications:

Patients with chronic and acute respiratory dysfunction may be taught to use the abdominal muscles and diaphragm as the primary structures for facilitating and maximizing the ventilatory attempts of the lungs.

Procedural guidelines[38,51]:

1. Ensure that nasal passage and trachea are free of secretions and congestion. If necessary, suction, use aerosol, encourage coughing, or perform postural drainage before teaching diaphragmatic breathing.
2. Assist patient to attain position of comfort, either sitting or in semi-Fowler's position in bed. Abdominal muscles should be relaxed and knees and hips flexed.
3. Instruct patient to inhale deeply through nose (keep mouth shut). As patient inhales, the focus should be to pull the diaphragm down and to force the abdominal wall outward. If a hand is placed on the patient's abdomen, the hand should rise.
4. Instruct patient to pause slightly after a deep and even inspiration and then, using a pursed-lip technique, to exhale quietly and naturally.
5. Encourage patient to use the abdominal muscles during expiration to remove all air from the lungs.

6. Explain that expiration should last two to three times longer than inspiration.
7. After the technique is mastered, place a 5-pound (2.25 kg) weight on the patient's abdomen to further strengthen the abdominal muscles.
8. Have patient practice the diaphragmatic breathing technique 10 to 20 minutes at least every 4 hours until ability and willingness to implement the technique are demonstrated.

Pursed-Lip Breathing

Indications:

This technique is used to control expiration and to facilitate maximum emptying of the alveoli. It functions to maintain a positive pressure in the airways and thus keep them open longer. In this way more air may be exhaled.

Procedural guidelines:

1. Assist patient to a position of comfort.
2. Instruct patient to inhale deeply through the nose (with mouth shut) and to pause slightly at end of inspiration.
3. Instruct patient to exhale slowly through pursed lips so a blowing effect occurs.
4. Explain that exhalation should be slow and purposeful.
5. As the technique is practiced and used on a continual basis, patient anxiety and anxiety-related dyspnea should decrease.

Deep Breathing, Coughing, and Splinting

Indications:

This technique is most frequently used during the first 48 hours after surgery to loosen secretions and force them to be expelled. The deep breathing dilates the airways, stimulates surfactant production, and expands the lung tissue surface, thereby increasing the area for respiratory gas exchange.[54] Coughing is used to force collected and consolidated secretions to be expelled. Splinting of the chest wall is used to produce stabilization, which in turn decreases discomfort.

Procedural guidelines:

1. Position patient to facilitate deep inspiration and coughing.
2. The incision area may be splinted with a pillow and hand pressure from the nurse. As the patient coughs, firmly assist the patient to stabilize the incisional area.
3. Instruct patient to take a slow, deep inspiration. If patient is postoperative, pain medications may need to be administered 20 to 30 minutes before initiating procedure.
4. Instruct patient to quickly close glottis and forcefully expel an explosive current of air.
5. Provide patient with tissues to collect expelled sputum.

Incentive Spirometers

Indications:

The incentive spirometer may be used postoperatively to encourage deep breathing. While it may provide assistive deep breathing exercises, it should not replace other deep breathing and coughing interventions.

Procedural guidelines:

1. Position patient in seated or semi-Fowler's position.
2. Instruct patient to seal mouth around mouthpiece and to inhale or exhale so as to activate the spirometer. Each brand of spirometer functions slightly differently. Some are operated by exhalation into the system; others are activated by inspiration. In either case the deeper the ventilatory effort, the more successful the use of the spirometer. Carefully inspect the operation of a specific unit before instructing the patient.
3. Instruct the patient to hold a deep breath for a few seconds before exhaling. This will help prevent pulmonary complications.
4. After the spirometer is used, wash the mouthpiece and tubing. They should not be used for any other patient.
5. The incentive spirometer should be used at least every 3 or 4 hours during the postoperative period until the patient is ambulatory and initiates effective deep breathing and coughing on his own.

Evaluation

All of the breathing techniques have similar evaluation criteria.

Patient Outcome	Data Indicating That Outcome is Reached
Optimum movement of air in and out of the lungs occurs.	Airway is clear, and breathing occurs without obstruction. Patient is able to inhale deeply and exhale effectively. There is no evidence of dyspnea or hypoxia.
Airway is patent.	There is no evidence of pulmonary congestion, or condition is optimal for patient; if sputum is present, patient is able to demonstrate productive sputum cough.
Clear breath sounds are heard in all areas.	Bronchovesicular breath sounds are heard throughout, or optimum breath sounds for patient. No areas of decreased breath sounds or consolidation are heard.
Patient is comfortable during coughing and deep breathing.	Patient is able to ask for splinting assistance or splints self during deep breathing and coughing exercises.

Figure 2-31 Positions for postural drainage. **A,** Anterior apical segment; sitting. **B,** Posterior apical segment; sitting. **C,** Anterior segment; lying flat on back. **D,** Right posterior segment; lying on left side. **E,** Left posterior segment; lying on right side. **F,** Right middle lobe; lying on left side. **G,** Left lingula; lying on right side. **H,** Anterior segments; lying on back. **I,** Right lateral segment; lying on left side. **J,** Left lateral segment; lying on right side. **K,** Posterior segments; lying on stomach. **L,** Superior segments; lying on stomach.
From Hirsch.[38]

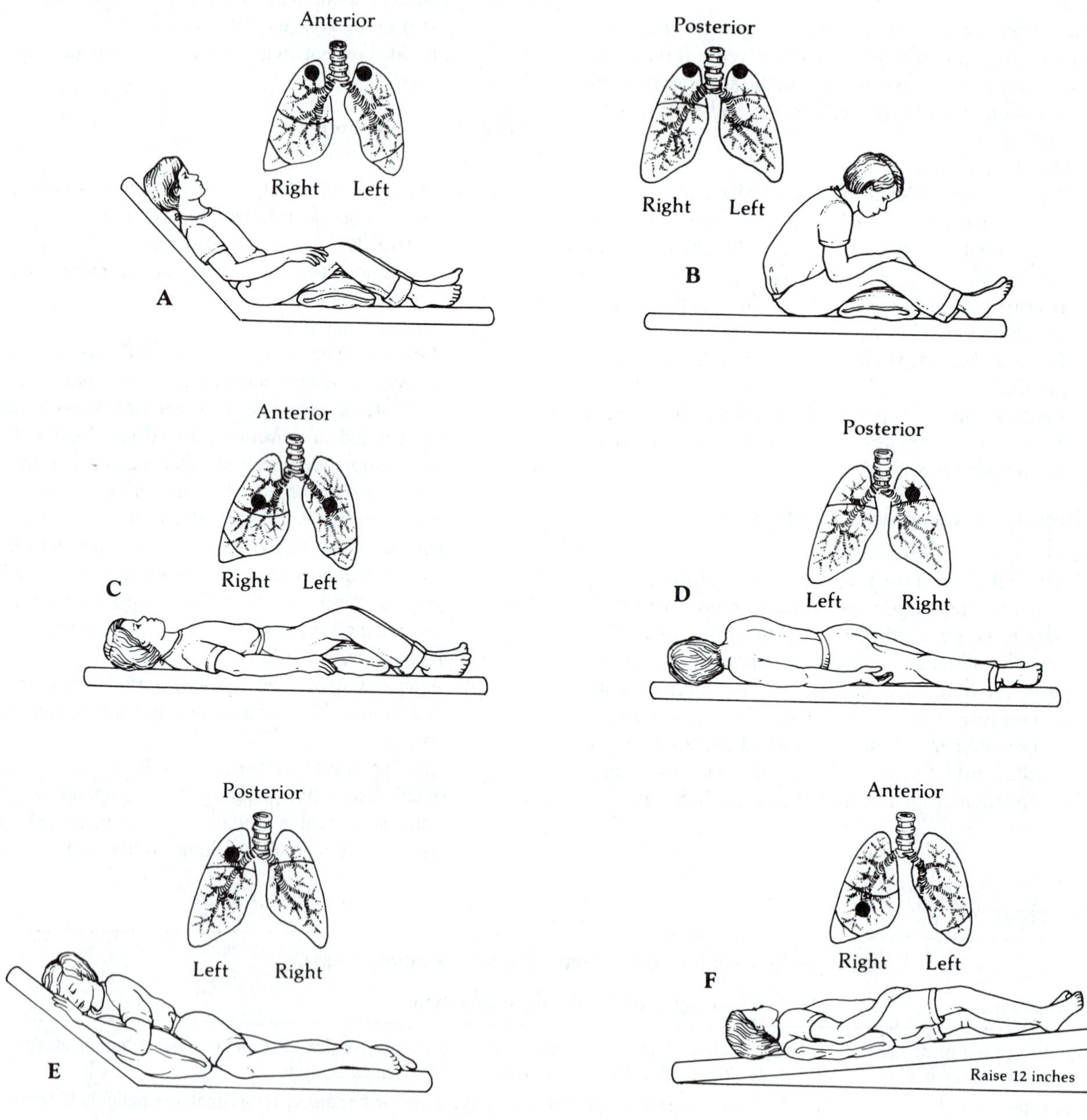

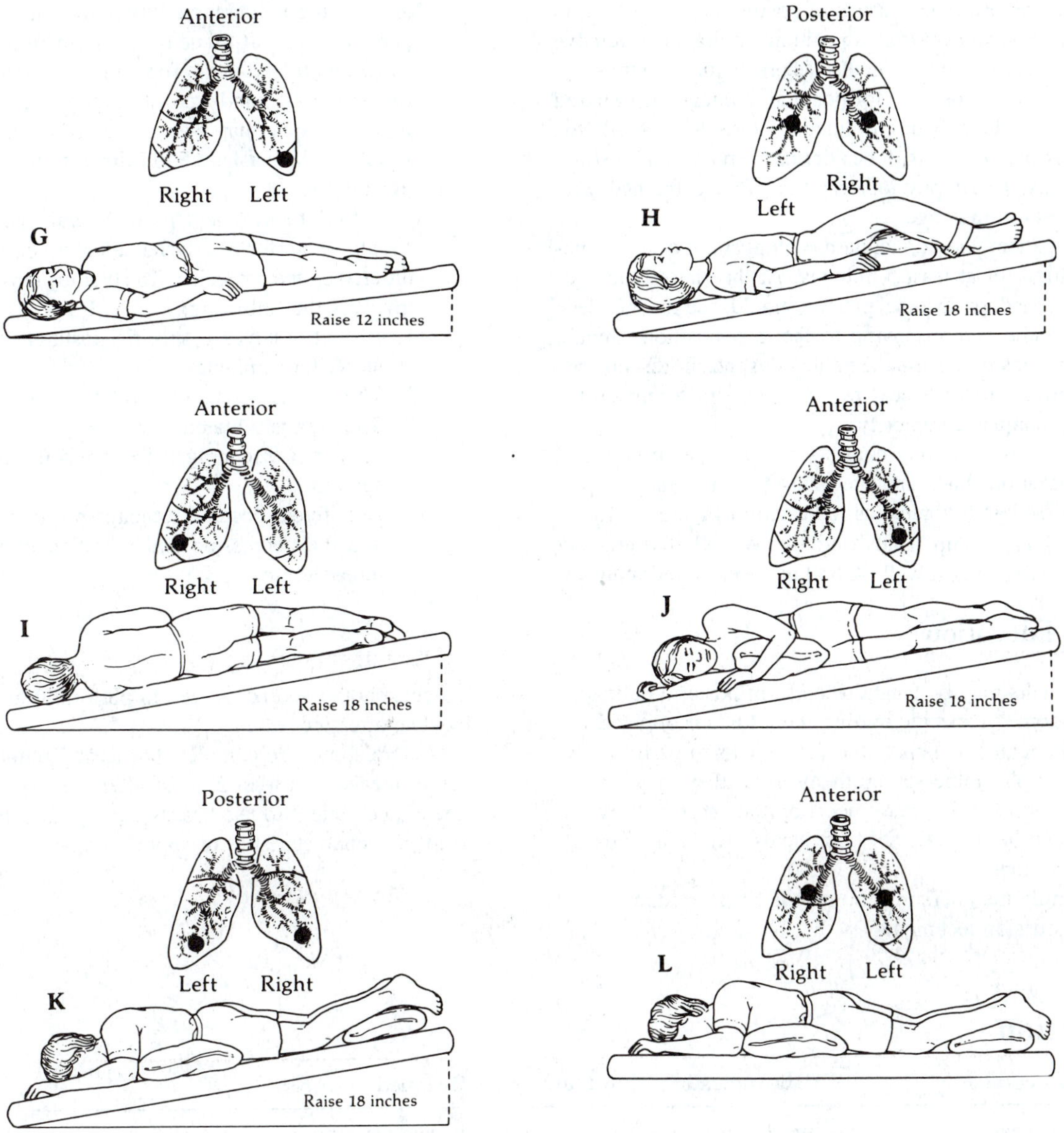

G
Anterior
Right Left
Raise 12 inches

H
Posterior
Left Right
Raise 18 inches

I
Anterior
Right Left
Raise 18 inches

J
Anterior
Right Left
Raise 18 inches

K
Posterior
Left Right
Raise 18 inches

L
Anterior
Right Left

Chest Physiotherapy and Postural Drainage

Postural drainage, chest percussion, and vibration are effective methods for loosening and moving secretions when patients are unable to loosen and cough up secretions on their own. The nursing diagnosis most frequently indicated is airway clearance, ineffective.

Specifically, these techniques are helpful for preoperative or postoperative patients who have large amounts of sputum, patients with cystic fibrosis or other types of lung diseases in which copious secretions are produced, and patients who have difficulty coughing up sputum.

Contraindications:

1. Cyanosis or dyspnea caused by the techniques
2. Increased pain or discomfort with the techniques
3. Suction equipment not available for:
   a. Patients with copious sputum
   b. Patients with prolonged bleeding and clotting times
   c. Extremely obese patients
   d. Patients with history of predisposition to pathologic fractures

Procedural guidelines:

Postural drainage consists of positioning the patient in specific and controlled positions to drain and remove secretions from particular segments of the lungs.

The various positions for postural drainage differ based on the lobes being drained. Figure 2-31 details the various positions, lobes drained, and special instructions. Chest physiotherapy is often combined with postural drainage.

The patient should maintain each postural drainage position for at least 5 minutes. At the end of each positioned period the patient should cough and deep breathe before moving to the next position. Should one position cause the patient dyspnea or discomfort, move on to the next position. Do not terminate the techniques completely.

Chest physiotherapy consists of chest percussion and vibration. Each indicated lung lobe area may be percussed and vibrated as indicated in Figure 2-31.

To *percuss,* cup hands and lightly and rhythmically strike the chest wall. A hollow, deep sound indicates that the technique is being performed correctly. Each area should be percussed for 1 to 2 minutes. Do not percuss over soft tissue or areas where the technique causes increased pain. To vibrate the area, gently but firmly vibrate hand against the thoracic wall directly over the area that was percussed. This technique should be done at least 5 to 7 times during the patient's expiration.

Chest physiotherapy and postural drainage techniques should be performed systematically and routinely as ordered by the physician. The therapy most frequently involves the following:

1. Patient assumes a specific postural drainage position for 5 minutes.
2. The area is percussed for 1 to 2 minutes.
3. The area is vibrated.
4. Patient is encouraged to cough up and spit out sputum.
5. A different postural drainage position is attained, and the percussion and vibration techniques are repeated.

Patient Education

1. Patients may be taught to perform postural drainage at home; a specific routine should be encouraged.
2. Although it is impossible for patients to perform chest physiotherapy on themselves, they may perform tapping movements on the chest wall by using the fingertips of both hands. This may loosen secretions.
3. Family members may be taught vibratory and percussion techniques.
4. Patients should be encouraged to perform oral hygiene after procedure.
5. Procedure should be completed at least 30 minutes before meals or at least 2 hours after the last meal.
6. Encourage patient to use tissues during coughing and to inspect characteristics of sputum.

Evaluation

Patient Outcome	Data Indicating That Outcome is Reached
Airways are clear.	Breath sounds are clear bilaterally following techniques.
Chest physiotherapy and postural drainage are maintained at a therapeutic level.	Patient tolerates procedures, and procedures appear to be beneficial to patient.
Productive sputum specimen is produced.	Patient is able to expectorate sputum after each postural drainage position.

Chest Tubes and Chest Drainage Systems

Description and Rationale

Chest tubes with attached drainage systems are placed in the pleural cavity to drain fluid, blood, or air from the pleural cavity and to reestablish a negative pressure that will facilitate expansion of the lung. Chest tubes may be inserted postoperatively, as an emergency procedure following chest trauma, or therapeutically as a disease treatment modality. Following are chest tube insertion sites:

Pneumothorax: usually in second and third intercostal space (anterior)

Hemothorax: usually in seventh, eighth, or ninth intercostal space (posterior)

Thoracotomy: one tube generally inserted in second or third intercostal space (anterior) and another in lower posterior axillary line

Chest tubes may be terminated when x-ray examination determines that the lung is reexpanded and when the drainage has slowed to less than 75 ml/day.[37]

Cautions

Chest tubes are inserted by a physician and sutured into place. Cautions specific to chest tubes and drainage systems include the following:

Sterility must be maintained so as not to introduce infection into pleural cavity.

The system must remain patent: the tubing must not become blocked; if this occurs, a tension pneumothorax may result.

If the drainage tubing becomes dislodged from the patient or a drainage bottle breaks, cross-clamps should be quickly applied to the tube(s) nearest the patient until the system's integrity can be reestablished.

If the chest tube becomes dislodged from the patient's chest, the patient should exhale forcefully, and the chest wall incision should be quickly covered with a petrolatum jelly gauze.

Preprocedural Nursing Care

Carefully assess patient's preprocedural condition including respiratory rate and quality. Note evidence of dyspnea, labored breathing, tachypnea, tachycardia, quality and distribution of breath sounds, mediastinal shift, subcutaneous emphysema, and crepitus.

Set up drainage equipment appropriately for the type of system being used.

Single-bottle system (Figure 2-32, *A*)

1. Unwrap bottles and tubing; maintain sterility.
2. Fill bottle with sterile water until the long glass tubing is submerged 2 cm. This bottle is called the water-seal bottle.
3. The short glass tubing (air vent) should never be covered with water
4. The long glass tubing is connected to the patient's chest tube, and the short tubing air vent may be open to the air or connected to gravity drainage.

Double-bottle system (Figure 2-32, *B*)

1. Prepare first bottle as described for the single-bottle system.
2. Prepare the second bottle (the suction control or manometer bottle) by running a tube from the air vent of the first bottle to an air vent in the second bottle. This is the bottle that regulates the amount of vacuum in the system.
3. Fill the second bottle with sterile water to the designated depth.
4. The second bottle contains a long glass middle tube that acts as the air vent. The length of the large tube submerged under water determines the amount of negative pressure required to drain the chest. A common depth of water is 10 to 20 cm.
5. The suction control or manometer bottle is generally connected to a suction device such as an Emerson or Stedman pump.

Figure 2-32 Bottle chest drainage systems. **A,** Single-bottle system. **B,** Double-bottle system. **C,** Triple-bottle system.

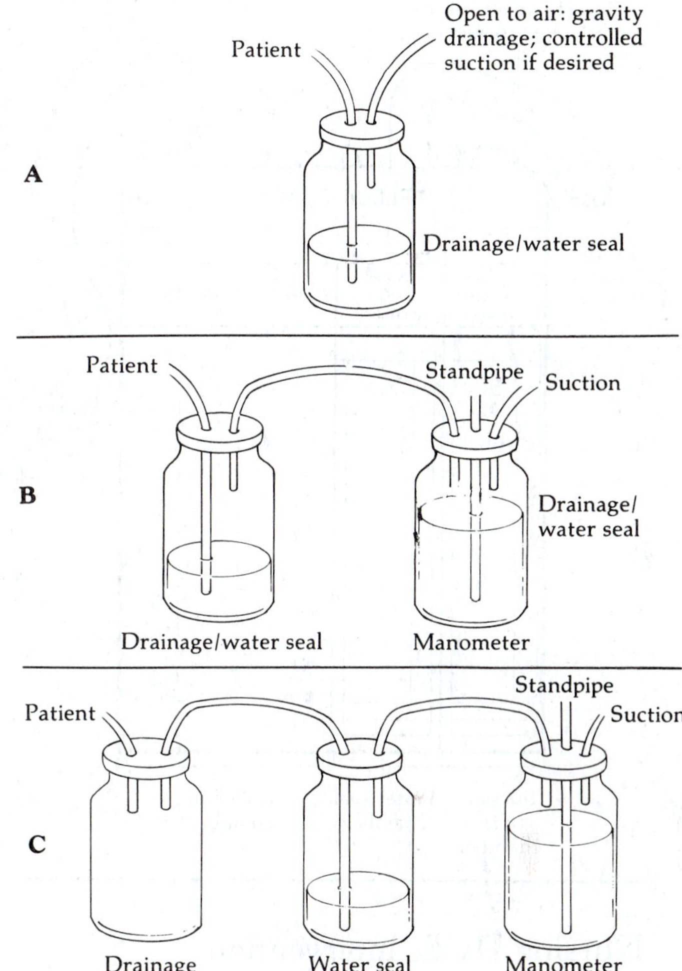

Triple-bottle system (Figure 2-32, *C*)

1. Prepare first two bottles as previously described.
2. A third bottle is prepared for a position closest to the patient. This bottle acts entirely as a drainage collection bottle.

Commercial disposable three-chamber units (Figure 2-33)

1. Pleur-Evac and Thoraseal are two common brands.
2. These systems function like the three-bottle systems.
3. Setup and operation directions are provided with the sterile units.

Figure 2-33 Commercial chest drainage system.

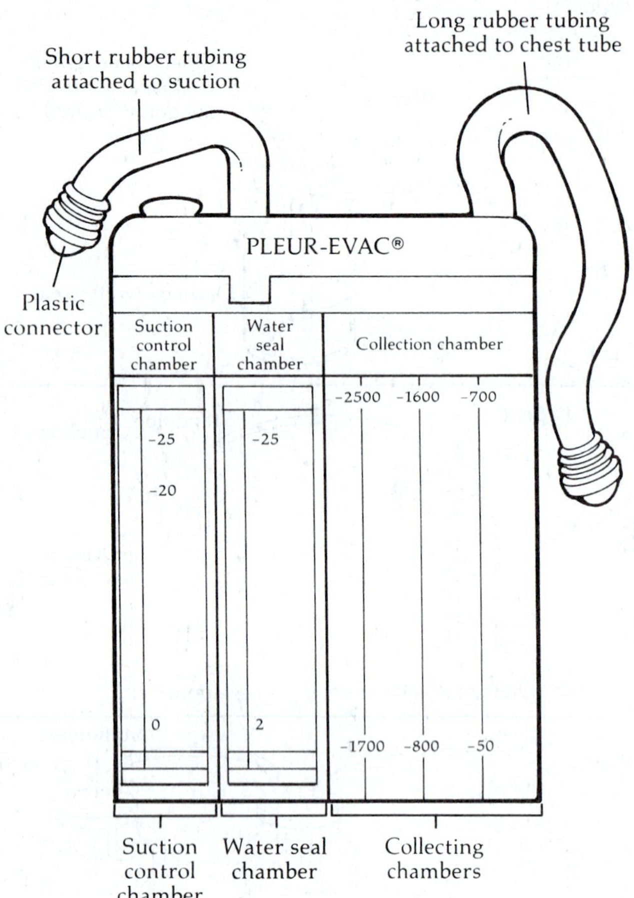

NURSING CARE

Nursing Assessment

System Functioning Properly[37]

Water in the water-seal bottle should fluctuate slightly when suction is applied to the patient's chest

There should be no bubbling in the water-seal bottle with expiration; *continuous bubbling suggests an air leak*

Potential Atelectasis from Hypoventilation

Dyspnea, evidence of consolidation on chest roentgenogram

Increased Accumulation of Air in the Pleural Space

Check for air leaks in the system

Assess to make sure chest tubes are securely placed and patent

Clinical signs include increased evidence of dyspnea, tachypnea, tachycardia, anxiety, and restlessness

Infection

Higher WBC, increased temperature, evidence of purulent drainage

Nursing Dx & Intervention

Nursing Diagnosis	Nursing Intervention/Rationale
Ineffective breathing pattern	• Assess and ensure patency of chest tubes by stripping and milking chest tubes every hour *to keep them clear of clots;* observe for tube kinking. • Observe for signs of intrapleural fluid accumulation such as decreased breath sounds on affected side, increased dyspnea, and mediastinal shift. • Always keep chest tube drainage system lower than patient's chest. • Observe volume, shade, color, and consistency of drainage from lung and record findings regularly. • Observe for "tidaling" or fluctuation of fluid in the water-seal bottle; this should rise and fall with breathing; if fluctuation is not seen, carefully evaluate the patency of the tubing. • Assure that all tubing connections are securely attached and taped. • Have at the bedside two rubber-shod clamps to cross-clamp the chest tube near the patient *should the water-seal drainage system become disconnected or break.* • Assist patient to cough, deep breathe, and change position at least every 2 hours. • Observe special positioning if indicated because of special technique or surgery. • Auscultate breath sounds at least every 2 to 4 hours *to assess quality of breath sounds.*
Fatigue	• Assess patterns of fatigue. • Assess factors related to fatigue and strategies for dealing with them. • Assess support systems and available resources. • Administer treatments or medications to relieve discomfort. • Enhance patient's ability to rest between specified activities.

Nursing Diagnosis	Nursing Intervention/Rationale
Pain	• Provide splinting to chest tube area when encouraging patient to cough or deep breathe; if necessary, administer medications as ordered to relieve pain associated with chest tubes; monitor and report patient response. • Place padding around chest tube when assisting patient to turn or move. • Make sure chest tubes are adequately taped to patient's chest *so they may not be pulled with moving or turning*.
Impaired skin integrity	• Assess chest tube site for redness or irritation when providing wound care. • Provide wound care around chest tube site; use sterile technique to clean area at least daily. • Change dressing around chest tube daily.
Potential for infection	• Assess for signs of infection, including increased temperature, purulent drainage, odor, or increased WBC.
Impaired physical mobility	• Provide passive and active range of motion to arm and shoulder of affected side. • Encourage patient to exercise lower legs to prevent venous stasis. • Ambulate patient as ordered.
Fear	• Carefully and completely explain all procedures to patient. • Assure patient that splinting and support will be provided to decrease discomfort. • Provide patient with opportunities to participate in own care.

Removal of Chest Tubes

Chest tubes may be removed after the lung has been reinflated for 24 hours to several days. Indications for removal are usually confirmed by chest x-ray examination. Removal procedures include the following:

1. Place patient in semi-Fowler's position or on side.
2. Physician instructs patient to take a deep breath and hold it.
3. The chest tube suture is clipped and the tube is quickly removed.
4. A pressure dressing with antibiotic ointment or petrolatum jelly gauze is placed over chest wall wound.
5. Patient is instructed to breathe normally, and the pressure dressing is taped securely.
6. Careful patient assessment should follow on a continuing basis, including rate of respirations, quality of breath sounds, any drainage from chest tube dressing, sudden chest pains, or shortness of breath.

Evaluation

Patient Outcome	Data Indicating That Outcome is Reached
Chest tube drainage system is intact and operational.	System remains intact. Water fluctuates in water-seal container. Drainage accumulates in drainage bottle.
Lungs reexpand.	Roentgenograms confirm lung reexpansion. Breath sounds are bilaterally equal and clear. Blood gases are within normal limits for patient. There is no atelectasis, consolidation, or associated infection.

Mechanical Ventilation[37,38,51,59,63]

Mechanical ventilation is indicated for patients who are unable to maintain adequate ventilation on their own. The ventilator does not cure; it is a temporary support that merely "buys time" for correction of the underlying situation.

There are currently three categories of ventilators in use: volume-cycled ventilators, pressure-cycled ventilators, and external body ventilators. Each of these is discussed separately.

Volume-Cycled Ventilators

Volume-cycled (volume-preset) ventilators terminate inspiration after delivering a preset volume of gas. The desired volume of gas is delivered regardless of the required pressure to do so. The ventilator continues to deliver a constant tidal volume regardless of the changes in the airway resistance or in compliance of the lungs and thorax.

The volume remains the same unless excessively high peak airway pressures are reached, in which case safety release valves stop the flow. The safety release pressure is usually set about 10 cm H_2O above the peak inspiratory pressure.

Inspiratory time is determined by adjusting the flow rate of gas to be delivered (more rapid the flow, shorter the inspiratory time; slower the flow, longer the inspiratory time).

Expiratory time is most commonly determined by setting

the respiratory rate. The operator must preset the following:

Tidal volume
Inspiratory pressure
Rate of breaks per minute
Peak flow
Degree of sensitivity required by patient to trigger inspiration
Frequency of sighs per hour
Sigh volume—or amount of gas to be delivered during a sigh
Sigh pressure limit during a sigh inspiration
Oxygen percent concentration to be delivered

Pressure-Cycled Ventilators

Pressure-cycled (pressure-preset) ventilators terminate inspiration when a preset pressure is achieved. When the pressure is reached, the gas flow stops and the patient passively exhales. The largest patient variable is that varying degrees of resistance interfere with gas flow. Thus the delivered volume may vary as the degree of resistance varies.

These ventilators are most commonly used for patients whose ventilatory resistance has not changed (e.g., drug overdose). They are not appropriately used for patients whose resistance may have changed (e.g., postoperative status or patients with severe respiratory infections). These respirators have only a low peak pressure capability (30 to 40 cm).

External Body Ventilator

External body ventilators function by applying intermittent subatmospheric pressure to the thorax and trunk of the body, thus assisting the patient to breathe.

NURSING CARE

Nursing Assessment

Preprocedural

Alveolar-arterial difference ($P[A\text{-}a]_{O_2}$) >400 mm Hg when patient receiving 100% oxygen
Pa_{CO_2} >55 mm Hg
Pa_{O_2} <60 mm Hg
pH <7.35
Dead space to total volume (V_D/V_T) >0.60
Inspiratory force (IF) <25 cm H_2O
Tidal volume (V_T) <5 ml/kg
Vital capacity (VC) <10 ml/kg
Expiratory force <60 cm H_2O

Procedural Problems[38]

Pa_{O_2} >110 mm Hg
- Determine FIO_2; report FIO_2 setting and Pa_{O_2} to physician (make sure FIO_2 was not left on 100% oxygen)
- Note patient's position; diaphragm movement and blood flow and ventilation ($\dot{V}/\dot{Q}$) relationships are affected by gravity and position

Pa_{O_2} <50 to 90 mm Hg depending on patient's underlying disease
- If patient shows signs of cyanosis, tachycardia, arrhythmias, restlessness, or decreased sensorium, remove patient from ventilator and bag breathe patient with 100% oxygen until physician's help and further assessment are possible
- Assessment of problem should include:
  - Machine or tubing malfunction
  - Patient's need for suctioning
  - Diminished patient lung functioning owing to pneumothorax or atelectasis
  - Malplaced endotracheal tube

Pa_{CO_2} >45 mm Hg or patient's baseline if the patient has COPD
- Verify that patient is connected to ventilator and that ventilator tubing is clear of obstruction or water accumulation
- Suction airway if necessary and determine position and patency of endotracheal tube
- Evaluate patient for metabolic acidosis
- If patient is on low, intermittent mandatory ventilation, determine whether patient has recently received respiratory depressing sedation, which would affect respiratory status

Pa_{CO_2} <35 mm Hg (unless desired control of cerebral blood flow)
- Assess patient's respiratory rate and depth
- Assess for metabolic acidosis

Nursing Dx & Intervention

Nursing Diagnosis	Nursing Intervention/Rationale
Ineffective airway clearance	• Secure endotracheal tube in place (see associated procedure in airway maintenance section). • Ensure 100% humidification and warming (between 32° and 36° C) of inspired gases as ordered. • Suction and clean tube as indicated *to maintain patency*. • Because patient is disconnected from ventilator before suctioning: Warn patient. Deliver high concentrations of oxygen for several minutes before and after suctioning *to prevent hypoxia and cardiac arrhythmias*. • Wait 20 minutes after suctioning to measure arterial blood gases. • Monitor airway pressure (should remain constant or <20 cm H_2O) frequently; empty water from tubing.

Nursing Diagnosis	Nursing Intervention/Rationale
Ineffective breathing pattern	• Consistently evaluate ventilatory pattern for rate, quality, signs of respiratory distress, or inappropriate inspiratory/expiratory ratio (should be at least 1:1). • Monitor patient signs of fighting the ventilator, which indicate that the patient's respiratory cycle is inconsistent with the mechanical cycle; may be due to pain, hypoxemia, secretions, fear, and anxiety; to correct, clear airways as indicated or give sedatives as ordered. • Ensure that the alarm on the ventilator is turned to the ON position whenever the patient is left alone. • Carefully check all connections of the ventilator tubing regularly to ensure that they are tightly secured. • Positive end-expiratory pressure (PEEP) may be used *to prevent alveolar collapse and thereby increase tidal volume. The major goal of PEEP is to enhance oxygen transport.* • Continuous positive airway pressure (CPAP) functions similar to PEEP but is intended for patients who are breathing spontaneously.
Impaired gas exchange	• Position patient so all lobes of lungs are adequately ventilated and perfused. • Reposition patient every 30 to 60 minutes; rotate positioning from right and left lateral positions to a semi-Fowler's position. • Carefully monitor ventilator pressure readings and the patient's breath sounds for presence and quality; pneumothorax, pneumomediastinum, and subcutaneous emphysema may be signs of barotrauma secondary to a high mechanical ventilator pressure. • Pneumothorax may be anticipated by seeing an abrupt rise in the peak inspiratory pressure for a constant tidal volume. • Carefully monitor all ventilator settings, as well as patient's arterial blood gas response.
Potential for aspiration	• Avoid triggering gag mechanism when performing caretaking activities, including mouth care. • If swallowing reflex is diminished, elevate head of bed when performing mouth care. • Assess and document amount of secretions present, patient's level of consciousness, and patient's ability to swallow secretions effectively. • Administer suction when necessary to remove secretions and maintain patent airway. • If secretions are thick or inspissated, ensure adequate humidification to help liquefy secretions. • For patients with reduced level of consciousness, ensure head of bed is elevated, unless contraindicated.
Fatigue	• Assess patterns of fatigue. • Assess factors related to fatigue and strategies for dealing with them. • Assess support systems and available resources. • Administer treatments or medications to relieve discomfort. • Enhance patient's ability to rest between specified activities.
Decreased cardiac output	• Decreased cardiac output may be due to hyperventilation or hypoventilation; therefore carefully assess ventilatory rate, rhythm, and quality; *$Paco_2$ may cause a transient alkalosis.*
Potential for infection	• Because of warm, moist nature of the ventilator equipment, the patient is prone to nosocomial infections. • Every 24 hours, change all parts of the ventilator equipment that come in contact with the patient. • Send sputum specimens to the laboratory for analysis as ordered. • Carefully monitor patient's temperature and characteristics of sputum.
Fear	• Assure patient that he will not be left alone. • Provide call-bell button for immediate access. • Assure patient that adequate ventilation is being provided.
Impaired verbal communication	• Provide Magic Slate or other mechanism by which patient may communicate.

Weaning from the Ventilator

Physiologic guidelines:

1. Vital capacity at least 10 to 15 ml/kg body weight
2. Alveolar-arterial oxygen tension difference ($P_{A\text{-}a}O_2$) measured with patient receiving 100% oxygen (should be less than 300 to 500 mm Hg)
3. Maximum inspiratory force greater than 20 cm H_2O
4. Tidal volume greater than 5 ml/kg
5. Resting minute ventilation greater than 10 l per minute
6. $Paco_2$ within stable range
7. Pao_2 greater than 70 to 80 mm Hg on 0.5 FIO_2
8. Pao_2 on 100% oxygen greater than 300 mm Hg
9. Shunt fraction less than 15%

If the patient is not completely ready to be weaned from the ventilator, intermittent mandatory ventilation (IMV) or intermittent demand ventilation (IDV) may be initiated.

IMV allows the patient's own reasonable breathing pattern to be maintained with positive-pressure breaths intermittently delivered by the ventilator. The positive-pressure breaths are completely independent of the patient's own breathing pattern.

Because mechanical ventilatory assistance leaves the patient's respiratory muscles weakened, it may be helpful to transfer the patient to IMV for gradual transition weaning.

IDV allows the patient to breathe a controlled atmosphere at a reasonable, spontaneous pattern, with intermittent positive augmentation in phase with the patient's own breathing pattern (on demand).

When disconnected from the ventilator, the patient should be in a sitting position and humidified oxygen should be readily available by mask.

Evaluation

Patient Outcome	Data Indicating That Outcome is Reached
Pulmonary system with assistance of mechanical ventilator has the power to maintain physiologic ventilation.	Breath sounds are heard in all lobes of lungs. Bilaterally equal lung expansion occurs. Tidal volume is >5 ml/kg. Vital capacity is >10 ml/kg. Inspiratory force is >25 cm H_2O. Dead space to tidal volume ratio is <0.60.
Effectiveness of ventilation or oxygenation is maintained.	$Paco_2$ is 35 to 45 mm Hg. Pao_2 is <80 mm Hg with FIO_2 0.4 or above. pH is >7.35. There are no clinical signs of dyspnea, restlessness, or cyanosis.
Myocardial work is decreased by diminishing ventilatory effort and improving ventilatory efficiency.	Blood pressure and pulse are within normal limits for patient. Patient appears rested without signs of agitation or hypoxia.

Oxygen Therapy

Description and Rationale

The goal of oxygen therapy is to provide sufficient amounts of oxygen to the tissues so that normal metabolism can occur. Clinically this means to provide oxygen at the lowest fractional inspired oxygen (FIO_2) to maintain a Pao_2 of at least 55 mm Hg. Therapy is indicated when the patient is unable to maintain an adequate Pao_2 by his own ventilatory efforts.

Spearman, Sheldon, and Egan[76] give the following clinical objectives for oxygen therapy:

- To reduce or correct arterial hypoxemia and tissue hypoxia
- To reduce or correct the need for physiologic compensatory mechanisms to hypoxemia

Hypoxemia may be caused by a variety of factors. Following are the most common:

- Reduced alveolar oxygen: results from either low ambient Pao_2 or hypoventilation
- Impaired alveolar-capillary diffusion: occurs secondary to pathologic changes such as fibrosis, increased connective tissue, interstitial edema, or tumors
- Hemoglobin deficiencies: may be either absolute owing to anemia or relative as in patients with carbon monoxide ingestion
- Ventilation/perfusion ratio imbalance: anatomic shunting that occurs secondary to congenital defects, disease or trauma, or physiologic shunting
- Circulatory failure: occurs secondary to decreased cardiac output or hypovolemia

Contraindications and Cautions

The following discussion of precautions regarding oxygen therapy is based primarily on Spearman, Sheldon, and Egan[72] and Holloway.[39] Following are risks and precautions regarding the use of therapeutic oxygen:

1. Oxygen-induced hypoventilation: when the arterial carbon dioxide tension is greater than 50 mm Hg, the risk of oxygen-induced hypoventilation increases. It is therefore advised, especially for patients with chronic lung diseases, to maintain oxygen therapy so the arterial oxygen tension remains about 50 to 60 mm Hg.

   To prevent this problem use low concentrations of oxygen if the patient is not mechanically ventilated. Observe ventilatory pattern and quality.
2. Atelectasis: the collapse of alveoli may occur secondary to high concentrations of oxygen in inspired air, which causes malfunctioning pulmonary surfactant.

   To prevent this complication, if possible limit the duration of 100% inspired oxygen to no more than 20 minutes; maintain patent airway; sigh the patient if on a ventilator; and provide high tidal volumes.
3. Oxygen toxicity: the lungs can normally handle oxygen concentrations of 21%. Although it is not clear exactly what fractional inspired oxygen (FIO_2) percent causes oxygen toxicity, it is most probable that an FIO_2 of over 50% administered for longer than 24 hours increases the risk (see assessment section for additional nursing guidelines).

Preprocedural Nursing Care: Assessment of Need for Supplemental Oxygen

- Hypoxia
  - Hypotension
  - Cyanosis
  - Dyspnea
  - Disorientation
  - Anxiety
  - Nausea
- Nasal flaring
- Retractions
- Atelectasis
- Pulmonary edema
- Central nervous system depression
- Muscle weakness
- Altered blood gas states
  - PaO_2 <55 mm Hg
  - $PaCO_2$ >42 mm Hg
  - Bradycardia
  - Cardiac arrhythmias
  - Tachypnea
  - Drowsiness
  - Headache
  - Poor judgment
  - Shortness of breath
- Pneumonia
- Emphysema
- Airway obstruction

Medical Plan

Oxygen therapy equipment may be divided into two major types: low-flow and high-flow systems

Low-flow systems do not apply all of the inspired gases that the patient breathes. This means that the patient breathes some room air along with the oxygen. For the system to be effective, the patient must be able to maintain a normal tidal volume, have a regular ventilatory pattern, and be able to cooperate. As the patient's ventilatory pattern changes, so does the concentration of inspired oxygen. Examples of low-flow systems include nasal cannula, simple oxygen mask, partial rebreathing mask with reservoir bag, and nonrebreathing mask with reservoir bag.

High-flow systems supply all gases at a preset FIO_2. These systems are generally not affected by changes in ventilatory pattern. The Venturi mask is the most common example of the high-flow system.

In addition to these two main types of systems there are blended-type systems that may use either high-flow or low-flow techniques. Examples of this type include oxygen hoods, Isolettes, T-tubes, and oxygen tents.

Table 2-14 summarizes the major types of oxygen therapy systems, their benefits, problems, and precautions.

NURSING CARE

Nursing Assessment

Respiratory Status

- Ventilatory pattern
- Tachypnea
- Retractions
- Work of breathing
  - Accessory muscle use
  - Posturing

Tissue Oxygenation

- Restlessness
- Irritability
- Disorientation
- Confusion

Cardiovascular

- Hypotension
- Sudden hypertension
- Tachycardia
- Cardiac arrhythmia

Predicting Effects of Oxygen Therapy

When the $P(A\text{-}a)O_2$ gradient is known, the FIO_2 may be calculated

$$FIO_2 = \frac{P(A\text{-}a)O_2 : \text{Desired } PaO_2}{760} \times 100\%$$

Oxygen analyzer may be used to monitor concentrations given (especially useful when oxygen hood is used)

Mucosa Hydration

Nasal and mucous membranes

Skin Integrity

- Protect bony prominences against pressure sores
- Dry skin from oxygen contact

Absorption Atelectasis

- This can occur when oxygen washes out nitrogen in the alveoli; without nitrogen the residual volume decreases and the alveoli collapse
- Patients at risk for developing:
  - Low tidal volume
  - Normal tidal volume without sighing
  - Airway trapping such as in chronic lung disease
- Problem may be prevented by:
  - Limiting 100% oxygen delivery to no more than 20 minutes at a time
  - Patent airway
  - Mobilizing secretions
  - Encouraging sighing
  - Providing continuous high tidal volume

Oxygen Toxicity

- Clinical signs that may occur after:
  - 6 hours of 100% oxygen therapy:
    - Sharp chest pain
    - Dry cough
  - 18 hours: decreased pulmonary function
  - 24-48 hours: ARDS occurs
- Guidelines to prevent oxygen toxicity:
  1. Limit use of 100% oxygen to brief periods
  2. As early as possible reduce FIO_2 to lowest possible level to maintain oxygenation
  3. Up to 70% oxygen may be used safely for 24 hours

Table 2-14
Oxygen Therapy Systems

Type of System	Description	Flow Rate (L/min)*	Approximate Oxygen Concentration Delivered (%)	Benefits	Problems	Nursing Care
Low-Flow Systems						
Nasal cannula		1 2 3 4 5 6	22-24 26-28 28-30 32-36 36-40 40-44	Comfortable, convenient method of delivering concentration of oxygen ranging from 22%-44% If minute ventilation is relatively low and constant, FIO_2 delivered approaches the percentages presented Major advantages of this method are low cost of equipment, allowance for patient mobility, ability to deliver oxygen and still permit patient to eat and talk, and lack of necessity for humidification of inspired gas mixture Practical system for long-term therapy Mouth breathing will not affect concentration of delivered oxygen	Unable to deliver oxygen concentration over 44% Assumes an adequate breathing pattern Equipment may not be used if patient has nasal problem or if unable to tolerate nasal prongs Patient must be able to cooperate to keep prongs in place Requires tight face seal similar to regular mask Must be removed for eating and talking If liter flow is maintained below 4 L/min, CO_2 may build up in the reservoir bag Bag may kink or twist	Clean equipment Evaluate for pressure sores over ears and cheek areas Lubricate nasal prongs before inserting into nose Liter flow above 6 L/min will *not* increase the FIO_2 Must maintain flow sufficient to keep reservoir bag from completely deflating during inspiration All other functions as with simple mask To initially fill bag, apply mask as patient exhales
Partial rebreathing mask with reservoir bag	Masks similar to simple face mask with addition of a reservoir oxygen bag; the purpose of the rebreathing mask is to conserve oxygen by permitting it to be rebreathed from the reservoir bag	8 10-12	40-50 60	The bag makes possible delivery of oxygen concentration between 40% and 60% provided that the reservoir is kept full by a continuous flow of oxygen	Requires tight face seal Impractical for long-term therapy Must be removed for eating and talking May lead to signs of oxygen toxicity	Arterial blood gases should be monitored Check mask for leaks around face; FIO_2 may decrease if mask is not tight fitting All other functions as with simple mask

Nonrebreathing mask with reservoir bag	Similar to rebreathing bag, but this mask has one-way expiratory valve that prevents rebreathing of expired gases	6 8 10 12-15	55-60 60-80 80-90 90	Effective as short-term therapy May deliver oxygen concentration up to 90%	Requires tight face seal Impractical for long-term therapy Must be removed for eating and talking May lead to signs of oxygen toxicity	Arterial blood gases should be monitored Check mask for leaks around face; FIO_2 may decrease if mask is not tight fitting All other functions as with simple mask
Simple face mask		5-6 6-7 7-8	40 50 60	If patient's ventilatory needs exceed flow of gas, holes on sides of mask allow for entry of room air Permits higher oxygen delivery than nasal cannula System does not tend to dry out mucous membranes of nose or mouth	Mask must be removed prior to patient's eating May not be operated at flow less than 5 L/min A tight face mask seal may cause facial irritation Face mask may increase anxiety in some patients, especially children Not practical for long-term therapy May feel hot and confining for some patients	Do not operate at flow less than 5 L/min (will not flush out accumulated CO_2) If FIO_2 above 60% is desired, patient must be switched to partial rebreathing mask with reservoir bag Should not be used for patients with chronic lung diseases Powdering may be necessary along bony prominence of face Equipment should be removed and cleaned several times each day
High-Flow Systems						
Venturi mask	Works on Bernoulli principle of air entrainment: for each liter of oxygen that passes through a fixed orifice, a fixed proportion of room air will be entrained; by varying size of orifice and flow of oxygen, precise FIO_2 is maintained The system operates by actually setting FIO_2	3 6 8	24 24 28 30 35 40	Delivers exact concentration FIO_2 remains constant regardless of the patient's ventilatory pattern FIO_2 may be measured directly by an oxygen analyzer FIO_2 dial may be changed and set to deliver a calculated oxygen concentration	May irritate face skin Interferes with eating and drinking Tight face seal must be maintained Condensation may collect within system If greater than 40% concentration is desired, must switch to different oxygen delivery system	Arterial blood gases should be monitored Check mask for leaks around face; FIO_2 may be altered if system not properly fitting All other functions as with simple face mask

*Normal breathing patterns are assumed.

Continued.

Table 2-14—cont'd
Oxygen Therapy Systems

Type of System	Description	Flow Rate (L/min)*	Approximate Oxygen Concentration Delivered (%)	Benefits	Problems	Nursing Care
Oxygen hood	Most convenient method to provide oxygen therapy to infants	10-12	Oxygen analyzer should be used to determine level of concentration	Hood covers head only, leaving rest of body available for patient care May be used in conjunction with high-flow Venturi system May be used in conjunction with Isolettes, which provide temperature and humidity regulation	Oxygen between 10 and 12 L/min may be necessary to keep oxygen concentrations steady (dependent on size of oxygen hood)	Make sure oxygen is warmed and humidified Active infants must be carefully observed; they may dislodge hood Pad edges of hood with towels or foam Condensation in tubing will build and must be emptied frequently Heat nebulizer should be maintained between 34.4° C (94° C) and 35.6° F (96° C)

4. Up to 50% oxygen may be used safely for 2 days
5. After 2 days an FIO_2 above 40% is potentially toxic
6. Prolonged use of FIO_2 below 40% rarely causes oxygen toxicity[39]

Equipment

Patency of tubing and bags
Cleanliness
Humidification
Correct size for the patient

Safety

While oxygen is in use, prohibit smoking in the area

Nursing Dx & Intervention

Nursing Diagnosis	Nursing Intervention/Rationale
Ineffective airway clearance	• Assess patient to identify inability to move secretions, *which would interfere with oxygenation.* • Assist patient to maintain proper body positioning *to ensure maximal airway availability.* • Carefully and frequently auscultate chest for quality of breath sounds and adventitious sounds *that could indicate complications of oxygen therapy.*
Ineffective breathing pattern	• Assess ventilation to include evaluation of breathing rate, rhythm, and depth, chest expansion, presence of respiratory distress such as dyspnea, shortness of breath, nasal flaring, pursed-lip breathing and prolonged expiratory phase, and use of accessory muscles. • Observe for signs of oxygen-induced hypoventilation. • Suction if necessary *to remove secretions.* • Assess patient for tiring in relation to attempts to breathe. • Assess to make sure that oxygen therapy equipment is not interfering with patient's attempts to breathe.
Impaired gas exchange	• Assess patient to identify signs such as restlessness, confusion, and irritability, *which may indicate the body's response to altered blood gas states.* • In collaboration with physician, monitor arterial blood gases; report increases or decreases of $Paco_2$ of more than 10 mm Hg. • In collaboration with physician consultation, administer oxygen *to maintain* Pao_2 *above 55 mm Hg.* • Assess patient to determine which oxygen therapy system is best to maintain the required Pao_2 level. • Assess for signs of oxygen toxicity and absorption atelectasis. • Monitor electrocardiogram and cardiac status *for arrhythmias secondary to alterations in blood gases.* • Monitor serum electrolytes, which may change *owing to alterations in oxygenation and metabolism.* • Carefully observe effectiveness of selected oxygen equipment *to maintain determined* FIO_2 *levels.* • Clean equipment several times daily.
Altered oral mucous membrane	• Assess and care for drying of mucous membranes of the nose and mouth secondary to oxygen therapy.
Altered nutrition: less than body requirements	• Assess patient's ability to remove oxygen equipment during periods of eating and respiratory response. • If mask system is being used for oxygen therapy, assess need for nasal cannula therapy during mealtime.
Impaired verbal communication	• Observe for signs of frustration secondary to hypoxia that is causing fatigue as patient attempts to communicate; provide alternative communication techniques. • Observe for signs of frustration secondary to wearing oxygen mask; provide alternative communication techniques.
Anxiety	• Assess patient's level of anxiety *related to the need to have oxygen therapy.* • Assess patient's level of anxiety *related to feeling of air hunger.*
Defensive coping	• Determine patient's ability to cooperate with health care providers regarding intervention strategies.
Potential for aspiration	• Avoid triggering gag mechanism when performing caretaking activities, including mouth care. • If swallowing reflex is diminished, elevate head of bed when performing mouth care. • Assess and document amount of secretions present, patient's level of consciousness, and patient's ability to swallow secretions effectively.

Nursing Diagnosis	Nursing Intervention/Rationale
	• Administer suction when necessary to remove secretions and maintain patent airway. • If secretions are thick or inspissated, ensure adequate humidification to help liquefy secretions. • For patients with reduced level of consciousness, ensure head of bed is elevated, unless contraindicated.

Patient Education

1. Assess the patient's knowledge and skills regarding the use of oxygen equipment.
2. Teach the patient the purpose and process of the selected type of oxygen equipment.
3. Teach importance of not smoking (and not permitting others in the area to smoke) during administration of oxygen.
4. Provide the patient and family with information regarding the care, cleaning, and maintenance of oxygen equipment being used in the hospital or to be used at home.

Evaluation

Patient Outcome	Data Indicating That Outcome is Reached
Optimum movement of air in and out of lungs occurs.	Vital capacity measurements including FEV_1, FVC, TLC, RV, and FRC are optimum for patient's status.
Airway is patent.	Blood gas values are within normal limits. Airways are clear, and breathing occurs without obstruction.
Patient and family have sufficient information to comply with oxygen therapy plan.	Therapy plan is maintained.

Thoracic Surgery

Description and Rationale[51]

Thoracotomy. Thoracotomy refers to a surgical incision of the chest wall. Many times an exploratory thoracotomy is performed to obtain a biopsy specimen or locate a source of bleeding. During the procedure the ribs are spread and the pleura is opened. Closed chest drainage is generally required postoperatively.

Pneumonectomy. Pneumonectomy refers to surgical removal of an entire lung. The surgeon severs and sutures off the main arteries, veins, and the mainstem bronchus at the bifurcation. The major indication for pneumonectomy is lung cancer. Closed chest drainage is generally not done postoperatively. It is desirable for the thoracic cavity on the affected side to fill with serous exudate. The exudate eventually consolidates. The phrenic nerve on the affected side may be severed by the surgeon. This permits the diaphragm to assume an elevated position, which also assists to fill the empty thoracic space.

Lobectomy. Lobectomy refers to removal of a lobe of the lung. Major indications for this procedure include isolated tumors, cysts, tuberculosis, abscess, or localized injury. Closed chest drainage is used following a lobectomy.

Segmental resection. Segmental resection refers to the removal of one or more segments of the lung lobe. Indications for the procedure include tuberculosis, bleb, localized abscess, or bronchiectasis. Closed chest drainage is used following this procedure.

Wedge resection. Wedge resection refers to the removal of a small, wedge-shaped localized area near the lung surface. Indications for the procedure include biopsy and removal of a small area of tuberculosis. The resected area is sutured off before removal. There is generally little disruption of overall lung function. Closed chest drainage is used after the procedure.

Decortication. Decortication refers to the stripping off of a thick fibrous membrane that may develop over the visceral pleura secondary to empyema or the prolonged presence of blood or fluid in the pleural space. Closed chest drainage is required postoperatively.

Thoracoplasty. Thoracoplasty refers to a surgical procedure intended to remove select portions of the ribs with the intent of reducing the overall size of the thoracic cavity.

Contraindications and Cautions

The following complications of surgery should be anticipated:

Respiratory insufficiency
Tension pneumothorax
Cardiac failure or myocardial infarction

Thrombosis or pulmonary embolism
Atelectasis
Bronchopleural fistula
Pulmonary edema
Subcutaneous emphysema
Infection

Preprocedural Nursing Care

Carefully determine preoperative status of patient including the following:

- Baseline pulmonary function studies
- Electrocardiogram
- Arterial blood gases
- Electrolytes
- Other existing medical problems
- Current respiratory status: amount and extent of dyspnea, cough, and respiratory distress
- General nutrition and hydration state

Provide preoperative teaching to include the following:

- Need to stop smoking preoperatively
- Coughing and deep breathing techniques
- Need for and technique of suctioning and closed chest drainage postoperatively
- Overview of equipment and procedures that will most likely occur postoperatively
- Listen preoperatively to patient and family questions and concerns; provide information and clarification when indicated
- Assure patient that pain medication will be available postoperatively to assist with discomfort
- Teach patient the need for postoperative range of motion and leg exercises

NURSING CARE

Nursing Assessment

Blood Gases

pH, Pa_{O_2}, Pa_{CO_2}, HCO_3^- to monitor ventilator assistance or patient's ability to ventilate self

Chest Tube Drainage

Amount of drainage, characteristics of drainage, patency of closed drainage system

Incision Status

Suture line characteristics; lack of signs of infection

Respiratory Status

Lung expansion status, lack of signs of atelectasis, consolidation, infection, pulmonary edema, pulmonary embolus, mediastinal shift, paradoxical motion

Cardiovascular Status

Electrocardiogram changes, hypovolemia, pulmonary edema, venous stasis, cardiac arrhythmias, central venous pressure within normal limits for patient

Pain

Pain management that facilitates patient's activities of turning, coughing, deep breathing, and range of motion

Fluid and Electrolyte Balance

Fluid intake managed in manner to facilitate adequate nutritional and electrolyte requirements
Adequate urinary output
Electrolytes remain within normal limits

Infection

Increased WBC, fever, purulent drainage, redness around incision area

Nursing Dx & Intervention

Nursing Diagnosis	Nursing Intervention/Rationale
Ineffective airway clearance	• Maintain patent airway by suctioning and adequate position; if patient has endotracheal tube, see p. 216 for additional strategies. • Assess for signs of airway obstruction including restlessness, inadequate chest expansion, stridor, noisy respirations, cyanosis, or dyspnea (atelectasis may be preventable with proper nursing care). • Evaluate for signs of atelectasis that may result secondary to airway obstruction; signs include increased respiratory rate, rapid pulse, increased temperature, cyanosis, and diaphoresis.
Ineffective breathing pattern	• Carefully monitor status of closed chest drainage system; note fluctuation or tidaling in the water-seal chamber and the drainage tubing near the patient; see closed-chest drainage system for additional strategies. • If patient is on mechanical ventilator, see pp. 225 to 228 for specific nursing strategies. • When patient is ventilating independently, carefully assess respiratory rate, depth, and quality; note signs of dyspnea and respiratory distress, hemoptysis.

Nursing Diagnosis	Nursing Intervention/Rationale
	• Administer intermittent positive-pressure breathing (IPPB) as ordered; evaluate and record response. • Encourage coughing and deep breathing on a regular basis until patient is able to maintain procedure by self; observe and record response. • Carefully auscultate lungs at least every 2 hours; note quality of breath sounds, rate and depth of respirations, presence of adventitious sounds, presence of paradoxic respirations, mediastinal shift. • Observe for chest wall movement and potential splinting *secondary to pain*. • Observe for signs of pulmonary embolism, which include dyspnea, fear, hemoptysis, symptoms of right-sided heart failure, hypoxia, engorgement of neck veins, tachycardia, hypotension, apprehension, sense of impending doom, nausea, sweating. • Observe for signs of gastric distention that may occur *secondary to anesthesia and swallowing air;* if this occurs, it may cause ventilatory compromise, which will further complicate the postoperative period; if gastric distention is noted and confirmed by x-ray examination, the physician may elect to insert a nasogastric tube until gastrointestinal mobility returns.
Potential for aspiration	• Avoid triggering gag mechanism when performing caretaking activities, including mouth care. • If swallowing reflex is diminished, elevate head of bed when performing mouth care. • Assess and document amount of secretions present, patient's level of consciousness, and patient's ability to swallow secretions effectively. • Administer suction when necessary to remove secretions and maintain patent airway. • If secretions are thick or inspissated, ensure adequate humidification to help liquefy secretions. • For patients with reduced level of consciousness, ensure head of bed is elevated, unless contraindicated.
Fatigue	• Assess patterns of fatigue. • Assess factors related to fatigue and strategies for dealing with them. • Assess support systems and available resources. • Administer treatments or medications to relieve discomfort. • Enhance patient's ability to rest between specified activities.
Pain	• Administer pain medications approximately 30 minutes before deep breathing, coughing, and ambulation. • Provide adequate splinting before coughing and deep breathing.
Impaired gas exchange	• Monitor arterial blood gases as ordered; report alterations. • Maintain oxygenation as ordered; monitor patient response. • Reposition patient frequently *to facilitate aeration of the lung*. • Move lobectomy patient from supine to side-lying position (place rolled towel around chest tubes to protect them from collapse).
Fluid volume deficit	• Assess for signs of circulatory insufficiency secondary to hypovolemia; *this circulatory insufficiency may cause clinical signs such as hypotension, tachycardia, tachypnea, hypoxia, acidosis, and ischemia to vital organs*. • Maintain accurate intake and output records. • Provide intravenous fluids as ordered and monitor patient's cardiovascular and urinary output response. • Observe for signs of fluid overload such as pulmonary congestion.
Impaired physical mobility	• Initiate passive and encourage active range of motion throughout the postoperative period. • The patient is at risk for developing stiffness and ankylosis of the shoulder on the side with the chest tubes; encourage range of motion for that shoulder on a regular schedule. • Encourage passive and active range of motion of the legs *to decrease the potential for thrombosis*. • Ambulate patient as soon as possible and in accord with patient's ability to tolerate ambulation.
Impaired skin integrity	• Provide sterile technique wound care of incision according to physician's orders. • Assess and record condition of suture line. • Observe and record amount and characteristics of drainage including color and odor. • Observe for elevated temperature or fever, which may be an indication of infection; report observations to physician.
Fear	• Assure patient that nursing assistance is constantly available. • Provide reassurance and explain all procedures before they are performed.

Nursing Diagnosis	Nursing Intervention/Rationale
Impaired verbal communication	• If patient is unable to communicate verbally because of mechanical ventilation, endotracheal tube, or tracheostomy, provide a Magic Slate or similar writing material to facilitate communication. • Make sure call button is conveniently placed for patient's use.

Evaluation

Evaluation criteria are based on the individual procedure performed and the underlying disease state.

References

1. A.C.C.P.-A.T.S. Joint Committee on Pulmonary Terms and Symbols: Chest 67:583, 1975.
2. American Lung Association: Chronic obstructive pulmonary disease, New York, 1981, The Association.
3. American Lung Association: Occupational lung diseases: an introduction, New York, 1983, The Association.
4. American Thoracic Society: A statement by the Committee on Diagnostic Standards for Nontuberculosis Respiratory Diseases, Am Rev Respir Dis 85:762, 1962.
5. American Thoracic Society: Surveillance for respiratory hazards in the occupational setting, Am Rev Respir Dis 126(5):932, 1982.
6. American Trauma Society: Definitions and classifications of chronic bronchitis, asthma, and pulmonary emphysema, Am Rev Respir Dis 85:762, 1962.
7. Berkow R, editor: Merck manual of diagnosis and therapy, ed 14, Rahway, NJ, 1982, Merck, Inc.
8. Bernard GR: Adult respiratory distress syndrome: diagnosis and management, Heart Lung 15(3):250, 1986.
9. Brandstetter RD: The adult respiratory distress syndrome, Heart Lung 15(2):155, 1986.
10. Brown M and Andrews J: How to manage adult respiratory distress syndrome, Geriatrics 34:39, 1979.
11. Budassi SA and Barber JM: Mosby's manual of emergency care, ed 2, St Louis, 1984, The CV Mosby Co.
12. Burkhart C: After pneumonectomy, Am J Nurs 83:1563, 1983.
13. Burrows B: An overview of obstructive lung diseases, Med Clin North Am 65:455, 1981.
14. Canobbio M: Chest x-ray film interpretation, Focus Crit Care 11(2):18, 1984.
15. Carrieri V, Murdaugh C, and Jason-Bjerklie S: A framework for assessing pulmonary disease categories, Focus Crit Care 11(2):10, 1984.
16. Celentano NL: Mechanical ventilation strategies in adult respiratory distress syndrome, Crit Care Nurse 6(4):71, 1986.
17. Cherniack RM: Current therapy of respiratory disease, ed 2, Philadelphia, 1986, BC Decker, Inc.
18. Chin R and Pesce R: Practical aspects in management of respiratory failure in chronic obstructive pulmonary disease, Crit Care Q 6(2):1, 1983.
19. Clancy GT: Blood gas monitoring and management of neonates with respiratory distress, Perinatal Neonatal Nurs 1(1):72, 1987.
20. Cronin LR and Carrizosa A: The computer as a communication device for ventilator and tracheostomy patients in the intensive care unit, Crit Care Nurs 4:72, 1984.
21. D'Agostino JS: Teaching tips for lung with COPD at home, Nursing 84 14(2):57, 1984.
22. Ellis EF: Asthma in childhood, J Allergy Clin Immunol 72:526, 1983.
23. Erikkson S: Pulmonary emphysema and alpha-1-antitrypsin deficiency, Acta Med Scand 175:197, 1964.
24. Farzan S: A concise handbook of respiratory diseases, Reston, Va, 1985, Reston Publishing Co.
25. Ferris BG: Epidemiology standardization project respiratory questionnaires, Am Rev Respir Dis 118:7, 1978.
26. Fishman AP, editor: Pulmonary diseases and disorders, New York, 1980, McGraw-Hill Book Co.
27. Fletcher CM et al: The significance of respiratory symptoms and the diagnosis of chronic bronchitis in a working population, Br Med J 2:257, 1959.
28. Fowler AA, Hamman RF, and Zerbe GO: Adult respiratory distress syndrome: prognosis after onset, Am Rev Respir Dis 132:472, 1985.
29. Fries JF and Ehrlich GE: Prognosis: contemporary outcomes of disease, Bowie, Md, 1981, The Charles Press Publishers.
30. Fuchs P: Streamlining your suctioning techniques. I. Nasotracheal suctioning, Nursing 84 14(5):55, 1984.
31. Fuchs P: Streamlining your suctioning techniques. II. Endotracheal suctioning, Nursing 84 14(6):46, 1984.
32. Fuchs P: Streamlining your suctioning technique. III. Tracheostomy suctioning, Nursing 84 14(7):39, 1984.
33. Gaensler EA et al: Epidemiology standardization project III. Recommended standardized procedures for pulmonary function testing. Am Rev Respir Dis 118(suppl):55, 1978.
34. George RB, Light RW, and Matthay RA, editors: Chest physiology, New York, 1983, Churchill Livingstone.
35. Guenter CA and Welch MH: Pulmonary medicine, Philadelphia, 1977, JB Lippincott Co.
36. Harber P: Value based interpretations of pulmonary function tests, Chest 88(6):874, 1985.
37. Harper RW: A guide to respiratory care: physiology and clinical approaches, Philadelphia, 1981, JB Lippincott Co.
38. Hirsch J and Hannock L, editors: Mosby's manual of clinical nursing practice, St. Louis, 1981, The CV Mosby Co.
39. Holloway NM: Nursing the critically ill adult, ed 2, Menlo Park, Calif, 1984, Addison-Wesley Publishing Co.
40. Hopp L: Ineffective breathing pattern related to decreased lung expansion, Nurs Clin North Am 22(1):193, 1987.
41. Janson-Bjerklie S: Defense mechanisms: protecting the healthy lung. Heart Lung 12:643, 1983.
42. Johanson BC et al: Standards for critical care, St. Louis, 1981, The CV Mosby Co.
43. Karnes N: Don't let ARDS catch you off guard, Nursing 87 17(5):34, 1987.
44. Kim MJ: Ineffective airway clearance and ineffective breathing patterns: theoretical and research base for nursing diagnosis, Nurs Clin North Am 22(1):125, 1987.
45. Kinney MR et al, editors: AACN's clinical reference for critical-care nursing, New York, 1981, McGraw-Hill Book Co.
46. Kirilloff LH and Tibbals SC: Drugs for asthma: a complete guide, Am J Nurs 83:55, 1983.
47. Kirsh MM and Shoan H: Blunt chest trauma: general principles of management, Boston, 1977, Little, Brown & Co.
48. Lakshminarayan S and Hudson LD: Pulmonary function following the adult respiratory distress syndrome, Chest 74:489, 1978.
49. Landis K and Smith S: The mechanically ventilated patient: a comprehensive nursing care plan, Crit Care Q 6(2):43, 1983.
50. Larson JL: Ineffective breathing patterns related to respiratory muscle fatigue, Nurs Clin North Am 22(1):207, 1987.
51. Luckmann J and Sorenson K: Medical-surgery nursing: a psychophysiological approach, ed 2, Philadelphia, 1980, WB Saunders Co.

52. Martin L: Pulmonary physiology in clinical practice: the essentials for patient care and evaluation, St Louis, 1987, The CV Mosby Co.
53. Matthay MA, editor: Symposium on pulmonary edema, Clin Chest Med, vol 6, 1985.
54. McDonald BR: Validation of three respiratory nursing diagnoses—ineffective airway clearance, ineffective breathing pattern, and impaired gas exchange, Nurs Clin North Am 20(4):697, 1985.
55. Miller LG and Kazemi H: Manual of clinical pulmonary medicine, New York, 1983, McGraw-Hill Book Co.
56. Morbidity and Mortality Weekly Report 32:463, Sept 9, 1983.
57. Pelty TL: ABC of simple pulmonary function assessment, Nurse Pract 11(6):50, 1986.
58. Phipps W, Long B, and Woods N: Medical-surgical nursing: concepts and clinical practice, St Louis, 1983, The CV Mosby Co.
59. Price SA and Wilson LM: Pathophysiology clinical concepts of disease processes, ed 2, New York, 1982, McGraw-Hill Book Co.
60. Rakel RE: Conn's current therapy, Philadelphia, 1987, WB Saunders Co.
61. Reynolds HY and Merrill WW: Airway changes in young smokers that may antedate chronic obstructive disease, Med Clin North Am 65:667, 1981.
62. Rhodes M: Update on chest trauma, Crit Care Q 6(2):59, 1983.
63. Rifas E: Teaching patients to manage acute asthma: the future is now, Nursing 83 13(4):77, 1983.
64. Robinson S and Russo P, editors: Providing respiratory care: nursing photobook, Springhouse, Pa, 1979, Intermed Communications.
65. Rokosky JS: Assessment of altered respiratory function, Nurs Clin North Am 16(2):198, 1981.
66. Rosen P, editor: Emergency medicine: concepts and clinical practice, St Louis, 1983, The CV Mosby Co, pp 774-789.
67. Ross MC: Healing under pressure, Am J Nurs 86(10):1118, 1986.
68. Sexton D: The supporting cast: wives of COPD patients, J Gerontol Nurs 10(2):82, 1984.
69. Shapiro B: Clinical application of blood gases, Chicago, 1979, Year Book Medical Publishers.
70. Smith L and Thier S: Pathophysiology: the biological principles of disease, Philadelphia, 1981, WB Saunders Co.
71. Snider GL: Pathogenesis of emphysema and chronic bronchitis, Med Clin North Am 65:647, 1981.
72. Spearman C, Sheldon R, and Egan D: Egan's fundamentals of respiratory therapy, ed 4, St Louis, 1982, The CV Mosby Co.
73. Thorn GW et al, editors: Harrison's principles of internal medicine, ed 10, New York, 1983, McGraw-Hill Book Co.
74. Tinits P: Oxygen therapy and oxygen toxicity, Ann Emerg Med 12:89, 1983.
75. Tisi GM: Pulmonary physiology in clinical medicine, Baltimore, 1980, The Williams & Wilkins Co.
76. Topics in clinical nursing: breathing and breathlessness, Germantown, Md, 1980, Aspen Systems Corp.
77. Traver GA: Ineffective airway clearance: physiology and clinical application, Dimen Crit Care Nurs 4(4):198-208, 1985.
78. Tucker SM et al: Patient care standards, ed 3, St Louis, 1984, The CV Mosby Co.
79. Ulrich SP, Canale SW, and Wendell SA: Nursing care planning guides: a nursing diagnosis approach, Philadelphia, 1986, WB Saunders Co.
80. Vaughn VC, McKay RJ, and Behrman RE, editors: Nelson's textbook of pediatrics, ed 12, Philadelphia, 1983, WB Saunders Co.
81. Vincent JE: Medical problems in the patient on a ventilator, Crit Care Q 6(2):33, 1983.
82. Waldbott G: Health effects of environmental pollutants, ed 2, St Louis, 1978, The CV Mosby Co.
83. Weilbrel ER: Morphometry of human lung, New York, 1963, Academic Press, Inc.
84. Weiss EB: Bronchial asthma, Clin Symp 27:39, 1975.
85. Weiss EB and Segal MS, editors: Bronchial asthma, Boston, 1976, Little Brown & Co.
86. West J: Respiratory physiology: the essentials, Baltimore, 1979, The Williams & Wilkins Co.
87. Whitcomb ME: The lung, normal and diseased, St Louis 1982, The CV Mosby Co.
88. York K: Clinical validation of two respiratory nursing diagnoses and their defining characteristics—ineffective airway clearance and ineffective breathing patterns, Nurs Clin North Am 20(4):657-667, 1985.

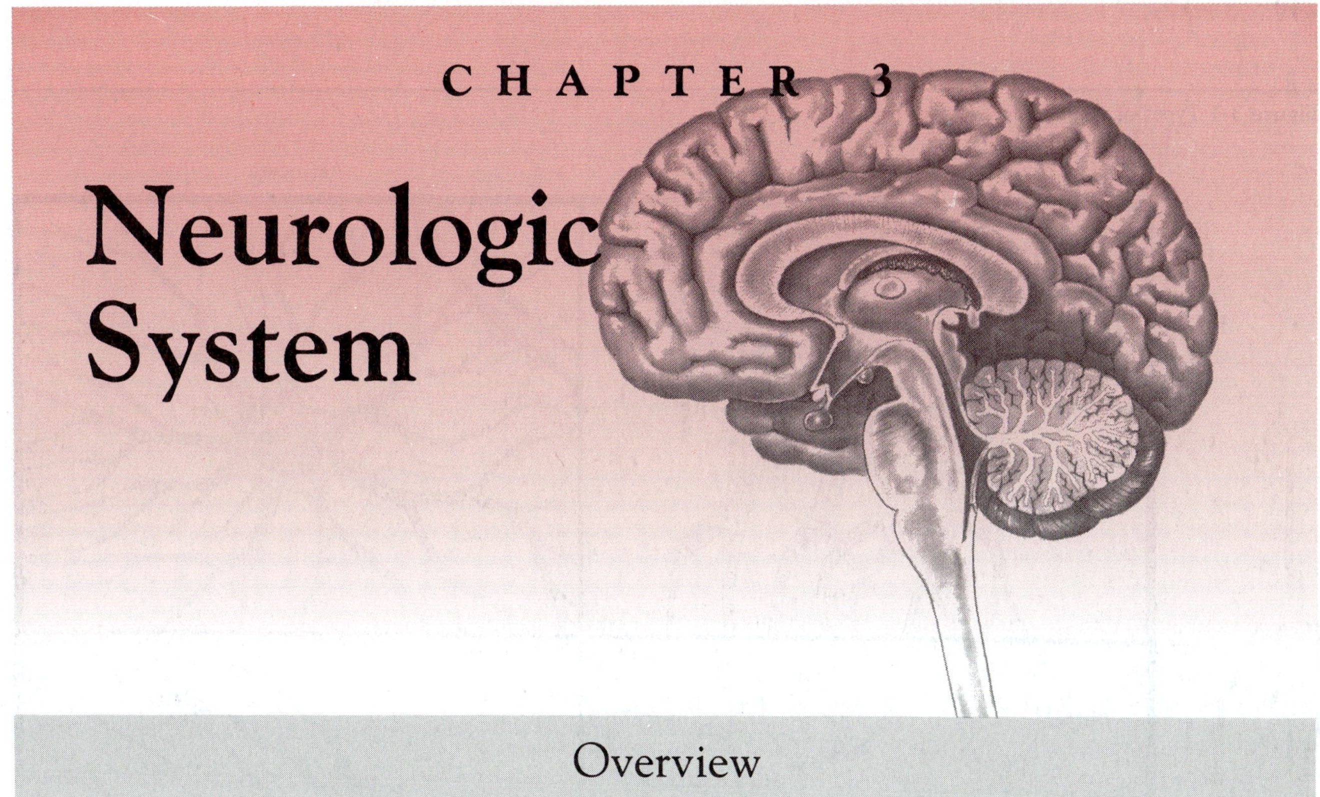

CHAPTER 3
Neurologic System

Overview

The human nervous system consists of complex structures and processes that provide an intricate circuit board through which the various functions of the body are integrated. Because these functions are integrative, the physiologic and psychologic ramifications of a neurologic dysfunction can be devastating for both patients and their families.

Anatomy, Physiology, and Related Pathophysiology

The nervous system is divided into two fairly distinct structural categories: the central nervous system (CNS), which consists of the brain and spinal cord, and the peripheral nervous system (PNS), which is made up of 12 pairs of cranial nerves, 31 pairs of spinal nerves, and the sympathetic and parasympathetic subdivisions of the autonomic nervous system. Functionally, the central and peripheral nervous systems are interdependent in that each is made of millions of shared neurons and neuroglia cells. The neuron is the basic unit of the nervous system. The neuroglia cells support the neuron.

Neuroglia Cells

About 40% of the structures of the brain and spinal cord are neuroglia cells. These cells protect, support, and nourish the cell bodies and processes of the neurons. There are four distinct types of neuroglia cells: astrocyte, ependyma, microglia, and oligodendroglia (Figure 3-1). All of these cells, except the microglia, come from the embryonic ectoderm. Unlike neurons, neuroglia cells can divide and multiply by mitosis and are a main source for nervous system tumors.

Astrocyte cells (astroglia) look like stars because of the many processes extending from their cell bodies. Their functions include helping to conduct impulses, helping to supply nutrition, storing information, supporting the neuron's structures, and helping to maintain the blood-brain barrier. Astrocytes are further divided into fibrillary astrocytes, which are found in white matter, and protoplasmic astrocytes, which are found in gray matter.

Ependymal cells are found within the epithelial lining of the cerebral ventricles, the choroid plexuses, and the spinal cord's central canal. Their main function is to help produce cerebrospinal fluid.

Microglia are stationary cells scattered throughout the central nervous system, mainly in white matter. These cells come from the embryonic mesoderm. The function of microglia is phagocytosis, during which the microglia become mobile and ingest and digest tissue debris.

Oligodendroglia cells synthesize a lipid-protein complex that forms myelin sheaths around the axonal projections of neurons in the central nervous system. Functions of the myelin sheath include holding nerve fibers together, providing insulation, promoting ionic flow, and transmitting nerve impulses (saltatory conduction). Oligodendroglia begin forming at about the fourth fetal month and continue until about 20 years of age. Unlike Schwann cells, the oligodendroglia cannot regenerate. Instead, damaged neuronal structures are replaced with astrocytes, forming a gliotic scar that can disrupt the neuronal tissue.

Neurons

Neurons (Figure 3-2) come in many sizes and shapes, and each transmits specific nervous stimuli. The neurons have

Figure 3-1 Types of neuroglia cells.

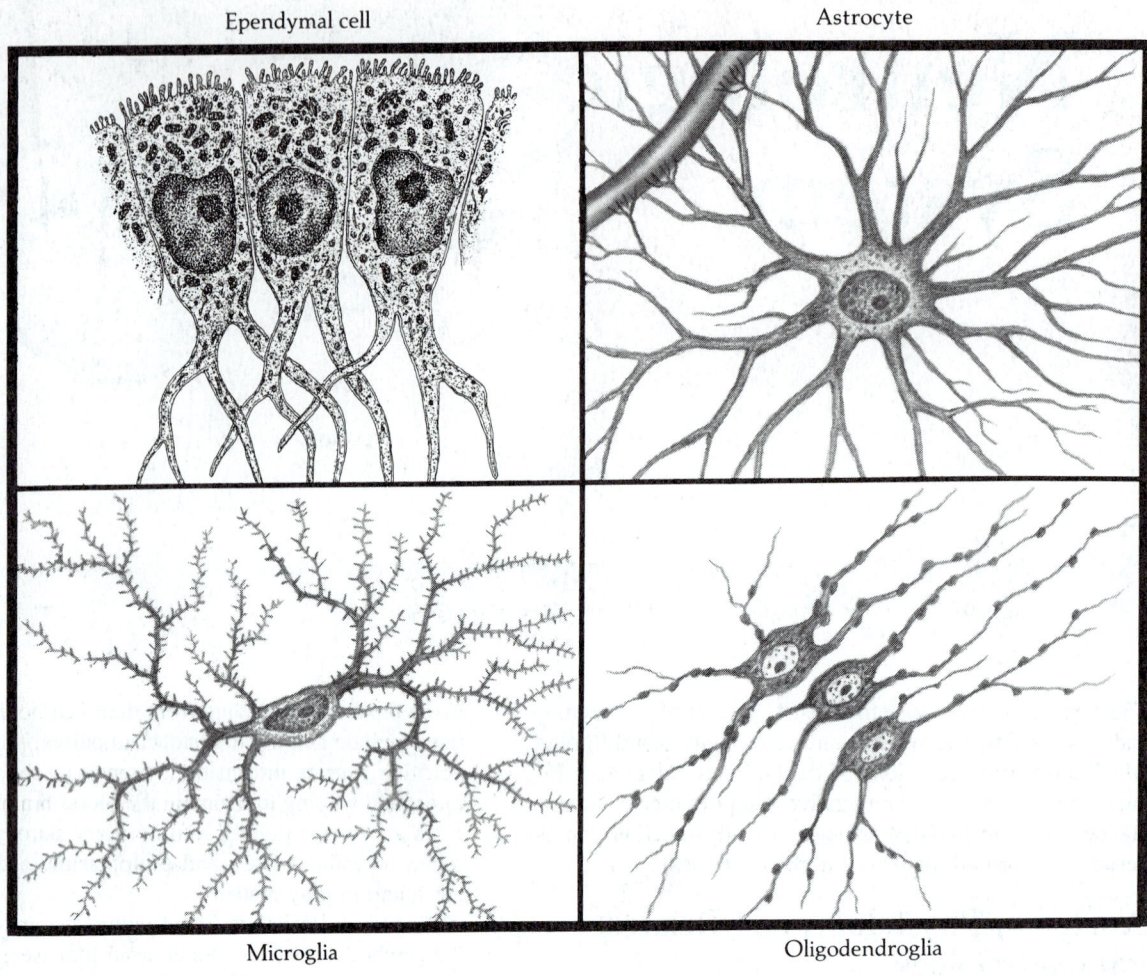

Ependymal cell

Astrocyte

Microglia

Oligodendroglia

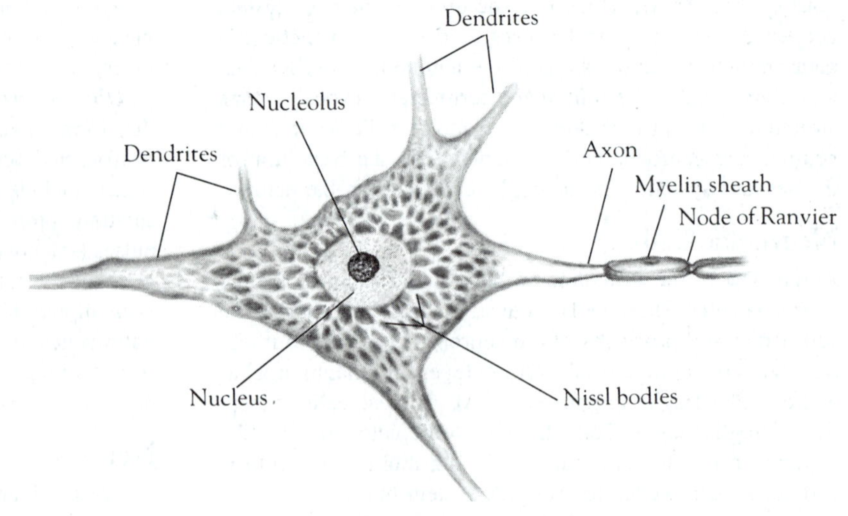

Figure 3-2 Diagram of neuron with composite parts.
From Rudy.[52]

properties of excitation and electrical-chemical conductivity. In the central nervous system, groups of neurons are called nuclei; in the peripheral nervous system they are called ganglia.

Cytologic features. The neuron is made of a *cell body,* or perikaryon; *prosections,* called dendrites; and an axon. The nerve cell body is the gray matter of the nervous system.

Each neuron contains only one centrally located *nucleus*. The nucleus is a large, double-membraned structure containing deoxyribonucleic acid (DNA). Inside the nucleus is a single nucleolus containing ribonucleic acid (RNA). Surrounding the nucleus is granular *cytoplasm* containing many organelles, including Nissl bodies, mitochondria, the Golgi complex, neurofilaments, and microtubules. Nissl bodies help to synthesize protein. *Mitochondria* are rod-shaped organelles that regulate the cell's respiratory metabolism. Metabolic energy is stored as adenosine triphosphate (ATP). The *Golgi complex,* located in the cytoplasm, condenses and stores substances needed to transmit impulses. Dense neurofilaments are found throughout the cytoplasm and in the axonal and dendritic processes. Neurofilaments are made of structures called neurotubules or microtubules. Together, they form the neurofibril, which is involved in axoplasmic transport within cells.

Processes. Extending from the cell body is a long, smooth projection called the *axon,* or *axis cylinder* (Figure 3-2). The axon originates from the neuron's cell body at a point called the axon hillock. The myelin around the axon protects and insulates it. Axons, which carry efferent impulses away from cell bodies, form the white matter of the central nervous system. Terminal branches of the axon are called terminal filaments, or boutons (axon telodendria).

Extending from the cell body to the immediate surrounding areas are short receptive processes, or *dendrites*. The branch-like dendrites have no myelin sheath and lie with the cell body in the gray matter. The dendritic branches increase the surface area from which neuronal impulses can be picked up. Dendrites transmit afferent impulses toward the cell body. Rootlike terminal endings of the dendrite, or dendritic spines, help to transmit synapses.

Classification. Structurally, neurons can be subdivided according to the number of processes and the axon lengths (Figure 3-3).

Unipolar neurons have only one process or pole, which divides close to the cell body. One branch of this division, called the peripheral process, carries afferent impulses toward the cell body. The other branch, the central process, conducts efferent impulses away from the body. *Bipolar* neurons have two processes: one axon and one dendrite. Bipolar neurons are found in the spinal ganglia, the nasal mucous membrane, and the rod and cone cells of the retina. *Multipolar* neurons make up most of the central nervous system, including all association (internuncial) and motor neurons. Multipolar neurons consist of a cell body, one long projection, and one or more shorter branches.

Neurons can also be classified by the axon length. Subdivisions within this classification are Golgi type I and Golgi type II (Figure 3-3). *Golgi type I* neurons are large and have long axons. They are found in the long fiber tracts located in the cerebral cortex, cerebellum, and spinal cord. *Golgi type II* neurons are small cells that are found between larger neurons and that establish complex circuits in the nervous system. These neurons are found throughout the brain and spinal cord. Golgi type II neurons have short axons that branch repeatedly and end near the cell body.

Figure 3-3 Structural and functional neuron classification.

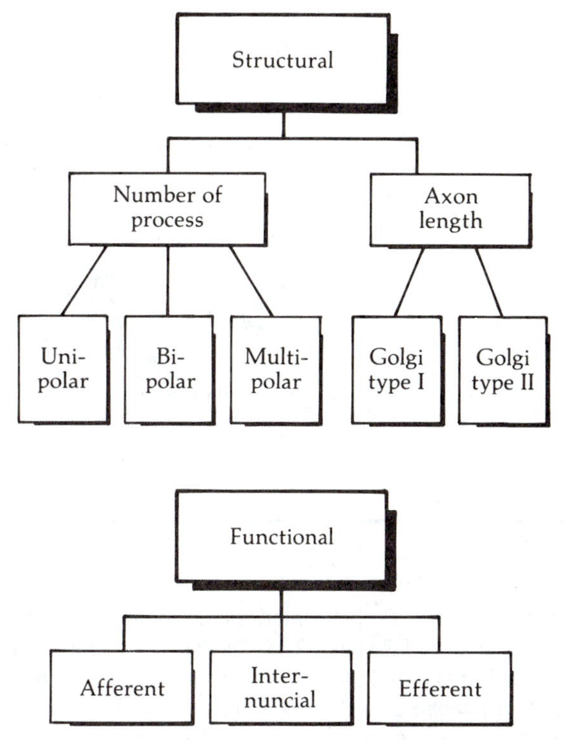

Functionally, the neurons are classified as afferent, internuncial (association), or efferent (Figure 3-3). *Afferent* (sensory) neurons conduct impulses to the central nervous system. *Internuncial* (association) neurons are in the central nervous system and conduct afferent and efferent impulses. *Efferent* (motor) neurons transmit impulses to effector organs and tissue.

Nerves

In the peripheral nervous system the neuron carries impulses to and from the central nervous system via the chainlike grouping of neuron cell fibers into *nerves* (Figure 3-4). (The term "nerve" applies only to cell fibers in the peripheral nervous system. In the central nervous system these are called *fiber tracts.*)

The axon is the part of the nerve that conducts impulses. The myelin sheath around the axon insulates, protects, and

Figure 3-4 Peripheral nerve.

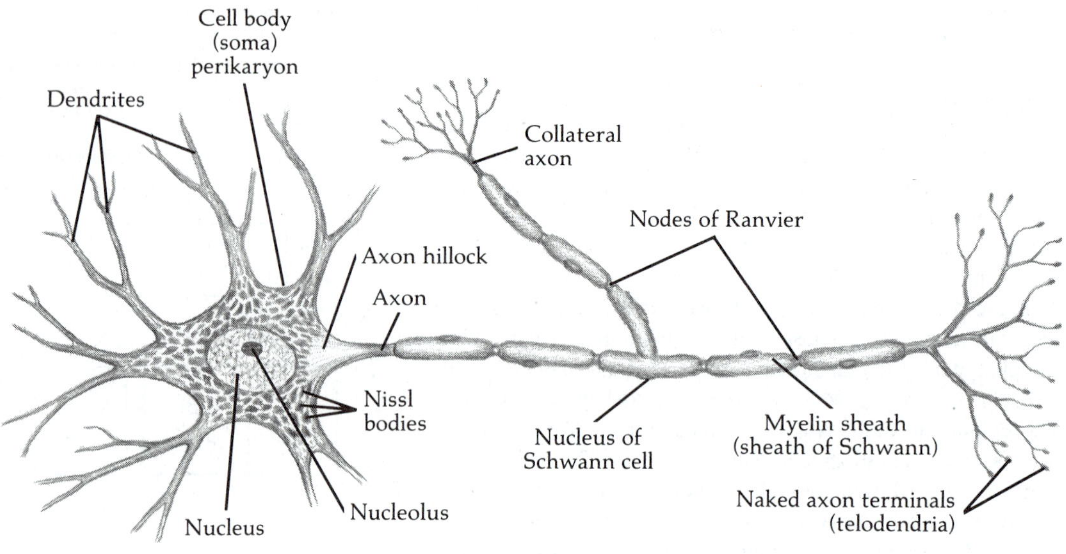

nourishes the axon. Periodic interruptions of the myelin sheath are called *nodes of Ranvier*. These nodes allow action potentials to skip from node to node, increasing impulse conduction. *Neurilemma* is a thin membrane formed by Schwann cells. The neurilemma membrane wraps spirally around the segmented myelin sheaths of myelinated nerve fibers or the axons of unmyelinated nerves. Functions of the neurilemma membrane include protection and support of the nerve processes. It provides a basic structure for the regeneration of nerve processes. The myelin, nodes of Ranvier, and neurilemma are sometimes referred to as the neurilemma cells.

Surrounding the nerve fibers are three layers of connective tissue coverings (Figure 3-5). The *endoneurium* surrounds the neurilemma cells. Next to the endoneurium is the *perineurium,* which surrounds groups of nerve fibers (fascicles). The *epineurium* is an outer covering that binds the groups of fascicles together.

The nerve fibers in the peripheral nervous system are clas-

Figure 3-5 Peripheral nerve trunk and coverings.

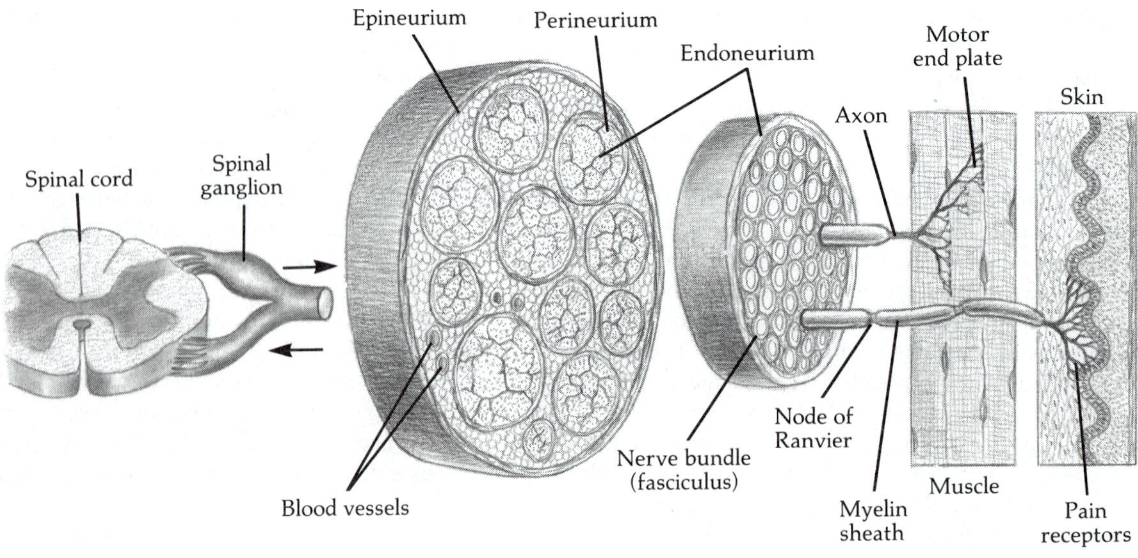

sified according to their function: afferent, internuncial (association), or efferent.

Nerve impulse. Nerve fibers are charged (polarized) in their resting state. In this state the cells have a resting membrane potential of −70 mV, which means the inside of the cell membrane has a negative charge in relation to the outside. There is a high concentration of sodium (Na^+) ouside the cell and a high concentration of potassium (K^+) in the cell. This results in unequal electrical charges across the cell membrane. This difference is the result of the relative impermeability of the cell to sodium and the sodium-potassium pump mechanism whereby sodium is pumped continuously out of the cell and potassium is pumped in.

When a strong enough stimulus (referred to as the threshold intensity) begins, there is a rapid, marked change in the cell membrane permeability. This change results in a gain of sodium and a loss of potassium in the cell. With the gain of sodium the cell becomes positive relative to the interstitial space, and an action potential or depolarization results. The depolarization stimulus excites one area, which then excites other parts of the cell membrane (conduction), until the entire membrane is stimulated at the same intensity. Thus the wave of depolarization moves cyclically along the entire length of the nerve process. Following depolarization, the ionic flow reverses. Sodium is pumped out as potassium is pumped back into the cell. This is the repolarization process whereby the membrane is returned to its resting potential. During depolarization and one third of the repolarization process, the neuron cell cannot be restimulated with another action potential. This time interval (or *absolute refractory period*) prevents repeated excitation of the neuron. Figure 3-6 illustrates this process.

The speed of impulse conduction depends on whether the nerve has a myelin sheath. In the unmyelinated nerve the action potential must travel the entire length of the nerve fiber. In myelinated nerves the axon is exposed only at the nodes of Ranvier; therefore the action potential is not transmitted along the entire axon membrane. Instead, the action potential "skips," discontinuously, from one node of Ranvier to the next. With this node-to-node conduction, termed *saltatory transmission,* the action potential travels faster. This increases the speed of the impulses and decreases the demand for energy.

Synapse. Because neurons occur in chainlike pathways, impulses must travel from one cell to another via functional junctions called *synapses.* Actual synaptic transmission is a chemical process that occurs because of the release of neurotransmitters. In addition, synapses are polarized so the impulse flows in one direction only (e.g., from the axon of one neuron to the axon, dendrites, or cell body of another neuron in a pathway).

The anatomic structures of the synapse consist of presynaptic terminals, the synaptic cleft, and the postsynaptic membrane (Figure 3-7). The presynaptic terminals (also called presynaptic knobs) contain hundreds of very small circular vesicles that store excitatory or inhibitory neurotransmitters.

Figure 3-6 Stages in impulse propagation.
From Schottelius.[53]

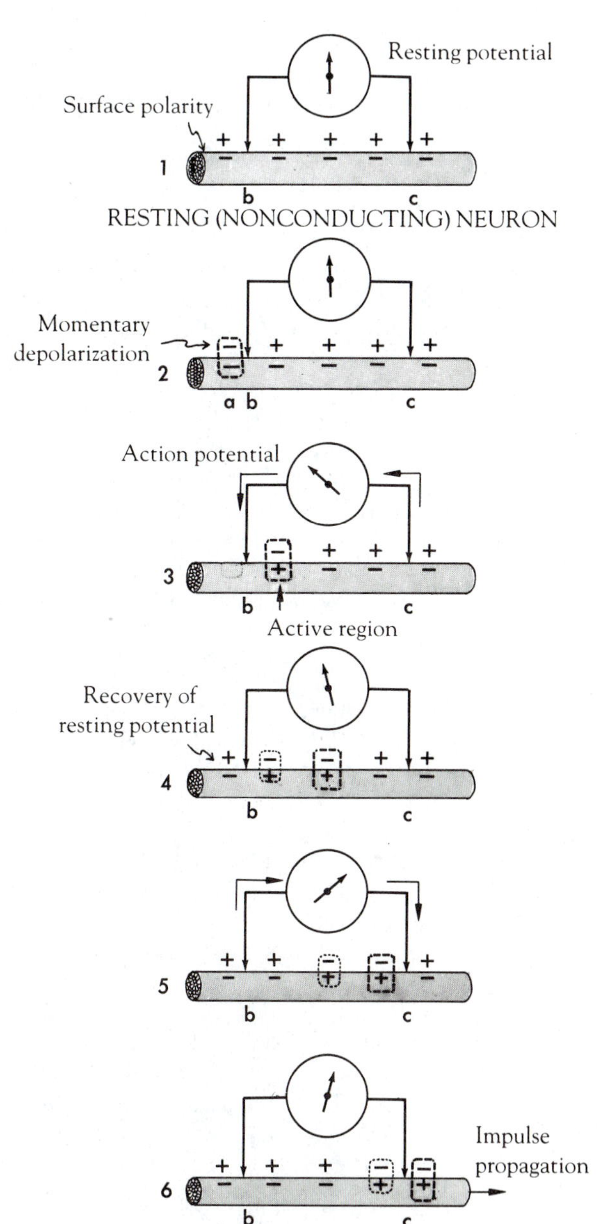

There are three types of interneuronal synapses: *axosomatic,* in which the axon of one neuron contacts the cell body of another neuron; *axodendritic,* in which the axon of one neuron contacts the dendrites of another nerve cell; and *axoaxonic,* in which one axon contacts with another axon.

Neurotransmitters

At least 30 different neurotransmitters can affect chemical transmission of an impulse at the synapse. When an impulse

Figure 3-7 Functional relationship between two neurons in pathway. Electrical impulse travels along axon of first neuron to synapse. Chemical transmitter is secreted into synaptic space to depolarize membrane (dendrite or cell body) of next neuron in pathway. Cell A represents unipolar cell; cell B represents multipolar cell.

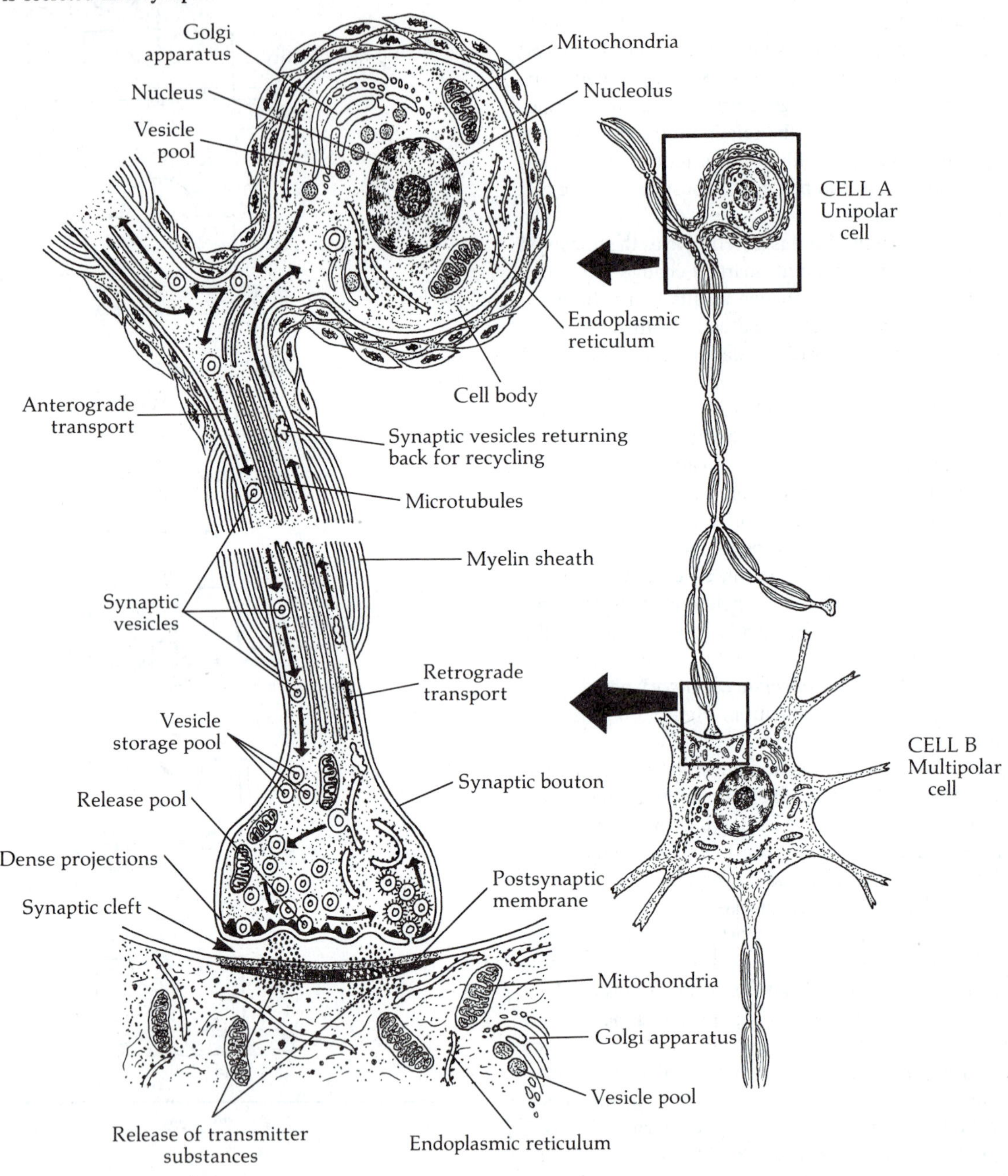

stimulates the presynaptic terminals, they secrete neurotransmitters into the synaptic cleft. This changes the permeability of the postsynaptic membrane. Neurotransmitters either excite or inhibit activity in the postsynaptic cell.

Excitatory neurotransmitters react with receptor sites on the postsynaptic membrane to enhance the membrane's permeability to sodium, potassium, and choride ions. The influx of sodium lowers the membrane potential (depolarization). Because of this lower membrane potential, an excitatory postsynaptic potential (EPSP) develops and stimulates the postsynaptic neuron toward an action potential. Acetylcholine is the principal excitatory neurotransmitter of the voluntary nervous system and the parasympathetic division of the autonomic nervous system. Other central excitatory neurotransmitters are norepinephrine, dopamine, serotonin, L-aspartate, and glutamic acid. Norepinephrine is the major postsynaptic excitatory neurotransmitter in the sympathetic division of the autonomic nervous system.[16]

Inhibitory neurotransmitters decrease the permeability of the postsynaptic membrane to sodium but increase its permeability to potassium and choride ions. The potassium ion flows out and chloride flows in, hyperpolarizing (the opposite of depolarizing) the postsynaptic cell membrane and forming an inhibitory postsynaptic potential (IPSP). The formation of the IPSP is called direct inhibition. Another type of inhibitory action is presynaptic inhibition, which occurs when the excitatory presynaptic terminals are stimulated by an inhibitory neuron. In presynaptic inhibition there is partial depolarization of the excitatory presynaptic terminals so that less excitatory neurotransmitters are released from these endings. This decreases the amplitude of the action potential as it arrives at the presynaptic terminals and decreases end-excitation of the neuron. Inhibitory neurotransmitters include γ-aminobutyric acid (GABA) (presynaptic) and glycine (postsynaptic).

The number of neurotransmitters depends on the rate and number of impulses that stimulate the presynaptic terminals. Therefore, to form an action potential on the postsynaptic membranes, one presynaptic terminal may have to depolarize repeatedly (referred to as temporal summation) or many presynaptic terminals may have to depolarize and release neurotransmitters (spatial summation).

To prevent overstimulation of the postsynaptic membrane, the neurotransmitter is inactivated chemically after synaptic transmission. The neurotransmitter is inactivated by enzyme degradation (i.e., acetylcholine is inactivated by acetylcholinesterase), retaken up by presynaptic terminals (i.e., dopamine, serotonin, and GABA), or diffused from the postsynaptic membrane.

Central Nervous System

Skull. The brain is protected by the bony structure of the skull (Figure 3-8). The skull is divided into two primary sections, the cranium and the skeleton of the face. The cranial portion of the skull is made up of eight relatively flat and irregular bones joined together by a series of fixed joints called sutures. These bones are composed of three layers: the solid *outer table,* the spongy middle *diploë,* and the solid *inner*

Figure 3-8 Lateral view of skull.
From Anthony.[1]

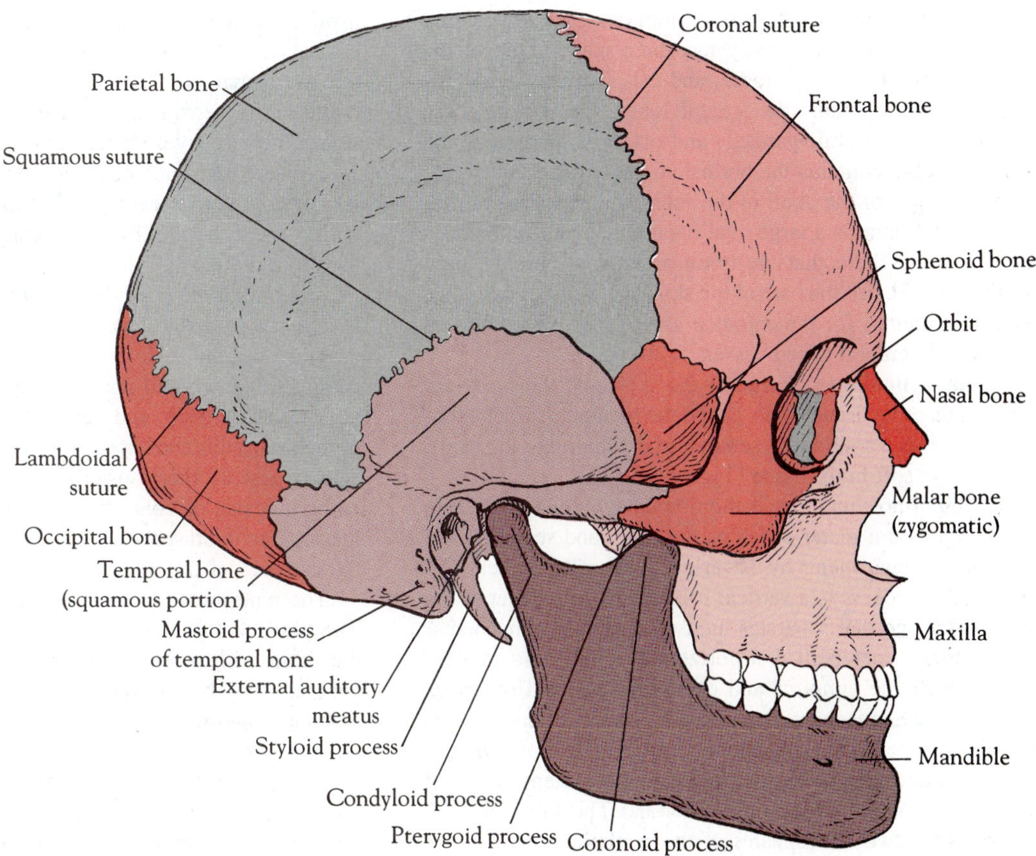

Figure 3-9 Meninges of brain.

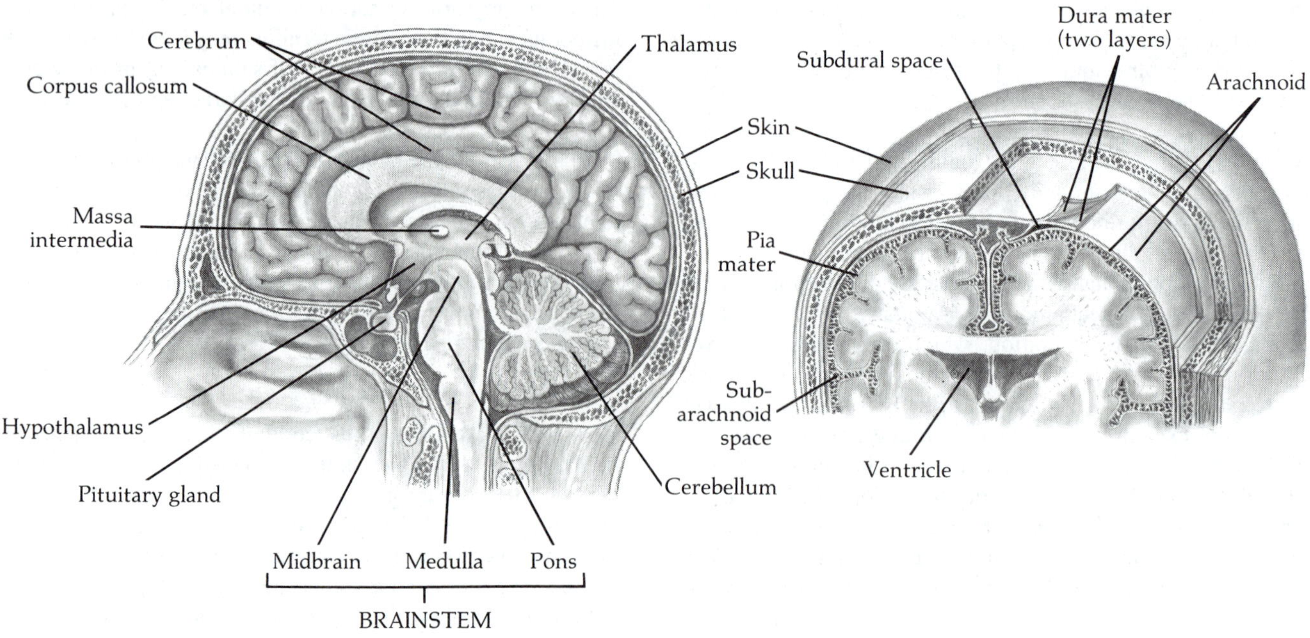

table. The inner table of the skull forms a cavity filled with ridges and convolutions that are custom designed for holding the brain. This internal cavity has three major regions: the anterior fossa, the middle fossa, and the posterior fossa. The anterior fossa contains the frontal lobes; the middle fossa contains the temporal, parietal, and occipital lobes; and the posterior fossa contains the brainstem and cerebellum.[16]

At the base of the skull in the inferior anterior portion of the occipital bone is a large oval opening called the foramen magnum. It is here that the brain and spinal cord become continuous. Also at the base of the skull is a series of openings (called foramina) for the entrance and exit of paired cranial nerves and cerebral blood vessels.

Cranial meninges. Between the skull and the brain are three connective tissue layers called the meninges. Each meningeal layer is a continuous separate sheet that, like the skull, protects the soft brain tissue (Figure 3-9).

The outermost meninge is the fibrous double-layered *dura mater*. This dura mater envelops the brain and separates the skull into compartments by its various folds or processes. The falx cerebri process is a vertical fold of the dura mater at the midsagittal line that separates the two cerebral hemispheres. The tentorium cerebelli is a horizontal double fold of dura that supports the temporal and occipital lobes and separates the cerebral hemispheres from the brainstem and the cerebellum. (The tentorium provides an important line of division. Structures above the tentorium are called supratentorial, and those below it are called infratentorial.) The falx cerebelli separates the two hemispheres of the cerebellum.

The cranial dura mater differs significantly from spinal dura mater in the following ways: the cranial dura is attached firmly, but the spinal dura is not attached to the vertebrae; cranial dura is made of two layers, periosteal and meningeal, but the spinal dura has only one meningeal layer; and the cranial dura separates in places and forms venous sinuses, which the one-layer spinal dura does not.[13]

Between the dura mater and the middle meningeal layer is a narrow serous cavity called the subdural space. Vessels within the subdural space have few support structures and therefore are easily injured.

The middle layer of the meninges is called the arachnoid. It is made of a two-layered, fibrous, elastic membrane that crosses over the folds and fissures of the brain, creating the spongy subarachnoid space. Within the subarachnoid space are cerebral arteries and veins of different sizes. At the base of the brain, dilations in the subarachnoid space form cisterns. The largest of these cisterns is the cisterna magna, which communicates or connects with the fourth ventricle. It is in the subarachnoid space that cerebrospinal fluid circulates over the surfaces of the brain.

The innermost layer of meninges is called the pia mater. The pia mater is rich in small blood vessels, which supply the brain with a large volume of blood. It is also in direct contact with the external structure of the brain tissue. The arachnoid and pia membranes are collectively called the leptomeninges.

Brain. Next to the pia mater is the brain. The brain is only about 2% (about 3 pounds) of the total body weight of an adult but receives about 20% of the cardiac output and requires 20% of the body's oxygen use.[48]

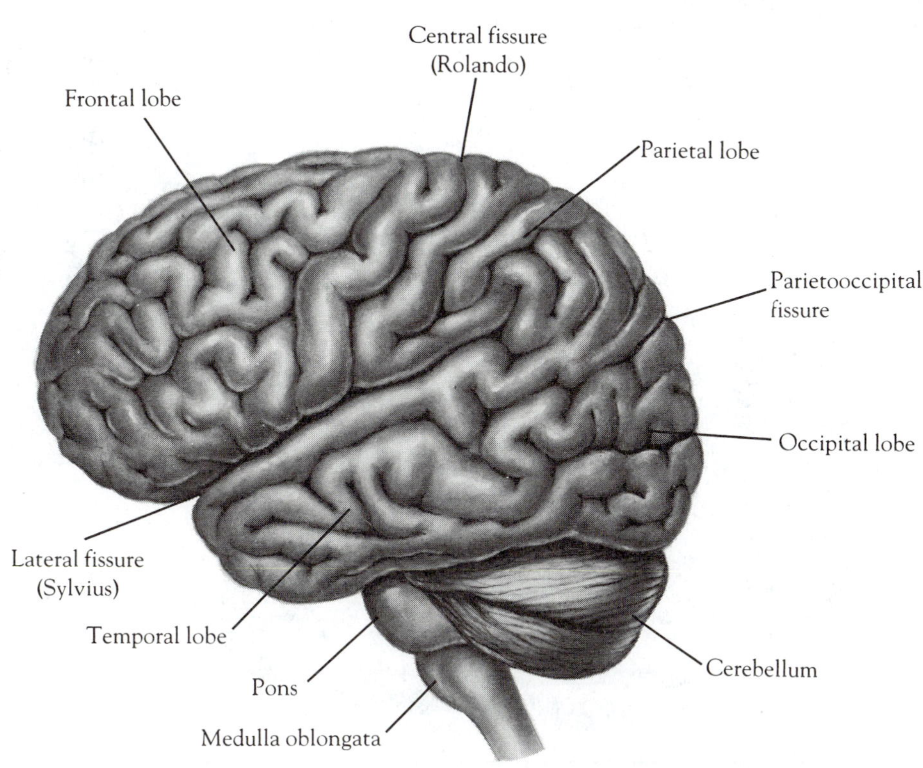

Figure 3-10 Lateral view of cerebral hemisphere (showing lobes and principal fissures), cerebellum, pons, and medulla oblongata.
From Rudy.[52]

The surface of the brain has many convolutions separated by shallow folds. Sulci and fissures are the deeper folds or grooves that divide the brain into lobes and hemispheres.

The brain (encephalon) is divided into three major anatomic areas: the cerebrum, the cerebellum, and the brainstem.

Cerebrum. The cerebrum is the largest anatomic portion of the brain and is covered with several layers of gray cells that make up the cerebral cortex. It consists of cerebral hemispheres, the rhinencephalon, the internal capsule and basal ganglia, and the diencephalon (i.e., thalamus and hypothalamus). The internal white matter of the cerebrum consists of many myelinated nerve fibers and neuroglia cells. The cerebrum is divided lengthwise into symmetric right and left sides by the longitudinal fissure. Each half is called a lateral cerebral hemisphere. The hemispheres are joined lengthwise by a large tract of white commissural fibers, the corpus callosum, that serves as the communication link between the hemispheres. The major folds of the cortex divide each lateral hemisphere into four lobes, or cerebral hemispheres, which are named for the overlying cranial bones: frontal, parietal, occipital, and temporal (Figure 3-10).

Certain areas of the cerebral cortex are responsible for specific functions of the cerebrum. Probably the best-known classification of these areas is *Brodmann's map*. On the basis of histologic studies, Brodmann developed a map of 47 different areas of the cerebral cortex (Figure 3-11) and classified them as primary function areas or association areas.

Primary function areas are those in which the movement or perception of movement occurs. *Association areas* surround the primary function areas. They provide higher levels of integration (i.e., memory, learning) for sensory experiences.

The *frontal lobe* is located in the anterior fossa and extends from the anterior portion of each hemisphere to the central sulcus (fissure of Rolando) posteriorly. The inferior border is the lateral cerebral fissure (fissure of Sylvius). The frontal lobe controls psychic and higher intellectual functions. It also contains higher-level centers for autonomic functioning, such as cardiovascular responses and gastrointestinal activity. Broca's area, which assists in the formation of words, is also located in the frontal lobe.

The *parietal lobe* is located in the middle fossa in the area between the central sulcus (fissure of Rolando) and the parieto-occipital fissure. The major functions of the parietal lobe are position sense, touch, and motor movement.

The *occipital lobe* is a pyramidal structure in the middle fossa, behind the parieto-occipital fissure and just above the cerebellum. The occipital lobe contains the primary vision centers (primary vision cortex).

The *temporal lobe* also is located in the middle fossa. It lies inferior to the lateral cerebral fissure (fissure of Sylvius) and extends posteriorly to the parieto-occipital fissure. Primary functions of the temporal lobe are memory storage and hearing. Wernicke's area, the auditory association area, is found in the temporal lobe.

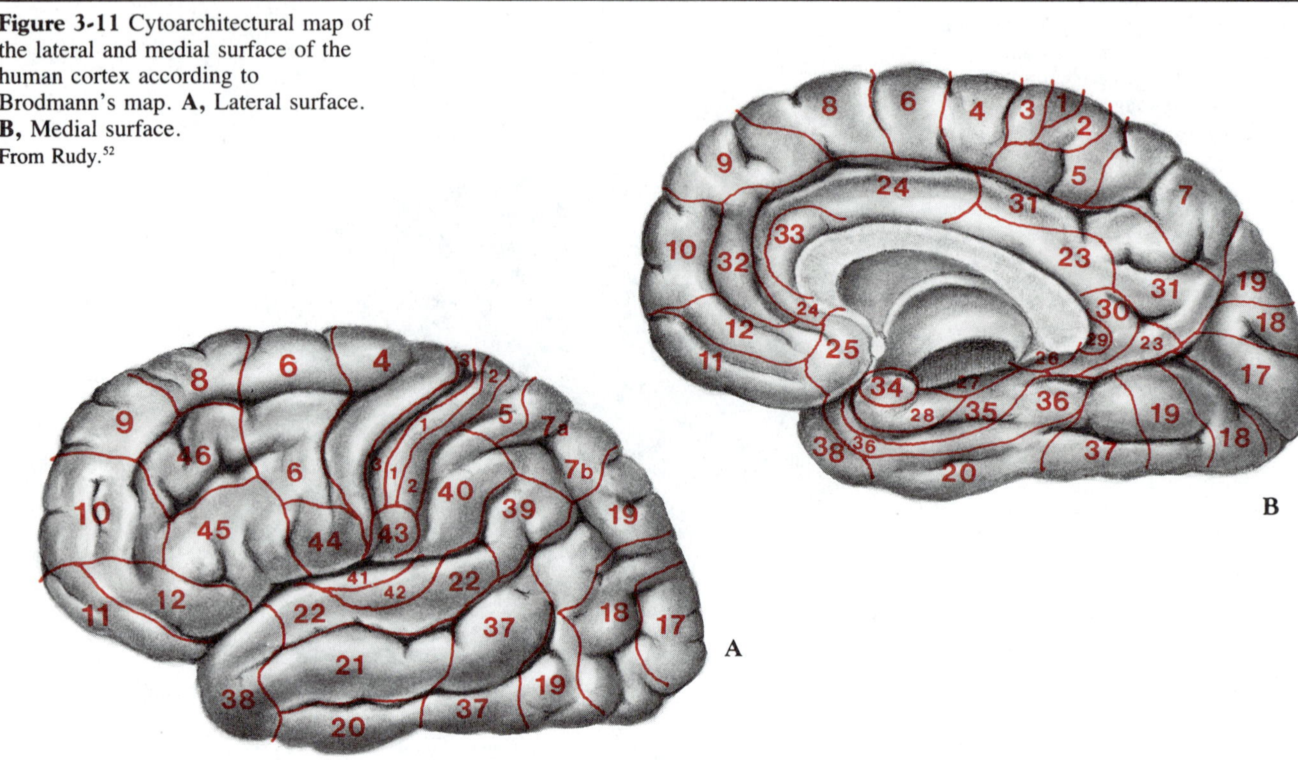

Figure 3-11 Cytoarchitectural map of the lateral and medial surface of the human cortex according to Brodmann's map. **A,** Lateral surface. **B,** Medial surface.
From Rudy.[52]

The *rhinencephalon* (limbic lobe) is anatomically part of the temporal lobe but has different functions. It consists of cortical and subcortical structures that form the border of the lateral ventricles of each cerebral hemisphere. The functions of the rhinencephalon involve self-preservation, visceral activities, instincts, feeling states, and moods.

The *basal ganglia* are gray nuclei located deep within the white matter of each cerebral hemisphere. They consist of the paired anatomic structures of the lenticular nucleus, caudate nucleus, amygdaloid body, and claustrum. The lenticular and caudate nuclei together are called the corpus striatum. Functions include motor control of fine body movements, particularly in the hands and lower extremities.

The internal capsule, located in the thalamic-hypothalamic area, is a massive bundle of white matter. It consists of afferent and efferent fiber tracts that transmit impulses from the cerebrum to the brainstem and spinal cord.

The oval *diencephalon* forms the rostral (toward the head) end of the brainstem and consists of gray matter.[34] The diencephalon contains pathways for visceral, sensory, somatic, and motor impulses and consists of the epithalamus, thalamus, hypothalamus, and subthalamus. The epithalamus, located in the most dorsal aspect of the diencephalon, is made of the pineal body, habenula, habenular commissure, posterior commissure, and striae medullares. The pineal body is the most important structure of the epithalamus and is composed primarily of neuroglia cells. It plays a role in growth and sexual development. The thalamus consists of two connected oval masses of gray matter in the dorsal portion of the diencephalon. Each half of the thalamus is located deep within the corresponding cerebral hemisphere.[34] The thalamus functions as a relay and integration station for cerebral, cerebellar, and brainstem activity. The hypothalamus lies inferior to the thalamus, forming the floor and portions of the walls of the third ventricle. Functions of the hypothalamus are indicated in Table 3-1. The subthalamus is situated between the tegmentum of the midbrain and the dorsal aspect of the thalamus. Its functions are part of the extrapyramidal system of the autonomic nervous system.

Cerebellum. The cerebellum (Figure 3-12) is approximately one fifth the size of the cerebrum and consists of two lateral hemispheres and a medial portion, the *vermis*. It is separated from the cerebrum by the tentorium cerebelli. The cerebellum has an outer cortex of gray matter and an internal medulla of white matter. Embedded deep within the white matter are four pairs of nuclei: dentate, emboliform, globose, and fastigial. The midbrain connects the cerebellum to the cerebral cortex. The cerebellum attaches on each side of the brainstem by three large bundles of nerve fibers, the *cerebellar peduncles*. The cerebellum also connects with the semicircular canals, or organs of balance. It is involved primarily in coordinating movement, equilibrium, muscle tone, and position sense. Each of the cerebellar hemispheres controls movement coordination for the same side of the body (ipsilateral).

Neuroanatomic Classification	Functional Classification	Principal Connections: Afferent Fibers	Principal Connections: Efferent Fibers	General Functions
Anterior nuclei				
Anteromedial	Nonspecific projection	From hypothalamus via mammillothalamic tract (of Vicq d'Azyr); higher-order olfactory neurons	To cingulate gyrus of cerebral cortex	Part of circuit involved in limbic system, convey olfactory impulses
Anterodorsal	Nonspecific projection			
Anteroventral	Nonspecific projection			
Midline nuclei				
Cell groups beneath lining of wall, third ventricle	Nonspecific projection	From spinothalamic, trigeminothalamic tracts, medial lemniscus, reticular formation, other thalamic nuclei, hypothalamus	To hypothalamus and cortex (few to anterior rhinencephalon); basal ganglia (?); other thalamic nuclei	Center for integrating crude visceral and somatic sensations
Massa intermedia	Nonspecific projection			
Medial nuclei				
Scattered cells in internal medullary lamina (intralaminar nuclei)	Nonspecific projection	From prefrontal cortex, septal areas, basal ganglia, and other thalamic nuclei	To prefrontal cortex	Integrate somatic and visceral sensory impulses before projecting information to cortex; association center for synthesis of crude somatic sensations
Dorsomedial	Nonspecific projection	From thalamic nuclei, prefrontal cortex, basal ganglia	To prefrontal cortex	
Centromedian	Nonspecific projection	From putamen, caudate nucleus, other thalamic nuclei	To basal ganglia, other thalamic nuclei (?)	Intrathalamic integrating center (?)
Lateral nuclei				
Anterior ventral	Nonspecific projection	From globus pallidus via thalamic fasciculus	To corpus striatum; cortex (frontal lobe)	Part of circuit involved in voluntary motor functions
Lateral ventral	Specific projection	From cerebellum via superior cerebellar peduncle; globus pallidus via thalamic fasciculus	To cerebral cortex (premotor areas) via posterior limb of internal capsule	Relays sensory impulses from trunk and limbs*
Posterolateral ventral	Specific projection	Termination of spinothalamic tracts, medial lemniscus	To sensory areas of cortex (postcentral gyrus) via posterior limb of internal capsule	
Posteromedial ventral	Specific projection	Termination of secondary trigeminal and taste fibers		Relays sensory impulses from face†
Dorsal lateral	Specific projection	From other thalamic nuclei; parietal lobe of cerebral cortex	To cerebral cortex (parietal lobe)	Primary sensory relay nuclei
Posterior lateral	Specific projection			Functions controversial
Reticular	Nonspecific projection	From entire cerebral cortex, other thalamic nuclei, reticular formation of brainstem	To other thalamic nuclei, tegmentum of midbrain	
Posterior nuclei				
Pulvinar	Specific projection	From other thalamic nuclei, cerebral cortex (parietal, temporal, occipital lobes)	To cerebral cortex (parietal, temporal, occipital lobes)	Integrates auditory, visual, somatic impulses (?)
Medial geniculate†	Specific projection	From brachium of inferior colliculus	To auditory cortex via sublenticular portion of internal capsule (bilateral projection)	Audition
Lateral geniculate†	Specific projection	From optic tract (cranial nerve II)	To ipsilateral striate cortex via retrolenticular portion of internal capsule	Vision

From Jensen.[34]

*The posterolateral ventral and posteromedial ventral nuclei of the thalamus are of major physiologic significance, since these structures provide the principal thalamic relay system for somesthetic afferent fibers.

†The medial and lateral geniculate bodies sometimes are classed together as the *metathalamus*.

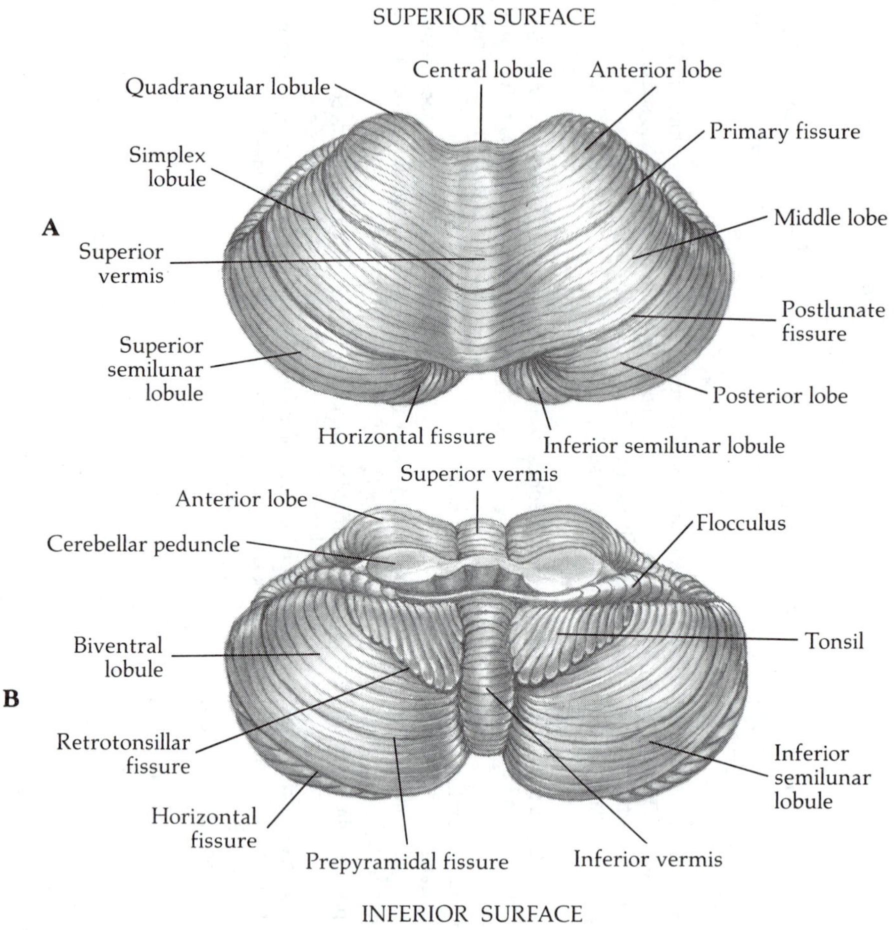

Figure 3-12 Cerebellum. **A,** Superior surface. **B,** Inferior surface.

Brainstem. The brainstem (Figure 3-13) consists of the midbrain (mesencephalon), the pons, and the medulla oblongata. The overall functions of the brainstem are to maintain involuntary reflexes for vital functioning of the body.

The *midbrain* (mesencephalon) forms a junction between the diencephalon and the pons. The lower surface contains two bundles of fibers, crura cerebri, which are made of the corticospinal, corticopontine, and corticobulbar tracts of the voluntary nervous system carrying descending motor fiber tracts from the cerebral cortex to the pons. The upper surface of the midbrain consists of four rounded elevations called the corpora quadrigemina. The rostral pair of elevations is the superior colliculi (eye tracking), and the caudal pair is the inferior colliculi (auditory reflexes). The major function of the midbrain is to relay stimuli dealing with muscle movement, visual reflexes, and auditory reflexes from the spinal cord, medulla oblongata, and cerebellum and to the cerebrum.

The *pons* (metencephalon; Figure 3-13) connects the midbrain to the medulla oblongata and relays impulses to the brain centers and to the lower spinal centers of the nervous system. Sensory and motor nuclei of the trigeminal (cranial V), abducens (cranial VI), facial (cranial VII), and acoustic (cranial VIII) nerves originate in the pons. The corticobulbar and corticospinal tracts make up the white matter of the pons.

The *medulla oblongata* (myelencephalon; Figure 3-13) contains the reflex centers for controlling involuntary functions such as breathing, sneezing, swallowing, coughing, salivation, vomiting, and vasoconstriction. The medulla also provides points of origin for the glossopharyngeal (cranial IX), vagus (cranial X), spinal accessory (cranial XI), and hypoglossal (cranial XII) nerves.

Reticular formation. The reticular formation is a scattered, interconnected complex of sensory nerve fibers extending from the upper spinal cord through the midventral portion of the medulla, pons, midbrain, and diencephalon. Located in the reticular formation are centers that regulate respiration, blood pressure, heart rate (medulla), and vegetative functions (Figure 3-14).

Reticular activating system. The reticular activating system (RAS) is a polysynaptic, nonspecific sensory pathway considered to be an integral regulatory center of the central nervous system. It extends from the superior level of the

Figure 3-13 Brainstem. **A,** Posterior view. **B,** Lateral view.

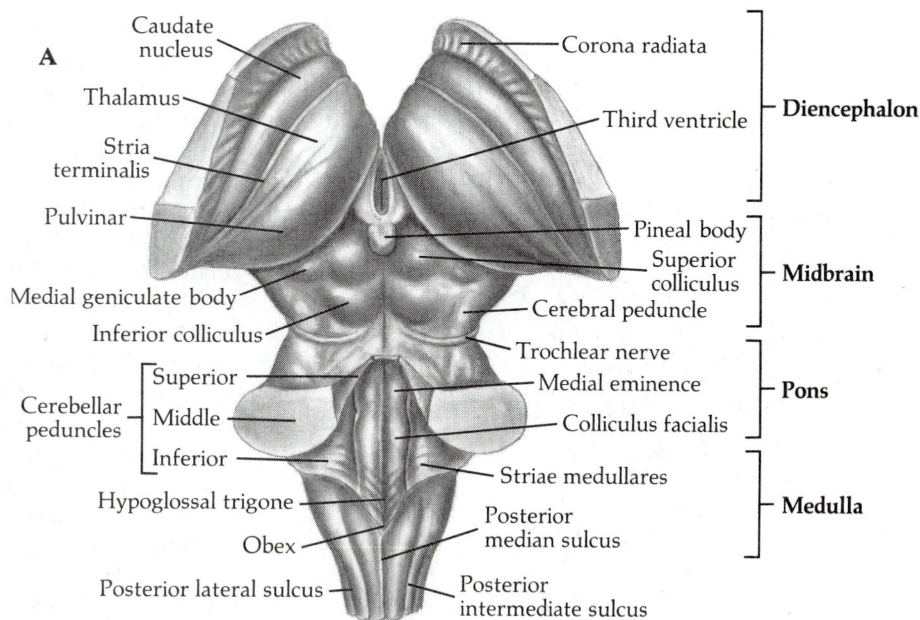

brainstem to the cerebral cortex. Most of the RAS is excitatory and is involved in maintaining attention, the sleep-awake cycle, regulation of visceral functions such as respiration and vasomotor tone, consciousness, perception of sensory input, regulation of temperature, emotional states, learning, conditioned reflexes, and regulation of skeletal muscle tone and activity.[34]

Spinal vertebrae. The vertebral column (Figure 3-15, *A*) is made up of 33 vertebrae divided into five anatomic and functional regions: cervical, thoracic, lumbar, sacral, and coccygeal. Vertebrae are joined together by numerous ligaments and intervertebral discs that provide strength and flexibility.

There are seven *cervical* vertebrae. C1 is a highly developed vertebra called the atlas because it supports the head. The atlas is different from other cervical vertebrae because it does not have a vertebral body or spinous process. C2, called the axis, forms a pivot on which the skull and atlas rotate. The axis also is different in that its vertebral body has a perpendicular toothlike projection, the odontoid process, on which the atlas articulates.

The 12 *thoracic* vertebrae progressively enlarge as they descend. The thoracic vertebral body is made of four costal facets, two inferior and two superior, that provide articulation for the heads of the ribs. Because of rib articulation, the vertebral column is least free for movement and rotation in the thoracic region.

The five *lumbar* vertebrae allow great freedom of movement. L5 and the base of the sacrum together form the lumbosacral angle.

The *sacrum* in the adult is a wedge-shaped bone formed by the fusion of the five sacral vertebrae. The sacral canal, containing the cauda equina and filum terminale, originates in this region.

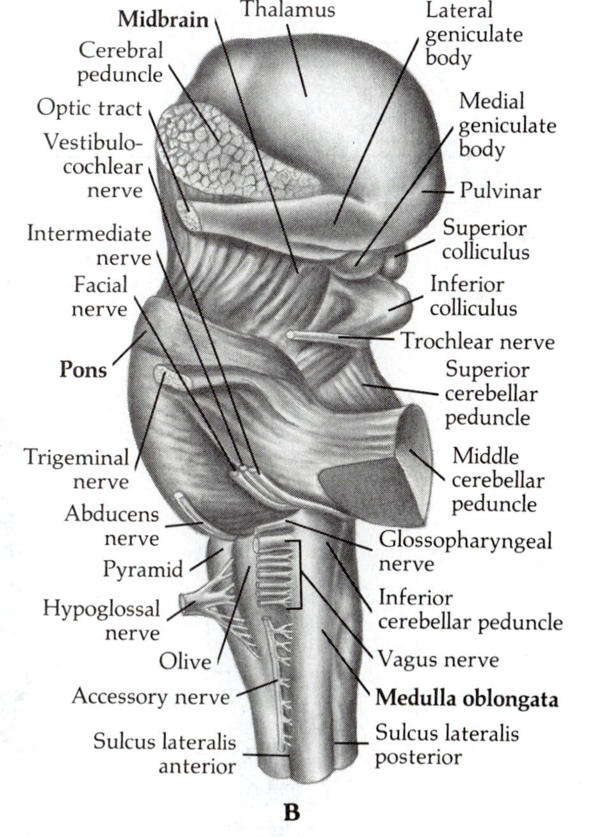

Figure 3-14 Reticular activating system.

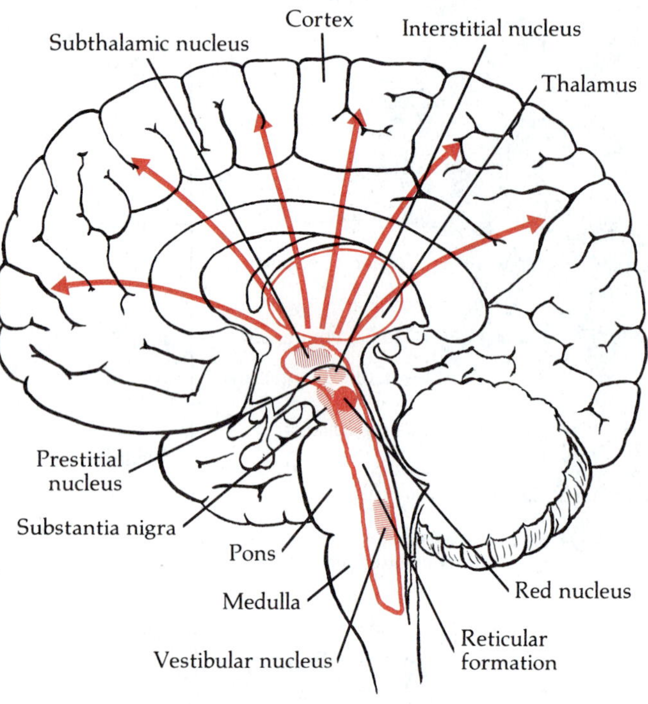

The *coccyx* in the adult is also a fused bone consisting of three to five coccygeal vertebrae.

The typical vertebra (Figure 3-15, *B*) found in the cervical, thoracic, lumbar, or sacral regions has several important anatomic characteristics. The vertebral body is the cylindric weight-bearing ventral portion. It is separated from the vertebral bodies above and below it by cartilage and fibrous tissue called intervertebral discs. The dorsal portion of the vertebra is the vertebral arch, which is formed by two laminae and two pedicles. In the center of the vertebra is the vertebral foramen. In conjunction with other vertebrae, it forms the vertebral canal containing the spinal cord and spinal meninges. The vertebral notch forms a part of the vertebral foramen from which spinal nerves and blood vessels exit the spinal cord. Finally, the vertebral processes (one spinous, two transverse, two superior articular, and two inferior articular) are sites for attachment of muscles and ligaments and for articulation with adjacent vertebrae.

Protective structures: meninges. The spinal cord, like the brain, is enveloped by the three layers of meninges: dura mater, arachnoid, and pia mater. Between the lining of the vertebral canal and the spinal dura mater is the epidural space. The epidural space contains areolar tissue, fat, and a number of venous plexuses. Adjacent to the epidural space is the spinal dura mater. The spinal dura mater extends from the

Figure 3-15 Vertebral column and anatomic structure of vertebrae.
From Rudy.[52]

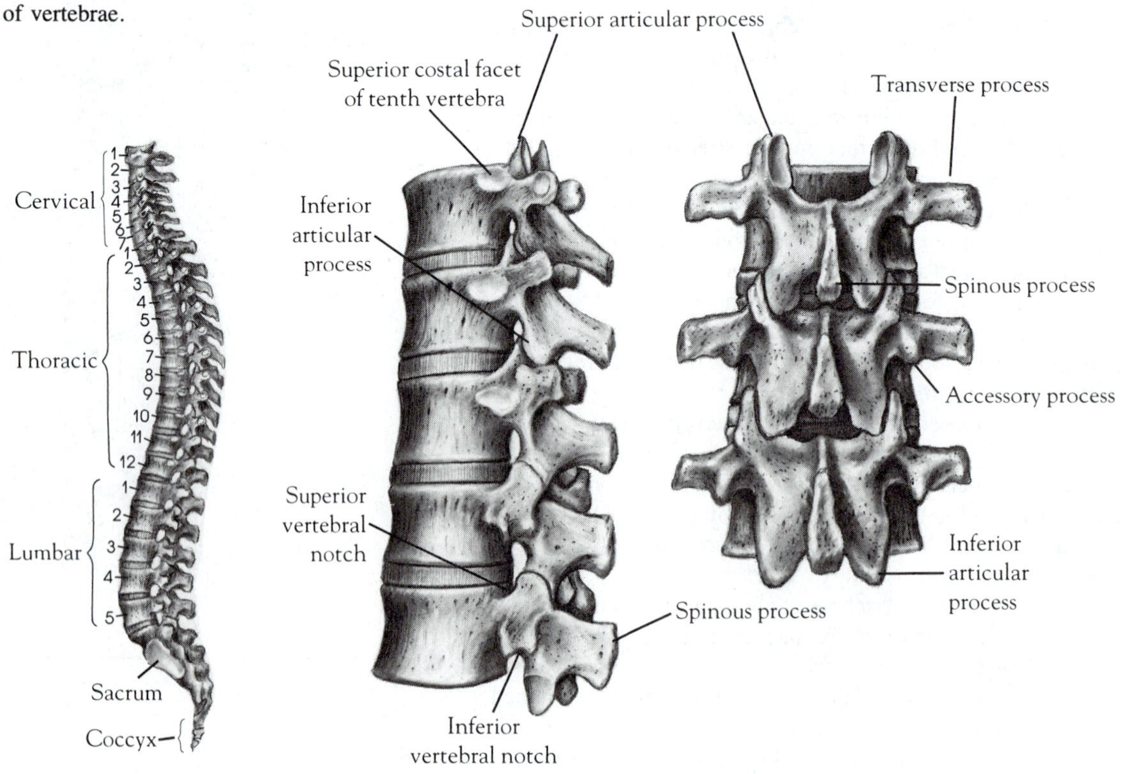

foramen magnum, where it is continuous with the cranial dura, to the second sacral vertebra, where it blends with the filum terminale. Laterally, the dura continues over the roots of the spinal nerves, forming dural root sleeves. Between the dura mater and the intermediate meningeal layer is the subdural space. The subdural space contains a small amount of fluid, which decreases friction between opposing surfaces.

The second meningeal layer, the spinal arachnoid, extends superiorly from the foramen magnum, to the inferior surfaces of the cauda equina and filum terminale. Laterally, the spinal arachnoid encloses the spinal nerve roots to the point of exit from the vertebral canal. The space between the arachnoid and the pia mater is the subarachnoid space, which contains cerebrospinal fluid.

The innermost layer, the spinal pia mater, extends downward to the filum terminale, where it is connected by the denticulate ligaments to the spinal dura mater between the ventral and dorsal spinal nerve roots.

Spinal cord. The spinal cord (Figure 3-16) originates at the foramen magnum and ends at the superior border of L2. It is a continuation from the medulla oblongata. The cord tapers in the lower thoracic area into a cone-shaped structure called the *conus medullaris*. Extending inferiorly from the conus medullaris is a thin prolongation, the *filum terminale,* that anchors the spinal cord to the coccyx. The spinal cord consists of 31 segments, each giving rise to a pair of spinal nerves.

Microscopically, the spinal cord consists of gray (unmyelinated) and white (myelinated) matter. The *gray matter* integrates the cord reflexes and is concentrated into an internal core. When this internal core is viewed in cross section, it resembles a butterfly (Figure 3-17). The paired gray matter projections forming the front "wings" of the butterfly are the anterior, or ventral, horns. The pair of projections forming the back "wings" is called the posterior, or dorsal, horns. The ventral horn consists of multipolar neuron structures (e.g.,

Figure 3-16 Spinal cord within vertebral canal and exiting spinal nerves. **A,** Posterior view of brainstem and spinal cord in situ with spinal nerves and plexuses. **B,** Anterior view of brainstem and spinal cord. **C,** Lateral view showing relationship of spinal cord to vertebrae. **D,** Enlargement of caudal area showing termination of spinal cord (conus medullaris) and group of nerve fibers constituting the cauda equina.
From Rudy.[52]

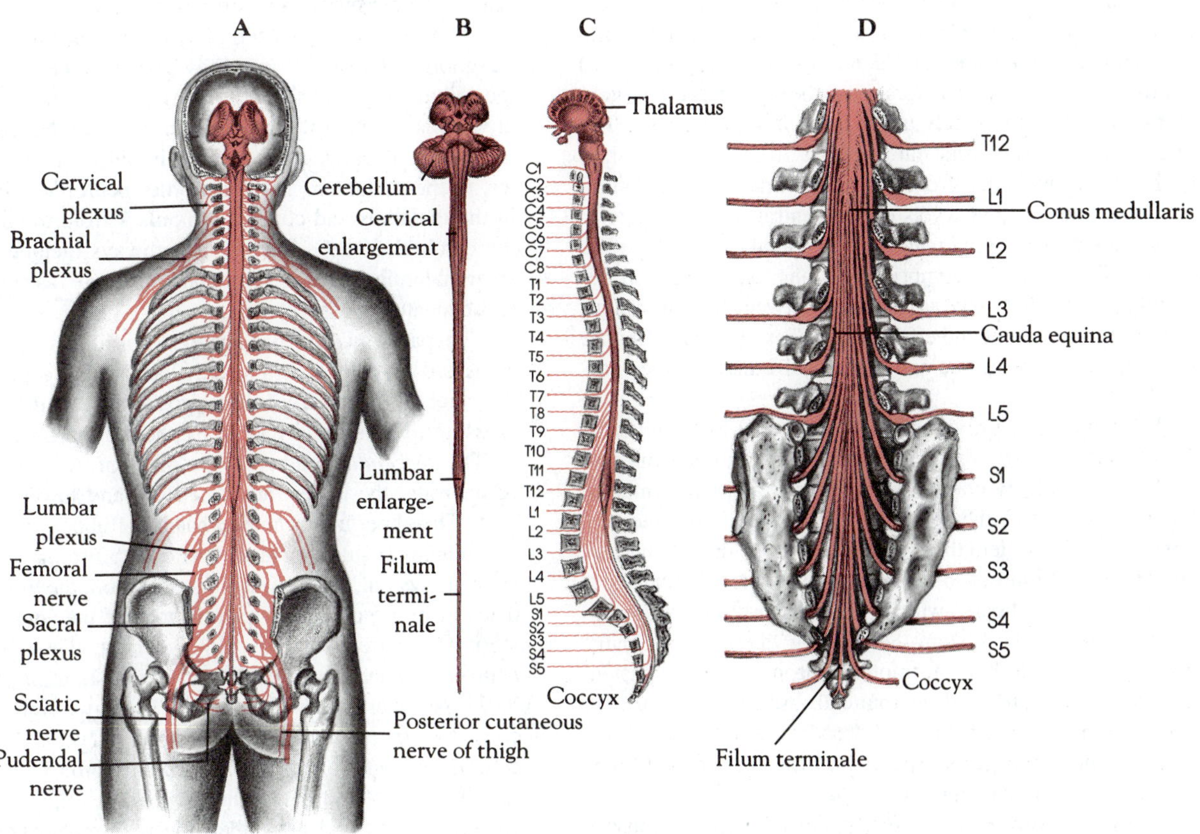

Figure 3-17 Cross section of spinal cord illustrating subdivisions of white and gray matter.
From Rudy.[52]

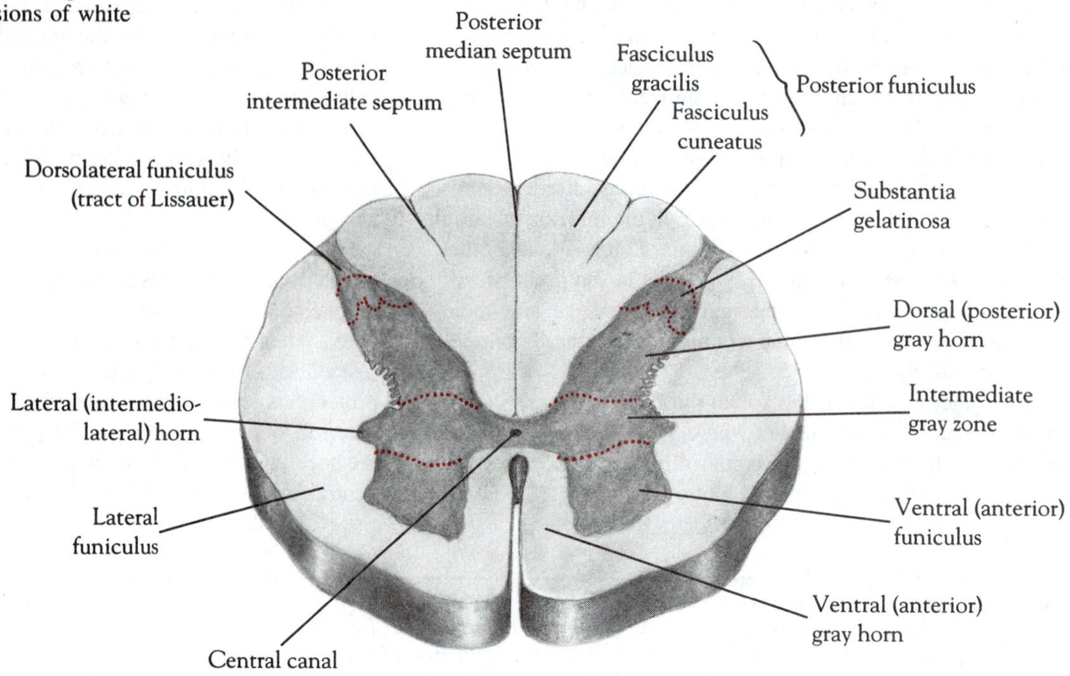

cell bodies, dendrites) that together form the motor efferent neurons of the ventral roots and spinal nerves. The dorsal horn contains cell bodies and dendrites of sensory (afferent) neurons and sensory receptors from the periphery. The gray matter also contains internuncial (association) neurons. The internuncial neurons transmit impulses from one lateral half of the cord to the other, from the dorsal portions to the ventral portions, and to other levels of the central nervous system.

Surrounding the gray matter of the spinal cord is the *white matter* (Figure 3-17), comprised of long ascending and descending tracts that serve as pathways between the spinal cord and brain for afferent and efferent impulses. The white matter is grouped into anatomic and functional bundles called fasciculi.

The spinal cord is divided into lateral halves by the *anterior fissure* and the *posterior sulcus*. Each lateral half is connected to the other half by commissures of gray and white matter. Each lateral half of the spinal cord is divided into three sections that run the length of the spinal cord: dorsal, lateral, and ventral. Within each of these divisions are distinct fiber tracts: ascending fibers, which bring sensory information to the central nervous system; descending fibers, which carry impulses from the brain to motor neurons of the brainstem and the spinal cord; and internuncial (association) neurons, which form short ascending and descending tracts that travel between spinal segments. These short tracts are called intersegmental tracts or pathways.

The neurons in the *ascending* pathways transmit sensory information from peripheral receptors to the spinal cord and brain. The sensory chain consists of a three-neuron pathway. The first-order neuron's cell body originates in the dorsal root ganglion and conducts impulses from peripheral receptors to the spinal cord. The second-order neuron's cell body is found at various levels of the gray matter of the spinal cord and the brainstem. These neurons conduct impulses, in the white matter, to the thalamus. The third-order neuron's cell body lies in the thalamus and conducts impulses from the thalamus to the cerebral cortex. Ascending pathways include the lateral spinothalamic, ventral spinothalamic, and fasciculi gracilis and cuneatus.

The pathways are organized according to body surface areas and cross in the brain so that sensory information enters the cerebral cortex from the opposite side of the body. This crossing over is usually done by the second-order neuron.

The *descending* pathways are made of two principal types of neurons, the upper motor neurons and lower motor neurons. The upper motor neuron has its cell body in the cerebral motor areas or subcortical areas (i.e., brainstem) of the central nervous system. It transmits impulses from the brain to motor neurons in the anterior (ventral) horn of the spinal cord and to motor neurons in the cranial nerves. The lower motor neuron begins in the central nervous system and terminates in the peripheral nervous system. The lower motor neurons consist of motor nuclei of the cranial nerves and the motor cells in the anterior horn of the spinal cord. The two major subdivisions of the descending pathways originate from the cerebral cortex and are called the pyramidal and extrapyramidal tracts.

Figure 3-18 Schematic drawing to show decussation of pyramids at level of medulla.
From Rudy.[52]

Figure 3-19 Extrapyramidal descending tracts. Upper motor neurons originate below level of cortex and converge on lower motor neurons (final common pathway) along with upper motor neurons of pyramidal tracts. Rubrospinal tract originates in red area.

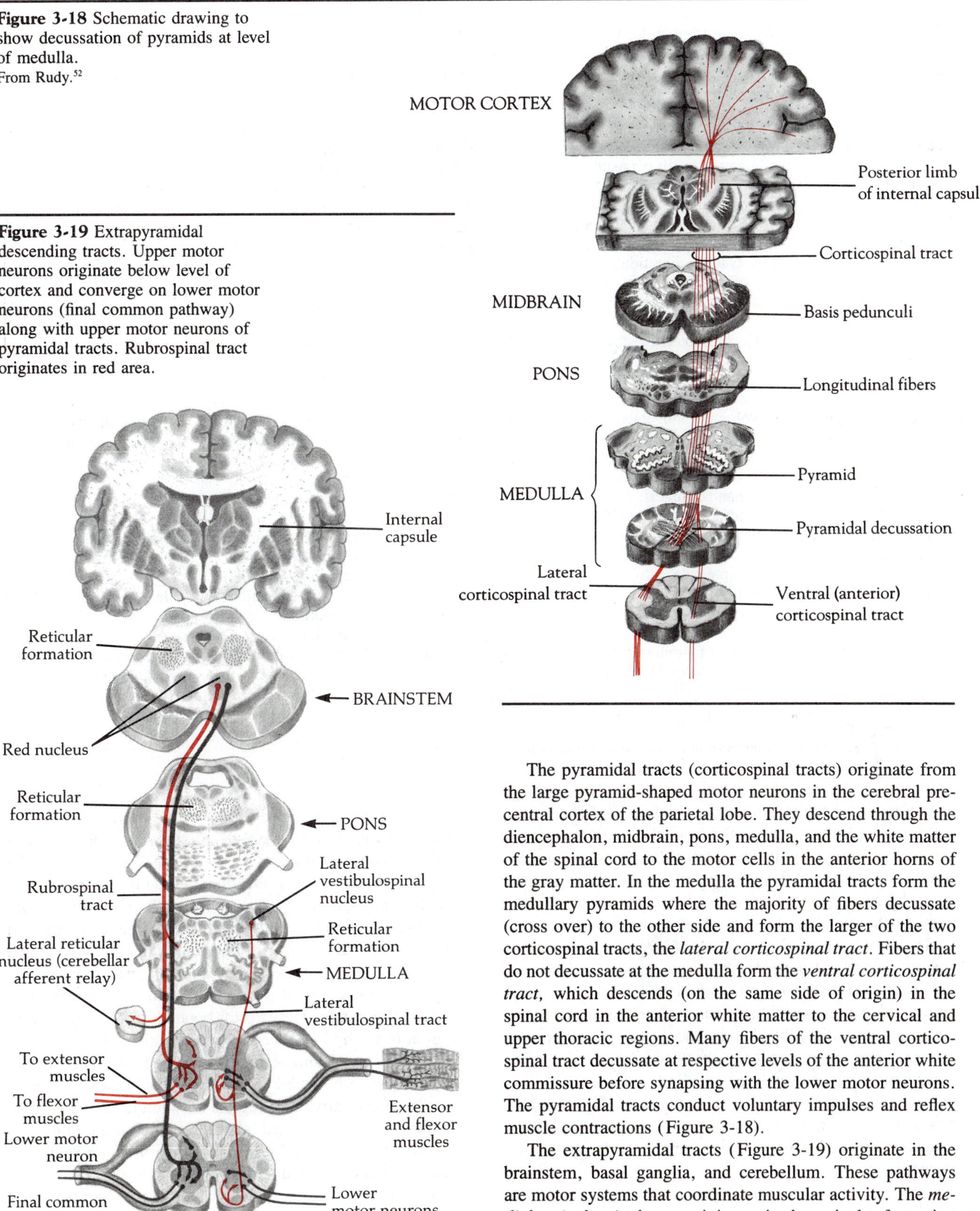

The pyramidal tracts (corticospinal tracts) originate from the large pyramid-shaped motor neurons in the cerebral precentral cortex of the parietal lobe. They descend through the diencephalon, midbrain, pons, medulla, and the white matter of the spinal cord to the motor cells in the anterior horns of the gray matter. In the medulla the pyramidal tracts form the medullary pyramids where the majority of fibers decussate (cross over) to the other side and form the larger of the two corticospinal tracts, the *lateral corticospinal tract*. Fibers that do not decussate at the medulla form the *ventral corticospinal tract,* which descends (on the same side of origin) in the spinal cord in the anterior white matter to the cervical and upper thoracic regions. Many fibers of the ventral corticospinal tract decussate at respective levels of the anterior white commissure before synapsing with the lower motor neurons. The pyramidal tracts conduct voluntary impulses and reflex muscle contractions (Figure 3-18).

The extrapyramidal tracts (Figure 3-19) originate in the brainstem, basal ganglia, and cerebellum. These pathways are motor systems that coordinate muscular activity. The *medial reticulospinal* tract originates in the reticular formation of the brainstem and descends uncrossed. It stimulates flexor

Table 3-2
Major Ascending and Descending Spinal Cord Tracts

Name	Function	Location	Origin*	Termination†
Ascending				
Lateral spinothalamic	Pain, temperature, and crude touch opposite side	Lateral white columns	Posterior gray column opposite side	Thalamus
Ventral spinothalamic	Crude touch, pain, and temperature	Anterior white columns	Posterior gray column opposite side	Thalamus
Fasciculi gracilis and cuneatus	Discriminating touch and pressure sensations, including vibration, stereognosis, and two-point discrimination; also conscious kinesthesia	Posterior white columns	Spinal ganglia same side	Medulla
Spinocerebellar	Unconscious kinesthesia	Lateral white columns	Posterior gray column	Cerebellum
Descending				
Lateral corticospinal (or crossed pyramidal)	Voluntary movement, contraction of individual or small groups of muscles, particularly those moving hands, fingers, feet, and toes of opposite side	Lateral white columns	Motor areas of cerebral cortex (mainly areas 4 and 6) opposite side from tract location in cord	Intermediate or anterior gray columns
Ventral corticospinal (direct pyramidal)	Same as lateral corticospinal except mainly muscles of same side	Lateral white columns	Motor cortex but on same side as tract location in cord	Intermediate or anterior gray columns
Lateral reticulospinal	Mainly facilitatory influence on motorneurons to skeletal muscles	Lateral white columns	Reticular formation, midbrain, pons, and medulla	Intermediate or anterior gray columns
Medial reticulospinal	Mainly inhibitory influence on motorneurons to skeletal muscles	Anterior white columns	Reticular formation, medulla mainly	Intermediate or anterior gray columns

Modified from Thibodeau.[60]
*Location of cell bodies of neurons from which axons of tract arise.
†Structure in which axons of tract terminate.

responses and inhibits extensor responses. The *lateral reticulospinal* tract also originates from the brainstem and is primarily uncrossed. The lateral tract stimulates extensor responses and inhibits flexor responses to maintain posture. Table 3-2 summarizes the principal ascending and descending tracts of the spinal cord and their respective functions.

The *extrapyramidal system* is a functional unit, not an anatomic one, and depends on an intact pyramidal system. This system consists of extrapyramidal areas of the cerebral cortex, the corpus striatum, thalamic nuclei connected to the corpus striatum, the subthalamus, and the rubral and reticular systems. The extrapyramidal system coordinates associated movements and changes in posture and integrates functions of the autonomic nervous system.[34] The system has fibers that originate from the cerebral cortex and project to the basal ganglia. The basal ganglia of the extrapyramidal system act to coordinate movement.

Reflexes

The reflex arc (Figure 3-20) is the basic functional unit that maintains body integrity by automatically conducting impulses from sensory receptors (afferent) to efferent neurons. In the reflex arc or loop a sensory nerve ending is stimulated and then conveys the impulse via sensory (afferent) neurons to gray matter nuclei in the spinal cord. In the gray matter the afferent neuron may synapse directly with lower motor neurons, or it may synapse with one or more internuncial (association) neurons, which transfer the impulse to the lower motor neuron. The lower motor neurons (efferent) carry the impulse via the ventral roots of the spinal cord to the neuroeffector junction. The effector organ then responds to stimulation (e.g., by muscle contraction or glandular secretion). An example of a simple reflex involving only two neurons and one synapse is the knee-jerk (patellar) reflex. When the knee is tapped, afferent receptors are stimulated and send the impulse to the spinal cord. In the spinal cord the impulse is directly relayed to the lower motor neuron. As a result, the quadriceps muscles contract and jerk the leg.

Unlike the knee-jerk reflex, which is the only monosynaptic reflex in the body, most reflex pathways involve numerous synaptic connections (polysynaptic). Reflex response time increases proportionately with the number of synapses.

Figure 3-20 Three-neuron reflex arc.

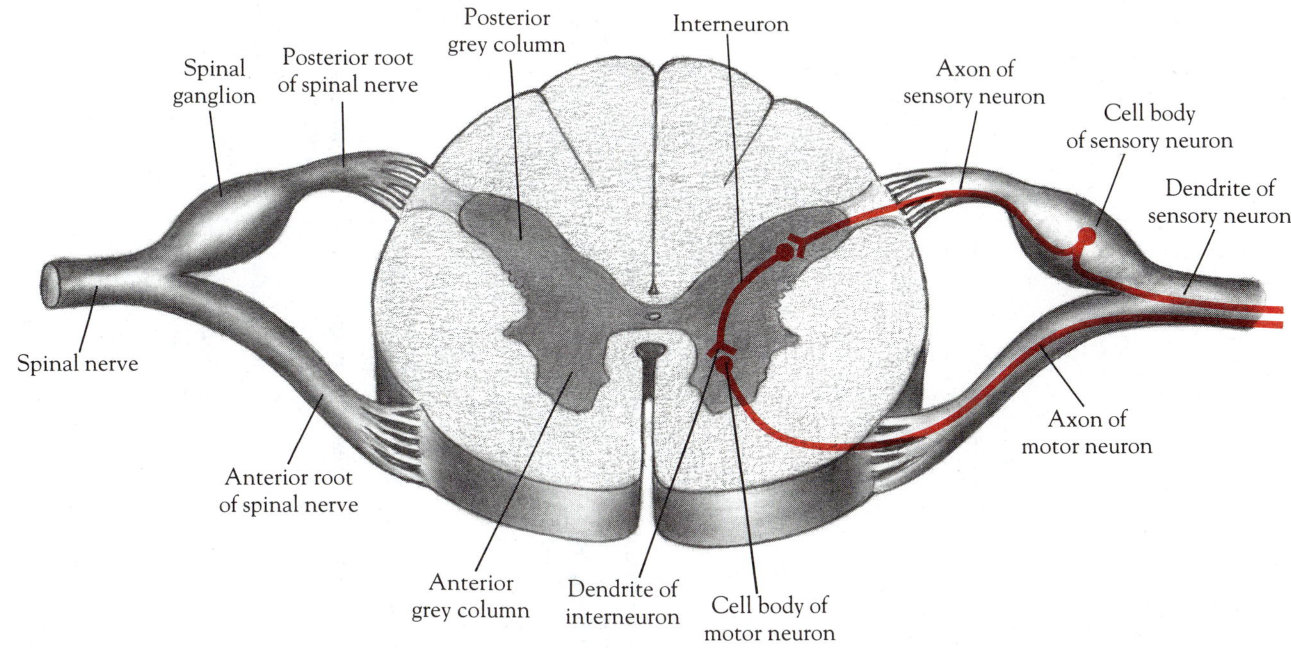

Some reflexes involve only one half of the body (e.g., flexor reflex) and are called ipsilateral reflexes. Other reflexes cross over, eliciting responses on the opposite side of the body (e.g., crossed extensor reflex). These are called contralateral reflexes. For example, when someone steps on a tack, there is a reflex flexion in one leg to move away from the tack, while in the opposite leg there is extension to maintain body balance.

Finally, both the brain and the spinal cord contain reflex centers that provide important data about level of functioning. Pupillary response, cardioregulatory mechanisms, and the medullary vasomotor mechanisms are all brain reflexes. Reflexes controlled predominantly by the spinal cord include emptying of the bowel and bladder, withdrawal from painful stimuli (known as a nociceptive reflex), increased blood flow to the skin, and stretch reflexes that maintain normal posture and position. Specific reflexes and responses elicited are discussed in the section on normal findings of the neurologic system.

Peripheral Nervous System

Cranial nerves. The 12 pairs of cranial nerves (Table 3-3) form the peripheral nerves of the brain. Some have only motor fibers (five pairs), some have only sensory fibers (three pairs), and the rest (four pairs) have both sensory and motor fibers. The cranial nerves "correspond to the spinal nerves serving common sensation, voluntary control of muscles, and autonomic functions in the head; in addition, they include the mechanism for the special senses of vision, hearing, smell, and taste."[31]

Table 3-3 summarizes origin, functional class, and primary functions of the cranial nerves. Assessment of their functions is in the section on neurologic assessment.

Spinal nerves. The 31 pairs of spinal nerves arise from different segments of the spinal cord. Each pair of spinal nerves is formed by the union of anterior and posterior roots attached to the spinal cord. Each pair of spinal nerves and its corresponding part of the spinal cord constitute a *spinal segment*. Individual spinal segments in turn innervate specific body segments.

Some spinal nerves join at the anterior rami to form a complex network of nerve fibers called a plexus. The *cervical* and *brachial plexuses* provide peripheral nerves for innervation to the upper extremities. The lower extremities are innervated by peripheral nerves from the *lumbar* and *sacral plexuses*. Unlike the cervical and thoracic spinal nerves, the lumbar and sacral nerves do not exit from the intervertebral foramen at right angles. Instead, these nerves extend obliquely and inferiorly and form a large bundle of nerve fibers called the *cauda equina*.

Table 3-4 summarizes the spinal nerves, corresponding plexuses, and peripheral innervation (see also Table 3-5).

Dermatomes. Each spinal nerve root innervates a specific area, or dermatome, of the body surface for superficial or cutaneous sensation. Although there is a great deal of overlap in the spinal nerves, knowledge of the distribution of dermatomes (Table 3-4) is useful for assessment and evaluation purposes.

Table 3-3
Cranial Nerves

Nerve*	Sensory Fibers†			Motor Fibers†		Functions‡
	Receptors	Cell Bodies	Termination	Cell Bodies	Termination	
I Olfactory	*Nasal mucosa*	*Nasal mucosa*	Olfactory bulbs (new relay of neurons of olfactory cortex)			*Sense of smell*
II Optic	*Retina*	*Retina*	*Nucleus in thalamus (lateral geniculate body): some fibers terminate in superior colliculus of midbrain*			*Vision*
III Oculomotor	*External eye muscles except superior oblique and lateral rectus*	?	?	**Midbrain (oculomotor nucleus and Edinger-Westphal nucleus)**	**External eye muscles except superior oblique and lateral rectus; fibers from Edinger-Westphal nucleus terminate in ciliary ganglion and then to ciliary and iris muscles**	**Eye movements, regulation of size of pupil, accommodation,** *proprioception (muscle sense)*
IV Trochlear	*Superior oblique*	?	?	**Midbrain**	**Superior oblique muscle of eye**	
V Trigeminal	*Skin and mucosa of head, teeth*	*Gasserian ganglion*	*Pons (sensory nucleus)*	**Pons (motor nucleus)**	**Muscles of mastication**	**Eye movements,** *proprioception*
VI Abducens	*Lateral rectus*					*Sensations of head and face,* **chewing movements,** *muscle sense*
VII Facial	*Taste buds of anterior two thirds of tongue*	*Geniculate ganglion*	*Medulla (nucleus solitarius)*	**Pons** **Pons**	**Lateral rectus muscle of eye** **Superficial muscles of face and scalp**	**Abduction of eye,** *proprioception* **Facial expressions, secretion of saliva,** *taste*
VIII Acoustic						
1 Vestibular branch	*Semicircular canals and vestibule (utricle and saccule)*	*Vestibular ganglion*	*Pons and medulla (vestibular nuclei)*			*Balance or equilibrium sense*

2 Cochlear or auditory branch	*Organ of Corti in cochlear duct*	*Spiral ganglion*	*Pons and medulla (cochlear nuclei)*			*Hearing*
IX Glossopharyngeal	*Pharynx; taste buds and other receptors of posterior one third of tongue*	*Jugular and petrous ganglia*	*Medulla (nucleus solitarius)*	**Medulla (nucleus ambiguus)**	**Muscles of pharynx**	*Taste and other sensations of tongue,* **swallowing movements, secretion of saliva,** *aid in reflex control of blood pressure and respiration*
	Carotid sinus and carotid body	*Jugular and petrous ganglia*	*Medulla (respiratory and vasomotor centers)*	**Medulla at junction of pons (nucleus salivatorius)**	**Otic ganglion and then to parotid gland**	
X Vagus	*Pharynx, larynx, carotid body, and thoracic and abdominal viscera*	*Jugular and nodose ganglia*	*Medulla (nucleus solitarius), pons (nucleus of fifth cranial nerve)*	**Medulla (dorsal motor nucleus)**	**Ganglia of vagal plexus and then to muscles of pharynx, larynx, and thoracic and abdominal viscera**	*Sensations and* **movements** *or organs supplied; for example,* **slows heart, increases peristalsis, and contracts muscles for voice production**
XI Spinal accessory	?	?	?	**Medulla (dorsal motor nucleus of vagus and nucleus ambiguus)**	**Muscles of thoracic and abdominal viscera and pharynx and larynx**	**Shoulder movements, turning movements of head, movements of viscera, voice productions,** *proprioception?*
				Anterior gray column of first five or six cervical segments of spinal cord	**Trapezius and sternocleidomastoid muscle**	
XII Hypoglossal	?	?	?	**Medulla (hypoglossal nucleus)**	**Muscles of tongue**	**Tongue movements,** *proprioception?*

From Thibodeau.[60]

*The first letters of the words in the following sentence are the first letters of the names of the cranial nerves. Many generations of anatomy students have used this sentence as an aid to memorizing these names. It is "On Old Olympus' Tiny Tops, A Finn and German Viewed Some Hops." (There are several slightly differing versions of this mnemonic.)

†Italics indicate sensory fibers and functions. Boldface type indicates motor fibers and functions.

‡An aid for remembering the general function of each cranial nerve is the following 12-word saying: "Some say marry money but my brothers say bad business marry money." Words beginning with "S" indicate sensory function. Words beginning with "M" indicate motor function. Words beginning with "B" indicate both sensory and motor functions. For example, the first, second, and eighth words in the saying start with "S," which indicates that the first, second, and eighth cranial nerves perform sensory functions.

Table 3-4
Spinal Nerves and Peripheral Branches

Spinal Nerves	Plexuses Formed from Anterior Rami	Spinal Nerve Branches from Plexuses	Parts Supplied
Cervical 1, 2, 3, 4	Cervical plexus	Lesser occipital; Great auricular; Cutaneous nerve of neck; Anterior supraclavicular; Middle supraclavicular; Posterior supraclavicular; Branches to numerous neck muscles	Sensory to back of head, front of neck, and upper part of shoulder, motor to numerous neck muscles
Cervical 5, 6, 7, 8; Thoracic (or dorsal) 1, 2	Brachial plexus	Phrenic (branches from cervical nerves before formation of plexus; most of its fibers from fourth cervical nerve)	Diaphragm
		Suprascapular and dorsoscapular	Superficial muscles* of scapula
		Thoracic nerves, medial and lateral branches	Pectoralis major and minor
		Long thoracic nerve	Serratus anterior
		Thoracodorsal	Latissimus dorsi
		Subscapular	Subscapular and teres major muscles
		Axillary (circumflex)	Deltoid and teres minor muscles and skin over deltoid
		Musculocutaneous	Muscles of front of arm (biceps brachii, coracobrachialis, and brachialis) and skin on outer side of forearm
		Ulnar	Flexor carpi ulnaris and part of flexor digitorum profundus; some of muscles of hand; sensory to medial side of hand, little finger, and medial half of fourth finger
		Median	Rest of muscles of front of forearm and hand; sensory to skin of palmar surface of thumb, index, and middle fingers
		Radial	Triceps muscle and muscles of back of forearm; sensory to skin of back of forearm and hand
		Medial cutaneous	Sensory to inner surface of arm and forearm
Thoracic 3, 4, 5, 6, 7, 8, 9, 10, 11, 12	No plexus formed; branches run directly to intercostal muscles and skin of thorax		
		Iliohypogastric (Sometimes fused)	Sensory to anterior abdominal wall
		Ilioinguinal (Sometimes fused)	Sensory to anterior abdominal wall and external genitalia; motor to muscles of abdominal wall

From Thibodeau.[60]
*Although nerves to muscles are considered motor, they do contain some sensory fibers that transmit proprioceptive impulses.
†Sensory fibers from the tibial and peroneal nerves unite to form the *medial cutaneous* (or sural) *nerve* that supplies the calf of the leg and the lateral surface of the foot. In the thigh the tibial and common peroneal nerves are usually enclosed in a single sheath to form the *sciatic nerve*, the largest nerve in the body with its width of approximately ¾ inch. About two thirds of the way down the posterior part of the thigh, it divides into its component parts. Branches of the sciatic nerve extend into the hamstring muscles.

Autonomic Nervous System

The autonomic nervous system (ANS) is considered part of the peripheral nervous system. It regulates the body's internal environment in close conjunction with the endocrine system. It is responsible for the unconscious moment-to-moment functioning of all internal systems, including visceral organs (e.g., digestive, urogenital), involuntary muscle fibers (e.g., smooth muscle), and glandular functions (e.g., adrenal medulla, islets of Langerhans in the pancreas). The autonomic nervous system is activated by centers in the hypothalamus, brainstem, and spinal cord. It is characterized by a two-neuron chain consisting of a preganglionic neuron and a postganglionic neuron.

Preganglionic neurons have cell bodies in the central ner-

Table 3-4—cont'd
Spinal Nerves and Peripheral Branches

Spinal Nerves	Plexuses Formed from Anterior Rami	Spinal Nerve Branches from Plexuses	Parts Supplied
Lumbar 1, 2, 3, 4, 5; Sacral 1, 2, 3, 4, 5; Coccygeal 1	Lumbosacral plexus	Genitofemoral	Sensory to skin of external genitalia and inguinal region
		Lateral cutaneous of thigh	Sensory to outer side of thigh
		Femoral	Motor to quadriceps, sartorius, and iliacus muscles; sensory to front of thigh and medial side of lower leg (saphenous nerve)
		Obturator	Motor to adductor muscles of thigh
		Tibial† (medial popliteal)	Motor to muscles of calf of leg; sensory to skin of calf of leg and sole of foot
		Common peroneal (lateral popliteal)	Motor to evertors and dorsiflexors of foot; sensory to lateral surface of leg and dorsal surface of foot
		Nerves to hamstring muscles	Motor to muscles of back of thigh
		Gluteal nerves, superior and inferior	Motor to buttock muscles and tensor fasciae latae
		Posterior cutaneous nerve	Sensory to skin of buttocks, posterior surface of thigh, and leg
		Pudendal nerve	Motor to perineal muscles; sensory to skin of perineum

vous system and efferent fibers that terminate in the autonomic ganglia. *Postganglionic* neurons have cell bodies outside the central nervous system in the autonomic ganglia and innervate the target, or effector, organ (e.g., cardiac muscle). The purpose of the postganglionic neuron is to relay impulses beyond the ganglia.

The autonomic nervous system has two major subdivisions (sympathetic and parasympathetic), and both consist of autonomic ganglia and nerves. Generally each effector organ has both sympathetic and parasympathetic innervation. The subdivisions differ in the type of neurotransmitters released, distribution of nerve fibers, and effects on organs innervated, in that the subdivisions produce antagonistic physiologic responses.

The *sympathetic* (thoracolumbar) subdivision is activated during internal and external stress situations (the flight-fight phenomenon). During those stressful situations, sympathetic responses include increases in blood pressure and heart rate and vasoconstriction of peripheral blood vessels. The sympathetic division is also called *adrenergic* because the transmitter substance norepinephrine (noradrenalin) is secreted by its postganglionic nerve terminals.

The preganglionic fibers of the sympathetic system are located in the intermediolateral columns of the thoracic and

Table 3-5
Cranial Nerves Contrasted with Spinal Nerves

	Cranial Nerves	Spinal Nerves
Origin	Base of brain	Spinal cord
Distribution	Mainly to head and neck	Skin, skeletal muscles, joints, blood vessels, sweat glands, and mucosa except of head and neck
Structure	Some composed of sensory fibers only; some of both motor axons and sensory dendrites; some motor fibers belong to somatic nervous system, some to autonomic	All of them composed of both sensory dendrites and motor axons; some of latter somatic, some autonomic
Function	Vision, hearing, sense of smell, sense of taste, eye movements	Sensations, movements, and sweat secretion

From Anthony.[2]

first two lumbar segments in the spinal cord (i.e., T1 to T2); thus this system is sometimes called the thoracolumbar system. After leaving the spinal nerves, the small, myelinated, preganglionic, sympathetic fibers enter the sympathetic trunk via the white ramus. The sympathetic trunk is a chain of ganglions extending from the base of the skull to the coccyx on either side of the spinal cord.

Most axons of sympathetic neurons synapse in the sympathetic trunk or travel up and down the trunk before synapsing. Some axons do not synapse within the sympathetic trunk; instead they exit to synapse in collateral ganglia nearer to the organ of innervation. Acetylcholine is the neurotransmitter at all preganglionic nerve terminals of the sympathetic division. Norepinephrine is the neurotransmitter at all postganglionic nerve terminals of the sympathetic system. Because of the sympathetic chain ganglia, the nerve fibers of the sympathetic system generally have short and long postganglionic fibers. Fibers terminate on two receptor sites (α or β), which determine the effects of the neurotransmitters. β receptors are divided into β and β_2 receptors because some drugs affect some, but not all, β receptors.

The adrenal medulla is a functional extension of the sympathetic nervous system. Its postganglionic neurons are specialized secretory cells. Epinephrine and norepinephrine are secreted by the adrenal medulla at the same time the sympathetic nerves are stimulating afferent organs and have almost the same effect as direct sympathetic stimulation. As a result, body tissues are stimulated simultaneously, directly by the sympathetic nerves and indirectly by the hormones of the adrenal medulla. After their release, the hormones are rapidly metabolized, primarily by the liver. Approximately one half of the catecholamines are excreted in the urine as free or conjugated normetanephrine and metanephrine. Daily normal urinary output of the catecholamines equals approximately 6 mg of epinephrine and 30 mg of norepinephrine.[29,34] Chapter 9 gives further detail on the adrenal medulla and the catecholamines.

The *parasympathetic* (craniosacral) subdivision of the autonomic nervous system consists of preganglionic fibers arising from cell bodies in cranial nerves III, VII, IX, and X, as well as sacral spinal nerves II through VII. This division is activated when an individual is at rest or relaxed, protecting and restoring the body's resources. It works slower than the sympathetic division, has a more discrete effect, and dominates control over the sympathetic subdivision during nonstressful conditions. Parasympathetic fibers in the cranial and sacral nerves form synaptic connections only with terminal ganglia located near the organs innervated. Therefore in the parasympathetic division, preganglionic fibers are long and postganglionic fibers are short. Both preganglionic and postganglionic fibers secrete the neurotransmitter *acetylcholine;* therefore the parasympathetic subdivision is called *cholinergic*.

The organs innervated and effects of stimulation by sympathetic and parasympathetic subdivisions are summarized in Tables 3-4 and 3-5.

Vascular Supply to Brain and Spinal Cord

Maintaining adequate blood supply to the brain and spinal cord is vital for proper functioning of the nervous system. The blood removes metabolic waste products and supplies the cells with nutrients.

Brain. The blood supply to the brain comes principally from two pairs of arteries, the internal carotid and the vertebral arteries. The *internal carotid* arteries arise from the common carotid artery at the level of the thyroid cartilage. They supply approximately 80% of the blood to the brain. The internal carotid arteries then give rise to the anterior and middle cerebral arteries at about the level of the optic chiasm. The *anterior cerebral artery* supplies portions of the medial surfaces of the frontal and parietal lobes, nuclei of the basal ganglia, caudate putamen, and portions of the internal capsule and corpus callosum. The *middle cerebral artery* supplies lateral surfaces of the parietal, frontal, and temporal lobes. It is the major source of blood supply to the precentral (motor) and postcentral (sensory) gyri. The vertebral arteries arise from the right and left *subclavian arteries* and provide the remaining 20% of cerebral blood supply. The vertebral arteries join at the base of the brain and form the basilar artery. The *basilar artery* enters the skull at the foramen magnum and ascends to the midbrain. Branches of the vertebral and basilar arteries supply the brainstem and cerebellum. In the midbrain the basilar artery splits into the pair of *posterior cerebral arteries*. The posterior cerebral arteries supply portions of the temporal and occipital lobes of each hemisphere, the vestibular organs, and the cochlear apparatus. Figure 3-21 illustrates the vessels supplying the brain tissue.

At the base of the brain the cerebral arteries are connected, by their communicating branches, into an arterial circle called the *circle of Willis* (Figure 3-22). More specifically, the posterior cerebral artery is connected to the middle cerebral artery by the posterior communicating branches. The anterior cerebral arteries are connected by the anterior communicating branches. The purpose of the circle of Willis is to ensure circulation if one of the four main blood vessels is interrupted.

Branches of cerebral arteries extend throughout the brain. These branches are called end arteries because they have few branching connections. This lack of branching results in decreased potential for collateral circulation.

Dense networks of capillaries are found in the gray matter of the brain. These capillaries are surrounded by a protective membrane formed by the end-feet of *astrocyte cells*. The capillary blood enters the deep veins, which then empty into the superficial venous plexuses and dural sinuses (principally the superior longitudinal sinus). The venous blood is drained from these sinuses by the internal jugular veins, which return the blood to the general circulation (a small volume of blood drains via the *pterygoid* and ophthalmic venous sinuses).

The anterior, middle, and posterior meningeal arteries provide an abundant blood supply to the cranial meninges.

Spinal cord. The arterial blood supply to the spinal cord comes from three main vessels: the one spinal artery and the two radicular arteries. The *spinal artery* arises from branches

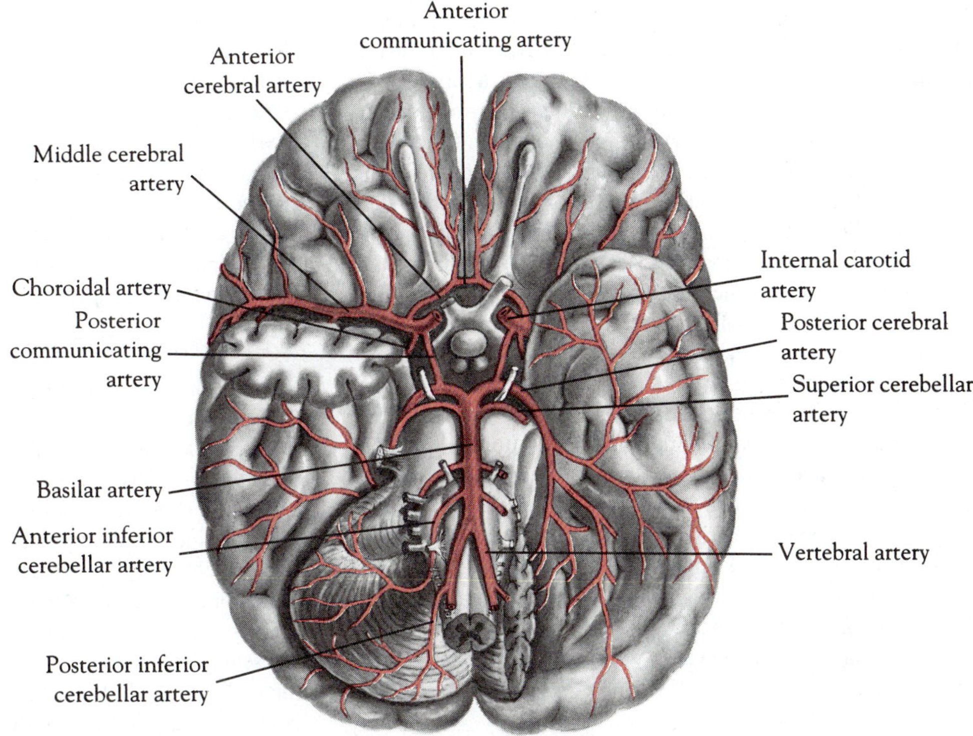

Figure 3-21 Blood supply of the brain.
From Rudy.[52]

of the vertebral arteries at the level of the foramen magnum. It then divides into one anterior and two posterior branches. These branches then enter the vertebral canal with the dorsal and ventral nerve roots. The *radicular* artery arises from the thoracic and abdominal aorta and divides into anterior and posterior branches that enter the spinal cord at the intervertebral foramina. At the spinal segments the radicular arteries connect with the spinal arteries to form an extensive vascular plexus around the entire spinal cord.

The spinal venous system is extensive, with many intradural veins exiting from the ventral median fissure. There also are numerous extradural veins that form a dense venous plexus in the pia mater. Venous blood is drained from the plexus by veins accompanying roots of the spinal nerves.

Figure 3-22 Anatomic diagram of circle of Willis.

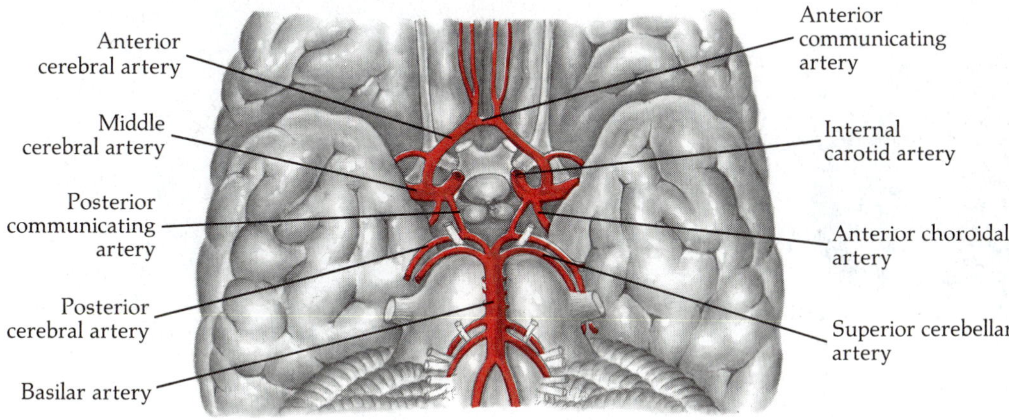

Brain barriers. The neuronal tissues of the brain are extremely sensitive to any changes in the ionic concentration of their environment. Therefore the composition of the brain's internal environment must be delicately balanced to ensure normal functioning. The *blood-brain barrier* is a physiologic mechanism that helps maintain and protect this homeostatic balance by way of selective capillary permeability. Since substances from the blood enter the brain either through capillaries into the cerebrospinal fluid or through capillaries into the extracellular fluid, there are actually two barrier mechanisms. The blood-brain and blood-cerebrospinal barriers function together to protect the neuronal brain tissue. The complex of intermembranes that form these barriers is found in most regions of brain parenchyma, the choroid plexus, and the vasculature of the brain. Unlike most capillaries in the body, these capillaries are surrounded by astrocyte end-feet that form tight junctions of the endothelial cells. It is thought the tight junctions and glial end-feet affect capillary permeability. Both the blood-brain and blood-cerebrospinal barriers are permeable to oxygen, carbon dioxide, and water. They are slightly permeable to electrolytes (e.g., Na^+, K^+, Cl^-) but are impermeable to fixed acids and bases and many drugs. These barriers develop in the postnatal period; thus the cerebral capillaries of the newborn are far more permeable than those of the adult.

Cerebral Ventricular System

The cerebral ventricular system is a series of four ependymal-lined cavities (Figure 3-23). The ventricles are interconnecting structures that originate from the single cavity of the embryonic neural tube. The two largest cavities, the lateral ventricles, are located within each cerebral hemisphere. Each lateral ventricle consists of a body and anterior (frontal), inferior (temporal), and posterior (occipital) horns. The lateral ventricles in each hemisphere are separated from each other by a thin layer called the septum pellucidum. Each of these ventricles communicates, via the interventricular foramen of Monro, with a central cavity. This central cavity is the third ventricle, which is a small cleft space between the thalamic structures of the diencephalon. In the midbrain the third ventricle communicates with the fourth ventricle via the aqueduct of Sylvius. The rhomboid fourth ventricle is located posterior to the pons and anterior to the cerebellum, extending down to the central canal of the upper cervical portion of the spinal cord. The fourth ventricle is connected by three foramina to the subarachnoid space.

Cerebrospinal Fluid

Parts of the lateral, third, and fourth ventricular structures are lined with dense networks of capillaries called the *choroid plexus* (tela choroidea). The choroid plexus secretes cerebrospinal fluid (CSF), which is a colorless, clear, and odorless fluid that contains glucose, electrolytes, oxygen, water, carbon dioxide, small amounts of protein, and a few leukocytes. The cerebrospinal fluid removes metabolic wastes, provides nutrition, performs some mechanical function (i.e., shock absorber), and participates in maintaining normal intracranial pressure. In 24 hours the choroid plexuses secrete approximately 500 to 750 ml of cerebrospinal fluid; however, only about 125 to 150 ml is present in the system at any one time.

From the choroid plexuses in the lateral ventricles, the cerebrospinal fluid passes through the foramen of Monro to the third ventricle. From there, it slowly flows through the aqueduct of Sylvius to the fourth ventricle. The fluid then leaves the fourth ventricle through the single medial foramen of Magendie (located in the roof of the fourth ventricle) and the paired foramina of Luschka (located in the lateral portion of the fourth ventricle). After leaving the fourth ventricle, the

Figure 3-23 Cerebral ventricles. **A,** Lateral view. **B,** Superior view.

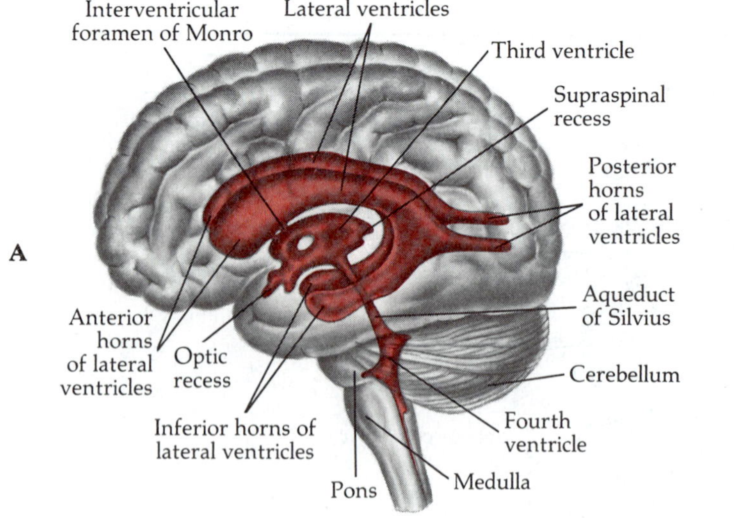

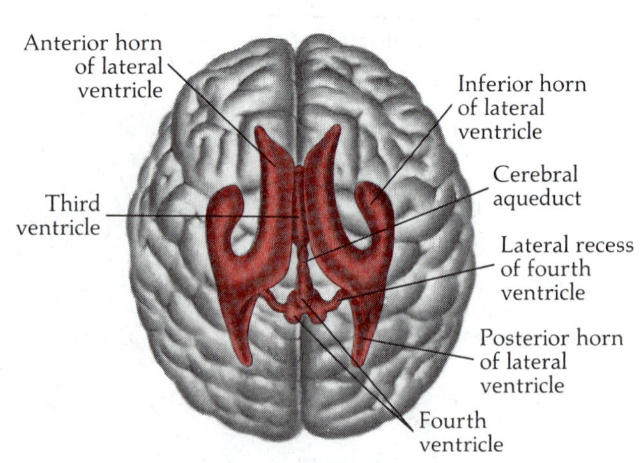

cerebrospinal fluid enters the subarachnoid space, where it fills the spinal cisterns and slowly diffuses upward over the convexities of the brain. The fluid is slowly absorbed from the subarachnoid space by the arachnoid villi, which are clusterlike protrusions extending into the superior sagittal sinus. The cerebrospinal fluid diffuses from the arachnoid villi into the intradural venous sinuses, where it is reabsorbed into the venous system.

Intracranial Pressure: Normal Dynamics

Approximately 88% of the contents of the cranial cavity is brain tissue, 2% is intravascular blood, and the final 10% is cerebrospinal fluid. These three components are the essential elements of intracranial pressure (ICP) dynamics. Intracranial pressure equals the volume of brain tissue (BTV) plus the volume of blood (BV) plus the volume of cerebrospinal fluid (CSFV).

$$ICP = BTV + BV + CSFV$$

The normal intracranial pressure in the recumbent position is about 0 to 15 mm Hg (110 to 140 mm H_2O). Standing decreases intracranial pressure, whereas such activities as sitting, sneezing, coughing, isometric exercises, sexual intercourse, and the Valsalva maneuver cause a transient rise in intracranial pressure. Because the skull limits brain expansion, these activities are normally compensated for by a redistribution of cerebrospinal fluid to the spinal subarachnoid space or by partial collapse of the cisterns and cerebral ventricles. (The skull of a young child is not rigid, so expansion is not so severely limited.)

Another important determinant in the dynamics of intracranial pressure is the autoregulation of cerebral blood flow. This blood flow is generally expressed as cerebral perfusion pressure (CPP) and is maintained by the regulation of resistance vessel diameters. The cerebral perfusion pressure equals the mean arterial blood pressure (MABP) minus the mean intracranial pressure (MICP).

$$CPP = MABP - MICP$$

The normal range of cerebral perfusion pressure is 80 to 100 mm Hg. Cerebral perfusion pressure must be at least 50 mm Hg for the brain to receive an adequate blood supply. To maintain normal cerebral perfusion, the blood vessels constrict or dilate and therefore directly affect intracranial pressure.

The last component in intracranial pressure is the actual brain tissue. The compensatory mechanism of brain tissue displacement or shifting is not usually considered a part of normal dynamics.

Any activity or condition that causes a sustained increase in one of the essential elements listed above must be compensated for by a decrease in one or both of the other two essential elements. This principle is known as the Monro-Kellie doctrine and must be understood in relation to normal dynamics of intracranial pressure as well as pathologic states that lead to increased intracranial pressure.

Variations in Older Adult

Like other systems in the body, the neural structures undergo significant changes as a person ages. Understanding these anatomic and physiologic changes assists the practitioner to establish realistic normative behaviors for the elderly population.

Brain. The neuronal cells of the central nervous system (brain and spinal cord) of all adults are postmitotic and therefore do not regenerate once destroyed. Studies indicate that the aging process causes a loss of brain cells, and that cells not destroyed may undergo significant structural changes. Brain cells decrease in number at a rate of about 1% a year after 50 years of age. However, this rate of loss is not consistent throughout the brain, so that certain areas may lose cells at a faster (e.g., cortex) or slower (e.g., brainstem) rate than others. Other cells, such as the neurons of the prefrontal neocortex, undergo structural changes that result in a progressive decline in dendritic interconnections. In addition, neuronal cells of the elderly contain the age pigment *lipofuscin* in the storage granules, as well as senile plaques and neurofibrillary tangles.

Cerebral blood flow studies indicate there is a change with age in cerebral blood flow and oxygen utilization. Cerebral blood flow showed a decline from 79.3 ml/min/100 g of brain tissue at the mean age of 17 to 46 ml/min/100 g at the mean age of 80, a net loss of 33.3 ml/min/100 g of brain. The rate of cerebral oxygen consumption declined from 3.6 ml/min/100 g of brain tissue at the mean age of 17 to 2.7 ml/min/100 g at the mean age of 80.[13]

Nerve conduction velocity of the individual over 50 years also differs from that of younger adults. By 80 to 90 years of age, conduction velocity equals about 50 m/sec, whereas a young adult has a conduction velocity of approximately 60 m/s. This loss of conduction velocity appears to be slightly greater in aging women. Nerve conduction velocity in the elderly is also affected by an increased synaptic delay and a change in neurotransmitters. Recent studies indicate that in the human brain, monoamine oxidase (MAO) and serotonin increase with age while norepinephrine decreases. This reciprocal increase may explain the depression and apathy often associated with aging.[13]

Vertebrae. The vertebral column may show advancing kyphosis in the thoracic region of the elderly patient. This degenerative change is the result of osteoporosis, vertebral collapse, or changes in vertebral cartilage. As the vertebral cartilage calcifies, there is decreased mobility of the vertebral column.

Spinal cord. The basic reflex arc does not change with the aging process. However, the spinal cord may show changes in sensory conduction because of decreased vascularity of the white matter in the cord. Therefore diminished reflexes in the distal portion of the lower extremities (i.e., ankle) are not uncommon. Degenerative changes in the peripheral nerves are responsible for the loss of vibratory sense at the ankles. Reflexes of the upper extremities should be intact in the healthy elderly individual.

Normal Findings

"Normal" behaviors must be evaluated in terms of the patient's baseline pattern, as well as significant variables (i.e., anxiety) affecting the assessment process. One way to establish the patient's baseline is through a careful and thorough health history. Whenever the health history or the physical examination provides data indicating a deviation from normal, that symptom or complex of symptoms requires a comprehensive symptom analysis.

Normative behaviors of the geriatric patient may vary from source to source. Therefore it is recommended that the examiner cross reference the assessment findings with the patient's previous patterns of behavior. The examiner also must carefully consider the effect on behavior of such variables as physical illness, displacement, examiner approach, change in self-image, and physiologic changes (i.e., diminished sense of hearing or vision).

Area of Concern	Normal Adult Findings
General Cerebral Functions	
Appearance and behavior	Age, height, weight; body proportionate in size in terms of body parts; clean; groomed; dressed appropriate to age, sex, peers, and background *Older adult:* Length of trunk decreased in relation to extremities
Posture	Shoulders back and relaxed; arms rest at sides; feet rest on floor (if applicable); stands with narrow base *Older adult:* May assume posture with slight semiflexion at principal joints; stands with narrow to medium base; may exhibit kyphosis in thoracic spine region with accompanying backward tilt of head
Gestures	Smooth; coordinated; deliberate
Movements	Coordinated; smooth; deliberate; able to change positions with smooth, even movements *Older adult:* Changes position with slow, even movements
Facial expression	Facial features symmetric; establishes eye contact; acknowledges examiner presence; uses eye contact throughout interview
Attention	Able to complete thought processes (i.e., able to repeat series of numbers forward and backward); has continuity of ideas
Level of consciousness	Responds appropriately to visual, auditory, tactile, and painful stimuli; oriented to person, place, time; able to carry out simple and complex commands; opens eyes spontaneously; extraocular eye movement present *Older adult:* May respond slower, appropriately to visual, auditory stimuli; may demonstrate diminished response to tactile and painful stimuli; able to carry out simple and complex commands, with slower response time
Intellectual functions	
Memory	
Immediate	Able to repeat a series of numbers (e.g., 12, 9, 5, 1, 6)
Recent	Able to repeat correct series of numbers after 5 min
Remote	Able to state correct birthplace; able to correctly state personal and vocational history
Abstract reasoning	Able to describe meaning of simple proverbs such as "A stitch in time saves nine," or "Rome wasn't built in a day"
Insight	Demonstrates consistent awareness of reality and perception of self *Older adult:* May demonstrate increased resistance to "new" ideas
Specific Cerebral Functions	
Sensory interpretation	
Visual	Recognizes objects; differentiates between size and shape
Auditory	Able to identify sound made by ringing bell
Tactile	Able to recognize familiar objects through use of touch (stereognosis) *Older adult:* Longer response time
Cortical	
Motor integration	Able to carry out a skilled act such as protruding tongue, using a comb
Comprehension	Able to answer questions correctly throughout history, interview, and examination
Judgment	Able to discuss plans for future
Language and speech	Smooth, flowing; easily able to formulate words; varied inflections; demonstrates ability to read appropriate to educational level; able to write letters and numbers to dictation *Older adult:* Flow may be slightly decreased

Area of Concern	Normal Adult Findings
Emotional status	
Affect	Appropriate to verbalization; body behaviors indicative of mild to moderate anxiety
Mood	Consistent with conversation; cooperates with examiner
Thought processes	
Content	Spontaneous, natural, logical, and free flowing *Older adult:* Thought patterns become more concrete; thought patterns increase in orderliness
Cranial Nerves	
Olfactory	Able to identify aromatic, volatile, nonirritating substances (e.g., lemon, peppermint) with each nostril *Older adult:* May demonstrate diminished sense of smell; able to identify changes in aromatic substances with each nostril
Optic	See Chapter 6
Oculomotor Trochlear Abducens	Eyelids symmetric and not drooping; pupils equal in size, regular in outline, with prompt and equal reaction (direct and consensual) to light stimulus; conjugate gaze; smooth conjugate eye movements intact through six cardinal positions of gaze; prompt accommodation to distant and near objects; bilaterally, equal corneal light reflex *Older adults:* Eyelids appear less elastic; eye movements intact with some limitation of upward gaze; eyes may be unable to converge
Trigeminal	
Sensory	Bilateral blink when limbus of cornea touched with cotton wisp; symmetric tickling sensation when cotton wisp touched to anterior scalp, paranasal sinuses, and jaws; symmetric pressure and pain sensation when alternating blunt and sharp ends of a safety pin are touched to anterior scalp, paranasal sinuses, and jaws; symmetric warm and cold sensation felt when tested for temperature over anterior scalp, paranasal sinuses, and jaws
Motor	Bilaterally strong contractions of temporal and masseter muscles
Facial	
Sensory	Able to correctly identify sweet, sour, salty, and bitter substances placed on anterior tongue
Motor	Symmetry of facial movements such as smiling, frowning, closing eyes, raising eyebrows, showing teeth, and puffing out cheeks
Acoustic	
Cochlear division	Bilateral ability to hear whispered voice (from distance of 1-2 ft); able to hear watch ticking (from distance of 1-2 in)
Weber test	Sound heard equally in both ears
Rinne test	Sound heard twice as long by air conduction as by bone conduction
Vestibular division (tested only with history of vertigo)	
Bárány test	Demonstrates a feeling of nausea, slow horizontal nystagmus toward side irrigated, with past pointing and falling
Bárány chair rotation	Nystagmus, past pointing, and postural deviation in direction of chair movement; vertigo and sensation of continued movement in opposite direction of chair movement
Electronystagmography	No displacement of corneal-retinal potential bilaterally
Glossopharyngeal and vagus	Immediate contraction of pharyngeal muscles, with or without gagging, with lateral, upper, lower, and posterior stimulation; speech smooth, without hoarseness; able to identify tastes of sweet, salty, sour, and bitter on posterior third of tongue
Spinal accessory	Able to turn head against resistance: sternocleidomastoid muscle bilaterally equal in strength and symmetry; able to shrug shoulders against resistance with bilaterally equal strength of upward movement
Hypoglossal	Able to protrude tongue in midline; able to move tongue in and out of mouth rapidly; able to wiggle tongue from side to side
Proprioception; Cerebellar and Motor Function	
Gait	Maintains upright posture of trunk; walks unaided with narrow base, weight shifts from one extremity to another, pelvis approximately at right angle to weight-bearing extremity; maintains balance; opposing arm swing *Older adult:* Maintains upright posture of trunk (if no kyphosis); walks with narrow to medium base

Area of Concern	Normal Adult Findings
Romberg test	Slight swaying, but upright posture and narrow foot stance maintained
Tandem walk	Able to walk heel to toe in straight line
One-foot balance	Able to maintain position for at least 5 sec; bilaterally equal response with eyes open and eyes closed
Hop in place	Able to maintain balance, hop on one foot, and stay in place: bilaterally equal response
Knee bends	Able to perform knee bends while maintaining balance
Upper extremity testing	Able to rapidly pronate and supinate hands with bilaterally equal timing, purposeful movement; able to touch nose repeatedly with alternate index finger in rhythmic fashion (eyes open and eyes closed); able to rapidly and purposefully touch each finger to thumb; able to move index finger from nose to examiner's finger in coordinated fashion (each hand tested)
Lower extremity testing	Able to purposefully run heel down contralateral shin with bilaterally equal coordination
Muscle strength and tone	See Chapter 4
Sensory Functions	
Primary	
Light touch	Able to perceive light or tickling sensation; able to identify location touched correctly
Pain	Able to perceive pain sensation as sharp or dull; able to identify area touched correctly
Temperature	Able to perceive sensation as hot or cold
Vibration	Able to perceive sensation of vibration
Discriminating sensation	
Stereognosis	Able to identify common objects (e.g., key, pencil) by handling it
Two-point discrimination	Able to distinguish whether touched by one or two objects; palms, 8-12 mm; dorsum of hands, 20-30 mm; fingertips 2.8-5 mm; dorsa of fingers, 4-6 mm; chest and forearm, 40 mm; back, 40-70 mm; upper arms and thighs, 75 mm; shins, 30-40 mm *Older adult:* May evidence diminishment from normal adult findings
Graphesthesia	Able to recognize traced letter or number on hand, back, etc.
Double simultaneous sensation	Able to distinguish if touched on one or two sides of body (at same level) *Older adult:* May not be able to distinguish
Kinesthetic	Able to identify change in position of fingers as up or down
Reflexes	
Superficial	
Upper abdominal (T8, T9, T10)	Upward movement of umbilicus toward area of stimulus *Older adult:* May be diminished or absent
Lower abdominal (T10, T11, T12)	Downward movement of umbilicus toward area of stimulation *Older adult:* May be diminished or absent
Cremasteric (T12, L1)	Elevation of ipsilateral testicle as cremaster muscle contracts (males only)
Gluteal (L4 to S3)	Contraction of anal sphincter
Deep tendon	
Biceps (C5, C6)	Flexion of arm at elbow
Triceps (C6, C7, C8)	Extension of arm at elbow and contraction of triceps muscles
Finger flexion (C7 to T1)	Fingers flexed
Brachioradialis (C5, C6)	Flexion at elbow and pronation of forearm
Patellar (L2, L3, L4)	Extension of leg at knee and contraction of quadriceps *Older adult:* May be diminished
Achilles (S1, S2)	Plantar flexion of foot at ankle *Older adult:* May be absent
Pathologic	
Plantar (Babinski) (L4, L5, S1, S2)	Dorsal flexion of great toe with fanning of other toes
Chaddock (L4, L5, S1, S2)	Dorsal flexion of great toe with fanning of other toes
Clonus	No movement of foot

Normal Laboratory Data

Indications for obtaining cerebrospinal fluid include all the following:

1. To measure or reduce pressure within the subarachnoid space (i.e., subarachnoid block from a neoplasm, vertebral fracture, or dislocation)
2. To assist in the diagnosis of bacterial or viral infections (e.g., meningitis)
3. To administer anticancer drugs
4. To administer antibiotics (not commonly used)
5. To assist in the diagnosis of demyelinating diseases, a subarachnoid hemorrhage, an intracranial hemorrhage, and brain abscesses

Samples of the cerebrospinal fluid are most commonly collected via the lumbar puncture. If the lumbar site is infected or deformed, the cerebrospinal fluid can be aspirated by a cisternal or ventricular puncture.

Laboratory Test	Normal Adult Values
Appearance	Crystal clear, colorless
Pressure (lateral recumbent)	50-180 mm H_2O
Protein	
Lumbar	6 mo and up: approximately 15-50 mg/dl Ventricular CSF protein is generally lower
Cisternal	15-25 mg/dl
Ventricular	6-15 mg/dl
Cell count	No RBCs 0-5 WBCs 0-10 cells/mm^3 (all lymphocytes and monocytes)
Glucose	50-80 mg/dl (60%-70% of plasma glucose)
A/G rates	8:1 (albumin to globulin)
Serologic studies	
Complement fixation	Nonreactive
Treponema pallidum immune adherence	Nonreactive
Treponema immobilization test	Nonreactive
Gram stain	Negative for organisms
Culture and sensitivity	No growth of organisms
Electrolytes	
Sodium	141 mEq/L
Potassium	3.3 mEq/L
Chloride	110-125 mEq/L
Bilirubin	Negative
Cholesterol	0.2-0.6 mg/dl
Creatinine	0.5-1.2 mg/dl
Urea	7-15 mg/dl
Urea nitrogen	10-15 mg/dl
Uric acid	0.5-4.5 mg/dl
pH	7.32-7.35

Laboratory Test	Normal Adult Values
Specific gravity	1.007
Glutamine	6-15 mg/dl (enzymatic)
IgG index	0.3-0.7
IgG	0-11% of total protein
Lactic acid	Control group with no CNS disorder: 0.6-2.2 mEq/L (0.6-2.2 mmol/L; 10-20 mg/dl)
LDH	Fluid LDH activity normally much less than plasma LDH activity; normal spinal fluid LDH levels are about 10% of serum levels
Myelin basic protein	<4 ng/ml CSF is normal
Oligoclonal bands	Normal CSF: no demonstrable oligoclonal bands
Protein electrophoresis (normal range depends on methodology)	
Gamma	3%-13%
Beta	7.3%-17.9%
$Alpha_2$	3%-12.6%
$Alpha_1$	1.1%-6.6%
Albumin	56.8%-76.9%
Prealbumin	2.2%-7.1%
CSF albumin	13.4-23.7 mg/dl
Total protein	15-50 mg/dl
Beta-gamma ratio	1.67-2.3
Oligoclonal bands	Absent
FTA-ABS	Nonreactive
Cryptococcal antigen titer	Negative
VDRL	Nonreactive
Mycobacteria culture	No growth
Counterimmunoelectrophoresis	Negative
India ink preparation	No *Cryptococcus* identified

Conditions, Diseases, and Disorders

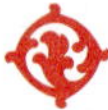

Brain Abscess

A brain abscess is a suppurative infection consisting of a collection of pus within the parenchyma of the brain.

The incidence of brain abscesses is site specific, depending on such factors as the size of the area and the amount of cerebral blood flow. As a result, 80% of the abscesses are found in the cerebrum, and 20% are found in the cerebellum. Statistics indicate that 5% to 20% of brain abscesses occur in more than one site. The individual with a brain abscess presents a difficult clinical situation, since a 30% to 60% mortality is associated with the disorder. Surgical intervention may reduce the mortality, but this depends on accessibility of the abscess and the general condition of the patient. Morbidity following a brain abscess presents continued difficulties. Individuals surviving brain abscesses may experience different types of neurologic deficits including paralysis and seizures.

Pathophysiology

The majority of brain abscesses result from extension of chronic middle ear, sinus, or mastoid infections. The bacteria of these infections can invade the cranial vault directly through the bone, through spinal dura mater, across the subdural and subarachnoid spaces, or along venous channels as in the extension of a septic thrombophlebitis. Suppuration from the ear accounts for one third to one half of all brain abscesses and produces disease either in the ipsilateral cerebellar hemisphere or in the temporal lobe. Extended infections from the frontal sinuses primarily affect the anteroinferior parts of the frontal lobes. Sphenoidal sinusitis may extend to the frontal or temporal lobes, and ethmoid sinusitis may extend to the frontal lobes.

Penetrating head injuries, compound skull fractures, and osteomyelitis of the skull also may lead to the formation of a brain abscess. Patients with right-to-left cardiac shunts are susceptible to the formation of brain abscesses because of polycythemia, which causes cerebral ischemia and necrosis. Most abscesses disseminated through the bloodstream are multiple and found in the white matter, particularly in areas distal to those perfused by the middle cerebral artery.

Organisms commonly isolated as the cause of brain abscesses include streptococci, aerobic Enterobacteriaceae, and the staphylococci. Anaerobic bacteria (i.e., *Bacteroides fragilis*) and aerobic Enterobacteriaceae (i.e., *Escherichia coli, Klebsiella*) are found in suppurative ear infections. Anaerobic and microaerophilic streptococci, *Bacteroides, Fusobacterium,* and *Veillonella* species are found in suppurative lung infections. Staphylococci frequently are associated with penetrating head injuries and endocarditis. In patients with impaired host resistance, disseminated fungal infections (e.g., candidiasis) may also result in brain abscesses.

Following the initial implantation of bacteria there is a localized inflammatory reaction (i.e., cerebritis or encephalitis), which is characterized by local edema, hyperemia, leukocyte infiltration, and parenchymal softening. Several days to weeks after bacterial invasion of the brain tissue, there is central liquefaction and necrosis of brain tissue that produces a cystic mass of pus. The cystic mass is encapsulated by a wall of granulated tissue from migration of fibroblasts. Continued fibroblastic activity and gliosis result in replacement of granulation tissue of the abscess wall by collagenous connective tissues. The encapsulation process usually is completed within about 3 weeks. The abscess wall generally is thinnest on the ventricular side, predisposing this side to rupture. Infiltration of the leptomeninges (subarachnoid and pia mater) may lead to low-grade cerebrospinal fluid pleocytosis (greater than normal number of cells in cerebrospinal fluid). When the infection extends toward the cortex, meningitis results; when it extends toward the ventricles, ventriculitis results.

Diagnostic Studies and Findings

Lumbar Puncture

Contraindication: May precipitate brain herniation if intracranial pressure is elevated severely

Roentgenograms: Skull, Sinuses, Mastoid Processes, Chest

Helpful in locating associated suppurative processes

CT Scan

Locates well-formed and encapsulated abscesses
Visualizes ventricle size and midline displacement

Brain Scan

Locates abscesses over 1 cm in size
Sensitive in early cerebritis when local alteration in permeability of blood-brain barrier can be visualized

CSF Studies (If Done)

Slight increase in pressure
Increase in WBC

Increased protein
Normal glucose levels
CSF cultures nonspecific unless abscess has ruptured

Carotid Arteriography

Locates temporal lobe abscesses
Posterior circulatory arteriography used to locate cerebellar abscesses

Magnetic Resonance Imaging (MRI)

Same as CT scan without radiation

Electroencephalogram (EEG)

Marked slowing at sites of abscess

Medical Plan

Surgery

Aspiration or complete excision and evacuation of abscess (method depends on site and accessibility)

Medications

Anti-infective agents; course of therapy may be 6 wk
- Penicillin G, 20 million units IV qd
- Chloramphenicol (Chloromycetin), 50 mg/kg/d in divided doses q6h IV
- Nafcillin (Unipen), 500 mg IV q4h
  - Semisynthetic, resistant penicillin used if *Staphylococcus aureus* isolated
- Metronidazole (Flagyl)
  - Loading: 15 mg/kg IV over 1 h
  - Maintenance: 7.5 mg/kg IV over 1 h q6h
  - Used if anaerobic bacteria such as *Bacteroides fragilis* are isolated
- Dexamethasone (Decadron), 6-12 mg IV q6h

General Management

Serial-order CT scans or brain scans
Support of vital functions (e.g., ventilator) if indicated
Physical therapy
Nutritional services

NURSING CARE

Nursing Assessment

Pain

Headache (70% of patients) that becomes increasingly severe
Activation
- Increased pulse
- Increased blood pressure
- Increased respiratory rate
- Dilated pupils
- Pallor
- Increased muscle tension
- Cold perspiration
- Raised hairs on some parts of body

Rebound phase
- Blood pressure lower than before pain experience
- Pulse rate slower than before pain experience

Adaptation phase
- Pain occurring frequently or for long duration: pulse rate and blood pressure not increased as much as in activation phase

Stress reaction
- Pain persisting for many days
- Increased production of 17-ketosteroids
- Increased production of eosinophils
- Increased susceptibility to other infections

Vocalizations
- Grunt
- Whimper
- Groan
- Sob
- Cry
- Gasp

Facial expressions
- Clenched teeth
- Eyes open wide or tightly shut lids
- Wrinkled forehead
- Biting lower lip

Other
- May withdraw
- May not initiate conversation

Level of Consciousness

Lethargy
Irritability
Confusion or coma

Increased Intracranial Pressure

Nausea, vomiting
Changing level of consciousness (see p. 311 for additional signs and symptoms of increased intracranial pressure)
Papilledema (late sign)

Meningeal Irritability

Nuchal rigidity (25% of patients)

Seizure Activity

Generalized or focal (30% of patients)
Preconvulsive (preictal) stage
- Aura: flash of light; sense of loss, fear; weakness; dizziness; peculiar taste, smell, and sounds
- Cry or scream
- Fall to floor
- Loss of consciousness
- Tachypnea

- Convulsive stage
  - Tonic: rigid body; flexed jaws; clenched fists; extended legs; cyanosis; holding breath
  - Clonic: urinary and/or fecal incontinence; jerking of facial muscles and extremities; biting tongue; frothing at mouth
- Postconvulsive (postictal) stage
  - Altered level of consciousness
  - Headache
  - Nausea and/or vomiting
  - Malaise
  - Muscle soreness
  - Aspiration
  - Breathing difficulty, choking, cyanosis, decreased breath sounds, tachycardia, tachypnea

Other

- Selective aphasia (if temporal lobe involved)
- Homonymous upper quadrantic or hemianopic defects in visual fields
- Weakness of lower facial muscles
- Ataxia, nystagmus, incoordination of extremities, and occasionally intention tremors (cerebellar abscess)
- Impaired two-point discrimination, altered position sense, astereognosis, visual inattention, and impaired opticokinetic nystagmus (parietal lobe abscess)

Anxiety

- Appearance
  - Increased perspiration, clammy skin
  - Fatigue
  - Increased muscle tension (rigidity)
  - Skin blanches; pale
  - Increased small motor activity (i.e., tremors, restlessness)
- Behavior
  - Decreased attention span
  - Increased immobility
  - Decreased ability to follow directions
- Other
  - Increased rate or depth of respirations
  - Increased heart rate
  - Rapid shifts in body temperature, blood pressure
  - Urinary urgency
  - Diarrhea
  - Dry mouth
  - Decreased appetite
  - Pupillary dilation

Nursing Dx & Intervention

Nursing Diagnosis	Nursing Intervention/Rationale
Ineffective airway clearance	• Assess patient's ability to handle secretions. • Maintain patent airway; avoid flexion of neck if patient is comatose. • Suction as needed *to prevent obstruction.* Assist ventilation as per protocol. • Monitor vital signs and neurologic status every 1 to 2 hours. • Keep emergency drugs and ventilator at bedside. • Maintain nothing-by-mouth status *to prevent risk of choking and aspiration.*
Ineffective breathing pattern	• Maintain patent airway; intubation and assisted ventilation may be indicated. • Assess arterial blood gases as per protocol *to monitor changes in oxygen and carbon dioxide levels:* Report decrease of Po_2 of 10 to 15 mm Hg. Report increase of Pco_2 greater than 10 to 15 mm Hg. • Note respiratory rate, depth, and level of consciousness every 15 to 30 minutes and as needed. • Check blood pressure, temperature, and pulse rate every 1 to 2 hours and as needed *to monitor cardiovascular status.* • Administer medications as per protocol. • Limit fluid intake as ordered; may include titrating according to pulmonary artery pressure, central venous pressure, or pulmonary capillary wedge pressure.
Altered cardiopulmonary tissue perfusion	• Take and record ECG rhythm strips every 2 to 4 hours and as needed, noting rate and rhythm. • Measure intake and output. Report hourly output less than 30 ml *to prevent potential hypotension or fluid overload.* • Monitor hemodynamics (central venous pressure, arterial pressure, pulmonary artery pressure, pulmonary capillary wedge pressure) as per protocol. • Monitor intracranial pressure (if monitoring device is used) every 30 minutes to 1 hour *to monitor neurologic status.* • Monitor vital signs every 1 to 2 hours and as needed.

Nursing Diagnosis	Nursing Intervention/Rationale
Altered cerebral tissue perfusion	• Assess arterial blood gases, blood chemistry, and electrolytes. • Maintain head of bed at 20- to 30-degree elevation. • Maintain body alignment. • Monitor intake and output every 1 to 2 hours or as condition indicates *to prevent fluid overload or dehydration.* • Monitor ECG rhythm and arterial pulses.
Pain	• Assess and document patient's degree of pain. • See general intervention strategies listed on p. 1720.
Potential impaired skin integrity	• Assess skin turgor and pressure points for signs of breakdown when turning patient and providing skin care. • Administer skin care every 2 to 4 hours *to stimulate circulation.* • Turn patient every 2 hours *to minimize pressure points on the skin.* • Use air mattress or egg-crate mattress. • Use sandbags or footboard *to prevent footdrop.* • Keep skin dry.
Impaired physical mobility	• Perform passive range of motion (ROM) exercises to all extremities every 4 hours *to reduce stiffness and to prevent contractures and muscle atrophy.*
Sensory/perceptual alterations	• Assess and record patient's orientation and ability to understand. • Keep side rails up at all times when patient is alone. Maintain patient safety at all times. • Maintain quiet environment, reducing external stimuli to a minimum. • Reorient patient frequently to time, place, and person. Introduce yourself each time you reorient patient. • Repeat explanations frequently and simply *to facilitate understanding.* • Have family bring in familiar objects. • Maintain planned rest periods *to allow sufficient time for REM sleep.* • Use day and night lighting appropriately. • Stimulate senses of touch, taste, and position.
Personal identity disturbance	• See general intervention strategies listed on p. 1754. • Avoid facial expressions that may indicate rejection. • Perform care in a quiet, unhurried manner.
Potential for trauma	
Preconvulsive	• Assess and record patient's level of consciousness. • Have oral airway at bedside *to prevent airway obstruction.* • Have suction equipment available at bedside. • Pad side rails, if indicated, *to prevent injury if patient is restless.* • Administer oxygen per protocol. • Identify auras if possible.
Convulsive	• Maintain patent airway. • Support and protect head; turn to side if possible. • Prevent injury. • Ease to floor if patient is in chair. • Place pillows along side rails if patient is in bed. • Remove surrounding furniture. • Loosen clothing *to prevent constriction.* • Provide privacy as necessary. • Stay with patient; remain calm. • Note frequency, time, involved body parts, and length of seizure *to establish the type of seizure activity.*
Postconvulsive	• Maintain patent airway. • Suction as indicated. • Check vital signs and neurologic status every 15 minutes. • Administer oxygen per protocol. • Reorient patient to environment *to minimize sensory-perceptual alteration.* • Provide emotional support *to minimize fear and anxiety.* • Place patient in position of comfort; turn head to side. • Administer oral hygiene as necessary for secretions and bleeding. • Prepare for diagnostic tests if ordered: CT scan, skull series, arteriogram, EEG.

Patient Education

1. Make certain the patient and family know and understand the following:
   a. Nature of a brain abscess, treatments, and procedures; explain as they occur
   b. Need to ambulate as tolerated
   c. Importance of maintaining planned rest periods
   d. Names of medications, dosages, frequency of administration, purposes, and toxic or side effects
   e. Need to avoid taking over-the-counter medications without consulting physician
   f. Possible residual effects such as headaches, sensory or motor deficits, seizures
2. Teach the patient and the family to recognize seizure activity and appropriate course of action:
   a. Sit or lie down.
   b. Avoid trying to stop seizure or restraining patient.
   c. Protect patient from injury.
   d. Observe and record body parts involved and duration of seizure activity.
3. Ensure that the patient and family understand importance of ongoing outpatient care (i.e., physician's visits and physical therapy).
4. Teach the patient and family the importance of maintaining a well-balanced diet.

Evaluation

Patient Outcome	Data Indicating That Outcome is Reached
Patient demonstrates effective airway clearance.	Breath sounds are normal. Chest excursion is symmetric. Rate and depth of respirations are normal. Cough is effective. There are no subjective or objective findings of shortness of breath, air hunger, or dyspnea on exertion.
Patient demonstrates an effective breathing pattern.	Patent airway is maintained. Chest excursion is symmetric. Breath sounds are normal, or there is no increase in adventitious sounds. Arterial blood gas values are within normal ranges or consistent with patient's baseline. Vital signs are within normal ranges or consistent with patient's baseline. Hemoglobin levels are 14 to 18 g/dl (male) and 12 to 16 g/dl (female). Intake and output are stable. There are no signs of respiratory distress. Resonance of all lobes is evident on percussion. Skin color is without cyanosis.
Patient maintains adequate cerebral and spinal tissue perfusion.	There is no change in level of consciousness. There is no evidence of neurologic deficits. Pattern of electrolytes is stable. There is no seizure activity.
Patient demonstrates an optimal level of mobility.	Skin integrity is maintained. The patient remains free of contractures and deformities. Level of mobility is appropriate to physiologic status. Intake and output pattern is stable. Nutritional status is adequate. Patient remains free of thrombophlebitis. Patient remains free of local infection.
Patient experiences minimal alterations in comfort.	Patient openly verbalizes feelings of discomfort when they occur. Patient is able to use measures to decrease discomfort. Patient verbalizes a decrease in subjective feelings of discomfort. There is a decrease in objective findings of pain.
Patient demonstrates minimal complications of sensory-perceptual alterations.	Patient maintains optimal level of mobility. Patient remains free of injury. Skin integrity is maintained. Nutritional status is adequate. Patient demonstrates minimal self-care deficits. Patient demonstrates social participation appropriate to physiologic status.
Patient demonstrates intact self-concepts.	Patient openly verbalizes feelings of grief, loss, etc. Patient verbalizes positive feelings about self. Patient acknowledges actual change in self-image. Patient focuses on present and future appearance and function. Patient verbalizes feelings of hopefulness and helpfulness.
Patient remains free of traumatic injury.	Safety measures appropriate to level of physiologic status are used. Skin integrity is maintained. Skin is free of bruises, burns, abrasions, redness, etc. Environment is safe. Patient is free of nosocomial infections.

Hydrocephalus

Hydrocephalus is characterized by an abnormal accumulation of cerebrospinal fluid within the cranial vault with subsequent dilation of the cerebral ventricles.[48]

Hydrocephalus has an incidence of 4 per 1000 births through the age of 3 months, but can occur at any age. In infants it is considered a primary disease, whereas in later life it occurs as a complication of other diseases.

Hydrocephalus has several known causes, which can be categorized as congenital or acquired. Congenital abnormalities obstruct the flow of cerebrospinal fluid; 70% of these obstructions result from stenosis of the aqueduct of Sylvius. Other anomalies causing or associated with hydrocephalus are the Arnold-Chiari malformation, Dandy-Walker syndrome, and spina bifida cystica.[44] Flow and absorption of cerebrospinal fluid also can be affected by fibrosis of meninges and obstruction of the aqueduct and basal cisterns caused by inflammatory lesions.

Causative mechanisms of hydrocephalus are (1) excessive secretion of cerebrospinal fluid as a result of a choroid plexus papilloma, (2) obstruction of cerebrospinal fluid flow in the ventricles or subarachnoid space, (3) obstruction by pacchionian granulations, and (4) hemodynamic production. Common sites for obstruction of cerebrospinal fluid are the third ventricle, the fourth ventricle, the foramina of Monro, and the aqueduct of Sylvius. Each site may be obstructed by a mass within or outside the lumen. Pacchionian granulations caused by inflammatory processes and fibrosis can occlude the arachnoid villi, preventing the escape of cerebrospinal fluid from the subarachnoid space and resulting in hydrocephalus.

Although most causes of hydrocephalus are associated with intraventricular hypertension, there are two types in which intraventricular pressure is not elevated. *Hydrocephalus ex vacuo* results in ventricular dilation to fill spaces caused by a decreasing neural mass (e.g., Alzheimer's disease and stroke). *Normal pressure hydrocephalus* is characterized by dilated ventricles, normal neural tissue mass, and normal intracranial pressure. The etiology and pathology of normal pressure hydrocephalus remain to be elucidated.

Communicating vs. Noncommunicating Hydrocephalus

A *communicating* or extraventricular hydrocephalus occurs when the obstruction is outside the ventricular system; therefore flow between the ventricles is not blocked. Excessive cerebrospinal fluid accumulates in the ventricles because the fluid is not adequately absorbed from the cerebral subarachnoid space. The *noncommunicating,* or intraventricular, hydrocephalus results in an accumulation of cerebrospinal fluid from a block of the normal flow at some point in the ventricular system. The cerebral ventricles proximal to the block then dilate.

Pathophysiology

When there is an obstruction in the ventricular system or in the subarachnoid space, the cerebral ventricles dilate, causing the ventricular surface to stretch, disrupting its ependymal lining. The underlying white matter atrophies and may be reduced to a thin ribbon. There is selective preservation of the gray matter, even when the ventricles have attained enormous size. The dilation process may be an insidious or acute process and may be selective, depending on the site of blockage. The acute process may cause a medical emergency. In the infant and young child the cranial sutures split and widen to accommodate the increasing cranial mass. If the anterior fontanel is not closed, it bulges and feels tense to palpation. Aqueductal stenosis, a sex-linked familial disease, causes a marked dilation of the lateral and third ventricles. This dilation gives the head a characteristic dominant frontal brow appearance. The Dandy-Walker syndrome occurs when there is an obstruction of the exit foramina of the fourth ventricle. Consequently the fourth ventricle dilates, with the posterior fossae becoming prominent and bossing below the tentorium. This type of hydrocephalus gives the patient generalized symmetric enlargement of the cerebrum, and the face appears disproportionately small.

In the older individual the cranial sutures have closed; therefore the space is fixed and limits expansion of the brain mass. As a result the older person usually exhibits the signs and symptoms of increased intracranial pressure before the cerebral ventricles become greatly enlarged.

Defects of cerebrospinal fluid absorption and circulation in hydrocephalus are not complete. Formation of cerebrospinal fluid exceeds the capacity of the normal ventricular system every 6 to 8 hours, and a total lack of reabsorption is incompatible with life. Ventricular dilation causes a disruption of the normal ependymal lining of the walls of the cavities, permitting increased absorption. If the collateral route is adequate to prevent progressive ventricular dilation, a state of compensation may exist.[12]

Diagnostic Studies and Findings

Angiography

Detection of vessel abnormalities caused by stretching
Vascular lesions

CT Scan

Detection of variations in tissue density
Presence of cysts or masses
Visualization of the ventricular system

Lumbar Puncture

Diagnosis of communicating hydrocephalus
Contraindication:
Elevated intracranial pressure

Subdural/Ventricular Puncture

As for lumbar puncture

Ventriculography

Visualization of ventricular system configuration
Shows ventricular dilation with hydrocephalus

Magnetic Resonance Imaging (MRI)

Same as CT scan

Medical Plan

Surgery*

Correction of CSF obstruction such as resection of cyst, neoplasm, or hematoma
Ventricular bypass into normal intracranial channel (i.e., Torkildsen procedure where CSF is shunted from lateral to cisterna magna) in noncommunicating hydrocephalus
Ventricular bypass into extracranial compartment (i.e., ventriculoperitoneal or ventriculoatrial shunt)
Reduction of CSF production as in third or fourth ventriculostomy or endoscopic choroid plexus extirpation (plexectomy or electric coagulation)

Medications

Acetazolamide (Diamox), 8-30 mg/kg in divided doses, IV
Mannitol (Osmitrol), in initial management of severe increased intracranial pressure
Dexamethasone (Decadron), 6-20 mg q6h IV

General Management

Intracranial pressure monitoring
Cardiac monitoring
Respiratory monitoring

NURSING CARE

Nursing Assessment

Head Circumference

Severely enlarged head
Bulging fontanels after pulsation

*Therapy of choice.

Fixed downward gaze of eyes with visible sclera above (sunset gaze)
Visible, distended scalp veins
Radiation of light throughout accumulated cerebrospinal fluid with translumination

Vomiting

More frequent in older patient
Likely to occur in morning (frequency may increase with increased intracranial pressure)

Seizures

Focal or general tonic-clonic seizures
May assume opisthotonic position

Behavioral Changes

Feeds poorly
Lethargy
Irritability when stimulated

Alterations in Vital Signs (with Increased Intracranial Pressure)

Decreased pulse
Increased systolic blood pressure
Irregular and decreased respirations

Muscle Tone

Alteration of muscle tone in extremities

Later Assessment Findings

Physical and/or mental development lag
Prominence of forehead
Scalp shiny, with scalp veins prominent
Optic atrophy, strabismus, nystagmus, exposed sclera

Nursing Dx & Intervention

Nursing Diagnosis	Nursing Intervention/Rationale
Ineffective breathing pattern	• Assess arterial blood gases as ordered: Report decrease of Po_2 of 10 to 15 mm Hg. Report increase of Pco_2 greater than 10 to 15 mm Hg. • Maintain patent airway. Have intubation and assisted ventilation equipment at bedside. • Suction as needed. Auscultate breath sounds before and after suctioning *to determine effectiveness of secretion removal.* • Position for maximum lung expansion; elevate head of bed slightly (10 to 20 degrees). • Note respiratory rate and depth and level of consciousness every 15 to 30 minutes and as needed. • Check pulse rate, temperature, and blood pressure every 1 to 2 hours and as needed. • Administer medications as per protocol. • Limit fluid intake as per protocol; include titrating according to intracranial pressure. • Measure and record intake and output; report hourly output less than 30 ml. • Administer tube feedings per protocol *to ensure adequate nutrition.*

Nursing Diagnosis	Nursing Intervention/Rationale

Fluid volume excess

- Assess intracranial pressure continuously if being monitored.
- Provide preoperative nursing care for patient who will have shunt implantation:
  - Monitor vital signs and neurologic status every 15 minutes to 1 hour and as needed.
  - Suction or aspirate mucus as needed *to prevent airway obstruction.*
  - Observe for signs and symptoms of shock.
  - Administer medications (i.e., antibiotics and anticonvulsants).
  - Turn every 2 hours and provide skin care every 2 hours.
  - Insert nasogastric tube for abdominal decompression, if indicated.
  - Avoid hyperthermia and hypothermia.
- Provide postoperative nursing care after shunt implantation:
  - Position patient and punp shunt per protocol *to maintain maximum effectiveness.*
  - Compress valve specified number of times at regular intervals.
  - Accurately measure intake and output and record on flow sheet.
  - Administer parenteral fluids per protocol.
  - Administer feedings per protocol *to provide adequate nutrition.*
  - Monitor for signs of complications, such as dehydration and infection.

Altered cerebral tissue perfusion

- Assess values and waveforms of intracranial pressure line, if appropriate:
  - Maintain patency and sterility of system.
  - Monitor effects of treatments on intracranial pressure.
  - Correlate neurologic status with intracranial pressure values, and notify physician if inconsistent.
- Assist with drainage of cerebrospinal fluid from system, if indicated, *to prevent or control intracranial hypertension.*
- Intervene *to prevent increased intracranial pressure:*
  - Administer medications, treatments, and intravenous lines per protocol.
  - Maintain elevation of head of bed per protocol *to maximize venous drainage.*
  - Accurately record intake and output.
  - Monitor serum electrolytes, blood count, and arterial blood gases for abnormalities.
- Intervene to monitor or prevent seizures:
  - Assess seizure history of patient.
  - Institute seizure precautions *to minimize potential for injury to the patient:*
    - Padded tongue blade and airway at bedside
    - Bed height at lowest level
    - Side rails up at all times and padded
    - Oxygen and suction equipment at bedside
    - Emergency medications at bedside
  - Administer anticonvulsants as per protocol:
    - Monitor effects and side effects.
    - Monitor serum for therapeutic levels of anticonvulsant.

Sensory/perceptual alterations

- Assess and record patient's level of orientation.
- Have side rails up at all times when patient is alone. Maintain patient safety at all times.
- Judiciously use soft restraints; monitor patient's response.
- Involve family in aspects of care as appropriate.
- Frequently reorient patient to time, person, and place. Reintroduce yourself each time you reorient patient.
- Have family bring in familiar objects.
- Allow family to stay with patient.
- Maintain planned rest periods *to allow sufficient time for REM sleep.*
- Use day and night lighting appropriately.
- Stimulate patient's sense of touch, taste, and position.

Potential impaired skin integrity

- Assess patient's skin condition for redness when turning or providing skin care.
- See general intervention strategies listed on p. 1646.
- Prevent pressure sores and contractures:
  - Keep scalp dry and clean.
  - Reposition every 2 hours, and turn head frequently. Rotate head and body together *to prevent strain on neck.*
  - Provide passive ROM exercises, especially to lower extremities, every 4 hours and as needed *to prevent contractures.*

Altered nutrition: less than body requirements

- Assess patient's nutritional level in consultation with nutritionist.
- Offer small, frequent feedings *to encourage adequate intake.*
- Complete nursing care before feeding times.

Nursing Diagnosis	Nursing Intervention/Rationale
	• Allow ample time for feeding. • Position patient in a semisitting position. Support head. • Encourage a high-protein diet. • Accurately measure and record intake on a flowsheet *to establish if intake is adequate.* • Administer parenteral fluids as per protocol. • Administer tube feedings as per protocol. • Position patient on his side after feeding *to prevent aspiration.* • Elevate head *to prevent aspiration.*

Patient Education

1. Make certain the patient and family know and understand the following:
   a. Nature of hydrocephalus, treatments, and procedures; explain as they occur
   b. Care of shunt devices if indicated
   c. Need to ambulate as tolerated
   d. Importance of maintaining planned rest periods
   e. Names of medications, dosages, frequency of administration, purposes, and toxic or side effects
   f. Need to avoid taking over-the-counter medications without consulting physician
   g. Possible residual effects such as headaches, sensory or motor deficits, seizures
2. Teach the patient and the family to recognize seizure activity and the appropriate course of action:
   a. Assist patient to sit or lie down.
   b. Avoid trying to stop seizure or restraining patient.
   c. Protect patient from injury.
   d. Observe and record body parts involved and duration of seizure activity.
3. Ensure that the patient and family understand the importance of ongoing outpatient care (i.e., physician's visits and physical therapy).
4. Teach the patient and family the importance of maintaining a well-balanced diet.

Evaluation

Patient Outcome	Data Indicating That Outcome is Reached
Patient demonstrates an effective breathing pattern.	Patent airway is maintained. Chest excursion is symmetric. Breath sounds are normal or there is no increase in adventitious sounds. Arterial blood gas values are within normal ranges or consistent with patient's baseline. Vital signs are within normal ranges or consistent with patient's baseline. Hemoglobin levels are 14 to 18 g/dl (male) and 12 to 16 g/dl (female). Intake and output are stable. There are no signs of respiratory distress. Resonance of all lobes is evident on percussion. Skin color is without cyanosis.
Patient maintains adequate cerebral tissue perfusion.	There is no change in level of consciousness. There is no evidence of neurologic deficits. Pattern of electrolytes is stable. There is no seizure activity.
Patient demonstrates minimum complications of sensory-perceptual alterations.	Optimum level of orientation is maintained. The patient remains free of injury. Skin integrity is maintained. Nutritional status is adequate. Self-care deficits are minimal. Social participation is appropriate to physiologic status.
Patient demonstrates skin integrity.	Skin is intact. Nutritional status is adequate. Electrolyte balance is maintained. Patient remains free of pressure sores and contractures.
Patient experiences minimum alterations in comfort.	Patient openly verbalizes feelings of discomfort when they occur. Patient is able to use measures to decrease discomfort. Patient verbally validates a decrease in subjective feelings of discomfort. Objective findings of pain are decreased.
Patient demonstrates intact self-concepts.	Patient openly verbalizes feelings of grief and loss. Patient verbalizes positive feelings about self. Patient acknowledges actual change in self-image. Patient focuses on present and future appearance and function. Patient verbalizes feelings of hopefulness, helpfulness, and powerfulness.
Patient demonstrates adequate nutritional status.	Weight pattern is stable: normal for height, age, sex, and previous baseline. Intake and output are balanced and stable. Diet is appropriate to age. Skin turgor is good. There is fluid and electrolyte balance. Dietary supplements are used as appropriate.

CRANIAL AND PERIPHERAL NERVE DISORDERS

Bell's palsy

Bell's palsy (facial paralysis) is the paralysis of the facial nerve (cranial nerve VII), resulting in a sudden loss of ability to move the muscles of expression of the face.

Any or all of the three branches of the facial nerve may be affected. The disorder can be unilateral or bilateral, transient or permanent. Generally the disorder appears static for about 10 days to 2 weeks, at which time muscle tone begins to reappear. Voluntary movement of the muscles may appear within 3 or 4 weeks. However, some individuals manifest no recovery for almost 6 months, and maximum recovery (which may not be complete) may occur in approximately a year. More than 80% of the patients with Bell's palsy recover without residual neurologic deficits.[16]

Pathophysiology

The pathogenesis and pathophysiology of Bell's palsy are unclear. One hypothesis is that a viral infection of the geniculate ganglion is responsible for the disorder. Other possible mechanisms include local ischemia and edema or emotional trauma and the resulting vasoconstriction.[23]

The disorder can occur at any age but most frequently occurs in individuals between 20 to 60 years. Men and women are affected about equally. The diagnosis of Bell's palsy is made by clinical features and a characteristic history.

Medical Plan

Medications

Corticosteroids
- Prednisone (Deltasone), 20-60 mg/d po; dosage is gradually reduced

Analgesics as required

General Management

Electrical stimulation of nerve
Warm, moist heat
Massage
Facial sling to prevent muscle stretching and to facilitate eating (by improving lip alignment)
Facial exercises (i.e., wrinkling brow, forcing eyes closed, puffing out cheeks) for 5 minutes three or four times daily, as muscle tone returns

NURSING CARE

Nursing Assessment

Pain

Usually begins behind the ear
May or may not be accompanied by herpetic vesicles in the external ear

Paralysis

Drawing sensation on affected side, followed by complete paralysis of affected side of face: all muscles powerless and flaccid (i.e., cannot smile, wrinkle forehead, or close eye; drooling of saliva; constant eye tearing)

Taste

Loss of taste sensation over anterior two thirds of tongue on affected side

Eating and Drinking Difficulties

May see anorexia and weight loss

Nursing Dx & Intervention

Nursing Diagnosis	Nursing Intervention/Rationale
Pain	• Establish baseline and ongoing assessment of patient's perception of discomfort. • Provide gentle massage as needed. • Provide warm moist heat per protocol. • Provide for electrical stimulation per protocol. • Apply facial sling as needed *to prevent muscle stretching and facilitate eating.* • Administer pain medications per protocol. • Provide eye care every 1 to 2 hours and as needed *to prevent corneas from drying and injury.* • Apply eye pads as indicated. • Teach patient to perform facial exercises three or four times daily for 5 minutes *to promote muscle tone:* Wrinkling brow Grimacing

Nursing Diagnosis	Nursing Intervention/Rationale
	Whistling Puffing out cheeks Forcing eyes closed • Provide patient with sunglasses as needed *to prevent eye strain.*
Altered nutrition: less than body requirements	• Assess patient's ability to chew and swallow. • Offer patient frequent, small feedings. • Maintain soft diet as indicated. • Avoid hot fluids and foods *to prevent burns to insensitive areas.* • Provide patient with privacy at mealtimes *to minimize anxiety and embarrassment.* • Provide patient with adequate time for eating meals. • Teach patient to take foods on unaffected side. • Apply facial sling *to improve lip alignment.* • Teach patient to chew food on unaffected side. • Provide meticulous mouth care before and after meals. • Provide dietary supplements as indicated.
Impaired verbal communication	• See general intervention strategies listed on p. 1784.
Anxiety	• See general intervention strategies listed on p. 1743. • Assist patient to deal with anxiety about the disorder, discomfort, changes in self-image, and fear of recurrence. Explain possible causes and treatments for the disorder: State explanations simply and monitor reactions. Repeat explanations as indicated.
Body image disturbance	• See general intervention strategies listed on p. 1751.
Social isolation	• See general intervention strategies listed on p. 1767.

Patient Education

1. Instruct regarding possible causes, involvement, symptoms, treatments, and usual course of Bell's palsy (explain procedures as they occur).
2. Instruct regarding signs of complications and progression of the disorder.
3. Teach special techniques such as the use of facial slings, massage, dietary adjustments, and exercise program to minimize discomfort.
4. Stress importance of continued eye care.
5. Instruct regarding safety measures for minimizing trauma to insensitive areas.
6. Instruct regarding name of medications, dosage, frequency of administration, purpose, and toxic or side effects of the medication.
7. Stress importance of ongoing outpatient care: physician's visits, physical therapy and exercise program, and support groups.

Evaluation

Patient Outcome	Data Indicating That Outcome is Reached
Patient and family demonstrate adequate knowledge of Bell's palsy.	Patient is able to explain possible causes of Bell's palsy. Patient is able to explain treatment modalities for the disorder. Patient is able to explain the usual course of the disorder.
Patient demonstrates a low level of anxiety.	Patient openly verbalizes concerns and feelings of grief, loss, and discomfort. Open verbalization of feelings is supported by the health care professionals and family.
Patient demonstrates minimal discomfort.	Patient is able to use measures such as facial sling and warm massage as needed. Patient openly expresses feelings of discomfort when they occur. Patient is able to perform facial exercises as indicated.
Patient does not demonstrate the complications of impaired communication.	

Patient Outcome	Data Indicating That Outcome is Reached
Patient demonstrates adequate nutritional status.	Weight pattern is stable: normal for height, age, sex, and previous baseline. Intake and output are balanced and stable. Diet is appropriate to age. Skin turgor is good. There is fluid and electrolyte balance. Dietary supplements are used as appropriate.
Patient demonstrates an intact, realistic body image.	Patient openly verbalizes feelings of grief and loss. Patient verbalizes positive feelings about self. Patient acknowledges actual changes in self-image. Patient focuses on present appearance and function. Patient verbalizes feelings of hopefulness, helpfulness, and powerfulness.
Patient demonstrates social participation.	Patient can state the importance of interpersonal relationships. Patient can relate to self and others. Patient participates in unit or group activities. Patient participates in family activities as appropriate to his condition.

Guillain-Barré syndrome

Guillain-Barré syndrome is an acute syndrome characterized by widespread inflammation or demyelination of ascending or descending nerves in the peripheral nervous system.

Guillain-Barré syndrome has an incidence of 1.7 per 100,000 persons. Eighty-five percent of individuals affected by the Guillain-Barré syndrome have complete functional recovery. The recovery period usually extends over several weeks, but it may last months or even years. The remaining 15% of affected individuals experience some degree of permanent neurologic deficit.

Guillain-Barré syndrome is also known as acute idiopathic polyneuritis, acute polyradiculoneuropathy, postinfectious polyneuritis, Landry-Guillain-Barré-Strohl syndrome, infectious neuronitis, infectious polyneuritis, acute polyradiculitis, acute idiopathic polyradiculoneuritis, and acute inflammatory polyradiculoneuropathy.

Pathophysiology

The pathogenesis of Guillain-Barré syndrome is thought to be related to the sensitization of peripheral nerve myelin and is characterized by infiltration of mononuclear cells at all levels of the peripheral nervous system. Over half of individuals affected have had a nonspecific infection 10 to 14 days before the onset of Guillain-Barré symptoms, suggesting that sensitized lymphocytes may produce demyelination. A significant number of persons have developed symptoms characteristic of Guillain-Barré syndrome after being inoculated for the swine flu. The syndrome occurs in both sexes and can affect persons of any age.

Morphologic alterations that characterize Guillain-Barré syndrome include (1) widespread monocytic inflammatory infiltrate around blood vessels throughout the cranial and spinal nerves, including nerve roots, ganglia, and distal nerves; (2) segmental demyelination of peripheral nerves; and (3) in severe cases, axon destruction with resultant axonal reaction and wallerian degeneration. Anterior horn cells and neurons in dorsal root ganglia occasionally show central chromatolysis. If the axon loss is severe, denervation group atrophy can be seen in distal muscles. Electron microscopic studies have shown a breakthrough of the basement membrane of the Schwann cell by phagocytic cells that insinuate themselves beneath the myelin layers and are then stripped away.[50]

Diagnostic Studies and Findings

CSF Sampling

Albuminocytologic dissociation: decreased protein initially (15 to 45 mg); then increases as high as 600 mg; followed by return to normal
Lymphocyte count normal

Electromyography (EMG)

Reduced nerve conduction velocity when tested near peak of illness (usually 4 to 8 weeks after onset)
Low voltage potentials
Fibrillations and positive sharp waves (more common in late stages)

Medical Plan

Surgery

Tracheotomy (see Chapter 7)

Medications

Pituitary hormones
- Corticosporin (ACTH), 25-40 U IM or subcutaneously tid (possibly valuable if given early in course of the disorder; dosage and frequency individually determined)

Corticosteroids
- Prednisone (Deltasone), 5-80 mg/d in divided doses

Anti-infective agents
- Prophylactic antibiotics

General Management

Cardiac monitoring
Mechanical ventilation
Plasmapheresis (plasma exchange)
Chest physiotherapy
Arterial blood gas monitoring
Nutritional maintenance (e.g., IV or nasogastric feedings)
Special eye care

NURSING CARE

Nursing Assessment

Autonomic Function

Hypertension
Sinus tachycardia or bradycardia
Postural hypotension
Chest and abdominal tightness
Profuse diaphoresis
Urinary and rectal incontinence
Paroxysmal facial flushing

Cranial Nerve Function

Cranial nerve VII most commonly involved; abnormal testing response elicited

Motor Function

Weakness following paresthesia
Most common type of weakness is ascending (i.e., lower to upper limbs to trunk)
Equal involvement of proximal and distal muscles
Atrophy possible

Reflex Status

Deep tendon reflexes absent or diminished

Sensory Function

Usually less severe than motor involvement
Superficial or deep sensory involvement: usually stocking-glove distribution

Nursing Dx & Intervention

Nursing Diagnosis	Nursing Intervention/Rationale
Ineffective breathing pattern	• Auscultate breath sounds every 1 to 2 hours; assess quality and any increase in adventitious sounds. • Maintain patent airway. Intubation, tracheostomy, and mechanical ventilation may be indicated.
Potential for aspiration	• Suction as needed *to prevent airway obstruction and aspiration*. Hyperinflate lungs with 100% oxygen for 1 minute before and 1 minute after suction, unless contraindicated. Maintain aseptic technique. • Monitor mechanical ventilation, if used: Ensure that tidal volume, rate, mode, and oxygen concentration are set as ordered. Ensure that ventilator alarms are on and functional. • Monitor arterial blood gases per protocol *to check for signs of respiratory failure:* Report decrease in Po_2 of 10 to 15 mm Hg. Report increase in Pco_2 greater than 10 to 15 mm Hg. • Note respiratory rate, depth, and level of consciousness every 15 to 30 minutes and as needed. • Check blood pressure, temperature, and pulse rate every 1 to 2 hours and as needed based on patient's condition *to monitor for signs of autonomic dysfunction*. • Assist and teach patient to cough and deep breathe every 2 hours *to improve respiratory functioning*. • Administer medications per protocol. • Limit fluid intake per protocol: may include titrating fluids according to pulmonary artery, pulmonary capillary wedge, or central venous pressure. • Measure and record intake and output; report hourly output less than 30 ml. • Monitor hemodynamics (central venous pressure, arterial pressure, pulmonary artery pressure, pulmonary capillary wedge pressure) per protocol.
Pain	• See general intervention strategies listed on p. 1720.
Impaired physical mobility	• See general intervention strategies on p. 1687.
Feeding, bathing/hygiene, dressing/grooming, and toileting self-care deficit	• Assess patient's abilities to provide self-care and intervene as appropriate. • Avoid giving oral feedings; administer IV or nasogastric feedings per protocol. • Administer oral hygiene every 2 hours and as needed. • Provide daily hygiene care *to promote cleanliness and self-esteem*. • Provide eye care every 2 hours: Cleanse eyes and remove crust. Apply eye shields or tape eyes closed *to protect cornea*. Administer artificial tears or eye drops per protocol *to provide lubrication*. • Maintain bowel function with regular evacuation.

Nursing Diagnosis	Nursing Intervention/Rationale
Anxiety	• Assess and document patient's anxiety level. • Deal realistically and honestly with patient's anxiety about the disorder, the discomfort, and the change in self-image. • Explain potential treatments for the disorder: State simply and monitor patient's reactions. Repeat explanations, as indicated. • Teach basic relaxation techniques. Reinforce teaching, as indicated. • Teach the essential aspects of care, as indicated by the patient's condition. • Assist the patient to participate in making decisions about care, as indicated by patient's condition. • Alert staff to possible emotional changes; expect mood swings.
Body image, self-esteem, and personal identity disturbances	• See general intervention strategies listed on pp. 1751, 1754, and 1756.

Patient Education

1. Encourage open verbalization regarding fears of permanent disability, loss of function, and dying, as well as changes in body image.
2. Stress importance of avoiding individuals who have upper respiratory infections.
3. Emphasize importance of maintaining planned rest periods.
4. Stress need for independence and socialization:
   a. Encourage self-care.
   b. Encourage patient to eat meals with family.
5. Instruct regarding name of each medication, dosage, frequency of administration, purpose, and toxic or side effects.
6. Stress need to check with physician before taking any over-the-counter medication.
7. Emphasize need to exercise to tolerance level and avoid fatigue.
8. Stress need for high-caloric, high-protein diet; progress from soft to solid as tolerated.
9. Emphasize need to arrange utensils and food so they are easily managed by the patient.
10. Teach need to maintain fluid intake at 2000 ml daily, unless contraindicated.
11. Stress need to avoid constipation:
    a. Drink fluids.
    b. Use stool softeners (as approved by physician).
    c. Eat foods and fruits high in roughage.
12. Emphasize need for diversional activities (e.g., watching television, reading, listening to radio).
13. Stress importance of ongoing outpatient care: physician's visits, physical therapy, and occupational therapy.
14. Ensure the patient or family demonstrates the following: speech exercises, active and/or passive ROM exercises with massage to all extremities, and exercises that increase strength and mobility of fingers (e.g., squeeze toys, balls, clay).
15. Teach importance of warm baths to alleviate pain and stiffness.

Evaluation

Patient Outcome	Data Indicating That Outcome is Reached
Patient demonstrates a low level of anxiety.	Patient openly verbalizes concerns and feelings of grief, loss, and discomfort. Patient openly verbalizes feelings, supported by health care professionals and significant others. Patient verbalizes essential aspects of care. Patient is able to demonstrate relaxation techniques when feelings of anxiety begin.
Patient demonstrates an effective breathing pattern.	Airway remains patent. Chest excursion is symmetric. Vesicular, bronchial, and bronchovesicular breath sounds are normal with no adventitious sounds. Arterial blood gas values are within normal ranges or consistent with patient's baseline. Vital signs are within normal limits or consistent with patient's baseline. Hemoglobin levels are 14 to 18 g/dl (male) and 12 to 16 g/dl (female). Intake and output are stable. There are no signs of respiratory distress (i.e., nasal flaring, increased pulse rate, air hunger). All lobes are resonant on percussion. Skin color is not cyanotic.

Patient Outcome	Data Indicating That Outcome is Reached
Patient demonstrates a minimum level of discomfort.	Patient openly verbalizes feelings of discomfort when they occur. Patient is able to use measures to decrease discomfort. Patient is able to verbally validate a decrease in subjective feelings of discomfort. Objective findings of pain are decreased.
Patient demonstrates minimum complications of impaired physical mobility.	Skin integrity is maintained. Contractures and deformities do not form. Level of mobility is appropriate to physiologic status. Intake and output pattern is stable. Nutritional status is adequate. There are no signs or symptoms of thrombophlebitis. There are no signs or symptoms of local infection.
Patient demonstrates minimum self-care deficits.	Outcome criteria stated for impaired physical mobility are met. Level of self-care is appropriate to physiologic status. Diet is high in calories and protein. Physical and occupational therapy is given as indicated.
Patient demonstrates intact self-concept.	Patient openly verbalizes feelings of grief and loss. Patient verbalizes positive feelings about self. Patient acknowledges actual change in self-image. Patient focuses on present and future appearance and function. Patient verbalizes feelings of hopefulness, helpfulness, and powerfulness.

Trigeminal neuralgia

(Tic douloureux)

Trigeminal neuralgia, or tic douloureux, is a neurologic condition that affects the sensory distribution of the trigeminal facial nerve (cranial nerve V) and is characterized by flashing, stablike paroxysms of pain radiating along the course of a branch of cranial nerve V from the angle of the jaw.[63]

Trigeminal neuralgia is caused by degeneration of or pressure on the nerve. Any of the three branches of the nerve may be affected. Attacks of lancinating pain, caused by trigeminal neuralgia, often cause the person to wince with facial contractions, thus the term "tic douloureux."

Pathophysiology

The etiology of trigeminal neuralgia is unknown. The term "neuralgia" is used because there is no demonstrable structural lesion along the course of the nerve. A similar syndrome can occur in cases of multiple sclerosis, gasserian ganglion tumor, cerebellopontine tumor, or brainstem infarction.[35]

The idiopathic form of trigeminal neuralgia affects 15,000 individuals in middle adult to late adulthood each year. There is slightly higher incidence in women. Although any of the nerve's three branches can be affected, the second and third divisions are most commonly involved. Neuralgia of the first division results in pain over the forehead and around the eyes. Neuralgia of the second division results in pain in the nose, cheek, and upper lip, and when it occurs in the third division it causes pain in the lower lip and on the side of the tongue. Episodes of the pain recur over weeks or months, although there may be spontaneous remissions. Tender areas (trigger zones) and any mechanical activity such as smiling, talking, or touching the face can set off an attack.[35] These trigger points are the parts of mucous membrane or skin that are close to the involved nerve. Common trigger points are:

First division: supraorbital notch
Second division: infraorbital foramen close to the junction of the cheek and nose
Third division: side of the tongue or the mental foramen

The diagnosis of trigeminal neuralgia is based on the characteristic history and clinical presentation of the disorder.

Medical Plan

Surgery

Microvascular decompression procedure for selective cutting of fibers within the trigeminal nerve
Radio frequency retrogasserian rhizotomy (surgical lesions, made at selected points on the trigeminal nerve, by radio frequency current)
Avulsion of the peripheral branches of the trigeminal nerve
Intracranial division of the sensory root of the trigeminal nerve

Medications

Carbamazepine (Tegretol), 400-1000 mg/d po or IV
Phenytoin (Dilantin), 200-400 mg/d po or IV
Absolute alcohol: injected into gasserian ganglion in very small amounts (i.e., 1 ml)
Glycerol: injection of small amounts percutaneously into subarachnoid spaces around gasserian ganglion
Analgesics

General Management

Semisolid, fluid diet
Psychosocial counseling

NURSING CARE

Nursing Assessment

Pain

Severe, shooting pain, starting at a particular point with a repetitive tic and increasing in severity to where it shoots violently and with explosive force through the face on the affected side

Apprehension

Protects face from any stimulation

Personal Identity

Actual change in function of facial nerve
Protection of face from any form of stimulation
Change in social involvement
Verbalization of:
 Negative feelings about self
 Preoccupation with change or loss
 Focus on past appearance and function
 Change in life-style
 Fear of rejection by others
 Feelings of powerlessness, helplessness, hopelessness
 Refusal to acknowledge actual change

Social Isolation

Preoccupation with own thoughts and meaningless, repetitive activities
Dull, sad affect
Hostility projected in voice and behavior
Seeks to be alone
Withdrawn, uncommunicative, no eye contact
Activities and interests inappropriate for developmental stage and age
Verbalizes feelings of rejection
Verbalizes interests inappropriate for developmental stage and age
Insecurity in public
Expresses feeling different from others
Inability to meet others' expectations
Absence of, or insecurity in, significant purpose in life

Nursing Dx & Intervention

Nursing Diagnosis	Nursing Intervention/Rationale
Anxiety	• See general strategies on p. 1743.
Pain	• Assess what precipitates the pain *to assist patient to avoid these factors* by decreasing noxious stimuli. • Promote rest and relaxation. • Modify anxiety associated with the pain experience. • Provide other sensory input. Administer medications per protocol. • Remain with the patient. • Improve effectiveness of pain relief measures by using them before the pain becomes intense.
Altered nutrition: less than body requirements	• Assess food for proper temperature and consistency. • Offer small, frequent feedings *to encourage adequate intake*. • Complete nursing care before feeding times. • Allow ample time for feeding. • Encourage a high-protein diet. • Accurately measure and record intake on a flowsheet *to establish if intake is adequate*. • Administer parenteral fluids per protocol. • Administer tube feedings per protocol.
Potential for aspiration	• Elevate head *to prevent aspiration*. • Teach patient to chew food on the unaffected side.
Body image, self-esteem, and personal identity disturbances	• See general intervention strategies listed on pp. 1751, 1754, and 1756. • Assist patient to become involved in self-care. • Assist patient to become involved in unit activities.

Social isolation	• Allow the patient to express perceptions regarding the illness. Offer support and clarification.
	• Foster a sense of relatedness to self.
	• Foster a sense of relatedness to family:
	  Provide for physical closeness of family member.
	  Include family in care as appropriate.
	  Have patient teach family about the disorder.
	• Encourage patient to personalize the environment. Allow personal items to be brought from home.

Nursing Diagnosis	Nursing Intervention/Rationale
	• Use touch as therapeutic intervention. • Encourage patient to verbalize needs met through interpersonal relationships. • Encourage group activities. • Encourage patient to maintain good grooming habits *to promote self-esteem*.

Patient Education

1. Instruct regarding involvement, symptoms, treatments, and usual course of trigeminal neuralgia (explain procedures as they occur).
2. Instruct regarding signs of complications and progression of the disorder.
3. Teach measures for minimizing stimulation of affected areas and trigger zones.
4. Instruct regarding name of medications, dosage, frequency of administration, purpose, and toxic or side effects of the medication.
5. Stress the importance of ongoing outpatient care and physician's visits.
6. Refer patient to support groups.
7. Teach family members about possible dietary alterations.

Evaluation

Patient Outcome	Data Indicating That Outcome is Reached
Patient and family demonstrate adequate knowledge of trigeminal neuralgia.	Patient is able to explain treatment modalities for the disorder. Patient is able to explain the usual course of the disorder.
Patient demonstrates a low level of anxiety.	Patient openly verbalizes concerns and feelings of grief, loss, and discomfort. Patient openly verbalizes feelings, supported by health care professionals and family. Patient verbalizes essential aspects of care.
Patient demonstrates minimum discomfort from the disorder.	Patient openly expresses feelings of discomfort when they occur. Patient is able to use measures to decrease discomfort such as decreasing stimuli to affected areas and judicious use of analgesics.
Patient demonstrates adequate nutritional status.	Weight pattern is stable. Intake and output pattern is stable. Skin turgor is good. There is fluid and electrolyte balance. Dietary supplements are taken as appropriate.
Patient demonstrates an intact, realistic body image.	Patient openly verbalizes feelings of grief and loss. Patient verbalizes positive feelings about self. Patient acknowledges actual changes in self-image. Patient focuses on present appearance and function. Patient verbalizes feelings of hopefulness, helpfulness, and powerfulness.
Patient demonstrates social participation.	Patient states the importance of interpersonal relationships. Patient experiences a sense of relatedness to self and to others. Patient participates in unit or group activities. Patient participates in family activities, as appropriate to patient's condition.

DEGENERATIVE DISORDERS

Alzheimer's disease

Alzheimer's disease is a chronic neurologic disorder that is characterized by progressive and selective degeneration of neurons in the cerebral cortex and certain subcortical structures.

Alzheimer's disease was originally described in 1907 by a German neuropsychiatrist named Alois Alzheimer. At that time Alzheimer published a brief report that depicted the pathologic and clinical manifestations of a 55-year-old institutionalized woman who experienced unexplained "premature aging." Although the woman's motor function, gait, muscle strength, coordination, and reflexes remained fairly normal, she experienced severe and progressive deterioration in mental functions. At autopsy Alzheimer found that the woman's brain had widened sulci and small gyri and was smaller than those of other 50-year-old women.[6]

Alzheimer's disease is the fourth leading cause of death among elderly persons in the United States.[47] An estimated 4.4% of individuals over 65 years of age demonstrate the manifestations of moderate to severe dementia syndromes, and two thirds of this group are believed to have Alzheimer's disease.[22] Both men and women may be affected, but the incidence is higher in women. Current research efforts indicate that Alzheimer's disease is age related; it is uncommon in young persons and rare in middle age. However, as age increases, so does the incidence of the disorder such that its prevalence in individuals over the age of 80 is estimated at greater than 20%.[7]

To date, only genetics and female gender have been identified as risk factors for Alzheimer's disease. The genetic factor is believed to be inherited in the form of an autosomal dominant trait.[68] The risk associated with female gender has been attributed to two factors. First, Alzheimer's disease is age related and women live longer than men. Second, it is believed that development of Alzheimer's disease is sometimes related to a gene on the X chromosome.[6]

The onset of Alzheimer's disease is usually subtle and insidious. The duration and rate of progression vary, but for the well-cared-for patient, the average survival rate from onset is approximately 8 to 9 years.[6]

Pathophysiology

Grossly, the primary pathologic feature of Alzheimer's disease is the degeneration and loss of selective neuronal cells in the cerebral cortex that ultimately results in symmetric and extensive convolutional atrophy, particularly in the frontal and medial temporal regions. This cerebral atrophy is accompanied by an enlargement of the cerebral ventricles, which is not severe unless concomitant hydrocephalus exists.[7]

Characteristic microscopic lesions in the brain tissue of persons with Alzheimer's disease include neuritic plaques, neurofibrillary tangles, granulovacuolar degeneration, and Hirano bodies. Neuritic plaques consist of degenerated intracortical foci of clustered and thickened neurites (axons and dendrites) that surround a spherical deposit of amyloid (starch-like protein) fibrils.[7] These plaques usually are found most prominently in the frontal cortex and hippocampus. Neurofibrillary tangles (neurofibrils) consist of masses of twisted and tangled intracellular protein that are deposited primarily in the cytoplasm of neuronal cell bodies. These neurofibrils are found primarily in the hippocampus and adjacent areas of the temporal lobe and are most abundant in areas of severe neuronal loss. Granulovacuolar degeneration consists of membrane-bound vacuoles containing finely granular material that is found most prominently in the pyramidal neurons of the hippocampus. Hirano bodies are found in the neuropil and consist of intracytoplasmic eosinophilic rods.[6] Cell loss in the hippocampus is believed to correlate with the memory loss of Alzheimer's disease.

Characteristic cell loss found in the brain of an individual with Alzheimer's disease includes both cortical and subcortical structures. Cell loss in the cortex includes the larger cells of the association cortex and cholinergic cells at the rostal portion of the reticular activating system (RAS). The loss of cholinergic cells results in reduced levels of the neurotransmitter acetylcholine. Recent studies have suggested that deficiencies in cholinergic transmission may lead to a breakdown of neuronal structures and play a role in the clinical expression of Alzheimer's disease.[68] Cell loss in subcortical structures includes noradrenalin cells in the locus ceruleus and dopamine-secreting cells of the pars compacta of the substantia nigra.[6]

The basic pathophysiology processes of brain damage occurring with Alzheimer's disease are not known. One proposed etiology is related to chronic aluminum toxicity. However, recent studies indicate that while aluminum apparently does accumulate in tangle-bearing neurons, it does not appear that such an accumulation is a necessary condition for Alzheimer changes in the cell. Further, epidemiologic data does not indicate a higher incidence of Alzheimer's disease in individuals who chronically ingest aluminum (i.e., antacids).[6]

One possible reason that brain cells degenerate and die may be the reduced rate in overall cerebral metabolism in Alzheimer's disease. This cerebral metabolic reduction is approximately 25% compared to age- and sex-matched cognitively intact controls.[6] Another possibility regarding the pathophysiology of Alzheimer's is that it may be linked to some type of generalized membrane abnormalities or abnormal cellular calcium metabolism.[6]

As previously stated, the pathophysiology of Alzheimer's is not known. However, many current research efforts are targeted at unraveling the mystery of this devastating disease.

Diagnostic Studies and Findings

CT Scan (Serial)

Cerebral ventricular and subarachnoid space enlargement because of diffuse brain atrophy (later stages)

Magnetic Resonance Imaging (MRI)

Same as CT scan

Electroencephalogram

Diffuse slowing of brain waves and diminished voltage (advanced stages)

Comprehensive History

Identification of symptoms listed in the assessment section for this disorder; family history of similar disorders; careful attention to medication history

Psychometric and Behavioral Rating Scales

Mini Mental State (MMS)
Mental Status Questionnaire (MSQ)
Haycox behavior scale
Hamilton depression scale

Medical Plan

Medications

Psychotropic agents
- Haloperidol (Haldol), 2-4 mg/d po (NOTE: Haloperidol has reported risk of inducing dyskinesia tarda[6])

Chloral hydrate, 0.5-1 g po
Lorazepam (Ativan), 2-6 mg/d po in divided doses
Diazepam (Valium), 2-20 mg/d po in divided doses
Alprazolam (Xanax), 0.75-1.5 mg/d po in divided doses
Tricyclic agents (NOTE: Agents have anticholinergic side effects that may impair cognitive function)
Nortriptyline (Aventyl), 75-100 mg/d po
Amitriptyline (Elavil), 25-100 mg/d po

General Management

Electroconvulsive therapy
Cardiac monitoring
Support of vital functions (i.e., ventilator) if indicated
Nutritional support: soft or liquid diet
Social services consult
Physical therapy
Psychologic counseling and support
Community referrals
Occupational therapy
Home nursing services
Extended care facility referrals

NURSING CARE

Nursing Assessment

The literature has described three stages of Alzheimer's disease.[67]

Initial Stage (2 to 4 Years)

Absentmindedness
Lack of spontaneity
Time and spatial disorientation
Loss of memory and emotional control
Changes in affect
Depression
Diminished ability to concentrate
Perceptual alterations
Neglectfulness in appearance
Careless actions
Judgment mistakes
Delusions (transitory) of persecution
Muscle twitching
Epileptiform seizures

Middle Stage (2 to 12 Years)

Nocturnal restlessness
Apraxia (impaired ability to perform purposeful activity)
Alexia (inability to comprehend written words)
Asterognosia (inability to identify objects by touch)
Auditory agnosia (total or partial inability to recognize familiar objects by the sense of sound)
Agraphia (inability to write)
Hypertonia
Increased aphasia
Hyperorality
Complete disorientation
Unsteady gait
Progressive memory loss
Increase in socially unacceptable behaviors
Decreased ability to comprehend
Preservation phenomenon (i.e., repetitive actions such as chewing, tapping)

Terminal Stage (Up to 1 Year)

Seizures (rare)
Marked weight loss; emaciation
Decreased appetite
Bulimia
Apraxia
Visual agnosia
Incontinence (bowels and/or bladder)
Hyperorality
Paraphasia
Hypermetamorphosis
Increased irritability
Feelings of helplessness
Bedridden
Unresponsive or comatose

Anxiety

Appearance
Increased perspiration, clammy skin
Fatigue
Increased muscle tension (rigidity)
Skin blanches: pale
Increased small motor activity (i.e., tremors, restlessness)
Behavior
Decreased attention span
Increased immobility
Decreased ability to follow directions
Other
Increased rate or depth of respirations
Increased heart rate
Rapid shifts in body temperature, blood pressure
Urinary urgency
Diarrhea
Dry mouth
Decreased appetite
Pupillary dilation

Seizure Activity

Generalized or focal
Preconvulsive (preictal) stage
Aura: flash of light; sense of loss, fear; weakness; dizziness; peculiar taste, smell, and sounds
Cry or scream
Fall to floor
Loss of consciousness

Tachypnea
Convulsive stage
Tonic: rigid body; flexed jaws; clenched fists; extended legs; cyanosis; holding breath
Clonic: urinary and/or fecal incontinence; jerking of facial muscles and extremities; biting tongue; frothing at mouth
Postconvulsive (postictal) stage
Altered level of consciousness
Headache
Nausea and/or vomiting
Malaise
Muscle soreness
Aspiration
Breathing difficulty, choking, cyanosis, decreased breath sounds, tachycardia, tachypnea

Nursing Dx & Intervention

Nursing Diagnosis	Nursing Intervention/Rationale
Sensory/perceptual alterations	• Assess and document patient's level of orientation. • Keep side rails up at all times when patient is alone. Maintain patient safety at all times. • Maintain quiet environment, reducing external stimuli to a minimum. • Reorient patient frequently to time, place, and person. Introduce yourself each time you reorient patient. • Repeat explanations frequently and simply *to facilitate understanding*. • Have family bring in familiar objects. • Maintain planned rest periods *to allow sufficient time for REM sleep*. • Use day and night lighting appropriately. • Stimulate senses of touch, taste, position.
Feeding, bathing/hygiene, dressing/grooming, and toileting self-care deficit	• Assess patient's ability to provide self-care and intervene where necessary. • Assist with feeding, as indicated; use IV or nasogastric feedings per protocol. • Administer oral hygiene every 2 hours and as needed *to remove secretions and promote comfort*. • Assist with daily hygiene care as indicated. • Administer eye care every 2 to 4 hours if indicated. • Perform intermittent urinary catheterization per protocol. • Maintain bowel function with regular evacuation *to prevent constipation*.
Potential impaired skin integrity	• Assess patient's skin condition for redness when turning or providing skin care. • Prevent pressure sores and contractures: Keep skin dry and clean. Reposition every 2 hours; massage pressure areas after turning. Provide passive ROM exercises every 4 hours and as needed: Perform ROM exercises gently, slowly, and rhythmically. Repeat each ROM exercise three times, every 4 hours. Use footboard or Spence boots *to prevent footdrop*. • Maintain high-protein, low-calcium diet *to prevent muscle wasting*.
Potential for trauma related to seizures	• Assess and document patient's potential for injury; institute safety measures. • Maintain bed in low position at all times unless side rails are up or when nurse is with the patient. • Provide the patient with a call light within easy reach. • Maintain side rails in up position at bedtime, after sedation, when patient is confused, and as needed. • Maintain wheelchairs and stretchers in locked position when transferring patient. • Pad side rails if patient is overactive.
Preconvulsive	• Have oral airway at bedside. • Support and protect head; turn to side if possible *to prevent aspiration*. • Prevent injury: Ease to floor if in chair. Place pillows along side rails if in bed. Remove surrounding furniture. Loosen constrictive clothing. • Provide privacy as necessary *to protect patient's dignity*. Stay with patient; remain calm. • Note frequency, time, involved body parts, and length of seizure *to determine type of seizure*.
Postconvulsive	• Maintain patent airway. • Suction as indicated. • Check vital signs and neurologic status. • Administer oxygen per protocol *to minimize cerebral hypoxia*.

Nursing Diagnosis	Nursing Intervention/Rationale
	• Reorient patient to environment *to minimize perceptual alteration.* • Place patient in position of comfort; turn head to side *to prevent aspiration.* • Administer oral hygiene as necessary for secretions and bleeding.
Impaired physical mobility	• Assess and document patient's level of mobility. Change position slowly *to prevent orthostatic hypotension.* Position in proper body alignment. • Use firm mattress or bed board *to support back and spine.* • Apply antiembolus stocking to lower extremities *to promote venous return.* • Administer anticoagulation therapy per protocol *to prevent embolus formation.*
Potential for disuse syndrome	• Encourage self-care activities to tolerance. • Plan all activities and maintain planned rest periods *to avoid fatigue.* • Obtain physical therapy referral.
Altered patterns of urinary elimination	• Assess characteristics of patient's voiding pattern (frequency, amount). • Perform intermittent catheterization per protocol. • Monitor intake and output. Maintain fluid intake at 2000 ml/day unless contraindicated. • Assess urine for sediment, concentration, color, and odor. • Acidify urine with foods such as orange juice and cranberry juice *to minimize potential for infection.* • Administer urinary tract germicides (e.g., methenamine mandalate [Mandelamine]) as ordered.
Altered nutrition: less than body requirements	• Assess food for proper temperature and consistency. • Offer small, frequent feedings *to encourage adequate intake.* • Complete nursing care before feeding times. • Allow ample time for feeding. • Encourage a high-protein, low-calcium diet. • Accurately measure and record intake on a flowsheet *to establish adequate intake.* • Administer parenteral fluids per protocol. • Administer tube feedings per protocol. • Elevate head *to prevent aspiration.*
Anxiety	• See general intervention strategies listed on p. 1743. • Support the family: Provide for ongoing contact. Give appropriate referrals to support groups. • Assist patient to deal realistically and honestly with anxiety about inability to predict course of the disorder and change in self-image and self-esteem.
Powerlessness	• Assist patient to reestablish as much physiologic control as condition allows: Share information about physiologic functioning with the patient. Focus on functions that remain intact. • Assist patient to reestablish some means of psychologic control: Encourage patient to express feelings as long as possible. Encourage patient to participate in care as long as able to do so. Encourage patient to become an active decision maker about care and immediate environment.
Body image and personal identity disturbances	• See general intervention strategies listed on pp. 1751 and 1754.
Social isolation	• See general intervention strategies listed on p. 1767.
Impaired adjustment	• Encourage patient to express feelings and fears regarding disease and disabilities. • Recognize possibility of emotional responses such as anxiety, depression, withdrawal, anger, helplessness, powerlessness, and crying. • Assist patient to examine own responses to the threatening situation. • Avoid judgment, criticism, or belittling of feelings and ideas. • Encourage focus on remaining strengths and intact roles. • Support patient's spiritual beliefs. • Encourage a sense of control: Include patient in specific aspects of care as appropriate. Share observations with patient regarding physical status and progress. • Teach patient to understand and manage feelings of anger and helplessness. • Assist patient to develop problem-solving skills regarding disappointments and dissatisfactions. • Assist patient to develop a stress management plan with simple relaxation exercises, self-monitoring activities, and use of imagery.

Nursing Diagnosis	Nursing Intervention/Rationale

Altered family processes

- Assist family to identify and understand what is occurring as specifically as possible *to focus on the situational factors.*
- Assist family to redefine situation in favorable terms.
- Support family in efforts to clarify family interactions.
- Assist family to express ideas assertively *to resolve the problem or situation.*
- Assist family in exploring alternatives for problem solution.
- Provide family with information about family dynamics *that enhance family's problem-solving skills.*
- Assist family in identification of consequences of proposed options for resolutions of the problem.
- Support family members in efforts to implement problem resolution.
- Assist family in evaluating effectiveness of problem solving.

Sleep pattern disturbance

- Assess patient's current sleep pattern as compared with usual sleep patterns.
- Assess for factors that interfere with sleep *to determine potential causes for inadequate sleep.*
- Encourage patient to express concerns when unable to sleep.
- Assess medication regimen *to determine whether it is factor in sleep pattern disturbance.*
- Assess patient's daytime habits and activities:
  - Assist in planning of daytime activities.
  - Discourage daytime napping if it negatively affects nighttime sleep patterns.
- Provide comfortable environment *to promote rest or sleep.*
- Teach patient simple relaxation techniques *to promote rest or sleep.*
- Decrease fluid intake before bedtime.
- Discourage intake of food or caffeine at bedtime.
- Discourage strenuous mental or physical activity before bedtime.
- Assist patient to maintain a normal day-night pattern to facilitate sleeping at night.
- Provide sedation per protocol if necessary. Evaluate effectiveness and side effects of sedatives.

Anticipatory grieving

- Encourage patient and family to identify and describe their perceptions of potential loss.
- Encourage patient and family to verbalize fears and concerns *to determine need for appropriate information.*
- Recognize the following factors as influencing coping behaviors: previous experiences with life-threatening situations, socioeconomic background, spiritual beliefs, cultural beliefs, educational background.
- Identify current sources of social support to the patient and family, as well as disruptions in present life-style related to anticipated loss such as finances or living arrangements.
- Identify grieving stage the patient and family are experiencing. Recognize patient and family may differ in stages of grieving.
- During stage of shock and disbelief, provide quiet environment *to minimize noxious environmental stimuli.*
- Allow for use of denial and other defense mechanisms. *To avoid false hope,* do not reinforce denial.
- Do not confront patient or family members who have distorted perceptions.
- Facilitate expression of emotions.
- Provide assurance that intense feelings and reactions are normal.
- Enlist support from other sources of support to patient and family *to encourage appropriate use of support resources.*
- During stage of developing awareness:
  - Provide family with ongoing information regarding patient's progress, care, and prognosis.
  - Encourage family to express need for information and desires in caring for the patient.
  - Facilitate family participation in patient's care as appropriate *to decrease feelings of isolation and loss.*
  - Arrange flexible visiting hours *to promote family interactions.*
  - Assist patient and family to share feelings, concerns, and fears with each other.
  - Assist family members to maintain own self-care needs *to promote and maintain physical health.*
  - Evaluate need for referral to resources such as the social services department.
- During period of mourning before patient's death:
  - Promote expression of what family expects when death occurs.
  - Discuss indicators of impending death as appropriate.
  - Provide comfort measures for the patient.
  - Encourage family to maintain verbal communication and touch with patient even though patient may not respond.
  - Provide privacy *to protect patient and family dignity.*

Patient Education

1. Instruct regarding name of medication, dosage, time of administration, purpose, and side effects.
2. Reinforce physician's explanation of medical management.
3. Emphasize need to avoid taking over-the-counter medications without notifying the physician.
4. Emphasize need for adequate nutritional status:
   a. Give diet as tolerated.
   b. Offer small, frequent feedings.
   c. Instruct to chew thoroughly and eat slowly and in small pieces.
5. Emphasize need for activity and exercise to tolerance:
   a. Plan activities of daily living.
   b. Maintain rest periods as planned.
   c. Do active and passive ROM exercises.
   d. Get at least 8 hours of sleep at night, if possible.
6. Encourage independent activities, as possible:
   a. Alert patient to limitations.
   b. Avoid overprotection.
   c. Stress need for supportive devices as indicated.
7. Emphasize importance of ongoing outpatient care.
8. Give outpatient, home nursing care or extended care facility referral as appropriate.
9. Emphasize safety measures: side rails, ramps, shower chairs, walkers, and canes.

Evaluation

Patient Outcome	Data Indicating That Outcome is Reached
Patient demonstrates minimal complications of sensory-perceptual alterations.	Level of orientation is optimum. Patient is free of injury. Patient demonstrates skin integrity. Self-care deficits are minimum. Social participation is appropriate to physiologic status.
Patient demonstrates minimal self-care deficits.	Outcome criteria listed for impaired physical mobility are met. Level of self-care activities is appropriate to physiologic status. Patient participates in physical and occupational therapy.
Patient demonstrates skin integrity.	Skin is intact. Nutritional status is adequate. Electrolyte balance is maintained. Patient is free of pressure sores and contractures.
Patient remains free of traumatic injury.	Safety measures are appropriate to physiologic status. Skin integrity is maintained. Skin is free of bruises, burns, abrasions, and redness. Environment is safe. Patient is free of nosocomial infections.
Patient demonstrates an optimum level of mobility.	Skin integrity is maintained. Patient remains free of contractures and deformities. Level of mobility is appropriate to physiologic status. Intake and output pattern is stable. Nutritional status is adequate. Patient is free of thrombophlebitis. Patient is free of local infection. Patient participates in an ongoing physical therapy program.
Patient demonstrates minimum complications from alterations in urinary elimination patterns.	Intake and output pattern is stable. Urine is clear, yellow to amber in color, and without sediment. Skin in perineal area is clean and dry. Urine is acidic (pH 6.0). Patient is free of urinary tract infections. Patient is free of bladder distention. Patient or family can describe symptoms of urinary tract infections that require medical intervention.
Patient demonstrates minimum complications of bowel incontinence.	Skin in perineal area is clean and dry. Dietary intake is adequate. Fluid intake is adequate (2000 ml daily, unless contraindicated). Intake and output patterns are stable. There is no fecal impaction. Bowel evacuation pattern is regular.
Patient demonstrates adequate nutritional status.	Weight pattern is stable. Intake and output pattern is stable. Diet is appropriate to physiologic status. Skin turgor is good. Fluid and electrolyte balance is maintained. Patient takes dietary supplements, as appropriate.
Patient demonstrates a low level of anxiety.	Patient openly verbalizes concerns and feelings of grief, loss, and discomfort. Patient openly verbalizes feelings, supported by health care professionals and family. Patient verbalizes essential aspects of care. Patient identifies methods to effectively deal with anxious feelings.
Patient demonstrates minimal feelings of powerlessness.	Optimum level of physiologic control, as possible for current health status, is maintained. Optimum level of psychologic control, as possible, is maintained. Patient participates, as possible, in decision making about care. Patient participates, as possible, in self-care.
Patient demonstrates intact self-concepts.	Patient openly verbalizes feelings of grief and loss. Patient acknowledges actual change in self-image. Patient verbalizes positive feelings about self. Patient focuses on present and future appearance and function. Patient verbalizes feelings of hopefulness, helpfulness, and powerfulness.

Patient Outcome	Data Indicating That Outcome is Reached
Patient demonstrates social participation.	Patient states importance of interpersonal relationships. Patient relates to self and others. Patient participates, as possible, in unit and group activities. Patient participates, as possible, in family activities.
Patient demonstrates optimum level of adjustment.	Patient actively involves self in future goal setting that is consistent with changed health status. Patient seeks and cooperates with assistance provided by competent caregivers. Patient demonstrates active self-care practices as appropriate to health status. Patient uses strengths and potentials to engage in maximally independent and constructive life-style.
Patient's family demonstrates intact family processes.	Family demonstrates role congruence. Family demonstrates clear communication. Family demonstrates constructive interactions. Family achieves resolution to the problem situation. Family learns and utilizes new approaches to problem solving.
Patient and family demonstrate constructive anticipatory grief work.	Patient and family demonstrate ability to discuss thoughts and feelings about impending loss. Patient and family verbalize needs for information. Patient and family demonstrate appropriate use of available resources. Patient's family demonstrates ability to meet ongoing self-care needs. Patient (as appropriate) and family participate in mutual decision making regarding anticipated loss. Patient and family demonstrate constructive interactional patterns.
Patient demonstrates minimum sleep-pattern disturbances.	Actual and potential causes of disturbances for inadequate sleep are identified. Management plan to correct or minimize causes of inadequate sleep is developed. Patient verbalizes feelings of being rested or refreshed.

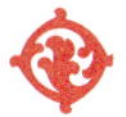

Amyotrophic lateral sclerosis

(Lou Gehrig's disease)

Amyotrophic lateral sclerosis (ALS) is a rapidly progressive degenerative disease of the motor neurons. It is characterized by atrophy of the muscles of the hands, forearms, and legs that eventually spreads to involve most of the body.[63]

Amyotrophic lateral sclerosis, also called Lou Gehrig's disease, is the most common variant of motor neuron disease. The cause and the cure of amyotrophic lateral sclerosis remain unknown.

Amyotrophic lateral sclerosis usually occurs between the ages of 40 to 70 years, but it also may occur in the very aged. The disorder has an incidence of 2 to 7 cases per 100,000 persons in the United States. In the United States, 95% of the cases are sporadic, and 5% are familial. Approximately two to three men are affected with amyotrophic lateral sclerosis to each woman. The disorder usually is fatal within 2 to 3 years after diagnosis, but one fifth of the patients may survive for between 5 and 20 years. A clustering of cases occurs in the western Pacific regions of Guam and Mariana Islands, where a form of amyotrophic lateral sclerosis is perhaps 50 to 100 times more common than in other regions.

The cause of amyotrophic lateral sclerosis is unknown. Virologic studies have not revealed any disease-specific abnormality, and most ultrastructural studies for virus material have been inconclusive or negative. Immunologic factors have been suggested by the finding of immune complex deposition in the glomeruli of some patients with the disease and the cytotoxicity of amyotrophic lateral sclerosis serum to anterior horn cells in tissue culture.[35] Epidemiologic studies in Guam support a genetic or external agent as a possible causative agent. Other proposed causes include metabolic disturbances (i.e., metal imbalances), inappropriate nutrition, and systemic stimuli responses (i.e., infection, trauma).

Pathophysiology

Amyotrophic lateral sclerosis is characterized by the deterioration of the anterior horn cells. Atrophy of the cortex, particularly of the precentral gyrus, may be grossly apparent in the cerebrum. Other pathologic changes include reduced numbers and size of the Betz cells of the motor cortex. In the brainstem there is loss of the motor neurons except for those serving the extraocular muscles. In the spinal cord there is a loss of large motor neurons and degeneration of the corticospinal tract.[35] The surviving motor neurons are atrophic and show pyknotic nuclei. The loss of the anterior horn cells results in denervation of the muscle fibers.

Diagnostic Studies and Findings

Serum

Creatinine phosphokinase may be twice normal value

CSF Sampling

Mild elevation of total protein with a normal IgG concentration and normal cell count

Myelography

Normal or shrunken spinal cord

CT Scan (Brain)

Normal; shows cerebral atrophy

Muscle Biopsy

Abnormalities and changes of denervation

Electromyography

Remarkable fibrillations indicating muscle wasting and denervation

Useful in confirming diffuse process in monoparetic or unilateral forms of the disease

Medical Plan

No specific treatment for amyotrophic lateral sclerosis has been established. Present modalities are aimed at treating symptoms when they occur.

Surgery

Cricopharyngeal myotomy to alleviate dysphagia

Cervical esophagostomy

Transtympanic neurectomy to control neural supply to parotid glands

Medications

Antianxiety agents (used for muscle relaxant effect)

- Diazepam (Valium), 5 mg po bid to tid

Muscle relaxants

- Baclofen (Lioresal), 5 mg po tid; up to 15-25 mg po tid (therapy initiated at low dosage and increased gradually until optimum results are achieved)

General Management

Cardiac monitoring

Mechanical ventilation

Prosthesis to support weakened muscles

Physical therapy

Psychosocial counseling and support

Nutritional support: soft or liquid diet

Community referrals

NURSING CARE

Nursing Assessment

Symptoms of amyotrophic lateral sclerosis vary, depending on which motor neuron cells are affected.

Muscle Functioning

Fasciculation of muscles; may be accompanied by weakness

Upper extremity (usually unilateral)

Atrophy evident in palms and both sides of thumbs

Loss of dexterity for fine hand movements

Lower extremities

- Spasticity and progressive weakness until flaccidity and atrophy occur
- Footdrop

Sensory Function

Not affected

Bulbar Palsy

Fasciculations and atrophy of the tongue

Dysphagia

Dysphonia

Dysarthria

Excessive drooling

Reflexes

Progressive decrease

Increase in pathologic reflexes

Mental Faculties

Not affected

Fear

Subjective statements of feeling fearful about health status and future life-style

Nursing Dx & Intervention

Nursing Diagnosis	Nursing Intervention/Rationale
Ineffective airway clearance; potential for aspiration	• Assess patient's ability to handle secretions and swallow. • Maintain patent airway; avoid flexion of the neck if patient is comatose. • Auscultate for breath sounds every 1 to 2 hours; report any changes. • Suction as needed *to prevent obstruction and manage secretions.* • Assist ventilation per protocol. • Monitor vital signs every 1 to 2 hours; monitor neurologic status every 1 to 2 hours. • Keep emergency drugs at the bedside. • Maintain nothing-by-mouth status *to prevent risk of choking or aspiration.* • Maintain quiet, nonstressful environment whenever possible *to minimize anxiety and fear.*
Ineffective breathing pattern	• See general intervention strategies on p. 1704.
Altered nutrition: less than body requirements	• Assess patient's nutritional needs. • Offer patient frequent, small feedings *to promote adequate nutrition and fluid intake.*

Nursing Diagnosis	Nursing Intervention/Rationale
	• Maintain soft or liquid diet as indicated. • Have suction equipment at bedside at all times *to prevent aspiration.* • Have patient eat and drink in an upright position with neck flexed. • Apply soft cervical collar if patient is unable to hold head upright. • Avoid mucus-producing foods such as milk *to control secretion production.* • Institute IV, nasogastric, or gastric feedings per protocol *to minimize risk of aspiration.*
Impaired physical mobility	• Use braces (hand splint; ankle-foot braces) *to maintain function.* • Teach family turning, positioning, and transfer techniques. • Turn and reposition patient every 2 hours and as needed *to reduce potential for spasticity* that occurs as a result of spinal cord involvement.
Feeding, bathing/hygiene, dressing/grooming, and toileting self-care deficit	• See general intervention strategies on p. 1692.
Anxiety	• See general intervention strategies on p. 1743.
Impaired verbal communication	• Assess and document patient's ability to communicate. • Develop a means of communication with patient: When patient is restricted to eye or eyelid movement, develop a code with the patient. Reinforce the techniques established. • Assist patient and family to identify other outlets for communication. • Continue to use sense of touch and nonverbal forms of communication.
Powerlessness	• Assess physiologic control and assist patient to reestablish as much control as condition allows: Share knowledge of physiologic functioning with the patient. Focus on functions that remain intact. • Assist patient to reestablish some means of psychologic control: Encourage patient to express feelings as long as possible. Encourage patient to participate in care as long as able to do so. Encourage patient to become an active decision maker about care and immediate environment.
Body image and personal identity disturbances	• See general intervention strategies on pp. 1751 and 1754.
Social isolation	• See general intervention strategies on p. 1767.

Patient Education

1. Encourage open verbalization of feelings and fears about loss of function, changes in body image, and dying.
2. Emphasize importance of maintaining planned rest periods.
3. Stress need for independence and socialization:
   a. Encourage self-care to tolerance.
   b. Encourage family to eat meals together for as long as possible.
4. Emphasize need to exercise to tolerance levels.
   a. Tell the patient to avoid fatigue.
   b. Teach the patient and family active exercises and ROM exercises.
5. Instruct regarding name of each medication, dosage, frequency of administration, purpose, and toxic and side effects.
6. Stress need to check with physician before taking any over-the-counter medications.
7. Emphasize need to maintain fluid intake at 2000 ml daily, unless contraindicated.
8. Teach proper techniques for turning, positioning, and transfer.
9. Stress importance of ongoing outpatient care:
   a. Physician's visits
   b. Physical therapy
   c. Occupational therapy
   d. Home nursing care, if indicated
   e. ALS Foundation referral
10. Ensure that the patient and family demonstrate application of hand splints and ankle-foot braces.

Evaluation

Patient Outcome	Data Indicating That Outcome is Reached
Patient demonstrates adequate airway clearance.	Airway remains patent. Breath sounds can be auscultated in all lobes. Chest excursion is symmetric during respiratory cycle. There are no signs of respiratory distress.
Patient demonstrates a low level of anxiety.	Patient openly verbalizes, as possible, concerns and feelings of grief, loss, and discomfort. Patient openly verbalizes, as possible, feeling of being supported by health professionals or significant others. Patient verbalizes, as possible, essential aspects of care.
Patient demonstrates an effective breathing pattern.	Airway remains patent. Chest excursion is symmetric. Vesicular, bronchial, and bronchovesicular breath sounds are normal. Arterial blood gas values are within normal limits or consistent with patient's baseline. Vital signs are within normal limits or consistent with patient's baseline. Hemoglobin levels are 14 to 18 g/dl (male) or 12 to 16 g/dl (female). Intake and output are stable. There are no signs of respiratory distress. Skin tone is appropriate to racial background. All lobes are resonant on palpation.
Patient demonstrates minimum impaired verbal communication.	Patient verbalizes feelings as long as physically able to do so. Patient develops alternative methods of communication.
Patient experiences a minimum level of impaired physical mobility.	Skin integrity is maintained. Patient remains free of contractures or deformities. Patient demonstrates a level of mobility appropriate to physiologic status. Intake and output are stable. Nutritional status is adequate. There are no signs or symptoms of local infection.
Patient demonstrates adequate nutritional status.	Weight pattern is stable. Intake and output pattern is stable. Diet is appropriate to physiologic status. Skin turgor is good. There is fluid and electrolyte balance. Dietary supplements are taken, as appropriate.
Patient demonstrates minimum feelings of powerlessness.	Patient maintains optimum level of physiologic control, as possible for current physiologic status. Patient maintains optimum level of psychologic control, as possible for current physiologic status. Patient participates, as possible, in decision making about care. Patient participates, as possible, in self-care.
Patient demonstrates minimum self-care deficits.	Outcome criteria listed for impaired physical mobility are met. Level of self-care is appropriate to physiologic status. Patient participates in physical and occupational therapy.
Patient demonstrates intact self-concepts.	Patient verbalizes, as possible, positive feelings about self. Patient acknowledges actual change in self-image. Patient verbalizes, as possible, feelings of grief, loss of functioning, and dying.
Patient demonstrates social participation, as possible.	Patient states importance of interpersonal relationships. Patient relates to self and others. Patient participates, as possible, in unit and group activities. Patient participates, as possible, in family activities.

Multiple sclerosis

Multiple sclerosis (MS), or disseminated sclerosis, is a chronic progressive neurologic disease that is characterized by disseminating demyelination of nerve fibers of the brain and spinal cord.[63]

Multiple sclerosis is the most prevalent of the human demyelinating diseases, with an incidence of 40 to 60 per 10,000 persons in the United States and Canada. Women are affected with the disorder slightly less often than men. The onset of symptoms occurs between 20 and 40 years of age in 75% of the cases. Incidence of the disease is rare in childhood, and the onset of symptoms rapidly decreases in old age. The severity, duration, and prognosis of multiple sclerosis vary. The survival rate of individuals with multiple sclerosis is approximately 85% of that for the general population. The diagnosis of this disorder is made on the presence of multiple lesions in the central nervous system and dissemination over time.

Studies show an association between the prevalence of multiple sclerosis and distance from the equator. Multiple sclerosis is most prevalent in western Europe, southern Canada, southern Australia, and New Zealand.[35] Within the United States, the prevalence of multiple sclerosis is higher in the Great Lakes region, the northern Atlantic states, and the Pacific Northwest.

The cause of multiple sclerosis is unknown. Etiologic hypotheses include genetic, virologic, epidemiologic, and immunologic features.

Studies indicate that first-degree relatives of a family member with multiple sclerosis have a 15 times greater incidence of multiple sclerosis than the general population. A person who has an identical twin affected with multiple sclerosis has a 20% risk of the disease, 300 times greater than in the general population.

Individuals with multiple sclerosis have elevated (i.e., up to twofold) serum and cerebrospinal fluid titers of antibodies to many viruses including herpes simplex type I, parainfluenza, rubella, mumps, measles, and Epstein-Barr virus.

The prevalence of multiple sclerosis is very low in warm climates and increases in temperate and colder climates. Studies have shown that persons who move from areas of higher prevalence to areas of lower prevalence after 15 years of age retain the risk of multiple sclerosis at the level of their previous environment. Individuals below 15 years of age acquire the risk prevalence of the new environment.[35]

Approximately 90% of individuals affected with multiple sclerosis have abnormalities of the cerebrospinal fluid, particularly increased IgG and oligoclonal bands. Suppressor lymphocyte function is altered, and acute deteriorations are accompanied or perhaps preceded by defective immunoregulation, allowing unimpeded damage to the myelin membrane and oligodendrocytes. Remission is accompanied by a rebound elevation in suppressor function.[35]

Pathophysiology

The neuropathologic changes in multiple sclerosis include multifocal plaques of demyelination distributed randomly within the white matter of the brainstem, spinal cord, optic nerve, and cerebrum. In the acute stages, perivenular cuffs of inflammatory cells have been noted. The active changes include three essentially concurrent processes: breakdown of myelin structure, lysis of oligodendrocytes, and activation of astroglial processes.[23] Within the cerebrum there is a predilection of plaques in the periventricular areas, particularly around the third and fourth ventricles. A mild lymphocytic meningitis mainly in deep sulcal recesses may accompany the parenchymal changes. The external surface of the brain appears normal. Brain weight may be diminished, and the ventricles may be enlarged. The most characteristic feature of the chronic lesions is a proliferation of astrocytic processes, which transform the lesion into a glial scar. As lesions age, the lipid products of myelin breakdown are phagocytosed.[23]

During the demyelination process (termed primary demyelination), the myelin sheath and the myelin sheath cells are destroyed. The demyelination process leads to four significant central disturbances: a decrease in nerve conduction velocity, nerve conduction block (frequency related), differential rate of transmission of impulses, and complete failure of impulse transmission. These disturbances account for the variety of clinical signs and symptoms. Symptom remission occurs when demyelinated areas are healed by sclerotic tissue. However, when the nerve fiber degenerates, symptoms become permanent.[32]

Diagnostic Studies and Findings

CSF Sampling

Elevated CSF γ-globulin
Normal or low CSF protein
Negative VDRL
Increased WBC count
Abnormal colloidal gold curve (in absence of neurosyphilis)
Presence of myelin basic pattern

CT Scan

May show ventricular enlargement and cerebral atrophy (with long-term disease)
Areas of low attenuation around cerebral ventricles

Positron Emission Tomography (PET)

May show altered locations and patterns of cerebral glucose metabolism

Medical Plan

Surgery

Contralateral thalamotomy
Rhizotomy

Medications

- Corticosteroids
  - Prednisone, 40-60 mg/d po for 8 d (dosage is reduced gradually)
  - Dexamethasone (Decadron), initial dose of 0.75-9 mg/d; maintenance dose individually adjusted to maintain an adequate clinical response
- Pituitary hormones
  - Corticotropin (ACTH, Athcar), 40-50 U bid for 7-10 d
- Muscle relaxants
  - Dantrolene sodium (Dantrium), initial dose of 25 mg po qid; maintenance dose up to 400 mg/d po
- Psychotherapeutic agents
  - Chlorpromazine (Thorazine), 10 mg po tid
- Muscle relaxants
  - Baclofen (Lioresal), 15-25 mg po tid
- β-Adrenergic blocking agents
  - Propranolol (Inderal), 40-240 mg/d po
- Potassium supplements if ACTH is administered

General Management

Braces
Splints
Wheelchair, walker, cane
Nutritional consultation
Physiotherapy
Occupational therapy
Home nursing services
Extended care facility referrals
Hydrotherapy
Speech therapy

NURSING CARE

Nursing Assessment

Sensory Symptoms

Numbness and tingling of involved extremity or face
Loss of joint sensation and proprioception (generally accompanies extremity edema)
Loss of sense of position, shape, texture, and vibration (50% of patients)

Ocular Symptoms

Optic neuritis (pain with eye movement, visual clouding, decrease in visual field)
Nystagmus (70% of patients)
Diplopia
Marcus-Gunn phenomenon (dilation of affected pupil when light is shone into eye)
Swinging-flashlight sign (dilation of affected pupil when light is moved from intact eye to eye with defect)

Motor Symptoms

Weakness in lower extremities (initially)
Decline in motor function after hot bath or shower (Uhthoff's phenomenon)
Incoordination
Intentional tremors of upper extremities and ataxia of lower extremities
Staggering gait and spastic weakness of speech muscles
Facial palsy

Vestibular/Auditory Functions

Vertigo

Mental/Behavioral Symptoms

Irritability
Inattentiveness
Emotional lability
Mild depression
Poor judgment
Later: memory deficits; depression; confusion; disorientation

Other

Hyperactive reflexes
Positive Babinski's sign
Ankle clonus (50%)
Impotence
Loss or impairment of sphincter control
Loss of abdominal reflexes (80%)
Lhermitte's phenomenon
Charcot triad (intentional tremors, nystagmus, and staccato speech) with brainstem involvement
Urine and fetal incontinence
Respiratory failure

Nursing Dx & Intervention

Nursing Diagnosis	Nursing Intervention/Rationale
Ineffective airway clearance	• Auscultate for breath sounds every 1 to 2 hours and as needed; report changes in breath sounds. • Maintain patent airway, and avoid flexion of the neck if patient is immobile. • Suction as needed *to prevent obstruction.* • Assist ventilation as indicated. • Monitor vital signs every 1 to 2 hours; monitor neurologic status every 1 to 2 hours. • Keep emergency drugs at bedside. • Maintain nothing-by-mouth status *to prevent risk of choking or aspiration.*
Potential for aspiration; ineffective breathing pattern	• See general intervention strategies listed on pp. 1635 and 1704.
Potential for injury	• See general intervention strategies listed on p. 1620.
Pain	• Decrease the noxious stimuli, whenever possible, by assessing precipitating factors and assisting patient to modify or avoid these factors. • Assist patient to modify the anxiety associated with the pain experience. • Provide other sensory input (e.g., gentle back rub). • Administer medications as per protocol: analgesics and muscle relaxants *to control pain and spasticity.*
Anxiety	• Assess patient's anxiety level. • Assist patient to deal realistically with anxiety about inability to predict course of the disorder, discomfort from spasticity, and change in self-image and self-esteem. • Explain potential treatments for the symptoms of the disorder: State in basic terms and monitor patient's response. Repeat explanations as needed. • Alert other health care professionals and family to potential emotional changes.

Nursing Diagnosis	Nursing Intervention/Rationale
Bathing/hygiene, dressing/ grooming, feeding, and toileting self-care deficit	• Assess patient's degree of deficit and intervene as necessary. • Assist with feeding, as indicated: Use of hand braces Use of IV or nasogastric feedings, as ordered • Administer oral hygiene every 2 hours and as needed. • Assist with daily hygiene care, as indicated. • Administer eye care every 2 to 4 hours. • Perform intermittent catheterization as per protocol *to maintain adequate bladder elimination and prevent infection.* • Maintain bowel function with regular evacuation.
Potential for disuse syndrome	• Assess patient's mobility level. • Encourage self-care activities to tolerance. • Plan all activities and maintain rest periods *to avoid fatigue.* • Obtain physical therapy referral.
Sensory/perceptual alterations	• See general intervention strategies listed on p. 1728.
Altered nutrition: less than body requirements	• See general intervention strategies listed on p. 1630.
Altered patterns of urinary elimination	• See general intervention strategies listed on p. 1666.
Impaired verbal communication	• Develop means of communication with the patient: pad and pencil, Magic Slate. • Teach patient to speak in a slow, unhurried manner. • Obtain referral for speech therapy. Reinforce techniques established. • Assist patient and family to identify other outlets for communication. • Continue to use sense of touch and other nonverbal forms of communication.

Patient Education

1. Instruct regarding nature of multiple sclerosis and treatment modalities (explain procedures as they occur).
2. Stress importance of routines for activities of daily living.
3. Emphasize importance of avoiding fatigue, overwork, and emotional stress.
4. Stress importance of regular exercise and planned rest periods.
5. Emphasize importance of diversional activities.
6. Stress importance of speech therapy, physical therapy, and occupational therapy.
7. Encourage verbalization about feelings.
8. Emphasize need for socialization with significant others.
9. Stress need for independence and self-care to level of tolerance:
   a. Support the patient when ambulating.
   b. Help the patient to walk with a wide base.
10. Instruct regarding symptoms of disease progression and flu or cold to report to the physician.
11. Emphasize need to avoid persons with upper respiratory infections.
12. Stress need to avoid extremes of hot and cold.
13. Teach name of medication, dosage, frequency of administration, purpose, and toxic or side effects.
14. Emphasize importance of avoiding over-the-counter medications.
15. Stress importance of ongoing outpatient care:
    a. Physician's visits
    b. Physical therapy
    c. Speech therapy
    d. Occupational therapy
    e. Home nursing services
    f. MS Society referral
16. Ensure that the patient and family demonstrate the following:
    a. Active and/or passive ROM exercises
    b. Proper techniques of ambulation
    c. Proper techniques for turning, positioning, and transfer
    d. Application of hand splints and braces
    e. Methods for maintaining patient safety
17. Teach the patient about factors that exacerbate symptoms of multiple sclerosis
    a. Overexertion
    b. Hot baths
    c. Fever
    d. Emotional stress
    e. Cold
    f. High humidity
    g. Pregnancy

Evaluation

Patient Outcome	Data Indicating That Outcome is Reached
Patient and family demonstrate adequate knowledge of multiple sclerosis.	Patient and family state that the disorder is not hereditary. Patient and family state the nature of the disease in basic terms. Patient and family can identify possible treatment modalities. Patient and family can identify symptoms of progression.
Patient demonstrates a patent airway.	Breath sounds are normal. Chest excursion is bilateral and symmetric. Rate and depth of respiration are normal. Cough is effective. There are no subjective or objective findings of shortness of breath, air hunger, or dyspnea on exertion.
Patient demonstrates a low level of anxiety.	Patient openly verbalizes concerns and feelings of grief, loss, and discomfort. Patient openly verbalizes feelings, supported by health care professionals and family. Patient verbalizes essential aspects of care. Patient identifies methods to deal effectively with anxious feelings.
Patient demonstrates minimum complications of bowel incontinence.	Skin in perineal area is clean and dry. Dietary intake is adequate. Fluid intake is adequate (2000 ml daily, unless contraindicated). Intake and output patterns are stable. There is no fecal impaction. Bowel evacuation pattern is regular.
Patient demonstrates an effective breathing pattern.	Airway is patent. Chest excursion is symmetric. Breath sounds are normal, or there is no increase in adventitious sounds. Arterial blood gas values are within normal ranges or consistent with patient's baseline. Hemoglobin levels are 14 to 18 g/dl (male) or 12 to 16 g/dl (female). Intake and output are stable. There are no signs of respiratory distress. All lobes are resonant on percussion. Skin color is not cyanotic.
Patient experiences minimum alterations in comfort.	Patient openly verbalizes feelings of discomfort when they occur. Patient can use measures to decrease comfort. Patient verbally validates a decrease in subjective feelings of discomfort. Objective findings of pain are decreased.
Patient remains free of traumatic injury.	Safety measures are appropriate to level of physiologic status. Skin integrity is maintained. Skin is free of bruises, burns, abrasions, and redness. Environment is safe. The patient is free of nosocomial infections.
Patient demonstrates minimum impaired verbal communication.	Patient verbalizes feelings for as long as physically able to do so. Patient develops alternative methods of communication.
Patient demonstrates social participation.	Patient states importance of interpersonal relationships. Patient relates to self and others. Patient participates, as possible, in unit and group activities. Patient participates, as possible, in family activities.
Patient demonstrates minimum complications from alterations in urinary elimination patterns.	Intake and output patterns are stable. Urine is clear, yellow to amber in color, and without sediment. Skin in perineal area is clean and dry. Urine is acidic (pH 6.0). Patient remains free of urinary tract infections. Patient remains free of bladder distention. Patient can describe symptoms of urinary tract infections that require medical intervention.
Patient demonstrates minimum complications of sensory-perceptual alterations.	Level of orientation is optimum. Patient remains free of injury. Skin integrity is maintained. Nutritional status is adequate. Self-care deficits are minimum. Social participation is appropriate to physiologic status.

Parkinson's disease

(Paralysis agitans)

Parkinson's disease is a chronic and slowly progressive degeneration of the brain's dopamine neuronal systems that is characterized by the clinical symptoms of mask-like facies, trunk-forward flexion, muscle weakness and rigidity, shuffling gait, resting tremors, finger pill-rolling, and bradykinesia.

The progressive, degenerative course of Parkinson's disease varies from individual to individual. Approximately 30% of persons with Parkinson's disease experience dementia.

The cause of Parkinson's disease includes known genetic, viral, vascular, and toxic factors and many unknown factors. Parkinson's disease occurs throughout the world in all racial and ethnic groups. Population surveys indicate an incidence of about 130 per 100,000 standard population. The disorder is uncommon in individuals under 40 years of age, with the mean age of onset at 60 years. The prevalence of Parkinson's disease increases with age, and statistics indicate that 1% of the population over 60 years of age are afflicted with the disorder. Family studies indicate that approximately 2% of the adult siblings of individuals with Parkinson's disease also have the disorder.

Pathophysiology

Parkinson's can be divided into three major types in terms of pathophysiologic mechanisms: parkinsonism-dementia complex, Lewy body Parkinson's disease, and neurofibrillary tangle Parkinson's disease. Parkinsonism-dementia complex is unique to certain Pacific islands and is often associated with amyotrophic lateral sclerosis. The pathologic characteristics of this complex include neurofibrillary tangles found throughout the neuraxis, atrophy of the thalamus and temporal and frontal lobes, and granulovascular degeneration in structures such as the hippocampus.

Lewy body Parkinson's disease involves the degeneration of the pigmented neurons of the substantia nigra and locus ceruleus. Other melanin-bearing neurons of the brainstem and spinal cord also degenerate, such as the dorsal motor nucleus of the vagal nerve, and paravertebral ganglia. The surviving melanin-bearing cells contain structures known as Lewy bodies, which are cytoplasmic inclusions consisting of a central core of filamentous proteins. Radiating from the central core is a less dense array of tubules that may represent excess axoplasmic transport material or degenerated storage granules.[39]

Neurofibrillary tangle parkinsonism demonstrates the following pathologic changes: atrophy of the cerebral cortex with an increased subarachnoid space and narrow gyri, depigmentation (usually) of the substantia nigra, and the presence of neurofibrillary tangles in the surviving neuronal cells of the substantia nigra. These neurofibrillary tangles consist of helically twisted pairs of filaments and result from proliferation of the neurofilaments. Studies suggest a possible relationship between this form of Parkinson's disease and viral encephalitis.

Iatrogenic parkinsonism, which closely resembles Parkinson's disease, may be induced by different drugs, such as the major tranquilizers or, rarely, methyldopa, α-methyl-para-tyrosine, and reserpine. These agents interfere with the synthesis or the storage of dopamine or block the striatal dopamine receptors.[35] The effects of chemical-induced parkinsonism are reversible within 1 to 2 weeks after discontinuation of the offending agent.

Progression of Parkinson's disease and resultant disabilities may be evaluated by the use of the following classification system:

- Stage I: Unilateral involvement
- Stage II: Bilateral involvement
- Stage III: Mild to moderate impairment; impaired postural reflexes
- Stage IV: Marked impairment; fully developed, severe disease
- Stage V: Confined to bed or wheelchair

Diagnostic Studies and Findings

Serum Examination

Mild microcytic anemia

Chest Roentgenograms

Slight scoliosis

CT Scan, Skull Films

Normal results (CT scan may show cerebral atrophy, with history of chronic dementia)

Electroencephalogram (EEG)

Normal results or shows minimum slowing and/or disorganization

With marked dementia and bradykinesia, may show moderate to marked slowing and diffuse disorganization

Cineradiographic Study of Swallowing (see Part Two)

Abnormal pattern: delayed relaxation of cricopharyngeal muscles

Gastrointestinal Studies (see Part Two)

Hypomotility

Delayed emptying of stomach

Varying degrees of large bowel distention (frank megacolon in patients with severe constipation)

Medical Plan

Surgery

Stereotactic thalamotomy: produces small lesion in ventrolateral nucleus of thalamus to alleviate contralateral tremor and rigidity

Medications

- Antiparkinsonism agents
  - Carbidopa (Sinemet), 10-25 mg po tid or qid
  - Trihexyphenidyl (Artane), 2-5 mg po tid or qid
  - Benztropine mesylate (Cogentin), 0.5-6.0 mg/d po
  - Amantadine (Symmetrel), 100 mg/d po for 5-7 d
  - Ethopropazine (Parsidol), 20-600 mg/d po
  - Bromocriptine mesylate (Parlodel), 2.5 mg po bid or tid
  - L-Dihydroxyphenylalanine (levodopa), 100-250 mg po tid or qid
  - Orphenadrine (Disipal), 50 mg po tid
- Antidepressant agents
  - Amitriptyline (Elavil), 75-150 mg/d po
- Antihistamine
  - Diphenhydramine (Benadryl), 10-50 mg po q6h prn

General Management

Heat massage

Walkers, canes, wheelchairs

Physiotherapy

Bowel and bladder program

Nutritional program

Occupational therapy

Extended care facility referral

Speech therapy

Resources available (National Parkinson Foundation)

NURSING CARE

Nursing Assessment

Initial Symptoms

Weakness, tendency to tremble (usually in one hand)
Slowness or awkwardness of affected limb
Some loss of facial expression
Deliberate quality of speech
Tendency to posture arm flexed at elbow
May progress to other side of the body after 1 to 2 years

Autonomic Dysfunction

Increased secretion of sebum resulting in scaly erythematous eruptions of skin (particularly by ears and eyebrows and in scalp and nasolabial folds)
Intermittent, profuse diaphoresis
Chronic constipation
Urgency and hesitancy in micturition
Orthostatic hypotension
Dysphagia

Equilibrium

Festination (leaning of the trunk farther and farther with each step):
- Propulsion (forward stepping with leaning of trunk)
- Retropulsion (backward stepping with leaning of trunk)
- Lateropulsion (sidewise stepping with leaning of trunk)

Face

Masklike facies
Decreased eye blinking

Gradual Dementia

Initial
- Forgetfulness
- Minor confusional episodes
- Depression

Later
- Irritability
- Paranoia and visual hallucinations
- Frank delirium

Hands

Fingers extended with metacarpophalangeal joints flexed approximately 30 degrees

Handwriting

Letters becoming progressively smaller (micrographia)
Tremulous writing

Nutrition

Impaired deglutition
Drooling
Weight loss
Failure of cricopharyngeal muscles to relax

Posture and Rigidity

Shuffling gait without arm swing
Akathisia (most evident in spinal musculature)
Hypertonicity

Speech

Involuntary repetition of sentences
Decreased amplitude
Soft, rapid monotone

Toes

Toe flexion with dorsiflexion of proximal phalanges
Great toe may assume continuous dorsiflexion position

Tremors

Lips, jaws, tongue, facial muscles, axial muscles, and limb muscles
Usually resting tremors (most apparent when affected area is at rest)

Nursing Dx & Intervention

Nursing Diagnosis	Nursing Intervention/Rationale
Ineffective airway clearance; potential for aspiration	• Auscultate for breath sounds every 1 to 2 hours and as needed. • Maintain patent airway, and avoid flexion of the neck if patient is immobile. • Suction as needed *to prevent obstruction.* • Assist ventilation as indicated. • Monitor vital signs every 1 to 2 hours; monitor neurologic status every 1 to 2 hours. • Keep emergency drugs and ventilator at bedside. • Maintain nothing-by-mouth status *to prevent risk of choking or aspiration.*
Ineffective breathing pattern	• Auscultate breath sounds every 1 to 2 hours; note quality and any increase in adventitious sounds. • Suction as needed. Hyperinflate lungs with 100% oxygen for 1 minute before and 1 minute after suctioning, unless contraindicated *to minimize hypoxia.* • Maintain patent airway. Intubation/tracheostomy and mechanical ventilation may be indicated.

Nursing Diagnosis	Nursing Intervention/Rationale
	• Monitor mechanical ventilator, if used: Ensure that tidal volume, rate, mode, and oxygen concentration are set as ordered. Ensure that ventilator alarms are on and functional *to prevent accidental disconnection.* • Monitor arterial blood gases, as ordered: Report decrease in Po_2 of 10 to 15 mm Hg. Report increase in Pco_2 greater than 10 to 15 mm Hg. • Note respiratory rate, depth, and level of consciousness every 15 to 30 minutes and as needed based on the patient's condition. • Check blood pressure, temperature, and pulse rate every 1 to 2 hours and as needed based on the patient's condition. • Turn every 2 hours and as needed *to prevent stasis of secretions and pulmonary complications.*
Pain	• See general intervention strategies on p. 1720.
Constipation	• Assess and document presence of bowel sounds. • Provide high-residue diet *to promote gastrointestinal motility.* • Maintain activity level to tolerance. • Maintain regular bowel evacuation with stool softeners, rectal suppositories, mild cathartics, and natural laxatives such as prune juice.
Potential for trauma	• See general intervention strategies on p. 1620. • Provide the patient with a call light within easy reach. • Maintain side rails in up position at bedtime, after sedation, when patient is confused, and as needed. • Pad side rails if patient is overactive. • Assist patient to change positions slowly *to prevent orthostatic hypotension.* • Keep walkways clear *to minimize physical dangers.*
Sensory/perceptual alterations	• See general intervention strategies on p. 1728.
Impaired physical mobility; potential for disuse syndrome	• Assess patient's level of mobility and intervene as necessary. • Institute gait-retraining program if indicated *to maintain balance and to improve walking.* • Apply splints and braces as indicated. • Continue with physiotherapy program. • Encourage outdoor ambulation (avoid extremes of hot and cold). • Encourage patient to dress daily *to promote self-esteem.* Avoid shoes with laces or snaps. Avoid clothes with buttons; use zippers. Place head of bed or chair on blocks *to facilitate getting up.* Provide raised toilet seat and side rails *to facilitate sitting and standing.*
Self-care deficit	• Assess self-care deficits and intervene as follows. • Perform range-of-motion exercises to prevent stiffness, muscle wasting, and contractures. • Assist with feeding, as indicated: Use of hand braces Use of IV or nasogastric feedings, as ordered • Administer oral hygiene every 2 hours and as needed *to control drooling.* • Assist with daily hygiene care, as indicated. • Administer skin care every 2 to 4 hours and as needed *to remove skin oil and perspiration.* • Administer eye care every 2 to 4 hours *to remove crustations.* • Perform intermittent urinary catheterization per protocol *to maintain adequate bladder elimination and to prevent infection.*
Anxiety	• See general intervention strategies on p. 1743. • Support the family: Provide for ongoing contact. Give appropriate referrals to support groups. • Assist patient to deal realistically and honestly with anxiety about inability to predict course of the disorder, discomfort from spasticity, and change in self-image and self-esteem. • Explain potential treatments for the symptoms of the disorder: State in basic terms and monitor patient's response. Repeat explanations as needed. • Alert other health care professionals and family to potential emotional changes. • Instruct family that patient is intellectually normal, despite physical disability.

Nursing Diagnosis	Nursing Intervention/Rationale
Impaired verbal communication	• Assess patient's ability to communicate and develop means of communication with the patient, such as pad and pencil, Magic Slate, call light. • Teach patient to speak in a slow, unhurried manner. Provide electronic amplifiers as needed *to augment decreased amplitude of speech.* • Obtain referral for speech therapy. Reinforce techniques established. • Assist patient and family to identify other outlets for communication. • Continue to use sense of touch and other nonverbal forms of communication.
Altered nutrition: less than body requirements	• Assess patient's nutritional status and ability to chew and swallow. • Offer small, frequent feedings *to minimize risks of dysphagia and aspiration.* • Complete nursing care before mealtimes. • Apply braces to minimize tremors. • Encourage a high-bulk, high-roughage diet. Provide supplements as needed. Control protein intake *to minimize blocking of effects of L-dopa.* • Allow ample time for eating, and keep food warm. Place utensils within easy reach. Cut foods for patient. Use blender for thick foods. • Use bib or straw as indicated.
Body image, self-esteem, and personal identity disturbances	• Provide an ongoing assessment of the patient's interpersonal strengths. Focus on strengths and potential. • Reorient to time, person, and place as appropriate. • Carefully explain what you are doing and why you are doing it. • Answer questions simply and honestly. • Correct misinformation. • Protect the patient's privacy. • Provide gentle physical care in a caring environment. • Assist patient to become involved in self-care. • Assist patient to become involved in unit activities.
Social isolation	• See general intervention strategies on p. 1767.
Altered patterns of urinary elimination	• Assess characteristics of patient's voiding pattern (frequency, amount). • Perform intermittent catheterization per protocol. • Monitor intake and output. Maintain fluid intake at 2000 ml/day unless contraindicated. • Assess urine for sediment, concentration, color, and odor. • Acidify urine with foods such as orange juice and cranberry juice *to minimize potential for infection.* • Administer urinary tract germicides (e.g., methenamine mandalate [Mandelamine]) as ordered.

Patient Education

1. Instruct regarding causes, symptoms, and treatment modalities for Parkinson's disease (explain procedures as they occur).
2. Stress importance of verbalization about loss of self-esteem, sexuality, and body functions.
3. Emphasize importance of verbalization about feelings.
4. Encourage social participation.
5. Emphasize capabilities.
6. Encourage independence and self-care; avoid overprotection.
7. Stress need for daily exercise program.
8. Emphasize need for high-calorie, soft diet; instruct the patient to eat slowly and take small bites.
9. Stress need for diversional activities.
10. Teach safety measures to prevent injury.
11. Emphasize need for speech therapy.
12. Stress need for frequent skin care and oral hygiene.
13. Emphasize need for bowel and bladder programs.
14. Instruct regarding name of medication, dosage, frequency of administration, purpose, and toxic or side effects.
15. Instruct the patient to take medications with food to reduce gastric irritation and nausea.
16. Stress importance of ongoing outpatient care:
    a. Physician's visits
    b. Physical therapy
    c. Home nursing care
    d. Parkinson's Disease Information Center; Parkinson's Foundation

Evaluation

Patient Outcome	Data Indicating That Outcome is Reached
Patient and family demonstrate adequate knowledge of Parkinson's disease.	Patient and family state the nature of the disease in basic terms. Patient and family can identify possible treatment modalities. Patient and family can identify symptoms of progression.
Patient demonstrates a patent airway.	Breath sounds are normal. Chest excursion is bilateral and symmetric. Rate and depth of respiration are normal. Cough is effective. There are no subjective or objective findings of shortness of breath, air hunger, or dyspnea on exertion.
Patient demonstrates minimum complications of bowel incontinence.	Skin in perineal area is clean and dry. Dietary intake is adequate. Fluid intake is adequate (2000 ml/day unless contraindicated). Intake and output patterns are stable. Patient remains free of fecal impaction. Patient demonstrates a regular bowel evacuation pattern.
Patient demonstrates a low level of anxiety.	Patient openly verbalizes concerns and feelings of grief, loss, and discomfort. Patient openly verbalizes feelings, supported by health care professionals and family. Patient verbalizes essential aspects of care. Patient can identify methods to effectively deal with anxious feelings.
Patient demonstrates an effective breathing pattern.	Airway is patent. Chest excursion is symmetric. Breath sounds are normal, or there is no increase in adventitious sounds. Arterial blood gas values are within normal ranges or consistent with patient's baseline. Vital signs are within normal ranges or consistent with patient's baseline. Hemoglobin levels are 14 to 18 g/dl (male) or 12 to 16 g/dl (female). Intake and output are stable. There are no signs of respiratory distress. All lobes are resonant on percussion. Skin is not cyanotic.
Patient experiences minimum alterations in comfort.	Patient openly verbalizes feelings of discomfort when they occur. Patient can use measures to increase comfort. Patient verbally validates a decrease in subjective feelings of discomfort. Objective findings of pain are decreased.
Patient demonstrates minimum impaired verbal communication.	Patient verbalizes feelings for as long as physically able to do so. Patient develops alternative methods of communication.
Patient remains free of traumatic injury.	Patient uses safety measures appropriate to level of physiologic status. Skin integrity is maintained. Skin is free of bruises, burns, abrasions, and redness. Environment is safe. Patient is free of nosocomial infections.
Patient demonstrates optimum level of mobility.	Skin integrity is maintained. There are no contractures and deformities. Patient's level of mobility is appropriate to physiologic status. Intake and output pattern is stable. Nutritional status is adequate. There is no thrombophlebitis. There is no local infection. Patient participates in an ongoing physical therapy program.
Patient demonstrates adequate nutritional status.	Weight pattern is stable. Intake and output pattern is stable. Diet is appropriate to physiologic status. Skin turgor is good. Fluid and electrolyte balance is maintained. Patient takes dietary supplements, as appropriate.
Patient demonstrates minimum self-care deficits.	Outcome criteria listed for impaired physical mobility are met. Level of self-care activities is appropriate to physiologic status. Patient participates in physical and occupational therapy.
Patient demonstrates minimum complications of sensory-perceptual alterations.	Optimum level of orientation is maintained. Patient remains free of injury. Skin integrity is maintained. Nutritional status is adequate. Self-care deficits are minimum. Social participation is appropriate to physiologic status.
Patient demonstrates intact self-concepts.	Patient openly verbalizes feelings of grief and loss. Patient verbalizes positive feelings about self. Patient acknowledges actual change in self-image. Patient focuses on present and future appearance and function. Patient verbalizes feelings of hopefulness, helpfulness, and powerfulness.
Patient demonstrates social participation.	Patient states importance of interpersonal relationships. Patient relates to self and others. Patient participates, as possible, in unit and group activities. Patient participates, as possible, in family activities.
Patient demonstrates minimum complications from alterations in urinary elimination patterns.	Intake and output pattern is stable. Urine is clear, yellow to amber in color, and without sediment. Skin in perineal area is clean and dry. Urine is acidic (pH 6.0). Patient is free of urinary tract infections. Patient is free of bladder distention. Patient can describe symptoms of urinary tract infections that require medical intervention.

Myasthenia gravis

Myasthenia gravis is a neuromuscular disease involving lower motor neurons and muscle fibers that is characterized by abnormal fatigue and motor weakness of skeletal muscles that increases with effort and improves with rest.

Voluntary muscles most commonly affected in myasthenia gravis include the oculomotor, facial, laryngeal, pharyngeal, and respiratory muscles.

The cause of myasthenia gravis is unknown, although considerable data suggest that it is a systemic autoimmune disease. Myasthenia gravis is not a hereditary condition, but 15% of infants born to myasthenic mothers manifest transitory symptoms lasting from 7 to 14 days after birth. The incidence of myasthenia gravis is 3 to 6 per 100,000 individuals. There are two characteristic ages of onset: between the ages of 20 and 30 years and in late middle age. When the disorder begins in the second or third decade, women are more commonly affected than men. When the disorder begins in late middle age, men are affected more often than women. Epidemiologic studies have not produced any specific socioeconomic or racial factors. Clinical studies have indicated that 80% of the patients with myasthenia gravis have thymic abnormalities (10% have a thymoma, and 70% have thymic hyperplasia). The role of the thymus in the pathogenesis is unclear. Mortality for individuals with myasthenia gravis is 15 times greater than for the general population.

Pathophysiology

Regardless of the cause, the basic physiologic defect in myasthenia gravis is that nerve impulses do not pass onto the skeletal muscle at the myoneuronal junction. This defect appears to result from either a deficiency in release of acetylcholine from the presynaptic terminals or a deficiency (i.e., blockage or reduced numbers) in the postsynaptic membrane receptor sites. Biopsy studies of myasthenic patients have shown that small end-plate potentials are normal in frequency but have markedly decreased amplitudes. Postsynaptic potentials are slightly smaller than normal but contain the normal number of acetylcholine quanta.[23]

Research pursuing the prospect that myasthenia gravis is produced by an autoimmune mechanism has shown that a major feature in the pathogenesis is an attack on end-plate acetylcholine receptors by circulating antibodies.[23] The reasons that these antibodies to acetylcholine receptors develop remains to be elucidated.

There is no evidence in myasthenia gravis of central or peripheral nervous system disease. Involved skeletal muscles usually do not atrophy, and there is no loss of sensation. The primary signs are extreme fatigability and weakness of voluntary muscles.

Diagnostic Studies and Findings

Chest Roentgenogram, CT Scan of Chest

May indicate presence of thymoma

Edrophonium Chloride (Tensilon) Test

Intramuscular injection of 2 mg of edrophonium chloride (Tensilon); if no symptoms occur, an additional 8 mg is injected and the patient is observed for improvement in muscle tone; in 30 seconds to 1 minute, patients with myasthenia gravis demonstrate marked improvement in muscle tone that lasts 4 to 5 minutes

Electromyogram (EMG)

Muscle fiber contraction with progressive decremental response

Curare Test

Myasthenia gravis patient will be curarized with 1/32 of the normal curare dose; done by a neurologist with anesthesia at the bedside, ready to intubate; done only if all the other findings are normal or questionable; frequently seen as the ultimate diagnostic technique for myasthenia gravis

Medical Plan

Surgery

Tracheotomy (see Chapter 7)
Thymectomy
- Suprasternal approach
- Transsternal approach

Medications

Cholinergic agents
- Neostigmine (Prostigmin), 7.5-45 mg q2-6h
- Pyridostigmine (Mestinon), individualized size and frequency of dosage (range 15-90 mg/d po)
- Ambenonium chloride (Mytelase), 10-25 mg po tid or qid

Corticosteroids
- Prednisone, 100 mg po qod (dose gradually reduced)

Diphenoxylate hydrochloride (Lomotil), prn

Pituitary hormones
- ACTH, 100-160 U/d for 10 d (rarely used)

General Management

Mechanical ventilation, if indicated
Plasma exchange (plasmapheresis)
Bronchoscopy (see Part Two for additional information)
Physical therapy
Occupational therapy

NURSING CARE

Nursing Assessment

Eye Muscles (Usually Affected First)

Ocular palsy
Ptosis (unilateral or bilateral)
Diplopia

Facial Muscles

Masklike expression and mobility (weakness) of face
Weak voice that may fade to a whisper
Dysphagia
Choking
Aspiration
Drooling
Nasal speech

Neck Muscles

Head bobbing up and down

Respiratory Muscles

Breathlessness
Respiratory weakness
Respiratory failure, reduced tidal volume, and vital capacity

Other Muscles

Stress incontinence
Anal sphincter weakness

Reflexes

Normal or brisk

Myasthenia Gravis Crisis

Respiratory distress
Tachypnea
Increased muscular weakness
Extreme fatigue
Anxiety
Restlessness
Irritability
Facial weakness
Dysphagia
Inability to chew
Elevated temperature
Ptosis
Speech impairment

Cholinergic Crisis

Respiratory distress
Vertigo
Blurred vision
Sweating
Lacrimation
Salivation
Anorexia
Dysarthria
Dysphagia
Abdominal cramps
Nausea and vomiting
Muscular spasms or cramps
Generalized weakness
Dyspnea and wheezing

Nursing Dx & Intervention

Nursing Diagnosis	Nursing Intervention/Rationale
Ineffective airway clearance; potential for aspiration	• Auscultate for breath sounds every 1 to 2 hours, and report any changes to the physician. • Maintain patent airway, and avoid flexion of the neck if patient is comatose. • Suction as needed *to prevent obstruction*. • Assist ventilation as indicated. • Monitor vital signs every 1 to 2 hours; monitor neurologic status every 1 to 2 hours. • Keep emergency drugs and ventilator at the bedside. • Maintain nothing-by-mouth status *to prevent risk of choking or aspiration*.
Ineffective breathing pattern	• See general intervention strategies listed on p. 1704. • If patient has a thymectomy, assess for signs of pneumothorax: restlessness, tachycardia, respiratory distress, cyanosis, diaphoresis. • Maintain patency of chest tubes. • Provide chest physiotherapy *to mobilize secretions*. • Monitor tidal volume and vital capacity every hour in acute stage.
Impaired physical mobility	• See general intervention strategies on p. 1687.
Feeding, bathing/hygiene, dressing/grooming, and toileting self-care deficit	• See general intervention strategies on p. 1692.

Nursing Diagnosis	Nursing Intervention/Rationale
Altered nutrition: less than body requirements	• Assess patient's nutritional status and ability to chew and swallow. • Offer small, frequent feedings. • Encourage a high-protein, high-bulk, high-roughage diet. • Administer medications 30 minutes before eating *to maximize muscle strength needed for chewing and swallowing of food.* • Allow ample time for eating. Stay with patient. • Accurately measure and record intake on a flowsheet. • Administer parenteral fluids per protocol *to ensure adequate fluid intake.* • Monitor the patient's weight pattern, and report any significant changes. • Obtain nutritional services consultation.
Constipation	• See general intervention strategies on p. 1658. • Assess patient for impaction every 1 to 2 days.
Impaired verbal communication	• Assess patient's ability to communicate. • Develop means of communication with patient: pad and pencil, Magic Slate, call light. • Teach patient to speak in a slow, unhurried manner *to avoid voice strain.* • Obtain referral for speech therapy. Reinforce technique established. • Assist patient and family to identify other outlets for communication. • Continue to use sense of touch and other nonverbal forms of communication.
Powerlessness	• See general intervention strategies on p. 1748.

Patient Education

1. Instruct regarding name of medication, dosage, time of administration, purpose, and side effects. For anticholinesterase medications:
   a. Stress importance of dosage.
   b. Instruct patient to take at scheduled times.
   c. Instruct patient not to skip doses.
   d. Instruct patient to avoid taking with fruit, tomato juice, coffee, or other medications.
   e. Instruct patient to take medications with food to minimize gastric irritation and nausea.
   f. Inform patient of toxic side effects (i.e., diarrhea, abdominal cramping, muscular weakness).
2. Stress need to avoid taking over-the-counter medications without notifying the physician.
3. Teach symptoms of progression or recurrence to report to physician.
4. Emphasize need to wear medical alert tag.
5. Stress importance of avoiding individuals with upper respiratory infection.
6. Teach symptoms of upper respiratory infection to report to physician (i.e., chills, cough, low-grade temperature).
7. Stress need to avoid alcohol, tobacco, and prolonged exposure to heat or cold.
8. Emphasize need for adequate nutritional status:
   a. Give diet as tolerated.
   b. Arrange food and utensils so they can be managed by patient.
   c. Instruct to chew thoroughly, and eat slowly and in small pieces.
9. Stress need for activity and exercise to tolerance:
   a. Plan activities of daily living.
   b. Maintain rest periods as planned.
   c. Do active and passive ROM exercises.
   d. Get at least 8 hours of sleep at night.
10. Emphasize need for diversional activities.
11. Stress importance of avoiding physical and emotional stress.
12. Emphasize need for speech therapy.
13. Stress importance of avoiding constipation.
14. Emphasize importance of ongoing outpatient care.
15. Give available agencies for reference (e.g., Myasthenia Gravis Foundation).
16. Give outpatient or home nursing care referrals.

Evaluation

Patient Outcome	Data Indicating That Outcome is Reached
Patient and family demonstrate adequate knowledge of myasthenia gravis.	Patient states the nature of the disorder in basic terms. Patient can identify treatment modalities. Patient can state treatment regimen. Patient can identify symptoms of progression.

Patient Outcome	Data Indicating That Outcome is Reached
Patient demonstrates a patent airway.	Breath sounds are normal. Chest excursion is bilateral and symmetric. Rate and depth of respirations are normal. Cough is effective. There are no subjective or objective findings of shortness of breath, air hunger, or dyspnea on exertion.
Patient demonstrates an effective breathing pattern.	Airway is patent. Chest excursion is symmetric. Breath sounds are normal, or there is no increase in adventitious sounds. Arterial blood gas values are within normal ranges or consistent with patient's baseline. Vital signs are within normal ranges or consistent with patient's baseline. Hemoglobin levels are 14 to 18 g/dl (male) or 12 to 16 g/dl (female). Intake and output are stable. There are no signs of respiratory distress. All lobes are resonant on percussion. Skin is not cyanotic.
Patient demonstrates an optimum level of mobility.	Skin integrity is maintained. Patient is free of contractures and deformities. Level of mobility is appropriate to physiologic status. Intake and output pattern is stable. Nutritional status is adequate. Patient remains free of thrombophlebitis. Patient remains free of local infection.
Patient demonstrates minimum self-care deficits.	Outcome criteria stated for impaired physical mobility are met. Level of self-care is appropriate to physiologic status. Diet is high in calories and protein. Patient participates in physical and occupational therapy as indicated.
Patient demonstrates minimum impaired verbal communication.	Patient verbalizes feelings for as long as physically able to do so. Patient develops alternative methods of communication.
Patient experiences minimum feelings of fear.	Patient has no subjective feelings of fear. Patient has no objective findings of fear.
Patient demonstrates minimum feelings of powerlessness.	Optimum level of physiologic control, as possible for current health status, is maintained. Optimum level of psychologic control, as possible, is maintained. Patient participates, as possible, in decision making about care. Patient participates, as possible, in self-care.
Patient demonstrates minimum complications of bowel incontinence.	Skin in perineal area is clean and dry. Dietary intake is adequate. Fluid intake is adequate (2000 ml daily, unless contraindicated). Intake and output pattern is stable. Patient remains free of fecal impaction. Patient demonstrates a regular bowel evacuation pattern.

TUMORS

Intracranial tumors

(Brain tumors)

Intracranial tumors include both benign space-occupying (primary) and malignant (metastatic) lesions. Intracranial tumors can occur in any structural area of the brain and in all age groups. Growth rates range from the rapid growth of glioblastomas to the almost imperceptible changes of some meningiomas.[35]

Brain tumors are named according to the tissues from which they arise. Primary brain tumors include oligodendrogliomas, ependymomas, astrocytomas and glioblastomas, medulloblastomas, and meningiomas. Secondary or metastatic tumors include metastatic carcinoma or sarcoma. (See Chapter 16 for a discussion of malignant brain tumors.)

Oligodendrogliomas form in the oligodendroglia cells that are responsible for the formation of the central nervous system myelin sheaths. These tumors evolve slowly and may be detected on a routine skull roentgenogram because of intracranial calcification. The most common site for oligodendrogliomas are the frontal and temporal lobes. This type of tumor makes up only 5% or less of all intracranial tumors. There is a high incidence of this tumor among young adults who have a childhood history of temporal lobe epilepsy.[39]

Ependymomas are fairly rare in the general adult population and make up only 5% of all intracranial tumors. They are more commonly found in young children and adolescents and account for 20% of brain tumors in this age group. Ependymomas form in the ependymal cells and astrocytes that line the walls of the cerebral ventricular system and most commonly affect the fourth ventricle.

Astrocytomas form in astrocyte cells at any level of the central nervous system. In the adult they are usually lateral and supratentorial, whereas astrocytes in children are in or near the midline.[39] Cerebellar astrocytomas, which constitute 30% of all pediatric brain tumors, are usually located just lateral to the midline in the cerebellar hemisphere. Simple surgical excision provides a long survival rate. Brainstem astrocytomas primarily affect school-aged children, who have a high mortality because of destruction of the local cranial nerve nuclei and the long tracts.

Cerebral astrocytomas are classified by grade (Table 3-6). Cerebral astrocytomas are common between 30 and 50 years of age, making up 30% of the brain tumors for this age group. These tumors have a growth rate proportional to their grade. For example, grades I and II grow slowly, whereas grades III and IV grow rapidly.[39]

Medulloblastomas constitute 20% of brain tumors in children and occur most frequently in children under 10 years of age. The tumor eventually obstructs the flow of cerebrospinal fluid from the aqueduct, resulting in hydrocephalus and cerebellar signs. Without irradiation, the tumor is fatal; with irradiation there is a 30% survival rate.

Meningiomas are adult tumors arising from the cells of vessels, pia-arachnoid, and surrounding fibroblasts. Meningiomas make up 15% of all adult tumors of the central nervous system and its coverings. They occur more frequently in women and are found in approximately 40% to 50% of patients with von Recklinghausen's disease (neurofibromatosis). The symptoms of a meningioma are manifested as the tumor indents a local area of the brain and raises the intracranial pressure.

Pathophysiology

An *oligodendroglioma* can be seen microscopically as small round cells with spheric nuclei. Many of these tumors have an astrocytic component; therefore recurrence of the tumor may have astrocytic characteristics.

An *ependymoma* has several variants. The *myxopapillary ependymoma* is a special variant occurring in adolescents. It develops in the fifth ventricle (ventriculus terminalis), formed by the caudal opening of the central canal of the spinal cord.[39] Generally symptoms of increased intracranial pressure are manifested when the ependymoma fills the fourth ventricle, blocking the flow of cerebrospinal fluid.

An *astrocytoma* of low grade (I or II) is gelatinous and frequently indistinguishable from cerebral gliosis. This type of tumor is slow growing and infiltrative. Astrocytomas commonly arise in the white matter. Their cellularity is almost normal.[39] Astrocytomas of grades III and IV are rapid-growing tumors characterized by a high degree of macroscopic necrosis. An astrocytoma of this grade is not confined to white matter and may grow into areas of the subarachnoid space and the brainstem. These tumors are very cellular, pleomorphic, and necrotic and demonstrate marked endothelial proliferation.[39]

A *medulloblastoma* arises in the caudal cerebellar vermis and is markedly cellular. The cells in the tumor have little cytoplasm and are undifferentiated. When medulloblastomas occur beyond the first decade of life, they arise more rostrally and laterally in the cerebellar hemispheres.[39]

A *meningioma* may have one of several cell types, each with a different prognosis depending on the cellular variety. The tumor cells are commonly uniform and may form characteristic whorls.[35] Frequent locations for these tumors include the ethmoid regions, parasagittal region, sphenoid ridge, and the dorsal roots of the spinal cord.

Regardless of the pathologic type of intracranial tumor, signs and symptoms reflect progressive neurologic deficits caused by focal disturbances and increased intracranial pressure. Focal disturbances are caused by increasing compression of brain tissue and the infiltration or direct invasion of brain parenchyma resulting in destruction of neural tissue.[48] Cerebral blood supply may also be altered by the tumor's compression of blood vessels, resulting in necrotic cerebral tissue or seizures. Approximately 30% of adults with intracranial tumors develop focal or generalized seizure activity. Increased intracranial pressure may result from regional edema, alterations in cerebrospinal fluid circulation, and an increase in tissue within the skull. Hydrocephalus results from disruption in the circulation of cerebrospinal fluid from the cerebral ventricles to the subarachnoid spaces.

The size and location of the specific tumor can cause shifts of brain tissue with associated brain herniation syndromes. If left untreated, herniation can lead to infarction and hemorrhage in the upper pons and the midbrain, resulting in pontomedullary decompensation.[23]

Table 3-6
Grades of Astrocytoma

Grade	Growth Rate	Prognosis
Astrocytoma		
Grade I	Slow	Good; 15-20 yr after surgery
Grade II	Slow	Good; 10-15 yr after surgery
Glioblastoma		
Grade III	Rapid, invasive	Poor; less than 2 yr without therapy
Grade IV (glioblastoma multiforme)	Rapid, invasive	Very poor; 6-9 mo without surgery

Diagnostic Studies and Findings

Skull Roentgenograms

Erosion of posterior clinoid process or presence of intracranial calcifications

Chest Roentgenograms

Detection of primary lung tumor or metastatic disease

CT Scan

Identification of vascular tumors
Shifts in midline structures
Changes in cerebral ventricular sizes

Electroencephalogram (EEG)

Marked focal slowing (with rapidly developing tumors)
Rhythmic, periodic, and high-voltage slowing (with increased intracranial pressure)

Dural Sinus Venography

May indicate narrowed sinuses and interference with cranial drainage

Echoencephalogram

Shifts in midline structures

Ophthalmoscopic Examination

Papilledema

Brain Scan

Increased uptake of isotope in the tumor

Pneumoencephalogram

Tumor localization
Contraindicated if increased intracranial pressure is suspected

Cerebral Angiography

Cerebral vascularity
Blood vessel deviations

Magnetic Resonance Imaging (MRI)

Same as CT scan, without radiation

Positron Emission Tomography (PET)

Same as CT scan, but also details sites of glucose metabolism in the brain under various conditions

Medical Plan

Surgery

Intracranial pressure monitoring
Tumor excision; craniotomy
Shunting procedure
Laser therapy

Medications

Corticosteroids
- Dexamethasone (Decadron), 20-40 mg/d po

Anticonvulsants
- Phenytoin (Dilantin), 100 mg po tid

Analgesic/antipyretics
- Acetaminophen, gr X po q4h prn

Laxatives
- Docusate sodium (Colace), 100 mg po bid or tid

Histamine receptor antagonist
- Cimetidine (Tagamet), 300 mg po qid

Antacids
- Magnesium hydroxide (Maalox), 30 ml po qid

Alkalating agents
- Triethylene thiophosphoramide (Thiotepa), 0.2 mg/kg IV for 5 d; repeat q4 wk as necessary
- Carmustine (BCNU), 200 mg/m^2 (single dose or divided doses of 100 mg/m^2) IV q6 wk

Antimetabolites
- Floxuridine (FUDR), 0.1-0.6 mg/kg/d intra-arterial infusion or 0.4-0.6 mg/kg/d via hepatic artery
- Fluorouracil (5-FU), 12.5 mg/kg/d IV for 3-5 d; repeat q4 wk as necessary

Other
- Procarbazine (Matulane), 100-150 mg/m^2 po for 10 d
- Vincristine (Oncovin), 1-2 mg/m^2 IV q wk

General Management

Radiation therapy
Mechanical ventilation, if indicated
Cardiac monitoring
Nutritional consultation
Physical therapy

NURSING CARE

Nursing Assessment

Focal Neurologic Disturbance

Gradually increasing weakness
Subtle sensory loss
Adult-onset seizures not always relieved by medications

Mentation

Personality changes (i.e., loss of emotional restraints)
Insidious decrease in mentation
Depression
Memory deficits
Judgment deficits

Pain

Headaches with steady, persistent, or intractable dull pain
Changes in character of headaches
Stress-induced headaches

Increased Intracranial Pressure

Restlessness, lethargy
Changes in level of consciousness
Changes in vital signs
Pupillary changes (i.e., mydriasis)
Impaired pupillary reflex
Papilledema (70%-75% of patients)
Vomiting (may be projectile)
Fluctuations in temperature
Seizures
Worsening of focal neurologic signs
Changes in respiratory patterns

Seizure Activity

Initial symptom in 15% of patients
Preconvulsive (preictal stage)
- Aura: flash of light; sense of loss; fear; weakness; dizziness; peculiar taste, smell, and sounds
- Cry or scream
- Fall to floor
- Loss of consciousness
- Tachypnea

Convulsive stage
- Tonic: rigid body; fixed jaws; clenched fists; extended legs; cyanosis; holding breath
- Clonic: urinary and/or fecal incontinence; jerking of

facial muscles and extremities; biting tongue; frothing at mouth

Postconvulsive (postictal stage)

Altered level of consciousness

Headache

Nausea or vomiting

Malaise

Muscle soreness

Aspiration: breathing difficulty, choking, cyanosis, decreased breath sounds, tachycardia, tachypnea

Pituitary Dysfunction

Cushing's Syndrome

Acromegaly

Giantism

Hypopituitarism

Nursing Dx & Intervention

Nursing Diagnosis	Nursing Intervention/Rationale
Ineffective airway clearance	• See general intervention strategies listed on p. 1702.
Ineffective breathing pattern	• See general intervention strategies listed on p. 1704.
Altered cerebral tissue perfusion	• Establish baseline and ongoing neurologic assessment every 1 to 2 hours and as needed as indicated by the patient's condition, level of consciousness, motor or sensory deficits, cranial nerve functioning, auditory functioning, nausea and vomiting, reflex status, pupillary size, reaction, behavior and personality changes, posturing spontaneously, or stimulus response. • Intervene *to monitor and prevent increased intracranial pressure:* Administer medications, treatments, and IV lines per protocol. Maintain elevation of head of bed per protocol *to facilitate venous drainage.* Accurately record intake and output *to monitor for imbalance.* Monitor serum electrolytes, blood count, and arterial blood gases for abnormalities. • Monitor values and wave forms of intracranial pressure line, if appropriate: Maintain patency and sterility of the system. Monitor effects of treatments of intracranial pressure. Correlate neurologic status with intracranial pressure values; notify physician if inconsistent. Assist with drainage of cerebrospinal fluid from the system *to lower intracranial hypertension.* • Intervene *to monitor and prevent seizures.* Assess seizure history. Institute seizure precautions: padded tongue blade and airway at bedside, bed height at lowest level, side rails up at all times and padded, oxygen and suction equipment at bedside, emergency medications at bedside. Administer anticonvulsants as per protocol: Monitor effects and side effects. Monitor serum for therapeutic levels of the anticonvulsant. Administer corticosteroids *to control cerebral edema.*
Potential altered body temperature	• Assess temperature q2h and prn *to prevent sudden elevations of temperature.* • Administer steroids per protocol *to reduce cerebral edema.* • Administer antipyretic agents per protocol. • Administer IV fluids at room temperature *to promote adequate fluid intake and prevent chilling.* • Monitor vital signs q2h and prn. • Adjust environmental temperature as indicated. • Adjust patient temperature as indicated, using cooling blanket, heat mattress, or warm blankets.
Sensory/perceptual alterations	• Assess patient's level of orientation. • Maintain quiet environment *to reduce external stimuli to a minimum.* • Reorient patient frequently to time, place, and person. Introduce yourself each time you reorient patient. • Repeat explanations frequently and simply. • Assist patient in judgments, perceptions, and reorientation as needed. • Have family bring in familiar objects. • Maintain planned rest periods *to allow sufficient time for REM sleep.* • Use day and night lighting appropriately. • Stimulate senses of touch, taste, and position.
Potential for trauma related to seizures	• Assess and document potential for and strategies to prevent injury. • Maintain bed in low position at all times unless side rails are up or when nurse is with the patient. • Provide the patient with a call light within easy reach.

Nursing Diagnosis	Nursing Intervention/Rationale
	• Maintain side rails in up position. • Pad side rails if patient is overactive. • Monitor for occult bleeding (gastric, stools, urine). • Assess for nosebleeds, bruising, and petechiae.
Preconvulsive	• Have oral airway at bedside. • Support and protect head; turn to side if possible. • Prevent injury: Ease patient to floor if in chair. Place pillows along side rails if in bed. Remove surrounding furniture. Loosen constrictive clothing. • Provide privacy as necessary. Stay with patient; remain calm. • Note frequency, time, involved body parts, and length of seizure.
Postconvulsive	• Maintain patent airway. • Suction as indicated *to prevent airway obstruction.* • Check vital signs and neurologic status. • Administer oxygen per protocol *to minimize cerebral hypoxia.* • Reorient patient to environment. • Place patient in position of comfort; turn head to side. • Administer oral hygiene as necessary *to remove or control secretions and blood.*
Impaired physical mobility	• See general intervention strategies listed on p. 1687.
Self-care deficit	• Assess self-care deficit and intervene as necessary. • Assist with feeding as indicated. Use IV or nasogastric feedings per protocol. • Assist with daily hygiene care as indicated. • Administer eye care every 2 to 4 hours if indicated *to prevent crustation and infection.* • Maintain bowel function with regular evacuation.
Potential impaired skin integrity	• See general intervention strategies listed on p. 1646. • Provide frequent skin care. • Monitor for signs of phlebitis. • Protect skin from tape application, sunlight, and friction.
Pain	• Assess and document patient's degree of pain. • Modify anxiety associated with the pain experience. • Provide other sensory input. • For patients receiving radiation or chemotherapy: Explain procedure or medication before implementing. Administer antiemetics and antidiarrheal medications as needed *to prevent nausea or control diarrhea.*
Altered oral mucous membrane	• Assess integrity of oral mucous membranes when providing mouth care. • Provide frequent mouth care and apply topical agents to mucous membranes *to minimize discomfort of stomatitis.* • Monitor patient's laboratory values for decreased RBC, WBC, or platelet levels *to detect bleeding and infection.* • Maintain planned rest periods. • Offer frequent, small feedings *to combat anorexia and discomfort of nausea.*
Powerlessness	• See general intervention strategies listed on p. 1748.
Altered nutrition: less than body requirements	• Assess patient's nutritional status in consultation with nutritionist. • Offer small, frequent feedings *to encourage adequate intake.* • Complete nursing care before feeding times. • Allow ample time for feeding. • Encourage a high-protein diet. • Accurately measure and record intake on a flowsheet *to establish whether intake is adequate.* • Administer parenteral fluids per protocol. • Administer tube feedings per protocol.
Potential for aspiration	• Position patient on his side after feeding *to prevent aspiration.* • Elevate head *to prevent aspiration.*

Nursing Diagnosis	Nursing Intervention/Rationale
Constipation	• See general intervention strategies listed on p. 1658.
Diarrhea	• See general intervention strategies listed on p. 1663.
Altered patterns of urinary elimination	• See general intervention strategies listed on p. 1666.

Patient Education

1. Involve the family in care, as possible; teach essential aspects of care.
2. Reinforce the physician's explanation of medical management.
3. Stress importance of ongoing outpatient care and follow-up visits.
4. Encourage independent activities, as possible:
   a. Alert the patient to limitations.
   b. Avoid overprotection.
   c. Stress need for supportive devices as indicated.
5. Stress need for a regular exercise program. Teach ROM exercises to family.
6. Stress importance of diet as ordered:
   a. Offer supplemental feedings.
   b. Offer small portions, and instruct the patient to chew slowly.
7. Stress importance of safety measures: side rails, ramps, shower chairs, and walkers and canes.
8. Instruct the patient regarding name of medication, dosage, time of administration, and toxic or side effects.
9. Instruct the patient regarding need to avoid over-the-counter medications without first consulting physician.
10. Encourage socialization with friends and family.
11. Stress importance of verbalization of feelings about anxiety, fear, and body image changes.
12. Teach the patient and family about seizures: safety measures and whom to contact.

Evaluation

Patient Outcome	Data Indicating That Outcome is Reached
Patient demonstrates a patent airway.	Breath sounds are normal. Chest excursion is bilateral and symmetric. Rate and depth of respirations are normal. Cough is effective. There are no subjective or objective findings of shortness of breath, air hunger, or dyspnea on exertion.
Patient demonstrates an effective breathing pattern.	Airway is patent. Chest excursion is symmetric. Breath sounds are normal, or there is no increase in adventitious sounds. Arterial blood gas values are within normal ranges or consistent with patient's baseline. Vital signs are within normal ranges or consistent with patient's baseline. Hemoglobin levels are 14 to 18 g/dl (male) or 12 to 16 g/dl (female). Intake and output are stable. There are no signs of respiratory distress. All lobes are resonant on percussion. Skin color is not cyanotic.
Patient maintains adequate cerebral tissue perfusion.	Level of consciousness is unchanged. There is no evidence of neurologic deficits. Pattern of electrolytes is stable. There is no seizure activity.
Patient demonstrates adequate body temperature regulation.	Vital signs are within normal range for patient. Serum electrolytes and fluid balance are within normal limits. Patient's body temperature is maintained between 35.8° and 37.3° C (96.4° and 99.2° F). Patient remains free of symptoms of hypothermia or hyperthermia including flushing or cyanosis, irritability, and seizures.
Patient demonstrates minimal complications of sensory-perceptual alterations.	Level of orientation is optimum. Patient is free of injury. Patient demonstrates skin integrity. Self-care deficits are minimum. Social participation is appropriate to physiologic status.
Patient remains free of traumatic injury.	Safety measures are appropriate to physiologic status. Skin integrity is maintained. Skin is free of bruises, burns, abrasions, and redness. Environment is safe. Patient is free of nosocomial infections.
Patient demonstrates an optimum level of mobility.	Skin integrity is maintained. Patient remains free of contractures and deformities. Level of mobility is appropriate to pnysiologic status. Intake and output pattern is stable. Nutritional status is adequate. Patient is free of thrombophlebitis. Patient is free of local infection. Patient participates in an ongoing physical therapy program.

Patient Outcome	Data Indicating That Outcome is Reached
Patient demonstrates minimum self-care deficits.	Outcome criteria listed for impaired physical mobility are met. Level of self-care activities is appropriate to physiologic status. Patient participates in physical and occupational therapy.
Patient demonstrates skin integrity.	Skin is intact. Nutritional status is adequate. Electrolyte balance is maintained. Patient is free of pressure sores and contractures.
Patient experiences minimum alterations in comfort.	Patient openly verbalizes feelings of discomfort when they occur. Patient can use measures to decrease discomfort. Patient can verbally validate a decrease in subjective feelings of discomfort. There is a decrease in objective findings of pain.
Patient demonstrates minimum feelings of powerlessness.	Optimum level of physiologic control, as possible for current health status, is maintained. Optimum level of psychologic control, as possible, is maintained. Patient participates, as possible, in decision making about care. Patient participates, as possible, in self-care.
Patient demonstrates adequate nutritional status.	Weight pattern is stable: normal for height, age, sex, and previous baseline. Intake and output are balanced and stable. Skin turgor is good. There is fluid and electrolyte balance. Dietary supplements are used as appropriate. Nausea and vomiting are controlled or absent.
Patient demonstrates minimum complications of bowel alteration.	Skin in perineal area is clean and dry. Dietary intake is adequate. Fluid intake is adequate (2000 ml/day unless contraindicated). Intake and output patterns are stable. There is no fecal impaction. Bowel evacuation pattern is regular. Diarrhea is controlled or absent.
Patient demonstrates minimum complications from alterations in urinary elimination patterns.	Intake and output patterns are stable. Urine is clear, yellow to amber in color, and without sediment. Skin in perineal area is clean and dry. Urine is acidic (pH 6.0). Patient remains free of urinary tract infections. Patient remains free of bladder distention. Patient can describe symptoms of urinary tract infections that require medical intervention.

Spinal tumors

Spinal tumors, although less common than intracranial tumors, are similar in pathologic types. They can arise from spinal nerve roots, the meninges, parenchyma of the cord, vertebral column, or the spinal vascular network.

Spinal tumors frequently affect young and middle-aged adults, and most involve the thoracic (50%), cervical (30%), and lumbosacral (20%) areas. The tumors are rare in children and elderly persons. Spinal tumors are classified according to their location; those occurring within the spinal cord tissue are called *intramedullary*, and those outside the spinal cord are called *extramedullary*. Extramedullary tumors are further categorized as intradural, extradural, or extravertebral. Spinal lesions constitute approximately 1% of all tumors in the general population. Men and women are affected about equally, except that meningiomas affect women more frequently. Approximately 85% of intraspinal tumors are benign.

Pathophysiology

Intramedullary tumors within the tissue of the spinal cord arise primarily from astrocyte or ependymal cells. Expanding intramedullary lesions may compress the spinal cord and nerve roots and destroy the parenchyma. Extramedullary tumors can be inside or outside the dural sac and produce spinal cord and spinal nerve root compression. Lesions outside the dural sac are called *extradural* and include herniated vertebral discs, acute and chronic infectious processes, metastatic lesions, meningiomas (5% to 10%), schwannomas (25% to 30%), and epidural hemorrhages. Tumors located within the dural sac but outside the spinal cord and nerve roots are called *extramedullary intradural* and include several types of glial tumors (e.g., ependymoma), most meningiomas and schwannomas, hemorrhages, and embryonic or congenital lesions. *Extramedullary extravertebral* tumors are commonly associated with bony destruction of vertebrae.[31]

Schwannomas are the spinal tumors most commonly arising from the nerve sheath and can be found in all portions of the spinal cord. These tumors appear as a firm, encapsulated, rounded mass that contains many small cysts. Schwannomas consist of interlacing bands of cells with parallel intracellular fibrils and elongated nuclei that are usually arranged in parallel rows. There are also a number of star-shaped cells resembling astrocytes loosely arranged in the microscopic structure. Small foci of degeneration with cysts are common. First, the schwannoma compresses as the spinal nerve root in the foramen of the canal, producing localized nerve root symptoms. As the lesion progresses, it further compresses other nerve roots and the spinal cord, producing neurologic findings of cord compression. Symptoms are usually asymmetric. Extradural schwannomas are often hourglass or dumbbell in shape with a portion in the spinal canal attached by a narrow band of tumor through the foramen to a part outside the spinal canal. This type of tumor can compress cervical, mediastinal, or abdominal tissue.[4]

Meningiomas constitute approximately 22% of all primary spinal tumors. Most meningiomas are extramedullary. Eighty percent of meningiomas affect women, usually in the fourth, fifth, or sixth decade of life. These tumors can appear anywhere in the spinal canal but are most common in the region of the nerve roots, particularly in the thoracic region (two thirds of meningiomas occur in this region). They appear as small, rounded, nodular masses that frequently attach to the insertion of the denticulate ligament and extend dorsally or ventrally. Meningiomas consist of groups of elongated cells with round or oval nuclei. There is a tendency toward the formation of whorls, and calcification frequently is present in the center of the whorls. Symptoms are initially produced by traction or irritation of the nerve roots (i.e., radicular pain) and progress to long motor tract signs (i.e., spasticity) as a result of compression. Meningiomas can undergo malignant changes.[4]

Ependymomas make up approximately 13% of all spinal cord tumors. They arise from the lining of the internal spaces of the central nervous system and are usually intramedullary. Ependymomas are found throughout the spinal cord but commonly are located caudally in the conus medullaris and the filum terminale (cauda equina ependymoma). They are more common in men, generally appearing in the fourth or fifth decade of life. These tumors occur as loculated masses in the spinal canal, frequently with fusiform swelling. Microscopically, an ependymoma appears as a crowded mass of polygonal-type cells. In the filum it appears as a central core of connective tissue and blood vessels that is surrounded by a single layer of ependymal cells. Ependymomas may extend to 10 vertebral spaces in length and produce symptoms resulting from cord compression.[4]

Astrocytomas and *oligodendrogliomas* are similar clinically. The oligodendroglioma is a rare type of spinal cord tumor. Astrocytomas are less common than ependymomas, generally intramedullary, and more common in men. Astrocytomas appear as elongated, fusiform swellings of the spinal cord. (See Table 3-6 for grading of astrocytomas.) Symptoms result from compression of the long tracts of the spinal cord.

The pathologic processes occurring with any spinal tumors can result from spinal cord destruction and infiltration, spinal cord displacement and compression, spinal nerve root irritation and compression, disruption in spinal blood supply, or disruption of cerebrospinal fluid circulation.[31]

Most benign lesions produce neurologic symptoms by compression and displacement of the spinal cord and by irritation and compression of the spinal nerve roots rather than by invasion and destruction of the spinal cord. The severity of neurologic symptoms depends on the degree of compression and how rapidly it develops. With slower-growing tumors, the spinal cord can accommodate the mass by compressing itself into a slender, ribbonlike tissue. Such a slow-growing tumor may produce minimum deficits. Fast-growing tumors can produce sudden cord compression, edema, and severe neurologic deficits.[28]

Diagnostic Studies and Findings

Roentgenograms

Determine presence of vertebral column lesions and bony destruction

Myelography (with Contrast)

Identifies size, boundaries, and level of tumor (with incomplete blockage of subarachnoid space)

CSF Sampling

Elevated protein levels

Froin's syndrome (xanthochromatic CSF with large amounts of protein, rapid coagulation, and absence of an increased number of cells) noted if CSF collected below level of tumor

Contraindication: If elevated intraspinal pressure is suspected

Electromyogram (EMG)

Assistive in differential diagnosis

Queckenstedt Test

Positive

CT Scan

Lesion location identified

Spinal Angiograms

Differentiates vascular lesions from tumors

Positron Emission Tomography (PET)

Lesion location identified

Medical Plan

Surgery

Tumor excision
Decompression laminectomy
Tracheotomy, if indicated
Spinal fusion
Lumbar puncture

Medications

Corticosteroids (for control cord edema)
- Dexamethasone (Decadron), 10-40 mg IV qid

Antacids
- Maalox, 15-30 ml po or nasogastric q4h

Histamine antagonist
- Cimetidine (Tagamet), 300 mg po or IV

Analgesic/antipyretics
- Acetaminophen, gr X po q4h prn

General Management

Radiation therapy
Mechanical ventilation, if indicated
CT scans
Soft cervical collar, if indicated
Spinal prostheses
Physiotherapy
Nutritional consultation

Psychosocial counseling and support
Extended care facility referral, if appropriate

NURSING CARE

Nursing Assessment

General Signs

- Sensory impairment
  - Slow, progressive numbness or tingling, and coldness in an extremity
  - Hyperesthesia at level of lesion
  - Loss of touch, vibration, and position sense (later signs)
- Motor impairment
  - Weakness, spasticity, and clumsiness: spreading contralaterally or homolaterally
  - Hyperactive reflexes
  - Hypotonia and ataxia (cerebellar signs)
  - Spasticity
  - Positive Babinski's reflex
  - Paresis
- Pain
  - Intermittent nerve root (radicular) pain, aggravated by straining, movement, and coughing
  - Persistent back pain
- Sphincter disturbances
  - Urinary urgency
  - Difficulty in initiating urination
  - Retention and overflow incontinence
  - Decreased sphincter control (later sign)
- Other
  - Brown-Séquard syndrome
  - Contralateral loss of temperature and pain
  - Ipsilateral motor loss
  - Ipsilateral loss of vibration, touch, and position sense

Cervical Tumors

- C4 and above
  - Sensory
    - Vertigo
  - Motor
    - Quadriparesis
    - Atrophy of sternocleidomastoid muscles
    - Dysphagia
    - Dysarthria
    - Tongue deviation
    - Respiratory insufficiency
    - Respiratory failure
  - Other
    - Occipital headaches
    - Nuchal rigidity
    - Down-beat nystagmus
    - Papilledema
- C4 and below
  - Sensory
    - Paresthesia
    - Horner's syndrome (ipsilateral pupillary constriction, ptosis, and anhidrosis)
  - Motor
    - Weakness
    - Muscle fasciculations
    - Muscle atrophy
  - Other
    - Shoulder and arm pain

Thoracic Tumors

- Sensory
  - Hyperesthesia band immediately above level of lesion
- Motor
  - Spastic paresis of lower extremities
  - Positive Babinski's sign
  - Lower motor neuron deficits
- Other
  - Sphincter impairment

Lumbar Tumors

- Sensory
  - Localized loss in legs and saddle area
- Motor
  - Footdrop
  - Diminished or absent patellar and Achilles reflexes
- Other
  - Severe low back pain with radiation down legs
  - Perineal and bladder discomfort
  - Decreased libido
  - Impotence
  - Bladder disturbances

Nursing Dx & Intervention

Nursing Diagnosis	Nursing Intervention/Rationale
Ineffective airway clearance; potential for aspiration	• Auscultate for breath sounds every 1 to 2 hours and as needed. • Maintain patent airway, and avoid flexion of the neck if patient is immobile. • Assist ventilation as indicated. Keep Ambu bag at bedside. • Monitor vital signs every 1 to 2 hours; monitor neurologic status every 1 to 2 hours. • Keep emergency drugs and ventilator at bedside. • Maintain nothing-by-mouth status *to prevent risk of choking or aspiration, if indicated.*

Nursing Diagnosis — **Nursing Intervention/Rationale**

Ineffective breathing pattern

- Auscultate for breath sounds every 1 to 2 hours. Assess quality and any increase in adventitious sounds *to prevent pulmonary complications:*
  - Suction as needed *to prevent airway obstruction and secretion stasis.*
  - Hyperinflate lungs with 100% oxygen for 1 minute before and 1 minute after suctioning, unless contraindicated, *to minimize hypoxia during suctioning.*
- Monitor mechanical ventilation, if used:
  - Ensure that tidal volume, rate, mode, and oxygen concentration are set as ordered.
  - Ensure that ventilator alarms are on and functional.
- Monitor arterial blood gases per protocol *to minimize risks of respiratory insufficiency and failure:*
  - Report decrease in Po_2 of 10 to 15 mm Hg.
  - Report increase in Pco_2 greater than 10 to 15 mm Hg.
- Check blood pressure, temperature, and pulse rate every 1 to 2 hours and as needed.

Altered cerebral and/or spinal tissue perfusion

- Establish baseline and ongoing neurologic assessment every 1 to 2 hours and as needed.
- Intervene *to monitor or prevent increased intracranial pressure:*
  - Administer medications, treatments, and IV lines per protocol.
  - Maintain elevation of head of bed per protocol *to facilitate cerebral venous drainage.*
  - Accurately record intake and output *to monitor for imbalance.*
  - Monitor serum electrolytes, blood count, and arterial blood gases for abnormalities.
  - Monitor values and waveforms of intracranial pressure line.
  - Maintain patency and sterility of the system.
  - Monitor effects of treatments on intracranial pressure.
  - Correlate neurologic status with intracranial pressure values; notify physician if inconsistent.
  - Assist with drainage of cerebrospinal fluid from the system *to decrease intracranial hypertension.*
- Intervene *to monitor or prevent seizures.* Institute seizure precautions:
  - Padded tongue blade and airway at bedside
  - Bed height at lowest level
  - Side rails up at all times and padded
  - Oxygen and suction equipment at bedside
  - Emergency medications at bedside
- Administer anticonvulsants per protocol:
  - Monitor effects and side effects.
  - Monitor serum for therapeutic levels of the anticonvulsant.
- Maintain balance between hyperthermia and hypothermia.

Sensory/perceptual alterations (kinesthetic, tactile)

- See general intervention strategies listed on p. 1728.

Potential for trauma related to seizures

- Assess and document patient's potential for injury and strategies used *to prevent injury.*
- Maintain bed in low position at all times unless side rails are up or nurse is with patient.
- Provide patient with a call light within easy reach.
- Maintain side rails in up position at bedtime, after sedation, when patient is confused, and as needed.
- Maintain wheelchairs and stretchers in locked position when transferring patient.
- Pad side rails if patient is overactive.

Preconvulsive

- Have oral airway at bedside.
- Support and protect head; turn to side if possible.
- Prevent injury:
  - Ease patient to floor if in chair.
  - Place pillows along side rails if patient is in bed.
  - Remove surrounding furniture.
  - Loosen constrictive clothing.
- Provide privacy as necessary. Stay with patient; remain calm.
- Note frequency, time, involved body parts, and length of seizure *to determine type of seizure.*

Postconvulsive

- Maintain patent airway.
- Suction as needed, as indicated.
- Check vital signs and neurologic signs.
- Administer oxygen per protocol *to minimize cerebral hypoxia.*
- Reorient patient to environment.
- Place patient in position of comfort; turn head to side *to prevent aspiration.*
- Administer oral hygiene as necessary for secretions and bleeding.

Nursing Diagnosis	Nursing Intervention/Rationale
Potential impaired skin integrity	• Assess skin integrity for potential breakdown every 2 hours. • Administer skin care every 2 hours *to prevent breakdown and decubitus ulcers.* Turn patient every 2 hours and as needed, unless contraindicated: Change position slowly. Position in proper body alignment. Massage pressure points every 2 hours *to stimulate circulation;* give gentle back rubs every shift and as needed. Keep skin dry and clean. Provide passive ROM exercises every 4 hours and as needed: Perform ROM exercises gently, slowly, and rhythmically. Repeat each ROM exercise three times, every 4 hours. • Maintain high-protein, low-calcium diet.
Impaired physical mobility	• Assess patient's mobility level and document the following interventions: Use firm mattress or bed board *to support back and spine.* Use footboard or Spence boots *to prevent footdrop.* Apply antiembolus stockings to lower extremities. Administer anticoagulation therapy per protocol. Encourage self-care activities to tolerance. Plan all activities and maintain planned rest periods *to avoid fatigue.* Obtain physical therapy referral.
Feeding, bathing/hygiene, dressing/grooming, and toileting self-care deficit	• Assess patient's degree of deficit and intervene as necessary. • Assist with feeding, as indicated; use IV or nasogastric feedings per protocol. • Administer oral hygiene every 2 hours and as needed. • Assist with daily hygiene care as indicated. • Administer eye care every 2 to 4 hours if indicated. • Perform intermittent urinary catheterization per protocol. • Maintain bowel function with regular evacuation.
Pain	• Assess and document patient's degree of pain. • Modify anxiety associated with the pain experience. • Provide other sensory input. • For patients receiving radiation or chemotherapy: Explain procedure or medication before implementing. Administer antiemetic and antidiarrheal medications as needed *to prevent nausea and control diarrhea.* Provide frequent skin care. Monitor for signs of phlebitis.
Altered oral mucous membrane	• Assess oral mucous membranes for signs of stomatitis. • Provide frequent mouth care and apply topical agents to mucous membranes *to minimize discomfort of stomatitis.* • Monitor patient's laboratory values for decreased RBC, WBC, or platelet levels *to detect bleeding and infection.* • Maintain planned rest periods. • Offer frequent, small feedings *to combat anorexia and discomfort of nausea.*
Body image, self-esteem, and personal identity disturbances	• Assess degree of orientation and ability to communicate. • Provide for a safe, comfortable, secure environment. • Reorient to time, person, and place, as appropriate *to maintain sense of personal identity.* • Carefully explain what you are doing and why you are doing it. • Answer questions simply and honestly. • Correct misinformation. • Protect the patient's privacy. • Provide gentle physical care in a caring environment.

Patient Education

1. Involve family in care, as possible; teach essential aspects of care.
2. Reinforce physician's explanation of medical management.
3. Stress importance of ongoing outpatient care and follow-up visits.
4. Encourage independent activities, as possible:
   a. Be alert to limitations.
   b. Avoid overprotection.
   c. Stress need for supportive devices as indicated.
5. Stress need for regular exercise program: teach ROM exercises to family.
6. Stress importance of diet as ordered:
   a. Offer supplemental feedings.
   b. Give small portions, and instruct patient to chew slowly.
7. Stress importance of safety measures:
   a. Side rails
   b. Ramps
   c. Shower chairs
   d. Removal of scatter rugs
   e. Walker, canes
8. Instruct regarding name of medication, dosage, time of administration, and toxic or side effects.
9. Stress need to avoid over-the-counter medications without first consulting physician.
10. Encourage socialization with friends and family.
11. Stress importance of verbalization of feelings about anxiety, fear, and body image changes.
12. Teach patient and family about seizures (i.e., safety measures and whom to contact).

Evaluation

Patient Outcome	Data Indicating That Outcome is Reached
Patient demonstrates a patent airway.	Breath sounds are normal. Chest excursion is bilateral and symmetric. Rate and depth of respirations are normal. Cough is effective. There are no subjective or objective findings of shortness of breath, air hunger, or dyspnea on exertion.
Patient demonstrates an effective breathing pattern.	Airway is patent. Chest excursion is symmetric. Breath sounds are normal, or there is no increase in adventitious sounds. Arterial blood gas values are within normal ranges or consistent with patient's baseline. Vital signs are within normal ranges or consistent with patient's baseline. Hemoglobin levels are 14 to 18 g/dl (male) and 12 to 16 g/dl (female). Intake and output are stable. There are no signs of respiratory distress. All lobes are resonant on percussion. Skin color is not cyanotic.
Patient maintains adequate cerebral and spinal tissue perfusion.	Level of consciousness is unchanged. There is no evidence of neurologic deficits. Electrolyte pattern is stable. There is no seizure activity.
Patient demonstrates minimal complications of sensory-perceptual alterations.	Level of orientation is optimum. Patient remains free of injury. Patient demonstrates skin integrity. Nutritional status is adequate. Self-care deficits are minimum. Social participation is appropriate to physiologic status.
Patient remains free of traumatic injury.	Safety measures are appropriate to level of physiologic status. Skin integrity is maintained. Skin is free of bruises, burns, abrasions, and redness. Environment is safe. Patient is free of nosocomial infections.
Patient demonstrates an optimum level of mobility.	Patient exhibits skin integrity. Patient is free of contractures and deformities. Level of mobility is appropriate to physiologic status. Nutritional status is adequate. Intake and output pattern is stable. Patient is free of thrombophlebitis. Patient is free of local infection. Patient participates in an ongoing physical therapy program.
Patient demonstrates minimum self-care deficits.	Outcome criteria listed for impaired physical mobility are met. Level of self-care activities is appropriate to physiologic status. Patient participates in physical and occupational therapy.
Patient demonstrates skin integrity.	Skin is intact. Nutritional status is adequate. Electrolyte balance is maintained. Patient is free of pressure sores and contractures.
Patient experiences minimum alterations in comfort.	Patient openly verbalizes feelings of discomfort when they occur. Patient can use measures to decrease discomfort. Patient verbally validates a decrease in subjective feelings of discomfort. Patient verbally validates a decrease in objective findings of pain.
Patient demonstrates intact self-concepts.	Patient openly verbalizes feelings of grief and loss. Patient acknowledges actual change in self-image. Patient verbalizes positive feelings about self. Patient focuses on present and future appearance and function. Patient verbalizes feelings of hopefulness, helpfulness, and powerfulness.

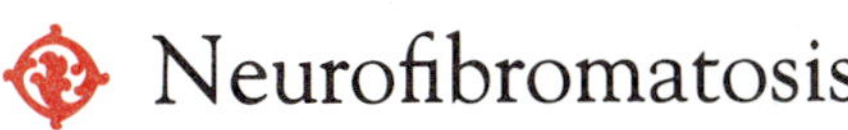

Neurofibromatosis

(Von Recklinghausen's disease)

Neurofibromatosis, also called multiple neuroma, neuromatosis, and von Recklinghausen's disease, is a genetic disorder transmitted as an autosomal dominant trait by either parent.

The disorder is characterized by numerous fibromas of spinal or cranial nerves and skin, café au lait spots, and developmental anomalies of bone, muscles, and viscera. It has an estimated frequency of 1:2500 to 1:3000 live births and sometimes is associated with spina bifida, meningocele, or epilepsy. Approximately 50% of the cases of neurofibromatosis are sporadic and demonstrate no familial history. Men are more commonly affected than women. There is malignant degeneration in 2% to 5% of the cases of neurofibromatosis. Mental retardation occurs in 10% of the patients.

Neurofibromatosis can be classified according to central or peripheral involvement. The *central* form is characterized by various combinations of gliomas, meningiomas, neurofibromas, and schwannomas that affect the intraspinal and intracranial nervous systems.[39] *Peripheral* neurofibromatosis shows little evidence of central nervous system involvement and primarily affects the peripheral nerve. The *visceral* form is characterized by involvement of the viscera and autonomic nervous system. The clinical symptoms of neurofibromatosis usually appear in later childhood or adolescence and continue to develop with age.

Pathophysiology

In neurofibromatosis Schwann cells or fibroblasts proliferate, resulting in a tortuous interlacing of tissue cords that manifests as circumscribed or poorly defined tumors in multiple areas.[39] These tumors vary in size from minute to several centimeters. The majority of the lesions are soft or firm and smoothly rounded or lobulated and occur as nodules scattered along the course of involved peripheral, intracranial, or intraspinal nerves. Often the superficial dermal tumors (cutaneous neurofibromas) sink into the subcutaneous fat on gentle pressure ("button-holing"). Most subcutaneous neurofibromas occur over the trunk and are asymptomatic. Along with neuromas, there may be tumors of the meninges (meningiomas) and tumors of the glia cells (astrocytomas, ependymomas, glioblastomas, etc.), as well as small, gliotic or glial nodules within the central nervous system.[42]

The café au lait macule is made of melanin located deep in the epidermis. Usually it is a uniformly pale brown macule, unevenly round to ovoid, ranging from 0.5 to 15 cm or more in diameter. Five or more café au lait macules of at least 1.5 cm diameter (Crowe's sign) are sufficient to establish a diagnosis even without the neurofibromas. The macules are frequently found in the axilla (axillary freckles), over the trunk, and over the pelvis. Because of giant melanosomes in pigment epithelial cells, the pigmented areas become even more evident with age.

Diagnostic Studies and Findings

CSF Sampling

Elevated protein levels

Myelography

Determination of presence of spinal cord tumors

CT Scan

Determination of presence of intracranial tumors

Skull Roentgenograms

Bone erosion from tumor growth

Medical Plan

Surgery

Tumor excision
Shunting procedures for hydrocephalus

General Management

Intracranial pressure monitoring if indicated
Genetic counseling
Psychosocial counseling
Support groups

NURSING CARE

Nursing Assessment

Skin

Multiple cutaneous neurofibromas
Café au lait, pigmented skin lesions with regular, sharp borders in axilla, pelvis, and trunk
Skin bronzing
Sacral hypertrichosis
Nevus anemicus
Macroglossia
Cutis verticus gyrata
Large, hairy, pigmented nevi

Endocrine System

Hyperparathyroidism
Cretinism
Acromegaly
Myxedema
Precocious puberty
Pheochromocytoma

Skeletal System

Lordosis
Kyphosis
Scoliosis
Spina bifida
Pseudarthrosis
Spontaneous fractures
Dislocations
Osteitis fibrosa cystica

Cranial Nerves

Facial numbness or weakness
Visual loss
Deafness
Optic nerve atrophy
Hydrocephalus
Increased intracranial pressure
Vertigo
Atrophy of muscles of mastication

Pain

Paresthetic or neurologic discomfort
Tumors possibly painful to pressure

Spinal Nerves and Spinal Cord

Paralyses
Brown-Séquard syndrome (with large fibromas in cervical or thoracic areas of the spinal cord)

Other

Ipsilateral cerebellar signs (with cerebellopontine angle meningiomas)
Elephantiasis neuromatosa (diffuse fibrosis and proliferation of affected part)
Mental retardation
Epilepsy
Visceral hypertrophy

Nursing Dx & Intervention

Nursing Diagnosis	Nursing Intervention/Rationale
Potential impaired skin integrity	• Assess skin and pressure points every 2 hours for signs of breakdown. • Keep skin clean and dry. • Assist with active and/or passive ROM exercises *to promote circulation and prevent muscle wasting*. • Maintain adequate nutritional status. • Monitor fluid and electrolyte balance: Monitor weights. Maintain intake and output. Monitor laboratory values (i.e., electrolytes).
Altered peripheral tissue perfusion	• Assess for signs of increased intracranial pressure or neurologic deficits every 2 to 4 hours and as needed. • If tumors are surgically excised: Monitor vital signs and neurologic status per protocol. Maintain patent airway and effective breathing pattern. Check incision site frequently *to prevent hemorrhage*. Administer parenteral fluids as ordered *to maintain fluid balance*. Administer medications as ordered. Maintain pain management. Keep patient warm and dry. Stay with patient, if restless.
Anxiety	• See general intervention strategies listed on p. 1743.
Pain	• Establish a baseline and ongoing assessment of the patient's pain and response to the pain experience. • Promote rest and relaxation. • Decrease noxious stimuli, whenever possible. • Assist patient to modify the anxiety associated with the pain experience. • Test or evaluate other sensory input (e.g., gentle back rub) *as means to minimize pain*. • Use behavior modification if indicated. • Administer medications (analgesics) per protocol. • Teach patient ways to modify precipitating and environmental factors.
Body image, self-esteem, and personal identity disturbances	• Provide an ongoing assessment of patient's interpersonal strengths. Focus on strengths and potential. • Reorient to time, person, and place as appropriate. • Explain what you are doing and why you are doing it.

Nursing Diagnosis	Nursing Intervention/Rationale
	• Listen to the feelings the patient expresses. • Answer questions simply and honestly. • Correct misinformation. • Protect patient's privacy *to minimize anxiety and embarrassment.* • Provide gentle physical care in a caring environment. • Provide positive feedback for achievement of daily goals. • Assist patient to become involved in self-care.
Social isolation	• See general intervention strategies listed on p. 1767.

Patient Education

1. Instruct regarding cause of the disorder, signs, and symptoms of progression.
2. Stress importance of genetic counseling.
3. Emphasize need for open expression of feelings of anxiety, fear, and changing body image.
4. Stress need for continued interactions with family and friends.
5. Teach methods of controlling physical discomfort.
6. Teach methods of controlling anxiety.
7. Instruct regarding name of medication, dosage, time of administration, purpose, and side effects.
8. Emphasize need to avoid over-the-counter medications without first consulting physician.
9. Stress importance of ongoing patient care.

Evaluation

Patient Outcome	Data Indicating That Outcome is Reached
Patient demonstrates skin integrity.	Skin is intact. Nutritional status is adequate. Electrolyte balance is maintained. Patient is free of pressure sores and contractures.
Patient demonstrates adequate tissue perfusion.	Criteria listed for skin integrity are met. Patient is free of signs of increased intracranial pressure. Present neurologic status is maintained. Patient is free of infections and complications.
Patient demonstrates a low level of anxiety.	Patient openly verbalizes concerns and feelings of grief, loss, and discomfort. Patient openly verbalizes feelings supported by health care professionals and family. Patient verbalizes essential aspects of care. Patient can identify methods to deal effectively with anxious feelings.
Patient experiences minimal alterations in comfort.	Patient openly verbalizes feelings of discomfort when they occur. Patient can use measures to decrease discomfort. Patient can verbally validate a decrease in subjective feelings of discomfort. Patient can verbally validate a decrease in objective findings of pain.
Patient demonstrates intact self-concepts.	Patient openly verbalizes feelings of grief and loss. Patient verbalizes positive feelings about self. Patient acknowledges actual change in self-image. Patient focuses on present and future appearance and function. Patient verbalizes feelings of hopefulness, helpfulness, and powerfulness.
Patient demonstrates social participation.	Patient can state importance of interpersonal relationships. Patient relates to self and others. Patient participates, as possible, in unit and group activities. Patient participates, as possible, in family activities.

VASCULAR DISORDERS

Aneurysm

(Cerebral aneurysm)

An intracranial aneurysm is a localized dilation that develops secondary to a weakness of the arterial wall.

Cerebral aneurysm is the fourth most frequent cerebrovascular disorder, with an incidence of 9.6 cases per 100,000 in the general population. The peak incidence is in the 35- to 60-year-old age group, and women are affected slightly more often than men. Cerebral aneurysms rarely occur in children and adolescents. Saccular aneurysms are associated with an increased incidence of congenital polycystic disease of the kidney and coarctation of the aorta.[45] Hypertension is found more frequently in persons who have aneurysms than in the average population; however, aneurysms also occur in normotensive individuals.

Ruptured cerebral aneurysm is the most common cause of nontraumatic subarachnoid hemorrhage. At least 28% of individuals with ruptured cerebral aneurysm die immediately. Of individuals who survive the initial hemorrhage but are not treated, approximately 50% experience rebleeding within a year. Approximately one third of individuals who survive ruptured cerebral aneurysms demonstrate some residual paralysis, headaches and mental changes, or epilepsy. Aneurysmal rupture often is associated with physical exertion (e.g., sports or coitus), severe emotional excitement, and a sudden rise in blood pressure, but it can also occur during sleep.

Pathophysiology

No single mechanism has been identified in the pathogenesis of intracranial aneurysm. Possible causes are congenital structural defects in the media and elastica of the vessel wall, incomplete involution of embryonic vessels, and secondary factors such as arterial hypertension, atherosclerotic changes, hemodynamic disturbances, and polycystic disease. Intracranial aneurysms also may result from the shearing forces produced during craniocerebral trauma. These shearing forces may weaken the arterial wall, which expands or dilates with each arterial pulsation until bleeding or symptoms occur.

Aneurysms are generally classified according to their predominant characteristics into (1) saccular, or berry; (2) fusiform, or atherosclerotic; and (3) mycotic. *Saccular* aneurysms constitute 95% of all ruptured aneurysms. They appear as small, thin-walled "berries" protruding from arteries primarily at points of bifurcations and branchings. Because of the local weakness in the vessel, the intima bulges outward and the sac slowly enlarges until finally wall dissolution and rupture occur.[23]

Fusiform (giant) aneurysms are spindle-shaped dilations of the entire circumference of an artery for several centimeters. They are characterized by degenerative changes in the elastic fibers and deposits of cholesterol in the intima and by fibrous replacement of smooth muscle.[3] These aneurysms most commonly occur along the trunk of the basilar artery. They infrequently rupture and generally produce symptoms by compression of adjacent cerebral tissue or cranial nerves. When rupture does occur, the atherosclerotic or fusiform aneurysm is often fatal.

Mycotic aneurysms are rare and can result when a septic embolus from acute or subacute bacterial endocarditis or other infectious process causes arterial necrosis that may lead to thrombosis or aneurysm formation. Mycotic aneurysms usually arise in a characteristic location along the distal branches of the middle and anterior cerebral arteries.[68] They tend to be multiple.

The majority of ruptured aneurysms are saccular, or berry, aneurysms. Saccular aneurysms characteristically occur at specific locations in the intracranial circulation. Approximately 85% of berry aneurysms are found in the anterior portion of the circle of Willis, and 15% are situated in the vertebral or basilar arteries. Within the anterior portion, there are three main sites of rupture: termination of the internal carotid artery (25%), the anterior communicating artery (23%), and the middle cerebral artery bifurcation (16%).[50] Aneurysms of the internal carotid are frequently large and may be situated either in the angle formed by the internal carotid and the posterior communicating artery or at the site of bifurcation of the internal carotid into the anterior and middle cerebral arteries. Aneurysms of the middle cerebral artery usually are located approximately 2 to 3 cm from the vessel's origin, at the site of origin of the first main branches.[27] Multiple aneurysms, often bilateral and symmetric, may be found in 15% to 20% of cases.

Most saccular cerebral aneurysms have a definable neck, and many are multilobular. Thickening, thrombosis, and wall calcification frequently are seen.[17] The aneurysms may vary from 2 mm to 5 cm in diameter. Most aneurysms are at least 10 mm in diameter at the time of rupture. Larger aneurysms may result in erosion of the bones of the skull and compression of cerebral tissue and adjacent cranial nerves.[17] Histopathologic examination shows thinning of the arterial wall with fragmentation of internal elastica and degeneration or absence of its smooth muscle wall.

Aneurysmal rupture occurs when the pulse pressure tears a very small hole in the fundus of the aneurysm, which results in direct hemorrhage into the leptomeningeal compartment (subarachnoid hemorrhage) under arterial pressure. Such a hemorrhage spreads rapidly, producing localized changes in the underlying cortex and focal irritation of the cranial nerves and arteries.[24] The bleeding commonly is stopped by the formation of a fibrin-platelet plug at the point of rupture and by tissue compression. Within approximately 3 weeks the hemorrhage undergoes *resorption*. Resorption occurs by the arachnoidal villi after the leukocytes and macrophages have begun their scavenging.[24] There is a serious risk of recurrent rupture 7 to 10 days after the original hemorrhage.

Massive hemorrhage (i.e., 30 to 50 ml) may produce rapid filling of the ventricular system and vasal cisterns or produce a hematoma that locally distorts the subarachnoid space and brain tissue. Aneurysms of the anterior communicating artery lying next to the medial surfaces of the frontal lobes and aneurysms of the middle cerebral artery within the sylvian fissure next to the frontal and temporal lobes are particularly prone to rupture into the parenchyma of the brain. Aneurysms of the anterior communicating artery may rupture into the frontal lobes. Aneurysms of the basilar artery may rupture into the midbrain or diencephalon. Secondary rupture into the cerebral ventricles can occur because these intracerebral hemorrhages commonly extend through the brain tissue.[17] Aneurysmal rupture may include bleeding in nearby cranial nerves. The most commonly affected cranial nerve is the oculomotor, or cranial nerve III, because of rupture of an aneurysm at the origin of the posterior communicating artery from the internal carotid artery. The optic nerve frequently is involved with ophthalmic artery aneurysms. Carotid aneurysms in the cavernous sinus involve cranial nerves III, IV, and VI, which act on the muscles and the first division of the trigeminal nerve. Increased intracranial pressure results in distortions that can produce unilateral or bilateral sixth nerve palsies. Most of the cranial nerve palsies that develop result from hemorrhage in the nerve and not from compression of the nerve by the aneurysm.[17]

Increased intracranial pressure is frequently a sequela of acute subarachnoid hemorrhage and occurs because of several mechanisms. First, an expanding hematoma acts as a rapidly enlarging space-occupying lesion that compresses or displaces adjacent brain tissue. Second, blood in the basal cistern may impede or interrupt the flow of cerebrospinal fluid. Last, if the pacchionian granulations become distended with blood, the spinal fluid resorption is impeded.[23] The increased intracranial pressure may retard subsequent hemorrhage.

Cerebral vasospasms are a frequent complication of subarachnoidal hemorrhage and occur in 35% to 40% of individuals with ruptured intracranial aneurysms. The pathophysiology of vasospasms is not clearly understood, but it is believed that certain substances, such as prostaglandins, serotonin, catecholamines, and methemoglobin, are released by the blood into the subarachnoid space. These vasoactive substances are thought to precipitate the vasospasms.[23] Edema, media necrosis, and proliferation of the intima have been described as sequelae to the initial vasospasms. Cerebral vasospasms usually appear 4 to 10 days after the hemorrhage and are characterized by measurable constriction or reactive narrowing of the cerebral arteries. The vasospasms are most evident in arteries adjacent to the site of hemorrhage and tend to be lessened when bleeding is minimal. Vasospasms can produce focal neurologic deterioration, cerebral ischemia, and infarction. Angiography shows severely constricted cerebral vessels and confirms the diagnosis.

Subarachnoid hemorrhages are graded according to their severity and clinical status. In one method for grading hemorrhages, individuals in grades I and II are managed medically for an average of 10 days and then treated surgically to prevent recurrent bleeding. Individuals in grades III and IV are managed medically for 3 to 4 weeks to stabilize them for surgery. Individuals in grade V are not surgical candidates unless they have life-threatening complications. The complete cerebral aneurysm classification system is listed in Table 3-7.

Table 3-7
Cerebral Aneurysm Rupture Classification System

Grade	Criteria
I (minimal bleed)	Asymptomatic: alert, minimal headache and minimum nuchal rigidity; no neurologic deficits
II (mild bleed)	Mild to severe headache; alert; nuchal rigidity; minimum neurologic deficits
III (moderate bleed)	Lethargic or confused; severe headache; nuchal rigidity; mild focal neurologic deficits
IV (moderate to severe bleed)	Stuporous, nuchal rigidity; mild to severe hemiparesis; may exhibit decerebrate posturing
V (severe bleed)	Comatose; decerebrate posturing

Diagnostic Studies and Findings

Lumbar Puncture

NOTE: Should be done with caution
Increased opening pressures
Elevated protein content (80 to 130 mg/dl)
Increased WBC count
Slightly decreased glucose
Bloody cerebrospinal fluid with xanthochromia (hemolyzed RBCs)

CT Scan (Serial)

Demonstration of blood in the subarachnoid space
Displaced midline structures
Localized blood clots

Magnetic Resonance Imaging (MRI)

Same as CT scan

Cerebral Arteriogram

Identification of local or general vasospasm
Outlining of cerebral vasculature

Skull Roentgenograms

May reveal calcified wall of aneurysm and areas of bone erosion

Echoencephalogram

Shifts in midline structure

Brain Scan

May indicate the presence of local diminution of flow

Serum Tests

Electrolyte imbalances
Changes in bleeding parameters (i.e., prothrombin time, partial thromboplastin time, and platelet count)

Regional Cerebral Blood Flow (rCBF)

Mean flow values for both hemispheres and determination of status of cerebral vasospasm

Medical Plan

Surgery

Tracheostomy or endotracheal intubation
Intracranial pressure monitoring
Ventriculoatrial shunting (hydrocephalus)
Clipping of aneurysm
Ligating of aneurysm
Wrapping of aneurysmal sac
Trapping of aneurysm with bypass grafting
Embolization of aneurysm
Evacuation of intracerebral clot

Medications

- Anticonvulsants
  - Phenytoin (Dilantin), 100 mg po or IV tid or qid (do not exceed 50 mg/min IV to prevent hypotension and cardiac arrhythmias)
  - Phenobarbital, 50-100 mg po in 2 or 3 divided doses
- Antihypertensive agents
  - Hydralazine (Apresoline) as ordered
  - Methyldopa (Aldomet), 250-500 mg IV q6h
- Antifibrinolytic agents
  - Aminocaproic acid (Amicar), 24-36 g/d IV for 3 wk (not given with coagulopathies)
- Corticosteroids
  - Dexamethasone (Decadron), 6-10 mg IV q6h
- Analgesic/antipyretics
  - Acetaminophen (Tylenol), gr X po or rectal suppository q4h prn
- Pituitary hormone
  - Vasopressin injection (Pitressin), 5-10 U IM or subcutaneously tid or qid (treatment of diabetes insipidus)
- Narcotic analgesics
  - Acetaminophen with codeine, 30 mg po or IV q4-6h prn
- Stool softeners
  - Docusate sodium (Colace), 100 mg po or nasogastric bid
- Psychotherapeutic agents
  - Chlorpromazine (Thorazine), dosage individualized (for shivering)
- Agents to control vasospasms
  - Antihistamine (antiserotonin effect)
    - Methysergide maleate (Sansert), 4-8 mg/d po
    - Phenoxybenzamine (Dibenzyline), 10-40 mg po bid or tid
  - Reserpine (Serpasil), 0.1 mg subcutaneously qid
  - Kanamycin sulfate (Kantrex), 1 g po tid
  - Calcium-blocking agents
    - Nifedipine (Procardia), 10-20 mg po tid (dosage titrated)

General Management

- Ventilatory support
- Hypothermia blanket
- ECG; cardiac monitoring
- Arterial blood pressure monitoring
- Elevation of head of bed
- Serial arterial blood gases
- Subarachnoid precautions
- Strict intake and output
- Intermittent catheterization
- Seizure precautions
- Antiembolus stockings

NURSING CARE

Nursing Assessment

Assessment findings depend on the location of the hemorrhage.

Level of Consciousness

- Varies from brief loss of consciousness to persistent coma

Meningeal Irritation

- Nuchal rigidity
- Positive Kernig's sign
- Positive Brudzinski's sign
- Fever
- Irritability
- Restlessness
- Later stages: seizures and blurred vision

Visual Disturbances

- Blurred vision
- Double vision
- Visual field defects: unilateral blindness

Cranial Nerve Involvement

- Ptosis and dilation of pupil
- Inability to move eye upward or inward
- Papilledema
- Photophobia

Autonomic Function

- Diaphoresis
- Chills
- Heart rate changes
- Changes in blood pressure
- Slight temperature elevation (37.8° to 38.9° C; 100° to 102° F)
- Altered respiratory rhythm

Motor Function

- Onset and worsening of hemiparesis
- Aphasia
- Dysphagia
- Hemiplegia
- Unilateral or bilateral transient paresis of lower extremities

Increased Intracranial Pressure

- Restlessness and lethargy
- Changes in level of consciousness
- Changes in vital signs (i.e., Cushing response with increased systolic blood pressure, wide pulse pressure, and decreased pulse rate)
- Pupillary changes (i.e., mydriasis)
- Impaired pupillary reflex
- Papilledema (late symptom)
- Vomiting

Fluctuations in temperature
Seizures
Worsening of focal neurologic signs
Changes in respiratory patterns

Seizure Activity

Preconvulsive (preictal stage)
- Aura: flash of light; sense of loss; fear; weakness; dizziness; peculiar taste, smell, and sounds
- Cry or scream
- Fall to floor
- Loss of consciousness
- Tachypnea

Convulsive state
- Tonic: rigid body; fixed jaws; clenched fists; extended legs; cyanosis; holding breath
- Clonic: urinary and/or fecal incontinence; jerking of facial muscles and extremities; biting tongue; frothing at the mouth

Postconvulsive (postictal) stage
- Altered level of consciousness
- Headache
- Nausea or vomiting
- Malaise
- Muscle soreness
- Aspiration: breathing difficulty, choking, cyanosis, decreased breath sounds, tachycardia, tachypnea
- Pneumonia

Pain

Sudden onset of a violent headache usually beginning as localized frontally or temporally and then generalizing to involve entire head

Vasospasms

Drowsiness followed by hemiplegia or hemiparesis
Aphasia
Focal neurologic deficits

ECG Abnormalities

Q waves
Elevated ST segments
ST and T wave changes

Other

Dizziness, nausea, and vomiting frequent
Cranial bruits may sometimes be auscultated on affected side
Babinski's sign

Nursing Dx & Intervention

Nursing Diagnosis	Nursing Intervention/Rationale
Ineffective airway clearance	• See general intervention strategies on p. 1702.
Ineffective breathing pattern	• See general intervention strategies on p. 1704.
Altered cerebral tissue perfusion	• Assess neurologic status every 15 to 30 minutes as needed. • Report any changes to physician. • Monitor closely for signs of increased intracranial pressure. • Main patency and sterility of intracranial pressure monitoring device, if used: Use surgical asepsis for all dressing changes. Monitor intracranial pressure responses to care and treatments. • Administer medications per protocol: anticonvulsants, steroids, antibiotics, antifibrinolytics (monitor prothrombin time, partial thromboplastin time, and platelet count), analgesics, and agents to control vasospasms. • Elevate head of bed 30 to 40 degrees, unless contraindicated, *to facilitate venous return.* • Maintain strict intake and output (1500 to 1800 ml/24 hours). • Observe for signs of dehydration or overhydration. • Maintain balance between hyperthermia and hypothermia per protocol. • Institute subarachnoid precautions, if appropriate: Provide private room with controlled lighting (i.e., dim artificial lighting). Maintain complete bed rest *to keep physical activity and exertion to a minimum.* Provide *all* nursing care for the patient. Limit visitors to immediate family members. Have patient wear elastic stockings or sequential compression devices *to prevent venous stasis.* Maintain dietary restrictions (no stimulants such as coffee, tea, or soda). Administer stool softeners *to prevent straining during bowel movement.* Instruct patient on need to avoid coughing and sneezing *to prevent sudden increases in intracranial pressure.* Instruct patient not to watch television, listen to radio, or read.

Nursing Diagnosis	Nursing Intervention/Rationale
Sensory/perceptual alterations (kinesthetic, tactile)	• See general intervention strategies listed on p. 1728.
Potential for trauma related to seizures	• Assess patient's potential for injury and document intervention strategies. • Maintain bed in low position at all times unless side rails are up or nurse is with patient. • Provide patient with a call light within easy reach. • Maintain side rails in up position at bedtime, after sedation, when patient is confused, and as needed *to prevent falls*. • Maintain wheelchairs and stretchers in locked position when transferring patient.
Preconvulsive	• Maintain seizure precautions: Have oral airway at bedside. Have suction equipment available at bedside *to prevent aspiration*. Pad side rails, if indicated. • Administer oxygen per protocol *to prevent cerebral hypoxia*. • Establish means of communication. Identify auras if possible.
Convulsive	• Maintain patent airway. • Support and protect head; turn to side if possible *to maintain airway*. • Prevent injury: Ease patient to floor if in chair. Place pillows along side rails if patient is in bed. Loosen constrictive clothing. • Provide privacy as necessary; stay with patient. • Note frequency, time, involved body parts, and length of seizure *to provide accurate description of seizure activity*.
Postconvulsive	• Maintain patent airway. • Suction as indicated. • Check vital signs and neurologic status. • Administer oxygen per protocol *to prevent hypoxia*. • Reorient patient to environment *to minimize sensory-perceptual alteration*. • Place patient in position of comfort, and turn head to side. • Administer oral hygiene as necessary *to remove secretions and bleeding*.
Impaired physical mobility	• See general intervention strategies listed on p. 1687. • Encourage mobility to tolerance, unless contraindicated by subarachnoid hemorrhage precautions. • Encourage self-care activities to tolerance unless contraindicated by subarachnoid hemorrhage precautions. • Plan all activities to avoid fatigue; maintain planned rest periods. • Obtain physical therapy referral.
Potential impaired skin integrity	• See general intervention strategies on p. 1646.
Altered patterns of urinary elimination	• See general intervention strategies on p. 1666.
Anxiety	• See general intervention strategies on p. 1743.
Impaired verbal communication	• Assess ability to communicate care and develop a means of communication with the patient: pencil, Magic Slate, or call light within easy reach. Reinforce the techniques established. • Assist patient and family to identify other outlets for communication. • Continue to use sense of touch and nonverbal forms of communication.

Patient Education[62]

1. Involve family in patient care, as possible; teach essential aspects of care.
2. Reinforce physician's explanation of medical management.
3. Stress importance of ongoing outpatient care and follow-up visits.
4. Stress need for regular exercise program:
   a. Teach ROM exercises to family.
   b. Instruct patient or family to perform ROM exercises to all body joints every 2 to 4 hours.
5. Encourage independent activities, as possible:
   a. Be alert to limitations.

   b. Avoid overprotection.
   c. Instruct regarding need for supportive devices as indicated (wheelchair, braces, walker, canes, overhead trapeze).
6. Stress importance of diet as ordered:
   a. Offer supplemental feedings.
   b. Offer small portions, and instruct patient to chew slowly.
   c. Arrange food and utensils within easy reach.
   d. Avoid foods such as soft breads, mashed potatoes, semicooked vegetables, and large pieces of meat that can cause choking.
7. Stress importance of safety measures:
   a. Side rails
   b. Ramps
   c. Shower chains
   d. Removal of scatter rugs
   e. Walker, canes, flat shoes
8. Instruct patient regarding name of medication, dosage, time of administration, and toxic or side effects.
9. Instruct patient regarding need to avoid over-the-counter medications without first consulting physician.
10. Encourage socialization with friends and family.
11. Stress importance of communication:
    a. Speak slowly and distinctly.
    b. Use one-word commands and short sentences. Repeat as needed.
    c. Use gestures and touch when giving directions. Maintain eye contact.
    d. Implement speech exercises twice a day.
12. Stress importance of verbalization of feelings about anxiety, fear, and body image changes.
13. Teach patient and family about seizures (i.e., safety measures and whom to contact).

Evaluation

Patient Outcome	Data Indicating That Outcome is Reached
Patient demonstrates a patent airway.	Breath sounds are normal or no increase in adventitious sounds. Chest excursion is bilateral and symmetric. Rate and depth of respirations are normal. Cough is effective. There are no subjective or objective findings of shortness of breath, air hunger, or dyspnea on exertion.
Patient demonstrates an effective breathing pattern.	Airway is patent. Chest excursion is symmetric. Breath sounds are normal, or there is no increase in adventitious sounds. Arterial blood gas values are within normal ranges or consistent with patient's baseline. Vital signs are within normal ranges or consistent with patient's baseline. Hemoglobin levels are 14 to 18 g/dl (male) and 12 to 16 g/dl (female). Intake and output are stable. There are no subjective or objective signs of respiratory distress. All lobes are resonant on percussion. Skin color is not cyanotic.
Patient maintains adequate cerebral tissue perfusion.	Level of consciousness is unchanged. There is no evidence of neurologic deficits. Pattern of electrolytes is stable. There is no seizure activity.
Patient demonstrates skin integrity.	Skin is intact. Nutritional status is adequate. Electrolyte balance is maintained. Patient remains free of pressure sores and contractures.
Patient demonstrates a low level of anxiety.	Patient openly verbalizes concerns and feelings of grief, loss, and discomfort. Patient openly verbalizes feelings, supported by health care professionals and family. Patient verbalizes essential aspects of care. Patient can identify methods to effectively deal with anxious feelings.
Patient demonstrates minimum impaired verbal communication.	Patient verbalizes feelings for as long as physically able to do so. Patient develops alternative methods of communication.
Patient demonstrates minimum complications of bowel incontinence.	Skin in perineal area is clean and dry. Dietary intake is adequate. Fluid intake is adequate (2000 ml/day unless contraindicated). Intake and output pattern is stable. Patient is free of fecal impaction. Patient demonstrates a regular bowel evacuation pattern.
Patient demonstrates minimum complications of sensory-perceptual alterations.	Level of orientation is optimum. Patient remains free of injury. Skin integrity is maintained. Nutritional status is adequate. Self-care deficits are minimum. Social participation is appropriate to physiologic status.
Patient remains free of traumatic injury.	Safety measures are appropriate to level of physiologic status. Skin integrity is maintained. Skin is free of bruises, burns, abrasions, and redness. Environment is safe. Patient is free of nosocomial infections.
Patient demonstrates optimum level of mobility.	Skin integrity is maintained. Patient remains free of contractures and deformities. Level of mobility is appropriate to physiologic status. Nutritional status is adequate. Intake and output pattern is stable. Patient remains free of thrombophlebitis. Patient remains free of local infection. Patient participates in an ongoing physical therapy program.

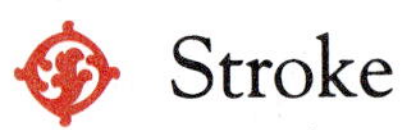

Stroke

(Cerebrovascular accident)

In stroke, or cerebrovascular accident (CVA), the cerebral vessels are occluded by an embolus or cerebrovascular hemorrhage, resulting in ischemia of the area of the brain normally perfused by the damaged vessels.[63]

The sequelae of a stroke depend on the extent and the location of the ischemia. Stroke is the third leading cause of death in the United States and accounts for approximately 200,000 deaths annually. Furthermore, stroke is the second leading cause of chronic disability and illness, with approximately 200,000 individuals experiencing some degree of disability from the residual effects. Statistics from 1980 indicate that stroke has an incidence of 196 per 100,000 general population. Persons 25 to 64 years of age are affected, but incidence increases rapidly from age 35 upward. The greatest increase in frequency occurs between 75 and 85 years of age.[31] Epidemiologic studies indicate variations in incidence in different geographic areas in the United States and in other parts of the world.

Certain risk factors may predispose an individual to a stroke; hypertension is the major risk factor. Risk factors showing some familial tendencies include diabetes mellitus, hypertension, cardiac disease, subclavian steal syndrome, and high serum cholesterol level. Obesity, sedentary life-style, cigarette smoking, stress, and high serum levels of cholesterol, lipoprotein, and triglycerides make the individual a high-risk candidate for stroke. In women the use of oral contraceptives and cigarette smoking increase the risk of stroke. Combinations of risk factors put the individual at a greater risk.[16]

Pathophysiology

The pathologic mechanisms of stroke are commonly listed as hemorrhagic, thrombotic, and embolic in the most recent vascular literature. Hemorrhage may be subarachnoid from rupture of the subarachnoid artery or intraparenchymal from rupture of an intraparenchymal artery. Embolic occlusion stems from tumors, valvular cardiac diseases, and, most commonly, plaques released from cerebral vessels that produce infarction. Thrombotic arterial occlusion produces various ischemic or hypoxic insults.[39]

Cerebral Hemorrhage

The pathogenesis of hypertensive cerebral hemorrhage is not completely understood. However, several facts are known: the hemorrhage usually occurs in relation to some mild exertion, and it occurs in individuals who have experienced significant increases in systolic-diastolic pressures for several years. Some researchers theorize that microaneurysms, known as *Charcot-Bouchard aneurysms*, in small arteries or arteriolar necrosis may precipitate the bleeding. The major sites of bleeding in hypertensive cerebral hemorrhage include the putamen (55%), cortex and subcortex (15%), thalamus (10%), pons (10%), and cerebellar hemisphere (10%).[50]

Hypertensive vascular disorders primarily affect the smaller arteries and arterioles, causing thickening of vessel walls, increase in cellularity of some vessels, and hyalinization, possibly with necrosis.[50]

Resolution of the hemorrhage occurs via resorption and begins when macrophages and reactive fibrillary astrocytes appear. After the tissue has been cleared of blood by the macrophages, there is a cavity surrounded by dense, fibrillary gliosis and hemosiderin-laden macrophages.[50]

Cerebral Infarction

Cerebral infarction occurs when a local area of brain tissue is deprived of blood supply because of vascular occlusion. Several hypotheses regarding the pathogenesis of cerebral infarcts include: abrupt vessel occlusion (e.g., embolus) that results in tissue infarction in the distribution supply of the occluded vessel; gradual vessel occlusion (e.g., atheroma), which may not result in an infarction if collateral blood supply is sufficient; and vessels that are stenosed but not completely occluded. This may precipitate an infarction if the collateral blood supply to the hypoxic area becomes comprised.[50]

Common causes of vascular occlusions are cerebral thrombi and cerebral emboli. Thrombi usually occur in larger vessels (e.g., internal carotid arteries) and are associated with localized damage to the vessel wall at the point of occlusion. Atherosclerosis and hypotension are important underlying processes, but other types of vascular injury (e.g., arteritis) can initiate thrombosis. Emboli usually affect smaller vessels and are commonly found at points of narrowed vessel lumen and bifurcation. The sources of cerebral emboli vary, but the most common is a mural thrombus in the left atrium or ventricle. Septic emboli may originate from bacterial endocarditis. Cerebral infarcts from embolic occlusions frequently are hemorrhagic, whereas thrombotic infarcts are bland or ischemic. Emboli occur most frequently in the middle cerebral artery.

A cerebral infarction may be ischemic or hemorrhagic. *Ischemic* infarctions usually are not demonstrable on gross examination for 6 to 12 hours. The initial change of the affected area is a slight discoloration and softening, with the gray matter taking on a muddy color and the white matter losing its normal fine-grained appearance.[50] After 48 to 72 hours, infarction, necrosis, circumlesional swelling, and mushy disintegration of the affected area are evident. Eventually there is liquefaction and formation of a cyst surrounded by a firm glial tissue.

Histologic changes after an infarction include cell body changes, interruption and disintegration of the myelin sheath and axis cylinder, and loss of oligodendroglia and astrocytes. Polymorphonuclear leukocytes begin to appear 48 hours after infarct. At 78 to 96 hours, macrophages appear about blood vessels.

Hemorrhagic infarctions usually occur in the cerebral cortex and result from a reflow of blood into the infarcted area. This reperfusion is caused by a fragmentation or lysis of the embolus or a reduction of vascular compression and reestablishment of blood flow.[50] Hemorrhagic infarcts therefore are ischemic in origin.

Diagnostic Studies and Findings

CT Scan

Infarct: appears initially (24 hours) as area of decreased density surrounded by area of intermediate density; shifts in midline structures and ventricular system
Older infarct: area of low density extending toward cortex or shift in ventricular system toward lesion

Magnetic Resonance Imaging (MRI)

Same as CT scan
Hemorrhage: rounded shape and uniformly high density

Lumbar Puncture

NOTE: Perform with caution in presence of intracranial hypertension
Increased pressure
Bloody spinal fluid

Electroencephalography

May show focal slowing around area of lesion

Brain Scan

Diminished perfusion
Detection of infarction, encapsulated hemorrhage, hematoma, and arteriovenous malformations

Cerebral Angiography

Shows occlusion or narrowing of large vessels, particularly carotid artery occlusions

B Mode Ultrasound

Outlines with ultrasound the flow of blood through large neck vessels

Skull Roentgenogram

Pineal body position
Intracranial calcifications

Echoencephalography

Shifts in midline structures
Displaced ventricles

Doppler Ultrasonography

Direction and velocity of blood flow through vessels

Medical Plan

Surgery

Carotid endarterectomy
Anastomosis of superior temporal artery and middle cerebral artery (STA-MCA anastomosis)
Intracranial pressure monitoring
Endotracheal intubation or tracheostomy
Evacuation of intracerebral clot or hematoma

Medications

Anticoagulants
- Warfarin sodium (Coumadin), loading doses: 40-60 mg (adult), 20-30 mg (elderly); maintenance dose: 5-10 mg

Antihypertensives
- Diazoxide (Hyperstat), 5 mg/kg IV

Diuretic
- Furosemide (Lasix), 40-80 mg IV, 30-60 min before each dose of diazoxide

Corticosteroids
- Dexamethasone (Decadron), 10 mg initially, then 4 mg q4-6h IV or IM

Anticonvulsants
- Phenytoin (Dilantin), 100-600 mg/d

Narcotic analgesic
- Codeine, 30-60 mg q3-4h

Analgesic/antipyretics
- Acetaminophen, gr X q4h po or rectal suppository

Antacids

General Management

Mechanical ventilation
Hypothermia blanket
ECG and cardiac monitoring
Subarachnoid precautions
Strict intake and output
Bed rest
Elevation of head of bed
Nasogastric tube
Foley or indwelling catheter
Elastic stockings
Serial arterial blood gases
Seizure precautions

NURSING CARE

Nursing Assessment

The following table summarizes assessment findings and diagnostic studies in seven types of strokes.

	Intracerebral Hemorrhage	Subarachnoid Hemorrhage	Subdural Hemorrhage
Onset	Rapid; minutes to 1-2h	Sudden; varied progression	Insidious; occasionally acute
Duration	Permanent if lesion is large; small lesions are potentially reversible	Variable; complete clearing may occur in days or weeks	Hours to months
Relation to activity	Usually occurs during activity	Most commonly related to head trauma	Usually related to head trauma
Contributing or associated factors	Hypertensive cardiovascular disease; coagulation defects	Intracerebral arterial aneurysm; trauma; vascular malformations	Chronic alcoholism
Sensorium	Coma common	Coma common	Generally clouded
Nuchal (neck) rigidity	Frequently present	Present	Rare
Location of cerebral deficit	Focal; arterial syndrome not common	Diffuse aneurysm may give focal sign before and after	Frontal lobe signs; ipsilateral pupil may dilate
Convulsions	Common	Common	Infrequent
Cerebrospinal fluid	Bloody unless hemorrhage entirely intracerebral	Grossly bloody; increased pressure	Normal to slightly elevated protein
Skull roentgenograms	Pineal shift, edema, hemorrhage, or hematoma	Normal or calcified aneurysm	Frequent contralateral shift of pineal gland

Nursing Dx & Intervention

Nursing Diagnosis	Nursing Intervention/Rationale
Ineffective airway clearance	• See general intervention strategies on p. 1702.
Ineffective breathing pattern	• See general intervention strategies on p. 1704.
Altered cerebral tissue perfusion	• Assess neurologic status every hour and as needed. • Monitor closely for signs of increased intracranial pressure. • Maintain patency and sterility of intracranial pressure monitoring device, if used: Use surgical asepsis for all dressing changes. Monitor intracranial pressure responses to care and treatments. • Administer medications per protocol: anticonvulsants, steroids, antibiotics, antifibrinolytics (monitor prothrombin time, partial thromboplastin time, and platelets), analgesics, and agents for control of vasospasms. • If steroids are being administered: Check stools *to detect occult blood.* Test urine for glucose and acetone *to detect glycosuria.* Administer phytonadine, MSD (Aquamephyton) intramuscularly daily or every other day *to control tendency for bleeding.* Administer antacids per protocol *to decrease or prevent gastric irritation.* • Elevate head of bed 30 to 40 degrees, unless contraindicated, *to facilitate cerebral venous drainage.*

Extradural Hemorrhage	Focal Cerebral Ischemia	Cerebral Thrombosis	Cerebral Embolism
Rapid; minutes to hours	Rapid; seconds to minutes	Minutes to hours	Sudden
Initially fluctuating; then steadily progressive	Seconds to minutes	Permanent if lesion is large; potentially reversible if lesion is small	Rapid improvement may occur depending on collateral flow
Almost always related to head trauma	Occurs during activity if related to decreased cardiac output	Usually occurs at rest	Unrelated to activity
Any condition that predisposes to trauma	Peripheral and coronary atherosclerosis; hypertension	Peripheral and coronary atherosclerosis; hypertension	Atrial fibrillation; aortic and mitral valve disease; myocardial infarct; atherosclerotic plaque
Rapidly advancing coma	Usually conscious	Usually conscious	Usually conscious
Rare	Absent	Absent	Absent
Temporal lobe signs; ipsilateral pupil may dilate; high intracranial pressure	Focal; or arterial syndrome	Focal; or arterial syndrome	Focal; or arterial syndrome
Common	Rare	Rare	Rare
Increased pressure; color and cells usually normal	Usually normal	Usually normal	Usually normal
Frequently fracture across middle meningeal artery groove	May show calcification of intracranial arteries	Possible arterial calcification and pineal shift from edema	Usually normal

Nursing Diagnosis	Nursing Intervention/Rationale
	• Maintain strict intake and output (1500 to 1800 ml/24 hours). Observe for signs of dehydration and overhydration. • Maintain balance between hyperthermia and hypothermia per protocol. • Institute subarachnoid precautions, if appropriate: Provide private room with controlled lighting (i.e., dim artificial lighting). Maintain complete bed rest *to keep physical activity and exertion to a minimum.* Provide *all* nursing care for the patient. Limit visitors to immediate family members only. Have patient wear elastic stockings at all times *to prevent venous stasis.* Maintain dietary restrictions (no stimulants such as coffee, tea, or soda). Administer stool softeners *to prevent straining during bowel movement.* Instruct patient on need to avoid coughing and sneezing *to prevent sudden increases in intracranial pressure.* Instruct patient not to watch television, listen to radio, or read.
Sensory/perceptual alterations (visual, auditory, kinesthetic, gustatory, tactile, olfactory)	• See general intervention strategies listed on p. 1728.

Nursing Diagnosis	Nursing Intervention/Rationale
Potential for trauma related to seizures	• Assess and document potential for injury and strategies instituted for prevention. • Maintain bed in low position at all times unless side rails are up or nurse is with patient. • Provide patient with a call light within easy reach. • Maintain side rails in up position at bedtime, after sedation, when patient is confused, and as needed. • Maintain wheelchairs and stretchers in locked position when transferring patient.
Preconvulsive	• Maintain seizure precautions: Have oral airway at bedside *to provide for adequate oxygenation.* Have suction equipment available at bedside *to prevent aspiration.* Pad side rails if indicated. Administer oxygen per protocol *to prevent cerebral hypoxia.* Establish means of communication; identify auras if possible.
Convulsive	• Maintain patent airway. • Support and protect head; turn to side if possible. • Prevent injury: Ease patient to floor if in chair. Place pillows along side rails if patient is in bed. Loosen constrictive clothing. • Provide privacy as necessary. Stay with patient. • Note frequency, time, involved body parts, and length of seizure.
Postconvulsive	• Maintain patent airway. • Suction as needed. • Check vital signs and neurologic status. • Administer oxygen per protocol. • Reorient patient to environment *to minimize sensory-perceptual alteration.* • Place patient in position of comfort, and turn head to side. • Administer oral hygiene as necessary *to remove secretions and bleeding.*
Impaired physical mobility	• Assess condition of skin and pressure point when providing skin care. • Administer skin care every 2 hours. Turn patient every 2 hours and as needed, unless contraindicated, *to prevent skin breakdown and to prevent respiratory complications.* Change position slowly *to prevent potential orthostatic hypotension.* Position in proper body alignment. Keep skin dry; administer perineal care as needed. Massage pressure points every 2 hours *to stimulate circulation;* give gentle back rubs every shift and as needed. Use air mattress *to prevent pressure points.* Use firm mattress *to provide support for the patient's back.* Perform active or passive ROM exercises every 2 to 4 hours *to prevent contractures.* • Perform dorsiflexion of quadriceps muscles and ankles every 2 to 4 hours unless contraindicated. • Assist patient out of bed to chair two or three times daily unless contraindicated. • Use footboard or Spence boots *to prevent footdrop.* • Apply elastic stockings *to prevent thrombus and embolus formation.* • Administer anticoagulation therapy per protocol: Monitor serum coagulation studies. Check stool for occult bleeding. Check urine for occult bleeding. Monitor for signs of thrombophlebitis and deep vein thrombosis including redness, tenderness, localized swelling, warmth, and upward red streaking on an extremity. • Monitor nutritional status. • Encourage mobility to tolerance unless contraindicated by subarachnoid hemorrhage precautions. • Encourage self-care activities to tolerance unless contraindicated by subarachnoid hemorrhage precautions. • Plan all activities and maintain planned rest periods *to avoid fatigue.* • Obtain physical therapy referral. • Encourage diversional activities if appropriate.
Feeding, bathing/hygiene, dressing/grooming, and toileting self-care deficit	• Assess degree of self-care deficit and institute the following: • Assist with feeding, if indicated; use IV or nasogastric feedings, as ordered. • Administer oral hygiene every 2 hours and as needed *to keep mucous membranes moist.* • Assist with daily hygiene care as indicated *to promote self-esteem.* • Administer eye care every 2 to 4 hours if indicated.

Nursing Diagnosis	Nursing Intervention/Rationale
	• Insert indwelling urinary catheter or perform intermittent urinary catheterizations per protocol. • Maintain bowel function with regular evacuation.
Potential impaired skin integrity	• See general intervention strategies on p. 1646.
Body image, self-esteem, and personal identity disturbances	• See general intervention strategies on pp. 1751, 1754, and 1756.
Altered patterns of urinary elimination	• See general intervention strategies on p. 1666.
Powerlessness	• Assist patient to reestablish as much physiologic control as possible. Share knowledge of physiologic functioning with patient and family. • Assist patient to reestablish some means of psychologic control: Encourage patient to express feelings. Encourage patient and family to participate in care. Encourage patient to become an active decision maker about care and immediate environment.
Impaired verbal communication	• Assess patient's ability to communicate. • Develop a means of communication with patient: pencil, Magic Slate, or call light within easy reach. Reinforce the techniques established. • Assist patient and family to identify other outlets for communication *to minimize frustration*. • Continue to use sense of touch and nonverbal forms of communication.

Patient Education

1. Involve the family in care, as possible. Teach essential aspects of care.
2. Reinforce the physician's explanation of medical management.
3. Stress importance of ongoing outpatient care and follow-up visits.
4. Stress need for regular exercise program:
   a. Teach ROM exercises to family.
   b. Perform ROM exercises to all body joints every 2 to 4 hours.
5. Encourage independent activities, as possible:
   a. Be alert to limitations.
   b. Avoid overprotection.
   c. Emphasize need for supportive devices as indicated (wheelchair, braces, walker, canes, overhead trapeze).
6. Stress importance of diet as ordered:
   a. Offer supplemental findings.
   b. Offer small portions, and instruct patient to chew slowly.
   c. Arrange food and utensils within easy reach.
   d. Avoid foods such as soft breads, mashed potatoes, semicooked vegetables, and large pieces of meat that can cause choking.
7. Stress importance of safety measures: side rails; ramps; shower chains; removal of scatter rugs; and walker, canes, and flat shoes.
8. Instruct regarding name of medication, dosage, time of administration, and toxic or side effects.
9. Stress need to avoid over-the-counter medications without first consulting physician.
10. Encourage socialization with friends and family.
11. Stress importance of communication:
    a. Speak slowly and distinctly.
    b. Use one-word commands and short sentences. Repeat as needed.
    c. Use gestures and touch when giving directions. Maintain eye contact.
    d. Implement speech exercises twice a day.
12. Stress importance of verbalization of feelings about anxiety, fear, and body image changes.
13. Teach the patient and family about seizures (i.e., safety measures and whom to contact).

Evaluation

Patient Outcome	Data Indicating That Outcome is Reached
Patient demonstrates a patent airway.	Breath sounds are normal, or there is no increase in adventitious breath sounds. Chest excursion is bilateral and symmetric. Rate and depth of respirations are normal. Cough is effective. There are no subjective or objective findings of shortness of breath, air hunger, or dyspnea on exertion.
Patient demonstrates an effective breathing pattern.	Airway is patent. Chest excursion is symmetric. Breath sounds are normal, or there is no increase in adventitious sounds. Arterial blood gas values are within normal ranges or consistent with patient's baseline. Vital signs are within normal ranges or consistent with patient's baseline. Hemoglobin levels are 14 to 18 g/dl (male) or 12 to 16 g/dl (female). Intake and output are stable and balanced. There are no signs of respiratory distress. All lobes are resonant on percussion. Skin color is not cyanotic.
Patient maintains adequate cerebral tissue perfusion.	Level of consciousness is maintained or improved. There is no evidence of neurologic deficits. Electrolyte pattern is stable. There is no seizure activity.
Patient demonstrates minimal complications of sensory-perceptual alterations.	Optimum level of orientation is maintained. Patient remains free of injury. Patient demonstrates skin integrity. Nutritional status is adequate. Self-care deficits are minimum. Social participation is appropriate to physiologic status.
Patient remains free of traumatic injury.	Safety measures are appropriate to physiologic status. Skin integrity is maintained. Skin is free of bruises, burns, abrasions, and redness. Environment is safe. Patient is free of nosocomial infections.
Patient demonstrates an optimum level of mobility.	Skin integrity is maintained. Patient remains free of contractures and deformities. Level of mobility is appropriate to physiologic status. Intake and output pattern is stable. Nutritional status is adequate. Patient remains free of thrombophlebitis. Patient remains free of local infections. Patient participates in an ongoing physical therapy program. Patient demonstrates minimum self-care deficits. Outcome criteria listed for impaired physical mobility are met. Level of self-care activities is appropriate to physiologic status. Patient participates in physical and occupational therapy.
Patient demonstrates skin integrity.	Skin is intact. Nutritional status is adequate. Electrolyte balance is maintained. Patient remains free of pressure sores and contractures.
Patient demonstrates minimum complications of bowel incontinence.	Skin in perineal area is clean and dry. Dietary intake is adequate. Fluid intake is adequate (2000 ml/day unless contraindicated). Intake and output pattern is stable. Patient remains free of fecal impaction. Patient demonstrates a regular bowel evacuation pattern.
Patient demonstrates intact self-concepts.	Patient openly verbalizes feelings of grief and loss. Patient verbalizes positive feelings about self. Patient acknowledges actual change in self-image. Patient focuses on present and future appearance and function. Patient verbalizes feelings of hopefulness, helpfulness, and powerfulness.
Patient demonstrates minimum feelings of powerlessness.	Optimum level of physiologic control, as possible for current health status, is maintained. Optimum level of psychologic control, as possible, is maintained. Patient participates, as possible, in decision making about care. Patient participates, as possible, in self-care.
Patient demonstrates minimum impaired verbal communication.	Patient verbalizes feelings for as long as physically able to do so. Patient develops alternative methods of communication.
Patient demonstrates minimum complications from alterations in urinary elimination patterns.	Intake and output pattern are stable. Urine is clear, yellow to amber in color, and without sediment. Skin in perineal area is clean and dry. Urine is acidic (pH 6). Patient remains free of urinary tract infections. Patient remains free of bladder distention. Patient can describe symptoms of urinary tract infections that require medical intervention.

TRAUMA

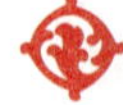

Craniocerebral trauma

Craniocerebral trauma is severe physical injury to the brain or structures within the cranium.

Trauma is the leading cause of death for individuals between 1 and 35 years of age. Craniocerebral trauma is a major factor in half the deaths resulting from physical injuries and is the second most common cause of neurologic deficits. In addition to the 77,000 individuals who die each year in the United States from traumatic brain injury, 50,000 to 60,000 individuals survive head injuries with varying levels of permanent deficit. Injury to the brain is the most serious complication of head trauma.

General effects of moderate to severe head injuries include

cerebral edema, sensorimotor deficits, and increased intracranial pressure. After the initial brain injury, secondary damage can result from brain herniation, cerebral ischemia, and hypoxemia. Leading causes of craniocerebral trauma include falls, industrial accidents, vehicular accidents (70% of victims sustain head injuries), assaults, sport accidents (e.g., football, boxing, diving), and intrauterine and birth injuries.

Pathophysiology

Craniocerebral injuries can result from primary or secondary trauma to the head. Primary trauma occurs when traumatic forces directly impact the head, setting into action the mechanisms of injury. The mechanisms of primary trauma that produce actual brain deformation include acceleration-deceleration with cavitation, as well as rotation of the skull and its cranial contents. These forces can occur simultaneously or in succession and damage the brain by compression, shearing, or tension. Acceleration injuries result when the head is struck by a moving object and set in motion. The slower-moving brain tissue is damaged by sudden contact with the edges of the dural membrane or the bony prominences of the skull. As a result of acceleration forces, there may be bruising or contusion of the undersurfaces of the occipital lobes, the brainstem, the superior surface of the cerebellum at the edge of the tentorium, or the tips of the frontal and temporal lobes. Another factor in the acceleration mechanism is the effect of positive and negative pressure waves traversing the skull. At the point of impact, a high-pressure wave (positive) occurs, while a low-pressure wave (negative) occurs opposite the site of impact. If the negative pressure reaches vapor pressure, theoretically it may produce cavitation and a contrecoup injury (injury in area opposite the site of impact).

Deceleration occurs when the moving head strikes a solid, immovable object (as when the head hits a windshield). There is rapid deceleration of the skull, but the brain decelerates more slowly (20 msec), and the brain tissue may travel 2 to 3 cm in that time period.

Acceleration-deceleration movements from lateral flexion, hyperflexion, hyperextension, and turning movements during the injury cause the cerebrum to rotate about the brainstem and produce shearing, straining, and distortion of neural tissue. Microscopically, the stretching or tension causes fracture of axons in the longitudinal bundles of the cerebrum and the long axons in the brainstem. This rotational mechanism is a major cause of contrecoup lesions and may account for most of the contusions to the brain tissue. Areas most frequently injured during rotation are the frontal and temporal lobes.

Primary trauma to the head may be followed by secondary injury that increases the morbidity and mortality of head-injured patients. Secondary trauma to the head may result when tension strains and shearing forces are transmitted to the cranium by extreme torsion and stretching of the neck, as in a hard fall on the buttocks. Other factors such as sustained intracranial hypertension, sustained cerebral edema, hypercapnia, hypoxemia, systemic hypotension, infections, and respiratory trauma and its complications may contribute to secondary injury to the brain.

Head injuries can be classified as open or closed. *Open* head injuries result from skull fractures or penetrating wounds. The velocity, mass, shape, and direction of impact are the major determinants of brain injury. With an open head injury there is some type of skull fracture, such as linear, comminuted, depressed, or perforated.

A linear fracture is a simple break in bone continuity that produces an inbending of the bone at the point of impact and an outbending of the skull in the surrounding area. A comminuted skull fracture occurs when two or more communicating breaks divide the bone into two or more fragments. Depressed fractures result when the bone is forced below the line of normal contour from impact with a moving object. Compound fractures may be linear, comminuted, or depressed.

Another and serious type of skull fracture is the basal fracture, which can be linear, comminuted, or depressed. Structures most commonly damaged with this type of fracture include the internal carotid artery and cranial nerves I, II, VII, and VIII. Basal skull fractures usually traverse the paranasal sinuses (frontal, maxillary, or ethmoid). The fragility of the bones and the close adherence of the dura account for the frequency of this type of fracture and the subsequent leakage of cerebrospinal fluid through the dural tear.[31]

With open head injuries there can be high- or low-velocity impacts. The higher the velocity of impact, the greater the explosive effect within the cranium. For example, in high-velocity impacts, such as with gunshot wounds, there is laceration at the entry site, cerebral edema, hemorrhage into the destroyed area, and remote contusions (secondary to tissue displacement).[59] Lower-velocity impacts usually result in distortion and linear fractures of the skull.

A *closed*, blunt head injury can produce the pathologic signs of cerebral concussion, contusion, or laceration. A *concussion* is a transient neurologic dysfunction of paralysis and is the least serious type of brain injury. With a concussion there may be immediate and transitory disturbances in equilibrium, consciousness, and vision. *Contusions* result in bruising of brain tissue, usually accompanied by hemorrhages of surface vessels. *Lacerations* are the actual tearing of the cortical surface. Contusions and lacerations result in microscopic hemorrhages around blood vessels with destruction of surrounding brain tissue.

A contusion or laceration directly beneath the site of impact is a *coup* lesion; those occurring opposite the site of impact are *contrecoup* lesions. The two major factors that determine the distribution of coup and contrecoup lesions are the ability of cerebrospinal fluid to act as a shock absorber and shifts of the intracranial contents. With a coup lesion the impact causes greater displacement of the skull than the brain. At the site of impact the cerebrospinal fluid is squeezed out from between the brain and skull, and the skull hits the brain at the point of impact.[39] Contrecoup lesions occur because of dissipation of the cerebrospinal fluid between the trailing edge of the brain and the trailing surface of the skull and because of a compensatory increase in the volume of cerebrospinal fluid between the leading edge of the brain and the leading surface of the skull.[39] The coup or contrecoup lesion may be accompanied by cavitation, which is the release of dissolved gases from cerebrospinal fluid, blood, or brain tissue. The release of these gases produces microscopic bubbles that extensively disrupt neural tissue, primarily in cerebrospinal pathways and near blood vessels.

Secondary responses to craniocerebral trauma may include the formation of an epidural, subdural, or intracerebral hematoma, a subarachnoid hemorrhage, cerebral edema, and brain herniation. An *epidural* hematoma usually occurs when there is a linear fracture of one of the skull's membranous bones, such as the temporal area near the meningeal artery and vein. After rupture the arterial blood forms a convex mass that indents the brain. If the hemorrhage continues, the hematoma may break periosteal attachments and the dural collagen.

A *subdural* hematoma may result from cerebral hemorrhage in the temporal, frontal, or midline region or in any region where there is a laceration of brain tissue or its parenchymal vessels. Because the subdural hematoma is venous, symptoms appear much later than with the arterial epidural hematoma and therefore can be classified as acute, subacute, or chronic. *Acute* subdural hematomas usually manifest symptoms within 24 to 48 hours after severe trauma. Symptoms of *subacute* subdural hematoma may develop anywhere from 48 hours to 2 weeks after severe head injury. *Chronic* subdural hematomas develop weeks, months, and possibly years after an apparently minor head injury. The chronic type of subdural hematoma is most common for those individuals in the 60- to 70-year age group because atrophy of the brain permits more room for expansion.

An *intracerebral hematoma* is a collection of blood within the actual brain tissue that usually occurs in the temporal or frontal region. Extensive removal of the hematoma and surrounding necrotic brain tissue generally is necessary to prevent further brain injury.

Subarachnoid hemorrhage is a frequent complication of head trauma. The pathologic processes of subarachnoid hemorrhage are presented in the discussion of vascular lesions.

Cerebral edema after craniocerebral trauma can occur locally around the injury and throughout the brain. Cerebral edema that develops after a traumatic head injury is not a single clinical or pathologic entity but exists in three forms: vasogenic, cytotoxic, and ischemic.[39] Vasogenic edema results from an increase in capillary permeability, which then permits transudation of plasma out of the cerebral vessels and into the compliant brain tissue. Cytotoxic edema occurs with impairment or failure of the cation pump, allowing infiltration of water and sodium into the intracellular space. Ischemic edema encompasses both previous types. Mechanisms of ischemic cerebral edema are initiated by the infiltration of water and sodium into the intracellular space (cytotoxic edema). This intracellular edema then affects the tight junction of the endothelial cell, with resultant infiltration of plasma across the damaged capillaries into the extracellular space (vasogenic edema).[39]

The mechanisms of traumatic cerebral edema are significant factors affecting both an individual's physiologic responses and survival after a severe head injury. If untreated or uncontrolled, cerebral edema produces a cycle of intracranial hypertension, reduced cerebral perfusion, and increased cerebral hypoxia. These mechanisms then produce more cerebral edema, and results are often fatal.[23]

The peak of cerebral edema is usually around 72 hours after the traumatic injury. Responses to the cerebral edema include increased intracranial pressure and the cerebral herniation syndromes.

Brain herniation is a secondary complication that can develop as a result of a primary head injury. The main types of brain herniation syndromes are uncal, transtentorial, and cerebellar. *Uncal* (lateral transtentorial) herniation involves displacement of the medial portion of the temporal lobe across the tentorium into the posterior fossa, compressing the midbrain and brainstem. *Transtentorial* (central) herniation involves downward displacement of the cerebral ventricles through the diencephalon against the midbrain. *Cerebellar* herniation results when the cerebellar tonsils move downward through the foramen magnum and compress the medulla.

Diagnostic Studies and Findings

Skull Roentgenograms

Detection of calvaria fractures (simple, compound, depressed, or comminuted)
Visualization of bone fragments

Cervical Roentgenogram

To confirm or rule out cervical spinal injury (assume neck injury until proven negative)

Chest Roentgenogram

Indicates presence of aspiration, chest injuries, and atelectasis
Indicates placement of endotracheal tube

CT Scan

May indicate subdural hematoma, intracerebral hematoma, or shift and distortion of cerebral ventricles

Magnetic Resonance Imaging (MRI)

Same as CT scan

CSF Sampling

May be contraindicated with increased intracranial pressure
Normal in cerebral edema and brain concussion
Increased pressure and blood with laceration and contusion

Cerebral Angiography

May indicate intracerebral or subdural hematoma by showing avascular areas with displacement of surrounding vessels

Pneumoencephalogram

Demonstration of cerebral ventricular shift, distortion, or dilation

Electroencephalogram (EEG) (Done Serially)

Appearance or development of pathologic waves
Determination of brain death

Cisternogram

Identification of dural tear site with basal skull fracture

Echoencephalogram

Detects shifts in midline structures

Serum Osmolarity

Hyperosmolar state (i.e., diabetes insipidus and syndrome of inappropriate secretion of antidiuretic hormone [SIADH])
Hypo-osmolar state

Serum Electrolytes

Natriuresis
Hypernatremia
Elevated plasma cortisol
Increased serum lactic dehydrogenase

Urine Osmolarity

Dilute urine

Arterial Blood Gases

Hypoxemia
Hypercapnia

Medical Plan

Surgery

Suturing of head and scalp lacerations
Debridement of wounds
Ventricular catheter, subarachnoid bolt, and epidural sensor
Ventriculostomy
Cranioplasty
Shunting procedures for hydrocephalus
Craniectomy
Craniotomy
Tracheostomy
Skull trephine (burr holes)

Medications

Diuretics
- Mannitol 20% (osmotic diuretic), 0.25 mg/kg IV q4-6h
- Furosemide (Lasix) (Loop diuretic), 20-40 mg IV q6-8h

Anticonvulsants
- Phenytoin sodium (Dilantin), 18 mg/kg; then maintenance dose of 5 mg/kg/d
- Phenobarbital sodium, 30-120 mg/d in 2 or 3 individual doses
- Carbamazepine (Tegretol), 200 mg bid initially; gradually increased up to 800-1200 mg/d in divided doses

Corticosteroids (to control cerebral edema)
- Dexamethasone (Decadron), 4-10 mg IV q6h

Histamine antagonist
- Cimetidine (Tagamet), 300 mg IV q6h

Analgesic/antipyretics
- NOTE: Avoid morphine sulfate because of medullary depressant effects
- Acetaminophen, 325-650 mg po or rectal suppository q4h prn

Antacids
- Maalox, 30 ml po or nasogastric q2h

Artificial tears, prn

Stool softeners
- Colace, 100 mg po tid

Muscle relaxants and paralyzers
- Pancuronium (Pavulon), 1-4 mg IV q4h
- Pentobarbital (Nembutal) for barbiturate coma; loading dose 3-5 mg/kg IV by slow push; maintenance dose 1-3 mg/kg IV by continuous infusion

Antibiotics
- Broad-spectrum agents used to prevent or control infections

General Management

Controlled mechanical ventilation
Hyperventilation to control intracranial hypertension
Cervical collars
Central venous pressure line
Arterial pressure line
Intracranial pressure monitoring
Hypothermia-hyperthermia balance
Incentive spirometry
Cardiac monitoring
Salem sump, nasogastric tube
Swan-Ganz catheterization
Glasgow Coma Scale
Endotracheal intubation
Nutritional support (i.e., enteral feedings, intravenous hyperalimentation)
Physical therapy program
Warm or cold compresses for periorbital edema and ecchymosis
Indwelling urinary catheter

Speech therapy, if indicated
Psychosocial counseling
Seizure precautions

NURSING CARE

Nursing Assessment

Cranial Nerve Palsies

- Bilateral anosmia
- Agnosia (less common)
- Paralysis of ocular movements: diplopia, nystagmus
- Partial or complete blindness
- Vertigo
- Deafness
- Numbness, paresthesias, or neuralgia of areas supplied by trigeminal nerve
- Strabismus

Level of Consciousness

- Mental changes
  - Irritability
  - Restlessness
  - Confusion
  - Delirium
  - Stupor
  - Coma
- Posttraumatic amnesia (loss of day-to-day memory after the injury)
- Retrograde amnesia (loss of memory regarding events immediately preceding the injury)

Pain

- Headache

Motor Function

- Concussion
  - Transitory extensor spasms
- Contusion
  - Weakness
  - Paresis
  - Paralysis
  - Decorticate (flexor) posturing: upper extremity flexion, lower extremity extension
  - Decerebrate (extension) posturing: extension and internal rotation of upper extremities, extension of lower extremities
  - Areflexia

Meningeal Irritability

- Nuchal rigidity
- Positive Kernig's sign
- Positive Brudzinski's sign

Skull Fracture

- Linear
  - No bone displacement
  - Possible epidural hematoma
- Depressed
  - Focal neurologic deficits
  - Cranial nerve injuries
- Basilar
  - Conjunctival hemorrhage
  - CSF rhinorrhea (drainage from nose)
  - Bilateral periorbital ecchymosis (raccoon eyes)
  - CSF otorrhea (drainage from ear)
  - Mastoid bone ecchymosis (Battle's sign)
  - Hearing impairments
  - Positive halo sign (drainage of blood encircled by CSF)

Cerebral Edema/Increased Intracranial Pressure

- Changes in level of consciousness
- Slow, labored respirations
- Changes in arterial blood pressure and pulse pressure (later sign)
- Bradycardia
- Anorexia
- Pupillary dysfunction
- Papilledema (late sign)
- Changes in motor function (i.e., posturing)
- Nausea and vomiting (may be projectile)
- Positive Babinski's sign (usually contralateral to lesion)
- Visual abnormalities (i.e., diplopia, visual blurring, decreased visual acuity)
- Monoparesis or hemiparesis (usually contralateral)

Brain Herniation

- Uncal
  - Decreased level of consciousness with almost simultaneous rapid motor function changes (decerebrate or decorticate posturing) and rapid changes in pupillary equality
  - Respiratory acidosis or alkalosis
  - Loss of oculocephalic reflex
- Transtentorial
  - Decreased level of consciousness
  - Nuchal rigidity
  - Headache
  - Unilateral or bilateral pupil dilation
  - Elevated blood pressure
  - Bradycardia
  - Cheyne-Stokes respiration
  - Cardiac arrhythmias
  - Decerebrate or decorticate posturing
- Cerebellar
  - Pupils constricted and nonreactive
  - Decreased level of consciousness
  - Apnea or ataxic respiration

Hemorrhage

Epidural hematoma
- Transient loss of consciousness
- Increasing intracranial pressure (rapid development)
- Ipsilateral dilated pupil

Subdural hematoma
- Increasing lethargy
- Headache
- Increasing intracranial pressure
- Seizures
- Minimal dilation of unilateral pupil

Intracerebral hematoma
- Increasing intracranial pressure
- Sensory and motor deficits

Reflexes

Pupils dilated
Loss of cutaneous and tendon reflexes (concussion)
Babinski's reflex positive (with increased intracranial pressure)

Vital Signs

Decreased blood pressure
Pulse slow (associated with intracranial hypertension) or rapid and feeble (associated with hemorrhage)
Respirations shallow or temporary cessation (concussion)
Hyperventilation
Cheyne-Stokes, apneustic, ataxic, or cluster respirations (dependent on level of function)
Hyperthermia associated with hypothalamic injury
Widening pulse pressure with hypertension and bradycardia (Cushing's syndrome) associated with intracranial hypertension and cerebral ischemia

Other

Punch-drunk encephalopathy: memory impairment, dysarthria, ataxias, tremors, parkinsonian manifestations
Postconcussion syndrome: headache, insomnia, nervousness, fatigability, giddiness
Dehydration
Polyuria
Shock

Extracranial Complications

Cervical fracture not diagnosed
Chest injuries
Fat emboli
Gastrointestinal hemorrhage
Hypoxia
Hypercapnia
Anemia
Hypotension

Nursing Dx & Intervention

Nursing Diagnosis	Nursing Intervention/Rationale
Ineffective airway clearance	• Assess patient's ability to clear secretions. • Maintain patent airway; avoid flexion of the neck until cervical films rule out neck injury. • Auscultate for breath sounds every 1 to 2 hours and as needed. Suction as needed *to remove secretions and blood.* • Monitor vital signs every 1 to 2 hours; monitor neurologic status every 15 to 30 minutes until stable, then every 1 to 2 hours. • Keep emergency drugs and ventilator at bedside. • Maintain nothing-by-mouth status, if indicated, *to prevent risk of choking or aspiration.* • Maintain neck in neutral position.
Ineffective breathing pattern	• Auscultate breath sounds every 1 to 2 hours; note quality and any increase in adventitious sounds. Suction as needed. Hyperinflate lungs with 100% oxygen for 1 minute before and 1 minute after suctioning, unless contraindicated. Limit suctioning to less than 15 seconds *to prevent suction-induced hypoxemia.* • Maintain patent airway. Intubation/tracheostomy and mechanical ventilation may be indicated. • Monitor mechanical ventilator, if used: Ensure that tidal volume, rate, mode, and oxygen concentration are set as ordered. Ensure that ventilator alarms are on and functional. • Monitor arterial blood gases per protocol: Report decrease in P_{O_2} of 10 to 15 mm Hg. Report increase in P_{CO_2} greater than 10 to 15 mm Hg. • Check blood pressure, respirations, and pulse rate every 1 to 2 hours and as needed based on patient's condition. • Administer muscle relaxants per protocol.
Altered cerebral tissue perfusion	• Establish baseline and ongoing neurologic assessment every 15 to 30 minutes and as needed as indicated by patient's condition. • Intervene *to monitor or prevent increased intracranial pressure:* Administer medications, treatments, and IV lines as per protocol.

Nursing Diagnosis	Nursing Intervention/Rationale
	• If steroids are being administered: Check stools *to detect occult blood.* Test urine for sugar and acetone *to detect glycosuria.* Administer phytonadine, MSD (Aquamephyton) intramuscularly daily or every other day *to control tendency for bleeding.* Administer antacids per protocol *to decrease or prevent gastric irritation.* • Maintain elevation of head of bed as per protocol *to facilitate cerebral venous drainage.* • Accurately record intake and output; monitor for imbalance. • Test urine pH every two hours *to detect onset of diabetes insipidus.* • Post fluid restriction chart that clearly indicates amount of fluid permitted for a 24-hour period and how restriction is allocated for each work shift. • Monitor serum electrolytes, blood count, and arterial blood gases for abnormalities. • Monitor values and waveforms of intracranial pressure line if appropriate: Maintain patency and sterility of the system. Monitor effects of treatments on intracranial pressure. Correlate neurologic status with intracranial pressure values; notify physician if inconsistent. Assist with drainage of cerebrospinal fluid from the system *to control intracranial hypertension.* Prevent initiation of Valsalva maneuver *to prevent increase in intrathoracic pressure.* • Intervene to monitor or prevent seizures: Monitor serum levels of anticonvulsant agents. Administer anticonvulsant agents per protocol. Monitor effects and side effects. Maintain seizure precautions.
Sensory/perceptual alterations (visual, auditory, gustatory, kinesthetic, tactile, olfactory)	• Assess patient's level of consciousness and degree of orientation. • Keep side rails up at all times when patient is alone. • Maintain patient safety at all times. • Avoid sedative agents, if possible. • Maintain quiet environment, reducing external stimuli to a minimum. • Reorient patient frequently to time, place, and person. Introduce yourself each time you reorient the patient. • Repeat explanations frequently and simply. • Have family bring in familiar objects. • Maintain planned rest periods, allowing sufficient time for REM sleep. • Use day and night lighting appropriately. • Stimulate senses of touch, taste, and position. • Support family members to understand what is happening as a result of perceptual alterations.
Potential for trauma related to seizures	• Assess and document potential for injury and strategies for prevention. • Maintain bed in low position at all times unless side rails are up or nurse is with patient. • Provide patient with a call light within easy reach. • Maintain side rails in up position at bedtime, after sedation, when patient is confused, and as needed. • Maintain wheelchairs and stretchers in locked position when transferring patient.
Preconvulsive	• Maintain seizure precautions: Have oral airway at bedside *to provide for adequate oxygenation.* Have suction equipment available at bedside *to prevent aspiration.* Pad side rails if indicated. Administer oxygen per protocol *to prevent cerebral hypoxia.* Establish means of communication; identify auras if possible.
Convulsive	• Maintain patent airway. • Support and protect head; turn to side if possible. • Prevent injury: Ease patient to floor if in chair. Place pillows along side rails if patient is in bed. Remove surrounding furniture. Loosen constrictive clothing. • Provide privacy as necessary; stay with patient • Note frequency, time, involved body parts, and length of seizure.
Postconvulsive	• Maintain patent airway. • Suction as needed, as indicated. • Check vital signs and neurologic status. • Administer oxygen as per protocol.

Nursing Diagnosis	Nursing Intervention/Rationale
	• Reorient the patient to environment. • Provide emotional support. • Place patient in position of comfort; turn head to side. • Administer oral hygiene as necessary for secretions and bleeding.
Impaired physical mobility	• Assess skin condition and pressure points when administering skin care. • Administer skin care every 1 to 2 hours: Turn patient every 2 hours and as needed, unless contraindicated. Change position slowly *to prevent orthostatic hypotension.* Position in proper body alignment; may need to use log-roll technique when turning. Massage pressure points every 2 hours *to stimulate circulation;* give gentle back rubs every shift and as needed. • Use firm mattress or bed board *to support back and spine.* • Use footboard or Spence boots *to prevent footdrop.* Instruct patient not to push against footboard *to prevent Valsalva maneuver.* • Apply antiembolus stockings or sequential compression devices to lower extremities *to promote venous return.* • Administer anticoagulation therapy per protocol *to prevent thrombus or embolus formation:* Monitor serum coagulation studies. Check stool *to detect occult bleeding.* Check urine *to detect occult bleeding.* Monitor for signs of thrombophlebitis and deep vein thrombosis including redness, tenderness, localized swelling, warmth, and upward red streaking on an extremity. • Monitor nutritional status. • Encourage mobility to tolerance or per protocol. • Avoid isometric exercises. • Encourage self-care activities to tolerance. • Plan all activities to avoid fatigue; maintain planned rest periods. • Obtain physical therapy referral.
Feeding, bathing/hygiene, dressing/grooming, and toileting self-care deficit	• Assess degree of deficit and institute necessary interventions. • Assist with feeding as indicated. • Use IV or nasogastric feedings per protocol. • Administer oral hygiene every 2 hours and as needed. • Assist with daily hygiene care as indicated. • Administer eye care every 2 to 4 hours if indicated *to prevent drying of corneas.* • Maintain bowel function with regular evacuation.
Potential impaired skin integrity	• See general intervention strategies on p. 1646.
Pain	• See general intervention strategies on p. 1720.
Body image, self-esteem, and personal identity disturbances	• Assess and document patient's degree of concern and confusion. • Provide for a safe, comfortable, secure environment. • Reorient the patient to time, person, and place, as appropriate. • Carefully explain what you are doing and why you are doing it. • Answer questions simply and honestly. • Correct misinformation. • Protect patient's privacy.
Anxiety	• See general intervention strategies listed on p. 1743. • Assist patient to reestablish as much physiologic control as condition allows. • Share knowledge of physiologic functioning with the patient and family. • Assist patient to reestablish some means of psychologic control. • Encourage patient to express feelings. • Encourage patient and family to participate in care. • Encourage patient to become an active decision maker about care and immediate environment.
Impaired verbal communication	• Assess patient's ability to communicate. • Develop a means of communication with the patient: pencil, Magic Slate, or call light within easy reach. • Reinforce the techniques established. • Assist patient and family to identify other outlets for communication. • Continue to use sense of touch and nonverbal forms of communication.

Patient Education

1. Involve family in care, as possible; teach essential aspects of care.
2. Reinforce physician's explanation of medical management.
3. Stress importance of ongoing outpatient care and follow-up visits.
4. Encourage independent activities, as possible:
   a. Alert to limitations
   b. Avoid overprotection.
   c. Stress need for supportive devices as indicated.
5. Emphasize need for regular exercise program. Teach ROM exercises to family.
6. Stress importance of diet as ordered:
   a. Offer supplemental feedings.
   b. Offer small portions; instruct patient to chew slowly.
7. Stress importance of safety measures: side rails; ramps; shower chairs; walker, canes.
8. Instruct patient regarding name of medication, dosage, time of administration, and toxic or side effects.
9. Stress need to avoid over-the-counter medications without first consulting physician.
10. Encourage socialization with friends and family.
11. Emphasize importance of verbalization of feelings about anxiety, fear, and body image changes.
12. Teach patient and family about seizures (i.e., safety measures and whom to contact).

Evaluation

Patient Outcome	Data Indicating That Outcome is Reached
Patient demonstrates a patent airway.	Breath sounds are normal. Chest excursion is bilateral and symmetric. Rate and depth of respirations are normal. Cough is effective. There are no subjective or objective findings of shortness of breath, air hunger, or dyspnea on exertion.
Patient demonstrates an effective breathing pattern.	Airway is patent. Chest excursion is symmetric. Breath sounds are normal, or there is no increase in adventitious sounds. Arterial blood gas values are within normal ranges or consistent with patient's baseline. Vital signs are within normal ranges or consistent with patient's baseline. Hemoglobin levels are 14 to 18 g/dl (male) or 12 to 16 g/dl (female). Intake and output are stable. There are no signs of respiratory distress. All lobes are resonant on percussion. Skin color is not cyanotic.
Patient maintains adequate cerebral and spinal tissue perfusion.	Level of consciousness is unchanged. There is no evidence of neurologic deficits. Electrolyte pattern is stable. There is no seizure activity.
Patient demonstrates minimum complications of sensory-perceptual alterations.	Optimum level of orientation is maintained. Patient remains free of injury. Patient demonstrates skin integrity. Nutritional status is adequate. Self-care deficits are minimum. Social participation is appropriate to physiologic status.
Patient remains free of traumatic injury.	Safety measures are appropriate to level of physiologic status. Skin integrity is maintained. Skin is free of bruises, burns, abrasions, and redness. Environment is safe. Patient is free of nosocomial infections.
Patient demonstrates on optimum level of mobility.	Patient exhibits skin integrity. Patient remains free of contractures and deformities. Level of mobility is appropriate to physiologic status. Intake and output pattern is stable. Nutritional status is adequate. Patient remains free of thrombophlebitis. Patient remains free of local infection. Patient participates in an ongoing physical therapy program.
Patient demonstrates minimum self-care deficits.	Outcome criteria listed for impaired physical mobility are met. Level of self-care activities is appropriate to physiologic status. Patient participates in physical and occupational therapy.
Patient demonstrates skin integrity.	Skin is intact. Nutritional status is adequate. Electrolyte balance is maintained. Patient remains free of pressure sores and contractures.
Patient experiences minimum alterations in comfort.	Patient openly verbalizes feelings of discomfort when they occur. Patient can use measures to decrease discomfort. Patient verbally validates a decrease in subjective feelings of discomfort. Objective findings of pain are decreased.
Patient demonstrates intact self-concepts.	Patient openly verbalizes feelings of grief and loss. Patient verbalizes positive feelings about self. Patient acknowledges actual change in self-image. Patient focuses on present and future appearance and function. Patient verbalizes feelings of hopefulness, helpfulness, and powerfulness.
Patient demonstrates a low level of anxiety.	Patient openly verbalizes concerns and feelings of grief, loss, and discomfort. Patient openly verbalizes feelings supported by health care professionals and family. Patient verbalizes essential aspects of care. Patient identifies methods to effectively deal with anxious feelings.

Patient Outcome	Data Indicating That Outcome is Reached
Patient demonstrates minimum feelings of powerlessness.	Patient maintains an optimum level of physiologic control, as possible for current health status. Patient maintains an optimum level of psychologic control, as possible. Patient participates, as possible, in decision making about care. Patient participates, as possible, in self-care.
Patient demonstrates minimum impaired verbal communication.	Patient verbalizes feelings for as long as physically able to do so. Patient develops alternate methods of communication.

Spinal cord trauma

Spinal cord trauma is physical injury to the spinal cord caused by violent or disruptive action.

Injuries to the spinal cord constitute approximately 10% of traumatic injuries to the nervous system. Approximately 10,000 spinal cord injuries occur each year in the United States, and spinal cord trauma from vehicular accidents accounts for one half to two thirds of the total incidence. Approximately one third of the individuals with spinal cord injuries die before reaching an acute care facility. About 80% of individuals sustaining a spinal cord injury are between the ages of 18 and 25 years, and most are male. Causes of spinal cord trauma include assaults (e.g., bullet wounds), falls, sport injuries (e.g., diving accidents), industrial accidents, birth injuries, degenerative changes (e.g., vertebral disk deterioration), and vehicular accidents. At present over 100,000 individuals in the United States are paralyzed as a result of spinal cord trauma.

The most common sites of injury are the lower cervical region (C4-7 and T1) and the thoracolumbar junction (T12, L1, and L2). Trauma to the spinal cord causes concussion, contusion, laceration, hemorrhage, transection (partial or complete), or impairment in the spinal vascular supply.

Pathophysiology

As with craniocerebral trauma, the spine (and spinal cord) can be injured by direct or indirect forces. Direct injuries such as falls on the head or buttocks can cause spinal cord lesions from fractured vertebrae or direct compression of the cord by depressed bone fragments. Indirect injuries (the major type of spinal cord injuries) can occur when excessive forces accelerate the cranium in relation to the trunk (i.e., whiplash injury) or when the trunk is suddenly decelerated in regard to the lumbar spine. Whether the forces are direct or indirect, the subsequent fractures of vertebrae seriously injure the neural elements of the spinal cord.

Vertebral Injuries

The primary mechanisms of vertebral injury, occurring alone or in combination, include hyperextension, hyperflexion, vertical compression trauma, and rotation.[31]

Hyperextension injuries (commonly termed *whiplash*) are common in the cervical region, and damage results from the forces of acceleration-deceleration and the sudden reduction in the anterior-posterior diameter of the spinal canal. Since the spinal canal is full of neural tissue in the cervical area, injury can produce profound disability. With a hyperextension injury the cord can be compressed between the body of one vertebra and the leading edge of the laminal arch of adjacent vertebrae, causing complete or partial transection. In addition, the ligamentum flavum may be torn or bulge inward, and intervertebral disks may tear. Severe hyperextension injuries can produce complete transverse fracture of the vertebral body. With the compression and shearing forces of a hyperextension injury, gray matter of the cord is destroyed and microcirculation at and around the level of the injury is disrupted.

Hyperflexion injury results in an overstretching, compression, and deformation of the spinal cord from a sudden and excessive force that propels the neck forward or an exaggerated lateral movement of the neck to one side or another. Hyperflexion injuries can occur with wedge or compression fractures of the vertebral body with or without dislocation, fracture of the pedicle with or without dislocation of intraspinal ligaments, or fracture of the vertebral body and rupture of the intervertebral discs.

Vertical compression trauma primarily occurs around the area of the thoracolumbar junction (T12 to L2) and results from a force applied along an axis from the top of the cranium through the vertebral bodies. With compression injuries the vertebral body bursts, compressing the spinal cord and damaging nerve roots with bony fragments.

Rotation can involve all portions of the vertebral body including pedicles, ligaments, and the articulation. Fracture of the pedicles or locked facets of the vertebrae can rupture ligaments and shear spinal cord tissue.

Vertebral injuries can be classified as simple fractures, compressed or wedged fractures, comminuted fractures, and vertebral dislocation.[31] A *simple* fracture is a single break usually affecting transverse or spinous processes. Vertebral alignment usually remains intact, and compression of the spinal cord is not usually present.

Compressed, or *wedged,* vertebral fractures occur when the vertebral body is compressed anteriorly. Spinal cord compression may or may not be present with a wedged fracture.

Comminuted, or *burst,* fractures can cause serious injury to the spinal cord. The vertebral body shatters into multiple fragments, and these fragments may penetrate the spinal cord. Burst fractures occur at the cervical, thoracic, and lumbar regions.

Dislocation of a vertebra may rupture the ligamentum flavum, resulting in dislocation of the vertebral facets, which can be unilateral or bilateral. This dislocation disrupts alignment of the vertebral column, and injury to the spinal cord may or may not be present. Partial dislocation of the spinal cord is called *subluxation*.

Spinal Cord Injuries

The neural elements of the spinal cord and spinal nerve roots are injured by compression from bone, disc herniation, hematoma, and ligaments; edema following compression or concussion; overstretching or disruption of neural tissue; and disturbances in spinal circulation.[23]

The sequence of pathologic processes following impact injury to the spinal cord are localized hemorrhaging, which advances from the gray to the white matter; reduced vascular perfusion and production of ischemic areas and decreased oxygen tension in tissue at the site of injury; edema; cellular and subcellular alterations; and tissue necrosis. Several minutes after the traumatic injury, microscopic hemorrhages appear in the central gray matter and in the pia-arachnoid. They increase in size until the entire gray matter is hemorrhagic and necrotic. Hemorrhaging and peritraumatic edema progress to the white matter, forming vacuolation and wedge-shaped foci that impair the microcirculation to the spinal cord. This impairment produces ischemia or vascular stasis.

Circulation in the white matter returns to normal within approximately 24 hours, but circulation in the gray matter remains altered.

Changes in the chemistry and metabolism of the traumatized regions include a transitory increase in tissue lactate, a rapid decrease in tissue oxygen tension within 30 minutes of the injury, and increased norepinephrine concentration. Increased concentrations of norepinephrine released to the cord tissue may produce ischemia, vascular rupture, or necrosis of neuronal tissue.[4]

Localized ischemia of neural tissue may result from compression on the vasculature of the cord or nerve roots by bony fragments or herniated disks. If the flow of blood from the vertebral artery to the anterior spinal artery or to the branches of the radicular arteries is impaired, severe cord ischemia results. Hemorrhage, other than with contusion and edema, usually does not produce significant neural impairment. Epidural and subdural hematomas rarely are large enough to cause serious compression. Although subarachnoid bleeding is usual, it is of little clinical significance. Larger intramedullary hematomas, on the other hand, may produce a tubular hematomyelia that can cause partial or complete interruption in spinal cord functioning.[23]

After the necrosis that occurs immediately after the injury, a phase of resorption and organization begins. This state is characterized by the appearance of phagocytes within 36 to 48 hours after injury, proliferation of microglial and mesenchymal cells, and changes in astroglias. Blood gradually is removed from the tissue by disintegration of red cells and resorption of hemorrhages. Macrophages engulf degenerating axons in the first 10 days after injury.[4]

The traumatized section of the cord is removed in the third to fourth week after the injury and gradually replaced with connective scar tissue or glial fibers. Injured segments of the spinal cord are replaced with connective scar tissue or glial fibers. Injured segments of the spinal cord are replaced with acellular collagenous tissue, which connects the meninges to the cord and central canal. Scarring in the injured area consists mainly of thickened meninges and connective tissue.

Spinal Shock

Spinal shock at the area of transection occurs after complete or incomplete severing of the spinal cord. It causes a complete loss of sensory, motor, autonomic, and reflex functioning below the level of the lesion. Spinal shock results from the loss of inhibition from descending tracts, continued inhibition of supraspinal impulses, and axonal degeneration of the interneurons.

Autonomic Hyperreflexia

Autonomic hyperreflexia may occur after spinal shock has been resolved and reflex activity has returned. The syndrome is associated with a massive uncompensated cardiovascular response to stimulation of the sympathetic division of the autonomic nervous system.[16] Individuals most likely to be affected with autonomic hyperreflexia have lesions at the level of T6 or above. If symptoms of autonomic hyperreflexia are not treated, serious damage and possibly even death can result (see Part Three).

Cord Syndromes

Trauma to the spinal cord results in several syndromes that develop from the specific area of cord damaged and vary in severity depending on the amount of cord compression or transection.

The *anterior* cord syndrome occurs after an acute flexion injury to the cervical area and is the most common syndrome. Damage to the anterior spinal artery, the ventral portion of the spinal cord, or both accounts for the loss of upper and lower motor function.

The *posterior* cord syndrome, although rare, is associated with cervical hyperextension trauma.

Central cord syndrome may result from hyperextension injuries or flexion injuries. The central cord syndrome is characterized by central edema of the spinal cord and compression on the anterior horn cells. Neurologic deficits include mixed upper and lower motor neuron loss (disproportionately more impairment in upper extremities) and spasticity below the level of injury.

The *Brown-Séquard* syndrome results from rotation-flexion injuries where subluxation or dislocation of the fracture occurs by unilateral pedicle-laminar injuries.[16] Neurologic deficits include ipsilateral paresis, loss of proprioception, and contralateral loss of pain and temperature sensations.

The *herniated disc* syndrome is one of the most common spinal cord syndromes. Degenerative changes with the fraying and tears of the anulus fibrosus predispose the intervertebral discs to posterior displacement through a laceration of the anulus fibrosus and the posterior longitudinal ligament. The extrusion of fibrocartilaginous material may occur spontaneously or in response to activity (e.g., lifting) or slight injury. The severity of symptoms depends on quantity of herniated disc tissue, number of involved discs and amount of nerve root compression, and amount of spinal canal narrowing.[31] Herniated discs most frequently (90%) affect the lower lumbar and lumbosacral regions.

Motor Neurons

Motor neurons are the nerve cell responsible for transmitting impulses from the brain or spinal cord to muscular or glandular tissue. Spinal cord trauma can cause varying degrees of motor neuron impairment, so it is important to understand the difference between the upper and lower motor neurons. *Upper* motor neuron lesions result from damage in the corticobulbar or corticospinal tract. *Lower* motor neuron lesions result in the loss of reflex and voluntary responses of muscles because of destruction of anterior horn cells, peripheral nerves, or ventral nerve roots or motor fibers.[31]

Diagnostic Studies and Findings

Roentgenograms (Anterior-Posterior and Lateral)

Vertebral fractures

Serum Chemistry

Hypoglycemia or hyperglycemia
Electrolyte imbalance
Possibly decreased hemoglobin and hematocrit

CT Scan

Spinal cord edema

Magnetic Resonance Imaging (MRI)

Spinal cord edema and compression

Spinal Puncture

Establishes presence or absence of spinal block

Myelography

Establishes presence of spinal block

Medical Plan

Surgery

Laminectomy
Tracheostomy or endotracheal intubation (nasal)
Spinal fusion for stabilization
Wound debridement; suturing of lacerations
Cervical tongs (i.e., Cone, Vinke, Crutchfield, Gardner-Wells)
Halo traction
Halo with femoral traction
Body casts
Spinal cord cooling
Myotomies, tenotomies, neurectomies, rhizotomies, and muscle transplants (treatment for spasticity)
Harrington rod insertion for stabilization of thoracic deformities

Medications

- Antianxiety agents
  - Diazepam (Valium), 2-10 mg tid or qid po
  - Meprobamate (Equanil), 1200-1600 mg/d po in divided doses
  - Corticosteroids (to control cord edema)
    - Dexamethasone (Decadron), 5-10 mg qid po
  - Anticoagulants
    - Heparin, 5000-7000 U subcutaneously q12h
- Antihypertensive agents
  - Diazoxide (Hyperstat),* 1-3 mg/kg, up to 150 mg, IV, repeated at intervals of 5-15 min until blood pressure reduced
  - Hydralazine (Apresoline),* 20 mg in slow IV push
- Muscle relaxants
  - Baclofen (Lioresal), 15-80 mg/d po in divided doses
  - Dantrolene sodium (Dantrium), 25 mg tid to 200 mg qid
- Anti-infective agents
  - Sulfisoxazole (Gantrisin), 2-4 g initially, then 4-8 g/d in divided doses
- Methenamine mendelate (Mandelamine), 1-2 g qid
- Laxatives
  - Glycerin or bisacodyl (Dulcolax), as rectal suppository
- Antacids
  - Magnesium hydroxide and aluminum hydroxide (Maalox T.C.), 20 ml po q4h

General Management

Mechanical ventilation
Stryker or Foster frame bed
Skeletal traction
Vital capacity and tidal volume measurements
Splints and braces
Phrenic nerve stimulator
Bed board and firm mattress
Cardiac monitoring
Intermittent urinary catheterization
Intake and output recording
Dietary consultation
Sex counseling

*Treatment for autonomic hyperreflexia.

- Psychosocial counseling for individual and family
- Cervical collar (soft or hard)
- Immobilization of part with sandbags
- Serial measurement of arterial blood gases
- Urine sugar and acetone; guaiac
- Antiembolus stockings or sequential compression devices
- Nasogastric tube

NURSING CARE

Nursing Assessment

Spinal Shock

- Complete transection
  - Flaccid paralysis below level of lesion
  - Loss of proprioception, pain, temperature, touch, and pressure below level of lesion
  - Loss of all spinal reflexes below level of lesion
  - Loss of vasomotor tone
  - Loss of visceral and somatic sensations below level of lesion
  - Loss of ability to perspire below level of lesion
    - Dysfunction of bowel and bladder
  - Possible priapism[31]
- Partial transection
  - Asymmetric flaccid paralysis below level of lesion
  - Asymmetric loss of reflexes below level of lesion
  - Some senses of proprioception, pain, temperature, touch, and pressure intact below level of injury
  - Some visceral and somatic sensations intact below level of lesion
  - Less vasomotor instability
  - Less bowel and bladder dysfunction
  - Possible priapism

Autonomic Hyperreflexia

- Paroxysmal hypertension
- Pounding headache
- Diaphoresis above level of lesion
- Flushing above level of lesion
- Cutis anserina below level of lesion
- Nasal stuffiness
- Nausea
- Bradycardia

Muscle Function According to Level of Spinal Cord Injury

C4 and above	Loss of all muscle function including respiratory (usually fatal)
C5	Quadriplegia with poor respiratory functioning
C6-C8	Quadriplegia with sparing of some arm and hand muscles
T1-T3	Quadriplegia with loss of muscle function below nipple line
T4-T10	Paraplegia with some chest and trunk muscles intact
T11-L2	Paraplegia with muscles intact through upper thigh
L3-S1	Paraplegia with muscles of chest, trunk, thigh, and most of leg intact; loss of voluntary bowel and bladder control
S2-S4	Loss of voluntary bowel and bladder control

Herniated Disc Syndrome

- Lumbar
  - Pain in lower back with radiation down back of one leg
  - Restricted spinal mobility
  - Walking painful
  - Back appears straight with loss of lumbar curve
  - Spastic paravertebral muscles
  - Impaired sensation of affected leg and foot
  - Less active ipsilateral ankle jerk may be present
  - Pain aggravated by jugular compression
- Cervical
  - Stiffness of neck
  - Pain radiating down arm to fingers

Pain

- Hyperesthesia immediately above level of lesion
- Intense tingling and burning pain below level of lesion (in paraplegia)

Spasticity

- Partial or complete loss of voluntary control
- Exaggerated deep tendon reflexes

Sexual Function Irregularities

- Varies from normal function to complete impotence
- Menstrual irregularies for short time after injury

Trophic Skin Changes

- Trophic ulcers
- Skin and nail changes

Nursing Dx & Intervention

Nursing Diagnosis	Nursing Intervention/Rationale

Ineffective airway clearance; potential for aspiration

- Auscultate for breath sounds every 1 to 2 hours as needed.
- Maintain patient airway, and avoid flexion of the neck.
- Suction as needed *to remove secretions and prevent aspiration.*
- Assist ventilation as indicated. Keep Ambu bag at bedside.
- Monitor vital signs every 1 to 2 hours; monitor neurologic status every 15 to 30 minutes.
- Maintain nothing-by-mouth status if indicated *to prevent risk of choking or aspiration.*

Ineffective breathing pattern

- Auscultate for breath sounds every 1 to 2 hours; note quality and increase in adventitious sounds:
  - Suction as needed. Hyperinflate lungs with 100% oxygen for 1 minute before and 1 minute after suctioning, unless contraindicated, *to prevent hypoxemia.*
- Maintain patent airway. Intubation/tracheostomy and mechanical ventilation may be indicated.
- Monitor mechanical ventilator, if used:
  - Ensure tidal volume, rate, mode, and oxygen concentration are set as ordered.
  - Ensure ventilator alarms are on and function *to prevent accidental disconnection.*
- Monitor arterial blood gases, as ordered:
  - Report decrease in Po_2 of 10 to 15 mm Hg.
  - Report increase in Pco_2 greater than 10 to 15 mm Hg.
- Check blood pressure, temperature, and pulse rate every 1 to 2 hours and as needed based on patient's condition.

Altered cerebral and spinal tissue perfusion

- Perform neurologic assessment every 15 to 30 minutes and as needed.
- Ensure immobilization vertebral column:
  - Maintain skeletal traction.
  - Maintain cervical skeletal traction:
    - *Crutchfield tongs:*
      - Check traction and orthopaedic frame every 4 hours.
      - Make sure tongs are secure.
      - Ensure weights hang freely.
      - Assess tong sites every 4 hours and as needed.
      - Provide tong site skin care: clean with hydrogen peroxide, and then apply povidine-iodine solution *to prevent sepsis.* Cover with sterile dressing.
    - *Halo traction:*
      - Assess traction pins to ensure they are tight and secure.
      - Assess fiberglass cast jacket for proper fit (should be able to insert index finger between cast and skin).
      - Assess cast edges for roughness and crumbling; petal rough edges:
        - Provide routine cast care.
        - Provide pin site skin care: clean site with hydrogen peroxide, and then apply povidone-iodine solution *to prevent infection.*
        - Cover with sterile dressing.
    - *Stryker frame:*
      - Inspect pressure points (face, chin, scapula, coccyx, and heels) every 2 to 4 hours *to prevent skin breakdown.*
      - Administer skin care every 2 to 4 hours *to prevent breakdown.*
      - Secure all bolts before turning patient.
      - Assess pulse and respirations before and after turning.
      - Check position of canvas under patient after turning.
      - Use armrests *to maintain alignment.*
      - Establish method of elimination.
  - Maintain *strict* body alignment; keep body straight and head flat:
    - Do not move head or spinal column.
    - Use sandbags, if needed, *to maintain alignment.*
  - Administer medications as ordered:
    - Give steroids *to control cord edema.*
    - When steroids are being administered:
      - Check stools *to detect occult blood.*
      - Test urine for sugar and acetone *to detect glycosuria.*
      - Administer phytonadine, MSD (Aquamephyton), intramuscularly daily or every other day *to control tendency for bleeding.*
      - Administer antacids per protocol *to decrease or prevent gastric irritation.*
  - Avoid injection below the level of the lesion.

Nursing Diagnosis	Nursing Intervention/Rationale
	Maintain parenteral fluids per protocol. Measure intake and output every hour. Immediately report urine output of less than 30 ml/hour.
Sensory/perceptual alterations (visual, auditory, kinesthetic, gustatory, tactile, olfactory)	• See general intervention strategies listed on p. 1728.
Potential for trauma	• Assess and document potential for injury and strategies for prevention. • Maintain bed in low position at all times unless side rails are up or nurse is with patient. • Provide patient with a call light within easy reach. • Maintain side rails in up position at bedtime, after sedation, and as needed. • Maintain stretchers in locked position when transferring patient. • Pad side rails if patient is overactive.
Impaired physical mobility	• Assess skin condition for signs of breakdown when administering skin care. • Administer skin care every 2 hours: Turn patient every 2 hours and as needed, unless contraindicated, *to prevent respiratory complications.* Change position slowly *to prevent orthostatic hypotension.* Position in straight body alignment; use log-roll technique when turning. • Keep skin dry; give perineal care as needed. • Massage pressure points every 2 hours *to stimulate circulation;* give gentle back rubs every shift and as needed. • Use heel and elbow guards as needed *to prevent skin irritation and breakdown.* • Use firm mattress. • Perform active or passive ROM exercises every 2 to 4 hours *to promote circulation and improve muscle tone.* • Use footboard or Spence boots *to prevent footdrop.* • Apply antiembolus stockings or sequential compression devices to lower extremities. • Administer anticoagulation therapy per protocol: Monitor serum coagulation studies. Check stool *to detect occult bleeding.* Check urine *to detect occult bleeding.* Monitor for signs of thrombophlebitis and deep vein thrombosis including redness, tenderness, localized swelling, warmth, and upward red streaking on an extremity. • Encourage mobility to tolerance or per protocol. • Encourage self-care activities to tolerance. • Plan all activities to avoid fatigue. Maintain planned rest periods. • Obtain physical therapy referral.
Feeding, bathing/hygiene, dressing/grooming, and toileting self-care deficit	• See general intervention strategies listed on p. 1692.
Bowel incontinence	• Assess pattern of bowel elimination. • Maintain fluid intake of 2000 ml/day, unless contraindicated. • Monitor intake and output. • Provide patient with diet that is high in roughage, protein, and bulk. • Keep patient's skin clean and dry. • Check patient for impaction every 1 to 2 days. • Institute a regular bowel evacuation program: Begin bowel retraining program *to prevent constipation.* Instruct patient to take 8 to 10 ounces of prune juice 12 hours before time set for defecating; insert glycerin suppository high in rectum 15 to 20 minutes before set time; then place patient on bedpan, toilet, or commode. Insert lubricated glycerin suppository 2 hours before set time, and position patient in sitting position or transfer to bedpan or commode at set time. Instruct patient to drink 4 to 8 ounces prune juice each night. Instruct patient to drink a warm drink (water, coffee, milk) 30 minutes before set time. Insert laxative suppository for 2 to 4 days, then glycerin suppository for 2 to 4 days; note length of time between insertion and defecation; place patient on bedside commode at appropriate time; if no bowel movement, give small tap water enema.[62]

	Nursing Intervention/Rationale
Altered patterns of urinary elimination	• Assess the characteristics of the patient's voiding pattern (frequency, amount). • Observe for bladder distention every 2 to 4 hours. • Perform intermittent catheterization per protocol. • Perform catheter care every shift: Maintain closed system. Tape catheter to thigh *to prevent pulling and tension* (female). Tape catheter to lower abdomen *to prevent pulling and tension* (male). • Monitor intake and output. Maintain fluid intake of 2000 ml daily unless contraindicated. • Assess urine for sediment, concentration, color, and odor. • Acidify urine with foods such as cranberry juice. • Administer urinary tract germicides (e.g., Mandelamine) as ordered. • Begin bladder retraining program: *Upper motor neuron bladder:* Administer fluids between 7 AM and 7 PM. Remove urinary catheter at 7 AM. Force fluids (i.e., 240 ml) every hour. After approximately 3 or 4 hours, trigger area (i.e., digital stimulation of rectum) until stimulated and attempt to void is made; if patient is able to void, residual urine is immediately checked: Residual urine of less than 100 ml is needed to continue with training. Residual urine of greater than 100 ml requires catheter reinsertion. Bladder retraining is then resumed another day. *Lower motor neuron bladder:* Administer fluids between 7 AM and 7 PM. Remove urinary catheter at 7 AM. Force fluids (i.e., 240 ml) every hour. After approximately 3 to 4 hours, patient attempts to void by Valsalva maneuver, Credé maneuver of bladder, or contraction of abdominal muscles. If patient is able to void, residual urine is immediately checked: Residual urine of less than 50 to 75 ml is needed to continue with training. Residual urine of greater than 75 ml requires catheter reinsertion. Retraining is then resumed on another day.
Potential impaired skin integrity	• See general intervention strategies listed on p. 1646.
Body image, self-esteem, and personal identity disturbances	• Assess and document degree of concern and confusion. • Provide a safe, comfortable, secure environment. • Carefully explain what you are doing and why you are doing it. • Listen to the feelings the patient expresses (i.e., feelings of grief and loss). • Answer questions simply and honestly. • Correct misinformation. • Protect the patient's privacy. • Provide gentle physical care in a caring environment. • Provide an ongoing assessment of the patient's interpersonal strengths. Focus on strengths and potential. • Assist the patient to become involved in self-care. • Assist the patient to become involved in unit activities.
Anxiety	• See general intervention strategies listed on p. 1743.
Powerlessness	• See general intervention strategies listed on p. 1748.

Patient Education

1. Instruct regarding name of medication, dosage, time of administration, purpose, and side effects.
2. Avoid over-the-counter medications without first checking with physician.
3. Teach muscle-building exercises: rubber balls, clay, trapezes, pulleys, squeeze toys, and sit-ups.
4. Stress importance of bladder retraining:
   a. Avoid food low in calcium.
   b. Force fluids to 2000 ml daily unless contraindicated.
   c. Maintain an acidic urine by drinking cranberry juice and taking ascorbic acid if ordered.

   d. Avoid alcoholic beverages, coffee, and tea.
   e. Maintain mobility as tolerated.
   f. Stress that rehabilitation may be a long process.
   g. Instruct regarding signs of full bladder.
   h. Avoid use of penile clamp to control incontinence.
   i. Avoid persons with infections, especially upper respiratory infections.
   j. Instruct regarding care of indwelling catheter.
   k. List symptoms to report to physician: urinary tract infection, kidney stone, upper respiratory infection, or skin lesions.
5. Ensure that the patient or family demonstrates:
   a. Bladder exercises every 2 to 4 hours:
      (1) Tighten rectum or vaginal vault.
      (2) Hold contraction for 5 seconds; then relax.
      (3) Continue tightening and relaxing for 5-min period.
   b. Credé maneuver for manual bladder stimulation:
      (1) Apply manual pressure over suprapubic region.
      (2) Contract abdominal muscles.
   c. Palpation of bladder distention
   d. Intake and output measurement
   e. Recording of time and amount of fluid intake
   f. Recording of time and amount of urine voided
   g. Testing of urine for pH
   h. Application of condom catheter if necessary
   i. Self-catheterization
6. Instruct regarding importance of bowel retraining program:
   a. Encourage patient participation in developing program.
   b. Evaluate previous bowel habits.
   c. Establish regular bowel habits: (1) time of day that will be convenient for patient once discharged (e.g., after breakfast) and (2) development of program to have bowel evacuation at same time of day or every 3 days.
   d. Teach exercises that will help to develop abdominal muscles and tone: pushing up, bearing down, and contracting abdominal muscles.
   e. Ensure privacy.
   f. Provide bedside commode rather than bedpan when possible: encourage sitting position rather than lying position.
   g. Keep equipment easily available at bedside.
   h. Teach the patient to recognize signals that may indicate full bowel: goose pimples, perspiration, rising of hair on arms or legs, and sense of fullness.
   i. Instruct the patient to develop exercise or signals that may help to stimulate urge to defacate: (1) pressure on inner thigh, (2) stroking anus, (3) digital rectal stimulation, (4) drinking coffee, and (5) massaging abdomen downward or side to side.
   j. Instruct the patient to respond to signals promptly.
   k. Discuss importance of establishing well-balanced diet that includes bulk and roughage.
   l. Discuss foods to avoid: bananas, beans, and cabbage.
   m. Instruct the patient to recognize impaction: (1) no formed stool for 3 days, (2) semiliquid stools, and (3) restlessness and increased feeling of discomfort.
   n. Discuss treatment for impaction: (1) laxative suppository, (2) tap water or oil retention enema, or (3) manual clearing of bowel followed by enema.
   o. Stress importance of reporting symptoms of autonomic hyperreflexia to physician immediately.
   p. Discuss posibility of accidental incontinence once program has been established.
   q. Instruct the patient to relate incontinence to change in diet or daily routine.
7. Stress importance of ongoing outpatient care such as physician's visits and physical therapy.
8. Refer to Spinal Cord Injury Foundation.

Evaluation

Patient Outcome	Data Indicating That Outcome is Reached
Patient demonstrates a patent airway.	Breath sounds are normal. Chest excursion is bilateral and symmetric. Rate and depth of respirations are normal. Cough is effective. There are no subjective or objective findings of shortness of breath, air hunger, or dyspnea on exertion.
Patient demonstrates an effective breathing pattern.	Airway is patent. Chest excursion is symmetric. Breath sounds are normal, or there is no increase in adventitious sounds. Arterial blood gas values are within normal ranges or consistent with patient's baseline. Vital signs are within normal ranges or consistent with patient's baseline. Hemoglobin levels are 14 to 18 g/dl (male) or 12 to 16 g/dl (female). Intake and output are stable. There are no signs of respiratory distress. Skin color is not cyanotic.

Patient Outcome	Data Indicating That Outcome is Reached
Patient demonstrates adequate spinal tissue perfusion.	Neurologic and vital signs are stable. Spinal column is immobilized via appropriate method. Straight body alignment is maintained. Intake and output are adequate.
Patient demonstrates minimum complications of sensory-perceptual alterations.	Level of orientation is optimum. Patient remains free of injury. Nutritional status is adequate. Skin integrity is maintained. Self-care deficits are minimum. Social participation is appropriate to physiologic status.
Patient remains free of traumatic injury.	Safety measures are appropriate to level of physiologic status. Skin integrity is maintained. Skin is free of bruises, burns, abrasions, and redness. Environment is safe. Patient is free of nosocomial infections.
Patient demonstrates an optimum level of mobility.	Skin integrity is maintained. Patient remains free of contractures and deformities. Level of mobility is appropriate to physiologic status. Intake and output pattern is stable. Nutritional status is adequate. Patient remains free of thrombophlebitis. Patient remains free of local infection. Patient participates in an ongoing physical therapy program.
Patient demonstrates minimum self-care deficits.	Outcome criteria listed for impaired physical mobility are met. Level of self-care activities is appropriate to physiologic status. Patient participates in physical and occupational therapy.
Patient demonstrates skin integrity.	Skin is intact. Nutritional status is adequate. Electrolyte balance is maintained. Patient remains free of pressure sores and contractures.
Patient demonstrates minimum complications of bowel incontinence.	Skin in perineal area is clean and dry. Dietary intake is adequate. Fluid intake is adequate (2000 ml/day unless contraindicated). Intake and output pattern is stable. Patient remains free of fecal impaction. Patient demonstrates a regular bowel evacuation pattern.
Patient demonstrates intact self-concepts.	Patient openly verbalizes feelings of grief and loss. Patient verbalizes positive feelings about self. Patient acknowledges actual change in self-image. Patient focuses on present and future appearance and function. Patient verbalizes feelings of hopefulness, helpfulness, and powerfulness.
Patient demonstrates a low level of anxiety.	Patient openly verbalizes concerns and feelings of grief, loss, and discomfort. Patient openly verbalizes feelings supported by health care professionals and family. Patient verbalizes essential aspects of care. Patient identifies methods to effectively deal with anxious feelings.
Patient demonstrates minimum feelings of powerlessness.	Patient maintains optimum level of physiologic control, as possible for current health status. Patient maintains optimum level of psychologic control, as possible. Patient participates, as possible, in decision making about care. Patient participates, as possible, in self-care.

Headache

(Vascular, tension, traction-inflammatory)

Headache, or cephalalgia, is any ache or pain in the head that results from the stimulation of pain-sensitive structures in the cranium or the extracranial tissues in the head and neck.

Approximately 30 million individuals in the United States seek health care for recent or recurring headaches. Headaches range in severity from a benign and transient discomfort to a severe, incapacitating pain. They may be the symptom of some potentially destructive pathologic process such as cerebral hypoxia, head trauma, inflamed meninges, cerebral hemorrhage, or expanding cranial mass. Therefore headaches, and particularly *recurring* headaches, require thorough investigation, including a complete history and neurologic examination.

Headaches may be classified as vascular, muscle contraction, and traction-inflammatory. Vascular headaches include migraine, cluster, and hypertensive headaches, as well as headaches from secondary responses (e.g., to infectious process). Muscle contraction headaches may occur from psychogenic problems, such as response to trauma or as a result of medical disorders such as cervical arthritis. Traction-inflammatory headaches may result from infection, intracranial or extracranial lesions, occlusive vascular disorders, diseases of facial structures, and medical disorders such as arteritis.[16]

Pathophysiology

Afferent pain fibers carry sensory stimuli to the tissue of the central nervous system by the three divisions of the trigeminal nerve, the first three cervical nerves, and cranial nerves IX (glossopharyngeal) and X (vagus). Intracranially, the trigeminal nerve supplies structures in the anterior and middle fossae of the skull above the tentorium. Trigeminal innervation extracranially includes all or most of the nervous supply to the facial skin; the subcutaneous tissues, and especially the blood vessels in this region; the eyes, nose, sinuses, and teeth; and most of the ear and external auditory canal.[4] The first three cervical nerves serve structures in the posterior fossae and the infradural region. Cranial nerves IX and X also supply portions of the posterior fossae and refer pain to the throat and ear.

Head pain can be caused by distention, dilation, or traction of intracranial or extracranial arteries; traction, compression, or disease states affecting sensory cranial or spinal nerves; meningeal irritation and increased intracranial pressure; displacement or traction of large intracranial veins or their dural envelopes; and voluntary or involuntary spasms and possible interstitial inflammation or traction of cervical and cranial muscles.

Extracranial causes of headaches include emotional tension, disorders of extracranial arteries, sinusitis, and inflammatory lesions of the bone and its coverings. Pain results from chronic sustained contractions of skeletal muscles, changes in intracranial pressure, vessel dilation and stretching of surrounding tissue, or a combination of the preceding factors.

Intracranial causes of headaches, such as mass lesions, produce pain from the compression, inflammation, distortion, or traction of the pain-sensitive blood vessels and meninges at the base of the brain.

Headaches of diffuse meningeal irritation are most likely caused by the chemical irritation of nerve endings and the stretching of pain-sensitive structures by dilation and congestion of inflamed meningeal vessels. This type of headache typically is throbbing because of the transmission of arterial pulsation to cerebral tissues already under increased tension.[55]

Vascular Headaches

Migraine headaches. Migraine headache generally begins in childhood, adolescence, or early adult life and is found in approximately 5% of the general population. It is frequently familial. Young women appear most susceptible, particularly just before or during the menstrual period. Migraine is characterized by a paroxysmal, throbbing, unilateral head pain that frequently is accompanied by autonomic symptoms such as nausea and vomiting. Attacks generally decrease in frequency and intensity with advancing age.

The exact pathogenesis of migraine is unknown. The initial physiologic change is that of vasospasm in the intracranial and extracranial arteries and their branches on one side of the head. Ten to 30 minutes later, dilation of the same vessels occurs. The constriction of the arteries is responsible for the symptoms of the aura, while vessel dilation produces the headache part of the syndrome. In headache-free intervals the cranial vessels of the migraine patient are hypersensitive to inhalation of carbon dioxide and intravenously administered histamine.[45]

Recent studies indicate that serotonin levels rise during the prodromal phase and drop during the headache phase. Also, the urinary excretion of 5-hydroxyindoleacetic acid (5-HIAA), a metabolite of serotonin, is increased during the migraine episodes. Platelet aggregability, which increases just before a migraine attack, is thought to be responsible for the release of serotonin.[35]

Agents and circumstances thought to precipitate migraine attacks include emotional stress and tension, menstruation, too much or too little sleep, and dietary agents such as tyramine, nitrate, and glutamate. However, none of these affect all individuals or consistently produce attacks in the same individual.[15] There is no evidence to support allergy or autonomic disorders as responsible for migraine attacks.

Cluster headaches. Cluster headaches (Horton's syndrome, histamine headache, migrainous neuralgia, or paroxysmal nocturnal cephalalgia) are intense repetitive vascular events. Cluster headaches are four times more common in men and generally occur in the third and fourth decades of life.[35] They are characterized by a distinct episode of excruciating pain, usually unilateral, which lasts from ½ to 1 hour, and is accompanied by ipsilateral lacrimation, nasal stuffiness, and drainage.[15] Usually, the same side of the head is involved in the cluster of attacks. There is no prodrome and usually only slight nausea. The attack may occur at any time (generally they are nocturnal), and multiple attacks are common.

Headaches may occur in an episodic or chronic pattern. The episodic pattern of cluster headaches is characterized by recurring headaches for several weeks to months, followed by months to years during which no headaches occur.

Chronic cluster headaches are either primary or secondary in type. The primary chronic pattern is characterized by persistent, repetitive attacks for years at a time. The secondary chronic type occurs when the episodic attacks evolve into chronic, unremitting attacks.[15]

The exact mechanism of cluster headaches is unknown. Increased histamine with resultant vasodilation has been implicated.

Tension Headaches

Muscle contraction headaches. Muscle contraction headaches are the most common type of head pain. Research studies indicate a preponderance of muscle contraction headaches in women and a higher incidence in adults from 20 to 40 years of age. This headache is usually bilateral and may be diffuse or confined to the frontal, temporal, parietal, or occipital area. The onset of an attack is more gradual than with a migraine, and duration is highly variable, but it may last for several days up to several months or years.

Muscle contraction headaches are frequently accompanied by contraction of skeletal muscles of the face, jaw, and neck. Concurrent arterial vasodilation may contribute further to the discomfort. There are no structural changes in the involved muscle groups.

Traumatic headaches. The posttraumatic, or postconcussion, headache, which consists of a dull, generalized pain, may develop after head injury and may be coupled with other symptoms such as lack of concentration, giddiness, or dizziness. Symptoms are much the same whether the head injury is mild or severe. Traumatic headaches usually are nonfocal, appearing for at least part of every day and persisting over days, weeks, or months. The headache is made worse by coughing and straining, which raises the pressure in both intracranial and extracranial venous systems.

Posttraumatic headaches are thought to be caused by vascular dilation, muscle contraction, or direct injury to the scalp.

Traction-Inflammatory Headaches

Traction headaches. Traction headaches may result from increased intracranial pressure, cerebral hemorrhage, decreased intracranial pressure (e.g., lumbar puncture), and inflammatory processes (e.g., encephalitis, meningitis). The discomfort produced with traction headaches occurs because of referred pain when the pain-sensitive structures (cranial nerves, arteries, etc.) are stretched or displaced by a mass lesion.

Temporal arteritis. Temporal arteritis, also called cranial arteritis or giant cell arteritis, generally affects individuals over 60 years of age. This headache usually is located in the temporal area and may be accompanied by visual loss, which is caused by ophthalmic artery involvement.[35]

Temporal arteritis is thought to result from an autoimmune mechanism and is included in the group of collagen-vascular diseases. The temporal arteries may be palpated as firm, tender cords or may be seen as tortuous, enlarged vessels.

• • •

Other clinical types of headaches include those from angioma and aneurysm, chronic subdural hematoma, brain tumor, and medical disorders such as hypothyroidism, Cushing's disease, fevers of any cause, chronic lung disease with hypercapnia, hypertension, acute anemia, chronic nitrate or ergot exposure, corticosteroid withdrawal, carbon monoxide exposure, adrenal tumors producing aldosterone, and sometimes Addison's disease.

Diagnostic Studies and Findings

Cervical and Skull Roentgenograms

Detection of abnormalities at base of brain

Funduscopic Eye Examination

Possible irritation of iris and ciliary body

Serum

Increased sedimentation rate
Anemia (lithium serum level *not* to exceed 1 mEq/L)

CT Scan

Possible intracranial lesions

Magnetic Resonance Imaging (MRI)

Same as CT scan

Cerebral Angiography

Detection of vascular abnormalities

Neurologic History and Examination

Identification of precipitating influences
Effects on activities of daily living
Neurologic deficits

Medical Plan

Medications

- Analgesic/anti-inflammatory agents
  - Ergot preparations (Table 3-8)
- Adrenergic agents
  - Isometheptene mucate (Midrin, Octinum), 1-2 capsules at onset of headache; followed by 1-2 capsules 1 h later
- Psychotherapeutic agents
  - Chlorpromazine (Thorazine), 25 mg IM, po, or rectal suppository
  - Promethazine (Phenergan), 25 mg IM or rectally; 50 mg po
  - Hydroxyzine (Vistaril), 75 mg IM or 50-100 mg po
  - Lithium carbonate (Lithane; others), initial dose of 300 mg po bid to qid; *must* be monitored by serum levels
  - Analgesic/antipyretics
    - Acetaminophen (Tylenol), 600 mg po q4h prn
  - Narcotic analgesics
    - Meperidine (Demerol), 50-75 mg IM q4-6h prn
  - Corticosteroids
    - Dexamethasone (Decadron), 8-12 mg IM
  - β-Adrenergic blocking agent
    - Propranolol (Inderal), initial dose 20 mg po bid or tid; titrated gradually up to 80-200 mg/d in divided doses
  - Antihistamines
    - Methysergide maleate (Sansert), 2 mg tid or qid; for up to 5-6 mo; followed by mandatory discontinuance for at least 1 mo
    - Cyproheptadine (Periactin), 4 mg po bid-qid
  - Antidepressants
    - Phenelzine (Nardil), 10-15 mg po bid-qid
  - Antihypertensive agents
    - Clonidine hydrochloride (Catapres), 0.2 mg po bid-tid
  - Antianginal agents
    - Dipyridamole (Persantine), 25-50 mg po tid or qid
  - Nonsteroidal anti-inflammatory agents
    - Sulfinpyrazone (Anturane), 200 mg po bid-qid
  - Antidepressants
    - Amitriptyline (Elavil), 25-100 mg po qid

General Management

- Application of heat or cold to affected areas
- Dietary counseling to eliminate food items that may provoke headaches: vinegar, chocolate, pork, onions, excessive caffeine, citrus fruits, bananas, yogurt, sour cream, alcohol, canned figs, ripened cheeses, herring, doughnuts, cured sandwich meats, chicken livers, broad bean pods, fermented or marinated foods, avocados, and MSG
- Psychologic counseling for behavioral modification, stress management, and biofeedback

Table 3-8
Drugs Used in the Treatment of Vascular Migraine Headaches

Drug	Use	Dose	Action	Side Effects
Methysergide maleate (Sansert)	For prophylactic treatment of vascular headaches such as migraine, cluster, and others which have been difficult to control; not effective for an acute attack; a serotonin antagonist *Alert:* Patient must be under medical supervision because this drug has such serious side effects	2 mg orally tid with meals; after taking drug for 5 mo, it should be discontinued for 3-4 wk to reduce the incidence of serious side effects; dosage should be reduced gradually to prevent rebound headache	The action is not clear, but it decreases the frequency of headache in patients who have a few headaches weekly and are difficult to control with other drugs	Fibrotic changes in the retroperitoneal and pleuropulmonary tissue and in the mitral and aortic valves are the most serious complications; any of the following symptoms should be reported at once: urinary tract obstruction, dysuria, back pain, peripheral vascular insufficiency, cold, numb, or painful extremities and diminished pulse, dyspnea, and chest pain *Contraindications:* Cardiac conditions, severe hypertension, pregnancy, peripheral vascular disease, and atherosclerosis
Ergotamine tartrate (Gynergen)	Treatment of vascular migraine headaches A single dose of ergotamine (1 or 3 mg by injection at bedtime) is effective for *cluster headaches*	2 mg orally 2 mg sublingually, initially to be followed by 2 mg every 30 min until the headache subsides, or until 6 mg have been taken (Some texts suggest that up to a total of 9 mg may be taken.) 0.25-0.5 mg *subcutaneously* or *IM* at onset; dose may be repeated hourly up to 1.0 mg in 24 h 0.25 mg intravenously at onset; no more than 0.5 mg/24 h; rarely given IV 2-4 mg by *rectal suppository* at onset; 2 mg may be repeated hourly, up to 6-8 mg	Ergot alkaloids result in cerebral vasoconstriction, which decreases the amplitude of the pulsations of the cranial arteries; in addition to its powerful vasoconstrictive property, it constricts the smooth muscles of the uterus; however, the major use of ergot alkaloids is for the treatment of migraine headaches	Has a *cumulative action,* so it must be taken sparingly and as ordered or ergotism will develop (*Ergotism:* numbness and tingling of fingers and toes, muscle pain and weakness, gangrene, and blindness) *Contraindications:* Diabetes mellitus, sepsis, hepatorenal disease, peripheral and coronary disease, hypertension, and pregnancy
Ergotamine with caffeine (Cafergot)	Same as ergotamine	Each tablet contains 1 mg of ergotamine tartrate and 100 mg of caffeine; usual dose is 1-2 tablets at onset and another tablet in 30 min, not to exceed 6 tablets per attack (also available in suppositories if vomiting occurs)	The caffeine increases the effectiveness of the ergotamine by its vasoconstrictive action	Same as ergotamine

From Hickey.[31]

Table 3-8—cont'd
Drugs Used in the Treatment of Vascular Migraine Headaches

Drug	Use	Dose	Action	Side Effects
Dihydroergotamine (DHE 45)	Treatment of migraine headaches which tend to be severe	1 mg IM or IV at onset; repeat in 1 h	Action is not clear, but a majority of patients receive relief in 15 min to 2 h after administration	Less toxic and fewer side effects than ergotamine; less likely to cause vomiting than ergotamine
Ergotamine tartrate, 0.3 mg Phenobarbital, 20 mg Belladonna alkaloid, 0.1 mg (Bellergal)	Reduces the number of attacks in patients who have one or more weekly	Give 2 or 3 times daily for a few weeks	Vasoconstriction, sedation, and reduction of spasm	Same as ergotamine, along with dryness of mucous membrane and drowsiness *Contraindications:* In addition to those of ergotamine, do not give to patients with glaucoma
Others				
Analgesics Codeine sulfate, 30 mg or Meperidine (Demerol), 50 mg	Either drug may be given for severe pain once the headache has become full-blown; narcotics are avoided unless the pain is very severe, and precautions should be taken to avoid addiction			
Aspirin, 0.6 g Butalbital (Fiorinal), 2 tablets	These drugs may be tried for less severe pain			
Diuretics Hydrochlorothiazide (Esidrix) or acetazolamide (Diamox)	These drugs are given 1 wk before menstruation if premenstrual tension predisposes the individual to headaches; in addition, mild tranquilizers and analgesics such as aspirin may be given			
Antihistamines Diphenhydramine (Benadryl) and others	May be helpful in cluster headaches			

NURSING CARE

Nursing Assessment

Migraine

- Classic migraine
  - Prodrome
    - Visual scotoma
    - Aphasia
    - Hemiparesis
    - Altered mood, hunger, and taste
    - Drowsiness
  - Pain
    - Throbbing, high-intensity, unilateral discomfort in temporal area, upper cranium, or lower hemicranium (rare)
  - Other
    - Photophobia
    - Nausea and vomiting
    - *Ergotism:* tingling and numbness of toes and fingers; muscle weakness and pain; gangrene; blindness
- Common migraine
  - Prodrome
    - None
  - Pain
    - Throbbing intense pain progressing to generalized, nonthrobbing head pain
  - Other
    - Photophobia
    - Nausea and vomiting
    - Irritability

Cluster

- Pain
  - Sudden, intense unilateral head pain beginning in area of nostril and spreading to area of adjacent eye and sometimes forehead

Other
- Flushing of skin
- Nose and eyes water
- Homolateral Horner's syndrome with ptosis and pupillary constriction
- Steady, nonpulsating, unilateral or bilateral head pain in temporal, frontal, parietal, or occipital areas

Posttraumatic

Pain
- Generalized, dull, aching head pain

Other
- Personality changes
- Insomnia
- Fatigue
- Giddiness
- Unsteadiness
- Concentration difficulties
- Nausea and vomiting

Hypertensive

Throbbing pain that is predominantly occipital

Traction

Deep, dull, steady ache usually worse in morning and aggravated by coughing or straining

Cerebral Arteritis

Variable intensity of unilateral or bilateral head pain in temporal, occipital, or fronto-occipital regions; may be accompanied by tenderness of painful areas

Lumbar Puncture Headache

Dull, pulsating occipital-nuchal discomfort and frontal pain after rising from a recumbent position

Nursing Dx & Intervention

Nursing Diagnosis	Nursing Intervention/Rationale
Anxiety	• See general intervention strategies listed on p. 1743.
Pain	• Assess and document degree of pain and effect of medication administered. • Promote rest and relaxation. • Decrease noxious stimuli. • Modify anxiety associated with the pain experience. • Provide other sensory input. • Administer medication per protocol. • Remain with patient *to reduce anxiety.* • Use whatever measures the patient believes will alleviate the pain. • Teach patient about his discomfort. • Use other professionals, as appropriate. • Improve effectiveness of pain relief measures by using them before the pain becomes intense.

Patient Education

1. Reinforce physician's explanation of medical management.
2. Instruct regarding name of medication, dosage, time of administration, and toxic or side effects.
3. Instruct regarding proper use of ergot drugs:
   a. Take medication at earliest symptom of a headache.
   b. Dosages greater than 10 mg/week can lead to ergotism and cumulative effects.
   c. Lie in quiet, dark room after taking the medication.
4. Stress need to avoid over-the-counter medications without first consulting physician.
5. Emphasize need for regular exercise program.
6. Instruct regarding possible food causes of headaches.

Evaluation

Patient Outcome	Data Indicating That Outcome is Reached
Patient experiences minimal alterations in comfort.	Patient openly verbalizes feelings of discomfort when they occur. Patient can use measures to decrease discomfort. Patient verbally validates a decrease in subjective feelings of discomfort. Objective findings of pain are decreased.
Patient demonstrates a low level of anxiety.	Patient openly verbalizes concerns and feelings of grief, loss, and discomfort. Patient openly verbalizes feelings, supported by health care professionals and family. Patient verbalizes essential aspects of care. Patient identifies methods to deal effectively with anxious feelings.

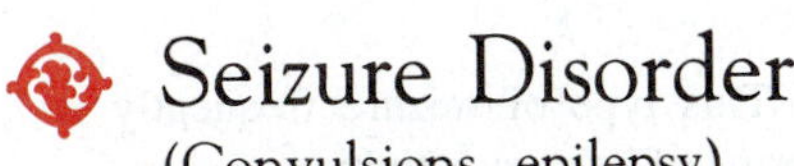

Seizure Disorder

(Convulsions, epilepsy)

Seizures, or convulsions, are paroxysmal episodes in which there are sudden and violent involuntary contractions of a group of skeletal muscles and disturbances in consciousness, behavior, sensation, and autonomic functioning.

Seizures may be tonic or clonic, focal, and unilateral or bilateral. The term "epilepsy" denotes a group of neurologic disorders characterized by the repeated occurrence of any of the various forms of seizures. Approximately 2 to 4 million Americans are affected with epilepsy, and many of this number are children. The social consequences of a seizure disorder are many, including possible loss of driving or educational privileges. Of all persons with epilepsy, 25% have recurrent seizures while receiving medication, 10% are institutionalized, and 5% are home-bound invalids.[39]

Pathophysiology

Seizure disorders can be classified as resulting from pathologic processes, endogenous or exogenous poisons, metabolic disturbances, fever, and idiopathic. *Pathologic processes* include formation abnormalities (e.g., vascular anomalies), space-occupying lesions (e.g., brain abscess, tumors, hematomas), craniocerebral trauma, acute cerebral edema (e.g., secondary to acute renal failure), infection (e.g., encephalitis), degenerative changes (e.g., leukodystrophies), vascular lesions (e.g., embolus, cerebrovascular accidents, and hemorrhages), and neuronal injury (e.g., anoxia from deficient oxygen).

Toxic endogenous substances (e.g., uremia) or *exogenous* substances such as certain medications (e.g., phenothiazines), lead ingestion, and alcohol intoxication or sudden withdrawal may precipitate seizure activity.

Metabolic disturbances (i.e., electrolyte imbalances) that cause an interference with crucial substances such as oxygen, glucose, or calcium being delivered to cerebral tissues can result in seizures.

Individuals with decreased neuronal thresholds may experience a seizure secondary to a *febrile* state.

Finally, *idiopathic* seizures may occur without any identifiable cause. The basis of idiopathic seizure disorders may be a biochemical imbalance.

These causative agents are either genetic factors or acquired factors. *Genetically,* epilepsy is rarely a predictable, inherited entity. The only well-defined inherited seizure pattern is that of the classic 2.5 to 3/s spike-and-wave pattern on the electroencephalogram (EEG).[35] Therefore, although inheritance may be a risk in developing seizures, environmental risk factors (e.g., trauma) play a significant role. *Acquired* factors include pathologic processes (e.g., infection), trauma that produces epileptogenic lesions, toxic substances, metabolic disturbances, and febrile states.

Traditionally, seizures have been classified as grand mal, petit mal, psychomotor (temporal lobe), and focal motor (jacksonian). With advanced technology it became evident that many neurologic manifestations of seizures did not fit into these categories. In 1969 the International League Against Epilepsy formulated a revised classification that incorporated pathophysiologic principles of all types of seizure activity.

Partial seizures start with a localized activation of neurons and generally do not involve the whole brain or significantly impair consciousness or memory. Partial seizures with simple symptoms produce symptoms of which the individual is aware, including autonomic, sensory, or focal motor symptoms. Simple partial seizures start with focal motor symptoms (jacksonian seizures), generally in the contralateral precentral gyrus. Symptoms first occur in the part of the body controlled by that brain area and then can spread to involve the entire limb and frequently the entire half of the body. The seizure ends with a gradual reduction of clonic, jerking movements. Seizure activity that occurs usually in the hand or face and is continuous, clonic, and localized is called *epilepsia partialis continua*. Simple sensory seizures are uncommon, but when present, they originate from hyperexcitable neurons in the postcentral gyrus. Symptoms of a partial sensory seizure include various degrees of numbness and paresthesias. Autonomic seizures result from hyperexcitable neurons of the frontal, temporal, mesial, orbital, or insular cortices. These seizures may begin with disturbances in gastric motility, which may progress to nausea and vomiting, tenesmus, or sudden bowel evacuation.[23] Partial seizures with only autonomic symptoms are rare.

Partial seizures with complex symptoms generally produce some type of episodic loss of consciousness. This type of seizure may include cognitive, affective, psychosensory, or psychomotor symptoms. Events that trigger the seizure occur within the structures of the temporal lobe. Complex partial seizures begin with various types of auras such as sensory illusions, déjà vu, or unusual smells. The individual may recognize these auras, or memory of them may be lost in postictal amnesia. In complex partial seizures, EEG abnormalities are localized in temporal or frontotemporal areas, including rhinencephalic structures. Complex partial seizures are characterized by purposeful behavior that is inappropriate for the time and place.[4] Automatisms such as lip smacking, walking aimlessly, or picking at one's clothing are common. The individual with this type of seizure usually cannot remember the seizure, but consciousness is not lost totally.

Psychomotor seizures in children can be confused with absence attacks because of the relative paucity of memory patterns in the temporal lobe of the young child. Complex partial attacks in children can be distinguished from absence attacks by the fact that the psychomotor attacks occur much less frequently and are of longer duration.

Generalized seizures begin locally but almost immediately result in bilateral involvement of the corticoreticular and reticulocortical systems of the diencephalon. Generalized seizures are usually petit mal (absence seizures) or grand mal (tonic-clonic) in nature. Petit mal seizures usually affect children after the age of 4 years and before puberty,[31] and although rare, they can occur in adults up to 70 years of age. Petit mal seizures consist of a sudden cessation of conscious activity without convulsive motor activity or loss of postural control.[45] These absence attacks usually last for seconds or minutes. The brief lapses of consciousness may be accompanied by minor motor manifestations (e.g., eyelid flickering and isolated myoclonic jerks). After a petit mal seizure the individual quickly regains consciousness or awareness and usually experiences no postictal confusion.

Grand mal seizures are one of the most common epileptic paroxysms and may be generalized seizures or the result of secondary generalization of partial seizures. Grand mal seizures usually occur without warning and follow a common pattern: (1) *tonic* phase; forceful contraction of axial and appendicular muscles, loss of postural control, epileptic cry, cyanosis; usually lasts 2 or 3 minutes; (2) *clonic* phase, characterized by gradual transition from tonic contractions to intermittent bilateral brisk clonic movements; this phase represents recurring inhibition phases interrupting the initial tonic phase; (3) *postictal* phase: amnesia of seizure and possibly even retrograde amnesia.

Generalized seizures also can result from secondary generalization of focal cortical discharges and are identical to primary generalized seizures. These facts make it difficult to distinguish secondary generalized seizures from primarily generalized tonic-clonic seizures. With secondary generalized seizures, however, there are usually diffuse cerebral pathologic findings.[4]

Generalized seizures such as myoclonic seizures, tonic seizures, infantile spasms, and atonic seizures usually occur during childhood and generally are associated with some type of genetic, perinatal, or metabolic brain disease. *Myoclonic* seizures may occur alone or coexist with other types of seizures. Individuals with severe and generalized myoclonus demonstrate evidence of disturbances in function of the reticular substance in relevant areas of the sensory cortex.

Tonic seizures are a less common type of primary generalized seizure marked by sudden rigid posturing of trunk and extremities, frequently with deviation to one side of the head and eyes. Tonic seizures are frequently of a shorter duration than tonic-clonic seizures and are not followed by a clonic phase. These seizures usually indicate a lesion in the area of the midbrain and are sometimes seen in individuals with severe cerebral palsy.

Infantile spasms (hypsarhythmia) are generalized seizures occurring between birth and approximately 12 months of age. They consist of brief synchronous contractions of the neck, torso, and arms.[45] Infantile spasms rarely occur in an apparently normal infant; rather, they usually occur in children with an underlying neurologic disorder (e.g., anoxic encephalopathy). Approximately 90% of children with infantile spasms develop mental retardation.

Atonic seizures consist of brief loss of consciousness and postural tone; these symptoms are not associated with tonic muscular contractions.[45] This type of seizure frequently is accompanied by other forms of seizure activity.

Unilateral seizure is a type of seizure in which clinical signs usually occur on one side of the body and the EEG discharges are recorded over the contralateral cerebral hemisphere.[4] Unilateral seizures may shift from one side to another but generally do not become symmetric.

The microscopic changes leading to pathologic processes occurring during the different types of seizure activities are essentially the same. The major alteration in the physiologic state is a hypersynchronous discharge in a localized area of the brain.[45] This localized area of hypersynchronized discharge is called the *epileptogenic focus,* producing a large, sharp EEG waveform known as the spike discharge.

Metabolic changes occurring within the cerebrum during the epileptic discharges include release of unusually large amounts of neuropeptides and neurotransmitters during the seizure, increased cerebral blood flow to primary involved areas, increased extracellular concentrations of potassium and decreased extracellular concentrations of calcium, changes in oxidative metabolism and local pH, and increased utilization of glucose.

Termination of seizure activity appears to be related to the large and lasting hyperpolarization of the neuronal cell membrane. This hyperpolarization is possibly generated by an electrogenic sodium pump. As the hyperpolarization is sustained, the neuronal cells cease firing and the surface potentials of the brain are suppressed.[23]

Diagnostic Studies and Findings

CT Scan

Structural changes

Magnetic Resonance Imaging (MRI)

Structural changes

Skull Roentgenogram

Evidence of fractures
Shift of calcified pineal gland
Bony erosion
Separated sutures

Echoencephalogram

Possible midline shifts of brain structures

Cerebral Angiography

Possible vascular abnormalities
Evaluation of a subdural hematoma

Electroencephalogram (EEG)

Grand mal: high, fast voltage spiked in all leads
Petit mal: 3/s, rounded spike wave complexes in all leads
Psychomotor (temporal lobe): square-topped 4-6/s spike wave complexes over involved lobe

Delta waves: usually associated with destroyed brain tissue
Theta waves: not always abnormal

Urine Screening

Indicates presence and levels of certain medications

Serum Chemistry

Hypoglycemia
Electrolyte imbalance
Increased blood urea nitrogen
Blood alcohol levels

History and Neurologic Examination

Pattern of onset and characteristics of seizure activity
Precipitating factors

Medical Plan

Surgery

Excision of epileptogenic focus
Stereotactic lesions

Medications

Anticonvulsants
- Grand mal, simple partial, and complex partial
  - Phenytoin (Dilantin), 100 mg po or IV tid or qid
  - Phenobarbital, 2-5 mg/kg/day
  - Primidone (Mysoline)
    - Day 1-3: 100-125 mg po hs
    - Day 4-6: 100-125 mg po bid
    - Day 7-9: 100-125 mg po tid
    - Day 10 and maintenance: 250 mg po tid
  - Carbamazepine (Tegretol), initially 200 mg po bid; increase dosage gradually until desired response is obtained (should not exceed 120 mg/d)
- Petit mal
  - Ethosuximide (Zarontin), initially at 3-6 yr of age, 250 mg/d po; 6 yr and older, 500 mg po qd; maintenance dose, individually determined according to patient's response

General Management

Emergency equipment at bedside
Serum chemistry monitoring (complete blood count, platelet count)
Routine urinalysis
Dietary therapy (i.e., ketogenic diet)
Serum drug levels (e.g., Dilantin, phenobarbital)
Seizure precautions

NURSING CARE

Nursing Assessment

Simple Partial Seizures

Motor signs
- Involuntary recurrent contractions of muscles (e.g., face, hand, arm, finger) of one body part; may be confined to one body area or spread to contiguous ipsilateral body parts (spread of activity such as left thumb to left hand to left arm to left side of face is known as jacksonian march)

Behavioral manifestations
- Sensory: auditory or visual hallucinations; paresthesias; vertigo
- Autonomic and psychic: sensation of déjà vu; complex hallucinations; illusions; unwarranted feelings of anger or fear; pupillary dilation; sweating

Level of consciousness
- No loss of consciousness

Complex Partial Seizures

Onset
- May consist of variety of auras (e.g., sensory hallucinations, déjà vu, unusual smells)

Motor activity
- Compulsive patting or rubbing of body parts, lip smacking, walking aimlessly, swallowing, picking at clothing (termed automatisms)
- Unconscious performance of highly skilled acts

Level of consciousness
- Episodic loss of conscious contact with environment

Postictal amnesia
- Amnestic for seizure events
- May be amnestic of auras

Generalized Seizures

Petit mal
- Transient loss of consciousness for few seconds to minutes
- May be accompanied by flickering eyelids or intermittent jerking movements of hands

Grand mal
- See findings listed on pp. 271 and 272

Myoclonic
- Sudden brief contraction of muscle groups producing rapid jerky movements in one or more extremities or entire body
- May be accompanied by violent fall without loss of consciousness

Tonic
- Sudden assumption of an abnormal dystonic posture for a few seconds to minutes
- Consciousness usually retained
- Head and eyes may deviate toward one side

Infantile spasms
Brief synchronous contractions (usually flexion) of both arms, neck, and trunk
Mental retardation
Atonic "drop attacks"
Brief loss of consciousness and postural tone without associated tonic muscular contractions

Unilateral Seizures

Clonic, tonic, or tonic-clonic seizures affecting only or predominantly one side of body
May be with or without impairment in level of consciousness
Seizures may shift from one side to another (usually not symmetric)

Unclassified Seizures

Any atypical seizure activity

Nursing Dx & Intervention

Nursing Diagnosis	Nursing Intervention/Rationale
Ineffective airway clearance	• See general intervention strategies listed on p. 1702.
Ineffective breathing pattern	• See general intervention strategies listed on p. 1704.
Sensory/perceptual alterations (visual, auditory, kinesthetic, gustatory, tactile, olfactory)	• See general intervention strategies listed on p. 1728.
Potential for trauma related to seizures	• Assess and document potential for injury and strategies for prevention. • Maintain bed in low position at all times unless side rails are up or nurse is with patient. • Provide the patient with a call light within easy reach. • Maintain side rails in up position at bedtime, after sedation, when patient is confused, and as needed *to prevent accidental falls.* • Maintain wheelchairs and stretchers in locked position when transferring patient.
Preconvulsive	• Maintain seizure precautions: Have oral airway at bedside. Have suction equipment available at bedside *to prevent aspiration.* Pad side rails, if indicated. Administer oxygen per protocol *to prevent cerebral hypoxia.* Establish means of communication. Identify auras if possible.
Convulsive	• Maintain patent airway. • Support and protect head; turn to side if possible *to maintain airway.* • Prevent injury: Ease patient to floor if in chair. Place pillows along side rails if patient is in bed. Loosen constrictive clothing. • Provide privacy as necessary; stay with patient. • Note frequency, time, involved body parts, and length of seizure *to provide accurate description of seizure activity.*
Postconvulsive	• Maintain patent airway. • Suction as indicated. • Check vital signs and neurologic status. • Administer oxygen per protocol *to prevent hypoxia.* • Reorient patient to environment *to minimize sensory-perceptual alterations.* • Place patient in position of comfort, and turn head to side. • Administer oral hygiene as necessary *to remove secretions and bleeding.*
Anxiety	• See general intervention strategies listed on p. 1743.
Social isolation	• See general intervention strategies listed on p. 1767.

Patient Education

1. Instruct regarding nature of the seizure disorder and need to adopt positive attitude.
2. Stress importance of verbalizing feelings of shame, humiliation, anxiety, and fears regarding seizure disorder. Assist in clarifying common fears and myths about epilepsy (i.e., not a form of insanity).
3. Emphasize need to avoid overprotection.
4. Stress need to continue with normal work and recreation routines. Assure the patient that activity may inhibit seizure activity.
5. Emphasize need to avoid excessive stress or emotional excitement.
6. Teach importance of wearing a medical alert band or carrying a medical alert card at all times.
7. Stress importance of well-balanced diet and avoidance of excessive use of stimulants such as alcohol.
8. Emphasize importance of identifying aura and course of action to take.
9. Instruct regarding name of medication, action, side effects, dosage, and frequency of administration.
10. Stress need to avoid taking over-the-counter medications without first consulting physician.
11. Emphasize importance of ongoing outpatient care.

Evaluation

Patient Outcome	Data Indicating That Outcome is Reached
Patient demonstrates a patent airway.	Breath sounds are normal. Chest excursion is bilateral and symmetric. Rate and depth of respirations are normal. Cough is effective. There are no subjective or objective findings of shortness of breath, air hunger, or dyspnea on exertion.
Patient demonstrates an effective breathing pattern.	Airway is patent. Chest excursion is symmetric. Breath sounds are normal, or there is no increase in adventitious sounds. Arterial blood gas values are within normal ranges or consistent with patient's baseline. Vital signs are within normal ranges or consistent with patient's baseline. Hemoglobin levels are 14 to 18 g/dl (male) or 12 to 16 g/dl (female). Intake and output are stable. There are no signs of respiratory distress. All lobes are resonant on percussion.
Patient remains free of traumatic injury.	Safety measures are appropriate to physiologic status. Skin integrity is maintained. Skin is free of bruises, burns, abrasions, and redness. Environment is safe. Patient is free of nosocomial infections.
Patient demonstrates a low level of anxiety.	Patient openly verbalizes concerns and feelings of grief, loss, and discomfort. Patient openly verbalizes feelings, supported by health care professionals and family. Patient verbalizes essential aspects of care. Patient can identify methods to effectively deal with anxious feelings.
Patient demonstrates social participation.	Patient can state importance of interpersonal relationships. Patient relates to self and others. Patient participates, as possible, in unit and group activities. Patient participates, as possible, in family activities.

Medical Interventions and Related Nursing Care

Chordotomy

Description and Rationale

A chordotomy is a surgical procedure in which the lateral spinothalamic tract of the spinal cord is divided to relieve pain. The lesion is created on the contralateral side, approximately two to three spinal segments above the desired level of anesthesia, which then severs the pain pathways. If the pain is midline, the lesions must be made bilaterally. The preferred surgical technique is the *percutaneous chordotomy*.

The procedure consists of stereotactic insertion of a spinal lumbar puncture needle laterally between C1 and C2 (at the cervical level). A wire electrode then is inserted into the anterior quadrant, and a lesion is made by use of a radiofrequency generator at a designated site to destroy ascending pain fibers. The percutaneous chordotomy may be repeated if pain recurs or the level of anesthesia falls. The other method for performing a chordotomy consists of a *surgical thoracic resection approach*. Following exposure of the spinal cord, the dendate ligament is divided at the level selected for the chordotomy.

Following a chordotomy, the patient may experience an

interruption in respiratory reflex pathways causing periods of apnea or respiratory arrest, temporary paralysis, permanent loss of temperature sensation, and loss of bowel and bladder control.

Medical Plan

Surgery

Tracheotomy, if indicated
Swan-Ganz catheterization

Medications

Local anesthesia (percutaneous chordotomy)
General anesthesia
Regional anesthetic blocks (preoperatively)

General Management

Radio-frequency generator (percutaneous chordotomy)
Mechanical ventilator, if indicated (i.e., high cervical chordotomy)
Pulmonary function testing (preoperatively and postoperatively)
Cardiac monitoring
Counseling and support regarding coping effectively with diffuse pain
Occupational therapy
Physical therapy

NURSING CARE

Nursing Assessment

Pain

Discomfort at puncture or incision site

Complications

Paralysis
- Leg weakness
- Temporary paralysis

Bowel/bladder control
- Temporary (i.e., several weeks) urine retention
- Incontinence

Respiratory function
- Periods of apnea
- Respiratory arrest (with cervical chordotomy)

Sensation
- Permanent loss of temperature sensation below level of interruption
- Paresthesias
- Decreased position sense

Other
- Postural hypotension

Nursing Dx & Intervention

Nursing Diagnosis	Nursing Intervention/Rationale
Ineffective breathing pattern	• Maintain patent airway; intubation/tracheostomy and mechanical ventilation may be indicated: Suction as needed. Hyperinflate lungs with 100% oxygen for 1 minute before and 1 minute after suctioning, unless contraindicated, *to prevent hypoxemia.* • Maintain aseptic technique during suctioning *to prevent infection.* • Monitor mechanical ventilator, if used: Ensure that tidal volume, rate, mode, and oxygen concentration are set as ordered. Ensure that ventilator alarms are on and functional. • Monitor arterial blood gases as ordered: Report decrease in Po_2 of 10 to 15 mm Hg. Report increase in Pco_2 greater than 10 to 15 mm Hg. • Note respiratory rate, depth, and level of consciousness every 15 to 30 minutes and as needed. • Stay with patient in acute distress *to monitor and minimize feelings of anxiety.*
Altered spinal tissue perfusion	• Perform neurologic assessment every 1 to 2 hours and as needed: Check level of consciousness. Assess pupillary size, reaction, and equality. Check for extraocular eye movements. Note motor and sensory deficits (i.e., color and strength of extremities). Report any increase in deficits immediately to the physician. • Administer medications as ordered (e.g., steroids *to control cord edema.*) • If steroids are being administered: Check stools *to detect occult blood.* Test urine for sugar and acetone *to detect glycosuria.*

Nursing Diagnosis	Nursing Intervention/Rationale
	Administer phytonadine, MSD (Aquamephyton), intramuscularly daily or every other day *to control tendency for bleeding*. Administer antacids per protocol *to decrease or prevent gastric irritation*. • Maintain parenteral fluids as ordered. • Measure intake and output every hour. Immediately report urine output of less than 30 ml/hour.
Sensory/perceptual alterations	• See general intervention strategies listed on p. 1728.
Impaired physical mobility	• Administer skin care every 2 hours: Turn patient every 2 hours and as needed unless contraindicated: Change position slowly. Position in straight body alignment. Use log-roll technique when turning. Keep skin dry; give perineal care as needed. Massage pressure points every 2 hours *to stimulate circulation;* give gentle back rubs every shift and as needed. • Use heel and elbow guards as needed. • Use firm mattress or bed board. • Perform active or passive ROM exercises every 2 to 4 hours. • Apply antiembolus stocking to lower extremities *to prevent thrombus and embolus*. • Administer anticoagulation therapy as ordered: Monitor serum coagulation studies. Check stool *to detect occult bleeding*. Check urine *to detect occult bleeding*. Monitor for signs of thrombophlebitis and deep vein thrombosis including redness, tenderness, localized swelling, warmth, and upward red streaking on an extremity. • Monitor nutritional status. • Encourage mobility to tolerance or as ordered. • Encourage self-care activities to tolerance. • Plan all activities to avoid fatigue. Maintain planned rest periods. • Obtain physical therapy referral.

Patient Education

1. Stress need to continue with physical and occupational therapy as ordered.
2. Teach methods of avoiding injury (e.g., burns) to lower trunk and legs.
3. Teach methods and routine for inspecting lower portion of the body and feet for infection and breaks in the skin.
4. Instruct regarding care of surgical incision (with thoracic approach chordotomy).
5. Emphasize importance of ongoing outpatient care by physician.

Evaluation

Patient Outcome	Data Indicating That Outcome is Reached
Patient demonstrates a patent airway.	Breath sounds are normal. Chest excursion is bilateral and symmetric. Rate and depth of respirations are normal. Cough is effective. There are no subjective or objective findings of shortness of breath, air hunger, or dyspnea on exertion.
Patient demonstrates an effective breathing pattern.	Airway is patent. Chest excursion is symmetric. Breath sounds are normal or there is no increase in adventitious sounds. Arterial blood gas values are within normal ranges or consistent with patient's baseline. Vital signs are within normal ranges or consistent with patient's baseline. Hemoglobin levels are 14 to 18 g/dl (male) or 12 to 16 g/dl (female). Intake and output are stable. There are no signs of respiratory distress. All lobes are resonant on percussion. Skin color is not cyanotic.
Patient demonstrates adequate cerebral tissue perfusion.	Level of consciousness is unchanged. There is no evidence of further neurologic deficits. Pattern of electrolytes is stable. There is no seizure activity. Vital signs are stable.

Patient Outcome	Data Indicating That Outcome is Reached
Patient demonstrates minimum complications of sensory-perceptual alterations.	Level of orientation is optimum. The patient remains free of injury. Skin integrity is maintained. Nutritional status is adequate. Self-care deficits are minimum. Social participation is appropriate to physiologic status.
Patient remains free of traumatic injury.	Safety measures are appropriate to physiologic status. Skin integrity is maintained. Skin is free of bruises, burns, abrasions, and redness. Environment is safe. Patient is free of nosocomial infections.
Patient demonstrates an optimum level of mobility.	Skin integrity is maintained. Patient remains free of contractures and deformities. Level of mobility is appropriate to physiologic status. Intake and output pattern is stable. Nutritional status is adequate. Patient remains free of thrombophlebitis. Patient remains free of local infection. Patient participates in an ongoing physical therapy program.
Patient demonstrates minimum self-care deficits.	Outcome criteria listed for impaired physical mobility are met. Level of self-care activities is appropriate to physiologic status. Patient participates in physical and occupational therapy.
Patient demonstrates skin integrity.	Skin is intact. Nutritional status is adequate. Electrolyte balance is maintained. Patient remains free of pressure sores and contractures.
Patient experiences minimum alterations in comfort.	Patient openly verbalizes feelings of discomfort when they occur. Patient uses measures to decrease discomfort. Patient verbally validates a decrease in subjective feelings of discomfort. There is a decrease in objective findings of pain.
Patient demonstrates a low level of anxiety.	Patient openly verbalizes concerns and feelings of grief, loss, and discomfort. Patient openly verbalizes feelings, supported by health care professionals and family. Patient verbalizes essential aspects of care. Patient can identify methods to effectively deal with anxious feelings.

Craniotomy

Description and Rationale

A craniotomy is a surgical procedure in which an opening is made into the cranium for removal of a tumor, control of bleeding, or relief of intracranial pressure. A flap is created by leaving the bone attached to the muscle so that the tissue can be turned down.[16] Next the dura is incised in the opposite direction so its base is near the midline. After the surgery's purpose is accomplished, closure is done in layers (i.e., dura, muscles, fascial, galea, and scalp).[5] Craniotomies can be classified into two major categories: supratentorial and subtentorial.

Supratentorial craniotomy refers to a surgical procedure performed on the brain structures located above the tentorium for removal of space-occupying lesions in the frontal, temporal, parietal, and occipital lobes. The incision usually is made behind the hairline. *Subtentorial* craniotomy is performed to relieve the discomfort of trigeminal neuralgia and for tumor removal from the cerebellum or cerebellar-pontine angle.[31] The incision usually is made slightly above the nape of the neck.

Complications following a craniotomy can include any or all of the following: increased intracranial pressure, seizures, meningitis, respiratory distress, cardiac arrhythmias, wound infection, diabetes insipidus, thrombophlebitis, visual disturbances, personality changes, bowel or bladder dysfunction, periocular edema, motor and sensory disturbances, headache, and postoperative hydrocephalus.

If part of the cranium is removed without replacement (i.e., to provide decompression from cerebral edema), the procedure is termed a *craniectomy. Cranioplasty* is the surgical repair of a cranial defect to reestablish the integrity and normal contour of the skull. The area of cranial defect is repaired through the use of substitute bone materials (i.e., tantalum, vitallium, or plastic).

Medical Plan

Surgery

Intracranial pressure monitoring

Medications

- Corticosteroids
  - Dexamethasone (Decadron), 20-40 mg/d po (dosage gradually tapered)
- Anticonvulsants
  - Phenytoin (Dilantin), 100 mg po tid
- Stool softener
  - Docusate sodium (Colace), 100 mg po bid or tid
- Histamine-blocking agents
  - Cimetidine (Tagamet), 300 mg po qid
- Antacids
  - Magnesium hydroxide (Maalox), 30 ml po or NG qid
- Anti-infective agents
  - Organism specific

General Management

- Mechanical ventilation, if indicated
- Cardiac monitoring
- Nutritional consultation
- Physical therapy

NURSING CARE

Nursing Assessment

Focal Neurologic Disturbance

- Gradually increasing weakness
- Subtle sensory loss
- Adult-onset seizures not always relieved by medications

Mentation

- Personality changes
- Insidious decrease in mentation
- Depression
- Memory deficits
- Judgment deficits

Pain

- Headaches with steady, persistent, or intractable dull pain
- Changes in character of headaches
- Stress-induced headaches

Increased Intracranial Pressure

- Restlessness, lethargy
- Changes in level of consciousness
- Changes in vital signs (i.e., Cushing response with increased systolic blood pressure, wide pulse pressure, and decreased pulse rate)
- Pupillary changes (i.e., mydriasis)
- Impaired pupillary reflex
- Papilledema
- Vomiting
- Fluctuations in temperature
- Seizures
- Worsening of focal neurologic signs
- Changes in respiratory patterns

Seizure Activity

- Preconvulsive (preictal) stage
  - Aura: flash of light; sense of loss; fear; weakness; dizziness; peculiar taste, smell, and sounds
  - Cry or scream
  - Fall to floor
  - Loss of consciousness
  - Tachypnea
- Convulsive stage
  - Tonic: rigid body; fixed jaws; clenched fists; extended legs; cyanosis; holding breath
  - Clonic: urinary or fecal incontinence; jerking of facial muscles and extremities; biting tongue; frothing at mouth
- Postconvulsive (postictal) stage
  - Altered level of consciousness
  - Headache
  - Nausea and/or vomiting
  - Malaise
  - Muscle soreness
  - Aspiration
    - Breathing difficulty
    - Choking
    - Cyanosis
    - Decreased breath sounds
    - Tachycardia
    - Tachypnea
  - Pneumonia

Diabetes Insipidus

- Marked polyuria
- Marked polydipsia
- Anorexia
- Weight loss
- Dehydration
- Dry skin
- Poor turgor
- Headache
- General weakness
- Irritability
- Apathy
- Laboratory studies
  - Urinary specific gravity of 1.001 to 1.005
  - Electrolyte imbalance
  - Increased plasma osmolality

Other

- Periocular edema
- Thrombophlebitis

Nursing Dx & Intervention

Nursing Diagnosis	Nursing Intervention/Rationale
Ineffective airway clearance	• See general intervention strategies on p. 1702.
Ineffective breathing pattern	• See general intervention strategies on p. 1704.
Altered cerebral tissue perfusion	• Establish baseline and ongoing neurologic assessment every 15 to 30 minutes and as needed. • Assess level of consciousness and motor or sensory deficits: Cranial nerve functioning Auditory functioning Nausea and vomiting

Nursing Diagnosis	Nursing Intervention/Rationale
	Reflex status Pupillary size and reaction Behavior and personality changes Posturing spontaneously or stimuli response • Intervene to monitor and prevent increased intracranial pressure: Administer medications, treatment, and IV lines as ordered. • If steroids are being administered: Check stools *to detect occult blood* Test urine for glucose and acetone *to detect glycosuria.* Administer phytonadine, MSD (Aquamephyton) intramuscularly daily or every other day *to control tendency to bleeding.* Administer antacids per protocol *to decrease or prevent gastric irritation.* • Maintain elevation of head of bed as ordered *to facilitate venous return.* • Accurately record intake and output; monitor for imbalance. • Monitor serum and urine osmolarity *to detect onset of diabetes insipidus.* • Monitor urine specific gravity. • Administer replacement fluids per protocol. • Monitor serum electrolytes, blood count, and arterial blood gases for abnormalities. • Monitor values and waveforms of intracranial pressure line if appropriate: Maintain patency and sterility of system. Monitor effects of temperature on intracranial pressures. Correlate neurologic status with intracranial pressure values; notify physician if inconsistent. Assist with drainage of cerebrospinal fluid from the system. • Intervene to monitor and prevent seizures: Assess patient's seizure history. Institute seizure precautions: Padded tongue blade and airway at bedside Bed height at lowest level Side rails up at all times and padded *to prevent injury* Oxygen and suction equipment at bedside *to prevent hypoxia and aspiration* Emergency medications at bedside Administer anticonvulsants as ordered: Monitor effects and side effects. Monitor serum for therapeutic levels of the anticonvulsant.
Impaired skin integrity	• Maintain head elevation at 30 to 45 degrees if supratentorial approach used *to promote cerebral venous return.* • Keep head of bed flat with infratentorial approach *to prevent pressure on brainstem;* avoid neck flexion *to prevent stress on suture line.* • Check head dressing every hour and as needed. Report any new or increased drainage. Measure and mark all drainage. • Change head dressing as needed *to prevent infection.* • Maintain patency of ventricular drainage system if used. • Provide wound care every shift and as needed when head dressing is removed. • Monitor laboratory results for elevated white blood cell count.
Sensory/perceptual alterations	• Keep side rails up at all times when patient is alone. Maintain patient safety at all times. • Maintain quiet environment, reducing external stimuli to a minimum. • Reorient patient frequently to time, place, and person. Introduce yourself each time you reorient the patient. • Repeat explanations frequently and simply. • Set realistic goals. • Assist patient in judgments, perceptions, and reorientation as needed. • Have family bring in familiar objects. • Maintain planned rest periods, allowing sufficient time for REM sleep. • Use day and night lighting appropriately. • Stimulate senses of touch, taste, and position. • Support family members to understand what is happening as a result of perceptual alterations.
Potential for trauma related to seizures	• Maintain bed in low position at all times unless side rails are up or when nurse is with patient. • Provide patient with a call light within easy reach. • Use restraints judiciously. • Maintain side rails in up position at bedtime, after sedation, when patient is confused, and as needed.

Nursing Diagnosis	Nursing Intervention/Rationale
	• Maintain wheelchairs and stretchers in locked position when transferring patient. • Pad side rails if patient is overactive.
Preconvulsive	• Maintain seizure precautions: Have oral airway at bedside *to provide for adequate oxygenation.* Have suction equipment available at bedside *to prevent aspiration.* Pad side rails if indicated. Administer oxygen per protocol *to prevent cerebral hypoxia.* Establish means of communication; identify auras if possible.
Convulsive	• Maintain patent airway. • Support and protect head; turn to side if possible. • Prevent injury: Ease patient to floor if in chair. Place pillows along side rails if patient is in bed. Remove surrounding furniture. Loosen constrictive clothing. • Provide privacy as necessary *to protect patient's dignity.* • Note frequency, time, involved body parts, and length of seizure.
Postconvulsive	• Maintain patent airway. • Suction as needed, as indicated *to prevent aspiraton.* • Check vital signs and neurologic status. • Administer oxygen as ordered *to prevent hypoxia.* • Reorient patient to environment *to minimize sensory-perceptual alteration.* • Place patient in position of comfort; turn head to side. • Administer oral hygiene as necessary *for secretions and bleeding.*
Impaired physical mobility	• See general intervention strategies listed on p. 1687.
Self-care deficit	• Assist with feeding as indicated; use IV or nasogastric feedings as ordered. • Administer oral hygiene every 2 hours and as needed. • Assist with daily hygiene care as indicated *to promote self-esteem.* • Administer eye care every 2 to 4 hours if indicated. • Perform intermittent urinary catheterization as ordered.
Pain	• Promote rest and relaxation. • Modify anxiety associated with the pain experience. • Provide other sensory input. • Remain with patient. • Improve effectiveness of pain relief measures by using them before the pain becomes intense. • For patients receiving radiation or chemotherapy: Explain procedure or medication before implementing. Administer antiemetics and antidiarrheal medications as needed. Provide frequent skin care. Provide frequent mouth care *to promote comfort.* Monitor patient's laboratory values for depressed red blood cells, white blood cells, or platelets. Report to physician. Maintain planned rest periods. Offer frequent, small feedings *to combat anorexia and discomfort of nausea.*
Body image, self-esteem, and personal identity disturbances	• See general intervention strategies listed on pp. 1751, 1754, and 1756.

Patient Education

1. Involve family in care, as possible; teach essential aspects of care.
2. Reinforce physician's explanation of medical management.
3. Emphasize the importance of ongoing outpatient care and follow-up visits.
4. Encourage independent activities, as possible:
   a. Alert the patient to limitations.
   b. Avoid overprotection.
   c. Stress need for supportive devices as indicated.
5. Explain the need for regular exercise program. Teach ROM exercises to family.
6. Teach the importance of diet as ordered:
   a. Offer supplemental feedings.
   b. Offer small portions; instruct the patient to chew slowly.

7. Teach the importance of safety measures: side rails, ramps, shower chairs, removal of scatter rugs, walker, and canes.
8. Explain name of medication, dosage, time of administration, and toxic or side effects.
9. Explain need to avoid over-the-counter medications without first consulting physician.
10. Encourage socialization with friends and family.
11. Teach the importance of verbalization of feelings about anxiety, fear, and body image changes.
12. Teach the patient and family about seizures (i.e., safety measures and who to contact).

Evaluation

Patient Outcome	Data Indicating That Outcome is Reached
Patient's airway is patent.	Breath sounds are normal. Chest excursion is bilateral and symmetric. Rate and depth of respirations are normal. Cough is effective. There are no subjective or objective findings of shortness of breath, air hunger, or dyspnea on exertion.
Patient's breathing pattern is effective.	Airway remains patent. Chest excursion is symmetric. Breath sounds are normal, or there is no increase in adventitious sounds. Arterial blood gas values are within normal ranges or consistent with patient's baseline. Vital signs are within normal ranges or consistent with patient's baseline. Hemoglobin levels are 14 to 18 g/dl (male) or 12 to 16 g/dl (female). Intake and output are stable. There are no signs of respiratory distress. All lobes are resonant on percussion. Skin color is not cyanotic.
Cerebral tissue perfusion is adequate.	Level of consciousness is unchanged. There is no evidence of neurologic deficits. Pattern of electrolytes is stable. There is no seizure activity.
Patient experiences minimum complications of sensory-perceptual alterations.	Patient maintains an optimum level of orientation. Patient remains free of injury. Skin integrity is maintained. Nutritional status is adequate. Self-care deficits are minimum. Social participation is appropriate to physiologic status.
Patient remains free of traumatic injury.	Safety measures are appropriate to level of physiologic status. Skin integrity is maintained. Skin is free of bruises, burns, abrasions, and redness. Environment is safe. Patient is free of nosocomial infections.
Patient's level of mobility is optimum.	Skin integrity is maintained. Patient remains free of contractures and deformities. Level of mobility is appropriate to physiologic status. Intake and output pattern is stable. Nutritional status is adequate. Patient remains free of thrombophlebitis. Patient remains free of local infection. Patient participates in an ongoing physical therapy program.
Self-care deficits are minimum.	Criteria listed for impaired physical mobility are met. Level of self-care activities is appropriate to physiologic status. Patient participates in physical and occupational therapy.
Alterations in comfort are minimum.	Patient openly verbalizes feelings of discomfort when they occur. Patient can use measures to decrease discomfort. Patient verbally validates a decrease in subjective feelings of discomfort. There is a decrease in objective findings of pain.
Patient maintains intact self-concepts.	Patient openly verbalizes feelings of grief and loss. Patient verbalizes positive feelings about self. Patient acknowledges actual change in self-image. Patient focuses on present and future appearance and function. Patient verbalizes feelings of hopefulness, helpfulness, and powerfulness.

 Intracranial Pressure Monitoring

Description and Rationale

Intracranial pressure (ICP) monitoring devices now make it possible to reliably measure the parameters of intracranial dynamics such as volume-pressure relationships, pressure waves, and cerebral perfusion pressures. Indications for intracranial pressure monitoring include any of the following: head trauma; cerebral hemorrhage; massive brain lesions; encephalitis; congenital hydrocephalus; hydrocephalus resulting in an alteration of cerebrospinal fluid production or absorption; and symptoms of increased intracranial pressure such as change in level of consciousness, headache, vomiting, or deterioration in respiratory status and motor function.[30] Intracranial pressure can be measured continuously via three basic monitoring systems: the ventricular catheter, the subarachnoid bolt, and the epidural sensor (Figure 3-24).

The *ventricular* catheter consists of a cannula that is implanted, via burr holes, into the anterior horn of the lateral ventricle of the nondominant cerebral hemisphere. The catheter then is connected by pressure-resistant, fluid-filled tubing

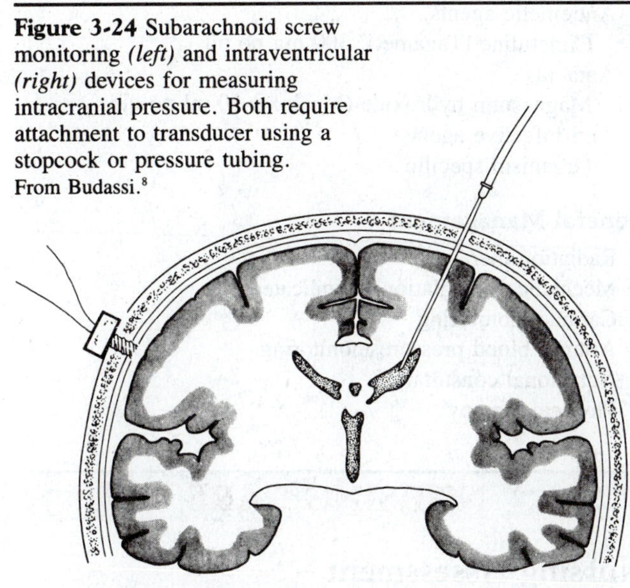

Figure 3-24 Subarachnoid screw monitoring *(left)* and intraventricular *(right)* devices for measuring intracranial pressure. Both require attachment to transducer using a stopcock or pressure tubing.
From Budassi.[8]

to a transducer and recording instrument.[16] (NOTE: Continuous flushing devices are not used for intracranial pressure measurement.) The transducer is positioned so the dome is at the level of the foramen of Monro. The external anatomic landmarks for this position are the tragus of the ear or the edge of the brow. An error of approximately 2 torr exists for each inch of discrepancy between the level of the transducer and the pressure source.

Advantages of the ventricular catheter include accurate measurement of intracranial pressure; instillation of a contrast medium; evaluation of pressure/volume responses; and ability to drain large amounts of cerebrospinal fluid, if needed.

Disadvantages of the ventricular catheter are that catheter placement may be difficult if the lateral ventricle is displaced, swollen, or collapsed; the catheter is the most invasive type of monitoring and can provide another route for infection; excessive cerebrospinal fluid drainage can occur if stopcock is not positioned properly; brain tissue or blood may occlude the catheter; false pressure readings may occur if the ventricle collapses and compresses the catheter; and frequent recalibration of the transducer and monitor is necessary for accurate readings.

The *subarachnoid bolt* method of intracranial pressure measurement began in the early 1970s. The device consists of a metal screw with a sensor tip that is inserted through a twist drill hole into the subdural or subarachnoid space. Although the cerebrum is not penetrated, the intracranial pressure is measured directly from the cerebrospinal fluid. The bolt is connected to a transducer and recording device via pressure-resistant, fluid-filled tubing. Here, as with the intraventricular catheter, continuous flushing devices are contraindicated. Indications for use of the subarachnoid bolt are to provide a means to measure and monitor intracranial pressure and to provide access for sampling of the cerebrospinal fluid.

Advantages of the bolt are that intracranial pressure is measured directly and accurately from cerebrospinal fluid; it provides access for cerebrospinal fluid sampling and drainage; it provides access for volume-pressure responses; and it can be placed quickly without penetrating the cerebrum.

Disadvantages of the bolt are that it may become occluded with tissue or blood; the infection rate is comparable to that of the ventricular catheter; it requires a closed skull; and frequent recalibration of the transducer and monitor is necessary for accurate readings.

The *epidural sensor* consists of placement of a fiber-optic sensor, radio transmitter, or tiny balloon with radioisotopes in the epidural space through a burr hole in the skull. The sensor cable then plugs directly into the monitor.

Advantages of the sensor are that it is less invasive; it can be easily placed; and it cannot become occluded.

Figure 3-25 Intracranial pressure waves. Composite drawing of A (plateau) waves, B waves, and C waves.

Reprinted by permission from Holloway, N.M.: Nursing the critically ill adult, p. 521. Copyright © 1979 by Addison-Wesley Publishing Co., Inc.

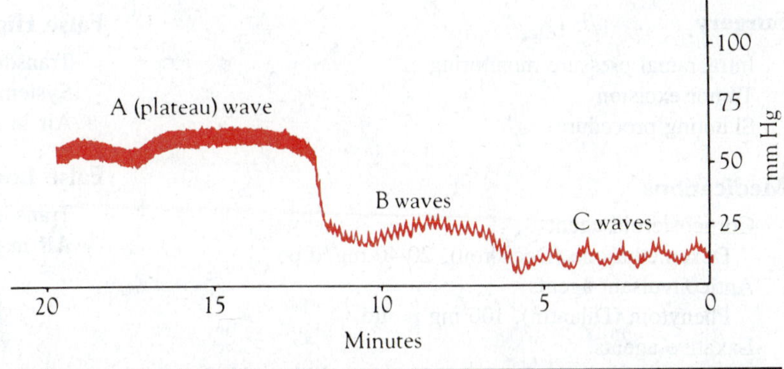

The major disadvantage of the sensor is its questionable reliability. Other disadvantages are that the system cannot be recalibrated if the sensor is affected by pressure or heat; cerebrospinal fluid sampling and drainage are not possible; and volume/pressure responses cannot be evaluated.

Pressure waves. Intracranial pressure's dynamic state is reflected by the pressure waves produced. These waveforms are most commonly known as A-waves, B-waves, and C-waves (Figure 3-25).

A-waves (or plateau waves), which occur at variable intervals, are spontaneous, rapid increases in pressure between 50 to 200 torr. Plateau waves usually occur in patients with moderate intracranial pressure elevations and last 5 to 20 minutes, falling spontaneously. Factors that can trigger plateau waves include REM sleep, emotional stimuli, isometric muscle contractions, the rebound phase of the Valsalva maneuver, hypercapnia, hypoxemia, sustained coughing and sneezing, arousal from sleep, and certain positions such as neck flexion or extreme hip flexion. A-waves are known to cause cerebral ischemia and brain damage and can produce paroxysmal or transient symptoms of change in level of consciousness, headache, nausea and vomiting, altered motor function, abnormal pupillary reactions, changes in vital signs (i.e., increased blood pressure, widened pulse pressure, and decreased pulse rate), and respiratory patterns (i.e., ataxic breathing and central neurogenic hyperventilation).[16] Because of the ischemia and previously stated symptoms, A-waves are the most clinically significant intracranial pressure waveforms and require immediate intervention to prevent further brain injury.

B-waves appear as sharp, rhythmic, sawtooth waves that occur every ½ to 2 minutes and have pressures up to 50 torr. B-waves correlate to changes in respiration, such as Cheyne-Stokes respirations. B-waves can also occur in patients with normal intracranial pressure.

C-waves are small, rapid, rhythmic waves that occur at a rate of approximately 4 to 8 per minute and increase pressures up to 20 torr. C-waves are also called Traube-Herring-Mayer waves. These waveforms correspond to normal changes in the systemic arterial pressure and are not clinically significant.

Medical Plan

Surgery

Intracranial pressure monitoring
Tumor excision
Shunting procedure

Medications

Corticosteroid agents
  Dexamethasone (Decadron), 20-40 mg/d po
Anticonvulsant agents
  Phenytoin (Dilantin), 100 mg po tid
Laxative agents
  Docusate sodium (Colace), 100 mg po bid or tid
Antiemetic agents
  Cimetidine (Tagamet), 300 mg po tid
Antacids
  Magnesium hydroxide (Maalox), 30 ml po qid
Anti-infective agents
  Organism specific

General Management

Radiation therapy
Mechanical ventilation, if indicated
Cardiac monitoring
Arterial blood pressure monitoring
Nutritional consultation
Physical therapy

NURSING CARE

Nursing Assessment

The reader is referred to the appropriate disorder for specific physical assessment findings.

Loss of Intracranial Pressure Waveform

Transducer may be incorrectly connected
Monitoring device could be occluded
Air may be between pressure source and transducer diaphragm

Low Intracranial Pressure

Cerebral ventricles may have collapsed
Transducer may have been incorrectly zeroed and calibrated

High Intracranial Pressure

Excessive activity
Body posture with neck or extreme hip flexion
Use of positive end-expiratory pressure (PEEP)
Hyperthermia
Respiratory distress
Fluid and electrolyte imbalances
Infection
Blood pressure changes

False High Intracranial Pressure

Transducer too low or incorrectly balanced
System incorrectly calibrated
Air in system

False Low Intracranial Pressure

Transducer too high
Air in system

Nursing Dx & Intervention

Nursing Diagnosis	Nursing Intervention/Rationale
Altered cerebral tissue perfusion	• Maintain sterility of the intracranial pressure monitoring equipment: Maintain strict sterile technique *to prevent infection.* Change equipment (i.e., tubing) daily or as ordered. • Maintain patency of intracranial pressure monitoring device: Keep all stopcock ports capped *to keep system closed to air.* *Never* flush the system. Observe for cerebrospinal fluid leaks and blood in the tubing. • Obtain accurate pressure measurements: Place patient in baseline position. Obtain measurements when patient is at rest—not when moving, coughing, sneezing, etc. Level the transducer. Recalibrate the transducer according to the manufacturer's instructions. Obtain measurements and record. Report significant changes in intracranial pressure to physician immediately.

Evaluation

Patient Outcome	Data Indicating That Outcome is Reached
Patient maintains adequate cerebral tissue perfusion.	Level of consciousness is unchanged. There is no evidence of neurologic deficits. Pattern of electrolytes is stable. There is no seizure activity. Vital signs are stable.

References

1. Anthony CP and Kolthoff NJ: Textbook of anatomy and physiology, ed 9, St Louis, 1975, The CV Mosby Co.
2. Anthony CP and Thibodeau GA: Textbook of anatomy and physiology, ed 10, St Louis, 1979, The CV Mosby Co.
3. Anthony CP and Thibodeau GA: Structure and function of the body, ed 7, St Louis, 1984, The CV Mosby Co.
4. Baker AB, editor: Clinical neurology, ed 2, New York, 1983, Harper & Row, Publishers, Inc.
5. Bates B: A guide to physical assessment, ed 3, Philadelphia, 1983, JB Lippincott Co.
6. Blass J: Alzheimer's disease, DM 31:4, 1985.
7. Braunwald E et al, editors: Harrison's principles of internal medicine, ed 11, New York, 1983, McGraw-Hill Book Co.
8. Budassi SA and Barber JM: Emergency nursing: principles and practice, St Louis, 1981, The CV Mosby Co.
9. Burns KR and Johnson PJ: Health assessment in clinical practice, Englewood Cliffs, NJ, 1980, Prentice-Hall, Inc.
10. Burrell O and Burrell ZL Jr: Critical care, ed 4, St Louis, 1982, The CV Mosby Co.
11. Cahill M: Diagnostics, ed 2, Springhouse, Penn, 1986, Springhouse Corp.
12. Caird FI and Judge TG: Assessment of the elderly patient, ed 3, California, 1977, Pitman Medical Publishing Corp.
13. Carnevali DL and Patrick M: Nursing management for the elderly, Philadelphia, 1979, JB Lippincott Co.
14. Carotenuto R and Bullock J: Physical assessment of the gerontologic client, Philadelphia, 1980, FA Davis Co.
15. Conn HF and Conn RB Jr: Current diagnosis, Philadelphia, 1980, WB Saunders Co.
16. Conway-Rutkowski, BL: Carini and Owens' neurological and neurosurgical nursing, ed 8, St Louis, 1982, The CV Mosby Co.
17. Crowell RM and Zervas NT: Management of intracranial aneurysm, Med Clin North Am 63:695, 1979.
18. Davis GT and Hill PM: Cerebral palsy, Nurs Clin North Am 15:35, 1980.
19. Davis JE and Mason CB: Neurologic critical care, New York, 1979, Van Nostrand Reinhold Co.
20. Demyer W: Technique of the neurologic examination: a programmed text, ed 3, New York, 1980, McGraw-Hill Book Co.
21. DeYoung S: The neurologic patient: a nursing perspective, Englewood Cliffs, NJ, 1983, Prentice-Hall, Inc.
22. Dietsche L and Pollman J: Alzheimer's disease: advances in clinical nursing, J Gerontol Nurs 8:2, 1982.
23. Eliasson SG et al, editors: Neurological pathophysiology, ed 2, New York, 1978, Oxford University Press.
24. Escourolle R and Poirier J: Manual of basic neuropathology, ed 2, Philadelphia, 1978, WB Saunders Co.
25. Geffner ES, editor: Compendium of drug therapy, New York, 1983, Biomedical Information Corp.
26. Go KG et al: Interpretation of nuclear magnetic resonance tomograms of the brain, J Neurosurg 59:574, 1983.
27. Groer MW and Shekleton ME: Basic pathophysiology: a conceptual approach, ed 2, St Louis, 1983, The CV Mosby Co.
28. Grundy JH: Assessment of the child in primary health care, New York, 1981, McGraw-Hill Book Co.
29. Guyton A: Textbook of medical physiology, ed 5, Philadelphia, 1976, WB Saunders Co.
30. Hazinski MF: Nursing care of the critically ill child, St Louis, 1984, The CV Mosby Co.
31. Hickey J: The clinical practice of neurological and neurosurgical nursing, Philadelphia, 1981, JB Lippincott Co.
32. Hickey J: The clinical practice of neurological and neurosurgical nursing, Philadelphia, 1986, JB Lippincott Co.
33. Hudak CM et al: Critical care nursing, ed 3, Philadelphia, 1982, JB Lippincott Co.
34. Jensen D: The principles of physiology, ed 2, New York, 1982, Appleton-Century-Crofts.
35. Kaye D and Rose LF: Fundamentals of internal medicine, St Louis, 1982, The CV Mosby Co.
36. Kim MJ, McFarland GK, and McLane AM, editors: Pocket guide to nursing diagnosis, ed 2, St Louis, 1987, The CV Mosby Co.
37. Kinney MR, editor: AACN's clinical reference for critical-care nursing, New York, 1981, McGraw-Hill Book Co.
38. Kintzel K, editor: Advanced concepts in clinical nursing, ed 2, Philadelphia, 1977, JB Lippincott Co.
39. Leech RW and Shuman RM: Neuropathology: a summary for students, New York, 1982, Harper & Row, Publishers, Inc.
40. Malasanos L et al: Health assessment, ed 2, St Louis, 1981, The CV Mosby Co.

41. McElroy DB: Hydrocephalus in children, Nurs Clin North Am 15:23, 1980.
42. Merrit HH: A textbook of neurology, ed 6, Philadelphia, 1979, Lea & Febiger.
43. Nikas DL, editor: The critically ill neurosurgical patient: contemporary issues in critical care nursing, vol 3, New York, 1982, Churchill Livingstone, Inc.
44. Passo S: Malformations of the neural tube, Nurs Clin North Am 15:5, 1980.
45. Petersdorf RG, editor: Harrison's principles of internal medicine, ed 10, New York, 1983, McGraw-Hill Book Co.
46. Phipps WJ, Long BC, and Woods NF: Shafer's medical-surgical nursing, ed 7, St Louis, 1980, The CV Mosby Co.
47. Pluckhan M: Alzheimer's disease: helping the patient's family, Nursing 86, Nov 1986.
48. Price SA and Wilson LM: Pathophysiology: clinical concepts of disease processes, ed 2, New York, 1982, McGraw-Hill Book Co.
49. Ramirez B: When you're faced with neuro patients, RN 42:67, 1979.
50. Robbins SL and Cotran RS: Pathologic basis of disease, ed 2, Philadelphia, 1977, WB Saunders Co.
51. Robinson J, editor: Coping with neurologic problems proficiently, Nursing Skillbook Series, Springhouse, Penn, 1982, Intermed Communications, Inc.
52. Rudy EB: Advanced neurological and neurosurgical nursing, St Louis, 1984, The CV Mosby Co.
53. Schottelius BA and Schottelius DD: Textbook of physiology, ed 18, St Louis, 1978, The CV Mosby Co.
54. Selzer P: Understanding NMR imaging with the aid of a simple mechanical model, Med Times 114:1, 1986.
55. Smith LH and Thier SO: Pathophysiology: the biological principles of disease, Philadelphia, 1981, WB Saunders Co.
56. Steinberg, FU: Cowdry's the care of the geriatric patient, ed 5, St Louis, 1976, The CV Mosby Co.
57. Stub RL and Black FW: The mental status examination in neurology, Philadelphia, 1977, FA Davis Co.
58. Swaiman KF and Wright FS: The practice of pediatric neurology, ed 2, St Louis, 1982, The CV Mosby Co.
59. Taylor JW and Ballinger S: Neurological dysfunctions and nursing interventions, New York, 1980, McGraw-Hill Book Co.
60. Thibodeau GA: Anatomy and physiology, St Louis, 1987, The CV Mosby Co.
61. Thompson JM and Bowers AC: Clinical manual of health assessment, St Louis, 1980, The CV Mosby Co.
62. Tucker SM et al: Patient care standards, ed 3, St Louis, 1984, The CV Mosby Co.
63. Urdang L, editor: Mosby's medical and nursing dictionary, St Louis, 1983, The CV Mosby Co.
64. Urosevich PR: Coping with neurologic disorders, Nursing Photobook Series, Springhouse, Penn, 1981, Intermed Communications, Inc.
65. Walleck C: Head trauma in children, Nurs Clin North Am 15:115, 1980.
66. Whaley LF and Wong DL: Nursing care of infants and children, ed 2, St Louis, 1983, The CV Mosby Co.
67. Williams L: Alzheimer's: the need for caring, J Gerontol Nurs 12:2, 1986.
68. Wyngaarden JB and Smith LH, editors: Cecil's textbook of medicine, Philadelphia, 1985, WB Saunders Co.

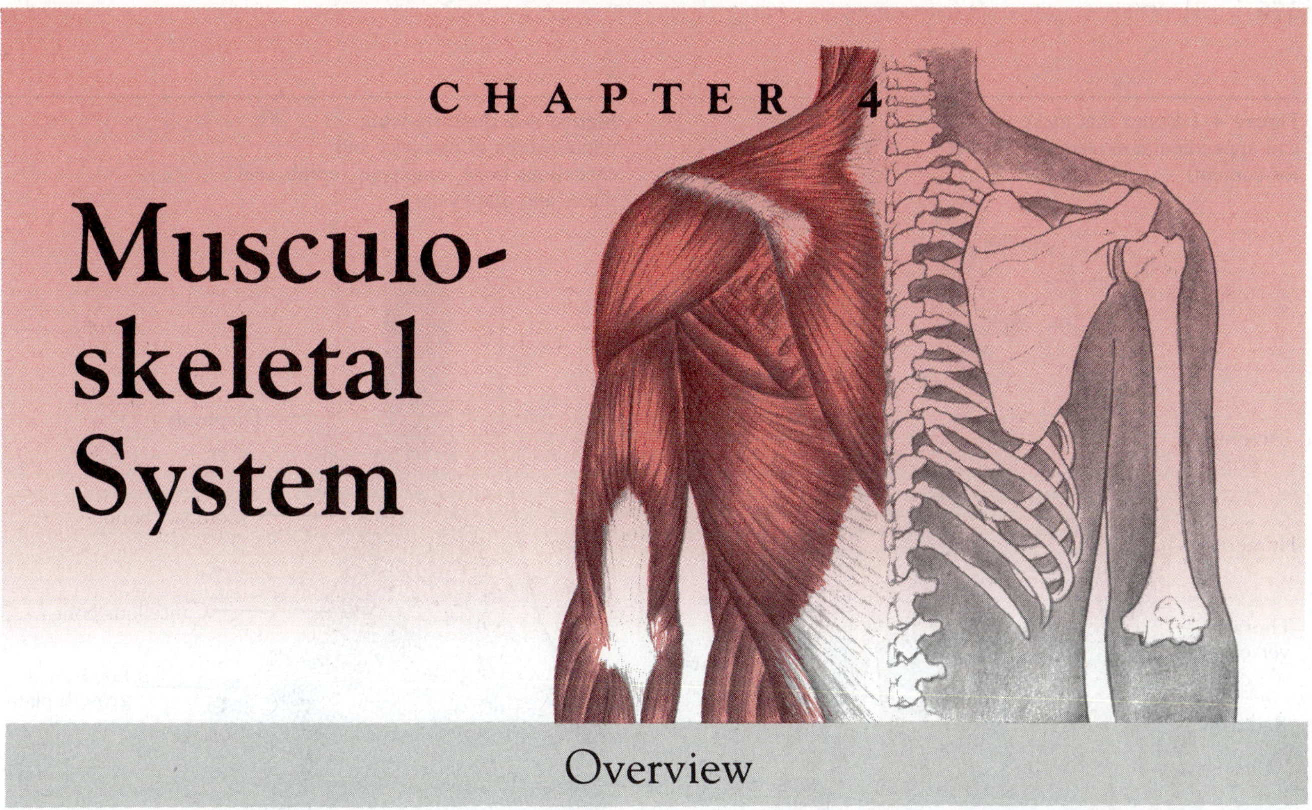

CHAPTER 4

Musculoskeletal System

Overview

The tissues of the musculoskeletal system are the framework for the rest of the body and provide the means for easy, comfortable movement. Because of their many important structures and functions, they greatly affect the body's general health when they are inflamed, injured, or anomalous. Musculoskeletal anomalies and birth injuries affect newborns and lead to disability in growth, development, and productivity throughout life. Injuries from sports or physical fitness activities are major factors in the health of young to middle-aged adults. Formerly, most musculoskeletal injuries occurred in men, but with more women participating in sports and physical fitness programs, the gender gap is narrowing. Trauma, primarily from automobile accidents, is the number one cause of death among people aged 16 to 24 years. Inflammatory, rheumatic, and degenerative diseases of the musculoskeletal tissues are significant causes of death among young adults and account for a large portion of the illness and disability of middle-aged and elderly adults. Billions of dollars are spent yearly for care and treatment of people of all ages with musculoskeletal conditions. The economic cost is a major health care problem.

Anatomy, Physiology, and Related Pathophysiology

Skeleton

According to Wolff's law, the 206 bones of the skeleton are shaped according to their function. They may be long (arm or leg), short (wrist or ankle), flat (sternum or scapula), irregular (vertebrae), or rounded (patella). The skull, face and auditory ossicles, vertebrae, ribs, sternum, and hyoid bone make up the axial skeleton; the appendicular skeleton consists of the bones in the upper and lower extremities, shoulders, and pelvis (Figure 4-1).

Bones support the body, enabling it to stand erect; protect internal organs and other soft tissues; assist movement by leverage and in coordination with muscles; make blood cells within the red bone marrow; and provide for storage of minerals, particularly calcium and phosphorus.

Structure of bone tissue. Long bones of the extremities and thorax consist of a long shaft, the diaphysis, and two ends, the epiphyses. The epiphyses are covered with articular cartilage and are separated from the shaft by the growth plate and nutrient arteries of the metaphysis (Figure 4-2). The outer surface (cortex) of a bone is hard, dense tissue called compact bone. Approximately 99% of the calcium in the body is contained in bone, with the remainder circulating in the blood plasma and interstitial fluid. The ends of long bones, the flat bones, and the ridges or crests of the ilium and tibia contain cancellous bone, which is soft and spongy and has cavities containing the red bone marrow for hematopoiesis. Red bone marrow depletions are replaced by fat cells of the yellow bone marrow, which is found in the shafts of long bones.

The periosteum is the tough outer membrane of connective tissue that covers each bone and provides protection and nutrition. Blood vessels in the inner layer of the periosteum bring nutrients and remove wastes. The periosteal blood vessels communicate with vessels in the central canal of the haversian system, which is the microscopic unit of compact bone.

The haversian system contains layers or plates of compact

Figure 4-1 Bones that make up axial and appendicular skeletons (see text for content).

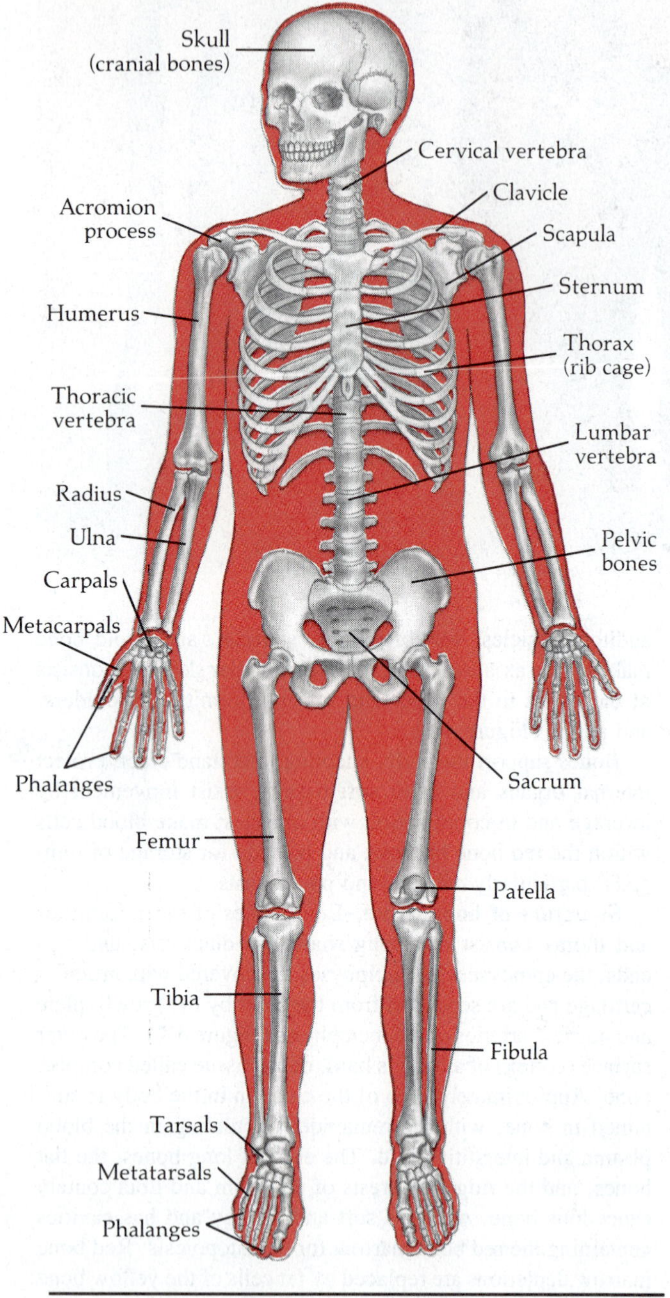

Figure 4-2 Bone showing relationships of compact and cancellous bone, epiphysis, epiphyseal plate, and diaphysis.

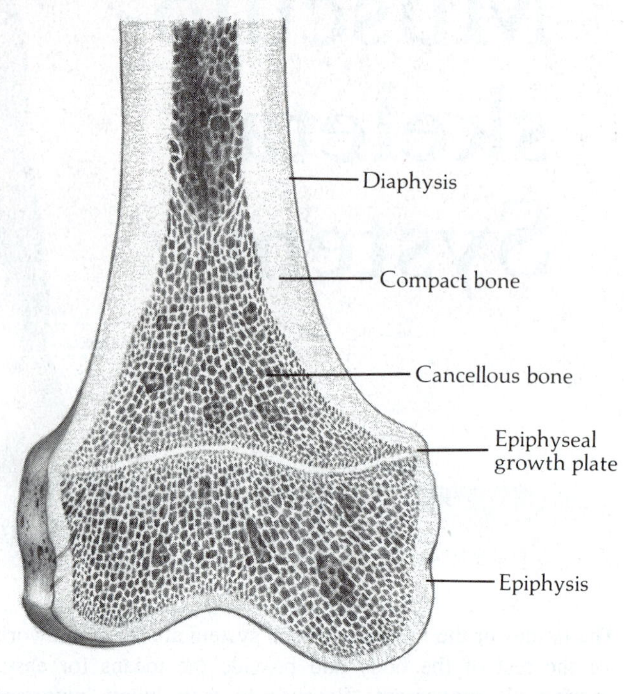

bone cells called lamellae. These lamellae surround the haversian canal, which contains two blood vessels and a nerve. The lamellae are aligned parallel to the shaft of the bone and encompass the lacunae, which are small cavities filled with bone cells and tissue fluids. The lacunae are connected to the blood vessels in the haversian canal by smaller canals, the canaliculi (Figure 4-3). The haversian canal provides nutrients to osteocytes for bone building and removes wastes and debris from bone growth and resorption. Osteocytes, the major bone-forming cells, develop from osteoblasts, which are spindle-shaped cells found beneath the periosteum and in the inner region of bones, the endosteum. Osteoblasts remain dormant until needed for bone growth, when they mature into osteocytes. A third type of cell, the osteoclast, also is needed for shaping and remodeling bone. It is used for resorption of unneeded or necrotic bone cells.

Bones are in a constant process of resorption counterbalanced by new bone formation. This process prevents bones from becoming excessively thick or heavy from new bone formation or from becoming thinner or weakened from resorption. The formation and resorption process is related to calcium and phosphate levels and metabolism in the body.

Extracellular calcium and phosphate concentrations are regulated by secretions of parathyroid hormone from the parathyroid glands, by absorption in the intestinal tract, and by retention or excretion by the kidneys so that relatively stable concentrations are maintained. Low calcium levels stimulate parathyroid hormone production, which stimulates osteoclasts to break down bone structure. The breakdown of bone frees calcium phosphate crystals to be available to increase serum

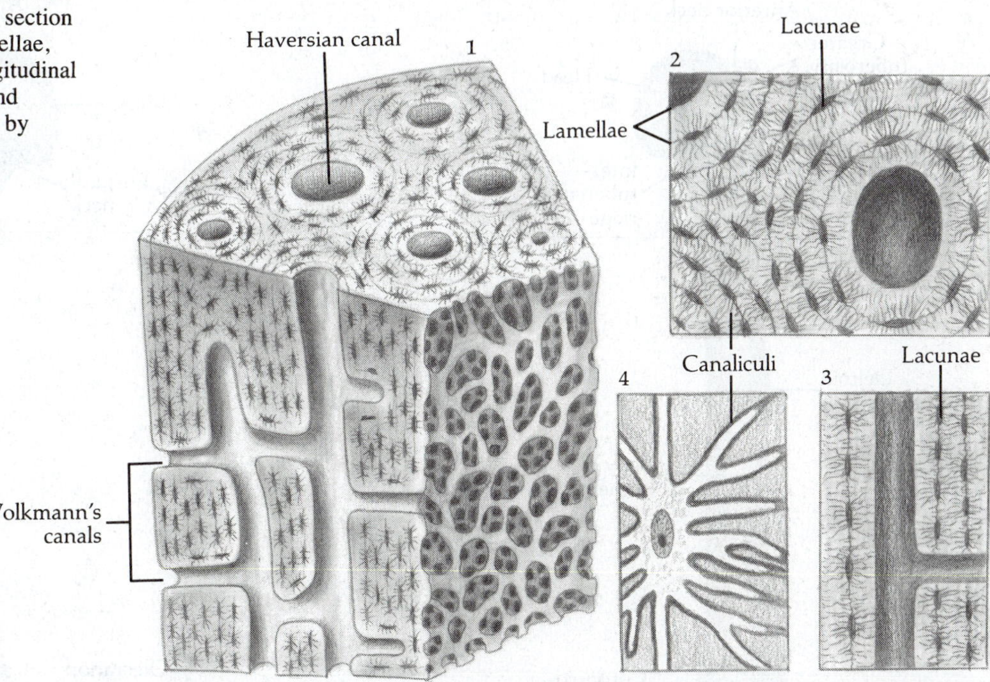

Figure 4-3 *1*, Three-dimensional view of compact bone; *2*, transverse section of compact bone depicting lamellae, lacunae, and canaliculi; *3*, longitudinal section of bone with lacunae and canaliculi; *4*, lacunae occupied by osteocyte.

calcium concentrations. The gastrointestinal ion transport system absorbs calcium and moves the ion from the gut lumen to the blood. Resorption of calcium increases in the renal tubules to raise serum calcium levels, which concurrently reduces the resorption of phosphate. Through these processes, calcium levels remain relatively constant in healthy people, and bone remains strong with relatively stable calcium concentration through formation and resorption.

Bone strength, formation, and resorption are affected by the amount and metabolism of vitamin D, which facilitates the absorption of calcium and phosphorus from the intestine. A deficiency of either vitamin D or sunshine (needed to activate sterol precursors to vitamin D in the skin) will cause changes in bones, known as rickets in children and osteomalacia in adults. Osteomalacia is discussed on p. 414.

The skeleton begins to develop from mesenchymal cells in the first prenatal month and is completely formed by the third month. Bones form through two basic processes: intramembranous and endochondral formation. In both processes, the first stage involves formation of cancellous or spongy bone tissue, which later becomes compact bone through deposition of bone matrix. The bone matrix then becomes calcified. Bone formation occurs where blood vessels supply minerals, oxygen, and nutrients. Where cancellous bone tissues predominate, the blood vessels are transformed into hemopoietic cells.[26]

In intramembranous bone formation, mesenchymal cells differentiate into osteoblasts. The osteoblasts align themselves into a preliminary framework of osteoid tissue containing large endoplasmic reticulum and are surrounded by a bone matrix; they are then called osteocytes. Although the newly formed bones are derived from type I collagen (see p. 388 for collagen types), the major form of collagen in the bone matrix is type III. Calcification of the osteoid tissues depends on the supply of minerals and nutrients from the adjacent capillaries. Mineral deposits align into the bone trabeculae, which become surrounded by lamellae. The lamellae eventually replace the initial trabeculae with lamellar compact bone. The bones of the skull and other flat bones are formed through intramembranous pathways.

Bones formed endochondrally develop within a preformed cartilage framework. The cartilage is gradually resorbed as the bones develop through the activity of osteoblasts. All long bones are formed from endochondral tissues and ossify from the center in the middle of the diaphysis. The chondrocytes align themselves in long, parallel columns, hypertrophy, and eventually die while initiating the synthesis of type I collagen laid down on the inner sides of their lacunae. As the lacunae enlarge, their intervening matrix decreases in quantity and becomes irregularly calcified. At the same time, intramembranous bone formation begins at the periphery of the diaphysis and is mediated through cells of type I and type III collagen molecules. The collagen molecules eventually transform this portion of the bone into the periosteum. The remaining cartilaginous mold cells are resorbed. The type III collagen molecules infiltrate the newly formed bone trabec-

Figure 4-4 **A**, Anterior and, **B**, posterior views of right humerus. **C**, Anterior and, **D**, posterior views of right femur.

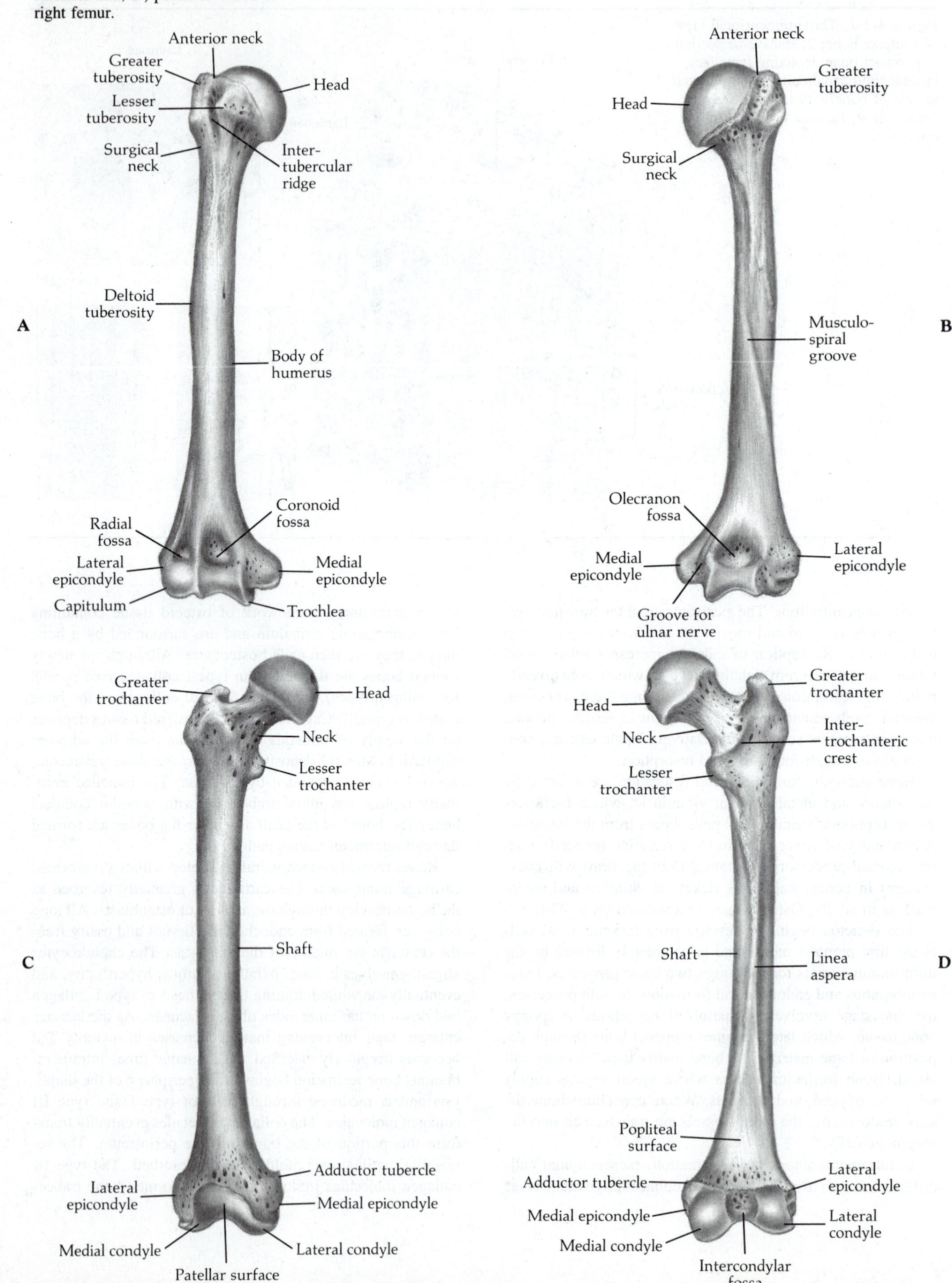

ulae and extend the mineralization and ossification toward both ends of the bone. After birth, secondary centers for ossification develop in the epiphyseal regions. The cartilage that remains in this region becomes the epiphyseal plate. The growth or proliferation of the columnar cartilage cells in this region results in the increased length of bones as the body grows. When the bone has reached its final size, these growth zones are resorbed and replaced by bone. As the bone grows longer, its outer diameter increases slightly. The volume in the bone marrow cavity also increases. New bone is continuously deposited on the outer surfaces with resorption from the inner surfaces, until the final bone shape is achieved. The shape of each bone maximizes its load-bearing ability and minimizes its mass or weight. Bone growth and ossification generally continue longitudinally until 15 years of age in girls and 16 years of age in boys. Bone maturation and shaping, however, continue until 21 years in both sexes and are so regular that a person's age can be fairly accurately determined by x-ray examination of the bones.

As shown in Figure 4-4, many processes (prominences) project outward from the surfaces of bones. Tendons or ligaments attach themselves to the bones at these processes. Bony prominences may be rounded and knucklelike (condyles); small, rounded projections (tubercles); large processes (trochanters); or narrow ridges or crests (frontal bone and iliac crests). Projections may be transverse (transverse processes of vertebrae and ear), or they may project posteriorly (posterior spinous processes) or anteriorly (nasal cartilages). Bones also contain alveoli (sockets), fossae (depressions), fissures (narrow slits), foramina (openings for nerves, muscles, and blood vessels), sinuses (cavities), and sulci (grooves).

Muscles

Muscle contraction. Muscles move the body through tightening and shortening of their fibers (contraction) brought about through the motor unit. Each motor unit has 100 to 200 muscle fibers innervated by a single motor nerve axon that stimulates the motor unit and sends the contraction through the muscle body. The muscle responds either entirely or not at all to the stimulus. The strength of the muscle contraction is determined by the number of motor units contracting and by the number of times per second each motor unit is stimulated. A stimulus strong enough to bring about contraction is called a liminal stimulus; a less intense stimulus is called subliminal. A phenomenon known as treppe occurs when a second stimulus takes place at the apex of a preceding one. The additive effects of the rapid subliminal stimuli increase the strength of the contraction.

Muscle contraction results from a series of interactions at the myoneural junction in the muscle tissue. The stimulus travels along the motor nerve to the motor end-plate (myo-

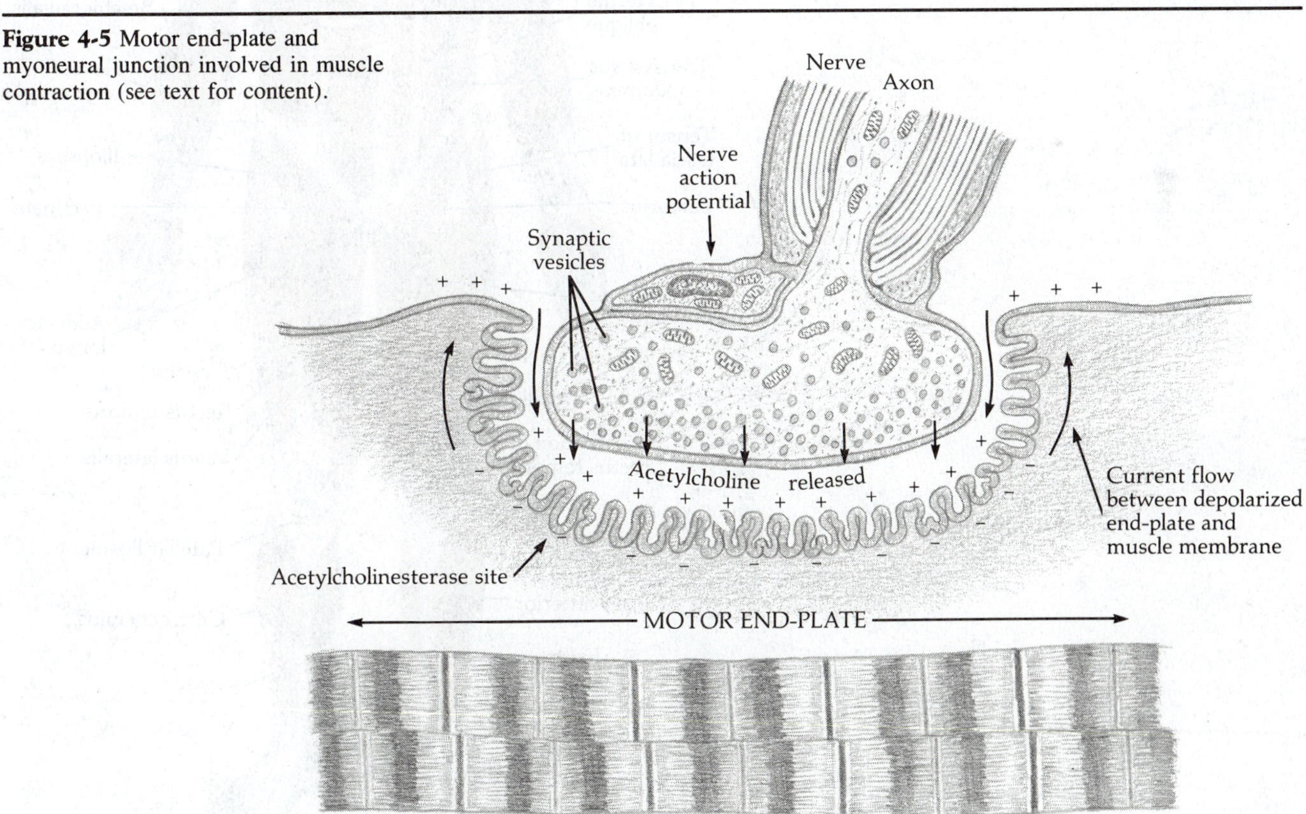

Figure 4-5 Motor end-plate and myoneural junction involved in muscle contraction (see text for content).

neural junction) of the muscle fiber. Acetylcholine is produced at this synapse (junction) and released. It causes the muscle to contract by depolarizing the sarcolemma. Depolarization permits interstitial calcium ions to enter the muscle membrane to aid the contraction. The wave of depolarization travels through the muscle fiber until it is deactivated by the enzyme acetylcholinesterase. The fiber is then ready for reactivation. The positive calcium ions catalyze an energy-releasing reaction to cause the actin to slide along the myosin, which results in contraction and shortening of the muscle (Figure 4-5).

The energy for muscle contraction comes from the hydrolysis of ATP into ADP + phosphate + energy. Additional energy sources are phosphocreatine, a protein-energy source found only in muscle tissues, and oxygen, which aids contraction by oxidizing the lactic acid that results from the anaerobic hydrolysis of the high-energy ATP bonds.

Muscle spasm is an involuntary contraction of one muscle

Figure 4-6 Muscles of body. **A,** Anterior view. **B,** Posterior view.

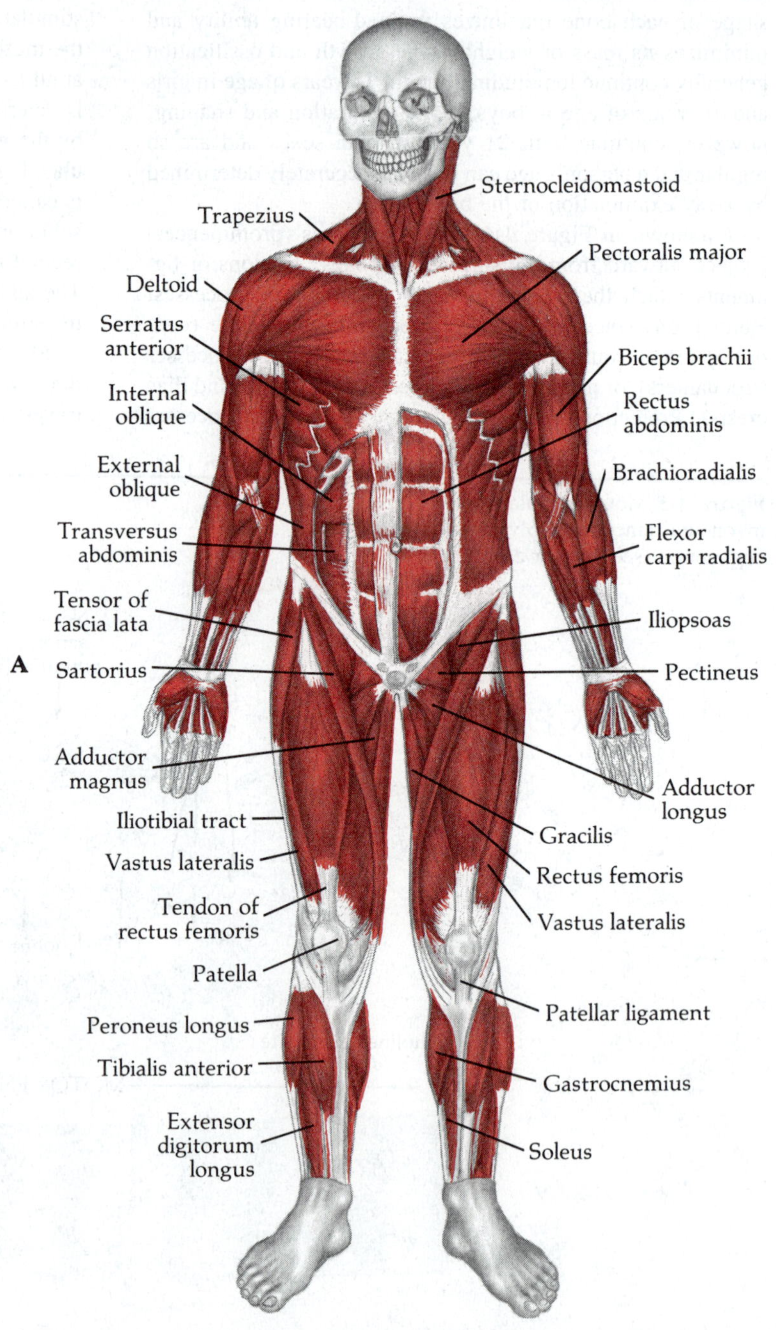

or a group of muscles caused by repetitive activation of entire motor units from the repetitive firing of a motor nerve. Tetanus is a sustained contraction caused by a repetitive series of stimuli conducted along the sarcolemmal membrane.

Muscles also have the ability to relax. A relaxing factor called relaxin acts by rendering ATP inactive until the next stimulus reaches a particular fiber, thereby keeping the muscle relaxed.

Muscle twitch. A muscle twitch occurs when a liminal stimulus is attained. All muscle fibers associated with the stimulated nerve contract and then relax.

An isotonic twitch causes the muscle to change length when constant tension is applied throughout its contraction. An isometric twitch is one in which the muscle remains or retains a constant length even with a sudden increase in muscle tension.

Muscle tone. Tone in muscles provides resistance to passive elongation or stretch and ensures a rapid reaction to an

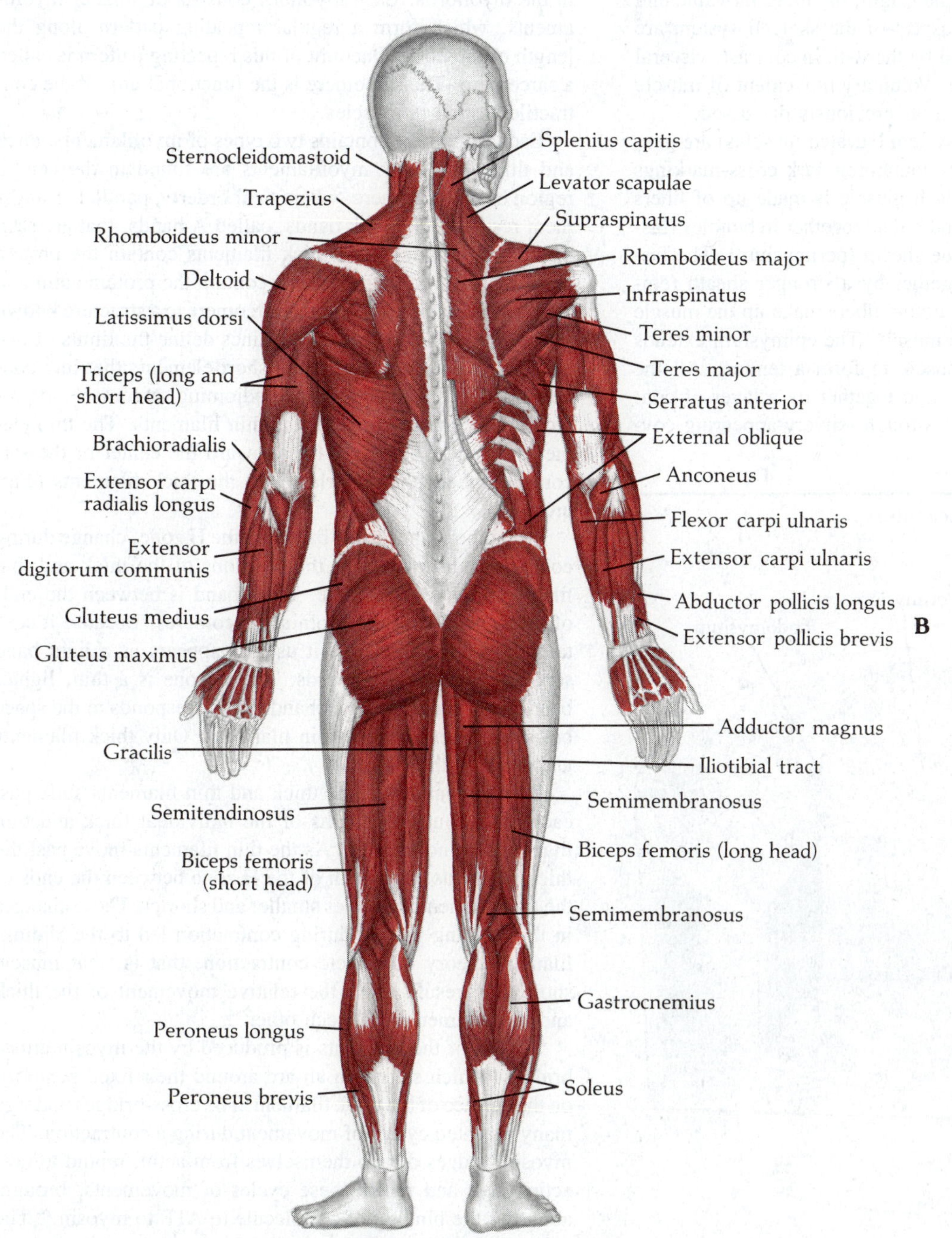

external stimulus. It results from a continuous flow of stimuli from the spinal cord to each motor unit. Muscle tone can be increased or decreased depending on the activity within the nervous system. Tone is increased in anxiety states and decreased during restful periods.

Structure of skeletal muscles. Skeletal muscles make up 40% to 45% of the body's weight (Figure 4-6). Through their contractions, they move the whole body or just parts of it. They cover the skeletal bones and help produce the contours of the body. Muscles are attached at each end to a bone, ligament, tendon, or fascia. One end of the muscle, the more fixed end, is referred to as the origin; the more movable end is the muscle insertion. Muscles of the skeletal system are voluntary muscles controlled by the will; in contrast, visceral muscles move involuntarily. Voluntary movement of muscle requires electrical stimulation as previously discussed.

Muscles of the skeletal system (striated muscles) are generally long, slender bundles containing dark cross-markings or lines called striations. Each muscle is made up of fibers enclosed in a sarcolemma and bound together in bundles (fasciculi) by a connective tissue sheath (perimysium). The fasciculi are further bound together by a stronger sheath (epimysium). These bundles of bound fibers make up the muscle belly, the fleshy part of the muscle. The epimysium extends beyond the belly of the muscle to form a tendon. All the muscles of the limbs are bound together by a layer of connective tissue called fascia, a tough, silvery-appearing covering.

Figure 4-7 Structure of muscle fibers and their coverings.

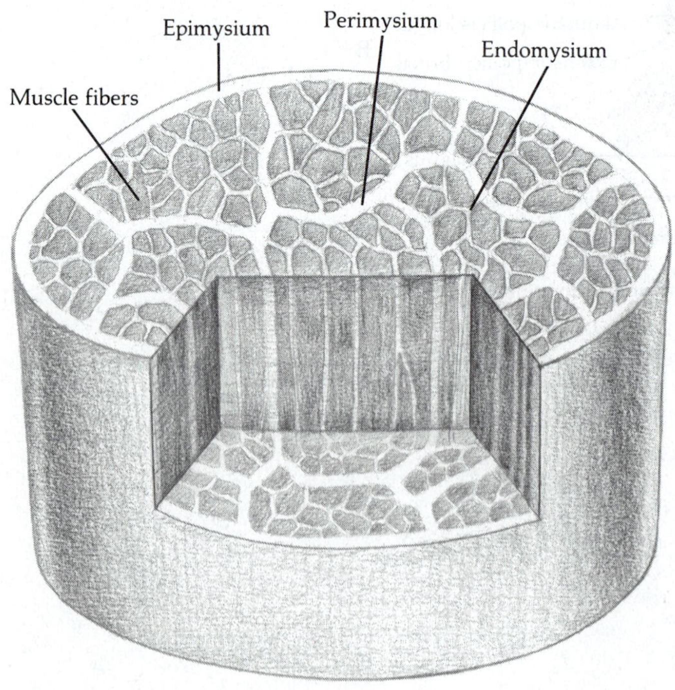

Skeletal muscles vary in length, width, diameter, and color (red or white). Red muscle gets its color from the pigment myoglobin. Being closely related to hemoglobin, myoglobin acts as a temporary oxygen store for the muscle. White muscle fibers contain less myoglobin. White muscles react rapidly when stimulated, whereas red muscles carry out slower, sustained movements (Figure 4-7).

The striations of skeletal muscles result from bands of muscle fibers made up of cylindric cytoplasmic elements called myofibrils. Myofibrils form the longitudinal striation of the muscle; transverse striations form the banding patterns in the myofibrils. Each myofibril consists of smaller myofilaments, which form a regular repeating pattern along the length of the fibril. One unit of this repeating pattern is called a sarcomere. The sarcomere is the functional unit of the contractile system in muscles.

Each sarcomere contains two types of myofilaments: thick and thin. The thick myofilaments are found in the central region of the sarcomere, where their orderly, parallel arrangement results in the dark bands, called A bands, that are seen in striated muscles. The thick filaments contain the protein myosin. The thin myofilaments contain the protein actin and are attached at either end of the sarcomere to a structure known as the Z line. Two successive Z lines define the limits of one sarcomere. The Z lines contain short elements that interconnect the thin filaments from two adjoining sarcomeres to provide an anchoring point for the thin filaments. The thin elements extend from the Z lines toward the center of the sarcomere, where they overlap with the thick filaments (Figure 4-8).

Two other bands, the I band and the H zone, change during contraction in relation to the positions of the thick and thin filaments in the sarcomere. The I band is between the ends of the A bands in two adjoining sarcomeres. Because it contains only thin filaments, it usually appears as a light band separating the dark A bands. The H zone is a thin, lighter band in the center of the A band that corresponds to the space between the ends of the thin filaments. Only thick filaments are found in the H zone.

During contraction the thick and thin filaments slide past each other, but the lengths of the individual thick and thin filaments do not change. As the thin filaments move past the thick filaments, the width of the H zone between the ends of the thin filaments becomes smaller and shorter. These changes in the banding pattern during contraction led to the sliding-filament theory of muscle contraction, that is, that muscle shortening results from the relative movement of the thick and thin filaments past each other.[84]

Sliding of the filaments is produced by the myosin cross-bridges, which swivel in an arc around their fixed positions on the surface of the thick filament. The cross-bridges undergo many repeated cycles of movement during a contraction. The myosin bridges detach themselves from actin, rebind to new actin sites, and repeat these cycles of movements, brought about by the binding of a molecule to ATP to myosin.[84] The process of binding ATP appears to break the linkage between

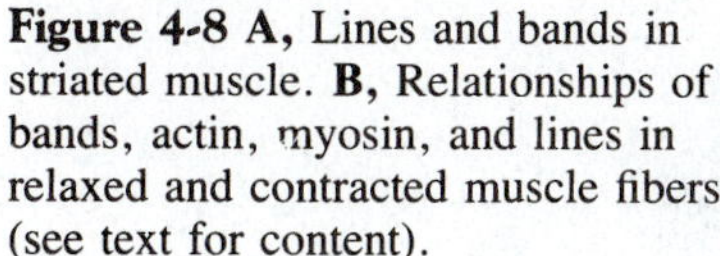

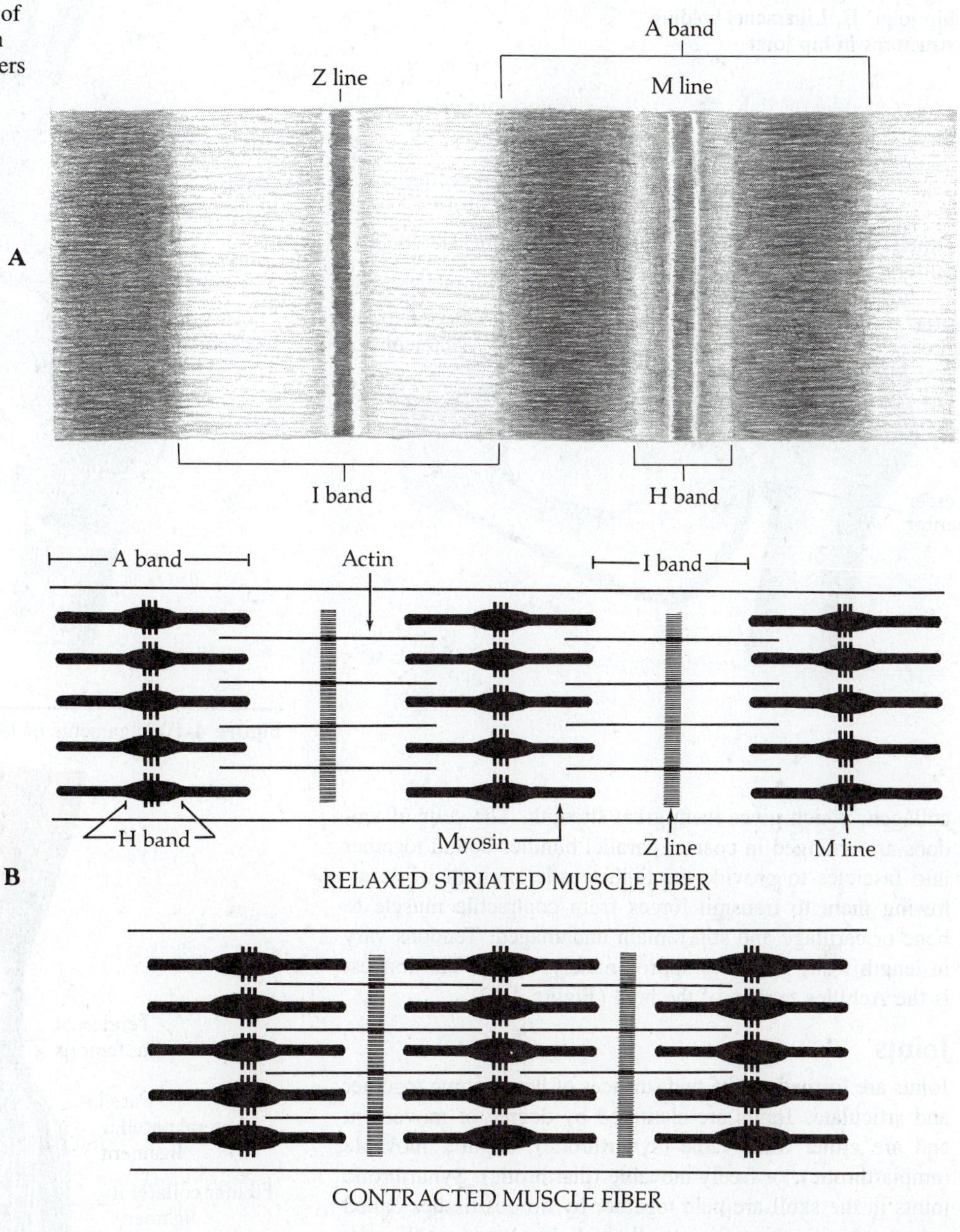

Figure 4-8 A, Lines and bands in striated muscle. **B,** Relationships of bands, actin, myosin, and lines in relaxed and contracted muscle fibers (see text for content).

actin and myosin. The reaction returns the bridge to its initial state so it can repeat the cycle of bridge movement.

Ligaments

Ligaments hold bones to bones. They may encircle a joint to add strength and stability, as they do around the hip joint (Figure 4-9), or they may hold obliquely or parallel to the ends of bones across the joint, as they do in and around the knee joint (Figure 4-10). Ligaments are relatively long bands. They are made up of tough bands of collagen fibers arranged in parallel bundles of fibers to add strength. Type I collagen produces these large, densely packed fibers (see pp. 387 to 388 for discussion of collagen structure and types). Type I collagen gives ligaments great tensile strength with limited extensibility. When ligaments are taut, they provide the greatest stability to the specific joint. Ligaments allow movement in some directions while restricting movement in other directions.

Tendons

Tendons hold muscles to bones (Figure 4-11). They form at the ends of muscles into strong, nonelastic cords of type I

Figure 4-9 A, Ligaments surrounding hip joint. **B,** Ligaments holding structures in hip joint.

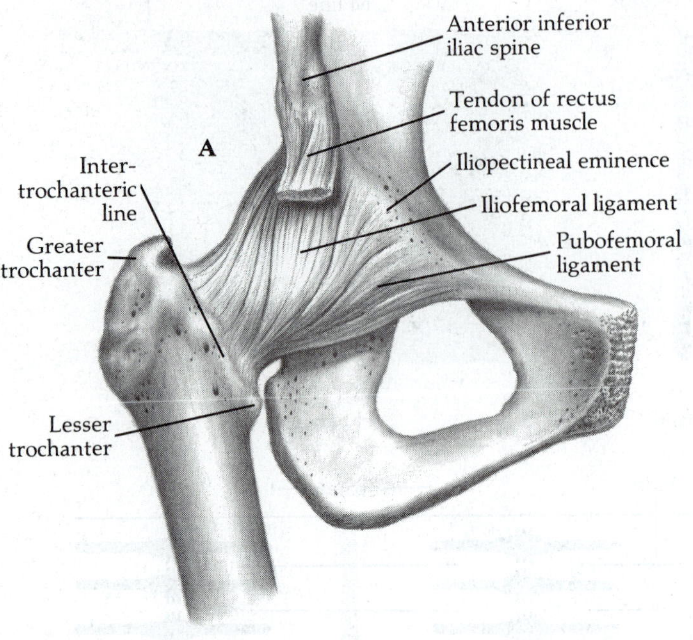

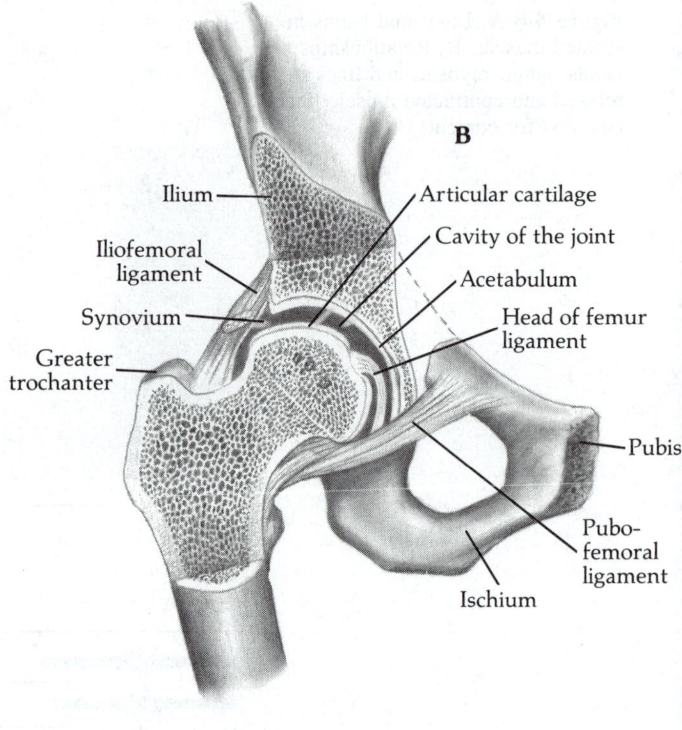

collagen, which gives them great strength. The cells of tendons are arranged in coarse, parallel bundles bound together into fascicles to provide the high tensile strength while allowing them to transmit forces from contractile muscle to bone or cartilage and still remain undamaged. Tendons vary in length from 1 inch to approximately 1 foot. The longest is the Achilles tendon of the heel (Figure 4-12).

Joints

Joints are formed where two surfaces of bones come together and articulate. Joints are classified by degree of movement and are either immovable (synarthrotic), slightly movable (ampiarthrotic), or freely movable (diarthrotic). Synarthrotic joints in the skull are held together by fibrous tissues called sutures. Ampiarthrotic joints allow slight movement through their fibrocartilage disc, such as in the symphysis pubis, or by a fibroligament, as in the radioulnar articulation.

Most joints are diarthrotic. They are also called synovial joints because they are lined with synovial membranes. Other components of diarthrodial joints are bones, articular cartilage, synovial fluid, nerves, lymphatics, and blood vessels. All these components are encased in the joint capsule, which is made up of ligaments and tendons encircling or surrounding the joints (Figure 4-13).

Diarthrodial joints are named for their major form of movement, such as ball and socket (hip, shoulder), hinge (elbow, knee), pivot (atlas, axis), condyloid (wrist), saddle (first metacarpal, trapezium), and gliding (intervertebral).

Figure 4-10 Ligaments of knee joint.

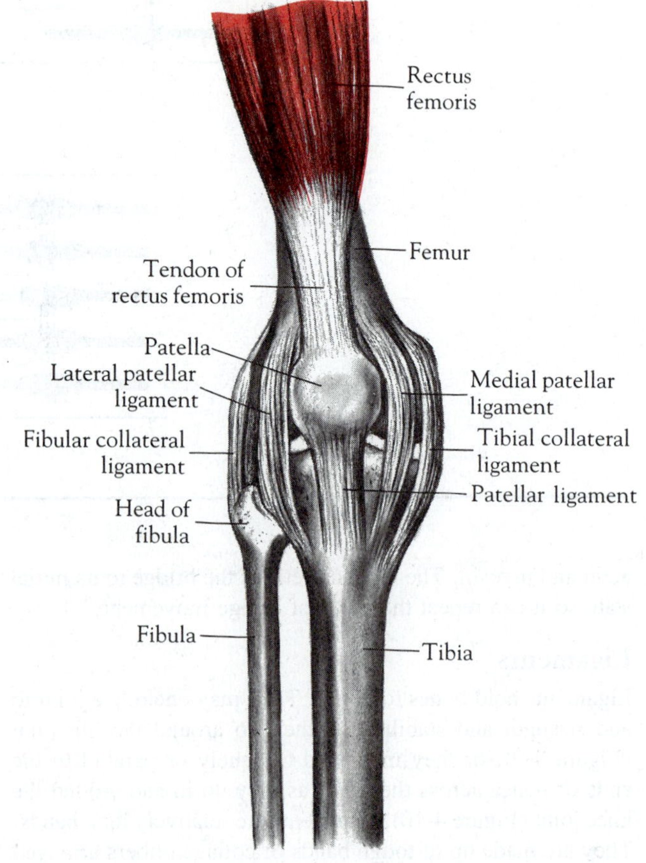

The degree of movement of a joint is called its range of motion. Joints have one or more of the movements listed below:

flexion Bending forward; shortening that decreases the angle between two bones.
extension Bending backward or lengthening that increases the angle between two bones or straightens the joint.
abduction Moving away from the midline of the body.
adduction Moving toward the midline.
rotation Moving around a central axis, perpendicular to the axis.
circumduction Making a conical movement, exemplified by winding up to throw a ball.
supination Turning the palm upward and forward.
pronation Turning the palm downward and backward.
eversion Turning the sole of the foot outward.
inversion Turning the sole of the foot inward.
dorsiflexion Pulling the foot and toes upward and forward.
plantar flexion Pushing the foot and toes downward and backward.
elevation Lifting upward.
depression Lowering.
protraction Moving a part forward.
retraction Moving a part backward.
apposition Moving the thumb toward the little finger to touch together.

When joints cannot or do not maintain their usual ranges of movement, they affect all musculoskeletal tissues and other body tissues, as noted later. Table 4-1 gives ranges of motion of major joints.

Synovium

The synovium is a membrane that completely lines the inner surfaces of the joint (Figure 4-13). It forms from mesenchymal cells within the inner layer of the joint capsule. The membrane has villous folds that contain the blood vessels and lymphatics. The membrane is made up of cells derived primarily from type I collagen molecules, although the blood vessels are derived from type III collagen (see later discussion of collagens).

The villous folds of the synovial membrane are filled with

Figure 4-11 Tendons and muscles around knee joint (anterior view).

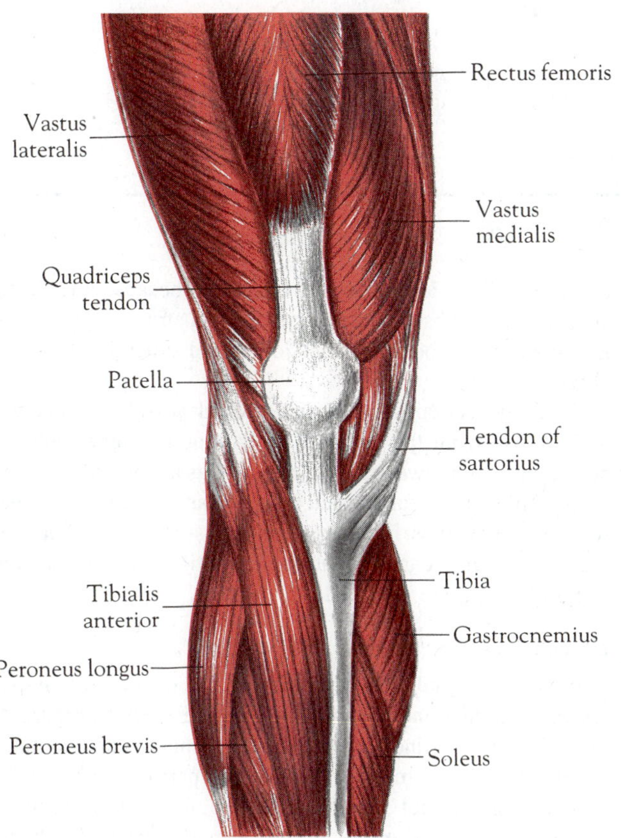

Figure 4-12 Achilles tendon in leg.

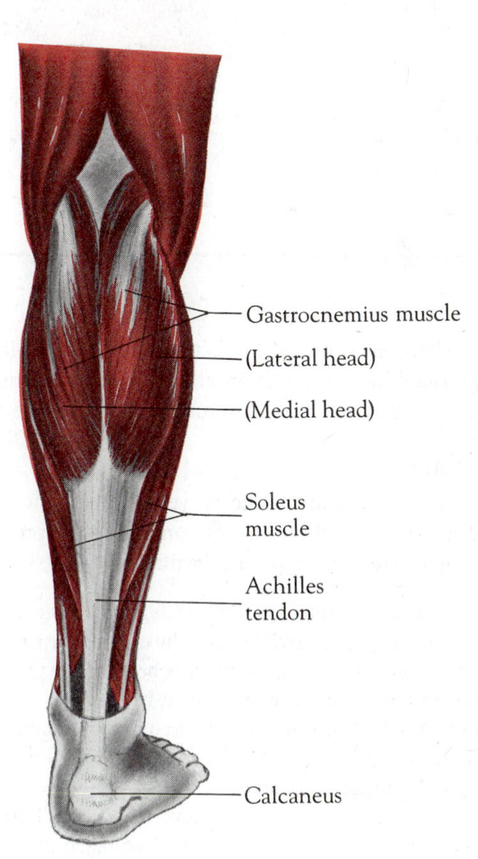

Figure 4-13 Knee joint (synovial joint).

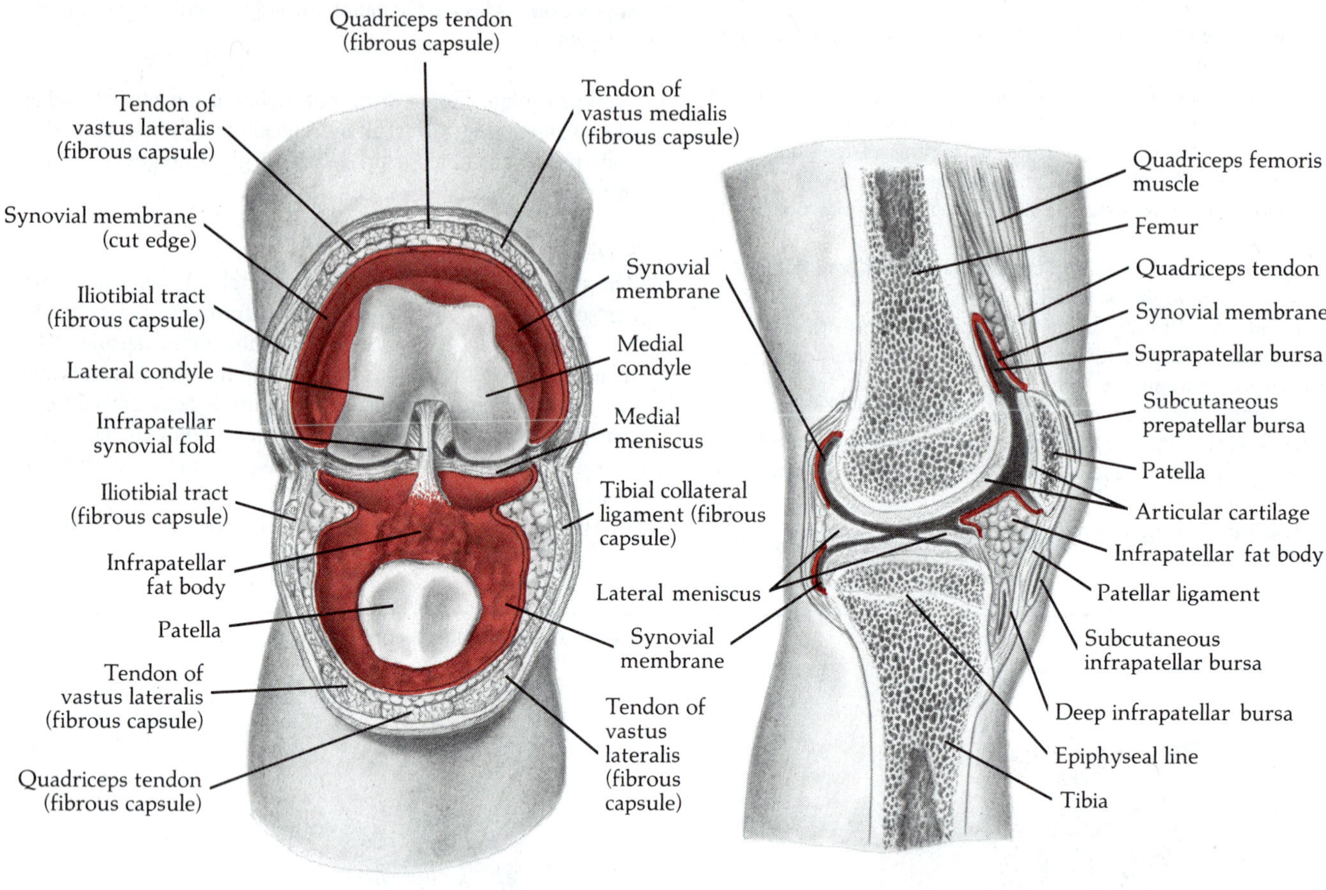

fluid, called the synovial fluid, that bathes the articular cartilage to facilitate articulation and provide nutrients, phagocytes, and other immunologic functions within the joints.

Cartilage

Cartilage is a smooth, white or yellow, resilient supporting tissue made up of elastic fibers containing the protein chondrin. There are three types of cartilage:

hyaline Bluish white, elastic cartilage covering the ends of bones making up synovial joints, the ends of the ribs, the nasal septum, and the walls of the trachea; made up of type II collagen molecules with some type I cells.

fibrous White fibers that are particularly resistant to tension and are found in the symphysis pubis and the knee; made up of type I collagen molecules.

yellow Elastic yellow fibers found in the epiglottis and the pinna (outer ear); made up of type I collagen molecules.

Cartilage serves as a smooth surface for articulating bones (Figure 4-13). It also absorbs weight and, because it is elastic and moldable, absorbs shock, stress, and strain to prevent or lessen injury to bones within joints and other joint tissues (Figure 4-13).

Cartilage contains no intrinsic blood vessels. It receives its nutrition from the synovial fluids that are forced into its porous cellular network by the movements and weight bearing of the joints. Therefore, when a particular joint ceases to bear weight or develops limitations of its usual range of movements, articular cartilage atrophies until joint motion and weight bearing are resumed.

Bursa

A bursa is a small sac or cavity in the connective tissues (usually the tendons) surrounding or near a joint (Figure 4-14). The bursa is lined with synovial membrane and contains synovial fluid. Normally the bursa is a part of the musculoskeletal tissues, but a bursa can also form as a result of pressure or friction over a prominent part. Just such a bursa

Table 4-1
Range of Motion of Major Joints

Joint	Movements	Average Ranges (in Degrees)*
Cervical spine	Flexion	35-45 (older adult 35)
	Extension	35 (older adult may have pain and some stiffness)
	Lateral bending	45
	Rotation	45
	Hyperextension	45
Thoracic and lumbar spine	Flexion	80-90
	Extension	30
	Lateral bending	28-35
	Rotation	35-38 (older adult 30)
	Hyperextension	30
Shoulder	Flexion	90 (some stiffness in older adult)
	Backward extension	44-55
	Abduction	90
	Adduction	45-50
	Circumduction	360 (older adult may have crepitation)
Elbow	Flexion	145-160 (older adult may only be able to flex 135 degrees)
	Hyperextension	0
Forearm	Pronation	70-90
	Supination	85-90
Wrist	Extension	70 (older adult may have soreness or stiffness)
	Flexion	73-90
	Ulnar deviation	33-55
	Radial deviation	19
Thumb	Abduction	58
Fingers	Flexion	Decreased (in older adult may be caused by Heberden's or Bouchard's nodes)
	Distal joint	80
	Middle joint	100
	Proximal joint	90
	Extension	
	Distal joint	0
	Middle joint	0
	Proximal joint	45
Hip	Flexion	120-135 (decreased in older adult because of degenerative changes)
	Extension	28
	Abduction	45-48
	Adduction	20-30
	Rotation	
	In flexion	
	Internal rotation	45
	External rotation	45
	In extension	
	Internal rotation	35
	External rotation	48
	Abduction in 90-degree flexion	45-60
Knee	Flexion	120-130 (same or decreased in older adult but with soreness and stiffness; may have crepitation)
	Hyperextension	10
Ankle	Flexion	48-50
	Extension	18-20
Forefoot	Inversion	30-33 (same or decreased in older adult because of hallux valgus or degenerative changes)
	Eversion	18-20
	Dorsiflexion	20
	Plantar flexion	45-50

*Zero degrees is the extended position; movement is measured by degrees in the specific directions in which the joint moves.

forms to become a bunion in hallux valgus deformity.

The bursa reduces friction between tendons and bones or between tendons and ligaments by lubrication with synovial fluid from the bursal sac. New bursae can develop as a result of increased pressure or friction. Their formation may increase the pressure and cause pain.

Collagen

The protein collagen is the principal supporting element in connective tissues. It makes up approximately half the total body protein in fully developed adults. Collagen also plays an active role in developmental processes, cell attachment, chemotaxis, and the binding of antigen-antibody complexes. Thus collagen is more than an inert structural protein.

The collagen molecule is an asymmetric, rigid, rodlike structure made up of three individual polypeptide strands that are aligned colinearly throughout the molecule. The three individual strands of collagen are tightly coiled together in the form of a left-handed helix (the minor helix). They are then coiled around a common central axis to form a right-handed helix (the major helix). This coiled-coil configuration is stabilized by interchain hydrogen bonds.

Collagen strands are made up of many amino acid residues, approximately 23% of which are proline plus hydroxyproline

Figure 4-14 Bursae of shoulder joint.

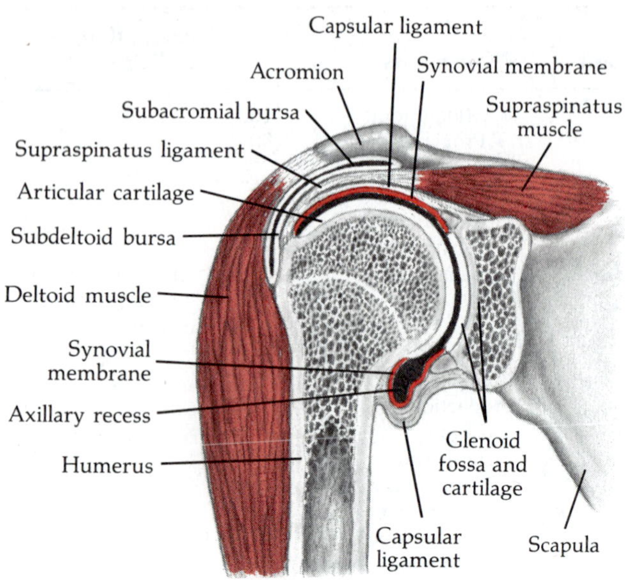

and 33% of which are glycine. Other amino acids are glutamic acid, alanine, and hydroxylysine. Collagen also contains lesser amounts of amino acids such as methionine, isoleucine, tyrosine, and histidine.

Collagen molecules are referred to as type I, II, or III; these types make up the most extensively occurring molecules. They are also called interstitial collagens, because fibers from these types are found predominantly in spaces between the cellular elements of a tissue or organ.

Fibers from type I collagen molecules are found in all major connective tissues and in the stroma of several organs. Tissues such as bone, tendon, and dentin and fibrocartilage appear to be formed exclusively of type I collagen molecules. Type I molecules play a major role as supporting elements in tissues that normally exhibit very little distensibility under mechanical stress. It also appears that type I collagen molecules can be synthesized by the connective tissue cells in which they are found.

Type I collagen molecules are made up of two identical α-1 strands and a different but homologous α-2 chain. Type II is made of three α-1 chains, found primarily in hyaline cartilage, where they lend their special properties to the mechanical strengths of the cartilage. Type III collagen molecules, which are also made up of three identical α-1 chains, are found in tissues that are the most distensible, such as the skin, blood vessel walls, and the uterine wall, and in several organs. Type III fibers coexist as fine reticular networks with type I molecules with larger fibers in the same tissues.

Differences in the three chains can be seen by electron microscopy. The α-2 chain contains more basic amino acid residues than the other chains. The α-chain of type II collagen contains significantly higher levels of threonine and glutamic acid than do the other chains, and it has markedly increased levels of hydroxylysine and glycosylated hydroxylysine. The α-1 chain of type III collagen contains relatively high levels of 4-hydroxyproline, glycine, and cysteinyl residues.[26] Each chain yields a unique set of peptides when examined, and each type of collagen develops from or under the control of separate and distinct structural genes. Thus the specific chain type and arrangement gives the particular collagen the strength and distensibility most suited to its specific tissue and distribution within the connective tissues of the body.

Normal Findings

The orthopaedic examination should take into account both the history and the physical examination.

The history should include any past and present orthopaedic problems as well as patterns of local and systemic signs and symptoms with review of all systems; social, marital, employment (occupational), and psychologic state; and habits or hobbies.

The physical examination includes an overall general inspection; observance of gait, posture, and movements while walking, sitting, and standing; assessment of bilateral symmetry, size and shape of musculoskeletal tissues, muscular development, generalized or localized edema, range of movements of each joint, condition of skin of body and of fingers and toes (with presence or complaints of Raynaud's phenomenon), lesions, rash (color and site), pain at rest or with movement in one or more joints, temperature of skin over and around joints, texture of skin and nails, nodules in or around joints, hair growth and distribution, and evidence of bruises, hemorrhage, bone or joint deformity, congenital defects or deformities, condition of blood vessels, peripheral pulses, color of tissues, lymph nodes, leg length equality, and "point" tenderness.

The following equipment is needed: goniometer to measure range of movements, percussion hammer, pin, cotton, sphygmomanometer, thermometer, tourniquet, tape measure, and stethoscope.

The following principles should be kept in mind in performing an orthopaedic examination:

Normal tissues are examined before injured, inflamed, or otherwise involved ones.

Local signs and symptoms are assessed with systemic findings.

Bilateral local and systemic observations are made.

Palpation is gently performed while observing facial or other reactions to note tenderness or sensitivity within the tissues.

Movements are assessed within norms for ranges of movements; differences between the right and left sides are noted.

Physical examination is but one part of the orthopaedic examination, along with the history and radiologic, serologic, surgical biopsy or exploratory, and consultative examinations.

Area of Concern	Normal Adult Findings
Skeleton	
Posture	Stands upright; head perpendicular to shoulders and pelvis; shoulders and pelvis aligned; convex curve to thoracic spine; concave curve to lumbar spine; arms hang freely from shoulders; feet aligned with toes pointing straight ahead *Older adult:* Stance less upright with head and neck more forward; thoracic curvature more pronounced; lumbar curvature less pronounced; shoulders may be hunched or rolled forward; angle of head of femur into acetabulum changes, leading to varus planting or placement of thighs, legs, and feet
Stature	Long, slender bones varying to short, thick bones; bone maturation ceases approximately age 21 *Older adult:* Height may decrease because of curvature changes; upper extremities appear longer and out of proportion to rest of body; calcium losses from bones also affect stature from osteoporosis
Symmetry	Slight differences in upper extremities because of handedness; hands may appear larger in larger people
Gait	Smooth, coordinated, easy, rhythmic with push off and swing through; arms move freely at sides; easy acceleration and deceleration; can stand still without swaying or tilt *Older adult:* Gait slow to initiate and stop; gait may be shuffling at times with less knee and ankle lifts; more stiffness of hips, knees, and back; steps may be shorter and more rapid but cover less overall distance
Muscles	
Shape and contour	"Full-bellied"; firm and supple; muscle mass in overall conformity with body build; tapered at either end of muscle mass *Older adult:* Shape and contour decrease, with less belly and mass common
Strength	Peak of muscle strength is 25-30 years; able to perform work of movements on demand and to maintain work activity over time; very smooth and firm when contracted; loose when relaxed; strong grip/push/pull strength *Older adult:* Initial work energy strong, but strength lessens over time (gradual 10% loss in muscle strength between 30-60 years); movements may be somewhat uncoordinated and jerky; grip/push/pull strength weaker than young adult
Range of movements	Able to move bones and joints through movements required or permitted by the bone/joint structures; movements are smooth and sustained if necessary; muscle action begins smoothly without jerking; usual length is regained when muscle is relaxed; paired opposing actions are smooth; there should be no limitation of movement (see Table 4-1) *Older adult:* All muscles can be put through passive range of movement slowly; active range of movement may be slower or limited in one or more joints either symmetrically or asymmetrically; slight to moderate tenderness or pain may accompany movement
Joints	
Shape and contour	Depends on specific type and position in body; bones of joint should articulate without deformity on one another in alignment; joint is firm and strong *Older adult:* Joints appear larger than surrounding tissues; contour may be irregular in one or more joints; bones may glide over one another with slightly audible click or sound; joint is stiffer than younger adult
Movements	Bones should move quietly and freely over one another; no clicks, crepitation, or pain should occur; movements should be smooth and coordinated according to particular type of joint; active range of movements should be pain free *Older adult:* Movements slower and more deliberate; balance may be harder to maintain; joints may be somewhat limited in range of movements; movements may be jerky and slightly painful
Temperature	Warmth around joint should be same as surrounding tissues
Swelling/edema	None *Older adult:* May have slight edema

Area of Concern	Normal Adult Findings
Ligaments, Cartilage, and Tendons	
Shape and contour	Taut, elastic, and firm; permit weight bearing *Older adult:* Taut but may be tighter and less elastic; may limit bone/joint contour
Movements	Easily moves through range of motion and holds joints and muscles according to place or function; movements of joints can be sustained without deformity or curvature; weight bearing is pain free *Older adult:* Less ease and range of movements; joints are stiffer; may have some joint laxity and weakness; weight bearing may cause some soreness or pain

Special Assessment Techniques

Examination or Test	Site	Normal Findings	Abnormal Findings
Joint range of movements	Any or all joints	Specific range of motion (ROM) as per Table 4-1; no soreness or pain; no edema or elevated temperature in or around joints	Limitation of range of movements in one or more spheres; pain, soreness, muscle weakness, edema, elevated temperature in or around joint or joints
Straight leg raising (Lasègue's)	Legs (one at a time)	No pain or soreness in back, buttocks when leg is raised while fully extended at knee; patient lies on back	Pain, soreness, or radiation of pain from low back to buttocks; may spread down leg to toes
McMurray's	Knee	No excessive or palpable pop or click in knee noted when ankle is grasped to turn knee medially and laterally, and while moving knee backward and forward from full flexion to extension	Click or pop felt or heard; pain or local tenderness is positive for meniscal damage or tears
Fabere-Patrick	Knee and hip	Knee can be flexed and brought to almost horizontal position to body with heel resting on opposite knee	Knee cannot be brought to horizontal position; limitation may be in hip, knee, or back (usually hip disease prevents knee rotation to horizontal position)
Drawer	Knee	Knee has slight forward or backward movement while flexed on tibia and fibula	Knee has more movement forward or backward (direction indicates tear of either anterior or posterior cruciate ligaments)
Trendelenburg's	Pelvis and gluteus muscles	With weight on one leg, pelvis on opposite side will be slightly elevated (observed posteriorly)	With weight on one leg, pelvis will drop (due to weakness or pain in hip joint or its muscles) on opposite side
Thomas'	Hip, knee, and lumbar spine	With patient on back, hip and knee are flexed to abdomen without flexion simultaneously occurring in lumbar spine	When patient flexes knee and hip to abdomen, lumbar spine will flex if there is a pathologic condition of the hip, and opposite leg will rise from table
Phalen's	Wrists	No tingling of fingers with wrists maximally against each other and held for 1 minute	Tingling felt in thumb, the index finger and the middle and lateral half of the ring finger
Tinel's	Carpal tunnel of wrist	No tingling into thumb, index, and middle fingers when median nerve is tapped at the wrist	Tingling felt as above for Phalen's test
Brudzinski's	Back and neck	With patient lying on back, no pain is felt in neck or back when head is passively flexed to chest	Pain in back and neck felt with passive flexion of head; knees and hips involuntarily flex to relieve pain (sign of meningeal irritation)
Kernig's	Back and leg	No back or leg pain felt when leg is extended (patient lies on back with hip and knee flexed)	Pain is felt in lower back, neck and/or head when leg is extended from flexed position (sign of meningeal irritation)

Normal Laboratory Data

Laboratory Test	Normal Adult Values
Serum calcium	Normal range slowly descends Up to 30 yr: 8.2-10.5 mg/dl *Older adult:* Decreases very slightly with age
Serum calcium (ionized)	4.75-5.2 mg/dl
Serum calcium (ionized, calculated, blood)	3.9-4.8 mg/dl
Serum phosphorus	2.5-4.5 mg/dl
Alkaline phosphatase*	3-13 King-Armstrong units or 1.5-4 Bodansky units
Acid phosphatase	Method dependent; up to 0.8 IU/L, ACA
Creatinine (24-h urine)	Adult male: 1-2 g/24 h Adult female: 0.8-1.8 g/24 h *Older adult:* Creatinine excretion decreases with advanced age as muscle mass diminishes
Creatinine clearance	Adult male: 85-125 ml/min/1.73 m^2 Adult female: 75-115 ml/min/1.73 m^2
BUN/creatinine ratio	6-20; mean about 10:1
Creatinine (serum)	Adult males: up to 1.2 mg/dl Adult females: up to 1.1 mg/dl There are slight differences between the sexes with males higher, since the range relates to the amount of muscle mass present.
Uric acid (serum)	Adult males: 3.4-7 mg/dl or slightly more Adult females: 2.4-6 mg/dl or slightly more
Uric acid (urine)	Approximately 250-750 mg/24 h
Serum glutamic pyruvic transaminase (SGPT)	3-30 IU/L (method dependent)
Serum glutamic oxaloacetic transaminase (SGOT)	8-42 IU/L
Creatine phosphokinase (CPK)	0-50 IU (method dependent)
Aldolase	1.5-7.2 mM/min/L
Erythrocyte sedimentation rate (ESR): Westergren method	Males <50 yr: 0-15 mm/h Males >50 yr: 0-20 mm/h Females <50 yr: 0-25 mm/h Females >50 yr: 0-30 mm/h
Zeta sedimentation ratio	<50 yr: <55% 50-80 yr: 40%-60%

*In nonpregnant subjects, percent residual activity >25% favors hepatic origin; <10% favors bone origin.

Conditions, Diseases, and Disorders

INFLAMMATORY CONDITIONS

Inflammatory conditions can affect one or more muscles, tendons, ligaments, bones, and structures in and around the joints. Because of the interaction of the structures, diagnosis and treatment of specific tissue inflammations may be difficult. Overlapping therapy may be needed to ensure relief of the condition. Treatment methods for many specific musculoskeletal inflammatory conditions are identical. Also, inflammatory or degenerative effects in one musculoskeletal tissue may have long-term effects on contiguous tissues. Therefore inflammatory conditions must be considered serious alterations even if only one small area of localized inflammation is noted.

Ankylosing spondylitis

Ankylosing spondylitis is a localized inflammatory condition that begins with low back (lumbar) pain and progresses throughout the spinal column, eventually resulting in hardening (ankylosis) and severe deformity of the vertebral column and adjacent tissues.

Ankylosing spondylitis (formerly Marie-Strümpell disease) progressively inhibits mobility. This disease affects men at a ratio of 8:1 or 9:1 over women; it occurs between 20 and 40 years of age and rarely occurs after 50 years of age. A marked hereditary factor, histocompatibility antigen HLA-B27, is associated with ankylosing spondylitis.

Pathophysiology

The exact pathologic condition in ankylosing spondylitis is unknown; the disease appears to begin in the sacroiliac bones and joints. The intervertebral discs become inflamed and are infiltrated by vascular connective tissue that then ossifies. The peripheral portions of the anulus fibrosus are the major areas initially affected, but as the disease progresses, the entire anulus, intervertebral ligaments, and the vertebrae themselves undergo similar inflammatory and ossifying changes. The disease gradually moves up the entire spinal column. The vertebral calcifications are called "bamboo" spines because the x-ray signs look like bamboo canes. The disease may also involve the hips, knees, and shoulders, but the primary site is the spine and sacroiliac joints.

Diagnostic Studies and Findings

Physical Examination of Back and All Musculoskeletal Tissues

Local or systemic limitations and pain
- Reiter's syndrome of conjunctivitis with uveitis, urethritis, and arthritis may be the complaint of patients with ankylosing spondylitis, along with morning stiffness and backache

Roentgenograms

Inflammatory or degenerative changes referred to as "bamboo" spine

Serologic Examination

Positive test for histocompatibility antigen HLA-B27, present in more than 90% of patients with ankylosing spondylitis but in less than 10% of general population

Rheumatoid factor is negative in most patients

Erythrocyte Sedimentation Rate

Elevated during the disease activity (normal elevations [male, 0 to 9 mm/h; female, 0 to 20 mm/h] increase to 10 to 15 mm/h and 20 to 25 mm/h respectively)

Medical Plan

Surgery

Total hip replacement to correct postinflammatory fixed flexion of hip joints

Osteotomy of the midlumbar vertebrae, only if patient cannot see straight ahead because of kyphosis

Cervical spinal fusion to aid in maintaining upright position in neck

Medications

Analgesic-antipyretic agents
- Salicylate analgesics (aspirin), 600 mg q4h

Nonsteroidal anti-inflammatory agents
- Indomethacin (Indocin), 25 mg tid; may be increased to a maximum of 200 mg/d
- Phenylbutazone (Butazolidin), 200-400 mg/d, given last because of multiple side effects, although it is very effective as an anti-inflammatory medication

General Management

Occupational therapy for identification and learning of modifications in activities of daily living (ADLs), employment, and changes in life-style necessary because of rigidity and curvature of spinal column

Consultations with social service and community nursing personnel to plan for long-term care and follow-up

Exercises to maintain mobility, including swimming and walking (rest is not beneficial in ankylosing spondylitis)

Physical therapy for exercises of the entire back, specific joint and muscle exercises, and deep-breathing exercises

A firm mattress and bed with only a small pillow

Occasionally, use of a back brace

Occasionally, use of cervical or pelvic belt traction

NURSING CARE

Nursing Assessment

Lumbar Area of Back

Pain (may alternate side to side and is usually worse on getting up or when rising in the morning)

Stiffness

Limitation of motion

Radiation to buttocks

Systemic Responses

Polyarthritis (asymmetric and of the large joints of the lower limbs)

Malaise, fatigue, weight loss, vague chest pains

Reiter's syndrome possible (Table 4-2)

Limitation of respiratory functions

Spread

Throughout spinal column as disease progresses and to sacroiliac, hips, knees, and shoulder joints

Psychosocial Concerns

Self-concept and body image concerns from limitation of social interactions and loss of mobility and independence

Table 4-2
Syndromes Associated with Arthritic Diseases

Syndrome	Patterns	Associated Diseases
Reiter's	Triad of conjunctivitis, urethritis, and arthritis; oral, genital, and mucocutaneous lesions (stomatitis, ulcerations, papules)	Ankylosing spondylitis; rheumatoid arthritis
Behçet's	Triad of iritis, oral lesions, and genital lesions; cutaneous lesions; phlebitis; colitis; polyarthritis	Polyarthritis of unknown etiology
Sjögren's	"Sicca" patterns of dryness (sicca) of conjunctiva and salivary glands; arthritis; swelling of parotid gland; Raynaud's phenomenon in some patients	Connective tissue diseases such as systemic lupus erythematosus (SLE), progressive systemic sclerosis (PSS), polymyositis
Stevens-Johnson (variant of erythema multiforme)	Stomatitis with ulcerations of oral mucosa; high fever; genital ulcerations; erythematous skin eruptions; arthritis	Erythema multiforme; erythema nodosum; rheumatic fever; rheumatoid arthritis and juvenile rheumatoid arthritis; ulcerative colitis

Nursing Dx & Intervention

Nursing Diagnosis	Nursing Intervention/Rationale
Impaired physical mobility (actual and potential) related to spinal inflammatory condition	• Assess for extent of impaired joint movements. • Observe movements for signs of relief or progressive impairment *to note patient's condition.* • Assist with range of motion (ROM) exercises *to maintain joint mobility.* • Encourage performance of prescribed exercises (swimming and walking) *to maintain mobility.* • Massage back as needed *to relieve tense or tired muscles.* • Assist with immersion in Hubbard tank *to lessen muscle spasms and strengthen extensor muscles.* • Teach deep-breathing exercises *to maintain respiratory functions and to aid peripheral oxygenation.*
Pain related to muscle/joint limitation of movements	• Assess patient for the presence, amount, and severity of pain. • Administer analgesic and anti-inflammatory medications as ordered *to relieve pain.* • Observe patient's movements for increasing ease and frequency *to note effects of medications.* • Listen for patient's verbalization of pain relief or continuing pain *to determine if changes are needed.* • Observe all involved points *to note abatement or continuation of inflammation.* • Encourage proper use of pillow and mattress *to prevent additional trauma and pain.* • Observe for side effects of medications (e.g., gastric irritation or burning; changes in complete blood count [CBC] and erythrocyte sedimentation rate [ESR]; diarrhea or constipation) *to note reactions to medications.*
Body image disturbance and altered role performance related to severe kyphosis and rigidity of spine	• Assess for implicit and expressed concerns. • Encourage socialization with family and friends *to maintain usual roles.* • Encourage team recreational activities and games, such as team swimming and walking with others, *to maintain patient's inclusion in activities.* • Encourage compliance with treatment regimen *to prevent severe deformity.* • Encourage patient to continue seeing physician for continuity of care and for current or recent developments in treatment of ankylosing spondylitis *to aid in maintaining long-term healthy status.*

Patient Education

1. Reiterate explanations of inflammatory processes and rationale for medical care to ensure that patient and family understand.
2. Explain rationale for exercise as opposed to rest of affected tissues: rest is harmful in ankylosing spondylitis.
3. Explain actions and side effects of salicylates and other anti-inflammatory medications. The patient should understand and be alert to the many side effects of ordered medications.
4. Explain skin reactions (reasons for and signs of) if radiotherapy is administered, to lessen the patient's concern if skin reaction occurs.
5. Teach (or reiterate explanations for) deep-breathing, ROM, and joint mobility exercises to encourage patient to comply.
6. Include family members in evaluation, practice, and performance of ADLs as necessary for home care continuity.

Evaluation

Patient Outcome	Data Indicating That Outcome is Reached
Patient retains adequate vertebral mobility and satisfactory curvature.	Patient's inflammation abates without ankylosis or severe curvature.
Patient maintains independence, social interactions, and self-care activities.	Patient continues own ADLs and usual employment activities, interactions, and recreation.
Patient complies with medical regimen.	Patient continues prescribed daily medication, rest, and exercise regimens.

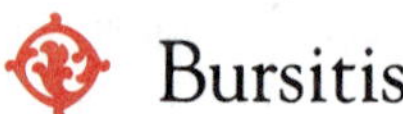

Bursitis

Bursitis is the inflammation of a bursa.

Since the bursa is an enclosed sac situated between muscles or tendons and bony prominences, the inflammation may spread to certain structures or may simply be an inflammation of the bursal fluid and sac.

One or more bursae can become inflamed, but the most common sites are the subdeltoid and subacromial bursae of the shoulder (Figure 4-14), the olecranon (elbow) bursa, the greater trochanteric bursa lateral to the hip, and the anserine bursa in the medial aspect of the upper tibia.

Pathophysiology

Bursitis usually results from constant friction between the skin and musculoskeletal tissues around the joint. Bursitis from friction would be sterile or aseptic without pathogenic organisms. Rarely, bursitis results from a foreign body or microorganism invasion. The area around the bursa becomes exquisitely tender. Motion is either partially or greatly limited by the swollen, enlarged sac, which causes pressure and pain when the tissues are moved. The area may be reddened, hot, and edematous with only point tenderness (the patient can point to the spot or area of greatest tenderness) or with soreness radiating to the tendons at the site. Tendinitis may also occur, further limiting motion and prolonging recovery. Calcium may be deposited in the sacs in long-standing or recurring bursitis.

Diagnostic Studies and Findings

Physical Examination

Localized inflammation
Point tenderness
Limitation of motion of one or more bursae and involved joints

Roentgenograms

May or may not show calcified deposits

Medical Plan

Surgery

Open removal of the calcified deposits
Aspiration of fluid within the sac (infrequently) for persistent edema and pressure
Removal of the bursal sac (rarely)

Medications

Analgesic-antipyretic agents
- Salicylates (aspirin), 600-1000 mg q4h

Nonsteroidal anti-inflammatory agents
- Indomethacin (Indocin), 25 mg bid, tid, or qid

If the bursa is infected, antibiotics specific for the offending organism following culture

Injections of steroids into the sac to relieve the inflammation; dosage is individualized

General Management

Avoidance of activities (such as kneeling) that cause pressure

Avoidance of constant friction movements (such as throwing or hitting a ball) that cause the inflammatory reaction

Moist heat applications every 4 hours to the inflamed area

ROM exercises to help regain or maintain motion

Wrapping with elastic bandages, if bursa is accessible, to reduce edema

NURSING CARE

Nursing Assessment

Inflammatory Process

Heat
Redness
Swelling
Tenderness
Limitation of motion

Systemic Response

Similar responses in one or more joints/bursae
Fever and malaise if pathogen is involved

Psychosocial Concerns

Limitation of use of muscles and joint possibly curtailing income or livelihood

Nursing Dx & Intervention

Nursing Diagnosis	Nursing Intervention/Rationale
Impaired physical mobility (limitation of motion) related to inflammation of bursa	• Assess degree of limitation of movement of involved joint. • Encourage exercise to maintain ROM as prescribed *to maintain functions*. • Caution against continuing activities that may cause recurrence *to lessen chance of chronicity*. • Observe for edema, pain, and redness related to limiting or increasing motion *to note progression*. • Apply compresses every 4 hours as ordered *to aid resolution or easing of inflammation*. • Remove bandages, observe site, and rewrap bandages (if used) *to prevent disarrangement or tightening*.
Pain related to inflammation of bursa	• Assess amount, severity, and duration of pain. • Administer medications as ordered *to relieve pain*. • Note continuation or relief of pain, tenderness, or inflammation *to note efficacy of medications*. • Observe for side effects of medications *to note presence or need for other medications*. • Handle inflamed tissues gently *to prevent additional trauma*.

Patient Education

1. Instruct the patient in ROM exercises to lessen possibility of bursa inflammation.
2. Instruct the patient about side effects of medications.
3. Alert the patient to the possibility that pain may increase temporarily after injection of steroids (1 to 24 hours), to be followed by noticeable pain relief and increasing ROM.
4. Caution the patient to avoid activities that could cause exacerbation until inflammation is resolved (4 to 6 weeks).

Evaluation

Patient Outcome	Data Indicating That Outcome is Reached
Pain in joint is relieved.	Patient states that pain, soreness, and stiffness are no longer present.
Patient regains ROM of affected joint.	Patient can engage in usual activities with affected joint.
Patient no longer needs medication.	Patient feels no pain with ROM actions or when using joint for usual activities.

Epicondylitis and tendinitis
(Tenosynovitis)

Epicondylitis is an inflammation of the tendons of the medial or lateral epicondyles of the radius, ulna, or other bones. Tendinitis (tenosynovitis) is an inflammation of the tendons and their sheaths.

Epicondylitis and tendinitis may occur together and, with some variations, the treatments are similar for both. The local sites of inflammation are next to one another, which makes proper diagnosis more challenging.

Lateral epicondylitis, commonly called tennis elbow, is caused by repetitive twisting and swinging movements of the elbow that accompany, among other activities, swinging a tennis racket or using a hammer or other tools. Inflammation affects the tendons that originate in the medial or lateral epicondyles of the radius or ulna. The tendons and their sheaths may both become inflamed (tendinitis and tenosynovitis, respectively). Medial epicondylitis is called golfer's elbow.

Pathophysiology

Repetitive trauma damages and tears the fibers of the common extensor tendon. Extravasation of tissue fluids sets up inflammatory reactions, and healing produces scar tissue and adhesions that limit the range of motion of the elbow joint. The joint can then become inflamed by repetitive trauma to the scarred, inelastic fibers. The inflammation can spread to the tendon sheath, with fibrosis binding the sheath to the tendon and thus further limiting joint movements. Classic symptoms of epicondylitis include tenderness (frequently point tenderness), pain, and edema. Pronation or supination of the hand when the elbow is in 45 degrees of flexion causes severe medial and epicondylar pain.

Diagnostic Studies and Findings

History

Elbow flexion and rotation and repetitive ROM actions from occupational or sports activities resulting in localized elbow pain, tenderness, and limitation of motion in involved joint

Physical Examination

Point tenderness and increased pain with supination and pronation of hand

Edema and tenderness radiating along the tendon and its sheath

Weak grasp

Medical Plan

Surgery

Removal of calcium deposits from the inflammatory processes occasionally required

Removal of a degenerated (scarred and bound-down) tendon sheath for chronic, persistent synovitis of a shoulder, elbow, or heel because of calcium deposits from repeated trauma

Medications

Corticosteroids orally in individualized doses

Injection of steroids into the inflamed area to relieve pain; may need to be repeated at intervals for complete pain relief; dosage and type individualized

Analgesic-antipyretic agents

Salicylates (aspirin), 600 mg q4h for mild conditions

General Management

Moist heat applications to area every 4 hours

Rest to the part or parts

Occasionally, splint applied to the forearm and elbow

NURSING CARE

Nursing Assessment

Inflammatory Process

Localized pain and pain radiating to forearm

Tenderness

Edema in elbow area

Range of Motion

Pain increased with supination and pronation of hand

Psychosocial Concerns

Concern for ability to earn a living if in an occupation requiring full elbow ROM (such as carpenter or sports professional)

Nursing Dx & Intervention

Nursing Diagnosis	Nursing Intervention/Rationale
Impaired physical mobility related to limitation of joint functions and pain	• Assess degree and amount of joint movements. • Encourage exercises *to maintain ROM as prescribed.* • Caution against continuing activities that may cause recurrence. • Observe for edema, pain, and redness related to limiting or increasing motion *to note progression of symptoms.* • Apply compresses every 4 hours as ordered *to relieve inflammation.*
Pain related to inflammation of tendons	• Assess amount, severity, and type of pain. • Administer medications as ordered *to relieve pain.* • Note continuation or relief of pain, tenderness, or inflammation *to assess effect of medications.* • Observe for side effects of medications *to note problem that may need treatment.* • Handle inflamed tissues gently *to avoid additional pain.*
Altered role performance related to presence and severity of condition	• Assess for evidence of concerns. • Encourage expression of concerns; seek guidance to resolve concern about employment or recurrence of condition. • Encourage patient to comply with treatment regimen and to continue medical care *to note recovery.*

Patient Education

1. Explain inflammatory processes and effects of repetitive trauma to lessen painful episodes and inflammation.
2. Instruct the patient about side effects of medications.
3. Alert the patient to the possibility that pain may increase temporarily after injection of steroids (1 to 24 hours), to be followed by noticeable pain relief and increasing ROM.
4. Caution the patient to avoid activities that could cause exacerbation until inflammation is resolved (4 to 6 weeks).
5. Instruct the patient about the effects of application of heat or cold.

Evaluation

Patient Outcome	Data Indicating That Outcome is Reached
Inflammation is resolved.	Patient has normal temperature and no pain or edema in elbow area.
Patient regains joint mobility without limitation.	Patient can put joint through normal ROM without pain or limitation.
Patient returns to employment as before.	No restrictions are necessary on employment activities.

Gouty arthritis

Gout is a metabolic condition of improper production of uric acid (hyperuricemia), which must be excreted through the kidneys. Some of the uric acid crystals may be deposited in joints, setting up an inflammation, or gouty arthritis.

Gouty arthritis must be included in inflammatory conditions of musculoskeletal tissues. Men constitute nearly 95% of patients with gout.

Pathophysiology

Arthritis associated with gout results from the deposition of sodium biurate crystals within the joint cartilage. The crystals are very irritating and cause the inflammatory response that is arthritis. The skin overlying the joint becomes red and hot; the joint is swollen and very tender, forcing the patient to attempt to hold it still. The biurate crystals can also be deposited in bone, resulting in cystlike, punched-out, translucent areas under the cartilage that can be seen on x-ray examination.

Severe, excruciating pain results from the inflammation. Acute attacks usually last 3 to 5 days. Although any joint can be affected, the metatarsophalangeal joint of the great toe is most commonly affected. The ankle and knee joints also are commonly affected.

When biurate crystals are deposited in other tissues, such as the ear cartilage or fingers, these deposits are referred to as tophi, a physical diagnostic feature of gout.

Diagnostic Studies and Findings

History

Severe pain localizing in joint of great toe or other joint
History of gout

Physical Examination

Inflamed joint or joints
Tophi possible

Serum Uric Acid

Elevated (normal levels: men, 3.9 to 7.8 mg/dl; women, 2.5 to 6.8 mg/dl)

Microscopic Examination of Aspirated Fluid

Characteristic biurate crystallizations

Medical Plan

Medications

Antigout agents
- Colchicine (Colsalide), 0.5-1 mg every hour during acute pain episode; continue administration of 1 mg/h until patient experiences nausea, vomiting, or diarrhea (stop administration because therapeutic blood level has been achieved [administer a maximum of 8-10 tablets])[58]
- Probenecid (Benemid), 0.5 g/d, with gradual increases to total dose of 2-3 g/d; decreases incidence of acute attacks and controls serum uric acid levels

Nonsteroidal anti-inflammatory agents
- Indomethacin (Indocin); dosages vary for acute attacks to maximum of 200 mg/d
- Phenylbutazone (Butazolidin), 400-600 mg/d; given in divided doses for several days during acute attacks, with gradually decreasing doses over 6-8 days
- Allopurinol (Zyloprim), 50-100 mg bid; reduces serum uric acid levels by reducing uric acid formation; dosage gradually increased in increments of 100 mg every 2-4 wk until total daily dose is 300-600 mg and serum uric acid is at normal level[58]

Analgesic-antipyretic agents
- Mild analgesics such as aspirin (for pain relief) in 600-1000 mg doses q4h

General Management

Application of cold via ice bags to decrease inflammatory processes; allow affected joint to rest on ice bag so pain is not increased
Gentle ROM exercises when the acute pain has subsided

NURSING CARE

Nursing Assessment

Inflammatory Processes

Exquisite pain in joint
Tenderness
Swelling
Heat
Redness

Systemic Processes

Tophi (deposits of monosodium urate): may be found in ear cartilages, small joints of fingers
Serum uric acid levels: may be elevated
Low-grade fever
Hypertension
Nephritis

Psychosocial Concerns

Loss of social interaction from pain and enforced immobility

Nursing Dx & Intervention

Nursing Diagnosis	Nursing Intervention/Rationale
Pain related to biurate deposits in joints	• Assess amount, duration, and severity of pain. • Do not allow patient to bear weight on involved joints *to lessen pain*. • Apply ice bags *to decrease inflammation*. • Administer ordered medications *to relieve pain*. Observe for side effects of medications (particularly colchicine) and for therapeutic blood levels and then discontinue (for acute attacks). • Apply splint to affected joint if ordered *to aid muscle relaxation*. • Keep bedding and pressure off affected joint or joints *to lessen pain*.

Nursing Diagnosis	Nursing Intervention/Rationale
Impaired physical mobility related to deposits in joints and pain	• Assess amount, type, and severity of pain. • Perform gentle ROM exercises after acute pain has subsided *to increase joint mobility.* • Encourage ambulation when pain relief has been achieved *to increase independence.* • Encourage return to normal activities *to aid in maintaining usual roles.*
Knowledge deficit related to condition	• Assess knowledge of disease processes *to aid in planning care.* • Explain treatment regimen *to aid in compliance.* • Clarify learning as needed *to increase understanding.*

Patient Education

1. Explain rationale for hourly administration of medications during acute attacks to achieve desired blood levels.
2. Explain side effects of each medication used during acute attacks and as maintenance medications; have the patient list them for reference.
3. Encourage the patient to maintain physician visits for medication or dosage change to control systemic aspects of gout.

Evaluation

Patient Outcome	Data Indicating That Outcome is Reached
Gout is controlled with medications.	Patient can maintain usual activities with no or infrequent acute attacks of pain; infrequent attacks can be relieved with intensified medication dosages.
Patient experiences no side effects of maintenance medications.	Patient has no nausea, vomiting, leukopenia, or pruritus.
Patient has correct information about gout.	Patient explains condition, medication and dosages needed, and side effects of medications.

Rheumatoid arthritis

Rheumatoid arthritis is a chronic systemic disease characterized by inflammation of the connective tissues throughout the body.

This severely disabling chronic disease is one of the major rheumatic diseases. Although the disease is a systemic disorder, this discussion concerns the local effects on the tissues in and around the joints.

Rheumatoid arthritis is thought to be an autoimmune disease (see Chapter 14 for discussion of autoimmune diseases), but the exact etiology has not been established. Women are affected four times as often as men, and there is a marked familial tendency. Most patients develop rheumatoid arthritis between 25 and 55 years of age, although the disease also occurs in children between 8 and 15 years old, when it is referred to as juvenile rheumatoid arthritis or Still's disease.

Pathophysiology

The disease begins in the synovial membrane within the joint, usually in one of the smaller joints of the wrist, fingers, or hand. However, bilateral symmetric joint involvement is a characteristic finding. The synovial membrane becomes inflamed from the autoimmune antigen-antibody effects, and the membrane becomes swollen, irritated, and painful. Fibrotic changes and hypertrophy of the synovial membrane occur. These changes are called pannus formation. The inflammatory reaction spreads to other joint tissues, including the cartilage, and eventually the bones. Ligaments and tendons also are involved; they are scarred and shortened, which eventually contributes to deformities, subluxations (partial dislocations), and contractures. Cartilage degeneration results in pain and grating with weight bearing and movements. As the cartilage erodes and degeneration continues, the bone ends are exposed and also develop erosions, bone cysts, or fissures. Eventually bone spurs and osteophytes develop, further limiting joint mobility and use. The entire joint and its structures remain inflamed, edematous, and painful. Also, collections of fibroblasts in collagen tissues near joints enlarge into rheumatoid nodules, a classic feature of rheumatoid arthritis.

Characteristically, rheumatoid arthritis affects smaller joints symmetrically before involving the larger weight-bearing joints. Bouchard's nodes are the classic enlargements of the proximal phalangeal and metacarpophalangeal joints.

Eventually the local disease in the joints involves major

organ systems in the remainder of the body, including the heart, kidneys, lungs, and skin.

Diagnostic Studies and Findings

History

Monoarticular or polyarticular inflammation

Physical Examination

Criteria for the diagnosis of rheumatoid arthritis have been established by the American Rheumatism Association (ARA); presence of 10 of the following confirms the diagnosis:
- Morning stiffness on arising; pain and tenderness in at least one joint
- Swelling in at least one and possibly two joints
- Symmetric joint swelling bilaterally
- Fatigue, malaise, and weight loss
- Paresthesias of hands or feet
- Raynaud's phenomenon of fingers and toes
- Development of subcutaneous nodules
- Involvement of major organs such as heart and kidney
- Pericarditis; valvular lesions; vasculitis
- Pneumonitis; fibrosis
- Tenosynovitis; ankylosis of joints
- Felty's syndrome (splenomegaly and leukopenia)
- Deformities of joints; ulnar drift of wrists

Serologic Examination

Rheumatoid factor (a large immune globulin)
- Positive in 95% of patients with rheumatoid arthritis

Erythrocyte sedimentation rate (ESR)
- Elevated (moderate to severe elevation [to 15 mm/h in males and 25 mm/h in females]); normal: 0-9 mm/h in males and 0-20 mm/h in females

C-reactive protein
- Present during acute phases

Red cell count
- Anemia, primarily hypochromic (normocytic is common)

White cell count
- Elevated over all cell types

Serum complement decreased

Synovial Fluid Aspiration and Analysis

May reveal immune complexes and elevated white cell counts

Synovial Membrane Biopsy

Positive for pannus formation and inflammatory changes

Roentgenograms

Rarefaction of bones, plus erosions of involved bone, as disease progresses

Subluxation (partial dislocation) of bones from joints

Medical Plan

Surgery

Synovectomy of inflamed synovial membranes to relieve pain and maintain muscle and joint balance

Repair of ruptured or fibrotic tendon sheaths to prevent deformity and subluxations

Total joint replacement to increase mobility

Arthrodesis (fusion of a joint): may be done to decrease deformity and joint instability; spinal fusion may be required to treat subluxation

Osteotomy to change weight-bearing surfaces and relieve pain

Medications

Analgesic-antipyretic agents
- Aspirin, divided doses up to 5 g/d

Nonsteroidal anti-inflammatory agents
- Ibuprofen (Motrin), single oral dose of 400 mg
- Fenoprofen (Nalfon), single oral dose of 200 mg
- Tolmetin (Tolectin), initially 400 mg tid to reach optimum daily dose of 600-1800 mg/d
- Naproxen (Naprosyn), 250-375 mg bid for chronic state; 250 mg tid for acute inflammatory attack

Antirheumatic agents
- Gold thiomaleate (Myochrysine), 20-50 mg/wk IM, or auranofin (Ridaura), 6 mg/d po, to decrease inflammation
- Penicillamine (Cuprimine, Depen), 125-250 mg/d increased to 500-750 mg/d; may be used as a substitute for patients sensitive to gold

Immunosuppressive agents
- Azathioprine (Imuran), 3-5 mg/kg/d initially; then 1-2 mg/kg/d maintenance dose

Antineoplastic agents
- Cyclophosphamide; dosage is individualized

Corticosteroids
- Primarily prednisone (Deltasone, others) or prednisolone (Delta-Cortef, others) in titrated doses of 2-10 mg/d, used after other medications for anti-inflammatory effects
- Hydrocortisone (Cortef, others), 100 mg, injected into the joint to reduce inflammation

General Management (Table 4-3)

Immersion in paraffin "glove"

Immersion in whirlpool

Application of splints to inflamed joints to maintain proper position

Moist warm applications to joints

Applications of cold alternating with heat

ROM exercises to maintain motion

Prescribed rest periods in morning and afternoon

Well-balanced diet; avoidance of obesity because of increased joint stress

Providing knowledge about the disease to ease patient's fears and increase compliance with treatment regimen

Table 4-3
Levels of Treatment in Management of Rheumatoid Arthritis*

First	Second	Third	Fourth	Fifth
Education for patient and family Heat Therapeutic exercises Rest Salicylates at therapeutic doses	Occupational and physical therapy Orthotic devices Nonsteroidal anti-inflammatory drugs Analgesic drugs	Gold Low-dose glucocorticoids Hydroxychloroquine Intra-articular glucocorticoids	High-dose glucocorticoids Hospitalization Reconstructive surgery	Immunosuppressive drugs, such as azathioprine Cytotoxic drugs, such as cyclophosphamide

*Treatment of rheumatoid arthritis generally includes each of the above modalities during the course of the disease process.

NURSING CARE

Nursing Assessment

Local Inflammatory Processes in Joint

Edema
Pain
Heat
Redness
Limitation of motion

Systemic Processes

Malaise
Fever
Elevated erythrocyte sedimentation rate
Multiple joint involvement
Subcutaneous rheumatoid nodules
Weight loss
Later, inflammatory changes within major organs

Psychosocial Concerns

Concerns with self-concept, body image disturbances, loss of mobility because of chronicity
Eventual death from major organ involvement

Economic Concerns

Major costs for treatments over extended periods of time

Nursing Dx & Intervention

Nursing Diagnosis	Nursing Intervention/Rationale
Activity intolerance related to anemia and disease state	• Assess levels of energy, tiredness, and fatigue. • Provide rest periods in morning and afternoon *to maintain strength.* • Provide 8 to 10 hours for uninterrupted nighttime sleep *to help maintain strength.* • Alternate activities with rest periods *to prevent fatigue.*
Pain related to inflammatory process	• Assess presence, amount, and severity of pain. • Administer medications as ordered *to relieve pain.* • Have patient sleep and rest on a firm mattress with a small pillow *to prevent deformities.* • Massage back *to ease tightness and pressure of muscles and joints.* • Encourage patient to be active during periods of pain relief *to maintain usual roles.* • Encourage patient to express thoughts and feelings about pain, disease, and loss of independence *to ease concerns.* • Encourage diversionary activities *to decrease focus on pain.* • Encourage patient to participate actively and positively in each type of treatment *to increase comfort.*
Impaired home maintenance management	• Assess ability and strength to carry out homemaking activities. • Use occupational therapists to teach modifications in home environment *to lessen joint stress.* • Use community health nurses *for home evaluation and continuity of care.* • Have patient practice with and use implements and utensils *to gain skill and independence.* • Encourage self-care and modify with utensils and learning experiences *to gain skills.*
Impaired physical mobility	• Assess degree and amount of joint movements or limitations. • Assist with treatment regimen (such as heat, cold, paraffin) *to maintain joint mobility.* • Provide ROM exercises as able *to prevent stiffening of joints.*

Nursing Diagnosis	Nursing Intervention/Rationale
	• Provide splints and walking aids such as cane or crutch *to lessen joint stress.* • Turn and position the patient every 2 to 4 hours *to prevent joint deformity.*
Sleep pattern disturbance	• Assess sleep patterns over time. • Prepare patient for rest with massage and straightening of bed linens *to aid relaxation.* • Position *to prevent contractures.* • Administer medications *to relieve pain and inflammation.* • Give warm milk or snack *to induce sleep.* • Maintain a quiet environment *to promote and maintain sleep periods.*
Body image disturbance and altered role performance	• Assess concerns about condition and role performance. • Encourage active participation in usual roles as able *to maintain self-concept.* • Allow patient to ventilate feelings about deformities and limitation of movements. • Offer support and encouragement *to help maintain a positive attitude about the disease and its treatment.* • Encourage family members to maintain open communication with the patient *to help maintain usual roles.* • Employ team concept (occupational therapy, physical therapy, medicine, and nursing) to discuss plan of care *to provide continuity of care and to build trust relationships with patient and family.*
Knowledge deficit related to disease and progression	• Assess knowledge and understanding of disease. • Explain inflammatory process *to increase understanding.* • Explain the different treatments and their purposes *to increase compliance.*

Patient Education

1. Reiterate explanations of chronicity and controllability of rheumatoid arthritis and its symptoms to aid understanding.
2. Reiterate necessity for patient compliance with treatment regimen for maximum benefits.
3. Teach patient and family members about each medication and common side effects to be aware of and to report to the physician.
4. Encourage patient to participate actively and fully in each aspect of the disease, its treatments, and alternatives for long-term care.
5. Explain the necessity for cooperative family relationships in the patient's care and treatments to maintain self-worth and role relationships.
6. Teach foods needed for a balanced diet.

Evaluation

Patient Outcome	Data Indicating That Outcome is Reached
Patient continues with localized disease for long periods.	Patient can maintain ADLs with mild restrictions of mobility and strength and minimum deformity of tissues.
Systemic organ involvement responds to medical regimen.	Patient has symptoms of cardiac or renal involvement controlled with minimum arrhythmias, no signs of congestive failure, mild edema, and no proteinuria or fever.
Surgical corrective procedures restore joint mobility and relieve pain and deformity.	Patient regains joint strength and structure and has tolerable pain and relief of deviation or deformity.
Patient retains or returns to social interactions over long periods of time.	Patient maintains roles in family and society.
Patient adheres to medication regimen over time without undue side effects.	Patient has minimum nausea, vomiting, bleeding disorders, gastrointestinal burning or pain, and anemia.
Patient engages in prescribed programs of physical therapy.	Patient participates actively in rest and activity periods, exercises, and joint mobility programs as prescribed.

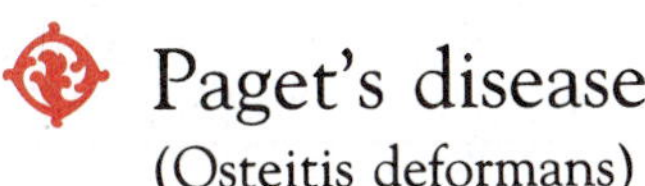

Paget's disease

(Osteitis deformans)

Paget's disease is a chronic inflammatory disease of bones that results in thickening, softening, and eventual bowing of the bones.

Paget's disease (osteitis deformans) is a fairly common disease affecting 3% of people over 40 years of age. It is inflammatory because of the increased warmth over the rapidly changing bone, although it is also a metabolic condition because of the high rates of bone formation and resorption. Men are affected about twice as often as women.

Pathophysiology

The cause of Paget's disease is unknown. It is very rare in Norway and Japan, for unknown reasons. This disease is characterized by high rates of bone resorption and bone formation occurring in several stages. In the so-called vascular stage, spaces left by bone absorption fill with vascular fibrous tissue. New osteoid bone tissue forms on both sides of the cortex, but it is not completely converted to mature bone. Thus even though the bone is thick, it is soft and bendable. The newly formed lamellae are not regularly layered as in correctly formed bones. During the later (sclerotic) stage, the bone is easily broken even though the lamellae calcify and become thick and sclerosed. The disease may begin in one bone only and remain localized for years. The most common sites for Paget's disease are the pelvis and tibia, followed by the femur, skull, spine, and clavicle. When only a single bone is involved, it becomes painful and deformed from bending. The pain is a dull ache that worsens at night. As the disease becomes more generalized, other signs become more evident, including deafness, deformities, stiffness, limb pain, fractures, headaches, and possibly even heart failure. Deafness results from otosclerosis; enlargement of the skull bones increases the head size, and pressure on the optic nerve may produce blindness. Kyphosis may be pronounced, with the patient becoming shorter and appearing apelike with bent legs and arms hanging in front of the trunk. The legs become bowed, and the patient experiences backache with nerve root pressure pain. Fractures become more common as the disease becomes systemic. In a small percentage of patients (5%), a malignant tumor may develop in the involved bone.

Diagnostic Studies and Findings

History and Physical Examination

Tenderness and increased warmth over involved sites
Pain worse at night; may be dull or sharp
Backache
Involvement of special senses
Signs of heart failure
Bones easily bendable
Possibility of fracture
Later in disease, possibility of malignant tumor

Roentgenograms

Thickened, bent bone, its density possibly decreased in the vascular stage and increased in the sclerotic stage
Coarse and widened trabeculae of bone, with a honeycomb appearance
Fine periosteal cracks as a result of stress

Serum Alkaline Phosphatase and Hydroxyproline

High; urinary excretion of hydroxyproline increased

Medical Plan

Surgery

Fracture reduction by closed or open manipulation
External casts or splints to maintain reduction and to help straighten bone

Medications

Thyroid hormones
- Calcitonin (Calcimar), 50-100 IU, injected qd for 3-6 mo; then given 3 times weekly for 6 more mo
- Diphosphonates, po; dosages not fully established to date
- Glucagon and mithramycin may also be used during high disease activity; dosage according to need
- Etidronate in individualized dosage

NURSING CARE

Nursing Assessment

Inflammatory Processes

Increased warmth over affected bone site or sites
Dull pain, may be sharp at times
Stiffness and limitation of motion (although bone may be easily manipulated and bent)

Systemic Processes

Headache
Back and limb pain
Heart failure signs
Hearing loss or deficit and visual changes possible

Psychosocial Concerns

Body image because of enlarged bones of head and legs
Progressive nature of disease (possibility of development of sarcoma and easy fracturing of bones)

Nursing Dx & Intervention

Nursing Diagnosis	Nursing Intervention/Rationale
Pain related to pressure on nerves	• Assess for presence, site, amount, and severity of pain. • Note complaints of bone pain, headache, joint pain and stiffness, dyspnea and edema from congestive heart failure. • Encourage active exercise and range of motion to unaffected musculoskeletal tissues *to maintain functions*. • Administer medications as ordered: calcitonin and etidronate lower osteoclastic (bone reabsorption) activity and serum alkaline phosphatase, thereby *strengthening bones and lessening pain and deformity*. • Note responses to medication: pain relief, increased bone and joint strength, less edema and dyspnea *to note effects of and responses to treatment*.
Potential for injury related to fracture	• Assess, record, and report patient's complaints of sudden increase in pain, hearing or sensing bone crack, or experiencing inability to bear weight or use bone normally. • If fracture occurs and is treated with manipulation, perform necessary nursing care (see p. 451 for care of a person in a cast or having open reduction with internal fixation) *to facilitate recovery*.
Impaired physical mobility related to backache and weakened bones	• Assess effects of pain and weakened bones on mobility. • Arrange for physical therapy for proper joint and muscle use and exercises *to increase mobility*.
Body image disturbance and altered role performance related to thick but weak bones and changing physical appearance	• Assess effects of condition on the patient. • Encourage patient to ventilate feelings about bone "brittleness" and deformity and loss of bone, joint strength, and mobility as desired *to ease concerns*. • Arrange for consultation with occupational therapist *to maintain customary roles with necessary modifications*. • Arrange for consultation with hearing and vision specialists *to maintain or regain adequate functions of these senses when possible*. • Instruct family members about possible role changes necessitated by the progressive nature of this disease *to aid continuity of care*.

Patient Education

1. Reiterate explanations of bone formation and reabsorption to ensure patient understands.
2. Explain purposes of drug therapy and side effects of medication.
3. Caution the patient to use care when moving to lessen probability of fracture.
4. Encourage patient and family activities to maintain independence and social roles.

Evaluation

Patient Outcome	Data Indicating That Outcome is Reached
Disease is controlled over long periods without systemic effects.	Patient experiences no progression of pain, deformity, fracture, or loss of bone strength and no joint or other organ involvement.
Pain is relieved with medications without side effects.	Patient has long pain-free periods, and if pain occurs, it is controlled with medications. Patient experiences no nausea, vomiting, or constipation.
Patient has no fracture.	Patient can use bones and move about at will.

BACTERIAL INFECTIONS

 Osteomyelitis

Osteomyelitis is an infection of bones.

Osteomyelitis is of great concern in any patient with an open wound, sore throat, or pneumonia because it may smolder undiagnosed for extended periods. Its long-term effects on bones and their contiguous tissues demand constant monitoring to prevent recurrence, bone damage, and eventually, even amputation. Although the incidence of osteomyelitis may not be high, even one occurrence should be prevented or avoided whenever possible because of the destructive nature of this infection.

Osteomyelitis is usually a direct invasion into bone tissues from an open wound or bone fracture. It may also be caused by an infection in distant organs in the body, such as streptococcal sore throat or bacterial pneumonia. The major pathogens are staphylococci and streptococci, but *Escherichia coli* and tubercle bacilli may also be involved. Children develop osteomyelitis from throat infections, and hematogenous spread is a major factor in childhood osteomyelitis. In adults, infection more often results from direct invasion following trauma. No sex or age group is immune.

Pathophysiology

The invading organisms travel to the site within the metaphysis (part of the bone between the shaft and epiphyseal area) by direct invasion or indirectly by hematogenous spread. The metaphysis provides a secluded, warm, well-nourished area for the organisms to grow and multiply. The pathogens produce pus, which at first remains localized and confined. As more purulent matter is produced, the enlarging mass eventually spreads out of the confined area, through the cortex of the bone, and into contiguous tissues. If untreated, the purulent mass will spread to the surface of the skin through a sinus tract. The purulent matter also continues to spread around and along the bone shaft and into more soft tissues. Bone cells are destroyed, and the dead bone, called sequestrum, becomes dense and walled off. New bone begins to form from the deeper layers of periosteal cells; this new bone is called involucrum. As the infection progresses, the affected bone weakens and may fracture, giving the first evidence of the existence of the infection. If the soft tissues around the infected bone become tense from accumulated purulent matter, the patient may experience soreness, tenderness, increased warmth at the site, and sometimes edema. Occasionally the patient may experience severe pain that is not relieved by rest. This pain may cause the patient to stop using the extremity (most commonly the lower extremity around the knee). With the soft tissue spread, the patient may experience high, spiking temperatures and appear toxic and ill.

Brodie's abscess is an indolent staphylococcal infection of bone as a result of osteomyelitis.

Diagnostic Studies and Findings

History

Antecedent infection or open trauma in previous 3 to 4 weeks

Physical Examination

Area of tenderness, edema, warmth, redness, and possibly mass or drainage in ends of long bones
Increased pain with movement
Spiking fevers in 39° to 40° C (103° to 104° F) range intermittently noted, chills and diaphoresis
Headache and nausea

Culture of Mass or Drainage

Infecting pathogenic organisms

White Cell Count

Elevated with increased levels of polymorphonuclear nuetrophils (PMNs) indicative of bacterial infection

Erythrocyte Sedimentation Rate

Increased

Roentgenograms

Initially may not reveal the destructive processes but will later show rarefaction of the involved bone with evidence of formation of sequestrum and involucrum

Serum cultures

Pathogenic organism, most commonly *Staphylococcus aureus*

Medical Plan

Surgery

Aspiration of abscess for culture purposes only
Following "sterilization" of abscess, sequestrum is removed and replaced by bone grafts
Saucerization is performed: involved bone is scraped to remove all necrotic cells, following which bone regenerates; if the defect is pronounced, bone grafts may be applied or metallic fixation may be applied (never used in infected areas or if uncertainty exists about the possibility of lingering pathogens remaining)
External fixation devices such as Hoffman apparatus (pp. 453-455) may be used to hold bones weakened from the initial infection or saucerization
Amputation of limb (done less frequently now because of improved treatment modalities)

Medications

Anti-infective agents: according to culture and sensitivity results and patient sensitivity or allergy

Aqueous penicillin, 500,000 to 1 million U, IV q6h continuously for 30 d or longer, up to 6 wk
Erythromycin (Erythrocin), 1-2 g, IV q6h (for penicillin-sensitive patients)
Ampicillin (Omnipen), 1 g IV q6h
Cephalosporin (cephalothin or Keflin), 1 g q6h IV for penicillin-resistant organisms

General Management

Splints to decrease joint pain
Bed rest to conserve energy
Sling for the arm
Cast to prevent a fracture of weakened bones; should have "windows" for dressing changes, if needed

NURSING CARE

Nursing Assessment

Inflammatory Processes

Increased warmth at site
Edema
Tenderness
Mild to severe pain
Affected part may not be used

Systemic Processes

Fever and chills; diaphoresis
Malaise
Weakness
Headache and nausea

Spread

Local tissues
Distant sites, where infection continues

Psychosocial Concerns

Body image
Disability from long-term disease processes

Nursing Dx & Intervention

Nursing Diagnosis	Nursing Intervention/Rationale
Pain related to presence of abscess in bone	• Assess for amount, site, severity, and duration of pain. • Maintain bed rest or limited activity *to lessen stress on involved tissues.* • Administer analgesics if ordered *to relieve pain.* Aspirin, 300 to 600 mg, is usually the medication ordered. • Handle affected limb gently *to lessen pressure and pain.* Use sling when appropriate. • Administer intravenous antibiotics in collaboration with physician *to clear infection and thereby lessen pain.* Monitor patient's response. • Encourage activities to divert attention from condition (e.g., with children, take child to playroom, outside, etc.) • Use care when initiating intravenous therapy per physician order and during therapy *to preserve venous integrity for long-term need.* Use care to maintain asepsis of all equipment *to prevent nosocomial infection.*
Impaired physical mobility related to bone involvement	• Assess effects on mobility and joint use. • Encourage ROM to unaffected joints *to decrease tiredness and prevent weakening.* • Encourage self-care *to maintain muscle strength.* • Encourage hobby and diversionary activities *to maintain motion and strength in all uninvolved joints.* • Use wheelchair or crutches *to aid ambulation and increase socialization.*
Altered peripheral tissue perfusion related to surgery	• Perform postoperative neurovascular checks *to determine tissue perfusion in affected tissues.*
Impaired skin integrity related to incision and surgery	• Assess skin surfaces over body. • Remove splint for care and *to check skin condition.* • Change dressings as needed *to remove drainage and to lessen odor and skin maceration.* • If surgical procedures are performed, perform thorough skin preparation and "scrub" *to lessen postoperative wound infections.*
Body image disturbance related to pathology	• Assess concerns related to condition or treatments. • Explain rationale for long-term therapy: *to clear disease.*

Nursing Diagnosis	Nursing Intervention/Rationale
	• Assess equipment (splint, Hoffman apparatus, etc.) for proper functioning, as well as patient's responses, *to monitor effects of treatments.* • If amputation is required, do preoperative preparation, allowing patient to talk about concern over loss of body part. Following amputation, do necessary care to promote wound healing and prevent complications (see p. 439). • Encourage patient and family interaction *to maintain relationships and usual roles.*

Patient Education

1. Reiterate need for prompt medical attention to local or systemic infections to prevent recurrence.
2. Explain rationale, purposes, and expected outcomes for long-term antibiotic therapy to increase understanding and compliance.
3. Explain side effects of long-term antibiotic therapy.
4. Explain purposes for continuing ROM exercises to maintain strength and mobility.

Evaluation

Patient Outcome	Data Indicating That Outcome is Reached
Infection is cleared without local or systemic extension or recurrence.	Patient's temperature is normal; patient has no pain, tenderness, or edema at site and no limitation of mobility; bone heals without loss of length and without sequestrum or involucrum following treatments.
Patient resumes social interactions and returns to employment activities.	Patient returns to family, social, and employment roles as before illness.

CONNECTIVE TISSUE DISORDERS

Connective tissue diseases can affect the musculoskeletal tissues directly or can indirectly cause musculoskeletal damage by affecting tissue such as muscles, arteries, skin, and joints, all of which contain collagen tissues. Connective tissue diseases used to be known as collagen diseases.

Collagen is the most prevalent protein in the body; it constitutes approximately half the total protein in adults. Collagen also is the principal supporting element in the connective tissues, and it is active in developmental processes, cell attachment, chemotaxis, and the binding of antigen-antibody complexes.

Another characteristic of collagen tissues is that interstitial collagens, as well as their biosynthetic precursors (procollagens), are "now recognized as distinct antigens capable of eliciting significant humoral and cellular immune responses."[26] Another correlation of connective and musculoskeletal tissues is that some of the major arthritides are thought to be of autoimmune origin. Rheumatoid arthritis, lupus erythematosus, and ankylosing spondylitis are diseases of specific connective tissues.

Specific types of collagen make up the connective tissues of bones, tendons, cartilage, and other connective tissues, including skin, muscles, uterine wall, and blood vessel walls.

This section concerns only progressive systemic sclerosis as a prototypical connective tissue disease.

NOTE: With all connective tissue diseases, compliance with medication regimens over extended periods is a basic necessity for control of these disabling chronic disorders. A major goal is to achieve maximum patient compliance, not only with the intake of all the requisite medications, but also with every part of the therapeutic regimen. Patient compliance is a nursing and medical concern with the connective tissue diseases because the various forms of treatment are symptomatic and noncurative.

Progressive systemic sclerosis
(Scleroderma)

Progressive systemic sclerosis is a chronic inflammatory disease of the collagen (connective) tissues.

The name "progressive systemic sclerosis" has replaced the term "scleroderma" because it more accurately reflects the progressive effects of this disease on multiple organs and other connective tissues throughout the body. Although progressive systemic sclerosis is a rare disease, it merits discussion because of its extensive involvement of the connective tissues.

Pathophysiology

In the early stages of progressive systemic sclerosis, the skin may be edematous and doughy. As the inflammation proceeds to fibrous tissue formation, large amounts of collagen are deposited and the skin becomes thickened, leathery, and bound to the subcutaneous connective tissues. In the later stages, atrophic changes are noted in the dermis and fat tissues, with thin, translucent skin stretched tightly over the subcutaneous structures. The face is pinched, nonexpressive, and stiff. The sclerosis (hardening) and fibrosis also occur in the gastrointestinal tract, heart, lungs, and kidneys. Arterial walls develop thickened intima and thickened basement membranes. This thickening leads to ischemic changes characterized as Raynaud's phenomenon, a classic sign of progressive systemic sclerosis. The disease proceeds slowly, and complications arise in specific areas. Complications include bowel obstruction; congestive heart failure; nephrosclerosis; esophageal thickening, leading to dysphagia; and lung fibrosis, causing respiratory problems.

Diagnostic Studies and Findings

Physical Examination

- CREST syndrome
  - C = calcinosis, hardening
  - R = Raynaud's phenomenon
  - E = esophageal dysfunction; dysphagia
  - S = sclerodactyly (hardening, thinning of fingers and skin)
  - T = telangiectasis (dilation of superficial capillaries, commonly called spider nevi)

Biopsy and Angiography

- Capillaries
  - Large dilated capillary loops with loss of capillaries from adjacent areas, leading to marked avascularity (seen in more than 80% of patients with progressive systemic sclerosis)
- Skin, subcutaneous tissues, fascia, and muscle
  - Collagen hypertrophy with cellular infiltrates and inflammatory changes

Medical Plan

Surgery

- Joint arthroplasty for ankylosis
- Bowel resection for bowel obstruction; occasionally, colostomy may be required

Medications

- Corticosteroids
  - Prednisone (Deltasone, others), 40-60 mg/d in divided doses for 8-12 wk
- Nutritional supplements
  - Potassium para-aminobenzoate (Potaba), 12 g/d in divided doses, for cutaneous changes; dose reduced as response is noted
- Cholinergic agents
  - Bethanechol (Urecholine), 5-10 mg 30 min before meals for dysphagia
- Analgesic-antipyretic agents
  - Aspirin, 600-1000 mg qd for joint symptoms
- See Chapters 1 and 11 for pharmacologic treatment of associated hypertension and renal dysfunction

General Management

- Individualized exercise programs to maintain ROM of joints affected are vital to prevent contractures
- Planned rest programs in morning and afternoon to prevent overtiring
- Wearing warm clothing and gloves and, in extreme cases, moving to a warmer climate for patients with pronounced Raynaud's phenomenon
- Avoidance of exposure to cold
- Forcing fluids lessens bowel and renal concerns
- Diet nutritious, well balanced, and high in bulk-forming foods

NURSING CARE

Nursing Assessment

Inflammatory Processes (Localized to Skin and Joints)

- Edema
- Tenderness
- Weakness and limitation of movements
- Raynaud's phenomenon in fingers and hands
- Tough and hardened feeling to skin
- Skin rash (may be localized to hands and feet)
- Taut and shiny appearance to skin as disease progresses with loss of skin folds

Systemic Responses to Inflammation (Vary with Particular Patient)

- Esophageal: dysphagia
- Respiratory
  - Dyspnea
  - Repeated respiratory infections
- Intestinal
  - Bowel distention
  - Constipation
  - Obstruction
- Renal
  - Hematuria
  - Decreased urinary output (late pattern)
  - Hypertension
- Musculoskeletal: multiple joint involvements with deformity and ankylosis

Psychosocial Concerns

Body image changes and disturbances
Progressive nature of condition

Nursing Dx & Intervention

Nursing Diagnosis	Nursing Intervention/Rationale
Impaired physical mobility related to muscle and joint involvement	• Assess joint functions and mobility. • Perform ROM exercises to joints *to maintain function.* • Help ambulate four times daily *to maintain strength.* • Provide rest periods *to retain or maintain strength.*
Impaired physical mobility related to other involved organs/tissues	• Assess swallowing *to note dysphagia.* • Check for bowel movement; note characteristics of stool *to determine intestinal competence.* • Check for peripheral edema, hypertension, or cardiac involvement *to note cardiac functions.* • Assist with ADLs as requested while maintaining patient's independence *to maintain activity levels.* • Provide nutritious diet high in bulk *to aid elimination.*
Altered patterns of urinary elimination related to disease process	• Assess urine and urinary output with renal involvement *to note remaining functions.* • Force fluids if possible and required *to aid renal function.*
Altered peripheral tissue perfusion related to Raynaud's phenomenon	• Assess fingers, hands, and toes, particularly for evidence of Raynaud's phenomenon: blanching, cyanosis, then redness (pattern is white to blue to red). • Assess for tingling and paresthesia in fingers and toes. • Observe for unusual reactions to cold *as a sign of arterial involvement.* • Note thinning, tightness, and shininess of skin (patient has a "pinched," expressionless facies); fingers appear more pointed, and tips are thin and fragile looking; tips may develop ulcers.
Body image disturbance related to appearance	• Assess effects of condition on patient's body image and self-esteem. • Encourage social interactions *to maintain self-esteem.* • Arrange for consultations with physical therapist *to maintain ROM to joints and muscles.*
Impaired gas exchange related to pulmonary involvement of the disease	• Assess respiratory rates, depth, presence of dyspnea, cough, or shortness of breath. • Teach deep-breathing exercises *to maintain pulmonary function.* • Listen to breath sounds in all lobes *to note condition and possible respiratory complications.*

Patient Education

1. Reiterate progressive nature of progressive systemic sclerosis.
2. Encourage the patient to maintain ADLs and social roles to prevent or lessen complications.
3. Explain patterns indicative of specific organ involvement: signs of congestive heart failure, hypertension, dysphagia, bowel obstruction and urinary/renal hematuria, and oliguria, if pertinent.
4. Explain side effects of medications.
5. Encourage patient and family interactions for clarifications as needed.

Evaluation

Patient Outcome	Data Indicating That Outcome is Reached
Patient maintains mobility for extended periods.	Patient is able to do self-care and ADLs and to move about adequately without undue limitations.
Patient experiences no skin breakdown or circulatory deficits.	Patient has no ulcers, numbness, tingling, or Raynaud's phenomenon; skin thickening or hardening is minimum.
Patient complies with treatment regimen.	Patient takes medications as ordered, does deep-breathing exercises, and rests as required.

DEGENERATIVE CONDITIONS

As people age, they experience some musculoskeletal conditions resulting from degeneration. Even though such conditions may begin in a specific tissue, such as the cartilage or bone, they affect not only that tissue but also other musculoskeletal tissues because of their anatomic and physiologic interrelationships. Therefore these conditions have local and systemic effects, as do the conditions previously discussed.

Hallux valgus

Hallux valgus is deviation of the great toe toward the other toes.

Figure 4-15 Hallux valgus (bunion). **A,** External view. **B,** Anatomic view.

A

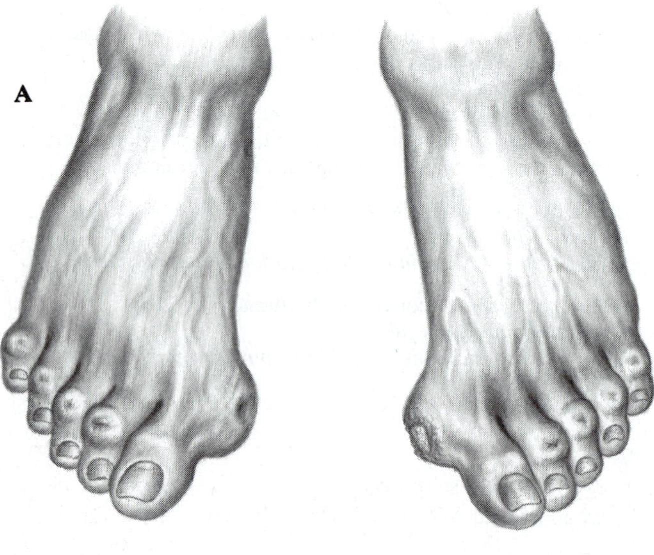

B

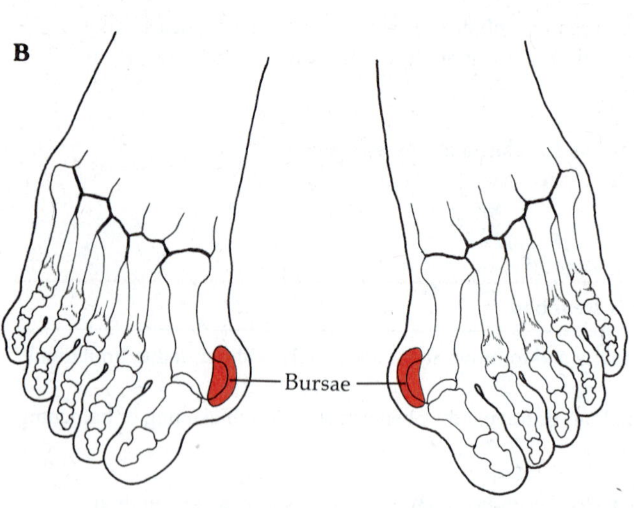

In hallux (great toe) valgus, the great toe deviates toward the other toes either from congenital abnormality or from degeneration caused by increasing weight and weight-bearing activities. The forefoot becomes splayed, allowing the first metatarsal bone to deviate into a more varus position (Figure 4-15).

Pathophysiology

Hallux valgus is most obvious from the increasing prominence and deformity of the first metatarsal bone, with this bone's shaft deviated medially away from the second metatarsal. The head of the first metatarsal bone develops a protective bursa (bunion) wherever it rubs against a shoe. As the valgus deformity of the proximal phalanx of the great toe increases, the second toe is crowded and may also become deformed.

Usually hallux valgus is bilateral, with one side more prominent and symptomatic than the other. It is most commonly noted in women during the sixth decade with a strong familial tendency. Adolescents also may have hallux valgus (valgus refers to lateral deviation away from the midline).

Diagnostic Studies and Findings

Physical Examination

Valgus deformity of great toe, with or without bursa development (bunion), hammer toe, corns, calluses, and bilaterality

Roentgenograms

Deformities described above

History

Familial occurrence

Medical Plan

Surgery

- Osteotomy to realign bones, such as Mitchell osteotomy
- Arthroplasty: Keller operation; Stone procedure (Figure 4-16)
- Arthrodesis, such as Lapidus operation
- Bunionectomy

Medications

- Analgesic-antipyretic agents
  - Aspirin, 600-1000 mg qid
  - Acetaminophen, 600-1000 mg qid

General Management

- Taping pad under metatarsal heads to change weight-bearing pressure
- Changing shoe style to wider, open-toed shoe with soft upper portions
- Foot exercises to lessen splayfoot
- Application of ice bag to site of bunion

Figure 4-16 One type of operative repair of hallux valgus.

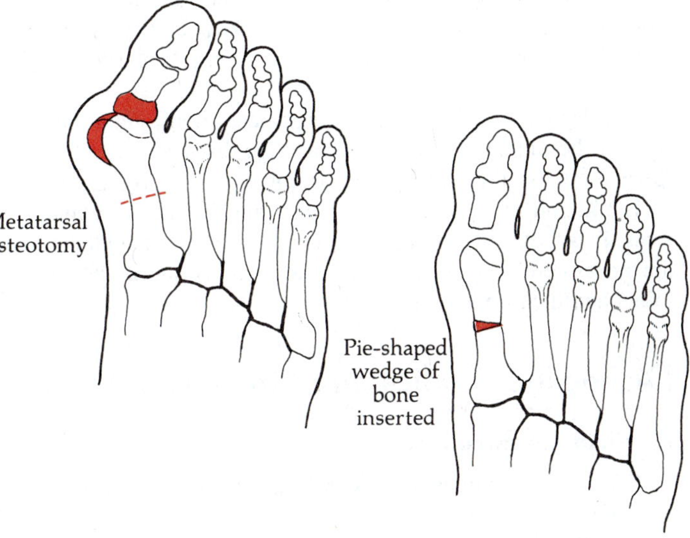

NURSING CARE

Nursing Assessment

Signs of Degeneration

Valgus (away from midline) deformity of great toe and varus deformity of first metatarsal bone
Presence of bunion
Corn development from pressure on other toes
Deformity or crowding of second toe
Hammer toe possible in other toes
Callus possible under metatarsal heads of other toes

Other Accompanying Signs

Presence of inflamed bursa, producing tenderness and often exquisite pain in and around joint (metatarsophalangeal of great toe)
Condition usually bilateral

Psychosocial Concerns

Concern with body image from deformity and pain

Nursing Dx & Intervention

Nursing Diagnosis	Nursing Intervention/Rationale
Body image disturbance related to deformities	• Assess concerns about presence of hallux valgus. • Encourage wearing of well-fitted footwear *to lessen progression.* • Encourage consulting with physician for possible surgical removal *to aid in positive feeling.* • Encourage exercises *to lessen progressive deformity.*
Pain related to bunion and inflammation	• Assess amount, duration, and severity of pain. • Administer ordered medication *to ease discomfort.* • Apply ice bag to inflamed bursa *to lessen edema and pain.* • Encourage temporary cessaton of weight bearing when pain is acute *to increase comfort.*
Impaired physical mobility related to pain and deformity	• Assess effects of condition on mobility. • Encourage use of padding in shoes *to change weight-bearing sites.* • Encourage usual activities when pain is relieved *to increase mobility.* • Encourage consulting with physician to remove bursa if necessary *to relieve condition and increase mobility.*

Patient Education

1. Clarify bunion as accompanying hallux valgus, not being only condition.
2. Instruct about preventive measures with proper footwear and exercises.
3. Explain surgical options previously discussed with physician, if necessary, for clarity.

Evaluation

Patient Outcome	Data Indicating That Outcome is Reached
Patient walks without pain or deformity of toe joint.	Patient uses orthotic devices as ordered, wears well-fitted shoes, applies ice during acute inflammation, and rests the joint. Patient undergoes surgical correction if necessary to relieve deformity and regain painless mobility.

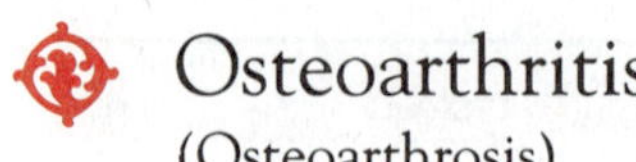

Osteoarthritis
(Osteoarthrosis)

Osteoarthritis is a degenerative condition of the articular cartilage, primarily within the major weight-bearing joints although other joints are also affected.

Currently there is disagreement about whether osteoarthritis or osteoarthrosis is the more accurate term. Sentiment appears to be swinging toward osteoarthritis at this time, so that term is used throughout this chapter.

Osteoarthritis is a disease of older adults. It usually begins after middle age and is the major cause of loss of joint mobility and increasing pain episodes in those affected. Although biochemical changes occur in the joints with age, aging alone does not account for the degeneration of the cartilage. The main cause of the degeneration is a discrepancy between the strength of the cartilage and the forces to which it is subjected. If the load to which the cartilage is subjected is too great, the cartilage gives way. It may also give way with normal loads if it has been weakened by damage or disease or if it is unsupported by normal bone. Osteoarthritis is slightly more common in women than men. Obesity is a major factor contributing to the development of osteoarthritis.

Pathophysiology

Early changes in the normal, whitish, smooth hyaline cartilage include an increase in its water content and a decrease in the amount of proteoglycan (complex protein-carbohydrate molecules). The cartilage looks irregular, pitted, and softer. It undergoes fibrillation, and cartilage flakes (detritus) are shed into the joint. This shedding rubs away the cartilage, primarily from sites where the maximum load is greatest. Repeated wear and erosion thin the cartilage.

Although the cartilage is not rubbed away or thinned in nonstress areas, it is unhealthy from undernourishment. Cartilage is nourished during compression by synovial fluid and transudates from subchondral vessels. This pumping action does not occur in nonstress areas, so there is undernourishment. The subchondral vessels hypertrophy and invade the cartilage, which calcifies and later ossifies, forming osteophytes. The hyperemia spreads into the bone beneath the stress area, but pressure in this area prevents the vessels from penetrating into the cartilage. The cartilage continues to be rubbed away, exposing the underlying bone, which becomes dense and hard. Stress (fatigue) fractures occur in the subchondral trabeculae, and cysts develop where pressure is greatest.

During cartilage erosion, detritus is deposited on the synovial lining, which then hypertrophies. Flakes of cartilage also penetrate into the subsynovial layer, where they induce fibrosis that extends into the capsule. The capsule becomes thickened and inelastic. The fibrous tissue shrinks as it matures, thereby limiting joint movement.

This restriction of movement resulting from fibrosis is the main feature of osteoarthritis. Symptoms appear early in joints such as the hip, where full extension is required for walking. Since the hip joint capsule is well supplied with pain fibers, slight restriction is noted by pain with attempts at full extension. Thus major weight-bearing joints show earlier symptoms. Weight bearing continues as an aggravation in osteoarthritis.

Besides the hip and knee the carpometacarpal joint at the base of the thumb, the vertebrae, and the distal joints of the fingers are also affected by osteoarthritis.

Limitation of movements and pain are the major symptoms. Pain frequently occurs after a night's rest. Usually there are no systemic signs, just the local signs confined to the joints and their contiguous tissues.

Diagnostic Studies and Findings

Physical Examination

Enlarged edematous joint with some stiffness and deformity
Usually only one joint has most pronounced signs, although more than one can be involved
If hip is involved, patient may hold it flexed, adducted, and externally rotated
Joint may be tender but rarely feels hot
Movements of joint limited
Crepitus common
Heberden's nodes may be present in distal interphalangeal joints of fingers, and Bouchard's nodes occur in the proximal interphalangeal joints

Roentgenograms

Decreased or diminished joint space
Sclerotic bone
Bone cysts
Osteophytes and lipping in some joints

Medical Plan

Surgery

Arthroplasty to repair the joint
Total joint replacement to replace diseased tissues
Osteotomy to change weight-bearing surfaces
Arthrodesis to limit joint movements (done to abolish pain)
Spinal fusion to maintain posture and eliminate pain

Medications

Analgesic-antipyretic agents
  Aspirin, 600-1000 mg 3-4 times daily
Nonsteroidal anti-inflammatory agents
  Ibuprofen (Motrin), 300-400 mg 3-4 times daily
  Naproxen (Naprosyn), 250-375 mg bid
  Tolmetin (Tolectin), 200-400 mg 3-4 times daily
  Indomethacin (Indocin), 25-50 mg 3-4 times daily

Sulindac (Clinoril), 150-200 mg bid
Phenylbutazone (Butazolidin), 300-400 mg/d, for short-term use only
Feldene, 20 mg/d

General Management

Moist heat applications with diathermy, hot water bottles, and radiant heat
Rest and modified weight-bearing activities beneficial
Canes, crutches, or walkers to aid walking and decrease joint stress
Soft collar and cervical traction to lessen pain
Back brace or support to lessen pain and maintain posture
Ace bandage to wrist or knee for support

NURSING CARE

Nursing Assessment

Local (Joint) Signs of Degeneration

Limitation of full extension, pain on arising and on weight bearing in joint
Pain disturbing sleep as disease progresses
Joint stiffness and deformity from fibrosis, shrinkage, and muscle imbalance
Limp
Joint feels unstable and may give way
Edema in superficial joints

Systemic Signs

None

Psychosocial Concerns

Body image changes
Pain
Limitation of movement

Nursing Dx & Intervention

Nursing Diagnosis	Nursing Intervention/Rationale
Impaired physical mobility related to joint pathology and pain	• Assess ROM and mobility limitations. • Encourage and assist with ambulation as needed *to maintain joint functions.* • Assist with ADLs as needed *to aid in completing activities.* • Use ambulatory aid as ordered *to facilitate walking.* • Assist with ambulation after pain is relieved with heat or medication *to increase distances.*
Pain related to joint pathology and pressure on contiguous tissues	• Assess amount and severity of pain. • Administer ordered analgesic or anti-inflammatory medications *to lessen pain.* • Assess effects of medications for pain relief *to note efficacy.* • Use heat and diathermy as ordered *to relieve pain.* • Stress proper posture when walking, standing, or sitting *to aid in proper muscle use.* • Encourage weight loss *to decrease joint stress.* • Apply traction or collar if necessary and ordered *to lessen muscle pain.*
Body image disturbance and altered role performance related to progressive degenerative condition	• Assess effects of condition on ADLs. • Encourage patient to perform usual activities and ADLs *for self-esteem.* • Encourage patient to comply with plan of medical care *to lessen joint deformity and decrease pain.* • Encourage planned rest *to maintain strength.* • If surgery is contemplated, review and clarify options previously discussed by physician with patient *to lessen anxiety.*

Patient Education

1. Clarify understandings of degenerative nature of this disease and effects on mobility.
2. Explain side effects of medications.
3. Caution about effects of heat on less sensitive tissues.

Evaluation

Patient Outcome	Data Indicating That Outcome is Reached
Patient walks with minimum limitation of motion or pain.	Patient maintains self-care, ADLs, and employment for as long as desired without experiencing uncontrollable pain or joint movement limitations or deformity.
Patient will comply with medication regimen without distressing side effects.	Patient takes medications as ordered without nausea, vomiting, gastrointestinal burning, bleeding, or pain, and no hematologic changes. Pain is relieved with medications, and joint mobility is enhanced.
Patient returns to social interactions.	Patient returns to usual family, social, and employment roles.

DEFICIENCY DISEASES

Osteomalacia

Osteomalacia is a disease of adults characterized by increasing softening, brittleness, flexibility, and deformity of bones.

Osteomalacia is the adult equivalent of rickets in children; both result from a vitamin D deficiency, which leads to reduced absorption of calcium and phosphorus. The vitamin D deficiency may be from inadequate dietary intake, insufficient sunshine, malabsorption in the intestines, or defective metabolism of vitamin D.

Pathophysiology

Without vitamin D, the amount of calcium and phosphorus available for bone calcification is inadequate to maintain strong bones. Defective growth and replacement of rigid bones are noted first in immature skeletal bones at sites of growth and in mature bones at points of stress, where turnover is most rapid. The physiologic balance of bone growth and reabsorption is disrupted. Defective replacement at the sites mentioned is noticed first because of the increased demand for new bone formation. Failure of mineralization and the bones' resultant inability to resist stress because of lack of rigidity are evident through the patient's symptoms and by x-ray examination.

Diagnostic Studies and Findings

History

Decreased intake or absorption of vitamin D, from unfortified milk, following gastrectomy, or other cause

Physical Examination

Bone pain, muscle weakness, and general malaise

Serum Calcium Levels

Lower than normal (4.5 to 5.5 mEq/L)

Serum Alkaline Phosphatase

Elevated above 13 King-Armstrong units

Sedimentation Rate

May be slightly elevated

Roentgenograms

General decalcification of bones
Pseudofractures (Looser's zones): incomplete fractures in various stages of healing

Biopsy of Iliac Crest

Excessive uncalcified bones

Renal Osteodystrophy (Chronic Renal Failure)

From lack of completion of vitamin D metabolism

Medical Plan

Medications

Nutritional supplements: vitamin D, 400-600 USP units, po or IV, daily, until deficiency is corrected

General Management

Supplying well-balanced diet with fortified milk and sources of vitamin D (egg yolks, tuna, cod liver oil, and salmon)

NURSING CARE

Nursing Assessment

Skeleton: Bone Growth, Maturation

Bone pain present and severe
Strength of bone impaired; fractures common
May have backache and muscle weakness
Deformation of bones that are not able to bear normal weights

Systemic Processes

General weakness throughout body; may have malaise and fatigue

Psychosocial Concerns

Body image disturbances

Nursing Dx & Intervention

Nursing Diagnosis	Nursing Intervention/Rationale
Impaired physical mobility related to weakened, deformed bones	• Assess musculoskeletal tissues *to note deformities.* • Position to support affected tissues; use pillows appropriately *to aid in maintaining positions.* • Assist with ambulation if no fracture is present *to increase mobility.* • Prevent additional injury through maintenance of a safe environment: side rails, nonskid surfaces, and clean, dry areas *for safety.*
Altered nutrition: less than body requirements, related to inadequate or inappropriate intake	• Assess intake of milk and other foods containing calcium and vitamin D. • Administer medications (vitamin D) per physician's order *to correct deficiency.* • Explain how therapy will improve patient's condition *to increase compliance.* • Supply well-balanced diet high in vitamin D foods; explain how this will affect condition *to aid compliance and relieve condition.*
Body image disturbance related to deformities	• Assess presence of deformities. • Listen to patient ventilate feelings of deformity *to ease concerns.* • If surgery is contemplated, discuss purposes (to correct deformity and prevent later degenerative changes) *to lessen anxiety.*

Patient Education

1. Instruct about sources of vitamin D and need for adequate intake.
2. Explain surgical treatment and recovery processes.

Evaluation

Patient Outcome	Data Indicating That Outcome is Reached
Patient regains and maintains adequate vitamin D levels.	Patient has normal serum levels of vitamin D.
Patient regains and maintains normal calcium levels and strength of bones without deformity.	Patient has normal serum calcium levels. Bones regain proper calcification, and roentgenograms show increased density and minimum or no deformity.

Osteoporosis

Osteoporosis is a systemic condition of overall reduction in bone mass or density in which bone resorption has outstripped bone formation, thereby upsetting the normal balance.

The disease is most common in postmenopausal women, probably because of endocrine involution and inactivity. Younger people may develop osteoporosis after severe injuries. In these cases paralysis and long periods of immobility can lead to osteoporosis. People with rheumatoid arthritis and liver disease may also develop osteoporosis. Men can develop osteoporosis but do so less frequently than women (ratio is 1:4).

Pathophysiology

Patients with osteoporosis have normal bones but less overall bone quantity. The remaining bone becomes weakened from the demands of weight bearing. Fractures can occur with little force, especially in the lower radius, femoral neck, and vertebrae. The vertebral column's overall mass is diminished, leading to increasing kyphosis (dowager's hump) and loss of height. Backache is common and can radiate down the legs. Dull, constant pain is common in the back and chest.

Diagnostic Studies and Findings

History

Prolonged immobility
Menopause
Decreased activity

Physical Examination

Increased kyphosis
Backache or neck ache with radiation to legs and arms
Few other symptoms

Roentgenograms

Soft vertebral bodies that are indented by the discs and become biconcave
Vertebrae possibly wedged from fractures
Thoracic vertebral curvature increased

Blood Serum Study

Low levels of alkaline phosphatase

Medical Plan

Medications

Nutritional supplements
- Calcium carbonate (Os-Cal or Os-Cal-Fluor), 1 g/d
- Vitamin D, 50,000 IU once or twice per wk
- Estrogens for postmenopausal women who have undergone hysterectomy; because of increased risk of endometrial cancer and cardiovascular complications, use of estrogens for osteoporosis is controversial; however, estrogen/progesterone combinations are now advocated as estrogen 0.625 mg/d; progesterone may be added to the estrogen (estrogen taken for 25 d/mo, combined with progesterone for days 16-25, then both stopped for rest of month)
- High-protein diet

General Management

Application of back corset or neck support to prevent stress fractures

Ambulation and maintaining active exercises to hold calcium in bones

NURSING CARE

Nursing Assessment

Skeletal Tissues

Degree of strength
Presence of increased kyphosis
Loss of height
Fracture of hip and compression fractures of vertebrae

Other Tissues

Backache
Neck pain
Pain radiating to legs and arms

Psychosocial Concerns

Self-concept: disturbances in self-esteem and body image
Alteration in physical mobility
Pain

Nursing Dx & Intervention

Nursing Diagnosis	Nursing Intervention/Rationale
Self-esteem disturbance and altered role performance related to kyphosis and pain	• Assess ability to carry out self-care, ADLs, and usual roles. • Explain or clarify the processes accompanying menopause as normal and natural *to ease concerns.* • Encourage usual ADLs and other activities *to maintain bone mass.* • Encourage fashion consultation for clothing to lessen evidence of increased kyphosis *to increase self-esteem.*
Impaired physical mobility related to decreased bone mass and pain	• Assess pain as it affects mobility. • Administer medications if ordered; monitor response *to correct condition.* • Perform ROM exercises actively and passively if necessary *to maintain muscle and joint strength.* • Use ambulatory aid (cane or crutch) if needed *to lessen stress on bones.* • Apply back corset or neck collar *to lessen pain and increase mobility* (use is controversial because they limit muscle movements).
Impaired gas exchange related to kyphosis	• Assess respiratory rates, depth, and breath sounds *to evaluate effects of kyphosis.* • Encourage attempts to maintain upright posture *to aid ventilation.*

Patient Education

1. Refute popular perception of osteoporosis as "thin" bones; bone mass is decreased, but bones are not thinner in this disease.
2. Instruct patient and family about advantages of activity to maintain bone mass and calcium in bones.
3. Clarify effects of increased calcium intake and reiterate need for serial examinations of serum calcium levels.
4. Encourage a program of active exercises to maintain strength of muscles and bones.

Evaluation

Patient Outcome	Data Indicating That Outcome is Reached
Patient maintains or regains bone calcification.	Patient has normal serum calcium levels; roentgenograms show normal bone densities.
Patient maintains pain-free ambulation and joint mobility.	Patient maintains self-care, ADLs, and mobility as desired without pain.
Osteoporosis is not progressively debilitating.	Patient's disease is controlled by medication, calcium intake, or activity. Patient has no major loss of bone density.

TRAUMA

Musculoskeletal trauma occurs in all age groups. One in five emergency department visits is associated with musculoskeletal trauma, and one in four patient visits to physicians correlates with musculoskeletal conditions. Among older people, musculoskeletal conditions and trauma rank second only to respiratory conditions as reasons for hospital admission. Because of our fast-paced life-styles, the injured person may suffer injuries not only to the musculoskeletal tissues but to other tissues as well. Even when these injuries are not fatal or life threatening, they may require long periods of hospitalization and recovery. Also, there is no assurance that there will be no future disability or pain, and periods of decreased mobility are likely.

Contusions, strains, and sprains

A contusion is a bruise without an external break in the skin.

A strain is a "pull" in a muscle, ligament, or tendon caused by excessive stretch.

A sprain is a tear in a muscle, ligament, or tendon; it may be mild to severe.

Trauma to the musculoskeletal tissues may involve one specific tissue, such as one ligament, one tendon, or a single muscle mass, although injury to single tissues is rare. Injury to several tissues is more common, such as multiple fractures of bones, with many fracture fragments associated with skin, nerve, and blood vessel trauma. Such injuries frequently are life threatening.

Less serious injuries comprise bruises or contusions of the skin; strain (stretch) of tendon or ligament fibers; and sprains (tearing) of some, many, or all tendons, ligaments, or even bones in and around a joint. These three conditions (contusion, strain, and sprain) have similar initial signs, require similar assessments, and have similar treatment.

Pathophysiology

Contusions are bruises from sudden external pressure that tear the subcutaneous circulatory veins and capillaries. Bleeding occurs in the injured subcutaneous tissues and is noted by bluish discoloration of the injured tissues, with edema or swelling accompanying the vessel or tissue injury. Depending on the extent or severity of the contusion, the edema and discoloration begin to abate in 48 to 72 hours. A charleyhorse is a contusion of a muscle.

A strain is caused by an undue force applied to muscles, ligaments, or tendons. It stretches the fibers, causing a temporary weakness, numbness, and some bleeding if the veins or capillaries within the injured tissues are excessively stretched. The weakness may last 24 to 72 hours, but the numbness usually disappears within hours. Bleeding may continue for 30 minutes or longer unless pressure or cold is applied to stop it. A strained muscle, ligament, or tendon can regain its full function following conservative treatments, which are discussed later. Muscles that are frequently strained are the hamstring and pectineus (hamstring and groin pull, respectively).

A sprain is a partial or full tearing off or away (avulsion) of one or more ligaments or tendons or portions of the bone in and around a joint. Sprains are caused by undue force, twisting, or pull exerted during sports or work activities. Most sprains occur in the ankles, wrists, fingers, and toes. Other joints can be sprained if undue force, pressure, or pull is applied without relief.

Sprains are classified as first degree (some tearing of fibers with some bleeding); second degree (moderate tearing and more extensive bleeding or hemorrhage); and third degree (full tearing or avulsion of the tendon or ligament from its bony attachment, with or without some bone attached, accompanied by marked hemorrhage, pain, edema, and loss of function).

Diagnostic Studies and Findings

History

Pressure
Undue force
Pull without relief (if strain or sprain)

Physical Examination

Skin, circulatory, and musculoskeletal signs as described on pp. 389-390

Medical Plan

	Contusion	Strain	Sprain
Surgery			
Open reduction and repair of torn or avulsed tissues	None	None	May be needed for full joint function; ligament or tendon may be reattached or may need to be removed
Medications			
Analgesics	None	Aspirin, 300-600 mg qid prn; or acetaminophen, 300-600 mg qid prn	Aspirin, 300-1000 mg q4h to relieve pain and inflammation
Narcotics	None	None	Codeine, 30-60 mg po q4-6h for severe pain
General Management			
Cold application	Ice bag for 24 h*	Ice bag for 24 h	Ice bag for 24 h or longer
External wrap	None	Ace wrap or sling	Ace wrap or cast; sling
Elevation	None	Elevate if extremity*	Elevate if extremity*
Exercises (ROM)	Gentle exercises after 48 h	Gentle exercises and use as able after 48 h	No exercises while severe edema and bleeding present; gentle exercises may be begun after 7-10 d, depending on tissue injured
Weight bearing	Full use	As able; full use	Cessation of weight bearing with crutch use for 7 d or longer depending on tissues involved*

*Part of treatment of musculoskeletal injuries referred to as RICE.

R = Rest for injured part. May be temporary nonuse or more prolonged non–weight bearing depending on injury.

I = Ice. Applications of ice lessen bleeding and edema. Ice is needed for 24 to 72 hours or longer depending on the injury.

C = Compression. Elastic bandages or at times a circular cast may be used for compression. Compression is to be of the *venous* vessels; therefore the wrapping should be applied only snugly enough that it does not compromise the *arterial flow*. Application of the bandages or cast should be from distal to proximal on the limb to aid venous constriction and venous return.

E = Elevation. The injured part is elevated to heart level to aid venous return and thereby lessen edema. Elevation of the part too high (or above the patient's central venous pressure) should be avoided, since too high elevation could impede arterial flow and increase rather than decrease edema. Normal central venous pressure (CVP) ranges from 6 to 13 cm H_2O pressure. Elevation should not exceed 5 inches above the heart level (2.5 cm = 1 inch; 5 inches = 13 cm), assuming the patient has the highest CVP. Accurate elevation can be achieved if the patient has a CVP line in place. If not, elevation to heart level is safest.

NURSING CARE

Nursing Assessment

	Contusion	Strain	Sprain
Specific tissue or tissues	Skin and subcutaneous tissue	Tendon, ligament, bone, and entire joint	Same as with strain
Local processes	Bluish discoloration and edema; skin openings; pain; soreness	Weakness, numbness, bleeding noted by discoloration; assess for skin opening; joint mobility, stability, or laxness; pain; edema; ability to bear weight or use joint normally	Same as with strain only more pronounced: more edema, bleeding, and discoloration; inability to use joint, muscles, or tendons normally; cannot bear weight; pain more severe and constant
Systemic processes	Other bruises or contusions possibly present	Distant joints possibly sore from initial injury	Same as with strain
Psychosocial concerns	Minor discomfort; no major concerns	Temporary (24-72 hours) impairment of mobility	Mobility impaired for varying periods (10 days to 3 or more weeks); may develop posttraumatic arthritis later

Nursing Dx & Intervention

Nursing Diagnosis	Nursing Intervention/Rationale
Impaired physical mobility related to specific injury	• Assess injured area *to determine condition.* • Handle injured tissues gently *to avoid further trauma.* • Apply ice bag *to decrease edema and bleeding.* • Elevate injured part or parts *to decrease edema and increase venous return.* • Assist with ROM exercises when allowed; perform as able *to increase mobility.* • Use sling for upper extremity injury *to lessen pain and increase comfort.* • Perform neurovascular checks as ordered *to determine condition and to note possible complications.* • Assist with crutch walking as needed; assess crutches for proper length *to provide for safety.* • Administer analgesics *to lessen pain and aid in relief of inflammation.* • Assist with personal hygiene as needed *to maintain healthy tissues.* • Assess concerns with immobility.
Altered role performance related to injury	• Assure patient that full function should be regained following treatment *to ease concerns.* • Encourage resumption of ADLs and usual activities as able *to enhance self-concept.* • Caution about possibility of reinjury if self-care is not learned.

Patient Education

1. Be sure the patient knows the nature and extent of injury.
2. Instruct the patient in use of crutches if necessary.
3. Instruct the patient or family in use of medications, dressing changes, and need for limited mobility if necessary.
4. Instruct the patient or family in signs or symptoms that would require physician's attention.

Evaluation

Patient Outcome	Data Indicating That Outcome is Reached
Patient recovers ROM of affected joints and tissues without limitations.	Patient experiences no pain, tenderness, limitation of motion, edema, or loss of function of tissues.
Patient returns to social interactions.	Patient returns to usual family, social, and employment roles.

Dislocation

A dislocation is a displacement of a part, usually a bone, from its normal anatomic position within a joint.

Dislocations may be complete or partial (called subluxations). They usually result from a blow, force, or pull strong enough to cause the bone to be forced or pulled from the joint. For some people, repeated dislocations are common because of repetitive or chronic trauma to a joint, which weakens ligaments, tendons, or muscles. Some joints, such as the shoulder, elbow, fingers, and knee, are more commonly dislocated than others.

Subluxations are more common in people with long-standing rheumatoid arthritis because fibrosis shortens the tendons, forcing the bones to subluxate; this is referred to as a swan-neck or boutonniére deformity.

Pathophysiology

The major signs of dislocation are deformity and inability to use the part or joint normally. Tendons or ligaments can become interposed, making reduction and replacement of the dislocated part into the joint difficult or impossible without open surgical reduction. Reduction and replacement within the joint space without surgery is more commonly impossible in cases of subluxations associated with rheumatoid arthritis because of the shortening of the tendon.

Diagnostic Studies and Findings

History

Repetitive trauma, such as throwing or hitting a ball
Presence of rheumatoid arthritis

Physical Examination

Head or other part of bone out of the normal anatomic position
Tendon shortening
Deformity
Inability to use joint normally

Roentgenograms

Dislocated parts

Medical Plan

Surgery

Open reduction of the dislocated bone
Tendon transplant for swan-neck and boutonniére deformities

General Management

Manual closed reduction of the dislocated bone into the joint
Application of a sling for the upper extremity to lessen stress
Adhesive or Ace wrap of lower extremity joint

NURSING CARE

Nursing Assessment

Joint and Bones of Joint

Palpation of dislocated part out of usual position
Deformity
Inability to use joint normally
Tenderness, soreness, or pain

Psychosocial Concerns

Self-concept
Disturbances of role expectations
Impaired mobility

Nursing Dx & Intervention

Nursing Diagnosis	Nursing Intervention/Rationale
Role performance disturbance related to injury or condition	• Assess patient's statements of limitations. • Assure that full ROM should be regained after reduction and healing *to lessen concerns*. • Assist with hygiene and ADLs as needed *to lessen patient stress*. • Provide postoperative care as needed *to aid recovery*.
Impaired physical mobility related to dislocation	• Assess effects of dislocation on patient's mobility. • Apply sling or elastic wrap *to maintain reduction*. • Perform ROM to all unaffected joints *to maintain strength*. • Assist with ambulation four times daily *to maintain strength*.

Patient Education

1. Explain how repetitive trauma weakens joint supports and predisposes to repeated dislocations.
2. Explain that prompt treatment lessens long-term effects of repetitive dislocations.

Evaluation

Patient Outcome	Data Indicating That Outcome is Reached
Patient has reduction of dislocation without recurrence.	Patient's bones are in normal anatomic positions.
Patient has normal ROM of affected joint.	Patient performs ADLs and ROM exercises without pain, limitation, or recurrence of dislocation.

Fractures

A fracture is a discontinuity or break in a bone.

Fractured bones cause major trauma to musculoskeletal tissues. Not only is the most vital part (bone) unable to perform its normal functions, but all the surrounding tissues also are unable to function. The cumulative effects may or may not be in direct relationship to the severity of the injury because of the interrelationship of these tissues.

The type of fracture is usually related to the source or force of the blow (Table 4-4). Only minor force may be needed for a greenstick fracture of one bone cortex, whereas more powerful forces cause comminuted fractures with associated soft tissue trauma. Anyone is susceptible to fractures; however, younger children and elderly people may suffer fractures from minor forces. Young and middle-aged adults have stronger musculoskeletal tissues; therefore greater force is required to fracture a bone, and there is more associated soft tissue trauma.

Pathophysiology

Bones are held relatively firmly in their normal anatomic positions by their shape, bony projections and processes, and the strong ligaments and tendons that hold them in their joints. Muscles surrounding the bones along their shafts also provide protection. However, either direct or indirect forces against the bone that are superior to the strength of the bone, muscles, tendons, or ligaments cause the tissues to "give in." Bones break when they cannot continue to resist the strength, duration, or repetitive nature of the applied forces.

Table 4-4
Classification of Fractures

Type of Fracture	Age of People Affected	Description	Force or Power Causing Fracture
Greenstick	Children and older adults	Break in one cortex (covering) of bone	Minor direct or indirect force
Transverse	All ages	Horizontal break across both cortices	Direct or indirect moderate force with angulation toward bone
Spiral	Young and older adults	Fracture curves around both cortices, which may twist out of place (become displaced)	Twisting force, direct or indirect
Oblique	All ages	Fracture at oblique angle across both cortices with or without displacement	Force is twisting and angulating, with axial compression
Comminuted	Young and older adults	Fracture has more than two pieces with much soft tissue trauma	Crushing force directly to tissues
Compression	All ages	Bone squeezed or wedged together at one cortex	Axial compressive force, directly applied to superior skeleton
Pathologic	Older adults	Transverse, oblique, or spiral fracture	Minor direct or indirect force through bone weakened by tumor
Open	All ages	Bones fractured, skin is opened, and there may be much soft tissue trauma	Moderate to severe force suddenly applied without relief; exceeds tissue tolerances
Avulsed	Children and young adults	Fracture pulls bone away from its normal attachments and place (occurs frequently at knee and elbow with patella or olecranon being avulsed from joints)	Force is direct or indirect with resisted extension of knee or elbow muscles causing pulling away of bone involved; muscles may also avulse from bones or tendons from resisted actions
Stress	Young and older adults	Crack in one cortex of a bone (scaphoid, lunate, or hamate in wrist) and others	Repetitive application of force (as striking a lever); also may result from steroids causing osteoporosis
Closed	All ages	Bone fractured, but skin over site remains intact	Minor, as with greenstick or pathologic fractures

A fractured bone can no longer maintain its normal length unless the two fragments impact into each other at the time of the fracture. Usually there will be shortening of the tissues around the fractured bone because of muscle contraction and spasms as the muscles respond to the stimulus of trauma. As the muscles contract and shorten, they move the distal fragment upward (cephalad). The distal fragment is less stable and more movable than the proximal fragment, which is held more firmly from the muscles' originations (the origins of muscles are less movable than their insertions). The shortening of the muscles and the displacement of the distal fragment result in deformity, a characteristic sign of a fracture. The deformity can generally be noted on physical examination as a deviation from the normal appearance of the tissues. Displacement of the distal fragment is significant, because the distal fragment must be replaced in continuity with the proximal fragment for healing and bone union. The amount of displacement and the angulation and rotation of the distal fragment are caused by the loss of the bone's continuity and the severity or strength of the muscle spasms and contraction. Force must be applied to the distal fragment and to the muscles to overcome the muscle contraction so that the two or more fracture fragments can again become aligned. Terms used to describe the position of the distal fragment include varus or valgus displacement, rotation, and medial, lateral, anterior, or posterior displacement.

When a bone is fractured, many or all of the following processes occur. These processes begin immediately with the injury and continue for weeks, months, and in some situations, even years before they are completed:

Hematoma formation. Blood and blood cells move into the injured tissues from vessels broken or bruised at the time of injury and from the inflammatory response to release of histamine, bradykinins, and serotonin into the injury site. Bleeding into the tissues causes a hematoma to form. Blood cells, especially thrombocytes, begin to work with fibroblasts to form a fibrin (clot) meshwork within the hematoma. Usually the hematoma is well formed in 24 to 48 hours, and frank or continued bleeding slows or ceases completely. There appears to be an optimum-size hematoma to facilitate bone union. Healing is delayed or prevented by hematomas that are too small or too large, although the exact favorable size is still undetermined.

Consolidation. Fibroblasts continue to invade the hematoma, firming up the fibrin meshwork. Mucopolysaccharides brought to the area help the fibrils adhere to each other. White cells brought to and circulating in the injured tissues wall off and surround the hematoma. They add strength while also localizing and removing wastes from the inflammatory responses. The fibrin meshwork is very fragile at this stage, so it is important to keep the fractured bones immobile. This period of consolidation lasts 10 days to 3 weeks.

Granulation. Osteoblasts (bone-forming cells) move into the meshwork, firming it and intertwining it with collagen connective tissue fibers to form strong scar tissues and to form new bone to bridge the gap between the fractured ends. Capillary buds develop into new blood vessels, which bring more nutrients and calcium molecules into the area to form bone callus. The granulation period lasts 3 to 6 weeks or longer.

Callus formation. This is probably the most vital period for bone healing for two reasons. First, enough nutrients must be present and in continuous supply to carry bone formation to completion. Oxygen is a major nutrient, along with sufficient amounts of vitamins A, B, C, and D, carbohydrates, proteins, minerals, and water. Second, callus formation is enhanced by the "right" amount of compression of the fractured fragments. Too little compression may result in pseudobone (false bone), and too much compression may decrease oxygen supply and tension, resulting in bone-end absorption and creating too large a gap for the collagen fibers to bridge. This decreases or prevents formation of strong callus. Osteoclast activity is greater when compressive forces are too great, because osteoclasts act to absorb or resorb bone cells, while osteoblasts aid formation. The balance is disrupted between the two cells, and callus or new bone formation is decreased. This period lasts 3 to 6 months or longer, depending on the type of fracture and the above conditions.

Remodeling. If present, excess bone is resorbed during this period. The collagen fibers and fibrous tissues are aligned to form trabeculae along the lines of stress according to Wolff's law, which states that bone will respond to stress by becoming thicker and stronger and that the structure of a bone depends on its function. Osteoclasts resorb the excess callus or poorly aligned trabeculae until they are firm and strong.

Bone healing, then, depends on several *local* factors, including the severity of the injury, nutrient supply, amount of bone bridge or gap, degree of immobilization, infection or necrosis of bone cells, and type of bone fractured. Cancellous bone fractures heal more quickly than fractures of compact bone because of the presence of blood and blood cells in greater quantities than in compact bone. *Systemic* factors influencing bone healing include the patient's age (children heal more quickly), concomitant diseases such as diabetes, hormonal balances (growth hormones aid healing while excess corticosteroids delay healing), and stress, immobility, or mobility at the fracture site. Application of electric current aids bone healing and has become a valuable adjunct in recent years.

Diagnostic Studies and Findings

History

Sudden, unexpected trauma; chronic, repetitive forces rather than sudden force usually cause stress fractures

Microvascular Repair and Replantation

Although not thoroughly discussed here, major advances in the care of patients with severe musculoskeletal trauma have been made with the development of microvascular surgical techniques. These include replantation of completely amputated body parts and revascularization of crush, avulsion, and other soft tissue injuries.

Before replantation or microsurgical repair, data are gathered and evaluated to determine whether functional return is possible, particularly if the injuries involve an upper extremity. Functional return is more likely when the injury is to a finger or fingers or low on the forearm because of the shorter distances for nerve regeneration. Repair or replantation should be performed as soon as possible after the injury, since ischemic tissues must be reperfused within 12 hours for function to be regained. Necrosis of tissues may preclude functional return if tissues are ischemic longer than 24 hours.

Surgical repair or replantation is done under a microscope and usually follows a pattern of stabilization of fractured bones followed by repair of arteries for restoration of blood flow. With circulation restored, nerves, veins, tendons, and ligaments are repaired, and skin closure, which may necessitate placement of a skin graft, is done. Nerves may not be repaired during the initial surgery but may be repaired 2 to 3 weeks later because the injuries or scarring from inflammatory processes and healing may delay or preclude nerve regeneration.

Postoperatively, nursing observations and care are critical for the success of the repair or replantation. Tissue pressure monitoring may be required in crush injuries to detect rising interstitial pressures, which may signal the development of compartment syndrome (see Figure 4-35). The digits are monitored closely for evidence of capillary refill and arterial flow through the use of Doppler detectors, arteriography, and plethysmography. Tissue temperatures are checked with thermometers, and edema, skin color, and turgor are closely assessed. Bleeding is carefully monitored, especially if anticoagulants are being administered. The external fixator or splint is checked for proper position and function. Dressings are changed as required to aid healing, and antibiotics are administered to prevent infection.

The patient, relatives, visitors, and all health care personnel in contact with the patient are not permitted to smoke because the nicotine in the tobacco could lead to vasospasm, vasoconstriction, and ischemia, which could threaten the integrity of perfusion and healing processes.

Initial outcomes after repair or replantation vary with the extent of trauma, the adequacy of tissue repairs, the degree of inflammatory responses, scarring, and absence of complications of arterial and venous occlusion and infection. Long-term success depends greatly on physical therapies and psychosocial rehabilitation.

Physical Examination

- Local deformity
- Edema or a mass
- Distal tissues held at abnormal angles or positions
- Limitation of use of part
- Crepitation
- Pain or tenderness at or around the site
- Subjective signs of numbness, tingling, weakness, or inability to use part normally
- Distal tissues cooler than proximal
- Peripheral pulses should be palpable
- Skin over injury site open or intact

Roentgenograms

- Complete break in bone continuity or in one cortex
- Rarely, may fail to reveal fracture initially
- Repeat in 10 days for certainty, since bone absorption at fracture site makes diagnosis easier

Medical Plan

Surgery

- Open reduction of the fracture with internal fixation of the fracture fragments with pins, nails, screws, staples, plates, intramedullary nails, or wire
- Arthroplasty with replacement with prosthesis
- Total joint replacement for crush injuries
- Amputation for severe crush injuries
- Microvascular surgery (see box)
- Application of external apparatus such as the Hoffman or Ace-Fischer device

Medications

- Narcotic analgesics
  - Meperidine (Demerol), 50-100 mg q3h IM for acute pain
  - Morphine, 5-20 mg q4h, subcutaneously, or hydromorphone (Dilaudid), 2-4 mg q4h subcutaneously, for acute pain
- Analgesic-antipyretic agents
  - Aspirin (ASA), 600-1000 mg q4h between narcotic administration times
  - Acetaminophen (Tylenol), 600-1000 mg q4h between narcotic administration
- Tranquilizers
  - Hydroxyzine (Vistaril), 25-50 mg IM, with narcotic as a narcotic potentiator
  - Diazepam (Valium), 2-10 mg q4-6h po, for muscle relaxant effects
- Anti-infective agents specific to the invading organisms (noted by culture) if the skin is open; commonly prescribed antibiotics include:

Figure 4-17 Examples of casts for upper extremity injuries.

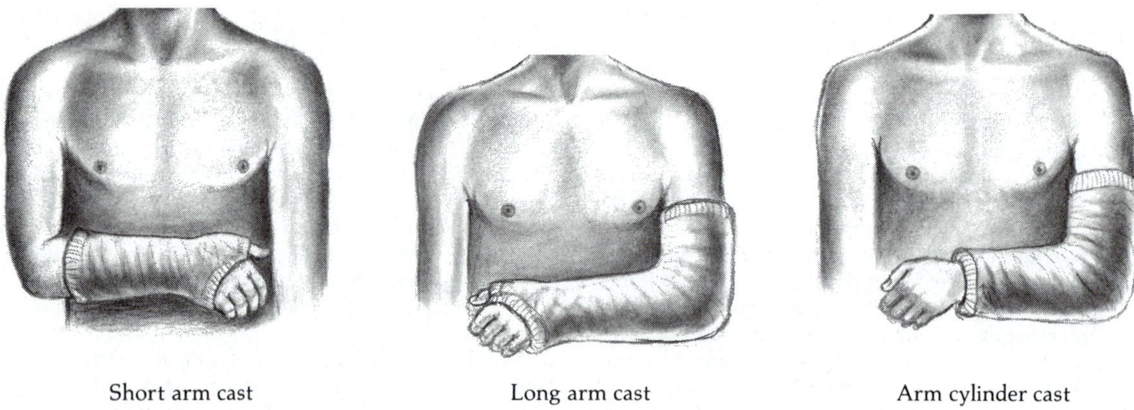

Figure 4-18 A, Plaster body jacket cast. **B,** Body jacket with halo apparatus attached.

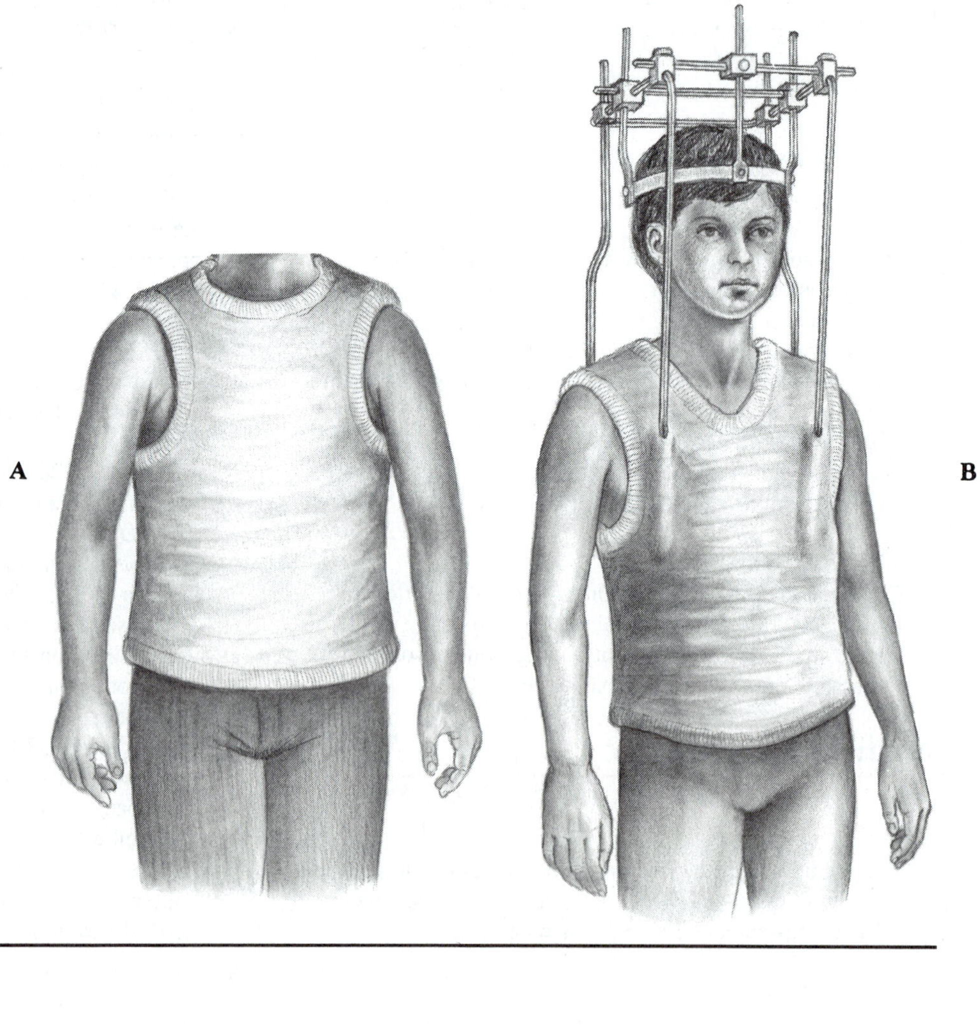

A

B

Figure 4-19 Spica casts. **A,** Shoulder spica (bivalved). **B,** Unilateral hip spica. **C,** One and one-half hip spica. **D,** Bilateral long leg hip spica.

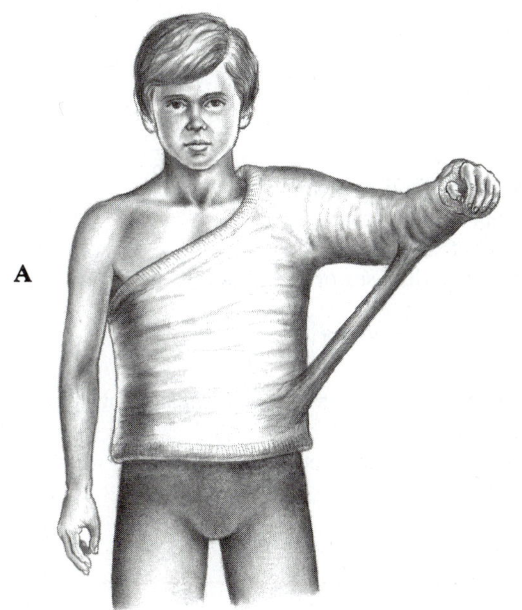

Ampicillin (Amcill, others), 1-2 g q6h IV and later, po
Cefamandole (Mandol), 500-1000 mg q4-8h IM or IV
Cephalexin (Keflex), 500-1000 mg po

Sedative-hypnotics
Phenobarbitol (Luminal), 15-30 mg 2-3 times daily
Flurazepam (Dalmane), 15-30 mg hs
Glutethimide (Doriden), 250-500 mg hs

General Management

Reduction of the fracture through closed, manual manipulation or open, direct manipulation of the fractured bones if fragments are displaced; if no displacement is present, reduction is not done

Application of an anterior and posterior splint for undisplaced or well-reduced, stable fractures of the radius, ulna, or wrist bones

Application of circular cast (see Figures 4-17 to 4-19 for types of casts and p. 451 for nursing concerns)

Wrapping injured tissues with elastic wraps for temporary immobilization (primarily for undisplaced stress fractures of wrist bones)

Placing patient in one or another type of traction (see Table 4-6 for traction forms and p. 455 for specific care)

RICE (see p. 418)

Application of a sling or splint to lessen stress on contiguous tissues

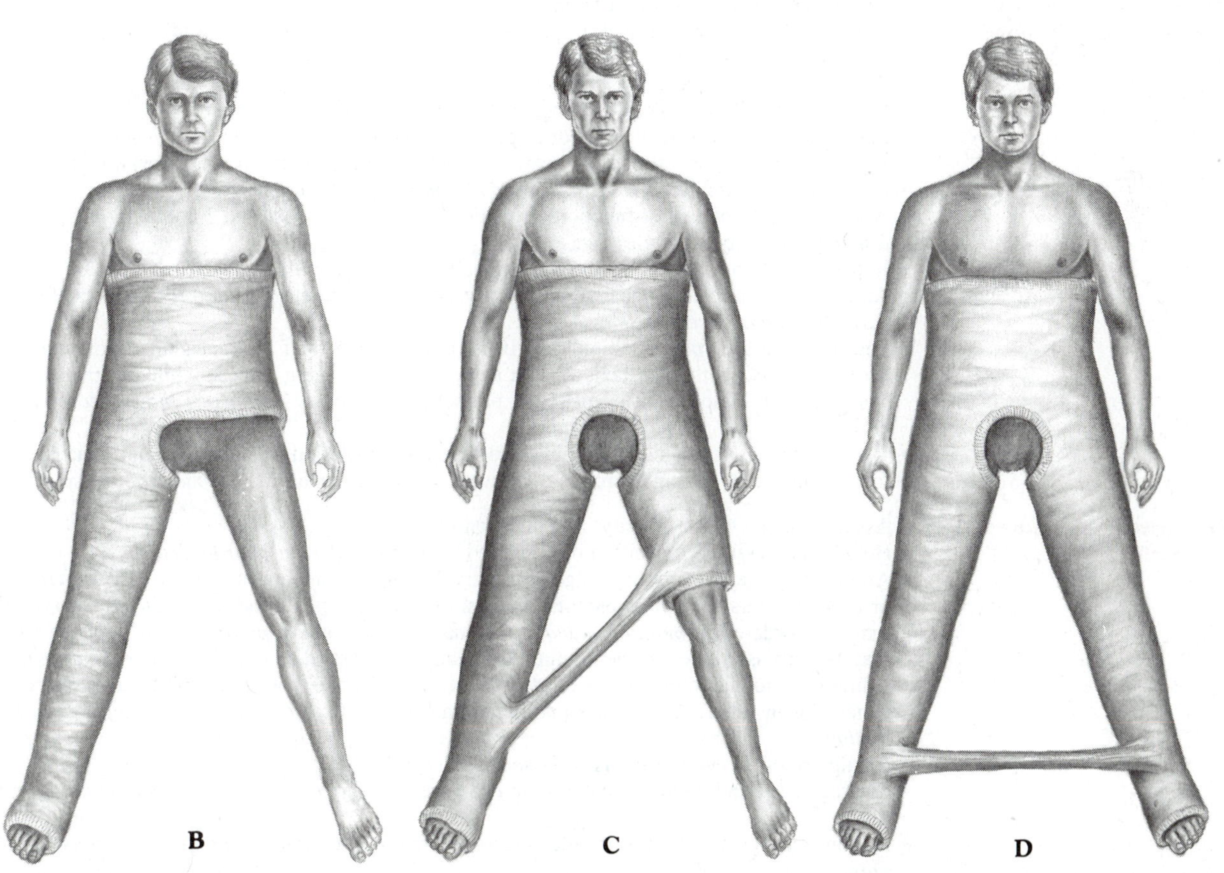

Placing on bed rest, if feasible
Ensuring patient does not bear weight on affected bone and joints; have patient use cane, crutches, or walker to avoid bearing weight on injured extremity
Well-balanced diet high in vitamins, proteins, carbohydrates, and minerals
Forcing fluids
Concurrent treatment of systemic diseases if present

NURSING CARE

Nursing Assessment

Fracture Site and Surrounding Tissues

Edema
Color changes
Deformity
Paresthesia with numbness and tingling
Pain
Limitation of movement or inability to use part
Skin closed or open
Crepitation (movement of parts normally not movable)
Bruising
Bleeding or hematoma (noted by mass)
Presence or absence of pulses distal to injury

Systemic Concerns

Pallor
Confusion
Dyspnea
Shock
Changes in blood pressure
Sweating or perspiring
Fear and anxiety
Concomitant diseases or other injuries to distant organs

Psychosocial Concerns

Self-concept
Disturbances in body image and impairment of physical mobility
Alteration in comfort, acute pain

Nursing Dx & Intervention

Nursing Diagnosis	Nursing Intervention/Rationale
Impaired physical mobility related to fractured bone and soft tissue trauma	• Assess area around fractured bone. • Gently handle injured tissues by supporting joint above and below site *to prevent additional injury and lessen pain*. • Apply ice bags to site *to lessen edema formation*. • Elevate extremity as ordered; support with pillows *to aid venous return*. • Put patient on bed rest, if ordered, *to put body and part at rest*. • Explain purposes for rest and not bearing weight on injured extremity *to ease patient's concerns*. • Perform neurovascular checks *to note condition of affected tissues*. • Assess integrity of cast or function of traction or wrapping every 1 to 2 hours initially, then every 4 hours *to note condition or functions*. • Explain position required for maximum healing *to aid compliance*. • Assist to proper position; change position every 2 hours or help patient position himself or herself correctly *to ease tired muscles*. • Teach patient the "post position" for lifting himself or herself (patient plants [posts] unaffected foot flat on bed with knee bent at right angle; lifts body using trapeze while pushing down with foot and leg). Help by lifting patient's buttocks if needed *to encourage independence and self-care*. • Teach exercises to maintain strength and facilitate resolution of inflammation; quadriceps, buttocks, and triceps setting exercises done every 4 hours when allowed *to maintain muscle strength*.
Pain related to pressure on nerve endings	• Assess amount, type, severity, and duration of pain. • Help patient assume a position of comfort if possible *to lessen pain or discomfort*. • Administer ordered narcotic analgesics: every 3 hours for meperidine (action is lost after 3 hours) or every 4 hours for opiate narcotics. Administer narcotics around the clock for 3 to 5 days or longer as ordered *to maintain adequate blood levels to relieve pain*. Periods between narcotics may be increased after the acute muscle spasms are relieved *to lessen dependence on narcotics*. • Administer nonnarcotic analgesics as ordered every 4 hours between narcotic administrations to enhance pain relief. Aspirin has additional anti-inflammatory effect *to aid resolution of inflammation*. • Change position every 2 hours *to lessen muscle fatigue*. • Massage back and buttocks *to decrease pressure and fatigue and to increase circulation in those areas*. • Administer muscle relaxant or sedatives as ordered *to aid reduction of muscle spasms and lessen pain*.

Nursing Diagnosis	Nursing Intervention/Rationale
Body image disturbance and altered role performance related to temporary loss of independence	• Assess self-concept and dependency concerns. • Maintain privacy while helping patient perform ADLs and hygienic care *to aid personal cleanliness and self-esteem.* • Offer oral hygiene and back care frequently *to maintain healthy tissues.* • Explain that proper positioning and prolonged immobility are required *to facilitate bone healing.* • Encourage patient to express feelings about enforced immobility and displacement from familiar surroundings *to foster comfort.* • Arrange for physical therapy and occupational therapy consultations *to maintain muscle strength and self-esteem.* • Encourage family members to interact with patient *to maintain customary roles and esteem.* • Help patient comply with high-nutrient diet *to lessen weight loss (a patient in skeletal traction may lose up to 20 pounds) and maintain positive body image.*
Altered tissue perfusion related to impaired circulation from trauma	• Assess condition of affected tissues. • Perform all parts of neurovascular checks every hour initially. Check color; temperature; peripheral pulses; edema; presence, amount, and type of pain; motor functions (patient should be able to move parts distal to injury; sensory functions (complaints of numbness, tingling, or pins and needles indicate sensory compromise); and capillary refill (compress nail of middle finger or toe, release; nail should pink up in 2 to 4 seconds for normal capillary refill; 4 to 6 seconds is abnormal and should be reported); compare the injured area with the same tissues on the opposite side of the body. Another critical finding, along with prolonged capillary refill, is increased pain on passive movement of the fingers or toes, which could signify that the patient may be developing compartment syndrome. Increased anoxia caused by the stretching of the muscle with the passive movement causes the increased pain (see Figure 4-35). Report abnormal findings to physician.
Potential impaired skin integrity related to immobility, presence of a cast, or traction equipment	• Assess skin surfaces for signs of pressure, such as redness, blistering, soreness, or open lesion. • Reposition patient every 2 hours *to relieve pressure.* • Turn to side if permitted *to distribute pressure to other areas and to relieve tired or sore muscles.* • Massage around bony prominences *to increase circulation.* • Use foam or lamb's wool bed pads *to distribute pressure.* • Encourage patient to eat adequately from a high-protein, high-carbohydrate, high-vitamin diet *to maintain healthy cellular tissues.* • Be sure patient gets at least 3000 ml of fluid daily *to maintain skin turgor.* • Teach patient how to move himself or herself in bed *to lessen friction and shearing forces and maintain healthy skin surfaces.*

Patient Education

1. Reiterate reasons for immobility and not bearing weight on injured limb (anxiety may prevent the patient from hearing or understanding initial explanations).
2. Explain reasons for weight loss and how the patient can lessen it through exercise and diet.
3. Explain measures for dealing with acute pain and changes in using medications as pain decreases.
4. Explain bone healing processes to elicit the patient's complete cooperation.
5. Explain turning and moving techniques to prevent skin breakdown.
6. Explain purposes and techniques for neurovascular checks.

Evaluation

Patient Outcome	Data Indicating That Outcome is Reached
Bone union occurs in anatomic position.	Roentgenograms reveal union of bones. Patient can use part without limitation or pain.
Patient resumes walking and bearing full weight on limb without limitation or discomfort.	Patient feels no discomfort or pain when walking or bearing weight on limb.

Patient Outcome	Data Indicating That Outcome is Reached
Patient has healthy skin turgor without developing pressure areas.	Patient has pink, well-nourished skin with good turgor.
Patient resumes social interactions and roles.	Patient returns to family, social, and employment roles.
Patient has normal tissue perfusion.	Patient has normal color, temperature, capillary refill, motor and sensory functions, and no edema of healed tissues.

CURVATURES OF THE SPINAL COLUMN

The spine develops its characteristic curves during fetal growth (Figure 4-20). Both prenatally and postnatally the curves may become abnormal because of defective bone, muscle, nerve, or other growth factors. The abnormal curves are called kyphosis (excessive curvature of thoracic spine), scoliosis (lateral or rotary curvature of thoracic spine), and lordosis (excessive curvature of lumbar spine) (Figure 4-21).

Kyphosis

Kyphosis is excessive curvature of the thoracic vertebrae.

Kyphosis can occur in various age groups. When it occurs in young children, it is usually congenital. It may become apparent in the adolescent years, when it is referred to as juvenile kyphosis, or Scheuermann's disease. Occasionally kyphosis may develop to compensate for lumbar lordosis. Kyphosis is also a classic symptom of ankylosing spondylitis. When kyphosis occurs in postmenopausal women, it is called senile kyphosis.

Pathophysiology

Since the thoracic vertebrae have a physiologic posterior curve normally, the curvature becomes pathologic only when it becomes excessive or exaggerated.

In young children the abnormal curvature may be the only pathologic sign without a specific cause. As children become adolescents, the curvature may become quite pronounced, especially with Scheuermann's disease, which produces irregular epiphyseal plate growth and ossification. These factors place undue strain on the anterior portion of the vertebral bodies. The irregular growth and additional strain lead to the excessive curvature.

In older people with kyphosis, some degenerative changes usually occur in the intervertebral cartilages. These changes lead to the excessive curvature. In postmenopausal women kyphosis is commonly associated with osteoporosis and degeneration in the anulus fibrosus rings between the vertebrae.

Diagnostic Studies and Findings

Physical Examination

- Excessive thoracic spinal curvature
- Rounded shoulders
- Occasional low back pain (40% of adolescents with Scheuermann's disease have back pain)
- Easy fatigability

Roentgenograms

- Forward curvature of thoracic spine
- Geriatric patients: possible osteoporosis
- Wedging and narrowing of anterior portions of thoracic vertebral bodies (T6 to T10)

Histocompatibility Testing

- Serum HLA-B27 antigen present in young adults with ankylosing spondylitis

Medical Plan

Surgery

- Spinal fusion for severe kyphosis

Medications

- Older adults may have hormonal treatment or mineral administration
- Young adults with ankylosing spondylitis receive several drugs (p. 391) for treatment of their disease

General Management

- Milwaukee brace for adolescents
- Back corset for older adults
- Orthotic devices (canvas/metal splint) for adolescents
- Teaching patient to stand up as straight as possible
- Exercise program to strengthen muscles and ligaments

Figure 4-20 Normal spinal alignment and abnormal spinal curvatures associated with scoliosis. **A,** Normal. **B,** Mild. **C,** Severe. **D,** Rotation and curvature of scoliosis.

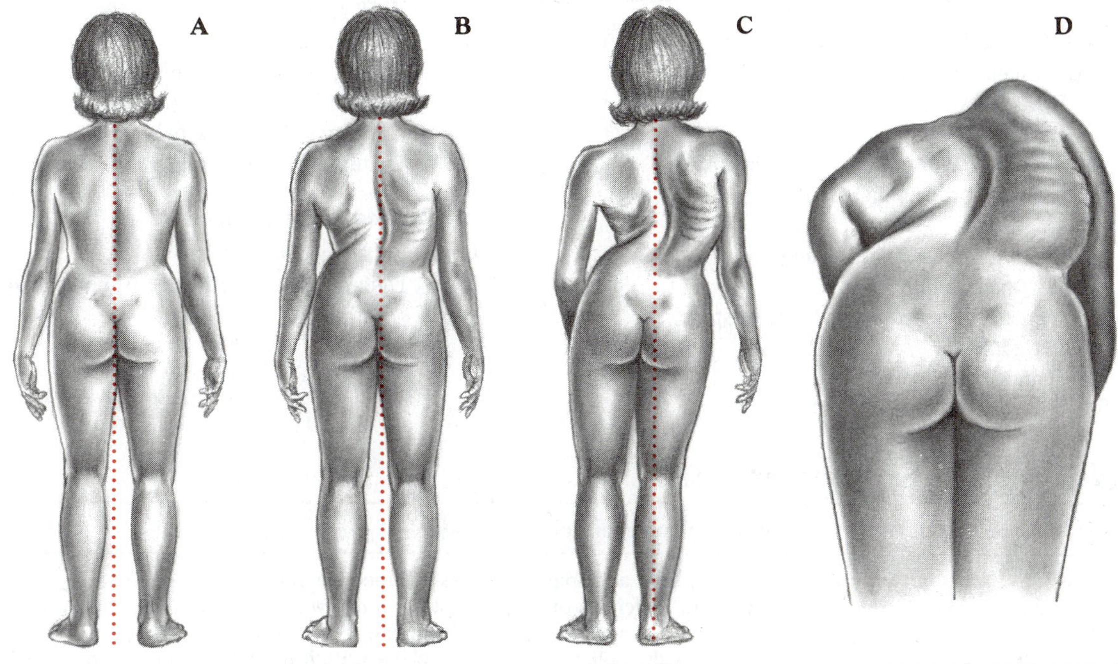

Figure 4-21 **A,** Normal spinal alignment and curvatures. **B,** Kyphosis. **C,** Lordosis.

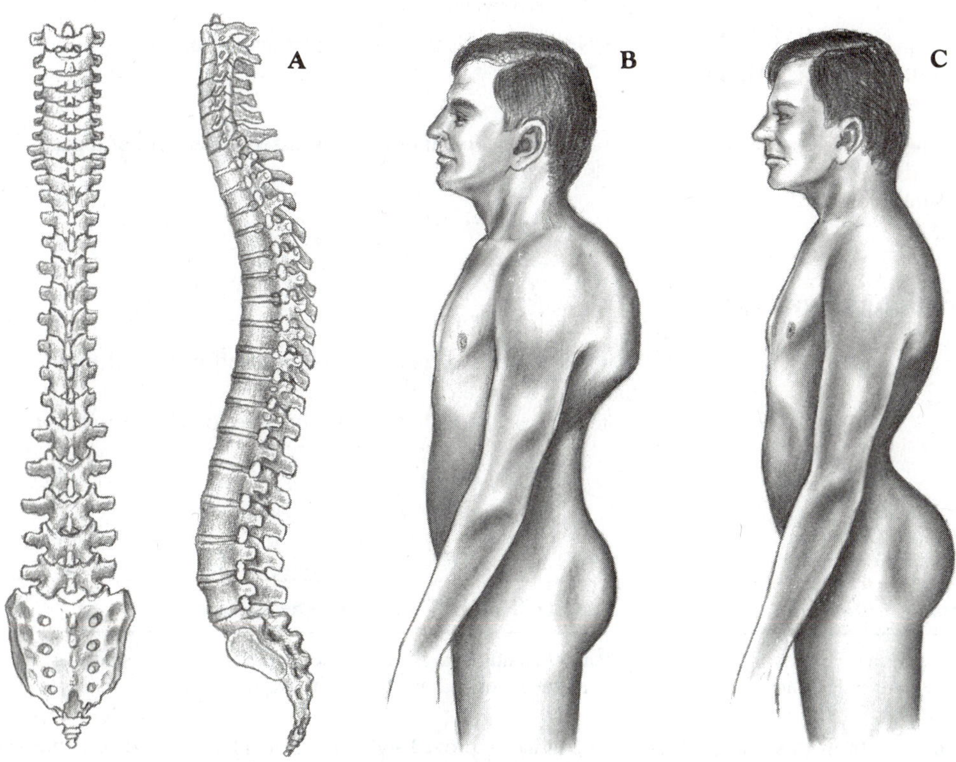

NURSING CARE

Nursing Assessment

Thoracic Spine

Adolescent
- Rounded shoulders
- Backache
- Excessive curvature of thoracic spine
- Lumbar lordosis increased

Young adult
- Stiff, sore back when rising on awakening
- Low back pain
- Increasing curvature of thoracic spine

Older adult
- Female
- Postmenopause
- Loss of height
- Excessive curvature of thoracic spine

Systemic Processes

Young adult
- Positive HLA-B27 histocompatibility antigen
- Reiter's syndrome (conjunctivitis, uveitis, genital lesions, low back pain)
- Pulmonary compromise

Psychosocial Concerns

Self-concept

Disturbances in self-esteem, body image, and role expectations

Nursing Dx & Intervention

Nursing Diagnosis	Nursing Intervention/Rationale
Self-esteem and body image disturbances and altered role performance related to spinal deformity	• Assess back and spine for excessive thoracic curvature. • Discuss principles of proper posture *to aid in maintaining upright posture.* • Explain that condition is not life threatening *to ease concern.* • Assist with application of brace, if used, until patient can do it alone *to aid compliance.* • Discuss clothing to make brace less obvious *to increase self-confidence.* • Discuss exercises to strengthen back muscles. • Discuss patient's life goals and review need for possible alteration (patient should set goals so as to be able to do what he or she desires without many limitations; see p. 392 for limitations with ankylosing spondylitis).
Impaired physical mobility related to back pain and deformity	• Nursing care is discussed under ankylosing spondylitis, p. 391.
Impaired gas exchange related to pulmonary compromise	• Nursing interventions are discussed under care of a person in a cast, p. 451.

Patient Education

1. Reiterate that the patient can help himself or herself through exercises, posture changes, and using a brace or splint.
2. Reiterate that the patient should be able to achieve life's goals even with kyphosis.

Evaluation

Patient Outcome	Data Indicating That Outcome is Reached
Posture has improved and curvature is lessened after treatment.	Patient stands straighter with less curvature and/or rotation, hips and shoulders are more normally aligned, respiratory functions are regained, and mobility is improved.
Patient returns to social interactions and roles.	Patient has improved self-concept and body image, is better able to regain family and social roles, and is positive about self and the future.

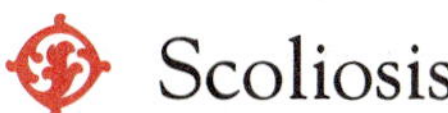

Scoliosis

Scoliosis is lateral curvature of the vertebral column.

Scoliosis may be noted in babies, young children, and adolescents. Infants may have two types of scoliosis, resolving and progressive, both of which are idiopathic. A familial genetic factor is associated with scoliosis, but the exact factor or factors have not yet been determined. Some hormonal and metabolic factors may be involved, affecting general skeletal growth of the trunk and upper limbs and leading to skeletal asymmetry in the upper body, but these factors have not yet been proved as causes of idiopathic scoliosis. The curvature may be minimum and barely noticeable in infants and young children.

As the child grows toward adolescence, the curvature becomes more pronounced and noticeable because of the laterality, rotation of the spine, and uneven shoulder and hip levels. Generally curvatures beyond 20 degrees require treatment.

Pathophysiology

The curvatures of scoliosis may be mild to severe and may also be associated with rotation of the spinal column. The curve is convex, and the vertebral bodies usually rotate toward the convexity of the curve, although the spinous processes and neural arches rotate toward the concave part of the curve. Both the curves and rotation are likely to increase with growth and stop as spinal growth ceases with maturity.

Scoliosis affects more girls than boys, although the exact ratio is difficult to determine.

Infantile scoliosis may have spontaneous resolution of the curvature in 80% of patients, with the remaining 20% having progressive deformity in their juvenile or adolescent years.[68]

Diagnostic Studies and Findings

History

- Asymmetry of shoulders or hips
- Uneven hemlines, pant length, or waistline

Physical Examination

- Lateral deviation with or without rotation of vertebrae
- Curvature may become more pronounced when patient bends forward
- Rotation may also be more noticeable when patient bends forward
- When hands of examiner are placed on hips, one hand is higher than other when patient is standing upright
- Examination of leg length reveals one leg shorter, and when patient sits, the curvature disappears
- Rib angles may protrude, and one hip may stick out
- Asymmetric shoulder levels
- Prominence of one shoulder

Roentgenograms

- Curvature and angle of curvature, plus rotation

Medical Plan

Surgery

- Straightening of curve with Harrington or Luque rod internal fixation with bone grafts to fuse spine
- Dwyer procedure involves removal of wedges of vertebral bodies containing intervertebral discs and their adjoining end-plates; staples and screws are fixed to the vertebral bodies, and a cable is inserted through the screw heads; tightening the cable closes the vertebral wedges and straightens the curve

General Management

- Use of Milwaukee (or similar) brace or orthotic device
- Application of distraction plaster cast to permit gradual straightening of curve (Figure 4-22)
- Application of Cotrel's traction (Figure 4-23) or halo-femoral traction
- Use of a neuromuscular stimulator

Figure 4-22 Types of casts for correcting scoliosis. **A,** Risser localizer cast. **B,** Turnbuckle cast.

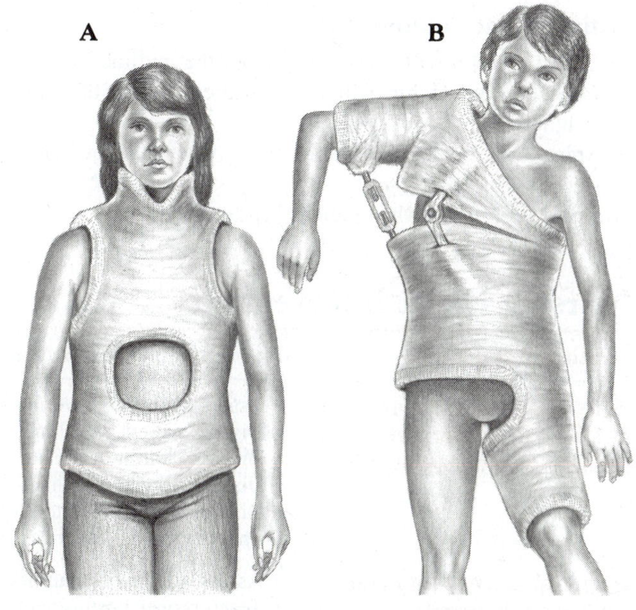

Figure 4-23 Cotrel's traction for scoliosis.

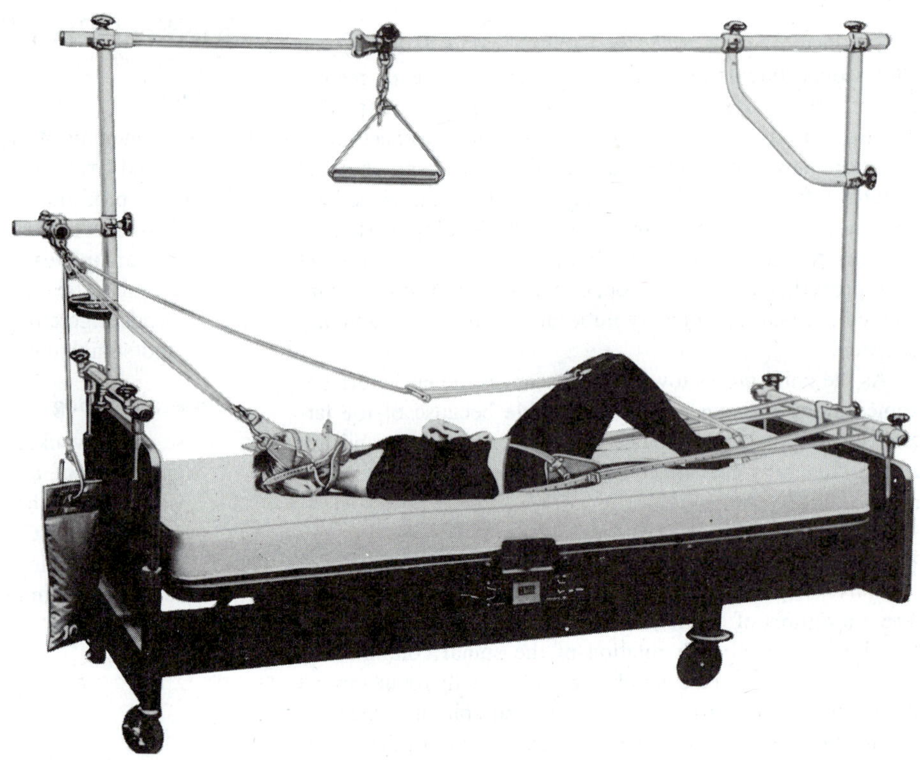

NURSING CARE

Nursing Assessment

Entire Spinal Column

Spinal column will curve away from the midline

One shoulder or hip will be a different height than the other

Spine will have a noticeable hump when patient bends over

Spine will rotate when patient bends over

Systemic Concerns

Patient may have muscle weakness through body

Cardiac or respiratory signs such as pulse rate or rhythm changes, dyspnea, or shortness of breath may be noted in more severe scoliosis

Psychosocial Concerns

Self-concept

Alteration in body image and role expectations

Impaired physical mobility

Nursing Dx & Intervention

Nursing Diagnosis	Nursing Intervention/Rationale
Body image disturbance and altered role performance related to spinal deformity	• Assess degree or severity of curvature. • Discuss patient's feelings of inadequacy because of deformity *to aid in ventilation of feelings.* • Discuss clothing to make brace less noticeable *to ease concerns.* • Discuss need to continue wearing brace *to prevent increase in rotation or lateralization.* • Discuss adjustments to clothing hemlines and so on *to negate effects of scoliosis.* • Encourage usual peer relationships and activities *to aid psychosocial development.*
Potential activity intolerance related to deformity	• Assess effects of condition on activities. • Teach proper posture and back-strengthening exercises *to prevent progression.*

Nursing Diagnosis	Nursing Intervention/Rationale
Impaired physical mobility related to deformity	• Assess effects of condition on mobility. • Discuss purposes of bed rest and Cotrel's or halo-femoral traction (Figure 4-23). • Change patient's position every 2 to 3 hours *to maintain tissue integrity.* • Discuss need to limit activities to maintain traction or brace use *to increase compliance.* • If surgery is performed, discuss need for bed rest *to permit healing.* (See p. 467 for nursing care for spinal fusion.) • Encourage patient to maintain peer visits and interactions while movement is restricted *to foster personal growth and esteem.* • Arrange for tutoring *to help patient keep up with schoolwork.* • Arrange for occupational therapy and physical therapy consultations *to maintain muscle strength and keep spirits up.* • Provide well-balanced diet *to promote healing after surgery.*
Impaired gas exchange related to pulmonary compromise	• Nursing care is discussed under fracture/cast care, p. 451.

Patient Education

1. Clarify inexorable progression of lateralization without treatment.
2. Encourage continuity of medical care to monitor status of scoliosis.
3. Reiterate need to wear brace at all times to prevent progression of scoliosis.
4. After surgery, explain bone healing processes.

Evaluation

Patient Outcome	Data Indicating That Outcome is Reached
Posture has improved and curvature is lessened after treatment.	Patient stands straighter with less curvature and rotation, hips and shoulders are more normally aligned, respiratory functions are regained, and mobility is improved.
Patient returns to social interactions and roles.	Patient has improved self-concept and body image, is better able to regain family and social roles, and is positive about self and future.

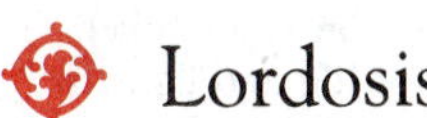

Lordosis

Lordosis is a normal curvature of the lumbar spine.

Lordosis may become exaggerated during pregnancy or in cases of large abdominal tumors or obesity, when overcorrection may be necessary to maintain balance when upright. Structural changes do not occur, and the condition is relieved with delivery, removal of the tumor, or weight loss.

Hyperlordosis, or "swayback," is fairly common in young children, especially girls, before puberty. The cause is thought to be rapid skeletal growth without appropriate stretching of the posterior soft tissues, such as the lumbar fascia and paraspinal muscles.[68]

Permanent hyperlordosis, although very rare, can occur from degenerative conditions (e.g., osteoporosis) of the lumbosacral discs or vertebral bodies. Treatments for hyperlordosis include use of a brace or lumbar belt, spinal fusion, or osteotomy.

PERIPHERAL NERVE INJURIES

During a difficult delivery the baby may be injured around the neck and shoulder because of the force required for delivery through a tight pelvis and vagina. The injuries may be traction injuries to the nerves of the brachial plexus, but the results of such injuries are musculoskeletal from weakness and atrophy. Table 4-5 presents several injuries that can occur at birth or develop later in life from trauma. Nerve damage at any time of life causes significant musculoskeletal defects.

Without stimuli, muscles become weakened and flaccid and eventually shrink and atrophy. As muscles atrophy, they pull the tendons, ligaments, bones, and skin with them. Since the flexor muscles are generally stronger than the extensors, flexion contractures usually result. Adduction is frequently more noted than abduction, although either may be present. Rotation and pronation of the muscles and joints are also common. Changes may also accompany the motor losses.

Table 4-5
Musculoskeletal Effects of Nerve Injuries

Nerve	Site of Injury	Cause of Injury	Effects of Injury
Brachial plexus	Cervical roots of C5-7	Traction to arm or shoulder during delivery; gunshot wound; avulsion of nerves from excess traction accidentally applied	Erb's palsy: affected arm, forearm, and hand internally rotated and pronated. Injury may cause temporary weakness and palsy; if severe, it will cause permanent paralysis with contracture of lower forearm, wrist, and fingers; sensory loss to outer arm
Brachial, axillary, and musculocutaneous	Cervical roots of C8 and T1	Breech delivery with arm above head; gunshot wound	Klumpke's palsy: intrinsic muscles of hand and flexor muscles of fingers are paralyzed; some sensory loss may be present in ulnar forearm and hand; permanent effects: a claw hand develops in a flaccid, weak limb
Radial	Shoulder or elbow	Leaning on crutches in axillae; elbow: fracture; other: cutting of nerve	Radial weakness from leaning on crutches with axillary pressure is fully reversible; elbow lesions: may have paralysis of wrist extensor and supinator muscles; eventually may need tendon transplants to wrist and fingers
Ulnar	Shoulder to elbow and to forearm	Open wounds (cut); fracture of medial epicondyle or lateral condyle; osteoarthritic changes	Ring and little fingers may be temporarily or permanently held in hyperextended positions while rest of the hand is clawed; sensation is lost over ring and little fingers; there is muscle wasting of intrinsic muscles of hand
Median	Wrist under transverse carpal ligament	Trauma; pregnancy; rheumatoid arthritis; postmenopausal state	Wasting of palmar thenar prominence (base of thumb); edema of hand; heavy, "clumsy" hand; sensory loss over radial 3½ fingers; if median nerve is severed without repair, paralysis of middle finger or index finger causes it to point ahead while other fingers are held in flexion; muscle wasting of hand (see below for carpal tunnel syndrome)
Peroneal	Neck of fibula	Pressure of splint; traction with leg in external rotation	Patient cannot dorsiflex or evert foot and toes; outer side of leg is wasted; footdrop is present; sensation is lost over front and outer half of leg and dorsum of foot and toes; posterior tibial nerve injuries may cause tarsal tunnel syndrome (p. 435)

 Carpal tunnel syndrome

Carpal tunnel syndrome is a cluster of symptoms affecting the functions of the wrist, hand, and fingers. It is caused by compression of the median nerve.

Carpal tunnel syndrome results from compression of the median nerve in the tendon sheath under the transverse ligament on the ventral surface of the wrist (Figure 4-24). Because the tissues in this part of the wrist normally fit closely together, any swelling will usually bring on the compressive symptoms. The syndrome usually develops after trauma and subsequent fibrosis and scarring of the tendon sheath. However, no previous trauma may be noted. Curiously, pregnant women may develop carpal tunnel syndrome during their last trimester. The reasons for this have not yet been determined, although fluid retention and edema may be contributing factors.

More women than men develop carpal tunnel syndrome. Menopausal women and people with rheumatoid arthritis also show a higher incidence of the condition.

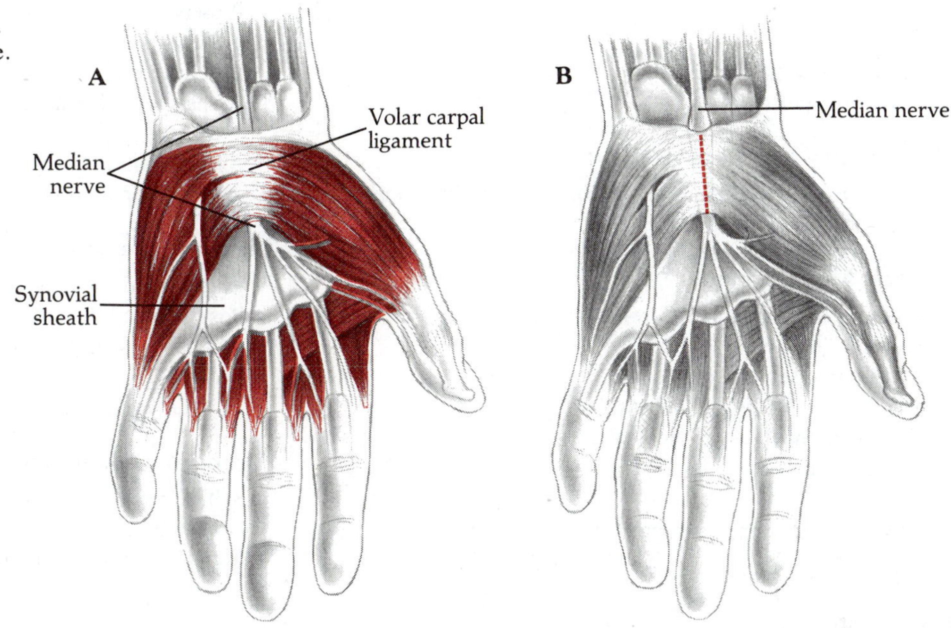

Figure 4-24 A, Wrist structures affected in carpal tunnel syndrome. **B,** Decompression of median nerve.

Pathophysiology

Pain is one of the first symptoms of carpal tunnel syndrome. It often occurs at night, waking the patient with burning, tingling, and numbness. The fingers feel swollen, and the hand feels heavy. The patient must usually hang the arm over the bed or get up and walk around to relieve the pain.

During the day the patient has few symptoms except when doing things that require turning the wrist, such as knitting and crocheting. The hand is weaker and feels clumsy, and sometimes pain may radiate up the arm.

Either one hand or both hands may be involved.

A condition similar to carpal tunnel syndrome can occur in one or more other peripheral nerves, including the radial and ulnar tunnels in the upper extremity. Tarsal tunnel syndrome, which is also similar to carpal tunnel syndrome, may occur in the lower extremity. Radial nerve weakness can temporarily occur from improper use of crutches. This clears when the person stops resting on the shoulder supports of the crutches. Ulnar nerve injuries frequently accompany elbow trauma. When severe, such upper extremity nerve injuries can cause clawing of and loss of sensation in the ring and little fingers.

Trauma to the posterior tibial nerve or entrapment in the transverse tunnel over the Achilles tendon can cause tarsal tunnel syndrome. The symptom patterns are the same as those of carpal tunnel syndrome, but the symptoms appear in the foot and ankle instead of the hand and wrist. Treatments for tarsal tunnel syndrome are the same as those for other entrapment syndromes and are specific to the particular nerve, ligament, and tendon sheath involved.

Diagnostic Studies and Findings

History

- Sensory changes
- Paresthesia and numbness
- Pain waking patient at night
- Motor changes, with clumsiness, heaviness of hand, and edema
- Pain, possibly radiating up arm
- Correlation with pregnancy, rheumatoid arthritis, postmenopausal state, diabetes, thyroid dysfunction
- Similar symptoms in lower extremity with tarsal tunnel syndrome

Physical Examination

- Deficits in sensory mapping along median nerve innervation pathways
- Positive Tinel's sign; increased tingling with gentle tap over tendon sheath on ventral surface of central wrist
- Edema of fingers noted
- Thenar surfaces of palm thinner than normal (wasting)
- Holding wrist in forced palmar flexion for 1 minute can elicit sensory changes of numbness and tingling—positive Phalen's test

Electromyogram

- Weakened muscle response

Medical Plan

Surgery

Release of carpal ligament and tendon to relieve compression (Figure 4-24)

Medications

Injection of hydrocortisone (dosage varies) into tendon sheath to relieve inflammation

General Management

Use of a cock-up splint to relieve pressure
Elevation to relieve edema
ROM exercises to lessen sense of clumsiness
Restriction of twisting and turning activities of wrist
Continuation of usual medical care for systemic illness (rheumatoid arthritis) if present

NURSING CARE

Nursing Assessment

Wrist, Hand, and Fingers (Both Extremities)

Inability to use hands and fingers through normal ranges of motion
Movements limited
Presence or absence of edema, numbness, tingling, pain
Assessment of time when pain is present, severity, and activities that increase or decrease pain
Assessment of palmar thenar (base of thumb) surfaces for atrophy
Assessment of distribution of paresthesia (if present) into fingers or up arm

Systemic Concerns

Rheumatoid arthritis
Postmenopausal state
Pregnancy in last trimester
Diabetes
Thyroid dysfunction

Psychosocial Concerns

Self-concept, disturbance in: body-image, role performance
Impaired physical mobility

Nursing Dx & Intervention

Nursing Diagnosis	Nursing Intervention/Rationale
Altered peripheral tissue perfusion related to compression and edema	• Assess circulatory status of limb by neurovascular checks (p. 427).
Impaired physical mobility related to pain, edema, and motor changes	• Assess effects of condition on wrist and hand ROM. • Explain inflammatory processes to correlate need to limit activities of wrist and hand *to ease concerns or anxiety.* • Assist with and teach proper splint application; assist with hygienic care if necessary *to increase independence and compliance.* • Elevate hand and wrist if edema present *to aid venous return.* • Assist with ROM exercises if ordered *to maintain functions.* • Continue care for concomitant illnesses *to relieve symptoms.* • Observe and assess site for relief of symptoms after injection of hydrocortisone, if used, or after surgical release *to note effects of treatment.* • Encourage continuing follow-up medical care until recovery is complete *to aid resolution of condition.*
Pain related to edema and compression of nerve	• Assess amount, type, and severity of pain. • Administer pain medication as ordered; monitor and report patient's response *to note efficacy.* • Apply ice bags *to decrease edema.*

Patient Education

1. Reiterate explanations of inflammatory processes as bases for symptoms.
2. Teach about activities to lessen stress on inflamed tissues.
3. Reassure about relief of symptoms after surgical release or injection of steroids that follows reduction of edema and healing of involved tissues.
4. If patient is pregnant, discuss probable relief of symptoms after delivery.

Evaluation

Patient Outcome	Data Indicating That Outcome is Reached
Patient regains joint ROM and muscle strength over time.	Patient performs self-care and regains strength after incision heals.
Patient experiences pain-free wrist and hand functions.	Patient has no pain, edema, numbness, or tingling when using wrist and hand.

Sciatic nerve injury

Sciatic nerve injury is a pathologic condition caused by external trauma to the nerve.

Injury to the sciatic nerve may be primary, from a gunshot wound, stabbing, fall, or other cause, or it may result from pressure from rupture of an intervertebral nucleus pulposus. The nucleus pulposus exerts pressure on the spinal nerves as they exit the spinal cord and traverse the sciatic nerve. The intervertebral discs that most often rupture (95%) are at L5-S1 and L4-L5 interspaces. Cervical intervertebral discs rupture less frequently.

The following discussion focuses on pathologic findings in the sciatic nerve resulting from herniation (rupture) of one or more lumbar intervertebral nuclei pulposi.

Pathophysiology

The nucleus pulposus is a semigelatinous mass inside the cartilaginous anulus (disc) between the bodies of each vertebra. When the cartilage of the anulus cracks or degenerates, it allows the nucleus pulposus to rupture through the cracks. A ruptured disc is a twofold process of degeneration of the anulus with herniation of the nucleus pulposus material.

Rupture of the anulus is generally caused by degenerative changes in the cartilaginous structures of the anulus. As the disc (anulus) ages, it loses elasticity, partly from changes and decreases in its collagen fibers and partly from decreases in its fluid content. These changes weaken the disc, making it unable to tolerate even usual body weight. The disc flattens or bulges, and additional pressure from lifting, straining, increased weight, or a sudden twist, turn, or sharp bending of the back may cause the anulus to bulge backward or tear. The nucleus pulposus can then extrude through the crack. The mass can extrude anteriorly toward the cord, laterally toward the lamina and facets, or posteriorly toward the posterior spinous processes. The extruded mass presses on the dura mater or nerve roots or both, causing pain in the back that radiates to the sciatic nerve. The presence of the extruded mass plus the pressure cause edema to develop, which also increases pain. At times, if the entire nucleus mass has not extruded, it may move back inside the disc when the edema subsides. If the mass stays extruded, it can adhere to the nerve roots or their dural sheaths, adding to the scarring and pain. Eventually the prolapsed material can also disturb the functioning of the facets of the vertebrae, leading to further degeneration of these joints.

The incident that causes the acute rupture can be as trivial as a sneeze or cough while the person is bent forward. Usually it is brought about by lifting something while the body is not in optimum lift position or if the load is unexpectedly heavy. Excessive pressure is referred from tensed abdominal and back muscles to the anulus and then to the nucleus, which ruptures through the weakened, cracked anulus. Signs of sciatic nerve pressure follow the rupture.

Diagnostic Studies and Findings

History

Sudden acute pain in low back

Physical Examination

- Loss of normal lordotic curve
- "List" or tilt to side
- Tense, tight back muscles
- Tenderness in low back that may radiate to buttocks
- ROM movements limited in forward flexion, in lateral flexion, and sometimes in extension
- Pain radiating down (usually) one leg to foot and toes
- Straight leg raising limited by pain
- Pain increased with foot dorsiflexion
- Sensations impaired on outer thigh, calf, and foot
- Paresthesia with numbness and tingling
- Knee and ankle reflexes possibly diminished or absent (knee reflex rarely lost)

Roentgenograms of Back

- Tilt
- Diminished disc space (not necessarily diagnostic)

Myelogram

Location of rupture revealed by impaired dye flow (see p. 1575 for myelography)

CT Scan

Ruptured disc

Magnetic Resonance Image (MRI)

Ruptured disc shows clearly

Medical Plan

Surgery

Hemilaminectomy with removal of extruded nucleus and degenerated anulus
Spinal fusion
Fenestration to open nerve root exit sites

Medications

Analgesic-antipyretic agents
- Aspirin (ASA), 600-1000 mg q4h
- Acetaminophen (Tylenol), 600-1000 mg q4h

Antianxiety agents
- Diazepam (Valium), 2-10 mg po q4-6h

Narcotic analgesics
- Oxycodone (Percodan), 30-60 mg q4h for severe pain uncontrolled by aspirin
- Meperidine (Demerol), 50-150 mg IM q3h

General Management

Application of skin traction (pelvic belt)
Williams' position in bed (head of bed and knee gatch each elevated 45 degrees)
Diathermy to low back three or four times daily; ice massage
Application of canvas back support or metal back brace
Physical therapy with specific exercises to strengthen back and abdominal muscles
Bed rest on firm mattress
Cessation of lifting and stooping
Back massage after diathermy

NURSING CARE

Nursing Assessment

Vertebral Column, Lumbar Back, and Sciatic Nerve Dermatomes

Degree of lumbar lordotic curve
Range of movements of back (forward, backward, lateral to each side)
"List" or tilt to either side
Tenderness
Pain in back or buttocks, radiating down posterior thighs and legs to feet and toes
Assessment of muscles for spasm, tenseness, or tightness
Leg-raising assessments
Sensory functions "around" thigh, leg, and foot (bilaterally)
Strength or absence of knee and ankle reflexes
Bowel or bladder function changes

Systemic Concerns

Concomitant systemic diseases
- Rheumatoid arthritis
- Ankylosing spondylitis
- Osteoarthritis

Psychosocial Concerns

Body image disturbance and altered role performance
Impaired physical mobility
Acute pain in lower back with radiation

Nursing Dx & Intervention

Nursing Diagnosis	Nursing Intervention/Rationale
Impaired physical mobility related to back and leg pain and muscle spasms	• Assess ability to move and limitations of movements. • Explain purposes of hospitalization, bed rest, and traction *to increase compliance.* • Explain use of firm mattress and bed position (Williams' position) *to relax spasm of back muscles.* • Prepare patient for physical therapy, diathermy, and massage; assist with hygienic care to have patient ready and to lessen strain on back *to aid compliance.* • Help apply back support, brace, or belt; teach self-application *to increase independence.* • Place in skin traction belt; observe responses; remove traction while sleeping *to lessen muscle spasms.*
Body image disturbance and altered role performance related to condition	• Assess condition's effects on usual roles and self-concept. • Encourage to discuss usual roles and temporary adjustments needed with family members *to ease patient's concerns.*
Pain in back and legs related to condition	• Assess amount, sites, and severity of pain. • Keep patient on bed rest *to relieve inflammation with acute low back pain.* • Administer analgesics around the clock as ordered *to maintain an adequate blood level for first 2 or 3 days.* • Administer muscle relaxants as ordered *to relieve spasms.* • Assess effect of Williams' position *in relieving spasms and pain.* • Offer back massage *to relax muscles and relieve inflammation.* • Assess relief of pressure signs on sciatic nerve by determining relief of paresthesia, numbness, etc. *to note resolution of symptoms.* • Perform "laminectomy checks" *to note progression of symptoms.*

Nursing Diagnosis	Nursing Intervention/Rationale
	• Report continued presence of pain, paresthesia, and muscle spasms to physician. • Use dietary measures, high fluid intake, and medication *to prevent constipation (straining increases pain).*
Impaired gas exchange related to bed rest	• See general intervention strategies, p. 1706.

Patient Education

1. Teach bed positions to relieve pain and inflammation.
2. Teach proper lifting postures, when feasible.
3. Teach exercises to strengthen muscles.

Evaluation

Patient Outcome	Data Indicating That Outcome is Reached
Back pain and muscle spasms are relieved.	Patient uses back for ADLs without pain, numbness, radiation to legs, or muscle spasms. Patient has no limitations in ROM.
Patient resumes social interactions and roles.	Patient returns to usual family, social, and employment roles and activities.

Medical Interventions and Related Nursing Care

Amputation

Description and Rationale

An amputation is the removal of all or part of a specific tissue or organ. Musculoskeletal tissues are frequently amputated because of crush injuries, severe sepsis, malignant tumors, or gangrene resulting from loss of arterial or venous circulatory integrity. Less frequently a limb may be amputated because of intractable pain from paralysis or because of multiple recurrent flare-ups of osteomyelitis that threaten not only the limb but also the individual's life.

The following terms refer to amputations involving the extremities:

forequarter Removal of entire arm, forearm, and hand; extremity disarticulated at shoulder joint.
arm Amputation above elbow or along forearm.
hemipelvectomy Removal of thigh, leg, and foot; also referred to as hindquarter amputation.
thigh Amputation above the knee (AKA).
lower leg Amputation below the knee (BKA).
foot Amputation of toes and part of foot at metatarsal joints.
finger or toe Amputation of part or all of one or more fingers or toes.

The three types of amputations are *provisional,* which is done when primary healing is unlikely, *definitive end-bearing,* which is done when weight will be borne through the end of the stump, and *definitive non-end-bearing,* which is done when weight will not be borne at the end of the stump. When weight will be borne through the end of the stump, the incision is not made at the end but is cut through or near a joint; if weight will not be borne at the end of the stump, the incision can be terminal (at the end of the stump). Also, the incision may be cut perpendicularly to the bone through all the tissues, called a guillotine incision, with little or no incisional closure and only loosely applied dressings. The guillotine incision is used in grossly infected tissues. The more frequently used incision is closed and snugly dressed after the tissues are amputated; it is commonly done in noninfected tissues.

During the surgical procedure, bleeding is controlled through application of a tourniquet unless there is arterial insufficiency. Skin flaps are made, usually of equal length for upper limb or above-knee amputations and with a longer posterior flap for below-knee amputations. The muscles are divided distal to the intended site of bone resection, and later opposing muscle groups are sutured over the bone end to each other and to the periosteum to provide better muscle control and circulation. Nerves are divided proximal to the bone end. After the bone is cut, all vessels and bleeders are ligated carefully and the skin flaps are sutured closed (unless tissues are infected), drains are inserted, and the stump is firmly dressed.

Contraindications and Cautions

1. If the amputation is to be done to remove a malignant tumor, metastasis to distant sites is usually a contraindication.
2. Lack of arterial circulation requires that the amputation be proximal to the gangrenous or necrotic tissues.
3. Enough tissues must be left on and over the stump for fitting of a prosthesis when possible.

Preprocedural Nursing Care

1. Meticulous skin cleansing with antiseptic solutions removes transient and some resident bacteria.
2. Determine presence of peripheral pulses (may be absent in "dry" gangrene).
3. Compare edema, color, temperature, skin condition, and pain (when present) with tissues on the opposite side of the body. Edema may be pronounced in venous obstruction associated with "wet" gangrene.
4. Observe the skin for open or draining areas.
5. Check vital signs for evidence of systemic infection and to monitor the patient's general condition.
6. With crush injuries, observe the patient for hemorrhage and possible shock.
7. If the patient is a child or older adult, determine factors related to age and developmental or educational level that could affect recovery and self-care after the amputation.
8. A rehabilitated person with a similar amputation may visit the patient preoperatively when possible.

Medical Plan

Surgery

Wound suction continuously
Change of dressings as needed

Medications

Anti-infective agents
Cephalothin sodium (Keflin), 500-1000 mg IV q4-6h for 48-72 h (or longer, if ordered)
Narcotic analgesic agents
Meperidine (Demerol), 50-100 mg IM q3h for pain
Intravenous fluid replacement with 5% dextrose in 0.45 normal saline, 2000-3000 ml for 24 h

General Management

Stump elevated for 24 hours, then kept flat and extended (order for elevation depends on presence or amount of edema in stump)
Adduction exercises of amputated extremity, 10 times per hour after 24 hours
For lower extremity amputation, turning to prone position four times daily
Thigh (hamstring) tightening exercises in prone position begun after 24 hours (10 times every 4 hours)
Up with crutches three times daily on second postoperative day
Physical therapy consultation for exercise regimen and to assist with ambulation
Regular diet as desired
Stump wrapping after fifth postoperative day (or after sutures are removed)
Orthotic technician (prosthetist) to measure stump for prosthesis
Stump check every hour for first 24 hours to note color, drainage, edema, bleeding, sutures (wound), and pulses proximal to incision site
Tourniquet always present at bedside
Up in chair after 12 to 24 hours
Pulmonary deep breathing and coughing every 4 hours

NOTE: Some patients may return from surgery with a prosthesis already in place, held to the stump with plaster (an immediate postsurgical fitting). It is usually left in place up to 10 days, after which it is removed, the sutures are removed, and a new cast is applied. This fitting lessens edema and pain, although the rigidity of the plaster delays the shaping of the stump into a conical shape. However, the immediate postsurgical prosthesis does permit earlier ambulation and discharge, particularly in younger patients.

NURSING CARE

Nursing Assessment

Site of Amputation (Stump)

Drainage or bleeding scant and serosanguineous
Edema slight
Dressing intact without constriction
Pain may be sharp and acute in incisional area
If Penrose drain is present, drainage may be scant to moderate, although still serosanguineous
Tourniquet should be at bedside

Entire Extremity

Extremity should remain extended
Range of motion of muscles and joints may be slightly limited by pain or stiffness
Only incisional area edema or erythema unless infection develops

Psychosocial Concerns

Concern with alteration in body image and appearance
Presence of phantom pain

Alteration in mobility and ability to maintain livelihood and income

Other Complications

Hemorrhage, wound infection, or dehiscence
Development of contractures
Persistence of phantom pain
Development of neuromas
Excessive scar formation
Inability to use prosthesis for ADLs and mobility

Nursing Dx & Intervention

Nursing Diagnosis	Nursing Intervention/Rationale
Body image disturbance related to loss of limb	• Assess effects of amputation on body image. • Allow and encourage patient to express feelings of mutilation, grief, anger, and loss, as well as avoidance of looking at stump, *to aid adaptation processes*. • Encourage patient to help with dressing changes and wrapping of stump as able. Teach family member wrapping techniques if necessary *to increase competence and independence*. • Encourage family members to walk with patient *to maintain strength and social contacts*. • Encourage grooming and wearing of personal clothing *to maintain individuality and personality*. • Encourage activities for self-care and ambulation *to maintain positive outlook and maximum strength*. • Encourage or arrange for social service consultation *for economic and employment aid*. • Arrange for follow-up care referral *to aid rehabilitation*.
Impaired physical mobility related to loss of limb	• Assess ability to use remaining limbs. • Turn and position on side, back, and abdomen (after 24 hours) *to maintain muscle and joint ROM*. • Teach adduction and extension exercises and help patient perform them every 4 hours *to prevent abduction and flexion contractures*. • Assist with sitting in chair and ambulation with aid as able *to maintain muscle strength*. • Prepare patient for physical therapy, transportation for exercises, and stump wrapping if appropriate. Encourage family members to learn wrapping (Figure 4-38). • Encourage family members to walk with patient during initial ambulation periods, accompanied by health professionals, *to increase independence*. • Teach purposes of prone and extension positions *to prevent contractures*. • Assist prosthetist with prosthesis measurements and fitting as needed *to aid rehabilitation*.
Pain (nerve trauma following surgery) related to surgical transection	• Assess type, amount, and severity of pain. • Administer narcotics as ordered every 3 hours for first 24 to 48 hours until surgical trauma is lessened; then administer as needed *to aid pain relief*. • Explain causes for phantom pain sensations and techniques to overcome them *to ease concerns*. • Administer antibiotics as ordered to prevent infection, thereby *lessening pain and scarring*.

Patient Education

1. Teach the patient and family proper positions, exercises, and ambulation techniques.
2. Teach the patient and family stump-wrapping techniques.
3. Teach the patient and family that prolonged phantom pain experiences are unusual and should receive medical attention.
4. Teach the patient and family skin care to prevent stump irritation or breakdown.
5. Teach the patient and family signs of a wound infection.

Evaluation

Patient Outcome	Data Indicating That Outcome is Reached
Skin and incision heal.	Scar is well approximated with no excess scarring.
Patient and family demonstrate ability to perform care.	Patient can wrap stump correctly and walk with crutches or prosthesis.
Alteration in body image and self-concept is achieved.	Patient has positive outlook about condition and can take up personal and employment roles after convalescence.

ARTHROPLASTY

Arthroplasty refers to repair or refashioning of one or both sides, parts, or specific tissues within a joint. Parts of a joint repaired during an arthroplasty include bones, cartilage, synovium, ligaments, and tendons. Bursae are outside a joint, but they may be removed during an arthroplastic procedure.

Arthroplasties are described as *interpositional arthroplasty,* in which a metal barrier is interposed between the bones after reshaping one or both bone ends (e.g., cup arthroplasty, currently done to preserve as much bone as possible, particularly the head of the femur), *gap arthroplasty,* in which one of the bones in the joint is excised (e.g., Girdlestone arthroplasty, now performed mainly to remove infected bones), *partial joint replacement arthroplasty,* in which one joint bone end is replaced with a prosthesis (e.g., Moore prosthesis of head of femur), and *total joint replacement arthroplasty,* in which both bone ends are replaced (e.g., total hip or knee replacement). Synovectomy is an example of an excisional arthroplasty, as is a meniscectomy with removal of the meniscus within the knee joint.

Refashioning or repairing a joint usually follows trauma, degeneration, or inflammation of one or more tissues within the joint. The surgery may be performed within hours of a traumatic injury, such as a hip fracture or meniscus tear, or it may be done after years of inflammation in a joint, such as occurs with rheumatoid arthritis or after degenerative erosions accompanying osteoarthritis from restrictive joint movements.

An arthroplasty, therefore, is usually performed to relieve restrictive movements of a joint, to relieve pain, to remove loose or torn tissues (ligaments, cartilage, or calcium), to reshape one or both bone ends to make a joint perform more smoothly, or to remove overgrown, hypertrophied tissue (synovium) or atrophic, avascular tissue (avascular head of femur).

Contraindications and Cautions

The age of a specific patient may be a contraindication to a particular arthroplasty. Arthroplasties are performed infrequently in children because they may damage the growth epiphyses and the immature cartilage and bones. Surgical repair of childhood conditions such as Legg-Perthes disease is undertaken only after more conservative medical treatments fail to resolve the condition. Adolescents with large, unsightly bunions may have an arthroplasty to correct them, but often surgical correction is required again in later years. Older adults with rheumatoid arthritis or degenerative osteoarthritis may have their surgical procedures delayed to correct a concurrent endocrine, cardiac, or respiratory condition, as also will those patients having arthroplastic surgery following trauma.

Bunionectomy: Keller or Mayo arthroplasty

Description and Rationale

Keller arthroplasty is one of the most commonly performed corrective procedures for hallux valgus and bunions. It involves excision of the proximal part of the proximal phalanx plus trimming of the prominent portion of the metatarsal head. Mayo procedure involves excision of the first metatarsal head and trimming of the prominent portion of the proximal phalanx. Both procedures are examples of gap arthroplasty; the gap is usually filled with a Silastic implant. The bunion (enlarged bursa and knob of bone) is also removed during the arthroplasty. A plaster toe cap or splint is then applied to some patients.

Contraindications and Cautions

1. Hallux valgus in an adolescent is primarily unsightly and deforming; surgical correction may be delayed until the patient is older, since osteotomy is a fairly radical procedure at this age.
2. Surgery may be delayed or avoided in some patients through careful attention to properly fitted footwear. Padding may protect the bunion to lessen pain. Exercise and use of a metatarsal arch support may lessen splayfoot.
3. Surgery may not be entirely successful or satisfactory. Bunions can recur, and surgery may weaken the foot slightly.

Medical Plan

Surgery

Arthroplasty
Bunionectomy

Medications

Narcotic analgesics
- Meperidine (Demerol), 75-100 mg IM q3h for 24-48 h for severe pain
- Codeine (codeine sulfate or phosphate), 30-60 mg
- Oxycodone (Percodan), 5-10 mg po

Analgesic-antipyretic agents
- Aspirin, 600-1000 mg po q4h for minor pain

General Management

Up with crutches when edema lessens, usually in 2 days (depends on whether surgery is bilateral)
Check cast or splint for tightness, intactness, and drainage
Assess wound for edema, pain, and drainage
Elevate foot (feet) on pillows
Elevate foot of bed
Keep patient on bed rest for 24 to 48 hours and then up in chair without weight bearing
Apply ice bags to operative site continuously

Assess motor and sensory functions in toes and foot postoperatively

NURSING CARE

Nursing Assessment

Preoperative

Area of great toe (bilateral)
- Presence of deformity
- Swelling over first metatarsal head (bursa)
- Pain
- Limitation of movement of joint with or without pain
- Presence of hallux valgus deviation
- Hammer toe
- Crowding of second toe
- Splayfoot
- Calluses or corns

Foot
- Varus or valgus deviation of one or both feet usually noted

Shoes
- Condition
- Type
- Evidence of wear
- Softness
- Data indicative of footwear contributing to hallux condition

Systemic
- Evidence of gout
  - Tophi
  - Elevated serum uric acid levels
  - Pattern of acute pain

Postoperative

Great toe or toes and incisional site
- Assessment of plaster cast or splint for intactness
- Visible portions of toe
  - Color
  - Edema
  - Pain
  - Pulses proximal or distal to incision (if able to locate in toe)
  - Drainage
  - Bleeding
- Dressing
  - Tightness
  - Drainage
- Amount of sensation and motion in operative area (cast may limit movement)

Psychosocial concerns
- Alteration in body image, comfort, and mobility
- Possibility of recurrence or lack of wound healing

Other complications
- Excessive scarring or recurrence of bursa
- Weakening of foot joint or joints of or near one or more toes

Nursing Dx & Intervention

Nursing Diagnosis	Nursing Intervention/Rationale
Pain related to corrective procedures	• Assess amount, type, and severity of pain. • Put bed cradles on bed to cover feet without pressure of linens *to aid comfort*. • Keep foot of bed and feet elevated *to lessen edema*. • Administer narcotics as ordered *for acute pain relief*. • Administer analgesics after acute pain is relieved *to continue pain relief*. • Apply ice bags as ordered *to lessen bleeding and edema*. • Assist with position changes and skin care; do back massage as needed *to relieve tired muscles*. • Instruct patient about analgesic and anti-inflammatory effects of aspirin and ice *to increase compliance*.
Impaired physical mobility related to foot surgery	• Assess limitations on mobility. • Help patient up in chair when able *to increase mobility*. • Assist with use of crutches when able *to aid mobility efforts*. • Encourage activities as strength and cast or splints permit *to maintain mobility*. • Encourage return to social activities "in spite of" cast, splint, or crutches *to lessen isolation*. • Help with fitting of soft shoes if or when cast is removed (to lessen pressure or rubbing on tender tissues) *to prevent additional injury*.
Altered peripheral tissue perfusion related to surgery or cast	• Assess neurovascular functions. • Remainder of nursing care is discussed on pp. 451 to 452.

Patient Education

1. Explain wound healing and signs of wound dehiscence to report to physician.
2. Teach principles and examples of proper footwear. Explain that friction and pressure of snug footwear can precipitate recurrence.
3. Teach bone and wound healing for long-term follow-up.

Evaluation

Patient Outcome	Data Indicating That Outcome is Reached
Incisional area and bones and joints operated on regain healing and functions.	Deformity has been removed; ROM is normal; scar formation is not excessive; pain in and around joint is gone.
Self-concept is positive and enhanced.	Patient returns to usual activities with unassisted, pain-free mobility. Footwear is comfortable. Patient feels better about body image.

Total joint replacement arthroplasty

Description and Rationale

Work done since the late 1950s and early 1960s has made it possible to repair and replace both bone surfaces of many joints. Initially, work with total replacement of hip joints has led to the ability to totally replace many joints, including ankles, knees, shoulders, elbows, wrists, and joints of the fingers and toes. Not all prosthetic materials or arthroplastic procedures work entirely satisfactorily in the joints with more and varied movements, such as the elbow, wrist, knee, and ankle. To date more successful replacements have been achieved in the ball and socket joints, primarily the hip. Research and design changes continue to perfect the prostheses and the techniques for all total arthroplastic procedures.

Replacement of both joint surfaces is required primarily in inflammatory or degenerative conditions within the joint, such as those accompanying rheumatoid arthritis or osteoarthritis from degeneration of the synovium or cartilage. As one or more of the normal joint tissues deteriorate or degenerate, the bone ends are exposed, causing pain and limitation of joint movements. Joint stiffness and muscle atrophy follow, further increasing pain and limiting movement and mobility, both locally in the involved joint and systemically as other joints become involved. Exposed bone surfaces will lead to bone growth that may eventually adhere to the opposing bone ends, causing bony ankylosis and loss of joint movements. Therefore replacement of the deteriorated or degenerated tissues and bones restores movement and relieves pain.

Total joint replacements involve removal of some or all of the synovium, cartilage, and bone in both sides of the joint. One of the joint bone surfaces is then replaced with a metallic prosthesis while the other surface is replaced with a ceramic or plastic, silicone-lined prosthesis. This metallic-plastic approximation is necessary to prevent metal-to-metal wear, friction, and possible electrolytic reactions from the interactions and intermingling of joint fluids. Individual physicians prefer specific combinations of prostheses for particular joints according to the patient's condition. Also, the timing for total joint replacement varies with physician and patient, since this procedure is usually elective except in situations of trauma.

Currently each prosthetic replacement on both sides of the joint may be secured with methyl methacrylate, a pliable polymer that hardens to hold the prostheses firmly. Through research and development, ceramic and metallic components have been designed that are self-adhering and immovable and do not require methacrylate adherence. These self-adhering replacements currently are being used in many centers, and they may become more widespread as the technique for their insertion is learned and the differences in postoperative recovery and rehabilitation are accepted. Patients take longer to start walking and use crutches or other aids for a longer time with the self-adhering replacements because the bone particles used as the natural interfacing material must granulate and ossify for solid adherence to the prosthetic replacements. Obviously, using the patient's own bone for the interface with the prostheses is desirable, since methyl methacrylate sets up an inflammatory response that may eventually lead to loosening or instability within the joint.

Total joint replacement involves special operative tables, instruments, and positions of patient and physicians. Expert anesthetic administration is required to prevent hypotension as the methyl methacrylate and prostheses are inserted; the temperature of the methyl methacrylate and the substance itself may cause a temporary and sudden drop in blood pressure as it is inserted, and communication between the surgeon and anesthesiologist prevents the hypotension from being prolonged or sufficient to lead to other complications. Total joint replacements require careful extensive physician-patient contact and consultation before and after surgery. When successful, as the great majority of joint replacements are, this surgery provides the patient with welcome relief from pain, increased mobility, and freedom not available with more conservative procedures. However, revisions of total joint replacements account for as many as 1500 reoperations for the hip and knee yearly.

Contraindications and Cautions

1. Joint infection with or without an associated systemic infection is the major deterrent to total replacement. Infection loosens components, prevents healing, and may eventually lead to osteomyelitis.
2. Active flare-up of a chronic rheumatic or other inflammatory disease is another deterrent. Flare-ups of such disorders as rheumatoid arthritis, ulcerative colitis, or systemic lupus preclude surgery until the condition is controlled or becomes quiescent.
3. Respiratory diseases and limitations from chronic conditions may preclude surgery. Methyl methacrylate is excreted through the lungs; this may set up a pneumonitis that could severely limit respiratory reserves.
4. Chronic renal conditions or mild failure may also preclude replacement, since hypotension could lead to acute renal shutdown.
5. Bleeding or clotting disorders would usually preclude surgery unless special care is taken to prevent hemorrhage.
6. Insertion of the femoral component into the femoral shaft during total hip replacement causes pressure changes in the venous system, which can lead to thrombophlebitis and pulmonary or fat embolization.
7. Limb length inequality can occur from inadequate muscle strength or improper operative fit. If limbs are unequal in length preoperatively, the inequality can possibly be corrected with the surgical procedure.
8. Porous-coated prostheses used for noncemented total joint replacements must be "press fit" for bioingrowth to occur.

Preprocedural Nursing Care

1. Begin skin cleansing procedures preoperatively; these include shampoo, shower, and local scrub of operative site with antiseptic antibacterial solutions.
2. Take roentgenograms and measure the limbs bilaterally to ensure use of the best-fitting prostheses.
3. If total hip replacement is to be done, teach the patient the proper position for postoperative lifting of body.
4. Begin respiratory care preoperatively, including deep-breathing and coughing exercises, respiratory therapy (intermittent positive-pressure breathing [IPPB]), and use of respiratory aids such as Triflow or Respirex apparatus or incentive spirometry.
5. Begin antibiotics intravenously preoperatively to establish a therapeutic blood level.
6. Occasionally skin traction may be applied preoperatively to relieve muscle spasms.

Medical Plan

Medications

Anti-infective agents
- Cefamandole (Mandol), 500-1000 mg q4-8h IM or IV
- Cefazolin (Ancef), 250-1000 mg q4-6h IV for 7 d
- Cephalexin (Keflex), 250-500 mg q6h po when IV antibiotics are discontinued

Narcotic analgesic agents
- Meperidine (Demerol), 50-100 mg IM q3h for pain

Antianxiety agents
- Hydroxyzine (Vistaril), 25-50 mg IM with meperidine

Anticoagulants
- Heparin, 2000-3000 units subq q12h

Sedative-hypnotics
- Flurazepam (Dalmane), 15-30 mg at bedtime

Cathartic or laxative agents
- Bisacodyl (Dulcolax), 1-2 tablets or rectal suppository prn

Analgesic-antipyretic agents
- Acetaminophen (Tylenol), 600 mg q4h prn for elevated temperature

If rheumatic or inflammatory disease is present, antirheumatic or anti-inflammatory medications are begun postoperatively as soon as patient can tolerate oral intake

General Management

Empty and record suction drainage every 4 hours, if ordered; otherwise, empty as needed

Give oxygen at 2 to 3 L per nasal cannula for 24 hours, then as needed

Perform respiratory therapy with IPPB every 4 hours, or instruct patient in use of incentive spirometer every 2 to 4 hours

Help patient do deep breathing and coughing every 2 hours

Record intake and output

Maintain bed rest for 24 to 48 hours (varies with specific joint replaced, the security of the replacement prostheses, and physician's choice)

Change dressing after 24 to 48 hours; may reinforce dressing if necessary

Give nothing by mouth for 24 hours; then clear liquids and advance to regular diet as tolerated

Perform neurovascular checks every hour for 24 hours, then every 2 hours for 24 hours, and then every 4 hours

Check vital signs every 4 hours

Maintain position of operative area with sling, splint, abduction pillow, immobilizer, brace, or elastic wrappings (varies with specific joint replaced)

Patient should be up but bearing no weight on operative limb after bed rest order expires (may be after 24, 48, or 72 hours, depending on joint replaced and whether cemented or noncemented replacement was done); some physicians may permit touch-down weight bearing

Begin physical therapy exercises on second postoperative day; exercises and schedule vary with joint replaced; exercises are either active or passive to all joints, excluding the operated joint, and include quadriceps setting, straight leg raising, flexion and extension, or other individually prescribed exercises for the particular joint replaced

Patient should be up with walker or crutches four times daily; ambulation should increase as patient is able with up to 25 pounds weight to operative limb, gradually increasing to full weight bearing with crutches

Patient should sit in chair for 10 to 15 minutes only (after hip replacement), two or three times daily for first week; then may sit in chair 20 or 30 minutes four times daily

Patient should wear antiembolism hose

Encourage fluid intake and high-fiber foods (if tolerated) to prevent constipation; administer rectal suppository if needed to empty rectum

Patient should use toilet riser for toilet (prevents hyperflexion of hip after total replacement)

NURSING CARE

Nursing Assessment

Joint and Incisional Area

Presence, amount, and type of drainage
Edema
Color of tissues and capillary refill
Presence, type, and tightness of dressing or bandages
Presence of peripheral pulses
Pain in incision or distal to operative site
Presence of immobilizing device, splint, or pillow to maintain proper position of prosthesis within joint

Systemic Concerns

Respiratory functions
- Excursion
- Dyspnea
- Orthopnea
- Pain in chest or lung areas
- Cough
- Decreased lung sounds

Urinary
- Presence of indwelling catheter
- Intake and output

Psychosocial Concerns

Concern with body image
Acute pain
Regaining mobility and weight bearing

Other Complications

Pneumonitis
Pneumonia
Wound infection (superficial or deep)
Limb inequality or limp
Urinary tract infection
Dislocation of prostheses

Nursing Dx & Intervention

Nursing Diagnosis	Nursing Intervention/Rationale
Impaired physical mobility related to surgical and soft tissue trauma	• Assess ROM of unaffected joints. • Maintain bed rest as ordered *to promote recovery*. • Begin ambulation with ambulatory aid and weight-bearing restrictions as ordered *to aid early rehabilitation and to prevent complications*. • Encourage performance of active and passive ROM exercises, isometric exercises, and other specific ordered exercises *to aid muscle strength*. • Encourage use of trapeze to assist with lifting, turning, and positioning *to increase independence*.
Impaired skin integrity related to incision through to joint structures	• Assess condition of all skin surfaces. • Reinforce and then change dressing with strict aseptic technique: note wound edge approximation, redness, edema, hematoma, or unusual tenderness of wound *as signs of possible wound infection*.
Altered peripheral tissue perfusion related to surgery and immobility	• Assess circulatory condition of operative limb. • Apply ice bags to operative site *to lessen edema and bleeding*. • Do circulation checks and record findings; note presence or absence of pain in calf and positive Homans' sign *as signs of thrombophlebitis*. • Check drainage in suction apparatus and record. Report unusual amounts *as signs of hemorrhage*. • Remove antiembolism hose twice daily; check color, presence of pulses, and skin condition; replace hose after 1 hour off *to aid circulation*. • Check vital signs; note presence of hypotension and elevated pulse or temperature; record and report *as signs of infection or sepsis*. • Maintain proper and ordered flexion, extension, and/or abduction of operative tissues according to specific joint replaced *to aid recovery and increase mobility*.

Nursing Diagnosis	Nursing Intervention/Rationale
Pain related to tissue trauma	• Assess amount, type, and severity of pain. • Administer narcotics with potentiator as ordered every 3 hours for first 24 hours; then use as needed for pain relief *to increase comfort*. • Turn, raise, or adjust position *to prevent pressure and lessen fatigue*. • Administer medications for concomitant disease as ordered *to relieve symptoms and pain*. • Administer sedative at bedtime as ordered *to provide for restful sleep*. • Assess bowel and bladder output; may need laxative, suppository, or enema *to aid elimination*. • Convalescent care: encourage self-care and return to ADLs as able *to aid recovery*. • Stress alternatives to medication for restful sleep (activity to become tired, reading, warm milk, snack) *to lessen dependence on medications*.
Impaired physical mobility related to bed rest and bone surgery	• Assess ROM of unaffected tissues. • Encourage walking as able *to aid recovery*. • Assist with ROM exercises *to maintain muscle strength*. • Monitor use of crutches or walker *to ascertain proper amount of weight bearing*. • Complete continuity of care referral for home care follow-up *to foster continuity of care*. • Stress compliance with prescribed rehabilitation program after discharge *for full recovery*. • Encourage continued contact with physician for follow-up care *for safety*.
Potential for injury related to displacement of prosthesis(es)	• Assess postoperative position for required position *to maintain prostheses inside joint*. • Reiterate preoperative instructions *to prevent dislocation:* avoid adduction of legs and not to cross ankles; keep head of bed below 90 degrees *to prevent unsafe hip flexion;* keep operative leg abducted by using abduction pillow or 2 to 3 pillows placed between legs; use the knee immobilizer *to prevent knee flexion, which could cause hip flexion;* keep leg abducted when turned to side. • Teach the "post" position *to prevent dislocation:* patient bends knee of unoperative leg and firmly plants (posts) foot on mattress, then grasps trapeze, stiffens back and pelvis and lifts body from bed by pushing on posted foot and leg while pulling up. • Maintain patient on bed rest for 1 to 3 days, then help patient up in a chair, cautioning to avoid adduction of the operative limb and to avoid 90-degree flexion of the hip. • Listen to patient's complaints of increased pain in operative area and observe position of the limb—if it is held in external or internal rotation, could indicate dislocation.
Potential for injury related to development of deep vein thrombosis	• Assess for complaints of pain or soreness in calf, redness, or edema along vein channels. • Remind patient to do dorsiflexion and plantar flexion exercises every 4 hours *to prevent venous stasis*. • Administer heparin, 3000 to 5000 U subcutaneously twice a day, *to lessen possibility of deep vein thrombosis*. • Monitor bleeding and clotting times while patient is receiving heparin (therapeutic range of partial thromboplastin time is up to 1½ times normal—normal is 30 seconds). • Monitor stools, urine, and emesis for blood and skin areas for bruising or ecchymosis while patient is receiving heparin.
Potential for infection related to wound or joint infection	• Assess wounds for signs of infection. • Perform wound care aseptically *to prevent introduction or transfer of organisms*. • Observe wound for redness, edema, abscess, or purulent drainage *as signs of infection*. • Monitor patient's vital signs and note elevations *as signs of possible infection*. • Listen to patient's complaints of deep, dull, aching pain in hip operative area *as signs of possible joint infection;* report findings to physician.

Patient Education

1. Stress that rehabilitation of muscles and joint tissues, locally and systemically, will require daily practice over time.
2. Stress compliance with medication regimen for chronic disease if present.
3. Stress that joint ROM and mobility should be regained after recovery and rehabilitation are accomplished.

Evaluation

Patient Outcome	Data Indicating That Outcome is Reached
Incision heals well.	Wound edges are well approximated; there is no edema or drainage.
Patient regains joint mobility and ROM.	Patient walks with crutches (if lower extremity) and performs prescribed exercises with comfort and assistance if required; discomfort is eased with analgesics only.
Self-concept is positive.	Patient returns to family and social roles when able.

Arthroscopy

Description and Rationale

With the advent and development of the arthroscope, startling changes have occurred in operative examination and treatment of pathologic joint conditions. Although the knee joint is still a major focus, nearly all joints can be examined with the arthroscope. The multiple benefits of early arthroscopic treatment with specialized techniques and instruments in the hands of a skilled practitioner include lessened inflammation, degeneration, and posttraumatic arthritis. Patients can usually return to their daily activities sooner with full use of the involved joint following arthroscopic examination and repair.

Arthroscopy is most frequently done for diagnosis and treatment of knee injuries, primarily torn or damaged menisci. The menisci, C-shaped rings of cartilage covering the ends of the tibia within the knee joint, are subject to degeneration, tears, and wear. Cartilage has no intrinsic blood supply, and if torn, worn, or degenerated, it rarely heals without developing unsatisfactory fibrocartilage. Trauma to the meniscus is greatest among athletes who suffer tears from external forces, such as a tackle, or from internal forces when a load exceeds the compressibility and resiliency of the cartilage; this may occur in a single incident or over time from repeated stressors. The meniscal tear may cause slight, partial, or complete avulsion from adjoining bone tissues.

The discussion that follows focuses on the knee because it is the joint most commonly examined and treated arthroscopically.

Loose or torn pieces of menisci 1 inch or slightly larger in size can be removed arthroscopically. One or more small incisions may be required for full visualization of the joint. Incisions or "ports" for arthroscopic procedures are on the mediolateral or posterolateral surfaces of the knee joint superior to the patella.

Contraindications and Cautions

1. Arthroscopy requires skilled practitioners, as well as more specialized techniques than more extensive arthrotomy procedures.
2. Using more than one port for visualization of the joint may lead to infection.
3. Small pieces of torn or loose cartilage may be missed if hidden under other joint tissues.
4. Hemorrhage must be prevented to lessen posttraumatic arthritis.
5. Scar formation may predispose to future tears in ligaments or cartilage.
6. Postoperative physical therapy and individualized exercise programs must be prescribed and performed to maintain or regain the joint's mobility, stability, and strength.

Medical Plan

Medications

Finish IV fluids; then attach IV needle to heparin well
Narcotic analgesics
- Meperidine (Demerol), 50-100 mg IM q3h as needed for 3 d
- Oxycodone (Percodan), 30-60 mg po q4h prn after 3 d

Anti-infective agents
- Cephazolin (Ancef), 250-1000 mg q6-8h IM
- Cephalexin (Keflex), 500 mg po q6h

General Management

Bed rest until patient is fully alert; then can be up with crutches four times daily
Check of vital signs every 2 hours for 6 hours; then every 4 hours
Neurovascular checks every hour for 24 hours
Ice bags to knee continuously
Change dressing as needed
Advancement to regular diet as tolerated
Physical therapy consultation for knee exercises

NURSING CARE

Nursing Assessment

Neurovascular Status of Knee Joint and Lower Extremity

Color: may be slightly paler, but capillary refill and perfusion should be within 2 to 4 seconds
Temperature: slightly cooler
Peripheral pulses: should be present
Movement: should be normal in ankle; knee should be able to be flexed with moderate discomfort
Sensations: should be normal

Psychosocial Concerns

Concern with regaining knee mobility to return to usual ADLs and activities without impairment

Complications

Hemorrhage
Thrombus formation
Posttraumatic degeneration and arthritis
Infection

Nursing Dx & Intervention

Nursing Diagnosis	Nursing Intervention/Rationale
Altered peripheral tissue perfusion related to use of tourniquet during arthroscopy	• Assess neurovascular status as ordered *to determine current status.* • Apply ice bags to knee continuously *to lessen bleeding and edema.*
Impaired physical mobility related to knee arthroscopy	• Assess effects of surgery on mobility. • Assist to positions of comfort; assist to ambulate as needed *to maintain strength.* • Assess drainage and change dressing as needed (drainage should be scant, serosanguineous) *to note condition of wound and healing.* • Assist with physical therapy exercises as needed *to regain joint functions.* • Teach walking up and down stairs *to regain joint motion.*
Pain related to removal of meniscus and arthroscopy	• Assess site, amount, and severity of pain. • Administer medications as ordered for pain *to aid comfort.* • Help patient stand to void (easier while standing). • Assist with and prepare tray for meals *to aid intake of food and fluids.* • Elevate leg as ordered *to aid venous return.* • Apply ice bags *to lessen edema* and thereby *decrease pain.*

Patient Education

1. Instruct the patient in physical therapy exercises as needed to gradually increase strength and mobility.
2. Instruct the patient in signs or symptoms that would require return to see physician.
3. Instruct the patient in appropriate use of pain medications and adequate diet to promote healing.

Evaluation

Patient Outcome	Data Indicating That Outcome is Reached
Patient regains joint motion.	Patient has full ROM without pain or limitation, has returned to usual activities, and does not have degenerative changes.

Chemonucleolysis

Description and Rationale

Chemonucleolysis is the chemical reduction by an enzyme of a ruptured or herniating disc. The enzyme used is chymopapain, obtained from the papaya plant. It acts similarly to a meat tenderizer to alter the fluid content of collagen fibers by "breaking" the disc into its biochemical constituents of sugars, amino acids, and water; this softens the disc and lessens its pressure. Scar tissue then replaces the disc tissues as the inflammatory processes resolve.

Chymopapain was first used in 1964; it was approved by the U.S. Food and Drug Administration (FDA) in 1975, but the approval was withdrawn because statistics showed no statistical differences in patients' symptom relief following its injection when compared to those treated with a placebo. Researchers disputed these data because the placebo was found to contain an enzyme. In November 1982 the FDA reapproved the use of chymopapain for relief of pain associated with disc herniations.

Chemonucleolysis is being done less often than in the past because of less than satisfactory results for some patients; however, it is still an option for selected patients.

Contraindications and Cautions

1. Allergic history, reactions to meat tenderizers, and other allergens are contraindications.
2. Pregnancy and prior injection with chymopapain are also contraindications.
3. Chymopapain is also not used in progressive nerve deficits, whether motor or sensory, or bowel or bladder dysfunction.
4. Postoperative muscle spasms are a common occurrence.
5. Some patients may still require operative disc removal; surgery is more difficult following chemonucleolysis because of scar tissue formation.
6. Discs treated with chymopapain age more rapidly because they lose water.
7. If the sedimentation rate is elevated above 20 mm in women, chemonucleolysis is contraindicated because anaphylactic reactions may occur.
8. Some physicians order preoperative diphenhydramine (Benadryl) and cimetidine (Tagamet) to lower histamine receptors and steroids (methylprednisolone) to lessen inflammation or anaphylactic reaction.
9. Morphine, urecholine, and meperidine should not be administered in the 24 hours preceding surgery.

Preprocedural Nursing Care

1. Obtain a detailed history of allergies.
2. Perform meticulous skin care.
3. Initiate intravenous infusion.
4. Insert a heparin well.

Medical Plan

Medications

Adrenergic agents
- Epinephrine (Adrenalin), 1:100,000, on hand

Antihistamines
- Diphenhydramine (Benadryl), 50 mg on hand

Narcotic analgesic agents
- Meperidine (Demerol), 50-100 mg q3h for severe pain for postoperative use only

Tranquilizers
- Diazepam (Valium), 2-5 mg IM q4-6h for muscle spasms

Intravenous, 1000 ml 5% D/.45 N/S at 75-100 ml/h for 12 h; then to "keep open" rate

General Management

Check vital signs every hour for 4 hours, then every 2 hours for four times, and then every 4 hours

Observe for development of signs of anaphylaxis: wheezing, dyspnea, anxiety, rash, vital sign changes, flushed skin

Give nothing by mouth until patient is fully awake; then give clear liquids and advance to regular diet as tolerated

Patient should be up in morning and then three times daily

Help patient to deep breathe and cough every 2 hours

Do laminectomy checks every hour for 4 hours, then every 2 hours for four times, and then every 4 hours

Monitor voiding and input and output

Discharge after physician visits (discharge varies per physician and patient's progress)

Nursing Dx & Intervention

Nursing Diagnosis	Nursing Intervention/Rationale
Pain related to ruptured disc or surgery	• Assess type, amount, and severity of pain. • Observe for presence and amount of muscle spasms (some physicians order ice applications; others order heat) *to note presence.* • Administer analgesics and/or muscle relaxants as ordered; see that patient has prescriptions for home medications *for continuity of care.* • Perform laminectomy checks every 2 to 4 hours *to note resolution or progression of symptoms.* • Help patient stand to void. • Assist with ambulation as needed *to increase independence.* • Change bed position as desired (lying prone is contraindicated) *to ease tired muscles.*
Patient problem: anaphylactic reaction to chymopapain	• Assess for rash, hives, or swelling of lips or eyes. • Monitor vital signs as ordered; observe for changes in pulse, decrease in blood pressure, dyspnea, wheezing, or anxiety (most commonly in first 2 to 4 hours). • Explain anaphylactic reaction signs to patient *to ease concerns.*

Patient Education

1. Discuss anaphylaxis signs to report to physician (can occur as late as 1 week after procedure).
2. Stress that relief of symptoms may not occur for several weeks or longer.
3. Instruct the patient to comply with physician's follow-up visit in 1 week.

Evaluation

Since the use of and experience with chymopapain are still new, data are not available to fully evaluate this treatment. It is still a controversial treatment.

Patient Outcome	Data Indicating That Outcome is Reached
Patient experiences no anaphylaxis.	Patient has no rash, blood pressure or pulse changes, wheezing, or dyspnea.
Patient is relieved of neurologic impairment.	Patient experiences tolerable muscle spasms initially with easing over time; motor and sensory changes are reversed: peripheral pulses are present; color is pink; temperature is warm; patient is able to move with normal ROM, void easily, and walk with upright posture with ease.

FIXATION FOR IMMOBILIZATION OF BONES (EXTERNAL)

Casts

Description and Rationale

Casts are hard structures of plaster, fiberglass, or plastic materials used to immobilize musculoskeletal tissues following injuries. Although plaster (gypsum) is still the most frequently used material for casts, newer fiberglass, plastic, and cast-tape casts are being used more often. Each of the particular materials requires specific application techniques and has advantages and disadvantages, such as being heavy, cumbersome, or expensive or requiring special drying procedures and care to prevent skin breakdown. The use of a particular material is determined by the patient's injury, length of time needed for immobilization, and the physician's preference (Figures 4-17 to 4-19).

Preparation for encasement in a cast varies from simply explaining its application and purpose to complete physical preparation, including an enema, bath, and skin cleansing with antiseptic solutions. Explanations and care should be geared to the patient's level of comprehension and need to prevent undue fear or anxiety. Handling the patient gently, especially the parts to be encased in a cast, alleviates tension and facilitates application without additional trauma.

Depending on the type of cast and the materials used, all supplies should be assembled and assistance for positioning and holding arranged for in advance. Privacy is required when the skin is exposed, and breast and genital areas should be covered for the patient's ease of mind. Padding may be used over bony prominences before the cast is applied.

Once a cast is applied, drying times vary with the material used, the amount of plaster used, the areas of the body put into the cast, and the weather conditions. Plaster casts dry more slowly in damp, high-humidity conditions and can take 3 or 4 days to dry thoroughly. While drying, the areas in a cast must remain uncovered for drying to proceed from inside out. Drying is also facilitated by using fans (except with open reductions) and heat lights with low-wattage bulbs.

During the drying periods, care must be taken to avoid making finger indentations in the cast, which would be reflected inward and cause a pressure area on the skin under the indented area. Pressure is also eased by turning the patient every 2 hours while the cast is drying to prevent molding and deformation. Propping or elevating with pillows helps maintain proper positioning. The pillows used should not have a plastic or rubber covering, since the heat given off by the cast material will be trapped by the rubber or plastic and reflected back to the tissues in the cast, causing injury or even a burn. Plastic and rubber also delay drying of plaster.

Contraindications and Cautions

1. Open fractures may not be treated with casts initially because of the need to observe the injury site over an extended period.
2. Plaster casts must be kept dry to prevent disintegration and weakening of the cast.
3. Fiberglass, plastic, and cast-tape casts can become wet without weakening; however, the skin under the cast must be dried if it becomes very wet to prevent maceration under the cast.
4. Abdominal distention should be treated before placing a patient in a spica cast, because the distention may increase, causing respiratory or circulatory compromise.

Preprocedural Nursing Care

1. The skin areas to be encased must be clean, dry, and free of open lesions.
2. Roentgenograms are taken to ascertain the extent of trauma.
3. All equipment and supplies must be assembled before the procedure is begun for ease and safety of application without unnecessary delay.
4. Sufficient skilled personnel should be present to assist with the application; two or three people may be needed to assist the physician with a spica or body cast.
5. A sedative, narcotic, or anesthetic may be given before cast application.

Medical Plan

Medications

Narcotic analgesic agents
- Meperidine (Demerol), 25-100 mg IM q3h (exact dosage varies with age and trauma)

Analgesic-antipyretic agents
- Aspirin, 300-600 mg po or rectally (if NPO) for moderate pain q4h prn

Sedative-hypnotics, nonbarbiturate
- Flurazepam (Dalmane), 30 mg po at hs, prn

General Management

Ice bags to site (would be ordered to a specific site)
Bed rest until cast is dry
Elevation of cast (extremity) on pillows
Neurovascular checks every hour for 24 hours, then every 2 hours for 24 hours, and then every 4 hours
For open reduction, recording and reporting amount of drainage or bleeding
Forcing of fluids

NURSING CARE

Nursing Assessment

Cast and Contiguous Tissues

Neurovascular condition of tissues around cast
Position of tissues in cast (e.g., in flexed or extended position)
Condition of cast (damp or dry)
Temperature of cast and tissues around cast
Ice bags: ice melted or still frozen

Nursing Dx & Intervention

Nursing Diagnosis	Nursing Intervention/Rationale
Impaired physical mobility related to presence of the cast	• Assess ROM of unaffected muscles. • Teach isometric exercises as feasible, such as quadriceps and gluteus setting exercises. If fracture is below knee, quadriceps setting exercises of affected leg are vital *to retain muscle strength and prevent atrophy.* • Assist with ambulation as needed *to increase mobility.* • Teach techniques for walking with crutches *for safety.* • Apply sling to hold cast snugly; teach patient to allow cast to lie in sling with shoulder loose *to prevent shoulder pain or "freeze" of muscles.*
Pain related to cast or trauma	• Assess presence and degree of pain. • Stress that return of pain after pain-free period should be reported to physician (may indicate loss of reduction or other complication). • Administer narcotic or analgesic as necessary and ordered *to relieve pain.* • Note increase in pain, numbness, or tingling and decrease or absence of pulses as indicative of compartment syndrome or that cast may be too tight; report promptly to physician, since cast may need to be cut (bivalved). • Stress need to elevate extremity if edema recurs after discharge *to relieve edema.* • Note signs of increasing anxiety, dyspnea, nausea or vomiting, or eructation or complaints of abdominal distention; may be caused by "cast syndrome" from excessive aerophagia (air swallowing) or from kinking of the superior mesenteric artery, leading to gastric or intestinal distention and ileus; cast may need to be bivalved, and a nasogastric tube may be inserted *to relieve ileus and vascular compromise.* • Consult occupational therapist and physical therapist for activities *to relieve boredom and maintain muscle strength.*
Constipation (potential) related to bed rest	• Assess bowel sounds and bowel elimination. • Stress importance of well-balanced, nourishing meals, high in residue and bulk *to prevent bowel problems (when patient resumes a full diet).*
Altered patterns of urinary elimination (potential) related to decreased intake and bed rest	• Assess intake and output every shift. • Force fluids *to maintain urinary functions.*
Impaired physical mobility related to edema and muscle weakness after cast removal	• Assess for presence of edema and muscle function after cast is removed. • Explain that affected tissues may develop edema and tenderness with reuse *to ease concern.* • Caution patient to resume usual activities slowly *to lessen edema and soreness.*

Patient Education

1. Explain techniques to keep cast clean and dry.
2. Explain need for well-balanced meals and adequate fluids.
3. Explain proper crutch and walking techniques.
4. Explain skin care after cast removal: gently cleanse skin with cold-water wash containing enzymes; allow to soak into skin for 20 to 30 minutes; then flush with clear water; dry carefully and apply a lubricating lotion to prevent cracking or drying of the skin.
5. Explain that the patient should report persistent pain, weakness, and edema to the physician (usually all symptoms are relieved in 3 or 4 days after cast removal, although muscle weakness may persist longer); at times special exercises may be prescribed.

Evaluation

Patient Outcome	Data Indicating That Outcome is Reached
Patient regains mobility and ROM.	Patient uses muscles and joints normally and without limitation or edema and has minimum initial postremoval pain and discomfort.

External fixation devices

Description and Rationale

Several types of externally applied fixation devices are currently used for immobilization of bones, including the Wagner, Roger Anderson, Murray, Hoffman, and Ace-Fischer apparatuses. The Hoffman apparatus consists of pins placed at right angles to the long axis of a bone and held by the clamps and screws of the device. The Ace-Fischer device has pins placed in oblique and vertical angles to the long axis of the bone and then attached to the retaining device. The latter device has only recently become available, whereas the Hoffman device has been in use for approximately 20 years. The use of one or another device depends on the patient's condition and physician choice as with any medical treatment (Figure 4-25).

Externally applied fixation is used in many sites and for many conditions. Sites where such fixation may be applied include bones of the face, jaw, upper and lower arm or leg, pelvis, ribs, and fingers or toes. Pins used vary in number, length, and thickness according to the bones or area to be treated. The major reasons for use of these devices are that they allow increased use of contiguous joints while maintaining the local immobility, they permit the patient's discharge to home, they hold unstable fractures or reductions and weakened muscles while allowing ambulation, and they hold bones with tissue or bone infection (pins are above and below the infected areas).

Contraindications and Cautions

1. Severely comminuted bone fractures may be a contraindication because the multiple pins needed may cause more fractures or weakening. Comminution with good alignment may be an indication for use.
2. Severe or spreading osteomyelitis may be another contraindication, since the multiple sites can be sources for progressive infection.
3. Overuse or excessive muscular movements may cause loosening or pin movements.
4. The multiple pin entrance and exit sites can be sources of skin and bone infection.
5. Following removal of the pins, bones can be refractured because of the multiple tracts through the bones; patients must be cautioned to increase activities slowly to prevent reinjury.

Preprocedural Nursing Care

1. Meticulous skin cleansing and preparation are required.
2. Roentgenograms must be taken.
3. Antibiotics are given intravenously.

Medical Plan

Surgery

Pin care every 4 hours or as needed (see below)

Medications

Narcotic analgesic agents
- Meperidine (Demerol), 50-100 mg IM q3h (dosage varies with age and trauma)

Anti-infective agents
- Cefamandole (Mandol) or cefazolin (Ancef), 250-1000 mg IV q6h for 7 d
- Cephalexin (Keflex), 500 mg q6h po after IV antibiotic is discontinued

Analgesic-antipyretic agents
- Aspirin, 600 mg q4h po, for moderate pain or temperature above 38.3° C (101° F)

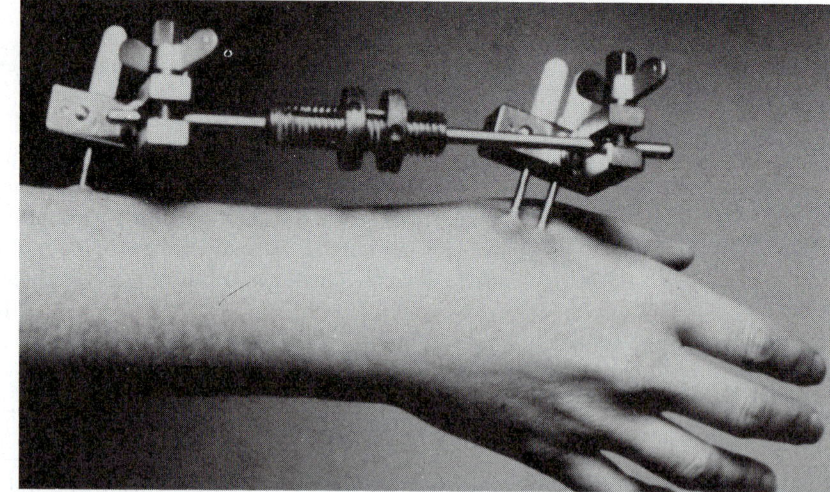

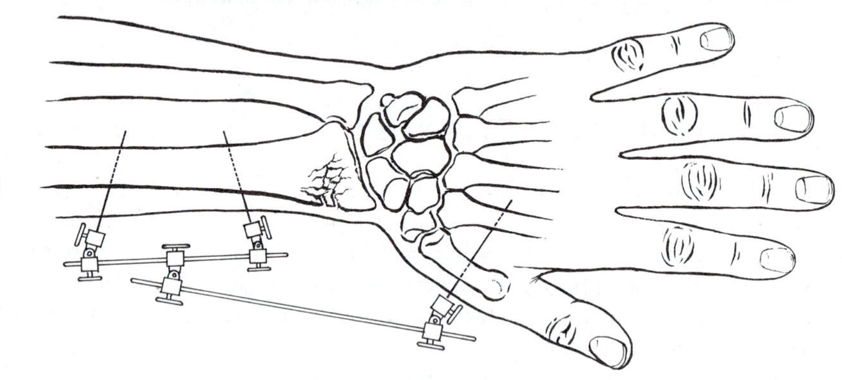

Figure 4-25 External fixation apparatuses. **A,** Hoffman. **B,** Roger Anderson.

General Management

- Neurovascular checks every hour for 24 hours, then every 2 hours for 24 hours, and then every 4 hours
- Ice bags to site continuously
- Elevation of extremity on pillows
- Up with sling (if upper extremity) or with crutches and no weight bearing (if lower extremity; after recovery from anesthetic)
- ROM to unaffected joints and muscles

NURSING CARE

Nursing Assessment

Site of Injury and External Apparatus

- Assessment of each pin entrance and exit site
  - Color
  - Temperature and edema of tissues
  - Drainage
  - Peripheral pulses
- Ability to move contiguous muscles and joints (unless ordered to be held immobilized)
- Pain, numbness, or tingling

Systemic Concerns

- Temperature and other vital signs
- Nausea
- Headache or other pain

Psychosocial Concerns

- Concern with body image
- Degree of mobility/immobility
- Acute pain
- Possibility of infection

Other Complications

- Nonunion or malunion
- Infection
- Muscle or nerve damage or injury
- Compartment syndrome

Nursing Dx & Intervention

Nursing Diagnosis	Nursing Intervention/Rationale
Impaired physical mobility related to trauma and fixation device	• Assess ROM of unaffected tissues. • Maintain bed rest until recovered from anesthesia *to aid recovery*. • Ambulate as ordered with sling or crutches *to enhance mobility*. • Turn and alter bed position as needed *to prevent development of pressure areas*.
Body image disturbance related to external apparatus	• Assess implicit or expressed concerns. • Clarify purposes of multiple pins and external device *to increase understanding*. • Stress positive aspects of use of external devices *to increase self-concept and body image*. • Explain that pins can be removed in physician's office when union has been achieved as determined by roentgenograms *to ease concern*.
Impaired skin integrity related to multiple pins, skin openings, and trauma	• Assess skin areas for signs of pressure or inflammation. • Wound care as needed. Pin care: clean each site with hydrogen peroxide–soaked swabs; remove drainage with normal saline; then dry. Topical antibiotic ointment may or may not then be lightly applied, depending on physician or institutional policy. (Pin care may not be done or is stopped if sites are clean, dry, and without drainage.) • Clean all sutures if present with antiseptic and redress if drainage is present. Sutures may be left open to air if unit policy.
Pain related to trauma or fixation apparatus	• Assess site and amount of pain (may initially be acute, sharp pain at pin insertion sites on skin) *to determine current status*. • Administer narcotics and analgesics as needed and ordered *to relieve pain or discomfort*. • Stress that recurrence of pain at site is a sign to be reported to physician—may indicate a developing problem. • Stress that acute pain episodes will lessen in 24 to 48 hours and that all pain will be relieved in approximately 7 to 10 days *to ease concern*. • Note localization of pain to one site (may be sign of infection or inflammation); continue hourly neurovascular checks *to note early changes*. • Note change in sensation or numbness and tingling as signs of circulatory pressure; report increases in either sign, as these may signify beginning compartment syndrome. • Apply ice bags as ordered *to lessen edema and pain*.

Patient Education

1. Teach the patient and family pin care techniques to continue at home if needed.
2. Stress the need to increase movements and weight bearing slowly after the pins are removed to lessen tenderness and to permit the muscles to regain strength.

Evaluation

Patient Outcome	Data Indicating That Outcome is Reached
Patient regains mobility and ROM.	Patient uses muscles and joints normally, without limitation or edema, and with minimum initial postremoval pain and discomfort.
Wound sites remain free of infection.	No drainage, redness, or erythema is noted at pin sites.

Traction

Description and Rationale

Traction is the application of force to the skin, muscles, and bones to aid in reduction of fractures, hold the reduced bones in alignment for healing, relieve muscle spasms and pain, and exert sufficient pull on muscles and bones to relieve pressure on peripheral spinal nerves. Traction can be applied to the skin and thus indirectly to the bones and muscles, or it can be applied directly to the bones through skeletal pins inserted through the skin and bones with the pins then being attached to ropes, pulleys, and weights. The particular type of skin or skeletal traction applied is determined by the physician with regard to the patient's injury or condition, the purpose of the traction, the age of the patient, the weight of the patient, the condition of the skin tissues to be placed in traction, and the length of time the patient will need to be kept in traction. Table 4-6 summarizes the various types of

Text continued on p. 460.

Table 4-6
Traction

Type	Patient's Age	Amount of Weight	Purposes and Principles	Considerations for Care
Buck's extension (one or both legs) (Figure 4-26, *A*)	Any age; most commonly used in adults	5-8 lb/leg	Applied preoperatively for hip fractures; for "pulling" contracted muscles; for relieving muscle spasms of legs or back; patient usually lies in recumbent position; may be turned to either side if no fracture is present; if there is a fracture, patient is turned to unaffected side	Skin of older patients is more "friable" and subject to loosening because of less subcutaneous fat; patient's complaints of burning under tape, moleskin, or traction boot should be assessed; traction may be removed for skin care even in presence of fracture
Russell's (one or both legs) (Figure 4-26, *B*)	Children 5 years or older to older adults	2-5 lb/leg	Applied for "pulling" contracted muscles; preoperatively for hip fractures; uses principle that "for every force in one direction, there is an equal force in the opposite direction" for the pulley placement and amount of weight used, because weight pull is doubled	Patient is positioned on back for most effective pull; knee sling can be loosened for skin care and checking pulses in popliteal area
Pelvic belt or girdle (abdomen and pelvis are enclosed) (Figure 4-26, *C*)	Adults or older adolescents	20-35 lb	Relieve muscle spasms and pain associated with "disc" conditions; pull is from iliac crests to relieve spasm	Patient may be positioned in Williams' position, which permits 45 degrees of flexion of the knees and hips to relax the lumbosacral muscles; orders usually state to be "in traction 2 hours, out 2 hours" and out of traction at night; traction straps should not put pressure over sciatic nerves
Pelvic sling (under pelvis and buttocks like a hammock)	Adults	20-35 lb	For holding fractured pelvic bones; buttocks must be slightly off bed	Patients are very comfortable in the sling even with extensive pelvic bruising; they may become quite dependent on being in the sling, and gradual "weaning" may be required; the sling should be kept clean and dry, and the patient can be removed from the sling for care and toileting, if institutional policies permit
Cervical head halter (under chin, around face, head, and back of head)	Adults	5-15 lb	For relieving muscle spasms caused by degenerative or arthritic conditions in or of the cervical vertebrae; halter should be applied so pull comes from occipital area, not through chin portion	Patients may be in low or high Fowler's position depending on the purpose of the traction; halter is usually incorrectly positioned if the patient complains of pain of chin, teeth, or temporomandibular joint; the side straps usually should be adjusted to relieve these complaints; patients should be removed from the traction for sleeping; patients may also use this type of traction at home for cervical arthritic conditions

Table 4-6—cont'd
Traction

Type	Patient's Age	Amount of Weight	Purposes and Principles	Considerations for Care
Cotrel's (cervical head halter and pelvic belt to pelvis)	Adolescents	5-7 lb to head halter and 10-20 lb to pelvic belt	For stretching muscles preoperatively for scoliosis; principle is to pull muscles and joints apart	Patient is put in this traction to relax muscles and curvature; should be in traction except for sleeping; rarely, patient may be placed in Cotrel's postoperatively, too, although less frequently because of newer operative techniques such as Harrington or Luque rod insertion
Dunlop's (lower humerus and forearm)	Children to adults	5-7 lb to humerus; 3-5 lb to forearm	For realigning fractures of the humerus; body is used for countertraction by slightly elevating side of bed of arm in traction; forearm is merely held at right angles to the humerus for comfort, by using Buck's extension to the forearm	Dunlop's can be totally skin traction by Buck's extension to the humerus or can be skeletal with a Steinmann pin inserted through the distal humerus; use of either depends on the patient's injury; traction to the *forearm* should be removed daily for skin care, pulse checks, and ROM exercises, since the forearm traction is merely a means to keep the forearm vertically at a right angle to the humerus; patients must have assistance during ADLs because they are held flat on their backs; they can turn enough for back care only
Cervical via skull tongs (skull bones bilaterally)	Any age (most commonly young adults)	20-30 lb (depends on weight of patient)	To realign fractures of cervical vertebrae and to relieve pressure on cervical nerves; patient must be on a special bed or frame such as a Circ-Olectric bed or Stryker frame to facilitate care; traction weights must never be "lifted"; traction must be continuous	Patients with this traction may be severely injured, having either upper or lower spinal cord injury or complete transection, making them quadriplegics or paraplegics; neurovascular checks and "craniotomy" checks are required hourly to assess progression or relief of symptoms; patients also may develop paralytic ileus (therefore are given nothing by mouth), may have a nasogastric tube inserted to suction, and have an indwelling urinary catheter; pin care is done every 4 hr: soak sterile applicators in a half-strength solution of hydrogen peroxide and normal saline; apply to each pin site; allow to stand 5-10 min; use soaked applicators to remove drainage; dry sites; apply antibiotic or antiseptic ointment to pin sites if ordered

Table 4-6—cont'd
Traction

Type	Patient's Age	Amount of Weight	Purposes and Principles	Considerations for Care
Halo-pelvic (pins inserted into skull in four areas to hold halo part and pins inserted through iliac pelvic bones for pelvic part)	Adolescents and adults	None; bars extending between skull and pelvic portions hold body in desired positions	For preoperative straightening of scoliosis curvature; straightening is accomplished by overcoming muscle contractions through tightening the bars	This traction is "comfortable" after a few days to recover from the insertional trauma; however, dressing is very complicated because of the vertical bar placements that interfere with most clothing; children with this traction are usually hospitalized; traction may remain in place postoperatively to be replaced by a brace or cast; halo-pelvic traction is a variant of halo-femoral traction, in which the pins are inserted through the distal femurs instead of the pelvic bones and the skull pins pull away from the femoral pins, thereby bringing about straightening
Balanced suspension to femur (Steinmann pin or Kirschner wire inserted through upper tibia; thigh and leg are suspended in a splint and leg attachment) (Figure 4-27)	Any age from 3 yr	20-35 lb	For realignment of fractures of the femur; to overcome muscle spasms associated with fractures of the femur; suspension of the thigh and leg is "balanced" by countertraction to the top of the thigh splint	Patients in this traction should be recumbent for best effects; they can turn approximately 30 degrees to either side briefly for back care or can lift themselves using the trapeze and by using the uninjured leg and foot; neurovascular checks are vital to assess circulatory status and to prevent compartment syndrome; tissue pressure monitoring is done (Table 4-7)

Table 4-7
Tissue Pressure-Monitoring Procedures for Detection of Compartment Syndrome

Steps	Purpose and Interpretation
1. Cleanse skin over site with antiseptic.	To lessen chance of infection.
2. Insert needle-tipped catheter into muscle to be assessed; attach catheter to stopcock and syringe filled with normal saline; attach to tubing of mercury manometer.	
3. Open stopcock; depress plunger of syringe to inject saline.	
4. Observe pressure readings on manometer. 5. Remove saline; close stopcock. 6. Record findings; report increasing pressures to physician.	Normal tissue pressures are 0-30 mm Hg; rising pressures that approach patient's diastolic blood pressure readings may indicate compartment syndrome. Patient may need fasciotomy.
7. Check distal peripheral pulses bilaterally; compare. 8. Measure site (usually thigh, calf, arm, or forearm) *bilaterally* to assess presence of, amount of, or increase in edema formation.	Rising venous pressures may exceed arterial tissue perfusion; peripheral pulses may be weak or nonpalpable; edema may be pronounced.

Figure 4-26 Types of skin traction. A, Buck's extension. B, Russell's. C, Pelvic belt.

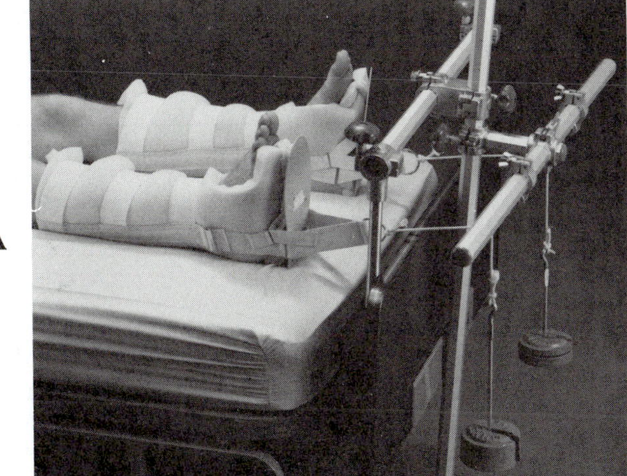

A

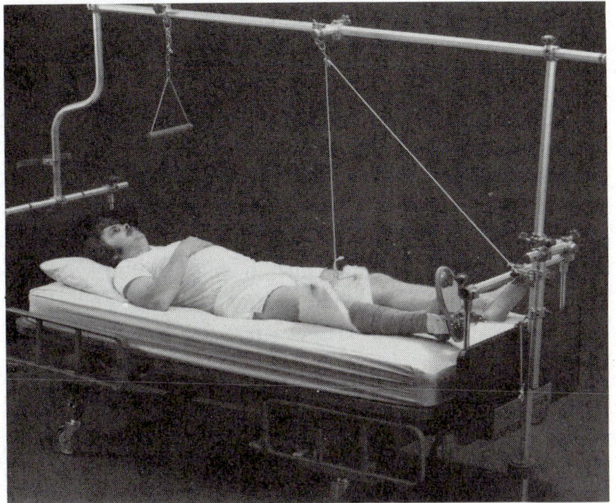

B

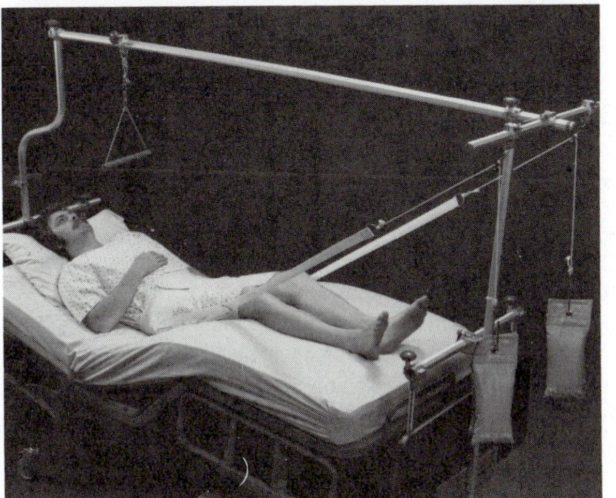

C

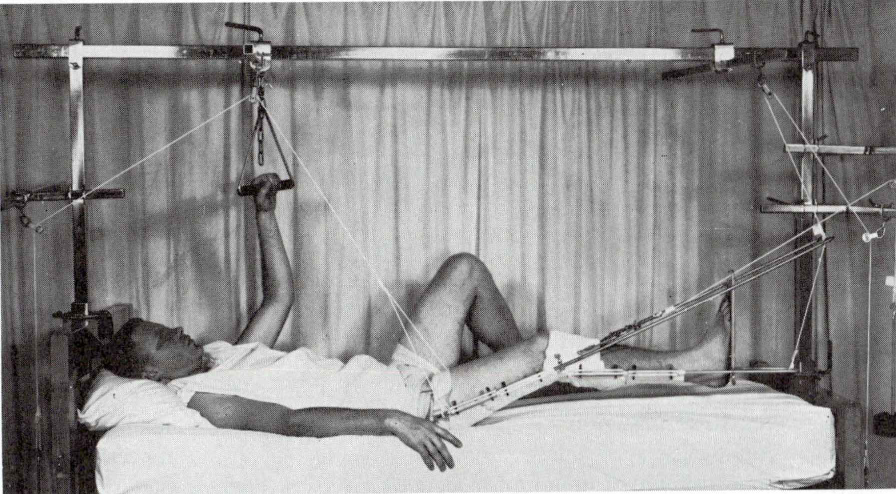

Figure 4-27 Balanced suspension skeletal traction to the femur. From Brashear.[11]

skin and skeletal traction and the specific points pertinent to each type of traction (Figures 4-26 and 4-27).

Because time is required to overcome muscle spasms, bone overriding, angulation, and shortening, patients may be in traction for as short a time as 24 to 48 hours or as long as 10 weeks or more. Generally, patients in traction must remain hospitalized for the entire time because of the specialized care and equipment required (except for patients being treated with home cervical traction with a head halter, or in rare instances in other types of traction). Since hospitalization in traction is extensive and also expensive, patients may be placed in traction for periods only to achieve relief of muscle spasms and to correct fracture overriding or angulation; once alignment is regained, the patient may be taken to surgery to have internal metallic fixation. Therefore although traction is still frequently required for specific treatment of an individual patient's injuries, the traction may be removed sooner than in the past because metallic implants may be used to maintain the reduction.

Contraindications and Cautions

1. Age is a restriction for the application of one or more types of skin or skeletal traction (Table 4-6). Because of lack of muscle mass or strength, a newborn baby or an elderly adult may not benefit from traction.
2. Open draining wounds or lesions are also contraindications to the use of either skin or skeletal traction, since such wounds predispose to infection.
3. The amount of weight applied must be determined by the physician, who will consider the amount of muscle spasm, the degree of overriding and angulation, and the specific purposes of the treatment. The weight may be increased or decreased as roentgenograms indicate the need for weight changes.

Preprocedural Nursing Care

1. Reiterate or clarify upcoming events for patient's traction.
2. Assess local and systemic physical condition for indications or contraindications to placement in traction (such as open lesions, drainage, deep calf pain).
3. Assist with hygienic self-care for clean, dry skin surfaces.
4. Assist with positioning for roentgenograms.
5. Administer preprocedural medication if ordered.
6. Assemble all equipment for application of specific traction.

Medical Plan

Medications

- Narcotic analgesic agents
  - Meperidine (Demerol), 50-100 mg IM q3h for 72 h
  - Morphine, 10-15 mg IM q4h
- Analgesic-antipyretic agents
  - Aspirin, 600-1000 mg q4h prn for moderate pain
- Tranquilizers
  - Diazepam (Valium), 2-10 mg po q4-6h

General Management

- Application of skin or skeletal traction (Table 4-6)
- Diathermy to back (lumbar area) twice daily
- Bed rest: specific position or positions as per Table 4-6
- Neurovascular checks every hour for 24 hours, then every 2 hours, and then every 4 hours
- Monitoring of tissue pressure if ordered
- Ice bags to affected tissues (site always ordered for application)
- Diet: high protein, high vitamin, low fat; force fluids
- Physical therapy for ROM and isometric exercises
- Pin care twice daily for skeletal traction

NURSING CARE

Nursing Assessment

Area of Body in Traction*

- Tissues
  - Color
  - Edema
  - Signs of pressure around traction
  - Pain
- Amount of weight
- Direction of pull

Systemic Concerns

- Patient
  - Pressure areas over bony prominences
  - Muscle strength or weakness
  - Weight loss
  - Position in bed
- Traction (entire traction setup)
  - Ropes
  - Pulleys
  - Weights
  - Knots
  - Pins
  - Slings
  - Belts
  - Each part of setup (Table 4-6)

Psychosocial Concerns

- Concern with changes in body image
- Immobility and loss of livelihood
- Acute pain

Other Complications

- Nonunion
- Malunion
- Embolic phenomena
- Pin necrosis
- Skin lesions or pressure areas

*See Table 4-6 for specific tissues.

Nursing Dx & Intervention

Nursing Diagnosis	Nursing Intervention/Rationale
Pain related to trauma and traction	• Assess pain experiences to determine extent, etiology, and patient's reactions. • Monitor tissue pressures every hour (Table 4-7) *to note early increases of pressure.* • Help patient alter position within traction limitations *to relieve muscle and joint stiffness or soreness.* • Administer narcotic analgesics as ordered to relieve acute pain and non-narcotic analgesic (aspirin) *to relieve inflammation.* • Assess patient's entire pain experiences: *local* pain at site of injury and *systemic* spread (e.g., chest pain, dyspnea, calf pain, headache, confusion); *may be indications of pulmonary, circulatory, neurologic, or other complications.* • Assess for evidence of fat embolism with symptoms of mental confusion, dyspnea, chest pain, and vital sign changes. A petechial rash may also develop over upper chest and neck with fat emboli. • Assess and perform Homans' procedure to determine possible cause of calf pain; could indicate thrombophlebitis if positive Homans' sign. • Assess degree of muscle spasms in injury site; clarify causes of and measures *to relieve spasms through traction and muscle-relaxant medications.* • Clarify use of ice bags and apply ice bags *to help relieve muscle spasms.* • Assist with ROM exercises *to maintain strength in unaffected muscles.* • Assess affects of diathermy *in relieving pain and muscle spasms* if pertinent to injury. • Perform pin care (Table 4-6) if needed *to remove secretions and to lessen possibility of infection.*
Body image disturbance related to weight loss and weakness	• Assess effects of injury on body image and self-concept. • Explain purposes of traction repeatedly, since patient's anxiety and pain may preclude hearing or full understanding. • Explain reasons for bed rest, weakness, and anorexia. Encourage patient to eat more as appetite returns *to help regain weight.* Patients can lose 20 to 30 pounds in skeletal traction because of decreased muscle activity over time. • Explain purposes of position changes: *to maintain healthy tissues.* • Assess appetite and intake and output *to note current status.*
Impaired physical mobility related to traction, hospitalization, and loss of livelihood	• Assess effects of injury and traction on mobility. • Clarify use of traction as one part of treatment regimen for patient's specific injury *to increase understanding and compliance.* • Encourage patient and family communications with physician for "timetable" of plans for overall treatment *to aid compliance.* • Seek consultations (per physician's order) for occupational therapy and physical therapy *to assist patient's recovery and adjustment to treatment regimen and hospitalization.* • Seek consultation with social service personnel to help patient and family plan and prepare for possible economic needs *to regain livelihood* (may lose employment while hospitalized). • Encourage patient's self-care activities *to maintain mobility within traction limits.* • If surgical repair follows traction use, assist to ambulate as ordered *to regain mobility.*

Patient Education

1. Ensure that patient and family can apply traction correctly if it is to be used in the home.
2. Instruct patient and family in use of muscle relaxants and pain medications if prescribed for home use.
3. Ensure that patient and family recognize when to contact physician if symptoms recur.

Evaluation

Patient Outcome	Data Indicating That Outcome is Reached
Patient regains mobility and ROM.	Patient uses muscles and joints normally without limitation or edema and with minimum initial postremoval pain and discomfort.

NOTE: One or another form of skin or skeletal traction may be applied as the major treatment for a specific musculoskeletal condition, as has been indicated throughout this chapter. Traction also can be used before surgical repair or replacement within a cast. Other nursing care concerns are discussed in those areas of the chapter and in Table 4-6.

FIXATION FOR IMMOBILIZATION OF BONES (INTERNAL)

Surgical implantation of metallic pins, nails, screws, plates, and other devices for immobilizing or repairing traumatized or damaged bones and joints is a major orthopaedic treatment. With the development in the early 1930s of nonreactive metal alloys, surgical repair has provided markedly decreased hospitalization periods, a more rapid return to home and social and employment opportunities, and a more rapid regaining of mobility. Surgical repair requires the concurrent administration of antibiotics to prevent infection, the major hazard and deterrent to use of more orthopaedic surgical and metallic implants for a wider range of injuries. However, in most instances the advantages of internal metallic fixation far exceed the disadvantages; therefore surgery is a major viable treatment for orthopaedic trauma.

Fractures of bones may be immobilized by (1) screws attached to a compression plate, (2) nails or pins, as in a hip nailing, (3) a rod or nail placed within the intramedullary canal (intramedullary rod) or parallel to the bones (Harrington or Luque rod), (4) screws or staples to hold fracture fragments together, or (5) natural bone grafts to fill in gaps in bones or to fuse two bone surfaces together, as in a spinal fusion.

This section will focus on three procedures representative of internal fixation procedures: hip nailing or pinning, spinal fusion by Harrington or Luque rods, and spinal fusion by natural bone grafts.

Internal fixation with hip nails or pins

Description and Rationale

The patient's specific injury, general physical and mental condition, and the physician's choice from the many available metallic nails and pins determine which type will be used for the particular patient. The injury may be a fairly stable fracture that requires only a single nail, such as a compression screw or a sliding compression nail. Unstable fractures may require multiple pins, such as Knowles pins, or use of a nail with a side plate.

The type of internal fixation used is also determined by the particular fracture type and site. Hip fractures are referred to as intracapsular or extracapsular. Intracapsular fractures are those of the femoral head or neck that are contained within the hip capsule (Figure 4-9). Intracapsular fractures may disrupt the blood supply to the head of the femur, with subsequent development of avascular necrosis of the head of the femur. Therefore fractures of the head or proximal femoral neck may be treated with insertion of a femoral prosthesis. Subcapital or distal neck fractures may heal without avascular necrosis; thus these latter fractures may be nailed or pinned.

Extracapsular fractures are those around or through the trochanters and are referred to as intertrochanteric or subtrochanteric fractures. These fractures heal well with the use of compression screws or nails because the blood supply to the

Figure 4-28 A, Internal fixation with cortical bone grafts. **B,** Grafts held with plate and screws.

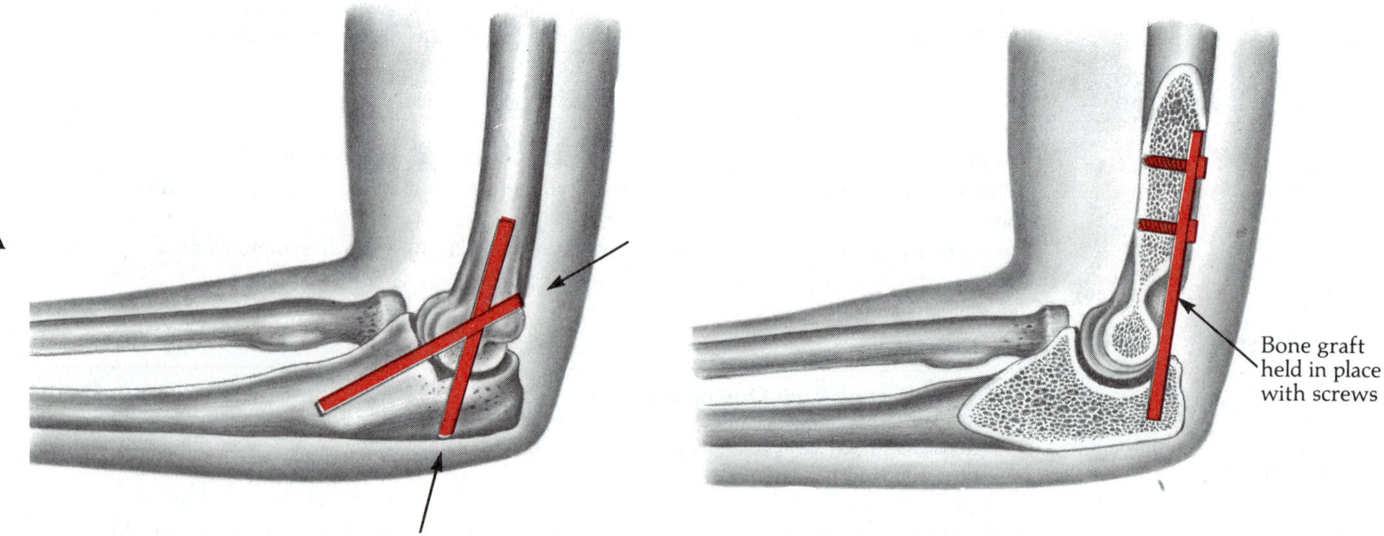

Figure 4-29 A, Type of hip nail. **B,** Prosthesis replacing head of humerus. **C,** Femoral head prosthesis.

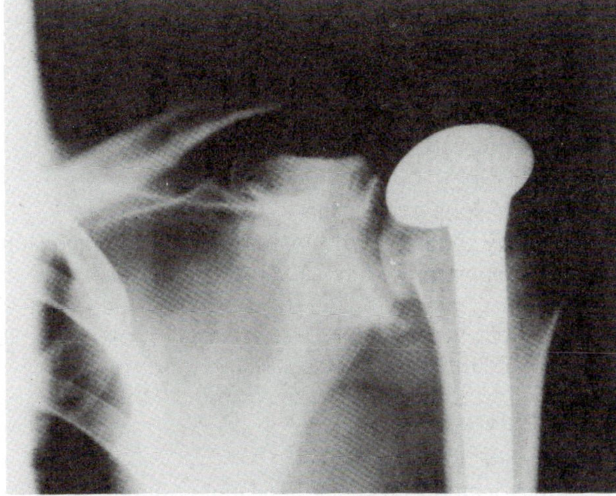

B

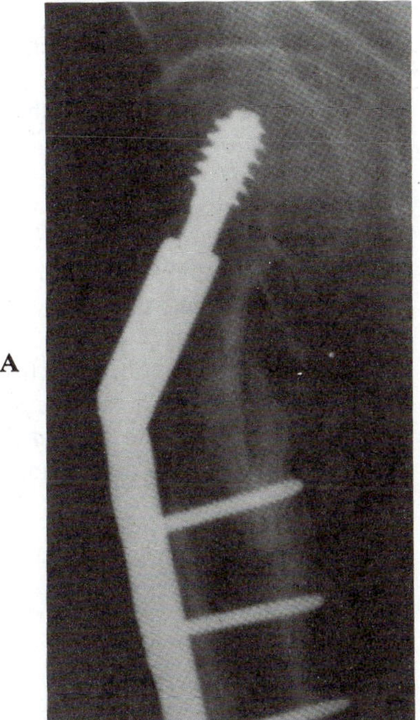

A

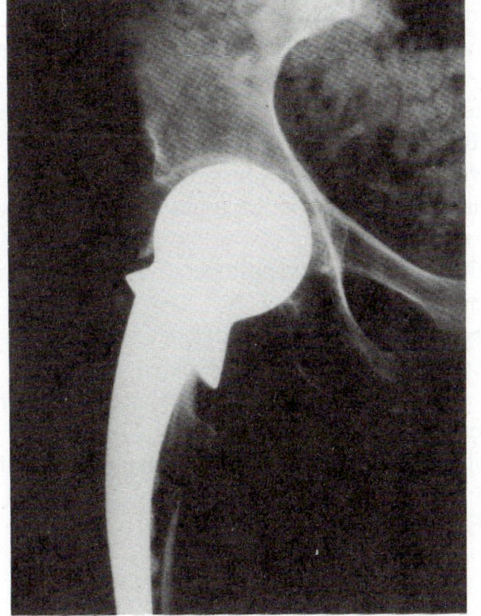

C

fracture site comes from the surrounding vessels outside the capsule. Side plates attached to the nails help maintain a stable reduction while healing progresses (Figure 4-29).

Finally, the patient's physical and mental condition may also help determine which type of internal fixation is performed. The weak or confused patient would benefit from a compression interlocking nail, which can withstand some weight bearing; a single nail with or without a side plate would be appropriate for a stable fracture in a mentally clear patient who could be cautioned and expected to walk with only minimum or touch-down weight bearing.

Thus the specific internal fixation and repair require careful evaluation and assessment by the surgeon and other health professionals for the patient's greatest benefit.

Preprocedural Nursing Care

1. The patient is placed in traction, usually Buck's extension or Russell's, while preparations for surgery are completed.
2. Chest and injury site roentgenograms are evaluated.
3. An enema is given, if needed, and an indwelling catheter may be inserted.
4. An electrocardiogram is done to determine cardiovascular status.
5. Serologic studies are done for chemistry analysis; urinalysis is done.
6. Skin cleansing is done to decrease organisms in the operative site.
7. Preoperative medication is administered.
8. Intravenous therapy is initiated for fluid intake.

Medical Plan

Medications

- Anti-infective agents
  - Cefazolin (Ancef), 250-1000 mg IV q6h
- Narcotic analgesic agents
  - Meperidine (Demerol), 50-75 mg q3h for 24 h, then q3h prn
- Analgesic-antipyretic agents
  - Aspirin, 600 mg rectal suppository q4h for temperature elevation above 38.3° C (101° F) and for moderate pain
- Intravenous 1000 ml 5% D/.2N/S at 125 ml/h; add 20 mEq KCl to each liter

General Management

- Pulmonary IPPB every 4 hours
- Bed rest with operative leg in neutral position
- Turning to unoperative side and back every 2 hours
- Change of dressing as needed; reinforcement as needed
- Record of input and output; separate record of suction drainage
- Deep breathing and coughing every 2 hours; Respirex (or Triflow) 10 times every hour
- Vital signs every 15 minutes for four times, every 30 minutes for four times, every hour for four times, then every 4 hours
- Up in chair three times on first postoperative day with no weight bearing
- Up with walker on second postoperative day; weight bearing on operated leg is specifically ordered
- Clear liquids after nausea has subsided; advance to regular diet as tolerated
- CBC, electrolytes, and CO_2 measurements in morning and daily for 4 days
- Physical therapy to help with walking

NURSING CARE

Nursing Assessment

Hip and Upper Thigh Incisional and Wound Area

- Assessment
  - Dressing
  - Drainage
  - Wound suction equipment
  - Drainage in container
- Presence of edema at wound site
- Position of thigh and leg
- Complaints of pain
- Color of tissues

Systemic Concerns

- Respiratory and circulatory status
- Vital signs
- Mental state and recovery from anesthesia
- Muscle strength or weakness
- Urinary output and catheter-drainage setup
- Intravenous fluid type, amount, and rate

Psychosocial Concerns

- Concern with body image
- Immobility
- Confusion
- Acute pain

Other Complications

- Loss of reduction and/or dislocation
- Thrombophlebitis
- Avascular necrosis of femoral head
- Pneumonia
- Cardiac arrhythmias
- Wound infection

Nursing Dx & Intervention

Nursing Diagnosis	Nursing Intervention/Rationale
Body image disturbance related to trauma	• Assess concerns. • Maintain bed rest; clarify need for bed rest, if needed *to aid compliance*. • Massage back *to aid comfort and circulation*. • Help walk with walker and weight bearing as ordered (may continue either no weight bearing or partial weight bearing for up to 1 month, gradually increasing to full weight by 3 months).
Impaired physical mobility related to modification in weight bearing	• Assess ability to understand instructions and limitations. • Assist to dangle at bedside on first postoperative day, then to pivot to chair with no weight on operative leg, or touch-down weight if allowed. • Stress that operative foot should be placed on floor but weight should be borne on unoperative leg (refer to limb as either left or right leg so patient has a clear understanding) *to maintain safety in care*. • Turn every 2 hours; prop with pillows between legs or back *to maintain position*. • Assist with ROM exercises *to maintain muscle strength*. • Help physical therapist walk patient with walker and limited weight to operative limb (if assistance is needed) *for comfort and safety*.

Nursing Diagnosis	Nursing Intervention/Rationale
	• Encourage patient and family members to walk together *for patient's safety.* Instruct family about weight-bearing techniques *for clarity and safety.*
Pain related to trauma and surgery	• Assess wound for evidence of resolution of surgical trauma and inflammation. • Assess patient's complaints of pain; clarify site, type, and amount of pain. • Administer analgesics judiciously because of patient's age; dosage should be sufficient to relieve pain without causing confusion (may need to vary dosage within ordered ranges) *for safety in care.* • Turn or reposition patient and massage back *to increase comfort.* • Perform Homans' test to determine development of thrombophlebitis, which could lead to pulmonary embolism. Observe for chest pain, dyspnea, and changes in vital signs, which *could indicate pulmonary embolism, atelectasis, or pneumonia.* • Assist with meal and food selections *to aid in healing, resolution of inflammation, and enhancement of bone calcification.* • Force fluids *to aid digestion and bowel and bladder elimination.*

Patient Education

1. Clarify need for weight-bearing restrictions for bone union.
2. Clarify signs to report to the physician: increased soreness or pain at operative site, fever, decreased urine output or burning with urination.
3. Reiterate techniques for use of walker or crutches.
4. Teach patient and family necessity to continue eating a well-balanced diet and drinking plenty of fluids for healing, circulation, and elimination.

Evaluation

Patient Outcome	Data Indicating That Outcome is Reached
Patient regains mobility.	Patient walks with progressive weight bearing as healing occurs, with minimum discomfort and satisfactory ROM.
Fracture has united.	Patient has no pain in fracture site. Muscle and joint strength is regained.

Internal fixation with Harrington or other rods

Description and Rationale

Harrington rods are long metallic implants attached posteriorly to the vertebral column following corrective repair and fusion as treatment for scoliosis. The rod or rods (they may be bilaterally used) hold the vertebrae in the corrected alignment to permit the bone grafts to heal and fuse the vertebrae solidly. The rods may remain in the site for extended periods or may be removed (rarely done) after roentgenograms indicate there is sound, solid fusion. In the early postoperative period some patients may wear a fitted brace to help the rods maintain spinal immobility if the curvature was marked preoperatively and multiple grafts were implanted during surgery. The brace is worn during waking hours and is removed for sleep.

Luque rods are another kind of metallic implant used for corrective spinal surgery. Luque rods are used on both sides of the spinal column with multiple attachments to each spinal segment to add corrective forces throughout the deformity. Additionally, Luque rods are contoured to aid in correcting the deformation.

Contraindications and Cautions

1. Harrington and other rods are foreign bodies, as are all metallic implants; thus they may cause a severe inflammatory reaction, which may necessitate their removal.
2. Open surgery may predispose to local wound infection or may lead to meningeal infections.
3. One or more bone grafts may be needed to maintain the correction of the curvature; parts of or whole grafts may not unite firmly, which may necessitate prolonged wearing of a brace, encasement in a plaster cast, or even reoperation.
4. The spinal attachments holding the rods may loosen, allowing the rods to move. Major movement of either end of the attachments would necessitate reoperation.

Preprocedural Nursing Care

1. The patient may be placed in Cotrel's or halo-femoral traction (Table 4-6) or a Risser cast (Figure 4-19) before surgery to stretch contracted muscles.

2. Meticulous skin cleansing is done to remove organisms to prevent infections.
3. Roentgenograms determine respiratory and spinal conditions; respiratory therapy with IPPB and a respiratory aid is done every 4 hours.
4. Serologic and urologic studies are done.
5. An enema is administered to clear the lower bowel.
6. An indwelling catheter is inserted into the urinary bladder.
7. A full-length bed pad or alternating pressure mattress is placed on mattress.

Medical Plan

Medications

Narcotic analgesic agents
- Meperidine (Demerol), 50-100 mg IM q3h
- Morphine, 10-15 mg IM q4h

Analgesic-antipyretic agents
- Aspirin, 600 mg rectal suppository for moderate pain q4h prn; or for temperature over 38.3° C (101° F)

Anti-infective agents
- Cefazolin (Ancef) or cefamandole (Mandol), 250-500 mg q6h IV

Intravenous 1000 ml 5% D/.45N/S at 75 ml/h with 10 mEq KCl in every other liter

General Management

IPPB every 4 hours
Maintain patient flat in bed
Do log roll every 2 hours
Help patient deep breathe and cough every 2 hours; use respiratory aid 10 times every hour
Do not change dressing; reinforce if needed
Do laminectomy checks every hour
Give clear liquids after patient has had nothing by mouth for 24 hours; advance to regular diet as tolerated
Force fluids after intravenous line is discontinued
Do ROM exercises to arms and legs every 4 hours
Keep cast uncovered until dry or keep brace on at all times (if ordered and used)
Consult physical therapist for ROM and isometric exercises

NURSING CARE

Nursing Assessment

Vertebral Column, Incisional Wound Site

Check of alignment and position of back and entire patient
Check of wound
- Drainage (may have suction drainage)
- Edema
- Dressing
- Presence of brace or plaster cast with open window in back portion

Skin condition of formerly contracted tissues
Respiratory excursions; depth, rate, and character of respirations
Site and amount of pain

Systemic Concerns

Assessment of motor and sensory functions by laminectomy checks or neurovascular checks
Catheter drainage
Intravenous fluid infusion site, solution, and rate
Presence of nausea or vomiting
Abdominal distention/ileus

Psychosocial Concerns

Self-concept and body image
Immobility
Acute pain
Length of convalescence

Other Complications

Shock
Hemorrhage
Wound infection
Nonunion
Loss of reduction
Pneumonia
Urinary tract infection
Meningitis

Nursing Dx & Intervention

Nursing Diagnosis	Nursing Intervention/Rationale
Body image disturbance related to deformity and dependence because of bed rest and surgery	• Assess patient's concerns with self-concept and image. • Stress patient's improved appearance following fusion *to aid positive self-concept.* • Encourage self-care as able; help with placement and removal of supplies *to maintain an esthetic atmosphere.*
Impaired physical mobility related to prolonged convalescence and muscle weakness and spasms	• Assess ROM of unaffected tissues. • Turn, with assistance of another health professional, by log rolling every 2 hours. (Teach family log-rolling technique if possible, and use their assistance.) Do not let patient turn himself or herself; log rolling cannot be accomplished safely this way because patient would twist. Twisting

Nursing Diagnosis	Nursing Intervention/Rationale
	could disrupt fibrin meshwork (see pp. 421 to 422 for bone healing), thereby delaying or preventing bone union and fusion. Brace will hold back sufficiently rigid after discharge so patient can safely turn or get up unassisted. • Encourage deep-breathing and leg exercises *to increase self-activities and independence and promote healing and circulation.* • Perform laminectomy checks every hour; that is, observe and compare in all four extremities: color, temperature, edema; ROM; grip, push, and pull strength; sharp and dull discrimination; and presence and type of pain, radiation, numbness, and tingling *to note signs of pressure.* • Massage exposed areas of shoulders, neck, back, and buttocks *to relieve tiredness and muscle spasms.* • Assist with stretching exercises if needed *to relieve skin restrictions from preoperative curvature limitations.*
Pain related to surgical trauma and muscle stretching	• Assess patient's complaints of pain; clarify site, type, and amount of pain. • Administer medication (dosage adjusted to age, if younger child or adolescent, and severity of pain) as ordered *to maintain therapeutic levels.* • Assess wound as pain source; note signs of resolution of inflammation and surgical trauma. Report continued edema, redness, and increased drainage *as untoward signs.* • Help patient increase amount and time of walking (when allowed up) *to help resolve muscle soreness and weakness and to lessen soreness and pain in operative site.* • Change dressings over incision (after initial dressing change by physician) as needed; note lessening of soreness and acute pain as healing proceeds *to note resolution of inflammation.* • Check bowel sounds, abdominal distention, passage of flatus (ileus may be source of pain).

Patient Education

1. Teach the patient and family how to put on brace.
2. Clarify that muscle stiffness, weakness, and soreness may increase with increase in activities but will last for brief periods only.
3. Reiterate stages of bone healing for strong union; stress need for caution against sudden position changes and need to continue wearing the brace.
4. Stress that the patient must eat a well-balanced diet to regain muscle strength and promote healthy bone growth.
5. Explain that sudden or gradually increasing pain should be reported to physician.

Evaluation

Patient Outcome	Data Indicating That Outcome is Reached
Patient has regained satisfactory spinal curves.	Patient has satisfactory posture and curvatures without spinal rotation.
Patient regains independence, mobility, and spinal motion with limited flexion.	Patient moves freely without muscle weakness, discomfort, or pain and has learned to use muscles of lower extremities and hips to assist lumbar muscles when stooping or bending (must kneel or bend from hips rather than from lumbar area).
Self-concept is positive.	Patient resumes social contacts.

Spinal fusion with bone grafts

Spinal fusion with natural autogenous bone grafts is done as treatment of a herniated nucleus pulposus. Nursing care of patients following spinal fusion for treatment of a ruptured disc is very similar to that discussed above, with the addition of assessing relief of sensory pressure signs, numbness, and tingling as surgical wound healing progresses. Autogenous bone grafts usually provide solid union without the problems associated with metallic implants, such as foreign body reactions, loosening, or infections.

Nursing care for spinal fusion is the same as for internal fixation with Harrington rods.

Hemilaminectomy

Description and Rationale

Hemilaminectomy is the partial removal of the lamina to gain access to the intervertebral space to remove a ruptured disc. The pathophysiology leading to disc degeneration and rupture is discussed on p. 437.

Contraindications and Cautions

1. Determination of the cause and location of one or more degenerated or ruptured discs requires physiologic and psychologic diagnostic profiles before surgery.
2. Removal of a degenerated or ruptured disc may not relieve the patient's complaints of pain.

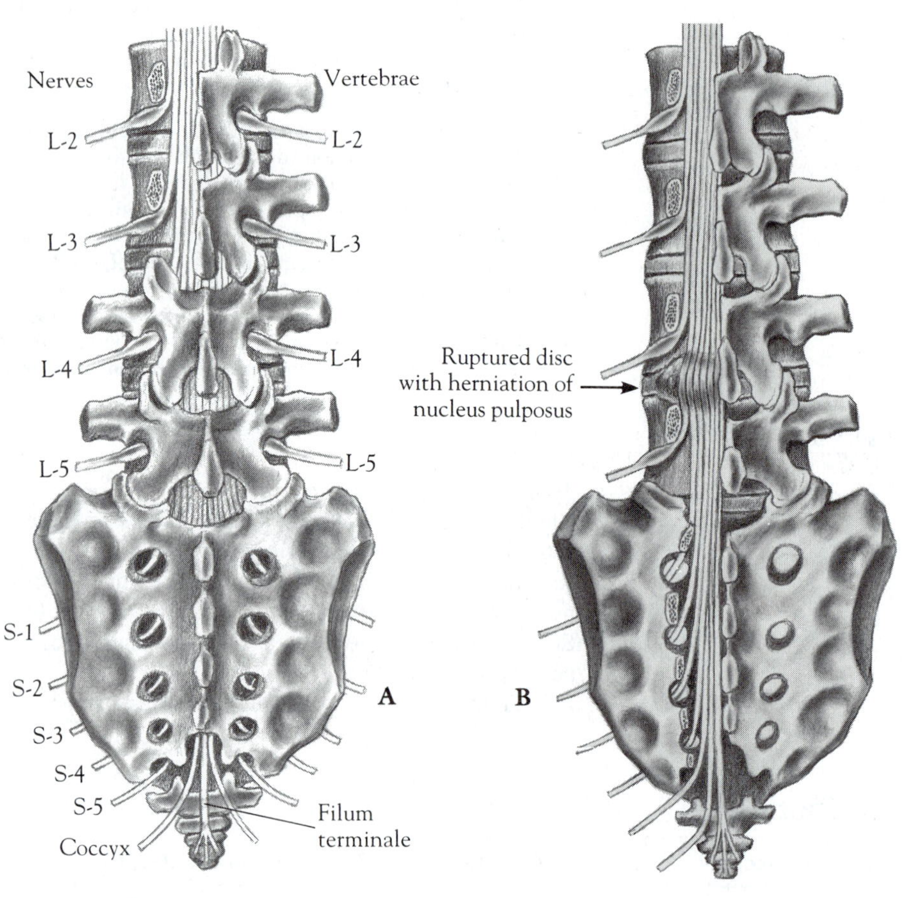

Figure 4-30 **A,** Spinal nerves exiting from cord. **B,** Herniated nucleus pulposus; note pressure on nerve.

Figure 4-31 Mechanisms that can cause degeneration of the anulus leading to herniation of the nucleus pulposus. **A,** Axial pressure. **B,** Lateral pressure. **C,** Posterior pressure.

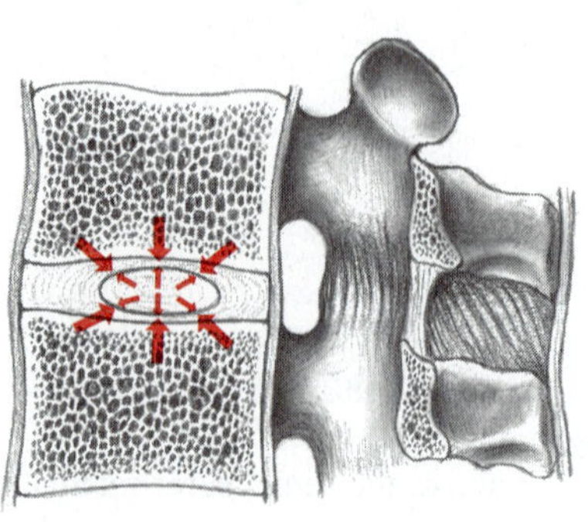

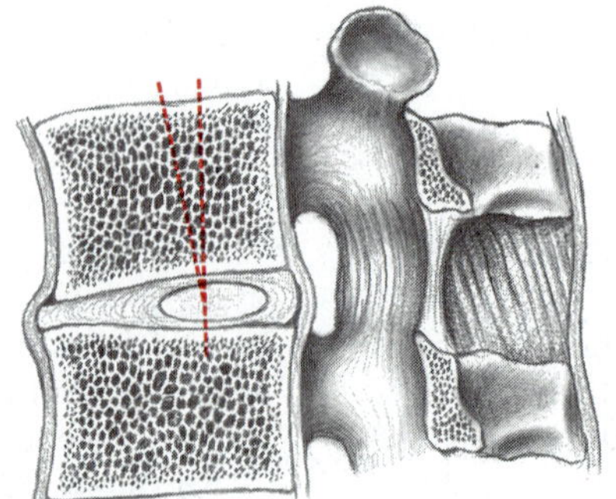

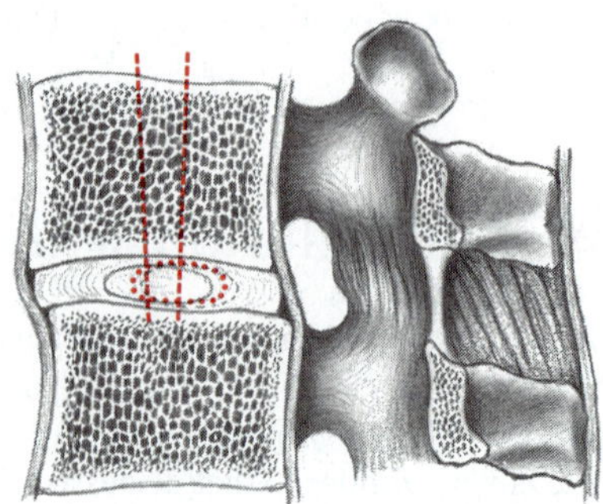

Figure 4-32 Laminectomy for herniation of nucleus pulposus. **A,** Area of lamina removed during a hemilaminectomy. **B,** Herniated nucleus pulposus.

Figure 4-33 A, Anterior and, **B,** posterior views of sensory dermatomes. L4, L5, and S1 = 95% of all ruptured discs. C1 to C7 = 5% of all ruptured discs.

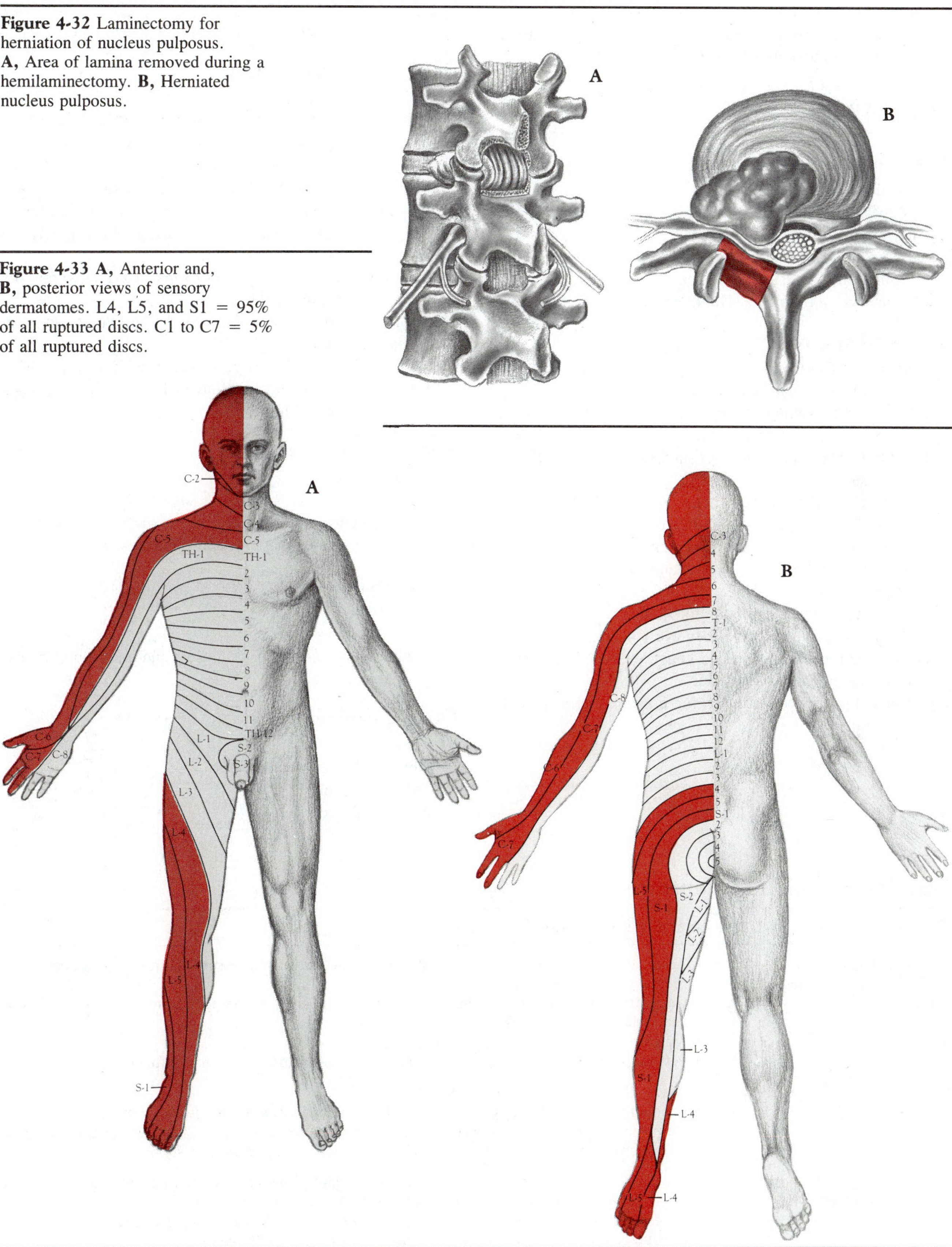

3. Postoperative rehabilitation requires the patient's cooperation and performance of daily exercises to strengthen the spinal and abdominal muscles.

Medical Plan

Medications

Narcotic analgesic agents
  Meperidine (Demerol) 50-100 mg q3-4h for pain
Anti-infective agents
  Cefazolin (Ancef) or cefamandole (Mandol), 250-500 mg q6h IV
Intravenous, 1000 ml 5% D/.45N/S at 75-100 ml/h

General Management

Nothing by mouth until morning; then clear liquids and advance to regular diet
Bed rest until evening of surgery
Turn side to side every 2 hours
Patient up at bedside evening of surgery and up three times daily thereafter
Laminectomy checks every hour for 4 hours, then every 2 hours for four times, and then every 4 hours
Patient may stand to void if necessary
Reinforce dressing if needed; change dressing after 24 hours
Check vital signs every hour for 4 hours, then every 2 hours for four times, and then every 4 hours
Have patient deep breathe and cough every 2 hours; use Respirex 10 times every hour
Physical therapy consultation for exercise regimen and program

NURSING CARE

Nursing Assessment

Incisional Area of Lumbar Back or Cervical Area

Assessment of motor strengths and sensory condition of feet and legs or arms and hands bilaterally (usually are within normal limits for push, pull strength; may have some remaining sensory changes such as lingering numbness or decreased sensitivity to sharp pinpricks)
All peripheral pulses palpable
Skin temperature of feet, legs, arms, and hands: may be slightly cool and pale
Drainage on dressing scant to moderate amount and serosanguineous
Pain mild to moderate in operative area with some radiation to shoulders and occipital area (if cervical) and to hips and buttocks (if lumbar)

Systemic Concerns

Headache
Nausea
Abdominal distention
Urinary retention (may need to stand to void)

Psychosocial Concerns

Acute pain
Lingering chronic pain
Limitation of neck or back muscle and joint mobility and strength

Other Complications

Hemorrhage
Motor and sensory weakness
Continued pain
Wound infection

Nursing Dx & Intervention

Nursing Diagnosis	Nursing Intervention/Rationale
Pain related to pressure on the nerve and surgical trauma	• Assess degree, site, type, and amount of pain; medicate as necessary. Turn or adjust position *to relieve fatigue and discomfort.* • Get patient up to change position and ease pain. Instruct on proper techniques to turn, sit up, and walk *to maintain safe care.* • Increase up time as able *to increase activity.* • Perform laminectomy checks. Report any decreases in motor or sensory functions.
Impaired physical mobility related to surgery	• Assess ROM of unaffected tissues. • Encourage physical therapy as ordered and prescribed *to increase muscle strength.* • Note and assess muscle spasms or limitation of movements when moving and doing wound care or hygienic care *to note current conditions or continuation of pain or soreness.*
Potential impaired skin integrity related to infection	• Assess incisional area for relief of inflammation and evidence of wound healing (approximation of wound edges, no drainage and, later, removal of sutures or staples). • Assess vital signs for fluctuations *that could indicate inflammation or infection.* • Encourage fluid and food intake of regular diet *to aid wound healing.*

Patient Education

1. Reiterate need to do exercises to regain muscle strength following surgery.
2. Clarify and stress normal motor and sensory functions as evidence of regaining full functions with relief of inflammation.
3. Explain lingering numbness as sign of former nerve pressure that may or may not completely abate.
4. Clarify physician's home care limitations in lifting and driving for 3 to 6 weeks or longer (individualized based on specific condition). Stress follow-up visit to physician to determine recovery.
5. Explain signs of fever, continued pain, and wound drainage as reportable to physician.

Evaluation

Patient Outcome	Data Indicating That Outcome is Reached
Neck or back pain is relieved.	Patient has little residual motor or sensory impairment and little or no pain, locally or systemically.
Patient has satisfactory ROM without muscle spasms or weakness.	Patient can move about comfortably and easily, can do prescribed exercises well, and returns to family, social, and employment activities.

Meniscectomy

Description and Rationale

Traditional meniscectomy for removal of larger portions of damaged or degenerated cartilage from the knee joint is still required at times, although the incidence of this more extensive procedure will surely lessen as arthroscopic techniques and skilled practitioners become more available. The techniques and equipment have been in use in the United States only since 1974, but the knowledge and understanding gained in the past 15 years are revolutionizing the thinking and surgical treatment of meniscal lesions. Open meniscectomy is still required for many patients, however, and some nursing care differs from that of closed arthroscopy (Figure 4-34).

Contraindications and Cautions

1. Small pieces of torn or loose cartilage may be missed if hidden under other joint tissues.
2. Hemorrhage must be prevented to lessen posttraumatic arthritis.

Figure 4-34 Meniscus of knee joint.

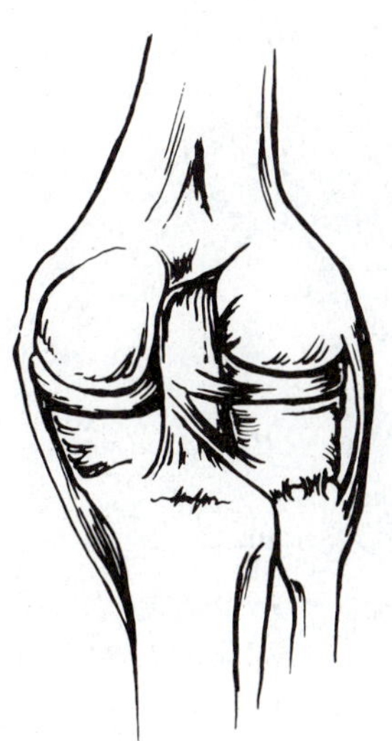

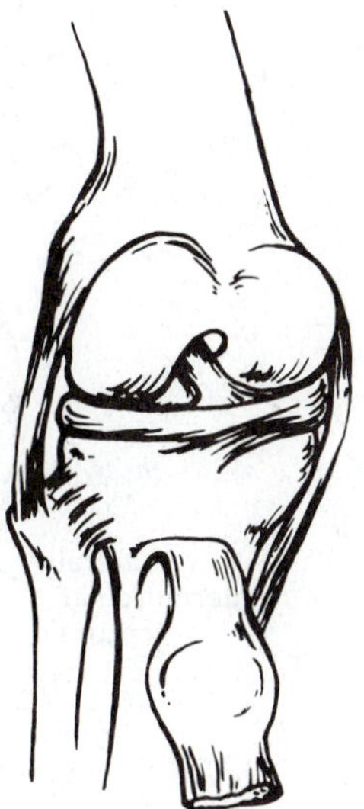

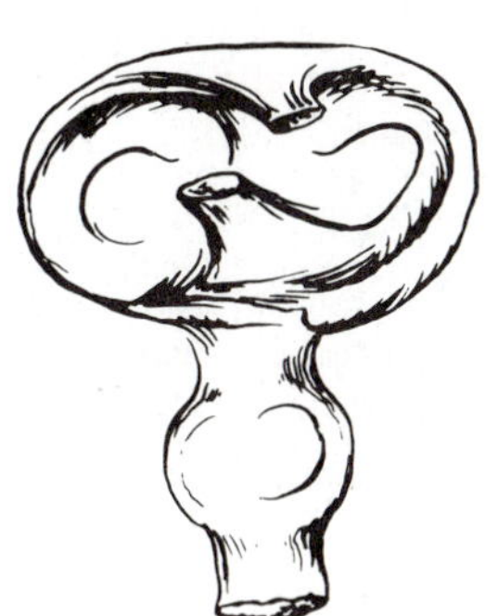

3. Scar formation may predispose to future tears of ligament or cartilage.
4. Postoperative physical therapy and individualized programs of exercises must be prescribed and performed to maintain or regain the joint's mobility, stability, and strength.
5. The long-term effects of loss of cartilage are not yet fully understood.

Medical Plan

Medications

Narcotic analgesic agents
- Meperidine (Demerol), 75-100 mg IM q3h for severe pain

Antianxiety agents
- Hydroxyzine (Vistaril), 25-50 mg IM q3h with meperidine for narcotic potentiation

Analgesic-antipyretic agents
- Aspirin, 600-1000 mg po q4h prn

Anti-infective agents
- Cefazolin sodium (Ancef) or cephalothin sodium (Keflin) (or other cephalosporin), 500-1000 mg q6-8h for 48-72 h, or longer as individually required
- Cephalexin (Keflex), 250-500 mg q6h po, after IV antibiotic is discontinued

General Management

Crutch walking with partial weight bearing; varies with specific procedure but may begin as early as 24 to 48 hours postoperatively

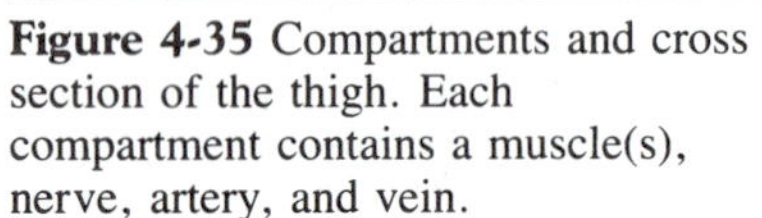

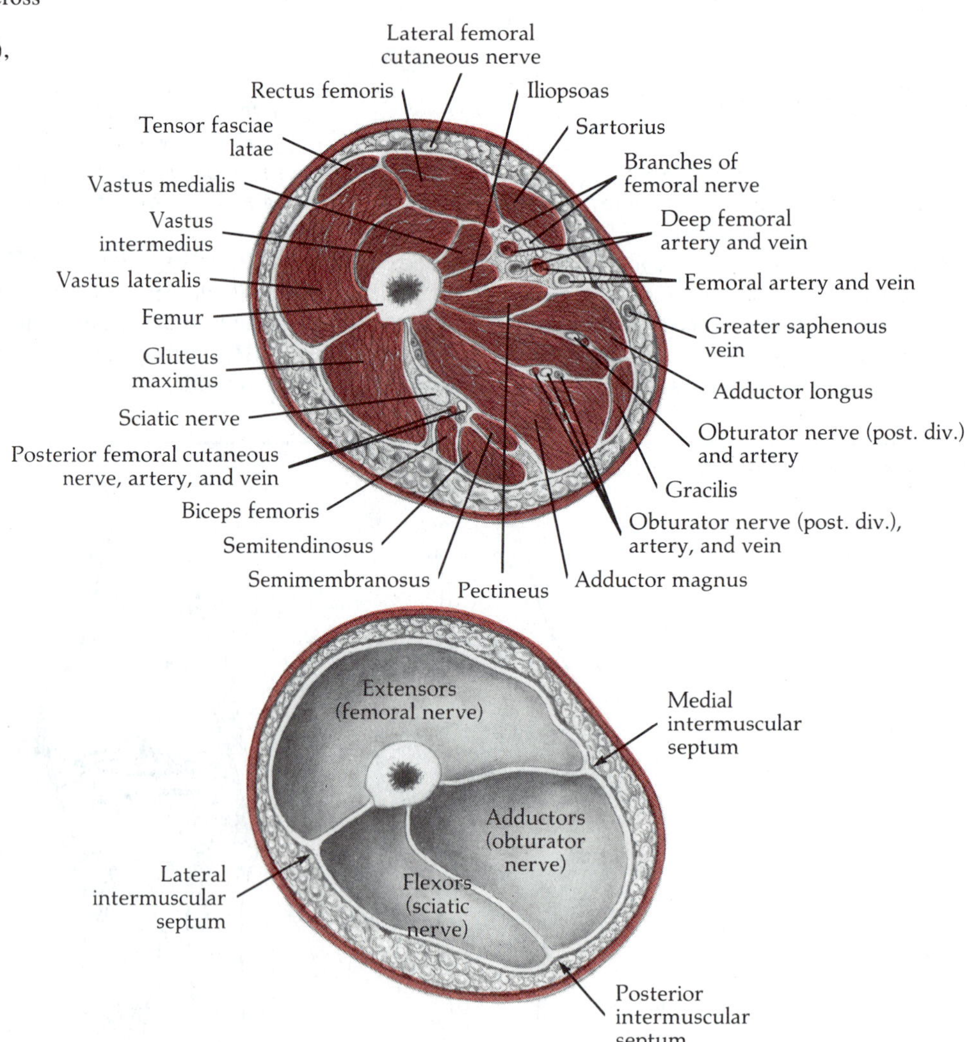

Figure 4-35 Compartments and cross section of the thigh. Each compartment contains a muscle(s), nerve, artery, and vein.

Knee immobilizer splint applied between exercise periods
Maintain postoperative dressing and immobilization as ordered (varies with specific procedure; for meniscectomy, 24 hours and then up with crutches four times daily)
Check peripheral pulses every 2 hours with neurovascular checks
Elevate leg and foot of bed
Apply ice bags to incisional area
On second or third postoperative day, begin straight leg–raising (SLR) exercises
Begin active and passive ROM knee exercises in physical therapy on third to fifth postoperative day (varies with procedure and patient need, but specific program will be prescribed)

NURSING CARE

Nursing Assessment

Knee Joint and Incisional Area

Presence, amount, and type of drainage (usually is scant, serosanguineous)
Skin color (paler than unoperative knee)
Edema and pain (increasing edema and pain are untoward signs of excessive bleeding)
Ability or inability to move leg with knee extended

Psychosocial Concerns

Alteration in or concerns with body image and ability to return to usual activities and sports (if an athlete)
Limitation of mobility over time

Other Complications

Development of hematoma or thrombus in or distal to knee or calf
Instability of knee joint
Recurrence of pain with or without degeneration or reinjury of tissues of knee joint
Compartment syndrome also possible (ischemia of muscles leading to necrosis of tissues)

Nursing Dx & Intervention

Nursing Diagnosis	Nursing Intervention/Rationale
Altered peripheral tissue perfusion related to surgery and use of tourniquet	• Assess color and temperature of operative limb. • Perform neurovascular checks every 2 hours, including check of color, edema, temperature, pain, sensory or motor changes, ability to use or lift leg, peripheral pulses, extension of inflammation to contiguous tissues above or below knee, and comparison of operative leg characteristics with unoperative leg *to note current status*. • Report changes in findings; may require removal of constricting dressings or additional surgery if pulses are absent *to aid perfusion and relieve pressure*. • Elevate leg and foot of bed *to increase venous return*. • Apply ice bags to site *to decrease edema*. • Continue checks every 4 to 6 hours *to note changes early*.
Impaired physical mobility related to surgery	• Assess ROM of unaffected joints. • Maintain bed rest as ordered *to aid recovery*. • Begin SLR exercises as ordered *to regain strength*. • Encourage performing quadriceps setting exercises every 2 hours *to maintain strength*. • Encourage setting of gluteus muscles every 2 hours when ordered *to maintain functions*. • Help patient up in a chair without weight bearing initially. Then progress as ordered to help patient walk with crutches as needed. Monitor patient's response *to note progress*. • Emphasize necessity to continue exercise program at home *to aid recovery*. • Teach patient how to put on knee immobilizer, splint, or brace if required *to aid independence and self-care*. • Assist with ADLs as required *to increase independence*. • Encourage weight lifting of operative leg as ordered *to regain full function*.
Altered patterns of urinary elimination related to bed rest	• Assess intake and output every shift. • Help patient stand to void. Check adequacy of voiding three times *to note progress or problems*. • Monitor intake and output *to determine if normal*.

Nursing Diagnosis	Nursing Intervention/Rationale
Impaired skin integrity related to surgical incision	• Assess condition of wound or incision. • Change dressings of wound as needed *to aid healing*. • Observe drainage characteristics and amount; report findings to physician if drainage cloudy or odorous—may be sign of infection.
Pain related to surgical procedure	• Assess presence of, amount, type, and severity of pain. • Administer narcotics per order every 3 hours with potentiator. Increase time between administration of narcotics or analgesics as acute pain abates *to lessen need*. • Administer aspirin between narcotics (enhances pain relief and relief of inflammation). Encourage use of aspirin as anti-inflammatory drug if ordered (patients are usually discharged with either aspirin or acetaminophen "prescription" to buy over the counter) *to substitute for narcotics*. • Encourage position changes *to lessen pressure and fatigue*. • Report continuing severe pain, change in peripheral pulses, or increasing edema as signs *indicative of ischemia, thrombus formation, or developing compartment syndrome** (Figure 4-35).

*A compartment contains one or more muscles, along with at least one artery, vein, and nerve held enclosed in a covering of inflexible fascia. The interstitial pressure rises with edema and bleeding into injured muscles. The pressure rises because the fascia does not allow the muscle to swell with the edema and bleeding. Unless the fascia is opened, the muscle will die in 6 to 12 hours from ischemia as the elevated venous and interstitial pressure or slow arterial inflow of blood delay removal of wastes.

Patient Education

1. Clarify recovery program and exercise and leg-raising activities to aid recovery.
2. Clarify rationale for each part of neurovascular check to gather thorough information about tissues.
3. Reiterate the need for continuing the exercise and walking programs prescribed for long-term recovery.
4. Encourage return to social contacts to regain mobility and comfort even though using crutches and having only partial weight bearing.
5. Stress need to refrain from sports activities that could retraumatize unhealed tissues until physician permits resumption.

Evaluation

Patient Outcome	Data Indicating That Outcome is Reached
ROM of knee joint is regained.	Patient has 90-degree flexion and full extension of knee without pain.
Patient engages in usual ADL as desired.	Patient returns to sports activities or usual ADLs with protective knee covering, if required. Patient does not experience posttraumatic arthritis.

References

1. Adams JC: Outline of orthopaedics, ed 10, New York, 1986, Churchill Livingstone.
2. Allen MJ et al: Intracompartmental pressure monitoring of leg injuries: an aid to management, J Bone Joint Surg 67[B]:53, 1985.
3. Andriacchi TP et al: Knee biomechanics and total knee replacement, J Arthrop 1:211, 1986.
4. Ball GV and Koopman WJ: Clinical rheumatology, Philadelphia, 1986, WB Saunders Co.
5. Bassett AL: Pulsed electromagnetic fields, a noninvasive therapeutic modality for fracture nonunion, Orthop Rev 15:781, 1986.
6. Bennett JB et al: Management of lateral epicondylitis, Contemp Orthop 13:53, 1986.
7. Bergfeld JA et al: Symposium: management of acute ankle sprains, Contemp Orthop 13:83, 1986.
8. Berquist TH: Imaging of orthopedic trauma and surgery, Philadelphia, 1986, WB Saunders Co.
9. Blankstein A et al: Hand problems due to prolonged use of crutches and wheelchairs, Orthop Rev 14:735, 1985.
10. Booth RE: Uncemented hips pose unanswered questions, Orthop Today 4:1, 1984.
11. Brashear RH Jr and Raney RB Sr: Shands' handbook of orthopaedic surgery, ed 10, St Louis, 1986, The CV Mosby Co.
12. Brumfield RH: Carpal tunnel syndrome in rheumatoid arthritis, Orthop Rev 12:69, 1983.
13. Callahan J: Compartment syndrome, Orthop Nurs 4:11, 1985.
14. Carpenter S and Karpoti G: Pathology of skeletal muscle, New York, 1984, Churchill Livingstone.
15. Chipman E, editor: Emergency department orthopedics, Rockville, Md, 1982, Aspen Systems Corp.
16. Colin A: Diagnosis and management of rheumatoid arthritis, Menlo Park, Calif, 1983, Addison-Wesley Publishing Co.
17. Cornell CN et al: A clinical and radiographic analysis of loosening of total knee arthroplasty components using a bilateral model, J Arthrop 1:157, 1986.
18. Crenshaw JH, editor: Campbell's operative orthopaedics, ed 7, vols 1 and 2, St Louis, 1987, The CV Mosby Co.

19. Cuomo F and Nicholas JA: Overview of strains and sprains. 1. Upper extremity, Pain Analgesia 1:3, 1985.
20. Doheny MR: Porous-coated femoral prosthesis: concepts and care considerations, Orthop Nurs 4:43, 1985.
21. Eisenberg RL: Diagnostic imaging in surgery, New York, 1987, McGraw-Hill, Inc.
22. Emery SE and Gifford JF: 100 years of tennis elbow, Contemp Orthop 12:53, 1986.
23. Engh CA et al: Porous-coated hip replacement, J Bone Joint Surg 69[B]:45, 1987.
24. Evarts CM: Surgery of the musculoskeletal system, vols 3 and 4, New York, 1983, Churchill Livingstone.
25. Fraser RD: Exacerbation of back pain after chemonucleolysis, Alternatives Spinal Surgery 3:5, 1986.
26. Gay S and Miller EJ: Collagen in the physiology and pathology of connective tissue, New York, 1978, Gustav Fischer Verlag.
27. Gillespie WJ et al: Subacute pyogenic osteomyelitis, Orthopedics 9:1565, 1986.
28. Gleit CJ and Graham BA: The role of calcium and estrogen in osteoporosis, Orthop Nurs 4:13, 1985.
29. Goldstein TB: Chemonucleolysis: still controversial but worthwhile for skeletal patients, J Musculoskel Med 3:21, 1986.
30. Graham RA: Carpal tunnel syndrome: statistical analysis of 214 cases, Orthopedics 6:1283, 1983.
31. Hadlen NM: Medical management of the regional musculoskeletal diseases, Orlando, Fla, 1984, Grune & Stratton.
32. Harper A: Initial assessment and management of femoral neck fractures in the elderly, Orthop Nurs 4:55, 1985.
33. Harper MC: Open and closed intramedullary nailing of the femur, Contemp Orthop 13:31, 1986.
34. Harris WH: No room for complacency in cemented total hip arthroplasty, Orthop Today 4:18, 1984.
35. Harris WH, editor: Advanced concepts in total hip replacement, Thorofare, NJ, 1985, Charles B Slack, Inc.
36. Harter MM: Arthroscopic surgery: anatomical factors in meniscal injuries, Contemp Orthop 9:13, 1984.
37. Hendee WR and Davis KA: Magnetic resonance imaging. II. musculoskeletal applications, Contemp Orthop 11:45, 1985.
38. Henning JH et al: Preparation for the Luque procedure: patient education booklet, Orthop Nurs 3:50, 1984.
39. Hughes J: Techniques of bone imaging. In Silberstein EB, editor: Bone scintigraphy, Mount Kisco, NY, 1984, Futura.
40. Inglis AE: Total joint replacement of the upper extremity, St Louis, 1982, The CV Mosby Co.
41. Johnson L: Arthroscopic surgery, ed 3, vols 1 and 2, St Louis, 1986, The CV Mosby Co.
42. Kalisman M and Millendorf JB: Managing osteomyelitic wounds of the lower extremity, Infect Surg 2:321, 1983.
43. Khan MA and Khan NK: Diagnostic value of HLA-B27 testing in ankylosing spondylitis and Reiter's syndrome, Ann Intern Med 96:70, 1982.
44. Kim MJ et al: Pocket guide to nursing diagnoses, ed 2, St Louis, 1986, The CV Mosby Co.
45. Lane JM and Vigorita VJ: Current concepts review: osteoporosis, J Bone Joint Surg 65[A]:274, 1983.
46. LeNoir JL: Subacromial-subdeltoid bursitis of the shoulder, Orthop Rev 15:730, 1986.
47. Liddle D: An in-depth look at osteoporosis, Orthop Rev 14:23, 1985.
48. Livingston RD Jr: Meniscal vasculature and repair, Contemp Orthop 8:39, 1984.
49. McCaffery M: Nursing management of the patient with pain, Philadelphia, 1983, JB Lippincott Co.
50. McCulloch JA: Alternatives in spinal surgery, New York, 1984, The Williams & Wilkins Co.
51. McGovern JJ and Tiller DJ: Shock: a clinicopathological correlation, New York, 1980, Masson.
52. Marshall JL et al: Anterior cruciate ligament, the diagnosis and treatment of its injuries, Orthop Rev 12:35, 1983.
53. Mears DC and Rubash HE: Pelvic and acetabular fractures, Thorofare, NJ, 1986, Charles B Slack, Inc.
54. Mears DC: External skeletal fixation, Baltimore, 1983, The Williams & Wilkins Co.
55. Meinhart NT and McCaffery M: Pain: a nursing approach to assessment and analysis, Norwalk, Conn, 1983, Appleton-Century-Crofts.
56. Modic MT et al: Nuclear magnetic resonance imaging of the spine, Radiology 148:752, 1983.
57. Moon K et al: Musculoskeletal application of nuclear magnetic resonance, Radiology 147:161, 1983.
58. Moskowitz RW et al: Osteoarthritis diagnosis and management, Philadelphia, 1984, WB Saunders Co.
59. Munson M: Operative treatment for subtrochanteric fractures, Orthopedics 6:874, 1983.
60. Nordby EJ: Managing low back pain: when to use chymopapain, J Musculoskel Med 1:27, 1984.
61. Pigg JS, Driscoll PW, and Caniff R: Rheumatology nursing: a problem-oriented approach, New York, 1986, John Wiley & Sons.
62. Potter RA and Perry AG: Fundamentals of nursing, St Louis, 1985, The CV Mosby Co.
63. Pradka L: Use of the wick catheter for diagnosing and monitoring compartment syndrome, Orthop Nurs 4:17, 1985.
64. Ramsey RG: MRI shows spinal defects without artifacts, Diagnostic Imaging 8:74, 1986.
65. Ranawat CS: Total-condylar knee arthroplasty, New York, 1985, Springer-Verlag.
66. Rand J: The role of arthroscopy in the management of knee injuries in the athlete, Mayo Clin Proc 59:77, 1984.
67. Reicher M et al: Meniscal injuries: detection using MR imaging, Radiology 159:753, 1986.
68. Renshaw TS: Pediatric orthopedics, Philadelphia, 1986, WB Saunders Co.
69. Richardson JD et al: Preventing pelvic fracture complications, Complications Orthopedics 1:113, 1986.
70. Riggs GK and Gall EP: Rheumatic diseases rehabilitation and management, London, 1984, Butterworth Publishers, Inc.
71. Rockwood CA Jr and Green DP: Fractures in adults, ed 2, vols 1 and 2, Philadelphia, 1984, JB Lippincott Co.
72. Sakellarides HT: The management of carpal tunnel syndrome, Orthop Rev 12:77, 1983.
73. Scoles PV: Pediatric orthopedics in clinical practice, Chicago, 1982, Year Book Medical Publishers, Inc.
74. Seidel HM et al: Mosby's guide to physical examination, St Louis, 1987, The CV Mosby Co.
75. Seligson D and Pope M: Concepts in external fixation, New York, 1982, Grune & Stratton.
76. Silberstein EB, editor: Bone scintigraphy, Mount Kisco, NY, 1984, Futura.
77. Snyder M, editor: A guide to neurological and neurosurgical nursing, New York, 1983, John Wiley & Sons.
78. Spiegel PC: Topics in orthopaedic trauma, Baltimore, 1984, University Park Press.
79. Stewart JR and Thorne RP: Complications of metrizamide (Ampaque) myelography, Orthop Nurs 4:53, 1986.
80. Sutter JS: Rehabilitation of the knee following arthroscopic surgery, Contemp Orthop 11:27, 1985.
81. Taylor AG et al: How effective is TENS for acute pain? Am J Nurs 83:1171, 1983.
82. Turek SL: Orthopaedic principles and their application, ed 4, vols 1 and 2, Philadelphia, 1984, JB Lippincott Co.
83. Tyler E et al: Transcutaneous electrical nerve stimulation: an alternative approach to the management of postoperative pain, Anesth Analg 61:449, 1982.
84. Vander AJ, Sherman JS, and Luciano DS: Human physiology, ed 2, New York, 1975, McGraw-Hill, Inc.
85. Waldron VD: Technique of hip nailing, Orthop Rev 12:45, 1983.
86. Wong S et al: The pathogenesis of osteoarthritis of the hip: evidence for primary osteocyte death, Clin Orthop 214:305, 1987.
87. Yates JW: Current status of meniscus surgery, Phys and Sportsmed 12:51, 1984.

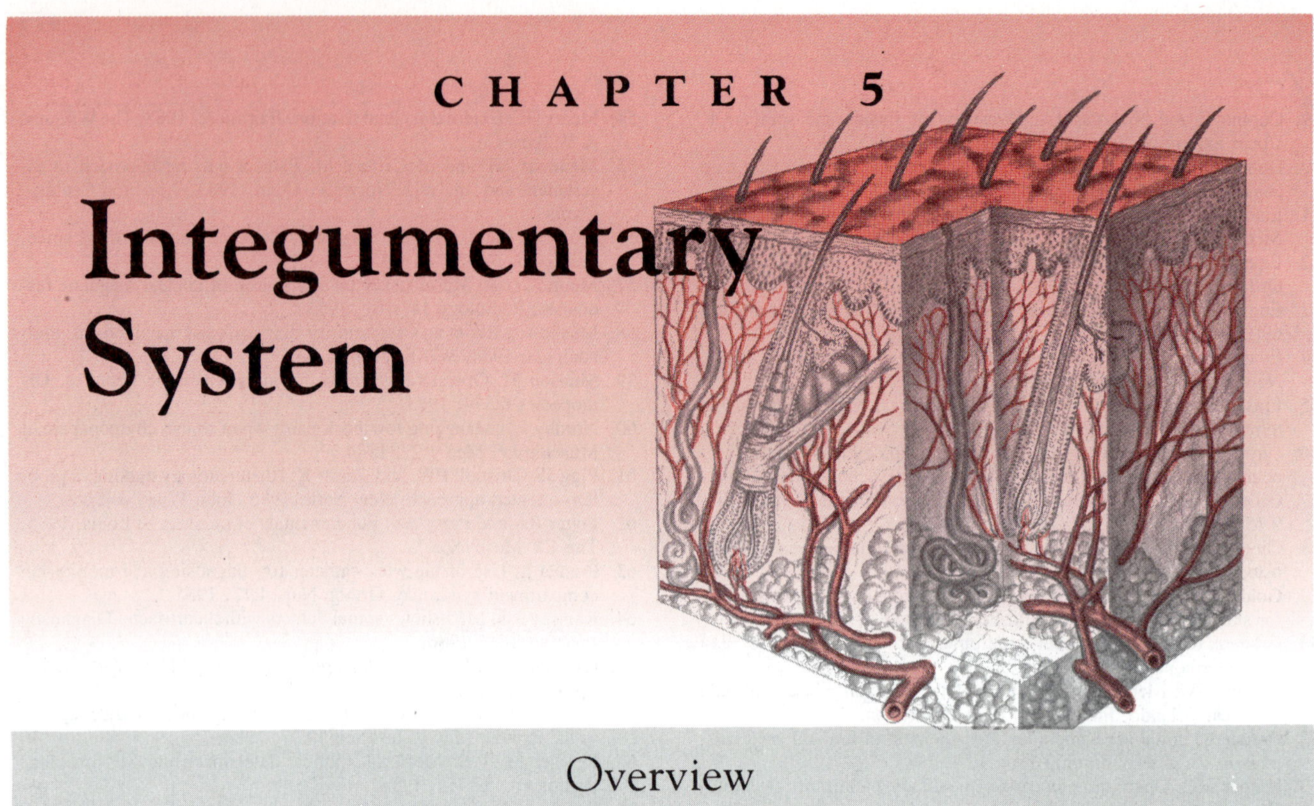

CHAPTER 5

Integumentary System

Overview

The integument, or skin, is the largest organ of the body. It is a protective barrier between the internal structures of the body and the external environment. It is tough, resilient, and virtually impermeable, but it is also affected by changes within the body. The condition of the skin can indicate a great deal about a person's health and how the environment affects that person.

According to the National Health and Nutrition Examination Survey, almost one third of the people in the United States have a skin disease requiring treatment. However, the true extent of skin disorders is difficult to determine, because many people with such disorders treat themselves rather than seek medical care. An estimated 60.6 million people between the ages of 1 and 74 years have one or more significant skin diseases. Of these approximately 3.4% have a disorder severe enough to be a handicap to employment or other activities of daily living. The economic cost of skin diseases is substantial.[55]

Anatomy, Physiology, and Related Pathophysiology

Structure

The skin comprises two principal layers: an outer layer, called the epidermis, and an underlying connective tissue layer, called the dermis. Beneath the dermis is the hypodermis (subcutaneous tissue), which technically is not part of the skin. The hypodermis is composed of loose connective tissue and fat cells that provide a layer of insulation. Specialized structures of the epidermis include glands, hair, and nails.

The anatomy of the skin varies from one part of the body to another, so the diagram of the skin in Figure 5-1 shows only the main parts and their approximate relationships. The pathologic conditions that arise in skin disorders occur in one or more of the various layers. The variation in anatomy often accounts for the distribution of skin diseases.

Epidermis. The epidermis is composed of stratified squamous epithelium. Two cell types, keratinocytes and melanocytes, make up most of the epidermal cells. The epidermis is composed of two major sublayers, the stratum corneum, which protects the body against harmful environmental substances and restricts water loss, and the cellular stratum, where keratin cells are synthesized. The basement membrane lies beneath the cellular stratum and connects the epidermis to the dermis. The epidermis has no blood and lymph channels and depends on the underlying dermis for its nutrition.

The *stratum corneum* is the outer horny layer of closely packed dead squamous cells that contain the waterproofing protein keratin and form the protective barrier of the skin. The variation in skin thickness (0.5 mm in the eyelids to 4 mm in the palms and soles) is due mostly to differences in the thickness of the stratum corneum.

The *cellular stratum* is composed of three or four layers; from the most superficial to the deepest they can be identified as follows:

Stratum lucidum. This is a thin translucent layer of protein-filled cells found only in the thicker skin of the palms and in the soles. The cells of this layer are filled with

Figure 5-1 Structures of skin.

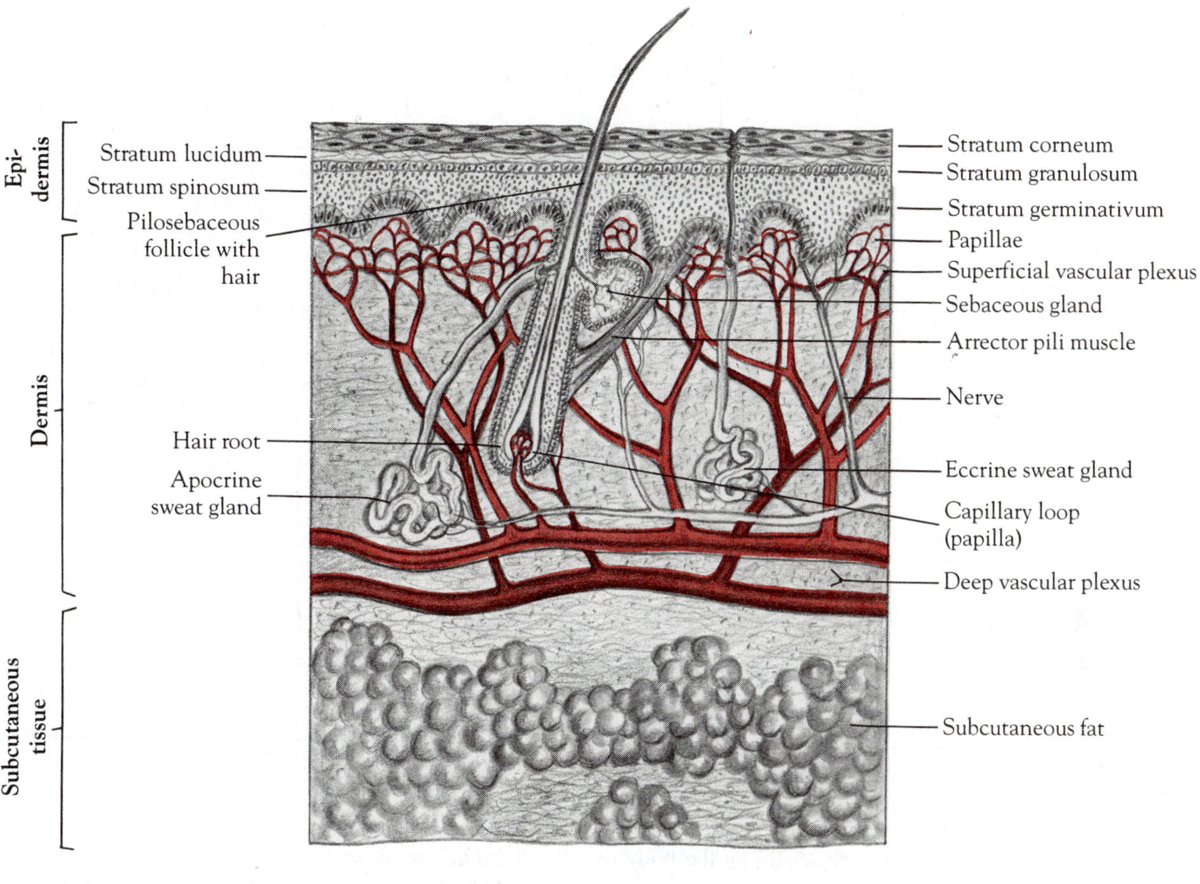

a transparent substance that appears to be a precursor of keratin.

Stratum granulosum. This granular layer is composed of cells containing granules of keratohyalin, an intermediate in keratin formation.

Stratum spinosum. This is the prickle cell layer, where cells begin to flatten and precursors of keratin appear.

Stratum germinativum. This is the basal cell layer, where mitotic activity occurs to replace the cells in the upper epidermal layer. The basal layer also contains the melanocytes, which synthesize the melanin that gives the skin its color.

The keratinocytes in the basal layer evolve into cells of the stratum corneum as they mature (keratinize) and make their way to the surface, where they are eventually desquamated. The transit time of basal layer cells to the final stage of desquamation is approximately 28 days.

Appendages. The epidermis invaginates into the dermis and forms eccrine sweat glands, apocrine sweat glands, sebaceous glands, hair, and nails.

The *eccrine sweat glands* are small, convoluted secretory coils that extend from the dermis and open directly on the surface of the skin. Only humans have eccrine glands. They are distributed throughout the body except for the lip margins, eardrums, nail beds, inner surface of the prepuce, and glans penis. The main function of the sweat glands is regulation of body temperature through water secretion. The eccrine sweat glands are innervated by sympathetic cholinergic nerve fibers, and heat is the primary stimulus for their secretion. Muscle exertion and emotional stress also stimulate secretion of water, chlorides and other electrolytes, and waste products such as lactate and urea.

The *apocrine sweat glands* are special structures found only in the axilla, nipple and areola, anogenital area, eyelids, and external ear. They do not develop fully until puberty. These glands are much larger and located deeper than the eccrine glands. The secretory duct of an apocrine sweat gland enters the hair follicle above the entrance of the sebaceous duct. The apocrine glands are adrenergic, and they secrete a white fluid containing water, salt, protein, carbohydrate, and other substances in response to emotional stimulation. Secretions from these glands are initially odorless, but bacteria on the skin decompose the organic components of sweat and cause distinctive body odors.

Figure 5-2 Structures of nail.

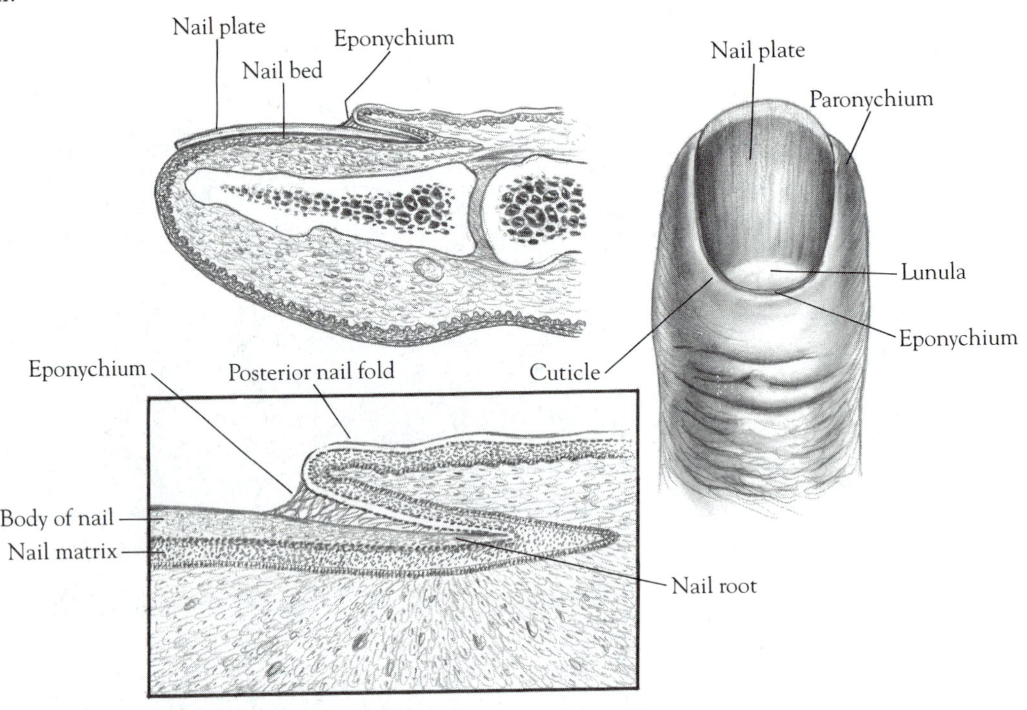

The *sebaceous glands* occur everywhere on the body except the palms and soles. They are continuous with and secrete into a pilosebaceous follicle, which may or may not contain a hair. They occasionally open directly onto the skin. Sebaceous glands secrete sebum, a lipid-rich substance that helps keep the skin and hair from drying out. These glands are stimulated by sex hormones, primarily testosterone, and their action varies according to hormonal levels throughout life.

Hair is formed by epidermal cells that invaginate into the underlying dermal layers. Hair consists of keratin that is synthesized by cells in the papilla at the base of the hair shaft. The papilla provides nourishment for mitosis, which causes the hair to grow. The hair shaft projects above the skin surface and at an acute angle with the hair root. Hair goes through cyclic changes: growth (anagen), atrophy (catagen), and rest (telogen), after which the hair is shed. Normal hair loss is not noticeable because neighboring follicles have differently timed cycles. Hair grows on most of the body except for the palms, soles, and parts of the genitalia. Men and women have about the same number of hair follicles, which are stimulated to differential growth by hormones. Melanocytes in the hair shaft give the hair its color. Hair follicle muscles, called arrectores pilorum, are immediately beneath the sebaceous glands. When innervated by adrenergic fibers, they elevate the hair to a more vertical position and indent the surrounding skin, producing "goose bumps."

The *nails* (Figure 5-2) are epidermal cells converted to hard plates of keratin. The nail root lies beneath the skin; the nail body (plate) is the visible part lying on the nail bed. The nail bed is highly vascular, giving the transparent nail body a pink color. The white crescent-shaped area extending beyond the proximal nail fold (lunula) marks the end of the matrix. This is the site of mitosis and nail growth. The stratum corneum of the skin covering the nail root is the cuticle, or eponychium, which pushes up and over the lower part of the nail body. The paronychium is the soft tissue surrounding the nail border. Nails protect the toes and fingers.

Dermis. The dermis is the connective tissue layer of the skin that supports the epidermis and separates it from the cutaneous adipose tissue. The dermis is highly vascular and provides nutrition for the epidermis. The vascular structure also controls body temperature and blood pressure. The appendages of the epidermis are located in the dermis.

The dermis is composed of two parts, the papillary layer and the reticular layer. The *papillary layer* contains blood vessels and some nerve elements that respond to stimuli applied to the skin. This layer is folded into ridges, or papillae, that extend into the upper epidermal layer. This folding produces ridges on the surface of the skin, most notably on the palms of the hands. The papillae also nourish the living epidermal cells and maintain a strong attachment between the dermis and epidermis.

The *reticular layer* contains elastin fibers for resilience, collagen fibers for strength, and reticulin fibers for stability.

This connective tissue portion also contains blood vessels, lymphatics, nerves, matrix, and various cells. Collagen forms the greatest part of the dermis.

The skin is actually the body's major sensory organ. The sensory fibers in the dermis form a complex network to provide the sensations of pain, touch, and temperature. The dermis also contains autonomic motor nerves that innervate blood vessels, glands, and the arrectores pilorum muscles.

Hypodermis (subcutaneous tissue). The dermis is connected to underlying organs by a layer of subcutaneous tissue that is composed mainly of loose connective tissue filled with fatty cells. This layer of adipose tissue provides heat, insulation, shock absorption, and a reserve of calories. Both sensory and autonomic motor nerve fibers are also located in the subcutaneous tissue.

Function

The skin provides several functions that are integral to the functioning of the entire body.

Protection. An intact stratum corneum creates a physical barrier against invasion by bacteria and foreign substances and minor physical trauma. Glandular secretions wash microorganisms from the pores, and colonies of nonpathogenic bacteria on the skin retard the growth of pathogens. Hairs in the nose, ears, anogenital areas, eyebrows, and eyelids act as barriers against the entry of foreign materials. Sebaceous gland secretions, along with the skin, prevent absorption of water during immersion. The skin reduces potential damage to deoxyribonucleic acid (DNA) from ultraviolet radiation through thickening of the stratum corneum that disperses radiation and through melanin production that forms a protective cap over the nucleus of the cell.

Retardation of body fluid loss. The skin acts as a barrier to minimize loss of internal content and to prevent the internal fluid environment from leaking out.

Excretion. The skin acts as a minor organ of excretion. Some urea and lactic acid are lost through the skin, along with sweat and sodium chloride.

Regulation of body temperature. The skin controls body temperature by four processes: *radiation* of heat energy from the body surface; *conduction* of heat from the skin to other objects or the air; *convection* or removal of heat by air currents; and *evaporation* of perspiration stimulated by the sympathetic nervous system when the body is overheated.

Blood vessels of the skin help control body temperature by dilating in warm environments to promote heat loss through radiation and by constricting in cold environments to help conserve heat. If the skin is directly exposed to temperatures below 15° C (59° F), blood vessels begin to dilate to prevent the tissues from freezing.

Blood pressure regulation. During strenuous exercise, anxiety, or hemorrhage, constriction of skin blood vessels through sympathetic stimulation reduces blood flow to the skin, promotes increased venous return, increases cardiac output, and thereby increases blood pressure.

Tissue repair. The skin maintains itself and repairs its own wounds through exaggeration of the normal process of replacement of desquamated stratum corneum and formation of scar tissue.

Vitamin D production. The skin provides an area for irradiation of vitamin D precursors. Through catalytic action, ultraviolet light converts the precursor found in the skin to vitamin D_3, which is reabsorbed into blood vessels. Vitamin D is necessary in the metabolism of calcium and phosphorus.

Sensory perception. Free nerve endings and special receptors in the skin function alone or together to detect environmental stimuli, including pain, touch, heat, cold, pressure, vibration, tickle, itch, wetness, oiliness, and stickiness.

Expression. Feelings such as anxiety, fear, and anger may be visible on the skin through sweating, pallor, or flushing. Because of its visibility, skin is also closely connected with an individual's body image.

Normal Findings*

Area of Concern	Normal Adult Findings
Skin	
Color	
Tone	Deep to light brown in blacks; whitish pink to ruddy with olive or yellow overtones in whites *Older adult:* Skin of whites tends to look paler and more opaque
Uniformity	Sun-darkened areas; areas of lighter pigmentation in dark-skinned people (palms, lips, nail beds); labile pigmented areas associated with use of hormones or pregnancy; callused areas appear yellow; crinkled skin areas darker (knees and elbows); dark-skinned (Mediterranean origin) people may have lips with bluish hue; vascular flush areas (cheeks, neck, upper chest, or genital area) may appear red, especially with excitement or anxiety; skin color masked through use of cosmetics or tanning agents *Older adult:* More freckles; uneven tanning; pigment deposits; hypopigmented patches
Moisture	Minimum perspiration or oiliness felt; dampness in skin folds; increased perspiration associated with warm environment or activity; wet palms, scalp, forehead, and axilla associated with anxiety *Older adult:* Increased dryness, especially of extremities; decreased perspiration

*Modified from Bowers.[10]

Area of Concern	Normal Adult Findings
Surface temperature	Cool to warm
Texture	Smooth, even, soft; some roughness on exposed areas (elbows and soles of feet) *Older adult:* Flaking and scaling associated with dry skin, especially on lower extremities
Thickness	Wide body variation; increased thickness in areas of pressure or rubbing (hands and feet) *Older adult:* Thinner skin, especially over dorsal surface of hands and feet, forearms, lower legs, and bony prominences
Turgor	Skin moves easily when lifted and returns to place immediately when released *Older adult:* General loss of elasticity; skin moves easily when lifted but does not return to place immediately when released; skin appears lax; increased wrinkle pattern more marked in sun-exposed areas, in fair skin, and in expressive areas of face; pendulous parts sag or droop (under chin, earlobes, breasts, and scrotum)
Hygiene	Clean, free of odor
Alterations	Striae (stretch marks) usually silver or pinkish; freckles (prominent in sun-exposed areas); some birthmarks *Older adult:* Nevi often become lighter or disappear; seborrheic keratoses (pigmented, raised, warty, slightly greasy lesions most often found on trunk or face); senile (actinic) keratoses on exposed surfaces, first seen as small reddened areas and then as raised, rough, yellow to brown lesions; senile sebaceous adenomas (yellowish flattened papules with central depressions); cherry adenomas (tiny, bright, ruby red, round; may become brown with age)
Nails	
Configuration	Nail edges smooth and rounded; nail base angle 160 degrees; nail surface flat or slightly curved *Older adult:* Toenails may be thickened and distorted
Consistency	Smooth, hard surface; uniform thickness *Older adult:* Fingernails may be more brittle or peel
Color	Variations of pink; pigment deposits in nail beds of dark-skinned individuals *Older adult:* Toenails may lose translucence and luster and become yellow
Adherence to nail bed	Nail base feels firm when palpated
Hair	
Surface characteristics	Scalp smooth; hair shiny; vellus hair short, fine, inconspicuous, and unpigmented; terminal hair coarser, thicker, more conspicuous, and usually pigmented *Older adult:* Sebaceous hyperplasia may extend into scalp
Distribution and configuration	"Normal" varies with individual; hair present on scalp, lower face, nares, ears, axillae, anterior chest around nipples, arms, legs, back, buttocks; female pubic configuration forms inverted triangle; hairline may extend up linea alba; male pubic configuration is upright triangle with hair extending up linea alba to umbilicus *Older adult:* Increased facial hair (especially in women), bristly quality; men may have coarse hair in ears, nose, and eyebrows; decreased scalp hair; symmetric balding in men (most often frontal or occipital); decreased pubic and axillary hair
Texture	Scalp hair may be fine or coarse; fine vellus hair over body; coarse terminal hair in pubic and axillary areas *Older adult:* Facial hair coarse; body hair fine
Color	Wide variation from pale to black; color may be masked or changed with rinses or dyes *Older adult:* Graying; whitening; hairs that do not lose pigment often become darker
Quantity	"Normal" varies with individuals; gradual symmetric balding of scalp hair in some men *Older adult:* General decrease of body and scalp hair

Descriptions and Characteristics of Skin Lesions

Primary Skin Lesions

Primary skin lesions occur as initial spontaneous manifestations of an underlying pathologic process.

Lesion

Macule—flat; nonpalpable; circumscribed; less than 1 cm in diameter; brown, red, purple, white, or tan in color
Examples: Freckles; flat moles; rubella; rubeola; drug eruptions

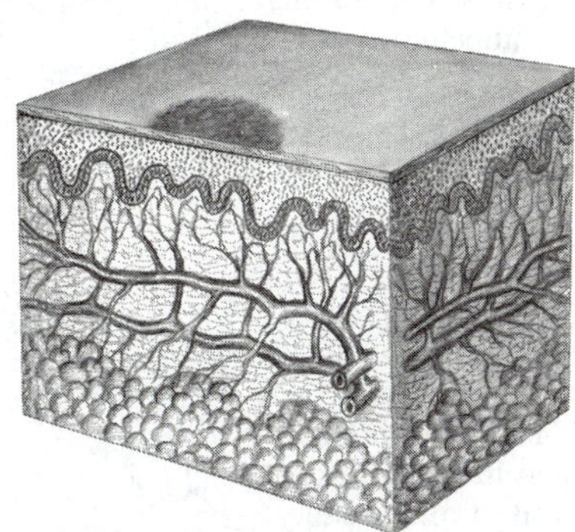

Patch—flat; nonpalpable; irregular in shape; macule greater than 1 cm in diameter
Examples: Vitiligo; port-wine marks

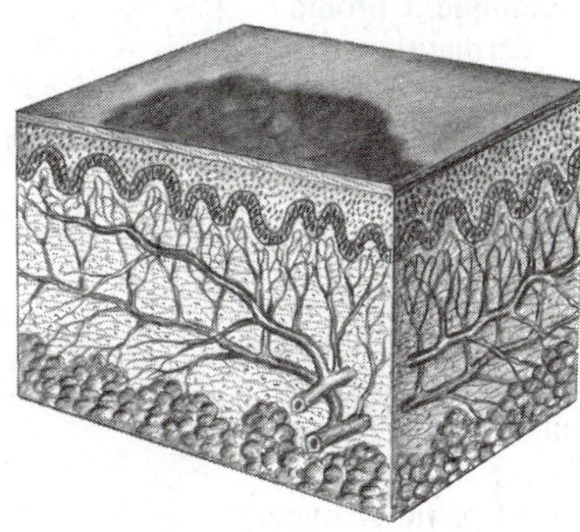

Papule—elevated; palpable; firm; circumscribed; less than 1 cm in diameter; brown, red, pink, tan, or bluish red in color
Examples: Warts; drug-related eruptions; pigmented nevi; eczema

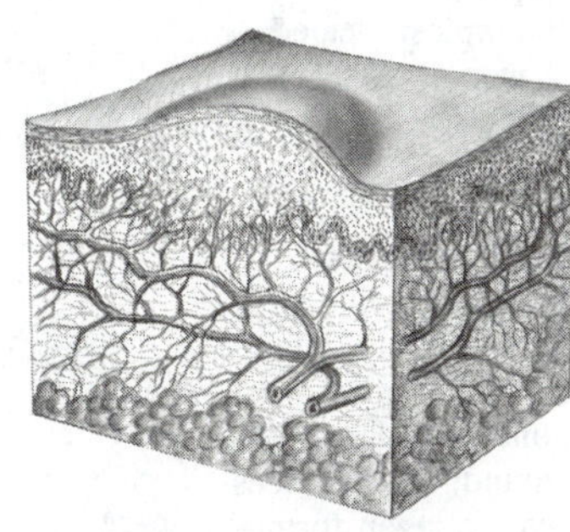

Plaque—elevated; flat topped; firm; rough; superficial papule greater than 1 cm in diameter; may be coalesced papules
Examples: Psoriasis; seborrheic and actinic keratoses; eczema

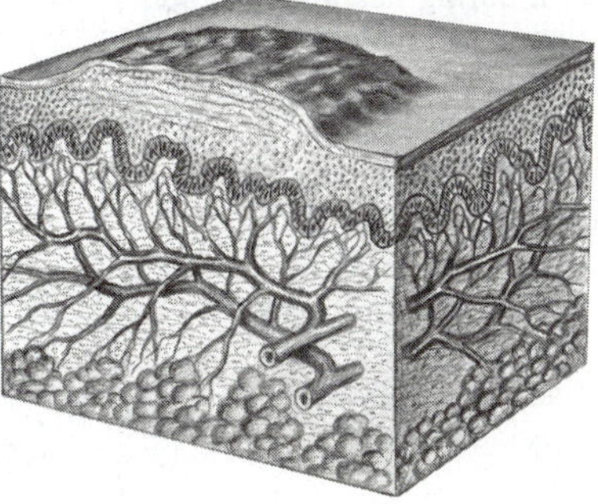

Lesion

Wheal—elevated, irregular-shaped area of cutaneous edema; solid, transient, changing; variable diameter; pale pink in color
Examples: Urticaria; insect bites

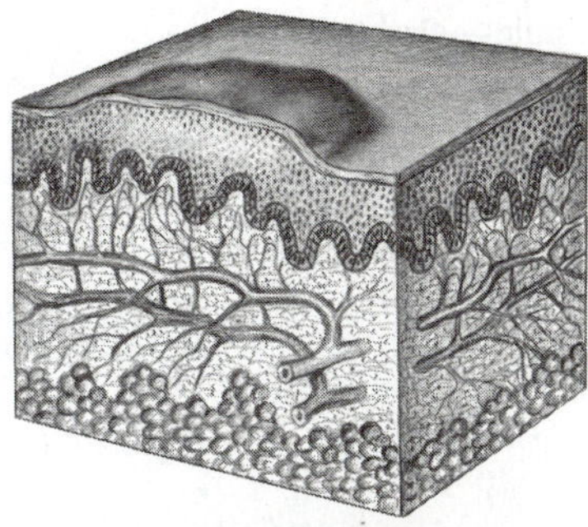

Nodule—elevated; firm; circumscribed; palpable; deeper in dermis than papule; 1 to 2 cm in diameter
Examples: Erythema nodosum; lipomas

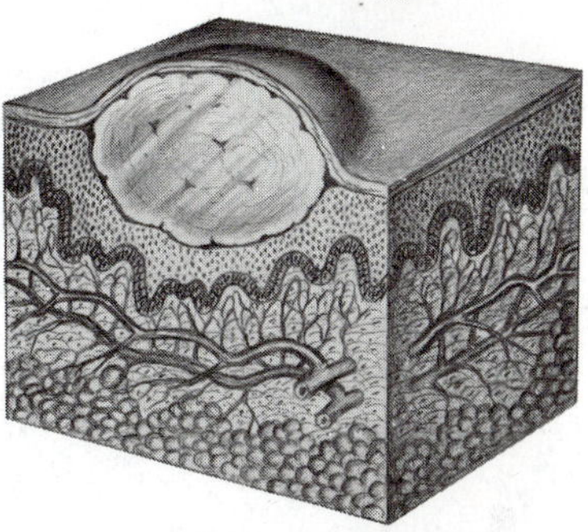

Tumor—elevated; solid; may or may not be clearly demarcated; greater than 2 cm in diameter; may or may not vary from skin color
Example: Neoplasms

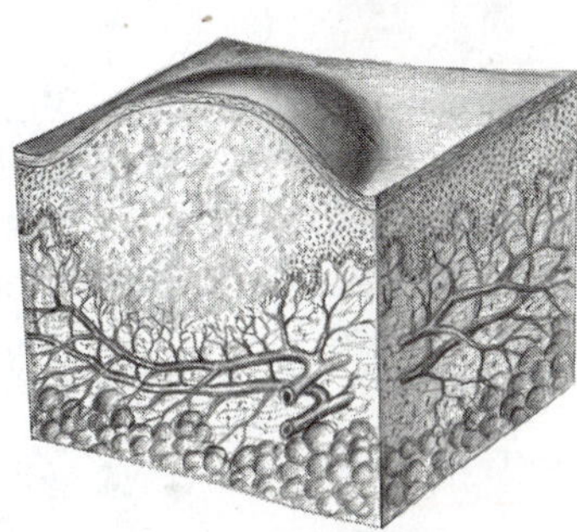

Vesicle—elevated; circumscribed; superficial; filled with serous fluid; less than 1 cm in diameter
Examples: Blister; varicella

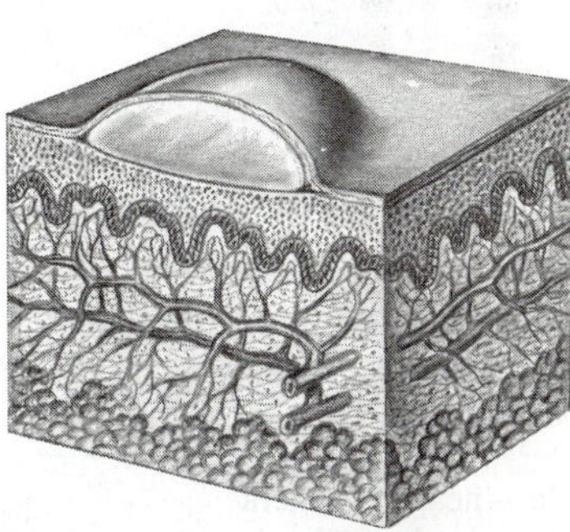

Bulla—vesicle greater than 1 cm in diameter
Examples: Blister; pemphigus vulgaris

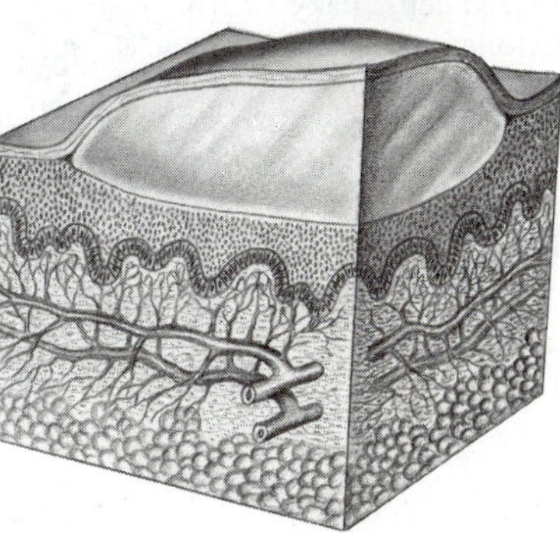

Lesion

Pustule—elevated; superficial; similar to vesicle but filled with purulent fluid
Examples: Impetigo; acne; variola; herpes zoster

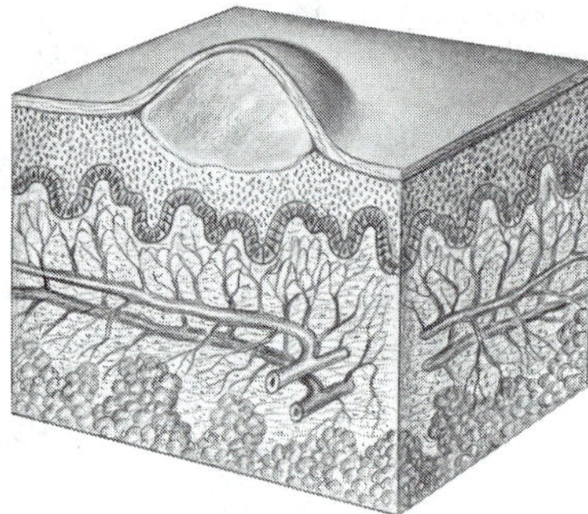

Cyst—elevated; circumscribed; palpable; encapsulated; filled with liquid or semisolid material
Example: Sebaceous cyst

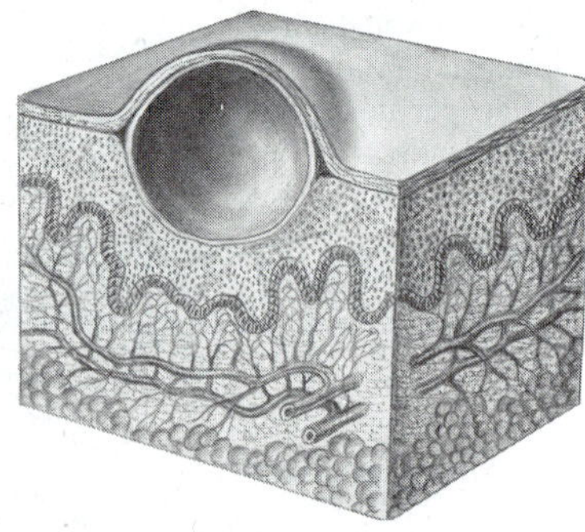

Telangiectasia—fine, irregular red line produced by dilation of capillary
Example: Telangiectasia in rosacea

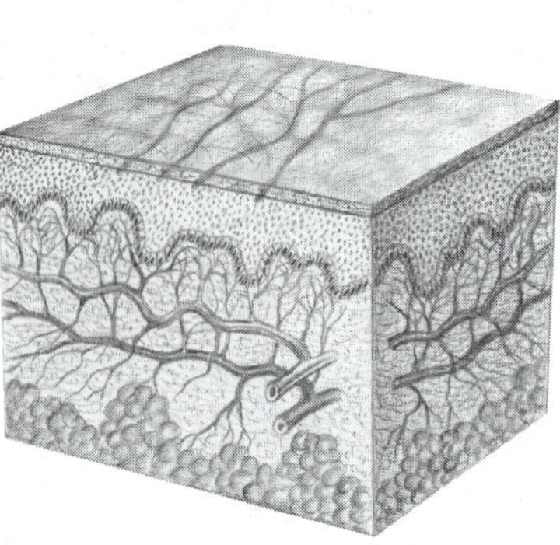

Secondary Skin Lesions

Secondary lesions are a result of later evolution of a primary lesion or are induced by external trauma to the primary lesion.

Lesion

Scale—heaped-up keratinized cells; flaky exfoliation; irregular; thick or thin; dry or oily; varied size; silver, white, or tan in color
Examples: Psoriasis; exfoliative dermatitis

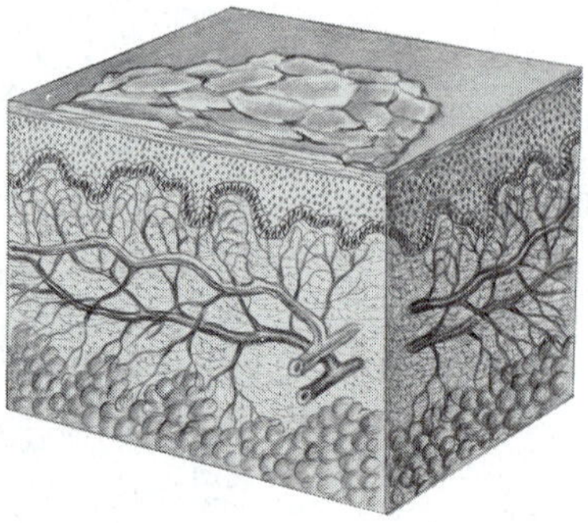

Lesion

Crust—dried serum, blood, or purulent exudate; slightly elevated; size varies; brown, red, black, tan, or straw in color
Examples: Scab on abrasion; eczema; impetigo

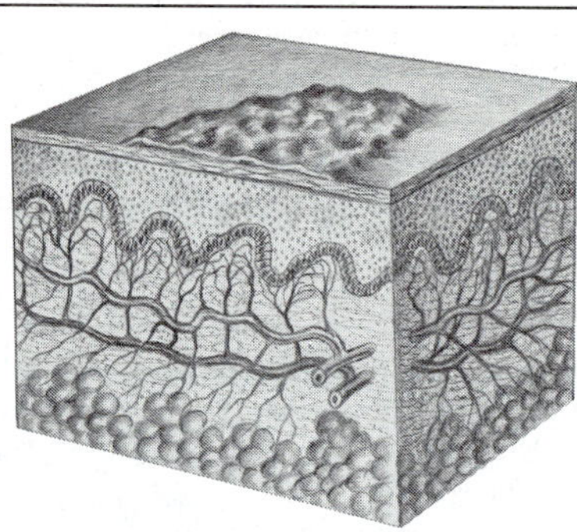

Lichenification—rough, thickened epidermis; accentuated skin markings due to rubbing or irritation; often involves flexor aspect of extremity
Example: Chronic dermatitis

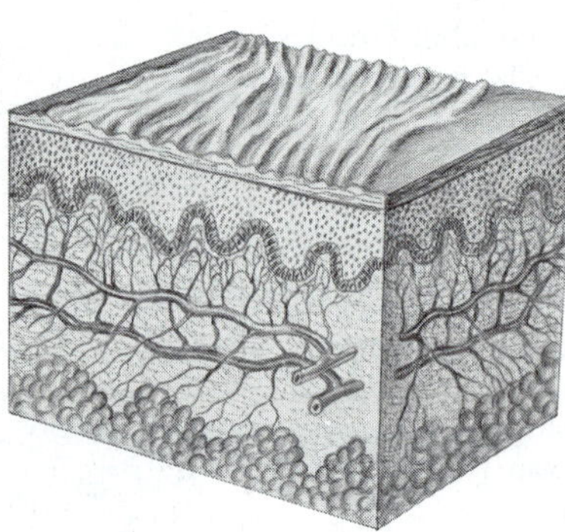

Scar—thin to thick fibrous tissue replacing injured dermis; irregular; pink, red, or white in color; may be atrophic or hypertrophic
Examples: Healed wound or surgical incision

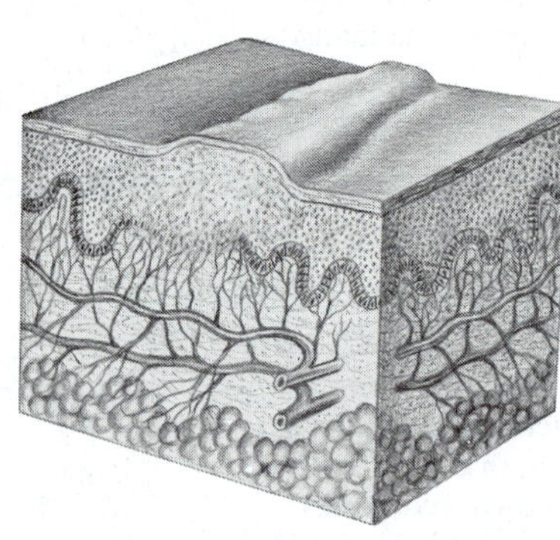

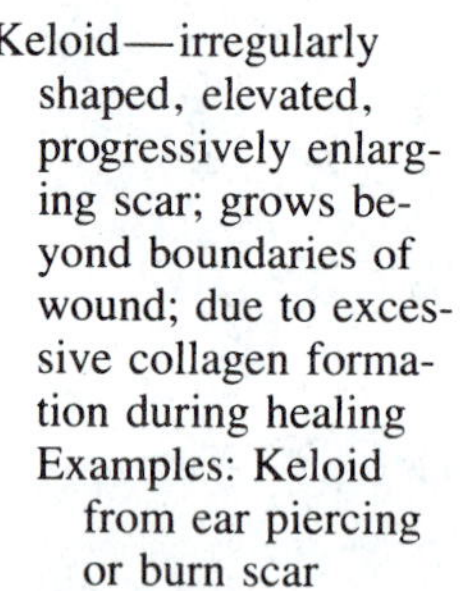

Keloid—irregularly shaped, elevated, progressively enlarging scar; grows beyond boundaries of wound; due to excessive collagen formation during healing
Examples: Keloid from ear piercing or burn scar

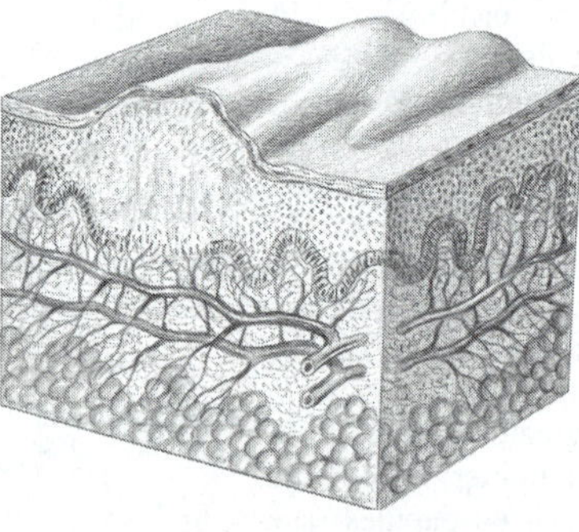

Excoriation—loss of epidermis; linear or hollowed-out crusted area; dermis exposed
Examples: Abrasion; scratch

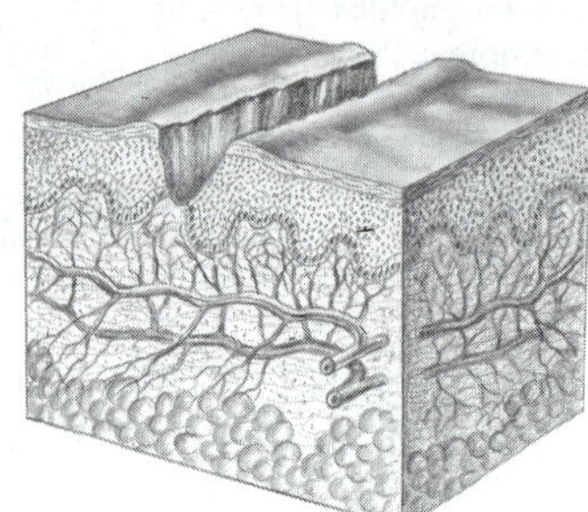

Lesion

Fissure—linear crack or break from epidermis to dermis; small; deep; red
Examples: Athlete's foot; cheilosis

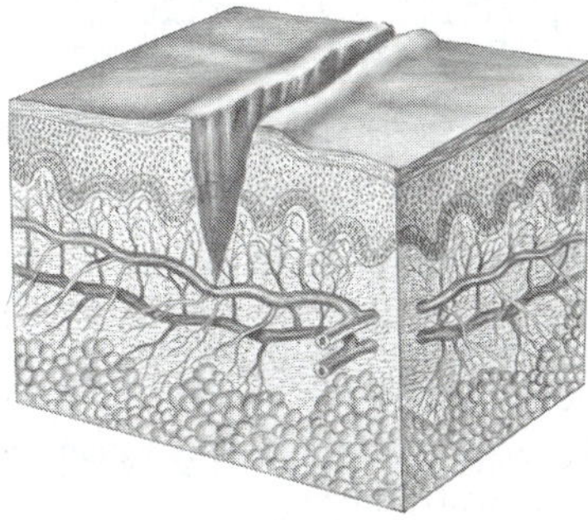

Erosion—loss of all or part of epidermis; depressed; moist; glistening; follows rupture of vesicle or bulla; larger than fissure
Examples: Varicella; variola following rupture

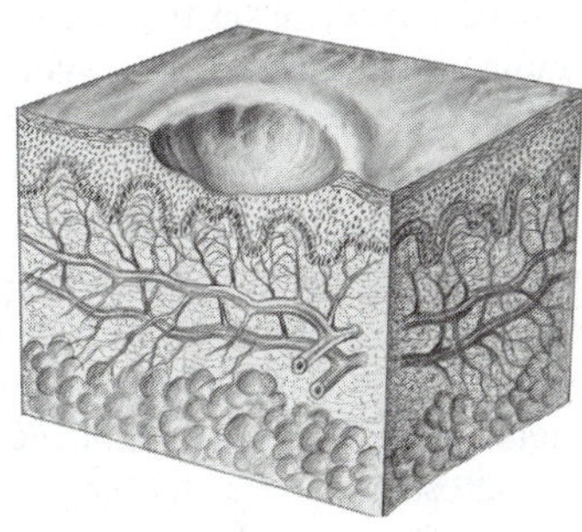

Ulcer—loss of epidermis and dermis; concave; varies in size; exudative; red or reddish blue
Examples: Decubiti; stasis ulcers

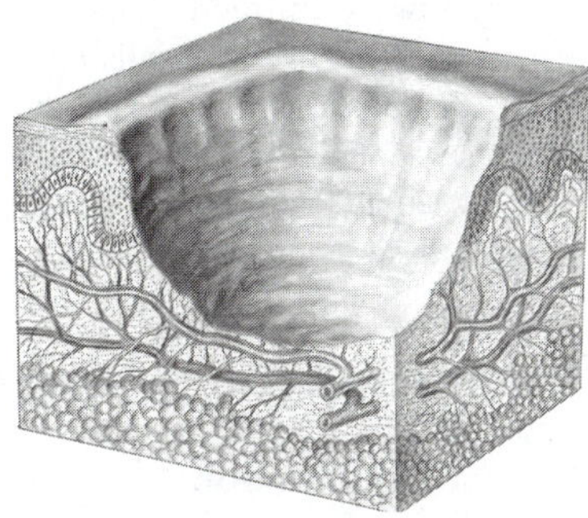

Atrophy—thinning of skin surface and loss of skin markings; skin translucent and paperlike
Examples: Striae; aged skin

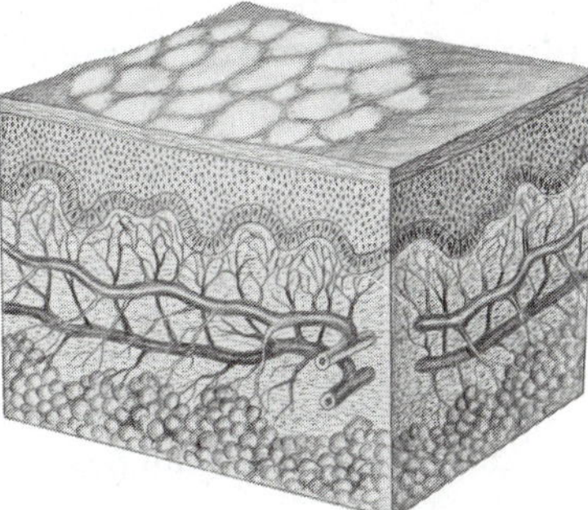

Patterns of Arrangement and Distribution

The patterns of arrangement of skin lesions often have diagnostic value. These patterns can sometimes be explained by their pathogenesis. There are three common patterns of arrangement:

Annular. The formation of rings indicates extension of the lesions from the initial location to the periphery with clearing in the center. The skin may revert to normal appearance or may be scarred. Annular configuration can also result from an allergic process in which the central area becomes refractory. Annular patterns are commonly seen in pityriasis rosea, tinea corporis, tinea cruris, urticaria, and erythema annulare.

Grouped. This pattern is the localization of numerous small primary lesions in one area. It may be from mechanical factors (as in insect bites) or from a predisposition of a particular body area to a specific lesion, as in herpes simplex.

Linear. This arrangement may be caused by external factors such as trauma or may occur in contact dermatitis. It may also be determined by developmental origins of the lesions, as in herpes zoster.

Skin disorders may appear as either generalized or localized lesions. The distribution of lesions may also provide diagnostic clues. Generalized lesions may indicate an underlying systemic disorder, as in erythema multiforme; an allergic response, as with drug reactions; or a genetic disorder, as with lamellar ichthyosis. Localized lesions occur frequently as the result of a primary irritant or allergic eczematous dermatitis. Many disorders produce lesions in specific regions of the body. For example, erythema nodosum produces nodules that are limited to the legs and thighs. Acne vulgaris produces lesions on the face, chest, back, and shoulders. Candidal infections usually manifest in intertriginous areas. Tinea cruris produces lesions in the perineal region. Pityriasis rosea may be distinguished from tinea corporis by the absence of lesions on the face and scalp. Pediculosis corporis is characterized by lesions along clothing lines, while scabies lesions are found in interdigital webs along the fingers and on the wrist and penis. In contrast, lesions from flea bites are limited to the ankles and lower legs.

In assessing skin lesions the following characteristics should be considered and described:

- Characteristics of the lesion
  - Size
  - Shape or configuration
  - Color
  - Elevation or depression
- Pattern of arrangement
  - Annular
  - Grouped
  - Linear
- Location and distribution
  - Generalized or localized
  - Region of the body
  - Discrete or confluent

Conditions, Diseases, and Disorders

BACTERIAL CONDITIONS

Furuncles and carbuncles

A furuncle is an acute localized staphylococcal infection that is initially limited to a hair follicle but spreads rapidly to the surrounding dermis and subcutaneous tissue. A carbuncle is a group of furuncles combined as one larger lesion and involving adjoining hair follicles.

Furuncles and carbuncles usually occur in areas exposed to friction, pressure, or plugging, such as sweat glands in the axilla. These skin lesions tend to develop in people who are debilitated, malnourished, fatigued, or obese. They also develop in people who have altered immune mechanisms, diabetes mellitus, severe acne, or seborrheic dermatitis. Poor personal hygiene is another predisposing factor.

Furuncles occur most frequently on the neck, breasts, face, and buttocks. The condition may be recurrent and troublesome (furunculosis) and often occurs in healthy young adults.

Carbuncles develop more slowly than single furuncles. They occur most frequently on the nape of the neck in men.

Figure 5-3 Furuncle.
Courtesy Jaime A. Tschen, M.D., Department of Dermatology, Baylor College of Medicine, Houston.

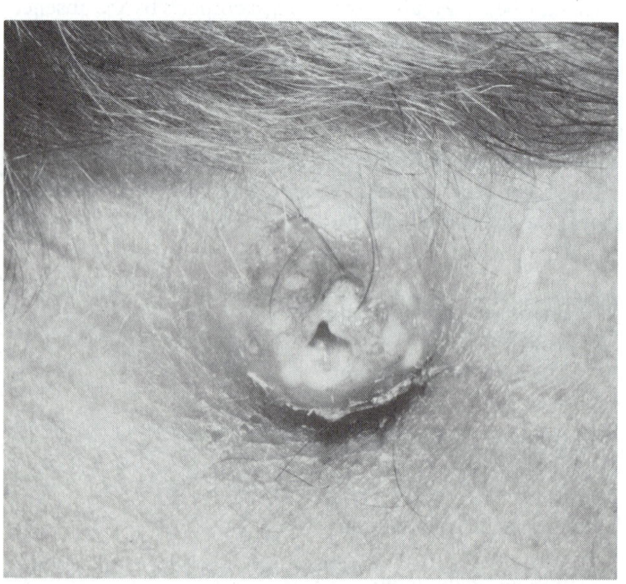

Pathophysiology

A furuncle develops as a small perifollicular abscess that ordinarily destroys the hair and follicle during its early stages. A carbuncle involves more than one pilosebaceous unit and may involve many.

The invading organism is *Staphylococcus aureus,* which is found anywhere on the body. It usually gains entry after trauma causes a break in the skin. The organism produces an acute inflammatory process around the hair follicle. The initial nodule becomes a pustule that is 5 to 20 mm in diameter at the base of the hair follicle. The surrounding skin becomes red, hot, and tender. Local edema occurs in 3 to 5 days. The center of the lesion fills with yellow pus and forms a core that may rupture spontaneously or require surgical incision (Figure 5-3). The initial drainage is purulent and progresses to a serosanguineous discharge. Healing occurs gradually, usually with residual scarring.

The infection is usually walled off by local defense mechanisms. However, if the inflammatory process spreads to the deeper structures of the dermis and subcutaneous tissue (cellulitis), the bacteria may reach the dermal vascular plexus and cause septicemia. This complication is more likely to occur in people with altered immune status and in infants, whose defense mechanisms are less efficient.

Diagnostic Studies and Findings

Physical Examination

Characteristic lesion

Culture of Lesion Discharge

Presence of infecting organism *(Staphylococcus aureus)*

Medical Plan

Surgery

Incision to promote drainage after lesion has become localized and filled with pus

Medications

- Anti-infective agents
  - Systemic antibiotics even for cutaneous lesions only
    - Penicillinase-resistant penicillin for 4-6 wk to prevent subsequent development of new lesions
    - Cloxacillin (Cloxapen, Tegopen), 250-500 mg po q8h
    - Dicloxacillin (Dycill, Dynapen, Pathocil, Veracillin), 125-250 mg po q6h

Nafcillin (Nafcil, Unipen), 250-1000 mg po q4-6h
Cephalexin (Keflex) for patients allergic to penicillin, 250-500 mg po q6h
Topical antibiotics once the lesions begin to drain, bacitracin or Neosporin applied locally tid or qid
Analgesics if lesions are extensive or pain is severe

General Management

Warm, moist compresses to promote suppuration
Nutritional therapy for underlying malnourishment, obesity, or debilitation
Appropriate therapies for underlying disease

NURSING CARE

Nursing Assessment

Inflammatory Process

Tenderness; pain; swelling; redness around infected follicle

Systemic Response to Infection

Malaise; fever; regional lymphadenopathy; increased white blood count; increased eosinophils; decreased neutrophils; increased lymphocytes; increased erythrocyte sedimentation rate

Spread of Infection

Personal hygiene; family hygiene

Psychosocial Concerns

Concern with body image

Nursing Dx & Intervention

Nursing Diagnosis	Nursing Intervention/Rationale
Impaired skin integrity	• Assess for inflammation, drainage, and signs of systemic infection. • Use meticulous handwashing *to prevent spread of infection.* • Apply hot, moist compresses *to promote suppuration.* • Change sterile dressings frequently after spontaneous drainage or surgical incision; properly dispose of contaminated articles *to prevent spread of infection.* • Teach importance of not picking or squeezing lesions *to decrease the spread of infection and the risk of scarring.* • Instruct patient in correct use of antibiotic therapies.
Potential impaired skin integrity	• When drainage begins, eliminate compresses *to prevent skin maceration and infection.* • Teach meticulous handwashing and proper hygiene practices *to prevent autoinoculation.*
Potential for infection	• Instruct patient to bathe daily with bacteriostatic soap and to avoid using oily preparations *to reduce risk of recurrence.* • Address predisposing factors such as altered nutritional status and obesity; patient should modify intake of fats and sugars.
Body image disturbance	• Assess for presence of defining characteristics. • Recognize importance of body image in growth and development. • Teach importance of not picking or squeezing lesions *to decrease the risk of scarring.* • See p. 1751 for additional strategies.
Pain	• Assess for discomfort. • Apply warm, moist compresses. • Instruct patient in use of analgesics.

Patient Education

1. Instruct the patient or family members to make sure that:
   a. The patient bathes daily with a bacteriostatic soap
   b. The patient uses towels, linens, and clothing separate from the rest of the family
   c. The patient's clothing, linen, and towels are changed and washed daily
   d. A clean washcloth is used each time lesions are cleaned or soaked; lesions should be washed gently, not scrubbed
2. Teach the patient and family how to apply warm compresses and to change dressings using aseptic technique.
3. Teach the patient and family the need to maintain the correct regimen of antibiotic therapy.

Evaluation

Patient Outcome	Data Indicating That Outcome is Reached
Therapeutic effect is achieved.	Existing lesions heal. Skin is intact and free of infection. Scarring is minimal. Pain is alleviated.
Hygiene measures to prevent spread or recurrence are instituted.	Lesions do not recur. Infection does not spread to family members.
Patient evaluates appearance in a realistic manner.	Patient engages in usual activities and relationships.

Folliculitis

Folliculitis is a superficial or deep bacterial infection and irritation of the hair follicle usually caused by *Staphylococcus aureus.*

The bacterial infection can be limited to the hair follicle, resulting in its destruction, or the process can extend deeper to involve all of the hair follicle and the surrounding dermis.

Newborns have multiple lesions of the forehead, face, and neck. In adults the lesions are found in hairy areas such as the thigh, face, scalp, groin, or axilla.

Folliculitis may become chronic where the hair follicles are deep in the skin, as in the bearded area. Stiff hairs in the bearded area may emerge from the follicle, curve, and reenter the skin, producing a chronic low-grade irritation without significant infection (pseudofolliculitis). Pseudofolliculitis occurs most often in black men.

Pathophysiology

Folliculitis is a variable condition, with lesions ranging from minute, white-topped pustules in newborns to large, yellow, tender, pus-containing lesions in adults.

The primary lesion is a small pustule 1 to 2 mm in diameter located over the pilosebaceous orifice. It is sometimes perforated by a hair. The pustule may be surrounded by inflammation or nodular lesions. A crust develops after the pustule ruptures.

Predisposing factors include superficial damage to the skin, exposure to certain chemicals, solvents, and greases, and the presence of staphylococci. Other bacteria can also cause folliculitis, especially after antibiotic therapy. Gram-negative folliculitis occurs in patients who receive long-term tetracycline or erythromycin therapy for acne.

Diagnostic Studies and Findings

Physical Examination

Characteristic lesions

Culture of Lesion

Presence of infecting organism: gram-positive *Staphylococcus aureus* or gram-negative organisms

Medical Plan

Medications

Anti-infective agents
- Systemic antibiotics
  - Erythromycin (Delta-E, E-Mycin, Ery-Tab, Eryc, others), 250 mg po q6h for 10 d
  - Penicillin V (Pen-Vee-K, V-Cillin K), 125-500 mg po q6h for 10 d
  - Penicillinase-resistant penicillins
    - Cloxacillin (Cloxapen, Tegopen), 250-500 mg po q6h
    - Dicloxacillin (Dycill, Dynapen, Pathocil, Veracillin), 125-250 mg po q6h
  - Cephalexin (Keflex), 250-500 mg po q6h
- Topical antibiotics
  - Bacitracin or Neosporin, applied locally tid or qid

NURSING CARE

Nursing Assessment

Inflammatory Process

Tenderness; pain; swelling; redness around infected follicle

Spread of Infection

Personal hygiene; presence of precipitating factors such as exposure to oils, greases, and solvents

Nursing Dx & Intervention

Nursing Diagnosis	Nursing Intervention/Rationale
Impaired skin integrity	• Assess for inflammation. • Use meticulous handwashing *to avoid spread of infection.* • Apply hot, moist compresses *to promote suppuration.* • Prevent maceration of skin *to avoid delay in healing.* • Instruct patient to use antibacterial soap. • Instruct patient in correct use of antibiotic therapies. • Assess predisposing factors.
Potential impaired skin integrity	• Teach meticulous handwashing and proper hygiene practices *to avoid autoinoculation.* • Help patient identify and eliminate precipitating factors such as skin maceration and exposure to oils, greases, and solvents *to prevent occurrence of new lesions.* • Encourage men with chronic folliculitis or pseudofolliculitis in bearded area to grow a beard *to prevent occurrence of new lesions.*
Body image disturbance	• Assess for presence of defining characteristics. • Recognize importance of body image in growth and development. • Help patient express feelings about body and body appearance *to begin process of realistic assessment.* • See p. 1751 for additional strategies.

Patient Education

1. Instruct the patient or family members to make sure that:
   a. The patient bathes daily with a bacteriostatic soap
   b. The patient uses towels, linens, and clothing separate from the rest of the family
   c. The patient's clothing, linen, and towels are changed and washed daily

Evaluation

Patient Outcome	Data Indicating That Outcome is Reached
Lesions heal.	Skin is intact and free of infection.
Hygienic measures to prevent spread or recurrence are instituted.	Lesions do not spread; no new lesions develop. Lesions do not spread to family members.
Precipitating factors are avoided.	
Patient evaluates appearance in a realistic manner.	Patient engages in usual activities and relationships.

Impetigo and ecthyma

Impetigo (impetigo contagiosa) is a superficial vesiculopustular infection. Ecthyma is an ulcerative form of impetigo.

Impetigo and ecthyma occur primarily in infants, children, and the elderly. They are highly contagious among newborns in nurseries and young children and less contagious in older people.

The arms, legs, and face are more susceptible to impetigo and ecthyma than unexposed areas, although lesions may occur anywhere. Impetigo occurs most commonly on the face. It usually appears first around the nose and mouth. Ecthyma occurs most often on the legs, the posterior aspect of the thighs, and the buttocks.

Impetigo occurs most frequently during the late summer and early fall. Biting insects, mosquitoes, and flies appear to be the most frequent transmitters. Predisposing factors include poor hygiene, anemia, and malnutrition. The infection spreads easily among family members and from one child to another in a classroom or playgroup.

Pathophysiology

Impetigo is produced by coagulase-positive staphylococci and β-hemolytic streptococci. The bacteria may be found alone or in combination. Staphylococci are usually seen in very early lesions, but streptococci predominate in chronic lesions.

The infectious process is located beneath the corneum. The initial lesion is a small erythematous macule that changes into a vesicle or bulla with a thin roof. In streptococcal impetigo the vesicle becomes pustular in a matter of hours. A characteristic thick, honey-colored crust forms when the vesicle ruptures. In staphylococcal impetigo the thin-walled bulla breaks and a thin clear crust forms from the exudate. Both forms usually produce pruritus, burning, and regional lymphadenopathy. Autoinoculation from scratching may cause satellite lesions to form. Since the process is very superficial, healing can occur spontaneously in the center of the lesion. This results in the formation of annular or circinate patterns.

A serious complication that develops in 2% to 5% of patients is acute glomerulonephritis from a nephritogenic strain of β-hemolytic streptococci. Impetigo in adults may have a more serious prognosis than impetigo occurring during childhood.

Ecthyma is a deeper infection than impetigo. It often develops in neglected superficial abrasions or from the scratching of insect bites. The inflammatory process is deeper and involves both the dermis and epidermis, so scarring results.

Ecthyma is characterized by localized thick, adherent crusted plaques with underlying ulceration and purulent exudate. The early lesions may appear as a vesicle or pustule surrounded by an area of erythema. Itching is common, and autoinoculation from scratching can transmit ecthyma to other parts of the body.

Diagnostic Studies and Findings

Physical Examination

Characteristic lesion

Gram Stain

Indentification of infecting organism (gram positive or gram negative)

Culture

Identification of infecting organism (coagulase-positive staphylococci; β-hemolytic streptococci)

Medical Plan

Medications

Anti-infective agents
- Systemic antibiotics
  - Penicillin V (Pen-Vee-K, V-Cillin K), 125-500 mg po q6-8h for 10-14 d
  - Benzathine penicillin G (Bicillin, Permapen), 1.2 million U IM as single injection
  - Erythromycin (Delta-E, E-Mycin, Ery-Tab, Eryc, others), 250-500 mg po q6h for 10-14 d
  - Cloxacillin (Cloxapen, Tegopen) if initial treatment fails, 250-500 mg po q6h
  - Cephalexin (Keflex) if initial treatment fails, 250-500 mg po q6h
- Topical antibiotics
  - Bacitracin or Neosporin applied locally tid or qid
- Antihistamines for itching

General Management

Crust removal through soap and water washing and cool, moist compresses

Nutritional therapy for underlying malnourishment or debilitation

Appropriate therapies for underlying disease

NURSING CARE

Nursing Assessment

Lesion

Vesicle, bulla, exudate, crust, or ulceration; satellite lesions; itching

Spread of Infection

Personal hygiene, particularly fingernails; family hygiene; contact with others; presence of lesions in other family members

Psychosocial Concerns

Concern that others may react to highly contagious disease; concern with body image

Nursing Dx & Intervention

Nursing Diagnosis	Nursing Intervention/Rationale
Impaired skin integrity	• Assess lesions for characteristics. • Use meticulous handwashing *to prevent spread of infection.* • Remove crusts: clean lesion with bactericidal soap and water; apply compresses of Burow's solution and cool water *to soften crust;* gently scrub crust; dispose of contaminated articles properly *to prevent spread of infection.*

Nursing Diagnosis	Nursing Intervention/Rationale
	• Apply topical antibiotics to area of lesion for 2 days after lesion disappears. • Cut patient's fingernails short *to minimize damage to lesion and to prevent autoinoculation from scratching*. • Assess for symptoms of glomerulonephritis.
Potential impaired skin integrity	• Cut patient's fingernails short *to prevent autoinoculation and new skin breaks*. • Teach patient and family meticulous handwashing *to prevent autoinoculation and spread to family members*. • Have patient and family bathe daily with bactericidal soap *to reduce recurrences and prevent spread to family members*.
Potential for infection	• Check family members for lesions *for early detection and treatment*. • Address predisposing factors such as insect control and nutrition.
Body image disturbance	• Assess for presence of defining characteristics. • Recognize importance of body image in growth and development. • Encourage patient to express feelings about body appearance and fear of reaction or rejection by others *to begin process of realistic self-evaluation*. • See p. 1751 for additional strategies.

Patient Education

1. Instruct the patient or family members to make sure that:
   a. The patient and all family members bathe daily with bacteriostatic soap
   b. The patient or any family member with lesions uses towels, linens, and clothing separate from the rest of the family
   c. The patient's clothing, linen, and towels are changed and washed daily
   d. A clean washcloth is used each time lesions are cleaned or soaked
2. Teach the patient and family how to remove the crust from the lesions: apply cool compresses of water and Burow's solution to soften the crust and then scrub the crust gently.
3. Instruct parents to check other family members, particularly other children, for lesions and have infected family members treated.
4. Teach the patient and family the need to maintain the correct regimen of antibiotic therapy even though the skin lesions have healed.

Evaluation

Patient Outcome	Data Indicating That Outcome is Reached
Lesions resolve.	Skin is intact and free of infection.
Hygienic measures are instituted.	Lesions do not spread to other areas of the body; lesions do not recur.
Measures to prevent spread of infection are instituted.	Infected family members are treated. Infection does not spread to noninfected family members.

Cellulitis and erysipelas

Cellulitis is a diffuse, acute streptococcal or staphylococcal infection of the skin and subcutaneous tissue. Erysipelas is a rarer form of streptococcal cellulitis.

Cellulitis occurs most frequently in the lower extremities, usually from bacterial invasion through a wound in the skin or an open lesion. The infection may also spread through the lymphatic system from an existing infection site, but often there is no predisposing condition or site of entry.

Erysipelas occurs on the face (bilaterally), ears, arms, and legs. Recurrences in the same area are not uncommon.

Pathophysiology

Cellulitis is most commonly caused by group A β-hemolytic *Streptococcus* or *Staphylococcus aureus*. Diffuse spread of the infection occurs because enzymes produced by the organism break down cellular components that would otherwise localize the inflammatory process. Areas of skin trauma, ulceration, or lymphedema are especially susceptible to developing cellulitis.

The area of infection is diffuse and involves all layers of the skin and subcutaneous tissue, with ill-defined borders. The skin is red, hot, indurated, and tender. Sometimes pitting is evident with pressure. Irregular lymphangitic streaks (seen as red streaks) may extend from the periphery, and regional lymphadenopathy may be present. The skin frequently has an infiltrated surface resembling the skin of an orange (peau d'orange). Breakdown of the infected area can occur with purulent discharge. Local abscesses form occasionally and require surgical incision.

Erysipelas occurs at the dermal level of the skin. It is caused specifically by group A β-hemolytic streptococci. The inflammatory process is acute with sudden onset. The area of infection is characterized by an erythematous, hot, and tender raised plaque with well-defined, sharply demarcated margins. Burning and pain, which may be severe, are common at the lesion site. Vesicles and bullae may develop and rupture, occasionally with necrosis of the involved skin. There is a great deal of exfoliation of the overlying skin as erysipelas heals.

Both cellulitis and erysipelas may be accompanied by systemic symptoms.

Diagnostic Studies and Findings

Physical Examination

Characteristic lesion

Culture of Lesion

For infecting organisms (group A β-hemolytic *Streptococcus* or *Staphylococcus aureus*); organism difficult to isolate unless drainage is present

Blood Culture

For infecting organism: only occasionally positive

Medical Plan

Surgery

Incision and drainage of localized abscesses
Debridement of devitalized structures

Medications

Anti-infective agents
- Systemic antibiotics
  - Should be continued for 1 wk after infection has cleared; may need to be prolonged for several wks for erysipelas
  - Penicillin V (Pen-Vee K, V-Cillin K), 125-500 mg po q6h for 10 d
  - Penicillin G or benzathine (Bicillin, Permapen), 1.2 million U IM in single dose
  - Erythromycin (Delta-E, E-Mycin, Ery-Tab, Eryc, others), 250-500 mg po q6h for 10-14 d
  - For severe infections requiring hospitalization: penicillin G aqueous, 400,000-1.2 million U IV q6h followed by oral therapy after 36-48 h

Analgesics
- Aspirin (ASA) or acetaminophen (Tylenol), alone or combined with codeine

General Management

Immobilization and elevation of affected limb to reduce edema
Hospitalization for patients with severe infections or systemic symptoms
Cool compresses for discomfort alternated with warm compresses or soaks to increase circulation
Appropriate therapies for underlying disease

NURSING CARE

Nursing Assessment

Inflammatory Process

Cellulitis: tenderness; pain; redness; heat; swelling; lymphangitic streaks; peau d'orange skin; purulent discharge; abscesses
Erysipelas: tenderness; pain; redness; heat; swelling; raised plaque; vesicles; bullae; purulent exudate

Systemic Response to Infection

Regional lymphadenopathy; fever; chills; tachycardia; headache; hypotension; malaise; increased white blood count; decreased neutrophils; increased eosinophils; increased lymphocytes; increased erythrocyte sedimentation rate

Nursing Dx & Intervention

Nursing Diagnosis	Nursing Intervention/Rationale
Impaired skin integrity	• Assess for inflammatory process. • Elevate and immobilize affected area for 2 to 3 days *to decrease edema and increase circulation for healing.* • Use meticulous handwashing *to prevent spread of infection.*

Nursing Diagnosis	Nursing Intervention/Rationale
	• Observe for signs of systemic infection (see "Nursing Assessment"). • Instruct patient in correct use of antibiotic therapies *to obtain maximum benefit*.
Pain	• Assess for discomfort. • Elevate and immobilize affected area *to promote lymphatic drainage*. • Apply cool wet compresses alternated with warm compresses or soaks. • Instruct patient in use of analgesics.
Impaired physical mobility	• Elevate affected area *to decrease edema and pain*. • Explain need to maintain elevation and immobility for at least 2 to 3 days. • Discuss with patient options to maximize elevation and immobility depending on patient's situation and severity of infection: bed rest, sling, crutches, or leg propped above heart level.

Patient Education

1. Explain the need to elevate and immobilize the affected area for at least 2 to 3 days or until redness and edema decrease.
2. Instruct the patient to wash an open or draining wound gently with clean washcloth and soap and water and to change dressings using aseptic technique.
3. Instruct the patient to apply a cool compress for discomfort alternating with a warm compress or warm soak to increase circulation.

Evaluation

Patient Outcome	Data Indicating That Outcome is Reached
Infection resolves.	Lesions heal. Skin is intact and free of infection.
Pain is relieved.	Symptoms of pain, burning, and discomfort are alleviated.
Mobility is regained.	Patient engages in usual activities.
Systemic infection does not occur or is quickly resolved.	Laboratory values are normal; temperature is normal.

Acne vulgaris

Acne vulgaris is an inflammatory disease of the pilosebaceous follicles characterized by comedones, pustules, papules, or nodular lesions.

Acne occurs during puberty, although lesions may occur as early as 8 years of age and continue through the twenties and thirties. The peak incidence appears to be around 14 years of age for girls and 16 years for boys. Acne occurs more frequently in boys but tends to be more severe and prolonged in girls. Almost all adolescents experience some degree of acne, and about 80% have substantial lesions that range from superficial noninflammatory comedones to cysts and scars. Only a small percentage of these people seek medical attention; most treat themselves with over-the-counter preparations that may be ineffective.

Acne lesions occur most frequently on the face, neck, upper back, and chest. The precise cause of acne is unknown. Research now centers on hormonal dysfunction and oversecretion of sebum as primary causes.[24] The course and severity of the disease seem to be genetically determined. Dietary factors have little or no influence on the development of the disease, although certain foods may aggravate the condition in some patients.[24] Predisposing factors include the use of cosmetics, steroids, oral contraceptives, and certain drugs (iodides, bromides, phenytoin, phenobarbital, trimethadione, isoniazid, ethionamide, rifampin, and lithium); exposure to heavy oils, greases, and tars; friction or occlusion from clothing such as sweatbands, shoulder straps, and football shoulder pads; emotional stress; hyperalimentation; or an unfavorable climate. Acne seems to improve during the summer and worsen in the fall and winter. This is probably because exposure to sunlight lessens the severity of acne during the summer months. However, a hot, humid climate can produce severe acne in some people.

Pathophysiology

The sebaceous gland increases in size and produces more sebum because of androgenic activity. This is accompanied by abnormal keratinization of the middle third of the hair follicle, which results in obstruction of the pilosebaceous unit. This blockage prevents the normal flow of sebum to the skin surface, causing retention of cells, lipids, fatty acids, hair, and focal masses of *Corynebacterium acnes (Propionibacterium acnes)*. Comedones then form either as open comedones (blackheads) or closed comedones (whiteheads). Open comedones have a raised opening that allows the contents to escape to the skin surface. The black appearance is due to oxidation of the keratinous material or by melanin granules. Closed comedones have a skin covering that prevents extrusion of the contents and promotes further retention of keratin and sebum. The open or closed comedones can remain free of inflammation, despite the presence of bacteria. As the contents of the structure continue to accumulate, the enlarging comedone becomes visible. This process may take weeks, months, or a year. If the wall of the upper third of the hair follicle becomes disrupted, its contents are discharged onto the epidermis and a pustule develops.

An enlarged follicle can eventually rupture and discharge its contents into the surrounding dermis. The result is the development of the inflammatory papule, nodule, or cyst. There is usually a combination of acute inflammation and foreign body reaction induced by keratin and hair in the dermis. Rupture of the follicle can occur spontaneously because of the inflammatory effects of the bacteria or can be caused by trauma such as squeezing the comedone. The deeper the lesions, the more severe the potential for and degree of scarring.

The regeneration of the ruptured follicular wall is accomplished by proliferating keratinizing epidermis, but cystic structures with surrounding fibrosis can form in the process. These can develop into deep cystic processes with interconnecting channels, gross inflammation, and abscess formation. Chronic, recurring lesions produce distinctive acne scars.

Diagnostic Studies and Findings

Physical Examination

Characteristic lesions and scarring

Medical Plan

Surgery

- Surgical removal of fibrotic cysts that have not responded to intralesional injections or liquid nitrogen therapy; excision should not be performed on actively inflamed acne cysts[24]
- Intralesional injections of corticosteroids (triamcinolone [Aristocort, Kenalog]) into cysts, 2.5-5 mg/ml of injectable steroid in saline or lidocaine, 0.1-0.3 ml in each cyst

Medications

- Vitamins
  - Oral retinoids[24,48,60]
    - Isoretinoin (Accutane), 1-2 mg/kg/d po in 2 divided doses for 15-20 wk; initial dose individualized for patient's weight and severity of disease, with dosage adjusted after 2 wk according to response of disease; second course may be initiated for persistent acne after 2 mo without therapy
  - Topical
    - Vitamin A acid (retinoic acid) (Retin-A) gel or cream, 0.01-0.1% applied nightly 30 min after washing face and 1 h before bedtime
- Anti-infective agents
  - Systemic antibiotics (for severe acne)
    - Tetracycline, 250-500 mg po qid for 4 wk then decreased to lowest maintenance dose that gives good response; ibuprofen (Motrin) 2.4 g/d will enhance the effect of 1 g of tetracycline daily[61]
    - Erythromycin (Delta-E, E-Mycin, Ery-Tab, Eryc, others), 250-500 mg po qid; same regimen as with tetracycline, if response to tetracycline is poor
  - Topical antibiotics
    - Clindamycin 1%, apply tid or qid to lesions
    - Erythromycin 2%, apply tid or qid to lesions
    - Tetracycline, apply tid or qid to lesions
- Keratolytic agents
  - Salicylic acid gel, apply nightly to affected areas
  - Benzoyl peroxide 2.5%-20%, 3-4 h/d for 4 d, then overnight if tolerated; patient establishes own level of tolerance for strength and time
- Estrogens (for women)
  - Mestranol, 0.075-0.1 mg or equivalent po in cyclic monthly routine

General Management

- Cryotherapy—liquid nitrogen applied with cotton-tipped applicator or fine spray onto cysts
- Expression of comedones by means of Schamberg or other extractor
- Ultraviolet light in increasing doses at least once a week
- Well-balanced diet to eliminate foods known to aggravate condition; foods will be specific to each individual

NURSING CARE

Nursing Assessment

Lesion

Presence of comedones (open or closed), pustules, papules, nodules, cysts, pitting scars on face, neck, shoulders, upper back, or chest; seasonal or monthly pattern and history of past inflammatory lesions; evidence of picking or squeezing lesions

Inflammatory Process

Tenderness; pain; swelling; redness around infected follicle

Psychosocial Concerns

Concern with body image and social relationships

Nursing Dx & Intervention

Nursing Diagnosis	Nursing Intervention/Rationale
Impaired skin integrity; potential for infection	• Assess for inflammatory process. • Encourage patient to seek medical attention when acne develops. • Stress importance of adhering to therapeutic regimen; assist in setting up overall schedule for managing regimen on daily basis. • Plan schedule for facial hygiene: clean skin with acne soap or mild soap once or twice a day, keep skin clean and dry, and avoid abrasive soaps. • Give written instructions for use of peeling agents such as benzoyl peroxide or retinoic acid. Alternating the creams can give better results. Never apply the two together. • Discourage squeezing, picking, and rubbing of lesions *to prevent infection*. • Teach patient how to use comedone extractor. Set up criteria for which comedones can be removed. Establish limited schedule for removal *to prevent further tissue damage*. • Apply hot packs to cystic lesions *to promote circulation and suppuration*. • Encourage frequent shampooing and hair-style that keeps hair off face. • Analyze diet and help patient identify foods that cause flare-ups. • Help patient deal with stress; help patient label feelings, identify alternative courses of action, and set reachable goals. • Identify and eliminate predisposing factors. • Dispel myths that sexual activity or abstinence causes or affects acne. • Instruct patient in correct use of antibiotic therapies.
Situational low self-esteem; body image disturbance	• Recognize importance of body image in growth and development. • Assess patient's perception of his or her appearance. • Teach importance of not picking or squeezing lesions, *to decrease risk of scarring*. • Encourage patient to express feelings about body, body appearance, or fear of reaction or rejection by others *to begin process of realistic self-evaluation*. • Encourage patient to develop interests and other attributes *to support positive self-image, feelings of self-worth, and self-confidence*. • Help patient evaluate facial scarring in realistic perspective *so it does not become focal point of existence*. • Advise patient of availability of tinted acne lotions that can mask lesions and scars. • Arrange for individual or group therapy *if patient is unable to adjust to appearance*.

Patient Education

1. Provide written instructions regarding:
   a. Side effects of systemic antibiotics and oral retinoids (isotretinoin should not be given to women of childbearing potential, since fetal abnormalities have been reported with use of this drug)
   b. Need for and schedule of follow-up laboratory work for long-term antibiotic therapy or with oral retinoids
   c. Untoward effects of topical preparations:
      (1) For increased redness and peeling, reduce time and strength of preparation until symptoms subside, then increase slowly
      (2) Photosensitizing properties of retinoic acid: use only at bedtime; do not go out into sunlight with it on
   d. Safe use of ultraviolet lamp: eyes covered, timed exposure with backup timer, and measured distance
2. Teach good hygiene practices to prevent secondary infection.
3. Teach the patient how to maintain a well-balanced diet and get adequate rest.
4. Instruct the patient to go out into the sunlight unless contraindicated.
5. Discuss with the patient and family that successful therapy requires the patient's full cooperation and patience and that therapy is long-term and results may not be immediate.
6. Instruct the patient to continue local lesion care even after the lesions have resolved.

Evaluation

Patient Outcome	Data Indicating That Outcome is Reached
Disease condition improves.	Patient has fewer comedones, pustules, papules, nodules, or cysts.
Acne lesions improve.	Lesions heal with as little scarring as possible. There is no secondary infection.

Patient Outcome	Data Indicating That Outcome is Reached
Inflammatory process recedes.	There is no pain, tenderness, swelling, or redness around affected follicle.
Side effects or untoward effects of medications are recognized and treated quickly.	Patient seeks medical attention for untoward or side effects.
Patient has realistic self-concept.	Acne disorder is not used as excuse for unsuccessful interpersonal relationships. Patient has realistic perception of his or her appearance.

Rosacea

Rosacea is a chronic inflammatory disorder involving the central area of the face, which is characterized by erythema, telangiectasia, papules, and pustules.

Rosacea tends to occur in people who blush easily and sunburn easily. It appears most often in white women in their forties and fifties. When it occurs in men, it is usually more severe and is often associated with rhinophyma. Rhinophyma is characterized by thickened red skin on the nose that can be disfiguring.

The cause of rosacea is unknown, although alcohol, coffee, spicy foods, stress, and sun exposure may precipitate or exacerbate it in some people. Physical activity, infection, endocrine abnormalities, use of tobacco, and extreme heat or cold—anything that produces flushing—can also aggravate rosacea. The use of fluorinated steroid creams can also cause rosacea.

Pathophysiology

The main pathologic processes of rosacea are instability of the superficial blood vessels, which results in persistent erythema and telangiectasia; overgrowth of normal bacteria, which results in pustules; and a granulomatous inflammation, which results in papular localization.

Rosacea develops gradually, beginning with periodic flushing across the forehead, nose, chin, and cheeks. The redness is intermittent at first but later becomes permanent. Telangiectasia develops along with pustules and papules. The inflammatory process causing the papules is granulomatous, differentiating it from the papules of acne. The pustules of rosacea appear similar to those of acne but do not have the characteristic comedones of acne. Rhinophyma is seen in advanced cases, where there is marked hyperplasia of the sebaceous glands of the nose. Rhinophyma develops on the lower half of the nose and produces red, thickened, bulbous skin with dilated follicles.

Rosacea is sometimes associated with ocular symptoms of keratitis, corneal vascularization and blepharitis, and uveitis.

Rosacea usually spreads slowly and does not subside without treatment.

Diagnostic Studies and Findings

Physical Examination

Characteristic vascular flushing and acneform lesions without comedones of acne vulgaris; rhinophyma

Medical Plan

See Chapter 6 for treatment of eye symptoms.

Surgery

Excision of excess tissue in rhinophyma

Medications

- Anti-infective agents
  - Systemic antibiotics
    - Tetracycline, 250-500 mg po qid initially for 1- to 2-wk periods to prevent pustules; decrease doses as symptoms subside
  - Topical erythromycin 2% or clindamycin 2% alternated with hydrocortisone cream
- Corticosteroids (topical preparations)
  - Sulfur 20% in hydrocortisone cream 1% applied bid
  - Hydrocortisone cream 1% applied bid

General Management

Electrolysis for large dilated blood vessels
Cryotherapy for rhinophyma

NURSING CARE

Nursing Assessment

Inflammatory Process

Erythema, telangiectasia, papules, and pustules across forehead, nose, chin, and cheeks; rhinophyma

Extension of Inflammation

Ocular symptoms of keratitis, conjunctivitis, uveitis, and vascular dilation

Precipitating Factors

Erythema in response to sunlight, hot beverages, spicy foods, vegetables, vinegar, alcohol, physical activity, and stress

Psychosocial Concerns

Concern with body image

Nursing Dx & Intervention

Nursing Diagnosis	Nursing Intervention/Rationale
Impaired skin integrity	• Assess for inflammatory process. • Instruct patient not to squeeze or pick pustules *to prevent infection.* • Instruct patient to keep skin clean and oil free but to avoid excessive dryness and irritation *to prevent aggravation of condition.* • Instruct patient to shampoo hair often *to avoid oiliness.* • Instruct patient in correct use of antibiotic and medication therapies *to maximize therapeutic benefit.*
Potential impaired skin integrity	• Help patient identify factors that cause exacerbations, and work with patient to eliminate them.
Body image disturbance; situational low self-esteem	• Assess patient's perception of his or her appearance. • Encourage patient to express feelings about body, body appearance, and fear of reaction or rejection by others *to begin process of realistic self-evaluation.* • Help patient evaluate his or her appearance in a realistic manner.
Impaired tissue integrity	• Assess for ocular symptoms of keratitis, conjunctivitis, uveitis, vascular dilation. • See Chapter 6 for nursing interventions.

Patient Education

1. Instruct the patient to eliminate factors leading to facial hyperemia: consuming hot beverages, spicy foods, or alcohol; exposure to external irritants; and extremes of environmental heat or cold.
2. Instruct the patient to avoid excessive sun exposure.
3. Teach the patient about the effects of long-term antibiotic therapy and to report untoward reactions.

Evaluation

Patient Outcome	Data Indicating That Outcome is Reached
Pustular lesions resolve.	Skin is intact with no papules or pustules.
Exacerbations are not triggered by avoidable factors.	Patient avoids factors leading to facial hyperemia.
Side effects or untoward reactions from long-term antibiotic therapy are recognized and treated.	Patient seeks medical attention for untoward or side effects.
Patient evaluates appearance in a realistic manner.	Patient engages in usual activities and relationships.

BENIGN SKIN CHANGES

Corns and calluses

A corn (clavus) is a painful circumscribed area of hyperkeratosis caused by external pressure. A callus is a superficial area of hyperkeratosis that forms at the site of repeated pressure or friction.

A corn is a flat or slightly elevated circumscribed lesion with a smooth hard surface. "Soft" corns are caused by the pressure of a bony prominence. They appear as whitish thickenings usually between the fourth and fifth toes. "Hard" corns have a sharply defined conical appearance. They appear most frequently over bony prominences, such as the interphalangeal joints of the toes at the site of pressure from footwear. Hard corns are usually quite painful. The pain may be dull and constant or sharp when pressure is applied, like the sensation of stepping on a pebble.

Calluses are not well demarcated and may be quite large. They are elevated, with a normal pattern of skin ridges running over the surface. Calluses usually occur on the weight-bearing areas of the feet, overlying bony prominences. Calluses may form over plantar warts and must be differentiated from them. They are also very common on the palmar surface of the hands, particularly in people who work with their hands. Calluses are usually not tender, but pressure may produce dull pain.

Pathophysiology

A corn contains a localized pinpoint accumulation of keratin that forms an elongated hard plug in the horny layer of the epidermis with thinning of the underlying epidermis. The plug presses downward on the dermal structures.

In callus formation the epidermis reacts to repeated friction with an increased mitotic rate that results in hyperkeratosis and thickening of the stratum corneum.

The severity of a corn or callus depends on the degree and duration of the trauma that caused it to form.

Diagnostic Studies and Findings

Physical Examination

Characteristic lesion consistent with history of chronic pressure or friction

Medical Plan

Surgery

Excision of superficial cornified layer of corn

Medications

Keratolytics
- 40% salicylic acid plaster or ointment

Corticosteroids
- Injection of triamcinolone (Kenalog, Aristocort), 10 mg/ml at base of corn to relieve pain

General Management

Orthopaedic correction of weight-bearing mechanics through use of bars and support devices

Corn pads to redistribute weight and relieve pressure

NURSING CARE

Nursing Assessment

Lesion

Thickened skin; may be tender to touch

Pain

Location, duration, and intensity

Nursing Dx & Intervention

Nursing Diagnosis	Nursing Intervention/Rationale
Impaired skin integrity	• Assess lesion for characteristics. • Teach patient how to apply keratolytic substance and to avoid normal skin *to prevent tissue damage*. • Demonstrate proper application of corn pads.
Pain	• Assess for pain and tolerance. • Teach patient use of corn pads to relieve pressure.
Knowledge deficit related to cause and prevention	• Teach patient that most corns and calluses on feet are caused by tight, ill-fitting shoes and that new lesions can be avoided by wearing shoes that fit properly. • Show patient potential areas of pressure and how shoes should fit.

Patient Education

1. Instruct the patient not to pare away existing corns and calluses.
2. Give the patient instructions for use of keratolytic plaster: apply sticky side to skin, making sure plaster is large enough to cover affected area; cover the plaster with adhesive tape and leave in place for designated period of time (overnight to 7 days); after the plaster is removed, soak the area in warm water and rub the soft macerated skin with a rough towel or pumice stone; reapply the plaster and repeat the process until all hyperkeratotic skin is removed.

Evaluation

Patient Outcome	Data Indicating That Outcome is Reached
Source of pressure is relieved.	Shoes fit properly. Orthopaedic correction is used. Corn pads redistribute weight. New lesions do not form.
Existing lesions resolve.	Symptoms of pain are alleviated. Thickened areas disappear.

Sebaceous, epidermal, and dermoid cysts

Sebaceous, epidermal, and dermoid cysts are slow-growing, benign, cystic, intradermal, or subcutaneous tumors.

Cysts are classified into three basic types depending on their histopathology: (1) epidermal cysts, (2) pilar or trichilemmal cysts (sebaceous cysts), and (3) dermoid cysts.

Epidermal cysts are usually found on the face, scalp, neck, and back. Epidermal cysts include milia, acne cysts, and traumatic inclusion cysts. Only a few lesions are usually present unless the patient has had severe acne, in which case multiple lesions may be present.

Pilar or trichilemmal cysts (wens) occur most frequently on the scalp but may also occur elsewhere. These cysts are usually referred to as sebaceous cysts. However, this is a misnomer. True sebaceous cysts are seen only in steatocystoma multiplex, a relatively rare inherited condition.

Dermoid cysts are usually found at birth. They are located deep in the subcutaneous tissue and may adhere to the periosteum.

Cystic lesions vary in size from 1 mm to several centimeters. Most cysts are less than 3 cm in diameter but can enlarge to the size of an orange. On palpation the mass is firm, movable, round, globular, and nontender unless infected.

Pathophysiology

The wall of the epidermal cyst is composed of keratinizing epidermis. The cyst contains keratin in laminated layers. The wall of the pilar cyst is made up of epidermal cells from the central part of the hair follicle. The contents of the pilar cyst are homogeneous rather than in laminated layers. The walls of the dermoid cyst are composed of keratinizing epidermis containing hair follicles, sebaceous glands, and sweat glands.

Cyst formation may occur after inflammation, trauma, or rupture of closed comedones. A person may also have a genetic predisposition to cyst formation. The contents of the cyst are the result of the obstructed hair follicle, and the exact nature depends on the level of the obstruction. The contents are soft and yellow-white and have a rancid odor.

Diagnostic Studies and Findings

Physical Examination

Characteristic lesion

Medical Plan

Surgery

Excision of cyst, including wall, to prevent recurrence
Incision and drainage of infected cysts

Medications

Corticosteroids
- Triamcinolone (Aristocort, Kenalog) by intralesional injection

NURSING CARE

Nursing Assessment

Lesion

Size; location; number; presence of tenderness, inflammation, or infection; on palpation, firm, movable, round, globular, and nontender

Psychosocial Concerns

Concern about body image

Nursing Dx & Intervention

Nursing Diagnosis	Nursing Intervention/Rationale
Impaired skin integrity	• Assess for number, size, location, and characteristics of lesions. • Teach importance of not picking or squeezing lesions, *since this may lead to infection of cyst.*
Body image disturbance	• Assess for presence of defining characteristics. • Recognize importance of body image in growth and development. • Teach importance of not picking or squeezing lesions, *which may lead to infection and result in scarring.* • Encourage patient to express feelings about body, body appearance, and fear of reaction or rejection by others, *to assist in process of realistic self-evaluation.*

Patient Education

1. Instruct the patient in dressing changes and suture care after excision of the cyst.

Evaluation

Patient Outcome	Data Indicating That Outcome is Reached
Nonexcised lesions do not become infected.	There is no redness, swelling, tenderness, pus, or fever; scarring is minimal.
Excised lesions heal.	Skin is intact and smooth.
Patient evaluates appearance realistically.	Patient engages in usual activities and relationships.

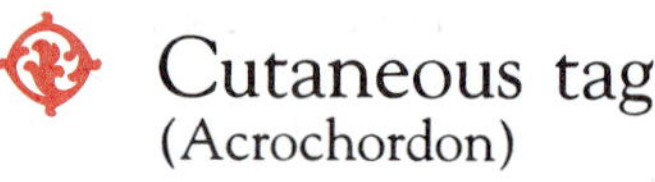

Cutaneous tag
(Acrochordon)

Cutaneous tags are common, small, flesh-colored or pigmented pedunculated lesions.

Acrochordons are found most often in middle-aged and elderly people. The number increases with pregnancy and menopause. The lesions occur most frequently around the neck, upper chest, axilla and groin and with seborrheic keratoses. They may occur singularly or in the hundreds. Although the lesion is benign, it may cause concern because of cosmetic embarrassment or irritation by clothing.

Pathophysiology

The cutaneous tag consists of an outpouched core of loose connective tissue and dilated capillaries covered by normal epidermis. The papilloma is pedunculated and varies in size from 12 mm in diameter to considerably larger, soft, baglike, fibrous lesions.

Diagnostic Studies and Findings

Physical Examination

Characteristic lesion

Medical Plan

Surgery

Removal with scalpel or scissors, with electrocoagulation of central vessel if needed

General Management

Removal through electrodesiccation or cryotherapy

NURSING CARE

Nursing Assessment

Lesion

Location; number; size; presence of irritation, tenderness, and inflammation

Psychosocial Concerns

Concern about body image

Nursing Dx & Intervention

Nursing Diagnosis	Nursing Intervention/Rationale
Potential impaired skin integrity	• Assess for location, number, and size of lesions and presence of irritation, tenderness, or inflammation. • Evaluate with patient the potential for irritation of tags through friction from clothing or rubbing against other body parts.
Body image disturbance	• Assess for presence of defining characteristics. • Encourage patient to express feelings about body, body appearance, or fear of reaction or rejection by others *to assist in process of realistic self-evaluation.*

Patient Education

1. Instruct the patient in the benign nature of the lesions.
2. Instruct the patient that lesions can be removed relatively easily for cosmetic purposes or if tags become irritated.

Evaluation

Patient Outcome	Data Indicating That Outcome is Reached
Patient evaluates lesions in realistic manner.	Patient seeks treatment for lesions that are irritated or inflamed. Lesions are removed if they become irritated or if patient is embarrassed.

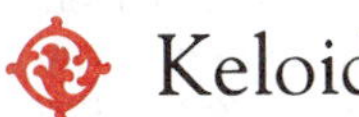

Keloid

A keloid is an overgrowth of fibroelastic tissue that occurs spontaneously or at the site of dermal trauma.

The factors that trigger keloid formation are unknown. There appears to be a genetic predisposition and a regional susceptibility because keloids commonly occur on the sternum, chest, upper back, and earlobes and where an injury crosses normal flexion creases. Keloids occur predominantly in children or young adults, particularly in dark-skinned persons (Figure 5-4).

Figure 5-4 Keloid.
Courtesy of Stephen B. Tucker, M.D., Department of Dermatology, University of Texas Health Science Center at Houston.

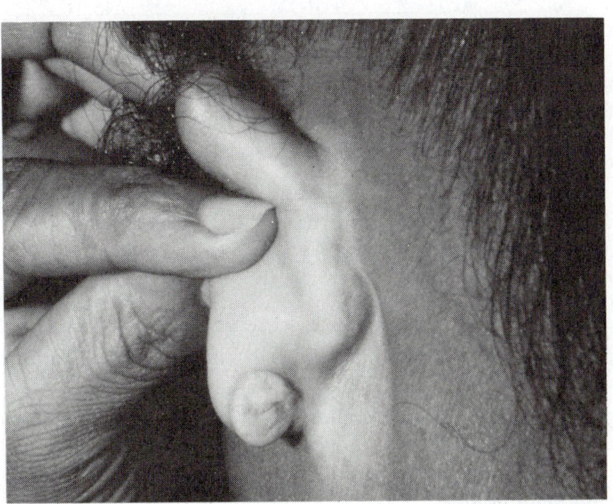

Pathophysiology

In susceptible people keloids form after any skin trauma, or they may arise spontaneously. Keloids are an abnormal progressive deposition of collagen that exceeds the requirements for wound repair. This may be the result of immune activity. The lesions are soft and pink in the early stages and then become firm and white. Keloids are raised, smooth, or ridged, extend beyond the edges of the initial wound, and may continue to grow for many months or years to form large irregular lesions. Keloid scars are frequently tender and pruritic.

Diagnostic Studies and Findings

Physical Examination

Characteristic lesion; clinical differentiation from hypertrophic scar not possible in first 3 months of lesion, but thereafter any continued increase in size and sensitivity of firm, indurated scar is indicative of keloid formation

Medical Plan

Keloids may become worse as the result of treatment; therefore the need for intervention must first be carefully assessed. Small keloids are often best left untreated. Many keloids gradually soften and flatten out over a period of years even without treatment.

Surgery

Surgical or carbon dioxide laser excision combined with radiation therapy or intralesional injection of steroids for large keloids—surgical excision alone will result in the formation of new and larger keloids

Medications

Corticosteroids

Triamcinolone (Aristocort, Kenalog), 20-40 mg/ml by intralesional injection; may require repeated injections at monthly intervals until keloid remains flattened and asymptomatic

General Management

Solid carbon dioxide or liquid nitrogen applied topically at 2-week intervals

NURSING CARE

Nursing Assessment

Lesion

Size; location; color; tenderness; pruritus

Psychosocial Concerns

Concern about body image

Nursing Dx & Intervention

Nursing Diagnosis	Nursing Intervention/Rationale
Impaired skin integrity	• Assess lesion for size, location, color, tenderness, pruritus. • Discuss nature of keloid formation and help patient find skilled practitioners for therapeutic intervention. • Inform patient that optimum time for treatment is within first few months of scar formation, while lesions are still vascular and growing, and that older keloids may be resistant to treatment. • Instruct patient not to scratch keloid that itches *to avoid skin trauma that could cause further keloid formation.*
Potential impaired skin integrity	• Discuss safety habits *to avoid injury that leads to keloid formation:* protective clothing, proper equipment, and so on.
Body image disturbance; situational low self-esteem	• Assess patient's perception of his or her appearance. • Help patient express feelings about body, body appearance, and fear of reaction or rejection by others *to assist in process of realistic self-evaluation.*

Patient Education

1. Discuss with the patient the nature of keloid behavior and the need to evaluate therapeutic intervention carefully with practitioners familiar with and skilled in treating keloids.
2. Inform the patient that many keloids gradually soften and flatten out over a period of years even without treatment.

Evaluation

Patient Outcome	Data Indicating That Outcome is Reached
Patient is knowledgeable about keloid therapies and risks.	Patient seeks intervention early and from practitioners familiar with and skilled in keloid treatment. Patient avoids surgical excision of keloids.
Patient takes measures to prevent injury that would result in keloid formation.	Patient uses safety measures, such as protective clothing and use of proper equipment, to avoid injury. Patient refrains from scratching or irritating scar tissue.
Patient evaluates appearance in a realistic manner.	Patient engages in usual activities and relationships.

Seborrheic keratoses

Seborrheic keratoses are common, benign, superficial, epithelial, pigmented tumors.

The cause of seborrheic keratoses is unknown. They occur most frequently after 40 years of age. They most commonly occur on the back, central chest, face, and scalp. In blacks the lesions tend to be more numerous and smaller and to occur earlier. The lesions are inherited as a dominant trait.

Seborrheic keratoses vary in color from yellow to brownish black. They are elevated plaques with sharply circumscribed borders and appear to be stuck on the skin. The size of the lesion varies from a few millimeters to several centimeters. They almost always occur in multiples rather than singly. These lesions do not become malignant, but a sudden increase in the number and degree of itching of the lesions can occur in association with an internal malignancy.

Pathophysiology

Immature keratinocytes accumulate, causing formation of seborrheic keratoses. Keratinization eventually occurs, causing the lesions to become warty, dry, and fissured. The surface of the lesions often appears greasy, with pits filled with keratotic material. These represent invaginations of the epidermis. There is also a papular variant of the lesion that has a smooth surface. Epidermal thickening is associated with an increase of dermal papillae and the formation of the verrucous surface. The lesions grow slowly and are round or oval.

Seborrheic keratoses are usually asymptomatic unless they become irritated. They may itch occasionally. Irritation of the lesions by physical or chemical trauma results in tenderness, itching, erythema, and an increase in the size of the lesion.

Diagnostic Studies and Findings

Physical Examination

Characteristic lesion

Biopsy

Done if squamous cell carcinoma is suspected

Medical Plan

In most instances small, asymptomatic seborrheic keratoses require no treatment. Treatment is instituted for lesions that itch, are irritated, or are cosmetically embarrassing.

Surgery

Shave ablation or curettage using local anesthesia

General Management

Liquid nitrogen cryotherapy at 2- to 3-week intervals

Carbon dioxide pencil applied with light to moderate pressure for 12 to 20 seconds

NURSING CARE

Nursing Assessment

Lesion

Location; size; number; appearance; color; surface characteristics; borders; pruritus; changes in characteristics

Irritation of Lesion

Erythema; tenderness; increased pruritus

Psychosocial Concerns

Concern with body image

Nursing Dx & Intervention

Nursing Diagnosis	Nursing Intervention/Rationale
Impaired skin integrity	• Assess lesions for characteristics. • Reassure patient that this lesion has no potential for malignancy. • Have patient identify lesions that itch, are irritated, or are cosmetically embarrassing *for potential treatment.* • Evaluate with patient lesions that are likely to become irritated from clothing or rubbing against other body parts *to identify for potential treatment.*
Body image disturbance; situational low self-esteem	• Assess patient's perception of his or her appearance. • Encourage patient to express feelings about body, body appearance, or fear of reaction or rejection by others *to assist in process of realistic self-evaluation.* • Inform patient that bothersome lesions can be removed, usually with minimum or no scarring.

Patient Education

1. Inform the patient that the lesion has no potential for malignancy.
2. Instruct the patient to seek medical therapy for lesions that become irritated or bothersome or that are cosmetically embarrassing.

Evaluation

Patient Outcome	Data Indicating That Outcome is Reached
Treated lesions heal.	Skin is intact with minimum scarring and is free of infection.
Patient evaluates lesions realistically.	Patient seeks treatment for lesions that itch, are irritated, or are cosmetically embarrassing.
Patient evaluates appearance realistically.	Patient engages in usual activities and relationships.

BULLOUS DISEASES

Pemphigus

Pemphigus is an uncommon, chronic, and potentially fatal skin disease that is characterized by the formation of intraepidermal bullae on apparently healthy skin and mucous membrane.

Pemphigus occurs most often in middle-aged people of Jewish descent and Mediterranean extraction. It often affects debilitated individuals and occurs equally in men and women. Pemphigus may occur at any age, although it is rare in children.

Mortality from untreated pemphigus is high. The disease may be fatal even with treatment; 50% of patients die within 6 months to 10 years of onset of the disease. Corticosteroid therapy has decreased mortality by two thirds.

In *pemphigus vulgaris* and *pemphigus vegetans,* erosion of the buccal mucosa is the first indicator of disease in approximately 50% of cases. The erosions are painful and persistent. Other cutaneous membranes such as the conjunctiva, esophagus, vulva, and rectal mucosa may be involved.

Cutaneous lesions can occur anywhere on the body as tense, fluid-filled bullae that become flaccid and rupture easily, leading to painful denuded erosions that bleed, ooze, and crust. Large areas of denuded skin result in substantial loss of body fluid, protein, and electrolytes and predispose the patient to secondary bacterial infection. Intact skin surfaces are easily damaged and separated from the dermis by light rubbing or friction (Nikolsky's sign). The lesions heal slowly, but when healing does occur, there is no scar because the lesion is intraepidermal.

Lesions are common in pressure areas, axillae, groin, face, and scalp. Generalized eruptions develop in 6 to 12 months from the onset of early lesions.

Pemphigus foliaceus is characterized by extensive generalized eruptions with a moist, red, edematous, exfoliating appearance. The buccal mucosa is rarely involved. In *pemphigus erythematosus* the lesions are localized to the face and chest and are red, moist, and crusted over. Both are benign forms of pemphigus.

Pathophysiology

The basic mechanism of pemphigus is an antigen-antibody reaction or an autoimmune response that destroys the mucopolysaccharide protein complex of the intercellular cement. The epidermal cells lose their cohesion, which results in splitting and separation of the normal intercellular contact between epidermal cells (acantholysis) and the formation of bullae. The basal cells remain attached to the basement membrane, and the bullae that form contain detached, rounded, epidermal cells.

The clinical appearance of pemphigus depends on the level and type of acantholysis. Thin-walled bullae and eruptions develop in pemphigus vulgaris and pemphigus vegetans, in which the acantholysis is predominantly suprabasal. Erythema and scaling occur in pemphigus foliaceus and pemphigus erythematosus, in which the acantholysis occurs higher in the epidermis.

Diagnostic Studies and Findings

Physical Examination

Characteristic lesion; positive Nikolsky's sign: lateral pressure on skin separates epidermis from dermis

Complete Blood Count

Eosinophilia

Immunofluorescence (IF)

Presence of IgG antibodies in serum (direct IF) or on epidermal or epithelial cell surfaces (indirect IF)

Biopsy

Suprabasal cell separation

Cytology

Tzanck smear: acantholytic cells stain blue with Wright's or Giemsa stain

Medical Plan

Medications

Corticosteroids
- Systemic
  - Prednisone, 150-300 mg/d po for 6-8 wk, then decreasing doses when no new lesions appear for 7-10 d, continued for 4-6 mo
- Topical
  - Fluocinonide (Lidex, Topsyn) 0.05% tid or qid; triamcinolone (Aristocort, Kenalog) 0.025%-0.1%, tid or qid

Antineoplastic agents (used for immunosuppressive effect)
- Methotrexate, azathioprine, and cyclophosphamide in individualized doses

Analgesics if lesions are extensive or pain is severe

General Management

Cool compresses or soaks
Wet Dakin's dressings
Potassium permanganate baths (see p. 564)
Intravenous therapy for fluid and electrolyte balance
Blood and plasma transfusions for fluid and protein loss
Nutrition—high-protein, high-calorie diet to support healing and reepithelization and to replace protein loss through extensive bullae

NURSING CARE

Nursing Assessment

Lesion

Raw, round, weeping lesions; pruritus; burning; odor; bullae with little or no inflammation; location and number of lesions; extent of body covered

Systemic Involvement

Anorexia; weight loss; weakness; fever; eosinophilia

Fluid and Electrolyte Balance

Weight loss; weakness; dry mucous membrane; hydration status; lowered serum sodium, chloride, and potassium levels

Secondary Infection

Inflammation; pus; odor; increased white blood count; increased eosinophils; increased lymphocytes; increased erythrocyte sedimentation rate; decreased neutrophils

Nutrition

Inability to eat because of mouth sores

Psychosocial Concerns

Concern with body image; concern about dying

Nursing Dx & Intervention

Nursing Diagnosis	Nursing Intervention/Rationale
Impaired skin integrity; potential for infection	• Assess location, number, and status of lesions. • In collaboration with physician, provide cool baths and soaks, Dakin's dressings, and potassium permanganate baths using aseptic technique *to promote healing and prevent infection.* • In collaboration with physician, use Stryker frame or CircOlectric bed *to relieve pressure and decrease painful movement on raw surfaces.* • Use meticulous hygiene *to prevent infection.* • Observe for signs of septicemia. • Assess for and prevent secondary infection; reverse isolation as needed. • Use room deodorizer. • Test urine for glucose and albumin when patient is receiving high doses of corticosteroids.
Altered oral mucous membrane	• Assess for buccal lesions. • Provide mouth care with saline or alkaline mouthwash *to prevent infection.* • Provide soft, bland diet *to prevent tissue trauma.* • Avoid acidic and astringent fluids *to promote comfort.* • Have patient use viscous lidocaine mouthwash *to promote comfort.*
Potential fluid volume deficit	• Assess hydration status. • Provide adequate hydration by mouth and intravenously. • Monitor intake and output. • Weigh daily *to monitor fluid loss.* • Monitor vital signs and hydration status. • Observe for adverse reaction after administration of blood or blood components.
Altered nutrition: less than body requirements	• Assess nutritional status. • Provide high-protein, high-calorie diet *to promote tissue healing and replace protein loss.* • Provide small, frequent feedings *to promote adequate nutrient intake.* • Provide snacks between meals *to promote adequate nutrient intake.*

Nursing Diagnosis	Nursing Intervention/Rationale
Pain	• Assess for discomfort. • Apply cool compresses or soaks. • Use Stryker frame or CircOlectric bed *to prevent pressure.* • Use talcum powder liberally on bedsheets *to prevent friction.* • Provide soft, bland foods *to prevent tissue trauma and promote comfort.* • Offer nonacidic, nonastringent fluids *to prevent tissue trauma and promote comfort.*
Body image disturbance; situational low self-esteem	• Assess for defining characteristics. • Help patient express feelings about body, body appearance, or fear of reaction or rejection by others *to assist in process of realistic self-evaluation.* • Spend time with patient *to reassure him or her that appearance or odor is not repulsive.* • Prepare visitors for patient's appearance. • Encourage self-esteem by showing interest in patient and being attentive to patient's needs.
Powerlessness	• Assess for presence of defining characteristics. • Observe for signs of depression and apathy. • Involve patient in decision making *to increase sense of power and control.* • Encourage patient to express dissatisfaction and frustration. • Accept feelings of anger. • Provide support for patient who is dying.
Anticipatory grieving	• Assess for presence of defining characteristics. • Encourage patient to express distress, anger, sorrow, and fear *to assist in movement through stages of grief.*

Patient Education

1. Instruct the patient in the effects of long-term, high-dose corticosteroid therapy.
2. Teach the patient who is at home to apply cool compress and Dakin's dressings and to prepare potassium permanganate baths (see p. 564).
3. Instruct the patient in aseptic technique.
4. Teach the patient the signs and symptoms of secondary infection and to seek medical attention if they occur.
5. Teach the patient the importance of a high-calorie, high-protein diet and provide specific diet instructions.

Evaluation

Patient Outcome	Data Indicating That Outcome is Reached
Disease condition improves.	Bulla formation decreases. Denuded areas are reepithelized. Skin and mucosa heal. Pain is alleviated.
Fluid and electrolyte balance is maintained.	Mucous membrane is moist. There is no dry skin or weight loss. Blood values are normal: pH 7.35 to 7.45, sodium 136-145 mEq/L, potassium 3.5-5 mEq/L, and chloride 100-106 mEq/L.
Nutritional requirements are satisfied.	Weight is maintained. Patient eats diet high in protein and calories. Lesions heal.
Secondary infection does not develop.	There is no pus, redness, swelling, or fever.
Patient works through psychosocial concerns.	Patient expresses dissatisfaction, frustration, anger, distress, sorrow, and fear. Patient moves through stages of grief.

Epidermolysis bullosa

Epidermolysis bullosa is a group of hereditary bullous disorders caused by abnormalities of the epidermis and dermoepidermal junction.

Pathophysiology

The six disorders of epidermolysis bullosa have varying characteristics and degrees of severity. They are classified as simple, recurrent, lethal, dystrophic dominant, dystrophic recessive, and dystrophic acquired.

Simple and recurrent epidermolysis bullosa. These two forms are inherited dominant disorders that are relatively mild. The blisters are caused by disintegration of the intraepidermal cells in the basal and subbasal layers. The clinical features are tense clear bullae that first appear in infancy with the normal trauma from bedsheets or crawling. Lesions occur on the feet, on the extensor aspects of the extremities, and over joints. Bullae are more numerous during the summer months because of exposed skin surfaces. The lesions heal without scarring.

Recurrent epidermolysis bullosa may not become apparent until early adulthood. Lesions are superficial and precipitated by trauma from footwear and warm weather exposure. These lesions also heal without scarring.

Lethal epidermolysis bullosa. This is an inherited recessive disorder. Blistering occurs at the basement membrane. It is extensive and nonscarring, with the mucous membrane affected. Death usually occurs shortly after birth because of involvement of the mucous membrane in the gastrointestinal and respiratory tracts.

Dystrophic dominant, recessive, and acquired epidermolysis bullosa. These are the deepest forms of the disorder and produce scars and chronic mucocutaneous erosions.

In the dominant form the abnormality is within the basal lamina of the dermoepidermal junction; bullae are subepidermal. The blisters leave atrophic or hypertrophic scars.

In the recessive form bullae occur within the upper dermis rather than in the immediate subepidermis. Large areas of erosion and scarring develop. The oral and esophageal mucosa may also be involved. The condition progresses to gross hypertrophic scarring of the fingers and toes with adhesions between the digits. All nails are dystrophic. One feature of this form is the presence of milia within the epidermis.

The acquired variant is not hereditary. The mechanism of acquisition is not known. The disease follows the course of the hereditary dystrophic forms of epidermolysis bullosa.

Diagnostic Studies and Findings

Physical Examination

Characteristic lesions that occur spontaneously or as result of trauma

Biopsy

Bulla formation in basal layer, basement membrane zone, and dermis

Medical Plan

Medications

Corticosteroids
- Systemic glucocorticoids such as prednisone; dosage determined by type and severity of disease

Vitamin derivatives
- Vitamin E, 200-3200 IU po qd; use controversial; effect at best limited to selected cases[24]

Anti-infective agents
- Systemic antibiotics for secondary infection; specific drug and dosage dependent on infecting organism

General Management

Permanent or long-term hospitalization for disabilities

NURSING CARE

Nursing Assessment

Lesion

Bullae or scars on extremities, hands, feet, and mucous membranes; number, size, and location of bullae; degree of involvement

Secondary Infection

Redness; swelling; tenderness; pus or purulent exudate; odor

Systemic Response to Infection

Regional lymphadenopathy; fever; chills; tachycardia; headache; hypotension; malaise; increased white blood count; increased eosinophils; increased lymphocytes; decreased neutrophils; increased erythrocyte sedimentation rate

Psychosocial Concerns

Concern with body image; loss of family member; fear of having other children with disease

Nursing Dx & Intervention

Nursing Diagnosis	Nursing Intervention/Rationale
Impaired skin integrity	• Assess location, number, and status of lesions. • Use meticulous hygiene and handwashing *to prevent secondary infection.* • Use antibacterial soap *to prevent secondary infection.* • Assess for and prevent secondary infection; provide reverse isolation if required.

Nursing Diagnosis	Nursing Intervention/Rationale
	• In collaboration with physician, provide Stryker frame or CircOlectric bed *to relieve pressure and decrease painful movement in eroded areas.*
Altered oral mucous membrane	• Assess for presence of defining characteristics. • Provide mouth care with saline or alkaline mouthwash *to prevent infection.* • Avoid astringent or acidic fluids *to promote comfort.* • Provide soft, bland diet *to prevent tissue trauma.*
Body image disturbance	• Assess for presence of defining characteristics. • Encourage patient to express feelings about body, body appearance, or fear of reaction or rejection by others.
Impaired physical mobility (scarring and disabilities); potential for disuse syndrome	• Assess for presence of defining and risk characteristics (see pp. 1686 and 1689). • Maintain skin integrity and circulation. • Implement passive and active range of motion exercises *to prevent contracture.* • In collaboration with physician, provide Stryker frame or CircOlectric bed. • Refer patient to physical therapy.
Powerlessness	• Assess for presence of defining characteristics. • Observe for signs of depression and apathy. • Involve patient in decision making *to increase sense of power and control.* • Assist patient in expressing dissatisfaction and frustration. • Assist family in expressing fear and anxiety regarding future children; assist in seeking genetic counseling.
Anticipatory grieving	• Assess for presence of defining characteristics. • Assist in expression of distress, anger, sorrow, and fear *to assist in movement through grief process.*

Patient Education

1. Instruct the patient and family in meticulous hygiene and handwashing to prevent secondary infection.
2. Instruct the patient and family in aseptic technique for dressing changes required for oozing or infected lesions.
3. Instruct the patient and family in signs and symptoms of secondary infection and to seek medical attention if they occur.
4. Instruct the patient and family in the importance of preventing trauma that can cause blister formation.
5. Assist in identifying ways to eliminate potential trauma, such as protective footwear, long sleeves, and long pant legs.
6. Instruct patients with dystrophic forms who are at home to perform range of motion exercises to minimize disability from scarring at the joints.

Evaluation

Patient Outcome	Data Indicating That Outcome is Reached
Existing lesions heal.	Bullae resolve. Skin and mucous membranes heal.
There is no secondary infection.	There is no redness, swelling, or pus in healing lesions.
Systemic response to infection resolves.	There are no systemic indicators: lymphadenopathy, fever, tachycardia, hypotension, or malaise. Laboratory values are normal: white blood count, 5000-10,000/mm^3; eosinophils, 50-400/mm^3; lymphocytes, 1000-4000 mm^3; neutrophils, 3000-7000/mm^3; and erythrocyte sedimentation rate normal (depends on method).
External trauma to skin is minimized.	Patient wears protective clothing and footwear. Patient avoids activities conducive to skin trauma.
Disability from scarring is minimized.	Patient performs active and passive range of motion exercises. Range of motion of joints is preserved.
Psychosocial needs are recognized and addressed.	Patient is involved in decision making. Patient and family express dissatisfaction, frustration, fear, anger, and sorrow. Patient and family move through grief process. Parents seek genetic counseling.

Erythema Multiforme

Erythema multiforme is an acute inflammatory eruption characterized by symmetric erythematous, edematous, or bullous lesions precipitated by numerous factors.

The cause and pathogenesis of erythema multiforme are unknown. The mechanism of response seems to be an allergic hypersensitivity.

The disease is associated with herpes simplex, bacterial and other infections, endocrine changes, and internal malignancies. Almost any drug can cause erythema multiforme; penicillin, sulfonamides, salicylates, and barbiturates are the most commonly implicated drugs. Bacterial and viral infections are often implicated in children and young adults, but association with drugs and malignancy is more common in adults. Attacks sometimes last for 2 to 4 weeks and recur in the fall.

Pathophysiology

In mild cases of erythema multiforme, eruption occurs only in cutaneous lesions of erythematous macules, papules, and plaques located predominantly in the distal portion of the extremities and face and symmetrically distributed. The classic lesion (target or iris lesion) is a dark, urticarial plaque with elevated circular borders and a depressed inner ring (Figure 5-5). After a few days the central area of erythema develops a dusky purplish discoloration that can become bullous.

In more severe cases fever, coryza, malaise, and arthralgia may also occur. In these cases the lesions are predominantly vesiculobullous and involve mucous membranes as well as skin. In children and young adults a severe and sometimes fatal form of erythema multiforme known as Stevens-Johnson syndrome can develop. In this syndrome mucous membrane lesions are present and may or may not be accompanied by cutaneous lesions. Vesicles and ulcerations develop on the mucous membrane of the lips, mouth, nasal passages, eyes, and genitalia. Conjunctival and corneal lesions are present in 90% of the cases.

Genitourinary lesions in erythema multiforme can compromise bladder function, and the inflammatory process can involve the kidneys with consequent hematuria and renal tubular necrosis. Mucous membrane ulceration can extend into the pharynx, esophagus, larynx, trachea, and bronchi.

The variety of histologic changes in erythema multiforme depends on the site of involvement and the degree of the inflammatory process. The blood vessels are dilated and are surrounded by lymphohistiocytic infiltrate with substantial edema of the papillary dermis. Edema of the upper dermis leads to the formation of bullae that are subepidermal without acantholysis. Epidermal necrosis occurs primarily in the center of the lesion, the site of the dusky iris (target) lesion.

Figure 5-5 Erythema multiforme (target lesion).
Courtesy of Stephen B. Tucker, M.D., Department of Dermatology, University of Texas Health Science Center at Houston.

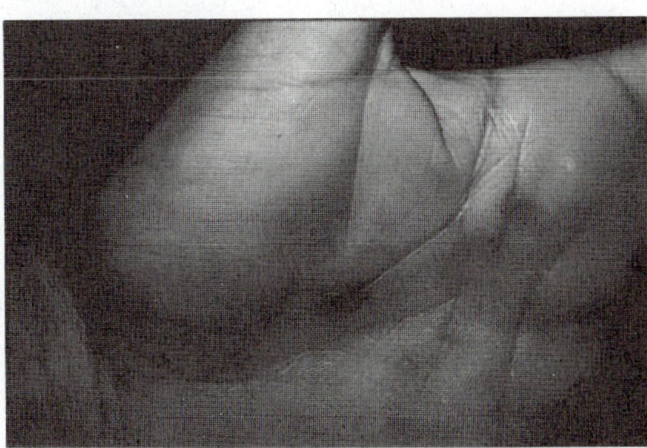

Diagnostic Studies and Findings

Physical Examination

Characteristic lesion, particularly iris or target lesion; lesions fixed and do not fade or change location; absence of itching

Complete Blood Count

Increased white blood count, increased erythrocyte sedimentation rate

Urinalysis

Red blood cells and albumin in urine if genitourinary lesions are present

Antistreptolysin Titer

Elevated if disease occurs after streptococcal infection

Medical Plan

Mild erythema multiforme clears spontaneously and may require no treatment other than elimination of the precipitating factor. For treatment of eye symptoms see Chapter 6.

Medications

- Anti-infective agents
  - Systemic antibiotics for underlying infection or to control secondary infection; specific drug and dosage depends on infection, its severity, and age of patient
- Corticosteroids
  - Systemic glucocorticoids (controversial)[70]
    - Prednisone, 60-80 mg po qd in divided doses, then decreased
- Local anesthetic agents
  - Viscous lidocaine (Xylocaine) swish for mouth lesions

Analgesics
Aspirin (ASA), 300 mg po q4-6h

General Management

Wet dressings to debride crusted lesions
Bed rest; hospitalization for severe cases
Bland diet for mouth lesions
Intravenous fluids for hydration in severe cases

NURSING CARE

Nursing Assessment

Lesion

Erythematous macules, papules, vesicles, or bullae at distal aspect of extremities and face; target or iris lesion; vesicles or ulcerations of mucous membranes

Systemic Involvement

Fever; coryza; arthralgia; malaise; chest pain; vomiting; diarrhea; hematuria; albuminuria; increased erythrocyte sedimentation rate; increased white blood count; radiologic changes in lungs

Nutrition

Inability to eat because of mouth ulcerations

Psychosocial Concerns

Concern about body image

Nursing Dx & Intervention

Nursing Diagnosis	Nursing Intervention/Rationale
Impaired skin integrity	• Assess lesions for characteristics. • In collaboration with physician, apply wet dressings to debride lesions (see p. 564). • Scrub crusted lesions gently with antibacterial soap *to promote healing and prevent infection.* • Teach meticulous handwashing and good hygiene *to prevent secondary infection.*
Altered oral mucous membrane	• Assess for presence of lesions. • Provide soft, bland diet *to prevent tissue damage.* • Avoid astringent or acidic liquids *to promote comfort.* • Provide mouth care with alkaline or saline mouthwash *to promote comfort and prevent infection.* • Instruct patient in use of viscous lidocaine mouth swish *to promote comfort.*
Pain	• Assess for discomfort. • Apply cool compresses or soaks. • Encourage bed rest. • Instruct patient in use of analgesics.
Altered nutrition: less than body requirements	• Assess nutritional status. • Provide soft, bland diet *to promote comfort while eating.* • In collaboration with physician, offer viscous lidocaine mouth swish 15 minutes before eating *to promote comfort.*
Body image disturbance	• Assess for defining characteristics. • Help patient express feelings about body, body appearance, or fear of reaction or rejection by others *to assist in process of realistic self-evaluation.*

Patient Education

1. Instruct the patient and family in the application of cool compresses or soaks using aseptic technique.
2. Instruct the patient and family in the need for follow-up urinalysis to detect the presence of renal tubular necrosis.
3. Instruct the patient and family in signs and symptoms of secondary infection and to seek medical attention if they occur.
4. Help the patient identify potential precipitating factors and to eliminate those factors when possible.

Evaluation

Patient Outcome	Data Indicating That Outcome is Reached
Existing lesions heal.	Lesions resolve. Ulcerations and erosions reepithelialize. Skin and mucous membrane heal. Discomfort is alleviated.
Secondary infection is avoided.	There is no swelling, redness, or pus in healing lesions.
Nutritional status is adequate.	Weight is maintained. Lesions heal.
Systemic involvement resolves.	There are no red blood cells or protein in urine. White blood count is 5000-10,000/mm^3. Erythrocyte sedimentation rate is normal (depends on method).
Complications are recognized early.	Patient has follow-up urinalysis. Patient seeks medical attention for vision changes.
Patient evaluates appearance in a realistic manner.	Patient engages in usual activities and relationships.

Erythema Nodosum

Erythema nodosum is an acute inflammatory nodular eruption that involves primarily the lower extremities and is precipitated by various factors.

Erythema nodosum is found equally in boys and girls but is more common in adults, particularly young women. It occurs more commonly from January to June.

There are many precipitating factors including various infections, drugs, diseases, and pregnancy. Erythema nodosum frequently follows an infection of the upper respiratory tract, especially from streptococci. In adults streptococcal infections and sarcoidosis are the most common causes. An underlying systemic cause is identifiable in more than 50% of cases. The remainder of the cases occur in apparently healthy young adults.

The prodromal symptoms may be fever, chills, malaise, and arthralgia, which occur a few days or several weeks before the onset of the eruption. Some of the prodromal symptoms may be from the underlying condition.

Pathophysiology

Erythema nodosum is a vascular reaction pattern, most likely a hypersensitivity response involving both cellular and humoral mechanisms (see Chapter 14).

The eruption is sudden with discrete, erythematous, hot, and very tender nodules on the shins, knees, ankles, thighs, buttocks, and sometimes lower arms. The nodules are bright red initially, but change to a purplish color and finally become a flat brown pigmentation that slowly fades completely. The total evolution of lesions takes 3 to 4 weeks.

The nodules vary in size from 6 to 8 mm and are usually bilaterally symmetric. There may be only a few lesions or many appearing in crops. New crops may occur periodically. Edema of the ankles and general aching of the legs are common and are aggravated by ambulation.

Cellular changes are probably due to the immunologic processes. Deep dermal inflammation extends down into subcutaneous tissue. Small blood vessels experience mild vasculitis and inflammatory infiltrate with partial obstruction of blood flow.

Diagnostic Studies and Findings

Physical Examination

Characteristic lesion; history consistent with possible precipitating factors

Complete Blood Count

Increased erythrocyte sedimentation rate; platelet estimate

Biopsy

Deep excision biopsy including subcutaneous tissue; shows histologic changes described previously

Diagnostic Studies to Isolate Underlying Disorders

Antistreptolysin titer; throat culture; tuberculosis test; rheumatoid factor; antinuclear factor

Medical Plan

Management of the disease is aimed at identifying and treating the precipitating factor or underlying disorder.

Medications

Analgesics
- Aspirin (ASA), 300 mg po q4-6h

Anti-infective agents
- Systemic antibiotics for underlying infection; may require long-term therapy; specific antibiotic depends on the underlying infection

Corticosteroids
- Intralesional injection of triamcinolone (Aristocort, Kenalog), 5 mg/ml

General Management

Bed rest
Cool compresses applied to nodules
Support stockings or elastic bandages

NURSING CARE

Nursing Assessment

Lesions

Red, hot, tender nodules (initially) on anterior aspect of lower extremities

Systemic Involvement

Fever; chills; malaise; arthralgia; ankle edema; aching legs

Underlying Disorder

Complete blood count; urinalysis; antistreptolysin titer; tuberculosis test; rheumatoid factor; throat culture; antinuclear factor

Psychosocial Concerns

Concern about body image

Nursing Dx & Intervention

Nursing Diagnosis	Nursing Intervention/Rationale
Pain	• Assess for discomfort. • Encourage bed rest and elevation of legs *to alleviate aching.* • Have patient use support hose and elastic bandages *to prevent venous pooling.* • Apply cool compresses.
Body image disturbance	• Assess for defining characteristics. • Encourage patient to express feelings about body, body appearance, or fear of reaction or rejection by others *to begin process of realistic self-evaluation.* • Assure patient that lesions heal without scarring.

Patient Education

1. Help the patient identify potential precipitating factors and eliminate them when possible (such as with drugs).
2. Instruct the patient in the effects of long-term antibiotic therapy if indicated.
3. Instruct the patient in management of symptoms: elevation of legs, rest, use of support hose or elastic bandages, and application of cool compresses.

Evaluation

Patient Outcome	Data Indicating That Outcome is Reached
Nodules resolve.	Discomfort is alleviated. Skin integrity is restored.
Underlying condition is identified and treated.	Symptoms of underlying disorder improve and resolve.
Precipitating factors are eliminated when possible.	Condition does not recur.
Patient evaluates appearance in realistic manner.	Patient engages in usual activities when possible and in usual relationships.

INFESTATIONS AND PARASITIC DISORDERS

Pediculosis

Pediculosis is an infestation by lice of the head (pediculosis capitis), the body (pediculosis corporis), or the genital area (pediculosis pubis).

Pediculosis is a highly pruritic and often secondarily infected disorder that results from two species of lice: *Pediculus humanus*, which affects the head and body, and *Pthirus pubis*, which infects the pubic area, the lower abdomen, and sometimes the eyebrows, eyelashes, and scalp.

Pediculosis capitis occurs most frequently in schoolchildren and is easily transmitted by personal contact and by objects such as combs and hats. Itching and excoriation are present. The posterior aspect of the scalp commonly shows the most involvement. The posterior occipital nodes may be enlarged and tender.

Pediculosis corporis is characterized by pruritus and parallel linear excoriations that are frequently secondarily infected. The infesting lice live in the seams of clothing and move onto the skin to feed frequently. Lesions are most common on the shoulders, buttocks, and abdomen. Infestation is associated with unhygienic living conditions ("vagabond's disease").

Pediculosis pubis is transmitted by close personal contact, usually through sexual contact. Infestation is usually in the pubic hair but may occur in the chest or axillary hair, eyebrows, or eyelashes. A sign of infestation is the presence of reddish brown specks on undergarments as a result of the excreta of lice.

Pathophysiology

In pediculosis capitis, injection of saliva from the lice during feeding produces severe pruritus. Scratching causes excoriation, and secondary infection is common. Each day the female louse lays seven to 10 eggs that hatch in 8 days. The eggs (nits) are cemented to the hair shaft and cannot be dislodged.

In pediculosis corporis the primary lesion is an urticarial papule, which is often obscured by secondary excoriation and infection. With prolonged infestation the skin becomes dry, scaly, and hyperpigmented.

Pediculosis pubis is manifested primarily by itching. The lice ova are commonly attached to the skin at the base of the hair follicle. Discrete, small, 1 to 3 cm, gray-blue macules can be seen on the trunk, thighs, and axillae. These lesions are due to a reaction of the lice's saliva with bilirubin, converting it to biliverdin. Excoriation and secondary infection are uncommon.

Diagnostic Studies and Findings

Physical Examination

Presence of lice or eggs; presence of nonspecific lesion with characteristic distribution

Wood's Light

Fluorescence of adult louse

Microscopic Examination

Examination of hair shaft for eggs

Medical Plan

Medications

Anti-infective agents
- Lindane (Kwell) shampoo, cream, or lotion, applied qd for 2 d; application repeated in 10 d; used with caution with young children because of neurotoxicity
- Ophthalmic preparation of yellow mercury oxide qd for infested eyelashes

Cholinergic agents
- Physostigmine (Eserine) 0.25% ophthalmic ointment qd for infested eyelashes

General Management

Rinsing with white vinegar diluted with equal amounts of water followed by washing to remove residual nits from hair

Lice removed from eyelashes with forceps

Body lice eliminated from clothing and bedding by thorough washing, hot ironing, boiling, and steaming

NURSING CARE

Nursing Assessment

Local Response to Infestation

Pruritus; excoriation; secondary infection

Infestation

Location and distribution of lesions or local responses

Psychosocial Concerns

Concern that others may react to transmissible infestation

Nursing Dx & Intervention

Nursing Diagnosis	Nursing Intervention/Rationale
Impaired skin integrity	• Assess for presence of lice, eggs, and lesions. • Isolate patient until treatment is complete *to prevent transmission.* • Instruct patient in use of lindane *to kill parasite.* • Instruct patient to comb hair with fine-toothed comb *to remove eggs after preparation is used.* • Instruct patient to remove lice from eyelashes with cotton-tipped applicator. • Instruct patient in good hygiene, meticulous handwashing, and need for short fingernails *to avoid secondary infection.*
Potential impaired skin integrity	• Teach patient how to decontaminate sources of infestation. • Treat all family members and sexual partners.

Nursing Diagnosis	Nursing Intervention/Rationale
	• Advise patient that recurrence is common. • Teach patient importance of not borrowing personal items such as combs.
Situational low self-esteem	• Assess for defining characteristics (see p. 1756). • Encourage patient to express feelings about the infestation, embarrassment, or fear of rejection by others *to begin the process of realistic self-evaluation.* • Assure patient and family that infestation can be treated successfully.

Patient Education

1. See "Nursing Dx & Intervention."
2. Instruct the patient that prolonged use of lindane may result in dermatitis.

Evaluation

Patient Outcome	Data Indicating That Outcome is Reached
Infestation is cleared in patient and affected family members and partners.	Pruritus subsides. No new areas of itching or excoriation develop. There are no lice or eggs on examination.
Lesions heal.	Excoriations resolve. Skin is intact.
Secondary infection is resolved or avoided.	Lesions heal without redness, swelling, or pus.
Infestation does not spread to unaffected family members or intimate contacts.	Associates of patient do not develop symptoms. Hair and skin are free of lice or eggs. All family members and sexual partners receive treatment.

Scabies

Scabies is a transmissible parasitic infestation characterized by burrows, pruritus, and excoriations with secondary infection.

Scabies is caused by the *Sarcoptes scabiei* mite. The infestation and lesions occur most commonly on the finger webs, the flexor surfaces of the wrist, and the elbows and axillary folds, along the belt line, and on the lower buttocks. The areolae in women and the genitals in men are particularly susceptible. Lesions do not extend to the face in adults but may do so in infants.

Scabies is transmitted readily by personal contact. It characteristically spreads to other family members, to intimate contacts, and between schoolchildren. It is not transmitted by clothing, bedding, or inanimate objects. Infestation can occur from cats, dogs, and other small animals, but the animal scabies mite does not burrow, only feeds.

Pathophysiology

The impregnated female mite burrows into the stratum corneum and forms a small tunnel that is seen as a fine, wavy, dark line. The burrow is a few millimeters to 1 cm long with a minute papule at the open end. The mite extends the burrow daily and deposits eggs and feces in it (Figure 5-6).

Figure 5-6 Scabies burrow.
Courtesy of Stephen B. Tucker, M.D., Department of Dermatology, University of Texas Health Science Center at Houston.

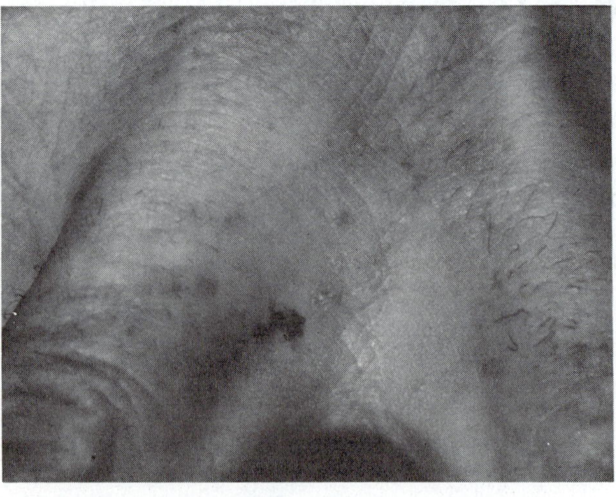

The lesions are at first asymptomatic. After several weeks, the person becomes sensitized to the mite and itching becomes noticeable. The itching is intense and more severe at night. The itching intensifies over a period of several weeks. The burrows and papules are often obscured by secondary excoriation, bacterial infection, crusting, and lichenification. A fine rash is present that consists of papules of various sizes.

Diagnostic Studies and Findings

Physical Examination

Burrows; nonspecific excoriations; papules with characteristic distribution; intense itching that worsens at night

Scrapings

Taken from burrow and placed in oil; presence of mite on microscopic examination

Medical Plan

Medications

Anti-infective agents

Benzyl benzoate topical emulsion 20%-25%; applied to entire cutaneous surface from neck down; left on 12-24 h, and then washed off; procedure repeated after 2 d; third treatment may be necessary in 2 wk

Lindane (Kwell) 1% cream or lotion applied according to above instructions; not used for young children because of neurotoxicity; not recommended during pregnancy

Sulfur ointment 5%-10% applied as above; used for infants

Crotamiton (Eurax) applied with benzyl benzoate; less irritating than benzyl benzoate

Corticosteroids

Fluorinated corticosteroid ointment 1% applied topically bid, tid, or qid for persistent itching

NURSING CARE

Nursing Assessment

Lesion

Linear gray-brown burrows a few millimeters in length; excoriation; secondary infection; crusting; papules; vesicles; lichenification

Local Response to Infestation

Intense itching out of proportion to visible signs; itching worse at night

Psychosocial Concerns

Concern that others may react to transmissible infestation

Nursing Dx & Intervention

Nursing Diagnosis	Nursing Intervention/Rationale
Impaired skin integrity	• Assess lesions for characteristics. • Isolate patient until treatment is completed *to prevent transmission.* • Instruct patient in meticulous handwashing and good hygiene *to avoid secondary infection.* • Have patient's fingernails cut short *to avoid excoriation from scratching.* • Instruct patient in use of treatment lotion; all skin surfaces except face must be covered.
Potential impaired skin integrity	• Have all family members and sexual partners treated.[24] • Have patient notify sexual contacts. • Instruct patient and family in modes of infestation and transmission.
Situational low self-esteem	• Assess for defining characteristics. • Prepare patient and family for potential reaction of others to transmissible infestation. • Encourage patient to express feelings about the infestation, embarrassment, or fear of rejection by others *to begin the process of realistic self-evaluation.* • Assure patient and family that infestation can be treated successfully.

Patient Education

1. Tell the patient and family that treatment irritates the skin and does not quickly reduce the pruritus; discomfort may persist for a few weeks.
2. Instruct the patient in the use of cool soaks and compresses to reduce itching after treatment is complete.
3. Stress the importance of the correct use of treatment lotion to avoid neurotoxicity and undue irritation.
4. Advise that all family members and sexual partners be treated.

Evaluation

Patient Outcome	Data Indicating That Outcome is Reached
Infestation is cleared in patient and affected family members and partners.	No new papules, burrows, or areas of itching develop.
Lesions heal.	Excoriations resolve. Skin is intact.
Secondary infection is resolved or avoided.	Lesions heal without redness, swelling, crusts, or pus.
Infestation does not spread to seemingly unaffected family members or sexual partners.	These people do not develop symptoms of infestation, or they seek treatment if symptoms develop.

Arachnid and Hymenoptera bites

Arachnids are ticks, spiders, and scorpions; Hymenoptera are bees, wasps, yellow jackets, and ants. Their bites cause toxic and allergic reactions as a result of the injection of a venom or toxin.

Tick bites. Tick bites are common in woods and fields throughout the United States. The tick attaches itself to a passing animal or person and after biting remains attached to the skin for several days or longer. Ticks transmit Rocky Mountain spotted fever, Q fever, relapsing fever, and Lyme disease. The tick bite is initially painless but begins to itch after several days. Infiltration and erythema develop around the bite with formation of firm, discrete, intensely pruritic nodules that may be present for several months or longer.

Systemic symptoms attributed to a toxin include fever, malaise, headache, and abdominal pain. Several species of ticks inject a salivary neurotoxin that causes paralysis. Paresthesia and pain in the lower extremities, weakness, and incoordination develop. The condition may progress to respiratory failure and death from bulbar involvement. Symptoms clear dramatically once the tick is removed.

Spider bites. The most important spider bites are caused by the black widow and brown recluse spiders. The black widow is common throughout the United States and southern Canada. It lives in old lumber, unused sheds, and outdoor toilets and may be found in attics, drawers, and closets. Only the female bites and only in self-defense. The female is recognized by her coal black coloring with an hourglass-shaped red or orange marking on the underside of the abdomen.

The black widow bite results from the injection of a neurotoxic venom through a clawlike appendage. The bite, which may go unnoticed, is felt as a pinprick followed by a dull numbing pain. Local necrosis may cause a small ulcer at the site. Within 10 to 60 minutes muscle spasms occur locally and then spread to include all extremities and the trunk. Excruciating pain is felt in waves. The attack subsides after several hours.

Systemic symptoms may include restlessness, vertigo, sweating, chills, pallor, hyperactive reflexes, hypertension, tachycardia, thready pulse, nausea and vomiting, headache, eyelid edema, urticaria, pruritus, and fever. Ascending paralysis, severe hypotension, circulatory collapse, convulsions, and death may result. Mortality is less than 1%.

The brown recluse spider is common in the south-central United States and is usually found in dark areas such as drawers and closets. It commonly bites people when they are asleep. The spider is small and light to dark brown, with a light violin-shaped mark on its head. The female is more dangerous than the male. Most bites occur between April and October.

Brown recluse venom is coagulotoxic. Pain and local symptoms develop 2 to 8 hours after the bite. Localized vasoconstriction causes ischemic necrosis at the site. The area is red with blisters and blebs surrounded by ischemia. After several days the center becomes dark and hard. After 2 weeks it becomes depressed, demarcated, and necrotic, and a large open ulcer forms. The ulcer may take several weeks to heal and may require grafting.

Systemic symptoms include fever, chills, malaise, weakness, arthralgia, nausea, vomiting, petechiae, hemolysis, and thrombocytopenia.

Scorpion bites. Scorpions are found throughout the United States but are most common in the southern United States and Mexico. The two deadly species are found in the southwest United States.

Scorpions are nocturnal and photophobic. They sting by means of a hooked caudal stinger that discharges venom. Most stings occur during the warmer months. Nonlethal bites cause local swelling, tenderness, pain, a sharp burning sensation, skin discoloration, paresthesia, regional lymphadenopathy, and, rarely, anaphylaxis. Lethal bites are neurotoxic and result in pain, hyperesthesia followed by hypoesthesia, drowsiness, itching of the nose, mouth, and throat, slurred speech, incontinence, vomiting, and convulsions. Symptoms last 24 to 48 hours. Death may follow cardiovascular or respiratory failure. Mortality is less than 1%.

Bee, wasp, hornet, yellow jacket, and ant stings. All female Hymenoptera have an egg-laying organ (stinger) that can be used for defense or offense. The venom of bees, hornets, wasps, and yellow jackets contains four to six distinct chemical compounds, each of which can produce an allergic reaction. The venoms of all stinging Hymenoptera are closely related and therefore cross-sensitizing.

Local reactions include swelling, pain, erythema, urticaria, and pruritus. Generalized allergic reactions include nausea, vomiting, diarrhea, urticaria, pruritus, and anaphylaxis, with shortness of breath, tightness in the chest, difficulty swallowing, anxiety, convulsions, or unconsciousness. Delayed reaction (serum sickness) occurs 1 to 4 weeks after the sting and is characterized by fever, malaise, lymphadenopathy, rash, urticaria, and arthralgia.

Pathophysiology

The local or systemic response to injection of a venom occurs as a result of direct action of the venom on susceptible cells, IgE-mediated humoral immune response (type I), and immune complex humoral response (type III).

The arthropod or Hymenoptera venom is toxic to all humans. The biologically active venom works directly on susceptible cells (such as nerve cells and blood cells). The protein component of the venom may contain enzymes that cause cell lysis, histamine release, anticoagulation, or interference with neuromuscular transmission.

The IgE-mediated immune response occurs in people who are sensitive to the protein component of the venom, which acts as an antigen. These people have come in contact with the allergen in the past and have become sensitized rather than immunized. Sensitization triggers the synthesis of specific antiallergenic IgE antibodies. On subsequent contact with the allergen, the person responds with a type I immune reaction.

IgE immunoglobulins are bound to mast cells and basophils. Mast cells are found in all body tissues, close to blood vessels, and in abundance in the skin. Basophils circulate as leukocytes in the blood. Both mast cells and basophils contain potent pharmacologically active substances such as histamine, bradykinin, serotonin, and other vasoactive amines. The venom (antigen) becomes bound to the IgE on the surface of the cell, creating degranulation of the cell that releases the active agents. These mediators cause increased vascular permeability and smooth muscle contraction. Histamine seems to be the most important agent. Its release causes peripheral vasodilation, increased permeability of capillaries with subsequent loss of plasma from the circulation, smooth muscle constriction (as in the bronchi), and increased mucous gland secretion. If the agents remain confined to the area of the bite, the tissue reaction remains localized (local anaphylaxis) with tissue swelling, wheal formation, and itching. If the mediators are released systemically, systemic anaphylaxis (anaphylactic shock) may result. The widespread response to histamine release causes profound bronchoconstriction and vasodilation with subsequent circulatory collapse. The severity of the reaction depends on the amount of the sensitizing dose, the amount and distribution of the IgE antibodies, and the dose of toxin that causes the reaction.

A type III (immune complex) reaction, or serum sickness, can develop 1 to 3 weeks after the antigen is injected. The antigen initiates an immune response, and antibodies are formed. The response is mediated by IgG or IgM and complement. The immune complexes are deposited in joints, blood vessels, kidneys, and the heart. Platelet aggregation is caused by the collection of immune complexes and complement along blood vessel walls. Anaphylatoxins are released during activation of the complement system, causing a severe inflammatory response.

Diagnostic Studies and Findings

Physical Examination

Puncture wound with characteristic symptoms

Complete Blood Count

Eosinophilia in type I reaction

Direct Immunofluorescence

Presence of antigen, immunoglobulin, or complement in type III reaction

Medical Plan

Surgery

Skin grafting—split-thickness graft to close brown recluse spider bite

Medications

- For anaphylaxis
  - Bronchodilators
    - Epinephrine (Adrenalin), 1:1000 for allergic reactions, 0.3-0.5 ml subcutaneously or IM for mild or severe reactions repeated q5-20 min as needed; 0.1-0.2 ml subcutaneously injected into site to decrease absorption of antigen; 0.25-0.5 ml IV in 10 ml saline repeated in 5-10 min for severe anaphylaxis with cardiovascular involvement
    - Epinephrine 1:200 aqueous suspension, 0.3 ml subcutaneously; long-acting for severe reactions without cardiovascular involvement after edema has subsided
    - Aminophylline (Aminodur, Lixaminol, Phyllacontin, Somophyllin) for bronchospasm, 6 mg/kg IV over 10-20 min followed by 0.5 mg/kg/h IV
  - Antihistamines
    - Diphenhydramine (Benadryl), 50-100 mg IV
- Adrenergic agents
  - Isoproterenol (Isuprel, Proterenol), 1 mg diluted in 500 ml D5W infused at rate of 0.5-1 ml/min for myocardial insufficiency

Vasoconstrictors for prolonged hypotension
Norepinephrine (Levophed, Levarterenol), 8-12 μg/min IV of 4 μg/ml dilution, titrated
Metaraminol (Aramine), 15-100 mg/500 ml D5W IV, titrated, for adults; 0.4 mg/kg IV for children
Corticosteroids
Hydrocortisone, 100 mg IV for prolonged symptoms
Oral antihistamines
Diphenhydramine (Benadryl), 25-50 mg po qid for mild reaction
For toxins
Antivenin, 1 ampule IV in 10-50 ml saline for black widow and scorpion bites
Anticonvulsant muscle relaxants
Calcium gluconate 10% 10 ml IV slowly q4h
Methocarbamol (Delaxin, Forbaxin, Metho-500, Robaxin, others), 300 mg/min IV to total of 3 g/d
Orphenadrine (Flexon, Flexoject, Norflex, others), 60 mg IV q12h
For convulsions from scorpion bites
Phenobarbital, 30-60 mg/min IV up to 600 mg
Corticosteroids
Dexamethasone (Decadron, Hexadrol), 4 mg IM q6h for brown recluse spider bites during acute phase, then in decremental doses
Antihistamines
Diphenhydramine (Benadryl), 25-50 mg po qid
Anti-infective agents
Bacitracin or Neosporin applied tid or qid as topical antibiotic for brown recluse spider bite
Immunologic agents
Tetanus prophylaxis as indicated with tetanus toxoid, 0.5 ml IM
Intravenous infusion with D5W or lactated Ringer's solution

General Management

Scraping to remove stinger if present; do not squeeze or pinch, since retained venom sacs discharge residual venom
Application of meat tenderizer paste (containing proteolytic enzyme) to sting site
Hospitalization for observation or ventilator support

NURSING CARE

Nursing Assessment

Local Response

Presence or absence of stinger; pain; itching; edema; blister; ulceration; tissue necrosis

Systemic Response

Anxiety; feeling of doom; fever; malaise

Respiratory

Respiratory distress; tightness in chest; shortness of breath; wheezing; dyspnea

Cardiovascular

Tachycardia; bradycardia; hypotension; imperceptible pulse; pallor

Musculoskeletal

Cramping; pain; rigidity; weakness

Gastrointestinal

Nausea; vomiting; diarrhea; cramping; constipation

Skin

Flushing; diffuse erythema; urticaria; pruritus

Delayed Response

One to 4 weeks after sting: fever; malaise; lymphadenopathy; arthralgia; rash; urticaria

Psychosocial Concerns

Concern about body image as result of disfigurement, depending on severity of tissue damage; fear of insects, spiders, bees, and scorpions

Nursing Dx & Intervention

Nursing Diagnosis	Nursing Intervention/Rationale
Ineffective breathing pattern	• Assess for shortness of breath, wheezing, dyspnea. • Maintain airway. • In collaboration with physician, perform oropharyngeal suctioning as needed *to clear secretions*. • Provide oxygen by cannula or mask. • Position *for ease of respiration*. • Administer drugs as indicated *for control of symptoms*.
Decreased cardiac output; fluid volume deficit (1)	• Monitor vital signs *to detect circulatory compromise*. • Initiate intravenous line in collaboration with physician *to provide vascular access for fluids and medications*.

Nursing Diagnosis	Nursing Intervention/Rationale
	• Administer drugs as indicated *to control symptoms.*
Impaired skin integrity	• Apply meat tenderizer or paste *to neutralize venom.* • Apply ice packs *to decrease pain and swelling and to limit venom absorption.* • Keep patient quiet *to limit venom circulation.* • Remove stinger by scraping *to prevent further discharge of retained venom by squeezing.* • Remove tick; do not pull since head and mouth may remain embedded; apply heat to body and tick will back out, or cover with oil, which blocks its breathing and causes it to withdraw. • Clean bite with antiseptic *to prevent infection.* • Clean brown recluse bite with 1:20 Burow's solution *to prevent infection.*
Pain	• Assess for discomfort. • Apply ice packs to area *to reduce swelling.* • Apply meat tenderizer paste *to neutralize venom.*
Fear (of arachnids and Hymenoptera)	• Assess for defining characteristics. • Encourage patient to express fears. • Help patient develop preventive measures (see "Patient Education").
Body image disturbance	• Assess for presence of defining characteristics. • Encourage patient to express feelings about body, body appearance, or fear of reaction or rejection by others *to begin process of realistic self-evaluation.* • Reassure patient with disfiguring ulcer that skin grafting can improve appearance.

Patient Education

1. Instruct patients sensitive to stings to carry an emergency kit that has an antihistamine and epinephrine. Teach the patient or a family member or friend how to inject epinephrine.
2. Instruct patients who are sensitive to wear or carry medical alert information and identification.
3. Refer the patient to an allergist for desensitization.
4. Instruct the patient in the removal of ticks and stingers.
5. Instruct the patient and family in general preventive measures such as wearing protective clothing when outdoors, spraying areas of spider infestation with creosote every 2 months, inspecting clothing before putting it on in infested areas, and not wearing bright colors or scents that attract bees when outdoors.
6. Instruct the patient and family to keep the site of the bite clean by washing two or three times daily with warm soapy water or water with hydrogen peroxide; apply antibiotic ointment as needed.
7. Instruct the patient in changing the dressing if needed.

Evaluation

Patient Outcome	Data Indicating That Outcome is Reached
Local toxic reaction is minimized.	Stinger or tick is removed correctly, and treatment is initiated immediately. Areas of ulceration and necrosis are limited. Pain is alleviated.
Systemic response is avoided or resolved.	Cardiovascular, neurologic, musculoskeletal, or gastrointestinal symptoms are avoided or resolved. Respirations are regular and easy. Pulse rate is 60 to 100 and regular. Blood pressure is within patient's usual limits. Reflexes, sensation, and motion are intact. Patient has urinary continence and bowel function. There is no malaise, fever, lymphadenopathy, arthralgia, rash, or urticaria after delayed response.
Lesions heal.	Areas of necrosis, ulceration, and blistering reepithelialize. Skin is intact and free of infection.
Sensitized patients institute precautionary measures.	Patient carries medical alert information and identification. Patient carries emergency kit. Patient, family member, or friend demonstrates injection of epinephrine. Patient arranges to see allergist for desensitization.
Psychosocial concerns are addressed.	Patient expresses feelings about body appearance. Patient with disfiguring ulcer has opportunity to seek surgical interventions.

Lesions caused by beetles and caterpillars

Toxic reactions to beetles and caterpillars occur from contact with the toxin on the skin.

Blister beetles produce local irritation and blistering if they are crushed while on the skin surface. Damage to the beetle causes release of a toxic substance in the insect's body fluids.

More than 50 species of caterpillars possess spines that contain a venom capable of producing dermatitis on human skin. These caterpillars are widely distributed throughout the United States and Canada. Contact with the venom occurs from direct contact with the insect or its nest or from wind-blown hairs. Papular lesions or urticaria may develop at the site or elsewhere on the body. The venom produces a stinging sensation followed by swelling and erythema. Symptoms can occur systemically, depending on the species and the amount of venom the person receives. Painful and persistent nodules are formed if the toxin comes in contact with the conjunctiva.

Pathophysiology

The venom produces a direct toxic response to human tissue. The caterpillar's venom is biologically very active and causes histamine release, anticoagulation, fibrinolysis, and plasminogen activity. The toxins are capable of producing impaired cellular activity or cellular destruction.

Diagnostic Studies and Findings

Physical Examination

Lesion consistent with history of beetle or caterpillar contact

Medical Plan

Medications

Corticosteroids
- Topical corticosteroid for skin inflammation: hydrocortisone 1% applied tid
- Ophthalmic corticosteroid and analgesic for eye injury: cortisporin ophthalmic solution, 1-2 drops qid

NURSING CARE

Nursing Assessment

Local Reaction

Pain; swelling; blister; papule; urticaria; necrosis

Systemic Reaction

Widespread papular lesions; urticaria

Nursing Dx & Intervention

Nursing Diagnosis	Nursing Intervention/Rationale
Impaired skin integrity	• Assess for lesions. • Flush skin with copious amounts of water and scrub gently with soap and water *to remove toxin*. • Irrigate eye with copious amounts of normal saline *to remove toxin*.

Patient Education

1. Instruct the patient to avoid crushing beetles.
2. Teach the patient how to flush the skin and eye.
3. Teach the patient to keep the site clean by washing two or three times a day with soap and water.
4. Instruct the patient in the use of eye drops.

Evaluation

Patient Outcome	Data Indicating That Outcome is Reached
Lesions heal.	Urticaria, blisters, or papules resolve. Necrotic areas reepithelialize. Pain is alleviated. Skin is intact and free of infection. Eye symptoms or visual disturbances resolve.

Lesions caused by fleas, flies, and mosquitoes

Toxic reactions to fleas, flies, and mosquitoes occur as a result of saliva that is injected during feeding.

Fleas. Any of the human or domestic animal fleas will attack humans. Adult fleas are attracted to moving objects and leap to attack them. Thus flea bites are often found on the ankles or lower legs. The bites are characteristically found in groups of three on the ankles, legs, or waist. The flea penetrates the skin, feeds, and then crawls to a higher location until stopped by constrictive clothing.

A flea bite usually results in a small wheal with a hemorrhagic puncture at the center. In susceptible persons the flea bite produces larger wheals, urticaria, intensely pruritic papules, bullae, and small necrotic ulcers. Flea bites are usually harmless but can produce a severe reaction in sensitive persons.

Flies. There are innumerable biting flies in the United States. Most common are the blackflies, houseflies, deer flies, gadflies, and dog or stable flies. Most flies feed during the day or at dusk and attack in swarms on exposed parts of the body such as the face, neck, and arms. Fly-transmitted tularemia occurs in the central and western United States.

Fly bites are painful and pruritic for several days. Urticaria may occur as a result of a protein in the fly's saliva.

Mosquitoes. Mosquitoes are important because they transmit viral encephalitis, dengue fever, yellow fever, malaria, and filariasis. Lesions are produced on the skin when the mosquito feeds and deposits droplets of saliva. These lesions commonly occur on exposed areas of the hands, arms, face, and legs.

Mosquitoes are attracted by lights, dark clothing, and the presence of warm-blooded creatures. In most species the female mosquito is the bloodsucking biter.

The usual mosquito bite produces transient local irritation and pruritic erythematous papules. Large numbers of bites can produce intense pruritus. Urticaria and serum sickness can develop in sensitive people.

Pathophysiology

For an explanation of toxic reactions and antigen-antibody reactions see p. 515.

Diagnostic Studies and Findings

Physical Examination

Puncture wound with characteristic symptoms

Medical Plan

For treatment of systemic reactions see p. 515.

Medications

Corticosteroids
- Glucocorticoid ointment (e.g., hydrocortisone 1%) with 0.5% menthol and 0.5% phenol applied topically to lesions q1-2h

Anti-infective agents
- Topical antibiotics
  - Bacitracin or Neosporin applied qd or bid

NURSING CARE

Nursing Assessment

Local Response

Puncture wound with any of the following: pain, pruritus, wheal, urticaria, erythematous papule, bullae, or small necrotic ulcer; secondary infection: pain, swelling, tenderness, exudate

Systemic Response

See p. 516

Serum Sickness

Fever; malaise; lymphadenopathy; arthralgia; rash; urticaria

Nursing Dx & Intervention

Nursing Diagnosis	Nursing Intervention/Rationale
Impaired skin integrity	• Assess for lesion, pain, and pruritus. • Apply ice to puncture wound *to decrease pain and swelling.* • Trim patient's fingernails *to decrease damage and prevent secondary infection from scratching.* • Instruct patient in good hygiene and handwashing *to prevent secondary infection.*
Potential impaired skin integrity	• Instruct patient in personal and prophylactic environmental control; see "Patient Education."

Patient Education

1. Teach the patient how to keep the lesion clean by washing two or three times a day with soap and water.
2. Teach the patient how to change the dressing for infected lesions.
3. Instruct the patient in the correct use of appropriate insect repellents:
   a. For flies: repellent should contain at least 20% *N,N*-diethyl-*m*-toluamide; reapply every 1 to 2 hours or after swimming.
   b. For mosquitoes: repellent should contain at least 20% *N,N*-diethyl-*m*-toluamide, indalone, or dimethyl pthalate; reapply every 1 to 2 hours or after swimming.
4. Instruct the patient in controlling fleas in the environment and animals.
   a. Environment: apply dimpylate 1%, lindane 1%, malathion 3%, methoxychlor 5%, ronnel 1%, or trichlorfon 1% in kerosene; use according to instructions on container.
   b. Animals and furniture: dust with malathion 4% powder, rotenone 1% powder, or methoxychlor 10%; use according to instructions on container. Repeat procedure at 2-week intervals to eliminate newly hatching fleas.

Evaluation

Patient Outcome	Data Indicating That Outcome is Reached
Lesions heal.	Puncture wound resolves. Pain disappears. Skin is intact and free of infection.
Systemic responses resolve.	There is no fever, malaise, lymphadenopathy, arthralgia, rash, or urticaria. Cardiovascular, neurologic, gastrointestinal, and musculoskeletal symptoms are also resolved.
Patient takes precautionary measures and uses environmental control.	No new lesions occur.

DERMATITIS

Eczematous dermatitis

(Eczema)

Eczematous dermatitis is a superficial inflammation of the skin that is characterized by vesicles, redness, edema, oozing, crusting, scaling, and itching.

Eczematous dermatitis is a reaction pattern of the skin. Several forms of dermatitis occur, including primary contact dermatitis, allergic contact dermatitis, atopic dermatitis, diaper dermatitis, and seborrheic dermatitis. The common feature of the various forms is the breakdown of the epidermis, usually as a result of intracellular vesiculation. Eczematous dermatitis is the model for understanding the other forms of dermatitis.[36,70] The treatments are similar, and the nursing care is virtually the same. Individual differences are identified in the following discussion when appropriate.

Pathophysiology

Eczematous dermatitis can be classified as acute, subacute, or chronic. The skin responds to a wide variety of noxious stimuli with a limited number of changes, including vasodilation, edema of the upper dermis, inflammatory cell infiltration of the upper dermis and epidermis, and breakdown of epidermal cells. Vesicles or bullae form when fluid accumulates between epidermal cells (spongiosis) or when there are changes within the cell itself.

The result of this inflammatory process is a skin surface that is erythematous (from vasodilation), edematous, exudative, or eroded (from vesicle formation), and crusted or scabbed (from infection or an accumulation of serous exudate). Thickening and scaling occur from attempted or exaggerated repair efforts (hyperkeratosis or parakeratosis).

Table 5-1 summarizes the clinical features and changes occurring in eczematous dermatitis. Acute dermatitis becomes subacute as it heals, as a result of either treatment or natural repair processes. Subacute eczematous dermatitis can resolve or become chronic if exposure to noxious stimuli persists. Acute, subacute, and chronic eczematous dermatitis may occur simultaneously.

Diagnostic Studies and Findings

See discussions of contact dermatitis, atopic dermatitis, and seborrheic dermatitis.

Table 5-1
Clinical Features and Changes in Eczematous Dermatitis

	Acute	Subacute	Chronic
Clinical features	Erythema; exudate; weeping vesicles; crusts; pruritus	Less erythema; involuting vesicles; excoriation; some scaling; pruritus	Dryness; scaling; lichenification; pruritus
Microscopic changes	Vasodilation; edema; inflammatory infiltrates; spongiotic vesicles	Less vasodilation, inflammatory infiltrates, and vesiculation; parakeratosis; hyperkeratosis; acanthosis	Hyperkeratosis; no frank vesicles; acanthosis

Table 5-2
Summary of Treatments for Eczematous Dermatitis

	Acute	Subacute	Chronic
Chemotherapeutic	Antihistamines; systemic corticosteroids; topical corticosteroids (water miscible); topical antibacterials; topical antifungals	Topical corticosteroids in emollient base	Keratolytic agents; tars; topical corticosteroids
Supportive	Wet dressings (Burow's, saline, or tap water)	Oil-in-water compresses; emollient creams	Oil soaks or compresses; occlusive dressings; hydration

Physical Examination

Characteristic eruption; history congruent with specific forms of eczematous dermatitis

Medical Plan

Table 5-2 summarizes the specific treatment measures for the different classes of eczematous dermatitis.

Medications

- Antipruritic agents
  - Antihistamines
    - Cyproheptadine (Cyproheptadine, Periactin), 12-16 mg/d po in divided doses
    - Trimeprazine (Temaril), 2.5 mg po qid
  - Antianxiety agents
    - Hydroxyzine (Atarax, Vistaril), 25-100 mg po tid or qid
- Corticosteroids
  - Systemic
    - Prednisone, 40-80 mg po in divided doses; dosage depends on severity of condition
  - Topical
    - Hydrocortisone (Cort-Dome, others) 1% tid or qid
    - Betamethasone valerate (Valisone) 0.1% tid or qid
- Anti-infective agents
  - Systemic—for secondary infection; specific drug and dosage depends on infecting organism and severity of condition
  - Topical antibacterials
    - Bacitracin or Neosporin applied tid or qid
  - Topical antifungals
    - Nystatin (Mycostatin, Nilstat, others), miconazole (Monistat-Derm), or clotrimazole (Lotrimin, Mycelex), applied bid
- Keratolytics
  - Salicylic acid, 3%-5% added to topical corticosteroid
  - Urea 10%-20% added to topical corticosteroids

General Management (see pp. 564 to 565)

- Wet Burow's dressings, saline, and plain water dressings
- Occlusive dressings
- Oil-in-water compresses
- Hydration

NURSING CARE

Nursing Assessment

Eruption

Clinical features as described in Table 5-1

Secondary Infection

Purulent drainage; fever; tenderness; regional lymphadenopathy

Psychosocial Concerns

Concern with body image; inability to sleep because of pruritus

Nursing Dx & Intervention

Nursing Diagnosis	Nursing Intervention/Rationale
Impaired skin integrity	• Assess for characteristics of lesions (Table 5-1). • Instruct patient in handwashing and good hygiene *to prevent secondary infection.* • Instruct patient to cut fingernails short *to decrease trauma and secondary infection.* • Apply dressings: wet, oil, or occlusive, as indicated (see pp. 564 to 565). • Scrub crusted lesions gently with antibacterial soap *to debride.* • Establish realistic therapeutic regimen with patient *to alleviate patient's frustration.* • Instruct patient in use of medications.
Patient problem: pruritus	• Assess for discomfort. • Apply cool compresses for wet skin or oil compresses for dry skin *to soothe itching and discomfort.* • Instruct patient in use of antipruritics *to relieve itching.*
Body image disturbance	• Assess patient's perception of personal appearance. • Encourage patient to express feelings about body, body appearance, or fear of reaction or rejection by others *to begin process of realistic self-evaluation.* • Encourage development of other interests *so skin condition does not become focal point of patient's existence.*

Patient Education

1. Instruct the patient in the application of compresses, soaks, and scrubs using aseptic technique.
2. Instruct the patient in the use and side effects of medications.
3. Inform the patient and family that successful therapy requires patience, that therapy may be long term, and that results may not be immediate.
4. Teach the patient the signs and symptoms of secondary infection and to seek medical treatment if they occur.

Evaluation

Patient Outcome	Data Indicating That Outcome is Reached
Eruption improves.	Erythema, exudate, crusts, dryness, scaling, and pruritus are decreased. Excoriated areas reepithelialize.
Pruritus is alleviated.	There are fewer areas of excoriation. Patient is able to sleep.
Secondary infection is avoided.	Lesions heal without purulent exudate. Temperature is normal.
Patient evaluates his or her appearance in a realistic manner.	Patient engages in usual activities and relationships.

Contact dermatitis

Contact dermatitis is an acute or chronic inflammation of the skin caused by external factors (primary irritant dermatitis) or specific sensitizers (allergic contact dermatitis).

Contact dermatitis is a form of eczematous dermatitis (see p. 520). Primary irritant dermatitis is caused by irritation from various chemical and biologic substances, including acids, alkalies, solvents, detergents, oils, salts, secretions, and excretions. Chronic hand dermatitis ("housewife's eczema") and industrial dermatoses are common primary irritant dermatoses. The degree of irritation depends on the physical and chemical characteristics of the substance and the degree and time of exposure. The amount of inflammation varies from person to person and depends on factors such as race, degree and pH of perspiration, type of skin, preexisting disease, and family history. People with little skin pigmentation are more susceptible to the effects of irritants.

Allergic contact dermatitis is a manifestation of delayed hypersensitivity. The allergen is an environmental substance to which the person has become sensitized. Genetically predisposed people and those who have had a previous episode of allergic contact dermatitis are more likely to experience episodes of the disorder. The most common causes of allergic contact dermatitis are chemicals that have a high sensitizing index, including certain plants (tulips and chrysanthemums), plant oils (poison ivy, oak, and sumac), nickel, chrome, rubber, and paraphenylenediamine (an ingredient in many dyes).

The severity of the reaction depends on how long and frequent the contact is. Since allergic contact dermatitis is enhanced by friction and pressure, the addition of these factors to simple exposure produces a more severe reaction.

Pathophysiology

The irritating substances of primary irritant dermatitis cause damage to the stratum corneum, alter its elasticity, and change the physical features of the skin's lipid film. This impairs the barrier function of the skin and allows absorption of the irritating substance and the subsequent changes of eczematous dermatitis. The basic features of primary irritant dermatitis are the same as those of eczematous dermatitis (see pp. 520 to 521). The condition can be acute, subacute, or chronic. Primary irritant dermatitis is frequently complicated by secondary bacterial infection.

Allergic contact dermatitis is a cell-mediated, type IV immune response (see Chapter 14). The sensitizing chemical (hapten) enters the epidermis through the stratum corneum and combines with epidermal proteins to form a new molecule (hapten-protein or hapten-carrier complex) that has antigenic potential. This molecule enters the local cutaneous lymphoid tissue, where specific committed lymphocytes are developed and selectively directed against the antigen. Subsequent exposure to the hapten results in release of the committed lymphocytes around the capillary endothelial cells with the development of inflammation and eczematous dermatitis.

Nursing Dx & Intervention

See p. 522.

Diagnostic Studies and Findings

Physical Examination

Characteristic history of contact with irritating or sensitizing substance; detailed history essential

Patch Test (see Part Two)

Usually positive to allergen in allergic contact dermatitis; should not be performed if patient has active acute dermatitis

Medical Plan

Management is directed toward identification and elimination of the precipitating factor (see also p. 522).

NURSING CARE

Nursing Assessment

Eruption

Erythema; exudate; vesicles; crusts; scaling; dryness; lichenification; pruritus; location and distribution of eruption; history of eruption; site of initial eruption; history of contact with irritating or sensitizing substances; pattern of flare-ups

Secondary Infection

Purulent drainage; fever; tenderness; regional lymphadenopathy

Psychosocial Concerns

Concern with body image; inability to sleep

Patient Education

1. Instruct the patient to eliminate or avoid the precipitating factors (also see p. 522).

Evaluation

Patient Outcome	Data Indicating That Outcome is Reached
Precipitating factor is identified and avoided.	There are no recurrent episodes of dermatitis.

Atopic dermatitis

Atopic dermatitis is a chronic, superficial, pruritic, inflammatory response of the skin that is often associated with other atopic diseases (asthma, hay fever, and allergic rhinitis).

Atopy refers to a type I immunologic response that is hereditary (see Chapter 14). Patients with atopic dermatitis usually have high serum levels of IgE. Patients with atopic dermatitis experience vasomotor changes, great susceptibility to environmental irritants, and susceptibility to bacterial and viral infections. Atopic dermatitis is associated with ichthyosis and xerosis and with numerous abnormalities of humoral and cell-mediated immunity.

Patients with atopic dermatitis have dry, highly sensitive skin with a lowered threshold to pruritus, so that a minor stimulus causes exaggerated itching. Scratching leads to epidermal breakdown and damage to nerve endings, which in turn increase the itch sensation. This itch-scratch cycle is characteristic of atopic dermatitis.

Atopic dermatitis can begin at any time. There are usually three phases: an infantile phase (3 or 4 months to 2 years of age), the childhood phase (4 to 10 or 12 years), and the adolescent and young adult phase. The condition gradually improves.

This section addresses only the adolescent and young adult phase.

Pathophysiology

The disease is the result of a type I immunologic response. The findings are the same as those of eczematous dermatitis and may be acute, subacute, or chronic (see discussion of eczematous dermatitis).

There is a great tendency toward vasoconstriction of superficial blood vessels, decreased response to cooling and warmth, increased sweat production in flexor areas, and a blanch phenomenon on stroking (white dermographism). Cold and low humidity are poorly tolerated. Heat and high humidity are also poorly tolerated; vasodilation increases the inflammatory response, thereby aggravating the dermatitis and causing increased itching. Psychologic and emotional factors do not play a causative role but do modify symptoms. Food allergies may exacerbate the skin disease in some patients, and a good history is extremely important.

Diagnostic Studies and Findings

Physical Examination

Characteristic eruption with typical distribution; personal or family history of allergies

Immunofluorescence

Serum IgE may be elevated

Medical Plan

Atopic dermatitis presents the whole range of the eczematous process from acute to chronic, and treatment must be directed accordingly. The focus of therapy is to interrupt the itch-scratch cycle.

Medications

- Adolescent and young adult phases
  - Corticosteroids
    - Topical steroids with menthol or camphor 0.25%-0.5% applied bid or tid
    - Systemic
      - Prednisone (Deltasone, Orasone, others), 60-80 mg/d as single morning dose for 1-2 wk
  - Keratolytics
    - Coal tar 2% (Alphosyl, Tar-Doak) applied topically at bedtime
  - Antihistamines
    - Diphenhydramine (Benadryl), 25-50 mg po tid or qid
    - Tripelennamine (Pyribenzamine, PBZ), 100 mg po bid or tid
  - Anti-infective agents
    - Systemic antibiotics for secondary infection; drug and dosage dependent on causative organism and severity of infection

General Management

- Burow's dressings and saline compresses (see pp. 564 and 565)
- Oatmeal and oil baths (see pp. 564 and 565)
- Occlusive dressings (see pp. 564 and 565)
- Allergy diet (controversial)[23,61,70]
- House humidified
- Light, cotton clothing

NURSING CARE

Nursing Assessment

Eruption

Lichenification; excoriation; subacute papular eruptions; generalized erythema; pruritus

Location

Face; neck; upper chest; flexor surfaces; wrists, feet; upper back; generalized

Special Disease Manifestations

Chronic hand eczema; nummular eczema

Secondary Infection

Purulent drainage; fever; tenderness; regional lymphadenopathy

Psychosocial Concerns

Concern with body image; inability to sleep because of pruritus; exacerbations caused by stress

Patient Education

1. Teach the patient and family that the patient should avoid:
   a. Heat, high humidity, and rapid changes of temperature
   b. Sweating
   c. Excessive bathing
   d. Strong soaps and detergents that can irritate skin
   e. Emotional stress
   f. Wools, coarse synthetic fabrics, and tight-fitting clothing
   g. Primary irritants
2. Teach the patient and family that the patient should:
   a. Keep skin well lubricated
   b. Wear light, loose, cotton clothing that "breathes"
   c. Bathe in lukewarm, not hot, water
3. Teach the patient and family the signs and symptoms of secondary infection and to seek medical attention if they occur.
4. Explain to the patient and family that therapy requires patience and results may not be immediate.
5. Teach the adolescent/young adult to manage the skin condition as soon as possible.

Nursing Dx & Intervention

See p. 522.

Evaluation

Patient Outcome	Data Indicating That Outcome is Reached
Known causative agents are avoided.	Eruption subsides. Exacerbations are limited.
Pruritus is relieved.	Scratching decreases. Excoriations heal. Patient is able to sleep.
Secondary infection is avoided.	Eruption is free from tenderness and purulent exudate. There is no fever or lymphadenopathy.
Patient assesses appearance in realistic manner.	Patient engages in usual relationships and activities when possible.

 Seborrheic dermatitis

Seborrheic dermatitis is a chronic, recurrent, erythematous scaling eruption that is localized in areas where sebaceous glands are concentrated.

In infants, seborrheic dermatitis may develop on the scalp, back, and intertriginous and diaper areas. The scalp lesions are scaling, adherent, thick, yellow, and crusted. Lesions elsewhere are erythematous, scaling, and fissured.

After puberty lesions tend to occur in the scalp, eyebrows, eyelids, nasolabial areas, postauricular areas, and presternal and intertriginous areas (Figure 5-7). Lesions may be mild or severe and vary from dry, greasy scales to erythema, excoriation, and crusting. Secondary bacterial or fungal infection may occur. Genetic factors seem to affect the incidence and severity of the disease. The disorder is worse during the winter months.

Pathophysiology

The cause of seborrheic dermatitis is unknown. Histologic changes include vasodilation and discharge of inflammatory cells into the epidermis from the capillary loops. Epidermal inflammation and eczema may be present. Scales are produced as a result of an increased mitotic rate and an accumulation of corneocytes. Despite the name, the composition, production, and flow of sebum are normal.

Diagnostic Studies and Findings

Physical Examination

Characteristic lesions and distribution

Figure 5-7 Seborrheic dermatitis.
Courtesy of Stephen B. Tucker, M.D., Department of Dermatology, University of Texas Health Science Center at Houston.

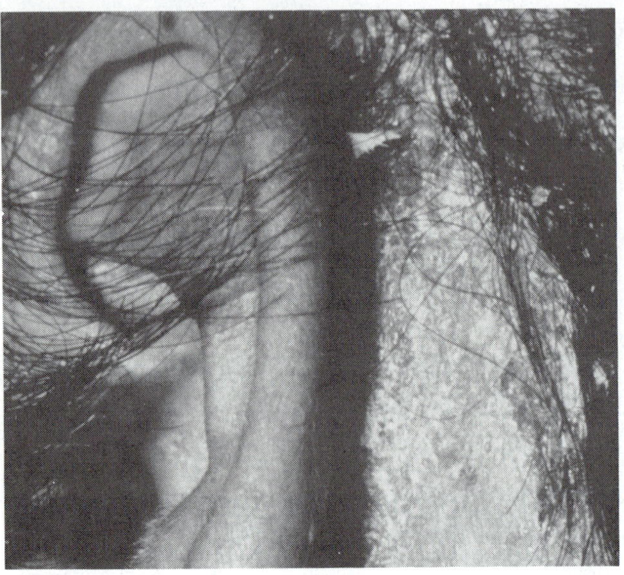

Medical Plan

Medications

Corticosteroids
- Topical
  - Hydrocortisone (Cort-Dome, others) 0.1% bid or tid in nonhairy areas
  - Betamethasone (Valisone) 0.05% bid in hairy areas

Antiseborrheic shampoos
- Zinc pyrithione 1%-2% (Head & Shoulders) qd
- Selenium sulfide (Selsun suspension) qd

Anti-infective agents
- Topical antibiotics for secondary infection
  - Neomycin 0.1% bid or tid
  - Chloramphenicol (Chloromycetin cream) 0.1% bid or tid

Keratolytics
- Salicylic acid 1%-3% topically bid
- Precipitated sulfur 1%-5% topically bid
- Tar cream 4% topically bid

General Management

Oils—castor, mineral, and olive, rubbed into scalp lesions and left overnight
Frequent shampooing
Burow's solution for weeping lesions

NURSING CARE

Nursing Assessment

Eruption

Erythema; scaling; fissures; inflammation; pruritus

Secondary Infection

Purulent discharge; fever; tenderness; increased inflammation; regional lymphadenopathy

Psychosocial Concerns

Concern about body image

Nursing Dx & Intervention

Nursing Diagnosis	Nursing Intervention/Rationale
Impaired skin integrity	• Assess for characteristics and distribution of lesions. • Instruct patient in use of medications and topical preparations. • Instruct patient to shampoo daily *to alleviate scaling and crusting*. • Instruct patient not to scratch or rub lesions, *since that will prolong course of disease*.
Body image disturbance	• Assess for defining characteristics. • Encourage patient to express feelings about body, body appearance, or fear of reaction or rejection by others *to begin process of realistic self-evaluation*. • Assure patient that treatment can be successful.

Patient Education

1. Instruct the patient in the use of medications and preparations.
2. Explain the care regimen to the patient.
3. Instruct the patient in the signs and symptoms of secondary infection and to seek medical care if they occur.
4. Instruct the patient to avoid external irritants, excessive heat, and excessive perspiration.

Evaluation

Patient Outcome	Data Indicating That Outcome is Reached
Eruption resolves.	Erythema and inflammation disappear. Scaling decreases. Fissures heal. Pruritus is relieved. Skin is intact.
Secondary infection is resolved or prevented.	There is no purulent discharge, fever, or lymphadenopathy.
Patient evaluates his or her appearance in a realistic manner.	Patient engages in usual activities and relationships.

Herpes Zoster

Herpes zoster is an acute cutaneous vesicular eruption caused by the varicella-zoster virus.

Herpes zoster, also known as shingles, occurs in approximately 3% of the population.[32] The condition results from reactivation of a dormant varicella virus. Reactivation can occur at any time. Older adults are more likely to develop the condition because of their diminishing immunologic functioning.

The eruption is generally limited to the skin of a single dermatome, although one or two adjacent dermatomes may be involved. Pain, itching, and burning along the dermatome precede the eruption by 4 to 5 days. The pain is often mistaken for pleurisy, myocardial infarction, or appendicitis, and diagnosis may be difficult until the characteristic eruption occurs. The eruption begins with erythematous plaques of various size that involve all or part of a dermatome. Purulent, fluid-filled vesicles arise in clusters from the erythematous base. Successive crops continue to appear for 7 days. The vesicles either involute or rupture and then heal in 10 to 14 days, frequently with residual scarring.

Postherpetic neuralgia, the most common complication, is a dermatomal pain syndrome that persists beyond the time of complete cutaneous healing. Pain can persist in a dermatome for months or years after the lesions have disappeared. Most cases do resolve in a few months. The pain is often severe, intractable, and exhausting. The incidence of postherpetic neuralgia increases with the age of the patient.

Pathophysiology

Herpes zoster occurs as a result of reactivation of the varicella virus that entered the cutaneous nerves during an earlier episode of acute infection with the virus. The virus remains dormant in the sensory root ganglia for the lifetime of the patient and can be reactivated at any time. Reactivation can be triggered by local trauma, acute illness, a compromised immunologic state, fatigue, emotional upsets, or chronic debilitation. Once reactivated the virus travels down the sensory nerve and infects the skin of the affected ganglion.

Diagnostic Studies and Findings

Physical Examination

Characteristic lesion: clusters of painful, itching vesicles along a single dermatome

Cytologic Smear

Direct identification of multinucleated cells

Culture

Vesicular fluid to determine presence of virus

Medical Plan

Medications

- Analgesic agents
  - ASA (Aspirin), 300 mg po q4h for mild pain
  - Acetaminophen (Tylenol, Datril), 250 mg po q4h for mild pain
  - Codeine po in dosages sufficient for more severe pain relief during eruptive phase or for postherpetic neuralgia
- Tranquilizers
  - Chlorpromazine (Thorazine), 25 mg po qid for severe postherpetic neuralgia
- Antiviral agents
  - Acyclovir (Zovirax), 400-800 mg po 5 times/d for 7-10 d during eruptive phase
- Systemic steroids
  - During eruptive phase for prevention of postherpetic neuralgia; use is controversial[32,61]
  - Prednisone, 20 mg po tid for 7 d, followed by 20 mg po bid for 7 d, followed by 20 mg each morning for 7 d

General Management

- Cryosurgery (for postherpetic neuralgia)
  - Affected area sprayed with refrigerant (freon, Frigiderm) until blanching occurs, repeated every 2 weeks for three to six treatments; if relief occurs, it is rapid and limited to specific area treated; produces relief in about 50% of affected patients[32]

NURSING CARE

Nursing Assessment

Lesions (Eruptive Phase)

Location and characteristics; crusting; scarring with healing

Secondary Infection (Eruptive Phase)

Erythema, swelling, purulent drainage from lesions

Discomfort (Eruptive Phase)

Pain, burning, itching of lesions; intensity

Discomfort (Postherpetic Phase)

Intensity and location; interference with activity

Nursing Dx & Intervention

Nursing Diagnosis	Nursing Intervention/Rationale
Impaired skin integrity	• Assess for lesion characteristics and location. • Apply wet compresses with Burow's solution for 20 minutes three times a day *to macerate vesicles, remove serum and crust, and suppress bacterial growth.* • Assess for secondary infection from scratching. • Trim fingernails short *to prevent secondary infection.*
Pain	• Assess for pain, itching, and burning during eruptive phase. • Assess for pain during postherpetic phase. • As physician directs, provide analgesic medications. • Provide empathy, understanding, and emotional support for patient with persistent pain. • Investigate alternate means of pain management with patient and physician, e.g., biofeedback, transcutaneous nerve stimulation.

Patient Education

1. Instruct patient in course of disease process.
2. Instruct in correct use of analgesics.
3. Instruct in application of wet compresses with Burow's solution (p. 564).

Evaluation

Patient Outcome	Data Indicating That Outcome is Reached
Eruption improves.	Lesions resolve; secondary infection does not occur.
Pruritus is alleviated.	Areas of excoriation resolve or do not occur.
Pain is relieved.	Patient is able to resume usual activities without fear of triggering paroxysms of pain.
Patient successfully manages intractable pain.	Patient engages in usual activities and maintains interpersonal relationships; is not withdrawn or suicidal.

Ichthyosis

Ichthyosis is a common inherited keratinization disorder that is characterized by varying degrees of dryness, scaling, and exfoliation.

Several genetic keratinization abnormalities result in dry, scaly skin. The most common condition is ichthyosis vulgaris, an autosomal dominant inherited disease that occurs in 1 in 1000 people. The other forms of ichthyosis are rarer.

Pathophysiology

In ichthyosis vulgaris the mitotic rate is decreased and the stratum corneum fails to desquamate normally. The granular layer is reduced or absent, and sweat and sebaceous glands may be reduced. The follicular orifices are hyperkeratotic and are often plugged with keratin. The ability of the stratum corneum to retain water is decreased. Aggravation during the winter months and improvement during the summer are common. The other forms of ichthyosis show similar pathologic changes.

Table 5-3 summarizes the clinical, pathologic, and genetic features of the four patterns of inherited ichthyosis (Figure 5-8).

Table 5-3
Summary of Ichthyosis Disorders

Disorder	Inheritance Pattern	Age of Onset	Prognosis	Histopathology	Type Scale	Distribution
Vulgaris	Dominant	Childhood (1 to 4 years)	Improves during adult years	Increased mitotic rate; retained stratum corneum; decreased granular layer; plugged follicular orifices	Fine, small, thin, light	Back and extensor surfaces; flexures spared; increased markings on palms and soles
Male, sex-linked	Recessive X-linked	Birth	Persistent	As above; increased plugging	Large, brown	Neck and trunk; total extremities; flexures spared; normal markings
Lamellar nonbullous	Recessive	Birth	Persistent	Increased mitotic rate; granular layer present; acanthosis; hyperkeratosis; plugged follicular orifices	Large, coarse, yellow, raised corners	Generalized; thick palms and soles
Bullous epidermolytic hyperkeratoses	Dominant	Birth	Persistent; very severe forms may cause death in early infancy from secondary infection	As above; vacuolation of epidermal cells	Thick, gray-brown, coarse, warty, vesicular, and bullous lesions	Patchy or generalized; flexures affected

Diagnostic Studies and Findings

Physical Examination

Characteristic lesion

Medical Plan

Medications

- Emollients (apply to moist skin bid after bathing)
  - Propylene glycol 40%-50%
  - Propylene glycol 60%, ethanol 2%, and salicylic acid 6% in gel base under occlusive dressing for 1-4 d and then every third night
  - Hydrophilic petrolatum
  - Water-miscible bath oil
- Keratolytics (apply after bathing to moist skin or 3-7 times/wk)
  - Salicylic acid 5% in emollient base
  - Urea 10% in water-miscible base
  - Sodium chloride 10% and salicylic acid 5%
- Vitamins
  - Tretinoin (Retin-A) 0.1% (vitamin A, retinoic acid), applied topically for lamellar ichthyosis
  - Oral synthetic retinoids, still under testing[15,24]

Figure 5-8 Lamellar ichthyosis.
Courtesy of Stephen B. Tucker, M.D., Department of Dermatology, University of Texas Health Science Center at Houston.

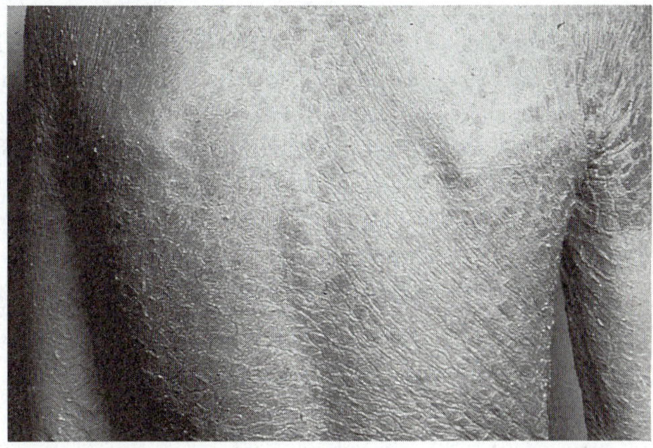

NURSING CARE

Nursing Assessment

Lesions

Type of scale and distribution as in Table 5-3; severity

Secondary Infection

Redness; tenderness; swelling; exudate; odor

Comfort and Mobility

Discomfort from dry, cracked skin; limitation on mobility

Psychosocial Concerns

Concern about body image

Nursing Dx & Intervention

Nursing Diagnosis	Nursing Intervention/Rationale
Impaired skin integrity	• Assess for distribution and severity of lesions. • Instruct patient and parent in use of topical preparations. • Stress importance of good hygiene *to prevent secondary infection.*
Chronic pain; impaired physical mobility	• Instruct patient in use of emollients *to decrease dryness.* • Instruct patient not to use soap or to use it sparingly while bathing *to prevent drying and cracking of skin.* • Instruct patient to maintain humidity in living environment *to prevent drying and cracking of skin.*
Body image disturbance	• Assess patient's or parents' perception of patient's appearance. • Encourage patient to express feelings about body, body appearance, and fear of reaction or rejection by others *to begin process of realistic self-evaluation.* • Encourage patient to develop interests and other attributes *to support positive self-image, feelings of self-worth, and self-confidence.* • Help patient evaluate appearance in a realistic manner *so it does not become focal point of existence.* • Inform parents that condition may improve as child matures.

Patient Education

1. Instruct the patient and family in the use of emollients and keratolytics.
2. Instruct the patient in the signs and symptoms of secondary infection and to seek medical care if they occur.
3. Inform the patient and family that successful therapy requires the patient's full cooperation and patience, that therapy is long term, and that results may not be immediate.

Evaluation

Patient Outcome	Data Indicating That Outcome is Reached
Dryness decreases.	Discomfort is relieved. Cracks and fissures improve. Limitations on mobility lessen.
Secondary infection is avoided.	There is no redness, tenderness, swelling, or purulent exudate.
Patient makes successful adaptations in self-concept.	Patient develops interests and participates in activities compatible with degree of mobility. Patient engages in satisfying relationships. Patient does not use disorder as excuse for unsuccessful relationships.

Lichen Planus

Lichen planus is a chronic pruritic inflammatory eruption of the skin and mucous membrane. It is characterized by small angular papules that may combine to form larger plaques.

Lichen planus occurs most frequently in adults. The onset may be gradual or abrupt. The average duration of the disease is 15 to 24 months, but it may persist or recur for years. Healing is followed by residual pigmentation that eventually fades.

Pathophysiology

The cause of lichen planus is unknown. However, certain drugs and chemicals used in developing color photographs can cause an eruption.

Inflammation occurs primarily at the dermal level with lymphocytic infiltrate. There are hyperkeratosis and prominence of the granular layer. Vacuolation, degeneration, and inflammatory changes occur in the basal layer. Fibrin and IgM are deposited in the papillary dermis.

Cutaneous lesions are pruritic, flat-topped, reddish violet, angular papules that are 0.5 to 5 mm in diameter. The papules have a sheen on cross-lighting. Whitish gray lines (Wickham's striae) are seen on the skin. The individual papules can combine to form larger plaques, becoming more scaly and verrucous. The lesions are usually symmetrically distributed and occur most commonly on the flexor surfaces of the wrist, forearm, and ankles and on the abdomen and sacrum. The face, palms, and soles are rarely affected. Eruption can occur at the site of minor trauma (Köbner's phenomenon).

Lesions of the buccal mucosa are present in 50% to 60% of the cases. These gray lacy lesions may ulcerate and be painful. Malignant degeneration occurs in about 1 in 100 cases.

Clinical variants of lichen planus include annular, bullous, hypertrophic, and atrophic lesions. Nails can be involved, with pitting, thinning, and increase in longitudinal ridging. In severe cases the nail may be shed completely.

Diagnostic Studies and Findings

Physical Examination

Characteristic lesion

Biopsy

Characteristic histologic changes

Immunofluorescence

IgG deposits in papillary dermis

Medical Plan

Medications

- Corticosteroids
  - Topical
    - Hydrocortisone (Cort-Dome, others) 0.1% or triamcinolone (Aristocort, Kenalog, others) 0.1% in occlusive dressing at bedtime; must be maintained until all signs of lesions disappear
    - Triamcinolone 0.1% in dental paste (Kenalog in Orabase) applied q3-5h for mouth lesions
  - Intralesional injection
    - Triamcinolone (Aristocort, Kenalog), 5 mg/ml (see p. 567)
  - Systemic corticosteroids for very severe or generalized lesions
    - Prednisone, 40-60 mg/d po, then decreasing doses
- Vitamins
  - Tretinoin (Retin-A) 0.1% applied with cotton-tipped applicator at night followed by triamcinolone 0.1% tid
- Local anesthetics
  - Viscous lidocaine (Xylocaine) mouth swish before meals
- Antipruritics
  - Anti-anxiety agents
    - Hydroxyzine (Atarax, Orgatrax, Vistaril), 25-100 mg po tid or qid
  - Antihistamines
    - Cyproheptadine (Cyproheptadine, Periactin), 4 mg po tid
    - Terfenadine (Seldane), 60 mg po bid

General Management

Withdrawal of all current medications and replacement with substitutes

NURSING CARE

Nursing Assessment

Lesion

Angular papules; bullous, hypertrophic, and atrophic lesions; coalesced plaques, mucosal plaques, or ulceration; distribution of lesions

Discomfort

Pruritus; pain from buccal ulceration

Nutrition

Inability to eat because of buccal ulceration

Psychosocial Concerns

Concern with body image

Nursing Dx & Intervention

Nursing Diagnosis	Nursing Intervention/Rationale
Impaired skin integrity	• Assess for location and characteristics of lesions. • Instruct patient in good hygiene and need for short fingernails *to prevent secondary infection.*

Nursing Diagnosis	Nursing Intervention/Rationale
	• Apply cool compresses *to relieve itching.* • Instruct patient in use of occlusive dressing (see p. 564) *to promote healing.*
Altered oral mucous membrane	• Instruct patient in use of viscous lidocaine (Xylocaine): 15 minutes before eating, swish in mouth *to promote comfort.* • Instruct patient to avoid astringent and acidic fluids *to avoid tissue trauma.* • Provide mouth care with alkaline or saline mouthwash *to promote comfort and prevent infection.*
Pain	• Assess for discomfort. • Provide soft diet *to prevent mechanical irritation.* • Provide bland foods *to prevent mechanical irritation.*
Body image disturbance	• Assess patient's perception of his or her appearance. • Encourage patient to express feelings about body, body appearance, or fear of reaction or rejection by others *to begin process of realistic self-evaluation.*

Patient Education

1. Instruct the patient in the treatment regimen, medications, and dressings.
2. Instruct the patient in the side effects of medications.
3. Teach the patient the signs and symptoms of secondary infection and to seek medical treatment if they occur.
4. Discuss the long-term nature of the disorder and the fact that treatment requires persistence and patience.
5. Instruct the patient to avoid precipitating drugs and chemicals.

Evaluation

Patient Outcome	Data Indicating That Outcome is Reached
Eruption improves.	Papules, bullae, and plaques resolve. Ulcerations reepithelialize. Pruritus resolves. Secondary infection does not occur.
Discomfort from buccal lesions is alleviated.	Patient is able to eat and does not lose weight.
Pruritus is alleviated.	Areas of excoriation resolve or do not recur.
Patient evaluates appearance in realistic manner.	Patient engages in usual activities and relationships.

PIGMENTED DISORDERS

Pigmented nevi, blue nevi, and mongolian spots

Pigmented nevi, blue nevi, and mongolian spots are benign skin lesions that are caused by accumulation of pigment in the dermis.

Pigmented nevi occur in various forms that vary in size and degree of pigmentation. Nevi are present on most persons and may occur anywhere on the body. They may be flat, slightly raised, dome shaped, smooth, rough, or hairy. Their color ranges from tan, gray, and shades of brown to black.

The blue nevus usually occurs as a single nodular lesion on the dorsal surface of the hands, face, or buttocks. The nevus is present at birth and remains unchanged through life.

Mongolian spots have a dusky blue color and blend into the surrounding normal skin. The spots occur primarily in Oriental and dark-skinned infants, usually in the lumbosacral area. The spots vary in diameter from 1 cm to several centimeters. They cause no symptoms and usually disappear during childhood.

Pathophysiology

The lesions occur as the result of nevus cells that migrate to the dermis during embryonic development. The nevus cells have the same origin as melanocytes and are closely asso-

Table 5-4
Features and Occurrence of Various Types of Pigmented Nevi

Type	Features	Occurrence	Comments
Halo nevus	Sharp, oval, or circular; depigmented halo around mole; may undergo many morphologic changes; usually disappears and halo repigments (may take years)	Usually on back in young adult	Usually benign; biopsy indicated because same process can occur around melanoma
Intradermal nevus	Dome shaped; raised; flesh to black color; may be pedunculated or hair bearing	Cells limited to dermis	No indication for removal other than cosmetic
Junction nevus	Flat or slightly elevated; dark brown	Nevus cells lining dermoepidermal junction	Should be removed if exposed to repeated trauma
Compound nevus	Slightly elevated brownish papule: indistinct border	Nevus cells in dermis and lining dermoepidermal junction	Should be removed if exposed to repeated trauma
Hairy nevus	May be present at birth; may cover large area; hair growth occurring after several years		Should be removed if changes occur

ciated with them. The nevus cells contain melanin pigment, which gives the lesions their color. The blue color of the blue nevus and the mongolian spots is caused by the concentration of melanin and its depth below the epidermis.

Table 5-4 summarizes the features of the various types of pigmented nevi.

Diagnostic Studies and Findings

Physical Examination

Characteristic lesion

Biopsy

Shows histologic configuration

Malignant Changes

Some changes in preexisting nevi may indicate malignancy. Moles that exhibit any of the following changes or irregularities should receive medical evaluation:

- Change in color, size, or thickness
- Bleeeding or crusting
- Formation of a depigmented halo around the nevus
- Notching or indentation of the border with pigment streaming from the eye
- Various shades of brown and black plus red, white, or blue and the half tones of pink or gray

Medical Plan

Most nevi do not require any treatment. Surgical removal may be indicated for cosmetic purposes or if changes occur in the nevus. Mongolian spots require no treatment.

Surgery

- Shave ablation with electrodesiccation of base for intradermal nevus
- Excisional or punch biopsy removal of junction nevus
- Excision of hairy nevus with full-thickness skin grafting (see p. 567)

NURSING CARE

Nursing Assessment

Lesion

Location; size; color; shape

Lesion Changes

Enlargement; darkening; crusting; bleeding; inflammation; ulceration; appearance of satellite lesions

Psychosocial Concerns

Concern about body image

Nursing Dx & Intervention

Nursing Diagnosis	Nursing Intervention/Rationale
Body image disturbance	• Assess for presence of defining characteristics. • Encourage patient to express feelings about body, body image, or fear of reaction or rejection by others *to begin process of realistic self-evaluation.*

Patient Education

1. Instruct the patient about the benign nature of the lesions.
2. Instruct the patient about changes that might indicate malignancy and to seek medical attention if they occur.

Evaluation

Patient Outcome	Data Indicating That Outcome is Reached
Patient seeks treatment for changes in lesions.	Patient seeks medical attention if color or size of nevus changes, if it bleeds, or if it is exposed to repeated trauma.
Patient evaluates appearance in realistic manner.	Patient seeks removal if lesion is cosmetically embarrassing.

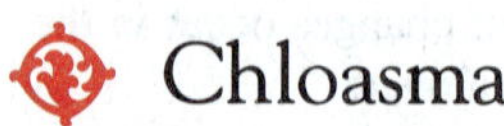

Chloasma

Chloasma is a diffuse, mottled brown pigmentation that appears over areas of the face and forehead.

Pathophysiology

Chloasma is a blotchy brown pigmentation that involves the forehead, malar prominences, and preauricular areas. The distribution is usually symmetric. Chloasma occurs primarily in women during and after childbearing years. Increased activity of melanocytes and the increase in melanin deposits in the basal cells of the epidermis can occur with pregnancy or from the use of anovulatory hormones. Exposure to sunlight exaggerates the pigmentation. It fades somewhat after childbirth or after the hormones are discontinued. Rarely, chloasma occurs idiopathically in dark-skinned men.

Diagnostic Studies and Findings

Physical Examination

Characteristic pigmentation and distribution; in women, history congruent with pregnancy or anovulatory hormones

Medical Plan

Medications

Topical depigmenting agents
- Hydroquinone (Eldopaque, Eldoquin), 2%-4% applied sparingly bid
- Compound of retinoic acid 0.1%, hydroquinone 5%, and dexamethasone 0.1% applied sparingly bid[61]

Sunscreen—para-aminobenzoic acid (PABA) 5% (Pabanol, Sunbrella) in ethyl alcohol 95%, applied twice a day and after swimming and bathing

General Management

Discontinuation of anovulatory hormones

NURSING CARE

Nursing Assessment

Pigmentation

Severity and extent of pigmentation; questioning to determine if woman is pregnant or taking anovulatory hormones

Psychosocial Concerns

Concern about body image

Nursing Dx & Intervention

Nursing Diagnosis	Nursing Intervention/Rationale
Body image disturbance	• Assess patient's self-perception. • Encourage patient to express feelings about body, body image, or fear of reaction or rejection by others *to begin process of realistic self-evaluation.* • Inform patient that pigmentation fades in time. • Instruct patient in use of medications.

Patient Education

1. Instruct the patient to avoid sun exposure, which will worsen the condition.
2. Instruct the patient to use sunscreens.
3. Instruct the patient in the side effects of depigmenting agents.

Evaluation

Patient Outcome	Data Indicating That Outcome is Reached
Existing pigmentation fades.	Blotchy brown areas become less noticeable.
Patient avoids sunlight and use of anovulatory hormones.	New areas of pigmentation do not occur.
Patient evaluates appearance in realistic manner.	Patient seeks treatment for areas that are cosmetically embarrassing. Patient engages in usual activities and relationships.

Depigmentation: albinism and vitiligo

Albinism and vitiligo are depigmentation that results from a congenital or acquired decrease in melanin production.

Albinism is a rare inherited disease that may be complete or partial. Partial albinism is autosomal dominant. The affected areas are usually linear and unilateral. The same area may be affected in more than one family member. A small area on the scalp with a streak of white hair is frequently seen.

Complete or universal albinism is autosomal recessive or irregularly dominant. There is no pigmentation in the skin, hair, and eyes. (Some pigmentation may occur with increasing age.) The skin is pale, the hair white, and the iris pink or red. Nystagmus and errors of refraction are common. Skin cancer and premature actinic keratosis are common.

Vitiligo is localized areas of depigmentation that are caused by the disappearance of previously active melanocytes. Vitiligo is fairly common, occurring in 1% of the world's population. It is a familial trait and can occur at any age. It has been associated with autoimmune and endocrine disorders. The depigmentation can also result from exposure to phenols, thiols, and quinones. Initial lesions frequently develop in areas exposed to the sun. The process may remain stable for years and involve only small areas, or it may progress to affect more extensive areas or the entire skin surface and hair. The eyes do not lose their pigment.

The lesions are completely depigmented and have well-demarcated borders that may be hyperpigmented. Vitiligo usually develops symmetrically and may follow trauma to the area. The hands, axillae, perineum, and periorbital areas are usually involved. The surface of the depigmented skin is normal except for the absence of pigmentation. There is no scaling. Some spontaneous repigmentation occurs in about 10% of patients, but complete repigmentation is rare.

Vitiligo is associated with thyroid dysfunction, diabetes mellitus, Addison's disease, and pernicious anemia.

Pathophysiology

In partial albinism melanocytes are not present in the depigmented area because they failed to migrate to the skin during embryonic development. In complete albinism melanocytes are present in the dermis, but they are unable to synthesize pigment because of a block in the formation of melanin from its precursor.

The cause of vitiligo is unknown. It is considered an autoimmune process that causes destruction of preexisting melanocytes. The melanocytes are abnormal and in various stages of cell death at the periphery of the lesions. Repigmentation is thought to result from the migration of melanocytes from residual areas of melanocytic activity within hair follicles.

Diagnostic Studies and Findings

Physical Examination

Distinctive lesions with characteristic configuration and distribution

Medical Plan

There is no treatment for albinism other than protection from sun exposure and actinic damage. The treatment for vitiligo is protracted and has mixed results.

Medications

Photosensitizers
- Psoralen therapy with 8-methoxypsoralen or methoxsalen (Oxsoralen, Trisoralen) to repigment
  - Psoralen, 40-50 mg po 2 h before sun exposure; sun exposure time initially 20 min then gradually increased
  - Psoralen, 40-50 mg po with long-wave ultraviolet light (PUVA), exposure time gradually increased[24,61] (see p. 568)

Sunscreens
- Para-aminobenzoic acid (PABA) 5% (Pabanol, Sunbrella) as protection against sunburn, applied topically q3h and after swimming

Skin dyes containing dihydroxyacetone (Vitadye); stain stratum corneum; applied topically several times a week

Corticosteroids
- Oral glucocorticoids or topical glucocorticoids used in occlusive dressings to repigment

Depigmenting agents
- For surrounding area in extensive vitiligo
  - 20% monobenzyl ether or hydroquinone

NURSING CARE

Nursing Assessment

Lesions

Location and distribution; extent of involvement

Psychosocial Concerns

Concern about body image

Nursing Dx & Intervention

Nursing Diagnosis	Nursing Intervention/Rationale
Potential impaired skin integrity	• Instruct patient *to protect against skin exposure* to sun through use of protective clothing and hats. • Instruct patient to use PABA as sunscreen *to protect skin from actinic damage.*
Body image disturbance; situational low self-esteem	• Assess patient's perception of his or her appearance. • Encourage patient to express feelings about body, body image, or fear of reaction or rejection by others *to begin process of realistic self-evaluation.* • Encourage development of interests and other attributes *to support positive self-image and feelings of worth and self-confidence.* • Help patient evaluate appearance in realistic way *so it does not become focal point of patient's existence.* • Advise patient of cosmetic products (Covermark) available for use on small areas. • Facilitate initiation of counseling if patient is unable to adjust to appearance.

Patient Education

1. Instruct the patient to protect against exposure to the sun to prevent premature actinic damage.
2. Instruct in the use and side effects of medications and preparations.
3. Inform the patient that treatment for vitiligo is protracted and results vary.

Evaluation

Patient Outcome	Data Indicating That Outcome is Reached
Actinic damage is avoided.	Epidermis is not dry or fissured. There are no actinic keratoses. Skin remains smooth and elastic.
Patient evaluates appearance in realistic manner.	Disorder is not used as excuse for unsuccessful interpersonal relationships. Patient develops interests and relationships so appearance is not focal point of existence.

Pityriasis Rosea

Pityriasis rosea is a self-limiting inflammation of unknown etiology.

The disease peaks in spring and fall. It is less likely to occur on tanned skin, and sunlight apparently hastens the course. Onset is sudden, with occurrence of a herald patch followed 1 to 3 weeks later by a generalized eruption. New lesions continue to appear for about a week after onset of the generalized eruption. A gradual involution follows. Total duration is 4 to 12 weeks with rare recurrence. The disease is not infectious or contagious.

Pathophysiology

The cause of pityriasis rosea is unknown. The primary (herald) patch is a single oval or round plaque with fine superficial scaling. The remainder of the lesions are smaller but similar in configuration to the primary lesion. The lesions develop on the trunk and extremities. The palms and soles are not involved, and facial involvement is rare. The lesions are characteristically distributed in parallel alignment following the direction of the ribs in a Christmas tree–like pattern. An inverse pattern can occur, with concentration of the lesions on the extremities and few lesions on the trunk. The lesions are usually pale, erythematous, and macular with fine scaling, but they may be papular or vesicular. Pruritus may be present.

Microscopic examination reveals nonspecific inflammation of the dermis, perivascular infiltrates, and localized epidermal changes with spongiosis and focal parakeratosis.

Diagnostic Studies and Findings

Physical Examination

Characteristic lesion with distinct distribution and congruent history

VDRL or Rapid Plasma Reagin (RPR) Test

Done to rule out secondary syphilis

Medical Plan

Treatment is usually unnecessary.

Medications

- Antipruritic effects
  - Antipruritic agents
    - Menthol 0.25% in cream base applied topically bid or tid
  - Antihistamines
    - Cyproheptadine (Cyproheptadine, Periactin), 4 mg po tid
  - Antianxiety agents
    - Hydroxyzine (Atarax, Orgatrax, Vistaril), 25-100 mg po tid or qid
- Corticosteroids
  - Prednisone, 10 mg po qid for severe pruritus until itching subsides, then in decremental doses over 14 d

NURSING CARE

Nursing Assessment

Lesion

Pale, erythematous macules with fine scaling or papules and vesicles; herald patch larger than new lesions; characteristic distribution

Psychosocial Concerns

Concern with body image

Nursing Dx & Intervention

Nursing Diagnosis	Nursing Intervention/Rationale
Impaired skin integrity	• Assess for lesions and pruritus. • Lubricate skin with emollient and water-miscible bath oil *to alleviate dryness and scaling.* • Stress importance of good hygiene *to avoid secondary infection.* • Have patient cut fingernails short *to avoid tissue trauma from scratching.*

Nursing Diagnosis	Nursing Intervention/Rationale
Body image disturbance	• Reassure patient that lesions will clear in 4 to 12 weeks. • Encourage patient to express feelings about body, body appearance, or fear of reaction or rejection by others *to begin process of realistic self-evaluation.*

Patient Education

1. Instruct the patient that the disease is self-limiting and will resolve.
2. Instruct the patient that exposure to sunlight may hasten the course of the disease.
3. Teach the patient the signs and symptoms of secondary infection and to seek medical attention if they occur.
4. Instruct the patient in the use and side effects of medications.

Evaluation

Patient Outcome	Data Indicating That Outcome is Reached
Lesions resolve.	Macules, papules, vesicles, and scaling disappear. Pruritus is relieved. Skin is intact.
Secondary infection is resolved or avoided.	There is no tenderness, swelling, purulent discharge, or fever.
Patient evaluates appearance in realistic manner.	Patient engages in usual activities and relationships.

Psoriasis

Psoriasis is a chronic and recurrent disease of keratin synthesis that is characterized by dry, well-circumscribed, silvery, scaling papules and plaques.

Psoriasis occurs in 3% to 5% of the population. Onset is usually between the ages of 10 and 40 years. A family history of psoriasis is common.

The onset of the disease is slow, and the course is characterized by periods of inactivity and exacerbation. Emotional stress may cause exacerbations. Spontaneous remission may occur. Psoriasis characteristically involves the back, buttocks, and extensor surfaces of the extremities, particularly the knees and elbows, and the scalp. The nails, axillae, umbilicus, eyebrows, and anogenital areas may be affected. Generalized eruptions can occur. Approximately 5% of people with psoriasis have associated arthritis. Lesions may develop at sites of recent epidermal injury.

The characteristic lesions of psoriasis are raised, erythematous, sharply demarcated papules covered with overlapping, silvery or shiny scales. The papules may combine as large plaques. When the scales are removed, a deep red base, covered with a thin membrane that bleeds, is revealed.

Pathophysiology

The basic defect in psoriasis is in the control of the growth of epidermal cells. This defect may be genetic, biochemical, or immunologic. The three main components of the psoriatic process are increased mitotic rate that results in rapid cellular turnover and shortened transit time of the epidermal cell from the basal layer to the epidermis (4 to 7 days versus the normal 28 days), faulty keratinization of the horny layer, which desquamates readily and affords little protection to the underlying skin, and dilation of upper dermal vessels and intermittent discharge of polymorphonuclear leukocytes into the dermis.

The three processes occur in different degrees that result in varying forms of psoriasis with differing clinical features. If the increased mitotic rate predominates, the result is a thick silvery scale because of the separation of corneocytes and the presence of air between them. If vasodilation predominates, the result is diffusely red, hot, slightly scaling skin.

The forms of psoriasis and their clinical features are summarized in Table 5-5.

Diagnostic Studies and Findings

Physical Examination

Characteristic lesions

Table 5-5
Clinical Features and Distribution of the Various Forms of Psoriasis

Clinical Pattern	Clinical Features	Distribution
Localized plaques	Erythematous plaques with silver scales; nails pitted, thickened, discolored, and crumbling beneath free edge	Extensor aspect of extremities; elbows; knees; scalp; nails
Generalized plaques	As above	Disseminated
Guttate	Tiny plaques (0.5-2 cm); sudden onset usually after streptococcal infection; may progress to other types; may itch	Disseminated
Pustular	Pustular lesions covered by thin scale	Palms and soles only or generalized
Erythrodermic exfoliative	More inflammatory; skin red and hot; deep erythema with massive shedding of scales; usually follows overly aggressive therapy; can cause temperature and fluid imbalances	Generalized

Medical Plan

Medications

- Corticosteroids
  - Topical nonfluorinated corticosteroids for lesions on face and intertriginous areas
    - Hydrocortisone (Cort-Dome, others) 2%-3% applied sparingly bid
  - Topical fluorinated corticosteroids for lesions on scalp, body, and extremities
    - Fluocinolone (Fluonid, Synalar) 0.025%-0.01% applied sparingly bid, tid, or qid
    - Betamethasone (Valisone) 0.05%-0.1% applied sparingly bid, tid, or qid
    - Triamcinolone (Aristocort, Kenalog) 0.05%-0.1% applied sparingly bid, tid, or qid
  - Topical corticosteroids in conjunction with tar preparations or in occlusive therapy (see p. 564)
  - Intralesional injections of corticosteroids
    - Triamcinolone (Kenalog), 10 mg/ml
  - Systemic corticosteroids—individualized treatment regimen; rarely used[24,25,61]
- Keratolytics
  - Coal tar preparations (Alphosyl, Psorigel, Balnetar) added to bath oil or shampoo or applied sparingly to lesions
  - Dianthrol compounds[45,74]
    - Anthralin (Anthra-Derm) 0.1%-1% applied sparingly at bedtime or bid; very irritating and stains clothing permanently; cannot be used simultaneously with corticosteroids
  - Phenol-saline mixture (P & S liquid) massaged into scalp and left for 3-4 h for scalp lesions, followed by tar shampoo
- Photosensitizing agents
  - Psoralen (Trisoralen, Oxysoralen), 0.6 mg/kg 2-4 h before exposure to ultraviolet light; used as photoactivator in combination with long-wave ultraviolet light therapy (see p. 568)
- Vitamins
  - Oral retinoids
    - Etretinate, 25 mg/kg; still under testing[21,24,37,61,75]
- Antineoplastic agents (used for antimetabolite effect)
  - Methotrexate in individualized treatment regimen for very severe disease; use is controversial[23,24,61]
- Anti-infective agents
  - Penicillin (Pen Vee-K, V-Cillin, others), 250 mg po qid for 10 d for underlying streptococcal infection in guttate psoriasis

General Management

- See p. 568
- Exposure to short-wave ultraviolet light (UV-B)—one to three times weekly with increasing UV-B exposure; kept below level that would cause erythema
- Goeckerman therapy—UV-B therapy in combination with coal tar applications that are photosensitizing; coal tar ointment applied and left on for several hours and then washed off; UV-B therapy then administered in doses to account for photosensitization; tar finally reapplied[45,51,61]
- Long-wave ultraviolet light (UV-A) in combination with psoralen as a photosensitizer (PUVA therapy)—psoralen administered in initial dose of 0.6 mg/kg; UV-A irradiation delivered 2 to 4 hours after psoralen administration; dosage and exposure determined by individual response; special equipment and careful monitoring required, so therapy is usually provided in special treatment centers; long-term effects remain controversial; treatment usually reserved for chronic, severe, refractory psoriasis[19,23,24,61]
- X-ray therapy and Grenz-ray therapy—used to provide temporary clearing of stubborn plaques; of limited value as therapeutic tools in psoriasis therapy[23]
- Peritoneal dialysis—mechanism for antipsoriasis effect unknown; therapy experimental[23,73]
- Occlusive dressings with topical corticosteroids or tar preparations or both (see p. 564)

Day care treatment centers for psoriasis—patients with severe psoriasis can undergo treatment regimens that are intensive or that require special equipment and supervision[51]

NURSING CARE

Nursing Assessment

Lesions

Characteristics and distribution as in Table 5-5

Psoriatic Arthritis

Pain; tenderness; stiffness in small distal joints (early); larger joints involved later

Environment

Presence of mechanical injury that can exacerbate lesions; stress factors

Nursing Dx & Intervention

Nursing Diagnosis	Nursing Intervention/Rationale
Impaired skin integrity	• Assess for lesion characteristics, distribution, and severity. • Explain disease process regarding exacerbations and remissions. • Stress importance of adhering to therapeutic regimen; help patient set up overall schedule for managing regimen on daily basis *to maximize therapeutic value.* • Give written instructions for use of topical preparations, tar baths, and shampoos. • Instruct patient in application of occlusive dressings. • Instruct patient to scrub scales gently during daily bath with soft brush and to apply medications after removing scales *to maximize absorption and therapeutic value.* • Instruct patient not to apply keratolytics and tar to unaffected areas, *since they may precipitate new lesions.* • Explore stress factors affecting patient and alternatives for dealing with stress *to help prevent exacerbations.*
Body image disturbance	• Recognize importance of body image in growth and development. • Assess patient's perception of his or her appearance. • Encourage patient to express feelings about body, body appearance, or fear of reaction or rejection by others *to begin process of realistic self-evaluation.* • Encourage patient to develop interests and other attributes *to support positive self-image, feelings of worth, and self-confidence.* • Facilitate initiation of individual or group therapy *if patient is unable to adjust to appearance.*
Social isolation	• Involve family members in treatment regimen. • Stress that psoriasis is not communicable. • Refer patient for counseling *if patient is socially disabled by disease.*
Powerlessness	• Assess for presence of defining characteristics. • Observe for signs of depression and apathy. • Involve patient in decision making *to increase sense of power and control.* • Encourage patient to express dissatisfaction and frustration.

Patient Education

1. Instruct the patient in the treatment regimen and the use of medications.
2. Instruct the patient in the side effects of medications.
3. Inform the patient that anthralin (Dithranol) stains skin, sheets, and clothing. Skin discoloration resolves in a few weeks as the stratum corneum is shed.
4. Evaluate the patient's ability to carry out home care and reteach procedures as necessary.
5. Instruct the patient in good hygiene to avoid secondary infection.

Evaluation

Patient Outcome	Data Indicating That Outcome is Reached
Lesions improve.	Scaling, pustules, erythema, and size of plaques decrease.
Exacerbating factors are avoided.	Patient takes precautions against skin trauma. Patient avoids or tries alternative strategies for reducing stress factors.
Untoward effects from therapies are minimized.	Patient seeks medical attention for untoward or side effects from medications or therapies.
Patient copes with disorder in an effective manner.	Patient engages in satisfying relationships. Patient seeks counseling when feeling overwhelmed by disease. Patient does not use disorder as excuse for failures in life or in relationships. Patient participates actively in treatment regimen.

Pruritus

Pruritus is a localized or generalized itching sensation that elicits the desire to scratch.

Pruritus may occur as a primary disorder or may be a symptom of a systemic disorder. Pruritus may result from inflammations caused by various factors including irritation, infection, infestations, and allergic reactions. It may be the result of systemic disease, malignancy, and altered physiologic states.

Three areas of the body are most frequently affected by pruritus: the anus (pruritus ani), vulva (pruritus vulvae), and ear (otitis externa). These are body orifices that have an abundance of sensory nerve endings.

Pruritus ani occurs primarily in men. It is caused by many factors and is associated with various diseases. Perianal erythema and scratches or gross excoriation are evident. Lichenification or fissures occur in long-term cases. The entire gluteal fold may be involved. Aggravating factors include contact dermatitis, anatomic abnormalities, infection, and systemic disorders. Common irritating factors include feces, irritation from toilet tissue, tight clothing, sweating, and long periods of sitting. The itching is often associated with tension, irritability, and depression.

Pruritus vulvae is caused by many factors and is associated with various diseases. Pruritus vulvae begins with intermittent episodes that can develop into unremitting pruritus. Erythema develops in the labia majora, with lichenification in longstanding disease. The perianal region may also be affected. Tight clothing, heat, perspiration, motion, sitting, and lying down aggravate the condition.

Otitis externa occurs in the external ear usually as a result of trauma, moisture in the ear, and bacterial colonization. The distal third of the external canal and the meatal skin develop a scaling erythema that becomes moist and oozing as the condition worsens. Itching is the main complaint. Otitis externa is aggravated by heat, humidity, moisture, and overzealous cleansing (see Chapter 7).

Generalized pruritus can signify a systemic disorder. Diabetes mellitus, drug reactions, biliary obstruction, renal disease, malignancy, and pregnancy are common causes of generalized pruritus.

Pathophysiology

The exact mechanism of pruritus is undetermined. The itch sensation seems to arise from nerve endings just below the epidermis and in the dermis. Itching may be a result of repetitive, low-frequency stimulation of C fibers that are similar to but distinct from those that transmit pain.[31]

Persistent scratching may produce erythema, urticarial papules, excoriation, and fissures. Prolonged scratching and rubbing may produce lichenification and pigmentation. Many factors, including personality, determine whether itching will be ignored, rubbed, or scratched and excoriated.

Diagnostic Studies and Findings

Physical Examination and History

To determine underlying cause or systemic disorder

Laboratory Studies with Generalized Pruritus

To determine possible systemic cause: complete blood count, blood urea nitrogen, serum bilirubin, serum iron, blood glucose, sulfobromophthalein retention, stool for occult blood, and parasites

Biopsy

To determine histopathologic changes

Medical Plan

Treatment is aimed at the specific underlying cause (see specific diseases for treatments) and at eliminating aggravating factors (see "Patient Education").

Medications

Topical preparation: combination of menthol 0.5%, phenol 0.5%, and betamethasone 0.1% applied sparingly tid

Anti-infective agents
- Topical antibiotics if pruritus has bacterial etiology; gentamicin (Garamycin) or polymycin, applied tid

Antianxiety agents (used for antipruritic effect)
- Hydroxyzine (Atarax, Orgatrax, Vistaril), 25 mg po at bedtime or q6h for localized itching

Antihistamines (used for antipruritic effect)
- Trimeprazine (Temaril), 5 mg po at bedtime or q6h for localized itching
- Terfenadine (Seldane), 60 mg po in the morning, with diphenhydramine (Benadryl), 50-100 mg po at bedtime

Psychotherapeutic agents (used for antipruritic effect)
- Chlorpromazine (Thorazine), 10-25 mg po q6-8h for severe generalized itching

General Management

Sitz baths
Burow's compresses
Emollients for dry skin

NURSING CARE

Nursing Assessment

Pruritus

Severity; localization; diurnal or seasonal patterns; distribution

Lesion

Erythema; scaling; excoriation; fissures

Environment

Aggravating factors; stress, tension; depression; irritability

Nursing Dx & Intervention

Nursing Diagnosis	Nursing Intervention/Rationale
Impaired skin integrity	• Instruct patient in good hygiene *to prevent secondary infection.* • Instruct patient to cut fingernails short *to avoid tissue damage from scratching.*
Pain	• Help patient identify and eliminate potentially aggravating factors (see "Patient Education"). • Help patient identify stress factors and alternative approaches to dealing with stress *to avoid aggravating the condition.* • Apply cool compresses and Burow's compresses *to alleviate itching.* • Offer sitz baths *to alleviate itching.* • Apply emollients *to prevent dry skin.* • Instruct patient in use of medications.

Patient Education

1. Instruct the patient to avoid aggravating factors:
   a. Heat and humidity
   b. Rubbing and friction from clothing
   c. Tight clothing
   d. Wool and rough fabrics
   e. Fabrics that do not allow ventilation
   f. Excessive perspiration
   g. External irritants (such as soap)
   h. Dry skin
   i. Temperature changes
2. Instruct the patient in the use and side effects of medications.
3. Instruct the patient in the use of compresses (see p. 564).
4. Instruct the patient in the signs and symptoms of secondary infection.

Evaluation

Patient Outcome	Data Indicating That Outcome is Reached
Aggravating factors are avoided.	Pruritus decreases. Exacerbations do not occur.
Underlying disease is identified and treated.	Erythema, scaling, excoriation, and fissures resolve. Pruritus is alleviated.

Patient Outcome	Data Indicating That Outcome is Reached
Secondary infection is resolved or avoided.	There is no tenderness, swelling, or purulent exudate in resolving lesions.
Discomfort is alleviated.	Scratching and excoriations decrease. Patient is able to sleep.

Tinea

(Dermatophytosis)

Tinea is a group of superficial fungal infections.

Dermatophytes (ringworm fungi) cause various superficial fungal infections through invasion of the stratum corneum, nails, or hair. The disorders are usually classified according to the anatomic location, since treatment of most superficial fungal disorders is the same and the clinical appearance of the eruption is not always related to the species of fungus. The disorder varies from mild inflammation to acute vesicular infection. Remissions and exacerbations may occur. Itching is usually present. The condition is transmissible from other persons or from animals.

Pathophysiology

The local response to fungal invasion is inflammation, scaling, erythema, and pruritus. A cell-mediated immunologic response may develop, with the production of further erythema, spongiosis, vesicles, and oozing. Table 5-6 summarizes the features of tinea.

Diagnostic Studies and Findings

Physical Examination

Characteristic lesion and distribution

KOH (Potassium Hydroxide) Scraping

Presence of branching mycelia or spores

Table 5-6
Summary of Tinea

Type	Distribution	Occurrence	Clinical Features
Tinea corporis	Nonhairy parts of body; face; neck; extremities	More common in hot and humid climates; more common in rural than in urban settings; occurs in both adults and children	Pruritus; papulosquamous annular lesions with raised borders; lesions expand peripherally with central clearing
Tinea cruris	Groin; inner thigh; scrotum or labia not involved	More common in adult men; tends to recur; flare-ups common in summer; aggravated by tight clothes, perspiration, and physical activity	Pruritus; hypopigmented; well-demarcated lesions; dryness and scaling; pustules present at margins; central clearing sometimes present; secondary bacterial or candidal infection and maceration common
Tinea capitis	Scalp	More common in children; contagious	Lesions vary: small gray scaly patches with short broken hairs; mild erythematous papules; raised, boggy, inflamed nodules dotted with perifollicular abscesses; thick, yellow, suppurative lesions; lesions may be small, coalesced, or cover entire scalp; hairless patches
Tinea pedis	Feet; begins in third and fourth interdigital spaces and spreads to involve plantar surface; may involve nails	Rare in children; not transmitted by simple exposure	Lesions vary: maceration, scaling, fissuring of interdigital space; vesicular scaling, erythema of plantar surface; chronic, noninflamed, diffuse scaling; nails brittle, discolored; pruritus
Tinea unguium	Toenails and (less commonly) fingernails	—	Nails thickened, lusterless, and discolored; subungual debris; nail plate crumbling or absent

Fungal Culture

Infecting organism

Wood's Light

Affected hairs fluoresce

Medical Plan

Medications

Anti-infective agents
- Griseofulvin (Fulvicin, Grifulvin, Grisactin, Gris Owen, Gris-Peg) for tinea capitis and severe cases of other tineas, 1 g po in divided doses with meals; may require more than 4 mo therapy; continue therapy for 2 wk after last sign of clinical activity
- Topical antifungals rubbed in bid for 3 wk
  - Tolnaftate 1% (Aftate, Tinactin)
  - Miconazole 2% (Monistat-Derm)
  - Clotrimazole 1% (Lotrimin, Mycelex)
  - Econazole 1% (Spectazole)
  - Ciclopiroxolamine 1% (Loprox)

Keratolytic agents (for noninflammatory scaling)
- Salicylic acid 3% and benzane acid 6% in ointment or alcohol

NURSING CARE

Nursing Assessment

Lesion

For description and distribution see Table 5-6

Secondary Infection (Bacterial or Candidal)

Itching; exudate; inflammation; odor; tenderness; maceration

Environment

Aggravating factors; hygiene; contacts

Nursing Dx & Intervention

Nursing Diagnosis	Nursing Intervention/Rationale
Impaired skin integrity	• Assess for lesion characteristics and distribution. • Decrease moisture in affected areas. • Stress importance of good hygiene and handwashing *to prevent secondary infection.* • Have patient's fingernails cut short *to avoid tissue trauma from scratching.* • For tinea capitis remove scales with shampoo and gently scrub before medication is applied *to maximize absorption of medication.* • Instruct patient in use of medications and preparations *to avoid recurrence.*
Potential for infection	• Inform patient that contacts should be screened and referred for treatment if symptoms appear *to avoid reinfection.* • Instruct patient that pets should be checked and treated for fungal infection *to avoid reinfection.* • Instruct patient and family to protect themselves and others by not sharing towels or personal articles and by wearing protective footwear in public showers.
Pain	• Assess for discomfort and itching. • Instruct patient to avoid tight clothing *to avoid aggravating the condition.* • Instruct patient to wear cotton next to skin *to avoid aggravating the condition.* • Instruct patient to stay in areas of decreased humidity *to avoid aggravating the condition.* • Instruct patient in use of medications and preparations as prescribed.

Patient Education

1. Teach the patient and family about the transmission, recurrence, and reinfection of the disease.
2. Instruct the patient to avoid aggravating factors: tight clothing, moist skin, and excessive humidity.
3. Stress the importance of following the therapeutic regimen to avoid recurrence and reinfection.
4. Instruct the patient and family in the side effects of medications.
5. Instruct the patient and family in the signs and symptoms of secondary infection and to seek medical attention if they occur.

Evaluation

Patient Outcome	Data Indicating That Outcome is Reached
Eruption clears up.	Papules, scaling, pustules, erythema, vesicles, and pruritus resolve. Nails resume smooth texture.
Secondary infection is avoided or resolved.	There is no tenderness, swelling, or purulent exudate.
Spread of infection is contained.	Contacts are notified and treated if symptoms appear. Personal articles and items are not shared.
Aggravating environmental factors are avoided.	Eruption clears. Exacerbations do not recur. Pruritus is alleviated.

Urticaria

Urticaria is a reaction pattern characterized by hives or wheals.

Urticaria is a common disorder that can occur at any age. It can be acute, chronic, or physical. Most cases are acute, lasting from hours to a few weeks. This condition is self-limited, and most people do not seek medical treatment. Patients who have a history of hives lasting 6 weeks or longer are considered to have chronic urticaria. The course of chronic urticaria is unpredictable and may last for months or years, followed by spontaneous resolution. The physical urticarias include dermographism, pressure urticaria, and cholinergic urticaria. Hives are elicited by physical stimuli to the skin; the attacks are brief and transient.

Drugs, foods, and environmental antigens are common causes of acute and chronic urticaria. Emotional stress should also be considered in the evaluation of chronic urticaria.

Pathophysiology

A hive or a wheal is a nonpitting edematous plaque that results from localized capillary vasodilation followed by transudation of protein-rich fluid into the surrounding tissue. The hive may be erythematous or white with irregular borders that extend or recede during the evolution of the hive. The hive resolves when the fluid is reabsorbed.

Histamine is the primary chemical mediator of urticaria. Histamine induces vascular changes resulting in vasodilation and pruritus. It also causes endothelial cell contraction, which allows vascular fluid to leak between the cells through the vessel wall. A variety of immunologic, nonimmunologic, physical, and chemical stimuli may cause release of histamine from the mast cells. Other factors that contribute to vascular dilation include alcohol ingestion, emotional stress, endocrine factors, exercise, fever, and heat.

Diagnostic Studies and Findings

Physical Examination

Characteristic lesion, location, pattern, and history; inducement of hive by physical stimuli to determine physical urticaria

Sinus and Dental Radiographic Examination

For chronic urticaria; a percentage of these patients exhibit sinusitis[32]

Change of Environment

For chronic urticaria; separation from the home and work environment for a 1- to 2-week trial period

Food Challenge

For chronic urticaria, foods containing salicylate, azo dyes, and benzoic acid preservative; to elicit hive development

Biopsy

For chronic urticaria; to rule out urticarial vasculitis

Laboratory Tests

For specific suspected causes in internal diseases such as hyperthyroidism, systemic lupus erythematosus, and carcinomas

There are no routine laboratory studies for acute urticaria

Medical Plan

Treatment is aimed at identifying and eliminating known causes or aggravating factors.

Medications

For symptom control
- Epinephrine 1:1000, 0.2-1 ml subcutaneously or IM for severe urticaria and laryngeal edema

Antihistamines
- Hydroxazine (Atarax, Vistaril), 10 mg q4h, then increase dosage as required to 25-100 mg q4h
- Cyproheptadine (Periactin), 4 mg qid

NURSING CARE

Nursing Assessment

Lesion

Edematous plaques of 1-3 mm; erythematous or white in color either uniformly or varied; approximately round or oval with borders that extend and recede; new hives appear as old ones resolve; duration varies from hours to weeks; generalized distribution with inhalants, ingestions, and internal disease; localized distribution with contact urticaria

Pruritus

Intensity and interference with activities

Secondary Infection

Erythema, excoriation, purulent exudate from scratching

Nursing Dx & Intervention

Nursing Diagnosis	Nursing Intervention/Rationale
Impaired skin integrity	• Assess for lesion characteristics and distribution.
Pain	• Assess for excoriation and secondary infection from scratching. • Trim fingernails short *to prevent secondary infection*. • Apply cool compresses to localized lesions or use cool baths for generalized eruption *to soothe pruritus*.

Patient Education

1. Instruct the patient in possible causes of condition and help identify and eliminate precipitating or aggravating factors: foods, drugs, emotional stress, exercise, heat, pressure or physical stimuli, other vasodilating factors.
2. Instruct the patient in diet free of salicylates, azo dyes, and benzoic acid preservatives if indicated.
3. Instruct the patient in use of antihistamines.
4. Instruct the patient with chronic urticaria in nature of disorder, that evaluation may be lengthy and unrewarding, and that in most cases the disorder resolves spontaneously.

Evaluation

Patient Outcome	Data Indicating That Outcome is Reached
Eruption improves.	Hives resolve and do not recur.
Pruritus is alleviated.	Areas of excoriation resolve or do not occur.

VASCULAR DISORDERS OF CUTANEOUS BLOOD VESSELS

Hemangiomas

Hemangiomas are congenital vascular lesions of the skin and subcutaneous tissue.

Pathophysiology

The three common types of hemangiomas are nevus flammeus, capillary hemangiomas, and cavernous hemangioma.

Nevus flammeus (port-wine stain) is a flat purple-red lesion that is present at birth and is caused by a mass of mature, dilated, congested capillaries in the dermis. The color depends on whether the superficial, middle, or deep dermal vessels are involved. The lesion does not disappear or fade over time, does not enlarge, and may develop a thickened nodular surface.

The occipital area of the scalp is the most common site of occurrence. The lesion may occur elsewhere and is frequently seen on the face. The lesions are usually unilateral and tend to follow the course of a cutaneous nerve. There is no satisfactory treatment for hemangiomas.

Capillary hemangioma (strawberry mark) is a very common, raised, bright red lesion that usually appears in the third to fifth week of life. It consists of a proliferation of endothelial cells arranged in strawberry-like lobules. It may occur anywhere on the body. It may enlarge for the first several months but rarely enlarges after the first year. It involutes spontaneously and is usually completely regressed by 3 to 5 years of age. Involution begins with an area of fibrosis in the center. The lesion may leave a brownish pigmentation or scarring and wrinkling of the skin as it involutes. No treatment is required unless the lesion is massively disfiguring or is near the eye or a body orifice where it might interfere with body functioning.

Cavernous hemangioma is a large vascular pool lined with mature epithelial cells that are located in the subcutaneous tissue of the dermis. It is deeper than the other types of hemangiomas and may contain many arteriovenous shunts and vascular formations.

The lesion, which is present at birth, is reddish blue and round and may be elevated and compressible. It can occur on any part of the body. Most lesions eventually involute at least partially.

Diagnostic Studies and Findings

Physical Examination

Characteristic lesion and congruent history

Medical Plan

No treatment for nevus flammeus currently exists. Laser techniques are under development.[1,2,11,13] For capillary or cavernous hemangiomas, treatment is as follows.

Surgery

Used for capillary or cavernous hemangiomas only if lesion does not involute; may leave more scarring than spontaneous resolution

Excision with grafting

Cryosurgery (see p. 565)

Medications

Corticosteroids

Prednisone, 10 mg po bid or tid with decremental doses until lesion resolves

Intralesional injection of triamcinolone (Kenalog, Aristocort); may cause scar formation

General Management

Electrocoagulation for small lesions; may leave scars

NURSING CARE

Nursing Assessment

Lesion History

Present or absent at birth; rate of growth or involution

Lesion

Size; color; texture; elevation; location; secondary trauma or bleeding

Nursing Dx & Intervention

Nursing Diagnosis	Nursing Intervention/Rationale
Potential impaired skin integrity	• Assess lesion for characteristics. • Instruct patient in ways to protect lesions from scratching (cut nails short) and trauma *to avoid tissue damage and bleeding and secondary infection.* • Stress importance of good hygiene *to avoid secondary infection.* • Advise patient that it is better to wait for involution of capillary and cavernous hemangiomas *to avoid complications and scarring through early treatment.*
Body image disturbance	• Assess for defining characteristics. • Advise patient of excellent prognosis for involution of capillary and cavernous hemangiomas but warn that lesion may grow before it involutes. • Use accurate measurements or photographs *to show progress of involution.* • Assess patient's self-perception or parents' perception of child's appearance. • Encourage patient to express feelings about body, body image, and fear of reaction or rejection by others *to begin process of realistic self-evaluation.* • Help patient or parent evaluate appearance in realistic manner *so lesion does not become focal point of existence.*

Patient Education

1. Inform the patient and family of the likelihood of involution.
2. Advise the patient and family of the hazards of unnecessary treatment.

Evaluation

Patient Outcome	Data Indicating That Outcome is Reached
Secondary trauma and infection are minimized.	Lesion remains intact and free of bleeding, crusting, excoriation, and purulent exudate.
Unnecessary scarring is avoided.	Family waits for spontaneous involution in capillary and cavernous hemangiomas before seeking treatment.
Patient and parents evaluate appearance in realistic manner.	Patient develops interest and attributes and engages in activities so hemangioma is not focal point of existence. Lesion is not used as excuse for unsuccessful interpersonal relationships.

Telangiectasia and hereditary hemorrhagic telangiectasia

Telangiectasia is a network of dilated superficial dermal capillaries and venules.

Pathophysiology

Essential telangiectasia is a disorder that is characterized by a network of small dilated veins on the thighs and calves of adult women. The condition is localized and often symmetric. The vessels involved are the superficial venous plexuses. The condition affects the appearance only, not the health, of the person.

Telangiectasia is also a component of certain systemic diseases, such as lupus erythematosus and scleroderma, and certain hereditary disorders. Hereditary hemorrhagic telangiectasia (Rendu-Osler-Weber disease) is a rare, autosomal dominant, inherited disorder. Telangiectatic lesions of the skin, mucous membranes, and internal organs are present in this disease. Lesions occur most commonly after puberty and increase throughout adult life. The small, red to violet lesions consist of thin, dilated vessels that blanch with pressure and tend to bleed spontaneously or with minor trauma. Bleeding may also occur from lesions in the mouth, pharynx, and gastrointestinal and genitourinary tracts. Anemia may result from continued oozing. Bleeding tends to become more severe with age. Systemic problems may arise from associated pulmonary arteriovenous fistulas and cerebrovascular malformations.

Diagnostic Studies and Findings

Physical Examination

Characteristic lesions

Complete Blood Count

Iron deficiency anemia

Medical Plan

For treatment of anemia see Chapter 15. For treatment of underlying systemic disorders see the specific diseases.

Medications

- For Rendu-Osler-Weber disease
  - Estrogens
    - Cyclic therapy to decrease bleeding tendency
  - Corticosteroids
    - Nasal spray to control bleeding
  - Hematinic agents
    - Iron po for iron loss through repeated bleeding

General Management

- For localized lesions
  - Electrolysis—free hydrogen via electric current to obliterate vessels
- Blood transfusion for acute hemorrhage

NURSING CARE

Nursing Assessment

Lesion

Number, location and bleeding tendency; symptoms of anemia (see Chapter 15)

Nursing Dx & Intervention

Nursing Diagnosis	Nursing Intervention/Rationale
Impaired skin integrity	• Assess lesions for characteristics. • Instruct patient *to avoid trauma to lesions;* wear protective clothing and cut fingernails short.

Nursing Diagnosis	Nursing Intervention/Rationale
Altered oral mucous membrane	• Instruct patient to eat soft foods *to avoid mechanical trauma.* • Instruct patient to use soft toothbrush *to avoid mechanical trauma.*
Body image disturbance	• Assess for defining characteristics. • Encourage patient to express feelings about body, body image, or fear of reaction or rejection by others *to begin process of realistic self-evaluation.* • Advise patient of availability of covering makeup (Covermark).

Patient Education

1. Instruct the patient in protective measures to avoid trauma that may cause bleeding (see "Nursing Dx and Intervention").
2. Instruct the patient in the use and side effects of medications.
3. Instruct the patient to seek medical attention if unable to stop a bleeding episode.

Evaluation

Patient Outcome	Data Indicating That Outcome is Reached
Trauma is minimized.	Bleeding episodes are less frequent.
Patient assesses self-concept in realistic manner.	Patient engages in activities compatible with limitations of disorder. Patient engages in interpersonal relationships. Patient employs protective measures and seeks medical attention as needed.

Vasculitis

Vasculitis is a range of cutaneous lesions associated with inflammation of the wall of blood vessels of the skin and subcutaneous tissue.

Vasculitis is a general term for a large number of disorders that cause skin lesions as a result of inflammation of the walls of cutaneous blood vessels. The diseases range in severity from mild to fatal. The cutaneous lesions appear as erythematous papules and plaques, nodules, urticaria, purpuric or hemorrhagic papules and vesicles, and pustular and necrotic lesions.

Lesions, which tend to develop in crops, occur most commonly on the legs, thighs, and buttocks, Some lesions begin as erythematous papules or plaques and progress to ulcerations that heal slowly. In severe ulcerative forms, lesions are progressive and involve other body organs. There is currently no universal or satisfactory classification system for the vasculitis disorders.

Pathophysiology

Vasculitis involves intravascular and extravascular changes. The sequence of events occurs as a result of damage to the vessel that is precipitated by numerous factors and modified by the body's response to noxious stimuli.

The inflammatory process of the vessel includes increased permeability; epithelial shedding; increased deposition of fibrin, platelets, and leukocytes; changes in endothelial cells during repair; and thrombosis. The cutaneous changes that occur as a result of the inflammation processes depend on the degree of inflammation and the size of the involved vessel.

The pathogenesis of vasculitis can be summarized as follows:

- Intravascular component
  - Deposition of circulating antigen-antibody complexes with chemotaxis of leukocytes and release of mediators of inflammation
  - Direct toxic effect of circulating chemicals, drugs, and bacterial antigens
  - Bacterial emboli and reaction to products of bacterial breakdown
- Vascular wall component
  - Endothelial proliferation in reparative attempt
  - Infiltration by lymphocytes and polymorphonuclear leukocytes
  - Fibrinoid necrosis and scarring from fibrin deposits
  - Granulomatous infiltrates
- Extravascular component
  - Leakage of red blood cells and fibrin into surrounding tissue
  - Deposition of inflammatory infiltrates
  - Thrombosis of small vessels with secondary tissue; ischemia
  - Increased fibrosis
  - Venous stasis

Diagnostic Studies and Findings

Physical Examination

Lesions and history as described in "Nursing Assessment"

Biopsy of Blood Vessel

Immunofluorescence shows cellular changes as described above; will determine type and severity of vasculitis

Further Studies to Determine Systemic Involvement and Underlying Conditions

Complete blood count
Antinuclear factor, serum protein, and rheumatoid factor
Serum fibrinolytic activity
VDRL test or rapid plasma reagin test
Culture and antistreptolysin titer
Urinalysis for red blood cells and casts
Serum complement and cryoglobulin
Roentgenograms of chest, sinuses, and teeth
Roentgenograms of gastrointestinal tract if symptoms indicate

Medical Plan

Specific treatment is aimed at the particular clinical condition or underlying disease process.

Medications

Antihypertensive agents
  If needed to minimize small vessel damage
Anti-infective agents
  Agent-specific to clear infection
Corticosteroids
  Systemic glucocorticoids for deep tender nodular lesions
Nonsteroidal anti-inflammatory agents
  Aspirin, potassium iodide, indomethacin (Indocin), ibuprofen (Motrin), phenylbutazone (Butazolidin, Azolid)

NURSING CARE

Nursing Assessment

Lesion

Erythematous papules, plaques, or nodules; persistent urticaria; purpuric papules and vesicles; pustules; necrotic lesions

Surrounding Tissue

Abnormal vascular patterns; abnormal reactions to cold

History

Precipitating factors; infection; food and drug allergies or sensitivity

General Medical Problems

Diabetes mellitus; arthritis; cardiovascular diseases; respiratory diseases; connective tissue diseases

Nursing Dx & Intervention

Nursing Diagnosis	Nursing Intervention/Rationale
	Nursing interventions other than those listed depend on the symptoms produced by the particular clinical condition and disorder.
Impaired skin integrity	• Assess lesions for characteristics. • Instruct patient in good hygiene and handwashing *to prevent secondary infection.* • Apply dressings on open or draining lesions.
Potential impaired skin integrity	• Encourage elevation of affected part *to promote lymphatic drainage.* • Initiate range of motion exercises *to maintain blood flow.* • Protect affected area from cold *to prevent vasoconstriction.*
Pain	• Assess for defining characteristics. • Encourage patient to rest affected area. • Apply cool compresses to hot, nodular lesions.

Patient Education

1. Teach the patient how to change dressings, if indicated, using aseptic technique.
2. Teach the patient how to use cool compresses as needed.
3. Instruct the patient in the use of medications and their side effects.
4. Instruct the patient in the signs and symptoms of secondary infection and to seek medical attention if they occur.

Evaluation

Patient Outcome	Data Indicating That Outcome is Reached
Clinical disorder is identified and treated.	Inflammatory response is not exacerbated or does not recur.
Cutaneous lesions improve.	Erythema and lesions resolve. Necrotic areas reepithelialize. Discomfort is alleviated. Skin is intact.
Secondary infection is resolved or avoided.	There is no swelling, purulent exudate, fever, or lymphadenopathy.

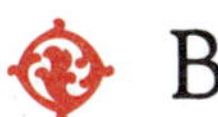

Burns

(Thermal, chemical, and electrical)

Thermal burns are caused by exposure to flames, hot liquids, and radiation. Chemical burns are caused by contact, ingestion, inhalation, or injection of acids, alkalies, or vesicants. True electrical burns occur when electrical current passes through the body to the ground. Electrical current can also cause secondary flash or flame burns.

More than 2 million people in the United States are burned each year. Although most of these burn injuries are minor, approximately 3% to 5% are life threatening. Burn injury is the second leading cause of death among young children and is the fourth overall cause of accidental death for people of all ages.[56]

Pathophysiology

Thermal and chemical injury disrupts the normal protective barrier function of the skin, causing a wide range of sequelae. In electrical injury heat is generated as the electricity passes through tissues. The thermal energy released is the cause of the injury.

The extent and depth of the burn injury determine the extent and severity of burn sequelae. Injury to the stratum corneum results in evaporative heat and water loss as a result of the loss or disruption of the lipid-water barrier of that layer. Injury to the stratum germinativum results in delayed or absent reepithelization and healing. Injury to the deeper structures results in scarring and tissue damage that may require skin grafting.

Vascular changes are caused by direct cellular damage or inflammatory processes. During the first few hours after the burn, vasoactive substances are released from the injured cells and vasoconstriction occurs. Vasodilation then occurs as a result of kinin release. During this period histamine causes increased capillary permeability, which allows plasma to leak into the burn area.

There are three zones of associated tissue damage.[65]

Zone of coagulation. This is the area of greatest destruction, where coagulation and irreversible cellular death occur. The area remains white because all viable tissue has been destroyed. Leukocytosis is inhibited or totally blocked. The zone can extend deeply into the tissue structures, causing full-thickness skin destruction.

Zone of stasis. This area surrounds the zone of coagulation and involves the vasculative dermis. Shortly after the burn, leukocytes and platelets aggregate in underlying capillaries, causing thrombosis. This, combined with the vasoconstriction, causes decreased circulation and transient ischemia to the area. With appropriate protection and treatment, circulation to the area can be restored, and the tissue saved. However, the tissue in this area is very fragile, and any further trauma because of rough handling or infection can convert this zone to one resembling the zone of coagulation.

Zone of hyperemia. This area, which is the least affected, forms the border of the burn wound. Vascular integrity is maintained with no cellular death. The area is bright red and blanches with pressure. The inflammatory processes are present.

In electrical injury, vessel wall changes occur that are characterized by cellular disintegration of the media of the arteries and arterioles and by severe arterial spasm.

Vascular changes and tissue loss cause fluid shifts. The first of these shifts, the hypovolemic stage, occurs during the first 24 to 48 hours. It is characterized by a rapid shift of fluid and protein from the vascular compartment into the interstitial spaces, causing blisters, edema, and fluid escape. Deep in the wound, sodium is translocated into skeletal muscle and other tissues and pulls water with it, which results in hyponatremia and hyperkalemia. This fluid shift, along with evaporative fluid loss from the surface of the wound, causes an abrupt decrease in the circulating blood volume resulting in hypovolemic shock. In turn hypovolemic shock causes decreased cardiac stroke volume, decreased blood pressure, increased peripheral resistance, decreased tissue perfusion, and circulatory collapse. Anuria, renal failure, and death result if treatment is delayed or inadequate.

Uninjured cells may become dehydrated as a result of this fluid shift. Hypoproteinemia develops from continued loss of protein as a result of increased capillary permeability. Nitrogen is lost through renal catabolism, and a negative nitrogen balance develops. Metabolic acidosis can occur as a result of decreased tissue perfusion, anaerobic metabolism, and retained acid end products.

Within 18 hours after the burn injury, the sodium and water

Figure 5-9 Estimation of adult burn injury: rule of nines. **A,** Anterior view. **B,** Posterior view.

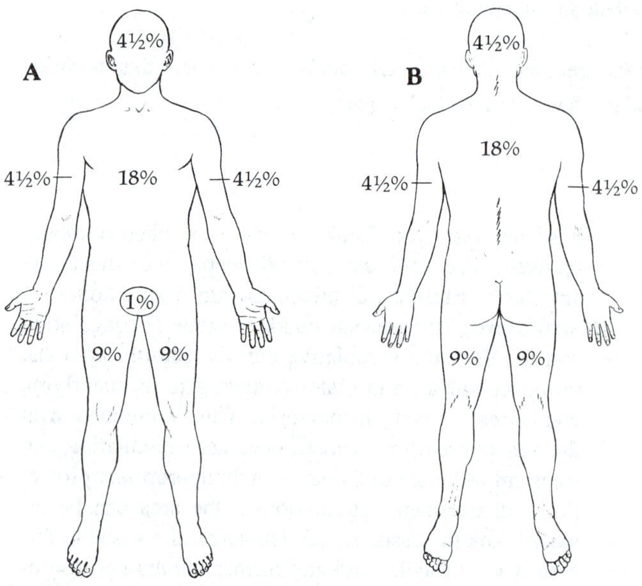

shunting reverse. Within 48 to 72 hours of the burn, a second fluid shift occurs in the opposite direction that causes fluid to return to the vascular compartment. In this phase the rapidly increasing blood volume causes diuresis and hemodilution that may result in dehydration, hyponatremia, and hypokalemia. Metabolic acidosis may occur because of bicarbonate loss in the urine and the catabolic state. Protein continues to be lost through the burn wound. Hypovitaminosis and weight loss also occur.

The evaporative fluid loss that occurs after the burn may be five to 19 times the normal loss. Associated with this fluid loss are tremendous heat loss and hypermetabolism that cause enormous caloric expenditure and hypothermia.

Erythrocyte hemolysis and a decrease in red cell mass occur as a result of direct damage and a decreased half-life of damaged red cells. Platelet function and half-life are also diminished. Hemoconcentration occurs as a result of fluid loss from the vascular system, which causes hematocrit values to rise.

Patients who have been injured in a fire may also have carbon monoxide poisoning from inhaling the gas that results from incomplete burning of some materials. Poisoning occurs becauses carbon monoxide has 200 times the affinity of oxygen to combine with hemoglobin.

Diagnostic Studies

Physical Examination

Determination of extent of injury using rule of nines (Figure 5-9); Lund and Browder charts (Figure 5-10); determination of degree of injury (Tables 5-7 and 5-8)

Figure 5-10 Estimation of burn injury: Lund and Browder chart. Areas designated by letters (*A*, *B*, and *C*) represent percentages of body surface area that vary according to age. The accompanying table indicates the relative percentages of these areas at various stages in life.
From Sabiston.[66]

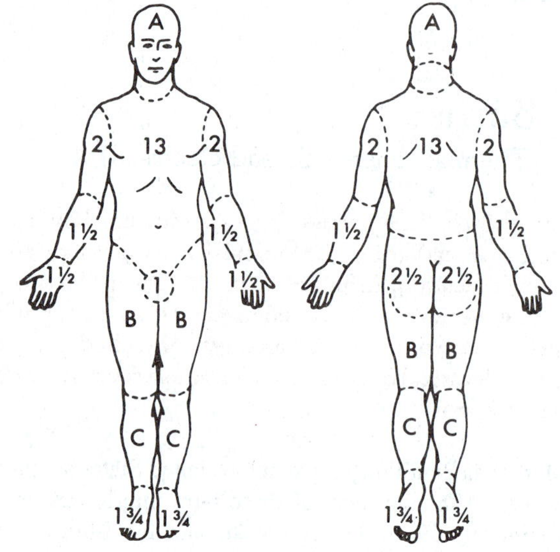

Relative percentages of areas affected by growth (age in years)

	0	1	5	10	15	Adult
A: half of head	9½	8½	6½	5½	4½	3½
B: half of thigh	2¾	3¼	4	4¼	4½	4¾
C: half of leg	2½	2½	2¾	3	3¼	3½

Second degree ________ and
Third degree ________ =
Total percent burned——

Determination of Mechanism of Injury

Thermal, chemical, or electrical

Baseline Laboratory Studies

Complete blood count
Serum electrolytes
Blood urea nitrogen
Creatinine
Arterial carboxyhemoglobin
Arterial blood gases
Bilirubin
Phosphorus
Alkaline phosphatase
Urine for myoglobin and hemoglobin levels

Fiberoptic Bronchoscopy

Inspection of major and proximal airways to determine upper airway injury

Table 5-7
Assessment of Burn Injury

Degree	Depth	Characteristics
Superficial (first degree)	Epidermis only; devitalization of epidermis and dilation of intradermal vessels	Pain; erythema; blanching with pressure; normal texture
Partial-thickness (second degree)	Destruction of epidermis and part of dermis	Erythema; blisters; pain; blanching with pressure; firm texture
Full-thickness (third and fourth degree)	Destruction of all layers of skin extending into subcutaneous tissue, muscle, nerves, and bone	Dryness; pale, white, brown, or red color; charring; no capillary refill; no pain; firm and leathery texture

Table 5-8
American Burn Association Classification of Burn Injury

Class	Description
Major	Full-thickness burns over 10% or more of body surface area (BSA)
	Partial-thickness burns over 25% of BSA
	All burns on face, hands, eyes, ears, feet, or perineum
	All inhalation and electrical burns
	All burns complicated by trauma
	All burns in poor-risk patients
Moderate	Full-thickness burns over 2%-10% of BSA
	Partial-thickness burns over 15%-25% of BSA
Minor	Full-thickness burns over less than 2% of BSA
	Partial-thickness burns over less than 15% of BSA

Xenon Lung Scan

Determination of small airway and parenchymal burns; bolus of xenon is injected; as xenon gas is expired from lungs, injured areas trap gas and show high-density levels

Medical Plan

Short-Term Care of Major Burns

Surgery

Escharotomy—may be needed for circumferentially burned extremities or chest

Fasciotomy—may be needed for electrical injuries

Medications

Narcotic analgesics
- Meperidine (Demerol) for pain, 20-25 mg IV

Immunologic agents
- Tetanus immunization
  - 0.5 ml IM for immunized patients
  - 0.5 ml IM plus 250 U tetanus immune globulin (Hyper-tet) for nonimmunized patients

Anti-infective agents
- Aqueous penicillin G for prophylaxis against gram-positive organisms, 1.2-2 million U IV in divided doses

General Management

Airway maintenance; intubation if needed

Humidification with 10% oxygen for inhalation injuries

Emergency treatment of musculoskeletal injuries or hemorrhage

Fluid replacement
- Parkland (Baxter formula)—2-4 ml lactated Ringer's solution/kg/% of BSA burned/24 hr; give one half of total amount in first 8 hours and one half during next 16 hours
- Brooke formula (after first 24 hours)—colloids (plasma, plasmanate, or dextran) 0.5 ml/kg/% of BSA burned plus 2000 ml of dextrose in water
- Electrical and inhalation injuries require more fluids

Urethral catheterization

Nasogastric tube insertion

Wound cleansing with povidone-iodine (Betadine), saline, or hydrogen peroxide

Central venous line insertion

Swan-Ganz catheter to monitor pulmonary arterial and capillary wedge pressures

Long-Term Care of Major Burns

Surgery

Skin grafts (see p. 567)
- Split-thickness—autograft from unburned area; postage stamp or strip application
- Mesh graft—split-thickness graft meshed with special instrument to cover large areas; held in place by dressing or sutures
- Homograft—skin from deceased person; used as temporary cover for about 10 days; may survive 4 to 5 weeks
- Heterograft—pigskin or synthetic substitute; acts as biologic dressing

Table 5-9
Comparison of Topical Burn Agents

Agent	Advantages	Disadvantages
Mafenide acetate (Sulfamylon)	Penetrates rapidly; not inactivated by pus or body fluids; softens wound, allowing better mobility; more effective in established infection	Painful; sulfa sensitivities; acidosis with renal or pulmonary impairment; antibacterial activity lasts 4-6 hours
Silver sulfadiazine (Silvadene)	Penetrates slowly; not inactivated by pus or body fluids; minimum systemic absorption; painless; antibacterial activity lasts up to 48 hours	Sulfa sensitivities; not as effective in established infection
Silver nitrate	Wet dressings retain heat, moisture, and reduce evaporation; no sensitivities	Painful; staining

Autologous cultured human epithelium—epidermal cells from unburned area cultured into sheets in flask; cultured sheets then attached to petrolatum gauze squares and sutured in place in wound; petrolatum gauze removed 7 to 10 days later[29]
Amputation of limb severely injured from electrical injury

Medications

Anti-infective agents
Topical (Table 5-9)
Mafenide acetate 10% (Sulfamylon); sterile application of amounts sufficient to just cover wound; wound left open to air; reapplied bid after washing off previous application and debriding wound
Silver sulfadiazine 1% (Silvadene) cream applied tid or qid; left open or covered with mesh gauze dressing; washed off before application, but no wound debridement done
Silver nitrate solution 0.5%; saturated thick gauze pads replaced q12-24h
Narcotic analgesics
Codeine, meperidine (Demerol), methadone (Dolophine); dosage determined on individual basis

General Management

Wound debridement (see p. 566)
Hydrotherapy (see p. 564) once or twice daily for 20 to 30 minutes for dressing removal and debridement
Dressings, wet or dry (see p. 564 for wet dressings)
Dry dressing—single layer of nonadherent fine mesh gauze held in place by coarse gauze wrap
Nutrition
2 to 4 g protein/kg/day
3500 to 5000 calories daily
Vitamin and iron replacement
Total parenteral nutrition (hyperalimentation) if needed
Physiotherapy

Care of Minor Burns

Medications

Immunologic agents
Tetanus immunization, 0.5 ml IM for immunized patients, 0.5 ml IM plus 250 U tetanus immune globulin (Hyper-tet) for nonimmunized patients
Anti-infective agents
Topical (applied with sterile tongue blade to completely cover wound with ⅛-inch thickness)
Mafenide acetate (Sulfamylon) 5%
Silver sulfadiazine (Silvadene) 1%
Povidone-iodine (Betadine)
Polymyxin B, bacitracin, Neosporin
Narcotic analgesics
Codeine, 30-60 mg po or subcutaneously q4-6h
Morphine, 8-10 mg subcutaneously
Meperidine (Demerol), 50-100 mg po q4-6h
Analgesic-antipyretics
Aspirin, 650 mg po q4-6h

General Management

Wound cleansed with one-half-strength Betadine solution
Wound debridement (see p. 566)
Dressing—innermost layer of nonadherent, porous, fine mesh gauze (fine enough to prevent epithelialization into gauze); second layer of bulky, fluffed coarse mesh gauze to absorb exudate; outer layer of semielastic coarse mesh to apply even pressure and hold dressing in place; change once or twice daily

NURSING CARE

Nursing Assessment

Wound

Degree and extent of injury; see Tables 5-7 and 5-8; mechanism of injury (thermal, chemical, or mechanical)

First Fluid Shift and Hypovolemic Shock

Vital signs: decreased blood pressure, increased pulse; urinary output (desirable: 50 ml/hour); monitoring of central venous pressure; potassium levels increased

Second Fluid Shift

Hyperpnea; blood pH less than 7.35; CO_2 combining power less than 21 mEq/L; $Paco_2$ less than 40 mm Hg

Airway

Pulmonary edema (see Chapter 2); singed nasal hair; soot in mouth or nose; darkened septum; rales, cough, or cyanosis; dyspnea or stridor

Carbon Monoxide Poisoning

Vomiting; chest pain; tachycardia; confusion; agitation; decreased coordination

Neurologic

Changes in level of consciousness

Cardiovascular

Vital signs; dysrhythmias; fluid shifts; cyanosis; capillary refill; pulses

Musculoskeletal

Fractures; decreased mobility; deformities; exposed bone or muscle

Hypermetabolism and Heat Loss

Body temperature; weight loss

Hemopoietic

Increased hematocrit; hemoglobinuria

Gastrointestinal

Mouth injuries; nausea and vomiting; blood in gastric contents; bowel sounds; paralytic ileus; stress ulcer

Renal

Renal failure resulting from hypovolemic shock; oliguria; anuria; desirable output 50 ml/hour for adults, 1 ml/kg/hour for children; myoglobinuria; hemoglobinuria; diuresis (second phase)

Pain

Presence or absence; location; intensity; severity

Psychosocial

Body image

Infection

Inflammation; exudate; odor

Nursing Dx & Intervention

Nursing Diagnosis	Nursing Intervention/Rationale
Impaired skin integrity	• Assess for degree and extent of injury. • Handle wound gently *to avoid converting zone of stasis to zone of coagulation.* • Implement isolation precautions *to prevent infection.* • Use sterile technique in wound care: debridement, topical preparations, and dressing changes *to prevent infection.* • Provide hydrotherapy *to debride burn.* • Provide wound care to graft donor site *to promote healing.* • Use sterile linen *to prevent infection.* • Use bed cradles *to prevent pressure to injured tissue.* • Assess for signs and symptoms of first and second fluid shifts.
Fluid volume deficit (2)	• Observe patency of urinary catheter. • Monitor input and output. • Replace fluids to achieve output of 50 ml/hour. • Monitor vital signs. • Monitor urine specific gravity. • Monitor central venous pressure.
Altered renal, cardiopulmonary, gastrointestinal, and peripheral tissue perfusion	• Maintain adequate fluid replacement *to maintain circulating volume.* • Maintain optimum mobility *to promote circulation.* • Provide adequate nutrition *to promote tissue healing.*
Impaired physical mobility; potential for disuse syndrome	• Provide active and passive range of motion exercises *to prevent muscle wasting and contractures.* • Use CircOlectric bed per physician order. • Refer patient for physiotherapy *to establish therapeutic regimen of motion and exercise.* • Apply splints *to prevent contractures.* • Have patient participate in water exercises *to maintain limb mobility.* • See pp. 1687 and 1689.

Nursing Diagnosis	Nursing Intervention/Rationale
Altered nutrition: less than body requirements	• Assess for nutritional status and weight loss. • Monitor protein intake: 2 to 4 g/kg/day. • Monitor caloric intake: 3500 to 5000 calories daily *to meet necessary requirements and promote healing*. • Monitor vitamin replacement. • In collaboration with physician, institute total parenteral nutrition *to replace or supplement oral intake*. • Provide high-protein powdered milk preparations. • Encourage self-feeding. • Offer favorite foods *to stimulate appetite*. • Avoid performing painful procedures near mealtime. • Offer snacks.
Constipation	• Assess for defining characteristics. • Give nothing by mouth until bowel sounds return. • Provide bulk foods *to promote peristalsis*. • Provide fruit juices *to promote peristalsis*. • Administer stool softeners *to aid elimination*.
Hypothermia	• Keep patient warm through control of environmental temperature *to prevent heat loss*. • Maintain adequate caloric intake (see Nutrition) *to provide energy and heat replacement*.
Pain	• Assess for pain. • Administer analgesics as ordered. • Position patient for comfort. • Provide or refer patient for hydrotherapy. • Instruct in relaxation techniques. • Refer patient for biofeedback training.
Body image disturbance; situational low self-esteem	• Assess for defining characteristics. • Encourage patient to express feelings about body, body appearance, or fear of reaction or rejection by others *to begin process of realistic self-evaluation*. • Spend time with patient *to reassure patient that appearance is not repulsive*. • Prepare visitors for patient's appearance *to reduce overt negative reactions*. • Encourage self-esteem by continued interest in patient and attentiveness to patient's needs.
Anticipatory grieving	• Assess for defining characteristics. • Encourage patient to express distress, anger, sorrow, guilt, and fear *to assist patient in movement through stages of grieving*.
Powerlessness	• Observe for signs of depression or apathy. • Involve patient in decision making *to increase sense of control*. • Encourage patient to express dissatisfation and frustration. • Accept patient's feelings of anger.

Patient Education

1. Instruct the patient in the care of minor burns:
   a. Cleanse wound with one-half-strength Betadine using sterile gauze; rub gently to remove existing topical agent.
   b. Apply topical agent thickly enough to cover wound with ⅛ inch of agent to provide healing and prevent bandage from adhering.
   c. Apply nonadherent fine mesh gauze (fine enough not to be epithelialized), then fluffed bulky coarse gauze to trap exudate; hold in place with semielastic net to exert even pressure.
2. Instruct the patient in the care of healed burns:
   a. Wash skin gently, rinse well, dry thoroughly, and apply cream.
   b. Avoid exposure to sunlight, harsh detergents, fabric softeners, and irritation by rubbing of clothing.
3. Instruct the patient to watch for signs of infection and to seek early treatment to avoid further complications.
4. Instruct the patient that increased calories and protein may be required until healing is complete.
5. Advise the patient of available support groups and community resources to assist in the resumption of usual activities and relationships.

Evaluation

Patient Outcome	Data Indicating That Outcome is Reached
State of homeostasis exists.	Normal blood values include the following: pH of 7.35-7.45; $Paco_2$ of 40-43; CO_2 combining power of 21-28 mEq/L; sodium 136-145 mEq/L; potassium 3.5-5 mEq/L; chloride 100-106 mEq/L. Nitrogen is in balance. Fluids are in balance.
Burn area heals.	Reepithelialization occurs. Skin is intact and free of infection.
Nutrition is adequate.	Patient eats diet high in protein, calories, minerals, and vitamins. Patient does not lose weight. Wounds heal.
Patient is free of contractures.	Patient has full extremity flexion and extension.
Patient resocializes and evaluates appearance in realistic manner.	Patient returns or plans to return to former activities if possible. Patient develops interests and activities compatible with degree of limitation. Patient engages in satisfactory interpersonal relationships.
Home care is satisfactory.	Healing remains uninterrupted. New tissue is free of irritation or infection. Scar tissue remains soft and pliable.
Complications are recognized and treatment is sought.	Patient seeks medical attention for infection, weight loss, contractures, or changes in scar tissue.

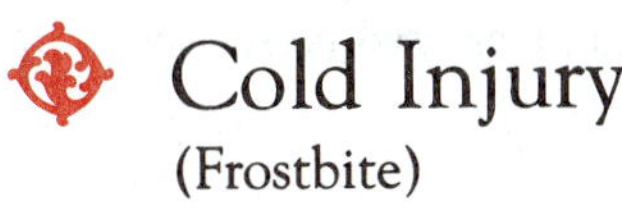

Cold Injury
(Frostbite)

Frostbite is a localized cold injury caused by exposure to freezing temperatures.

Several predisposing factors are associated with the occurrence of frostbite. People who are not acclimated to the cold and those from warmer climates have more vasospasm and less heat production in their extremities when exposed to cold temperatures; thus their risk of cold injury is increased. A racial predisposition of blacks to cold injury has been noted.[65] Fatigue, hunger, young or old age, circulatory disorders, fear, use of alcohol, and hypoxia increase the risk of cold injury. Factors that promote heat loss such as contact with metal, wet skin, and high wind velocity contribute to the occurrence and severity of frostbite injuries.

Pathophysiology

Cellular injury in frostbite is caused by direct freezing of cells at the time of injury or by inadequate tissue perfusion resulting from vascular spasm and occlusion of small vessels in the injured area.

With direct freezing of cells (crystallization), ice crystals form in extracellular fluids and osmotically draw intracellular fluid, thereby causing cell dehydration. Vascular changes include vasoconstriction, decreased capillary perfusion, and increased viscosity of the blood with sludging and thrombus formation.

After thawing, vascular stasis occurs in the injured area as a result of obstruction in the vascular bed. Edema occurs in the injured area and peaks 2 to 3 days after thawing. Thrombi, interstitial hemorrhaging, and leukocyte infiltration are present. Tissue necrosis occurs and becomes more prominent as the edema resolves. It may take 60 to 90 days before the necrotic tissue becomes fully evident.

The extent of the injury is determined by the amount and rate of heat loss from the skin. Frostbite is classified as superficial or deep. Superficial injury involves the skin and subcutaneous tissue. The injured area is white, waxy, soft, and anesthetic. Capillary refill is absent. On thawing the area becomes flushed, edematous, and painful and then may turn mottled or purplish. Large blisters may develop within 24 hours and resolve in about 10 days, leaving a hard dark eschar. After 3 to 4 weeks the eschar separates, leaving sensitive new epithelium. Throbbing and burning pain last for several weeks. The area is sensitive to heat and cold for months, and the frostbitten part may perspire excessively.

Deep frostbite injures the skin, subcutaneous tissue, muscle, tendon, and neurovascular structures. The injured part is hard and solid and remains cold, mottled, and blue or gray after thawing. Blisters may be absent or may form after several weeks at the point where viable and nonviable tissue meet. Edema occurs in the entire limb and may take months to resolve. When the blisters dry, blacken, and slough off, a line of demarcation remains where the viable tissue separates and retracts from the dead tissue.

Diagnostic Studies and Findings

Physical Examination

Characteristic findings with congruent history

Medical Plan

Surgery

Escharotomy
Sympathectomy for severe vasospasm and pain

Debridement after retraction of viable tissue (13 weeks to 4 months after injury)
Amputation of nonviable extremity after retraction of viable tissue and medical intervention; may be several months after injury

Medications

Immunologic agents
- Tetanus immunization, 0.5 ml IM for immunized patients, 0.5 ml IM plus 250 U tetanus immune globulin (Hyper-tet) for nonimmunized patients

Plasma expanders
- Low–molecular weight dextran 40, 20 ml/kg IV q24h to decrease sludging; this therapy is controversial[65]

Anti-infective agents
- Tetracycline or ampicillin (Amcill, Omnipen, others) for prophylaxis, 250 mg po q6h

Narcotic analgesics
- Morphine, up to 15 mg IM q3h

Analgesic-antipyretics
- Aspirin, 650 po q3h

General Management

Rapid rewarming by immersion for 20 minutes in water at 38° to 45° C (100° to 112° F)
Protective isolation of patient or extremity
Whirlpool baths three times a day at 32° to 37° C (90° to 98° F)

NURSING CARE

Nursing Assessment

Injured Area

Color of skin; resilience of tissue; extent of limb involvement; duration of contact with cold; superficial injury: white, waxy, soft, no capillary refill; deep injury: hard, solid, mottled, blue or gray

Healing Process

Pain; edema; color; blister formation; eschar formation; line of demarcation between viable and nonviable tissue

Infection

Pus; odor; redness; heat; fever

Complications

Vasospasm; pain; hyperesthesia; increased perspiration

Nursing Dx & Intervention

Nursing Diagnosis	Nursing Intervention/Rationale
Altered tissue perfusion	• Assess injured area for characteristics. • In collaboration with physician, initiate rapid rewarming in water at 38° to 45° C (100° to 112° F) for 20 minutes. • Completely immerse affected area in water, avoiding contact of skin with container. • Instruct patient not to smoke *to avoid vasoconstriction.*
Impaired skin integrity	• Use sterile sheets *to prevent infection.* • Isolate patient or extremity if necessary *to prevent infection.* • Use bed cradle *to prevent mechanical trauma to injured tissue.* • Keep blisters intact *to avoid introducing pathogens.* • Keep extremity exposed to air *to prevent maceration.* • Avoid debridement *to prevent further tissue injury.*
Impaired physical mobility	• Assess for impaired mobility. • Elevate extremities periodically *to promote venous return and prevent stasis.* • Initiate range of motion exercises *to promote circulation and prevent contractures.*
Pain	• Assess for pain. • Keep sheets off extremity *to avoid pressure.* • Administer analgesics as ordered. • Instruct patient in relaxation techniques. • Refer patient for biofeedback training.
Body image disturbance	• Assess for defining characteristics. • Encourage patient to express feelings about body, body appearance, or fear of reaction or rejection by others *to begin process of realistic self-evaluation.*

Nursing Diagnosis	Nursing Intervention/Rationale
Anticipatory grieving	• Encourage patient to express distress, anger, sorrow, guilt, and fear about potential loss of extremity part or function *to assist in movement through stages of grieving*.
Powerlessness	• Observe for signs of depression and apathy. • Inform patient that healing process is long-term, slow, and uncertain; provide accurate information about healing. • Encourage patient to express dissatisfaction and frustration. • Involve patient in decision making *to increase sense of control*. • Accept patient's feelings of anger.

Patient Education

1. Instruct the patient to protect the extremity from temperature extremes and rapid changes in temperature, since the tissue is sensitive to temperature changes and refreezing will cause tissue loss.
2. Instruct the patient to avoid tight, constrictive clothing or pressure to an area that might decrease circulation.
3. Instruct the patient in the application of dry, sterile dressing to small, open areas.
4. Instruct the patient to avoid smoking to reduce vasoconstriction.
5. Instruct the patient in preventive measures to avoid future episodes or reinjury of the frostbitten part: protective, multilayered, warm, nonconstrictive clothing; avoidance of fatigue, hunger, and use of alcohol when exposed to the cold.

Evaluation

Patient Outcome	Data Indicating That Outcome is Reached
Maximum tissue is preserved.	Initial rapid thawing with no refreezing of tissue occurs. Tissue is free of infection. Healing is allowed to occur without premature surgical intervention.
Joints are functional.	Patient has full extension and flexion of joints.
Patient evaluates self in realistic manner.	Patient resumes former activities if possible. Patient develops interests and activities compatible with degree of limitation. Patient engages in satisfactory interpersonal relationships.
Patient prevents further injury to area.	Patient avoids tight, constrictive clothing or pressure to area. Patient does not smoke.
Patient prevents further episodes of cold injury.	Patient wears protective clothing and avoids hunger, fatigue, and use of alcohol when exposed to cold.

DISEASES OF THE NAILS

Fungal infections

See "Tinea."

Paronychia

Paronychia is an acute or chronic inflammation of the proximal nail fold.

Erythema, induration, and swelling of the nail folds and consequent pain and tenderness are the primary features of paronychia. Staphylococci, streptococci, and sometimes *Candida* are the organisms usually responsible for the infection. One or more fingers or toes may be involved. Paronychia may be acute or chronic. Acute paronychia usually results from minor trauma or a hangnail. Chronic paronychia occurs in people whose hands are exposed to chronic irritation and moisture.

Pathophysiology

In acute paronychia organisms enter through a break in the epidermis. The infection may follow the nail margin or extend beneath the nail and suppurate. Purulent exudate may drain from beneath the nail fold. The eponychium remains attached to the nail plate. This separation creates a space in which foreign material and inflammatory exudate accumulate. Such an environment is conducive to bacterial and yeast growth.

Chronic paronychia usually leads to nail ridging, distortion, and discoloration.

Diagnostic Studies and Findings

Physical Examination

Characteristic lesion

Culture

Growth of infecting organism

Medical Plan

Surgery

Incision and drainage of purulent pocket

Medications

Anti-infective agents
- Systemic antibiotics; depending on infecting organism
- Anticandidal solutions or lotions applied topically tid, clotrimazole (Lotrimin, Mycelex), miconazole (Monistat-Derm)
- Thymol 4% in chloroform solution, 1 drop tid to affected area

NURSING CARE

Nursing Assessment

Inflammatory and Infectious Processes

Erythema; swelling; heat; tenderness; pain; purulent exudate; nails ridged, distorted, and discolored

Environmental Factors

Constant moisture and trauma to hands or feet; history of previous infections

Nursing Dx & Intervention

Nursing Diagnosis	Nursing Intervention/Rationale
Impaired skin integrity	• Assess nail folds for inflammation and infection. • Apply hot soaks *to promote suppuration and drainage.* • Instruct patient in proper handwashing *to reduce existing pathogens.* • Instruct patient to scrupulously dry hands and feet, especially around nails, and to use hot air drying rather than towel when possible *to prevent a wet environment that predisposes to infection.*
Potential impaired skin integrity	• Instruct patient to protect hands and feet from moisture by wearing cotton socks and rubber gloves with cotton liners when hands are in water. • Discuss with patient role of environmental factors such as moisture and trauma, and explore ways to eliminate them.
Pain	• Offer hot soaks *to decrease swelling.* • Elevate affected limb *to prevent throbbing.*

Patient Education

1. Instruct the patient regarding handwashing, drying, protection from moisture, and trauma (see "Nursing Dx & Intervention").
2. Instruct the patient in the use of medications and their side effects.
3. Instruct the patient in aseptic dressing changes if needed for draining lesions or after incision and drainage.

Evaluation

Patient Outcome	Data Indicating That Outcome is Reached
Inflammation subsides, and infection resolves.	There is no erythema, swelling, heat, tenderness, pain, or purulent exudate.
Chronic moisture and trauma are avoided.	Paronychia does not recur.

DISEASES OF THE HAIR

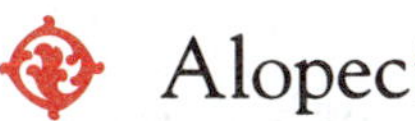

Alopecia

Alopecia is a partial or complete loss of hair.

Alopecia may occur as a result of genetic factors, the aging process, or local or systemic disease. Alopecia can be scarring or nonscarring and localized, patterned, or diffuse. The biologic dysfunctions of hair have little clinical importance, but the psychologic and social importance is substantial (Figure 5-11).

Pathophysiology

Table 5-10 summarizes the clinical features and pathophysiology of the various types of hair loss.

Figure 5-11 Alopecia areata.
Courtesy of Stephen B. Tucker, M.D., Department of Dermatology, University of Texas Health Science Center at Houston.

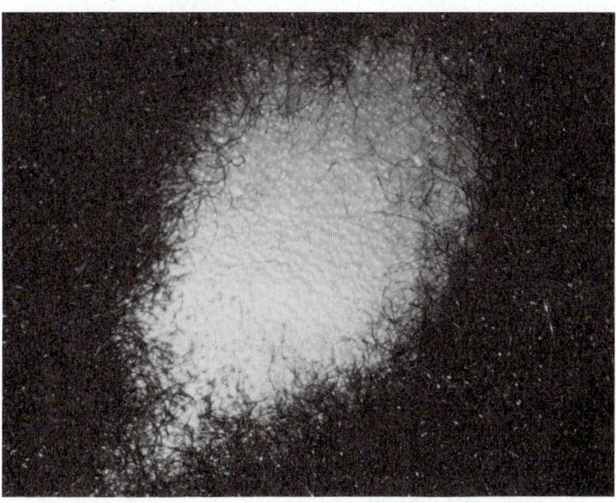

Table 5-10
Clinical Features and Pathology of Various Forms of Alopecia

Disease	Type	Features	Pathology
Areata	Nonscarring; localized or general	Occurs on any part of body; associated with family incidence; skin soft, smooth, not inflamed; one or several patches of loss; loss sudden; regrowth may occur with fine, light hair; hair pigments eventually	Inflammatory infiltrate around hair bulb; retraction in anagen hair; abnormal keratinization; loss of melanin and melanocytes; increased number of hair follicles in telogen phase
Androgenic	Nonscarring; patterned	Occurs on scalp; in men frontal and temporal loss; thinning over vertex in women; mild, severe, or complete loss; familial trait	Androgens cause hair follicles to become smaller in size; terminal hair no longer formed; most hair follicles eventually disappear
Mechanical and chemical	Nonscarring; localized	Acute or chronic; attributable to hairdressing procedures or habitual hair pulling; skin may show trauma from tight braids or curlers	Trauma to hair shaft; localized breakage of hair
Telogen effluvium	Nonscarring; diffuse	Occurs 6 to 16 weeks after precipitating episode; hair loss seen on shampooing or brushing; occurs as diffuse thinning; common precipitating factors are pregnancy, hormone therapy, stress, surgery, fever, and illness	Increased percentage of hairs in resting phase and subsequently in normal process of shedding
Drug related	Nonscarring Diffuse	Caused by antimitotic drugs (anagen hair loss) or by oral contraceptives, anticoagulants, propanolol (telogen hair loss); usually temporary	Antimitotic drugs cause decreased mitosis and decreased number of anagen hairs; hair shaft constricted; cause increase in percentage of hairs in telogen phase and subsequently in normal process of shedding
Scarring	Scarring	Due to systemic diseases such as lupus erythematosus, scleroderma, lichen planus, folliculitis decalvans; regrowth does not occur	Follicle destroyed by infection or scarring

Diagnostic Studies and Findings

Physical Examination

Hair loss distribution, characteristics, and history

Biopsy

Reveals hair phase and structural damage

Culture

Infecting bacteria or fungus

Medical Plan

Surgery

Hair transplant for androgenic hair loss

Medications

Corticosteroids
- Intralesional injection of 1-2 ml of triamcinolone (Kenalog), 10 mg/ml
- Topical glucocorticoids under occlusive dressing (see pp. 564 to 565)
  - Betamethasone (Valisone) 0.1%
  - Fluocinolone (Fluonid, Synalar, Fluosyn, Synemol, Minoxidil) 0.025%

For scarring alopecia, treatment directed at eliminating cause

NURSING CARE

Nursing Assessment

Lesion

As described in Table 5-10; location; distribution; scarring

Precipitating Factors

Trauma; drugs; family history; systemic diseases

Psychosocial Concerns

Concern about body image

Nursing Dx & Intervention

Nursing Diagnosis	Nursing Intervention/Rationale
Body image disturbance; situational low self-esteem	• Assess patient's self-perception. • Encourage patient to express feelings about body, body appearance, or fear of reaction or rejection by others *to begin process of realistic self-evaluation.* • Advise patient that regrowth will occur in certain temporary conditions. • Discuss use of wigs and hairpieces.

Patient Education

1. Advise the patient that commercial preparations will not restore hair or encourage hair growth.
2. Instruct the patient in the cause and course of the disease.
3. Instruct the patient in the use of glucocorticoids under an occlusive dressing when indicated (see pp. 564 to 565).

Evaluation

Patient Outcome	Data Indicating That Outcome is Reached
Underlying cause of hair loss is diagnosed and treated.	There is no new hair loss. Hair regrowth occurs in some conditions.
Patient evaluates appearance in realistic manner.	Patient does not use commercial hair restorative preparation. Patient uses wigs or hairpieces. Patient engages in satisfactory interpersonal relationships.

Hypertrichosis and hirsutism

Hypertrichosis refers to nonspecific hair growth of all types. Hirsutism is excessive hair growth induced by androgens in women.

Pathophysiology

Hypertrichosis occurs as a result of increased activity of the hair follicle with the production of a coarse terminal hair. Localized hypertrichosis can be the result of persistent trauma that causes chronic hyperemia and inflammation of the dermis. Hypertrichosis can also be caused by systemic disorders, including severe infection, gross malnutrition, and gluten enteropathy.

Hirsutism occurs as a result of increased androgen activity and simulates the male pattern of hair distribution, with increased coarse terminal hair on the face, areolae, midline of the abdomen, and extremities. Hirsutism may be familial. Onset usually occurs slowly with no other symptoms of virilization. It may occur after menarche. Sudden onset of hirsutism may be from increased androgen production from adrenal, ovarian, or pituitary sources or by certain drugs such as systemic steroids, androgens, testosterone, progesterone, norethindrone, and phenytoin.

Diagnostic Studies and Findings

Physical Examination

Distribution of hair with congruent history

Screening for Adrenal, Ovarian, and Pituitary Disorders

Medical Plan

For treatment of adrenal, ovarian, or pituitary disorders, see the specific diseases. Generally, tumors are removed surgically; glucocorticoids are used for adrenal hyperplasia.

General Management

Electrolysis—hair follicle destroyed by passage of galvanic electric current

Diathermy—tissue destroyed through electrocoagulation; not recommended, since it may cause scarring[23]

Depilatories (wax or chemical)—chemicals can be irritating

Shaving

Bleaching with hydrogen peroxide and ammonia to depigment hair

NURSING CARE

Nursing Assessment

History

Onset; menstrual history; drug history; family history of hirsutism

Hair Characteristics

Description of hair; type; distribution and pattern

Systemic Features

Signs of virilization; size of ovaries and clitoris; uterine development

Psychosocial Concerns

Concern about body image

Nursing Dx & Intervention

Nursing Diagnosis	Nursing Intervention/Rationale
Body image disturbance; situational low self-esteem	• Assess patient's self-perception. • Encourage patient to express feelings about body, body image, and fear of reaction or rejection by others *to begin process of realistic self-evaluation.* • Advise patient of treatments available for hair removal or bleaching.

Patient Education

1. Advise the patient of the advantages and disadvantages of the methods to remove or bleach the hair.
2. Instruct the patient in the cause and course of the disorder.

Evaluation

Patient Outcome	Data Indicating That Outcome is Reached
Underlying or systemic disorders are diagnosed and treated.	Hair growth diminishes or ceases.
Patient chooses acceptable method for removing or bleaching hair.	Patient is satisfied with method and appearance.
Patient evaluates appearance in realistic manner.	Patient engages in usual activities and relationships.

Medical Interventions and Related Nursing Care

Common Therapeutic Interventions and Topical Preparations and Medications

	Therapeutic Effect	Nursing Care/Patient Education
Common Therapeutic Interventions		
Balneotherapy	Treat large areas of body or widely disseminated lesions	Fill tub half full (20 to 25 gallons) at room temperature. Keep water from cooling. Bathe for 10 to 15 minutes. Use safety mat, since medications make tub slippery. Keep room warm. Remove loose skin and crusts after bath. Apply medications while skin is still moist. Blot dry. Have patient dress in light, loose clothing.
Tap water	Antipruritic cooling; anti-inflammatory	
Colloid, oatmeal, 1 cup	Antipruritic; nondrying	
Colloid, cornstarch, 2 cups	Antipruritic; drying	
Tar, commercial preparations, 2 teaspoons	Antipruritic; nondrying	
Carbonis detergens liquor, 1 ounce	Antipruritic; nondrying	
Oil (Alpha-Keri, Domol, Lubath, Jeri-Bath, etc.)	Lubrication	
Burn hydrotherapy May add prescribed amounts sodium chloride, potassium chloride, calcium hypochlorite, or detergent	Facilitate dressing change and debridement	Immerse in water at temperature of 100° F (37.8° C) for 20 to 30 minutes. Stay with patient. Administer pain medications. Plug catheter. Shave and debride as needed. Use aseptic technique.
Occlusive dressings	Increased absorption and penetration of topical preparations; produces moisture retention, skin maceration, and decreased evaporation to increase effect of topical preparations	Apply airtight plastic film over medicated skin. Remove for 12 of 24 hours to prevent complications. Watch for complications: bacterial and candidal infections, sweat retention, folliculitis, and side effects of medications.
Shampoos		Lather sufficiently. Gently work into scalp. Avoid contact with eyes.
Selenium sulfide	Antiseborrheic	
Betadine	Antibacterial	
Zinc pyrithione 2%	Antiseborrheic	
Carbonis detergens liquor, 5%	Antiseborrheic Antipruritic	
Triethanolamine sulfate 40%	Bland (can add medications)	
Wet dressings and compresses	Cool and dry acute inflammation through evaporation	Soak compress to point of dripping. Keep at room temperature. Remoisten every few minutes. Apply for 15 minutes every 2 to 3 hours. Do not rub or blot. Do not treat more than one third of the body at one time. Keep patient warm and covered. Advise patient that potassium permanganate stains skin, clothing, and tub. Instruct patient to use soft towels or cotton sheeting for home care to avoid irritating skin. Instruct patient to use clean towel or sheet each time compress is used, to keep them separate from rest of family linens, and to launder between each use.
Tap water or normal saline	Antipruritic; anti-inflammatory used in acute oozing dermatoses	
Aluminum acetate (Burow's)	As above; also antibacterial	
Potassium permanganate 1:10,000 solution; 5 grains/3 quarts water	As above; also antifungal and antibacterial	
Dry burn dressing		Cleanse wound with one-half strength Betadine using sterile gauze; rub gently to remove existing topical agent. Apply topical agent thick enough to cover wound with ⅛ inch of agent to provide healing and prevent bandage from adhering. Apply layers of dressing: fine gauze, bulky coarse gauze; semielastic mesh. Change dressing one or two times daily.
Nonadherent, porous, fine mesh gauze	First layer; nonadherent; fine enough to prevent epithelialization into gauze	
Bulky, fluffed, coarse, mesh gauze	Second layer; absorbs exudate	
Semielastic coarse mesh	Outer layer; applies even pressure; holds dressing in place	

	Therapeutic Effect	Nursing Care/Patient Education
Topical Preparations		
Creams and ointments Petrolatum, mineral oil, lanolin, Eurin, Qualatum, Unibase, Dermabase	Lubrication; protection; vehicle for medications; decrease water loss; ointments greasy with oil base; creams lighter and water washable	Rub into skin by hand. Cover ointments with light dressing to protect clothing. Apply frequently. Wash off before reapplication.
Gels Contain propylene glycol and carboxymethylene	Like creams and ointments; clear and nongreasy; may be used on hairy areas	Apply with fingers. Avoid rubbing, since they are thixotropic agents (become thinner with rubbing). Apply frequently.
Lotions With 0.5% menthol and 0.25% phenol	Liquid vehicles for medications; lubrication; cooling through evaporation Antipruritic; drying	Apply with cotton gauze. Lotions are usually not washed off between applications.
Pastes	Stiff vehicle of powder and ointment; porous and less occlusive than ointments; protective	Apply with tongue depressor. Wash off between applications. Scrub gently if paste is difficult to remove.
Powders Talc, zinc, oxide, cornstarch	Absorbent; hygroscopic (take up water); reduce friction	Apply with shaker. Avoid accumulation in intertriginous areas.
Topical Medications		
Antiseptic agents Chlorhexidine, povidone-iodine, hexachlorophene	Treat carriers of pathogens; reduce overall skin bacterial count	Observe for sensitivities. Do not use hexachlorophene for infants and children.
Antibacterial agents	Like antiseptic agents	Observe for sensitivities. Cover with light dressing to protect clothing. Apply two to four times a day. Wash off before reapplication. With sulfamylon debride wound before reapplication.
Neomycin	For gram-negative and gram-positive organisms	
Bacitracin	For gram-negative organisms and *Pseudomonas*	
Silver sulfadiazine (Silvadene)	For burns; for gram-negative and gram-positive organisms and yeast	
Sulfamylon	For burns; bacteriostatic only; for gram-negative and gram-positive organisms	
Precipitated sulfur 3%	Antiseborrheic	Observe for irritation.
Salicylic acid 3%-5%; urea 10%-20%	Keratolytic; increases absorption of other medications	Observe for irritation.
Corticosteroids Hydrocortisone 1%; fluocinolone 0.01%; triamcinolone 0.025%-0.1%; betamethasone	Decrease inflammation through vasoconstriction and direct action on leukocytes; decrease prostaglandin synthesis; decrease mitotic rate of epidermal cells	Apply sparingly to skin or apply in occlusive dressing. When used for prolonged periods, especially under occlusive dressings, watch for thinning of skin, striae formation, telangiectasia, and follicular hyperkeratosis.

Cryosurgery

In cryosurgery tissue is frozen to remove hyperkerolytic growths (such as warts) or to cause involution of cysts.

Contraindications and Cautions

1. Overfreezing can cause scarring and hyperpigmentation.
2. Application of liquid nitrogen can be painful and is not well tolerated by children.

Procedure

1. Liquid nitrogen is applied with a cotton-tipped applicator and is held in place for 10 to 20 seconds.
2. Carbon dioxide is applied via CO_2 pencil, which is held in place with moderate pressure for 20 to 30 seconds.

Nursing Interventions

1. Inform patient before treatment of possibility of scarring or hyperpigmentation, and help patient evaluate the benefit/risk trade-off.
2. Instruct patient in the procedure.
3. Observe for blister formation immediately with CO_2 or in 5 to 10 hours with liquid nitrogen.
4. Instruct patient to prevent infection by keeping area clean and dry, not puncturing blister, and not picking at scab.
5. Instruct patient to observe for signs of infection and to seek medical attention if they occur.

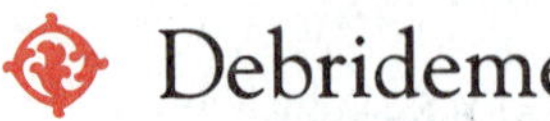

Debridement

In debridement dead tissue or eschar is removed to facilitate healing or in preparation for skin grafting.

Procedure

Surgery

Surgical excision—large areas removed down to fascia

Tangential excision—layers of eschar removed with dermatome or scalpel to point of capillary bleeding; edge of tissue picked up with forceps and necrotic tissue cut with scissors; margin of 0.5 cm left to avoid cutting viable tissue; debridement limited to area of 10 cm; bleeding controlled by direct pressure; topical agent applied

Medications

Proteolytic enzymes applied with saline to erode and consume eschar

Mechanical

Removal through mechanical action in dressing changes, hydrotherapy, and showers

Nursing Interventions

1. Describe procedure to patient.
2. Administer analgesics 20 minutes before debridement.
3. After procedure, assess area for exudate, color, sensation, bleeding, and size of area debrided.
4. Assess patient's response: pain, stress, or fear.

Dissection, Blunt

This technique is an office surgical procedure for removal of epidermal tumors, using a blunt dissector. Normal tissue is not disturbed, and scarring does not usually occur.

Procedure

1. Before procedure, the patient is given systemic analgesics if lesions are such that postoperative pain is anticipated, such as with large plantar or periungual warts.
2. Local anesthesia with lidocaine is provided via needle injection or jet injector.
3. The plane of dissection is established by inserting the tip of blunt-tipped scissors between the lesion and the normal skin and cutting the skin circumferentially.
4. The blunt dissector is then inserted into the opened plane, which is separated from the normal underlying tissue with short firm strokes.
5. After the lesion is removed, the dissector is drawn back and forth over the exposed surface of the bed to remove tissue fragments.

Nursing Interventions

1. Instruct patient in the procedure.
2. After procedure cover wound with Band-Aid. Advise patient to change it daily for 3 to 4 days and thereafter to leave wound exposed to air.
3. Advise patient that moderate to intense pain may occur for 30 minutes to 2 hours after blunt dissection of periungual and plantar warts.

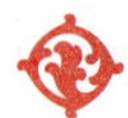

Electrodesiccation and Curettage

In electrodesiccation an electric current is used to remove superficial lesions. In curettage a dermal curette with round or oval sharp surfaces is used to remove superficial lesions. The procedures may be used together or separately.

Procedure

Fulguration

1. The surface to be treated is cleaned so it is dry and free of blood.
2. The pointed electrode is held slightly away from the tissue surface, and the unit is activated.
3. A sparking occurs resulting in tissue dehydration and charring of immediate surrounding area.

Desiccation

1. The pointed electrode is placed in contact with the skin surface or inserted slightly in the tissue, and the unit is activated.
2. The resulting tissue char is produced by fulguration.

Electrocoagulation

1. The bipolar setting is used.
2. The active electrode is placed in contact with the tissue, and the unit is activated.
3. Tissue necrosis is more extensive than with fulguration or desiccation.

Curettage

1. The area is anesthetized with lidocaine via needle injection or jet injector.
2. The skin around the lesion is supported with the fingers of the hand not holding the instrument.
3. With several smooth strokes, the curette is drawn through the tissue.

Nursing Interventions

1. Instruct patient in the procedure.
2. Clean surrounding skin with antibacterial agent.
3. If oozing occurs after procedure, cover with sterile gauze.

4. Area may be left exposed to air or covered with light dressing.
5. Encourage daily washing with soap and water.

Intralesional Injections

Intralesional injections are injections of a corticosteroid into a lesion. The anti-inflammatory action helps clear lesions and reduce the size of cysts.

Contraindications and Cautions

1. Injection into subcutaneous tissue can result in transient or permanent atrophy and local tissue depression.

Procedure

1. Aqueous suspension (usually triamcinolone, 5-10 mg/2 ml) is injected intracutaneously into the lesion or cyst with a fine-gauge needle. The more superficial the injection, the better the result.

Nursing Interventions

1. Inform the patient before treatment of the possibility of atrophy and help the patient evaluate the benefit/risk tradeoff.
2. Instruct the patient to observe for side effects of treatment: bleeding, hemorrhaging, pigmentation, and atrophy; adrenal suppression may occur with multiple injections.
3. Instruct the patient to observe for desired effects: cyst decreases in size and lesion clears.
4. Instruct the patient to keep the area clean to avoid secondary infection.

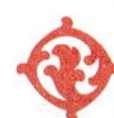

Skin Graft

In a skin graft a section of skin tissue that is separated from its blood supply is transferred to a recipient site to provide tissue for epithelization.

split-thickness graft Composed of epidermis and superficial layers of dermis.
full-thickness graft Composed of epidermis and all layers of dermis.
homograft (allograft) Skin from a deceased person that is used as temporary cover for about 10 days, and may survive for 4 to 5 weeks.
heterograft (xenograft) Pigskin or synthetic substitute that acts as biologic dressing.
autograft Skin from another part of the patient's own body.
mesh graft Split-thickness graft meshed with a special instrument to cover large areas and held in place by a dressing or sutures.
autologous cultured human epithelium Unburned epidermal cells cultured into sheets in a flask. The cultured sheets are then attached to petrolatum gauze squares and sutured in place in the wound. The petrolatum gauze is removed 7 to 10 days later.[29]

Procedure

1. The donor site is prepared by surgical scrub. The recipient site is debrided and cleansed.
2. A split- or full-thickness graft is taken from the donor site with a dermatome. The graft is cut as "postage stamps" or strips or is meshed and is placed on recipient sites.
3. The graft is held in place by a pressure dressing or sutures.
4. The donor site is covered with nonadherent gauze held in place by a gauze dressing.

Nursing Interventions

Donor Site

1. Remove the outer dressing in 24 hours.
2. Inspect the site daily.
3. Assess for bleeding, pain, and infection.
4. Leave nonadherent gauze in place until it separates spontaneously.
5. If infection occurs, treat it with medicated wet dressing.

Recipient (Graft) Site

1. Inspect the site daily.
2. Assess for edema, hematoma formation, fluid collection, infection, and viability of graft tissue.
3. Immobilize the affected part to avoid disrupting the graft.
4. Elevate the grafted extremity for 7 to 10 days.
5. Protect the graft from scratching by the patient.
6. If infection occurs, treat it with a medicated wet dressing.
7. The heterograft acts as a biologic dressing; expect it to slough off in 10 days to 5 weeks.

Healing Phase

1. Inform the patient about the changing hues of graft scar tissue: pale, then pink, then red, then fading to resemble surrounding skin; a full-thickness graft may remain deeply red for several months.
2. Anticipate skin scaling with a full-thickness graft.
3. Lubricate the donor site with lanolin or cocoa butter to keep the tissue soft and pliable.
4. Apply mineral oil or lanolin to the graft site after the second or third week to remove superficial crusts, moisten the graft, and stimulate circulation.
5. Instruct the patient who will be at home to avoid overexposure of the graft site to the sun, since the site is sensitive to the sun and can burn easily.
6. Encourage the patient to express feelings about body, body appearance, or fear of reaction or rejection by others.

Systemic Steroid Therapy

In systemic steroid therapy parenteral or oral glucocorticoids are used for their anti-inflammatory action.

Contraindications and Cautions

1. Hypertension and diabetes mellitus can be exacerbated.
2. Concurrent infections can be masked.
3. Therapy is used with caution in patients who are predisposed to peptic ulceration, thrombophlebitis, adrenal suppression, and mood swings.

Procedure

The dose and duration of treatment depend on the severity of the disease and the patient's response. The patient should receive a dose sufficient to produce a therapeutic response and then be maintained with a minimum effective dose; the dose should be tapered slowly after the lesions have cleared.

Approximate equivalent doses of various steroids are:

Betamethasone, 0.5 mg	Methylprednisolone, 4 mg
Dexamethasone, 0.75 mg	Prednisolone, 5 mg
Fludrocortisone, 2 mg	Prednisone, 5 mg
Hydrocortisone, 20 mg	Triamcinolone, 4 mg

Nursing Interventions

1. Inform the patient about the side effects to watch for and to seek medical attention if they occur: euphoria, gastrointestinal pain or bleeding, bruising, thrombophlebitis, hypertension, moon face, cushingoid features, acne, hirsutism, osteoporosis, and mood swings.
2. Instruct the patient to take medication with milk or antacids to decrease gastric irritation.
3. Instruct the patient to increase protein intake to combat osteoporosis.

Ultraviolet Light Therapy

Short-wave ultraviolet light (UV-B) is used for the treatment of psoriasis and acne.

In Goeckerman therapy ultraviolet light therapy is used in combination with coal tar applications that are photosensitizing; it is used for the treatment of psoriasis.

In PUVA therapy long-wave ultraviolet light (UV-A) is used in combination with psoralen, which is a photosensitizer (P + UV-A = PUVA); it is used for treating psoriasis.

Procedure

Short-Wave Ultraviolet Light

1. The patient is exposed one to three times per week.
2. The exposure time is increased to keep skin just below erythema level.

Goeckerman Therapy

1. Coal tar ointment is applied, left on for several hours, and then washed off.
2. UV-B therapy is given in doses to account for photosensitization.
3. The skin is kept just below erythema level.
4. Coal tar ointment is reapplied after UV-B exposure.

PUVA Therapy

1. Psoralen is administered in an initial dose of 0.6 mg/kg.
2. UV-A irradiation is delivered 2 to 4 hours after psoralen administration.
3. Dosage and exposure are determined by individual response.
4. Therapy is usually provided in specific treatment centers, since specialized equipment, careful calibration, and close monitoring are required.

Contraindications and Cautions

PUVA Therapy

1. Long-term effects of PUVA therapy remain controversial, and treatment is usually reserved for chronic, severe, refractory psoriasis.[23,24]

Nursing Interventions

1. Instruct the patient in the procedure.
2. Assist the patient in setting up a schedule to maintain the therapeutic regimen.
3. Instruct a patient who is using short-wave ultraviolet light therapy at home to:
   a. Use a lamp with an automatic timer to shut off
   b. Use a backup timer
   c. Measure the distance from the lamp carefully and maintain the correct distance
   d. Increase exposure time slowly and keep the skin below erythema level
   e. Wear an occlusive protective eye covering
4. Advise a patient who is using concomitant photosensitizing agents to avoid lengthy exposure to sunlight.
5. Advise a patient who is receiving PUVA therapy of the undetermined long-term effects, and assist the patient in evaluating the risk/benefit trade-off.

References

1. Apfelberg D et al: The role of the argon laser in the management of hemangiomas, Int J Dermatol 21:579, 1982.
2. Arndt K: Treatment technics in argon laser therapy, J Am Acad Dermatol 11:90, 1984.
3. Ashton R et al: Anthralin: historical and current perspectives, J Am Acad Dermatol 9:173, 1983.
4. Barkin R and Rosen P, editors: Emergency pediatrics, St. Louis, 1984, The CV Mosby Co.
5. Baron M: The skin and wound healing, Top Clin Nurs 5:11, 1983.
6. Bates B: A guide to physical examination, ed 4, Philadelphia, 1987, JB Lippincott Co.
7. Berliner H: Aging skin. Part I, Am J Nurs 86:1138, Oct 1986.
8. Berliner H: Aging skin. Part II, Am J Nurs 86:1259, Nov 1986.

9. Bickers D: Position paper: PUVA therapy, J Am Acad Dermatol 8:265, 1983.
10. Bowers A and Thompson J: Clinical manual of health assessment, ed 2, St. Louis, 1984, The CV Mosby Co.
11. Buecker J, Ratz J, and Richfield D: Histology of port-wine stain treated with carbon dioxide laser, J Am Acad Dermatol 10:1014, 1984.
12. Camp R: Generalized pruritus and its management, Clin Exp Dermatol 7:557, 1982.
13. Carruth J and McKenzie J: The argon laser in dermatology: safety aspects, Clin Exp Dermatol 7:247, 1982.
14. Clayton B: Mosby's handbook of pharmacology in nursing, ed 3, St. Louis, 1984, The CV Mosby Co.
15. Coskey R: Dermatologic therapy: December, 1982, through November, 1983, J Am Acad Dermatol 11:25, 1984.
16. Cronin E: The management of allergic contact dermatitis, Clin Exp Dermatol 7:281, 1982.
17. Dawber R: Alopecia and hirsutism, Clin Exp Dermatol 7: 177, 1982.
18. Delancy V and North C: Skin assessment, Top Clin Nurs 5:5, 1983.
19. Diette K et al: Role of ultraviolet A in phototherapy for psoriasis, J Am Acad Dermatol 11:441, 1984
20. Dimick A: The burn at first sight, Emerg Med 15:130, 1983.
21. Ellis C et al: Isotretinoin therapy is associated with early skeletal radiographic changes, J Am Acad Dermatol 10:1024, 1984.
22. Elton R: Complications of cutaneous cryosurgery, J Am Acad Dermatol 8:513, 1983.
23. Epstein E: Common skin disorders: a physician's illustrated manual, ed 2, Oradell, NJ, 1983, Medical Economics Books.
24. Epstein E, editor: Controversies in dermatology, Philadelphia, 1984, WB Saunders Co.
25. Farber E, Abel E, and Charuworn A: Recent advances in the treatment of psoriasis, J Am Acad Dermatol 8:311, 1983.
26. Fischbach FT: A manual of laboratory diagnostic tests, Philadelphia, 1980, JB Lippincott Co.
27. Fitzpatrick T and Parrish J: PUVA in perspective. In Epstein E, editor: Controversies in dermatology, Philadelphia, 1984, WB Saunders Co.
28. Galles E: Identifying dermatological conditions in blacks, J Emerg Nurs 4:56, 1978.
29. Gallico G et al: Permanent coverage of large burn wounds with autologous cultured human epithelium, N Engl J Med 311:448, 1984.
30. Graham J and Jouhar A: The importance of cosmetics in the psychology of appearance, Int J Dermatol 22:153, 1983.
31. Guyton A: Human physiology and mechanisms of disease, Philadelphia, 1982, WB Saunders Co.
32. Habif T: Clinical dermatology: a color guide to diagnosis and therapy, St Louis, 1985, The CV Mosby Co.
33. Heng M, Kloss S, and Haberfelde G: Pathogenesis of papular urticaria, J Am Acad Dermatol 10:1030, 1984.
34. Henwood B and MacDonald D: Caterpillar dermatitis, Clin Exp Dermatol 8:77, 1983.
35. Huff JC, Weston W, and Tonnesen M: Erythema multiforme: a critical review of characteristics, diagnostic criteria, and causes, J Am Acad Dermatol 8:763, 1983.
36. Jones RR: The histogenesis of eczema, Clin Exp Dermatol 8:213, 1983.
37. Kaplan R, Russell D, and Lowe N: Etretinate therapy for psoriasis: clinical responses, remission times, epidermal DNA and polyamine responses, J Am Acad Dermatol 8:95, 1983.
38. Kim MJ, McFarland G, and McLane A: Pocket guide to nursing diagnosis, ed 2, St. Louis, 1987, The CV Mosby Co.
39. Korting G: Geriatric dermatology, Philadelphia, 1980, WB Saunders Co.
40. Kravis T and Warner CG, editors: Emergency medicine: a comprehensive review, St. Louis, 1983, The CV Mosby Co.
41. Lane A, Wachs G, and Weston W: Once-daily treatment of psoriasis with topical glucocorticosteroid ointments, J Am Acad Dermatol, 8:523, 1983.
42. Lawlis G and Achterberg J: Acne: the disease and stress, Top Clin Nurs 5:23, 1983.
43. Lever R and Mackie R: The use of oral sodium cromoglycate in young adults with severe chronic atopic dermatitis, Clin Exp Dermatol 9:143, 1984.
44. Leverne G: The treatment of pemphigus and pemphigoid, Clin Exp Dermatol 7:643, 1982.
45. Lowe N et al: Coal tar phototherapy for psoriasis reevaluated: erythemagenic versus suberythemagenic ultraviolet with a tar extract in oil and crude coal tar, J Am Acad Dermatol 8:781, 1983.
46. Lowe N et al: Anthralin for psoriasis: short-contact anthralin therapy compared with topical steroid and conventional anthralin, J Am Acad Dermatol 10:9, 1984.
47. Luckmann J and Sorensen K: Medical-surgical nursing: a psychophysiologic approach, ed 2, Philadelphia, 1980, WB Saunders Co.
48. Lyell A: Review of significant progress in clinical dermatology since 1977, J Am Acad Dermatol 6:195, 1982.
49. Malseed R: Quick reference to drug therapy and nursing considerations, Philadelphia, 1983, JB Lippincott Co.
50. Marks R: Chronic idiopathic urticaria, Int J Dermatol 21:19, 1982.
51. Menter A and Cram D: The Goeckerman regimen in two psoriasis day care centers, J Am Acad Dermatol 9:59, 1983.
52. Monroe E: Urticaria, Int J Dermatol 20:32, 1981.
53. Moynahan E: The treatment and management of epidermolysis bullosa, Clin Exp Dermatol 7:665, 1982.
54. Nater J and DeGroot A: Unwanted effects of cosmetics and drugs used in dermatology, Princeton, NJ, 1983, Excerpta Medica.
55. National Center for Health Statistics: Prevalence of dermatological disease among persons 1-74 years of age: United States, Advance Data from Vital and Health Statistics 572(4), Public Health Service, Washington, DC, Jan 26, 1977, US Government Printing Office.
56. National Safety Council: Accident facts: 1987 edition, Chicago, 1987, The Council.
57. Phipps W, Long B, and Woods N, editors: Medical-surgical nursing, ed 2, St. Louis, 1983, The CV Mosby Co.
58. Pillsbury DM and Heaton CL: A manual of dermatology, ed 2, Philadelphia, 1980, WB Saunders Co.
59. Price S and Wilson L: Pathophysiology: clinical concepts of disease processes, New York, 1982, McGraw-Hill Book Co.
60. Pye R: Prospects for the treatment of acne vulgaris and rosacea, Clin Exp Dermatol 7:195, 1982.
61. Rakel R, editor: Conn's current therapy, Philadelphia, 1987, WB Saunders Co.
62. Rand R and Baden H: The ichthyoses: a review, J Am Acad Dermatol 8:285, 1983.
63. Rentoul J: Management of the hirsute woman, Int J Dermatol 22:265, 1983.
64. Robertson D and Maibach H: Topical corticosteroids, Int J Dermatol 21:59, 1982.
65. Rosen P et al: Emergency medicine: concepts and clinical practice, St. Louis, 1983, The CV Mosby Co.
66. Sabiston DC Jr, editor: Textbook of surgery: the biological basis of modern surgical practice, ed 11, Philadelphia, 1977, WB Saunders Co.
67. Samman P: Management of disorders of the nails, Clin Exp Dermatol 7:189, 1982.
68. Seidel H et al: Mosby's guide to physical examination, St. Louis, 1987, The CV Mosby Co.
69. Steinberg, F, editor: Care of the geriatric patient, ed 6, St. Louis, 1983, The CV Mosby Co.
70. Vasarinsh P: Clinical dermatology: diagnosis and therapy of common skin diseases, Woburn, Mass, 1982, Butterworth Publishers.
71. Verbov J: Pruritus ani and its management: a study and reappraisal, Clin Exp Dermatol 9:46, 1984.
72. Verbov J and Morley N: Color atlas of pediatric dermatology, Philadelphia, 1983, JB Lippincott Co.
73. Ward R and Wathen R: Principles of dialysis: utilization in nonuremic psoriatic subjects, Int J Dermatol 21:154, 1982.
74. Williamson D: Treatment of chronic psoriasis by Psoradrate (0.1% dithranol in a 17% urea base) applied under occlusion, Clin Exp Dermatol 8:287, 1983.
75. Wolska H, Jablonska S, and Bounameaux Y: Etretinate in severe psoriasis, J Am Acad Dermatol 9:883, 1983.

CHAPTER 6

The Eye

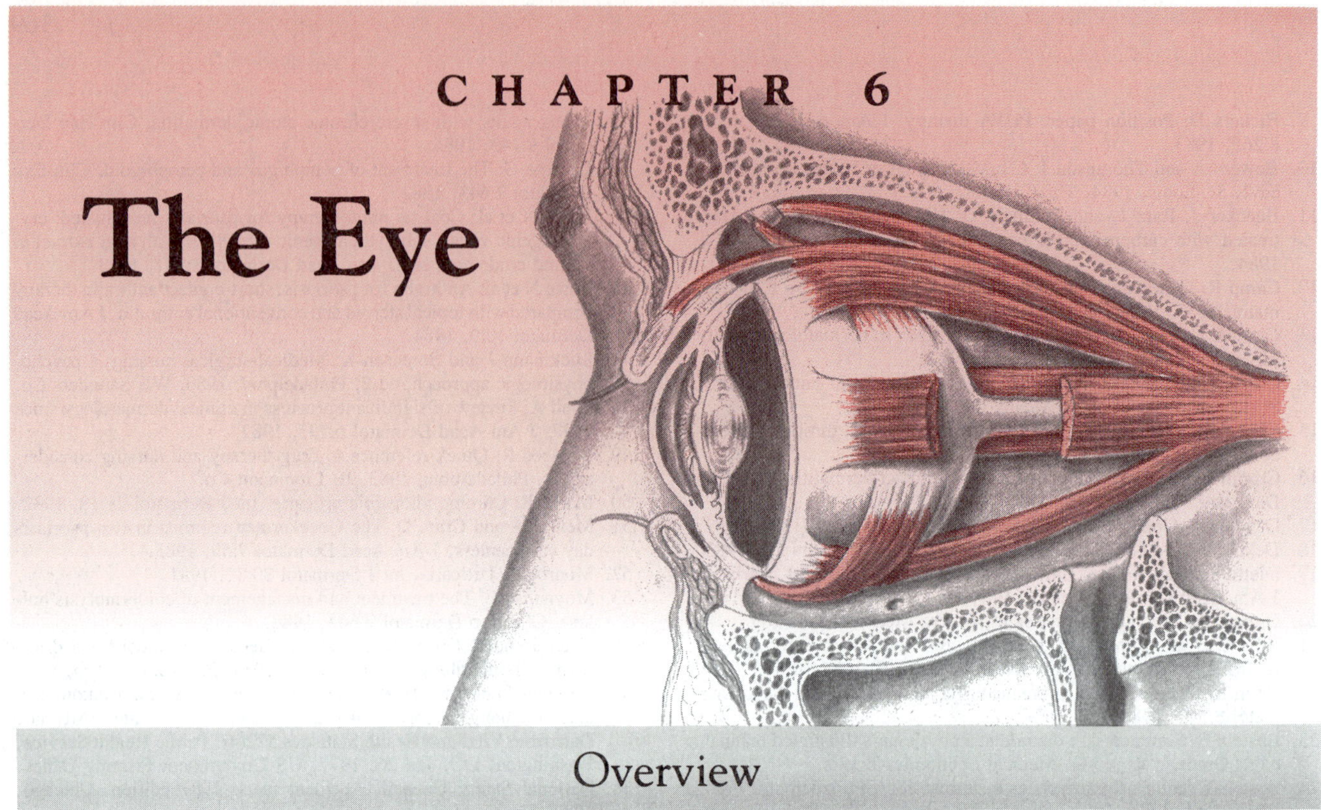

Overview

Preserving vision and preventing blindness are important to everyone. A recent poll found that Americans fear blindness more than any other disorder except cancer.[12] The American Academy of Ophthalmology's Committee on Eye Care for the American People reports that "approximately 500,000 Americans are legally blind, more than 11.4 million are visually impaired because of chronic or permanent defects, 80 million have a disease in one or both eyes, and additional millions need eyeglasses or contact lenses to see clearly."[12] Eye care has become the focus of more attention in recent years because expanding knowledge and technology have increased the opportunity for early diagnosis and successful treatment of eye disorders. Technologic advances include microsurgical techniques, laser surgery, contact lens refinement, development of an intraocular lens, and corneal replacement. Screening programs offered by schools and community agencies have enhanced public awareness of eye disorders and preventive eye care. This greater awareness of the need for periodic eye examinations, of specific measures for preventing eye injuries, and of the early signs or symptoms of eye disorders has contributed to the prevention of visual impairment. Major eye disorders include cataract, corneal impairments and injuries, glaucoma, retinal diseases, strabismus, and amblyopia. All these impairments can cause blindness, but most of them are partially or fully treatable if diagnosed early. Nurses can contribute significantly to the prevention of visual impairment by becoming knowledgeable about the cause and prevention of eye disorders and by urging patients to follow through with self-care and health promotion measures. For example, the American Academy of Ophthalmology's Committee on Eye Care has made the recommendations in the box at right.

Guidelines for Eye Examinations for Adults and the Elderly

All adults with decrease in visual acuity for distant or near objects should have an ophthalmologic eye examination or refractive eye examination.

All adults should have an eye examination by a family physician, internist, or other health care professional as a component of regular health care.

Adults with risk factors such as a family history of glaucoma, cataract, retinal detachment, or significant degenerative eye disease should have an ophthalmologic eye examination early in adult life and at medically appropriate intervals thereafter.

Adults with diabetes mellitus should have an ophthalmologic eye examination at the time of diagnosis and at medically appropriate intervals thereafter.

Adults with systemic disease and/or medical treatment known to be associated with increased risk of eye disease should have an ophthalmologic eye examination at time of diagnosis and/or treatment onset.

All adults 65 or more years of age should have an ophthalmologic eye examination at least every 2 years.

Adults should participate in vision screening programs conducted by eye care and health care professionals, industry representatives, or volunteer organizations annually or every 2 years.

From Eye care for the American people.[12]

Anatomy, Physiology, and Related Pathophysiology

External Structures

Orbit and its contents. The human eye is approximately 24 mm in diameter. It rests within a fatty cushion in a bony orbit of the skull.[25] The orbit comprises six bones forming a cavity that converges into two major posterior openings, the optic foramen and the superior orbital fissure (Figure 6-1). Through these openings run blood vessels and nerves that connect the eyeball to the brain and the body's blood supply. The ophthalmic artery, the optic nerve, and sympathetic nerves from the carotid plexus enter the orbit through the optic foramen. The oculomotor nerve (CN III), trochlear nerve (CN IV), abducent nerve (CN VI), and ophthalmic branch of the trigeminal nerve (CN V) pass through the superior orbital fissure.[41]

The orbit contains the eyeball, which is cradled in the anterior portion; six oculomotor muscles, which surround and insert into the eyeball; a muscle for elevating the eyelid; and fat, ligaments, and connective tissue in the posterior section that cushion and support the eyeball and the extrinsic muscles. The anterior orbital walls are relatively thick and provide good protection for the eye. The medial wall, which separates the orbit from the ethmoid sinus, is extremely thin and vulnerable to ethmoid sinus infection.[41] The medial wall also contains a fossa for the lacrimal sac, which extends downward through the nasal lacrimal duct into the nose. The lateral posterior wall is also very thin and separates the orbit from the temporal lobe.

The anterior roof of the orbit contains the fossa for the lacrimal gland. The floor of the orbit is supported primarily by the orbital plate of the maxilla, which contains the infraorbital fissure. The maxillary branch of the trigeminal nerve (CN V) passes through this infraorbital fissure. The posterior wall of the orbit contains a fibrous sheet that encircles the optic foramen and is the origin for the extrinsic muscles, which stretch forward to encircle and insert into the anterior and medial aspects of the eyeball (Figure 6-2). The orbital contents are supported and separated from the bone

Figure 6-1 Right bony orbit.

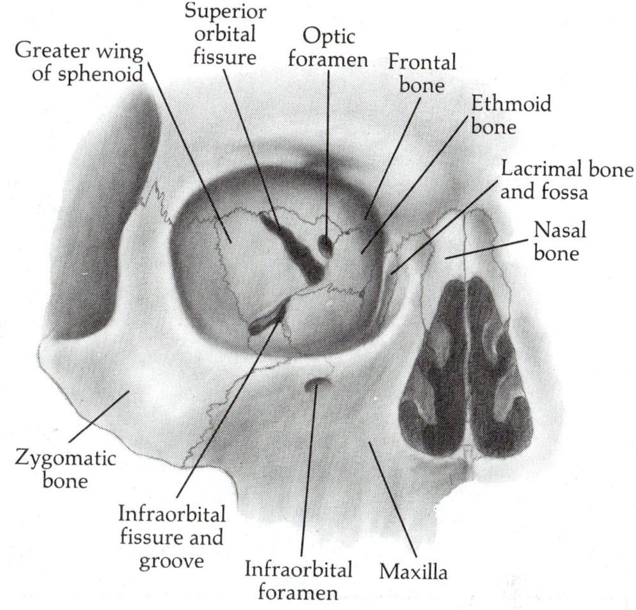

Figure 6-2 Diagrammatic section of orbit.

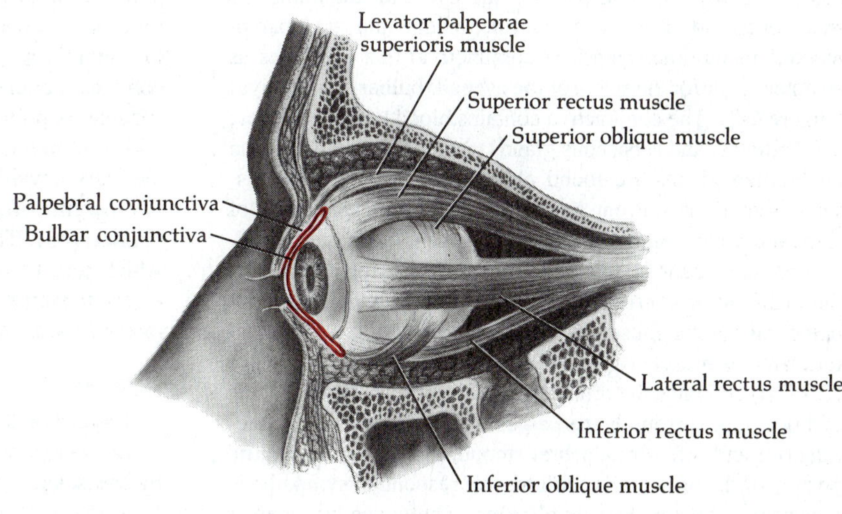

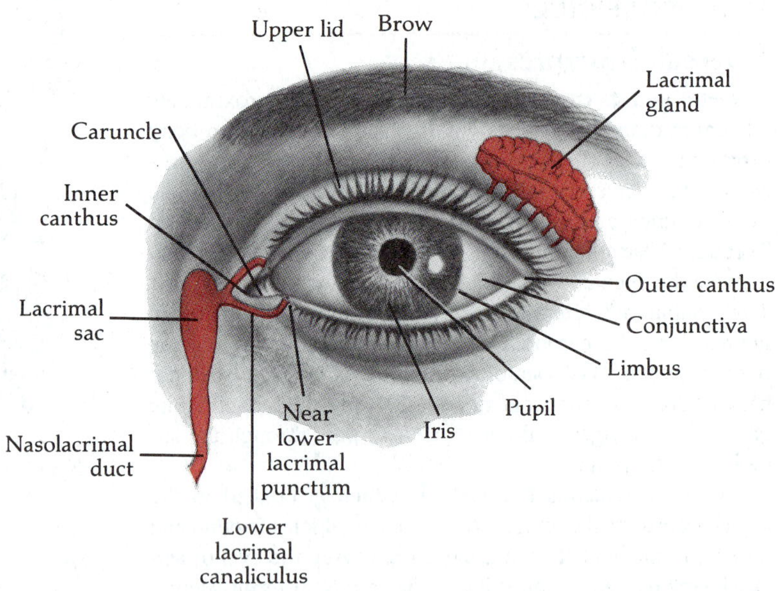

Figure 6-3 Visible surface of eye.

by a periosteal lining and fascial tissue that form the eye socket in which the eyeball rests.

Eyelid. The exposed part of the eye is protected by a lid that serves as a shield from external injury and exposure to excessive light. As the upper lid blinks, it distributes tears over the surface of the eye to keep it moist. When the lids are open, they form the palpebral fissure (the elliptic opening). As a result, the upper lid covers part of the iris (Figure 6-3). The lids meet at the medial (inner) canthus and fold over a small elevation, called the lacrimal caruncle. This caruncle contains large sebaceous glands. The inner canthus is sometimes obscured by a vertical skin fold (epicanthus) in Oriental people and young children.[4] The central portion of the upper and lower lid is thickened with a firm connective tissue (tarsal plate) that protects the eye and maintains the shape of the lid. The eyelids are lined with a thin, transparent mucous membrane (palpebral conjunctiva) that continues as an outer cover for the sclera of the eyeball (bulbar conjunctiva) (Figure 6-2). The conjunctiva contains blood vessels, nerves, hair follicles, and sebaceous glands (meibomian glands). The meibomian glands are found along the margin of the lids. Their secretions prevent rapid evaporation and overflow of tears and create an airtight seal when the eyelids are closed.

Lid movement is supplied from the superior division of the oculomotor nerve (CN III), which activates the superior palpebral levator muscle for upper lid elevation and the inferior rectus muscle for lower lid retraction. The facial nerve (CN VII) activates the orbicularis oculi muscle, an oval sheet of fibers that surrounds the palpebral fissure, for lid closure. Superior and inferior palpebral smooth muscles and a central portion of the orbicularis oculi muscle respond to sympathetic innervation for involuntary blinking. The upper lid receives its sensory innervation from the ophthalmic division of the trigeminal nerve (CN V), and the lower lid is innervated by the maxillary branch of the trigeminal nerve.

The eyelids are the only portion of the eye that has a lymphatic system. The medial portions of the upper and lower lids drain into the submaxillary nodes, and the lateral aspects drain into the preauricular nodes.[41]

Lacrimal apparatus. The lacrimal apparatus secretes and drains a fluid that moistens and lubricates the anterior surface of the eye. Tears are produced in the lacrimal gland, which is located in the anterior lateral fossa of the orbit. Smaller accessory glands scattered throughout the palpebral conjunctiva also secrete fluid. Lacrimal fluid is normally clear and does not overflow unless reflex or mental-emotional stimuli produce excessive tearing. Sebaceous gland secretions and a thin mucin layer combine with the aqueous portion of tears to maintain a constant film over the cornea. Lacrimal fluid contains immunoglobulins, lymphocytes, phagocytes, and lysozyme as protective substances.[41]

Lid blinking helps distribute tears over the eye and draws the tears inward to the puncta, which are small openings in the margins of the upper and lower lids at the inner canthus (Figure 6-3). The puncta empty into the lacrimal canaliculi, which join to form the nasolacrimal sac (Figure 6-3). The adjacent lacrimal duct empties into the nasal cavity in the inferior nasal meatus.[40]

Eyeball

Layers of the eye

Outer layer: cornea and sclera. The eyeball is surrounded by the sclera, the "white" of the eye. It is a tough fibrous layer that covers the posterior five sixths of the eye.

The cornea covers the anterior one sixth of the eye. It is transparent, avascular, and richly innervated with sensory nerves (trigeminal [CN V]). The anterior surface of the cornea is convex, and irregularities of the curvature cause astigmatism. Since the cornea is avascular, it depends on the atmosphere, tears, and aqueous humor for oxygenation and nourishment. The cornea has three layers: the superficial epithelial layer, which is continuous with the bulbar conjunctiva; the substantia propria, which constitutes 90% of corneal thickness; and an endothelial layer.[40,60]

The epithelial layer is a regenerative multilayered barrier. If its cells are injured, uninjured cells migrate to the traumatized area and form a new barrier one cell thick within an hour of the injury.[41] Total repair of the corneal epithelium takes approximately 6 weeks. Because of its dependence on exposure to tears, corneal epithelium is subject to edema if deprived of oxygen. (The implications for contact lenses are discussed later.) The substantia propria is lined anteriorly with a collagenous membrane (Bowman's membrane) that resists infection and trauma. If Bowman's membrane is destroyed, it reforms with scarring and irregular cell formation that contribute to astigmatism. The endothelial layer pumps fluid from the other corneal layers into the aqueous humor. A relatively diminished fluid volume is necessary for corneal transparency.[1] If the endothelium is destroyed, it does not regenerate, and the remaining corneal layers become edematous.

The sclera and cornea merge at a junction called the limbus (Figure 6-3). The corneoscleral limbus has a rich vascular supply that encircles and nourishes the outer edges of the cornea. In the limbus, corneal cells are mixed with conjunctival and scleral layers. Bowman's membrane ends abruptly at this junction. The posterior inner surface of the limbus adjoins the trabecular meshwork and the canal of Schlemm, which drain aqueous fluid from the anterior chamber.[60]

The sclera is the outer layer that surrounds most of the eye. It is adjacent to the second layer, the uveal tract, which includes the choroid layer, the ciliary body, and the iris (Figure 6-4). The sclera has three layers. The outermost is the episclera, which merges with fascial tissue at the limbus; it is vascular and dense, and the minute vessels can be seen through the conjunctiva. The middle layer, the scleral stroma, is composed of tough collagenous fibers that create the white appearance of the sclera. The innermost layer, the lamina fusca, contains melanocytes that may contribute to a yellow-brown scleral hue in dark-skinned people. The lamina fusca contains collagenous fibers that filter into the choroid layer for adherence. The oculomotor muscles attach to the sclera at various points near the midsection of the eyeball (Figure 6-2). The sclera also has numerous openings through which nerves and blood vessels pass. The two major openings are the posterior foramen, which admits the optic nerve into the eye, and the anterior foramen, where the ciliary muscle adjoins at the limbus in the anterior chamber.

Middle layer: choroid, ciliary body, and iris. The middle layer of the eyeball (the uveal tract) comprises the choroid, a vascular layer; the ciliary body, which contains smooth muscles attached to the lens and an epithelial portion for secreting aqueous humor; and the iris, which surrounds the pupil (Figure 6-4).

Figure 6-4 Cross section of eye.

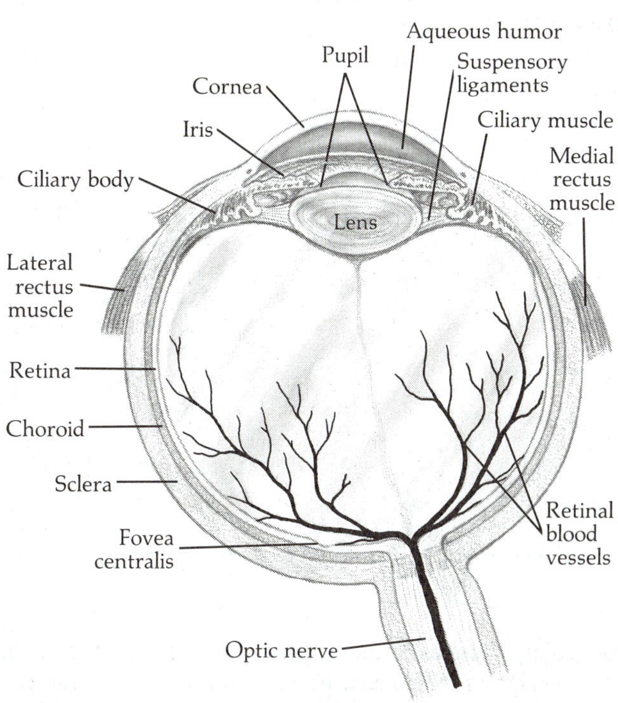

The choroid adheres to the sclera at the entrance point of the optic nerve and extends anteriorly to the ciliary body. It has five layers. The outer layer, the suprachoroid, contains melanocytes, smooth muscle fibers, and ciliary arteries that nourish a portion of the choroid. The three middle layers contain veins and arterioles that feed into the ciliary body, the iris, and the outer portion of the retina. The inner layer of the choroid is called Bruch's membrane. It is multilayered and collagenous and contains cells from the adjacent retinal and choroid layers.

The ciliary body has both a muscular and a secretory function. The ciliary muscles expand from the choroid and extend anteriorly and medially toward the lens (Figure 6-5). The body forms a ring of smooth ciliary muscle that surrounds the lens and parallels the overlying sclera. There are three groups of ciliary muscles. Muscles in the outer division are longitudinal and parallel and adjacent to the sclera. Contraction of these fibers opens the canal of Schlemm, a thin-walled vessel that encircles the eye and drains aqueous fluid from the anterior chamber. The canal of Schlemm is located at the inner aspect of the sclerocorneal junction (limbus) (Figure 6-5). The middle layer of ciliary muscles is a meshwork of fibers that connects the longitudinal muscles to the inner circular fibers. The circular fibers are directed medially toward the lens. A series of delicate ligaments (zonular fibers) attach

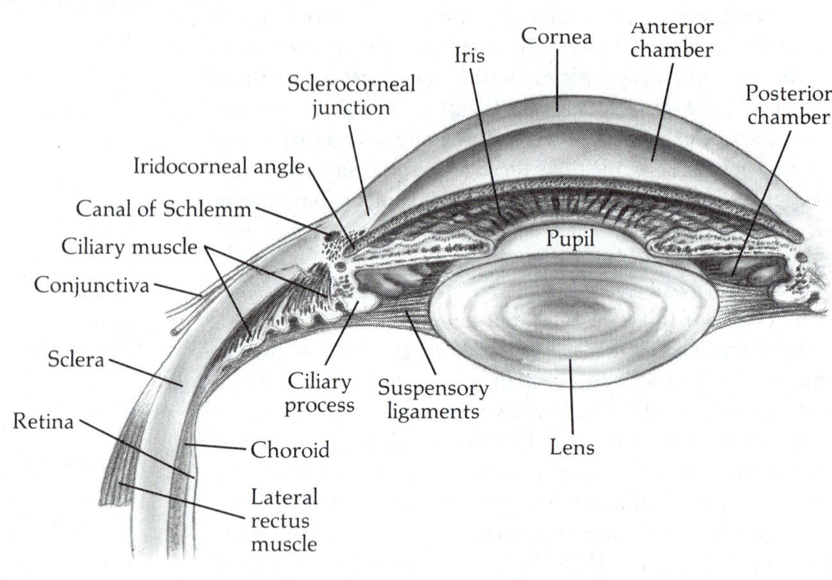

Figure 6-5 Close-up view of ciliary body, zonules, lens, and anterior and posterior chambers.

the ciliary muscles to the equator of the lens (Figure 6-5). The tension of the zonular fibers suspends the lens and stabilizes its position. The zonular tension relaxes with ciliary circular muscle contraction to increase the convexity of the lens for accommodation.[41]

The ciliary body ends in ciliary processes behind the peripheral portion of the iris. The processes are lined with non-pigmented epithelium that secretes aqueous humor. The non-pigmented epithelial cells extend into the sensory portion of the retina. The retina also joins the inner lining of the ciliary epithelium (the pars plana) at a serrated structure called the ora serrata, which corresponds in shape to the ciliary processes (Figure 6-6).[25]

Figure 6-6 Posterior view of ciliary body and surrounding structures. (Retina and ciliary body join at ora serrata.)

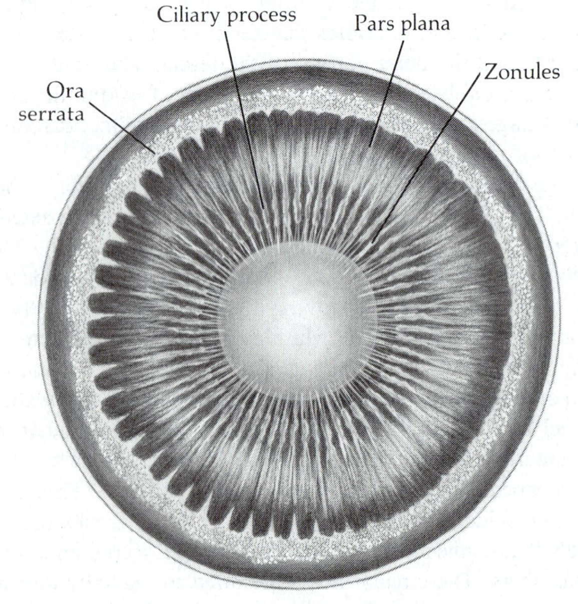

The iris is a circular muscular membrane that surrounds the pupil. The pupil is a hole (aperture) that appears black because light cannot be seen behind it. The iris separates the anterior and posterior eye chambers and rests in front of the lens (Figure 6-5). The iris has two layers: the stroma, which is the anterior surface, and the pigmented epithelium. The amount of melanin in the stroma determines the color of the eyes; the more melanin in the stroma, the darker the iris. The iris sphincter surrounds the pupil, and its contraction decreases pupil size. The pigmented epithelium layer contains the dilator pupillae muscle, which dilates the pupil when contracted. Pupillary response is described in more detail in the discussion of the nervous system of the eye.

The iris is located at the medial portion of the iridocorneal angle (Figure 6-5). This angle separates the canal of Schlemm and the trabecular meshwork beneath it from the iris. If the iris inserts at the anterior edge of the ciliary body, the angle may become narrow. Pupillary dilation also thickens the iris, which may affect the width of the angle. The effects of iris location and shape on the iridocorneal angle are discussed in the section on glaucoma.

Inner layer: retina. The retina is an extension of the central nervous system. This inner layer of the eye begins posteriorly at the optic nerve, coats the inside of the sphere, and ends at the ora serrata, where it joins the ciliary body (Figures 6-4 and 6-6). The retina is normally transparent. It has 10 layers and contains rods and cones (photoreceptor cells), which are connecting cells that synapse with ganglion cells in a peripheral layer. Optic nerve fibers (axons) pass into the optic nerve (Figure 6-7). The pigmented epithelium (adjacent to the choroid surface) contains enzymes and protein binding sites for vitamin A. These protein sites are necessary for the photochemical visual process. The rods and cones are elongated cells that respond to light and convert it into electrical energy. They pass through the next four layers. Both types of cells contain light-sensitive pigments that undergo chemical changes necessary for neural transmission of light. Rods are light sensitive in low levels of light (scotopic vision). Cones perceive images and color in higher levels of light (photopic vision). Rods and cones are so named because of their microscopic appearance; rods are more cylindric and generally more elongated. Rods and cones connect with each other in the plexiform layer and synapse with a variety of cells that ultimately reach the ganglion cells. The ganglion cells transmit electrical discharges through their axons to the midbrain.[25]

Rods and cones are scattered throughout the retinal surface. If the retina were laid out on a flat surface, its center would be the fovea centralis. The fovea is a small depression that contains no rods but is densely packed with cones. Each cone synapses with more than one foveal photoreceptor and ganglion cell but with fewer of these cells than elsewhere in the retina. Visual acuity is sharpest in this area if enough light is available for photopic vision. The fovea is surrounded by the macula lutea, a pigmented area about 4.5 mm in diameter. Rods are densely packed in the periphery of this region (approximately 150,000 rods/mm^2) and become less dense as they extend toward the periphery. Cones average about 4500/mm^2 and also become sparse in the periphery.[41] The optic disc (the head of the optic nerve) perforates the retina about 3 mm toward the nose from the fovea. The disc is approximately 1.5 mm in diameter and contains no rods or cones. This results in a small blind spot for each eye located about 15 degrees laterally from the center of vision. The viewer is not aware of this because the other eye compensates for the loss. The periphery of the retina contains primarily rods. When viewed through the ophthalmoscope, the fovea appears as a small pinpoint of light surrounded by a yellow-brown pigmented area (the macula). The head of the optic nerve appears as a pink or cream-colored circle with a white

Figure 6-7 Layers of retina.

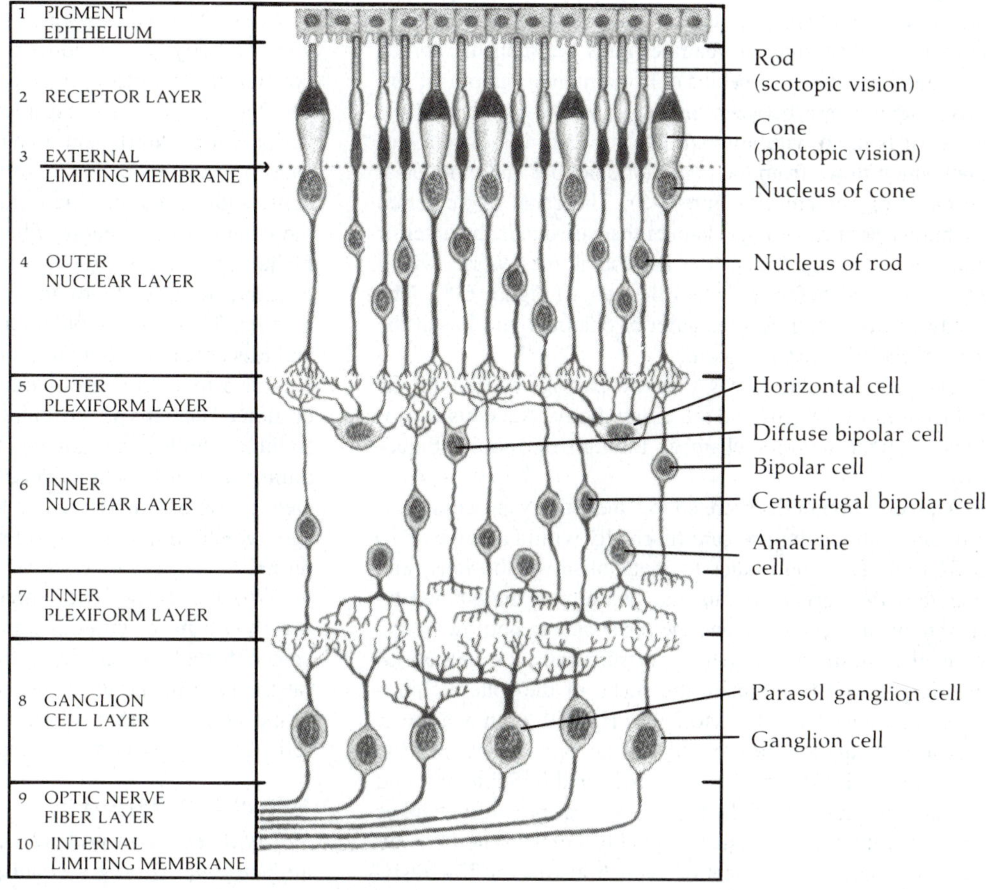

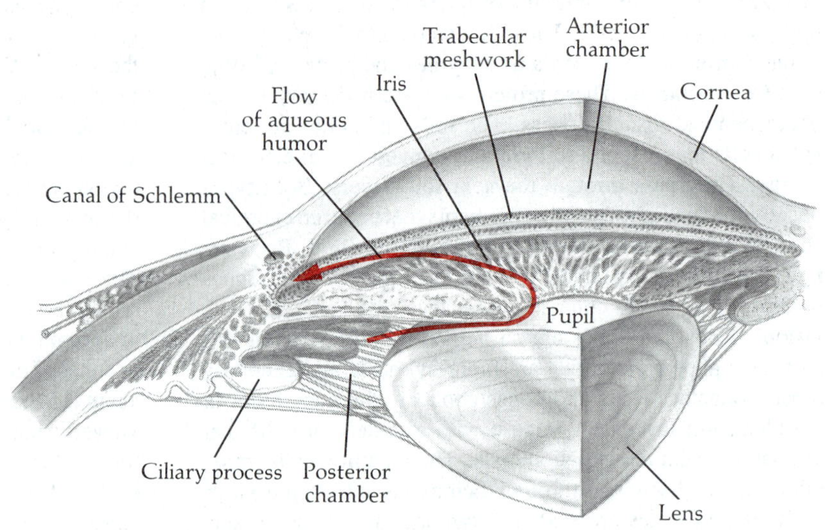

Figure 6-8 Close view of trabecular meshwork and flow of aqueous humor.

depression in the center. This depression is where the central retinal artery and central vein bifurcate, emerge, and feed into smaller branches throughout the retinal surface.

Chambers, fluids, and inner structures of the eye

Aqueous fluid and intraocular pressure. The eye contains three chambers: the anterior, the posterior, and the vitreous body. The anterior chamber rests between the cornea (in front) and the iris (behind). It maintains a depth of approximately 3 mm between the center of the cornea and the pupil.[4] It is filled with approximately 0.2 ml of aqueous humor, which flows from the posterior chamber and empties at the canal of Schlemm (Figure 6-5). The canal of Schlemm is a highly permeable oval channel that surrounds the anterior chamber. It is adjacent to the trabecular meshwork, which filters the fluid before it enters the canal (Figure 6-8). The meshwork also encircles the anterior chamber and lies at the apex of the iridocorneal angle.

The posterior chamber is a narrow passage behind the iris and in front of the lens and the ciliary body. Aqueous humor flows into the anterior chamber through the pupil (Figure 6-8).

Aqueous humor is secreted by the ciliary processes. It maintains intraocular pressure (normally within a range of 10 to 22 mm Hg), contributes to metabolism of the lens, and nourishes the cornea. Intraocular pressure is maintained by the rate of fluid secretion and the resistance to outflow by the trabecular meshwork. Eyeball pressure must exceed atmospheric pressure to maintain the shape of the sphere. Intraocular pressure fluctuates 1 to 2 mm Hg with each heartbeat. Pressure fluctuations are based on the pressure within the episcleral veins, which connect to the canal of Schlemm, and the osmotic pressure of the blood. Normal pressure changes (up to 5 mm Hg) are usually quickly compensated for by trabecular meshwork distention, which lowers outflow resistance.[41] The Valsalva maneuver (bearing down to complete a bowel movement) increases venous pressure and so greatly increases intraocular pressure, which quickly returns to normal when the maneuver ends. Drinking large quantities of water or receiving saline intravenous fluids causes a slight increase in intraocular pressure.

Lens. The lens separates the posterior chamber from the vitreous body. It is biconvex and transparent and is held in position by suspensory ligaments attached to the ciliary body. The lens comprises a capsule that encases it, a cortex (the peripheral portion), and a central core. It is transparent because most of its cells do not have a nucleus. Newly formed cells, with nuclei, originate at the periphery and move toward the center, where mature fibers have lost their nuclei. New fibers are formed throughout the life span of the lens and continue to migrate to the center core and become compressed. Therefore an older lens is larger, denser, less elastic, and less able to contract to accommodate for near vision. The lens also maintains transparency by avoiding excessive hydration. The lens is surrounded by media that are high in sodium. The lens membrane is relatively impermeable to sodium, and lens metabolism pumps out sodium, which decreases osmotic activity. The lens becomes yellow in middle age, which diminishes the intensity of blue-toned light on the retina.[25]

Vitreous body. The vitreous cavity contains approximately 4.5 ml of vitreous humor, which is a gelatinous substance that adheres firmly to the retina, the ciliary epithelium (at the base of the lens), and the margin of the optic nerve. If the vitreous humor diminishes in volume or degenerates, retinal tears may occur because of traction on the retina.

Image Formation

Light reception and refraction. The receptors of the eye are sensitive to only a small portion of the light spectrum. Light in wavelengths less than 400 nm or greater than 700

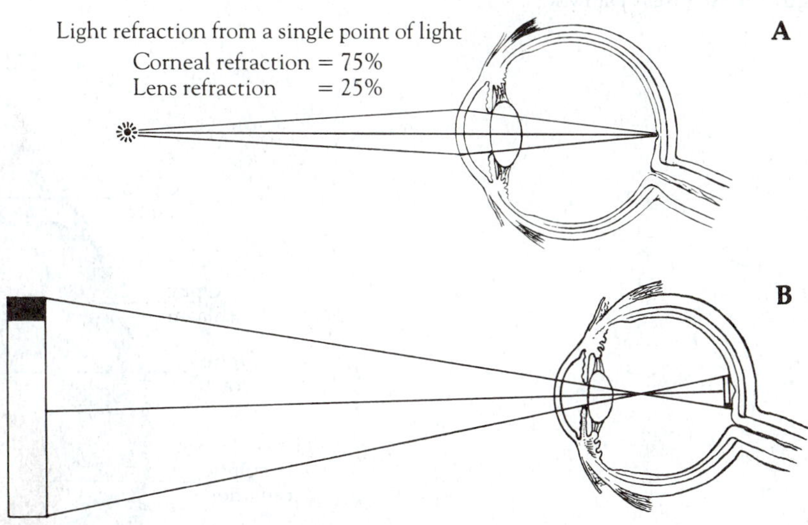

Figure 6-9 A, Light refraction from single point of light. **B,** Light refraction from object with more than one point of light.

nm is not absorbed by rods and cones and therefore not seen.[35]

To reach the retina, light must pass through the clear media of the cornea, aqueous fluid, the lens, and the vitreous body. Light rays are emitted in all directions from any source. These light rays pass through the optic system, which focuses them at a specific point to achieve image accuracy.

A ray of light that passes from one clear medium into another is affected by the density of the medium. The density of the cornea slows the light ray, and the curvature of the cornea bends it. This process is known as refraction. The surface of the cornea is curved so light rays hit the surface at different angles but are bent to redirect them to the lens. The lens further bends and directs them to a single point on the retina (Figure 6-9, *A*). When a person focuses on an object, the light waves from that object are directed to the fovea centralis for image identification and clarity (called focal vision). Most objects have more than one point of focus. As different points of focus from an object reach the retina, they form an image that is upside down and reversed (Figure 6-9, *B*). Light waves also enter the eye from a wide visual field (approximately 170-degree arc for each eye) that surrounds the object of focus. These peripheral sources focus on the outer areas of the retina (ambient vision) and help with spatial sense.[41]

The anterior surface of the cornea is the primary refractive area of the eye. The more a surface bends light rays, the greater the refractive power. The shift in the direction of light when it moves through the corneal surface is greater than the second shift at the lens surface.

Accommodation. Accommodation is the process by which the lens alters its shape for visual clarity when the eye is viewing an object at close range. In other words, the lens surface increases its refractive power by becoming thicker and more convex to accommodate near objects. Normally the lens is somewhat flattened and held tight by the ligaments that attach to the circular ciliary muscle. When these muscles contract, the ligaments relax and release their tension on the lens. The lens contracts and becomes more spheric. The lens is constantly adjusting to stimuli at different distances. Ciliary branches of the oculomotor nerve respond to brain signals for this automatic response.

Binocular vision and vergence. Normal eyes are aligned in their orbits so that they can direct light rays to the fovea centralis of each eye. The visual axis is an imaginary line drawn from each fovea centralis to a fixation point. When a three-dimensional object is focused on the back of both eyes, there is a slight difference in the horizontal placement of the two images. This slight difference sets up two images in the brain, which permits the binocular viewer (using both eyes) to experience the visual sensation of depth (stereopsis).

Vergence is a visual reflex of simultaneous eye movements. When distant objects are viewed, the visual axes of the eyes become more parallel and the eyes are rotated outward (divergence). As the object draws nearer, the medius rectus muscles contract and pull the eyes inward (convergence).[40] This reflex is necessary to prevent diplopia (double vision). If a person holds a finger about 10 inches in front of his nose and focuses on the finger, he sees one finger. If he suddenly shifts his focus to a distant object, he sees two fingers because the parallel visual axes do not meet at the finger.

Image Interpretation

Visual pathway. We are able to see because refracted light rays stimulate retinal photoreceptors and are changed into electrical energy. This energy is transmitted to different cerebral cortical areas for interpretation. Light rays constantly stimulate photoreceptors. Rods and cones contain specific pigments (opsins) that combine with a form of vitamin A to absorb light and convert it to an electrical potential. These photoreceptors synapse with second- and third-order neurons

Figure 6-10 Visual pathway.

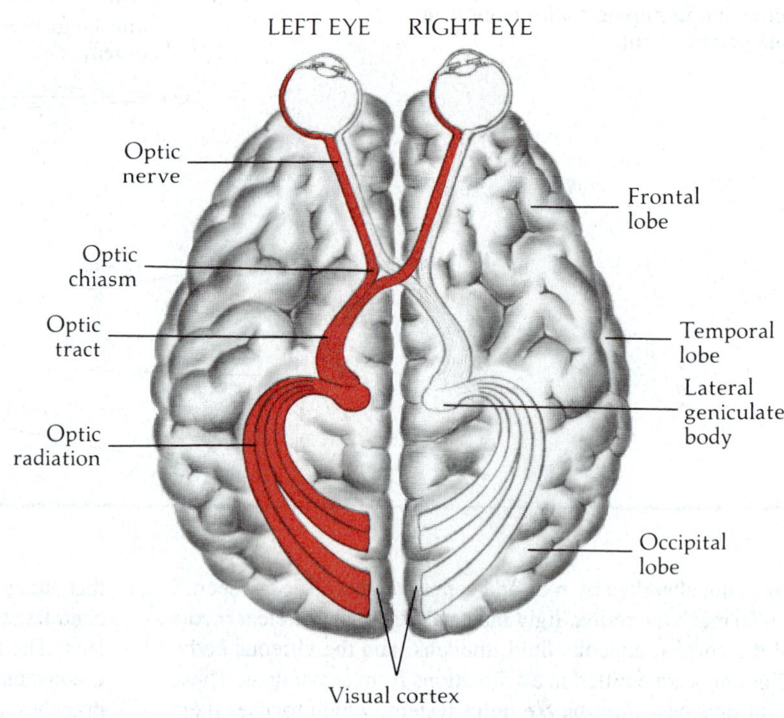

within the retina, which converge into fibers that enter the optic nerve. The optic nerve forms the optic disc and exits the eyeball at the posterior region. The choroid and all the retinal layers except the nerve fiber layer end at the edge of the disc.

The optic nerve contains more than 1 million fibers (axons of ganglion cells) that control vision, eye movement, and pupillary reflexes. As the optic nerve exits the sphere, it is encased in dura mater, an arachnoid sheath, and pia mater. It forms an S-shaped curve that allows it to stretch when the eye is moved. The orbital portion of the nerve is about 30 mm long. The optic nerve also contains the central retinal artery and vein, which bifurcate and branch into the eyeball near the head of the nerve (the disc). The central artery and vein exit the optic nerve about 12 mm behind the eyeball.[41]

The optic nerves from each eye pass through the optic foramen and meet at the optic chiasm, which lies above and in front of the pituitary gland. Optic tracts emerge from the chiasm and encircle the hypothalamus. They terminate in the lateral geniculate bodies in the temporal lobes (Figure 6-10). Cells in the lateral geniculate bodies send fibers (optic radiation) to the occipital lobe of each cerebral hemisphere. The visual cortex in the posterior aspect of the occipital lobe receives most of the visual fibers representing central vision (stimuli from the fovea centralis and the surrounding macula). Adjacent occipital lobe areas receive fibers representing the more peripheral portions of the retina. Reversed images are righted when perceived in the cortex.

Objects in the visual field stimulate the opposite side of the retina. When nerve fibers pass into the optic nerve, the nasal (closest to the nose) and temporal (closest to the side of the face) fibers are separate within the sheath. Temporal fibers pass on the temporal side of the nerve, nasal fibers are on the nasal side, and central (foveal) fibers are in the center of the nerve. When the nerves merge at the chiasm, nasal fibers cross (decussate) to the opposite optic tract. Temporal fibers do not cross but continue in the optic tract on the same side as the nerve that conveys them to the chiasm (Figure 6-11). Therefore the pathway of vision for an object seen on a person's right side would be through nasal receptors in the right eye and then through the nasal side of the optic nerve to the chiasm, where it would cross to the left optic tract and proceed to the left cerebral occipital lobe. Visual field defects can often be traced to disorders in specific anatomic locations because of the arrangement of nerve fibers. A left or right optic nerve lesion would cause a corresponding defect in the left or right eye. Chiasm lesions can cause a variety of defects depending on the location of the lesion. A common defect is bitemporal hemianopia, which results from a pituitary tumor. A left optic tract lesion would result in a bilateral right visual field deficit. These defects are depicted in Figure 6-12.

Light and dark adaptation. The concentration of pigment in the photoreceptor cells of the retina determines the sensitivity of these cells to light. Photoreceptive pigments are constantly being used and replaced through chemical changes in the retina. When the eyes are exposed to bright light, the

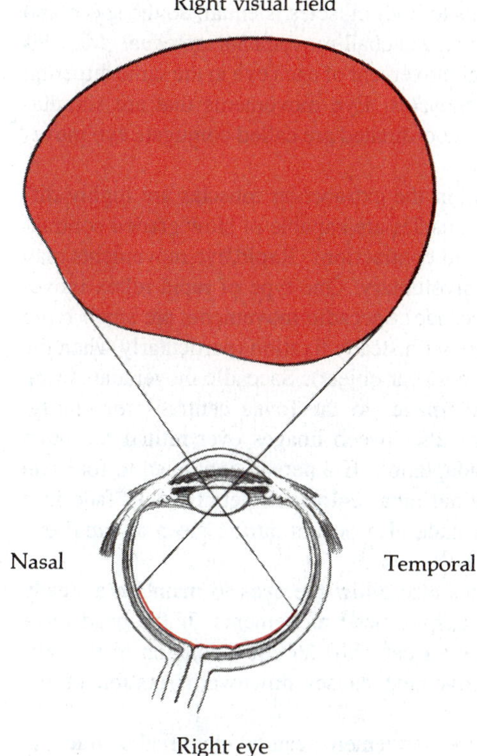

Figure 6-11 Image placement on retina.

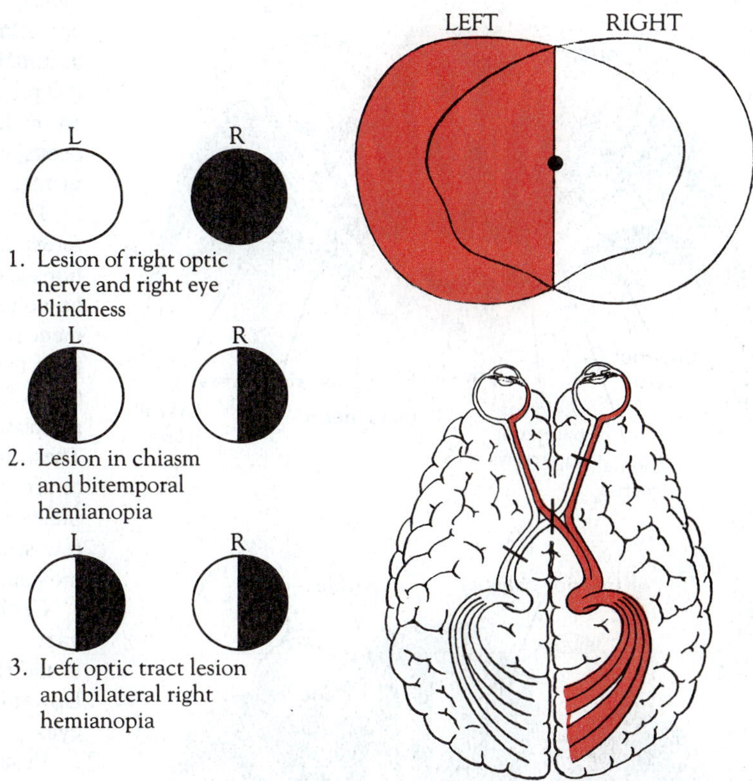

Figure 6-12 Visual pathway defects.

pigments become bleached and the sensitivity of the photoreceptors diminishes. Bright light causes discomfort for several minutes until breakdown of the photopigments produces a gradual rise of the visual threshold. Together with pupillary constriction, decreased rod and cone sensitivity to light protects the retinal cells in bright light. This is called light adaptation.[25]

Exposure to darkness tends to increase photopigment regeneration to increase sensitivity to light. Rhodopsin, the photopigment in rods, is particularly sensitive to dim light and enables a person to visualize dim forms and shapes in near darkness. Rhodopsin does not absorb color wavelengths, so color is not perceived in dim light.

Color perception. Light waves do not contain color. Color is perceived according to the wavelength (frequency) of a light ray. Colors are determined by hue (the standard recognition of a particular shade) and saturation (the intensity of a color). A less intense color contains larger amounts of white and appears relatively pale. Any object that reflects all visible light rays evokes a sensation of white. The absence of light rays is perceived as black.

The retina contains three types of cones, and each has a different photopigment that absorbs light waves of different frequencies. Each type of cone responds to a primary color: red, green, or blue. If all of the cones are equally stimulated, white is perceived. Rods do not perceive color.[25]

Eye Movement

The movement of each eye is controlled by six muscles. Four of these (the recti) originate behind the eyeball, move forward around the sphere, and insert into the sclera about 7 mm behind the limbus (Figure 6-13, *A*). The superior oblique muscle begins at the posterior orbit, passes forward to the anterior orbital rim, loops through the trochlea (a fibrocartilaginous structure) to return to the eyeball, and inserts into the sclera under the belly of the superior rectus muscle (Figure 6-13, *B*). The sixth muscle, the interior oblique, originates at the nasal side of the orbit and passes under the eyeball to attach at its lateral surface (Figure 6-13, *B*). The oculomotor nerve (CN III) supplies the medial, inferior, and superior rectus muscles and the inferior oblique muscle. The trochlear nerve (CN IV) supplies the superior oblique muscle, and the abducent nerve (CN VI) supplies the lateral rectus muscle (Figure 6-14).[40]

Contraction of an eye muscle turns the eye toward that muscle. All six muscles are constantly coordinating stretch and contraction functions to permit full and continuous eye movement.

Figure 6-13 Extraocular muscles.

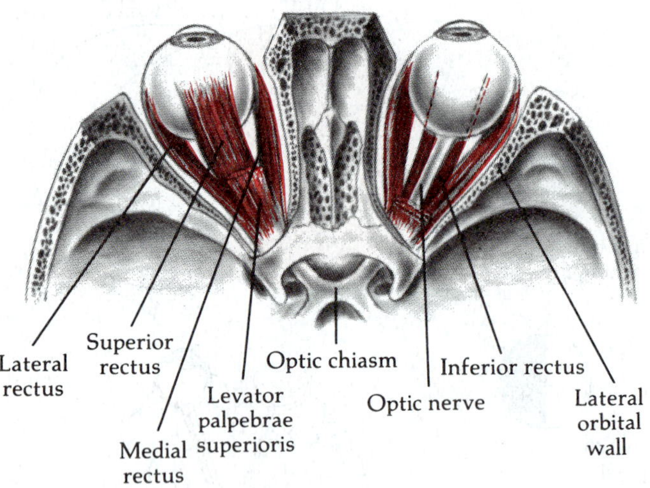

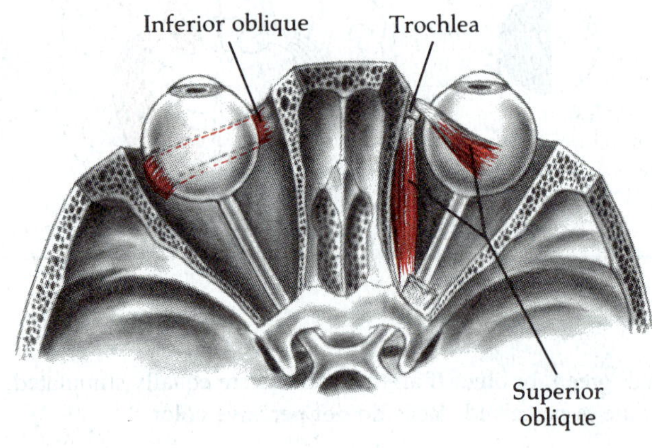

Both eyes must move together to maintain a clear focus. When a person looks to the right, the right lateral rectus muscle and the left medial rectus muscle contract. The innervation stimulus to both muscles is equal, so the speed and destination of the two eyeball movements are equal. Muscles that produce equal movement of each eye in the same direction are called yoke muscles. Eye movements that are simultaneous, equal, and coordinated are called conjugate eye movements.

The fibers within the extraocular muscles are highly differentiated. Eye muscles are capable of slow graded contractions and very rapid contractions. Rapid eye movements may be voluntary or involuntary. One type of rapid reflex movement is called saccade. Saccadic movements are small rapid jerks that alternate with steady fixation (particularly when the eye is focusing on a near object). Saccadic movements bring peripheral retinal images to the fovea centralis for clarity. These movements also sweep images over retinal receptors to prevent light adaptation. If a person continued to focus an image in one retinal area, color and detail would fade in a few seconds. Saccade also occurs during sleep as rapid eye movement (REM).[35]

Certain reflexes also allow the eyes to maintain a steady gaze of fixation despite head movements. If the head turns to the right, the eyes can shift an equal rotation to the left. Upward head movement causes downward rotation of the eyes.

In summary, eye movements can be classified as tracking (slow, smooth, coordinated rotations for maintaining the image of an object on the fovea centralis); vergence (slow, smooth movements that rotate the eyes inward or outward to track an object as being near or far); saccadic movements (rapid reflexes that alternate with fixation to keep the image clear and steady); and compensatory movements (reflexes that coordinate head movement with object fixation and steady gaze). Table 6-1 summarizes the major nervous system mechanisms of the eye.

Figure 6-14 Innervation and movement of extraocular muscles.

Table 6-1
Summary of Major Nervous System Mechanisms of the Eye

Function	Mechanism
Lid movement	
Oculomotor (CN III)	Innervates levator palpebrae superioris and inferior rectus
Facial (CN VII)	Innervates orbicularis oculi
Sensation (trigeminal [CN V])	Ophthalmic division for upper lid; maxillary division for lower lid
Reflex response	Sympathetic fibers from superior cervical ganglion innervate palpebral muscles
Tears	Normal moisture maintained by secretory function of palpebral accessory glands; excess tears mediated through stimulation of facial nerve (CN VII) and trigeminal nerve (CN V)
Corneal sensation	Trigeminal nerve (CN V)
Pupil	
Constriction	Light stimulates retina and afferent fibers that pass through optic nerve (CN II) and chiasm and then deviate from tract to area of midbrain (superior colliculus); axons leave this area and connect to nucleus of oculomotor nerve (CN III), which sends efferent fibers to ciliary ganglion (between optic chiasm and posterior orbit); parasympathetic fibers leave ciliary ganglion and enter eye to stimulate iris sphincter
Consensual response	Both pupils constrict when only one is stimulated; oculomotor nucleus responds to afferent fibers from one eye and sends signals through its fibers and parasympathetic fibers to both iris muscles
Dilation	Reduction of parasympathetic tonic flow to iris sphincters in dim light; sympathetic stimulation of fibers from carotid plexus occurs with startle or pleasure responses
Lens accommodation	Oculomotor nerve (CN III) mediates parasympathetic stimulation for ciliary muscle contraction and resultant lens convexity
Vision	Light focuses on retinal receptors; axons pass into optic nerve (CN II), chiasm, optic tracts, lateral geniculate bodies, and optic radiation to occipital lobe and visual cortex
Eye movement	Conjugate movements occur because nuclei of CN III, IV, and VI connect in fiber tract in midbrain
Oculomotor nerve (CN III)	Innervates superior rectus, medial rectus, inferior rectus, and inferior oblique muscles
Trochlear nerve (CN IV)	Innervates superior oblique muscle
Abducent nerve (CN VI)	Innervates lateral rectus muscle

Data from Jensen[25]; Newell[41]; and Vaughan.[60]

Normal Findings[4,57,58]

Area of Concern	Normal Adult Findings
Eyelids	Blink response to light or corneal touch; frequent involuntary bilateral blinks (average 15-20/minute); lid margins rest over inferior and superior borders of cornea
Eyeball	Anterior-posterior diameter 22-27 mm Caucasian: Eyeball does not protrude beyond supraorbital bridge of frontal bone Negroid: Eyeball may protrude slightly beyond ridge
Lacrimal function	Eyeball surface moist; excess tears in response to emotion or noxious atmospheric stimuli; puncta nontender and without discharge on palpation *Older adult:* Over 50 years: Diminished reflex response for excess tearing
Conjunctivae	Palpebral: Pink with uniform small vessels showing no discharge Bulbar: Clear, tiny, red vessels may be visible *Older adult:* Bulbar: May lack luster of young adult
Sclera	White; slight overall yellowish cast or black dots (pigmentation) in dark-skinned individuals
Cornea	Transparent; smooth surface; convex curvature *Older adult:* Arcus senilis (gray ring of lipid deposit around limbus)
Iris	Rounded; consistent, bilateral coloration *Older adult:* Bilateral irregularity of pigment density (color may appear paler)
Pupil	Equal; round; reacts to light and accommodation; consensual response *Older adult:* Often miotic with slower dilation reaction to dark
Anterior chamber	Clear; approximately 3.3 mm between cornea and iris *Older adult:* Becomes slightly shallower with aging

Area of Concern	Normal Adult Findings
Internal eye	Full, round, bilateral red reflex
Retina	Uniform pink and granular texture (negroid surface uniformly more pigmented); choroid layer may be visible showing linear light orange vessels *Older adult:* May appear slightly paler
Vessels	Central vein and artery emerge on nasal side of physiologic cup within disc, and each immediately breaks into two branches; arteries light red and 25% narrower than dark red veins; narrow band of light may appear at center of arteries; vessel caliber regular and uniformly decreases as vessel branches toward periphery; venous pulsations more prominent in young adults *Older adult:* Arteries slightly narrower; arterial light reflex may be widened; arterial caliber may be slightly irregular
Disc, cup	Whitish, cream, or pink; vertically oval or round with distinct border (nasal side may be slightly less demarcated and temporal border may appear as grayish crescent); approximately 1.5 mm diameter (magnified 15 times through ophthalmoscope); cup is small, white or pale depression in center of disc and occupies approximately half of disc diameter *Older adult:* Disc may appear slightly smaller and more opaque
Macula, fovea	Macula is darker area two disc diameters temporally from disc; fovea is pinpoint bright light in center of macula
Visual acuity	
Distant vision	20/20 (able to read designated size letter on standardized chart at 20 feet distance) *Older adult:* 20/20-20/30
Near vision	Able to read newsprint at 14 inches *Older adult:* Presbyopic owing to loss of lens refractive power (average person over 60 years cannot focus more closely than 3 feet without corrective lenses)
Peripheral vision	Temporal vision 90 degrees from central visual axis Upward: 50 degrees Nasalward: 60 degrees Downward: 70 degrees *Older adult:* May be slightly diminished but usually not measurable with confrontation testing
Eye movement, coordination, and interpretation	Both eyes demonstrate coordinated, parallel movements in six cardinal fields of gaze; physiologic nystagmus (mild rhythmic twitching if eye held in extreme gaze); eyes converge and diverge in smooth coordinated fashion as person focuses on near and far objects; tracking, saccadic, and compensatory movements enable person to perceive objects clearly in depth and accurately in terms of distance and surrounding space
Color perception	Able to identify all colors accurately when tested with series of pictures or cards that present mutlicolored field for color differentiation *Older adult:* Brightness of colors may be dimmed; yellow overcast to hues owing to aging lens

Conditions, Diseases, and Disorders

DISORDERS OF THE EYELID

Lid disorders are extremely common and varied. Since the lids are responsible for tear maintenance and dispersion, structure and position defects can result in excess tears or drying of the eyeball surface. Deformities and movement abnormalities interfere with the lid's vital protective function and with vision. Structure and movement malfunctions alter facial expression and appearance and create cosmetic concerns. Many pain receptors are near the lid margin, and stretching and inflammation of the tissue result in acute discomfort. Since the palpebral conjunctiva is adjacent to the lid margin, disorders in this area can produce acute and diffuse redness of the eye.

Two types of lid disorders are covered: those involving position, structure, and movement and inflammatory disorders. Most disorders of lid structure and function require surgical intervention if localized nerve or muscle malfunction is diagnosed as the causative factor. Inflammatory disorders can affect the glands in the eyelids, the eyelid margins, and the meibomian glands. The skin of the eyelids may also be involved in a variety of inflammations because of the skin's looseness, its exposed position, and the secondary involvement of the eye. Contact dermatitis is common in the eye area because of use of cosmetics and frequent rubbing of the eyes.[5,41]

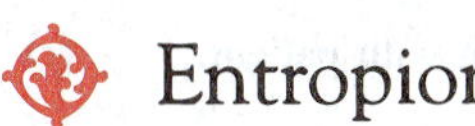

Entropion

Entropion is an abnormal turning inward of the margin of the eyelid.[49]

Pathophysiology

The lower lid is most commonly involved. Involution of the lid can be caused by atrophy of the lower lid retractor muscle (atonia), spasms of the orbicularis oculi muscle, or scarring and deformity of the tarsal plate resulting from trauma or chemical or inflammatory assaults. Atonia is relatively common in the elderly and can occur in varying degrees of severity. If the lashes are turned inward, corneal and conjunctival inflammation may occur. Spastic entropion results from chronic or acute irritation of the horizontal muscle. Corneal inflammation, conjunctivitis, and ocular surgery are common causes of spasm. Congenital entropion occurs with a deformity of the tarsal plate.[41,60]

Medical Plan

Surgery

Orbicularis procedure—small section of orbicularis oculi muscle is resected to tighten remaining muscle farthest from lid margin, which results in peripheral lid eversion

Tarsal resection—wedge of tarsal plate is removed, which prevents lid margin from rotating inward

Mucosal graft—scarred, atrophied conjunctiva may be replaced with section of mucous membrane from mouth[41,60]

General Management

For entropion (spasm from irritation), remove irritation (such as eye dressing) to reduce or relieve spasms; stabilize lower lid with pressure patch or tape lower lid to cheek for temporary relief

NURSING CARE

Nursing Assessment

Eyelid and Lashes

Lashes turned inward; possible tear spillage

Cornea and Conjunctiva

Possible conjunctivitis; secondary corneal infection

Nursing Dx & Intervention[5,31,36]

Nursing Diagnosis	Nursing Intervention/Rationale
Potential for injury: cornea and conjunctiva, related to entropion spasms or inverted eyelashes	• Assess conjunctiva and cornea for inflammatory signs. • Remove irritation if possible (e.g., by removing eye dressing). • Splint or stabilize everted lid by taping to cheek *to reduce spasms.* • Place pressure patch over eye.
Potential for injury: cornea and conjunctiva, related to inadequate tearing	• Assess eye for symptoms of dryness. • Administer artificial tears, sustained-release tear insert, or lubricating ointment as ordered. • Be certain that lid is closed when applying dressing.
Anxiety	• Assess patient's level of anxiety. • Listen to patient's concerns. • Provide supportive counseling.
Sensory/perceptual alterations (visual) related to use of unilateral eye patch	*Before surgery:* • Warn patient that depth perception will be lost and that 50% of peripheral vision will be lost on affected side. *After surgery:* • Help patient with ADLs. • Caution patient to bring hand forward slowly to touch objects (especially containers of hot liquid and containers receiving poured liquids) *to ensure safety.* • Explain that patient should turn head fully toward affected side to view objects or obstacles. • Teach patient to use up and down head movements to judge stair dimensions and oncoming objects when walking and to proceed slowly.

Nursing Diagnosis	Nursing Intervention/Rationale
Sensory/perceptual alterations (visual) related to use of bilateral eye patches	*Before surgery:* • Warn patient that eyes will be patched. • Orient patient to bedside equipment and room arrangement. • Arrange for placement of personal belongings in advance and review plan with patient. • Warn patient that side rails will be raised for safety. *After surgery:* • Raise side rails *to ensure safety.* • Address patient by name from doorway and identify yourself *to reduce anxiety.* • Complement voice stimulation with touch *to notify patient of your proximity.* • Reorient patient to equipment (such as call light) and personal belongings at bedside by directing patient's hand. • Encourage patient to perform self-care with personal hygiene *to maximize independence.* • Ensure patient's privacy, and assure patient that privacy is provided. • Provide patient with television set or radio *to encourage mental and memory stimulation.* • Engage patient in discussions about news or other items heard. • Provide patient with clock that can be felt and remind patient of date. • Discourage napping, which patient may want to do as he or she loses track of time. • Help patient with meals: Read menu selections. Guide hand to utensils and food on tray. Describe food on tray in clock terms (e.g., coffee is at 2 o'clock, knife and spoon are at 3 o'clock). Help with cutting meats, removing lids from containers, buttering bread, and so on. • Help with walking: Walk slowly and slightly ahead of patient; patient's hand should rest on your arm at elbow. If possible, allow patient to trace progress by running the dorsal aspect of his or her free hand along a wall. Describe surroundings as you proceed. Warn of steps, turns, and narrow passageways in advance. Allow patient to feel chair, toilet, or bed before turning to sit.
Pain (postoperative) related to eyelid surgery	• Assess patient's level of discomfort. • Give pain medication as ordered.
Potential for injury to surgically repaired lid, related to nausea or vomiting	• Assess patient's feelings of nausea. • Request order for antiemetic and administer if needed.
Potential for infection	• After removal of patch(es), administer antibiotic ointment as ordered.

Patient Education

1. Teach the patient to avoid rubbing or picking at the eyes.
2. Teach the patient to apply prescribed ointment to eye(s).

Evaluation

Patient Outcome	Data Indicating That Outcome is Reached
Cornea and conjunctiva are healthy.	Cornea is transparent, smooth, glossy, and moist. Palpebral conjunctiva is homogeneous pink color, and bulbar conjunctiva is clear. There is no burning or itching.
Surgically repaired eyelid maintains proper position and movement.	Lid margins are flush against eyeball surface. Eyelids close completely. Lid margins rest over inferior and superior borders of cornea. There is no tear spillage.
Patient is able to care for abnormally positioned lid that is not surgically repaired.	Patient administers prescribed medications successfully. Patient is able to monitor condition of eye and report conjunctival or corneal irritation in early stage.[4]

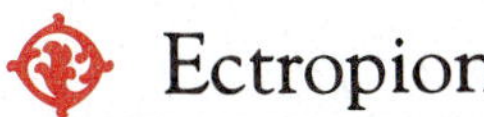

Ectropion

Ectropion is an abnormal outward turning of the margin of the eyelid.[49]

Pathophysiology

Ectropion occurs in two main forms, atonic and cicatricial. Only the lower eyelid is involved in the atonic type, which is the more common. Older adults are frequently subject to the atonic type from the bulbar conjunctiva owing to relaxation of the orbicularis oculi muscle. This condition can occur in all degrees of severity and may cause corneal drying and irritation and conjunctivitis. Paralysis of the orbicularis oculi muscle (CN VII) also results in atonic ectropion. Cicatricial entropion can affect either the upper or lower eyelid and follows burns, lacerations, and infections of the eyelid skin.[5]

Medical Plan

Surgery

Ectropion repair—wedge of skin, muscle, and tarsal plate removed to tighten lower lid(s)[40]

Skin grafting—replacement of scar tissue that relieves constriction of inferior part of lower lid

General Management

Monitoring of exposed conjunctiva for infection and drying

Lubricating ointment as needed

NURSING CARE

Nursing Assessment

Eyelid

Possible tear spillage

Cornea and Conjunctiva

Corneal drying; conjunctivitis

Nursing Dx & Intervention[5,36,57]

Nursing Diagnosis	Nursing Intervention/Rationale
Potential for injury: cornea and conjunctiva, related to inadequate tearing	• Assess eye for symptoms of dryness. • Administer artificial tears, sustained-release tear insert, or lubricating ointment as ordered. • Be certain lid is closed when applying dressing.
Body image disturance related to eyelid deformities	• Assess patient's concerns. • Assist family members with being supportive. • See p. 1751.
Knowledge deficit	• Educate patient about disorder. • Discuss alternative care plans, rationale, and consequences.
Anxiety	• Assess patient's level of anxiety. • Listen to patient's concerns. • Provide supportive counseling.
Sensory/perceptual alterations (visual) related to use of unilateral eye patch	*Before surgery:* • Warn patient that depth perception will be lost and that 50% of peripheral vision will be lost on affected side. *After surgery:* • Help patient with ADLs. • Caution patient to bring hand forward slowly to touch objects (especially containers of hot liquid and containers receiving poured liquids) *to ensure safety.* • Explain that patient should turn head fully toward affected side to view objects or obstacles. • Teach patient to use up and down head movements to judge stair dimensions and oncoming objects when walking and to proceed slowly.
Sensory/perceptual alterations (visual) related to use of bilateral eye patches	*Before surgery:* • Warn patient that eyes will be patched. • Orient patient to bedside equipment and room arrangement. • Arrange for placement of personal belongings in advance and review plan with patient. • Warn patient that side rails will be raised for safety.

Nursing Diagnosis	Nursing Intervention/Rationale
	After surgery: • Raise side rails *to ensure safety.* • Address patient by name from doorway and identify yourself *to reduce anxiety.* • Complement voice stimulation with touch *to notify patient of your proximity.* • Reorient patient to equipment (such as call light) and personal belongings at bedside by directing patient's hand. • Encourage patient to perform self-care with personal hygiene *to maximize independence.* • Ensure patient's privacy, and assure patient that privacy is provided. • Provide patient with television set or radio *to encourage mental and memory stimulation to prevent withdrawal.* • Engage patient in discussions about news or other items heard. • Provide patient with clock that can be felt and remind patient of date. • Discourage napping, which patient may want to do as he or she loses track of time. • Help patient with meals: Read menu selections. Guide hand to utensils and food on tray. Describe food on tray in clock terms (e.g., coffee is at 2 o'clock, knife and spoon are at 3 o'clock). Help with cutting meats, removing lids from containers, buttering bread, and so on. • Help with walking: Walk slowly and slightly ahead of patient; patient's hand should rest on your arm at elbow. If possible, allow patient to trace progress by running the dorsal aspect of his or her free hand along a wall. Describe surroundings as you proceed. Warn of steps, turns, and narrow passageways in advance. Allow patient to feel chair, toilet, or bed before turning to sit.
Pain (postoperative) related to eyelid surgery	• Assess patient's level of discomfort. • Give pain medication as ordered.
Potential for injury to surgically repaired lid related to nausea or vomiting	• Assess patient's feelings of nausea. • Request order for antiemetic and administer if needed.
Potential for infection	• After removal of patch(es), administer antibiotic ointment as ordered.

Patient Education

1. Teach the patient to avoid rubbing or picking at the eyes.
2. Teach the patient to apply prescribed ointment to eye(s).

Evaluation

Patient Outcome	Data Indicating That Outcome is Reached
Cornea and conjunctiva are healthy.	Cornea is transparent, smooth, glossy, and moist. Palpebral conjunctiva is homogeneous pink color, and bulbar conjunctiva is clear. There is no burning or itching.
Surgically repaired eyelid maintains proper position and movement.	Lid margins are flush against eyeball surface. Eyelids close completely. Lid margins rest over inferior and superior borders of cornea. There is no tear spillage.
Patient is able to care for abnormally positioned lid that is not surgically repaired.	Patient administers prescribed medications successfully. Patient is able to monitor condition of eye and report conjunctival or corneal irritation in early stage.[4]

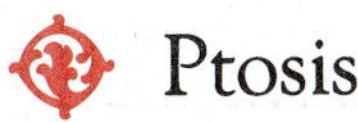

Ptosis

Ptosis is a drooping of the upper eyelid.[5]

Pathophysiology

Ptosis can be bilateral or unilateral, constant or intermittent, and congenital or acquired.[59] Congenital deformity usually involves malfunction of the levator muscle and is often accompanied by limited eye movement associated with superior rectus muscle failure. Acquired ptosis is mechanical, neurogenic, or myogenic in origin. Mechanical factors usually stem from abnormal weight of the eyelid imposed by such conditions as chronic edema, tumor, or excess tissue. Malfunction of the oculomotor nerve (CN III) interferes with lid elevation, eye movement, and pupillary constriction. Carotid aneurysms and diabetic neuropathy are common causes of CN III degeneration. Interruption of the sympathetic innervation of the smooth muscle that maintains lid tone and dilates the pupil causes ptosis. Horner's syndrome (a miotic pupil and drooping lid) occurs with sympathetic pathway lesions such as goiter, cervical lymph node enlargement, or apical bronchogenic carcinoma.[41] Unilateral ptosis is frequently the first sign of myasthenia gravis, which is characterized by fatigability of striated muscles. Bilateral involvement with progressive diminished eye movement may ensue. Aging eyes lose muscle tone of the lid elevator and the smooth muscle within the lid, and a general mild lid sag may occur.[41]

Medical Plan

Surgery

Resection of levator palpebrae superioris muscle—if functioning, muscle is reattached to tarsus at shorter length to increase muscle strength and lid-raising capacity

Upper eyelid suspension—when levator muscle is not functioning, supportive band of material is threaded within lid and attached to frontalis muscle to provide sling effect; lid movement is not affected, but cosmetic effect is improved[41,60]

General Management

Glasses with "crutch" can be worn to suspend inoperable lid

Treatment of systemic disorder (such as treatment of myasthenia gravis or removal of sympathetic pathway lesion) may relieve lid drooping[41]

NURSING CARE

Nursing Assessment

If both lids are involved, head may be thrown back and forehead constantly furrowed.

Nursing Dx & Intervention

Nursing Diagnosis	Nursing Intervention/Rationale
Body image disturbance related to eyelid deformities	• Assess patient's concerns. • Assist family members with being supportive. • See p. 1751.
Anxiety	• Assess patient's level of anxiety. • Listen to patient's concerns. • Provide supportive counseling.
Pain (postoperative) related to eyelid surgery	• Assess patient's level of discomfort. • Give pain medication as ordered. • Apply ice compresses as ordered *to decrease swelling*.
Potential for infection	• Administer antibiotic ointment as ordered.

Patient Education

1. Educate patient about disorder.
2. Discuss alternative care plans, rationale, and consequences.

Evaluation

Patient Outcome	Data Indicating That Outcome is Reached
Cornea and conjunctiva are healthy.	Cornea is transparent, smooth, glossy, and moist. Palpebral conjunctiva is homogeneous pink color, and bulbar conjunctiva is clear. There is no burning or itching.

Patient Outcome	Data Indicating That Outcome is Reached
Surgically repaired eyelid maintains proper position and movement.	Lid margins are flush against eyeball surface. Eyelids close completely. Lid margins rest over inferior and superior borders of cornea. There is no tear spillage.
Patient is able to care for abnormally positioned lid that is not surgically repaired.	Patient administers prescribed medications successfully. Patient is able to monitor condition of eye and report conjunctival or corneal irritation in early stage.[4]

Lagophthalmos

Lagophthalmos is inadequate closure of the eyelids.

Lagophthalmos may result from facial nerve (CN VII) weakness or enlargement or protrusion of the eyeball.[41]

Medical Plan

Surgery

Immediate surgical closure of lids may be necessary to prevent corneal drying and trauma; upper and lower eyelid adhesions can be temporarily or permanently created[57]

General Management

When only small portion of central cornea is exposed:
- Lubricating ointment instilled at bedtime for protection during sleep
- Soft contact lens worn or artificial tears administered several times a day
- Sustained-release tear insert in each eye once a day[41]

NURSING CARE

Nursing Assessment

Cornea

Corneal drying; secondary keratitis

Nursing Dx & Intervention[5,36,57]

Nursing Diagnosis	Nursing Intervention/Rationale
Potential for injury: cornea and conjunctiva, related to inadequate tearing	• Assess eye for symptoms of dryness. • Administer artificial tears, sustained-release tear insert, or lubricating ointment as ordered. • Be certain lid is closed when applying dressing.
Body image disturbance related to eyelid deformities	• Assess patient's concerns. • Assist family members with being supportive. • See p. 1751.
Knowledge deficit	• Educate patient about disorder. • Discuss alternative care plans, rationale, and consequences.
Anxiety	• Assess patient's level of anxiety. • Listen to patient's concerns. • Provide supportive counseling.
Sensory/perceptual alterations (visual) related to use of unilateral eye patch	*Before surgery:* • Warn patient that depth perception will be lost and 50% of peripheral vision will be lost on affected side. *After surgery:* • Help patient with activities of daily living. • Caution patient to bring hand forward slowly to touch objects (especially containers of hot liquid and containers receiving poured liquids) *to ensure safety.* • Teach patient to turn head fully toward affected side to view objects or obstacles. • Tell patient to use up and down head movements to judge stair dimensions and oncoming objects when walking and to proceed slowly.
Sensory/perceptual alterations (visual) related to use of bilateral eye patches	*Before surgery:* • Warn patient that eyes will be patched. • Orient patient to bedside equipment and room arrangement. • Arrange for placement of personal belongings in advance and review plan with patient. • Warn patient that side rails will be raised for safety.

Nursing Diagnosis	Nursing Intervention/Rationale
	After surgery: • Raise side rails. • Address patient by name from doorway and identify yourself *to reduce anxiety.* • Complement voice stimulation with touch *to notify patient of your proximity.* • Reorient patient to equipment (such as call light) and personal belongings at bedside by directing patient's hand. • Encourage patient to perform self-care with personal hygiene *to maximize independence.* • Ensure patient's privacy, and assure patient that privacy is provided. • Provide patient with television set or radio *to encourage mental and memory stimulation to prevent withdrawal.* • Engage patient in discussions about news or other items heard. • Provide patient with clock that can be felt and remind patient of date. • Discourage napping, which patient may want to do as he or she loses track of time. • Help patient with meals: Read menu selections. Guide hand to utensils and food on tray. Describe food on tray in clock terms (e.g., coffee is at 2 o'clock, knife and spoon are at 3 o'clock). Help with cutting meats, removing lids from containers, buttering bread, and so on. • Help with walking: Walk slowly and slightly ahead of patient; patient's hand should rest on your arm at elbow. If possible, allow patient to trace progress by running the dorsal aspect of his or her free hand along a wall. Describe surroundings as you proceed. Warn of steps, turns, and narrow passageways in advance. Allow patient to feel chair, toilet, or bed before turning to sit.
Pain (postoperative) related to eyelid surgery	• Assess level of discomfort. • Give pain medication as ordered.
Potential for injury to surgically repaired lid related to nausea or vomiting	• Assess patient's feelings of nausea. • Request order for antiemetic and administer if needed.
Potential for infection	• After removal of patch(es), administer antibiotic ointment as ordered.

Patient Education

1. Teach the patient to administer eye drops, lubricant, or tear insert if ordered; tell the patient to wash hands before and after the procedure.
2. Caution the patient to avoid rubbing or picking at the eyes.
3. Tell the patient to avoid noxious odors or fumes such as cigarette smoke.
4. Suggest that the patient use a humidifier in the home if the atmosphere is dry.
5. Show the patient how to monitor the eye for signs and symptoms of dryness or irritation.

Evaluation

Patient Outcome	Data Indicating That Outcome is Reached
Cornea and conjunctiva are healthy.	Cornea is transparent, smooth, glossy, and moist. Palpebral conjunctiva is homogeneous pink color, and bulbar conjunctiva is clear. There is no burning or itching.
Surgically repaired eyelid maintains proper position and movement.	Lid margins are flush against eyeball surface. Eyelids close completely. Lid margins rest over inferior and superior borders of cornea. There is no tear spillage.
Patient is able to care for abnormally positioned lid that is not surgically repaired.	Patient administers prescribed medications successfully. Patient is able to monitor condition of eye and report conjunctival or corneal irritation in early stage.[4]

Blinking disorders

Blinking disorders may occur as excessive blinking or a diminished rate of blinking.

Pathophysiology

Blinking is both a voluntary and an involuntary action. The rate of involuntary blinking varies among individuals, but blinking occurs frequently enough to spread tears over the surface of the eye. Reflex blinking increases in response to conjunctival or corneal irritation or pain in the eye. Chronic irritation may result in a continuous clonic response that is sustained until the stimulus is removed. Rapid blinking also accompanies anxiety and may become a prolonged pattern with chronic stress. Spasms of the orbicularis oculi muscle (blepharospasm) sometimes occur in elderly people.[60] These spasms are involuntary, tonic, spasmodic, usually bilateral contractions. They range from an annoying tic to a dangerous level during which the person cannot see. They are also unattractive. Causes include irritation of the eyes, facial nerve lesions, fatigue, and anxiety. Absence or diminishment of blinking may accompany parkinsonism or hyperthyroidism.

Medical Plan

Blinking disorders are usually relieved when the cause (systemic origin, anxiety, or local irritation) is treated or removed.

NURSING CARE

Nursing Assessment

Blinking Disorder

Rapid bilateral blinking
- Multiple anxiety behaviors

Tics
- Anxiety; statements of stress

Cornea and Conjunctiva

Diminished blinking
- Conjunctival drying and irritation or corneal drying; keratitis

Nursing Dx & Intervention[36,57]

Nursing Diagnosis	Nursing Intervention/Rationale
Potential for injury: cornea and conjunctiva, related to inadequate tearing	• Assess eye for symptoms of dryness. • Administer artificial tears, sustained-release tear insert, or lubricating ointment as ordered. • Be certain lid is closed when applying dressing.
Knowledge deficit	• Educate patient about disorder. • Discuss alternative care plans, rationale, and consequences.
Anxiety	• Assess patient's level of anxiety and stressors. • Listen to patient's concerns. • Provide supportive counseling.

Patient Education

1. Teach the patient to administer eye drops, lubricant, or tear insert if ordered; tell the patient to wash hands before and after the procedure.
2. Caution the patient to avoid rubbing or picking at the eyes.
3. Tell the patient to avoid noxious odors or fumes such as cigarette smoke.
4. Suggest that the patient use a humidifier in the home if the atmosphere is dry.
5. Teach the patient to monitor the eye for signs and symptoms of dryness or irritation.

Evaluation

Patient Outcome	Data Indicating That Outcome is Reached
Cornea and conjunctiva are healthy.	Cornea is transparent, smooth, glossy, and moist. Palpebral conjunctiva is homogeneous pink color, and bulbar conjunctiva is clear. There is no burning or itching.
Lid movement is normal.	Open and closure movement of lid is not excessive. Vision is not obscured. Source of nervous mannerisms or local irritant has been removed.[4]

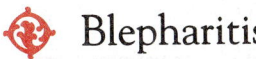

Blepharitis

Blepharitis is an inflammation of the eyelid margins.

Pathophysiology

Blepharitis is a chronic condition that can be caused by organisms (chiefly *Staphylococcus*), associated with seborrheic dermatitis, or aggravated by allergies. Often the causative factors are inseparable. Other conditions commonly associated with chronic blepharitis are diabetes, gout, anemia, and rosacea.[41] Infections of the nose and mouth can be transferred to the eyes and lids by frequent eye rubbing. Staphylococcal lesions usually ulcerate and often involve the conjunctiva and meibomian glands. Chalazions and hordeola (styes) may develop and recur. Seborrheic blepharitis is frequently accompanied by dermatitis of the scalp, eyebrows, and external ears. Some people first have this chronic condition in childhood and continue to have intermittent exacerbations throughout life.[57]

Medical Plan

Medications[31,41,57,60]

Anti-infective agents
- Ointment applied locally qd or bid, usually at bedtime if infection is present
  - Sulfacetamide sodium (Sulamyd, others), 10%-30% solution or 10% ointment
  - Bacitracin (Baciguent), 500 U/1 g ointment
  - Neomycin sulfate (Myciguent), 0.5% ointment
- Systemic medication
  - Tetracycline (Achromycin), 250 mg bid
- Selenium sulfide shampoo and soak for brows, eyelids[36]

General Management

Warm compresses to soften and remove crusts and scaling, 10 to 20 minutes twice a day
Oil to soften crusts
Mild baby shampoo to clean lids

NURSING CARE

Nursing Assessment

Eyelids and Lashes

Red lid margins; flaking and scaling around lashes; localized discomfort; loss of lashes; ingrown lashes; thickening and eversion of lid margins; tear spillage; in ulcerative staphylococcal blepharitis, pus, multiple lesions and crusting at lid margins, development of ulcers, lids glued shut by dried drainage

Cornea and Conjunctiva

Light sensitivity; possible chronic conjunctivitis; possible corneal inflammation[41]

Nursing Dx & Intervention

Nursing Diagnosis	Nursing Intervention/Rationale
Impaired skin integrity; potential impaired skin integrity	• Assess lids and conjunctivae for crusting, inflammation. • Use oil to soften crusts *to prevent lid injury at time of cleansing.* • Apply warm compresses with clean cloth for 10 to 20 minutes two or three times a day. • Soften crusts and clean lids, lightly stroking toward lid margin with cotton applicator.[36]
Potential for infection	• Assess patient's self-care and hygiene habits (e.g., handwashing, avoidance of rubbing eyes). • Instruct patient in self-care *to prevent reinfection.* • Demonstrate and instruct patient in self-administration of ointment *to prevent injury and contamination.*

Patient Education

1. Instruct the patient in the application of warm compresses and antibiotic ointment if ordered.
2. Instruct the patient in hygiene practices related to self-care of the eye, such as washing hands before and after self-care and avoiding fumes and smoke.
3. If the patient is a woman, tell her to avoid using eye makeup during the acute phase of lid infection, since makeup is a common allergen.

Evaluation

Patient Outcome	Data Indicating That Outcome is Reached
Eyelids are normal.	Lid margins are smooth and without scaling.
Conjunctiva is normal.	Palpebral conjunctiva is homogeneous pink color, and bulbar conjunctiva is clear. There is no excessive tearing.[4]

Meibomianitis

Meibomianitis is excessive secretion and inflammation of the meibomian glands.

Pathophysiology

Meibomianitis most often occurs in middle adulthood. It may accompany acute blepharitis or recur periodically without infection.[60] Mild compression over the lid margins expresses an oily, yellowish discharge that contains no organisms.

Medical Plan

Medications[41,57,60]

Anti-infective agents
- Ointment applied locally qd or bid, usually at bedtime if infection is present
- Sulfacetamide sodium (Sulamyd, others), 10%-30% solution or 10% ointment
- Bacitracin (Baciguent), 500 U/1 g ointment
- Neomycin sulfate (Myciguent), 0.5% ointment

General Management

Warm compresses and clean cloth two or three times a day

Tarsal massage—mild compression at lid margin to express gland contents twice a day

NURSING CARE

Nursing Assessment

Eyelids

Red-rimmed eyes; localized burning and discomfort; prominent meibomian glands; continuous frothy, yellowish discharge

Conjunctiva

Possible chronic conjunctivitis

Nursing Dx & Intervention

Nursing Diagnosis	Nursing Intervention/Rationale
Impaired skin integrity; potential impaired skin integrity	• Demonstrate tarsal massage (light compression over lid margin to express gland contents) and instruct patient to perform it twice a day. (This is difficult to do to oneself because the lid must be elevated to massage it well.[28]) • Demonstrate and instruct patient in application of warm compresses.

Patient Education

1. Instruct the patient in the application of warm compresses and antibiotic ointment if ordered.
2. Instruct the patient in hygiene practices related to self-care of the eye, such as washing hands before and after self-care and avoiding fumes and smoke.
3. If the patient is a woman, tell her to avoid using eye makeup during the acute phase of lid infection, since makeup is a common allergen.

Evaluation

Patient Outcome	Data Indicating That Outcome is Reached
Eyelids are normal.	Lid margins are smooth, without crusting.
Conjunctiva is normal.	Palpebral conjunctiva is homogeneous pink color, and bulbar conjunctiva is clear. There is no excessive tearing.[4]

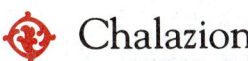

Chalazion

Chalazion is a granulomatous inflammation of a meibomian gland.[5]

Pathophysiology

A chalazion forms on the conjunctival aspect of the upper or lower eyelid as glands in both are affected. It begins as a nontender swelling and may take several weeks to develop. It does not appear inflamed unless a secondary infection occurs. If large enough, the nodule can compress the eyeball and cause an astigmatism. A large nodule also produces discomfort as the upper lid closes, causing pressure on the cornea. Some chalazia disappear in a few months without ever causing symptoms. Chronic chalazia tend to subside partially and reactivate periodically.[41,60]

Medical Plan

Surgery

Localized excision of chronic chalazion with patient under local anesthesia; antibiotic eye drops administered three or four times a day before and after surgery

Medications

Anti-infective agents
- Ointment applied locally 4 times/d postoperatively
  - Sulfacetamide sodium (Sulamyd, others), 10%-30% solution or 10% ointment
  - Bacitracin (Baciguent), 500 U/1 g ointment
  - Neomycin sulfate (Myciguent), 0.5% ointment

NURSING CARE

Nursing Assessment

Eyelids

Small, nontender, noninflamed lump on outer lid; lid eversion reveals nodule that points toward conjunctiva; secondary infection produces redness, pain, and suppuration; sensitivity to light

Nursing Dx & Intervention

Nursing Diagnosis	Nursing Intervention/Rationale
Potential for infection	• Assess entire lid for inflammatory signs. • Apply warm compresses with clean cloth for 10 to 20 minutes two or three times a day after excision of chalazion *to expedite healing*.

Patient Education

1. Instruct the patient in hygiene practices related to self-care of the eye, such as washing hands before and after self-care and avoiding fumes and smoke.
2. If the patient is a woman, tell her to avoid using eye makeup during the acute phase of lid infection, since makeup is a common allergen.
3. Teach the patient how to administer ointment.
4. Teach the patient how to apply warm compresses to eyes.

Evaluation

Patient Outcome	Data Indicating That Outcome is Reached
Eyelids are normal.	Lid margins are smooth, without lesions.
Conjunctiva is normal.	Palpebral conjunctiva is homogeneous pink color, and bulbar conjunctiva is clear. There is no excessive tearing.[4]

Hordeolum

A hordeolum (sty) is an acute infection of an eyelash follicle or the glands of Moll or Zeis (sebaceous glands).

Pathophysiology

The offending organism is usually *Staphylococcus*. The lesion becomes a pustule that eventually points and may rupture. Multiple pustules may occur along adjacent lash follicles because of reinfection.[59]

Medical Plan

Medications

Anti-infective agents (ointment applied locally 2-4 times/d)
Sulfacetamide sodium (Sulamyd, others), 10%-30% solution or 10% ointment
Bacitracin (Baciguent), 500 U/1 g ointment
Neomycin sulfate (Myciguent), 0.5% ointment

General Management

Warm compresses with clean cloth for 10 to 20 minutes two or three times a day
Local incision of pustule if rupture is not spontaneous

NURSING CARE

Nursing Assessment

Eyelids

Initial tenderness with localized redness and swelling that forms pustule at lid margin; may be multiple pustules; generalized lid edema; pain that increases as pustule enlarges and ceases with rupture

Nursing Dx & Intervention

Nursing Diagnosis	Nursing Intervention/Rationale
Potential for infection	• Assess patient's hygiene practices (e.g., handwashing before touching the eye) *to prevent spread of infection.* • Assess the patient for *Staphylococcus* infections or lesions elsewhere on the body *to monitor potential or presence of systemic staphylococcal infection.*
Impaired skin integrity; potential impaired skin integrity	• Apply warm compresses with clean cloth for 10 to 20 minutes two or three times a day *to expedite healing.*

Patient Education

1. Instruct the patient in the application of warm compresses and antibiotic ointment if ordered.
2. Instruct the patient in hygiene practices related to self-care of the eye, such as washing hands before and after self-care and avoiding fumes and smoke.
3. If the patient is a woman, tell her to avoid using eye makeup during the acute phase of lid infection, since makeup is a common allergen.

Evaluation

Patient Outcome	Data Indicating That Outcome is Reached
Eyelids are normal.	Lid margins are smooth, without lesions.
Conjunctiva is normal.	Palpebral conjunctiva is homogeneous pink color, and bulbar conjunctiva is clear. There is no excessive tearing.[4]

LACRIMAL APPARATUS DISORDERS

Patients with lacrimal disorders usually complain of "dry eyes," excessive tearing, or pain and swelling of the lacrimal duct. Inadequate tearing can result in drying and severe damage to the cornea. Excessive tearing can be caused by overproduction of tears by the lacrimal gland or a faulty drainage system that results in tear spillage. Tear accumulation can interfere with vision and irritate the eyeball. Inflammation of the lacrimal sac and adjacent canaliculi can be associated with conjunctivitis, nasal disease, or drainage obstruction.

 Dry eye syndrome

Dry eye syndrome is a condition in which tear production is inadequate.

Pathophysiology[31,41,60]

Dry eye syndrome occurs for three primary reasons: lacrimal gland malfunction, mucin deficiency, and mechanical abnormalities that interfere with the spread or maintenance of tears over the eyeball surface. Lacrimal gland malfunctions can be congenital or acquired. The most common congenital disorders are lacrimal gland aplasia, ectodermal dysplasia, and trigeminal nerve (CN V) malfunction, which disrupts sensory stimulation to the upper lid. Acquired disorders that affect lacrimal gland function can be systemic, infectious, or related to trauma. Common systemic disorders that may be associated with diminished tear production are rheumatoid arthritis (Sjögren's syndrome), leukemia, lymphoma, sarcoidosis, and systemic sclerosis. Facial nerve (CN VII) palsy inhibits tearing. Mumps and some forms of conjunctivitis may obstruct tear flow. Chemical burns and irradiation may reduce lacrimal gland function. Some medications such as antihistamines, atropine, and β-adrenergic blockers decrease tear production. Even if the lacrimal gland is not functioning, accessory glands in the palpebral conjunctiva may secrete sufficient tears to prevent severe corneal damage.

A layer of mucin, produced by goblet cells in the lid, maintains a homogeneous tear spread over the eyeball surface. The absence of mucin causes the tear film to break up, leaving "dry holes" over the cornea. Mucin deficiency is commonly associated with some forms of chronic conjunctivitis, vitamin A deficiency, and medications such as antihistamines and β-adrenergic blockers.

Mechanical defects that contribute to dry eyes include abnormalities of eyelid structure and function (see p. 582), protrusion of the eyeball (proptosis), and use or misuse of contact lenses (see p. 643).

The symptom most commonly associated with inadequate tearing is keratoconjunctivitis sicca (KCS). The person experiences burning, itching, and a foreign body sensation in the eyes. The cornea and conjunctiva may show inflammation, erosion, or keratinization. The signs and symptoms may occur in any age group but are most common in women 50 to 60 years old. Untreated or severe KCS can result in blindness.

Diagnostic Studies and Findings[31,41,57,60]

Rose Bengal Staining

Drop of 1% or 2% solution placed in conjunctival sac; 2% solution demonstrates loss of corneal and conjunctival epithelium in keratoconjunctivitis sicca; 1% solution valuable in demonstrating conjunctival and corneal epithelial cell loss and degeneration; patients with deficiency of aqueous portion of tears have punctate staining of lower two thirds of cornea and bright red staining of bulbar conjunctiva in area corresponding to palpable aperture

Schirmer's Test

Strip of filter paper, 3.5 × 0.05 cm, placed in conjunctival cul-de-sac of lower lid for 5 minutes; 10 to 15 mm length of paper wetted with tears considered normal; more than 25 mm moistened paper indicates excessive tearing

Basic Secretion Test

Topical anesthetic administered to eyeball before filter paper inserted; anesthesia reduces lacrimal output to allow measurement of tear production of accessory glands in eyelid

Medical Plan[5,31,41]

A correlation does not always exist between the failure of tear production and inflammatory or degenerative changes on the surface of the eye. The mechanisms that connect tear and mucin production to ocular surface maintenance are not fully understood. Depending on the cause and severity of the condition, the examiner may select from or combine the following therapeutic approaches.

- Restoration or stimulation of tears
  - Estrogen replacement therapy has been associated with relief of dry eye symptoms in some postmenopausal women[5,31]
  - Elimination of systemic medications that have created the problem
  - Treatment and resolution of eyelid or conjunctival inflammation
  - Alteration in contact lens prescription or patient's self-care methods
- Preservation of existing tears
  - Surgically induced punctal occlusion
  - Eyelid repair (ectropion) or lid closure repair
  - Wearing of airtight goggles to prevent tear evaporation

Tear replacement
Maintenance and treatment of ocular surface
  Antibiotic ointments
  Lubricating ointments
  Some studies have reported success with the use of topical vitamin A preparations in the maintenance of healthy conjunctival tissue[31]

Surgery

Occlusion of puncta to conserve tears
Surgical repair of lid position or movement abnormalities

Medications

Anti-infective agents
  Ointment applied locally for existing inflammation
  Polysporin Ophth. Oint. (Polymixin, 10,000 U; Bacitracin, 500 U), 2-4 times/d
Tear substitute
  Adsorbobase hydroxylethyl Cellulose Thimeros 1 0.002%, edetate disodium 0.05% (Tears Naturale), 1-2 drops tid prn
  Duasab Polymeric system with Dextran, benzalkonium chloride 0.01%, edetate disodium 0.05% (Tears Naturale), 1-2 drops prn
Ointment to lubricate and protect the eyes
  White petroleum and mineral oil (Duolube, Akwa Tears), instill in conjunctival sac prn

General Management

Humidifier in environment
Airtight goggles or eye shield

NURSING CARE

Nursing Assessment

Dry Eyes

Burning; itching; foreign body sensation; sensitivity to light; blurred vision; lack of tears; loss of glossy appearance of cornea; tear film interspersed with mucus strands

Nursing Dx & Intervention[5,36,57]

Nursing Diagnosis	Nursing Intervention/Rationale
Potential for injury: cornea and conjunctiva, related to lack of tears	• Assess eye for signs and symptoms of irritation (itching, burning, and loss of glossy appearance of eyeball surface). • Administer artificial tears, sustained-release tear insert, or lubricating ointments as ordered *to prevent tissue damage to ocular surface.*
Sensory/perceptual alterations (visual) related to bilateral eye patches or lid closure	• Raise side rails. • Address patient by name from doorway and identify yourself. • Complement voice stimulation with touch *to notify patient of your proximity.* • Orient patient to bedside equipment (such as call light, bed control, and side rails) and personal belongings at bedside by directing patient's hand over objects. • Encourage patient to perform self-care with personal hygiene *to maximize independence.* • Provide support and supervision with ADLs. • Provide patient privacy, and assure patient that privacy is provided. • Help with meals. (Patients may become so frustrated at mealtime that they may not eat without this assistance.) Read menu selections. Guide hand to utensils and food on tray. Describe food on tray in clock terms. Teach patient to "trail," that is, to use dorsal aspect of index and middle fingers to find objects on food tray. Fill glasses only half full, since patient may spill easily. Help patient with cutting meat, removing lids from cartons, buttering bread, and so on. • Help with walking. Walk slowly and slightly ahead of patient. Patient's hand should rest on your arm at your elbow. If possible, allow patient to trace progress by running the dorsal aspect of his or her free hand along a wall. Describe surroundings as you proceed. Allow patient to feel chair, toilet, or bed before turning to sit.
Pain related to localized inflammation	• Assess patient's degree of discomfort. • Provide analgesics as ordered.

Patient Education

1. Teach the patient how to administer eye drops, lubricant, or a tear insert; stress the importance of washing hands before and after the procedure.
2. Instruct the patient to avoid rubbing or picking at the eyes.
3. Instruct the patient to avoid noxious odors or fumes and to use a humidifier in the home if the atmosphere is dry.
4. Teach the patient how to monitor the eye for signs and symptoms of dryness or irritation.

Evaluation

Patient Outcome	Data Indicating That Outcome is Reached
Cornea and conjunctiva are healthy.	Cornea is transparent, smooth, glossy, and moist. Palpebral conjunctiva is homogeneous pink color, and bulbar conjunctiva is clear. There is no burning or itching.[4]

Excessive tears

Excessive tears can occur from overproduction or inadequate drainage of tears.

Pathophysiology[5,41,60]

Tear spillage most commonly occurs because the drainage system is faulty (epiphora). The puncta can be occluded because of congenital absence of an opening or because of infection in the lacrimal sac. Lid abnormalities, such as ectropion, cause abnormal alignment of the lacrimal tear pool and the puncta. An accumulation of tears in the inner canthus is an irritant that stimulates more tear production. Obstructions may also occur in the lacrimal duct or the meatus in the nasal cavity.

Lacrimation (excessive tear production) occurs most commonly with reflex stimulation of the lacrimal gland. Corneal injury, eye pain, noxious odors, eyestrain, bright light, and allergies are examples of sensory stimuli affecting the trigeminal nerve (CN V). Glaucoma often stimulates tear production because of trigeminal irritation. Facial nerve (CN VII) irritation during vomiting or laughter also stimulates tear production. Abnormal regeneration of the facial nerve following Bell's palsy causes "crocodile tears," a phenomenon of excess tearing that occurs during eating. Parasympathetic stimulants (cholinergic drugs) and some endocrine disorders (such as hyperthyroidism) can also increase tearing.

Diagnostic Studies and Findings

Dye Disappearance

Cul-de-sac of lower lid flooded with 2% fluorescein solution; fluorescein normally disappears from cul-de-sac in 1 minute

Dacryocystography

Radiopaque medium injected into lacrimal sac before roentgenography; shows patent lacrimal passage

Dacryoscintography

Isotope instilled in cul-de-sac and traced with gamma camera; irrigation of lacrimal sac before dacryoscintography will stain mucosal lining a readily identifiable blue color; shows patent lacrimal passage

Medical Plan

Surgery

Repair of lid structure abnormalities to enhance punctal access to tear pool

Probing of obstructed punctum

Construction of tube connecting conjunctival cul-de-sac to nasal cavity

General Management

Related to removal of cause of lacrimation

NURSING CARE

Nursing Assessment

Excessive Tears

Tear spillage; blurred vision; puncta red and swollen; puncta may exude purulent material on mild compression over lacrimal sac; conjunctivitis (reddened conjunctiva)

Nursing Dx & Intervention[57]

Nursing Diagnosis	Nursing Intervention/Rationale
Potential for infection	• Assess eye for amount of lacrimation or increased symptoms of irritation or infection. • Encourage patient to maintain excellent hygiene.

Patient Education

1. Instruct the patient in hygiene practices related to self-care of the eyes, such as washing hands before and after self-care and keeping hands away from the eyes.

Evaluation

Patient Outcome	Data Indicating That Outcome is Reached
Lacrimal drainage system is patent.	There is no excess tearing. Inner canthus of eye is homogeneous pink color. When eye is compressed at medial infraorbital rim, punctum does not exude any material.[4]
Underlying endocrine cause, if any, is corrected.	Amount of tears produced is not excessive.

Dacryocystitis

Dacryocystitis is an inflammation of the lacrimal sac.

Pathophysiology

Dacryocystitis can be acute or chronic and is usually caused by obstruction of tear drainage from the punctum or lacrimal sac.

Normal newborns often do not have patent nasolacrimal ducts. The duct usually opens about the third week of life. If the duct fails to open, tearing occurs and eventually purulent material exudes from the punctum. The condition often corrects itself by 3 to 6 months of age. Lacrimal probing may be performed if spontaneous patency does not occur. Surgical construction of a duct is rarely needed, but if necessary it is performed when the child reaches 3 or 4 years of age.[41]

Chronic dacryocystitis most often occurs in middle-aged adults. Spontaneous punctum obstruction is followed by bacterial infection with a mucopurulent discharge. The nasolacrimal duct can also be obstructed by injury or nasal lesions, causing an inflammatory response.

Acute dacryocystitis has a rapid onset with marked swelling and tenderness of surrounding tissue.[60]

Medical Plan[41,60]

Surgery

Incision and drainage of abscess

Dacryocystorhinostomy for construction of passage between lacrimal sac and nasal cavity

Medications

Anti-infective agents

- Systemic antibiotics for acute, severe infection
- Instillation of antibiotic or sulfonamide eye drops 4-5 times/d until infection subsides

General Management

Daily massage of lacrimal sac to rid it of purulent material

Warm compresses over affected eye during acute phase

Lacrimal probing with graduated sizes of probe while patient is under local anesthesia

Temporary lacrimal drainage splint

NURSING CARE

Nursing Assessment

Lacrimal Inflammation

Tear spillage; purulent material exuding from punctum on compression; punctum swollen, and surrounding tissue may be reddened; localized pain

Nursing Dx & Intervention

Nursing Diagnosis	Nursing Intervention/Rationale
Potential for infection	• Assess punctum and surrounding tissue for inflammation. • Apply warm compresses over affected eye for 10 or 20 minutes three or four times a day. • Lightly massage lacrimal sac at medial infraorbital rim *to rid sac of accumulated purulent material.* • Administer antibiotic or sulfonamide eye drops or ointment as ordered. • Wash hands thoroughly before and after care of affected eye.

Patient Education

1. Instruct the patient in hygiene practices related to self-care of the eyes, such as washing hands before and after self-care and keeping hands away from the eyes.

Evaluation

Patient Outcome	Data Indicating That Outcome is Reached
Cornea and conjunctiva are healthy.	Cornea is transparent, smooth, glossy, and moist. Palpebral conjunctiva is homogeneous pink color. Bulbar conjunctiva is clear. There is no burning or itching.[4]
Lacrimal drainage system is patent.	There is no excess tearing. Inner canthus of eye is homogeneous pink color. Punctum does not exude any material when eye is compressed at medial infraorbital rim.[4]

CONJUNCTIVAL DISORDERS

The bulbar conjunctiva is a protective coating for the scleral portion of the eyeball. It can be affected by many injuries or infections from the environment. It adjoins the palpebral conjunctiva in the lid cul-de-sac and is susceptible to infection because it is close to the eyelid. The conjuctiva also responds to internal infections or diseases such as measles, diabetes mellitus, or riboflavin deficiency. This outer layer contains blood vessels that dilate rapidly and pain receptors that register mild to moderate discomfort in response to inflammation. The conjunctiva is adjacent to the cornea and can be an avenue for spreading infection to this vital area.

 Conjunctivitis

Conjunctivitis is an inflammation or infection of the conjunctiva.

Conjunctival tissue can become inflamed by dust, smog, tobacco smoke, noxious fumes, wind, sun, and airborne allergens. Conjunctivitis is common and easily spread, particularly in crowded environments such as schools and nursing homes.

Pathophysiology[5,41,44,60]

Conjunctivitis varies in severity. Vascular dilation and engorgement can be a response to external irritants such as smog, hair sprays, or noxious fumes. The person may experience lacrimation and a foreign body sensation, but no discharge or progressive infectious process appears. Generalized hyperemia and burning are initial responses to insufficient tearing, and a secondary infection can follow rapidly. Allergic responses may be seasonal and include vascular injection, moderate tearing, and severe itching.

Viral conjunctivitis is characterized by generalized hyperemia, profuse tearing, and little exudate. Preauricular nodes are commonly associated with viral infections. Some adenoviruses invade the upper respiratory or gastrointestinal systems, causing fever and acute systemic signs along with the conjunctivitis. Viral infections may be mild and self-limited or may quickly invade the cornea and surrounding tissue and cause severe ocular surface and periorbital pain. Type 1 herpes simplex conjunctivitis has been diagnosed more often in recent years with fluorescent antibody staining of corneal scrapings. Herpes conjunctivitis often invades the cornea with inflammation, erosion, and ulceration. Usually only one eye is involved initially, but both may be affected eventually. Recurrent eye lesions that may cause scarring and diminished vision can be brought on by stress, immunosuppression, menstruation, fever, or exposure to ultraviolet light.

Bacterial conjunctivitis, the most common type, is frequently called pinkeye. Almost any bacterium can be involved, but *Pneumococcus, Staphylococcus,* and *Streptococcus* organisms are common. The infection usually begins in one eye and is transferred to the other eye through contamination. The onset is acute, with a mucopurulent exudate, tearing, generalized hyperemia, and moderate discomfort. This form of conjunctivitis is highly contagious.

Some organisms rapidly invade the cornea and the conjunctiva and lead to corneal ulceration and perforation. Two of the most virulent organisms are *Neisseria gonorrhoeae* and *Chlamydia trachomatis*. Ophthalmia neonatorum, a conjunctivitis that occurs in newborns, is commonly transmitted from the mother with acute gonorrheal urethritis during birth. Ophthalmia neonatorum occurs within the first 10 days of life and is characterized by a rapid progression of signs from mild inflammation to marked redness, swelling, and purulent exudate. Corneal involvement is common and severe. *Chlamydia trachomatis* organisms can also be transmitted during a newborn's passage through the vagina. The early symptoms are similar to those of gonococcal conjunctivitis, but the incubation period is slightly longer (5 to 14 days). *Chlamydia* organisms do not respond to silver nitrate, which has been traditionally administered prophylactically to newborns. Since 1980, erythromycin has been more commonly used because it is effective against both *N. gonorrhoeae* and *Chlamydia*. Both gonococcal and chlamydial organisms (which are transmitted venereally) can invade adult conjunctivae and cause severe, acute, purulent infection.

The conjunctival infections that have been described are generally acute and can be successfully treated. Some persons have a chronic recurrent conjunctivitis characterized by periodic eye discomfort, redness, and discharge. Repeated inflammatory episodes can cause thickening of the conjunctiva and lid margins. The causes are numerous, but the most common are contact allergens (such as cosmetics or chlorine), airborne allergens, excessive meibomian gland secretions, and chronic blepharitis. Trachoma (a chronic *Chlamydia trachomatis* conjunctivitis) has been described as the leading cause of blindness in the world. It is prevalent in warm climates where living conditions are crowded and hygienic practices are poor. Insects may transmit the disease. In some cases the disease heals spontaneously, but in other cases it leads to conjunctival scarring and loss of vision if left untreated.

Diagnostic Studies and Findings[5,41,60]

Microscopic Examination of Stained Conjunctival Scrapings

Numerous polymorphonuclear neutrophils in bacterial infections; monocytes in viral infections or trachoma; eosinophils and basophils in allergies

Culture of Exudate or Conjunctival Scrapings

Organism identification

Medical Plan[11,41,60]

Medications

- Anti-infective agents (medication varies with causative organism)
  - Sulfacetamide sodium (Sulamyd, Bleph 10), 10%-30% solution or 10% ointment for 3-7 d
  - Erythromycin (Ilotycin), topical 0.5% ointment for 3-7 d
  - Gentamicin sulfate (Garamycin, Genoptic), topical, 3 mg/ml solution or 3 mg/g ointment for 3-7 d
- Antiviral agents
  - Idoxuridine (IDU, Dendrite Herplex), 0.1% solution, 1 drop q1h during day and q2h at night
  - Adenine arabinoside (Ara-A, Vira-A), 3% ointment instilled 5 times/d
  - Trifluridine (TFT, Viroptic), 1% solution, 1 drop q2h during waking hours during epithelial healing, then 1 drop q4h for 7 d
  - For gonococcal or chlamydial conjunctivitis or severe purulent conjunctivitis
    - Tetracycline (Achromycin, Terramycin), 250-500 mg po qid for 21 d
    - Erythromycin (E-Mycin, others), 250 mg qid for 21 d
  - Prophylactic dose within first hour of life for newborns
    - Erythromycin ophthalmic ointment, 0.5%, in each eye
    - Tetracycline ophthalmic ointment, 1% in each eye

General Management

- Saline irrigations for purulent discharge
- Warm compresses for discomfort and inflammation, 10 to 15 minutes two or three times a day
- Cold compresses for allergic itching, 10 to 15 minutes two or three times a day
- Oil or shampoo swabbing for softening, loosening, and removing crusts on eyelids[41,55]

NURSING CARE

Nursing Assessment

Allergic and General Irritant Responses

Lacrimation; generalized hyperemia; gritty, sandy sensation; severe itching (with allergies)

Viral Inflammation

Lacrimation; minimum mucopurulent discharge; generalized hyperemia; possible preauricular nodes; some lid swelling; moderate discomfort; possible photophobia

Bacterial Inflammation

Purulent discharge; lid swelling; generalized hyperemia; moderate discomfort; possible photophobia; complaints of blurred vision (owing to excess exudate over eye surface); blurring may disappear with blinking

Severe (Corneal) Involvement

Moderate discomfort that becomes severe

Nursing Dx & Intervention

Nursing Diagnosis	Nursing Intervention/Rationale
Potential for infection	• Assess patient's eyes for presence of mucopurulent discharge *to confirm presence of bacterial, possible gonococcal, or chlamydial infection.* • Isolate patient from others (in institutional setting) and use isolation precautions *to prevent spread of infection.* Administer prescribed topical ointments or systemic antibiotics.
Potential for injury	• Administer saline irrigations for excessive discharge *to expedite healing and prevent crusting.* • Cleanse lids and lashes with mild shampoo and applicators *to remove crusts.*
Pain	• Apply warm compresses to eyes *to increase comfort.* • Administer analgesics as ordered.

Patient Education

1. Teach the patient to perform saline irrigation of the eye.
2. Teach the patient to apply warm compresses with a clean cloth or cold compresses (ice should not be applied directly to eyelids).
3. Instruct the patient to wash hands thoroughly before and after treating each eye.
4. Tell the patient to keep the hands away from the face.
5. Instruct the patient to avoid crowded environments when possible.
6. Instruct family members to avoid touching their faces and to wash hands thoroughly when contact has occurred.[40]
7. Tell the patient to avoid noxious fumes and smoke.
8. Instruct the patient not to wear contact lens during the suppuration period.

Evaluation

Patient Outcome	Data Indicating That Outcome is Reached
Conjunctiva and cornea are healthy.	Palpebral conjunctiva is homogeneous pink color. Bulbar conjunctiva is clear and glossy. Cornea is clear and glossy. There is no eye discomfort, lacrimation, or discharge.[4]

Subconjunctival hemorrhage

Subconjunctival hemorrhage is a common phenomenon caused by the rupture of a blood vessel. It appears suddenly as a well-defined, bright red area on the surface of the eyeball and gradually disappears in 2 to 3 weeks. A large hemorrhage may be darker in color and expand for the first few days. The patient feels no discomfort but is usually quite alarmed. The ruptured vessel is usually the result of localized increased pressure (following severe coughing, vomiting, or sneezing) or minor trauma. Often a cause cannot be found, and no treatment exists. In rare instances blood dyscrasias, hypertension, or viral conjunctivitis is associated with this hemorrhage.[41,60]

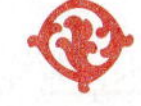

Conjunctival discoloration and growths

The conjunctiva is subject to a large variety of growths, tumors, and discolorations. Bilirubin is absorbed in the conjunctiva with jaundice and gives the underlying sclera a yellow coloring. This discoloration is different from the normal yellowish pigmentation that occurs with increased melanin deposits in dark-skinned people.

Two of the most common benign growths are pterygium and pinguecula. A pterygium is a triangular growth of connective tissue that usually advances from the nasal side of the conjunctiva and encroaches on the cornea. It occurs more commonly among people who are frequently exposed to the sun and wind. It is not surgically removed unless it creates a cosmetic concern or threatens to involve the central cornea. A pinguecula is common in older adults and appears as a yellow nodule on either side of the cornea at the limbus. It usually involves both eyes. It may be periodically inflamed but does not invade the cornea and is usually not treated unless the patient is concerned about its appearance.

DISORDERS OF THE CORNEA AND SCLERA

The cornea is the main exterior protector of vision. Visual clarity depends on uniformity, smoothness, and transparency throughout the corneal layers. The avascular central cornea depends on its periphery (the limbus) for nourishment and on its epithelial (outer layer) and endothelial (inner layer) activity for hydration stability. Because the cornea is exposed to the external environment, it is more vulnerable to trauma and infection. Injury to the outer epithelial layer exposes Bowman's membrane and the substantia propria (stromal layer) to infection. If untreated infection perforates the cornea, the eye may be lost. The epithelial layer regenerates rapidly without scarring, but the deeper layers form opacities that may cause astigmatism or mild to severe visual loss.

Recently developed surgical techniques for corneal transplantation involving new microscopic and illuminating systems have greatly improved the prognosis for patients needing new corneas.[23] Corneal transplant and implications for nursing are covered in the last section of this chapter (p. 649).

The sclera surrounds the eyeball and is adjacent to the uveal tract (including the choroid layer). It opens posteriorly to admit the optic nerve and other nerves and vessels into the eye. Scleral inflammation and disease are often associated with systemic connective tissue disorders.

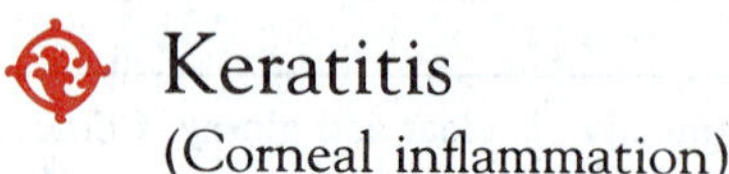

Keratitis

(Corneal inflammation)

Keratitis is an inflammation of the cornea.

Pathophysiology[5,41,44,45,60]

The cornea can be injured by exposure (drying), ischemia, nutritional deficiency, microbe invasion, anesthesia (sensory interruption), and trauma. Keratitis (corneal inflammation) may be superficial (epithelial), invade the stroma (subepithelial), or eventually break through the inner layer (Descemet's membrane) to the endothelium. Most organisms require a break in the epithelium before they can enter the cornea. The epithelium can be damaged by hypersensitivity to conjunctival inflammation, corneal drying, mechanical injury, or chemical irritants. Since the epithelium is richly innervated, superficial inflammation causes moderate to severe pain. Epithelial erosions may appear in the form of tiny pits or small or coarse lesions scattered over the surface. Central ulcers (or craters) may invade deeply into the underlying layers. Some of the medical treatments prescribed for therapy or relief of discomfort may facilitate bacterial invasion. People whose immune systems have been suppressed are more vulnerable to infection; the misuse of local corticosteroid therapy increases the tissue destruction activity of collagenase, which is produced when epithelial cells are injured. Immunosuppression also makes a person more vulnerable to invasion by fungi, which easily penetrate Descemet's membrane. Fluorescein solution, which is used to stain and detect epithelial damage, is easily contaminated and can inoculate the epithelium with organisms. A patient who is given local anesthetics (particularly for use at home) can further abrade the cornea without knowing it. Besides inhibiting the protective corneal reflex, anesthesia of the eye interrupts epithelial regeneration.

Almost any bacterium can invade the cornea. *Pneumococcus, Staphylococcus, Streptococcus,* and *Pseudomonas* organisms are the most common. Fungal infections have become much more common since the introduction of topical corticosteroids and antibiotics. Chronic debilitating disease increases vulnerability to fungal infections. Viral infections, most commonly caused by herpes simplex, are also prevalent.

Herpes zoster can also invade the eye through inflammatory lesions of areas served by the trigeminal nerve. The lesions, in the form of scattered erosions or plaques, may be superficial or embedded in the deeper corneal layers. Residual corneal stromal infiltrates and scarring may ensue. The acute phase of herpes zoster keratitis resolves in 4 to 6 days. Treatment is primarily aimed at relieving the symptoms. Topical and systemic steroids and some newly approved antiviral topical medications speed recovery.

Recent reports have created concern about the increasing incidence of *Acanthamoeba* keratitis. *Acanthamoeba* is commonly found in fresh water, soil, and airborne dust. The organisms have been recovered from the nose and throat of seemingly healthy individuals, suggesting that they can be inhaled as well as acquired through contaminated water. The amebae are resistant to freezing, to most antimicrobial agents, and to levels of chlorine used to disinfect swimming pools, public drinking water, and hot tubs. Most people who have this infestation are contact lens wearers who use distilled or tap water to clean or rinse their lenses. The organism is devastating because it is resistant to most antimicrobials, it is often misdiagnosed as herpes simplex keratitis and treated without success, and it tends to cause recurrent epithelial breakdown. A large percentage of patients with this disorder have had to undergo a corneal transplant to regain useful vision.

The severity of corneal destruction depends on the virulence of the organism, the degree of corneal destruction, the accuracy and promptness of therapy, and the immunocompetence of the host. *Pneumococcus* and *Pseudomonas* organisms tend to spread rapidly and form ulcers that penetrate deep into the stroma. Herpes keratitis can be recurrent; it is triggered by stress, exposure to ultraviolet light (sunlight), or by other illness. It is relatively asymptomatic because it attacks the trigeminal nerve (CN V) and diminishes pain. Corneal ulceration and optic atrophy develop rapidly in neonates contaminated with herpesvirus at birth. Adults with recurrent herpes keratitis may heal with or without scarring.[28] Herpesvirus is also activated with the use of topical steroids. Some virus forms are highly contagious and cause outbreaks, especially in schools, institutions, and eye clinics. Chronic disabling illness increases an individual's vulnerability to corneal damage, as do certain diseases, such as diabetes mellitus, leukemia, chronic alcoholism, severe vitamin A deficiency, and autoimmune diseases.

Diagnostic Studies and Findings[5,41,60]

Fluorescein Stain (2%)

Sterile paper strips most commonly used; breaks in epithelium are stained green

Ulcer Scrapings for Microscopic Viewing (Gram or Giemsa Stain)

Organism identification

Ulcer Scrapings for Culture

Organism identification

Medical Plan[5,11,41,45]

Surgery

Corneal transplantation (see p. 649)
Enucleation (or evisceration) (see p. 647)

Medications

Mode, frequency, and duration of therapy depend on identified organism and degree of corneal penetration[28,40]

- Anti-infective agents
  - Topical
    - Erythromycin, 5 mg/g
    - Gentamicin, 3-8 mg/ml
    - Penicillin G, 10,000-20,000 U/ml
    - Bacitracin, 10,000 U/ml
    - Sulfacetamide sodium, 10% solution
    - Amphotericin B, 1.5-3 mg/ml
    - Idoxuridine, 0.1% solution or 0.5% ointment
  - Subconjunctival injections of antibiotics for acute, severe central ulcerations
  - Systemic antibiotics (IV or po) for acute severe central ulcerations, if sclera is involved, or if perforation threatens
- Antiviral agents
  - Idoxuridine (IDU, Dendrite Herplex), 0.1% solution, 1 drop q1h during day and q2h at night
  - Adenine arabinoside (Ara-A, Vira-A), 3% ointment, instill 5 times/d
  - Trifluridine (TFT, Viroptic), 1% solution, 1 drop q2h during waking hours during epithelial healing, then 1 drop q4h for 7 d
- Mydriatic-cycloplegic agents
  - Atropine, 1% solution bid or tid for painful inflammation of iris and inflammatory constriction of pupil
- Mucolytics
  - Acetylcysteine, 10%-20% solution for inhibiting collagenase
- Analgesics (for severe pain)
  - Acetaminophen (Tylenol), 650 mg po q4h prn
  - Acetaminophen (Tylenol 650 mg) with codeine (30 mg), 1-2 tablets po q4h prn
  - Codeine, 30-60 mg po q4h prn

General Management

Supportive therapy according to cause and severity of condition
Hospitalization for extensive central ulcer (over 2-3 mm diameter or penetrating deep into stroma)
Pressure dressings (often over both eyes) for discomfort
Loose epithelium mechanically removed with applicator and local anesthetic for viral keratitis
Warm compresses for 10 to 15 minutes two or three times a day for discomfort and inflammation
Therapeutic soft contact lenses for recurrent corneal erosion or other chronic keratopathy

NURSING CARE

Nursing Assessment

Corneal Epithelium

Moderate to severe pain; blurred vision; haloes seen around lights; lacrimation; generalized hyperemia; fluorescein stains green on corneal surface; possible photophobia; possible purulent exudate, especially with accompanying conjunctivitis

Scarring

Opacity or irregular light reflection may be visible on corneal surface; diminished vision if opacity in visual axis

Edema

Cornea appears dull and uneven; visual loss (blurring)

Ulceration

Ulcers vary in appearance and size; whitish gray opacity with overhanging margins; fungous ulcer may be white, fluffy, and elevated; severe pain with epithelial damage or iritis; lacrimation and possible purulent discharge; generalized hyperemia

Nursing Dx & Intervention

Nursing Diagnosis	Nursing Intervention/Rationale
Potential for infection	• Assess eye for purulent exudate. If purulent exudate is present, isolate patient (in institutional setting) and practice isolation precautions *to prevent spread of infection*. • Administer topical and systemic medications as ordered for infection.
Potential for injury	• Assess cornea for epithelial disruption with inspection and with fluorescein stain. • Instill mydriatic-cycloplegic topical solutions as ordered *to prevent inflammatory constriction of pupil and iritis*.
Pain	• Administer topical anesthetic if ordered. • Apply pressure bandage to eye; be certain eye is closed before covering (one or both eyes may be covered). • Apply warm compresses for 10 to 15 minutes two or three times a day *to relieve discomfort*. • Provide systemic analgesic as ordered. • Ensure comfort and safety of hospitalized patient.
Sensory/perceptual alterations (visual) related to use of bilateral eye patches	• Raise side rails *to ensure safety*. • Address patient by name from doorway and identify yourself. • Complement voice stimulation with touch *to notify patient of your proximity*. • Orient patient to bedside equipment (such as call light, bed control, and side rails) and personal belongings at bedside by directing his or her hand over objects. • Encourage patient to perform self-care with personal hygiene. • Provide patient's privacy, and assure patient that privacy is provided. • Help with meals. Read menu selections. Guide hand to utensils and food on tray. Describe food on tray in clock terms. Help with cutting meat, removing lids from cartons, buttering bread, and so on. • Help with walking. Walk slowly and slightly ahead of patient. Place patient's hand on your arm at your elbow. If possible, allow patient to trace progress by running the dorsal aspect of his or her free hand along a wall. Describe surroundings as you proceed. Allow patient to feel chair, toilet, or bed before turning to sit.

Patient Education

1. Teach the patient self-care of corneal abrasion.
2. Teach the patient how to apply eye drops or ointments as ordered.
3. Teach the patient the application of warm or cold compresses.
4. Instruct the patient to wear dark glasses if a cycloplegic drug is ordered.
5. Tell the patient to wash hands before and after treating each eye.
6. Instruct the patient to keep hands away from the face and eyes except when treating condition.
7. Instruct the patient not to use a soiled handkerchief or tissue on the eyes.
8. Instruct the patient to avoid noxious fumes and smoke.
9. Teach the patient to monitor the eye for increased pain or change in discharge.
10. Explain visual changes (increased blurring) or visual blockage.

Evaluation

Patient Outcome	Data Indicating That Outcome is Reached
Cornea is healthy.	Cornea is clear and glossy. There is no eye discomfort, lacrimation, or discharge.[4]

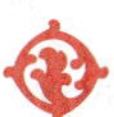

Corneal injuries

Corneal injuries are injuries to the surface epithelium or deeper layers of the eye in the form of contusions, abrasions, perforations, lacerations, burns, or damage from chemical irritants.

Pathophysiology*

Contusions result from blows that do not penetrate the corneal surface. Frequently the protective lid suffers the most damage, with edema and bruising. A subconjunctival hemorrhage may result, which looks alarming but usually heals spontaneously over 2 to 3 weeks without residual effects. The anterior chamber should be examined for repository blood, which gravitates to the lower segment and is absorbed within a few days, leaving no aftereffects. If the entire chamber is filled with blood, normal intraocular pressure is threatened and surgical evacuation through an incision at the corneal margin may be required. Severe blows may dislocate the lens, which causes visual distortion and possible ciliary spasms that are extremely painful. Surgical intervention with lens removal may be necessary. Retinal hemorrhages may occur; they are usually self-limited and without complications unless the macula is the site of bleeding. A large retinal hemorrhage might invade the vitreous, permanently obscuring vision, and increase the risk of a retinal tear.

Corneal abrasion is the disruption of cells and the loss of the superficial epithelium. This outer surface is easily separated from the underlying layers and can be injured or destroyed by exposure (lack of moisture), chemical irritants that dissolve in the protective tear film, and scrapes from foreign bodies. Drying of the surface occurs with structural or functional alterations of the eyelids, which normally blink and spread tears to maintain moisture. Some studies have shown that eye surface irritation is a risk with individuals who work with computer visual display terminals (VDTs) for prolonged periods. There is some evidence that the rate of blinking is reduced during the intense staring at the VDTs, and heated or air-conditioned offices with low humidity contribute to drying and irritation of the eye surface. Contact lenses, eyelashes, dust and dirt particles, fingernails, and crusted matter from purulent eye drainage are among the most common offenders for scraping the corneal surface. The industrial disaster in Bhopal, India, in 1984 is an example of an irritant, methyl isocyanate (MIC), causing edema and permanent destruction of the exposed epithelial surface of the eyes of thousands of victims.

The epithelium heals quickly (within 24 to 48 hours) and leaves no scarring or residual damage. However, severe pain occurs with even minor abrasions because of the numerous pain receptors in the epithelium. Lacrimation and photophobia accompany the pain. Short-acting anesthetic drops may be administered to provide immediate relief and ease the eye examination, but the drops are not given after the examination because the anesthetic slows epithelial repair. The extent of the abrasion can be viewed with fluorescein dye. Foreign bodies are often spotted during examination of the surface. If no foreign bodies are found, the upper eyelid may need to be everted and examined. Even with removal of the foreign body and rapid healing, the eye surface must be monitored (and is often treated) for possible secondary infection because epithelial breaks invite a variety of bacteria that cannot normally invade an intact epithelium.

Lacerations and perforations are serious emergencies because of invasion and disruption of the underlying stroma, endothelium, lens, and vitreous. The eye should be patched or shielded (if a foreign body is protruding) until surgery is performed. The iris may fall forward to close a corneal wound and may need to be partially excised before the wound is closed. Lens perforations usually result in cataract formation and therefore must be repaired. After surgical repair the eye is treated for potential massive infection and monitored for uveitis (see p. 608), vitreous clouding, scarring, and changes in vision. Mydriatic-cycloplegic agents may be given to maintain pupil dilation and thus prevent adhesions from forming on the underlying lens.

Many perforations occur in industrial settings, where flying metal flakes or particles are produced by high-speed drilling, riveting, and grinding. Workers are encouraged to wear protective goggles to prevent such injuries. Foreign bodies with iron or rusted particles may leave a deposit in the form of a rust ring. This deposit can be surgically removed after the epithelium has healed if it is superficially deposited. Deeply dispersed iron particles may interfere with an individual's vision in the future. Some foreign bodies, such as glass, are inert and can remain embedded in the eye tissue for years without harmful effects.

Chemical irritants, depending on the substance, can burn and destroy the underlying corneal layers. Regardless of the substance, the eye should be irrigated with copious amounts of water or sterile saline. Alkaline substances (such as ammonia, lime and cement dust, and sodium hydroxide) penetrate the tissues rapidly and continue to burn into the cornea unless they are removed. Acids coagulate the protein and often result in relatively superficial reversible damage. Local anesthetic drops may be used initially to provide comfort and ease irrigation and examination, but they are not used more than twice because they obstruct the healing process of the epithelium.

Ultraviolet burns (or irritation) can occur with sun exposure and are a risk for welders who are not protected from welding flashes. Epithelial irritation, swelling, and possible desquamation may occur. Desquamation is usually repaired without visual loss or changes.

Diagnostic Studies and Findings

Fluorescein Stain (2%)

To identify corneal surface disruption

*References 5, 8, 18, 41, 52, 56.

Slitlamp Examination

To view deeper layers of the cornea and anterior eye

Ophthalmoscopy

To view eye surface, anterior chamber, vitreous, and retina

Medical Plan

Surgery

Removal of foreign objects
Removal of damaged or prolapsed eye tissue
Repair of wounds

Medications

Mode, frequency, and duration of therapy depend on degree of corneal penetration and potential for secondary infection

- Topical anesthetics (administered once or twice for pain relief during examination or removal of foreign body)
  - Proparacaine (Alcaine, Ophthetic), 0.5% solution, 1-2 drops in injured eye; onset within 2 min; duration, 20 min
  - Tetracaine (Pontocaine), 0.5% solution or ointment, 1-2 drops in injured eye; onset within 1 min; duration, 20 min
- Anti-infective agents (type and duration of medication depend on extent of injury)
  - Topical
    - Erythromycin (Ilotycin), 1% ointment applied qd or bid in conjunctival cul-de-sac
    - Combination of Bacitracin 400 U, Polymixin B 5000 U, and Neomycin 0.25% (Neosporin) ointment, applied tid or qid in conjunctival sac
    - Tetracycline (Achromycin), 1% suspension or ointment, 1-2 drops bid or qid
- Mydriatic-cycloplegic agents (may be given to prevent inflammatory pupillary constriction, uveitis)
  - Scopolamine hydrobromide (Isopto Hyoscine), 0.25% solution, 1-2 drops in injured eye; duration, 48-72 h
- Systemic antibiotics may be prescribed for severe invasive trauma
- Systemic analgesics may be prescribed for severe invasive trauma

General Management

Protective eye patch or shield applied until patient is examined
Eye irrigation—boric acid solution (2%) may be used as irrigating solution; sterile water or normal saline are commonly used
Pressure dressing often prescribed for 24 hours to promote rest and reduce discomfort
Tinted glasses to reduce discomfort of photophobia

NURSING CARE

Nursing Assessment

Corneal Epithelium

Moderate to severe pain; blurred vision; lacrimation; photophobia; generalized redness; fluorescein stains green on disrupted corneal surface; presence of foreign body

Surrounding Conjunctivae

Generalized redness, bleeding, excoriation, presence of foreign body; evert upper lid to inspect for foreign body if discomfort persists and foreign body is not present on eye surface

Anterior Chamber

May be partially or completely filled with blood

Surrounding Eye Tissue

A portion of the iris may prolapse through open corneal wound

Nursing Dx & Intervention

Nursing Diagnosis	Nursing Intervention/Rationale
Pain	• Assess patient's level of discomfort. If discomfort is severe, delay visual testing or other assessment until topical or systemic anesthetic or analgesic has been ordered and has taken effect. • Administer medications as ordered immediately *to relieve discomfort*. • After treatment, apply pressure bandage to eye *to relieve discomfort* (be certain eye is closed before applying bandage). • Apply a warm compress for 10 to 15 minutes as ordered *to relieve discomfort and inflammation*. • Apply a cool compress for 10 to 15 minutes as ordered for burns. • Administer cycloplegic medication as ordered *to prevent pain from inflammatory pupil constriction and iritis*. • Ensure the safety and comfort of hospitalized patient.
Potential for injury	• Assess surface of eye for foreign body. If foreign body is not visible on surface, evert upper eyelid and assess conjunctival surface for foreign body. • Assess eye for surface injury. • Assess eye for corneal epithelial breaks with fluorescein stain. • Apply bandage or shield to eye until patient can be examined.

Nursing Diagnosis	Nursing Intervention/Rationale
	• Warn patient not to touch eye for duration of topical anesthetic *to avoid self-injury.*
Potential for infection	• Administer topical and systemic medications as ordered *to prevent infection.*
Fear related to discomfort and uncertainty about present and future visual loss	• Relieve discomfort as quickly as possible. • Assess patient for signs of fear. • Provide comfort and realistic reassurance. • Keep patient informed about all procedures as they occur *to alleviate as much uncertainty as possible.*
Sensory/perceptual alterations (visual) related to use of unilateral eye patch	• Warn patient that depth perception will be lost and 50% of peripheral vision will be lost on affected side. • Caution patient to bring hand forward slowly to touch objects (especially containers of hot liquid and containers receiving poured liquids) *to ensure safety.* • Explain that patient should turn head fully to affected side to view objects or obstacles. • Teach patient to use up and down head movements to judge stair dimensions and oncoming objects. • Teach patient to proceed slowly with all movement.
Sensory/perceptual alterations (visual) related to use of bilateral eye patches	• Assess patient for level of fear or disorientation related to sudden loss of vision. • Review events since injury and present situation with patient *to reorient patient and to maximize patient's capacity to deal with present circumstances.* • Raise side rails *to ensure safety.* • Address patient by name and identify yourself *to reduce anxiety.* • Complement voice stimulation with touch *to notify patient of your proximity.* • Orient patient to equipment (such as call light) and personal belongings at bedside by directing patient's hand. • Encourage patient to perform self-care with personal hygiene *to maximize independence.* • Ensure patient's privacy, and assure patient that privacy is provided. • Provide patient with television set or radio *to encourage mental and memory stimulation.* • Provide patient with a clock that can be felt and remind patient of date. • Continue to assess patient for evidence of sensory deprivation signs (e.g., withdrawal, anxiety, depression). • Balance privacy and quiet with stimulation events. • Help patient with meals. Read menu selections. Guide hand to utensils and food on tray. Describe food on tray in clock terms (e.g., coffee is at 2 o'clock, knife and spoon are at 3 o'clock). Help with cutting meats, removing lids from containers, buttering bread, and so on. • Help with walking. Walk slowly and slightly ahead of patient; patient's hand should rest on your arm at elbow *to maximize patient's capacity to maintain balance and assurance of attending support.* • If possible, allow patient to trace progress by running the dorsal aspect of his or her free hand along a wall. • Warn of steps, turns, and narrow passageways in advance. • Allow patient to feel chair, toilet, or bed before turning to sit.

Patient Education

1. Teach the patient how to apply eye drops or ointment as ordered.
2. Teach the patient how to apply warm or cold compresses as ordered.
3. Tell the patient to wash hands well before treating eye(s).
4. Instruct the patient to wear dark glasses if a cycloplegic drug is ordered.
5. Tell the patient to keep hands away from face and eyes except when treating condition.
6. Instruct the patient not to use a soiled handkerchief or tissue on the eyes.
7. Instruct the patient to avoid noxious fumes and smoke.
8. Teach the patient to monitor the eye for increased pain and for blood or discharge from the eye or on the dressing.
9. Interpret any temporary or permanent visual alterations the patient might experience (e.g., blurring with corneal healing, swelling, blurring with ointment over eye surface, blurring and photophobia with pupil dilation).
10. Review with patient the need for eye protection at work (e.g., protective goggles) or at other times (e.g., care of contact lenses—see p. 643)

Evaluation

Patient Outcome	Data Indicating That Outcome is Reached
Cornea is healthy.	Cornea is clear and glossy. There is no discomfort, visual loss, or distortion.

Scleritis

Scleritis is an inflammation of the sclera.

Scleral inflammations are uncommon. The sclera has a poor blood supply and a low metabolism that does not encourage infection. Deep-seated aching and tenderness to touch without loss of vision are early indicators of the disease. An ocular muscle may contract and turn the eye if the inflammation is near its insertion. Because of the proximity of the sclera to the uveal tract, secondary choroiditis or retinal detachment may occur.

The episclera (located anteriorly) is more vascular than the rest of the sclera, and infections in this area may be worse. Infection is usually unilateral, has a sudden onset, and is accompanied by marked generalized hyperemia and pain. The cause is not always apparent, and the inflammation often subsides spontaneously.

Chronic or recurrent scleritis may result in scleral thinning with a localized outward bulging of the choroid layer. Perforation may occur.

DISORDERS OF THE UVEAL TRACT AND PUPIL

The uveal tract comprises the iris, ciliary body, and choroid layer. The iris surrounds the pupil and controls its size; the ciliary body secretes aqueous humor and controls accommodation; and the vascular choroid nourishes the anterior uveal tract and part of the retina. The location and extent of uveal lesions determine the variety and severity of signs, symptoms, and visual alterations. Deep corneal inflammation often spreads to the iris and results in a painful contraction of the iris and ciliary body. Iris abnormalities or inflammation can alter the shape of the pupil, disrupt the pupillary light reflex, or form adhesions to the cornea or lens to cause glaucoma. Ciliary body lesions can interfere with accommodation or cause anterior chamber or vitreous clouding with exudates, which diminishes visual acuity. Choroidal inflammation can spread to the sensory retinal layer and destroy central or peripheral vision. Retinal detachment may occur because of vitreous pull on the retina.[28]

Uveitis

Uveitis is an inflammation or infection of the uveal tract.

Uveitis is the most common uveal lesion. Organisms can be identified if the inflammation is peripheral enough to give the examiner access to infected tissue for staining or culture. Often the cause is unknown, and the inflammation is treated on the basis of the presumed cause. Some inflammatory processes are associated with endogenous causes or chronic conditions that can be diagnosed and treated systemically. Acute inflammations vary in severity and may subside without residual alterations. The uveal tract is also subject to congenital or developmental lesions that may or may not affect vision.

Pathophysiology[5,41,60]

Inflammation of the uveal tract can be acute or chronic, can be mild or severe, and can involve primarily the anterior tract (iris, ciliary body, and anterior choroid), the posterior choroid, or the entire eye. The most common form of uveitis is acute anterior inflammation. The onset is sudden, and the symptoms of pain and visual loss appear abruptly and are sometimes severe. The arteries of the anterior ciliary body become engorged and dilated, creating a purplish discoloration around the limbus (circumcorneal flush). The iris and the ciliary body release an exudate that increases protein and inflammatory cells in the anterior chamber. The protein causes clouding of the chamber (aqueous flare), and the cells form in clumps that adhere to the posterior cornea (keratic precipitates). Keratic precipitates, a diagnostic determinant, can be viewed with a slitlamp and occasionally with the ophthalmoscope if the deposits are large enough. A massive production of cells forms pus in the anterior chamber (hypopyon). The ciliary body also releases exudate into the vitreous to cause clouding and cell production. The iris is usually constricted (miotic pupil) and does not respond to light. The constriction is painful, and pain intensity increases with light stimulation. If the pain is severe, it is difficult to open the lid for examination. If the iris remains constricted, it quickly forms adhesions to the underlying lens (posterior synechiae) that may obstruct aqueous flow and cause a pupillary block glaucoma. With anterior inflammation the iris, ciliary body, and anterior choroid are usually all involved because of a common blood supply.

Posterior uveitis is usually confined to the posterior choroid and quickly spreads to the sensory retina. The vitreous becomes clouded with cells and exudate that can be viewed with an ophthalmoscope. Chorioretinal lesions can also be seen as irregular gray-white areas on the retinal surface. Vision impairment is the chief symptom of posterior choroiditis. Often there is no pain, redness, or photophobia. The degree of visual impairment depends on the extent of vitreous clouding and the location of retinal sensory layer inflammation. If the macula is involved, central vision is severely impaired. Retinal inflammations often leave scars that permanently impair vision.

Acute uveitis results from external infection, trauma (laceration, puncture, or contusion), or chemical burns. Herpes simplex, herpes zoster, and fungal infections are common causes of iritis. There are many endogenous sources. Rubella, rubeola, or mumps may cause a mild, transient uveitis. A hypermature cataract may release exudate into the anterior chamber and cause severe inflammation. Systemic diseases such as rheumatoid arthritis, regional enteritis, ankylosing spondylitis, and collagen disorders may contribute to uveitis. Many uveitis exacerbations are idiopathic and treated symptomatically. Acute uveitis can recur, particularly if the cause is endogenous and chronic.

Chronic uveitis is usually a continuous and progressive inflammation that involves cell production in the anterior and posterior chambers, frequent posterior synechia formation, retinal involvement, minimum exterior inflammatory signs or pain, and residual scarring of inflammatory sites. Some organisms invade and remain in the uveal tract. Tuberculosis, herpes zoster, and some forms of fungi are common causes of chronic inflammation. Systemic diseases such as sarcoidosis, rheumatoid arthritis (Still's disease), and histoplasmosis may be implicated. Some of the chronic syndromes are caused by local eye degenerative reactions. Chronic infections resulting from the degenerative changes in blind eyes may force a decision to perform enucleation for relief. Pars planitis is a chronic inflammation of the posterior choroid that involves vitreous opacites with a chief complaint of "floaters," retinal inflammation, and scarring. The cause is unknown, and the disease extends over 5 to 10 years.

In severe infections the entire inner eyeball may become inflamed (panophthalmitis). Pyogenic bacteria may penetrate to the uvea with trauma, through rupture of a corneal ulcer, or through endogenous sources such as septicemia, meningitis, or bacterial endocarditis. *Staphylococcus aureus, Pseudomonas,* and *Proteus* are commonly involved organisms. Suppurative panophthalmitis is acute and severe. Severe pain, visual loss, and necrosis of the sclera may be followed by rupture of the globe. Sometimes the infection does not invade the sclera but remains confined to the inner eyeball (endophthalmitis). In this case the onset and course are less severe and the infection is more responsive to treatment.

Diagnostic Studies and Findings[41,60]

Staining and Culture of Scrapings

Performed if uveitis is associated with peripheral inflammation or ulceration; organism is identified through culture and Gram stain

Slitlamp (Binocular Microscope) Examination

Focuses on thin sections of cornea, anterior chamber, lens, or anterior vitreous; presence and extent of inflammatory cells or pus in anterior chamber and anterior vitreous can be viewed

Gonioscopy

Corneal contact lens (goniolens) is placed over anesthetized cornea to permit viewing of anterior chamber angles with microscopic lens; cellular debris and adhesions are seen in anterior chamber; angles can be viewed

Ophthalmoscopy

Vitreous opacities and chorioretinal lesions can be viewed

Diagnostic Studies to Rule Out or Identify Systemic Disease

Medical Plan[11,41,60]

Acute uveitis is often treated symptomatically because the cause cannot be identified.

Surgery

Enucleation for ruptured globe or marked eye degeneration (see p. 647)

Lens extraction for lens-induced uveitis

Medications

Mydriatic-cycloplegic agents (duration of administration depends on severity of infection)

- Atropine sulfate (Atroprisol, Isopto Atropine), 1% solution bid or tid to maintain full pupillary dilation

Corticosteroids—topical (often the choice with anterior uveitis)

- Instilled as frequently as q1-2h initially for severe inflammation, or bid or tid; to reduce inflammation and prevent iritic adhesions; patient response must be carefully supervised since herpes simplex and fungal organisms increase in activity and growth with steroid therapy; immunosuppression may increase host susceptibility to secondary infection; since open-angle glaucoma is a common complication of topical steroid treatment, ocular tension must be carefully monitored
- Dexamethasone alcohol suspension (Maxidex), 0.1% suspension, 1-2 drops 4-6 times/d
- Fluorometholone suspension (FML Liquifilm), 0.1%, 1-2 drops 4-6 times/d

Corticosteroids—subconjunctival injections (sometimes administered along with topical medication; administration and dosage determined by physician)
- Dexamethasone sodium phosphate (Decadron phosphate, Hexadrol), 4 mg/ml
- Hydrocortisone acetate (Hydrocortone Acetate, Cortef Acetate), 25 mg/ml or 50 mg/ml

Topical anti-infective agents (type and duration of medication depend on severity of infection)
- Erythromycin (Ilotycin), 1% ointment applied qd or bid in conjunctival sac
- Combination of Bacitracin 400 U, Polymixin B 5000 U, and Neomycin 0.25%, (Neosporin) ointment, applied tid or qid in conjunctival sac
- Tetracycline (Achromycin), 1% suspension or ointment, 1-2 drops bid or qid

Systemic medications
- Analgesics
  - Acetaminophen (Tylenol), 650 mg po q4h prn
  - Acetaminophen (Tylenol), 650 mg with codeine (30 mg), po q4h prn
- Corticosteroids
  - For posterior uveitis and inflammations that do not respond to local treatment

NURSING CARE

Nursing Assessment

Anterior Uveitis

Moderate pain; severe pain if associated with keratitis; intense photophobia; no visual change, possible blurred vision if eye chambers clouded with exudate, or possible blurred distant vision with ciliary spasm; circumcorneal flush (purplish coloration); pupillary constriction

Posterior Uveitis

Minimum or no pain; blurred vision from vitreous opacities or sensory retina inflammation (may be central [macular] or peripheral depending on extent and location of inflammation); ophthalmoscopy may reveal vitreous opacities as black dots

Nursing Dx & Intervention

Nursing Diagnosis	Nursing Intervention/Rationale
Pain related to acute anterior iridocyclitis	• Assess patient for degree of discomfort. • Administer cycloplegics as ordered *to reduce painful pupillary constriction.* • Apply warm compresses for 10 to 15 minutes two or three times a day as ordered. • Administer systemic analgesics as ordered. • Instruct patient to wear dark glasses or avoid light *to reduce photophobic discomfort.*
Potential for injury: adhesions and increased intraocular pressure, related to iridocyclitis	• Administer cycloplegics as ordered *to prevent adhesions from iris to lens.* • Assess patient for signs of increased intraocular pressure, increased haziness of vision (corneal edema), extreme pain, nausea, vomiting, or onset of conjunctival injection.
Potential for infection	• Administer topical and systemic medications (steroids, anti-infective agents) as ordered.

Patient Education

1. Teach the patient how to apply eye drops and ointments.
2. Teach the patient to apply warm compresses.
3. Instruct the patient to wear dark glasses.
4. Teach the patient to monitor the eye for increased pain, visual changes (increased blurring), and inflammatory signs.
5. Warn the patient that vision will be blurred because the pupil will be dilated.

Evaluation

Patient Outcome	Data Indicating That Outcome is Reached
Uveal tissue is healthy.	Cornea is clear and glossy. There is no photophobia, eye discomfort, inflammation (corneal, circumcorneal, or conjunctival), or discharge.
Vision is restored.	There is no blurring at close or distant range.

Uveal tract deformities

Uveal tract deformities range from minor defects to severe impediments to visual functioning.

A coloboma is a localized absence of uveal tissue. An absence of a portion of the iris may cause a pupil shape defect (see p. 613) with no visual defects. If the choroidal coloboma is large, the overlying retina is deprived of blood supply in that area, which affects sensory vision. Aniridia is absence or diminishment of the iris. The pupil appears greatly enlarged, and no iris is showing. Photophobia and severe reduction of visual acuity follow. Aniridia may be inherited or associated with other chromosomal disorders such as mental retardation, Wilms' tumor, and urogenital abnormalities. The iris can atrophy over a period of years, leaving a misshapen pupil or holes (looking like additional pupils) over the visible surface of the iris. The presence of holes can cause diplopia. Atrophy can follow severe eye inflammation or trauma or occur as a primary disease. Choroid atrophy can be a benign disorder or result in marked retinal degeneration. Some forms of choroid atrophy cause progressive night blindness and diminished visual acuity.

The size of the pupil is controlled by dilator and constrictor muscles in the iris. There are no disorders of the pupil, but its size, response to light (accommodation), uniformity of shape, and symmetric responses with the corresponding eye are indicators of iris, eye, or systemic disorders.[37,41,43] Following is a summary of pupil abnormalities (Table 6-2).

Glaucoma

Glaucoma incorporates a variety of diseases that exhibit all or at least one of the following abnormalities: increase in intraocular pressure, degeneration of the optic nerve (disc), and visual field losses that may lead to total loss of vision.

Glaucoma is detected in a variety of ways. Simple tonometry testing reveals intraocular pressure (IOP) that exceeds the normal range of 10 to 22 mm Hg. Only 5% to 10% of persons with IOP over 21 mm Hg have visual defects or optic nerve changes.[32] A variety of variables (discussed later) determine whether an unaffected person with a high IOP will only be monitored or will be treated for glaucoma. When screening methods include ophthalmoscopy or perimetry testing for visual field defects, some patients with a normal IOP exhibit optic nerve degeneration or visual field losses. Approximately one third of the visual defect population have a normal IOP when first examined.[32] The prevalence of glaucoma is difficult to determine because of the different screening methods and criteria for diagnosis among physicians and regions of the world. An estimated 1.5% of persons over 40 years of age have glaucoma, and approximately 67,500 persons in the United States are blind as a result of this disease.[12] Tonometry alone is not an adequate screening method for detecting glaucoma, and higher incidences are reported when persons are more thoroughly examined.

Glaucoma occurs because aqueous fluid cannot be drained adequately from the anterior chamber to maintain a normal IOP. Excessive pressure results in optic nerve degeneration.

Primary glaucomas (from an unknown cause) include open-angle, closed-angle, and glaucoma "suspect" disorders. Open-angle glaucoma is the more common and generally affects adults over 40 years of age. The onset is insidious and asymptomatic, and the disease progresses slowly. Many elderly persons with glaucoma are successfully treated with medications and retain vision. Closed-angle glaucoma occurs because of eye structure defects or changes and results in a mechanically blocked drainage system. The onset is usually acute and dramatic. The category of glaucoma "suspect" disorders includes individuals with an elevated IOP (above 24 mm Hg) who exhibit no ocular changes and persons with normal IOP levels (low tension) who show abnormal optic disc and peripheral field changes. Secondary glaucomas can be caused by inflammation, trauma, corticosteroid administration, systemic disorders, or local eye changes. In addition, a number of congenital syndromes include glaucoma.

Glaucoma can be classified as follows[41]:

- Primary
  - Chronic open-angle
  - Glaucoma "suspect"
    - Low-tension
    - Ocular hypertension
  - Closed-angle
    - Pupillary block
    - Plateau iris
      - Ciliary body block
- Secondary open-angle
  - Pretrabecular
  - Foreign cells within trabecular meshwork
  - Trabecular meshwork abnormality
  - Increased venous pressure
- Secondary closed-angle
  - Membrane contracture
  - Pupillary block
  - Angle shift
- Developmental glaucoma
  - Primary
  - Secondary

Pathophysiology*

Open-Angle Glaucoma

Approximately 90% of cases of primary glaucoma are of the open-angle type. The incidence of this disease increases with age. Population studies have shown that less than 1% of

*References 11, 32, 33, 41, 55, 60.

Text continued on p. 614.

Table 6-2
Pupil Abnormalities

Abnormality	Contributing Factors	Appearance
Bilateral		
Miosis (pupillary constriction; usually less than 2 mm in diameter)	Iridocyclitis; miotic eye drops (such as pilocarpine given for glaucoma)	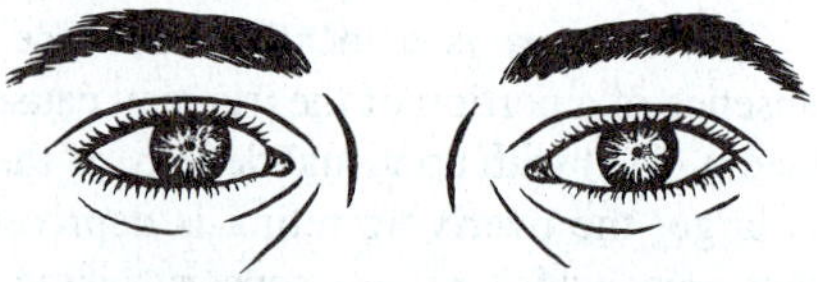
Mydriasis (pupillary dilation; usually more than 6 mm in diameter)	Iridocyclitis; mydriatic or cycloplegic drops (such as atropine); midbrain (reflex arc) lesions or hypoxia; oculomotor (CN III) damage; acute-angle glaucoma (slight dilation)	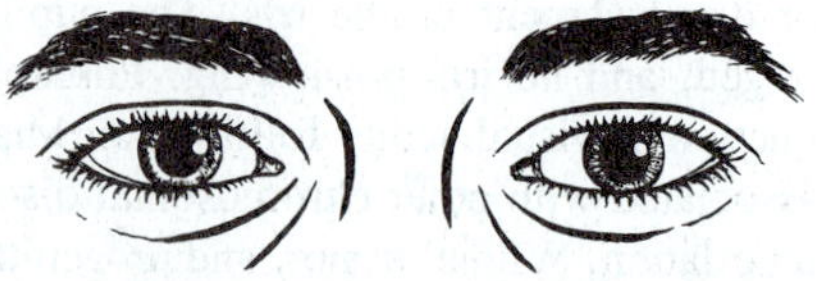
Failure to respond (constrict) with increased light stimulus	Iridocyclitis; corneal or lens opacity (light does not reach retina); retinal degeneration; optic nerve (CN II) destruction; midbrain synapses involving afferent pupillary fibers or oculomotor nerve (CN III) (consensual response is also lost); impairment of efferent fibers (parasympathetic) that innervate sphincter pupillae muscle	
Argyll Robertson pupil	Bilateral, miotic, irregular-shaped pupils that fail to constrict with light but retain constriction with convergence; pupils may or may not be equal in size; commonly caused by neurosyphilis or lesions in midbrain where afferent pupillary fibers synapse	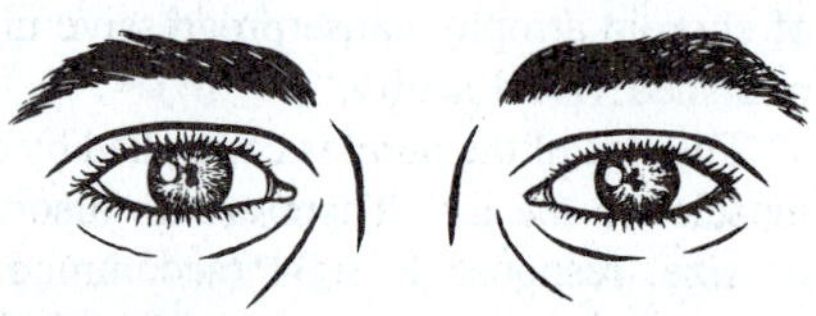
Oval pupil	Sometimes occurs with head injury or intracranial hemorrhage; transitional stage between normal pupil and dilated, fixed pupil with increased intracranial pressure (ICP); in most instances returns to normal when ICP is returned to normal	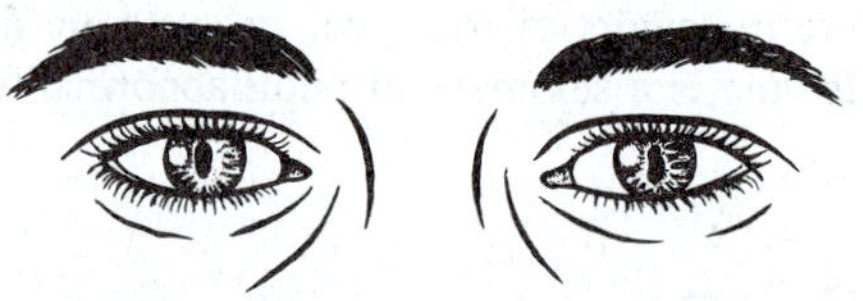
Unilateral		
Anisocoria (unequal size of pupils)	Congenital (approximately 20% of normal people have minor or noticeable differences in pupil size, but reflexes are normal) or caused by local eye medications (constrictors or dilators), amblyopia, or unilateral sympathetic or parasympathetic pupillary pathway destruction (NOTE: Examiner should test whether pupils react equally to light; if response is unequal, examiner should note whether larger or smaller pupil reacts more slowly [or not at all], since either pupil could be abnormal size)	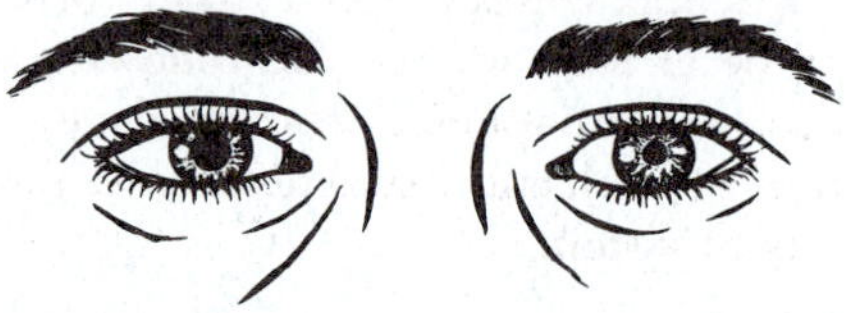
Iritis constrictive response	Acute uveitis is frequently unilateral; constriction of pupil accompanied by pain and circumcorneal flush (redness)	Normal eye / Affected eye 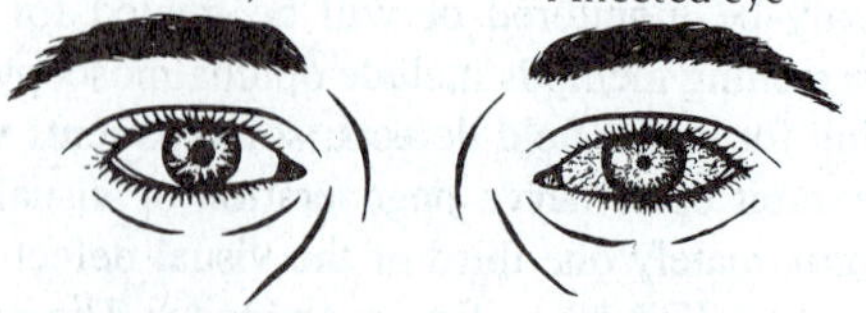
Oculomotor nerve (CN III) damage	Pupil dilated and fixed; eye deviated laterally and downward; ptosis	Normal eye / Affected eye 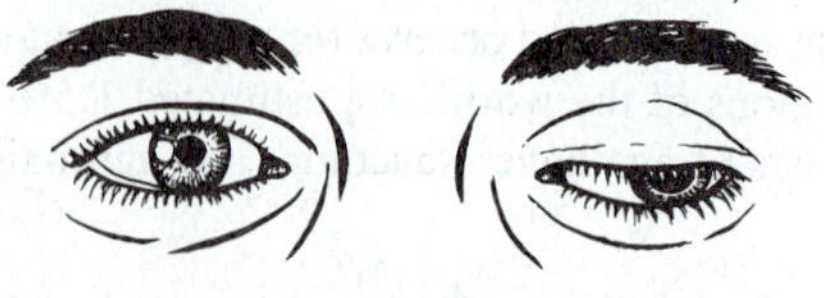

Table 6-2—cont'd
Pupil Abnormalities

Abnormality	Contributing Factors	Appearance
Horner's syndrome	Miotic pupil; ptosis; interruption of sympathetic nerve supply to dilator pupillae muscle; may be caused by goiter, cervical lymph enlargement, apical bronchogenic carcinoma, or surgical injury to neck	Normal eye / Affected eye
Adie's pupil (tonic pupil)	Affected pupil dilated and reacts slowly or fails to react to light; response to convergence normal; caused by impairment of postganglionic parasympathetic innervation to sphincter pupillae muscle or ciliary malfunction; often accompanied by diminished tendon reflexes (as with diabetic neuropathy or alcoholism)	Normal eye / Affected eye
Other Irregularities		
Iridectomy	Sector iridectomy	
	Peripheral iridectomy Surgical excision of portion of iris usually done in superior area so upper lid will cover additional exposure	
Coloboma (localized absence of portion of iris)	Congenital absence of area of iris; remaining iris shows normal light response	
Iridodialysis (circumferential tearing of iris from scleral spur)	Blunt trauma; more than one "pupil" in eye can cause diplopia	

persons under 65 years of age have glaucoma and that approximately 3% of the population over 75 years of age have this disorder.[32] Other risk factors for open-angle glaucoma have been identified. Nonwhites have a much higher incidence and frequently exhibit an earlier onset and a more rapid eye degeneration. Hypertension has been linked to glaucoma, as have the hypotensive episodes associated with treatment for hypertension. Approximately 20% to 25% of glaucoma patients have a family history of this disease. Persons with myopia and diabetes are reported to have a higher incidence of glaucoma.

Increased IOP occurs because of degenerative changes of unknown cause in the trabecular meshwork and the canal of Schlemm. Excess fluid cannot be emptied from the anterior chamber.

IOP is not static but normally varies 2 to 5 mm Hg with increased heart rate, activity, or excitement. One high reading does not constitute a basis for diagnosis. Some persons exhibit visual field defects and optic nerve changes with normal or near-normal IOP, whereas others are able to tolerate elevated IOP without eye damage. Elevated IOP without ocular damage is called ocular hypertension. Some physicians believe that this elevation is a precursor of glaucoma, but others think that a mildly elevated IOP (20 to 24 mm Hg) is a normal state. The risk for eye damage increases with age, a family history of glaucoma, diabetes, and systemic vascular disorders.

Early open-angle glaucoma may be difficult to diagnose because it is asymptomatic. Even persons with visual field defects do not usually perceive them until they become extensive. There is no pain or blurred vision, and the outer eye does not appear inflamed or abnormal to the examiner. Tonometry usually shows an elevated IOP. The Schiötz tonometer is less accurate in higher pressure ranges and consistently shows lower pressures than applanation or noncontact tonometers. Direct ophthalmoscopy may reveal the earliest finding if the examiner is sufficiently skilled. The physiologic cup (a depression in the center of the disc) may be larger in one eye than the other. As the disease progresses, the cup widens and extends toward the disc temporal margin. The temporal vessels appear to drop (or bend) abruptly into the cup. The large vessels become displaced and crowded toward the nasal side of the disc. The temporal disc border atrophies and loses its pink coloration to appear a flat white. The cup widens and deepens (excavation) as the surrounding optic nerve margin diminishes and atrophies.

Visual field testing often shows the most tangible alterations. Visual field testing by confrontation does not measure early or limited defects. The Goldmann perimeter measures both central and peripheral losses. Characteristic defects (blind areas or scotomas) appear and enlarge as the disease progresses. Nerve fiber bundles originating from the optic nerve cease to function as the nerve head atrophies. The nasal visual field is often first affected, and eventually the periphery is diminished. The person may retain only a small portion of central vision with acuity of the unaffected area.

Many older adults are treated successfully with medication. Parasympathomimetic agents (miotic eye drops) increase the outflow of fluid by enlarging the area around the trabecular meshwork. β-Adrenergic blocking agents (eye drops) and orally administered carbonic anhydrase inhibitors decrease aqueous production. These drugs are given in various combinations. Miotic drops disturb vision because of pupillary constriction and may cause ciliary spasms. β-Blockers must be administered cautiously to asthmatic patients. Epinephrine drops are sometimes prescribed to increase outflow, but their use should be evaluated carefully because of potential systemic effects (tachycardia) and occasional local effects (macular edema). Diuretics deplete potassium and may cause thirst and drinking of large amounts of fluids, which could increase pressure. Patient receiving medication need careful and continuous supervision.

If IOP cannot be controlled through medication, laser trabeculoplasty (creating openings in the trabecular meshwork with laser beams), laser iridotomy, or surgery may be performed. Surgery usually involves the creation of an opening between the anterior chamber and the subconjuctival space. Many physicians prefer laser therapy because it is less damaging to the eye (see p. 651). Success rates for laser and surgical therapies are variable. The openings or filter systems may not remain patent. Invasive therapy for open-angle glaucoma is a last resort for eyes that do not respond to chemotherapeutic regimens.

Closed-Angle Glaucoma

Closed-angle glaucoma occurs because mechanical blockage of the anterior chamber angle results in accumulation of

Figure 6-15 A, Normal anterior chamber. **B,** Shallow anterior chamber. Shallow chamber shows forward displacement of iris and narrow anterior angle.

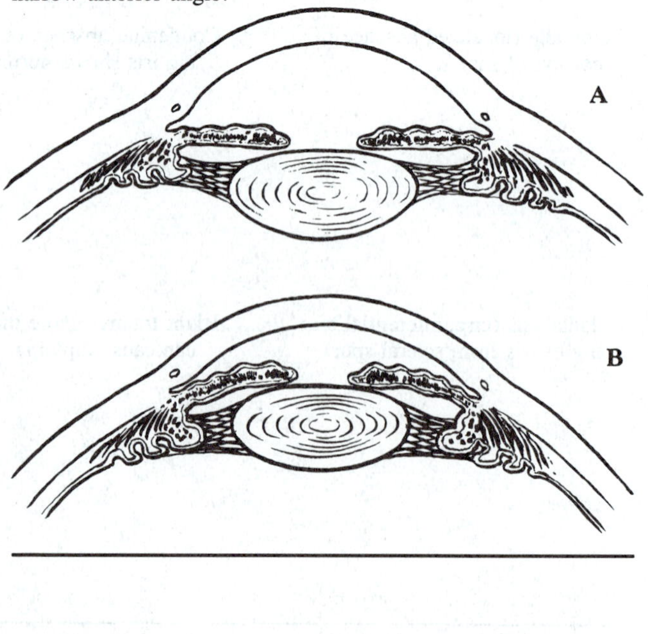

A

B

aqueous fluid and increased IOP. Most persons with closed-angle glaucoma have shallow anterior chambers (less than 3 mm depth between the iris and the posterior corneal surface), which is often a familial trait. These persons do not exhibit IOP elevations unless the angle is closed and obscures the trabecular meshwork, which ordinarily drains fluid from the anterior chamber. The shallow chamber is often accompanied by narrowed anterior angles (Figure 6-15). Narrow angles are more vulnerable to other physiologic events that cause further crowding of the angles.

Angle closure occurs because of pupillary dilation or forward displacement of the iris. In some instances pupillary dilation (physiologic or induced) causes the iris to crowd into the anterior angle, resulting in obstruction. Forward displacement of the iris occurs with enlargement of the lens, which normally thickens with aging. The iris can also be pushed forward with physiologic pupillary block. In a shallow anterior chamber the iris may press against the lens and obstruct aqueous flow from the posterior chamber to the anterior chamber. As fluid accumulates posteriorly, it bulges forward against the iris. A bulging iris can be viewed by an examiner with a penlight aimed obliquely at the cornea. The bulge casts a shadow on the opposite side of the light source (Figure 6-16).

Angle closure can occur in a subacute, acute, or chronic form. Subacute episodes often precede an acute attack. These episodes may involve transient angle obstruction with symptoms of blurred vision, mild to severe pain, and haloes seen around lights. Persons with subacute angle closure may not exhibit increased IOP during an examination, but provocative testing with rapid drinking of water, sitting in a dark room to cause pupil dilation, or induced mydriasis may elicit an increased IOP (see descriptions of methods on p. 616).

Acute angle closure causes a dramatic response. A sudden onset of blurred vision, severe ocular pain, and haloes seen around lights is followed by a progression of symptoms as the pressure increases. Ciliary injection (a purplish red coloration around the limbus), profuse lacrimation, a mildly dilated, nonreactive pupil (5 to 6 mm in diameter), and nausea and vomiting may occur. Corneal edema causes the cornea to appear hazy. An acute episode constitutes a medical emergency. If the pressure is not relieved within several hours, eye damage occurs. Adhesions (anterior synechiae) begin to form between the iris and the cornea, which eventually closes the angle. Within a few days the iris and ciliary body begin to atrophy, the cornea shows permanent changes because of chronic edema, and optic atrophy and deterioration of nerve fibers occur. Total loss of vision is the result.

Emergency medical treatment consists of oral or intravenous administration of carbonic anhydrase inhibitors to suppress aqueous humor secretion, miotic eye drops to pull the iris away from the inner angle, osmotic agents to reduce pressure, and systemic analgesics to reduce pain. Surgical treatment (usually iridotomy) follows as soon as ocular pressure is stabilized. Although usually only one eye is affected at a time, surgery is eventually performed on the other eye as a preventive measure.

Chronic episodes of increased IOP can occur when anterior angles are sufficiently narrowed to partially obstruct outflow. The patient may have minimum symptoms (hazy vision, mild pain) or none, and the IOP is usually elevated when measured. Subacute and chronic forms of angle closure are often treated medically or surgically to prevent insidious eye damage, such as slow formation of anterior adhesions.

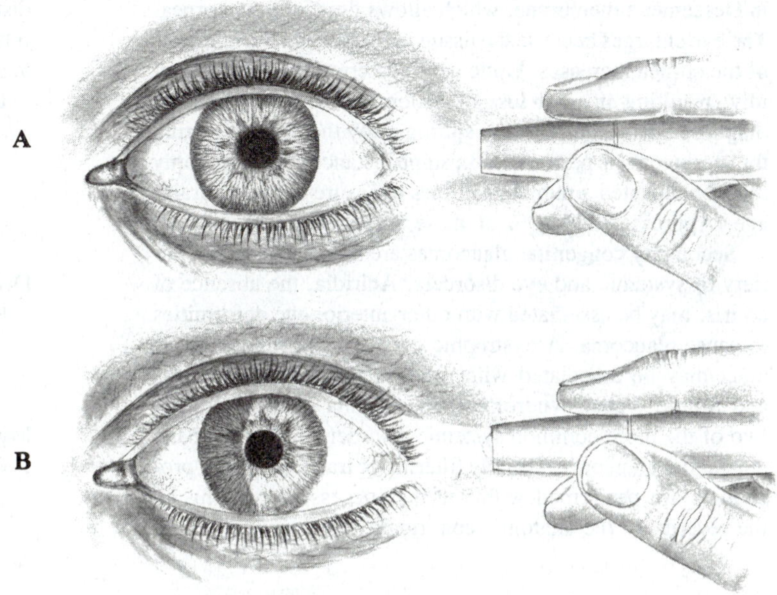

Figure 6-16 A, Normal anterior chamber: iris is flat. **B,** Shallow anterior chamber: iris is bulging, and crescent shadow appears on far side. From Seidel.[54]

Secondary Glaucomas

Trabecular meshwork obstruction or closed-angle glaucoma can occur because of eye deformities, inflammation, or trauma (surgical or accidental). Corticosteroid therapy increases IOP; this may be transient or may cause permanent eye damage.

A displaced, enlarged, hypermature, or ruptured lens can result in a crowding of the angle, an associated trabecular meshwork obstruction, or uveitis. Uveitis may cause a pupillary block with ciliary spasms or posterior synechiae (adhesions of the iris to the lens), which ultimately obstructs angle drainage. Trabeculitis with resultant scarring and damage may follow iridocyclitis when inflammatory cells and fibrous material are deposited in the anterior angles. Eye contusions elevate IOP, usually temporarily. If hemorrhage or edema of the iris or ciliary body ensues, the IOP increase is sustained and the angle flow may be compromised. If the anterior eye is traumatized through surgery or laceration, the iris root may reform or adhere to the ciliary body to obstruct the anterior angle.

Congenital Glaucoma

Primary congenital glaucoma is a hereditary disease. It occurs when the structures of the anterior chamber angle do not fully develop at about the fifth month of fetal life. A thin remnant of iris tissue inserts into the trabecular meshwork and partially or fully covers it. The IOP increases, and corneal and optic nerve destruction ensues. Boys are affected more often than girls, and the disease is most commonly diagnosed at birth or within the first 2 years of life. The disease is most often bilateral. The earlier the symptoms, the less favorable the prognosis because earlier onset indicates a greater anatomic abnormality. Other systemic congenital defects may accompany primary congenital glaucoma. Early symptoms are excessive tearing and photophobia. A hazy cornea eventually becomes opaque because of edema and stretching with breaks in Descemet's membrane, which allows fluid into the cornea. The eye enlarges because the tissue is elastic, and the diameter of the cornea increases. Optic nerve deterioration occurs rapidly, resulting in total loss of vision. If the symptoms are diagnosed early, goniotomy (cutting away the tissue covering the meshwork) is performed. In some instances the goniotomy must be repeated a number of times to ensure adequate drainage. Approximately 80% of these surgeries are successful.

Secondary congenital glaucomas are associated with a variety of systemic and eye disorders. Aniridia, the absence of an iris, may be associated with other anterior eye deformities to cause glaucoma. A dystrophic cornea or a congenital cataract may be associated with glaucoma. Neurofibromatosis and Sturge-Weber syndrome (hemangioma of the face) are two of the more common systemic disorders that accompany congenital glaucoma. Usually filtering or trabeculoplasty procedures are performed with varying success, depending on the severity of the anatomic abnormality.

Diagnostic Studies and Findings

Tonometry (Schiötz, Applanation, or Contact Methods)

Test for intraocular pressure; normal range 10 to 22 mm Hg

Visual Field Studies

Central field tangent screen

Central vision covers approximately 50 degrees of patient's central vision, 25 degrees in each direction from central fixation point; black screen 1 m^2 is placed 1 m from eye; blind spots are outlined by using 1 to 3 mm white target placed on board; normal blind spot is 13 to 18 degrees temporal from central fixation; abnormal isolated spots (scotomas) or confluent areas can be identified; nasal areas are usually lost first

Automated perimetry

Various automated machines (such as Goldmann perimeter) measure both central and peripheral fields

Gonioscopy

Corneal contact lens (goniolens) placed over anesthetized cornea to permit viewing of anterior chamber angles with microscopic lens; cellular debris and adhesions in anterior chamber angles can also be viewed

Ophthalmoscopy

See pp. 1560

Provocative Tests

Used for patients with mildly elevated IOP, those who have optic nerve changes or field defects without elevated IOP, and those with shallow anterior chambers and compromised anterior angles; results not definitive but may distinguish potentially glaucomatous persons from others

Water drinking test

In morning, fasting patient drinks approximately 1 L of water as fast as possible (within 2 to 4 minutes); IOP is measured before and at 15-minute intervals for 45 minutes; normal eyes show IOP increase of 3 to 5 mm Hg; increase of 8 mm Hg is indicative of glaucoma

Dark room test (for narrow-angle glaucoma)

Patient sits in dark room for 60 minutes to dilate pupils; IOP increase of 7 to 8 mm Hg is indicative of iris bunching into and blocking anterior angle flow

Mydriatic testing

One eye is dilated at a time (under careful supervision), and pupil is constricted when test is ended; IOP increase of 8 mm Hg is indicative of glaucoma

Medical Plan

Open-Angle Glaucoma

Surgery

Surgery performed if medications do not control pressure

Laser trabeculoplasty—may be done on outpatient basis; 100 to 120 laser impacts aimed evenly spaced around anterior portion of trabecular meshwork through goniolens; resultant scarring thought to increase tension within meshwork to maintain openings; success rate not fully determined[33]; see p. 654

External trabeculectomy—favored over other filter device procedures because it does not disrupt anterior chamber and adhesions do not form between iris and posterior canal; portion of meshwork is removed through scleral flap incision; flap is replaced over surgical site to keep anterior chamber intact; procedure performed in hospital with patient under general anesthesia[28]

Medications

β-Adrenergic–blocking agents

- Timolol maleate (Timoptic), 0.25%-0.5% solution, 1 drop in each eye, usually bid; reduces aqueous production; serious side effects include bradycardia, palpitation, bronchial asthma, hypotension, and congestive heart failure; these necessitate discontinuation in 5%-10% of patients
- Betaxolol (Betopic), 0.5% solution, 1 drop in each eye qd; reduces aqueous production; side effects are similar to Timolol, but air flow obstruction responses may be less common

Miotics

- Pilocarpine (Isopto carpine, Pilocar), 0.25%-8% solution, 1-2 drops 2-6 times/d
- Pilocarpine continuous-release insert device (Ocusert)—Device is placed in conjunctival sac and releases medication over 7-day period; reduction in IOP is same as with drops; some patients have difficulty removing and inserting
- Anticholinesterase drops (long-acting, strong miotics) for aphakic glaucoma; these agents should not be used for narrow-angle glaucoma because pupillary block may occur
  - Echothiophate iodide (Phospholine, Echodide), 0.03%-0.25% solution, 1 drop qd or bid

Adrenergic agents (to increase aqueous outflow)

- Epinephrine drops (Epifrin, Glaucon), 0.25%-2% solution bid (possible side effect of tachycardia and extrasystole may occur)
- Dipivefrin (Propine), 0.1% solution, 1 drop bid in each eye

Diuretics

- Acetazolamide (Diamox) to suppress aqueous production, 125-250 mg po, qid

Closed-Angle Glaucoma

Surgery

Laser iridotomy—lens placed over anesthetized cornea; argon laser aimed at iris for approximately 50 deliveries to penetrate iris and create opening for aqueous flow; laser sessions repeated several times if necessary; ultimately both eyes usually treated; see p. 654

Peripheral iridectomy—3 to 4 mm incision made at limbus or parallel to limbus over cornea; iris prolapses through limbus, or forceps is inserted into anterior chamber to pull portion of iris outward so small wedge or piece of iris can be excised; remaining iris is massaged back into chamber, and pupil is constricted to assure therapist that it is intact and round surrounding excised wedge; incision is then closed; pupil is dilated postoperatively, and steroid eye medication is given for few days so inflamed iris will not form adhesions; iridectomy opens channel between anterior and posterior chambers and creates opening in anterior angle for aqueous flow

Medications

In acute attacks, medications given to lower and control IOP so surgery can be performed

Hyperosmotic agents

- Glycerin (Glycerol, Osmoglyn), 50% solution, 1.5 g/kg body weight po; duration, 4-6h
- Mannitol (Osmitrol), 20% solution, 2 g/kg body weight, IV

Carbonic anhydrase inhibitors

- Acetazolamide (Diamox), 250 mg po bid or qid, or 500 mg followed by 250 mg IV q4h; should be given immediately to abort acute attack

Narcotic analgesics

- Meperidine (Demerol), 100 mg IM q4-6h prn

Miotics

- Pilocarpine hydrochloride (Isopto carpine, Pilocar), 0.25%-8% solution, 1-2 drops q4-6h

Congenital Glaucoma

Surgery

Goniotomy—knife inserted near limbus to penetrate anterior chamber and reach area of trabecular meshwork in anterior angle; special goniolens used to scrutinize angle while knife tears away tissue covering meshwork; procedure may be repeated a number of times to ensure patency of drainage system

Medications

Medications not usually given; surgery necessary for alleviation; miotics sometimes given in preparation for surgery

NURSING CARE

Nursing Assessment

Open-Angle Glaucoma

Asymptomatic (no blurring, pain, or inflammatory signs, early visual defects not perceived by patient); outer eye appears normal

Tonometry

IOP usually elevated (more than 24 mm Hg) but may be within normal limits (under 22 mm Hg)

Optic disc

Cupping and disc atrophy

Initially one cup larger than other; enlarged cup occupies more than half of disc diameter; cup widens and extends toward temporal disc border; temporal disc border loses translucence and appears flat white; crowding of disc vessels toward nasal border

Visual fields (perimetry)

Typical central blind spots (scotomas) identifiable; nasal vision usually lost before peripheral vision

Closed-Angle Glaucoma

Excessive lacrimation; acute, severe ocular pain (usually bilateral); blurred vision; haloes seen around lights; pupil in mild dilation (5 to 6 mm diameter); corneoscleral flush (purplish red coloration at limbus); cornea may appear hazy; possible nausea and vomiting

Tonometry

IOP usually markedly elevated (may be over 50 mm Hg)

Congenital Glaucoma

Excessive lacrimation; photophobia; hazy opaque cornea; affected eye enlarged (both eyes may be affected); affected cornea enlarged in diameter

Tonometry

IOP usually elevated but elastic eye tissue may stretch and give false low reading

Nursing Dx & Intervention[4,5,57]

Nursing Diagnosis	Nursing Intervention/Rationale
Open-Angle Glaucoma	
Noncompliance related to side effects of eye medications	• Assess patient's needs and response to medications *to see if negative responses are occurring* (physician may be able to change medication if side effects are severe). • Assess patient's knowledge about disease and its insidious progress unless treated to anticipate noncompliance. • Be certain patient can read medication labels. • Explain that number of medications and number of administrations can be confusing, inconvenient, and easy to forget. Enlist patient's assistance and understanding in devising medication schedule that patient can meet *to reduce noncompliance*. • Discuss with patient that medications do not relieve any symptoms and may cause unpleasant side effects. • Ensure that patient is aware of possible side effects: Miotics—blurred vision for 1 to 2 hours after administration, diarrhea Timolol—fatigue, weakness, depression Diamox—numbness, tingling of extremities and lips, decreased appetite or nausea, impotence
Potential for injury related to side effects of medications	• Instruct patient with new prescription that frequent checkups by physician are needed *to detect side effects and other symptoms such as increased IOP, sudden blurred vision, and inflammation of eyes*. • Teach patient about possible side effects: Miotics—pupillary block, myopia from excessive accommodation Timolol—keratitis, asthma, bradycardia Epinephrine—eye irritation, periorbital edema, tachycardia Diamox—hypokalemia, confusion, urinary calculi • Inform patient that examination (tonometry, health history, ophthalmoscopy, gonioscopy, and perimetry) will be needed every 2 to 3 months until physician determines that IOP is stable and there is no further optic nerve damage or visual field loss. Examination should be performed annually thereafter. • Demonstrate correct method for administration and storage of eye drops. Have patient repeat demonstration *to ensure proper technique*.
Sensory/perceptual alterations (visual)	• Assess and review patient's family and support system for assistance in dealing with visual loss. • Assess patient's feelings about visual loss or changes. • Review patient's life-style and suggest adjustments to blurred vision associated with miotics. • Offer support for feelings of loss and helplessness.

Nursing Diagnosis	Nursing Intervention/Rationale
Potential for injury related to diminished peripheral vision	• Inform patient that diminished peripheral vision is a great safety hazard and that peripheral vision may be markedly reduced with advanced glaucoma. • Explain that patient must learn to turn head to visualize either side *to ensure safety.* • Ask patient to reduce clutter in home (such as electrical cords, loose rugs, and items on floor) *to prevent falls.* • Inform patient that home should be well lighted (especially stairways) and that night light in bathroom is helpful. • Warn patient that seeing at night, at dusk, or in dim lighting will be difficult *because miotic pupils do not dilate to admit more light to retina in subdued lighting or darkness.*
Laser Trabeculoplasty	
Knowledge deficit	• Describe procedure carefully to patient and family members, including discussion of equipment, length of procedure, nature of procedure, and postoperative events. • Educate patient about administering eye medications and necessity for maintaining prescribed therapy, since iris may become inflamed postoperatively and IOP may be increased: Glaucoma medications—resumed until inflammatory process subsides and then discontinued or adjusted Topical steroid drops—often prescribed for approximately 1 week after surgery; reduce inflammation but may raise IOP • Inform patient that IOP may rise postoperatively and needs to be carefully monitored. • Educate patient about necessity for keeping appointments for monitoring IOP. • Educate patient about self-monitoring for symptoms (especially sudden onset): Excessive lacrimation Photophobia Severe ocular pain • Advise patient that vision will be blurred for first day or two after procedure.
Anxiety related to uncertainty about discomfort and outcome of laser procedure	• Assess patient's level of anxiety. • Offer support, comfort and information *to ease anxiety.* • Administer anesthetic eye drops immediately before procedure as ordered. • Inform patient that headache and blurred vision may occur for first 24 hours after procedure.
Pain	• Administer systemic analgesics as ordered for headache that may occur a day or two after procedure. • Apply eye patch for a few hours postoperatively *to avoid discomfort associated with light exposure.*
Peripheral Trabeculectomy	
Knowledge deficit related to lack of information about the procedure	• Describe procedure carefully to patient and family members, including discussion of equipment used, length of procedure, nature of procedure, and postoperative events.
Anxiety	• Assess patient's level of anxiety. • Offer support and comfort. • Orient patient to surroundings and inform patient that affected eye will be patched postoperatively. • Explain to patient that damaged vision cannot be restored, but further damage probably will be prevented.
Potential for injury	• Assess patient's vital signs until stable. • Observe eye dressing for excessive bleeding (small amount of serosanguineous drainage may be present). • Inform patient that periodic tonometry measurements are usually performed *because IOP may temporarily increase postoperatively.* • Administer antiemetics as ordered for nausea *to avoid elevated IOP associated with emesis.* • Administer mydriatics as ordered; pupil of affected eye is dilated immediately or within 2 or 3 days postoperatively *to prevent formation of iris adhesion.* • Administer glaucoma medications as ordered for unoperated eye.
Sensory/perceptual alterations (visual) related to unilateral eye patch	*Before surgery:* • Warn patient that depth perception will be lost and 50% of peripheral vision will be lost on affected side. *After surgery:* • Help patient with activities of daily living. • Caution patient to bring hand forward slowly to touch objects (especially containers of hot liquid and containers receiving poured liquids).

Nursing Diagnosis	Nursing Intervention/Rationale
	• Teach patient to turn head fully toward affected side to view objects or obstacles. • Tell patient to use up and down head movements to judge stairs and oncoming objects and to go slowly.
Pain	• Assess patient for postoperative discomfort and give systemic analgesics as ordered.
Closed-Angle Glaucoma	
Pain	• Assess patient's level of discomfort. • Give medications as ordered *to reduce discomfort* (meperidine may not be ordered for some patients because it tends to cause nausea and vomiting). • Administer osmotics or carbonic anhydrase inhibitors as ordered *to reduce aqueous production*.
Anxiety	• Assess patient's level of anxiety. • Offer comfort and support. • Give realistic assurance about maintenance of vision if IOP is brought under control quickly. • Keep patient informed of progress and planned medical and surgical interventions. • Describe impending surgical procedures, including equipment, length of procedure, nature of procedure, and postoperative events.
Laser Iridotomy	
Pain	• During procedure, help patient to hold still (head is stabilized on chin rest). Offer reassurance and support. • Administer topical anesthetic as ordered. • Administer systemic analgesics as ordered if headache and mild eye pain continue for day or two. • Eye patch is usually applied for a few hours postoperatively *to avoid discomfort associated with light exposure*.
Knowledge deficit	• Educate patient about necessity of maintaining prescribed therapy. • Educate patient about necessity of keeping appointments for monitoring IOP. (This procedure may be done on outpatient basis, and patient compliance is a vital factor.) • Educate patient about self-monitoring for symptoms (especially sudden onset): Excessive lacrimation Photophobia Severe ocular pain • Advise patient that vision will be blurred for first day or two after procedure. • Advise patient that procedure may have to be repeated several times to ensure patency of angle.
Potential for injury	• Assess patient's vital signs until stable. • Observe eye dressing for excessive bleeding. • Observe patient for sudden onset of severe pain in operated eye and administer medications as ordered *to avoid eye injury related to elevated IOP*. • Inform patient that tonometry measurements will probably be performed periodically. • Administer antiemetics as ordered for nausea *to avoid elevated IOP*. • Administer mydriatics and steroid drops for operated eye as ordered *to avoid inflammation and adhesions*. (Unoperated eye may need to be maintained with glaucoma medications if patient has previously received them.)
Sensory/perceptual alterations (visual) related to unilateral eye patch	*Before surgery:* • Warn patient that depth perception will be lost and 50% of peripheral vision will be lost on affected side. *After surgery:* • Help patient with activities of daily living. • Caution patient to bring hand forward slowly to touch objects (especially containers of hot liquid and containers receiving poured liquids). • Teach patient to turn head fully toward affected side to view objects or obstacles.[24] • Tell patient to use up and down head movements to judge stairs and oncoming objects and to go slowly.
Pain	• Assess patient for postoperative discomfort and give systemic analgesics as ordered.

Patient Education

Specific knowledge needs are described in "Nursing Dx & Intervention" because glaucoma is commonly managed on an outpatient basis.

1. Inform the patient that glaucoma is not curable but can be controlled.
2. Explain to the patient that medications *must* be taken regularly.
3. Instruct the patient to visit the physician regularly as prescribed.
4. Explain that the patient must monitor himself or herself for side effects (see p. 618) and report any to the therapist, since therapy may be changed according to the patient's response to medications (either undesirable side effects or ineffective therapy).
5. Tell the patient to watch for sudden changes, including severe eye pain, inflamed eye, excessive lacrimation, marked photophobia, and visual field losses (inability to use peripheral vision), which may be noted because of bumping into obstacles from the side or at the patient's feet.
6. Remind the patient of any existing limited vision and related safety concerns.
7. Warn the patient of factors that may increase IOP, such as constrictive clothing around the neck or torso, constipation (straining), heavy exertion or lifting, and sneezing or coughing (upper respiratory infection).
8. Explain that family members should be examined regularly because glaucoma and shallow anterior chambers are often familial.

Evaluation

Patient Outcome	Data Indicating That Outcome is Reached
IOP is under control.	Tonometry shows IOP of less than 24 mm Hg.
Eye damage is not present or not increasing.	There are no visual field defects, or existing field defects are not increasing. Eye examination shows normal findings. Eyeball surface is moist without excessive tearing. Conjunctiva is clear without injection. Cornea is clear, and no redness appears at limbus. Pupil may be constricted because of medication. Red reflex is full and round. Retinal surface is pink, granular, and uniform in color and consistency. Optic disc is pinkish white and translucent with physiologic cup that occupies no more than half of disc diameter. Both optic cups are same size. Central vessels emerge evenly from optic disc and are not crowded toward nasal side.

DISORDERS OF THE LENS[6,25]

The lens is a 4 mm (sagittal diameter) by 9 mm (equatorial diameter), transparent structure between the anterior chamber and the vitreous body. Its transparency and biconvex shape enable it to focus light rays on the retina through refraction. The lens is suspended by fibers (zonule) that attach to the ciliary muscles, and it is stabilized behind the iris. The elasticity of the lens enables it to increase its spheric shape in response to ciliary contraction for near vision (accommodation). Loss of elasticity with aging results in diminished refractive power for near vision (presbyopia).

Diseases of the lens result in either opacity or dislocation of the lens. Because the lens contains no pain fibers or blood vessels, usually the only symptom is blurred vision without discomfort.

Lens dislocation[41,60]

The lens can be dislocated by trauma (a blow to the eye), systemic congenital disorders, or deformities of the lens itself.

In most instances the lens loses the full support of the zonular fibers and is either partially dislocated or fully detached and floating in the vitreous. Iritis and glaucoma are common complications of a lens in the vitreous. The detached lens may be surgically removed to prevent further eye damage, although complications may ensue because of disruption and loss of vitreous. Partially dislocated lenses are often successfully treated with glasses to correct blurred vision.

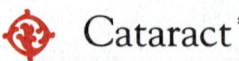

Cataract*

Cataract is an opacity of the lens.

No one has perfectly transparent lenses. Minor imperfections do not impair vision and are not apparent with gross examination. Gradual opacification of the lens is a physiologic process; if all people lived long enough, they would develop cataracts. The diagnosis of cataract is usually confirmed when a patient reports visual impairment. Considerable opacification may occur before the patient notices visual changes. The prevalence of the disease is difficult to determine because in some studies cataracts are defined as lens changes, whereas in others the disease is reported when vision is altered or the lens must be surgically removed. A summary of available data states that visible lens changes occur in 42% of the 52- to 64-year-old population and that 5% of these people demonstrate some visual impairment. Between 60% and 91% of the 65- to 85-year-old group show senile lens opacities, and approximately 25% to 46% of these people demonstrate visual impairment.[33] Cataracts are the third leading cause of blindness.

Congenital cataracts are relatively rare and occur in all degrees of severity. Newborns can exhibit total or minimum opacification. Surgery may be performed in infancy, or the eyes may be observed and surgically treated at a later time. In many instances opacification does not impair vision sufficiently to warrant surgical removal.

The only therapy for lens opacities that impair vision is surgical removal of the lens. Surgical procedures for the eye have changed dramatically in the last 20 years. Fine suture materials, the operating microscope, microsurgical instruments, improved general anesthetic procedures, and ultrasonic probes for lens emulsification and lens suction have all contributed to an improved prognosis and rapid recovery from surgery.[10,42] In the past, patients had to wait for the cataract to become "ripe" (develop marked edema and liquefaction) before surgery was possible. Newer techniques permit the decision to be made jointly by the patient and physician on the basis of visual impairment and the patient's need for visual clarity. Extended-wear soft contact lenses and, in some instances, surgically implanted lenses allow monophakic persons (those with one lens removed) to enjoy binocular vision. Over 95% of surgically treated cataract patients can now look forward to restored useful vision.

Pathophysiology

Acquired cataracts can occur because of trauma, heat, toxins, intraocular inflammation, systemic disease, or aging. Aging is considered the primary risk factor for cataract formation. Senile cataracts occur because of protein alterations, accumulation of water, increasing edema, and migration and disruption of normal fibers within the lens. The exact cause for these changes is unknown. Cataracts are usually bilateral but progress more rapidly in one eye than the other.

Opacities occur in different formations and in different areas of the lens (Figure 6-17). The central part of the lens (nucleus) is harder and denser than the periphery (cortex) because newly formed fibers continuously migrate toward and pack together in the central nucleus. The lens is surrounded by the capsule, a semipermeable membrane. The most common type of senile cataract occurs in the posterior subcapsular area. These opacities tend to obscure central vision relatively early. Cortical (or peripheral) cataracts, called soft cataracts may cause marked opacification without interfering with vision. Eventually the opacities encroach on the visual axis and decrease visual acuity. Nuclear (or hard) cataracts occur in the central area of the lens. As the central lens changes, it enlarges and increases its spheric shape, which permits some persons to enjoy "second sight," an increase in near vision. This diminished presbyopia is a temporary improvement and is followed by increased opacities that ultimately reduce vision. Opacities may develop very slowly and form different configurations. An early symptom may be glare (especially at night) because the opacities reflect light rays inefficiently. In some instances central opacities split light rays and cause a monocular diplopia. This symptom disappears as the opacity increases. Vision may improve in dim light (or with pupil dilation) because the person has more pupil available to see around the opacity. Some patients are able to "see" the dark spots, which remain fixed in the visual field, unlike floaters (debris in the vitreous) that move around.

If the cataract is not removed, it may eventually cause the entire lens to be opaque. This can be seen with gross observation as a whitish discoloration of the entire pupil. Less advanced opacities may be seen through the ophthalmoscope as dark spots, patches, or networks of lines that disrupt the red reflex.

Decision for removal of the lens is usually based on the patient's need to see. Vision is evaluated by examining both eyes. If one eye enables the patient to maintain adequate vision, the failing eye is often not surgically treated. In some instances the lens swells and encroaches on the anterior chamber angle to cause glaucoma. Hypermature cataracts may release toxic products that cause a secondary uveitis or glaucoma or both. Surgical intervention is sometimes undertaken to prevent eye damage regardless of visual acuity.

Risk factors other than age have been identified as possible sources for cataract formation. Women over 65 years of age are reported to have a higher rate of cataract formation than men. Some studies have shown that people living in warm, sunny climates have a significantly higher incidence of cataracts. The correlation between cataract formation and ultraviolet light exposure is under further investigation. The lens is susceptible to heat because its avascular tissue does not transfer heat efficiently.

High-dose radiation has been proved to cause cataracts. Survivors of atomic bomb explosions have exhibited a high prevalence of this disease. Study findings of the effects of

*References 2, 5, 6, 14, 33, 37, 41, 62.

Figure 6-17 Various types of senile cataracts. **A,** Nuclear sclerosis. **B,** Nuclear sclerosis and posterior subcapsular cataract. **C,** Nuclear sclerosis and anterior and posterior cortical cataracts.
From Newell.[41]

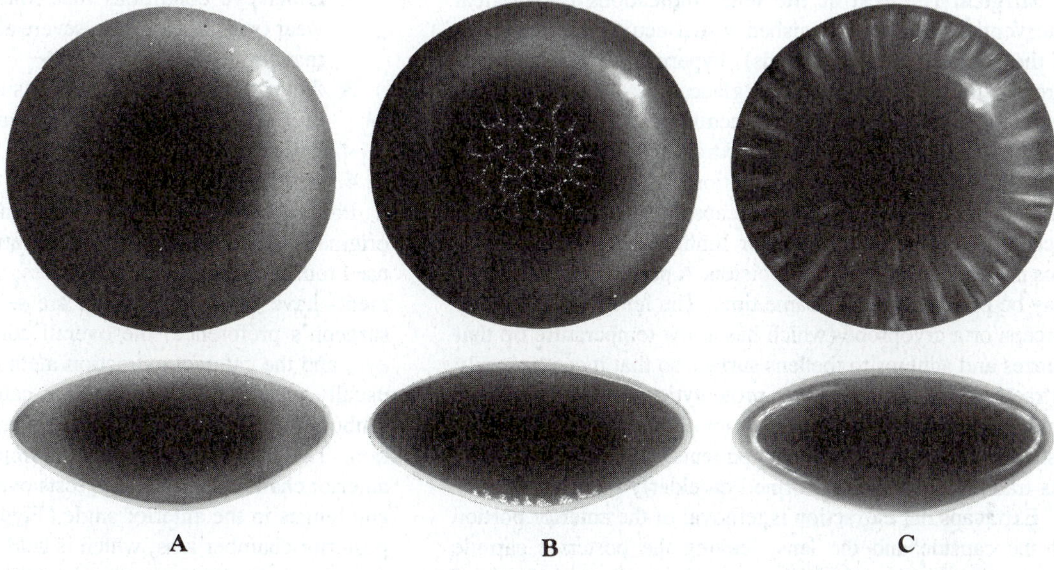

exposure to low doses of radiation over a prolonged period are not conclusive. Some concern has been raised about computed tomography scans of the skull as a direct source of radiation to the eyes.[33]

Some drugs are reported to be associated with early cataract formation. Corticosteroids, phenothiazines, and some cancer chemotherapy agents are commonly used medications cited in clinical and animal studies.

Diabetes is associated with an earlier onset of cataracts. Young adults with poorly controlled diabetes may rarely exhibit fulminating bilateral cataracts. Sorbitol, a by-product of excessive glucose, is known to accumulate in and damage the lens. Hypertensive patients also have a higher incidence of cataracts.

Blunt trauma (contusion) to the eye may result in opacification of the lens that occurs several months after the injury. If the trauma is invasive, localized opacification occurs as a response to rupture of the lens capsule.

Congenital cataracts may be associated with multiple systemic disorders or other eye deformities, or they may occur in the absence of other signs or symptoms. Maternal rubella in the first trimester often results in infant cataracts that may be accompanied with other signs of deformity. Down's syndrome is commonly associated with cataracts, which usually do not progress sufficiently to impair vision. Infants with identifiable cataracts should be examined and monitored for other physical abnormalities, developmental delay, impaired hearing, and mental retardation.[64]

Most infants and children with cataracts do not exhibit enough opacification to interfere with normal vision. If a newborn has dense opacities, surgery is often performed shortly after birth to prevent permanent sensory loss from disuse of the eye. Foveal stimulation must occur in both eyes in the first 4 months of life to allow normal visual development. Long-wearing contact lenses may be prescribed for monophakic infants if the parents are able to manage the care involved. Children with slowly progressive cataracts have a better prognosis for normal binocular vision if surgery can be delayed until 10 to 12 years of age.

Congenital cataracts can be detected at birth if severe opacification is present. Marked density can be seen with gross observation. The newborn normally manifests a full round red reflex when examined with an ophthalmoscope. Lens opacities interrupt the red reflex and require further examination with a gonioscope. In some instances the parent may notice that the infant is not responding visually at home. The family of the affected child should be examined for cataracts.

Diagnostic Studies and Findings

Cataracts are identified through ophthalmoscopy or slit-lamp examination. Visual acuity is measured periodically to assess visual function in both the impaired eye and the less impaired eye.

Medical Plan[5,6,41,60]

Surgery

Surgical removal of the lens. Indications for surgical intervention include diminished visual acuity (by definition of the patient's life-style needs), hypermature cataracts that threaten to cause eye damage (glaucoma, uveitis), and the necessity to treat or view the structure behind the lens.

Two procedures are used for extraction: intracapsular and extracapsular. Intracapsular extraction is removal of the entire lens, including its surrounding capsule. An 18 to 20 mm incision is made at the superior limbus arc, and the entire lens is extracted through the incision. A peripheral iridectomy may be performed at the same time. The lens is extracted by forceps or a cryoprobe (which has a low temperature tip that freezes and adheres to the lens surface so that it can be easily extracted). Chymotrypsin, a proteolytic enzyme, is sometimes briefly instilled in the anterior chamber to dissolve resistant zonular fibers in younger patients. Total lens extraction has traditionally been performed on elderly patients.

Extracapsular extraction is removal of the anterior portion of the capsule and the lens, leaving the posterior capsule intact. An incision at the limbus provides access to the anterior capsule, which is mechanically disrupted so the lens nucleus can be removed. The remaining lens cortex is irrigated and suctioned out, leaving the posterior capsule in place. This procedure is often used with younger adults and children because the posterior lens capsule adheres to the vitreous until about 20 years of age. Leaving the capsule in place avoids disruption and loss of vitreous. This method is also favored by some surgeons to accommodate placement of a lens implant. Occasionally the posterior capsule becomes opaque and has to be removed at a later date.

With younger adults, ultrasonic fragmentation (phacoemulsification) is used to disintegrate the lens so it can be aspirated. A rapidly vibrating needle powered by ultrasonic energy breaks up the lens tissue. This method is not used with older adults because the lens nucleus is hardened and resistant to emulsification. The incision for this procedure is only 3 mm, and the patient is usually able to leave the hospital the following day.

The lens can be removed with either general or local anesthesia. General anesthesia is usually used if a lens is implanted. Postoperative care is usually uncomplicated, and the patient is ambulatory on the first or second day. An eye patch may be applied to the operative eye for a brief period, or longer if the physician prefers. An eye patch is not worn after phacoemulsification. A metal eye shield is applied to the eye at night for several weeks to prevent accidental rubbing or injury. The postoperative phase requires patient precautions to avoid increased intraocular pressure, as well as adjustments to distorted vision (see p. 627) unless a lens is implanted in the eye.

Lens implantation. Indications for lens implantation include the following[37]:

1. Persons who cannot manage the care and insertion or removal of extended-wear or regular contact lenses (e.g., because of mental impairment or limited manual dexterity)
2. Other eye conditions that contraindicate contact lens wear (such as dry eyes, severe allergies, or severe astigmatism)
3. Adverse work environment (such as presence of dust or fumes) that does not permit tolerance of contact lenses
4. Only one eye affected

Polymethylmethacrylate (Plexiglas), the lens material originally discovered to be nonirritating to the eyes, is still used today. A wide variety of sizes, shapes, and lens placements have been devised and are selected according to the surgeon's preference, the overall condition of the patient's eye, and the cataract extraction method used. The implant is usually placed at the time of the cataract removal, and the limbus incision may have to be enlarged to allow implantation. The two common types of implant lenses are (1) the anterior chamber lens, which rests over the pupillary opening and lodges in the anterior angle (Figure 6-18, *A*) and (2) the posterior chamber lens, which is held in position either in the capsule of the lens or sutured to the iris (Figure 6-18, *B*).

Mydriatic drops are usually prescribed for anterior chamber lenses to avoid the development of adhesions and secondary glaucoma. The lens may be sutured in place or stabilized with clips or hooks.

Lens implantation offers many advantages over the use of spectacles and is particularly useful for patients with good vision in the unoperated eye. Binocular vision is rapidly restored, with improved depth perception and good distant and near visual acuity. The lens implant provides accurate distant vision, and glasses are often prescribed to correct near vision difficulties. However, many patients are not good candidates for implantation because of potential postoperative complications. Patients with severe myopia, a history of chronic iritis, retinal detachment, diabetic retinopathy and glaucoma, congenital cataracts, or complications during surgery would not be advised to receive an implant. The rate of surgical complications is reported to be 2% to 5% of implantations performed, and complications include corneal edema, secondary glaucoma, iritis, hemorrhage, retinal detachment, and lens displacement.[28,37,65]

Some surgeons believe that implants should be used only if the patient cannot tolerate contact lenses. The long-range durability of the lenses is uncertain, and in most instances they are used only for patients over 65 years of age. Some surgeons believe that extended-wear lenses will eventually replace lens implants as methods for the manufacture and use of contact lenses improve.

Medications[6,41,59,60]

A wide variety of preoperative and postoperative medications are ordered according to the surgeon's preference, the patient's condition, and the nature of the procedure.

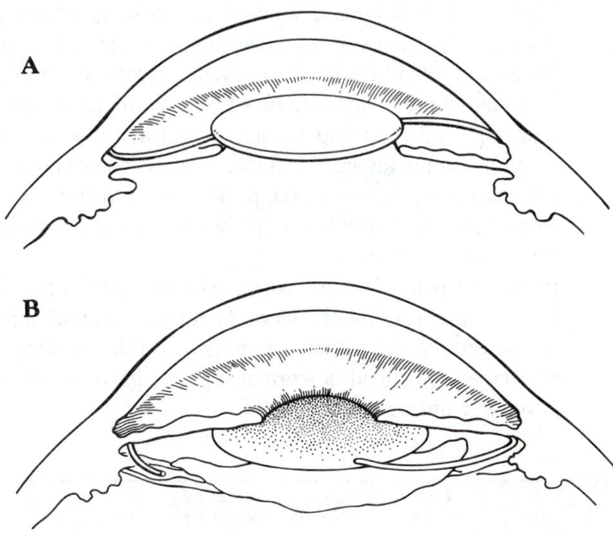

Figure 6-18 A, Anterior chamber intraocular lens that is held in position with loop of nylon (haptics) placed in anterior chamber angle. **B,** Posterior chamber lens placed in lens capsule from which most of anterior portion has been excised.
From Newell.[41]

Preoperative
- Topical anti-infective agents (usually prescribed 1 wk before surgery)
  - Gentamicin sulfate (Genoptic, Garamycin), 3.0 mg/ml, 1-2 drops q4h
- Mydriatic-cycloplegic agents (usually prescribed 2h before surgery)
  - Atropine sulfate (Atroprisol, Isopto Atropine), 1% solution 1 drop
  - Cyclopentolate (Cyclogyl), 1 drop of 1% solution or 2 drops of 0.5% solution q5 min for 15 min
- Hyperosmotic agents
  - Glycerin (Glycerol Osmoglyn), 50% solution, 1.5 g/kg body weight, po
  - Mannitol, IV 500 mg by slow drip
- Sedative-hypnotics
  - Secobarbitol (Seconal), 100 mg po
- Antiemetics
  - Promethazine (Phenergan), 25 mg IM
- Narcotic analgesics
  - Meperidine (Demerol), 50-100 mg IM

Postoperative
- Mydriatic-cycloplegic agents (not used with lens implant)
  - Atropine sulfate 1%, 1 drop bid for 2-6 wk after surgery
- Corticosteroids
  - Prednisolone suspension (Metimyd, others), 1 drop of 0.2%-0.5% suspension qid
  - Hydrocortisone acetate (Cortef, others), 1 drop of 0.5%-2.5% suspension qid
- Analgesics
  - Acetylsalicylic acid with codeine (Empirin #3), po q4h prn
  - Acetaminophen (Tylenol), 650 mg po q4h prn

General Management

Corrective lenses may be prescribed for aphakic patients. The removal of the lens causes a severe hyperopia because of loss of accommodative powers and a marked magnification of visual objects. Adults must receive some type of corrective lens to maintain visual function. Based on the patient's overall condition, the physician prescribes spectacles or contact lenses or performs lens implantation. Aphakic infants must have corrective lenses to permit development of vision in the first 6 months of life.

Spectacles are still commonly prescribed for elderly patients who cannot tolerate contact or implanted lenses. Adjusting to spectacles is difficult because image magnification of approximately 30% is still present and peripheral vision and depth perception are obscured. Binocular vision is not possible with a unilateral cataract removal unless contact lenses are prescribed. Corrective lenses are usually trifocal or bifocal, and the prescription may have to be changed several times over a period of months until the most effective visual correction is attained.

Contact lenses are usually the prescription of choice for adults and infants if the wearer can tolerate them. Increased depth perception, less image magnification (approximately 7%), and binocular vision are attained.

Many elderly patients who cannot remove and insert lenses visit a physician weekly and later monthly or quarterly for removal and cleansing of extended-wear lenses and examination of the eyes. Parents of infants receiving contact lenses must be capable of removing, inserting, and cleansing the lenses and monitoring the eyes for complications. For further discussion of contact lens care and precautions see p. 643. A permanent corrective lens can usually be prescribed within 4 to 6 weeks after surgery.

A protective patch is worn postoperatively for 24 to 72 hours. Dark glasses are worn to relieve photophobic discomfort, if the patient's pupil(s) are dilated, and a protective eye shield is worn at night to prevent injury to the eye during sleep.

NURSING CARE

Nursing Assessment

Cataract

Opacities usually not visible on gross examination but may be seen as dark spots, clusters, or linear networks against retinal background with ophthalmoscope; glare at night and in bright light; blurred vision; peripheral vision may diminish before central vision; near vision may improve temporarily (with nuclear cataract); monocular diplopia if central opacity splits visual axis

Advanced Cataract

Pupil cloudy and white on gross examination; total blindness

Aphakia with Spectacle Correction

Thick lenses; 30% magnification of images; clear vision perceived only when looking through center of lens; diminished and distorted peripheral vision; good near vision; monocular aphakic patient unable to use binocular vision (diminished depth perception)

Aphakia with Contact Lens Correction

7% to 10% magnification of images; peripheral vision intact; monocular aphakic patient able to experience binocular vision (improved depth perception); improved near and far visual acuity; reading glasses may be needed

Aphakia with Implanted Lens Correction

Most often used for monocular aphakia and useful in unoperated eye; full binocular vision restored; minimum magnification; peripheral vision intact; improved near and far visual acuity; reading glasses may be needed

Nursing Dx & Intervention[5,6,37,57]

Nursing Diagnosis	Nursing Intervention/Rationale
Sensory/perceptual alterations (visual) related to cataract formation	• Assess patient's visual acuity. • Review patient's life-style needs and suggest possible alterations for adjustment to blurred vision or reduced peripheral vision. • Assess patient's family and support system *to provide assistance in dealing with visual loss.* • Review with patient and family safety measures in home and community and necessary life-style changes and resultant feelings *to clarify decisions about surgery to remove cataract(s).*
Fear related to anticipation of eye surgery	• Assess patient for fears regarding blindess, pain, and surgical procedure. • Discuss with patient concerns about cataract surgery and correct any misconceptions, such as that the remaining eye will deteriorate faster after surgery or that total immobilization is necessary postoperatively for a prolonged period. • Assess patient for visual acuity, other physical problems, frailty, knowledge about condition, and available support system. • Offer support and comfort. • Orient patient to room and surroundings (if admitted to hospital). • Describe procedure carefully to patient and family members, including equipment, length of procedure, nature of procedure, and postoperative events, *to reduce fear.*
Potential for trauma related to lack of preoperative measures	• Tell patient to refrain from squeezing eyelids shut or touching eyes postoperatively. • Encourage older patient to wear glasses during day as reminder not to rub eye. • Teach patient to avoid heavy lifting, straining, or bending over at the waist, *since this might cause dizziness and precipitate a fall.* • Administer preoperative medications as ordered (antibiotic drops or ointments, mydriatic or cycloplegic drops, ocular hypotensive agents, and preanesthetic medications).
Potential for injury: postoperative complications related to cataract surgery	• Position head of bed at 30-degree elevation. • Observe dressing for excessive drainage or bleeding. • Assess patient for marked temperature elevation or sudden onset of severe pain.

Nursing Diagnosis	Nursing Intervention/Rationale
	• Report temperature elevation or pain increase to physician *to avoid eye injury from inflammation or increased ocular pressure.* • Help patient avoid nausea, vomiting, sneezing, coughing, straining with elimination, and touching operated eye *to avoid increased ocular pressure.* • Help patient to turn to unoperated side. • Approach patient from unoperated side. • Help patient walk the night of surgery. • Maintain eye patch in place (usually for first or second day). • Apply eye shield at night. • Give postoperative medications as ordered (mydriatic drops, miotic medication [lens implant], antibiotic or steroid drops *to prevent infection,* laxative as needed, and antiemetic as needed).
Sensory/perceptual alterations (visual) related to unilateral eye patch	*Before surgery:* • Help in measuring visual acuity of unoperated eye preoperatively. • Have patient's glasses available for immediate use postoperatively. • Warn patient that depth perception will be lost and 50% of peripheral vision will be lost on affected side. *After surgery:* • Help patient with activities of daily living. • Caution patient to bring hand forward slowly to touch objects (especially containers of hot liquids and containers receiving poured liquids). • Teach patient to turn head fully toward affected side to view objects or obstacles *to avoid falls.* • Tell patient to use up and down head movements to judge stairs and oncoming objects and to go slowly.
Pain related to surgery	• Assess patient for postoperative discomfort (which is usually mild) and itching and administer analgesics as ordered *to prevent patient from inadvertently rubbing eye.*

Patient Education

1. Instruct the patient to avoid heavy lifting, straining with elimination, and strenuous exercise for 6 weeks, since increased intraocular pressure should be avoided until the eye is healed.
2. Teach the patient to wear an eye shield at night for 2 to 6 weeks to avoid injury to the eye.[36]
3. Inform the patient that dark glasses may be worn during the day to avoid pupil constriction and glare associated with mydriatic medication. The eye is sensitive to light after surgery, and tearing or squinting may occur in bright natural or artificial light.
4. Teach the patient the correct procedures for instilling eye drops and ointments and applying an eye shield (without touching or applying pressure on the eyeball) to avoid self-inflicted injury.
5. Instruct the patient and family that the patient's life-style must be altered to deal with continued diminished vision in one or both eyes, since final prescription spectacles or contact lenses take 4 to 8 weeks to attain.
6. Explain to a patient receiving spectacles that images will be magnified 30%, peripheral vision will be obscured and distorted, and the lenses will probably be bifocal or trifocal. Therefore life-style changes and safety concerns will need to be assessed; for example, the patient must learn to judge distances when descending stairs or viewing oncoming objects and must turn the head from side to side to see the peripheral environment. Several recent studies have shown an association between loss of peripheral vision and driving performance. A few states require some form of visual field testing before awarding or renewing a driver's license, but most do not.[26] The visual acuity testing that is ordinarily performed does not usually pick up peripheral loss. Patients with peripheral loss will need to be evaluated and counseled about their driving potential. Losing the ability to drive is a huge alteration for most people. Follow-up in the form of support is necessary to assure compliance with the driving ban, continued access to the community, and maintenance of the patient's well-being in the face of this loss of independence.
7. Explain to a patient receiving contact lenses that images will be magnified 7% to 10%, peripheral vision will be intact, and reading glasses may also be prescribed. Therefore the patient must learn to care for, insert, and remove lenses (see p. 646) or arrange to visit a physician routinely for removal, cleansing, and reinsertion of extended-wear lenses (see p. 646).
8. Warn the patient that it will be necessary to adjust to mild magnification when performing daily activities.
9. Alert the patient and family to signs and symptoms of complications to watch for and report: sudden onset of eye pain, redness and watering of eyes, photophobia, and sudden onset of visual changes.

Evaluation

Patient Outcome	Data Indicating That Outcome is Reached
Patient with cataracts has adjusted to visual changes.	Life-style needs are not hampered by diminished vision. Patient is able to participate in activities requiring near and far vision. Patient understands cause of visual changes and recognizes that further changes will ensue. Patient expresses feeling of self-control in terms of participating in future decisions about cataract surgery. Patient is not endangering himself or herself with activities requiring more vision than patient has, such as driving, venturing into community without assistance, home maintenance, self-care activities (self-administering medication), or working at a job.
Patient with cataract removal has adjusted to visual correction with spectacles.	Patient recognizes and avoids safety hazards, does not trip or fall, and does not feel physically insecure. There is no eye pain, further marked visual change, eye redness, lacrimation, or photophobia.
Patient with cataract removal has adjusted to visual correction with contact lenses.	Patient can demonstrate insertion, removal, and cleansing of lens or reports regular visits to practitioner for lens care. Peripheral vision is intact. Binocular vision is intact. There is no eye pain, further marked visual change, eye redness, lacrimation, or photophobia.
Patient with cataract removal has adjusted to visual correction with lens implant.	Peripheral vision is intact. Binocular vision is intact. There is no eye pain, marked visual change, eye redness, lacrimation, or photophobia.

DISORDERS OF THE RETINA[41,60]

The retina, the inner lining of the eyeball, is a multilayered extension of the central nervous system that receives images and transmits them to the brain. Lesions or disorders affecting this surface result in altered vision without pain because sensory fibers do not exist in this area. The degree and type of diminished vision depend on the extent and location of the lesions. Central retinal lesions encroach on the macula and the fovea centralis, severely reducing central vision, near vision, and color differentiation. Peripheral (rod) lesions affect peripheral vision, causing isolated blind spots, night blindness, or gradual peripheral loss until the person is reduced to tunnel (or tubular) vision. Retinal diseases can be congenital or acquired through inflammation, trauma, vascular insufficiency, or aging. The diseases vary in severity from total blindness at birth or a slowly deteriorating condition to minor defects that are unnoticed by the person. The cause and cure for many of these diseases are unknown. Photocoagulation can sometimes arrest the pathologic process, but treatment is difficult if the lesion is in the macular area because photocoagulation causes scarring and further vision reduction. Alterations in the configuration of the retina can cause traction, hole formation, and tearing that are surgically treatable.

Retinal vascular occlusion

Occlusion of the retinal artery or vein can cause loss of vision.

Pathophysiology

Retinal arterial occlusion causes a sudden, unilateral, painless loss of vision. The severity of vision diminishment ranges from total loss with an occluded central artery to a visual field defect that corresponds to blockage of a branch. Emboli associated with atherosclerosis, valvular heart disease, and blood hyperviscosity are among the most common causes. Emboli sometimes form in elderly patients with carotid plaques. Retinal arterial spasms cause transient vision losses that often progress to a permanent loss. Treatment for occlusion must be swift (within 2 hours) to restore vision. Massage of the eyeball (intermittent moderate pressure on the globe) may dislodge an embolus and send it to a more peripheral branch. Evaluation and treatment of the systemic disorder that led to the retinal artery occlusion follow emergency treatment.

Retinal vein occlusion results in a more gradual loss of vision, occurring over several hours in contrast to the abrupt loss with arterial blockage. Venous blockage usually occurs in only one eye, and the degree of vision interruption depends on whether the central vein or one of its branches is occluded. Vein occlusion is associated with systemic vascular disease, venous stasis, arterial hypertension, and blood hyperviscosity. Branch occlusion is more common than central blockage and is sometimes successfully treated with photocoagulation. Photocoagulation does not cure the vascular or systemic disease but deters localized hemorrhage and neovascularization (formation of new vessels). When retinal veins are obstructed, they become engorged and tortuous, and neovascularization occurs in the retina and iris and may extend into the vitreous. The new vessels leak protein and blood. Hemorrhage from dilated veins, retinal edema, and neovascularization may result in anterior synechia formation (adhesions at the anterior angle) and acute glaucoma. Some patients recover from venous stasis retinopathy without treatment. Others respond to photocoagulation. Some patients are left with irreversible visual defects.

Diagnostic Studies and Findings[16,41,59,60]

Direct Ophthalmoscopy

Venous dilation and tortuosity; arterial narrowing or obliteration; opacities; hemorrhage; microaneurysms; neovascularization; retinal pallor, detachment, breaks, and folds

Fluorescein Angiography

Abnormal placement of vessels (crowding, shunts, obliteration); vessel leakage; microaneurysms; neovascularization

Medical Plan[41,60]

Retinal Artery Occlusion

Surgery

Anterior chamber paracentesis—with patient under local anesthesia, needle is injected through limbus into anterior chamber; 1 or 2 drops of aqueous fluid is removed to cause sudden lowering of intraocular pressure, which might dislodge embolus

Medications

Anticoagulant agents (may be prescribed in early phases of occlusion)
- Heparin, IV loading dose of 5000-10,000 U followed by 5000-10,000 U q4-6h for adult[11]

General Management

Intermittent massage of eyeball—physician applies moderate pressure to globe for 5 seconds, releases pressure for another 5 seconds, and then repeats maneuver in attempt to dislodge embolus to more peripheral branch

Oxygenation—95% oxygen for 10 minutes each hour over period of hours[28]

Evaluation and treatment of systemic cardiovascular dysfunction

Retinal Vein Occlusion

Recovery may be spontaneous, and no curative therapy exists. Therapy is given to prevent further retinopathy in the affected eye and occlusive responses to the other eye.

Surgery

Photocoagulation (see p. 651) to burn small or new vessels

Medications

Anticoagulant agents
- Heparin, for adult, IV loading dose of 5000-10,000 U followed by 5000-10,000 U q4-6h, followed by bishydroxycoumarin (Dicumarol), 25-150 mg/d as maintenance dose
- Acetylsalicyclic acid (aspirin), for adult, 200 mg every third day; may be given for antithrombotic effect as preventive measure for remaining eye

Corticosteroids
- Prednisone (Deltasone, others), 30 mg qd in divided doses for retinal edema

General Management

Monitoring of eye for increased intraocular pressure

NURSING CARE

Nursing Assessment

Central Retinal Artery Occlusion

Monocular event; sudden (within seconds), painless loss of vision; pale posterior retina; opaque posterior retina; fovea cherry red in contrast to surrounding whiteness; narrowed arteriole columns; no pupil constriction response; consensual response present

Central Retinal Vein Occlusion

Usually monocular event; gradual (within hours), painless loss of vision; retinal veins dilated and tortuous; optic disc swollen; neovascularization; cotton wool patches; visible hemorrhages

Nursing Dx & Intervention

Nursing Diagnosis	Nursing Intervention/Rationale
Sensory/perceptual alterations (visual) related to sudden unilateral loss	• Assess extent of visual impairment. • Offer support and comfort. • Keep patient informed of status, progress, and events during emergency care.
Anxiety related to threat of further visual loss	• Assess patient's level of anxiety. • Inform patient of related systemic disease and its effect on present and future visual dysfunction *to reduce anxiety.* • Be realistic in describing health status assessment and prognosis to patient. • Offer continuing support and comfort to patient and family.
Patient problem: bleeding related to anticoagulant therapy	• Assess patient for spontaneous bleeding, such as hematuria, tarry stools, bleeding gums, or bruising.

Nursing Diagnosis	Nursing Intervention/Rationale
	• Observe patient for allergic responses (pruritus, rash, or wheals). • If medication is continued at home, educate patient concerning dosage, frequency, signs of bleeding, necessity for keeping appointments with physician, drug interactions, and necessity for keeping laboratory appointments for prothrombin time monitoring.

Patient Education

1. Teach the patient about the systemic disease that contributes to the vascular problem.
2. Explain the degree of visual loss (usually unilateral) and its effect on the patient's life-style.

Evaluation

Outcomes vary from a fully restored healthy retina with fully functional vision to total loss of central or peripheral vision, or both, with marked retinal destruction.

Patient Outcome	Data Indicating That Outcome is Reached
Vision returns.	Vision returns to or approaches previous acuity.
Condition of retina is normal for patient.	Appearance of retina returns to normal or shows improvement.
Patient has adjusted to partial or complete loss of vision.	Patient is fully informed about present visual status and prognosis. Patient is able to draw on effective support system to supplement self-care. Patient is aware of safety measures to use at home or in the community related to visual changes or loss.

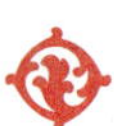

Diabetic retinopathy[1,41,49,59]

Diabetic retinopathy is a vascular disorder that occurs in patients with diabetes.

Diabetic retinopathy is one of the leading causes of blindness in the Western world. The prevalence of retinal pathology is directly related to the length of time that diabetes has been present.[49] Newell states that 7% of diabetics who have had the disease less than 10 years have retinopathy, as do 26% of those with diabetes of 10 to 14 years' duration and 63% of those with diabetes for 15 years or more.[41] These figures are estimates because the onset of non-insulin-dependent diabetes is not easily determined. The incidence of retinopathy is increasing as diabetics receive better treatment and live longer. Retinopathy is also related to the degree of control of diabetes in the early years of the disease.[59]

Pathophysiology[5,17,41,59,60]

Diabetic retinopathy exists in all degrees of severity, and the loss of visual acuity depends on the location of the lesion rather than its extent. An early lesion in the central retina (macular area) can obliterate central vision. Multiple scattered lesions throughout the periphery may not affect visual acuity. Clinicians divide retinopathy into background retinopathy and proliferative retinopathy on the basis of severity. Both conditions involve the same lesions of deterioration, but proliferation is marked by the onset of neovascularization and greater tissue destruction.

Initially the venous capillaries lose vascular tone, dilate, and develop permeable microaneurysms that contribute to ischemia and edema of the surrounding retinal tissue. Hard yellow exudates (lipid deposits) form in the edematous tissue as the fluid is being reabsorbed. The remaining retinal veins become dilated, tortuous, and irregular in caliber. Soft deposits (cotton wool patches) also form in response to vascular insufficiency. These small, white, fluffy patches indicate microinfarction in the nerve fiber area of the retina. Hemorrhages within the layers of the retina appear as small red dots that eventually are reabsorbed and disappear. Larger hemorrhages also occur between the vitreous and the retina. Opacities and hemorrhages obscure vision to the extent that they occur in the visual axis. A preretinal hemorrhage might suddenly obliterate vision as it spills into the vitreous.

The formation of new vessels (neovascularization) marks the onset of proliferative retinopathy. A network of fine, permeable vessels, venous in origin, leaks protein and blood into the surrounding tissue, which becomes edematous and opaque in appearance. More hard and soft deposits form in the retina in response to edema and vascular insufficiency. The tiny vessels spread out over the inner surface of the retina and contribute to further hemorrhage and vitreous detachment from the retina. Eventually the vessels and surrounding tissue become fibrous and the vitreous contracts and fully detaches.

The course of retinopathy varies greatly. The pathologic

changes may take many years to develop, and the patient may or may not lose functional vision.

Photocoagulation of the vascular abnormalities frequently slows the progress of microaneurysm formation and neovascularization. However, photocoagulation cannot be used in the macular area. Control of diabetes after retinopathy has begun is less effective in reducing retinal damage than careful control at the onset of diabetes.

Diagnostic Studies and Findings

Indirect Ophthalmoscopy

Venous dilation and tortuosity; arterial narrowing or obliteration; opacities; hemorrhage; microaneurysms; neovascularization

Slitlamp Examination (Biomicroscopy)

Magnification of lesions

Medical Plan

Surgery

Photocoagulation (see p. 651) to destroy neovascularization sites, prevent retinal edema, and seal small leaking vessels

Vitrectomy—if portion of vitreous is clouded with blood or fibrous membrane, opacities can be removed with fine probe passed through anterior scleral incision; fiberoptic light attached to probe permits direct viewing of vitreous and retina with microscope and special contact lens; cannulated probe cuts and removes vitreous fragments; removed vitreous is replaced with a basic salt solution; simultaneous infusion and aspiration maintain intraocular pressure during surgery; after surgery, gas (sulfhexafluoride) or air may be introduced into the eye to stabilize the retinal layer until the vitreous is expanded; silicone oil may also be used as a vitreous replacement[5,14]

Medications

For vitrectomy
- Cycloplegic agents (prescribed before and for 4-6 wk after surgery)
  - Atropine sulfate (Atroprisol, Isopto Atropine), 1% solution bid or tid
- Topical anti-infective/steroid agent (to prevent inflammation and secondary infection)
  - Combination of dexamethasone alcohol 0.1%, neomycin 3.5 mg, polymixin B, 6000 U (Maxitrol), suspension or ointment, 1-2 drops qid for 4 wk
- Systemic analgesics
  - Acetaminophen (Tylenol), 650 mg po q4h prn
  - Acetaminophen (Tylenol), with codeine (30 mg) po q4h prn

General Management

Vitrectomy
- Pressure patch to operative eye immediately after surgery
- Ice packs to operative eye as ordered to reduce inflammation
- For 4 to 5 days, patient must spend most of the time on abdomen or sitting forward with unoperative side of the head resting on a table (to permit air in eye to float against retina); this positioning is not necessary if oil is injected into the eye
- Dark glasses worn postoperatively to reduce discomfort from photophobia
- Assessment and careful control of diabetes; some think this is more effective in preventing or delaying retinopathy during first 5 years of disease, although this is controversial

NURSING CARE

Nursing Assessment

Background Retinopathy

General Factors

Visual loss may be total, partial, or absent; may not correspond to number or severity of lesions seen; possible complaints of glare; absence of pain; visible retinal changes

Microaneurysms

Small, round, red dots; usually located away from visible vessels; may turn white (hyalinized)

Hard Yellow Exudates

Yellow, waxy, confluent deposits that surround microaneurysm area

Cotton Wool Patches

Fluffy, white soft deposits scattered over retinal surface

Subretinal Hemorrhages

Small, round, red spots, less circumscribed and usually larger than microaneurysms

Preretinal Hemorrhages

Larger, blotchy, red spots

Dilated Retinal Veins

Enlarged and tortuous; may appear "beaded" (irregular in caliber)

Proliferative Retinopathy

General Factors

Visual loss still may not correspond to number or severity of lesions seen; visible retinal changes

Neovascularization

Minute network of fine vessels (often at arteriovenous crossing)

Retinal Opacification

Increased clouding or whitening of area surrounding neovascularization

Vitreous Hemorrhage

Large, red blotches (may obscure much of retina); patient may "see" vitreous hemorrhage as red shower over eyes or multiple floaters, or vision may suddenly be obscured; lesions described in background retinopathy may also be present

Nursing Dx & Intervention[5,14,37,57,60]

Nursing Diagnosis	Nursing Intervention/Rationale
Sensory/perceptual alterations (visual) related to bilateral gradual loss of vision	• Assess visual acuity and review activities of daily living that are affected or diminished because of loss of vision. • Be alert for patient's feelings of guilt about lack of self-care. (Patient may express misconceptions and blame himself or herself for present condition.) • Devise strategies for carrying out activities of daily living with patient *to maximize patient independence*. • Assess patient's support system at home and encourage full use of it. • Give realistic encouragement for maintenance of independent functioning.
Knowledge deficit related to self-care and monitoring of diabetes mellitus	• Assess patient's knowledge of disease status and self-care practices.
Potential for injury related to self-care and safety threatened by diminished vision	• Help patient to adopt self-care practices to visual handicaps. • Review activities that require close vision and color differentiation (such as urine testing, reading medication labels [use large print], and administering insulin injections). • Review patient's support system and encourage full use of it. • Help patient identify resources available in community for other assistance as needed.
Anxiety related to hospitalization and uncertainty about outcome of vitrectomy	• Assess patient's level of anxiety, which may be increased because of poor vision. • Assess patient for present visual acuity, other physical problems, frailty, knowledge about condition, and available support system. • Offer support and comfort. • Orient patient to room and surroundings. • Ensure that small personal items are within easy reach. • Describe procedure and warn patient that one or both eyes may be patched after surgery and that operative eye will be swollen and bruised for a period of time. • Explain that patient will not be totally immobilized for a long period. Bathroom privileges are usually permitted by second day. • Inform patient that outcome for functional vision depends on condition of retina. • Patient should be able to learn his or her visual status from physician (to the extent that physician can offer prognosis). • Inform patient that decision for using general or local anesthetic will be made by physician.
Potential for injury (postoperative) related to vitrectomy	*Before surgery:* • Administer antibiotic, cycloplegic eye drops as ordered. *After surgery:* • Assess patient's vital signs until stable. • Be alert for fever. • Help patient assume and maintain position on abdomen or sitting forward with unoperated side of head resting on table if ordered *to permit air injected in eye to float against retina*. • If position of head is not stipulated, semi-Fowler's position or side-lying position with operated eye upward is favored. • Check dressing for excessive bleeding (swelling and serous drainage will exist for first 24 to 48 hours). • Give postoperative eye drops as ordered (cycloplegic, antibiotic, and anti-inflammatory). • Assess patient for nausea, coughing, excessive restlessness, and disorientation. • Give narcotics and antiemetics as ordered *to prevent excessive restlessness, bumping head, sneezing, coughing, and vomiting to avoid increased intraocular pressure*. • Report any signs of upper respiratory infection to physician. • Encourage patient to do periodic deep breathing *to avoid respiratory infection associated with bed rest*.

Nursing Diagnosis	Nursing Intervention/Rationale
Sensory/perceptual alterations (visual) related to monocular vision with postoperative eye patch	*Before surgery:* • Be sure patient's glasses are available for immediate use postoperatively. • Warn patient that depth perception will be lost and 50% of peripheral vision will be lost on affected side. • Notify patient that no reading will be permitted while operative eye is patched *to prevent eye movement* but watching television may be permitted. *After surgery:* • Help patient with activities of daily living. • Caution patient to bring hand forward slowly to touch objects (especially containers of hot liquids and containers receiving poured liquids). • Teach patient to turn head fully toward affected side *to view objects or obstacles.* • Tell patient to use up and down head movements to judge stairs and oncoming objects and to go slowly.
Sensory/perceptual alterations (visual) related to binocular patches	• Assess patient for restlessness, anxiety, depression, or disorientation. • Keep side rails up at all times *to ensure safety.* • Identify yourself when entering room; touch patient as you approach and identify yourself and what you are doing *to maintain patient orientation.* • Put note at door instructing all who enter to identify themselves and explain reason for being there (e.g., cleaning staff). • Help with feeding and hygienic measures as needed. (Patient may have entered hospital with severely diminished vision and may have some self-care skills.) • Place call bell and all personal articles within reach; have patient locate them with hand. • Maintain patient's independence as much as possible. • Describe events and nursing activities as they occur. • Visit patient frequently and offer backrubs, deep breathing, range of motion exercises, and conversation *to provide stimulation.*

Patient Education

1. Maintain the patient's awareness of the diabetic state and self-care needs.
2. Inform the patient of the need for regular visual examinations.
3. Teach the patient to monitor visual responses and changes at home and to report any sudden changes to the physician:
   a. Sudden loss of vision (usually unilateral; loss may be within seconds or persist over a day or two)
   b. Increase in floaters or persistent floaters
   c. Flashes of light
   d. Sharp pain in or around eyes
4. Tell the patient to be aware of any changes in visual status, especially changes in peripheral vision (as evidenced by running into large objects, "blind" spots on either side of central vision, or changes in ability to differentiate colors).
5. Inform the patient that visual changes may be very gradual (over many years). Give the patient realistic reassurance to help him or her continue an independent life-style to the fullest extent and develop ways to adapt to diminishing vision.
6. If the patient has had a vitrectomy:
   a. Cycloplegic, antibiotic, and anti-inflammatory eye drops will be continued at home. Review the procedure for administering eye drops and emphasize the importance of maintaining the prescribed dosage. Tell the patient to wash hands before administering drops.
   b. Tell the patient to avoid constipation (straining), sneezing, coughing, heavy lifting (more than 5 pounds), rapid or jarring head movements, and heavy exercise the first week or two at home.
   c. Watching television or reading is acceptable.
   d. Have the patient make an appointment with the physician for a week after discharge.
   e. Visual function should be restored to the extent that the retina is intact. Tell the patient to review visual prognosis with the physician.

Evaluation

Outcomes vary from a healthy retina with fully functional vision to total loss of central and or peripheral vision with marked retinal destruction.

Patient Outcome	Data Indicating That Outcome is Reached
Condition of retina is optimal for patient.	Changes in retinal appearance are slowed or stopped.
Patient has adjusted to partial or complete loss of vision.	Patient is fully informed about present visual status and prognosis. Patient is able to draw on effective support system to supplement self-care. Patient is aware of safety measures to use in home or in community related to visual changes or loss.

Retinal degeneration[5,41,57,60]

Degenerative changes in the retina cause a partial or complete loss of vision.

Pathophysiology

Retinal degeneration may occur because of genetic defects, inflammation, vascular insufficiency, or aging. In many instances the cause of the disorder is unkown; the defect is often familial. Some defects occur at birth, with total blindness, whereas others develop insidiously and lead to severe visual loss. Some degenerative changes only minimally affect vision or are considered harmless. The extent, spread, and location of the deterioration and ensuing lesions determine the effect on visual acuity. Lesions that encroach on the macula often diminish vision dramatically.

Senile macular degeneration occurs because layers of the choroid thicken and the capillaries of the choroid are sclerosed and deprive the fovea centralis of nourishment. The onset is slow, involving both eyes, but deterioration may progress faster in one eye than the other. Near and central vision diminishes over a period of years, but some of the peripheral vision remains intact.

Many forms of senile macular degeneration are not treatable because photocoagulation over the area of the macula is as destructive to (central) vision as the disease is. However, a treatable form of senile degeneration involves a serous detachment of the pigment epithelium, followed by neovascularization, hemorrhaging, and eventual scarring of the overlying retina. Photocoagulation disrupts the neovascular network and may restore some vision or delay visual loss if the macula is not destroyed in the process. Most elderly adults with macular degeneration experience gradual (bilateral) loss of central vision and are eventually classified as legally blind.

Diagnostic Studies and Findings[5,41,60]

Indirect Ophthalmoscopy

Opacities; hemorrhage; microaneurysms; neovascularization; retinal pallor, detachment, breaks, and folds

Slitlamp Examination (Biomicroscopy)

Magnification of lesions

Fluorescein Angiography

Retinal vessel irregularities, vessel leakage, and detached pigment epithelium

Medical Plan

Surgery

Photocoagulation (see p. 651) used when degenerative site is not over macula to destroy neovascularization sites, prevent retinal edema, and seal small leaking vessels

NURSING CARE

Nursing Assessment

Senile Macular Degeneration

Bilateral event (pathologic progress usually not the same in both eyes); gradual diminishment of vision over months or years

Drusen

Hyaline bodies associated with choriocapillaris sclerotic changes; ophthalmoscopy may show cluster (or coalescence) of yellowish dots in macular area[30]; retinal field may show minimum changes in contrast to visual changes

Nursing Dx & Intervention[5]

Nursing Diagnosis	Nursing Intervention/Rationale
Sensory/perceptual alterations (visual) related to bilateral gradual loss	• Assess visual acuity and review activities of daily living that are affected or diminished because of loss. • Devise strategies for carrying out activities of daily living. • Assess patient's support system at home and encourage full use of it. • Give realistic encouragement for maintenance of independent functioning. • See p. 1728.

Patient Education

Education depends on the extent of visual changes (usually bilateral) and whether the prognosis indicates that further changes will occur.

1. Inform the patient or family that the patient should have regular visual examinations.
2. Provide full information to the patient or family about visual status and prognosis (realistic reassurance about a gradual loss may help the patient maintain an independent life-style).

Evaluation

Outcomes vary from mild to severe loss of vision.

Patient Outcome	Data Indicating That Outcome is Reached
Patient has adjusted to loss of vision.	Patient is fully informed about present visual status and prognosis. Patient is able to draw on effective support system to supplement self-care. Patient is aware of safety measures to use in the home or community.

Retinal holes, tears, and detachment

Retinal holes and tears are breaks in the continuity of the retina. Detachment is a separation of the sensory layers of the retina from the pigmented epithelium.

Pathophysiology[5,14,41,60]

The retina is a smooth, unbroken, multilayered surface that attaches to the hyaloid membrane of the vitreous on its inner aspect. The posterior retinal lining (pigmented epithelium) attaches to Bruch's membrane of the choroid layer on its outer aspect. Breaks in the continuity of the retina can occur in the form of small holes caused by degeneration or tearing (tears are U shaped with flaps over the holes).

Degenerative holes usually occur in the retinal periphery and are the result of retinal thinning that often parallels the ora serrata. Multiple holes form a row of latticework that is fluid filled and covered by vitreous that adheres to either side of the series of holes. Latticework degeneration occurs in about 8% of the population in all age groups and contributes to about 30% of hole-formation retinal separations.[60] The holes are often missed during general ophthalmoscopic inspection and can be seen only with scleral depression and an indirect ophthalmoscope. Many of these patients are asymptomatic, and retinal detachment does not occur. They are carefully monitored for further degeneration or tearing throughout their lifetimes.

Retinal tears occur most often because of vitreous traction. The vitreous degenerates with age and falls forward, resulting in fluid-filled cavities and collagenous areas that tug on the inner lining of the retina. The vitreous also contracts with fibrous band formations associated with retinal degeneration or diabetic retinopathy. Aphakic and myopic persons are at a higher risk for separation because the posterior chamber space is enlarged, which increases vitreous pull. A tear may be small or large, and underlying tissue bulges through it. Holes and tears may lead to detachment, a pulling away of the sensory retinal layers from the pigmented epithelium. The inner layers buckle or fold into the vitreous.

Holes and tears in the retina do not cause pain. Visual diminishment does not occur unless the retinal break is in the macular area. Vitreous pull often stimulates a sensation of lightning flashes or bright streaks of light that are momentary and unilateral. The light sensation may be a harmless phenomenon or may signal potential retinal damage. If the retina breaks or tears with vitreous pull, the patient may experience a shower of floaters (black spots or dots) because minute capillary hemorrhages send particles floating through the vitreous within the visual axis.

Retinal detachment occurs because of traction holes or breaks in the retina (rhegmatogenous) or because fluid, blood, or a mass separates the sensory portion from the pigmented epithelium (exudative) (Figure 6-19). Inflammation, hemorrhage, and tumors are common contributors to retinal separation.

Detachment often begins in the periphery and continues to spread posteriorly. The circumferential spread may occur over a few hours or may continue for several years. A relatively rapid separation gives the sensation that a curtain is being pulled over the eyes. A slow separation may offer no symptoms until the macular area is invaded or the person closes the unaffected eye and notes decreased vision in the affected eye.

Examination with an ophthalmoscope shows the detached portion of the retina as a gray bulge, ripple, or fold in contrast to the pink attached retina. If holes or tears are within the examiner's visual range, the choroid layer shows through as a contrasting cherry red spot.

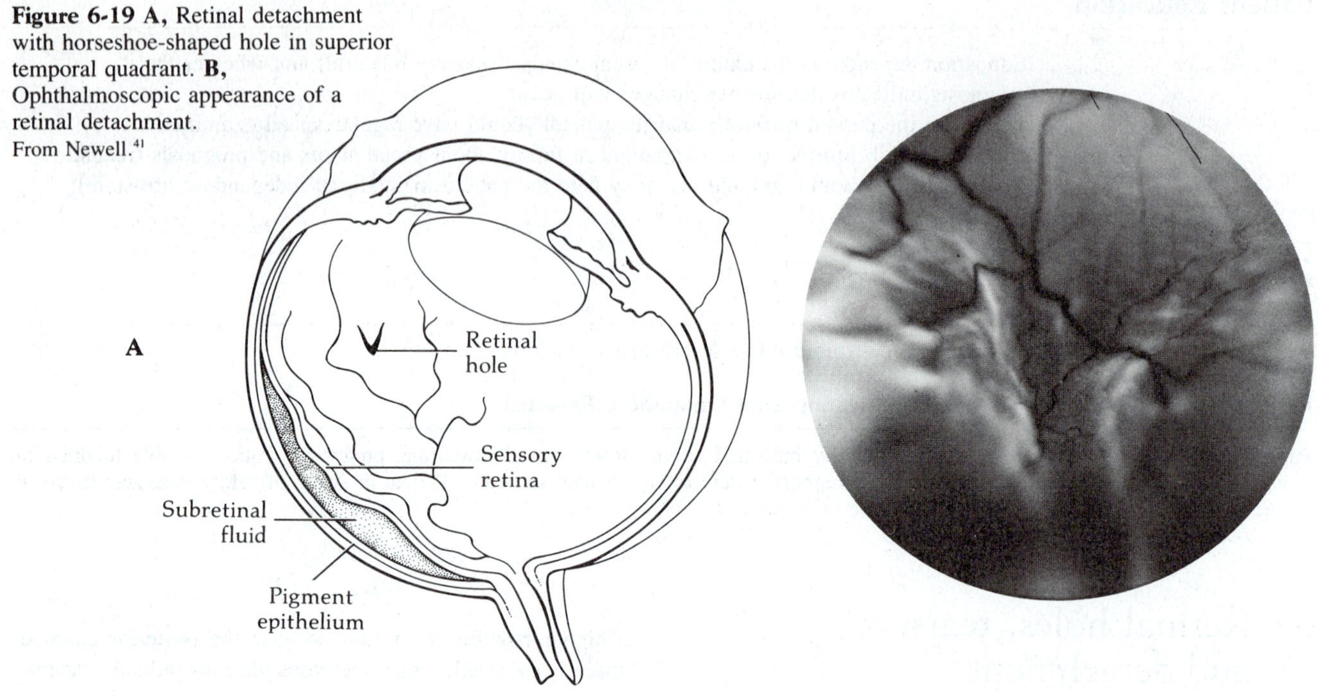

Figure 6-19 A, Retinal detachment with horseshoe-shaped hole in superior temporal quadrant. **B,** Ophthalmoscopic appearance of a retinal detachment.
From Newell.[41]

Diagnostic Studies and Findings[41,59,60]

Indirect Ophthalmoscopy

Retinal pallor, detachment, breaks, and folds

Slitlamp Examination (Biomicroscopy)

Magnification of lesions

Three-Mirror Gonioscopy

Magnified view of retinal lesions

Medical Plan

The use and type of surgical therapy depend on the extent and location of the retinal detachment.

Surgery

Photocoagulation (see p. 651)—used to burn and eventually seal localized tears or breaks in posterior portion of eyeball

Cryothermy—frozen-tipped probe placed on sclera directly over area of retinal hole; borders of hole are "frozen," inflammatory response ensues, and eventual scarring seals hole

Diathermy—heat applied by means of ultrasonic probe to scleral surface directly over site of retinal break; resultant burn causes inflammatory response with eventual scarring and sealing

Scleral buckle—sclera indented by means of local implant or encircling strap so it is flattened against retinal tissue that has fallen away from inner surface; conjunctiva pulled back to expose scleral surface; indirect ophthalmoscopy and diathermy probe used to identify areas of detachment; partial thickness of sclera is incised and pulled back to form flaps that eventually hold implant in place; rectus muscles tied with sutures so eyeball can be rotated to expose equator; detached area may be treated with diathermy before implant is put in place; encircling rod or strap often used if multiple retinal holes exist; implant sutured in place, and subretinal fluid drained from site of detachment; air, other gases such as sulfur hexafluoride, or liquids such as silicone oil may be injected into vitreous to flatten detached retina against choroid surface; air or liquid is absorbed and eventually replaced with vitreous fluid

Medications

Adrenergic-mydriatic agents

Phenylephrine (Neo-Synephrine) 2.5%-10%, 1-2 drops instilled for preoperative pupil dilation

Mydriatic-cycloplegic agents

Cyclopentolate (Cyclogyl), 1 drop of 1% solution or 2 drops of 0.5% solution preoperatively and postoperatively, frequency and duration of postoperative dosage vary with degree of inflammation

Anti-infective agents (postoperative eye drops to prevent uveitis complications)
- Gentamicin sulfate (Garamycin), 3 mg/ml topical solution, 1-2 drops qid
- Neomycin sulfate and prednisolone sodium phosphate, neomycin 3.5 mg/ml and prednisolone 5 mg/ml, frequency and duration of prescription vary according to physician's order, usually 1 drop tid or qid for 4-6 wk

General Management

Postoperative monocular or binocular eye patches (according to physician's preference) to rest eyes for day or two (usually bilateral patches because operated eye may move when unoperated eye moves)

If air is injected into vitreous cavity, head positioned so air bubble will rise and remain flush against detached retinal segment; physician specifies optimum head position and duration for positioning (usually 4 to 5 days); usual position is face down or angled to unoperated side; pillows or rubber or plastic ring used to support head; pillows under abdomen for support

Dark glasses to reduce discomfort from photophobia

NURSING CARE

Nursing Assessment

Visual Symptoms Reported by Patient

Flashing lights (unilateral, may be repeated over a period of days, months, or years); shower of floaters (black dots within visual field); sensation of curtain folding over eyes

Appearance of Retina

Detached portion grayish and less transparent than surrounding retina; retinal folds may be visible; vessels over detached portion dark red in color; holes or breaks within detached area cherry red, in contrast to the grayish area

Nursing Dx & Intervention[5,57]

Nursing Diagnosis	Nursing Intervention/Rationale
Anxiety related to sudden loss of unilateral vision	• Assess patient's level of anxiety. • Offer comfort, support, and realistic reassurance (about 90% of retinal detachment repairs are successful). • Inform patient that both eyes may be patched postoperatively.
Potential for injury related to preoperative status: detached retina	• Supervise limited activities or bed rest as ordered. • Maintain bilateral eye patches if ordered. • Keep room dark. • Keep patient supine. • Keep side rails up if patient is bedfast. • Assist with walking and avoid jarring, bumps, or falls *to prevent further detachment*. • Administer cycloplegic drops as ordered.
Sensory/perceptual alterations (visual) related to preoperative or postoperative binocular patching	• Assess patient for disorientation and agitation. • Identify yourself when entering room; touch patient as you approach and identify yourself *to notify patient of your proximity*. • Instruct others to identify themselves and state purpose of entering room. • Help with feeding, hygienic measures, and walking as needed. • Provide frequent sensory stimulation with visits and conversation postoperatively.
Potential for injury related to postoperative status	• Assess patient's vital signs until stable. • Position patient as ordered. (If gas or air has been injected into vitreous, head position may need to be maintained for 4 to 5 days.) • Supervise bed rest or limited activities as ordered (bathroom privileges are usually ordered on second day.) • Keep patient's head parallel to floor when patient is out of bed for brief periods. • Check dressing for excessive bleeding. • Report sudden severe pain. • Assess and document marked swelling and serous drainage, which is present for first 24 to 48 hours. • Initiate deep-breathing exercises four times a day *to prevent respiratory infection*. • Administer cycloplegic, mydriatic, antibiotic, and anti-inflammatory eye drops as ordered. • Assess patient for nausea, coughing, excessive restlessness, and disorientation.

Nursing Diagnosis	Nursing Intervention/Rationale
	• Administer antiemetics as ordered *to prevent elevated intraocular pressure.* • Avoid excessive restlessness, jarring or bumping head, sneezing, coughing, and vomiting.
Pain related to postoperative status	• Monitor patient's pain (which is usually moderate) and administer narcotics according to physician's orders.

Patient Education

1. Inform the patient that cycloplegic and antibiotic eye drops will be continued at home. Review the procedure for administering eye drops and emphasize the importance of maintaining the prescribed dosage and washing the hands thoroughly before administration.
2. Tell the patient to avoid constipation (straining), sneezing, jarring head movements, and heavy exercise for the first 4 to 6 weeks at home.
3. Inform the patient that television watching is permitted but reading should generally be avoided for the first week (physician will specify).
4. If the patient's occupation is sedentary, work may be resumed after the second week at home (physician will specify).
5. Tell the patient to be aware of visual changes or sensation and to report sudden loss of vision, severe pain in the eyeball, a heavy shower of floaters, or flashing lights to the physician. (Usually some floaters are seen for a period of weeks postoperatively, but they should be reported.)
6. Have the patient schedule an appointment with the physician a week after hospital discharge.[36]
7. With the patient and physician, review and ensure that the patient understands visual status, including the possibility of recurrence of detachment in the affected eye, ultimate visual acuity and macular damage, and potential for retinal detachment or holes in the other eye.

Evaluation

Outcomes vary from a fully restored healthy retina with fully functional vision to total loss of central or peripheral vision, or both, with marked retinal destruction.

Patient Outcome	Data Indicating That Outcome is Reached
Vision returns.	Vision returns to or approaches previous acuity.
Condition of retina is optimal for patient.	Appearance of retina returns to normal or shows improvement.
Patient adjusts to partial or complete loss of vision.	Patient is fully informed about present visual status and prognosis. Patient is able to draw on effective support system to supplement self-care. Patient is aware of safety measures to use in home or community.

Visual impairment

(Blindness)

Visual impairment is a state of diminished visual acuity that ranges from low vision (partial vision) to total blindness.

Legal blindness was defined in the United States in the 1920s and 1930s as a means to identify people who could not function in society without official assistance. The legally blind category, still used today, includes individuals with a maximum acuity of 20/200 (with optimum correction) and/or a visual field that is reduced to a range of 20 degrees (rather than the normal range of 180 degrees). This definition is unique to the United States and does not reflect the universal visual status and complementary needs for visual assistance that people present to the health professions.

The World Health Organization and a variety of experts have attempted to define and standardize categories of visual impairment to serve as guidelines for research and reporting. Table 6-3 is adapted from the International Classification of Diseases, published by the World Health Organization in 1977.

Pathophysiology

The categories of impairment are helpful to health professionals but still do not incorporate the vast array of visual

Table 6-3
Categories of Visual Impairment

Category	Visual Acuity (with Optimum Correction)	Visual Field Radius
Low Vision Status		
1	20/70	Not defined
2	20/70 to 20/200	Not defined
Blindness Status		
3	Able to count fingers at 3 m; 20/200 to 20/400	Radius reduced to 5-10 degrees regardless of visual acuity status
4	Able to count fingers at 1 m; 20/400 to 20/1200 (5/300)	Radius reduced to 5-10 degrees regardless of visual acuity status
5	No light perception	—

Modified from Vaughan.[60]

alterations that must be assessed, managed, or prevented. Regardless of the specific disorder or the degree of impairment, most visual alterations are frightening, immobilizing, and handicapping to an individual. Uncorrected myopia can seriously hamper a person's performance in school. A lack of near vision can cause the loss of a job. Visual field loss can contribute to an automobile accident or a disastrous fall at home. Even a minor transient incident such as a mild corneal abrasion arouses fear of further visual loss and temporarily incapacitates the patient. Nurses are called upon to provide comfort, education, and skilled care whether a patient has a symptom, a specific disease, a concern, or simply healthy vision that can be maintained with knowledgeable health promotion practices. The purpose of this section is to present some of the major causes of blindness or visual impairment throughout the world and to identify the major disorders that are treatable, correctable, and preventable.

More than 79.5 million Americans have a disorder of one or both eyes, not including the millions who have refractive errors. The chief causes of blindness in the United States are retinal degeneration, glaucoma, cataract, and amblyopia. With the exception of amblyopia, most of these diseases are associated with aging and are increasing in incidence as the American population grows older. Laser therapy has helped slow or stop visual deterioration associated with retinal degeneration in recent years. Macular degeneration is still often untreatable as are some forms of congenital retinal disorders. Some research has shown a correlation between poor control of diabetes mellitus in the first 5 years of the disease and the incidence of diabetic retinopathy, indicating that rigorous control of the disease may prevent or deter the onset of visual complications. However, as more diabetic individuals survive early and middle adulthood because of better care, the number of visually handicapped people is likely to increase. At present, about 413,000 people in this country have visual impairments, and 192,500 are legally blind because of retinal diseases. Further research is in progress in the areas of diabetic care, laser therapy, and other forms of retinal therapy. Genetic counseling and research are expected to reduce the incidence of some disorders. Early detection and careful monitoring of a number of systemic diseases, especially diabetes and cardiovascular disorders, will eliminate or slow visual complications. In addition, rehabilitative services for the visually handicapped continue to improve the quality of life for these individuals.

Cataract, another disease associated with aging, is usually treatable with surgery (removal of the lens), and vision is usually restored so the individual can function satisfactorily. The surgical procedure has become more available and simpler since patients no longer have to wait for surgery until they are severely handicapped and they do not have to endure long recovery periods. The incidence of cataract is increasing because Americans are living longer. One study reported that 18% of the group between the ages of 65 and 74 years showed a decrease in vision to 20/30 or less, and 46% of those between 75 and 85 years of age showed the same effect; in both sets the effect was related to cataract. Yet even with improved and simplified treatment, about 71,500 people in this country are legally blind because of cataract.

Glaucoma is still a leading cause of blindness in this country, but it is becoming less so because detection and early care have enabled people to control intraocular pressure and prevent optic nerve deterioration. Vision screening, compliance with prescribed care, and familial screening and counseling are major issues with this disorder.

Blindness from amblyopia can be prevented with comprehensive eye examination of infants and acuity screening and follow-up with preschool children.

The World Health Organization estimates that 10 million people throughout the world are totally blind and that millions more have incapacitating impairments. The leading worldwide causes of blindness are trachoma, leprosy, onchocerciasis, and xerophthalmia. Trachoma, a form of chronic keratoconjunctivitis caused by *Chlamydia trachomatis,* currently affects about 400 million people. It exists primarily in rural areas of the Middle East, Africa, and Asia, where poverty, crowding, flies, lack of sanitation, and malnutrition dominate. It can be cured with sulfonamides and tetracyclines, but if it is not treated, recurrent scarring leads to total blindness. In the United States, the disease exists among Indians in the Southwest and in some rural areas. Leprosy (Hansen's disease) affects about 15 million people throughout the world. Chronic eyelid inflammation, keratoconjunctivitis, and iritis result in granuloma formation and eventual blindness. The disease is treated systemically, and topical rifampin is used with severe corneal involvement. Because international reporting systems are vague, the estimates of the percentage of eye involvement from the systemic disease range from 6% to 90%. The disease is uncommon in the United States. Onchocerciasis (river blindness) is transmitted by black fly bites. Infected larvae are deposited in clear running streams in Central Africa, Mexico, and Central and South America. Microfilariae from the adult female enter the eyes and cause corneal opacification, inflammation and atrophy of the iris, and eventual destruction of the eyes. Treatment is not very effective, and attempts are being made to rid areas of the fly with insecticides. It is estimated that this disease affects about 40 million people. Xerophthalmia (dry eye) is caused by protein, calorie, and vitamin A deficiency. If the cornea is not protected with moisture, it softens, becomes vulnerable to fungal and bacterial invasion, or becomes necrotic. Eventually retinal deterioration and destruction of the optic nerve result in blindness. In countries where malnutrition is common (India, Bangladesh), infants with this disorder frequently die of infection or pneumonia before reaching adulthood. Supplemental vitamin A (along with anti-infective agents) can reverse early eye complications and prevent blindness.

Besides the most common causes of blindness, other disorders contribute greatly to visual impairment. Corneal diseases and infestations are not the major contributors to blindness that they are in other parts of the world because Americans have better access to a higher quality of care. However, herpes simplex virus is being reported and treated increasingly in the United States. The treatments are partially successful, and new antiviral agents are being explored, but the disease tends to recur or reactivate and threatens the corneal structure. Some corneal problems have occurred because of use or misuse of contact lenses (see p. 643). The cornea is also vulnerable to damage from exposure to toxic agents (in vapor, spray, dust, or liquid form) such as ammonia, butanol, lime and cement dust, some forms of detergents and pesticides, and other concentrated liquid alkalies or acids. People must be educated and counseled about early symptoms of eye irritation or inflammation and measures to protect the eyes.

Safety regulations need to be explored and put into practice to assist the public with eye protection. Protective goggles should be worn in some work settings and while traveling on vehicles in the open air. Some sports activities require eye protection. The scrutiny of children's toys and the laws that some states have passed regulating the sale of BB guns have helped reduce eye injuries.

Many other varieties of eye diseases threaten visual functioning. Most are treatable if detected early and followed by skilled therapy. The American Academy of Ophthalmology's Committee on Eye Care states, "Despite the fact that an increasing number of people seek out and utilize eye care services, approximately a third of all new blindness is potentially avoidable if only Americans had access to or could take full advantage of existing and available technology . . . ."[12]

NURSING CARE

Nursing Assessment

Signs and Symptoms for Further Evaluation or Referral

Blurred vision (uncorrectable with lenses; uncorrectable by wiping film from eyes); double vision; sudden loss of vision; alternating dimming and clearing of vision; red eye; traumatized eye; eye pain; loss of side vision; haloes (colored rays or circles around lights); crossed, turned, or wandering eye; twitching or shaking eye; flashes or streaks of light; floaters (dots, streaks, or strands, especially in showers or large numbers, or a floater that does not go away); a sense of pressure or "pulling" within the eye; discharge, crusting, or excessive tearing; swelling of any part of the eye; bulging of one or both eyes; difference in size of eyes or pupils

Emotional Reactions

Fear, immobilization (physical and emotional), anxiety, disorientation, altered self-esteem, altered body image

Chronic Visual Impairment

Possible unsafe living conditions, possible isolation, possible nutritional deficit (related to self-care), possible general ineffective coping (with activities of daily living, earning income, maintaining support system, intellectual stimulation, or recreational activities)

Nursing Dx & Intervention

Nursing Diagnosis	Nursing Intervention/Rationale
Potential for injury related to sudden onset of alteration in eye or vision	• Assess eye surface and lid for signs listed above. • Assess patient for visual symptoms listed above. • Apply pressure patch or shield (with trauma) *to protect from further injury.* • Refer patient to physician *to secure medical diagnosis, care, and prognosis.* • Provide wheelchair, put up side rails, or assist with walking by offering arm for patient's hand *to ensure safety while transporting patient.*
Fear related to sudden onset of alteration in eye or vision	• Assess patient's level of fear. • Orient patient to surroundings, people in the vicinity, and procedures taking place *to alleviate as much uncertainty as possible.*

Nursing Diagnosis	Nursing Intervention/Rationale
	• Constantly reassure patient that he or she is being cared for: speak in a soothing voice and use touch as a comfort. • Avoid lengthy and complicated explanations *to avoid sensory overload.* • Maintain a quiet atmosphere.
Pain	• Administer topical analgesic as soon as ordered. • Apply eye patch after treatment as ordered *to alleviate discomfort from photophobia.* • Administered cycloplegics as ordered *to reduce painful pupillary constriction.* • Administer systemic analgesics as ordered.
Potential for infection	• Administer topical and systemic anti-infectives as ordered.
Sensory/perceptual alterations (visual) related to use of unilateral eye patch	*Before surgery or treatment:* • Warn patient that depth perception will be lost and 50% of peripheral vision will be lost on affected side. *After surgery:* • Help patient with activities of daily living. • Caution patient to bring hand forward slowly to touch objects (especially containers of hot liquids and containers receiving poured liquids) *to ensure safety.* • Explain that patient should turn head fully toward affected side *to view objects or obstacles.* • Teach patient to use up and down head movements to judge stairs and oncoming objects and to proceed slowly *to compensate for loss of three-dimensional vision.*
Sensory/perceptual alterations (visual) related to use of bilateral eye patches	*Before surgery or treatment:* • Warn patient that eyes will be patched. • If possible, orient patient to bedside equipment and room arrangement *to avoid or reduce disorientation.* • Arrange for placement of personal belongings in advance, and review plan with patient. • Warn patient that side rails will be raised for safety. *After surgery:* • Assess patient's level of anxiety and disorientation. • Reorient patient to equipment (such as call light) and personal belongings at bedside by directing patient's hand. • If necessary review immediate past events and procedures with patient *to assist in reorientation.* • Raise side rails *to ensure safety.* • Address patient from doorway and identify yourself. • Complement voice stimulation with touch *to notify patient of your proximity.* • Help family members and other staff to use vocal and touch approach *to reduce patient's anxiety.* • Encourage patient to perform self-care with personal hygiene. • Ensure patient's privacy, and assure patient that privacy is being provided. • Provide patient with television set or radio *to encourage mental and memory stimulation.* • Provide patient with clock that can be felt and remind patient of date. • Help patient with meals. Read menu selections. Guide hand to utensils and food on tray. Describe food on tray in clock terms (e.g., coffee is at 2 o'clock, knife and spoon are at 3 o'clock). Help with cutting meats, removing lids from containers, buttering bread, and so on. • Assist with walking. Walk slowly and slightly ahead of patient; patient's hand should rest on your arm at elbow. If possible, allow patient to trace progress by running the dorsal aspect of his or her free hand along the wall. Describe surroundings as you proceed. Warn of steps, turns, and narrow passageways in advance. Allow patient to feel chair, toilet, or bed before turning to sit.
Knowledge deficit related to cause of visual loss and ways to prevent further loss or maintain present vision	• Assess patient's knowledge about events and localized or systemic causes for visual alteration. • Assess patient's level of knowledge about the treatment prescribed. • Assess patient's capacity and motivation for further learning *to avoid patient education that is not usable* (because of anxiety, inability to take in too much or too complicated information at one time, or because patient cannot read directions or labels). • Plan to extend elaborate teaching beyond hospital stay *to avoid sensory overload.*
Impaired adjustment related to irreversible loss of vision	• Assess patient's personal reactions to present level of visual functioning. • Assess patient's reactions to anticipated discharge from hospital and functioning at home.

Nursing Diagnosis	Nursing Intervention/Rationale
	• Help patient identify specific fears in terms of self-care. • Provide specific information about visual capacity and changes that will have to be made at home.
Potential for trauma related to self-care at home with impaired vision	• Assess patient's visual functioning in relation to self-care potential (e.g., ability to drive an automobile, maneuver in home, maneuver in community, support system available to assist, access to community). • Help patient and family identify specific changes that must be made to ensure safety (e.g., driving prohibited, placing furniture in home in familiar locations) *to prevent falls and increase independence.* • Plan for assessment and counseling beyond hospital stay *to monitor safety and deal with problems as they arise at home.*
Self-esteem disturbance related to irreversibly impaired vision	• Assess patient's feelings about himself or herself in the context of living and functioning with visual loss. • Assess family's perception of patient's ability to function with impaired vision. • Identify specific self-care capabilities in the hospital and encourage patient to exercise self-care *to help patient achieve a sense of independence.* • Encourage patient to make as many decisions as possible about daily routines *to enhance competence.*
Family coping: potential for growth	• Assess family's reaction to patient's altered visual status. • Discuss family's changed perceptions with family members *to make them more aware of altered behavior toward patient.* • Encourage family to help patient toward independent living as quickly as possible. • Recognize that family dynamics will change over a long period of time and that continued counseling should be available.

Patient Education

1. Describe the anatomy and function of the normal eye.
2. Describe the alterations in visual function that have occurred.
3. Clarify the prognosis so that the patient understands the time frame and degree of recovery or the degree of irreversible visual impairment.
4. While the patient is in the hospital, teach and help him or her practice self-assistance skills to maximize independence:
   a. Exploring and mapping out furniture, steps, and doorways in the room through guidance and touch
   b. Using another's arm to serve as a guide when walking
   c. Tracing the wall (or rail) with free hand to orient to perimeters of the room while walking
   d. Using a lightweight walking stick when walking alone to identify obstacles
   e. Exploring food, containers, liquids, and utensils with touch before eating
   f. Feeling chairs or toilet before turning to sit
   g. Obtaining assistance for selection of clothing before dressing and approval and support of appearance afterward
   h. Placing articles for grooming and hygiene near bed and arranging them so they can be retrieved whenever patient wishes
5. On discharge, review specific hazards in the home with patient and family:
   a. The patient's room arrangement and living quarters should not be altered once the patient is familiar with the placement of furniture and furnishings.
   b. The patient should proceed slowly and with assistance in exploring living arrangements.
   c. The family must evaluate and maintain living quarters for a clutter-free environment (e.g., loose throw rugs, loose articles on floor or stairways, electric cords).
   d. Exploration of the outdoors must proceed carefully and with assistance (uneven ground, steps, loose gravel, and icy sidewalks are some of the additional hazards of the outdoors).
   e. Exploration of the community must proceed slowly and with assistance.
6. Warn the patient and family that progress will be slow; they must allow for frustration and should seek additional support from community or health agencies.
7. Encourage the family to explore the future for increased independence when the patient has made initial adjustments to impaired vision. The state agency for the blind should be contacted immediately upon discharge; this agency can give early assistance and provide support for future concerns (e.g., computer-assisted reading, talking books, time and temperature devices, rehabilitation for future employment, acquisition of new skills).

8. In collaboration with the physician, teach the patient to care for eye(s) at home:
   a. Administering drops or ointment as prescribed
   b. Keeping eye(s) free of infection by washing hands, not contaminating dropper, using clean tissues or cloth to wipe eyes, and gently wiping from inner to outer canthus
   c. Monitoring eye(s) for signs and symptoms of infection (pain, itching, redness, swelling, discharge)
   d. Monitoring eye(s) for signs and symptoms of the specific disorder

Evaluation

Patient Outcome	Data Indicating That Outcome is Reached
Patient adjusts to visual impairment.	Patient reports no signs or symptoms of infection or disease. Patient reports no accidents in the home or community. Patient reports satisfaction with self-care abilities. Patient reports progress with (or mastery of) selected visual handicap aids. Patient reports ability to earn income or is seeking or getting employment training. Patient reports interpersonal relationships are satisfactory. Patient reports resumption of old recreational or diversional skills or acquisition of new ones. Patient exhibits confidence in caring for himself or herself and in relating to others.

Medical Interventions and Related Nursing Care

Contact Lenses

Description and Rationale

Contact lenses are rounded plastic discs that are curved and shaped to fit over the cornea and beneath the eyelid. As methods for producing them improve, they are being used increasingly as a substitute for eyeglasses to correct refractive errors.

Contact lenses, introduced in the 1940s, are available in many forms and serve a multitude of purposes. Hard lenses were originally used to correct refractive errors and high astigmatism associated with corneal irregularities.[60] The introduction of soft lenses in 1971 and extended-wear lenses in 1981 has expanded the benefits of contact lenses and the indications for their use.[39] Some of the major indications for contact lenses are cosmetic preference over eyeglasses, monocular aphakia, marked difference in refractive error between eyes (anisometropia), active occupation or sports participation, and severe corneal irregularities.

A major concern with all types of lenses is to maintain an adequate oxygen supply to the corneal surface. The cornea receives most of its oxygen from precorneal tears. Contact lenses float on the precorneal tear film and act as foreign bodies that interrupt normal tear flow.

Hard or rigid lenses often cover only the corneal surface (7 to 9 mm in diameter).[41,57] Blinking action pumps tear fluid under the lens to keep the corneal surface moist. The corneal lens is small enough to shift during blinking so tears can be pumped under the lens and debris can be carried away from the cornea. Some hard lenses are fashioned to cover the cornea and part of the sclera. A buffer solution is then required to keep the chamber between the cornea and the lens full of fluid.[57] Scleral lenses are less comfortable than corneal lenses and more difficult to wear. Hard lenses are still prescribed for correction of marked corneal irregularities because their shape does not conform to the corneal surface as readily as soft lenses and they provide better peripheral vision. Hard lenses can be worn only for a limited time (10 to 14 hours) and are not worn during sleep. They eventually change the shape of the corneal surface and therefore cannot be worn alternately with eyeglasses.

Soft lenses are made of hydrophilic plastics that increase access of fluid to the cornea. They are usually larger in diameter and more easily tolerated than hard lenses and can be worn longer. They are regarded as a medical device and are regulated by the Food and Drug Administration. Soft lenses absorb medications, cleaning solutions, and chlorinated water from swimming pools and gradually release them into the tear film.[41] This can cause local irritation and systemic side effects. Soft lenses are removed every day for cleansing and are not worn during sleeping hours to allow the cornea to recover.

Extended-wear lenses are designed to provide continuous oxygen to the cornea. One type of lens is ultrathin and permits absorption of oxygen through it. The other type is thicker but has a higher concentration of water (70% to 80%), which continuously bathes the corneal surface.[7] Extended-wear lenses can be worn for periods ranging from a few days to several months, depending on patient tolerance, self-care habits, and the patient's eye condition. The effects of extended wear and the development of new materials are the subjects of considerable research.[3]

Contact lenses are successfully worn by many people but are definitely contraindicated in some instances. Corneal infection and damage can occur if lenses are not handled appropriately. People who wear lenses must have a clear understanding of how to insert, remove, and care for them. Misuse can result in severe eye damage and loss of vision.

Contraindications

Chaotic or disorganized life-style
Lack of motivation to monitor eye responses and care for lenses
Manual dexterity problems or any condition that interferes with daily removal and insertion and lens care (Daily-wear lenses can sometimes be replaced with extended-wear lenses that are monitored, removed, and cleaned by a professional.)
Poor blinking or lid function
Diminished corneal sensation
Chronic blepharitis or conjunctivitis
Occupation or life-style that involves heavy fumes or dust in the environment
High astigmatism (contraindicated for soft and extended-wear lenses)[4,5]

Medical Plan[39,60]

The patient is evaluated for indications and contraindications for lens wearing and the appropriate type of lens. After the lenses are prescribed and fitted, the patient is closely followed for signs of complications. The major complications are corneal abrasion, corneal edema, infection, ulceration, tight lens syndrome, and giant papillary syndrome.

Corneal Abrasions

Corneal abrasions occur when hard lenses are left in too long (overwear syndrome) and drying of the corneal surface results in minute epithelial breaks. Abrasions also form if foreign bodies lie between the lens and the cornea or if the corneal surface is scraped during insertion or removal. A fluorescein stain can be used to identify epithelial breaks. The patient experiences severe pain and usually seeks care immediately. Epithelial abrasions can heal in 24 to 48 hours.

Medications

Anti-infective agents
- Sulfisoxazole (Gantrisin) 4% ointment applied to each eye before 24-h patching
- Sulfacetamide sodium (Sulamyd) 10% ointment applied to each eye before 24-h patching

Anesthetics
- Proparacaine (Ophthaine) 0.5% solution, 1-2 drops in each eye, gives relief for 10-15 min

Mydriatic-cycloplegic agents
- Tropicamide (Mydriacyl) 0.5%-1% solution, 1-2 drops bid or tid for 24 h

General Management

Binocular tight patches for 24 hours (if patient has someone to care for him or her) or monocular patch on more painful eye and mydriatic drops in open eye to reduce ciliary spasm and pain (see above for dosage); reexamination of patient in 24 hours[39]

Corneal Edema

Corneal edema most commonly occurs with soft or extended-wear lenses because of a more gradual oxygen deprivation to the cornea. The epithelium becomes edematous, and vision becomes blurred. There is usually no pain, but slight redness of the eye may be evident.

General Management

Removal of contact lens reverses condition; lens prescription may have to be changed

Corneal Ulceration and Infection

Corneal ulceration and infection occur if corneal abrasions or edema are not successfully treated. A secondary uveitis may ensue and require intensive emergency care to prevent loss of vision (see pp. 608 to 610 for pathophysiology and interventions). Infection also occurs if insertion, removal, and lens care are not managed hygienically by the patient.

Medications

Anti-infective agents
- Sulfacetamide sodium (Sulamyd) 10% or 30% solution, 1-2 drops several times/d for 3-7 d (varies with severity of infection)
- Sulfisoxazole (Gantrisin) 4% solution, 1-2 drops several times/d (varies with severity of infection)

General Management

Warm compresses for discomfort and inflammation for 10 to 15 minutes two or three times a day

Tight Lens Syndrome

Tight lens syndrome occurs in soft lens wearers. The lens tends to change in shape and become more curved and less mobile over the cornea. The change may take place within hours after the fitting or within several days (with extended-wear lenses). The wearer experiences decreased visual acuity and conjunctival congestion.[10]

General Management

Removal of lens reverses process; wearer may have to be refitted with new prescription

Giant Papillary Syndrome

Giant papillary syndrome occurs after several months or years of lens wearing and manifests itself as a cobblestone-appearing inflammation of the inner lining of the upper lid. Redness, tearing, and discharge accompany the tissue inflammation. The cause is unknown, and the treatment is removal of the lens.[60]

NURSING CARE

Nursing Assessment[3,39,41,60]

Corneal Abrasion (Epithelial)

Moderate to severe pain; blurred vision; halo seen around lights; generalized hyperemia; lacrimation; fluorescein stains (green) on corneal surface; patient unable to open eyes (owing to pain)

Corneal Edema

Blurred vision; absence of pain; dull appearance of cornea; slightly reddened conjunctiva

Corneal Ulceration

Ulcers varying in appearance and size; whitish gray opacity with overhanging margins; severe pain associated with epithelial damage; iritis; lacrimation and possible purulent discharge; generalized hyperemia

Localized Infection

Purulent discharge; generalized hyperemia; moderate discomfort; possible photophobia; crusting around lids; eyes may be "stuck together" in morning (or on awakening); complaints of blurred vision (owing to excessive exudate over eye surface), which disappears with blinking

Tight Lens Syndrome

Eye discomfort; decreased visual acuity (onset may be sudden [within hours] or more gradual); patient unable to remove lens; conjunctival congestion with some redness

Giant Papillary Syndrome

Bilateral cobblestone appearance of inner lining of upper eyelids; slow onset over months or years; lacrimation; conjunctival redness; discharge may be present

Nursing Dx & Intervention

Nursing Diagnosis	Nursing Intervention/Rationale
Knowledge deficit related to care of contact lenses	• See "Patient Education" for specific instructions. • Deficit exists with new prescription or if medical problems arise after lenses are fitted.
Potential for injury related to epithelial damage to cornea with potential for stroma injury	• Assist with identification of epithelial breaks with fluorescein stain as ordered. • Instill medications as ordered, such as topical antibiotics and cycloplegic drops.
Pain related to corneal epithelial damage	• Apply pressure bandage to eye(s) as ordered, being certain that covered eye is closed *to reduce blinking and eye movement.* • Apply topical anesthetic as ordered. • Apply warm compress as ordered for 10 to 15 minutes for inflammation or discomfort. • Administer systemic analgesic as ordered and document response. • Discourage patient from reading *to reduce eye movement.*
Sensory/perceptual alterations (visual) related to total loss of vision with binocular patches	• Raise side rails *to ensure safety.* • Address patient by name from doorway and identify yourself and reason for presence. • Complement voice stimulation with touch *to notify patient of your proximity.* • Orient patient to bedside equipment (such as call light, bed control, and side rails) and personal belongings at bedside by directing his or her hand over objects. • Encourage patient to perform self-care with personal hygiene *to maximize independence.* Provide support and supervision. • Provide privacy, and ensure patient that privacy is provided. • Help with meals. Read menu selections. Guide hand to utensils and food on tray. Describe food on tray in clock terms. Assist with cutting meat, removing lids from cartons, and so on. • Help with walking. Walk slowly and slightly ahead of patient with patient's hand resting on your arm at your elbow or on your shoulders.

Nursing Diagnosis	Nursing Intervention/Rationale
	If possible, allow patient to trace progress by running the dorsal aspect of his or her free hand along the wall. Describe surroundings as you proceed. Allow patient to feel chair, toilet, or bed before turning to sit. • Visit frequently to be certain patient is sufficiently stimulated *to avoid withdrawal.* • Be certain that someone will be at home to supervise patient's activity after discharge. • Review above safety and comfort measures with caretaker.[36]
Sensory/perceptual alterations (visual) related to blurred vision with corneal edema or tight lens	• Assure patient that condition is temporary. • Review activities of daily living (such as driving, preparing food, housekeeping, personal hygiene, toileting, and maneuvering around house) and responsibilities at work *to be certain that they can be performed safely by patient or with assistance from someone else.*

Patient Education[3,39,41,60]

1. Caution the patient to wash hands and dry well before inserting and removing lenses.
2. Tell the patient that eyelashes and face should be thoroughly cleaned before lenses are inserted.
3. Inform the patient that instructions for care and follow-up should be carried out meticulously.
4. Explain the care of hard contact lenses.
   a. Encourage the patient to monitor himself or herself for sudden onset of pain, excessive eye redness, sudden decrease in vision, mucus discharge, or foreign body sensation. Tell the patient to remove the lenses and report to the physician.
   b. Inform the patient that adjustment to new lenses may take 2 to 3 weeks and that mild photophobia, tearing, and lid edema may occur.
   c. Inform the patient that hard lenses are not recommended for wearing alternately with glasses or on a part-time basis after initial adjustment and that wearing time will increase to 10 to 14 hours after the adjustment period.
   d. Inform the patient that hard lenses should not be worn when engaging in contact sports.
   e. Tell the patient that lenses must be removed at night or before sleeping.
   f. Explain that lenses must be cleaned after each removal according to the manufacturer's directions and stored in their case.
   g. Explain that the lens is wetted with an approved wetting solution before being placed over the cornea.
   h. Review the insertion and removal procedure with the patient and have the patient demonstrate it to ensure competence.
   i. Inform the patient of the importance of consistently applying one lens before the other to avoid mixing the lenses. If vision is blurred immediately after application, the lenses may be reversed.
   j. Tell the patient to check the lenses daily for scratches, tears, loose debris, or clouding. Tell the patient to report to the physician if unable to wash the lenses clear.
   k. Emphasize the need to keep appointments with the physician. Eyes may change shape, or refractory error may cause changes. Lenses should be replaced regularly (usually every 1 to 2 years).
5. Explain the care of soft and extended-wear lenses.
   a. Encourage the patient to monitor himself or herself for sudden onset of pain, excessive eye redness, sudden decrease in vision, mucus discharge, or foreign body sensation. Tell the patient to remove the lenses and report to the physician.
   b. Inform the patient that the adjustment time for soft lenses is usually shorter and involves less eye irritation than with hard lenses.
   c. Inform the patient that soft lenses are less likely to pop out.
   d. Tell the patient that soft lenses can be alternated with glasses.
   e. Caution the patient not to wear soft lenses while swimming, applying eye medications, or using hair or body sprays because soft lenses absorb chemicals easily.
   f. Explain that soft lenses are usually removed at night and that the wearing time will increase to 12 to 14 hours after adjustment time.
   g. Tell the patient that lenses must be cleaned after each removal according to the manufacturer's instructions and stored in a specified solution. Soft lenses should not be permitted to dry out.
   h. Explain that the storage solution must be changed as directed.
   i. Inform the patient soft lenses are fragile and can be damaged by exposure to makeup, creams, or mascara or nicked by fingernails.

j. Tell the patient that lenses should be checked daily for scratches, tears, loose debris, or clouding. Tell the patient to report to the physician if unable to wash the lenses clear.
k. Explain that the lens must be wetted with an approved wetting solution before being placed in the eye.
l. Review the insertion and removal procedure with the patient and have the patient demonstrate it to ensure competence.
m. Inform the patient of the importance of consistently applying one lens before the other to avoid mixing the lenses. If vision is blurred immediately after application, the lenses may be reversed.
n. Stress the need to keep appointments with the physician, since the eyes and lenses should be checked regularly.

Evaluation

Patient Outcome	Data Indicating that Outcome is Reached
Cornea is healthy.	Cornea is clear and glossy without eye discomfort, redness, or discharge.
Contact lenses are successfully worn.	Visual acuity is 20/20 OD, OS, and OU. Near vision is clear at 14 inches.[4]

Enucleation

Description and Rationale

Enucleation, or surgical removal of the eyeball, is performed when other treatment of the eyeball is insufficient to prevent pain, disfigurement, or spread of malignant disease. Indications include severe infections, malignancies such as melanoma and retinoblastoma, large and infiltrating tumors, extensive trauma to the eye, blindness when severe eye pain is also present, and end-stage glaucoma, when the patient is blind with no light perception and has increased intraocular pressure. Enucleation may also be performed for cosmetic improvement of a blind eye and as a prophylactic measure when sympathetic ophthalmia is likely to occur. Sympathetic ophthalmia is a rare granulomatous inflammation that usually develops within 3 months of an injury to one eye and involves the entire area. The injured eye is called the exciting eye, and the other eye (the sympathizing eye) can also become inflamed with uveitis unless the exciting eye is enucleated before the inflammation spreads.

Enucleation can be performed with the patient under local or general anesthetic. During surgery a 360-degree peritomy is performed at the limbus, opening the conjunctiva and allowing Tenon's fascia to be separated between the rectus muscles. The rectus muscles are separated, hooked, and cut with scissors near their insertion into the sclera. The inferior oblique muscle and superior oblique tendons are hooked and cut, the medius rectus muscle is clamped, and enucleation scissors are placed between the sclera and Tenon's capsule. The optic nerve is then cut as far behind the globe as possible, and the eye is removed.[55] After adequate hemostasis is obtained at the socket, the muscles may be sutured to each other around a plastic or Teflon sphere to build up the eye and provide a more acceptable cosmetic appearance.

After the enucleation a "conformer" is placed in the socket until postoperative edema subsides and an artificial eye can be placed, usually 10 to 14 days after enucleation.

Two relevant surgical procedures are evisceration and exenteration. In evisceration the entire contents of the eyeball and sometimes the cornea are removed but the sclera remains. This procedure may be used when panophthalmitis, an inflammation of the entire inner eye including the sclera, is present. Exenteration is a more radical procedure in which the eyelids, eyeball, and orbital contents are removed, usually in cases of malignancies of the lacrimal gland, extension of eyelid malignancies in the orbit, malignant melanoma of the conjunctiva, or melanoma or retinoblastoma that has invaded the orbit.

Contraindications and Cautions

Panophthalmitis is a contraindication to enucleation because the risk of postoperative meningitis is increased after removal of an actively infected eyeball.

Medical Plan

Surgery

Removal of the eyeball as described previously

Medications

Narcotic-analgesic agents
- Meperidine (Demerol), 50-75 mg IM q4-6h prn for severe pain

Acetaminophen with codeine (Tylenol with Codeine), 30-60 mg po q4-6h prn for less severe pain

General Management

Firm pressure dressing applied to operative site for 24 to 48 hours
Activity progression without restrictions as tolerated
Progressive diet as tolerated

NURSING CARE

Nursing Assessment

Eye Socket

Pain at enucleation site; headache on side of enucleation; no fever or bleeding

Nursing Dx & Intervention

Nursing Diagnosis	Nursing Intervention/Rationale
Pain	• Administer pain medications as ordered by physician and document response. • Notify physician if pain or headache persists, *since this may indicate infection.* • Notify physician if temperature is elevated.
Potential for injury	• Assess dressing at operative site frequently for signs of oozing or frank bleeding. • Document absence of blood or amount if present. • Maintain firm pressure dressing at operative site until removal is ordered by physician. • Monitor and document patients' vital signs according to protocol, and report any change in pulse and blood pressure.
Sensory/perceptual alterations (visual)	• Help patient walk as tolerated. • Ensure that patient's call light and personal belongings are close by on unaffected side. • Help patient with meals as needed.
Body image disturbance	• Assess patient for depression and anxiety. • Assure patient that appearance will be quite normal when patient is fitted with artificial eye and that satisfactory visual adjustment usually occurs. • Listen to patient's fears and concerns in comforting, supportive manner. • Assure patient that period of depression is normal after procedure such as removal of eye.

Patient Education

1. Teach the patient how to care for the eye socket. These instructions are usually given on an outpatient basis.
2. Teach the patient and family how to care for, insert, and remove an artificial eye if one is used. The artificial eye is fitted after the patient leaves the hospital and the wound has healed.
3. Ensure that the patient is aware of the need to protect the vision in the remaining eye. Some physicians recommend that a patient wear safety glasses for protection.
4. Educate the patient regarding the signs and symptoms of infection, abscess, and meningitis.
5. Discuss the limited field of vision and the need to exaggerate head movement to achieve a full visual field, for example, when driving. Discuss the changes in depth perception.

Evaluation

Patient Outcome	Data Indicating That Outcome is Reached
There is no infection.	Patient and family demonstrate ability to care for eye socket and artificial eye after discharge from hospital. Patient verbalizes signs and symptoms of possible infection: pain, headache, drainage, and elevated temperature.
Body image is adequate.	Patient is fitted with and wears artificial eye, if appropriate, to improve appearance after discharge from hospital. Patient verbalizes understanding of need for eye removal and expresses concerns and frustrations regarding disease process and body image.

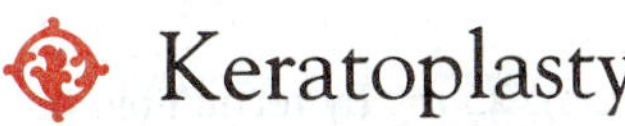

Keratoplasty

Description and Rationale

Keratoplasty, or corneal transplant, is the excision of corneal tissue and its replacement by a cornea from a human donor.[41] This procedure may be performed to replace a corneal opacity, which is a lack of corneal transparency resulting from injury or inflammation, or to correct a variety of corneal abnormalities called corneal dystrophies. Certain bilateral hereditary disorders may be present at birth but usually develop during adolescence and progress through adulthood. Some do not affect vision, but many do. The success of corneal transplantation as a treatment for these dystrophies depends on the type and extent of the corneal abnormality. The dystrophy may possibly recur in the donor graft. One of the dystrophies for which keratoplasty is particularly successful is keratoconus, a condition in which the symmetric curvature of the cornea is distorted by an abnormal thinning and forward bulging of the central portion of the cornea. A penetrating corneal transplant restores useful vision with a 95% success rate.[41] Corneal perforation, which is usually a complication of a corneal ulcer, is a serious condition that may destroy vision if not treated rapidly. Keratoplasty may be performed if there is imminent danger of perforation of a corneal ulcer.

There are two types of keratoplasty: lamellar and penetrating. Lamellar or nonpenetrating keratoplasty is a partial-thickness graft in which the surgeon removes and replaces a superficial layer of cornea without entering the anterior chamber. In a penetrating keratoplasty the entire thickness of cornea is removed and replaced by donor corneal tissue. This is the traditional type of keratoplasy and can be either complete or partial, depending on whether the entire cornea is excised.

Donor eyes are obtained from cadavers of noninfected people who have died as a result of injury or acute disease or from patients whose eyes have been surgically removed for some reason but whose corneas are normal. Ideally the donor is between 25 and 35 years of age. Corneas should not be used from patients who were ill for a long time before death or who had such diseases as leukemia, sepsis, hepatitis, HIV positivity, or certain tumors of the eye.

If it is known when a patient dies that the eyes are to be donated, the lids should be closed and covered with small ice bags. Nothing should touch the corneas themselves. The donor eyes should be enucleated within an hour after death, but up to 5 hours is acceptable if ice bags have been placed on the eyes at death. Ideally corneas are transplanted into the recipient immediately after removal, but many eye banks can now safely store corneas for longer periods. Whole eyes can be stored from 24 to 48 hours if refrigerated; corneal tissue can be kept longer if removed with a 3 mm rim of scleral tissue attached. Corneas must not be folded during storage, because this damages the endothelium. They must be stored at a temperature of 4° C (39° F) in a modified tissue culture medium.[41]

Transplantation is usually performed with the patient under topical and retrobulbar anesthesia. The surgeon removes the cornea from the donor's eye with a trephine and then removes the impaired areas from the recipient eye using another trephine the same size or slightly larger. The donor cornea, called the donor button, is sutured into place with continuous or interrupted sutures to align and graft and ensure a watertight wound (Figure 6-20).

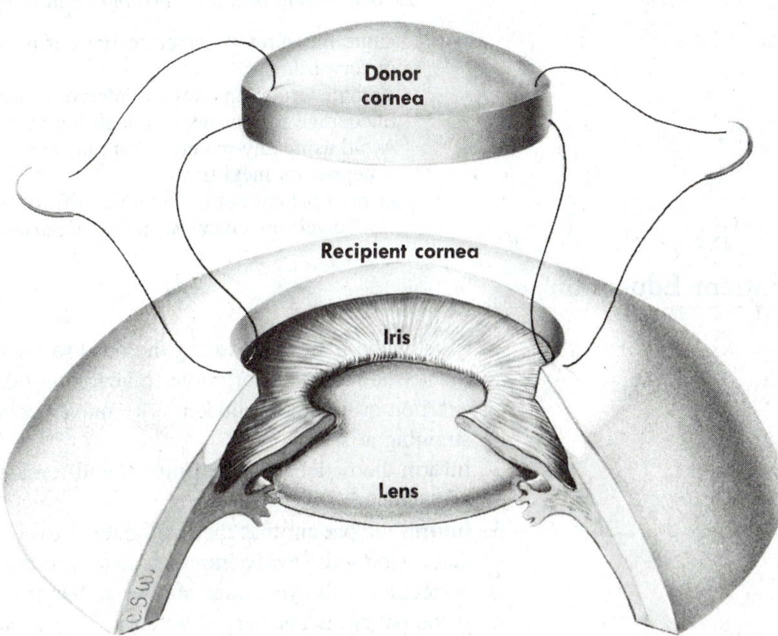

Figure 6-20 Keratoplasty. Excised central portion of cornea is being replaced with clear donor cornea. From Newell.[41]

Contraindications and Cautions

Light perception and projection must be normal before surgery will be considered.

There is the possibility that some corneal dystrophy will recur in the transplanted cornea.

Corneal graft rejection may occur. This starts 3 weeks or more after keratoplasty and is limited to the donor cornea, since there are no blood vessels or lymphatics to sensitize the recipient. The inflammatory process begins at the graft margin and spreads to involve the entire graft.

Medical Plan

Surgery

Lamellar or penetrating keratoplasty as described previously

Medications

Narcotic analgesic agents
- Meperidine (Demerol), 50-100 mg IM q4h prn for pain

Antiemetic agents
- Prochlorperazine (Compazine), 25 mg by rectum bid or 5-10 mg IM q4-6h for nausea

Corticosteroids
- Pred-Forte eye drops, 1 drop qid

Laxatives
- Docusate sodium (Colace), 240 mg po to prevent straining during bowel movement

General Management

Unilateral eye patch for 24 hours

Activity and diet progress as tolerated

NURSING CARE

Nursing Assessment

Cornea

Wound edema; inflammation; photophobia; decreased vision; clouding caused by vascularization as result of graft rejection

Nursing Dx & Intervention

Nursing Diagnosis	Nursing Intervention/Rationale
Sensory/perceptual alterations (visual)	• Ensure that eye patch remains securely in place for at least 24 hours. • Help patient with walking postoperatively, since patient may be unsteady and must be prevented from falling and injuring eye. • Ensure that call light is in place, side rails are up, and items at bedside are in familiar place for patient *to ensure safety*. • Administer eye drops as ordered by physician.
Pain	• Administer pain medication as ordered, particularly on first postoperative night, *to decrease discomfort and promote rest and healing of eye*.
Potential for injury	• Institute measures designed to prevent increases in intraocular pressure that might push healing graft forward. Administer antiemetics as ordered *to prevent vomiting*. Encourage patient not to cough but to breathe deeply often *to increase lung expansion*. Avoid using any material that may cause sneezing: talcum powder, perfumes, room sprays, or pepper on meal trays. Instruct patient not to lean over, lift, or push heavy objects and to avoid straining when having a bowel movement *to avoid increased intraocular pressure*.

Patient Education

1. Instruct the patient regarding the need to prevent increases in intraocular pressure, since eye tissue requires more time to heal than other tissue. Warn the patient to avoid extreme exertion or emotion, sudden jerky movements, lifting or pushing heavy objects, or straining at stool.
2. Inform the patient that the sutures will remain in the eye for as long as a year to ensure adequate healing.
3. Inform the patient that the photophobia experienced after surgery will gradually decrease, that vision will slowly improve, that dark glasses may be worn if needed, and that further correction with eyeglasses may be necessary.
4. If the patient is discharged with eye drops, ensure that the patient or family can demonstrate the appropriate technique of instillation.

5. Instruct the patient and family in the signs and symptoms of graft rejection (inflammation, clouding, drainage, and pain at graft site), and tell them to notify the physician immediately so treatment can begin promptly.

Evaluation

Patient Outcome	Data Indicating That Outcome is Reached
Corneal graft heals adequately.	Wound edema and inflammation dissipate. Photophobia decreases. Vision improves slowly. No evidence of graft rejection occurs. No injury is caused to the graft from increase in intraocular pressure.

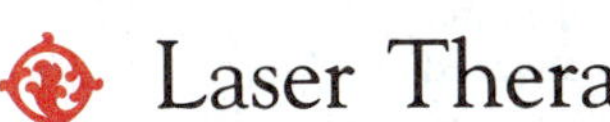

Laser Therapy

Description and Rationale

The word "laser" is an acronym for *l*ight *a*mplification by *s*timulated *e*mission of *r*adiation. Experimentation with the effect of light on the retina began in the 1800s after the invention of the ophthalmoscope, when ophthalmologists began noticing solar burns in patients' eyes after solar eclipses. Early investigators used the effects of the sun or the carbon arc to produce a lesion in the retina.[34] Since that time, research with laser therapy has refined and broadened its use, and lasers are now the treatment of choice for a wide variety of ophthalmic disorders. Laser therapy produces excellent results (Table 6-4). Types of laser used today include argon, xenon arc, ruby, dye, carbon dioxide, and krypton.

A basic principle of laser therapy is that the light absorbed by pigment is converted to heat energy. When enough heat is generated to coagulate the protein in the tissue, a thermal burn, called photocoagulation, ensues. The retinal pigment epithelium and the uveal pigment within the eye are ideal for this absorption of light.[57] Two other types of laser therapy, less widely used than photocoagulation, are photoradiation therapy and photovaporization therapy. Photoradiation therapy is the use of photosensitizing drugs and a dye laser to treat malignant tumors such as melanomas of the eye, and photovaporization therapy is the use of carbon dioxide laser radiation to vaporize malignant intraocular and extraocular tumors in a very precise manner. When repeated surface impacts are made with the carbon dioxide laser, carbon dioxide radiation is highly absorbed by ocular tissue, with almost complete absorption and conversion to heat within a tissue depth of 100 μm.[34]

Photocoagulation provides a nonsurgical approach to many ophthalmic disorders and can usually be performed on an outpatient basis. The goal of photocoagulation therapy is to maintain the hemodynamics, fluid dynamics, and physiologic structure of the macular region. In cases of anatomic barrier breakdown, photocoagulation is used to destroy the offending tissue elements or retinal vessels in an effort to seal the abnormal area and prevent leakage from a retinal or choroidal vascular system into the sensitive sensory retina. In cases of neovascularization, photocoagulation is used to obliterate the newly vascularized areas to prevent further deterioration of the involved regions.[34] It has offered new hope to patients with diabetic retinopathy. Although photocoagulation does not increase vision, it can prevent further loss of vision by cauterizing the newly formed, fragile vessels of the retina with an intense minuscule light beam, thereby diverting blood to the already established sturdy vessels on the retina and eliminating the most likely areas of stress and hemorrhage.[48]

Photocoagulation has also become useful in the treatment of glaucoma to control intraocular pressure. A procedure called laser goniophotocoagulation can control pressure successfully in about 85% of cases, especially in eyes with wide angles and slight pigmentation of the trabecular meshwork.

Laser therapy is also useful in treating chronic primary closed-angle glaucoma. The aim of therapy is to prevent the pressure in the posterior chamber from exceeding that of the anterior chamber by creating an opening that eliminates the accumulation of aqueous humor in the posterior chamber. The surgeon performs a laser iridotomy in which a localized area of the midperipheral iris is caused to bulge forward by means of mild laser burns. The central portion of this area is then perforated by a laser beam of much higher energy. Many applications of the beam may be necessary.[41]

Contraindications and Cautions

Before photocoagulation therapy each segment of the eye must be closely examined for factors that would diminish the effectiveness of therapy, as described in Table 6-5.

Table 6-4

Results of Treatment of Various Ocular Abnormalities by Argon, Xenon Arc, Ruby, Dye, Carbon Dioxide, and Krypton Lasers

Disease	Argon Laser	Xenon Arc	Ruby Laser	Dye Laser	Carbon Dioxide Laser	Krypton Laser	
						Red	Green-Yellow
Peripheral Retinal Structural Abnormalities							
Retinal tears	Excellent*	Excellent	Excellent	Excellent	None	Excellent	Excellent
Retinal degenerations	Excellent*	Excellent	Excellent	Excellent	None	Excellent	Excellent
Retinal detachments	Excellent—requires absorbent pigment*	Excellent—effective with slightly elevated retinas, meridional folds, tears	Good—effective if retina attached	Excellent	None	Good—effective if retina attached	Excellent
Retinoschisis	Good—use limited to delimiting bulla,* possibly barrage	Good—used to barrage* or delimit bulla; with encircling element*	Fair—to delimit bulla after collapse by surgery	Good	None	Fair—to delimit bulla after collapse by surgery	Excellent
Peripheral Retinal Vascular Abnormalities							
Eales' disease	Excellent*	Excellent	Poor	Excellent	None	Poor	Excellent
Leber's disease	Excellent—especially for macular lesions*	Excellent	Poor	Excellent	None	Poor	Excellent
Coats' disease	Excellent	Excellent*	Poor	Excellent	None	Poor	Excellent
Proliferative sickle retinopathy	Excellent*	Excellent	Poor	Excellent	None	Poor	Excellent
Retrolental fibroplasia	Equivocal*	Equivocal	Poor	Equivocal	None	Poor	Excellent
Diabetic Retinopathy							
Nonproliferative	Excellent*	Excellent	Poor	Excellent	None	Good	Excellent
Proliferative	Excellent—especially for epipapillary, peripapillary, papillovitreal, and retinovitreal neovascularization*	Excellent—especially for surface neovascularization*	Fair—ablation technique only	Excellent	None	Good—ablation technique only	Excellent

From L'Esperance.[34]
*Preferred method of treatment.

Table 6-4—cont'd

Results of Treatment of Various Ocular Abnormalities by Argon, Xenon Arc, Ruby, Dye, Carbon Dioxide, and Krypton Lasers

Disease	Argon Laser	Xenon Arc	Ruby Laser	Dye Laser	Carbon Dioxide Laser	Krypton Laser	
						Red	Green-Yellow
Peripheral Chorioretinal Tumors							
Retinoblastoma	Fair	Good*	Poor	Excellent*	None	Poor	Poor
Malignant melanoma	Good—6 disc diameters	Good*—<6 disc diameters	Poor	Excellent*	None	Poor	Poor
Angiomatosis retinae	Excellent	Excellent*	Poor	Excellent*	None	Poor	Excellent
Macular Serous Abnormalities							
Serous detachment of pigment epithelium	Excellent*	Excellent	Good	Excellent	None	Good	Excellent
Central serous choroidopathy	Excellent*	Excellent	Excellent	Excellent	None	Excellent*	Excellent
Macular Hemorrhagic Abnormalities							
Hemorrhagic detachment of the pigment epithelium	Excellent	Excellent	Poor	Excellent	None	Excellent*—especially in foveolar avascular zone	Excellent—especially in foveolar avascular zone
Hemorrhagic detachment of the sensory retina	Good*	Good	Poor	Excellent	None	Excellent*	Excellent
Choroidal neovascularization and secondary exudative maculopathy	Excellent	Excellent	Poor	Excellent	None	Excellent—especially for perifoveal and macular area*	Excellent
Macular Intraretinal Abnormalities							
Branch retinal vein occlusion	Excellent*	Excellent	Good—ablation technique only	Excellent	None	Excellent*	Excellent
Central retinal vein occlusion	Excellent*	Good	Good—ablation technique only	Excellent	None	Excellent*	Excellent
Miscellaneous Macular Diseases							
Macular hole, penetrating	Fair*	Fair	Good	Excellent	None	Excellent	Excellent
Preretinal fibrosis	Equivocal*	Equivocal	Equivocal	Equivocal	None	Equivocal	Equivocal

*Preferred method of treatment.

Continued.

Table 6-4—cont'd
Results of Treatment of Various Ocular Abnormalities by Argon, Xenon Arc, Ruby, Dye, Carbon Dioxide, and Krypton Lasers

Disease	Argon Laser	Xenon Arc	Ruby Laser	Dye Laser	Carbon Dioxide Laser	Krypton Laser	
						Red	Green-Yellow
Toxoplasmic retinochoroiditis	Good(?)*	Good(?)	Good(?)	Good	None	Equivocal	Equivocal
Toxocara canis infestation	Equivocal(?)	Equivocal(?)*	Poor	Equivocal	None	Equivocal	Equivocal
Pigment epitheliopathy	Good	Good	Fair	Excellent	None	Excellent*	Excellent
Angioid streaks	Good	Good	Poor	Excellent	None	Excellent*	Excellent
Anterior Segment Abnormalities							
Iris defects							
Deformed pupils	Excellent*	Good	Poor	Excellent	None	Good	Excellent
Iris cyst	Excellent*	Excellent	Poor	Excellent	None	Good	Good
Iridocyclitic membrane	Excellent*	Good	Poor	Excellent	None	Poor	Excellent
Glaucoma							
Laser photomydriasis	Excellent—especially if lens present*	Good	Poor	Excellent	None	Excellent	Excellent
Laser iridotomy	Excellent*	Good	Excellent—Q-switched only	Excellent	None	Good	Good
Laser trabeculoplasty	Excellent*	Poor	Good—Q-switched	Good	None	Good	Excellent
Laser gonioplasty	Excellent*	Good	Poor	Excellent	None	Excellent	Excellent
Laser goniophotocoagulation	Excellent*	Poor	Poor	Excellent	None	Poor	Excellent
Laser trabeculostomy	Good(?)	Poor	Poor	Poor	Excellent*	Poor	Poor
Laser trabeculosclerostomy							
Internal							
External	Good*	Poor	Poor	Excellent	None	Poor	Good
	Poor	Poor	Poor	Poor	Excellent*	Poor	Poor
Laser cyclocautery							

*Preferred method of treatment.

Table 6-4—cont'd

Results of Treatment of Various Ocular Abnormalities by Argon, Xenon Arc, Ruby, Dye, Carbon Dioxide, and Krypton Lasers

Disease	Argon Laser	Xenon Arc	Ruby Laser	Dye Laser	Carbon Dioxide Laser	Krypton Laser	
						Red	Green-Yellow
Transpupillary	Excellent*	Excellent	Poor	Excellent	None	Poor	Good
Trans-scleral	Poor(?)	Poor(?)	Good—Q-switched only*	Poor	None	Poor	Poor

*Preferred method of treatment.

Table 6-5

Factors Affecting Photocoagulation

Eye Segment	Consideration	Caution
Cornea	Defects in epithelium; embedded foreign bodies; disruptions of Bowman's membrane; stromal haze, maculas, or opacities	Could cause scatter, deflection, or absorption of laser beam
Corneal endothelium	Increase in guttata; pigment deposition; breaks, doubling, or rolling of Descemet's membrane; accumulations of red or white cells or keratotic precipitates on posterior surfaces	Could decrease effectiveness of laser beam and introduce complications
Anterior chamber	Presence of cells; protein accumulation; blood, pigment flecks, or other unusual particles	Could decrease effectiveness of photocoagulation and visualization of posterior segment
Iris	Should dilate to at least 4 mm in diameter	To permit adequate visualization of areas of retina
Lens	Wedgelike cortical opacities	Could decrease impact power of beam by occlusion of segment as beam passes through opacity
	Presence of nuclear or posterior subcapsular cataracts	Could refract beam in various directions and diminish or negate effectiveness of procedure
	Presence of anterior and posterior polar cataracts	Presents problem if pupil cannot be dilated; beam must be channeled eccentrically through outer portion of pupillary sphere to avoid central opacification
Vitreous	Blood clots; opacities; pigment accumulation; collagen condensations and membranes	Could decrease effectiveness of beam and cause further deterioration or damage
Retina	Areas of hemorrhagic activity; edema or exudate; retinoschisis; serous accumulations beneath sensory retina; increase in sensory retinal edema	Would require change in later approach or increase in energy to ensure adequate coagulation of underlying neovascularization

Modified from L'Esperance.[34]

Medical Plan[34]

	Argon Laser	Xenon Arc	Ruby Laser
Energy source	Electrically pumped gaseous discharge tube	High-pressure xenon arc bulb	Ruby crystal pumped by xenon flash
Tissue reaction	Absorption primarily at pigmented areas, such as melanin, xanthophyll, and hemoglobin; heat production and coagulum formed, resulting in eventual pigment and glial proliferation	Coagulation with sufficient absorption of any wavelength (400 to 1600 nm); edema, exudation, pigment proliferation, gliosis, and atrophy	Absorption primarily at pigmented areas, with production of heat; late result similar to light coagulation
Anesthesia	Topical anesthesia required; occasionally retrobulbar akinesia and anesthesia necessary	Occasionally preoperative sedation, retrobulbar and lid akinesia and anesthesia; topical anesthesia necessary	None required
Ancillary equipment	Low-vacuum or three-mirror contact lens for retinal photocoagulation; occasionally cooling contact lens for anterior segment therapy	Contact lens for correcting high ametropia, lid speculum, and constant saline corneal lavage; forceps manipulation of eye may be necessary	None required
Hospitalization and aftercare	None required	Monocular patch for 12 hours	None required
Hazards	No danger to operator; overall hazards to patient minimal because of minute total energy transmitted through refractive media	Accidental retinal burn of operator; overheating of anterior chamber, thermal cataract, vitreous hemorrhages, secondary retinal necrosis and tears; secondary exudative retinal detachment, and macular deterioration	Accidental retinal burn of operator more probable because of coherence and energy density of stray laser beam; similar ocular complications; less total energy transmitted through media

NURSING CARE

Nursing Assessment

Vision

Constriction of peripheral fields; temporary decrease in central vision; slight decrease in night vision; headache from bright laser light.

Nursing Dx & Intervention

Nursing Diagnosis	Nursing Intervention/Rationale
Knowledge deficit	• Explain purpose of laser therapy. • Assure patient that procedure causes little pain and that topical anesthetic (eye drops) will be administered *to alleviate anxiety.*

Dye Laser	Carbon Dioxide Laser	Krypton Laser
Dye pumped by argon laser	Gaseous discharge tube pumped electrically	Gaseous discharge tube pumped electrically
Absorption in various portions of ocular tissues depending on dye used and wavelength generated; heat production and coagulum formed, resulting in pigment and glial proliferation; certain wavelengths useful in phototherapy and photosensitization of tumors	100% absorption by all ocular and extraocular tissues within 100 μm of surface impact; solid tissue vaporized to water vapor and smoke instantaneously; absorption independent of pigmented material; beam hemostatic, bacteriostatic, lymphostatic; tissue response, slight char and minimum injury; healing excellent	Absorption primarily at pigmented areas such as melanin (red, yellow, and green beams), xanthophyll (violet and blue beams), and hemoglobin (blue, green, and yellow beams); heat production and coagulum formed, resulting in eventual pigment and glial proliferation
Topical anesthesia required; occasionally retrobulbar akinesia and anesthesia necessary	Topical anesthesia required as well as local infiltration anesthesia for external lesions; retrobulbar akinesia and anesthesia necessary for intraocular therapy; occasionally general anesthesia required	Topical anesthesia required; occasionally retrobulbar akinesia and anesthesia necessary
Low-vacuum or three-mirror contact lens for retinal photocoagulation; stereotaxic manipulator for delivery and distribution of laser beam by fiberoptic cables	Low reflective instruments necessary; positive pressure nitrogen flow and/or vacuum apparatus for smoke and vapor; glasses for operating room personnel	Plano–low-vacuum or three-mirror contact lens for retinal photocoagulation; occasionally other specialized lenses for anterior segment therapy
None usually required; phototherapy and photosensitization procedures may require brief hospitalization	May be required for intraocular and extraocular dissections	None required
No danger to operator; minimum hazards to patient possible with phototherapy procedures	Mild danger to operator and operating room personnel; ordinary glasses should be worn; nonreflective instruments and noninflammable draperies should be used; constant monitoring by technician of instrumentation and personnel necessary	No danger to operator; overall hazards to patient minimal because of minute total energy transmitted through refractive media

Nursing Diagnosis	Nursing Intervention/Rationale
	• Describe procedure to patient and family. Explain that patient will be awake and sitting up in a chair and may have special contact lens placed on eye. • Describe bright lights caused by laser beam that patient will see during procedure. • Explain that procedure may take 15 to 40 minutes. • Tell patient that family member or friend should accompany patient and drive home, *since patient's eyes will be dilated and vision may be temporarily blurred.*
Pain	• Explain to patient that headache may develop after treatment because of bright laser light. Suggest acetaminophen *to relieve discomfort*. Warn patient not to use aspirin *because of its anticoagulant effect*.

Patient Education

1. Emphasize the importance of not increasing the venous pressure in the head, neck, and eyes, particularly with the Valsalva maneuver. Instruct the patient to keep the head up and to move slowly and not to bend over or make sudden movements.
2. Caution the patient not to lift anything heavier than 5 pounds and not to strain for any reason, as when having a bowel movement. Encourage the patient to take a stool softener to avoid constipation.

3. Instruct the patient to avoid strenuous activities such as athletics and sexual intercourse for approximately 3 weeks, but encourage the patient to participate in mild forms of exercise such as walking.
4. Explain that spots may be seen before the eyes for 24 to 48 hours after treatment. Inform the patient that there may be some discomfort around the eye for about 3 weeks; the lid may be black and blue, the eye may be bloodshot, the vision may be somewhat blurred temporarily, and night vision may be temporarily decreased.
5. Instruct the patient to sleep with the head of the bed elevated 15 to 20 degrees to decrease the pressure in the eyes.
6. Advise the patient to avoid coughing and sneezing and not to blow the nose vigorously. (However, sneezes should not be stifled, since this raises the pressure in the eyes.)
7. Teach the patient not to rub the eyes.
8. Caution the patient to avoid altitudes above 8000 feet. The patient may fly on commercial airlines, however, since the cabins are pressurized.
9. Instruct the patient to avoid medications that contain epinephrine, such as nose drops or sprays, since these may raise the blood pressure.

Evaluation

Patient Outcome	Data Indicating That Outcome is Reached
Vision is restored or improved.	Blurred vision decreases after about 3 weeks, and normal vision returns.

Figure 6-21 Location of incisions in radial keratotomy. Central 3 to 4 mm optical zone of cornea is not incised, and incisions do not extend beyond corneoscleral limbus. Four, eight, or 16 radial incisions are made.
From Newell.[41]

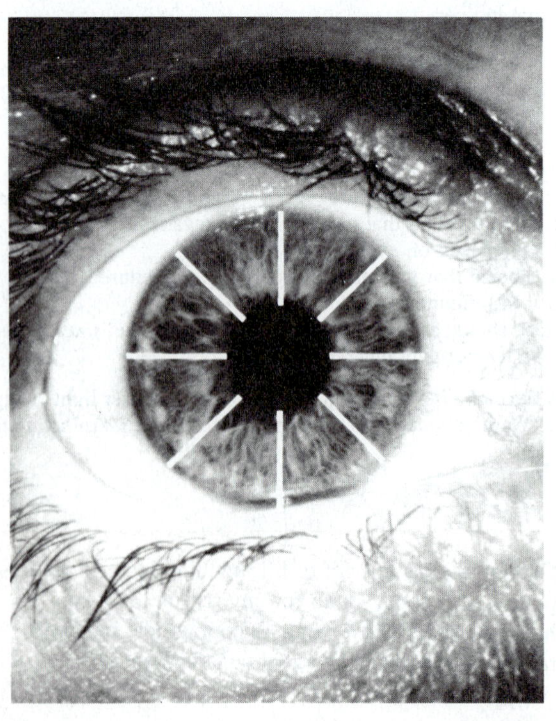

 Radial Keratotomy

Radial keratotomy is a newly approved and somewhat controversial procedure designed to correct or modify mild myopia (nearsightedness). Radial incisions, like the spokes of a bicycle wheel, are made around the periphery of the cornea, ultimately resulting in a flattening of the cornea (Figure 6-21). The flattened cornea redirects the light rays to a more appropriate level on the surface of the retina to reduce the myopia. A calibrated diamond knife is used to make anywhere from four to 16 equally spaced incisions in the corneal surface. The central portion of the cornea (a 3 to 4 mm diameter) is left untouched so resultant scarring does not cause glare or interfere with central vision.

Candidates for this procedure are mildly or moderately myopic patients who usually attain 20/40 vision without further correction following the surgery. However, some patients may still need eyeglasses to attain maximum correction.

The procedure is controversial because a variety of unknowns can cause problems after surgery. For example, the cornea heals and reshapes differently in each patient, and the visual acuity is not fully predictable in any individual. While the procedure does not threaten vision, the outcome may be increased astigmatism for some patients and less-than-expected reduction in myopia for others. The danger of perforating the cornea and cutting into the anterior chamber is always present during the procedure. Slight perforations heal quickly with no complications; deeper perforations cause loss of the pressure stability in the chamber and may delay the completion of surgery for a month or so. Fluctuating chamber pressures cause visual impairment until healing is complete.

In some patients the corneal scars may become pigmented and visible in 6 to 12 months. Long-term follow-up research is still being done.

The procedure has been approved for outpatient therapy and is accomplished with the use of a topical anesthesia. The eye is pressure patched for 24 hours after the procedure, and the patient may experience foreign body sensations for the first 12 to 24 hours.

References

1. Allweiss P et al: Guidelines for diabetic disease control—Kentucky, Morbidity Mortality Weekly Report, Mass. Medical Society 36:93, 1987.
2. Bernth-Petersen P: A change in indications for cataract surgery? A 10 year comparative epidemiological study, Acta Ophthalmol 59:206, 1981.
3. Binder PS: The physiologic effects of extended wear soft contact lenses, Am Acad Ophthalmol 87:745, 1980.
4. Bowers AC and Thompson J: Clinical manual of health assessment, St Louis, 1988, The CV Mosby Co.
5. Boyd-Monk H: Nursing care of the eye, Norwalk, Conn, 1987, Appleton & Lange.
6. Carver JA: Cataract care made plain, AJN 87:626, 1987.
7. Cavanagh HD, Bodner BI, and Wilson LA: Extended wear hydrogel lenses, Am Acad Ophthalmol 87:871, 1980.
8. Denyer B: Reducing the incidence of eye injuries, Occup Health 38:112, 1986.
9. Driebe, WT: Contact lenses, Ophthalmology 94:1355, 1987.
10. Eichenbaum JW, Feldstein M, and Podos SM: Extended-wear aphakic soft contact lenses and corneal ulcers, Br J Ophthalmol 66:663, 1982.
11. Ellis PP: Ocular therapeutics and pharmacology, ed 7, St Louis, 1985, The CV Mosby Co.
12. Eye care for the American people (supplement to Ophthalmology), Am Acad Ophthalmol 94, April 1987.
13. Fine, S and Patz, A: Ten years after the diabetic retinopathy study, Ophthalmology 94:739, 1987.
14. Foulds WS: The changing pattern of eye surgery, Br J Anaesth 52:643, 1980.
15. Gardner TW and Schoch DE: Handbook of ophthalmology: a practical guide, Norwalk, Conn, 1987, Appleton & Lange.
16. Gilman AG, Goodman LS, and Gilman A, editors: The pharmacological basis of therapeutics, ed 6, New York, 1980, MacMillan Publishing Co, Inc.
17. Goldberg MF: Knowledge of diabetic retinopathy before and 18 years after the Arlie House symposium on treatment of diabetic retinopathy, Ophthalmology 94:741, 1987.
18. Grimstone D: Nursing care of the eye, Occup Health 38:115, 1986.
19. Groër MW and Shekleton ME: Basic pathophysiology: a conceptual approach, St Louis, 1983, The CV Mosby Co.
20. Hedges TR: Consultation in ophthalmology, Toronto, 1987, BC Decker, Inc.
21. Helveston EM and Ellis FD: Pediatric ophthalmology practice, St Louis, 1980, The CV Mosby Co.
22. Hillis A, Flynn JT, and Hawkins BS: The evolving concept of amblyopia: a challenge to epidemiologists, Am J Epidemiol 118:192, 1983.
23. Hirst LW, Smiddy WE, and Stark WJ: Corneal perforations: changing methods of treatment, 1960-1980, Ophthalmology 89:630, 1982.
24. Jampol LM: Lasers—past, present, and future, Sight Saving 53:10, 1984-85.
25. Jensen D: The principles of physiology, ed 2, New York, 1980, Appleton-Century-Crofts.
26. Keltner JL and Johnson, CA: Visual function, driving safety and the elderly, Ophthalmology 94:1180, 1987.
27. Kim M, McFarland G, and McLane A: Pocket guide to nursing diagnoses, St Louis, 1987, The CV Mosby Co.
28. Kornzweig AL: New ideas for old eyes, J Geriatr Soc 28:145, 1980.
29. Kovalesky A: Nurses' guide to children's eyes, Orlando, Fla, 1985, Grune & Stratton, Inc.
30. Krupin T et al: Intraocular pressure the day of argon laser trabeculoplasty in primary open-angle glaucoma, Ophthalmology 91:361, 1984.
31. Lemp MA: Recent developments in dry eye management, Ophthalmology 94:1299, 1987.
32. Leske MC: The epidemiology of open-angle glaucoma: a review, Am J Epidemiol 118:166, 1983.
33. Leske MC and Sperduto RD: The epidemiology of senile cataracts: a review, Am J Epidemiol 118:152, 1983.
34. L'Esperance FA: Ophthalmic lasers, ed 2, St Louis, 1983, The CV Mosby Co.
35. Luciano DS, Vander AJ, and Sherman JH: Human function and structure, New York, 1978, McGraw-Hill Book Co.
36. Luckmann J and Sorensen KC: Medical-surgical nursing: a psychophysiologic approach, Philadelphia, 1980, WB Saunders Co.
37. Marshall LF: The oval pupil: clinical significance and relationship to intracranial hypertension, J Neurosurg 58:566, 1983.
38. McCoy K: Cataracts and intraocular lenses: from cloudy to clear, Nurs Clin North Am 16:405, 1981.
39. Melamed M: Complications of contact lenses, Emerg Med 12:218, 1982.
40. Moses RA and Hart WM, editors: Adler's physiology of the eye: clinical application, ed 8, St Louis, 1987, The CV Mosby Co.
41. Newell FW: Ophthalmology: principles and concepts, ed 6, St Louis, 1986, The CV Mosby Co.
42. Newton C et al: Acanthamoeba keratitis associated with contact lenses—United States, Morbidity Mortality Weekly Report, Mass. Medical Society 35:405, 1986.
43. Norman S: The pupil check, Am J Nurs 82:588, 1982.
44. Parlato C et al: Acanthameoeba keratitis associated with contact lenses—United States, Morbidity Mortality Weekly Report, Mass. Medical Society 35:405, 1986.
45. Pavan-Langston D: Promising therapy for herpes infections of the eye, Sight Saving 53:12, 1984-1985.
46. Pearson LJ and Kotthoff ME: Geriatric clinical protocols, Philadelphia, 1979, JB Lippincott Co.
47. Pesci BR: When the patient's problem is really poor vision, RN 49:22, 1986.
48. Perrin ED: Laser therapy for diabetic retinopathy, Am J Nurs 80:664, 1980.
49. Pizzarello LD: The dimensions of the problem of eye disease among the elderly, Ophthalmology 94:1191, 1987.
50. Price SA and Wilson LM: Pathophysiology: clinical concepts of disease processes, ed 2, New York, 1982, McGraw-Hill Book Co.
51. Randolph SA: Contact lens survey, AAOHN 35:7, 1987.
52. Resler M and Tumulty G: Glaucoma update, Am J Nurs 83:752, 1983.
53. Salmon AG: Eye injuries from industrial chemicals, Occup Health 28:125, 1986.
54. Seidel HM et al: Mosby's guide to physical examination, St Louis, 1987, The CV Mosby Co.
55. Shields JA: Diagnosis and management of intraocular tumors, St Louis, 1983, The CV Mosby Co.
56. Silver J: Can VDU's affect your vision? Occup Health 18:122, 1986.
57. Smith JF and Nachazel DP: Ophthalmologic nursing, Boston, 1980, Little, Brown & Co.
58. Steinberg FU, editor: Care of the geriatric patient, ed 6, St Louis, 1983, The CV Mosby Co.
59. Straatsma BR: The aging eye, Transition, p. 18, 1984.
60. Vaughan D and Asbury T: General ophthalmology, ed 10, Los Altos Calif, 1983, Lange Medical Publications.
61. Von Noorden GK: Practical management of amblyopia, Int Ophthalmol 6:7, 1983.
62. Waring GO, editor: Pars plana lensectomy by ultrasonic fragmentation, Surv Ophthalmol 27:96, 1982.
63. Waring GO: Shaping the eye for better vision: refractive corneal surgery, Sight Saving 53:21, 1984-1985.
64. Whaley LF and Wong DL: Nursing care of infants and children, ed 3, St Louis, 1987, The CV Mosby Co.
65. Yanoff M: Cataract surgery—when and how, Geriatrics 37:71, 1982.
66. Yanoff M: "Magnetic" views of the eye and brain, Sight Saving 53:16, 1984-1985.

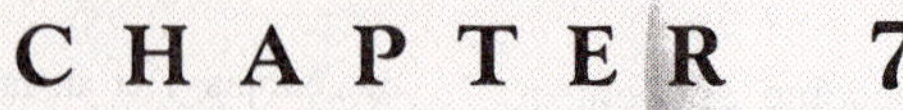

CHAPTER 7

Ear, Nose, and Throat

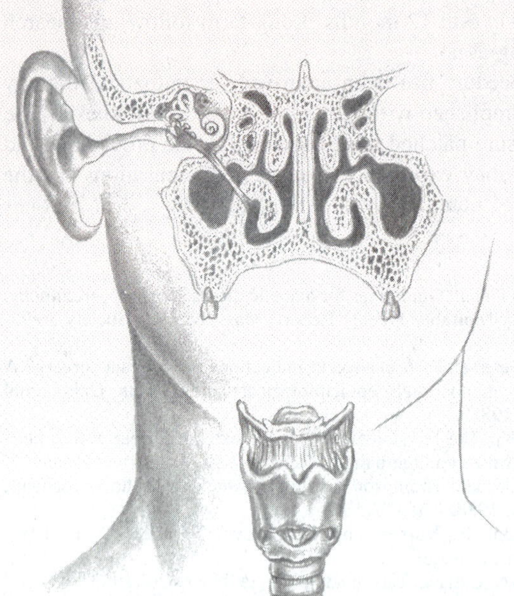

Overview

The ears, nose, and throat (ENT) are responsible for many of the body's senses, such as sound, smell, and taste, and for balance and speaking. Health professionals who care for patients with disorders affecting these areas must be highly sensitive and skilled in assessing the symptoms of disorders that may have a great impact on a patient's life or self-perception.

Few ENT disorders prove fatal (with the exception of neoplastic diseases, which are discussed in Chapter 16), but they can cause painful, incapacitating illnesses and major disruptions in communication, appearance, eating, swallowing, and breathing.

Since many ENT disorders are treated on an outpatient basis, patient and family education is a focus of this chapter.

The development of antibiotics and new surgical techniques have greatly reduced the impact of ENT diseases. Hearing loss was once a common occurrence after severe or repeated ear infections, but now it has been nearly eliminated in the United States. Other diseases that once were life threatening are now considered minor if treated early. Surgical techniques such as microsurgery, stapedectomy, cochlear implant, and tympanoplasty have greatly improved the treatment of hearing loss.

Anatomy, Physiology, and Related Pathophysiology

Ear

The ears are responsible for both hearing and equilibrium. The ear is divided into three anatomic sections: the external ear, the middle ear, and the inner ear (Figure 7-1).

External ear. The function of the external ear is to receive sound waves and direct them to the tympanic membrane. The external ear includes the outer projection (known as the auricle or pinna) and a passageway called the external auditory meatus, or the external auditory canal. The auricle is attached to the head by muscles innervated by the facial nerve. It is composed of cartilage and covered by skin. However, the ear lobe contains no cartilage (Figure 7-2). The auricle is highly susceptible to frostbite because it has little subcutaneous fat to protect it and only one layer of blood vessels. The sensory nerve supply of the auricle is provided by the great auricular nerve, the lesser occipital nerve, the auricular branch of the vagus nerve, the auriculotemporal nerve, and the fifth, seventh, and tenth cranial nerves.

The external auditory meatus or canal has a slight downward curve; it ends at the tympanic membrane. The outer half is cartilaginous, and the inner half is bony except in infants, in whom ossification has not yet occurred. The skin that lines the cartilaginous portion of the canal is thick and contains fine hairs, large sebaceous glands, and ceruminous glands. Cerumen (earwax), the combined secretion of the sebaceous and ceruminous glands, may accumulate so much that it obstructs sound transmission. The epithelium that lines the bony half of the external canal is very thin and does not contain hair or glands. In adults the external canal is approximately 24 mm long, and the bony portion is slightly longer than the cartilaginous portion (Figure 7-3).

The temporomandibular joint is anterior to the ear canal. Diseases of this joint can cause referred pain to the ear.

Tympanic membrane. The tympanic membrane, which

Figure 7-1 Relationship of external, middle, and inner ear.

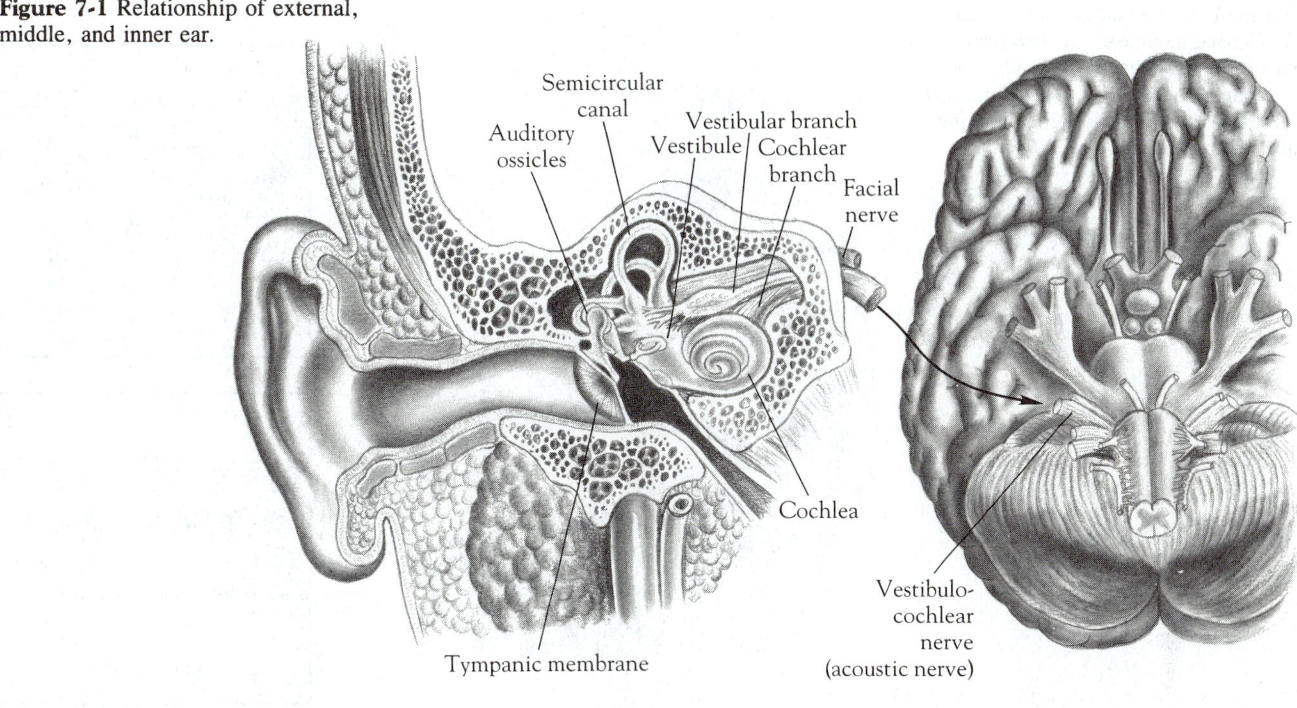

Figure 7-2 Anatomic structures of the external ear.
From Seidel.[47]

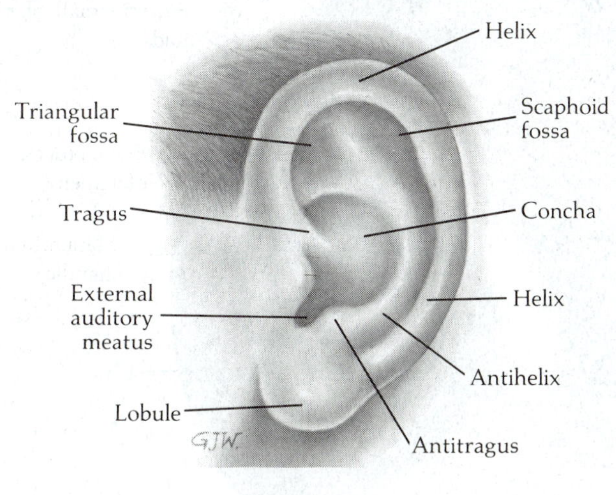

separates the external ear from the middle ear, is composed of two layers of epithelium—the outer layer squamous and the inner cuboidal—and a middle layer of fibrous collagen tissue. New cells of the tympanic membrane are produced in the periphery and migrate toward the center of the drum. The drum is somewhat conical and slightly inclined; the concavity of the drumhead (umbo) and its position in relation to the ear canal vary and may be greatly altered during disease.

The fibers of the tympanic membrane condense into an incomplete, dense, fibrous ring called the anulus, which fits into the tympanic sulcus. The anulus contains a superior break, the notch of Rivinus, between the anterior and posterior malleolar ligaments. The portion of the tympanic membrane closing this area is the pars flaccida, so named because it does not contain a fibrous collagen layer.

The tympanic membrane is described as a translucent window through which the middle ear may be viewed. The color is usually a translucent pearl gray, although this may vary slightly in normal membranes (Figure 7-4).

Middle ear. The middle ear, or tympanic cavity, is covered by the tightly stretched tympanic membrane. It is a small, roughly oblong, flattened space that is lined with nonciliated, single-layered mucous membrane and contains bony walls. During an infection the membrane becomes ciliated and multilayered. This area holds air and three small bones, or ossicles: the malleus, the incus, and the stapes (Figure 7-5).

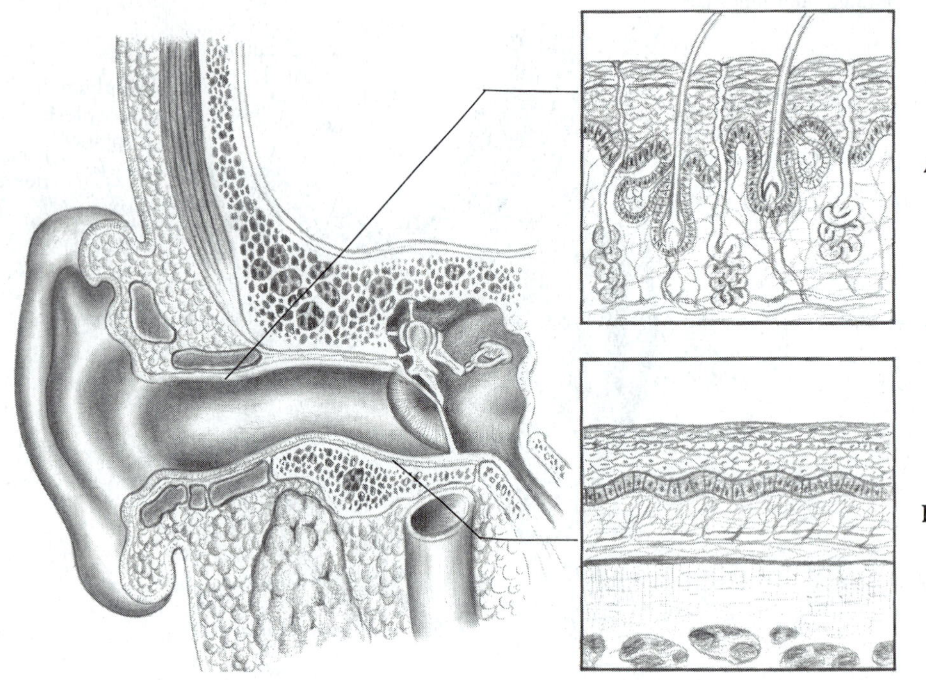

Figure 7-3 External auditory canal. **A,** Cartilaginous ear canal showing hair follicles, sebaceous glands, and ceruminous glands. **B,** Bony ear canal with thin epithelial lining, containing no hair or glands.

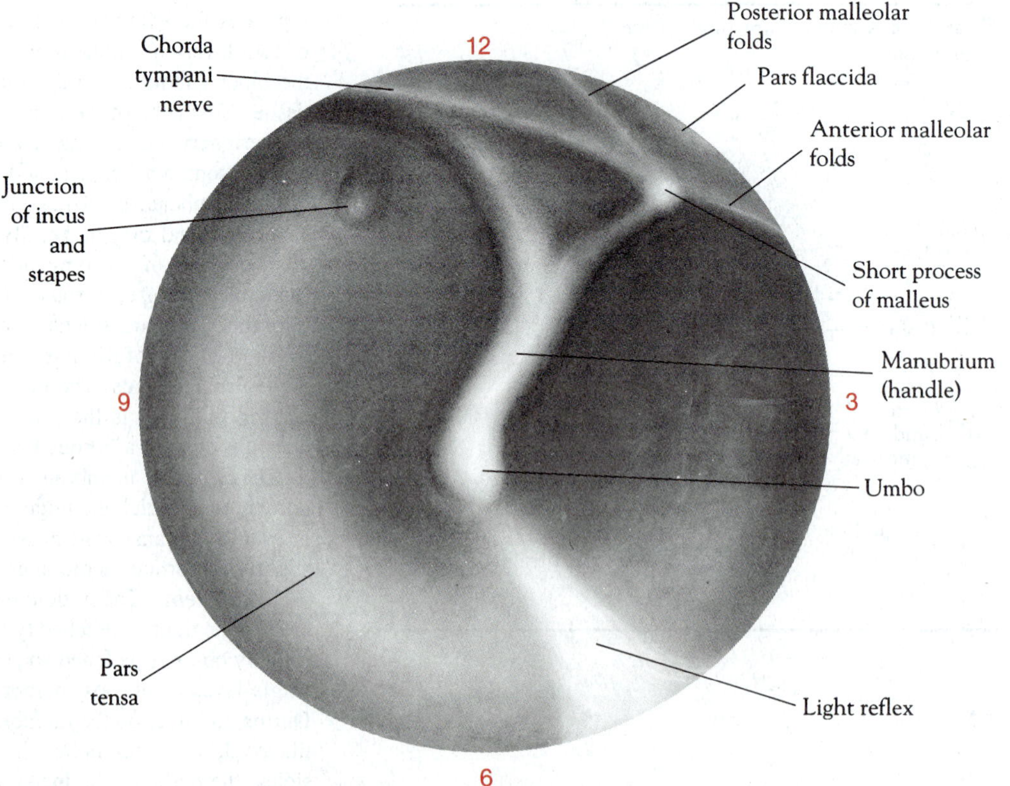

Figure 7-4 Normal tympanic membrane.
From Whaley.[59]

Figure 7-5 Ossicles of right middle ear.

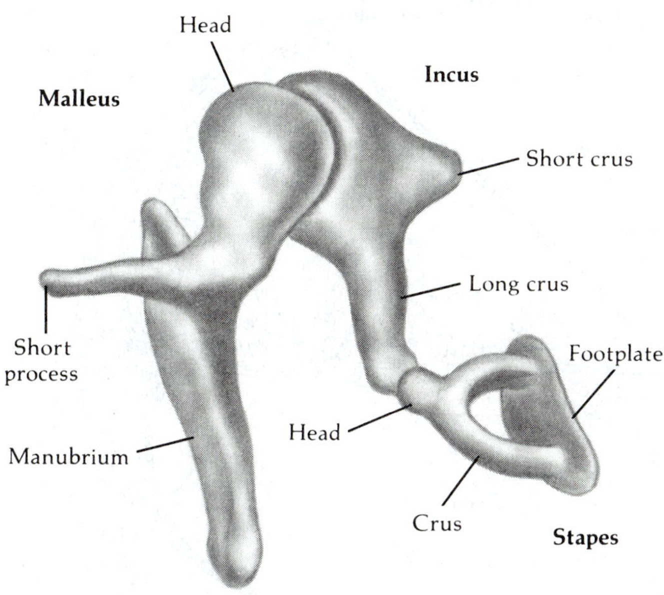

Figure 7-6 Bony labyrinth and membranous inner labyrinth.
From Ganong.[12]

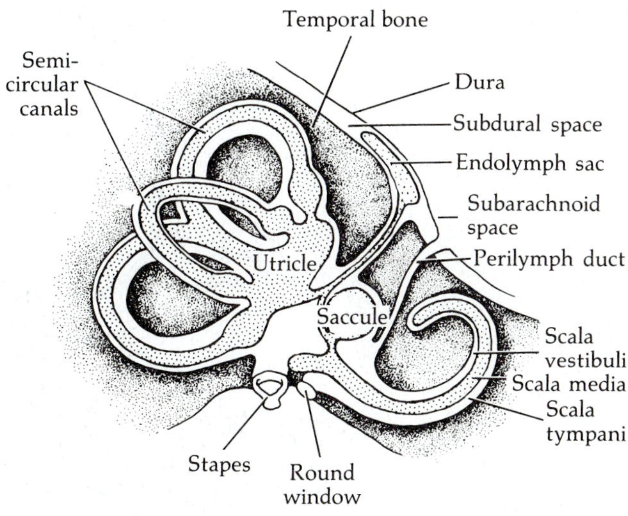

The ossicles connect the tympanic membrane with the oval window and represent the normal pathway of sound transmission across the middle ear space. The first bone is the malleus (hammer); it has a head, neck, handle, and short process. The manubrium (handle) and the short process attach to the tympanic membrane, and the headlike portion connects to the second bone, the incus or anvil, to form a true joint. The incus connects to the third bone, the stapes (stirrup). The footplate of the stapes fits into the oval or vestibular window, which is a small opening in the wall between the middle and inner ear.

The major function of the middle ear is to transfer sound waves from the outer ear to the fluid-filled inner ear. Since the fluid in the inner ear is more difficult to move than air, the pressure waves must be increased. The bony ossicles are joined so they amplify sound waves received by the tympanic membrane and transmit these waves to the inner ear by a lever action of their freely movable joints. The oval window's membrane vibrates and conducts sound waves to the fluid in the inner ear. In otosclerosis the joints of the ossicles are no longer freely movable, resulting in decreased sound transmission. Two small skeletal muscles attached to the ossicles affect the transmission of sound waves. The tensor tympani muscle pulls the malleus inward to tense the tympanic membrane, which attenuates high-pitched sounds. The stapedius muscle pulls the footplate of the stapes outward, possibly making low-frequency sounds more audible.

The middle ear communicates directly with the nasopharynx by means of the eustachian tube. This tube, which leads downward and medially to the nasopharynx, carries air into the middle ear to equalize pressure on both sides of the tympanic membrane. The mucosal lining of the middle ear is continuous with that of the nasopharynx via the eustachian tube. Normally the eustachian tube is passively closed; it opens by action of the tensor and levator muscles of the palate, usually, although not always, during swallowing, yawning, or sneezing to equalize middle ear pressure with atmospheric pressure. The eustachian tube is a direct route for infection to reach the middle ear from the upper respiratory tract.

A third structure of the middle ear is the collection of mastoid air cells. These are air-filled spaces in a portion of the temporal bone in the skull. They communicate posteriorly with the middle ear. They are present at birth but are small and filled with diploic bone and loose osseous tissue between the two tables of cranial bones. Between the ages of 2 and 6 years the diploic bone is gradually replaced by air cells that bud off from the mastoid antrum, which is the first and largest air cell and connects directly to the middle ear.

Inner ear. The end organs for hearing and equilibrium are housed in the inner ear. The inner ear, or labyrinth, is composed of two portions, one inside the other (Figure 7-6). The bony labyrinth is a series of channels within the petrous portion of the temporal bone. Lining the bony labyrinth is the membranous labyrinth, which is the same shape as the bony channels. Inside the bony channels is fluid called perilymph, which surrounds the membranous labyrinth. The membranous labyrinth is filled with fluid called endolymph. There is no communication between the fluid-filled spaces.[12]

Components of the inner ear include the cochlea for hearing, the semicircular canals for equilibrium, that is, rotational

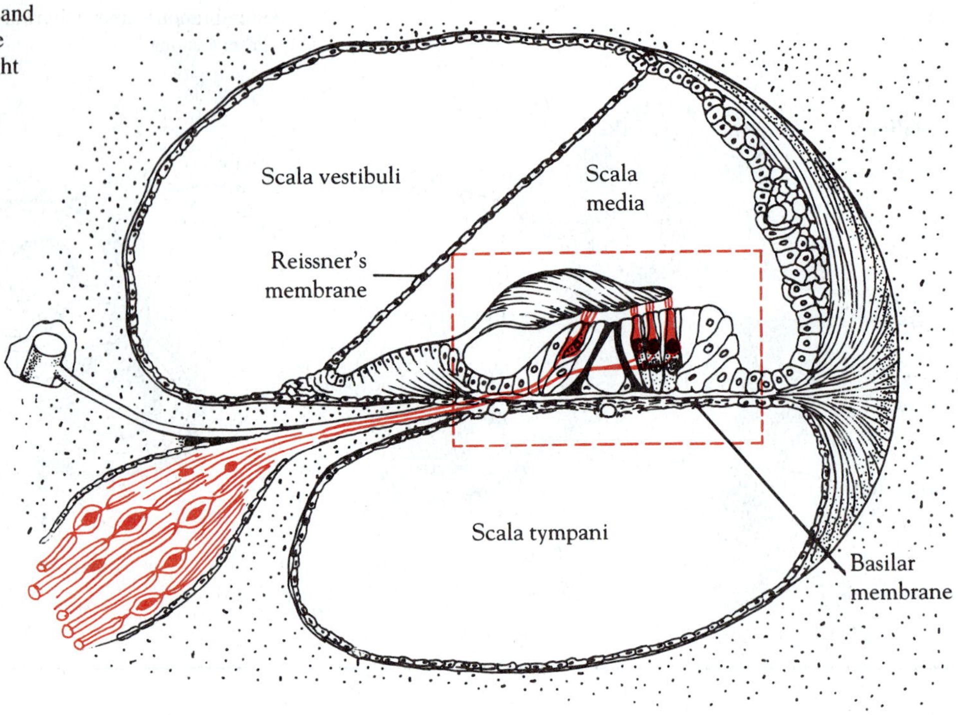

Figure 7-7 Scalae of the cochlea, separated by Reissner's membrane and basilar membrane. *X* and *Y* indicate orientation vis-a-vis drawing on right in Figure 7-9.
From Berne.[3]

and angular acceleration, and the vestibule, which houses the utricle and saccule responsible for sensing changes in gravity and linear and angular acceleration. The vestibule is a space that opens onto the oval window and serves as the entrance into the inner ear. It communicates anteriorly with the cochlea and posteriorly with the semicircular canals and utricle.

Cochlea. The cochlea is a snail-shaped bony tube that contains the organ of Corti, which is the neural end organ for hearing. The cochlea is about 3.5 cm long with about 2¾ spiral turns. Throughout its length, the basilar and Reissner membranes separate it into three tubes or chambers called scalae (Figure 7-7).[3]

The upper scala vestibuli and the lower scala tympani contain perilymph and communicate with each other through the helicotrema, a small opening at the apex of the cochlea. The scala vestibuli at the base of the cochlea ends at the oval window, where the footplate of the stapes is attached. The scala tympani ends at the base of the cochlea into or at the round window, which is an opening enclosed by a secondary tympanic membrane. The round window bulges outward to dissipate the pressure waves that are set up in the inner ear fluid during sound transmission. The scala media, or the middle cochlear chamber, contains endolymph and does not communicate with the other two scalae (Figures 7-8 and 7-9).[3]

The organ of Corti is located on the basilar membrane and contains the receptors of hearing (Figure 7-10). It extends from the base of the cochlea to the apex and has a spiral shape. The receptors for hearing are hair cells arranged in two rows. There are 3500 inner and 20,000 outer hair cells, and their tips are embedded in the tectorial membrane (see Figure 7-10, *B*). When these hair cells are bent or distorted by pressure waves, sound is changed (transduced) into electromechanical impulses. These impulses are carried by the afferent neuron to the spiral ganglion in the bony core of the cochlea. The axons of these nerves form the auditory division of the eighth cranial nerve (vestibulocochlear nerve) and terminate in the dorsal and ventral cochlear nuclei of the medulla oblongata. From the cochlear nuclei, axons carry auditory information to the inferior canaliculi for reflexes associated with hearing, such as turning the head to locate a sound. The fibers then pass to the medial geniculate body in the thalamus and to the primary auditory cortex, Brodmann areas 41 and 42, which are located in the superior portion of the temporal lobe.[41]

Semicircular canals. The semicircular canals are perpendicular to each other on each side of the head. Three canals are on each side: a superior, posterior, and horizontal canal; they are so oriented to sense changes in the three planes of space. Inside the bony canals are the membranous canals suspended in the perilymph. Near the end of each canal is an enlargement called the ampulla, which houses the crista ampullaris, or the vestibular receptors. The hair cells of the crista ampullaris are stimulated with rotation. The pattern of stimulation varies with the direction and plane of rotation. Nerve fiber tracts compose the vestibular portion of the vestibulocochlear nerve, or cranial nerve VIII, to the vestibular nuclei

Figure 7-8 Middle ear, showing relationship of ossicles and cochlea. Communication between scala vestibuli and scala tympani is shown. Arrows indicate displacement of liquid inside bony cochlea and round window from movement of stapedial footplate and displacement of oval window.

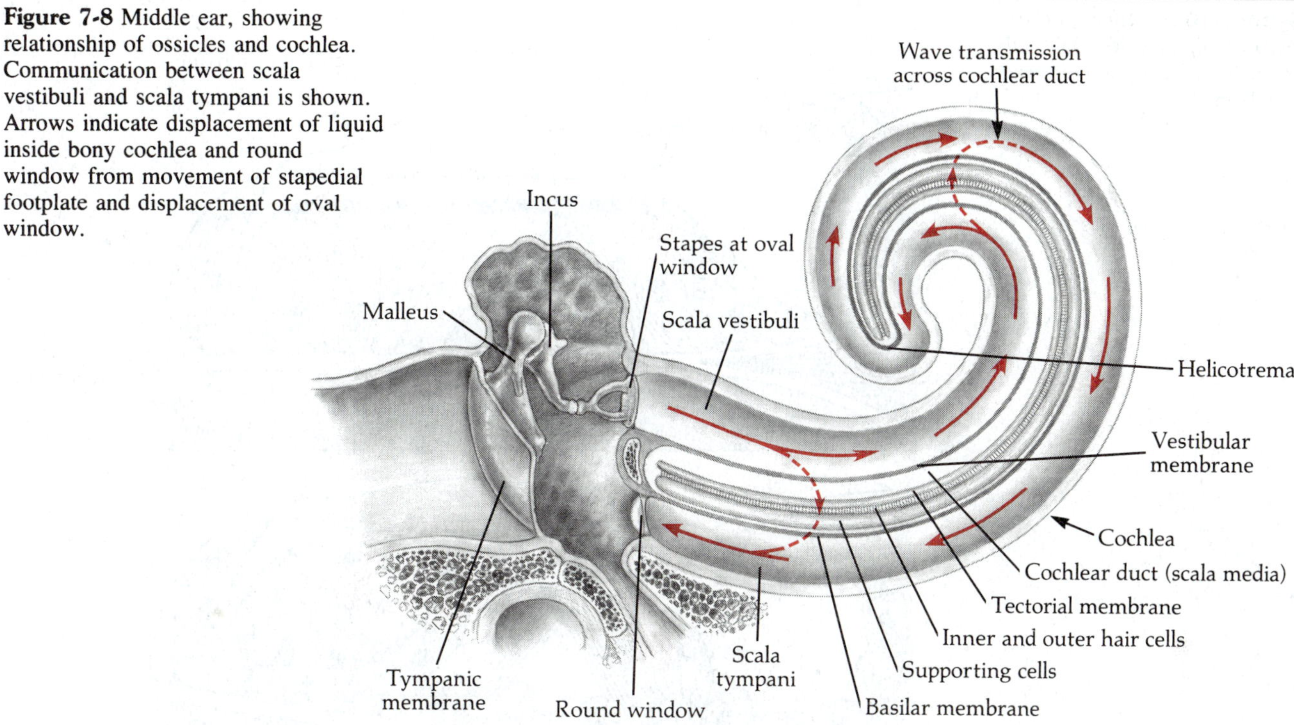

Figure 7-9 Coiled structure of cochlea showing relationships of oval window, scala vestibuli, scala media, and scala tympani. Arrows indicate path of continuous flow from scala vestibuli through helicotrema to scala tympani.

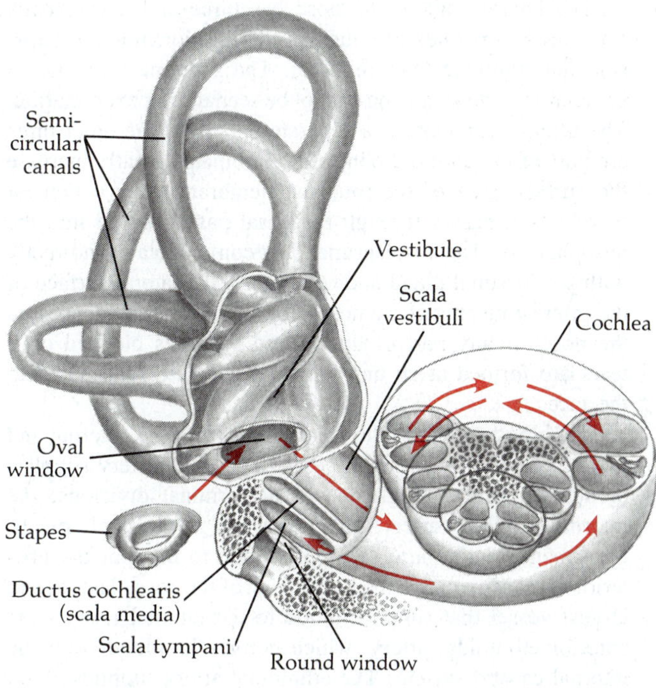

and terminate the four vestibular nuclei at the level of the pons and medulla in the brainstem. Tracts that descend from the vestibular nuclei into the spinal cord are responsible for head-righting reflexes and changes with muscle tone associated with rotation. Ascending fibers from the vestibular nuclei are concerned with eye movements, that is, nystagmus associated with rotation.

Utricle and saccule. Housed within the vestibule are the utricle and saccule, which are responsible for sensing changes in gravity and forward and backward movement. Hair cells in the macula of the utricle and saccule are stimulated by head tilting and by jumping or falling, respectively. Both macular structures are sensitive to forward and backward movement. Fibers from the utricle and saccule compose portions of the vestibular division of cranial nerve VIII, which is the vestibulocochlear nerve. The vestibular division is important for the control of posture and the maintenance of balance. The cochlear division is responsible for hearing.

Nose

The nose is composed of bone in the upper third segment and cartilage in the lower two thirds. The midline point where the nose joins the forehead is called the nasion. The bridge of the nose is called the dorsum, and the base, which includes the nares (nostrils), is the point where the nose joins the upper lip.[34] The two nares are separated by columella and allow air to enter and pass posteriorly to the nasopharynx. The nose is separated in the middle by the septum, which is composed of both cartilage and bone (Figure 7-11). The septum is usu-

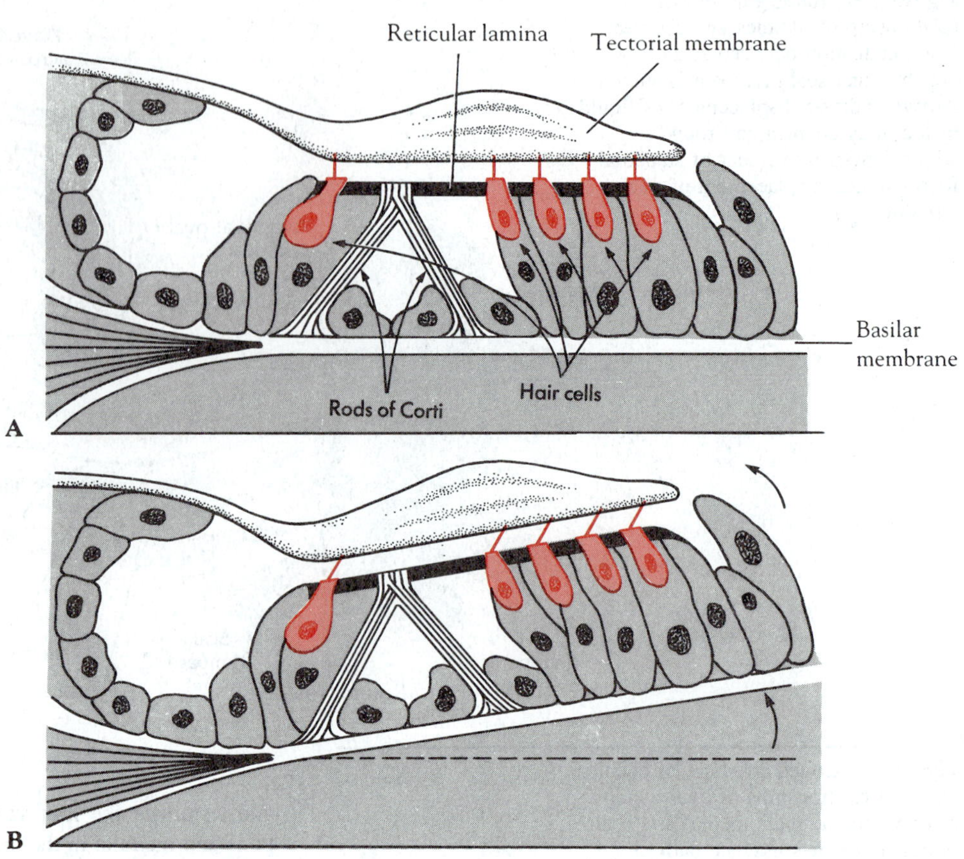

Figure 7-10 A, Organ of Corti on basilar membrane. **B,** Hair cells embedded in tectorial membrane. From Berne.[3]

ally straight at birth but becomes deformed or deviated in almost every adult; it can appear dislocated into one nasal vestibule. The septum maintains the shape of the external nose by acting as a strut that prevents the roof from collapsing. The anterior cartilaginous portion melds into the medial margins of the lateral cartilage and holds them in place.[34]

The nasal cavity is an irregularly shaped space that extends from the bony palate, which separates the nose and mouth cavities, upward to the frontal ethmoid and sphenoid bones of the cranial cavity. The walls of the nasal cavity are made of bone covered with mucous membrane.

Definite relationships have been established between geographic regions and nasal configurations. In warm climates with high absolute humidity, noses tend to be flat; in areas with low absolute humidity, noses are narrow and protrude farther from the face. This latter configuration probably improves the air-conditioning efficiency of the nose.[6]

The vestibule of the nostril is lined with skin containing vibrissae, or nasal hairs, and some sebaceous and sweat glands. The nose is lined with respiratory mucosa, except for the skin in the vestibule and the olfactory epithelium. Mucus secreted by the mucosa is carried back to the nasopharynx by the cilia of the mucosa. The nasal mucosa is extremely vascular, which makes it appear redder than the oral mucosa.

The lateral wall of the nose has three and occasionally four nasal turbinates or conchae: the inferior, middle, superior, and supreme (Figure 7-12). The supreme turbinate, if present, is quite small and cannot be seen during examination. The inferior turbinate is a separate bone, but the other three are part of the ethmoid bone. The turbinates greatly increase the surface area of the mucous membrane over which air travels as it passes through the nasal passages and into the nasopharynx. The nasolacrimal duct communicates indirectly with the lacrimal gland and opens onto the lateral surface of the inferior meatus of the nose. Tears drain continuously into the nose. If any part of the system becomes blocked or if tears are formed at an unusual rate, the fluid runs out onto the face.

The blood supply to the nose comes from the external and internal carotid arteries. The external carotid artery supplies blood primarily through one of its terminal divisions, the internal maxillary artery. This artery and its terminal branch, the sphenopalatine artery, supply blood to most of the posterior nasal septum and the lateral wall of the nose. The second largest vessel that supplies blood to the internal nose is the anterior ethmoidal artery, which derives its blood from the internal carotid system. The ethmoidal artery supplies blood to the anterosuperior part of the septum and the lateral wall

Figure 7-11 Nasal septum.

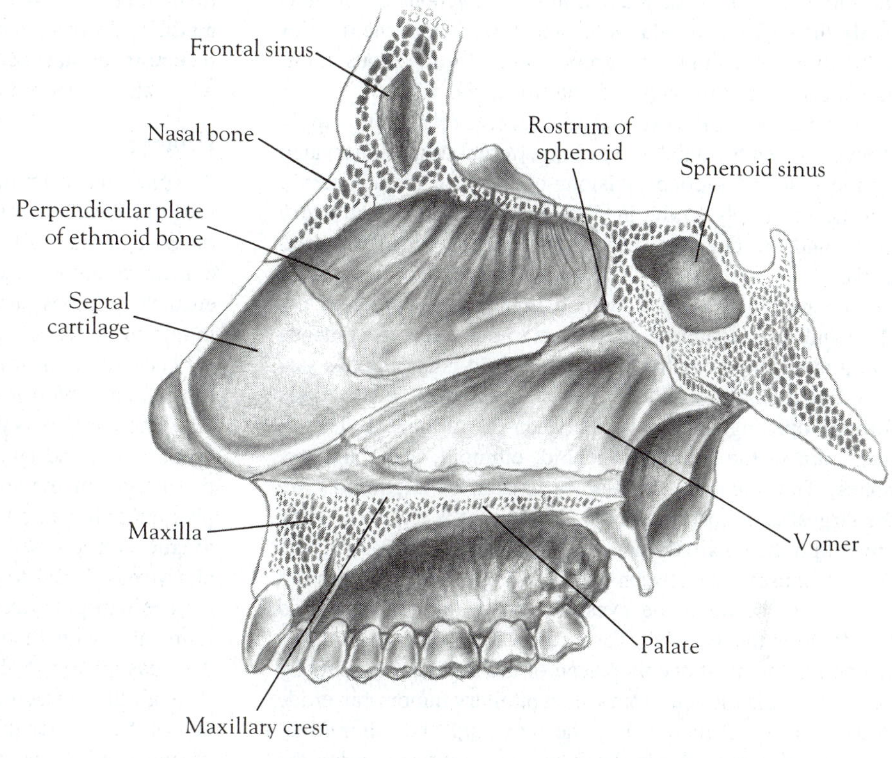

Figure 7-12 Lateral wall of nose.

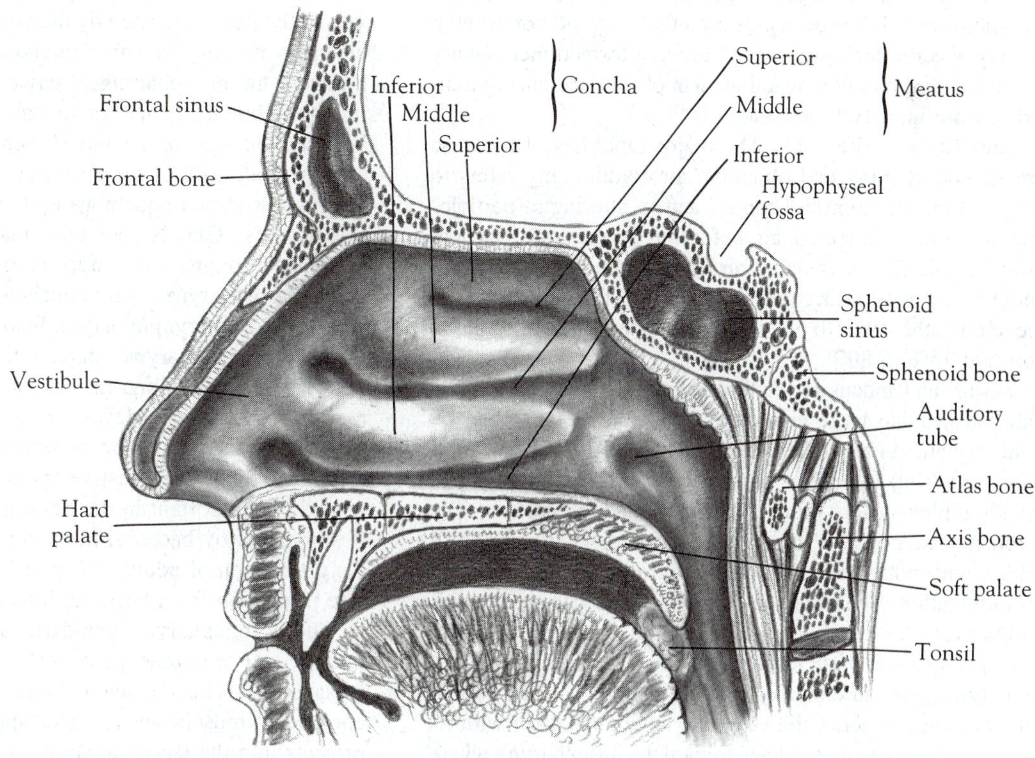

of the nose. The external nose receives blood mostly from the same arteries as the internal nose; but venous drainage is partly through the angular vein, which leads into the inferior ophthalmic vein and the cavernous sinus. Most venous drainage is downward through the anterior facial vein.

The muscles of the external nose receive their nerve supply from the seventh cranial nerve. The external skin is innervated by the first and second divisions of the fifth cranial nerve. The nerve supply to the internal nose is from the olfactory nerve and the first and second divisions of the fifth cranial nerve.

The paranasal sinuses, which lighten the weight of the skull and give resonance and timbre to the voice, are mucous membrane–lined cavities in the facial and cranial bones surrounding the nasal cavities. They drain into the nasal cavities through openings in grooves between the turbinates. The sinuses are in the frontal, sphenoid, ethmoid, and maxillary bones. The maxillary sinuses (or antrum of Highmore) are the largest and most accessible if treatment is required. They are within the maxillary bones on either side of the nose. The frontal sinuses are between and above the eyes, the ethmoid sinuses are between the eyes and nose, and the sphenoid sinuses lie at the rear of the nasal cavity. The sphenoid sinuses, which are the most deeply placed of the sinuses, are directly below the sella turcica, from which pituitary tumors can erode downward to fill them. Only the maxillary and ethmoid sinuses are present at birth; the frontal sinuses form during the second year of life, and the sphenoid sinuses form during the third year.

The normal physiologic functions of the paranasal sinuses are unknown.[34] It has been proposed that they did not develop for any specific biologic reason but were formed incidentally to the forward and downward growth of the face during transition from infancy to adulthood.[34,42]

Functions of the nose. The major functions of the nose are air conditioning and olfaction; air conditioning refers to temperature and humidity control and to filtering of particles and bacteria in inspired air before it reaches the trachea, bronchi, and lungs. Inspired air reaches the nasopharynx in about ¼ second; during this short period, the temperature of the air reaches 97° to 98° F and the humidity becomes a constant 75% to 80%.

Serum and mucus cover the surface of the nasal mucosa and can provide large amounts of water to be absorbed by cold, dry air. As much as 1 L of moisture can evaporate from the nose during 24 hours of normal breathing; the submucosal glands replenish this moisture as the water evaporates. The turbinates are covered with erectile tissue that can rapidly fill with blood, which allows greater control of temperature and humidification. The nose, sinuses, pharynx, trachea, bronchi, and bronchioles are covered by a continuous mucous blanket to which airborne particles cling on contact. The blanket contains lysozyme, an enzyme that causes most bacteria to disintegrate on contact. Cilia carry the mucous blanket with its trapped particulate matter back toward the nasopharynx where it is swallowed. Residual bacteria are then destroyed by hydrochloric acid and gastric juices.

The olfactory sense organs are located in the olfactory membrane that covers the roof of the nose and is reflected medially downward over the superior turbinate. The olfactory receptors are hair cells or chemoreceptors that are stimulated when air is inspired through the nose.

Pharynx

The pharynx, from the Greek word for throat, is the muscular tube that is behind the oral cavity and extends downward from the base of the skull to the larynx. The pharynx is a somewhat conical chamber. It conducts air between the nasal cavities, eustachian tubes, and larynx and conducts food from the mouth to the esophagus.

The structures of the pharynx include the uvula, epiglottis, tonsils, and anterior and posterior tonsillar pillars (Figure 7-13). The pharynx is divided into three sections: nasopharynx, oropharynx, and laryngopharynx. The nasopharynx is above the margin of the soft palate posterior to the nose; the oropharynx is the area behind the mouth that is visible when the tongue is depressed with a tongue blade; and the laryngopharynx is dorsal to the larynx.

The nasopharynx lies behind the nasal cavities and communicates with them through the posterior nasal apertures. The nasopharynx also communicates with the middle ear through the eustachian tube about 1 cm behind the posterior end of the inferior turbinate. Near these openings are patches of lymphoid tissue called the pharyngeal tonsils, which lie in the mucous membrane at the junction of the posterior wall and roof. (Hypertrophied pharyngeal tonsils are adenoids.) The nasopharyngeal space opens inferiorly into the oropharynx so the floor is formed by the dorsal part of the soft palate, which is its only movable boundary. At birth the mucosal lining of the nasopharyngeal cavity is columnar ciliated epithelium, but this changes to patchy squamous epithelium between the ages of 10 and 80 years. Squamous epithelium covers about 80% of the posterior wall, and surface mucosa becomes stratified squamous epithelium after about the age of 10 years. Glands secreting mucus and serous fluid are scattered throughout the mucous membrane.

The oropharynx communicates with the nasopharynx above and the laryngopharynx below to the level of the epiglottis. The oropharynx contains the palatine tonsils, which with the pharyngeal and lingual tonsils (on the dorsum of the tongue) comprise Waldeyer's ring. This ring is a protective barrier of lymphoid tissue between the mouth and throat and the respiratory and digestive tracts. This lymphoid tissue is considered important in the development of immune bodies. If stimulated by bacterial infection, immune bodies promote the production of additional immune factors that provide future protection from bacterial infection.[9]

The laryngopharynx boundaries are the superior constrictor muscle and vertebrae posteriorly, the larynx and piriform fossa below, and the hyoid bone, base of the tongue, and constrictor muscle above. The upper end of the epiglottis projects into the laryngopharynx.

The oropharynx and laryngopharynx are spaces surrounded by muscles that provide support to the surrounding tissue and

Figure 7-13 Structures of pharynx.
A, Uvula, epiglottis, and tonsils.
B, Hypopharynx (posterior view).

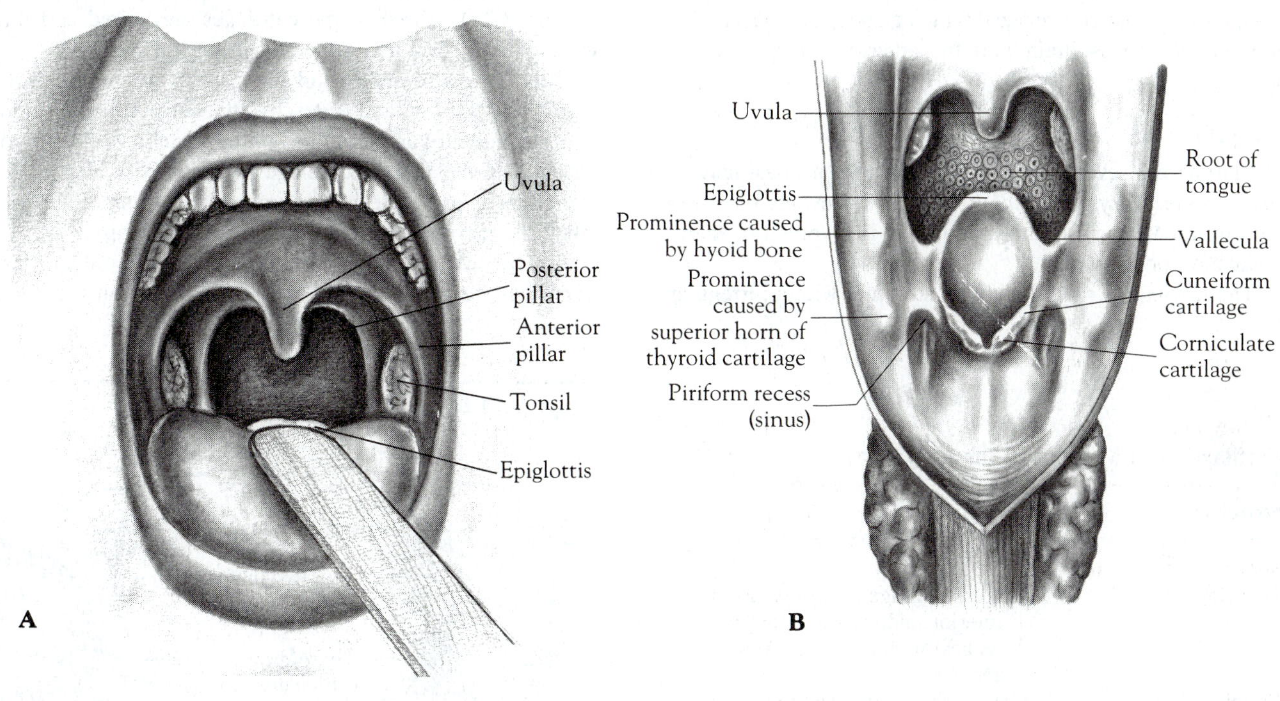

a passageway through which air, food, and fluids can be ingested. Swallowing is accomplished by the action of the constrictor muscles in the pharynx and by the suprahyoid and infrahyoid muscles. Action of these muscles and their nerves is also responsible for the gag reflex, which protects the air and food passages from the entrance of any unwanted material. Two cranial nerves are responsible for the gag reflex: the glossopharyngeal nerve (cranial nerve IX) and the vagus nerve (cranial nerve X). The glossopharyngeal nerve has sensory and motor divisions. The sensory division supplies sensation to the pharynx, and the motor division innervates the posterior wall of the pharynx. The vagus nerve innervates all of the thoracic and abdominal viscera and conveys impulses from the walls of the intestines, the heart, and the lungs.[41]

Tonsils. The tonsils are small masses of primarily lymphoid tissue. They are covered by mucous membrane and contain small openings that deliver phagocytes to the mouth and pharynx.

In the past, removal of the tonsils and adenoids was commonplace, but it is now known that the lymphoid tissue of the pharynx plays an important role in the immune system of

Table 7-1
Tonsils

Structure	Description
Pharyngeal tonsil or adenoid	Mass of lymphoid tissue in nasopharynx; extends from its roof almost to free end of soft palate; present in all infants and children; starts to regress just before puberty; normally absent in adults
Lateral pharyngeal bands	Extend down lateral wall of pharynx from adenoids; located behind posterior tonsillar pillar; gradually become thinner until they disappear below level of faucial tonsil
Faucial (palatine) tonsil	Located laterally at junction of oropharynx and oral cavity; composed of large lymphoid follicles; contains numerous crypts lined with squamous epithelium; supplied by tonsillar and palatine arteries, which come from external carotid artery
Lingual tonsils	Two masses of lymphoid tissue located on dorsum of tongue; extend from circumvallate papillae of tongue to epiglottis

the body, and they are not removed as frequently (Table 7-1).

The lymphatic tissues of Waldeyer's ring drain into the lymph nodes of the neck. The adenoids in the nasopharynx drain into the posterior cervical lymph glands, and the palatine and lingual tonsils drain into the anterior cervical lymph nodes.

Larynx

The larynx has several functions: (1) it is the air passageway between the pharynx and the lungs; (2) it prevents food and fluid from entering the lungs; and (3) it is involved in sound production or phonation.

The larynx is a roughly tubular structure with an irregular shape. It is somewhat wider at the top where it is attached to the pharynx and narrower below where it attaches to the trachea. The larynx is composed of cartilages, ligaments, and muscles that keep its walls from collapsing on inspiration (Figure 7-14). Three of the cartilages are paired and three are unpaired, for a total of nine cartilages (Table 7-2).

Cartilages and muscles of the larynx. The larynx is protected on its front and sides by thyroid cartilage (thyroid means shieldlike) and from behind by vertebrae. The thyroid cartilage is the largest cartilage of the larynx. Its midline prominence forms the hard bump in the front of the neck called the laryngeal prominence, or "Adam's apple."

Just below the thyroid cartilage lies the cricoid cartilage, which can be palpated in normal necks and can usually be

Table 7-2
Cartilages and Muscles of the Larynx

Structure	Description
Unpaired Cartilages	
Thyroid	Largest cartilage of larynx; forms anterior midline shield called laryngeal prominence or Adam's apple
Cricoid	Only complete cartilaginous ring in respiratory tract; located just below thyroid cartilage
Epiglottis	Leaf shaped; projects upward at base of tongue and guards opening of larynx
Paired Cartilages	
Arytenoid, corniculate, and cuneiform	Serve as attachment for vocal ligaments; movement of cartilages controls tension of vocal ligaments
Intrinsic Muscles	
Thyroarytenoideus	Tilts arytenoid cartilages toward thyroid; results in shortening and relaxation of vocal cords
Arytenoideus	Approximates arytenoid cartilages and closes glottis
Cricothyroideus	Lifts anterior section of cricoid cartilage; results in increased tension on vocal cords
Posterior	
Cricoarytenoideus	Produces lateral rotation of arytenoid cartilages; results in separation of vocal cords and opening of glottis
Lateral	
Cricoarytenoideus	Produces medial rotation of arytenoid cartilages; results in approximation of vocal cords and closing of glottis

Figure 7-14 Larynx. **A,** Cartilages and ligaments.

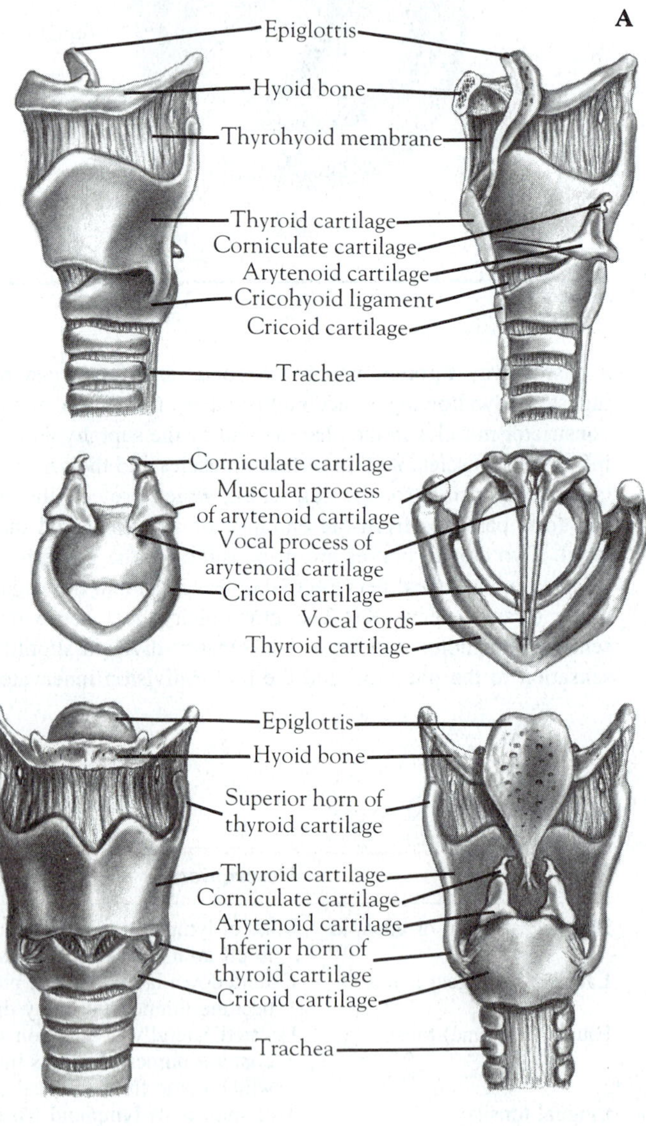

seen in people with thin necks. The cricoid (ring-shaped) cartilage is the only complete ring of cartilage in the respiratory tract. Structurally it resembles a signet ring, with the signet portion located posteriorly. The cricoid cartilage articulates with the thyroid and arytenoid cartilages. The cricoid and thyroid cartilages are attached by the cricothyroid membrane.

The arytenoid, corniculate, and cuneiform cartilages are the paired cartilages of the larynx and serve as attachments for the vocal ligaments. The arytenoid cartilages swing in and out. This action opens or closes the space between the vocal cords, since the posterior end of each vocal cord is attached to an arytenoid cartilage and thus must move with it.

The epiglottis is a leaf-shaped cartilaginous structure that is attached to the thyroid cartilage by ligaments and projects upward and posterior to the base of the tongue to guard the opening of the larynx.

The larynx contains extrinsic and intrinsic striated muscles. The extrinsic muscles connect the larynx to adjacent structures of the neck (the hyoid and sternum) and assist in swallowing. The five intrinsic muscles (Table 7-2) connect the laryngeal cartilages and alter the shape of the laryngeal cavity by contracting. The intrinsic muscles act as constrictors, dilators, and tensors so they are important in sound production or phonation. A branch of the vagus nerve, the recurrent laryngeal nerve, supplies the intrinsic muscles except for the cricothyroid muscle, which is supplied by the superior laryngeal nerve. This innervation becomes particu-

B, Neck muscles.

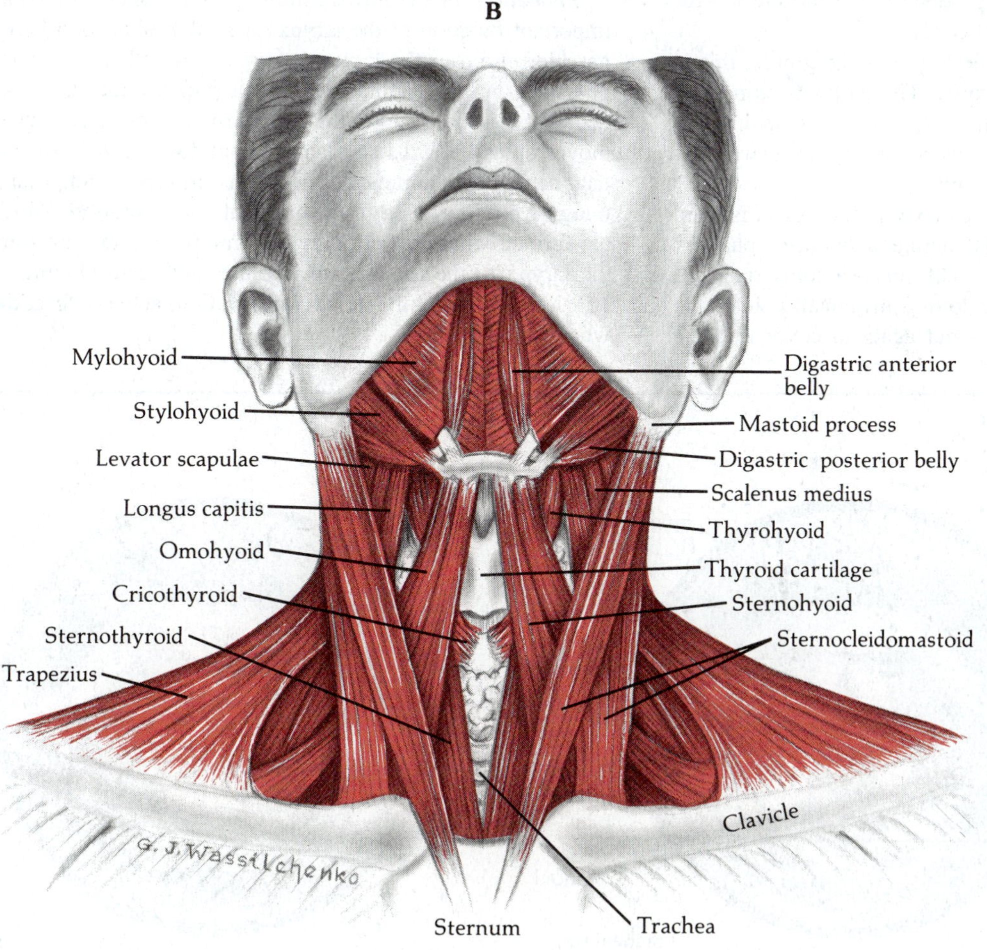

larly significant during endotracheal intubation; mechanical manipulation of the vocal cords and musculature may result in bradycardia from vagal stimulation.

Internal structures of the larynx. The internal structures are protected by the thyroid cartilage in front and include the vestibule, the false vocal cords, the true vocal cords, the laryngeal ventricle, and the glottis.

The inlet to the larynx lies in the anterior wall of the pharynx and is bordered by the epiglottis and arytenoid cartilages. From the inlet the larynx expands into a wide vestibule that ends below at the level of the true vocal folds.

Inside the larynx are two pairs of shelflike folds that project inward from the lateral walls of the larynx. The superior folds, or false vocal cords, are attached to the cartilage anteriorly and the arytenoid cartilage posteriorly. They do not move. Just under the false vocal cords are the true vocal cords. The true vocal cords are joined anteriorly where they attach to the inner surface of the thyroid cartilage. This is a fixed point at which the cords are held immobile, but they attach posteriorly to the movable arytenoid cartilages, which allow them to adduct and abduct.

The laryngeal ventricle, a fold of mucous membrane between the true and false cords, extends up under the thyroid cartilage. Glands in the upper portion of the ventricle secrete mucus that lubricates the vocal cords.

The narrowest portion of the larynx is the glottis; this is the space between the vocal cords. The glottis is somewhat larger in men than in women. It is very small in infants, thereby causing much greater danger when the airway becomes edematous as with laryngitis.

Additional structures of the larynx. The larynx is lined with mucous membrane that is continuous with the pharynx above and the trachea below. The mucosa folds over the false cords beneath the epiglottis, invaginates into the laryngeal ventricle, and comes out again to cover the true vocal cords before descending into the trachea.

Most of the blood supply to the larynx is provided by the superior and inferior thyroid arteries through their branches, the superior and inferior laryngeal arteries.

Lymphatic drainage is provided by lymph nodes in the middle and upper cervical chains along the internal jugular vein. All parts of the extrinsic larynx and the arytenoid area contain a somewhat rich lymphatic network, but the true vocal cords have a sparse supply of lymphatic vessels. Most carcinomas of the larynx develop in the true vocal cords.

Functions of the larynx. The most important function of the larynx is to form an airway between the pharynx and the trachea. The larynx is not merely a tube, as is the trachea. It is an organ with sphincter functions that help prevent aspiration and assist in coughing. During swallowing the aryepiglottic folds, the arytenoids, and the tubercle of the epiglottis fold inward, close the larynx, and prevent food from entering the trachea. Other actions close the glottis when a foreign body enters the throat and assist in expelling it by increasing intrathoracic pressure when coughing. The cough reflex is an important protective mechanism and is set off whenever the highly sensitive laryngeal mucosa is touched by a foreign body.

Phonation, or the formation of speech sounds, is also an important function of the larynx. Although phonation is not its chief purpose, the larynx is sometimes called the "voice box." During phonation, tracheal air pressure increases and decreases; as the edges of the cords firm and relax, the larynx moves up and down so the air columns above and below are lengthened and shortened. The larynx creates sounds (humming or buzzing) as a result of vocal cord vibration. Words are formed when the vibrating column of air comes up from the larynx to the tongue, lips, palate, and teeth (Figure 7-15). Movements of the mouth (articulation) actually form the words.

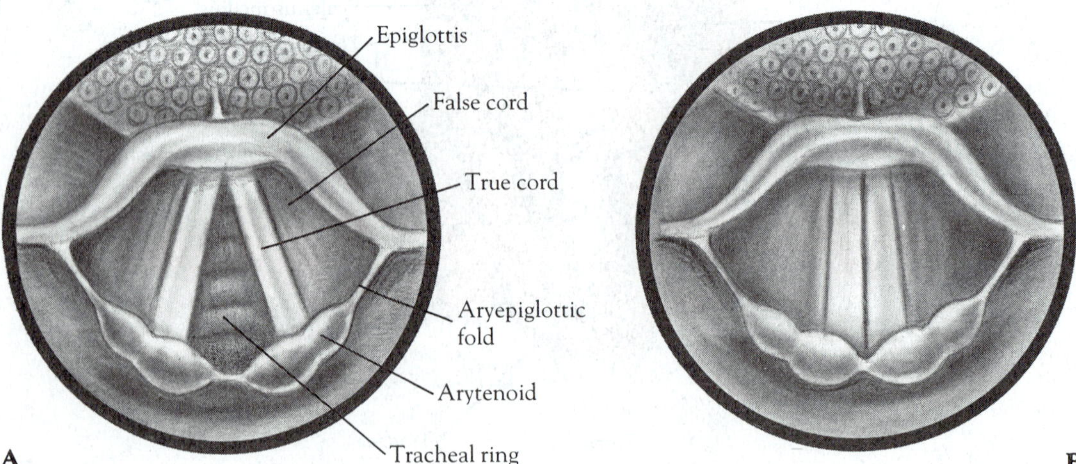

Figure 7-15 Larynx. **A,** In quiet respiration. **B,** In phonation.

Normal Findings

Area of Concern	Normal Adult Findings
Ear	
External ear	Height and size equal; skin clean; no evidence of injury or trauma *Older adult:* Earlobes may appear pendulous
Auricle	Moves freely without causing pain *Older adult:* May be more prominent
Tympanic membrane	Drumhead slightly conical, quite shiny, and pearl gray in color; oblique position when viewed with otoscope; cerumen color varying from black to brown to creamy pink; cerumen waxy or flaky; depending on translucency, should be possible to visualize following in normal drumhead: malleus, anterior and posterior malleolar folds, anulus (whiter and denser than rest of drumhead), long process of incus (frequently seen posterior to manubrium of malleus), occasionally chorda tympani nerve seen crossing transversely behind drumhead at about level of short process of malleus *Older adult:* Some landmarks may appear more pronounced because of atrophied or sclerotic tympanic changes; cerumen may appear very dry as fewer sebaceous glands are active
Eustachian tube	Eardrum moves with Valsalva maneuver if tube is patent
Vestibulocochlear nerve (cranial nerve VIII)	Patient able to hear whisper from distance of 2 feet; tuning fork placed in middle of head heard equally well in both ears *Older adult:* Presbycusis (hearing loss from senile degenerative changes) may be present
Nose	
Nares	Oval and symmetric
Mucosa	Nose mostly lined with respiratory mucosa that is deep pink and glistening *Older adult:* May be somewhat drier
Septum	Septum usually not straight but deviates from midline; posterior two thirds bony, anterior one third cartilaginous *Older adult:* Usually deviates
Turbinates	Turbinates deep pink and similar in color to rest of nasal mucosa, firm consistency
Sinuses	No tenderness, swelling, or purulent secretions from sinuses
Olfactory nerve (cranial nerve I)	Patient able to identify odor of substances such as lemon or coffee *Older adult:* Sense of smell may be somewhat depressed
Pharynx	
Oropharynx	Soft palate pink, showing fine vessels under mucosa; hard palate white, more irregular, showing rugae running transversely; ducts of mucous glands may be seen in back of hard palate; uvula may vary greatly in size and may be bifid or "split"; tonsils same color as rest of oral mucosa, with crypts of whitish epithelium showing; small irregular red or pink spots of lymphoid tissue commonly seen in mucosa of posterior pharyngeal wall; gag reflex induced by touching posterior wall of pharynx
Nasopharynx	Superior, middle, and inferior turbinates can be seen and may vary greatly in appearance; orifice of eustachian tube seen, usually pale, yellowish, and small; orifice normally closed but opens during yawning and swallowing; adenoids seen growing from roof and posterior wall if not surgically removed, usually small
Hypopharynx	Circumvallate papillae in inverted V, may vary greatly in size; lingual tonsils on either side of tongue, may vary in size; small white spots that are debris in tonsillar crypts frequently seen; valleculae seen as cup-shaped spaces between tongue and epiglottis, may have large veins; epiglottis varies in size, shape, and color, free edge thin and slightly curved
Larynx	
External (by visual examination)	Thyroid cartilage (Adam's apple) protrudes, more obvious in men; laryngeal crepitation should occur when thyroid cartilage is grasped between thumb and forefinger and is moved from side to side; cricoid cartilage can be seen in thin persons with head extended and can be easily palpated; hyoid bone palpable above thyroid cartilage; cricoid cartilage drawn upward when patient says high-pitched E-E-E as normal cricothyroid muscle contracts *Older adult:* Thyroid cartilage may be very noticeable

Area of Concern	Normal Adult Findings
Internal (via indirect laryngoscopy)	Cords move only slightly during normal respiration; phonation causes adduction of cords, which should approximate perfectly; true vocal cords appear white and sharp edged, although they are actually pink with rounded edges; a few tracheal rings sometimes seen all the way to carina; false vocal cords appear dull pink and thicker than true vocal cords; arytenoids dull red, mobile, and swing in and out with phonation; they appear as small mounds at posterior end of glottis *Older adult:* Musculature control decreases, producing characteristic hoarseness and quavering voice; atrophy of muscles and mucosa in trachea; fatty infiltration of trachea
Normal variations in pregnancy	Increased vascularity of upper respiratory tract from elevated estrogen levels; nasal stuffiness, epistaxis, fullness in ears, and impaired hearing may result from engorgement of capillaries of nose, pharynx, and eustachian tubes[47]

Conditions, Diseases, and Disorders

EAR DISORDERS

Benign tumors

Benign tumors affecting the ear are nonmalignant growths such as keloids, nodules, sebaceous cysts, polyps, and exostoses.

Nonmalignant tumors may develop on the external ear or anywhere in the ear canal. They rarely become malignant, but they may occlude the ear canal and cause retention of cerumen and a conductive hearing loss. The prognosis is excellent with proper diagnosis and treatment.

Pathophysiology

Keloids are large overgrowths of hypertrophied scar tissue that result from surgery or trauma. They are much more common in blacks than in whites. In the ear keloids commonly form as a result of ear piercing, but other trauma to the auricle can also cause them. The treatment is excision followed by repeated injections of a long-lasting steroid.

Nodules may form along the superior rim of the auricle and become indurated or painful. The cause is unknown. Treatment is excision or injection of a long-lasting steroid such as methylprednisolone or triamcinolone (Kenalog).

Sebaceous cysts are sebaceous glands that become obstructed with sebum, a soft, cheesy material. These cysts may occur in the meatus of the canal or just behind the earlobe. They are normally painless, but can enlarge quickly and become painful if infected. Acute sebaceous cysts are incised and drained, and hot, moist compresses are applied.

Exostoses are small, hard, bony lumps covered with normal epithelium. They arise from the osseous ear canal near the tympanic membrane and are attached to the posterior wall. The bases of these exostoses are close to the facial nerve. Exostoses are usually bilateral and frequently occur in multiples. They rarely occur during childhood and are more common in men than in women. They are usually asymptomatic and seldom cause an obstruction of the canal. It is believed that exostoses form from an irritation of the periosteum as a result of swimming in cold water. Treatment is usually unnecessary, although removal may be indicated if they grow to a large size.

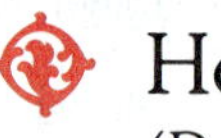

Hearing impairment

(Deafness)

Hearing impairment is a state of diminished auditory acuity that ranges from partial to complete loss of hearing.

Hearing loss can be partial or total and can occur in low, medium, or high frequencies or in combination. Hearing is measured in decibels (dB), which is a ratio that compares the relationship between two sound intensities.

The American Medical Association's formula for hearing loss is that hearing is impaired 1.5% for every decibel that the pure tone average exceeds 25 dB. A hearing loss of 40 dB in both ears, or a 22.5% hearing impairment, usually impairs a person's ability to function normally in social situations and requires the use of a hearing aid unless it can be medically or surgically treated. True deafness, however, is defined as 85 to 90 dB below normal. Hearing losses can occur in one or both ears, depending on the etiology, and may imply only a partial loss of function, depending on the severity.

Pathophysiology

The six types of hearing loss are sensorineural, conductive, mixed, congenital, simulated, and central.

Sensorineural hearing loss. Sensorineural hearing loss is the result of disease within the cochlea, the cochlear nerve, or the brain. It usually results from trauma, an infectious process, a degenerative process such as presbycusis, a senile degenerative change in the hair cells in the organ of Corti, a congenital abnormality, or exposure to ototoxic substances such as certain drugs. Intense noise may destroy cochlear hair cells, thereby causing a sensorineural hearing loss. Injury to the organ of Corti may also destroy cochlear hair cells. This may also be called perceptive or nerve-type hearing loss. Patients with sensorineural hearing losses are often unable to use hearing aids satisfactorily.

Conductive hearing loss. Conductive hearing loss is also called transmission hearing loss. It occurs in disorders of the external or middle ear such as otitis media, otosclerosis, or a perforated eardrum. These patients have a normal inner ear, but sound waves are prevented from reaching the inner ear normally. If sound is amplified, these patients may be able to hear very well, and therefore a hearing aid can be beneficial. With the exception of otosclerosis in which the drumhead usually appears normal, disorders that cause conductive hearing loss also cause changes in the normal appearance of the drumhead, such as thickening or retraction.

Mixed hearing loss. Some patients have both conductive and sensorineural hearing losses.

Congenital hearing loss. Congenital hearing loss is present from birth or early infancy. "Neonatal" causes may be anoxia, trauma during delivery, or Rh incompatibility. Other causes may be maternal exposure to syphilis or rubella during pregnancy or the use of ototoxic drugs during pregnancy. Infants with serum bilirubin levels above 20 mg/dl may also incur hearing losses from the toxic effect of high bilirubin levels on the brain.[33]

Simulated hearing loss. Simulated hearing loss is also called functional, psychogenic, or nonorganic hearing loss. It means that an apparent hearing loss is not the result of an organic cause and may represent malingering or a functional disorder.

Central hearing loss. Central hearing loss is caused by damage to the brain's auditory pathways, as in a cerebrovascular accident.

Diagnostic Studies and Findings

Weber Test

Lateralization of sound to deaf ear in conductive hearing loss; lateralization of sound to better ear in sensorineural hearing loss

Rinne Test

Bone conduction heard longer than or equal to air conduction in conductive hearing loss; air conduction heard longer but not twice as long as bone conduction in sensorineural hearing loss

Schwabach Test

Patient hears longer than examiner in conductive hearing loss; examiner hears longer than patient in sensorineural hearing loss

Audiometric Tests

Speech and impedance audiometry, tympanometry, and electrocochleography to differentiate between types of hearing loss and to identify degree of impairment

Medical Plan

Surgery

Depending on the type of hearing impairment, a variety of surgical interventions may be appropriate

Stapedectomy—see p. 720

Cochlear implant—complex procedure in which inferior aspect of the basal scala tympani is exposed; bone is removed from inferior margins of scala tympani for distance of approximately 4 to 5 mm from round window; surgeon then negotiates tip of Silastic-sheathed multielectrode around first turn of basal cochlea in bony groove in posterior canal wall, which is then covered with cortical bone and temporalis fascia[45]; device electrically stimulates intact auditory nerves in people who cannot hear; electronic "heart" of device is small processor that can be carried on belt and can receive sound through microphone and electronically break signal into four channels; a tiny transmitter, which is mounted behind ear, sends signal to receiver implanted under skin; from internal receiver, fine wire leads to electrode, which is implanted against auditory nerves in cochlea

General Management

Hearing aids—amplifier or transducer type hearing aids prescribed depending on nature of hearing impairment

NURSING CARE

Nursing Assessment

Stares blankly; asks to have things repeated; gives irrelevant answers to questions; may not participate in conversations; withdraws; may hear much better when watching speaker's face; inattentive; daydreams; scholastic performance below apparent ability (if school age); delayed speech and language development (if small child); may complain of sound distortion; intolerant of loud noise

Nursing Dx & Intervention

Nursing Diagnosis	Nursing Intervention/Rationale
Sensory/perceptual alterations (auditory)	• Assess patient's degree of hearing impairment and concomitant ability to communicate with others. • Ensure that other health-care providers are aware of patient's hearing impairment—place a note on Kardex, on door, and at intercom at nursing station. • When conversing speak slowly and distinctly and face patient directly *so patient can see your face*. • Ensure that patient has heard and understood everything said. • Ascertain whether patient hears better from one ear than from the other and speak toward that ear when talking with patient. • Obtain speaker phone or pocket talker and a pillow speaker for television set *so patient can use telephone and television comfortably*. • Discuss with family members any strategies used at home to assist patient with hearing. • If patient is hospitalized for problem unrelated to hearing impairment, ascertain whether patient has been evaluated for hearing problem and discuss with physician, patient, and family the possibility of audiology consultation and follow-up, if appropriate. • If patient is completely deaf, provide Magic Slate or notepad *so patient can communicate in writing*. • If patient wears a hearing aid at home, encourage patient to wear it in the hospital also. • If patient is being fitted for a hearing aid, encourage and assist patient to wear it for progressively longer periods of time and assure patient that any discomfort is temporary. • If patient is hospitalized for ear surgery to improve or stabilize hearing, provide patient with appropriate preoperative and postoperative care and assess and record any improvements in hearing after operation.

Patient Education

1. Inform the patient of proper use and maintenance of hearing aid, if prescribed.
2. Ensure that the patient and family are aware of any postoperative instructions, if appropriate.
3. Encourage the patient to ask people to speak more slowly or clearly or to repeat statements so the patient does not feel left out of conversations.

Evaluation

Patient Outcome	Data Indicating That Outcome is Reached
Patient recovers uneventfully (if surgery performed).	Hearing level is improved to normal. Patient verbalizes ear care regimen and any symptoms to be reported to physician.
Patient copes well with hearing impairment.	Patient verbalizes and demonstrates use and maintenance of hearing aid (if used). Hearing level is improved with use of hearing aid. Patient has learned to use strategies, such as lip reading or sign language.

External otitis

External otitis is a general term used to describe inflammatory diseases of the auricle and the external auditory canal.

External otitis may be acute or chronic and may be localized as with furunculosis, or diffuse, involving the entire canal. The disorder may be caused by either infections or dermatosis or by a combination of the two. It is more common in summer and is sometimes called swimmer's ear. External otitis varies in severity; there is occasionally no infection, and it may result from either contact or seborrheic dermatitis. Either bacteria or fungi may produce infectious external otitis. Bacterial causes are usually attributed to *Pseudomonas, Proteus, Streptococcus,* and *Staphylococcus*. Fungi, which are most common in the tropics, are usually *Aspergillus* and *Candida*. Predisposing factors include allergies that may increase the likelihood of external otitis; irritants such as hair sprays, hair dyes, or dust that cause the person to scratch the ear canal, resulting in excoriation; cleaning or scratching the ear canal with a foreign object, such as a cotton swab, bobby pin, or finger, which causes irritation and possible introduction of infectious organisms; continual use of earphones, earplugs, or earmuffs, which trap moisture in the ear, thereby creating a medium for infection; and swimming in contaminated water, which is absorbed by the wax in the ear, macerates the skin of the canal, and allows the introduction of organisms.

Pathophysiology

Acute external otitis is frequently caused by *Pseudomonas,* which can be cultured from the auditory canal. The infection begins in the external auditory canal, usually after minor trauma. It may spread from the canal through Santorini's fissures in the conchal cartilage, after involving the perichondrium. It then invades the periauricular tissue, including the parotid gland, temporomandibular joint, and soft tissues at the base of the skull. The infection can progress along the base of the skull, causing paralysis of the seventh cranial nerve at the stylomastoid foramen, the ninth, tenth, and eleventh cranial nerves at the jugular foramen, and the hypoglossal nerve at the hypoglossal canal. The jugular vein may become thrombosed, progressing to a lateral sinus thrombosis. The infection could also progress from the external auditory canal, through the tympanic membrane, and into the middle ear, and through the mastoid air cells and into the petrous apex and brainstem. Mortality is 67% among patients with facial nerve paralysis and 20% for those with other cranial nerve involvement.[46]

Acute external otitis can range from mild to severe. In the mild stage, pain is moderate to severe and is aggravated by traction on the auricle or pressure on the tragus. The patient may have a low-grade fever and a sticky, yellow discharge from the ear canal. There may be a partial loss of hearing or the feeling of a blocked ear if the ear canal is swollen or obstructed with debris.

Pain is more intense during the severe stage of external otitis. Often the entire side of the head aches, and the patient cannot tolerate examination of the auricle. There is usually a sticky, yellow discharge from the ear canal, hearing may be diminished, and the ear feels blocked. The patient's temperature may be as high as 40° C (104° F). The external auditory canal is swollen or entirely closed, and the tragus and external meatus are also swollen. The epithelium of the canal is usually soggy and pale. Desquamated epithelium and wax are often present in the canal. However, the canal may be reddened rather than pale, or the epithelium may be dry instead of wet. Patients may also have lymphadenopathy anterior to the tragus, behind the ear, or in the upper neck. If the auricle is involved, the skin is crusted and oozing. Pustules may be present and the ear swollen and tender. If the infection did not originate on the face or scalp, it may spread to these areas. The eardrum frequently cannot be seen well in acute external otitis because the ear canal is so swollen. An infected canal usually causes much more pain than if the auricle alone is affected because the epithelium of the ear canal cannot stretch much without causing pain.

With chronic external otitis, itching rather than pain is the usual complaint. There is no pain even with manipulation of the auricle or tragus. The epithelium is thickened and red, and the canal and drumhead are insensitive to pressure from cotton applicators. A discharge is usually present.

A rare, lethal type of external otitis, which is called malignant external otitis, is caused by *Pseudomonas;* it is a fulminant bone-destroying infection. It occurs mostly in patients with diabetes. It quickly involves all contiguous structures and has a mortality of 50% to 75% unless recognized early and treated with potent parenteral antibiotics.[30]

In fungally caused external otitis, a characteristic mass (black or grayish with *Aspergillus niger*) forms in the ear canal. Its removal reveals a hyperemic, edematous epithelium that may be denuded. Fungal infections may be asymptomatic, since frequently the growth is found only on wax or other debris in the ear and has not invaded the tissue.

Furunculosis is a localized type of external otitis in the outer half of the ear canal. Glands and hair follicles in this area may become infected and form boils or furuncles. The onset of a furuncle may be acute; the patient may notice a feeling of fullness in the ear, loss of hearing, adenopathy, and swelling behind the ear. The area is reddened. It may be very swollen and may obstruct the entire canal. Pain is intense; even a small furuncle causes severe pain until it is surgically drained or breaks spontaneously. Movement of the auricle and tragus causes pain, as does chewing if the furuncle is on the canal floor or anterior wall.

Diagnostic Studies and Findings

Culture of Discharge

Identification of causative organisms; usual organisms are *Pseudomonas, Proteus, Streptococcus, Staphylococcus, Aspergillus,* and *Candida*

Medical Plan

Surgery

Surgery not performed unless furuncle needs incision and drainage

Medications

Narcotic analgesics
- Analgesic for pain is codeine, 30 mg po q4h

Corticosteroids
- A wick is inserted into the ear canal; 1% hydrocortisone is sometimes used to reduce swelling and to allow penetration of antibiotics

Anti-infective agents
- Antibiotic or antifungal ear drops may be prescribed, which usually contain 0.5% neomycin or 10,000 U/ml of polymyxin
- Systemic antibiotics may be prescribed if infection is severe; specific drug depends on causative organism

General Management

Careful cleansing of ear canal to remove debris and impacted cerumen

Heat therapy to external ear for pain relief

NURSING CARE

Nursing Assessment

Infection of External Ear

Acute

Moderate to severe pain in the ear, which is exacerbated by chewing and manipulation of the auricle or tragus; headache; fever; feeling of fullness or blockage in ear; foul-smelling, yellow, sticky discharge from ear (black if from fungal infection); hearing normal or decreased; tinnitus; localized swelling; erythema; lymphadenopathy behind ear and in upper neck; persistent granulation tissue on floor of external auditory canal near junction of bony and cartilaginous portions

General Ear

Chronic

Chief complaint itching rather than pain; discharge usually present; thickened, red epithelium; canal and drumhead insensitive to pressure

Nursing Dx & Intervention

Nursing Diagnosis	Nursing Intervention/Rationale
Pain	• Assess need for pain medication and in collaboration with physician, provide medication as required *for pain relief;* evaluate and document effectiveness. • Monitor vital signs, especially temperature. • If chewing is painful, arrange for soft or full-liquid diet.
Impaired skin integrity	• Assess ear canal and auricle for swelling, crusting, scabs, pustules, and discharge. • Keep ear canal clean: Cleanse gently with cotton swab soaked with Burow's solution and also apply directly to auricle. Dry gently and completely. • Administer antibiotics as ordered. • Instill medicated ear drops as ordered. • Observe and record amount of aural drainage.
Sensory/perceptual alterations (auditory)	• Assess degree of hearing impairment. • If patient's hearing is diminished, be sure that adequate method of communication is used. • Speak slowly and clearly and stand directly in front of patient when speaking. • Instruct patient and family about factors contributing to development of external otitis and encourage patient to keep foreign objects such as bobby pins out of ears. • Encourage patient to use earplugs when swimming and to minimize amount of water that gets into ears when showering and shampooing.

Patient Education

1. Inform the patient and family of the necessity of completing the prescribed course of medication, whether antibiotics or ear drops, to avoid inadequate treatment or possible recurrence.
2. Teach the patient and family the proper way to instill ear drops.
3. If Burow's soaks are done, give instructions in the proper method.

Evaluation

Patient Outcome	Data Indicating That Outcome is Reached
Inflammation of external ear and canal is cleared.	There is no pain in the ear. Patient's temperature is within normal limits. There is no discharge from ear canal. Hearing is within normal limits for patient. There is no cervical lymphadenopathy.
Patient and family verbalize increased knowledge of disease and its treatment.	Patient and family verbalize understanding of cause of, contributing factors to, and ways to prevent recurrence of disease. Patient and family verbalize understanding of necessity of completing prescribed course of antibiotics.

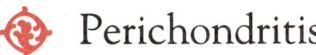

Perichondritis

Perichondritis is an inflammation of the auricular cartilage.

Perichondritis may follow a skin infection, but it more usually follows exposure of the cartilage from infection or trauma, which allows bacteria to enter.

Pathophysiology

Perichondritis may be initiated by trauma, insect bites, or incision of superficial infections of the pinna, which causes pus to accumulate between the cartilage and the perichondrium. The causative organism is usually a gram-negative rod, frequently *Pseudomonas*. Perichondritis can cause a loss of blood supply to the cartilage, resulting in breakdown and necrosis of the cartilage. The pinna appears enlarged, inflamed, and shiny. Pain is usually severe, and localized fluctuant areas may be present on the auricle. Perichondritis must be treated early and aggressively to prevent a lengthy, destructive course.

Diagnostic Studies and Findings

Culture of Purulent Material

Identification of causative organism

Medical Plan

Surgery

Incision and drainage of any purulent material; removal of any necrotic cartilage

Medications

Anti-infective agents
- Systemic parenteral antibiotic therapy, depending on cultured organism; local irrigations with antibiotic solutions (usually polymyxin B [10,000 U/ml], bacitracin, neomycin 0.5%, or a combination)

Narcotic analgesics or analgesic/antipyretic agents
- Analgesia for pain relief; aspirin or acetaminophen (Tylenol), 650 mg, with codeine, 30 mg po q4h

General Management

Small polyethylene tube inserted into area beneath nonpressure dressing to facilitate irrigation

Local heat applications for relief

NURSING CARE

Nursing Assessment

Auricular Cartilage

Inflammation and swelling of the cartilage, usually with pus; fluctuant areas on auricle; severe pain; history of trauma, insect bite, or incision of superficial infection on pinna

Nursing Dx & Intervention

Nursing Diagnosis	Nursing Intervention/Rationale
Pain	• Assess need for pain medication and provide analgesic medications for pain relief as ordered. Evaluate and document effectiveness.
Sensory/perceptual alterations (auditory)	• Assess patient's hearing ability before and during treatment with ototoxic drugs. • Administer antibiotics as ordered. • Perform irrigations as ordered with room-temperature antibiotic solution. • Be aware that irrigating solution contains potentially ototoxic drugs. • Monitor vital signs, especially temperature.
Impaired skin integrity	• Assess auricular cartilage for inflammation, swelling, and presence of pus. • Perform wound care of affected area if incision and drainage have been done. • Apply local heat for comfort as ordered.

Patient Education

1. Instruct the patient and family in the necessity of completing the prescribed course of antibiotics to avoid recurrence or complications.
2. If wound care is being done, be sure that the patient and family know the procedures to change the dressing and aseptic techniques to avoid wound contamination.

Evaluation

Patient Outcome	Data Indicating That Outcome is Reached
Inflammation of auricular cartilage is absent.	There is no pain or drainage from affected ear. Temperature is within normal limits for patient. There are no fluctuant areas on auricle. Patient and family demonstrate ability to change dressing properly using aseptic technique.
Patient and family verbalize and demonstrate knowledge of treatment.	Patient and family verbalize understanding of necessity of completing prescribed course of antibiotics to prevent recurrence of infection.

Infectious myringitis

Infectious or bullous myringitis is an inflammation of the tympanic membrane.

Vesicles in the tympanic membrane and at the end of the external auditory canal appear hemorrhagic and rupture spontaneously, which is revealed by serosanguineous fluid in the external ear. The cause is either viral or bacterial, and the disorder sometimes occurs after acute otitis media. It is common in children.

The patient experiences severe ear pain and some tenderness over the mastoid area. Occasionally fever and mild hearing loss are present. Treatment consists of pain management with aspirin or other analgesics, local heat for comfort, and either local or systemic antibiotic therapy to prevent secondary infection. Infectious myringitis usually resolves spontaneously within 3 days to 2 weeks.

Otitis media

Otitis media is an inflammation of the middle ear and can be classified as acute and suppurative or subacute (otitis media with effusion).

Acute Otitis Media

Acute suppurative otitis media is very common in young children and is usually the result of a bacterial or viral infection of the upper respiratory tract. Organisms travel from the nasopharynx to the middle ear via the eustachian tube. Infants and children have shorter, straighter eustachian tubes than do adults; this easier access to the middle ear is probably the reason otitis media is common in children. Another contributing factor is that children have not developed immunities to the organisms that cause the infection. Children also have a large mass of adenoid tissue which usually disappears during adolescence. If this lymphoid tissue is swollen, it can obstruct the opening of the eustachian tube and contribute to the development of otitis media by preventing equalization of the atmospheric pressure in the ear, thereby causing a vacuum and effusion of the middle ear.

Most episodes of recurrent acute otitis media occur between 6 and 36 months of age and in the winter and early spring. Prophylactic antibiotics, prescribed and used appropriately, may be helpful in protecting children during this period.[23]

Otitis Media With Effusion (Subacute)

Otitis media with effusion results from incomplete resolution or inadequate treatment of acute otitis media. The most recent evidence indicates that in a large number of cases, bacteria or bacterial products are trapped in the middle ear as a result of poor tubal muscular function. This situation causes a high negative pressure in the middle ear and produces transudation of fluid from the blood vessels in the membranes of the middle ear. Ciliostasis may be another factor; it causes stagnation of the collected effusion. Yet another factor may be failure to clear the bacteria and bacterial products by dysfunctional phagocytes or inadequate host-immune response to eradicate bacteria. These trapped bacteria in the middle ear may initiate a host response that causes tissue injury leading to otitis media with effusion.[37] Otitis media with effusion can also be caused by allergies that produce edema in the lumen of the eustachian tube or by barotrauma that results from external pressure markedly exceeding lowered pressure of the middle ear, as during diving or the descent of an airplane. It is common in children.

Patients feel a fullness in their ears but have no pain or fever. A conductive hearing loss may occur, especially in chronic otitis media with effusion. Otoscopic examination reveals mild retraction of the tympanic membrane with a clear transudate from the blood vessels. The tympanic membrane is immobile and amber colored, and a fluid level or air bubbles may be seen through the tympanic membrane. The meniscus of the fluid may appear as a thin black hair or line across the tympanic membrane. If blood is present, as with barotrauma, the fluid may appear blue-black.

Treatment consists of inflation of the eustachian tube, a Valsalva maneuver (in which the patient inspires, holds the breath, and bears down as though having a bowel movement) several times a day, myringotomy to drain fluid from the middle ear, or antihistamine therapy to improve eustachian tube function. A small plastic tube may be left in place for several weeks to promote drainage and equalize air pressure; this is most commonly done in children but also occasionally in adults.

Chronic otitis media with effusion that results from inadequate treatment of acute otitis media or from overgrowth of the lymphoid tissue in the nasopharynx caused by nasal sinus infections or allergies poses a serious threat to the patient's hearing. There are few symptoms; a fluctuating hearing loss or a feeling of heaviness on one side of the head is most common. Treatment is directed at the underlying cause and the removal of fluid by myringotomy. A small tube is frequently inserted during myringotomy to equalize pressure on both sides of the eardrum and is left in place for 8 to 9 months, when it usually falls out by itself. These tubes may need to be replaced. Patients should be instructed not to swim while a tube is in place.

Not to be overlooked as a cause of chronic otitis media with effusion in adults is carcinoma of the nasopharynx; if the effusion is unilateral, a thorough workup must be done to eliminate carcinoma.[9]

Chronic otitis media caused by repeated attacks of acute otitis media and acute mastoiditis may result in a permanent perforation of the tympanic membrane. Chronic changes such as thickening and scarring of the mucosa eventually occur in the middle ear, and the ossicles may be destroyed. These permanent tympanic perforations result in a slight conductive hearing loss. If the ossicles are involved, the hearing loss may be greater.

There are two types of perforations, central and marginal. In central perforations, the margin of the eardrum is not involved; in marginal perforations, the anulus or margin of the drum is destroyed. Central perforations are more benign than marginal ones and less likely to result in cholesteatomas. Cholesteatomas occur when the marginal perforation of the eardrum allows squamous epithelium of the external auditory canal to grow into the middle ear, which then becomes lined with squamous epithelium. As the epithelium grows, it desquamates and the debris collects inside the middle ear. Cholesteatomas enlarge slowly, expand into the mastoid antrum, and destroy adjacent structures.

The most common symptom of chronic otitis media is a constant, painless, serous discharge from the ear, which varies from foul smelling to nearly odorless. The discharge becomes much worse when the patient has an infection of the upper respiratory tract, and it occasionally causes slight discomfort in the ear.

Treatment consists of thoroughly cleaning the ear and instilling a solution of 0.5% acetic acid with 1.0% hydrocortisone three times a day for 5 to 7 days. Severe cases require systemic antibiotic therapy. Tympanoplasty can also be performed to restore and reconstruct the mechanisms of the middle ear (see p. 727).

Pathophysiology

The usual pathogens of acute otitis media are gram-positive cocci; *Streptococcus* is cultured from approximately 30% of effusions, but *Haemophilus influenzae* is also frequently found (20% of cases).[23] The inflammation usually results from an infection that ascends via the eustachian tube and involves the lining of the whole middle ear. This has several effects. Exudate and edema interfere with ciliary action in the eustachian tube so its efficiency as a barrier to infection is lost. The opening of the tube is also abnormal, since edema has decreased the size of the lumen and inflammation has caused hyperemia of the mucosal lining of the middle ear, which results in increased oxygen absorption. This leads to decreased aeration, development of a partial vacuum, retraction of the tympanic membrane, and serous exudation. This stage is common in viral infections of the upper respiratory tract, but the infection does not progress if the middle ear is reaerated. However, if there is bacterial superinfection, the exudate becomes purulent and causes bulging of the tympanic membrane as the pus collects behind it. This is called purulent otitis media.

Diagnostic Studies and Findings

Culture of Purulent Organism

Identification of causative organisms

Medical Plan

Surgery

Myringotomy—to drain pus and fluid from middle ear (see p. 719)

Medications

Anti-infective agents
- Amoxicillin (Amoxil, Larotid), 500 mg po tid for 10 d
- Sulfamethoxazole (Septra or Bactrim), 1 tab po bid or qid (if allergic to penicillin)
- Penicillin G or V, 250-500 mg po q6h for 10 d for patients older than 8 yr
- Ampicillin (Amcil, others), 50-100 mg/kg/d for 10 d for children under 8 yr because of frequency of *H. influenzae* infections in this age group
- If patient is allergic to penicillin, erythromycin (E-Mycin, others), 250 mg po for adults and older children; combination of erythromycin and sulfisoxazole for children younger than 8 yr

Analgesic/antipyretic or narcotic analgesics
- Codeine, 30 mg po q4h (for severe pain); sedatives sometimes given to small children

Antihistamines
- Chlorpheniramine (Chlor-Trimeton), 4 mg po q4-6h for 7-10 d for adults; 0.35 mg/kg qid for children

Bronchodilators
- Pseudoephedrine (Sudafed), 30 mg po q4-6h for adults

NURSING CARE

Nursing Assessment

Tympanic Membrane

Severe, deep, throbbing pain behind tympanic membrane; pain may disappear if eardrum ruptures; feeling of fullness in ears; partial loss of hearing

Infectious Process

Fever that may be as high as 40° C (104° F); chills; malaise, weakness and dizziness; nausea and vomiting; tympanic membrane appears red, inflamed, and bulging; if it is perforated, pulsating purulent material can be seen coming through drum after ear is cleaned of pus and debris

Nursing Dx & Intervention

Nursing Diagnosis	Nursing Intervention/Rationale
Pain	• Assess need for pain medication and provide analgesia as ordered; evaluate and document effectiveness. • Administer sedatives, if ordered, to young children as needed, *to assist with relaxation and sleep.* • Instruct parents in appropriate dosages of medication to give child at home. • Encourage bed rest if patient is weak, complains of malaise, or has nausea and vomiting.
Impaired skin integrity	• Assess patient's outer ear for purulent drainage. • If patient has had myringotomy, keep ear clean and dry. • Place sterile cotton in outer ear *to absorb drainage and prevent possible contamination of outer ear, which leads to development of external otitis media.* • Monitor vital signs, especially temperature, and report any changes.
Sensory/perceptual alterations (auditory)	• Assess patient for symptoms of hearing deficit. • If patient is child, ask parents if they have noticed any signs of hearing loss: inattentiveness, blank stares, lack of response to questions, or pulling at affected ear. (Ear pain is frequently so severe that hearing loss is not noticed.) • Administer antibiotics as ordered and instruct patient and family about appropriate dosages. • Instruct patient or family to monitor level of hearing (it should return to normal with appropriate antibiotic therapy).

Patient Education

1. Instruct the patient and family of the necessity for completing the entire course of antibiotics to prevent a recurrence or complications.
2. Instruct the parents to feed children in an upright position and not lying down to prevent reflex of nasopharyngeal flora through the eustachian tube into the middle ear.
3. Instruct the patient not to blow the nose forcefully, which forces contaminated material into the eustachian tube.
4. If the patient has had a myringotomy, instruct the patient and family how to change the cotton in the outer ear at least twice a day.

Evaluation

Patient Outcome	Data Indicating That Outcome is Reached
Otitis media is resolved.	There is no purulent drainage from tympanic membrane. Tympanic membrane appears normal with no bulging, redness, retraction, or inflammation. Hearing is normal for patient. Patient is afebrile. Patient's activity level is normal.
Patient and family have increased knowledge of treatment.	Patient and family verbalize understanding of necessity for completing prescribed course of antibiotics.

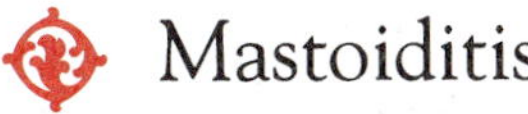

Mastoiditis

Mastoiditis is an inflammation of the air cells of the antrum.

Usually of bacterial origin, mastoiditis is the result of the extension of a middle ear infection. It was quite common before the discovery of antibiotics but is now found only in patients whose otitis media was untreated or inadequately treated.

Pathophysiology

Mastoiditis occurs when pus is left in the middle ear from otitis media, and infection progresses into the bony portion of the mastoid antrum and cells. This can cause bony necrosis of the mastoid process and breakdown of its bony structure. If untreated, the infection can lead to formation of subperiosteal abscesses and other complications, including meningitis, facial paralysis, brain abscesses, and sigmoid sinus thrombosis.

With mastoiditis, large amounts of thick purulent material usually fill the external auditory canal, which indicates perforation of the tympanum. The soft tissue that is next to the eardrum may be ruptured and sagging. Roentgenograms of the mastoid are needed to determine the extent of involvement. Findings vary from clouding of the air cells and some decalcification of the bony walls to complete coalescence of the air cells. If early decalcification is present, intense antibiotic therapy and myringotomy can usually cure mastoiditis; if it has progressed to further destruction, simple mastoidectomy is necessary.[9]

Diagnostic Studies and Findings

Mastoid Roentgenograms

May show cloudy air cells and decalcification of cell walls

Medical Plan

Surgery

Mastoidectomy if necessary; involves removing involved bone and cleansing area; can be performed through postaural or endaural incision

Myringotomy to drain fluid and pus from middle ear (see p. 719)

Medications

Anti-infective agents

- Penicillin G procaine suspension (Wycillin, Duracillin), 600,000-1,200,000 U IM
- Penicillin G aqueous, 1.5 million U q4-6h for severe infections
- Other agents specific to organism

NURSING CARE

Nursing Assessment

Tympanic Membrane

Thick purulent discharge; membrane appears dull, thickened, and edematous, and otoscopic examination reveals that it is ruptured; dull aching behind ear; low-grade fever; auricle may be pushed out from head by erythema or edema; conductive hearing loss

Nursing Dx & Intervention

Nursing Diagnosis	Nursing Intervention/Rationale
Pain	• Assess need for pain medication, and administer analgesics as ordered. Evaluate and record effectiveness of pain relief. • Administer antibiotics as ordered.
Impaired skin integrity	• Assess dressings and reinforce as necessary after mastoidectomy. • Place gauze between ear and head *to avoid crushing ear against head and to promote adequate circulation.* • Record amount and color of wound drainage and patient's temperature.
Sensory/perceptual alterations (auditory)	• Assess patient's hearing before and after mastoidectomy and myringotomy. • If patient experiences hearing loss, speak slowly and clearly when talking with patient. • Ensure that family and other staff members are aware of hearing loss and use appropriate methods of communication. • Assist patient with standing and ambulation initially, *since patient may experience some vertigo.*

Patient Education

1. Inform the patient and family of the necessity of completing the prescribed course of antibiotics to prevent recurrence or complications.

Evaluation

Patient Outcome	Data Indicating That Outcome is Reached
Inflammation of mastoid is cleared.	There is no pain in ear. There is no drainage in external canal. If mastoidectomy was performed, wound is well healed. Temperature is within normal limits for patient. Hearing is normal for patient.
Patient and family verbalize knowledge of treatment of mastoiditis.	Patient and family verbalize understanding of necessity for completing the prescribed course of medication.

Labyrinthitis

Labyrinthitis is an inflammation of the labyrinth of the inner ear.

Labyrinthitis is quite rare, and it is usually classified into four types: paralabyrinthitis, serous, purulent, and viral. Because the membranous labyrinth is protected by bone, it is difficult for microorganisms to enter the area unless the bony labyrinth is eroded, as it is with cholesteatoma formation in chronic otitis media. However, organisms can gain entry through the oval and round windows during acute otitis media or through the cochlear aqueduct during meningitis. Symptoms are usually severe vertigo and nystagmus, followed by total sensorineural hearing loss on the affected side.

Paralabyrinthitis causes the least serious symptoms of the four types of labyrinthitis. A fistula between the bony and membranous labyrinths is caused by erosion of the bone from granulation or cholesteatoma formation, but there is no inflammation or infection. There is no spontaneous nystagmus, and vertigo may be present only because the membranous labyrinth is exposed when exogenous stimulation occurs. A diagnosis is usually made when alternating positive and negative pressures are applied to the external meatus: applying positive pressure may induce nystagmus toward the affected ear, and negative pressure has the opposite effect. Nystagmus is not always produced, however, and the presence of vertigo usually assists in making the diagnosis. Treatment consists of surgically exteriorizing the fistula.

In *serous labyrinthitis* the membranous labyrinth is inflamed and direct labyrinthine stimulation occurs, probably by a direct effect on the nerve endings. This stimulation produces nystagmus on the affected side. Nystagmus may also result from the caloric effect caused by the hyperemia. The patient experiences severe vertigo and nausea and vomiting, characteristically lies quietly with the affected side down, and looks up in an attempt to decrease the nystagmus. The patient may experience some deafness. Any type of movement may worsen the vertigo, and an attempt to stand results in a fall. Heavy sedation, bed rest, and systemic antibiotics in high doses are indicated. If the patient's hearing returns, the labyrinthitis was serous rather than purulent.

Purulent labyrinthitis causes destruction of the labyrinth and cochlea, resulting in permanent deafness in the affected ear. Symptoms and treatment are the same as for serous labyrinthitis; massive doses of antibiotics are administered to prevent the spread of infection and pus and resultant meningitis. Drugs such as ampicillin are usually prescribed because penicillin does not easily cross into the labyrinth. Patients may require intravenous hydration and administration of antivertigo drugs such as meclizine.

Viral labyrinthitis may be suspected after infections of the upper respiratory tract or if sudden unilateral deafness occurs in a young patient with no concomitant infection of the middle ear. The mumps virus is commonly associated with sudden deafness in young children. Rubella in the mother during the first trimester of gestation may cause congenital deafness. Infants born of these mothers have elevated rubella titers. The best prevention is prophylactic vaccination of young women during their childbearing years.

Nursing care is aimed at preventing falls. Bed rails are kept up, and the patient is instructed to lie quietly and not to get out of bed without assistance. Antiemetic and antivertigo medications are administered for patient comfort. Antibiotics are given if ordered. The patient's intake and output are monitored for symptoms of dehydration, and intravenous fluids are given if ordered.

If not hospitalized, the patient should stay in bed at home and request assistance from a family member before getting up.

The patient and family should be informed that recovery from the symptoms may take up to 6 weeks, and the patient should be cautioned about activities that may cause vertigo, such as climbing or working in high places.

Obstruction

Obstruction of the ear canal is usually caused by excessive secretion or impaction of cerumen or by foreign bodies, including insects.

Young children put various objects, such as beads, pebbles, beans, and small toys, into their ears. An obstruction of the ear canal can lead to infection and to conductive hearing loss if auditory function is disrupted.

Pathophysiology

Cerumen is normally produced in small amounts and dries in the ear, where it is forced out bit by bit during chewing and talking. Some people, however, have overactive glands that produce excessive amounts of cerumen that can completely occlude the ear canal. Others have narrow or tortuous ear canals that can become impacted with cerumen.

Insects occasionally fly into the ear, which causes an unpleasant sensation as they beat their wings.

Foreign objects, which children frequently put into their ears, may not cause symptoms or may cause intense pain if deep in the canal. Physicians occasionally find foreign objects in children's ears during a routine examination.

Diagnostic Studies and Findings

Otoscopic Examination

Visualization of obstructing object

Medical Plan

Surgery

Surgical removal of foreign object with patient under anesthesia may be necessary if patient, who is often a child, is unable to remain still during removal

Medications

Carbamide peroxide 6.5% (Debrox drops), 5-10 gtt in ear canal to soften cerumen

General Management

Removal of cerumen by irrigation or with cerumen spoon

If insect is cause of obstruction, it is smothered with drops of oily substance and removed with forceps

Other foreign objects removed with forceps if possible

NURSING CARE

Nursing Assessment

Auditory Function

Ear feels occluded; some tinnitus or "buzzing" may be present; pain in ear; slight hearing loss; canal may be completely occluded by cerumen; may be insect or foreign body in canal

Nursing Dx & Intervention

Nursing Diagnosis	Nursing Intervention/Rationale
Sensory/perceptual alterations (auditory)	• Assess degree of hearing impairment or tinnitus. • Instill ear drops or perform irrigation if ordered. Use solution at room temperature *to avoid stimulating a caloric response*. • Warn patient and family not to put foreign objects in ears.
Pain	• Assess need for pain medication and provide instruction about safe analgesic medications.

Patient Education

1. For patients who produce excessive cerumen, suggest a method for preventing impaction or obstruction: Once a week put 1 or 2 drops of an oily substance in the ears at night. In the morning put 1 or 2 drops of hydrogen peroxide in the ears and clean gently with a soft cotton wick.

Evaluation

Patient Outcome	Data Indicating That Outcome is Reached
Obstruction is removed.	There is no feeling of occlusion, tinnitus, or pain in ear. Hearing is normal for patient.

Otosclerosis

Otosclerosis is a disease of the bone in the bony labyrinth, or the otic capsule, in which normal bone is replaced by the formation of highly vascular, "spongy" otosclerotic bone.

Otosclerosis most commonly (85%) occurs at the oval window and eventually causes a conductive hearing loss. Most patients have the disease in both ears, although not to the same degree. It is unilateral in about 10% to 15% of patients.[33]

Otosclerosis is present to some degree in about 10% of whites. It is not found as frequently in Orientals and blacks but is reported as common in southern India. About half of patients with otosclerosis have a family history of the disease. Women are apparently affected more often than men, and although the etiology is unclear, pregnancy frequently triggers a rapid onset of this condition. It is usually noticed first in the late teens or early twenties.[9]

Pathophysiology

The precise pathophysiologic process that causes otospongiotic and otosclerotic disease is still unclear. It is not thought to have any relationship to previous ear infections. During the process, however, normal bone in the otic capsule is gradually replaced by otosclerotic bone that is highly vascular and described as spongy. Although it is controversial, one theory postulates that the destructive process causes the release of proteolytic enzymes, which destroy the capsular bone, freeing other destructive enzymes. As these enzymes enter the labyrinthine fluid, they may affect the neural elements of the inner ear, causing vestibular and cochlear functional impairment. The second stage of this process is the body's natural reaction to heal the involved area by calcification. The calcification causes local expansion of the bone and leads to progressive fixation of the stapes with physical intrusion into labyrinthine spaces and virtual immobilization of the footplate in the oval window.[37] This produces a conductive hearing loss, since sound pressure vibrations can no longer be transmitted to the fluid media. Patients may also experience a mixed or sensorineural hearing loss if the cochlea is involved.

In otosclerosis the eardrum usually appears normal, although a pink blush called Schwartz's sign can occasionally be seen through the eardrum. This indicates a high degree of vascularity in active otosclerotic bone.

Diagnostic Studies and Findings

Rinne Test

Bone conduction lasts longer than air conduction in affected ear

Weber Test

Reverse is true in normal hearing

Audiometric Tests

Hearing loss ranges from 60 dB in early stages to total loss in later stages; sound lateralizes more to affected ear

Medical Plan

Surgery

Stapedectomy (see p. 720)

Stapedotomy—minimal (0.4 mm) opening of oval window; ribbon-shaped, platinum Teflon prosthesis is crimped to long process of the incus through opening into footplate before rather than after disrupting the incudostapedial joint and breaking off the stapes arch; this causes less trauma to inner ear, prevents migration of prosthesis, and produces better hearing results[37]

Medications

Sodium fluoride, 40 mg/d po for 1-2 yr to stabilize cochlear otosclerosis and improve hearing[37]

Anti-infective agents

Tetracycline (Achromycin), 250 mg po q6h for 10 d (after surgery)

General Management

Air conduction hearing aid if stapedectomy is not indicated

NURSING CARE

Nursing Assessment

Auditory Function

Slowly progressive conductive hearing loss; low- to medium-pitched tinnitus; tympanic membrane normal on examination with otoscope

Nursing Dx & Intervention

Nursing Diagnosis	Nursing Intervention/Rationale
Potential activity intolerance related to bed rest and vertigo after stapedectomy	• Assess patient for pain, nausea, or dizziness. • Encourage activity level within physician's protocol. (Some patients can be up the day of surgery, others require bed rest for at least a day.) • Instruct the patient to lie flat with head turned to side and operated ear facing upward *to maintain position of inserted prosthesis.*

Nursing Diagnosis	Nursing Intervention/Rationale
	• Point out to the patient that vertigo, pain, nausea, and vomiting may occur. • Administer pain medication as needed. • Keep side rails up *to prevent fall from bed.* *Convalescent care:* Assist patient to begin ambulation gradually *to minimize vertigo.*

Patient Education

1. Instruct the patient not to cough, sneeze, or blow his nose for at least 1 week to prevent bacteria from entering the eustachian tube and to prevent dislodging the prosthesis and graft over the oval window.
2. Instruct the patient to avoid loud noises, although there is no evidence that any damage is caused.
3. Inform the patient that a decrease in hearing may occur after surgery because of increased fluid in the middle ear.
4. Tell the patient to ask the physician when flying will be permitted, since pressure changes may cause injury to the prosthesis and graft. This varies greatly from physician to physician and can range from 2 to 3 days after surgery to 1 to 2 months after surgery.

Evaluation

Patient Outcome	Data Indicating That Outcome is Reached
Patient recovers uneventfully from stapedectomy.	Patient experiences no vertigo. Patient experiences no pain. Hearing is improved to normal (remember that patient may experience decrease in hearing after surgery until blood in middle ear is reabsorbed).
Patient and family verbalize understanding of stapedectomy.	Patient verbalizes understanding of importance of completing antibiotic regimen and knowledge of convalescent care.

Acoustic neuroma

Neuromas are benign lesions that arise from the neurilemma or Schwann cell sheath in the covering of the axon of a neuron.

Acoustic neuromas actually arise from the vestibular portion rather than from the cochlear portion of the eighth cranial nerve; the origin is only occasionally found to be the acoustic nerve. Thus these tumors are also called vestibular schwannomas, tumors of the eighth cranial nerve, or cerebellopontine angle tumors. Since most of these neuromas arise within the internal auditory meatus, early effects may be from pressure on the meatus, the cochlear division of the eighth cranial nerve, and the vestibular nerve. Initially patients usually have tinnitus, unilateral hearing loss, and nystagmus.[37] Although these tumors can affect people at any age, most patients are 40 to 50 years of age, with women affected slightly more frequently (60%) than men. Acoustic neuromas comprise approximately 8% to 10% of all intracranial tumors.[4]

During the past 20 years, advances in diagnosis and techniques for removal of these tumors, such as the use of lasers and microsurgery, have greatly reduced morbidity and mortality.

Pathophysiology

The neuroma is a well-defined, fleshy, lobulated mass that is soft and cystic in some areas. It has a variegated appearance that may be caused by areas of old hemorrhage, although the tumor itself is quite avascular. Small, white, patchy areas of calcification may also be present.

The tumor usually arises in the internal auditory meatus. It is called an intracanalicular tumor if it lies entirely within the auditory canal and is considered an ear tumor. Small tumors measure between 2 and 5 cm, and large tumors have a minimum diameter of 5 cm.[58] As the tumor increases in size, it grows into the cerebellopontine angle and may begin to erode the wall of the internal meatus above and below. After the tumor grows out of the bony canal, it can expand medially, anterosuperiorly, and posteroinferiorly. As it grows medially, the tumor encroaches on the brainstem in the region of the pons. By this time the neuroma is usually about 2.5 cm in diameter and may be in contact with the anterior inferior cerebellar artery, which is responsible for the blood supply to the side of the pons and medulla. Continued enlargement medially compresses and distorts the pons and aqueduct, producing brainstem signs and causing an obstructing hydrocephalus.

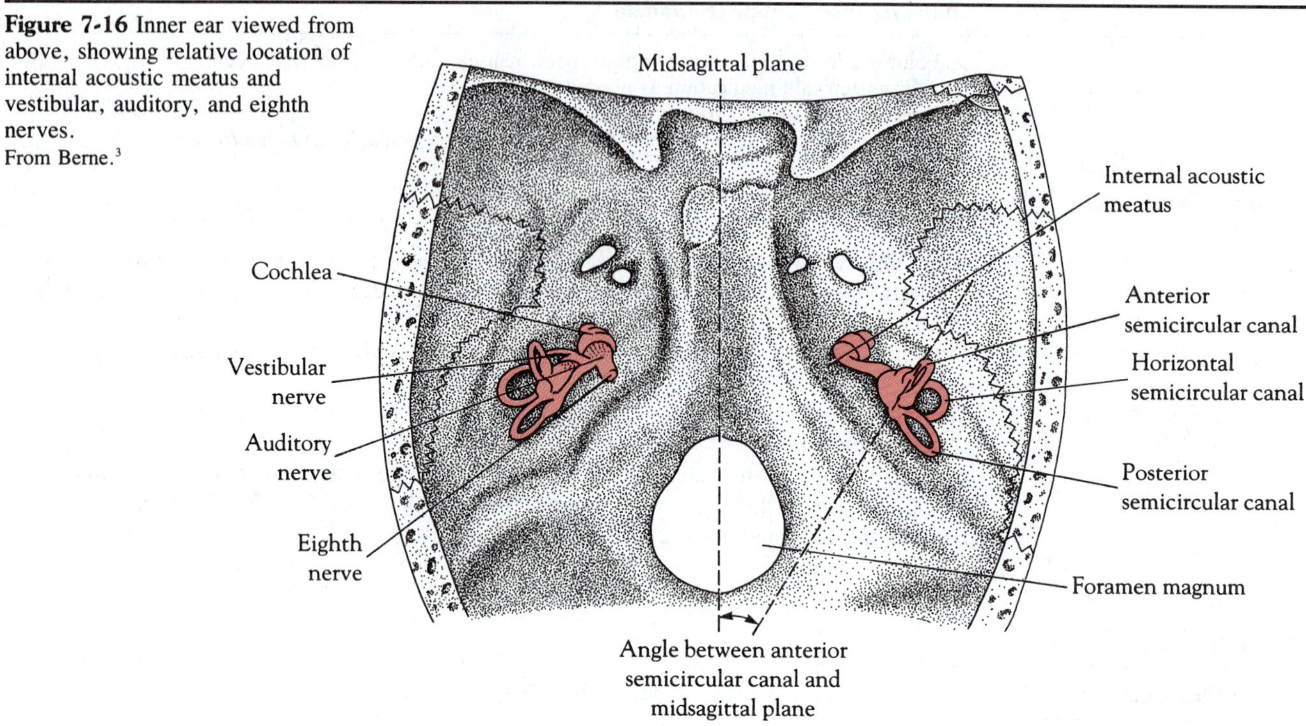

Figure 7-16 Inner ear viewed from above, showing relative location of internal acoustic meatus and vestibular, auditory, and eighth nerves.
From Berne.[3]

As the tumor expands anterosuperiorly, it displaces the facial nerve and stretches it over the surface of the tumor. Although it may adhere to the facial nerve, the tumor can usually be separated from the nerve at surgery because the tumor does not normally wrap itself around the nerve. As the tumor extends farther, it usually involves the trigeminal nerve, lifting it up from below, causing facial numbness, pain, and decreased corneal sensation.

If the tumor extends inferiorly and posteriorly, it may compress the middle cerebellar peduncle and the cerebellum. It also stretches the ninth, tenth, and eleventh cranial nerves as it approaches the foramen magnum.

Most acoustic neuromas grow within the subarachnoid space. They are usually considered slow growing, although this can vary from patient to patient. Tumors seem to grow fairly rapidly in young adults and more slowly in the elderly.

Substantial cochlear and labyrinthine changes occur with these space-occupying lesions of the internal meatus (Figure 7-16), causing abnormalities of the cochlear and eighth cranial nerves. There may be chemical alterations, such as high concentrations of protein in the perilymph, and the sense organs themselves may be destroyed, although the hair cells of the organ of Corti often remain quite normal.

Von Recklinghausen's disease, or neurofibromatosis, can also cause acoustic neuromas that are usually bilateral and expand within the nerve rather than against the nerve, such as in isolated neuromas.[58]

Diagnostic Studies and Findings

Audiology, Electrocochleography, and Brainstem Response to Audiometry

Performed to evaluate degree of hearing loss and to differentiate between conductive and sensorineural hearing losses

Cerebral Arteriography

Used less frequently in recent years but may be performed to diagnose aneurysms, to outline size and location of tumors, and to determine location and deviation of major vessels (see Part Two for description)

Computed Tomography (CT) and Magnetic Resonance Imaging (MRI) Scan

Can indicate presence of tumor, pinpoint location, and show evidence of enlarged ventricles (see Part Two for description)

Lumbar Puncture

Cerebrospinal fluid examined for increased protein; should not be performed if increased intracranial pressure is suspected to prevent herniation of cerebellar tonsils through foramen magnum or uncal herniation through tentorial notch[58] (see Part Two for description)

Tomograms

Can show flaring of internal acoustic canal along medial aspect and erosion of posterior wall of canal[54]

Roentgenograms of Petrous Pyramid of Temporal Bone

May show erosion of petrous portion of temporal bone or internal acoustic meatus by tumor[54]

Medical Plan

Surgery

Surgery is treatment of choice, since these tumors do not respond well to chemotherapy or radiation; objective is to remove tumor completely while saving facial nerve; surgery can last from 9 to 14 hours and is done with patient in sitting position; suboccipital or transpetrosal approach usually used; for suboccipital approach, small portion of hair at base of neck is shaved; some surgeons prefer translabyrinthine approach: one institution reports that all acoustic neuromas, regardless of size, can be removed with this approach, although there may be technical problems with very large tumors; translabyrinthine approach associated with lower mortality, better facial nerve function, less postoperative ataxia, and much less postoperative hydrocephalus than with suboccipital approach but greater loss of hearing[37]; advantage is avoidance of pressure on cerebellum[55]

If tumor is large and adheres to facial nerve, total removal of tumor may necessitate sacrifice of facial nerve; if possible, end-to-end anastomosis of nerve stumps is done at time of surgery and should result in return of nerve function[58]

Ventriculostomy—sometimes performed during surgery so intracranial pressure can be monitored after surgery

Medications

Corticosteroids

Dexamethasone (Decadron), 4-6 mg IV q4h to decrease cerebral edema

Antihypertensives

Propranolol (Inderal), 160 mg po over 24 h before operation for prophylaxis, then nitroprusside (Nipride) during operation and after operation as needed

General Management

Cardiac and intracranial pressure monitoring; intubation with mechanical ventilation during and immediately after surgery; oxygen administered via face mask after extubation

Nothing by mouth and intravenous feedings until patient is able to eat; tube feedings necessary in some patients until gag reflex or ability to chew returns

Physical therapy and possibly speech therapy after surgery

NURSING CARE

Nursing Assessment

Symptoms are dependent on size and location of tumor.

Auditory Function

Sensorineural hearing loss, usually unilateral and slowly progressive; tinnitus; dizziness and transient unsteadiness; true vertigo (sense of rotation, nausea, and vomiting) in some patients; otalgia (ache within ear or mastoid); tension or neck pain on same side as otalgia; occasional facial numbness; occasional tic douloureux

Visual Function

Depression of corneal reflex; delayed blink reflex; decreased tear production; eyes feel dry and gritty; nystagmus, with eye movement slower and coarser toward side of tumor[17]; with large tumors, diplopia, ataxia, headaches, papilledema, loss of vision

Gustatory Function

Diminished sense of taste on anterior two thirds of tongue; difficulty chewing

Motor Function

Poor coordination and gait disturbances; patient leans toward affected side; impairment of fine movements[17]

Nursing Dx & Intervention

Nursing Diagnosis	Nursing Intervention/Rationale
Altered cerebral tissue perfusion	• Establish neurologic baseline and assess neurologic status and vital signs every 15 minutes until stable, then every 1 hour, then every 4 hours. • Monitor and record amount of and describe ventricular drainage, if used. • Assess for signs of increasing intracranial pressure: widening pulse pressures, decreased level of consciousness, papilledema, seizures, hyperactive deep tendon reflexes, complaints of headache, vomiting. • Administer dexamethasone as ordered *to decrease cerebral edema.*

Nursing Diagnosis	Nursing Intervention/Rationale
	• Observe for symptoms of hydrocephalus from edema or bleeding into ventricles, which is possible after surgery. • Assess for presence of cerebrospinal fluid leak. • Observe cardiac monitor *to detect any arrhythmias* resulting from cerebral edema or vagal stimulation during surgery. • Keep head of bed elevated 45 degrees *to promote venous drainage and limit cerebral edema.*
Altered peripheral tissue perfusion related to rebound hypertension	• Assess patient's blood pressure frequently; be alert for hypertension, which could be significant after surgery. • Monitor Nipride drip per protocol.
Ineffective breathing pattern related to decreased gag reflex, mechanical ventilation	• Assess patient's arterial blood gases and chest expansion for adequate ventilation. • Maintain ventilator settings and suction airway as needed (patient will be mechanically ventilated for 1 or 2 days after surgery). • Observe patient after extubation for return of gag reflex and ability to cough effectively. • Provide oxygen via face mask as ordered after extubation. • Continue suctioning or physical therapy of the chest as needed.
Potential fluid volume deficit related to dehydration necessary to decrease congestion in vasculature and to minimize effects of postoperative swelling[17]	• Assess skin turgor and lung sounds *to monitor fluid status.* • Maintain and record intravenous infusions at ordered rate. Titrate *to maintain serum osmolarity between 300 and 310 mOsm/L.* • Permit nothing by mouth initially. • Maintain strict intake and output records. • Monitor electrolyte levels, *since patients are given diuretics to decrease brain bulk during surgery.* Perform care of Foley catheter *to prevent urinary tract infection;* patient will have catheter until able to void normally. • Provide frequent mouth care; patient may suck on lollipops.
Pain	• Assess for pain and give medication as needed *to minimize pain, nausea, and vomiting.*
Altered nutrition: less than body requirements	• Administer antacids *to decrease increased gastric acidity and prevent stress ulcers.* • Begin offering patient soft or pureed foods when gag reflex has returned, feeding on unaffected side if patient experiences difficulty or facial numbness. • Evaluate need for dietary consultation.
Impaired swallowing related to decreased gag reflex	• Maintain by mouth until gag reflex has returned. • Provide tube feedings in collaboration with physician until gag reflex returns, if appropriate. • Provide excellent mouth care.
Impaired skin integrity	• Assess dressing for drainage and bleeding and reinforce or change as needed. • Remove dressing 3 to 5 days after surgery. Observe for redness, inflammation, drainage, or puffiness near operative site. Puffiness may be from accumulation of subgaleal fluid, since dura was entered; fluid should be reabsorbed in few days. Position patient comfortably and change position frequently until patient is mobile *to prevent skin breakdown.* • Provide adequate support to head and back when positioning, *since neck muscles are weakened.*
Impaired tissue integrity	• Assess corneas for excessive dryness. • Provide artificial tears to patient's eyes as needed (every few hours) *to maintain normal lubrication because of loss of corneal reflex and decreased secretions.* • Place eye bubble over the affected eye *to collect moisture and protect the cornea.*

Patient Education

1. Instruct the patient and family regarding signs and symptoms of wound infection.
2. Instruct the patient and family regarding signs and symptoms of hydrocephalus, which in rare cases occurs several weeks after surgery.
3. Instruct the patient and family regarding the need for continued physical therapy rehabilitation and possible speech therapy.
4. Instruct the patient and family regarding maintenance of nutrition, especially if a chewing or swallowing deficit remains. If the patient is discharged but will continue tube feedings, be sure that the patient or a family member can perform the procedure safely.
5. Ensure that the patient and family understand that deficits may take several months to resolve or may not resolve at all; assess family's coping mechanisms and the possible need for assistance in dealing with these deficits.

Evaluation

Patient Outcome	Data Indicating That Outcome is Reached
Preoperative symptoms are improved or absent.	Hearing is improved or normal. Tinnitus is absent. Dizziness or unsteadiness has improved or disappeared. Facial numbness, tickling, and pain have improved or disappeared (this may take 3 to 6 months). Headaches and vomiting are absent. Gait and coordination difficulties are improved.

Ménière's disease

Ménière's disease, also called endolymphatic hydrops, is a labyrinthine dysfunction associated with dilation of the membranous labyrinth.

The dilation causes three typical symptoms: severe vertigo, tinnitus, and a sensorineural hearing loss, which is usually initially of low tones. Although never fatal, Ménière's disease is nonetheless quite incapacitating during attacks, which occur periodically between intervals of remission. As hearing decreases, the attacks become less frequent, and they may stop altogether when the patient's hearing loss is almost total. The acute attacks usually last for several hours, but between attacks the patient may have no symptoms except for tinnitus and a gradually progressive hearing loss. In severe or untreated cases, however, the patient may have daily attacks, although with periods of complete relief from vertigo between attacks.

Adults between the ages of 30 and 60 years are usually affected. Although it can occur at any age, Ménière's disease is rare in children (it has been seen in a 6-year-old). It is distributed equally by sex; the condition is more often unilateral than bilateral, although the likelihood of bilaterality increases as patients grow older. Half of those who developed the disease in the second ear did so within 2 years of onset in the first ear, and another 27% developed it after 5 years or longer.[37]

A likely cause has been found in approximately 25% of those affected, and a positive family history noted for 10% to 20%, so that genetic Ménière's disease remains a possibility.[37]

Some researchers believe that the incidence of Ménière's disease may have increased since World War II, possibly because of a correlation between the disease, current living habits, and environmental conditions, such as increased stress and increased salt intake.

Pathophysiology

The most widely accepted theories regarding the cause of Ménière's disease are (1) an overproduction of endolymph from some disturbance in the formation of fluid in the inner ear and (2) a decreased absorption of endolymph from a disturbance in the sac, which leads to an accumulation of endolymph.

Many other theories have been postulated, but few have been widely accepted. Endolymphatic hydrops, however, is thought to cause degeneration of the neural end organ of the labyrinth and cochlea. Some researchers believe that fluid disturbances are caused by sodium retention, allergies, or vascular spasm. Small vesicles may form in the walls of the endolymphatic system, and the sudden rupture of these vesicles may cause acute attacks of vertigo. The cause of the formation of these vesicles is unclear. Premenstrual edema precipitates attacks in some women.

The principal cause appears to be failure of the resorption mechanisms of the endolymphatic sac, resulting in slow accumulation of endolymph with distention and rupture of the membranous labyrinth. Potassium-rich neurotoxic endolymph may then enter the perilymphatic space, causing temporary paralysis of sensory and neural structures. As the disease progresses, there are permanent morphologic changes in sensory and neural structures and persistent losses in auditory and vestibular function.[37]

These patients have hypocellular mastoid processes and deficiencies of the vestibular aqueduct. Trautmann's triangle is often small or distorted, primarily because of the anatomy of the lateral sinus, which is displaced anteriorly and more medially in most patients.

A fundamental problem seems to be malabsorption in the duct or sac. All forms of Ménière's disease develop after some inciting cause that may have occurred years earlier. Known or inciting factors include infection, trauma, otosclerosis, and syphilis, although the disease may be idiopathic. The syndrome is probably related to developmental abnormalities of the endolymphatic duct or sac, hypodevelopment of Trautmann's triangle, anterior displacement of the lateral sinus, and sometimes vascular anomalies, especially in venous drainage. Thus the quality of the endolymph is affected.[37]

Characteristically, in advanced Ménière's disease, endolymphatic hydrops is seen in the scala media and saccule. It fills the vestibule and scala vestibuli in many cases. Because of the displacement of perilymph in advanced disease, the radial fluid flow decreases and longitudinal fluid flow becomes dominant. Less often, the utricle or cochlear duct extends to occupy the vestibule. Stagnation of outflow can occur, and such distention can interfere with traveling waves and alter cochlear function.[37]

Diagnostic Studies and Findings

Audiology

Tuning fork test
- Shows sensorineural deficit

Rinne test
- May be false positive if there is severe unilateral hearing loss

Pure tone test
- Shows sensorineural loss involving low tones

Electrocochleography

Used frequently to aid in differential diagnosis of auditory diseases

Caloric Tests

5 ml ice water instilled into each ear with patient's head elevated 30 degrees to cause acute attack with nausea, vomiting, vertigo, and nystagmus; response is occasionally hypoactive in involved ear and sometimes in both ears

Roentgenograms of Petrous Bones

Internal auditory meatus examined carefully; patients with Ménière's disease usually have shorter, straighter vestibular aqueducts than do patients without Ménière's disease

Injection of Intravenous Acetazolamide

Causes temporary increase in pure tone and speech audiometric thresholds, which suggest temporary increase in preexisting hydrops, possibly from transient reduction in plasma osmolality (many patients with Ménière's disease have moderately elevated serum osmolality)[5]

Medical Plan

Goals are preservation of hearing and control of vertigo.

Surgery

Recent increased interest in surgical therapies because medical therapy has failed to halt hearing losses; if medical therapy has failed, two surgical procedures may be performed
- Decompression of endolymphatic sac—done by inserting Teflon endolymphatic subarachnoid shunt or by incision in sac kept patent by muscle flap or Teflon sheet; has some benefit in about two thirds of patients
- Destruction of end organ and neural connections by labyrinthectomy or vestibular neurectomy; labyrinthectomy performed only as last resort when vertigo is persistent and little or no hearing is left, since cochlear function is destroyed; vertigo disappears in almost every case, but tinnitus may remain; vestibular neurectomy may be regarded as operation of choice; middle cranial fossa approach is used; 90% of patients have relief from vertigo, some with improvement in hearing; in one study 16% of 52 patients had improvement in hearing and 64% had stabilization of hearing loss; in another study 32% of 78 patients had improvement in hearing at least 2 years after neurectomy[54]

Medications

Vasodilators (used for histamine effect)
- Histamine (Diphosphate), 2.75 mg given in 200-500 ml of 5% glucose; drip over 1 h (in remission); based on theory that labyrinthine ischemia is cause of disease; most have not been found to be effective, but β-histamine may improve vertigo, hearing, and tinnitus[7]

Vestibular suppressants
- Acetyl-D-leucine, 500 mg po q12h
- Prochlorperazine (Compazine), 10 mg po q6h
- Droperidol (Inapsine), 25-50 mg/d IV
- Haloperidol (Haldol), 5 mg IV q8h
- Diazepam (Valium), 2.5-5 mg po q6h
- Lorazepam (Ativan), 0.5-1 mg po q4-6h prn

Diuretics (used as vestibular compressant)
- Hydrochlorothiazide (Hydrodiuril), 25-200 mg/d

Cholinergic blocking agents
- Atropine, 0.01 mg/kg to maximum of 0.04 mg/kg subcutaneously or IM

Adrenergic agents
- Epinephrine, 0.2-0.5 mg IV may be administered to stop an attack; sedatives and antiemetics such as meclizine (Antivert), 25 mg po qid, and prochlorperazine (Compazine), 10 mg po q6h may be used

General Management

- Bed rest maintained during acute attack
- To prevent attacks, Furstenberg diet (neutral ash and salt free)
- Restriction of salt and water intake
- Avoidance of tobacco, alcohol, caffeine, and high triglycerides

NURSING CARE

Nursing Assessment

During Acute Attack

Balance
- Sudden onset of acute vertigo

Auditory function
- Tinnitus described by patient as a persistent background hum

Visual function
- Nystagmus

General
- Nausea and vomiting; sweating; abdominal pain; diarrhea; and bradycardia

Between Attacks

Auditory function

Gradually progressive sensorineural hearing loss; tinnitus; loudness intolerance; some patients describe a fullness, pressure, or dull ache in ear; normal tympanic membranes

Nursing Dx & Intervention

Nursing Diagnosis	Nursing Intervention/Rationale
Potential for trauma	• Assess patient for vertigo, nystagmus, nausea and vomiting. • Keep side rails of bed up *to prevent a fall*. • Encourage patient to lie quietly and *not* to get up without assistance during attack. • Instruct patient to avoid sudden head movements or position changes, since *attacks may begin without warning*. • Administer antiemetics and sedatives *to help prevent vomiting and promote rest*.
Sensory/perceptual alterations (auditory)	• See p. 1728.

Patient Education

1. Instruct the patient in theories about the etiology of the disease and acute attacks.
2. Ensure that the patient is aware that there may be a progressive hearing loss unless treatment is successful.
3. Inform the patient of ways to minimize tinnitus if the patient is bothered by it.
4. Inform the patient that the attacks will last a few hours and will stop on their own, but that treatment is available to diminish or stop them if necessary.
5. Ensure that the patient understands the danger of trying to walk unassisted during an attack because of vertigo.
6. Instruct the patient and family in dietary or medical regimen if used or inform them about surgical interventions if used.

Evaluation

Patient Outcome	Data Indicating That Outcome is Reached
Patient has increased knowledge of Ménière's disease.	Patient verbalizes understanding that attacks will eventually stop of their own accord. Patient verbalizes understanding that sudden movements and hazardous tasks should be avoided because of sudden onset of vertigo. Patient expresses knowledge of side effects of medical regimen if ordered or of surgical intervention if used. Patient expresses understanding of possibility of hearing loss.

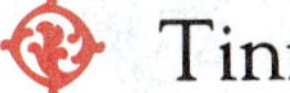

Tinnitus

Tinnitus is the perception of sound in the absence of an acoustic stimulus.

Tinnitus is usually described as a ringing in the ears, although it may also be perceived by the patient as roaring, sizzling, whistling, or humming. Although usually a subjective experience, tinnitus occasionally can be heard as a blowing sound or bruit by the examiner.

The intensity of tinnitus varies greatly from patient to patient. It is often slight and is noticed by the patient only at night when other sounds are minimal. At other times it can be loud and continuous to the point that some patients may even consider suicide. It can be intermittent or continuous and may be accompanied by a hearing loss. It may also be unilateral or bilateral.

Although the mechanism that produces tinnitus is not thoroughly understood, it can be a symptom of nearly all ear disorders. In many cases it is the first or only symptom of disease, and any patient complaining of tinnitus must have a thorough examination to determine the cause.

Pathophysiology

The exact mechanism that causes tinnitus is unknown. However, it is known that tinnitus can be caused by a disturbance anywhere in the ear, as well as in the acoustic nerve, brainstem, or cortex (Figure 7-17). Two disorders with tinnitus as a major symptom, Ménière's disease and acoustic neuroma, are discussed separately in this section.

External ear causes include obstruction of the canal by foreign bodies or cerumen; patients usually describe the sound as low pitched, muffled, and intermittent. These patients may perceive their own voices as having a hollow sound.

Most middle ear disorders can also cause tinnitus. Otosclerosis is usually accompanied by tinnitus, which is described by patients as a ringing or whistling. It is constant, and some patients experience more than one sound. Infectious or inflammatory processes usually produce tinnitus, which is described as pulsating. This type of tinnitus usually ends when the infection is cleared.

Acoustic trauma caused by very loud noises frequently produces high-pitched tinnitus and may be associated with a temporary hearing loss. These symptoms should warn the patient that the ears should be protected before future exposure to loud noises or a permanent hearing loss may result. The pitch of tinnitus in these patients is usually near the frequency where their hearing loss is the greatest.

Tinnitus is commonly caused by certain drugs. Quinine, salicylates, some diuretics, and aminoglycoside antibiotics frequently cause tinnitus and can also cause a hearing loss. These drugs damage the cochlea and the eighth cranial nerve; the tinnitus is usually high pitched and may or may not continue after the drug is stopped.

Other causes of tinnitus include anemia and hypotension. This tinnitus usually resolves when the underlying condition is corrected. Cardiovascular diseases, such as arteriosclerosis and hypertension, may also produce a tinnitus that may fluctuate with the patient's blood pressure.

Audible or objective tinnitus can be heard by another person. It is better understood, and the cause usually is easily diagnosed. If a patient complains of a blowing sound that coincides with respirations or complains of clicking sounds, the physician should suspect audible tinnitus and may be able to hear it by placing an ear or a stethoscope over the patient's ear. An abnormally patent eustachian tube is usually the cause of blowing tinnitus, and this is quite annoying to patients. Luckily it may be of short duration, and patients can improve the condition somewhat by performing repeated Valsalva maneuvers to increase the negative pressure in the nasopharynx

Figure 7-17 Areas where tinnitus may occur.

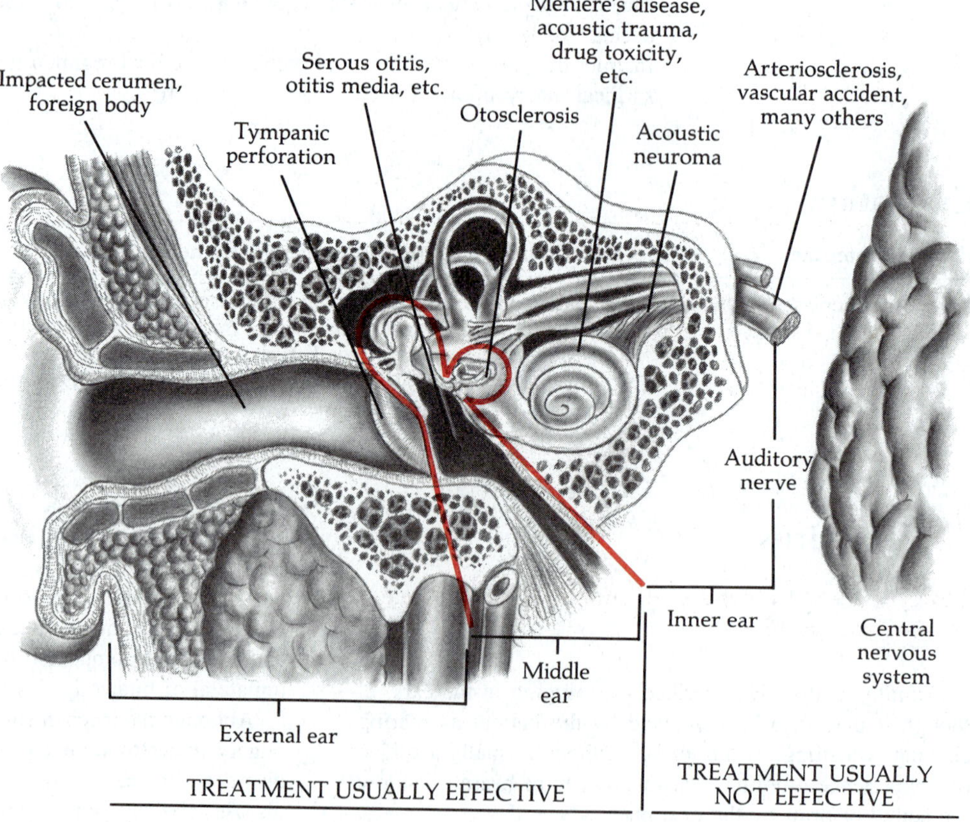

or equalize the pressure in the middle ear with the atmosphere. The clicking noises are fairly rare, are usually intermittent, and are produced by tetanic contractions of the muscles of the soft palate. The cause of this condition is unknown, but it is a reflex action, and the palate can be seen to contract, sometimes 175 to 200 times a minute. This is usually treated with injections of lidocaine on the involved side to stop the contraction of the palate.

Diagnostic Studies and Findings

Audiology

Presence or absence of concurrent hearing loss; any diagnostic study may be performed to rule out the presence of systemic or ear diseases known to produce tinnitus

Pitch—the patient manipulates the frequency of tone until the pitch is equal to the most prominent pitch of the tinnitus

Loudness—can be evaluated by adjusting the level of pure tone until it has the same loudness as tinnitus; if a profound hearing loss is present, the measurement may be only a few decibels sensation level, whereas in regions of normal hearing, the measurement may be 40 dB sensation level

Pure tone masking—measures the minimum level of a pure tone required to mask the tinnitus as a function of the masker frequency[37]

Medical Plan

Surgery

None, unless surgery is indicated for particular disorder that is found to be cause of tinnitus

Medications

Hypocholesterolemic agents

Nicotinic acid (Niacin), 50-200 mg/d po to vasodilate blood vessels that supply inner ear; its efficacy is questionable

Antianxiety agents (used for sedative effect)

Diazepam (Valium), 5 mg po q4-6h

Anticonvulsants (used for sedative effect)

Carbamazepine (Tegretol), 200 mg po bid for 1 d, then maintenance dose of 800 mg-1.2 g qd

Phenytoin (Dilantin), 100 mg po tid

Primidone (Mysoline), 100-125 mg/d at bedtime for 3 d, then 250 mg tid or qid, and carbamazepine in combination; have helped in some cases, but exact mechanism is unknown

General Management

Feedback helpful in some cases; radios or masking units to drown out tinnitus or to make it less noticeable to patient

NURSING CARE

Nursing Assessment

Auditory Function

Patient describes sound in one or both ears as ringing, sizzling, whistling, roaring, humming, or hissing; may be intermittent or continuous; may be high pitched; history of acoustic trauma, that is, exposure to loud noise; history of ototoxic drugs; hearing may be normal to decreased

Nursing Dx & Intervention

Nursing Diagnosis	Nursing Intervention/Rationale
Sensory/perceptual alterations (auditory)	• Assess patient for hearing impairment or degree of tinnitus • Encourage use of background noise, that is, radios or masking units *to present a more pleasant noise*. • Ensure that use of any ototoxic substances is discontinued, if possible. • Assist with any procedures necessary for diagnosis or treatment.

Patient Education

1. Inform the patient that tinnitus is usually a symptom of a systemic or ear disease and that a thorough examination should be performed.
2. Warn the patient against exposure to loud noises that may cause acoustic trauma.
3. Inform the patient about the ototoxic effects of some drugs. If the patient must take an ototoxic drug, be sure that periodic audiologic testing is performed to detect any hearing loss.

Evaluation

Patient Outcome	Data Indicating That Outcome is Reached
Patient's understanding of cause of tinnitus is increased.	Patient verbalizes understanding of cause of tinnitus if known. Patient verbalizes understanding that tinnitus can be side effect of certain drugs. Patient understands that loud noises may be damaging and cause tinnitus and hearing loss. Patient verbalizes knowledge of various ways to diminish or minimize the tinnitus, that is, radios or masking units.

NOSE DISORDERS

Epistaxis

Epistaxis is bleeding from the nose caused by irritation, trauma, coagulation disorders, hypertension, or chronic infection.

Epistaxis is thought to have occurred at least once in over 10% of the normal population. It is either a primary disorder or secondary to another condition such as hemophilia or leukemia and many cases are idiopathic.

In children, who are twice as likely to have epistaxis as adults, the bleeding is usually mild and tends to originate from the anterior nasal septum. In older adults bleeding is more likely to originate from the posterior septum so that the bleeding point is more difficult to locate and the bleeding may be profuse.[41] Epistaxis is more common in men than in women and occurs more frequently in winter, probably because of the dryness of the air.

Although epistaxis is a frightening experience for the patient, it generally looks and feels worse than it actually is. The blood is usually bright red and the patient may swallow some of it, which is an unpleasant sensation. Although adults can lose up to 1 L per hour during severe bleeding, the mortality is extremely low. When the patient bleeds enough to show signs of shock, the nosebleed usually stops because of low blood pressure. Some deaths are thought to have been caused by coronary ischemia from blood loss.[41]

Pathophysiology

The most common cause of epistaxis is trauma to the nasal mucosa from damage by a foreign object, picking crusts from the nasal septum, or dryness of the nasal mucosa. Nosebleeds are fairly common in patients with coagulation defects such as hemophilia, leukemia, and purpura. Infection, tumors, and some drugs and toxins may cause nosebleeds; in many instances, however, the cause is simply not identified or is considered idiopathic.

There may be some relationship between menstruation and epistaxis. It may be that in some women with premenstrual syndrome the nasal mucosa becomes congested at the time of menstruation, setting the stage for epistaxis.[53]

The incidence of epistaxis is no higher in hypertensive patients than in normotensive patients. However, hypertensive patients may bleed more profusely, partly because of the direct effect of the increased pressure and also because the small nasal arteries and arterioles of hypertensive patients tend to have much of their muscular walls replaced by fibrous tissue and are incapable of contracting adequately to attain hemostasis.[34]

Children experience frequent nosebleeds from the anteroinferior part of the septum known as Little's area or Kiesselbach's plexus (Figure 7-18). The etiology is not clear, but the area is richly vascular, and children have hyperemic and congested upper respiratory tracts. Children also pick and rub their noses in the area where the mucosa is stretched over cartilage and bone.

Intractable nose picking is another cause of anterior nosebleeds. Some patients cannot stop picking their noses, either because of a nervous habit or because crusts are present from an earlier ulceration or perforation. Constant nose picking can cause septal ulceration or even a perforation, which leads to epistaxis.

A hereditary disease that is an unusual cause of epistaxis is Rendu-Osler-Weber disease or hemorrhagic hereditary telangiectasia. This disease is gene dominant and may be passed from either parent to a child of either sex. Epistaxis is usually the initial symptom, but telangiectasis is commonly found in

Figure 7-18 Kiesselbach's plexus.
From DeWeese.[9]

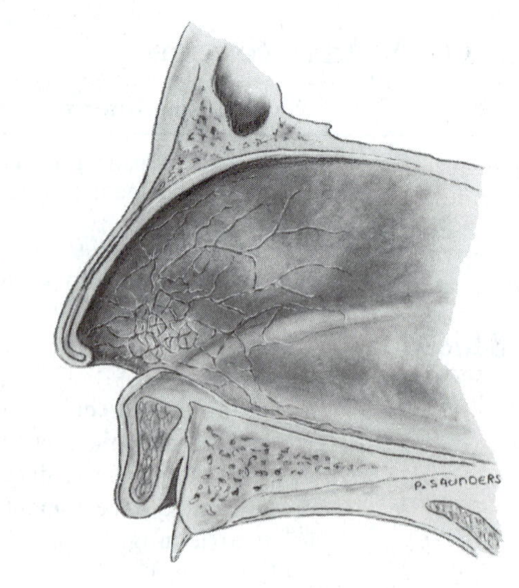

other mucous membranes or anywhere on the external surface of the body. Bleeding usually occurs from the nose and gastrointestinal tract because mucosa in those areas is very fragile, whereas other areas have protective layers of squamous epithelium.

Most nosebleeds in the anterior part of the nose originate from Kiesselbach's plexus, the highly vascular network in the anterior nasal septum. It is also anatomically closer to the rapid inspiratory air flow, which may dry the normal mucus flow, especially in cold, dry weather.[34] Since the vessels are fairly small and easily accessible, these nosebleeds are the easiest to treat. If bleeding is from the posterior part of the nose, the exact source of bleeding is more difficult to locate, since it is sometimes impossible to see and bleeding is more profuse. Usually just one source on one side of the nose bleeds, although bleeding frequently originates from both sides in patients with blood dyscrasias.

Diagnostic Studies and Findings

Hematocrit, Hemoglobin, Platelets, Prothrombin Time, Partial Thromboplastin Time, Reticulocyte Count, and Differential

Done to rule out coagulation defect; results usually normal; bleeding from other parts of body likely in patients with hematologic disorders

Rhinoscopy

To detect and localize site of bleeding

Medical Plan

Surgery

Arterial ligation if proper packing fails to control nosebleed

Septal dermoplasty for Rendu-Osler-Weber disease—skin graft is placed in nose to cover anterior parts of septum and floor and walls of nose anteriorly to provide protective covering over fragile mucosa

Medications

Fibrinolytics

- Vitamin K (Aquamephyton), 10 mg/d po or IM; useful in some cases of epistaxis, but packing remains therapy of choice

Anti-infective agents

- Penicillin, 1.5 million U IV q6h recommended for infection prevention because packing obstructs drainage of paranasal sinuses

General Management

Nosebleed from anterior part of nose

- Easiest to treat; source of bleeding located, and clots and fresh blood aspirated with suction; cotton ball

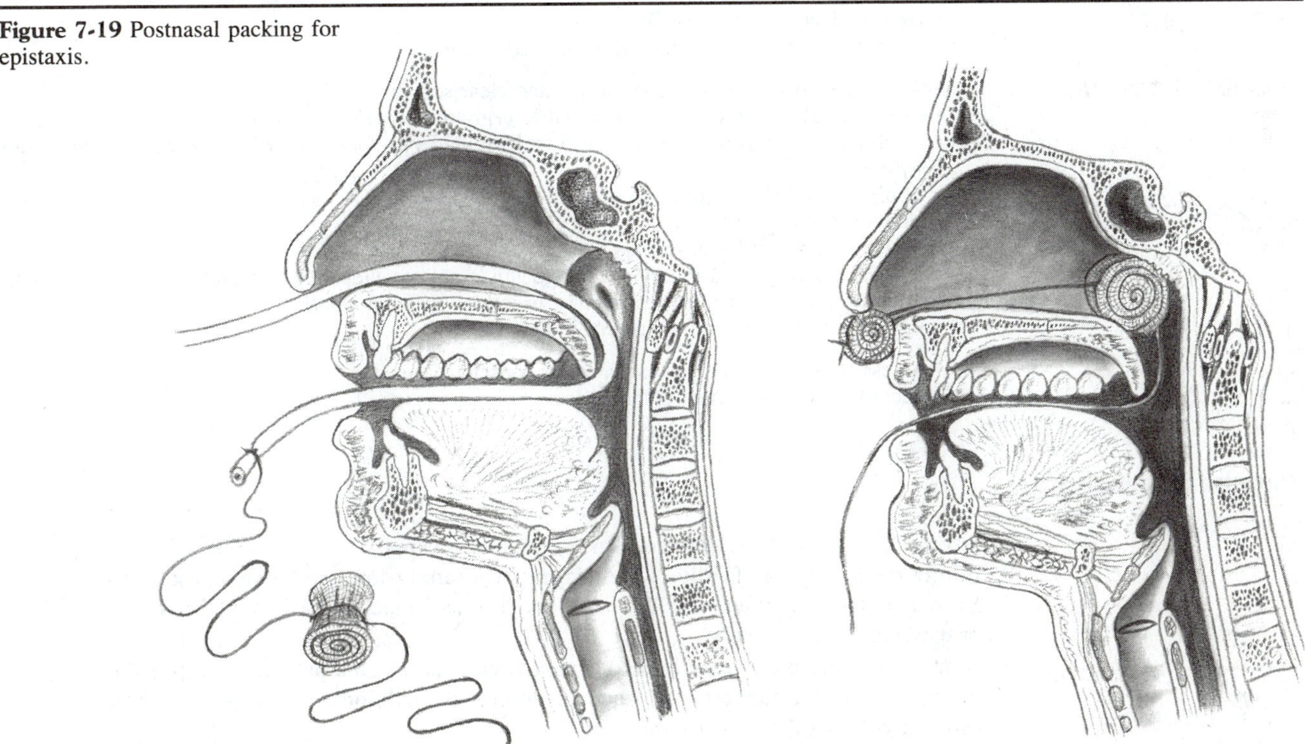

Figure 7-19 Postnasal packing for epistaxis.

saturated with 1:1000 epinephrine inserted into bleeding nostril, and strong pressure applied to compress cotton ball against septum for several minutes; after cotton ball is removed, cauterization performed by means of silver nitrate or electric cautery; packing unnecessary if bleeding is controlled with cauterization; pressure alone may control bleeding

Intractable nose picking

Both sides of nose packed with antibiotic-saturated cotton ball and nose taped completely shut for 7 to 10 days to facilitate healing of mucous membranes

Epistaxis from posterior part of nose

Postnasal packing: with patient sitting to prevent aspiration of blood, bleeding site located by advancing strong suction tip until nose fills with blood when suction tip has passed; large postnasal pack introduced through mouth by attaching it to catheter that is inserted into nostril and out mouth (Figure 7-19); catheter pulled through nose, lodging pack in posterior part of nose and providing compression to bleeding site; packing remains in place 48 to 96 hours; if both choanae occluded because of large size of pack, patient must be checked daily for ear or eustachian tube symptoms; patient will have some difficulty swallowing

NURSING CARE

Nursing Assessment

Nasal Bleeding

Bright red blood comes from the nares; patient may also swallow or expectorate blood; history of trauma, nose picking, hypertension, or other known cause; inspection of anterior part of nose with the patient seated and using bright light (if bleeding spot seen, treatment may begin; if patient continues to swallow blood and no source is located, bleeding may be from posterior source); examination of patient's body for bruises or petechiae that may indicate underlying hematologic disorder

Nursing Dx & Intervention

Nursing Diagnosis	Nursing Intervention/Rationale
Fear	• Assess patient's emotional state. • Reassure patient that amount of blood lost looks worse than it probably is. • Encourage patient not to swallow blood *to prevent nausea and vomiting.* • Have patient breathe through mouth. • Have basin nearby for patient *to expectorate blood.*
Potential for aspiration	• Assess patient's ability to expectorate and clear secretions. • Elevate head of bed or have patient sit *to prevent aspiration of blood.* • Pinch patient's nostrils together for 5 to 10 minutes *to compress soft portion of nostril against septum.* • Apply ice or cold compress to nose *to help stop bleeding.* • Notify patient's physician. • Assist with packing if necessary. • If nasal packing is in place, encourage fluids and provide frequent oral hygiene *to decrease mucosal dryness, since patient will be breathing through mouth.* • Inspect oropharynx for presence of blood.
Altered cerebral and cardiopulmonary tissue perfusion	• Assess patient's vital signs and level of consciousness. • Record color and amount of blood loss.

Patient Education

1. Inform the patient of the inherent dangers in nose picking.
2. Inform the patient and family of the dangers of inserting foreign objects into the nose.
3. Encourage the patient and family to seek medical assistance immediately if nasal infection or epistaxis occurs.
4. If epistaxis is from dryness of mucous membranes, inform the patient about possible benefits of using a humidifier or vaporizer to provide additional humidity in the home, especially during the winter months.

Evaluation

Patient Outcome	Data Indicating That Outcome is Reached
Epistaxis is well controlled.	Bleeding is absent. Patient's hematocrit value and hemoglobin level are normal. Mucous membranes are healed if bleeding is from picking or ulceration. Patient verbalizes understanding of cause of epistaxis, if known, and ways to prevent bleeding in future.

Nasal fractures

A nasal fracture is a traumatic injury to the nasal bones.

Nasal fractures occur quite commonly and more often than fractures of the other facial bones. Common causes are accidents, sports injuries, and assaults. In children, falls are the most common cause of nasal fractures. They occur more commonly in men.[34] However, when nasal fractures are diagnosed, it is essential to rule out fractures of associated facial bones such as zygomatic or mandibular fractures, since facial injuries or trauma may also damage these bones.

Even a nasal fracture that appears simple usually has associated damage to the mucosal lining of the nose. If a patient has suffered a facial trauma that causes epistaxis, damage to the bone-cartilage structures of the nose is likely.

Pathophysiology

A nasal fracture occasionally occurs in the birth canal during delivery. These are usually "greenstick" fractures, and the baby's nose inclines slightly to one side. The nose can be grasped at the tip and pulled toward the midline to realign it in these cases.

Nasal fractures can be classified as unilateral, bilateral, or complex. A unilateral fracture may produce little or no displacement and may appear as a simple crack on a roentgenogram. Bilateral fractures, which are the most common, may be caused by a swinging punch or blow that pushes both nasal bones to one side or by a frontal blow that depresses the nasal bones and gives a flattened look to the nose. The entire nose may be deviated, and the nose may have a C or S deformity.

Complex fractures are usually caused by powerful frontal blows. Such blows may shatter the nasal pyramid and frequently the frontal bones as well, causing a marked depression of the nasal and facial bones.

The usual findings are epistaxis, a noticeable facial deformity, and a history of trauma. Edema occurs quickly at the injury site and depending on the severity may include periorbital swelling. Ecchymosis is common, the nose is exquisitely tender, and nasal obstruction occasionally occurs. Complex fractures of the nose and face may result in diplopia or subscleral hemorrhage.

Diagnostic Studies and Findings

Roentgenograms of Face and Nose

Show fractures and depressed areas of facial and nasal bones; done to complement clinical, visual evaluation

Ophthalmoscopy

Performed to rule out eye injury such as corneal abrasion or laceration, also to check lacrimal apparatus and orbit

Medical Plan

Surgery

Reduction and fixation of the fractures as quickly as possible after injury (within first hour or two before swelling begins, or after 3 or 4 days when swelling has decreased) because fragments tend to stabilize quickly; bilateral nasal packing usually done during surgery to maintain stability and position of nasal structure; wiring or splinting may be required for complex fractures

Medications

Narcotic analgesics or analgesic/antipyretics
- Acetaminophen (Tylenol), 325-650 mg q4-6h
- Acetylsalicylic acid (aspirin) with codeine, po q4h prn

General Management

Simple thumb pressure on convex side of the nose occasionally enough to push bones back together

NURSING CARE

Nursing Assessment

Facial Swelling

Deformity; ecchymosis; epistaxis; nose very tender; history of trauma to face and nose; possible accompanying lacerations; possible bony crepitus; if leak of cerebrospinal fluid is present, clear fluid dripping from nose and ears

Respiratory Status

Difficulty in breathing; mouth breathing

Nursing Dx & Intervention

Nursing Diagnosis	Nursing Intervention/Rationale
Pain	• Assess need for pain medication and provide adequate analgesia for pain relief; evaluate and document effectiveness.
Ineffective breathing pattern related to nasal obstruction and swelling	• Assess for shortness of breath, dyspnea from nasal obstruction, or difficulty in swallowing. • Apply ice to face and nose *to minimize swelling and bleeding without pressure to nose.* • Monitor amount and color of epistaxis and record. • Keep head of bed elevated, even when sleeping, *to prevent aspiration of blood or secretions.* • Prevent patient from swallowing blood or aspirating; encourage patient to breathe through mouth. • Have basin nearby for patient *to expectorate blood.* • Provide frequent oral hygiene and encourage intake of oral fluids. • Monitor vital signs and level of consciousness.
Sensory/perceptual alterations (visual)	• Assess for eye swelling; apply ice *to minimize edema.* • Observe for scleral hemorrhage and periorbital edema. • If eyes are not completely closed, assess patient's ability to see.

Patient Education

1. Ensure that the patient knows to keep head elevated, even while sleeping.
2. Instruct patient in timing of pain medication.
3. Instruct patient to seek medical assistance immediately if there is a decrease in vision, level of consciousness, or ability to breathe.

Evaluation

Patient Outcome	Data Indicating That Outcome is Reached
Nasal fracture is well healed.	There is no facial deformity. There is no nasal obstruction; patient can breathe normally through nose. Sclera is clear without redness or swelling.

Nasal polyps

Polyps are benign growths that appear as soft, pale gray, nontender masses and gradually form from recurrent localized swelling of the sinuses or nasal mucosa (Figure 7-20).

Polyps are seen in about 90% of patients with chronic maxillary sinusitis. Polyps may become quite large. They are usually bilateral, occur in multiples, and may cause actual distention and enlargement of the bony structures of the nose. Even after surgical removal, some nasal polyps recur. Although rare in children, polyps are occasionally found in children with cystic fibrosis and allergies and in those with Peutz-Jeghers syndrome. The symptoms of this syndrome include pigmented spots on the skin, especially around the mouth, and polyposis of the gastrointestinal tract.

Many patients with polyps have anosmia or hyposmia.[34]

Pathophysiology

The etiology of nasal polyps is not clear. They are often pedunculated and suspended in the nasal cavity by stalks of varying lengths. The polyps and stalks usually originate in the paranasal sinuses, particularly the ethmoid sinuses, and pass into the middle meatus of the nose through the ostia connecting them to the nasal cavities. They are often called pseudotumors. Their pathogenesis is thought to be the result of focal mucosal edema that causes a polypoid swelling. Because of the polyp's weight, the swelling tends to enlarge and eventually becomes suspended on a stalk.[34]

Polyps are usually found in the middle meatus near the openings of the sinuses and occasionally in the roof of the nose. They are never found on the septum or in the lower meatus; the reason for this is not known.[33]

Polyps were once commonly thought to be a consequence of allergies, but evidence does not support a relationship between allergies and polyps.[34] In a 1979 study reported by Settipane and associates,[48] 4986 adults with asthma or chronic rhinitis were studied and only 4.2% had polyps. Only 0.1% of 1051 children with asthma or chronic rhinitis had polyps.

An interesting phenomenon that occurs in some patients with asthma and nasal polyposis is an intolerance to aspirin, indomethacin, and some coal tar dyes. This intolerance is severe and can cause respiratory arrest if these substances are

Figure 7-20 Nasal polyps.

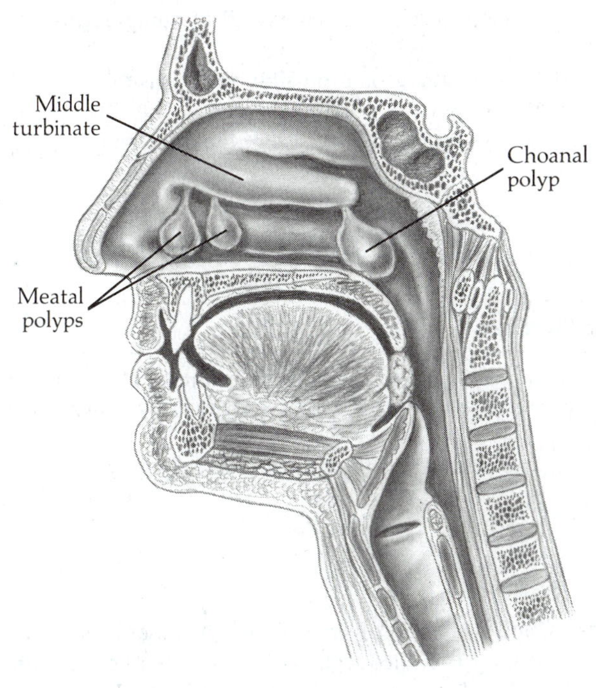

ingested. This is thought to be related to the inhibitory action of these substances on prostaglandin synthesis.[33]

Diagnostic Studies and Findings

Roentgenograms of Sinuses

Shadows over affected areas; ethmoid sinuses and sometimes maxillary sinuses appear cloudy

Medical Plan

Surgery

Polypectomy—each polyp avulsed with wire snare
Caldwell-Luc procedure—may be performed if polyps are caused by chronic maxillary sinusitis

Medications

Corticosteroids
- Betamethasone (Celestone), 0.6-4.8 mg/d causes polyps to disappear
- Cortisone not recommended for long-term use; local sprays such as beclomethasone (Vanceril Inhaler) may be useful, since they are effective in treating asthma (0.1 mg/spray, 2 sprays in each nostril bid or tid)

Antihistamines (to treat allergy symptoms)
- Chlorpheniramine (Chlor-Trimetron), 4 mg po q4-6h prn

Adrenergic agents (for antihistamine effect)
- Pseudoephedrine (Sudafed), 30 mg po q4-6h prn

Anti-infective agents
- Agent-specific antibiotics if infection is present

NURSING CARE

Nursing Assessment

Nasal Obstruction

Feeling of fullness in face or nose; shortness of breath; nasal discharge; anosmia; other symptoms of allergic rhinitis, such as sneezing, watery eyes, eczema, and asthma; grayish growths visible on examination with nasal speculum

Nursing Dx & Intervention

Nursing Diagnosis	Nursing Intervention/Rationale
Ineffective airway clearance related to bleeding and swelling of the nasal mucosa	• Assess patient's ability to clear secretions. Assess amount of bleeding and swelling. • After polypectomy, elevate head of bed, and apply ice compresses to nose *to minimize swelling and bleeding.* • Change nasal drip pad as indicated and record amount and consistency of drainage. • Encourage patient not to swallow blood or secretions but to expectorate into basin *to prevent nausea.* • Monitor patient's vital signs. • Instruct patient not to blow nose *to prevent tissue trauma and promote healing.* • *Convalescent care:* Observe for bleeding, especially after packing has been removed (1 to 2 days after surgery). • If patient is still hospitalized, notify physician, elevate head of bed, check vital signs, and compress outside of nose against septum. • If bleeding persists, pack if necessary.
Sensory/perceptual alterations (olfactory)	• Assess patient's ability to smell. • Assure patient that sense of smell should return postoperatively after packing is removed and swelling is decreased.

Patient Education

1. Ensure that the patient knows how to reach the physician immediately if bleeding begins after the patient has been discharged.
2. Instruct the patient with allergies to avoid known allergens if possible and to take antihistamines early to minimize allergic reactions.
3. Instruct the patient to use nose drops and sprays cautiously because of the rebound effect on the mucous membranes.

Evaluation

Patient Outcome	Data Indicating That Outcome is Reached
Patient's knowledge of polyps is increased.	Patient verbalizes understanding of possible causes and ways to prevent recurrence of nasal polyps. Patient seeks early treatment for sinusitis or minimizes severity of allergies by taking antihistamines.
Patient's recovery from polypectomy is unremarkable.	There is no bleeding, nasal obstruction, shortness of breath, or anosmia after surgery.

Septal deviation and perforation

A deviated septum is a shift of the septum from the midline, which is common in many adults. It is either S or C shaped.

Although the septum is usually straight at birth, it may shift from one side to another as a result of trauma or injury.

A septal perforation is a hole in the nasal septum between the nostrils, which is usually in the anterior or cartilaginous septum but may occasionally occur in the bony septum. A small perforation, which can be caused by infections, nasal crusting, or nose picking, is often asymptomatic, although a slight whistle may be heard as the patient breathes. Larger perforations may produce rhinitis, nasal crusting, or epistaxis.

Pathophysiology

The nasal septum is usually straight. The septum is occasionally bent during birth, and the infant may have a twisted-appearing nose. This can usually be corrected when first noticed by placing light pressure on the convex side of the nose. There is no need for packing or a splint. Minor degrees of deviation go unrecognized in the newborn period.[34]

With aging, the septum has a tendency to become deviated or to form a hump. There is frequently no history of injury to account for the deviation. As a result, few adults have a totally straight septum. Trauma during childhood may also contribute to septal deviation in the adult.

Although there are frequently no symptoms associated with a deviated septum, some patients have moderate to severe degrees of nasal obstruction. Other, less well-defined symptoms include headaches, which occur in some patients who have a septal spur impinging on the inferior turbinate; epistaxis; and symptoms of sinusitis, which are rare but may be influenced by a deviated septum that obstructs a sinus opening.

Septal perforations may be small or large. They may be asymptomatic or may cause annoying symptoms such as crusting, a watery discharge, or a whistling noise as the patient breathes. Small perforations are usually caused by repeated irritation of the nose, such as picking it; they are also often caused by septal surgery. Less frequent causes are repeated cauterizations because of epistaxis, snorting cocaine, and chronic nasal infections. Once quite common, perforations resulting from syphilis and tuberculosis are now rare. Approximately 25% to 30% of perforations are of unknown etiology.[39] Ninety percent of perforations are in the anterior cartilaginous portions of the nose, less than 10% are in the posterior or superior bony portions. The margins of many are lined by smooth, shiny, flat mucosa; others have elevated edges of granulation tissue and crusted edges. These latter types should be fully evaluated for the presence of serious underlying disease.[34]

Diagnostic Studies and Findings

Facial Roentgenograms, Examination with Otoscope

Show a shift of the septum

Medical Plan

Surgery

For deviation

Submucous resection—may be performed to reposition septum and relieve nasal obstruction

Rhinoplasty—may be done to correct nasal structure deformity
Septoplasty to replace septum in midline—may be done to relieve nasal obstruction and to enhance external appearance of nose
For perforation
Bilateral nasal packs—used for 24 to 48 hours to hold mucosa and septum in place
Surgical closure—possible but not always successful; a Silastic "button" prosthesis may be inserted to close perforation[39]

Medications

Analgesic/antipyretics
Acetylsalicylic acid (aspirin), 600 mg po q4-6h to relieve headache if present (for deviation)
Antihistamines (to decrease secretions and congestion)
Chlorpheniramine (Chlor-Trimeton), 4 mg po q4-6h
Adrenergic agents
Pseudoephedrine (Sudafed), 30 mg po q4-6h (for perforation)
Anti-infective agents
Antibiotics topically applied to prevent infection; bacitracin (Baciquent), 500 U/g in petrolatum base

General Management

Local application of lanolin or petrolatum twice a day to prevent crusting (for perforation)
Irrigate nose with normal saline or a dilute solution of sodium bicarbonate two or three times a day to keep the nasal mucosa hydrated (for perforation)
Packing to control bleeding if present (for deviation)

NURSING CARE

Nursing Assessment

Nasal Obstruction

Irregularities or deformity of external nose; examination with bright light and nasal speculum shows septal deviation from midline, which is sometimes S shaped with a greatly reduced airway; feeling of facial fullness, headaches, epistaxis, or sinusitis

Nursing Dx & Intervention

Nursing Diagnosis	Nursing Intervention/Rationale
Ineffective breathing pattern	• Assess and record respiratory status. • Postoperative care includes explanation to patient that facial and periorbital edema will be present and that nasal packing will be in place for 24 to 48 hours. • Instruct patient to breathe through mouth during this time.
Impaired skin integrity	• Keep head of bed slightly elevated *to prevent edema and promote drainage*. • Use ice packs on face *to decrease edema, pain, and bleeding*. • Use cool vaporizer *to assist in liquefying secretions*. • Point out that patient will experience difficulty swallowing while nasal packs are in place. • Change drip pad as necessary, recording color, consistency, and amount of drainage. • Provide meticulous mouth care, *since the patient is breathing through mouth*.
Potential for injury	• Assess and report presence of excessive bleeding, swallowing, or purulent drainage. • Caution patient against attempting to blow nose, *which may cause bruising and edema*. • Caution patient not to smoke for at least 2 days and to limit physical activity for 2 to 3 days *to prevent irritation or trauma to tissues*.

Patient Education

1. To prevent tissue trauma, remind the patient not to smoke or blow the nose.
2. Remind the patient to avoid overexertion for several days.

Evaluation

Patient Outcome	Data Indicating That Outcome is Reached
Nasal obstruction is lessened.	The patient breathes comfortably. There is no epistaxis, headache, or infection. If the septum was perforated, the area is well healed without evidence of infection.

Sinusitis

Sinusitis is an inflammatory process caused by bacterial, viral, fungal, or allergic conditions that change the mucosa of a sinus.

Sinusitis is frequently blamed for such symptoms as headaches or nasal problems, but actually it is present in less than 10% of patients who consult an otolaryngologist. The types of sinusitis are acute, subacute, suppurative, chronic suppurative, allergic, and hyperplastic.

The changes in the sinus mucosa caused by sinusitis produce definite signs and symptoms, most of which can be assessed during physical examination or on roentgenograms.

An attack of sinusitis may follow a common cold (0.5% of the time) as infection spreads from the nasal passages to the sinuses; excessive or forceful nose blowing may also force infected material into the sinuses. Since the sinuses normally drain secretions through their normal routes into the meatus, any condition that obstructs these openings and forces the secretions to back up into the sinuses may cause sinus infection. These conditions may include the presence of nasal polyps, a deviated nasal septum, or edema of the turbinates resulting from an allergic disorder.[18]

The maxillary sinus (antrum) is the one most frequently affected with acute sinusitis, although the entire anterior group of sinuses may be involved. These are the maxillary, frontal, and anterior and middle ethmoid, all of which drain into the middle meatus of the nose. The posterior group of sinuses, the posterior ethmoid and sphenoid, are usually affected with chronic sinusitis only when the anterior group is also involved.

The prognosis for sinusitis is usually good with identification and treatment if necessary, but some complications may result from sinusitis if the infection spreads. These complications include septicemia, periorbital abscesses, brain abscesses, and osteomyelitis.

Regardless of the type of sinusitis, patients should avoid cold, damp conditions and maintain a constant room temperature and humidity. Air conditioning aggravates sinusitis, and so does smoking because smoke irritates the mucous membranes and inhibits their normal self-cleansing ciliary action.

Pathophysiology

Acute suppurative sinusitis may follow a common cold or may be caused endemically by a specific organism after a sudden drop in temperature. In addition, during swimming or diving, infected water may be forced into the nose and cause a bacterial infection.

Bacteria that are commonly responsible include gram-positive cocci, such as *Streptococcus, Staphylococcus,* and *H. influenzae*. Other organisms are less commonly responsible.

Swimming and diving may cause an acute onset of sinusitis; otherwise the symptoms occur gradually as the involved sinus becomes more inflamed. The nasal mucosa appears red and swollen, and purulent discharge is obvious in the middle meatus. The discharge increases, may be blood tinged in the first 24 to 48 hours, and may cause an inflamed, sore throat from the postnasal discharge. As fluid fills the sinuses, they become opaque to transillumination and an actual fluid level may be seen on roentgenograms of the sinus.

Pain varies from low-grade to intense as the oxygen in the sinus is absorbed into the blood vessels. This creates negative pressure in the sinus and allows it to be filled with transudate, which produces a painful positive pressure. Tenderness is also present over the involved sinus.

Most cases of acute sinusitis are cured with conservative treatment; antibiotics are unnecessary. Purulent secretions are present for 3 to 4 days and then slowly resolve over the next 10 days to 2 weeks. In a few cases, however, a purulent nasal discharge persists, and the patient may continue to complain of nasal congestion and vague discomfort over the sinuses or face. This is classified as subacute sinusitis. These patients may have persistent pus in the nose for more than 3 weeks after the acute infection. Since antibiotic therapy may be needed, a culture of the exudate should be obtained and roentgenograms taken to determine if more than one sinus is involved.

Frontal sinusitis can cause severe intracranial complications because these sinuses are in close physical relationship with the orbits and are separated from them by thin bony walls. Infection spreads easily from these sinuses to the orbits either through dehiscences in the bones or via infected thrombophlebitic veins. Spread of the infection is made easier by the rich plexus of valveless veins passing between the frontal and ethmoid sinuses and the orbits.[18] Fungal sinusitis may occur both in healthy persons and in persons who are compromised by immunosuppression, debilitation, diabetes, or malignancies being treated with cytotoxic drugs. Depending on the particular fungus and the health of the affected person, fungal sinusitis may be fatal. Healthy individuals may be infected and respond well to treatment.

The most common infecting agent is *Aspergillus*. Patients usually have a unilateral infection of the maxillary sinus after a long-standing sinus infection. Similar infections may be caused by *Alternaria, Petriellidum,* or *Paecilomyces,* all commonly found soil organisms.[23]

Patients with persistent subacute sinus infections may have an allergy; recognition of this obviously aids in treatment.

If sinus infections are neglected or a patient has repeated attacks, the mucosal lining of the sinus may become permanently damaged. This is known as chronic suppurative sinusitis. Often the only symptom is continued purulent nasal discharge. If the patient seems unable to overcome the infection, the physician must look for systemic conditions that may lower resistance to infection, such as anemia, malnutrition, or hypometabolism.

Allergic sinusitis occurs only in conjunction with allergic rhinitis. The symptoms are the same, and the sinus mucosa undergoes the same changes as the nasal mucosa. Patients

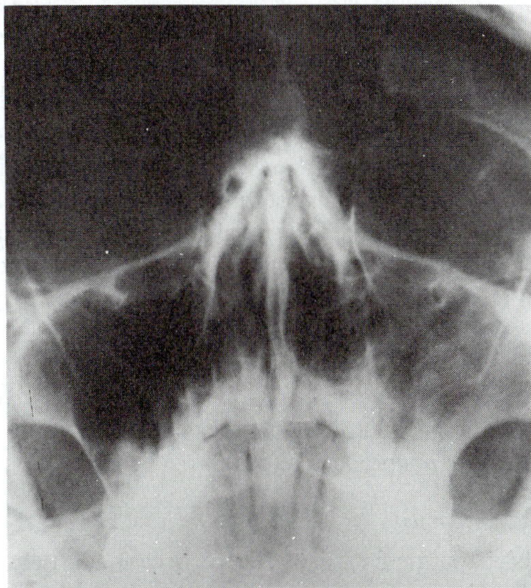

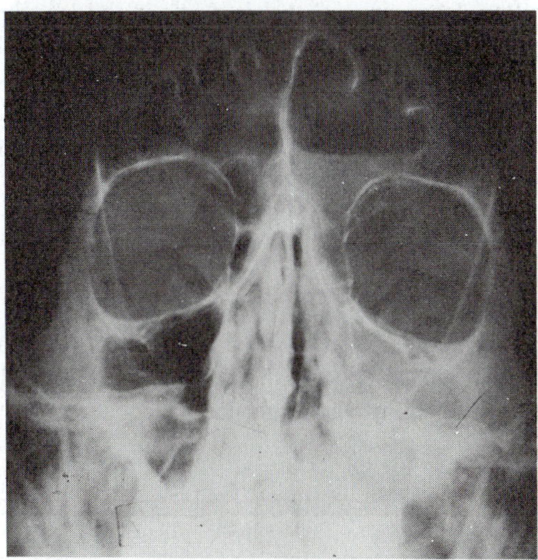

Figure 7-21 Sinus films showing clouding and fluid level from sinusitis. From DeWeese.[9]

with allergic rhinitis probably also have allergic sinusitis; polyps, which are common with allergic rhinitis, also occur with regularity in the mucosal lining of the sinuses.

Purulent sinusitis superimposed on allergic rhinitis and sinusitis is called hyperplastic sinusitis. The lining of the mucosa and submucosa becomes chronically thickened, and nasal polyps tend to form and recur even after surgical removal. These polyps may block the natural openings to the meatus and obstruct drainage of purulent material. Tissue swelling remains severe, and the nasal tissue does not respond to the usual shrinking solutions. The nose feels plugged most of the time, and a frontal headache is common.

Diagnostic Studies and Findings

Transillumination

Examiner shines bright light in patient's mouth with lips closed around bulb; involved sinus appears dark whereas normal sinus transilluminates

Sinus Roentgenograms

Involved sinuses appear clouded or actual fluid level may be seen (Figure 7-21)

Culture of Sinus Discharge

To identify causative organism

Medical Plan

Surgical

- For acute maxillary sinusitis
  - Creation of nasal window—to open sinus and allow pus and secretions to drain through nose
- For chronic maxillary sinusitis
  - Caldwell-Luc procedure (radical antrum operation) through incision under lip to remove diseased mucosa and periosteum
- For chronic ethmoid sinusitis
  - Ethmoidectomy—to remove infected tissue through incision into ethmoid sinus
- For chronic frontal sinusitis
  - Creation of osteoplastic flap—involves incision across skull and behind hairline to drain sinuses
  - Frontoethmoidectomy—allows removal of infected frontal sinus tissue through external ethmoidectomy
- For sphenoid sinusitis
  - External ethmoidectomy—performed through incision that begins under eyebrow and extends along side of nose, allowing removal of infected sinus tissue
- For fungal sinusitis
  - Aggressive local surgical debridement of diseased tissue

Medications

- Anti-infective agents
  - Penicillin G or V, 250 mg po q6h for 10 d
  - Erythromycin (E-Mycin), 250 mg po q6h for 10 d
  - Amoxicillin (Amokil, Larotid), 500 mg po tid for 10 d
  - Sulfamethoxazole (Bactrim, Septra), 1 tab po bid or qid
  - Cephalexin (Keflex), 500 mg po qid
  - Ampicillin, 500 mg po q6h (for chronic sinusitis)
  - Tetracycline 500 mg po q6h (for chronic sinusitis)
  - Amphotericin (Fungizone), 1 mg in 250 D5W over 2-4 h, or 0.25 mg/kg daily by slow infusion over 6 h; increase gradually as patient's tolerance develops, to a maximum of 1 mg/kg d; dosage must not exceed 1.5/mg/kg/d; premedicate patient with acetaminophen (Tylenol) and diphenhydramine (Benadryl) as a prophylactic measure to avoid some of the unpleasant side effects

Narcotic analgesics (used to relieve headache from acute sinusitis)
- Codeine, 30-60 mg po q4-6h
- Meperidine (Demerol), 50 mg po q4-6h

Antihistamines (used to decrease secretions and congestion)
- Azatadine (Optimine), 1 or 2 mg po q12h

Adrenergic agents
- Pseudoephedrine (Sudafed), 30 mg po q4-6h prn
- Aerosol bacitracin (for chronic sinusitis)

Vasoconstrictors
- Nose drops or nasal spray containing vasoconstrictor to keep the nose open; Afrin (1 spray in each nostril q12h) is commonly prescribed

General Management

Drainage of involved sinus if usual therapy fails

Antral puncture (puncture of medial wall of maxillary sinus) to provide means of irrigation (may also be done to collect specimen for diagnosis)

Steam inhalation to encourage drainage and promote vasoconstriction

Hot, wet packs applied locally for relief of pain and congestion at least four times a day

NURSING CARE

Nursing Assessment

Acute Sinusitis

Malaise; anorexia; nasal congestion; purulent nasal discharge; cough; sore throat; fever, usually low grade; pain over sinus areas that worsens as patient lowers head; pressure over involved areas and upper teeth; orbital or facial edema; constant, severe headaches; enlarged turbinates; pus apparent in nasal cavity and nasopharynx when examined with nasopharyngeal mirror; loss of vocal resonance, hyposmia; halitosis

Subacute Sinusitis

Stuffy nose; vague intermittent discomfort in involved areas; fatigue; pus in nose more than 3 weeks after acute infection; nonproductive cough

Chronic Sinusitis

Persistent purulent nasal discharge; occasional slight headache (from edema of nasal tissue or allergic rhinitis, and not from sinuses) that is worse in the morning and relieved slightly during the day; postnasal drip; halitosis

Allergic Sinusitis

Nasal stuffiness; symptoms of allergic rhinitis: watery eyes, eczema, and asthma; itching and burning of nose; sneezing; frontal headache; thin nasal discharge; presence of nasal polyps

Hyperplastic Sinusitis

Severe tissue edema; mucosal polyps; thickened mucosal lining of sinuses; poor response of nasal tissue to shrinking solutions; low-grade frontal headache

Nursing Dx & Intervention

Nursing Diagnosis	Nursing Intervention/Rationale
Pain	• Assess and document level of comfort. • Encourage bed rest with head of bed slightly elevated *to promote drainage of secretions*. • In collaboration with physician, give analgesics and antihistamines as needed for relief. Assess and document effectiveness. • Administer antibiotics if ordered. • Apply warm, moist compresses locally at least four times a day *for pain relief and promotion of drainage*. • Monitor vital signs, especially temperature. • Watch for and report increase in headaches, blurred vision, periorbital edema, chills, or vomiting.
Sensory/perceptual alterations (olfactory)	• Assess patient's ability to smell. • Administer antihistamines and nose drops or spray in collaboration with physician *to relieve nasal congestion*. • Reassure patient that condition is temporary.
Sleep pattern disturbance	• Assess patient's comfort and relaxation level at bedtime. • Give analgesic medications per physician's orders before patient goes to bed *to minimize headaches*. Administer antihistamines or nose drops at bedtime *to clear nasal passages*. • Make sure that patient understands importance of using nose drops as prescribed *to prevent rebound effect on mucous membranes if they are used over long period of time*.

Nursing Diagnosis	Nursing Intervention/Rationale
Potential ineffective breathing pattern	• Assess and document patient's respiratory status frequently. • Inform patient before surgery that nasal packing will be in place for 12 to 48 hours, that breathing through the mouth will be necessary, and that nose blowing cannot be performed postoperatively *to prevent tissue trauma.*
Patient problem: potential bleeding after surgery	• Assess patient for bleeding after surgery. • Monitor vital signs and watch for frequent swallowing, which may indicate hemorrhaging and swallowing of blood.
Impaired skin integrity	• Assess surgical site every 1 to 2 hours. • Place patient in semi-Fowler's position *to prevent edema and promote drainage.* • Use iced compresses *to minimize swelling and bleeding for first 24 hours.* • Apply cool or warm vapor inhalations as ordered. • Provide meticulous mouth care, since *patient will be breathing through mouth and may have copious bloody secretions.* • Change dressing or nasal drip pad and record amount and color of drainage. (There will normally be small amounts of bright red blood with some clots.) • Inform patient that some numbness of upper lip and teeth may be present after Caldwell-Luc procedure and that black eye and some swelling of operative area are not uncommon for about a week after sinus surgery. • Instruct patient not to brush teeth in this area during this time *to prevent tissue trauma.*

Patient Education

1. Instruct the patient not to smoke for 2 to 3 days after surgery to minimize irritation of the mucous membranes.
2. Tell the patient to watch for bleeding after the nasal packing is removed and to notify the physician immediately if it occurs.
3. Instruct patient about the early signs and symptoms of sinusitis so prompt treatment can be sought.

Evaluation

Patient Outcome	Data Indicating That Outcome is Reached
Signs and symptoms of sinusitis are improved.	There is no headache, nasal congestion, or purulent discharge.
There are no surgical complications if a procedure was performed.	There is no excessive bleeding or postoperative infection; the wound is completely healed.
Patient's knowledge of sinusitis is increased.	Patient verbalizes understanding of causative factors of sinusitis, signs and symptoms of infection, and when to seek medical assistance.

THROAT DISORDERS

Abscesses

Throat abscesses are infections in the fascial spaces.

The most common throat abscesses are peritonsillar (quinsy), retropharyngeal, and pharyngomaxillary. These abscesses form after tonsillitis or an infection of the upper respiratory tract. A peritonsillar abscess forms in the space between the tonsil and the fascia that covers the superior constrictor muscle; a retropharyngeal abscess forms between the posterior pharyngeal wall and the prevertebral fascia; and a pharyngomaxillary abscess forms in the deep space between the fascia of the parotid gland, the internal pterygoid muscle, and the superior constrictor muscle (Figure 7-22).

Pathophysiology

A peritonsillar abscess usually forms after a patient has had tonsillitis for a few days and appears to improve. Peritonsillar abscesses are usually caused by group A β-hemolytic streptococci or occasionally anaerobic organisms. They are rare in children but fairly common in young adults.

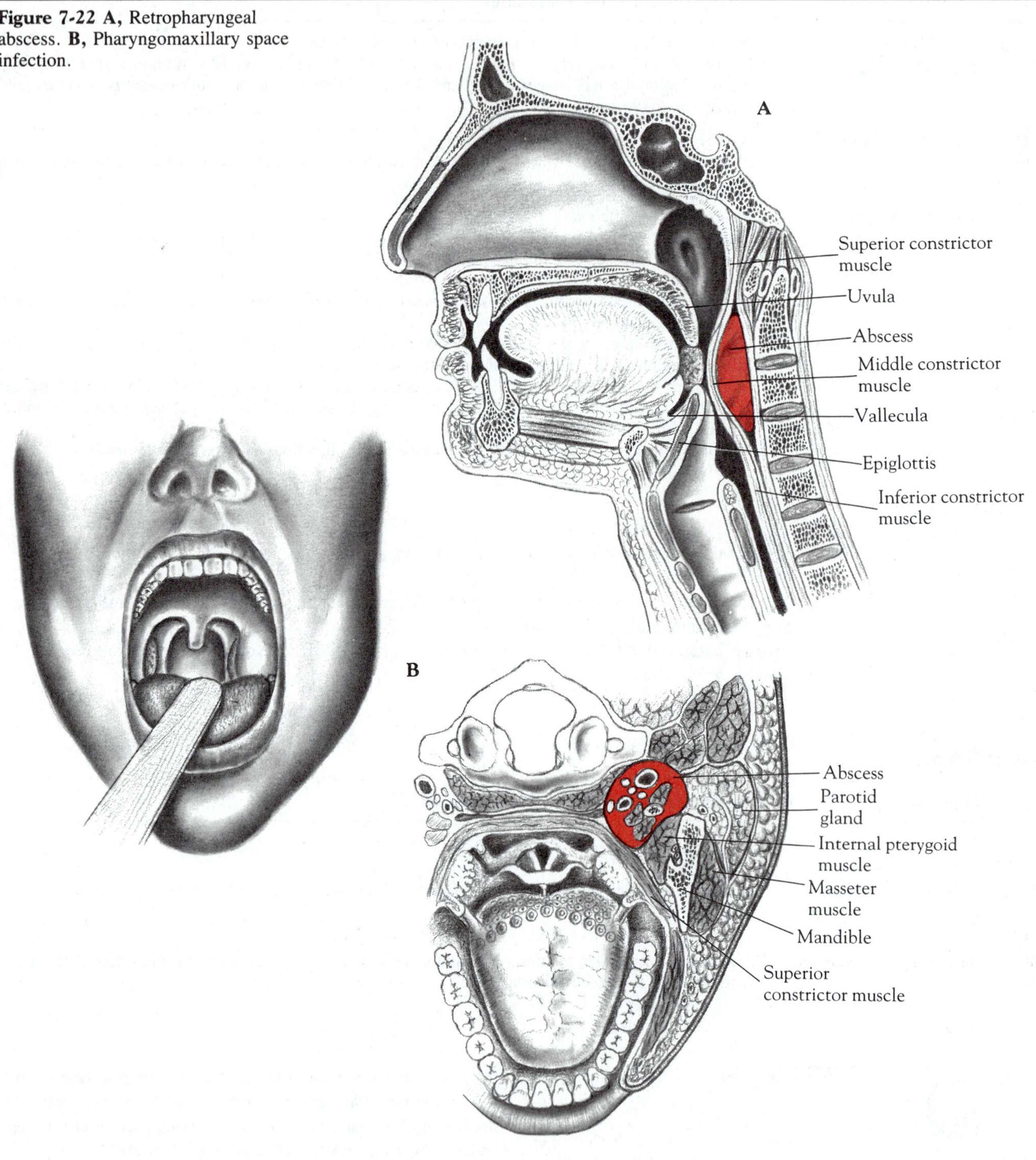

Figure 7-22 A, Retropharyngeal abscess. **B,** Pharyngomaxillary space infection.

Retropharyngeal abscesses are found almost exclusively in infants and young children because the lymph nodes in the retropharyngeal space have usually disappeared by young adulthood. These are usually found as complications of infections that have spread from the pharynx, sinuses, adenoids, or ears to the retropharyngeal lymph nodes.

Pott's disease, or tuberculosis of the cervical spine, can also cause a "cold" retropharyngeal abscess that may appear at any age.

Pharyngomaxillary abscesses are less common than peritonsillar abscesses but more common than retropharyngeal abscesses. Pharyngomaxillary abscesses usually occur as a result of direct contamination with a needle or by the spread of an adjacent infection.

Diagnostic Studies and Findings

Roentgenograms of Neck Area

Larynx appears pushed forward; mass shows in posterior pharynx with retropharyngeal abscesses

Culture of Abscess

To identify causative organism

Medical Plan

Surgery

Incision and drainage of abscess with or without local anesthetic

Tonsillectomy about 1 month after peritonsillar abscess has healed to prevent recurrence

Medications

Anti-infective agents

Penicillin G aqueous, 1-2 million U q4h IV or another broad-spectrum antibiotic for 7-10 d

NURSING CARE

Nursing Assessment

Peritonsillar Area

Severe sore throat; difficulty in swallowing; trismus; drooling; muffled voice; thick secretions; fever, chills, nausea, and malaise; tonsil appears pushed toward midline, forward, and downward; uvula may rest against tonsil or palate

Retropharyngeal Area

Stridor and nasal obstruction; muffled cry; child lies with head extended; fever; posterior pharyngeal wall soft, red, and bulging

Pharyngomaxillary Area

Fullness behind jaw; trismus

Nursing Dx & Intervention

Nursing Diagnosis	Nursing Intervention/Rationale
Pain	• Assess and record amount of pain experienced, and need for pain medication. • Administer analgesic and antipyretic agents as ordered. • Assess and document effectiveness. • Administer hot saline gargles or irrigation *for comfort*.
Ineffective breathing pattern	• Observe airway until abscess has been drained. • Assess for dyspnea, restlessness, stridor, and cyanosis.
Potential for aspiration	• Before abscess is drained, assess patient closely for signs of spontaneous rupture of abscess and possible asphyxiation from pus. (When abscesses are drained, it is not unusual for pus to pour out.) • Keep patient upright with strong suction applied continuously through mouth *to prevent aspiration of pus that would result in suffocation*. • After incision and drainage, administer antibiotics as ordered. • Monitor and document vital signs, skin color, and presence of bleeding. • Ensure adequate fluid intake; intravenous therapy will probably be ordered.

Patient Education

1. Instruct the patient or family about the necessity of continuing antibiotic therapy for the entire prescribed course to prevent recurrence or complications.
2. Inform the patient that peritonsillar abscesses are likely to recur and that a tonsillectomy will probably be performed about a month after the abscess has healed to prevent recurrence.

Evaluation

Patient Outcome	Data Indicating That Outcome is Reached
Throat abscess is well healed.	There is no pain in throat. Temperature is within normal limits for patient. Trismus and drooling are absent. Incised area is healing well.
The patient and family understand course of treatment for abscess.	Patient and family verbalize understanding about completing prescribed course of antibiotic therapy.

Ludwig's angina

Ludwig's angina is a virulent, rapidly spreading cellulitis of the floor of the mouth that occurs in both the sublingual and submaxillary spaces (Figure 7-23).

Ludwig's angina is actually not an abscess, although it resembles one, and there is no lymphatic involvement. Over 80% of cases develop in patients with dental disease such as gingivitis, tooth extraction, or trauma (fractures of the mandible, peritonsillar abscess, or lacerations of the floor of the mouth).[9]

Figure 7-23 Ludwig's angina. *A* and *B* indicate spaces in which infection may start.

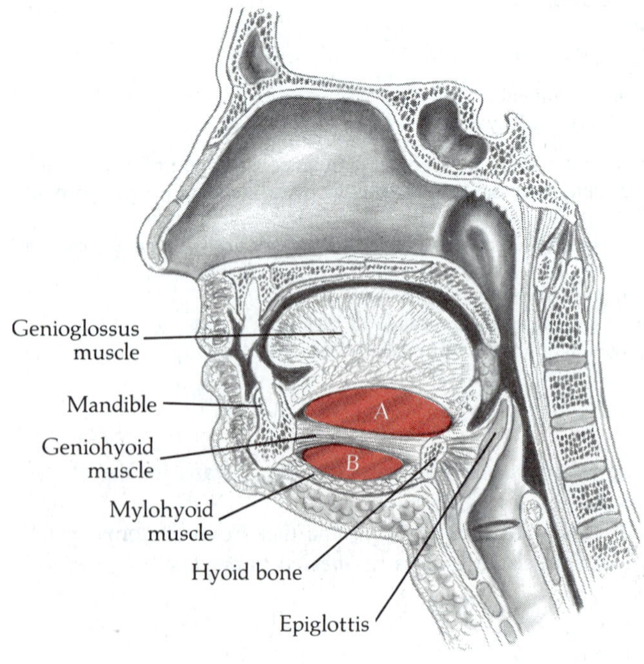

Pathophysiology

These patients' lower molars oddly have the roots closer to the inner than to the outer side of the jaw, and the tips of the roots may extend below the mylohyoid line. The infection usually begins around a tooth root that drains into the submaxillary space rather than into the sublingual space because of root placement. The usual causative organisms are *Streptococcus viridans* and *Escherichia coli*.

The infection spreads rapidly to the sublingual space, which causes the floor of the mouth to become very swollen. It may involve all the tissues under the mandible and usually one or both submaxillary spaces. The swelling may extend all the way down to the clavicle. Since the tongue is elevated in the back of the mouth, airway obstruction is a danger. The patient has a fever and systemic signs of illness.

Pus is seldom found if an incision and drainage are performed, although they must occasionally be done to drain fluid and relieve the pressure on the swollen tissues.

Tracheotomy must often be performed, since the patient's airway is greatly compromised from both swelling and excessive secretions.

Diagnostic Studies and Findings

Identification of Causative Organism

Culture of exudate; visual examination

CT Scan

Indicates presence of and pinpoints location of abscess

Medical Plan

Surgery

Incision and drainage—to relieve pressure
Tracheotomy if airway is impaired

Medications

Anti-infective agents
- Penicillin G aqueous, 1-2 million U q4h IV
- Cefotaxime (Claforan), 1-2 g q6-8h IM or IV (given if patient is allergic to penicillin)

NURSING CARE

Nursing Assessment

Infectious Process in Mouth

Severe pain in involved tooth area; trismus (difficulty opening mouth); dysphonia; patient unable to eat; excessive secretions and drooling; tongue elevation from swelling of the floor of the mouth

Respiratory Function

Dyspnea and stridor from laryngeal edema

Nursing Dx & Intervention

Nursing Diagnosis	Nursing Intervention/Rationale
Ineffective airway clearance	• Assess patient for signs of airway obstruction. • Perform usual tracheostomy care and frequent suctioning; assist patient in handling secretions. • Observe vital signs and symptoms of dyspnea and stridor.
Pain	• Assess level of pain experienced and need for pain medication. • Provide adequate analgesia for pain relief; assess and document effectiveness. • Perform wound care gently but thoroughly if incision and drainage were performed.
Fear	• Provide reassurance that patient is being closely monitored. • Explain tracheostomy procedure and suctioning, and assure patient it will assist with breathing.
Altered nutrition: less than body requirements	• Assess and document patient's fluid and nutrition status. • Ensure adequate fluid intake *to prevent dehydration.* • Monitor intravenous line closely. • As soon as patient can take food and fluids orally, have nutritionist visit patient to plan diet *to provide needed caloric intake.*

Patient Education

1. Stress the importance of good dental hygiene to prevent recurrence of Ludwig's angina or other oral or dental problems.

Evaluation

Patient Outcome	Data Indicating That Outcome is Reached
Cellulitis is well healed.	Airway is patent without respiratory difficulty. Tracheostomy stoma is healing well. There is no swelling in the floor of mouth. Tongue is not elevated. Temperature is within normal limits. There is no pain. Wound is healed if incision and drainage were performed. Nutritional status is adequate for patient.
Patient's knowledge base is increased.	Patient verbalizes understanding of importance of prophylactic dental care and early treatment of any oral inflammation.

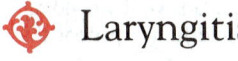

Laryngitis

Laryngitis, or inflammation of the larynx, is a common disorder that may be either acute or chronic.

Acute laryngitis may be found as part of a viral or bacterial infection of the upper respiratory tract, or it may be an isolated infection limited to the vocal cords. Trauma such as abuse of the voice may also cause acute laryngitis.

Chronic laryngitis implies inflammatory changes in the laryngeal mucosa. It can be progressive and may lead to a serious voice disability.

Pathophysiology

Acute laryngitis is often found in combination with viral or bacterial infections of the upper respiratory tract. Viral infections are the most common, but organisms such as β-hemolytic streptococci and *Streptococcus pneumoniae* are also causative agents. Laryngitis may occur with colds, bronchitis, pneumonia, or influenza.

Noninfectious causes include excessive use of the voice, such as by public speakers or singers, inhalation of toxic or irritating fumes, or aspiration of caustic chemicals.

Chronic laryngitis can be caused by frequent attacks of acute laryngitis, chronic abuse of the voice, and smoking. Chronic tonsillitis and adenoiditis, allergies, or hypermetabolic states may occasionally cause chronic laryngitis.

Diagnostic Studies and Findings

Laryngoscopy, Direct or Indirect

Shows abnormalities in true cords, reddened mucosa, and secretions on vocal cords

Medical Plan

Surgery

None unless tracheotomy is required because of severe laryngeal edema

Medications

Anti-infective agents
- Penicillin G; 250 mg po q6h for 10-12 d

Analgesic/antipyretics
- Acetaminophen (Tylenol), 600 mg po q4-6h prn

Analgesics
- Throat lozenges (Chloraseptic or Cepacol) if necessary for throat pain

Antitussive agents
- Guaifenesin (Robitussin), 100-400 mg q4h to relieve cough

General Management

Voice rest

Steam inhalation

NURSING CARE

Nursing Assessment

Laryngeal Function

Acute
- Hoarseness to aphonia; nonproductive cough; rough, scratchy throat; edema, stridor, and dyspnea in very severe cases; fever or malaise; true vocal cords appear red rather than white with rounded rather than sharp edges as determined by indirect laryngoscopy; entire laryngeal area erythematous; bilateral swelling of cords; drops of secretions in trachea or on vocal cords

Chronic
- Progressive hoarseness, if present, is worse in morning because of dried secretions in larynx; voice improves during day and deteriorates again toward evening; usually no throat pain; nonproductive cough; laryngeal mucosa uniformly reddened but smooth; usually no swelling; in some cases polypoid growths, which are called chronic polypoid laryngitis

Nursing Dx & Intervention

Nursing Diagnosis	Nursing Intervention/Rationale
Pain	• Assess level of pain experienced. • Administer analgesics, throat lozenges, or antitussives *for comfort.* • Administer antibiotics as ordered. • Provide for inhalation of warm steam *for symptomatic relief.*
Impaired verbal communication	• Assess patient's understanding of need for voice rest. • Encourage complete voice rest. • Provide Magic Slate or paper and pencil *to facilitate communication.* • Anticipate patient's needs as much as possible *to eliminate need for patient to talk.* • Encourage family and friends to assist patient by asking questions patient can answer by nodding. • If patient is hospitalized, mark on intercom that patient cannot respond and notify patient that someone will come to room when light is turned on.

Patient Education

1. Ensure that the patient understands possible sequelae of constant voice abuse and smoking and encourage improvement of these habits.

Evaluation

Patient Outcome	Data Indicating That Outcome is Reached
There is no inflammation of larynx.	There is no hoarseness, and voice is normal for patient. Raw, tickling feeling in throat is gone. Cough and throat pain are absent. Temperature is within normal limits for patient. There is no inflammation or swelling in laryngeal mucosa or vocal cords.
Patient's understanding of laryngitis is increased.	Patient verbalizes understanding of causes of laryngitis and preventive measures: no smoking, no voice abuse, early treatment of colds, and recognition of symptoms of bronchitis.

Pharyngitis

Pharyngitis is an acute or chronic inflammation of the pharynx.

Pathophysiology

Pharyngitis is the most common of the throat disorders. It frequently precedes or accompanies the common cold and is characterized by a mild sore throat, difficulty and pain in swallowing, and a low-grade fever. In more than 50% of cases pharyngitis is viral in origin.[23] The bacterial cause is usually *Streptococcus,* especially in children. Unless complicated by other bacteria, pharyngitis usually resolves in 4 to 6 days. It is communicable for 2 to 3 days after the initial symptoms appear.

If follicular pharyngitis develops, usually from infection by β-hemolytic streptococci, the mucous membrane becomes severely inflamed and studded with white or yellow follicles. If these follicles are present, most are on the tonsils; if the tonsils have been removed, the follicles appear on the lymph areas in the posterior pharynx and also on the lingual tonsil and in the nasopharynx.

In approximately 10% of cases, pharyngitis is a result of infection with adenovirus. Primary infections occur during childhood; summer epidemics may result from waterborne vectors. In winter the mode of transmission is mainly respiratory. This can cause a severe and rapidly infectious diffuse respiratory infection known as acute febrile respiratory disease, often accompanied by primary atypical pneumonia.[23]

Diagnostic Studies and Findings

Throat Culture

Taken to rule out streptococcal infection

Medical Plan

Medications

Anti-infective agents
- Penicillin G or V, 250 mg po q6h for 10 d (if pharyngitis has bacterial cause)

Analgesic/antipyretics
- Acetylsalicylic acid (aspirin), 300-600 mg po q4-6h

General Management

Bed rest
Humidification
Warm saline throat irrigations
Adequate fluid intake; if throat is so painful and swollen that adequate fluids cannot be taken orally, the patient is often hospitalized for intravenous fluid intake for 24 to 72 hours or until inflammation subsides

NURSING CARE

Nursing Assessment

Infectious Process in Throat

Sore throat, with slight difficulty swallowing, especially saliva; mild fever; headaches, malaise, and joint pain; cervical lymphadenopathy; pharynx reddened and inflamed; blisters or follicles on tonsils or lymph areas

Nursing Dx & Intervention

Nursing Diagnosis	Nursing Intervention/Rationale
Pain	• Assess level of pain experienced. • Administer antibiotics and analgesics as ordered. • Assess and document effectiveness. • Provide warm saline throat irrigations *for comfort.* • Encourage bed rest.

Nursing Diagnosis	Nursing Intervention/Rationale
Potential fluid volume deficit	• Assess patient's fluid intake, skin turgor, and urine output. • Encourage a fluid intake of at least 2500 ml/day. • Monitor intake and output, observe for signs of dehydration (dry skin, cracked lips, and decreased urine output). • If intravenous fluid is ordered, maintain adequate flow rate. • Assist patient with frequent oral hygiene; patient may be mouth breathing, which adds to discomfort. • Monitor patient's temperature and report abnormalities.

Patient Education

1. Instruct the patient and family about the necessity of completing the prescribed course of antibiotics to prevent complications or recurrence of infection.
2. Inform the patient and family of possible irritants (smoking and lack of humidity) and ways to prevent inflammation.

Evaluation

Patient Outcome	Data Indicating That Outcome is Reached
Pharyngitis is resolved.	Sore throat is gone. Patient is afebrile. Activity level is normal for patient. Fluid and nutritional status are adequate for patient. There is no swelling or infection in throat. Cervical lymphadenopathy is absent.
Patient verbalizes knowledge of treatment.	Patient verbalizes understanding of necessity of completing prescribed course of antibiotics.

Tonsillitis

Tonsillitis is an inflammation of the palatine tonsil.

Tonsillitis may be acute or chronic. It usually remains localized in the tonsillar tissue and is considered mildly contagious. It is characterized by a sore throat, but the patient may experience referred pain to the ears.

Tonsillitis is usually an airborne or foodborne bacterial infection. It can occur at any age but is most frequently found in children between the ages of 5 and 10 years. If uncomplicated, it usually resolves after 5 to 7 days. Treatment makes the patient more comfortable and may prevent serious complications such as arthritis, glomerulonephritis, or chronic tonsillitis. A less common cause of tonsillitis is viral infection; epidemics of viral tonsillitis have occurred among military recruits.[2]

Several years ago the role of the tonsils and adenoids in the immune system was not as well known as it is today, and surgical removal of the tonsils and adenoids was common. However, these procedures are performed less today because the importance of this lymphoid tissue to the body's immune system has been established.

Pathophysiology

Tonsillitis begins as a sore throat accompanied by fever, chills, headache, myalgia, joint pain, and anorexia. The patient may also have enlarged and tender anterior cervical lymph nodes. The tonsils appear enlarged, reddened, and inflamed with pus or exudate projecting from between the pillars of the fauces or in the crypts. Some of the exudate can be pulled away from the tonsil, which causes bleeding. The white blood cell count is frequently increased to 10,000 to 20,000/mm^2.

A throat culture should be obtained to identify the infecting organism. *Streptococcus* (β-hemolytic streptococci group A) is the most common organism. If this is the cause, the tonsils appear studded with yellow follicles. Other causative agents are *Pneumococcus* and gram-negative organisms *(Proteus, Pseudomonas,* or coliforms), which have steadily increased as infective agents over the past 10 years.

Diagnostic Studies and Findings

Throat Culture

Identification of causative organism

Medical Plan

Surgery

Tonsillectomy, if indicated, after acute infection has subsided (see p. 722)

Medications

Analgesic/antipyretics
- Acetylsalicylic acid (aspirin) or acetaminophen (Tylenol), 600 mg po q4-6h for adults

Anti-infective agents
- Penicillin V (PenVee), 125 mg po q6h
- Penicillin G (Bicillin), 600,000-1,200,000 U IM

NURSING CARE

Nursing Assessment

Infectious Process in Throat

Moderate to severe sore throat; pain referred to ears; anterior cervical lymphadenopathy; fever and chills; headache; muscle and joint pain; anorexia; increased secretions from throat; enlarged, reddened, inflamed tonsils; pus or exudate on tonsils; edematous or inflamed uvula; white blood count of 10,000 to 20,000/mm^2

Nursing Dx & Intervention

Nursing Diagnosis	Nursing Intervention/Rationale
Pain	• Assess level of pain experienced and need for pain medication. • Provide adequate analgesia *for relief of throat pain;* assess and document effectiveness. • Administer antibiotics as ordered. • Perform throat irrigations; provide hot saline gargles or ice collar as comfort measures. • Maintain bed rest during acute phase and emphasize importance of rest while convalescing.
Potential fluid volume deficit	• Assess skin turgor, intake and urine output, and ability to swallow fluids. • Encourage increased fluid intake keeping in mind that children can become dehydrated very quickly. Note that the child may like ice cream, sherbet, or flavored drinks; avoid juices, *since they may burn throat.* • If patient is hospitalized, monitor intravenous intake *to ensure adequate intake of fluid.*
Altered nutrition: less than body requirements	• Assess patient's nutritional status and ability to eat. • Ensure that patient has adequate intake of soft, nourishing foods. • Encourage patient to eat foods that are minimally irritating to throat and provide adequate caloric intake, that is, soups and milkshakes.

Patient Education

1. Stress to the patient and family the importance of completing the prescribed course of antibiotics to prevent complications or recurrence.

Evaluation

Patient Outcome	Data Indication That Outcome is Reached
Patient recovers uneventfully from attack of tonsillitis.	Patient is afebrile. Tonsils are normal in size and free of pus and exudate. There is no pain in throat. Lymph nodes are not enlarged, although this might persist after other symptoms have disappeared. White blood count is within normal limits. Patient and family verbalize understanding of necessity of completing the required course of medication.

Vocal cord paralysis

Vocal cord paralysis is the loss of nerve and motor supply to the vocal cords resulting in fixation and abnormal position of one or both cords.

Paralysis of the vocal cords is the result of either disease or injury to the superior laryngeal nerve or the recurrent laryngeal nerve, which is the branch of the vagus nerve that provides the entire motor supply to the larynx.

Vocal cord paralysis may be unilateral or bilateral. The quality of the voice depends on whether one or both cords are affected, as well as the position and tenseness of the affected cords. Paralysis of the vocal cords may also be described as complete versus incomplete or abductor versus adductor. Lesions of the central nervous system, such as multiple sclerosis, syringomyelia, brain tumors, and vascular accidents, produce paralysis of the vocal cords.

Pathophysiology

The left recurrent laryngeal nerve, which follows a longer path, is paralyzed in over 70% of cases in contrast to about 15% for the right recurrent laryngeal nerve. Men are affected about 10 times more commonly than women, and the most common age is in the seventies. The most common cause is malignant disease, possibly because of an increased incidence of smoking and cancer of the lung and larynx. One in four recurrent laryngeal nerve paralyses is caused by cancer.[33]

Peripheral causes are also common. These include stretching of the nerve, as occurs with aortic aneurysms and mitral stenosis. Stretching causes enlargement of the left auricle and also stretches the left recurrent laryngeal nerve. The nerve can be infiltrated or stretched by lung or bronchial tumors. Thyroid carcinomas may cause paralysis, and tumors of the larynx itself eventually cause fixation of one or both cords.

Probably 10% of the cases of vocal cord paralysis are unexplained and are called idiopathic. These cases may be from viral infections that remain undiagnosed. In many of these cases the function of the vocal cord recovers spontaneously; this is probably true in 80% of the patients with vocal cord paralysis if recovery has begun before 6 months has passed. The high incidence of infections of the upper respiratory tract suggests a viral cause in many cases. Improved methods of diagnosis should decrease the number of cases labeled idiopathic.[33]

The most common form of paralysis is unilateral: one cord is paralyzed and the other remains normal. If the affected cord is paralyzed in the midline, the normal cord can usually approximate it and the patient may have a normal voice. However, if the paralyzed cord is abducted, the normal cord cannot meet it and the patient has a husky, "breathy" voice.

Dyspnea is not associated with unilateral cord paralysis because the laryngeal airway is adequate; the good cord abducts enough for the airway. However, bilateral cord paralysis affects the airway more seriously. The cords are usually paralyzed in the adducted position. The cords may be within 2 to 3 mm of the midline, and the patient suffers both stridor and dyspnea on exertion.

Diagnostic Studies and Findings

Laryngoscopy

Shows paralyzed condition of cords

Bronchoscopy and Esophagoscopy

Done as part of malignancy workup

Skull Roentgenograms, Thyroid Scan, Upper Gastrointestinal Series, and Complete Neurologic Examination

Performed to rule out other causes

Medical Plan

Surgery

- For unilateral paralysis
  - Injection of measured amounts of Teflon into paralyzed cord under direct laryngoscopy; enlarges or swells cord and brings it closer to midline so normal cord can better approximate it; strengthens voice and prevents aspiration
- For bilateral paralysis
  - Tracheotomy may be needed because of inadequate airway
  - Alternative therapy is arytenoidectomy in which one arytenoid cartilage is removed and glottis is opened posteriorly
  - King procedure is another alternative in which suture is passed around arytenoid cartilage and through adjacent cricoid cartilage; arytenoid is rotated and fixed laterally; improves airway patency but may adversely affect quality of voice; many patients decide to conserve their voices and keep tracheotomy tube
  - Lateralization of vocal cords; used in 22 patients with paralysis of bilateral abductor cord; consists of segmental removal of thyroarytenoid muscle fibers that are adjacent to vocal ligament down to conus elasticus medially and thyroid cartilage laterally; excision made by microcautery, and surgical defect closed after vocal cord is lateralized with two sutures, one into endolarynx superiorly and other into vocal ligament inferiorly; voice becomes whispery and coarse, but procedure negates need for tracheotomy[33]

NURSING CARE

Nursing Assessment

Voice

Vocal weakness; hoarse, breathy quality

Respiratory Function

Stridor and dyspnea on exertion if paralysis is bilateral

Nursing Dx & Intervention

Nursing Diagnosis	Nursing Intervention/Rationale
Impaired verbal communication	• Assess and document quality of patient's voice before and after operation. • Ensure that patient understands Teflon procedure. • Indicate to patient that voice will be improved but may not be completely normal.
Ineffective breathing pattern	• Assess patient closely for excessive secretions and need for suctioning. • Provide usual postoperative care after tracheotomy is performed. • After assessing patient's readiness, teach patient to care for tracheotomy tube: suctioning, cleaning, and changing tube.

Patient Education

1. Remind the patient that speaking can be accomplished normally by using a tracheotomy plug or by occluding the lumen of the tracheotomy with a finger.
2. Advise the patient to wear a Medic-Alert bracelet indicating that a tracheotomy is present.

Evaluation

Patient Outcome	Data Indicating That Outcome is Reached
Vocal cord paralysis has resolved.	Airway is patent. Voice maintains good quality.
Patient demonstrates ability to care for tracheotomy tube.	Patient demonstrates ability to suction, clean, and humidify tracheotomy tube.

Vocal cord polyps and nodules

Polyps usually develop on the vocal cords from chronic abuse of the voice, allergies, or chronic inhalation of irritants, which frequently starts during an acute infection of the upper respiratory tract. Polyps are edematous masses of mucous membrane that attach to the vocal cords by either broad or narrow bases. Most have a broad base so there is permanent interference with voice production; however, some polyps are pedunculated, hang under the vocal cord, and cause only intermittent symptoms. Polyps are usually unilateral and may appear anywhere on the cord. They are common in adults who smoke, have allergies, or live in very dry climates. Polyps are far more common in men and rarely found in children. Since the cords are inhibited from approximation, painless hoarseness is the only symptom.

Polyps are gelatinous and telangiectatic, but mainly transitional types of polyps can be seen. Examination may show a change in the permeability of blood vessels, allowing extravasation of fluid, fibrin, or erythrocytes. After this, reactive processes develop and labyrinthine vascular spaces form. This process is similar to the formation of a thrombus. The polyps develop at the site of maximum muscular and aerodynamic forces exerted during phonation and are considered a sequela of phonotrauma.[28]

Vocal cord nodules, also called singer's, teacher's, or screamer's nodules, are caused by chronic voice abuse, such as singing, screaming, or constantly speaking outside the natural voice range. Nodules occur at any age and usually in girls and women, although they are sometimes found in young boys who scream and shout excessively.

The nodules are benign growths that first appear red and raised above the vocal cord surface. They later change into small white lumps that touch when the cords approximate. Since they are raised, the cords are kept apart and produce a characteristic hoarse, breathy voice (Figure 7-24).

Conservative treatment of nodules and complete voice rest often cause even large nodules to disappear. After voice rest, speech therapy may be indicated to prevent recurrence of the nodules and restore a normal voice. In contrast, polyps usually require surgical removal; they do not disappear with voice rest. Direct laryngoscopy is performed, and the polyps are excised. If a patient has bilateral polyps, the excision should be done in two stages, since doing both sides at the same time may cause a laryngeal web to form between the two raw surfaces.

Figure 7-24 Vocal cord nodules.
A, During respiration. **B,** During phonation.

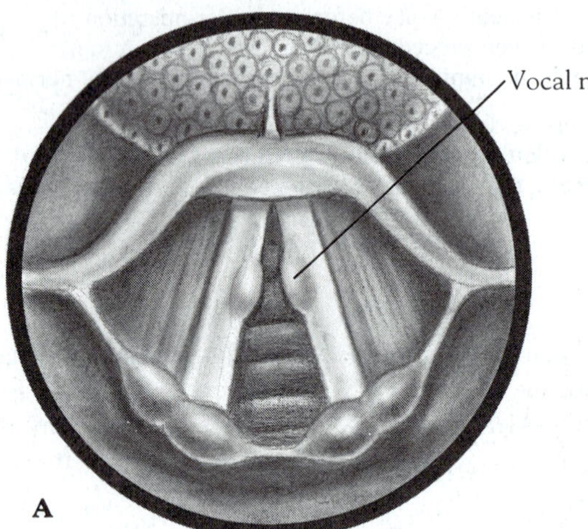

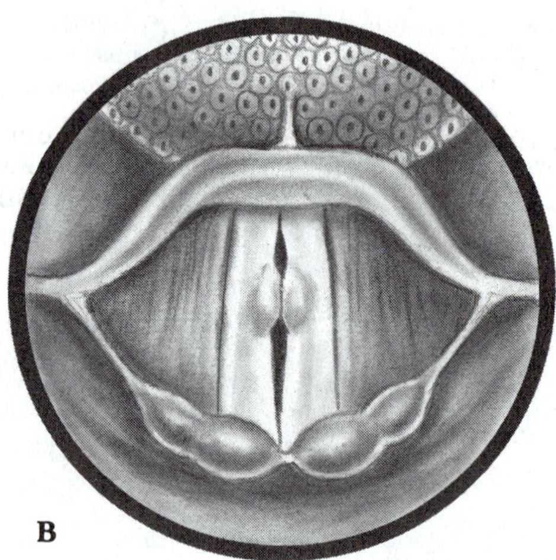

Nursing Dx & Intervention

Nursing Diagnosis	Nursing Intervention/Rationale
Impaired verbal communication	• Assess patient's understanding of need for voice rest. • Ensure that patient does not speak during period of voice rest; provide patient with Magic Slate or paper and pencil *to encourage nonverbal written communication.* • Remind visitors and staff members that patient is not to speak; attempt to anticipate patient's needs so patient will not have to speak. • Use humidifier in room *to provide adequate moisture in air and decrease throat irritation.* • Discourage patient from smoking during recovery from polyp removal *to keep tissue from exposure to irritants.*

Patient Education

1. Refer the patient to a speech therapist after discharge to prevent recurrence of nodules or polyps.
2. Discourage the patient from smoking, since exposure to irritants such as smoke predisposes patients to polyp formation.
3. Instruct the patient about the importance of adequate humidification in the home to prevent throat irritation.

Evaluation

Patient Outcome	Data Indicating That Outcome is Reached
Patient recovers uneventfully from removal of nodules or polyps.	There are no nodules or polyps on vocal cords. Patient is able to speak in a normal voice. Patient verbalizes understanding of stresses on voice and how to minimize these: no smoking, avoidance of allergens, and no excessive shouting or screaming.

Medical Interventions and Related Nursing Care

Myringotomy

Description and Rationale

Myringotomy is an incision of the tympanic membrane, usually to drain pus or fluid from the middle ear. Myringotomy was once performed routinely for ear infections such as otitis media, but the advent of antibiotics has greatly decreased the need for it.

A local or general anesthetic may be used, although the procedure is relatively painless. A curved incision is made in the posteroinferior portion of the drumhead with a very sharp myringotomy knife. The physician wears a head mirror and uses an aural speculum to visualize the drumhead to avoid injuring the ossicles.

Myringotomy may also be performed by touching a heated wire loop to the drumhead for 1 second to produce a 2 mm hole. This small opening stays open for about 3 to 4 weeks and heals without scarring.[2,15]

After the drumhead is incised, pus may pour out or suction may be used to remove fluid. Cotton is then placed in the ear to absorb the drainage, which may continue for several days.

A myringotomy incision heals quickly with only minimal scarring and does not disrupt hearing.

Contraindications and Cautions

When making the incision the physician must carefully avoid injuring the ossicles and cutting too deep. A deep incision may cut the mucous membrane covering the promontory, causing bleeding and pain. If it is cut, however, the injury is not serious. The drumhead can be easily visualized posteriorly and inferiorly, which is where the incision should be made to avoid injury to the medial wall of the middle ear and the ossicles.

There are no apparent contraindications to myringotomy if the disease process requires its performance.

Medical Plan

Surgery

Incision of eardrum with sharp myringotomy knife for evacuation of pus and fluid

Medications

Anti-infective agents
- Tetracycline (Achromycin), 250 mg po q6h
- Polmyxin B sulfate (Neosporin) ear drops

Analgesics
- Acetaminophen (Tylenol), 600 mg with codeine q4-6h prn

General Management

Cotton in ear to absorb drainage

NURSING CARE

Nursing Assessment

Tympanic Membrane

Drainage from eardrum; bleeding and pain at incision site; no impairment of hearing

Nursing Dx & Intervention

Nursing Diagnosis	Nursing Intervention/Rationale
Pain	• Assess degree of discomfort. • Provide analgesia as needed for pain relief; assess and document effectiveness. • Administer antibiotics and ear drops as ordered. • If patient is child, instruct parents in treatment regimen and proper instillation technique for ear drops.
Impaired tissue integrity	• Assess amount of drainage from ear. • Change cotton as needed. • Teach technique to patient or to parent. • Since drainage is usually infected, wash hands well after handling drainage and teach patient or parents to do same *to prevent contamination.* • Keep external ear dry and clean. • Assess for and report symptoms such as headache, nausea, fever, or increased ear pain.

Patient Education

1. Instruct the patient and family of the necessity for completing the prescribed course of antibiotics to prevent recurrence or complications.
2. Instruct the patient or family to monitor for hearing loss or increased ear pain. Myringotomies occasionally need to be performed again for reaccumulation of fluid.

Evaluation

Patient Outcome	Data Indicating That Outcome is Reached
Patient recovers uneventfully from myringotomy.	Myringotomy incision is healed well with no evidence of pus or fluid behind eardrum. There is no drainage from eardrum. Patient is afebrile. Patient does not experience hearing loss.

Stapedectomy

Description and Rationale

Attempts to reverse hearing losses that result from otosclerosis have been made for almost 100 years. Stapedectomy is the result of refinement of these various attempts and is now the operation of choice in many patients with hearing losses from otosclerosis. One author states that the conductive component of stapedectomy is better understood than the sensorineural component.[49] Preliminary results of studies indicate that the sensorineural component of otosclerosis may be an autoimmune response to the primitive cartilage in the fissula ante fenestrum and otic capsule in which the otosclerotic process begins.[49] During stapedectomy the surgeon partially or completely removes the footplate and the stapes and replaces them with a prosthesis that allows the reestablishment of normal sound pathways. The prostheses are usually made of tissue or plastic.

If patients are appropriately selected for the procedure and the surgeon has the necessary skills, 90% of patients experience an improvement in the level of hearing and in many instances hearing is almost normal.

Patients who may benefit from stapedectomy include those with a negative Rinne test of at least 572 Hz with a vibrating tuning fork and an air-bone gap of at least 20 dB for speech frequencies. Patients with otosclerosis and accompanying tinnitus may experience relief from tinnitus after stapedectomy.

Since the "worst" ear is the one operated on, patients selected for this surgery must have one ear functioning at a fairly adequate level. The operative ear must have a mobile malleus and a normally situated tympanic membrane.

Contraindications and Cautions

Active external otitis or otitis media must be well healed before stapedectomy will be considered

Severe vertigo from Ménière's disease

Occupation that requires frequent or large changes in barometric pressure, that is, divers, pilots, and those who work at heights

"Dead" or nonfunctioning ear on one side, unless patient has reached stage at which hearing aid can no longer be satisfactorily used

Patients younger than 25 years of age, since otosclerosis may still be in an active stage

Older patients assessed carefully for general health status and adequate sensorineural reserve and for evidence of vestibular damage; caution exercised in patients with any vestibular damage and poor sensorineural reserve because results may not be satisfactory

Medical Plan

Surgery

With patient under local anesthetic surgeon turns eardrum back on itself like omelette; microscope used to magnify bones of middle ear; stapes and footplate removed by means of various picks and sometimes electric drill; when footplate is removed, open oval window sealed with fascial graft from temporal muscle, and prosthesis connected to incus to restore normal sound conduction; several types of prostheses used; one end attached to the incus and other to graft or plug in oval window; external ear canal packed to ensure healing of tympanum; packing left in place 5 or 6 days

Medications

Narcotic analgesics
- Meperidine (Demerol), 50-100 mg IM q4h prn

Antiemetic agents
- Prochlorperazine (Compazine), 10 mg IM q6h prn
- Meclizine (Antivert) for vertigo effect, 25 mg po ½ h ac and hs

Sedative agents
- Sedation, such as pentobarbital (Nembutal), 60-100 mg po before surgery
- Phenobarbital, 60-100 mg po before surgery

Anti-infective agents
- Tetracycline (Achromycin), 250 mg po q6h for 10 d

General Management

Bed rest for 24 hours (may vary with physician) with operative side facing upward to maintain position of prosthesis and graft

NURSING CARE

Nursing Assessment

Infectious Process

Fever or other symptoms of infection; pain in operated ear

Auditory Function

Hearing ability; vertigo

Gustatory Function

Ability to taste with anterior tongue

Reparative Granuloma

Occurs in about 1% of stapedectomies; cause is unknown, but it may be related to contamination of the implant or trauma to the tissue; can be recognized if the flap and tympanic membrane still appear reddened and inflamed and there has been no hearing improvement 1 week after surgery; granuloma can fill much of middle ear and must be completely removed along with prosthesis; different type of prosthesis must then be inserted

Nursing Dx & Intervention

Nursing Diagnosis	Nursing Intervention/Rationale
Impaired physical mobility	• Assess patient's understanding of need for bed rest and immobility. • Enforce bed rest as ordered; patient should lie flat with operative side up *to maintain position of prosthesis and graft*. • Do not turn patient. • Keep side rails up *to prevent falls*. • When patient is allowed to be up, assist patient, since *vertigo may be present*. • Begin movement and ambulation gradually and provide medication for pain or dizziness as needed.
Sensory/perceptual alterations (auditory)	• Assess patient's hearing levels before and after operation. • Improvement in hearing may not be noticeable immediately because of packing in ear and bleeding. Make sure that patient is aware of this fact *to avoid disappointment immediately after surgery*.
Potential impaired skin integrity	• While patient is hospitalized, assess for excessive bleeding, drainage, fever, and ear pain and report any symptoms immediately. • Inform patient that after usual 5- to 6-day packing a piece of cotton may be placed in ear for few days *to provide protection*. • Instruct patient in appropriate technique of changing cotton and tell patient to do it once or twice a day.
Pain	• Assess patient's degree of pain and report excessive ear pain immediately. • Administer pain medication and antiemetics as needed; assess and document effectiveness. • Encourage patient to move gradually, avoiding sudden movement, *to minimize pain at operative site*.

Patient Education

1. Inform the patient to avoid sneezing or nose blowing for at least 1 week to protect the eustachian tube from contaminated material and to prevent dislodgment of the prosthesis and graft.
2. Ensure that the patient is aware of the necessity for careful ear care both immediately before surgery and on an ongoing basis.
3. Inform patient that the ear must not become wet (as by shampooing) while deep external packing remains in place.
4. Inform the patient that smoking is contraindicated after stapedectomy.

Evaluation

Patient Outcome	Data Indicating That Outcome is Reached
Patient recovers uneventfully from stapedectomy.	Activity level is normal for patient; no weakness or vertigo is present. There is no pain or excessive drainage from operated ear. Hearing is improved to normal. Patient verbalizes understanding of ear care regimen and symptoms to report to physician.

Tonsillectomy

Description and Rationale

Tonsillectomy is the surgical removal of the tonsils and usually the adenoids (adenoidectomy). The rationale for this procedure is usually the removal of chronically infected tissue. A general anesthetic is used; the most common method for removal of the tonsils is dissection and snare, since it can be used for all sizes of tonsils whether they are in shallow or deep fossae. Although it has disadvantages, the guillotine method is chosen by some physicians. Injury to the tonsillar pillar is more common with this method, and it is not suitable for deeply recessed tonsils. It may also not reach the base of the tonsils and will leave a tonsil tag. Adenoids are removed with an adenotome; a curette may also be used to remove residual adenoid tissue.

Contraindications and Cautions

Presence of any acute infection, especially tonsillitis
Active tuberculosis
Presence of hematologic disorders, such as hemophilia, leukemia, or aplastic anemia

Medical Plan

Surgery

Tonsil and adenoidal tissue removed to secure all bleeding points

Medications

Narcotic analgesics
- Acetaminophen (Tylenol), 600 mg with codeine, po q4-6h prn (avoid aspirin because of possibility of bleeding)

General Management

Intravenous fluids until nausea has subsided and patient is drinking well
Soft or liquid diet
Bed rest

Postoperative Instructions for Tonsillectomy and Adenoidectomy

1. For the next 7 to 10 days there may be pain and soreness in the throat and ears.
2. Small amounts of bleeding occur during this period. If bleeding persists, call the physician immediately.
3. If signs and symptoms of infection occur, such as purulent exudate or increase in pain or fever, call the physician immediately.
4. Keep the fluid intake high for the first few days after surgery, which will help keep the temperature down.
5. The diet should consist of soft bland foods, gelatin, cooked cereals, ice cream, soft-boiled eggs, custard, broth, mashed potatoes, and noncitrus juices for about 1 week. Apple and grape juice are the best liquids. Carbonated beverages may be taken if the patient tolerates them. Well-ground meat should be added as soon as tolerated.
6. Activity should not cause overexertion for the next 7 to 10 days. If tolerated, the patient may go outside after the second day. Persons with acute infections should be kept away. Bathing may be carried out in the usual manner.
7. Acetaminophen (Tylenol) (if patient is not allergic) may be taken by mouth, 650 mg every 4 hours for pain, especially ½ hour before meals. If the patient is given medications to take home from the hospital, they may be substituted for Tylenol.
8. The patient should not gargle but only gently rinse mouth.
9. If you have any questions or concerns, call your physician to discuss these areas.

Courtesy Ruth Weddle, RN, and Eden Rivera, RN, University of California, San Francisco.

NURSING CARE

Nursing Assessment

Postoperative Status

Vital signs stable; no fever; pulse and blood pressure normal for patient; skin warm and dry; level of consciousness appropriate for recovery from anesthesia; no bleeding at operative site; if adenoidectomy is done, there may be some nasopharyngeal trickling down back of throat

Complications

Bleeding from failure to secure bleeding points during surgery; airway obstruction from blood or secretions; aspiration of blood or secretions

Nursing Dx & Intervention

Nursing Diagnosis	Nursing Intervention/Rationale
Pain	• Assess patient's degree of pain. • Provide adequate pain relief; assess and document effectiveness. • Provide hot saline rinses *for comfort.* • Ensure adequate fluid intake. • Monitor intravenous intake at prescribed rate until discontinued and then provide soothing fluids *to prevent dehydration.* • Do not offer juices, *which would cause a burning feeling in the throat.* • Offer ice chips to suck *to encourage fluids and provide comfort.* • Monitor vital signs, level of consciousness, and presence of bleeding and report any change immediately.
Potential for aspiration	• Maintain patent airway; keep patient on bed rest lying on side as much as possible *to prevent aspiration.* • Observe for vomiting of dark brown fluid because of "swallowed" blood during surgery. • Watch for frequent swallowing, which may indicate bleeding; check frequently with flashlight *to see if blood is trickling down back of throat if adenoidectomy was done.*

Patient Education

1. Instruct the patient not to clear the throat, to watch for bleeding, and to call the physician immediately if any symptoms occur. They may occur on about the fifth day after surgery when the scab sloughs from the operative area.
2. Since most patients are hospitalized for only a short time, give the patient a preprinted list of instructions for postoperative care at home (see box on opposite page).

Evaluation

Patient Outcome	Data Indicating That Outcome is Reached
Patient recovers uneventfully from tonsillectomy.	There is no bleeding from operative site. Patient is afebrile and takes fluids and food well. Activity level is normal for patient. Patient verbalizes understanding of necessity of watching for late postoperative bleeding and calling physician immediately. Patient verbalizes knowledge of when to return to physician for postoperative visit.

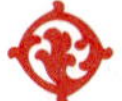

Tracheotomy

Description and Rationale

A tracheotomy is an incision into the trachea to form a temporary or permanent opening, which is called a tracheostomy. The incision is made through the second, third, or fourth tracheal ring, and a tube is usually inserted through the opening to allow passage of air and the removal of tracheobronchial secretions.

Except in the cases of head, neck, and face trauma, a tracheotomy is rarely performed as an emergency procedure. If immediate airway control is needed and the patient is hospitalized, endotracheal intubation is usually performed; a tracheotomy is performed as an elective procedure if an artificial airway is necessary longer than an endotracheal tube should be left in place.

Aside from tracheotomy performed to reduce anatomic dead space (by approximately 150 cc) in patients with chronic pulmonary disease or to aid in mechanical ventilation of an unconscious patient, most tracheotomies are performed on patients in two categories. Patients in the first group have an obstruction at or above the level of the larynx, such as foreign body obstruction, carcinoma of the larynx, severe infection (such as Ludwig's angina), trauma to the tongue or mandible, or stenosis from prolonged intubation. Patients in the second group have no actual obstruction but are unable to raise their own secretions and are in danger of anoxia if secretions accumulate and are not removed from the chest. These patients include those with paralysis of the chest muscles and diaphragm (as in Guillain-Barré syndrome), patients who are unconscious or semiconscious with head injuries, and patients with fractured ribs or other chest injuries causing severe pain that inhibits them from coughing. Tracheotomy is an excellent way to provide access to the trachea when a patient needs frequent suctioning. Other indications include patients with smoke inhalation or severe burns around the head and neck and patients who are at risk of bleeding from thyroidectomy or radical neck dissection.

Contraindications and Cautions

Caution exercised in infants because of extremely small size of their tracheas and small size of tube that must be used[10,13]

Caution exercised if surgical incision in neck would increase risk of infection

Medical Plan

Surgery

Vertical incision in midline of neck from lower border of thyroid cartilage to slightly above suprasternal notch; soft tissue and muscle layers divided and isthmus of thyroid exposed and divided between clamps or retracted upward, which exposes rings of trachea; vertical incision made, usually between third and fourth rings, secretions thoroughly aspirated, and tracheostomy tube of correct size for patient inserted; first tracheal ring should not be cut (Figure 7-25); complete hemostasis ensured after procedure; if procedure is elective, endotracheal tube left in place and tracheotomy performed over tube; endotracheal tube can be removed after airway is secured

Medications

Drugs prescribed depending on reason for tracheotomy, that is, infection or laryngeal edema

General Management

Tracheobronchial suctioning

Humidification of inspired air

Figure 7-25 Correct area of trachea for incision and insertion of tracheotomy tube.

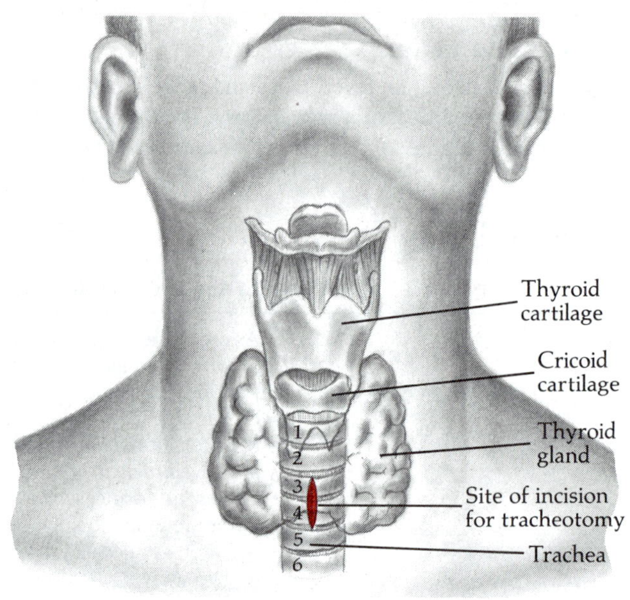

NURSING CARE

Nursing Assessment

Respiratory Function

Respiratory rate; amount and color of tracheal secretions; need for and frequency of suctioning; anxiety level; arterial blood gases; presence of bleeding at tracheostomy site (should be absent); no excessive coughing after suctioning; adequate humidification provided to tracheostomy (mucus is thin and without thick plugs); breath sounds audible in all lobes after suctioning; tracheostomy ties securely fastened

Pneumomediastinum

No dyspnea, crepitus, or edema of face and neck

Pneumothorax

No cough, anxiety, sharp chest pain, or tachycardia

Cardiac Tamponade

No increase in central venous pressure, narrowed pulse pressure, paradoxic pulse, decreased pressure, dyspnea, or decreased level of consciousness

Nursing Dx & Intervention

Nursing Diagnosis	Nursing Intervention/Rationale
Ineffective airway clearance; potential for aspiration; impaired gas exchange	• Assess for and report any symptoms suggesting pneumomediastinum, pneumothorax, cardiac tamponade, hemorrhage, or subcutaneous emphysema. • Suction airway as often as necessary *to maintain patent airway and remove secretions*. This can be done as frequently as every 5 to 10 minutes immediately after surgery to every 3 to 4 hours after tracheostomy has been in place awhile. Use catheter that is no greater than half diameter of tracheostomy tube. Preoxygenate and hyperinflate patient using Ambu bag before suctioning. Give patient five sigh breaths. Do not suction for more than 5 to 10 seconds, *since suctioning decreases alveolar oxygen pressure by 30 mm Hg*. Keep bypass port open on catheter while inserting it *to minimize oxygen removal*. Gentle twisting motion of catheter should be used while suctioning. • Stop suctioning immediately if any signs of respiratory distress occur, *since there may be mucus blockage and patient may quickly become hypoxic*. Postoxygenate patient after suctioning by giving five sigh breaths with Ambu bag to reopen small airways. Maintain adequate humidification *to keep secretions loose and minimize difficulty in secretion removal*. (Sputum is 95% water and mucous membranes dry out easily without proper hydration.) If necessary, 5 to 10 ml of sterile saline can be instilled into tracheostomy tube before suctioning *to facilitate removal of secretions*. • Clean inner cannula (if present) of tracheostomy tube every 4 hours or as necessary. • If appropriate, ensure that patient receives chest physiotherapy depending on condition and reason for tracheotomy. • Document suctioning, patient response, result of chest assessment, and all treatments. • If patient is receiving ventilation assistance or intermittent positive pressure breathing treatments, a cuffed tracheostomy tube will be used. The cuff pressure should be maintained at level that just occludes trachea. Pressure should be less than 20 mm Hg. • *Convalescent care:* Observe for any frank bleeding from tracheostomy or pulsation of cannula. *(Innominate artery is in close proximity, and tracheostomy tube may erode through the artery wall.)* • Ensure that tracheostomy ties are secured at all times *to prevent tube from falling out or becoming dislocated*. • When tracheotomy has just been performed, change ties with assistance *so tracheostomy tube is held in place while ties are replaced*. Institutional policy may vary regarding whether nurses may change tracheostomy ties within first 48 hours after surgery. • Avoid using aerosol sprays, talcum powder, or tissue or gauze containing cotton *to prevent patient from inhaling foreign particles*. • Use precut tracheostomy gauze or unlined gauze opened full length and folded into U shape.
Anxiety	• Assess patient's level of anxiety and carefully explain suctioning procedure to patient. • Provide assurance that patient will be closely observed for respiratory distress or need for suctioning and that call light will be answered promptly.
Impaired verbal communication	• Assess patient's understanding of inability to communicate verbally. • Provide patient with Magic Slate or pen and paper *to facilitate communication*. • Use word cards with commonly used phrases *to decrease patient frustration*. • *Convalescent care:* Instruct patient to occlude tracheostomy opening with finger or plug *to allow verbal communication*. • If condition warrants, a fenestrated tracheostomy tube may be used to allow patient to speak without occluding the trachea.
Impaired skin integrity	• Assess stoma during every shift and note any bleeding, purulent drainage, and condition of surrounding tissue. • Check skin under tracheostomy dressing and note areas of breakdown. • Wear gloves to change dressing when soiled or on every shift. • Clean wound thoroughly when changing dressing. • Clean inner cannula of tracheostomy tube during every shift or as necessary. • Ensure that sterile technique is maintained while suctioning. • Make sure that patient is turned at least hourly if condition warrants and that areas of breakdown are noted and treatment begun promptly.
Altered nutrition: less than body requirements	• Assess closely for signs of dehydration and malnutrition and report immediately. • Monitor intravenous or tube feedings as necessary and document appropriately. • Weigh patient daily. • *Convalescent care:* Assess patient's ability to swallow.

Nursing Diagnosis	Nursing Intervention/Rationale
	• If patient is eating, has a cuffed tracheostomy tube, and is prone to aspiration, inflate cuff while patient eats and deflate after meals. • Consult nutritionist to plan attractive, nourishing meals. • Provide high-calorie snacks if needed. • Provide attractive, clean environment at meals and meticulous mouth care before meals, since *patient may experience loss of taste because of decreased sense of smell.* • Weigh patient daily and maintain accurate record of intake and output. • If patient is receiving tube feedings, ensure that they are of sufficient caloric value *to maintain weight and promote wound healing.* • Monitor patient's hydration and nutritional status. • Follow established guidelines for tube feedings; that is, check for placement in stomach and residual before next tube feeding. • Replace residual, and hold feeding if greater than 100 ml. • Feed patient with head of bed elevated *to prevent aspiration.* • Assess patient's bowel activity.
Impaired home maintenance management	• *Convalescent care:* If patient will be discharged with tracheostomy, ensure that patient and family have been instructed in and understand management of tracheostomy at home, including suctioning, cleaning, wound care, humidification, changing tracheostomy ties, and tube feeding if necessary. • Ensure that family and patient know where to purchase supplies and when to return to see physician. *To prepare tracheostomy tube for decannulation:* • Assess patient's ability to breathe and cough effectively, gag reflex, and swallowing reflexes. • Report any symptoms of distress to physician immediately. • "Plug" tracheostomy tube intermittently and increase length of time for occlusion as patient tolerates. • Remove tracheostomy tube or assist physician with removal of tube when patient tolerates occlusion well. • Apply Steri-Strips or tape *to approximate wound edges.* • Check and cleanse wound site daily. • Observe for signs of infection; opening should heal within few days. • Make referral to visiting nurse or public health nurse.

Patient Education

1. Inform the patient that there will be frequent suctioning, a loss of speech, and decreased ability to smell and that he will not be breathing through the nose or mouth while the tracheostomy is present.
2. Refer the patient to a speech therapist, if appropriate, to learn esophageal or alternative method of speech.

Evaluation

Patient Outcome	Data Indicating That Outcome is Reached
If short-term tracheostomy is used, respiratory status is within normal limits.	Patient has no excess secretions and tracheostomy stoma is healed without signs of infection. Patient does not experience dyspnea or shortness of breath.
If long-term tracheostomy is needed, patient and family demonstrate ability to care for all aspects of tracheostomy at home.	Patient or family demonstrates suctioning and cleaning techniques, wound care, changing ties, and methods for humidification. Visiting or public health nurse assists patient or family if necessary.
Nutritional status is maintained.	Weight and caloric intake are normal for patient. Patient eats regularly, or patient and family demonstrate ability to administer tube feedings as necessary.

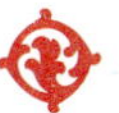 Tympanoplasty

Description and Rationale

Tympanoplasty is a reconstructive or reparative procedure of the middle ear that is usually performed to correct conductive hearing loss caused by chronic suppurative otitis media. The procedure involves rebuilding the structures of the middle ear or replacing them with prostheses. Tympanoplasty may also be occasionally performed to close a perforation of the tympanic membrane (myringoplasty or type I tympanoplasty) or to assist with clearing infections in patients with chronic suppurative otitis media and a sensorineural (rather than conductive) hearing loss. There is no chance of correcting the hearing loss in these patients. Tympanoplasty may also be indicated in patients with ossicular problems such as dislocation of the incus from trauma, congenital middle ear problems, or tympanosclerosis, in which the malleus is fused to the incus. In these cases metal or plastic prostheses, autogenous material, or cadaveric ossicles are commonly used. Since these patients have no concomitant infection, the results are often good.[9]

The principal rationale for tympanoplasty is to improve hearing in patients with conductive hearing loss but intact nerve function or cochlear reserve. The greatest improvement is seen in patients with bilateral disease and a large difference between air and bone measurements. In chronic otitis media the tympanic membrane, malleus, and incus are frequently damaged or destroyed. If this occurs, sound waves can enter the oval and round window with equal intensity and cancel each other, since the tympanic membrane is not there to protect the round window from sound pressure. Chronic otitis media also disrupts the areal ratio, or the tympanic membrane—footplate ratio, thereby negating the transformer action of the middle ear.

Tympanoplasty, of which there are five types described below, improves hearing by reestablishing two important middle ear functions: restoring the areal ratio and creating sound protection for the round window.

Contraindications and Cautions

Presence of infection; procedure to clear infection must be performed before tympanoplasty

Patients with poor nerve function as determined by bone conduction tests

Hearing loss from otosclerosis or serous otitis media rather than chronic suppurative otitis media

Medical Plan

Surgery (Figure 7-26)

Postaural or endaural approach; with operating microscope at high magnification, surgeon performs one of five types of tympanoplasty, using either temporal fascia or tissue from nearby vein as graft; tympanic membranes from human cadavers sometimes used as graft, although this technique is still being evaluated; Teflon or stainless steel wires also used occasionally

Type I (myringoplasty)—performed for closure of perforation; epithelium removed from edge of perforation and graft of autogenous tissue, usually fascia or vein placed under tympanic membrane; areal ratio and round window sound protection restored

Type II—performed when malleus is eroded; perforation closed with graft against incus or what remains of malleus; enough ossicular chain must remain to create new areal ratio

Type III—also restores both areal ratio and sound protection of round window by means of autogenous graft; performed when tympanic membrane and ossicular chain are destroyed but normal stapes remains; graft is placed in contact with stapes

Type IV—areal ratio cannot be restored, but round window sound protection is provided; only footplate remains intact, and air pocket is placed between round window and graft to provide sound protection

Type V—only round window sound protection provided; footplate is fixed and fenestration into inner ear must be performed

Medications

Narcotic analgesics
- Meperidine (Demerol), 50 mg IM q4h prn
- Acetaminophen (Tylenol), 600 mg with codeine q4-6h prn

Anti-infective agents
- Tetracycline (Achromycin), 250 mg po q6h, or penicillin G, 250-500 mg po q6h

Antiemetics (for antivertigo effect)
- Meclizine (Antivert), 250 mg po ½ h ac and hs

General Management

Bed rest until next morning with head of bed elevated 40 degrees and operative side facing upward

NURSING CARE

Nursing Assessment

Middle Ear Function

Bleeding; amount, color, and consistency of drainage; temperature and dizziness when getting out of bed or with sudden movement; nausea; vertigo

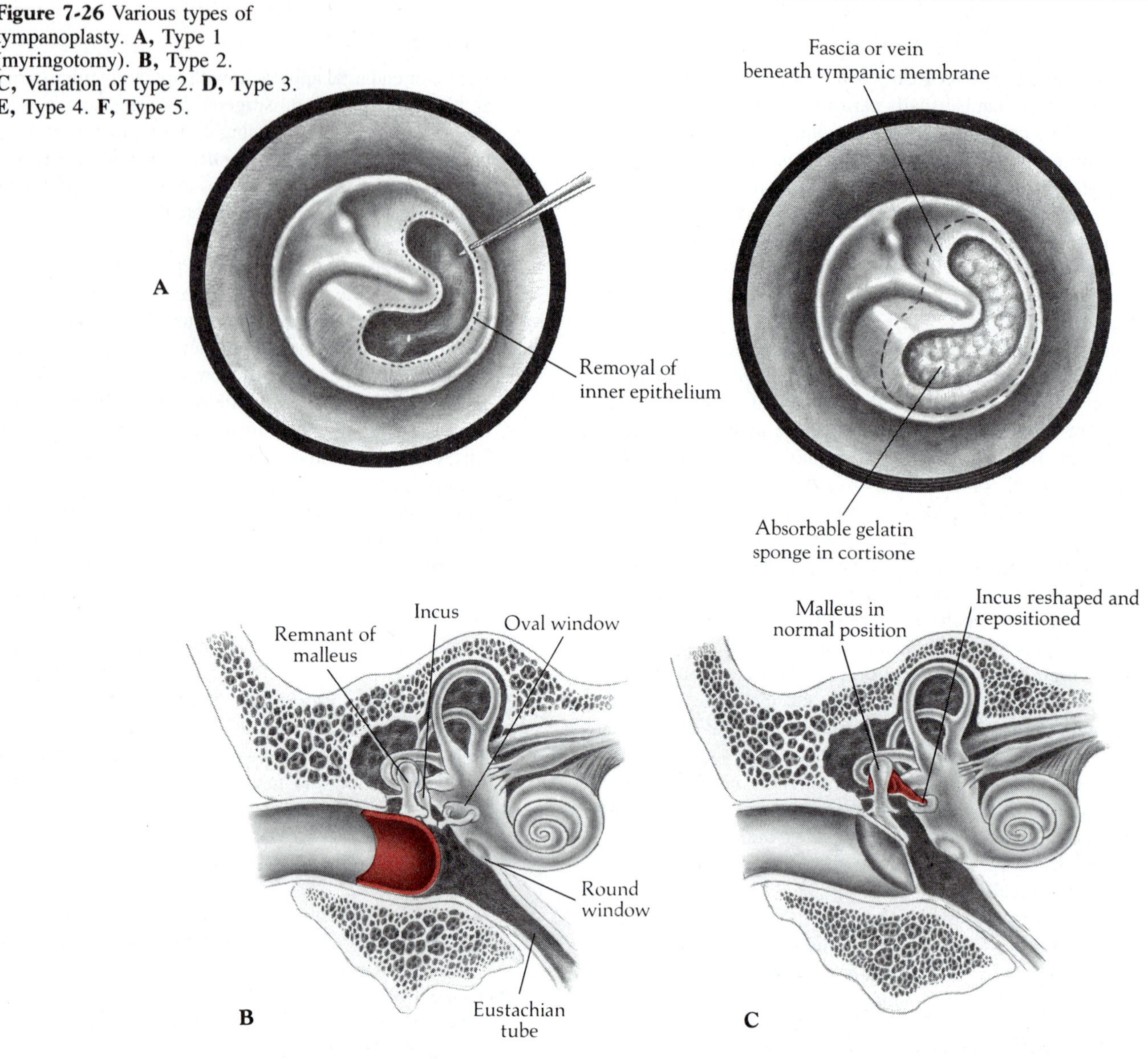

Figure 7-26 Various types of tympanoplasty. **A,** Type 1 (myringotomy). **B,** Type 2. **C,** Variation of type 2. **D,** Type 3. **E,** Type 4. **F,** Type 5.

Nursing Dx & Intervention

Nursing Diagnosis	Nursing Intervention/Rationale
Potential for injury	• Assess, record, and report unusual bleeding or drainage from operative site. • Encourage patient to maintain bed rest until first morning after surgery. • Keep patient from lying on operative side *to prevent pressure on graft.* • Elevate head of bed 40 degrees. • Assist with ambulation when patient is allowed to get up.
Sensory/perceptual alterations (auditory)	• Assess patient's hearing ability before and after operation. • Reassure patient that hearing improvement, if expected, will not be noticed until edema and drainage at operative site have decreased.

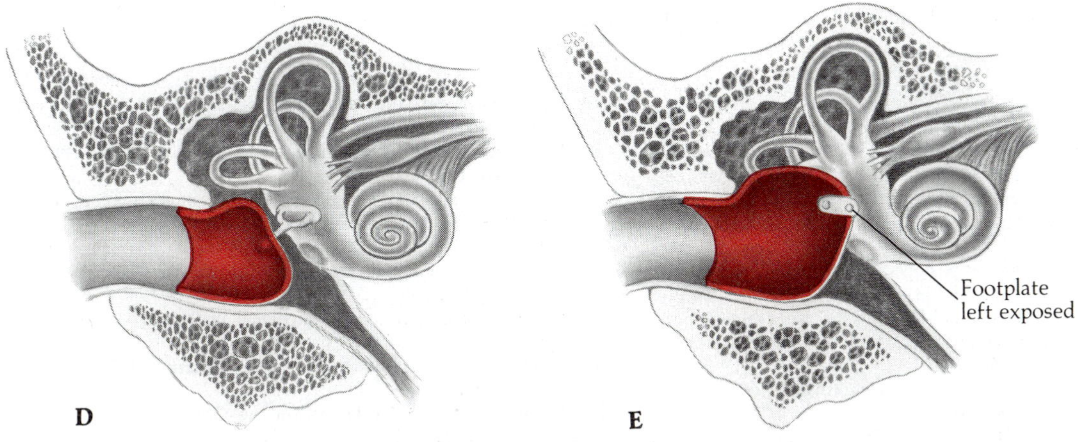

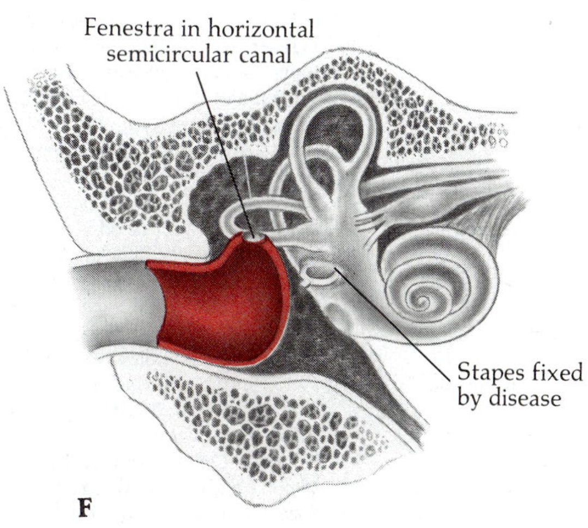

Patient Education

1. Instruct the patient to avoid showering or shampooing until permitted by the physician to prevent contamination of the ear canal.
2. Instruct the patient to notify the physician immediately if there is evidence of fever, bleeding, increased drainage, or dizziness after discharge.
3. Instruct the patient to use Antivert for about 1 month after surgery to minimize dizziness.
4. Instruct the patient to avoid blowing the nose with force.

Evaluation

Patient Outcome	Data Indicating That Outcome is Reached
Graft heals well.	There is no fever, excessive drainage, or dizziness.
Hearing is improved if this was reason for procedure.	Increased hearing is verified by audiometric testing.

References

1. Bauth R and Baker S: Epiglottitis in children: review of 24 cases, Otolaryngol Head Neck Surg 90:157, 1982.
2. Berkow R, editor: The Merck manual of diagnosis and therapy, ed 14, Rahway NJ, 1982, Merck, Sharpe & Dohme Laboratories.
3. Berne RM and Levy M: Physiology, ed 2, St Louis, 1988, The CV Mosby Co.
4. Blanco KM: Acoustic neuroma: postoperative nursing care and rehabilitation, J Neurosurg Nurs 13:153, 1981.
5. Brooks GB et al: Acetazolamide in Meniere's disease: evaluation of a new diagnostic test for reversible endolymphatic hydrops, Otolaryngol Head Neck Surg 90:358, 1982.
6. Carey JW and Steegman AT: Human nasal protrusion, latitude and climate, Am J Phys Anthropol 56:313, 1981.
7. Chiu RTK et al: Meniere's disease at the University of Iowa, 1973-1980, Otolaryngol Head Neck Surg 90:482, 1982.
8. Cole P: The extra thoracic airways, J Otolaryngol 5:74-85, 1976.
9. DeWeese DD and Saunders WH: Textbook of otolaryngology, ed 7, St Louis, 1988, The CV Mosby Co.
10. Diseases—the nurse's reference library, Nursing 82 Books, Springhouse, Pa, 1982, Intermed Communications, Inc.
11. Dohlmann GF: Mechanism of the Ménière attack, ORL J Otorhinolaryngol Rel Spec 42:10, 1980.
12. Ganong WF: Review of medical physiology, ed 12, Los Altos, Calif, 1985, Lange Medical Books.
13. Gerson CR and Tucker GF: Infant tracheotomy, Ann Otol Rhinol Laryngol 91:413, 1982.
14. Geurkink N: Nasal anatomy, physiology and function, J Allergy Clin Immunol 72:123, 1983.
15. Goode RL and Schulz W: Heat myringotomy for the treatment of serous otitis media, Otolaryngol Head Neck Surg 90:764, 1982.
16. Gray LP: Deviated nasal septum: incidence and etiology, Ann Otol Rhinol Laryngol (suppl 50):3, 1978.
17. Gruppi LA: Acoustic neuromas: nursing management during the acute postoperative period, Crit Care Nurs 7(5):16, 1987.
18. Gwaltney JM et al: Etiology and antimicrobial treatment of acute sinusitis, Ann Otol Rhinol Laryngol 90:68, 1981.
19. Havener WH et al: Nursing care in eye, ear, nose and throat disorders, ed 4, St Louis, 1979, The CV Mosby Co.
20. Hirsch JE and Hannock LA, editors: Mosby's manual of clinical nursing procedures, St Louis, 1981, The CV Mosby Co.
21. Hughes GB et al: Cerebrospinal leaks and meningitis following acoustic tumor surgery, Otolaryngol Head Neck Surg 90:117, 1982.
22. Jazbi B: Subluxation of the nasal septum in the newborn: etiology, diagnosis and treatment, Otolaryngol Clin North Am 10:125, 1977.
23. Johnson JT, editor: Antibiotic therapy in head and neck surgery, New York, 1987, Marcel Dekker, Inc.
24. Jongkees LBW: Some remarks on Ménière's disease, ORL J Otorhinolaryngol Rel Spec 42:1, 1980.
25. Kim MJ and Moritz DA: Classification of nursing diagnoses, Proceedings from third and fourth national conferences, New York, 1982, McGraw-Hill Book Co.
26. Kirchner FR: Endoscopic rehabilitation of the airway in laryngeal paralysis, Ann Otol Rhinol Laryngol 91:382, 1982.
27. Kitahara M et al: Experimental study on Ménière's disease, Otolaryngol Head Neck Surg 90:470, 1982.
28. Kleinsasser O: Pathogenesis of vocal cord polyps, Ann Otol Rhinol Laryngol 91:378, 1982.
29. Leonidas JD: Radiologic diagnosis in pediatric otorhinolaryngology, Otolaryngol Clin North Am 10:1, 1977.
30. Lucente FE et al: Malignant external otitis: a dangerous misnomer, Otolaryngol Head Neck Surg 90:266, 1982.
31. Luckmann J and Sorensen K: Medical-surgical nursing: a psychophysiologic approach, ed 2, Philadelphia, 1980, WB Saunders Co.
32. Malasanos L et al: Health assessment, ed 3, St Louis, 1986, The CV Mosby Co.
33. Maran AGD and Stell PM, editors: Clinical otolaryngology, Oxford, Eng, 1979, Blackwell Scientific Publications, Inc.
34. Marshall KG and Attia EL: Disorders of the nose and paranasal sinuses: diagnosis and management, Littleton, Mass, 1987, PSG Publishing Co, Inc.
35. Michaels L: Ear, nose and throat histopathology, London, 1987, Springer-Verlag.
36. Moran WB: Nasal trauma in children, Otolaryngol Clin North Am 10:95, 1977.
37. Myers E, editor: New Dimensions in Otorhinolaryngology, Head and Neck Surgery, Proceedings of the XIII World Congress, vols 1 and 2, Amsterdam, 1985, Excerpta Medica.
38. Nordmark MT and Rohweder AW: Scientific foundations of nursing, ed 3, Philadelphia, 1975, JB Lippincott Co.
39. Pallanch JF et al: Prosthetic closure of nasal septal perforations, Otolaryngol Head Neck Surg 90:448, 1982.
40. Parisier SC: Surgical therapy of chronic mastoiditis with cholesteatoma, Otolaryngol Head Neck Surg 90:767, 1982.
41. Price S and Wilson L: Pathophysiology: clinical concepts of disease processes, New York, 1982, McGraw-Hill, Inc.
42. Proetz AW: Essays on the applied physiology of the nose, ed 2, St Louis, 1953, Annals Publishing Co.
43. Rejowski J et al: Nasal polyps causing bone destruction and blindness, Otolaryngol Head Neck Surg 90:505, 1982.
44. Saxton DF et al: The Addison-Wesley manual of nursing practice, Menlo Park, Calif, 1983, Addison-Wesley Publishing Co.
45. Schindler RA and Merzenich MM, editors: Cochlear implants, New York, 1985, Raven Press.
46. Schlossberg D, editor: Infections of the head and neck, New York, 1987, Springer-Verlag, Inc.
47. Seidel HM et al: Mosby's guide to physical examination, St Louis, 1987, The CV Mosby Co.
48. Settipane GA and Chafee FH: Nasal polyps and rhinitis: a review of 6037 patients, J Allergy Clin Immunol 59:17, 1977.
49. Shea JJ: Stapedectomy—a long term report, Ann Otol Rhinol Laryngol 91:516, 1982.
50. Sheehy JL: Diffuse exostoses and osteomata of the external auditory canal: a report of 100 operations, Otolaryngol Head Neck Surg 90:337, 1982.
51. Silverstein H and Norrell H: Retrolabyrinthine vestibular neurectomy, Otolaryngol Head Neck Surg 90:778, 1982.
52. Thompson JM and Bowers AC: Clinical manual of health assessment, ed 2, St Louis, 1988, The CV Mosby Co.
53. Toppozada H et al: The human nasal mucosa in the menstrual cycle: a histochemical and electron microscopic study, J Laryngol Otol 95:1237, 1981.
54. Tortorelli BA: Acoustic neuroma: an overview of the disorder and nursing care for these patients, J Neurosurg Nurs 13:170, 1981.
55. Tos M and Thomsen J: The price of preservation of hearing in acoustic neuroma surgery, Ann Otol Rhinol Laryngol 91:240, 1982.
56. Tucker SM et al: Patient care standards, ed 4, St Louis, 1988, The CV Mosby Co.
57. Ward P and Berci G: Observations on so-called idiopathic vocal cord paralysis, Ann Otol Rhinol Laryngol 91:558, 1982.
58. Wehrmaker SL and Wintermute JR: Case studies in neurological nursing, Boston, 1978, Little, Brown & Co.
59. Whaley LF and Wong DL: Nursing care of infants and children, ed 3, St Louis, 1986, The CV Mosby Co.

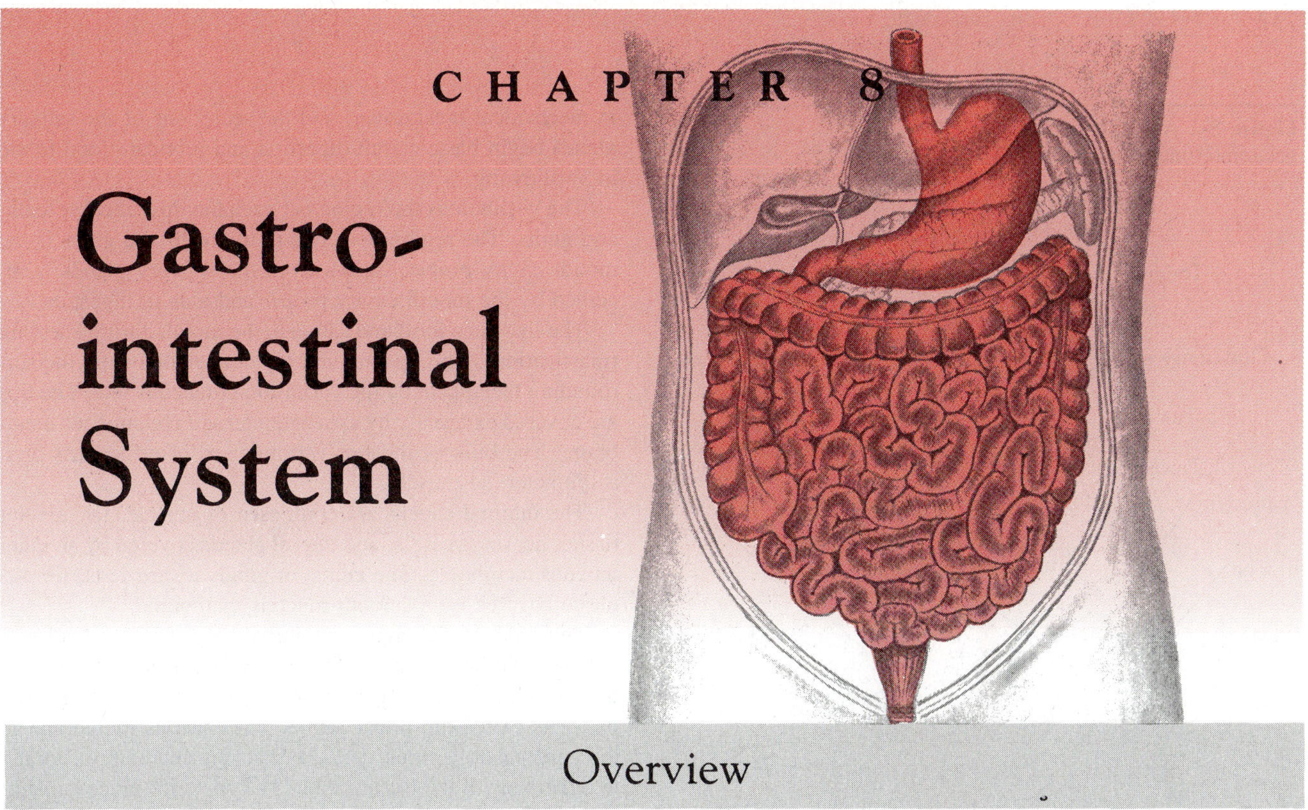

CHAPTER 8

Gastro-intestinal System

Overview

Disorders or inflammation of any organs in the gastrointestinal system are commonly called digestive diseases. Examples of digestive diseases are reflux esophagitis, peptic ulcer disease, ulcerative colitis, pancreatitis, and cancer. The diagnosis, treatment, and management vary with each digestive disease.

More Americans are hospitalized with disorders of the digestive system than any other group of disorders. The National Digestive Disease Advisory Board (NDDAB) reports that 20 million people are chronically ill with digestive diseases and are absent from work as a result of digestive problems.[54] The NDDAB also reports an annual cost of $50 billion in lost wages, disability payments, health care expenditures, and lost tax revenues associated with digestive diseases. Approximately 200,000 people die each year from digestive diseases, including malignancies. Thus this group of diseases may have devastating long-term personal, social, and economic effects. The NDDAB is only one national group concerned with digestive diseases. There are 25 lay organizations and 18 professional associations involved in digestive disease programs and education. This reflects the national concern with the management of digestive diseases.

The importance of digestive diseases and their implications for health care have often been minimized. The group of diseases involving the gastrointestinal tract may vary from mild to severe. The chronicity of the diseases and the symptoms can affect the person's ability to maintain a desired lifestyle. Psychosocial stressors often intensify the symptoms.

The National Digestive Disease Advisory Report[54] also showed that research involving the gastrointestinal tract is relevant to the study of acquired immunodeficiency syndrome (AIDS). The immune dysfunction damages the gastrointestinal tract, and this damage contributes to the malnutrition and wasting syndrome observed in AIDS. The latest research on neuropeptides found in the intestine indicates that these substances may modulate immune function. This finding may have significance for future research.[54]

Anatomy, Physiology, and Related Pathophysiology

The gastrointestinal tract is a series of connected organs and accessory organs whose overall purpose is to break down food products that can be used by the body as a source of energy. Three key processes are associated with the gastrointestinal tract: digestion, absorption, and metabolism. Digestion is the mechanical and chemical breakdown of food into amino acids, glucose, and fatty acids that can be used by the body for cellular functions. Absorption is the passage of the digested food products (essential nutrients) from the lumen of the gastrointestinal tract into the blood and lymphatic system. Metabolism is the utilization of the basic food product by the cell. Digestion and absorption can be affected by infections, inflammatory diseases, surgery, or other alterations of the gastrointestinal tract. To adequately assess the effects of digestive diseases, the nurse must have a basic understanding of the alimentary, or gastrointestinal, system.

The gastrointestinal system consists of the mouth, pharynx, esophagus, stomach, and small and large intestines. Accessory organs include liver, gallbladder, and pancreas. The accessory organs in the mouth are the teeth and salivary glands (Figure 8-1).

The gastrointestinal system produces both exocrine and

Figure 8-1 Anatomy of gastrointestinal system.

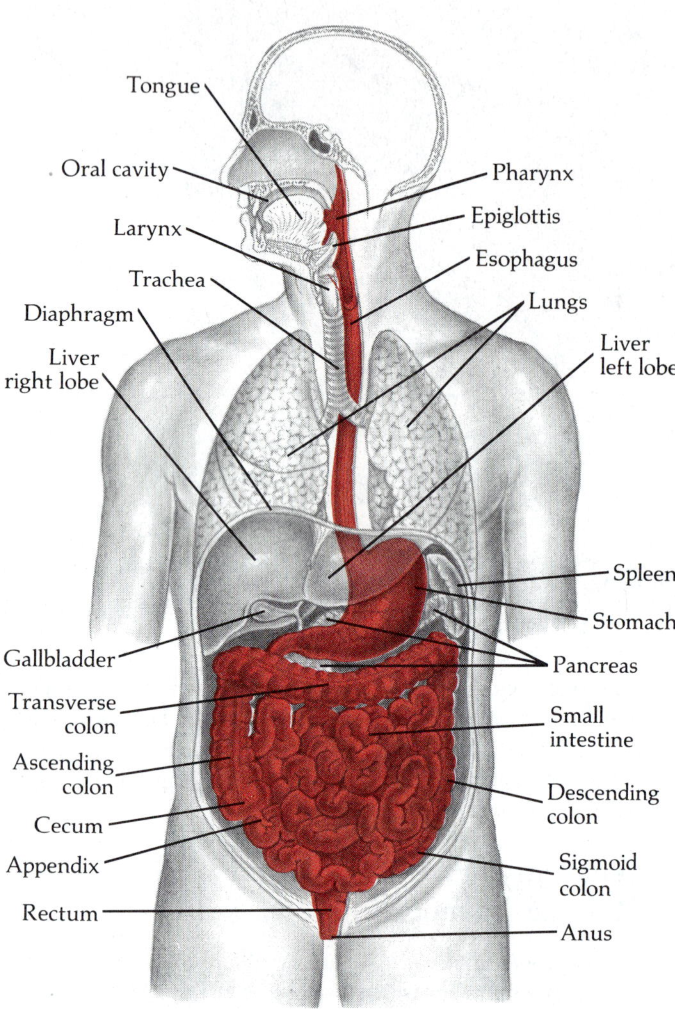

endocrine secretions. Exocrine secretions prepare food for absorption by diluting it to the osmolality of plasma (isotonic), altering the pH for hydrolysis, and hydrolyzing complex foods. The exocrine secretions also protect the mucosa from physical and chemical irritants. Endocrine secretions are important in the control and coordination of secretory and motor activities involved in the digestion and absorption of food. The types and functions of the secretions are discussed as they appear in the gastrointestinal tract.

Mouth

The mouth, also called the buccal cavity or oral cavity, is the beginning of the gastrointestinal tract. Mechanical and chemical digestion begins in the mouth. The teeth and tongue aid in mechanical breakdown, and the secretions of the salivary glands begin basic starch digestion and lubricate food to aid in swallowing.

The vestibule is the region between the lips, cheeks, teeth, and gums. The region posterior to the teeth and gums is the mouth cavity proper. Saliva from the salivary glands is received by the mouth cavity proper and aids in digestion.

The lips keep food and saliva in the mouth during chewing (mastication). The lips are sharply demarcated from the surrounding facial skin by the vermilion-cutaneous line. The lips are covered externally by skin and internally by mucous membrane. The bulk of the lips is composed of orbicularis oris, a sphincterlike muscle.

The internal cheeks are composed of muscle, fat, areolar tissue, nerves, vessels, and buccal glands covered by an inner mucous membrane. The gums, or gingivae, are dense fibrous tissue covered by a smooth mucous membrane.

The roof of the mouth is formed by the hard and soft palates. The hard palate is formed by two palatine bones and parts of the superior maxillary bone. The midline of the hard palate is called the linear raphe. The mucous membrane of the hard palate is thick, pale, and corrugated anterior to and to either side of the linear raphe. The posterior mucous membrane is thin, smooth, and a deeper pink. Attached to the posterior portion of the hard palate is the soft palate. The soft palate forms the partition between the mouth and nasopharynx. In a relaxed position the anterior surface of the soft palate is concave and continuous with the roof of the mouth while the posterior surface is convex and continuous with the nasal cavities. The uvula is the conical fingerlike projection of the posterior border of the soft palate. During swallowing the soft palate moves upward, closing off the nasopharynx and preventing foods and fluids from entering the pharynx.

The tongue is a muscular organ anchored to the hyoid bone and the mandible and covered with a mucous membrane. The frenum, or frenulum, is a fold of mucous membrane under the tongue that attaches the tongue to the floor of the mouth. Mucous membrane also attaches the tongue to the epiglottis, soft palate, and pharynx. The tip of the tongue is the apex.

The tongue contains mucous and serous glands. The mucous glands are behind the apex and secrete mucin. The serous glands, also called Ebner's glands, are found in the back of the tongue. Ebner's glands assist in the distribution of substances to be tasted over the tongue.

The muscles of the tongue are divided into lateral halves by a median fibrous septum. The two groups of muscles can be identified by their role in the tongue's functions. The muscles that assist the tongue in protrusion, retraction, elevation, and depression during mastication are the genioglossus, hyoglossus, chondroglossus, styloglossus, and palatoglossus. The muscles that are responsible for altering the shape of the tongue (shortened, curved, narrowed) include the longitudinalis superior, longitudinalis inferior, transversus, and verticalis. These movements are important in the enunciation of different letters and words.

The four types of papillae that contain taste buds are located on the anterior two thirds of the dorsum of the tongue. They are papillae vallatae, papillae fungiformes, papillae filiformes, and papillae simplices. Papillae vallatae, or circumvallate papillae, form an inverted V on the posterior dorsal surface of the tongue. These are the largest papillae and are round and flattened. The taste buds are found on their lateral surfaces.

Papillae filiformes are numerous and arranged in tight parallel rows. They contain thick, dense epithelium and appear white on the tongue's surface. The filiform papillae also contain elastic fibers.

The papillae fungiformes are found mainly at the apex and sides of the tongue. They are large and deep red.

The papillae simplices are similar to papillae of the skin and cover the entire mucous membrane of the tongue. The papillae simplices play a minor role in taste sensation.

Taste buds are concentrated in the circumvallate and fungiform papillae. Adults have approximately 10,000 taste buds, and children have a few more.[34] As a person ages, the taste buds begin to degenerate and perception of taste becomes less acute.

The four primary sensations of taste are sweet, sour, salty, and bitter. Taste buds detecting a primary taste tend to be localized in certain areas of the tongue. Sweet taste is primarily on the anterior surface and the tip of the tongue; sour taste on the two lateral sides; bitter taste on the papillae vallatae; and salty taste over the entire tongue. Taste buds respond in varying degrees to all four taste sensations. A taste bud may be very sensitive to one or two tastes but respond moderately to the other taste sensations.

Since taste buds respond to taste sensations with a different degree of sensitivity, the brain determines the taste based on the degree of stimulation of various taste buds. The sense of smell also affects the sense of taste. Odors from food stimulate the olfactory system. When the sense of smell is decreased, the degree of taste is often reported as diminished. Taste preference is used by animals and humans to regulate diet.

Adults have 32 teeth, and children have 20. Teeth serve as an accessory to digestion by cutting and mixing food. Mixing the food with saliva begins some chemical digestion and lubricates the food for swallowing.

Chewing involves the stimulation of jaw muscles. Much of the chewing process is innervated by the motor branch of the fifth cranial nerve. There is also a chewing reflex. The presence of food in the mouth causes a reflex inhibition of the muscles of mastication, which allows the lower jaw to drop. This drop initiates a stretch reflex in the jaw muscles, leading to a rebound contraction: raising the jaw and closing the teeth. The closure of the teeth on the bolus of food inhibits the jaw muscles, allowing the jaw to drop and rebound. This is then repeated.

Since digestive enzymes work only on the surface of food particles, chewing increases the surface area exposed to the enzymes. Chewing food also increases the ease with which food is swallowed and affects the ease of emptying of food from the stomach into the small intestine.

Salivary Glands

The salivary glands are the parotid, submaxillary, and sublingual glands. Some small salivary glands are found in the lips, buccal mucosa, and palate. These are exocrine glands that secrete a mixture of serous and mucous fluid into the oral cavity.

The parotid gland is anterior to the external ear and wraps around the mandible. The parotids are the largest of the salivary glands; each weighs approximately 14 to 30 g. The parotid (Stensen's) duct enters the mouth at its papillae opposite the second maxillary molar tooth. The parotid gland produces ptyalin (salivary amylase), which begins the chemical breakdown of starches. But the action of ptyalin in the mouth breaks down only 5% to 10% of the starches. The action of the enzyme continues in the stomach for 30 minutes to several hours, until the pH falls, rendering the enzyme inactive.

The submaxillary gland is smaller, weighing 7 to 10 g, and is located inferior to the mylohyoid muscle. It lies adjacent to the body of the mandible. The submaxillary (Wharton's) duct opens on the floor of the mouth adjacent to the base of the frenulum of the tongue. The secretory motor fibers originate in the chorda tympani nerve. The submaxillary gland produces a mixture of mucous and serous secretions.

The sublingual glands are located beneath the floor of the mouth and weigh approximately 3 g. The sublingual glands consist of predominantly mucous acini with a few serous acini. The primary purpose of the sublingual gland secretions is lubrication.

Approximately 1000 to 1500 ml of saliva is produced by the salivary glands in 24 hours. The pH of the saliva is between 6.0 and 7.0. The superior and inferior salivatory nuclei are located in the brainstem and may be stimulated by taste and tactile sensations from the tongue and mouth. Pleasant taste stimuli result in more salivation than unpleasant tastes, and smooth-textured foods stimulate more saliva production than rough-textured foods. Less salivation may result in less lubrication of food and more difficulty in swallowing. More saliva is produced when a person is eating a food he or she likes than when eating a disliked food. Thus salivation may be divided into three phases: psychic, gustatory, and gastrointestinal. The psychic phase occurs when the mouth is preparing itself to receive food. It is stimulated by thoughts or smells of pleasant foods. The gustatory phase occurs while one is chewing or swallowing food. The saliva is stimulated to aid in mastication and lubricate the food for swallowing. The gastrointestinal phase occurs when one has eaten irritating foods. The salivation is a response to reflexes originating in the stomach or upper intestines. The swallowed saliva dilutes or neutralizes the irritant.

Oropharynx

The oropharynx is the midpoint of the upper respiratory tract and digestive tract. The superior boundary is at a horizontal line that would connect the soft palate with the second cervical vertebra. The inferior line would connect horizontally the tip of the epiglottis and the base of the tongue. The nasopharynx lies between the oropharynx and the hypopharynx (see Chapter 7).

The oropharynx is lined by a mucous membrane of stratified squamous epithelium that is continuous with the lining of the mouth, nasal cavities, and larynx. The contents of the oropharynx include the soft palate, the uvula, the tonsils and their pillars, and the base of the tongue.

Esophagus

The esophagus is a hollow muscular tube approximately 25 cm (10 inches) long. It begins in the neck at the lower border of the fifth cervical vertebra and connects the hypopharynx to the cardia of the stomach. On each side of the esophagus are the thyroid lobes and parathyroids. The recurrent laryngeal nerves run directly in front of the esophagus. In the thorax the esophagus is found to the left of the midline with the pericardium and left atrium in front. The arch of the aorta crosses the lateral aspect of the esophagus at the level of the fourth thoracic vertebra. The descending aorta runs laterally and slightly posterior to the esophagus. At the level of the tenth thoracic vertebra the esophagus passes through the diaphragm into the abdominal cavity.

The esophagus narrows slightly at three points: near its origin in the region of the cricoid cartilage, at the arch of the aorta, and as it passes through the diaphragm. The esophagus is more vulnerable to perforation and trauma in these areas.

The arterial blood supply of the esophagus comes from the inferior thyroid artery in the neck, from branches of the descending aorta, and from the left gastric artery. The esophageal veins join the vena azygos, which joins the superior vena cava and the systemic circulation. The veins at the lower end of the esophagus communicate freely with the tributaries of the left gastric vein that join the portal vein. The upper part of the esophagus drains into the superior vena cava; the middle part drains into the azygos system; and the bottom third drains into the portal system via the gastric veins. There is no connection here of the portal and systemic venous systems. The hepatic vein drains the liver and empties into the superior vena cava, which is the connection between the two systems. When there is increased pressure in the portal system, there is increased pressure in the esophageal veins, leading to the development of esophageal varices.

The wall of the esophagus has all the characteristics of the gastrointestinal tract except for the serosa. This lack of serosa becomes important when esophageal surgery (i.e., anastomosis) has been performed, since there may be an increased chance for leakage postoperatively. The innermost, or mucous, membrane is composed of a stratified squamous epithelium that is continuous with the oral cavity and pharynx. At the lower end of the esophagus the mucous membrane changes to a simple columnar (transitional) epithelium that merges with the gastric mucosa in the cardiac portion of the stomach.

The submucosa layer underlying the squamous epithelium contains the blood vessels, nerves, mucous cells, and connective tissues. The mucous cells secrete mucus to further lubricate the food and protect the wall of the esophagus. The secretions are amphoteric, neutralizing both acid and base.

The muscle layer is composed of an internal circular and outer longitudinal layer. It differs from the remainder of the alimentary tract in several ways. First, the longitudinal layer is thicker than the inner circular layer. Second, the upper third of the esophagus is striated muscle. This portion of the esophagus receives its innervation from lower motor neurons and is dependent on cholinergic mechanisms. If these nerves are cut, flaccid paralysis of the upper esophagus will occur.[78] The middle third of the esophagus is mixed muscle tissue, and the lower third is primarily smooth muscle. The innervation of the smooth muscle found in the lower two thirds of the esophagus is preganglionic fibers of the autonomic nervous system. No flaccid paralysis develops if these nerves are cut.

Swallowing

Deglutition (swallowing) can be divided into several phases. In the voluntary phase the tongue moves upward and backward, forcing a bolus of food into the pharynx. The next phases are involuntary phases and involve transfer and transport. Transfer results in changes in the pharyngeal and upper esophagus, while transport involves the middle and lower esophagus.

During the voluntary stage of swallowing, the bolus of food stimulates swallowing receptors around the pharynx. The impulses pass to the brainstem, resulting in a series of autonomic pharyngeal muscular contractions. First, the soft palate rises to meet the posterior pharyngeal wall, closing the nasopharynx. Second, contraction of the suprahyoid muscles elevates the larynx and trachea, which increases the diameter of the pharynx. Third, the epiglottis bends backward and the vocal cords come together, further blocking the respiratory tract.

As the bolus enters the pharynx, the cricopharyngeal muscle relaxes, permitting the bolus to enter the esophagus. This stimulates rapid peristaltic waves. These actions increase the size of the pharynx, pull the pharynx up to receive the food, and close the larynx to prevent aspiration. The nerve impulses of the pharynx, which are stimulated by the bolus of food, travel the trigeminal nerve to the medulla oblongata, where the swallowing center is located. Nerve impulses then travel back along the glossopharyngeal and vagus nerves to move the bolus into the esophagus.

The esophageal phase of swallowing moves the bolus from the pharynx to the stomach by peristalsis. There are three types of esophageal peristalsis: primary, secondary, and tertiary. Primary peristalsis is a continuation of the movement begun in the pharynx. If a person is upright, downward gravity also affects the travel time through the esophagus. If primary peristalsis fails to move all the food that has entered the esophagus into the stomach, secondary peristalsis is stimulated from the distention of the esophagus by the retained bolus. The only difference is that primary peristalsis is initiated in the pharynx and secondary peristalsis is initiated in the esophagus at the level of the aortic arch.

Tertiary contractions may occur in some individuals, particularly after middle age. These are nonperistaltic contractions and do not assist in transport of food through the esophagus.

Approximately 1 to 3 cm above the junction of the esophagus and stomach is a segment, called the lower esophageal sphincter, that has a higher resting pressure than that in the body of the esophagus and that in the stomach. Under normal circumstances this area relaxes with primary or secondary peristalsis. The purpose of this high-pressure area is to prevent reflux of acid gastric contents into the esophagus. Certain factors* increase or decrease this high-pressure zone:

- Increase high-pressure zone
  - Gastrin
  - Cholinergic agents
    - Methacholine (Mecholyl)
    - Bethanechol (Urecholine)
  - Metoclopramide
  - Prostaglandin F_2
  - Gastric alkalinization (antacids)
  - α-Adrenergic agonists
  - Protein meal
  - Nonfat milk
  - Ethanol (low dose)
  - Bombesin
- Decrease high-pressure zone
  - Secretin
  - Cholecystokinin
  - Glucagon
  - Anticholinergics
  - Gastric inhibitory polypeptide
  - Vasoactive intestine peptide
  - Verapamil
  - Prostaglandins E, E_2, A_2
  - Gastric acidification
  - α-Adrenergic antagonists
  - Fat meal
  - Whole milk
  - Ethanol (high dose)

Peritoneal Cavity

The abdomen is the largest cavity in the human body. It contains the stomach, small intestine, kidneys, adrenal glands, uterus in women, liver, colon, gallbladder, pancreas, and major vessels. The abdomen is bordered anteriorly by the abdominal muscles and iliacus, posteriorly by vertebral column and lumbar muscles, inferiorly by the plane of the superior aperture of the lesser pelvis, and superiorly by the diaphragm.

The structures in the cavity are protected and covered by peritoneum, which is made up of serous membrane composed of mesothelium and a thin layer of irregular connective tissue. The parietal peritoneum is the tissue that lines the abdominal wall. The mesentery is a double fold of parietal peritoneum that is fan shaped and encircles the jejunum and ileum (segments of the small intestines) attaching them to the posterior abdominal wall. The blood vessels and nerves of the small intestine pass through the mesentery. The greater omentum is an apron-shaped double fold of peritoneum that hangs loosely over the intestines. The greater omentum is attached to the upper border of the duodenum, the lower edge of the stomach, and the transverse colon.

A small amount of serous fluid separates the space between the parietal and visceral peritoneum. The fluid provides lubrication between the organs and the abdominal wall.

Stomach

The function of the stomach is to alter the consistency and the composition of ingested foods. The ingested foods are liquefied into chyme as the stomach mixes the material with gastric secretions. The chyme is then released in a regulated manner into the duodenum for further digestion and absorption.

The stomach connects to the esophagus 3 cm below the diaphragm. The stomach lies obliquely beneath the cardiac sphincter of the esophagus, above the pyloric sphincter next to the small intestine, and under the left lobe of the liver and diaphragm. The size, shape, and position of the stomach vary depending on body size, posture, degree of gastric retention, degree of gastric muscle development, and effects of pressures from adjacent organs. Its normal capacity is 1 to 2 L. The stomach functions as a reservoir where mechanical and chemical breakdown of food continues.

The stomach is divided into the cardia, fundus, body, antrum, and pylorus (Figure 8-2). The cardia is the proximal portion of the stomach. The lesser curvature of the stomach extends from the cardiac orifice to the pyloric opening in a downward curve. Attached to this border is the lesser omentum, or gastrohepatic ligament. The greater curvature is almost four times longer than the lesser curvature, and the greater omentum is attached to it.

The fundus is the uppermost portion of the stomach. Although the fundus is distal to the cardia, it is superior to the cardia anatomically. The body of the stomach extends distally from the fundus to the level at which the gastric lumen assumes a transverse direction. The antrum is the peristaltic portion of the stomach and is distal to the body. The motor activity and mucosal surface are different in the antrum. The pylorus is the portion just before the duodenum.

The wall of the stomach is composed of four layers: (from the innermost lining layer out) the mucosa, the submucosa, the muscle layer, and the serosa. The mucosa layer is separated from the submucosa by the muscularis mucosa and is

*Adapted from Bolt, R.J., et al.: The digestive system, New York, 1983, John Wiley & Sons.

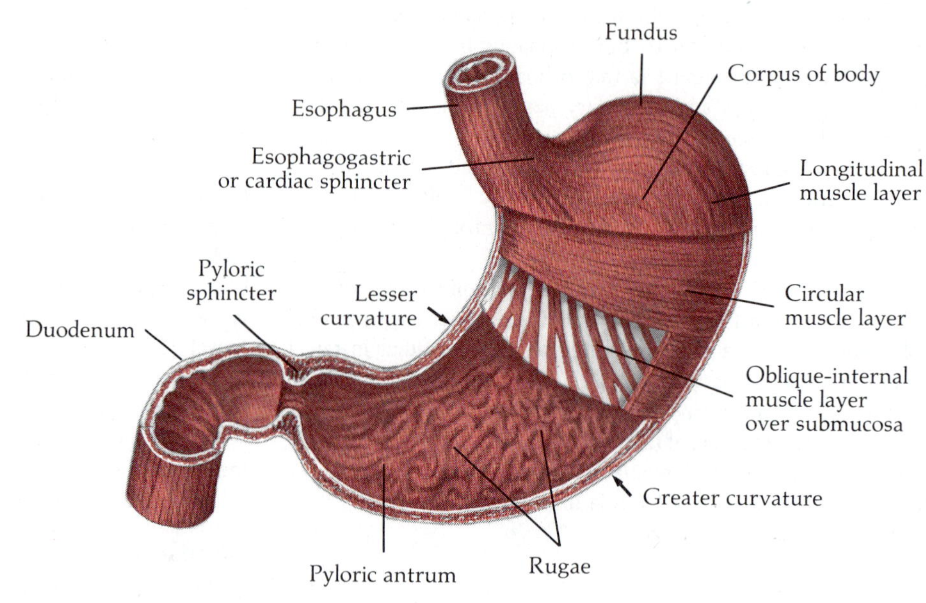

Figure 8-2 Gross anatomy of stomach.

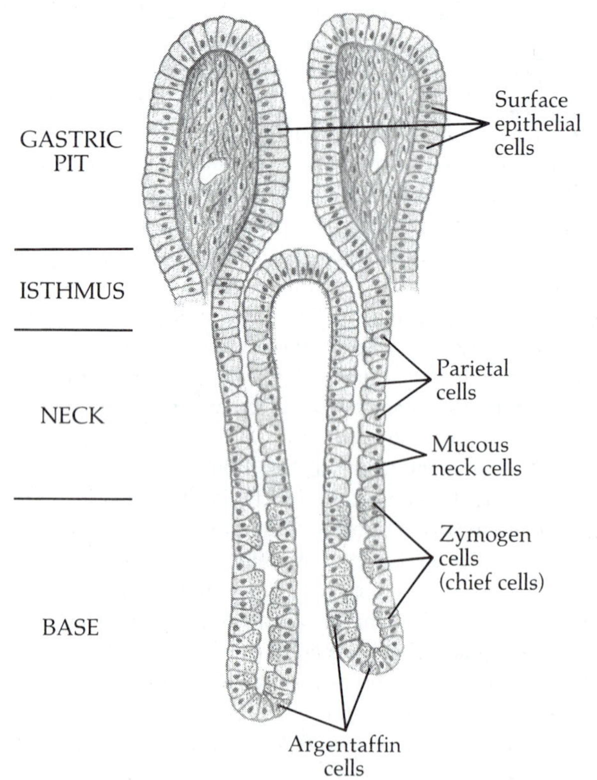

Figure 8-3 Human gastric mucosa. Diagram of tubular gland from fundic area of stomach.

composed of gastric epithelium. The mucosa is arranged in longitudinal folds called rugae found most predominantly in the fundus and body regions of the stomach. The rugae are low and flat in the lesser curvature and are sometimes absent in the antrum.

The cells of the mucosa are tall and columnar and contain mucus. The gastric epithelial layer invaginates to form gastric pits or foveolae, which communicate with deeper gastric glands (Figure 8-3). The gastric glands secrete into the gastric lumen via the gastric pit.

There are three distinct areas of cells within the stomach: the cardia, the oxyntic, and the antral, or pyloric. The mucosa of the cardia is columnar epithelium that secretes mucus. This zone or area has also been referred to as the transitional or junctional mucosa.

The glands of the fundus and body are straight, closely packed, and tubular. These glands contain neck cells, parietal (oxyntic) cells, chief (zymogen) cells, and argentaffin cells. Mucous neck cells are most numerous and play a role in mucosal cell renewal. Parietal cells are located at the upper portion of the gland. Parietal cells produce hydrochloric acid (HCl) and intrinsic factor. Chief cells are most abundant in the deeper portion of the gland and secrete pepsinogen (type I). Argentaffin cells are in the deeper portion of the gland and produce serotonin.

The fundus and body are often referred to as the acid-pepsin secreting area. The pepsinogen is activated in a pH below 5.0. The optimum level of pH is 1.8 to 3.5. The hydrochloric acid provides the acidity necessary for the pepsinogen to convert to its active form, pepsin.

The antrum mucosa is thinner than the oxyntic, and the

foveolae are deeper. The glands are tubular and coiled. Gastrin-producing G cells are located in the mucosa adjacent to the tubular glands. The tubular glands secrete mucus and pepsinogen II.

The submucosa is composed of loose areolar and elastic tissue. It contains vascular and lymphatic channels and an intrinsic nerve plexus, Meissner's plexus. The muscle layer is thick and is composed of three separate strata of smooth muscle. The outer, longitudinal layer extends downward from the esophagus along the greater and lesser curvatures to the pyloric sphincter. The middle circular muscle forms a uniform layer over the entire stomach. There is a second nerve plexus found between the two muscle layers, Auerbach's plexus. The inner oblique muscle layer is continuous with the circular muscle of the esophagus and is thickest in the fundus region. It extends to the pyloric sphincter. The outermost layer is the serosa and is an extension of the peritoneum.

The blood supply to the stomach is from large branches of the celiac artery. There may be variation in the branching pattern of the celiac axis. In approximately one fourth of all people, the left hepatic artery arises in part or totally from the left gastric artery. Gastrectomy in this group of patients may lead to necrosis of the left lobe of the liver unless the surgeon first assesses the pattern of arterial blood flow.[5] Arterial branches passing through the muscle layer form an extensive plexus of blood vessels in the submucosa. These vessels then enter the mucosa and subdivide to form a capillary network in the lamina propria surrounding the gastric glands and pits. Blood can be shunted from one area of the stomach to another or from one layer of the stomach to another by submucosa anastomoses and numerous submucosa arteriovenous communications. Mucosal ischemia can be caused by a redistribution of blood flow from vasoconstrictor activity of the sympathetic nervous system and by vasoconstrictor drugs. Bolt and co-workers[5] state that it is not clearly understood whether the vagus nerve is capable of directly mediating vasodilation of the gastric vascular supply. Venous blood from the stomach, the right and left gastric veins, empties directly into the portal vein.

The vagus and splanchnic nerves innervate the stomach. Branches of the left and right vagus nerves join to form the anterior esophageal plexus, and branches of the right vagus form the posterior esophageal plexus. At the distal esophagus they join to form the anterior and posterior vagal trunk. The anterior trunk provides the anterior gastric and hepatic divisions. The anterior gastric division goes along the lesser curvature to the pyloric sphincter with branches to the anterosuperior wall of the stomach. The hepatic division supplies the gallbladder, biliary tree, and proximal duodenum.

The posterior trunk of the vagus nerve divides into the posterior gastric and celiac divisions. The posterior gastric division goes along the lesser curvature with branches to the posteroinferior wall of the stomach. The celiac division descends with the left gastric artery through the celiac plexus to the superior mesenteric plexus, supplying the small intestine and ascending and transverse colon to the splenic flexure.

The splanchnic nerves contain sensory fibers and postganglionic sympathetic fibers (whose transmitters are catecholamines). The vagi contain sensory fibers, preganglionic parasympathetic fibers (cholinergic), and purinergic fibers (adenosine triphosphate receptors).[5] These fibers synapse with the ganglion cells of the myenteric (Auerbach's) plexus and the submucosal (Meissner's) plexus. The postganglionic fibers end in the gastric glands and muscle fibers stimulating gastric secretion and muscle contraction.

The reservoir function of the stomach is the capacity of the stomach to accommodate a meal. A vagal-mediated reflex relaxes the body of the stomach so that it accepts the ingested meal with minimal increase in intragastric pressure. Once swallowing is completed, the gastric wall tension increases and intragastric pressure is proportional to the volume ingested. This also helps to determine gastric emptying. If the normal vagal reflex activity is inhibited or if the capacity of the stomach is reduced, the reservoir function is altered. People with significantly compromised reservoir functions need to eat frequent, smaller meals to avoid or minimize symptoms such as early satiety, postprandial epigastric pain, and nausea and vomiting.

Gastric secretions include mucus, pepsinogen, hydrochloric acid, intrinsic factor, and the hormone gastrin. Gastric mucus is composed of proteins, glycoproteins, mucopolysaccharides, and blood group substances. The principal component is glycoprotein. Gastric mucus is a thin layer of mucus adherent to the cell surface. The role of gastric mucus in the mucosal barrier is not well defined. The gastric mucosal barrier helps separate acid in the lumen from bicarbonate on the epithelial cell surface. The mucosal barrier prevents diffusion of hydrogen ions from lumen to mucosa and diffusion of sodium ions from mucosa to lumen.

The surface mucous cells are stimulated by vagus nerve and acetylcholine in response to chemicals (i.e., ethanol) and physical contact and friction from roughage in the diet. They protect the mucosa with an alkaline layer of lubricant.

Pepsinogen is secreted by the chief cells of glands in the body and fundus with a small amount secreted by neck cells and by Brunner's glands in the duodenum (the first portion of the small intestine). Pepsinogen is converted to active pepsin at a pH less than 6.0. The optimum pH of pepsin is 1.8 to 3.5 with no activity above pH of 5.0. Pepsinogen is stimulated by both vagal stimulation and a local reflex activity. Pepsinogen secretion is increased by the presence of gastrin, calcium, histamine, and secretin.

Hydrochloric acid is secreted by the parietal cells. Endogenous stimuli for hydrochloric acid production is acetylcholine, gastrin, and histamine. The basal secretion of hydrochloric acid is lowest between 5 and 11 AM and highest between 2 PM and 1 AM.[38]

The production of intrinsic factor by the parietal cells is an essential function of the stomach. Intrinsic factor is a mucoprotein that binds with vitamin B_{12} and is absorbed at specific receptor cells. This complex attaches to special cells in the terminal ileum. The stimuli that increase secretion of

Figure 8-4 Mechanisms for stimulation of acid secretion. From Johnson.[38]

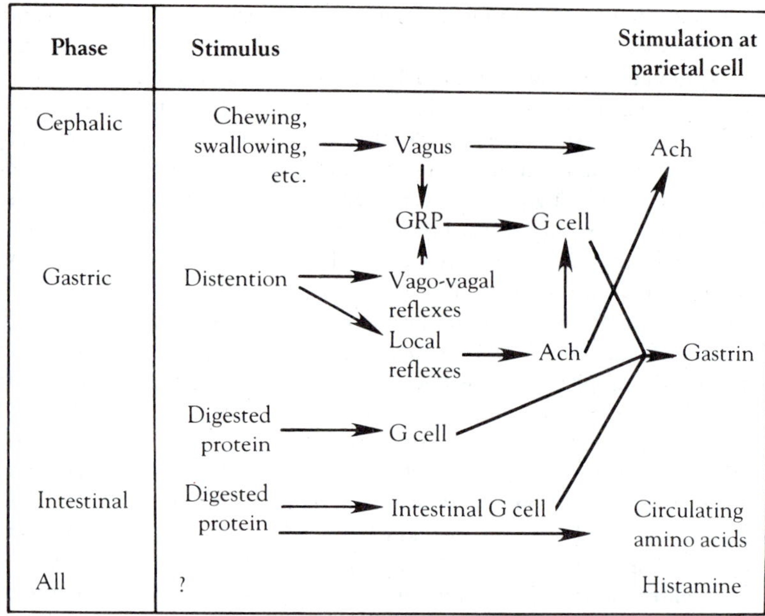

intrinsic factor are the same as those stimulating hydrochloric acid production. The failure to secrete intrinsic factor is associated with achlorhydria and the absence of parietal cells. The condition results in vitamin B_{12} deficiency and subsequent pernicious anemia.

The hormone gastrin is secreted by the antral G cells and is the primary mediator of gastric acid secretion. Gastrin is also secreted by cells in the duodenum, pancreatic islets, and jejunum. Vagal stimulation, gastric distention, and the presence of amino acids and peptides stimulate the secretion of antral gastrin. Antral gastrin then circulates in the blood system with the parietal cells as the target organ. Calcium ions will also stimulate antral gastrin. When the gastric pH is below 1.5, gastrin release is inhibited. Duodenal gastrin is secreted in response to distention and protein.

Gastric secretion has been divided into three phases (cephalic, gastric, and intestinal) that occur almost simultaneously. The cephalic phase includes the sight, smell, taste, thought, and chewing of food, as well as conditional reflexes and intracellular hypoglycemia. The vagus nerve releases acetylcholine by postganglionic fibers in the gastric mucosa, causing the secretion of hydrochloric acid, intrinsic factor, and pepsinogen. The gastric phase constitutes the major physiologic stimulus for gastric secretion and is activated by the presence of food in the stomach. The intestinal phase serves mainly to inhibit gastric secretions. Duodenal gastrin that is released in response to protein digestion products and distention functions in the same way as antral gastrin (Figure 8-4).

Inhibition of gastric secretions in the intestinal phase is related to the actions of cholecystokinin (CCK), secretin, gastric inhibitory polypeptide (GIP), vasoactive intestinal peptide (VIP), glucagon, and prostaglandins (Figure 8-5). CCK is stimulated by L-amino acids and fatty acids in the duodenum. When CCK and gastrin are both present, a competitive inhibition of gastrin occurs because both have the same active terminal tetrapeptide. Thus the secretory function of gastrin is inhibited. Hydrogen ions in the duodenum stimulate the release of secretin. Secretin inhibits acid output and blocks the secretory effects of gastrin and histamine. Secretin stimulates pepsinogen output. Both CCK and secretin stimulate pancreatic secretion of bicarbonate.

Gastric inhibitory polypeptide (GIP) is composed of 43 amino acids and is found throughout the intestinal tract, although it is concentrated in the duodenum. GIP has a wide range of functions, including inhibition of food-stimulated release of gastrin, gastric acid secretion, and pepsinogen secretions. VIP and glucagon inhibit gastric secretion and stimulate intestinal electrolyte secretion.

Prostaglandins are a group of cyclic fatty acid compounds with 20 carbon acids. Approximately 20 subtypes have been identified, of which several inhibit gastric secretagogues, including gastrin, histamine, food, acetylcholine, hypoglycemia, and reserpine.

Enterogastrone is a general term often used to designate hormones released from duodenal mucosa in response to acid, fatty acids, and hyperosmotic solutions that inhibit gastric acid secretions.[78] There are still unanswered questions regarding gastric inhibition. Future research should answer many of the uncertainties in the understanding of hormonal inhibition of gastric secretion.

Gastric motility can be divided into tonic, mixing, and peristaltic contractions. Gastric tone controls luminal volume

Figure 8-5 Mechanisms for inhibition of acid secretion.
From Johnson.[38]

Region	Stimulus	Mediator	Inhibit gastrin release	Inhibit acid secretion
Antrum	Acid (pH < 3.0)	Somatostatin	+	
Duodenum	Acid	Secretin	+	+
		Nervous reflex		+
	Hyperosmotic solutions	Unidentified enterogastrone		+
Duodenum and jejunum	Fatty acids	GIP	+	+
		Unidentified enterogastrone		+

and maintains a relatively constant pressure despite changes in volume. The fundus and body serve as a receptacle and the antrum as a pump. The antrum portion mixes gastric contents and empties the contents into the duodenum in a controlled fashion. Circular muscle contractions in the body of the stomach mix the food with the gastric secretions. Contractions in the antrum are stronger and produce considerable mixing motions as well as propulsion.

Antral peristaltic contractions force the chyme (liquefied food) into the pyloric canal and then into the duodenum. The pyloric sphincter is a high-pressure zone that relaxes with antral peristalsis and contracts in response to acids, fats, amino acids, and nonisotonic solutions in the duodenum. Gastric distention stimulates stretch receptors, which results in increased gastric peristalsis and increased gastric emptying. The stimulus for rapid gastric emptying is gastric distention.

There are three receptors in the duodenum that release substances inhibiting gastric emptying: osmoreceptors, acid-sensitive receptors, and fat-sensitive receptors. Hormones released in the duodenum (gastrin, CCK, secretin, pancreatic polypeptide, gut glucagon, GIP, VIP, calcitonin, prostaglandins, and bulbogastrone) inhibit gastric emptying. The complete physiologic role of the hormones is not understood.[5,38]

Gastric emptying can be impaired by drugs, diseases, and surgery. Incomplete emptying may result in early satiety, postprandial epigastric pain, and vomiting. Rapid gastric emptying may occur with duodenal ulcers and following surgery for peptic ulcers.

In summary, the primary function of the stomach is mixing and liquefaction of food to a suitable consistency for the duodenum. The intrinsic factor is an essential substance secreted by the stomach necessary for vitamin B_{12} absorption in the terminal ileum.

Small Intestine

In the small intestine, ingested food is mixed, digested, and absorbed. The small intestine is divided into three segments: duodenum, jejunum, and ileum. The first portion is the duodenum; at 20 to 30 cm (8 to 12 inches) long, it is the shortest segment. The ligament of Treitz is the dividing point between the duodenum and jejunum, although histologic changes cannot be demonstrated. The jejunum is 2.5 m (8 feet) long, and the ileum is 3.5 m (11⅓ feet) long. The jejunum and ileum have no specific anatomic division (Figure 8-6).

The small intestine is 6.5 to 7 m (21 to 22¾ feet) long and is divided into four layers: mucosa (innermost layer), submucosa, muscularis externa, and serosa (outer layer). As in outer segments of the gastrointestinal tract, the mucosa is separated from the submucosa by the muscularis mucosae. The submucosa contains the connective tissue, lymphatics, blood vessels, and nerves. Meissner's plexus is in the submucosa. The muscularis externa consists of an inner circular layer and an outer longitudinal layer. Auerbach's (myenteric) plexus lies between the two muscle layers.

The duodenum is C shaped. The first portion of the duodenum lies behind and below the right and caudate lobes of the liver and gallbladder and in front of the common bile duct and portal vein. This portion is suspended from the lesser omentum and lies within the peritoneal cavity. The remaining duodenum is located retroperitoneally. The second portion of the duodenum descends vertically to the level of the fourth lumbar vertebra and lies in front of the vena cava, right ureter,

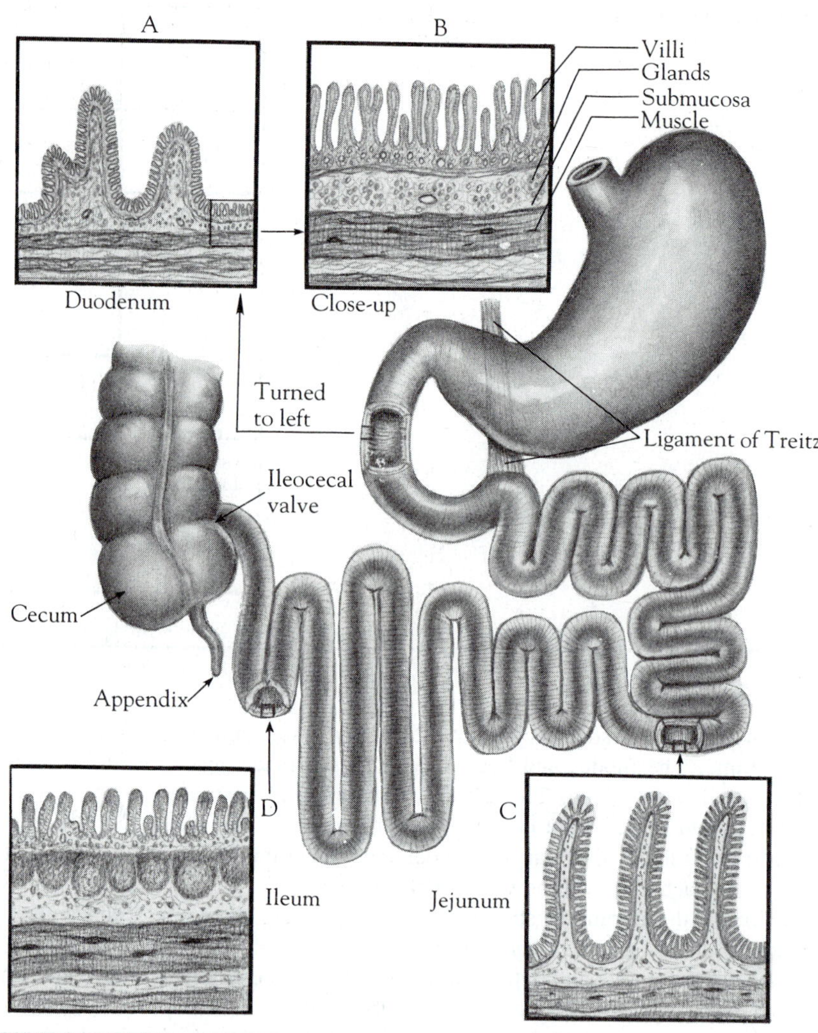

Figure 8-6 Clinical anatomy of small intestine.

and psoas muscle. Ventrally, the second portion is related to the right lobe of the liver, transverse colon, and small intestine. The common bile duct and main pancreatic duct empty into the duodenum at the ampulla of Vater, 7 to 10 cm distal to the pyloric sphincter.

The third portion, or horizontal segment, crosses the third and fourth lumbar vertebrae, vena cava, and aorta. The superior mesenteric vessel crosses this segment anteriorly. The fourth segment ascends along the left side of the aorta, turns sharply anteriorly, and then descends caudally as the jejunum. The ligament of Treitz, a suspensory ligament of the duodenum, is a band of fibers and muscle tissue originating in the right crus of the diaphragm. The portion of the duodenum proximal to the ampulla of Vater receives its blood supply from the celiac axis. The remainder is supplied by the superior mesenteric artery.

The duodenum contains Brunner's glands in the submucosa, which secrete an alkaline fluid containing pepsinogen. The hormones secreted in the duodenum include gastrin, CCK, secretin, GIP, VIP, and enterogastrone.

The jejunum and ileum have a greatly increased mucosa and submucosa surface area for absorption. Three characteristic features of this portion of the small intestine are a large series of circular folds of mucosa and submucosa; minute, fingerlike projections of the mucosa called villi; and microvilli, or brush border. Mucosal crypts at the base of the villi extend into the wall of the small intestine to the muscularis mucosae. Epithelial cells migrate from the crypts to extrude from the tip of the villi. As an epithelial cell migrates to the tip of the villus, its absorptive capacity increases. The brush border (microvilli) is covered with a glycocalyx (mucopolysaccharide) cover that contains many of the digestive enzymes of the small intestine. Also found in the microvillus-calyceal area are receptors for vitamin B_{12}.[78] The surface epithelial cells and the microvillus brush border constitute the digestion-absorption unit. Several enzymes are found in this unit including alkaline phosphatase, folic acid, folic acid conjugase, and a number of disaccharides and peptidases, as well as adenylcyclase and the "active pump" for sodium.[5,78] In addition to surface epithelial cells, goblet cells (mucin secreting), crypt cells (fluid and electrolyte secreting), and enteroendocrine cells (hormonal) are found in the small intestine.

The mesentery of the small intestine is fixed to the left of the second lumbar vertebra and goes downward and to the right to approximately the level of the right sacroiliac joint. The vascular supply of the entire jejunum and ileum (except for the terminal portion of the ileum) arises from the left border of the superior mesenteric artery. The vessels are contained within the mesentery. The terminal ileum is supplied by the ileocolic artery from the right side of the superior mesenteric artery. Venous drainage is through the superior mesenteric vein to the portal vein.

The small intestine has both sympathetic and parasympathetic stimulation. In addition to the autonomic nervous system, the enteric nervous system also regulates small bowel activities. The enteric nervous system involves purinergic, peptidergic, and serotonergic neurotransmitters. The complexity and interrelatedness of the two systems' regulation of intestinal motility are being studied. The autonomic nervous system stimulation can be interrupted with vagotomy and sympathectomy without significant alteration in intestinal motility. The intactness of the enteric nervous system may be more important for peristalsis than autonomic innervation.

The primary function of the motility of the small intestine is to facilitate the digestive-absorptive process. Two motions are found in the small intestine: mixing, or segmental, and propulsive, or peristaltic. The mixing movements bring the chyme in contact with pancreatic and biliary secretions. The musculature constricts at the rate of 11 to 12 contractions per minute, resulting in segmentation so it resembles links. Segmentation also increases the contact of the chyme with the intestinal villi and microvilli, enhancing absorption. Peristalsis propels chyme forward at a rate of 2 to 20 cm/minute. This appears as a progressive moving ring. The myenteric plexus supplies the sympathetic and parasympathetic stimulation for segmentation and peristalsis.

The terms "digestion" and "absorption" emphasize two phases of a single continuing process. The digestion of dietary lipids, carbohydrates, and proteins is initiated in the lumen of the duodenum and proximal jejunum and is completed at the glycocalyx and microvilli plasma membrane of enterocytes (jejunal absorptive cells). Most absorption occurs in the jejunum. Vitamin B_{12} is absorbed in the terminal ileum, and bile salts are reabsorbed by active transport in the terminal ileum. Otherwise, minimum absorption occurs in the ileum unless the jejunum is nonfunctioning or diseased. The processes of absorption in the small intestine are passive absorption and active transport. Passive absorption resembles diffusion of a substance through a membrane, and the rate of movement depends on a higher concentration in the lumen than in the bloodstream. Active transport is more rapid, more complex, and more efficient and requires energy.

Carbohydrate absorption requires conversion of starches to monosaccharides. Starch digestion by pancreatic amylase yields oligosaccharides and disaccharides. Active absorption of sugars occurs primarily in the brush border and at the apex of the epithelial cell. Brush border enzymes include lactose, sucrose, maltose, isomaltose, and trehalose. Lactose is hydrolyzed to glucose and galactose, sucrose to fructose, and dextrins, maltotriose, and maltose to glucose. Disaccharides are further hydrolyzed by brush border enzymes. Disaccharides, sucrose, and lactose are not dependent on pancreatic amylase but are hydrolyzed by the brush border enzymes. Glucose and galactose are transported through a sodium-dependent ATPase process into the epithelial cells. Fructose appears to be absorbed by a nonactive facilitated diffusion transport process.[5] Carbohydrate absorption is in the duodenum and jejunum.

Dietary fat consists of long-chain triglycerides that are insoluble in water. In the stomach, fat is shaken into a very fine emulsion. Gastric pepsin strips fat of its protein wrapper. Lipase secreted from mouth and tongue remains active in digesting fats in the stomach. In the duodenum and jejunum, pancreatic lipase breaks down triglycerides to diglycerides, then to monoglycerides, and finally to glycerol and fatty acids. Glycerol is absorbed into the epithelial cell and capillaries directly. Monoglycerides, fatty acids, and conjugated bile salts form the micelle. At the brush border the micelle breaks up, allowing the monoglyceride and free fatty acid to enter the cells. The bile salts return to the intestinal lumen, where they are reabsorbed in the terminal ileum. Bicarbonate from the pancreas is also important because efficient lipolysis occurs in an alkaline pH. At the surface epithelial cell, the conjugated bile salt separates, permitting fatty acids and β-monoglycerides to be absorbed. The bile salts remain in the lumen and are reabsorbed in the terminal ileum. (Reabsorbed bile salts are cycled through the liver and reexcreted in the bile.)

The absorbed fatty acids and β-monoglycerides are resynthesized to triglycerides, are enclosed in a protein covering, forming chylomicrons, are transported through the lymphatics and thoracic duct, and finally reach the blood. Some medium-chain triglycerides do not depend on micelle formation and after hydrolysis can be absorbed by the epithelial cell as fatty acids and transported directly into the portal venous system.

Although gastric pepsin begins protein digestion, it is not essential for protein digestion. Pancreatic proteases include trypsinogen, chymotrypsinogen, procarboxypeptidases A and B, leucine aminopeptidase, and nucleases. The hormone cholecystokinin (CCK) is the primary stimulator of the pancreatic acinar cells. CCK is released in the duodenum and jejunum in the presence of amino acids and fatty acids. The presence of hydrogen ions, or a low pH, stimulates the release of the hormone secretin. Secretin stimulates the bicarbonate and fluid responses of the pancreas. The activation of the pancreatic enzyme trypsinogen depends on the intestinal secretion of the enzyme enterokinase. Thus pancreatic functioning depends on the presence and functioning of a normal proximal small bowel.

The intraluminal protein digestion by-products are peptides of two to six amino acids. The brush border and intracellular enzymes further break down these products to free amino acids, dipeptides, and some tripeptides that can enter the epithelial cell. The enterocyte has at least three carrier-mediated transport systems, including one for neutral amino acids, one for basic amino acids, and one for peptide-linked amino acids. In the cell the small peptides are hydrolyzed into free amino acids, which are absorbed into the capillary, where further protein breakdown occurs.

Vitamin B_{12} binds with intrinsic factor (gastric secretion) to protect it from gastric digestion and bacterial digestion in the small bowel. The intrinsic factor also is essential for attachment of vitamin B_{12} to receptors of the glycocalyx membrane of the ileal absorptive cell. Calcium, magnesium, and pH greater than 5.6 are also necessary for the attachment of vitamin B_{12} and the transport through the cell. The vitamin B_{12} is then transported in the portal blood bound to a carrier (transcobalamin). Pancreatic insufficiency is also associated with a vitamin B_{12} deficiency. This is because R binders found in saliva, gastric secretions, bile, and intestinal secretions can bind with vitamin B_{12} rather than the intrinsic factor. Pancreatic proteases degrade the R binders, making it possible for vitamin B_{12} to bind with the intrinsic factor. Intestinal microflora is capable of synthesizing vitamin B_{12}. When oral vitamin B_{12} is reduced, the use of antibiotics may alter intraluminal flora, resulting in vitamin B_{12} deficiency. The body stores of vitamin B_{12} may be adequate for years. Thus clinical signs of vitamin B_{12} deficiency are unusual.

Calcium absorption is highest in the upper small intestine where the pH is lowest. Its absorption and transport are enhanced by vitamin D. Calcium is transported against a concentration gradient. Passive absorption occurs when intraluminal concentrations are greater than 6 mM/L. Calcium absorption is decreased by phosphate ingestion, anticonvulsant drugs, alcohol, and steroids.

Dietary folate is composed of multiple glutamyl units, and the linkage is broken by the mucosal epithelium to monoglutamate. Absorption occurs primarily in the proximal small bowel. The transport mechanism is unclear. Folate enters the portal circulation and functions as a cofactor in many enzyme systems.

Iron absorption depends on the physiologic demands of the body. When iron stores are low or when red blood cells are being rapidly formed, iron absorption is increased. Iron absorption occurs primarily in the duodenum and proximal jejunum against a concentration gradient. Iron is absorbed in the ferrous form, bound to globulin (transferrin), then released into the portal circulation or stored within cells as apoferritin.

One of the major functions of the small intestine is fluid and electrolyte shifts from gastrointestinal lumen to blood and from blood to lumen. In a 24-hour period, approximately 9 L of fluid enters the lumen of the small intestine. Approximately 7.5 to 8.2 L is endogenous secretions (saliva, gastric, intestinal, pancreatic, and bile). Another 1 to 1.5 L is exogenous. Most of the fluid is reabsorbed, and only 500 to 1000 ml passes through the ileocecal valve into the colon. The duodenum and jejunum are primarily responsible for the large amounts of absorption of fluids, electrolytes, and nutrients because of large pores that allow rapid flow of solutes and water in both directions. Isomolarity in the lumen is rapidly attained and maintained throughout the small intestine. Several factors help prevent osmotic disequilibrium, including the relative impermeability of gastric mucosa, the regulation of gastric emptying, the fact that nutrients are largely macromolecules with low osmotic activity, and rapid absorption of products of macromolecule digestion or breakdown. Fat is high in most diets, but since its osmotic potential is low, it does not impede osmotic equilibrium. Maintaining osmolarity requires rapid flow of salt and water through the intestinal membrane. The direction of the flow is determined by hydrostatic and osmotic forces.

Sodium absorption is a major function of the small intestine, with approximately 1145 mEq being reabsorbed every 24 hours. Sodium absorption plays a part in regulating cellular absorption of electrolytes and water. The brush border contain a carrier that binds sodium and glucose. When intraluminal glucose is present, sodium is actively reabsorbed by the shared carrier. Sodium is also absorbed from the lumen by a sodium-hydrogen exchange mechanism. A sodium pump at the basolateral border of epithelial absorbing cells transports sodium from intracellular to intercellular spaces by means of a sodium-potassium ATPase activity. The decrease of intracellular sodium concentration enhances the sodium-glucose carrier mechanism.

In the ileum a chloride-bicarbonate exchange mechanism is present. The bicarbonate concentration in the ileum is much higher than in the jejunum. Potassium is absorbed based on sodium-potassium ATPase and hydrostatic and osmotic forces.

Water transport is passive and depends on osmotic and hydrostatic pressures. Increased solute concentration in the intercellular space (e.g., from sodium pump activity) provides osmotic forces for water absorption. As water flows through the pores it brings small solutes with it. This is referred to as solvent drag. Hydrostatic forces from the serosa layer will restrict passive water and solute absorption. Water from the interstitial fluid will enter the lumen when solutes accumulate in the lumen. The flow continues until osmotic equilibrium exists.

The secretory function of the intestinal epithelium appears to be the result of electrogenic activity. If the secretory function is greater than the absorption function, significant fluid and electrolyte loss can occur. This is frequently seen in diseases or abnormal states (malabsorption syndromes).

Immunologic function of the small bowel through Peyer's patches and lymphoid cells is not clearly documented. Peyer's patches are found in the submucosa and contain small lymphocytes from the mesenteric nodes. Lymphoid cells differing from Peyer's patches are found in the lamina propria. IgA is

Table 8-1
Gastrointestinal Hormones and Their Actions

Hormone	Location	Primary Action	Secondary Action
Gastrin	Antrum, duodenum, proximal jejunum	Stimulates gastric acid secretion	Trophic effect on gastrointestinal mucosa
Cholecystokinin	Throughout small intestine, but primarily found in jejunum	Stimulates contraction of gallbladder Stimulates secretion of pancreatic enzymes	Motility of stomach and small intestine
Secretin	Throughout gastrointestinal tract, except colon; primary sites are duodenum and jejunum	Stimulates pancreatic bicarbonate secretions	Numerous interactions with other gastrointestinal hormones
Gastric inhibitory peptide	Small intestine, primarily jejunum	Increases release of insulin from pancreas	Decreases gastric acid secretion Increases intestinal secretion
Enteroglucagon	Primarily lower ileum and colon	Inhibits motility	May be trophic for mucosa
Vasoactive intestinal peptide	Esophagus to rectum	Increases intestinal and pancreatic secretions	Decreases gastric acid secretion Increases insulin secretion Causes peripheral vasodilation

the prominent immunoglobulin found in the small bowel, but IgM, IgG, IgD, and IgE are also present. The IgA found in the small bowel differs from serum IgA. An infant is born without secretory or serum IgA. The secretory IgA appears first and reaches adult levels sooner. The secretory IgA has antiviral and antibacterial activities. The immune system of the small bowel appears to be complex, and further investigation may reveal its precise role.

Enzyme activity in the small intestine is located in the brush border of the villi and within the absorbing epithelial cell cytoplasm. The only enzyme secreted by the small intestine with luminal activity is enterokinase. The old concept of succus entericus, luminal intestinal enzymes, is no longer accepted.

Hormonal function of the small intestine is of great interest. The small intestine may be the body's largest and most diffuse endocrine organ. Bolt and associates[5] provide the following criteria for a gut hormone:

- Production of a biologic response in another organ
- Production of a response with no innervation between the gut and another organ
- Similar response in the organ when an extract of the gut tissue is given
- Occurrence of biologic response when pure or synthetic exogenous hormone is given

Four hormones meet these criteria: secretin, gastrin, cholecystokinin (CCK), and gastric inhibitory polypeptide (GIP). Hormone candidates include substances that do not necessarily meet all four criteria. Some of the hormone candidates have known structures, while the structures of others have yet to be identified:

- Known structure
  - Vasoactive intestinal peptide
  - Motilin
  - Pancreatic polypeptide
  - Somatostatin
  - Neurotensin
  - Substance P
  - Urogastrone
  - Enkephalins
- Unknown structure
  - Chymodenin
  - Bombesin-like peptides
  - Gut glucagon–like immunoreactants
  - Gastrozymin
  - Anticholecystokinin peptide
  - Incretin
  - Villikinin
  - Entero-oxyntin
  - Bulbogastrone
  - Pancreatone

The actions of the hormones are complex, and many have more than one action. The activity may be as a paracrine agent, a neuroendocrine or neurotransmitter substance, or an exocrine agent. Based on amino acid sequence and pharmacologic and physiologic action, two categories of hormones in the small intestine can be identified. Family 1 includes gastrin and CCK. The terminal amino acids in the last four positions are the same in gastrin and CCK. Family 2 includes secretin, enteroglucagon, vasoactive intestinal peptide (VIP), and GIP. Numerous amino acids in similar positions can be found in each of the family 2 hormones.

Table 8-1 summarizes small intestinal hormones and their activities.

Large Intestine (Colon) and Rectum

The colon is approximately 150 cm (4½ to 5 feet) long. The terminal ileum joins the colon at the ileocecal valve. The appendix arises from the cecum medially, about 2 cm below the junction of the ileum and cecum. The cecum is continuous with the ascending colon, which goes from the cecum to the undersurface of the right lobe of the liver. The colon bends to the left, forming the hepatic flexure. The colon then extends to the left, becoming the transverse colon. The transverse colon has a mesentery and therefore a wide range of movement. The cecum, ascending colon, and proximal half of the transverse colon are derived from the midgut. The innervation and vascular supply are shared with the small intestine.

The transverse colon continues to the left and slightly upward, forming the splenic flexure. The splenic flexure is slightly higher than the hepatic flexure and is in front of and above the left kidney. As the colon turns downward, it becomes the descending colon. The sigmoid colon begins at the point where the descending colon crosses the iliac artery at the rim of the pelvis. The mesentery of the sigmoid colon attaches it to the posterior (retroperitoneal) wall of the pelvis. Near the midsacrum, the sigmoid colon becomes the rectum. The rectum descends in front of the sacrum and coccyx. The rectum becomes the anal canal approximately 2 cm anterior to the tip of the coccyx. The upper portion of the rectum is in the peritoneal cavity, but the distal 12 to 15 cm has no peritoneal covering. This area lies behind the bladder in the male with the seminal vesicles on either side. In the female the distal 12 to 15 cm is posterior to the uterus. The rectal ampulla is the lowest part of the rectum and is anterior to the posterior aspect of the prostate in the male. In the female the rectal ampulla is attached to the posterior wall of the vagina.

The distal half of the transverse colon, splenic flexure, descending sigmoid, and rectum are derived from the hindgut. The inferior mesenteric artery supplies this portion of the large intestine and rectum. The nervous innervation is from the sacral parasympathetic fibers.

The wall of the colon is divided into the same four layers as the small intestine: mucosa, submucosa, muscularis externa, and serosa. There are no villi in the large intestine. The simple columnar epithelial surface is flat and is broken into polygonal units by clefts. Goblet cell openings occur on the epithelial surface. In the center of polygonal units are crypts of Lieberkühn. These crypts are lined with goblet cells and extend into the muscularis mucosae. At the bottom of the crypts are proliferating undifferentiated epithelial cells and occasionally argentaffin cells. Cell renewal begins in the crypts. The cells then migrate upward to the surface and extrude into the lumen. The renewal time is approximately 3½ to 4 days.

The mucosa, submucosa, and circular muscle layer form semilunar folds (plicae semilunares) dividing the haustra (sacculations). The semilunar folds are crescent shaped and extend one third of the way around the wall of the intestine. The longitudinal muscle layer is incomplete in the large colon. It is called teniae coli and is the noticeable band in the colon wall. Fatty tags (appendices epiploicae) project from the serosa coat of the colon; this is another difference between the large and small intestines.

The musculature of the rectum is a continuation of the colonic muscular layers. The outer longitudinal layer spreads from the teniae of the sigmoid colon to form a continuous even coat. The superficial fibers insert into the perianal body and merge with the levator ani muscles of the pelvic floor. The deep fibers insert into the perianal skin. The circular muscle forms the internal sphincter surrounding the anal canal. The pectinate line marks the boundary between the anal canal and rectum. At this anorectal junction, the lining layer changes from columnar to squamous epithelial cells. The external sphincter is striated muscle and lies outside the internal sphincter. The external sphincter encircles the terminal portion of the anal canal.

The mesenteric attachments of the colon permit considerable mobility of the ileocecal junction and sigmoid colon. Two potential problems are a volvulus, or twisting of the bowel upon itself, and intussusception. The hepatic and splenic flexures, descending colon, and rectum are relatively fixed.

The major blood vessels of the large colon and rectum are the superior and inferior mesenteric arteries as previously stated. The superior rectal artery is a branch of the inferior mesenteric and branches as low as the proximal anal canal. The middle and inferior rectal arteries are branches of the internal iliac artery and supply the anal canal and subcutaneous perianal area. The superior hemorrhoidal vein empties into the inferior mesenteric vein, which drains into the portal system. The inferior hemorrhoidal veins drain into pudendal veins and the systemic venous system. Because of the venous relationship with the portal system, portal hypertension can lead to congestion and enlargement of the hemorrhoidal system and hemorrhoids.

The lymph nodes of the colon include epicolic nodes, found on the surface; paracolic nodes, found on the mesenteric border; and intermediate nodes, associated with superior and inferior mesenteric arteries. The lymphatics from the intermediate nodes join the lymph nodes adjacent to the abdominal aorta (Figure 8-7).

Nervous innervation includes external sympathetic and parasympathetic fibers and submucosal and myenteric nerve plexuses. Sympathetic innervation is from segments T2 to L2. These form the mesenteric hypogastric nerves. The parasympathetic fibers to the right colon are through the vagus nerve. The left colon parasympathetic fibers are from the second to fourth sacral segments by way of the pelvic nerves.

The integrated functions of the colon, rectum, and internal and external sphincters require both sensory and motor innervation. The sensory pathways for the anal canal and perianal skin go through the somatic nerves to S2, S3, and S4. Proprioceptive spindles are found in the striated muscle of the external sphincter. Autonomic sensory innervation for the rectum passes through the same segments (S2, S3, and S4), but through parasympathetic pathways. The pudendal nerve and coccygeal plexus originating in S2 to S5 form the motor fibers for the external sphincter. The hypogastric nerve provides excitatory motor stimuli of the parasympathetic fibers. The rectal sympathetic fibers are from L2 through L4 and the parasympathetic fibers are from S2 through S4.

The normal functions of the colon include controlling tran-

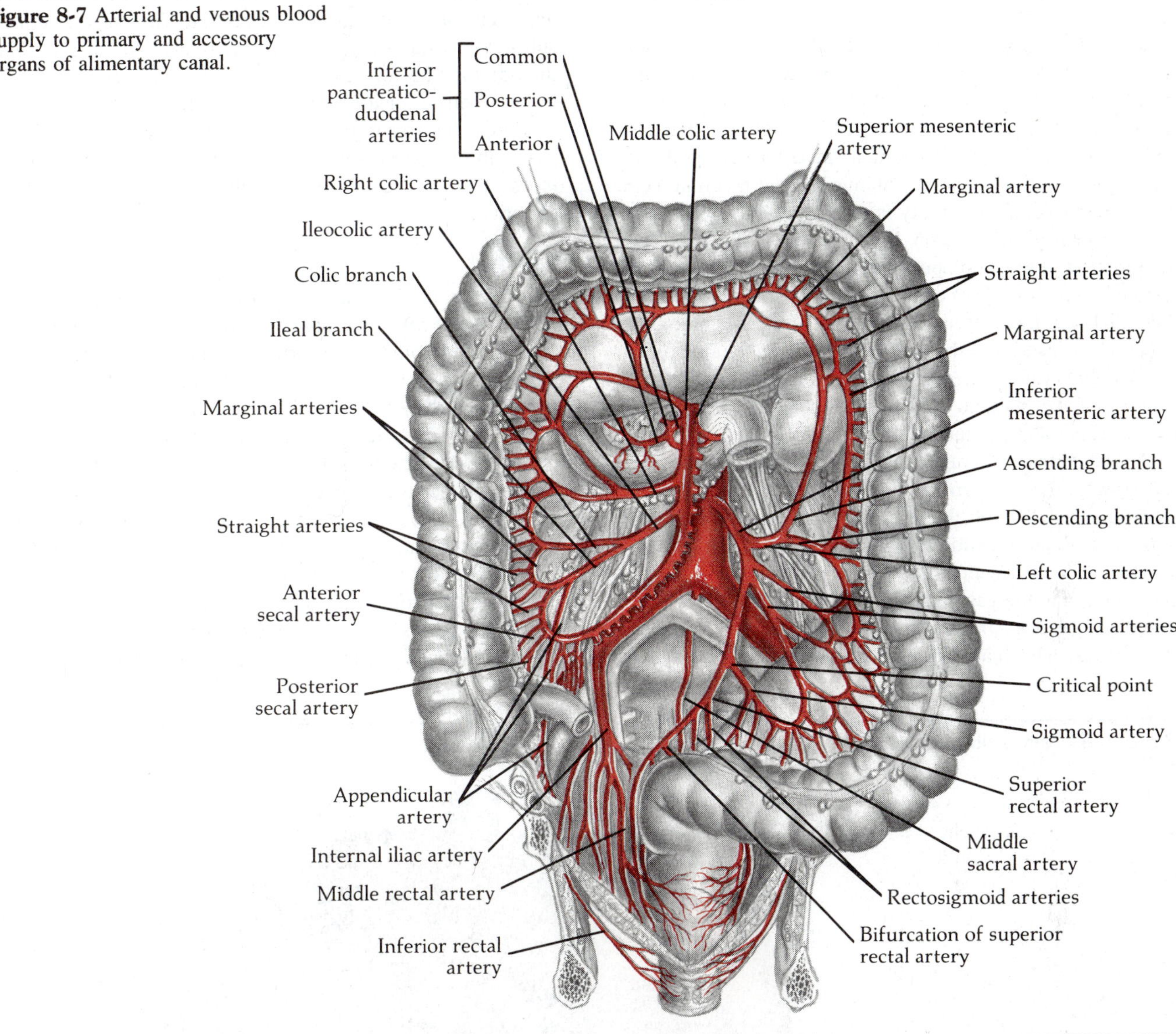

Figure 8-7 Arterial and venous blood supply to primary and accessory organs of alimentary canal.

sit of waste, absorption, and limited secretion. Defecation is the mechanism for eliminating metabolic waste and dietary residue. Colonic motor activity includes segmentation (mixing) and peristaltic movement. Segmentation occurs by alternate formation and relaxation of haustral folds. Peristalsis is a forward movement over longer segments of bowel. Colonic activities increase after a meal. There is an increase in ileal activity resulting in a slow filling of the cecum and ascending colon. The fluid contents of the right colon are moved back and forth (segmentation) over the absorptive epithelium. The proximal colon retains the contents longer than the distal colon.

Gradually the sigmoid colon fills, and the stool periodically passes into the rectum. Distention of the rectum causes an urge to defecate. Defecation can be a simple emptying of the rectal area, or it may stimulate mass propulsion and empty the distal half of the colon. Defecation in a continent person includes voluntary relaxation of external sphincters, relaxation of internal sphincters, increase in intra-abdominal pressure, tensing of the pelvic floor, and colon contraction.

Most absorption of fluid and electrolytes occurs in the right colon. The mechanism for water absorption is passive flow in response to an osmotic gradient. The osmotic gradient is produced by active absorption of sodium. The colon is sensitive to aldosterone and other mineralocorticoids, and the response of the colon is to increase sodium absorption and potassium secretion. Potassium is secreted into the colon lumen. The mucus secreted by the goblet cells can contain high quantities of potassium. If the luminal potassium concentration goes above 15 mEq/L, a shift occurs and potassium is absorbed. Chloride ion is absorbed as a pair with sodium bicarbonate secreted by the colon. The chloride and bicarbonate are related. As chloride is absorbed, bicarbonate is secreted.

The colon has a minimum digestive or synthetic function. Ingested cellulose is not digested and passes into the colon largely unaltered. In constipated people, when feces remain in the lumen for prolonged periods, the colon can digest and absorb the cellulose. The bacteria in the colon can synthesize folic acid, riboflavin, biotin, vitamin K, and nicotinic acid. The importance of this ability is unknown.

Enterohepatic circulation involving the colon has been identified. The urea-ammonia enterohepatic circulation is related to the hydrolysis of circulating blood urea in the colonic epithelial wall by bacterial ureases. This produces ammonia, which is absorbed into the blood. Any remaining ammonium ion that enters the lumen is converted to free ammonium as a result of the alkaline pH of the lumen. Free ammonium readily penetrates the mucosa and returns to the liver.

A wide variety of drugs can be administered by enema or suppository. The rectum has a poor absorptive capacity, so absorption depends on the level at which the preparation is in the colon and retention time in the colon.

The average amount of gas in the gastrointestinal tract is 100 ml. Gas in the gastrointestinal tract is made up of swallowed air, gas diffusing across the mucosa, and gas produced by bacteria. The major components of flatus are oxygen, nitrogen, carbon dioxide, methane, and hydrogen. Hydrogen and methane are produced by bacteria. The bacteria utilize substrate found within the lumen, related to diet. Carbon dioxide may be formed as a result of neutralization of acid by bicarbonate, or it may be swallowed. Bacterial utilization of oxygen may result in low concentrations of oxygen. Flatus passes through the colon more rapidly than liquid or semisolid feces, since resistance to flatus flow by haustration is less effective.

Liver

The liver is the largest organ in the body, weighing 1.4 to 1.8 kg (3 to 4 lb). It is a complex organ with many functions, including bile production, protein metabolism, carbohydrate metabolism, fat metabolism, coagulation, and detoxification and storage of certain minerals and vitamins.

The liver is located under the diaphragm in the upper right portion of the abdominal cavity (Figure 8-8). The superior surface of the liver is under the right and left halves of the diaphragm. The inferior surface is above (from right to left) the hepatic flexure of the colon, the upper pole of the right kidney, the first portion of the duodenum, the inferior vena cava, and the stomach. The liver normally extends from the fifth intercostal space to just below the right costal margin. The right lobe is normally palpable on inspiration 1 to 2 cm

Figure 8-8 Liver, gallbladder, and pancreas.

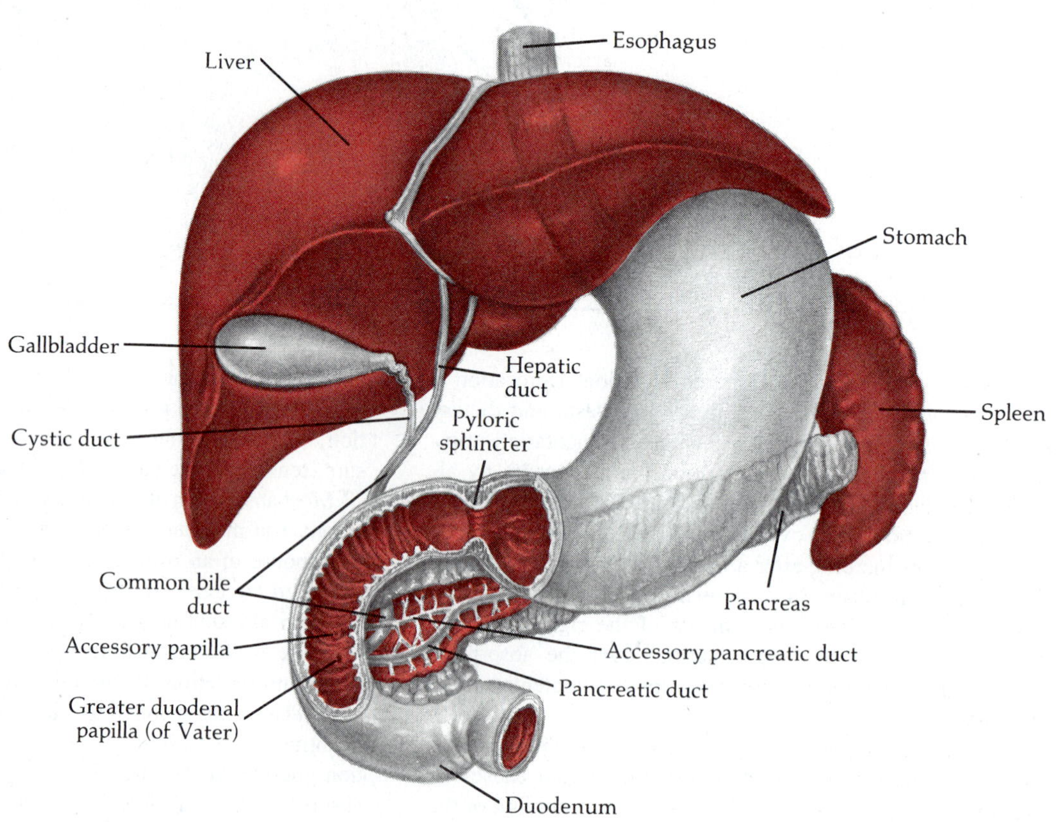

below the right costal margin. The left lobe is rarely palpable in the epigastric region of a healthy person.

The liver is divided into two lobes, with the right six times larger than the left in an adult and three times larger in infants. The falciform ligament separates the lobes. The right lobe is further subdivided into quadrate and caudate lobes. Riedel's lobe is a common accessory lobe on the right that is lateral to the gallbladder. This is a functional as well as anatomic division of the liver created by the falciform ligament. The division is determined largely by the liver's vascular supply.

The liver has a dual blood supply: the portal vein and the hepatic artery. The portal vein brings nutrients from the gastrointestinal system, and the hepatic artery provides the arterial circulation. The origin of the hepatic artery varies. In approximately 55% of individuals the hepatic artery originates from the celiac artery. The remainder have hepatic arteries arising from the left gastric or splenic artery. Off the hepatic artery is the gastroduodenal artery; then the hepatic artery enters the porta hepatis, divides into the right and left hepatic arteries, and enters the corresponding lobes of the liver. A middle hepatic artery originates from one branch and supplies the quadrate lobe. The possible variations in blood flow play an important role in surgical interventions in the gastrointestinal tract. Blood flow to the liver can be disturbed if the origin of the hepatic artery is not carefully noted. In 25% of individuals the left hepatic artery originates from the left gastric artery and this may be the only left hepatic artery present. Occasionally the right hepatic artery arises from the superior mesenteric artery. Another deviation is for the entire hepatic artery to arise from the superior mesenteric artery. In reading arteriograms, it is helpful to know of possible alternative patterns of blood flow. Arteriography can be useful before surgery. Also, for effective intra-arterial chemotherapy, a knowledge of possible anomalies of the hepatic arteries is necessary. The right, middle, and left hepatic arteries supply different areas and do not anastomose with each other to any significant degree.

Within the liver, branches of the hepatic artery, the portal vein, and bile ducts in the portal tract, described as the portal triad, accompany each other and empty into sinusoids. The portal vein is formed by the superior mesenteric vein at its junction with the splenic vein. The inferior mesenteric vein also empties into this system. The portal vein has several tributaries, of which the left gastric or coronary vein is the most important. The left gastric vein anastomoses with the esophageal veins, which empty into the vena cava.

The branches of the hepatic artery and portal vein are next to each other within the substance of the liver, with the portal vein emptying into the sinusoids. Approximately 1500 ml of blood passes through the liver every minute. Seventy percent of the blood flow is from the portal vein, which is derived primarily from the inferior and superior mesenteric veins, with one third or less coming from the splenic vein. The remaining 30% of the blood flow is from the hepatic artery.

Sinusoidal outflow is into central veins that flow into the hepatic veins. The three hepatic veins (right, middle, and left) enter the inferior vena cava separately. Normal portal pressure is 8 to 10 mm Hg. Arteriolar resistance, pressure in the aorta, and pressure in the inferior vena cava are important determinants of hepatic blood flow. Exercise, standing, or assuming an erect position reduces hepatic blood flow.

In the liver a superficial subcapsular lymphatic network communicates with the gallbladder and a deep lymphatic network that runs in portal triads with branches of the portal vein, hepatic artery, and bile ducts. The lymphatic drainage is primarily to the nodes at the hilum of the liver and eventually into the thoracic ducts.

The innervation of the liver is sympathetic (paravertebral ganglia, T7 to T10) and parasympathetic (vagus). The sympathetic fibers are distributed to the hepatic arterial branches and bile ducts. The parasympathetic fibers innervate the biliary tree. Although neuronal stimulation affects hepatic blood flow and biliary tree pressures, there are no known direct effects on parenchymal cell function.

The stroma is the connective tissue of the liver. It includes Glisson's capsule, which covers the liver and the connective tissue around the vascular and biliary branches. A reticular framework extends into the lobules and lies between the liver plates and sinusoidal lining cells.

The liver is composed of a complex circulatory system involving the hepatic artery, portal vein, sinusoids, central vein, and hepatic vein. The biliary system includes the bile canaliculi, ductules (or cholangioles), hepatic duct, and common duct.

Several cell types are present in the liver. The parenchymal cell, or hepatocyte, is the most important. The chemical actions that occur in the liver take place in the parenchymal cells. Kupffer (reticuloendothelial) cells line the sinusoids.

The flow of bile is in the opposite direction of the flow of blood through the liver. The bile canaliculi carry the bile from the central vein area to the portal triads. The bile canaliculi are small, intercellular channels between parenchymal cells. The canaliculi join the bile ductules, which are lined by columnar epithelium. The ductules join together to form the bile ducts, which form part of the portal triad with the hepatic artery and portal vein. The bile ducts go toward the hilum of the liver and join, forming the right and left hepatic ducts. The common hepatic duct joins the cystic duct from the gallbladder to form the common bile duct.

The common bile duct is joined by the pancreatic duct, and the two combined ducts form the ampulla of Vater on the duodenal mucosa. Oddi's sphincter at the opening regulates the one-way flow of bile and pancreatic secretions into the duodenum.

Heme, a source of bile pigments, is an end product of the breakdown of hemoglobin and accounts for 80% to 90% of the bilirubin produced daily in adults.[5] Hemoglobin is broken down into globin, iron, and protoporphyrin heme. The metabolic process for the conversion of protoporphyrin heme to bilirubin is poorly understood. It has been suggested that heme is converted to bilirubin by microsomal heme oxygenase found in reticuloendothelial cells of the spleen and liver. This is a multistep process that begins with the oxidation of heme to carbon monoxide and verdoheme. Verdoheme loses its iron to yield biliverdin, which is then reduced to bilirubin. The bilirubin is taken up by the parenchymal cells (hepatocytes) by active transport. This is unconjugated bilirubin, a lipid-soluble pigment that cannot be excreted by the liver unless it is conjugated, increasing its water solubility. Within the parenchymal cell the bilirubin is conjugated. The enzyme located on the endoplasmic reticulum, glucuronyl transferase, stimulates this process.

Conjugated bilirubin is not absorbed from the intestine or gallbladder. In the colon, bacteria hydrolyze conjugated bilirubin to urobilinogen. Urobilinogen is found in feces, bile, and urine. It is partially absorbed and reexcreted by the liver and kidneys. Most urobilinogen is found in the feces.

In the kidneys, urobilinogen is secreted by the proximal tubules and partially reabsorbed. The amount of reabsorption is increased in acid urine. Urine urobilinogen is influenced by the amount of hemolysis of red cells: an increase in hemolysis increases urine urobilinogen. In the presence of decreased bowel motility and stagnation of the small bowel contents, small bowel bacterial colonization and hence bacterial activity are increased. This increases the formation of urobilinogen from bilirubin. Absorption in the small bowel is more efficient, and the absorbed urobilinogen is excreted by the kidney, increasing urine urobilinogen. Hepatocellular disease or transhepatic shunting of portal blood increases the amount of urobilinogen in the systemic circulation, increasing excretion by the renal system. In the presence of biliary tract obstruction, less bilirubin enters the intestines, decreasing both fecal and urine urobilinogen.

The formation of bile is a major function of the liver. Hepatic bile has a specific gravity of 1.009 and an alkaline pH. It contains approximately 97% water, cholesterol, bile salts, phospholipids, mucin, conjugated bilirubin, electrolytes (sodium, potassium, chloride, and bicarbonate), calcium, and many enzymes. The liver secretes approximately 700 ml of bile per day. Although bile is secreted continuously, a meal augments the rate of secretion. The volume of bile produced by the liver is determined by the amount of bile salts synthesized. Conjugated bile salts are secreted by the hepatocytes, and this provides an osmotic pressure for the movement of water into bile. The volume of bile increases as it flows through the biliary tree because of active secretion of an electrolyte solution high in bicarbonate by the biliary epithelium.

Secretion of bile is increased by vagal stimulation and by the action of secretin, cholecystokinin-pancreozymin, vasoactive intestinal peptide, gastrin, and glucagon. Vagal stimulation and cholecystokinin-pancreozymin cause relaxation of the sphincter of Oddi. Exogenous agents that increase hepatic bile secretion and contraction of the gallbladder include bile salts, acetylsalicylic acid, pilocarpine, acetylcholine, choline, histamine, and insulin.

Bile is composed of bile acid, phospholipids, cholesterol, and bile pigments. Bile salts are necessary for micellular solubilization of dietary lipids and to maintain biliary cholesterol in solution. Two primary bile salts are cholic (trihydroxy) and chenodeoxycholic (dihydroxy). They are synthesized in the liver from cholesterol, are conjugated with glycine and taurine, and then form salts with sodium and potassium. Most bile salts are reabsorbed in the terminal ileum by an active transport process. Bile salts entering the colon are deconjugated and dehydroxylated by bacterial enzymes to form secondary bile acids. Cholic acid is broken down to deoxycholic (dihydroxy) acid, which is absorbed, conjugated in the liver, and secreted into bile. Chenodeoxycholic acid gives rise to lithocholic (monohydroxy) acid, which is poorly absorbed. Bile salts are formed when potassium and sodium combine with conjugated bile acids, of which 80% are cholic and chenodeoxycholic acids, with the largest percentage of the remaining bile salts being deoxycholic.

There is approximately 5 g of bile salts with a half-life of 3 to 5 days; these salts are recirculated six to 10 times a day. New bile acids account for 10% of the total amount each day, replacing the amount lost in the feces.

The formation of bile is only one function of the liver. Protein, carbohydrate, and lipid metabolism is an additional function. The liver is the source of albumin, which is 50% to 60% of the total plasma protein. For protein synthesis the liver uses dietary amino acids, amino acids formed by endogenous protein catabolism, and amino acids formed during carbohydrate and fat metabolism. Deamination of amino acids in the liver releases nitrogen, which is converted to urea. The liver also converts ammonia formed in other parts of the body to urea. Other functions related to protein metabolism include uric acid formation from nucleoprotein, creatine formation from glycine, and synthesis of methionine and arginine. Other proteins of importance to coagulation include haptoglobin, C-reactive protein, several glycoproteins, transferrin, serum enzymes, and ceruloplasmin.

Albumin has two major functions. First, it helps maintain the plasma colloid osmotic pressure because of its small molecular size and high charge. About one third of the body's albumin (4.5 to 5 g/kg) is intravascular, and the rest is extravascular. Second, albumin plays a role in active transport.

Carbohydrate metabolism involves the liver's ability to store glycogen within the hepatocyte. The liver converts glucose, fructose, and galactose to glycogen. If a diet is low in carbohydrates, or in the presence of prolonged fasting, the liver can convert protein and fat to glycogen. This is referred to as gluconeogenesis. Glucose not stored as glycogen or aminated to amino acid is converted to fatty acids, carbon dioxide, and water.

A normal blood glucose level depends on the liver's ability to remove glucose from the blood, store glucose as glycogen, break glycogen into glucose, and release glucose into the blood. Glycogenolysis (breaking glycogen to glucose) is increased by a decreased blood glucose, exercise, glucagon, and epinephrine. In a fasting state, glycogen stores can be significantly depleted in approximately 12 hours. In hepatocellular disease, glycogen stores may be reduced, resulting in hypoglycemia. This may also occur during stress and exercise.

Dietary lipid enters the liver in the form of chylomicrons. Triglycerides are hydrolyzed to glycerol and fatty acids. The liver also takes up fatty acids mobilized from fat depots and synthesizes fatty acids from carbohydrates and amino acids. The fatty acids are used in oxidation for energy production, resynthesis of triglycerides, formation of cholesterol esters, and conversion to phospholipids. Hepatic triglyceride accumulation, or fatty liver, may be the result of an excess of fatty acids, reduced lipid oxidation, or decreased lipoprotein formation.

Cholesterol is synthesized in the liver from acetate. Other sources of cholesterol are kidneys, adrenals, and small bowel mucosa. The liver removes cholesterol from the blood and excretes cholesterol into bile, forming a bile acid. Cholesterol may also combine with fatty acids to form cholesterol esters. Serum cholesterol is kept in solution by phospholipids.

The liver plays a major role in coagulation in that it is the site of production of coagulation factors I, II, VI, VII, VIII, IX, and X. Vitamin K is required for the synthesis of factors II, VII, IX, and X. Natural vitamin K is lipid soluble. There are synthetic forms of vitamin K that are water soluble. Vitamin K is stored in the liver. Oral anticoagulants such as coumarin interfere with the action of vitamin K within the parenchymal cell. The liver also removes active clotting factors from the circulation, contributing to coagulation homeostasis.

Plasminogen (profibrinolysin), the inactive form of plasmin (fibrinolysin), is believed to be synthesized by the liver. Plasminogen levels may be decreased in hepatocellular disease. Antiplasmin, a proteinase inhibitor found in plasma and serum, is also formed in the liver.

Clotting abnormalities may accompany almost any type of liver disease. The severity of acquired clotting problems associated with hepatic disease depends on the extent of hepatocellular damage. Vitamin K deficiency is uncommon, since vitamin K is found in food and is synthesized by colonic bacteria. Vitamin K deficiency may be seen in chronically ill people with limited oral intake who are taking broad-spectrum antibiotics. Chronic alcohol abusers may be vitamin K depleted because of their diets and liver disease. Also, patients on long-term total parenteral nutrition develop clotting abnormalities if their diet is not supplemented with vitamin K. Malabsorption of vitamin K may result from problems that cause a decrease in lipid absorption; for example, biliary obstruction. Coagulation problems seen in hepatocellular damage are usually caused by increased utilization of clotting factors, decreased production of clotting factors, production of abnormal clotting factors, or platelet abnormalities.

The liver also plays a role in detoxification of many materials, particularly drugs. Basically, the liver process involves making the substance water soluble for excretion in bile or urine. Enzymes from the smooth endoplasmic reticulum oxidize, reduce, hydrolyze, and conjugate foreign compounds. The enzymes have a low substrate specificity and readily detoxify substances. The processes that determine whether a compound is excreted in the urine or the bile are multiple and not always understood. Substances that are highly polar and those with molecular weights over 200 are excreted in the bile. Substances with smaller molecular weights are excreted in the urine.

The effectiveness of lipid-soluble drugs may be altered by their conversion in the liver to a water-soluble state. Some drugs, such as phenylbutazone, become more potent after conversion in the liver to oxyphenylbutazone. However, oxidation of barbiturates decreases their effect and may produce a toxic by-product. Some drugs require metabolic transformation in the liver for production of a therapeutic action. In a patient with liver disease it is important to know the effects of a drug. Certain medications should be avoided, and others should be given in reduced dosages.

Gallbladder

The gallbladder (Figure 8-8) is a pear-shaped sac 6 to 8 cm (3 to 4 inches) long and attached to the inferior surface of the liver. It is joined to the biliary tree by the cystic duct at the point where the hepatic duct becomes the common bile duct.

The mucosa of the gallbladder is columnar epithelium overlying a lamina propria. The mucosa is in multiple, irregular folds that increase its absorptive area. The fibromuscular layer forms the framework of the sac. It is a mixture of longitudinal smooth muscle fibers and dense fibrous tissue. The fibromuscular layer is covered by a subserous adventitia. The serous layer is continuous with the serosa of the liver.

The gallbladder is supplied by the superior and inferior cystic artery, which branches off the hepatic artery. The venous system consists of capillary plexuses that drain into superficial veins on the gallbladder surface. These superficial veins empty directly into the liver. The gallbladder also has an extensive lymphatic system that connects with the lymphatic channels draining the liver. This system then combines with the lymphatics of the cystic duct and proximal sections of the extrahepatic ductal system and drains into the nodes at the porta hepatis.

Innervation of the gallbladder and biliary tree is from the sympathetic and parasympathetic systems. Parasympathetic stimulation causes contraction of the gallbladder. Sympathetic stimulation is inhibitory. Preganglionic sympathetic fibers are from the seventh or tenth thoracic segment, and postganglionic fibers from the celiac ganglia.

The hepatic division of the vagal nerve supplies parasympathetic preganglionic fibers that synapse with postganglionic fibers in the gallbladder wall. Afferent fibers travel with the splanchnic nerves and the right phrenic nerve. Right referred shoulder pain in gallbladder disease is related to this shared course with the right phrenic nerve.

The function of the gallbladder is to concentrate and store bile. The organ stores 30 to 50 ml of bile. In the presence of cholecystokinin-pancreozymin the gallbladder contracts, forcing bile through the cystic duct into the common bile duct and hence the duodenum (see discussion of bile under "Liver").

Pancreas

The pancreas (Figure 8-8) is an important accessory organ of digestion. It is located transversely across the posterior wall of the abdomen. It is about 20 cm (10 inches) long and weighs 60 to 160 g. The head of the pancreas is situated in the concavity of the duodenal loop on the right side of the vertebral column at the level of the first lumbar vertebra. The body of the pancreas extends leftward and superiorly to the hilum of the spleen. The terminal portion of the pancreas is the tail.

The pancreas resembles the salivary glands histologically. The difference between the two is the presence of islets of Langerhans within the pancreas. The pancreas has both exocrine and endocrine functions. Acinar cells secrete the exocrine products, bicarbonate and pancreatic enzymes, and the endocrine secretions of insulin, glucagon, and gastrin are from the alpha, beta, and delta cells of islets of Langerhans.

The blood supply of the pancreas is from the superior and inferior pancreaticoduodenal arteries and from branches of the splenic artery. The venous flow from the body and tail of the pancreas is through the splenic vein, and the head empties directly into the portal vein. The lymphatic system drains through the pancreaticoduodenal nodes to the celiac nodes.

The innervation of the pancreas is sympathetic and parasymphathetic. The sympathetic fibers follow the arterial blood vessels and play a part in regulating blood flow to the pancreas. The parasympathetic fibers terminate at the acinar cells, the islet cells, and the smooth muscle cells and regulate pancreatic secretion.

The pancreas is divided into lobules, and each lobule empties into a branch of the main pancreatic duct. The individual lobule is a group of acini formed from acinar cells, drained by a ductule that forms intralobular ducts that empty into the pancreatic duct. In the acinar cells are dark zymogen granules that are the precursors of pancreatic enzymes. The acini are continuous with the excretory ducts and are composed of an epithelial lining layer on a basal membrane.

The exocrine secretion of the pancreas is approximately 2000 ml per day. The secretions are aqueous fluid, rich in bicarbonate, enzymes, and electrolytes. The enzymes formed in the acinar cells are secreted into the ducts. Water and electrolytes are secreted by the ductular epithelium. The major pancreatic exocrine function is digestion and absorption in the small intestines. The bicarbonate, calcium, and magnesium in the pancreatic secretions are necessary for creating an optimum environment for enzyme activity. Interference with the exocrine function may lead to severe malabsorption of the dietary fats, fat-soluble vitamins, protein, and carbohydrates in starch form.

The hormones involved in the regulation of pancreatic exocrine secretions are gastrin, secretin, and cholecystokinin-pancreozymin. Gastrin is released by the antral mucosa in response to the presence of food in the stomach, distention, a decrease in hydrogen ion concentration, and vagal stimulation. In the duodenum, gastrin release is stimulated by distention and the presence of protein. Cholecystokinin-pancreozymin is secreted by the duodenal and proximal jejunal mucosa by the presence of L-amino acids, long-chain fatty acids, and hydrogen ions. The response of the pancreas to gastrin and cholecystokinin-pancreozymin is the secretion of enzyme-rich fluid. There is a minimum increase in volume in bicarbonate output, and chloride concentration decreases slightly. Calcium and magnesium secretions parallel enzyme output. Secretin is released from duodenal and proximal jejunal mucosa in response to hydrogen ion. Secretin stimulates large volumes of pancreatic secretions, which are high in bicarbonate, with little increase in enzyme output. The concentration of cations (sodium and potassium) remains relatively constant. Anion concentration varies with the flow rate. As bicarbonate concentration increases, chloride concentration decreases. Secretin does interact with gastrin and cholecystokinin-pancreozymin to augment the secretory response.

Vagal stimulation augments the hormonal stimulation of the exocrine secretions. The sight, smell, and taste of food stimulate the vagus. Also, gastric distention stimulates the vagus nerve. Vagal stimulation of the pancreas results in the secretion of pancreatic enzymes with a minimum increase in bicarbonate concentration or volume.

Any disease process that obstructs the duct system or destroys the acinar cells reduces the secretion of enzymes and bicarbonate and progresses to malabsorption and damage of the duodenal mucosa from unneutralized hydrochloric acid. In the presence of pancreatic disease, secretory functions can be decreased by limiting or eliminating food ingestion, minimizing vagal stimulation with anticholinergics, and reducing acids by nasogastric suctioning and use of cimetidine or antacids. A pancreas that is not secreting properly may be partially compensated for by an increase in fat and protein in the diet, use of medium-chain triglycerides, or administration of pancreatic enzyme extracts.

The islets are spheric cells that are outgrowths from the walls of the pancreatic duct during embryonic life. The hormones released from the islets directly enter the circulation.

The endocrine functions are the secretion of glucagon (alpha cells), insulin (beta cells), and gastrin (delta cells). Glucagon causes glycogenolysis in the liver. A blood glucose level below 60 to 80 mg/dl stimulates the alpha cells to release glucagon, causing the breakdown of glycogen to glucose in the liver. A normal blood glucose level "turns off" the alpha cells.

The beta cells of the islets of Langerhans secrete insulin, which increases glucose utilization. It carries glucose by active transport through the cellular membrane. An increased blood glucose level, usually following a meal, stimulates the beta cells to release insulin. The insulin carries the glucose across the cell membrane, reducing the blood level to normal.

Normal Findings

Area of Concern	Normal Adult Findings
Mouth	
Temporomandibular joint	Mobility: smooth jaw excursion; 3.5-4.5 cm Tenderness: absent on palpation Crepitus: absent Referred pain: absent on closing jaw
Occlusion	Top back teeth rest directly on lower teeth; upper incisors slightly override lowers *Older adult:* May change because of missing teeth Marked overclosure may be associated with edentulous patient Individuals who stoop and thrust head forward tend to habitually protrude lower jaw
Lips	Color: pink Symmetry: vertical and lateral symmetry at rest and on movement Moisture: smooth and moist Surface characteristics: slight vertical linear markings *Older adult:* Decreased saliva production may contribute to drier lips and difficulty swallowing foods Vertical markings increased "Purse-string" appearance associated with edentulism or overclosure of jaws
Inner lips and buccal membrane	Color: pale coral, pink; increased pigmentation, general or localized, in dark-skinned individuals Landmarks: parotid duct; pinpoint red marking; may be slightly elevated Surface characteristics: where teeth meet, occlusion line may appear on adjacent mucosa; clear saliva over surface *Older adult:* Surface characteristics: mucosa becomes thinner and less vascular; may appear shinier than in younger adults Fordyce's granules common
Gums	Color: pink, coral Surface characteristics: slightly stippled, clearly defined, tight margin at tooth; patchy brown pigmentation in dark-skinned individuals Hypertrophy may appear during puberty or pregnancy If inflammation (gingivitis) appears, refer to dentist *Older adult:* Color: may be slightly paler Surface characteristics: stippling may be decreased
Teeth	Number: 32 (adult); upper and lower third molars may be absent Color: white, yellowish, or grayish hues Form: smooth edges Surface characteristics: smooth; dental restorations Movement: none or slight movement *Older adult:* Color: may appear more yellowish or slightly darker Form and surface characteristics: teeth may appear elongated as more root surface or neck of tooth is exposed with resorption of supporting bone
Tongue	Symmetry and movement: forward thrust smooth and symmetric; tongue appears symmetric Color: pink Surface characteristics: dorsal and lateral is moist and glistening, with papillae; elongated vallate papillae; fissures; smooth, even tissue Ventral surface: pink and smooth with large veins *Older adult:* Papillae may appear slightly smoother and shinier Epithelium is thin and loosely attached Veins may be varicosed
Floor of mouth	Frenulum is centered Submaxillary duct opening can be found Color: pale, coral pink

Adapted from Bowers, A.C., and Thompson, J.M.: Clinical manual of health assessment, ed. 3, St. Louis, 1988, The C.V. Mosby Co.

Area of Concern	Normal Adult Findings
Hard and soft palate	Color: hard palate: pale; soft palate: pink Surface characteristics Hard palate: immovable, irregular transverse rugae; midline exostosis (torus palatinus) may be present Soft palate: movable, symmetric elevation; smooth
Mouth odor	Absent or sweet
Oropharynx	Landmarks: anterior and posterior pillars symmetric; uvula midline; tonsils Color: posterior wall pink Surface characteristics: smooth; tonsils may be cryptic; slight vascularity on posterior wall
Abdomen	
Inspection	On inspection the following are normal findings Skin color: may be pale in comparison to body parts that are more exposed Surface characteristics: smooth, soft, silver-white striae Scars: configuration, location, and length Venous network: very faint, fine network Umbilicus: centrally located; usually shrunken, but may protrude slightly; should be smooth and noninflamed Contour: flat, rounded, or concave (scaphoid) Symmetry: evenly rounded with maximum height of convexity at umbilicus Surface motion: peristalsis usually not visible but may be visible in thin people; pulsations in upper midline may be visible in thin people Movement with respirations: smooth and even; female primarily exhibits costal movements while males evidence primarily abdominal movements Contour remains smooth and symmetric when patient takes a deep breath and holds it Rectus abdominis muscles are prominent; on tightening muscle, midline bulge may appear *Older adult:* Contour: geriatric patients may have an increase in fat deposits over abdominal area even though subcutaneous fat over extremities is decreased
Auscultation	Bowel sounds: usually 5-34/min; irregular; gurgles, clicks, and quality vary greatly; all four quadrants Absence of vascular sounds Absence of friction rub
Percussion	
Four abdominal quadrants	Tone: general distribution of tympany depending on amount of air and solid material in bowel; suprapubic dullness over distended bladder
Liver percussion	Lower border: usually at costal margin or slightly below Upper border: begins in fifth to seventh intercostal space Midclavicular liver span: 6-12 cm (2½-4½ inches); liver span usually greater in men than women; liver span greater in taller individuals Right midaxillary liver: liver dullness; may be heard in fifth to seventh intercostal space Midsternal liver span: 4-8 cm (1½-3 inches) Liver descent with deep inspiration: lower border should move inferiorly by 2-3 cm (¾-1 inch) *Older adult:* Lower border: in elderly patient with distended lungs, liver border is 1-2 cm (½-¾ inch) into abdominal cavity Upper border: with distended lung may descend 1-2 cm (½-¾ inch) Deep inspiration may be difficult for elderly individual
Spleen percussion*	Left posterior midaxillary line: small area of splenic dullness at sixth to tenth rib, or tone may be tympanic (colonic) Left intercostal space in anterior axillary line: tympanic Left lower rib cage: gastric "bubble"; tympanic; varies in size
Palpation	
Four abdominal quadrants	
Light and moderate palpation	Tenderness: none Muscle tone: abdomen relaxed; muscular resistance may be seen in anxious patients Surface characteristics: smooth, consistent tension opposed to localized area of rigidity (increased tension)

*If an enlarged spleen is suspected, it may be advisable to perform palpation before percussion.

Area of Concern	Normal Adult Findings
	Masses: none
	Older adult:
	Muscle tone: often more lax
Deep palpation	Tenderness: often present in midline near xiphoid process over cecum, over sigmoid colon
	Masses: aorta often palpable at epigastrium and pulsates in forward direction; can palpate borders of rectus abdominis muscles; feces may be palpated in ascending or descending colon; sacral promontory may be palpable
	Umbilicus: check for bulges, nodes, and umbilicus ring; normal findings include umbilicus ring with no irregularities or bulges; umbilicus may be inverted or slightly everted
	Older adult:
	Muscle tone: often more lax
Liver	Liver border and contour: liver often not palpable; liver may "bump" against fingers on inspiration, especially in thin people
	Liver border surface: smooth
	Tenderness: none
	Older adult:
	Liver commonly palpated 1-2 cm (½-¾ inch) below costal margin in patients with distended lungs, emphysema, and lowered diaphragm
Spleen	Spleen not normally palpable
Kidney	Occasionally lower pole of kidney may be palpable in thin individuals; right kidney most often palpable
	Contour: smooth, firm
	Tenderness: none
Inguinal nodes	Note presence of nodes: small, mobile; none tender; nodes often present
	Contour: smooth or nonpalpable
	Consistency: soft or nonpalpable
Assessment for abdominal fluid	None should be found
	Techniques for assessment include flank bulging and fluid shift
Rectal-Anal Region	Skin and surface characteristics: smooth, clear
	No tenderness in coccygeal area
	Anus: surface characteristics include increased pigmentation, coarse skin
	Sphincter muscle: tightens evenly around finger with minimal discomfort for patient
	Anal muscular ring: smooth, even pressure on finger
	Rectal wall: continuous, smooth surface (examination should cause minimal discomfort for patient)
	Stool: brown, soft

Normal Laboratory Data

Laboratory Test	Normal Adult Values
Albumin	
Whole blood, serum, or plasma	Serum quantitative (1-31 yr): 3.5-5 g/dl with A/G ratio greater than 1; after age 40, normal range gradually decreases 4-5.5 g/dl (electrophoresis)
Urine	Qualitative: random sample negative Quantitative: less than 20 mg/dl
Ammonia	
Whole blood, serum, or plasma	Varies somewhat between laboratories; 11-35 μmol/L
Urine	Ammonia nitrogen: 20-50 mEq/24 h (500-1200 mg/24 h)
Amylase	Method dependent
Ascorbic acid (vitamin C)	
Serum or plasma	0.2-2 mg/dl
Urine	Random sample: 1-7 mg/dl 24 h: >50 mg/24 h
Bicarbonate	Arterial: 21-28 mEq/L Venous: 22-29 mEq/L
Bile acids	
Whole blood, serum, or plasma	Positive: >10 cholesterol monohydrate or calcium bilirubinate crystals per slide Suspicious: 1-9 cholesterol monohydrate or calcium bilirubinate crystals per slide
Urine	Negative
Bilirubin	
Serum	Direct (conjugated): up to 0.4 mg/dl

Laboratory Test	Normal Adult Values
	Indirect (unconjugated): 0.1-1 mg/dl Total: 0.3-1 mg/dl
Urine	Qualitative: random sample negative
Calcium	
Serum	Ionized: 3.9-4.8 mg/dl for one formula available Total (up to 30 yr): 8.2-10.5 mg/dl; decreases very slightly in older years
Urine	Qualitative (Sulkowitch; random): 1+ turbidity Quantitative: varies with diet; based on average calcium intake of 600-800 mg/24 h: 100-250 mg/24 h (average diet); <150 mg/24 h (low calcium diet); 250-300 mg/24 h (high calcium diet)
Chloride	
Serum	97-107 mEq/L
Urine	24-h collection: 110-250 mEq/24 h in adults; lower values in infancy and childhood; results depend on ingestion of chloride
Cholesterol	
Serum	See footnote*
Coagulation	
Bleeding time (Ivy)	2-7 min
Bleeding time (Duke)	5 min
Clot reaction	Half in the original mass in 2 h
Dilute blood clot lysis time	Clot still intact after 2 h is "normal"
Euglobin clot lysis time	Lysis time >90 min
Partial thromboplastin time	25-39 s, usually stated to be within 10 s of control; kaolin activated: 35-50 s
Prothrombin time	10-13 s
Venous clotting time	8-15 min
Whole blood clot lysis time	None in 24 h
Creatine as creatinine	
Serum or plasma	Male: 0.1-0.4 mg/dl Female: 0.2-0.7 mg/dl
Urine	Creatine excretion decreases with advanced age as muscle mass diminishes Male: 0-40 mg/24 h Female: 0-100 mg/24 h (higher in pregnancy)
Creatinine	
Serum	Men: up to 1.2 mg/dl Women: up to 1.1 mg/dl There are slight differences between the sexes with males higher since range relates to amount of muscle mass present
Urine	Male: 1-2 g/24 h Female: 0.8-1.8 g/24 h
Creatinine clearance (endogenous)	Male: 85-125 ml/min/1.73 sq m Female: 75-115 ml/min/1.73 sq m
Fatty acids	
Serum	Total (free and esterified): 9.5 mM
Plasma	Free (nonesterified): 300-480 μEq/L
Urine	Fat (qualitative): random sample negative
Fibrinogen	
Plasma	200-400 mg/dl
Folate	
Whole blood, serum, or plasma	>2 ng/ml
Fructose	
Urine	24-h collection: 30-65 mg/24 h
Galactose	
Whole blood	None
Urine	<10 mg/dl
Gamma globulin	
Serum	0.5-1.6 g/dl
Globulins (total)	
Serum	2.3-3.5 g/dl
Urine	No monoclonal gammopathy detected
Glucose	
Fasting	
Serum or plasma	60-115 mg/dl (normal range increases with age over 50)
Whole blood	60-100 mg/dl
Oral glucose tolerance (serum or plasma)	Fasting: 60-115 mg/dl (normal range increases with age over 50) 30 min: 30-60 mg/dl above fasting 60 min: 20-50 mg/dl above fasting 120 min: 5-15 mg/dl above fasting 180 min: fasting level or below
2-h postprandial	0-50 yr: 70-140 mg/dl 50-60 yr: 70-150 mg/dl 60 yr and up: 70-160 mg/dl

*Sharp inconsistencies are obvious when one studies published normal ranges of serum cholesterol in the United States. Although 100-210 mg/dl would be regarded as a low normal range for American adults, an increase between ages 25 and 45 of about 25 mg/dl is recognized. Levels above 180 are not desirable but are commonplace in the United States, and adult normal ranges over 300 mg/dl are offered.

Laboratory Test	Normal Adult Values
Intravenous glucose tolerance (serum or plasma)	Fasting: 70-110 mg/dl 5 min: maximum of 250 mg/dl 60 min: significant decrease 120 min: <120 mg/dl 180 min: fasting level
Random glucose	Dependent on time and content of last meal
Urine	Qualitative: random sample negative Quantitative (24 h): copper reducing substances: 0.5-1.5 g/24 h Glucose: up to 100 mg/24 h
Glucose-6-phosphate dehydrogenase (G6PD)	140-280 U/billion cells
Gamma glutamyl transferase	
Serum	5-40 IU/L
Haptoglobin	
Serum	40-180 mg/dl but values are method dependent
Hematocrit	Male: 40-47 ml/dl Female: 37-42 ml/dl
Hemoglobin	
Whole blood, serum, or plasma	Male: 15.5 ± 1.1 g/dl Female: 13.7 ± 1 g/dl
Urine	Random sample, negative
Immunoglobulins	
Serum	IgG: 564-1765 mg/dl IgA: 85-385 mg/dl IgM: 53-375 mg/dl IgD: 0-40 mg/dl IgE: 0.01-0.04 mg/dl
Iron	
Serum	Total: 42-135 μg/dl Binding capacity: 218-385 μg/dl Saturation: 20%-50%
Ketone bodies	
Serum	Negative
Urine	Random sample negative
17-Ketosteroids	
Plasma	25-125 μg/dl
Urine	Male: 6-22 mg/24 h Female: 4-17 mg/24 h (with decrease in advancing years)
Lactose	
Lactic acid (lactate)	Venous: 5-20 mg/dl Arterial: 3-7 mg/dl
Lactose intolerance	Increase of blood glucose <20 mg/dl over fasting level, with symptoms, is considered abnormal; evidence for lactase deficiency; >30 mg/dl is normal
Urine	14-40 mg/24 h
Lipase	Method dependent
Lipids	
Serum	Total: 400-800 mg/dl Cholesterol* Triglycerides† Phospholipids: 150-380 mg/dl Fatty acids (free): 9-15 mM/L (300-480 mEq/L) Phospholipid phosphorus: 8-11 mg/dl
Feces	
Macroglobulins, total‡	
Whole blood, serum, or plasma	53-375 mg/dl
Magnesium	
Serum	1.2-1.9 mEq/L (may be expressed in mg/dl)
Urine	5-16 mEq/24 h
Mean corpuscular volume	Male: 80-100 μ^3 Female: 79-98 μ^3
Mucoprotein	
Serum	80-200 mg/dl
Mucin	
Urine	100-150 mg/24 h
Osmolality	
Serum	280-300 mOsm/kg H_2O
Urine	Random sample: 250-900 mOsm/kg H_2O
pH	
Whole blood	Arterial: 7.35-7.45 Venous: 7.32-7.43
Serum or plasma	Venous: 7.35-7.45
Urine	Random sample: 4.8-7.8
Phenylalanine	
Serum	>3 mg/dl
Phospholipid phosphorus	
Serum	8-11 mg/dl
Phospholipids	
Serum	150-380 mg/dl
Phosphorus, inorganic	
Serum	2.5-4.5 mg/dl

*Sharp inconsistencies are obvious when one studies published normal ranges of serum cholesterol in the United States. Although 100-210 mg/dl would be regarded as a low normal range for American adults, an increase between ages 25 and 45 of about 25 mg/dl is recognized. Levels above 180 are not desirable but are commonplace in the United States, and adult normal ranges over 300 mg/dl are offered.

†Different ranges are in use. Moderate increases from childhood occur. At the 95th percentile: white males, 25-29 yr: up to 250 mg/dl; 35-54 yr: up to 320 mg/dl; 55-64 yr: up to 290 mg/dl; 65 yr and over: up to 260 mg/dl; white females, 35-39 yr: up to 195 mg/dl; 55-64 yr: up to 250 mg/dl.

‡Immunoglobulin M now replaces this; values are for immunoglobulin M.

Laboratory Test	Normal Adult Values
Urine	Random sample: 0.9-1.3 g/24 h (dependent on dietary intake)
Potassium	
Plasma	3.5-5 mEq/L; add approximately 0.2 to normal ranges if serum is sampled rather than plasma
Urine	40-80 mEq/24 h
Platelet count	
Whole blood, serum, or plasma	150,000-400,000/mm^3
Protein	
Serum	Total: 6-8 g/dl Albumin: 3.5-5 g/dl witl A/G ratio >1 Globulin: 2.3-3.5 g/dl Electrophoresis Albumin: 58%-74%* 4 5.5 g/dl† Alpha-1: 2%-3.5%; 0.15-0.25 g/dl Alpha-2: 5.4%-10.6%; 0.43-0.75 g/dl Beta: 7%-14%; 0.5-1 g/dl Gamma: 8%-18%; 0.6-1.3 g/dl
Urine	Qualitative random sample negative 24 h: 30-150 mg/24 h (method dependent)
Prothrombin time	10-13 sec
Sodium	
Serum or plasma	135-145 mEq/L
Urine	27-287 mEq/24 h (varies markedly with dietary intake of sodium); there is also diurnal variation (output lower at night)
Transferases	
Serum	Aspartate aminotransferase (AST or SGOT): levels in infancy are two to three times those found in adults; ranges decrease during childhood years; SMA method: 16 yr and up: 8-42 U/L Alanine aminotransferase: slightly increased ranges in infancy compared to adult normal range; adult: 3-30 IU/L depending on method Gamma glutamyl transferase (GGT): 5-40 IU/L at 37° C
Triglycerides	
Whole blood, serum, or plasma	Different ranges are in use; moderate increases from childhood occur; at 95th percentile: white males: 25-29 yr: up to 250 mg/dl; 35-54 yr: up to 320 mg/dl; 55-64 yr: up to 290 mg/dl; 65 and over: up to 260 mg/dl; white females: 35-39 yr: up to 195 mg/dl; 55-64 yr: up to 250 mg/dl
Urea nitrogen	
Blood	1-40 yr: 5-20 mg/dl; gradual slight increase subsequently occurs
Urine	6-17 g/24 h
Urea clearance	
Serum and urine	Maximum: 64-99 ml/min Standard: 41-65 ml/min or >75% of normal clearance
Uric acid	
Serum	Male: 3.4-7 mg/dl or slightly higher Female: 2.4-6 mg/dl or slightly higher
Urine	Approx. 250-750 mg/24 h
Urobilinogen	
Urine	2-h collection Male: 0.3-2.1 mg/2 h Female: 0.1-1.1 mg/2 h Can be expressed in Ehrlich units (1 mg urobilinogen = 1 EU) 24-h collection: 0.05-2.5 mg/24 h or 0.5-4 Ehrlich units/24 h
Vitamin A	
Serum	15-60 μg/dl Vitamin A tolerance: fasting 3 h or 6 h after 5000 U: 15-60 μ/dl Vitamin A/kg/24: 200-600 μg/dl; fasting values are higher
Vitamin B_{12}	
Serum	160-950 pg/ml Unsaturated vitamin B_{12} binding capacity: 1000-2000 pg/ml
Vitamin C	
Serum or plasma	0.2-2 mg/dl
Urine	Random sample: 1-7 mg/dl 24 h: >50 mg/24 h (as ascorbic acid)
Zinc	
Whole blood, serum, or plasma	0.66-1.1 μg/ml
Urine	0.15-1.2 mg/24 h

*Percentage of total protein.
†Concentration.

Conditions, Diseases, and Disorders

ORAL CAVITY DISORDERS

Glossitis

Glossitis is a chronic or acute inflammation of the tongue.

Glossitis is manifest as a reddened, inflamed, smooth, and sore tongue, which is usually due to one of several causes:

1. Ulcerations, from stomatitis, lichen planus, or carcinomas of the tongue, can cause glossitis.

2. Anemia (usually iron deficiency or pernicious anemia) is one of the most common causes of glossitis. Other vitamin B group deficiencies can also produce glossitis, as can the presence of candidiasis.

3. Sometimes a patient's tongue appears normal, but the patient complains of soreness. In these cases anemia must be ruled out, but depression and other psychogenic causes or factors have been known to cause a painful tongue.

4. Geographic tongue, the cause of which is unknown, is manifest as irregular, smooth, red areas with sharply defined borders that heal and then reappear in a few days. Examination reveals thinning of the epithelium in the middle of the lesion with mild hyperplasia and hyperkeratosis around the edges. Some chronic inflammatory cells can be found in the underlying tissue. Most patients are asymptomatic, but some complain of soreness and hypersensitivity to certain foods.

A variation of geographic tongue is hairy tongue, in which the filiform papillae become elongated and resemble hair. The papillae can vary in length and color; the cause is unknown, but usually only adults are affected. Some drugs, for example, clindamycin, can also cause these papillae.

Treatment for glossitis consists of correction of the underlying cause if known, pain relief, meticulous mouth care, and a bland diet if necessary for patient comfort.

Leukoplakia

Leukoplakia is persistent white patches in the oral mucosa that cannot be removed by the patient.

Increased keratin production is known to cause the whitish appearance, but its development can be the result of many factors. A small percentage of leukoplakias (about 5%) undergo malignant change and become squamous cell carcinomas. Biopsies should be done on all leukoplakias to determine the probable cause.

Pathophysiology

The causes of leukoplakia vary. Friction from cheek biting or prolonged denture wearing can cause lesions that are initially pale and translucent and later become white and thick with a rough surface. Smoking, usually pipe smoking, causes a lesion that is probably formed from both chemical components of the smoke and irritation from the heat.

Tertiary syphilis (which is rare today) produces a characteristic leukoplakia on the dorsum of the tongue.

Another uncommon cause is white sponge nevus, a familial disorder characterized by large, soft thickening of the superficial epithelial layers. The entire inner surface of the mouth can be affected by the thick, white plaque. Although untreatable, this is a benign condition.

Patients who have chronic candidal infections in their mouths have plaque formed from epithelial overgrowth. This is another uncommon cause and is treated with local or systemic antifungal agents.

Most commonly, leukoplakias are of unknown etiology. In these patients the degree of hyperkeratinosis ranges from simple to severe. Treatment of choice may be local excision of the leukoplakia. However, recurrence is common, so many physicians simply choose to see the patient frequently to observe for any changes in the appearance of the leukoplakia; if changes do occur, they perform periodic biopsies to assess for malignancy.

There are three types of leukoplakia: simplex, verrucous, and erosive, depending on its degree and likelihood of malignant transformation. Leukoplakia simplex, which is the smooth and nonindurated type, rarely results in malignant change, while erosive leukoplakia more commonly becomes malignant.

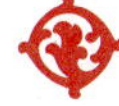

Periodontal disease

The term "peridontal disease" refers to diseases of the supporting tissues of the teeth that are usually inflammatory.

The characteristic feature of chronic periodontitis is the destruction of these supporting tissues; almost every case begins with chronic gingivitis, which, if not treated properly, progresses to the irreversible chronic periodontitis, loosening, and loss of teeth.

Acute Gingivitis

Acute ulceromembranous gingivitis, also called trench mouth, is usually seen in young adults who have neglected oral hygiene but is also frequently seen in parts of Africa where malnutrition, anemia, and malaria are rampant.

Although the exact cause is unclear, two particular organisms, *Bacteroides vincenti* and *Fusobacterium fusiforme,* are thought to be implicated in this infection that may also require lowered host resistance. The inflammation starts at the tips of the interdental papillae and progresses quickly to involve the gingival membranes and periodontal tissues. Crater-shaped ulcers with erythematous, edematous edges are characteristic, with a thick yellowish or grayish material over the surface of the ulcer. Bleeding occurs if this material is removed.

The infection remains localized, although the mouth is very sore and the gums bleed; the patient experiences no fever, malaise, or lymphadenopathy.

Treatment is with antibiotics for the specific organism and oral hygiene measures to reduce the acute oral infection. The patient and family must also be given explicit instructions in the performance of meticulous oral hygiene.

Chronic Gingivitis

Almost everyone has a degree of chronic gingivitis. It is probably caused by the accumulation of plaque around the neck of the tooth, which if not removed adequately by toothbrushing, involves the epithelium and progresses to the periodontal membrane and alveolar bone, causing osteoporotic loss of bone and finally loss of the teeth. Gingivitis can develop in 2 days if plaque is allowed to accumulate, and there is a correlation between the amount of plaque and the severity of the gingivitis.

Although the exact relationship between gingivitis and the destruction of the supporting tissues is not clearly understood, it is probable that the bacteria present in the plaque begin an inflammatory response that is assisted by interactions between antibodies, complement, neutrophils, lymphocytes, and macrophages. Immunologic responses have also been implicated.

As plaque begins to collect at the neck of the teeth, inflammatory changes occur in the gingiva. The epithelium becomes hyperplastic, blood vessels dilate, and some extend almost to the surface, causing the gums to appear darker than normal, even purplish, as a result of congestion. These inflammatory cells spread so that the gingiva appears edematous, soft, and slightly glazed. The gums bleed easily, and there is usually a collection of calculus, or calcified plaque, above the gingival margins.

Chronic gingivitis, if it has not progressed further than the gingiva, will subside if meticulous oral hygiene is begun and followed strictly. Part of the treatment must be aimed at teaching the patient and family about oral hygiene, diet principles, and the progression of the disease if these instructions are not followed.

Periodontitis

Acute periodontitis is quite uncommon and usually does not last long. It can be caused by trauma, most often from biting on a hard object, which may produce some minor damage that heals quickly; a periodontal abscess, which is a complication of periodontal disease; or progression from ulceromembranous gingivitis if untreated.

However, chronic periodontitis is very common and is also important because it is the main reason for loss of teeth in adults. As discussed in the section on chronic gingivitis, periodontitis is usually a continuation of that process, since untreated infection of the gingiva leads to progressive inflammation and destruction of the supporting structures of the teeth.

The four main features of chronic periodontitis are destruction of periodontal membrane fibers, resorption of alveolar bone, migration of the epithelial attachment along the root toward the apex, and formation of pockets around the teeth.[12]

The pocket formation is characteristic of periodontitis; these pockets form a closed space where bacteria (and possibly anaerobic bacteria) grow. The infected material cannot drain, and these bacteria irritate the tissues.

Clinical symptoms include bleeding from the gums, a bad taste in the mouth, and foul-smelling breath; later there is gum recession and loosening of the teeth. The gingiva appears purplish and swollen, and plaque and calculus are evident.

The best treatment is prevention; regular and thorough toothbrushing and removal of plaque would make any further treatment or surgery unnecessary. However, surgery is necessary when the disease has been neglected, pockets have formed, and the gingiva cannot be restored to normal without surgical intervention.

Patients who are considered for surgery must realize that they will have to expend some effort to maintain their teeth during the postoperative period. The rationale for surgery includes debridement and removal of plaque and calculus and restoring soft tissue and bone to its normal contour and state of health.

Several surgical procedures may be carried out, depending on the severity of the periodontal disease. A local anesthetic is used in most cases, and patients rarely require hospitalization. Patient education remains a vital part of the overall treatment because, if a patient is unaware of or fails to comply with meticulous oral hygiene measures, the disease will undoubtedly recur or progress. When the disease has reached the point where surgery would not be useful, the teeth must be extracted and the patient will have to wear dentures.

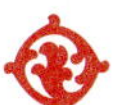

Salivary gland disorders

Disorders or inflammation can occur in the parotid, sublingual, or submaxillary glands.

Salivary gland disorders can be classified into several categories: inflammation, as in mumps and acute and chronic sialadenitis; obstruction, as in calculi; and degenerative diseases and neoplasms, which are not discussed here. Dry mouth (xerostomia), which may be caused by damaged salivary glands, is an unpleasant problem and can be the result of local or systemic causes as well as chronic anxiety states.

Pathophysiology

Inflammation of the salivary glands is most commonly caused by mumps. Mumps is discussed further in Chapter 13.

Less common infections are acute ascending parotitis and chronic sialadenitis. Acute ascending parotitis is the result of dehydration and inattention to oral hygiene, sometimes during or immediately after surgery in which an endotracheal tube has been used and placed pressure on the salivary ducts. This has also occurred in patients who have nasogastric tubes, swelling, and severe throat infection, resulting in painful swelling of the glands with fever and malaise. Purulent material can be expressed from the duct. This disorder can be prevented by proper hydration, good oral hygiene, and care taken during surgery to avoid trauma to the duct orifices.

Chronic sialadenitis is usually caused by chronic duct obstruction, which may be due to mucus plugs or other causes. It is usually unilateral, and the patient experiences painful swelling of the gland accompanied by an inflamed duct and purulent discharge from the orifice. Treatment is removal of the obstruction or excision of the gland.

Obstructions of the salivary glands are usually caused by calculi, although mucoceles and cysts may also form, and these must be excised. Calculi formation is quite common, and most (80%) of them form in the submandibular gland and Wharton's duct. About 10% to 12% form in the parotid gland or Stensen's duct, and the rest are in the sublingual and minor salivary glands. Although salivary calculi occur at any age, they are uncommon in children. Men are affected twice as often as women.

These stones are composed mainly of calcium and phosphate and tend to form more frequently in the submandibular gland because its saliva has a high pH and is viscous because of a high mucin content. This gland also may be irritated by the teeth during chewing, and it is larger in diameter and longer than the parotid duct.

Usually pain and swelling occur suddenly during eating and subside within a short time. Symptoms may not occur with every meal, and sometimes the patient is asymptomatic until the stone enlarges, moves along the duct, and can be felt in the mouth. Usually there is no inflammation, but occasionally a gland or duct becomes infected, indicated by increased swelling and tenderness over the gland and purulent discharge from the orifice. Pain and fever accompany this infection.

Dry mouth can result from a variety of transient and chronic causes. Fear and acute anxiety are the most common causes of transient dry mouth. Chronic conditions can be caused by mouth breathing, heavy smoking, some drugs such as antihistamines and sympathomimetics, chronic anxiety states, and treatment with radiation to the head and neck, which causes damage to the salivary glands. Salivary calculi do not cause xerostomia.

Diagnostic Studies and Findings

Roentgenograms of Lateral and Oblique Views of Jaw and Upper Neck

May demonstrate large stones

Roentgenograms Using Dental Film to Project through Floor of Mouth from Below

Demonstrate small stones

Medical Plan

Surgery

Surgical removal if stone cannot be removed by manual manipulation

Medications

Narcotic analgesics
- Meperidine (Demerol), 50-75 mg IM q4-6h as needed for pain relief
- Tylenol with codeine, 30-60 mg q4-6h as needed for pain relief

General Management

Many stones can be removed by manipulation of duct

NURSING CARE

Nursing Assessment

Inflammation

Localized swelling
Fever; malaise
Purulent discharge from orifice of duct
Dehydration

Obstruction

Pain and swelling related to chewing; may be transient or infrequent
Palpation of stone in gland or duct

Nursing Dx & Intervention

Nursing Diagnosis	Nursing Intervention/Rationale
Pain	• Assess degree of discomfort. • Provide analgesia for pain relief and assess and document effectiveness. • Provide hard sour candies for patient to suck.
Altered oral mucous membrane	• Assess for signs of infection in opened or excised duct, if stone has been surgically removed. • Instruct patient in meticulous mouth care and ways *to prevent or minimize dry mouth (e.g., mouthwash, toothettes, or hard sour candies).*

Patient Education

1. Instruct the patient in oral hygiene measures.
2. Inform the patient of the symptoms of inflammation and calculi, and encourage the patient to seek medical treatment when these occur.
3. Inform the patient that calculi tend to recur in some people.

Evaluation

Patient Outcome	Data Indicating That Outcome is Reached
Inflammation is resolved.	There is no localized pain, swelling, or fever. Patient verbalizes understanding of symptoms of inflammation and calculi and when to seek medical treatment. Patient verbalizes understanding of oral hygiene measures.

Stomatitis

Stomatitis is ulceration in the mouth that may be on the gums or the oral mucosa.

Stomatitis may be a single lesion, as from a local injury, or widespread, caused by systemic factors. Stomatitis is mainly inflammatory, and there are several types: viral, bacterial, noninfective, and drug related. It may result from excessive smoking, spicy foods, poor nutrition, poor oral hygiene, or allergic responses. All types of stomatitis are usually quite painful and therefore may inhibit food ingestion; this can be a major problem in an already debilitated patient.

Pathophysiology

Herpetic stomatitis is the most common form of viral stomatitis; after an initial infection, usually in infancy or childhood, it begins with vesicle formation. After the rupture of the vesicles and the shedding of the cells, an ulcer is visible. These ulcers are usually scattered over the mucous membranes and are circular and about 3 to 4 mm in diameter. The gingivae are swollen and inflamed, and the local lymph nodes are usually swollen. The patient may have an elevated temperature, increased salivation, and severe mouth pain. These lesions usually clear in 7 to 10 days.

After the primary infection, many people are subject to recurrent infections. These are usually not within the mouth but affect the skin around the lips at the mucocutaneous junctions. These infections, known as herpes labialis, are caused by the herpes simplex virus and are discussed further in Chapter 13.

Angular stomatitis, which is the result of iron deficiency anemia, causes inflammatory changes at the angles of the mouth that vary from reddening to ulcerated, crusting fissures. More common in elderly patients with full dentures, it can cause deep folds at the corners of the mouth, where infection can spread if not treated, making the condition much more extensive. Lack of vitamins such as niacin and riboflavin can cause cellular weakening, since cell growth, oxidation, and metabolism are impaired.

Denture stomatitis is caused by occlusion of the mucous membranes by a tight-fitting denture for a long time. This creates a closed environment in which organisms can grow. Although the patient may be asymptomatic, there is normally a reddened, erythematous area corresponding to the area covered by the denture. These patients should leave their dentures out, at least at night, to allow the mucous membranes to heal.

Aphthous stomatitis is one of the more common diseases affecting the mucous membranes. The underlying cause of these small, yellowish, very painful ulcers is unclear, although several factors have been implicated (virus, allergy, gastrointestinal disease, psychosomatic causes). Women are affected slightly more often than men. The disease is most troublesome in adolescence or early adult life and often clears up by early middle age. The first sign of aphthous stomatitis is usually a pricking feeling in the mucous membrane, followed soon after by eruption of painful ulcers that may appear alone or in groups. They resemble craters with red, raised margins, and they usually heal in a week or so without scarring.

Thrush, or oral candidiasis, is one of the most common types of stomatitis. This mycotic stomatitis is characterized by white plaques on the oral mucous membrane, gums, and tongue. It is frequently seen in patients who are malnourished, diabetic, or taking antibiotics (since they destroy the normal oral flora) and in oncology patients.

Although *Candida* is part of the normal mouth flora, some weakening of the body's resistance can permit an increase in its growth (usually *C. albicans* or *C. tropicalis*). Fungal spores lodge between the epithelial cells and cause a gradual separation of the layers, spreading the infection to the surface of the mucous membrane and the rest of the mouth. White patchy growths appear in several areas of the mucous membrane and spread so a continuous membrane forms.

One of the more distressing types of stomatitis appears as a result of drug treatment. It is frequently seen in patients who have been taking systemic antibiotics for long periods and who have bacterial overgrowth in the mucous membranes or in patients receiving chemotherapy for cancer treatment, and it may be quite debilitating since the patient may already have a lowered resistance to infection. In a severely leukopenic patient, necrotizing ulceration of the mucous membranes, gums, and throat may occur, which can in turn cause septicemia. Usually, these ulcers appear on the mucous membranes in any number and are very painful. They may cause increased salivation and prevent the patient from eating normally.

Medical Plan

Medications

Anesthetic agents
- Topical anesthetic (viscous lidocaine [Xylocaine] as needed)

Vitamins
- Vitamin replacement if caused by underlying deficiency

Anti-infective agents
- Nystatin (Mycostatin) oral suspension or lozenges for *Candida* every 6 hours

General Management

Well-balanced diet; bland if necessary; high in protein, calories, and needed vitamins

Mild mouthwashes for comfort

NURSING CARE

Nursing Assessment

Oral Mucous Membrane

Painful, ulcerated areas on oral mucous membranes that may appear yellowish with reddened, raised edges

Increased salivation

Halitosis

General Well-Being

Fever and lymphadenopathy with primary herpetic stomatitis

Malaise

Nutritional Status

Sensitivity to spicy foods and discomfort when eating

History of dietary habits; recent or current chemotherapeutic or antibiotic regimen; debilitated physical appearance

Presence of dentures in angular and denture stomatitis

Nursing Dx & Intervention

Nursing Diagnosis	Nursing Intervention/Rationale
Pain	• Assess patient for discomfort related to eating. • Provide analgesia as prescribed, especially before meals. Topical anesthetic agents such as viscous lidocaine (Xylocaine) may be helpful in relieving the discomfort.
Altered oral mucous membrane	• Assess oral mucous membrane for indications of ulcerations. • Provide mouthwashes, avoiding those with alcohol since they are irritating, and assist patient with thorough but gentle mouth care. • Keep lips lubricated *to prevent drying and further irritation.* • Administer nystatin (Mycostatin) if ordered. Freezing nystatin may make it more tolerable for patient. • Offer ice or ice chips to suck *for a numbing effect.*
Altered nutrition: less than body requirements	• Assess patient's nutritional status. • Assess patient's oral intake and make note of any decrease in intake associated with discomfort when eating.

Nursing Diagnosis	Nursing Intervention/Rationale
	• Provide dietary consultation *to produce a palatable, nourishing diet that is high in protein, calories, and vitamins*. Instruct patient to avoid hot, spicy foods. A bland or full liquid diet may be more tolerable. • Maintain needed level of hydration, intravenously, as prescribed.

Patient Education

1. Teach the patient the importance of continued meticulous mouth care.
2. Instruct the patient and family in maintenance of a proper diet.
3. If stomatitis is herpetic, inform the patient of its infective nature and instruct in isolation and handwashing techniques.

Evaluation

Patient Outcome	Data Indicating That Outcome is Reached
Stomatitis is resolved.	Oral mucous membranes do not have painful lesions. Patient's weight and hydration are maintained at normal levels. Patient understands infective nature of herpetic lesions and necessity of handwashing and isolation techniques.

ESOPHAGEAL DISORDERS

Achalasia

Achalasia is a neuromuscular disorder of the esophageal motility that is characterized by failure of the lower esophageal sphincter to relax, esophageal dilation, and hypertrophy.

Achalasia is normally found in adults but may be seen in children and even in infants. In a geriatric patient, achalasia may be related to cancer of the lower end of the esophagus. In a very young individual, achalasia may be associated with familial glucocorticoid deficiency. Trauma of the tissues during vagotomy may result in a transient condition simulating achalasia.

The cause of achalasia is unknown. Although there are reports of several cases in one family, it has not been classified as hereditary. Emotional factors may exaggerate or trigger a latent defect. Achalasia appears to be of neurogenic origin, but how, where, and why are unknown.

Pathophysiology

There are three pathophysiologic changes in achalasia: elevated lower esophageal sphincter pressure, residual pressure after swallowing because of poor relaxation of the lower esophageal sphincter, and aperistalsis of the body of the esophagus.

The esophageal sphincter pressure is elevated to approximately 50 mm Hg (twice normal level). This high pressure does not relax with swallowing. In a normal situation the lower esophageal sphincter pressure drops to the level of the stomach pressure. In achalasia the pressure drops but not enough to permit unrestricted passage of food into the stomach.

The lower esophageal sphincter is sensitive to the stimulatory effects of gastrin and cholinergic drugs. Gastrin is responsible for the normal tone of the sphincter. There is some suggestion that oversensitivity to endogenous gastrin results in achalasia. When endogenous gastrin activity is inhibited by infusion of acid into the stomach, lower esophageal sphincter pressure drops in the achalasia patient. Exogenous gastrin in achalasia leads to a significant increase in pressure. This reaction is considered to be the result of denervation of the sphincter. The denervation is the key abnormality, and the sensitivity to gastrin is the reason for the high pressure.

Motility disturbances in the body of the esophagus mean that the peristalsis is weak and ineffectual in pushing a bolus of food through the closed sphincter. Aperistalsis may be located throughout the length of the esophagus. The esophagus may empty only when the hydrostatic pressure of its contents is great enough to overcome the pressure resistance in the lower esophageal sphincter. Since esophageal emptying depends on gravity in this case, emptying is improved if the person is sitting rather than lying down.

In the early stages the body of the esophagus is dilated symmetrically. In later stages the esophagus dilates considerably, lengthens, and curves. The body of the esophagus may bend and rest on the diaphragm. A dilated esophagus in achalasia may hold 1 to 2 L of fluid.

Diagnostic Studies and Findings

Splash-Down Time

Length of time between swallowing and reaching the stomach, normally 8 to 10 seconds, is lengthened or not heard at all

Radiography Studies: Chest Roentgenogram, Barium Swallow

Possible aspiration pneumonia
Presence of food in esophagus

Manometry: Pressure Readings

Elevated lower esophageal sphincter pressure (50 mm Hg or above) and residual pressure after swallowing

Radionuclide Scans for Esophageal Emptying

Decreased or delayed esophageal emptying

Endoscopy

Particularly in geriatric patient, to rule out cancer
Aperistalsis of body of esophagus
Possible presence of tumor

Video or Line Esophagram

Barium is swallowed and followed on tape

Medical Plan

Surgery

May be required when dilation cannot be done or is unsuccessful

Surgical procedure used is an esophagomyotomy, which divides muscle fibers enclosing esophagus, allowing mucosa to pouch out through divisions in muscle layers; when this surgery includes the cardiac end of the stomach, it is referred to as a cardiomyotomy

Medications*

Sublingual isosorbide dinitrate (Isordil), 5 mg
Oral isosorbide dinitrate (Isordil), 10 mg
Slow channel blocking drugs (calcium ion antagonist): verapamil (Isoptin) or nifedipine (Procardia capsules); dosage varies in clinical studies, and overall benefits are still uncertain

*Used with varying benefits.

General Management

Forceful dilation of esophagus is primary treatment and is done to decrease ability of sphincter to react to stretch

Bougienage: simple passage of a mercury-filled bougie; normally the swallowed bougie reaches lower esophageal sphincter and after a pause drops into stomach to prove absence of a tight sphincter

Carcinoma following treatment remains a possibility, and diagnosis may be more difficult because of lack of early symptoms; a tumor in the dilated esophagus may be large before obstructive symptoms develop; pain and dysphagia associated with carcinomas may be assumed to be part of the primary diagnosis of achalasia

Pulmonary problems may still develop after dilation from overflow at night, and patient instruction should include refraining from oral intake 1 to 2 hours before bedtime

NURSING CARE

Nursing Assessment

Digestion

Dysphagia, without pain; apparent abrupt onset

Gradual symptoms and adaptation techniques of patients include fullness after meals; swallowing water or bicarbonate of soda after a meal; and using a modified Valsalva maneuver after a meal

Regurgitation of retained material can be recognized as food eaten hours earlier; nocturnal regurgitation may be severe

Dysphagia becomes continuous and annoying with difficulty first with liquids and later with solids

Little belching because of tonic condition of lower esophageal sphincter

Chest pain may be associated with esophageal spasm or esophageal irritation from retained food

Nocturnal regurgitation may be associated with overflow of food and fluids into bronchi, with development of pulmonary disease or aspiration pneumonia

Carcinoma of esophagus more frequent in patients with achalasia

Nutritional Status

Gradual weight loss

Vomiting (overflow from esophagus): does not have "sour" characteristics of emesis from stomach (usually undigested or stale food)

Nursing Dx & Intervention

Nursing Diagnosis	Nursing Intervention/Rationale
Altered nutrition: less than body requirements	• Assess patient to determine which foods patient can and cannot swallow. • Provide diet that avoids alcohol, spicy foods, or foods at temperature extremes, *since these items may be irritating to the esophagus.*

Nursing Diagnosis	Nursing Intervention/Rationale
	• Instruct patient to eat slowly, chew food thoroughly, and arch the back while swallowing *to facilitate swallowing.* • Instruct patient to eat sitting upright and remain sitting after completion of the meal, *since emptying of the esophagus is improved if patient is sitting.* • Request nutritional consultation. • Administer medications as ordered *to relieve discomfort, thus promoting appetite.*
Potential for aspiration	• Elevate head of bed while patient sleeps *to avoid regurgitation or aspiration.*
Anxiety	• Allow patient to express concerns and frustration regarding disruption of mealtimes and inability to participate in social functions involving food. • See nursing diagnoses on p. 1743.

Patient Education

1. Instruct the patient to avoid eating or drinking for at least 2 hours before bedtime. Using more than one pillow, with head and shoulders slightly elevated, may also be indicated.
2. Teach the patient how to perform the Valsalva maneuver to increase hydrostatic pressure in the esophagus and relax the lower esophageal sphincter.
3. Instruct the patient in preparation of liquid foods to maintain nutritional status if solid foods cause dysphagia.
4. Inform the patient of signs and symptoms of pneumonia or other pulmonary problems.
5. Inform the patient of the relationship between achalasia and a slightly higher incidence of esophageal cancer and of the difficulty of distinguishing between the symptoms.

Evaluation

Patient Outcome	Data Indicating That Outcome is Reached
Nutritional status is adequate.	Patient maintains healthy status.
There are no pulmonary problems.	Patient verbalizes an understanding of the relationship between eating, lying down, and pulmonary problems and verbalizes strategies to prevent aspiration. Patient continues to have medical follow-up for managing achalasia and for regular assessments for esophageal cancer.

Esophageal diverticulum

An esophageal diverticulum is a hollow outpouching of the esophageal wall.

A true diverticulum contains all layers of the esophageal wall, while a false diverticulum lacks a muscular coat. Diverticula in the esophagus are also defined as pulsion or traction. A pulsion diverticulum is pushed out of the esophagus into adjacent structures. This effect is called tubercupressure.[78] A traction diverticulum is pulled out of the esophagus by adjacent inflammatory tissue. A diverticulum in the posterior pharynx is known as Zenker's diverticulum, and although not esophageal, it is considered in discussions on esophageal diverticulum. Zenker's diverticulum is three times more common than esophageal diverticula and is more common in men than in women. Esophageal diverticula are rare.

Pathophysiology

The only diverticula of consequence are those that retain food or fluid. Zenker's diverticulum is related to a developmental weakness of the muscular coat of the posterior portion of the pharynx. A small hernia of the esophageal wall is pushed out with swallowing and forms a diverticulum. Zenker's diverticulum can enlarge and obstruct the esophagus.

Most diverticula are found in the middle section of the esophagus. Tuberculosis has been associated with inflammation, which results in traction diverticula. Epiphrenic diverticula are located just above the cardioesophageal junction, are rare, and are associated with motility disorders such as esophageal spasm.

Diverticula may obstruct and perforate the esophagus.

Diagnostic Studies and Findings

Barium Swallow

Herniation of esophageal wall

Endoscopy

Herniation of esophageal wall (not always recommended since there is an increased incidence of perforation of the diverticulum)

Medical Plan

Surgery

Epiphrenic diverticulum: removed with esophagomyotomy; advised if motility problems are also present

Zenker's diverticulum: one-stage procedure, along the left sternocleidomastoid muscle

Surgery indicated when other management does not prevent nocturnal regurgitation

General Management

Patient taught to empty diverticulum before going to bed at night to prevent aspiration

Careful assessment of patient so that other esophageal diseases are not overlooked in managing esophageal diverticulum

NURSING CARE

Nursing Assessment

Zenker's Diverticulum

Regurgitation of food eaten hours earlier

Aspiration at night may lead to chronic pulmonary disease

Dysphagia, late symptom, indicates obstruction of esophagus

Bad taste in mouth

Foul odor to breath

Sloshing of fluid in diverticulum heard as gurgling noises

Esophageal Diverticulum

Regurgitation of food eaten hours earlier

May have other esophageal disease

Tracheoesophageal fistula

Pulmonary symptoms

Bleeding (rare)

Abscess formation (rare)

Nursing Dx & Intervention

Nursing Diagnosis	Nursing Intervention/Rationale
Potential for aspiration	• Assess patient closely for signs of pulmonary problems (i.e., choking or aspirating). • Keep head of bed elevated. • Encourage patient to sleep with head and shoulders elevated on at least two pillows *to prevent aspiration.* • Ensure that patient has emptied diverticulum before lying down (if ordered by physician) *to prevent aspiration.*
Altered nutrition: less than body requirements	• Assess nutritional status. • Weigh patient daily. • Monitor and record intake and output accurately. • Ensure that patient's knowledge of food preparation is adequate *to facilitate swallowing and emptying of diverticulum.*

Patient Education

1. Teach the patient to empty the diverticulum (if ordered by physician) by postural drainage. The patient should lie on the bed with head on the floor and hips flat on the bed and remain this way for 5 to 10 minutes. Make sure the patient's bed is on a frame and off the floor but not too far off the floor. This procedure drains the diverticulum and prevents regurgitation.

Evaluation

Patient Outcome	Data Indicating That Outcome is Reached
Nutritional status is maintained.	Patient's weight remains stable.
There are no pulmonary complications.	Airway is clear. There is no evidence of aspiration or other pulmonary complications.

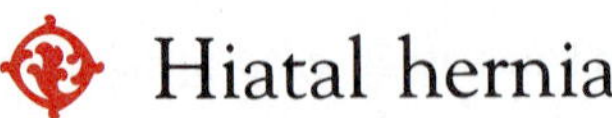

Hiatal hernia

Hiatal hernia refers to the presence in the chest, above the diaphragm, of a part of the stomach that has passed through the normal esophageal hiatus.

Hiatal hernia is very common, occurring in an average of 29.6% of people.[78] It is more common in women and much more common in elderly individuals. A hiatal hernia is clinically significant when it is accompanied by a reflux of acid.

Pathophysiology

Muscle weakness is a primary factor in developing a hiatal hernia. Loss of muscle tone in middle age or after a long illness weakens the muscles around the diaphragmatic opening, predisposing the person to hiatal hernia. Increased abdominal pressure helps to push the upper portion of the stomach through the large opening of the diaphragm.

Intra-abdominal pressure may be increased by the effort needed to evacuate firm stools associated with low-residue diets or constipation. Hiatal hernia is uncommon in countries where the diet is high in fiber. Obesity, pregnancy, and ascites are associated with hiatal hernia, as are the use of girdles and tight-fitting belts and clothes. Esophagitis may lead to secondary shortening of the esophagus and spasm, which may pull part of the stomach upward, creating a small hiatal hernia. Esophageal carcinomas may also pull upward on the stomach. This may cause problems in diagnosing the primary cause. Hiatal hernia is also seen with kyphoscoliosis.

Hiatal hernia may develop after surgical treatment for achalasia. After partial gastrectomy, hiatal hernia may be found because of the straightening and opening of the gastroesophageal junction angle and the elimination of the sphincter.

There are several forms of hiatal hernia, and they are difficult to distinguish clinically. Paraesophageal hernia involves the rolling of the cardia of the stomach up into the chest with the gastroesophageal junction remaining below the diaphragm. There is no acid reflux in this type. The complication in paraesophageal hernias is incarceration.

Congenital short esophagus is also referred to as a congenital hiatal hernia. The cause is probably a spasm rather than an actual short esophagus. The true congenital short esophagus is probably Barrett's esophagus. (Barrett's esophagus refers to an esophagus in which the lower portion is lined with columnar rather than squamous epithelium.)

Sliding hiatal hernia is the most common type. The lower edge of the esophagus and the cardia slide up into the chest through a loose esophageal hiatus. The result is reflux of acid and esophagitis.

Hiatal hernias interfere with normal protective mechanisms of the cardia or lower esophageal sphincter, allowing reflux of acid into the esophagus. Also, if the hiatal hernia is fixed above the diaphragm, congestion of the gastric mucosa may lead to gastritis and ulcerations in the herniated portion of the stomach. The size of the hiatal hernia does not matter in the development of esophagitis and the severity of the symptoms.

Diagnostic Studies and Findings

Laboratory Studies

Stool for diagnosing occult blood
Serum for diagnosing anemia

Chest Roentgenogram

Air shallow behind the heart: presence of pneumonia

Barium Swallow

Outpouching, depending on patient's position when test performed

Endoscopy and Biopsy

Assessment of degree of esophagitis

Motility Studies

Demonstration of reflux and low pressure in lower esophageal sphincter (not routinely done)

pH Monitoring of Lower Esophagus

Increase in acidity

Bernstein Test (Acid Perfusion Test)

Differentiation between cardiac chest pain and pain resulting from esophageal origin (patient has esophageal pain or heartburn if test is positive)

Radioisotope Scintiscan

Diagnosis of nocturnal aspiration

Medical Plan

Surgery

Conservative medical management usually successful; surgery is indicated in the following situations:
- Persistent symptoms not responding to medical treatment
- Reflux stenosis not responding to moderately frequent dilation
- Strangulation or incarceration

Types of procedures
- Nissen's fundoplication: surrounds entire esophagus with a pouch of the stomach
- Allison: reconstruction of angle of the stomach and esophagus, narrowing the hiatus posteriorly, and suturing phrenoesophageal ligament to underside of diaphragm
- Belsey's Mark IV: holds esophagus in place by plicating fundus around lower end of esophagus for about two thirds of its circumference
- Hill: narrows esophagus orifice, pulls gastroesophageal junction below diaphragm, and anchors stomach to median arcuate ligament (posterior gastropexy)

Medications

Antacids used hourly in acute phases with a bland diet
Histamine receptor antagonists
H_2 blockers (cimetidine [Tagamet], 300 mg qid, or ranitidine [Zantac], 100 mg qid, with meals and at bedtime) to relieve the heartburn of reflux esophagitis
Antiemetic agents (used to enhance gastric emptying)
Metoclopramide (Reglan), dopamine depletor, to relieve symptoms of reflux by stimulating gastric emptying and increasing lower esophageal sphincter pressure; neurologic side effects occur
Autonomic agents
Bethanechol (Urecholine), 25 mg qid, to increase lower esophageal sphincter pressure

General Management

Instruct patient to use 4-inch bed blocks so that he or she lies on an inclined plane
Pillows may double the patient in the middle, impeding gastric drainage
Bland diet, avoiding foods that are irritating for the individual
Avoidance of eating 1 to 2 hours before bedtime
Walking around after a meal
Chocolate, associated with relaxation of the esophageal sphincter, is contraindicated, as is smoking
Sipping half glass of water after a meal to cleanse the esophagus

NURSING CARE

Nursing Assessment

Digestion

Reflux esophagitis: symptoms include heartburn or pain made worse by lying down or stooping over; pain relieved by sitting up or by antacids; water brash (mouth filling with fluid from esophagus); and dysphagia
Epigastric pain
Contortions of neck and arms to reduce discomfort

Hematology Status

Upper gastrointestinal bleeding
Anemia from chronic ulcerations

Pulmonary Status

Chronic lung disease after nocturnal regurgitation and aspiration; may include hoarseness, chronic laryngitis, inflammation of the arytenoids, bronchitis, and pulmonary fibrosis
Incarceration: symptoms include sudden onset of vomiting, pain, and complete dysphagia

Nursing Dx & Intervention

Nursing Diagnosis	Nursing Intervention/Rationale
Altered nutrition: less than body requirements	• Assess patient's nutritional status. • Provide a bland diet, avoiding foods that are irritating. Chocolate is associated with relaxation of the esophageal sphincter and is contraindicated. • Avoid eating 1 to 2 hours before bedtime *to reduce the heartburn of reflux esophagitis.* • Have patient sip a half glass of water after a meal *to cleanse the esophagus.*
Pain	• Assess patient for symptoms of reflux esophagitis: heartburn or pain that increases when lying down, water brash (mouth filling with fluid refluxing from the esophagus), and dysphagia. • Provide 4-inch blocks for head of the bed (and help patient find out where they can be bought for home use); *this will maintain the patient in an inclined plane, reducing the abdominal pressure.* • Provide antacids at the bedside for frequent use during the acute phase. Administer antacids to patients with poor memory or who are confused. • Explain the relationship between food and the pain the patient is experiencing; that is, that the pain is related to reflux of gastric contents.

Patient Education

1. Instruct the patient on the relationship between hiatal hernia, reflux esophagitis, and the treatment plan.
2. Provide instructions on use of antacids. If the patient has other medical problems and is taking other medications, check with the pharmacist before choosing the antacid to be used.
3. Provide information on the use of 4-inch blocks under the head of the bed; the patient may also need help to prevent sliding out of the bed, as will the patient's partner, since it is difficult to sleep this way.
4. Other substances that reduce pressure in the lower esophageal sphincter and should be avoided include chocolate, peppermint, smoking, and anticholinergics.

Evaluation

Patient Outcome	Data Indicating That Outcome is Reached
Symptoms of esophagitis are absent.	Heartburn or pain from esophagitis is reduced. There is no perforation or bleeding.

Esophageal stricture

An esophageal stricture is a fibrotic process usually at the lower end of the esophagus.

An esophageal stricture is associated with reflux esophagitis. The interesting point is that it is difficult to determine when an esophageal stricture will occur. In some patients strictures develop after a short history of heartburn, while others have persistent reflux esophagitis for years before a stricture develops.

Pathophysiology

Esophageal stricture may be caused by changes following gastroesophageal surgery, in-lying nasogastric tube, prolonged vomiting, and ingestion of corrosive agents. Esophageal stricture is also associated with mucotaneous candidiasis and epidermolysis bullosa. The true esophageal stricture involves fibrosis through all layers of the esophagus. Narrowing of the esophageal lumen may also occur with edema and inflammation that stiffen the esophagus or with spasms secondary to inflammation.

Diagnostic Studies and Findings

Barium Studies

Show tapering

Endoscopy and Biopsy

Remove food plugs and help rule out a tumor

Medical Plan

Surgery

Simple antireflux procedures, with or without dilation of the strictured segment; procedures similar to those for reflux esophagitis

Medications

Acute dysphagia related to bolus of meat in the esophagus
- Solution of commercial meat tenderizer, 2 tsp in 8 oz water; instruct patient to swallow several spoonfuls, wait 30 min, swallow several sips of soda water, and bear down in modified Valsalva maneuver; use only when food impaction has been present less than 6 h

Vasodilating agents
- Sublingual nitroglycerin or nifedipine (Procardia) may be used to relax spasm around food, *or*

Hypoglycemic agent
- Glucagon, 0.25 to 1 mg IV

General Management

Esophagoscopy to remove food obstruction

Esophageal dilation can be done with mercury bougies, is usually successful, and prevents need for surgical intervention; if not successful, a guided bougienage (Eder-Puestow technique) may be used

Esophageal dilation can also be done through endoscope

NURSING CARE

Nursing Assessment

Digestion

History of heartburn

Difficulty in swallowing (solids, steaks, and apples are good tests of esophageal patency)

History of ingestion of caustic agents (lye, ammonia)

History of esophageal surgery

Nursing Dx & Intervention

Nursing Diagnosis	Nursing Intervention/Rationale
Pain	• Assess the patient for difficulty in swallowing solids, complaints of heartburn, or discomfort following eating. • Prepare and administer solution of meat tenderizer as prescribed *to relieve a food impaction* (duration should be less than 6 hours).

Nursing Diagnosis	Nursing Intervention/Rationale
Altered nutrition: less than body requirements	• Assess patient for weight loss. • Provide enteral nutrition high in calories as ordered until the esophageal dilation has relieved the underlying problem (the stricture or narrowing of the esophageal lumen). • Weigh the patient daily *to determine weight loss or gain if receiving enteral nutrition.*

Patient Education

1. Explain the problems related to meat, painful swallowing, and use of meat tenderizer solution. Prevention may involve less meat in diet, particularly steaks, or eating small pieces, chewing well, and waiting between bites.
2. Prepare the patient for various medical procedures.

Evaluation

Patient Outcome	Data Indicating That Outcome is Reached
There are no symptoms of esophageal stricture.	There are no dietary limitations. There is no dysphagia.

Esophageal varices

Esophageal varices are dilated blood vessels in the esophagus caused by portal hypertension.

Portal hypertension results in the enlargement of collateral blood vessels and the predisposition to ascites. Normally blood flows from the higher pressures of the portal system through the liver sinusoids and then through the hepatic vein to the lower pressure of the vena cava and the systemic venous system. As long as this normal flow is uninterrupted, the potential collateral circulation between the portal and systemic circulations remains closed. Potential collateral circulation exists at the cardioesophageal junction, in the lower rectum, and around the umbilicus. When the normal hemodynamics are disturbed by portal hypertension, the flow of blood that normally goes from the coronary veins into the splenic vein is reversed.[78] This forces open the collaterals between the esophagus and the gastric veins, leading to esophageal varices. Internal hemorrhoids and dilated veins around the umbilicus also occur.

Portal hypertension is the result of blockage or increased resistance to the inflow of blood into the liver or decreased outflow of blood from the portal system into the vena cava. Causes of portal hypertension include congenital obstruction of portal vein, thrombosis of splenic vein from acute pancreatitis, liver parenchymal disease, occlusion of the hepatic vein, and cirrhosis.

Pathophysiology

The veins from the small segment of the abdominal esophagus and the fundus and cardia of the stomach drain into the left coronary vein. These two venous systems are connected by small veins that lie in the esophageal submucosal plexus and normally remain closed. When these veins become dilated, they quickly become tortuous and variceal because of poor support in the esophageal submucosa. In portal hypertension the pressure of the portal system is transmitted through these collateral vessels, which dilate and then produce large esophageal varices. The focus of care is on the management of massive gastrointestinal hemorrhages that occur in these patients.

Diagnostic Studies and Findings

Endoscopy

Tortuous protrusions into lower end of esophagus
May show large amount of blood and possibly source of bleeding

Mesenteric Angiography

Demonstrates collateral circulation
May demonstrate bleeding site

Medical Plan

Surgery

Portacaval shunt: portal vein or one of its tributaries is connected to the inferior vena cava, and portal vein blood flow bypasses diseased liver; complication: hepatic encephalopathy
Splenorenal shunt: diverts portion of blood flow away from liver to reduce pressure; lower incidence of hepatic encephalopathy

Mesocaval shunt: unites high-pressure superior mesenteric vein of patient with portal hypertension to low-pressure inferior vena cava, directly or with a synthetic graft
Distal splenorenal shunt: uses spleen to conduct blood from high pressure of esophageal and gastric varices to low-pressure renal vein
Surgery recommended if patient has bled once, since 60% to 90% run a risk of further bleeding
May need to ligate the bleeders

Medications

Focus is on management of the massive gastrointestinal hemorrhages that occur
Correction of electrolyte imbalances; prevention of encephalopathy (e.g., lactulose)
Pituitary hormone
- Vasopressin (Pitressin), to reduce portal and mesenteric blood flow, given intravenously or during endoscopy or angiography; side effects include abdominal cramps, diarrhea, hyponatremia, peripheral vasoconstriction, hypertension, decreased cardiac output, angina, arrhythmias, and infarction of bowel; used as adjunctive treatment

Histamine receptor antagonist
- Cimetidine (Tagamet), 300 mg qid, or ranitidine (Zantac), 100 mg qid, at meals and bedtime

Antacids
- Maalox

Vitamins
- Vitamin K, IM

Antibacterial agents
- Neomycin (Mycifradin) or lactulose (Cephulac)

General Management

Sclerotherapy of varices may be done by a transhepatic approach or through an endoscope; involves injecting varices with agents that irritate them, causing thrombosis; complications include perforation of esophagus, aspiration pneumonia, pleural effusions, increased ascites, and ulceration of esophagus
Esophageal tamponade to control bleeding
- Sengstaken-Blakemore tube: gastric aspiration with two balloons (esophageal and gastric); need additional nasogastric tube to empty esophagus if patient is not alert
- Linton tube: two aspiration lumens (esophageal and gastric) and one balloon (gastric)
- Boyce's modified Sengstaken-Blakemore tube
- Complications of esophageal tamponade include rupture or erosion of esophagus, occlusion of airway by balloon, and aspiration of secretions

Blood transfusions
Removal of ascitic fluid (paracentesis)

NURSING CARE

Nursing Assessment

Gastrointestinal Bleeding

Massive hematemesis
Melena
Amount of blood loss

Nursing Dx & Intervention

Nursing Diagnosis	Nursing Intervention/Rationale
Altered cerebral, cardiopulmonary, gastrointestinal, and peripheral tissue perfusion	• Assess patient for signs and symptoms of hypovolemic shock related to GI bleeding: Postural changes in pulse and blood pressure Cool, clammy skin Increase in respiratory rate Change in mental status Decreased urine output Hemoglobin and hematocrit unchanged immediately but decreased within 24 hours • Start IV line with large-bore catheter and administer IV fluids as ordered by physicians *to begin fluid replacements and to facilitate possible blood transfusions.* • Assist with the insertion of Swan-Ganz or CVP catheter and perform ongoing hemodynamic monitoring. • Assess patient for possible blood transfusion reaction per protocol. • Perform gastric lavage with iced saline or water as ordered by physician. • Prepare patient for endoscopic procedures as ordered. • Assist with esophageal tamponade *to control bleeding* if ordered and monitor patient closely following insertion of the tube. • Assess for signs of complications associated with esophageal tamponade: rupture or erosion of the esophagus, occlusion of the airway by the balloon, and aspiration of secretions.
Constipation	• Assess amount, color, and consistency of stools. • Assess skin frequently for potential breakdown *caused by diarrhea associated with lactulose and neomycin, which is very irritating.*

Nursing Diagnosis	Nursing Intervention/Rationale
	• Assess patient for signs and symptoms of dehydration from diarrhea: skin turgor, elevated temperature. • Administer neomycin, lactulose, or neomycin enemas as ordered. These agents help eliminate blood from patient's gut; if untreated, hepatic encephalopathy could occur from by-products of protein metabolism produced by bacterial action in gut.[73,76] • Keep patient's skin clean and dry. • Evaluate patient for use of rectal pouch or rectal tube if diarrhea is uncontrollable. • Monitor intake and output.
Altered thought processes	• Assess patient closely for symptoms of hepatic encephalopathy: apathy, euphoria, asterixis (flapping), personality changes, confusion, disorientation, and stupor progressing to coma; document and report to physician immediately if any of these occur. • If confusion or disorientation occurs, frequently reorient patient to time, date, and place. • If patient is disoriented or combative, ensure patient's safety by placing side rails up or restraining patient if necessary. • Stay with patient or enlist assistance from family members *to keep patient from harming himself or herself.* • Continue to administer lactulose or neomycin as ordered by physician. • Provide usual care necessary for comatose patient if hepatic coma should occur.
Impaired skin integrity	• Assess skin around patient's perirectal area and sacrum frequently *since constant diarrhea can be very erosive.* • Cleanse skin thoroughly with warm water and a mild soap. • Rinse well and spray with a skin sealant; then coat the skin with a water-repellant ointment. • If skin breakdown has occurred, cleanse stool from skin gently with a cotton ball soaked in glycerin. • Apply a mixture of skin cream and ointment over the perirectal area.

Patient Education

1. Prepare the patient for all diagnostic procedures, treatments, or surgery so the patient will understand what will happen and what to expect.
2. Instruct the patient on the effects of high-protein diets and alcohol consumption in preventing future complications.
3. Inform the patient of the relationship of the esophageal varices to the primary diagnosis that resulted in portal hypertension.

Evaluation

Patient Outcome	Data Indicating That Outcome is Reached
There is no gastrointestinal bleeding.	Hematocrit and hemoglobin are normal for patient. Vomiting and diarrhea are not present. Vital signs are stable. Skin turgor is normal for patient.
Mental status is normal for patient.	Patient is alert and oriented to time, date, and place.
Skin integrity is maintained.	There is no skin breakdown in perirectal area or pressure points.

STOMACH DISORDERS

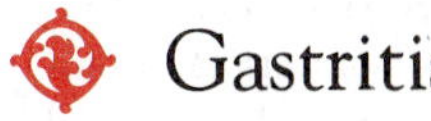

Gastritis

Gastritis refers to any diffuse lesion in the gastric mucosa that can be identified histologically as inflamed.

Gastritis may occur as an acute or a chronic disorder, and it is more common in elderly people. The reported incidence of chronic gastritis associated with gastrointestinal bleeding has fluctuated over the past few years from 40% to 10%.[78] This shift is probably related to successful use of endoscopic diagnostic procedures. The incidence of acute gastritis is undetermined except when associated with gastrointestinal bleeding. Acute gastritis is responsible for 10% to 30% of upper gastrointestinal bleeding.[26,78] Recent research has shown the presence of the bacterium *Campylobacter pylori* in patients with chronic gastritis.[54]

Pathophysiology

Acute gastritis is a brief inflammatory process affecting the stomach mucosa. It involves erosion of the mucosa. The mucosa is spotted with submucosal hemorrhages that resemble ecchymoses and may be round or linear. There may also be shallow erosions that appear as brown spots or red petechiae or small breaks in the mucosa. The hemorrhagic erosions usually involve only the glandular layer, are extremely shallow, and are found anywhere in the stomach. Acute gastritis is more common in gastric ulcer than duodenal ulcer. The difference between gastritis erosion and gastric ulcer is that in erosion the muscularis mucosa is uninvolved and healing leaves no scar.

Erosion and hemorrhage are caused by a back-diffusion of hydrogen ions and mucosal ischemia. The disruption of the gastric mucosal barrier allows the back-diffusion of the hydrogen ion, which stimulates the release of vasoactive substances, increased capillary permeability, and inflammation.

A number of drugs, stimuli, and circumstances are associated with acute gastritis, including aspirin, anti-inflammatory agents, alcohol, corticosteroids, major physiologic stress, and intense emotional reactions. The most common cause of acute superficial gastritis is alcohol.[75,78] Stress ulcers are a form of acute gastritis. The term "stress ulcer" is a misnomer because the lesions are not ulcers.

Steroids appear to potentiate the action of other factors in acute gastritis. Nonsteroidal anti-inflammatory agents used to treat rheumatoid arthritis probably affect gastric mucosa because they work by inhibiting prostaglandin synthesis. Prostaglandins have a cytoprotective function on the gastric mucosa. Apparently, patients taking both nonsteroidal anti-inflammatory agents and aspirin are at a greater risk for bleeding from acute erosive gastritis. In these cases the treatment for rheumatoid arthritis is not stopped, but the patient must be observed and treated for erosion as indicated.

Chronic gastritis is often referred to as a nonerosive, nonspecific gastritis that is further differentiated by the histologic appearance of the gastric mucosa into superficial gastritis, atrophic gastritis, or gastric atrophy.

Superficial gastritis is characterized by an inflammatory infiltration of the lamina propria. Lymphocytes, plasma cells, and eosinophils are found in the outer one third of the mucosa. The gastric glands are not involved.

Atrophic gastritis shows a loss of fundic glands, parietal cells, and chief cells. The muscularis mucosa is split and thickened, and marked inflammation is present.

Gastric atrophy refers to marked or total gland loss with minimum inflammation. The mucosa is thinned.

Two additional features, intestinal metaplasia and pseudopyloric metaplasia, may be seen in the three types of chronic gastritis. Intestinal metaplasia is the replacement of normal gastric cells by cells identical to those of the normal small intestine. Intestinal metaplasia is greater in more severe degrees of gastric atrophy. The surface of the normal stomach is columnar, whereas the small intestine has a prominent brush border and may contain goblet and Paneth's cells. When intestinal metaplasia occurs, the stomach acquires the appearance and absorptive capacity of the small intestine. Cancer is much more likely to develop in intestinalized gastric mucosa in comparison to the rare instances of carcinoma of the intestinal epithelium in the small intestine.

In pseudopyloric metaplasia the normal fundic glands are replaced by clear-staining mucous glands that cannot be distinguished from mucous glands in the antral gland or cardial gland mucosa. The replacement may be partial or total. Diagnosis of pseudopyloric metaplasia is made by biopsy. It is imperative that the location of the biopsy be carefully stated on pathology slips so the pathologist does not mistake normal antral gland mucosa for pseudopyloric metaplasia or vice versa.

Chronic gastritis has also been divided into type A and type B. Type A gastritis involves the fundus. There are circulating parietal cell antibodies and high serum gastrin levels. Pernicious anemia evolves almost exclusively from type A gastritis.[6,78] The relationship of the parietal cell antibodies and intrinsic factor lends support for the hypothesis that type A gastritis has an autoimmune background. Type B gastritis involves the fundus and the antrum. There is a lack of parietal cell antibodies, and approximately 10% of patients with type B gastritis have gastrin cell antibodies.[78]

In type A gastritis there is a marked reduction in acid secretion, hypergastrinemia, and eventually impaired vitamin B_{12} absorption. Type B has less reduction of acid secretions, normal gastrin levels, and only rare impairment of vitamin B_{12} absorption. As the mucosa of the stomach changes with atrophy, the acid secretion is reduced, resulting in achlorhydria or hypochlorhydria.

Atrophic gastritis and gastric atrophy are associated with an increase in gastric malignancies. There is a high rate of cell death and increased cell turnover in atrophic gastritis. Mucosal nuclear activity is increased during the premalignant state.[6] The highest mitotic rates are found in areas of intestinal metaplasia.

Although pernicious anemia is discussed at length in Chapter 15, the relationship between the intrinsic factor and vitamin B_{12} absorption should be briefly discussed here. Vitamin B_{12} refers to cyanocobalamin (CN-Cbl). Humans depend on dietary sources of vitamin B_{12} provided by foods of animal origin. The minimum daily requirement is 0.6 to 1.2 $\mu g/d$. The vitamin is stored in the liver. The liver stores of vitamin B_{12} are sufficient to last 3 to 5 years.

Under normal conditions of gastric acidity, dietary vitamin B_{12} enters the jejunum bound to proteins. Pancreatic proteases remove the protein, and the vitamin B_{12} binds with the intrinsic factor, secreted in the stomach by parietal cells. Intrinsic factor is crucial to protect vitamin B_{12} from bacterial destruction. In the distal ileum the intrinsic factor–vitamin B_{12} complex attaches to specific brush border receptors. A pH equal to or greater than 5.7 and the presence of divalent cations, particularly calcium, are required for binding (attachment). Once vitamin B_{12} enters the cell, it binds with transcobalamin (II), a transport protein, and is carried to the liver.

Vitamin B_{12} deficiency is difficult to detect early because of the liver stores that continue to supply it. Conditions associated with vitamin B_{12} deficiency include chronic gastritis, ileitis, surgical removal of the ileum, gastrectomy, or loss or deficiency of pancreatic enzymes. Prophylactic intramuscular injections of vitamin B_{12} may be used to prevent the sequelae associated with a vitamin B_{12} deficiency.

Diagnostic Studies and Findings

Acute Gastritis

Nasogastric Aspiration

Frank blood or heme-positive aspirate

Endoscopy

Erosions, superficial ulcerations, and diffuse oozing of blood when procedure is done during acute phase; after 3 days, lesions will begin to heal

Angiographic Visualization

To detect and treat lesions with infusion of vasopressin

Double-Contrast Barium Study

Superficial gastric erosions
Cannot be used to detect bleeding lesions

Chronic Gastritis

Serum Gastrin

Elevated: in a few patients with type B, the level will be normal or low

Serum Parietal Cell Antibodies

Presence suggests gastritis

Pentagastrin Stimulation

Normal gastric secretion for person's age and sex would indicate minimum likelihood of gastritis
Diminished gastric secretions increase likelihood of gastritis

Serum Pepsinogen I Levels

Elevated in superficial gastritis
Low level in atrophic gastritis reflects absence of chief cells

Schilling Test

Assessment of vitamin B_{12} absorption by measuring urinary excretion of an oral dose of radiolabeled vitamin B_{12}

Barium Swallow with Double Contrast

Appearance of a "bald fundus" and thinning of gastric rugae

Endoscopy with Biopsy and Cytology

Biopsy necessary to obtain a definitive diagnosis
Cytology of multiple biopsy sites through the stomach is used to rule out gastric carcinomas

Differential Diagnosis

Rule out Zollinger-Ellison syndrome vs. chronic gastritis; high serum gastrin and high serum pepsinogen levels are indicative of Zollinger-Ellison syndrome; may also indicate multiple poorly healed ulcers

Medical Plan

Acute Gastritis

Surgery

Partial gastrectomy, pyloroplasty, vagotomy, or total gastrectomy may be indicated for managing patients with major bleeding from erosive gastritis

Medications

- Histamine receptor antagonists
  - Ranitidine (Zantac), 100 mg po qid
  - Parenteral cimetidine (Tagamet), 300 mg q6h in 100 ml of D_5W over 20 min; dosage should maintain gastric pH at 7.0[78]
- Antacids
  - Antacids recommended to help maintain alkaline pH
  - Antacids (30 ml q2h) have been shown to be 80% to 90% effective in keeping pH above 4.0
- Fluid volume replacement
  - Intravenous fluid replacement during a bleeding episode to maintain volume
  - Blood replacement may be required when gastrointestinal hemorrhage is associated with acute gastritis
- Pituitary hormone
  - Vasopressin (Pitressin) per angiography or IV, 20 U in 100 U D_5W over 10 min, may be used in severe cases and may be repeated q3-4h if bleeding recurs; may lose efficacy after repeated doses

General Management

Ice water or saline lavage used in patient with gastrointestinal bleeding
Laser therapy with direct coagulation of bleeding spots through an endoscopic approach may be used
Removal of causative agents (alcohol, aspirin, nonsteroidal anti-inflammatory agents)
Withholding of food and fluids until vomiting and inflammation subside; then bland diet of medium temperature in acute gastritis without bleeding will assist healing process

Chronic Gastritis

Medications

Antacids to reduce or alleviate symptoms
Vitamins
 Vitamin C (ascorbic acid) to facilitate iron absorption in the patient with achlorhydria[76]
 Vitamin B_{12} injections (cyanocobalamin), 1 mg/ml (1000 μg)
Antibacterial agents to eradicate *Campylobacter pylori* may be indicated, based on recent research; further studies will define agents and dosages

General Management

Routine endoscopy to assess formation of gastric polyps and gastric carcinomas in patients diagnosed with atrophic gastritis and gastric atrophy
Routine Schilling tests or serum vitamin B_{12} levels to evaluate intrinsic factor deficiency

NURSING CARE

Nursing Assessment

Acute Gastritis

Stomach

Asymptomatic; or vague complaints of postprandial distress after a large meal; or vague ulcerlike distress, particularly relieved by food
Massive gastrointestinal hemorrhage
History of aspirin or alcohol intake
History of hematemesis or melena
Nasogastric aspirate or stool heme positive for blood (in hospitalized patient)

Chronic Gastritis

Stomach

Often asymptomatic
Diffuse, epigastric burning or pain that increases after eating large amounts; relieved by a small amount of antacid
Vomiting

Pernicious Anemia

May be first clinical sign of chronic gastritis
Weakness; numbness and tingling in extremities; fever; pallor; anorexia; weight loss
Smooth or beefy red tongue

Nursing Dx & Intervention

Nursing Diagnosis	Nursing Intervention/Rationale
Altered renal, cerebral, cardiopulmonary, gastrointestinal, and peripheral tissue perfusion	• Observe patient for early signs of gastrointestinal bleeding: hematemesis, melena, blood in nasogastric aspirate or stool. • Assess for signs of hypovolemic shock and initiate replacement of fluid volume. • Permit nothing by mouth; keep patient quiet if hemorrhage is considered a possibility. • Maintain intravenous fluids and blood as ordered and observe for transfusion reactions. • Prepare patients for endoscopy as a diagnostic or treatment procedure.
Altered nutrition: less than body requirements	• Assess patient's nutritional status, since dietary intake may be altered *because of symptoms related to eating*. • Monitor intake and output. • Record nausea and vomiting. • Administer antiemetics as ordered. • Provide frequent (approximately six) small feedings a day if acute gastritis *to relieve postprandial distress associated with large meals*.
Altered oral mucous membrane	• Assess patient's oral membrane *to identify a key symptom of pernicious anemia, the smooth or beefy red tongue*. • Assess patient for additional signs of pernicious anemia. • Administer cyanocobalamin as ordered.

Patient Education

1. Identify agents that irritate the gastric mucosa, including aspirin, aspirin-containing compounds, over-the-counter agents, alcohol, prescription drugs such as indomethacin, phenylbutazone, reserpine, nicotine, ibuprofen, sulindac, and naproxen.

2. Provide the patient with information related to the cause-and-effect relationship of the above agents and gastritis.
3. Identify need for an asymptomatic patient with chronic gastritis to continue to see physician regularly.
4. Discuss bland diets, amounts of food eaten, use of antacids, and their relationship to pain management.

Evaluation

Patient Outcome	Data Indicating That Outcome is Reached
Gastrointestinal hemorrhage ceases.	Blood pressure, pulse, and respirations are within normal limits. Hematemesis and melena are absent.
Laboratory studies are within normal limits.	Serum vitamin B_{12} level is within normal limits. Schilling test is normal (8% to 40% of original oral dose of radioactive vitamin B_{12} appears in a 24-hour urine specimen). Endoscopy demonstrates normal mucosa (acute episode) or absence of polyps and carcinoma (chronic gastritis).
There is no pain.	Patient reports eating frequent, small feedings of bland foods (chronic gastritis). Patient identifies possible causes in acute gastritis and omits these from his or her intake.

Dyspepsia

Dyspepsia is a vague gastric discomfort that occurs after eating. The person may complain of fullness, pain, heartburn, bloating, and nausea.

Many patients (30% to 55%) with dyspepsia do not have obvious pathologic findings in the gastrointestinal system.[75] Dyspepsia has also been divided into two classifications: ulcer-negative dyspepsia and functional dyspepsia.

Ulcer-negative dyspepsia involves classic symptoms of duodenal ulcers. The patient complains of epigastric pain 1 to 3 hours after eating and can obtain relief with antacids. This has also been referred to as Moynihan's disease.[75,78] Spiro[78] reports that 40% of patients with ulcerlike dyspepsia will have a gastric or duodenal ulcer, 40% will have duodenitis, and the remaining group will have a normal endoscopic examination or a gastric cancer. In addition, Spiro reports that patients with ulcer-negative dyspepsia have an increased likelihood of developing duodenal ulcers in the future.

Functional dyspepsia involves epigastric pain shortly after a meal, belching, bloating, and nausea. Antacids offer little if any relief.

Pathophysiology

Ulcer-negative dyspepsia may be part of a continuum of diseases involving duodenitis and peptic ulcer disease. The functional dyspepsia may be related to poor gastric emptying with gastric distention causing pain or discomfort.

Psychologic factors may play a role in both types of dyspepsia. Gomez and Dally[33] found that 80% of the patients with persistent or recurrent abdominal pain were diagnosed as chronically depressed, suffering from chronic tension, or having hysterical mechanisms. This may indicate a need for early psychologic evaluation of patients with vague recurrent abdominal pain. Although the origin may be psychosomatic, the symptoms are real.

Prescription and nonprescription drugs may also produce dyspepsia. The patient may have epigastric pain with or without nausea and vomiting. Anti-inflammatory agents, theophylline, and digitalis are known to produce dyspepsia. Other agents play a role in gastritis and ulcer formation.

Diagnostic Studies and Findings

Double-Air Contrast Barium Swallow

Negative for ulceration or early carcinoma

Endoscopy

Negative for duodenitis or ulceration

Medical Plan

Medications

Ulcer-negative dyspepsia
- Histamine receptor antagonists
  - Ranitidine (Zantac), 100 mg po bid
  - Cimetidine (Tagamet), 400 mg/d po
- Antacids
  - Antacids 1 and 3 h after meals and at bedtime

Antiulcer agents
Sucralfate (Carafate), 1 g po qid, on empty stomach (1 h before meals and at bedtime)
Pirenzepine in clinical trials is effective in relieving symptoms in ulcer-negative dyspepsia
Functional dyspepsia
Antiemetics (used to enhance gastric emptying)
Metoclopramide (Reglan), 10 mg po, 30 min before each meal and at bedtime

General Management

Low-fat diet

NURSING CARE

Nursing Assessment

Gastric

Symptoms of fullness, pain, heartburn, bloating, and nausea
Relationship of symptoms to eating
Use of effectiveness of antacids
History of prescribed medications and over-the-counter drugs that are ulcerogenic
History of ulcer disease
Assessment of emotional status, tension, and stress

Nursing Dx & Intervention

Nursing Diagnosis	Nursing Intervention/Rationale
Pain	• Assess pain: note description, location, and patient's previous efforts to relieve the pain *to identify comfort measures*. • Administer medications for symptomatic relief as ordered.
Ineffective individual coping	• Assess with patient life-style, work-related tension, depression, and history of nonprescription drug use *to manage the discomfort*. • Discuss with patient how stress and emotion are related to symptoms of dyspepsia. • Recommend or refer for stress management strategies as appropriate.

Patient Education

1. The patient should be able to identify prescribed medications, dosage regimen, and interactive effects. (For example, antacids cannot be taken 30 minutes before or after sucralfate or they will inactivate sucralfate.)

Evaluation

Patient Outcome	Data Indicating That Outcome is Reached
There is no dyspepsia, pain, or discomfort.	Patient has no complaints of fullness, pain, heartburn, bloating, or nausea following a meal.
Patient verbalizes sources of psychosocial stress and tension.	Patient is able to verbalize sources of stress and tension and is able to identify coping or adaptation skills.

Gastric ulcers

A gastric ulcer is a well-defined break in the gastric mucosa that extends into the muscularis mucosae.

A gastric ulcer must be differentiated from a duodenal ulcer and from gastric erosion. Often gastric ulcers are included with duodenal ulcers and discussed under the classification of peptic ulcer disease. However, the cause, incidence, and pathophysiology of gastric and duodenal ulcers are not the same. Duodenal ulcers are three to four times more common than gastric ulcers.[78] In gastric erosions, commonly seen in gastritis, healing occurs without the formation of the scar tissue formed when gastric ulcers heal.

The incidence of gastric ulcers is high in middle-aged and elderly persons, predominantly men. Gastric ulcers are strongly correlated with aspirin and alcohol abuse.* Other

*Aspirin abuse is considered to be the ingestion of 15 or more aspirins per week.[78]

causative drugs or agents are those that damage the gastric mucosal barrier.

It is also interesting that gastric ulcers are more common in people with type A blood (type O is more common in people with duodenal ulcers). Gastric ulcers also occur within family groups. Patients with gastric ulcers also have an increased chance of developing a gastric malignancy. The relationship of gastritis to gastric ulceration has also been examined.

Pathophysiology

Gastric ulcers are generally found at the junction of the fundic with the pyloric mucosa. Ulcers in the antrum are usually smaller than those in the proximal part of the stomach. Gastritis is more common in patients with gastric ulcers and is often seen around the ulceration. The relationship of gastritis and gastric ulcer can be stated as follows: it appears that a gastric ulcer is more than a localized lesion and that gastritis contributes to the hyposecretion of gastric ulcers and to the susceptibility of the mucosa to ulcerate.

Patients with gastric ulcers have normal to below normal gastric acid secretion. If gastritis is also present, this will contribute to the hyposecretion of acid. An exception to the decreased acid production occurs when the gastric ulcer is close to the pylorus or is associated with a duodenal ulcer, in which case hypersecretion of acid occurs.

There are two proposed processes involved in the formation of gastric ulcers: back-diffusion of acid and pyloric dysfunction. The normal gastric mucosa maintains a barrier against back diffusion by the tight junctions of epithelial cells that mechanically prevent reflux. The plasma membrane of the surface epithelial cells is made up of layers of lipids and contributes to the mucosa barrier.

Agents that are barrier breakers (e.g., aspirin, alcohol, and indomethacin) disrupt the tight junctions, and acid flows back into the mucosa. Detergents, such as bile salts, and toxic agents can destroy the lipid plasma membrane. When the mucosal barrier is damaged, acid diffuses back from the stomach into the mucosa. Histamine is released, stimulating more acid production, vasodilation, and increased capillary permeability. Bleeding may develop. Protein loss may occur, and an increased sodium content may be found in the stomach.

Bile is generally prevented from contact with the gastric mucosa by a competent pyloric sphincter. In gastric ulcer disease the pylorus does not respond normally to secretin or cholecystokinin and increase the pressure preventing reflux. Bile is allowed to reflux into the stomach.

Antral motility is also decreased in a patient with a gastric ulcer. The delay in gastric emptying may be observed during barium studies. The effect on antral motility appears to be more common in patients with gastric ulcers near the pylorus. The motility returns to normal when healing occurs.

The four layers of a peptic ulcer include the superficial layer, which lines the ulcer with a white fibrinous coat composed of leukocytes and erythrocytes; a second layer of fibrinoid necrosis; the next layer, inflammatory granulation tissue containing blood vessels; and the fourth layer, a dense scar of fibrous tissue lacking elastic tissue. The dense scar forms the base of the ulcer and extends beyond the margins of the mucosal defect. In a rapidly developing ulceration, massive bleeding may develop in asymptomatic patients when the vessel wall erodes. When the ulceration develops at a slower rate, inflammatory responses, thrombosis, and endarteritis occur and inhibit massive bleeding, and the patient experiences symptoms of peptic ulcer disease.

Ulcers heal slowly because of the scarred avascular tissue. The scarred mucosa over a healed ulcer contains patches of atrophic epithelium and scattered glands. The more scar tissue present, the thinner the mucosal layer. Endarteritis is frequent, and the muscularis mucosae is interrupted and may be partially obliterated. The mucosa and glands that develop are often a simple pyloric type with areas of intestinalization, rather than gastric glands of the fundic type.

Diagnostic Studies and Findings

Double-Contrast Barium Study

Detection of a gastric ulcer; when present, radiologist must determine if lesion is a gastric ulcer or a gastric carcinoma

Gastric Analysis

Normal to decreased presence of acid

Gastric Cytology

Abnormal findings would indicate gastric carcinoma

Endoscopy and Biopsy (Esophagogastroduodenoscopy)

May be used as a first procedure in most actively bleeding patients

May identify gastric ulcers too shallow to detect with barium studies

Biopsy to rule out gastric cancer

Endoscopy repeated in 2 weeks for evaluation of treatment

Serum Gastrin Levels

Normal or slightly elevated

Stool for Guaiac

Often positive

Medical Plan

Surgery

Partial gastrectomy and vagotomy (used to treat complications of gastric ulcers: persistent bleeding, perforations)

Medications

Histamine receptor antagonists
- Cimetidine (Tagamet), 300 mg po qid
- Ranitidine (Zantac), 100 mg po bid

Antiulcer agents
- Sucralfate (Carafate), 1 g po qid on an empty stomach (primary agent in duodenal ulcer, but may be ordered for gastric ulcer)

Antacids
- Antacids, prn

General Management

Esophagogastroduodenoscopy (EGD) to manage bleeding
Ice water or saline lavage if massive hemorrhage
Arteriography with intra-arterial vasopressin
Bland diet of six meals per day
Elimination of barrier breakers (aspirin, steroids, alcohol)
Elimination of smoking
Bed rest

NURSING CARE

Nursing Assessment

Gastric Pain

Complaints of heartburn and dyspepsia
Note absence of duodenal pattern of pain; pain occurs closer to intake of food
Note relief of pain with a few ounces of antacids
Location of pain in left midepigastric area or pain radiating to the back (ulcer on posterior wall)
Vomiting, fullness, and distention may indicate delayed gastric emptying
Weight loss

Upper Gastrointestinal Bleeding

Hematemesis; melena
Change in vital signs; weakness; dizziness

Perforation

Sudden onset of severe, diffuse abdominal pain

Nursing Dx & Intervention

Nursing Diagnosis	Nursing Intervention/Rationale
Altered renal, cerebral, cardiopulmonary, gastrointestinal, and peripheral tissue perfusion	• Assess patient for gastrointestinal bleeding: monitor vital signs, central venous pressure, Swan-Ganz catheter pressure, laboratory values, urinary output, early signs of hypovolemic shock. • Maintain intravenous fluids and blood replacements as ordered to replace fluid volume loss. • Prepare patient for endoscopic procedures: permit nothing by mouth, explain procedure, and administer preprocedural medications as ordered. • Institute ice-water lavage if ordered for gastrointestinal bleeding not controlled by endoscopy.
Altered nutrition: less than body requirements	• Assess nutritional history, note any weight loss (associated with abdominal pain, distention after eating, and patient's limitation of intake) or gain. *(Some patients may eat more in an attempt to decrease the pain.)* • Provide six small meals a day, *since pain may be relieved by eating small amounts.* • Monitor intake and output. • Record complaints of fullness, nausea, and vomiting, *since these symptoms may indicate delayed gastric emptying.* • Administer antiemetics as ordered.
Pain	• Assess patient for location of pain, relief of pain with antacids, or sudden onset of severe, diffuse abdominal pain *to plan appropriate management and to determine if perforation occurs.* • Provide antacids as needed, *since pain is often relieved by small amounts of antacids.*

Patient Education

1. Teach the patient about the relationship of causative agents to the development of gastric ulcers, recurrence rate (approximately 40%), and repeat of endoscopy.
2. Provide written information on medication regimen, and ensure that the patient can identify the drugs and when each is to be taken, which require empty stomach or should be taken after a meal, and so forth.

Evaluation

Patient Outcome	Data Indicating That Outcome is Reached
Gastric ulcer heals.	Findings on endoscopy are normal. There is no pain.
Patient adheres to plan of care.	Patient resumes a normal diet, avoids causative agents, and continues medical regimen as ordered for prophylaxis against recurrence.

INTESTINAL DISORDERS

Duodenal ulcers

A duodenal ulcer is a chronic circumscribed break in mucosa extending through the muscularis mucosae that leaves a residual scar with healing. The duodenal ulcer is the most common form of peptic ulcer disease.

The incidence of duodenal ulcers has been decreasing since the 1950s. At this writing, approximately 300,000 to 500,000 new cases of duodenal ulcer will develop each year.[75,78] Approximately 4 to 8 million Americans have active or recurrent ulcers.[75] The ratio of men to women is approximately 2:1. The decrease in duodenal ulcers has been attributed to changing environmental factors such as dietary habits and changing stress levels related to various historical occurrences. For example, urbanization at the beginning of the twentieth century was new and may have been a source of stress that has less effect in the 1980s. A profile of the person who develops duodenal ulcers has also changed. The incidence has declined in young women and increased in older women.

More efficient diagnostic techniques and treatment may also have a role in the decline of duodenal ulcers. The duodenal ulcer can be differentiated from dyspepsia, duodenitis, and gastric ulcer. Medical treatment with H_2 receptor antagonists has been successfully used, and patients often undergo diagnostic techniques and treatment as outpatients. Surgery is used only to manage complications of duodenal ulcers such as perforation.

There are also regional differences in duodenal ulcers. For example, prevalence is higher in Scotland and northern England than southern England. In India, duodenal ulcers are more common in the south. Occupational factors have also been associated with duodenal ulcers. The common myth that duodenal ulcers occur in high-pressured professionals and executives is not true.[54,75] Duodenal ulcers are more common in unskilled laborers and assembly-line workers. Duodenal ulcers are more common in lower-income families and in persons with a low level of education.[63]

Pathophysiology

The duodenal ulcer usually is less than 1 cm in diameter and is located 0.5 to 2 cm from the pylorus. Duodenal ulcers occur on both the anterior and posterior walls. The ulcers on the anterior wall appear to have a greater incidence of perforation. Posterior wall ulcers tend to be larger. The four layers of a peptic ulcer are as follows:[76]

1. Superficial layer lining the ulcer with a white fibrinous coat composed of leukocytes and erythrocytes
2. Zone of fibrinoid necrosis
3. Inflammatory granulation tissue
4. Layer of dense fibrotic tissue without elastic tissue (scar), forming the base of the ulcer and extending beyond the margins

Patients with duodenal ulcers secrete more gastric acid than normal in basal states and in response to stimuli. The increased acid production may be the result of an increased capacity to secrete hydrochloric acid because of increased parietal cell mass, or heightened vagal activity increasing the response to stimuli to overproduce acid, or a decreased ability to stop or "turn off" gastric secretions.

The nervous system phase of gastric secretions includes impulses from the cortex (limbic system and hypothalamus) to the vagal nerve. Vagal stimulation acts directly on the parietal cells and indirectly on the antral G cells to release gastrin. Pepsin and hydrochloric acid secretions are stimulated. The stimuli to the nervous system may include food in the mouth (tactile), thoughts and anticipation of food, or the sight of food.

Gastric activity also affects the regulation of secretions. The person with a duodenal ulcer secretes a larger amount of gastric juices and may be unable to stop the release of gastrin in response to normal hormonal stimuli. The concentration of acid in the duodenum is higher than normal. Hypersecretion of acid, in and of itself, does not result in a duodenal ulcer. If one or more members of one's immediate family have an ulcer, a person has an increased possibility of developing an ulcer. This relationship appears to be both genetically and environmentally related. The emotional aspects of the duodenal ulcer patient must also be considered. Ulcer patients as a group tend to repress external expressions of emotions and feelings. It may be that psychosocial stressors and increased susceptibility to stressful life events plus familial or environmental factors may be related to duodenal ulcers.

The more rapid the development of the ulcer, the more likely that blood vessels in the ulcer will show inflammatory changes, medial hypertrophy, or endarteritis. Blood vessels adjacent to the ulcer will have arteriosclerotic changes. The blood vessels 5 cm away from the ulcer will appear normal. In rapidly developing ulcers, bleeding is more common and may be massive because the blood vessel wall may erode in an asymptomatic patient. In instances where the duodenal ulcer develops slowly, thrombosis, endarteritis, and inflammatory changes result in an avascular, scarred area that heals slowly.

In addition to upper gastrointestinal bleeding, other complications of duodenal ulcer disease include gastric outlet obstruction, perforation, and intractable pain. Obstruction of the gastric outlet may be caused by spasms, edema, or scarring. Protracted vomiting may indicate outlet obstruction.

Perforation is a life-threatening event. Perforation occurs in 2% to 5% of all duodenal ulcers. The overall incidence has been decreasing.

Intractability may develop from other complications of duodenal ulcers, stresses in patients' lives, and other disorders. Primarily, the patient no longer responds to medical management, or recurrences interfere with activities of daily living. Posterior penetration of the ulcer through the duodenal wall and into the pancreas will alter the pain. An increase in pain, loss of antacid relief, and radiation of pain to the back are the primary symptoms. Acute pancreatitis is rare but may occur.

Diagnostic Studies and Findings

Double-Contrast Barium Studies

- Presence of a crater or scar in duodenum
- Delayed gastric emptying of barium (gastric outlet obstruction)
- No evidence of marked scarring and minimal deformity of duodenal bulb (posterior penetration)

Abdominal Films

- Free air under diaphragm (perforation)

Endoscopy

- Presence of an ulcer; degree of healing

Gastric Analysis

- Hypersecretion of gastric acid (also used to evaluate effectiveness of vagotomy in reducing acidity)
- Nocturnal acid
- Presence of blood in gastric analysis (may indicate bleeding)

Hematocrit and Hemoglobin

- Decreased (bleeding; microcytic anemia)

Stool for Occult Blood

- Melena (may indicate bleeding)

Pepsinogen Levels in Blood

- High levels associated with duodenal ulcers

Serum Amylase

- Increased with posterior penetration

Medical Plan

Surgery

- Removal of a portion of gastrin-producing portion of stomach (antrectomy or partial gastrectomy) with attachment of duodenum to stomach (Billroth I) or attachment of stomach to jejunum (Billroth II) and vagotomy
- Rarely indicated except for management of complications; there are many postsurgery problems: diarrhea, dumping syndrome, and recurrent ulcers

Medications

- Antacids
  - Antacids (aluminum-magnesium regimen), po: provide 144 mEq buffering capacity 1 and 3 h after a meal and at bedtime (amount required varies based on commercial antacid used; Table 8-2)
- Histamine receptor antagonists
  - Cimetidine (Tagamet), 300 mg qid po for 4-8 wk; with meals and at bedtime; prophylactic treatment: 400 mg at bedtime
  - Ranitidine (Zantac), 150 mg bid po
- Antiulcer agents
  - Sucralfate (Carafate), 1 g qid on an empty stomach for 4-8 wk; avoid antacids 30 min before and after dose

General Management

- Stop smoking
- Abstain from use of aspirin-containing compounds
- Abstain from coffee (caffeinated and decaffeinated [stimulates gastric acid production])
- Small, frequent meals recommended, with no bedtime snacks

Table 8-2
Relative Potency of Liquid Antacids

Antacid	Potency*
Concentrated aluminum and magnesium hydroxides	
Delcid	100
Maalox Therapeutic Concentrates	75
Mylanta II	75
Gelusil II	60
Regular aluminum and magnesium hydroxides	
Maalox	45
Mylanta	40
Gelusil	40
Riopan	40
Aluminum hydroxide	
Alternagel	40
Amphojel	20

Modified from Sleisenger.[75]
*Millimoles of neutralizing capacity per 15 ml.

Milk is not used as therapy (calcium and protein content stimulates gastric acid)

Avoid calcium carbonate antacids (rebound effect because of calcium content, hypercalcemia, renal stones) and sodium bicarbonate antacids (alkalosis, fluid retention)

NURSING CARE

Nursing Assessment

Pain

Well-localized epigastric pain occurring when stomach is empty (11 AM, 4 PM, 11 PM, 2 AM), relieved by food or antacids

Bowel Habits

Constipation (may be related to diet and drugs)

Diarrhea (may be present from antacid therapy)

Abdominal Tenderness

Physical examination; palpation denotes tenderness (anterior duodenal ulcers)

Upper Gastrointestinal Bleeding

Hematemesis

Melena

Dizziness or syncope

Decreased blood pressure and increased pulse

Decreased hematocrit

Perforation of Duodenum

Sudden, severe, diffuse upper abdominal pain

Referred pain to shoulder

Rigid, boardlike abdomen

Rebound tenderness

Rapid, shallow respirations

Pyloric Outlet Obstruction

Protracted vomiting

Posterior Penetration

Increased pain

Pain radiating to back

Loss of antacid relief

Nursing Dx & Intervention

Nursing Diagnosis	Nursing Intervention/Rationale
Altered renal, cerebral, cardiopulmonary, gastrointestinal, and peripheral tissue perfusion	• Assess patient for gastrointestinal bleeding: monitor vital signs, central venous pressure, Swan-Ganz catheter pressure, laboratory values, urinary output, and early signs of hypovolemic shock. • Maintain intravenous fluids and blood replacements as ordered *to replace fluid volume loss*. • Prepare patient for endoscopic procedures: permit nothing by mouth, explain procedure, administer preprocedural medications as ordered. • Institute ice water lavage if ordered for gastrointestinal bleeding not controlled by endoscopy.
Pain	• Observe patient for changes in nature, location, and relief of pain that would denote impending complications. • Provide frequent small meals and antacids at the bedside *to relieve well localized epigastric pain associated with an empty stomach*.
Noncompliance (medical therapy)	• Assess patient's compliance with medical (drug) regimen and treatment plan; look for reasons for noncompliance, such as the cost of the medication or side effects. • Provide patient information and education *to facilitate compliance*. • Initiate social service consultation if cost of treatment is a contributing factor.

Patient Education

1. Provide instructions (verbal and written) on medication regimen; ensure that the patient can identify drugs and when each is to be taken, which requires an empty stomach or should be taken after a meal, and so forth.
2. Provide information on relationship of duodenal ulcers and smoking, alcohol, coffee, aspirin-containing compounds, milk, and various antacids.

Evaluation

Patient Outcome	Data Indicating That Outcome is Reached
Duodenal ulcer heals.	Endoscopic examination reveals normal findings and scar. There is no pain.

Patient Outcome	Data Indicating That Outcome is Reached
Patient adheres to plan of care.	Patient resumes a normal diet; avoids coffee, alcohol, aspirin, and smoking; and continues prophylactic medicines as ordered.

Appendicitis

Appendicitis is the inflammation of the vermiform appendix; it may be classified as simple, gangrenous, or perforated. Simple appendicitis involves an inflamed and intact appendix, whereas in gangrenous appendicitis the appendix may have focal or extensive necrosis with microscopic perforations. Gross disruption of the appendix wall occurs in perforated appendicitis.

Acute appendicitis is one of the most common indications for emergency abdominal surgery. The rate of appendicitis is 1 to 2 per 1000, and the disorder is more common in adolescents and young adults. The diagnosis is difficult to determine in very young and elderly individuals. A very young child is often unable to describe the symptoms that are key clues to the diagnosis. In an elderly person the symptoms are vague and may cause the person to delay seeking medical assistance, and then the physician may not consider appendicitis as a possibility. The abdominal tenderness in the elderly may be mild, making diagnosis more difficult. Acute appendicitis is more common in some families than others. Statistics show acute appendicitis to be slightly more common in males than females.

Pathophysiology

Appendicitis can be compared to a closed loop obstruction in which obstruction occurs first and inflammation and infection second. In acute appendicitis the long narrow tube of the appendix is obstructed, hypoxia develops, the mucosa ulcerates, and bacteria invade the wall. The lumen of the appendix may be obstructed by a kinking of the appendix (this is uncommon), edema of the lymphoid tissue, or a fecalith. The lymphoid hyperplasia or edema may develop in response to a viral or bacterial infection. A fecalith is a formed, hard mass of feces. Fecaliths are associated with diets deficient in fiber. After the lumen becomes obstructed, the mucosa continues to secrete fluid until the intraluminal pressure exceeds the venous pressure. Hypoxia develops because blood flow is impeded. The mucosal wall ulcerates, and bacterial invasion occurs. The infection results in more edema, which further impedes blood flow. Gangrene and perforation occur in 24 to 36 hours. Perforation of the appendix creates serious complications, including periappendiceal abscess, pelvic abscess, or peritoneal inflammation.

Atypical appendicitis refers to situations in which the symptoms do not follow the classic presentation of appendicitis. The position of the appendix (retrocecal, pelvic, retroileal, preileal, subcecal), the age of the patient, and pregnancy may affect the symptoms of appendicitis, making diagnosis more difficult.

Diagnostic Studies and Findings

White Blood Cells

Elevated, with shift to the left; 10,000 to 16,000/mm^3; 75% neutrophils

Abdominal Films

Appearance of fecalith in right lower quadrant or localized ileus

Barium Enema (Under Low Pressure)

Nonfilling of the appendix and a mass (useful in atypical cases and infants); not commonly used in routine cases

Intravenous Pyelogram (IVP)

To differentiate appendicitis from suspected urinary tract disease

Urinalysis

Small number of erythrocytes and leukocytes

Medical Plan

Surgery

Appendectomy

Medications

Anti-infective agents
- Metronidazole (Flagyl) or cefamandole (Mandol) as a single prophylactic dose before surgery or for a period postoperatively (to prevent wound infection or pelvic abscess)

NURSING CARE

Nursing Assessment

Abdominal Pain

Pain in epigastrium or periumbilical area that is colicky, peaks in 4 hours, and subsides

Pain reappears in right lower quadrant, is progressively severe, and is exacerbated by movement

Gastrointestinal Functioning

May vomit once or twice; anorexia present
Constipation and failure to pass flatus

Physical Examination

- Temperature
  - Low-grade fever, does not usually exceed 39° C (102° F)
- Abdomen
  - Patient can point to localized pain at McBurney's point (midway between iliac crest and umbilicus)
  - Coughing or moving abdominal wall up and out will reproduce or exacerbate pain
  - Rebound tenderness; muscle rigidity (palpate abdomen with *one* finger)
  - Pain on palpation or percussion can be localized to a spot
- Rectum
  - May be normal; if tenderness present, may be sign of obscure or atypical appendicitis
- Respirations
  - Shallow, rapid
- Positioning
  - Knees bent to reduce tension on abdominal muscles

Atypical Appendicitis

- Retrocecal or retroileal
  - Pain less intense (no discomfort with walking or coughing) and poorly localized
  - Urinary frequency (irritation of ureter)
- Pelvic
  - Very severe, constant pain
  - Localized pain on left
  - Urge to urinate and defecate
  - Tenderness on rectal examination
  - Absence of muscle rigidity and abdominal tenderness
- In infants
  - Lethargy, irritability; anorexia
  - Localized tenderness by abdominal and rectal examinations (done under sedation)
  - May be complication of necrotizing enterocolitis
- In elderly persons
  - Symptoms vague; pain minimal
  - Pain
- In pregnancy
  - Late in gestation, diagnosis more difficult because of displacement of cecum by uterus

Nursing Dx & Intervention

Nursing Diagnosis	Nursing Intervention/Rationale
Pain	• Assess patient's description of the pain type, duration, changes in, and location, since these data are important to the diagnosis. • Help patient reduce pain by having him or her lie still and avoid sudden movements, such as coughing. • Administer analgesics as ordered after the diagnosis has been established.
Altered renal, cerebral, cardiopulmonary, gastrointestinal, and peripheral tissue perfusion	• Assess patient carefully for signs of perforation and peritonitis: Fever Sudden relief of pain, followed by increased diffuse pain, rebound tenderness, and abdominal guarding Increasing abdominal distention Tachycardia Rapid, shallow breathing • Prepare patient for surgery as ordered: give anti-infective agents, shave and prepare the abdomen, and remove dentures. • Provide preoperative teaching, keeping in mind that patient will be unable to practice turn, cough, and deep-breathing exercises because of acute abdominal pain.
Fear	• Assess patient and family for increased tension, apprehension, and other characteristics associated with fear. • Provide emotional support for patient and family, since the pain is acute and frightening and surgery is imminent. • Reassure patient during physical examination of the abdomen, since the procedure is extremely painful; limit the number of abdominal examinations performed.
Ineffective individual coping	• Assess patient's developmental level and previous coping patterns *to plan care (occurs most often in adolescents and young adults).* • Encourage family members to remain with patient as appropriate before surgery *to reduce the amount of separation from sources of support.*

Patient Education

1. Wound or incisional care instructions should be provided.
2. A pattern of increasing activities (i.e., walking, driving) should be provided as recommended by the physician.

Evaluation

Patient Outcome	Data Indicating That Outcome is Reached
Abdominal incision heals.	There is no abdominal pain. Incision heals with scar and without wound exudate, inflammation, or opened edges.
Activity level is normal.	Patient returns to presurgical activities, diet, and interests.

Diverticular disease

Diverticulosis is an out-pocketing or herniation of the mucosa of the large colon through the muscle layers. At first the diverticulum is reducible, but it becomes fixed as the thin covering of longitudinal muscle fibers is lost. In prediverticular disease the pathologic, physiologic, and clinical features are similar to those of diverticulosis without the presence of diverticula.

Diverticulitis is the result of an inflammatory process and localized peritonitis following the perforation of a single diverticulum.

It is often difficult to distinguish between diverticulosis and diverticulitis based on symptoms and diagnostic findings. Spiro[78] recommends the use of a generic descriptive term: diverticular disease of the colon.

The incidence of diverticular disease has increased, and the disorder is more common in Western countries. Australia, the United States, the United Kingdom, and France have high rates of diverticular disease, whereas African, Asian, and Third World countries have low rates. Diverticular disease is related to low-fiber diets; when a Western diet is adopted by blacks in Africa, diverticular disease develops.[73,78]

Diverticular disease is uncommon in persons under 30 years and increases in frequency with age. Approximately one third of individuals over 60 years have diverticular disease, and less than 5% of people with diverticular disease are under age 40.[73] Autopsy studies demonstrate that the disease occurs about equally in both sexes.[78] Diverticula are most often found in the sigmoid colon.[75] Bleeding from diverticular disease is one of the most common causes of lower gastrointestinal hemorrhage.[75]

Pathophysiology

The development of diverticula is related to muscle activities and intraluminal pressures. Normal intraluminal pressure is less than 10 mm Hg in the sigmoid colon. The normal pressure can be increased significantly when the bowel is divided into segments by the muscular contraction rings. The muscular activities in the localized segments can exert enough pressure to increase intracolonic pressure to 90 mm Hg, and this high pressure may push out diverticula.

The outer longitudinal muscle layer in the colon forms a continuous sheath around the colon and is concentrated into three narrow bands, or teniae. The diverticula are usually found between the mesenteric teniae and the antemesenteric teniae. When the circular muscle layer is prominent, the neck of the diverticulum will be narrow.

The muscular weakness that develops with age may result in simple asymptomatic diverticulosis, in which the mucosa slips through a weakened musculature. The hernias, or outpockets, are not fixed and may move back and forth, disappearing on occasion. Muscular hypertrophy in the sigmoid colon may cause thick, prominent longitudinal muscles as well as a thick, corrugated circular muscle layer in the colon. The bowel lumen is constricted by the muscular thickening and the redundant folds. No diverticula are present, but clinical symptoms and radiologic studies often lead to a diagnosis of diverticulosis. This disorder is commonly referred to as prediverticulitis.

Constipation has also been associated with diverticular disease. More pressure is required to move hard, dry fecal material through the lumen. Moist, soft stools and multiple bowel movements each day are associated with high-fiber diets. The decrease in segmentation and intracolonic pressure with high-fiber diets may lessen diverticular disease.

Whether colonic motility is normal is a key issue in examining diverticular disease. Normal colonic motility has been defined as an absence of abdominal pain, whereas pain is present with abnormal colonic motility.[78] The person with abdominal pain with other symptoms of diverticulosis and without radiologic indications of diverticula may still be classified as having diverticular disease based on colonic motility assessments.

The blood flow to the large colon runs from the mesentery around the bowel and divides into branches that go subserosally. These vessels enter the circular muscle obliquely from the mesenteric side of the bowel between the mesenteric and lateral teniae. There is a rich submucosa plexus around the circumference of the colon. The diverticulum that pushes out under the muscular coat has a prominent vasculature over the dome of the diverticulum and at the antemesenteric border of the orifice of the diverticulum. Major bleeding in diverticular disease is associated with the large vessel over the dome. Localized inflammation at the base of the diverticulum with vascular granulation tissue may be the source of minor bleeding from diverticula.

Previously, diverticulitis was believed to be inflammation or abscess formation with a diverticulum that progressed to ulceration and perforation. It is now thought that diverticulitis is the result of a single perforating diverticulum leading to free perforation or a localized pericolic abscess. Perforation of the diverticulum may also be caused by intracolonic pressures and abrasions by fecal material. During episodes of increased intracolonic pressure, fecal abrasions may progress to small diverticular perforations. Fecal material may irritate the mucosa, causing inflammation at the apex or neck of the diverticulum and leading to perforation. Localized peritonitis is more common when the perforation has occurred gradually.

Diagnostic Studies and Findings

Barium Enema

Demonstrates diverticulum and shortening, narrowing, and haustral deformity of the intestine

Ultrasonography

May demonstrate mass or abscess

Sigmoidoscopy or Colonoscopy

Orifices of the diverticula may be visible (high risk of perforation if instrument enters a diverticulum)

Intravenous Pyelogram

To rule out a mass on the left ureter or a colonic vesical fistula

White Blood Cells

Elevated with a shift to the left in diverticulitis

Urinalysis

A few red cells may be found in urine if left ureter is affected

Medical Plan

Surgery*

Sigmoid myotomy (allows colon to resume its width and length)

Bowel resection with or without temporary diverting colostomy

Intestinal obstruction: diverting colostomy in transverse colon

Bladder fistula: resection of fistula, portion of bladder and colon removed, reanastomosis of bladder wall, reanastomosis of colon with or without temporary diverting colostomy

Surgical resection if bleeding uncontrolled by medical management

*Most cases are treated medically; surgery is used only in acute diverticulitis with perforation.

Medications

- Diverticulosis
  - Bran, 10 to 25 g/d in divided doses (must slowly increase to develop tolerance; will help relieve abdominal pain; lowers intraluminal pressure)
  - Laxatives
    - Hydrophilic colloid laxatives (rather than bran in acute phases may be better tolerated; slowly decrease amount as bran and fiber in diet increase)
- Diverticulitis
  - Intravenous fluid therapy
  - Narcotic analgesic
    - Meperidine (Demerol) for analgesia (dose calculated for patient)
  - Anti-infective agents
    - Ampicillin (Amcill), 2 g, *or*
    - Cephalexin (Keflex), 1-4 g/d parenterally in divided doses (mild diverticulitis)
  - Anti-infective agents
    - Gentamicin (Garamycin) or tobramycin (Nebcin), 5 mg/kg/d, and clindamycin (Cleocin), 1.6-2.4 g/d parenterally in divided doses (severe diverticulitis or perforation)
    - Chloramphenicol (Chloromycetin), 4 g/d tapering to 2 g/d (severe diverticulitis)
    - Cefoxitin (Mefoxin), 4-6 g/d parenterally in divided doses
    - All anti-infective agents continued for 7-10 d; not all listed would be used

General Management

Nasogastric tube inserted if nausea, vomiting, and abdominal distention are severe

Radiographic studies and ultrasonography used to evaluate the response to therapy (i.e., resolution of abscess)

Carcinoma: difficult to detect in bowel with narrowed areas and partial obstruction; use colonoscopy procedures to distinguish between acute diverticular disease and carcinoma following an acute episode

Bleeding; angiographic injection of vasopressin, 0.5 to 1 ml/min

High-fiber diet for managing diverticulosis

Give nothing to eat initially in acute diverticulitis; slowly resume diet; when inflammation has resolved and bowel functioning returns to normal, resume high-fiber diet

For acute diverticulitis, bed rest

NURSING CARE

Nursing Assessment

Pain

Aching pain in left lower quadrant, tenderness; suprapubic pain may be reported; referred pain from lower colon is to the back

Pain more intense with acute diverticulitis

Urinary System

Dysuria; frequency

Passage of gas or stool through urethra (colovesical fistula)

Abdominal Examination

Diverticulosis: tenderness in left lower colon; palpable colon

Diverticulitis: palpable colon, tenderness in left lower quadrant, distended and tympanic abdomen, decreased bowel sounds

Obstructed lumen: increased bowel sounds (if partial) may become an ileus (if total), abdominal distention

Nursing Dx & Intervention

Nursing Diagnosis	Nursing Intervention/Rationale
Altered renal, cerebral, cardiopulmonary, gastrointestinal, and peripheral tissue perfusion	• Assess patient for lower gastrointestinal bleeding, a complication of diverticular disease. • Assess patient for signs and symptoms of sepsis, a complication of diverticulitis. • Maintain intravenous fluids, monitor vital signs, intake, and output if complications occur *to prevent intravascular fluid imbalance*.
Pain	• In acute phase, provide low-fiber diet *to allow bowel inflammation to resolve*. (Patients with acute and chronic disease should avoid nuts and popcorn.) • In diverticulosis, provide bran or other good fiber source with instructions on slowly increasing the amount *to promote soft, moist stools*. • Discuss with patient efficacy of increasing fiber, fluids, and activity *to prevent constipation*. • Provide analgesic as ordered.
Constipation	• Provide bran or hydrophilic colloid laxative, increase oral fluid intake, and increase patient's activity level *to reduce constipation (dry stool)*. • Initiate dietary consultation or provide information on high-fiber diets. • See p. 860 for management of temporary colostomy and interventions related to care and adaptation.

Patient Education

1. Dietary instructions on high-fiber diet should be provided. Teach the patient ways to make bran more palatable (e.g., muffins, use on cereals).
2. Discharge instructions should include relationships of diet to diverticular disease, assessment of bowel movements to evaluate dietary intake of bran and fluids, and signs of complications of acute diverticular disease.
3. Instruct the patient in bowel training, that is, to set aside a time daily without anxiety or interruption to have a bowel movement.
4. See p. 862 for colostomy care instructions.

Evaluation

Patient Outcome	Data Indicating That Outcome is Reached
Body functioning is normal.	Bowel movements are soft and occur at least once a day. There is no abdominal pain, nausea, vomiting, or anorexia. Temperature is normal. Temporary colostomy, if performed, is closed. Patient is able to describe high-fiber diet, plan meals, and describe medications and relationship of foods and drugs to disease.
Diagnostic findings are normal.	White blood cell count is within normal range. There is no evidence of acute disease or carcinoma on radiologic study or colonoscopy.
Abdominal incision (if surgical intervention required) heals.	There is no abdominal pain; incision heals with scar and without wound exudate, inflammation, or open edges.

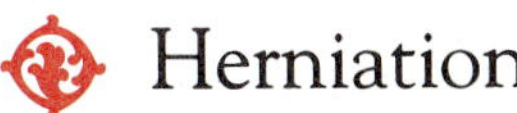

Herniation

A hernia is a protrusion of an organ (usually bowel) through an abnormal opening in the muscle wall. Hernias may be congenital (failure of certain structures to close after birth) or acquired when muscle weakens (associated with obesity, surgery, or illness or from increased abdominal pressure secondary to straining or ascites).

Hernias may be found in any age group. There is a common association between heavy lifting and hernia formation. Regardless of whether the hernia is congenital or acquired, the primary concern is the possibility of obstruction of the bowel lumen, ischemia to the segment, or decrease in blood flow, and loss of blood leading to necrosis and perforation. Congenital internal hernias may be diagnosed because of the complication of intestinal obstruction.

Pathophysiology

Internal congenital hernias are associated with a failure of the intestine to rotate in the usual sequence in the fetus. There are three stages of rotation. Initially the intestine is an unattached, mobile tube; during gestation, as the loop of bowel forming the midgut elongates, it migrates into the umbilicus cord and rotates 180 degrees counterclockwise with the mesenteric vessels as an axis. As the intestines return to the peritoneal cavity, rotation 90 degrees counterclockwise occurs. The cecum will move from the left side of the abdomen over the superior mesenteric vessels toward the right lower quadrant. The duodenum, descending colon, and the mesentery of the small intestines are fixed to the posterior abdominal wall. The mesentery of the bowel follows an oblique path across the abdomen from the ligament of Treitz (upper left) to the lower right quadrant. When this series of events does not occur, complications develop. The infant may be born with an omphalocele, nonrotation, reversed rotation, or malrotation. The results are abnormal adhesions, fixations, and bands that lead to obstructions, volvulus, and internal hernias.

Internal hernias are associated with malrotation. Paraduodenal hernias develop when the mesentery is not fixed. Left-sided paraduodenal hernias are more common than right-sided paraduodenal hernias. The left paraduodenal hernia forms when the rotation of the midgut is reversed; the duodenum lies posterior to the descending colon and is separated from the rest of the peritoneum. Paracecal hernias are also associated with malrotation.[78]

External hernias include inguinal, femoral, umbilical, and incisional hernias. The inguinal hernia is the most common. It is a weakness in the abdominal wall where the spermatic cord (men) or the round ligament (women) emerges. In an indirect inguinal hernia the herniation protrudes through the inguinal ring and follows the round ligament or spermatic cord. A direct inguinal hernia goes through the posterior inguinal wall. Inguinal hernias are more common in men.

A femoral hernia, or protrusion through the femoral ring into the femoral canal, is seen as a bulge below the inguinal ligament. It occurs more frequently in women. Femoral hernias strangulate easily.

The umbilical hernia is more common in children and occurs when the umbilical opening fails to close after birth.

Ventral and incisional hernias are associated with muscle weakness from abdominal incisions. Hernias after surgery are more common in obese persons, those with ascites, and those who have had wound infections or wounds healed by secondary intention.

Medical Plan

Surgery

Herniorrhaphy (surgical repair of hernia) or hernioplasty (reinforcement of weakened area with wire, fascia, or mesh)

Temporary colostomy (for complications of intestinal obstruction or strangulation of hernia)

General Management

Binder or truss (to reduce hernia and to prevent protrusion; danger: strangulation if not reduced properly)

NURSING CARE

Nursing Assessment

Physical Examination of Abdomen

Examine patient supine and sitting

Can often see hernia "bulge" or protrude as person changes position, coughs, or when children cry or laugh (many patients have a history of being able to reduce their own hernias before seeking repair)

Palpate weakened muscle area

Abdominal distention, nausea, and vomiting may be early signs of intestinal obstruction

Pain of increasing severity, fever, tachycardia, and abdominal rigidity are signs of strangulations

Nursing Dx & Intervention

Nursing Diagnosis	Nursing Intervention/Rationale
Altered renal, cerebral, cardiopulmonary, gastrointestinal, and peripheral tissue perfusion	• Assess patient for signs of impending intestinal obstruction or strangulation and ischemia of the herniation (see pp. 793 and 798). • Provide preoperative teaching *if surgery is required to reduce the hernia or to manage complications.* • Assess postoperatively for complications related to anesthesia and surgery: hemorrhage, shock, and respiratory distress. • Ambulate patient per physician's order. • Apply scrotal support for inguinal hernia repairs. • Use ice packs *to reduce or prevent scrotal edema following surgery.*
Altered patterns of urinary elimination	• Assess bladder for distention, *since patient may have difficulty voiding postoperatively.* • Help male patient stand to void.
Impaired gas exchange	• Assess respiratory function after surgery. • Have patient turn and deep breathe after surgery; caution patient to avoid coughing, *since it increases pressure or strain on the surgical repair.* • Teach patient to splint incision with hands or pillows if necessary to cough or sneeze *to provide incisional support.*
Potential impaired skin integrity	• Assess patient's skin for irritation *from binders or truss.* • Evaluate the binder for size, pressure points, and effectiveness in maintaining a reduced hernia.

Patient Education

1. Inform the patient of the need to lose weight if the patient is obese.
2. The patient should avoid heavy lifting for 6 to 8 weeks unless otherwise specified by the physician.
3. If the patient will use a binder at home, provide correct instructions for application. Teach the patient to observe the skin for irritation and to evaluate the effectiveness of the system.

Evaluation

Patient Outcome	Data Indicating That Outcome is Reached
Patient recovers from surgical procedures.	Hernia or bulge is absent. Incision heals with scar and without wound infection, open edges, or exudate. Patient returns to presurgical activity, with delayed return to lifting objects.

Hirschsprung's disease

Hirschsprung's disease is a congenital disorder in which the autonomic nerve ganglia in the smooth muscle of the colon are absent. The aganglionic segment may be limited or occasionally involve the entire colon. There is absence of peristalsis in the involved narrowed segment progressing to stasis of stool and dilation of the proximal colon, which is commonly referred to as congenital megacolon.

Hirschsprung's disease is a familial disease, occurring in approximately 1 of 5000 live births. It is more common in males than females, with a ratio of 3.8:1.[7,78] Long-segment disease is more common in females and has a greater incidence among siblings. Approximately 75% of patients with Hirschsprung's disease have aganglionosis in the rectum and lower sigmoid colon extending proximally above the anorectal junction. In short-segment Hirschsprung's disease, aganglionosis extends to and below the anorectal junction. Ultrashort-segment Hirschsprung's disease is limited to the anal canal. The entire colon is aganglionic in 5% to 8% of the cases.[75,78]

Hirschsprung's disease is associated with Down syndrome. Although congenital megacolon and Down syndrome occur in approximately 2% of the cases, Hirschsprung's disease is also associated with other anomalies, such as megalocystis and megaureter, hydrocephalus, ventricular septal defect, cystic deformities of the kidney, imperforate anus, Meckel's diverticulum, and familial polyposis.

Although Hirschsprung's disease is more commonly diagnosed and treated in children, occasionally adults will have previously undiagnosed disease. The older individual generally has a history of chronic constipation and regular use of enemas. Fecal masses may be palpable in the colon.

Pathophysiology

The primary problem in Hirschsprung's disease is the absence of ganglion cells in the submucosa (Meissner's plexus) and intramuscular (Auerbach's plexus) layers of the bowel wall. The aganglionosis develops when the caudal migration of cells from the neural crest fails. Although the cause is unknown, congenital susceptibility and an ischemic episode (before or after birth) may be responsible for Hirschsprung's disease. Anoxia of the bowel for 4 hours has been found to destroy intramural ganglion cells in the colon of mice and is postulated as a part of the cause of Hirschsprung's disease.[37]

The aganglionic segment is narrowed, strictured, and permanently contracted. The bowel proximal to the aganglionic segments hypertrophies and dilates, hence the term "megacolon." The bowel contents fail to enter the aganglionic segment, and a functional obstruction occurs.

The relaxation of the internal anal sphincter is a normal response to rectal distention, but this response is absent in Hirschsprung's disease. Rather than relaxing, the internal sphincter contracts. The internal sphincter represents the distal end of the circular smooth muscle, and the aganglionic portion of the colon adjacent to the internal anal sphincter also contracts rather than relaxing. Resting pressure in the internal sphincter is normal or slightly elevated in Hirschsprung's disease, with the inappropriate contraction as a response to rectal distention.

The rectal wall in Hirschsprung's disease has an increased resistance to stretch that has been related to the prognosis of clinical symptoms. The more resistance present, the more severe the clinical symptoms.[3] Acetylcholinesterase has been found in excessive amounts in aganglionic segments. The enzyme is used in nerve impulse transmissions. The presence of acetylcholinesterase in serum and red blood cells and in superficial biopsy specimens may be used as a diagnostic test for Hirschsprung's disease. In Hirschsprung's disease the enzyme cannot be used by the aganglionic segments, resulting in higher levels.

Diagnostic Studies and Findings

Full-Thickness Biopsy of Bowel Wall

Biopsy should be obtained at least 3 cm proximal to pectinate line

Absence of ganglion cells indicates Hirschsprung's disease

Mucosal Suction Biopsy

Presence of ganglia in Meissner's plexus excludes Hirschsprung's disease

Absence of ganglia cells does not establish diagnosis and is followed by full-thickness biopsy

Barium Enema

Narrowed distal rectal or rectosigmoid segment with dilated proximal colon is indicative of Hirschsprung's disease (exception: infants in whom narrowed segment will not have had time to develop significantly)

Retention of barium enema at 24 hours is suggestive of Hirschsprung's disease

Proctosigmoidoscopy

Normal empty rectum with no evidence of organic obstruction indicative of Hirschsprung's disease

Manometry

Loss of normal relaxation response of internal anal sphincter (test is recommended in older children and is supportive but not diagnostic by itself; false negative or false positive in 10% of cases)

Staining Biopsy Specimens for Acetylcholinesterase

Elevated levels in Hirschsprung's disease

Differential Diagnosis of Acquired Megacolon or Habitual Constipation

Stool present in rectum and fecal soiling more common in acquired megacolon

History of constipation for several weeks

Medical Plan

Surgery

Diverting temporary colostomy for proximal decompression

Definitive surgery involves removal of the aganglionic segment and a pull-through procedure of the ganglionic bowel to the anus (commonly used pull-through procedures: Swenson, Duhamel, and Soave)

General Management

Enemas may be used for decompression before surgery but are not recommended for long-term treatment

NURSING CARE

Nursing Assessment

Infant

Abdomen
- Abdominal distention
- Functional bowel obstruction
- Vomiting
- Gas and fluid-filled loops of small intestine on x-ray examination

Rectum
- Initial passage of meconium delayed
- Absence of stool in rectum (following rectal examination there may be a gush of meconium and a temporary decompression of bowel)

Enterocolitis
- Bloody diarrhea
- Fever
- Explosive, watery diarrhea
- Rapid onset of dehydration
- Perforation
- Pericolic abscess
- Septicemia

Young Child: Abdominal Examination and History

- Persistent abdominal distention; recurrent fecal impaction and constipation
- Fecal mass may be palpable in left colon
- Growth and mental retardation
- History of congenital anomalies

Adult: Abdominal Examination and History

- Chronic intermittent constipation requiring enemas
- Abdominal distention

Nursing Dx & Intervention

Nursing Diagnosis	Nursing Intervention/Rationale
Constipation	• Assess the abdomen of newborn who has not passed meconium in the first 48 to 72 hours for signs of intestinal obstruction. • Report presence of abdominal distention, repeated vomiting, and constipation or diarrhea (diarrhea may be early sign of associated enterocolitis). • Monitor intake and output. • Replace fluid losses as ordered. • Give enemas as ordered; observe patient carefully for complications of procedure. Amount is determined according to body size: Tap water enemas (greater than 2 L): readily absorbed in dilated, hypertrophied colon; assess for water intoxication Soapsuds enemas: carry risk of causing soapsuds colitis Mineral oil enemas: may be valuable in lubricating very dry stool in colon Saline enemas: shock has been reported from absorption of water from excessive quantities of isotonic saline enemas Hypertonic phosphate enemas: in infants and young children may be a problem; large quantities of water move into colon while sodium or phosphate or both are absorbed; central nervous system changes related to sodium concentrations; tetany related to hyperphosphatemia and hypocalcemia • Assess colostomy stoma for mucocutaneous junction, stoma color, and bowel functioning. • Apply skin barrier and pouch *to protect the skin and contain the stool* (see p. 862 for colostomy care).
Actual and potential altered parenting	• Provide parents with an opportunity to nurture and care for the child during initial and subsequent hospitalizations. • Provide ongoing support for families during hospital and outpatient experiences. • Coordinate an interdisciplinary approach including the patient, family, primary physician, surgeon, ET nurse, primary nurse, and social worker.
Potential impaired skin integrity	• Provide skin protection from colostomy effluent with solid-form skin barriers and open-ended drainable pouches. • Provide skin protection for the perineal area following the pull-through procedures (diarrhea is a common postoperative problem and can progress to extremely denuded or severely irritated perineal skin). • Use a combination of perineal skin cream and a perineal ointment if diarrhea or incontinence occurs postoperatively.

Patient Education

1. Prepare the parents to care for the colostomy (p. 862).
2. Teach young child to empty his or her pouch and progress to self-care as appropriate to child's age level.

Evaluation

Patient Outcome	Data Indicating That Outcome is Reached
Body functioning is normal.	Patient is continent for bowel elimination. There is no diarrhea, constipation, or skin irritation.

Intestinal obstruction

An intestinal obstruction occurs when the contents of the intestines fail to propel forward through the lumen. Intestinal obstructions may be mechanical or functional.

Mechanical obstructions are caused by a blockage of the bowel lumen by adhesion, hernia, volvulus, tumor, inflammation (as in Crohn's disease), impacted feces, or intussusception. Functional obstructions, also referred to as ileus, occur when there is a loss of propulsive peristalsis associated with abdominal surgery, hypokalemia, intestinal distention, peritonitis, severe traumas, spinal fractures, ureteral distention, or the effects of some narcotic drugs and diphenoxylate (Lomotil).

Intestinal obstructions are more common in persons who have undergone abdominal surgery or who have had congenital abnormalities of the bowel. An intestinal obstruction, if untreated, can progress to a life-threatening disorder. The severity and types of symptoms vary according to the cause and location of the intestinal obstruction. Ninety percent of intestinal obstructions are the result of adhesions or incarcerated hernias. Intussusceptions are the most common cause of intestinal obstructions in children between the ages of 2 months and 5 years.[76]

Mechanical obstructions can be caused by factors that block the lumen of the bowel wall, in which case they are referred to as obturation obstructions. This category includes intussusception, large gallstones, feces, meconium, or bezoars. Intrinsic factors that may progress to mechanical obstructions include congenital atresia or stenosis, strictures associated with chronic inflammation or neoplasms, iatrogenic strictures following intestinal surgery or radiation therapy, and mesenteric vascular occlusion. Extrinsic factors that may lead to mechanical obstructions of the intestine are the most common cause of intestinal obstructions and include adhesions, hernias, neoplasms, abscesses, and volvulus.

Mechanical obstructions may be simple obstructions in the small bowel or colon or strangulation obstructions. The location of a mechanical obstruction is important in determining the sequelae. Simple mechanical obstructions may resolve medically, whereas strangulation obstructions require surgical intervention.

The paralytic ileus or functional obstruction commonly occurs in patients undergoing abdominal surgery. Prolonged intestinal distention, hypokalemia, peritonitis, narcotic use, and intestinal ischemia are associated with the development of an ileus.

Pathophysiology

An accumulation of fluid and gas proximal to an obstruction occurs in a simple mechanical obstruction of the small bowel. Initially, the pooled fluids include ingested foods and digestive enzymes. Intestinal gas, in obstruction, is primarily made up of swallowed air that has high concentrations of nitrogen and is not absorbed by the intestinal mucosa. The distention of the bowel by the trapped fluids and gases causes the small bowel to secrete water and electrolytes into the obstructed lumen.

The distention impedes venous return and inhibits the absorptive quality of the mucosa. The bowel wall becomes edematous. The bowel continues to secrete water, sodium, and potassium into the obstructed segment. As the obstruction continues, the intestinal distention is self-perpetuating. Distention increases the intestinal secretions of water and electrolytes into the lumen. As fluid and gas pour into the intestine, motility is further compromised and the distention enlarges proximally. Successive loops of proximal bowel distend, fill with fluid, and stop absorbing. Transudation of water through the wall of the obstructed segment may develop, leading to the development of peritoneal fluid. Distention may lead to pressure necrosis of the bowel wall.

Bacteria are not usually found in the small intestine, but during intestinal obstruction an abnormal bacterial flora that rapidly proliferates is found in the intestinal lumen. The bacteria produce some hydrogen or methane gas that contributes to the gaseous distention. Also, the small bowel contents become feculent during obstructions as a result of the bacterial proliferation.

The site and duration of intestinal obstruction affect the symptoms and potential metabolic effects. Obstructions in the upper jejunal area usually result in vomiting and little abdominal distention. Dehydration and electrolyte depletion occur.

In distal small bowel obstruction or ileal obstructions, constipation is an early symptom. Vomiting, which is not a prominent symptom, is less effective in reducing intestinal decompression. Reflex vomiting may result from intestinal distention. In distal small bowel obstruction, large quantities of fluid and electrolytes may become trapped in the intestinal lumen, resulting in nausea and passage of gas. As much as

8 L of fluids may be found in the lumen with untreated, prolonged obstructions.[78] The patient has classic signs and symptoms of circulatory shock (severe hypovolemia). Before the development of shock, dehydration and metabolic acidosis accompanied by oliguria, azotemia, and hemoconcentration occur. Early circulatory changes may be detected by tachycardia, low central venous pressure, and hypotension. Hypovolemic shock develops if the obstruction is not treated.

The intestinal distention can impair breathing because abdominal distention causes elevation of the diaphragm. The increased intra-abdominal pressure caused by the intestinal distention may impede venous return from the legs.

Death of the bowel wall (bowel necrosis) complicates intestinal obstructions. Shock can quickly develop when long loops of bowel are affected. Short-segment involvement progresses quickly to perforation and peritonitis.

Impaired circulation to the bowel wall during obstructions is referred to as a strangulation obstruction. The circulation may be impeded by a closed-loop obstruction that causes occlusion of the lumen at two points along the length of the bowel segment. Volvulus is an example of a closed-loop obstruction. The closed-loop obstruction progresses to strangulation more rapidly than a simple mechanical blockage of the lumen. The circulation to the bowel may also be impaired by a sustained increase in intraluminal pressure, as with intestinal distention.

When the circulation is impaired, the venous outflow is impaired and the mural veins become engorged. The bowel wall becomes ischemic. An arterial spasm follows, and the bowel responds to anoxia with increased peristalsis. Within 15 minutes, blood escapes from the engorged veins and infiltrates the submucosa and mucosa, resulting in a hemorrhagic infarction of the tissues. Venous thrombosis occurs, further compromising circulation. The necrosis develops from the mucosa outward. Small intravascular thrombi extend the area of necrosis. The lymph channels dilate and may carry bacteria from the lumen into the serosa. Initially, the fluid accumulating resembles plasma, and it gradually becomes bloody and contains bacteria and toxins.

Strangulation results in loss of blood and plasma from the affected segment. Shock occurs quickly if the patient has been dehydrated before strangulation developed. Gangrene may develop and progress to peritonitis. Perforation of the strangulated segment may occur. The toxic substance released during a strangulation obstruction into the peritoneum and the circulation is lethal when given to normal animals. The toxic material may be absorbed from the peritoneal cavity, producing systemic effects. Bacterial infection and toxemia are generally thought to be responsible for the shock that can quickly develop in strangulation obstructions.

In colonic obstructions the colon may become massively distended by gas. Fluid and electrolyte losses are not as significant as in small bowel obstructions and occur when the obstruction is prolonged. When the ileocecal valve is competent, there is little if any small bowel distention. However, a competent ileocecal valve may resist backward decompression enough to produce a closed-loop obstruction. If this develops, cecal distention may be significant and may progress to perforation of the cecum.

The most common cause of colon obstruction is cancer, and perforation during obstructive episodes is adjacent to the tumor. As in small bowel obstructions, the patient must be carefully observed for signs and symptoms of strangulation obstruction.

Diagnostic Studies and Findings

History and Physical Examination

Crampy abdominal pain, the onset of which is clearly recalled
Vomiting
Obstipation
Abdominal distention and tenderness
Peristaltic rushes

Serial Abdominal Roentgenograms

Abnormally large amounts of gas in the bowel
Films taken with patients standing or sitting, supine, and on left side

Barium Enema*

Barium will clear entire colon or stop at site of obstruction

Serum Electrolytes

Demonstrates electrolyte losses

White Blood Cell Count

Sudden rise greater than 10,000 indicates strangulation

Serum Amylase

Normal value rules out acute pancreatitis

Hemoglobin or Hematocrit

Raised values indicate hemoconcentration secondary to fluid losses

Medical Plan

Surgery

Used when cause of obstruction is thought to be adhesions, necrosis, tumor, or unresolved inflammatory lesions (e.g., strictures found in Crohn's disease)
Surgical resection of mechanical obstruction after patient's fluid and electrolytes are stabilized; strangulation obstructions are a surgical emergency
In colonic obstructions, a decompression colostomy to allow relief of the obstruction is the first stage; a cecostomy tube may be used rarely in patients with cecal distention

*Meglucamine diatrizoate (Gastrografin) used if perforation is suspected.

The second surgical procedure is resection and anastomosis
The third surgical stage is closure of colostomy

General Management

Nasogastric (for upper or jejunal obstruction) or intestinal suctioning (for distal obstructions); Cantor, or long, tubes used when obstruction is caused by infection or inflammation and can resolve with medical therapy (intravenous fluids and electrolytes; administration of blood or plasma)

NURSING CARE

Nursing Assessment

History

Abdominal pain
- Crampy pain with sudden onset in periumbilicus area, intermittent with pains associated with peristaltic waves (attempting to move the obstruction)
- Localized tenderness and continuous severe pain existing between colic attacks and indicative of strangulation

Vomiting
- Proximal jejunal obstructions: profuse vomiting unassociated with abdominal distention
- Distal small bowel obstruction: less vomiting, feculent odor (secondary to bacterial proliferation in obstructions)
- Colonic obstructions: vomiting after prolonged obstructions; usually secondary to pain; may contain fecal material

Constipation
- Obstipation and failure to pass gas are signs of a complete obstruction *after* the bowel distal to the obstruction has been evacuated

Previous surgeries
- Adhesions, malrotations, and hernias are common causes of mechanical obstructions

History of inflammatory bowel disease
- Crohn's disease, ulcerative colitis, diverticulitis, or symptoms of malignancy

Physical Examination

Abdomen
- Observe for presence of hernias
- Note amount of abdominal distention; girth measurements may be beneficial in observing the progress of an obstruction
- Mechanical obstruction: peristalsis is high-pitched, tingling sound with rushes
- Visible peristalsis: seen moving toward obstruction and reversing
- Paralytic ileus: absence of bowel sounds or low infrequent sounds
- Auscultate abdomen for full 5 minutes before palpating
- Localized tenderness, constant pain, guarding, and rebound tenderness are signs of strangulation obstructions

Additional physical findings
- Tachycardia and hypotension may indicate dehydration or peritonitis
- Fever and leukocytosis may indicate strangulation
- Loss of skin turgor and dry mucous membranes indicate dehydration
- Blood in stool may indicate cancer, intussusception, or infarction as obstructing lesions

Nursing Dx & Intervention

Nursing Diagnosis	Nursing Intervention/Rationale
Fluid volume deficit (1)	• Assess patient carefully for signs and symptoms of severe fluid and electrolyte loss, metabolic acidosis, and hypovolemic shock secondary to accumulation of gas and fluids and distention of intestine and sepsis (if perforation occurs). • Replace intravenous fluids and electrolytes, blood, and plasma *to replace and maintain fluid volume.* • Monitor vital signs, central venous pressure, blood pressure, urinary output, and nasogastric aspirations every hour. • Measure abdominal girth every 4 to 8 hours *to assess distention.* • Notify physician of changes in patient's status, since they generally indicate a decline in patient's stabilization for surgical intervention.
Ineffective breathing pattern	• Assess patient's pulmonary status, since abdominal distention and abdominal guarding can impair pulmonary ventilation, as can metabolic imbalances. • Elevate head of bed *to relieve pressure on the diaphragm.* • Provide oxygen therapy as ordered.
Pain	• Assess abdominal area for signs of perforation and peritonitis: increased severity and diffuseness of pain, rebound tenderness, guarding.

Nursing Diagnosis	Nursing Intervention/Rationale
	• Help patient assume a comfortable position (one that places minimum stress on the abdominal muscles); limit sudden movement and abdominal examination. • Provide analgesics as prescribed.
Patient problem: potential obstruction	• Assess bowel sounds: High-pitched, tingling sounds with rushes (mechanical obstruction) Absence of bowel sounds or low infrequent sounds (paralytic ileus) • Assess bowel movements: obstipation and failure to pass gas are signs of complete obstruction.

Patient Education

1. Do primary postoperative teaching if resection and anastomosis of small bowel obstruction were performed. This includes showering, activity progression, driving, and returning to work.
2. Colonic obstructions are often treated with a temporary diverting colostomy, and the patient requires instruction in colostomy care and plans for continued surgical interventions, and education about the primary cause of the obstruction (see p. 862).

Evaluation

Patient Outcome	Data Indicating That Outcome is Reached
Body functioning is normal.	Bowel elimination pattern is normal. Colostomy is closed, and patient returns to normal elimination functions.
Fluid balance is maintained.	Patient returns to normal hydration levels as assessed by skin turgor, skin color and mucous membrane, and blood pressure and pulse.
Laboratory studies are normal.	Serum electrolytes, hematocrit, and hemoglobin are within normal limits.
Sepsis is not present.	Patient is not febrile; white blood cell count is within normal limits.

Intestinal ischemia

Intestinal ischemia may develop when the mesenteric vascular supply is insufficient. Acute and chronic occlusion of blood flow to the splanchnic bed, thrombosis or embolus of the superior mesenteric artery, strangulation obstructions, chronic vascular insufficiency, anoxia, or hypotension may lead to intestinal ischemia.

Intestinal ischemia has in the past been difficult to diagnose. The symptoms initially do not correspond with physical examination and laboratory findings. As the ischemia progresses, the severity of the patient's condition becomes apparent, and perforation and peritonitis may have already occurred. Advances in angiography have assisted the physician in diagnosing intestinal ischemias. Awareness of intestinal ischemias is increasing, and angiography is being used to rule out acute occlusion of vessels when patients are seen with sudden onset of severe abdominal pain. Poor perfusion of the intestine is known to result in ischemia, and the syndromes of poor perfusion are gaining more attention. The frequency of thrombosis or embolus as the cause of mesenteric ischemia has been reported to be as high as 75%. Diagnosis of poor perfusion syndromes as the pathologic cause of the ischemic episode has decreased the incidence of occlusions of the large vessels to 25%.[78]

Advances in vascular surgery and advances in nutritional and fluid replacement following intestinal resections have allowed a more aggressive approach in the treatment of intestinal ischemias. Although vascular disorders of the intestines are more common in older persons with arteriosclerosis, cases have been reported in children and pregnant women.

Pathophysiology

The blood flow to the intestines may be affected by a variety of factors.[41] The following factors increase splanchnic blood flow:

- Presence of food
- Digestive hormones: gastrin, secretin, and cholecystokinin
- Metabolite-produced muscle activity
- Beta-stimulating sympathomimetic amines

The following factors decrease splanchnic blood flow:

- Physical activities
- Abdominal distention (marked intraluminal pressure)
- Alpha-stimulating sympathomimetic amines
- Cardiac glycosides (digitalis)

The response to the alteration in blood flow depends on the degree of obstruction of blood flow, the rapidity of onset, the duration of the process, and the efficiency of the collateral circulation. Disease processes may affect both large and small vessels. This section reviews the normal pattern of blood flow to the intestines; the cause of alteration of blood flow, including a variety of diseases that affect blood distribution to the bowel; and the pathophysiology of events.

The intestine receives its blood supply from the celiac, the superior mesenteric, and the inferior mesenteric arteries. These three major vessels arise from the abdominal aorta and subdivide into a complex collateral circulation. The celiac artery divides into the splenic, left gastric, and hepatic arteries; all three of these divisions supply the stomach. The splenic artery supplies the greater curvature, and the left gastric artery supplies the lesser curvature. The hepatic artery divides into the gastroduodenal, which divides to form the superior pancreaticoduodenal and right gastroepiploic arteries. The celiac axis is interconnected with the superior mesenteric through pancreaticoduodenal arcades.

The celiac artery originates from the aorta at the level of the first lumbar and twelfth thoracic vertebrae. It then passes to the median arcuate ligament of the diaphragm. In celiac compression syndrome, abnormal positioning of the artery and the ligament affects blood flow.

The superior mesenteric artery divides into the ileocolic, middle colic, and right colic arteries. The terminal ileum, cecum, and proximal ascending colon are supplied by the ileocolic artery. The ascending colon and hepatic flexure are supplied by the right colic artery. The middle colic vessel supplies the proximal portion of the transverse colon.

In addition to the above branches, the superior mesenteric artery divides into smaller arteries that supply the jejunum and ileum. The superior mesenteric artery connects with the celiac axis through the pancreaticoduodenal artery. In this way the small intestine receives its blood flow.

The vessels originating from the superior mesenteric artery ultimately enter the wall of the intestine as end arteries. Few anastomotic connections are found in the bowel wall. Vasculitis may result in the selective occlusion of the distal vessels and may lead to segmental infarction and small bowel ischemia and necrosis.

The superior mesenteric artery is susceptible to atherosclerotic changes and is a common site for thrombosis and embolus. The inverted Y shape of the superior mesenteric artery as it leaves the aorta provides a channel for emboli. Thromboses and emboli tend to occlude the superior mesenteric within 2 cm of its origin off the aorta.

The inferior mesenteric artery supplies blood to the distal transverse colon, the descending and sigmoid colon, and proximal portions of the rectum. The distal transverse colon and the splenic flexure appear to be more vulnerable to ischemia. A "watershed" area refers to branches of the inferior mesenteric artery anastomosing with the superior artery branches in the rectosigmoid area. The branches involved are the inferior mesenteric and the hypogastric.

Vascular occlusion may be the result of thrombosis or embolus to the superior mesenteric artery. The development of emboli is associated with atrial fibrillation in patients with subacute bacterial endocarditis and cardiac valve disease, mural thrombosis of myocardial infarct, and postintracardiac surgery. Thrombosis of mesenteric vessels is associated with polycythemia, sickle cell trait, intra-abdominal sepsis, pancreatic disorders, and blood dyscrasias. It may also occur after bowel surgery, other major surgery, or abdominal trauma, when there may be a decrease in blood flow to the mesentery. Infarction of the bowel results in a sudden onset of severe abdominal pain, distention, fluid loss, and shock.

Intestinal angina is an obstructive vascular disease involving atherosclerotic changes in two of the three major vessels. An increase in mesenteric blood flow is required to supply oxygen for the metabolic processes of digestion, absorption, and increased peristalsis. Abdominal pain occurs when the superior mesenteric artery supply is less than the demand of the smooth muscle activity in the intestine. Between meals, the patient is free of pain. Intestinal angina is a chronic problem. The patient may develop a fear of eating and begin losing weight. Diagnosis may be delayed because many physicians first test the patient for cancer, since weight loss and pain in older persons are associated with malignancies. Intestinal ischemia may progress to frank infarction of the intestine.

Nonocclusive intestinal ischemia has been reported with increasing frequency. The patient tends to be younger than those with obstructive ischemia. Patients with recent myocardial infarctions, severe congestive cardiac failure, shock, anoxia, or hypotension may develop a nonocclusive intestinal ischemia. An episode of inadequate cardiac output and poor tissue perfusion results in shunting of blood away from the gut to vital organs. The use of α-adrenergic vasoconstrictors in patients in shock adds to the effect of the increased secretions of endogenous catecholamines, further reducing mesenteric blood flow. The mucosa layer is the most sensitive to oxygen deprivation, since it has the highest energy requirement because of its high metabolic activity and rapid cell turnover. The mucosa undergoes hemorrhagic necrosis. As the anoxia continues, the necrosis becomes transmural (involving all layers of the bowel wall).

The patient who develops nonocclusive intestinal ischemia may have evidence of some degree of occlusive or atherosclerotic changes in smaller splanchnic vessels.

Digitalis has been associated with the development of poor perfusion syndromes. Digoxin constricts splanchnic vessels. In patients with early intestinal infarction, considerations should be made regarding discontinuation of digoxin therapy.[72]

Necrotizing enterocolitis of infancy is a variant of intestinal ischemia. In premature infants, anoxia and hypotension lead to poor perfusion of the intestines. Ischemic enterocolitis develops with its progressing sequelae.

Celiac axis compression by the median arcuate ligament of the diaphragm or by neurofibrous tissue of the celiac ganglion is associated with recurrent epigastric pain and an epi-

Table 8-3
Systemic Disorders Affecting Splanchnic Perfusion

Disorder	Definition	Gastrointestinal Implications
Periarteritis nodosa	A progressive, polymorphic disease of connective tissue characterized by numerous large, palpable or visible nodules in clusters along segments of medium-sized arteries	Segmental ischemia with ulceration, hemorrhage, or perforation to massive infarction of bowel; may also have hepatic artery thrombosis; nodules obstruct lumen of vessels
Lupus erythematosus	A chronic inflammatory collagen disease affecting many systems; includes severe vasculitis, renal involvement, and lesions of skin and nervous system	Segmental lesions of ischemia progressing to necrosis and perforation; involvement of submucosa and muscularis leads to protein-losing enteropathy; abdominal pain may be caused by serositis or acute pancreatitis; ulcerative colitis and Crohn's disease have been associated with lupus erythematosus; diagnosis of gastrointestinal involvement difficult to evaluate
Dermatomyositis	A disease of the connective tissue characterized by pruritic or eczematous inflammation of skin and tenderness and weakness of muscles	Vasculitis associated with ischemia of bowel; increased incidence of gastrointestinal cancers with this disorder
Rheumatoid arthritis	A collagen disease that affects the connective tissue by inflammation and fibrinoid degeneration	Vasculitis associated with intestinal ischemia; occurs with abdominal pain
Scleroderma	A relatively rare autoimmune disease affecting blood vessels and connective tissue; most common in middle-aged women	Bowel symptoms arise from fibrosis of the intestinal wall and loss of muscle; focal areas of vasculitis may lead to ischemia
Anaphylactoid purpura (Henoch-Schönlein syndrome)	A self-limited hypersensitive vasculitis that occurs primarily in young children; palpable purpuric skin lesions appear on lower abdomen, buttocks, and legs; arthritis and abdominal pain are also seen; occasionally seen in adults, whose prognosis is not as favorable as children	Colicky abdominal pain; surgery demonstrates submucosal and subserosal hemorrhages; may have upper or lower gastrointestinal bleeding; segmental ischemic bowel episodes may occur but do not generally progress to gross infarction or perforation
Degos' disease (malignant atrophic papulosis)	A rare syndrome of progressive occlusive vascular disease affecting small and medium-sized arteries; primarily involves the skin (malignant atrophic papulosis) and intestine; skin lesions usually precede gastrointestinal symptoms; primarily affects young men	Lesions (identical to skin lesion) are found in mucosa and serosa of bowel; weight loss and diarrhea develop; progresses to intestinal infarction and perforation

gastric bruit (which does not radiate to the lower abdomen). The celiac axis compression is more common in young women and is relieved by surgical division of the ligament or bands. The medical profession has challenged the validity of celiac axis compression as a disorder or a syndrome.[75,78] The cause of the pain and the absence of symptoms in many patients with stenosis of the celiac axis have raised unanswered questions.

Vasculitis has been associated with mesenteric infarction in approximately 3% of reported cases. However, the vasculitis associated with systemic disorders may be seen as intestinal angina or frank infarction. The systemic disorders include polyarteritis nodosa, lupus erythematosus, dermatomyositis, rheumatoid vasculitis, scleroderma, anaphylactoid purpura, and Degos' disease. Table 8-3 examines the bowel involvement that occurs as a result of systemic vasculitis.

Certain surgical procedures such as coarctation of the aorta, excision of abdominal aneurysms, and iliac or femoral grafts are associated with mesenteric vascular insufficiency.

The oxygenation of the bowel depends on patency of the major arterial vessels, arteriolar resistance, adequacy of perfusion pressure, arterial oxygen saturation, and oxygen need. Acute or chronic changes of any or all of the above affect the blood flow to the bowel.

The events of intestinal ischemia include structural changes in the cells within 5 minutes of the occlusion of the superior mesenteric artery. The epithelium becomes detached from the basement membrane at the villus tips, and subepithelial blebs form. Within 30 to 60 minutes, the villi are denuded of epithelium. The mucosa undergoes necrosis and ulceration with an inflammatory cell infiltration. A secondary bacterial invasion occurs. In acute ischemic necrosis, massive submucosa edema and bleeding into the mucous membrane develop because of an increase in capillary permeability followed by loss of capillary integrity.

The submucosal edema and hemorrhage are seen as the "thumbprint" pattern in radiographic studies. The exudation of protein-rich fluid, and later blood, found in the intestinal lumen is the result of the loss of epithelial and vascular integrity. Fluid loss and hypovolemia further compromise blood flow to the intestine.

The development of peritonitis indicates the involvement

of the muscle and serosa layer and that the perforation is imminent or has occurred. If the ischemic episode is self-limited and does not progress to perforation and resection, the acute inflammatory response resolves with granulation tissue, fibrosis, and scarring with potential for development of strictures.

In chronic or gradual reduction of blood flow, the anoxia damages the mucosa initially. The necrosis may be limited to the mucosa, in which event the mucosa will slough with regeneration occurring in 4 to 5 days. The villi may recover, but their shape and functioning abilities are affected and a temporary malabsorption develops that is seen clinically as enterocolitis. As the anoxia continues, the necrosis progresses. A microscopic examination of the bowel may reveal a coagulative necrosis of the inner two thirds of the wall with muscle and serosa uninvolved. A scar may form.

The bowel totally deprived of its blood supply ultimately becomes black and necrotic. The bowel perforates with leakage of intestinal contents. Bacterial invasion of the necrotic bowel produces gas cysts, massive sepsis, and shock. Repair cannot take place when this degree of injury has occurred, and bowel death usually results. If surgery is performed, it is usually a massive bowel resection.

Diagnostic Studies and Findings

Abdominal Films

Tonic contraction of bowel

Plain Films

Complete absence of small bowel air

Generalized distention (later sign)

Thickening of bowel wall with edema and fluid (ischemic colitis)

String or ring of gas outside lumen of bowel (marked necrosis)

Gas in portal vein (evidence of leak of bacteria from infarcted bowel)

Angiography

Abnormal vascular tree (intestinal angina)

Demonstrates site of arterial blockage or spasm (angiographic studies generally indicated only in patients with disorders predisposing to embolization but may be used when other tests are negative and patient is symptomatic; also used preoperatively to map vessels that are narrowed or occluded)

Barium Studies

Early stages find appearance of spasm and irritability with narrowing of bowel lumen and thumbprinting

Colonoscopy

Swollen folds and mucosa, dusky color, presence of ulcerations similar to those found in Crohn's disease

Hematocrit

In presence of necrosis, hemocentration (decreased fluid volume)

White Blood Cell Count

Leukocytosis (20,000 and higher)

Amylase and Lipase

Elevated (from leakage into peritoneum or from back-pressure secondary to development of intestinal obstruction)

Medical Plan

Surgery

Balloon angioplasty (intestinal angina) to improve blood flow

Bypass graft, embolectomy, endarterectomy, and reimplantation procedures have been used effectively

Resection of necrotic bowel segments with a second-look operation to observe bowel viability 12 to 36 hours after initial exploration

Resection, temporary colostomy or ileostomy, and subsequent reanastomosis (colonic ischemia)

Medications

Anti-infective agents

- Agent-specific antibiotics given to reduce bacterial flora of bowel and treat sepsis

Adrenergic agents

- Dopamine in low dosages may be used as a vasopressor if fluid replacement does not correct shock (alpha-stimulating sympathomimetic amines [e.g., norepinephrine] should be avoided)

Vasodilators

- Intra-arterial infusion of vasodilators (glucagon, isoproterenol, papaverine, histamine, and others) has been used, but effectiveness of this treatment has not been clearly documented[75,78]
- Anticoagulation with heparin followed by bishydroxycoumarin (dicumarol) (used in patients with mesenteric venous occlusion that tends to recur); dosages adjusted based on patient's coagulation time

General Management

Electromyography

Doppler ultrasonography

Injection of radioactive microspheres

Intraoperative fluorescein angiography (may be used during surgery to determine viability of bowel and evaluate mesenteric vessels)

Intravenous fluid replacements (low molecular dextran, albumin, fresh frozen plasma, blood)

Nasogastric or intestinal suctioning preoperatively

Hyperalimentation postoperatively

Elemental diets (intestinal angina)

NURSING CARE

Nursing Assessment

This section is divided primarily into assessments of chronic ischemia of the bowel (i.e., intestinal angina) and acute episodes of ischemia. The acute episodes are similar in progression of symptoms, and therefore not all causes are outlined. Acute occlusive ischemia is used as the example. Exceptions are noted. The assessment of abdominal pain is an example of an area where differences do exist in the acute episodes.

Abdominal Pain

Intestinal angina: severe crampy or colicky pain around umbilicus; radiates to back; lasts 2 to 4 hours; no pain between meals

Acute occlusive ischemia: severe colicky pain in the periumbilical area; as ischemia progresses, pain becomes more severe and poorly localized

Ischemic colitis: lower abdominal pain of abrupt onset

Mesenteric venous thrombosis: gradual progression of abdominal pain until it resembles acute occlusive ischemia

Gastrointestinal Response of Ischemia or Necrosis

Intestinal angina: nausea and vomiting; abdominal bloating; malabsorption with steatorrhea and diarrhea

Acute occlusive ischemia: copious vomiting and hematemesis indicate necrosis adjacent to ligament of Treitz; gross rectal bleeding

Enterocolitis symptoms: malabsorption; diarrhea, may be hemorrhagic (seen regardless of cause of ischemia, secondary to sloughing of mucosa and to bacteremia)

Abdominal Findings

Absence of significant abdominal findings intially; hyperperistalsis, with no tenderness or resistance

After necrosis occurs: classic signs of peritonitis with rebound tenderness, rigidity, abdominal distention, and ileus

Signs of Necrosis

Tachycardia

Fever

Hypotension (may have significant amounts of fluids in bowel lumen)

Changes in laboratory values

Nutritional Assessment

Intestinal angina: weight loss; fear of eating because of chronic malabsorption syndrome; malnutrition

Evidence of Poor Perfusion Episodes

Shock; hypotension; anoxia; severe congestive heart failure; recent myocardial infarction or some cause that results in shunting of blood away from the gut to "vital" organs

Nursing Dx & Intervention

Nursing Diagnosis	Nursing Intervention/Rationale
Fluid volume deficit (1)	• Assess patient carefully for signs and symptoms of severe fluid and electrolyte loss, metabolic acidosis, and hypovolemic shock *secondary to accumulation of gas and fluids and distention of intestine and sepsis* (if perforation occurs). • Replace intravenous fluids and electrolytes, blood, and plasma as ordered. • Monitor vital signs, central venous pressure, blood pressure, urinary output, diarrhea, and nasogastric aspirations every hour. • Measure abdominal girth every 8 hours *to assess distention*. • Notify physician of changes in patient's status, since they generally indicate a decline in patient's stabilization for surgical intervention.
Pain	• Assess abdominal area for signs of perforation and peritonitis: increased severity and diffuseness of abdominal pain, rebound tenderness, guarding. • Help patient assume a comfortable position; limit sudden movement and abdominal examination. • Provide analgesics as prescribed.
Diarrhea	• Assess patient for signs of steatorrhea and diarrhea (intestinal angina); gross rectal bleeding (acute occlusive ischemia); and hemorrhagic diarrhea (enterocolitis), which are diagnostic assessments of ischemia of the intestine.
Altered nutrition: less than body requirements	• Assess through careful history a "fear of eating" versus other causes of weight loss. • Provide enteral nutrition as tolerated. • Initiate and monitor hyperalimentation as ordered after operation for significant small bowel resections.

Patient Education

1. Help the patient understand the relationship of eating and pain in intestinal angina.
2. After surgery for venous thrombosis, the patient may need instruction regarding anticoagulant therapy.
3. In colonic ischemia a temporary colostomy may be performed. If so, the patient requires colostomy teaching and plans for surgical closure at a later date.
4. The patient who has had a massive bowel resection may be on home total parenteral nutrition. In these cases the patient and family require extensive discharge preparation (i.e., line care; management of total parenteral nutrition).
5. Help the patient deal with an increase in diarrhea, especially for the first 6 months postoperatively, caused by rapid transit time or varying degrees of malabsorption.

Evaluation

Patient Outcome	Data Indicating That Outcome is Reached
Body functioning is normal.	There is no pain or diarrhea; bowel function is normal. Colostomy is closed.
Fluid balance is maintained.	Patient returns to normal hydration levels as assessed by skin turgor, color, mucous membranes, blood pressure, and pulse.
Laboratory studies are normal.	Serum electrolytes, hematocrit, and WBC are within normal limits.
Nutritional status is normal.	Patient returns to "normal" body weight. Nutritional status is maintained through home hyperalimentation (major resection of small bowel).

Irritable bowel syndrome

Irritable bowel syndrome (IBS), or functional bowel syndrome, is a disorder of the large bowel that results in altered bowel habits, abdominal pain, and absence of detectable disease.

The patient may have diarrhea or constipation or both. Abnormal motor activity of the large bowel can be measured. It is believed that the small bowel may also be involved, but measurement of motor activity in the small bowel is not as easily accomplished.[75]

It is also important to recognize the mislabeling of IBS in the past. Nervous colon, spastic colon, and mucous colitis are incorrect terms. Nervous colon recognizes only one aspect of the possible cause of IBS. Spasticity is one sign or response of the colon to the altered motor activity. Inflammation is not present, making "colitis" a misnomer. IBS does not progress or predispose individuals to inflammatory bowel disease or cancer.

The incidence of IBS is considered high, but accurate data on the prevalance are not available. IBS does not lead to death and therefore does not appear on death certificates. Rarely does IBS require hospitalization. Cohen[15] states that it may be the most common disorder for which medical care is sought. IBS is a leading cause of absenteeism from work. Approximately 20% to 50% of referrals to gastroenterologists are for irritable bowel syndrome.[75,78] Many people with IBS do not seek medical attention because they have mild symptoms, making it more difficult to estimate the prevalence.

The incidence of IBS is higher in females than males with a 2.3:1 ratio. There is a higher incidence in whites than nonwhites and in Jews than non-Jews. Symptoms generally begin before the age of 35, and in many patients isolated instances of IBS during adolescence can be identified by the patients. A third of the patients can trace IBS to childhood.[27]

In children with IBS a high familial incidence has been reported. One or both parents and siblings will have reported IBS. The ratio of males to females is higher during childhood. As with adults, the incidence of IBS is higher in Jewish than non-Jewish children and in whites than nonwhites.

Pathophysiology

IBS is a functional disorder of gastrointestinal motility. The abdominal pain and altered bowel pattern are caused by the altered motility. Motility may be affected by emotions, food, neurohumoral agents, gastrointestinal hormones, toxins, prostaglandins, and colon distention.

Two patterns of IBS are identified: painful IBS with diarrhea, constipation, or both and IBS with painless diarrhea. The two types of IBS can be differentiated on observations of motility recordings. Patients with painful IBS have a characteristic response to rectal distention that is not found in painless IBS.

Segmental contractions are the predominant form of normal motor activity in the colon, consisting of 90% of recorded motor activity. Segmental contractions slow the forward progress of stool, promoting mixing, absorption, and dehydration. Segmental contractions appear as haustral markings on barium studies. Increasing segmental contractions produce constipation, whereas decreasing segmentation results in diarrhea.

A pattern of hypermotility with high-amplitude pressure waves is common in patients with painful IBS. Studies have also demonstrated that contractions over long segments of colon may be accompanied by abdominal pain.[16] Hypermotility in the small bowel is also associated with abdominal pain. Motility in the pain-free diarrheal-predominant IBS is normal or lower than normal.

Motility of the bowel may be affected by a variety of factors. For example, sleep lowers the motor activity in the colon. This may account for the infrequency of nocturnal symptoms. The presence of nocturnal symptoms usually indicates an organic etiology rather than the functional cause of IBS.

Anxiety, depression, fear, and hostility have been identified in IBS as well as other gastrointestinal disorders. Stress and emotions alone do not cause IBS but are related to the clinical course. Stress can be related to the onset of symptoms. Diarrhea can readily be associated with stressful situations such as test taking or job interviews. Constipation is not apparent for several days, and it may be more difficult to pinpoint the source of anxiety or generalized depression.

Meals, or the ingestion of food and caffeine, will stimulate colonic hypermotility in irritable bowel syndrome. The postprandial symptoms are related to this effect. Normally, a meal will lengthen segmental contractions, allowing for additional mixing and absorption, and the effect of the meal slows after approximately 50 minutes. In IBS the meal stimulation of segmental contractions is blunted and the effect continues postprandially, gradually becoming stronger.

The gastroileocolic response to food ingestion moves intestinal contents forward, emptying material in the distal colon and creating distention. Colon distention induces exaggerated spastic contractions in IBS. Patients with alternating diarrhea and constipation or diarrhea-predominant IBS often have a bowel movement after every meal. For some this may be the only symptom of IBS. Based on myoelectric studies, the gastrocolic reflex has been divided into two phases: early neurogenic myoelectric and motor reflex and a delayed hormonally mediated phase.

Smooth muscle cells of the bowel act as small electrical oscillators that produce myoelectrical activity.

The myoelectric activity in IBS is different from the myoelectric activity in normal colons. In IBS the myoelectric frequency is three cycles per minute. The three cycle per minute activity remains constant during symptomatic and asymptomatic periods, regardless of whether the predominant symptom is diarrhea or constipation, and is unaltered by successful treatment. Although researchers are continuing to debate the significance of the three cycles per minute in IBS, it may become a diagnostic marker for IBS. It should also be noted that three cycles per minute is also seen in neurotic personality disorders (with or without IBS), suggesting that this pattern is more characteristic of neurotic disorders than motor disorders.

Neurohumoral agents, such as cholinergic, anticholinergic, adrenergic, and adrenergic-blocking substances, produce hyperactivity of the colon in both normal bowels and in irritable bowel syndrome. In IBS, response to neurohumoral agents is more pronounced and occurs during both symptomatic and asymptomatic periods.

Anticholinergic agents affect colonic activity induced by meals. Anticholinergics suppress an early neurogenic myoelectric and motor reflex component of the gastrocolic reflex in normal subjects. In IBS the myoelectric and motor reflex is not suppressed, but anticholinergics inhibit the second, delayed component of gastrocolic reflex, which is hormonally mediated.

The gastrointestinal hormones that affect motility include cholecystokinin, gastrin glucagon, and vasoactive intestinal peptide. Cholecystokinin is associated with abdominal pain and colonic hypermotility when given through infusion. Since cholecystokinin is released following a meal, this may account for the postprandial pain in IBS. Also, the delayed hormonally mediated phase of the gastrocolic reflex is dependent on the fatty content of the meal. This indicates a relationship with cholecystokinin that produces colonic contractions.

Diagnostic Studies and Findings

Sigmoidoscopy

Spastic contractions that prevent passage of the instrument beyond 10 to 12 cm

Reproduction of symptoms with air insufflation

Mucosa free of ulcers, bleeding, friability, and masses

Do not use enemas or cathartics before sigmoidoscopy (may produce edema, obscuring the normal colon appearance)

Rectal Balloon Distention

Induces spastic contractions and pain

Manometric Studies

May be used to evaluate electric response to colon

Balloons are placed in rectosigmoidal colon (cephalad balloon) and rectum (caudad balloon), and 20 mm of air is instilled into the cephalad balloon every 20 minutes; balloon mimics presence of stool in the area; a graph recording is made of the bowel response to the stimulus

Response in a normal bowel is a brief contraction in rectosigmoid and rectum, with a rapid return to the prestimulus state; in patient with IBS, the distention produces a diffuse spastic contraction in rectosigmoid and rectum

Classically, patients with IBS and diarrhea do not experience significant weight loss as do patients with an inflammatory or viral origin to their diarrhea

Biopsy

To rule out other disorders; not helpful in diagnosing IBS

Stool Test for Guaiac

To rule out inflammatory bowel diseases and malignancy

Stool Stains

To rule out motile amebic trophozoites, leukocytes, and mucus

Stool Cultures

To rule out ova and parasites, specifically *Giardia*

Complete Blood Count

To rule out anemia and inflammation

Differential Blood Cell Count (Eosinophilia)

To rule out parasitosis, cytosis (suggests tuberculosis), and vacuolated cells (suggest inflammation)

Three-Day Trial on Lactose-Free Diet, Lactose Tolerance Test, or Breath Hydrogen Test

To rule out lactose insufficiency in patients with distention and bloating or diarrhea

Double-Contrast Barium Enema

Exaggerated haustral contractions or absence of haustrations; narrow lumen with pellet stones; lumen easily dilated

Cholecystogram or Ultrasonography of Gallbladder

To rule out gallbladder disease in presence of dyspepsia

Small Bowel Series

To rule out obstruction of bowel, if diarrhea and symptoms suggest obstruction

Colonoscopy

To rule out inflammatory bowel disease when clinically justified as in change in symptoms in patient with longstanding IBS; uncontrollable exacerbation of IBS

Thyroid Function

To rule out hyperthyroidism or hypothyroidism if constipation predominates

Carotene (Serum)

To rule out celiac sprue

Medical Plan

Surgery

Rarely colostomy may be done

Medications

Bulk-forming laxatives
- Psyllium preparations (Metamucil, Konsyl, L.A. Formula, Mitrolan) taken at meal times; in obese patients before meals and in thin patients after meals (hydrophilic properties bind water, preventing excessive dehydration of stool and excess liquidity)

Antidiarrheal agents
- Diphenoxylate (Lomotil), 2.5 to 5 mg q4-6h
- Loperamide (Imodium), 2 mg q6-8h
- Paregoric or opium tincture (Parelixir) has been prescribed
- Dependency on antidiarrheals can develop; slow withdrawal of medicines as coping abilities are developed is recommended

Cholinergic blocking agents
- Antispasmodics (for temporary relief of crampy pain related to intestinal spasm)
- For postprandial pain give one of the following 30 to 45 minutes before meals:
  - Dicyclomine (Bentyl), 20 mg
  - Propantheline (Pro-Banthine), 15 mg
  - Tincture of belladonna, 10 to 20 drops

General Management

Patient should be placed on high-fiber (12 to 16 g/d as 2 tablespoons of bran qid; gradually reduced), low-lactose, no caffeine diet before trying drug therapy

Low-fat diet (to reduce stimulation of cholecystokinin)

Avoid irritating foods (idiosyncratic)

Psychotherapy or counseling

Relaxation techniques

NURSING CARE

Nursing Assessment

History and Physical Examination

Presence of lower abdominal pain; small stools, alternating diarrhea and constipation, diarrhea, or constipation

Correlation of onset of symptoms with periods of stress and heightened emotional tension

Symptoms initially appeared during an intercurrent illness and persisted

Tense, anxious patient who may be unaware of features of tenseness

Autonomic lability: rapid, labile pulse; elevated blood pressure; sweaty palms; abdominal tympany

No evidence of weight loss

Palpable, tender sigmoid colon

Constipation

Episodic initially, becomes continuous, increasingly intractable to laxatives and later to enemas

Stools: hard, narrow

Objectively defined as passage of fewer than three stools per week; sometimes patient will have diarrhea following a week of constipation

Subjectively defined as difficult or painful evacuation

Diarrhea

Defined as loose, mushy, or watery stools

Urgency and tenseness in morning or after meals, followed by evacuation

Initial movement may be of normal consistency and is rapidly followed by a softer, unformed stool and then by increasingly loose stools

Abdominal pain relieved by bowel movement

Postprandial diarrhea correlating with quantity rather than type of food

Patients with diarrheal only–type IBS more likely to have explosive, watery stools; classically these patients experience no weight loss

Pain

Often patient locates pain by using the palm to describe a circular motion (rather than finger pointing to one discrete spot)

Pain often precipitated by meals

Pain often relieved by defecation

Abdominal Distention

Quantitative measures indicate that patients with IBS who complain about increased gas, bloating, and flatus produce a normal amount but have a decreased tolerance

Mucus

Amount produced varies

Cause of increased mucus production is unknown, although in the past it was associated incorrectly with inflammation

Nursing Dx & Intervention

Nursing Diagnosis	Nursing Intervention/Rationale
Constipation	• Assess history of bowel movements; in IBS patients often experience constipation followed by diarrhea—constipation may be defined as fewer than three stools per week; defecations described as painful or difficult.
Diarrhea	• Assess history of bowel movements; in IBS diarrhea is defined as loose, mushy, or watery stools; urgency after meals is common; abdominal pain is relieved by defecation.
Ineffective individual coping	• Assess for related factors that would increase stress, tension, or an emotional state. • Help patient recognize the role of emotions, stress, and diet in the symptoms of IBS. • Help patient and family understand that the symptoms are based on functional motility problems and that psychosocial stress accentuates rather than causes the symptoms. • Help patient identify irritating or troublesome foods *since diet may affect motility in IBS.* • Help patient identify sources of stress and counterbalancing relaxation techniques.

Patient Education

1. Provide information on irritable bowel syndrome. Patient education material is available through the National Digestive Disease Education Information Clearinghouse, NIH, 1555 Wilson Blvd., Suite 600, Rosslyn, VA 22209-2461.
2. Instruct the patient in necessary diet alterations. Inform patient that often it is possible to manage with diet and stress reduction without using any medications.
3. Provide written instructions for medications prescribed for the management of IBS by the physician. Ensure that the patient knows the names, amounts, and rationales for the treatment plan.

Evaluation

Patient Outcome	Data Indicating That Outcome is Reached
Psychosocial stress is reduced.	Patient can identify sources of stress and uses effective coping mechanisms.
Symptoms are managed so that life-style does not center around bowel elimination.	Combination of counseling, relaxation techniques, modification of diet (avoiding irritating foods), and medications is effective in relieving symptoms.
Bowel functioning is normal.	Diarrhea and constipation are relieved, and recurrences are managed through medical regimen and stress reduction.

 Lactose intolerance

Lactose intolerance results from a deficiency of the enzyme lactase. Lactase is necessary for the digestion or breakdown of the disaccharide lactose found in the brush border of the intestinal villi. Lactose is found in milk and milk products. Lactose intolerance is a common cause of diarrhea, nonspecific lower gastrointestinal symptoms, and abdominal pain.

Lactose intolerance in the United States is more frequent in blacks, Native Americans, Hispanics, Asians, and some Jews and Arabs.[56,74] Spiro[78] states that 10% to 20% of the white population of northern European ancestry has a lactase insufficiency and that three fourths of the blacks in Africa, as well as some Chinese, Indians, and Mediterranean inhabitants, have lactase insufficiency.

Age also plays a part in lactose intolerance. Primary disaccharidase deficiency refers to a congenital, hereditary absence of the lactase enzyme. The symptoms may be present from birth or may become apparent in middle life. By the age of 10 to 20 years, most persons with genetic tendencies for lactase deficiency have the same low level of lactase as adults. Primary lactase insufficiency is associated with a normal bowel mucosa and epithelial cells.

Secondary disaccharidase deficiency occurs when injury or disease damages the brush border of the intestinal mucosa. The secondary lactase deficiency may be temporary or permanent. Diseases or disorders associated with secondary lactase insufficiency include gastroenteritis, ulcerative colitis, Crohn's disease, operative procedures (partial gastrectomy, small bowel resection), and cholera.

Pathophysiology

The basis of the symptoms found in lactose intolerance is an excessive amount of sugar in the bowel lumen. Disaccharides form a large part of the dietary carbohydrate, and the three predominant forms are maltose (glucose), lactose (glucose and galactose), and sucrose (glucose and fructose). The disaccharides are not digested by enzymes in the lumen of the bowel but are taken into the brush border of the intestinal mucosal cell. The disaccharide is split by enzymes in the brush border into the simple sugars (glucose, galactose, and fructose), which can be further absorbed and metabolized. The enzymes of the brush border are lactase, sucrase, and a series of four enzymes that are called maltase.

The lactose absorption begins in the duodenum, and lactase activity is highest in the jejunum and nearly absent in the ileum. The process of lactose digestion is slower, normally, than sucrose and maltose. The blood sugar level after a meal of lactose will show little increase.

Lactase is present in the microvillus membrane of the columnar epithelial cells. Many intestinal bacteria also contain lactases. The two forms of lactase differ in their actions. Gut lactase splits the disaccharide, lactose, into glucose and galactose. Bacterial lactase results in the formation of hydrogen gas, carbon dioxide, and short-chain organic acids.

The diarrhea associated with lactose intolerance is caused by the osmotic effect of the lactose in the small bowel. The osmotic load of the lactose increases fluid secretion into the small bowel. The organic acids and fermentation products of the bacterial lactase in the colon impede colonic absorption. The pH of the stools in children may drop to 5.5 in response to the presence of organic acids.

The bloating and gaseous symptoms are the end products of bacterial lactase breaking down lactose.

Diagnostic Studies and Findings

Dietary Trial: 3 Weeks on a Lactose-Free Diet

Absence of gastrointestinal symptoms

Lactose Tolerance Test

Positive for lactose intolerance: blood sugar rise less than or equal to 20 mg/dl after lactose load of 50 g/m^2 in children or 50 g in adults; accompanied by characteristic symptoms

Hydrogen Breath Test

A rise of more than 20 parts per million is consistent with lactose intolerance (NOTE: Oral antibiotics can suppress bacteria that produce hydrogen; smoking increases breath hydrogen concentrations; small percentage of individuals do not normally produce hydrogen gas)

Stool pH

Drop from the normal pH of 7.0 or 8.0 to 5.5 (more common in children)

Small Bowel Biopsy

Used to determine whether lactose insufficiency is primary or secondary; epithelial abnormalities indicate secondary disorder

Medical Plan

Medications

Commercial lactase preparation can be used in milk for patients with limited tolerance to milk

Lactose-free diet

General Management

Low-lactose diet (is tolerated well by most individuals; lactose added until symptoms appear and then decreased until asymptomatic)

Calcium supplements (particularly in postmenopausal women)

NURSING CARE

Nursing Assessment

Clinical Symptoms

Excessive gas and flatus
Abdominal gurgling and pain
Persistent to profuse diarrhea
May vary from mild to extreme

Bone Disease

Osteoporosis from low intake of calcium

Nursing Dx & Intervention

Nursing Diagnosis	Nursing Intervention/Rationale
Diarrhea	• Assess for history of milk tolerance or intolerance *to determine onset*. • Assess for familial tendency for lactose intolerance. • Assess for relationship between foods and onset of abdominal symptoms. • Record amount, frequency, and consistency of bowel movements.
Altered nutrition: less than body requirements	• Assess patient for bone disease involvement caused by low intake of calcium and provide calcium supplements. • Refer mothers of infants with diarrhea and failure to thrive to physician *for evaluation of lactase deficiency versus other malabsorption syndromes*.

Patient Education

1. Provide oral and written instructions on lactose-free or low-lactose diets. Patients should be taught to read all labels to avoid packaged foods containing milk, milk products, milk solids, whey, lactose, milk sugar, curd, casein, galactose, and skim milk powder. Restricted foods include milk, yogurt, ice cream (also sherbets), cheese, desserts (made from milk and milk chocolate), sauces or stuffings (made with milk, cream, or cheese), and cream soups.

Evaluation

Patient Outcome	Data Indicating That Outcome is Reached
Bowel elimination is normal.	There are no symptoms with low-lactose or lactose-free diet.
Nutritional status is good.	Calcium level is normal; there are no signs of bone disease.

Celiac sprue

Celiac sprue can result in severe malabsorption. The mucosa of the small intestine is damaged by gluten-containing grains (wheat, barley, rye, and probably oats). The disease has the same clinical features, cause, pathology, and response to treatment in adults and children.

The most suitable names for this disease are celiac sprue and gluten-sensitive enteropathy. The seriousness of celiac sprue is the potential for severe malabsorption from the small bowel, resulting in marked malnutrition, debilitation, dehydration, and complications of nutrient and vitamin deficiencies.

Celiac sprue was first described in the literature in 1932. In 1950 a landmark study recognized the relationship of certain dietary grains to celiac sprue.[75] The incidence of celiac sprue is estimated at 0.03% of the general population. It appears that the estimate may be low, however, since asymptomatic celiac sprue patients have been identified during studies of familial and genetic tendencies of the disease.[48] The highest incidence of celiac sprue is in western Ireland, but there are cases of celiac sprue worldwide.[75] Celiac sprue is rare among blacks, Jews, and persons of Mediterranean descent. Women are affected more often than men. Celiac sprue is also more common in people with blood type O and less common in people with blood type A.

The onset of celiac sprue symptoms occurs at two peak periods. The first peak occurs when the infant's diet is changed to include cereals. There is a period during late childhood when the disease becomes asymptomatic; however, in the fourth and fifth decades the second onset of symptoms occurs. Unequivocal evidence of celiac sprue in childhood indicates a need to remain on a gluten-free diet indefinitely to avoid recurrent disease during adult life.

Pathophysiology

In celiac sprue the interaction of the water-soluble protein moiety (gluten) with the mucosa of the small bowel produces bloating, malaise, abdominal cramps, and diarrhea within a few hours. The fecal fat excretion increases. The mucosal changes of the intestinal segment exposed to gluten develop within 8 to 12 hours.[89] The intestinal absorptive cells are damaged. The dying absorptive cells are sloughed from the mucosal surface more rapidly than normal. The number of proliferating cells increases, and the crypts become hyperplastic to compensate for the excessive loss of absorptive cells. The mucosal layer of the small bowel appears flat, the villi are absent, and the intestinal crypts are markedly elongated and open onto a flat, absorptive surface. These structural changes decrease the amount of epithelial surface available for digestion and absorption. Many of the mucosal enzymes necessary for digestion and absorption are altered in the damaged mucosal cells. Thus the absorptive cells are reduced in number and functionally compromised. The crypt cells are increased in number, which accounts for the elongation of the crypts.

Celiac sprue may involve varying lengths of small intestine. The amount of involved bowel does correlate with the severity of the clinical symptoms. The proximal bowel is always involved and is usually more severely involved than the distal bowel. In mild cases of celiac sprue, some villous structure will remain even in the proximal bowel.

Treatment with a gluten-free diet results in significant improvements in the intestinal mucosa. The absorptive cells improve in days. The mucosa of the distal small intestine improves more rapidly than the proximal bowel, which was more severely involved. It may take months or years to reach its full recovery. Complete reversion to normal is uncommon. This may be in part related to inadvertent gluten ingestion.

The cause of gluten damage to the intestinal mucosa is not known. Three possible mechanisms are an immune reponse to dietary gluten, a genetic disorder, and a metabolic disorder. Circulating antibodies to gluten fractions have been found in patients with celiac sprue. However, there does not appear to be a correlation between the presence of the circulating antibodies and the severity of the disease. Researchers have also found that immunoglobulins synthesized by celiac sprue mucosa have antigluten specificity. Although evidence implicates the immune response theory, it is inconclusive at this time.

Genetic factors do play a role in celiac sprue. The incidence of disease in relatives is higher than in control populations. Approximately 80% of celiac sprue patients carry the histocompatibility antigen HLA-B8. HLA-DW3 antigen, which is associated with HLA-B8, is also found in over 80% of patients with celiac sprue. However, not all patients with HLA-B8 or HLA-DW3 have celiac sprue, nor do all patients with celiac sprue have these two antigens.[75]

In addition, antigens have been detected on the surface of B lymphocytes that are identified from antisera of celiac sprue patients. These antigens are present in most patients with celiac sprue and in all the parents of celiac sprue patients. This suggests a recessive inheritance.[61] It may be that the cause is a combined genetic and immune response.

Levels of some specific peptidases have been found to be reduced in the mucosa in untreated celiac sprue. These peptidases are important in the digestion of gliadin (a complex mixture of proteins obtained by alcohol extraction of wheat gluten). In the treatment of celiac sprue, the peptidase levels return to normal. If the lack of the peptidases caused celiac sprue, the deficiency would be apparent in treated as well as untreated celiac sprue. This does not support the theory of a metabolic disorder as a cause of celiac sprue.

Several factors contribute to the diarrhea in celiac sprue. The stool volume and osmotic load entering the colon are increased by the malabsorption in the small bowel. Water and electrolytes are secreted into the upper small bowel lumen rather than being absorbed. Cholecystokinin and secretin release is impaired in celiac sprue, decreasing pancreatic and biliary secretions and compromising digestion. Thus the digestion and absorption of nutrients and fluids and electrolytes is impaired in the small bowel, resulting in higher stool volume and the osmotic load. The diarrhea is aggravated by the presence of dietary fats and bile salts. The excessive dietary fat is broken down by the colon bacteria into hydroxy fatty acids, which are potent, irritating cathartics. If the terminal ileum is involved, conjugated bile salts are not absorbed and enter the colon. Bile salts have a direct cathartic action in the colon.

Esophageal cancer and intestinal lymphomas have been associated with celiac sprue. The incidence of carcinomas in celiac sprue patients is approximately 10%.[75] Patients who have been responding well to a gluten-free diet and who suddenly develop gastrointestinal systems (weight loss, malabsorption, abdominal pain, bleeding) should undergo diagnostic studies to rule out carcinoma. Before the diagnostic workup, it is necessary to ask the patient about adherence to the gluten-free diet. Any amount of gluten can damage the mucosa and create symptoms.

Refractory sprue is another complication. In refractory sprue, patients initially respond to a strict gluten-free diet and then relapse despite maintaining the diet. Some of these patients respond to corticosteroids. If patients do not respond, malabsorption becomes progressive and may lead to death. Since the advent of home total parenteral nutrition, however, death is less common.

Mucosal ulceration and intestinal strictures can develop in celiac sprue. The ulcers may perforate, with ensuing peritonitis. Intestinal strictures may lead to intestinal obstructions.

Diagnostic Studies and Findings

Quantitative Stool for Fat, 72- to 96-Hour Collection

Normal results: 2 to 7 g of fat per 24 hours while ingesting 100 g/d

Hemoglobin, Hematocrit, Folic Acid, and Vitamin B_{12} Levels

Anemia common in celiac sprue
Anemia may be related to folic acid or vitamin B_{12} deficiencies

Prothrombin Time

Prolonged if vitamin K deficiency present

Xylose Tolerance Test

Excretion in urine is decreased in severe, untreated celiac disease

Hydrogen Breath Test for Lactose Intolerance

Secondary lactase deficiency

Serum Electrolytes

Decreased
Metabolic acidosis present

Serum Calcium, Magnesium, Phosphorus, Zinc, Albumin, Globulins, Cholesterol, and Carotene

Decreased

Alkaline Phosphatase

Increased in patients with osteomalacia

Barium Contrast Studies: Barium Swallow

Dilation of small intestine
Marked coarsening of mucosal pattern or complete obliteration of mucosal folds
Fragmentation of barium
Delayed transit time of barium

Small Bowel Biopsy (Serial Sections)

Most valuable diagnostic procedure
Flat mucosal surface
Absence of villi
Elongated intestinal crypts

Gluten Challenge

Following response to gluten-free diet, rechallenge bowel to establish diagnosis unequivocally

Medical Plan

The major treatment is a gluten-free diet.

Medications

Used to manage effects of malnutrition and malabsorption
Hematinic agent
- Anemia: iron

Vitamins
- Anemia: folic acid, vitamin B_{12}
- Multivitamins daily to replace vitamins A, C, and E; thiamin; riboflavin; niacin; and pyridoxine
- Electrolyte and nutritional replacements
- Dehydration: intravenous fluid with potassium chloride added
- Calcium: tetany, 1 to 2 g IV calcium gluconate
- Magnesium: tetany, 0.5 g magnesium sulfate in dilute solution IV, *or* 100 mEq magnesium chloride po
- Osteomalacia: calcium gluconate or calcium lactate, 6 to 8 g/d and oral vitamin D

NURSING CARE

Nursing Assessment

Malabsorption

Diarrhea: watery, bulky, semiformed, light tan or grayish, greasy-appearing, rancid odor
Constipation: large quantities of "puttylike" stool
Weight loss (some patients lose little weight because of a tremendous intake of calories and enormous appetite until disease becomes severe)
Failure to gain weight and growth retardation in children
Weakness; lassitude; fatigue

Abdomen

Excessive amounts of malodorous flatus
Protuberant and tympanic
"Doughy" consistency
Ascites (hypoproteinemia)

Severe Anemia

Weakness; fatigue

Impaired Coagulability (Vitamin K Deficiency)

Purpura
Gastrointestinal, nasal, vaginal, or renal bleeding

Osteomalacia and Osteoporosis

Bone pain (low back, rib cage, pelvis)
Pathologic fractures (uncommon but may occur)

Calcium and Magnesium Depletion

Paresthesias, muscle cramps, tetany; positive Chvostek's or Trousseau's sign

Vitamin A Deficiency

Night blindness

Hypokalemia

Severe muscle weakness
Ileus

Secondary Hyperparathyroidism

Osteomalacia, bone pain, pathologic fractures

Adrenocortical Insufficiency

Sodium depletion: weakness, lassitude, dizziness
Increased skin and mucous membrane pigmentation

Hypotension

Decreased blood pressure, increased pulse (from fluid and electrolyte loss or adrenocortical insufficiency)

Integument

Clubbing of nails
Dry skin
Poor skin turgor
Edema (hypoproteinemia)
Skin pigmentation
Ecchymoses (hypoprothrombinemia)
Hyperkeratosis follicularis (vitamin A deficiency)
Pallor
Dermatitis herpetiformis

Mouth

Cheilosis and glossitis
Decreased papillation of tongue

Extremities

Loss of light touch, vibration, and position (peripheral neuropathy)

Nursing Dx & Intervention

Nursing Diagnosis	Nursing Intervention/Rationale
Altered nutrition: less than body requirements	• Do thorough nutritional assessment with a physical assessment. • Consult with nutritionist. • Weigh patient daily. • Provide dietary supplements as ordered; in severe malabsorption, hyperalimentation may be used during initial stabilization period. • Check dietary trays for foods containing gluten. • Support patient and family as they learn the implications of a gluten-free diet. • Evaluate patient's comprehension of dietary patient education. • Evaluate, in outpatient setting, patient's dietary intake and nutritional status (weight gain and stabilization); a diary may be helpful.
Potential fluid volume deficit	• Assess weight loss. • Monitor vital signs, intake and output (include stools), and daily weights. • Replace intravenous fluids and electrolytes, vitamins, and minerals as ordered. • Observe patient for signs and symptoms of specific deficiencies: anemia, calcium, and magnesium.
Diarrhea	• Assess frequency, volume, and consistency of bowel movements. • Assess history or pattern of diarrhea (i.e., onset and duration, symptoms as an infant or child, severity).

Patient Education

1. Provide written and oral instructions on a gluten-free diet.
2. Encourage the patient to buy a cookbook on gluten-free cooking.
3. Instruct the patient to read labels carefully. Wheat flour is often used as an extender in processed foods and is in many brands of ice cream, salad dressings, canned foods, instant coffee, catsup, mustard, and candy bars.
4. Provide consultation with a nutritionist to teach the patient about the presence of gluten in many foods.

Evaluation

Patient Outcome	Data Indicating That Outcome is Reached
Body functioning is normal.	Bowel elimination is normal with no steatorrhea; quantitative stool specimens for fat are within normal range of 2 to 7 g of fats per 24 hours on 100 g of fat per day diet. Patient gains weight.

Patient Outcome	Data Indicating That Outcome is Reached
	Blood pressure is within normal limits. Skin turgor is good. There is no edema or ascites. Intestinal biopsy shows recovery of mucosa.
Laboratory values are within normal limits.	Serum, whole blood, or plasma levels of calcium, magnesium, sodium, potassium, folate, zinc, cholesterol, and carotene are within normal limits. Prothrombin time is within normal limits. Hemoglobin level is within normal limits.

Short bowel syndrome

Short bowel syndrome refers to the severe diarrhea and significant malabsorption symptoms that develop following small bowel resections. The severity of short bowel syndrome is influenced by the amount of bowel resected and the portion of small bowel resected. Symptoms are related to the diarrhea (fluid and electrolyte losses) and malnutrition (mineral, vitamin, fat, carbohydrate, and protein deficiencies).

Catastrophic malabsorption may develop from massive resections of the small bowel. The total length of resected bowel and the bowel lost must be considered in establishing the prognosis and treatment. Forty percent of the small bowel may be resected and tolerated well, *if* the duodenum, proximal jejunum, distal half of ileum, and ileocecal sphincter are spared. In contrast, resection of 25% of the small bowel can result in severe diarrhea and malabsorption if the distal two thirds of the ileum and ileocecal valve are removed.[72] The advent of hyperalimentation has improved the survival rate of people who have lost significant amounts of small bowel.

Pathophysiology

The loss of small bowel affects the body's ability to absorb nutrients and vitamins. Intestinal ischemias that compromise the blood flow to the small bowel are the most common clinical conditions that require massive bowel resections. In children, volvulus of the small bowel, aganglionosis of the small bowel, meconium ileus, or necrotizing enterocolitis may lead to resections of large amounts of small bowel. Crohn's disease may also require repeated resections of small bowel. Neoplasms and traumas have also been associated with small bowel resections. Jejunal bypass procedures for obesity are no longer recommended because of the severe malabsorption associated with the surgery.

The pathophysiologic response to resections of small bowel varies depending on length and segments involved. The ileocecal valve plays an important role in reducing contamination of residual small bowel by colonic flora. The valve also increases transit time of the contents. When short bowel syndrome occurs, absorption of water, electrolytes, fat, protein, carbohydrates, vitamins, and trace elements is reduced. Fluid loss is greatest in the first few days after surgery. Fluid loss is also higher when all or part of the colon has also been resected.

The small bowel absorbs nutrients and vitamins in different segments. Resections of small portions of the midintestine do not generally create clinical problems. However, smaller resections involving proximal or distal segments result in more significant clinical symptoms. The duodenum is responsible for iron, folate, and calcium absorption. Resection or bypass of the duodenum may result in anemia. The distal or terminal ileum is responsible for bile salt and vitamin B_{12} absorption. Reduction or absence of the active absorptive sites for bile salts will disrupt the enterohepatic circulation of bile salts. Two forms of diarrhea may develop: cholerheic or steatorrheic. Cholerheic diarrhea is a watery diarrhea that is common if less than 100 cm of distal ileum is resected.[72] In cholerheic diarrhea the hepatic synthesis of bile salts compensates for the bile salts not being absorbed in the ileum. Fat digestion remains normal. The bile salts in the colon impair fluid and electrolyte absorption and stimulate further secretions of fluid into the colon. If more than 100 cm of distal ileum is removed, bile salt loss cannot be compensated by hepatic synthesis and fat digestion is impaired (this can be resolved by using an agent such as cholestyramine). Undigested fat in the colon also impairs fluid and electrolyte absorption and stimulates colonic secretions. Steatorrheic diarrhea contains water, electrolytes, bile salts, and undigested fats. After ileal resections, gallstones have been reported to be 25% to 32% higher than in the general population. This has been related to the depletion of the bile salt pool.[72]

Interestingly, the small bowel undergoes an adaptive process following bowel resections. The remaining villi enlarge and lengthen, increasing the absorptive surface area. The epithelial hyperplasia is associated with accelerated cell renewal and migration. It appears that exposure to nutrients (oral feedings), exposure to bile and pancreatic enzymes, and response to trophic gut peptides influence the adaptative process. Cholecystokinin and secretin support the adaptative process. The presence of oral feedings is necessary for adaptation to occur, but the oral intake should be gradually started and advanced. Clinically, the patient tends to improve in absorptive ability with time.

Gastric hypersecretion occurs in approximately half of the patients who have massive small bowel resections. This can impair intestinal absorption by damaging the mucosa. This is often a temporary effect and decreases to normal levels.

Diagnostic Studies and Findings

Double-Contrast Barium Films

Estimation of amount of small bowel remaining
Increase in caliber of remaining segment several weeks following surgery (adaptation)

Laboratory Studies: Folate, Iron, Vitamin B_{12}, Vitamin A, Calcium, Magnesium, Potassium, MCV, MCHC, MCH, Sodium, Carotene, Cholesterol, Zinc

Reduced

Prothrombin Time

Lengthened

Quantitative Stool Test for Fat

Steatorrhea
Normal: 2 to 7 g of fat per day on diet of 100 g of fat per day

Lactose Intolerance

Lactase deficiency (jejunal loss)

Xylose Tolerance

Excretion in urine decreased

Culture of Intestinal Fluid

Bacterial overgrowth

D-Lactate Levels (Serum)

Elevated

Medical Plan

Medications

- Parenteral replacement of fluid loss
- Antidiarrheal agents
  - Diphenoxylate (Lomotil), 2.5-5 mg q4h po
  - Loperamide (Imodium), 2 mg q6h po
  - Paregoric may be used; dosage varies with degree of resection and diarrhea
- Cholinergic blocking agents
  - Propantheline bromide (Pro-Banthine), 15-30 mg ½h ac
- Anti-infective agents
  - Tetracycline (Achromycin) or ampicillin (Amcill) for bacterial overgrowth, 1 g/d for 2 wk
- Histamine receptor antagonist
  - Cimetidine (Tagamet), 300 mg qid with meals and at bedtime (for gastric hypersection)
- Antilipemic agent
  - Ileal resections with cholerrheic diarrhea: cholestyramine, 8 to 12 mg/d
- Antacid
  - Aluminum hydroxide, 15-30 ml qid
- Vitamins
  - Cyanocobalamin (vitamin B_{12}), 1000 μg IM monthly
  - Folate, 1 mg po daily

General Management

Hyperalimentation for nutrition, especially immediately postoperatively
Gradual oral feedings: elemental diets initially; followed by polymeric supplements; add milk carefully (a low-lactose diet may be preferred)
High caloric intake; six meals per day
Home hyperalimentation

NURSING CARE

Nursing Assessment

Malabsorption: Caloric Deprivation

Severe weight loss
Fatigue
Lassitude
Weakness

Calcium and Magnesium Levels

Tetany; positive Chvostek's or Trousseau's signs
Osteomalacia; osteoporosis; bone pain; spontaneous fractures

Vitamin K

Purpura; generalized bleeding

Protein

Mild or moderate hypoalbuminemia

Iron, Folate, Vitamin B_{12}

Anemia

Bile Salts

Cholerheic or steatorrheic diarrhea
Gallstones

Dehydration

Poor skin turgor
Hypokalemia
Hyponatremia

Excessive Colonic Absorption of Oxalate

Calcium oxalate kidney stones

Lactic Acidosis (D-Lactate Levels)

Altered personality; confusion; stupor; ataxia (elevated D-lactate is the result of anaerobic colonic bacteria and unabsorbed carbohydrates)

Nursing Dx & Intervention

Nursing Diagnosis	Nursing Intervention/Rationale
Altered nutrition: less than body requirements	• Assess patient for signs of malabsorption: severe weight loss, fatigue, dehydration, osteoporosis, hypokalemia, hyponatremia. • Help patient design a nutritional plan to meet life-style and caloric needs. • Provide nutritional replacements as ordered *to prevent complications of malabsorption.* • Provide hyperalimentation: Observe catheter site (Broviac, Hickman, central line). Change dressing three times per week or per protocol. Observe for signs of infection (fever or redness at insertion site). • Monitor vital signs, intake and output, urine for sugar and acetone, and daily weights while receiving parenteral nutrition. • Record description of stools including frequency, characteristics, and odor.
Fluid volume deficit (1)	• Assess patient carefully for signs of fluid loss and shock: skin turgor, daily weights, intake and output, and blood pressure (sitting and lying). • Provide fluid replacement as ordered.
Diarrhea	• Assess stools for signs of cholerheic vs. steatorrheic diarrhea. • Provide antidiarrheal agents as ordered. • Record accurate description of stools and frequency. • Provide fluid replacements as ordered.

Patient Education

1. Provide information, oral and written, on dietary restrictions, dietary supplements, and medications regarding nutritional effects of malabsorption.
2. Teach the patient home hyperalimentation if necessary. Provide a home care referral to evaluate and assist patient and family.
3. Teach the patient signs and symptoms of key electrolyte, fluid, and nutritional losses and complications from increased acidity and oxalate stones.
4. Instruct the patient to notify the physician immediately if gastroenteritis develops, since the patient can become seriously dehydrated quickly.

Evaluation

Patient Outcome	Data Indicating That Outcome is Reached
Nutritional status is normal.	Dietary plans provide adequate nutrition for absorptive capacity of bowel. Degree of diarrhea is minimized. Patient gains weight.
Laboratory values are within normal limits.	Hemoglobin level, prothrombin times, MCV, MCHC, and MCH are within normal limits. Levels of calcium, magnesium, sodium, potassium, folate, zinc, cholesterol, and carotene are within normal limits.
Home hyperalimentation is performed.	Infusion at night is without incident. Line is free of infection.

Peritonitis

Peritonitis is the inflammation of the peritoneum. The inflammatory response may be localized or generalized.

The cause of peritonitis is contamination of the peritoneal cavity by bacteria or chemicals. Peritonitis is also classified as primary and secondary. Primary peritonitis is an acute or subacute bacterial infection of the peritoneum not associated with any underlying bowel disorder. It is often seen in children with underlying nephrotic syndromes and urinary tract infections. Cirrhosis with ascites has also been associated with primary peritonitis. Secondary peritonitis is the result of contamination of the peritoneum from perforation of the gastrointestinal tract (peptic ulcer, diverticulum, or appendix), gangrene of the bowel, salpingitis, traumatic injuries, and surgical contaminants. Peritonitis is a common complication of many diseases and can progress to perforation or rupture of the organs of digestion. In secondary peritonitis the inflammation is a result of bacterial and chemical irritation.

Secondary (generalized) peritonitis is a serious complication of an acutely ill patient. The mortality of generalized peritonitis is 50% even with the use of antibiotics and intensive support systems.[72] Three factors that negatively affect the prognosis are age, type of contamination, and tissue perfusion. An older patient is at a higher risk for a poor prognosis or poor response to treatment. Fecal contamination is the most serious. Poor tissue perfusion indicates a poor prognosis. Poor tissue perfusion is associated with hypotension, acidosis, hypokalemia, or respiratory difficulties. Perforated peptic ulcer, ruptured appendix, trauma, ischemic bowel disease, intestinal obstruction, pancreatitis, and perforated colon are common causes of a generalized peritonitis.

Primary peritonitis accounts for approximately 1% of the incidence of infectious peritonitis.[41] Primary peritonitis may be divided into idiopathic (or spontaneous) and tuberculous peritonitis. Spontaneous bacterial peritonitis is associated with 2% of all abdominal emergencies and 13% of diffuse peritoneal sepsis in children.[75]

Tuberculous peritonitis is caused by a reactivation of latent tuberculosis in the peritoneum. The patient may not have active pulmonary, intestinal, or genital tuberculosis. Peritonitis from fungi and parasites is uncommon. *Candida albicans* may cause severe peritonitis, but it requires a contamination of the peritoneum, usually from an occult gastrointestinal perforation. *Coccidioides immitis* may result in granulomatous peritonitis in 1% to 2% of patients with coccidioidomycosis. Parasitic infections rarely lead to clinical symptoms of peritonitis but may closely resemble peritoneal carcinomatosis or tuberculosis during laparotomy.

Pathophysiology

The peritoneum is a semipermeable membrane enclosing the abdominal viscera and mesentery. It forms a closed, saclike structure that is opened in the female at the fallopian tubes. The peritoneum is divided into visceral and parietal peritoneum. The visceral peritoneum covers the intraperitoneal organs and forms the mesenteries of these organs. The parietal peritoneum lines the abdominal wall, the undersurface of the diaphragm, the pelvic floor, and the retroperitoneal viscera (duodenum, ascending and descending colon, portions of the pancreas, kidney, and adrenals). The omentum is formed by a double layer of fused peritoneum and enclosed lymphatic vessels and blood vessels. The omentum plays a primary role in the peritoneal defense mechanism against impending perforations and small perforations.

The nervous innervation of the parietal peritoneum is from the same nerves that supply the abdominal wall. The irritation of the parietal peritoneum stimulates afferent nerves, which are transmitted through the intercostal nerves. The pain is perceived as somatic pain. No pain receptors are identified in the visceral peritoneum, and afferent stimulation is conducted through the visceral sympathetic nervous system. The different responses or symptoms of irritation are related to the nerve pathways. The symptoms of parietal peritonitis include a sharp, localized pain, whereas the pain in visceral peritonitis is poorly characterized and poorly localized.

The diaphragmatic peritoneum is innervated in the central portion from phrenic nerves and in the peripheral portion by branches of the intercostal nerves. Symptoms vary depending on the location of the pathologic process. The phrenic nerve stimulation would result in referred pain to either shoulder. Intercostal nerve stimulation may cause pain in the thoracic or the abdominal wall, as occurs in cholecystitis.

The peritoneal defense mechanism is the body's attempt to localize or wall off any contamination of the peritoneal cavity and prevent diffuse peritonitis. The first response is vascular dilation and increased capillary permeability. Large numbers of polymorphonuclear leukocytes pour into the area and through phagocytosis remove bacteria and foreign matter. Fibroplastic exudate is deposited and plasters the adjacent bowel, mesentery, and omentum to the inflamed area, forming a watertight seal. Thus the inflammation is enclosed as an abscess. Peritoneal injuries heal without fibrous adhesions unless infection, ischemia, or foreign bodies are associated with the peritonitis.

The body's response to secondary (acute bacterial) peritonitis includes removal of the bacteria through diaphragmatic lymphatics; phagocytosis and destruction of bacteria by opsonins, polymorphonuclear leukocytes, and macrophages; and localization by the omentum and fibroplastic exudate. Vascular dilation, hyperemia, and a fluid shift occur. The vascular dilation and hyperemia lead to an increase in polymorphonuclear leukocytes and macrophages. The absorption capacity of the peritoneum increases, facilitating the absorption of bacteria and toxins. A fluid shift occurs from the extracellular fluid compartment into the free peritoneal space, into the loose connective tissue (as edema), and into the lumen of the atonic gastrointestinal tract. The translocation of water, electrolytes, and protein into this third-space compartment depletes the circulating fluid volume. The rate of fluid shift is proportional to the degree of peritoneal involvement and the success of the body's peritoneal defense mechanism.

Early diagnosis and treatment are necessary to prevent severe shock from the loss of fluid into the peritoneal space. The principal complications of untreated peritonitis are septicemia, shock, ileus, and major organ failure including respiratory, renal, hepatic, and cardiac systems. The patient has symptoms of an acute condition in the abdomen, and it is necessary to rule out other causes of the symptoms.

Diagnostic Studies and Findings

Laboratory Studies

WBC: increased leukocytes
RBC: hemoconcentration
Metabolic acidosis
Respiratory alkalosis
Electrolytes: vary

Plain Abdominal Roentgenograms

Intestinal distention (small and large)
Air-fluid levels
Free air (perforations)

Peritoneal Aspiration

Identification of organisms (primary peritonitis)
Appearance of aspirate (cloudy, blood-tinged, etc.)

Medical Plan

Surgery

Operative procedure determined by primary cause

Objectives of surgery are to close perforation, to prevent septicemia, and to prevent abscess formation (or to drain abscess)

Medications

Adequate volumes of electrolytes and colloid solutions to correct hypovolemia

Analgesics to control pain

Antibiotic therapy to cover multiple bacterial flora contaminating the peritoneal cavity; usually includes aminoglycoside (aerobic gram negative), clindamycin or metronidazole (anaerobes), ampicillin (enterococci), and cephalosporins (broad spectrum)

General Management

Nasogastric suctioning

Monitoring: CBC, electrolytes, creatinine, arterial pH, Po_2, Pco_2

CVP or Swan-Ganz catheter

Oxygen (increased metabolic demand and respirations decreased because of pain and abdominal distention)

Continuous peritoneal lavage with antibiotics or antiseptic agents (in diffuse, poorly localized peritonitis to remove residual necrotic debris)

Respiratory assist devices or endotracheal intubation

Nutritional supplements: total parenteral nutrition (TPN), providing 3000 to 4000 calories per day (to avoid major catabolic losses)

NURSING CARE

Nursing Assessment

Abdomen

Abdominal pain; diffuse tenderness and rigidity
Diminished or absent bowel sounds
Abdominal distention
Nausea
Vomiting

Respirations

Shallow and rapid
Pain associated with deep respirations

Cardiovascular Concerns

Rapid, weak, thready pulse
Decreased blood pressure
Shock

Temperature

Fever
Septicemia

Kidney

Decreased urinary output

General Appearance

Lying quietly in bed with knees flexed

Guards abdomen against sudden movements or physical examination

Appears "ill"

Nursing Dx & Intervention

Nursing Diagnosis	Nursing Intervention/Rationale
Pain	• Assess abdominal area for signs of perforation and peritonitis: increased severity and diffuseness of abdominal pain, rebound tenderness, guarding. • Help patient assume a comfortable position (one that places minimum stress on the abdominal muscles); limit sudden movement and abdominal examination. • Provide analgesics as prescribed. (Some surgeons will not order analgesics, since they may mask signs and symptoms.)
Fluid volume deficit (1)	• Assess patient carefully for signs and symptoms of severe fluid and electrolyte loss, metabolic acidosis, and hypovolemic shock *secondary to accumulation of gas and fluids, distention of intestine, and sepsis.* • Replace intravenous fluids and electrolytes, blood, and plasma as ordered. • Monitor vital signs, central venous pressure, blood pressure, urinary output, and nasogastric aspirations every hour. • Notify physician of changes in patient's status, as they generally indicate a decline in patient's stabilization for surgical intervention.

Nursing Diagnosis	Nursing Intervention/Rationale
Ineffective breathing pattern	• Assess patient's pulmonary status, since abdominal distention and abdominal guarding may impair pulmonary ventilation, as can metabolic imbalances. • Elevate head of bed *to relieve pressure on the diaphragm.* • Provide oxygen therapy as ordered. • Observe for breathing difficulties: shallow, rapid respirations secondary to pain; assist with respiratory devices (e.g., incentive spirometer) as appropriate.
Altered nutrition: less than body requirements	• Provide nutritional replacements as ordered *to prevent complications of malabsorption.* • Provide hyperalimentation: Observe catheter site (Broviac, Hickman, central line). Change dressing three times per week or per protocol. Observe for signs of infection (fever or redness at insertion site). • Monitor vital signs, intake and output, urine for sugar and acetone, and daily weights while receiving parenteral nutrition. • Record description of stools including frequency, characteristics, and odor.

Patient Education

1. The patient manages any wounds, abscesses, or incisions that have not closed or continue to drain before and following discharge from the hospital.
2. The patient identifies purpose of discharge medications and appropriate method of administration, including times, route, and length of course of medications.

Evaluation

Patient Outcome	Data Indicating That Outcome is Reached
Body functions normally.	Pain, fever, and abdominal signs are absent. Urinary output is adequate, and normal bowel pattern is restored. Incision heals without any drains and stab wounds. Blood pressure and pulse are normal.
Laboratory studies are within normal limits.	WBC, hemoglobin, hematocrit, Po_2, Pco_2, and pH are within normal limits.

Polyps

The term "polyp" refers to a discrete tissue mass that is elevated above the mucosal surface. A polyp may be described according to histology, presence or absence of a stalk, and whether it is one of multiple similar protrusions in the gastrointestinal tract.

The histology of a polyp determines the tissue from which the polyp developed and the descriptive name. For example, adenoma develops from epithelium, myoma from smooth muscle, and hemangioma from blood vessels. The most common type of colonic polyp is an adenoma. Pedunculated polyps are attached to the mucosa by a stalk, while sessile polyps rest on a broad base of mucosa. Although polyps may occur throughout the gastrointestinal tract, the predominant site is in the distal 25 cm of the colon. Colonic polyps may be classified as neoplastic or nonneoplastic. Neoplastic polyps include adenomas and carcinomas. Categories of nonneoplastic polyps include mucosal polyps, hyperplastic polyps, pseudopolyps of inflammatory bowel disease, and juvenile polyps. Syndromes that involve multiple gastrointestinal polyps include familial polyposis, Gardner's syndrome, Turcot syndrome, Peutz-Jeghers syndrome, and juvenile polyps.

The frequency of colonic adenomas, although varying widely among populations, tends to be highest in North America and Europe. Autopsy surveys in the United States indicate that 50% of the population have at least one adenomatous colonic polyp. When age is considered as a variable, it is noted that two thirds of those over 65 years of age have colonic adenomas. Adenomas in the colon and rectum are more likely to become malignant. The diagnosis and removal of polyps play an important role in preventing colon and rectal cancers.

Familial polyposis, an inherited autosomal dominant trait, is characterized by progressive development of hundreds of polyps (adenomas) throughout the colon. Familial polyposis is a precancerous condition. The development of colon cancer in familial polyposis is inevitable without surgical intervention. The polyps begin to develop after puberty, and the patient may remain asymptomatic for several years. The presence of multiple cancers at the time of diagnosis is high. Family assessments and genetic counseling are important in reducing the rates of early death from colon cancer by identifying family members who have the gene for familial polyposis.

Gardner's syndrome is a variant of familial polyposis and consists of gastrointestinal polyposis, osteomas of the skull, mandible, and long bones, and soft-tissue tumors. Gardner's syndrome is inherited as an autosomal dominant trait. The gastrointestinal polyps appear in the small and large intestine and are precancerous.

Turcot syndrome describes the combination of familial polyposis and malignant central nervous system (CNS) tumors. The CNS tumors include glioblastomas and medulloblastomas.

Peutz-Jeghers syndrome involves mucocutaneous pigmentation of the mouth, lips, hands, and feet and multiple polyps in the small and large intestines. The polyps are hamartomas; that is, they develop from glandular epithelium supported by smooth muscle. The pigmentation generally fades after puberty with the exception of those found in the mouth.

Juvenile polyps are distinctive hamartomas found in the rectum of children. The polyps do not tend to be precancerous lesions but are removed because of the associated problems of bleeding, obstructions, and intussusception.

Pathophysiology

Colonic polyps or adenomas are composed of immature epithelial cells that continue to proliferate. Normally, the lower third of the colonic crypt is the site of cell division. As the cells move upward toward the lumen of the colon, they differentiate into colonic epithelium that secretes mucus. When the normal processes of cell proliferation and differentiation are altered, cells migrate to the surface, where they continue to synthesize DNA and divide. The surface epithelium of undifferentiated cells accumulates and leads to the formation of a polyp. The same steps are found in familial polyposis, where normal-appearing mucosa is found to be mature and differentiated epithelium and polyps are composed of proliferative cells.

Adenomatous polyps may develop as tubular adenomas, villous adenomas, or tubulovillous adenomas. Tubular adenoma is used to describe polyps that consist of densely packed colonic cells with some loss of goblet cell mucin, branching of glands, and varying degrees of nuclear atypia. Tubular adenomas are more common and usually smaller. Villous adenomas contain a proliferation of villi. Villous adenomas are larger than tubular adenomas. The polyps that contain villi and tubular epithelium are referred to as tubulovillous adenomas. The involvement of the villi is associated with a higher incidence of cancer.

The relationship between polyps and cancer has been developed through longitudinal observations. Dysplasia, in varying degrees, is found during histologic examination of polyps following biopsy. Evidence supporting the relationship between polyps and colon carcinomas is based on three major findings: location of clusters of cancers within adenomatous polyps, findings in patients with multiple polyposis, and epidemiologic studies. Although small, isolated colon carcinomas are rare, small groups of cancers are found within adenomatous polyps. The development of carcinomas in patients with colonic polyps is usually 10 to 15 years after the appearance of benign adenomas. Data supporting the time span are based on patients with familial polyposis. However, residual adenomatous tissue may be found surrounding malignant tissue in patients with early colon cancer lesions at diagnosis and surgery. The same population groups tend to have high rates of colon cancer and colonic adenomas, further supporting the relationship.

When a polyp is removed, cytology and histology studies are performed to carefully assess the patient for further medical or surgical intervention. Polyps may be associated with mild to severe degrees of dysplasia. When the polyp contains foci in which the nuclei are large and irregular, cells are crowded, polarity is lost, and cribiform glands are present, the cytologic appearance is malignant. The interpretation of the finding is then made by examining the entire polyp. If the foci do not extend into the muscularis mucosae, the polyp contains carcinoma in situ. If there is extension into the muscularis mucosae and submucosa (and thus lymphatic and blood supply), the polyp is considered invasive carcinoma.

The development of polyps in familial polyposis is through the alteration of the normal cell proliferation and differentiation as previously described. In familial polyposis, young people develop hundreds to thousands of colonic polyps. Cancer, in one or more polyps, generally develops before 40 years of age.

Studies of skin fibroblasts of patients with familial polyposis and Gardner's syndrome have demonstrated abnormal growth characteristics in culture. The cells have lost normal contact inhibition; they grow in multilayered, crisscrossed patterns and have decreased serum requirements for growth. The study of skin fibroblasts in patients to detect the familial polyposis trait may be a diagnostic tool for the future.[75]

In Gardner's syndrome, polyps may be found throughout the gastrointestinal tract. Duodenal polyps are more common than jejunal or ileal and are precancerous. Multiple polyps may also be found in the stomach. Interestingly, in Japan, gastric polyps are reported as associated with gastric carcinomas, but this is not true in the Western world.[86] Extracolonic manifestations include osteomas of the mandible, skull, and long bones (e.g., epidermoid cysts, fibromas, lipomas, and desmoid tumors), dental abnormalities (e.g., impacted teeth, mandibular cysts), and soft tissue tumors (e.g., carcinoma of the thyroid and adrenal glands).

Diagnostic Studies and Findings

Stool for Occult Blood

Positive for blood

Proctosigmoidoscopy

Visualization of bowel lumen (flexible fiberoptic sigmoidoscopy is better tolerated, but only 30 cm in length)

Colonoscopy

Visualization and polypectomy; biopsy (total excision of polyp is the accepted method of providing an accurate histologic diagnosis)

Radiography Studies

Osteomas found in Gardner's syndrome

Air-Contrast Barium Enema

Used to identify polyps above the rectosigmoid area

Medical Plan

Surgery

Colonic adenomas: require colon resection with wide margins for invasive carcinoma, sessile polyps, cancer in stalk, cancer at margin of resection by polypectomy, and undifferentiated cancer in any polyp

General Management

Colonic adenomas: colonic polypectomy by colonoscopy for benign polyp, pedunculated polyp, and carcinoma in situ when confined to head of polyp

Juvenile polyps: colonoscopy with polypectomy

Routine or periodic proctosigmoidoscopy or colonoscopy in patients at risk for developing familial polyposis or Gardner's syndrome

Genetic counseling

NURSING CARE

Nursing Assessment

Colonic Polyp

Intestinal symptoms
- Occult or overt rectal bleeding
- Constipation or change in caliber of stool (polyps decreasing lumen size)
- Diarrhea with hypokalemia and dehydration (villous adenoma)
- Crampy, lower abdominal pain (caused by intermittent intussusception)
- In presence of above symptoms, must rule out possibility of colon carcinoma

Familial Polyposis

History
- Family history used to identify asymptomatic individuals at risk

Intestinal symptoms
- Hematochezia (rectal bleeding)
- Diarrhea
- Abdominal pain

Gardner's Syndrome

History
- Family history to identify asymptomatic individuals at risk

Intestinal symptoms
- Bleeding
- Diarrhea
- Abdominal pain

Extracolonic manifestations (osteomas, soft tissue tumors)
- Careful examination for presence of sebaceous cysts, fibromas of the skin, and bony tumors

Juvenile Polyps

Intestinal symptoms
- Bleeding
- Crampy abdominal pain
- Constipation

Peutz-Jeghers Syndrome

Intestinal symptoms
- Observation for symptoms of intestinal obstruction, intussusception, and gastrointestinal bleeding

Extracolonic manifestations
- Macular lesions, brown to greenish black, around mouth, nose, lips, buccal mucosa, hands, feet, and occasionally in perianal and genital regions

Nursing Dx & Intervention

Nursing Diagnosis	Nursing Intervention/Rationale
Patient problem: potential altered bowel elimination	• Assess carefully patient's history regarding bowel patterns, changes in pattern, rectal bleeding, and abdominal pain. • Prepare patient through preprocedural teaching for colonoscopy examination, barium enemas, and proctosigmoidoscopy.
Personal identity disturbance	• Assess patient's level of understanding of genetic factor in familial polyposis and Gardner's syndrome. • Help patient learn about disease, treatment, and implications for future. • Provide genetic counseling. • Identify additional family members for workup for familial polyposis and Gardner's disease, since these have a genetic link.

Nursing Diagnosis	Nursing Intervention/Rationale
Body image disturbance	• Assess patient who is to undergo surgery for familial polyposis regarding verbal responses to the actual change in the structure of his or her body function; physical changes anticipated with surgery; and age, sex, and developmental level. • Assist patient by providing information on rationale of total colectomy for familial polyposis and available surgical procedures including conventional ileostomy, continent (Kock) ileostomy, and anal sphincter–saving surgeries. • Request a visit from a cured patient who has undergone the same surgical procedure selected by the patient. • Refer patient to ET nurse and ostomy organization for support.

Patient Education

1. Close follow-up should be planned because of recurrence rates. Evaluation will require barium enema, proctosigmoidoscopy, or colonoscopy. The pattern should be as follows:
   Benign colonic adenoma: every 2 to 3 years
   Carcinoma confined to polyp: in 6 months, then yearly
   Multiple polyps and family history of cancer: yearly
   Asymptomatic familial polyposis: every 6 months
   Familial polyposis, following surgery when rectal segment is left: every 6 months

   See p. 862 for instructions on ostomy care if appropriate.

Evaluation

Patient Outcome	Data Indicating That Outcome is Reached
Body functions normally.	There is no diarrhea, constipation, rectal bleeding, or abdominal pain.
Patient can care for ileostomy or continent ileostomy (familial polyposis).	For conventional ileostomy, patient is able to manage external pouch, skin is in excellent condition, and diet is normal. For continent ileostomy, patient is able to intubate pouch, and diet is normal.

Pseudomembranous enterocolitis

Pseudomembranous enterocolitis is an inflammation and necrosis of the bowel that primarily affects the mucosa and occasionally the submucosa. Pseudomembranous exudative plaques are found attached to the mucosal surface of the small bowel (enteritis), colon, (colitis), or both (enterocolitis).

In 1893, original reports on pseudomembranous colitis indicated intestinal ischemia as the basic cause. The advent of antibiotics resulted in a series of studies that implicated antibiotic use and *Staphylococcus aureus*. The widespread use of colonoscopy as a diagnostic procedure has improved the detection of pseudomembranous enterocolitis. Stool cultures have ruled out *S. aureus* as the cause. At this time, *Clostridium difficile* has been identified as the enteric pathogen responsible for pseudomembranous colitis following antibiotic therapy. Although many antimicrobial agents have been implicated in pseudomembranous colitis, the most common agents include clindamycin, lincomycin, cephalosporins, and ampicillin.

Risk factors for developing pseudomembranous enterocolitis, excluding antimicrobial agents, include surgery of the colon, stomach, or pelvis region complicated by shock during or following the surgery; spinal fractures; intestinal obstructions; Crohn's disease; neonatal necrotizing enterocolitis; and Hirschsprung's disease. Age also appears to be a risk factor in antibiotic-associated pseudomembranous enterocolitis, with older patients at higher risk.

Pathophysiology

Antibiotic-induced pseudomembranous colitis develops when the normal bowel flora is altered by antibiotic therapy. The *C. difficile* organisms multiply, producing two toxins. The toxins damage the membranes of the epithelial cells, leading to cell necrosis. Poor vascular perfusion to the mucosa may also progress to necrosis of the mucosal layer of the gut. Antibiotic-induced pseudomembranous enterocolitis tends to be primarily a disease of the colon, whereas studies of pseudomembranous enterocolitis not associated with antibiotics demonstrated lesions in the small bowel as well.

The pseudomembrane is composed of fibrin, mucin, sloughed epithelial cells, and inflammatory cells. The mildest form of pseudomembranous enterocolitis consists of focal necrosis. A characteristic "summit" lesion develops from a collection of fibrin and polymorphonuclear cells. As the disease progresses, the appearance changes to a "volcanic" lesion that includes glandular cell disruption and the typical pseudomembrane of elevated yellow-white plaques. As the necrosis worsens, there is an extensive involvement of the lamina propria and a thick overlaying of the pseudomembrane. If the pseudomembranes slough, the bowel is left with large denuded areas.

Pseudomembranous colitis can progress to a life-threatening illness. The symptoms may not develop for 4 to 7 weeks after the antibiotic therapy has been discontinued. Patients generally have severe diarrhea, abdominal tenderness, fever, and leukocytosis. As the bowel wall necrosis continues, the patient begins to lose fluids, electrolytes, and albumin. Toxic megacolon may develop. The colon may perforate, leading to the sequelae of peritonitis and sepsis.

Early diagnosis is important in initiating oral treatment and preventing the disorder from becoming fulminant or intractable to medical management. The medical management consists of antimicrobials that are effective against *C. difficile*. In patients with a less severe disease, an anion exchange resin (cholestyramine) has been used to bind the toxins produced by *C. difficile*. Cholestyramine should not be used in combination with antimicrobials, since the resin will bind the antimicrobial and reduce the drug levels in the colon.

Diagnostic Studies and Findings

Plain Films of Abdomen

Markedly edematous colon
Distorted haustral markings
Colon distention
Air fluid levels in toxic megacolon

Barium Air-Contrast Studies

Rounded filling defects outlining plaques

Colonoscopy

Yellowish white plaques
Erythema
Edema
Friable mucosa
Ulcerations
Hemorrhage

Stool Analysis

C. difficile toxin assay

Medical Plan

Surgery

Severely ill patients with fulminant or intractable symptoms may require colectomy or diverting ileostomy (rare)

Medications

Vancomycin, 500 mg to 2 g daily q7-14 d
Cholestyramine, 12 g/d q5d
Bacitracin, 2 g/d q7-10 d
Metronidazole, 1.2-1.5 g/d q7-15 d

General Management

Intravenous fluids; hyperalimentation
Bowel rest

NURSING CARE

Nursing Assessment

Bowel Habits

Diarrhea consisting of watery stools containing mucus; severity varies up to 30 loose stools per day; may begin during antibiotic therapy or after drug is discontinued

Physical Examination

Abdominal pain and tenderness on palpation
Signs of severe dehydration and electrolyte imbalance
Abdominal distention and decreased peristalsis (signs of toxic megacolon)

Blood Work

Peripheral leukocyte count of 10,000 to 20,000/cu ml or higher

Nursing Dx & Intervention

Nursing Diagnosis	Nursing Intervention/Rationale
Diarrhea	• Assess all patients receiving antibiotics for diarrhea, particularly those receiving clindamycin, ampicillin, and cephalosporins. • Report to physician patients experiencing loose, watery, frequent diarrheal stools. • Observe patient for signs and symptoms of fluid loss, electrolyte imbalance, abdominal pain or tenderness, and fever. • Document number, description, amount, and frequency of bowel movements. • Initiate enteric precautions to prevent infections transmitted by direct or indirect contact with feces: Private room may be indicated.

Nursing Diagnosis	Nursing Intervention/Rationale
	Gowns are indicated if patient is incontinent and soiling is likely. Gloves are indicated if handling infective material. Handwashing with an antiseptic is necessary after touching patient or contaminated articles. Contamination of the environment is more common when patients have frequent watery diarrhea and incontinence.
Altered renal, cerebral, cardiopulmonary, gastrointestinal, and peripheral tissue perfusion	• Assess patient for signs of toxic megacolon, colonic perforation, and intestinal ischemia. • Assess patient's blood pressure, pulse, temperature, and respirations, reporting any signs of shock. • Assess for presence of maroon stools and abdominal distention. • Maintain patient's intravenous fluids as ordered.
Potential impaired skin integrity	• Assess for skin breakdown and the need for pressure-relieving devices for patients who are not ambulatory. • Cleanse skin carefully after each bowel movement; warm sitz baths will help cleanse the skin and soothe irritated perianal skin.

Patient Education

1. Patients will be given oral medications, and it is important that the patient understand the rationale for the agent and the importance of compliance with the prescribed protocol.
2. If surgery is required for fulminating disease, the patient and family will require instructions in management of the diverting or permanent ileostomy. The surgery is rarely necessary.

Evaluation

Patient Outcome	Data Indicating That Outcome is Reached
Body functions normally.	Patient has no diarrhea, nor does diarrhea recur after discontinuation of treatment.
Fluid balance is maintained.	Patient returns to normal hydration levels as assessed by skin turgor, mucous membranes, color, blood pressure, and pulse.
Laboratory studies are normal.	Serum electrolytes, hematocrit, and WBC are within normal limits.

Crohn's disease

Crohn's disease, a chronic inflammatory disorder of the gastrointestinal tract, may occur in any part of the gastrointestinal tract from the mouth to the anus, but the most common sites are the terminal ileum and colon.

Crohn's disease, granulomatous colitis, regional enteritis, transmural colitis, and transmural ileitis all refer to the same disease process. Crohn's disease is segmental in nature, and normal mucosa will be found between diseased segments (skip lesions). Crohn's disease and ulcerative colitis are often called inflammatory bowel diseases (IBD), and differential diagnosis between the two diseases is important in planning treatment. A chronic disorder, Crohn's disease frequently recurs after surgical resection of diseased segments.

The overall incidence of Crohn's disease has increased by a factor of 1.4 to 4 over the past 20 years, with a prevalence range of 10 to 70 cases per 100,000 population.[75] The disease has also been increasing in the young.[78] It is hard to determine if the increase is in actual numbers of cases or whether it is related to an increased awareness of Crohn's disease and improved diagnostic techniques. Crohn's disease is more common among Jews than non-Jews and among whites than nonwhites. The age at onset of the disease is the early teens and early twenties, with a range of 15 to 30 years of age.[7,75] A positive family history for inflammatory bowel disease may be found in 20% to 30% of the patients.[75] The frequency among siblings is higher than with more distant relatives.

Crohn's disease is described by the anatomic location of the disease. Crohn's disease may be limited to the small bowel, involve both small bowel and colon (ileocolitis), be limited to the colon, or be present in the stomach or duodenum. A small group of patients may have Crohn's disease that is limited to the anorectal region. The majority of patients have Crohn's disease involving both the small bowel and colon.

The cause of Crohn's disease is unknown. Research funded through the National Foundation of Ileitis and Colitis (NFIC) and other digestive disease groups is directed toward discovery of the cause and cure for this chronic illness.

Pathophysiology

Although the cause of Crohn's disease is unknown, it has been hypothesized that an exogenous agent penetrates the intestinal epithelium, creating a cytopathic immune response in a susceptible individual. Factors that have been examined as possible causes include infectious agents (bacteria and viruses), altered host susceptibility, immune-mediated intestinal damage, psychologic factors, and dietary and environmental factors.

Psychologic factors that have been implicated in the cause of inflammatory bowel disease have not been documented in patients with Crohn's disease.[7,75,78] This is probably one of the continuing myths about Crohn's disease that is perpetuated in nursing literature. The effect of the chronic illness, its recurrence, and the potential of debilitating symptoms may result in psychologic or social problems. Stress has been associated with clinical exacerbations of the disease.

The role of infectious agents has been studied to identify a specific myobacteria or virus responsible for Crohn's disease. Recent studies have explored the possibility of cell wall–defective variants of enteric bacteria, while other research suggests a viruslike agent. Granulomatous lesions have been produced on the footpads of mice by injecting extracts from Crohn's lesions. The same results were discovered when injections were made from intestinal extracts from normal specimens. So far, studies have failed to document a specific cause in Crohn's disease.

Altered host susceptibility has been considered in the cause of Crohn's disease. Although a specific infectious agent has not been identified, some researchers suggest that an impaired immune or inflammatory response to an infectious agent might progress to Crohn's disease. Impairment of various manifestations of cell-mediated immunity has been found in a substantial portion of patients with Crohn's disease.[66] Genetic transmission of specific histocompatibility antigens has also been explored, without conclusive findings.

Immune mechanisms have been implicated in the cause of Crohn's disease because of the recurrent inflammatory process, presence of granulomatous lesions, systemic manifestations, and the positive response to corticosteroids. Studies have examined the following as possible immune causes: hypersensitivity reaction in the intestines, "autoimmune" antibody–mediated damage to intestinal epithelium, tissue deposition of antigen-antibody complexes, lymphocyte-mediated cytotoxicity, and impairment of cellular immune mechanisms.[7]

Sleisenger and Fordtran[75] identify three weaknesses in the immunity basis for inflammatory bowel disease. First, the cytotoxicity of lymphocytes disappears after surgical removal of the diseased bowel. Second, the antibody-dependent, cell-mediated damage to intestinal mucosa has not been demonstrated in the intact host. Third, it is not confirmed that the K cell–mediated cytotoxicity induced by lymphocytes is specific to inflammatory bowel disease.

Dietary and environmental factors have also been questioned in the cause of Crohn's disease. Chemical food additives, such as carrageenin, reduced dietary fibers, and increased refined sugars have been studied. No evidence firmly links dietary or environmental factors to Crohn's disease at this time.

In Crohn's disease the inflammatory process extends through the layers of the bowel wall, hence the term "transmural." Microscopically the following are found in the intestines: transmural inflammation, submucosal infiltration, submucosal thickening and fibrosis, ulceration through the mucosa, fissures, and focal granulomas. As the disease progresses, the bowel wall thickens and the lumen narrows. Stenosis is common. The mucosa shows skip lesions, with normal bowel between diseased segments. The mesentery thickens and may extend over the serosal surface toward the antimesenteric border of the bowel. The intestinal segment may become fixed as the mesentery becomes fibrotic and contracts. The mesenteric nodes are enlarged and firm and may come together to form an irregular mass. The lymphatic vessels dilate and may be visible in the involved mesentery and serosal layer of the bowel.

The mucosal layer in advanced Crohn's disease consists of deep mucosal ulcerations and nodular submucosal thickening, producing a cobblestone appearance to the surface layer. The ulcers usually extend into the submucosa, and two or more ulcers may coalesce to form deep longitudinal ulcers traversing long segments. These ulcers are often referred to as *rake* ulcers. As the disease progresses, the mucosa becomes denuded.

The inflammation of the serosa and mesentery leads to a characteristic tendency in Crohn's disease for involved loops of bowel to adhere to one another. Fissures extend through the entire wall of the bowel and erode into adjacent loops of bowel or bladder, forming a fistula. It is not unusual for a fistula tract to develop to the skin (enterocutaneous), the umbilicus, or the perineum. When the rectum is diseased, ulcers arising in the rectal crypts may end in the perirectal fat and form abscesses. Rectal abscesses may erode into the anal sphincter and the supporting muscles. Abscesses can occur anywhere in the peritoneum, retroperitoneal area, or pelvis.

The severity of the malabsorption depends on the severity of the Crohn's disease, the amount of gut involved, and the treatment regimen. Crohn's disease in the jejunum and ileum decreases the capacity of the small bowel mucosa to absorb multiple nutrients, including carbohydrates, amino acids, folate, water-soluble vitamins, fats, and fat-soluble vitamins. Disease in the terminal ileum may lead to vitamin B_{12} (cobalamin) malabsorption and bile salt reabsorption, resulting in increased diarrhea because of increased osmolality of bile salt in the colon and decreased fat absorption. Lactase deficiency may develop with small bowel disease. The presence of ulcerations in extensive disease may result in protein loss. Iron deficiency anemia may develop from a chronic, slow blood loss and decrease in iron absorption. Bleeding in Crohn's disease is often mild, and the stool color may not change. The characteristic changes of the lymphatic system in Crohn's disease contribute to an impaired fat absorption.

The strictures and internal fistulas common in Crohn's

disease may lead to stasis of intestinal contents in the bypassed segment, which results in bacterial overgrowth in the lumen; bacterial overgrowth impairs absorption of carbohydrates, fats, and vitamin B_{12} and alters bile salt metabolism, affecting fat absorption.

Therapy may also affect nutrition. Some patients impose dietary restrictions on themselves or limit their oral food intake. Patients should be tested for lactose intolerance before a lactose-free diet is imposed. Surgical resection of diseased segments of small bowel and colon may also affect nutrition. Resection or bypass of an intestinal segment may decrease the absorptive surface area. Resection of the terminal ileum may lead to vitamin B_{12} and bile salt malabsorption. The distal ileum is the site for reabsorption of conjugated bile salts, and the loss of ileum results in loss of bile salts through the colon, thereby decreasing the total bile salt pool and thus decreasing biliary secretion of bile salts, resulting in fat malabsorption. Unabsorbed bile salts stimulate the colon mucosal secretion and reduce the net absorption of water and electrolytes in the colon, and the patient experiences increased diarrhea.

Surgeries that result in enteroenterostomies (bowel anastomosis to bowel), surgical blind loops, and loss of ileocecal valve create conditions in which bacterial overgrowth frequently occurs. The effect of overgrowth of enteric microorganisms was discussed previously.

Folate deficiency is common in patients with Crohn's disease. Decreased dietary intake and decreased absorption affect folate levels. In addition, sulfasalazine (which is frequently used in treating Crohn's disease) impairs the absorption of folate. Patients with Crohn's disease may also have an increased requirement for folate because of increased catabolism and chronic blood loss.

Patients with Crohn's disease frequently have increased caloric and protein requirements because of the catabolic effects of the chronic inflammation and superimposed infections. This further depletes the patient's nutritional status. The consequences of the impaired absorption and nutritional deficiencies are more serious in children than adults. Growth retardation and delayed sexual maturation occur in 20% to 30% of young patients. The use of corticosteroids over a prolonged period also contributes to growth retardation.

Complications of Crohn's disease are either intestinal (e.g., small bowel obstructions, abscesses, cancer, perforation, or fistula formation) or systemic. Obstructions are usually the result of inflammation and edema in a strictured or narrowed segment of bowel. The typical obstruction tends to progress slowly to a complete obstruction. Sudden complete obstruction may occur if the bowel becomes kinked by adhesions.

Fistula formation is very common in Crohn's disease and is a characteristic that often distinguishes Crohn's disease from ulcerative colitis. Perianal and perirectal fistulas and fissures can be extremely severe and may cause more problems for the patient than other clinical symptoms. Enterocutaneous fistulas can also cause severe management problems for the patient. A fistula between the bowel and bladder is infrequent, but when it occurs, it leads to chronic urinary infections and if untreated may progress to irreversible renal damage. Free perforation is rare in Crohn's disease because of the more frequent fistula formation and walled-off abscesses.

Systemic manifestations include arthritis, iritis, erythema nodosum, ankylosing spondylitis, pyoderma gangrenosum, aphthous mouth ulcers, and occasionally liver disease. Arthritis is the most common systemic manifestation. Arthritic symptoms may be present several years before bowel symptoms appear. Children with arthritic symptoms should have tests done to rule out inflammatory bowel disease. The arthritis may be migratory arthritis involving large joints, sacroilitis, or ankylosing spondylitis. In Crohn's disease the arthritis does not seem to reflect the degree of intestinal disease. (However, in ulcerative colitis, arthritis tends to be more severe, and the patient experiences exacerbations or remissions depending on the intestinal state.)

Erythema nodosum and pyoderma gangrenosum are inflammatory disorders of the skin that may occur with Crohn's disease. Pyoderma gangrenosum is the more severe disorder and may be found during a recurrence of active Crohn's disease in a patient following a surgical resection. The lesion may develop before the bowel symptoms.

Although liver disease is unusual in patients with Crohn's disease, mild abnormalities of liver function may be observed in hospitalized patients. Sclerosing cholangitis occurs more frequently in patients with Crohn's disease than in the general population. Renal disorders may also be a complication of Crohn's disease. The infections related to enterovesical fistulas may lead to urinary tract infections. The ureters may also be affected by the bowel and mesenteric inflammation, leading to obstruction and hydronephrosis. Oxalate stones and hyperoxaluria have been associated with steatorrhea in patients with Crohn's disease.

Cancer of the colon occurs three times more often in patients with Crohn's disease than in the general population. This is less frequently than colon cancer is found in patients with ulcerative colitis. Crohn's disease may vary from a mild to severely debilitating disease. An individual may experience one acute episode and be asymptomatic for years. Medical management is the primary form of therapy; however, most patients will require surgery at some time to manage intestinal complications of the long-term effects of the disease. The recurrence of Crohn's disease following a surgical resection ranges from 75% to 90% in 15 years.[75]

Diagnostic Studies and Findings

Differential Diagnosis

Crohn's disease often diagnosed by ruling out other disorders with similar symptoms and clinical signs

Early, acute phase: small or large intestinal involvement

- Viral gastroenteritis
- Appendicitis
- *Yersinia* enterocolitis

Salmonella infection
Chronic, recurrent phase: small or large intestinal involvement
Giardiasis
Amebiasis
Intestinal tuberculosis
Intestinal lymphoma
Fungal infection
Pseudomembranous enterocolitis
Duodenal ulcer disease
Involvement limited to colon and rectum
Ulcerative colitis
Ischemic colitis
Cancer of colon
Diverticulitis

Stool Cultures

Negative (used to rule out infections)

Stool for Guaiac

Positive (slow blood loss)

Blood Work

Serum albumin
Low (protein loss through lesions and increase in protein catabolism)
Liver function
Abnormal (pericholangitis or fatty liver)
Serum cobalamin
Low (ileal disease)
Serum folic acid
Low (malabsorption)
Hemoglobin, hematocrit
Anemia

Lactose Tolerance Test

To rule out lactase deficiency

Sigmoidoscopy

Rectum: rectal mucosa may be free of disease; perianal or perirectal fissures, fistulas, or abscesses may be found
Distal colon: aphthous ulcers or erosions; deep longitudinal fissures with intervening edematous mucosa

Colonoscopy

Skip lesions; cobblestone mucosa

Biopsy

Presence of granulomas
Also aids in differentiation of pseudopolyposis, ulcerative colitis, adenomatous polyp, and cancer

Barium Studies

Upper small bowel, barium enemas
Asymmetric disease, skip lesions, pseudodiverticula, linear ulcerations, transverse fissures, cobblestone mucosa, strictures, fistulas (NOTE: routine preparation of colon should be omitted, since it may initiate an exacerbation of the disease; prepare patient with a clear liquid diet for 2 to 3 days)

Medical Plan

Surgery

Surgical resection of diseased segments of bowel (operative therapy reserved for complications of Crohn's disease or unequivocal failure to respond to medical management)
Total colectomy with ileostomy (when disease is limited to the colon and is not responsive to medical management or cancer is found)
Subtotal colectomy with temporary ileostomy or with ileorectal anastomosis (when the rectum is not involved)

Medications

Sulfasalazine (Azulfidine): acute phase: 3 to 4 g/d in divided doses tid; maintenance: 1 to 2.5 g/d tid
Prednisone: acute phase: 50 to 80 mg/d (intravenously in severely ill patient); maintenance: 5 to 15 mg/d po
6-Mercaptopurine (6-MP): acute phase: 1.5 mg/kg/d po; maintenance: 1.5 mg/kg/d po (has a steroid-sparing effect)
Metronidazole (Flagyl): 20 mg/kg/d in divided doses
Other antibiotics may be indicated in the acute phase
Diarrhea: loperamide, Lomotil, codeine; if diarrhea related to bile salt malabsorption: cholestyramine, aluminum hydroxide; metamucil may be used for watery stools in the chronic phase

General Management

Acute phase: intravenous fluids, nothing by mouth, bed rest or limited activity
Complication of small bowel obstruction: nasogastric suctioning
Stenosis or narrowing of lumen: avoid foods containing cellulose or those foods that are not readily digested
Nutritional support: vitamin replacement, folic acid, iron, total parenteral nutrition (TPN), enteral alimentation; lactose restrictions (if indicated); some institutions use peripheral amino acids, fat for 1 to 5 days, with bowel rest and then start food or TPN

NURSING CARE

Nursing Assessment

Gastrointestinal Concerns

Initially, diarrhea, abdominal cramping, and fever; as disease progresses, must observe patient for signs of complications

Diarrhea: when disease confined to ileum, five or six loose bowel movements per day; when colon involved, urgency and incontinence frequent
Abdominal cramping: mild to severe, lower quadrant, intermittent periumbilical colic experienced during bowel movements
Fever: low grade
Gastrointestinal complications
- Fistulas
  - Stool in urine
  - Passing gas via vagina
  - Fecal drainage through skin (enterocutaneous)
- Small bowel obstructions
- Toxic megacolon
- Cancer
- Free perforations (rare)
- Hemorrhage (infrequent)

Perianal Concerns

Presence of fissures, fistulas, or abscesses

Extracolonic Manifestations

Arthritis
Inflammation of eye, skin, or mucous membrane in form of iritis, pyoderma gangrenosum, erythema nodosum, or aphthous ulcers of mouth and tongue

Nursing Dx & Intervention

Nursing Diagnosis	Nursing Intervention/Rationale
Diarrhea	• Assess the frequency of bowel movements and the appearance of stools. • Note signs of steatorrhea or bleeding. • Check stools for occult blood. • Provide antidiarrheal medications as ordered.
Potential fluid volume deficit	• Assess patient's vital signs, intake, output, and daily weights. • Provide intravenous fluids as ordered.
Altered nutrition: less than body requirements	• Assess nutritional status. • Assist patient in identifying irritating foods. • Provide nutritional supplements as ordered. • Assess blood work for indications of anemia and compare serum levels of folate, vitamin B_{12}, and iron. • Assess patient for signs of magnesium deficit (associated with long-standing diarrhea).
Potential impaired skin integrity	• Assess perianal region for signs of fissures, fistulas, or abscesses. • Assess perianal region for irritation from chronic diarrhea. • Provide interventions or treatment for perianal fissures as ordered (e.g., sitz baths; keep area clean following bowel movements). • Protect perianal skin in patients with frequent bowel movements; use gentle cleansing solutions (Periwash, Uniwash, Tucks, witch hazel pads); if area is denuded, cleanse with cotton balls soaked in mineral oil, or use Nupercainal ointment or Anusol suppositories with or without hydrocortisone to decrease perianal pain. • Evaluate enterocutaneous fistula for amount and type of drainage. See p. 859 for specific management suggestions. • Protect skin from erosion from fistula drainage.
Pain	• Provide analgesic as ordered.
Family coping: potential for growth	• Assess patient and family needs regarding knowledge of Crohn's disease, compliance with medical treatment, and myths or misconceptions. • Help patient and family support each other as they learn to manage the effects of a chronic illness. • Provide opportunities for patient and family to express their feelings regarding the illness and to identify their perceptions for a successful outcome. • Assess the family background for inflammatory bowel disease. • Help parents and siblings cope with Crohn's disease and guilt implications if family history is positive. • Provide patients with information about support groups: National Foundation for Ileitis and Colitis and United Ostomy Association.
Altered sexuality patterns	• Assess patient's sexual history in relation to the presence of perianal or perirectal disease that may make sexual activity extremely painful. (Patient may avoid sexual activity because of painful experiences.) • Provide patient and partner opportunities to discuss their feelings regarding any actual or feared changes in sexual activities. (The fear of colectomy surgery may be an underlying theme related to changes in self-image and body image.)

Patient Education

1. Provide written schedule for medications and for "tapering" schedule for drugs as dosages are decreased.
2. Provide information on Crohn's disease and the relationship of stress and exacerbations.
3. Provide information on drug toxicities. For example, the patient taking metronidazole (Flagyl) may have an antiabuse reaction with alcohol; metronidazole is also related to peripheral neuropathy. Sulfasalazine is associated with rashes; the patient may be desensitized with small doses.
4. Provide specific instructions for procedures and allow return demonstrations: perianal care, fistula management, dietary instructions, TPN, central line care.

Evaluation

Patient Outcome	Data Indicating That Outcome is Reached
Disease is in remission.	There is no pain, diarrhea, fever, fistulas, or perianal disease. Patient participates in routine activities of daily living and working.
Nutrition is adequate.	Patient gains weight; there are no signs of malnutrition or vitamin deficiency. Nutrition is maintained by supplements: TPN, vitamins, and minerals.
Fluid balance is maintained.	Patient returns to normal hydration levels as assessed by skin turgor, color, mucous membranes, blood pressure, and pulse.

Ulcerative colitis

Ulcerative colitis is a chronic mucosal inflammatory disease limited to the colon and rectum.

The disease generally starts in the rectum and progresses uninterrupted through the colon. The mucosa and submucosa layers of the colon and rectum are affected by ulcerative colitis. It is often difficult to differentiate the symptoms of ulcerative colitis from Crohn's disease of the large colon. The distinction between the two diseases is important in planning treatment and long-term prognosis. Ulcerative colitis is cured by total proctocolectomy. The incidence of cancer associated with long-standing ulcerative colitis is four times greater than in Crohn's disease. Ulcerative colitis is characterized by bloody, frequent, watery diarrhea. Patients report as many as 20 to 30 diarrheal stools per day. Remissions and exacerbations of the disease are common.

The annual incidence of ulcerative colitis in the United States has been relatively stable, with six to eight cases per 100,000 persons per year.[7,75] The incidence of ulcerative colitis is more common among Jewish than non-Jewish populations and among whites than nonwhites. Interestingly, the incidence of ulcerative colitis is more common among European and American Jews than Jews living in Tel-Aviv.[30] Diagnosis of ulcerative colitis peaks in the third and fifth decades of life.

There is a higher frequency of additional cases of ulcerative colitis in families than in control populations. It is not uncommon to have family members with ulcerative colitis and Crohn's disease. A small percentage of patients may demonstrate features of both ulcerative colitis and Crohn's disease.

As with Crohn's disease, research continues to focus on discovery of the cause. Surgery is no longer considered a "last resort," and newer surgical techniques have improved the outlook for patients. Continent ileostomies (Kock pouch) and ileoanal reservoir procedures (Parks pouch) have eliminated the need for conventional ileostomies in selected patient populations.

Pathophysiology

The cause of ulcerative colitis is unknown. Proposed causes include infectious agents, genetic factors, immunologic mechanisms, and psychosomatic determinants. No specific bacterium or virus has been found to be the exogenous agent producing the inflammatory reaction seen in ulcerative colitis. The genetic hypothesis is suggested because of the familial tendency for the disease, the higher incidence in Jews, and the low incidence among nonwhites.

The immunologic mechanisms have been suggested to be the cause of ulcerative colitis or to contribute to the mucosal inflammation and extracolonic manifestations of the disease. Patients with ulcerative colitis have been found to have alterations of T and B cell lymphocytes, suggesting an immune-deficient state. In addition, the cell-free filtrates of disrupted lymphocytes from patients with ulcerative colitis are cytotoxic to normal colonic epithelium.

Some patients with ulcerative colitis have circulating antibodies to normal colon epithelium that cross react with specific enterobacterial antigens (e.g., *E. coli*).[7] Thus the components of bacteria could change the protein structure, altering the antigenic configuration to create an autoimmune reaction, and the inflammatory bowel disease results from the hypersensitivity to antigens of bacteria.

The association of ulcerative colitis with other autoimmune diseases, such as lupus erythematosus, hemolytic anemia, and vasculitis, strengthens the view that ulcerative colitis is an immunologic reaction.

Research has documented that psychosomatic factors are not the cause of ulcerative colitis. Controlled studies have shown that patients with ulcerative colitis have no higher incidence of psychiatric problems than a control group.[52] Less than 20% of the sample could document a traumatic emotional experience before the onset of the disease.[52] Social and occupational backgrounds of patients with inflammatory bowel disease do not differ from the general population.

Patients with ulcerative colitis have been labeled in the past with a "colitis personality." It is time to eliminate any reference to personality or psychosomatic mechanisms as the cause. The effects of chronic illness on a person's life should be explored. Twenty to 30 bowel movements per day with urgency and occasional incontinence may interfere with work, social, and sexual activities. A patient may need help in learning how to cope with the illness and symptoms. Stress and tension may influence the symptoms of ulcerative colitis and have been known to cause exacerbations.

Ulcerative colitis is an inflammatory disease confined primarily to the mucosa and to a lesser degree to the adjacent submucosa. The primary lesion appears to be crypt abscess formation in the crypts of Lieberkühn. Polymorphonuclear cells accumulate near the tip of the crypt, and degenerative changes occur in the crypt epithelial cells. As the crypt abscess progresses, frank necrosis of the crypt epithelium occurs and the polymorphonuclear infiltrate extends through the colonic epithelium. A more chronic inflammatory infiltrate composed of mast cells, lymphocytes, plasma cells, and eosinophils develops. Vascular engorgement appears in the submucosa. The microabscesses in the crypts are not visible to an unaided eye. However, as the microabscesses coalesce by lateral enlargement, they produce shallow ulcerations of the mucosa extending down to the lamina propria. In some areas the extensions of the abscesses undermine the mucosa on three sides, producing an area of ulceration adjacent to a hanging fragment of mucosa, which is referred to as a pseudopolyp during radiographic or endoscopic procedures.

The body attempts to heal itself even as the destruction of the mucosa is occurring. Highly vascular granulation tissue may develop in ulcerated, denuded areas. Collagen is deposited in the lamina propria. Fibrosis is minimal. In long-standing disease the muscularis mucosae may hypertrophy. The hypertrophy and spasms of the muscularis mucosae may result in shortening and narrowing of the colon, loss of haustral markings, and apparent stricture formation. All of these are reversible in ulcerative colitis, since they are not caused by fibrosis.

The two most prominent symptoms of ulcerative colitis are hematochezia and diarrhea. The bleeding is the result of the mucosal changes: ulceration, vascular engorgement, and highly vascular, friable granulation tissue. As the mucosa is destroyed or damaged, it loses its ability to absorb sodium and water, resulting in watery diarrhea. The absence of involvement of the muscularis and serosa layers accounts for the lack of localized abdominal pain, fistula formation, and well-defined peritoneal signs observed frequently in Crohn's disease.

Complications of ulcerative colitis include perforation, toxic megacolon, adenocarcinoma of the colon, massive hemorrhage, and extracolonic manifestations. Perforation of the colon may develop if the disease process extends through the muscle and serosa layers of the colon. Toxic megacolon is a severe and serious complication of ulcerative colitis. Toxic megacolon is associated with fulminant disease, in which the circular and longitudinal muscles have been destroyed. Damage to the myenteric ganglia in the wall of the colon produces a loss of contractibility, and peristalsis ceases with marked dilatation of the colon developing. The transmural inflammation may lead to necrosis and perforation. Narcotics, anticholinergics, and hypokalemia may precipitate toxic megacolon, since they produce atony of the smooth muscles of the colon.

Cancer of the colon and rectum occurs at a much higher rate in patients with ulcerative colitis than in the general population. Two factors appear to be related to the incidence of adenocarcinoma of the colon and rectum. First, the duration of the disease process has been related to the cancers. Ulcerative colitis of 10 years' duration increases the risk, and the risk continues to increase thereafter. Second, the extent of colonic involvement influences the risk of colorectal cancers. The more universal (affecting the entire colon and rectum) ulcerative colitis is, the higher the incidence of cancer. Patients with the disease limited to the rectum have no greater risk of colon cancer than persons of the same age and sex without ulcerative colitis. The cancerous lesions tend to be flat and infiltrative in nature and are multicentric. Early diagnosis is important. In patients with ulcerative colitis of 10 years or longer, double-contrast barium enemas alternating with pancolonoscopy yearly and proctoscopy or flexible sigmoidoscopy with rectal biopsies twice yearly are recommended. Even with close follow-up, colon cancer may be detected too late for curative therapy.

The question often arises of prophylactic colectomy after a duration of 10 years. Colectomy does cure ulcerative colitis and also prevents colon cancer. Of course, the person will have some type of diversional procedure (conventional ileostomy, continent [Kock] ileostomy, ileorectal pouch). One question of length of duration is the actual beginning of the disease. Patients may have ulcerative colitis for a year or two before diagnosis. The decision to have surgery is a serious one with which patients are faced. By the time a patient with long-standing disease is admitted for surgery, he or she has dealt with a variety of emotions and may be "ready" for surgery. Other patients prefer to wait until it is essential that surgery be done. While it is impossible to generalize and recommend surgical interventions for all patients, the nurse does play an important role in educating patients to the risk of cancer, the long-term effects of a disease, its treatments, and the need for consistent follow-up, even when the patient is asymptomatic.

A medical emergency for a person with ulcerative colitis is a massive hemorrhage, which occurs in approximately 4% of patients.[75] Patients with ulcerative colitis are often severely ill, with high temperatures, tachycardia, and fluid depletion. Massive fluid replacements are required to replace the circulating volume and maintain blood pressure. The hemorrhage usually subsides spontaneously. Surgical intervention (total proctocolectomy) is rarely necessary.

The mortality of an acute initial episode of ulcerative colitis is approximately 5%.[67] The prognosis is negatively affected by total colonic involvement, age at onset over 60 years, and presence of toxic megacolon.

Extracolonic manifestations can also be serious complications of ulcerative colitis. Arthritis, uveitis, and skin disorders reflect the disease process and will have remissions and exacerbations with the disease. The arthritis of ulcerative colitis involves the larger joints and is migratory. The joint is frequently swollen, erythematous, and tender.

Uveitis (iritis) is the most common eye lesion seen accompanying ulcerative colitis. The patient may experience blurred vision, eye pain, and photophobia. An acute attack of iritis may be followed by atrophy of the iris, anterior and posterior synechiae, and old pigment deposits on the lens.

The extracolonic skin disorders consist of erythema nodosum and pyoderma gangrenosum. Erythema nodosum consists of raised, tender, erythematous swellings of 2 to 3 cm on the arms and legs. The condition often develops during an exacerbation of the colitis and is frequently found when arthritis is associated with the exacerbation of the primary disease. Occasionally arthritis and erythema nodosum appear just before the first overt bowel symptoms of ulcerative colitis. Pyoderma gangrenosum is less frequent than erythema nodosum and is usually associated with severe ulcerative colitis. Pyoderma gangrenosum first appears as a pinpoint lesion, a boil, or an infected hair follicle. The lesion collects purulent drainage that contains few polymorphonuclear cells and no bacteria. The lesion may drain spontaneously. There is a characteristic purple border around the lesion. As the lesion becomes gangrenous, progressive necrosis of the dermis occurs and the area is deeply ulcerated. Healing of the lesions requires control of the ulcerative colitis through corticosteroids or surgical removal of the colon and rectum.

Liver diseases have also been associated with ulcerative colitis. The pathogenesis is not understood, and the incidence of liver disease is approximately 7%. Liver disease may range from minor abnormalities in one or more liver function tests to more serious changes in liver structure and function. Diseases of the liver associated with ulcerative colitis include fatty infiltrations, pericholangitis, chronic active hepatitis, postnecrotic cirrhosis, amyloidosis, and sclerosing cholangitis. The question remains as to the degree of improvement in liver diseases following colectomy.

Renal stone formation is associated with ulcerative colitis and is probably related to dehydration, inactivity of the patient, and changes in the composition of the urine.

Ulcerative colitis may range from mild to severe. The degree of involvement of the colon influences the severity. For many patients, ulcerative colitis will remain in remission for years after an acute phase of the illness. The treatment and the nursing interventions will be influenced by the degree of involvement and the severity of the colitis.

Diagnostic Studies and Findings

Differential Diagnosis*

- Mild ulcerative colitis with rectal bleeding
  - Hemorrhoids
  - Anal fissures
  - Rectal polyp
  - Carcinoma of rectum
  - Factitious proctitis
  - Crohn's colitis
- Mild ulcerative colitis without bleeding
  - Irritable bowel syndrome
- Moderate ulcerative colitis
  - Irritable bowel syndrome
  - Diverticular disease
  - Chronic small bowel diarrhea
  - Crohn's disease
- Severe ulcerative colitis
  - Acute infectious colitis (salmonellosis, shigellosis, or amebiasis)
  - Pseudomembranous colitis
  - Necrotizing colitis

Stool Cultures

- Negative

Laboratory Studies

- Hemoglobin, hematocrit
  - Anemia
- Liver function
  - Abnormal
- Serum albumin
  - Low

Sigmoidoscopy

- Submucosal inflammation and edema
- Subepithelial infiltration and edema

*The diagnosis of ulcerative colitis is often based on the combination of clinical symptoms and an inflamed, abnormal colonic mucosa. The clinical symptoms of ulcerative colitis (chronic, watery diarrhea with intermittent blood and mucus, weight loss, fatigue, and general debility) are associated with other diseases. The disorders listed should be considered in the differential diagnosis.

Microscopic mucosal erosions
Crypt abscesses
Granular appearance
Friable (bleeds easily)

Rectal Biopsy

Inflammatory changes in the mucosa
Helps to differentiate between ulcerative colitis and Crohn's colitis

Colonoscopy

Superficial mucosal changes in early disease: hyperemia, mucosal friability, fine granular pattern, shallow ulcerations
Late disease: coarse, granular appearance; deep mucosal ulcerations; pseudopolyps; shortening of colon; loss of haustrations
NOTE: colonoscopy should be avoided in acute situations because of danger of perforation

Roentgenography

Plain film of abdomen
Shortening of colon, loss of haustrations
Irregular mucosa caused by pseudopolyps, ulcerations, and mucosa tags
Midtransverse colon dilated with air in toxic megacolon

Double-Contrast Barium Enemas

Evaluates disease above the sigmoidoscopy level (preferred over colonoscopy)
Early disease: study may appear normal, or there may be a reticulated pattern denoting the denudation of the mucosa
Late disease: ulceration of mucosa, shortening of the bowel, pseudopolyps
NOTE: under no circumstances should a patient with ulcerative colitis be prepared with irritant cathartics; such treatment may worsen the disease[57]; barium enemas should be avoided in acute situations because of danger of perforation

Medical Plan

Surgery

Ulcerative colitis intractable to medical management: colectomy with rectal mucosal stripping and ileoanal reservoir; or proctocolectomy with ileostomy or with continent ileostomy
Surgery varies depending on the presence of complications
Perforation
First stage: subtotal colectomy and ileostomy
Second stage: rectal mucosal stripping and ileoanal reservoir (this surgery often requires additional surgical stages to complete) if possible; or abdominoperineal resection
Toxic megacolon
First stage: diverting ileostomy (loop stoma or ileostomy and mucous fistula) and a decompression, cutaneous colostomy
Second stage: total colectomy and proctocolectomy (in some patients it may be possible to consider an ileoanal reservoir)
Cancer: proctocolectomy and ileostomy or continent ileostomy

Medications

Corticosteroids
In mild disease (ulcerative proctitis), acute phase: hydrocortisone retention enemas (Contenema), 100 mg in 60 ml daily, should retain for 20 min
In mild disease, remission: hydrocortisone retention enemas several times per week slowly tapering down and discontinuing
In moderate disease, acute phase: prednisone, 40 to 60 mg/d po
In moderate disease, remission: taper off prednisone slowly
In severe disease, acute phase: prednisolone, 100 mg IV over 24 h (need intravenous potassium to prevent steroid-induced hypokalemia) q10-14d followed by prednisolone, 60 to 100 mg/d po (If patient does not respond, surgery may be indicated.)
Sulfasalazine (Azulfidine): acute phase, 3 to 4 g tid po; maintenance, 2 g po qid
For diarrhea:
Loperamide (Imodium), 4 mg/d and 2 mg after each unformed stool up to a maximum of 16 mg
Diphenoxylate hydrochloride (Lomotil), 5 mg qid (codeine and Lomotil used with caution since opiates and atropine in Lomotil can precipitate toxic megacolon)
Metamucil, 1 tsp qid (used to add bulk to watery stools; avoid in the very ill patient)

General Management

Acute phase: intravenous fluids, limited activity or bed rest, total parenteral nutrition (TPN) (for severe dehydration and cachexia); blood replacement usually required
Nutrition: no general restrictions; patients should avoid foods that they identify as irritating; usually a low-fiber diet advanced as tolerated with one food added at a time; milk can be a problem for some patients; need extra calories and protein

NURSING CARE

Nursing Assessment

Mild Disease

Gastrointestinal symptoms
Short episodes of anorexia
Mild lower abdominal cramping
Small amounts of rectal bleeding

Frequent stools, small in volume, without gross bleeding
Extracolonic manifestations
In absence of diarrhea and colonic bleeding

Moderate Disease

Gastrointestinal symptoms
Diarrhea: stools are frequent and loose, and contain blood
Abdominal cramping
General symptoms
Intermittent low-grade fever
Fatigue
Anorexia and weight loss
Extracolonic manifestations
Arthritis
Uveitis
Erythema nodosum
Pyoderma gangrenosum

Severe Disease

Gastrointestinal symptoms
Profuse diarrhea, rectal bleeding, tenesmus, anorexia, weight loss
Distended, tender, tympanitic abdomen without evidence of localized or generalized peritonitis
Bowel sounds decreased or absent
Systemic findings
High fever, unless on steroids, which may mask fever
Weakness
Pallor
Anemia
Hypoalbuminemia
Dehydration
Extracolonic manifestations
One or more extracolonic conditions may be present
Toxic megacolon
Severe abdominal distention
Increasing abdominal pain
Fever
Tachycardia
Sharp decrease in number of stools and in gas
Rectal bleeding
Hypoactive or absent bowel sounds

Nursing Dx & Intervention

Nursing Diagnosis	Nursing Intervention/Rationale
Diarrhea	• Assess the frequency and appearance of bowel movements. • Record amounts and presence of blood. • Provide antidiarrheal medications as ordered.
Potential fluid volume deficit	• Assess patient's vital signs, intake, output, and daily weights. • Provide intravenous fluids as ordered.
Altered nutrition: less than body requirements	• Assess nutritional status. • Identify irritating foods for the individual patient. • Provide nutritional supplements as ordered. • Assess blood work for indications of anemia. • Assess patient for signs of magnesium deficit associated with long-standing diarrhea. • Assess children for signs of growth retardation.
Potential impaired skin integrity	• Assess perianal region for signs of fissures, fistulas, or abscesses. • Assess perianal region for irritation from the chronic diarrhea. • Provide interventions or treatment for perianal fissures as ordered; sitz baths; keep area cleansed following bowel movements. • Protect perianal skin in patients with frequent bowel movements; use gentle cleansing solutions (Periwash, Uniwash, Tucks, witch hazel pads); if area is denuded, cleanse with cotton balls soaked in mineral oil; use Anusol suppositories or Nupercainal Ointment.
Pain	• Assess patient with severe disease receiving narcotics, opiates, and anticholinergics for early signs of toxic megacolon. • Provide analgesics as ordered.
Family coping: potential for growth	• Assess patient and family needs regarding knowledge of ulcerative colitis, compliance with medical treatment, or myths regarding disease. • Help patient and family support each other as they learn to manage the effects of a chronic illness in their lives. • Provide opportunities for patient and family to express their feelings regarding the illness and to identify their perceptions for a successful outcome. • Assess the family background for inflammatory bowel disease. • Help parents and siblings cope with ulcerative colitis and guilt implications if family history is positive.

Nursing Diagnosis	Nursing Intervention/Rationale
Altered sexuality patterns	• Assess patient's sexual history in relation to the presence of perianal or perirectal disease that may make sexual activity extremely painful. (Patients may avoid sexual activity because of painful experiences.) • Provide patient and partner opportunities to discuss their feelings regarding any actual or feared changes in sexual activities. (The fear of ileostomy surgery may be an underlying theme related to changes in self-image and body image.)

Patient Education

1. Provide written schedule for medications and tapering schedule for drugs as dosages are decreased.
2. Provide information on ulcerative colitis and the relationship of stress and exacerbations.
3. Provide information on drug toxicities. For example, sulfasalazine is associated with rashes, and patients may be desensitized with small doses.
4. Provide information on relationship between ulcerative colitis and colorectal cancers.
5. Provide information on various surgical options to patients with ulcerative colitis.
6. Provide specific instructions for procedures and allow return demonstrations: perianal care, ileostomy care, dietary instructions, TPN, central line care.

Evaluation

Patient Outcome	Data Indicating That Outcome is Reached
There is no active disease.	There is no diarrhea, rectal bleeding, or abdominal cramping. Patient returns to all activities of daily living. There are no signs of cancer of the colon or rectum.
Nutrition is adequate.	Patient gains weight and does not experience anorexia. Protein and calorie intake is adequate (serum albumin level is within normal range by electrophoresis).
Fluid balance is maintained.	Normal hydration levels return as assessed by skin turgor, color, mucous membrane, blood pressure, and pulse.

Benign tumors

The term "tumor" is used to refer to neoplasm, a new growth of tissue characterized by uncontrolled proliferation of cells. A tumor may be malignant or benign.

The benign tumors of the small and large intestines include colonic adenomas (polyps), villous or papillary adenomas, lipomas, leiomyomas, and lymphoid hyperplasia. Polyps have been discussed on p. 813. A villous adenoma is a rare tumor found most often in the rectosigmoid area; it may be benign or contain foci of carcinoma. Lipomas are smooth, round tumors found in the submucosal layer of the colon. Leiomyomas are found in the small intestine and are submucosal or subserosal growths that protrude intraluminally, extraluminally, or in both directions. Malignant tumors of the colorectal area are covered in Chapter 16.

Benign tumors in the intestines occur equally in men and women. The benign tumors are most often discovered between the ages of 50 and 80. Symptomatic benign tumors are commonly diagnosed between the ages of 30 and 60. Most benign tumors in the small and large intestines are asymptomatic and may be discovered during routine examinations or surgery. Symptoms, when present, are generally related to the size of the tumor. A benign tumor may block the lumen, resulting in obstruction or intussusception. If the mucosa covering a tumor is irritated and becomes ulcerated, the patient may have signs of intestinal bleeding.

The cause of isolated benign tumors of the small intestine is unknown. Benign tumors in the small bowel include adenomas, leiomyomas, lipomas, hamartomas (associated with Peutz-Jeghers syndrome), and neurogenic tumors. Pseudotumors may also be found in the small intestine, and surgical excision is required for histologic studies and differential diagnosis.

The most common benign tumor of the colon is the polyp (or colonic adenoma). Neurofibromas, leiomyomas, and lipomas are found, but the incidence is low. Histologic examination of the tissue is required to determine the type of tumor. Villous adenomas are polyps found in the rectosigmoid area, and they are associated with more symptoms than other tumors. Both colonic polyps and villous adenomas are associated with malignancies.

Pathophysiology

Adenomas in the intestines may be tubular, villous, or tubulovillous. Adenomas in the small intestine are generally found near the ileum. Villous adenomas are rare in the small intestine and when they occur are found in the duodenum. The villous adenoma is most often found in the rectosigmoid areas. The rectosigmoid villous adenoma appears as a "frondlike, velvety surface."[78] It tends to recur, to secrete large amounts of mucus, and to act as a site for development of cancer.

The primary symptoms of villous adenomas in the rectosigmoid area include increased colonic motility, diarrhea, and electrolyte loss. A villous adenoma higher in the gastrointestinal tract does not seem to have the electrolyte loss, probably because of the reabsorption capacity of the colon distal to the adenoma. Villous adenomas consist of branching papillary fronds lined with goblet cells. The villous adenoma secretes large amounts of mucus. If the villous adenoma is large, the amount of fluid lost through mucous secretions can be significant. Sodium and potassium are lost in the mucous diarrhea. The fluid and electrolyte imbalance may divert attention away from the presence of a villous adenoma as other conditions and causes are considered during diagnosis.

Lipomas may occur anywhere in the small and large intestines, but they are more common in the colon. Lipomas tend to be single lesions averaging 4 cm in diameter. Most lipomas are found incidentally during surgery. Symptoms are associated with intussusception, obstruction, or bleeding. Lipomas in the colon may be detected during water enemas when the returns contain fat. An enlargement of the ileocecal valve may be caused by lipomatosis or by a tumor in the cecum. Lipomatosis is more common, and differential diagnosis can be made by colonoscopy.

Leiomyomas in the small intestine are found in the jejunum and tend to produce more symptoms than other benign tumors of the small intestine. Ulceration of the mucosa is common, and patients' initial complaint is bleeding. Obstruction and intussusception are rare.

Lymphoid hyperplasia of the colon is found more often in children than adults. An enlarged lymphoid follicle may occur in the rectum. No intervention is required. When lymphoid hyperplasia appears in multiple numbers throughout the rectum and colon, it can be confused with familial polyposis. Differential diagnosis is important, since treatment is not indicated in lymphoid hyperplasia and total colectomy is used to treat familial polyposis.

Diagnostic Studies and Findings

Small Bowel

- Barium studies
  - Prograde enteroclysis or retrograde infusion through ileocecal valve
  - Small isolated tumors
  - Multiple small tumors
- Exploratory laparotomy
  - Biopsy and removal of tumor for histologic studies

Colon

- Sigmoidoscopy, colonoscopy
  - Visualization, biopsy, and removal of tumor
- Double-contrast barium enema
  - Villous adenoma: reticulated appearance
  - Presence of tumors in colon and rectum

Medical Plan

Surgery

- Laparotomy may be used for diagnosis and removal of tumors in small bowel when patient is symptomatic
- Villous adenoma
  - Above peritoneal reflection: resection of bowel containing villous adenoma
  - Below peritoneal reflection: local excision
  - With evidence of frank invasive carcinoma: abdominoperineal resection

NURSING CARE

Nursing Assessment

Abdomen

- Signs of intestinal obstruction: abdominal pain, distention, nausea and vomiting, absence of peristalsis, absence of bowel movements
- Large bowel or distal small bowel obstructions: fecal odor to emesis

Rectum

- Occult, blood-tinged, or black tarry stools

Nursing Dx & Intervention

Nursing Diagnosis	Nursing Intervention/Rationale
Constipation	• Assess patient for signs and symptoms of intestinal obstructions: abdominal pain, abdominal distention, decreased peristalsis, nausea, vomiting. • Determine if patient has regular bowel habits and if bowel pattern has changed. • Observe stool for shape, consistency, color, quantity, and odor. • Note and report any signs of blood-tinged stools. • Check stool for occult blood, an early sign of a bowel tumor.

Patient Education

1. Provide patient with information about the type of tumor and any impact regarding long-term care (e.g., following removal of villous adenoma, regular follow-up required if a focus of carcinoma is present).
2. Provide routine postoperative information on activity, diet, driving, and returning to work associated with any abdominal surgery.

Evaluation

Patient Outcome	Data Indicating That Outcome is Reached
Body functions normally.	Bowel elimination is adequate. Surgical wound heals.

Volvulus

A volvulus is a twisting of the bowel on itself. The two most common sites for the development of a volvulus are the cecum and the sigmoid colon.

The twisting or rotation of the bowel kinks the gut, producing a mechanical obstruction. When the blood supply is also involved, the strangulation leads to acute, early gangrene. The clinical symptoms, diagnosis, and management are similar to those related to any mechanical obstruction of the colon.

A cecal volvulus may occur any time from adolescence but is most common in the fifth decade. Sigmoid volvulus is more common in elderly persons and has been associated with chronic constipation.

Pathophysiology

A volvulus usually develops in an area where an underlying abnormality exists. A midgut volvulus may develop from a congenital malrotation of the mesentery. If the cecum and ascending colon are poorly fixed on mesentery rather than being retroperitoneal, the cecum may be mobile and able to twist, creating a volvulus. The twisting or torsion is commonly in a clockwise direction and points obliquely toward the left upper quadrant. A sigmoid volvulus develops when the sigmoid colon is long or redundant. It is easy for a long loop to twist about its leash, creating a closed-loop obstruction. A volvulus may also develop when adhesions produce an axis about which the sigmoid colon can twist.

When there is a sudden tight twisting of the mesentery impeding the blood flow to the bowel, gangrene, necrosis, and perforation may develop, resulting in an acute abdominal emergency. A closed-loop obstruction results in marked distention, aperistalsis, and pain. Intermittent, recurrent volvulus produces repeated episodes of abdominal pain, tenderness, and distention.

The reader is referred to the section on intestinal obstruction for the pathophysiology of intestinal obstructions.

Diagnostic Studies and Findings

Abdominal Roentgenograms

Cecal volvulus: marked distention of the cecum
Sigmoid volvulus: large dilated loop, from right to left side of abdomen; two fluid levels can be visualized

Barium Enema

Cecal volvulus: conical narrowing at the twist
Sigmoid volvulus: narrowing at the twist

Medical Plan

Surgery

Cecal volvulus: untwisting bowel; if viable, the cecum and ascending colon are anchored in place; if gangrene is present, bowel resection of involved parts
Sigmoid volvulus: resection of twisted segment if viability is questioned; resection of redundant mesentery or fixation to prevent recurrence

General Management

Reduction of volvulus; if reduction does not occur, colonoscopy will assist by releasing trapped gas and fluids (surgery may be advised following a reduction if the viability of mucosa is in doubt)

NURSING CARE

Nursing Assessment

Abdomen

Acute abdominal pain, guarding, distention, nausea and vomiting
Sigmoid loop volvulus may be palpable

General Physical Findings

Auscultation of abdomen for full 3 to 5 minutes before palpating

Signs of strangulation obstructions: localized tenderness, constant pain, guarding, vomiting, rebound tenderness, and absence of gas or bowel movement

Additional Physical Findings

Tachycardia and hypotension: may indicate dehydration or peritonitis

Fever and leukocytosis: may indicate peritonitis

Loss of skin turgor and dry mucous membranes: dehydration

Blood in the stool: may indicate cancer, intussusception, or infarction of obstructing lesions

Nursing Dx & Intervention

Nursing Diagnosis	Nursing Intervention/Rationale
Fluid volume deficit (1)	• Assess patient carefully for signs and symptoms of severe fluid and electrolyte loss, metabolic acidosis, and hypovolemic shock secondary to accumulation of gas and fluids, distention of intestine, and sepsis (if perforation occurs). • Replace intravenous fluids and electrolytes, blood, and plasma as ordered. • Monitor vital signs, central venous pressure, blood pressure, urinary output, and nasogastric aspirations every hour. • Measure abdominal girth every 4 to 8 hours as an assessment of distention. • Notify physician of changes in patient's status, since they generally indicate a decline in patient's stabilization for surgical intervention.
Altered renal, cerebral, cardiopulmonary, gastrointestinal, and peripheral tissue perfusion	• Assess patient carefully for signs of perforation and peritonitis: fever; sudden relief of pain, followed by increased diffuse pain, rebound tenderness, and abdominal guarding; increasing abdominal distention; tachycardia; rapid, shallow breathing. • Prepare patient for surgery as ordered: give anti-infective agents, shave and prepare the abdomen, remove dentures, etc. • Provide preoperative teaching, keeping in mind that patient will be unable to practice turn, cough, and deep-breathing exercises because of acute abdominal pain.
Ineffective breathing pattern	• Assess patient's pulmonary status, *since abdominal distention and abdominal guarding may impair pulmonary ventilation,* as can metabolic imbalances. • Elevate head of bed *to relieve pressure on the diaphragm.* • Provide oxygen therapy as ordered.
Pain	• Assess abdominal area for signs of perforation and peritonitis: increased severity and diffuseness of abdominal pain, rebound tenderness, guarding. • Help patient assume a comfortable position (one that places minimum stress on the abdominal muscles); limit sudden movement and abdominal examination. • Provide analgesics as prescribed.
Patient problem: potential altered bowel elimination	• Assess bowel sounds: high-pitched, tingling sounds with rushes (mechanical obstruction); absence of bowel sounds or low infrequent sounds (complete occlusion of the lumen). • Assess bowel movements: obstipation and failure to pass gas are signs of complete obstruction.

Patient Education

1. The patient should undertake primary postoperative progression if resection and anastomosis of the small bowel were performed. This includes showering, activity progressions, driving, and returning to work.
2. Colonic obstructions are often treated with a temporary diverting colostomy, and the patient requires teaching about colostomy care, plans for surgical closure, and education about the primary cause of the obstruction.

Evaluation

Patient Outcome	Data Indicating That Outcome is Reached
Body functions normally.	Pattern of bowel elimination is normal. Colostomy is closed, and normal elimination functions return.

Patient Outcome	Data Indicating That Outcome is Reached
Fluid balance is maintained.	Patient returns to normal hydration levels as assessed by skin turgor, skin color and mucous membranes, blood pressure, and pulse.
Laboratory studies are normal.	Serum electrolytes, hematocrit, and hemoglobin are within normal limits.
Sepsis is not present.	There is no fever; white blood cell counts are within normal limits.

ANAL AND RECTAL DISORDERS

Anorectal abscess

An anorectal abscess is a localized infection with pus found in the tissue spaces adjacent to and in the anorectal area.

Anorectal abscesses are classified according to location:
Perianal: beneath perianal skin
Ischiorectal: ischiorectal fossa
Submucosal: beneath the mucosa of the upper anal canal
High intramuscular: below the circular muscle layer
Intersphincteric: between internal and external sphincters
Pelvirectal or supralevator: above the levators ani and below the pelvic peritoneum

Anorectal abscesses are more common in men. Certain diseases and conditions increase the likelihood of developing anorectal abscesses. Anorectal abscesses are common in patients with Crohn's disease and in homosexual men who engage in traumatic anal intercourse. Hematologic and immune-deficient conditions have also been associated with anorectal abscesses.

Pathophysiology

Anorectal abscesses develop from infections beginning in an anal crypt and moving along anal ducts through the internal sphincter before spreading in different directions. An infection may also develop in anal fissures, prolapsed internal hemorrhoids, traumatic injuries, and superficial skin lesions that progress to form anorectal abscesses. Extension of the abscess formation is the most common complication. An abscess may eventually progress to an anorectal fistula.

Diagnostic Studies and Findings

Differential Diagnosis

Rule out pilonidal sinus, carcinoma, Bartholin's gland abscess, and inflammatory bowel disease (Crohn's disease, ulcerative colitis)

Studies used: sigmoidoscopy, barium enema, and small bowel series

Visual Inspection of Perianal Region

Tender, erythematous area that displaces the anus (superficial abscess)
Tender mass in an anatomic space may indicate a deep abscess

Anoscopy (Proctoscopy)

Visualization of lesions below the pectinate line

Medical Plan

Surgery

Surgical drainage of abscess, with or without excision of fistula tracts associated with anorectal abscesses

Medications

Antibiotic therapy based on causative organisms
Stool softeners: Docusate (Colace), 50 to 200 mg/d; dose based on individual's response

General Management

Sitz baths

NURSING CARE

Nursing Assessment

Anorectal Concerns

Throbbing, constant pain increased by walking or sitting (pain diminishes if abscess drains spontaneously)
Foul-smelling drainage

Systemic Concerns

Fever, malaise

Abdomen

Low abdominal pain may occur with a deep anorectal abscess

Nursing Dx & Intervention

Nursing Diagnosis	Nursing Intervention/Rationale
Patient problem: potential altered bowel elimination related to presence of infection	• Assess perianal region for signs of tender mass, purulent drainage, or erythema. • Determine patient's bowel habits and any recent change in the pattern (e.g., pain with defecation, purulent discharge, increased odor); also determine patient's last bowel movement and use of laxatives or stool softeners. • Keep the perianal area clean. • Provide sitz baths *for comfort and for cleansing purposes.* • Assess patient during sitz bath for hypotension secondary to dilation of the pelvic blood vessels. • Apply the dressing over the wound; change frequently, noting color and amount of drainage; dressing may be held in place with mesh "panties" available for use in incontinence management. • Keep the surgical wound clean; care is needed following urination and defecation; packing may be used to ensure that the wound heals from the inside out; following bowel and bladder elimination, it is necessary to check the dressing and replace if soiled. • Shave the perianal area weekly to keep hair from the wound *(hair will delay wound healing and is often the cause of infection or irritation).* • Irrigate the wound before packing with normal saline or irrigation solution as ordered.
Pain	• Provide analgesics as ordered. • Provide a thick pillow, cushion, or flotation pad for sitting (avoid air rings and rubber donuts, *since they tend to spread the buttocks apart*).
Altered patterns of urinary elimination	• Assess intake and output records for 24 hours, *since urinary retention may develop following surgery.* • Have patient stand or sit to void. • Pour warm water over pubic area or use sitz bath to help patient void by relaxing the bladder.

Patient Education

1. Teach the patient to irrigate the wound (Water Pik or shower massager may be used) and to reinsert dressing. Family member may need to assist the patient. The patient should comprehend the necessity of keeping the wound clean and free of fecal soiling.

Evaluation

Patient Outcome	Data Indicating That Outcome is Reached
Body functions normally.	Elimination is inadequate; there is no constipation or hard, formed stools. Wound heals. Temperature is normal.

Anorectal fistula

An anorectal fistula is a hollow, fibrous tunnel or tract with two openings.

The internal opening of an anorectal fistula is inside the anal canal or rectum and leads to the secondary, or external, opening. The external opening is in the perianal skin. Fistulas from the colon, small bowel, or urethra may exit through the perineum and be mistaken for anorectal fistulas.

Although an anorectal fistula may occur without predisposing conditions, it is more common to find anorectal fistulas associated with Crohn's disease in the large or the small bowel (regional enteritis). Anorectal fistulas are associated with the presence of an anorectal abscess. An anorectal abscess that is drained may reduce the discomfort and pain, but a fistulous tract may remain through which the abscess continues to drain.

Pathophysiology

The primary, or internal, opening of an anorectal fistula is usually at a crypt near the pectinate line. Infection in the crypt progresses to form an abscess that drains (spontaneously or with surgical drainage), and the tract is preserved as the abscess heals. Anorectal fistulas are associated with traumatic injury, fissures, Crohn's disease, cancer, and radiation therapy. Once the tract is fibrosed, it will not close on its own and surgical intervention is indicated. The terminal opening of the tract is in the perianal skin. Stool, pus, mucus, blood, and flatus may drain through the fistula. Patients may have single or multiple anorectal fistulas. The skin opening may seal over temporarily, but it will reopen spontaneously and drain.

Following treatment, recurrent fistulas in the anorectal area are associated with inadequate exposure of the tract, with primary openings not being identified, and with failure of the tract to heal from the inside out. When a patient has Crohn's disease, recurrent anorectal fistulas are associated with exacerbation of the inflammatory bowel disease.

Diagnostic Studies and Findings

Digital Rectal Examination

Palpate tract direction internally

Anoscopy (Proctoscopy)

May reveal the primary opening in a crypt

Sigmoidoscopy

Used to rule out other sources of fistula formation

Fistulography

Used if the tract is of questionable origin; rules out colonic, small bowel, and urethral fistulas

Medical Plan

Surgery

Fistulotomy or fistulectomy may be indicated depending on location and depth of the fistula tract

Medications

Antibiotics per sensitive organism

Stool softener: Docusate (Colace), 50 to 200 mg/d; dose based on individual's response

Metronidazole (Flagyl), 20 mg/kg/d in divided doses (for perianal disease associated with inflammatory bowel disease)

General Management

Sitz baths as needed and after defecation

NURSING CARE

Nursing Assessment

Anorectum

Raised, red papules

Drainage of pus, blood, mucus, or stool through the open skin lesions

Complaints of pain and discomfort; greater when lesions are sealed and not draining

Pruritus

Inundated, "cordlike" pattern may be palpated from cutaneous opening toward anus

History

Anorectal abscesses or inflammatory bowel disease

Nursing Dx & Intervention

Nursing Diagnosis	Nursing Intervention/Rationale
Patient problem: potential altered bowel elimination related to presence of infection or surgical incision	• Assess perianal skin for signs of fistula tracts and drainage. • Estimate amount of drainage; note color, odor, and consistency of drainage. • Determine patient's bowel habits and record date of last bowel movement, noting consistency of stool; record any changes in bowel habits, such as blood, pus, or odor. • Assess patient's use of laxatives, stool softeners, anal intercourse, or anal dilators (e.g., vibrators or other instruments). • Keep the perianal area clean following bowel movements with sitz baths and irrigation of the site. • Assess patient for hypotension secondary to vasodilation of the pelvic blood vessels during sitz bath. • Replace dressings as soiled and assess appearance of wound, signs of healings, and early signs of postoperative infection. • Irrigate the wound before packing or dressing. • Shave the perianal area regularly to prevent hair from irritating or infecting the wound as granulation tissue develops following surgery.
Pain	• Provide pain medication as needed. • Provide a thick foam cushion or pillow for patient to use in sitting (avoid air rings and rubber donuts, *since they tend to spread the buttocks apart*).

Patient Education

1. Teach the patient to irrigate the wound with a Water Pik or shower massager, to shave the perianal area, and to redress the wound.
2. Teach the patient to use a mirror to inspect the area and look for redness or firm reddened areas of increased itching and tenderness.
3. Mesh panties can be used to hold dressings in place, or sanitary pads or belts may be used in the underwear. Jockey shorts will be more effective than boxer shorts for managing dressings.
4. A family member's help may be needed.
5. Sitz baths can be used for cleansing and for comfort. (The sitz bath does not replace the irrigation procedure.)

Evaluation

Patient Outcome	Data Indicating That Outcome is Reached
Body functions normally.	Elimination is adequate; there is no constipation or hard, formed stools. Wound heals. Temperature is normal, and there is no purulent, odorous drainage.

Anal fissure

An anal fissure is a small tear in the lining of the anus. The tear resembles a slitlike crack and may extend from the anal verge to the pectinate line.

Fissures are most common in young and middle-aged adults. The posterior midline is the most common site, but occasional anal fissures will be found in the anterior wall. Fissures in other positions on the anal wall are usually associated with Crohn's disease or ulcerative colitis.

Pathophysiology

Anal fissures are usually caused by trauma from passing large, hard stools. Acute fissures are tears that may become chronic when the patient has an elevated resting anal pressure and contraction of the internal anal sphincter after rectal distention. Defecation stimulates spasms of the internal anal sphincter, which causes the edges of the sphincter to adhere, trapping any drainage. Edema and fibrosis of adjacent tissue develop and progress to hypertrophied anal papillae and a tag of skin at the anal verge.

Loss of elasticity of the anal canal may predispose a person to anorectal fissures. Laxative abuse, scarring from anal surgery, and chronic diarrheal diseases may lead to a loss of elasticity, as will frequent anal intercourse.

Diagnostic Studies and Findings

Differential Diagnosis

If fissure is not found in midline, rule out inflammatory bowel disease, carcinoma, tuberculosis, syphilis, herpes, and other venereal diseases

Digital Rectal Examination

Use topical anesthesia before digital examination to decrease pain from the procedure
Induration
Tenderness
Sphincter spasm
Hypertrophied anal papillae

Anoscopy (Proctoscopy)

Visualization of the anorectal fissure: a superficial tear that bleeds easily and has a reddish base

Medical Plan

Surgery

Lateral subcutaneous sphincterotomy (internal sphincter is divided up to the pectinate line, hypertrophied papillae and anal tag are excised, and fissure is left to heal)

Medications

Bulk agents
- Psyllium (Metamucil or Effersyllium), 1 tsp (7 g) 1-3 times per day

Emollient suppositories
Analgesic ointments
- Dibucaine (Nupercaine) prn

Tucks or witch hazel pads to cleanse

General Management

Topical application of silver nitrate solution or cautery with silver nitrate sticks
Sitz bath
Warm compresses

NURSING CARE

Nursing Assessment

Anorectum

Pain during evacuation; may be described as tearing or burning
Evacuation stimulates spasms, which result in prolonged, gnawing discomfort for extended periods
Presence of bright red blood following bowel movements
Rectal tag of skin
Rectal discharge
Pruritus

History

Patient may be able to identify the onset with the presence of constipation and pain with defecation
Bowel movements may be painful and associated with slight bleeding
Delayed onset of pain following a bowel movement
History of anal intercourse, use of laxatives, enema abuse, or diseases such as Crohn's disease or ulcerative colitis

Nursing Dx & Intervention

Nursing Diagnosis	Nursing Intervention/Rationale
Constipation	• Assess perianal region for tears. • Obtain a history of patient's bowel habits (e.g., constipation, use of laxatives, dietary history); following surgery, record consistency of stool and effectiveness of stool softeners. • Record date of last bowel movement. Patients often postpone or delay having bowel movements because of the pain. • Keep the postoperative site clean and free of stool by using sitz baths and careful cleansing following surgery. • Assess patient for hypotension secondary to vasodilation of pelvic blood vessels during sitz bath.
Pain	• Provide warm compresses, sitz baths, and analgesic ointments for pain and discomfort.

Patient Education

1. Provide the patient with information on natural methods of relieving or preventing constipation (i.e., diet high in bulk and fiber, increased fluid intake, avoidance of harsh laxatives and constipating medications such as codeine).

Evaluation

Patient Outcome	Data Indicating That Outcome is Reached
Body functions normally.	Elimination is adequate, and there is no constipation. Wound heals. There is no pain with evacuation or delayed pain.

Hemorrhoids

Hemorrhoids are masses of vascular tissue found in the anal canal.[75]

Internal hemorrhoids are found above the pectinate line, arise from the superior hemorrhoidal venous plexus, and are covered with mucosa. External hemorrhoids are found below the pectinate line, arise from the inferior hemorrhoidal venous plexus, and are covered by anoderm and perianal skin. Patients may have a combination of internal and external hemorrhoids.

Internal hemorrhoids may also be classified according to the degree of involvement:

First-degree: project slightly into the anal canal
Second-degree: prolapse with defecation and reduce spontaneously
Third-degree: prolapse with defecation and reduce manually
Fourth-degree: irreducible

The usual location of internal hemorrhoids is around the anal circumference, including right anterior, right posterior, and left lateral areas.[75]

The commonly accepted cause is that hemorrhoids are varicose veins. This cause has been recently questioned because of weaknesses in the original theory. The basis of the varicose vein theory of hemorrhoids is that increased pressure in the veins results in congestion. Certain occupations, the erect positions of humans, structural absence of valves in the veins, and increased abdominal pressure from straining at defecation, constipation, and pregnancy have been associated with the development of hemorrhoids. The varicose vein and increased pressure cause has been questioned because internal hemorrhoids may appear in early pregnancy before the uterus is large enough to create increased abdominal pressure and because the blood associated with hemorrhoidal bleeding is bright red, not dark as expected with the venous system.

A hypothesis is that the hemorrhoidal plexus is a rich vascular network with direct arteriovenous shunts. The vascular tissue slides easily and may be displaced downward with the evacuation of stool.[31,75,84] High resting anal pressures and failure of the internal sphincter to relax may contribute to the development of hemorrhoids in some people. In older patients, low resting anal pressures and sliding of tissues during bowel movements have been associated with hemorrhoids.

Pathophysiology

Based on Thompson's description[84] of the hemorrhoidal plexus as a vascular mound on a cushion, an internal hemorrhoid is a prolapse of normal vascular mounds or a prolapse of normal anal canal lining. The prolapse may be caused by spasms of the internal sphincter that require straining or increased pressure to push the stool through the internal sphincter and at the same time push out the hemorrhoid.

The complications associated with internal hemorrhoids include bleeding, prolapse, and thrombosis. Since the hemorrhoid is composed of spongy vascular tissue, bleeding tends to be an oozing of bright red blood. The blood may appear as a bright spot on toilet paper or on the surface of the stool. Blood may drip from the anus for a few minutes after the stool has been expelled. Iron deficiency anemia may develop if blood loss continues over a period of time.

Prolapse of hemorrhoids is first perceived as a mass of tissue that protrudes from the anus following a bowel movement. Initially, it slips back into the anal canal spontaneously. As the condition continues, the hemorrhoid will later need to be manually replaced and may become irreducible. A mucous discharge is associated with irreducible hemorrhoids because of the mucosal covering of the internal hemorrhoid. Protection of undergarments will be required. Pain is associated with prolapsed and inflamed hemorrhoids but is not a general symptom of internal hemorrhoids. Patients whose initial complaint is pain should be assessed for other anorectal conditions (fissure, abscess) and colorectal diseases.

Thrombosis of prolapsed hemorrhoids can create severe pain. This is also referred to as strangulated hemorrhoids. Ulceration and secondary infections can develop. One or all hemorrhoids may be affected.

A thrombosis of an external hemorrhoid is a blood clot within a hemorrhoidal vein. The pectinate line is visible and separate from the mass or lump that forms. Thrombosis of external hemorrhoids has been associated with heavy lifting, straining at defecation, and childbirth. The patient has a painful lump that appeared suddenly at the anus. Pain may be constant and is increased with sitting and defecation. It usually disappears in a week. The thrombosed external hemorrhoid should not be confused with prolapsed, thrombosed internal hemorrhoids. If the skin covering the clot becomes ulcerated, bleeding may be noted.

Diagnostic Studies and Findings

Complete Blood Count (CBC) and Iron Studies

To determine presence of anemia and if it is caused by iron deficiency

Digital Rectal Examination

Tone of internal sphincter; usually increased in young men with hemorrhoids; may be low in older patients and women with hemorrhoids

Palpation of third-degree internal hemorrhoids

Anoscopy

Visualization of hemorrhoids as instrument is removed

Sigmoidoscopy and Barium Enema

To rule out carcinoma and inflammatory disease

Particularly important in patients over 40 years

Medical Plan

Surgery

Injection of sclerosing solutions (5% phenol in vegetable oil) submucosally around hemorrhoid; complications: sloughing of overlying mucosa, infection, reaction to injected material

Rubber band ligation (placement of rubber band over base of hemorrhoid causes necrosis and sloughing of hemorrhoid in 7 days)

Cryosurgery (application of metal probe cooled by liquid nitrogen or carbon dioxide freezes hemorrhoid)

Lateral internal sphincterotomy (partial division of internal sphincter lowers anal pressure); seldom used unless an anorectal fissure is also present

Hemorrhoidectomy (surgical excision of the hemorrhoidal masses); complication: anal stenosis

Excision under local anesthesia of thrombosed external hemorrhoid if seen in a day or two of onset

Medications

Anesthetic ointments and suppositories

Nupercaine (Dibucaine) prn

Stool softeners

General Management

Manual dilation of anus (anus is dilated 4 cm regularly by patient with a special dilator); complication: incontinence

High-fiber diet, adequate hydration, and exercise to minimize constipation and straining

Warm sitz baths; compresses

NURSING CARE

Nursing Assessment

Inspection of Perianal Skin

External hemorrhoids visible in subcutaneous skin at anus; if hemorrhoids are thrombosed, tender, bluish spheric mass at anal verge

Prolapsed internal hemorrhoids: moist, red mucosa covering upper portion; presence of mucoid discharge or staining of undergarments

Nursing Dx & Intervention

Nursing Diagnosis	Nursing Intervention/Rationale
Pain	• Assess amount, character, and threshold of pain or discomfort; relate to bowel pattern. • Use thick foam pillows or pads under buttock; avoid air or rubber donuts *since they spread the buttocks apart.* • Promote the use of sitz baths *for comfort and for cleansing* after bowel movements. • Assess patient during sitz bath for hypotension secondary to vasodilation of pelvic blood vessels. • Provide analgesics as ordered. • Use ice packs as ordered *to reduce congestion and edema.* • Use warm compresses *to promote circulation* (also soothing).
Constipation	• Instruct patient to defecate promptly with the urge, to avoid sitting on the toilet for prolonged periods, and to avoid straining. • Provide adequate fluids *to maintain hydration.* • Encourage patient to exercise (mild at first). • Give patient medication before first bowel movement. • Encourage patient to have a bowel movement after surgery even though patient may be afraid of increased pain *(prevents formation of strictures and preserves lumen size of the anus).* • Assess patient during the first bowel movement for signs of weakness or dizziness.
Altered patterns of urinary elimination	• Assess intake and output for 24 hours, *since urinary retention may develop following surgery.* • Have patient stand or sit to void. • Pour warm water over pubic area *to relax bladder and aid voiding,* or use sitz bath.
Potential for injury (hemorrhage)	• Assess vital signs for signs of blood loss; if surgical ligatures slip, blood may collect unnoticed in the rectum. • Assess perianal area for signs of bleeding. • Check stools for blood. • Note frequent unrelieved sensation to defecate (sequestered blood may result in edema, which creates pressure and the urge to defecate).

Patient Education

1. Management and prevention of constipation with diet, fluids, and physical activities should be discussed with the patient.
2. The patient needs to respond to urge to defecate, to avoid straining, and to keep the stool soft and moist.

Evaluation

Patient Outcome	Data Indicating That Outcome is Reached
Body functions normally.	Elimination is adequate, there is no constipation, and stools are soft. Patient does not experience pain, bleeding, or prolapsed hemorrhoids.
Nutrition is adequate.	Patient eats a high-fiber diet with good hydration.

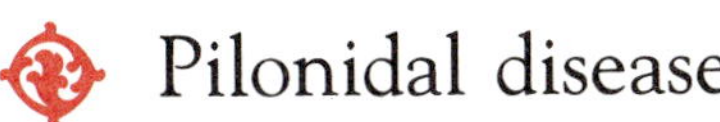

Pilonidal disease

Pilonidal disease occurs in the midline of the upper portion of the gluteal fold. A sinus channel develops that is lined with epithelium and hair.

The sinus channel may appear as a hairy dimple that is asymptomatic unless it becomes infected or inflamed. A cyst or abscess may develop, or the tract may open at the skin, creating a draining fistula. Differential diagnosis between pilonidal disease and anorectal fistula is important. In pilonidal disease the sinus tract does not connect with the anus or rectum.

Pathophysiology

Pilonidal disease occurs during embryonic development when a small amount of endothelial tissue is included beneath the skin. The penetration of hair beneath the skin and the enlargement of hair follicles irritate the skin, which becomes infected.

Diagnostic Studies and Findings

Refer to diagnostic studies on anorectal fistulas.

Differential Diagnosis

Rule out anorectal fistula

Medical Plan

Surgery

Incision and removal of hair and granulation tissue; wound may be closed or left open and packed

Medications

Antibiotic therapy to treat the infection per organism

General Management

Sitz baths

NURSING CARE

Nursing Assessment

Perineal Area

Hairy dimple in gluteal fold

Open, draining lesion in sacral region with hair protuding from sinus opening

Nursing Dx & Intervention

Nursing Diagnosis	Nursing Intervention/Rationale
Pain	• Assess perianal area for presence of inflammation of a sinus channel. • Apply hot moist compresses when an abscess is present. • Assist patient with sitz bath. • Assess patient during sitz bath for hypotension (related to vasodilation). • Position patient on abdomen or side.
Potential for infection	• Assess wound for signs of healing or infection. • Protect wound during urination and defecation. • Change dressing as needed if contaminated during elimination.

Patient Education

1. Prepare the patient or family member to change dressing as needed, to keep wound free of fecal and urinary contamination, and to cleanse wound as needed.

Evaluation

Patient Outcome	Data Indicating That Outcome is Reached
Body functions normally.	There is no infection or drainage. Wound heals. There is no pain and discomfort.

LIVER DISORDERS

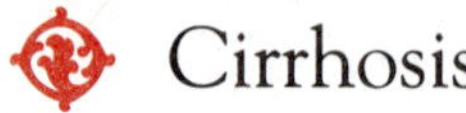

Cirrhosis

Cirrhosis is a chronic degenerative disease of the liver in which diffuse destruction and regeneration of hepatic parenchymal cells have occurred.

In cirrhosis the lobes are covered with fibrotic tissue, and the lobules are infiltrated with fat. The diffuse increase in connective tissue results in disorganization of the lobular and vascular structure of the liver, affecting the many functions of the liver and its blood flow. Cirrhosis is characterized by nodular regeneration, which is an attempt by the liver to heal itself by fibrosis or scar tissue. Cirrhosis is the end result of pathologic changes associated with liver disease.

A variety of conditions may progress or lead to cirrhosis of the liver and range from genetic disorders to alcohol abuse. The genetic disorders include galactosemia, alpha-1-antitrypsin deficiency, and Wilson's disease. Biliary atresia, a congenital malformation of bile ducts, may progress to cirrhosis. Chemical agents that are toxic to the liver include thorazine, ether, amitriptyline (Elavil), and various household cleansers (carbon tetrachloride). Infectious causes, such as viral hepatitis, syphilis, and schistosomiasis, may progress to cirrhosis. Alcoholic cirrhosis is the most common and accounts for approximately 80% of the liver disease in urban areas.

Cirrhosis develops in approximately 10% to 20% of alcoholics. Of interest to clinicians and researchers is why all individuals who abuse alcohol do not develop cirrhosis. One theory is that certain individuals have an increased ability to oxidize alcohol that may be familial or heredity based.[78] Thus alcohol ingestion in a susceptible host in the presence of an unknown factor may lead to cirrhosis of the liver.

Pathophysiology

The pathophysiology of cirrhosis will vary according to the initial cause (viral hepatitis, biliary obstruction, alcohol abuse). The symptoms and results of cirrhosis are the same. For this reason and because of the high incidence of alcohol abuse–related cirrhosis, the pathophysiology of the alcohol-induced cirrhotic changes will be described. Alcoholic cirrhosis is also referred to as portal cirrhosis, Laënnec's cirrhosis, and micronodular cirrhosis.

Several steps occur before the liver becomes cirrhotic. Initially, subcellular changes develop and may progress to a fatty liver. (Fatty livers are not limited to alcoholic cirrhosis.) The fatty liver is a reversible stage if alcohol intake is eliminated. The fatty liver can be recognized by its increased size and the marked degree of fatty infiltration seen microscopically. The fatty liver in the presence of continued alcohol ingestion may progress to alcoholic hepatitis. It is the continuing use of alcohol that causes the development of cirrhosis versus the progression from fatty liver to hepatitis to cirrhosis. These may not be related. The patient could have cirrhosis and develop acute hepatitis because of a drinking bout if the patient has cirrhotic changes. In alcoholic hepatitis the fatty infiltration is combined with liver cell necrosis, leukocytic inflammation, and fibrosis. As the disease progresses, the inflammatory changes decrease and fibrotic changes increase. Continued alcohol ingestion leads to chronic changes (i.e., alcoholic cirrhosis).

The microscopic changes in cirrhosis consist of degeneration and death of hepatocytes, proliferation of connective tissue, and regeneration of hepatocytes. The connective tissue spreads from the portal tracts and from the central veins throughout the liver, changing the normal lobular architecture. The extension of fibrous cords throughout the liver alters the relationship between the hepatic veins and the portal veins. Scar tissue and nodular regeneration of hepatocytes may compress small branches of the portal vein. The compression of the vessels leads to an increased alteration in the vascular system. The veins become engorged and dilated, and portal hypertension develops. The nodular regeneration of the hepatic cells produces postsinusoidal obstruction, which causes the portal system to become congested and contributes to portal hypertension.

The overall effects of the structural and vascular changes are seen in the resulting dysfunction of the liver and the changes in the portal circulation. The liver is a very complex organ and plays a major role in metabolism, detoxification, blood-forming functions, storage of iron, copper, and various vitamins, and formation of bile. As the liver functions are altered, various clinical manifestations develop, including bleeding disorders (decreased clotting factors), muscle wasting (decreased protein metabolism), hepatic coma (detoxification of ammonia), jaundice (inability to conjugate bilirubin), and peripheral edema (low serum albumin and an increase in hydrostatic pressure). The changes in the portal circulation result in portal hypertension, one of whose clinical manifestations is esophageal varices. Ascites and mesenteric congestion are other clinical manifestations.

Ascites in chronic liver disease has been associated with portal hypertension, low serum albumin, and abnormalities in the lymphatic system. The transudation of fluid between capillaries and tissue spaces is determined by the equilibrium of hydrostatic and osmotic forces in the two compartments. In the normal situation the hydrostatic pressure is higher at the arterial end of the capillary and promotes the passage of protein-free fluid into the pericapillary space. The hydrostatic pressure is lower than the osmotic pressure and the extravascular tissue pressure at the venous end of the capillary, and reabsorption of the fluid occurs.[69] The patient with advanced cirrhosis and portal hypertension has an increased intravascular hydrostatic pressure (portal hypertension) and decreased vascular osmotic pressure (low serum albumin). The combination of the changes in hydrostatic pressure and osmotic pressure leads to the loss of fluid into the peritoneal cavity, an extravascular space.[69] Abnormalities in the lymphatic system contribute to ascites formation. In cirrhosis with portal hypertension, the thoracic duct is enlarged and lymph flow is significantly increased. The high lymph flow may decompress the hepatic or splanchnic vessels. Lymph from the liver is generally high in protein. When the lymph flow is greater than the thoracic duct can manage, a hepatic venous outflow obstruction develops, with resultant ascites. The ascitic fluid in a venous outflow obstruction is high in protein. When the obstruction is an extrahepatic venous obstruction, the protein concentration is low in the fluid.[78]

The communication between the thoracic duct and the subclavian vein helps to determine the occurrence and severity of ascites. Thoracic duct drainage can decrease ascitic volume and portal pressure. Fluid exudes from the surface of the liver into the peritoneal cavity when the lymph system is unable to manage it.

The formation of ascites is not a simple reaction to increased hepatic venous outflow obstruction. Interrelated factors include aldosterone, antidiuretic hormone (ADH), and prostaglandins. The development of ascites results in a decreased blood volume, which stimulates aldosterone secretion. Reexpansion of blood volume stimulates ascites formation, reducing blood volume, restimulating aldosterone, and creating a cycle. This traditional hypothesis of the relationship between ascites and aldosterone has been challenged. It has been proposed that sodium retention occurs first followed by fluid retention and then ascites.

ADH has been found to be elevated in the serum and urine of patients with ascites from cirrhosis. The increase in ADH may be the result of a decrease in effective plasma volume. Effective plasma volume has been defined as the portion of the total plasma volume that effectively stimulates volume receptors.[69] ADH in patients with ascites may contribute to the retention of water, resulting in hyponatremia.

Prostaglandins have also been suggested in the complexity of the ascites formation in cirrhosis because of sodium retention. Prostaglandins may play a role in determining renal plasma flow and sodium retention in decompensated cirrhosis. Indomethacin, a potent inhibitor of prostaglandins, decreases renal flow and creatinine clearance in cirrhotic patients with sodium retention. Indomethacin also decreases plasma renin activity and aldosterone levels.[69]

There are three types of jaundice: obstructive jaundice, hemolytic jaundice, and hepatocellular jaundice. Obstructive jaundice develops in association with obstruction of the biliary ductal system. There is marked elevation of alkaline phosphatase, mild elevation of serum glutamic-oxaloacetic transaminase (SGOT) and lactate dehydrogenase (LDH), and significant bile in the urine. Hemolytic jaundice is associated with an increased load of bilirubin from hemolysis that a diseased liver is unable to manage. Large amounts of urobilinogen may be found in the urine. Anemia is generally associated with hemolytic jaundice. Hepatocellular jaundice develops because of a failure of the liver cells to metabolize bilirubin. In acute hepatocellular failure, the LDH and SGOT are markedly increased and urine contains both bile and urobilinogen. In chronic cirrhosis or hepatocellular failure, there may be no elevation of enzymes and the jaundice may not correlate with the severity of the liver disease. Its presence usually indicates acute disease, and in the patient with chronic cirrhosis the presence of jaundice indicates a poor prognosis. Severe hepatic parenchymal necrosis may develop in the absence of jaundice.[69] Hemolysis is common in cirrhosis and may contribute to jaundice. Biliary obstruction may also occur in cirrhosis.

Hepatic encephalopathy encompasses several stages of mental deterioration culminating in coma. The pathophysiology and treatment are presented on pp. 845 to 846. Bleeding esophageal varices are a major complication associated with portal hypertension and are discussed on p. 769.

The healthy liver plays a role in the metabolism of estrogens. In cirrhosis, hyperestrogenism develops, which includes an increase in sex hormone–binding globulin and other hormone-binding proteins and an increase in the secretion of prolactin.[69] Clinically, the patient shows signs of feminization, including gynecomastia, spider angiomas, palmar erythema, and testicular atrophy. The distribution of body hair changes, with less chest hair and axillary hair being noted. In women testosterone may accumulate, with some masculinization.

Hematologic disorders associated with cirrhosis include impaired coagulation and anemia. The liver is responsible for the synthesis of proteins needed for coagulation: fibrinogen, prothrombin, and various other clotting factors. The liver uses vitamin K to produce prothrombin. Vitamin K absorption is dependent on bile. Treatment of cirrhosis by wiping out intestinal bacteria will decrease the production of vitamin K.

Anemia in cirrhosis may be microcytic, hypochromic anemia secondary to gastrointestinal blood loss and iron deficiency; macrocytic anemia from folic acid deficiency, leukopenia, or thrombocytopenia; or hemolytic anemia. Hemolysis may be indicated by reticulocytosis, hyperbilirubinemia, or increased levels of serum LDH. Splenomegaly may be associated with leukopenia, thrombocytopenia, and hemolytic anemia.

A major complication of cirrhosis is hepatorenal syndrome. Hepatorenal syndrome occurs when a patient with decompensated cirrhosis develops an acquired, functional renal failure. The usual causes of renal insufficiency are present in hepatorenal syndrome, but the kidneys are normal. The patient has oliguria, azotemia, and a urine of high osmolality and low sodium content. Oliguria and azotemia will persist in hepatorenal syndrome even if blood volume and cardiac output are normal. Hepatorenal syndrome carries a very high mortality and does not respond well to medical management.

Hypotension in liver failure is common and may lead to oliguria, azotemia, hyponatremia, and changes in potassium levels. Clinically, the patient may have a high cardiac output and a low total peripheral resistance. Changes in the liver circulatory system may be responsible for this development, and treatment focuses on improving liver function. In addition, oliguria may be associated with a depletion of circulatory blood volume (decreased cardiac output) and decreased renal perfusion. Treatment requires volume expanders.

The patient with cirrhosis has a complex, interrelated group of clinical manifestations. The symptoms observed in cirrhosis can be correlated with a particular dysfunction in the liver or its vascular system. The nurse must be able to identify potential life-threatening complications of advanced liver failure.

Diagnostic Studies and Findings

Laboratory Studies

Serum bilirubin
- Elevated in jaundice

SGOT, SGPT, LDH
- Elevated (SGOT may be higher if alcoholic cirrhosis)

Serum albumin
- Decreased (tissue edema)

Prothrombin time
- Prolonged

Complete blood count
- Anemia, leukopenia, thrombocytopenia

Blood glucose
- Hypoglycemia (from impaired gluconeogenesis)

Serum ammonia
- Elevated (sign of impending hepatic coma)

Urinalysis
- Sodium and potassium levels; urine dark, bile colored; presence of urobilinogen

Bromsulfophthalein (BSP) Excretion Test

Elevated levels found in cirrhosis (test rarely done; has been replaced by liver enzyme studies and liver scan)

Endoscopic Retrograde Cholangiopancreatography (ERCP)

May show common bile duct obstruction

Esophagoscopy

Presence of esophageal varices

Percutaneous Liver Biopsy

Histologic changes found in cirrhosis of liver: fatty infiltration; degeneration and regeneration of hepatocytes (increase in connective tissue)

Ultrasonography

Differentiates biliary obstruction from nonobstructive, parenchymal jaundice

Liver Scans

Decreased uptake in liver (caused by intrahepatic shunts that bypass liver cells)

Cold spots of cirrhosis can be differentiated from hepatocellular carcinoma by gallium scans

Barium Contrast Esophagography

Documents esophageal varices

Angiography

Detects sites of upper gastrointestinal bleeding

Percutaneous Transhepatic Portography (Angiographic Study)

Visualization of portal venous system

Paracentesis

Clear, straw-colored fluid; decreased total protein

Medical Plan

Surgery

Refer to discussions of esophageal varices and hepatic coma

Ascites: peritoneovenous shunt (LeVeen valve, ascites drainage system implanted in abdominal wall and connected to peritoneal cavity and to venous system)

Medications

Diuretics (used to promote fluid loss; recommended weight loss slightly less than 2 pounds/d[69])
- Spironolactone (Aldactone, potassium-sparing diuretic), 100 mg/d (higher dosage may be used initially or given in combination with other diuretics)
- Hydrochlorothiazide (Esidrix) or furosemide (Lasix); dosage varies; given with spironolactone

Digestants
- Pancreatin (Panteric), 1 or 2 tablets po with meals; each tablet contains 2400 mg; use in presence of steatorrhea; promotes fat digestion

Vitamins
- Menadiol sodium diphosphate (Synkayvite; vitamin K), 5-15 mg IM, subcutaneously, or IV; repeat dosage in 12 h if no improvement or give 10 mg for 3 d
- Vitamin C (decreased vitamin C associated with gastrointestinal bleeding)
- Folic acid, 1 mg/d po (for anemia)

Cathartics and laxatives
- Stool softeners (to reduce straining and thereby reduce chance of bleeding from hemorrhoids); dioctyl (Colace), 50-200 mg/d

Antibiotics (as required for infections)

General Management

Paracentesis: indicated for diagnostic purposes, relief of abdominal pain, relief of dyspnea or orthopnea, reduction of intra-abdominal pressure; complications: perforation of abdominal viscera, hemorrhage, infection, shock, hyponatremia syndromes

Ascites reinfusion (as an albumin substitute for expanding plasma volume)

Oxygen and incentive spirometer if respiratory complications develop

Intravenous fluids

Fresh whole blood during acute bleeding episodes

Albumin replacement
Vitamin supplements including thiamine, iron, and vitamins K and C
Sodium restrictions
Salt substitutes
Fresh frozen plasma or platelets
Diet: high in protein (70 to 90 g), high in carbohydrates, approximately 3000 calories
Diet: with impending liver failure, restrict protein and fluids

NURSING CARE

Nursing Assessment

History

Dietary pattern; signs of malnutrition
Drug use, toxic substance ingestion, alcohol use
History of hepatitis or previous liver disease

Physical Signs of Liver Disease

Recent change in weight (loss or gain)
Fatigability
Jaundice
Ascites
Edema of lower extremities
Spider angiomas; spider telangiectasis
Palmar erythema
Nail changes (transverse pale bands)
Anorexia, nausea, vomiting
Fever (more common in alcoholic cirrhosis)
Signs of tissue wasting or loss of muscle mass (often seen in legs)

Estrogen-Androgen Imbalance

Loss of chest hair
Gynecomastia

Portal Hypertension

Splenomegaly
Edema of lower extremities
Distention of collateral circulation (esophageal varices, hemorrhoids)
Caput medusae (dilated veins around umbilicus; also develops around ileostomy, colostomy, and ileal conduit stomas when patient develops portal hypertension)

Urinary Output

Changes in volume of output; oliguria
Alteration in sodium and potassium levels; osmolality of urine
Color of urine: dark yellow, amber, mahogany

Psychosocial Concerns

Ability to give up alcohol ingestion (if alcoholic cirrhosis)

Gastrointestinal Symptoms

Esophageal varices
Change in bowel habits
Gastrointestinal bleeding

Mental Status

Changes in thinking and mental function secondary to increased serum ammonia levels; may progress to hepatic coma (serum ammonia levels do not always correlate with mental functions; that is, some patients with very high levels have minimum mental function alteration whereas others with low levels may progress to coma)

Nursing Dx & Intervention

Nursing Diagnosis	Nursing Intervention/Rationale
Potential for injury (hemorrhage)	• Assess patient for signs of bleeding: hematemesis, melena, signs of shock. • Monitor vital signs and laboratory studies. • Provide intravenous fluids as ordered. • Prepare patient for endoscopy for treatment and/or diagnosis of bleeding. • Maintain patency of nasogastric tube. • If ordered, perform cool saline or water lavage. • Assess intake and output, color, and characteristics of aspirate. • Provide medications as ordered: vitamin K, vasopressin, neomycin. • Monitor use of Sengstaken-Blakemore tube.
Potential for injury (altered clotting factors)	• Help patient minimize trauma (e.g., forceful nose blowing, harsh toothbrush, safety razors). • Assess for signs of bleeding. • Provide stool softener and remind patient not to strain during bowel movements. • Use small-gauge needles for injections and apply pressure following injections. • Record any indications of small bleeding sites. • Monitor platelet count and prothrombin time.

Nursing Diagnosis	Nursing Intervention/Rationale
Altered renal, cerebral, cardiopulmonary, gastrointestinal, and peripheral tissue perfusion	• Assess patient for alterations in cardiac output and decreased renal perfusion. • Monitor and record urinary output, urine osmolality, and sodium and potassium levels. • Weigh daily.
Fluid volume deficit (1)	• Assess for clinical signs of electrolyte imbalance, particularly sodium, potassium, and magnesium. • Maintain accurate intake and output records, reporting abnormalities. • Record daily weights. • Measure abdominal girth daily *to monitor ascites.* • Monitor serum and urine electrolytes. • Provide diuretics as ordered. • Restrict fluid intake if ordered. • Perform frequent mouth care.
Altered nutrition: less than body requirements	• Assess nutritional status. • Provide small frequent feedings high in calories, carbohydrates, and protein, low in fats, and low in sodium. • Provide salt substitutes if ordered.
Potential impaired skin integrity	• Assess patient for risk of developing pressure sores. • Assess patient for risk factors: edema, decreased movement or turning. • Provide pressure relief device appropriate for patient based on size of patient, bony prominences, and areas of continued stress. • Change linens regularly if patient is perspiring or tissues are weepy from edema (moisture contributes to skin breakdown). • Manage symptoms of pruritus with calamine lotion and baths. • Use preventive protocol for perianal area when patient is to be treated with neomycin or other agents, such as lactulose, that promote diarrhea. Use vanishing cream and skin sealant (Bard Protective Barrier Film) *before* skin breaks down. Repeat applications with each cleansing of perianal area. The skin may be cleansed with mineral oil and cotton balls *to reduce harshness of washcloths and toilet paper.* Cleansers are available that soften stool, reduce odors, and are gentle to the skin (Bard Cleanser, Uniwash).
Ineffective breathing pattern	• Assess lung fields for signs of congestion or infection. • Place patient in semi-Fowler's or high Fowler's position *to increase lung expansion compromised by ascites.* • Assess perianal area for signs of pressure sores associated with shearing forces. • Turn frequently from side to side. • Use pressure relief devices. • Monitor blood gases. • Monitor vital signs.
Altered thought processes	• Observe for early signs of mental changes: lethargy, confusion, drowsiness, and irritability. • Avoid use of sedatives or tranquilizers. • Refer to section on hepatic coma.

Patient Education

1. Stress the importance of avoiding alcohol and provide information on alcoholic cirrhosis.
2. Help the patient identify community resources available for alcohol rehabilitation.
3. Provide the patient with information on altered drug effects with cirrhosis and caution to use only physician-prescribed or -approved medications.
4. Provide written dietary instructions. Stress the role of nutrition in recovery. Include any restrictions required, specifically sodium.
5. Instructions should include the need for rest and diversional activities to prevent boredom.
6. Provide written instructions of signs and symptoms that warrant seeing a physician: increased abdominal girth, rapid weight gain or loss, edema, fever, blood in urine or stool, bleeding that does not cease with pressure in a short time (nosebleeds, cuts, gums), gross upper gastrointestinal bleeding, or tarry stools.
7. Instruct the family in all of the above plus signs of mental changes: confusion, untidiness, night wandering, personality changes, irritability, and sleeplessness.

Evaluation

Patient Outcome	Data Indicating That Outcome is Reached
Blood clotting factors are normal.	Hemorrhage is controlled and recurrence prevented. Platelet count is normal. Prothrombin time is normal.
Tissue perfusion is adequate.	Satisfactory urinary output is maintained.
Fluid volume is maintained.	Serum electrolytes (sodium, potassium, and magnesium) are normal. Fluid weight loss is slightly less than 2 pounds per day. Abdominal girth decreases. Peripheral edema is reduced.
Nutrition is adequate.	Patient does not experience anorexia, nausea and vomiting, indigestion, or muscle wasting. Calorie and protein intake is sufficient for healing. Patient does not drink alcohol.
Breathing pattern is normal.	Patient does not experience atelectasis or pneumonia. Ascites decreases or disappears; therefore lung expansion improves.
Skin integrity is maintained.	There are no signs of irritation, pressure, or broken areas.
Thought processes are normal.	Thought processes are not altered. Serum ammonia levels are controlled.

Hepatic coma

In acute and chronic liver diseases, a series of neuropsychiatric manifestations may develop that range from hepatic encephalopathy to precoma to hepatic coma. Hepatic coma is the end stage of the neuropsychiatric manifestations.

The pathophysiology of hepatic coma has become better understood and has been related to the presence of two factors: the shunting of blood around the liver so that substances toxic to the brain are no longer completely metabolized or cleared by the liver, and hepatic insufficiency. The syndrome is currently referred to as portal-systemic encephalopathy (PSE). PSE is characterized by recurrent changes in consciousness, impaired intellectual function, neuromuscular abnormalities, metabolic slowing of electroencephalogram, and elevated serum ammonia levels.[69]

The majority of patients who develop hepatic coma or PSE have cirrhosis. However, PSE may develop in fulminant liver failure, deficiency of urea cycle enzyme, and Reye's syndrome. PSE occurs in patients with cirrhosis who have portal hypertension or portal-systemic shunting. Hepatic coma also develops in half of those patients who have portacaval shunts.

Several clinical situations have been associated with the initiation of PSE and include azotemia; medications such as sedatives, tranquilizers, and analgesics; gastrointestinal bleeding; high dietary protein; and hypokalemic alkalosis. An iatrogenic cause occurs in approximately half of the cases of hepatic coma.

Pathophysiology

The vast majority of episodes of PSE are caused by ammonia intoxication. Ammonia is a by-product of nitrogen metabolism. Nitrogen is a by-product of amino acid digestion. The bacteria in the colon break down nitrogen to ammonia. The ammonia is absorbed and carried through the portal veins to the liver, where it is converted to glutamine, a nontoxic form. Glutamine is later synthesized by the liver into urea, which is excreted.

The colon, when in a fasting state, is a continuous source of ammonia. The colon bacteria responsible for ammonia formation may also be found in the small bowel of patients with cirrhosis.[78] When the portal vein flow bypasses the liver, such as with a portal-systemic anastomosis, the systemic blood ammonia levels increase to toxic levels.

The following equation refers to the ammonia and ammonia hydroxide balance:

$$NH_4OH \leftrightharpoons NH_4^+ + OH^-$$

Only ammonia hydroxide can cross the cell membrane and thus create toxic effects. The pH of the extracellular and intracellular compartments affects this equation. Abnormalities of acid-base balance, primarily alkalosis associated with hypokalemia, result in an increase in ammonia hydroxide and passage of the substance into the cells. Hypokalemia in alcoholic cirrhosis may be related to vomiting, diarrhea, diuretics, and secondary aldosteronism.

Ammonia is also released during muscle activities from the muscles of the extremities. Under normal resting conditions, a small quantity of ammonia uptake occurs. This uptake may increase when arterial levels of ammonia are increased.[69]

PSE may be initiated by conditions that increase nitrogen levels. Endogenous factors include azotemia, blood in the gastrointestinal tract, and constipation. Azotemia affects the kidney's ability to excrete nitrogen. Blood is a source of more ammonia than dietary protein, and the ammonia is liberated from the blood in the colon. Constipation may exaggerate other factors. In constipation the waste products remain in the colon for longer periods, providing more opportunity for colonic bacteria to convert nitrogenous products to ammonia.

Exogenous factors that contribute to the nitrogenous cause of PSE include dietary protein, ammonia salts, urea, cation exchange resins, amino acids, and diuretics. In addition, potassium depletion is associated with nitrogenous PSE.

Several noncirrhotic clinical conditions in which ammonia levels are associated with PSE include hereditary deficiencies of urea cycle enzymes and Reye's syndrome.

The blood ammonia levels do not correlate well with the clinical manifestations of PSE. Schiff and Schiff[69] have identified several reasons. Venous blood levels do not reflect what is delivered to the tissues. Arterial ammonia blood levels are recommended, and since individuals respond differently to various levels of ammonia, serial studies of ammonia levels would provide a better indication of the relationship of increasing symptoms to blood levels. Blood ammonia levels are also affected by potassium levels and food ingestion. Hypokalemia results in more tissue uptake of ammonia with a resultant low serum ammonia level. Serum levels of ammonia increase after meals and vary according to the amount of protein consumed. Fasting and serial arterial ammonia levels are more likely to correlate with the clinical symptoms of PSE.

Nonnitrogenous factors have also been associated with PSE and include sedatives, tranquilizers, analgesics, hypoxemia, hypoglycemia, fulminant viral hepatitis, and hypokalemia. Although these are not as common as other factors in the cause of PSE, it is important to identify the cause of PSE in order to appropriately treat the patient.

Diagnostic Studies and Findings

Arterial Ammonia Blood Levels (Fasting)

Elevated

Serum Electrolytes

Hypokalemia
Alkalosis

Blood Glucose

Hyperglycemia: iatrogenic hyperglycemia may cause coma; in cirrhosis there is little glycogen stored, so patients are usually hypoglycemic

Electroencephalogram (EEG)

- Paroxysms of bilateral, synchronous, symmetric slow waves at a rate of 1½ to 3/sec
- Four grades of EEG
  - Grade 0: normal
  - Grade 1: mild impairment
  - Grade 2: moderate impairment
  - Grade 3: severe impairment
  - Grade 4: coma
- Rule out other causes of coma such as subdural hematomas and nonnitrogenous causes of PSE

Medical Plan

Surgery

Colectomy (rare)
Ileosigmoidostomy (rare)

Medications

- Anti-infective agents (nonabsorbable)
  - To decrease bacterial action in colon
  - Neomycin (Mycifradin) or paromomycin (Humatin), 2 to 6 g/d
- Broad-spectrum antibiotics
  - Ampicillin (Cephulac)
- Ammonia detoxicants
  - Lactulose (synthetic disaccharide), 300 ml syrup diluted with 700 ml water by enema (retain 20 to 30 min), or 30 to 45 ml tid or qid po (acidifies contents of colon)

General Management

- Removal of blood from gastrointestinal tract: cathartics
- Gastric lavage with cool saline or water
- Cleansing enemas with dilute acetic acid or neomycin
- Discontinuation of any precipitating substance: dietary proteins, sedatives, diuretic therapy, analgesics
- Intravenous glucose (minimizes protein breakdown)
- Oxygen (respiratory or metabolic alkalosis)
- Correction of any electrolyte imbalances

NURSING CARE

Nursing Assessment

Fetor Hepaticus

Sweetish odor detected on breath and in urine

State of Consciousness

Hypersomnia, insomnia, or inversion of sleep pattern
Slow responses
Lethargy
Minimum disorientation
Somnolence
Confusion
Semistupor
Stupor
Unconsciousness (coma)

Neuromuscular Abnormalities

Metabolic tremor
Muscular incoordination
Impaired handwriting
Asterixis (liver flap)
Slurred speech
Hypoactive reflexes
Ataxia

Hyperactive reflexes
Nystagmus
Babinski's sign (clonus)
Rigidity
Dilated pupils
Opisthotonus (coma)

Intellectual Function

Subtly impaired computations (use number connection test [NCT] for assessment—it permits serial assessment of minimum changes)
Shortened attention span
Loss of time
Grossly impaired computations
Amnesia for past events
Loss of orientation to place
Inability to compute
Loss of orientation to self
No intellect (coma)

Personality Behavioral Changes

Exaggeration of normal behavior
Euphoria or depression
Garrulousness
Irritability
Decreased inhibitions
Overt changes in personality
Anxiety or apathy
Inappropriate behavior
Bizarre behavior
Paranoia or anger
Rage
None (coma)

Nursing Dx & Intervention

Nursing Diagnosis	Nursing Intervention/Rationale
Altered thought processes	• Assess for early signs of changes in consciousness, intellect, personality, behaviors, and neuromuscular activities. • Record indications of changes. • Have patient do simple arithmetic computations or use NCT. • Have patient do serial handwriting to compare differences. • Monitor arterial ammonia and potassium levels. • Assess for clinical signs of hypokalemia and alkalosis. • Provide sedatives, tranquilizers, and analgesics as ordered, note any delayed or prolonged reactions, and report immediately; avoid use of above if possible. • Protect the patient from injury as personality behaviors become more overt and inappropriate and as neuromuscular activities alter. • Identify personality and behavior changes and relate them to the progression of the disease and help family and staff understand and learn about the disease progression. • Document treatment ordered by physician as implemented (e.g., retention or cleansing enemas, gastric lavage, medications).
Potential impaired skin integrity	• Assess perianal skin. • Begin protective perianal skin care before beginning lactulose or neomycin orally or rectally. Diarrheal stools will be more acidic. Cleanse the skin with periwash (Sween), Uniwash (United), or another gentle, nondetergent solution. Cotton balls can be used rather than rough cloth or gauze. • Pat the skin dry or use a hair dryer on cool or warm; avoid hot settings. • Apply a vanishing cream. • Cover the area with a skin sealant (Bard Protective Barrier Film); spray forms are easiest to use. Allow to dry. Use ointment on top of protective film. Repeat with each bowel movement.
Impaired skin integrity	• Keep in mind that skin impairment is harder to treat than to prevent. • Cleanse perianal skin with Domeboro (aluminum acetate) solution and cotton balls; dry with hair dryer. • Apply vanishing cream and cover with thick ointment-based product. If skin is severely eroded, Karaya and glycerin can be combined to form a paste (commercial paste contains alcohol and will be painful), which should be thick, almost like cookie dough. The paste should be applied rather than the creams and ointments and should be a thin coat. A pectin-based wafer may be used. Be careful that stool does not become trapped underneath the wafer. Pouching the rectum or a rectal tube may help. • Repeat the procedure with each bowel movement.

Patient Education

1. Provide the family with written signs of changes in mental functions that are related to early PSE: confusion, untidiness, night wandering, and personality changes. They should notify the physician if symptoms occur.
2. Provide written dietary instructions for reduced protein intake.

Patient Outcome	Data Indicating That Outcome is Reached
Thought processes are not impaired.	Thought processes, personality, behavior, consciousness, and neuromuscular activities are not altered. Arterial ammonia levels are normal.
Skin integrity is maintained.	There are no signs of irritation or erosion.

GALLBLADDER DISORDERS

Cholecystitis with cholelithiasis (Gallstones)

Cholecystitis refers to the acute or chronic inflammation of the gallbladder.

Acute cholecystitis is associated with gallstones (cholelithiasis) in 90% of cases. Less than 10% of cases of acute cholecystitis are acalculous or unrelated to stone formation. Chronic cholecystitis refers to repeated attacks of acute cholecystitis and an abnormal-looking gallbladder. Pain often follows a meal in chronic cholecystitis.

Acute cholecystitis is common and accounts for one fourth of all gallbladder surgeries. Although it may occur in all ages, it is more common in middle age. The number of surgeries for acute cholecystitis may increase in the future. The current trend is toward early surgical intervention for cholecystitis.

Recent research has found that crystals of cholesterol, a major component of gallstones, form in 6 hours. The process can be visualized by video-enhanced, time-lapse photography. Physicians may be able to use this knowledge in the future to "test" bile samples of people at high risk for gallstones and initiate preventive measures.[54]

Pathophysiology

Acute cholecystitis consists of acute inflammation of the wall of the gallbladder. In calculous cholecystitis an obstruction of the cystic duct by a stone or from edema secondary to the passage of a stone is the underlying problem. The cystic duct is obstructed. The gallbladder distends, and the wall becomes edematous, compressing the capillaries and lymphatics and resulting in ischemia and inflammation. The inflamed mucosa allows bile salt to be reabsorbed, further damaging the mucosa. If the inflammation continues, the wall will become friable and necrosis may develop. Perforation of the gallbladder may occur. The perforation may be small and localized, forming an abscess. In severe acute cholecystitis, inflammation spreads to the serosal layer of the gallbladder and may progress to form inflammatory adhesions to adjacent structures. Bacteria may be found in the bile and is associated with secondary infections.

The gallbladder heals after the acute attack with scarring and decreased absorptive capacity. The mucosa of the gallbladder in a patient with chronic cholecystitis is also ulcerated and scarred. Chronic cholecystitis may develop from repeated intermittent episodes of cystic duct obstruction resulting in chronic inflammation. The gallbladder is contracted, white in color, and thick walled. The bile is turbid and filled with debris.

Acute cholecystitis in the absence of stones has been associated with sudden starvation and immobility. These are changes that affect the regular filling and emptying of the gallbladder. A patient hospitalized for cardiovascular disease, burns, traumas, or biliary surgery may develop acalculous acute cholecystitis. The patient on TPN may also develop cholecystitis secondary to gallbladder distention and biliary stasis.

The primary symptom associated with acute cholecystitis is pain. The pain of acute cholecystitis has been described as colicky. However, this is not a true colic pain that waxes and wanes. The pain of acute cholecystitis is abrupt in onset, reaches a peak intensity quickly, and remains at that level for 2 to 4 hours. Initially the pain may be poorly localized, but as it becomes more severe it localizes in the right upper quadrant epigastric region. The pain radiates around the midtorso to the right scapular area. Guarding and rigidity represent peritoneal involvement. Tenderness may be elicited at the tip of the ninth costal margin during inspiration (i.e., Murphy's sign). Jaundice may be found in acute cholecystitis. The jaundice may be related to edema of the ducts or to direct involvement of the liver by inflammation, since stones are not always found in patients with jaundice.

In acute cholecystitis it is important to rule out concomitant acute pancreatitis, peptic ulcer disease, pneumonitis, hepatitis, and acute appendicitis. In chronic cholecystitis one must rule out peptic ulcer disease, chronic pancreatitis, and hiatal hernia.

Diagnostic Studies and Findings

Acute Cholecystitis

Plain Films of Abdomen

Gallstones visualized

Ultrasound

Gallstones
Thickening of wall

Biliary Scintigraphy

Scans 15 to 30 minutes after IV injection of radionuclide show the ducts but not the obstructed gallbladder; recommend repeat scan 4 hours after injection to rule out late filling of gallbladder

Serum Amylase

Elevated may indicate concomitant acute pancreatitis; usually indicates common duct stone

White Blood Count

Leukocyte count of 12,000 to 15,000/mm^3

Chronic Cholecystitis

Double-Dose Oral Cholecystogram

Nonfunctioning gallbladder

Ultrasound

Presence of gallstones

Upper Gastrointestinal Series

Excludes peptic ulcer disease and hiatus hernia

Medical Plan

Acute Cholecystitis with Cholelithiasis

Surgery

Cholecystectomy with exploration of common bile duct
Cholecystotomy (in critically ill patient only a drain is inserted into the gallbladder to drain the abscess, to be removed later when the patient is stable)

Medications

Narcotic analgesics
For acute pain, meperidine hydrochloride (Demerol), 100 mg, and atropine, 0.6 mg, IM
Anti-infective agents
Agent-specific antibiotics for existing or impending secondary infections as indicated by a worsening of clinical condition or acute attack for 4-5 d without clinical improvement

General Management

Intravenous fluids to correct dehydration
Nasogastric tube; give nothing by mouth

Chronic Cholecystitis

Surgery

Cholecystectomy with exploration of common bile duct

NURSING CARE

Nursing Assessment

Acute Cholecystitis with Cholelithiasis

Jaundice

Mild jaundice of skin noted
Pruritus not commonly a problem

Pain

Severe right upper quadrant pain with referral to right scapula
Rebound tenderness; rigidity
Positive Murphy's sign
Gallbladder may be palpable

Gastrointestinal Symptoms

Anorexia
Vomiting

Temperature

Fever of 37° to 39° C (99° to 102° F)

Chronic Cholecystitis

Gastrointestinal Symptoms

Fat intolerance
Flatulence
Nausea
Anorexia

Pain

Nonspecific abdominal pain and tenderness in right hypochondrium

Nursing Dx & Intervention

Nursing Diagnosis	Nursing Intervention/Rationale
Pain	• Assess and document characteristics, location, and severity of pain. • Provide pain medication as ordered and record patient's response. • Allow patient to assume position that is least painful. • Provide patient with an opportunity to express feelings and fears.
Potential fluid volume deficit	• Assess patient for signs of dehydration: dry mouth and mucous membranes, dry skin. • Maintain careful intake and output records, including emesis and nasogastric aspiration. • Monitor serum electrolytes. • Provide intravenous fluids as ordered. • Maintain frequent oral hygiene.
Altered nutrition: less than body requirements	• Provide diet that is low fat, high carbohydrate, and high protein when acute phase is ended.
Potential impaired skin integrity	• Assess patient carefully for risk factors for developing pressure sores. • Provide mechanical relief of pressure points: turn patient following pain medication and assess for changes in skin. NOTE: Elderly patients are at high risk during episodes of acute pain when movement intensifies the pain. • Protect the skin from drainage around the T-tube insertion site using pectin-based wafers. If the insertion site leaks for prolonged periods following removal of the T tube, consider a sterile pouching system.

Patient Education

1. During the acute phase, the patient will need explanation of all procedures and may require pain medication before moving. The patient should be made aware that the nurse recognizes the severity of the pain during acute cholecystitis.
2. Following or during the resolution of the acute phase, the patient will need information about cholecystectomy in order to make an informed decision regarding surgery.
3. Patients electing medical management will need information on chronic cholecystitis; signs and symptoms of recurrence; signs of potential complications (recurrent attacks, jaundice, obstruction of common bile duct, cholangitis, pancreatitis, internal biliary fistula, carcinoma); and low-fat diets.

Evaluation

Patient Outcome	Data Indicating That Outcome is Reached
Body functions normally.	Patient does not experience jaundice, anorexia, vomiting, pain, or fever. Fluid and electrolyte balance is normal.
There is no infection.	There are no signs or symptoms of secondary infection; white blood count is normal, and there is no fever.

PANCREATIC DISORDERS

Pancreatitis

Pancreatitis is an inflammation of the pancreas that may be acute or chronic.

Acute pancreatitis involves a diffuse inflammation caused by premature activation of pancreatic enzymes into active, potent proteolytic enzymes. The acute pancreatitis is a process of autodigestion. The two types of acute pancreatitis are interstitial, or edematous, pancreatitis and hemorrhagic, or necrotizing, pancreatitis. It may be that the two forms are actually a continuum of the same process. Interstitial pancreatitis is milder and characterized by interstitial edema with exudation. As the disease progresses, frank necrosis develops with disruption and thrombotic occlusion of blood vessels. Bleeding, ischemic necrosis, and fat necrosis are found throughout the pancreas.

Complications of acute pancreatitis include hemorrhage, pseudocysts, pancreatic ascites, and abscesses. A pseudocyst occurs when an accumulation of tissue debris, blood, fat droplets, and pancreatic juice develops within confluent areas of necrosis. A pseudocyst may arise within or adjacent to the pancreas. Pancreatic ascites develops when the accumulation of active pancreatic enzymes and leukocytes imitates the peritoneal surfaces and fluid accumulates in the peritoneal cavity. The same process of irritation through the diaphragmatic lymphatics leads to pleural effusion. Abscesses result from secondary infection of necrotic tissue and fluid collection.

Chronic pancreatitis is progressive functional damage to the pancreas. Removal of the cause does not improve the pancreatic function. The primary clinical features are pain, malabsorption, diabetes mellitus, and intraductal calcifications. The primary causative factor is chronic excessive alcohol ingestion. Complications consist of loss of exocrine and endocrine function, pancreatic necrosis, hemorrhage, abscess, and pseudocysts.

Chronic excessive alcohol ingestion and gallbladder disease are associated with acute pancreatitis. The age and sex of the patient will vary according to the primary disease associated with the acute pancreatitis. Gallbladder disease is more common in middle-aged women. Alcohol as an associated agent is seen more often in men. Alcohol ingestion plays a major role in the development of chronic pancreatitis. The disease occurs more often in men than women, and the average age is 49. These patients tend to be overweight and have other signs of alcoholic disease such as hepatitis, cirrhosis, or fatty liver. The patient who has signs of malabsorption and diabetes mellitus usually is malnourished and has weight loss.

Pathophysiology

Acute Pancreatitis

Acute pancreatitis is a process of autodigestion, but the agent that triggers prematurely the activation of the enzymes is unknown. Several theories have been proposed, including obstruction of the pancreatic ducts, reflux of bile, reflux of duodenal contents, and the toxic effect of alcohol. Unfortunately, none of the proposed theories has proven to be the cause.

The process of enzyme activation regardless of the etiology is the basis of the disease process. Trypsinogen may undergo spontaneous activation to trypsin in the presence of an alkaline pH. Trypsin is inactivated by a specific trypsin inhibitor found in the pancreatic secretions and in the pancreatic tissue. However, the small amount of trypsin may activate other proteolytic enzymes. Phospholipase A and elastase have been proposed as the primary enzymes responsible for autodigestion. Phospholipase A, in the presence of bile, results in severe pancreatic parenchymal and adipose tissue necrosis. Elastase dissolves the elastic fibers of blood vessels and is implicated in the hemorrhage associated with necrotizing pancreatitis.

Many substances released from the injured pancreas will have systemic effects. Two low–molecular weight vasoactive peptides (kinins) are released and result in vasodilation and increase in vascular permeability, resulting in circulatory shock. Severe pulmonary edema and pain are also associated with the vasoactive peptides.

Hypocalcemia develops when a decreased binding of calcium to serum protein occurs secondary to a drop in albumin levels. In addition, a decrease in ionized serum calcium occurs in acute pancreatitis. Damage to the islet cells results in mild, transient hyperglycemia from release of glucagon and decreased release of insulin. The glucose levels are too high for the insulin production to control.

Patients with acute pancreatitis are at risk for developing adult respiratory distress syndrome (ARDS). Arterial hypoxia occurs when intrapulmonary right-to-left shunting develops. Pulmonary edema from disruption of the alveolar-capillary membrane is a serious complication. In addition, renal function may be altered during acute pancreatitis. Hypovolemia and shock are not always the causative factors in altered renal function. The blood flow may be reduced and the vascular resistance increased in the kidney in the absence of hypovolemia.

Another major potential complication of acute pancreatitis is disseminated intravascular coagulation (DIC), which involves the development of microthrombi and consumption of clotting factors. Mild DIC may play a role in the development of early hypoxia and renal impairment.

Chronic Pancreatitis

Chronic pancreatitis generally develops from an insidious sclerosing process in the pancreas; however, it may develop from repeated bouts of acute inflammation and necrosis. The histologic changes in the pancreas include irregularly distributed fibrosis, reduced number and size of acini and islet cells, and obstruction of the pancreatic ductal system.

The clinical signs of chronic pancreatitis include pain and functional impairment of the pancreas. The pain may be intermittent or chronic and affects the productivity of the patient and his or her activities of daily living. Nausea and vomiting often accompany the pain. The pain is described as steady, boring, dull, or sharp and radiates from the epigastrium to the back. The pain may be lessened by leaning forward from a sitting position. Eating or lying down may increase the pain.

Malabsorption and weight loss develop during the course of the chronic illness. Patients may limit food intake because of the pain. Secretions of pancreatic enzymes decrease in chronic pancreatitis, and fat and protein are poorly digested. Steatorrhea and azotorrhea are observed. Carbohydrate malabsorption is clinically not seen, since salivary amylase is unimpaired. Pancreatic amylase is highly efficient and in fact would have to be reduced by 97% before carbohydrate malabsorption would develop.[75]

Insulin response to glucose is impaired in chronic pancreatitis. Overt diabetes mellitus will occur in most of these patients. The ability of the pancreas to release glucagon is also affected.

Diagnostic Studies and Findings

Acute Pancreatitis

Differential Diagnosis

Perforated peptic ulcer
Acute cholangitis
Mesenteric infarction

WBC

Greater than 15,000/mm^3

Serum Glucose

Greater than 180 mg/dl with no prior history of hyperglycemia

BUN

Greater than 45 mg/dl after fluid volume replacement

Arterial Po_2

Less than 60 mm Hg

Serum Calcium

Less than 8 mg/dl (in patients with hyperparathyroidism and acute pancreatitis level may be within normal range)

Serum Albumin

Less than 3.2 g/dl

Serum LDH

Greater than 600 U/L

SGOT or SGPT

Greater than 200 U/L

Amylase

Serum: greater than 500 U/dl; highest levels 2 to 12 hours after onset, drop to normal (60 to 180 U/dl) within 48 to 72 hours
Urine: levels remain elevated for 3 to 5 days; amylase–creatinine clearance ratio (ACR) above 5% indicates acute pancreatitis
Lipase: elevated; may remain elevated for 5 to 10 days

Chronic Pancreatitis

Urinalysis

Glycosuria (diabetes mellitus)

Serum Glucose

Elevated

Amylase–Creatinine Clearance Ratio

Normal

Serum Amylase and Lipase

Normal
Increased in presence of pseudocysts and pancreatic ascites

Alkaline Phosphate

Increased five times normal for 4 weeks indicates common bile duct stenosis

Lactoferrin Levels

Increased (specimens obtained by endoscopic retrograde cannulation)

Exogenous Stimulation: Secretin-CCK

Decreased stimulation of pancreatic enzymes

Endogenous Stimulation: Perfusion and Feedings

Diminished function

Lundh Test Meal

Mean trypsin concentration decreased

Para-Aminobenzoic Acid (PABA) Test

Urinary recovery of PABA low in pancreatic insufficiency

Endoscopic Retrograde Cholangiopancreatography (ERCP)

Not indicated in acute pancreatitis or pseudocyst
Identifies ductal changes in chronic pancreatitis and presence of calculi

Both Acute and Chronic Pancreatitis

Plain Films of Abdomen

Peripancreatic, extraluminal gas bubbles indicating pancreatic abscess
Diffuse pancreatitis; calcification of chronic pancreatitis

Ultrasonography

Demonstrates presence of gallstones, pancreatic pseudocyst, pancreatic abscess, calcification of pancreatic ducts

Computed Tomography

Delineates spread of peripancreatic inflammation, pseudocyst, abscess, and localized hematoma formation; presence of calcification

Intravenous Cholangiography

Differentiates acute cholecystitis from acute pancreatitis

Upper Gastrointestinal Series

Used to rule out perforated duodenal ulcer
Demonstrates pancreatic enlargement and inflammation, widening of duodenal C-loop, and enlargement of ampulla of Vater
Stomach can be displaced by pseudocyst

Medical Plan

Acute Pancreatitis

Surgery

Surgical drainage of pancreatic pseudocyst may be indicated if it does not resolve spontaneously
Surgical drainage of pancreatic abscesses may be indicated
Laparotomy for common duct obstruction

Medications

Narcotic analgesics
 Meperidine (Demerol), 75-125 mg IM q4h or prn (hold analgesics until initial laboratory samples are drawn, since many will cause elevations in serum amylase and lipase)
Antacids
 Aluminum-magnesium preparation, 30-40 ml (clamp nasogastric tube for 15 min after dosage)
Histamine H_2 receptor antagonists
 Cimetidine or ranitidine, 300 mg IV qid if any evidence of upper gastrointestinal bleeding
Anti-infective agents
 Cephalothin (Keflin), 2 g q6h IV or with peritoneal lavage
 For abscess, chloramphenicol (chloromycetin), 0.5 g q6h IV, and penicillin G, 5-10 million U/d IV, *or* cefoxitin, 1 g q6h IV (used before cultures are known)
Adrenergic agents
 For hypotension, dopamine (Intropin), 2-5 μg/kg/min, diluted in solution and titrated as needed or isoproterenol (Isuprel) may be used

General Management

Continuous hemodynamic and arterial blood gas monitoring; Swan-Ganz or CVP catheter
Nasogastric suctioning
Peritoneal lavage for persistent hypotension (removes pancreatic exudate, which contains large amounts of vasoactive kinins)
ARDS: endotracheal intubation and controlled ventilation with positive end-expiratory pressure (PEEP)
Restoration and maintenance of intravascular volume including human serum albumin, low–molecular weight dextran 40
Correction of electrolyte imbalances: hypocalcemia, hypomagnesemia, hyperglycemia, hyperkalemia, and metabolic acidosis
Nutritional support with TPN or feeding jejunostomy

Chronic Pancreatitis

Surgery

Not primary treatment but may be used to treat intractable pain complications (e.g., pseudocysts or abscesses)
Drainage procedures
 Longitudinal pancreaticojejunostomy (modified Puestow procedure)
 Caudal pancreaticojejunostomy (Du Val procedure)
Resection
 Subtotal or total pancreatectomy
 Pancreaticoduodenostomy (Whipple procedure)
To preserve islet cell function
 Islet cell autotransplantation by infusion of islet cell preparations into portal system
 Segments of pancreas autotransplanted
 Insertion of closed-loop insulin infusion system

Medications

Analgesics
 Acetaminophen or narcotics prn for pain
Digestants
 Pancreatic enzyme supplements (use one of the following)
  Pancreatin (Viokase), 6 tablets with each meal
  Pancrelipase (Cotazym), 5 capsules with each meal
  Pancrelipase (Pancrease), enteric-coated, 2-3 capsules with each meal
Antacids and adsorbents
 Sodium bicarbonate or aluminum hydroxide antacids may be used with pancreatic enzyme supplements to improve results
Histamine H_2 receptor antagonists
 Cimetidine, 300 mg po 30 min before meals (may be used rather than above to improve effects of pancreatic enzyme supplements)
 Medium-chain triglycerides (MCT; Portagen) supplements
 Insulin therapy: does vary with individual (remember that glucagon deficiency is present and patient may have hypoglycemic reactions easily)

General Management

Enteral nutritional support or TPN as indicated by nutritional status and weight loss

NURSING CARE

Nursing Assessment

Acute Pancreatitis

Abdomen

Steady, dull, boring pain in epigastrium or left upper quadrant: poorly localized; reaches peak intensity within 15 minutes to 1 hour; radiates to lower thoracic vertebral area; worsens in supine position
Palpation: localized epigastric tenderness to deep palpation is intense
Soft abdomen (retroperitoneal location of pancreas means that signs of peritoneal irritation, rigidity, and rebound tenderness will not be present initially)
Mild abdominal distention and mild ascites

Gastrointestinal Symptoms

Nausea and vomiting; hematemesis
Intestinal ileus

General Concerns

Fever of 38° C (100° to 101° F)

Circulatory System

Tachycardia, hypovolemia, and hypotension: may progress to circulatory shock and coma

Grey Turner's Sign

Bluish brown discoloration of flanks

Cullen's Sign

Bluish brown discoloration in periumbilicus area

Jaundice

Seen in some patients; hyperbilirubinemia of 3 mg/dl

Pulmonary Concerns

Pleuritic pain; pleural effusion; pulmonary infiltrates
Impaired ventilation
Adult respiratory distress syndrome (ARDS) may develop

Diaphragm

Irritation results in hiccups and referred shoulder pain

Urine

Decreased output (oliguria); less than 400 ml/24 hours; associated with acute tubular necrosis

Pancreatic Pseudocyst

Fluid collection in pancreas: may be detected on ultrasound or CT scan
Palpable mass
Fever of 38° C (100° to 101° F)

Pancreatic Abscess

Fever above 38° C (101° F)
Increasing pain: palpable mass
Leukocytosis (above 10,000/mm^3)
Tachycardia
Chills
Hypotension

Pancreatic Cutaneous Fistula

Spontaneous drainage of pancreatic abscess through an abnormal tract to skin or following surgical drainage of an abscess

Chronic Pancreatitis

Malabsorption

Weight loss, steatorrhea, voluminous diarrhea, nausea and vomiting (associated with pain and with complications)

Pancreatic Endocrine Function

Signs and symptoms of diabetes mellitus
Reactive hypoglycemia to insulin therapy

Chronic Pain

Intermittent or chronic pain
Boring, dull, or sharp pain that is steady
Epigastric, right or left subcostal region, periumbilical region, or lower abdomen
Radiates to back
Patient observed sitting up and leaning forward to relieve pain

Nursing Dx & Intervention

Nursing Diagnosis	Nursing Intervention/Rationale
Potential fluid volume deficit	• Assess for signs of impending cardiac failure, *since circulatory shock is a possibility from the release of vasoactive peptides (kinin) from an injured pancreas (acute pancreatitis).* • Assess for signs and symptoms of electrolyte imbalance. • Assess intake and output, central venous pressure, Swan-Ganz catheter pressure, daily weights. • Assess vital signs and blood pressure every 4 hours, more often if indicated. • Monitor laboratory values, particularly hematocrit and hemoglobin, which will decrease after volume is restored. • Provide fluid volume replacement as ordered; intravenous fluids, dextran, fluid expanders.
Ineffective breathing pattern	• Assess patient carefully for signs of respiratory distress: breath sounds, cough, sputum, fluid accumulation, elevated diaphragm, shallow breathing, *since patients are candidates for ARDS.* • Monitor arterial blood gases.
Patient problem: potential altered bowel elimination	• Assess bowel for indications of paralytic ileus: adynamic, fluid accumulation, vomiting.
Potential for injury (complications)	• Assess for signs of pseudocyst: upper abdominal pain, mass, tenderness, fever, a general deterioration or no improvement in patient's condition.

Nursing Diagnosis	Nursing Intervention/Rationale
Potential impaired skin integrity	• Assess for indications of enterocutaneous fistula. • Monitor output of any fistula. • Provide skin protection for a pancreatic fistula with a clean or sterile skin barrier and pouch.
Pain	• Assess patient's pain: steady, dull, boring pain in epigastrium, worsens when supine. • Allow patient to assume a comfortable position; usually sitting up and leaning forward will help relieve pain. • Provide analgesics as ordered, since pain may be severe and steady; analgesics before procedures alleviate or minimize discomfort.
Altered nutrition: less than body requirements	• Assess patient's nutritional status. • Give patient nothing by mouth during acute pancreatitis episodes *to eliminate unnecessary secretion of pancreatic enzymes.* • Measure and record nasogastric output. • Provide frequent mouth care. • Monitor blood and urine glucose levels, since damage to islet cells may result in mild transient hyperglycemia. • Assess stools for diarrhea and steatorrhea, a sign of malabsorption of fats. • Provide insulin as ordered for endocrine dysfunction in chronic pancreatitis (note possibility of reactive hypoglycemia to insulin therapy).

Patient Education

1. Assist the patient in understanding the cause or causal relationships of pancreatitis with alcohol use or gallstones.
2. Plan an appropriate rehabilitation program if alcohol abuse is related to disease process.
3. Provide written dietary instructions.
4. Provide written medication instructions.
5. Teach the patient about diabetes mellitus: signs, symptoms, and insulin therapy.

Evaluation

Patient Outcome	Data Indicating That Outcome is Reached
Pain is absent.	Patient experiences no pain.
Fluid volume is normal.	Hydration and electrolyte balance are adequate.
Nutrition is adequate.	Weight is stable. Patient does not experience steatorrhea or diarrhea. Serum glucose is stabilized. Patient does not experience anorexia, nausea, or vomiting.
Respiratory function is normal.	There are no signs of respiratory distress. Arterial blood gas levels are within normal range.
Liver function studies are normal.	Laboratory values for SGPT, SGOT, alkaline phosphatase, gamma glutamyltransferase (GGT), isocitrate dehydrogenase (ICD), leukocyte alkaline phosphatase, 5′-nucleotidase (5′NT), ornithine carbamoyltransferase (OCT), lactate dehydrogenase (LDH_5; accounts for 2% to 11% of total LDH), bilirubin (total), albumin, and urobilinogen are within normal limits.

Medical Interventions and Related Nursing Care

Abdominal Surgeries for Selected Diseases of Gastrointestinal Tract

Description and Rationale

Abdominal surgeries involve an incision into the abdomen with the patient under general anesthesia. A variety of abdominal surgeries may be required under the broad scope of gastrointestinal diseases. Commonalities exist in the preoperative and postoperative patient care assessment and interventions that will be covered in this section. Examples of abdominal surgeries in which a portion of the gastrointestinal tract is surgically removed include appendectomy (appendix), cholecystectomy (gallbladder), colectomy (colon), and gastrectomy (stomach). An intestinal resection may be referred to as an ileotransverse colostomy (ileum is reanastomosed to transverse colon with removal or bypass of the ascending colon: in this case there is no externalization of the bowel even though the term "colostomy" is used).

Surgery is indicated in many gastrointestinal diseases when medical management is ineffective or when complications develop. In cholecystitis with cholelithiasis, surgery is the primary choice of treatment. Surgery may be palliative, as in the case of Crohn's disease, or curative, as with ulcerative colitis and familial polyposis.

Contraindications and Cautions

1. Patients with signs and symptoms of an acute condition in the abdomen or an emergency situation will need to be quickly stabilized with fluid and electrolyte replacements.
2. The surgical intervention in an emergency may be considered a first stage, diverting the problem, with a required second operation for definitive treatment.
3. For patients with permanent colostomies, ileostomies, continent ileostomies, and ileoanal reservoirs, recommend medical alert card stating: "No rectal temperatures, no rectal enemas, no rectal suppositories: the rectum has been removed." Provide definition of above procedures.

Preprocedural Nursing Care

1. Thorough bowel preparation is required for many abdominal surgeries including oral antibiotics and enemas. Caution must be used not to deplete weakened or elderly patients with multiple tap water enemas.
2. Drains and tubes, such as nasogastric tubes, T tubes, and gastrostomy tubes, are often used after surgery, and patients should be prepared for their presence.

Medical Plan

Medications

- Bowel preparation (for intestinal surgery); nonabsorbable anti-infective agents
  - Neomycin (Mycifradin), 500 mg qid
  - Erythromycin (E-Mycin), 500 mg qid
- Postoperatively, broad-spectrum antibiotic prophylaxis
  - Cefazolin (Ancef), 500-1000 mg q6-8h for 24-36 h IV
  - Cephapirin (Cefadyl), 500-1000 mg q4-6h for 24-36 h IV
- Narcotic analgesics
  - Meperidine (Demerol), 75-100 mg IM q3-4h for pain; then po q3-4h for pain
  - Acetaminophen with codeine phosphate (Tylenol with codeine), 1 or 2 tablets po q4h prn for pain

General Management

- Incentive spirometry
- Postural drainage
- Nasogastric drainage
- Gastrostomy tubes; T tubes
- Transcutaneous electrical nerve stimulation (TENS)
- Patient-controlled analgesia (PCA) pumps
- Intravenous fluids with electrolytes (particularly potassium)
- Total parenteral nutrition

NURSING CARE

Nursing Assessment

Abdomen

- Abdominal pain
- Abdominal distention
- Absence of bowel sounds, rigidity, rebound tenderness: paralytic ileus, intestinal obstruction, peritonitis; intestinal ischemia
- Adhesions

Abdominal Incision, Surgical Site

- Hemorrhage
- Drainage other than serosanguineous during first 24 hours

Signs of wound infection: redness, pain, edema, drainage
Wound dehiscence or evisceration
Fistula formation

Bowel Function

Routine of bowel activity, gas pains, bowel movement
Constipation, diarrhea

Circulatory System

Shock and circulatory failure associated with hemorrhage and fluid and electrolyte imbalance
Thrombophlebitis and pulmonary emboli associated with extensive pelvic surgery (i.e., abdominoperineal resection) and in elderly persons

Fluids and Electrolytes

Intestinal obstruction and paralytic ileus and fistulas associated with fluid and electrolyte loss
Nausea, vomiting, diarrhea, and nasogastric and intestinal suctioning may affect fluid and electrolyte balance

Mental Status

Evaluation of effects of narcotics: fluid and electrolyte imbalance, insomnia, fatigue

Emotional consideration varies with type of abdominal surgery and changes that result from that surgery (i.e., colostomy or ileostomy versus appendectomy)

Respiratory System

Hypoxia from respiratory depressants such as narcotics
Shallow breathing and inadequate coughing secondary to abdominal pain
Abdominal distention compromising lung expansion

Temperature

Low-grade fever first 24 to 48 hours common
Fever of 38° C (100° F) or fever that does not subside may indicate pulmonary complications, wound infection, urinary infection, or thrombophlebitis
Fever of 38.3° C (101° F) occurring suddenly and accompanied by chills, weakness, fatigue, rapid respirations, tachycardia, and sudden drop in blood pressure indicates septic shock

Urinary Tract

Decrease or cessation of urinary output reflects renal dysfunction
Voiding problems following indwelling catheter removal

Nursing Dx & Intervention

Nursing Diagnosis	Nursing Intervention/Rationale
Potential for infection	• Assess wound during postoperative period for redness, pain, edema, unusual drainage, odor, and separation of the suture line. • Observe wound dressing frequently for signs of bleeding. • Monitor vital signs every 2 hours until patient is stable and then every 4 hours.
Patient problem: potential altered renal, cardiopulmonary, gastrointestinal, and peripheral tissue perfusion	• Assess patient for signs and symptoms of alterations in tissue perfusion associated with major abdominal surgeries for complications of pancreatitis, cholecystitis, ulcerative colitis, and other diseases, including shock, circulatory failure, intestinal ischemia, and renal failure. • Monitor patient's vital signs and central venous pressure or Swan-Ganz catheter for changes in cardiac output and tissue perfusion. • Encourage patient to do leg exercises, and measure and apply elastic hose *to facilitate venous circulation.*
Ineffective breathing pattern	• Assess patient for shallow breathing, splinting with respirations, decreased breath sounds, and respiratory distress. • Auscultate lungs every 2 hours. • Encourage patient to turn, deep breathe, and cough every 2 hours. • Encourage use of incentive spirometer *to promote maximal inspiratory maneuvers.* • Provide pain medication and splint abdomen with pillow *to decrease abdominal pain associated with deep breathing and coughing.*
Potential fluid volume deficit	• Monitor intake and output including all drainage from nasogastric, gastric, intestinal, and T tubes as well as wound drainage or fistula output. • Weigh patient daily. • Assess patient's hydration status by mucous membrane, skin turgor, and blood pressure. • Monitor color, consistency, amount, and odor of any drainage; test drainage (i.e., nasogastric aspirate, stool, fistula) for blood or pH if indicated. Provide fluid replacement as ordered.
Pain	• Assess the location, type, and duration of pain, pattern of pain occurrence, effectiveness of medications, and positioning and alternative methods of pain relief. • Provide analgesics as ordered as needed *for pain.* • Encourage the patient to take the medication postoperatively; reassure the patient that narcotic addiction will not occur. PCA pumps allow patients to control analgesia.

Nursing Diagnosis	Nursing Intervention/Rationale
	• Monitor changes in pain associated with signs of abdominal distention, rigidity, and rebound tenderness and with temperature as a sign of complications.
Potential impaired skin integrity	• Assess patient for risks in developing pressure sores. • Protect the nares when nasogastric tube is to be left in place several days. • Change wound dressings frequently if output is high *to protect skin from moisture maceration.* • Apply a pectin-based (Stomahesive, Hollihesive) wafer to the skin and tape to the wafer rather than applying tape on the skin. Montgomery straps can be applied on top of the pectin-based wafer. Keep in mind that drainage from the gastrointestinal tract continues to contain very irritating digestive enzymes (bile, gastric, pancreatic, intestinal). • Evaluate patient with wound drainage for a wound pouching system to contain the drainage, protect the skin, allow for accurate measurement, and decrease cost of dressing changes (see box opposite). • Protect tubes from pulling by adequately taping and provide skin protection if there is leakage around a tube (see box below).
Altered oral mucous membrane	• Provide regular mouth care *to prevent problems associated with nasogastric tubes, limited oral intake for several days, and mouth breathing.* • Assist patient in brushing his or her teeth and rinsing the mouth with nonastringent solutions every 4 hours or more often *for patient comfort.* • Provide anesthetic lozenges or hard candy if not contraindicated *(use will result in saliva production and stimulate gastric secretions).*
Constipation; diarrhea	• Assess patient for first bowel movement after surgery. • Assess dietary and fluid intake as it relates to normal stool consistency. • Observe color, consistency, frequency, and amount of stools. • Evaluate pattern change following gastrointestinal surgery (e.g., diarrhea related to bile in colon following cholecystectomy or small bowel resection).
Bathing/hygiene self-care deficit	• Assist patient with activities of daily living following surgery. • Allow patient to participate in self-care as tolerated. • Encourage patient to assume primary responsibility for care as tolerated as nasogastric tube and IVs are removed.
Altered nutrition: less than body requirements	• Assess patient for signs of malabsorption: steatorrhea, diarrhea, weight loss. • Evaluate potential nutritional deficiency based on the gastrointestinal organs involved in the disease process and treatment or interventions. • Monitor TPN or enteral supplements as ordered.
Altered patterns of urinary elimination	• Assess for signs of urinary retention associated with anesthesia, pain, anxiety, and removal of indwelling catheter. • Observe and record intake and output. • Provide privacy and promote relaxation when patient needs to void. • Palpate bladder for distention if patient has not voided for 6 to 8 hours or if patient is voiding small amounts frequently (overflow voiding). • Catheterize patient if ordered.

Gastrostomy Tube Care

1. Use a pectin-based wafer (skin barrier) around the tube. Cut a small opening in the wafer ⅛ inch larger than the skin exit site.
2. Cleanse the skin with warm water and pat dry.
3. Apply the wafer, and seal to the skin.
4. Apply a paste (Karaya, Stomahesive) to any exposed skin around the tube. Use a thin coat of paste.
5. Anchor the tube to the wafer with the use of a baby bottle nipple. Cut open the end of the nipple large enough to accommodate the tube. Cut up through the side of the nipple (base to top), open the nipple, and wrap around the tube. Then tape the base of the nipple to the pectin-based wafer.
6. Tape the tube to the top of the nipple.
7. Remove the nipple daily and assess the exit site. If needed, gently cleanse around the tube exit site and dry, reapply paste, and replace nipple. If the skin barrier has drainage leaking under the seal, remove and replace. The wafer should be changed weekly otherwise.

Containment of Wound Drainage and Fistula Output

1. Determine whether a sterile or a clean system is required.
2. Make a pattern of the wound or fistula. The pattern opening should be back ¼ inch from the wound edge. Label the pattern carefully with the following: patient's name, date, patient's left, right, head, and feet, pouch side (the side of the pattern facing the nurse if the pattern is against the skin), and skin side (the side of the pattern that lies against the skin).
3. Select a pectin-based wafer (skin barrier) and an ostomy or wound pouch that will accommodate the pattern. The pouch should have a spout if the drainage is liquid or be able to be attached to a bedside bag.
4. Trace the pattern opening onto the wafer. Take care to place the pattern appropriately or you will cut the pattern inversely. One suggestion is to place the pattern against the patient's abdomen. Lay the wafer down on the pattern as it would be applied to the abdomen (i.e., paper-backing side to abdomen). Lift the two off the patient and turn them over together and trace the pattern.
5. Cut the opening in the pectin-based wafer.
6. Trace the pattern onto the pouch adhesive backing. The same method can be used to avoid inverting the pattern.
7. Cut the opening in the pouch adhesive ¼ inch larger than the line you traced.
8. Remove the paper backing from the pouch and apply the pouch to the "shiny" or top side of the wafer. Press firmly, sealing the two together.
9. Cleanse the patient's skin with warm water and pat dry.
10. Apply a thin coat of paste around the wound edges if the pouch has a spout and no access cap.
11. Remove packing from the skin barrier.
12. Center the pouching system and apply to the skin. Press and seal to the skin.
13. Apply paste to any exposed skin through the access cap or by going up through the bottom of the pouch.
14. Close the spout, and connect to bedside bag or clamp the bottom.
15. Check the system each shift for signs of leakage and change when necessary.
16. Empty according to amount of drainage. Pouch should not fill and pull down against the seal.

Patient Education

1. Instruct the patient on routine care following major abdominal surgery: ambulate at regular times, rest frequently, and slowly increase activities as tolerated; keep incision dry, and report any signs of redness, pain, or drainage of incision; avoid heavy lifting for 6 to 8 weeks, and splint abdomen when coughing or sneezing.
2. Provide written instructions on medications and medication schedule.
3. Identify with the patient the importance of regular follow-up care.
4. Provide information related to primary diagnosis, type of surgery, and expected outcomes.
5. Provide written instructions for any at-home care: wound, T tube, gastrostomy tube, and so on.

Evaluation

Patient Outcome	Data Indicating That Outcome is Reached
Body functions normally.	Abdominal incision heals with no drainage; bowel and bladder function normally.
Patient returns to activities of daily living.	Patient resumes activities at home and at work (e.g., driving, exercising).
Patient does not experience pain.	Abdominal pain is resolved; patient no longer requires mild pain medication.
Nutrition is adequate.	Patient tolerates a regular diet or special diet for type of disorder or surgery; patient gains weight.
Skin integrity is maintained.	There are no signs of skin irritation.

 Diversions: Colostomy and Ileostomy

Description and Rationale

A colostomy is a diversion involving the colon in which a segment of diseased or injured colon is bypassed or removed and an end or loop of colon is brought through a small opening in the abdominal wall and matured, forming a stoma. The anatomic location in the colon is an important description and influences the care. Ascending, transverse, and sigmoid colostomies may be performed. Transverse colostomies are most often loop ostomy stomas and are temporary. A loop means that the intact bowel has been brought through the abdominal wall, a rod placed under the bowel, the incision closed, and a cautery used to open the top wall of the bowel (the lower wall remains intact). The proximal opening will drain the stool while the distal opening may drain mucus and leads to the rectum. The patient may have bowel movements from the rectum that consist of stool in the bowel before surgery or mucus. The stool is semiformed, extremely odorous, and unpredictable.

The sigmoid colostomy is the most common permanent stoma and is indicated for cancer of the colon. The stool from the sigmoid colostomy is similar to normal bowel movements. Generally, stool is evacuated once or twice a day. A regular pattern before surgery is used to predict the possibility of regulation of the sigmoid colostomy with diet or with colostomy irrigations.

For patients with a sigmoid colostomy a new device that plugs the stoma is available. The two-piece system (Conseal) consists of a skin barrier flange or plate (which resembles the faceplate on several two-piece pouching systems) and a plug made of a soft, pliable material that fits into the stoma and then snaps to the flange. The system is indicated for people who have four or fewer bowel movements a day or who are irrigating the sigmoid colostomy.

The removal of the entire colon and rectum (total proctocolectomy) results in the ileum being brought through the abdominal wall, forming an ileostomy stoma. The stool from the ileostomy is liquid to semiformed and contains residual digestive enzymes. The drainage from the ascending colostomy is similar, and the nursing interventions are the same for both. Fluid and electrolyte imbalance is a potential problem with an ileostomy and may result in significant problems.

Contraindications and Cautions

1. Only a sigmoid colostomy should be irrigated to obtain regular bowel eliminations.
2. An ileostomy lavage for a food blockage refers to the insertion of 30 to 50 ml of normal saline through a small catheter using an Asepto syringe. *This is not a colostomy irrigation.*
3. Laxatives should *never* be given to a patient with an ileostomy. The results can be severe fluid and electrolyte imbalance.
4. Bowel preparation for a person with an ileostomy consists of clear liquids for 2 to 3 days.

Preprocedural Nursing Care

1. Consultation with an enterostomal therapy (ET) nurse is arranged.
2. A preoperative visit by a United Ostomy Association (UOA) trained visitor (rehabilitated person with an ostomy) is recommended.
3. Stoma site selection is marked by ET nurse for the surgeon. This is an important phase to ensure a good pouch seal after surgery.

NURSING CARE

Nursing Assessment

Perineum

Removal of rectum (abdominoperineal resection) results in large wound
Perineal infection: redness, tenderness, drainage

Intestine

Intestinal obstruction
Food blockage (ileostomy)
Perforation (colostomy irrigation)

Anemia

Vitamin B_{12} deficiency (ileostomy)

Stoma

Peristomal skin irritation or erosion
Parastomal hernias
Stomal stenosis
Stomal prolapse
Stomal retraction
Necrosis of stoma

Colostomy

Constipation
Diarrhea

Ileostomy

Diarrhea
Dehydration
Food blockage

Sexual Functioning

Wide resections in perineal area for cancer of rectum may damage nerves responsible for erection, ejaculation, and orgasm in male; no impairment or one or a combination of all functions may be affected

Physiologic effects on women have been poorly studied

Self-Concept and Body Image

Adjustment and integration of ostomy require time and support from family and health care providers

Complications: prolonged use of defense behaviors, noninvolvement in physical care, social isolation

Nursing Dx & Intervention

Nursing Diagnosis	Nursing Intervention/Rationale
Body image and self-esteem disturbances	• Assess patient's verbal and nonverbal responses to the alteration in bowel function and the physical change (presence of stoma). • Provide patient and family an opportunity to express their feelings regarding the ostomy preoperatively and postoperatively. • Remind patient that an ostomy is an alternative pattern of elimination, that it will take time to adjust to, both physically and emotionally, and that people are available to help. • Provide consistent management of the ostomy, control odor, and prevent leaking, giving patient a sense of control over the stoma. • Select a system that is invisible under clothing, is odorproof, and fits the body size. • Encourage patient to return to all presurgical activities as soon as possible. • Recommend a trained ostomy visitor of same age and sex as patient and preferably one who has had same type of ostomy procedure. • Allow patient to grieve for the loss of a body part and the loss of control of elimination. • Be realistic and positive: negative reactions will be picked up by patient and will make adjustment harder; most people adapt successfully to ostomy surgery.
Altered sexuality patterns	• Allow patient to discuss concerns and fears regarding sexual activities. Many patients fear rejection by spouse or significant other. • Discuss positions with patient: Back to belly: pouch is against bed and not as noticeable. Missionary: pouch should be empty to prevent leakage. Female on top: pouch is fully exposed. • Suggest material pouch covers; other patients have recommended crotchless panties for women and binders for men to hold pouch in place. • Remind patient that he or she must first be comfortable with self. Spouse or significant other is most often kind, gentle, and caring. Communication between partners is extremely important. • Refer men who have had nerve damage and are unable to obtain an erection to a urologist for information on penile prosthesis. • Refer to family and sexual counselors as indicated by poor coping or maladaptation.
Potential impaired skin integrity	• Assess the skin integrity with each pouch change. • Protect the peristomal skin with skin barriers: pectin-based wafers, paste, Karaya washers (Karaya protects skin but does not hold a pouch on and requires tape or belt). • Change pouching system whenever the pouch first begins to leak (an early sign is odor); *do not* tape a leaking pouch seal and plan on changing it later. Skin is damaged within minutes by trapped ileostomy effluent. Prevention is easier than treatment.
Impaired skin integrity	• Consult an ET nurse at first indication of skin irritation. • Treat skin reactions that are secondary to ileostomy drainage, stool, urine, glue, solvents, and soaps as follows: Remove the source of the irritation. Cleanse the skin with warm water and pat dry. A hair dryer on cool may be used. Expose the skin to air, light, and heat for 15 to 20 minutes. A hair dryer on cool and a 60-watt light 12 to 16 inches away may be used. Cover the irritated skin with a pectin-based wafer to which the patient is not sensitive. Apply a pouch. Repeat every 48 hours. • Treat skin that is eroded or ulcerated as follows: Cleanse skin with warm water and pat dry. Apply aluminum acetate (Burow's solution) compresses for 20 to 30 minutes. Expose skin to light, air, and heat for 15 to 20 minutes. Use hair dryer on cool and 60-watt bulb 12 to 16 inches away.

Nursing Diagnosis	Nursing Intervention/Rationale
	Cover with a pectin-based wafer and apply a pouch. Change every 24 to 48 hours. • Avoid mechanical injury to the skin by gentle removal of tape and skin barriers. • Empty pouches rather than changing and discarding pouches that are full. • Observe for monilial *(Candida albicans)* reactions associated with antibiotics and changes in normal bowel flora. Skin appears bright red with weepy papulae, satellite lesions, and secondary crusting. • Assess other sites for monilial infection: under arms, under breasts, and in groin. • Consult physician for order of nystatin (Mycostatin) powder. Powder used in peristomal area must be sealed in with a sealant or water (Bard Protective Barrier, Skin Prep). Ointments will keep pouch from sealing. • Prevent radiation dermatitis by not having any portion of the pouch or pouch adhesive in the field of radiation. If pouch must be removed daily for treatments use a Karaya-only backed pouch that is belted in place. • Avoid use of light when treating irradiated skin.
Patient problem: altered bowel elimination	• Assess output for color, consistency, frequency, and amount. • Select a pouching system that contains the stool, is easy to empty, is odorproof, and is invisible under the patient's clothing. • Clean the spout after each emptying to eliminate odor from a dirty spout. • Avoid pinholes in pouches that lead to constant odor release; either empty pouch of gas or use commercial gas release valves added or made into the pouching system.
Potential fluid volume deficit	• Assess patient for dehydration that may develop with high-volume ileostomy output. • Observe patient with ileostomy for diarrhea: high-volume, watery, hot drainage; pouch emptied every 20 to 30 minutes. • Monitor intake and output, vital signs, and daily weights.
Patient problem: potential altered nutrition	• Assess patient for sign of food blockage (ileostomy): history of high roughage in diet and not chewing well; no output and abdominal distention; nausea and vomiting. • Perform an ileostomy lavage: Remove pouch; stoma will become edematous. Apply irrigation sleeve. Have patient assume knee-chest position and massage abdomen under stoma; if blockage is removed, stop here and reapply pouching system; if not, continue. Insert catheter gently into stoma to level of blockage (usually at fascia level). Irrigate with 30 to 50 ml normal saline using Asepto syringe; allow to return. Repeat instillation of 30 to 50 ml of saline. Procedure may take 1 to 2 hours; may try knee-chest position between irrigations if patient is stable. Assess for dehydration; fluid becomes trapped behind food blockage, which acts as an intestinal obstruction. Provide intravenous fluids as ordered. NOTE: This procedure is *not* taught to patients. However, patient should be taught to recognize early signs and symptoms and seek medical assistance. Assist patient in returning to regular diet, avoiding only foods that give that person problems. • Instruct patient to chew food carefully and eat slowly.

Patient Education*

1. Colostomy and ileostomy care involves the following:
   a. Stomal and skin assessment: stoma should be red and moist; skin should be free of irritation.
   b. Management of frequently encountered skin problems:
      (1) Rash can be located under the tape, under the faceplate, and on any part of the skin where the pouch comes in contact with the skin. A generalized reddish appearance that covers an entire area, similar to a diaper rash, will be seen. Cause may be leaking appliance, perspiration, allergies to tape, or hair follicle irritation. Advise patient to use heat lamp or hair dryer to dry the skin. Patient should sprinkle a small amount of powder (Karaya, Stomahesive) on the skin, wipe off the excess, then blot with a skin sealant to seal the powder to the skin. Powder the skin on which the pouch lies after the pouch is applied. Patient should make or buy a pouch cover. Wearing a pouch belt too tight may break the seal.

*Portions reprinted with permission from Broadwell, D.C., and Sorrells, S.L.: Summary of your ileostomy care and Summary of your colostomy care, Atlanta, 1978 (revised 1988), Patient Education Booklets.

(2) Cement or solvent burns can be located anywhere under the faceplate but usually are found at the outside edges. Their cause is chemicals in the cement or solvent that were not allowed to evaporate off the skin surface before applying pouch or cement that was too thick and was unable to dry completely. Patient should apply heat lamp or hair dryer to the weeping skin, cover the burn with a pectin-based skin barrier and apply pouch in usual way (advise patient to try to leave the pouch on 24 to 48 hours), and omit using cement on skin or pouch.

(3) Ulcerated area on stoma may be caused by a stomal opening of the pouch that is too small or activities that caused the faceplate to rub or cut into the stoma. Patient should enlarge the size of the pouch opening, evaluate activities (a different size or shaped faceplate may be needed), and loosen belt. The skin should be protected by a skin barrier or paste.

(4) Infected or irritated hair follicles may be located under the faceplate. They are raised red areas (similar to acne) at the shaft of the hair follicle from not keeping the area under the faceplate shaved. Advise patient to let the irritation improve before removing any more hair by shaving or cutting, use hair dryer or heat lamp to dry the skin if oozing is present, and use a skin barrier between skin and faceplate until irritation improves.

(5) Remind patient that weeping skin may prevent a pouch or a skin barrier from adhering to the skin for long periods. If skin is severely irritated and weeping, it may be necessary to change pouch more frequently to prevent leakage and further damage.

(6) Remind patient that the hair under faceplate should be removed by an electric razor or a safety razor.

c. Principles of changing a pouching system should be accompanied by several opportunities for practicing the procedure.

(1) Instruct patient to assemble all equipment: cotton balls, tissues, toilet paper, wash cloths, towels, premoistened towelettes (to cleanse the skin); pouch; skin barriers; pouch closure; tape or belt; and equipment for cleansing or disposing of used pouches.

(2) A paper towel may be used to trace a pattern, which should hug the stoma but not ride up on it, and top should be labeled. Outer dimensions of the pattern (avoiding hip bones, pubic areas, ribs and folds at waist and navel) should be considered.

(3) For skin barrier (if applicable) wafer size will depend on size of stoma and abdomen. Instruct patient to round the corners or conform the wafer to the shape of the adhesive on the pouch, trace the stomal pattern on the paper side, cut hole on pattern line, and smooth sides of the opening.

(4) Pouch opening should be slightly larger than opening of skin barrier. Instruct patient to trace pattern on the paper side of the pouch, cut the hole larger than the line of the pattern, remove paper backing from the pouch, center the openings, and apply the shiny side of the skin barrier to the pouch.

(5) Empty and remove the pouch being worn. Cleanse and dry the skin.

(6) Patient should note any changes in skin or stoma (color, size, ulcerations, irritations), center and apply skin barrier and pouch, close end, and tape edges.

(7) Instruct patient to check supplies and reorder as necessary.

d. Dietary considerations should be discussed with the patient.

(1) Foods associated with odor are fish, eggs, asparagus, onions, garlic, and some spices.

(2) Foods associated with diarrhea are green beans, broccoli, spinach, raw fruits, highly seasoned foods, and beer.

(3) Foods used to manage diarrhea (low-residue diet) are strained bananas, peanut butter (without nuts), and applesauce.

(4) Foods used to manage constipation are high-fiber foods (bran, celery), increased raw fruits and vegetables, and increased fluid intake (water, fruit juices).

(5) Foods associated with gas are brussels sprouts, cabbage, beans, peas, mushrooms, carbonated drinks, onions, cucumbers, and beer.

(6) Patients are encouraged to eat all above foods in moderation, chewing well, and adding one new food at a time to evaluate tolerance.

e. Provide patient with written instructions for follow-up, and initiate home care referral if indicated.

2. Sigmoid colostomy patient teaching should also include a section on colostomy irrigation that includes adequate opportunity for return demonstrations. Colostomy irrigations are started after the patient has active bowel sounds and has progressed to a low-residue diet.

a. Define colostomy irrigation: an enema through the colostomy stoma that stimulates peristalsis and a bowel movement with the intent of emptying the colon so no further bowel movements occur until the next irrigation.

b. Remind patient that spillage is common for several weeks. Chemotherapy and radiation therapy will result in spillage and are indications for withholding the colostomy irrigation.

c. Below are general guidelines and tips for colostomy irrigation directed to the patient.
   (1) Assemble all equipment: water container and water, irrigating sleeve and belt, items to clean skin and stoma, way to dispose of old pouch, clean, cut pouch, and closure, and skin care items.
   (2) Remove old pouch and dispose of it.
   (3) Clean skin and stoma with water, and let dry. Observe condition and color of skin and stoma.
   (4) Apply irrigating sleeve and belt securely (but not too tight). If you use Karaya washer, dampen and apply this first.
   (5) Fill irrigating container with about 1 quart tepid water when you are ready to start.
   (6) Suspend the irrigating container so that the bottom of the container is even with the top of shoulder.
   (7) Remove air from the tubing (helps prevent the air from increasing gas pains). Do not use a large amount of irrigating water for this, or it will be necessary to refill irrigation container.
   (8) Gently insert irrigating cone into stoma, holding it parallel to the floor, and start the water slowly. If water does not flow easily, try or check the following:
      (a) Slightly change the position or the angle of the cone; cone opening may be blocked by a loop of your bowel.
      (b) Check for kinks in tubing from irrigating container.
      (c) Check height of irrigating container.
      (d) Relax and take some *deep* breaths to relax abdominal muscles.
      (e) Stool immediately under skin level may be slightly hard and blocking water flow. Instill *small* amounts of water to loosen it up.
   (9) The following are variations in water for irrigations:
      (a) People vary in the amount of water they can hold at one time.
      (b) The amount of water used can vary daily.
      (c) Do not get discouraged. Remember that you want to cleanse as much of the fecal matter out as possible: learn to pay attention to the full feeling and the feeling that you need to expel stool so you do not continue to force water into your bowel.
      (d) Do *not* force water into your bowel; if you are cramping, the flow of water stops, or water is forcefully returning around the irrigating cone or catheter.
      (e) If you feel bloated or constipated, you may irrigate with about ½ quart more water in the same day or take a mild laxative after consulting physician.
   (10) The majority of the stool will return in about 15 minutes. When you feel that you have expelled most of the stool, rinse the sleeve with water, dry the bottom edge, roll it up, close the end, and go about your activities for about 30 to 45 minutes to allow the bowel adequate time to finish emptying.
   (11) When you feel that you have obtained complete results, assemble and apply clean pouch and any skin barriers.
   (12) Rinse the irrigation sleeve with cold water, hang it up to dry, and put away other equipment.
   (13) Check supplies and reorder as necessary.
   (14) Try to irrigate within the same 2- or 3-hour period each day so that bowels become regulated; if possible, try to irrigate close to time bowels moved before surgery.

3. If you decide to use the colostomy plug (Conseal, by Coloplast), specific patient instructions will be needed. A 14-day bowel training program should be instituted to allow the bowel to adapt to the length of the time the plug can be left in place. The plug contains a carbon filter that allows flatus to pass odor free. The flange can accommodate irrigation sleeves, mini-caps, and pouches. If the patient develops diarrhea from the flu, antibiotic therapy, or foods, pouches should be used until the stool returns to a solid consistency. Please refer to the manufacturer's literature for forms that patients can use to record their progress during the 14-day period. The product has been available for a limited time, and not all complications and contraindications are known. Potential problems may be related to changes in colonic bacterial flora, mucosal pressure, increased mucus production, and increased peristalsis. Previous devices providing continence for colostomy patients have been unsuccessful because they required the implantation of parts of the system. The external flange provides a method of securing the plug and protecting the skin. The second advantage of this system is that the flange can be used with a pouching system if needed. Keep in mind that the device is intended for sigmoid colostomies.

4. Ileostomy patient teaching should include the following:
   a. Instruct patient about symptoms of food blockage and what to do if it occurs.
      (1) Discharge changes from semisolid to a thin liquid; lumen is blocked by food, but water passes around it.
      (2) Total volume of output increases and functions almost constantly; water is drawn from bloodstream in attempt to rid the bowel lumen of blockage and intestines become hyperactive.
      (3) There is an objectionable odor; bacterial overgrowth occurs at the blockage and causes fermentation of foodstuff.
      (4) Cramping occurs, usually followed by increase in watery output; this is caused by increased bowel activity to rid itself of blockage.
      (5) Abdomen is distended; the blockage traps gas and liquids in the bowel lumen.

(6) Vomiting occurs; this is a further attempt of body to rid itself of blockage by traveling in direction of least resistance.
(7) There is no ileostomy output because of complete blockage.
(8) Instruct patient to get into a knee-chest position for a few minutes or take a hot shower to relax and then try the knee-chest position.
(9) Many blockages relieve themselves; however, if the blockage persists more than 3 to 4 hours, contact physician.

b. Foods associated with blockage include celery, Chinese foods, corn, nuts, coleslaw, dried fruits, coconut, wild rice, popcorn, whole vegetable skins, and fibrous vegetables. Do not eliminate from diet. Eat in moderate amounts and chew well.

Evaluation

Patient Outcome	Data Indicating That Outcome is Reached
Patient returns to activities of daily living.	Patient returns to work and to social activities, including sex. Patient wears "normal" clothes.
Body functions normally.	Wound (abdominal and perineal) heals with no drainage.
Patient performs self-care.	Patient can care for colostomy or ileostomy. Patient can identify information related to stoma and skin, fluid and electrolytes, diet, and need for regular follow-up.
Personal adjustment is achieved.	Patient verbalizes feelings related to ostomy and external pouching system.

Diversion: Continent Ileostomy

(Kock pouch)

Description and Rationale

The continent ileostomy or Kock pouch was first described by Nils Kock in 1969.[45] The procedure involves the creation of an internal pouch constructed of ileum and of a nipple valve that maintains continency of stool and flatus. The patient has a stoma flush with the skin located in the lower right quadrant, which is intubated with a large-bore tube several times a day to evacuate the stool and flatus. The key to success of the continent ileostomy is the nipple valve.

The continent ileostomy may be recommended for people with emotional problems associated with a conventional ileostomy. Conversion from a conventional to a continent ileostomy may be important for patients who have been unable to cope. Patients do report sensitive reactions to the continent ileostomy. The lack of an external appliance is the major factor. Also, a flush rather than a protruding stoma is cited as an advantage by patients. Patients do not find the intubation or catheterization procedure bothersome once the pouch capacity increases.

The advantages of the continent ileostomy include the following[29]:

No appliance required
No noise or odor from stoma except during emptying
No skin irritation
Improved psychosocial adjustment

The continent ileostomy has a higher risk of complications than conventional ileostomies. Long-term problems are more common and may be associated with loss of continency.

The disadvantages of the procedure are associated with the high percentage of nipple valve dysfunction and the reoperative rate. Even with the high rate of reoperation, patients who have converted to a continent ileostomy state that it is a more satisfactory procedure.

The continent ileostomy is constructed from 45 cm of terminal ileum after the colectomy has been performed. The 45 cm section of ileum is brought through the abdominal incision, maintaining the blood supply to the loop of small bowel. The end 15 cm is left free and will ultimately be used to form the nipple valve. First, the surgeon loops the proximal 30 cm segment back on itself; each side is 15 cm. Then the loop is sutured along its antimesenteric border where the two segments touch. A long U-shaped incision is made around the 30 cm loop close to the suture line. The ileum then can be opened up into a cuplike shape. The small flaps of tissue on either side of the suture line are sutured together, forming a double suture line. The double suture line produces a smooth internal surface of the reservoir and provides a safeguard against intestinal leakage from the pouch. The nipple valve is then constructed by intussuscepting several centimeters of terminal ileum into the reservoir. The two layers of the valve are anchored by numerous sutures or staples. The pouch is then sutured closed and assessed for adequacy of the valve and the suture line by filling it with a saline solution and air. If no signs of leakage are noted from the valve or from the sutures, the pouch is inserted into the abdominal cavity and anchored. The end portion of the distal ileum is brought through the abdominal wall, and a flush stoma is constructed.

A catheter is placed in the reservoir during surgery and remains in the pouch for 3 to 4 weeks.

It should be noted that a similar pouch is being constructed for urinary diversions.

Contraindications and Cautions

1. The diagnosis must be familial polyposis or ulcerative colitis.
2. The patient needs medical alert cards, since the continent ileostomy is an uncommon procedure.
3. Obesity is considered a contraindication.

Preprocedural Nursing Care

1. There should be a preoperative consultation with an ET nurse regarding the possible surgical options: conventional ileostomy, continent ileostomy, and ileoanal reservoir.
2. A rehabilitated patient with a continent ileostomy should visit preoperatively.

NURSING CARE

Nursing Assessment

Continent Ileostomy Pouch

"Pouchitis": local crampy pain, diarrhea that may be bloody, fever, valve leakage, intubation difficulty

Leakage of nipple valve
Valve prolapse
Skin stricture
Pouch perforation

Intestine

Intestinal obstruction; adhesions
Perforation

Abdominal Incision

Wound infection

Perineum

Infection of perineal wound
Poor wound healing; drainage

Sexual Functioning

Potential dysfunction in males when rectum resected; rare when performed for inflammatory bowel disease

Body Image

Presence of stoma and no external pouch more positive; if valve leaks, requires external pouch (p. 861)

Nursing Dx & Intervention

Nursing Diagnosis	Nursing Intervention/Rationale
Body image disturbance	• Assess patient's response to presence of flush stoma and intubation. • Allow patient opportunity to explore feelings regarding surgery and loss of rectum. • Provide trained visitor for patient.
Potential impaired skin integrity	• Protect peristomal skin with skin sealant (Bard Protective Barrier, Hollister Gel) from moisture in mucus. • Cover stoma with small pad. • Protect skin from ileostomy drainage if nipple valve leaks (p. 861).
Potential fluid volume deficit	• Assess patient for dehydration that may develop with high-volume output. • Monitor intake and output, vital signs, and daily weights.
Patient problem: potential altered nutrition	• Instruct patient to chew foods well and eat slowly. There are no dietary restrictions (see p. 863 for foods associated with odor, gas, and diarrhea).

Patient Education

1. Intubation and irrigation of continent ileostomy involve the following:
   a. First 3 weeks (catheter in place)
      (1) Irrigate the internal continent ileostomy pouch; insert 30 ml water and allow to drain out by gravity; repeat three or four times; irrigate every 2 hours during day and once at night.
      (2) Attach bedside bag, leg bag, and flushing tubing.
      (3) Clean bedside and leg bags with soapy water; allow to dry; have two and alternate.
      (4) Eat a low-residue diet.
   b. Week 4
      (1) Catheter is removed in outpatient clinic, and patient is taught to intubate the continent ileostomy.
      (2) Intubate and irrigate every 2 hours during day.
      (3) Intubate with catheter to straight drainage at night; irrigate once at night.

c. Week 5
   (1) Intubate every 3 hours, and irrigate twice a day.
   (2) Connect to gravity drainage at night; irrigate once at night.
d. Week 6
   (1) Intubate every 4 hours and irrigate twice during day.
   (2) Intubate at night only if sign of fullness or uncomfortable.
e. Week 7 and thereafter
   (1) Intubate pouch four times each day.
   (2) Irrigate pouch once each day until return is clear.

2. The following procedure is employed for emptying and intubating the continent ileostomy:
   a. The patient sitting on the commode inserts a well-lubricated catheter into the stoma and through the nipple valve. Stool and flatus will drain through the catheter directly into the toilet. If the stool is thick, water can be inserted through the catheter to loosen the stool. The catheter may need to be removed and flushed if the lumen becomes blocked with undigested residue. Grape juice and prune juice are often used by patients to keep their stool "thin."
   b. Several types of catheters are available (Marlen, Atlantic). The patient should have at least two catheters and should know how to order additional ones. It is important to discard catheters when they become old. Hard, brittle catheters are more likely to damage the valve or the pouch.
3. The patient should be provided with written instructions on the signs and symptoms of "pouchitis" and procedures if he or she experiences difficulty intubating pouch or leakage of nipple valve develops.
4. The patient should be given instructions on low-residue diet and advancing to a regular diet.

Evaluation

Patient Outcome	Data Indicating That Outcome is Reached
Body functions normally.	Wound heals. Pouch functions, and nipple valve is continent. Patient empties pouch four times a day. Patient eats regular diet.
Patient returns to activities of daily living.	Patient returns to work, to social activities, and to sexual functioning.
Patient performs self-care.	Patient manages continent ileostomy with no or minimum assistance.
Personal adjustment is achieved.	Patient verbalizes positive feelings related to adjustment to continent ileostomy.

 Diversion: Ileoanal Reservoir

Description and Rationale

The ileoanal reservoir is the procedure that provides the most normal mechanism for maintaining continency and the most natural method of evacuation. The ileoanal reservoir may be the first choice for patients with familial polyposis or ulcerative colitis. However, the patient must be an appropriate candidate for the ileoanal reservoir. Factors that should be assessed when evaluating a patient for this procedure include normal anorectal sphincter mechanism, minimal disease of the rectal mucosa, no evidence of cancer of the colon or Crohn's disease, absence of perianal disease, good physical condition, motivation, maturity, and age. It is important that the patient understand that it is a two- or three-stage procedure and that close follow-up is important throughout. A temporary ileostomy requires that the patient learn stomal care. The patient must also be aware that diarrhea may be a problem for 6 months to 1 year following the closure of the ileostomy. During this time, incontinence may occur but is usually minimal and is more common at night.[65]

Four types of procedures may be done to preserve normal bowel elimination. Each involves removal of the rectal mucosa. The first step in constructing the ileoanal reservoir is the mucosal stripping of the rectal segment to form a muscular cuff through which to bring the ileum. The rectal mucosectomy removes the mucosa and submucosa of the rectum for 4 to 6 cm above the dentate line. The rectal muscle layers and the anal sphincters are left intact while the primary disease is removed. During the abdominal colectomy, the rectosigmoid is removed with care to preserve the autonomic nerves on the posterior and lateral pelvic walls.

When no reservoir is constructed, diarrhea and incontinence are major problems. In 1978, Parks and Nicholls[59] added an ileoanal reservoir to the previously described rectal mucosectomy and ileorectal pull-through. The reservoir provided an important addition, a means by which the liquid effluent could be held until evacuation was appropriate. Thus the patient undergoing total colectomy also has rectal mucosectomy, construction of an ileal reservoir, ileoanal anastomosis, and a temporary ileostomy during the first stage of the procedure. During the second stage, the ileostomy is closed. The ileoanal reservoir may be constructed in three configurations. It is constructed from 30 to 50 cm of terminal ileum. In the S reservoir, three loops of ileum, approximately 12 to 15 cm in length, are aligned side by side. The reservoir is constructed by suturing the limbs and opening the segments, creating a pouch. A remaining 5 cm of ileum forms a spout that is sutured to the dentate line, completing the ileoanal portion of the procedure.

The J reservoir consists of two loops of ileum. The ileum is brought down to the rectal cuff and one limb is looped upward, creating a J shape. The loops are anastomosed in a side-by-side fashion by use of a stapler. The portion where the ileum curves upward is sutured to the anus and opened.

In the isoperistaltic reservoir, a single lumen of 25 to 30 cm of ileum is brought down and through the rectal cuff. The distal end is sutured to the anus, and the proximal end is closed. An ileostomy is performed. In the second stage the ileostomy is taken down and a lateral side-to-side ileal anastomosis is performed to create the reservoir.

The advantages of the ileoanal reservoir include the following:

Avoidance of a permanent cutaneous stoma
Avoidance of repeated stomal catheterizations
Avoidance of body image alterations
Decreased incidence of sexual dysfunction
Provision of a near-normal pattern of defecation

The disadvantages of the procedure are as follows:

Possible residual rectal mucosa
Regeneration of rectal mucosa
Problems with differentiation of gas, fluids, and solids
Tenesmus or fecal urgency
Nocturnal incontinence
Diarrhea
Perianal skin denudation

Contraindications and Cautions

1. Crohn's disease or cancer of the rectum
2. Obesity
3. Short mesentery
4. Decreased sphincter control

Preprocedural Nursing Care

1. Manometric studies of sphincter muscles are done before first and second stages of the procedure.
2. Before second stage, Gastrografin studies of reservoir are performed.

NURSING CARE

Nursing Assessment

Perineum

Skin erosion from mucus, frequent bowel movements, incontinence, pruritus, and perianal pain

Ileoanal Reservoir

Anal stenosis
Ischemia of reservoir
Rectal cuff abscess
Nocturnal leakage
Fecal incontinence
"Pouchitis" (sudden onset of high-volume diarrhea, cramping, and bleeding)

Abdominal Surgery

Adhesions; intestinal obstructions
Wound infection
Pain

Medical Plan

Medications

Bulk-forming agents
  Psyllium (Metamucil), 1 tsp prn for diarrhea
Antidiarrheal agents
  Loperamide (Imodium), 1-3 capsules po per day for diarrhea
Dermatologic agents
  Balneol cleansing agent
Antifungal agents
  Clotrimazole (Mycelex cream) 1%, prn for pruritus

General Management

Sitz bath

Nursing Dx & Intervention

Nursing Diagnosis	Nursing Intervention/Rationale
Stage 1: Ileostomy; Ileoanal Reservoir Constructed	
Fluid volume deficit (1)	• Assess patient for signs and symptoms of dehydration: dry mucous membranes, poor skin turgor, dry skin, decreased urinary output. • Monitor fecal output from ileostomy; 800 to 1200 ml is not uncommon. • Replace fluid and electrolytes as ordered. • Monitor daily weights.

Nursing Diagnosis	Nursing Intervention/Rationale
Impaired skin integrity	• Assess perianal skin daily. • Provide perianal skin care, since mucus contains residual enzymes, is copious, and is odorous. • Use skin sealants and vanishing creams before skin breaks down. • Instruct patient in wearing absorbent pads at night. • Irrigate the reservoir daily *to remove mucous drainage.* • Protect peristomal skin and maintain pouch seal.
Stage 2: Ileostomy Closure; Ileoanal Reservoir Functioning	
Impaired skin integrity	• Assess perianal skin after each bowel movement initially. • Avoid irritants such as nylon underwear, harsh or deodorant soaps, and fragrant toilet papers. • Cleanse skin with water or Domeboro (aluminum acetate) solution and cotton balls; dry with hair dryer. • Apply vanishing cream and cover with skin sealant. • Protect skin because of frequency of bowel movements and the residual enzymes present in the stool. • Provide sitz baths, Balneol cleansing agents, or Tucks pads *to help with perianal cleansing and to reduce pruritus.*
Diarrhea; bowel incontinence	• Assess frequency of bowel movements and consistency of stools. • Expect 10 to 20 bowel movements per day in early postoperative period; frequency slows to 6 to 12 per day as diet increases and averages 3 to 4 per day after 1 year. • Provide a regular diet *to help manage diarrhea.* • Provide psyllium (Metamucil) or loperamide (Imodium) as ordered as needed for diarrhea.

Patient Education

The following list applies to stage 1.

1. Teach patient ileostomy management (p. 862).
2. Teach patient Kegel exercises. Patient is instructed to practice these exercises to increase sphincter tone before the second stage of the procedure. The patient can be instructed to (a) hold a coin between the buttocks and tighten the sphincter, (b) tape the buttocks together and tighten the sphincter, or (c) practice walking with (a) or (b). The exercises of squeezing and relaxing the perianal muscles can also be done when the patient irrigates the reservoirs, which helps to assess continency.
3. Intubation and irrigation are done daily to remove mucus, which is a source of irritation and odor.
4. Perianal skin care is essential. Mucous drainage through the anus is expected and may be irritating. The skin can be protected by the use of skin sealants and vanishing creams. Minipads may be worn at night to absorb the drainage. Bloody mucous drainage may occur approximately 10 to 14 days after surgery when the sutures are dissolving.
5. Approximately 6 to 8 weeks after surgery, a Gastrografin x-ray film is taken to assess the reservoir, ruling out anastomotic leaks and checking the anatomic position of the reservoir. Gastrografin is water soluble and easier to evacuate from the reservoir than barium would be. Following the Gastrografin study, the reservoir should be irrigated with 100 to 200 ml of tap water.
6. Manometric studies of the sphincter muscle are repeated postoperatively.

The following list applies to stage 2.

1. For perianal skin care:
   a. Avoid nylon underwear, harsh or deodorant soaps, and fragrant toilet papers.
   b. Cleanse the perianal skin with water or Domeboro solution and cotton balls and dry with hair dryer.
   c. Protect the skin with vanishing creams, skin sealants, or ointments.
   d. Manage pruritus with sitz baths, Balneol cleansing agents, or Mycelex cream.
2. Frequency of bowel movements will drop to 6 to 12 per day for first year and then decrease to 3 or 4 per day. Diarrhea associated with flu or viral infection will increase number and amount of bowel movements.
3. Irrigation of reservoir daily may be necessary to reduce incidence of "pouchitis."

Evaluation

Patient Outcome	Data Indicating That Outcome is Reached
Body functions normally.	Abdominal incision heals. There are no signs of infection. Patient has three or four bowel movements per day.
Perianal skin is normal.	Perianal skin is intact with no signs of irritation or pruritus.

Liver Transplantation

Description and Rationale

Orthotopic liver transplantation (OLT) has been performed since the early 1960s and has gained national publicity and interest in the last few years. The success rate of these transplants has improved since the introduction of cyclosporine (CSA) as an immunosuppressive agent in 1979.[80] The procedure involves the removal of the recipient's liver (hepatectomy) and the transplantation of a donor liver. Sometimes children's livers are left in place; this is called heterotopic transplantation. A person may be on a waiting list for a liver transplant for an extended period, and approximately 30% of transplant candidates die before compatible organs are donated.[55]

Many families of transplant candidates have used publicity to encourage organ donation. Organ donor programs have been developed to facilitate the process of locating suitable donors. The Omnibus Budget Reconciliation Act of 1986 states that hospitals participating in Medicare programs must establish protocols to identify potential donors. Families of potential donors must be assured information about the options for donation of organs and tissue, as well as the right to refuse consent. The law also encourages discretion and sensitivity concerning the circumstances, views, and beliefs of the donor family. This law encourages organ and tissue donation when appropriate criteria are met.

Diagnostic groups that the NIH Consensus Development Conference (1984) has identified as potential candidates for orthotopic liver transplantation include extrahepatic biliary atresia, chronic active hepatitis (excluding antigen positive hepatitis B), primary biliary cirrhosis, hepatic vein thrombosis, sclerosing cholangitis, primary hepatic malignancy, cryptogenic cirrhosis, alcohol-related cirrhosis (rare), fulminant hepatic failure, and inborn errors of metabolism. A patient with one of these diagnoses may become a candidate for surgery when spontaneous stabilization or remission is improbable, when death is imminent, when irreversible damage to the central nervous system is inevitable, and when the quality of life is unacceptable.[55]

Frequently the transplant recipient is very ill at the time of surgery. The surgical procedure is long, and postoperative complications can be multiple and varied. The liver is responsible for many vital body functions such as metabolism of nutrients, detoxification of drugs, excretion of bile, and synthesis of coagulation factors, and many of the complications reflect these functions. The anatomic structure of the liver influences the surgical requirements of transplantation: four vascular and one biliary anastomoses must be performed.

Size of the donor liver is an important consideration, unlike with other organs. Recent research has used ultrasound imaging and computer tomography scans to measure the weight and volume of the diseased livers of candidates for liver transplantation. The results were found to be accurate when compared to the actual size and weight of the diseased livers removed. This technique may prove useful in the future for matching liver sizes between donors and recipients.[55] Another consideration in matching livers to recipients include ABO compatibility testing, which is sometimes performed, although children sometimes receive total pheresis to change blood type. HLA matching is not done. Orthotopic liver transplantation in pediatric patients has been limited because of the size match needed between donor and recipient. Some surgeons now reduce the size of the donor liver for pediatric patients.[24]

Drug therapy for immunosuppression and treatment of rejection episodes will continue to affect all transplantations. As new drugs are made available, changes will become apparent in the long-term management of all transplant patients. Advances in drug therapy, particularly in the area of immunosuppression, have improved the national graft survival rate to 70% at 1 year.

Contraindications and Cautions

1. An extensive workup and evaluation by the transplant team is required before transplantation. It may include a complete history and physical examination to establish a primary diagnosis and prognosis, evaluation of the psychologic, financial and family situation, determination of portal vein and hepatic artery patency, which is essential, and extent of disease if hepatic tumor is suspected. Numerous laboratory and diagnostic procedures are performed, such as coagulation studies, liver function studies, electrolytes, bilirubin, Hct, WBC, HB_sAg, pulmonary function studies, urine studies, ultrasound, ERCP, and MRI.
2. Percutaneous transhepatic cholangiography with brushings may be used to rule out cholangiocarcinoma in patients with sclerosing cholangitis, since this is a contraindication to transplantation.
3. Patients and families should be provided with ongoing support and evaluations as they make the decision to undergo this major procedure, which requires a lengthy recovery. An evaluation of the educational needs is also made to provide the patient and family with the information needed to manage these life changes. Most transplant teams have nurse coordinators who follow patients and families from evaluation through transplantation and postoperatively.

Preprocedural Nursing Care

1. These patients usually are extremely ill and require expert nursing care to manage the primary diagnosis and any existing complications.
2. Inform patient about the specific procedure and the rationale for the diagnostic procedure.
3. Prepare patient for the intensive care unit and for any reverse isolation planned for the postoperative period (used if patient's WBC is less than 100).
4. Inform patient that drains and tubes will be present after surgery.

Medical Plan

Medications

Medication dosages are based on dry body weight in kilograms and vary based on physician and individual central protocol.

- Intraoperative
  - Ampicillin, 1 g IV (sometimes given)
  - Claforin, 1 g IV (sometimes given)
  - Cyclosporine, 0.5 mg/kg IV by continuous drip
- Postoperative
  - Cyclosporine, 2 mg/kg IV or nasogastric q8h; changed to po (based on GI function, T tube); bile refeeding may be done because 94% of cyclosporine is excreted in the bile
  - Solumedrol or methylprednisolone in daily decreasing IV doses, changed to po (based on GI function, T tube)
  - Ampicillin, 1 g IV q6h for 5 d
  - Claforin, 1 g IV q6h for 5 d
  - Mycostatin, 5 ml swish and swallow qid after nasogastric tube removed
  - Mycostatin vaginal suppository tid for female patients
- Clinical rejection (based on biopsy)
  - Solumedrol or methylprednisolone (dosage based on body weight); repeat postoperatively and taper
  - Antilymphocyte globulin (ATGAM), 10-30 mg/kg over several h, although Minnesota Anti-Lymphocyte Globulin (MALG) is used more frequently, for 10-14 d after test dose administered; premedicate patient with Benadryl 10-25 mg IM, methylprednisolone 25-50 mg, and Tylenol by suppository to reduce drug reaction
  - OKT-3 (Monoclonal antithymocyte globulin), 5-10 mg IV push, 1 ml over 1 min (OKT-3 is given only if patient has gained no more than 3 kg and has had a clear chest roentgenogram for 1 wk)

General Management

- Mechanical ventilation for 24 to 48 hours, then oxygen via mask or nasal prongs
- If patient has been encephalopathic preoperatively, intracranial pressure monitoring is done until patient is awake
- Endotracheal suction while ventilated as needed
- Central venous pressure or pulmonary capillary wedge pressure monitoring
- T tube
- Nasogastric drainage
- One or two Jackson-Pratt drains
- Intravenous fluids

NURSING CARE

Nursing Assessment

Circulatory System

- Shock and circulatory failure associated with the potential large volume of blood loss intraoperatively
- Monitor coagulation factors
- Hemorrhage

Fluid and Electrolytes

- Nausea, vomiting, diarrhea, and nasogastric suctioning may affect fluid and electrolyte balance; replacement K^+ is always given
- Serum potassium shifts in early postoperative period
- Glucose shifts in early postoperative period
- Monitor Ca^{++}, alkalosis (occasionally HCl drip is administered), acidosis

Abdominal Incision, Surgical Site

- Hemorrhage
- Drainage during first 24 hours (replaced with plasma)
- Signs of wound infection: redness, pain, edema, drainage
- Wound dehiscence or evisceration
- Clotted hepatic artery or portal vein

Bowel Function

- Assess bowel sounds, presence of gas, bowel movement
- Constipation, diarrhea

Mental Status

Monitor to evaluate liver function and evidence of increased cerebral pressure, since intracranial bleeding is a major complication. Notify physician of any of the following:

- Decreased intellectual function
- Altered state of consciousness
- Mild to moderate EEG abnormalities
- Altered behavior
- Asterixis
- Agitation
- Drowsiness
- Confusion

Respiratory System

- Right-sided pleural effusions and atelectasis may occur (even if thoracotomy is not performed during surgery) secondary to location of liver and concomitant surgical site
- Assess respiratory function: bilateral breath sounds, chest expansion during inspiration, unassisted respiratory rate
- Dyspnea and hypoxia (early signs of *Pneumocystis* pneumonia and cytomegalovirus [CMV])

Urinary System

Decrease or cessation of urinary output secondary to cyclosporine toxicity or acute renal failure

Voiding problems following removal of indwelling catheter

Dysuria, urgency, frequency, hematuria

Rejection

Only way to confirm rejection in this population is with biopsy

Malaise, fever (not always seen secondary to prednisone and cyclosporine), graft tenderness (rarely occurs), diminished graft function as evidenced by decreased bile output

Increased bilirubin and transaminase levels

T tube biliary drainage thinner and lighter in color

Infection

Assess carefully for early signs of infection: fever, herpes virus infections (oral, esophageal, or gastric), *Candida* or CMV, pulmonary infiltrate *(Legionella, Pneumocystis),* wound or urinary tract symptoms

Nursing Dx & Intervention

Nursing Diagnosis	Nursing Intervention/Rationale
Ineffective breathing pattern	• While endotracheal tube is in place (usually about 24 hours), suction every 2 hours or as needed. Turn every 2 hours and provide postural drainage *to decrease risk of pleural effusion and atelectasis postoperatively.* A right thoracotomy may be performed to provide adequate exposure of the liver and portal veins, but the patient is at risk even if thoracotomy is not performed. • Provide oxygen therapy as ordered. • Auscultate the chest for abnormal breath sounds and assess for adventitious sounds at least every hour. • Assist patient out of bed as soon as possible, within 24 hours. • Observe mucous membranes and nail beds *to assess for cyanosis.*
Altered renal, cerebral, cardiopulmonary, gastrointestinal, and peripheral tissue perfusion	• Monitor vital signs every 15 minutes until patient is stable and then every hour. Monitor intake and output every hour (include all drainage tubes: nasogastric, Jackson-Pratt [J-P], Foley, T tube). • Monitor and document any incisional drainage. • Monitor hourly central venous pressure, pulmonary artery pressures, pulmonary capillary wedge pressure, and right arterial pressure *because hemodynamic instability is a potential problem in the early postoperative period.* Intraoperative blood loss may be extensive. • Observe carefully for signs of transfusion reactions, since patients may receive multiple units of blood during and after surgery. Fresh frozen plasma may also be ordered. • Assess for signs of shock: hypotension, tachycardia, peripheral vasoconstriction, oliguria. • Weigh patient daily. • Monitor serum electrolytes, CBC, prothrombin time, partial thromboplastin time, platelets, BUN, creatinine, bilirubin (total/direct), SGOT, SGPT, alkaline phosphatase, and albumin daily. • Assess patient in early postoperative period for signs of hyperkalemia (T-wave elevation and widening of QRS complex on ECG) and hypokalemia (U-wave on ECG, ectopic beats, leg cramps). *Serum potassium levels shifts may occur during this period because (Collins) preservative solution in the transported donor liver is high in potassium and enters the recipient's body following revascularization. Although the liver is flushed completely and K^+ should not be high, patients receive diuretics to keep urine output high and sometimes the K^+ will decrease from increased urine output.* • Assess for signs of glucose shifts *resulting from the inability of the transplanted liver to control glucose metabolism in the early postoperative period and from steroid-induced diabetes and symptoms of hyperglycemia:* lethargy, decreased response to stimuli; hypoglycemia: glycosuria, osmotic diuresis, changes in mental status. • Test urine for glucose and ketones. • Monitor closely the urine output, serum creatinine level, and urine electrolyte levels, *since a change in renal function is an early sign of nephrotoxicity associated with cyclosporine use.*
Potential for infection	• Institute protective isolation if the WBC is less than 100, *since patient is immunosuppressed and will be unable to combat infections.* • Provide meticulous care of the mouth, skin, and perineal area *to prevent breakdown.* • Clean sites thoroughly with povidone-iodine when entering lines, especially central lines, *to prevent introduction of bacteria.* • Monitor body temperature. Do not take rectal temperatures, *since the mucous membranes are more fragile and can be irritated, leading to an infection* (although rectal probes may be used in some intensive care units). • Routine cultures of body fluids may be ordered. If the temperature increases (greater than

Nursing Diagnosis	Nursing Intervention/Rationale
	all drains, tubes, open wounds, and indwelling lines. Frequently the organisms cultured include cytomegalovirus, *Candida, Legionella,* or *Pneumocystis,* although any other viral or bacterial organism may be cultured. • Additional diagnostic tests for signs of infection include lumbar puncture, transhepatic cholangiogram or ERCP, hepatitis screen, ultrasonography, CT scan, and an indium scan, with tagged white cells most commonly used. • Observe wounds for erythema, purulent drainage, and odor. • Observe drains and tubes for increased or decreased drainage, changes in the type or color of drainage, and presence of odor.
Patient problem: potential rejection of donor organ	• Assess for signs of rejection: malaise, fever, graft tenderness, and diminished graft function (increased transaminases, increased bilirubin, elevated clotting times, decreased platelet counts, and jaundice). • Assess for signs of cyclosporine side effects: hypertension, hypertrichosis, and gingival hyperplasia. • Assess for signs of cyclosporine toxicity: tremulousness and nephrotoxicity. • Monitor serum cyclosporine levels every 1 to 3 days to maintain a level of 250 to 350 mg/dl.[79] • Assess patient for signs and symptoms of side effects of OKT-3 or other drugs used to treat rejection (ATGAM, MALG, prednisone): chills, fever, development of ARDS and anaphylaxis, hypotension, chest pain, nausea, vomiting, diarrhea, pulmonary edema (if patient is fluid overloaded, no OKT-3 should be administered), joint pains, shortness of breath, and hypotension. If acute respiratory symptoms occur, discontinuation of the drug is necessary.
Potential impaired skin integrity	• Assess patient's skin daily *to identify any areas of redness or potential breakdown.* • Provide pressure-relief mattress based on patient's body size and initial skin assessment: a foam pad may be inadequate, since the patient may be on bed rest for an extended period. • Turn at least every 2 hours and assist out of bed as soon as possible, at least within 24 hours, *to improve circulation.* • Use care in applying any tape to and removing it from the skin. A liquid skin barrier can be used before the application of tapes. A solid wafer barrier may be used around a wound and Montgomery straps applied to the wafer *to facilitate changing abdominal dressings.* Leaking drains or T tubes can be managed with a sterile pouching system if necessary *to protect the skin.*
Pain	• No pain medication may be ordered, *since the signs and symptoms of mental status changes with liver dysfunction may be masked by pain medication. In addition, the liver is responsible for detoxifying most drugs, and if the liver is not functioning well, the half-life of drugs may be prolonged.* If pain medication is ordered, carefully assess patient's neurologic status between sedations. Avoid use of opiates (morphine sulfate), *since morphine may cause vasodilation and decreased blood flow to the liver.* • Promote a calm, quiet environment and plan nursing care *to facilitate periods of rest.* • Provide diversion for patient *to assist in dealing with pain or discomfort.*
Patient problem: acceptance of donor organ; coping, family: potential for growth	• Encourage patient and family to discuss feelings regarding the transplantation. • Provide resources available to patient and family *to assist in the perioperative period.* This support will need to be continued after discharge from the hospital. Suggest participation in support groups.

Patient Education

Patient education can be done effectively on a one-to-one or a group basis.

1. Instruct the patient on routine care following any major surgery: ambulate at regular times; rest frequently; increase activities slowly; keep incision dry; report any signs of redness, pain, or drainage; avoid heavy lifting; keep appointments for follow-up visits.
2. Provide written instructions on medication schedule and side effects.
3. Provide written instructions on signs and symptoms that should be reported to the physician.
4. Provide written instructions on any procedures for at-home care. Make sure that the patient has had an opportunity to practice the procedures before discharge.

Evaluation

Patient Outcome	Data Indicating That Outcome is Reached
Respiratory function is normal.	Patient has unassisted ventilation with respiratory rate of 14 to 30 breaths/minute. There are bilateral equal breath sounds with clear lung fields.
Hemodynamic state is normal.	Vital signs are stable. Hematocrit is normal. Electrolyte levels are normal.
Renal function is normal.	Urine output is adequate. Renal function studies are within normal range.
Liver function is normal.	Liver function studies are within normal range. There are no signs of rejection. Coagulation studies are within normal limits.
There is no infection.	Abdominal incision is healed. There is no drainage or signs of infection. Cultures are negative.
Orthotopic liver transplantation is successful.	There are no signs or symptoms of rejection of the organ or of infection. Patient is maintained on low dosages of immunosuppressive drugs.
Skin integrity is maintained.	There are no signs of skin breakdown.

References

1. American Cancer Society: Cancer facts and figures, New York, 1985, The Society.
2. Appelbaum PC et al: Intestinal bacteria in patients with tropical sprue, S Afr Med J 57:1081, 1980.
3. Arhan P et al: Viscoelastic properties of the rectal wall in Hirschsprung's disease, J Clin Invest 62:82, 1978.
4. Beahrs OH et al: Indwelling ileostomy valve device, Am J Surg 141:111, 1981.
5. Bolt RJ et al: The digestive system, New York, 1983, John Wiley & Sons.
6. Brandt L: Gastrointestinal disorders of the elderly, New York, 1984, Raven Press.
7. Broadwell DC and Jackson BS: Principles of ostomy care, St Louis, 1982, The CV Mosby Co.
8. Buls JG and Goldberg SM: Surgical options in ulcerative colitis, Postgrad Med 74:175, 1983.
9. Bussey HJR: Familial polyposis coli, Baltimore, 1975, Johns Hopkins University Press.
10. Cancer statistics, Cancer 31:13, 1981.
11. Canty TG, Self T, and Bonaldi L: The lateral reservoir technique of ileal endorectal pull-through for ulcerative colitis and familial polyposis in children, J Pediatr Surg 18:862, 1983.
12. Cawson RA: Essentials of dental surgery and pathology, ed 3, London, 1978, Churchill Livingstone.
13. Chen Ch-L et al: Biliary sludge-cast formation following liver transplantation, Hepatogastroenterology 35:22, 1988.
14. Cohen S: Clinical gastroenterology: a problem-oriented approach, New York, 1983, John Wiley & Sons.
15. Cohen S: The facts about IBS, DDEIC publication, Bethesda, Md, 1984, National Institute of Health.
16. Connell AM, Jones FA, and Rowlands, EN: Motility of the pelvic colon: abdominal pain associated with colonic motility after meals, Gut 6:105, 1965.
17. Davenport HW: Physiology of the digestive tract, ed 5, Chicago, 1982, Year Book Medical Publishers.
18. Delpre G et al: HLA antigens in ulcerative colitis and Crohn's disease in Israel, Gastroenterology 78:1452, 1980.
19. Department of Health and Human Services: Organ transplantation, issues and recommendations, Report of the Task Force on Organ Transplantation, United States, Washington, DC, 1986, US Government Printing Office.
20. Donald PJ: The oral cavity. In Bolt JR et al: The digestive system, New York, 1983, John Wiley & Sons.
21. Dworken HF: Gastroenterology: pathophysiology and clinical applications, Boston, 1982, Butterworth.
22. Eastwood GL, editor: Core textbook of gastroenterology, Philadelphia, 1984, JB Lippincott Co.
23. Emond J et al: Liver transplantation and the management of fulminant hepatic failure, Gastroenterology, 94:A537, 1988.
24. Emond J et al: Application of reduced-sized liver transplants (RLT) in pediatric recipients, Gastroenterology 94:A538, 1988.
25. Esquivel C et al: Transplantation for primary biliary cirrhosis, Gastroenterology 94:1207, 1988.
26. Farmer RG, Achkar E, and Fleshler B: Clinical gastroenterology, New York, 1983, Raven Press.
27. Fielding JF: A year in outpatients with irritable bowel syndrome, Lancet 2:753, 1969.
28. Fonkalsrud EW: Endorectal ileoanal anastomosis with isoperistaltic after colectomy and mucosal proctectomy, Ann Surg 199:158, 1984.
29. Gerber A: The Kock continent ileal reservoir: an alternative to conventional urostomy, J Enterostomal Ther 12:15, 1985.
30. Gilat T et al: Ulcerative colitis in the Jewish population of Tel Aviv Jafo. I. Epidemiology, Gastroenterology 66:757, 1974.
31. Goldberg SM, Gordon PH, and Nivatvongs S: Essentials of anorectal surgery, Philadelphia, 1980, JB Lippincott Co.
32. Goldman SL and Rombeau JL: The continent ileostomy: a collective review, Dis Col Rect 21:594, 1978.
33. Gomez J and Dally P: Psychologically mediated abdominal pain in surgical and medical outpatient clinics, Br Med J 1:1451, 1977.
34. Guyton AC: Textbook of medical physiology, ed 6, Philadelphia, 1981, WB Saunders Co.
35. Guyton AC: Human physiology and mechanisms of disease, ed 3, Philadelphia, 1982, WB Saunders Co.
36. Hodgson HJF and Bloom SR: Gastrointestinal and hepatobiliary cancer, Boston, 1983, Butterworths.
37. Hukuhara T, Kotani S, and Sato G: Effects of destruction of intramural ganglion cells on colon motility: possible genesis of congenital megacolon, Jpn J Physiol 11:635, 1961.
38. Johnson LR, editor: Gastrointestinal physiology, ed 3, St Louis, 1986, The CV Mosby Co.
39. Joossens JV and Geboers J: Nutrition and gastric cancer, Proc Nutr Soc 40:37, 1981.
40. King SA: Quality of life: the continent ileostomy, Ann Surg 1982:29, 1975.
41. Kinney MD et al: AACN's clinical reference for critical care nursing, New York, 1981, McGraw-Hill Book Co.
42. Kirsner JB: Observations of the medical treatment of inflammatory bowel disease, JAMA 243:557, 1980.
43. Klein K, Stenzel P, and Katon RM: Pouch ileitis: report of a case with severe systemic manifestations, J Clin Gastroenterol 5:149, 1983.
44. Klipstein FA: Sprue and subclinical malabsorption in the tropics, Lancet 1:277, 1979.
45. Kock NG, Myrvold HE, and Nilsson LO: Progress report on the continent ileostomy, World J Surg 4:143, 1980.
46. Lauren P: The two histologic main types of gastric carcinoma: diffuse and so-called intestinal type carcinoma. An attempt at a histo-clinical classification, Acta Pathol Microbiol Scand 64:31, 1965.

47. Lindeman RJ et al: Ulcerative colitis and intestinal salmonellosis, Am J Med Sci 254:855, 1967.
48. MacDonald WC, Dobbins WO, and Rubin CE: Studies of the familial nature of celiac sprue using biopsy of the small intestine, N Engl J Med 272:448, 1965.
49. Mendeloff AI et al: Illness experiences and life stresses in patients with irritable colon and with ulcerative colitis, N Engl J Med 282:14, 1970.
50. Miller C et al: Orthotopic liver transplantation for massive hepatic lymphangiomatosis, Surgery 103:490, 1988.
51. Ming SC: Gastric carcinoma: a pathological classification, Cancer 39:2475, 1977.
52. Monk M: An epidemiological study of ulcerative colitis and regional enteritis among adults in Baltimore. III. Psychological and possible stress-precipitating factors, J Chron Dis 22:565, 1970.
53. Morowitz DA and Kisner JB: Ileostomy in ulcerative colitis: a questionnaire study of 1803 patients, Am J Surg 141:370, 1981.
54. National Institute of Arthritis, Diabetes, and Digestive and Kidney Diseases (NIADDK): Second annual report, DHHS, PHS, NIH Pub No 83-2493, Washington, DC, 1988, US Government Printing Office.
55. National Institutes of Health Consensus Development Conference Statement: Liver transplantation, Hepatology 4:107s, 1984.
56. Neurcomer AD et al: Tolerance to lactose deficiency in American Indians, Gastroenterology 74:44, 1975.
57. Nord HJ and Brady PG: Critical care gastroenterology, New York, 1982, Churchill Livingstone.
58. Oster J: Recurrent abdominal pains, headache, and limb pain in children, Pediatrics 50:429, 1972.
59. Parks AG and Nicholls RJ: Proctocolectomy without ileostomy for ulcerative colitis, Br Med J 2:85, 1978.
60. Pemberton JH et al: A continent ileostomy device, Ann Surg 197:618, 1983.
61. Pena AS et al: Genetic bases of gluten-sensitive enteropathy, Gastroenterology 75:230, 1978.
62. Postier RG, O'Malley V, and Pruitt L: Continent-preserving operations for ulcerative colitis and multiple polyposis, J Enterostomal Ther 11:237, 1984.
63. Prevalence of selected chronic digestive conditions, U.S., 1975. Vital health and statistics. National health survey, DHHS Pub No PHS 79-1558, Washington, DC, 1979, National Center for Health Statistics.
64. Ravitch MM and Sabiston DC: Anal ileostomy with preservation of the sphincter: a proposed operation in patients requiring colectomy for benign lesions, Surg Gynecol Obstet 84:1095, 1947.
65. Rolstad BS: Ileoanal reservoir: functional results and management, South Med J 77:1535, 1984.
66. Sachar DB, Auslander MO, and Walfish JS: Aetiological theories of inflammatory bowel disease, Clin Gastroenterol 9:231, 1980.
67. Sales DM and Kirsner JB: The prognosis of inflammatory bowel disease, Arch Intern Med 143:294, 1983.
68. Santulli TV, Kiesewetter WB, and Bill AH: Anorectal anomalies: a suggested international classification, J Pediatr Surg 5:281, 1970.
69. Schiff L and Schiff ER: Diseases of the liver, Philadelphia, 1982, JB Lippincott Co.
70. Schrock TR: Complications of continent ileostomy, Am J Surg 138:162, 1979.
71. Sernka TJ and Jacobson ED: Gastrointestinal physiology: the essentials, ed 2, Baltimore, 1983, Williams & Wilkins Co.
72. Shanbour LL and Jacobson ED: Digitalis and the mesenteric circulation, Am J Digestive Dis 17:826, 1972.
73. Shearman DJC and Finlayson NDC: Diseases of the gastrointestinal tract and liver, New York, 1982, Churchill Livingstone.
74. Simons FJ: New light on ethnic differences in adult lactose intolerances, Am J Dig Dis 18:595, 1973.
75. Sleisenger MH and Fordtran JS: Gastrointestinal disease, ed 3, Philadelphia, 1983, WB Saunders Co.
76. Smith L, Friend WG, and Medwel SJ: The superior mesenteric artery: the critical factor in pouch pull-through procedure, Dis Col Rect 27:741, 1984.
77. Soave F: A new surgical technique for the treatment of Hirschsprung's disease, Surgery 56:1007, 1964.
78. Spiro HM: Clinical gastroenterology, New York, 1983, Macmillan Publishing Co, Inc.
79. Spisso J, Clark B, and Wallace T: The postoperative liver transplant patient, Crit Care Nurse 8:53, 1988.
80. Starzl T et al: Homotransplantation of the liver in humans, Surg Gynecol Obstet 117:659, 1963.
81. Stroehlein JR and Romsdahl MM: Gastrointestinal cancer, New York, 1981, Raven Press.
82. Swenson O et al: Diagnosis of congenital megacolon, J Pediatr Surg 8:587, 1973.
83. Texter EC: The aging gut, New York, 1983, Masson Publishing Co.
84. Thompson WHF: The nature of hemorrhoids, Br J Surg 62:542, 1975.
85. Utsunomiya J et al: Total colectomy, mucosal proctectomy, and ileoanal anastomosis, Dis Col Rect 23:459, 1980.
86. Watanabe H et al: Gastric lesions in familial adenomatosis coli, Hum Pathol 9:269, 1978.
87. Watt R: The J-pouch, unpublished patient education material, Stanford, Calif, 1985, Stanford University Medical Center.
88. Weill FS: Ultrasonography of digestive diseases, St Louis, 1980, The CV Mosby Co.
89. Wolstenholme GEW and Cameron MP, editors: Intestinal biopsy, Boston, 1962, Little, Brown & Co.
90. Zakim D and Boyer TD: Hepatology: a textbook of liver disease, Philadelphia, 1982, WB Saunders Co.

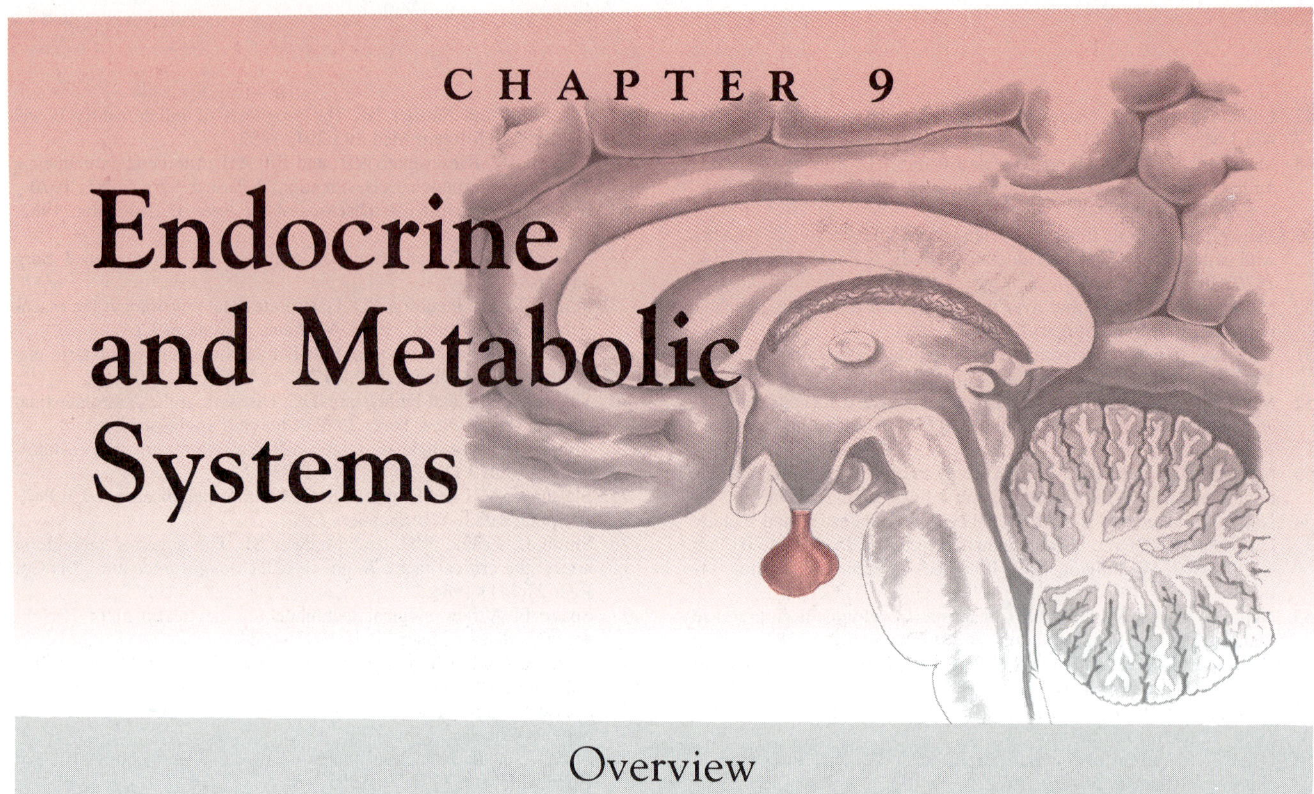

CHAPTER 9

Endocrine and Metabolic Systems

Overview

The endocrine system is a widely diversified system of glands, hormones, intermediate metabolites, and cellular responses. The functional responsibilities of this system include growth, development, reproduction, production of energy, fluid and electrolyte balance, and a response to stress. A single gland may hold primary responsibility for a particular function, but the interrelationships between and among glandular functions are called the endocrine and metabolic systems.

The hypothalamus and anterior pituitary gland work together to regulate the endocrine system. These two very small organs mediate essential functions such as growth, thyroid balance, and fertility. The hypothalamus coordinates central nervous system input with hormone release. It regulates the anterior lobe of the pituitary gland, which in turn directs target organ release of specific hormones (e.g., release of cortisol from the adrenal glands).

The posterior lobe of the pituitary gland is known as the neurohypophysis. It secretes two hormones, vasopressin (antidiuretic hormone) and oxytocin. These hormones are responsible for the control of water balance and the milk letdown reflex, respectively.[103]

The thyroid gland is one of the largest endocrine glands. A well-functioning and healthy thyroid gland is essential for normal growth and development and maintenance of metabolic stability in the adult.[32] Thyroid disease is relatively common.[32] Special diagnostic problems may occur because a multiplicity of metabolic processes are affected by the thyroid hormones. Thyroid hormones, for example, influence the concentration and activity of numerous enzymes, as well as the metabolism of substrates, vitamins, and minerals.[103] The secretion and degradation rates of all other hormones, as well as their target tissue responses, are also affected by the thyroid hormones. For these reasons, thyroid hormones affect all tissues and organ systems.[103]

Parathyroid glands regulate calcium exchange through three major hormones: parathyroid hormone, calcitonin, and $1,25(OH)_2D_3$ (vitamin D). Calcium is regulated by a negative-feedback mechanism involving the intestines, kidneys, bones, and mammary glands during lactation. Homeostasis of calcium ion concentration is essential for bone formation, transmission of nerve impulses, maintenance of cardiac and skeletal muscle contractility, and efficient blood clotting. Calcium levels are maintained in equilibrium with phosphate levels for storage and release of energy, metabolism of carbohydrates and lipids, and regulation of serum pH.

The adrenal glands are two of the major endocrine organs in the body. Although small, they are vital to human life.[26] The condition of the adrenal cortex determines how effectively the body can respond to stress, trauma, and infections, as well as perform carbohydrate, fat, and protein metabolism. The adrenal medulla is part of the sympathetic nervous system. Homeostasis is maintained during physical and emotional stress in part by the release of catecholamines from the chromaffin cells of the adrenal medulla. Catecholamines are hormones that evoke an adrenergic, metabolic, and glycemic response from the body systems. The central nervous system also secretes catecholamines, making survival possible without adrenal medullary activity.[45]

The pancreas functions primarily as an exocrine gland, secreting enzymes for the digestion of food. Two percent of the gland (islets of Langerhans) has an endocrine function, secreting glucagon, insulin, gastrin, and somatostatin. The endocrine role of the pancreas was first demonstrated in 1886 when Minkowski and Von Mering produced diabetes in a dog by total pancreatectomy.

The gonads are the endocrine glands responsible for production of the reproductive (sex) cells. They are also the body's major contributor of the sex hormones. The male gonads, the testes, secrete testosterone in utero, which is necessary for sex differentiation of the fetus. The female gonads, the ovaries, primarily secrete estrogen. Through direct stimulation by the pituitary gland, gonadal hormones initiate pubertal development. Likewise, they take the child through puberty into adulthood, sustaining the development of secondary sexual characteristics and fertility.[52]

Genetic disorders may result in a direct alteration in the formation of a gland or the release and effect of a hormone. More often, however, genetic alterations result in problems of intermediary metabolism.

Anatomy, Physiology, and Related Pathophysiology

Hypothalamus and Anterior Pituitary Gland

The hypothalamus is part of the cerebrum of the brain and is located beneath the cerebral hemisphere on each side of the third ventricle. It is connected to the thalamus above by neural tissue and to the pituitary gland below by the pituitary stalk (Figure 9-1).[74] The hypothalamus is approximately 6 cm in diameter.[65]

The pituitary gland is located in an indentation of the sphenoid bone, the sella turcica, at the base of the brain. The gland is ovoid and approximately 1 cm in diameter. It has two parts: the anterior lobe (75%) and the posterior lobe (25%). Phylogenetically, the anterior pituitary gland (the adenohypophysis) originates from an outpouching of the roof of the mouth.[74] It is the anterior pituitary gland that is involved in the regulation of the majority of endocrine functions.

The hypothalamus regulates autonomic nervous system and endocrine functions.[74] With neural regulation, it affects multiple diverse functions such as body temperature, sweating, gastrointestinal secretion and motility, blood pressure, sleep, and response to pleasure and pain. The hypothalamus influences fluid and electrolyte balance and cell metabolism by the production and release of hypothalamic hormones, which directly affect the pituitary gland. These hormones are known as releasing hormones (if a chemical structure has been identified) or releasing factors (if the chemical structure is unknown).[98] The hypothalamic-stimulating hormones are corticotropin-releasing hormone (CRH), growth hormone–releasing factor (GRF), thyrotropin-releasing hormone (TRH), and gonadotropin-releasing hormone (GnRH, LHRH). The hypothalamic-inhibiting factors and hormones are melanocyte-inhibiting factor (MIF), prolactin-inhibiting factor (PIF), and somatostatin (also known as growth hormone–inhibiting hormone).[43]

The hypothalamic hormones travel down the pituitary stalk through the portal blood supply to their target, the anterior pituitary gland. They cause the pituitary gland to release specific hormones: luteinizing hormone (LH), follicle-stimulating hormone (FSH), growth hormone (GH), prolactin (PRL), adrenocorticotropic hormone (ACTH), thyroid-stimulating hormone (TSH), and melanocyte-stimulating hormone (MSH). These hormones travel through the bloodstream to their target tissues.

Figure 9-1 Anatomy of the hypothalamus and pituitary.

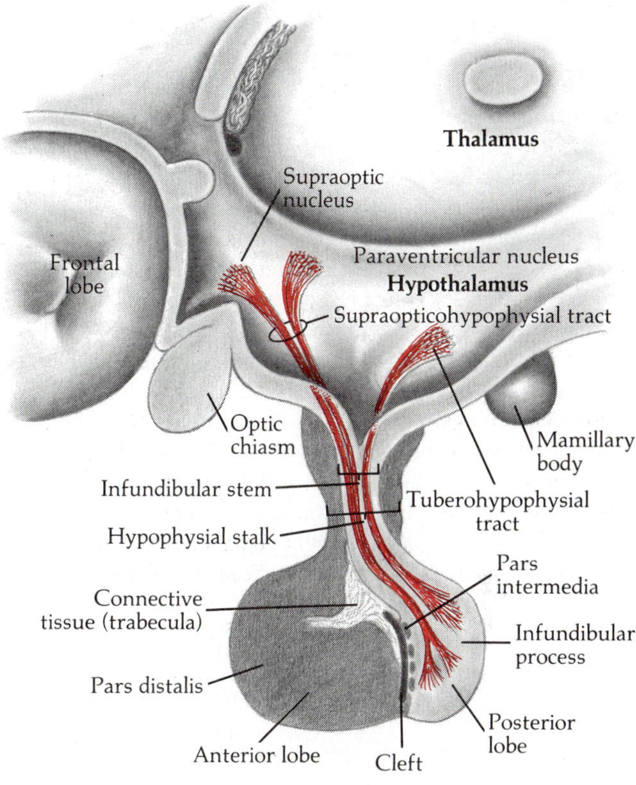

The physiologic effects of GH are multiple and diverse, whereas PRL, MSH, LH, and FSH cause more specific tissue responses. GH influences the body's growth and metabolism. It promotes bone growth, "stimulates protein anabolism, promotes lipolysis, enhances absorption of dietary calcium, and antagonizes the action of insulin."[45] PRL is responsible for breast development and lactation. MSH stimulates pigmentation activity in the skin. LH and FSH are responsible for the development of secondary sexual characteristics as well as fertility. LH and FSH are released in a cyclic, pulsatile fashion in both sexes; this release is necessary for normal gonadal function.

The three tropic hormones directly affecting gonadal function are FSH, LH, and PRL. In males, LH and FSH bind to specific receptors in the testes, Leydig's cells and Sertoli cells, respectively. LH stimulates maturation of Leydig's cells and stimulates synthesis and secretion of the gonadal steroid testosterone. Testosterone and FSH facilitate LH effects by helping develop LH receptors in Leydig's cells. Studies suggest that PRL and FSH may also help androgen synthesis in Leydig's cells.[32]

FSH was originally thought to be the hormone responsible for spermatogenesis. However, LH and testosterone both are needed for full spermatogenesis.[32] FSH is necessary for the conversion of spermatogonia into sperm, and testosterone is postulated to be necessary for final maturation.[59]

The gonadotropin release is regulated by a negative-feedback system from testicular secretions. Testosterone has a negative feedback on LH secretion. Estradiol, produced through testosterone, has also been found to inhibit LH secretion.[32] A testicular hormone, inhibin, produced in the Sertoli cells, has been identified as the negative feedback for FSH. These negative feedbacks appear not only at the pituitary level but at the hypothalamic level as well. Tissues in the hypothalamus have a high affinity for testosterone and estradiol, and these both inhibit GnRH secretion.[4]

Communication along the hypothalamus-pituitary-target tissue axis is maintained through feedback mechanisms to control the fluctuating hormone levels. The feedback system between the hypothalamus and pituitary gland is known as a short-loop, negative-feedback mechanism.[26] With this mechanism, high levels of pituitary hormones cause the hypothalamus to decrease the release of its hormones, which in turn causes levels of pituitary hormones to decrease. The target organs also communicate by a long-loop, negative-feedback mechanism to regulate hormone release from the pituitary gland and the hypothalamus (Figure 9-2).

Figure 9-2 Negative-feedback mechanism.
Adapted from information in Muthe[74] and Williams.[103]

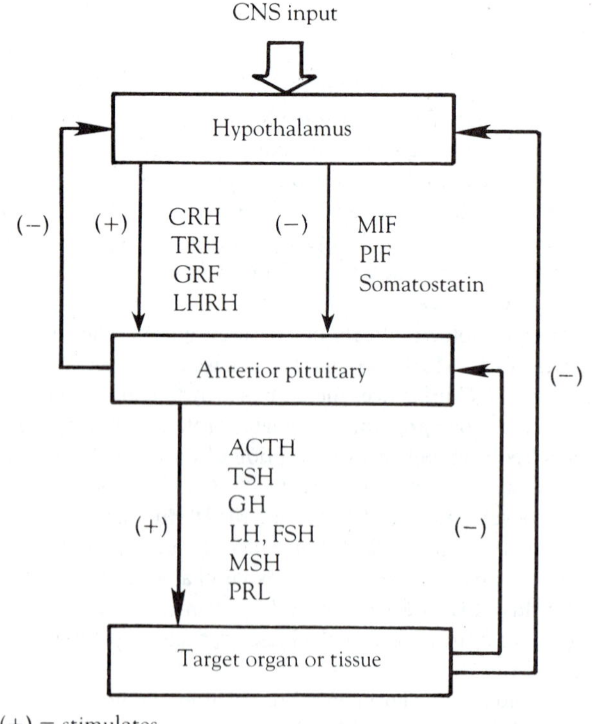

Another factor that affects circulating hormone levels is an intrinsic rhythm of the release of pituitary hormones. This is probably controlled by the central nervous system through the hypothalamus.[103] One example of this rhythmicity is the sharp release of GH, LH (during puberty), and PRL from the pituitary gland 1 hour after the onset of deep sleep.[103] Another example is the diurnal variation of ACTH secretion. The secretion of hypothalamic hormones is also affected by psychoneurologic components, such as stress.

The neurohypophysis secretes two hormones: vasopressin and oxytocin. Vasopressin is the primary regulator of water metabolism in human beings. Oxytocin is responsible for the milk letdown phenomenon and stimulates the contraction of uterine muscles in labor. Neurogenic reflexes from the nipple travel through the spinal cord and midbrain to the hypothalamus. The neurohypophysis then releases oxytocin, which stimulates contractions of mammary myoepithelium; this results in the ejection of milk. Both of these hormones are synthesized in the supraoptic and paraventricular nuclei of the hypothalamus. They are transported along the neurohypophyseal tract to the posterior lobe of the pituitary gland, where they are stored. Rapid release of these hormones occurs in response to a variety of stimuli.[103] Oxytocin may be inhibited by emotional stress, pain, or fright. Oxytocin release is stimulated by a crying baby, sexual excitement, and orgasm. Although oxytocin may be used to induce labor and control obstetric hemorrhage, its physiologic role in initiating and maintaining normal labor is unclear. Patients with complete hypophysectomy seem to progress through labor normally.[26,103]

Vasopressin conserves water in the renal collecting duct; thus it is also known as the antidiuretic hormone (ADH). ADH causes an increase in the permeability of the renal collecting ducts to water, thereby increasing water retention and decreasing urine output. The production of ADH in the hypothalamus and the release of ADH from the posterior pituitary gland are determined by plasma osmolality and extracellular fluid volume. The secretion of ADH is regulated by three factors:

Osmoreceptors in the median eminence of the hypothalamus respond to changes in plasma osmolality. Increases in osmolality stimulate the release of ADH; decreases in osmolality inhibit ADH release.

Volume receptors in the left atrium and great vessels inhibit ADH release when vascular volume is increased.

Baroreceptors in the carotid sinus and aortic arch stimulate ADH release when blood pressure is decreased.[103]

ADH secretion is stimulated by such factors as hemorrhage, a reduction in cardiac output, dehydration, and hypoalbuminemic states. The limbic system also plays a role in the stimulation of ADH during stress, trauma, heat, fear, and pain. Certain drugs also promote ADH secretion, such as morphine, nicotine, barbiturates, β-adrenergic agents, general anesthetics, vincristine, cyclophosphamide (Cytoxan), carbamazepine, and chlorpropamide. Inhibition of ADH occurs during states of hypervolemia and hypo-osmolality. Total body immersion in water and a sensation of cold also inhibit ADH secretion. Pharmacologic agents inhibiting ADH include morphine antagonists, α-adrenergic agents, and ethyl alcohol.[26]

Free water loss leads to concentration of the blood, and plasma osmolality rises. When plasma osmolality reaches about 288 mOsm/kg, two things occur. First, the osmoreceptors in the hypothalamus are stimulated and promote synthesis of ADH in the hypothalamic nuclei and release of ADH from the posterior pituitary gland. Second, a perception of thirst occurs, leading to the ingestion of water. ADH causes the kidney to increase water reabsorption, resulting in antidiuresis. As plasma osmolality returns toward normal, stimulation of osmoreceptors is reduced, and ADH secretion decreases. The sensation of thirst is reduced. Overhydration dilutes the blood, and plasma osmolality decreases. When it reaches about 282 mOsm/kg, the synthesis and release of ADH are inhibited. The kidneys decrease water reabsorption, and diuresis ensues. Serum osmolality returns toward normal.[32,64]

Thyroid Gland

The thyroid gland weighs approximately 20 g in a healthy adult. It is composed of two encapsulated lobes positioned on either side of the trachea and joined by the isthmus. The right lobe is larger and more vascular than the left. The recurrent laryngeal nerves run in the grooves beside the trachea and behind the lobes of the thyroid gland. The thyroid gland is located anteriorly just below the cricoid cartilage (Figure 9-3).

Embryologically, the thyroid gland begins as epithelial tissue in the pharyngeal floor. Deviations in normal embryonic development may consist of failure of lobe development, development of a lingual thyroid gland from remnants of the thyroglossal duct, thyroglossal cyst formation from duct remnants, or substernal goiter formation from resultant descent of the thyroid gland along the developmental path of the thymus into the thorax.[32,103]

Thyroid blood supply is well in excess of the kidney blood supply. This blood supply is furnished by two major pairs of arteries that account for the rich vascularity of the gland and for the increased risk of hemorrhage that may occur postoperatively. The presence of a palpable thrill or audible bruit over the gland or surrounding area is indicative of an increased blood flow.[103]

The thyroid gland is innervated by the adrenergic nervous system, from the cervical ganglia; the cholinergic nervous

Figure 9-3 Thyroid anatomy.

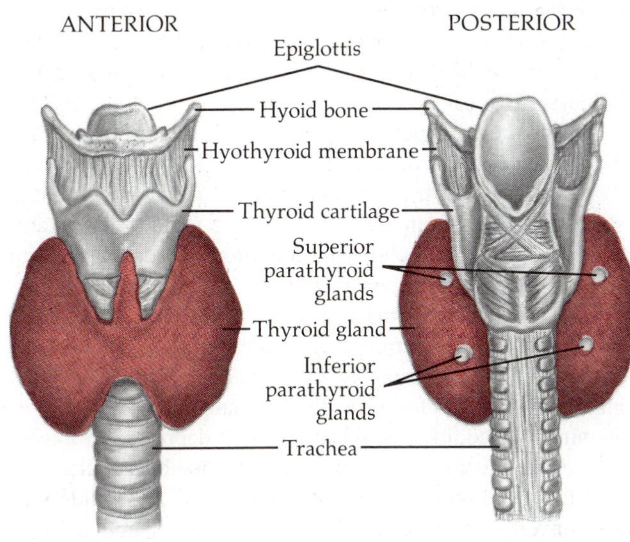

system, from the vagus nerve; and a network of adrenergic fibers that terminate near the basement membrane of the follicular walls.[103] Thyroid blood flow is regulated by neurogenic stimuli.

The thyroid is composed of follicular and parafollicular cells. The follicles are filled with proteinaceous colloid.[32] Colloid is the major constituent of total thyroid mass.

The function of the follicular cells is to secrete the two major thyroid hormones, thyroxine (T_4) and triiodothyronine (T_3). The parafollicular cells or C cells secrete a third hormone, thyrocalcitonin (calcitonin), a calcium-lowering substance. Parafollicular cells are located in the interfollicular connective tissue.[103]

The major component of thyroid hormones is iodine. Normal iodine balance depends on sufficient dietary intake. Seafoods and water are the major natural sources. Medications, diagnostic agents, dietary supplements, and the use of iodine by the food-processing industry and in the food given to animals have increased iodine ingestion in the more highly developed countries.[103] Normal daily dietary intake of iodine varies widely throughout the world primarily because of the varying iodine content of soil and water and because of cultural food preferences.[103] The minimum recommended daily requirement of iodide is about 150 μg (50 to 75 μg is required for adults to prevent goiter caused by iodine deficiency).[102] However, dietary intake of iodine ranges as high as 500 μg or more daily in most areas of the United States.[32]

Iodine is rapidly absorbed from the gastrointestinal tract, primarily as iodide, the form in which it is carried in the blood, and is largely confined to the extracellular fluid (ECF) compartment.[103] When absorbed in organic form, iodine is converted to iodide in the liver.[32] Small quantities of iodine are lost in the stool, in expired air, and through the skin.[103]

During lactation, more notable losses occur.[103] Primary removal from the ECF pool occurs by excretion of iodine into the urine and by transport of iodine into the thyroid gland.

Renal clearance of iodide is important because it determines the availability of iodide to the thyroid gland.[103] The kidneys are considered passive participants in iodide metabolism and are not a part of the body's defense mechanism for maintenance of thyroidal homeostasis.

Biosynthesis of the thyroid hormones occurs in sequential stages: iodide trapping; oxidation of the iodide ion; organification of thyroglobulin; and coupling of iodotyrosines to form the active hormones T_4 and T_3.

The first step in synthesis is iodide uptake by the follicular cells. This step is referred to as iodide transport or the iodide pump. Iodide is transported from the ECF into the thyroid glandular cells and follicles. TSH stimulates iodide transport activity.[103] In addition, iodide transport is depressed by excess iodide administration and increased by iodide deficiency.[32]

During the second phase of biosynthesis, the iodide ions are converted to an oxidized form of iodine capable of combining directly with tyrosine amino acids located within thyroglobulin. Thyroglobulin is a large glycoprotein molecule synthesized and secreted into the follicles.

The binding of iodine with the thyroglobulin molecule is called organification. Oxidized iodine combines with tyrosine to form the hormonally *in*active iodotyrosines, monoiodotyrosine (MIT) and diiodotyrosine (DIT). The coupling phase continues and results in the formation of the hormonally *active* iodothyronines. T_4 is formed when two molecules of DIT combine. T_3 results when one molecule of MIT couples with one molecule of DIT.

Thyroglobulin serves as a storage depot for the thyroid hormones and the precursors MIT and DIT. A 30-day supply of T_3 and T_4 and a 2-day supply of iodine stored as MIT or DIT are normally contained within the thyroglobulin.[20] The thyroid gland is therefore unique among the endocrine glands because of its large storage of hormones.

T_4 and T_3 enter the bloodstream directly after being cleaved from the thyroglobulin molecule. This process occurs in sequential steps. Most of the inactive iodotyrosines do not reach the circulation. Instead, their iodine is cleaved from them and reutilized in the thyroid gland.[102] This process is an important salvage mechanism for maintenance of iodothyronine synthesis.

T_4 is solely produced by the thyroid gland with a total daily production rate of 80 to 100 μg.[32] T_3 is secreted from the thyroid gland, but most of it is produced by extrathyroidal deiodination of T_4. Approximately 80% of the daily T_3 production (20 to 30 μg) is produced in this manner.[32] The half-life of T_4 in the circulation is 6 to 7 days.[32] T_3 has a half-life of 30 hours in the circulation.[32]

Upon entering the bloodstream, T_4 and T_3 are bound to circulating plasma proteins.[32] These proteins are thyroxine-binding globulin (TBG), a glycoprotein synthesized in the liver; thyroxine-binding prealbumin; and albumin. Any disorders producing changes in the serum-binding protein concentrations have major effects on serum T_4 and T_3 concentrations. Unbound T_4 and T_3 levels are reflected in measurements of serum-*free* T_4 and T_3.

Regulation of thyroid function is achieved through the hypothalamic-pituitary-thyroid axis (Figure 9-4) and an autoregulatory mechanism within the gland. Thyrotropin-releasing hormone (TRH) is synthesized by neurons in the hypothalamus and is transported to cells of the anterior pituitary gland that contain specific cell membrane receptors for TRH binding. Thyroid-stimulating hormone (TSH) in the anterior pituitary gland is stimulated by the secretion of TRH. Most of the thyroid gland's metabolic processes are regulated by TSH. However, the primary action of TSH is the production and secretion of the thyroid hormones. The thyroid hormones, on the other hand, inhibit TSH secretion at the level of the anterior pituitary gland. Small alterations in serum T_4 and T_3 concentrations result in reciprocal changes in both TSH secretion and TSH response to exogenous TRH. Serum thyroid hormone levels will override the pituitary gland's response to TRH if the T_4 and T_3 levels are high.[32]

Blockage or removal of TSH stimulation results in hypovascularity and atrophy of the thyroid gland.[103] The reverse effects occur when stimulatory doses of TSH are produced.

Figure 9-4 Thyroid negative-feedback mechanism.

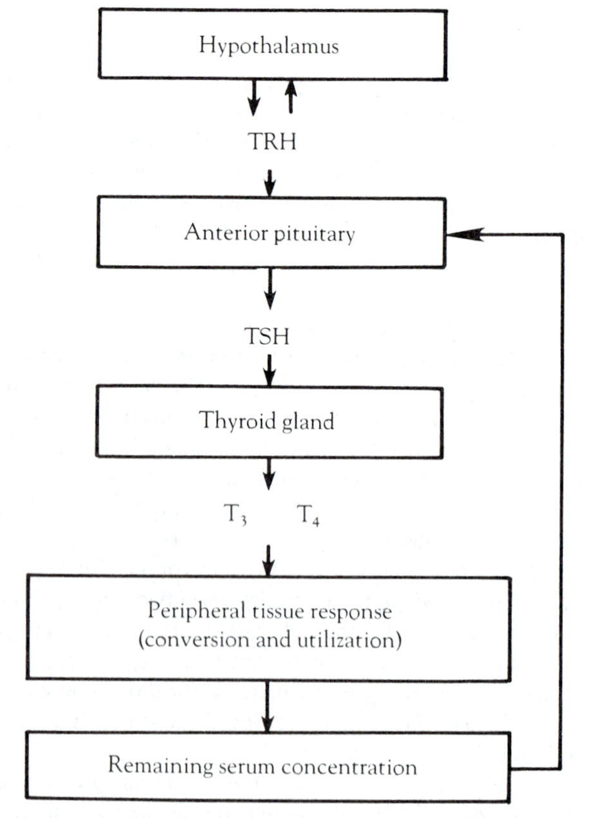

Secretion of TSH in serum is pulsatile in nature and is subject to a circadian rhythm. TSH secretion is characterized by fluctuations at 1- to 2-hour intervals and by a nocturnal surge before the onset of sleep.[103] The circadian variation does not appear to be determined by the cortisol rhythm or by fluctuations in serum T_4 and T_3 levels. If TSH secretion is completely destroyed (i.e., by hypophysectomy or suppression), there is a decreased activity of the thyroid iodide transport mechanism and organic binding is inhibited. The reverse effect occurs with administration of TSH.[103]

Many factors influence thyroid hormone function. For example, TSH secretion is affected by somatostatin, dopamine, and the catecholamines. Other factors that influence thyroid hormone functioning include sex and sex hormones; pregnancy; the newborn state; age; the glucocorticoids; environmental temperatures, especially exposure to extreme cold; alterations in nutritional states (i.e., starvation or overfeeding); and other nonthyroid illnesses, such as cirrhosis and chronic renal failure.

Parathyroid Glands

There are usually two pairs of parathyroid glands located near the posterior surface of the thyroid gland. However, there may be as few as three glands or as many as six, and their location may vary. These glands are sometimes found in the mediastinum, within the thyroid gland, or behind the esophagus. The usual size of a gland is 5 × 5 × 3 mm.

The parathyroid glands are made up of three types of cells: chief cells, which are the main source of parathyroid hormone (PTH); water clear cells, which increase in number as hormone secretion increases; and oxyphil cells, which may be involved in the synthesis and secretion of PTH. PTH is a polypeptide that regulates calcium and phosphate metabolism. Its functions include the regulation of bone metabolism, maintenance of calcium concentration, and regulation of vitamin D synthesis.

PTH has three target areas, which are affected by the amount of hormone secreted. The first of these areas is bone. PTH increases the activity of osteoclasts, which form a pool to inhibit osteoblasts from forming bone when serum calcium levels are low. This mechanism allows calcium resorption into the ECF. Increased serum calcium levels cause a decrease in PTH secretion, which causes the reverse effect (i.e., osteoblasts are stimulated to form bone and calcium resorption is decreased).

The second target area affected by PTH is the kidney. As PTH secretion is increased, there is an increase in renal tubular resorption of calcium and increased excretion of phosphate. This mechanism keeps calcium levels in equilibrium with phosphate.

The third target area is the gastrointestinal tract, where PTH stimulates $1,25(OH)_2D_3$ (vitamin D) to increase absorption of calcium in the small intestine. Vitamin D allows calcium to transfer from the intestinal lumen into the intestinal wall. There is evidence that vitamin D is also essential for PTH to act effectively on bone synthesis.

Adrenal Glands

The adrenal glands are located at the level of the eleventh thoracic rib, lateral to the first lumbar vertebra. Positioned suprarenally, the adult adrenal glands are one-thirtieth the size of the kidney. The left adrenal gland is larger than the right and weighs 4 to 6 g.[26] There are two structures making up the adrenal gland: the adrenal cortex and the adrenal medulla.

Embryonically, the *adrenal cortex* is of mesodermic origin and arises from the coelomic epithelium.[81] The cortex has three distinct zones containing specific cell types responsible for the production of the glucocorticoids, mineralocorticoids, and androgen. The zona glomerulosa is the chief producer of aldosterone (the major mineralocorticoid), while the glucocorticoids and androgens are produced by the zona fasciculata and zona reticularis.[26,81]

The mineralocorticoids are responsible for sodium conservation and potassium excretion via the renal tubules and for maintenance of adequate extracellular volume.[103] The secretion of aldosterone is regulated by potassium ion concentration, the renin-angiotensin system, and ACTH (although this is a weak regulator).[72] The renin-angiotensin system influences ECF volume by regulating aldosterone secretion.[93] When fluid volume or intra-arterial volume is decreased, renin is released from the renal juxtaglomerular cells. This results in the formation of angiotensin I, which then converts to angiotensin II. The cells of the zona glomerulosa produce aldosterone in response to angiotensin II. Sodium is reabsorbed, extracellular volume increases, and renin secretion is decreased.[72,93] Aldosterone secretion increases as serum potassium increases.[93] When ACTH is administered, a rise in aldosterone secretion is documented.

Cortisol is the principal glucocorticoid secreted in humans.[93] Cortisol is secreted in a circadian rhythm. The level is higher in the morning than the evening.[56] Carbohydrate, protein, and fat metabolism are regulated by cortisol. Gluconeogenesis is potentiated by cortisol.[93] Glucocorticoids exert a catabolic effect on protein cells except in the liver, where there is an anabolic effect.[56] The excretion of digestive enzymes, maintenance of emotional well-being, maintenance of normal excitability of the myocardium, and catecholamine action depend on the presence of glucocorticoids.[93] Studies have shown that without the existence of increased glucocorticoids in response to increased stress, death will occur.[93] The term "stress" is defined by Nelson to be "anything that exerts an effect upon the cell that disturbs its homeostatic balance beyond the cell's ability to compensate for that disturbance."[81] Glucocorticoids also exhibit an anti-inflammatory effect. Leukocytes are produced and neutrophils are increased along with a corresponding decrease in lymphocytes and eosinophils.[93] Capillary permeability is decreased.[37] The regulation of glucocorticoid release is via a negative-feedback system. The release of corticotropin-releasing hormone and ACTH does not depend on the source of cortisol. Exogenous forms of cortisol influence the negative-feedback system.

ACTH secretion regulates the release of androgens. Androgens are responsible for the masculinization present in

Figure 9-5 Steroid hormones of the adrenal cortex.

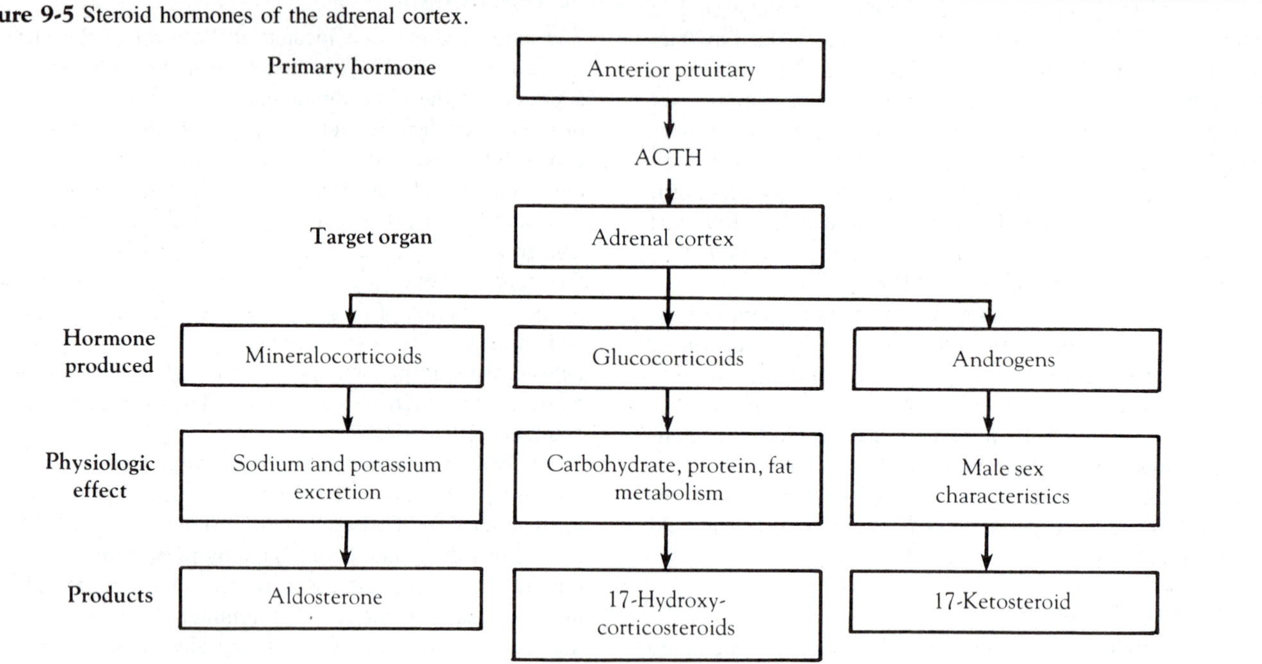

Figure 9-6 Catecholamine biosynthesis in the adrenal medulla. From Felig.[32]

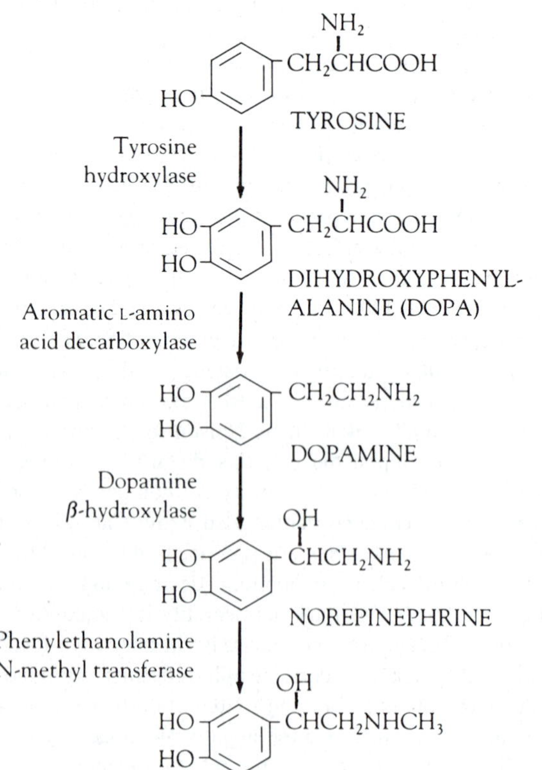

females (axillary and pubic hair) and supplement the major source of androgens in males (the testes) (Figure 9-5).[93]

The adrenal medulla is the middle portion of each adrenal gland; it is made up of chromaffin cells and arises from the neural crest in the embryo. The chromaffin cells, or pheochromocytes, are functional at birth. The medulla is normally dark red-brown and is 8% to 10% of total adrenal weight. Central nervous system stimulation of the medulla is provided by the splanchnic nerve. The medulla receives its vascular supply from blood that has flowed through the adrenal cortex, thus exposing the medulla to high levels of corticosteroids.[26]

The sympathetic nervous system innervates the adrenal medulla and on stimulation causes release of catecholamines. Catecholamines are both hormones (chemical substances that are released into the circulation and elicit a response from a target organ) and neurotransmitters (chemical substances released from nerve endings that have local effects).[32] Catecholamines are biosynthesized from tyrosine, an amino acid that comes from dietary sources, or from conversion of phenylalanine to tyrosine in the liver. Tyrosine is acted on by enzymes to initiate the catecholamine pathway (Figure 9-6).

Norepinephrine and *epinephrine* are the main products of the pathway. Medullary catecholamine secretions are approximately 15% norepinephrine and 85% epinephrine. It is thought that the steroid-rich blood supply of the adrenal medulla maintains the enzyme phenylethanolamine N-methyl transferase (PNMT) and thus promotes the conversion of norepinephrine to epinephrine (Figure 9-6). The medulla is the primary source of epinephrine production, whereas the central nervous system secretes norepinephrine almost exclusively.

Table 9-1
Catecholamine Functions

Class and Function	α-Adrenergic	β-Adrenergic	Dopaminergic
Agonist	Norepinephrine	Epinephrine	Dopamine
Antagonist	Phentolamine	Propranolol	Haloperidol
Actions			
Heart		Inotropic and chronotropic	Inotropic
Smooth muscle	Contracts	Relaxes	Mixed
Metabolic		Lipolysis Glycogenolysis Gluconeogenesis	
Molecular	Decreases cAMP	Increases cAMP	Increases cAMP

From Korenman.[57]

Epinephrine is 5 to 10 times more potent than norepinephrine, although norepinephrine has a longer duration of action.[32,74]

Norepinephrine and epinephrine are both α- and β-adrenergic agonists, but norepinephrine primarily stimulates the α-adrenergic receptors, and epinephrine stimulates the β-adrenergic receptors. The actions of these catecholamines are briefly summarized in Table 9-1.

Catecholamines are excreted in the urine as urinary epinephrine and norepinephrine and are metabolized by enzymes and excreted as urinary metanephrine and urinary vanillylmandelic acid (VMA) (Figure 9-7).

Pancreas

The pancreas lies behind the stomach to the left of the liver and is attached to the duodenum by ducts from the head and body section of the pancreas. It is through this duct that the pancreatic digestive enzymes enter the small intestine.

Each islet of Langerhans consists of a grouping of two to several hundred cells. The islets are scattered over the entire gland but are concentrated in the tail section of the pancreas. The islets contain at least three different types of cells. About 10% to 20% of islet cells are alpha (A) cells, which secrete glucagon; 60% to 70% of the cells are beta (B) cells, which produce and secrete insulin.[10] The delta (D) cells, which make up 2% to 8% of the islet cells, secrete somatostatin and gastrin.

The islet cells have a large blood supply and many nerve fibers. The central nervous system is linked to the islets through the autonomic nervous system's adrenergic and cholinergic fibers.[31] Stimulation of the sympathetic fibers in-

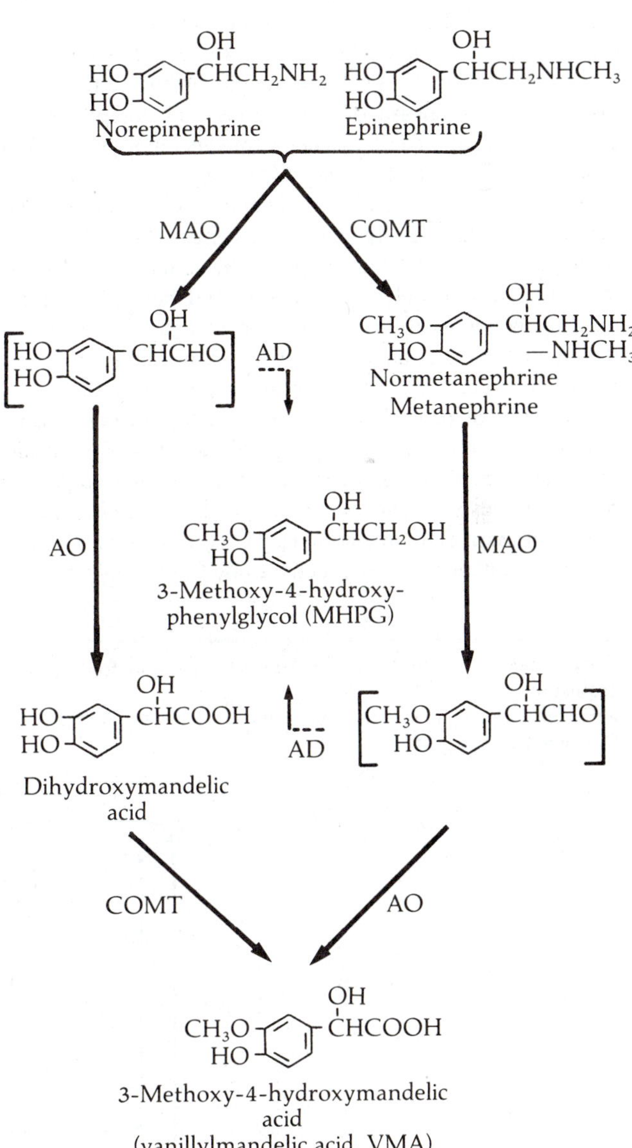

Figure 9-7 Catecholamine metabolism. *COMT*, Catechol-*O*-methyl transferase; *MAO*, monoamine oxidase; *AO*, aldehyde oxidase; *AD*, alcohol dehydrogenase.
Modified from Felig.[32]

creases blood glucose through stimulation of glucagon and inhibition of insulin.[31] Parasympathetic stimulation causes the opposite effect.[31] It is thought that various neurotransmitters (somatostatin, serotonin, and prostaglandins) may also affect the activity of the islet cells.[31]

Glucagon is produced chiefly by the alpha cells of the pancreas and is also found in the mucosa of the stomach and small intestine. Like insulin, glucagon plays an important role in the body's metabolism of nutrients. Details regarding the synthesis and secretion of glucagon are not completely known. Secretion of glucagon is stimulated by low blood sugar. The chief effects of glucagon are to trap amino acids in the liver and to increase gluconeogenesis, glycogenolysis, and lipolysis. The primary target organ of this hormone is the liver, where it attaches to a glucagon receptor on a liver cell.[58] Glucagon output from islet alpha cells varies inversely with blood glucose concentrations, in the presence of insulin. Stimulation of glucagon also stimulates release of insulin by either raising the blood sugar level or by directly stimulating beta cells to increase insulin secretion, or both.[74] Glucagon also stimulates release of epinephrine and norepinephrine from the adrenal medulla, causing conversion of glycogen to glucose, which further elevates blood sugar.

Insulin is synthesized in the endoplasmic reticulum of the beta cells, under the direction of messenger RNA. After the terminal connecting C-peptide fragment is removed (Figure 9-8), the insulin molecule is folded and held together by disulfide bonds. Both insulin and C-peptide are secreted into the circulation. C-peptide has little if any insulin activity and can be measured in the circulation by radioimmunoassay as an indicator of pancreatic beta cell function in persons receiving exogenous insulin.[31] The main stimulus for insulin secretion is glucose, although fats, proteins, and other carbohydrates also enhance secretion. Once secreted, insulin travels in the portal circulation to the liver and then into the general circulation. To be effective, insulin must first bind to cell membrane receptors on target tissues (liver, fat, and muscle cells).

In the fasting state, low insulin levels (and high glucagon levels) allow glycogenolysis and gluconeogenesis by the liver to maintain blood glucose levels and adequate glucose supply to the cells for energy. In the fed state, insulin levels may rise to between 30 and 80 μU/ml to prevent severe elevations in blood sugar by both suppressing liver production of glucose and stimulating glucose uptake by liver, fat, and muscle cells.[31] An estimated 25% of glucose ingested is used by non-insulin-dependent tissues (brain, eye, red blood cells) for energy.[32]

The net effects of insulin are growth promoting and are summarized in Table 9-2. In muscle tissues, insulin causes the uptake of glucose and amino acids, the formation of glycogen, and protein synthesis. In the liver, insulin increases fatty acid and glycogen synthesis through its effect on major enzyme systems. Gluconeogenesis is also inhibited. The action of insulin on fat metabolism involves increasing the uptake of fatty acids and inhibiting lipase activity within the fat cell. The end result is a stimulation of glucose uptake, fatty acid synthesis, enhanced triglyceride synthesis, and inhibition of fatty acid oxidation. Insulin also has a suppressive effect on circulating ketones.

While blood glucose regulation is mainly affected by insulin, at least four other counterregulatory hormones (including glucagon) interact with insulin to maintain a normal blood sugar at all times. Growth hormone, secreted from the anterior pituitary gland, has the effect of increasing blood sugar levels and accelerating anabolic processes in the body. Its secretion is enhanced by hypoglycemia, exercise, and amino acids; it is suppressed by hyperglycemia.[31] Insulin is secreted in response to hyperglycemia and has the effect of decreasing blood sugar, growth hormone, glucagon, and catecholamines. Finally, insulin lowers serum potassium through stimulation of potassium uptake by liver and muscle cells.[31]

Figure 9-8 Formation of insulin and connecting peptide from proinsulin.
Reprinted with permission from Imagimedic Productions, Practical Diabetology **2**(1):3, 1983.

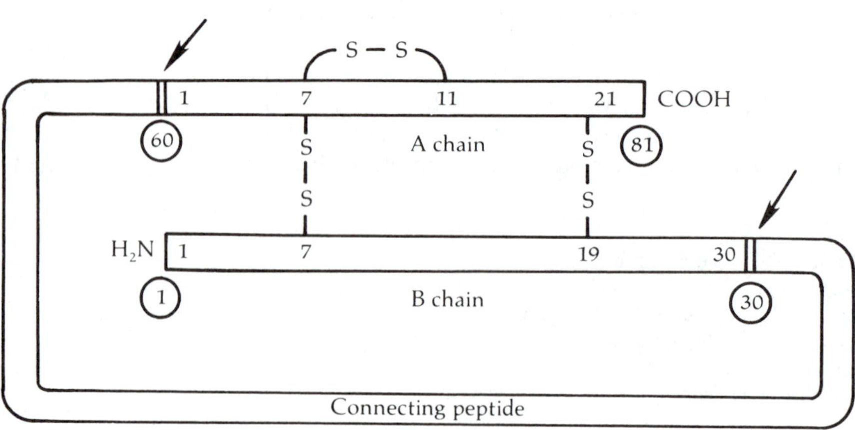

Table 9-2
Action of Insulin

	Liver	Adipose Tissue	Muscle
Anticatabolic effects	Decreased glycogenolysis Decreased gluconeogenesis Decreased ketogenesis	Decreased lipolysis	Decreased protein catabolism Decreased amino acid output Decreased amino acid oxidation
Anabolic effects	Increased glycogen synthesis Increased fatty acid synthesis	Increased glycerol synthesis Increased fatty acid synthesis	Increased amino acid uptake Increased protein synthesis Increased glycogen synthesis

From Ellenberg.[31]

Figure 9-9 Sexual differentiation in utero.

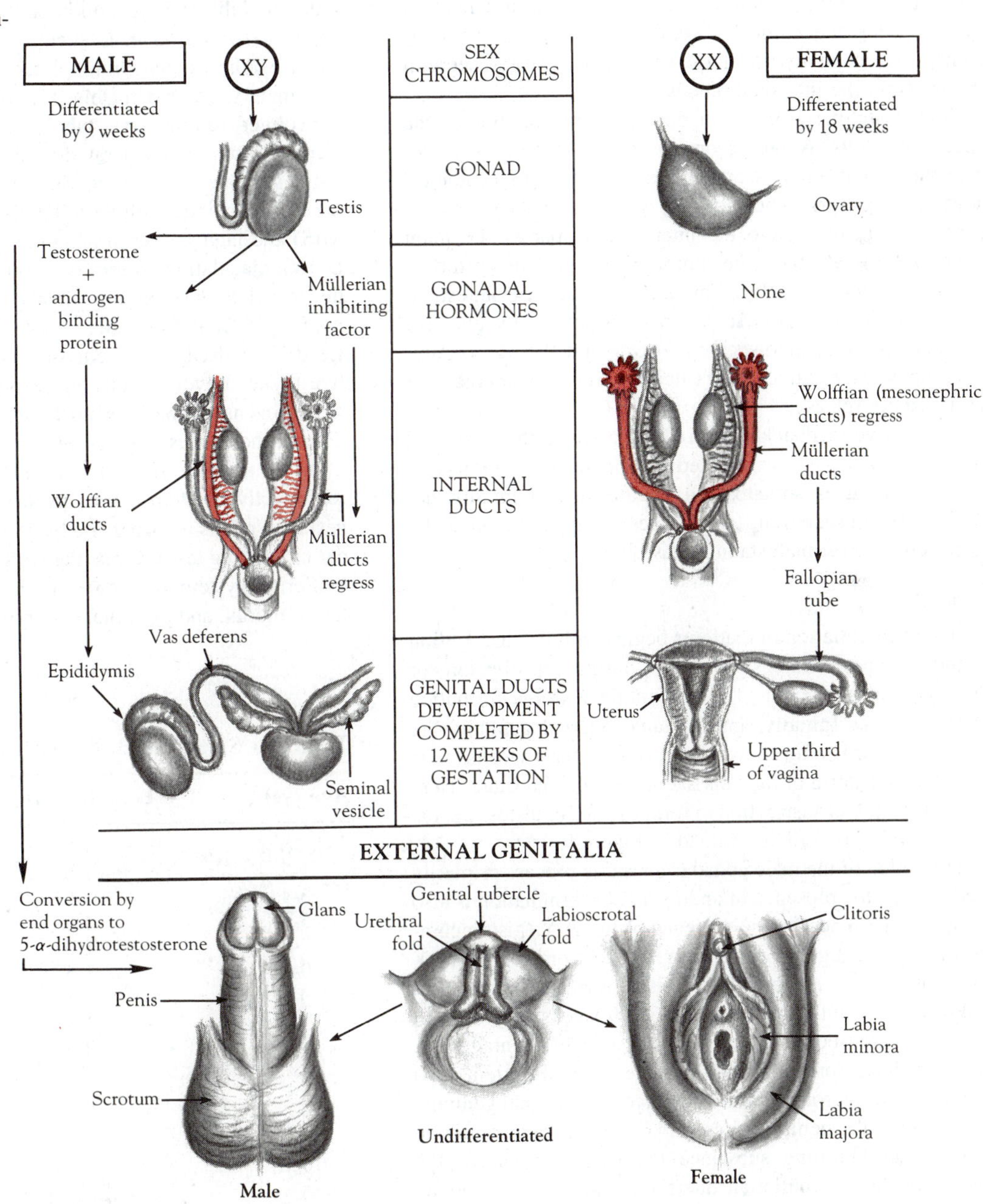

Gastrin is a polypeptide hormone secreted by pancreatic delta islet cells, as well as by the pyloric gland, proximal duodenum, and upper duodenum.[74] Release of gastrin may be stimulated by any of the following: mechanical distention of the antrum of the stomach; foods entering the stomach, especially those containing alcohol, amino acids, or calcium[74]; increased stomach acid; decreased blood sugar; and vagal stimulation.[59]

Once gastrin is released, it is carried in the circulation to the target tissues, the parietal cells of the stomach. Its actions are as follows[74]: increases gastrointestinal muscular tone (including stomach, large and small intestine, and gallbladder); increases digestive secretions from the stomach and pancreas (including insulin); promotes growth of the gastric mucosa by increasing the number of parietal cells, including their ability to secrete hydrochloric acid; and activates secretin release from the intestinal mucosa.

Somatostatin is formed in the secretory granules of the islet delta cells as preprosomatostatin, changed to prosomatostatin, and finally secreted as somatostatin in a calcium-dependent process. The secretory granules expel their contents (somatostatin) into the intercellular space. The main effects of somatostatin are inhibitory on growth hormone, thyrotropin, insulin, glucagon, and various gastrointestinal hormones. Somatostatin secretion is stimulated by glucose, arginine, leucine, ketoisocaproic acid, and β-hydroxybutyrate. Increases in extracellular calcium and potassium increase somatostatin release.[31]

A negative-feedback system exists between the alpha and beta cells of the islets mediated by somatostatin. Glucagon release stimulates somatostatin release, which in turn decreases insulin secretion. Insulin does not appear to have any direct effect on somatostatin release.[31]

Gonads

Sexual differentiation of the fetus begins with the distribution of the sex chromosomes, X and Y, during cell division, or meiosis, and is completed at conception with the formation of the zygote. Initially, internal and external genitalia are identical. Shortly after conception, primordial germ cells move from the endoderm of the yolk sac to the gonadal ridge. Here they await further instruction to form ovaries or testes. Sexual differentiation is further outlined in Figure 9-9.

Formation of the male gonad is an active process primarily mediated by the presence of androgens. Determination is also thought to be made by the presence of the H-Y (histoincompatibility-Y) antigen located near the centromere of the Y chromosome.[52] It is thought that this antigen directs the germ cell to proceed into the testes. By 6 to 9 weeks of gestation, the testes are secreting testosterone, which maintains the wolffian ducts (precursor of the male internal system) and converts to dihydrotestosterone to direct the external genitalia into forming the penis and scrotum.[52] The testes also secrete a müllerian-inhibiting substance (MIS), which causes the regression of the müllerian ducts (precursor of the female internal system), thereby preventing the formation of the female internal genitalia.

During the seventh to ninth months of gestation the testes descend from the posterior abdominal cavity to the scrotal sac. Because the scrotum temperature is approximately 2° C lower than the abdominal cavity, this descent is necessary to permit spermatogenesis during puberty. A tubelike structure projecting from the peritoneal cavity, the processus vaginalis, precedes the descending testis into the inguinal canal. Failure of the tube to shrink and close after proper positioning of the testis produces a congenital indirect inguinal hernia.[9] Varying degrees of cryptorchidism occur with incomplete or misdirected descent of the testis.

The testes are ovoid; their size varies with age and degree of sexual maturity. Age-related testicular dimensions are found in Table 9-3. In adulthood the mature testes can weigh between 10 and 45 g. Clinically, testicular volume is measured by the Prader Orchiometer and is expressed in cubic centimeters. Approximately 95% of the testes is made up of convoluted seminiferous tubules that are contained in septa (septate testis) and separated by the tunica albuginea. Figure 9-10 illustrates a crosscut view of the adult testis. In utero the tubule is lined with Sertoli cells (support cells that secrete MIS) and later by germinal epithelium that produces sperm. During ejaculation, sperm is emptied into the epididymis, to the vas deferens, passing finally into the urethra. The remaining 5% of the testis is interstitial tissue made up of Leydig's cells, lymphatic tissue, blood vessels, and connective tissue. Leydig's cells are responsible for the production of androgens, primarily testosterone.[34] Further information on gonadal hormones is given in Table 9-4.

In the absence of the Y chromosome and MIS, the female reproductive system begins to develop at 6 to 11 weeks of gestation and is recognizable by 18 weeks of gestation. Without circulating testosterone the wolffian ducts regress and the müllerian system progresses to form the internal fallopian tubes, uterus, and proximal one third of the vagina. Although

Table 9-3
Testicular Size from Birth to Maturity

Age (yr)	Length (cm)	Volume (ml)
Under 1	1.5	0.6
1-2	1.6	0.7
3-4	1.6	0.8
5-6	1.6	0.8
7-8	1.6	0.8
9-10	1.6	0.9
11	1.7	1.5
12	1.9	2.0
13	2.3	5.0
14	2.8	8.0
15	3.0	12.0
16	3.5	13.0
17	—	15.0
18-19	—	16.0-20.0
20-25	4.0-5.0	16.0-20.0

From Kaplan.[52]

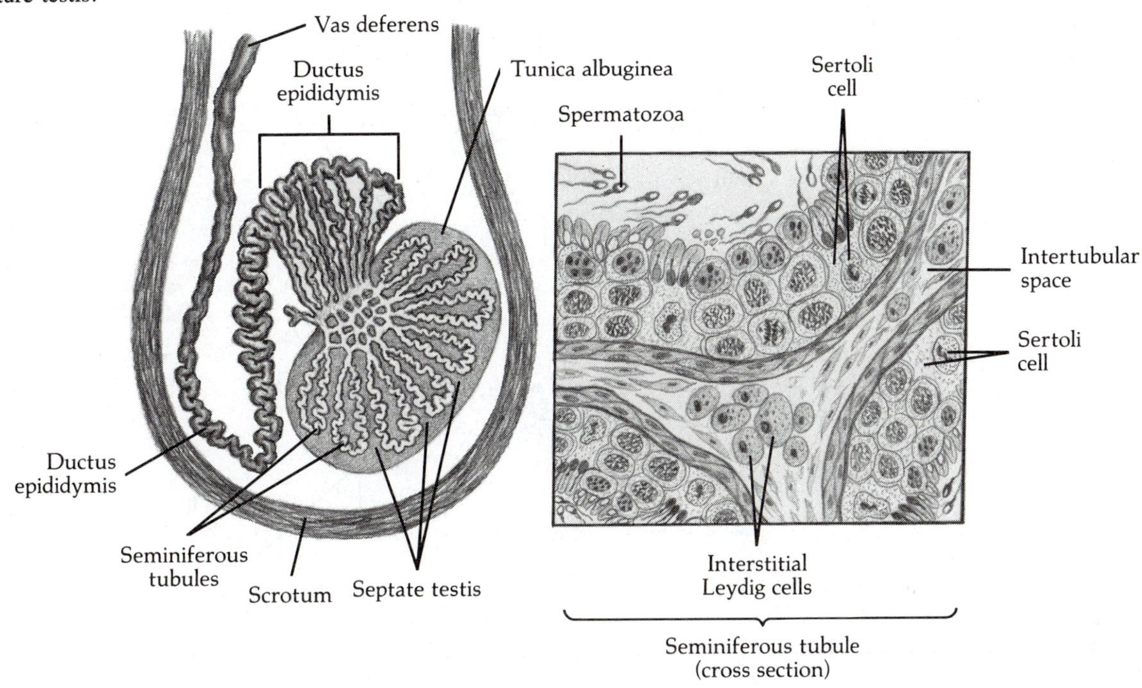

Figure 9-10 Mature testis.

development of the müllerian system is not maintained by ovarian function, further evolution of the ovary does depend on two normally structured X chromosomes.[52] At approximately the sixth month of pregnancy, primordial follicles form from meiotic oocytes. Here they await further maturation during puberty. Generally each ovary is whitish, flat and almond shaped, situated to either side of the uterus just posterior of the fallopian tube and held in place by the meso-ovarian ligament, a portion of the broad ligament. As in the male testes, size and weight depend on normal development and stage of maturation. Each ovary consists of a medulla and cortex similar to the adrenal gland, which shares a similar embryonic origin. Contained in the cortex are the maturing follicles, whereas the medulla supports tissues of the lymphatic, nervous, and circulatory systems. The entire unit is protected by the tunica albuginea and again by the germinal

Table 9-4
Gonadal Hormones

	Origin	Location	Appearance	Function
Male				
Sertoli cells	Surface epithelium; development of gonad and testis	Line seminiferous tubules	Fetal	Secrete MIS Provide support for developing spermatids
Leydig's cells	Mesenchyme	Interstitial tissue of testes	Fetal and pubertal	Secrete testosterone
Female				
Granulosa/follicular	Surface epithelium; rete ovary	Cortex of ovary	Early fetal	Houses maturing ova Secretes small amounts of nonaromatized testosterone (theca cells)
Corpus luteum	Postovulatory follicle	Cortex of ovary	Postovulatory	Secretes progesterone for support of pregnancy Produces 17OH progesterone Produces small amounts of estrogen and androgen

Figure 9-11 Ovary.

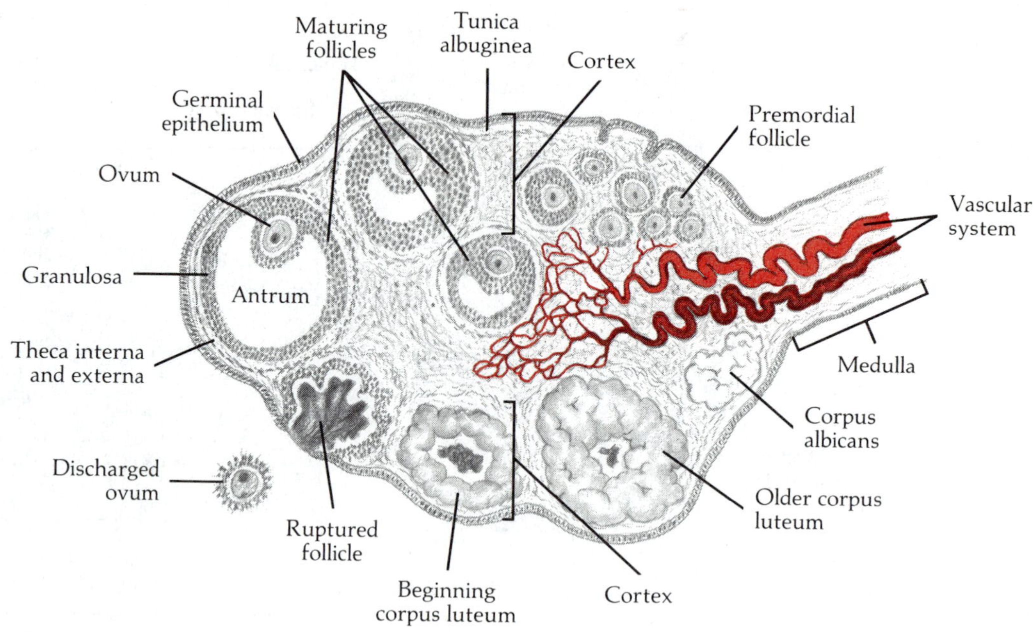

epithelium.[34] Figure 9-11 gives a crosscut diagram of the ovary. In response to pituitary secretion of LH and FSH, graafian follicles, each housing an ovum, begin maturing. Normally, the two ovaries contain an average total of 400,000 ova.[34] Following an LH surge and fall in estrogen, a mature ovum is released to be swept up the fimbrae of the fallopian tubes. The two primary ovarian hormones are given in Table 9-4. The primary hormone of the follicle, or granulosa, is estrogen, whereas the corpus luteum secretes progesterone. In the mature ovary, interstitial cells seem to have androgenic properties that are unclear at this time.[34]

Table 9-5

Summary of Hormonal Effects

Area of Concern	Hormonal Influence	Area of Concern	Hormonal Influence
Normal growth	Thyroid Insulin Growth hormone Gonadotropins Sex steroids	Muscle mass and contractility	Glucocorticoids Insulin Growth Hormone Androgens
Metabolic rate	Thyroid	Skin turgor	Mineralocorticoids, glucocorticoids
Protein, carbohydrate, and fat metabolism	Thyroid Glucagon Insulin Gastrin, glucocorticoids	Secondary sex characteristics	Gonadotropins Sex steroids
Cardiac contractility	Calcium, epinephrine	Lactation	Calcium Prolactin, oxytocin
Blood pressure; pulse rate	Glucocorticoids, mineralocorticoids Epinephrine, norepinephrine	Skin pigmentation	Melanocyte-stimulating hormone

Normal Findings*[52,69,70]

Tanner Stage and Mean Age	Normal Findings	
Male		
Tanner I	Prepubertal; less than 10 yr of age Nonmature genitalia; testes volume approximately 3 ml Vellus hairs over genitalia	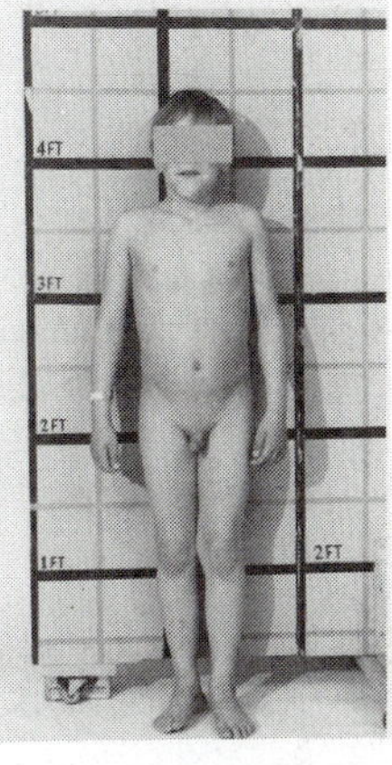
Tanner II (11.7 yr ± 1.3 [standard deviation, SD])	Increase in testicular size Few sparse terminal (pigmented) straight pubic hairs (difficult to appreciate in illustration) Testicular volume greater than 3 ml Scrotum somewhat reddened and thinning with increased rugae	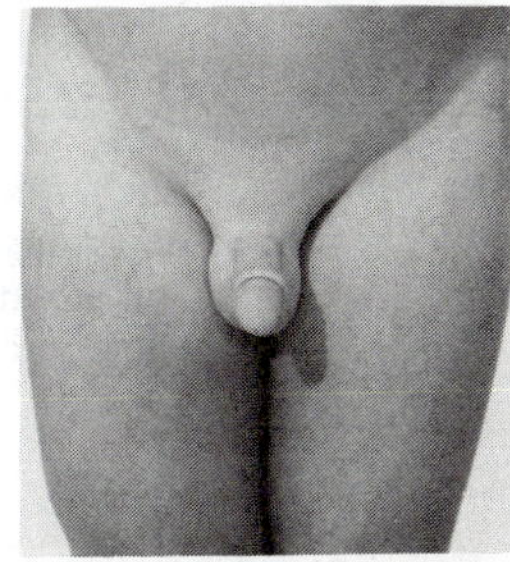
Tanner III (13.2 yr ± 0.8 [SD])	Further testicular growth Penile enlargement in length and circumference Increasing number of pubic hairs, at base of shaft (curled, coarse) Increased muscle bulk, acne and oil production, body odor	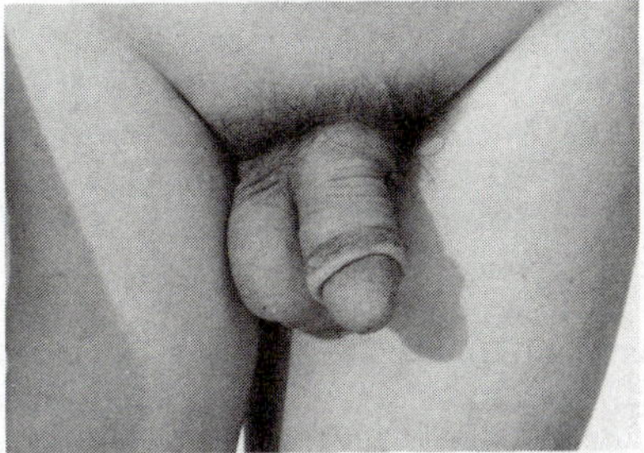
Tanner IV (14.7 ± 1.1 [SD])	Continued growth of testes, scrotum, and penis Development of glans penis Increased pigmentation of genital skin Developing libido Growth spurt at 13-14 yr Pubic hair over symphysis pubis Possible temporary gynecomastia (or earlier)	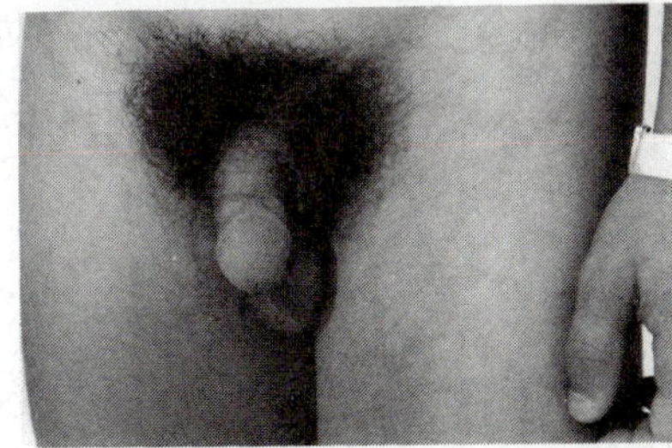

*Illustrations courtesy National Institutes of Health.

Tanner Stage and Mean Age	Normal Findings
Tanner V (15.5 yr ± 0.7 [SD])	Pubic hair extends to medial surfaces of thighs Mature genitalia Facial and axillary hair Adult height reached with epiphyseal closure Reproductive capability Libido

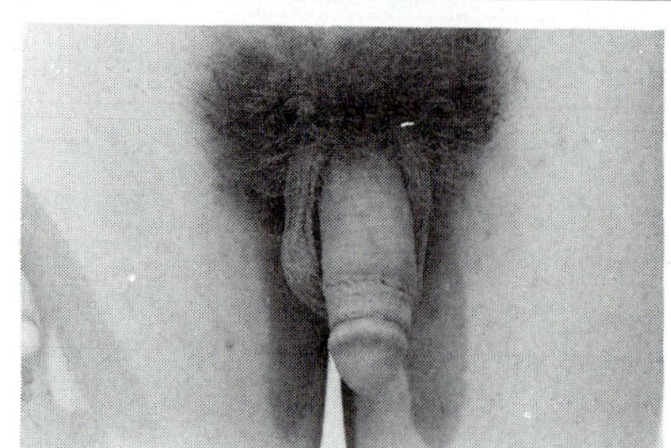

Female

Tanner Stage and Mean Age	Normal Findings
Tanner I	Immature genitalia Less than 9 yr of age Vellus hairs present No palpable breast tissue Mean areolar diameter of 11.9 mm

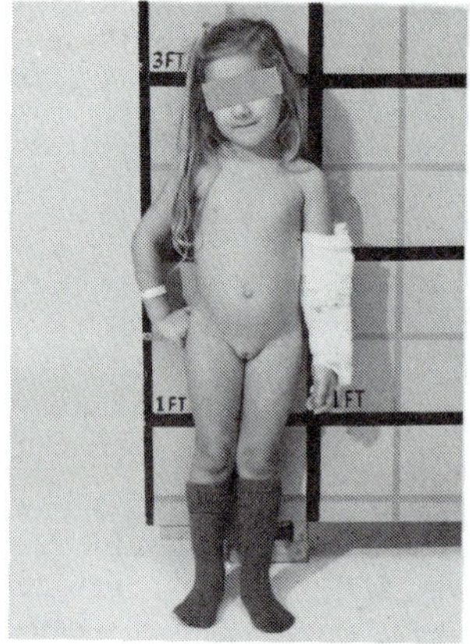

Tanner Stage and Mean Age	Normal Findings
Tanner II (10.08 yr ± 1.1 [SD])	Few terminal hairs along labia Beginning estrogen stimulation of breast tissue Small buttonlike mound (breast bud) over nipple Labia pinker and moist

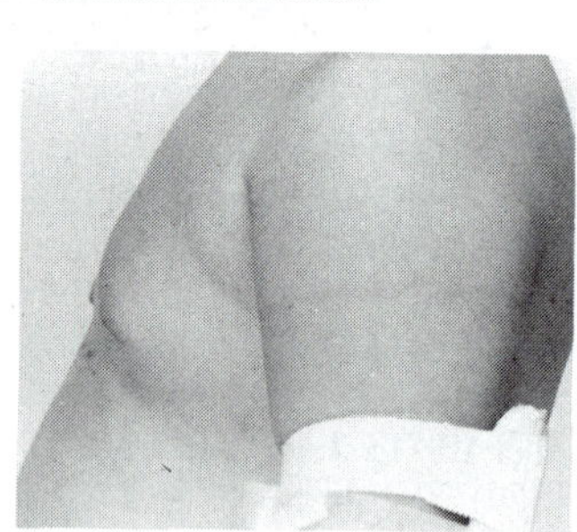

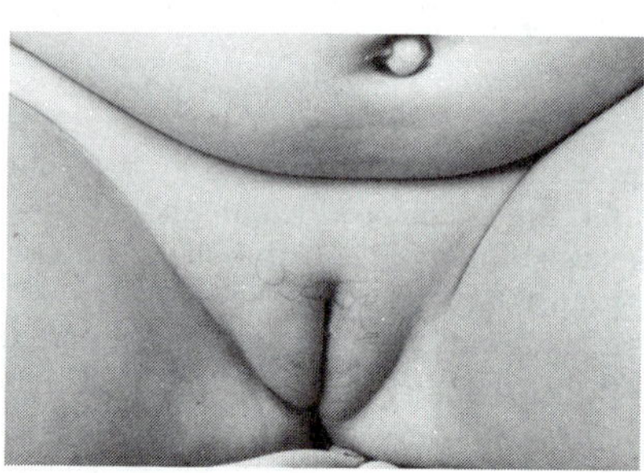

Tanner Stage and Mean Age	Normal Findings
Tanner III (12.0 yr ± 1.1 [SD])	Pelvic widening Pubic hair increased on mons Breast tissue extends beyond areola to form doughnut-shaped mound Asymmetry of breast development likely Menarche (mean age of 12.7 yr ± 1.0) Body odor, increased oil production, and acne

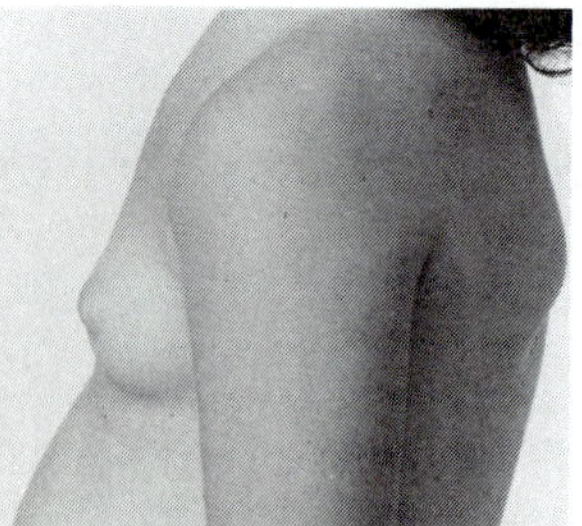

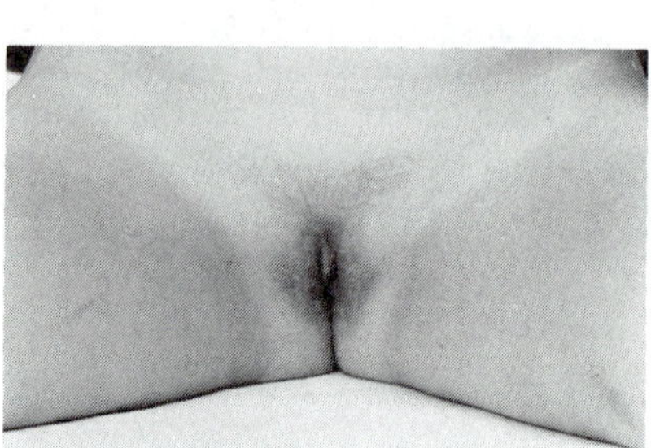

Tanner Stage and Mean Age	Normal Findings
Tanner IV (13.0 yr ± 2.2 [SD])	Pubic hair approaching feminine triangle Contour separation of areolar mound from breast Growth spurt at 11-13 yr Moderate amount of axillary hair
Tanner V (14.0 yr ± 1.2 [SD])	Pubic hair extending up on thighs and up linea alba Areola and breast as one; similar to Tanner stage III Asymmetry of breast development may persist Cyclic moodiness with monthly menses Conception possible with ovulation Adult height reached with epiphyseal closure

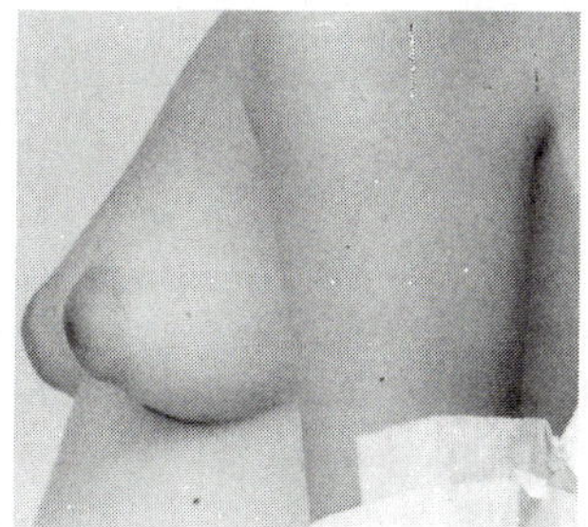

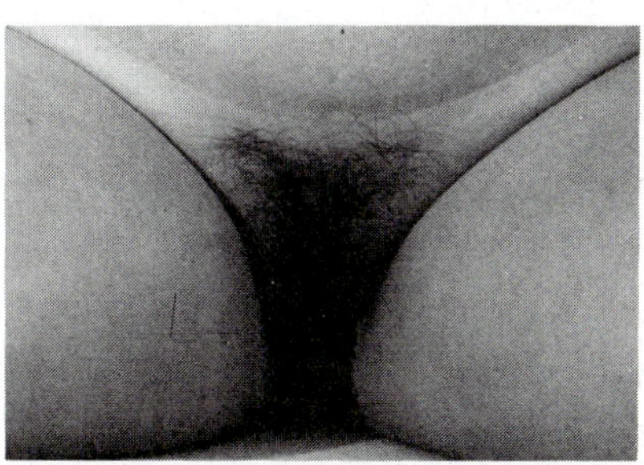

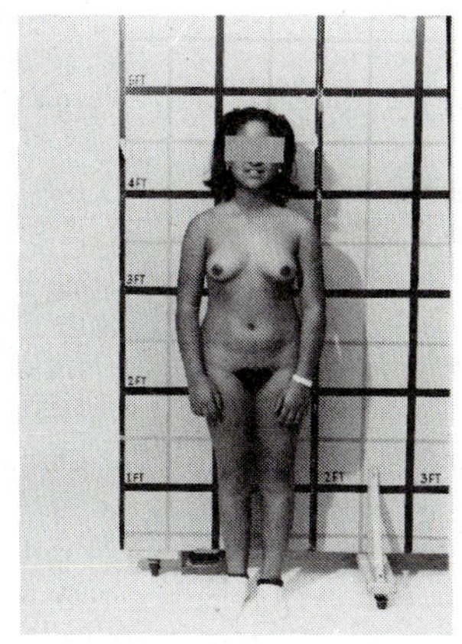

Normal Laboratory Data

Laboratory Test	Normal Adult Values
Blood or Serum	
Adrenocorticotropic hormone (ACTH)	8 AM: <140 pg/ml 4 PM: 10-50 pg/ml
Aldosterone	
Normal salt diet	
Supine	5.4-9.8 ng/dl
Upright	8.9-58 ng/dl
Low salt diet	2-4 times above values
Androstenedione	<250 ng/dl
Calcitonin	<150 pg/ml; usual basal fasting level is about 20-100 pg/ml, depending on assay
Calcium	
Serum	Up to 30 yr: 8.2-10.5 mg/dl; decreases very slightly in older years
Ionized serum	4.75-5.0 mg/dl
Calculated ionized	3.9-4.8 mg/dl
Catecholamines	
Supine	
Epinephrine	20-97 pg/ml
Norepinephrine	125-310 pg/ml
Standing	
Epinephrine	20-109 pg/ml
Norepinephrine	169-515 pg/ml
Cortisol	8 AM: 8-18 μg/dl 4 PM: 4-10 μg/dl
C-peptide	
Fasting	0.9-4.2 ng/ml
Nonfasting	1.5-9.0 ng/ml
Dehydroepiandrosterone (11-Deoxycortisol) (DHEA)	Adult male: 270-1400 mg/dl Adult female: 200-800 ng/dl
DHEA sulfate (serum)	Adult male: 130-550 μg/dl Premenopausal female: 60-340 μg/dl Postmenopausal female: <130 μg/dl
Estrogen	
Male	2-8 ng/ml
Female	6-40 ng/ml

Laboratory Test	Normal Adult Values
Follicle-stimulating hormone	Male: <22 IU/L Female: Midcycle: <40 IU/L Preovulation or postovulation: <20 IU/L *Older adult:* postmenopausal women: 40-160 IU/L
Free thyroxine	Approximately 0.7-1.8 ng/dl (varies among laboratories)
Gastrin	Fasting: 50-170 pg/ml Postprandial: 95-140 pg/ml; usually <250 pg/ml
Glucagon	20-100 pg/ml
Glucose	Adult: 70-120 mg/dl
Glycosylated hemoglobin	5.4%-7.6% (laboratory specific)
Growth hormone	<10 ng/ml
17-Hydroxycorticoids (during Metyrapone test)	Rise to at least 2 times basal levels, or 8-10 mg/24 h
Human chorionic gonadotropin	<3 mIU/ml (nonpregnant)
Insulin	Fasting level: up to 25 μU/ml with slight differences in upper limit of normal among laboratories
Karyotyping	Sex chromosomes: XX or XY
Luteinizing hormone	
Male	7-24 mIU/ml; normal ranges vary among laboratories
Female	Follicular phase: 6-27 mIU/ml Midcycle: 35-154 mIU/ml Luteal: 5-17 mIU/ml *Older adult:* postmenopausal: 29-96 mIU/ml
Osmolality, serum	280-295 mOsm/L
Osmolality, urine	50-1400 mOsm/L
Parathyroid hormone	Dependent on individual laboratory, calcium result; the calcium value is related to the parathyroid hormone value by some laboratories on a two-dimensional graph or nomogram to ascertain abnormality
Phenylalanine	<20 mg/dl
Progesterone	
Male	13-97 ng/dl *Older adult:* 7-33 ng/dl
Female	Follicular: 95 ng/dl Luteal: 1130 ng/dl
Progesterone receptor assay	<5 fmol/mg protein is negative
Prolactin	2-37 ng/ml
Renin*	
Supine	20-160 ng/dl/h
Upright	70-330 ng/dl/h
Somatomedin C	0.4-2.0 U/ml
Somatostatin	10-80 pg/ml
Testosterone	Male: 300-1100 ng/dl Female: 20-100 ng/dl
Triiodothyronine	Approximately 80 to 200-230 ng/dl with some variation among laboratories; increase occurs in pregnancy
Thyroglobulin	About 1-20 ng/ml; mean values of 5.1-9.5 ng/ml
Thyroid-stimulating hormone (TSH)	Upper limit of normal varies among laboratories from about 5.4 μU/ml to approximately 10 μU/ml
Thyroxine	5.5-11.5 μg/dl Pregnancy: approximately 5.5-16 μg/dl
Thyroxine-binding globulin	Variability among laboratories exists; 10-28 μg/ml; increased in pregnancy
Urine	
Aldosterone	3-19 μg/24 h
Calcium	Varies with diet; based on average calcium intake of 600-800 mg/24 h, excretion may be 100-250 mg/24 h On a diet of 400-800 mg of calcium daily, others set the upper limit at 200 mg calcium in a 24-h urine collection
Catecholamines	
Epinephrine	0-20μ/24 h
Norepinephrine	15-80 μg/24 h
Metanephrine	0.2-0.8 g/24 h
Dopamine	65-400 μg/24 h
Creatinine clearance	Male: 85-125 ml/min/1.73 m^2 Female: 75-115 ml/min/1.73 m^2
Free cortisol	Male: 11-84 μg/24 h Female: 10-34 μ/24 h
FSH	
Male	3-11 IU/24 h
Female	5-50 IU/24 h *Older adult:* Postmenopausal: 2-3 times adult values
HCG	<10 IU/24 h
Hydroxyprolines	See individual laboratory reference ranges; excretion on meat-free, gelatin-free diet is approximately 10-50 mg/24 h

*Varies between laboratories; depends on sodium intake, age, and posture and whether there has been stimulation (e.g., furosemide). Values from right and left renal veins should normally be equal. In arterial constriction, abnormal result is considered a ratio of greater than 1.5.

Laboratory Test	Normal Adult Values	Laboratory Test	Normal Adult Values
17-Ketosteroids	Male: 9-22 mg/24 h Female: 6-15 mg/24 h *Older adult:* Decrease in advancing years	17-Hydroxysteroids	Male: 3-10 mg/24 h Female: 2.5-10/24 h
		LH	Male: 5-25 IU/24 h Female: 8-90 IU/24 h *Older adult:* Postmenopausal: 2-3 times adult values
VMA	1.8-7 mg/24 h		

Conditions, Diseases, and Disorders

DISORDERS OF THE ADRENAL GLANDS

Adrenal insufficiency

Adrenal insufficiency can be defined as an abnormality of the adrenal glands with destruction of the adrenal cortex so that glucocorticoid production and mineralocorticoid production are impaired.

Primary adrenal insufficiency can be found in all age groups ranging from newborn to elderly. Men and women alike are affected, and there is no differentiation between races. Secondary adrenal insufficiency is most common among patients who have withdrawn from exogenous cortisol therapy.

In patients with idiopathic primary adrenal insufficiency the prognosis is favorable because of advances made in cortisol replacement therapy. Although the condition is lifelong, with appropriate management and an increased patient awareness, the disease is manageable.

Patients diagnosed with secondary adrenal insufficiency may have other causes for a reduction in ACTH secretion. These causes include pituitary tumors, hypophysectomy for pituitary tumors, postpartum pituitary necrosis, tumors of the third ventricle, trauma, and optic glioma.[45]

Adrenal crisis can occur in any patient deficient in adrenal steroids. Many times, the patient who is adrenally insufficient may not have the diagnosis made until a crisis occurs. Once the signs and symptoms are recognized and treatment initiated, response is encouraging.[26] Because of the life-threatening nature of adrenal crisis, response must be prompt.

Many factors can be the precipitating cause of adrenal crisis. Anything that causes additional stress in the adrenally insufficient patient may be significant, such as infection, surgery, or trauma (automobile accident). If the patient does not receive sufficient coverage with glucocorticoids, crisis ensues.

Pathophysiology

Sixty-six to eighty percent of cases of primary adrenal insufficiency have an idiopathic cause (most likely autoimmune). Causes of primary adrenal insufficiency include fungal infections and vascular and metastatic disease.[10]

Secondary adrenal insufficiency results from an impairment of the hypothalamic-pituitary-adrenal axis. Insufficient ACTH stimulation is responsible for the hypofunction of the adrenal gland. If the cause of the decreased ACTH production is a pharmacologic source of cortisol, the axis may recover; however, it may take months or even years.[45]

Primary adrenal insufficiency reflects both mineralocorticoid and glucocorticoid deficiency. Patients with secondary adrenal insufficiency have only glucocorticoid deficiency[103] because the regulation of mineralocorticoid secretion by the renin-angiotensin system is independent of ACTH secretion.

Adrenal insufficiency affects the balance of metabolic regulators. Muscle work capacity is diminished. Cardiac contractility and output decrease, and this may lead to circulatory collapse. Decreased cardiac output results in reflex tachycardia and increased secretion of ADH, which leads to water retention. Free fatty acid mobilization is impaired, which reduces free fatty acid levels. This in turn leads to increased utilization of glucose, resulting in hypoglycemia.[64] Decreased cortisol increases ACTH production causing hyperpigmentation,[17] and there is a decrease in gastrointestinal enzymes. The loss of diurnal cortisol causes a loss of mental acuity and vitality.[54] Mineralocorticoid deficiency is reflected by hyperkalemia and hyponatremia, which may be manifested by hypotension.[55] Androgen deficiency results in loss of body hair.[45]

Adrenal insufficiency is manifested only after 90% of the adrenal gland is not working. The onset is usually gradual, although one third of the cases diagnosed have a history of 3 months from wellness to insufficiency.[32] With the gradual onset, symptoms may not be readily apparent. Plasma steroids may, in fact, be within the normal range. With exposure to stress, however, the glands are unable to provide the appropriate response, and adrenal crisis may occur.[32]

Adrenal crisis is characterized by a worsening of the symptoms associated with adrenal insufficiency. Hypovolemic shock may develop as sodium is depleted and ECF volume decreases. Vomiting and diarrhea contribute to volume depletion. Fever may be present, either as a result of a precipitating infection or as a result of hypoadrenalism. The presence of hyperpigmentation may be the only clue to the diagnosis. Therefore examination of scars, buccal mucosa, and palmar surfaces should be included for any patient in unexplained shock.[32]

Diagnostic Studies and Findings

ACTH Stimulation

Primary adrenal insufficiency: little or no cortisol and 17-hydroxysteroid response

Secondary adrenal insufficiency: normal to intermediate cortisol and 17-hydroxysteroid response

Insulin Tolerance Test

Secondary adrenal insufficiency: abnormal response

Blood Chemistry and CBC Levels

Adrenal crisis: hyponatremia, hyperkalemia, lymphocytosis, and eosinophilia[32]; these findings are helpful for differentiating the diagnosis of a patient in shock

Urine Collection (24-Hour) for 17-Hydroxysteroids and 17-Ketosteroids

Decreased in both primary and secondary adrenal insufficiency

Medical Plan

Medications

Corticosteroids
- Hydrocortisone (Cortisol, Compound F), 20 mg in morning and 10 mg in evening
- Hydrocortisone acetate, 25 mg in morning and 12.5 mg in evening
- Prednisone (Deltasone), 5 mg in morning and 2.5 mg in evening
- Dexamethasone (Decadron, Dexasone), 0.5-0.75 mg/d
- Fludrocortisone (Florinef), 0.05-0.2 mg/d

These medications are considered life sustaining for the patient. This fact cannot be overemphasized.

Because of the ever-present potential of adrenal crisis, these patients need to be able to use the intramuscular injection of hydrocortisone or Solu-Cortef (hydrocortone phosphate) for times when oral medication is not tolerated. This injection should be carried with the patient at all times, and a family member or significant other should be taught how to use the intramuscular injection along with the patient.

Special Medication Complications

Incorrect dosage. It may take time to determine correct replacement.

Overtreatment with glucocorticoids may result in short stature and symptoms of Cushing's syndrome. Excess mineralocorticoids may result in fluid overload and hypertension.

NURSING CARE

Nursing Assessment

Circulation

Postural hypotension
Lightheadedness
Hypopyrexia or hyperpyrexia*
Shock*

Food and Fluid Needs

Salt craving
Weight loss
Nausea
Vomiting
Hyponatremia*
Hyperkalemia*

Elimination

Diarrhea
Renal shutdown*

Neurosensory Area

Lassitude
Coma*
Confusion*

Sleep and Rest

Tires easily

Mobility

Muscle aches
Muscle wasting
Muscle weakness

Comfort and Pain

Severe headache*
Severe abdominal pain*
Severe leg pain*
Severe lower back pain*

Hygiene and Skin Care

Hyperpigmentation
Decreased body hair

Sexuality

Amenorrhea
Decreased libido

*Characteristic of adrenal crisis.

Nursing Dx & Intervention

Nursing Diagnosis	Nursing Intervention/Rationale
Potential for infection	• Assess environment for stress inducers (lighting, warm temperature, noise level). • Encourage frequent rest. • Reinforce importance of medications to patient.
Altered nutrition: less than body requirements	• Assess dietary intake. • Encourage patient to choose foods high in sodium and low in potassium. • Take apical pulse to detect cardiac arrhythmias. • Employ means to combat nausea *to maintain nutritional balance and promote homeostasis.* • Maintain intake and output records.
Altered peripheral tissue perfusion	• Assess vital signs frequently (every 15 to 30 minutes). • Recognize early presyncopal signs (dizziness, lightheadedness, visual changes, etc.). • Have patient change positions (from lying to sitting to standing) slowly *to avoid fainting from orthostatic hypotension.* • Take lying and standing blood pressures and pulses. • Administer IV fluids as ordered *to maintain adequate hydration.* Monitor intake and output. • Explain rationale for IV therapy to patient.
Sleep pattern disturbance	• Assess quantity and quality of patient's sleep. • Do not disturb patient when sleeping. • Encourage methods of achieving relaxation (back rub, warm milk, dark room, etc.) *to promote sound sleep.* • Allow for period of uninterrupted rest during the day. • Decrease amount of external stimuli.
Fluid volume deficit (1)	• Assess skin turgor for signs of dehydration. • Monitor intake and output. • Observe for signs and symptoms of shock. • Monitor vital signs frequently and as indicated by patient's condition. • Maintain IV line. • Employ means to combat vomiting and diarrhea *to maintain fluid and electrolyte balance.*

Patient Education

1. Teach the patient the importance of avoiding obvious sources of infection such as persons with infections.
2. Teach the patient the importance of and how to take medication regularly and in emergency situations.
3. Teach the steps to follow when early symptoms of crises are noted.
4. Teach the importance of regular medical follow-up and wearing medical identification.

Evaluation

Patient Outcome	Data Indicating That Outcome is Reached
The patient is free of infection.	Temperature is within normal range. The patient has no signs or symptoms of infection. Glucocorticoid and mineralocorticoid levels are within therapeutic range.
Electrolytes are within the normal range.	Sodium and potassium blood levels are within normal limits.
Tissue perfusion is adequate.	The patient makes no statements concerning syncope. Peripheral pulses are adequate. Output equals intake. The patient adheres to activity limitations.
The sleep pattern is undisturbed.	The patient verbalizes and demonstrates methods of achieving relaxation. The patient verbalizes receiving an increased amount of sleep.
Hydration is adequate.	Urine output is greater than 40 ml/hour. Blood pressure is maintained within normal limits. Skin is intact, and turgor is normal.

Primary aldosteronism

Primary aldosteronism is defined by Biglieri and Baxter as "a condition in which there is increased and inappropriate production of aldosterone by the adrenal gland leading to a mineralocorticoid excess state."[31a]

Primary aldosteronism is not a common disease. When patients are first seen with hypertension, it is prudent to consider the diagnosis of primary aldosteronism, since the incidence of this syndrome ranges from 0.5% to 2% of the hypertensive population.[26] It occurs in women more frequently than men in a ratio of 3:1 and is more prevalent between 30 and 50 years of age.[26]

Pathophysiology

Primary aldosteronism is a disorder of the adrenal cortex. Causes include adrenal adenoma, idiopathic adrenocortical nodular hyperplasia, and adrenal carcinoma.[92] Sixty to seventy percent of patients diagnosed with primary aldosteronism have an adrenal adenoma.[26]

Excess aldosterone results in increased sodium reabsorption, increased total body sodium, and hypervolemia. Edema is rarely exhibited because of an "escape" mechanism, where proximal tubular sodium reabsorption is inhibited by the renal regulatory system.[26,45]

Arterial hypertension is present because of volume expansion, arteriolar sodium content, and vascular and sympathetic reactivity.[45] The degree of hypertension ranges from mild to severe.

Potassium depletion, both intracellular and extracellular, occurs because of increased renal tubular excretion of potassium.[45] Hypokalemia results in muscle weakness, fatigue, nocturnal polyuria (because of defective urinary concentration), altered electrical conductivity of the myocardium, and diminished glucose tolerance.[45]

Hydrogen ion secretion is increased with hyperaldosteronism, resulting in metabolic alkalosis. The alkalosis correlates to the degree of hypokalemia.[45] Marked alkalosis may be demonstrated by positive Chvostek's and positive Trousseau's signs.[72]

Plasma renin activity is suppressed. Laboratory values will reveal suppressed renin levels after the patient is exposed to conditions that will cause elevated levels in normal patients.[103] Simultaneous elevation of aldosterone secretion is also observed in these patients.

Diagnostic Studies and Findings

Diagnosis of primary aldosteronism is based on the following[103]:

- Observation of hypertension
- Presence of hypokalemia
- Suppressed renin levels
- Elevated aldosterone secretion

Renin and Aldosterone Levels

Measured after challenging the system with upright posture and restricted sodium and diuretic therapy; normally, renin levels would increase under this challenge; with primary aldosteronism, renin levels remain low[45,72]; aldosterone levels can be measured after volume expansion through salt loading; this can be accomplished by diet, infusion of normal saline, or administration of a mineralocorticoid; the failure to suppress aldosterone secretion occurs with primary aldosteronism[45]

CT Scans of Adrenal Gland

Used to detect the presence and location of an adenoma; because less radiation and time is involved than that with an iodocholesterol scan, it is a preferred diagnostic aid[32]

Venous Catheterization of Adrenal Glands with Measurement of Plasma Cortisol and Aldosterone

May be performed to distinguish between a unilateral and bilateral source of the hyperaldosteronism[56]

Medical Plan

Surgery

Adrenalectomy

Medications

Receptor blockade: spironolactone (Aldactone), 400-600 mg/d

General Management

Low-sodium diet

NURSING CARE

Nursing Assessment

Circulation

- Mild to severe hypertension
- Hypokalemia
- U waves and widened QT intervals on ECG
- Hypernatremia

Food and Fluid

- Polydipsia

Elimination

- Polyuria
- Nocturia

Neurosensory Area

- Positive Chvostek's sign
- Trousseau's sign

Sleep and Rest

Fatigue

Mobility

Muscle weakness

Comfort and Pain

Muscle aches

Frontal headache

Nursing Dx & Intervention

Nursing Diagnosis	Nursing Intervention/Rationale
Altered cardiopulmonary tissue perfusion	• Assess for presence of edema, increased skin turgor. • Obtain daily weight. • Provide rest periods. • Reinforce diet restrictions *to prevent fluid retention.*
Fluid volume excess	• Assess vital signs every 4 hours. • Monitor intake and output. • Check peripheral pulses. • Observe for edematous tissue. • Elevate any edematous area when possible.
Patient problem: acid-base imbalance	• Assess respiratory status and quality of respirations *to monitor for early acidosis.* • Reinforce low-sodium diet *to decrease fluid retention.* • Monitor laboratory data, especially potassium, sodium, and other electrolytes. • Assess for Chvostek's and Trousseau's signs *to monitor for early signs of alkalosis.*

Patient Education

1. With surgical intervention, see p. 949.
2. With chemotherapeutic intervention, teach the patient the importance of and how to take medication regularly and the side and toxic effects to report.
3. Explain rationale for diet and mobility restrictions.

Evaluation

Patient Outcome	Data Indicating That Outcome is Reached
Cardiopulmonary tissue perfusion is adequate.	Blood pressure is within the normal range. No dysrhythmias are present. Electrolytes are within the normal range.
Excess fluid is decreased or absent.	There is no edema. Output equals intake. Skin turgor is normal. Peripheral pulses are within the normal range.
Acid-base balance is normal.	Respirations are within the normal range. Chvostek's and Trousseau's signs are absent. Potassium and sodium blood levels are within the normal range.

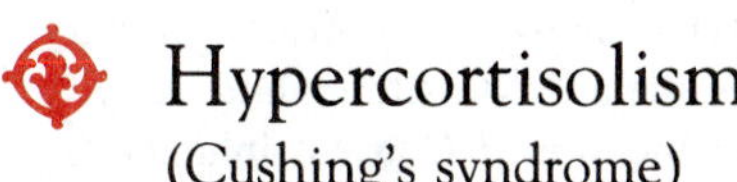

Hypercortisolism
(Cushing's syndrome)

Hypercortisolism is the overproduction of cortisol, the primary glucocorticoid, from the adrenal cortex. The numerous clinical features present in glucocorticoid excess are referred to as Cushing's syndrome.[56]

Cushing's syndrome is rare; approximately 10 cases per million population occur per year. Sex predominance and age predominance depend on the specific etiology of the disorder. Generally, there is a higher ratio of females to males affected (3:1). Hypercortisolism from adrenocorticotropic hormone (ACTH) secreting tumors of ectopic origin occurs more often in males. Cushing's syndrome in children is unusual.[56]

Scientific developments have been ongoing in the diagnosis of hypercortisolism, the search for pathologic causes, and treatment. Investigations are now under way to develop more accurate and more reliable methods to diagnose and identify the source of the hypercortisolism. Interventions such as petrosal sinus sampling for steroids and the corticotropin-releasing hormone (CRH) stimulation test are being instituted and tested in hopes of improving the accuracy of diagnosis.[33,50] Current research also includes the role of β-endorphins in the hypothalamic-pituitary-adrenal axis, cortisol production in association with endogenous depression, and the use of antiglucocorticoids as a new approach to treatment of hypercortisolism.[35]

Pathophysiology

In adrenocortical hyperfunctioning, hypercortisolism occurs in association with mineralocorticoid excess and hyperandrogenism.[56]

The etiology of hypercortisolism (Cushing's syndrome) falls into two major classifications: ACTH dependent and ACTH independent.

Pituitary hypersecretion of ACTH is called Cushing's disease and occurs in 70% of patients with Cushing's syndrome. Extrapituitary sources of ACTH secretion are referred to as ectopic ACTH syndromes (e.g., oat cell carcinoma of the lung). The amount of cortisol produced in these disorders depends on the amount of ACTH secreted. Elevated ACTH levels result in adrenal hyperstimulation and hyperplasia.[56]

Adrenal adenomas (benign) and adrenal carcinomas (malignant) involve pathologic conditions in the gland itself. Normal tissue transforms into neoplastic tissue and produces cortisol independently of ACTH. Levels of ACTH are low, owing to the negative feedback within the axis.

Hypercortisolism can also be a result of other conditions such as chronic alcoholism, endogenous depression, and factitious use of corticosteroids.[56] Hypothalamic disease resulting in hypercortisolism has been postulated as a cause in some cases of Cushing's disease.

High levels of cortisol have profound effects on many tissue and organ systems. Cortisol possesses sodium-retaining properties, increasing extracellular fluid volume and causing mild to moderate hypertension.[26]

Carbohydrate metabolism is affected by the ability of cortisol to (1) increase glucose formation from circulating amino acids, (2) stimulate gluconeogenesis, and (3) render muscle and fat cells insulin resistant. The resulting state of hyperglycemia, glucose intolerance, and glycosuria has been labeled "steroid diabetes." The severity depends on the individual's own predisposition to diabetes.[26]

The mechanism for the fat deposition and distribution in hypercortisolism is yet unclear. It has been suggested that the increased secretion of insulin (resulting from the hyperglycemia) stimulates lipogenesis.[26] Some individuals with simple exogenous obesity present with fat distribution typical of Cushing's syndrome without classic biochemical findings.

Catabolic effects of cortisol cause muscle atrophy, especially in the extremities, and muscular weakness. A mild hypokalemia, present in hypercortisolism, contributes to debilitation (Figure 9-12).

Figure 9-12 Forty-six-year-old woman diagnosed with Cushing's disease. Note classic cushingoid habitus with prominent supraclavicular fat pads and muscle wasting in extremities.
Courtesy National Institutes of Child Health, Bethesda, Md.

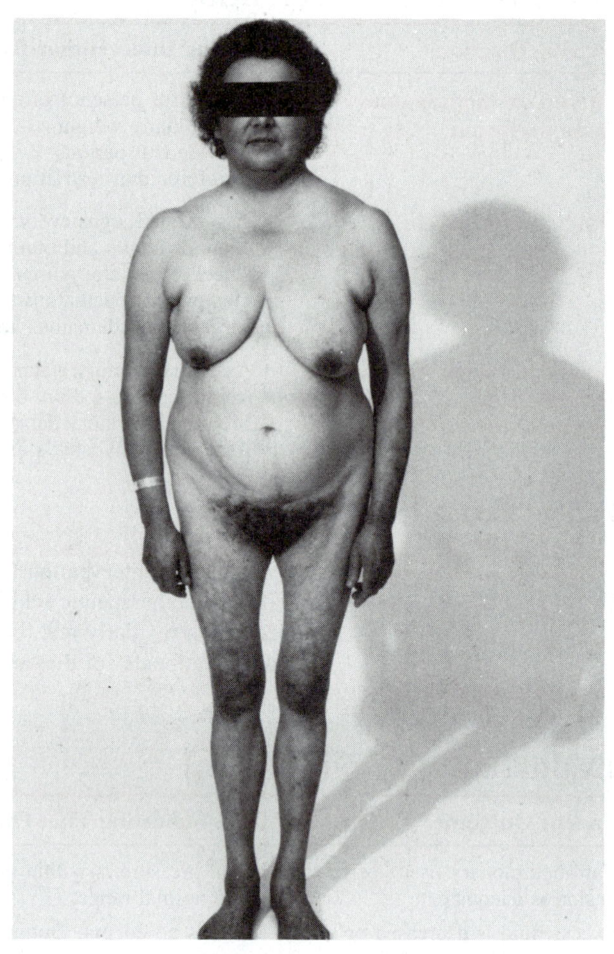

Atrophy of the epidermis and the inhibition of collagen formation are thought to be the result of excess cortisol. Increased susceptibility to infection is present, resulting in frequently observed fungal infections of the skin and nails. Hyperpigmentation is caused by the concomitant release of beta-lipotropic hormone (β-LPH) with ACTH from the pituitary or ectopic site. β-LPH has melanocyte-stimulating activity and results in darkening of the skin.[17] Cortisol inhibits the protein matrix in bone; calcium is abnormally absorbed. Demineralization and hypercalciuria occur. Subsequent osteoporosis in hypercortisolism of long duration and renal calculi may develop.[26] Inhibition of growth hormone by cortisol, as well as cortisol's direct effect on growth cartilage, causes growth retardation and delayed skeletal development in children with this disorder. Psychiatric disturbances are recognized in some patients with hypercortisolism. Loss of the

Figure 9-13 Preoperative and postoperative appearance of 23-year-old woman with adrenal carcinoma. Note moon facies, buffalo hump, supraclavicular fat pads, and mild hirsutism. **A,** Preoperative adrenal carcinoma with moon facies and hirsutism. **B,** Preoperative adrenal carcinoma with buffalo hump. **C,** Postoperative adrenal carcinoma with loss of moon facies and hirsutism. **D,** Postoperative adrenal carcinoma with loss of buffalo hump.
Courtesy National Institutes of Child Health, Bethesda, Md.

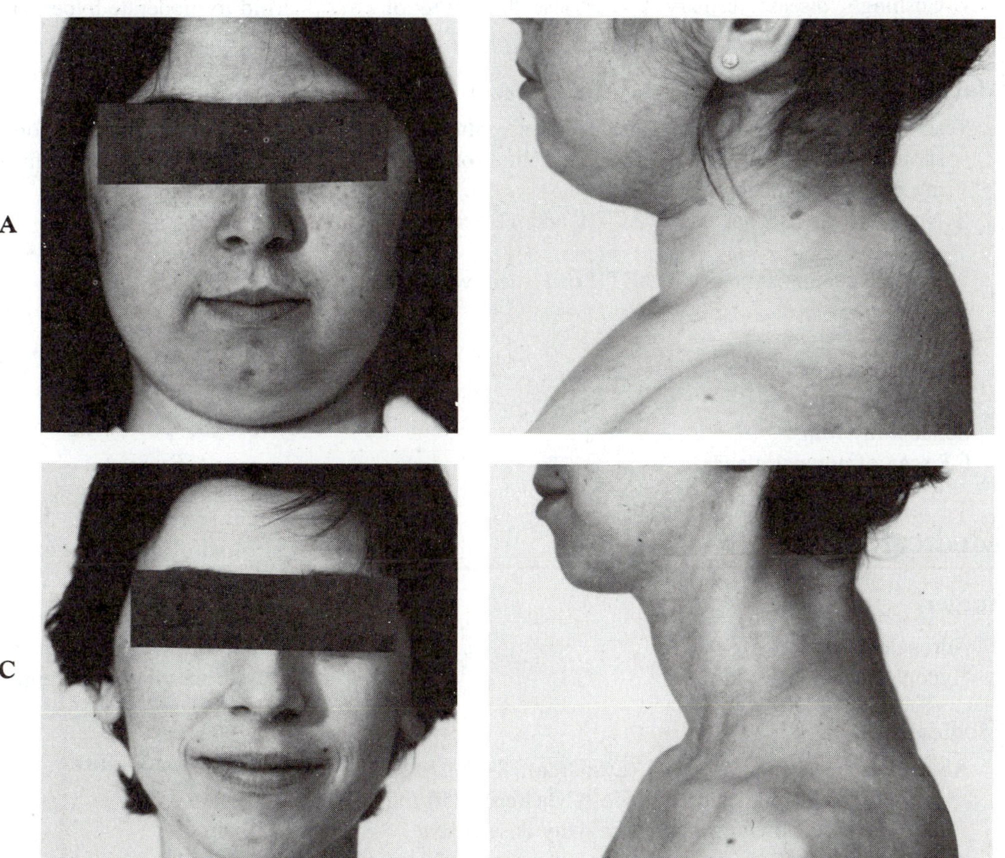

normal diurnal rhythm of cortisol release has been associated with insomnia.

Hyperandrogenism from adrenal hyperfunctioning in Cushing's syndrome causes menstrual irregularities (oligomenorrhea or amenorrhea). Mild to moderate hirsutism in females is seen depending on the amount of androgen secreted and the sensitivity of the hair follicle to androgen (Figure 9-13).

Diagnostic Studies and Findings

Blood

- Serum cortisol
  - Loss of diurnal rhythm; elevated at night
- Plasma ACTH
  - Elevated (ectopic syndromes); normal to slightly elevated (Cushing's disease); low to immeasurable (adenoma or carcinoma); loss of diurnal variation
- Potassium
  - Decreased concentration
- Eosinophil
  - Reduction in number

Urine

- Urinary free cortisol (UFC): 24 hours
  - Elevated; greater than 100 g/24 h
- Urinary 17-ketosteroids (17-KS): 24 hours
  - Elevated (age dependent)
- Urinary 17-hydroxysteroids (17-OH): 24 hours
  - Elevated

Endocrine

- Dexamethasone suppression test
  - Tests the state of negative feedback between the adrenal and the hypothalamic-pituitary unit; false positive readings may occur in depression, alcoholism, or patients receiving phenytoin and phenobarbital

Low dose (0.5 mg q6h for 2 d)
Normal response: suppression of ACTH; decreased production of urinary 17-0H
Cushing's disease: little or no effect
High dose (2 mg q6h for 2 d)
Cushing's disease: urinary 17-OH less than 50% of baseline

Metyrapone Test (750 mg q4h for six doses)

Tests hypothalamic-pituitary feedback response; altered response when patient has thyroid abnormalities or is taking estrogen or phenytoin
Normal response: increased ACTH and 11-deoxycortisol
Adrenal adenoma: no rise in ACTH or 11-deoxycortisol

Radiologic Tests

Chest tomograms
CT scan of sella
Sellar x-ray film
CT scan of adrenal glands

Medical Plan

Surgery

Adrenalectomy
Hypophysectomy (p. 956)

Medications

Antineoplastic agents: mitotane (Lysodren), 8-10 g/d in divided doses; aminoglutethimide (Cytadren), 250 mg q6h; increase slowly to maximum daily dose of 2 g

General Management

Pituitary irradiation (p. 961)

NURSING CARE

Nursing Assessment

Circulation

Mild to moderate hypertension

Nutrition

Moderate weight gain
Fat distribution: truncal obesity, supraclavicular fat pads, buffalo hump, moon facies
Hyperglycemia
Increased appetite

Elimination

Glycosuria
Proteinuria
Hypercalciuria

Neurologic Concerns

Impaired memory
Impaired concentration

Musculoskeletal Concerns

Fatigue
Muscle weakness
Inability to rise from squat position
Muscle wasting in extremities
Growth retardation (pediatrics)

Pain and Discomfort

Back pain
Rib pain

Skin

Blood vessel fragility: plethora and easy bruisability
Thin, translucent skin
Hyperpigmentation
Poor wound healing

Psychosocial Concerns

Irritability
Altered body image

Nursing Dx & Intervention

Nursing Diagnosis	Nursing Intervention/Rationale
Altered nutrition: less than body requirements	• Assess patient's stature alteration (via old pictures) resulting from disease onset. • Assess compliance to prescribed caloric, high-protein diet. • Record urine chemistry daily (i.e., sugar, acetone, and protein). • Administer insulin as prescribed.
Activity intolerance	• Assess patient's current activity tolerance. • Identify patient's priorities for energy expenditures. • Plan activity and rest periods with patient daily *to maximize energy and minimize fatigue.* • Discuss limitations with patient.
Impaired skin integrity	• Assess skin, especially areas of thinning and loss of integrity, *to identify areas of risk.* • Instruct patient concerning good skin hygiene: Wash and dry thoroughly. Use lotions as needed. Use antifungal cream as needed. Perform aseptic care to minor lacerations and abrasions. • Provide adequate pressure to venipuncture sites *to prevent subcutaneous hematoma.* • Instruct patient to avoid minor bumps and trauma. • Keep patient's room clear of obstructions (excess furniture, etc.) • Instruct patient in the use of protective clothing, especially shoes and socks, *to prevent trauma.*
Ineffective individual coping	• Assess emotional factors related to disorder. • Assess patient's current stressors, coping skills, and past successful adaptive strategies. • Give emotional support. • Identify sources of irritability and depression. • Assist patient with problem solving. • Collaborate with mental health nursing specialist or psychiatrist.
Body image disturbance	• Assess degree of body image change since onset of disease *to determine what aspects of body image change is related to disease onset.* • Discuss cushingoid features of the disorder with patient; give emotional support. • Discuss palliative treatment for hirsutism (i.e., shaving or depilatories).

Patient Education

1. Teach the importance of and how to administer chemotherapeutic medication and to report side or toxic effects.
2. Stress the importance of regular, lifelong medical follow-up.
3. Teach the importance of wearing or carrying medical alert information.

Evaluation

Patient Outcome	Data Indicating That Outcome is Reached
Nutrition is adequate.	Weight is proportionate to height and stature. Urine chemistry levels are within normal limits. Blood sugar is within normal limits. Patient verbalizes use of appropriate dietary regimen.
Activity tolerance increases.	Patient maintains maximum activity levels for physical limitations. Patient verbalizes realistic plan for alternating activities and rest based on limitations. Patient participates in recreational activities.
Skin is intact.	There are no breaks, cracks, ulcers, or ecchymosis. There is no infection. Wound healing is normal. Patient verbalizes a method for maintaining hygiene.
Patient copes effectively.	Patient verbalizes one or more sources of stress and a plan to prevent or decrease stress. Patient seeks assistance with coping when appropriate. Patient functions to maximum level of independence based on limitations.
Patient's self-concept improves.	Patient uses realistic self-care methods to enhance physical features. Patient is not preoccupied with negative aspects of physical appearance. Patient participates in age-related activities and groups. Patient maintains peer relationships. Patient expresses realistic expectations concerning physical abilities and appearance.

Pheochromocytoma

A pheochromocytoma is a chromaffin cell tumor of the sympathetic nervous system that produces excessive amounts of the catecholamines epinephrine and norepinephrine.

The incidence of pheochromocytoma is rare. Less than 0.5% of all patients with a recent diagnosis of hypertension have pheochromocytoma. The disorder has no predominance for sex or race and occurs more commonly in the third and fourth decades of life. Tumors in children are usually associated with a familial tendency, are frequently bilateral, and are often malignant. Familial tendencies are unusual and inherited as an autosomal dominant trait. Pheochromocytomas are often linked with medullary carcinoma of the thyroid and multiple endocrine neoplasias (MEN II syndromes).[26]

Pathophysiology

Ninety percent of tumors arising from the chromaffin system are found in the adrenal medulla and are called pheochromocytomas. The remainder are extra-adrenal and are classified as paragangliomas; they usually are found in the abdomen. Multiple pheochromocytomas occur in approximately 20% of cases and often in patients possessing the inherited trait. Pheochromocytomas can occur in pregnancy and lead to increased morbidity and mortality for mother and fetus. Malignant pheochromocytomas are a rarity and occur in 5% of patients. Metastatic sites include bone, lung, liver, and lymph nodes.[32]

Pheochromocytomas produce excessive amounts of epinephrine and norepinephrine; however, norepinephrine is more prevalent and is responsible for most of the clinical manifestations. Norepinephrine, an α-adrenergic agonist, primarily causes the hypertensive effects of the disorder and is the principal hormone seen in extra-adrenal tumors. Epinephrine, a β-adrenergic agonist, is responsible for hypertensive as well as hypermetabolic and hyperglycemic effects of the disorder.

Overproduction of norepinephrine causes sustained hypertension, the most outstanding clinical sign in patients. Excess epinephrine production can also bring about hypertension and postural hypotension. Blood pressure measurements can range from 200 to 300/150 to 175 mm Hg. Patients may have widely fluctuating blood pressures with or without paroxysmal hypertensive episodes. During a hypertensive crisis the patient may experience severe headaches, palpitations, profuse sweating, pupillary dilation, pallor, or flushing. Hypertensive episodes can be provoked by stimuli such as palpation of the tumor, emotional stress, or increased abdominal pressure (i.e., micturition). Extreme cases of hypertension may lead to cerebrovascular accidents that can be life threatening. Nephrosclerosis and retinopathy may accompany severe sustained hypertension. Myocarditis, dysrhythmias, and congestive heart failure are seen in patients who develop cardiomyopathies related to the direct effect of high levels of catecholamines on the myocardium.[32]

Elevated levels of circulating epinephrine and norepinephrine create a state of hypermetabolism similar to thyrotoxicosis.[26] The patient may have tachycardia, tacharrhythmias, weight loss, heat intolerance, tremors, and hyperreflexia. Sympathetic overstimulation can give rise to apprehension and emotional instability. Catecholamines suppress insulin secretion and stimulate the conversion of glycogen to glucose in the liver, resulting in hyperglycemia and glycosuria.[32]

Diagnostic Studies and Findings

Computerized Tomography (CT Scan)

Urine Studies for Metanephrines and Vanillylmandelic Acid (VMA)

Medical Plan

Surgery

Vena caval catheterization (p. 1589)
Excision of pheochromocytoma (p. 960)

Medications

α-Adrenergic blocking agents: used to lower arterial pressure and to increase vascular volume
- Phentolamine (Regitine), 0.5-5 mg IV and/or by continuous infusion at a rate of 0.25 to 1 mg/min; short acting (carefully monitor blood pressure)
- Phenoxybenzamine (Dibenzyline), 10-60 mg/d po; long acting

β-Adrenergic blocking agents*
- Propranolol (Inderal), 40 mg/d po; used for tumors that secrete epinephrine, which causes tachycardia and dysrhythmias

Tyrosine inhibitors
- Alphamethylparatyrosine (AMPT), 1-2 g/d po; interferes with catecholamine synthesis and decreases the amount of circulating catecholamines

NURSING CARE

Nursing Assessment

Respiratory Concerns

Increased respiratory rate
Dyspnea

Circulation

Increased heart rate
Palpitations
Postural hypotension

*β-Adrenergic blocking agents should be added only *after* alpha blockade has been achieved. β-Adrenergic blockade alone may exacerbate hypertension.

Sustained hypertension
Paroxysmal hypertension

Food and Fluid

Weight loss
Nausea
Anorexia
Hyperglycemia

Elimination

Glycosuria
Oliguria
Renal failure
Constipation

Neurosensory Concerns

Tremor
Hyperreflexia
Nervousness
Paresthesia

Comfort and Pain

Headache

Mobility

Muscle weakness

Sleep and Rest

Inability to sleep

Psychosocial Concerns

Anxiety

Hygiene and Skin

Sweating
Warmth (heat intolerance)

Nursing Dx & Intervention

Nursing Diagnosis	Nursing Intervention/Rationale
Altered cardiopulmonary and renal tissue perfusion	• Assess blood pressure and pulse (use same arm; routinely take measurements lying and either sitting or standing). • Monitor renal output *to monitor renal perfusion.* • In hypertensive crisis: Notify physician. Have emergency cardiac drugs available. Monitor neurologic status frequently. Monitor blood pressure and pulse electronically *to monitor for acute cardiovascular/neurologic changes.* • Perform actions *that minimize hypertension:* Do not palpate abdomen. Have patient avoid constrictive clothing. Elevate head of bed, restrict activity. Do not allow smoking. Eliminate beverages with caffeine. Have patient avoid Valsalva maneuver, straining at stools, etc.
Altered nutrition: less than body requirements	• Assess patient's current nutritional intake, including adequacy of total calories, protein, and vitamins. • Consult dietitian; provide nutritional meals, incorporating patient's food preference; make a daily calorie count if calories are inadequate. • Give medications for nausea, prior to meals. • Test urine for percentage of sugar, acetone, and protein. • Weigh daily *to monitor weight loss.*
Activity intolerance	• Assess current activity levels and patient's ability to tolerate inactivity. • Plan rest and activity schedule with patient daily. • Assist with gradual position change from lying or sitting to standing. • Limit activity if necessary *to prevent hypertensive events.*
Sleep pattern disturbance	• Assess quantity of sleep; inquire about quality of sleep. • Promote sleep and rest: private, darkened room; quiet, calm environment; and no disturbances while patient is asleep.
Ineffective individual coping	• Assess patient's coping skills (especially ability to tolerate limited activity), support systems, and adaptive skills, that have been successful in the past. • Collaborate with mental health nurse specialist or psychiatrist as necessary. • Provide patient with opportunities to verbalize concerns and fears. • Involve patient in plan of care *to decrease sources of powerlessness and loss of control.* • See also p. 1804.

Patient Education

1. Teach about medication action, schedule, dose, and side effects.
2. Teach the importance of regular visits to physician and lifelong follow-up.
3. Instruct the patient to carry or wear medical alert information.
4. Teach how to take and record blood pressure measurements.

Evaluation

Patient Outcome	Data Indicating That Outcome is Reached
Tissue perfusion is normal.	Blood pressure and pulse are within normal range, both lying and standing or sitting. Output is 30 ml/hour. There are no paresthesias, tremors, or palpitations.
Nutrition is adequate.	Patient verbalizes a decrease or absence of nausea. Patient maintains body weight in proportion to height and stature. There are no signs of dehydration. Urine chemistry levels are within normal limits.
Activity tolerance and sleep pattern improve.	Patient plans ADL schedule to alternate rest and activity. Patient participates in desired activities without fatigue. Patient verbalizes a feeling of well-being after sleep.
Patient copes effectively.	Patient identifies strengths and uses them in ADLs. Patient verbalizes ability to manage stressful situations or decrease their frequency. Patient maintains relationships with family and contemporaries. Patient participates in independent self-care.

DISORDERS OF THE PITUITARY GLAND

Hyperpituitarism

Hyperpituitarism is the overproduction of one or more anterior pituitary hormones. The most common cause is a pituitary tumor, but other causes, such as hypothalamic lesions or starvation, have been implicated.[26]

Current knowledge regarding hyperpituitarism has been expanded by many recent innovations, including (1) the development of bioassays to measure directly an increasing number of different hormones; (2) the use of sensitive radiologic techniques, especially CT scans, for earlier diagnosis; (3) the use of microsurgical techniques for pituitary surgery; and (4) the ability to synthesize an increasing number of hypothalamic hormones, which is important for diagnosis. Current research includes attempts at exact localization of the tumor (hypothalamic, pituitary, target organ, or ectopic source) and increasing the understanding of the complex rhythmicity of the hypothalamic-pituitary system.

Epidemiologically, pituitary tumors are far more common than is suggested clinically; one study involving autopsies reported an incidence in the general population of 22%,[32] the majority of which were asymptomatic. Among symptomatic patients, men and women are generally equally affected with pituitary tumors.[32] The most common age of the affected person is 35 to 40 years, although this may be decreasing as diagnostic techniques improve.[32] The disease is rare in children under 9 years of age.[26] Pituitary tumors make up 7% of all intracranial tumors.[32] Onset of the disease is often slow and insidious[32] and can be difficult to diagnose, especially in the early phase. A genetic component has been postulated because hyperpituitarism has been seen in more than one member of a single family, but this point remains controversial.

Pathophysiology

There is no known etiology of pituitary tumors.[26] These tumors are classified by identifying either the staining properties of the tumor or the hormones secreted in excess. There are four types of tumor according to the former method: basophilic—those that typically secrete adrenocorticotropic hormone (ACTH); eosinophilic—those that usually secrete growth hormone (GH); chromophobic—those formerly thought to be nonfunctioning but now believed to secrete prolactin[32]; and combinations of the other three types. This classification system is subject to controversy because of the variability of staining techniques.[105] It is being replaced by the second classification system, which uses terminology to indicate the hormone that is hypersecreted. With this classification, prolactinomas are most common, followed by GH-secreting tumors, ACTH-secreting tumors, and, finally, the more rare thyroid-stimulating hormone (TSH) and luteinizing hormone (LH), follicle-stimulating hormone (FSH) secreting adenomas.[100]

Two separate yet related disease entities deserve mention in a discussion of pituitary tumors. The first, Nelson syndrome, is a rare disorder that occurs after bilateral adrenalectomy is used to treat Cushing's disease. It is characterized by hyperpigmentation, caused by excessive production of

ACTH and melanocyte-stimulating hormone (MSH) by a pituitary tumor. It is believed that this tumor is the original cause of the Cushing's disease and that it enlarges after adrenalectomy because of the lack of negative feedback. Therefore there is an increase in the production of ACTH and, concurrently, MSH. The second disease entity is a type of tumor that occurs in the region of the pituitary but does not secrete hormones.[26] This tumor is called a craniopharyngioma; it is important in the differential diagnosis of any sellar tumor.

The extent of the pathophysiology caused by pituitary tumors is based on two factors: the size of the tumor and the hormone secreted in excess. In terms of the size, the tumors are classified as either microadenomas (diameter less than 10 mm) or macroadenomas (diameter more than 10 mm).[103] The larger tumors cause problems simply by their size; they impinge on the surrounding tissue, including normal pituitary tissue, which can cause varying degrees of hypopituitarism.[103] Other structures that may be affected by a large tumor include the bony sella turcica, which can be enlarged; the optic chiasm, which may be compressed, causing visual field defects; and the hypothalamus, which also may be compressed. The second factor that determines the extent of the pathophysiology is the hormone secreted in excess; the physical manifestations vary greatly (discussed in detail in the section on nursing assessment).

Diagnostic Studies and Findings

Radiologic Studies and Skull Roentgenograms, Sellar Tomograms, Head and Sellar CT Scans

Enlargement of the bony sella

Visualization of the adenoma within the sella or with suprasellar extension

Angiogram

Used to rule out a possible aneurysm

Ophthalmologic Examination

Visual field deficits; decreased acuity

Endocrine Function Testing

Inappropriate baseline hormone levels in blood or urine; inability to suppress or stimulate normal release of pituitary hormones (p. 1593)

Neurologic Examination

Cranial nerve deficits; unequal pupil size; inappropriate reaction to light

Medical Plan

Surgery

Removal of the pituitary tumor (intercranial or transsphenoidal approach) (p. 956)

Removal of the target organ (adrenal glands, thyroid; see target organ for discussion)

Medications

Dopamine receptor antagonist: bromocriptine mesylate (Parlodel), used to treat prolactinomas and GH-secreting tumors; usual dosage is 2.5-10 mg/d for prolactinomas; GH-secreting tumors typically require much higher doses, the upper limit being that of patient tolerance

General Management

Radiation therapy (p. 961)

NURSING CARE

Nursing Assessment

Macroadenomas

- Sensory and vision concerns
  - Bitemporal hemianopsia
  - Decreased acuity
  - Blurred vision
- Neurologic concerns
  - Chronic headaches, usually intermittent, of moderate intensity, and variably located; may be associated with nausea and vomiting
  - Possible neurologic changes, particularly those involving the third cranial nerve (unequal pupil size, inappropriate reaction to light)
- Endocrine concerns
  - Signs and symptoms of hypofunction (in regard to hormones other than those produced by the tumor)

Growth Hormone–Secreting Tumors

- Musculoskeletal concerns
  - Coarse facial features (thick ears, nose)
  - Prognathism causing chewing difficulties
  - Thick fingers and toes with concomitant increase in shoe or glove size
  - Atrophied skeletal muscle
  - Laryngeal hypertrophy causing voice to deepen
  - Arthritis, arthralgia, backaches
  - Osteoporosis
  - Mobility difficulties related to pain, fatigue
- Prepubertal concerns
  - Rapid increase in height, making patient considerably taller than classmates
- Hygiene and skin
  - Oily skin
  - Acne
  - Diaphoresis
  - Metabolic concerns
    - Glucose intolerance

Psychosocial concerns
- Irritability, hostility, and other psychologic manifestations
- Anxiety over "being different" from others
- Difficulty with social interactions, including sexual partner and family (acting fearful, hostile, withdrawn)
- Incongruity between self-concept and current self-image

Prolactin-Secreting Tumors

Gynecologic concerns
- Galactorrhea involving one or both breasts
- Irregular menses
- Oligomenorrhea or amenorrhea
- Infertility

Androgenic concerns
- Decreased libido
- Impotence
- Gynecomastia

Psychosocial concerns
- Anxiety about fertility, sexual performance, and self-image

Melanocyte-Stimulating Hormone–Secreting Tumors

Skin
- Hyperpigmentation, especially noticeable in skin folds, mucous membranes, and new scars

Past history
- Cushing's disease treated with bilateral adrenalectomy

Nursing Dx & Intervention

Nursing Diagnosis	Nursing Intervention/Rationale
Pain	• Assess patient for type, location, intensity, and frequency of pain, and ask about successful and unsuccessful measures used in the past for pain control. • Assess use and schedule of medications and other physical comfort measures (e.g., heat, cold, light massage). • Discuss factors that precipitate pain and restructure the environment accordingly *to decrease or eliminate these factors.* • Instruct patient regarding relaxation techniques (deep breathing, selective focusing). • Discuss realistic expectations about pain control.
Body image disturbance	• See p. 1751.
Ineffective individual coping	• Assess patient's coping behaviors, stresses, and adaptive skills. • Discuss with patient and family the relationship of psychologic manifestations to the disease process *to increase family understanding and support.* • Encourage family not to blame patient for inappropriate behavior. • See also p. 1804.
Sexual dysfunction	• Assess patient's and significant other's attitudes toward sexual expression and its importance in their relationship. • Establish trusting relationship with patient and sexual partner. • Encourage patient to verbalize feelings, with both health care provider and sexual partner. • Instruct patient and sexual partner regarding relationship between disease process and sexual dysfunction. • Provide patient and sexual partner with information about various methods to obtain sexual gratification *to maximize skills of sexual expression.*
Activity intolerance	• Assess patient's current activity levels and priorities for activity performance. • Thoroughly evaluate patient's abilities and limitations, both at home and in the community. • Discuss with patient alternate ways of performing limited activities. • Help patient structure time to allow for rest periods throughout the day, especially after activities. • Encourage patient to participate in care to maximum ability. • Assist patient to set realistic activity goals and to prioritize activities *to maximize patient satisfaction.*

Patient Education

1. Instruct the patient regarding methods for modifying pain control program for use at home (e.g., structuring a supportive physical environment and appropriate self-administration of analgesics).
2. Inform the patient about community mental health resources (support groups, individual therapists, etc.).
3. Instruct the patient regarding methods for modifying activity program for use at home.
4. Teach and encourage continued performance of range-of-motion exercises at home.

Evaluation

Patient Outcome	Data Indicating That Outcome is Reached
Comfort is increased.	Patient verbalizes a decreased frequency and amount of pain. Patient verbalizes pain-precipitating factors and means of decreasing or eliminating these factors. Patient demonstrates relaxation techniques. Patient follows a pain control program.
Body image improves.	Patient verbalizes acceptance of body changes. Patient maintains relationships with others. Behavior is appropriate during interactions. Patient maintains physical appearance appropriate to age. Patient verbalizes and expresses feelings and concerns about differences between ideal self and realistic self.
The patient copes effectively.	Patient can identify results of ineffective coping mechanisms. Patient uses strengths in planning home care. Patient discusses alternate home care methods and makes positive choices.
Sexual functioning improves.	Patient verbalizes feelings about sexual dysfunction. Patient expresses an understanding of the relationship between prolactinoma and sexual dysfunction or infertility. Patient verbalizes improvement in sexual functioning.
Activity tolerance improves.	Patient identifies increased number of activities performed independently. Patient demonstrates active range-of-motion exercises and performs these three times daily. Patient demonstrates an ability to structure day, including all ADLs and appropriate rest periods.

Diabetes insipidus

Diabetes insipidus is a transient or permanent disturbance of water metabolism that results in the excretion of a large volume of dilute urine. It may be pituitary, nephrogenic, or psychogenic in nature.

Central (or pituitary) diabetes insipidus results from a failure of vasopressin synthesis or release. Nephrogenic diabetes insipidus results from a deficiency of vasopressin receptors in the renal collecting ducts. Psychogenic diabetes insipidus (polydipsia) occurs following a large intake of fluid that may suppress antidiuretic hormone (ADH). All these causes result in the excretion of large volumes of dilute urine. Current research centers on the development of more effective and specific analogues of vasopressin, such as DDAVP, a vasopressin analogue with prolonged action.

Pathophysiology

The maintenance of water homeostasis is a function of the posterior pituitary gland and the kidney. The neurohypophysis secretes a polypeptide hormone with marked antidiuretic properties called antidiuretic hormone (ADH), or vasopressin. ADH acts on the collecting duct of the nephron and regulates its permeability to water. In the absence of ADH, an average adult will produce about 10 to 12 L of dilute (specific gravity = 1.001; osmolality = 100 mOsm/kg) urine daily. In the presence of maximal vasopressin concentrations, urine flow can be reduced to less than 0.5 L/d of very concentrated (specific gravity = 1.035; osmolality = 1000 mOsm/kg) urine.[64]

Central diabetes insipidus may be caused by head trauma, neurosurgery, hypothalamic tumors, or infiltrative diseases. Half of all cases are idiopathic. Diabetes insipidus is transient when the supraoptic hypophyseal tract is damaged below the median eminence, and it is permanent when damage is above the median eminence. Only 10% of the neurosecretory neurons need to be present to prevent diabetes insipidus. It may be corrected by vasopressin replacement therapy.[105]

Nephrogenic diabetes insipidus is inherited as an autosomal dominant trait and is therefore predominantly found in males. It may be acquired in association with disorders causing a decrease in glomerular filtration rate (chronic renal disease, electrolyte disturbances, pharmacologic agents, sickle cell disease, or dietary abnormalities). Treatment of nephrogenic diabetes insipidus is directed toward the primary disorder and may involve the use of diuretics to produce a paradoxical antidiuretic effect to enhance fluid reabsorption.

Psychogenic polydipsia results in the same clinical picture as central and nephrogenic diabetes insipidus. This disorder is dangerous only when intake exceeds renal capacity to excrete water. Treatment is directed at control of fluid intake.

Diagnostic Studies and Findings

Dehydration Test

Central diabetes insipidus (DI): urine remains dilute (low osmolality)
Nephrogenic DI: urine remains dilute
Psychogenic polydipsia: urine will become concentrated; if polydipsia is severe, urine may show limited concentration during test

Administration of Vasopressin Following Dehydration

Central DI: urine will become concentrated
Nephrogenic DI: no change
Psychogenic polydipsia: no change

Visual Field Testing

Defects suggest hypothalamic pituitary lesions

CT Scan and X-Ray Films of Sella Turcica

Useful for detection of hypothalamic pituitary lesions

Medical Plan

Medications

Pituitary hormones

- Vasopressin (Aqueous Pitressin), 2-5 U 2-4 times daily IM, subcutaneously, or IV; duration of drug: 2-8 h; used in acute settings or for initial emergency treatment; for close monitoring during transient episodes; too short acting for chronic use; used for differential diagnosis of diabetes mellitus
- Vasopressin (Pitressin Tannate in oil), 5-10 U q2-4d IM or subcutaneously; duration of drug: 48-72 h; longer duration, preferred for chronic therapy; used for differential diagnosis of diabetes insipidus
- Lypressin nasal solution (Diapid Nasal Spray; synthetic lysine), 1 or 2 sprays in one or both nostrils qid; onset: 1 h; duration of drug: 3-8 h; may be used alone or in conjunction with vasopressin tannate; if patient has nasal congestion, there will be decreased absorption of drug
- Desmopressin (DDAVP; synthetic arginine, vasopressin), 5-40 μg/d in 1-3 divided doses; administer by nasal insufflation (high in nose, not inhaled into throat); onset: 1 h; duration of drug: 8-20 h; drug of choice for chronic treatment because of its long duration and infrequent side effects

NURSING CARE

Nursing Assessment

Thirst

Polydipsia
Unquenchable thirst
Preference for cold or iced water

Urinary Function

Polyuria (output greater than 4 L/day)
Frequency
Nocturia
Low specific gravity (1.001 to 1.005)

Hydration Status

Poor skin turgor
Dry skin
Weight loss

Bowel Function

Constipation

Nursing Dx & Intervention

Nursing Diagnosis	Nursing Intervention/Rationale
Fluid volume deficit (1)	• Assess for signs and symptoms of dehydration: dry mouth, poor skin turgor, soft eyes, low blood pressure, fast pulse, output greater than intake, and weight loss. • Measure urine output. *With diabetes insipidus, urine output is usually greater than 4 L/day and may exceed 10 L/day if severe. Rule of thumb: patient voiding more than 200 ml/hour of dilute urine indicates presence of diabetes insipidus.* • Obtain accurate daily weight *to assess fluid loss.* • Specific gravity measurement is not necessary *because urine excretion rates of this magnitude can occur only with dilute urine except in case of diabetes mellitus.* • Measure urine glucose *to exclude diabetes mellitus as cause of polyuria* ("insipidus" means tasteless; "mellitus" means sweet). • Measure plasma osmolality. *If thirst mechanism is normal, plasma osmolality will be in high normal range. If thirst mechanism is abnormal, plasma osmolality will be above normal.*

Patient Education

1. Teach the patient how to measure and record intake and output.
2. Teach the patient to weigh self daily in the morning in the same clothes.
3. Teach the importance of why and how to administer vasopressin; side or toxic effects to report to physician; and parameters for as-needed administration based on output volume and characteristics.
4. Teach the patient how to check the urine's specific gravity.
5. Teach the importance of wearing a medical alert bracelet to identify the disorder.

Evaluation

Patient Outcome	Data Indicating That Outcome is Reached
Hydration is adequate.	Adequate hydration is evidenced by moist mucous membranes, good skin turgor, firm eyes, normal vital signs, stable weight, and intake approximate to output. Urine output is less than 4 L/day. Plasma osmolality is normal (285 to 290 mOsm/L).

Syndrome of inappropriate antidiuretic hormone

The syndrome of the inappropriate secretion of antidiuretic hormone is the continuous secretion of antidiuretic hormone when plasma osmolality is low, that is, at a time when ADH secretion should be inhibited.[103]

Syndrome of inappropriate antidiuretic hormone (SIADH) is one of the most common causes of hyponatremia. Etiologies include head trauma, central nervous system neoplasms, pulmonary diseases, certain endocrinopathies, and some pharmacologic agents such as morphine and barbiturates. The following outline provides a complete listing of conditions that may predispose a patient to SIADH[98,103]:

1. Central nervous system
   a. Brain tumor
   b. Head trauma
   c. Subarachnoid hemorrhage
   d. Infections
      (1) Meningitis
      (2) Encephalitis
      (3) Abscess
   e. Guillain-Barré syndrome
   f. Acute intermittent porphyria
   g. Cerebellar and cerebral atrophy
   h. Cavernous sinus thrombosis
   i. Neonatal hypoxia
   j. Rocky Mountain spotted fever
   k. Delirium tremens
2. Pulmonary disorders
   a. Pneumonia
   b. Tuberculosis
   c. Cystic fibrosis
   d. Cavitation (aspergillosis)
   e. Abscess
   f. Empyema
   g. Pneumothorax
   h. Asthma
   i. Positive pressure breathing
3. Hypovolemia and hypotension
   a. Sodium-losing renal disease
   b. Adrenal insufficiency
   c. Hemorrhage
4. Endocrinopathies
   a. Addison's disease
   b. Hypopituitarism
   c. Myxedema
5. Tumors producing ectopic ADH
   a. Mesothelioma
   b. Carcinoma of lung, duodenum, pancreas, ureter, bladder
   c. Thymoma
   d. Ewing's sarcoma
   e. Lymphoma
   f. Hodgkin's disease
   g. Prostatic carcinoma
6. Pharmacologic agents
   a. Drugs that increase tubular reabsorption of water
      (1) Vasopressin
      (2) Oxytocin
   b. Drugs that stimulate the release of ADH
      (1) Vincristine
      (2) Nicotine
      (3) Morphine
      (4) Barbiturates
      (5) General anesthesia
   c. Drugs potentiating the action of ADH
      (1) Chlorpropamide
      (2) Carbamazepine
      (3) Thiazide diuretics
      (4) Phenothiazines
7. Acute psychosis
8. Idiopathic causes

Antidiuretic hormone (ADH) can also be secreted by nonpituitary neoplasms such as oat cell carcinoma of the lung. The most common form of treatment is water restriction, but current research in the area is directed primarily at devising improved therapies. For example, lithium salts and demeclocycline have recently been shown to antagonize the effects of ADH and have found a place in the treatment of this syndrome.[64]

Pathophysiology

The syndrome of inappropriate antidiuretic hormone occurs when there is continuous synthesis and release of ADH in the presence of serum hypo-osmolality. Normally, when plasma osmolality drops, production and release of ADH are reduced, resulting in a diuresis. In SIADH, antidiuretic hormone continues to be released in the face of a subnormal serum osmolality. This also results in a simultaneous urine osmolality that is greater than that of serum. Dilutional hyponatremia occurs in SIADH from an increase in tubular reabsorption of water. The retention of water causes an expansion of plasma volume. This increase in intravascular fluid causes an increase in the glomerular filtration rate, and the reabsorption of sodium and water in the renal tubules is inhibited. The expansion of the plasma volume also inhibits the release of renin and aldosterone. This further increases the loss of sodium in urine and intensifies the dilutional hyponatremia. Because SIADH results in the retention of free water and not salt, edema is not a feature of this disorder.[103]

Diagnostic Studies and Findings

Serum Osmolality

Below normal (less than 285 mOsm/L)

Urine Osmolality

Above normal (greater than 150 mOsm/L)

Serum Sodium

Below normal (less than 135 mEq/L)

Medical Plan

Medications

Diuretics
- Furosemide (Lasix), 40-80 mg/d in divided doses, or 20-40 mg/d IV
- Hypertonic saline, dosage individually calculated

General Management

Fluid restriction (free water restriction)

NURSING CARE

Nursing Assessment

Fluids and Electrolytes

Decreased volume of urine
Increased specific gravity of urine
Increased weight
Abdominal and muscle cramping

Neurologic Changes

Early sign: change in level of consciousness, confusion
Disorientation; uncooperativeness
Hostility
Increased deep tendon reflexes
Drowsiness
Lethargy
Headache
Increased seizure potential

Gastrointestinal Changes

Anorexia
Nausea and vomiting
Diarrhea (from water intoxication)
Constipation (from fluid restriction and hyponatremia motility)

Psychosocial Changes

Anxiety
Frustration
Irritability
Uncooperativeness
Hostility

Nursing Dx & Intervention

Nursing Diagnosis	Nursing Intervention/Rationale
Fluid volume excess	• Assess for signs and symptoms of water intoxication: increased irritability, change in sensorium, headache, and hyperreflexia. • Maintain strict fluid limitations, especially free water intake and output *to prevent water intoxication.* • Monitor weight daily *to assess for fluid retention.* • Assess patient and visitor compliance with fluid restrictions; provide thorough explanations for restricting fluids. • Monitor environment *to control patient's access to fluids.*
Altered thought processes	• Check orientation to time, place, and person *to assess for confusion and level of consciousness.* • Set limits as necessary *to maintain stable and safe environment.* • Reduce confusing environmental stimuli. • Explain rationale for disturbances in thought processes to family members.

Patient Education

1. Teach the patient and family the rationale for fluid restrictions.
2. Teach the patient and family the importance of measuring intake and output; reinforce how to do intake and output measurements.

Evaluation

Patient Outcome	Data Indicating That Outcome is Reached
Fluid volume is normal.	Intake is approximately equal to output. Specific gravity is within normal limits. Vital signs are within normal limits. Weight of patient is stable.
Thought processes are normal.	Patient is oriented to time, place, and person. There is no injury to self, others, or property. Statements are reality oriented. Patient performs ADLs, within physical limitations, independently.

DISORDERS OF THE THYROID GLAND

Hyperthyroidism

Hyperthyroidism is the clinical and biochemical syndrome that results when tissues are exposed to excessive quantities of thyroid hormones.[32]

Hyperthyroidism produces multiple system abnormalities because the thyroid hormones affect all organs and metabolic processes. The clinical signs and symptoms may be mild to severe. The nature of the manifestations depend on the patient's age, the severity of the syndrome, the rate of onset, the presence or absence of concomitant abnormalities in various organ systems, and the additional clinical features presented by the causative agent. Hyperthyroidism is a common disorder and may be transient or permanent. Its exact prevalence in the United States is not known, although it is known to be more common in young women regardless of the underlying cause.

Pathophysiology

Unregulated production of excessive amounts of thyroid hormones may result from intrinsic thyroid disease; unregulated thyroid-stimulating hormone (TSH), or thyroid-releasing hormone (TRH) secretion; production of abnormal thyroid-stimulating hormones, such as thyroid-stimulating immunoglobulins or chorionic gonadotropin; destruction of thyroid tissue with release of hormones; or exogenous thyroid hormone replacement.[32] Varieties of hyperthyroidism are listed in Table 9-6. A brief review of these causes is outlined. Graves' disease is the most common cause of hyperthyroidism.

Graves' disease is defined as a multisystem disease characterized as consisting of one or more of the following: diffuse thyroid enlargement, hyperthyroidism, infiltrative ophthalmopathy, infiltrative dermopathy, and thyroid acropachy. Most patients with Graves' disease have both hyperthyroidism and goiter that develop concurrently. Thyroid disease and infiltrative phenomena may occur singly or concurrently and may run courses largely independent of one another.

There is evidence that hereditary factors predispose to the development of Graves' disease. Thyroid antibodies, abnormalities in thyroid regulation, and thyroid-stimulating immunoglobulins (TSIs) have been found in euthyroid family members of patients with Graves' disease.[32] Finally, there is an increased evidence of other autoimmune disorders, such as Hashimoto's disease and pernicious anemia, in these patients and their families.[103]

The exact cause of Graves' disease remains unknown. There is general agreement that the thyroid abnormalities result from the action on the gland of immunoglobulins that may be antibodies against components or regions of the thyroid plasma membrane[103] related to the TSH receptor. These autoantibodies, listed below, have been given various names on the basis of the assays used to detect them.

LATS	Long-acting thyroid stimulator
LATS-p	Long-acting thyroid stimulator protector
HTS	Human thyroid stimulator
HTACS	Human thyroid adenylate cyclase stimulator
TSab	Thyroid-stimulating antibody
TBII	Thyroid-binding inhibiting immunoglobulins
TDII	Thyrotropin displacement activity

These autoantibodies are now usually known as thyroid-stimulating immunoglobulins (TSIs).[32] TSIs bind to the thyroid cell and activate the TSH receptor, which in turn stimulates thyroid function and thyroid growth.[32] Possible mechanisms for TSI production are thyroid injury, an infectious or other agent that stimulates production of the antibodies, suppressed B-lymphocytes, and abnormal T-lymphocyte regulation of B-lymphocytes.[32]

The thyroid gland in Graves' disease is diffusely enlarged (diffuse toxic goiter). The gland has increased vascularity, and there is often infiltration to a varying degree with lymphocytes and plasma cells.[103]

The cause or causes of infiltrative ophthalmopathy, infiltrative dermopathy, and thyroid acropachy remain unknown. Hyperthyroidism may initially develop without these extrathyroidal manifestations, although approximately 20% to 40% of patients have clinical evidence of ophthalmopathy.[32]

Infiltrative dermopathy is an uncommon manifestation seen in approximately 5% to 10% of patients.[103] It usually occurs months or years after treatment for hyperthyroidism and in patients who have significant ophthalmopathy.[32] Thyroid acropachy is seen in patients who have previously treated hyperthyroidism, localized dermopathy, and ophthalmopathy.[32] Generally, no symptoms or deformities occur, but thyroid acropachy may produce contractures.[32]

Table 9-6
Varieties of Hyperthyroidism

Disorder	Incidence	Cause
Graves' disease (Basedow's disease; often referred to as toxic diffuse goiter)	More common in women during third and fourth decades of life; estimated to occur in 0.4% of US population	Believed to be an autoimmune disorder resulting from thyroid-stimulating immunoglobulins
Subacute thyroiditis (granulomatous, giant-cell, or de Quervain's thyroiditis)	Uncommon; more frequent in women; increased incidence during fourth and fifth decades; tendency for seasonal and geographic aggregations; mild hyperthyroidism in about 50% of cases	Probable viral infection of gland results in: Destruction of follicular epithelium Loss of follicular integrity Release of large quantities of preformed hormones and abnormal iodinated materials[103]
Painless thyroiditis	Increasing in general population; may occur in the postpartum period in over 50% of women with a history of Graves' disease	Subacute thyroiditis or an unusual manifestation of chronic autoimmune thyroiditis[32]
Radiation-induced thyroiditis	Rare; usually occurs 1-2 wk after therapy	^{131}I therapy resulting in follicular necrosis and inflammation
Toxic multinodular goiter (Plummer's disease)	Unknown; more frequent in women in the sixth or seventh decade; usually a long history of gradually increasing thyroid enlargement	Hyperfunctioning autonomous thyroid tissue
Toxic uninodular goiter (thyroid adenoma)	Female/male ratio: 3:1 to 6:1; US incidence: 5% of hyperthyroid patients; adults: all ages, especially in younger age group in 30s and 40s; occasionally seen in children	Adenoma functions autonomously With continued growth, the adenoma assumes a greater share of glandular function and ultimately results in atrophy and complete suppression of the remainder of the gland[103] Adenoma may infarct, resulting in a change from hyperfunctioning to hypofunctioning nodule with relief from hyperthyroidism[103]
Exogenous hyperthyroidism		
Iatrogenic		L-Thyroxine in doses of 0.3 mg/d or more L-Triiodothyronine in doses of 0.075 mg/d or more Desiccated thyroid in doses of 180 mg/d or more More likely to develop when T_3 or a combination of T_4 and T_3 is used[56]
Factitious (thyrotoxicosis factitia)	More common in women with background of underlying psychiatric disease, paramedical personnel with access to thyroid hormone, or patients for whom thyroid medications have been prescribed in the past[103]	Chronic ingestion of excessive quantities of thyroid hormone
Iodide-induced hyperthyroidism (jod-basedow)	Iodide-deficient populations (usually in patients with underlying thyroid disorders) or in multinodular goiter)	Administration of supplemental iodine to individuals with endemic, iodine-deficiency goiters; hyperthyroidism may be induced in patients with nonendemic goiter when large quantities of iodine are administered in the form of expectorants, x-ray contrast media, medications containing iodine, or any other form[103]
Ectopic hyperthyroidism (struma ovarii)	Very rare	Dermoid tumor or teratoma of ovary that contains a hyperfunctioning thyroid adenoma[32]
Thyroid carcinoma (follicular or mixed papillary follicular)	Uncommon; occurs predominantly after 40 yr of age; women are affected 2-3 times more commonly than men	Large, autonomously functioning thyroid tumor

Table 9-6—cont'd
Varieties of Hyperthyroidism

Disorder	Incidence	Cause
Pituitary thyrotropin (TSH)	Rare	Excessive TSH secretion from a pituitary tumor[32] or inappropriate TSH secretion caused by pituitary resistance to thyroid hormone[88]
Trophoblastic tumor		Tumors of trophoblastic origin: hydatidiform mole, choriocarcinoma or embryonal carcinoma of the testis with very high levels of chorionic gonadotropin
T_3 toxicosis	Unknown; more common in elderly population; occurs in association with Graves' disease, toxic multinodular goiter, toxic adenoma, or carcinoma	Preferential increase in thyroid secretion of T_3

In general, the actions of the thyroid hormones are stimulatory in nature. The excessive production of thyroid hormones produces a state of hypermetabolism. The manifestations of hyperthyroidism usually reflect increased functions of various organs or tissues and an inability of an organ system to meet the increased demands.[32] Less severe manifestations are seen when the onset is gradual. Hyperthyroidism is tolerated fairly well, especially in younger patients, but it tends to be more debilitating in the elderly.[32]

Excessive heat production, increased neuromuscular activity, and hyperactivity of the sympathetic nervous system account for most of the clinical manifestations.[74] Compensatory mechanisms are called into action to meet the demands of the hypermetabolic state. These changes include an increased cardiac output; an increased peripheral blood flow with dilation of superficial skin capillaries; an increased body temperature; an increased oxygen consumption, resulting in an increased respiratory rate; increased absorption of glucose by the gastrointestinal tract; increased cellular use of glucose; hyperinsulinemia; decreased supply of fats and carbohydrates; increased metabolism of vitamins, leading in extreme cases to significant vitamin deficiencies; increased mobilization of bone, leading to a state of hypercalcemia; and increased secretions of ACTH and MSH, leading to skin pigmentation changes.

Apathetic or masked hyperthyroidism may occur in the elderly patient whose hyperthyroidism is manifested primarily by cardiac failure, atrial fibrillation, muscle weakness, or weight loss.[32] These elderly patients do not exhibit the clinical manifestations that are commonly seen in younger patients, such as nervousness, heat intolerance, increased appetite, and general hyperactivity.[32]

Thyroid storm or thyroid crisis is a severe life-threatening form of hyperthyroidism. Thyroid storm is uncommon but is the most severe and dramatic form of hyperthyroidism. It generally occurs in association with Graves' disease but can be seen with toxic multinodular goiter.[103]

Diagnostic Studies and Findings

Thyroid Suppression Test

No suppression of radioiodine or serum T_4 uptake after T_4 or T_3 administration (no longer a common test)

Thyrotropin-Releasing Hormone (TRH) Stimulation Test

Little or no response of TSH to TRH stimulation (supersedes suppression test; an extremely sensitive test of pituitary suppression)

Laboratory Findings

Serum T_4
Increased
Serum T_3
Increased
Serum free T_4 and T_3
Increased
Radioactive T_3 uptake (RT_3U)
High
Thyroid radioiodine uptake and scan
Increased uptake in most patients with hyperthyroidism except patients with subacute thyroiditis, painless thyroiditis, and exogenous hyperthyroidism; should be used only to confirm a diagnosis of painless thyroiditis or exogenous hyperthyroidism
TSH
Suppressed and does not respond to TRH
Thyroid-stimulating immunoglobulins (TSIs)
Present in Graves' disease

Medical Plan

Surgery

Subtotal thyroidectomy

Medications[20]

Thioamides

Propylthiouracil (PTU), 50-300 mg/d in 3-4 doses po for adults; initially 300-600 mg/d; inhibits thyroid hormone synthesis but not release; used to lower thyroid hormone levels; clinical improvement of hyperthyroidism is delayed; agranulocytosis may occur in 1.4% of patients during first 2 mo of therapy; skin rashes occur in roughly 3% of patients

Methimazole (Tapazole) (MMI), 5-20 mg/d po in 2-3 doses for adults; initially 30-60 mg/d in 3-4 doses; inhibits thyroid hormone synthesis but not release; similar to PTU

Oral cholecystographic agents (Ipodate), experimental; adults: oral, 1.5-3 g; rapidly inhibits extrathyroidal T_3 production; may be useful for short-term therapy for the occasional patient in whom antithyroid drug treatment or ^{131}I is contraindicated[32]

β-Adrenergic blockers

Propranolol (Inderal), 40-240 mg/d po in divided doses for adults; 5 mg or less IV at 1 mg/min or more slowly for adults; controls symptoms of hyperthyroidism but does not lower T_3 and T_4 levels; controls palpitations, tremor, sweating, proximal muscle weakness, and cardiac symptoms of hyperthyroidism by competitively blocking β-adrenergic receptors; bronchospasm may occur in asthmatics; may precipitate frank heart failure in patient with heart function maintained by sympathetic tone; causes 10%-20% reduction in serum T_3 concentrations[74]

Iodines

Potassium or sodium iodide (Strong Iodine; Lugol's Solution), 0.1-0.3 ml po tid for adults; IV: 250-500 mg/d for adults in thyrotoxic crisis; produces short-term inhibition of thyroid hormone synthesis by direct action on thyroid; used as presurgical medication to reduce size of thyroid gland after thioamide therapy; used with thioamide and propranolol for hyperthyroid crisis; may produce iodism[20]

Radioactive iodine (^{131}I NaI or ^{125}I NaI)

Adults: 4-10 mCi as single dose for Graves' disease; for thyroid carcinoma, single doses of up to 150 mCi; smaller doses used for diagnostic purposes; concentrated in the thyroid and release radiation, which destroys thyroid tissue; used to destroy thyroid tissue without surgery for control of Graves' disease or thyroid carcinoma; hypothyroidism ultimately develops in most patients

Glucocorticoids

Inhibit extrathyroidal T_3 production when given in large doses; inhibits thyroid hormone secretion in patients with hyperthyroidism due to Graves' disease; toxicity precludes their use in all but emergency situations[32]

General Management

Treatment of Graves' disease ophthalmopathy (often no cure)

Palliative treatment

Corticosteroids

Surgical orbital decompression

Surgical correction of muscle imbalance

Radiation of orbit

0.5% methylcellulose eye drops for eye irritation and pain

Treatment of Graves' disease dermopathy (often no cure)

Palliative treatment for extensive bulbous or ulcerated lesions

0.2% fluocinolone or other corticosteroid cream

Diet

Control of environment

Psychotherapy

NURSING CARE

Nursing Assessment

Skin and Appendages

Warm and moist; smooth velvety texture; erythema

Increased body temperature (37.8° C or greater may indicate thyroid storm)

Increased sweating

Increased diffuse pigmentation

Localized myxedema

Eyes

Lid retraction and lag

Proptosis

Conjunctival irritation; lacrimation

Characteristic bright-eyed, frightened, or startled look

Cardiovascular Status

Increased systolic blood pressure; wide pulse pressure

Tachycardia

Presence of arrhythmias

Respiratory Status

Changes in rate or depth of respirations

Increased restlessness

Gastrointestinal Status

Weight loss or modest weight gain (especially if large food intake; seen in younger patients)

Polyphagia; increased food intake

Diarrhea

Muscular Status

Generalized muscular wasting and weakness

Hyperactive deep tendon reflexes

Noticeable tremor

Nervous System Status

Restlessness; irritability
Decreased ability to concentrate; memory loss; easily distracted
Insomnia

Mental and Emotional Status

Emotionally labile; irritable
Manic behavior
Family members report changes in performance

Renal Status

Polyuria; urgency and frequency of micturition
Polydipsia

Reproductive Status

Women
- Hypomenorrhea
- Amenorrhea

Men
- Reported loss of libido
- Decreased potency
- Gynecomastia

Nursing Dx & Intervention

Nursing Diagnosis	Nursing Intervention/Rationale
Patient problem: potential for increased cardiac output	• Assess pulse, blood pressure, color, and temperature *to evaluate cardiovascular status and effectiveness of treatment.* • Assess sleeping pulse *for more accurate assessment of tachycardia.* • Measure and record intake and output (I & O) *to detect fluid overload and impending heart failure.*
Ineffective breathing pattern	• Assess breathing pattern, including rate, depth, and character of respirations, and the presence of dyspnea, shortness of breath, nasal flaring, use of accessory muscles, and muscular retraction. • Auscultate breath sounds. • Record vital signs every 4 to 6 hours. • Provide scheduled uninterrupted rest *to maximize energy for respiratory effort.* • Allow minimal exertion during care *to minimize energy expenditure.*
Altered nutrition: less than body requirements related to hypermetabolic state	• Assess daily weight, daily food intake, and serum glucose levels. • Stress importance of avoiding coffee, tea, colas, and foods that increase peristalsis *to minimize hyperactivity and nervousness, and to decrease hypermotility of the bowel.* • Provide high-calorie, high-protein, high-carbohydrate vitamin B diet with between-meal nourishments *to counterbalance loss of calories, vitamins, glucose, and proteins from bowel hypermotility, increased vitamin metabolism, and increased mobilization of nutrients.* • Provide dietary consultation.
Hyperthermia (potential)	• Assess body temperature and serum electrolytes *to evaluate patient's heat intolerance and electrolyte loss and to identify impending thyroid storm.* • Regulate environmental temperature; place patient in cool and quiet room. • Have patient wear light clothing; change clothing twice daily. • Provide light bed linens (i.e., sheet only).
Altered thought processes	• Assess level of orientation to person, place, and time. • Avoid discrepancies in timing, activities, and methods of performing procedures. • Provide physically and emotionally safe environment. • Explain procedures slowly and carefully *to facilitate patient concentration.* • Repeat instructions. Limit number of instructions. • Limit number of care givers *to facilitate routines and decrease distractions.* • Decrease external stimuli *to minimize distractions and increase the hyperactive patient's ability to concentrate.*
Impaired skin integrity	• Assess skin daily. • Monitor for development of localized myxedema. • Keep skin and linens clean, dry, and wrinkle free. • Lubricate and massage around affected skin *to protect integrity of skin.* • Force fluids (3000 to 4000 ml/day, unless contraindicated by cardiovascular status). • Elevate legs *to reduce or prevent edema.*

Patient Education

1. Teach signs and symptoms for early recognition and adjustment of treatment of hyperthyroidism.
2. Teach medication administration: name, dosage, action, frequency of administration, side effects, and importance of taking medicines on schedule.
3. Teach the signs and symptoms of hypothyroidism and the necessity of reporting to physician.
4. Instruct the patient regarding high-calorie, high-protein, high-carbohydrate, vitamin B diet with between-meal nourishment.
5. Stress the importance of planned rest and avoidance of stress whenever possible.
6. Prepare the patient and family members for emotional outbursts and potential alterations in body image.
7. Stress the importance of and necessity for follow-up evaluations.

Evaluation

Patient Outcome	Data Indicating That Outcome is Reached
Cardiovascular function is normal.	Dysrhythmias are absent or less frequent. Cyanosis is absent or decreased. Skin remains warm and dry. Hourly urine output is 30 ml.
Respiratory function is normal.	Patient demonstrates adequate respiratory depth and effort. There is no cyanosis. Restlessness is absent or decreased. Dyspnea is absent or decreased.
Nutritional intake is adequate.	Patient demonstrates adherence to prescribed diet. Patient maintains stable weight and increases food intake. Patient verbalizes the importance of a well-balanced diet.
Comfort is increased.	Patient verbalizes a decrease in or relief from heat intolerance. Patient identifies and uses several techniques to control heat intolerance.
Thought processes are normal.	Patient demonstrates orientation to person, place, and time. There is no injury to self, others, or property. Patient validates thought processes with staff. Statements are reality oriented.
Skin is intact.	There are no breaks, cracks, or ulcers. There is no evidence of infection. Skin turgor is normal.

Hypothyroidism

Hypothyroidism is the clinical state resulting from deficient thyroid hormones.

Hypothyroidism is a common disorder affecting both sexes from birth through old age. It occurs more often in women between the ages of 30 to 60 years than in any other group. The incidence of hypothyroidism in infants is estimated to occur in 1 out of every 4000 to 5000 newborns.[103] Population studies have indicated that unrecognized hypothyroidism may be more common in the elderly population than previously thought.[103] Neonatal screening programs have made major contributions toward health care, and it is suggested that screening programs be extended to cover the elderly as well.

The clinical manifestations of hypothyroidism may range from mild, with few signs or symptoms, to severe, culminating in the life-threatening myxedema coma. The clinical manifestations depend on the degree of thyroid hormone deficiency.

Pathophysiology

Hypothyroidism results from inadequate peripheral tissue levels of thyroid hormones, usually caused by inadequate thyroid secretion.[32] Hypothyroidism may result from loss or atrophy of thyroid tissue (intrinsic disease), insufficient stimulation of an intrinsically normal gland (resulting from hypothalamic or pituitary disease), or association with compensatory goitrogenesis as a result of defective hormone biosynthesis.[103] Causes of hypothyroidism as well as defining characteristics are listed in Table 9-7.

Clinical manifestations of hypothyroidism are reflections of decreased metabolic processes. Pathophysiologic changes including excessive interstitial glycosaminoglycan deposition occur throughout all organ systems. Glycosaminoglycan is the highly hydrophilic substance causing the mucinous edema (myxedema) that accounts for the majority of clinical manifestations seen in hypothyroidism.

There are three main forms of hypothyroidism: cretinism, juvenile hypothyroidism, and adult hypothyroidism (myxedema). Cretinism is a state of severe hypothyroidism found in infants. Thyroid hormones are essential for physical and mental growth. They are essential for central nervous system development, as well as skeletal maturation. Cretinism is characterized by an interruption in the normal physical and mental development in the infant.[95] It occurs either during fetal life or in the first few months after birth.[95] It is treatable, and permanent retardation may be preventable if treatment begins early.[95] If it is untreated, however, irreversible cerebral

Table 9-7
Varieties of Hypothyroidism

Variety	Incidence	Cause
Chronic autoimmune thyroiditis Atrophic (nongoitrous)—previously called "idiopathic hypothyroidism" Hashimoto's disease (goitrous)	Unknown; most common cause of spontaneously occurring hypothyroidism in both children and adults[102] More common in women in their thirties or older[102] Strong hereditary risk factor (thyroid autoantibodies are found in up to 50% of siblings of patients)[102] Patients and their relatives have a higher incidence of other associated autoimmune disorders	Autoimmune disorder; probably results from both cell- and antibody-mediated thyroid injury Characterized by antithyroid microsomal and antithyroglobulin antibodies in serum, often in very high titer[102]
Transient autoimmune thyroiditis	Most often occurs in postpartum period; rare in other populations Usually appears 3-6 mo after delivery Recurrences following subsequent pregnancies are common[102]	Autoimmune disorder; characterized by development of modest thyroid enlargement, hypothyroidism, and high titers of antithyroid microsomal antibodies (all such findings subside within several months)[102]
Hypothyroidism after radioiodine therapy and external neck radiation therapy	Common occurrence within a year after therapy with ^{131}I for hyperthyroidism (thereafter it occurs at a rate of 0.5%-2%/yr) Frequency determined by degree of radiation given[102]	Radioiodine (^{131}I or ^{125}I) therapy; external neck radiation therapy using doses of 2500 rad or more[102]
Postoperative hypothyroidism	Following total thyroidectomy: almost immediate occurrence Following subtotal thyroidectomy: less predictable, ranges from 5%-30% prevalence rate and then continues to appear indefinitely at rate of 1%-2%/yr[32] Following subtotal thyroidectomy for hyperthyroid Graves' disease: 25%-75% occurrence in first year	Surgery with loss of thyroid tissue or damage to it
Transient hypothyroidism	Exact incidence unknown; occurs within several weeks or months following ^{131}I therapy, subtotal thyroidectomy for Graves' disease, subacute thyroiditis, or withdrawal of prolonged thyroid hormone therapy in patients who are euthyroid[102]	Low serum TSH concentration occurs because of preceding thyroid hormone–induced inhibition of TSH secretion or high serum TSH levels until remaining thyroid tissue mass grows large enough to maintain normal thyroid secretion[102]
Thyroid dysgenesis (sporadic nongoitrous cretinism)	Most common cause of hypothyroidism in newborn; occurs in 1 of every 4000-5000 births	Developmental defects of thyroid gland; cause is unknown
Hypothyroidism caused by iodine deficiency	Most common cause of hypothyroidism in many parts of world	Iodine deficiency resulting in decreased production of thyroid hormones; important contributing factors are dietary goitrogens, genetic factors, and water pollution
Hypothyroidism caused by antithyroid agents and iodide excess	Exact prevalence unknown; not an important cause of hypothyroidism	Ingestion of compound with antithyroid potency Drugs: thiocyanate, perchlorate, nitroprusside, sulfonamides, sulfonylureas, iodides, lithium, paraaminosalicylic acid Antithyroid drugs: PTU, MMI Goitrin plants: rutabaga, white turnips, soybeans, cabbage, peanuts
Hypothyroidism caused by hereditary defects in thyroid hormone biosynthesis	Rare	Defects caused by defective iodide transport Defective iodide organification caused by inadequate or defective thyroid peroxidase, thyroglobulin formation, or peroxide

Continued.

Table 9-7—cont'd
Varieties of Hypothyroidism

Variety	Incidence	Cause
		Defective or insufficient thyroglobulin biosynthesis and formation of abnormal iodoproteins Defective dehalogenation of iodotyrosines
Hypothyroidism caused by thyroid insensitivity to TSH	Rare; also in some patients with pseudohypoparathyroidism	Defect is not known; patients may have a TSH receptor or postreceptor defect[102]
Hypothyroidism due to thyroid injury from other causes	Incidence unknown Occurs occasionally in patients with hemochromatosis, amyloidosis, sarcoidosis, scleroderma, cystinosis, and frequently in those with fibrous invasive thyroiditis (Riedel's thyroiditis)	Thyroid tissue damage
Pituitary hypothyroidism	Rare; less than 5% of hypothyroidism	Deficiency of TSH caused by destruction of pituitary tissue: functioning or nonfunctioning pituitary macroadenomas, surgery, pituitary radiation, postpartum pituitary necrosis (Sheehan's syndrome), pituitary cysts, craniopharyngioma, carotid aneurysm, trauma, hemochromatosis, and infiltrative diseases such as metastatic tumor, tuberculosis, histiocytosis
Hypothalamic hypothyroidism	Rare; occurs predominantly in children[102]	TRH deficiency caused by cranial irradiation; traumatic, infiltrative, and neoplastic diseases of hypothalamus; pituitary lesions that interrupt hypothalamic-pituitary portal circulation[102]
Hypothyroidism caused by impaired peripheral sensitivity to thyroid hormones	Rare; partial generalized resistance may occur sporadically or cluster in families (cause not known)	Postulated theory: the kinetics of T_3 nuclear uptake may be impaired (postreceptor defect)[102]
Spontaneous hypothyroidism following Graves' disease	Generally occurs following remission of Graves' disease; not associated with antithyroid drugs	May result from concomitant chronic autoimmune thyroiditis that frequently occurs with Graves' disease[32]

brain damage occurs. If the patient is treated during the first 3 months after birth, a better mental prognosis is achieved.[95]

Juvenile hypothyroidism develops during childhood. It is most often caused by chronic autoimmune thyroiditis but may also be caused by medications or defects in thyroid hormone synthesis. Growth and sexual maturation are most often affected. The clinical manifestations usually resemble signs and symptoms similar to those seen in adult myxedema. Myxedema is the term often used to describe adult hypothyroidism.

Myxedema coma is a rare, life-threatening state of hypothyroidism. It is the end stage of neglected or undiagnosed hypothyroidism and has a 50% mortality. Myxedema coma normally requires several years for development, but it has been noted to occur after the administration of sedatives or other psychotropic drugs to patients with undiagnosed hypothyroidism. It is seen more commonly in elderly patients who have been without medical care and has been noted to occur more often during the winter months, suggesting that cold exposure may be a precipitating factor. Myxedema coma is characterized by coma, hypothermia in more than 80% of patients, cardiovascular collapse, hypoventilation, and severe metabolic derangements such as hyponatremia, hypoglycemia, and lactic acidosis. The comatose state is produced by complications such as carbon dioxide retention, reduction in cardiac output, and consequently increasing cerebral hypoxia.[32]

Diagnostic Studies and Findings

TRH Stimulation Tests

Primary hypothyroidism: TSH increases above normal basal level

Pituitary hypothyroidism: subnormal TSH response or no response to TRH

Hypothalamic hypothyroidism: normal TSH, but retarded response to TRH

TSH Stimulation Tests (Rarely Used)

Distinguishes between primary hypothyroidism and secondary hypothyroidism caused by TSH deficiency; normal gland responds by increasing iodine uptake and T_4 release

RAIU

Below normal uptake

Serum T_4

Decreased

Serum T_3

Decreased; neither a specific nor a sensitive test for hypothyroidism

Serum Free T_4 and T_3

Decreased

Serum TSH

Elevated (primary hypothyroidism, chronic autoimmune thyroiditis, after subtotal thyroidectomy, ^{131}I therapy) normal or undetectable (pituitary or hypothalamic hypothyroidism, nonthyroidal illnesses)

RT_3U

Below normal

Medical Plan

Medications[20]

Natural thyroid hormones
- Thyroid USP (Delcoid; Thyrar; Thyrocrine; Thyro-Teric); 60-180 mg/d po for adult maintenance; initial doses 15 mg qd; double the dose every 2 wk until appropriate maintenance dose is reached; impure mixture of thyroid components that includes T_3 and T_4; replacement therapy for hypothyroidism; overdose produces symptoms of hyperthyroidism; too large a dose at onset of therapy may cause vascular occlusion, especially in patients with arteriosclerosis
- Thyroglobulin (Proloid), 32-180 mg/d po for adult maintenance; initial doses are small and are gradually increased to maintenance levels; contains T_3 and T_4, as well as other iodine-containing compounds; replacement therapy for hypothyroidism; overdose produces same symptoms as seen with Thyroid USP

Synthetic thyroid hormones
- Levothyroxine sodium (Cytolen; Levoid; Levothyroid; Synthroid Sodium), 150-200 μg/d po for adult maintenance; initial doses are small and are gradually increased to maintenance levels; IV, adults, 0.5 mg with mannitol (Synthroid) or without (Levothroid); chemically pure form of T_4; replacement therapy for hypothyroidism; IV form used for myxedemic coma; peak effect 9 d after start of therapy; serum half-life about 11 d
- Liothyronine sodium (Cytomel, Cytomine), 25-75 μg/d po for adult maintenance; initial doses should be low and gradually increased to maintenance levels; chemically pure form of T_3; replacement therapy for hypothyroidism; peak effect in 2 d; serum half-life 4-6 d
- Liotrix (Euthroid; Thyrolar), 30 μg T_4 with 7.5 μg T_3 or 25 μg T_4 with 6.25 μg T_3 po for adults; doses may be gradually increased as needed; chemically pure T_4 and T_3 combined in a ratio of 4:1; replacement therapy for hypothyroidism

Adenohypophyseal hormones
- Thyroid-stimulating hormone (TSH) (Thytropar), 10 IU IM or subcutaneously qd or bid; extract of bovine anterior pituitary contains natural peptide, TSH; diagnostic agent to establish hypothyroidism; may cause release of thyroid hormones that can precipitate adrenal crisis in patient with secondary adrenal insufficiency; may also cause cardiovascular symptoms and rare allergic reactions
- Protirelin (thyrotropin-releasing hormone, TRH) (Relefact TRH; Thypinone) 400-500 μg IV for adults; synthetic preparation of natural hypothalamic tripeptide hormone; diagnostic agent to differentiate pituitary-induced hypothyroidism from other types of hypothyroidism; may transiently produce nausea, facial flushing, hypertension, and urge to micturate

General Management

Control of environment
Diet: high protein, high fiber, low calorie

NURSING CARE

Nursing Assessment

Skin and Appendages

Cool, pale, dry, coarse; yellowish tint
Rough, scaly skin
Puffy, masklike face
Periorbital edema
Hypothermia
Myxedema

Cardiovascular Status

Bradycardia; decreased blood pressure
Decreased exercise tolerance
Arrhythmias

Respiratory Status

Hypoventilation
Hoarseness
Sensitivity to narcotics, tranquilizers, sedatives, and anesthetics

Gastrointestinal Status

Anorexia
Modest weight gain
Constipation; fecal impaction
Abdominal distention; myxedema ileus

Muscular Status

Nonspecific fatigue; weakness
Slow muscle movement
Delayed relaxation of tendon reflexes

Nervous System Status

General slowing of all intellectual functions, including speech
Decreased hearing
Lethargy and somnolence
Impaired memory; inattentiveness
Loss of initiative

Mental-Emotional Status

Paranoia
Depression
Agitation

Skeletal Status

Aches and stiffness of joints

Renal System Status

Decreased urine output
Slightly impaired ability to concentrate urine

Reproductive Status

Women
- Diminished libido
- Failure of ovulation
- Amenorrhea

Men
- Diminished libido
- Impotence

Nursing Dx & Intervention

Nursing Diagnosis	Nursing Intervention/Rationale
Decreased cardiac output	• Assess pulse, blood pressure, color, and temperature *to determine cardiovascular stability.* • Measure and record intake and output; weigh daily *to evaluate fluid balance.* • Observe level of consciousness and orientation. • Monitor for potentiating effects of drugs (use lower doses of sedatives, narcotics, etc.) *to identify cardiovascular depression caused by drug accumulation resulting from lowered metabolic rate.*
Ineffective breathing pattern	• Assess rate, depth, and character of respirations *to identify respiratory depression.* • Assess breath sounds *to observe for early signs of infection and hypoventilation.* • Provide scheduled uninterrupted rest. • Allow minimum exertion during care. • Position *to maximize rest and minimize work of breathing.*
Altered thought processes	• Assess level of orientation to person, place, and time. • Provide tolerable activity schedule *to conserve energy.* • Provide physically and emotionally safe environment. • Explain procedures slowly and carefully *to support decreased concentration.* • Assist family in accepting patient's dullness and slowness. • Time nursing activities to patient's response level *to prevent further disorientation.* • Explain procedures slowly and simply, reinforcing them repeatedly, *to support the patient with lethargy, impaired memory, and inattentiveness.* • Schedule nursing activities around patient's activity cycles.
Impaired skin integrity	• Assess skin daily for increased edema, breakdown, signs of infection, and bleeding tendency. • Take measures to conserve body temperature (i.e., warm blankets, robes, socks, bed jacket) *to prevent further hypothermia.* • Utilize lubricants and protective gels *to prevent further skin breakdown.* • Provide safe environment *to protect patient with hypoactive reflexes, lethargy, and/or impaired memory.*
Constipation	• Assess frequency, color, consistency, and amount of stool. • Assess effectiveness of anticonstipation aids. • Provide high-protein, high-fiber, low-calorie diet in smaller, frequent meals. • Encourage increased fluid intake; record I and O *to monitor dehydration.* • Establish daily routine bowel training program. • Avoid use of enemas *to prevent fluid retention in a patient with myxedema.*

Patient Education

1. Teach the signs and symptoms of hypothyroidism and hyperthyroidism to report.
2. Teach the patient that thyroid hormones are essential for life and that treatment is therefore lifelong.
3. Teach medication administration: name, dosage, frequency of taking, and side effects.
4. Instruct the patient regarding maintenance of a well-balanced, high-fiber diet with adequate iodine and fluid intake.
5. Stress the importance of adequate rest alternating with increasing periods of exercise.
6. Stress the importance of avoiding over-the-counter medications without consulting the physician.
7. Emphasize the importance of and necessity for follow-up evaluations.

Evaluation

Patient Outcome	Data Indicating That Outcome is Reached
Cardiovascular function is normal.	Patient demonstrates normal sinus rhythm. Skin remains warm and dry. Patient remains alert and fully oriented. Patient maintains an hourly urine output of 30 ml.
Respiratory function is normal.	Respiratory depth and rate are adequate. Chest expansion is equal. There is no cyanosis.
Thought processes are normal.	Patient is oriented to person, place, and time. Patient validates thought processes with staff. Statements are reality oriented. Patient is interested in work, environment, friends, and family.
Skin integrity is normal.	Skin remains intact. Skin remains free of infection. Edema is absent or decreased. Patient verbalizes or demonstrates skin care measures.
Constipation is absent or decreased.	Bowel movements are regular and of normal consistency, color, and quantity. Patient verbalizes adherence to prescribed diet and fluid intake. Patient identifies high-fiber foods to use in diet plan.

DISORDERS OF THE PARATHYROID GLANDS

Hyperparathyroidism

Hyperparathyroidism is the hyperactivity of one or more of the parathyroid glands as a result of one of a number of primary or secondary causes.

Hyperparathyroidism is manifest as hypercalcemia. The disease occurs in adults between the ages of 30 and 70. Women have the disease more frequently than do men (2:1 ratio). Patients with hypercalcemia have chronic elevations in serum calcium levels (above 5.3 mEq/L).

Technical advances and research have created a greater awareness of parathyroid disorders. Symptoms are recognized earlier, and the means for making diagnoses have become more sophisticated in the past decade. New treatments for parathyroid disorders are being used with greater success rates, and diagnostic workups are being made with accuracy as a result of these advancements. Continued research and a strong focus on education of the health care team will ensure early detection and treatment as well as prevention of complications manifested by these disorders.

Pathophysiology

More than 80% of the patients with primary hyperparathyroidism have a single parathyroid adenoma (a neoplasm of the gland, which may be 2 to 200 times the size of a normal gland). The adenoma is an encapsulated tumor made of chief cells. Primary clear cell hyperplasia is a rare disorder in which all four glands become enlarged 30 to 100 times their normal size. Primary chief cell hyperplasia is more common than clear cell hyperplasia, but it is difficult to differentiate from an adenoma. Chief cell hyperplasia also occurs in patients with multiple endocrine neoplasias, types I and II.[66]

Parathyroid carcinoma occurs rarely. Its progress is more rapid and severe than most hyperparathyroid disorders. Surgical excision and radiation are usually ineffective in its treatment.

The etiology of primary hyperparathyroidism is unclear. It is felt that radiation to the neck might be a possible cause. Secondary hyperplasia may develop as a result of conditions causing a decrease in serum calcium levels, such as chronic renal disease, vitamin D deficiency, pregnancy, rickets, pyelonephritis or glomerulonephritis, hyperphosphatemia, and calcium deprivation.

Clinical manifestations of hyperparathyroidism are based on the effects of increased parathyroid hormone on the target areas: bone, kidney, and gastrointestinal tract. Increased serum calcium levels cause a decrease in parathyroid hormone secretion, resulting in the stimulation of osteoblasts to increase bone resorption. Cysts and fibrous tissue invade bones, causing pain and pathologic fractures. Calcifications form in renal tubules, causing obstructions that inhibit the concentration of urine. Renal colic, dull back pain, and hematuria are symptoms resulting from the formation of calculi.[26]

Other manifestations of increased serum calcium levels include decreased neuromuscular excitability caused by the polarization of cell membranes by high calcium levels and decreased motility of the gastrointestinal tract. Cardiac changes that occur as a result of hypercalcemia include decreased neuronal permeability, defects in conduction, and an increased threshold for stimulation.

Diagnostic Studies and Findings

Serum Calcium Levels

Greater than 5.3 mEq/L in adults; greater than 6 mEq/L in children

Serum PO_4

Less than 1.8 mEq/L

Urinary Calcium Levels

Less than 25 mEq/L

Urinary PO_4

Greater than 0.6 mEq/L

Creatinine Clearance

Decreased

Hydroxyproline

Increased

Urinary cAMP

Increased

Medical Plan

Surgery

Parathyroidectomy

Medications

Diuretic agents: furosemide (Lasix), 20-80 mg q1-8h, IV or po
Volume expansion up to 3000 ml/d IV or po
Phosphates, 1-3 g/d IV or po
Parathyroid hormone agents: calcitonin (Calcimar), 4-8 μg/kg of body weight, IM or subcutaneously

NURSING CARE

Nursing Assessment

Renal Concerns

Polyuria
Nephrolithiasis
Nephrosclerosis
Urinary tract infection

Gastrointestinal Concerns

Anorexia
Nausea
Vomiting
Weight loss
Constipation

Cardiovascular Concerns

Bradycardia
Cardiac irregularities (shortened Q-T interval)

Skeletal Concerns

Enlarged skull
Demineralization
Skeletal pain
Pathologic fractures

Central Nervous System

Personality disturbances
Disorientation
Paranoia

Disturbed Consciousness

Lethargy
Drowsiness
Stupor
Coma

Decreased Neuromuscular Excitability

Muscle weakness
Hypotonia
Uncoordination

Nursing Dx & Intervention

Nursing Diagnosis	Nursing Intervention/Rationale
Decreased cardiac output	• Assess for signs of hypoperfusion: mental status change, decreased urine output, etc. • Assess vital signs every 4 hours; check pulse for bradycardia. • Assess ECG strip every 4 hours (flattened or inverted T wave, P wave changes, and Q-T interval changes). • Monitor stools, urine, sputum, and emesis for blood *to determine possible causes of secondary anemia*. • Monitor for petechiae and bruising.
Potential fluid volume deficit	• Assess for dehydration. • Weigh daily. • Record intake and output. • Check skin turgor and turgor of tongue and mucosa *to identify early dehydration*. • Encourage fluids to 3000 ml/day. • Administer medications to reduce calcium.
Activity intolerance	• Assess patient for signs of pain with movement *to assess patient's tolerance for movement*. • Observe for steadiness on ambulation. • Assist the patient with ambulation when necessary. • Handle the patient gently; allow him or her to move slowly. • Identify with the patient environmental hazards at home and suggest alterations as necessary *to prevent injury*.
Pain	• Assess for indications of pain with movement, guarding, or protection of particular body parts. • Avoid extreme temperature changes. • Obtain physical therapy consultation. • Administer warm packs or soaks to painful areas. • Administer pain medications on schedule rather than as needed. • Emphasize good body alignment and posture *to maintain normal anatomic position*. • Splint ribs while the patient turns, coughs, and so on, when fractures are apparent *to decrease pain and prevent further injury*.
Ineffective individual coping	• Assess for precipitating factors causing stress. • Assess for life stressors, coping skills, and adaptive behaviors used successfully in the past. • Maintain a calm approach if the patient becomes agitated or irritable. • See also p. 1804.

Patient Education

1. Teach how to monitor and maintain adequate fluid intake.
2. Teach the method for checking urine for stones and hematuria.
3. Stress the importance of proper body alignment and mechanics and the need for increasing activity to tolerance.
4. Teach how to check pulse and to report changes.
5. Assist the patient in developing a plan for using alternate pain-relieving methods rather than relying on pain medication.
6. Teach the signs and symptoms for early recognition and treatment of hypocalcemia.
7. Ensure that the patient understands the importance of changing the home environment to prevent accidents.

Evaluation

Patient Outcome	Data Indicating That Outcome is Reached
Cardiac output is adequate.	ECG strip is normal. Vital signs are stable.
Fluid and electrolyte balance is maintained, and calcium levels are normal.	Sodium level is 137 to 145 mEq/L. Potassium level is 3.3 to 4.6 mEq/L. Chloride level is 100 to 110 mEq/L. Calcium level is 4.3 to 5.3 mEq/L. Phosphorus level is 1.8 to 2.6 mEq/L. Intake approximates output. Specific gravity is normal.
Comfort and activity level are increased.	Optimum level of mobility is maintained with little or no pain experienced. Patient follows plan for using alternate pain-relieving methods. Patient uses pain medications infrequently. Patient verbalizes increased feelings of well-being. Patient participates in desired activities.

Patient Outcome	Data Indicating That Outcome is Reached
Patient copes effectively.	Patient expresses feelings and uses effective coping mechanisms for problems surrounding illness. Patient is able to identify factors leading to increased stress and possible solutions to prevent these situations. Patient's affect is appropriate to the situation.

Hypoparathyroidism

Hypoparathyroidism is a condition in which the parathyroid glands secrete an inadequate amount of parathyroid hormone (PTH) to maintain normal levels of serum calcium.

Hypoparathyroidism is manifested by hypocalcemia. This condition may occur at any age and is usually the result of damage to the parathyroid glands during parathyroid or thyroid surgery.

Pathophysiology

Although hypoparathyroidism is usually caused by damage to the parathyroid glands during surgical procedures, the disease may also be idiopathic. Idiopathic hypoparathyroidism is a rare autoimmune disorder that usually occurs before 15 years of age. It is sometimes one of a number of endocrine disorders included in a polyendocrine syndrome called HAM (hypoparathyroidism, Addison's disease, and moniliasis). Hypoparathyroidism has been acquired, in a few rare cases, following treatment with ^{131}I therapy. It has also been associated with metastases of malignant tumors to the parathyroid glands.[32]

The signs and symptoms of hypoparathyroidism are associated with hypocalcemia resulting from the decreased level of PTH. Neuromuscular irritability is the most common and recognizable feature of hypocalcemia, causing symptoms that range from mild paresthesias to tetany and hypocalcemic seizures. These symptoms are caused by a decrease in resting ability and increased excitability of nerve and muscle membranes.[14,60]

Bone resorption decreases in hypoparathyroidism, causing a decrease in osteoclastic activity. Bones remain normal or slightly more dense in adults. New growth is suppressed and may cause dwarfism in children. Calcification of the basal ganglion, another clinical manifestation of hypoparathyroidism, results in a Parkinson-like syndrome with bizarre posturing and dystonic choreoathetoid movements.[14] Other characteristics of the disease include dental abnormalities caused by decreased calcium levels, cataracts resulting from a calcification of the lens, and hypotension caused by decreased cardiac contractility. Pseudohypoparathyroidism is a separate disease entity that is a familial disorder characterized by an atypical phenotype, chemical hypoparathyroidism, and increased circulating PTH levels.[32]

Diagnostic Studies and Findings

Serum Calcium

Less than 4.3 mEq/L

Urine Calcium

Greater than 200 mEq/24 h

Serum PO_4

Increased

Urinary PO_4

Decreased

Medical Plan

Medications

- Parathyroid hormone, 20-40 USP U q12h IM, IV, or subcutaneously
- Vitamins
  - Dihydrotachysterol, 0.25-1.75 mg/wk po
  - Vitamin D, 200-400 IU/d po
- Nutritional replenishers
  - Calcium gluconate, 5 g tid po (liquid)
  - Calcium glubionate, 10-60 ml po or IV
  - Calcium lactate, 4-10 g bid po (chewable tablet)

General Management

Dietary supplement of calcium

NURSING CARE

Nursing Assessment

Central Nervous System

- Personality disturbances
  - Anxiety
  - Depression
  - Irritability
- Increased neuromuscular excitability
  - Paresthesias
  - Tetany
  - Dysphagia
  - Chvostek's and Trousseau's signs

Headache
Retardation
Bilateral cerebral calcification

Cardiovascular System

Decreased contractility
Decreased cardiac output

Gastrointestinal System

Nausea
Vomiting
Diarrhea
Abdominal pain

Soft Tissue

Calcification (especially in eyes)

Ectodermis

Exfoliative dermatitis
Coarse, dry, scaly skin
Cutaneous pigmentation
Thin, patchy hair

Skeletal System

Dwarfism
Developmental abnormalities

Nursing Dx & Intervention

Nursing Diagnosis	Nursing Intervention/Rationale
Potential fluid volume deficit	• Assess intake and output, vital signs, and skin turgor *to identify early signs of fluid loss.* • Force fluid as ordered.
Potential for trauma	• Assess the patient for steadiness on ambulation, history of falls or trauma, and potential safety hazards in present environment. • Assist the patient when necessary. • Instruct the patient to use assistive devices or help when moving, as needed.
Altered nutrition: less than body requirements	• Assess current calcium intake of patient, and identify food preferences that are high in calcium. • Make high-calcium snacks available to patient at all times. • Have the dietitian discuss dietary calcium supplements with the patient. • Give calcium replacement medications on time *to enhance dietary intake of calcium.* • Monitor Chvostek's and Trousseau's signs *to identify early loss of calcium.*
Ineffective individual coping	• Assess patient's current coping skills, support systems, and history of adaptive behaviors that worked in the past. • Maintain a calm approach if the patient is agitated or irritable. • Observe for precipitating factors causing stress; intervene when possible *to decrease stressors.* • Observe for changes in mood and thought processes *to identify psychologic changes that may require medical interventions.* • See also p. 1804.
Decreased cardiac output	• Assess vital signs, mental status, and urine output for symptoms of hypoperfusion. • Check rhythm strip for Q-T interval changes and abnormal T wave and P wave changes *to identify hypocalcemia that is interfering with normal electrical activity of the myocardium.*

Patient Education

1. Teach the patient to monitor pulse and the importance of reporting irregularities.
2. Teach the patient to maintain fluid balance, especially when nausea, vomiting, and diarrhea are present.
3. Instruct the patient and family in the use of dietary calcium supplements and the reasons for the treatment.
4. Instruct the patient and family in the use and side effects of medications.
5. Teach early recognition and treatment of hypocalcemia.

Evaluation

Patient Outcome	Data Indicating That Outcome is Reached
Fluid intake is adequate.	Intake and output are within normal limits. Skin turgor is normal.
There is no injury.	There are no bruises or skeletal breaks. Patient states that environment is arranged for safety. Chvostek's and Trousseau's signs are negative.

Patient Outcome	Data Indicating That Outcome is Reached
Nutrition is adequate.	Patient verbalizes adherence to dietary plan. Calcium level is 4.3 to 5.3 mEq/L. Phosphorus level is 1.8 to 2.6 mEq/L. There are no signs or symptoms of hypocalcemia.
Cardiac output is adequate.	Vital signs are stable. Rhythm strip is normal.

METABOLIC DISORDERS

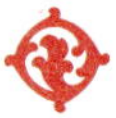

Insulin-dependent and non-insulin-dependent diabetes mellitus

Diabetes mellitus is a condition of relative or absolute lack of insulin, affecting carbohydrate, protein, and fat metabolism.

In 1985, 0.43 million persons in the United States had insulin-dependent diabetes mellitus (IDDM). In the same year, 5.07 million persons in the United States had non-insulin-dependent diabetes mellitus (NIDDM).[25]

The guidelines for classifying diabetes mellitus come from the NIH National Diabetes Data Group. Their classification of diabetes mellitus is as follows[75]:

Insulin-dependent
Non-insulin-dependent
Secondary (diabetes mellitus associated with certain conditions or syndromes)
Impaired glucose tolerance
Gestational diabetes mellitus
Previous abnormality in glucose tolerance
Potential abnormality in glucose tolerance

(This discussion is limited to the first two types.)

Pathophysiology

Insulin-dependent diabetes mellitus is a different disorder from non-insulin-dependent diabetes mellitus, although both share a common defect: relative or absolute lack of insulin (Table 9-8). Genetic predisposition for insulin-dependent diabetes mellitus seems to be conferred by a certain histocompatibility antigen, human leukocyte antigen (HLA), coded on chromosome 6.[31] Environmental factors may have a role in the development of insulin-dependent diabetes in the genetically susceptible individual. Viruses (coxsackie, mumps, rubella) may either cause direct destruction of the beta cells or induce an immunologic reaction to the beta cells of the pancreas.[31]

Initially, insulin dependence appears as insulitis and mononuclear cell infiltration of the pancreas, progressing to actual destruction of the functioning beta cells.[31] Islet cell antibodies, cell-surface antibodies, and cell-mediated immunity are present, suggesting the possible role of autoimmunity in the development of insulin-dependent diabetes.

Once beta cells are destroyed, metabolic compensation and the ability to maintain blood sugar within normal limits deteriorate steadily. Symptoms are the direct result of the lack of insulin and subsequent deterioration of body processes and metabolism associated with or requiring insulin.

Insulin deficiency causes hyperglycemia by decreasing glucose uptake by peripheral adipose and muscle tissues. The lack of restraining effect on the liver processes of glycogenolysis and gluconeogenesis causes the liver to overproduce glucose.[58] Glucose and amino acid uptake by muscle and fat tissue is impaired; synthesis of protein, glycogen, fat, DNA, RNA, and ATP is decreased.[58] Protein and fat are actually broken down, freeing up more substrate for the liver to use in out-of-control gluconeogenesis. Elevated levels of triglyceride and cholesterol bind to proteins in the blood. Since these lipoproteins cannot be metabolized in the peripheral tissues, they deposit under the skin.

Individuals with non-insulin-dependent diabetes are usually over 30 years of age at the time of diagnosis, and 80% are obese. Environmental etiologic factors are related to the urban life-style and include obesity, decreased exercise, and possible dietary factors.[31] A possible genetic component has not yet been identified.

Obesity is associated with insulin resistance or diminished sensitivity to insulin or both.[31] The exact cause of the defect is unknown, but it could occur at any step in the sequence of insulin action, from receptor binding to intracellular metabolism. Down regulation of receptors in response to hyperinsulinism has been demonstrated.[31] Therefore insulin resistance may begin as an adaptive mechanism to protect the body from hypoglycemia in the face of sometimes severe hyperinsulinemia. Hyperglycemia causes overactivity of the polyol pathway, causing sorbitol to accumulate in Schwann cells. This process damages myelin nerve covering, causing diabetic neuropathies.[58] Attachment of glucose to proteins (glycosylation) in the basement membranes of capillaries causes a thickening of the membranes and resultant diabetic microangiopathy. Microangiopathy is implicated in the development of retinopathy and nephropathy. Accelerated atherosclerosis in the heart and large arteries combined with decreased elasticity of arterial walls and the hypercoagulable state of diabetic blood result in high cardiac-related morbidity and mortality among the diabetic population.[31]

Other metabolic abnormalities associated with hyperglycemia, including elevated serum lipids, elevated plasma glucagon, and elevated growth hormone, may also have a contributory effect on the development of long-term complications. Glycosylated hemoglobin measurements are useful in

Table 9-8
Types of Diabetes and Characteristics

	Type I: Insulin-Dependent Diabetes (Juvenile Onset [JOD])	Type II: Non-Insulin-Dependent Diabetes (Maturity Onset [MOD])
Age of onset	<30 yr	>40 yr
Body weight	Normal or underweight	Overweight (80%)
Prevalence	0.5%	5%
Etiology	Unknown Heredity: associated with specific human leukocyte antigen (HLA) types but only 50% concordance in twins Autoimmune disease: 70% circulating islet cell antibodies Viral infections are possible trigger	Unknown Heredity: not associated with specific HLA types but 95% concordance in twins Autoimmune disease: 10% circulating islet cell antibodies No evidence for viral infections
Insulin	Early in disease, insulin secretion is impaired; late in disease, secretion may be totally absent	Insulin deficiency and/or insulin resistance Deficiency: insulin secretion sufficient to meet demands created by obese state; possible impairment in glucose receptor of the beta cell Resistance: in nonobese patients, there is hyperinsulinemia and a defect in tissue responsiveness to insulin; insulin resistance may be mediated by a decreased number of insulin receptors
Ketosis	Common	Rare
Complications	Frequent Microangiopathies Neuropathies Accelerated atherosclerosis	Frequent Accelerated atherosclerosis Microangiopathies Neuropathies
Leading cause of death	Microangiopathies (i.e., renal failure secondary to diabetic nephropathy)	Accelerated atherosclerosis (i.e., myocardial infarction)
Treatment	Diet and insulin	Diet (reduction) *or* Diet and oral hypoglycemic agents *or* Diet and insulin

From Kozak.[57]

assessing overall blood glucose control during the previous 3 to 4 months.[25] Although a number of these abnormalities return to normal with proper management of diabetes, none are causally related to the pathologic changes in the long-term complications of diabetes mellitus.

Diagnostic Studies and Findings

Fasting Blood Sugar

Venous plasma: ≥140 mg/dl
Venous whole blood: ≥200 mg/dl

Glucose Tolerance Test

2-Hour oral glucose tolerance test sample and one other sample after 75 g glucose
 Venous plasma: ≥200 mg/dl
 Venous whole blood: ≥180 mg/dl

Blood Insulin Levels

Absent in insulin-dependent diabetes
Normal to high in non-insulin-dependent diabetes

Plasma Proinsulin

Not applicable in insulin-dependent diabetes
Normal to high in non-insulin-dependent diabetes mellitus

Plasma C-Peptide

Absent in insulin-dependent diabetes
Normal to high in non-insulin-dependent diabetes

Medical Plan

Surgery

Interventions for complications (i.e., bypass grafts, eye surgery)

Medications

- Insulin preparations—doses are individually adjusted
  - Rapid-acting preparations
    - Regular
      - Iletin I, II (beef, pork)
      - Velosulin or Quick (pork)
      - Actrapid (pork)

Semilente
Iletin I (beef, pork)
Semitard (pork)
Human
Humulin R
Actrapid Human
Intermediate-acting preparations
NPH
Iletin I, II (beef, pork)
Insulatard NPH (pork)
Lentard (beef, pork)
Lente
Iletin I, II (beef, pork)
Monotard (pork)
Lentard (beef, pork)
Globin
Human
Humulin N
Monotard Human
Long-acting preparations
Utralente
Ultratard (beef)
Iletin I (beef, pork)
Protamine Zinc
Iletin I, II (beef, pork)
Oral hypoglycemic agents: sulfonylureas
First generation
Tolbutamide (Orinase), 500 mg to 2 g/d in divided doses
Chlorpropamide (Diabinese), 100-250 mg/d
Acetohexamide (Dymelor), 250 mg to 1.5 g/d in divided doses
Tolazamide (Tolinase), 100 mg to 1 g/d
Second generation
Glipizide (Glucotrol), 2.5-30 mg/d in divided doses
Glyburide (DiaBeta, Micronase), 1.25-20 mg/d in divided doses[36]

General Management

Open-loop infusion pumps (listing not inclusive)
Autosyringe: AS6C and AS6C-U100, AS6MP (Baxter-Travenol Laboratories, Inc.)
Beta 1 (Orange Medical Instruments)
Delta SP-250 (Delta Medical Industries)
Medix 209-100 (Medix Corp.)
Micromed (Pacesetter Systems, Inc.)
Betatron II, model 9200 (CPI-Lilly Co.)
CPI, model 9100 (Eli Lilly Co.)
Photocoagulation (see Chapter 6)
Penile prosthesis (see Chapter 12)
Kidney dialysis (see Chapter 11)
American Diabetes Association diet

NURSING CARE

Nursing Assessment

Food and Fluid

Hunger, thirst, nausea
Weight loss or obesity

Elimination

Frequent urination in large amounts
Nocturia
Diarrhea or constipation

Neurosensory Concerns

Decreased sensation to pain and temperature in feet
Blurred vision
Headaches, cataracts, halos around lights

Mobility

Muscle weakness
Tiredness
Wrist-drop
Ankle-drop

Skin

Infection (frequent skin boils and ulceration)
Rubeosis; dermopathy

Sexuality

Impotence
Vaginal discharge
Increased susceptibility to vaginal infection

Circulation

Cold extremities
Loss of hair on toes; skin shiny, thin, and atrophic
Orthostatic hypotension
Painful calves when walking
Numbness and tingling of lower extremities
Weak pedal pulse

Psychosocial Concerns

Verbalization of inability to cope
Verbalization of change in life-style
Negative feeling about body

Teaching and Learning

Lack of exposure to diabetes if newly diagnosed
Lack of recall
Misinformation
Inadequate demonstration of skills required (urine and/or blood testing, injection technique)
Lack of interest
Unfamiliarity with facts of management

Nursing Dx & Intervention

Nursing Diagnosis	Nursing Intervention/Rationale
Altered peripheral tissue perfusion	• Assess peripheral pulses and color, temperature, blanching, and tenderness of lower extremities *to determine circulatory status.* • Teach patient to prevent pressure at the back of the knees from crossing legs or sitting on a chair that is too high *to prevent venous stasis.* • Teach patient to avoid constricting garments on the lower trunk and extremities *to prevent venous stasis.* • Instruct patient regarding Buerger-Allen exercises *to develop collateral circulation.*
Potential fluid volume deficit	• Assess skin turgor for dehydration *to determine the presence of fluid deficit.* • Encourage patient to drink noncaloric fluids for hyperglycemia *to replace fluid loss resulting from polyuria.*
Altered nutrition: more than body requirements	• Assess for psychosocial concerns that may be related to overeating. • Arrange a dietary consultation. • Reinforce the meal plan as ordered. • Suggest support group such as Weight Watchers *to provide group and peer support.* • Allow patient to verbalize feelings regarding weight. • Positively reinforce patient's effort at weight loss.
Altered nutrition: less than body requirements	• Assess for factors that may influence diet preferences. • Arrange a dietary consultation. • Reinforce the meal plan as ordered. • Encourage patient to verbalize feelings about weight, body size, and eating behavior.
Potential impaired skin integrity	• Assess patient's feet every day for pressure areas and skin changes. • Ensure that patient maintains good hydration and nutritional status. • Instruct patient regarding proper foot care *to prevent injury and infections.*
Ineffective individual coping	• Assess personal strengths and weaknesses, current stressors, and stress-management skills. • Emphasize that daily management can become as routine as personal hygiene. • Encourage self-care to patient's maximum ability. • Encourage participation in diabetic support groups through local American Diabetes Association (ADA) and Juvenile Diabetes Foundation (JDF). • See p. 1804.

Patient Education

1. Teach the importance of and how to administer insulin or oral hypoglycemics; teach side or toxic effects to report.
2. Teach the method for monitoring blood sugar: regular urine testing or home blood glucose monitoring.
3. Teach the need for maintaining the prescribed diet and for regular, routine exercise and activity to maintain blood sugar control.
4. Teach early recognition and treatment of hypoglycemia and hyperglycemia.
5. Teach sick day management.
6. Teach personal hygiene, stressing specifics related to dental, foot, and skin care.
7. Stress the methods of care to prevent complications.
8. Teach the importance of regular medical care.
9. Provide adequate information about the disease process to permit informed decision making (e.g., about pregnancy).

Evaluation

Patient Outcome	Data Indicating That Outcome is Reached
Tissue perfusion is adequate.	Peripheral pulses are present. Skin is warm and moist. Turgor is normal. Capillary refill time is less than 3 seconds.
Nutrition is adequate.	Weight is within range for height and stature. Blood sugar is within individual target range set for fasting and postprandial levels. Output equals intake. Glycosylated hemoglobin is within normal limits.

Evaluation

Patient Outcome	Data Indicating That Outcome is Reached
Skin is intact.	There are no breaks, cracks, ulcers, or discoloration. There are no infections. Wound healing is normal.
Patient copes effectively.	Patient verbalizes coping with limitations imposed by required care. Patient expresses feelings of control. Patient accepts support from others as needed. Patient exhibits no destructive behavior. Patient functions independently in ADLs to maximum ability. Patient incorporates diabetic care into life-style.
Self-care is achieved.	Patient verbalizes understanding of and demonstrates the following: Insulin or oral hypoglycemic administration Urine or home blood glucose testing Procedures to follow for hypoglycemia, hyperglycemia, and other illnesses General personal hygiene and specific hygiene related to dental care, skin, and feet Prescribed diet, exercise, activity Disease process and related complications

Diabetic ketoacidosis and hyperglycemic hyperosmolar nonketotic coma

Diabetic ketoacidosis (DKA) is acute insulin deficiency that causes metabolic acidosis from ketone bodies (organic acids) as a result of fat breakdown.

Hyperglycemic hyperosmolar nonketotic coma (HHNC) is severe hyperglycemia and hypertonic dehydration without significant ketoacidosis.

DKA accounts for 14% of all diabetic hospital admissions.[31] It is estimated that 15% to 30% of all episodes of DKA occur during initial diagnosis, and 50% of all cases are related to the occurrence of a stressful event such as an infection.[31] There are many predisposing factors possible in the development of DKA: failure to take insulin, insufficient amount of insulin taken, infection, or physiologic or emotional stress. Frequently the cause is not clear.

Currently, HHNC accounts for approximately 5% to 15% of all hospital admissions for diabetic coma.[31] Serious hyperosmolarity is not restricted to the diabetic individual. Severe hyperglycemic hyperosmolarity has been observed in association with diabetes insipidus; central nervous system damage; gastrointestinal hemorrhage; intravenous therapy with large amounts of glucose solutions; dialysis of hyperosmolar dialysate; concentrated milk formula in feeding of infants; acromegaly; hypothermia; and drugs such as the thiazide diuretics, phenytoin, diazoxide, glucocorticoids, furosemide, propranolol, and cimetidine; and after the ingestion of large amounts of sugary beverages or high-protein gastric tube feedings.[31] About 80% of patients with HHNC have impaired renal function, a significant predisposing condition that contributes to the development of HHNC.[31]

Most victims are elderly and infirm, institutionalized, or mentally impaired.

Unfortunately, both hyperglycemia and hyperosmolarity are also present in the patient with DKA, making it very difficult to separate these entities entirely. Usually the precipitating factors are the same. Research is currently focused on explaining the exact biochemical basis for the nonketotic condition of HHNC and developing a recommendation on preferred rate of insulin and intravenous therapy.

Pathophysiology

The contribution of counterregulatory (stress) hormones to the extreme hyperglycemia of insulin deficiency can quickly cause the development of diabetic ketoacidosis (DKA). During stress, the secretion of these hormones (glucagon, catecholamines, growth hormone, and cortisol) increases. In the insulin-deficient individual the effects of these hormones are magnified because of both an exaggerated release and an enhanced responsiveness when insulin levels are below normal.[31] Specifically, catecholamines increase liver glycogenolysis; cortisol increases hepatic gluconeogenesis and blocks peripheral use of glucose; growth hormone stimulates lipolysis, freeing up fatty acids and glycerol to be used in gluconeogenesis; and glucagon stimulates glycogenolysis, gluconeogenesis, and lipolysis. Thus deficiency of insulin itself permits an out-of-control secretion and response to the secretion of counterregulatory hormones, which only serve to accelerate the development of DKA. Since the stress that precipitates the occurrence of DKA is prolonged, the effects of all four stress hormones are also prolonged. In addition, there appears to be a synergistic effect among all four stress hormones, which further increases blood sugar and causes a rapid deterioration of metabolic balance.[31]

The events of DKA are summarized in Figure 9-14. In the absence of adequate insulin, peripheral fat, muscle, and liver cells are unable to utilize glucose. Breakdown of fat and protein is accelerated, freeing up more substrate (fatty acids and amino acids) for use in gluconeogenesis affected by the counterregulatory hormones.

Excessive amounts of fatty acids are used by the liver (under the control of glucagon) for the formation of ketone bodies, β-hydroxybutyric acid, and acetoacetic acid.[58] Ace-

Figure 9-14 Diabetic ketoacidosis.

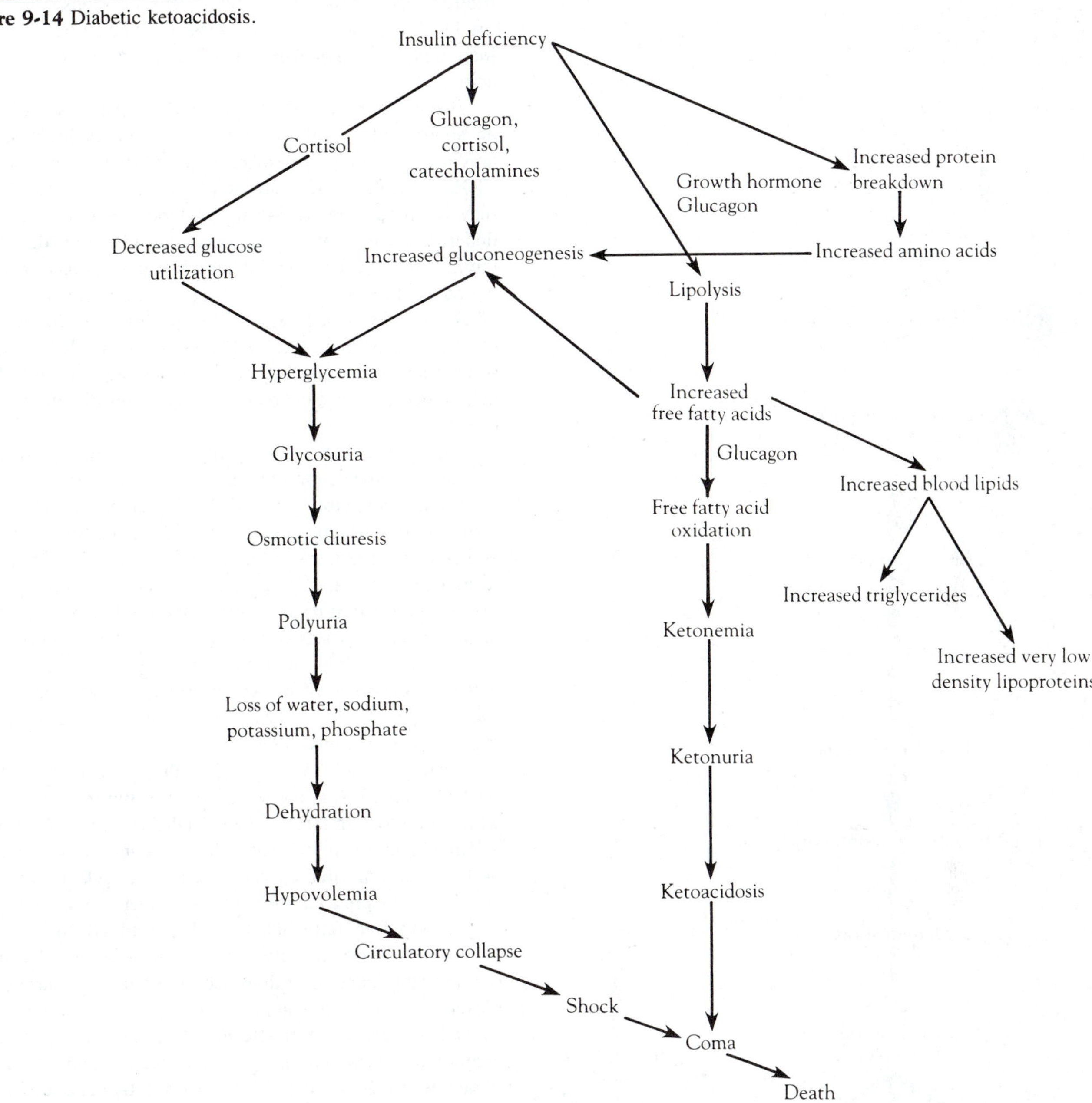

tone, responsible for the characteristic fruity breath in DKA, is formed from acetoacetic acid by a simple decarboxylation reaction.[58] The ketone bodies are produced faster than they can be metabolized or excreted. Acetoacetic acid and β-hydroxybutyric acid cannot be metabolized in the absence of insulin; therefore their levels also increase in the plasma.[58] These strong organic acids dissociate at body pH and provide 1 mEq of H+ cation and a ketoacid anion. Metabolic acidosis occurs when the body's buffer system and respiratory compensatory mechanisms are unable to maintain normal pH.

Hyperglycemia results in glycosuria with a large osmotic water and electrolyte loss through the kidneys.[40] In addition, the organic acids are excreted through the kidneys as anions, significantly decreasing potassium and sodium in the body. The acidotic state also creates a shift in electrolytes; extracellular H+ is exchanged for intracellular K+. Therefore serum K+ may be elevated as H+ moves intracellularly. Hypovolemia may seem to increase the degree of hyperkalemia, but eventually the loss of potassium through the kidneys seriously depletes body potassium. There are many con-

Figure 9-15 Pathophysiology of hyperosmolar coma.
Modified from Arieff.[6]

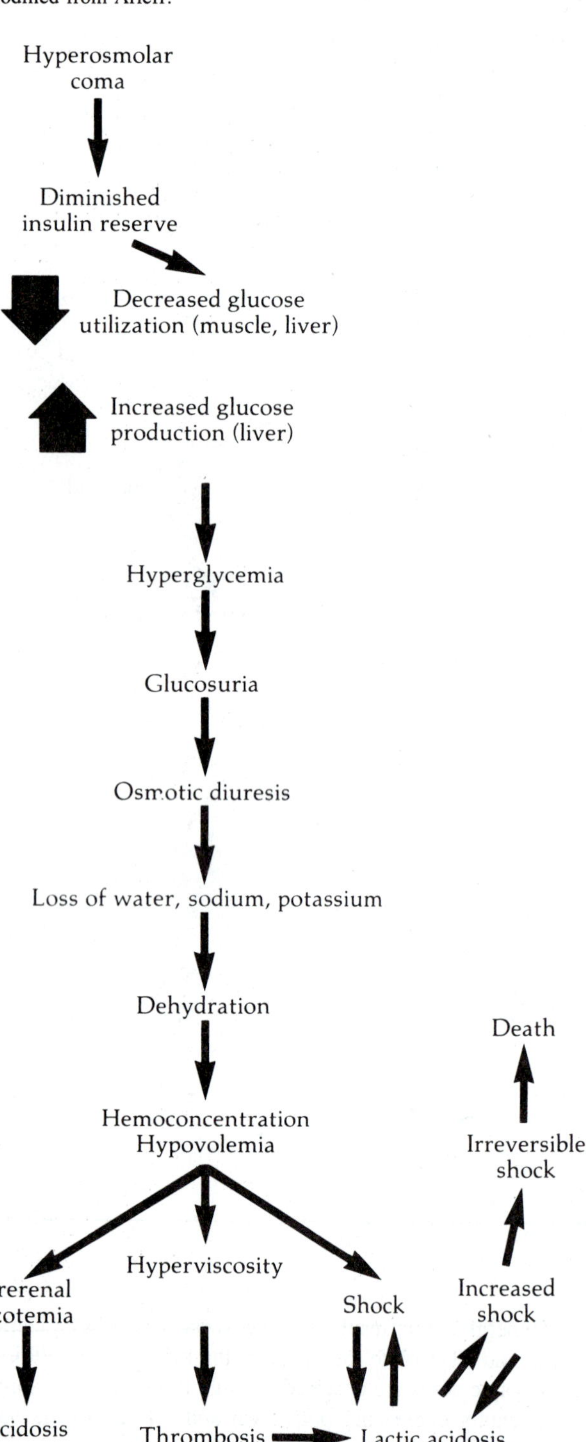

tributing factors to the changes in levels of consciousness in the DKA patient, such as decreased oxygenation of tissues, increased H+, hyperosmolarity, and increased acetoacetic acid.

Twenty to sixty-five percent of DKA patients experience an abnormality of plasma serum enzymes including serum amylase, creatine phosphokinase (CPK), transaminases (SGOT, SGPT), and lysosomal enzymes.[31] These changes may be directly related to the metabolic acidosis or to the underlying cause of the acidosis. Phosphorus deficiency is thought to be related to increased protein breakdown, impaired glucose use by the cells, and altered renal excretion of electrolytes in acidosis.[31] Magnesium is an intracellular cation lost in a manner parallel to potassium in DKA. Initially, serum magnesium may be normal or elevated, but a total body deficit may be recognizable only after insulin therapy has begun.

The initial step in the progression from non-insulin-dependent diabetes mellitus (NIDDM) to hyperglycemic hyperosmolar nonketotic coma (HHNC) begins with low serum insulin levels, which cause derangement in carbohydrate, fat, and protein metabolism (Figure 9-15). Blood sugar rises in response to decreased glucose use by the cells and increased glucose production by the liver in the total or partial lack of insulin. Osmotic water and electrolyte loss begins in response to glycosuria. Amino acid uptake and protein synthesis are halted. Breakdown of protein furnishes the liver with more substrate for gluconeogenesis. Fat is also broken down, causing an excess of fatty acids.

The most significant aspect of the disease that differentiates HHNC from DKA is the serum level of the free fatty acids, which are lower in HHNC than in DKA.[58] (See Table 9-9 for a comprehensive comparison of the two conditions.) This may be the most plausible explanation for the lack of ketosis in HHNC. There are a number of theories that attempt to explain why serum free fatty acids are lower in HHNC: there is decreased release of fatty acids from adipose cells and a concomitant decrease in their use by the liver because of the presence of small amounts of insulin in the circulation;[31] glucagon levels are higher in HHNC[31]; hyperosmolarity or severe dehydration itself inhibits fatty acid release and production of ketones by the liver[58]; and the excess fatty acids are instead utilized in other pathways, such as triglyceride synthesis.[50]

Serum concentrations of the counterregulatory hormones differ significantly from those in DKA: serum glucagon levels are higher and growth hormone and cortisol levels are lower in HHNC. The elevated glucagon levels appear to be primarily responsible for the severely elevated blood sugar values, a direct result of stimulation of liver gluconeogenesis by glucagon. The presence of renal impairment (80% of patients), either primary (kidney disease) or secondary to circulating volume depletion, also appears to play a significant role in elevating blood sugar levels in HHNC.[31] The kidneys are unable to rid the body of excess sugar or maintain water balance. Body water loss that is not replaced results in hyperosmolality and dehydration. Increased solutes increase os-

Table 9-9
Comparison of Hyperglycemic Hyperosmolar Nonketotic Coma (HHNC) and Diabetic Ketoacidosis (DKA)

Clinical Picture	HHNC	DKA
General	More dehydrated, not acidotic Frequently comatose No hyperventilation	More acidotic and less dehydrated Rarely comatose Hyperventilation
Age frequency	Usually elderly	Younger patients
Type of diabetes mellitus	Type II or non-insulin-dependent	Type I or insulin-dependent
Previous history of diabetes mellitus	In only 50%	Almost always
Prodromes	Several days duration	Less than 1 day
Neurologic symptoms and signs	Very common	Rare
Underlying renal or cardiovascular disease	About 85%	About 15%
Laboratory findings		
Blood sugar	Over 800 mg/dl	Usually less than 800 mg/dl
Plasma ketones	Less than large in undiluted specimen	Positive in several dilutions
Serum sodium	Normal, elevated, low	Usually low
Serum potassium	Normal or elevated	Elevated, normal, or low
Serum bicarbonate	Over 16 mEq	Less than 10 mEq
Anion gap	10-12 mEq	Over 12 mEq
Blood pH	Normal	Less than 7.35
Serum osmolality	Over 350 mOsm/L	Les than 330 mOsm/L
Serum BUN	Higher than DKA (↑ ↑ ↑ to ↑ ↑ ↑ ↑)	Not as high as in HHNC (↑ ↑)
Free fatty acids	Less than 1000 mEq/L	Over 1500 mEq/L
Complications		
Thrombosis	Frequent	Very rare
Mortality	20%-50%	1%-10%
Diabetes treatment after recovery	Diet alone or oral agents sometimes	Always insulin

From Kozak.[58]

motic pressure. The effective serum osmolarity (Eosm) is calculated as follows[31]:

$$\text{Esom} = 2(\text{Na} + \text{K [in mEq]}) + \text{Glucose}\,\frac{(\text{mg/dl})}{18}$$

When this value exceeds 320 mOsm/L, severe hyperosmolarity is present.[31] The hyperosmolarity of HHNC is a direct result of excessive blood sugar and increasing sodium concentration in dehydration.

Insulin output continues at a level to prevent ketosis. The steady loss of sodium, potassium, and water with hyperglycemia and glycosuria exacerbates the hyperosmolar state and ultimately results in hypovolemia and increased blood viscosity.[6] These two factors are primarily responsible for decreasing the blood flow to vital organs and resultant tissue hypoxia. Decreased circulation to brain cells combined with intracellular fluid and electrolyte shifts are responsible for the abnormal and confusing neurologic findings in HHNC.[6] Since most abnormalities resolve after therapy, it is suggested that the neurologic examination be repeated 48 hours after fluids and insulin therapy have been effective in restoring homeostasis.

Diagnostic Studies and Findings

Diagnostic Study	Diabetic Ketoacidosis (DKA)	Hyperglycemic Hyperosmolar Nonketotic Coma (HHNC)
Blood sugar	High (300 to over 800 mg/dl)	Over 800 mg/dl
Plasma ketones	Positive	Less than large
Serum sodium	Low	Normal, elevated, or low
Serum potassium	Elevated, low, or normal	Normal or elevated
Serum bicarbonate	Less than 10 mEq/L	Greater than 16 mEq/L
Blood pH	Less than 7.35	Normal
Serum osmolarity	Less than 330 mOsm/L	Greater than 350 mOsm/L
Free fatty acids	Over 1500 mEq/L	Less than 1000 mEq/L

Medical Plan

Medications

IV fluids
- DKA
  - Adult deficit is usually 6-12 L
- HHNC
  - Rapid IV fluid replacement
  - Plasma expanders:
    - Dextran 70 (Macrodex; others), 500-1000 ml of 6% solution, IV
    - Dextran 75 (Gentran 75; others), 500-1000 ml of 6% solution, IV
    - Dextran 40 (LMD; others), 10-20 ml/kg of 10% solution, IV

Insulin: regular insulin, U-40 or U-100
- Given at same rate for both DKA and HHNC, although less needed totally in HHNC
- Given until blood sugar reaches about 250 mg/dl

Electrolytes
- Sodium chloride, IV as required
- Potassium chloride, IV up to 10 mEq/h or up to 100-200 mEq/d
- Phosphate, IV as required
- Magnesium sulfate, up to 2 mEq/kg q4h

NURSING CARE

Nursing Assessment

Area of Concern	Diabetic Ketoacidosis (DKA)	Hyperglycemic Hyperosmolar Nonketotic Coma (HHNC)
Air	Rapid, deep respirations Acetone breath	
Circulation	Hypotension Tachycardia Weak, thready pulse ECG changes: elevated P wave, flattened T wave or inverted prolonged Q-T interval	Rapid, thready pulse Cool extremities Normal to low blood pressure Orthostatic hypotension 30% in frank shock[58]
Food and fluid	Extreme thirst Nausea and vomiting	Extreme thirst Weight loss Nausea and vomiting
Elimination	Nocturia Polyuria	Polyuria
Neurosensory concerns	Twitching and tremors Muscle weakness Drowsiness; lethargy; coma Headache Decreased reflexes	50% have impaired consciousness[58] Visual changes Increased or decreased reflexes Positive Babinski's sign Various abnormal neurologic findings such as aphasia, hemisensory defects, seizures, hemiparesis
Mobility	Decreased muscle tone Muscle wasting Muscle weakness	Muscle weakness
Comfort and pain	Abdominal bloating Abdominal cramping	Abdominal pain and cramping Leg cramping
Hygiene and skin	Hyperthermia Dried mucous membranes Sunken eyeballs Hot, dry flushed skin Parched tongue	Hypothermia Parched, dry lips and tongue Poor skin turgor Soft, sunken eyeballs Flushed face
Psychosocial concerns	Frightened Crying; restlessness Unable to care for self because of high levels of anxiety or decreased consciousness	Unable to care for self because of change in levels of consciousness

Nursing Dx & Intervention

Nursing Diagnosis	Nursing Intervention/Rationale
Fluid volume deficit (1)	• Assess skin turgor *to determine fluid balance*. • Assess pulse, temperature, and blood pressure every 30 to 60 minutes. • Monitor intake and output every hour and urine specific gravity as ordered *to assess changes in fluid balance*. • Administer intravenous fluids at prescribed rate *to replace fluid volume*. • Report signs and symptoms of circulatory collapse immediately. • Start and maintain patent peripheral IV line. • Provide mouth care every hour *to maximize comfort*. • Instruct patient and family about therapy ordered *to minimize anxiety*.
Altered nutrition: less than body requirements related to acid-base imbalance	• Assess respiratory status. • Monitor laboratory data *to assess fluid and electrolyte status*. • Administer insulin at times ordered. • Monitor and record changes in level of consciousness. • Monitor blood glucose levels by fingerstick as ordered *to monitor level of blood glucose control*. • Check urine for sugar and acetone as ordered *to monitor blood glucose indirectly and determine presence of acetone*. • Instruct patient and family about therapy ordered and results of laboratory tests *to decrease anxiety*.
Altered nutrition: less than body requirements related to electrolyte imbalance	• Check all voidings for sugar and acetone *to monitor presence of acidosis and blood sugar elevation*. • Instruct the patient and family about therapy ordered and results of laboratory tests. • Monitor blood glucose levels by fingerstick as ordered. • Assess patient for development of signs and symptoms of decreased serum electrolytes. • Administer electrolyte replacements as ordered.
Ineffective individual coping	• Explain all procedures to the patient and family. • Encourage the patient's participation in self-care *to maximum ability as soon as able*. • See p. 1804.

Patient Education

1. Teach the patient essential skills and concepts of diabetes mellitus education (p. 929), especially sick day rules.

Evaluation

Patient Outcome	Data Indicating That Outcome is Reached
Fluid balance is achieved, and cardiac output is normal.	Blood pressure is within normal limits. Pulse is within normal limits. Shock is not present. Circulation to peripheral tissues is adequate. There is no dehydration. Output equals intake. Skin turgor is normal.
Acid-base balance is achieved.	Blood pH is normal. Blood sugar is within normal limits. Patient is conscious and alert. Respiratory rate and character are normal.
Electrolyte balance is achieved.	Electrolytes are within normal level. ECG is at baseline.
Patient copes effectively.	Family and patient participate in care. Patient verbalizes concerns and fears. Behavior is calm and appropriate. Patient discusses potential causes of condition. Patient verbalizes methods to prevent recurrence.
Self-care is achieved.	Patient verbalizes understanding and demonstrates knowledge and skills required to control disease process (see discussion of diabetes mellitus, p. 929).

Galactosemia, hereditary fructose intolerance, and glycogen storage diseases

Galactosemia, hereditary fructose intolerance, and glycogen storage diseases are metabolic disorders of carbohydrate metabolism.

Galactosemia, hereditary fructose intolerance, and glycogen storage diseases are rare inborn errors of metabolism that usually first appear within the neonatal period or early childhood. Early and precise diagnosis of specific genetic metabolic defects is essential in providing a level of functioning for the patient and family.

Pathophysiology

Galactosemia is a disorder of galactose metabolism and may be classified into two types of enzyme deficiencies. Classic galactosemia is the result of the missing enzyme galactose-1-phosphate uridyl transferase. Galactokinase-deficiency galactosemia is a mild and rare form of the disorder. This form of galactosemia is the result of the deficient enzyme galactokinase. In both forms of the disorder, glyconeogenesis is impaired, and a toxic buildup of galactose-1-phosphate and galactitol accumulates in the enzyme-deficient cells. Toxicity may lead to cell death and impaired organ energy metabolism in the kidney, liver, brain, intestinal mucosa, and eyes. Symptoms of hypoglycemia occur as blood glucose decreases. Infants affected with classic galactosemia appear normal at birth and present signs and symptoms of genetic metabolic defect shortly after the ingestion of milk or other lactose products.[24] Lenticular cataracts may be the clinical finding for those individuals with galactokinase-deficiency galactosemia. Cataracts develop only after a long period of lactose ingestion. Consequently, the patient may not be diagnosed until later in life. Diagnosis of galactosemia can be assumed by clinical presentation, the presence of reducing substances in the urine, lesions in the lens nucleus, elevated liver enzymes, acinar formation in liver biopsy, and absence of galactose-1-phosphate uridyl transferase or deficiency of galactokinase in the red blood cells.[103]

Hereditary fructose intolerance is apparent when fructose-1-phosphate aldolase is deficient in the cells. A toxic buildup of fructose-1-phosphate occurs directly after fructose ingestion. Glyconeogenesis is impaired, and the liver is unable to replenish glucose supplies. The liver is unable to metabolize fructose properly after ingestion of foods containing fructose. Hepatomegaly occurs secondary to lipid accumulation. Nausea, vomiting, and diarrhea occur with rapid onset of hypoglycemia after fructose ingestion and the accumulation of fructose-1-phosphate. Following the ingestion of fructose, blood glucose drops and blood fructose rises. Elimination of fructose from the diet leads to a marked reversal of symptoms. Signs and symptoms of metabolic disorder usually appear in the neonate. Clinical manifestations may vary with age, and less severely affected individuals may not develop symptoms until later in childhood or early adulthood. The evaluation of fructose ingestion and fructose-1-phosphate leads to the diagnosis for this inborn error of metabolism.

The glycogen storage diseases may be broken down into hepatorenal, musculoskeletal, and generalized symptoms directly related to the accumulation and deposits of glycogen and fat in the affected individual. The corresponding enzyme deficiency is responsible for impeding glycogen metabolism and synthesis. Blood sugar and lactate levels as well as clinical manifestations may vary with each specific enzyme deficiency. Life-threatening hypoglycemia is present after a long period of fasting. Diagnosis can be confirmed with altered molecular structure or concentration of glycogen in body tissue, and the absence of a specific enzyme (Table 9-10).

Diagnostic Studies and Findings

Blood

Low blood glucose

Urine

Presence of reducing substances

Lens Examination (Ophthalmoscopic)

Lesions in nucleus

Liver

Elevated enzyme levels
Acinar formation identified by biopsy

Medical Plan

General Management

Dietary management

NURSING CARE

Nursing Assessment

Respiratory Status

Dyspnea

Circulation

Hemorrhagic manifestations
Hepatomegaly
Splenomegaly

Food and Fluids

Chronic vomiting and diarrhea
Failure to thrive

Table 9-10
Types of Glycogen Storage Diseases

Type	Disease Name	Defective or Deficient Enzyme	Organ Involvement	Prognosis
I	von Gierke's	Glucose-6-phosphate	Hepatorenal with kidney, liver, and intestine as primary sites	Guarded in infancy; variable in later life depending on severity of signs and symptoms
II	Pompe's	2-Acid glucosidase (acid maltase)	Generalized with blood cells, heart, liver, and muscle as primary sites	Poor: death within first 1-2 yr of life
III	Cori's (debrancher's)	Amylo-1,6-glucosidase (debrancher enzyme)	Generalized with blood cells, kidney, and liver as primary sites	Good: high probability for reaching adulthood
IV	Andersen's	2-1,4-Glucan: 2-1,4-glucan 6-glycosol transferase (brancher enzyme)	Generalized with liver and blood cells as primary sites	Poor: death usually within first 6-24 mo of life
V	McArdle's	Muscle phosphorylase	Musculoskeletal with blood cell involvement	Good: high probability for reaching adulthood
VI	Liver phosphorylase defect	Phosphorylase	Hepatorenal with blood cell, kidney, and liver as primary sites	Guarded in infancy, with probability for reaching adulthood
VII	Muscle phosphofructokinase defect	Phosphofructokinase	Musculoskeletal with blood cell involvement	Variable, depending on severity of signs and symptoms
VIII	Spencer-Peet	Fructose isomerase	Hepatorenal with liver as primary site	Guarded in infancy; probability for reaching adulthood
IX	Type IX	Phosphorylase kinase	Generalized with liver muscle and blood cells as primary sites	Variable, depending on severity of signs and symptoms
O	Lewis'	Glycogen synthase	Hepatorenal with blood cell, kidney, and liver as primary sites	Variable, depending on severity of signs and symptoms

Hypoglycemia
Food intolerances

Neurosensory Concerns

Decreased visual fields
Decreased intellectual functioning
Delayed developmental milestones

Neuromuscular Concerns

Progressive muscular atrophy, myopathy, hypotonia, pain

Psychosocial Concerns

Unresolved feelings related to growth retardation, short stature, degenerating disease, progressive signs and symptoms
Death during childhood in severe cases

Body Image Concerns

Enlarged abdomen
Short stature

Comfort and Pain

Frequent headaches

Family Coping

Prognosis
Management of chronic illness
Diagnosis of genetic defect

Nursing Dx & Intervention

Nursing Diagnosis	Nursing Intervention/Rationale
Fluid volume deficit (1)	• Assess skin turgor and other signs of dehydration. • Monitor intake and output. • Offer small, frequent feedings every 1 to 3 hours *to prevent hypoglycemia.* • Monitor urine specific gravity *to check for potential dehydration.* • Monitor patient for signs and symptoms of hypoglycemia. • Encourage fluid and electrolyte replacement.
Altered cardiopulmonary tissue perfusion	• Monitor patient for epistaxis, hematomas, and abdominal distention. • Monitor vital signs. • Encourage rehabilitation and physical therapy. • Provide comfort measures. • Monitor blood glucose levels at regular intervals.
Altered nutrition: less than body requirements	• Assess physical developmental stage. • Assess intellectual functioning. • Encourage calorie count daily. • Offer foods and fluids allowed every 1 to 3 hours *to maximize caloric intake and prevent hypoglycemia.* • Weigh daily at the same time with the same scale.
Body image and self-esteem disturbances	• Assess patient's strengths in intellectual and physical functioning; reinforce use of these strengths. • Encourage verbalization concerning delayed maturation. • Discuss and urge the practice of alternate methods of mental and physical functioning.
Ineffective family coping: compromised	• Assess family members' state of grieving and coping related to patient's illness. • Assess alterations in family roles related to patient's illness. • Encourage family to verbalize guilt related to the genetic defect. • Reinforce family's positive actions toward care giving and providing maximal functioning of patient. • Promote discussions about disappointment in patient's ability to achieve and function to expectations. • Support the family throughout its grieving process.

Patient Education

1. Teach a dietary plan for achieving maximal growth and development possible.
2. Teach how to assess hydration and calorie utilization.
3. Teach early recognition of signs and symptoms of exacerbation, and teach a plan to follow.
4. Stress methods of care to permit maximal independent functioning.
5. Teach the importance of support groups and psychologic assistance.

Evaluation

Patient Outcome	Data Indicating That Outcome is Reached
Hydration is adequate.	Intake equals output. There are no signs of dehydration. Episodes of vomiting and diarrhea decrease.
Tissue perfusion is normal.	Heart rate is within normal limits. Peripheral pulses are present. Hemorrhagic tendencies are absent.
Nutrition is adequate.	Weight is in proportion to height and stature. Blood sugar level is within normal limits. Patient verbalizes understanding of dietary restrictions.
Body image and self-esteem improve.	Patient participates in age-related activities. Patient maintains relationships with peers. Patient capitalizes on strong areas of functioning.
Coping improves.	Family verbalizes plans for maximizing independent functioning of patient, needed alterations in life-style consistent with required medical plan, and realistic developmental expectations.

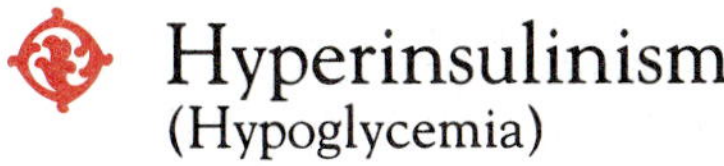

Hyperinsulinism
(Hypoglycemia)

Hyperinsulinism is a condition of excess serum insulin, which causes a reduction in blood sugar, producing symptoms of hypoglycemia.

One classification of hyperinsulinism is based on insulin levels in the fasting, postprandial, or induced hypoglycemic state. Some of the most frequent causes of hyperinsulinism are outlined as follows:

- Fasting
  - Insulin-producing islet cell tumor
  - Extrapancreatic neoplasm
  - Nesidioblastosis
  - Infants of diabetic mothers
  - Leucine-induced
- Postprandial
  - Reactive hypoglycemia
  - Early diabetes mellitus
  - Rapid gastric emptying
- Induced
  - Exogenous insulin
  - Miscellaneous drugs

The true prevalence of each entity is uncertain. However, insulin-producing islet cell tumors (arising from beta cell tumors or insulinomas) are the most frequently occurring of the islet cell tumors, with 80% showing excessive insulin secretion with measurable hypoglycemia.[10] These tumors vary in size with no relationship between the size of the tumor and severity of symptoms.[10] Ninety percent of insulinomas are benign, and 90% occur in individuals over the age 30.[32] Beta cell tumors can be present with other endocrine abnormalities, such as in the MEN I (multiple endocrine neoplasias, type 1) syndrome associated with adenomas of the pituitary and parathyroid tissue and the occurrence of Zollinger-Ellison syndrome.

Induced hypoglycemia is a condition brought about by various agents, most commonly by insulin use in the insulin-dependent diabetic and alcohol abuse in the adult population.[45] The following discussion is limited to hypoglycemia associated with hyperinsulinism.

Insulin abuse in the nondiabetic patient was first described in 1947, but it was not until the 1970s that C-peptide was recognized to be a marker of endogenous insulin production,[31] useful in determining whether the source of hyperinsulinemia was endogenous or exogenous. The possibility of self-injection of insulin in the nondiabetic patient, or surreptitious insulin use, should be considered in all cases of fasting hypoglycemia, particularly in health professionals and persons acquainted with or having contact with diabetes.[45] These persons often display no psychologic disorder and are ingenious in concealing their use of insulin. Sulfonylurea abuse has also been reported as a cause of factitious hypoglycemia, and together with surreptitious insulin abuse, factitious hypoglycemia may occur as frequently as insulinoma.[31]

Pathophysiology

Normally, varying concentrations of insulin are responsible for maintaining blood sugar in the normal range. In hyperinsulinemia, excess serum insulin disrupts this balance by increasing glucose use and inhibiting hepatic glycogenolysis, which results in a decreasing serum glucose level. The early subjective feelings associated with low blood sugar are associated with inhibition of glucose receptors in the ventromedial hypothalamic nucleus, which in turn stimulate the sympathetic fibers of the autonomic nervous system and epinephrine release in an attempt to restore blood glucose levels to normal. This adrenergic response is most noticeable when the blood sugar fall is rapid. A fall in blood sugar actually results in an increase in secretion of all four counterregulatory hormones (growth hormone, glucagon, cortisol, and catecholamines), although it appears that the catecholamines exert the major influence.[45]

The brain is most sensitive to disruption in normal blood sugar, since brain cells cannot utilize free fatty acids as an energy source. With a continued decline in blood sugar, brain cells are deprived of glucose and cerebral oxygen consumption is decreased.[45] The neuroglycopenic symptoms predominate when blood sugar decline is gradual. They are more severe and occur at a higher blood sugar level in the elderly than in the young.[31] It has been suggested that some irreversible brain damage, including decrease in intellectual function, impaired nerve function, and personality changes, may occur as the result of frequent or prolonged hypoglycemia.[31]

Insulin-secreting pancreatic tumors, as well as nesidioblastosis (in which exocrine cells are transformed to endocrine cells), produce absolute elevations of plasma insulin levels in the fasting state. Insulin levels are not responsive to changes in blood glucose levels, and the hypoglycemia results from elevated glucose uptake by insulin-dependent tissues and inhibition of glycogenolysis and gluconeogenesis mechanisms. Exercise intensifies hypoglycemic symptoms caused by increased use of glucose by muscle cells. Seventy-five to ninety percent of patients with insulinoma develop symptoms of hypoglycemia during the first 24 hours of a fast.[7]

In the patient with reactive hypoglycemia, adrenergic symptoms of hypoglycemia are usual, with neuroglycopenic symptoms only rarely occurring, because of the abrupt decline of blood sugar levels and shorter duration of symptoms.[32] These patients have no symptoms of hypoglycemia when fasting but experience hypoglycemic symptoms most commonly after a breakfast or lunch containing large amounts of carbohydrates.[45]

A similar pattern of postprandial hypoglycemia is seen in individuals with mildly impaired glucose tolerance or early non-insulin-dependent diabetes mellitus and obesity where the early rise in blood glucose related to inadequate insulin release is followed by a delayed but excessive insulin response resulting in a sudden drop of blood sugar and adrenergic symptoms of low blood sugar.

Rapid gastric emptying of carbohydrates into the small

intestine following gastrectomy, gastrojejunostomy, or vagotomy with pyloroplasty or with hyperthyroidism causes an early hyperglycemia that stimulates excessive insulin secretion resulting in alimentary hypoglycemia. Other gastric factors, such as secretin, enteroglucagon, and gastric inhibitory peptide, may also influence insulin secretion, perhaps even earlier than hyperglycemia.[31] Adrenergic symptoms usually predominate and may be severe, occurring 1½ to 3 hours postprandially.

Diagnostic Studies and Findings

Islet Cell Tumor

Blood sugar
  Low fasting level
Insulin
  Elevated fasting insulin level
Plasma proinsulin and C-peptide
  Elevated levels
Angiography
  Localization of islet cell tumor
72-Hour fast

Nesidioblastosis

Blood sugar
  Low-fasting level
Insulin
  Elevated fasting level
Plasma proinsulin and C-peptide
  Elevated levels

Leucine-Induced Hypoglycemia

Blood sugar
  Low fasting and postprandial levels
Insulin
  Elevated fasting and postprandial levels
Leucine tolerance test
  Positive for hypoglycemia

Reactive Hypoglycemia

Blood sugar
  Low level 1½ to 5 hours after glucose tolerance test load

Alimentary Hypoglycemia

Upper gastrointestinal series
  Rapid gastric emptying
Blood sugar
  Low postprandial values

Glucose Intolerance

Tolbutamide test
  Blood sugar values of more than 78% fasting value at 20 minutes
Insulin tolerance test
  Blood sugar drop of less than 50%
Plasma proinsulin and C-peptide
  Normal to elevated levels
Oral glucose tolerance test
  Elevated blood sugar 1½ to 5 hours after glucose load

Exogenous Insulin Use

Plasma proinsulin and C-peptide
  Low levels
Plasma insulin antibodies
  Present

Sulfonylurea Use

Plasma proinsulin and C-peptide
  Normal to high levels
Plasma or urine screen for sulfonylureas
  Positive

Extrapancreatic Neoplasm

Blood sugar
  Normal to low fasting levels
Insulin
  Normal to high fasting levels

Medical Plan

Surgery

Subtotal pancreatectomy
  Insulinoma resection

Medications

Diazoxide (Hyperstat) for insulinoma and nesidioblastosis: 200 mg tid first day, then 100 mg tid maintenance dose
Antineoplastic agents: streptozocin (Zanosar) for malignant islet cell tumor (see Chapter 16)

General Management

Diet

NURSING CARE

Nursing Assessment

Circulation

Tachycardia
Elevated blood pressure

Food and Fluid

Relief of symptoms with food intake
Hunger
Weight loss
Weight gain

Neurosensory Concerns

Tremor
Headache
Mental dullness
Confusion
Amnesia
Seizures
Unconsciousness
Paralysis
Paresthesias
Dizziness
Irritability
Visual disturbance

Psychosocial

Change in role performance
Resents enforced dependence
Unable to stay alone: related to episodes of loss of consciousness
Past history of destructive behavior

Nursing Dx & Intervention

Nursing Diagnosis	Nursing Intervention/Rationale
Altered nutrition: less/more than body requirements	• Assess symptoms patient normally experiences with hypoglycemia and whether or not patient is awakened by symptoms at night. • Assess patient for symptoms of low blood sugar, and check blood glucose by fingerstick using strip or meter determination: fasting, before and 2 hours after meals, at bedtime, and at 3 to 5 AM. • Check blood pressure, pulse, and respiration with occurrence of symptoms. • Provide patient with 3 AM snack if needed *to prevent nocturnal hypoglycemia.* • Arrange a dietary consultation.
Ineffective individual coping	• Assess patient's personal strengths and weaknesses and coping skills. • Remove potentially dangerous articles from patient's room (factitious use of insulin or sulfonylureas). • Encourage maximum independence. • Assist patient to communicate with others. • Discuss need for restrictions and precautions related to potential loss of consciousness *to maintain safety and prevent injury.* • Give information about disease *to enhance feeling of control.* • See also p. 1804.
Sleep pattern disturbance	• Assess patient's quality and quantity of sleep. • Discuss the importance of feeding during the night if indicated *to prevent early morning hypoglycemia.* • Suggest naps or early bedtime *to allow for increased quantity of sleep.* • Minimize other disturbances during sleeping time *to maximize quality of sleep.*

Patient Education

1. Teach signs and symptoms for early recognition and treatment of hypoglycemia.
2. Teach a 24-hour diet plan and the importance of adhering to it.

Evaluation

Patient Outcome	Data Indicating That Outcome is Reached
Hypoglycemia can be recognized and promptly managed.	There are no seizures or loss of consciousness. Patient verbalizes understanding of diet and signs, symptoms, and treatment of hypoglycemia.
Nutrition is adequate.	Patient complies with dietary prescription including restrictions and snacks. Blood sugar is within normal limits. Weight is in proportion to body height and stature.
Patient copes effectively.	Anxiety is decreased. Family verbalizes adapting to changes imposed by hypoglycemia. Patient accepts support from health professionals. Patient establishes and follows plan to minimize symptoms and maximize functioning. Maximum independence is maintained. There is no self-destructive behavior. Patient complies with the precautions and restrictions imposed.
Sleep patterns improve.	Patient verbalizes feeling rested. Total quantity of sleep is increased. Interruptions during sleep are minimized.

 Hyperlipidemia

Hyperlipidemia is the presence of abnormally high levels of lipids in the blood. Although in other disorders the term "abnormally high" refers to levels present in the upper 5% of the population (95th percentile), in most hyperlipidemias it refers instead to blood lipid levels associated with significantly increased risk of coronary artery disease.

The hyperlipidemias are a group of disorders of lipid metabolism. They vary in cause, severity, response to treatment, and prognosis. Hyperlipidemias occur in all ages and races and in both sexes. *Primary hyperlipidemias* are often hereditary disorders caused by deficiencies of certain mechanisms involved in lipid metabolism and excretion. *Secondary hyperlipidemias* occur in relation to renal or hepatic disorders (renal failure, nephrotic syndrome, obstructive liver disease), hormonal imbalances (hypopituitarism, hyperestrogenemia, and pregnancy), metabolic diseases (hypothyroidism, diabetes mellitus), and other disorders (hypogammaglobulinemia, myeloma, macroglobulinemia, lipodystrophy, dysproteinemia).

In addition, various medications such as β-adrenergic blockers, thiazide diuretics, corticosteroids, and oral contraceptives can cause blood lipid levels to increase significantly.

The most significant hyperlipidemias are those associated with an increased risk of coronary artery disease. Heart disease is the leading cause of death in the United States; it is responsible for more than 550,000 deaths per year—more than deaths from all forms of cancer combined. Elevated blood lipid levels are associated with the development of atherosclerosis and resultant coronary artery disease. Over 50% of the adult population in the United States has elevated lipid levels.

A very few types of hyperlipidemia do not carry an increased risk of coronary artery disease. In these specific disorders, recurrent severe pancreatitis tends to be the disease sequela.

Lipid Metabolism

Three major types of lipids circulate in the blood: cholesterol, triglycerides, and phospholipids. *Cholesterol* is absorbed from food, produced by the liver, and released from aging cells. It is used in the manufacture of cell membranes, hormones, vitamin D, and bile salts. *Triglycerides,* also absorbed from food, are composed of fatty acids and glycerol. The fatty acid components are used by the tissues for energy or are deposited into adipocytes, forming body fat. Blood lipids are transported as *lipoproteins*—large, complex molecules containing an inner core of lipid (cholesterol or triglyceride) encased in a thin membrane made of phospholipids, cholesterol, and proteins. These membrane proteins, termed *apoproteins,* act as enzyme cofactors, inhibitors, or transfer agents in lipid metabolism.

The four major lipoproteins are chylomicrons, very low density lipoprotein (VLDL), low density lipoprotein (LDL), and high density lipoprotein (HDL). A fourth lipoprotein, intermediate density lipoprotein (IDL), is a by-product of VLDL metabolism. *Chylomicrons* are normally present in the blood only after eating. They primarily contain triglycerides. VLDL is produced by the liver from fatty acids and carbohydrates and contains triglycerides. LDL carries two thirds to three fourths of the body's circulating cholesterol. LDL is also responsible for depositing cholesterol into arterial walls, forming atherosclerotic plaque. HDL carries one fourth of the body's circulating cholesterol and is a pivotal agent in cholesterol metabolism.

After a meal, fat and cholesterol are absorbed from the gut. Ingested fat is transported in the blood as chylomicrons (containing triglycerides) and carried to the tissues. There *apoprotein CII* activates an enzyme in the capillary endothelium, *lipoprotein lipase,* which leads to the removal of fatty acids from the triglycerides. These fatty acids are either used by muscle tissue for energy or stored as fat in the adipocytes. A chylomicron remnant containing apoprotein E is left over from this process and is transported to the liver. There *apoprotein E* interacts with the cell surface receptors to change the chylomicron remnant into LDL. LDL then binds to the surface receptors on the hepatocytes and is degraded, releasing cholesterol.

Cholesterol is also synthesized by the liver at a rate regulated by the enzyme *HMG CoA reductase*. The cholesterol is secreted by the liver as a constituent of VLDL. After its production and release, triglyceride is removed from the VLDL, resulting in the cholesterol-rich LDL. Tissues can then utilize the LDL cholesterol for cell membrane synthesis, hormone production, or vitamin D manufacture.

Aging cells are yet another source of cholesterol. In a process termed *reverse cholesterol transport,* aging body cells release cholesterol from their cell membranes. When this occurs, *apoprotein A-1* (from HDL) activates the enzyme *lecithin cholesterol acyltransferase* (LCAT), which binds the cholesterol to HDL. HDL then transports the cholesterol to LDL and VLDL, which in turn carry the cholesterol to the liver. The liver may use the cholesterol to manufacture bile salts or recycle it by releasing it back into the bloodstream.

The liver is active in other aspects of lipid metabolism. VLDL is produced in the liver from fatty acids and carbohydrates. After release from the liver, VLDL combines with apoprotein C-II in plasma. *Apoprotein C-II* activates lipoprotein lipase to allow the triglyceride from VLDL to be deposited into tissues.

The liver is also critical in regulation of LDL levels. LDL receptors on the liver cells recognize the *apoprotein B* component of LDL. Apoprotein B binds LDL to these receptors, permitting the liver cells to degrade LDL, which releases cholesterol. Excess LDL is also removed by circulating macrophages, or scavenger white blood cells. Despite these regulatory mechanisms, excess LDL may accumulate, depositing cholesterol into arterial walls to form atheromatous plaques.

Pathophysiology

There are several different types of hyperlipidemias. Some are hereditary, and others are associated with high fat and high cholesterol diets in combination with physical inactivity. In the past, hyperlipidemias were classified according to the clinical picture presented by the patient and the turbidity of the patient's plasma. Currently hyperlipidemias are categorized according to the pattern of lipid elevation and the metabolic defect. Overall, the biochemical bases of hyperlipidemias are deficient enzymes, deficient or defective cell receptors, and deficient, defective, or excessive apoproteins (which influence both enzymes and cell receptors).

Familial hypercholesterolemia (FH) is an inherited disorder in which the LDL receptors that break down LDL are deficient or defective. As a result, LDL accumulates in the blood. VLDL remnants also accumulate and in time are converted to LDL, further increasing LDL levels.

FH is an autosomal dominant disorder that has two forms. *Heterozygous FH* is a relatively common (1:500) and milder form of the disease in which one defective gene for LDL receptors is counterbalanced by one normal gene. Poor dietary habits and other life-style factors can greatly worsen this disease.

When both LDL receptor genes are defective, *homozygous FH* results. This form of FH is rare (1:1 million) and much more severe. FH homozygotes sometimes die of myocardial infarction in childhood. Because of the gravity of the disease if untreated, all siblings of children with FH must be tested for the disease.

Patients with FH have xanthomas (yellowish deposits of plaque in the skin) and corneal arcus (a white ring around the eye). Lipid profiles show elevated levels of LDL and cholesterol. VLDL profiles show elevated levels of LDL and cholesterol. VLDL levels may or may not be elevated.

The treatment of FH emphasizes a very low cholesterol, low fat diet and achievement of ideal body weight if needed. Cholestyramine, colestipol or lovastatin therapy may be added since diet alone is usually insufficient in reducing blood levels of LDL and cholesterol.

Familial combined hyperlipidemia is a common (1:200) hereditary disease that in its milder form is often associated with diabetes mellitus. For an as yet unknown reason, apoprotein B levels are elevated in this disorder, resulting in high levels of LDL and possibly VLDL, cholesterol, and triglycerides. Severe premature atherosclerosis is the result. Men with this disease have myocardial infarctions at the average age of 40 years. Cigarette smoking greatly increases the risk of myocardial infarction. Treatment includes very low cholesterol diets, avoidance of concentrated sweets, and achievement or maintenance of ideal body weight. Therapy with niacin, clofibrate, or gemfibrozil may be necessary.

Familial hypertriglyceridemia is the result of a metabolic defect that causes oversynthesis of VLDL and triglyceride by the liver. This disorder is common (1:300 to 1:200) and usually does not present a problem before 20 years of age. Familial hypertriglyceridemia does not carry an increased risk of coronary artery disease, is not associated with diabetes mellitus, and does not cause xanthomas. However, it can be worsened by poor diet and cigarette smoking as well as by obesity, alcohol, and drugs, which elevate triglyceride levels (estrogen, glucocorticoids). Asymptomatic persons do not require treatment but should avoid using drugs that increase triglyceride levels.

Defective lipoprotein lipase–related triglyceridemia is a very rare lipid disease in which lipoprotein lipase or its apoprotein CC-II is deficient. The deficiency results in inadequate breakdown of triglyceride. Patients with this disorder often show an intolerance to fatty foods in childhood. Additional symptoms are hepatosplenomegaly, abdominal pain, lipemia retinale, and xanthomas, especially of the elbows, knees, and buttocks. Patients are at very high risk for pancreatitis. Treatment focuses on low fat and low cholesterol diets and abstention from alcohol. Drugs are ineffective.

Familial dysbetalipoproteinemia or remnant removal disease is an inherited deficiency of apoprotein E2. This deficiency results in both an overproduction of VLDL and an insufficient breakdown of VLDL remnants. Familial dysbetalipoproteinemia is uncommon; estimates of its incidence range from 1:10,000 to 1:40,000. Patients with this disease exhibit xanthomas on the palms, Achilles tendons, and patellae, as well as corneal arcus. Lipid studies can vary widely in the same patient but generally reveal markedly elevated levels of VLDL and elevated levels of cholesterol and triglyceride. In addition, hyperglycemia and hyperuricemia may occur in these patients. Patients with familial dysbetalipoproteinemia have accelerated atherosclerosis and pancreatitis. Weight loss (if indicated) and a low cholesterol, low fat diet are an important part of treatment. Therapy with niacin or clofibrate may also be required.

Chylomicronemia syndrome, LCAT deficiency, apolipoprotein B deficiency, and *Tangier disease* are rare lipid disorders resulting in elevated triglyceride levels. These disorders may cause pancreatitis rather than coronary artery disease and also may require drug and dietary therapy. Plasmapheresis may be used to remove excess chylomicrons from plasma.

Diagnostic Studies and Findings

Lipid Profile

"Normal" and "elevated" levels vary among laboratories; numbers given are examples

Cholesterol

Normal to markedly elevated: 200->1000 mg/dl

Triglycerides

Normal to markedly elevated: 150->1500 mg/dl (even up to 29,000 mg/dl)

LDL
  Normal to elevated: 100-200 mg/dl
HDL
  Normal to low: 50-20 mg/dl
LDL/HDL ratio
  Normal to high: 2:1->4:1
VLDL
  Normal to elevated: 30->40 mg/dl

Liver Function Tests

To verify normal liver function before pharmacologic therapy; periodically thereafter to identify abnormalities necessitating discontinuation of medication

Uric Acid Level

To verify normal levels before pharmacologic therapy; periodically thereafter to identify abnormalities necessitating discontinuation of medication

Glucose Level

To verify normal levels before pharmacologic therapy; periodically thereafter to identify abnormalities necessitating discontinuation of medication

Ophthalmologic Examination

To establish baseline of lens opacity before pharmacologic therapy; periodically thereafter to identify abnormalities necessitating discontinuation of medication

Medical Plan

General Management

- Dietary management
  - Foundation of management of hypercholesterolemia
    - Reduction of total dietary fat to ≤30% of total calories
    - Reduction of saturated fat in diet to <10% of total calories
    - Increase in polyunsaturated fats in diet but not more than 10% of total calories
    - Reduction of dietary cholesterol to ≤250-300 mg/day
- Management of lipid levels
  - Cholesterol ≤200 mg/dl
  - Triglycerides ≤150 mg/dl
  - LDL ≤100 mg/dl
  - HDL ≥50 mg/dl
  - LDL/HDL ratio 2:1 or lower
- Ideal body weight
  - Engage in regular, moderate physical exercise
- Elimination of other risk factors
  - Cigarette smoking
  - Hypertension
  - Diabetes mellitus
  - Alcohol abuse

Medications

Pharmacologic therapy usually employed only after dietary management has proved inadequate in reducing blood lipids to prescribed levels; cholesterol-reducing medications are then added to dietary regimen

- Bile acid sequestrants
  - Cholestyramine
  - Colestipol
- Niacin (nicotinic acid, vitamin B_3)
- Probucol
- Fibric acids
  - Clofibrate
  - Gemfibrozil
- HMG CoA reductase inhibitors
  - Lovostatin

Special medication precautions: Since antilipemic drugs can greatly reduce the absorption of other drugs administered simultaneously, other drugs should be taken 1 hour before or 4-6 hours after the antilipemic medication. Cardiac glycoside (digoxin) levels should be monitored in patients also on antilipemic therapy. If the antilipemic drug is stopped, cardiac glycoside absorption may greatly increase, resulting in toxicity. Antilipemic drugs also interact with other medications: Oral contraceptives and rifampin may increase the effect of clofibrate. Probenecid antagonizes clofibrate's effect. Oral hypoglycemics may antagonize response to colestipol. Coumadin's anticoagulant effect is enhanced by colestipol and antagonized by cholestyramine if the two drugs are administered within 6 hours of each other.

NURSING CARE

Nursing Assessment

Circulation

Xanthomas
Corneal arcus
Lipemia retinale

Comfort and Pain

Abdominal pain*

Food and Fluid Needs

Obesity
Signs and symptoms of glucose intolerance
GI distress, nausea*

Elimination

Constipation*
Diarrhea*
Bloating, flatulence*

*Related to side effects of pharmacologic therapy.

Hygiene and Skin Care

Rash*

Neurosensory Area

Pruritus of head, neck, shoulders*
Cutaneous flushing*
Cataract formation*
Dizziness*

Mobility

Tired feeling in legs*
Myopathy*
Joint pain*

*Related to side effects of pharmacologic therapy.

Nursing Dx & Intervention

Nursing Diagnosis	Nursing Intervention/Rationale
Altered nutrition: more than body requirements	• Assess patient for psychosocial concerns that may be related to overeating. • Arrange a dietary consultation. • Encourage patient to choose foods that are low in fat, especially saturated fat and cholesterol, *to maintain nutritional balance and avoid elevating lipid levels.* • Reinforce meal plan as needed. • Suggest that patient join a support group such as Weight Watchers *to provide group and peer support.*
Altered coronary tissue perfusion (potential)	• Instruct patient in the signs and symptoms of reduced coronary artery blood flow and the need to notify health care worker immediately if symptoms occur.
Constipation related to drug therapy (potential)	• Encourage patient to increase fluid intake. • Encourage patient to increase fiber in diet. • Contact physician regarding need for bulk laxatives such as psyllium-containing compounds. • Encourage patient to take medications with antacids and/or meals *to decrease gastrointestinal discomfort, bloating, and flatulence and to promote compliance.*
Diarrhea related to drug therapy (potential)	• Assess fluid loss from diarrhea. Replace lost fluid and electrolytes *to prevent dehydration and electrolyte imbalance.* • Assess patient for symptoms of dehydration, hypokalemia, and hypomagnesemia. • Assess patient for perianal irritation. Contact physician if necessary.

Patient Education

1. Instruct the patient in dietary management of the disease.
2. Instruct the patient in the importance of achieving ideal body weight.
3. Instruct the patient in the importance of engaging regularly in moderate physical exercise.
4. Teach the patient the importance of eliminating other factors related to hyperlipidemia and coronary artery disease, such as cigarette smoking and hypertension.
5. Teach patient the name, action, dosage, schedule, and side effects of ordered medications.
6. Ensure that the patient understands the importance of regular reevaluations (follow-up medical care).

Evaluation

Patient Outcome	Data Indicating That Outcome is Reached
Hyperlipidemia is controlled.	Blood lipids are at prescribed levels. Patient maintains regular follow-up visits with health provider. Patient consistently maintains laboratory appointments for blood tests.
Ideal body weight is achieved.	Weight is in proportion to height and frame. Patient participates in regular, moderate physical activity.
Nutrition is adequate.	Patient verbalizes understanding of dietary restrictions. Patient complies with ordered diet.
Patient is knowledgeable about disease cause, symptoms, and treatment.	Patient and family verbalize understanding of disease, cause, symptoms, and treatment. Patient complies with medication regimen.

Zollinger-Ellison syndrome

Zollinger-Ellison syndrome (ZES) is gastric acid hypersecretion and recurrent peptic ulcer disease caused by excessive gastrin secretion from pancreatic delta islet cell tumors or gastrinomas.

Although ZES is uncommon, it is not rare. Multiple endocrine neoplasia, type 1 (MEN I) is present in 25% of patients with ZES. Between 30% and 50% of gastrinomas occur as a single pancreatic tumor, most commonly in the head and tail section of the pancreas.[101] Sixty percent of ZES patients are men, usually between 20 and 50 years of age.[101] Gastrinomas vary in size and location, and up to two thirds are malignant. Usual sites of metastasis are lymph nodes, liver, spleen, bone, skin, and peritoneum.[101]

The mortality from ZES is high, not so much from metastases of the malignant tumor as from the extreme effects of hypergastrinemia and complications of ulcers: perforation, fistula formation, and hemorrhage.[101] Until recently, total gastrectomy was the only relatively successful treatment for ZES. The development of histamine H_2-receptor blocking agents since 1978 has shown promising possibilities for the management of ZES.

Pathophysiology

The major effect of gastrin is the stimulation of hydrochloric acid secretion from parietal cells, possibly through stimulation of a histamine- or cyclic AMP–mediated process.[38] The continuous high serum gastrin levels found in ZES produce a state of constant gastric acid hypersecretion, which exceeds the duodenum's capacity to neutralize it. This accounts for the upper gastrointestinal ulcerations found in sites as far distal to the stomach as the jejunum[101] and the presence of large amounts of fluid in both stomach and duodenum even in the fasting state.[38] Parietal cell mass is increased because of the trophic effect of high serum gastrin levels, ultimately causing the development of prominent rugal folds in the stomach. The increased number of parietal cells in ZES is significant in the development of hyperacidity because a close relationship exists between the number of parietal cells and the amount of gastric acid secreted.[38]

The diarrhea of ZES is caused by a number of factors:

1. Large amounts of hydrochloric acid irritate the gastrointestinal mucosa and increase peristalsis.
2. Gastrin has a direct influence on increasing intestinal motility.
3. Pancreatic lipase is inactivated in the presence of low intestinal pH and fat breakdown, and absorption is not accomplished.[38]
4. Precipitation of bile salts in the acid environment of the small intestine also prevents fat absorption.
5. The direct effect of gastrin stimulates gastric, pancreatic, liver, and intestinal secretion of water and electrolytes.[38]
6. The malabsorption of a variety of substances is caused by inactivation of intestinal enzymes in the presence of acidity.

The ultimate results of these factors are diarrhea, steatorrhea, and the severe loss of potassium and magnesium that accompanies diarrhea in the ZES patient.

Gastrin is also known to cause moderate stimulation of pepsin release from gastric chief cells. In the presence of low pH in the proximal and distal duodenum and jejunum, pepsin contributes only to the development of mucosal ulcerations even at points as distal as the jejunum.

The secretion of gastrin by tumor tissue (gastrinomas) is not responsive to the normal inhibitory stimuli (low gastric pH and secretin), as is normal gastrin secretion. In the patient with ZES, secretin paradoxically stimulates gastrin release.

Gastrin also stimulates intrinsic factor secretin. However, in ZES, malabsorption of vitamin B_{12} is thought to result from the low intestinal pH, which may interfere with the action of intrinsic factor in facilitating the absorption of vitamin B_{12}.[101] This condition is not corrected by the administration of the intrinsic factor; only monthly vitamin B_{12} injections can ameliorate it.

Diagnostic Studies and Findings

Elevated Serum Gastrin

Level of 500 pg/ml virtually diagnostic of ZES after exclusion of other disorders with hypergastrinemia

Provocative Testing

Secretin
- Serum gastrin rises by 400 pg/ml over basal value

Calcium infusion
- Serum gastrin rises by 50% of basal value or by 500 pg/ml over basal value

Meal test
- Positive if meal fails to increase gastrin by more than 50%

Gastric Analysis

Basal acid concentration of greater than 15 mEq/hr in previously unoperated patient and greater than 5 mEq/hr in previously operated patients

Radiologic Findings

Irregular thick gastric mucosal folds with ulcers at usual and unusual sites; pancreatic D islet cell tumor demonstrated by angiography

Medical Plan

Surgery

Total gastrectomy
Partial pancreatectomy (tumor excision)

Medications

Histamine H_2–receptor blocking agents
- Cimetidine, 300-600 mg q6h
- Ranitidine, 150 mg qid or qid and hs

Streptozoticin, 5-FU, doxorubicin (see cancer section) for treatment of malignant tumors with metastases

NURSING CARE

Nursing Assessment

Circulation

Decreased blood pressure
Tachycardia
Cold, clammy skin

Food and Fluid

Burning, pain in epigastric region between meals
Coffee-ground or frank blood emesis
Thirst
Decreased appetite
Weight loss
Dry mouth

Elimination

Increased frequency of stools
Foul smelling, foamy stools
Abdominal cramping

Neurosensory

Restlessness
Impaired touch and temperature sensation and paresthesias of hands and feet
Unsteady gait
Hyperreflexia

Comfort and Pain

Severe upper abdominal pain, may be referred to top of shoulders
Abdomen rigid and tender
Sore mouth

Hygiene and Skin

Skin color sallow with lemon-yellow tint
Smooth, red, beefy tongue
Prematurely gray hair

Psychosocial

Feelings of helplessness
Decreased participation in outside-the-home activities because of diarrhea
Embarrassment

Teaching and Learning

Lack of exposure to information about or unfamiliarity with Zollinger-Ellison syndrome and associated symptoms

Nursing Dx & Intervention

Nursing Diagnosis	Nursing Intervention/Rationale
Potential fluid volume deficit	• Assess fluid balance (intake and output, daily weights, vital signs, signs of dehydration) *to identify dehydration early.* • Measure daily fluid loss in stools *to prevent undetected loss.* • Replace fluids with water, tea, carbonated beverages, gelatin, popsicles, and broth. • Instruct patient regarding need to include foods high in potassium and magnesium *to replace losses in diarrhea.*
Altered nutrition: less than body requirements	• Assess patient for symptoms of vitamin B_{12} deficiency. • Administer vitamin B_{12} injections as ordered. • Stress the importance of follow-up and vitamin B_{12} injections as ordered *to prevent deficiency.*
Diarrhea	• Assess fluid losses in diarrhea by daily measurement. • Check with physician about medication for perianal irritation from frequent stools. • Replace lost fluid and electrolytes *to prevent fluid and electrolyte imbalance.* • Observe patient for signs and symptoms of dehydration, decreased potassium, and magnesium.
Ineffective individual coping	• Assess patient's and family's coping skills and support systems, and adaptive skills successful in the past. • Encourage open communication between patient and family members. • Assist patient in identifying strengths and positive coping skills *to cope with current stressors.* • Offer suggestions as to how patient can cope with problem areas and function away from home.

Patient Education

1. Make the patient aware of serious complications or changes that require medical attention (gastric bleeding, vitamin B_{12} deficiency).
2. Teach the patient the importance of fluid and electrolyte replacement for diarrhea to prevent dehydration and changes in electrolyte balance.
3. Teach the patient the need for strict medication compliance to maintain the status of healed ulcers and avoid pain.
4. Teach the patient the dose, schedule, action, and side effects of the medication ordered, to ensure safe and effective use of medication.

Evaluation

Patient Outcome	Data Indicating That Outcome is Reached
Fluid and electrolyte balance is maintained.	There is no hemorrhage. There are no changes in blood pressure or pulse. Patient verbalizes understanding of and complies with fluid and electrolyte (potassium, magnesium) replacement with diarrhea. There is no dehydration.
Patient has normal vitamin B_{12} levels.	Patient verbalizes understanding of and complies with vitamin B_{12} injections as ordered.
Patient has adapted to limitations imposed by disease.	Patient and family demonstrate open communication and problem-solving capabilities. Patient participates in support group. Patient functions at highest level in ADLs.
Patient is knowledgeable about disease, symptoms, and treatment	Patient and family verbalize understanding of disease and the causes of symptoms and their treatment. Patient demonstrates compliance with medication regime.

Medical Interventions and Related Nursing Care

Adrenalectomy

Description and Rationale

Adrenalectomy is the removal of the adrenal gland. Unilateral adrenalectomy is the intervention for benign adrenal adenomas involving one gland. Adrenal carcinoma and ectopic adrenocorticotropic hormone (ACTH) producing tumors require bilateral adrenalectomy.

Contraindications and Cautions

1. Bilateral adrenalectomy dictates lifelong glucocorticoid and mineralocorticoid replacement.
2. Patients undergoing unilateral adrenalectomy will be adrenally insufficient immediately postoperative and will require glucocorticoid, but usually not mineralocorticoid, replacement for 6 months to 2 years or until the remaining adrenal recovers.
3. Hyperglycemia should be controlled before surgery.
4. Patients undergoing adrenalectomy may have hypoaldosteronism or hyperkalemia after surgery.

Preprocedural Nursing Care

Administration of preoperative steroids

NURSING CARE

Nursing Assessment

Skin

Poor wound healing
Surgical incision

Complications

Adrenal insufficiency (potential)
Unresolved hypertension from primary aldosteronism may require continued treatment with medication

Nursing Dx & Intervention

Nursing Diagnosis	Nursing Intervention/Rationale
Impaired skin integrity	• Assess wound for edema, redness, warmth, induration, and drainage *to observe for signs of healing or infection.*
Potential for infection	• Follow actions for adrenal insufficiency and for acute adrenal insufficiency when applicable.

Patient Education

1. Teach wound care.
2. Teach early recognition and treatment of adrenal insufficiency.
3. Teach how to use replacement steroids and emergency intramuscular injection of steroids.
4. Instruct the patient to wear or carry medical alert information.

Evaluation

Patient Outcome	Data Indicating That Outcome is Reached
The patient's wound is healed.	Patient's wound closed without redness, edema, warmth, or drainage.
The patient is adrenally sufficient.	Patient displays no symptoms of adrenal insufficiency.

Crisis Intervention for Adrenal Insufficiency

Description and Rationale

The patient experiencing adrenal crisis must receive adrenocorticosteroids. The response to IV cortisol can be dramatic. Nelson[26] has reported blood pressure response from an unobtainable diastolic reading to one of over 80 after the initial dose of cortisol was given. Therefore it is vital that the patient be treated with corticosteroids before other interventions, to enable the system to stabilize. The effects of corticosteroids on the electrolyte imbalance, hypovolemia, and blood pressure will become apparent quickly. An IV infusion of 5% dextrose in saline should be part of the therapy, since the patient will likely be hypoglycemic because of the vomiting, diarrhea, and lack of food. Dehydration also compounds the problem. Response to therapy is encouraging, and in fact, within 24 hours most patients are able to resume an oral course of corticosteroids.

Since most glucocorticoids exert some mineralocorticoid effect, additional mineralocorticoid is not always necessary.[26] Also, the sodium present in the IV fluid may be sufficient to restore a normal level.[103] However, if mineralocorticoid replacement is deemed necessary, desoxycorticosterone pivalate can be given intramuscularly.

Antibiotic therapy may also be necessary if the underlying cause of the adrenal crisis is infection.

Volume expanders may or may not be used, depending on how effective the steroid treatment and IV fluid are.

There is controversy in the literature regarding use of vasopressors to treat hypovolemic shock. Response to initial glucocorticoid infusion and IV therapy should be evaluated before employing the use of vasopressors.

Contraindications and Cautions

1. Complications associated with IV therapy
2. Danger of electrolyte imbalance as the potassium level responds to therapy

NURSING CARE

Nursing Assessment

Circulation

Hypotension
Shock
Hypovolemia

Food and Fluid

Vomiting
Hyponatremia
Salt craving

Elimination

Decreased urine output
Diarrhea

Neurosensory Concerns
Confusion
Restlessness

Mobility
Weakness

Psychosocial Concerns
Anxiety

Teaching and Learning
Lack of knowledge about medications and crisis

Nursing Dx & Intervention

Nursing Diagnosis	Nursing Intervention/Rationale
Potential for infection	• Assess patient's understanding of the risk of infection. • Keep patient in an environment as free from stress as possible (low lighting, warm temperature, reduced noise level) *to minimize environmental stress.* • Encourage frequent rest. • Reinforce importance of medications to patient.
Altered nutrition: less than body requirements related to potential for electrolyte imbalance	• Assess intake of electrolytes, especially potassium and sodium. • Encourage patient to choose foods high in sodium and low in potassium. • Take apical pulse *to detect cardiac dysrhythmias.* • Employ means *to combat nausea.* • Maintain intake and output records.
Altered peripheral tissue perfusion	• Assess for early presyncopal signs (dizziness, lightheadedness, visual changes). • Have patient change positions (from lying to sitting to standing) slowly *to prevent orthostatic hypotension.* • Take lying and standing blood pressures and pulses *to assess for hypovolemia.* • Administer IV fluids as ordered. • Monitor intake and output. • Monitor vital signs frequently (every 15 to 30 minutes). • Explain rationale for IV therapy to patient.
Sleep pattern disturbance	• Assess quantity and quality of patient's sleep; identify usual sleeping patterns and aids. • Do not disturb patient when sleeping. • Encourage methods of achieving relaxation (back rub, warm milk, dark room). • Allow for period of uninterrupted rest during the day. • Decrease amount of external stimuli.
Fluid volume deficit (2)	• Assess fluid balance via daily weights at the same time on the same scale. • Monitor intake and output. • Observe for signs and symptoms of shock. • Monitor vital signs frequently. • Maintain IV line. • Employ means to combat vomiting and diarrhea. • Assess skin turgor.

Patient Education

1. Teach the patient the importance of avoiding obvious sources of infection, such as persons with infections.
2. Teach the patient the importance of and how to take medication regularly and in emergency situations.
3. Teach the steps to follow when early symptoms of crises are noted.
4. Teach the importance of regular medical follow-up and wearing medical identification.

Evaluation

Patient Outcome	Data Indicating That Outcome is Reached
Patient is free of infection.	Temperature is within normal range. Patient has no signs or symptoms of infection. Glucocorticoid and mineralocorticoid levels are within therapeutic range.

Patient Outcome	Data Indicating That Outcome is Reached
Electrolytes are within the normal range.	Sodium and potassium blood levels are within normal limits.
Tissue perfusion is adequate.	Patient makes no statements concerning syncope. Peripheral pulses are adequate. Output equals intake. Patient adheres to activity limitations.
The sleep pattern is undisturbed.	Patient verbalizes and demonstrates methods of achieving relaxation. Patient verbalizes receiving an increased amount of sleep.
Hydration is adequate.	Urine output is greater than 40 ml/hour. Blood pressure is maintained within normal limits. Skin is intact, and turgor is normal.

Dietary Management for Select Diseases

Description and Rationale

The patient with impaired glyconeogenesis is unable to tolerate fasting and has frequent episodes of dehydration and hypoglycemia. Glycogen storage for tissue use is impaired.

Patients with galactosemia must eliminate milk, milk products, and lactose from the diet.

Patients with hereditary fructose intolerance must eliminmate fruit, fruit juices, invert sugars, sorbitol, and levulose from the diet.

Patients with glycogen storage diseases must eat small, frequent meals, often requiring nocturnal nasogastric feedings of high glucose content to restore blood glucose levels. They may also require high starch content approximately every 3 hours while awake. The amount of glucose and starch supplements needed varies according to severity of symptomatology and age and weight of the individual.[100,103]

Contraindications and Cautions

1. Prolonged fasting and limited fluids must be avoided in patients with glycogen storage diseases.

NURSING CARE

Nursing Assessment

Food and Fluids

Positive versus negative food-related behaviors
Satiety versus nonsatiety
Weight loss
Appropriate weight maintenance
Adequate hydration

Psychosocial Concerns

Positive versus negative self-esteem and body image

Growth and Development

Normal for age and sex

Family Coping

Dietary adherence or noncompliance
Management of diet and child's behavior

Body Secretions

Normal or abnormal odor to body secretions

Neurologic Status

Normal or abnormal blood values
Normal or abnormal reflexes

Skin

Maintenance or loss of skin turgor

Nursing Dx & Intervention

Nursing Diagnosis	Nursing Intervention/Rationale
Altered nutrition: more than body requirements	• For glycogen storage diseases: Give frequent feedings. Give nocturnal nasogastric feedings every 1 to 3 hours. Maintain fluid volume. Assess for hypoglycemia.

Nursing Diagnosis	Nursing Intervention/Rationale
Noncompliance	• Assess reason for noncompliance. • Assist with alternate methods of coping with undesired side effects of impaired glyconeogenesis.

Patient Education

1. Teach the prescribed diet to the patient or care giver.
2. Stress the importance of maintaining a diet and of reporting signs and symptoms of exacerbation of the condition.
3. Ensure that the patient or care giver knows community resources to assist with compliance.
4. Teach integration of exercise into the overall care program.
5. Instruct the patient or care giver in the method of administering nasogastric feedings (for patients with glycogen storage diseases).

Evaluation

Patient Outcome	Data Indicating That Outcome is Reached
Dietary compliance is achieved.	Weight is toward range of normal for nutritional requirements. Environment is safe. Patient is fed adequately. There is no hypoglycemia. Skin integrity is maintained. Blood values are normal. Growth and development are progressing at optimum level.

Exogenous Growth Hormone Injections

Description and Rationale

Patients with isolated growth hormone deficiency and short stature may be treated successfully with exogenous growth hormone. When this external supply of human growth hormone is maintained in the body, an increased growth rate equal to or greater than 5 cm per year is expected.

Indications for treatment include the following:

1. Height below the first percentile of average growth for chronologic age
2. Delayed bone age of 2 or more years
3. Psychosocial complications related to short stature
4. Euthyroid state

Treatment may continue until significant height is obtained, or bone epiphyses become fused and future bone growth is no longer possible.

Contraindications and Cautions

1. Somatomedin generation disorders
2. Short stature secondary to other physiologic or psychosocial disease
3. Abnormal thyroid function

NURSING CARE

Nursing Assessment

Mobility

Increased arm and leg span

Growth

Increased height
Attainment of physical and developmental milestones

Psychosocial Concerns

Improved ability to maintain independent ADLs
Improved age-appropriate physical appearance
Positive self-esteem
Appropriate onset of puberty
Appropriate size of genitalia

Other Complications Related to Injections

Difficulty maintaining injection schedule
Anxiety related to giving injection

Nursing Dx & Intervention

Nursing Diagnosis	Nursing Intervention/Rationale
Knowledge deficit (medical treatment)	• Assess the patient's level of knowledge regarding medications and treatments; identify motivational factors for patient learning. • Teach about the medication's action, dosage, and side effects to be reported *to maximize self-care.* • Teach injection technique, time schedule, site rotation, comfort measures after injection, equipment, and medicine storage *to promote safety and compliance with medical regimen.*

Evaluation

Patient Outcome	Data Indicating That Outcome is Reached
Exogenous growth hormone is successfully administered.	Two individuals demonstrate proper injection technique. The patient verbalizes no discomfort after injection. Injection site does not become infected. Growth continues at expected rate. Physical and developmental milestones are attained.

Fluid and Electrolyte Replacement

Description and Rationale

In diabetic ketoacidosis (DKA) and hyperglycemic hyperosmolar nonketotic coma (HHNC), restoration of circulatory volume is needed to ensure delivery of insulin to target tissues and to maintain cardiac output, blood pressure, and pulse and bring osmolarity back to normal.

Electrolytes lost in osmotic diuresis (in HHNC and DKA) must be replaced to prevent serious abnormalities in sodium, potassium, phosphorus, and magnesium.

Contraindications and Cautions

1. Cerebral edema
2. Overhydration
3. Elevated serum electrolytes as measured by laboratory analysis
4. Edema related to sodium excess

Medical Plan

Medications

Fluid replacement
- Diabetic ketoacidosis (DKA)
  - 1-2 L of 0.9% normal saline over first 2 to 4 h (rate: 500-1000 ml/h)
  - 4-5 L of 0.45% saline over next 24 h (rate: 175-250 ml/h)
  - After blood sugar brought to 250 mg/dl range, 5% dextrose in 0.45% saline is given (rate: 175-200 ml/h)
- Hyperglycemic hyperosmolar nonketotic coma (HHNC)
  - 1-2 L of 0.9% normal over first 2 h (rate: 500-1000 ml/h)
  - 4-6 L of 0.45% saline over next 24 h (rate: 175-250 ml/h)
  - After blood sugar brought to 250 mg/dl range, 5% dextrose in 0.45% saline is given (rate: 175-200 ml/h)

Electrolyte replacement
- Sodium: replaced as IV fluid (normal saline)
- Potassium: rate of administration is 20-30 mEq of potassium per liter of IV fluid
- Phosphorus: replaced as a potassium salt in the intravenous fluid

NURSING CARE

Nursing Assessment

Circulatory Concerns

Tachycardia
Venous distention; edema
Increased blood pressure
Coughing
Shock

Food and Fluids

Intestinal cramping
Nausea

Elimination

Diarrhea

Nursing Dx & Intervention

Nursing Diagnosis	Nursing Intervention/Rationale
Altered renal and cardiopulmonary tissue perfusion	• Assess blood pressure, pulse, and level of consciousness every 30 to 60 minutes *to prevent unobserved cardiovascular complications*. • Assess for signs of overhydration, and notify the physician immediately of venous distention, increased blood pressure, coughing, or shortness of breath. • Assess for signs of cerebral edema, and notify the physician immediately of headaches, convulsions, decreasing levels of consciousness, or varying abnormalities in vital signs *to prevent neurologic complications*.
Patient problem: electrolyte imbalance	• Assess patient for signs of increased or decreased serum electrolytes. • Monitor pulse and blood pressure every 30 to 60 minutes. • Monitor serum electrolyte levels.

Evaluation

Patient Outcome	Data Indicating That Outcome is Reached
Circulation is normal.	Patient is not dehydrated. Patient is not overhydrated. Blood pressure and pulse are normal. Patient is not short of breath. IV fluids are replaced at a rate of 6 to 12 L over 24 hours. Intake and output are balanced. Level of consciousness is unchanged.
Electrolyte balance is maintained.	Electrolyte balance is maintained. Baseline ECG is normal.

Gonadotropin Replacement Therapy

Description and Rationale

Human chorionic gonadotropin (HCG) is used to treat hypogonadal men interested in fertility. This drug is extracted from the urine of pregnant women; in men it acts like luteinizing hormone (LH) to stimulate androgen secretion by the testes. In partial gonadotropin deficiency only HCG is needed for testicular growth and spermatogenesis.

In complete gonadotropin deficiency, which occurs frequently in hypogonadotropic hypogonadism, the combination of FSH with HCG allows for complete spermatogenesis. After 18 to 24 months, if the patient remains azoospermic and testicular size has not increased, follicle-stimulating hormone (FSH) is added to HCG. This drug is extracted from the urine of postmenopausal women.

Testosterone enanthate is used to induce virilization in prepubertal boys with hypogonadotropic hypogonadism or adult men who are no longer concerned with procreation.

Contraindications and Cautions

HCG is generally not given in the presence of the following conditions:

- Precocious puberty
- Prostatic carcinoma
- Prior allergic reaction to HCG (rare)

FSH is generally not given in the presence of the following conditions:

- Normal gonadotropin levels
- Elevated gonadotropin levels indicating primary testicular failure

Testosterone is generally not given in the presence of the following conditions:

- Patients with prostatic cancer
- Patients with cardiac, renal, or hepatic disease

Medical Plan

Medications

- Pituitary hormones
  - Chorionic gonadotropin (human chorionic gonadotropin; HCG) for injection, 1000-10,000 U; dosages individualized
  - Menotropins (HMG; human menopausal urinary gonadotropin), 75 U of FSH and 75 U of LH daily for 9-12 d
- Androgenic agent: testosterone enanthate (Delatestryl), 200 mg IM q2-4 wk

NURSING CARE

Nursing Assessment

Testosterone

- Genitalia
  - Initial effects of treatment (4 to 6 months)
    - Increase in testicular size

Maximum effects of treatment (4 to 5 years)
- Increase in phallus size
- Increase in libido

Body hair
- Increase in Tanner stage in pubic area
- Increase in chest, facial, and axillary hair

Muscular concerns
- Muscle mass increase
- Postinjection induration

Bone
- Increase in size and strength

Vocal cords
- Voice deepens

Psychosocial concerns
- Initial (immediately)
  - Increase in libido
  - Increase in self-esteem
  - Increased confidence with both male and female peers
  - Improved body image

Human Chorionic Gonadotropin (HCG)

Testes
- Initial (4 months)
  - Increase in size
- Maximum (3 to 4 years)
  - Increase to 8 ml only if patient has complete hypogonadotropic hypogonadism; if partial hypogonadotropic hypogonadism, testicular size will exceed 8 ml

Leydig's cells
- Initial (monthly)
  - Increased plasma testosterone
- Minimum (8 to 12 months)
  - Sperm production
- Maximum (3 to 4 years)

Human Chorionic Gonadotropin (HCG) and Human Menopausal Gonadotropin (HMG)

Testes
- Intial (3 to 6 months)
  - Increase in size greater than 8 ml

Leydig's cells
- Initial (3 to 6 months)
  - Sperm production
- Maximum (3 to 4 years)

Chest
- Gynecomastia possible

Nursing Dx & Intervention

Nursing Diagnosis	Nursing Intervention/Rationale
Anxiety	• Assess with the patient areas causing anxiety and usual coping mechanisms. • Encourage open communications between patient and partner. • Explore alternative coping behaviors. • Provide patient education covering areas of concern. • Ask patient about any need for home health nurse visits for continued supervision of injections.

Patient Education

1. Teach name, dosage, action, schedule, side effects, and proper storage of medications.
2. Teach procedure for intramuscular self-injection, including preparation and site rotation.
3. Teach the method for collection of semen for analysis.
4. Stress the importance of follow-up medical care.

Evaluation

Patient Outcome	Data Indicating That Outcome is Reached
Anxiety decreases.	Patient discusses feelings surrounding need for treatment. Patient continues open communication with partner regarding body changes. Patient complies with medical treatment program.
Patient complies with intramuscular injection of gonadotropins.	Patient is able to prepare medication and perform self-injection without hesitance or difficulty. Partner demonstrates preparation of medication, injection, site rotation, and disposal of equipment.

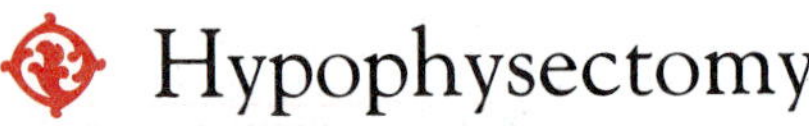

Hypophysectomy

Description and Rationale

Surgical resection of the pituitary gland (hypophysectomy) is often necessary to treat tumors of the pituitary gland and craniopharyngiomas and for the palliation of metastatic breast and prostate cancer.[105] Resection of pituitary microadenomas is often the treatment of choice for Cushing's disease and acromegaly. Emergency hypophysectomy is occasionally required to treat pituitary apoplexy.

The surgical approach to the pituitary gland is by the transsphenoidal or transfrontal approach. The transsphenoidal route is preferred because it provides direct access to the contents of the sella turcica, is relatively safe, and avoids disruption of intracranial structures. It is a well-tolerated procedure that produces no visible scarring. Transsphenoidal hypophysectomy is microscopic surgery performed with the patient in a semisitting position. A gum-line incision is made, a nasal speculum is introduced, and the surgeon has access to the pituitary gland through the sphenoid sinus and floor of the sella turcica.[105] Transfrontal craniotomy may be indicated if the tumor is inaccessible by the transsphenoidal route because of its geometry or because of anomalies of the carotid arteries obstructing access to the pituitary gland.

The indications for hypophysectomy include progressive deterioration of visual fields and increasing hydrocephalus in patients with sellar and parasellar tumors.

Contraindications and Cautions

1. Contraindications
   a. Sphenoidal or nasal infection
   b. Vascular anatomy preventing transsphenoidal approach (threat of damage to carotid arteries)
2. Complications
   a. Diabetes insipidus (40% of patients have transient diabetes insipidus following transsphenoidal hypophysectomy; 10% of patients have persistent diabetes insipidus following transsphenoidal hypophysectomy)[105]
   b. Cerebrospinal fluid (CSF) rhinorrhea
   c. Meningitis
   d. Hypothalamic damage (with visual changes)
   e. Uncontrollable hemorrhage (carotid)

Preprocedural Nursing Care

Provide explanations regarding diagnostic testing and procedures (skull roentgenograms, tomograms, angiograms, brain scans, urine collection, and blood work). Preoperative teaching specific to transsphenoidal hypophysectomy includes:

Presence of nasal packing postoperatively (2 or 3 days)
Mouth breathing while nasal packing is in place
Moustache dressing
Graft site on thigh (muscle plug removed from thigh for packing dura)
Expected decrease in sensation of smell and taste (few months)
No toothbrushing (2 weeks postoperative); mouth care with saline or peroxide solution
Avoidance of coughing, sneezing, nose blowing, and bending over, since these may affect muscle graft
Fluid restrictions possibly necessary
Possibly sent to ICU, surgical ICU, or neurosurgical ICU (variable with institution)

NURSING CARE

Nursing Assessment

Neurologic Status

Visual changes
Changes in level of consciousness
Disorientation
Change in extremity strength or coordination
Postnasal drip (CSF rhinorrhea)

Fluid and Electrolyte Balance

Foley catheter for urine output accuracy
Polydipsia; intake
High fluid intake
Polyuria (200 ml/hour)
Urine specific gravity (1.001 to 1.005)

Gum Line Incision

Redness, swelling, drainage

Thigh (Graft Site)

Redness, swelling, drainage

Psychosocial Concerns

Anxiety

Air Exchange

Difficulty breathing due to mouth breathing
Dry mouth

Nursing Dx & Intervention

Nursing Diagnosis	Nursing Intervention/Rationale
Impaired skin integrity	• Assess secretions from nasal drains; assess quality and quantity of drainage. • Question the patient about postnasal drip. • Perform frequent oral care with normal saline or half-strength H_2O_2 solution. Do not allow toothbrushing for 2 weeks, until sutures are healed. • Apply petroleum jelly *to prevent the patient's lips from cracking as a result of mouth breathing.* • Instruct the patient to avoid sneezing, coughing, nose blowing, straining, and bending over *to protect muscle graft.*
Potential fluid volume deficit	• Assess serum and urine osmolality and electrolytes. Check urine specific gravity *to identify early signs of diabetes insipidus.* • Closely measure and record intake and output.

Patient Education

1. Teach the patient and family about hormonal replacement, which may be indicated postoperatively.

Evaluation

Patient Outcome	Data Indicating That Outcome is Reached
Healing progresses normally, and there is no infection at the postoperative site.	There are no signs or symptoms of infection at operative sites (gum line, thigh). Signs and symptoms of meningitis (i.e., nuchal rigidity, fever, headache) do not develop.
Fluid balance is normal.	Intake approximates output; weight is stable. Urine output is less than 200 ml/hour. Specific gravity is 1.005 to 1.015.

Parathyroidectomy

Description and Rationale

Surgical removal of hyperactive parathyroid tissue is the treatment of choice. Surgical techniques vary with different etiologies. When an adenoma is evident, surgical removal of the entire gland is necessary (there may be more than one adenoma present). Hyperplasia usually affects more than one gland; therefore three glands are removed completely, and three fourths of the remaining gland is removed, leaving enough tissue to maintain normal serum calcium levels.

Contraindications and Cautions

1. Contraindications for surgery
   a. Inability to locate the glands
   b. Underlying medical conditions such as renal failure or severe cardiac disorders
   c. Hypercalcemia from nonparathyroid etiology
2. Complications
   a. Hypocalcemia
   b. Edema
   c. Airway obstruction
   d. Paralysis of vocal cords

NURSING CARE

Nursing Assessment

Renal Concerns

Adequate output

Cardiovascular Concerns

Blood pressure irregularities
Bleeding

Respiratory Concerns

Obstruction of airway
Edema of incisional area

Neuromuscular Concerns

Paresthesias
Dysphagia
Laryngeal spasm
Tetany

Pain

Incision
Shoulder
Throat

Gastrointestinal Concerns

Dietary tolerance
Calcium intake

Personality Disturbances

Anxiety
Depression
Psychoses

Nursing Dx & Intervention

Nursing Diagnosis	Nursing Intervention/Rationale
Potential fluid volume deficit	• Assess patient for dehydration. • Weigh patient daily. • Record intake and output *to monitor fluid balance*. • Check skin turgor. • Check urine for pH, glucose, and protein. • Monitor electrolytes.
Impaired physical mobility	• Assess patient for signs of pain on movement. • Observe for steadiness on ambulation *to maintain patient safety*. • Assist patient with ambulation when necessary. • Handle patient gently; allow patient to move slowly *to prevent injury*.
Pain	• Assess which type of pain is to be treated. • Administer pain medications as needed. • Provide ice chips for pain from sore throat. • Administer throat lozenges. • Support the neck when patient is turning or sitting *to protect incision and promote healing*. • When fractures are apparent, splint ribs while patient turns or coughs *to limit pain*.
Altered nutrition: less than body requirements	• Assess Chvostek's and Trousseau's signs *to identify symptoms of hypocalcemia*. • Make high-calcium snacks available to patient at all times. • Keep emergency calcium replacement medications available at bedside. • Have dietitian discuss high-calcium diet with patient.

Patient Education

1. Teach the signs and symptoms of hypocalcemia (paresthesias, muscle cramps in extremities, and tingling in fingers and around the mouth) to report.
2. Instruct the patient in incisional care.
3. Teach body mechanics and the importance of mobility, especially for patients with irreversible skeletal impairment.
4. Instruct the patient about dietary supplements containing calcium and their use in the treatment of hypocalcemia.
5. Instruct the patient about calcium replacement medications: actions, uses, side effects, and measures to use in case of emergencies.

Evaluation

Patient Outcome	Data Indicating That Outcome is Reached
Patient complies with medical plan.	Patient reports decreased incidence of paresthesias and other signs and symptoms of hypocalcemia. Calcium level is 4.3 to 5.3 mEq/L. Phosphorus level is 1.8 to 2.6 mEq/L.
Patient tolerates increased activity.	Patient resumes ADLs within limitations of underlying disease parameters.
Comfort increases.	There is no operative pain. Patient does not complain of a sore throat. Patient ambulates without statements of discomfort.

Partial Pancreatectomy: Insulinoma and Gastrinoma

Description and Rationale

Surgery is the treatment of choice for both insulinoma and gastrinoma. Preoperative localization of the tumor by CT scan or arteriography is preferable and increases the chance of successful surgery, but it is sometimes difficult. In the case of unsuccessful surgery or when the tumor has metastasized, symptoms should be controlled by medical means, diet and medication. In infants with nesidioblastosis, an 80% pancreatectomy usually relieves the hyperinsulinemia. Usually no more than 85% of the pancreas is resected to prevent malabsorption problems.

Contraindications and Cautions

1. With insulinoma, debilitated condition, extrapancreatic neoplasm, reactive hypoglycemia
2. With gastrinoma, active bleeding ulcer

NURSING CARE

Nursing Assessment

Circulation

Decreased blood pressure
Tachycardia
Pallor
Abdomen rigid and tender
Increasing abdominal girth

Food and Fluid

Dry mouth
Nausea
Gas pain

Comfort and Pain

Describes incisional pain
Splints, protects, or favors incisional area when moving

Skin

Redness, swelling at incision
Wound disruption
Drainage from incision

Nursing Dx & Intervention

Nursing Diagnosis	Nursing Intervention/Rationale
Decreased cardiac output	• Assess blood pressure, pulse, and respiratory rate every 2 to 4 hours. • Observe patient for signs or symptoms of bleeding or shock. • Check dressing and drainage tube every 1 to 4 hours postoperatively *to identify early signs of hemorrhage*.
Altered nutrition: less than body requirements (gastrinoma)	• Assess bowel sound every shift postoperatively. • Stop feeding if pain, vomiting, or nausea occurs.
Pain	• Assess type, location, character, and duration of pain. • Evaluate effectiveness of pain medication. • Report sudden increase in incisional pain or abdominal pain.
Impaired skin integrity	• Assess incision site every shift for redness, swelling, and drainage. • Report signs of wound infection or dehiscence immediately to physician.

Patient Education

1. Teach the patient the signs and symptoms of wound infection to ensure prompt recognition of infection and increase the chance of early treatment and less spread of infection.
2. Teach the patient proper wound care to decrease the chance of infection.
3. Teach the patient the signs and symptoms and treatment of hypoglycemia (if surgery is unsuccessful) to ensure correct management and no loss of consciousness (insulinoma only).
4. Teach the patient the correct dose, schedule, purpose, and side effects to ensure safe and effective use of medication.

Evaluation

Patient Outcome	Data Indicating That Outcome is Reached
Patient's normal nutrition requirements are met.	Patient progresses to a regular diet postoperatively. There is prompt recognition and correct treatment of hypoglycemia (insulinoma only). Patient's blood sugar is within normal limits (insulinoma only).
Patient has tolerable pain related to the incision, which allows for activity as needed.	Patient verbalizes a decrease in pain. Patient participates in or initiates coughing or deep breathing activity, as ordered. Patient requests pain medication as needed.
The incision heals without infection.	Patient has no redness, pain, swelling, or discharge from the incision. The wound edges are well approximated. Patient is afebrile.

Pheochromocytoma Excision

Description and Rationale

Resection of a pheochromocytoma may involve the removal of one or both adrenal glands.

Contraindications and Cautions

1. Alpha blockers or alpha and beta blockers in combination must be instituted preoperatively to control hypertension before and during the operative procedure.
2. Induction of anesthesia produces a release of catecholamines.
3. Intraoperative hypertension and hypotension occur during manipulation and removal of the tumor.

Preprocedural Nursing Care

Administer alpha and beta blockers

NURSING CARE

Nursing Assessment

Circulation

Hypotension
Reexpansion of peripheral circulation
Hypovolemia

Elimination

Oliguria

Complications

Postoperative shock

Nursing Dx & Intervention

Nursing Diagnosis	Nursing Intervention/Rationale
Altered cardiopulmonary tissue perfusion related to hypotension, hypovolemia	• Assess vital signs frequently. • Administer adrenergics by IV line *to maintain blood pressure in safe range*. • Note hypotensive effects of narcotics in the continued assessment of the patient. • Record intake and output *to maintain fluid balance*. • Administer routine postoperative care.

Patient Education

1. Teach the medication's action, schedule, dose, and side effects.
2. Teach the signs and symptoms of disorder and the need to report any change in health status.
3. Ensure that the patient understands the importance of regular reevaluations.
4. Stress that hypertension may persist after surgery until peripheral storage of catecholamines is depleted.

Evaluation

Patient Outcome	Data Indicating That Outcome is Reached
Tissue perfusion is normal.	Vital signs remain stable. Output approximates intake. There are no symptoms of shock.

 Radiation Therapy for Treatment of Pituitary Tumors

Description and Rationale

Radiation therapy is the use of 4500 to 5000 rads[32] of radiation in an attempt to destroy a pituitary adenoma and consequently reduce the elevated hormone levels in the blood to normal range. It is used as an alternative or adjunct to removal of the adenoma. Indications include a pituitary tumor with little or no suprasellar extension, incomplete removal of the tumor with hypophysectomy, or regrowth of the tumor. Typically, radiation therapy reduces tumor size, but hormone levels do not always return completely to normal. It may take up to 2 years to see clinical results of radiation therapy.

Contraindications and Cautions

1. Optimally, radiation therapy is not used with tumors large enough to mandate treatment faster than radiation therapy can provide (e.g., those causing pressure on the optic nerve with ensuing partial blindness).
2. Often there is an initial acute inflammatory response[32] with possible hydrocephalus and exacerbation of symptoms.
3. Destruction of normal tissue (pituitary, hypothalamus, or cranial nerves) is possible.[53]
4. Pituitary tumors occasionally turn out to be radioresistant.[32]

NURSING CARE

Nursing Assessment

Neurologic Concerns

Headache

Neurologic status changes: increased blood pressure, pulse, and respirations; unequal pupils; abnormal pupil reaction to light; disorientation to person, place, and time

Skin

Scalp alopecia

Skin changes: scalp and facial dryness, redness, flaking, itching

Psychologic Concerns

Level of anxiety initially and as therapy proceeds

Mobility

Decreased energy level

Nursing Dx & Intervention

Nursing Diagnosis	Nursing Intervention/Rationale
Altered cerebral tissue perfusion (potential)	• Assess neurologic signs every 4 to 8 hours *to identify evidence of increased intracranial pressure (especially important initially).* • Encourage patient to report headache immediately. • Provide analgesics and other supportive measures for headaches (quiet environment, cool compresses, etc.) *to minimize increased intracranial pressure.*
Impaired skin integrity	• Assess skin daily, observing for thinning, scaling, hair loss, etc. • Instruct patient regarding skin care measures, including use of gentle soaps and shampoos and nonirritating creams; exposure to the sun should be minimized. • If moist desquamation of the skin occurs, apply treatment (ointments, soaks) as ordered. • Encourage the use of wigs or scarves for patients with alopecia *to support a positive self-image.*
Anxiety	• Assess patient frequently for psychosocial and physiologic manifestations of anxiety. • Encourage the discussion of concerns and feelings regarding therapy, including the length of time needed to see the results of therapy, *to support realistic expectations.* • Instruct patient and family on the theory of radiation therapy, including safety measures taken to safeguard normal body tissues, length of time needed to see results, and possible side effects *to maximize self-care and safety.* • Instruct patient and family on specific details of therapy, including therapy schedule and the use of markings that cannot be washed off. • Instruct patient and family that skin changes, alopecia, and fatigue usually resolve once therapy is completed.
Activity intolerance	• Assess patient's activity tolerance and limitations; identify the patient's priorities regarding rest and activity. • Help patient to structure each day to include frequent rest periods. • Encourage patient to limit activities during the period of radiation therapy.

Patient Education

1. Instruct the patient on the importance of returning consistently for follow-up examinations.

Evaluation

Patient Outcome	Data Indicating That Outcome is Reached
Cerebral tissue perfusion is adequate.	Neurologic signs are within normal limits. Patient reports no headache or worsening of headache if it is present at baseline.
Skin integrity is unimpaired.	Patient uses appropriate skin care measures. Patient verbalizes a decision to use or not use cosmetic devices to disguise alopecia.
Anxiety decreases.	Patient verbalizes concerns regarding radiation therapy. Patient states general and specific facts about radiation therapy. Patient exhibits no observable signs of anxiety.
Activity tolerance improves.	Patient uses stress-reducing methods routinely. Patient structures each day to allow for rest periods and desired activities. Patient performs ADLs within limitations imposed by underlying disease state. Statements about "feeling tired" are reduced.

Radioactive Iodine Therapy

Description and Rationale

The goal of radioactive iodine (RAI) therapy is a reduction in the amount of functioning thyroid tissue. Preparations used for radiation treatment include ^{131}I and ^{125}I. ^{131}I is more often used because it is less expensive and normally requires only a single dose. Radiation treatment is less traumatic than surgery, causes no cosmetic disfigurement, and has fewer complications. The major disadvantages of this treatment are that a long period of time may be necessary before hyperthyroidism is ameliorated, hypothyroidism may develop, and there may be radiation effects to the body. RAI is the treatment of choice for Graves' disease, patients unable to tolerate antithyroid drugs, and patients whose Graves' disease recurs after thyroid surgery.

^{131}I is given to the patient after determination of the desired therapeutic dose. The dosage is determined by the severity of toxicity, size of the gland, and age of the patient. ^{131}I is available in a capsule form. Small doses may be given on an outpatient basis. Doses greater than 30 mCi (which are unusual) require hospitalization and radiation isolation. ^{131}I is readily taken up and stored in the thyroid gland, where it destroys its ability to synthesize hormones. ^{131}I also exerts a delayed effect on the ability of the thyroid cells to replicate. Full or conventional doses of RAI are recommended for patients over 50 years of age because of their limited life expectancy and their susceptibility to serious complications of hyperthyroidism such as thyrocardiac disease. Smaller doses are recommended for patients between 30 and 50 years of age. RAI is not recommended for use in infants and children because of its carcinogenic potential.

^{131}I therapy for young adults, adolescents, and children has not been recommended in the past for reasons concerning future fertility, birth defects, the development of neoplasms, and an increased incidence of hypothyroidism. Data on these areas is not clear, and this realm of treatment continues to be controversial.[102]

Contraindications and Cautions

1. ^{131}I crosses the placenta and can destroy the fetal thyroid. A pregnancy test should be performed on all women of childbearing age before treatment. Pregnancy is an absolute contraindication to its use.
2. Pregnant nursing personnel should be restricted from contact with patients receiving ^{131}I therapy.
3. Hypothyroidism is a consequence of RAI therapy. Rarer complications associated with RAI therapy include hypoparathyroidism, radiation thyroiditis, exacerbations of hyperthyroidism, and thyroid crisis.
4. Antithyroid drugs may be given before radiation therapy. Drug therapy must be discontinued 48 to 72 hours before the ^{131}I uptake is determined.
5. Iodides, iodide-containing drugs, and contrast agents should not be given before therapy.
6. After therapy, saliva, perspiration, urine, feces, vomitus, wound drainage, breast milk, and so on are radioactive.
7. Hyperthyroidism, increased swelling of the gland, pain, tenderness, and sore throat are signs of radiation thyroiditis. These signs may develop 1 to 2 weeks after therapy.

Preprocedural Nursing Care

1. Small doses of RAI are usually given on an outpatient basis. Special instructions are included in the section on patient education.
2. Large doses of radioiodine require hospitalization and radiation isolation
   a. Private room at least 6 feet away from other patients or traffic flow

b. Special protective measures for care givers and visitors: gowns, gloves, booties, dosimeter, radiation badges, and consultation by radiation safety branch of hospital
c. Special precautions regarding visitors (no children, pregnant women, etc.)

NURSING CARE

Nursing Assessment

Thyroid Gland

Increased swelling
Tenderness and pain with pressure
Difficulty swallowing

Respiratory Status

Dyspnea
Difficulty breathing

Psychosocial Concerns

Body image alteration
Social isolation
Fear
Anxiety

Nursing Dx & Intervention

Nursing Diagnosis	Nursing Intervention/Rationale
Ineffective individual coping related to anxiety, fear, social isolation	• Assess patient's coping skills, support systems, and history of the adaptive skills that were successful. • Listen attentively and provide an atmosphere of acceptance. • Reduce situations that might startle or frighten patient. • Avoid discrepancies in timing, activities, and methods of performing procedures. • Anticipate and provide for patient's needs. • Encourage expression and discussion of feelings. • Help patient clarify source(s) of anxiety. • Help patient identify strengths and resources. • Encourage patient to learn and use diversional activities. • Encourage use of telephone to communicate with family and friends. • Keep patient informed of daily reductions in radioactivity. • Remind patient that isolation is limited.
Knowledge deficit related to radiation isolation procedures	• Assess patient's knowledge regarding the need for radiation precautions. • Provide private room away from traffic flow; keep door closed. • Explain rationale for isolation and visitor limitations. • Explain purpose of gowns, gloves, booties, dosimeter, and radiation badges. • Explain all procedures for handling of secretions: Saving of urine in special containers or lead pig and flushing of toilet three times after use Use of disposable eating utensils; rinsing sink out after brushing teeth Special handling of linens Special handling of trash Special handling of emesis • Have patient handle own specimens if able. • Explain rationale for rotation of nursing personnel. • Explain rationale for use of Geiger counter. • Instruct patient concerning signs and symptoms to report. • Establish and practice procedures for communicating with nursing personnel. • Check on patient approximately every 2 hours or more often as determined by his or her physical and emotional state *to reduce social isolation*. • Establish patient's plan for diversional activities *to reduce boredom of isolation*.

Patient Education

1. For an outpatient, stress:
   a. The importance of urinating frequently during the first 24 hours
   b. The avoidance of contact with others (especially children) (Suggest sleeping alone for at least 2 nights following dose.)

c. The avoidance of sharing eating utensils, kissing, etc.
d. The importance of flushing the toilet three times after use
e. The avoidance of breast-feeding for 1 week, followed by testing of milk for RAI before resumption

2. For an inpatient or outpatient, explain:
   a. Signs and symptoms of hypothyroidism, hypoparathyroidism, and radiation thyroiditis
   b. Importance of follow-up care

Evaluation

Patient Outcome	Data Indicating That Outcome is Reached
Patient develops strategies for coping with anxiety, fear, or social isolation.	Patient demonstrates ability to cope with restrictions imposed by isolation. Patient verbalizes fears and concerns regarding radiation isolation. Patient identifies source(s) of anxiety and fears. Patient verbalizes decrease in or absence of anxiety and fear. Patient uses strategies to reduce anxiety and fear.
Patient understands radiation isolation procedure.	Patient verbalizes rationale for isolation, visitor restriction, and special radiation precautions. Patient verbalizes procedures for nursing personnel entering and leaving isolation room. Patient verbalizes or demonstrates procedures for handling of secretions. Patient verbalizes signs and symptoms to report. Patient verbalizes or demonstrates method(s) of communicating with nursing staff. Patient verbalizes diversional activities to be used during isolation.

Subtotal Thyroidectomy

Description and Rationale

Surgery results in a decrease in excessive quantities of thyroid hormones through permanent removal of thyroid tissue. A subtotal thyroidectomy involves the removal of about five sixths of the gland. The remaining one sixth of the gland is then capable of providing sufficient hormones.[74] Thyroidectomy may be used for patients with hyperthyroidism who do not follow the prescribed medical regimen; patients with large goiters; patients with drug reactions to antithyroid agents; women and men of childbearing age who want to avoid radiation exposure; and pregnant women whose disease cannot be managed with antithyroid drugs.

Contraindications and Cautions

1. Patients must be euthyroid at the time of surgery. Preoperative treatment is accomplished by antithyroid drugs for 1 to 2 months to bring the patient into a euthyroid state, and with iodine preparations for 7 to 10 days to reduce excessive vascularity of the gland.
2. Inadvertent removal or damage to the parathyroid glands may result in hypocalcemia and tetany.
3. Damage to the recurrent laryngeal nerves during surgery may result in aphonia or dysphonia because of vocal cord paralysis.
4. Permanent hypothyroidism following a subtotal thyroidectomy for Graves' disease develops in the first year after surgery in approximately 25% to 75% of patients.[102]

NURSING CARE

Nursing Assessment

Respiratory Status

Tachypnea
Abnormal breath sounds
Increased restlessness
Complaints of tightness in throat; inability to swallow; inability to get air; pressure or fullness in neck; dressing too tight
Change in level of orientation

Circulatory Status

Variations in pulse and blood pressure readings
Changes in skin condition: cool and clammy
Increased swelling in tissue surrounding incision
Decreased peripheral pulses
Excessive bleeding on surgical dressing
Hemorrhage

Electrolyte Imbalance

Dysphagia; laryngeal spasms
Headache
Positive Chvostek's or Trousseau's sign
Tetany: muscular twitching

Personality changes
Complaints of numbness and tingling of lips, fingers, and toes

Laryngeal Nerve Damage

Change in pitch and tone of voice
Aphonia
Hoarseness; weakness; "whispery" voice

Incision Site

Redness
Swelling
Drainage
Fever
Pain
Guarding behavior
Distraction behavior (restlessness, moaning)

Nursing Dx & Intervention

Nursing Diagnosis	Nursing Intervention/Rationale
Decreased cardiac output related to hemorrhage (potential)	• Assess serum electrolytes, hemoglobin, and hematocrit values *to identify early signs of bleeding*. • Monitor pulse, blood pressure, color, and temperature. • Monitor level of consciousness and orientation. • Check the dressing for evidence of excessive bleeding; watch for bleeding at the side of the neck and back of the head (immediately after operation, check every hour) *to identify signs of bleeding*.
Ineffective breathing pattern (potential)	• Assess rate, depth, and character of respirations *to identify early signs of tracheal compression from edema or hemorrhage*. • Monitor level of consciousness. • Monitor for apprehension, restlessness, and cyanosis. • Keep suction equipment and tracheostomy set at *bedside to use in case of sudden tracheal compression*.
Sensory/perceptual alterations (kinesthetic) related to electrolyte imbalance related to hypocalcemia	• Assess closely for signs and symptoms of hypocalcemia and tetany. • Check reflexes every 2 hours; check vital signs every 4 hours. • Check Chvostek's and Trousseau's signs every 2 hours. • Observe for changes in personality. • Have a 10% solution of calcium gluconate and equipment for IV administration at the bedside or readily available *to treat hypocalcemia*.
Pain	• Place patient in semi-Fowler's position *to promote ease in breathing*. • Monitor edema surrounding incision: apply an ice collar when appropriate. • Observe body language for evidence of pain *to ensure comfort despite impaired communication*. • Log-roll patient's head and chest *to prevent strain on sutures*. • Teach patient to support the head and neck with a folded towel during mobility *to support surgical site*.
Impaired verbal communication	• Assess pitch and tone of patient's voice every 1 to 2 hours postoperatively *to evaluate damage to recurrent laryngeal nerves (vocal cord paralysis)*. • Discourage talking *to prevent edema of vocal cords*. • Monitor for edema of glottis and surgical incision. • Establish alternate means of communication (i.e., pad and pencil). • Reassure patient that hoarseness (from edema or pressure) will subside in a few days.

Patient Education

1. Teach the signs and symptoms of hyperthyroidism, hypothyroidism, and hypocalcemia to report.
2. Teach the name, action, dosage, schedule, route of administration, and side effects of thyroid hormone replacement if ordered.
3. Teach care of the surgical incision.

Evaluation

Patient Outcome	Data Indicating That Outcome is Reached
Cardiovascular function is normal.	Serum electrolytes, hemoglobin, and hematocrit are normal. Patient's skin remains warm and dry. Patient's vital signs remain stable. Patient remains oriented to person, place, and time.
Respiratory function is normal.	Patient demonstrates adequate respiratory depth and rate. Patient does not demonstrate cyanosis, dyspnea, or restlessness. Patient remains oriented to person, place, and time.
Electrolyte balance is normal.	Serum calcium levels are normal. Chvostek's and Trousseau's signs are negative. Patient remains oriented to person, place, and time. There are no signs of tetany.
Comfort increases.	Patient verbalizes decreased pain or relief from pain. Signs of edema at surgical incision are decreased or absent. Patient demonstrates adequate support of head and neck during rest and mobility.
Communication is normal or adequate.	Pitch and voice tone are normal. There are no voice changes (i.e., hoarseness). Patient uses alternate means of communication to preserve voice.

References

1. Acostal PB and Wenz E: Diet management of PKU for infants and preschool children, DHEW Publ No (HSAO) 78-5209, Rockville, Md, 1978, US Government Printing Office.
2. Allen M and Makesh V, editors: The pituitary: a current review, New York, 1977, Academic Press.
3. Allison SK and Allison KL: Drug treatment of lipid disorders, US Pharmacist, December 1985.
4. Amelar R et al: Male infertility, Philadelphia, 1977, WB Saunders Co.
5. Anderson BJ: Antidiuretic hormone: balance and imbalance, J Neurosurg Nurs 11(2):71, 1978.
6. Arieff AI and Felts P, editors: Current concepts: hyperosmolar coma, Kalamazoo, Mich, 1974, A Scope Publication, Upjohn Co.
7. Avioli LV, editor: Fasting hypoglycemia in adults, Arch Intern Med 142:465, 1982.
8. Bashan N et al. Glycogenolysis due to liver and muscle PK deficiency, Pediatr Res 15:229, 1981.
9. Bergsma D, editor: Birth defects compendium, ed 2, New York, 1979, Alan R Liss, Inc.
10. Bloodworth JMB, Jr: Endocrine pathology—general and surgical, ed 2, Baltimore, Md, 1982, Williams & Wilkins.
11. Bondy PK and Rosenberg LE: Metabolic control and disease, ed 8, Philadelphia, 1980, WB Saunders Co.
12. Bone C, editor: Med Clin North Am 67:6, 1983.
13. Braunwald E, editor: Heart disease: a textbook of cardiovascular medicine, Philadelphia, 1988, WB Saunders Co.
14. Brickman AS: Diagnosis, classification and treatment of hypoparathyroid disorders, Nutley, NJ, 1982, Hoffman-LaRoche, Inc.
15. Brobeck J, editor: Best and Taylor's physiological basis of medical practice, ed 10, Baltimore, Md, 1979, Williams & Wilkins.
16. Brook CGD: Practical pediatric endocrinology, New York, 1978, Grune & Stratton, Inc.
17. Brown JD et al: Pituitary pigmentary hormones, JAMA 240(12):1273, 1978.,
18. Castelli WP et al: Incidence of coronary heart disease and lipoprotein cholesterol levels: the Framingham study, JAMA 256:2835, 1986.
19. Chiumello G and Laron L, editors: Recent progress in pediatric endocrinology, New York, 1977, Academic Press.
20. Clark J, Queener S, and Karb V: Pharmacologic basis of nursing practice, ed 2, St Louis, 1986, The CV Mosby Co.
21. Cockett A and Urry R, editors: Male infertility, New York, 1977, Grune & Stratton, Inc.
22. Comite F et al: Short term treatment of idiopathic precocious puberty with a long-acting analogue of leuteinizing hormone–releasing hormone, N Engl J Med 305(26): 1546, 1981.
23. Comite F et al: Luteinizing hormone–releasing hormone analog treatment of boys with hypothalamic hematoma and true precocious puberty, Clin Endocrinol Metab 59:888, 1984.
24. Cornblath M and Schwartz RT: Major problems in clinical pediatrics, vol 3. Disorders of carbohydrate metabolism in infancy, Philadelphia, 1976, WB Saunders Co.
25. Davidson JK, editor: Clinical diabetes mellitus: problem-solving approach, New York, 1986, Thieme, Inc.
26. DeGroot L, editor: Endocrinology, vols 1-3, New York, 1979, Grune & Stratton, Inc.
27. deGrouchy J and Turleau C: Clinical atlas of human chromosomes, New York, 1977, John Wiley & Sons, Inc.
28. Dillon RS: Handbook of endocrinology: diagnosis and management of endocrine and metabolic disorders, ed 2, Philadelphia, 1980, Lea & Febiger.
29. DiMauro S and Eastwood AB: Disorders of glycogen and lipid metabolism, Adv Neurol 17:123, 1977.
30. Duncan PD et al: The effects of pubertal timing and body image, school behavior, and deviance, Youth Adolescence 14:227, 1985.
31. Ellenberg M and Rifkin H, editors: Diabetes mellitus: theory and practice, ed 3, New York, 1983, Medical Examination Publishing Co.

31a. Felig P et al: Endocrinology and metabolism, ed 1, New York, 1981, McGraw-Hill Book Co.

32. Felig P et al: Endocrinology and metabolism, ed 2, New York, 1987, McGraw-Hill Book Co.
33. Findling JW: Selective venous sampling for ACTH in Cushing's syndrome, Ann Intern Med 94:647, 1981.
34. Frigley MS and Luttge WG: Human endocrinology: an interactive text, New York, 1982, Elsevier Biomedical.
35. Galliard RC et al: The antifertility steroid RU486 is an antiglucocorticoid depressing the pituitary-adrenal system in the human, The Endocrine Society, 1983 (Abstract).
36. Gerich JE: Sulfonylureas in the treatment of diabetes mellitus, Mayo Clin Proc 60:439, 1985.
37. Gotch PM: Teaching patients about adrenal corticosteroids, Am J Nurs 81:78, 1981.
38. Greenburgh NJ: Gastrointestinal diseases, ed 2, Chicago, 1981, Year Book Medical Publishers, Inc.
39. Grundy SM: Cholesterol and coronary heart disease, a new era, JAMA 256:2849, 1986.
40. Guthrie DW and Guthrie RA: DKA: breaking a vicious cycle, Nursing 78, p 54, June 1978.
41. Harris RB: Pheochromocytoma: medical review, Heart Lung 13:1, 1984.
42. Hauser ST et al: Family contexts of pubertal timing, Youth Adolescence 14(4):317, 1985.
43. Hazelton Assay Services, Hazelton Laboratories America, Inc.
44. Herbert P: Self care after hypophysectomy, J Neurosurg Nurs 11:118, 1979.
45. Hershman JM: Endocrine pathophysiology: a patient-oriented approach, ed 2, Philadelphia, 1982, Lea & Febiger.
46. Hoeg JM, Gregg RE, and Brewer HB Jr: An approach to the management of hyperlipoproteinemia, JAMA 255:512, 1986.

47. Holm VA and Laurnen EL: Prader-Willi syndrome and scoliosis, Dev Med Child Neurol 23:192, 1981.
48. Imagimedic Productions, Practical Diabetology 2(1):3, 1983.
49. Jackson LG and Schmike RN, editors: Clinical genetics: a source book for physicians, New York, 1979, John Wiley & Sons, Inc.
50. Joosten R et al: Hyperosmolar nonketotic diabetic coma, Eur J Pediatr 137:233, 1981.
51. Karpe B et al: LHRH treatment in unilateral cryptorchidism: effect on testicular descent and hormonal response, J Pediatr, 103:892, 1983.
52. Kaplan SA: Clinical pediatric and adolescent endocrinology, Philadelphia, 1982, WB Saunders Co.
53. Kelly PP and Tinsley, C: Planning care for the patient receiving external radiation, Am J Nurs 18:338, 1981.
54. Kelly S, editor: Metabolic, endocrine, and genetic disorders of children, vol 2, New York, 1974, Harper & Row.
55. Kempe CH, Silver HK, and O'Brien D: Current pediatric diagnosis and treatment, ed 7, Los Altos, Calif, 1982, Lange Medical Publications.
56. Kohler PO, editor: Clinical endocrinology, New York, 1986, John Wiley & Sons, Inc.
57. Korenman et al: Practical diagnosis/endocrine disease, Boston, 1978, Houghton-Mifflin Professional Publishers.
58. Kozak G, editor: Clinical diabetes mellitus, Philadelphia, 1982, WB Saunders Co.
59. Krieger DT and Bardin CW: Current therapy in endocrinology 1983-1984, Philadelphia and St Louis, 1983, BC Decker, Inc and The CV Mosby Co.
60. Krueger J and Ray J: Endocrine problems in nursing: a physiologic approach, St Louis, 1976, The CV Mosby Co.
61. Krupp MA and Chatton MJ: Current medical diagnosis and treatment, Los Altos, Calif, 1984, Lange Medical Publications.
62. Krupp MA, Chatton MJ, and Werdegar D, editors: Current medical diagnosis and treatment, Los Altos, Calif, 1985, Lange Medical Publishers.
63. Lave L et al: Precocious puberty associated with neurofibromatosis and optic gliomas, Am J Dis Child 139:1092, 1985.
64. Loriaux DL: Personal communication, 1983.
65. Luciano DS, Vander A, and Sherman J: Human function and structure, New York, 1978, McGraw-Hill Book Co.
66. Lukert BP: Hypercalcemia, Crit Care Q 3(2):11, 1980.
67. Management of newborn infants with phenylketonuria, DHEW Pub No (HSA) 79-5211, Washington, DC, 1979, US Government Printing Office.
68. Mansfield M et al: Long-term treatment of central precocious puberty with a long-acting analogue of luteinizing hormone–releasing hormone: effects on somatic growth and skeletal maturation, N Engl J Med 309(21):1286, 1983.
69. Marshall WA and Tanner JM: Variations in pattern of pubertal changes in girls, Arch Dis Child 44:291, 1964.
70. Marshall WA and Tanner JM: Variations in pattern of pubertal changes in boys, Arch Dis Child 45:13, 1970.
71. McKusick V: Mendelian inheritance in man: catalogs of autosomal dominant, autosomal recessive, and X-linked phenotypes, ed 6, Baltimore, Md, 1983, The Johns Hopkins University Press.
72. Miller P: Primary aldosterone: a review of assessment, nursing diagnosis, and intervention, Dimensions Crit Care Nurs, March-April 1984.
73. Money J and Walker PA: Psychosexual development, maternalism, nonpromiscuity, and body image in 15 females with precocious puberty, Arch Sex Behav 1(1):45, 1971.
74. Muthe NC: Endocrinology: a nursing approach, Boston, 1981, Little, Brown & Co.
74a. National Cholesterol Education Program: Report of the Expert Panel on Detection, Evaluation, and Treatment of High Blood Cholesterol in Adults, Washington, DC, 1988, National Institutes of Health.
75. National Diabetes Data Group: Classification and diagnosis of diabetes mellitus and other categories of glucose intolerance, Diabetes 28:1042, 1979.
76. National Diabetes Data Group, NIADDK, National Institutes of Health: The prevalence and incidence of diabetes in the United States, Bethesda, Md, 1982, National Diabetes Data Group.
77. National Heart Lung and Blood Institute: Facts about blood cholesterol, Washington, DC, US Dept of Health and Human Services, Public Health Service.
78. National Institutes of Health: Consensus Development Conference statement, Vol 5, No 7, Lowering blood cholesterol to prevent heart disease, Washington, DC, US Dept of Health and Human Services, Public Health Service.
79. National Institutes of Health: Fact sheet: hyperlipoproteinemia, No 81-734, Washington, DC, June 1981.
80. National Institutes of Health, Clinical Center: Clinical pathology cumulative survey, Bethesda, Md, Dec 1982, The Institutes.
81. Nelson DH: The adrenal cortex: physiological function and disease, vol 18, Philadelphia, 1980, WB Saunders Co.
82. Nevins SK: Pre and postoperative care of patients undergoing transphenoidal pituitary surgery, J Neurosurg Nurs 8(1):45, 1976.
83. O'Dorisio TM: Hypercalcemic crisis. Heart Lung 7:425, 1978.
84. Pang S et al: A pilot newborn screening for congenital adrenal hyperplasia in Alaska, J Clin Endocrinol Metab 55:413, 1982.
85. Pediatric laboratory sciences, Tarzana, Calif, 1981, Endocrine Sciences.
86. Pescovitz OH et al: The NIH experience with precocious puberty: diagnostic subgroup releasing hormone to short-term luteinizing hormone–releasing hormone analogue theory, J Pediatr 108(1):47, 1986.
87. Reindollar RH and McDonough PG: Delayed sexual development: common causes and basic clinical approach, Pediatr Ann 10(5):30 1981.
88. Robbins J: Personal communication, 1984.
89. Root AW and Reiter EO: Evaluation and management of the child with delayed pubertal development, Fertil Steril 27:745, 1976.
90. Rosenfield R: Low-dose testosterone effect on somatic growth, Pediatrics 77(6):853.
91. Rudolph A, Hoffman J, and Axelrod S, editors: Pediatrics, Norwalk, Conn, 1982, Appleton-Century-Crofts.
92. Russo L and Moore WV: A comparison of subcutaneous and intramuscular administration of human growth hormone in the therapy of growth hormone deficiency, J Clin Endocrinol Metab 55:1003, 1982.
93. Sanford SJ: Dysfunction of the adrenal gland: physiologic considerations and nursing problems, Nurs Clin North Am 15:481, 1980.
94. Schulte HM et al: The effect of corticotropin-releasing factor on the anterior pituitary function of stalk sectioned cyanomalgus macaques—dose response of cortisol secretion. J Clin Endocrinol Metab 55(4):810, 1982.
95. Sharkey PL and Meyer S: Hypothyroidism, Crit Care Update 8(6):5, 1981.
96. Sharkey PL and Meyer S: Hyperthyroidism, Crit Care Update 8(5):12, 1981.
97. Silver HK et al: Handbook of pediatrics, ed 13, Los Altos, Calif, 1980, Lange Medical Publications.
98. Solomon, BL: The hypothalamus and the pituitary gland: an overview, Nurs Clin North Am 15:435, 1980.
99. Stamler J, Wentworth D, and Neaton JD: Is the relationship between serum cholesterol and risk of premature death from coronary heart disease continuous and graded? Findings in 356,222 primary screenees of the multiple risk factor intervention trial (MRFIT), JAMA 256:2823, 1986.
100. Stanbury J et al: The metabolic basis of inherited disease, New York, 1983, McGraw-Hill Book Co.
101. Streisenger, MH and Fortran JS, editors: Gastrointestinal disease, ed 2, Philadelphia, 1978. WB Saunders Co.
102. Utiger, RD: The thyroid: physiology, hyperthyroidism, hypothyroidism, and the painful thyroid—endocrine and metabolism, ed 2, New York, 1987, McGraw-Hill Book Co.
103. Williams R, editor: Textbook of endocrinology, Philadelphia, 1985, WB Saunders Co.
104. Wyngaarden JB and Smith LH, editors: Cecil textbook of medicine, ed 18, Philadelphia, 1988, WB Saunders Co.
105. Youmans JR, editor: Neurological surgery, vol 6, ed 2, Philadelphia, 1982, WB Saunders Co.

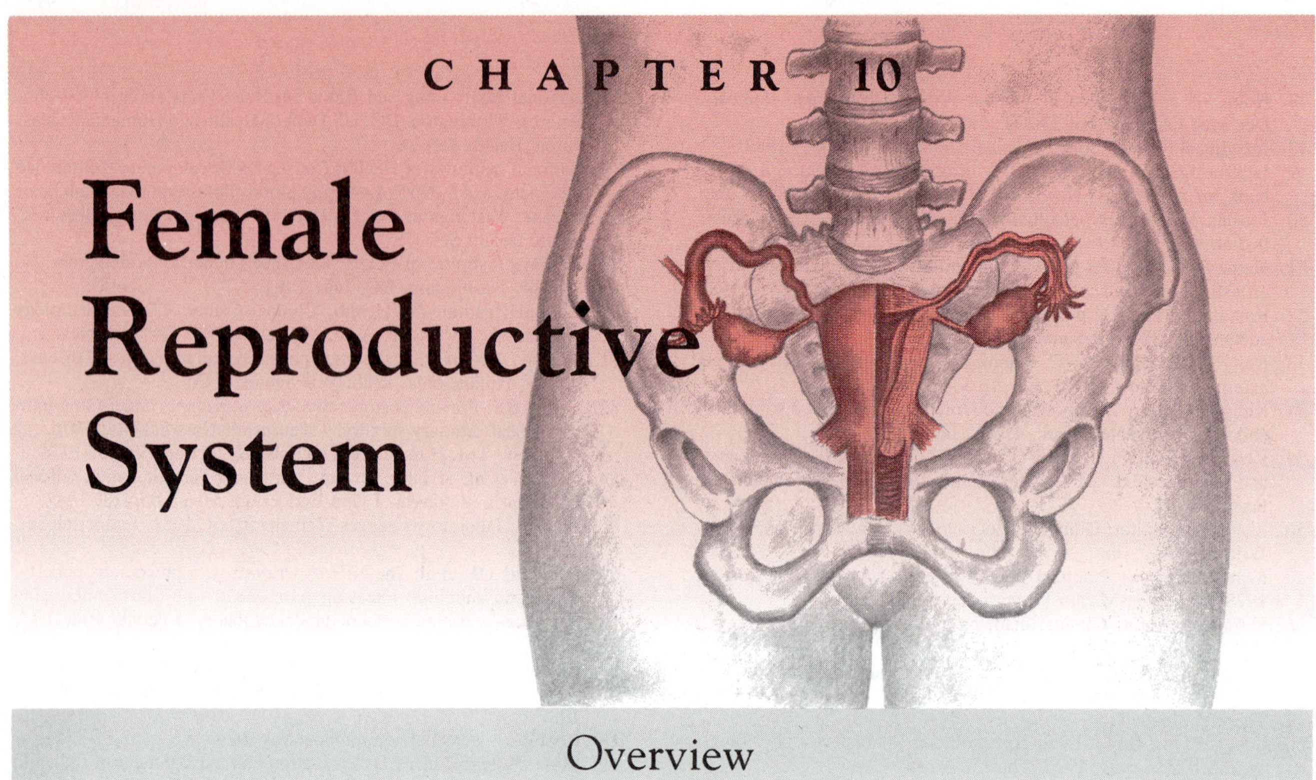

CHAPTER 10

Female Reproductive System

Overview

The major physiologic function of the reproductive system is the procreation of new life and perpetuation of the human species. This biologic process is primarily under endocrine control, but it is also influenced by neural and metabolic factors and human sexuality. Not merely a biologic phenomenon, human sexuality is the sum of physical, functional, and psychologic attributes that are expressed by a person's gender identity and sexual behavior. These factors interact when gynecologic and reproductive processes or conditions threaten, alter, or interfere with female sexual integrity. The focus of this chapter is the female organ system. Selected female organ dysfunctions, interventions based on the nursing diagnosis, and treatment of the patient's responses to actual or potential health problems are discussed, as well as anatomy and physiology.

The comparative incidences of cancers involving the female reproductive organs have changed considerably in recent years. Endometrial cancer has replaced cervical cancer as the most common gynecologic malignancy. Some 36,000 cases of endometrial carcinoma are diagnosed each year, compared with 14,000 cases of invasive cervical cancer.[15,62] Although endometrial cancer can occur at any age, it is most common in women past the age of 50 years, with the peak incidence occurring at about 55 years. In contrast, cervical cancer most often occurs between the ages of 40 and 49 for invasive cancer and at an average age of 35 years for preinvasive cancer.[62] Cancer of the endometrium occurs predominantly in middle- and upper-class women, and a major risk factor is long-term unopposed exposure to estrogen. The incidence of cancer of the cervix is higher in sexually active women who began coitus before the age of 20, particularly those who were in their early teens at the age of first coitus. Multiparity increases the occurrence, and a history of multiple sex partners seems to be an important factor.[15,62]

Breast cancer is the leading cause of death in women 40 to 55 years of age. One in 10 women will develop breast cancer during her lifetime. In 1986 more than 123,300 new cases were reported, and more than 39,900 deaths occurred from the disease. In a small percentage of women, breast cancer develops coincident with pregnancy, but most new cases occur in the decade before and the two decades after menopause (40 to 70 years of age).[11] Although little is known about the prevention of breast cancer, the chance for survival appears to be good if it is found early and treated promptly. The overall cure rate for breast cancer is 30% to 40%. It approaches 85% for mammographically diagnosed breast cancer when the cancer is minimal and discovered early. Several factors are associated with an increased risk of breast cancer. The most common are age over 40 years, a family history of breast cancer, nulliparity or first parity after age 34, previous cancer of one breast, and fibrocystic disease of a precancerous mastopathy type.

Anatomy, Physiology, and Related Pathophysiology

The female organ system consists of internal organs in the pelvic cavity and external organs in the perineum. The internal organs are the ovaries, fallopian tubes, uterus, and vagina. The external genitalia are the mons pubis, labia majora, labia minora, and the vestibule of the vagina (Figure 10-1).

Figure 10-1 External female genitalia.
From Bobak.[4]

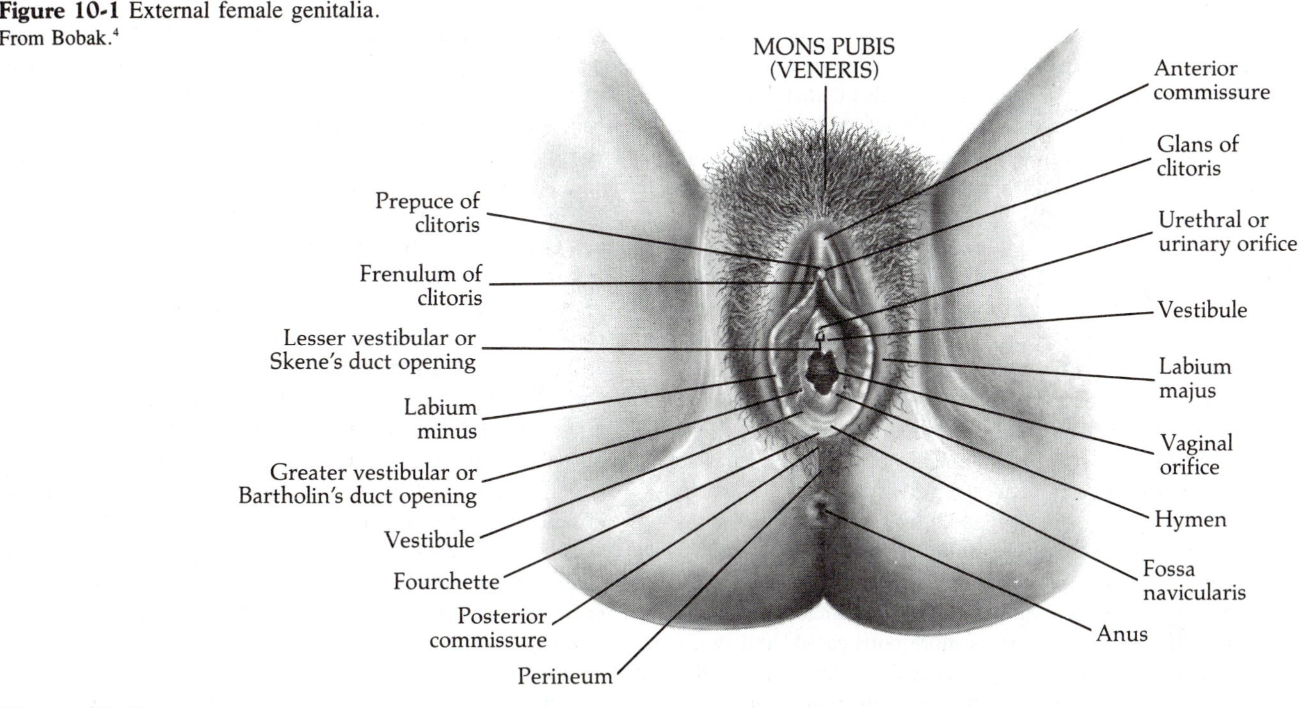

External Structures

The vulva includes all externally visible structures from the pubis to the perineum. These are the mons pubis, labia majora and minora, clitoris, vestibular glands, hymen, urethral opening, and perineum.

Mons pubis. The mons pubis or mons veneris is a cushionlike elevation of adipose tissue over the symphysis pubis. It is covered by pubic hair after puberty.

Labia majora. The labia majora are two rounded folds of adipose tissue with overlying skin that extend from the mons pubis downward and backward, encircle the vestibule, and merge into the perineum. The outer surfaces are covered by hair, and the inner surfaces containing sebaceous follicles are smooth and moist. The labia majora are homologous with the male scrotum.

Labia minora. The labia minora are two flat folds of skin medial to the labia majora. They are devoid of hair and usually in contact with each other. They come together anteriorly at the frenulum of the clitoris and posteriorly at the frenulum of the labia.

Clitoris. The clitoris, situated at the anterior end of the labia minora, is a small, cylindric, erectile body consisting of a glans, a body (corpus), and two crura. It is partially covered by the anterior ends of the labia minora and is very sensitive to tactile stimulation. It consists of two corpora cavernosa enclosed in a dense fibrous membrane that is made up of smooth muscle and elastic fibers. It is connected to the ischiopubic rami by two crura. The clitoris, which corresponds to the male penis, rarely exceeds 2 cm in length even in a state of erection during sexual arousal. The glans of the clitoris is covered by stratified epithelium that is richly supplied with free nerve endings within the fibers, terminating in small knoblike thickenings in or adjacent to the cells. Genital corpuscles, distributed in the glans and corpora, are considered the main mediators of erotic sensation.

Vestibule. The vestibule is the area between the labia minora. The hymen, vaginal orifice, urethral orifice, ducts of Bartholin's glands, and Skene's ducts are contained within the vestibule. The Bartholin's or greater vestibular glands secrete mucoid material during sexual excitement. They are on either side of the vaginal opening under the constrictor muscle of the vagina.

Urethral opening. The urethral opening or urinary meatus is in the midline of the vestibule posterior to the clitoris and anterior to the vaginal opening. The Skene's or paraurethral ducts open on the vestibule on either side of the urethra. Occasionally these openings are found on the posterior wall of the urethra just inside the meatus.

Hymen. The hymen is a fold of vascularized mucous membrane at the introitus of the vagina. It is not richly supplied with nerve fibers and has no glandular or muscular elements. The hymenal opening is usually very small in virgins who do not use tampons but is rarely imperforate, which would cause a retention of the menstrual discharge. During the first coitus or in certain other situations the hymen generally tears at several points. The edges of the tears soon cicatrize. Bleeding does not always occur when the hymen is ruptured.

Perineum. The perineum is a triangular area that is the inferior end of the trunk. It is situated dorsal to the pubic arch, superior to the tip of the coccyx, and lateral to the pubic and ischial rami. It supports and surrounds the distal portions of the urogenital and gastrointestinal tracts of the body. The central fibrous perineal body between the vagina and the anus divides the perineum into a posterior anal triangle and an anterior urogenital triangle.

Internal Structures

The internal organs include the ovaries, uterine (fallopian) tubes, uterus, and vagina.

Ovaries. The ovaries are two oval structures in the upper part of the pelvic cavity, between the uterus medially and the lateral pelvic wall. They are suspended from the posterosuperior surface of the broad ligaments by the mesovarium. During the childbearing years each ovary is 2.5 to 5 cm in length, 1.5 to 3 cm in breadth, and 0.6 to 1.5 cm in thickness. After menopause the ovaries diminish markedly in size.[15,51] In young women the ovary has a smooth, dull white surface through which glisten several small clear follicles. With advancing age the ovary becomes more corrugated, and in elderly women its exterior may appear convoluted. From the first stages of development until after menopause, the ovary undergoes constant change. From birth to puberty an estimated 200,000 to 400,000 oocytes are present.[28,49] It is evident that a few hundred ova suffice for reproduction, since ordinarily only one ovum is cast off during a menstrual cycle. The glandular elements of the ovaries are described as interstitial, thecal, and luteal cells. The interstitial glandular elements are formed from cells of the theca interna of degenerating follicles. The thecal glandular cells are formed from the theca interna of ripening follicles. Luteal cells are derived from granulosa cells of ovulated follicles and from undifferentiated stroma surrounding them.

The ovarian cycle and its hormones are discussed in greater detail later in the chapter.

Uterine (fallopian) tubes. The uterine (fallopian) tubes are two flexible, trumpet-shaped, muscular tubes that extend from the uterine cornua to the ovaries and provide the ova with access to the uterine cavity. They are approximately 10 cm in length in an adult and are suspended by a fold of the broad ligament called the mesosalpinx. The isthmus end of the tube opens into the uterine cavity. The ampulla is the dilated central part of the tube that is continuous with the infundibulum, the fimbriated funnel-shaped opening of the distal end of the tube. This fimbriated portion of the tube, which is adjacent to the ovary, draws the ovum into the tube, where fertilization may occur. The tubal musculature undergoes rhythmic contractions that transport the ovum into the uterus.

Uterus (Figure 10-2). The uterus is a pear-shaped, thick-walled, muscular organ suspended in the anterior part of the pelvic cavity above the bladder and in front of the rectum. It consists of two major but unequal parts: an upper triangular portion, the body or corpus, and a lower cylindric or fusiform

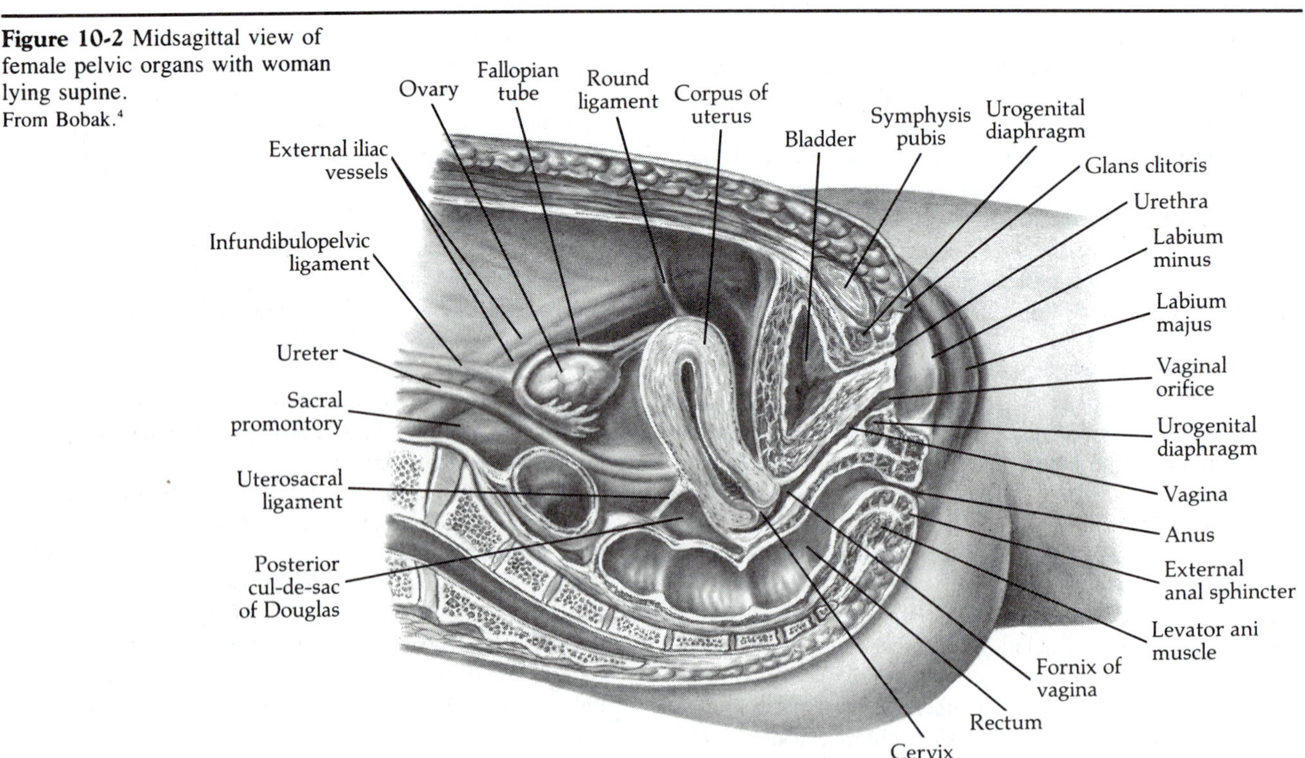

Figure 10-2 Midsagittal view of female pelvic organs with woman lying supine.
From Bobak.[4]

Figure 10-3 Cross section of uterus adnexa and upper vagina.
From Bobak.[4]

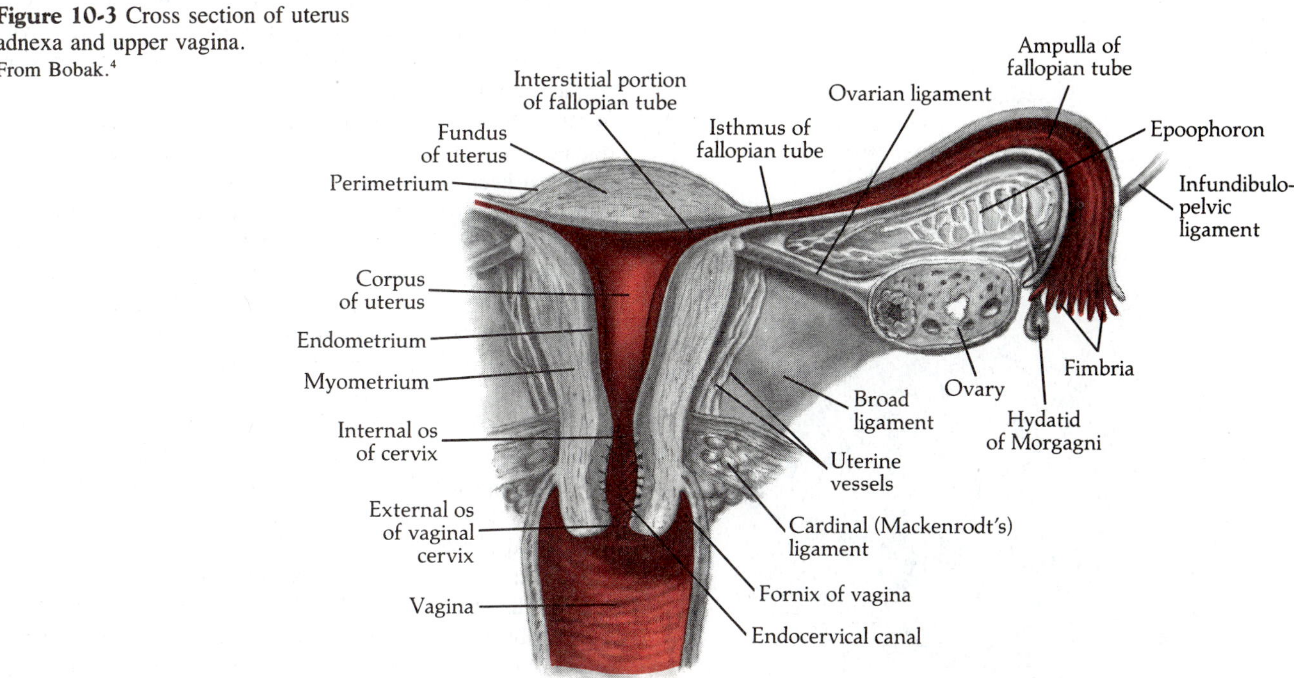

portion, the cervix (Figure 10-3). The isthmus divides these two portions. The uterine (fallopian) tubes emerge from the cornua of the uterus at the junction of the superior and lateral margins. The convex upper segment between the cornua is the fundus uteri. Before puberty the length of the uterus varies from 2.5 to 3.5 cm. In a mature nulliparous woman the uterus is 6 to 8 cm in length, as compared with 9 to 10 cm in a multiparous woman (Figure 10-4). The uterus is covered with a layer of peritoneum from which arise the broad ligaments that extend from the lateral margins of the uterus to the pelvic

Figure 10-4 Comparative sizes of prepubertal, adult nonparous, and multiparous uteruses.

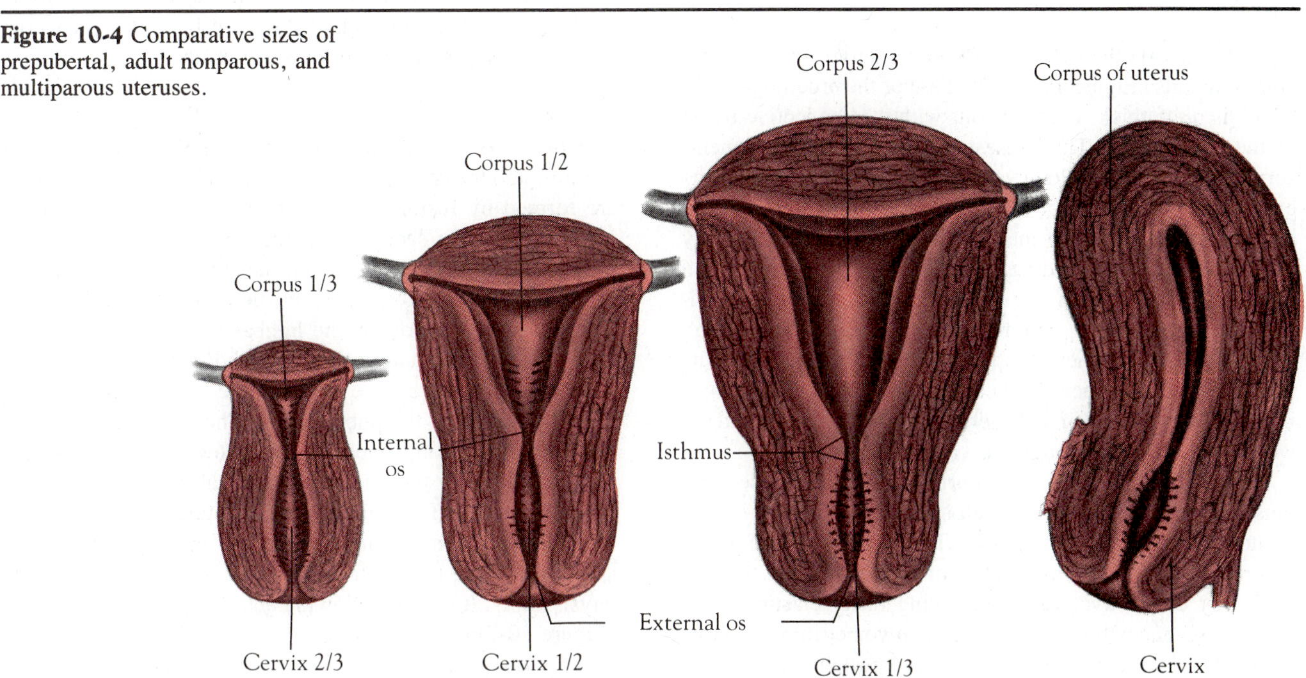

Figure 10-5 Female pelvic contents as viewed from above.

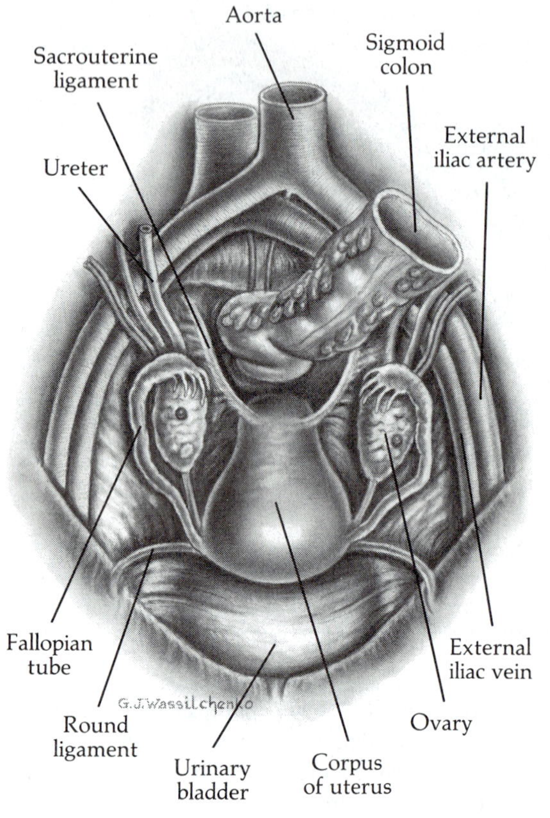

walls and divide the pelvic cavity into anterior and posterior compartments (Figure 10-5). The base of the broad ligament, which is quite thick, is continuous with the connective tissue of the pelvic floor. The densest portion (cardinal ligament) surrounds the uterine blood vessels. The two round ligaments extend from each side of the uterus below the uterine tubes and hold the organ in the anterior position. During pregnancy the round ligaments undergo considerable hypertrophy and increase in both length and diameter. The uterosacral ligaments extend from the sacrum around the rectum to the cervix of the uterus. They help support the uterus and maintain its position. The uterosacral and cardinal ligaments are the most important ligaments of the uterus; without them the uterus would tend to pass through the vagina, or prolapse.

The wall of the uterus comprises three layers: serosal, muscular, and mucosal. The serosal layer is formed by the peritoneum covering the uterus. The muscular portion, or myometrium, consists of bundles of smooth muscle that are united by connective tissue containing many elastic fibers. During pregnancy the thickness of the myometrium increases markedly. This occurs because of hypertrophy (actual enlargement of existing fibers) and addition of new fibers derived from transformation and division of mesenchymal cells. The innermost or mucosal layer that lines the uterine cavity in the nonpregnant state is the endometrium. It comprises surface epithelium, glands, and interglandular tissue. The uterine glands extend through the entire thickness of the endometrium to the myometrium and secrete a thin alkaline fluid that keeps the uterine cavity moist.

Two types of arteries supply blood to the endometrium. The straight basal arteries extend to the basal layer of the endometrium from the radial and arcuate arteries in the myometrium. The coiled or spiral arteries, which are a continuation of the radial and basal arteries, supply the superficial layer of the endometrium. The coiled arteries play an important part in the mechanism of menstruation.

The cervix is the lower part of the uterus. The entrance of the uterus is the cervical os or opening, which changes in size and shape depending on pregnancy or previous deliveries. Hormonal changes influence mucus production by the endocervical glands.

Vagina. The vagina is a tubular canal 10 to 15 cm in length, directed backward and upward and extending from the vestibule to the uterus. It is located between the bladder anteriorly and the rectum posteriorly. It is the female organ of copulation, the birth canal, and the excretory duct of the uterus through which the menstrual flow escapes. In an adult the anterior wall of the vagina is approximately 8 cm long and the posterior wall is 9 to 10 cm long. The difference is due to the projection of the cervix into the anterior aspect of the superior end of the vagina. The anterior, posterior, and two lateral fornices are produced by the cervix projecting into the vagina. The fornices are of clinical importance because the internal pelvic organs can be easily palpated through the thin wall. The mucous membrane lining the vagina forms thick folds so that the vaginal walls are in contact with each other and kept moist by cervical secretions.

Pelvis

The pelvis is composed of the two innominate bones, the sacrum, and the coccyx (Figure 10-6). The innominate bones are formed by fusion of the ischium, ilium, and pubis and are joined to the sacrum and each other at the symphysis pubis. The pelvis has two parts: the shallow, upper, or false pelvis and the lower, smaller, or true pelvis. The false pelvis is bounded posteriorly by the lumbar vertebrae, laterally by the iliac fossa, and anteriorly by the abdominal wall. The true pelvis is bounded by the sacrum, the inner surface of the ischial bones, and the pubic bones. The shape and diameter of the true pelvis are important in obstetrics because it must accommodate the fetal head in a vaginal delivery.

Pelvic inlet. The pelvic inlet is bounded posteriorly by the sacral promontory, laterally by the linea terminalis, and anteriorly by the horizontal rami of the pubic bones and symphysis pubis. It has the following anterior-posterior diameters (Figure 10-7):

True conjugate (conjugata vera), the distance from the upper margin of the symphysis to the sacral promontory

Figure 10-6 A, Right coxal bone, medial aspect. **B,** Articulated right coxal bone, sacrum, and coccyx, left oblique view.

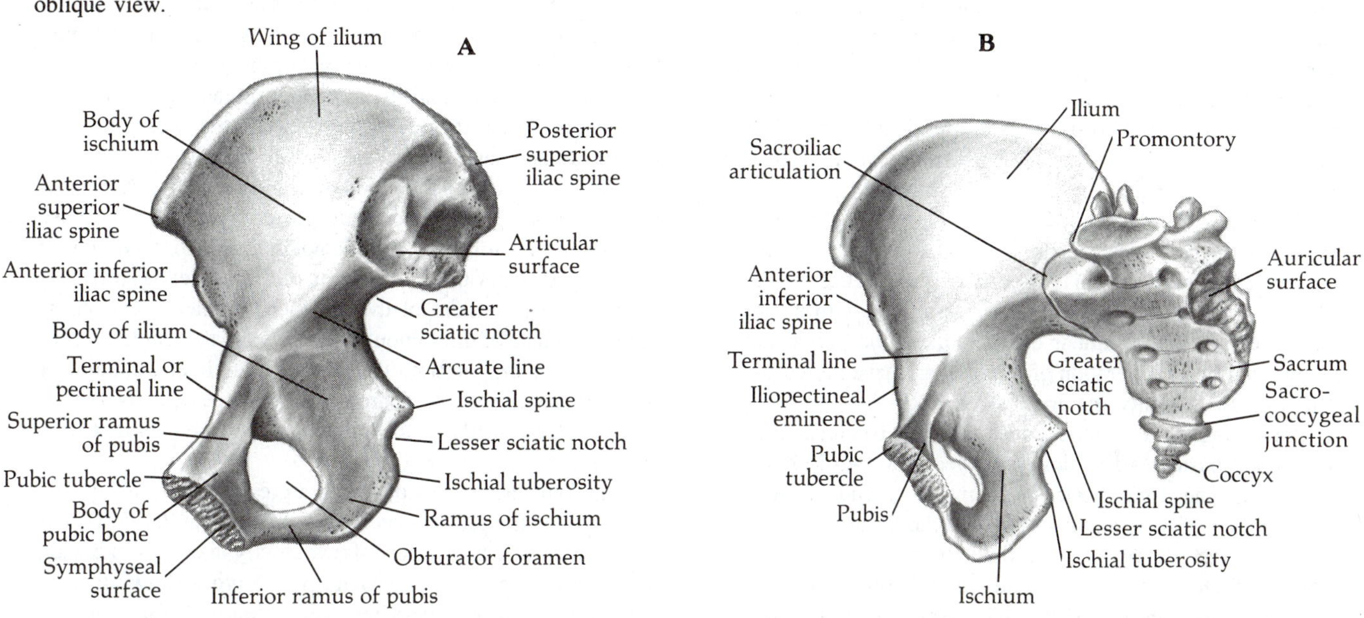

Obstetric conjugate, the distance from the most convex posterior surface of the symphysis to the sacral promontory; this is about 0.5 cm less than the true conjugate and is the shortest anteroposterior diameter through which the fetal head must descend

Diagonal conjugate, the distance from the lower border of the symphysis to the sacral promontory; this is the only anteroposterior measurement that can be obtained by clinical examination

The transverse diameter of the pelvic inlet is at a right angle to the obstetric conjugate and represents the greatest distance between the lineae terminales on either side. The oblique diameters extend from each sacroiliac synchondrosis to the opposite iliopectineal eminence.

Figure 10-7 Planes of pelvic inlet.

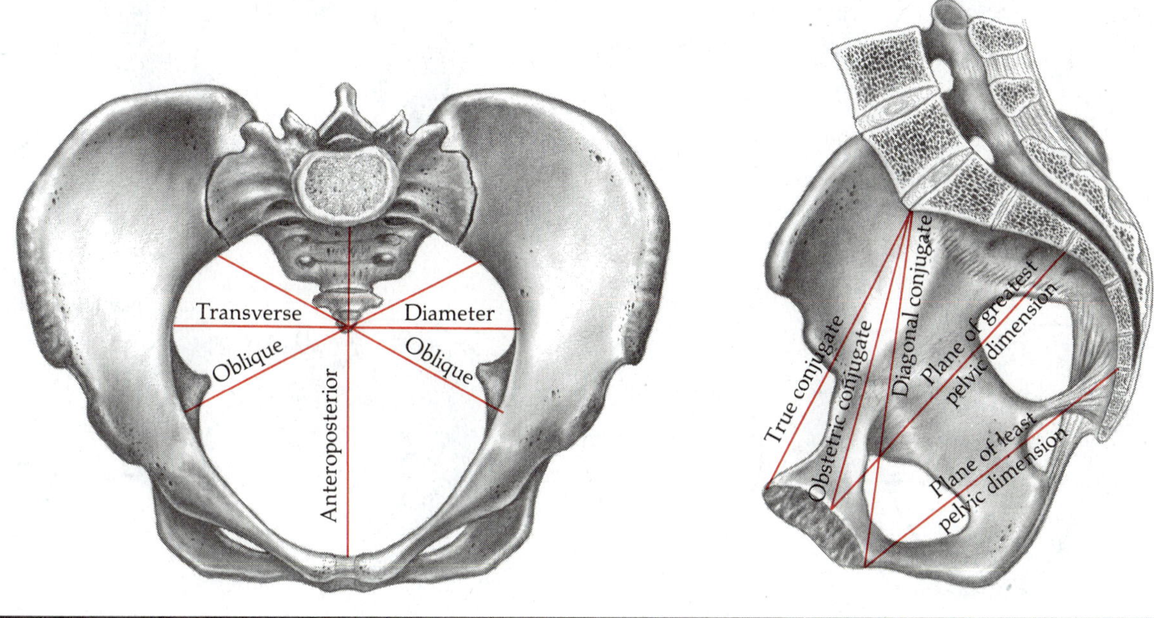

Midpelvis. The midplane of the pelvis is the roomiest portion of the pelvic cavity. It extends from the middle of the symphysis pubis to the junction of the second and third sacral vertebrae and passes laterally through the ischial bones over the middle of the acetabulum. The interspinous (bispinous) diameter of 10 cm or slightly more in an adult is usually the smallest diameter of the pelvis. The anteroposterior diameter at the level of the ischial spines is normally at least 11.5 cm. The posterior sagittal diameter of the midpelvis is normally approximately 4.5 cm.

Pelvic inclination. In a woman who is standing, the upper portion of the pelvis is normally directed downward and backward and the lower portion is directed downward and forward. The tilt of the pelvis, or inclination, is altered with posture. Straightening of the lumbar curve reduces the pelvic inclination, and an exaggeration of the lumbar curve increases it. This tilt can influence the progress of labor.

Pelvic outlet. The outlet consists of two triangles having a common base at a line drawn between the two ischial tuberosities. The anteroposterior diameter extends from the lower border of the symphysis pubis to the tip of the sacrum. The transverse diameter is the distance between the ischial tuberosities. This is also called the intertuberous or bi-ischial diameter. The posterior sagittal diameter extends from the tip of the sacrum to a right-angled intersection with a line between the ischial tuberosities.

Pelvic classification. Classification of the pelvis by Caldwell and Moloy in 1933 defined four basic shapes: gynecoid, anthropoid, platypelloid, and android.[42] The classification is based on the configuration of the inlet and the corresponding changes in the midpelvis and lower pelvis. The pelvic inlet is divided into a posterior segment behind a line of the widest transverse diameter and an anterior segment in front of it. The length of the transverse diameter and the anteroposterior length of each segment are assessed to classify the inlet.

The sacrosciatic notch is visualized laterally. A narrow notch indicates a reduced anteroposterior diameter because the sacrum lies forward. A wide notch means that the sacrum is displaced posteriorly. Evaluation of the midpelvis and outlet includes measurement of the bispinous diameter and observation of shape of the spinous processes and the length, width, and curve of the sacrum. The subpubic angle and contour of the arch are noted. The degree of divergence or convergence of the lateral walls is also noted when classifying pelvic shapes.

The four basic types of pelvis are evaluated to assess the adequacy of the pelvic structures for a vaginal delivery. It is uncommon for a pelvis to conform exactly in every dimension to any one type; most pelves are mixed types showing combinations of various characteristics (Figure 10-8).

Gynecoid pelvis. The gynecoid pelvis is characteristic of the normal female and is associated with the lowest incidence

Figure 10-8 Female pelvis—pure types.

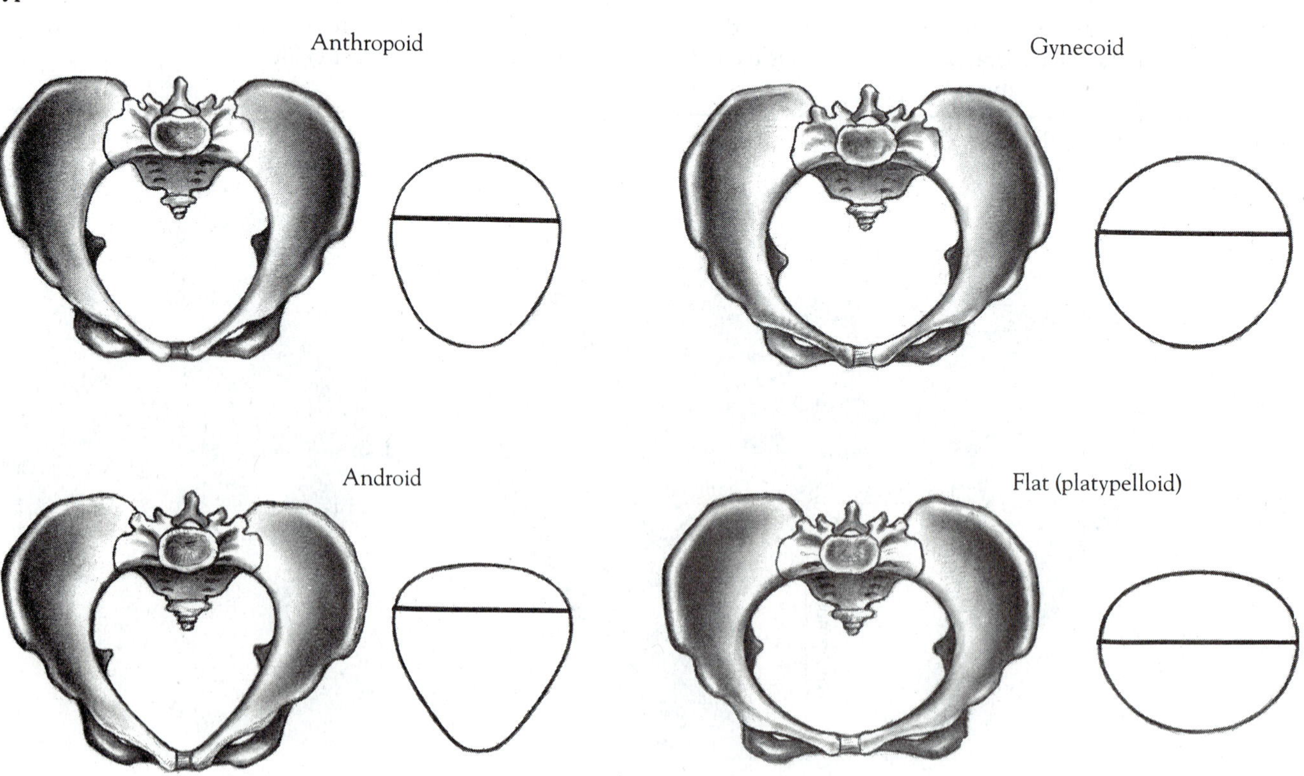

of fetopelvic disproportion. The inlet is nearly round. The sacrum is well curved and has average inclination. The sacrosciatic notch is of average size. The side walls are straight, and the ischial spines are not prominent. The subpubic arch is wide, and the transverse diameter is about 10 cm.

Android pelvis. The android pelvis is characteristic of the normal male. The posterior segment is wide and flat, and the anterior segment is narrow. The sacrum is straight and inclined forward. The sacrosciatic notch is narrow, and the side walls convergent. The ischial spines are prominent, and the subpubic arch is narrow. This is a typical "funnel pelvis."

Anthropoid pelvis. The anthropoid pelvis has a reduced transverse diameter as compared with the gynecoid pelvis, making it a long narrow oval with an elongated anterior-

Figure 10-9 Perineum. **A,** Superficial components. **B,** Deep components.

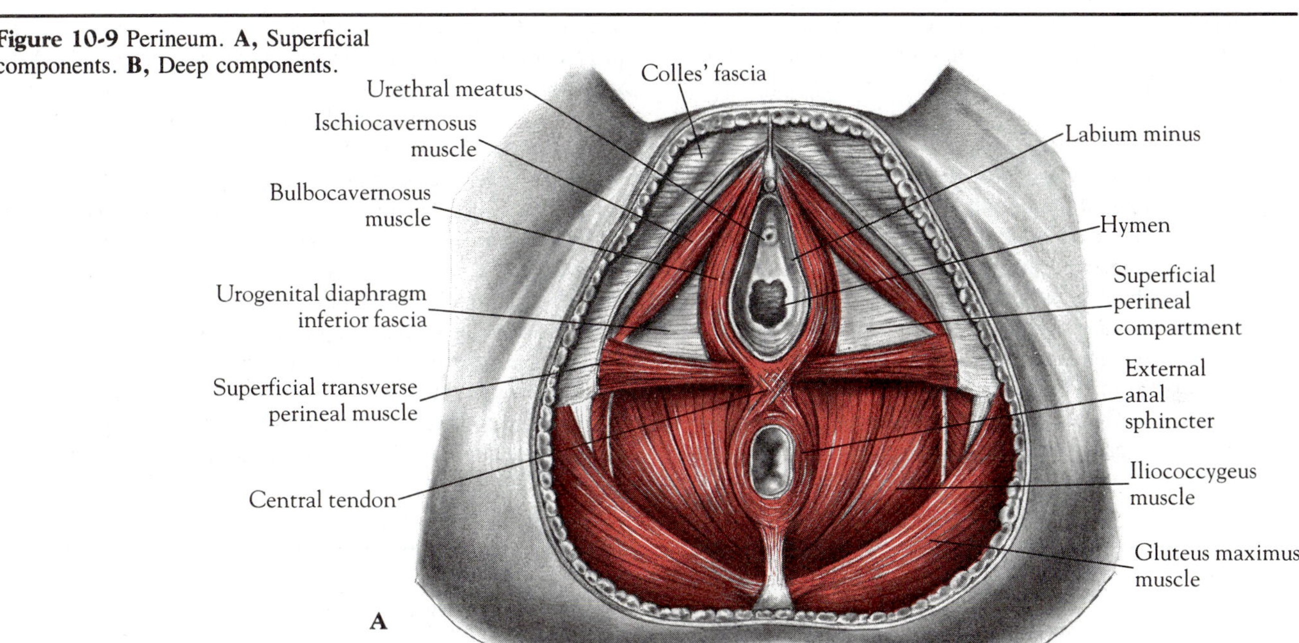

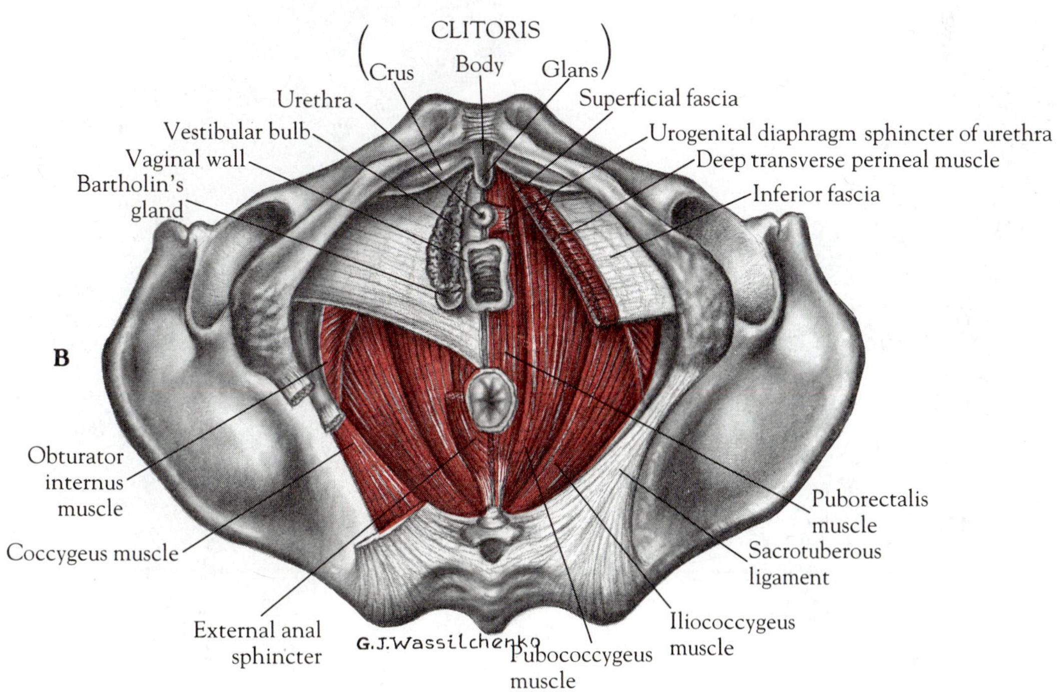

posterior segment and a slightly narrowed forepelvis. The sacrum is long and narrow with an average curvature posteriorly. The sacrosciatic notch is wide and shallow, and the side walls are straight. The ischial spines are prominent with a shortened bispinous diameter. The subpubic arch is narrowed.

Platypelloid pelvis. The platypelloid pelvis is similar to the gynecoid pelvis except for narrowing of the anterior-posterior diameters at all levels. The inlet appears as a wide transverse oval. The sacrosciatic notch is wide, and the side walls are straight. The ischial spines are prominent, and the subpubic arch is wide.

Pelvic Floor (Figure 10-9)

A number of tissue layers form the pelvic floor. From the inside outward toward the skin they are the peritoneum, subperitoneal connective tissue, internal pelvic fascia, levator ani and coccygeus muscles, external pelvic fascia, superficial muscles, and subcutaneous tissue.

The levator ani and the fascia close the lower end of the pelvic cavity and diaphragm and present a concave upper surface. On both sides the levator ani consists of a pubic and iliac portion. The fibers pass backward to encircle the rectum, and a few fibers pass behind the vagina. The posterior and lateral portions of the pelvic floor not covered by the levator ani are covered by the piriformis and coccygeus muscles on either side.

Three layers of fascia fill out the triangular space between the pubic arch and a line joining the ischial tuberosities. This is called the urogenital diaphragm; it forms a compartment in which lie the superficial perineal muscles.

Breasts (Figure 10-10)

The breasts or mammary glands are accessory organs of reproduction. They consist of a glandular epithelium and a duct system embedded in interstitial tissue and fat. They lie anterior to the pectoralis major muscle and are separated from it by a layer of fat that is continuous with the fatty stroma of the gland itself. They extend from the anterior border of the axilla to the lateral edge of the sternum. Each gland consists of a comma-shaped mass of fat and collagenous tissue. The tail of Spence extends toward the axilla. The position of the breasts is maintained by suspensory (Cooper's) ligaments, which are condensations of connective tissue. They are easily stretched, especially if the breasts are large. Lymph drainage is mainly toward the axillary lymph nodes, with some drainage directed toward the substernal and diaphragmatic nodes. Some women (as well as some men) have supernumerary

Figure 10-10 Anatomy of breast.

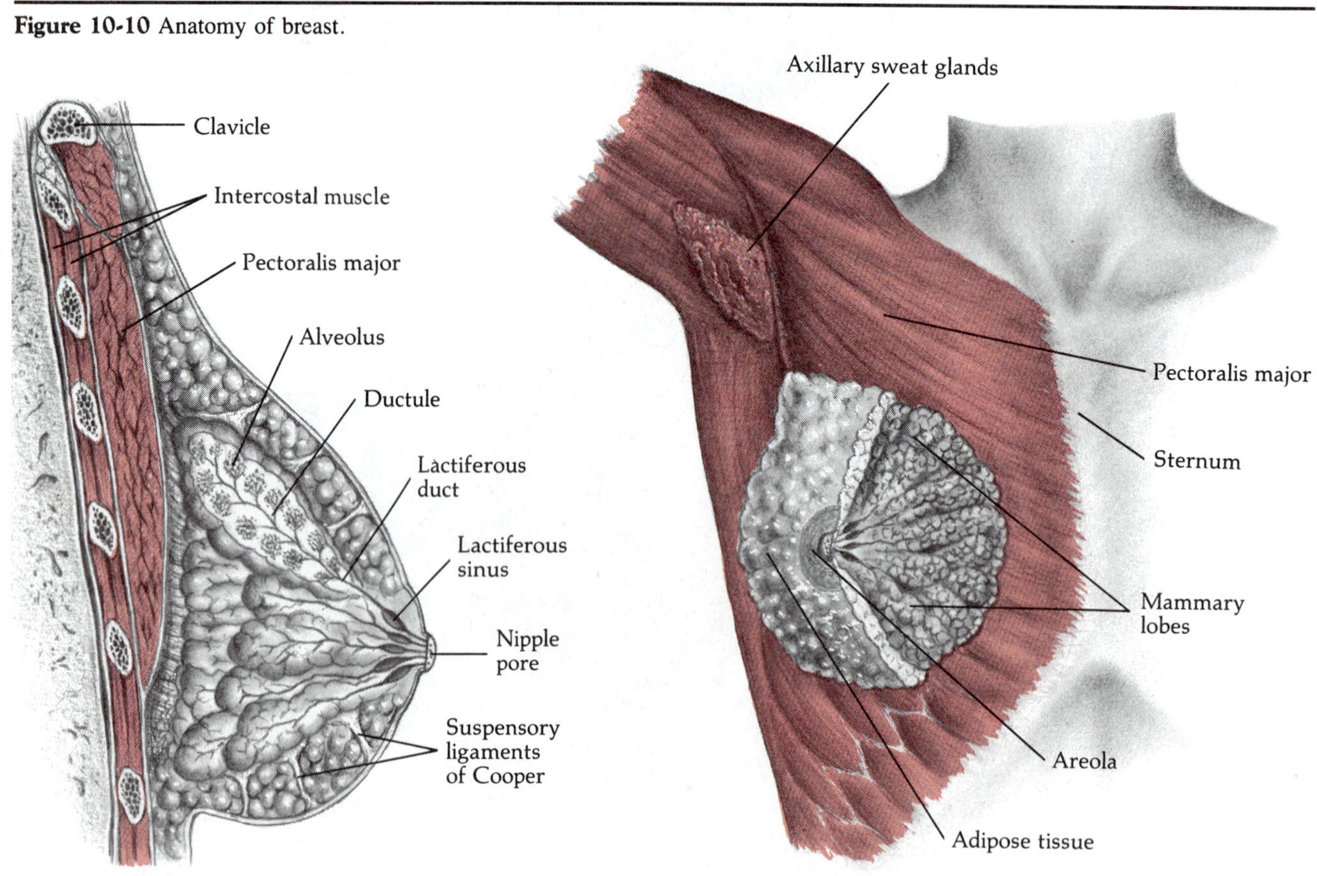

nipples or breast tissue that develops along the longitudinal ridges extending from the axilla to the groin, which existed during early embryonic development (Figure 10-11).

The center of the fully developed breast in an adult woman is the nipple, which is elevated above the breast. Bundles of smooth muscle fibers in the nipple have erectile properties. The areola that surrounds the nipple has a diameter of 1.5 to 2.5 cm. Small sebaceous glands located under the areola give it a rough appearance. Arranged radially under the areola are 15 to 20 lactiferous ducts. In a lactating woman these ducts drain milk from the lobes of glandular tissue embedded in the adipose tissue of the breast. The ducts enlarge slightly before reaching the nipple to form the short lactiferous sinuses in which the milk may be stored. From the sinuses the ducts extend toward the chest wall, uniting various lobules or acinar structures of the breast. Each lobule contains 10 to 100 alveoli or acini, and 20 to 40 lobules compose each of the 15 to 20 lobes that are distributed in each breast. The alveolus is lined by a single layer of milk-secreting epithelial cells, encased in a network of myoepithelial strands; it is surrounded by a dense capillary network.

Figure 10-11 Supernumerary nipples.

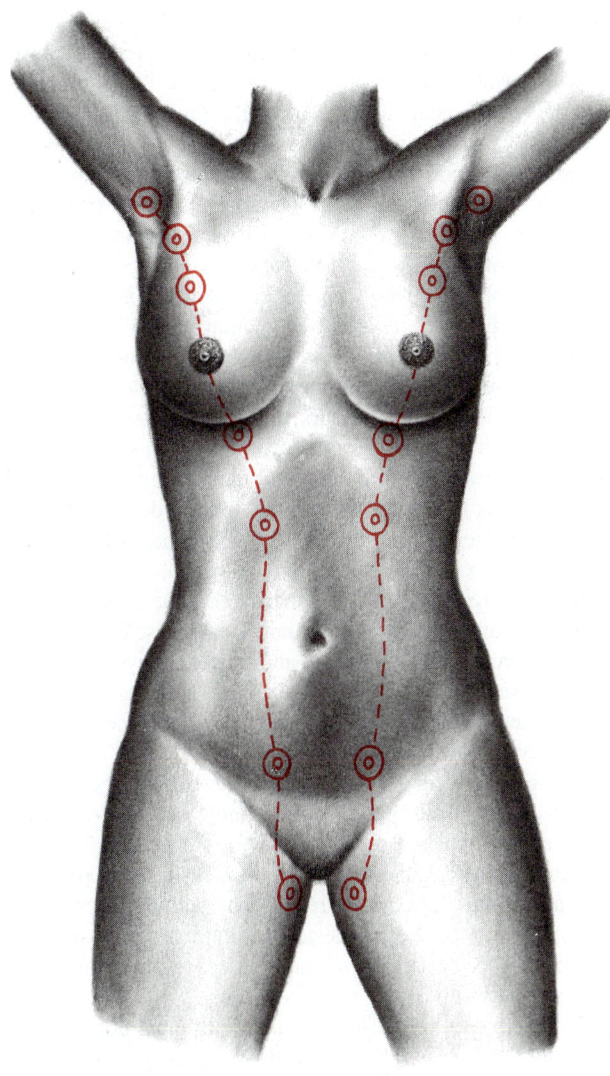

Secretory alveoli develop in pregnancy as a response to the rising estrogen and progesterone levels. Before puberty the breasts consist mostly of lactiferous ducts. Under the hormonal influence of puberty there are branching and growth of the duct system, as well as extensive distribution of fat. Small masses of cells are formed at the ends of the ducts that are the potential alveoli. During the first trimester of pregnancy a proliferation of the ducts creates a maximum number of epithelial structures for future alveolus formation. In the second trimester the ducts group together to form large lobules, and as the lumens dilate, the alveoli are formed and lined with cuboidal epithelium. In the third trimester the existing alveoli dilate in preparation for lactation. As glandular and duct tissue proliferates during pregnancy, the adipose tissue appears to diminish.[28,63]

Toward the end of pregnancy and until lactation begins 1 to 3 days after childbirth, the mammary glands form colostrum. It is produced at a much lower rate than milk and contains protein and lactose in amounts similar to milk but almost no fat.

Initiation and maintenance of lactation are achieved through a complex neuroendocrine process involving sensory nerves in the nipple and breast tissue, the spinal cord and hypothalamus, and the pituitary gland.

Ovarian Cycle and Hormones

The purpose of the ovarian cycle is to provide an ovum for fertilization, whereas the purpose of the endometrial cycle is to furnish a suitable site for the fertilized ovum to implant and develop.

Follicle development. Female primordial germ cells are derived from the germinal epithelium in the embryo. By mitotic division these form primitive ova, or oogonia, until the fifth or sixth month of gestation. Between the second month of gestation and the sixth month of life, some oogonia become primary oocytes through the prophase of meiosis. At birth some 2 million oocytes are in the ovary, decreasing through attrition to about 300,000 by the onset of puberty.

The first stage of follicle development occurs slowly during the childbearing years. The cells of the follicle divide, creating several layers of granulosa cells around the oocyte. Mucopolysaccharides secreted from the granulosa cells form a protective halo or zona pellucida around the oocyte (Figure 10-12). The primary oocyte, the surrounding layers of granulosa cells, and the outer basal lamina membrane make up the primary follicle.

The second stage of development occurs more rapidly, requiring 2 to 4 weeks for completion. During an ovarian cycle, approximately six to 12 primary follicles undergo growth and development but only one reaches maturity and ovulates. All others degenerate and become atretic follicles.

Figure 10-12 Oogenesis. Chromosome content of germ cell is shown at each stage, including sex chromosome shown after comma.

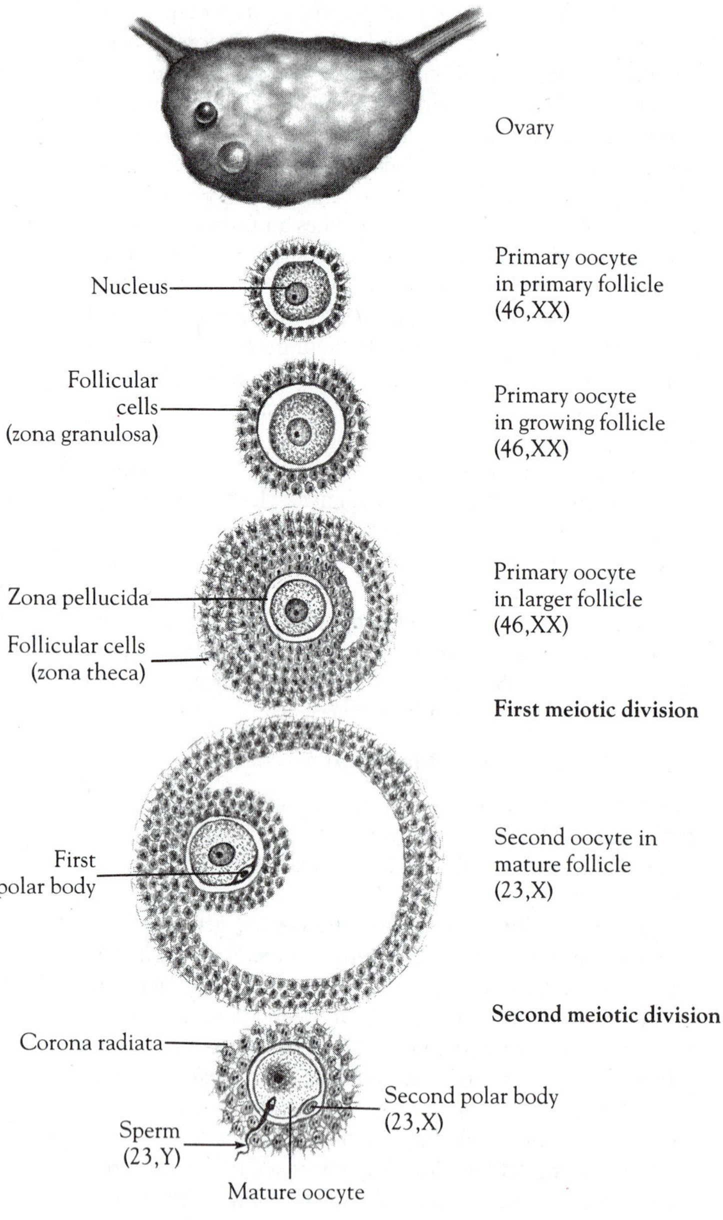

The proliferating granulosa cells are separated into two parts. The cavity or antrum is filled with follicular fluid that presses the oocyte to one side. Several cells known as the cumulus oophorus surround the oocyte, forming a stalk that projects into the antrum. The follicle distends with fluid and moves outward to the surface of the ovary. The theca cells surrounding the antrum proliferate, and those nearest the basal lamina are transformed into cuboidal steroid-secreting cells called the theca interna. Spinal cells from the stroma form around this, comprising the theca externa. At this point in development the entire complex is known as the graafian follicle.

The third and last stage of follicular development is complete within 48 hours. Before ovulation a single graafian follicle becomes dominant, and as the follicle ruptures, the oocyte is released into the peritoneal cavity. Since the initial meiotic division is complete at this time, this is called the secondary oocyte. Fertilization of this oocyte in the fallopian tube causes completion of the second meiotic division, resulting in a haploid ovum.[5]

Ovulation. Ovulation is the actual discharge of the secondary oocyte from the graafian follicle. This usually occurs at the midpoint of both the ovarian and the menstrual cycle. The time from the first day of the menstrual period to ovulation is the follicular phase or preovulatory period. The postovulatory period is the luteal phase.

Some women experience mittelschmerz, a lower abdominal discomfort at the time of ovulation. This is believed to be caused by peritoneal irritation from blood or follicular fluid that has escaped from the ruptured follicle. Another response to ovulation is an increase in basal body temperature caused by the thermogenic action of progesterone. Changes in the cervical mucus near the time of ovulation include decreases in viscosity and opacity, an increase in clarity, and an increase in sodium chloride content, which is demonstrated by arborization or ferning when mucus is allowed to dry on a glass slide. The signs and symptoms of ovulation are important both for women who wish to conceive during a particular cycle and for those who desire to avoid conception.

Corpus luteum. A yellow glandular mass formed at the site of the ruptured follicle is called the corpus luteum. It secretes large amounts of progesterone and lesser amounts of estrogen. If fertilization occurs, the corpus luteum increases in size, remains enlarged for about 3 months until the placenta takes over secreting functions, and then degenerates. If fertilization does not occur, the corpus luteum degenerates and shrinks. The yellow or "luteal" tissue then changes to a white fibrous tissue known as the corpus albicans.

Estrogens. Estrogen is a generic term for substances capable of producing the typical changes of estrus. The common estrogens are estradiol, estrone, and estriol. They are secreted by the developing ovarian follicle and subsequently by the corpus luteum. Estrogens are secreted by the placenta during pregnancy.

Estrogens are responsible for the development of the female secondary sex characteristics, increased growth of the uterus at puberty, and repair of the endometrium after menstruation. They tend to increase uterine sensitivity to oxytocin and uterine motility. In this respect the actions of estrogens are opposite to those of progesterone. Estrogens also increase bone matrix formation and slightly increase sodium and water reabsorption by the renal tubules.

Progesterone. Progesterone is the principal hormone secreted by the corpus luteum. During pregnancy it is secreted by the placenta. Progesterone prepares the uterine endometrium for the reception and development of the fertilized ovum by converting a proliferative endometrium to the secretory stage. It also inhibits the contractility of smooth uterine muscle, which is the opposite action of estrogen. Progesterone is responsible for the development of acini and lobules in the breast during pregnancy and inhibits the action of prolactin. Removal of the placenta, a source of massive progesterone production, removes the inhibitory effect on prolactin, thereby permitting lactation. Progesterone is also called luteo or progestational hormone.

Androgens. Androgens are substances that produce masculine characteristics such as hair growth, lowering of the voice, muscularity, and, in the male, development of the genital system. The major androgen secreted by the female ovary is androstenedione, a biologically weak compound but one that can undergo peripheral conversion to testosterone. The adrenal gland also secretes androgens, androstenedione and dehydroepiandrosterone (dehydroisoandrosterone). Dihydrotesterone is formed in peripheral tissue by the action of an enzyme on testosterone. In addition, testosterone, which is secreted by the embryonic testicular cells of Leydig, is required in the male fetus for the differentiation of the genital tubercle, swellings, folds, and urogenital sinus into the penis, scrotum, penile urethra, and prostate. Testosterone stimulates fetal differentiation of the wolffian ducts into the epididymis, vas deferens, and seminal vesicles.

Pituitary gonadotropic hormones. The basophils of the anterior pituitary gland secrete follicle-stimulating hormone (FSH) and luteinizing hormone (LH). The acidophils secrete prolactin, which is also called lactogenic or luteotropic hormone (LTH).

FSH stimulates ovarian follicle growth and maturation. The FSH level rises slightly before both ovulation and menstruation. This hormone is essential to the production of estrogen by the ovary. After menopause the level of FSH in the plasma and the amount excreted in the urine are increased.

LH induces ovulation and stimulates formation of the corpus luteum and progesterone secretion.

Prolactin serves as a luteotropic hormone in helping to maintain the corpus luteum. This hormone stimulates the mammary glands to develop secretory alveoli and secrete milk.

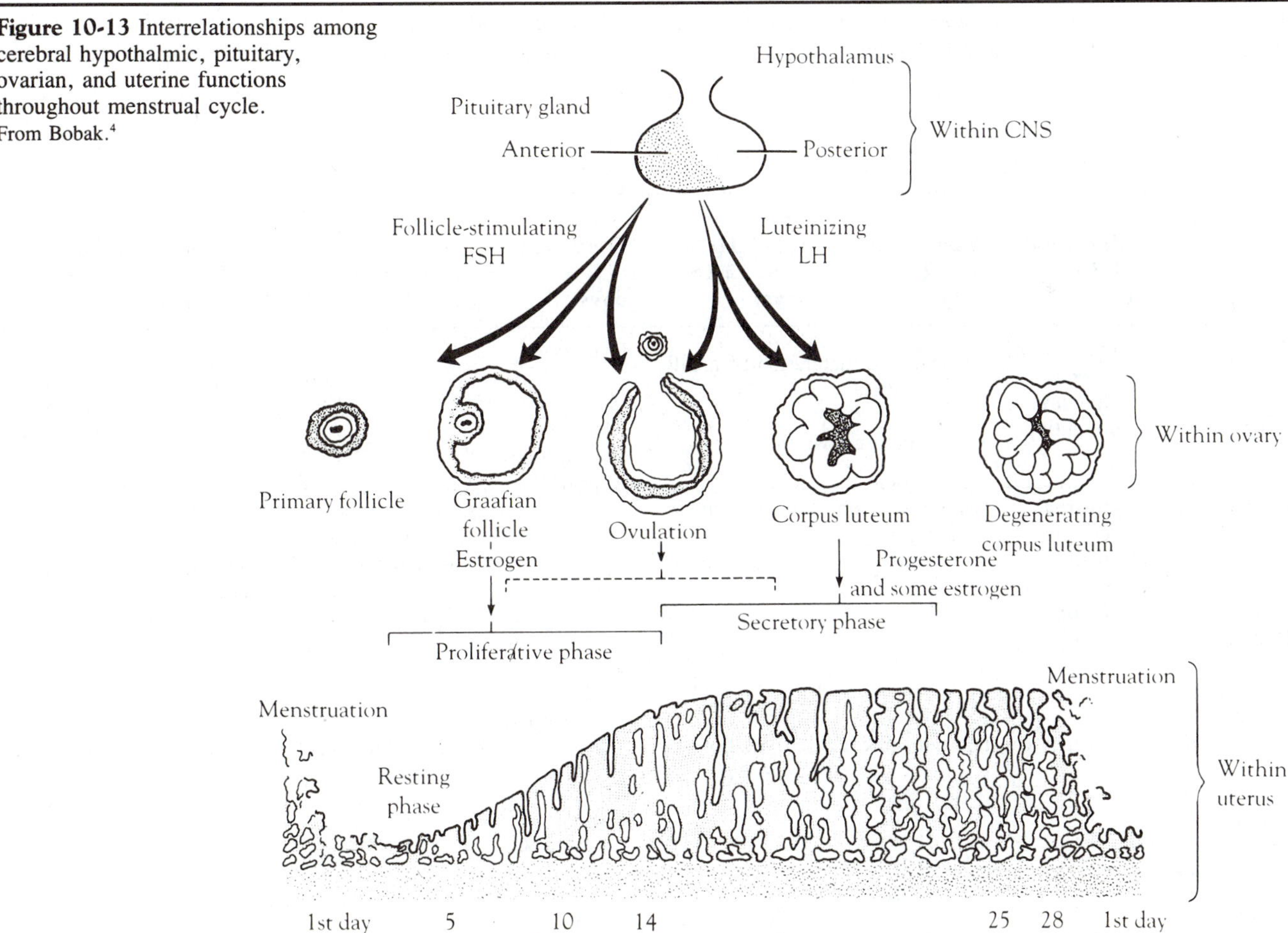

Figure 10-13 Interrelationships among cerebral hypothalmic, pituitary, ovarian, and uterine functions throughout menstrual cycle.
From Bobak.[4]

Menstrual Cycle (Figure 10-13 and Table 10-1)

The menstrual cycle begins at puberty and continues until menopause some 40 years later. The day of onset of menstrual flow is considered to be the first day of the cycle. The cycle ends on the last day before the next onset of menstruation. The cycle can vary from 22 to 35 days but is generally 28 days.

The proliferative or follicular phase begins about the fifth day of the cycle and extends through ovulation. It is also known as the postmenstrual or estrogenic phase. During this phase the uterine endothelium thickens as estrogen secretion rises.

The secreting phase occurs after ovulation. It is also called the postovulatory, luteal, or progestational phase. During this phase the three endometrial zones become well defined. The basal zone is adjacent to the myometrium; the compact zone lies immediately below the endometrial surface; and the spongy zone lies between the compact and basal layers. The endometrium becomes extremely vascular and rich in glycogen, an ideal environment for implantation of the fertilized ovum. The uterine spiral arteries become more coiled and tortuous during this period, growing almost to the surface of the endometrium. If implantation of a fertilized ovum does not occur, the corpus luteum loses functional activity and degenerates. If fertilization and implantation occur, the secretion of human chorionic gonadotropin by the placenta maintains the corpus luteum. This promotes the continued secretion of progesterone and estrogen and prevents menstruation.

The premenstrual phase occurs 2 to 3 days before menstruation with infiltration of the stroma by polymorphonuclear or mononuclear leukocytes. The reticular framework of the stroma in the superficial zone disintegrates, resulting in a loss of tissue fluid and thinning of the endometrium. Some 4 to 24 hours before the onset of menstruation, a vasoconstriction of the arterioles and coiled arteries causes anoxia and shriveling of the compact and spongy zones. After a period of constriction the coiled arteries relax and bleeding occurs from them or their branches. This marks the onset of menstruation.

The menstrual phase lasts from the first to about the fifth day of the cycle. As the coiled arteries rupture, hematomas form that distend and eventually rupture the superficial endometrium. Fissures develop in adjacent layers and tissues, become fragmented, and detach. The entire functional layer of the endometrium is eventually sloughed, leaving only the deep basal layer intact. Bleeding stops when the coiled arteries return to a state of constriction.

Physiologic Female Sexual Response

Vasocongestion and myotonia are responsible for the phenomena observed during the cycle of sexual response. Va-

Table 10-1
Correlation of Ovarian and Endometrial Cycles (Ideal 28-Day Cycle)

	Menstrual (1-3 to 5 days)	Early Follicular (4 to 6-8 days)	Advanced Follicular (9 to 12-16 days)	Ovulation (12-16 days)	Early Luteal (15-19 days)	Advanced Luteal (20-25 days)	Premenstrual (26-32 days)
Ovary	Involution of corpus luteum	Growth and maturation of graafian follicle		Ovulation	Active corpus luteum		Involution of corpus luteum
Estrogen	Diminution	Progressive increase		High concentration	Secondary rise		Decreasing
Progesterone	Absent			Appearing	Rising		Decreasing
Endometrium	Menstrual desquamation and involution	Reorganization and proliferation	Further growth and watery secretion		Active secretion and glandular dilation	Accumulation of secretion and edema	Regressive
Pituitary secretion							
Follicle-stimulating hormone (FSH)	Fairly constant until just before ovulation			Moderate increase just before	Rapid decrease in previous levels		
Luteinizing hormone (LH)	Same as above			Marked increase just before	Same as above		

From Pritchard.[49]

socongestion is a congestion primarily of venous blood vessels and is the major response to sexual stimulation. Myotonia is a secondary response to stimulation characterized by an increase in muscular tension.

In their classic work published in 1966 Masters and Johnson[35] described the female sexual response cycle as divided into four physiologic phases: excitement, plateau, orgasm, and resolution.

The excitement phase develops as a response to physical or psychic stimuli. The physiologic characteristics include clitoral tumescence, elongation, and widening; vaginal lubrication and expansion; partial uterine elevation; thickening of the labia majora in a multiparous woman; elevation and flattening of the labia majora in a nulliparous woman; erection of the nipples; engorgement of the areolae of the breasts; enlargement of the breasts; spreading of a maculopapular rash or "sex flush" over the epigastric area and breast; and increase in cardiac rate and blood pressure.

The plateau phase occurs if stimulation is maintained. During this period the clitoris retracts and vasocongestion in the labia major and the outer third of the vagina causes an increase in their size. This is referred to as the orgasmic platform. With elevation of the uterus, the cervix produces a tenting effect. The labia minora changes from bright red to wine color, a phenomenon known as "sex skin" that indicates an impending orgasm. A "sex flush" may cover the entire body. There are voluntary and involuntary contractions of the facial, abdominal, and intercostal muscles. Hyperventilation and transient tachycardia and hypertension occur during this phase.

The orgasm phase is characterized by an involuntary release of sexual tension. The primary response occurs in the orgasmic platform with contraction of the perineal, pubococcygeal, and bulbospongiosus muscles. Uterine contractions begin at the fundus and progress to the lower uterine segment. The intensity of the orgasmic experience is paralleled by the sex flush and by excursions of the contracting uterus. Respiratory rate, pulse rate, and blood pressure increase during this phase.

The resolution phase generally parallels the excitement phase in length. The uterus descends, the clitoris descends, and the vagina, labia majora, and labia minora return to their normal sizes. Normal coloring returns to the vaginal wall and the labia minora. The cervical os remains open for 20 to 30 minutes after orgasm. The nipples lose their erection, breast size decreases, and the sex flush disappears. Respiratory and pulse rates and blood pressure return to normal levels. Pelvic vasocongestion and myotonia decrease and eventually disappear.

Parallels between sexual response, birth, and breast feeding were described by Niles Newton in 1973. Labor has been compared with the excitement phase of sexual response and orgasm with birth. In addition, a close resemblance between the emotions experienced during breast feeding and sexual arousal has been described. Birth, breast feeding, and sexual response are all based on neurohormonal reflexes,[5] are sensitive to environmental stimuli,[6] and appear to elicit caretaking behaviors.[46]

Normal Findings

Area of Concern	Normal Adult Findings
External Genitalia	
Surface characteristics	Homogeneous
Hair distribution	Variable in adults; usually inverse triangle with base over pubis; some hair may extend up midline toward umbilicus *Older adult:* Pubic hair thinned, perhaps sparse, often gray
Inguinal and mons pubis skin surface	Smooth; clear
Labia and vestibule	
Labia majora, outer surface	Darker pigmentation; shriveled or full; gaping or closed; usually symmetric; skin surface smooth; may appear dry or moist *Older adult:* Labial folds flattened or may disappear into surrounding skin; decrease in subcutaneous fat in folds that usually corresponds to degree of loss of subcutaneous fat elsewhere on body; skin appears smooth, often shiny, and paler than in younger adult
Labia majora, inner surface	Dark pink pigmentation; moist; usually symmetric *Older adult:* Shiny; usually dry; paler than in young adult; fewer folds
Labia minora	Dark pink pigmentation; moist; usually symmetric
Vestibule surface	Dark pink pigmentation; moist; usually symmetric
Palpation of labia and vestibule	Soft, homogeneous consistency; nontender
Clitoris	
Size	2 cm length visible; 0.5 cm diameter *Older adult:* Slightly smaller than in younger adult

Area of Concern	Normal Adult Findings
Surface	Medial aspect covered by prepuce *Older adult:* Medial aspect covered by prepuce; pink
Urethral meatus and surrounding tissue surface	Irregular opening or slit; may be close to or slightly within vaginal introitus; usually located midline *Older adult:* Relaxed perineal musculature may result in meatus being situated more posteriorly; very near or within vaginal introitus
Milking of urethral duct	Nontender; no discharge
Vaginal introitus and surrounding tissue	
Surface	Thin vertical slit or large orifice with irregular edges (hymenal caruncles); moist tissue *Older adult:* May be smaller than in younger adult; multiparous client may manifest gaping introitus with vaginal walls rolling toward opening
Palpation of lateral and posterior introitus	Nontender; no discharge *Older adult:* Opening may be very narrow and admit only one finger
Vaginal tone	Nullipara: squeezes tightly around examiner's index and middle fingers; unipara or multipara: squeezes firmly but with less tone than nullipara; no bulging or urinary incontinence when bearing down or pushing *Older adult:* May be relaxed; client has difficulty squeezing examiner's finger with voluntary vaginal constriction; vaginal wall may roll slightly outward; no incontinence
Perineum	
Surface	Smooth; midline or mediolateral episiotomy scar may be visible *Older adult:* Smooth; midline or mediolateral episiotomy scar may be visible
Palpation between index finger and thumb	Nontender; nullipara: thick, smooth; unipara or multipara: thin, rigid, scarring *Older adult:* Thin; rigid
Anal surface	Increased pigmentation and coarse skin
Internal Genitalia	
Cervix	
Color	Pink color evenly distributed; bluish in pregnancy; symmetric, circumscribed erythema surrounding os may indicate normal condition of exposed columnar epithelium, but inexperienced examiners should consider any reddened appearance a problem for consultation *Older adult:* Paler than in younger woman; color evenly distributed
Position	Midline; cervix and os may be pointed in anterior or posterior direction; may project into vaginal tube 1 to 3 cm (resulting in 1 to 3 cm fornices surrounding cervix) *Older adult:* Cervix protrudes less into vaginal tube; may be flush against back of vaginal wall; surrounding fornices diminish or may disappear
Size	Usually 2.5 cm diameter *Older adult:* Cervix decreases in size with age
Surface	Smooth; firm; occasional visible squamocolumnar junction (symmetric reddened circle around os); nabothian cysts (smooth, round, small, yellowish raised areas) *Older adult:* Smooth; may appear paler than in younger woman; occasional visible squamocolumnar junction (symmetric reddened circle around os)
Contour	Evenly rounded or slightly ovoid *Older adult:* Nabothian cysts (smooth, round, yellowish, raised areas) common
Os	Nullipara: small, evenly round; unipara or multipara: slitlike, may be star shaped or irregular *Older adult:* Often very narrow or stenosed; may be obliterated
Cervical discharge	Mucus plug may be present at os; odorless; creamy or clear; thin, thick, or stringy; discharge often heavier at midcycle or immediately before menstruation *Older adult:* Often scanty; if present, should be clear or slightly opaque and odorless
Vagina	
Length	10 to 15 cm
Color	Pink *Older adult:* Shortens with aging Paler than in younger women
Surface	Transverse rugae (diminish after vaginal deliveries); moist; smooth *Older adult:* Less moisture; smooth (rugae diminish with aging); shiny
Consistency	Smooth; homogeneous
Secretions	Minimum to moderate amount; thin; clear or cloudy; odorless *Older adult:* May be absent or sparse; if present, should be clear or slightly opaque
Fornices	Pliable; smooth *Older adult:* Diminish and may disappear with aging; if palpable, should be pliable, smooth, and nontender

Area of Concern	Normal Adult Findings
Uterus	Mobile; nontender *Older adult:* Diminishes greatly; often not palpable
Position	Fundus anteverted; palpable at level of pubis *Older adult:* If palpated with internal hand, body of uterus should be smooth, firm, freely movable, and nontender
Contour of fundus	Rounded
Uterine wall	Firm consistency; smooth surface; pear shaped; 5.5 to 8 cm long
Ovaries	May not be palpable; slightly tender on palpation; firm; smooth; ovoid; mobile; diameter about 4 cm (size of walnut) *Older adult:* Atrophy with age and rarely palpable in aged women; fallopian tube palpable
Breasts	
Size	Varies *Older adult:* Increase in adipose tissue
Symmetry	Bilaterally equal; slight asymmetry; breasts hang equally when woman is seated and leaning forward; breasts appear symmetric when woman is seated and pushing hands into hips or pushing palms together
Contour	Smooth; convex; even
Skin color	Even throughout
Skin texture	Smooth; elastic; movable; striae
Venous patterns	Bilaterally similar

Pertinent Background Information

An additional consideration in assessment of the female organ system is a review of pertinent background information, including the following:

- Concurrent diseases or conditions
  - Menstruation
    - Age at onset
    - Length of cycles (duration)
    - Interval between cycles
    - Regularity of cycles
    - Amount and type of flow
      - Number of tampons or napkins used
      - Date of most recent douching
      - Type of contraceptive used
    - Date of last menstrual period (LMP)
    - Associated symptoms (such as dysmenorrhea, menorrhagia, or metrorrhagia)
    - Premenstrual syndrome (PMS)
  - Pregnancy
    - Number of pregnancies and outcome of each
    - Complications of pregnancy and delivery or abortion
  - Menopause
    - When occurred
    - Related symptoms
      - Hot flashes
      - Dry vaginal mucosa
  - Gastrointestinal (GI) system
    - Constipation
    - Hemorrhoids
  - Endocrine system
    - Hypothyroidism
    - Hyperthyroidism
    - Stein-Leventhal syndrome
    - Blood dyscrasias
    - Hypertension
- Previous surgery or illness
  - Gynecologic surgery
  - Other major surgery or illness (e.g., of abdomen or endocrine system)
- Family history
  - Cancer
  - Sickle cell disease
  - Thyroid disorder
  - Diabetes
  - Other diseases
  - Death from gynecologic-related condition
  - Maternal diethylstilbestrol (DES) usage
- Social history
  - Smoking
  - Sexual activity
    - Abnormal lesions or discharge in sexual partner
  - Contraception
- Medication history
  - Oral contraceptives
  - Estrogen therapy
  - Intrauterine contraceptive device (IUD)
  - Phenothiazines
  - Digitalis
  - Diuretics

Data from Brunham,[10] Thompson,[56] and Tucker.[58]

Area of Concern	Normal Adult Findings
Moles, nevi	Long history of presence; nonchanging; nontender
Areolae	
Size	Bilaterally equal
Shape	Round or oval
Surface characteristics	Smooth; bilaterally similar; Montgomery tubules
Nipples	
Direction	Bilaterally equal in pointing direction
Size and shape	Bilaterally equal; long-standing inversion (unilateral or bilateral)
Color	Homogeneous
Surface characteristics	Smooth or may be slightly wrinkled; skin intact
Discharge	Absent
Suspensory ligaments	Equal bilateral pull when woman is seated with arms abducted over head *Older adult:* Relaxed; breasts may appear elongated or pendulous
Palpation of breasts	
Tone	Bilaterally firm and equal; sagging of breast tissue may occur with aging or poor bra support
Tissue qualities	Smooth diffuse tissue bilaterally; nodular, bilateral granular consistency; premenstrual engorgement; elastic; nontender; firm mammary ridge along each breast at approximately 4 to 8 o'clock position *Older adult:* Decrease in grandular tissue
Lymph nodes (including supraclavicular, infraclavicular, central and lateral axillary, pectoral, subscapular, scapular, brachial, intermediate, and internal mammary chains)	Nonpalpable

Normal Laboratory Data

Laboratory Test	Normal Adult Values
Blood	
Clotting time (Lee-White)	8-15 min
Factor II	83%-117% of normal; term pregnancy 92%
Factor V	50%-150% of normal; term pregnancy 108%
Factor VII	50%-150% of normal; term pregnancy 170%
Factor VIII	50%-150% of normal; term pregnancy 196%
Factor IX	50%-150% of normal; term pregnancy 130%
Factor X	50%-150% of normal; term pregnancy 130%
Factor XI	50%-150% of normal; term pregnancy 69%
Factor XIII	Clot stable in 5M urea for at least 24 hr; if factor XIII deficiency is present, clot usually dissolves in 1-2 hr
Fibrinogen	200-400 mg/dl (quantitative); in pregnancy and early puerperium, 300-600 mg/dl
Partial thromboplastin time	25-39 sec (usually stated to be within 10 sec of control); slightly shortened in pregnancy
Prothrombin time	10-13 sec or 60%-100% of control; slightly shortened in pregnancy
Thrombin time	Less than 1½ times control value; term pregnancy 8 sec
Erythrocyte sedimentation rate	Westergren method Females Less than 50 yr 0-25 mm/hr Over 50 yr 0-30 mm/hr
Zeta sedimentation rate	Less than 50 yr 55% 50-80 year 40%-60%
Leukocytes	Females 3.9-5.9 $10^6/mm^3$; pregnancy 10,000-15,000/mm^3; may increase to as much as 25,000/mm^3 in labor and early puerperium

Laboratory Test	Normal Adult Values
Red blood cell (RBC) volume	1355 cells/mm^3 in nonpregnant state; 1790 cells/mm^3 in late pregnancy
α_1-Fetoprotein	Up to approximately 40 ng/ml for serum (interlaboratory differences exist); maternal serum increases to maximum of 500 ng/ml at wk 32, and ranges are stratified by weeks of gestation; normal ranges are available for amniotic fluid by wk
Androstenedione	Less than 250 ng/ml
Bilirubin	Total, 0.3-1 mg/dl; direct, up to 0.4 mg/dl; indirect, 0.1-0.8 mg/dl
Chorionic gonadotropin	3 IU/ml (nonpregnant); 60-70 IU/ml (late pregnancy); 50,000 mIU/ml about 65 days after implantation
Chorionic somatomammotropin	Varies with duration of gestation; may reach 10 μg/ml
Creatine	0.2-0.8 mg/dl; increased in pregnancy
Dihydrotestosterone	None detectable
Estradiol	Menstruating female Early cycle 20-170 pg/ml Midcycle 70-500 pg/ml Late cycle 45-340 pg/ml Patient taking oral contraceptives 12-50 pg/ml Postmenopausal female 1-5 ng/dl Adult male 13-42 pg/ml
Estriol	Nonpregnant female less than 0.5 ng/ml; pregnant female—estriol increases until term and then decreases: 30-32 wk 2-12 ng/ml 33-35 wk 3-19 ng/ml 36-38 wk 5-27 ng/ml 39-40 wk 10-30 ng/ml
Estrogens, total	Menstruating female 15-80 μg/24 hr Postmenopausal female Less than 20 μg/24 hr
Estrone	Menstruating female Early in cycle 50-300 pg/ml Midcycle 100-600 pg/ml Late cycle 80-450 pg/ml Menopausal female 0-30 pg/ml
Follicle-stimulating hormone (normal ranges vary among laboratories)	Menstrual female Before or after ovulation less than 20 IU/L Midcycle less than 40 IU/L Menopausal female 40-160 IU/L
17-Hydroxyprogesterone	Adult female Early cycle 100 ng/dl Late cycle 80-300 ng/dl
Luteinizing hormone	Midcycle 6-30 mIU/ml Follicular phase 2-30 mIU/ml Ovulatory peak 40-200 mIU/ml Luteal phase 0-20 mIU/ml Menopause 35-120 mIU/ml
Magnesium	1.2-1.9 mEq/L
Progesterone	Follicular phase 95 ng/dl Luteal phase 1130 ng/dl End of cycle less than 1 ng/ml Wk 20 of pregnancy up to 50 ng/ml
Prolactin	Normal range varies with laboratory
Testosterone	Female 20-100 ng/dl
T_3, triiodothyronine (total circulating)	Approximately 80 to 200-230 ng/dl with some variation among laboratories; increase during pregnancy
T_4, thyroxine (radioimmunoassay)	Cord T_4 and neonatal values much higher, falling over first months and years 10 yr and up approximately 5.8-11 μg/dl, varying somewhat among laboratories
Thyroid-binding globulin	10-26 μg/dl
Transferrin	Approximately 200-360 mg/dl with some variation among laboratories
Urea nitrogen (BUN)	1-40 yr 5-20 mg/dl; gradual slight increase thereafter
Uric acid	Adult female 2.4-6 mg/dl or slightly more
Urine	
Chorionic gonadotropin	Negative; positive in pregnancy
Creatinine	Adult female 0.8-1.8 g/24 hr; creatinine excretion decreases with advanced age as muscle mass diminishes
Estriol	Starting at wk 30, minimum of 9 mg/24 hr
Dehydroepiandosterone	Normal ranges usualy provided by laboratories doing such fractionation; ranges often stratified by age and sex
Estrogens	Menstruating female 15-80 μg/24 hr Postmenopausal female less than 20 μg/24 hr
Follicle-stimulating hormone	Follicular phase 5-20 IU/24 hr Luteal phase 5-15 IU/24 hr Midcycle 15-60 IU/24 hr Menopause 50-100 IU/24 hr
Luteinizing hormone	Follicular phase 2-25 IU/24 hr Ovulatory phase 30-95 IU/24 hr Luteal phase 2-20 IU/24 hr Postmenopausal 40-110 IU/24 hr
Pregnanediol	Proliferative phase 0.5-1.5 mg/24 hr Luteal phase 2-7 mg/24 hr Menopause 0.2-1 mg/24 hr 10-12 wk pregnant 5-15 mg/24 hr 12-18 wk pregnant 5-15 mg/24 hr 18-24 wk pregnant 15-33 mg/24 hr 24-28 wk pregnant 20-42 mg/24 hr 28-32 wk pregnant 27-47 mg/24 hr

Conditions, Diseases, and Disorders

UTERINE AND OVARIAN DISORDERS

Pelvic inflammatory disease

Pelvic inflammatory disease (PID) is an infectious process that may involve the fallopian tubes, ovaries, pelvic peritoneum, veins, or pelvic connective tissue.

The incidence of PID is difficult to estimate, since it is not a reportable disease and is not identified in a consistent manner. It is not always treated, especially when symptoms are mild. It most often occurs in sexually active women under 25 years of age and is the result of infection transmitted through sexual intercourse, use of an intrauterine contraceptive device (IUD)[2] or, less commonly, through childbirth or abortion. It has been directly or indirectly linked to approximately one fifth of all gynecologic problems. Specific risk factors include teenager (10 to 19), multiple sex partners, IUD, single marital status, contact with sperm, previous diagnosis of PID, and sexual contact with urethritis or gonorrhea.[55]

PID may be confined to one structure or involve the entire pelvis. Infections may be acute, subacute, recurrent, or chronic. PID in the fallopian tubes (the most common site) is referred to as salpingitis.

Pathophysiology

PID begins in the vulva or accessory glands and spreads upward through the entire genital tract. The principal pathogen is *Neisseria gonorrhoeae,* but gram-negative bacilli, gram-positive cocci, *Mycoplasma,* and viruses are also implicated as causative agents. Salpingitis resulting from tuberculosis has become rare. If PID follows childbirth or an abortion, anaerobic streptococci, staphylococci, coliform bacteria, or *Clostridium perfringens* is usually involved. Infections can also be caused by *Chlamydia trachomatis,* actinomycosis, schistosomiasis, leprosy, oxyurias, sarcoidosis, and foreign bodies (such as radiographic contrast media).

Gonococcal disease is characterized by an acute suppurative reaction with subsequent copious discharge of yellow pus. Hyperemia, edema, and tenseness occur in the involved structures, which are often bilaterally involved. The organisms spread over the mucosal surfaces, eventually involving the tubes and tubo-ovarian region. In an adult the vagina is resistant to the inflammation, but vulvovaginitis may develop in a child because of the more delicate mucosa. The nongonococcal infections spread upward through the lymphatics or venous channels rather than on the surface of the mucosa. As the lumen of the fallopian tube fills with purulent exudate, some leaks out of the fimbriae. Over the course of days or weeks the fimbriae may seal or become adherent to the ovary, causing salpingo-oophoritis. The collection of pus in the sealed tube causes distention of the tube and is referred to as pyosalpinx. In this form the infection may persist for months. The demise of the organisms and sterilization of the infection occur eventually owing to progressive anaerobiasis and increasing acidity. The pus then undergoes a slow proteolysis, and the exudate is transformed to a thin serous fluid in a condition known as hydrosalpinx.

Tubo-ovarian abscesses can occur when exudate collects where the tube is sealed against the ovary. This inflammatory process affects the most superficial layers of the ovary but spares the underlying ovarian tissue. Peritonitis resulting from spread of the exudate to the pelvic peritoneum is common. Infertility caused by mucosal destruction and tubal occlusion is a common sequel of salpingitis.[10,55]

In addition PID is implicated as the cause in as many as 50% of ectopic pregnancies, which are estimated to occur in one of every 20 pregnancies.[55]

Diagnostic Studies and Findings

Culture of Purulent Secretions

Identification of organism and sensitivity to antibiotics

White Blood Cell Count

Elevated

Erythrocyte Sedimentation Rate

Elevated

Laparoscopic Examination

Visualization of pelvic inflammation
Mild: erythema, edema, no obvious purulent exudate, tubes freely movable
Moderate: gross, purulent material evident; marked erythema and edema; tubes not always freely movable
Severe: pyosalpinx, severe inflammation, abscess[55]

Gram Stain of Secretions

Identification of gram-positive or gram-negative organisms

Ultrasonography

Visualization of abscess or inflammation

Needle Culdocentesis

White blood cells or nonclotting blood
Purulent material

Medical Plan

Surgery

Hysterectomy with bilateral salpingo-oophorectomy—may be required for patients with abscesses, hydrosalpinx, and tubal obstruction if antibiotic therapy is unsuccessful

Laparotomy with incision and drainage of abscesses and lysis of adhesions

Medications

Anti-infective agents

For *Neisseria gonorrhoeae*

Aqueous procaine penicillin, 2.4 million U IM in two separate sites, and probenecid (Benemid) 1 g po, or

Cefoxitin (Mefoxin), 1-2 g IM or 2 g IV q6h followed by doxycycline (Vibramycin) 100 mg po bid for 10-14 d

Tetracycline (Achromycin, others), 1.5-2 g/d po for 7-10 d; for severely ill patients with acute pain who are hypersensitive to penicillin, 500 mg IV qid for first 24-48 h, then 500 mg po qid to complete 10 d of therapy; should not be given to pregnant patients and those with renal failure

Crystalline penicillin (for severely ill patients with acute pain), 10-40 million U IV over first 24 h; continue treatment for 36-72 h as indicated, follow IV therapy with ampicillin (Amcill), 500 mg po qid for at least 10 d

For gram-negative organisms

Kanamycin (Kantrex), 7.5 mg/kg/12 h IM, *or* streptomycin, 1 g/d IM; kanamycin or streptomycin should be added to initial penicillin therapy and continued until sensitivity of identified pathogens is determined[10,37]

For gram-positive organisms and *Bacteroides*

Clindamycin (Cleocin), 300 mg po qid until organisms are identified and sensitivity is determined

For anaerobic infections

Clindamycin (Cleocin) or gentamicin (Garamycin)

General Management

Bed rest in semi-Fowler's position

Heat applied to abdomen

Warm douches

Parenteral fluids

Nasogastric suctioning if ileus is present

Removal of intrauterine device (IUD)

NURSING CARE

Nursing Assessment

Subjective Data

Abdominal and pelvic pain; low back pain; dyspareunia; menstrual irregularity; urinary discomfort; constipation; malaise; nausea and vomiting; diarrhea; vaginal drainage

Abdomen

Rebound tenderness; normal bowel sounds progressing to ileus in untreated persons

Cervix

Pain with movement; copious purulent discharge

Vulva

Pruritus; maceration

Temperature

Elevated >100.4° F (38° C)

Nursing Dx & Intervention

Nursing Diagnosis	Nursing Intervention/Rationale
Pain	• Maintain complete bed rest; semi-Fowler's position may be most comfortable. • Increase activity as tolerated. • Explain cause of pain *to allay any undue anxiety.* • Instruct patient to request analgesic before pain becomes severe *to avoid inconsistent control of pain.*
Potential fluid volume deficit	• Explain need to increase fluid intake during infectious processes. • Encourage fluid intake of 3000 ml daily unless contraindicated. • Monitor intake and output. • Explain cause of vaginal discharge and pruritus if present.
Impaired skin integrity	• Assist and teach patient to perform perineal care every 3 to 4 hours or as needed *to maintain skin integrity.* • Blot skin dry; do not rub *to prevent excoriation.* • Prevent excessive warmth in room; light covers over bed cradle may be indicated.

Nursing Diagnosis	Nursing Intervention/Rationale
Knowledge deficit	• Explain importance of handwashing before and after contact with perineal area and of wiping from front to back after elimination *to prevent contamination of vaginal area with cross-contaminants from anal area.* • Explain need to use perineal pads, which should be changed frequently according to amount of vaginal drainage. Instruct patient not to use tampons. • Explain that a shower is preferable to a tub bath.
Sexual dysfunction	• Encourage patient to share concerns regarding sexual partner as probable source of infection *to promote health-seeking behaviors of partner.* • Explain rationale for removal of intrauterine device (IUD) if this is ordered by physician.

Patient Education

1. Explain the need to avoid using tampons, having intercourse, or douching for at least 1 week after antibiotic therapy.
2. Explain methods to prevent venereal disease if the condition is caused by gonorrhea or *Chlamydia.*
3. Explain the importance of encouraging the patient's sexual partner to be examined and treated.
4. Explain alternative methods of conception control if the condition is related to an IUD.
5. Describe symptoms of recurrence that the patient should report to a physician.

Evaluation

Patient Outcome	Data Indicating That Outcome is Reached
Comfort is achieved. Pain is gone.	Patient reports that lower abdominal, low back, pelvic, or perineal pain is gone.
Skin and mucous membrane color is good.	There is no vaginal drainage or pruritus, inflammation, or maceration of vulva.
Body temperature is normal.	There is no fever. Temperature is within normal limits. Intake and output are within normal limits.
Infection and inflammation are controlled.	Patient showers rather than taking tub baths. Patient verbalizes intent to prevent venereal disease if condition is caused by gonorrhea or chlamydia. Patient verbalizes intent to avoid douching, intercourse, or use of tampons for at least 1 week after completion of drug therapy. Patient wipes front to back after elimination. Patient verbalizes intent to have sexual partner examined. Patient takes medications at time and dosage prescribed by physician. Patient describes symptoms of PID and expresses intent to notify health care provider in timely manner if they recur.

Toxic shock syndrome

Toxic shock syndrome (TSS) is an acute bacterial infection generally caused by *Staphylococcus aureus* and most frequently associated with the use of tampons during menses.

National attention was not directed to TSS until the fall of 1980, when some 300 cases were reported to the Centers for Disease Control. These cases occurred from January to September in 285 women, among whom 25 deaths were reported. The overall incidence appears to be about 1 in 20,000 menstruating women. Toxic shock syndrome is most common in women who use high-absorbency tampons, but it has occurred in newborns, children, and men. The incidence in women dropped precipitously in 1981 after widespread publicity and withdrawal of some vaginal tampons from the market.[65]

TSS is now associated with a variety of surgical situations unrelated to menses. It has been diagnosed in patients with surgical wounds, tubal ligation, hysterectomy, laparotomy, mastectomy, bladder suspension, orchidectomy, uterolithotomy, hip osteoplasty, and knee surgery. It has also been associated with septal reconstruction in which nasal packing was used. TSS apparently can occur in situations in which staphylococcal infection can be harbored, including cellulitis, infected skin bites, burns, and hidradenitis.[21]

Pathophysiology

Almost all cases of TSS have been caused by pyrogenic exotoxin-producing strains of phage group I *Staphylococcus aureus*. The organism has been found in the nasopharynx, vagina, and trachea, as well as sequestered in empyema and abscess sites. It is thought that mechanical factors associated with use of high-absorbency tampons by a woman with a preexisting *S. aureus* colonization of the vagina increase the risk. As the outflow of menses is obstructed by the tampon, bacterial exotoxins are able to enter the bloodstream through a mucosal break or enter the peritoneal cavity via the uterus. Adult respiratory distress syndrome, which is manifested as pulmonary and peripheral edema despite low central venous pressure, may be a cardiopulmonary complication of toxic shock syndrome.[65]

In postsurgical cases, TSS symptoms appear within 48 hours. Exceptions occur when packing is used to control bleeding, such as in nasal surgeries, and with postpartum or dilation and curettage procedures. A common factor in all cases of TSS is a disruption of the normal skin or mucous membrane barrier, allowing a localized *S. aureus* infection to transmit toxins systemically.[21]

Diagnostic Studies and Findings

White Blood Cell Count

Increased

Blood Urea Nitrogen

Increased

Creatinine

Increased

Bilirubin

Increased

Serum Glutamic Oxaloacetic Transaminase (SGOT)

Increased

Serum Glutamic Pyruvic Transaminase (SGPT)

Increased

Creatinine Phosphokinase (CPK)

Increased

Platelets

Decreased

Medical Plan

Medications

- Anti-infective agents
  - β-Lactamase-resistant agents
    - Cefoxitin sodium (Mefoxin), 1-2 g IV or IM q6-8h
    - Cefazolin sodium (Ancef), 250 mg to 1 g q6-8h IM or IV
    - Cephalothin sodium (Keflin), 500 mg to 1 g q4-6h IV or deep IM
  - Penicillinase-resistant agents
    - Methicillin sodium (Staphcillin), 1-1.5 g IM q4-6h
    - Oxacillin sodium (Bactocill), 500 mg q4-6h for at least 5 d
    - Cloxacillin sodium (Cloxapen), 500-1000 mg q4-6h
  - Antistaphylococcal agents
    - Penicillin G (Bicillin), 600,000 U IM at various intervals
    - Dicloxacillin sodium (Dycill, others), 125 mg po q6h
    - Methicillin sodium (Staphcillin), 1-1.5 g IM q6h
- Corticosteroids
  - Hydrocortisone sodium succinate (Solu-Cortef), 50-300 mg/d IV or IM

General Management

Septic shock treatment if indicated

Fluid intake of 3000 ml daily unless contraindicated

NURSING CARE

Nursing Assessment

Subjective Data

Sudden onset of high fever (102° to 105° F [39° to 40.5° C]); myalgia; vomiting; profuse watery diarrhea; sore throat; headache; profound tiredness

Extremities

Edema; impaired perfusion

Palms and Soles

Erythematous rash (sunburnlike); desquamation and sloughing within 1 to 2 weeks

Level of Consciousness

Disorientation; intermittent confusion

Blood Pressure

Rapid hypotension (within 48 hours); orthostatic syncope

Renal System

Diminished urine output

Conjunctiva

Nonpurulent inflammation

Oropharynx

Hyperemia; edema

Vagina

Hyperemia

Nursing Dx & Intervention

Nursing Diagnosis	Nursing Intervention/Rationale
Altered renal, cerebral, cardiopulmonary, gastrointestinal, and peripheral tissue perfusion	• For complete list of nursing diagnoses and interventions, see care of patient in septic shock in Chapter 1 and adult respiratory distress syndrome in Chapter 2 if applicable.
Potential for injury	• Instruct patient to use sanitary napkins rather than tampons during menses. • Closely monitor patients with packing in a body cavity for early signs of toxic shock syndrome.

Patient Education

1. Instruct the patient to avoid using tampons until vaginal culture findings are negative and clearance from a physician is obtained.
2. Instruct the patient to wash hands thoroughly before inserting a tampon.
3. Instruct the patient not to use high-absorbency, noncotton tampons.
4. Instruct the patient to change tampons frequently during the day, to wear sanitary napkins at night, and to avoid prolonged use of a single tampon.
5. Instruct the patient not to use tampons if she has a concurrent skin infection, since there is a possibility of reinfection with *S. aureus*.
6. Instruct the patient to report signs of recurrence to a physician immediately.

Evaluation

Patient Outcome	Data Indicating That Outcome is Reached
Tissue perfusion is adequate.	There are no symptoms of shock.
Infection is gone.	Vaginal culture findings are negative for causative organism. Patient does not have fever; hyperemia of oropharynx, conjunctiva, or vagina; myalgia; vomiting; diarrhea; sore throat; headache; or malaise.
Patient education is effective.	Patient demonstrates understanding of reasons for health education and expresses intent to maintain behaviors and health practices that will prevent reinfection.

Dysfunctional uterine bleeding

Irregular or excessive bleeding from the uterus is one of the most common gynecologic symptoms.

Abnormalities and variation in uterine bleeding are the most frequently encountered health care problems for women. Patients often think that uterine bleeding is life threatening or indicative of a major problem in reproductive or sexual functioning. Abnormal bleeding, varying from spotting to the passage of clots, may occur at any age and for a variety of reasons.

Dysfunctional uterine bleeding (DUB), which is almost always anovulatory and painless (whereas dysmenorrhea is associated with ovulatory cycles), can occur at any age from puberty through menopause. It generally occurs at the extremes of menstrual life, when disturbances in ovarian function are common. About 50% of dysfunctional bleeding occurs in premenopausal women (age 40 to 50), about 20% during the adolescent years, and about 30% during the reproductive period.[37,41]

The following terms are often used to describe variations in uterine bleeding:

dysfunctional uterine bleeding (DUB) abdominal uterine bleeding not associated with tumor, inflammation, pregnancy, trauma, or hormonal effects.

hypomenorrhea deficient amount of menstrual flow.

menorrhagia (hypermenorrhea) increased amount (≥60 ml each period) or duration of menstrual bleeding.

metrorrhagia intermenstrual bleeding.

metrorrhea any pathologic uterine discharge.

oligomenorrhea infrequent menstruation.

polymenorrhea increased frequency of menstruation (not consistently associated with ovulation).

postmenopausal bleeding bleeding from the reproductive tract occurring 1 year or more after menopause.

spotting small amounts of bloody vaginal discharge ranging from pink to dark brown.

Pathophysiology

The preceding terms used to describe abnormal bleeding do not indicate the cause of the abnormality or reason for bleeding. The following are the most common types of bleeding and their causes:

- Midcycle spotting—midcycle estradiol fluctuation associated with ovulation
- Delayed menstruation with excessive bleeding—anovulation or threatened abortion
- Frequent bleeding—chronic pelvic inflammatory disease, endometriosis, DUB, or anovulation
- Profuse menstrual bleeding—endometrial polyps, adenomyosis, DUB, submucous leiomyomas, or presence of intrauterine contraceptive device
- Intermenstrual or irregular bleeding—endometrial polyps, DUB, uterine or cervical cancer, or oral contraceptive use
- Postmenopausal bleeding—endometrial hyperplasia, estrogen therapy, or endometrial cancer

Other causes of bleeding include foreign bodies, lacerations, and systemic diseases such as leukemia, hypothyroidism, and blood dyscrasias. In addition, precocious puberty may warrant consideration as a cause, as may vaginal adenosis in young women with prenatal exposure to the synthetic estrogen diethylstilbestrol (DES).

DUB is most common before and after the reproductive years and occurs as painless, irregular, heavy bleeding (menometrorrhagia), midcycle spotting, oligomenorrhea, or periods of amenorrhea. In most cases the cause is anovulation, but bleeding may reflect defects in the follicular or luteal phase of the ovulatory cycle.

With anovulation, the persistent unopposed estrogen stimulation may be endogenous from an ovarian tumor such as a granulosa cell tumor, polycystic ovaries (Stein-Leventhal syndrome), or abnormal metabolism of estrogen as in liver disease. Exogenous estrogen taken by the patient can also result in anovulation. Unopposed estrogen stimulation causes endometrial hyperplasia; when the estrogen can no longer maintain the endometrium, sloughing and vaginal bleeding occur.

Follicular phase defects result from premature maturation of the ovarian follicle owing to pituitary hyperstimulation. The cycle is less than 22 days. Increased levels of follicle-stimulating hormone (FSH) and slightly elevated estradiol levels result in a progressively shortened proliferative phase that can cause spotting in perimenopausal women. Oligomenorrhea most commonly occurs in young women and may result from a prolonged proliferative phase.

Luteal phase defects may result in profuse and prolonged bleeding caused by delayed involution of the corpus luteum. A corpus luteum cyst or persistent corpus luteum can cause a delay in menses, with premenstrual spotting.[15,63]

The endometrium of women with menorrhagia has been found to have higher levels of prostaglandin E_2 and prostaglandin F_2 when compared with women with normal menses. In addition prostaglandin E_2 is associated with vasodilatory effects that contribute to bleeding.[60]

Diagnostic Studies and Findings

Complete Blood Count

To determine the degree of anemia and to detect abnormal leukocyte production

Thyroid Function Tests

To assess thyroid function

Dilation and Curettage with Cervical or Endometrial Biopsy

To assess endometrium and identify carcinoma or polyps

Hysterography

To identify presence of endometrial polyps, submucous myomas, adenomyosis, endometrial carcinoma, and adnexal lesions

Hysteroscopy

To identify intrauterine abnormalities such as submucous fibroids, endometrial polyps, and foreign bodies

Endocrine Profile

To assess functioning of the adrenal glands, ovaries, and pituitary glands

Tests Confirming Ovulation

- Endometrial biopsy
  - To demonstrate secretory or menstrual endometrium
- Basal body temperatures
  - Biphasic pattern is indicative of ovulation
- Cytologic examination of consecutive vaginal smears
  - To show shift from estrogen- to progesterone-dominated smears
- Examination of cervical mucus
  - To determine presence of ferning
- Serum or urine progesterone levels
  - To assess progesterone metabolites consistent with progestational phase of menstrual cycle

Measurement of Blood Loss

Weigh pads and tampons

Medical Plan

The plan of medical care selected is contingent on the cause of the bleeding.

Surgery

- Total abdominal hysterectomy with partial or complete bilateral salpingo-oophorectomy (TAH/BSO) (see p. 1016)
- Dilation and curettage (see p. 1015)
- Excision of polyps

Endometrial ablation

Done with a hysteroscopic resectoscope by applying a cauterizing current to the endometrium in women who are not candidates for hysterectomy, such as those with major medical diseases, severe heart disease, bleeding diatheses, and major respiratory difficulty[17]

Medications

Progesterone or progestin

Medroxyprogesterone (Provera, others), 2.5-10 mg/d po or 100-400 mg/d IM (may be given if patient is anovulatory and infertility is not a concern)

Estrogens

Conjugated estrogens (Premarin), 0.625-3.75 mg/d followed by high doses of estrogen-progestin combinations (given for excessive anovulatory bleeding)

Clomiphene citrate can be used when excessive bleeding is caused by inadequate luteal phase or to anovulation

Prostaglandin inhibitors

Meclofenamate sodium 100 mg po tid

NURSING CARE

Nursing Assessment

Variations depend on the cause of the bleeding.

Bleeding

Heavy menstrual flow; bleeding between periods; infrequent menstruation; increased frequency of menstruation; spotting

Pain

Menstrual cramps or pain with menses; low abdominal pain at midcycle*; uterine cramps at midcycle*

Vaginal Secretions

Wet mucoid vaginal secretion at midcycle*

Other Complications

Altered sexual function; psychosocial concerns; anemia

*Signs and symptoms suggestive of ovulation.

Nursing Dx & Intervention

Nursing Diagnosis	Nursing Intervention/Rationale
Situational low self-esteem	• Assess meaning of dysfunction for patient *to explore self-concept issues.* • Encourage patient to express her feelings. • Consider nursing interventions associated with loss and grief if results of diagnostic studies confirm anovulatory cycles and infertility.
Pain	• Assist in and teach patient pain-relieving techniques *to promote self-sufficiency in managing pain.*
Sexual dysfunction related to change	• Explain importance of sharing concerns with sexual partner *to come to an understanding of preferences, concerns, and behavior related to DUB.*

Patient Education

1. Explain the importance of recording dates, type of flow, and number of pads or tampons used.
2. Explain the importance of ongoing care.

Evaluation

Patient Outcome	Data Indicating That Outcome is Reached
Patient demonstrates adaptive responses related to self-concept.	Patient asks appropriate questions. Patient keeps record of bleeding, including type and date. Patient shows signs of grief if she learns of undesired infertility.
Comfort is achieved; there is no pain.	Patient uses pain-relieving techniques or medication as ordered.
Sexual adjustment is made.	Patient indicates that she has discussed concerns with partner.

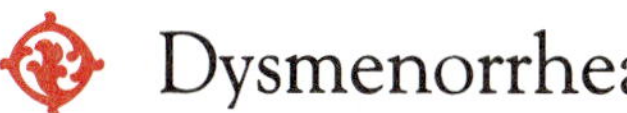

Dysmenorrhea

Dysmenorrhea is menstruation that is painful enough to limit normal activity or cause a woman to seek medical treatment.

Dysmenorrhea is a common gynecologic complaint. It occurs in approximately 10% of high school–age girls, keeping them home from school for 1 or 2 days, and it also affects many college students and young women in the work force. Dysmenorrhea is classified as primary or secondary. Primary dysmenorrhea is pain associated with menstruation during ovulatory cycles in the absence of organic disease. Secondary dysmenorrhea is due to a demonstrated disorder.

Pathophysiology

Primary dysmenorrhea usually develops 1 or 2 years after menarche, when ovulatory cycles are established. Increased amounts of prostaglandin are released from the endometrium under the influence of progesterone in the luteal phase of the cycle. Very little prostaglandin is produced during anovulatory cycles, which are almost never painful. Increased sensitivity of the myometrium and endometrium to prostaglandin F_2 can produce uterine contractions and ischemia, causing the cramping pain of dysmenorrhea.[15,41,63]

Secondary dysmenorrhea is associated with pelvic disorders such as endometriosis, adenomyosis, or chronic pelvic inflammatory disease. It may appear after years of normal menstruation, and it is characterized by cramping as large clots pass through the cervix.

Diagnostic Studies and Findings

Pelvic Examination

To rule out or confirm underlying disorders in secondary dysmenorrhea

Laparoscopy

To rule out or confirm underlying disorders in secondary dysmenorrhea

Dilation and Curettage

To rule out or confirm underlying disorders in secondary dysmenorrhea

Hysterosalpingography

To rule out or confirm underlying disorders in secondary dysmenorrhea

Medical Plan

Surgery

Total abdominal hysterectomy and bilateral salpingo-oophorectomy (TAH/BSO)—may be indicated for disorder associated with secondary dysmenorrhea

Presacral neurectomy (severance of nerve trunks in hypogastric plexus)—performed in rare cases when no underlying disorder can be found and there is no response to medications

Medications

Nonsteroidal anti-inflammatory agents
- Ibuprofen (Motrin), 400-600 mg po q4-6h as prostaglandin synthetase inhibitor

Analgesic/antipyretic agents
- Aspirin, 650 mg po q3-5h beginning 1-2 d before menses to control mild discomfort

Narcotic analgesics
- Meperidine (Demerol), 50-100 mg q4-6h prn
- Codeine phosphate and sulfate (Methylmorphine), 30-60 mg q4-6h prn (not for prolonged use)

Oral contraceptives—may be ordered for hormonal effect to relieve pain by suppressing ovulation

General Management

Adequate exercise

Balanced diet with increased consumption of fruits and vegetables

Adequate rest and sleep

Attention to personal hygiene

NURSING CARE

Nursing Assessment

Comfort

Colicky and cyclic pain, infrequently nagging and dull in low pelvis and often with radiation toward vulva, perineum, rectum, and down back of thighs; may be experienced 24 to 48 hours before menses or with start of menstruation; may be associated with symptoms of premenstrual tension, including nausea, vomiting, diarrhea, urinary frequency, chills, abdominal bloating, breast tenderness, irritability, or depression

Nursing Dx & Intervention

Nursing Diagnosis	Nursing Intervention/Rationale
Pain	• Identify and help patient use pain reduction methods, including relaxation techniques, heating pad, effleurage (abdominal massage), and orgasm (relieves cramps in some women). • Evaluate patient's use of pain control techniques and encourage use of those that reduce her pain.
Body image disturbance	• Encourage patient to express feelings about any self-perceptions, as well as how she believes she is viewed by others. • Explore patient's role and behaviors when dysmenorrhea is present *to identify effects on life-style.* • Evaluate support system and coping strategies *to determine their effects on body image.*

Patient Education

1. Instruct the patient about the prescribed dosage and frequency of doses of prostaglandin antagonists or other medications.

Evaluation

Patient Outcome	Data Indicating That Outcome is Reached
Comfort is achieved. Pain is gone.	Patient uses pain-relieving techniques or medications as ordered.

Endometriosis

Endometriosis is an abnormal growth of endometrial tissue outside the uterine cavity.

Endometriosis is a benign disease, but it has certain characteristics of a malignancy, including the ability to grow, infiltrate, and spread. The ectopic tissue is responsive to hormonal variations of the menstrual cycle and is subject to menstrual-like bleeding.

The incidence of endometriosis is unknown because it exists in many women without causing significant symptoms. Characteristic lesions are found in at least 20% of patients undergoing gynecologic surgery. Endometriosis is a significant finding in only about one third of these patients. Symptoms severe enough to require treatment generally occur between the ages of 25 and 35 years. Endometriosis is rare in women over 50 years of age. The greatest incidence of the disease seems to be in white women of higher socioeconomic levels, who tend to marry later and have fewer children. However, there is some question about the reliability of these impressions, since the greater demand for medical attention in this higher socioeconomic group may account for earlier and more frequent diagnosis of the condition. The fertility rate of patients with endometriosis is about 66%, compared with 88% for the general population. Endometriosis occurs in young women with congenital obstructions of the vagina or cervix that are associated with reflux menstruation.

Endometriosis is associated with infertility, pregnancy wastage, decreased fertilization, and decreased pregnancy rates with in vitro fertilization.[18] Recent studies suggest that endometriosis is associated with polyclonal B cell activation, which is a classic characteristic of autoimmune disease.[22]

Pathophysiology

Endometriosis has been identified in unusual sites in the body, but the majority of lesions are limited to the pelvis. The most common pelvic sites, in order of frequency, are the ovary, peritoneum of the cul-de-sac or pouch of Douglas, uterosacral ligaments, round ligament, oviduct, and peritoneal surface of the uterus. Endometriosis of the cervix occurs infrequently but is associated with diagnostic and therapeutic traumatizing cervical procedures such as colposcopy.[60] Isolated lesions in the appendix, bladder, ileum, cecum, cervix, or vagina are far less common. Endometriosis has been identified infrequently in laparotomy or episiotomy scars and in the umbilicus, arms, legs, lungs, kidneys, and nose.

Three major theories exist regarding the pathogenesis of endometriosis:

Transportation. Endometrium is regurgitated through the fallopian tubes during a normal menses. Following the retrograde flow, endometrial fragments implant on the ovary, peritoneal surfaces, and other areas.

Metaplasia or formation in situ. Celomic epithelium differentiates to endometrial epithelium by inflammatory or hormonal influence and alteration.

Induction. This is a combination of transportation and

metaplasia in which regurgitated endometrium liberates chemical-inducing substances that activate undifferentiated mesenchyme to form endometrial epithelium. This is thought to be the most likely pathogenesis of endometriosis.

The appearance of the lesions varies depending on the stage of the disease and its duration. The foci of endometrial tissue are under hormonal influence and bleed periodically. The foci appear as bluish red to yellow-brown nodules implanted on or lying beneath serosal surfaces. They may be microscopic or 1 to 2 cm in diameter. As individual lesions enlarge and coalesce, they can immobilize the affected structures and form adhesions. Endometriosis of the ovaries is characterized by endometriomas, cystic spaces 8 to 10 cm in size. Since they are filled with brown blood debris, they are also referred to as chocolate cysts.

Diagnostic Studies and Findings

Laparoscopy

To visualize foci and perform a biopsy of lesions

Biopsy of Lesions

To confirm histologic diagnosis by presence of glands, stroma, or hemosiderin pigment (an insoluble form of storage iron that indicates bleeding)

Fine Needle Aspiration of Cervix

To provide a relatively noninvasive method of confirmation of clinically and colposcopically suspicious endometriotic lesions of the cervix

Medical Plan

The treatment plan is directed toward producing maximum relief of symptoms and minimum interference with childbearing function in patients who desire children in the future.

Surgery

Total abdominal hysterectomy and bilateral salpingo-oophorectomy

Resection or cautery destruction of visible lesions

Laser laparoscopy to remove endometriotic implants, endometrioma capsules, and lysis of adnexal lesions

Medications

- Progestational steroids
  - Cyclic
    - Norgestrel (Lo/Ovral), 0.3-0.5 mg/d po
  - Continuous
    - Norethynodrel (Enovid), 5-15 mg/d po
  - Long-acting
    - Medroxyprogesterone acetate (Provera), 2.5-10 mg po for 5 d q2 mo
    - Hydroxyprogesterone (Delalutin), 125-250 mg IM q4 wk
- Antigonadotropic agents
  - Danazol (Danocrine), 100-800 mg/d in divided doses for 6-9 mo; produces hypoestrogenic state similar to menopause with eventual atrophy of endometrial lesions[25]
  - Gestrinone, 2.5 mg 2-3 times wk or 1.25 mg/d[9]

NURSING CARE

Nursing Assessment

Comfort

Pelvic pain with menstruation; vague aching, cramping, or bearing-down sensation in pelvis or lower back; dyspareunia; pain with defecation

Bimanual Pelvic Examination

Tender nodules along uterosacral ligaments; uterus may be immobile

Bleeding

Menses excessive or long or both

Nursing Dx & Intervention

Nursing Diagnosis	Nursing Intervention/Rationale
Pain	• Assist with and teach pain-relieving techniques. • Instruct patient to take analgesics as ordered.
Body image disturbance	• Explore meaning of condition with patient *to establish plan of care.* • Encourage patient to express feelings and to share these with partner.

Refer to nursing interventions for specific surgical procedure if done.

Patient Education

1. Instruct the patient about the importance of ongoing patient care.

Evaluation

Patient Outcome	Data Indicating That Outcome is Reached
Comfort is achieved.	Intervention has relieved pain, ended abnormal bleeding, and preserved fertility if desired.

Leiomyomas

Uterine leiomyomas are well-circumscribed, nonencapsulated, benign tumors also called myomas, fibromyomas, fibromas, or fibroids.

Leiomyomas can be found in at least one fifth of women past 30 years of age and are more common in black women.[62] The incidence of myomas in African blacks is reported to be very low, which implies causative factors other than heredity. An estimated 60% of pelvic laparotomies are performed for leiomyomas, although almost all leiomyomas are asymptomatic.[15]

Pathophysiology

Leiomyomas are classified according to their location in the uterus as follows:

- Intramural—central portion of the uterine wall
- Submucous—beneath the endometrium protruding into the intrauterine cavity; may become pedunculated with growth, protruding into the cervix or vagina
- Subserous—beneath the peritoneal covering and projecting into the abdominal cavity; may become pedunculated with growth
- Cervical—within the musculature of the cervix
- Intraligamentous—lateral tumor growth between the leaves of the broad ligament
- Wandering or parasitic—a subserous growth that has lost its connection to the uterus and receives blood from adjacent viscera, peritoneum, or omentum

Leiomyomas arise from smooth muscle within the myometrium, most commonly during the reproductive years. They increase in size during pregnancy, when estrogen production is high, and with the use of oral contraceptives. They generally regress after menopause.

As the tumor enlarges, it reduces the blood supply, resulting in degenerative changes. The most common type of degeneration is hyalinization, in which fibrous and muscle tissue is replaced by hyaline tissue that is smooth and soft and lacks the whorled fascicular pattern. Less commonly, cystic degeneration occurs, with the hyaline material breaking down further and undergoing liquefaction owing to a further decrease in blood supply. Calcification of the leiomyoma may occur after menopause because of calcium deposits. In a large tumor, areas of yellow-brown or red softening, referred to as red or carneous degeneration, may develop because of aseptic necrosis associated with hemorrhage into the tumor. Necrosis may also occur because of twisting or torsion of a pedunculated leiomyoma. Fertility may be impaired when leiomyomas occlude the endocervical canal.

Diagnostic Studies and Findings

Pregnancy Test

To confirm or rule out pregnancy as a cause of symptoms

Dilation and Curettage

To detect submucous leiomyomas

Laparoscopy

To visualize subserous myomas

Ultrasonography

To distinguish between adnexal inflammatory masses and endometriosis from pedunculated or subserous leiomyomas

Laboratory Studies

Leukocytosis with degenerating tumor

Medical Plan

Surgery

Myomectomy to preserve uterus for potential future childbearing in young women

Total hysterectomy

General Management

Pelvic examinations at regular intervals to monitor status of leiomyoma

NURSING CARE

Nursing Assessment

Pain

Dull ache, soreness, or colicky pain; acute pain if torsion or twisting of pedunculated leiomyoma has occurred; bilateral pelvic discomfort if large tumor causes pressure on adjacent viscera; cramping pain if uterus attempts to expel submucous tumor; dysmenorrhea from intramural tumors; pelvic heaviness; feeling of bearing down

Elimination

Constipation from pressure on rectum; urinary frequency and urgency if leiomyoma causes pressure on bladder

Abdomen

Firm, irregular nodules palpated in lower abdomen; irregular abdominal contour

Bleeding

Menses excessive or long or both

Temperature

Elevated with degenerating tumor

Nursing Dx & Intervention

Nursing Diagnosis	Nursing Intervention/Rationale
Body image disturbance	• Assess meaning of condition for patient. • Encourage patient to express her feelings.
Pain	• Assist and teach patient to use pain-relieving methods, including relaxation techniques and analgesics as ordered.

Patient Education

1. Instruct the patient about the importance of obtaining follow-up care and regular examinations to check for unusual growths or complications.

Evaluation

Patient Outcome	Data Indicating That Outcome is Reached
Comfort is achieved.	There is no pain. Menses is normal if myomectomy was performed. There are no subjective or objective signs or symptoms of leiomyomas if hysterectomy was performed.

Polyps

Polyps are benign neoplasms or protruding growths in the cervix or endometrium.

Cervical polyps are soft, red, pedunculated lesions protruding from the cervical os. Endometrial polyps are small, mostly sessile masses that project into the endometrium and may be pedunculated.

Polyps are usually asymptomatic and are often an incidental discovery during visual examination of the cervix, curettage, or hysterectomy. Because endometrial polyps frequently occur in association with leiomyomas and endometrial hyperplasia, specific symptoms are difficult to identify. The symptoms of cervical polyps are similar to those of chronic cervicitis with irregular bleeding. Polyps are the most common lesions of the cervix and occur most often during the reproductive years. Endometrial polyps can also occur at any age but are more common around the time of menopause. Polyps associated with the use of oral contraceptives tend to regress after the drug is discontinued.[51]

Pathophysiology

Cervical polyps most commonly arise from the lower end of the endocervix and vary from a few millimeters to 2 cm in diameter. The base of the pedicle is usually small. Polyps develop as a result of inflammatory hyperplasia of endocervical mucosa owing to hyperestrinism, chronic inflammation, or vascular congestion. Microscopic examination shows a surface covered by columnar epithelium with areas of metaplasia and ulceration. The stroma is often congested with blood and infiltrated by inflammatory cells. The polyps may bleed following trauma from coitus or douching.

Endometrial polyps develop as single or multiple soft tumors composed of hyperplastic endometrium. Most arise from the fundus or cornua, and some may protrude through the cervix. They are usually paler and firmer than cervical polyps. Most frequently the polyp is made up of endometrium similar to that of the basalis and therefore does not show secretory changes. Polyps protruding into the cervix may become necrotic or inflamed, particularly if they are long.[43,51]

Diagnostic Studies and Findings

Endometrial polyps are usually an incidental finding with curettage or hysterectomy, but it is possible to diagnose an endometrial polyp from a hysterosalpingogram. Cervical polyps are diagnosed by inspection of the cervix.

Medical Plan

Surgery

Curettage to remove endometrial polyps
Removal and cauterization of base of cervical polyps; can be performed in outpatient setting
Cryosurgery for cervical polyps (see discussion of cervical conization on p. 1582)

Uterine prolapse

Uterine prolapse (pelvic relaxation, pudendal hernia) is an abnormal protrusion of the uterus through the pelvic floor and vaginal outlet. Uterine prolapse cannot occur without vaginal prolapse.

Approximately half of all parous women have some degree of vaginal or uterine prolapse. One or two women in 10 have symptoms severe enough to warrant surgical intervention. Most cases of pelvic relaxation are associated with cystocele and rectocele.[1] A cystocele is a herniation of the bladder base into the upper portion of the vagina.[4] A rectocele is a herniation of the rectum into the vagina.[4] Uterine prolapse is commonly seen in multiparous Caucasian women during the postmenopausal period.[29]

Pathophysiology

Some authorities believe that probably all cases of vaginal or uterine prolapse are associated with some degree of endopelvic congenital weakness. The aforementioned incidence of varying degrees of uterine prolapse presents a strong argument for this belief.

A more accepted belief is that the most common cause of uterine prolapse is childbirth trauma.[1] Examples of trauma are an episiotomy extension, laceration of the vagina or cervix, or improper episiotomy repair. Pelvic support tissues are damaged by the normal stretching, tearing, and pressure of a vaginal delivery.[4] Other precipitating factors include these:

Pregnancy. Hormonal changes and the increased weight of the uterus during pregnancy contribute to softening or relaxation of uterine support structures.

Menopause. Decreased hormone levels following menopause contribute to atrophy of uterine support structures. If prolapse is present premenopausally, it will progressively worsen during this time.

Chronic pressure. Pelvic structures that are exposed to chronic pressure from asthma, chronic bronchitis, or obesity are weakened.

It appears that many factors contribute to progressive relaxation of uterine support structures, which eventually leads to varying degrees of uterine prolapse.

The amount of uterine descent into the vagina is measured in degrees:

A first-degree prolapse occurs when the cervix is between the ischial spines (normal placement is at the level of the ischial spines) and the vaginal opening.

A second-degree prolapse occurs when only the cervix, not the entire uterus, protrudes through the vaginal opening.

A third-degree prolapse occurs when the entire cervix and uterus extend beyond the vaginal opening. This is sometimes referred to as a procidentia. Some authorities use total procidentia as a fourth-degree classification.

Normally the pelvic floor supports the pelvic viscera and resists intra-abdominal pressure from daily straining, lifting, and coughing. A narrow opening in the central anterior portion of the pelvic floor allows the urethra, vagina, and rectum to enter the pelvic floor, thus creating a weakened area. Certain members of the levator muscle group, puborectalis, pubococcygeal, and iliococcygeal, act as a control mechanism for this narrow opening. The uterus usually forms an acute angle with the axis of the vagina, which prevents prolapse. When the cardinal or sacral ligaments relax, the relationship of the uterus to the vagina is altered, which contributes to prolapse. When the levator muscles or cardinal and sacral ligaments weaken or are injured, the uterus can descend through the weakened area, pulling the urethra and rectum through, which leads to uterine prolapse, cystocele, and rectocele. Both cystoceles and rectoceles can occur before uterine prolapse, depending on which pelvic support structures are weakened.

Diagnostic Studies and Findings

Pelvic Examinations

To determine the degree of uterine prolapse, cystocele, and rectocele

Medical Plan

Surgery

Vaginal hysterectomy—as indicated by symptoms associated with increased pelvic pressure
Anterior and posterior colporrhaphy—as indicated by symptoms
Colpocleisis (LeFort's procedure)—used for elderly, high-risk patients who are not sexually active

Medications

Hormones
Topical estrogen—Premarin vaginal cream inserted 2 times/wk for 6 wk; if effective, continued on a once-a-week basis; used to facilitate regeneration of support mechanism

General Management

Perineal exercise
Kegel exercises for relaxed vaginal outlet and minimum stress urinary incontinence

Pessaries

Devices worn in the vagina to support the uterus; once widely used, they are currently not the treatment of choice except for women who are poor surgical risks

NURSING CARE

Nursing Assessment

Subjective Data

A sense of heaviness or dragging in the low back or pelvis, a feeling of something falling out

Vagina

Dyspareunia, excess vaginal mucus and bleeding in post-menopausal period

Cervix

Depending upon degree of prolapse, may have constant irritation with tissue changes and cervical erosion

Bladder

Urinary tract infection, stress urinary incontinence

Bowel

Hemorrhoids from straining with constipation

Other Complications

Altered sexual function

Nursing Dx & Intervention

Nursing Diagnosis	Nursing Intervention/Rationale
Pain	• Assess patient's degree of discomfort. Responses are varied and relate to the gradual relaxation of the pelvic floor over time. Often patient has adjusted to the pressure changes.
Impaired skin integrity	• See "Patient Education."
Anxiety	• Explain all procedures.
Body image disturbance	• Assess meaning of dysfunction for patient. Encourage patient to express feelings.
Sexual dysfunction related to change	• Explain importance of sharing concerns with sex partner.

Patient Education

1. Instruct the patient about the need to change the pessary every 2 to 3 months and to douche once or twice a week to prevent vaginitis from the presence of the pessary.
2. Explain the importance of reporting any changes in vaginal secretions and elimination patterns to a physician.
3. Explain Kegel's perineal exercises. The Kegel exercises were designed to strengthen the pubococcygeus muscle. (This is the muscle that rims the vagina.) To firm up the pubococcygeus muscle, do this: When you urinate, try to stop in midstream. Then start again. Then stop again. When doing the exercise correctly, you will have the sensation of "pulling up" into the vagina with the buttocks squeezed together. The pubococcygeus muscle, which controls the starting and stopping, will be strengthened by this exercise. The muscles surrounding the vagina and rectum should be squeezed off when doing this exercise, which will create a sensation of pulling everything up into the vagina. Hold for 3 to 4 seconds, relax, and repeat 25 times in sequence each time the exercises are performed. These exercises should be performed at least four times daily.

Evaluation

Patient Outcome	Data Indicating That Outcome is Reached
Comfort is achieved.	Discomfort is relieved, abnormal vaginal discharge has stopped, and normal elimination patterns are achieved.
Patient demonstrates progress toward acceptance of altered body image and self-concept.	Patient shows adaptive response to changes in self-concept and movement toward acceptance of physiologic and psychologic changes associated with treatment regime, whether it is exercise or surgical correction.

Ovarian cysts

A cyst is a sac containing fluid or semisolid material. Ovarian cysts may develop at any time but are most common from puberty to menopause.

The ovary is the most frequent location of a pelvic mass. There are a variety of ovarian cysts, most being small and considered clinically unimportant. Only a few cysts require surgical removal. Most cyst enlargements disappear within a few months. However, malignancy must be considered when evaluating all pelvic masses.[1]

Ovarian cysts are classified as follows[4]:

Functional cysts are follicle and corpus luteum cysts that are normal transient physiologic structures.

Follicle cysts. These are common and appear on the ovary surface. They are usually asymptomatic and disappear spontaneously within 60 days.

Lutein cysts

Granulosa lutein cysts are found within the corpora lutea. They are nonneoplastic enlargements of the ovary caused by an unexplained increase in fluid secretion by the corpus luteum after ovulation or during early pregnancy. They are 4 to 6 cm in diameter, raised, brown, and filled with tawny serous fluid. They may cause local pain and tenderness with either amenorrhea or delayed menses. Most cysts disappear within 2 months in nonpregnant women and gradually decrease in size during the third trimester of a pregnancy. A small percentage of cysts may rupture, requiring surgery.

Theca lutein cysts can vary in size from minute to several centimeters in diameter and are filled with straw-colored fluid. They appear in association with hydatidiform mole, choriocarcinoma, and gonadotropin therapy. Few abdominal symptoms are present, but the patient may feel a sense of pelvic aching or weight. Pregnancy signs and symptoms continue, especially hyperemesis and breast tenderness. A small percentage of cysts may rupture, requiring surgery, but most disappear spontaneously following removal of the causative factor.

Inflammatory cysts. Cysts of the fallopian tube and ovaries can form after an acute infection, such as gonorrhea. Pain is persistent and severe in the pelvis and accompanied by hypermenorrhea. The white blood cell count is elevated, and a pregnancy test will be negative. Surgery is generally not required unless an ectopic pregnancy or acute appendicitis is suspected.

Endometrial cysts. Patients with endometriosis may have endometrium implant on the ovary that will bleed with hormonal stimulation, thus forming a cyst through alternate oozing and healing. These cysts vary in size from microscopic to 10 to 12 cm in diameter. The cysts are filled with thick, chocolate-colored old blood. Large endometrial cysts should be surgically removed, leaving as much functioning ovary as possible. Endometrial cysts are sometimes referred to as "chocolate cysts," although not all chocolate cysts are endometrial in origin.

Inclusion cysts. These cysts are most often microscopic in size and located just beneath the surface of the ovary. The cysts are filled with a minute amount of serous fluid and cause no discomfort. They occur after menopause or after an inflammatory state. No treatment is required.

Parovarian cysts. These cysts are located between the fallopian tube and ovary and are rarely larger than 4 cm in diameter. Found only in postpubertal females, these cysts are generally asymptomatic unless they grow in size to become palpable.

The most important consideration in evaluating an ovarian cyst is the patient's age. Perimenopausal and postmenopausal women with palpable ovarian cysts stand a greater chance of having malignancy.

Diagnostic Studies and Findings

Ultrasonography

To distinguish functional cysts from neoplastic cysts

Laparoscopy

Used when the diagnosis of endometriosis exists or polycystic ovaries can be diagnosed and managed completely by this procedure

Abdominal Roentgenograms

To distinguish functional cysts from neoplastic cysts, especially when calcified structures are present

Barium Enema

To determine if an adnexal mass is caused by a colonic disease; not done routinely

Pelvic and Rectal Examination

To determine location and size of ovarian cyst

Pregnancy Test

To determine if patient is pregnant, especially with suspected lutein cysts

Human Chorionic Gonadotropin Hormone

Increased in theca lutein cysts

Medical Plan

Surgery

Laparotomy to remove cysts, especially if they rupture and bleed, so as to control hemorrhage

General Management

Pelvic examinations at regular intervals to monitor reduction of cysts

NURSING CARE

Nursing Assessment

Pain

Dull ache, severe pain, local pain and tenderness depending upon the type of cyst; severe pain if cyst ruptures

Abdomen

Some cysts are palpable, bilaterally or unilaterally, in the lower abdomen

Bleeding

Menses excessive with inflammatory cyst

Nursing Dx & Intervention

Nursing Diagnosis	Nursing Intervention/Rationale
Body image disturbance	• Assess meaning of condition for patient. Encourage patient to express feelings.
Pain	• Assist with and teach patient to use pain-relieving methods, including relaxation techniques and analgesics as ordered.

Patient Education

1. Instruct the patient about the importance of obtaining follow-up care and regular examinations to check for growth or reduction of cyst.

Evaluation

Patient Outcome	Data Indicating That Outcome is Reached
Comfort is achieved.	There is no pain, and cyst has been reduced in size or removed by laparotomy.

HORMONAL DISORDERS

 Premenstrual syndrome

Premenstrual syndrome (PMS) may be defined as the cyclic recurrence, during the luteal phase of the menstrual cycle, of a combination of physical, psychologic, and behavioral changes severe enough to damage interpersonal relationships or interfere with normal activities.[54] It affects 9 to 12 million women in the United States.[52]

Premenstrual syndrome generally occurs in women in their late twenties and older and increases in incidence and severity as women near menopause. The various behaviors and symptoms described in epidemiologic studies can be placed in the three major categories of edema, emotionality, and headache. The symptoms generally appear 7 to 10 days before menses and sharply decrease with the onset of menses. The cause of PMS remains obscure.

Pathophysiology

The exact cause of premenstrual tension is unknown, but it is believed to be related to decreasing concentrations of estrogen and progesterone and related changes in electrolyte balance. Progesterone stimulates the production of aldosterone, which increases sodium retention and edema formation. Interestingly, no distinct differences in aldosterone levels have been shown between women with and those without premenstrual syndrome. The decrease in brain levels of monoamine oxidase that occurs as estrogen production falls before menses probably accounts for the feeling of depression. Fluctuation of monoamine oxidase and catecholamine levels in the brain may result in the frequently observed symptom of irritability. Studies have shown that carbohydrate metabolism and the adrenal production of corticosteroids change before menses. In addition serotonin levels are significantly lower during the last 10 days of the menstrual cycle in women with PMS. Decreased serotonin is known to be associated with depression in humans.[50] The treatment of PMS must be individualized for each woman, and practices vary. For example, there is concern that even low doses of vitamin B_6 may result in potentially toxic effects.[30] Premenstrual tension may well be caused by a variety of factors.[20,63]

Diagnostic Studies and Findings

There are no specific tests for diagnosis of premenstrual syndrome.

Medical Plan

Medications

Hydrochlorothiazide, 50-100 mg/d po during 7-10 d before cycle or 24-36 h before onset of expected symptoms
- Diazepam, 5-10 mg po bid
- Medroxyprogesterone (Provera), 10-20 mg/d po during last half of cycle
- Alprazolam, 0.25 mg po tid from cycle day 20 until second day of menstruation[54]
- Danazol, 200 mg po qd from onset of symptoms until onset of menses[52]

Vitamins
- Vitamin B_6, 200-800 mg/d
- Vitamin E, 600 U/d

General Management

Limitation of intake of salt, refined sugars, and animal fats

Emotional and psychologic support

NURSING CARE

Nursing Assessment

Hydration

Edema; weight gain; backache; breast tenderness; oliguria; palpitations; mastalgia

Gastrointestinal

Abdominal bloating; diarrhea or constipation; nausea; vomiting; food craving; compulsive eating

Affect and Behavior

Irritability; anxiety; lability; fatigue; depression; lethargy; agitation; insomnia; hypersomnia; difficulty in concentrating; decreased interest in usual activities

Neurologic

Headache; vertigo; fainting; migraine; paresthesias of head and feet

Respiratory

Increase in colds, asthma, or allergic rhinitis

Urologic

Cystitis; enuresis; urethritis

Ophthalmologic

Conjunctivitis; styes

Breasts

Tenderness; enlargement

Dermatologic

Recurrence of herpes; acne; urticaria; boils; easy bruising

Nursing Dx & Intervention

Nursing Diagnosis	Nursing Intervention/Rationale
Anxiety	• Reassure patient that her symptoms are temporary and not related to significant disease.
Pain	• See "Patient Education."
Altered health maintenance	• Help patient evaluate personal strengths and needs that affect health maintenance ability. • Encourage participation in group therapy and/or sharing of feelings with family or significant other. • Encourage patient to express her feelings. • Suggest that patient may wish to maintain a personal journal or diary *to describe feelings, strengths, and needs on a daily basis.* This should be reviewed on a regular basis *to identify any patterns or opportunities for changes in behavior.*

Patient Education

1. Explain that fatigue exaggerates symptoms and that adequate rest and sleep are needed during the premenstrual period.
2. Encourage the patient to avoid stressful activity during the premenstrual period.
3. Instruct the patient to avoid glucose fluctuation by taking small frequent feedings of a high-protein, complex carbohydrate diet and by decreasing sugar intake to less than 5 tablespoons daily.
4. Instruct the patient to reduce salt intake and to avoid foods with "hidden salt" such as soy sauce, salted crackers and bread, luncheon meats, dried meats, hot dogs, tomato juice, and cheeses.
5. Instruct the patient to avoid dairy products and animal fats.
6. Instruct the patient to restrict caffeine by decreasing intake of coffee, tea, cola, and chocolate.
7. Instruct the patient to restrict alcohol.

8. Instruct the patient to increase intake of leafy green vegetables and whole grain cereals.
9. Instruct the patient to take medications as prescribed and explain the reasons for taking specific medications. (For example, vitamin B_6 is taken to increase blood progesterone and promote diuresis, and vitamin E is taken to reduce breast tenderness.)

Evaluation

Patient Outcome	Data Indicating That Outcome is Reached
Comfort is achieved. There is little or no anxiety.	Patient describes feeling of well-being and absence of bloating, weight gain, edema, mastalgia, irritability, anxiety, and other symptoms of PMS.
Patient uses strengths to comply with plan of care.	Patient recognizes personal strengths and needs that are directed toward elimination or reduction of symptoms.
Patient establishes appropriate control of mood swings.	Patient verbalizes about mood and advises others of her particular sensitivities. Patient develops a support system with significant others. Patient demonstrates increased interest in social and occupational activities.

Menopause and climacteric

Menopause is the physiologic cessation of menses. The climacteric is the transitional period during which reproductive function diminishes and eventually ceases.

As the average life span has increased in the United States, so has the number of postmenopausal women. In 1970 there were 27.2 million women over 50 years of age, in 1979 there were 32 million, and in 2000 there will be an estimated 49 million. Postmenopausal women constitute one eighth to one sixth of the population. The average life span of women is 76 years, whereas that of men is only 68 years. As the ratio of men to women decreases with age, many women in the climacteric phase of life must cope with societal as well as physical changes.[15,62]

The normal decrease in ovarian function begins during the fourth decade, and the majority of women cease to menstruate between the ages of 45 and 55. The average age at which menses disappears is 51 years, although some women cease to menstruate as early as 35 years and others continue until 55 years or older.

Artificial or premature menopause is the cessation of ovarian function as a result of radiation, surgery, immunologic disease, or bacteriologic or viral agents. Although the signs and symptoms of natural and premature or artificial menopause are similar, the medical management may vary based on the patient's age.

Physiology

A notable event of the climacteric phase of life is menopause, the complete cessation of menses. Before the actual menopause there are usually gradual changes, such as a decrease in the amount of menses, lengthening of the interval between menses, periodic amenorrhea, and finally slight spotting. These events are due to a progressive decline in the ovarian secretion of estrogen. When too little estrogen is secreted to cause endometrial growth, bleeding stops permanently. Irregular menses followed by amenorrhea for more than 1 year is indicative of menopause.

With menopause the estrogen fractions change and estrone becomes more available than estradiol. Peripheral conversion of androstenedione, a product of the adrenal glands, to estrone occurs principally in the fat. Some women produce enough estrone to cause endometrial growth and shedding or bleeding. Since obesity is a common factor in women with endometrial cancer, it has been hypothesized that production of estrone in the adipose tissue may contribute to the genesis of a tumor.

Changes in reproductive structures are related directly to decreased estrogen. Labial fat is reabsorbed; the labia majora become flattened and the labia minora disappear. The vaginal mucosa becomes thinner, the vagina smaller, and the fornices shallower. The myometrium thins, causing the uterus to decrease in size until it resembles that of a prepubertal girl.

Hot flushes, the most characteristic symptom of menopause, coincide with a pulsatile release of luteinizing hormone. A slight increase in core body temperature and a higher increase in skin temperature occur. The sensation of heat is often accompanied by tachycardia, vertigo, palpitation, and a feeling of faintness.

The atrophic changes that result from estrogen deprivation may lead to dyspareunia owing to decreased precoital lubrication or constriction of the introitus or vagina.

Menopausal arthralgia, pain and stiffness in the joints in climacteric women, may be caused by changes in the soft tissues surrounding the joints or by lack of exercise of the muscles and tendons.

Nervousness and other psychologic symptoms are not a direct result of estrogen deficiency. The patient's personality and response to aging are the keys to promoting adaptation to the climacteric.

The use of hormonal therapy in the treatment of menopause is associated with a diminution of subjective complaints, a decrease in age-specific mortality for all categories of cause of death except cancer,[47] and a decrease in collagen loss and osteoporosis.[8,40]

Diagnostic Studies and Findings

Papanicolaou Smear

Decrease in estrogen effect noted in vaginal mucosa

Blood Chemistry

Estradiol, 1-5 ng/dl
Estrogen, 0-14 ng/dl
Estrone, 25-50 pg/dl
Luteinizing hormone, 35-120 mIU/ml
Follicle-stimulating hormone, 40-200 mIU/ml

Urine Chemistry

Estrogens, 1.4-19.6 μg/24 hours
Pregnanediol, 0.2-1 mg/24 hours
Luteinizing hormone, 40-110 mIU/24 hours
Follicle-stimulating hormone, 2-25 mIU/24 hours

Medical Plan

Medications

Estrogens

Sodium estrone sulfate, 0.3-25 mg/d po, or ethinyl estradiol (Estinyl, others), 0.05-0.2 mg/d po; initial doses should be lowest amount that will control symptoms; drug is taken for first 25 d of month; withdrawal should be gradual over several months to prevent recurrence of hot flushes

Indications: Treatment of hot flushes and senile atrophic vaginitis; prevention of osteoporosis

Contraindications: Presence or history of breast or genital cancer (except cervical cancer in some cases); history of thromboembolism; fluid retention owing to cardiac, renal, or hepatic disease; abnormal liver function

Cautions: Administration is closely monitored in women with uterine fibroids, endometriosis, hypertension, or insulin-dependent diabetes mellitus; annual endometrial biopsy needed for patient receiving long-term estrogen therapy to prevent osteoporosis

Estrogen creams applied to vagina are more effective than oral estrogen in treatment of atrophic vaginitis

Progestins or progestogens

Medroxyprogesterone acetate (Provera), 2.5-10 mg/d po in last 10 d of estrogen cycle

Indications: To prevent endometrial cancer, which may develop with unopposed estrogen stimulation

Cautions: May stimulate withdrawal bleeding; patients receiving long-term estrogen replacement therapy should have annual endometrial biopsies

NURSING CARE

Nursing Assessment

Subjective Complaints

Hot flushes; night sweats; diaphoresis; insomnia; headache; vertigo; syncope; numbness, tingling, or pain in joints; chilly sensation; lack of appetite or weight gain; constipation or diarrhea; nausea or vomiting; flatulence; fatigability; irritability; nervousness; depression or crying spells; fits of anger; forgetfulness; difficulty in concentrating; dyspareunia (resulting from vaginal atrophy)

Vulva

Decreasing labial fat; atrophy of muscle

Vagina

Decreased size with shallow fornices

Abdomen

Abdominal fat deposition

Cardiac Rate and Rhythm

Tachycardia; palpitations

Breasts

Reduction in size

Body Hair

Loss of pubic and axillary hair

Nursing Dx & Intervention

Nursing Diagnosis	Nursing Intervention/Rationale
Knowledge deficit	• Explain physiologic process of climacteric and menopause. • Explain importance of keeping fit and eating well-balanced diet, getting adequate rest and sleep, avoiding stress and fatigue, and continuing contraception until health care provider indicates it is safe to stop.

Nursing Diagnosis	Nursing Intervention/Rationale
	• Inform patient about side effects of estrogen replacement therapy, need to report any vaginal bleeding occurring 6 months or more after last menstrual period, and availability of water-soluble lubricants if needed before coitus.
Body image disturbance	• Encourage patient to express concerns about femininity, sexuality, and aging. • Reinforce correct information and provide factual information *to correct any misconceptions*.
Altered sexuality patterns	• Encourage patient to express her concerns regarding sexuality. • Encourage patient to discuss concerns with partner or significant other. • Provide information for patient to access group or individual counseling and education.

Evaluation

Patient Outcome	Data Indicating That Outcome is Reached
Patient has acquired knowledge about climacteric.	Patient expresses understanding of physiology and desired health behaviors. Patient relates understanding of prescribed medications including dosage, route of administration, frequency, and side effects.
Patient demonstrates progress toward acceptance of altered body image and self-concept.	Patient shows adaptive responses to changes in self-concept and movement toward acceptance of both physiologic and psychologic processes associated with climacteric.

Fertility control

Fertility can be controlled by natural, mechanical, chemical, hormonal, and surgical means.

Nearly 80 million infants are born worldwide each year, as compared with 10 million a year in the early 1900s. United Nations researchers project that the world population will grow from the current 4.2 billion to 6.35 billion by the year 2000. Continued population growth at current rates could have a negative impact on natural resources, food supply, and political stability, especially in Third World countries. The number of people the earth can sustain is unknown. It is known that poverty leads to high fertility, which in turn further increases poverty.[49]

Population growth in the United States is currently at a level just over replacement, with a rate of 0.8% or 1 million people per year.[48] Fertility rates are higher among the poor and less educated. The goal of every pregnancy occurring as a result of an informed decision and resulting in a wanted child is far from being achieved.

Many factors affect the selection of a fertility control method, including the person's perception of the risk of pregnancy, knowledge of fertility control methods, and willingness and ability to use them; social pressures; the attitude of health care providers; desires of the partner; and the cost and effectiveness of various methods. The methods most widely used in the United States in order of popularity are oral contraceptives, condoms, intrauterine devices (IUDs), rhythm, foam, diaphragm, and coitus interruptus.[49] The method of fertility control varies according to the duration of the relationship or marriage. Young couples often use oral contraceptives until their first child is born, change to the use of an IUD until their family is complete, and then select sterilization.

There has been a general decline in the use of oral contraceptives and a fourfold increase in those selecting sterilization in the last decade. Approximately equal numbers of men and women have undergone sterilization. More than 12 million Americans have already undergone voluntary sterilization, and approximately 1 million are sterilized annually.[49]

Abortion, although not a contraceptive technique, is a method of preventing unwanted children. In January 1973 the U.S. Supreme Court declared all restrictive abortion laws by individual states unconstitutional. As a consequence, abortion in both the first and second trimesters is legal in all states, with the decision made by the woman and her physician. States may develop regulations regarding who can perform second-trimester abortions and where they may be done. In some states third-trimester abortions are prohibited except to preserve the life or health of the woman.

Since the Supreme Court decision the numbers of illegal abortions and abortion-related deaths have fallen precipitously. A national trend toward increased abortions appears to have leveled off in 1981, the latest year for which figures are available. In that year 1,300,760 legal abortions were reported in the United States, an increase of 3154, or less than 1%, over the number reported in 1980. There were 11 abortion-related deaths, the lowest number since the Center for Disease Control in Atlanta began keeping records in 1972.[12]

The health care provider has a responsibility to provide information to women or couples choosing a method of contraception. The decision is a voluntary one based on explanation of the methods available, including their action, safety and effectiveness, expected effects, risks, and contraindications. The methods of fertility control can be divided into five major groups: natural or physiologic, mechanical, chemical, hormonal, and surgical.

Natural or Physiologic Methods

Rhythm. In the rhythm method, coitus is confined to phases in the menstrual cycle when conception is unlikely to occur. This can be determined by the calendar method, temperature method, or ovulation method. With the *calendar* method the fertile period is determined by recording the number of days of each menstrual cycle for a year, subtracting 18 days from the length of the shortest cycle to determine the beginning of the fertile period, and subtracting 11 days from the length of the longest cycle to determine the postovulatory safe period. The *temperature* method is based on abstinence from the end of the menses until 4 days after the rise in basal body temperature. The woman must take her temperature the first thing in the morning, since the basal body temperature is the lowest temperature reached by the body during the waking hours. The *ovulation* method is based on the recognition of characteristic changes in cervical mucus. Initially after menstruation there is little mucus and the introitus is dry. The mucus becomes sticky and cloudy as estrogen stimulation increases, and as ovulation occurs it becomes abundant, clear, and slippery and stretches without breaking, the spinnbarkheit phenomenon. Following ovulation and an increase in progesterone, the mucus becomes opaque and sticky again, with the woman experiencing a sensation of dryness. Coitus should be avoided from first recognition of the sticky mucus until after the watery discharge disappears.

Coitus interruptus. Withdrawal of the penis from the vagina before ejaculation is probably the oldest and most frequently used fertility control method throughout the world. It is associated with a fairly high failure rate, since live sperm may be present in the seminal fluid that leaks from the urethra during coitus.

Mechanical Methods

Condom. The condom or penile sheath must be applied over the erect penis, leaving space at the tip to contain the ejaculate. It must be removed before penile detumescence, with the rim held tightly to prevent leakage.

Diaphragm. The diaphragm is a latex dome-shaped cup that must be fitted to the patient to ensure that the cervix is covered. The woman must be instructed in its use and be able to demonstrate its application.

Cervical cap. The cervical cap is smaller than the diaphragm and made of thick rubber or plastic. It may be applied some time before intercourse and left in place for at least 8 hours after intercourse. It is more difficult to apply than the diaphragm, and some women object to the odor when it is left in place for a long time. Its use, except in a few research centers, is not approved by the Food and Drug Administration.

Intrauterine device (IUD). The IUD is a small plastic device connected to a string that protrudes into the vagina. IUDs are available in various sizes and shapes. A health care provider inserts the device into the uterus, usually during menses when the cervix is partially open.

Chemical Methods

Spermicidal jellies, creams, suppositories, or aerosol foams are placed in the vagina immediately before intercourse and act as a chemical barrier to the sperm. They are often used in conjunction with another method such as a natural or a mechanical method.

Hormonal Methods

The most popular form of hormonal contraception is the oral contraceptive ("the pill"). This is most commonly a combination of estrogen and progestin that inhibits ovulation and changes in the endometrium, cervical mucus, and probably tubal function. Oral contraceptives are extremely effective in preventing pregnancy but are known to affect every body system and may produce significant dangers with long-term use. Generally the benefits and effectiveness outweigh the risk in healthy women below 30 years of age. See Table 10-2 for a summary of current agents.

Diethylstilbestrol (the "morning-after pill") is the postcoital agent most commonly used in the United States. It is not for routine use but should be considered an emergency measure to be taken as soon as possible but no later than 72 hours after unprotected midcycle intercourse. The possibility of an established pregnancy must be ruled out before this drug is administered, since ingestion by the mother is known to cause vaginal adenosis and clear cell carcinoma in daughters.[13]

Surgical Methods

Abortion. First-trimester abortion is done by dilation and curettage, aspiration of intrauterine contents through a suction device, or menstrual extraction. Second-trimester abortion is achieved by dilation and evacuation, intrauterine drug instillation, or hysterotomy.

Dilation and curettage is a painful procedure requiring general anesthesia; a sharp metal curette is inserted into the uterus to remove products of conception.

Vacuum aspiration can be done following a cervical block. The cervix is prepared by instillation of laminaria, an absorbent dried seaweed, into the cervix to expand the cervical canal. After the laminaria is removed, the aspiration curette is inserted and the products of conception are removed.

Menstrual extraction is the aspiration of endometrium and intrauterine contents through a polyethylene catheter that has been inserted into the uterus through the cervix. The procedure seldom requires cervical dilation and is performed no later than 8 weeks after the last menstrual period. Uterine injury and bleeding and continuation of pregnancy are the major risks associated with this procedure, which should not be considered a substitute for contraception.

The cervix must be more dilated for dilation and evacuation than for curettage. Dilation is usually effected with laminaria. The intrauterine contents are evacuated through a crushing

Table 10-2
Summary of Methods of Conception Control

Method	Action	Safety-Effectiveness	Effects	Contraindications
Oral Contraceptive ("The Pill")				
Combination pill: each pill contains progestin and estrogen; schedule: one pill daily for 21 days, then discontinue for 7 days; placebo may be advised for last 7 days; pill cycle started and repeated on fifth day after onset of menstrual flow	Inhibits ovulation by suppression of pituitary gonadotropin Produces cervical mucus that is hostile to sperm Modifies tubal transport of ovum May have effect on endometrium to make implantation unlikely	100% effective if taken accurately Failure results from failure to take pill regularly If woman forgets to take pill one day, she can "make up" by taking two pills next day Chances of pregnancy increased if pill is missed for even 1 day Highly acceptable to users; easy to take Linked with mortality caused by thromboembolus phenomena Does not alter fertility	Useful Relief of dysmenorrhea in 60% to 90% of cases Relief of premenstrual tension Regulation of menstrual cycles Relief of acne in 80% to 90% of cases Improved feeling of well-being Minor side effects (usually decrease after third cycle) Weight gain Breast tenderness Headaches Corneal edema Nausea Breakthrough bleeding Hypertension Major side effects Thromboembolus disorders May decrease lactation in breast-feeding women	Undiagnosed vaginal bleeding Breast or pelvic cancer Liver disease Cardiovascular disease Renal disease Thyroid disease Diabetes Uterine fibroid tumors Use with caution if history of: Epilepsy Multiple sclerosis Porphyria Otosclerosis Asthma
Intrauterine Contraceptive Device (IUD or IUCD)				
Small objects of various shapes made of plastic, nylon, or steel inserted into uterus; most have nylon string attached that protrudes from cervix into vagina; inserted using aseptic technique; follow-up visits in 1 month, then individualized EXAMPLES ParaGard (Copper T380A) Progestesert	Unknown Probably modifies endometrium or myometrium to prevent implantation Probably hastens tubal transport of ovum	Easily inserted, highly effective: 97% to 99% Can be inserted any time during cycle; presence of menstrual flow rules out early pregnancy Can be inserted immediately postpartum, but expulsion rate is higher Can be left in place indefinitely Effectiveness highly dependent on knowing IUD remains in place; women need to be taught to feel for string after each period	Uterine cramping Heavy menstrual flow Irregular menses NOTE: Usually disappear in 2 to 3 months Problems Infection: usually minor and occurs soon after insertion Perforation of uterus: varies with types of device; highest rates in first 6 weeks postpartum; usually occurs at time of insertion	Current infection of reproductive tract Uterine fibroids Undiagnosed vaginal bleeding

Continued.

Table 10-2—cont'd
Summary of Methods of Conception Control

Method	Action	Safety-Effectiveness	Effects	Contraindications
		Spontaneous expulsion occurs most often during menstruation (expulsion rates: 10% to 20%) Failure rate (pregnancy) 1.5% to 3% during first year of use; rate declines thereafter Does not alter fertility		
Diaphragm (with Spermicidal Foam, Cream, Jelly)				
Rubber dome attached to flexible metal ring; inserted into vagina to cover cervix; available in various sizes (require careful fitting); self-inserted by user; inner surface of diaphragm coated with spermicide before insertion; inserted at least 2 hours before intercourse and left in place at least 6 hours after intercourse	Provides mechanical barrier to sperm Spermicidal preparation destroys large number of sperm	97% to 98% effective if fitted properly and used correctly Requires sustained motivation for repeated insertion and removal Refitting necessary after childbirth, abortion, surgery of cervix and vagina, or weight change of 10 pounds or more	None	Severe uterine prolapse
Cervical Cap				
A flexible natural rubber device available in various sizes (requires careful fitting); self-inserted by user; inserted before intercourse and left in place at least 8 hours (but no more than 48 hours) after intercourse	Provides mechanical barrier to sperm	82.6% to 93.6% effective if fitted properly and used correctly Requires 30-90 minutes' education time to learn insertion procedure Requires sustained motivation for repeated insertion and removal	Potential for Papanicolaou test conversion from normal to abnormal at 3 months' follow-up (use of cervical cap is discontinued if this occurs)	Cervical dysplasia with abnormal Papanicolaou test History of toxic shock syndrome Concurrent vaginal or cervical infection

Condom ("Rubber," "Safe," "Prophylactic")				
Thin, flexible plastic worn over penis; available without prescription; does not require medical supervision	Provides mechanical barrier to prevent sperm from entering vagina Prevents spread of venereal diseases	Effectiveness increased with use of diaphragm by woman Effectiveness decreased by tearing or slipping of condom during intercourse Failure rate 10% to 15%	None	None
Natural Family Planning (Ovulation, Symptothermal)				
Periodic abstinence from intercourse during fertile periods of menstrual cycle; days 12 to 16 before expected date of menstruation are possible ovulating days; because sperm can survive up to 48 hours, days 11, 17, and 18 added to fertile period	Sexual abstinence around time of ovulation	Safe 65% to 85% effective Fertile period varies; precise time of ovulation not known Effectiveness increased with calculation of fertile period, high motivation to prevent pregnancy, determination of basal body temperature, and observation of mucous secretions' consistency	Frustration Lack of sexual gratification during period of abstinence	Irregular menstrual cycles Medical contraindications to pregnancy
Chemical Contraceptive (Jellies, Creams, Foams, Suppositories)				
Applied inside vagina by means of plunger-type applicator or aerosol spray	Contains spermicidal ingredients Partial barrier to entrance of sperm into cervix	Effectiveness increased when used with diaphragm or condom Easily available without prescription Effectiveness depends on dispersion of substance within vagina	None	None

Modified from Phipps.[48]

instrument, followed by aspiration. The procedure is most frequently done in women who are 13 to 16 weeks pregnant.

Hypertonic saline solution is injected into the amniotic cavity to induce a second-trimester abortion. Complications are inadvertent infusion into the maternal bloodstream, producing salt intoxication; disseminated intravascular coagulation; and infection, especially if there is a long interval between instillation of the drug and uterine evacuation. Prostaglandin can be given by intra-amniotic or intraveous infusion or as a vaginal suppository. This method has virtually replaced use of hypertonic saline solution for abortion. Prostaglandins stimulate contractions of smooth uterine muscle and generally result in abortion within 24 hours. Side effects include nausea, vomiting, diarrhea, and abdominal cramping, which can be controlled with analgesics and antiemetics.[49]

Hysterotomy is a surgical incision into the uterus for the removal of products of conception. It is associated with morbidity and is used only rarely for midtrimester abortions.

Sterilization. Sterilization is the ultimate method of fertility control, rendering a person unable to reproduce. This is accomplished by vasectomy in men and tubal ligation or hysterectomy in women.

Vasectomy is a procedure for male sterilization involving the bilateral surgical removal of a portion of the vas deferens. It is most commonly performed on an outpatient basis with the patient under local anesthesia.

Tubal sterilization is the disruption of tubal patency to prevent the union of the ova and spermatozoa. It can be achieved through the vagina or by an abdominal approach through an incision or with laparoscopic visualization. A variety of techniques can be used:

Irving procedure. The oviduct is severed, and the uterine end is buried in the myometrium posteriorly and the distal or ovarian end is placed in the mesosalpinx.

Pomeroy procedure. A loop of oviduct is ligated and excised.

Parkland procedure. A segment of the fallopian tube is separated from the mesosalpinx and ligated proximally and distally, and then the midportion is excised.[49]

Fimbriectomy. The distal portion of the ampulla, including all of the fimbriae, is resected.

Tubal sterilization can be done at any time but is most convenient during the postpartum period because the uterine fundus is near the umbilicus and the fallopian tubes are readily accessible. Laparoscope sterilization is often referred to as "band aid" surgery, since it can be performed in an ambulatory surgical center with general or occasionally local anesthesia. A pneumoperitoneum is produced with carbon dioxide, and the oviduct is ligated and most commonly electrocoagulated. In a vaginal tubal sterilization the peritoneal cavity is entered through the posterior vaginal fornix (culdotomy, colpotomy) and a Pomeroy procedure or fimbriectomy is performed. The care of women undergoing tubal ligation is discussed on p. 1018.

A summary of the common methods of conception control is provided in Table 10-2.

 Infertility

Infertility is the inability to conceive during a period of 1 year of unprotected intercourse. Primary infertility exists when there has been no prior conception. Secondary infertility follows at least one normal pregnancy.

Infertility affects 10% to 15% of couples in the United States. About 25% of women who do not use contraception and who have coitus regularly conceive within 4 months, more than 60% do so within 6 months, and about 80% within 1 year. The incidence of infertility shows a progression with advancing age of the woman. Fertility peaks between 20 and 25 years of age and decreases after 30 years of age in women and 40 years of age in men.[62]

It is estimated that male factors are responsible for about 40% of infertility problems. The cause of infertility is not identifiable in 10% to 20% of cases. Female factors are responsible for the remaining cases. Of these around 20% to 30% are the result of disorders of the fallopian tubes, 10% to 15% lack of ovulation, and 50% cervical factors. It is believed that endometriosis is responsible for 30% to 40% of female infertility.[26]

About 40% of those who seek medical attention for infertility eventually conceive. The identified cause of infertility cannot be corrected in 40% of the couples, and the cause of infertility in the remaining couples is never identified.

Pathophysiology

Normal fertility is dependent on many factors, including normal ovarian function, endocrine preparation of the uterus for implantation of the fertilized ovum, cervical mucus favorable for transport of sperm, normal anatomic structures, lack of obstruction to sperm and ovum, and normally functioning fallopian tubes. The male partner must have a sufficient number of motile and mature sperm that can be ejaculated without any anatomic or physiologic obstruction and that are capable of penetrating the egg.

The causes of infertility are as follows[36]:

- Female factors
  - Vaginal abnormalities
    - Rigid hymen or small hymenal orifice; psychogenic vaginismus; hyperacidity of vaginal secretions
  - Cervical abnormalities
    - Obstructive lesions such as polyps, pedunculated fibroids, or congenital atresia; alterations in cervical mucus owing to bacteria or chemical agents; surgical destruction of endocervical glands
  - Uterine factors
    - Submucous myomas; structural malformations such as bicornuate or septate uterus; hypoplasia owing to endocrine disturbances; synechiae owing to endometritis; pelvic inflammatory disease
  - Tubal and peritoneal abnormalities
    - Peritubal and periovarian adhesions following peri-

tonitis; inflammatory damage owing to intrauterine devices, severe puerperal infections, and pelvic inflammatory disease; endometriosis

Ovarian abnormalities

Oligo-ovulation or anovulation owing to hypothalamic, pituitary, or ovarian deficits; hyperprolactinemia and galactorrhea associated with anovulation or luteal phase defects; faulty nutrition; metabolic dysfunction; luteal phase defects, which may be due to abnormal stimulation of the graafian follicle, hyperandrogen states, or increased prolactin levels; ovarian tumors (such as Stein-Leventhal syndrome)

Male factors

Sperm-related factors

Testicular hypoplasia; endocrine disorders such as hypopituitarism and hypothalamic disorders; cryptorchidism; varicocele; gonadal damage from trauma, surgery, or radiation; exposure of testicles to heat including wearing of tight shorts; systemic infections including mumps, tuberculosis, and syphilis; late descent of testicles; high viscosity of semen; autoimmunity as result of trauma, vasectomy, or infection; low volume

Ductal obstructions

Resulting from epididymitis or infection of ejaculatory ducts; congenital absence of ducts

Transport-related factors

Hypospadias; ejaculatory problems; impotence

Factors affecting either male or female

Stress

Physical or psychic; long-term psychiatric problems

Nutritional deficiencies

Malnutrition such as anorexia nervosa and starvation; vitamin, mineral, or fat deficiencies

Substances

Exposure to toxins including alcohol, nicotine, metals such as lead, dyes such as aniline dyes, drugs such as narcotics, quinine, hormonal agents, and antineoplastic drugs, radiation

Congenital anomalies

Chromosomal abnormalities (such as Turner's and Klinefelter's syndromes)

Disease processes

Dysfunctions or disturbances of thyroid, adrenal, or pituitary gland; diabetes mellitus; anemia; chronic nephritis; severe cardiac disturbances; infections; immune responses

Causes of infertility in the couple

Sexual problems

Unconsummated relationships; infrequent intercourse; sexual dysfunction; vaginismus; suboptimum technique

Other problems

Discordant relationships; immunologic reaction

Diagnostic Studies and Findings

Semen Analysis

Standards for fertility are volume of 2 to 6 ml semen per ejaculation; 20 to 300 million sperm/ml; 60% to 80% of sperm actively motile; 60% or more of sperm normally shaped[62]

Tubal Patency Determination

Hysterosalpingography

May indicate obstruction of tube if radiopaque dye fails to spill into peritoneum

Uterotubal insufflation (Rubin's test)

May indicate tubal obstruction if pressurized carbon dioxide cannot pass through tubes

Cervical examination in midcycle

Cervix not opened; lack of copious mucus; lack of spinnbarkheit and arborization

Laparoscopy or culdoscopy

Absence of direct observation of dye passing through fimbriated ends of fallopian tube; peritubal adhesions may be observed

Basal Body Temperature Graph

Absence of normal biphasic pattern with sustained rise of at least 1° F during last 2 weeks of cycle

Serum Progesterone

Level less than 10 ng/ml indicative of abnormal luteal function; concentration of less than 3 ng/ml suggestive of anovulation

Postcoital Test (Sims-Huhner)

Fewer than five highly motile sperm in mucus from upper cervix; inadequate spinnbarkheit and arborization suggestive of estrogen deficiency and secretory defect of cervical epithelium

Endometrial Biopsy

Findings inconsistent with cycle

Immunologic Compatibility Tests

Evaluation of sperm agglutination and immobilization

Ultrasound

Observation of ovarian follicle rupture

Medical Plan

Surgery

Removal of myomas
Polypectomy
Dilation and curettage
Unilateral or bilateral tuboplasty

Salpingostomy
Ovarian wedge resection (for patients with polycystic ovaries)

Medications

Anti-infective agents
- Therapy based on culture findings

Ovulatory stimulants
- Clomiphene citrate (Clomid), 50-100 mg for 5-7 d
- Human menopausal gonadotropin (HMG; Pergonal), 1 ampule IM for 9-12 d followed by 10,000 IU human chorionic gonadotropin 1 d after last dose of HMG
- GnRH (Factrel™) as ordered to treat hypothalamic amenorrhea[16]

Estrogens
- Estrone (Hormonin, others), 0.7-1.4 mg po qd cyclically
- Conjugated estrogens (Premarin), 0.625-3.75 mg qd po cyclically

Pituitary-related agents
- Bromocriptine (Parlodel), individually adjusted

General Management

In vitro fertilization
Artificial insemination
Psychotherapy
Improvement of coital technique
Use of condoms and avoidance of orogenital sex for 6 to 12 months to treat immunologic infertility

NURSING CARE

Nursing Assessment

Couple

Name; age; occupation; religion; ethnocultural influences; years of marriage; previous marriages; duration of involuntary infertility; habits; diet; health status; exposure to alcohol, nicotine, narcotics, quinine, hormones, antineoplastic agents, metals, dyes, and radiation; physical or psychic stress

Female

Health history
- Tuberculosis; venereal disease; endometriosis; tumors

Gynecologic history
- Menarche; frequency, duration, and amount of menstrual flow; menstrual irregularities; evidence of dysmenorrhea; mittelschmerz; increased midcycle discharge; pelvic inflammatory disease; previous surgical procedure including pelvic operation and appendectomy

Obstetric history
- Full-term deliveries; complications; abortions (reason, if elective) or premature deliveries

Conception control history
- Type of contraceptives used and duration of use

Sexual history
- Frequency of coitus; postcoital practices; libido; orgasm capacity; position during and after intercourse; use of lubricants; sexual involvement with other partners

Male

Health history
- Tuberculosis; venereal infection; mumps; orchitis; varicocele; previous surgical procedure including orchiopexy and herniorrhaphy; hydrocele; injury to genitals

Sexual history
- Frequency of coitus; technique and position; premature ejaculation; adequacy of erection; timing of coitus; sexual involvement with other partners

Male and Female Psychosocial Factors

Motivation for pregnancy; perception of and feelings related to inability to achieve conception; effect of sociocultural and familial factors related to desired pregnancy

Nursing Dx & Intervention

Nursing Diagnosis	Nursing Intervention/Rationale
Knowledge deficit regarding optimum sexual technique; sexual dysfunction related to lack of knowledge	• Ensure that both partners are aware of practices that promote conception, including: 1. Intercourse every 2 days during fertile period 2. Woman in supine position with man astride 3. Woman's hips elevated on pillow with thighs flexed 4. Avoidance of commercial lubricants 5. Penis maintained in vagina without thrusting for short time after ejaculation 6. Woman remaining in bed with hips elevated for approximately 30 minutes after coitus 7. Woman not urinating or douching for at least 1 hour after coitus
Anticipatory grieving	• Support couple's grief through listening and offering explanations about their reactions. • Promote cohesiveness; avoid laying "blame" on one person. • Help couple express their feelings when they find it difficult to do so.

Nursing Diagnosis	Nursing Intervention/Rationale
	• Help couple explore their feelings and eventually accept the normal ambivalence toward expectations of being a parent. • Promote grief work with responses to grieving process of denial, isolation, depression, anger, guilt, fear, and rejection.
Ineffective individual coping	• Assess both partners' coping mechanisms. • Explain consequences of prolonged stress. • Help couple problem solve in constructive manner. • Discuss alternatives to treatment. • See also p. 1804.
Body image disturbance	• Encourage patient to express feelings about the way patient views himself or herself. • Clarify misconceptions. • Promote sharing of feelings with partner. • Explore patient's personal strengths and resources. • Promote discussion regarding resolution of altered body image.

Evaluation

Patient Outcome	Data Indicating That Outcome is Reached
Realistic self-concept is achieved.	Patient exhibits adaptive responses to altered body image through verbal statements.
Grief is resolved.	Patient has expressed grief, shared concerns with partner, and planned constructively for future.
Knowledge of sexual functions is increased.	Patient indicates practice of optimum sexual technique. Patient relates valid information about sexual function.
Patient uses adaptive coping behavior.	Patient verbalizes feelings about infertility and can identify personal strengths. Patient follows through with decisions and appropriate actions.

BREAST DISEASE

Fibrocystic disease of the breast

Fibrocystic disease of the breast is the presence of singular or multiple cysts in the breast. The condition is also called mammary dysplasia or cystic hyperplasia.

Fibrocystic disease is the single most common disease of the breast, accounting for more than half of all surgical procedures on the female breast. It affects 10% to 25% of all women, but it is not always clinically apparent and frequently is undiscovered until postmortem examination. Fibrocystic disease occurs primarily in the menopause years and is a rare occurrence before adolescence and after menopause.[51]

Pathophysiology

Fibrocystic disease is thought to be caused by hormonal imbalance in the reproductive years, principally because of estrogen excess and progesterone deficiency during the luteal phase of the menstrual cycle. It is characterized by pain and tenderness of one or both breasts immediately before menses. The cysts may be unilateral or bilateral, firm, regular in shape, and mobile and are most common in the upper outer quadrant of the breasts. Their size may fluctuate during the cycle.

A wide variety of morphologic changes can be found, ranging from an overgrowth of fibrous stroma to a proliferation of epithelium. Four patterns of morphologic change are distinguishable: fibrosis, cyst formation, sclerosing adenosis, and duct epithelial hyperplasia.

Fibrosis is characterized by an overgrowth of stromal fibrous tissue. This type is usually unilateral and occurs most often in women from 30 to 35 years of age. The breast becomes larger before menses and then regresses with a recurrence of pain and tenderness in the next cycle.

Cystic disease is also known as Bloodgood's disease, Schimnelbusch's disease, and blue dome cyst. It is characterized by the formation of cysts, usually over 3 mm in diameter. It is thought to be caused by dilation of ducts and hyperplasia of ductal epithelium concurrent with the menstrual cycle. This type of disease is more common in women between 45 and 55 years of age. Multiple bilateral cysts are readily palpable and usually distinguishable from the characteristic solitary focus of carcinoma.[23,51]

The histologic characteristics of sclerosing adenosis are proliferation of small acini and intralobular fibrosis. It is most commonly unilateral and more common in women between 35 and 45 years of age.

Epithelial hyperplasia of the ducts is ill-defined masses found most commonly in women between 35 and 45 years of age. The more atypical the hyperplasia, the greater the risk of carcinoma.[23,51]

Biopsy and examination of the tissue is the only method of specifically differentiating fibrocystic disease from carcinoma.

Women with fibrocystic disease have a nearly threefold greater risk of developing carcinoma than women without it.

Diagnostic Studies and Findings

Biopsy

Fibrosis: Collagenous stroma engulfing epithelial structures and obliterating periductal and myxomatous stroma

Cysts: Overgrowth of stroma with cystic dilation of ducts filled with serous opaque fluid

Fibroadenosis: Proliferation and compression of small ducts and gland buds

Epithelial hyperplasia: Proliferation of epithelium lining duct, sometimes with solid masses of hyperplastic cells encroaching into lumen of duct

Needle Aspiration of Cyst

Varying histologic descriptions

Medical Plan

Surgery

Subcutaneous mastectomy in lieu of multiple diagnostic biopsies and associated discomfort

Medication

Progestins or progestogens

Progesterone (Proluton, others), 5-50 mg IM during second half of cycle

General Management

Local heat

Support bra

Avoidance of foods with methylxanthines, including tea, coffee, cola, and chocolate, which tend to stimulate cyclic adenosine monophosphate (AMP) and increase metabolic activity in breast[39]

NURSING CARE

Nursing Assessment

Breast

Palpation of discrete or diffuse nodules; asymmetry; nipple discharge; irregular firmness; cyclic pain of cystic area during premenstrual period

Nursing Dx & Intervention

Nursing Diagnosis	Nursing Intervention/Rationale
Anxiety	• Explain rationale for tests and procedures. • Encourage verbalization of concerns. • Answer patient's questions and explain disease process. • See also p. 1743.
Pain	• Encourage use of bra *to maintain adequate breast support.*

Patient Education

1. Ensure that the patient understands the method for breast self-examination (BSE) and can demonstrate this procedure.
2. Explain that only 10% to 15% of masses are malignant and that 90% of cancers confined to the breast are curable.
3. Outline a diet that avoids foods with methylxanthines.
4. Explain need to avoid film mammography if compression of breast during this procedure is painful. Xeromammography may be an alternative.
5. Explain importance of maintaining appointments for clinical examination and mammography.

Evaluation

Patient Outcome	Data Indicating That Outcome is Reached
Anxiety is diminished.	Patient demonstrates adaptive responses to knowledge about and prognosis related to fibrocystic disease.
Patient understands and monitors condition.	Patient demonstrates BSE and lists progression of signs and symptoms to report to health care provider, including increase in dimension of cyst, change in texture, lack of clearly defined margins, nipple discharge, severe pain, immobility of cysts, skin dimpling or retraction, and increasing asymmetry. Patient avoids foods with methylxanthines.

Medical Interventions and Related Nursing Care

Dilation and Curettage

Description and Rationale

Dilation and curettage is the expansion of the cervix and scraping of the uterine endometrium. It is performed for diagnostic or therapeutic purposes, such as the removal of retained products of conception after an incomplete abortion.

NURSING CARE

Nursing Assessment

Bleeding

Vaginal hemorrhage

Pain

Pelvic and low back pain

Signs of Infection

Foul odor of vaginal drainage; fever; hematuria

Nursing Dx & Intervention

Nursing Diagnosis	Nursing Intervention/Rationale
Altered renal, cerebral, cardiopulmonary, gastrointestinal, and peripheral tissue perfusion	• Monitor blood pressure, temperature, pulse, and respirations as indicated by condition until patient is stable.
Potential for infection	• Administer perineal care after elimination as necessary. • Explain importance of wiping from front to back after elimination. • Explain that shower is preferred to tub bath for 3 to 4 days. • If vaginal packing was used, ensure that it is removed by the physician as indicated in the medical plan of care.
Pain	• Administer analgesics as ordered.

Patient Education

1. Explain that spotting and bleeding may last a week and may be accompanied by cramping.
2. Explain signs and symptoms of infection that should be reported to the physician.
3. Inform the patient that coitus and douching should be avoided for 2 to 3 weeks.
4. Explain that minimum activity is preferred for 2 to 3 days.

Evaluation

Patient Outcome	Data Indicating That Outcome is Reached
Vital signs are within normal limits.	Temperature, pulse, respirations, and blood pressure are within normal limits.
There are no signs of infection.	Color and amount of urine are normal. Vaginal drainage decreases in amount and is not purulent.
Comfort is achieved.	Patient says that she is comfortable and does not have uterine cramping.

Salpingectomy

Description and Rationale

Salpingectomy is the removal of one or both fallopian tubes. It is performed for ectopic or tubal pregnancy, chronic salpingitis, and hydrosalpinx.

Nursing Care

The care of a patient undergoing salpingectomy is similar to that of a patient with total hysterectomy, with a few exceptions:

Anti-Rh globulin should be administered to an Rh-negative woman following a unilateral salpingectomy for tubal pregnancy.

The patient should understand the importance of preventing pregnancy for at least 2 months or as indicated by the physician and that reproductive ability is usually diminished, especially if a tubal pregnancy occurred as a result of acute or chronic salpingitis.

Her partner should be included in the discussion of feelings of loss and grief, especially if pregnancy was desired.

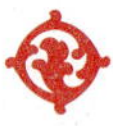

Total Abdominal Hysterectomy and Bilateral Salpingo-Oophorectomy

Description and Rationale

Surgical removal of the uterus, both fallopian tubes, and the ovaries is most commonly done to treat malignant neoplastic disease of the reproductive tract and chronic endometriosis. Other indications for hysterectomy are an enlarged myoma, adenomyosis, and hydrosalpinx. If possible, a portion of one ovary is left to prevent symptoms of sudden menopause. The patient is under general anesthesia during the procedure.

Contraindication and Cautions

Abdominal hysterectomy is preferred to vaginal hysterectomy when the diagnosis is in question and exploration is needed, when the uterus is excessively large, when an incidental appendectomy is to be done, and when there is a history of severe pelvic inflammatory disease.

Preprocedural Nursing Care

A douche with an antiseptic soluton is usually ordered the evening before or the morning of surgery, or both.

NURSING CARE

Nursing Assessment

Perineum

Vaginal hemorrhage; vaginal discharge other than serosanguineous; vaginal discharge with foul odor

Temperature

Fever

Abdomen

Redness, pain, swelling, or drainage at site of incision

Pelvic Area

Congestion as evidenced by fullness, pain, or thrombophlebitis of legs

Urinary Output

Retention of urine, with or without overflow; burning, urgency, and frequency of urination; vaginal leakage of urine

Other Complications

Paralytic ileus; pneumonia; ligation of ureter during surgery

Mental Status

Emotional investment in value of uterus; signs of depression; misconceptions about procedure

Nursing Dx & Intervention

Nursing Diagnosis	Nursing Intervention/Rationale
Altered renal, cerebral, cardiopulmonary, gastrointestinal, and peripheral tissue perfusion	• Provide routine measures for postanesthesia recovery. • Monitor blood pressure, temperature, pulse, and respiration every 4 hours for 24 hours, then four times a day for 2 days or as ordered. • Avoid placing patient in high Fowler's position and placing pressure under knees *to promote venous circulation in legs.* • Apply antiembolic stockings as ordered *to prevent thrombus formation in legs.* • Auscultate abdomen for bowel sounds every 6 to 8 hours. Permit nothing by mouth until bowel sounds are active *to prevent paralytic ileus.* • Assist with initial ambulation as needed *to support if faintness occurs secondary to orthostatic hypotension.*
Potential fluid volume deficit	• Administer parenteral fluids as ordered, progressing to 3000 ml of fluid orally daily. • Monitor intake and output *to ensure appropriate hydration and fluid balance.*
Ineffective breathing pattern	• Assist with turning, coughing, and deep breathing every 2 hours or as needed, decreasing frequency as patient increases general activity *to prevent stasis of pulmonary secretions and risk of pneumonia.* • Auscultate chest for breath sounds four times a day for 2 days and as needed thereafter *to ensure that breath sounds are clear.*
Impaired skin integrity	• Observe incision for drainage or hemorrhage every 2 to 4 hours, decreasing frequency as indicated. • Change or reinforce dressing as indicated.
Constipation	• Progress to high-protein or high-fiber diet as ordered *to promote adequate nutritional status for wound healing.* • Give Harris flush or insert rectal tube *for gas as indicated.* • Give stool softeners or mild laxatives as ordered *to prevent constipation and straining at stool.*
Altered patterns of urinary elimination	• Connect indwelling catheter to drainage bag. • Promote micturition when catheter is removed *to avoid the need for recatheterization.* • Monitor for signs of urine retention, such as small amounts of urine voided or a distended bladder. • Encourage voiding on commode rather than bedpan *to promote complete emptying of bladder.*
Bathing/hygiene self-care deficit	• Assist with bed bath, allowing patient to bathe or shower alone when indicated. • Administer catheter care twice a day or as needed until removed.
Body image disturbance	• Encourage patient's comments and questions about surgery, progress, and prognosis *to encourage understanding of same.* • Reinforce correct information and provide factual information *to correct any misconceptions.* • Encourage patient to talk about feelings with significant others. • Acknowledge the patient's feelings to support her in sharing this information with significant others.
Pain	• Administer analgesics as ordered. • Assist with moving and positioning *to promote comfort.*
Sexual dysfunction (potential)	• Encourage patient to express any concerns in a private setting. • Avoid premature responses and reassurances *to promote full expression of concerns.* • Be aware of own values regarding sexuality and body image *to avoid transference or overidentification with the patient.* • Consistently use terminology the patient understands.

Patient Education

1. Instruct the patient to avoid coitus or douching for 6 weeks or as indicated by physician to maintain integrity of the vaginal cuff, the healing process, and to prevent infection.
2. Instruct the patient to walk at regular intervals and to avoid sitting for prolonged periods at home or when traveling.
3. Explain incision care and signs of infection to report to the physician, including redness, swelling, pain, or discharge at the incision site, increase in vaginal drainage, or presence of foul odor.
4. Emphasize the need to avoid heavy lifting and vigorous activities for 6 to 8 weeks after surgery.

5. Instruct the patient to maintain regular outpatient gynecologic examinations.
6. If both ovaries have been removed, explain that surgical menopause will occur and that replacement estrogen may be ordered.
7. If both ovaries have been removed, explain that menstruation will no longer occur and that pregnancy is no longer possible.

Evaluation

Patient Outcome	Data Indicating That Outcome is Reached
Body functioning is normal.	Wound healing is normal. Vaginal drainage is absent. Bowel and bladder elimination are adequate. Ventilatory pattern has returned to presurgical state.
Patient resumes activities of daily living.	Patient walks with erect posture. Patient avoids prolonged sitting and heavy work until physician permits them.
There is no infection.	There is no evidence of inflammation, swelling, pain, or discharge at abdominal site, no fever, and no purulent or odorous vaginal discharge. Urinary elimination pattern is normal.
Comfort is achieved.	Patient says she has no lower abdominal, pelvic, or vaginal pain.
Patient demonstrates adaptive responses related to self-concept.	Patient asks appropriate questions. Patient gives correct information related to procedure and prognosis. Patient speaks appropriately about body parts that are present or absent.
Patient makes sexual adjustment.	Patient indicates that she has discussed concerns with partner. Patient expresses sexual concerns and is working toward resolution of any related problems.

Tubal Ligation

Description and Rationale

Tubal ligation is tying of the fallopian tubes. Usually the procedure includes excision of a portion of the tubes to ensure that their continuity is disrupted. The procedure is done to provide permanent sterilization. Generally the procedure is done through the laparoscope with the patient under a general or local anesthetic. However, it can be performed through an abdominal incision, as is often done in the immediate postpartum period.

NURSING CARE

Nursing Assessment

Pain

Abdominal pain

Signs of Infection

Inflammation at site of incision; fever

Other Complications

Abdominal distention; absence of bowel sounds; body image disturbances

Nursing Dx & Intervention

Nursing Diagnosis	Nursing Intervention/Rationale
Altered cardiopulmonary, gastrointestinal, and peripheral tissue perfusion	• Monitor blood pressure, temperature, pulse, and respirations as indicated until patient is stable.
Impaired skin integrity	• Observe site of incision for inflammation. • Keep dressing dry; patient should not shower for at least 24 hours.
Pain related to altered bowel motility	• Auscultate bowel sounds *to confirm peristalsis before giving food or fluids by mouth.* • Administer stool softeners as indicated. • Give Harris flush or insert rectal tube *to relieve abdominal distention.*
Pain related to incision	• Administer analgesics as ordered.

Nursing Diagnosis	Nursing Intervention/Rationale
Body image disturbance	• Encourage patient to express feelings and concerns. • Correct any misconceptions. Explain that hormonal therapy is not necessary, *because ovaries are not affected by this procedure.*

Patient Education

1. Explain that sterility is considered permanent and is rarely reversible.
2. Explain that libido will not be diminished and is often increased by removal of fear of pregnancy.
3. Inform the patient that ovarian function will continue, because the ovaries are not removed in this procedure.
4. Explain signs and symptoms of wound infection that should be reported to the physician.

Evaluation

Patient Outcome	Data Indicating That Outcome is Reached
Incision heals normally.	Site of incision shows no signs of inflammation or infection.
Patient has normal body functioning.	Vital signs are within normal limits. Bowel function is normal.
Patient has no disturbance in self-concept.	Patient does not report adverse changes in body image.

References

1. American College of Obstetricians and Gynecologists Precis III: An update in obstetrics and gynecology, Washington, DC, 1986, ACOG.
2. Aral SO, Mosher WG, and Cates W: Contraceptive use, pelvic inflammatory disease and fertility problems among American women: 1982, Am J Obstet Gynecol 157:1, 1987.
3. Babson S et al: Diagnosis and management of the fetus and neonate at risk, St Louis, 1980, The CV Mosby Co.
4. Benson R: Handbook of obstetrics and gynecology, Los Altos, Calif, 1980, Lange Medical Publications.
5. Berne RM and Levy MN: Physiology, St Louis, 1983, The CV Mosby Co.
6. Billings DM and Stokes LG: Medical surgical nursing: common health problems of adults and children across the life span, ed 2, St Louis, 1986, The CV Mosby Co.
7. Bobak IM and Jensen MD: Essentials of maternity nursing: the nurse and the childbearing family, ed 2, St Louis, 1987, The CV Mosby Co.
8. Brincat M et al: Skin collagen changes in postmenopausal women receiving different regimens of estrogen therapy, Obstet Gynecol 70:1, 1987.
9. Brosens IA, Verleyen A, and Cornillie F: The morphologic effect of short-term medical therapy of endometriosis, Am J Obstet Gynecol 157:1215, 1987.
10. Brunham RC: Therapy for acute pelvic inflammatory disease: a critique of recent treatment trials, Am J Obstet Gynecol 148:235, 1984.
11. Cancer Statistics, 1986, New York, American Cancer Society.
12. Centers for Disease Control: Statistics on abortion; 1981 end of year figures, Los Angeles Times, July 7, 1984.
13. Chez RA and Yuzpe AA: Postcoital contraception for unprotected intercourse, Contemp Ob/Gyn 20:79, 1982.
14. Creasy RK and Resnick R, editors: Maternal-fetal medicine, Philadelphia, 1984, WB Saunders Co.
15. Danforth D, editor: Obstetrics and gynecology, Philadelphia, 1983, Harper & Row Publishers Inc.
16. Davidson BJ: Current treatment of the anovulatory infertile woman, Am J Cont Educ Nurs 2:37, 1987.
17. DeCherney AH et al: Dysfunctional uterine bleeding, Obstet Gynecol 70:668, 1987.
18. El-Roeiy A et al: Correlation between peripheral blood and follicular fluid auto-antibodies and impact on in-vitro fertilization, Obstet Gynecol 70:163, 1987.
19. Fanaroff AA and Martin RJ: Behrman's neonatal-perinatal medicine, ed 4, St Louis, 1987, The CV Mosby Co.
20. Faratian B et al: Premenstrual syndrome: weight, abdominal swelling, perceived body image, Am J Obstet Gynecol 150:200, 1984.
21. Fridell S and Mercer LJ: Non-menstrual toxic shock syndrome, Obstet Gynecol 4:336, 1986.
22. Gleicher N et al: Is endometriosis an autoimmune disease: Obstet Gynecol 70:115, 1987.
23. Gompel C and Silverberg SG: Pathology in gynecology and obstetrics, Philadelphia, 1985, JB Lippincott Co.
24. Gordon M: Manual of nursing diagnosis, New York, 1982, McGraw-Hill Book Co.
25. Guzick DS and Rock JA: A comparison of danazol and conservative surgery for the treatment of infertility due to mild or moderate endometriosis, Fertil Steril 40:580, 1983.
26. Hammond MG and Tolbert LM: Infertility, Oradell, NJ, 1985, Medical Economics Co Inc.
27. Health United States 1979, DHEW Pub No 80-1232, Washington, DC, 1980, US Dept of Health, Education and Welfare, Public Health Service.
28. Jacobs SW and Francone CA: Structure and function in man, Philadelphia, 1982, WB Saunders Co.
29. Kase NC and Weingold AB: Principles and practice of clinical gynecology, New York, 1983, John Wiley & Sons.
30. Kendall KE and Schnurr PP: The effects of vitamin B_6 supplementation on premenstrual symptoms, Obstet Gynecol 70:145, 1987.
31. Kim MJ, McFarland GK, and McLane AM: Pocket guide to nursing diagnosis, ed 2, St Louis, 1987, The CV Mosby Co.

32. Loucks A: Pelvic inflammatory disease, Nurse Pract 8:13, 1983.
33. Malasanos L et al: Health assessment, ed 3, St Louis, 1986, The CV Mosby Co.
34. Martin L: Health care of women, Philadelphia, 1978, JB Lippincott Co.
35. Masters W and Johnson V: Human sexual response, Boston, 1966, Little Brown & Co.
36. McKenzie CA and Edlund B, editors: Nurs Clin North Am 17(1), 1982.
37. Merck manual, Rahway, NJ, 1982, Merck Sharp & Dohme Research Laboratories.
38. Methods of midtrimester abortion, Technical Bulletin of the American College of Obstetricians and Gynecologists, No 56, Washington, DC, 1979.
39. Minton JP et al: Caffeine, nucleotides and breast disease, Surgery 86:105, 1979.
40. Mishell DR: Menopause: physiology and pharmacology, Chicago, 1987, Yearbook Medical Publishers.
41. Mishell DR and Brenner PF: Management of common problems in obstetrics and gynecology, Oradell, NJ, 1983, Medical Economics Books.
42. Mosby's medical and nursing dictionary, ed 2, St Louis, 1986, The CV Mosby Co.
43. Mountcastle VB: Medical physiology, ed 14, St Louis, 1980, The CV Mosby Co.
44. National Center for Health Statistics: Monthly vital statistics report, Vol 33, No 6, Sept 20, 1984.
45. National Center for Health Statistics: Monthly vital statistics report, Vol 32, No 13, Sept 21, 1984.
46. Newton N: Interrelationships between sexual responsiveness, birth and breast feeding. In Zubin J and Money J, editors: Contemporary sexual behavior: critical issues in the 1970's, Baltimore, 1973, Johns Hopkins Press.
47. Petitti DB, Perlman JA, and Stephen S: Non-contraceptive estrogens and mortality: long-term follow-up of women in the Walnut Creek study, Obstet Gynecol 70:289, 1987.
48. Phipps WJ, Long BC, and Woods NF: Shafer's medical-surgical nursing, ed 7, St Louis, 1980, The CV Mosby Co.
49. Pritchard JA and MacDonald PC: Williams' obstetrics, New York, 1980, Appleton-Century-Crofts.
50. Rapkin AJ et al: Whole blood serotonin in premenstrual syndrome, Obstet Gynecol 70:533, 1987.
51. Robbins S and Cotran R: Pathologic basis of disease, Philadelphia, 1979, WB Saunders Co.
52. Sarno AP, Miller EJ, and Lundblad EG: Premenstrual syndrome: beneficial effects of periodic low dose danazol, Obstet Gynecol 70:33, 1987.
53. Smith ED: Women's health care: a guide for patient education, New York, 1981, Appleton-Century-Crofts.
54. Smith S et al: Treatment of premenstrual syndrome with alprazolam, Obstet Gynecol 70:37, 1987.
55. Thomason JL: Pelvic inflammatory disease: diagnosis and management, Female Patient 9:38, 1984.
56. Thompson JM and Bowers AC: Clinical manual of health assessment, St Louis, 1980, The CV Mosby Co.
57. Tilkian SM, Conover MB, and Tilkian AG: Clinical implications of laboratory tests, ed 4, St Louis, 1987, The CV Mosby Co.
58. Tucker SM et al: Patient care standards, St Louis, 1988, The CV Mosby Co.
59. US National Center for Health Statistics: Vital statistics of the United States, Washington, DC, 1982, US Government Printing Office.
60. Vargyas JM, Campeau JD, and Mishell DR: Treatment of menorrhagia with meclofenamate sodium, Am J Obstet Gynecol 157:944, 1987.
61. Viega-Ferreira MM et al: Cervical endometriosis: facilitated diagnosis by fine needle aspiration cytologic testing, Am J Obstet Gynecol 157:849, 1987.
62. Willson JR and Carrington ER: Obstetrics and gynecology, St Louis, 1983: The CV Mosby Co.
63. Wilson MA: Menstrual disorders: premenstrual syndrome, dysmenorrhea, amenorrhea, JOGN 13(suppl 2):11s, 1984.
64. Worthington-Roberts BS, Vermeersch J, and Williams SR: Nutrition in pregnancy and lactation, St Louis, 1984, The CV Mosby Co.
65. Wroblewski SS: Toxic shock syndrome, Am J Nurs 81:82, 1981.

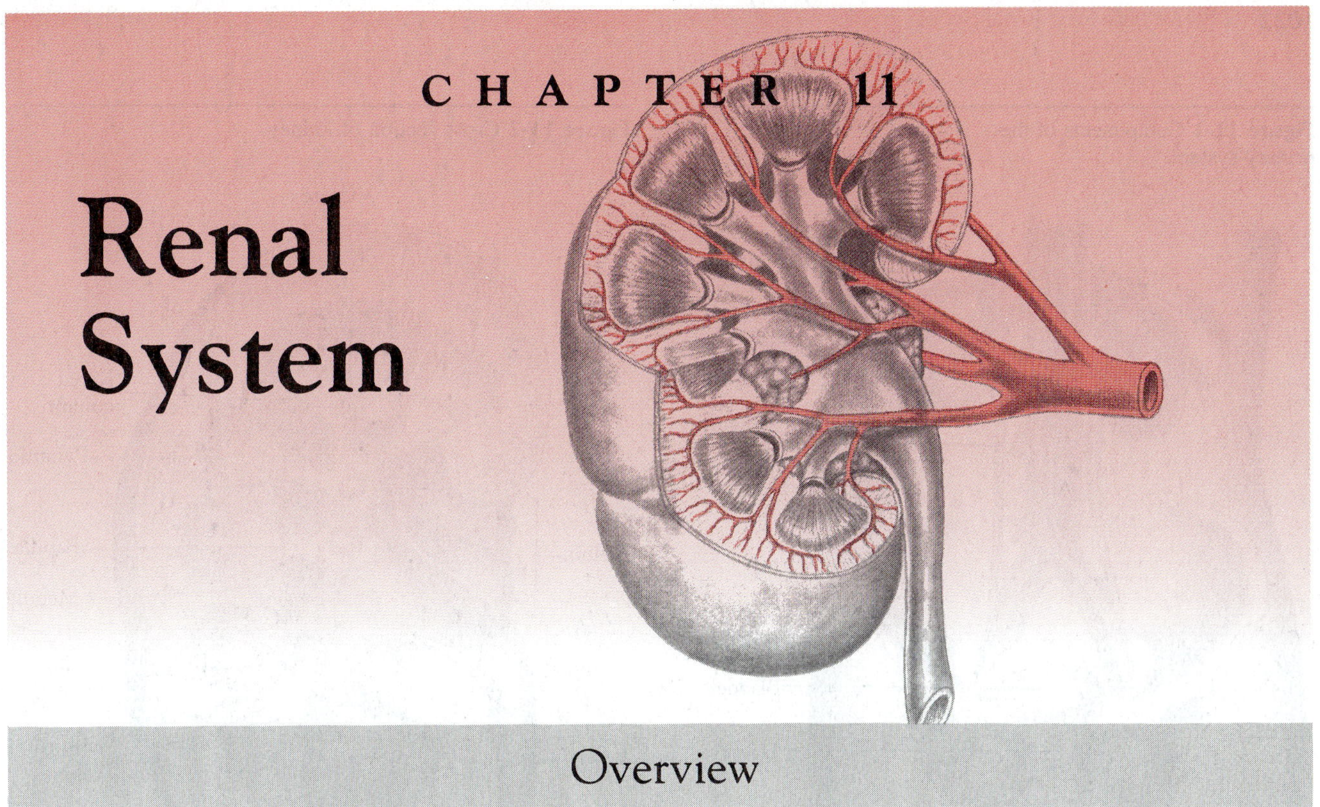

CHAPTER 11

Renal System

Overview

The kidneys are a major part of the urinary system, which also includes the ureters, urinary bladder, and urethra. These latter three components transport and store the urine formed by the kidneys and eventually expel it from the body.

Renal function depends on the normal and interrelated functioning of the cardiovascular, nervous, endocrine, and urinary collecting systems. The cardiovascular system delivers the blood to be filtered, sustains the hydrostatic pressure needed for filtration, and provides specialized capillaries that do the filtering. The nervous system helps regulate blood pressure, thus contributing to the first two functions.

An increase in blood pressure causes the kidneys to increase excretion of sodium and water to decrease extracellular fluid and return the blood pressure to normal. If blood pressure is lower than normal, the kidneys retain sodium and water to increase the extracellular fluid and return the blood pressure to normal. Increased blood pressure inhibits the secretion of renin.

The nervous system also controls the process of urination (see Chapter 12) and interacts with the activity of the endocrine system to affect renal function directly through aldosterone and antidiuretic hormone (ADH). The calyces, pelvis, ureters, urinary bladder, and urethra form the urinary collecting system. The urethra provides the exit for urine from the body.

Urine volume varies with food and fluid intake and extrarenal fluid losses through feces, perspiration, and respiration. A diurnal variation in volume that is associated with light-dark periods or sleep-wake patterns occurs.

The kidneys have excretory and nonexcretory functions vital to the regulation of substances essential to the human body.

Excretory functions are excretion of end products of metabolism (urea, creatinine, uric acid, phosphates, sulfates, nitrates, and phenols); excretion of excess normal fluid and electrolyte components (H_2O, Na^+, K^+, HCO_3^-, Cl^-, H^+), thus maintaining the volume and osmolality of the extracellular and intracellular fluids; and excretion of certain drugs and other substances (penicillin and metabolites of hormones).

Nonexcretory functions are secretion of renin, erythropoietin, kallikrein, and prostaglandins; metabolism of carbohydrates, lipids, plasma proteins, and peptide hormones such as insulin and glucagon; and regulation of vitamin D metabolism.

For additional information on the genitourinary system, see Chapter 12.

Anatomy, Physiology, and Related Pathophysiology

The kidneys are located in the posterior abdominal cavity in the retroperitoneal area to the right and left of the lumbar spinal column. Each kidney is covered by a tough capsule, surrounded by a cushion of fat, and supported by fascia. Each kidney is partially protected by the ribs. The lower end of each kidney extends below the ribs; the right one is lower than the left (Figure 11-1). The kidneys move downward during respiration as the diaphragm contracts.

Each kidney has an outer cortex, an inner medulla, and a pelvis, the area in which urine is collected (Figure 11-2). The fluid filtered from the blood travels through the nephron to

Figure 11-1 Components of the urinary system.

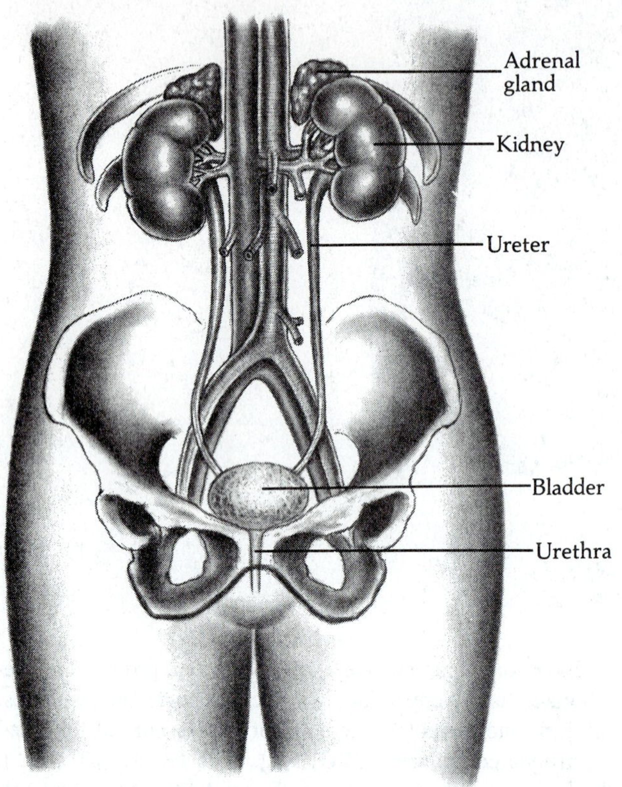

Figure 11-2 Cross section of kidney.

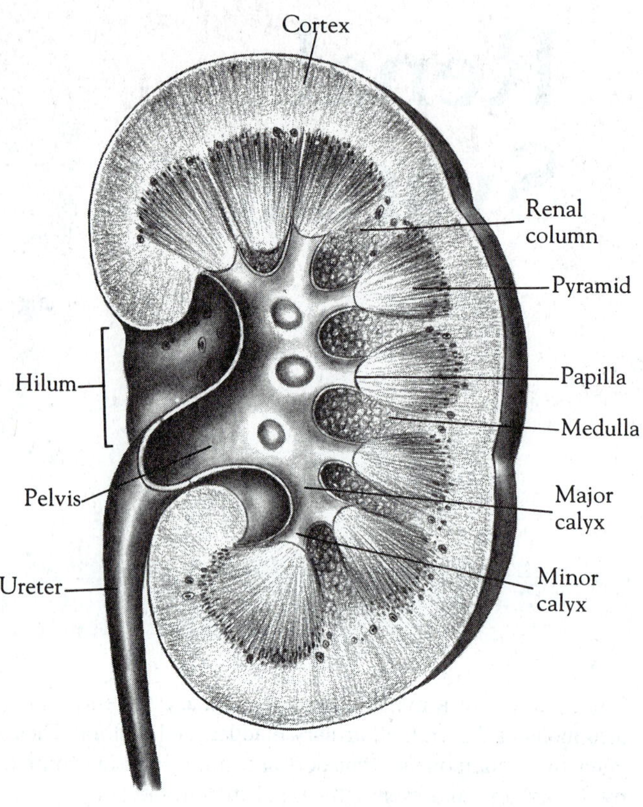

reach the large collecting ducts (ducts of Bellini) that form the renal pyramids in the medulla. The ducts empty into a calyx at the papilla. Interspersed between the pyramids is cortical tissue known as the "renal columns" (columns of Bertin). The glomerulus, proximal and distal tubules, and most of the loop of Henle are in the cortex. The deepest part of the loop of Henle and the collecting ducts are in the medulla.

Blood Supply

The renal artery and nerves enter and the renal vein and ureter leave the kidney at the hilum. The blood pumped to the kidneys with each heartbeat equals about one fourth to one fifth of cardiac output. Almost 90% of the blood flows rapidly through the cortex; the rest moves slowly through the medulla. The renal artery branches into interlobar, arcuate, and interlobular arteries (Figure 11-3). Veins draining the kidneys follow the same pattern as the arteries.

Nephrons are divided into superficial cortical and juxtamedullary nephrons. The efferent arteriole of the superficial cortical nephron divides to form a peritubular capillary network. The efferent arteriole of the juxtamedullary nephron branches to form a peritubular network and a series of vascular loops, the vasa recta, that form a capillary network around the collecting ducts and ascending limbs of the loop of Henle. Each nephron is perfused by peritubular capillaries arising from the efferent arterioles of many different glomeruli.

Each nephron can control the amount of blood that enters and leaves the glomerulus by means of the afferent and efferent arterioles. Such autoregulation permits the kidney to respond to variations in blood flow and pressure.

Autonomic nerve fibers are found in the kidneys. They are thought to mediate renal vasoconstriction.

The Nephron

The nephron is the functional unit of the kidney (Figure 11-4). Each nephron is composed of a glomerulus with afferent and efferent arterioles, Bowman's capsule, proximal tubule, loop of Henle, distal tubule, and a collecting duct.

The major functions of the nephron components are:

Glomerulus: filtration

Proximal tubule: reabsorption of Na^+, H^+, H_2O (antidiuretic hormone [ADH] not required), glucose, K^+, amino acids, Cl^-, HCO_3^-, $PO_4^=$, urea; secretion of H^+ and foreign substances

Henle's loop: countercurrent flow, concentration of urine; Na^+ is passively and Cl^- is actively reabsorbed; Ca^{++} is reabsorbed

Figure 11-3 Blood supply of nephron.

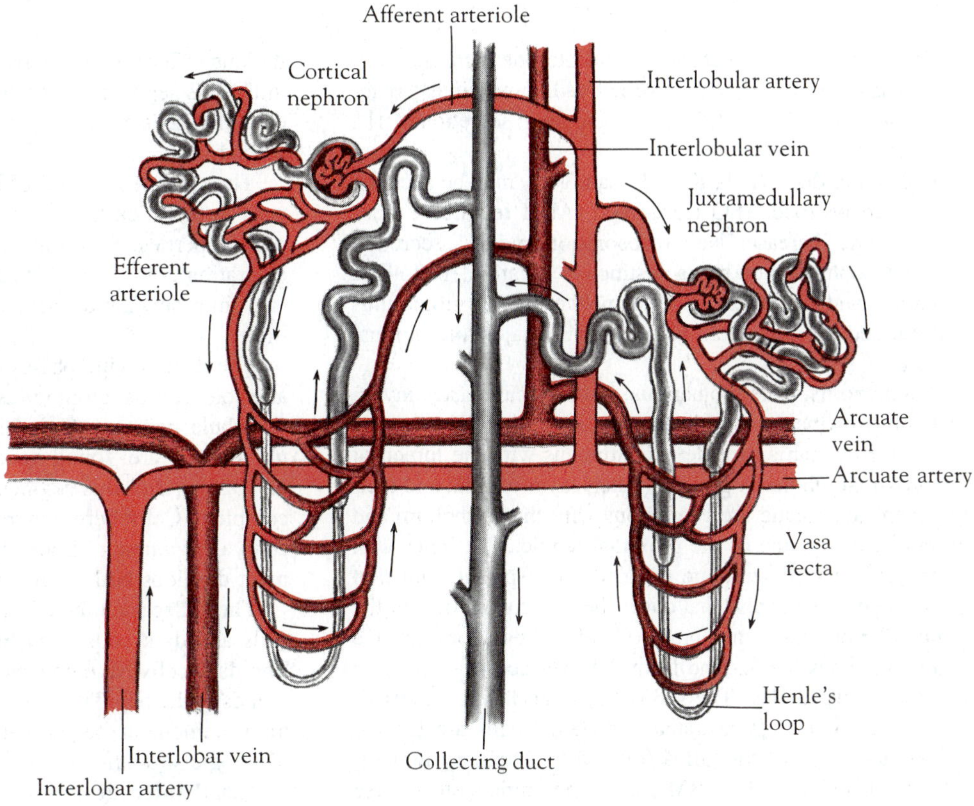

Figure 11-4 Components of nephron.

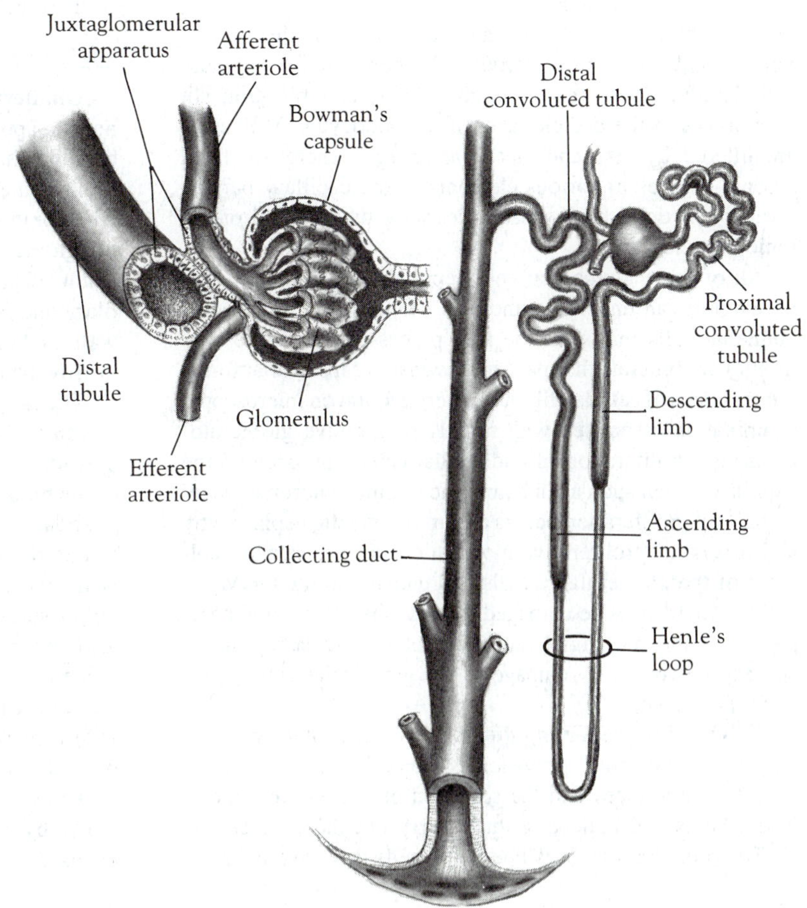

Distal tubule: Na^+ reabsorbed (aldosterone increases Na^+ reabsorption); H_2O reabsorbed (ADH required); reabsorption of Cl^-, HCO_3^-, K^+, and urea; secretion of H^+ and K^+

Collecting duct: Na^+, K^+, H^+, and NH_3 may be secreted or reabsorbed; H_2O reabsorbed (ADH required); aldosterone increases Na^+ reabsorption and K^+ secretion

Each nephron part has a distinctive location, histologic structure, and pattern of vascular network. The glomerulus is discussed in some detail because of its major role in renal disease.

Glomerulus. The glomerulus, a tuft of capillaries invaginated in Bowman's capsule, serves as the filter. The urinary space in Bowman's capsule is continuous with the lumen of the proximal tubule. A parietal (outer) layer of cells and their basement membrane are continuous with the epithelium and basement membrane of the proximal tubule. The inner wall of the cup-shaped structure is lined with special epithelial cells called "podocytes" that cover the external surface of the glomerular basement membrane (GBM). The podocytes have many processes that extend from their surfaces to form foot processes or pedicles. The GBM has three layers: external, middle, and inner. Fenestrated endothelial cells are located on the inner side of the GBM (toward the capillary lumen). Also on this side of the GBM are the mesangial cells. These irregularly shaped cells embedded in an amorphous matrix form a slender branching stalk of specialized connective tissue that supports the capillaries.

Thus the filtration barrier has numerous complex layers. Solutes and water move through the pores in the capillary endothelium, loose matrix of the GBM, and filtration slit membranes of the pedicle layer of the podocytes. Molecules are filtered by size and electrical charge. There are fixed anionic charges in various elements of the capillary barrier. Cationic particles have greater clearance than neutral or anionic particles.[33]

All of these glomerular cells (epithelial, endothelial, and mesangial) can undergo pathologic changes: proliferation of epithelial cells may fuse the foot processes (nephrotic syndrome) or obliterate the space in Bowman's capsule that forms the crescents of cellular-fibrous material found on microscopic examination associated with rapidly progressive glomerulonephritis. Proliferation of endothelial cells may occlude the capillary lumen such as in hemolytic uremic syndrome. Mesangial cell proliferation occurs as part of diabetic nephropathy and membranoproliferative glomerulonephritis, causing collapse of the glomerular vessels and damage to the GBM.

The GBM may be damaged by deposits of immune complexes in the mesangial, subendothelial, and subepithelial spaces, as well as by damage to the glomerular cells previously described.

Tubules and collecting ducts.[8] Since the filtering mechanism is nonspecific, provision is made for reabsorption of essential substances and the secretion of excess substances. The tubules and collecting ducts carry out these functions.

The proximal tubule is lined with cells that have interdigitations to increase their area and surfaces covered by microvilli. This segment has high transport capacity and low transepithelial resistance to the movement of molecules being reabsorbed.

The cells of the loop of Henle appear to be simpler, with cells in the thick limb having highly developed active transport properties. This limb can reabsorb sodium against a concentration gradient and is relatively water impermeable. The thin limb appears to lack the transport systems of the thick limb.

The distal tubule passes between the afferent and efferent arterioles of its glomerulus. In the region where the distal tubule lies near the arteriole, specialized cells, the macula densa, are found (see "Juxtaglomerular Apparatus," p. 1026). After this segment the tubular cells become more complex. Cells here can reabsorb sodium ions without an equivalent amount of negatively charged particles. This segment develops both ionic and electrical gradients.

The collecting tubule has two well-defined cell types, light cells and dark cells. The light cells have sparse microvilli. The dark cells have conspicuous microvilli. As the duct descends to the papilla, the number of dark cells decreases until there are none in the papillary region. The significance of this histologic structure is not clear.

Renal interstitium. Cells that form the interstitium lie between the nephrons and their blood supply. More interstitial cells are found in the medulla than in the cortex. The function of these cells is unknown.[5]

Urine Formation

Glomerular filtration. Total renal blood flow to both kidneys is approximately 1200 ml/min. Approximately 650 ml of this volume is plasma; of this amount about 125 ml filters through the glomerulus to Bowman's capsule. The renal arteries branch directly off the aorta. Therefore blood perfuses the glomerulus at a high pressure. The filtration force is the result of the pressure gradient between the glomerular capillary and Bowman's space, the permeability of the capillary wall, and the difference between the colloid osmotic pressure in Bowman's space and in the capillary lumen.

The rate of glomerular filtration is proportional to filtration pressure. The glomerular filtrate is an isotonic ultrafiltrate of plasma. Large molecules of protein and the cellular elements of the blood are not filtered. The pH of the glomerular filtrate is about 7.4, or equal to that of plasma. The volume of the filtrate decreases with systemic hypotension, localized renal ischemia, urine outflow obstruction, and changes in the filtering surface. Moderate reductions in glomerular filtration also occur with exercise, pain, and dehydration. Extreme reductions in glomerular filtration occur with severe hypotension. Glomerular filtration remains fairly constant even with a marked increase in arterial blood pressure owing to the kidney's autoregulatory mechanisms.

Solute reabsorption and secretion. Solutes and water move by active and passive membrane transport mechanisms.[22] They include simple diffusion—electrochemical potential gradient; convection—hydrostatic or osmotic pressure gradient; and mediated transport—facilitated diffusion, electromechanical potential gradient, and active transport, which requires free energy from metabolism.

"Transport maximum" refers to the amount of a substance that can be reabsorbed per minute. It is a constant value, and when the amount of a substance filtered exceeds this value, the excess is excreted in the urine.

The solutes in the glomerular filtrate are threshold and nonthreshold substances. Urea, sodium, potassium, and others are nonthreshold substances, since the urine always contains at least some of each. Glucose and phosphates are threshold substances, since a certain serum level must be reached before the glomerular filtrate will contain enough that the transport maximum of the substance will be exceeded and the excess will be excreted in the urine.

As the glomerular filtrate moves through the tubules, selective reabsorption of water and solutes and selective secretion of solutes occur. A large volume of isosmotic glomerular filtrate is converted into a small volume of hyperosmotic urine. The composition of the glomerular filtrate triggers appropriate activities in the tubular cells. In the tubules about 87% of the water and electrolytes, all of the glucose, and almost all of the amino acids are reabsorbed in the proximal tubules. The proximal tubule preserves metabolically important components and resists the reabsorption of nitrogenous wastes. It secretes foreign substances. The remaining 13% of the glomerular filtrate passes through the loops of Henle and the distal tubules where variable amounts of the water and electrolytes remaining are absorbed. The exact amounts depend on the needs of the body. The final quantity of urine is about 1 ml/min. The pH of the urine may vary from 4.5 to 8.0, and the osmolality may range from one fourth to four times that of plasma (50 to 1200 mOsm/kg). Urine specific gravity may range from 1.001 to 1.030. The usual range is 1.003 to 1.029 with a normal fluid intake.

Urine concentration and dilution. Obligatory water reabsorption occurs in the proximal tubule since active reabsorption of sodium is accompanied by passive reabsorption of water and anions. Facultative water reabsorption occurs in the distal tubule. Water and solutes are reabsorbed independently, depending on the body's needs. The urine becomes either concentrated, as water without solutes is reabsorbed, or dilute, as solutes without water are reabsorbed. Antidiuretic hormone controls the volume and concentration of the urine by regulating the reabsorption of water.

The medulla increases in hypertonicity with increasing distance from the cortex. The collecting ducts, the long capillary loops (vasa recta), the slower circulation in the medulla, and the impermeability to sodium of the ascending limb of the loop of Henle contribute to the countercurrent mechanism that permits the concentration of urine (Figure 11-5).

In the juxtamedullary nephrons, the loop of Henle serves as a countercurrent multiplier; that is, it returns sodium ions to the peritubular fluid of the medulla, creating hypertonic interstitial fluid. The back-diffusion of urea (possibly a legacy of an evolutionary stage) adds to the osmolality. The degree of hypertonicity depends on antidiuretic hormone, urine flow rate, and the amount and types of solutes in the tubular fluid in the loops of Henle. The osmotic concentration may become four times that of normal extracellular fluid. The vasa recta loops receive increasing amounts of sodium chloride as the blood flows downward and reaches 1200 mOsm/kg at the bottom of the loop. As the blood flows upward, sodium chloride diffuses into the interstitial fluid, thereby remaining in the medulla. The hypertonic interstitial fluid causes water to

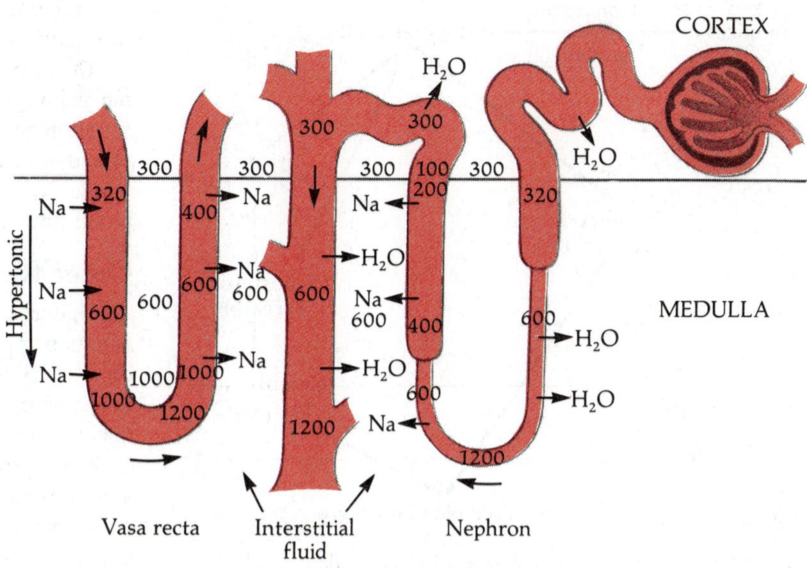

Figure 11-5 Countercurrent mechanism for concentrating urine. Numbers represent osmotic concentration (in mOsm/kg).

be absorbed by osmosis from tubular fluid in the presence of antidiuretic hormone by creating a concentration gradient. Osmoreceptors in the anterior hypothalamus regulate the secretion of antidiuretic hormone, which controls the permeability to water of the distal tubules and collecting ducts. Normally, 500 ml of concentrated urine removes the day's solutes. More than 2 L of water would be needed to excrete the same solute load in isotonic urine. Failure of the concentrating mechanism causes polyuria and especially nocturia.

Acid or alkaline urine. The kidneys excrete strong nonvolatile acids and excess alkali. They provide the third line of defense against changes in hydrogen ion concentration. Acid-base buffer systems in all body fluids and the respiratory system respond rapidly, while the kidneys require several hours to a day or more to readjust the balance. The kidneys excrete excess hydrogen ions and conserve bicarbonate ions. Chloride ions are excreted when bicarbonate ions are needed by the body. Almost all of the bicarbonate in the glomerular filtrate is reabsorbed. Excess bicarbonate ions are excreted when present, causing the urine to become alkaline.

Urine pH may range from 4.5 to 8.0. While the lungs remove the volatile acid, as in the following reaction

$$H^+ + HCO_3^- \rightleftharpoons H_2CO_3 \rightleftharpoons H_2O + CO_2 \uparrow$$

the kidneys excrete strong nonvolatile acids (sulfuric and phosphoric) and strong organic acids (ketone bodies). Hydrogen ions are buffered by bicarbonate ions. The anion base of the acid is balanced electrochemically by sodium ions (Na_2SO_4 and Na_2HPO_4). The tubular cells form bicarbonate ions that combine with the sodium ions of these salts and are reabsorbed. The tubular cell manufactures ammonia, which accepts a hydrogen ion and combines with the sulfate to form $(NH_4)_2SO_4$, which enters the urine. This mechanism permits excretion of hydrogen ions without lowering the urine pH. The Na_2HPO_4 accepts a hydrogen ion to become the acid salt, NaH_2PO_4, which is excreted. The other sodium ion is reabsorbed. Potassium and hydrogen ions compete for excretion in exchange for the reabsorbed sodium ions. The concentration of each ion is important. Acidosis and potassium depletion enhance hydrogen ion secretion. In chronic renal failure, the acid residues of nitrogen metabolism accumulate, and the tubules cannot meet the demand for hydrogen ion secretion. Since the tubular transport system is overwhelmed, potassium cannot be excreted and hyperkalemia results.

Figure 11-6 Renin-angiotensin mechanism.

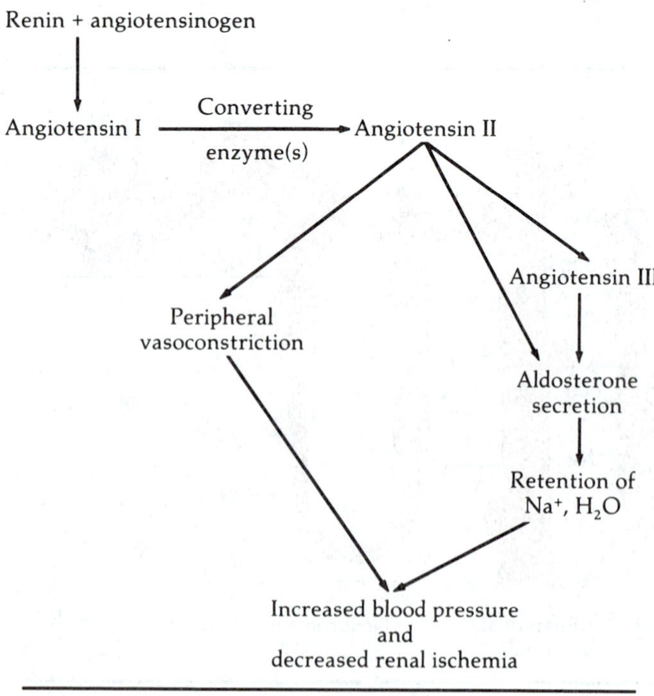

Juxtaglomerular Apparatus

The juxtaglomerular apparatus is composed of special epithelial cells (the macula densa cells) in the early distal tubule and special myoepithelial cells in the renal afferent arteriole near the glomerulus. These juxtaglomerular cells respond to renal ischemia, low sodium concentration, and activity of the renal sympathetic nerves by secreting renin, which initiates the process that results in the formation of the vasopressor substance, angiotensin II.

Renin is an enzyme that acts on angiotensinogen, a glycoprotein made in the liver, to form angiotensin I. A converting enzyme formed in the lungs changes it to angiotensin II. With the loss of an amino acid, angiotensin III is formed. These forms of angiotensin cause peripheral vasoconstriction and increased secretion of aldosterone. The first action elevates blood pressure by increasing peripheral resistance; the second action decreases salt and water loss and therefore increases extracellular fluid volume. Both actions cause an increase in arterial pressure, which relieves renal ischemia. The schema of the renin-angiotensin mechanism is outlined in Figure 11-6.[19]

The juxtaglomerular apparatus appears to play a role in the autoregulation of renal blood flow and the glomerular filtration rate (GFR) by responding either to the concentration of sodium ions or to the osmolality of the urine in the distal tubule. The conditions of the distal tubule appear to control blood flow in the afferent arteriole.

Other Renal Functions

The kidneys produce erythropoietin, which promotes differentiation, proliferation, and maturation of precursors of red blood cells in the bone marrow. Erythropoietin is produced in response to decreases in oxygen tension and renal perfusion that may arise from anemia, hypoxia, or renal ischemia.

Renal prostaglandins are synthesized in the renal cortex and medulla. They appear to be produced in response to both renal ischemia and vasoconstriction. Observations suggest that they participate in the maintenance of renal vascular resistance and glomerular filtration rate especially when renal hemodynamics are altered.[19] The complex relationships of renal prostaglandins are not yet clearly understood.

The kidneys have a role in the metabolism of vitamin D. Vitamin D_3 is formed in the skin, metabolized in the liver to 1-hydroxy D_3, and then metabolized by the kidney to an active form (1,25-dihydroxy D_3 and others). The 1,25-dihydroxy D_3 is produced in response to hypocalcemia or hypophosphatemia. It acts in conjunction with the parathyroid hormone to increase intestinal absorption of calcium and phosphate, mobilize calcium from bones, and increase renal tubular reabsorption of calcium and phosphate. The production of 1,25-dihydroxy D_3 is suppressed by hypercalcemia and hyperphosphatemia. Decreased production of 1,25-dihydroxy D_3 occurs in chronic renal failure and is considered significant in the development of renal osteodystrophy.

Concept of Clearance[19]

Since the kidneys' functions include clearing the plasma of unwanted materials, the concept of renal clearance of a substance is helpful in evaluating renal function. The rate at which a substance is excreted in terms of its plasma concentration is the clearance of that substance.

Clearance of creatinine is used to monitor renal function since it is an endogenous product from muscle creatine phosphate, and its production is relatively independent of protein anabolism and catabolism. The amount of creatinine produced depends on the lean body mass, and this variation is responsible for the differences in serum creatinine levels and creatinine clearances found in men and women. While a small part of the creatinine that appears in the urine is secreted by the tubules, the major portion is filtered by the glomerulus and is not reabsorbed. Creatinine clearance is a practical, clinically useful measure of glomerular filtration rate. Clearances show wide variations between subjects but are reproducible in the same subject. Serial clearance studies permit the following of a patient's clinical course. Creatinine clearance may be affected by the presence of high glucose concentration, acetone, acetoacetic acid, ascorbic acid, methyldopa, and levodopa in the urine. It may also be affected by a high-protein diet before the test and by strenuous exercise during the urine collection period.[31]

Because the total urine for a specified period is required for accurate determination, patients and staff must understand the procedure: (1) empty the bladder and mark the time; (2) save all urine; (3) void exactly 24 hours later (or the period specified) and save the specimen; (4) measure total volume; and (5) collect serum creatinine once during the 24-hour period.

$$\text{Creatinine clearance (ml/min)} = \frac{\text{Urine creatinine (mg/dl)} \times \text{Urine flow (ml/min)}}{\text{Serum creatinine (mg/dl)}}$$

Inulin clearance is clinically useful as a measure of glomerular filtration rate (GFR). Inulin is freely filtered by the glomerulus and is not reabsorbed or secreted by the tubules so that the amount filtered is the amount excreted. Inulin clearance is used when an exact measure of GFR is required.

$$\text{Inulin clearance (ml/min)} = \frac{\text{Urine inulin (mg/dl)} \times \text{Urine volume (ml/min)}}{\text{Plasma inulin (mg/dl)}} = \text{GFR}$$

Age and Renal Function

Differences in age are associated with differences in renal function that become clinically significant when a young or aged individual has an illness that places excessive demands on the kidneys.

The kidney is immature at birth. Renal blood flow and the glomerular filtration rate of infants are low compared with those of adults. The ability to excrete sodium, potassium, water, and acid loads is limited. The kidneys continue to develop until 1 year of age. Their combined weight continues to increase beyond adolescence (24 g at birth, 140 g at age 6 years, 183 g at age 12 years, and 300 g for adults).[16]

Renal blood flow decreases with age, which is partly related to a decrease in cardiac output.[27] The loss of renal mass and functioning nephrons also decreases the effective filtering surface and glomerular filtration rate. Creatinine clearance is stable until the fourth decade, when it begins to decrease.[28] Serum creatinine decreases with the decrease in muscle mass associated with aging. Therefore serum creatinine levels may overestimate glomerular filtration rate. To avoid overdoses of drugs in the elderly, creatinine clearance rate is used when dosage of such drugs as digoxin is determined. Also of note is the slower rate of response in elderly patients to acute changes in fluid and electrolyte balances associated with illness. The renin-aldosterone system becomes less responsive with lowered renin levels and an associated reduction in plasma level of aldosterone. The ability to conserve Na^+ and excrete K^+ is decreased. The decrease in renal response to antidiuretic hormone and in glomerular filtration rate contribute to the inability to conserve water and concentrate the urine.[27] The maintenance of Na^+, K^+, and water balance becomes exceedingly important in elderly patients.

Normal Findings

Area of Concern	Normal Adult Findings
General	
Temperature	Normal range
Blood pressure	Normal range
Weight	No marked increase (>2 kg)
Skin	Warm, dry and normal turgor; no pallor, yellowish color, excoriations, uremic snow, edema, petechiae, ecchymoses, or purpura
Eyes	No periorbital edema, redness, retinal hemorrhages, exudates, or papilledema
Ears	Hearing normal; no tophi in ear cartilages
Mouth	No odor of ammonia; no stomatitis: ulcers, exudate, or bleeding
Neck	Parathyroid glands not palpable
Chest	Normal breath sounds, rate, and rhythm; normal heart sounds, rate, and rhythm
Abdomen	Normal bowel sounds; no masses; no tenderness in flank, groin, or costovertebral angle on palpation or percussion; no bruit on auscultation
Neurologic examination	No change in cognitive function, level of consciousness, or behavior; no change in superficial or deep tendon reflexes; no change in muscle action or sensation
Extremities	No edema

Normal Laboratory Data

Laboratory Test	Normal Adult Values
Bicarbonate	21-28 mEq/L
Calcium	
Ionized	4.75-5.2 mg/dl
Ionized (calculated, blood)	3.9-4.8 mg/dl
Total	1-30 yr: 8.2-10.5 mg/dl; decreases very slightly with age
CO_2, total	
Arterial	22-29 mEq/L
Venous	23-30 mEq/L
Chloride	97-107 mEq/L
Cholesterol, total	20 yr and up: 100-210 mg/dl*
Creatinine	Men: up to 1.2 mg/dl; women: up to 1.1 mg/dl; there are slight differences between the sexes with males higher, since the range relates to the amount of muscle mass present
Glucose, fasting	2 yr-adult: 60-115 mg/dl; normal range increases with age over 50
Glucose tolerance test	Fasting: 60-115 mg/dl; 60 min: <184 mg/dl; 90 min: 100-140 mg/dl; 120 min: <138 mg/dl
Osmolality	280-300 mOsm/kg H_2O
pH	Venous: 7.32-7.43; arterial: 7.35-7.45
Protein (total serum)	6-8 g/dl
Albumin	1-31 yr: 3.5-5 g/dl; after age 40, normal range gradually decreases
Phosphorus	2.5-4.5 mg/dl
Potassium (plasma)	3.5-5 mEq/L; add approximately 0.2 to normal ranges if serum is sampled
Sodium	135-145 mEq/L
Blood urea nitrogen	1-40 yr: 5-20 mg/dl; gradual, slight increase subsequently occurs
Uric acid	Men: 3.4-7 mg/dl or slightly more; women: 2.4-6 mg/dl or slightly more
Hematology	
Hematocrit (%)	Men: 46 ± 3.1; women: 40.9 ± 3
Hemoglobin (g/dl)	Men: 15.5 ± 1.1; women: 13.7 ± 1
Platelet count	150,000-400,000/mm^3
Red blood cell count	Men: 4.6-6.2 million/mm^3; women: 3.9-5.9 million/mm^3
White blood cell count	4500-11,000/mm^3

*Sharp inconsistencies are obvious when one studies published normal ranges of serum cholesterol in the United States.

Laboratory Test	Normal Adult Values
Coagulation	
Bleeding time	Duke: 1-5 min; Ivy: 2-7 min
Clotting time (Lee-White)	8-15 min
Serology	
Antistreptolysin titer	<125 Todd U
Hepatitis associated antigen (HB_sAg)	Not detected
Urinalysis	
Calcium (24 h)	100-250 mg/d (diet dependent; based on average calcium intake of 600-800 mg/24 h)
Chloride	110-250 mEq/d
Creatinine	Men: 1-2 g/24 h; women: 0.8-1.8 g/24 h
Glucose	Up to 100 mg/24 h
Osmolality	250-900 mOsm/kg
Protein	30-150 mg/24 h (method dependent)
pH	4.5-8.0
Phosphorus	0.9-1.3 g/d (diet dependent)
Potassium	26-123 mEq/24 h (markedly intake dependent)
Sodium	27-287 mEq/24 h (diet dependent; output is lower at night)
Specific gravity	1.003-1.029 (range in SI units)
Urea nitrogen	6-17 g/d
Uric acid	250-750 mg/d
Volume	Men: 800-2000 ml/d; women: 800-1600 ml/d
Color	Pale to darker yellow
Clarity	Clear
Ketones	None
Red blood count	0-5/high-power field
White blood count	0-5/high-power field
Bacteria	None/occasional in voided specimen
Casts	0-4 hyaline casts/low-power field
Crystals	Interpreted by physician
Culture	Negative
Other	
Creatinine clearance	Men: 85-125 ml/min/1.73 m^2; women: 75-115 ml/min/1.73 m^2; geriatric: 96.9 ± 2.9 mg/min/1.73 m^2
Renal blood flow	600 ml/min/1.73 m^2; geriatric: 300 ml/min/1.73 m^2
Glomerular filtration rate	120 ml/min/1.73 m^2; geriatric: 65.3 ml/min/1.73 m^2
Plasma renin activity	Normal diet: supine 1.1 ± 0.8 ng/ml/h, upright 1.9 ± 1.7 ng/ml/h; low-sodium diet: supine 2.7 ± 1.9 ng/ml/h, upright 6.6 ± 2.5 ng/ml/h

Conditions, Diseases, and Disorders

Renal and Perinephric Abscess

A renal abscess is a localized infection found within the cortex of the kidney; a perinephric abscess extends into the fatty tissue around the kidney.

Multiple renal abscesses can occur in a normal or diseased kidney. They can be a complication of subacute bacterial endocarditis and systemic infections. Delay in treatment results in a high mortality for perinephric abscesses.

Pathophysiology

Renal abscesses may arise from diffuse pyelonephritis or hematogenous transport of bacteria that occur in a systemic infection. Staphylococcal bacteremia, for example, may cause multiple cortical abscesses. Frequently abscesses are caused by gram-negative organisms such as *Proteus* and *Escherichia coli*. Renal abscesses may extend into the tissues surrounding the kidney. When infection from the kidney spreads to the fatty and fascial tissues surrounding the kidney, it is known as a "perinephric abscess." Drainage collects at the lower pole of the kidney because of the effects of gravity. Such abscesses are frequently associated with renal calculi or urinary tract obstructions. The infection may extend through the fascia to nearby organs such as the pancreas, duodenum, and colon.

Diagnostic Studies and Findings

Intravenous Urogram

Renal mass and calyceal distortion or renal displacement are shown when radiopaque dye is injected, filtered by the kidneys, and excreted through the urinary tract

Renal Computed Tomography

Differentiates between a cyst and an abscess

Medical Plan

Surgery

Incision and drainage may be required if the renal abscess is localized; incision and drainage are usually required for perinephric abscesses

Intrarenal: percutaneous aspiration, instillation of antibiotics; less expensive and causes less discomfort than open drainage

Perinephric: percutaneous drainage, if possible; open surgical drainage more likely; specimen sent for culture and sensitivity determinations

Medications

Anti-infective agents

Sulfisoxazole (Gantrisin, Novosoxazole), po, 1-2 g initially followed by 1 g bid or tid

Ampicillin (Omnipen, Polycillin), po, patients ≥20 kg: 250-500 mg q6h; patients <20 kg: 50-100 mg/kg/d in equally divided doses q6-8h

Carbenicillin disodium (Geopen, Pyopen), IM, IV, 1-2 g q6h

Gentamicin (Garamycin, Apogen), IM, IV, 3-5 mg/kg/d q8h

General Management

Bed rest, adequate fluids (2500 to 3000 ml/day), and normal nutrition are important; a normal diet ensures protein, calories, and other nutrients sufficient to meet the needs of the individual's current stage of the life cycle; sterile dressing changes are needed after incision and drainage of abscesses

NURSING CARE

Nursing Assessment

Signs of Infection

Renal abscess

None with solitary abscess; chills and fever; increased white blood count; flank tenderness; nausea; vomiting; anorexia; malaise

Perinephric abscess

Chills and fever; increased white blood count; dull ache in flank; costovertebral angle tenderness on palpation; mass in flank; abdominal pain with guarding

Nursing Dx & Intervention

Nursing Diagnosis	Nursing Intervention/Rationale
Impaired skin integrity related to percutaneous or open surgical drainage	• Administer antimicrobial agents as ordered by physician. • Monitor temperature and report any changes. • Explain medications and their purposes. • Encourage oral fluids up to 3 L/day if not contraindicated *to flush out bacteria*. • Change wound dressing using sterile technique. Observe and document kind and amount of drainage and appearance of wound (redness, tenderness, swelling). • Follow isolation precautions if necessary.
Pain	• Assess patient's need for pain relief and administer analgesic drugs as ordered by physician; observe and document response.
Feeding and bathing/hygiene self-care deficit	• Assist as necessary with food and fluid intake, personal hygiene, and rest.

Patient Education

1. Explain the side effects and adverse reactions of pharmacologic agents used.
2. Explain care of the incision and teach dressing changes if necessary.
3. Explain the relationship between perinephric abscesses and pyelonephritis, renal calculi, and urinary tract obstruction.

Evaluation

Patient Outcome	Data Indicating That Outcome is Reached
Infection clears.	Temperature is in the normal range. Patient is pain free. White blood cell count is normal.
Incision heals.	There is no infection; wound is closed.
Patient demonstrates knowledge of renal or perinephric abscesses.	Patient can describe the nature of renal or perinephric abscess.

Renal Tuberculosis

Infection caused by *Mycobacterium tuberculosis* can occur in the kidneys.

Renal tuberculosis is much less frequent today than in the past; however, 3987 new cases of extrapulmonary tuberculosis were reported in the United States in 1986. Of these cases 476 were in the genitourinary system.[4] Prevention is important. About 4% to 9% of people with active pulmonary tuberculosis develop genitourinary involvement.[7] Contact with people with active pulmonary tuberculosis should be avoided, and early diagnosis is important.

Renal tuberculosis often occurs in older persons. Prophylactic care with isoniazid is ordered for susceptible persons (household members of patients with tuberculosis and persons with positive reactions to the tuberculin skin test).

Pathophysiology

The tuberculosis organism spreads by the bloodstream from the lungs or gastrointestinal tract. Renal tuberculosis is associated with primary pulmonary infection or occurs during reactivation many years later from infection previously seeded in the kidney. Tuberculosis occurs more frequently in men; the bladder, prostate, epididymis, and testicle may also be involved. An abscess in the cortex may erode into a calyx and spread to the pelvis and downward to the bladder. Early treatment of pulmonary tuberculosis may be reducing the number of patients who develop renal lesions.

The organism causes a low-grade inflammation and granuloma formation; healing causes fibrosis, calcification, and scarring, and thus destruction of renal tissue. Damage may obstruct the drainage system and impair the blood supply, causing hypertension.

Diagnostic Studies and Findings

Intravenous Urogram

Kidney appears "moth-eaten" when radiopaque dye is filtered through it; reveals strictures

Kidney, Ureter, Bladder Roentgenogram

Cavity formation is shown by irregular outline of kidney and calcification

Medical Plan

Treatment, as for tuberculosis, takes more than 6 months to 2 years (see p. 1198).

Medications

Anti-infective agents
- Isoniazid (INH, Isotamine), po or IM, 5 mg/kg/body weight up to 300 mg/d
- Rifampin (Rifadin, Rifampicin), po, 600 mg/d
- Streptomycin, IM, 1 g/d, reduce to 1 g 2-3 times/wk when sputum cultures become negative
- Ethambutol (Etibi, Myambutol), po, 15 mg/kg body weight/d
- Pyridoxine (Beesix, Vitabee-6), po, IM, or IV, for isoniazid-induced deficiency: 100-200 mg/d for 3 wk, then 25-100 mg/d maintenance

Surgery

May be necessary to remove nonfunctioning kidney, a continuing source of organisms or uncontrollable hypertension

Repair of sequelae, such as ureteral strictures, may be necessary

General Management

Bed rest is usually prescribed at first; ensure adequate nutrition; observe isolation precautions if sputum or urine is positive for tuberculosis bacilli; proper disposal of urine (flushed down toilet and not bedpan flusher) and other infected material (double-bagged and incinerated) is part of plan of care

NURSING CARE

Nursing Assessment

General

Fever; weight loss; flank pain; sweating

Urine

Asymptomatic pyuria; tuberculosis organism cultured; hematuria

For culture use the second-voided early morning specimen; rifampin may darken the urine

Other

Monitor liver function tests of patients receiving rifampin because it may cause hepatotoxicity

Nursing Dx & Intervention

Nursing Diagnosis	Nursing Intervention/Rationale
Altered renal tissue perfusion related to presence of infection	• Give antimicrobial agents as ordered and observe response. • Explain drugs and their purposes *to begin preparation for self-medication after discharge.* • Measure and record intake, output, weight, temperature, pulse, respirations, and blood pressure. Measure specific gravity *to monitor kidney's ability to concentrate urine.*
Impaired physical mobility; bathing/hygiene and toileting self-care deficit	• Maintain bed rest during acute phase. Implement nursing measures *to prevent adverse effects of bed rest* (such as pneumonia, deep vein thrombosis). • Assist with personal hygiene as needed.

Patient Education

1. Explain the nature of tuberculosis, its cause, spread, and treatment (see p. 1197).

Evaluation

Patient Outcome	Data Indicating That Outcome is Reached
Infection clears.	Urine culture is negative within 2 months. Temperature is in the normal range.
Renal lesions heal.	Follow-up roentgenograms reveal healing.
Patient complies with long-term drug therapy regimen.	Drugs are taken as directed.
Patient demonstrates knowledge of tuberculosis.	Patient can describe measures to prevent the spread of tuberculosis.
Patient's mobility and self-care capabilities improve.	There are no limitations of activities of daily living.

CONGENITAL ANOMALIES

A wide variety of anomalies related to the kidneys can occur. The abnormalities may be in number, volume, form, location, rotation, blood vessels, pelvis, or ureter. These errors in renal development result from failure to develop, abnormal division of the elements, fusion of the elements, or abnormal movement from the pelvis to the lumbar area. These anatomic deviations may range from minor to severe and from easily correctable to incompatible with life. Renal abnormalities are frequently associated with additional anomalies such as low-set ears, imperforate anus, genital anomalies, and abnormalities of the spinal cord and extremities.

Kidney displacement and supernumerary kidneys

Kidney displacement occurs occasionally when the kidneys do not ascend to their normal positions, or one may cross over, causing both kidneys to be on one side. A supernumerary, or extra, kidney, rarely occurs, although duplication of the renal pelvis is common.

Pathophysiology

The displaced kidneys may be normal except for their abnormal location or rotation. They have increased susceptibility to trauma because they are not protected as well as a kidney in its normal location. Obstruction may occur, as may infarction or infection if the normal blood supply and urinary channel are interrupted. The extra kidney may be small, dysplastic, and infected.

Diagnostic Studies and Findings

Intravenous Urogram

Abnormally located or rotated kidney; extra kidney(s) visualized when radiopaque dye filters through the kidney

Medical Plan

Surgery

Correction of obstruction to blood supply or urine elimination in displaced kidney and removal of extra kidney(s) may be indicated; function of remaining kidney tissue must be adequate

NURSING CARE

Nursing Assessment

Renal Function

Asymptomatic; signs of infection or obstruction

Nursing Dx & Intervention

Nursing Diagnosis	Nursing Intervention/Rationale
Potential for infection	• Observe for signs and symptoms of urinary tract infection. • Monitor temperature, pulse, and respirations and report any abnormalities.
Impaired skin integrity related to surgery	• Prepare for surgery. • Explain procedure, diagnostic studies, and postoperative care to be given to patient and family. • Prepare the area of skin for incision. • Bowel preparation may include enema and nothing by mouth after midnight. *Postoperative care:* • Monitor site of incision for drainage and signs of infection. • Keep any drainage tubes patent, unkinked, and anchored *to avoid inadvertent displacement.* • Monitor intake (intravenous and oral) and output. • Care for urethral catheter. Be alert for and report foul-smelling urine, blood, pus, etc.
Pain	• Assess patient's need for pain relief. • Relieve pain at incision site with analgesics as ordered.
Bathing/hygiene self-care deficit	• Assist with personal hygiene as needed immediately after surgery *when pain may interfere with self-care.*

Patient Education

1. Explain the location of the displaced or extra kidney(s).
2. Explain the signs and symptoms of possible problems (trauma to abdomen, urinary tract infections, or urinary tract obstruction).
3. Explain measures to prevent urinary tract infection: adequate fluid intake (to avoid dehydration), regular emptying of the bladder to avoid overdistention, and good perineal hygiene to prevent the entrance of microorganisms into the urinary tract.
4. Explain postoperative care, including care of the incision and self-monitoring skills (intake and output, weight, temperature, etc.).

Evaluation

Patient Outcome	Data Indicating That Outcome is Reached
Family knows kidney's location.	Family can describe the location of the displaced or extra kidney and its implications.
Incision heals.	No infection is present; wound is closed.
Family knows how to prevent urinary tract infections.	Family can describe measures to prevent urinary tract infections.

 Hypoplasia and dysplasia

Hypoplasia refers to having less than the usual number of nephrons. Dysplasia refers to areas of the kidney with underdeveloped structures. When on occasion both occur together, the term used is hypodysplasia.

Pathophysiology

The kidneys are small but normal in structure. They may be dysplastic with malformation of renal tissue. If both kidneys are severely malformed, death occurs during the neonatal period. One kidney usually has poorer function than the other.

Diagnostic Studies and Findings

Intravenous Urogram

Small, malformed kidney(s) are seen when radiopaque dye is filtered through the kidneys

Medical Plan

Surgery

Elective surgical removal of the dysplastic kidney is usually performed. Careful assessment of the contralateral kidney is essential. If chronic renal failure occurs, renal dialysis or transplantation may be undertaken if technically feasible (see pp. 1070 and 1079).

Medications

Anti-infective agents
- Parenteral agents (IM or IV)
  - Gentamicin (Garamycin, Apogen), 3-5 mg/kg/d q8h
  - Cephalosporins: Cefazolin sodium (Ancef, Kefzol), 250-1000 mg q6-8h
  - Penicillins
    - Sodium ampicillin (Omnipen-N, Polycillin-N), patients ≥40 kg: 250-500 mg q6h; <40 kg: 25-50 mg/kg/d in equally divided doses q6-8h
    - Carbenicillin disodium (Geopen, Pyopen), 1-2 g IM q6h
    - Penicillin G potassium (aqueous penicillin G), penicillin G sodium, 1-20 million U/d
- Oral agents
  - Sulfonamides: Sulfisoxazole (Gantrisin, Novosoxazole), 2-4 g initially followed by 1-2 g q4-6h
  - Tetracycline (Achromycin, Tetracyn), 250-500 mg q6h
  - Penicillins
    - Amoxicillin (Amoxil, Amoxycillin), patients ≥20 kg: 250-500 mg q8h; <20 kg: 20-40 mg/kg/d in divided doses q8h
    - Ampicillin (Omnipen, Polycillin), patients ≥20 kg: 250-500 mg q6h; <20 kg: 50-100 mg/kg/d in equally divided doses
    - Penicillin G, 200,000-500,000 U q6-8h
  - Erythromycin (Erythrocin, Ilotycin), 25 mg q6h
  - Sulfamethoxazole, trimethoprim (Septra and Bactrim), 2 tab q12h

General Management

See "Renal Dialysis," p. 1070

NURSING CARE

Nursing Assessment

Renal Function

May be asymptomatic; bilateral: uremia; unilateral: infection, hypertension, or renal failure

Nursing Dx & Intervention

Nursing Diagnosis	Nursing Intervention/Rationale
Potential for infection	• Observe for signs and symptoms of urinary tract infection (burning on urination, frequency, urgency, dysuria, hematuria, and nocturia). • Monitor temperature, pulse, and respirations; report any abnormalities.
Impaired skin integrity related to surgery	• Prepare for surgery. • Explain procedure, diagnostic studies, and postoperative care to be given to patient and family. • Prepare area of skin for incision. • Bowel preparation may include enema and nothing by mouth after midnight. *Postoperative care:* • Assess site of incision for drainage and signs of infection. • Monitor temperature, pulse, respirations, and blood pressure. *Be alert for shock or respiratory complications.* • Keep any drainage tubes patent, unkinked, and anchored *to avoid inadvertent displacement.* • Monitor intake (intravenous and oral) and output. • Care for urethral catheter. Watch for and report foul-smelling urine, *a sign of infection.* • Monitor bowel sounds. Patient may take nothing by mouth for 1 to 2 days. Start food and fluid by mouth as ordered and as patient tolerates.

Nursing Diagnosis	Nursing Intervention/Rationale
	• Assess patient's need for pain relief and give analgesics as ordered. • Implement nursing measures such as deep breathing, coughing, and turning *to prevent complications of bed rest,* such as pneumonia.

Patient Education

1. Explain the kidney abnormality.
2. Explain possible problems: urinary tract infection, renal failure, and their signs and symptoms.
3. Explain postoperative care if needed.
4. Explain renal dialysis and transplantation as likely future options in end-stage renal disease program.

Evaluation

Patient Outcome	Data Indicating That Outcome is Reached
Patient and family understand renal abnormality.	Patient and family can describe the renal abnormality and its implications.
Patient and family know how to prevent urinary tract infections.	Family can describe measures to prevent urinary tract infections.
Skin integrity is normal.	Incision, if any, has healed without complications.

Polycystic kidney disease

In polycystic kidney disease the kidney tissue is replaced by grapelike clusters of cysts.

Polycystic kidney disease (PKD) is a genetically transmitted disorder, autosomal dominant in adults. An infant form (autosomal, recessive) occurs; such children rarely live more than a year. The adult form has a similar onset, clinical course, and manifestations within a family.

Pathophysiology

The normal kidney tissue is replaced by grapelike clusters of cysts that destroy the surrounding tissue by compression. Why cysts are formed is not clear. In time they grow larger. They may be associated with cysts in the liver. Cysts may occur anywhere along the nephron. Fluid within the cysts may be yellow, brown, thick, and cloudy. It may contain urine components. Progressive fibrosis of the interstitial tissue occurs. Infection and renal stones often occur because of urinary stasis and compression. Ascending infection may form a persistent source of infection. These kidneys do not resist infection well and thus may harbor organisms. Poor perfusion may prevent antibiotics from reaching pockets of infection. A perinephric abscess may form; septicemia may occur. In these cases a nephrectomy may be necessary. Hypertension and renal failure follow the onset of symptoms within 5 to 15 years.[8]

Diagnostic Studies and Findings

Kidney, Ureter, Bladder, Roentgenogram

Kidney size, shape, and location are seen on roentgenogram

Intravenous Urogram

Renal function and presence of cysts, nephrocalcinosis, or obstruction of the collecting system is evaluated when radiopaque dye filters through the kidney and urinary tract

Medical Plan

No specific treatment is available. Medical goals concentrate on preventing hypertension and infection to preserve renal function. Instrumentation of the urinary tract, which is occasionally followed by a urinary tract infection, should be avoided. If patients do not have symptoms, creatinine clearance and urine cultures should be obtained twice a year. Genetic counseling may be suggested for families with polycystic kidney disease. Renal dialysis and transplantation may be indicated when chronic renal failure ensues.

NURSING CARE

Nursing Assessment

Renal Function

Intermittent hematuria; proteinuria; infection; hypertension; flank pain (dull or acute) or lateral abdominal pain; palpable kidneys; decrease in renal function tests

Nursing Dx & Intervention

Nursing Diagnosis	Nursing Intervention/Rationale
Altered renal tissue perfusion	• Assess and monitor intake, output, and weight if needed. • Monitor blood pressure. • Give antihypertensives, if needed, as ordered by physician. • Monitor laboratory tests reflective of renal function *to follow any decline in function.*
Potential for infection	• Avoid instrumentation of the urinary tract *to avoid nosocomial infection.* • Be alert to signs and symptoms of active urinary tract infections. See "Pyelonephritis," p. 1045.
Pain	• Assess patient's need for pain relief and administer analgesics as ordered by physician. Rest and application of external heat to lumbar area may help. The cysts may be enlarged and infected, thus causing discomfort.
Altered family processes (potential)	• Be alert to how the diagnosis of the family member affects others in the family. Help them seek genetic counseling if appropriate. Some people do not want to know this information.

Patient Education

1. Explain the nature of the kidney abnormality and the availability of genetic counseling.
2. Explain the need to monitor renal function and blood pressure.
3. Explain measures to prevent urinary tract infection: adequate fluid intake to avoid dehydration, regular emptying of the bladder to avoid overdistention, observation of urine, and good perineal care to prevent entrance of microorganisms into the urinary tract.
4. Explain signs and symptoms of urinary tract infections (see "Pyelonephritis," p. 1045).
5. Explain renal dialysis and transplantation as options for the future.

Evaluation

Patient Outcome	Data Indicating That Outcome is Reached
Early decreases in renal function are recognized.	Urinalysis and blood chemistries are performed every 6 months, and any change is noted.
Patient and family know how to prevent urinary tract infection.	Patient can describe measures to prevent urinary tract infections.
Infections will be treated promptly.	Patient seeks medical help when signs and symptoms of urinary tract infection occur.
Plans are made for long-term treatment.	Patient describes the anticipated course of the disease and the possible relationship of dialysis and transplantation for the future.

GLOMERULONEPHRITIS

A discussion of glomerulonephritis (GN) is difficult because of the confusion among the older definitions used before renal biopsy was introduced and the newer terms used since. One classification of GN uses clinical course (acute, rapidly progressive, and chronic), histopathology (membranoproliferative, for example), and pathogenetic mechanisms (immune complexes and antibodies against kidney antigens).[32]

The kinds of GN include acute poststreptococcal GN (APSGN) (immune complexes); Goodpasture's syndrome and rapidly progressive GN (antiglomerular basement membrane or anti-GBM antibodies); and membranoproliferative GN. A renal biopsy is necessary to differentiate among the various kinds of GN (see p. 1581). Only APSGN is discussed in this section.

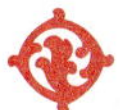

Acute poststreptococcal glomerulonephritis

Acute poststreptococcal glomerulonephritis (APSGN) is an inflammation of the glomeruli that occurs after a streptococcal infection elsewhere in the body.

Glomerulonephritis can follow a respiratory or skin infection. Several stains of group A β-hemolytic streptococci that cause GN have been isolated. In temperate zones the most common nephritogenic strain causing pharyngitis is M-type 12. Only about 5% of such infections are followed by APSGN. Children and young adults are affected most frequently. The incidence of APSGN decreases with age because many children (especially in urban areas) develop immunities to type 12 β-hemolytic streptococci before reaching adulthood. Renal problems occur abruptly 1 to 3 weeks after the infection. Most patients (95%) recover normal renal function within 2 months.[7,8] The others have irreversible damage that causes long-term problems. Whether prompt treatment of streptococcal infections prevents renal complications of APSGN is unclear.

Pathophysiology

Antibodies of the host react with circulating antigens that appear to arise from the toxic products of the infecting organism to form immune complexes that then become lodged in the glomeruli. Both kidneys are affected by an acute, diffuse, nonsuppurative inflammation that damages the glomerular basement membrane. The damage results in an acute interference with renal function.

Diagnostic Studies and Findings

Kidney, Ureter, Bladder Examination

Normal to slight bilateral kidney enlargement seen on plain roentgenogram

Medical Plan

The medical plan includes treating the symptoms, attempting to prevent cerebral and cardiac complications, and supporting the patient through a period of decreased renal functioning.

Medications

Antihypertensive agents
- Clonidine (Catapres, Dixarit), po, 0.1 mg bid or tid initially, then increase by 0.2-0.8 mg/d (maximum effective dose 2.4 mg/d)
- Diazoxide (Hyperstat IV, Proglycem), IV, 300 mg by bolus in 30 sec or 1-2 mg/kg up to 150 mg at 5-15 min intervals
- Hydralazine (Apresoline, Dralzine), po, 10 mg qid for 2-4 d; increase to 25 mg qid, then 50 mg qid; maintenance dose is lowest effective level; IM, IV, 10-40 mg repeated as needed (q4-6h)
- Methyldopa (Aldomet, Dopamet), po, 250 mg bid or tid for 48 h; then increase or decrease q2 d if needed; maintenance of 500 mg to 2 g in 2-4 divided doses (maximum of 3 g)
- Propranolol (Inderal, Novopranol), po, 40 mg bid at 6-8 h intervals; increase if needed to 160-480 mg/d in divided doses; 640 mg/d may be needed

Diuretics
- Furosemide (Lasix, Uritol), po, 20-80 mg followed by second dose in 6-8 h up to 600 mg; IM, IV, 20-40 mg given slowly over 1-2 min; high dose by IV not more than 4 mg/min
- Hydrochlorothiazide (Hydrodiuril, Esidrix), po, 25-100 mg/d or bid initially; then maintenance of 25-100 mg/d according to patient's response
- Spironolactone (Aldactone), po 25-200 mg/d in divided doses initially for 5 d, then adjust to maintenance level

Agents for treatment of hyperkalemia
- Sodium polystyrene sulfonate (Kayexalate, SPS), po or enema, 15 g qd-qid; give po dose in 45-60 ml of water, syrup, fruit juice, or soft drink
- Calcium gluconate (Kalcinate), IV, 1 g (90 mg Ca^{++}) in 10 ml
- Sodium bicarbonate, IV, 2-5 mEq/kg infusion over 4-8 h
- Glucose 50% IV, 25-50 g, and regular insulin, IV, 10-15 U

Antacids
- Aluminum carbonate (Basaljel), po, 30-40 ml 1 h after meals and at bedtime of regular strength (400 mg $Al[OH]_3$/5 ml); 15-20 ml 1 h after meals and at bedtime of extra strength (1000 mg $Al[OH]_3$/5 ml)
- Aluminum hydroxide, gel (Amphojel, Dialume), aluminum hydroxide gel, dried (Amphojel tab, Alu-Cap), po, 40 ml 1 h after meals and at bedtime; 8 tab 1 h after meals and at bedtime

Anticonvulsive agents
- Phenytoin (Dilantin, Novophenytoin), po, 100 mg tid up to 600 mg/d
- Diazepam (Valium, Novodipam), po, 2-10 mg bid-qid
- Phenobarbital (Luminal, Barbita), po, 50-100 mg/d

Anti-infective agents (if infection is still present)
- Infection is frequently a complication of acute renal failure
- Agents specific to microorganism cultured should be used
- Agents whose route of excretion is primarily renal need to be used in smaller doses or at lengthened intervals depending on glomerular filtration rate[7]; agents excreted by only the liver require no change; when partial excretion occurs via the kidneys, some adjustment is needed at low glomerular filtration rates

Cardiac glycosides (for congestive heart failure)
- Digoxin (Lanoxin, Novodigoxin), po, 1-1.5 mg/d in divided doses; IV, 0.75-1.25 mg initially, maintenance of 0.125-0.5 mg/d

General Management

Hemodialysis, peritoneal dialysis, or CAVH (see pp. 1067, 1071, and 1076)
Limit sodium intake to 500-1000 mg/day
Limit fluids to 500 ml plus amount equal to volume of urine for previous 24 hours
Limit potassium intake (if hyperkalemia) to 1500 mg/day
Limit protein intake (if uremic) to 60 g/day
Provide 2500-3500 calories/day
Prescribe bed rest during acute phase of illness

NURSING CARE

Nursing Assessment

Infection

Antistreptolysin O (ASO) titer: 200 to 2500 Todd U; fever and chills

Urine

Hematuria (dark brown or rust colored); red blood cell casts; proteinuria; oliguria

Cardiovascular

Hypertension; edema

Blood Chemistries

Increased blood urea nitrogen level; increased serum creatinine level

Hematology

Normal or decreased complement (C3); mild anemia

General

Headache; low back pain; malaise; nausea; vomiting

Nursing Dx & Intervention

Nursing Diagnosis	Nursing Intervention/Rationale
Altered renal tissue perfusion	• Assess and monitor renal functions: serum creatinine and blood urea nitrogen. • Limit protein and potassium intake *to decrease excretory load on kidney and the possible accumulation of H^+ and K^+.* • Observe urine for color and presence of blood and protein.
Fluid volume excess (potential)	• Assess and monitor intake, output, weight, blood pressure, pulse, and respirations. • If volume excess is severe, monitor pulmonary capillary wedge pressure, central venous pressure, neck veins, peripheral edema, and pulmonary status (e.g., dyspnea). • Limit sodium and fluid intake *to avoid increasing fluid overload.*
Potential for infection	• Assess and monitor temperature. • Observe for signs and symptoms of infection: burning on urination, dysuria, frequency, urgency, nocturia. • Avoid exposure to persons with infection.
Altered nutrition: less than body requirements	• Ensure adequate calorie intake from carbohydrates and fats *to prevent the use of tissue proteins for energy.* • Be alert to anorexia, nausea, and vomiting *to be aware of decreased intake or unusual losses.* • Offer small, frequent feedings.
Impaired physical mobility	• Help patient stay on bed rest. • Implement nursing measures such as deep breathing, coughing, and turning *to prevent complications of bed rest,* such as pneumonia.
Bathing/hygiene self-care deficit	• Assist with personal hygiene as needed *because of malaise, fatigue, or weakness.* Altered mental status may occur if uremia is present.

Patient Education

1. Explain the diagnosis of APSGN, its signs, symptoms, and the course of the disease.
2. Explain the medical regimen, if any, for discharge.
3. Explain follow-up care: monitoring of blood pressure and urinalysis (hematuria and proteinuria).

Evaluation

Patient Outcome	Data Indicating That Outcome is Reached
Patient has normal renal function.	Urine output balances with intake. Urine is clear. Edema is gone. Blood pressure is in normal range. Weight is stable. Blood urea nitrogen, serum creatinine, and complement levels return to normal range.
Patient feels well and returns to normal activities of daily living.	Malaise is gone.
Patient is knowledgeable about APSGN.	Patient can describe signs, symptoms, and course of the disease. Patient can describe his or her level of renal function and possible problems and can outline the medical regimen prescribed.

Hydronephrosis

Hydronephrosis is the dilation of the renal pelvis by the pressure of urine that cannot flow past an obstruction of the ureter.

Obstruction can be proximal to the bladder or occur below the level of the bladder. Hydronephrosis, which is usually on the right side, always occurs during pregnancy and for a time after delivery because of obstruction caused by the enlarged uterus.

Pathophysiology

Obstruction of the ureter that results in hydronephrosis may be caused by renal calculi, tumors, inflammation associated with infection, fibrous bands that obstruct the ureteropelvic junction, or prostatic urethral valves. The renal pelvis and ureters dilate and hypertrophy. The pressure of the urine, if prolonged, causes fibrosis and loss of function in affected nephrons. The duration and severity of the obstruction are significant. Compression causes ischemia and then atrophy of renal tissue. The kidney may be destroyed without pain.

Diagnostic Studies and Findings

Renal Ultrasonography

Dilation of collecting system

Intravenous Urogram

Calyceal clubbing is shown after injection of radiopaque dye

Medical Plan

Management is usually conservative if the condition is not severe.

Surgery

Surgical intervention is used to relieve the obstruction and preserve renal function; pyeloplasty may be indicated; repair of the ureteropelvic junction may be indicated; a nephrectomy may be indicated if the kidney is severely damaged; antimicrobial agents are used to treat infection if present

Medications

- Anti-infective agents if infection is present
- Parenteral agents (IM or IV)
  - Gentamicin (Garamycin, Apogen), 3-5 mg/kg/d q8h
  - Cephalosporins
    - Cefazolin sodium (Ancef, Kefzol), 250-1000 mg q6-8h
  - Penicillins
    - Ampicillin sodium (Omnipen-N, Polycillin-N), patients ≥40 kg: 250-500 mg q6h; <40 kg: 25-50 mg/kg/d in equally divided doses q6-8h
    - Carbenicillin disodium (Geopen, Pyopen), 1-2 g q6h
    - Penicillin G potassium (Aqueous penicillin G), Penicillin G sodium, 1-20 million U/d
- Oral agents
  - Sulfonamides
    - Sulfisoxazole (Gantrisin, Novosoxazole), 2-4 g initially, followed by 1-2 g q4-6h
  - Tetracycline (Achromycin, Tetracyn), 250-500 mg q6h

Penicillins
- Amoxicillin (Amoxil, Amoxycillin), patients ≥20 kg: 250-500 mg q8h; <20 kg: 20-40 mg/kg/d in divided doses q8h
- Ampicillin (Omnipen, Polycillin), patients ≥ 20 kg: 250-500 mg q6h; <20 kg: 50-100 mg/kg/d in equally divided doses

Erythromycin (Erythrocin, E-Mycin), 25 mg q6h

Sulfamethoxazole and trimethoprim (Septra, Bactrim), 2 tab q12h

NURSING CARE

Nursing Assessment

Renal

Hematuria; pyuria

Abdominal

Mass

General

Fever (with infection); pain; hypertension

Nursing Dx & Intervention

Nursing Diagnosis	Nursing Intervention/Rationale
Altered renal tissue perfusion (potential)	• Give antimicrobial drugs if ordered and observe the response and side effects. • Monitor intake and output. • Monitor urine for bleeding that may be present during the first hours after surgery.
Potential for infection	• Monitor temperature, pulse, and respirations *to assess for signs and symptoms of infection.*
Impaired skin integrity related to surgery	• Prepare for surgery. • Explain procedure, diagnostic studies, and postoperative care to be given to patient and family. • Prepare area of skin for incision. • Bowel preparation may include enema and nothing by mouth after midnight. *Postoperative care:* • Assess site of incision for drainage and signs of infection. • Keep any drainage tubes patent, unkinked, and anchored *to avoid inadvertent displacement.* • Monitor intake (intravenous and oral) and output. Care for urethral catheter. Watch for and report foul-smelling urine, a sign of infection. • Tubes may include a stent (a catheter inserted in the ureter), a nephrostomy tube, and an incisional drain. • Observe for flank pain and urine output in relation to intake after nephrostomy tube is removed. *Pain, fever, and decreased urine may indicate obstruction or urine leaking into the retroperitoneal space.* • Observe dressing. Drainage of urine may continue for some time. Keep area clean and dry *to avoid skin breakdown.*

Patient Education

1. Explain the kidney-ureter abnormality.
2. Explain possible problems: recurrent infection and obstruction.
3. Explain signs and symptoms of urinary tract infection and obstruction.
4. Explain measures to prevent urinary tract infection: adequate fluid intake to avoid dehydration, regular emptying of bladder to avoid overdistention, and good perineal hygiene to prevent entrance of microorganisms into the urinary tract.
5. Explain postoperative care, including care of the incision and self-monitoring skills as needed.
6. Explain plans for medical follow-up of renal function.

Evaluation

Patient Outcome	Data Indicating That Outcome is Reached
Obstruction is relieved.	Roentgenograms show that hydronephrosis is lessened or does not increase. K^+ level is normal.
Surgical incision heals.	Incision is closed; no signs of infection are present.
Renal function is not impaired.	Renal function tests are normal.
Patient knows how to prevent urinary tract infections.	Patient can describe the measures used to prevent urinary tract infection.
Patient seeks medical follow-up.	Continuing medical supervision is sought.

Interstitial Nephritis

Interstitial nephritis (IN) is renal disease that involves inflammatory interstitial tissue damage.

Damage to the cortical interstitial tissue is the second most common cause (after glomerular disease) of chronic renal failure. Causes of IN include infections (e.g., streptococcal) and drug use (antibiotics such as methicillin and ampicillin, sulfonamides, phenindione, and phenytoin). The cause may be idiopathic. Early detection of drug reactions, infections, and urinary tract obstruction is useful. It is important to be alert to the possibility that some patients may abuse the use of over-the-counter analgesics, especially those containing acetaminophen.

Pathophysiology

Acute inflammation of the interstitium may cause scarring and a rapid decline in renal function. As many as 10% to 15% of the cases of acute renal failure may be associated with acute interstitial nephritis.[19] The inflammatory process is usually diffuse and accompanied by interstitial edema. An immune response appears to cause acute IN that may involve both immune complex and anti-tubular basement membrane antibody deposition.

Chronic IN results in a shrunken kidney with an irregular outline caused by scarring and tissue destruction. It follows a slowly progressive course with few clinical manifestations. Changes in renal hormone activity may occur. Renin, erythropoietin, and vitamin D production may decline. Ability to concentrate urine also decreases. Common causes of chronic IN are anatomic abnormalities, such as obstruction in the urinary tract, analgesic use, hyperuricemia, and nephrosclerosis.

Diagnostic Studies and Findings

Intravenous Urogram

Decreased kidney size, irregular cortical outlines, calyceal cupping are seen after injection of radiopaque dye

Medical Plan

The cause of IN can be removed by treating infection, discontinuing the drugs associated with acute IN, and relieving obstruction. Renal function may gradually improve. Chronic IN requires monitoring as renal function decreases. Changes in the function of the glomeruli and tubules occur as the interstitial inflammation and scarring progress (see "Chronic Renal Failure," p. 1053).

Surgery

Relieve any obstruction

Medications

- Anti-infective agents
  - Parenteral agents (IM or IV)
    - Gentamicin (Garamycin, Apogen), 3-5 mg/kg/d q8h; 6-7.5 mg/kg/d q8h
    - Cephalosporins
      - Cefazolin sodium (Ancef, Kefzol), 250-1000 mg q6-8h
    - Penicillins
      - Ampicillin sodium (Omnipen-N, Polycillin-N), patients ≥40 kg: 250-500 mg q6h; <40 kg: 25-50 mg/kg/d in equally divided doses, q6-8h
      - Carbenicillin disodium (Geopen, Pyopen), 1-2 g IM q6h
      - Penicillin G potassium (Aqueous penicillin G), penicillin G sodium, 1-20 million U/d
  - Oral agents
    - Sulfonamides
      - Sulfisoxazole (Gantrisin, Novosoxazole), 2-4 g initially, followed by 1-2 g q4-6h
    - Tetracycline (Achromycin, Tetracyn), 250-500 mg q6h
    - Penicillins
      - Amoxicillin (Amoxil, Amoxycillin), patients ≥20 kg: 250-500 mg q8h; <20 kg: 20-40 mg/kg/d in divided doses q8h
      - Ampicillin (Omnipen, Polycillin), patients ≥20 kg:

250-500 mg q6h; <20 kg: 50-100 mg/kg/d in equally divided doses

Penicillin G, 200,000-500,000 U q6-8h

Erythromyin (Erythrocin, Ilotycin), 25 mg q6h

Trimethoprim and sulfamethoxazole (Septra, Bactrim), 2 tab q12h

General Management

Dialysis, if needed

Fluid intake to equal amount needed to replace measurable losses in urine, nasogastric drainage, wound drainage, and the like; avoid fluid overload; daily weights reflect fluid gain or loss

Nutritional support includes maintenance of body weight and positive nitrogen balance[7,26]

Calorie intake should include glucose 100 g/day

Protein intake may be maintained through parenteral administration of essential amino acids (50 to 85 g/L solution); oral intake is started as soon as possible (protein of 30 to 40 g/day with 75% having high biologic value)

Vitamin supplements needed, since 40 g protein diet is deficient in calcium and folic acid and is low in phosphorus and the B vitamins

Sodium intake of 1 to 2 g/day if edema or hypertension is present; potassium in the diet is restricted to 2 g/day if serum levels are more than 5 mEq/L

NURSING CARE

Nursing Assessment

Renal

Polyuria; nocturia; pyuria; white blood cells and tubular casts; microscopic hematuria; mild proteinuria

Blood Chemistries

Elevated blood urea nitrogen and serum creatinine levels; decreased creatinine clearance

Nursing Dx & Intervention

Nursing Diagnosis	Nursing Intervention/Rationale
Sensory/perceptual alterations (visual, auditory, kinesthetic) (potential); altered thought processes (potential)	• Provide a safe environment. • Assess orientation to time, place, and person. • Observe for behavioral changes. • Observe level of consciousness. • Be alert to possible convulsions.
Altered nutrition: less than body requirements	• Assess caloric intake: kinds and amount, amount of protein, and fluid intake. • Watch for nausea, vomiting, and anorexia *that decrease intake of food.* • Monitor weight.
Bathing/hygiene, feeding, and toileting self-care deficit	• Give assistance as necessary in feeding, bathing and hygiene, and toileting.
Impaired physical mobility	• If patient is on bed rest, give assistance as necessary in feeding, bathing and hygiene, and toileting. • Establish routine for changing position.
Altered renal tissue perfusion	• Give medications as ordered and monitor response. • Watch K^+ and Ca^{++} levels if diuretics, digitalis, or banked blood is given. Report K^+ levels greater than 5 mEq/L. • Watch for electrocardiographic changes: peaked T waves, prolonged PR interval, widened QRS complex, and cardiac standstill. • Watch for signs of hypocalcemia: tetany and Chvostek's and Trousseau's signs.
Potential fluid volume deficit; fluid volume excess (potential)	• Assess and monitor weight, intake and output, blood pressure, pulse, respirations, and breath sounds. • Observe neck veins and skin turgor. • Be alert to electrolyte losses in body fluid losses. Vomitus contains Na^+, K^+, H^+, Cl^-, and water. Diarrhea losses include K^+ and HCO_3^-. Fever and hyperpnea increase water losses. Transudates contain protein-rich fluid.
Potential for infection	• Assess for signs and symptoms of infection. Monitor temperature. • Give meticulous care to any wounds and incisions. • Avoid exposure to persons with infections. • Establish a routine for deep breathing, coughing, and turning. • Give mouth care at regular intervals.

Nursing Diagnosis	Nursing Intervention/Rationale
Knowledge deficit related to interstitial nephritis	• Help prepare patient to understand what is happening: diagnosis, treatment, bodily responses, and expected outcomes.
Altered family processes (potential)	• Help family understand what is happening to patient. Help family as needed in meeting the situation.

Patient Education

1. Explain the nature of interstitial nephritis and the cause in the individual patient.
2. Explain the patient's level of renal function.
3. Explain the need for periodic medical evaluation with tests of renal function.
4. Explain the likelihood of dialysis or transplantation in the future.

Evaluation

Patient Outcome	Data Indicating That Outcome is Reached
Patient is knowledgeable about interstitial nephritis.	Patient and family describe the nature and extent of interstitial nephritis, the need for follow-up, and implications for the future.
Renal function returns.	Fluid and electrolyte balances are within normal limits; serum creatinine and blood urea nitrogen (BUN) are normal.
Uremic signs and symptoms clear.	No alterations in sensory perception and thought processes remain.
Patient's mobility and self-care abilities improve.	Patient can walk and carry out activities of daily living without assistance.

Nephrotic Syndrome

Nephrotic syndrome (NS) encompasses a group of symptoms: proteinuria (primarily albuminuria), hypoalbuminemia, generalized edema, hyperlipidemia, and lipiduria. NS occurs in both adults and children.

NS may occur in various conditions: glomerulonephritis, glomerular lesions associated with such systemic diseases and conditions as diabetes mellitus, infections, circulatory diseases, reactions to allergens and drugs, pregnancy, and renal transplantation. NS is frequently idiopathic in children. Long-term studies are under way to determine the usefulness of corticosteroids and cyclophosphamide in children and adults.[8]

Pathophysiology

NS results from increased glomerular permeability. The albuminuria causes hypoalbuminemia because the liver cannot replace the losses rapidly enough. The resulting drop in oncotic pressure permits water to escape from the vascular compartment. Adaptive responses to the contraction of fluid volume include increased secretion of antidiuretic hormone and aldosterone, which contribute to the problem of fluid retention. The liver is stimulated to increase the synthesis of many proteins. It also increases production of lipoproteins, thereby causing the hyperlipidemia characteristic of NS.

The results of a renal biopsy in patients with NS may show minimum changes or marked changes. Most patients with NS who have minimum changes respond well to corticosteroid therapy. Patients with marked changes are usually unresponsive and progress to end-stage renal disease.

The decrease in plasma proteins may result in less binding proteins for drugs. The usual effect of a drug may occur with half the usual dose. The protein loss may also cause a decrease in vitamin D precursor, transferrin, T_3, and thyroid-binding globulin. Calcium may be required, but thyroid hormone usually is not. Iron may be needed if iron deficiency anemia occurs.

Diagnostic Studies and Findings

Renal Biopsy

To identify histologic features of lesion classified as:
- Minimum change—podocytes of epithelial cells appear to be fused together on electron microscopy
- Membranous change—predominantly thickening of the basement membrane and visible by light and electron microscopy
- Proliferative change—glomerular cells appear hypercellular
- Membranoproliferative change—there is both hypercellularity and basement membrane thickening

Medical Plan

Medications

Corticosteroids
- Prednisone (Deltasone, Orasone), po, 5-60 mg/d

Antineoplastic agents (used for immunosuppressive effect)
- Cyclophosphamide (Cytoxan, Neosar), po, 1-5 mg/kg/d; IV, 40-50 mg/kg/d initially; 10-15 mg/kg q7-10d, or 3-5 mg/kg twice wk, or 1.5-3 mg/kg/d maintenance
- Azathioprine (Imuran), po (highly individualized): 3-5 mg/kg/d initially; 1-2 mg/kg/d maintenance
- Chlorambucil (Leukeran), po, 0.1-0.2 mg/kg/d for 3-6 wk initially; 0.03-0.1 mg/kg/d maintenance

Plasma expanders and blood components
- Albumin human (Albuminate, Plasbumin), 5 g/dl or 25 g/dl, IV, 25 g initially; repeated in 15-30 min

Diuretics
- Furosemide (Lasix, Uritol), po, 20-80 mg followed by second dose in 6-8 h up to 600 mg; IM, IV, 20-40 mg given slowly over 1-2 min; high dose by IV not more than 4 mg/min
- Hydrochlorothiazide (Hydrodiuril, Esidrix), po, 25-100 mg/d or bid initially; then maintenance of 25-100 mg/d according to patient's response
- Spironolactone (Aldactone), po, 25-200 mg/d in divided doses initially for 5 d; then adjust to maintenance level

Protein diet supplements
- Meritene, 8-10 oz bid or tid
- Citrotein, 8 oz bid or tid

Immunosuppressive agents are used because they have been shown empirically to decrease or stop the proteinuria. Prednisone, the treatment of choice, is initially given as a single dose at breakfast and may be later given on alternate days. The other immunosuppressive agents are used if corticosteroids cannot be used. Diuretics are often used in conjunction with salt-poor albumin infusions to relieve massive edema. Thoracentesis or paracentesis may be needed if excess fluid accumulates in the chest or abdominal cavities. In minimum disease NS, corticosteroids are started and the responses noted. Often proteinuria clears rapidly. Repeat treatment with corticosteroids is indicated for those who have a relapse after therapy is discontinued.

General Management

Protein intake is increased to replace urinary protein losses.[26] If the glomerular filtration rate is normal, adults may have 1.5 to 2 g/kg body weight. If the glomerular filtration rate is decreased, protein intake is lowered. Sodium intake is limited (500 to 1000 mg/day) to control edema. Caloric intake must be sufficient to prevent muscle catabolism and provide energy. The amount varies with height, weight, age, sex, and daily activity. Adults need 35 to 45 kcal/kg ideal body weight/day. The help of a dietitian and the use of exchange lists make implementing these complex diets easier.

Changes in vascular volume are monitored carefully to prevent hypovolemic shock, as well as the hypokalemia and ototoxicity that can accompany diuretic use. Hospitalization is avoided unless the patient has severe generalized edema with ascites, significant hypertension, severe infection, hypovolemic shock, or a persistently low glomerular filtration rate. Bed rest is advised if complications are present. The level of proteinuria is monitored.

NURSING CARE

Nursing Assessment

Renal

Proteinuria (albuminuria) may be greater than 3 g/day; urine: foamy, deeper yellow color, oval fat bodies; oliguria

Blood Chemistries

Hypoalbuminemia less than 2.5 g/dl; hyperlipidemia

Cardiovascular

Edema: periorbital, external genitalia, peritoneal and pleural spaces, and extremities

Gastrointestinal

Anorexia; vomiting; diarrhea

General

Weight gain

Nursing Dx & Intervention

Nursing Diagnosis	Nursing Intervention/Rationale
Altered renal tissue perfusion	• Assess and monitor losses of protein in urine *to help determine replacement needed.* • Give medications as ordered and monitor response and side effects. • Monitor serum protein, blood urea nitrogen, and serum creatinine levels.
Fluid volume excess	• Assess and monitor weight, intake, output, blood pressure, pulse, and respirations *to recognize alterations in fluid status.* • Observe for edema. If edema is severe, monitor neck veins, central venous pressure, and pulmonary capillary wedge pressure.

Nursing Diagnosis	Nursing Intervention/Rationale
	• Be alert for side effects of diuretics used, especially those that cause excretion of potassium.
Impaired physical mobility	• Maintain bed rest during acute phase and if edema is excessive; otherwise encourage moderate activity. Implement measures *to prevent the complications of bed rest, such as pneumonia.*
Potential for infection	• Assess for signs and symptoms of infection. • Monitor white blood cell count altered by immunosuppressive drugs. • Avoid exposure to persons with infections. • Encourage good general health habits.
Potential impaired skin integrity	• Provide meticulous skin care of edematous body areas *to prevent excoriation, maceration, or infection.*
Altered nutrition: less than body requirements	• Encourage intake as ordered. Provide palatable meals, and consider patient's likes and dislikes. Protein diet supplements may be needed if urinary losses are excessive.
Body image disturbance	• See p. 1751. • Warn patient to expect alopecia as a side effect of cyclophosphamide and recurrence of edema and change in body appearance as side effects of corticosteroids.

Patient Education

1. Explain the nature of NS, its cause, and the possibility of relapse.
2. Explain the psychologic responses to NS and its treatment: massive edema, side effects of corticosteroids, and long-term effects of other immunosuppressive agents, which may include aspermia, ovarian fibrosis, and the increased likelihood of malignant tumors.
3. Explain follow-up medical care for monitoring changes in renal function.
4. Explain renal dialysis and transplantation as possible future options.

Evaluation

Patient Outcome	Data Indicating That Outcome is Reached
Symptoms of NS are absent.	Patient has normal serum albumin and lipid levels, stable weight, and no edema or gastrointestinal problems.
Renal function is normal.	Patient has normal urine without protein or lipids. Urine volume is normal and balances intake.
Patient is knowledgeable about NS.	Patient and family describe NS and its implications for long-term care in their particular situation.

Pyelonephritis

Pyelonephritis (PLN) is an infection of the kidney and pelvis. It is a major problem of the renal system.

Although urinary tract infections, including PLN, cause considerable morbidity, they do not progress to end-stage renal disease unless there is an underlying urinary tract problem such as obstruction. During pregnancy women should be screened for bacteriuria and treated to prevent the development of PLN.[18] Personal health habits should include adequate fluid intake (2500 to 3000 ml/day) and prompt emptying of the bladder.

Pathophysiology

The infection is caused by bacteria that spread by hematogenous or lymphatic routes or most commonly by ascending from the lower urinary tract. Obstructive uropathy, glomerulonephritis, polycystic kidney disease, diabetes mellitus, renal calculi, and analgesic abuse appear to lower the kidney's resistance to infection. Without treatment a significant number of pregnant women with asymptomatic bacteriuria will develop PLN.[18]

Damage to the kidneys is caused by inflammation, fibrosis, and scarring that occur because of the infection. Chronic PLN causes tissue destruction and contracted, small kidneys. The medulla is susceptible to the ascending spread of bacteria because of the hypertonic environment and slow blood flow there. Infection spreads through the collecting ducts to the interstitium. Papillary necrosis may be a complication of PLN, and detached pieces of tissue may block the ureters. Infection spreads to the cortex and eventually involves the nephron and blood vessels. The organism most frequently involved is *Escherichia coli*. Other organisms include *Proteus, Enterobacter, Pseudomonas, Klebsiella, Staphylococcus,* and *Streptococcus*.

Most infections are acute. A long-term, smoldering, chronic infection may occasionally occur. One or more of the factors previously mentioned contribute most often to a chronic infection of the kidney.

Diagnostic Studies and Findings

Intravenous Urogram

Small kidneys with an irregular outline and focal clubbing of the calyceal system are seen after injection of radiopaque dye

Medical Plan

Medications

Anti-infective agents
- Parenteral agents (IM or IV)
  - Gentamicin (Garamycin, Apogen), 3-5 mg/kg/d q8h
  - Cephalosporins
    - Cefazolin sodium (Ancef, Kefzol), 250-1000 mg q6-8h
  - Penicillins
    - Ampicillin sodium (Omnipen-N, Polycillin-N): patients ≥40 kg: 250-500 mg q6h; <40 kg: 25-50 mg/kg/d in equally divided doses q6-8 h
    - Carbenicillin disodium (Geopen, Pyopen), 1-2 g q6h
    - Penicillin G potassium (Aqueous penicillin G), penicillin G sodium, 1-20 million/d
- Oral agents
  - Sulfonamides
    - Sulfisoxazole (Gantrisin, Novosoxazole), 2-4 g initially, followed by 1-2 g q4-6h
  - Tetracycline (Achromycin, Tetracyn), 250-500 mg q6h
  - Penicillins
    - Amoxicillin (Amoxil, Amoxycillin), patients ≥20 kg: 250-500 mg q8h; <20 kg: 20-40 mg/kg/d in divided doses q8h
    - Ampicillin (Omnipen, Polycillin), patients ≥20 kg: 250-500 mg q6h; <20 kg: 50-100 mg/kg/d in equally divided doses
    - Penicillin G, 200,000-500,000 U q6-8h
  - Nalidixic acid (NegGram), 500-1000 mg q6h for 2 wk
  - Erythromycin (Erythrocin, Ilotycin), 25 mg q6h
  - Sulfamethoxazole and trimethoprim (Septra, Bactrim), 2 tab q12h

General Management

High normal (3500 to 4000 ml/day) fluid intake to dilute urine and decrease burning on urination, flush out urinary tract, and prevent dehydration (with normal renal function)

Bed rest is usual during acute phase

NURSING CARE

Nursing Assessment

General

Fever and chills; severe flank pain; weakness; anorexia

Renal

Hematuria; bacteriuria; pyuria; urine culture: significant growth; dysuria; nocturia; frequency

Nursing Dx & Intervention

Nursing Diagnosis	Nursing Intervention/Rationale
Altered renal tissue perfusion	• Give antimicrobial agents as ordered and observe response for side effects. • Explain drugs and their purpose. • Encourage high normal fluid intake; explain that this is *to flush kidney, but not to lower the drug concentration to ineffective levels.* • Measure intake, output, weight, temperature, pulse, respirations, and blood pressure *to assess volume status.*
Pain	• Assess need and give analgesics if ordered. • Provide external applications of heat, *which relieve pain.*
Impaired physical mobility	• Encourage bed rest during acute phase. Implement measures *to prevent complications of bed rest* (pneumonia, deep vein thrombosis) when needed.
Bathing/hygiene self-care deficit (potential)	• Assist with personal hygiene as needed; fatigue is common.

Patient Education

1. Explain pyelonephritis: its causes, signs, and symptoms.
2. Explain antimicrobial therapy: drugs, dosage, interval, side effects, and the need to complete course of treatment.
3. Explain the possibility of relapse or reinfection.
4. Explain measures to prevent urinary tract infection, including adequate fluid intake (2000 to 2500 ml/day for adults) to avoid dehydration, regular emptying of bladder to avoid overdistention, and good perineal hygiene for women to prevent the entrance of microorganisms into the urinary tract.

Evaluation

Patient Outcome	Data Indicating That Outcome is Reached
Signs and symptoms of pyelonephritis are clear.	Temperature, pulse, and respirations are normal, pain is gone, urine is clear of bacteria or pus cells, and problems in urination are gone.
Evaluation of urinary tract is completed.	Intravenous urogram is obtained to rule out any structural defect.
Patient is knowledgeable about pyelonephritis.	Patient can describe signs, symptoms, and any further treatment needed.

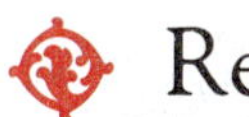

Renal Calculi

Renal calculi are stones formed in the kidney, primarily in the pelvis. Stones may be gravel like or formed in the shape of the pelvis, the so-called stag-horn calculus.

Renal stones are often associated with obstructions and infections of the urinary tract. They occur more frequently in men than in women. Geographic areas such as the southeastern United States have a particularly high incidence of renal calculi.

Pathophysiology

The formation of a stone is a physiochemical process involving a nidus of crystals or organic material around which the stone components form. The pH, temperature, ionic strength, and concentration of the urine affect the solubility of the stone-forming substances. The supersaturation of poorly soluble substances, the absence of crystalline inhibitors, and sources of seed crystals contribute to calculus formation.

The primary components of renal calculi include calcium salts, uric acid, cystine, and struvite (magnesium ammonium phosphate). The stones most frequently contain calcium or uric acid.

Hypercalciuria with or without hypercalcemia may be caused by hyperparathyroidism or osteoporosis or may be idiopathic. Calcium and phosphate are more soluble when pH is low. Bacterial infection by urea-splitting organisms causes the urine to become alkaline. Stones composed of struvite are called infection stones.

Hyperuricemia occurs with idiopathic gout, renal failure, blood dyscrasias, and the use of thiazide diuretics and alkylating agents. Uric acid is less soluble in high concentrations, low urine volume, and with low urine pH.

Diagnostic Studies and Findings

Kidney, Ureter, Bladder Examination

Radiopaque stone visualized on roentgenographic examination

Renal Ultrasonography

Stones identified

Medical Plan

The goals of medical care are to remove calculi, relieve effects of the calculi (pain and infection), resolve any causative factors (obstruction, infection, and metabolic abnormalities), and prevent future calculous growth.[8] The achievement of these goals should prevent permanent damage to the kidney and recurrence of calculi.

Surgery

Procedures used may include: pyelolithotomy, nephrolithotomy, ureterolithotomy, cystoscopy-basket extraction of calculi, and percutaneous fragmentation and extraction through a nephroscope; surgical intervention is a last resort with struvite stones because recurrence is so frequent

Additional procedures: extracorporeal shockwave lithotripsy, percutaneous lithotripsy (see p. 1138)

Medications

Anti-infective agents
- Parenteral agents (IM or IV)
  - Gentamicin (Garamycin, Apogen), 3-5 mg/kg/d q8h
  - Cephalosporins
    - Cefazolin sodium (Ancef, Kefzol), 250-1000 mg q6-8h
  - Penicillins
    - Ampicillin sodium (Omnipen-N, Polycillin-N), patients ≥40 kg: 250-500 mg q6h; <40 kg: 25-50 mg/kg/d in equally divided doses q6-8 h
    - Carbenicillin disodium (Geopen, Pyopen), 1-2 g q6h
    - Penicillin G potassium (Aqueous penicillin G), penicillin G sodium, 1-20 million U/d
- Oral agents
  - Sulfonamides
    - Sulfisoxazole (Gantrisin, Novosoxazole), 2-4 g initially, followed by 1-2 g q4-6h
  - Tetracycline (Achromycin, Tetracyn), 250-500 mg q6h
  - Penicillins
    - Amoxicillin (Amoxil, Amoxycillin), patients ≥20 kg: 250-500 mg q8h; <20 kg: 20-40 mg/kg/d in divided doses q8h
    - Ampicillin (Omnipen, Polycillin), patients ≥20 kg: 250-500 mg q6h; <20 kg: 50-100 mg/kg/d in equally divided doses
    - Penicillin G, 200,000-500,000 U q6-8h
  - Erythromycin (Erythrocin, Ilotycin), 25 mg q6h
  - Sulfamethoxazole and trimethroprim (Septra, Bactrim), 2 tab q12h

Diuretics
- Hydrochlorothiazide (Hydrodiuril, Esidrix) (to reduce idiopathic urinary calcium excretion), po, 25-50 mg bid

Analgesics
- Meperidine (Demerol, Pethadol), po, subcutaneously, IM, IV, 50-150 mg q3-4h
- Codeine sulfate (Methymorphine), oral, subcutaneously, IM 15-60 mg qid
- Morphine sulfate (Roxamol), po, subcutaneously, IM, 5-15 mg q4h prn

Electrolytes (used to ensure alkaline urine)
- Sodium bicarbonate, po, 300 mg to 1.8 g qd-qid not to exceed 16 g/d

Antirheumatic and anti-inflammatory agents
- Allopurinol (Zyloprim, Alloprin), decreases uric acid production, po, 200-800 mg in divided doses if more than 300 mg
- Penicillamine (Cuprimine, Depen) (combines with cystine to form a soluble compound), po, 250 mg qid

General Management

Low-calcium diets (less than 400 mg/day) and extra-high fluid intake (3500 to 4000 ml/day) are helpful but difficult to maintain; patients should avoid dehydration by drinking water rather than fluids that may be high in unwanted substances (such as tea with its high oxylate content); increased fluid intake should be spread out evenly over the 24-hour period, including once during the night; low purine diets may help decrease uric acid output; foods extremely high in purines (greater than 150 mg/100 g) are limited; oxalate intake is usually limited to less than 50 mg/day on low-oxylate diets

NURSING CARE

Nursing Assessment

Renal

Hematuria; crystalluria; passage of stone (strain urine); elevated 24-hour urine excretion of Ca^{++}, uric acid, or oxylate; urine pH increases or decreases; cystinuria; nocturia; urinary tract infection

Blood Chemistries

Variable levels of serum Ca^{++}, Cl^-, $PO_4^=$, pH, CO_2, uric acid, and creatinine

General

Fever; pain in flank that may extend to groin, labia, or testicle

Nursing Dx & Intervention

Nursing Diagnosis	Nursing Intervention/Rationale
Pain	• Note pattern of pain. • Assess need, give analgesic agents, and note responses. • Apply external heat to area *to relieve discomfort*. • Assist with increased fluid intake and walking, which *may help passage of the stone*.
Potential for infection	• Observe for signs and symptoms of urinary tract infection. • Monitor temperature. • Give antimicrobial drugs if ordered.

Nursing Diagnosis	Nursing Intervention/Rationale
Potential fluid volume deficit	• Assess and monitor blood pressure, pulse, respirations, intake, output, and weight. • Force fluids over the 24 hours to high normal level; avoid fluids that contain unwanted substances (such as tea with its high oxylate content).
Altered nutrition: more than body requirements	• Lower calcium intake with calcium stones (reduce intake of dairy products). • Lower purine intake with uric acid stones (reduce intake of organ meats, meat extracts, shrimp, and dried beans). • Lower intake of oxylate-containing foods (such as tea, chocolate, nuts, and spinach) *to prevent formation of oxylate stones.* • Avoid dehydration.
Impaired skin integrity related to surgery	• Prepare for surgery by explaining procedure and postoperative care and by preparing the skin and bowels. *Postoperative care:* • Monitor site of incision *for drainage and signs of infection.* • Monitor temperature, pulse, respirations, and blood pressure. • Keep any drainage tubes patent, unkinked, and anchored *to avoid inadvertent displacement.* • Monitor intake (intravenous and oral) and output. • Care for ureteral, urethral, and nephrostomy catheters, record output from each, and be alert for foul-smelling urine.
Bathing/hygiene self-care deficit (potential)	• Assist with personal hygiene as needed after surgery.

Patient Education

1. Explain the nature of renal calculi, their causes, and manifestations.
2. Explain medical management, including medications (purpose, dosage, interval, and side effects), diet (low calcium, purine, or oxylate), and fluid intake (amount, schedule, and kinds).
3. Explain medical follow-up to monitor the outcome of treatment.

Evaluation

Patient Outcome	Data Indicating That Outcome is Reached
Signs and symptoms of renal calculi are clear.	Urine is clear, no infection is present, and pain is gone.
Patient recovers from surgery.	Incision is closed. No infection is present.
Patient is aware of need for life-style changes.	Patient describes any medications, diet, or other instructions given to prevent recurrence of renal calculi.

RENAL FAILURE

Changes in renal function may be considered on a continuum from impairment to failure. Renal impairment may be revealed only by specific urine concentration or dilution tests. Renal insufficiency is revealed when the kidneys cannot meet the extra demands of dietary or metabolic stress. Renal failure occurs when the normal demands of the body cannot be met.

Health professionals can assist in the early detection of renal problems and the prevention of renal failure. Control of environmental factors such as nephrotoxic substances (drugs, organic solvents, insecticides, and cleaning agents) is important. Safe use and disposal of such agents in industry, agriculture, and the home must be encouraged. Avoidance of unnecessary urinary tract instrumentation could prevent infection. Elimination of predisease factors such as excessive or inadequate urination and fluid intake patterns, urinary tract problems, bacteriuria in pregnant women, and streptococcal infections should be supported. Renal function should be monitored in patients with hypertension or diabetes mellitus.

When some of the nephrons are damaged, the normal nephrons remaining are hyperperfused. If unchecked, progressive sclerosis of the glomerulus occurs, leading to end-stage renal disease. It is believed that restriction of dietary protein, if started early, will decrease the hyperperfusion and slow the progression of renal failure.[30] Being alert to prerenal problems in patients with surgery, burns, or trauma helps prevent complications. Genetic counseling may be indicated for some families.

Acute renal failure

Acute renal failure (ARF) is a sudden, severe impairment of renal function causing an acute uremic episode.

Major causes of ARF include acute tubular necrosis, acute glomerulonephritis, acute urinary tract obstruction, nephrotoxic agents, occlusion of the renal artery or vein, acute pyelonephritis, and bilateral cortical necrosis. A wide variety of substances may be nephrotoxic: antibiotics (aminoglycosides), anesthetics, iodinated radiographic contrast medium, organic solvents, heavy metals, endogenous toxins, and abnormal concentrations of physiologic substances. It is helpful to categorize the causes as prerenal, renal, or postrenal:

Prerenal: dehydration; hemorrhage; shock; burns; trauma

Renal: glomerulonephritis; acute pyelonephritis; occlusion of renal artery or vein; bilateral cortical necrosis; nephrotoxic substances; blood transfusion reactions

Postrenal: acute urinary tract obstruction

Prerenal causes result from a decrease in renal blood flow. Renal causes are those resulting from primary damage to the kidneys. Postrenal causes are those involving obstruction of the urinary tract distal to the kidneys. The mortality from ARF is more than 50%.[3] The prognosis depends on the cause and extent of renal failure. The very young and very old are particularly at risk.

ARF is frequently found in older patients in whom the common inciting events are more common. Dehydration is often a cause of ARF in the elderly or in young persons than in middle-aged adults. Elderly patients with multiple system problems or preexisting renal insufficiency are particularly at risk.

The five stages of ARF according to Muehrcke[23] are (1) onset: usually a short time from precipitating event to onset of oliguria or anuria; (2) oliguric-anuric: time during which output is less than 400 ml/24 hours (8 to 15 days; if longer, prognosis is poor); (3) diuretic, early: from the time when daily output is greater than 400 ml/day to the time that blood urea nitrogen (BUN) stops rising; (4) late or recovery: from the first day BUN falls to the day it stabilizes or is in the normal range; and (5) convalescent: from the day BUN is stable to the day the patient returns to normal activity; urine volume and BUN and normal; may take several months; some patients develop chronic renal failure.

Pathophysiology

The current explanations for the pathogenesis of ARF include leakage of tubular fluid from damaged tubules into the interstitial areas; tubular obstructions owing to an accumulation of intratubular debris or casts; glomerular abnormalities; and renal hemodynamic alterations, primarily excessive vasoconstriction.[3]

Damage caused by nephrotoxins appears to affect the proximal tubular epithelium and leave the tubular basement membrane intact. Damage caused by renal ischemia is more widespread and involves patchy areas of epithelial necrosis. Whatever the damage, the glomerular filtration rate decreases and urine formation is impaired.

In prerenal azotemia, urinary osmolality is high (greater than 900 mOsm/kg) and urinary sodium concentrations are low (less than 20 mEq/L), which is consistent with renal hypoperfusion and well-preserved tubular function. These findings reflect the physiologic response to hypovolemia or ineffective circulating blood volume. Urinary findings with parenchymal disorders reflect glomerular damage and inability to conserve Na^+ (urinary Na^+ greater than 27 mEq/L) or concentrate the urine (urine osmolality less than 250 mOsm/kg). In postrenal problems urinary osmolality and Na^+ levels may be normal.

Generally, the ratio of the blood urea nitrogen level to the serum creatinine level is 10:1. A ratio greater than that suggests dehydration, gastrointestinal bleeding, increased protein intake, decreased cardiac output, or antianabolic agents.

The management of fluid volume before, during, and after surgery helps protect renal function. The use of crystalloid and colloid volume replacement products and blood products helps prevent volume depletion and renal ischemia. When renal function is at risk, nephrotoxic agents such as the anesthetic methoxyflurane and antibiotics such as the aminoglycosides (gentamicin or kanamycin) should be avoided.

Diagnostic Studies and Findings

Kidney, Ureter, Bladder Roentgenogram and Renal Ultrasonography

Kidney size (normal or enlarged); presence or absence of obstruction

Medical Plan

Attempts are made to prevent decreased renal perfusion from progressing to ARF. Fluids and osmotic agents may be used. In any case, the cause of the ARF is determined if possible. The major complications of ARF in the oliguric phase include acidosis, hyperkalemia, infection, hyperphosphatemia, hypertension, and anemia. Hypovolemia and hypokalemia may be problems in the diuretic phase. Prompt and adequate management is essential to survival.

Medications

Electrolytes

Alkalinizing agents (for acidosis)

Sodium bicarbonate, po, IV, 1-4 g/d; 2-5 mEq/kg infused over 4-8h

Sodium citrate and citric acid (Shohl's solution),[11] po, 10-20 ml tid (1 mEq Na^+/ml)

Treatment for hyperkalemia

Sodium polystyrene sulfonate (Kayexalate, SPS), po or enema, 15 g qd-qid; give oral dose in 45-60 ml of water, syrup, fruit juice, or soft drink

Calcium gluconate (Kalcinate), IV, 1 g (90 mg Ca^{++}) in 10 ml

Sodium bicarbonate, IV, 2-5 mEq/kg infusion over 4-8h

Glucose 50%, IV, 25-50 g, and insulin-regular, IV, 10-15 units

Anti-infective agents

Infection is frequently a complication of ARF

Agents specific to the microorganism cultured should be used

Agents whose route of excretion is primarily renal should be omitted or used in smaller doses or at lengthened intervals depending on glomerular filtration rate

Agents excreted by only the liver require no change; when partial excretion occurs via the kidneys, some adjustment is needed at low glomerular filtration rates

Antacids (used as phosphate-binding agents)

Aluminum carbonate (Basaljel), po, 30-40 ml 1 h after meals and at bedtime of regular strength (400 mg Al $[OH]_3$/5 ml); 15-20 ml 1 h after meals and at bedtime of extra strength (1000 mg Al $[OH]_3$/5 ml)

Aluminum hydroxide gel, dried (Amphojel tab, Alu-Cap), 8 tab 1 h after meals and at bedtime

Antihypertensive agents

Clonidine (Catapres, Dixarit), po, 0.1 mg bid or tid initially, then increase by 0.2-0.8 mg/d (maximum effective dose, 2.4 mg/d)

Diazoxide (Hyperstat IV, Proglycem), IV, adults only: 300 mg by bolus in 30 sec or 1-2 mg/kg up to 150 mg at 5- to 15-min intervals

Hydralazine hydrochloride (Apresoline, Dralzine), po, 10 mg qid for 2-4 d, increase to 25 mg qid, then 50 mg qid; maintenance dose is lowest effective level; IM, IV 10-40 mg repeated as needed (q4-6h)

Methyldopa (Aldomet, Dopamet), po, 250 mg bid or tid for 48 hr, then increase or decrease q2d if needed; maintenance 500 mg-2 g in 2-4 divided doses (maximum 3 g)

Prazosin (Minipress), po, 1 mg bid-tid initially; maintenance may be increased slowly to a maximum of 20 mg/d in divided doses; up to 40 mg/d may be required

Propranolol (Inderal, Novopranol), po, 40 mg bid at 6-8 h intervals; increase if needed to 160-480 mg/d in divided doses; 640 mg/d may be needed

Diuretics

Furosemide (Lasix, Uritol), po, 20-80 mg followed by second dose in 6-8 h up to 600 mg; IM, IV, 20-40 mg given slowly over 1-2 min; high dose by IV not more than 4 mg/min

Hydrochlorothiazide (Hydrodiuril, Esidrix), po, 25-100 mg/d or bid initially, then maintenance 25-100 mg/d according to patient's response

Spironolactone (Aldactone), po, 25-200 mg/d in divided doses initially for 5 d, then adjust to maintenance level

Particular care is needed in all drug administration: dosage, interval between doses, and recognition of increased sensitivity because of altered renal function

General Management

Dialysis, either hemodialysis or peritoneal dialysis, is used to manage fluid volume and electrolyte imbalances (pp. 1071 and 1076); dialysis is particularly needed in pulmonary edema, hyperkalemia, uremic pericarditis, and convulsions; some nephrotoxic agents are dialyzable

Continuous arteriovenous hemofiltration is used to remove fluid in an unstable patient (see p. 1067)

Fluid intake must equal amount needed to replace measurable losses in urine, nasogastric drainage, wound drainage, and the like; avoid fluid overload; daily weights reflect fluid gain or loss

Packed red blood cells may be needed if there are symptoms associated with anemia

Nutritional support should include maintenance of body weight and positive nitrogen balance[7,26]

Calorie intake should include 100 g of glucose/day

Protein intake may be maintained through parenteral infusion of essential amino acids (50 to 85 g/L solutions); oral intake is started as soon as possible; protein intake is 30 to 40 g/day with 75% of high biologic value; high biologic value proteins are those that contain the essential amino acids in the proportions needed to promote growth, such as milk, eggs, and meat

Vitamin supplements are needed since a 40 g protein diet is deficient in calcium and folic acid and low in phosphorus and the B vitamins

Sodium intake is 500 to 1000 mg/day if edema or hypertension is present; potassium in the diet is restricted to 1500 mg/day if serum levels are over 5 mEq/L

NURSING CARE

Nursing Assessment

Cardiovascular

Prerenal: hypotension, flat neck veins, low central venous pressure, pulmonary capillary wedge pressure, dry mucous membranes, and decreased skin turgor

Renal: hypertension, edema, enlarged neck veins, elevated central venous pressure, elevated pulmonary capillary wedge pressure, and tachycardia

Cardiac arrhythmias

Respiratory

Shortness of breath; altered breath sounds; hyperventilation; infection

Gastrointestinal

Vomiting, anorexia, and nausea; hematemesis; melena; stomatitis

Renal

Urine volume in relation to intake: normal, oliguria, or anuria; infection; urinary sediment: normal or hematuria, proteinuria, bacteriuria, pyuria, casts (granular, pigment-stained hyaline, red blood cell; white blood cell), epithelial cells, and crystals; osmolality: hyperosmotic, isosmotic, or hyposmotic in relation to serum osmolality; urine pH lowered

Hematologic

Anemia; platelet deficiency

Blood Chemistries

Lowered pH, Na^+, Ca^{++}, and HCO_3^-; and elevated K^+, Cl^-, $PO_4^=$, and Mg^{++}; elevated blood urea nitrogen and serum creatinine; blood urea nitrogen: serum creatinine ratio greater than 10:1, in prerenal azotemia greater than 20:1, and in parenchymal disease less than 20:1 abnormal glucose tolerance curve

Neurologic

Changes in level of consciousness (somnolence or coma); changes in cognitive function or behavior; asterixis; convulsions

General

Septicemia; bruises; pruritus; dry skin; short-term weight changes

Nursing Dx & Intervention

Nursing Diagnosis	Nursing Intervention/Rationale
Altered renal tissue perfusion	• Give medications as ordered. • *Dosages of all medications may be less than usual, and the intervals between doses may be lengthened.* • Avoid nephrotoxic drugs *because of decreased ability to excrete drugs via the kidney.* • Monitor for responses and side effects. • Watch K^+ and Ca^{++} levels *if diuretics, digitalis, or banked blood is given.* • Watch for rapid changes in K^+ levels. • Report changes in K^+ levels less than 3.8 mEq/L or greater than 5 mEq/L. • Watch for electrocardiographic changes typical of hyperkalemia: peaked T waves, prolonged PR interval, widened QRS complex, and cardiac standstill. • Watch for acidosis: HCO_3^- less than 22 mEq/L or Kussmaul breathing. • Watch for signs of hypocalcemia (tetany): Chvostek's or Trousseau's signs.
Potential fluid volume deficit; fluid volume excess (potential)	• Assess and monitor weight, intake and output, blood pressure (sitting and lying), central venous pressure, pulmonary capillary wedge pressure, pulse, respirations, and breath sounds. Also check pulmonary status from chest roentgenograms and arterial blood gas studies. *Hypervolemia occurs in the anuric phase of acute renal failure.* • Observe neck veins, skin turgor. • Be alert to electrolyte losses in body fluid losses. *Vomitus contains Na^+, K^+, Cl^-, and water. Diarrhea losses include K^+ and HCO_3^-. Fever and hyperpnea increase water losses. Transudates contain protein-rich fluid.*
Potential for infection	• Observe for signs and symptoms of infection and fever. • Give meticulous care to any wounds or incisions *to avoid infection.* • Avoid exposure to persons with infections. • Establish a routine for deep breathing, coughing, and turning *to decrease possibility of pneumonia developing.* • Give mouth care at regular intervals.
Sensory/perceptual alterations (potential); altered thought processes (potential)	• Provide safe environment. • Assess patient's orientation to time, place, and person. • Observe for behavioral changes. • Observe level of consciousness. • Be alert to possible convulsions.
Altered nutrition: less than body requirements	• Assess caloric intake: kinds and amount. • Watch for nausea, vomiting, and anorexia *that increase losses of needed nutrients.* • Monitor weight.

Nursing Diagnosis	Nursing Intervention/Rationale
Self-care deficit (potential)	• Give assistance as necessary in feeding, bathing and hygiene, and toileting.
Impaired physical mobility	• If patient is on bed rest, give assistance with self-care. • Implement measures such as deep breathing, coughing, and turning *to prevent adverse side effects of bed rest, such as pneumonia.*
Knowledge deficit related to acute renal failure	• Help prepare patient to understand what is happening: diagnosis, treatment, bodily responses, and expected outcomes.
Altered family processes (potential)	• Help family understand what is happening to patient. Help family as needed in meeting the situation.
Ineffective individual coping (maladaptive; potential)	• Support patient's positive coping mechanisms. • Help patient develop new coping mechanisms. • See p. 1804.

Patient Education

1. Explain the cause of the episode of acute renal failure.
2. Explain the level of renal function after the acute phase is over.
3. Explain diet and fluid restrictions, which may continue or be lessened or discontinued.
4. Teach self-observational skills, such as the measurement of temperature, pulse, respirations, blood pressure, intake and output, daily weight, and record keeping.
5. Explain good personal hygiene.
6. Explain how to avoid infections.
7. Explain exercise and rest in the amounts advised.
8. Describe medications, if any, with name, purpose, dosage, time interval, and adverse reactions (by discussion and in writing).
9. Explain the schedule of medical follow-up.
10. Explain renal dialysis and transplantation if they are likely options for the future.

Evaluation

Patient Outcome	Data Indicating That Outcome is Reached
Renal functions return to normal.	There are stable blood urea nitrogen levels, no edema, normal blood pressure, normal urine volume, and normal activities.
Patient is knowledgeable about acute renal failure.	Patient and family can describe what has occurred and the implications for long-term follow-up of renal function.

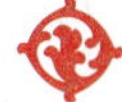 Chronic renal failure

Chronic renal failure (CRF) is a slow, insidious, and irreversible impairment of renal function. Uremia usually develops slowly.

Major causes of CRF include polycystic kidney disease, chronic glomerulonephritis, chronic pyelonephritis, chronic urinary obstruction, hypertensive nephropathy, diabetic nephropathy, and gouty nephropathy. Causes can be either primary renal disease or other systemic diseases:

Primary renal disease
  Glomerulonephritis; pyelonephritis; polycystic kidneys; hypernephroma
Secondary to systemic disease
  Hypertensive nephropathy; diabetic nephropathy; gouty nephropathy; lupus nephritis; renal amyloidosis; myeloma kidney; nephrocalcinosis; hereditary nephropathy

Levels of chronic renal failure are identified by changes in the glomerular filtration rate.[7] In early renal failure the rate is 30 to 10 ml/minute; in late renal failure it is 10 to 5 ml/minute; in the terminal stage it is 5 ml/minute. Symptoms are prominent in later renal failure and life threatening in terminal renal failure or end-stage renal disease (ESRD). Because patients vary greatly in their clinical picture, renal function, and performance capabilities, the Renal Section of the Council on Circulation of the American Heart Association developed criteria for the Evaluation of the Severity of Established Renal Disease.[7] These criteria take into account the severity of the signs and symptoms, the level of impairment of renal function (glomerular filtration rate and serum creatinine level), and the performance level (what the patient says he or she is able to do).

Pathophysiology

Nephrons are permanently destroyed by various processes that occur in the course of renal disease: ischemia, inflammation, necrosis, fibrosis, sclerosis, and scarring. The normal nephrons remaining may respond with hypertrophy and hyperplasia. A point is reached, however, when renal deficits become manifest. As many as 50% of the nephrons may be lost before renal deficits are discovered.[14] Such deficits include the inability to respond to excessive salt intake or decreased water or salt intake, decreased synthesis of substances such as erythropoietin by the kidney, and the inability to excrete the end products of metabolism. All the organ systems are eventually affected by renal dysfunction.

Diagnostic Studies and Findings

Kidney, Ureter, Bladder Roentgenogram and Renal Ultrasonography

Small, contracted kidneys

Medical Plan

The goal of therapy is to delay end-stage renal disease by conservative management and to begin dialysis or perform a renal transplant at the appropriate point in the course of the disease trajectory. Drug dosages and intervals must be modified when the kidney is involved in the drug's excretion. Rates of excretion, metabolism, and sensitivity to drugs may be altered.

Surgery

Renal transplantation (p. 1079); creation of an internal arteriovenous fistula for hemodialysis or insertion of a Tenckhoff catheter for peritoneal dialysis

Medications

- Electrolytes for acidosis
  - Sodium bicarbonate, po, 1-4 g/d; IV, 2-5 mEq/kg infused over 4-8 h
  - Sodium citrate and citric acid (Shohl's solution),[11] po, 10-20 ml tid (1 mEq Na^+/ml)
- Treatment for hyperkalemia
  - Sodium polystyrene sulfonate (Kayexalate, SPS), po or enema, 15 g qd-qid; give oral dose in 45-60 ml of water, syrup, fruit juice, or soft drink
  - Calcium gluconate (Kalcinate), IV, 1 g (90 mg Ca^{++}) in 10 ml
  - Sodium bicarbonate, IV, 2-5 mEq/kg infusion over 8 h
  - Glucose 50%, IV, 25-50 g, and regular insulin, IV, 10-15 units
- Anticonvulsant agents
  - Phenytoin (Dilantin, Novophenytoin), po, 100 mg tid up to 600 mg/d
  - Diazepam (Valium, Novodipam), po, 2-10 mg bid-qid
  - For status epilepticus, IM, IV, 5-10 mg initially; repeat if necessary at 10-15 min intervals, if necessary up to 30 mg; repeat in 2-4 h if necessary
  - Phenobarbital (Luminal, Barbita), po, 50-100 mg/d
  - Phenobarbital sodium, IV, 100-320 mg/d
- Antihypertensive agents
  - Clonidine (Catapres, Dixarit), po, 0.1 mg bid or tid initially; then increase by 0.2-0.8 mg/d (maximum effective dose 2.4 mg/d)
  - Diazoxide (Hyperstat IV, Proglycem), IV, adults only: 300 mg by bolus in 30 sec or 1-2 mg/kg up to 150 mg at 5-15 min intervals
  - Hydralazine (Apresoline, Dralzine), po, 10 mg qid for 2-4 d; increase to 25 mg qid, and then 50 mg qid; maintenance dose is lowest effective level; IM, IV, 10-40 mg repeated as needed (q4-6h)
  - Methyldopa (Aldomet, Dopamet), po, 250 mg bid or tid for 48 h, then increase or decrease q2d if needed; maintenance 500 mg-2 g in 2-4 divided doses/d (maximum of 3 g)
  - Prazosin (Minipress), po, 1 mg bid-tid initially; maintenance may be increased slowly to maximum of 20 mg/d in divided doses; up to 40 mg/d may be required
  - Propranolol (Inderal, Novopranol) (functions as β-adrenergic blocker), po, 40 mg bid to 6-8 h intervals; increase if needed to 160-480 mg/d in divided doses; 640 mg/d may be needed
  - Captopril (Capoten) (functions as an angiotensin converting enzyme inhibitor), po, 25 mg tid initially; increase of 50 mg tid in 2-3 wk if necessary; may be increased to 100 mg tid, then 150 mg tid
- Diuretics
  - Furosemide (Lasix, Uritol), po, 20-80 mg followed by second dose in 6-8 h up to 600 mg; IM, IV, 20-40 mg given slowly over 1-2 min; high dose by IV not more than 4 mg/min and repeat in 6-8 h
- Anti-infective agents
  - Infection is frequently a complication of chronic renal failure
  - Agents specific to the microorganism cultured should be used
  - Agents whose route of excretion is primarily renal should be omitted or used in smaller doses or at lengthened intervals depending on glomerular filtration rate[7]; agents excreted by only the liver require no change; if partial excretion occurs via the kidneys, some adjustment is needed at lower glomerular filtration rates
- Antacids (used as phosphate-binding agents)
  - Aluminum carbonate gel (Basaljel), po, 30-40 ml of regular strength (400 mg $Al[OH]_3$/5 ml) or 15-20 ml

of extra strength (1000 mg $Al[OH]_3$/5 ml) 1 h after meals and at bedtime
- Aluminum hydroxide gel (Amphojel, Dialume), po, 40 ml 1 h after meals and at bedtime
- Aluminum hydroxide gel, dried (Amphojel tab, Alu-Cap), po, 8 tab 1 h after meals and at bedtime

Androgenic agents
- Fluoxymesterone (Halotestin, Android-F), po, 10-30 mg/d
- Methandrostenolone (Dianabol), po, 5-20 mg/d
- Nandrolone (Deca-Durabolin, Anabolin-LA), IM, up to 300 mg/wk

Antiemetic agents
- Prochlorperazine (Compazine), po, 5-10 mg tid-qid
- Trimethobenzamide (Tigan, Ticon), po, 250 mg tid or qid; IM, 200 mg tid or qid
- Antihistamines (for antiemetic effect)
  - Cyproheptadine (Periactin, Cyprodine), po, 4 mg tid or qid not more than 0.5 mg/kg/d
- Phenothiazine (for antiemetic effect)
  - Trimeprazine tartrate (Temaril, Panectyl), po, 2.5 mg qid

Laxatives/stool softeners
- Methylcellulose (Methulose, Cologel), po, 5-20 ml tid
- Docusate sodium (Colace, DCS), po, 50-200 mg/d

Electrolytes, minerals, and nutritional replacements
- Calcium supplements
- Calcium carbonate (Titralac, Tums), po, 0.5-2 g 4-6 times daily
- Calcium gluconate (Kalcinate), po, 1-5 g tid
- Hematinic agents
  - Ferrous sulfate (Feosol, Fer-iron), po, 300 mg-1.2 g/d in divided doses
  - Iron-dextran injection (Imferon, Feostat), IM, IV, varies with weight and hemoglobin level
- Vitamins
  - Multivitamin supplements (water-soluble vitamins), daily requirements: thiamine, 1.5 mg/d; riboflavin, 1.8 mg/d; niacin, 20 mg/d; pantothenic acid, 5 mg/d; pyridoxine, 5 mg/d; vitamin B_{12}, 3 μg/d; vitamin C, 100 mg/d
  - Folic acid (Folvite, Folate sodium), po, subcutaneously, IM, IV, up to 1 mg/d
  - Vitamin D
    - Calcitrol (1,25 dihydroxycholecalciferol) (Rocaltrol), po, 0.25 μg/d; maintenance is 0.5-1 μg/d
    - Dihydrotachysterol (DHT, Hytakerol), 0.2-0.4 mg/d

General Management

Dialysis: peritoneal or hemodialysis (see pp. 1071 and 1076)

Fluid intake should balance output: about 400 to 600 ml (about the amount of insensible losses) plus an amount equal to 24-hour urine volume; avoid dehydration and volume excess

Nutritional modifications are made to achieve or maintain adequate nutritional status and to reduce work of diseased kidney[1]
- Protein: 0.6 g/kg body weight/day; glomerular filtration rate (GFR) 20 to 25 ml/min–90 g/day; GFR 10 to 15 ml/min–50 g/day; GFR 4 to 10 ml/min–40 g/day
- Sodium: 1000 to 2000 mg/day; the specific amounts depend on weight, blood pressure, serum creatinine, and 24-hour urine sodium excretion
- Potassium: 1500 to 2000 mg/day; no restriction is needed with normal urine output (at least 800 ml/day)
- Calories: 35 to 55 kcal/kg body weight; calories from fat and carbohydrates are used; adequate calories must accompany protein intake to prevent the use of protein for energy and weight loss
- Vitamins

NURSING CARE

Nursing Assessment

Urinary/Renal

Oliguria; anuria; infection; urine sediment may contain white blood cells, red blood cells, granular, hyaline, and broad and waxy casts; decreased creatinine clearance

Cardiovascular

Edema; hypertension; tachycardia; anemia; congestive heart failure; pericarditis; arrhythmias; cardiomegaly; atherosclerosis

Dermatologic

Pruritus; excoriations; yellow-tan or grayish color; uremic frost; pallor; bruises; dry skin; thin, brittle nails

Electrolytes

Increased K^+, H^+, Na^+, PO_4^-, and Mg^{++} and decreased HCO_3^- and Ca^{++}

Gastrointestinal

Urinous odor on breath; metallic taste; stomatitis and gingivitis; loss of sense of smell; anorexia; nausea; vomiting and hematemesis; esophagitis; gastritis; hiccoughs; melena; diarrhea or constipation; thirst

Metabolic

Increased blood urea nitrogen and serum creatinine levels; increased uric acid level; anion gap greater than 9 to 13 mEq/L; carbohydrate intolerance and altered glucose tolerance curve (delayed rate of decrease); altered insulin degradation (decreased renal extraction); hypertriglyceridemia (impaired removal of triglycerides by lipoprotein lipase activity); acidosis; tetany

Neurologic

Changes in cognitive function and behavior; altered levels of consciousness (drowsiness to coma and convulsions); changes in motor function and proprioception; peripheral neuropathy; nocturnal leg cramping; formication and other paresthesias of lower extremities; apathy, lethargy, and fatigue; headaches

Ocular

Retinal changes (hypertension); "red eyes" (calcification of conjunctiva); blurred vision

Reproductive

Infertility; impotence; amenorrhea; decreased libido; gynecomastia

Respiratory

Pulmonary edema; pneumonia; pleural effusions; hyperventilation; Kussmaul breathing; apnea

Skeletal

Renal osteodystrophy; soft tissue calcification; fractures; bone pain; increased alkaline phosphatase

General

Weight loss

Nursing Dx & Intervention

Nursing Diagnosis	Nursing Intervention/Rationale
Altered renal tissue perfusion	• Give medications as ordered by physician. • Be alert to altered dosages and schedules *needed because of altered renal function.* • Monitor response and side effects. • Watch K^+ and Ca^{++} levels. Watch for electrocardiographic changes typical of hyperkalemia: peaked T waves, prolonged PR intervals, widened QRS complex, and cardiac standstill. • Watch for signs of acidosis: HCO_3^- less than 22 mEq/L and Kussmaul breathing. • Watch for signs of tetany: Chvostek's and Trousseau's signs.
Fluid volume excess (actual or potential)	• Monitor weight, intake, output, blood pressure *(standing and sitting to detect postural hypotension),* pulse, and respiration. • Observe for thirst, tachycardia, dry mouth, venous jugular distention, and decreased skin turgor. • Observe for dyspnea and edema, and listen for rales. • Spread limited fluid intake over 24 hours. Cool liquids help quench thirst. • Be alert for electrolyte losses in body fluid losses: *Vomitus contains Na^+, K^+, H^+, Cl^-, and water. Diarrhea losses include K^+ and HCO_3^-. Fever and hyperpnea increase water losses.*
Potential for infection	• Observe for signs and symptoms of infection and temperature elevation. • *Note that a hypercatabolic state such as infection can cause life-threatening hyperkalemia.* • Give meticulous care to any wound or incision. • Keep patient away from persons with infections. • Establish a routine for deep breathing, coughing, and turning. • Give mouth care at regular intervals.
Sensory/perceptual alterations (potential); altered thought processes (potential)	• Provide safe environment. • Assess orientation to time, place, and person. • Observe for behavioral changes. • Observe level of consciousness. • Implement seizure precautions. • See p. 1728.
Impaired skin integrity	• Excoriations of the skin *may be related to pruritus.* • Relieve pruritus: oral drugs may help, as may vinegar or starch baths. • Keep fingernails trimmed. • Watch for infections. • Elevate edematous extremities. Avoid trauma. • Use bland soap. • Observe for bruises and petechiae, *which may occur because of bleeding abnormalities associated with uremia.*
Altered nutrition: less than body requirements	• Assess and monitor intake of food *to maintain protein, sodium, potassium, fluid, and high-calorie diet.* • Provide dietary supplements if ordered. • If nausea and vomiting interfere with meals, give antiemetics. Postpone meals. Serve foods the patient likes and present them attractively *to increase intake and prevent dehydration.*

Nursing Diagnosis	Nursing Intervention/Rationale
	• Provide mouth care *to help the bad taste in the mouth*. Sour candy balls and gum also help. • Monitor weight.
Self-care deficit (potential)	• Give assistance as necessary in feeding, bathing and hygiene, and toileting. Encourage independence.
Impaired physical mobility (potential)	• See interventions for self-care deficit. • If bed rest is needed, implement measures such as turning, coughing, and deep breathing *to prevent complications of bed rest*. • If patient is ambulatory, encourage physical activity to patient's tolerance. Fatigue may be a problem *because of anemia*.
Sleep pattern disturbance	• Provide time for rest and sleep. • *Be aware that uremia can reverse normal sleep-wake patterns.*
Knowledge deficit related to chronic renal failure	• Help prepare patient to understand what is happening: diagnosis, treatment, bodily response, and expected outcomes. • Teach diet, fluid restrictions, self-observational skills (temperature, pulse, respirations, blood pressure, and input and output), record keeping, avoidance of infection, personal hygiene, exercise-rest balance, and medications (dosage, purpose, interval, and adverse reactions).
Body image disturbance	• Observe patient's response to having a chronic illness, altered renal function, alteration in other body systems, or possibility of dialysis or transplantation in the future. • Recognize denial, guilt, aggression, fear, displacement, regression, resentment, disbelief, and anxiety in patient. • Recognize changes in psychosocial aspects of patient's life: change in social interaction, irritability, hostility, extreme dependence, fear of rejection, inability to work, loss of job, decreased financial stability, and altered hopes for the future. • Identify significant aspects of patient's cultural background and religion that may affect responses to chronic renal failure. • Help patient move through denial and discouragement, to acceptance of the condition, and to rehabilitation by sharing information needed, listening, and offering continuing emotional support. Refer patient to other professional resources as needed. • See p. 1751.
Sexual dysfunction	• Help patient and spouse understand physiologic basis of dysfunction. • Suggest positive aspects of closeness and touching without intercourse. • See p. 1794. • Refer patient and spouse for counseling, when appropriate.
Altered family processes (potential)	• Involve family from the beginning in all items under knowledge deficit and help them understand patient's responses. • Work with health team as they help family meet illness situation.

Patient Education

1. Explain the nature of chronic renal failure.
2. Explain the medical regimen and its rationale, including diet (restricted protein, sodium, and potassium intake), restricted fluid intake, and medications (purpose, dosage, interval, and adverse reactions).
3. Teach self-observational skills (temperature, pulse, respirations, blood pressure, intake and output, and weight) and record keeping.
4. Explain avoidance of infection.
5. Explain personal hygiene, rest, and exercise.
6. Explain when to call the physician.
7. Explain the plan for medical follow-up.
8. Explain renal dialysis and transplantation.

Evaluation

Patient Outcome	Data Indicating That Outcome is Reached
Patient is knowledgeable about CRF and its treatment.	Patient and family describe CRF, medical plan of care, and future options for renal dialysis or transplantation.

Patient Outcome	Data Indicating That Outcome is Reached
Conservative management of CRF is effective.	There is no uremia, glomerular filtration rate is greater than 15 ml/minute, and serum creatinine level is less than 10 mg/dl. Fluid and electrolyte values are stable. Diet restrictions are followed. Weight is stable; there is no weight loss or excessive weight gain.
Patient's mobility and self-care capacity improve.	Patient can walk and care for himself or herself with minimum help.
Patient shows positive acceptance of changes.	Patient recognizes changes secondary to CRF and their impact on life goals, activities.
If CRF progresses, dialysis or transplantation is instituted when needed.	There are persistent signs and symptoms of uremia, serum creatinine level is greater than 10 mg/dl, and glomerular filtration rate is less than 10 to 15 ml/minute.[8]

Renal Tubular Acidosis

Renal tubular acidosis (RTA) occurs when the kidney is unable to excrete an acid urine because of a defect in the tubules. Hyperchloremic acidosis ensues.

Both infants and adults may have tubular defects in acid handling. Causes of RTA may be hereditary or associated with cystinosis and hyperparathyroidism.

Pathophysiology

The tubular defect may be in the proximal tubule, which causes a failure in the usual reabsorption of bicarbonate ions. If the defect is in the distal tubule, acidification of the urine is impaired and hypokalemia occurs. Renal function is otherwise normal. A third type of RTA has defects in both parts of the tubule and a normal or elevated serum K^+ level. Renal calculi occur frequently in patients with distal RTA (see p. 1047).

Diagnostic Studies and Findings

Kidney, Ureter, Bladder Roentgenogram

Decrease in kidney mass, presence of renal calculi or intrarenal calcification

Medical Plan

Medications

Electrolytes (alkalinizing agents)
- Sodium bicarbonate, Shohl's solution, or Polycitra; for distal RTA: po, 1-3 mEq/kg/d; for proximal RTA: po, 5-10 mEq/kg/d
- The acidosis must be corrected slowly to avoid further lowering the potassium level

Diuretics (for proximal RTA)
- Hydrochlorothiazide (Hydrodiuril, Esidrix) (to decrease Ca^{++} excretion), 1.5-2 mg/kg/d
- Potassium supplement (for proximal RTA if serum K^+ <3 mEq/L) KCl (4 mEq K^+/5 ml), po, 20 mEq/kg/d in divided doses

NURSING CARE

Nursing Assessment

Renal

Distal: urine pH greater than 6.0; hypercalciuria greater than 4 mg/kg/day; nephrocalcinosis

Proximal: urine pH 4.5 to 8.0

Blood Chemistries

Hyperchloremic acidosis; hypokalemia less than 3 mEq/L

General

Weakness and lethargy; anorexia; bone pain

Nursing Dx & Intervention

Nursing Diagnosis	Nursing Intervention/Rationale
Patient problem: potential altered acid-base balance	• Monitor serum levels of H^+, HCO_3^-, Ca^{++}, K^+, and blood pH. • Monitor urinary calcium levels (Sulkowitch test), which become normal (2 to 3 mg/kg/day) *when adequate alkali is given for distant renal tubular acidosis.* Sulkowitch test: Add a special reagent to a urine sample taken after a meal. *Results give a qualitative measure of urine calcium: fine white cloud—normal Ca^{++}; clear solution—decreased Ca^{++}; heavy precipitation—excess Ca^{++}.* • Watch for tetany *caused by hypocalcemia:* Trousseau's or Chvostek's signs.

Patient Education

1. Explain the nature of the RTA.
2. Explain the treatment regimen: alkalinizing agent with dosage, interval, and side effects.
3. Teach the patient to check urine for pH and calcium.
4. Explain medical follow-up.

Evaluation

Patient Outcome	Data Indicating That Outcome is Reached
Patient is knowledgeable about RTA.	Patient and family describe RTA and medical management being instituted.
Acid-base imbalance is corrected.	Urine pH is 4.5 to 8.0. Urine calcium is 2 to 3 mg/kg/day. Serum HCO_3^- is 24 to 28 mEq/L. Serum chloride is 97 to 107 mEq/L. Serum potassium is 3.5 to 5.0 mEq/L. Serum pH is 7.32 to 7.43.
Nephrocalcinosis and renal calculi are prevented.	Roentgenograms reveal neither calcifications nor obstruction of urinary tract.

RENAL VASCULAR ABNORMALITIES

Renal artery occlusion or stenosis

Renal artery occlusion is a sudden complete blockage of the renal artery or a branch of it. Stenosis is a narrowing of the artery.

Pathophysiology

The complete cessation of arterial blood flow causes an infarct with coagulation necrosis in the kidney. If the person has a single kidney, acute oliguric renal failure ensues. Occlusion is most frequently the result of an embolism caused by mitral valve stenosis, subacute bacterial endocarditis, and mural thrombi after a myocardial infarction.

If a thrombus begins in the aorta and extends into the renal artery, percutaneous transluminal angioplasty is less successful than if only renal artery is involved.

Severe stenosis caused by atherosclerosis leads to ischemic atrophy and fibrosis. Decreased pressure in the arterioles stimulates the juxtaglomerular apparatus to produce an increase in renin secretion and can lead to renovascular hypertension.

Diagnostic Studies and Findings

Intravenous Urogram or Renal Arteriogram

Absence of function in all or part of the kidney is seen as radiopaque dye is filtered by the kidney

Medical Plan

A conservative approach is used. Patients usually have serious cardiac disease.

Surgery

Embolectomies are not usually performed for renal artery occlusion; renal damage usually has occurred by time diagnosis is made

Selected patients with renal artery stenosis may have surgical correction; percutaneous transluminal angioplasty may be used[7]

Aortorenal bypass; autogenous vascular graft

Medications

Anticoagulants (used for renal artery occlusion)
- Heparin sodium, IV, subcutaneously: 10,000-20,000 U initially (68 kg man); maintenance 8000-10,000 U q8h or 15,000-20,000 U q12h

Analgesics
- Meperidine (Demerol, Pethadol), po, subcutaneously, IM, IV, 50-150 mg q3-4h
- Codeine sulfate (Methylmorphine), po, IM, subcutaneously, 15-60 mg qid
- Morphine sulfate (Roxamol), po, subcutaneously, 5-15 mg q4h prn

Antihypertensive agents (used for renal artery stenosis)
- β-Blockers
  - Propranolol (Inderal, Novopranol), po, 40 mg q6h or q8h initially; increased to 160-480 mg/d in divided doses; up to 640 mg/d
- Angiotensin antagonists
  - Captopril (Capoten), po, 25 mg tid initially; may be increased to 50 mg tid after 1-2 wk then to 100-150 mg tid as needed

General Management

Dialysis may be needed (see p. 1070)
Relief of pain of renal artery occlusion
Monitoring of contralateral kidney function
Stabilization of cardiac function
Sodium and fluid restrictions for renal artery stenosis (see discussion of hypertension in Chapter 1)

NURSING CARE

Nursing Assessment

Renal Artery Occlusion

Renal
- Microscopic hematuria; few signs if infarct is small

General
- Pain in flank or upper abdomen; elevated white blood cell count; elevated lactic dehydrogenase (LDH) level

Renal Artery Stenosis

Cardiovascular
- Hypertension

Renal
- Increased plasma renin activity in renal vein; renal artery bruit

Nursing Dx & Intervention

Nursing Diagnosis	Nursing Intervention/Rationale
Altered renal tissue perfusion; fluid volume excess (potential)	• Assess and monitor intake and output, weight, blood pressure (standing and lying), and urine changes. • Monitor heart rate. • Monitor Na^+ and fluid intake if necessary. • Monitor neck veins, central venous pressure, and pulmonary capillary wedge pressure if necessary. • Give medications as ordered. Observe responses for side effects. • Assess for signs of hemorrhaging, injury, change in stools, localized bleeding, epistaxis, and bruises *to watch for side effects of anticoagulants*. • Give preoperative and postoperative care, if indicated.
Pain	• Assess level and pattern of pain. • Give analgesics as needed if ordered and monitor response.

Patient Education

1. Explain the nature of renal artery occlusion or stenosis.
2. Explain the treatment regimen and rationale.
3. Explain follow-up medical care.

Evaluation

Patient Outcome	Data Indicating That Outcome is Reached
Some function returns after renal artery occlusion.	Patient has improved renal function findings.
Medical therapy or surgery helps renal artery stenosis.	Hypertension is relieved or controlled.

Renal vein thrombosis

The renal vein or a branch of it can be blocked by an embolus or thrombus.

Renal vein thrombosis is most frequently associated with nephrotic syndrome (NS). It may also accompany a neoplasm that compresses the renal vein.

Pathophysiology

A sudden and complete occlusion of the renal vein causes an infarct. The kidney swells, pressing against the capsule. Slow development of an occlusion may permit the development of collateral venous circulation and cause less impairment of renal function.

Renal vein thrombosis may be associated with dehydration, sepsis, or hypercoagulable states.

Diagnostic Studies and Findings

Intravenous Urogram

Unilateral change in kidney function when radiopaque dye injected: enlargement, poorly visualized

Renal Venogram

Demonstrable clot

Medical Plan

The prevention of pulmonary emboli is vital. The underlying cause of the NS should be treated if possible (see "Nephrotic Syndrome"). Other disease states must be treated.

Medications

Anticoagulants

- Heparin sodium, IV, subcutaneously, 10,000-20,000 U initially (68 kg man); maintenance of 8000-10,000 U q8h or 15,000-20,000 U q12h
- Warfarin (Coumadin, Panwarfin), po, IM, IV, 10-15 mg/d for 2-3 days; then maintenance dose of 2-10 mg/d

NURSING CARE

Nursing Assessment

Renal

Gross hematuria; signs of nephrotic syndrome: proteinuria (albuminuria) >3 g/day, foamy, deep yellow urine, oliguria

Other

Pain in flank

Nursing Dx & Intervention

Nursing Diagnosis	Nursing Intervention/Rationale
Altered renal tissue perfusion	• Monitor urine losses of protein. • Monitor serum protein, blood urea nitrogen, and creatinine. • Give anticoagulants and watch for side effects: signs of hemorrhaging; bleeding caused by injury; change in urine, stools, and other body fluids; and bruises and ecchymoses.
Pain	• Assess patient's need for pain relief and give ordered analgesics as needed; observe patient's response.

Patient Education

1. Explain the nature of renal vein thrombosis.
2. Explain the medical regimen and rationale.
3. Explain the plan for medical follow-up.

Evaluation

Patient Outcome	Data Indicating That Outcome is Reached
Renal function returns if treatment is successful.	Renal function tests are normal.
Renal function is impaired if treatment is unsuccessful.	Renal function findings are abnormal.

Diabetic nephropathy

Diabetic nephropathy refers to glomerulosclerosis caused by lesions of the arterioles and glomeruli and associated with pyelonephritis and necrosis of the renal papillae.

Diabetic nephropathy (DN) or diabetic glomerulosclerosis is a very important complication of adult onset diabetes mellitus and the most important complication leading to death in juvenile onset diabetes.[8] The changes are related to the duration of the diabetic state. All insulin-dependent diabetic patients can expect the development of DN. Once proteinuria occurs, the renal changes invariably progress. Patients with diabetic nephropathy have increased morbidity and mortality. Although the survival of diabetic patients treated with dialysis or transplantation has improved somewhat in recent years, the outcomes are not nearly as good as in nondiabetic patients.[9] Diabetic patients have particular problems with atherosclerosis, coronary artery disease, peripheral vascular disease, retinopathy, and neurologic deficits. The likelihood of their successful rehabilitation is limited but has increased in recent years (see Chapter 9).

Pathophysiology

The glomeruli are affected by diffuse sclerosis and thickening of the basement membrane and mesangial areas. Nodular glomerulosclerosis may also occur. Both afferent and efferent arterioles are affected by thickened walls and hyaline deposits. The glomerular filtration rate decreases and azotemia occurs. The diabetic patient may appear clinically uremic at levels lower than the nondiabetic patient. This may be related to the diabetic patient's systemic vascular changes.[8]

Diagnostic Studies and Findings

Intravenous Urogram

Kidneys may be of normal size, swollen, or small and scarred (irregular cortical surface)

Renal Biopsy

Diffuse or nodular thickening of glomerular basement membrane and mesangial regions

Medical Plan

Some authorities believe that control of blood pressure and fluctuations in blood sugar levels slows the deterioration of renal function. Others believe that diabetic nephropathy follows an inexorable downhill course.[8]

Surgery

See "Renal Transplantation" (p. 1079). Diabetic patients who have a renal transplant have more complications, poorer rehabilitation, and a lower survival rate than nondiabetic patients with a renal transplant[8]; the underlying disease process cannot be corrected by transplantation

Medications

Insulin requirements may decrease as renal degradation of the hormone decreases or may increase as resistance to insulin's effects increases; antihypertensive drugs and diuretics may be needed

Electrolytes, minerals
- Alkalinizing agents (for acidosis)
  - Sodium bicarbonate, po, 1-4 g/d; IV, 2-5 mEq/kg infused over 4-8 h
- Treatment for hyperkalemia
  - Sodium polystyrene sulfonate (Kayexalate, SPS), po or enema, 15 g qd-qid; give po dose in 45-60 ml of water, syrup, fruit juice, or soft drink
  - Calcium gluconate (Kalcinate), IV, 1 g (90 mg Ca^{++}) in 10 ml
  - Sodium bicarbonate, IV, 2-5 mEq/kg infusion over 8 h
  - Glucose 50%, IV, 25-50 g, and regular insulin, IV, 10-15 U

Anticonvulsive agents
- Phenytoin (Dilantin, Novophenytoin), po, 100 mg tid up to 600 mg/d
- Diazepam (Valium, Novodipam), po, 2-10 mg bid-qid
- Phenobarbital (Luminal, Barbita), po, 50-100 mg/d

Antihypertensive agents
- Clonidine (Catapres, Dixarit), po, 0.1 mg bid or tid initially; then increase by 0.2-0.8 mg/d (maximum effective dose, 2.4 mg/d)
- Diazoxide (Hyperstat IV, Proglycem), IV, 300 mg by bolus in 30 sec or 1-2 mg/kg up to 150 mg at 5-15 min intervals
- Hydralazine (Apresoline, Dralzine), po, 10 mg qid for 2-4 d; increase to 25 mg qid then 50 mg qid; maintenance dose is lowest effective level; IM, IV, 10-40 mg repeated as needed (q4-6h)
- Methyldopa (Aldomet, Dopamet), po, 250 mg bid or tid for 48 h; then increase or decrease q2d if needed; maintenance 500 mg to 2 g in 2-4 divided doses/d (maximum 3 g)
- Prazosin (Minipress) (α-adrenergic blocker), po, 1 mg bid-tid initially; maintenance may be increased slowly to maximum of 20 mg/d in divided doses; up to 40 mg/d may be required
- Propranolol (Inderal, Novopranol) (β-adrenergic blocker), po, 40 mg bid at 6-8 h intervals; increase if needed to 160-480 mg/d in divided doses; 640 mg/d may be needed
- Captopril (Capoten) (angiotensin converting enzyme inhibitor), po, 25 mg tid initially; increase to 50 mg tid in 2-3 wk if necessary; may be increased to 100 mg tid then to 150 mg tid

Diuretics
- Furosemide (Lasix, Uritol), po, 20-80 mg followed by second dose in 6-8 h up to 600 mg; IM, IV, 20-40 mg given slowly over 1-2 min; high dose by IV not more than 4 mg/min and repeat in 6-8 h

Anti-infective agents
- Infection is frequently a complication of nephropathy/chronic renal failure
- Agents specific to the microorganism cultured should be used
- Agents whose route of excretion is primarily renal need to be used in smaller doses or at lengthened intervals depending on glomerular filtration rate; agents excreted by only the liver require no change; if partial excretion occurs via the kidneys, some adjustment is needed at lower glomerular filtration rates

Antacids (used as a phosphate-binding agent)
- Aluminum carbonate gel (Basaljel), po, 30-40 ml of regular strength (400 mg Al $[OH]_3$/5 ml), 15-20 ml 1 h after meals and at bedtime or extra strength (1000 mg Al $[OH]_3$/5 ml) at same dosage
- Aluminum hydroxide gel (Amphojel, Dialume), po, 40 ml 1 h after meals and at bedtime
- Aluminum hydroxide gel, dried (Amphojel tab, Alu-Cap), po, 8 tab 1 h after meals and at bedtime

Androgenic agents
- Fluoxymesterone (Halotestin, Android-F), po, 10-30 mg/d
- Methandrostenolone (Dianabol), po, 5-20 mg/d
- Nandrolone decanoate (Deca-Durabolin, Anabolin-LA), IM, up to 200 mg/wk

Antiemetic agents
- Prochlorperazine (Compazine), po, 5-10 mg tid-qid

Antipruritic agents
- Cyproheptadine (Periactin, Cyprodine) (antihistamine), po, 4 mg tid or qid not more than 0.5 mg/kg/d
- Trimeprazine tartrate (Temaril, Panectyl) (phenothiazine), po, 2.5 mg qid

Laxatives/stool softeners
- Methylcellulose (Methulose, Cologel), po, 5-20 ml tid
- Docusate sodium (Colace, DCS), po, 50-200 mg/d

Electrolytes, minerals
- Calcium (supplement): calcium carbonate (Titralac, Tums), po, 0.5-2 g 4-6 times daily
- Calcium gluconate (Kalcinate), po, 1-5 g tid

Hematinic agents
- Ferrous sulfate (Feosol, Fer-Iron), po, 300 mg-1.2 g/d in divided doses
- Iron-dextran injection (Imferon, Feostat), IV, IM, varies with weight and hemoglobin level

Vitamins
- Multivitamin supplements (water-soluble vitamins)
  - Thiamine, 1.5 mg/d
  - Riboflavin, 1.8 mg/d
  - Niacin, 20 mg/d
  - Pyridoxine, 5 mg/d
  - Vitamin B_{12}, 3 mg/d
  - Vitamin C, 100 μg/d
- Folic acid (Folvite), folate sodium, po, subcutaneously, IM, IV, up to 1 mg/d; maintenance: up to 0.3 mg/d
- Vitamin D
  - Calcitriol (1,25-dihydroxycholecalciferol) (Rocaltrol), po, 0.25 μg/d; maintenance: 0.5-1 μg/d
  - Dihydrotachysterol (DHT, Hytakerol), 0.2-0.4 mg/d

General Management

- See "Hemodialysis" and "Peritoneal Dialysis" (pp. 1071 and 1076); the underlying disease process cannot be corrected by dialysis; vascular complications of diabetes cause major problems in access to vascular system for hemodialysis
- Fluid intake should balance output: about 400 to 600 ml (about amount of insensible losses) plus amount equal to 24-hour urine volume; avoid dehydration and volume excess; specific amount determined by patient's dry weight (weight at which, after dialysis, patient has normal volume relationship)[21]
- Nutritional modifications are made to achieve or maintain adequate nutritional status and to reduce work of diseased kidney[1]
  - Protein, 0.6 g/kg body weight/day; glomerular filtration rate (GFR), 20 to 25 ml/minute to 90 g/day; GFR, 10 to 15 ml/minute to 50 g/day; GFR, 4 to 10 ml/minute to 40 g/day
  - Sodium, 1000 to 2000 mg/day; specific amounts depend on weight, blood pressure, serum creatinine, and 24-hour sodium excretion
  - Potassium, 1500 to 2000 mg/day; with normal urine output (at least 800 ml/day), no restriction is needed
  - Calories, 35 to 55 kcal/kg body weight/day; calories from fat and carbohydrate are used; adequate calories must accompany protein intake to prevent use of protein for energy and weight loss; control of protein intake takes priority in nutritional management; calories from fat and carbohydrates are increased

NURSING CARE

Nursing Assessment

Renal

Proteinuria; oliguria; anuria; infection; urine sediment may contain white and red blood cells, granular, hyaline, broad, and waxy casts

Cardiovascular

Hypertension; edema

Nursing Dx & Intervention

Nursing Diagnosis	Nursing Intervention/Rationale
Altered renal tissue perfusion	• Assess patient's need for pain relief and give medications as ordered; monitor response. • Be alert to altered dosage and schedules, *related to altered renal function.* • Watch K^+ and Ca^{++} levels. Watch for electrocardiographic changes: peaked T waves, prolonged PR intervals, widened QRS complex, and cardiac standstill. • Watch for signs of hypocalcemia (tetany) and Chvostek's and Trousseau's signs. • Radiocontrast medium in diagnostic tests should be avoided. *Diabetic patients with renal insufficiency are at risk for severe allergic reactions to the contrast medium.* Avoiding dehydration and decreasing the dosage do not appear to prevent renal damage.[9] • Avoid use of nephrotoxic agents.
Fluid volume excess or deficit (actual or potential)	• Assess and monitor weight, intake, output, blood pressure (standing and sitting *to detect postural hypotension*), pulse, and respirations. • Observe for thirst, tachycardia, dry mouth, venous jugular distention, and decreased skin turgor. • Observe for dyspnea and edema and listen for rales. • Spread limited fluid intake over 24 hours. Cool liquids help quench thirst. • Be alert for electrolyte losses in body fluid losses. *Vomitus contains Na^+, K^+, H^+, Cl^-, and water. Diarrhea losses include K^+ and HCO_3^-. Fever and hyperpnea increase water losses.*
Potential for infection	• Assess for signs and symptoms of infection and temperature. *Note that a hypercatabolic state such as infection can cause life-threatening hyperkalemia.* • Give meticulous care to any wound or incision. • Avoid exposure to persons with infections. • Establish a routine for deep breathing, coughing, and turning. • Give mouth care at regular intervals.
Sensory/perceptual alterations (potential); altered thought processes (potential)	• Provide a safe environment. • Assess orientation to time, place, and person. • Observe for behavioral changes. • Observe level of consciousness. • Implement seizure precautions.
Altered nutrition: less than body requirements	• Monitor intake of food *to maintain limited protein, sodium, potassium, fluid, and high-calorie diet.* • Dietary supplements may be ordered. • If nausea and vomiting interfere with meals, give antiemetics as ordered by physician. Postpone meals. Attractively served foods the patient likes increase intake. Prevent dehydration. • Provide mouth care *to help the bad taste in the mouth.* Sour candy balls and gum also help. • Monitor weight.
Feeding, bathing/hygiene, and toileting self-care deficit (potential)	• Give assistance as necessary in feeding, bathing and hygiene, and toileting. Encourage independence.
Impaired physical mobility	• Give assistance as necessary in feeding, bathing and hygiene, and toileting. Encourage independence. • Establish routine for changing positions. • If patient is ambulatory, encourage physical activity to patient's tolerance.
Sleep pattern disturbance	• Provide time for rest and sleep. • *Be aware that uremia can reverse normal sleep-wake patterns.*
Knowledge deficit related to diabetic nephropathy	• Help prepare patient understand what is happening: diagnosis, treatment, bodily response, and expected outcomes. • Develop an educational plan for end-stage renal disease. • Teach diet, fluid restrictions, self-observational skills (temperature, pulse, respirations, blood pressure, and intake and output), record keeping, avoidance of infection, personal hygiene, exercise-rest balance, and medications (dosage, purpose, interval, and adverse reactions).
Body image disturbance	• Observe patient's response to having a chronic illness, altered renal function, alteration in other body systems, and the possibility of renal dialysis or transplantation in the future. • Recognize denial, guilt, aggression, fear, displacement, regression, resentment, disbelief, and anxiety in patient. • Recognize changes in psychosocial aspects of patient's life: change in social interaction, irritability, hostility, extreme dependence, fear of rejection, inability to work, loss of job, decreased financial stability, and altered hopes for the future. • Identify significant aspects of patient's cultural background and religion *that may affect response to chronic renal failure.*

Nursing Diagnosis	Nursing Intervention/Rationale
	• Help patient move through stages of denial, discouragement, acceptance of the condition, and rehabilitation. Share information needed, listen, and offer continuing emotional support. Refer patient to other professional resources as needed. • See p. 1751.
Skin integrity, impaired	• Assess skin integrity. • Excoriations of the skin may be related to pruritus. • Relieve pruritus: oral drugs may help, as may vinegar or starch baths. Seek order in collaboration with physician. • Keep fingernails trimmed. • Watch for infections. • Elevate edematous extremities. Avoid trauma. • Use bland soap.
Sexual dysfunction	• Help patient understand physiologic basis for dysfunction. • Help spouse understand. • Suggest positive aspects of closeness and touching even without intercourse. • See p. 1794.
Altered family processes (potential)	• Involve the family from the beginning *to help them understand patient's responses.* • Work with health team as they help family meet illness situation.

Patient Education

1. Explain the nature of diabetic nephropathy and chronic renal failure. (See p. 1053.)
2. Explain the medical regimen and its rationale, including diet (restricted protein, sodium, and potassium), restricted fluid intake, and medications (purpose, dosage, interval, and adverse reactions).
3. Teach the patient self-observational skills (temperature, pulse, respirations, blood pressure, intake and output, and weight) and record keeping.
4. Explain avoidance of infection.
5. Explain personal hygiene, rest, and exercise.
6. Explain when to call the physician.
7. Explain the plan for medical follow-up.
8. Explain renal dialysis and transplantation.

Evaluation

Patient Outcome	Data Indicating That Outcome is Reached
Patient is knowledgeable about diabetic nephropathy and its treatment.	Patient and family describe diabetic nephropathy, medical plan of care, and future options for renal dialysis or transplantation.
Conservative management of nephropathy is effective.	There is no uremia, glomerular filtration rate is 15 ml/minute, and serum creatinine level is less than 10 mg/dl. Fluid and electrolyte values are stable. Diet restrictions are followed. Patient's weight is stable; there is no weight loss or excessive weight gain.
Patient's mobility and self-care capacity improve.	Patient can get about and care for himself or herself with minimum help.
Patient shows positive acceptance of changes.	Patient recognizes changes secondary to chronic renal failure and their impact on life goals and activities.
If nephropathy progresses, dialysis or transplantation is instituted when needed.	Signs and symptoms of uremia persist, serum creatinine level is greater than 10 mg/dl, and glomerular filtration rate is less than 10 to 15 ml/minute.[8]

Nephrosclerosis

Severe hypertension can cause deterioration in renal function. Nephrosclerosis is the damage to the renal arteries, arterioles, and glomeruli caused by prolonged elevated blood pressure.

Pathophysiology

A slow, variable progression of vascular changes can occur over the years. The process includes spasm, thickening, hypertrophy, and hyaline degeneration of the renal arterial system. In malignant hypertension renal changes are rapid and include fibrinoid necrosis.

Diagnostic Studies and Findings

Kidney, Ureter, Bladder Roentgenogram; Intravenous Urogram

Small kidneys, bilaterally

Medical Plan

Goals of therapy include aggressive control of blood pressure to slow renal deterioration, delay of end-stage renal disease by conservative management, and initiation of dialysis or performance of a renal transplant at the appropriate point in the course of the disease. Drug dosages and intervals must be modified when the kidney is involved in the drug's excretion. Rates of excretion and metabolism and sensitivity to drugs may be altered.

Surgery

Transplantation of donor kidney as described on p. 1079 may be needed; patient may be prepared with adequate dialysis for surgery (see "Hemodialysis," p. 1071); uremic problems are controlled before surgery

Medications

Antihypertensive agents

- Clonidine (Catapres, Dixarit), po, 0.1 mg bid or tid initially; then increase by 0.2-0.8 mg/d (maximum effective dose; 2.4 mg/d)
- Diazoxide (Hyperstat IV, Proglycem), IV, 300 mg by bolus in 30 sec or 1-2 mg/kg up to 150 mg at 5- to 15-min intervals
- Hydralazine (Apresoline, Dralzine), po, 10 mg qid for 2-4 d; increase to 25 mg qid, then 50 mg qid; maintenance dose is lowest effective level; IM, IV, 10-40 mg repeated as needed (q4-6h)
- Methyldopa (Aldomet, Dopamet), po, 250 mg bid or tid for 48 h; then increase or decrease q2d if needed; maintenance, 500 mg-2 g in 2-4 divided doses/d (maximum 3 g)
- Prazosin (Minipress), po, 1 mg bid-tid initially; maintenance may be increased slowly to maximum of 20 mg/d in divided doses; up to 40 mg/d may be required

Diuretics

- Ethacrynic acid (Edecrin), po, 50-100 mg initially; maintenance 50-100 mg/d or bid after meals (up to 400 mg) on continuous or intermittent schedule
- Furosemide (Lasix, Uritol), po, 20-80 mg followed by second dose in 6-8 h up to 600 mg; IM, IV, 20-40 mg given slowly over 1-2 min; high dose by IV not more than 4 mg/min and repeat in 6-8 h

General Management

Dialysis by home or in-center hemodialysis, home or in-center intermittent peritoneal dialysis, or continuous ambulatory peritoneal dialysis (CAPD) may be needed; see p. 1076

Fluid intake to balance output: about 400 to 600 ml (about the amount of insensible losses) plus amount equal to 24-hour urine volume; patient should avoid dehydration and volume excess

Nutritional modifications to achieve or maintain adequate nutritional status and to reduce work of diseased kidney[1]

- Protein: 0.6 g/kg body weight/day; glomerular filtration rate (GFR) 20 to 25 ml/min to 90 g/day; GFR 10 to 15 ml/min to 50 g/day; GFR 4 to 10 ml/min to 40 g/day
- Sodium: 1000 to 2000 mg/day; specific amounts depend on weight, blood pressure, serum creatinine, and 24-hour sodium excretion
- Potassium: 1500 to 2000 mg/day; with normal urine output (at least 800 ml/day), no restriction needed
- Calories: 35 to 55 kcal/kg body weight/day; calories from fat and carbohydrate used; adequate calories must accompany protein intake to prevent use of protein for energy and weight loss

NURSING CARE

Nursing Assessment

Renal

Urinary sediment: few white and red blood cells, few casts, and small amount of albumin; nocturia (urinating at night due to loss of ability to concentrate urine); oliguria; anuria; infection

Cardiovascular

Hypertension; see Chapter 1

Nursing Dx & Intervention

Nursing Diagnosis	Nursing Intervention/Rationale
Altered renal tissue perfusion	• Give medications as ordered by physician. Be alert to altered dosages and schedules. • Monitor response and side effects. • Watch K^+ and Ca^{++} levels. Watch for electrocardiographic changes typical of hyperkalemia: peaked T waves, prolonged PR intervals, widened QRS complex, and cardiac standstill. • Watch for signs of acidosis: HCO_3^- less than 22 mEq/L and Kussmaul breathing. • Watch for signs of tetany: Chvostek's and Trousseau's signs.

Patient Education

1. Explain the nature of chronic renal failure (see p. 1053).
2. Explain hypertension and its care (see Chapter 1).
3. Explain the medical regimen and its rationale, including diet (restricted protein, sodium, and potassium), restricted fluid intake, and medications (purpose, dosage, interval, and adverse reactions).
4. Teach self-observational skills (temperature, pulse, respirations, blood pressure, intake and output, and weight) and record keeping.
5. Explain avoidance of infection.
6. Explain personal hygiene, rest, and exercise.
7. Explain when to call the physician.
8. Explain the plan for medical follow-up.
9. Explain renal dialysis and transplantation as future options.

Evaluation

Patient Outcome	Data Indicating That Outcome is Reached
Progression of renal failure is delayed (refer to "Hypertension" in Chapter 1).	Renal function findings do not worsen.
Patient is knowledgeable about nephrosclerosis and its treatment.	Patient and family describe nephrosclerosis, medical plan of care, and future options for renal dialysis or transplantation.
Conservative management of nephrosclerosis is effective.	Uremia is not present, glomerular filtration rate is greater than 15 ml/minute, and serum creatinine level is less than 10 mg/dl.
If nephrosclerosis progresses, dialysis or transplantation is instituted when needed.	Signs and symptoms of uremia persist, serum creatinine level is greater than 10 mg/dl, and glomerular filtration rate is less than 10 to 15 ml/minute.[8]

Medical Interventions and Related Nursing Care

Continuous Arteriovenous Hemofiltration

Description and Rationale

Continuous arteriovenous hemofiltration (CAVH) is a process that removes excess water and controls azotemia in patients with uncomplicated acute oliguric renal failure, especially those who are unstable hemodynamically. It has been especially useful in critical care units. The continuous removal of water allows for less restriction of fluids needed for parenteral nutrition or medications. It is a safe, simple procedure that requires minimum priming volumes (18 to 60 ml). Fluid volumes and electrolyte concentrations change more slowly and thus cause fewer problems. For patients with a hypercatabolic state, hemofiltration can be alternated with hemodialysis to control the more complex azotemia, acid-base abnormalities, electrolyte excesses, and anemia, thus limiting the number of conventional hemodialysis treatments needed.[24]

Using a highly permeable, hollow fiber filter such as the Amicon Diafilter 20, plasma water and all unbound substances with molecular weights between 500 and 10,000 daltons can move from the vascular space and through the membrane of the fiber to form an ultrafiltrate (Figure 11-7).

Arterial and venous access sites are needed. The blood is propelled by the force of arterial blood pressure through an extracorporeal circuit, which includes the hemofilter (HF), and back to the patient. The tubing is kept as short as possible to decrease resistance to flow in the system. For the process to work successfully, the mean arterial pressure (MAP) must be 60 mm Hg and the hematocrit must be less than 40%. The filter has a large surface area, a high sieving coefficient, and low resistance so it can be used in patients with low mean arterial pressures. Since the volume in the circuit is small, unstable patients can tolerate CAVH treatments. Percutaneous cannulation of the femoral artery and vein is frequently used for access, but an arteriovenous shunt may be used.

Blood leaves the arterial cannula and enters the tubing

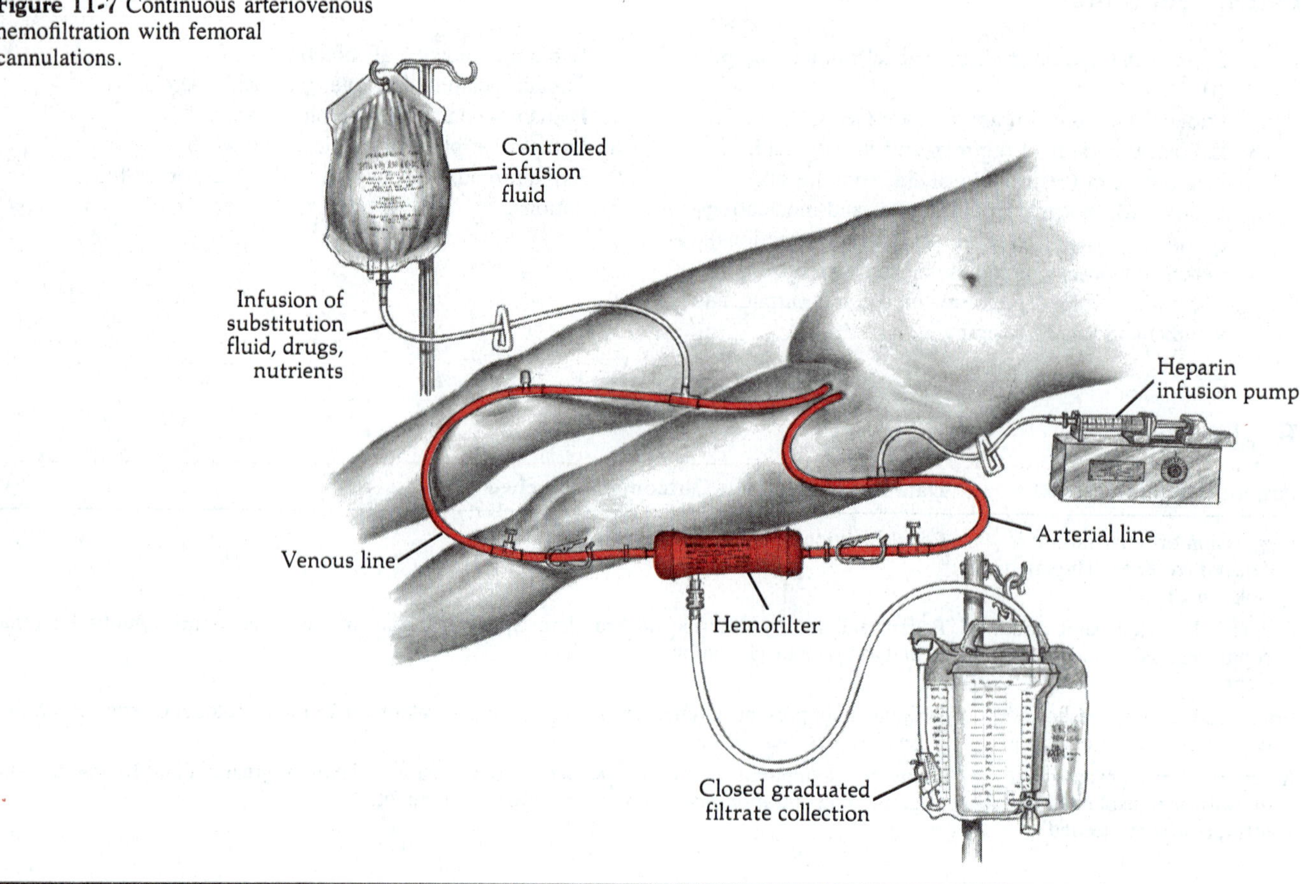

Figure 11-7 Continuous arteriovenous hemofiltration with femoral cannulations.

leading to the HF. A continuous infusion of heparin is added to the blood before it enters the HF to prevent clotting. The pressure difference in the HF (arterial pressure minus the oncotic pressure and the low pressure on the outer side of the hollow fibers) allows water and solutes to cross the membrane, forming an ultrafiltrate. The process is similar to the filtration process of the glomerular basement membrane in the kidney. The resulting ultrafiltrate is composed of water and solutes (Na^+, K^+, Cl^-, urea, glucose, creatinine, uric acid, $PO_4^=$); it drains into a collection device. The level of the collection device is important in determining the rate of ultrafiltration. Raising the level decreases the negative pressure and thus the rate of ultrafiltration, whereas lowering it increases the negative pressure and the rate of ultrafiltration. Generally, with adequate blood flow rates (30 to 120 ml/min), the ultrafiltration rate is 5 to 16 ml/min or 7 to 24 L/24 hours.[24] As the blood leaves the HF, it is rediluted with solutions that provide the water, electrolytes, and nutrition needed by the patient. Unwanted electrolytes are not replaced, and thus the patient's serum levels decline.

Indications for CAVH include overhydration unresponsive to diuretics; cardiovascular instability; the need for parenteral nutrition; elderly patients with serious cerebrovascular disease, coronary artery sclerosis, or uncomplicated acute renal failure; acute renal failure with multiple organ failure; and inability to tolerate conventional hemodialysis.

Contraindications and Cautions

A variety of conditions may be contraindications to the use of hemofiltration. They include hypercatabolic state; hyperkalemia; poisoning; low blood flow (MAP <60 mm Hg), shock, or low colloid oncotic pressure; congestive heart failure; and severe atherosclerosis. Because of hemofiltration's lower efficiency, it should not be used in situations requiring rapid removal of unwanted substances. At times a blood pump is used, requiring all the monitoring devices used with hemodialysis and specially trained dialysis nurses.

Excessive anticoagulation should be avoided. Patients with coagulation abnormalities may be treated without heparin. Procedures such as placing or removing central lines should be avoided during hemofiltration.

The procedure exposes the patient to large volumes of fluid needed to replace most of the filtrate removed. This means possible exposure to bacterial contamination, pyrogens, and trace elements.

Medical Plan

Medications

Anticoagulant agents

Heparin sodium: initial dose 500-2500 USP U; continuous infusion 500 USP U/h if no coagulation abnormalities; keep clotting time between 15 and 30 min; check prothrombin time and partial thromboplastin time as ordered

General Management

A portion of the fluid removed and discarded is replaced with water and solutes needed by the patient; typical replacement fluid contains Na^+ (140 mEq/L); K^+ (0 to 2 mEq/L); acetate (35 to 40 mEq/L); Mg^{++} (1.5 mEq/L); Ca^{++} (3.5 mEq/L); Cl^- (110 to 120 mEq/L); and dextrose (0 to 200 mg/dl)[10]; infusion rates range from 400 to 600 ml/hour

Nutritional needs can be met without fluid overload by infusing parenteral nutrition solutions with the replacement fluids

Mechanical Problems

Few problems occur with CAVH. Lines may kink or disconnect; the filter may crack, leak, or rupture. The ultrafiltrate collection device may be positioned too high or too low, thus causing negative pressure on the HF to be too low or too high. Replacement fluid can be added before the filter (predilution) or, as is usually the case, after the filter (postdilution).

If the hematocrit is too high (>40%), the blood may sludge and clot in the filter. In this situation prediluting the blood might be indicated. The blood flow rate, hydration status, and hematocrit all affect the amount of ultrafiltrate formed. Blood flow rates are better in percutaneous catheters than in arteriovenous shunts or fistulas.

A new filter must be rinsed well with sterile normal saline to remove the glycerin coating, the ethylene oxide used in sterilization, and all air bubbles.

NURSING CARE

Nursing Assessment

Cardiovascular

Vascular access problems: bleeding, infection, thrombosis, embolus; hypervolemia; hypovolemia

Nursing Dx & Intervention

Nursing Diagnosis	Nursing Intervention/Rationale
Knowledge deficit related to hemofiltration	• Explain procedure and its purpose.
Fluid volume excess related to too-rapid reinfusion of replacement fluid	• Assess intake, output, weight, pressure, pulse, respirations, cardiac output, pulmonary artery pressures, and pulmonary capillary wedge pressure *to evaluate volume status.*
Potential fluid volume deficit related to too-rapid fluid removal, bleeding	• Assess for bleeding, bruising, prothrombin time (PT), partial thromboplastin time (PTT), clotting times, platelet count; watch for clotting in filter, as evidenced by darkening of blood in circuit and a decrease by >20% in ultrafiltration rate *to evaluate the coagulation status.* • Check blood chemistries: blood urea nitrogen, creatinine, Na^+, K^+, and hematocrit *to evaluate hydration and effects of solute removal.* • Check level of ultrafiltrate collection device and ultrafiltration rate per hour. Note color of filtrate (pink or red means filter rupture) and presence of air bubbles (means air entering system, negative pressure too high, disconnected lines, leaks, cracks, clotting in filter).
Impaired skin integrity related to vascular access; potential for infection	• Assess cannula sites for redness, swelling, warmth, pain, and purulent drainage. • Use aseptic technique in site care. Do not take blood pressures or draw blood if arm is used. Watch for oozing of blood. Avoid trauma to catheter or shunt and apply prolonged pressure when they are removed.
Impaired physical mobility related to femoral arterial and venous catheters	• Maintain bed rest and stability of femoral catheters. Tape and secure all connections. • Restrain patient's movements, if necessary. Perform range of motion exercises; implement other measures to prevent complications of bed rest.

Patient Education

1. Explain purpose of hemofiltration, the equipment, and its role in life support.
2. Explain reasons for bed rest.

Evaluation

Patient Outcome	Data Indicating That Outcome is Reached
Patient and family understand purpose of hemofiltration.	Patient and family can describe the purpose of the process.
Fluid status and renal function are within normal limits.	Blood pressure, pulse, cardiac outout, pulmonary artery pressures, pulmonary capillary wedge pressure, intake, output, and serum chemistry measurements are within normal limits.

RENAL DIALYSIS

Dialysis is the differential diffusion of permeable substances through a semipermeable membrane separating two solutions. Hemodialysis and peritoneal dialysis are two forms of dialysis used clinically to treat patients with acute or chronic renal failure. The dialysate fluid contains electrolytes similar to those in normal blood plasma to permit diffusion of electrolytes into or out of the patient's blood. Glucose is added to the dialysate fluid to raise the osmolality and remove water from the blood channel.

Dialysis replaces some, but not all, of the kidney's functions. Fluid volume, electrolyte balance, acid-base balance, and nitrogenous wastes are controlled.

Dialysis options include home or in-center hemodialysis, home or in-center intermittent peritoneal dialysis, continuous cycling peritoneal dialysis (CCPD), and continuous ambulatory peritoneal dialysis (CAPD). Dialysis plays an important role in renal transplant programs by providing a backup for failed transplants and a pool of potential transplant recipients.

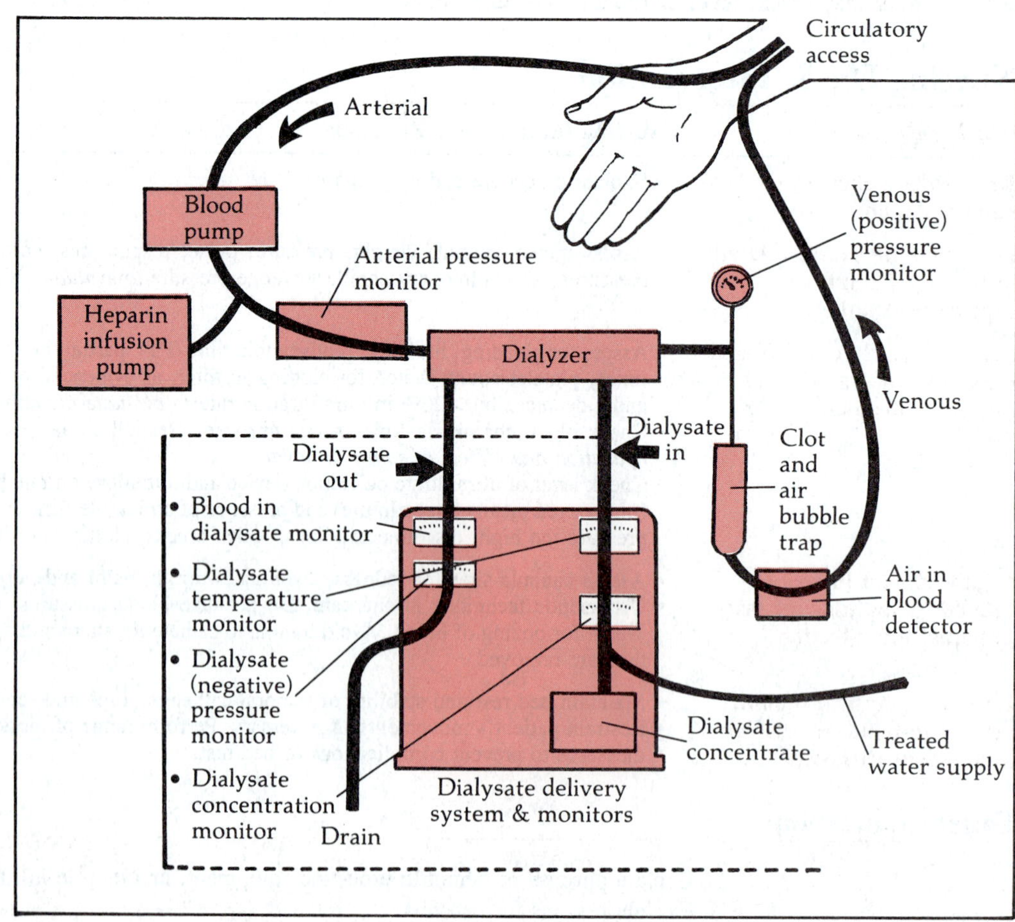

Figure 11-8 Components of typical hemodialysis system.
Modified from Lancaster.[19a]

Hemofiltration is an alternative to dialysis. This treatment uses a convective filtration process on a continuous rather than intermittent schedule. Pressure differences in the hemofilter force water and solutes through the highly permeable membrane in proportion to their concentrations in the blood. The ultrafiltrate formed is discarded, and depending on the patient's condition, most of the water and solutes removed are replaced. This procedure is used increasingly in the United States for acute renal failure; in Europe, it is used with a blood pump for patients with chronic renal failure. It is a simple system that uses a percutaneous access. A longer treatment time is required, thus avoiding peaks and valleys in blood chemistry values.

Hemodialysis

Description and Rationale

Hemodialysis involves circulating the patient's blood through semipermeable tubing that is surrounded by a dialysate solution in the artificial kidney (Figure 11-8).

The blood circuit includes an access device (cannula or internal arteriovenous fistula); arterial blood lines (with blood pressure monitor); a blood pump; a dialyzer, where diffusion, osmosis, and ultrafiltration occur; and venous lines with filter and monitors (for clots or air emboli and pressure), which return blood to the patient.

The dialysis circuit includes a supply of dialysate concentrate and a supply of treated water, which are combined by a proportioning pump so that the desired concentration is delivered to the dialyzer; monitors that detect the pressure, concentration, and temperature of the dialysate and stop the flow of dialysate if preset levels are not met; a dialyzer, where the dialysate accepts wastes, excess electrolytes, and water; dialysate exit lines, which may have a leak detector (blood-in-effluent lines) or are monitored using Hemastix to detect the presence of blood; a negative pressure gauge on the dialysate lines that controls ultrafiltration; and a bypass circuit (not shown in Figure 11-8) for diversion of dialysate that is not within the preset temperature, conductivity, or pressure limits.

The composition of the diluted dialysate solution is sodium, 130 to 145 mEq/L; potassium, 0 to 3 mEq/L; calcium, 2.5 to 4 mEq/L; chloride, 96 to 107 mEq/L; and acetate, 33 to 41 mEq/L.[8]

Blood access is achieved by means of an internal arteriovenous fistula created surgically with the patient's artery and vein, endogenous vein grafts, exogenous vein (bovine) grafts, or grafts made of artificial material such as expanded polytetrafluorethylene or by means of an external arteriovenous shunt or cannula (Figure 11-9).

Hemodialysis treatment schedules vary with the kind of machine used and the patient's condition. Treatments are usually scheduled three times a week for 3 to 6 hours each.

Major types of artificial kidneys are hollow fiber and flat plate. The hollow fiber kidney is increasingly used because it can be adapted to the size of the patient. In the hollow fiber

Figure 11-9 Circulatory access. **A,** Internal arteriovenous fistula. Needles are inserted into arterialized vein. **B,** External arteriovenous shunt, with circuit closed *(left)* and attached to tubing from artificial kidney *(right)*.

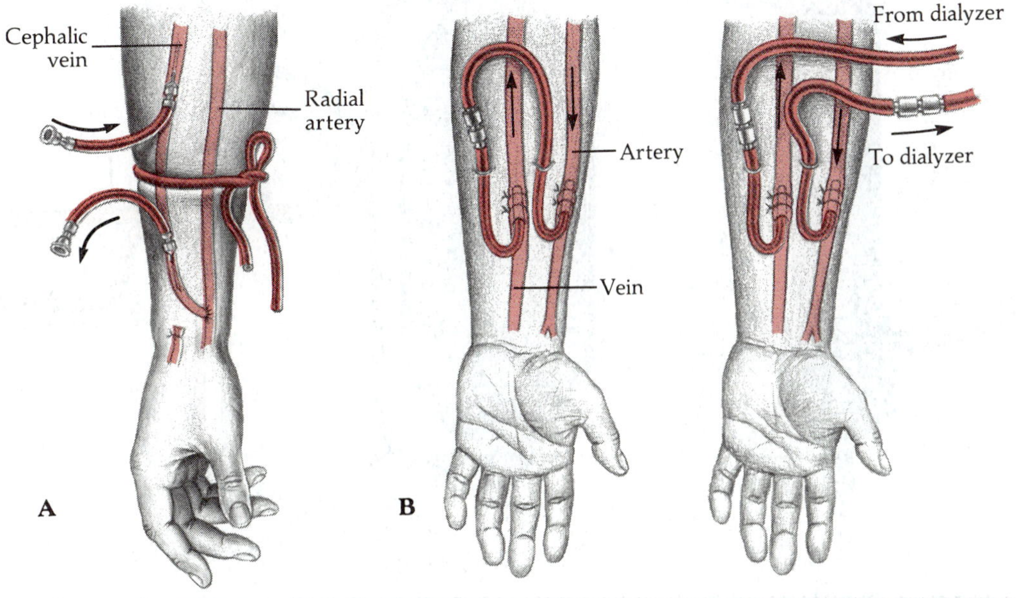

Figure 11-10 General scheme for dialyzer design.
Modified from Lancaster.[19a]

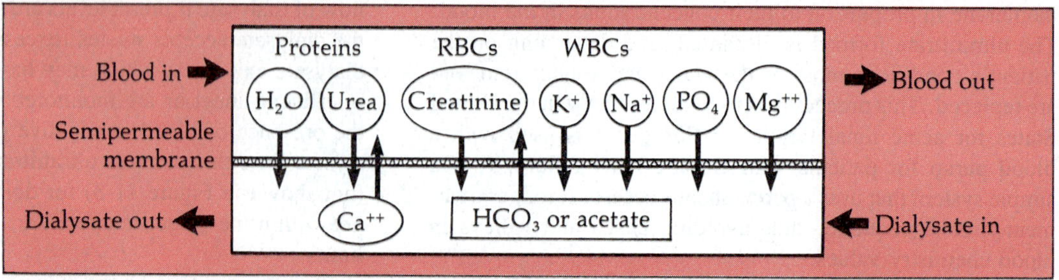

kidney the blood flows through narrow filaments that are surrounded by dialysate (Figures 11-10 and 11-11). In the flat plate kidney the blood and dialysate flow in opposite directions in alternate layers.

Indications for hemodialysis include need for rapid efficient treatment; acute poisoning (aspirin, methanol, or phenobarbital); acute renal failure; chronic renal failure; severe edema states; hepatic coma; metabolic acidosis; extensive burns with prerenal azotemia; transfusion reactions; postpartum renal insufficiency; and crush syndrome.

Figure 11-11 Kinds of dialyzers.
A, Hollow-fiber. **B,** Flat plate.

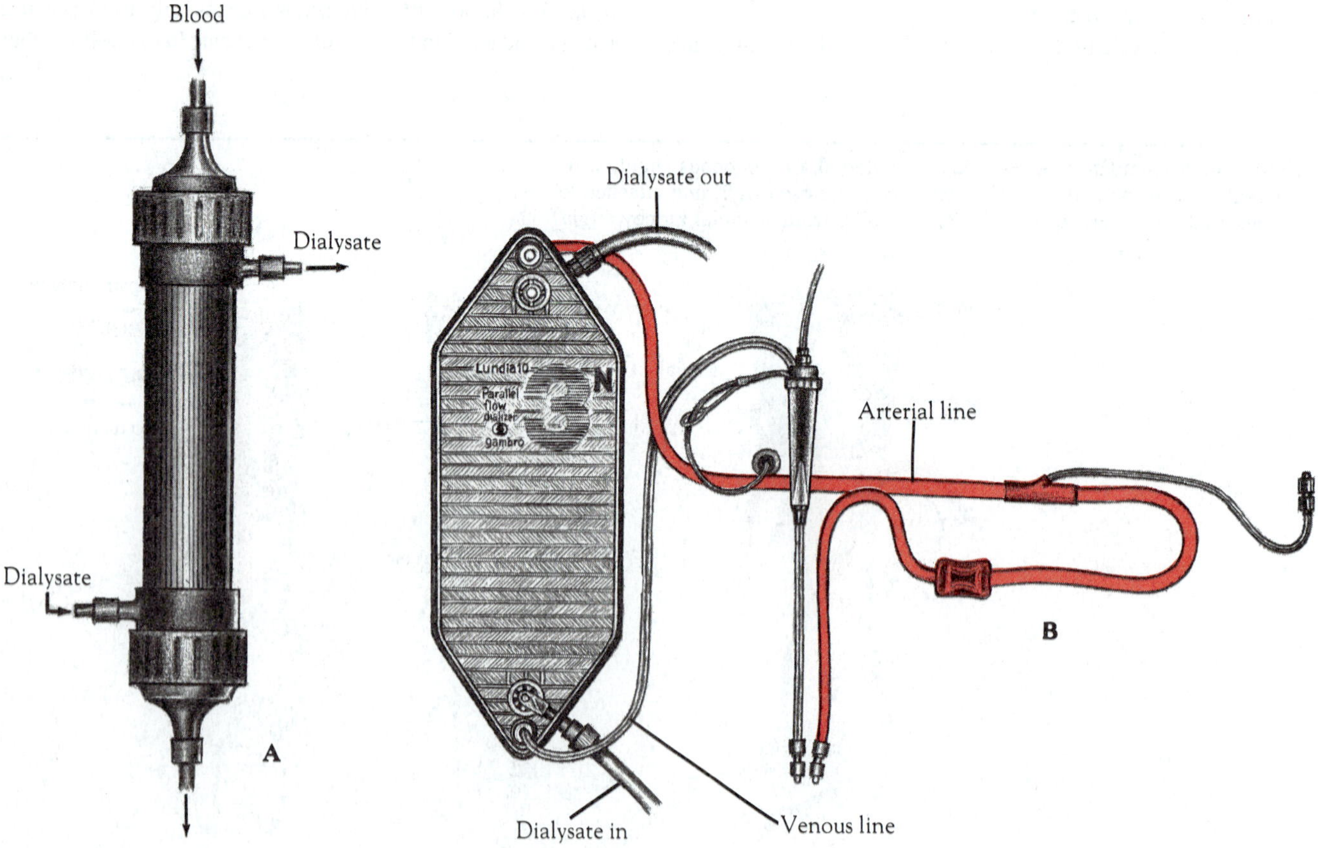

Contraindications and Cautions

1. Other major chronic illness
2. No vascular access
3. Hemorrhagic diathesis
4. Extremes of age
5. Inability to cooperate with treatment regimen

Medical Plan

Anemia, hypertension, infection, peripheral neuropathy, pericarditis, renal osteodystrophy, reproductive dysfunction, and psychosocial difficulties associated with uremia continue to require treatment (see "Chronic Renal Failure," p. 1053). The goal of therapy is to delay end-stage renal disease by conservative management and to begin diaylsis or perform renal transplant at the appropriate point in the course of the disease. Drug dosages and intervals must be modified when the kidney is involved in the drug's excretion. Rates of excretion and metabolism and sensitivity to drugs may be altered.

Surgery

Internal arteriovenous fistula created or shunt inserted to provide access to arterial and venous circulation

Medications

Anticoagulation agents

Heparin sodium, systemic: (1) intermittent IV injection, priming dose 100 mg/kg body weight with smaller doses repeated as determined by the clotting time, which should be 30-60 min; (2) continuous infusion by pump, 1000-2000 U/hr determined by the clotting time; regional: inject heparin into blood line to the dialyzer, add protamine to the exit blood line before blood is returned to patient

Antidotes (used as an antiheparin agent)

Protamine sulfate: amount and kind of heparin determine how much protamine is needed; each 1 mg of protamine sulfate neutralizes activity of about 90-115 U of heparin; keep patient's clotting time normal; monitor clotting time in machine and patient, watch for heparin rebound; this is return of anticoagulation up to 10 h later; more protamine sulfate may be needed

Antihypertensive agents: omit dosage on day of dialysis to prevent excessive hypotension during treatment

Vitamins (water-soluble) (lost in dialysate)

Daily requirements: thiamine, 1.5 mg/d; riboflavin, 1.8 mg/d; niacin, 20 mg/d; pantothenic acid, 5 mg/d; pyridoxine, 5 mg/d; vitamin B_{12}, 3 μg/d; vitamin C, 100 mg/d; folic acid, 1 mg/d

General Management

Medical management between dialyses includes: diet: low protein (1.0 g/kg/day, 50% high biologic value); low sodium (1500 to 2000 mg or 65 to 85 mEq/day); low potassium (1560 to 2760 mg or 40 to 70 mEq/day); calories (35 kcal/kg ideal body weight/day); fluids restricted (0.5 to 1 L/day); a specific amount is determined by patient dry weight (weight at which, after dialysis, patient has normal volume relationships)[20]

NURSING CARE

Nursing Assessment

Cardiovascular

Vascular access problems: bleeding, infection, and clotting; hypertension; hypotension; hypovolemia; hypervolemia; angina; arrhythmias; hemolysis; pyrogenic reaction

Neurologic

Headache; dialysis disequilibrium; dialysis dementia; subdural hematoma

Psychologic

Uncooperative; denial, depression, and anger

Other

Muscle cramps; pruritus; hepatitis B antigen and antibody

Mechanical Problems

Electrical outage; hypertonic dialysate; hypotonic dialysate; overheated dialysate; air infusion

• • •

Dialysis disequilibrium syndrome may occur near the end of dialysis or after it. The condition is related to the osmotic gradient produced across the blood-brain barrier by the efficient removal of urea from the blood, but not from the brain tissue. The urea draws in water from the extracellular fluid and causes cerebral edema. Other factors that may be involved are changes in serum pH, rapid ion shifts, and cardiovascular changes. The signs and symptoms of disequilibrium syndrome are headache, nausea, vomiting, agitation, twitching, confusion, and seizures.[14] This syndrome can be prevented by slowing the rate of solute removal by dialyzing at a slower blood flow rate (100 ml/minute) and for a shorter time, using a less efficient dialyzer, or using peritoneal dialysis.

Dialysis dementia, or progressive dialysis encephalopathy, is a syndrome that has emerged as experience with hemodialysis has increased. The clinical picture includes disturbed speech that occurs first during dialysis, myoclonus, dementia, or behavioral changes. It is a progressive condition that ends in death. A number of studies have implicated aluminum accumulation from the water supply or from aluminum hydroxide taken as a phosphate binder.[14]

Dialysis-associated hepatitis B is a major concern for patients (often active carriers of the hepatitis B virus), staff (at risk because of frequent exposure to patient's blood), and families (at risk because of close contact, especially sexual, and from environmental surfaces). It should be noted that special precautions with blood and other bodily fluids are needed to prevent spreading the hepatitis B virus (HBV). Health care professionals and patients in dialysis units are particularly at risk, because a patient with chronic renal failure receives frequent transfusions and may have a subclinical case of hepatitis B infection owing to impairment of the immune system.

The hepatitis B surface antigen (Hb_sAg) is a useful marker for active HBV infections.[6] Transmission occurs by way of some environmental surfaces (toothbrushes, razors, and needles) and by blood, blood products, and other bodily excretions or secretions. The primary sources are infected serum, saliva, and semen. Other sources of HBV can be feces, bile, sweat, tears, breast milk, vaginal secretions, cerebrospinal fluid, synovial fluid, and cord blood.

Programs to prevent the spread of HBV infections focus on identifying persons who are HB_sAg positive. Screening of all dialysis unit personnel and patients is done regularly. Such programs also include hygienic measures: safe, reliable procedures for handling laboratory specimens; procedures for hepatitis B precautions for hospitalized patients, including safe care of disposable materials, food handling, and laundry service; segregation of equipment used for patients who are HB_sAg positive; vigilant handwashing practices; sterilization measures appropriate to the material involved; no eating, smoking, or other hand-to-mouth activity in the dialysis unit or laboratory; use of protective clothing, such as masks, goggles, gloves, aprons, shoe covers, gowns, and caps; and policy of reporting and recording any unusual exposure to HBV.

Hepatitis B vaccine is used for active immunization for preexposure prevention in high-risk populations, such as dialysis unit personnel. Hepatitis B immune globulin is used for passive immunization after exposure to HBV.

Nursing Dx & Intervention

Nursing Diagnosis	Nursing Intervention/Rationale
Knowledge deficit related to hemodialysis	• Explain hemodialysis procedure and its purpose. Demonstrate safe aseptic cannula care.
Fluid volume excess (potential)	*Prehemodialysis care:* • Measure weight, temperature, pulse, respirations, and blood pressure (lying and standing) to have baseline data. • Record these prehemodialysis figures. • A patient should not gain more than 1.5 kg between treatments. • Review blood chemistry findings (blood urea nitrogen, creatinine, Na^+, K^+, and hematocrit).
Potential for infection	• Wear mask over nose and mouth and place mask over patient's nose and mouth while making connections with dialyzer tubing, wearing goggles *to prevent blood splash in eyes.* • Use sterile technique to initiate hemodialysis, needle insertions, or shunt connections. Anchor connections securely. • Use disposable gloves and plastic apron over clothes *to prevent direct contact with blood.* • Identify HB_sAg status of patient. Check HIV status, if known.
Potential fluid volume deficit	• Minimize blood loss, *since patient with chronic renal failure is anemic.* • Measure intake and output. • Check bleeding and clotting times. • Observe hemodialysis system monitors *to ensure patient safety* (flow rate, pressure, temperature, osmolality, clots, air emboli, negative pressure for ultrafiltration, and blood leaks). Watch for equipment or electrical failures. • Assess and monitor vital signs throughout procedure. Check patient's response to the procedure. • Infuse normal saline intravenously if patient is hypotensive (nausea and muscle cramps). • Check blood pressure, temperature, pulse, respirations, and weight. *Patient should weigh less, have lower blood pressure, and higher temperature than before dialysis treatment.* Check blood chemistries: *blood urea nitrogen, creatinine,* Na^+*, and* K^+ *levels should be decreased.*
Impaired skin integrity	*After hemodialysis:* • Permit no one to take blood pressure or to perform intravenous punctures in arm with fistula or shunt *(to prevent infection or clotting).* • Perform regular shunt care. Wear mask and goggles. Inspect exit sites *for infection.* Cleanse gently with hydrogen peroxide and applicator sticks using aseptic technique. Clean shunt with alcohol sponges, starting at exit site. Cover with dry sterile dressing and hold in place with paper tape and woven gauze bandage. • Avoid trauma to shunt. Check circulation (palpate thrill) on venous side and check for clots. Instruct patient to wear loose sleeves, avoid temperature extremes or lifting heavy objects, avoid prolonged immersion of arm in water (arm may be temporarily covered with plastic), and carry clamps *to stop bleeding if the shunt separates.*

Nursing Diagnosis	Nursing Intervention/Rationale
	• Provide fistula care. Apply direct pressure to needle sites for 5 minutes or until bleeding stops. Cover with Band-Aid. Pressure dressing may be used. • Watch for signs of bleeding, infection, ischemia of hand, or aneurysm formation. Watch for clotting and formation of scar tissue *from repeated venipunctures.*
Altered thought processes (potential)	• Watch for dialysis disequilibrium and dialysis dementia.
Body image disturbance	• Observe patient's response to having a chronic illness, altered renal function, alteration in other body systems, and the possibility of renal transplantation in the future. • Recognize patient's response to dependence on a machine. *Patient may feel helpless and hopeless, deny reality, and personalize machine or may accept it as necessary.* • Be aware of changes in social involvement: fewer social-recreational activities, life-style changes, and withdrawal because of being different. • Support patient's strengths: self-confidence, determination, and motivation to live. • Help patient develop or continue interests beyond dialysis and return to as normal a life as possible. • Be alert to excessive concern with losses, depression, self-neglect, and noncompliance with medical regimen and to possibility of suicide. • Be aware of effect loss of libido, impotence, and decreased orgasm has on the marital and sexual life of patient. • Try to help patient develop realistic expectations of dialysis. • Try to keep lines of communication open. • See p. 1751.
Altered family processes	• Recognize that chronic renal failure and hemodialysis can cause disruption, expense, and considerable alteration in time commitments in family. • Try to support family's willing cooperation in patient's care and help them look at ways to decrease domestic tension and unhappiness. • Help patient and spouse recognize demands of illness situation on spouse and patient's need for emotional support. Recognize spouse's fears. • See p. 1772.
Impaired home maintenance management	• Observe the home *to see that it is large enough, clean, and adequately supplied with electricity, water, and heat and has a phone to be suitable for home hemodialysis.* • Recognize patient's inability to continue family role of homemaker or breadwinner, and help patient accept this through discussion of alternatives. • In home dialysis recognize stresses that spouse faces and support spouse in learning about dialysis and carrying out hemodialysis in the home.

Patient Education

1. Explain function of normal and artificial kidney.
2. Explain principles of hemodialysis.
3. Explain aseptic technique for needle insertions or shunt care. Explain care of access sites.
4. Teach self-observational skills (temperature, pulse, respirations, blood pressure, intake and output, and weight) and record keeping.
5. Explain components of system with preparation, operation, cleaning, storage (repair and maintenance if home hemodialysis).
6. Explain initiating dialysis, monitoring during dialysis, and discontinuing dialysis.
7. Explain emergencies related to machine and to patient's medical condition.
8. Explain care while off machine: diet, fluid restrictions, medical complications, care of blood access route, medications, and prevention of infection.
9. Explain medical supervision, including help available from medical center, and schedule of return visits, and assistance from the local physician.
10. Review education plan for chronic renal failure (see p. 1057).

Evaluation

Patient Outcome	Data Indicating That Outcome is Reached
Dialysis is adequate.[15]	Patient and family describe principles of hemodialysis, plan of care, and correct use of hemodialysis machine: good general and nutritional status, normal blood pressure, clinically tolerated anemia, no osteodystrophy and calcifications on roentgenogram; no uremic polyneuropathy and encephalopathy; predialysis plasma concentrations of urea, creatinine, K^+ and Na^+ in desirable range; and good quality of life and rehabilitation.
Patient and family understand chronic renal failure and hemodialysis.	Patient and family describe chronic renal failure and medical plan of care.
Patient and family have adjusted to life on hemodialysis.	Patient and family have returned to work and social activities as are possible. Family continues to use support of health team.

Peritoneal dialysis

Description and Rationale

Peritoneal dialysis (PD) involves the introduction of dialysate fluid into the abdominal cavity, where the peritoneum acts as a semipermeable membrane between the dialysate and the blood in the abdominal vessels. A machine may be used, or the fluid may be instilled and drained manually from the peritoneal cavity.

Components of peritoneal dialysis solutions include varying amounts of glucose and electrolytes. Glucose at 1.3 mOsm/kg of water yields a 1.5% solution; 2.2 mOsm/kg yields a 4.5% solution; 3.86 mOsm/kg yields a 7% solution. Commonly used concentrations of electrolytes are sodium, 132 mmol/L; potassium, 0 mmol/L; calcium, 1.75 mmol/L; magnesium, 0.5 to 0.75 mmol/L; chloride, 96 mmol/L; and lactate, 35 to 40 mmol/L. The total osmolality is 346 mOsm/kg for the 1.5% solution, 396 mOsm/kg for the 4.5% solution, and 485 mOsm/kg for the 7% solution. The pH of the solution is 5.2. Volumes available range from 250 to 3000 ml per bag.

Additions may include potassium, 0 to 3 mEq/L, and heparin, 500 to 1000 U/L.

Continuous ambulatory peritoneal dialysis (CAPD) is an alternative to intermittent peritoneal dialysis for chronic renal failure. A permanent peritoneal dialysis catheter is inserted into the abdomen; a Luer-Lok titanium connector joins the transfer set to the bag of fluid (Figure 11-12).

CAPD usually involves four exchanges of 1-2 L each in 24 hours and dwell times of 4 to 8 hours.[31,32] Dialysate in plastic bags is used. When the solution is infused, the plastic bag is folded up and concealed under the person's clothes. When the fluid is drained, that bag is discarded and a new bag is attached, and its fluid is instilled for the next cycle. CAPD is self-administered and machine free.

Continuous cycling peritoneal dialysis involves connecting the peritoneal catheter to an automated peritoneal dialysis machine that performs three to seven cycles during the night while the patient sleeps. During the day one cycle of fluid is left in the abdomen. The person is free of dialysis activities during the day, and connections are less frequent than in CAPD.

Peritoneal dialysis is indicated when less rapid treatment is needed; equipment and staff for hemodialysis are not available; there is inadequate blood access; the patient is in shock or has had cardiovascular surgery; severe cardiovascular disease is present; and the patient refuses blood transfusions.

Contraindications and Cautions

1. Peritonitis
2. Abdominal adhesions
3. Recent abdominal surgery

Medical Plan

Surgery

The peritoneal catheter is inserted into the peritoneal cavity, generally under local anesthetic in the operating room; if the catheter is permanent, it has an internal Dacron cuff that lies between the peritoneum and the abdominal muscles; it has an external cuff that is 1 to 1.5 cm below the skin at the other end of a 3 to 4 cm subcutaneous tunnel.

Medications

Anticoagulants

Heparin may be added to dialysate to prevent fibrin formation and obstruction to the fluid flow; antimicrobial agents are used when peritonitis is diagnosed; they usually are given by the intraperitoneal route; vitamins (water-soluble) are lost and must be replaced (see "Hemodialysis," p. 1071)

General Management

Medical management of the continuing uremic problems is discussed in the section on chronic renal failure (p. 1053); the use of peritoneal dialysis causes an increased

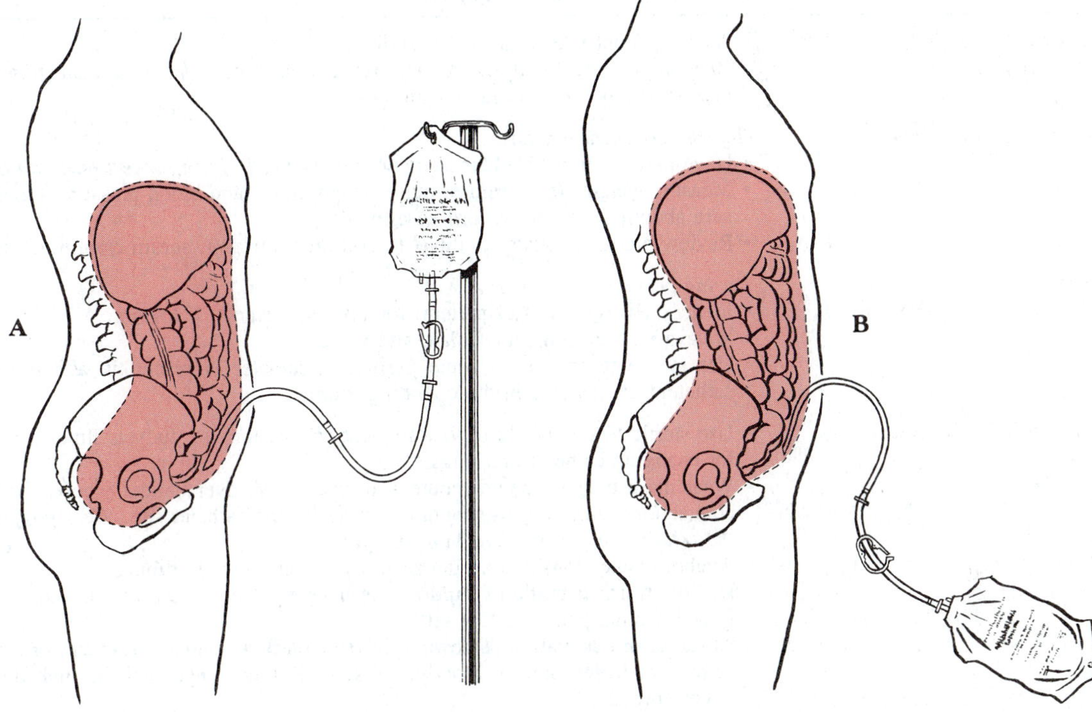

Figure 11-12 Peritoneal dialysis. **A,** Inflow. **B,** Outflow (drains to gravity).

loss of blood proteins and amino acids with the fluid in the outflow; a more generous protein intake is indicated to replace these losses (suggested intake: 1.2 to 5 g/kg/day, 50% of high biologic value); restrictions continue in sodium (1500 to 2000 mg/day) and potassium (2500 to 3500 mg/day); caloric intake may be partly supplied by the glucose in the peritoneal dialysis fluid; patients need 35 kcal/kg ideal body weight/day; fluid restriction ranges from 0.5 to 1 L/day

NURSING CARE

Nursing Assessment

Abdominal Cavity

Peritonitis; infectious or chemical (rebound abdominal tenderness, increase in white blood cells in effluent, and fever); peritoneal access problems (infection and obstruction); leakage of fluid into tissues, thoracic cavity, or scrotum; adhesions

Cardiovascular

Hypovolemia; hypervolemia

Neurologic

Hyperosmolar coma and convulsions

Respiratory

Tachypnea; pulmonary edema and effusions

Nursing Dx & Intervention

Nursing Diagnosis	Nursing Intervention/Rationale
Knowledge deficit related to peritoneal dialysis	• Assess patient's level of understanding. • Explain peritoneal dialysis, its purpose, and procedure. Plan for education about end-stage renal disease and peritoneal dialysis training.
Fluid volume excess	*Before peritoneal dialysis:* • Have patient empty bladder *to avoid puncturing it during insertion of an acute catheter.* • Measure weight, temperature, pulse, respirations, and blood pressure (lying and standing). Measure abdominal girth. Record baseline data. • Review blood chemistry findings (blood urea nitrogen, serum creatinine, serum Na^+ and K^+).
Impaired skin integrity related to the peritoneal dialysis catheter	*During peritoneal dialysis:* • Identify HB_sAg status of patient. Identify HIV status, if known. • Wear masks (patient, physician, and nurse). • Use sterile technique as acute peritoneal catheter is placed in abdominal cavity. Permanent catheters are inserted in the operating room.
Potential for infection	• Use sterile technique during subsequent connections of dialysis fluid to peritoneal catheter and for changing catheter dressings. • Wear mask over nose and mouth and place mask over patient's nose and mouth while making connections with dialysis tubing or caring for the catheter site. Wear goggles *to avoid splashing the returned dialysate fluid into the eyes.* • Anchor connections and tubing securely. Avoid kinks in tubing. • Dry off warmed bottle of fluid before hanging it up or use plastic bags of solution warmed in folded heating pad on a low setting. • Observe for perforation of bowel (dialysate outflow stained with feces or blood; watery diarrhea) or bladder (urine pink or bloody). First several exchanges will be pink tinged, but gross blood is not normal. • Observe for peritonitis. Collect samples of dialysate outflow for culture and sensitivity whenever it is turbid, bloody, or has an odor. • Observe for catheter tunnel site infection.
Fluid volume excess (potential)	• Measure intake, output (inflow, dwell, and outflow times), and weight, as well as temperature, pulse, respirations, and blood pressure regularly and record results. Keep accurate records of dialysis cycles. Record strength of solution used, additions made, and fluid balance (retained or lost). Outflow of dialysate may be obstructed by fibrin or omentum, constipation, or catheter malposition. • Observe for respiratory embarrassment (manifested by dyspnea and rales) *resulting from abdomen being too full of fluid or leakage of dialysate into the thoracic cavity through defect in diaphragm.*
Constipation related to use of phosphate binding agents	• Assess defecation routine and normal pattern *because constipation may interfere with drainage of dialysate.* • Assess need for and administer stool softeners and laxatives as ordered and monitor response.
Potential fluid volume deficit	• Do not prolong dwell times, especially with solutions of 4.5% glucose, *because water depletion can result.* A high concentration of glucose in the dialysate and a prolonged dwell time can result in excessive losses of body fluid. Watch for weight loss during the procedure.
Body image disturbance	• Observe patient's response to having chronic illness, altered renal function, alteration in other body systems, the necessity of renal dialysis, and transplantation as a probability in the future. • Recognize denial, guilt, aggression, fear, displacement, regression, resentment, disbelief, and anxiety in patient. • Recognize changes in psychosocial aspects of patient's life: change in social interaction, irritability, hostility, extreme dependence, fear of rejection, inability to work, loss of job, decreased financial stability, and altered hopes for future. • Identify significant aspects of patient's cultural background and religion *that may affect response to chronic renal failure and dialysis.* • Help patient move through stages of denial, discouragement, acceptance of the condition, and rehabilitation. Share information needed, listen, and offer continuing emotional support. Refer patient to other professional resources as needed. • Recognize patient's response to dependence on machine. *Patient may feel helpless or hopeless, deny reality, personalize the machine, or accept it as necessity.* • Support patient's strengths: self-confidence, determination, and motivation to live. • Help patient develop or continue interests beyond dialysis and return to as normal a life as possible.

Nursing Diagnosis	Nursing Intervention/Rationale
	• Be alert to excessive concern with losses, depression, self-neglect, noncompliance with medical regimen, and possibility of suicide. • Be aware of effect loss of libido, impotence, and decreased orgasm has on marital and sexual life of patient. • Try to help patient develop realistic expectations of dialysis. • Try to keep lines of communication open. • See p. 1751.
Altered family processes	• Recognize that chronic renal failure and dialysis can cause disruption, expense, and considerable alteration in time commitments in the family. • Try to support family's willing cooperation in patient's care, and help them look at ways to decrease domestic tension and unhappiness. • Help patient and spouse recognize demands of illness situation on spouse and patient's need for emotional support. Recognize spouse's fears. • Involve family from the beginning in all aspects and help them understand patient's responses. • Work with health team as they help family meet illness situation.

Patient Education

1. Explain the nature of chronic renal failure.
2. Explain the medical regimen and its rationale, including diet (restricted protein, sodium, and potassium), restricted fluid intake, and medications (purpose, dosage, interval, and adverse reactions).
3. Explain the function of normal and artificial kidneys and the principles of peritoneal dialysis.
4. Teach aseptic technique.
5. Explain components of the system, preparation, operation, cleaning, and storage (repair and maintenance if home dialysis).
6. Explain initiating dialysis, monitoring during dialysis, and discontinuing dialysis.
7. Explain emergencies related to the machine, if used, and to the patient's medical condition.
8. Explain care while off the machine: diet, fluid restrictions, medical complications, care of peritoneal access route, medications, and prevention of infection.
9. Teach self-observational skills (temperature, pulse, respirations, blood pressure, intake and output, and weight) and record keeping.
10. Explain ways to avoid infection.
11. Explain personal hygiene, rest, and exercise.
12. Explain when to call the physician.
13. Explain the plan for medical follow-up.

Evaluation

Patient Outcome	Data Indicating That Outcome is Reached
Dialysis is adequate.[15]	Patient has good general and nutritional status, normal blood pressure, clinically tolerated anemia, no osteodystrophy or calcifications on roentgenograms, no uremic polyneuropathy or encephalopathy, predialysis plasma concentrations of urea, creatinine, K^+, and Na^+ in desirable range, and good quality of life and rehabilitation.
Patient and family understand chronic renal failure and peritoneal dialysis.	Patient and family describe chronic renal failure and medical plan of care. Patient and family describe principles of peritoneal dialysis, plan of care, and correct use of peritoneal dialysis equipment.
Patient and family have adjusted to peritoneal dialysis.	Patient and family have returned to work and social activities as are possible. Family and patient continue to use support of health team.

Renal Transplantation

Description and Rationale

Renal transplantation (RT) is the surgical insertion of a human kidney from a living or cadaveric source into a patient with end-stage renal disease, thus replacing the lost renal function. A donor is sought when the patient's serum creatinine is around 5 mg/dl, serum blood urea nitrogen is greater than 70 mg/dl, and creatinine clearance is 15 ml/minute.[28] When successful, a transplant restores the recipient to a healthy, useful life. If a transplant is unsuccessful, the patient can return to dialysis or have a second transplant.

The donated kidney is placed in the retroperitoneal area in the iliac fossa on the contralateral side. Thus a donated

Figure 11-13 Renal transplant.

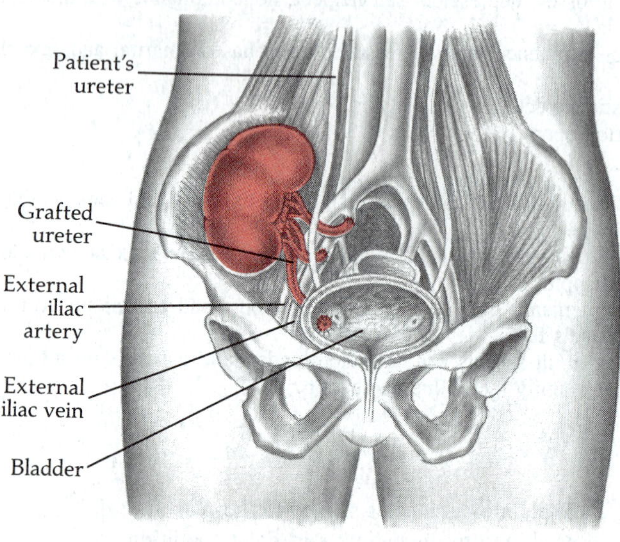

left kidney is placed in the recipient's right iliac fossa (Figure 11-13). The donor's artery is anastomosed end to end to the recipient's hypogastric artery.

The donor's vein is anastomosed to the recipient's internal iliac vein. The donor's ureter is implanted in the recipient's bladder.

The kidney from a living related donor is flushed with a cold solution and then placed in the recipient. A cadaveric kidney may be preserved by flushing followed by cold storage or by constant perfusion with a special solution.

Transplantation is usually the treatment of choice in children. Aging patients may have problems with transplantation because of atherosclerosis or other serious systemic disorders. Patients with diabetes are increasingly considered for transplantation, but the problems with the continuing diabetic condition increase complications such as infection. The use of corticosteroids exacerbates problems in glucose level control.

Indications for a renal transplant include end-stage renal disease, loss of a solitary kidney through trauma, and the inability to adjust to dialysis.

Contraindications and Cautions

1. Age younger than 5 years or older than 50 years
2. Malignancy
3. Acute uncontrollable infection
4. Hepatic disease
5. Presence of antikidney antibodies
6. Severe psychosis
7. Tuberculosis or peptic ulcer disease
8. Chronic respiratory insufficiency
9. Severe atherosclerosis
10. Severe myocardial dysfunction

Preprocedural Care: Preoperative Assessment

Recipient

Medical examination
- History and physical examination, including blood pressure and weight
- Renal-urologic: flat plate abdomen, urinalysis three times, urine culture three times, creatinine clearance two times, 24-hour urine protein and electrolyte excretion, and voiding cystoureterogram
- Hematologic: red and white blood cells with differential, platelets, hemoglobin, hematocrit, bleeding-clotting time, prothrombin time, partial thromboplastin time, and thrombin time
- Cardiovascular: chest roentgenogram (heart size), electrocardiogram, serum electrolytes, glucose, protein, blood pressure, and eye examination
- Respiratory: chest roentgenogram and pulmonary function tests
- Gastrointestinal: upper gastrointestinal series and liver function tests
- Skeletal: signs of hyperparathyroidism (serum Ca^{++}, $PO_4^{=}$, Mg^{++}, and alkaline phosphatase) and metabolic bone survey
- Neuromuscular: nerve conduction time
- Infectious: fungal skin tests; urine, blood, skin, nose, throat, and feces cultures
- Immunologic: serum electrophoresis, LE cell test, rheumatoid factor (RF) test, anti-streptolysin O (ASO) titer, complement, antinuclear factor, anti–glomerular basement membrane antibodies, blood type (ABO, Rh), tissue type (HLA), serial cytotoxic antibody determinations, HB_sAg, and HIV

Psychiatric examination
- Psychologic testing
- Evaluation for psychopathology
- Evaluation of metabolic encephalopathy

Socioeconomic evaluation
- Resources
- Family status
- Potential for return to preillness activities

Donor—Living Related

Medical examination
- History and physical, including blood pressure and weight
- Immunologic: blood type (ABO, Rh). tissue type, leukocyte cross-matching, antidonor antibody, VDRL, HB_sAg, and mixed lymphocytic culture (MLC) tests, HIV
- Renal-urologic: urinalysis, urine culture two times, creatinine clearance, renogram, intravenous urography, and renal arteriogram
- Hematologic: hematocrit, platelet count, white blood cells with differential, prothrombin time, partial thromboplastin time, and thrombin time

- Cardiovascular-respiratory: chest roentgenogram, electrocardiogram, blood chemistries, and electrolytes
- Endocrine: fasting blood sugar and glucose tolerance test

Psychiatric examination
- Emotional maturity and stability
- Motivation

Socioeconomic evaluation
- Resources
- Responsibilities

Donor—Cadaveric

No systemic disease such as infection, cancer, or advanced vascular disease including hypertension
No renal-urologic disorders
No prolonged hypoxia or hypotension before death
Relatively young (4 to 55 years old)
Renal function tests normal

Medical Plan

Surgery

The donor kidney is transplanted as described on p. 1079; the patient is prepared with adequate dialysis for surgery (see "Hemodialysis," p. 1071); the uremic problems are controlled before surgery

Medications

Antiemetics
- Prochlorperazine (Compazine), po, 5-10 mg tid or qid
- Trimethobenzamide (Tigan, Ticon), po, 250 mg tid or qid; IM, 200 mg tid or qid

Narcotic analgesics
- Meperidine (Demerol, Pethadol), po, subcutaneously, IM, IV, 50-150 mg q3-4h
- Codeine sulfate (Methylmorphine), po, subcutaneously, IM, 15-60 mg qid
- Morphine sulfate (Roxamol), po, subcutaneously, IM, 5-15 mg q4h prn

Anti-infective agents
- Parenteral agents (IM or IV)
  - Gentamicin (Garamycin, Apogen), 3-5 mg/kg/d q8h
  - Cephalosporins
    - Cefazolin sodium (Ancef, Kefzol), 250-1000 mg q6-8h
  - Penicillins
    - Ampicillin sodium (Omnipen-N, Polycillin-N), patients ≥40 kg: 250-500 mg q6h; <40 kg: 25-50 mg/kg/d in equally divided doses q6-8h
    - Carbenicillin disodium (Geopen, Pyopen), 1-2 g q6h
    - Penicillin G potassium (Aqueous penicillin G), Penicillin G sodium, 1-20 million U/d
- Oral agents
  - Tetracycline (Achromycin, Tetracyn), 250-500 mg q6h
  - Penicillins
    - Amoxicillin (Amoxil, Amoxycillin), 250-500 mg q8h
    - Ampicillin (Omnipen, Polycillin), 250-500 mg q6h
    - Penicillin G, 200,000-500,000 U q6-8h
  - Erythromycin (Erythrocin, Ilotycin), 25 mg q6h
  - Sulfamethoxazole and trimethoprim (Septra, Bactrim), 2 tab q12h

Antihypertensive agents
- Clonidine (Catapres, Dixarit), po, 0.1 mg bid or tid initially; then increase by 0.2-0.8 mg/d (maximum effective dose, 2.4 mg/d)
- Diazoxide (Hyperstat IV, Proglycem), IV, 300 mg by bolus in 30 sec or 1-2 mg/kg up to 150 mg at 5- to 15-min intervals
- Hydralazine (Apresoline, Dralzine), po, 10 mg qid for 2-4 d, increase to 25 mg qid then 50 mg qid; maintenance dose is lowest effective level; IM, IV, 10-40 mg repeated as needed (q4-6h)
- Methyldopa (Aldomet, Dopamet), po, 250 mg bid or tid for 48 h, then increase or decrease q2d if needed; maintenance, 500 mg to 2 g in 2-4 divided doses/d (maximum, 3 g)
- Prazosin (Minipress) (α-adrenergic blocker), po, 1 mg bid-tid initially; maintenance may be increased slowly to maximum of 20 mg/d in divided doses; to 40 mg/d may be required
- Propranolol (Inderal, Novopranol) (β-adrenergic blocker), po, 40 mg bid at 6-8 h intervals; increase if needed to 160-480 mg/d in divided doses; 640 mg/d may be needed
- Captopril (Capoten) (angiotensin converting enzyme inhibitor), po, 25 mg tid initially; increase to 50 mg tid in 2-3 wk if necessary; may be increased to 100 mg tid then 150 mg tid

Immunosuppressive agents[2,11,25]
- Azathioprine (Imuran), po, 100-150 mg/d; 1.7-2.5 mg/kg/d determined by white blood cell level
- Antilymphocyte globulin, IM, IV, 5-10 mg/kg depending on potency of preparation, qd for 5-21 d after surgery with intermittent doses for 4 mo
- Cyclophosphamide (Cytoxan, Neosar), po, 2 mg/kg/d as substitute for azathioprine in patients with liver dysfunction
- Cyclosporine (Cyclosporin A, Sandimmune), po, IV, 10-25 mg/kg/d
- Muromonab-CD3 (OKT3), IV bolus, 5 mg/kg/d for 10-14 d[30]

Corticosteroids (used as immunosuppressive agents[2,11,25])
- Prednisone (Deltasone, Orasone), po, 20-150 mg/d, 0.3-2.5 mg/kg decreasing to 10-15 mg/d by 4 mo; increase to 100-300 mg/d (up to 3 g) to treat rejection

Methylprednisolone (Solu-Medrol, A-MethaPred), IV, 250-1000 mg qd or alternate days for maximum dose of 3-5 g

Antacids (peptic ulcer disease may be a problem)

Aluminum carbonate gel, basic (Basaljel), po, 300 ml divided into 6 doses

Aluminum phosphate (Phosphajel), po, 180-360 ml divided into 4-12 doses

Insulin preparations (for hyperglycemia resulting from corticosteroid therapy): highly individualized according to blood and urine glucose determinations (see "Diabetes Mellitus," Chapter 9)

General Management

Dialysis may be needed (see p. 1070)

No dietary restrictions after gastrointestinal function returns; caloric intake may need to be restricted if appetite is increased by corticosteroids; if renal function is decreased or hypertension continues, restrictions may be needed:

Fluid intake should balance output: about 400 to 600 ml (about the amount of insensible losses) plus amount equal to 24-hour urine volume; patient should avoid dehydration and volume excess

Nutritional modifications to achieve or maintain adequate nutritional status and to reduce work of diseased kidney[1]

Protein: 0.6 g/kg body weight/day; glomerular filtration rate (GFR) 20 to 25 ml/minute to 90 g/day; GFR, 10 to 15 ml/minute to 50 g/day; GFR, 4 to 10 ml/minute to 40 g/day

Sodium: 1000 to 2000 mg/day; the specific amounts depend on weight, blood pressure, serum creatinine, and 24-hour sodium excretion

Potassium: 1560 to 2340 mg/day; with normal urine output (at least 800 ml/day), no restriction needed

Calories: 35 to 55 kcal/kg body weight/day; calories from fat and carbohydrate are used; adequate calories must accompany protein intake to prevent use of protein for energy and weight loss

Vitamins

Routine cultures of likely places for infection (urinary tract, wound, throat, and blood) may be done, since the immunosuppressive agents mask the signs and symptoms of infection. All immunosuppressive agents currently in use affect phagocytosis, cellular immunity, or humoral immunity. Liver function is monitored because azathioprine can cause cholestatic hepatitis. Cyclosporine may damage the kidney and liver. Muromonab-CD3 causes a flulike symptom complex.

The signs and symptoms of rejection are monitored. These include decreased urine production, hypertension, fever, weight gain, decreased creatinine clearance, increased serum creatinine level, increased blood urea nitrogen level, proteinuria, decreased urine sodium, decreased renal blood flow on renogram, increase in renal size, anxiety, apathy, lethargy, anorexia, and tenderness over the graft site. Rejection may be treated with high-dose steroids (methylprednisolone, 1 g/d for 3 days, and OKT3, 5 mg/day for 10 to 14 days). If rejection is not reversed, the graft is removed and the patient is returned to dialysis.

NURSING CARE

Nursing Assessment

Renal

Ischemic damage (acute renal failure, p. 1050); rejection: hyperacute, acute, and chronic (increase in serum creatinine greater than 0.3 mg/dl from previous level; increase in blood urea nitrogen level; proteinuria; hematuria; decrease in creatinine clearance; decrease in urinary sodium, urea, and creatinine; oliguria or anuria; fever and weight gain; edema; enlargement of the graft and decreased renal blood flow; tenderness of graft site; increase in blood pressure and pulse; and anxiety, apathy, and lethargy); spontaneous rupture of the graft (intense pain and shock); reappearance of primary renal disease

Urinary Tract

Bacteriuria; ureteral fistula or obstruction or hydronephrosis; obstruction of vascular graft and extravasation of urine as revealed by renal scan; perirenal hematoma or lymphocele (an accumulation of lymph from lymphatics cut during surgery that collects in a closed space); perinephric abscess; renal calculi

Cardiovascular

Arrhythmias; cardiac arrest; hypotension; hypertension; congestive heart failure; vascular calcification; renal artery stenosis; renal vein thrombosis

Respiratory

Pulmonary edema; pneumonia and other infections such as cytomegalovirus and *Pneumocystis carinii* pneumonia (fever, chills, productive cough, and pleuritic pain); pulmonary emboli; reactivated tuberculosis; adult respiratory distress syndrome

Hematopoietic

Leukopenia (related to azathioprine); neoplasms

Gastrointestinal

Hepatitis (related to azathioprine and HB_sAg positive); pancreatitis; peptic ulcer disease; infections: oral and esophageal (fungal)

Neurologic

Infection; changes in behavior

Skin and Mucous Membrane

Infection; purpura; striae; hirsutism; acne; alopecia; neoplasms; wound infection and delayed healing

Musculoskeletal

Hyperparathyroidism; osteoporosis; avascular necrosis of femur (pain in hip and limp); myopathy (muscular weakness)

Eyes

Infection; increased intraocular pressure; cataracts

Psychologic

Euphoria; excitability; psychosis; appearance changes

• • •

Most frequent complications are related to technical problems, effects of preexisting uremia, graft rejection, and side effects of immunosuppression.

Nursing Dx & Intervention

Nursing Diagnosis	Nursing Intervention/Rationale
Fluid volume excess; potential fluid volume deficit	• Measure temperature, pulse, respirations, and blood pressure every 15 minutes for 4 hours, then every half hour until stable, and then every 2 hours for 24 hours. • Measure central venous pressure. *Patients are sensitive to fluid volume changes.* • *Try to maintain patency of blood access device* by avoiding hypovolemia and blood pressure measurements or intravenous punctures in that arm (dialysis may be needed).
Impaired skin integrity related to surgery; potential for infection	• Provide aseptic wound care; *patients receiving immunosuppressive drugs have a greater risk of infection.* • Assess wound frequently; little drainage is expected. • Provide aseptic care to intravenous lines (peripheral and central venous pressure) and urinary catheters. • Watch for signs and symptoms of infection *that are masked by immunosuppressive drugs.* Temperature may not be elevated. • Provide a clean environment. • Have patient breathe deeply, cough, and turn (only to operative side) *to prevent respiratory complications. (Infections of the lungs by opportunistic organisms are serious complications and frequent causes of death.)* • Help patient with oral and personal hygiene *to prevent infection.*
Altered renal tissue perfusion (potential)	• Measure urine hourly and save *to determine urinary creatinine, urea, sodium, potassium, pH, specific gravity, and presence of blood and protein.* Report anuria or volumes less than 100 ml/hour. Urine flow starts in 2 to 10 minutes after revascularization at 5 to 10 ml/minute and returns to normal volume in 48 to 72 hours. • Review daily blood chemistries that reflect renal function: creatinine clearance, serum creatinine, and blood urea nitrogen levels, as well as hemoglobin, hematocrit, and white blood cell count. • Do not clamp urethral or ureteral catheters. Connect catheters to closed drainage system. Avoid kinks in tubing and anchor them securely. • Observe urine; it may be blood tinged or quite bloody at first. Sudden cessation of urine may be caused by clot. Urethral catheter irrigation by means of sterile technique may be necessary to dislodge it. Ureteral catheter irrigation is done with particular care when ordered to avoid damage to ureteral anastomosis. • When uretheral catheter is removed, patient should void frequently *to avoid overdistention of bladder.* • Patients may have bladder spasms *as unused bladder is distended with urine.*
Fluid volume excess; potential fluid volume deficit	• Measure intake (intravenous and oral fluids when started) and output. • Measure weight every day. Check pulmonary status (respiratory rate, dyspnea, breath sounds).
Impaired physical mobility; bathing/hygiene self-care deficit (potential)	• Maintain bed rest for first 24 hours with patient lying flat (head at 30-degree angle) or on operative side with knees straight *to prevent tension on the anastomoses.* • Ambulate in 24 hours. • Assist with personal hygiene as needed.
Pain	• Assess patient's need for pain relief and give analgesics as ordered; record response.
Altered nutrition: less than or more than body requirements (potential)	• Nothing by mouth or a nasogastric tube is ordered at first. • When bowel sounds return, liquids and food by mouth are begun: normal diet with or without restrictions (see "Chronic Renal Failure," p. 1053).

Nursing Diagnosis	Nursing Intervention/Rationale
Body image disturbance	• A major concern is incorporation of new part into body. • Acceptance by nurse of the patient's feelings of guilt and concern for donor is helpful. • Be aware that side effects of azathioprine (alopecia) and prednisone (e.g., moonface, acne, body fat redistribution) require marked adjustment. • See p. 1751.
Altered family processes	• Keep lines of communication open with family and assist in family-patient communication. • Deal sensitively with feelings of family members concerning transplantation. Family has become used to chronically ill person. Return to real health will modify family-patient expectations. Living related donor, a hero or heroine before transplantation, may feel forgotten afterward. Source of cadaver kidney may be a concern. Recipient may be perceived as too independent or not independent enough. Death of patient after transplant fails is very difficult. • Be sure family understands that side effects of corticosteroids can interfere with interpersonal relationships. • If family and patient do not already know others who have gone through this situation, offer to introduce them to a patient and family. • Refer family to other professional colleagues (social workers or psychologists) when they can better meet family's needs (financial concerns, occupational problems, and need for family counseling beyond nurse's expertise). • See p. 1772.

Patient Education

1. Preparation for discharge includes teaching the following:
   a. Self-observational skills (temperature, pulse, respiration, weight, intake and output, urine collection, and record keeping)
   b. Medications: name, dosage, strength, schedule, purpose, and side effects
   c. Diet: restriction, if any (patient should avoid becoming overweight)
   d. Fluids: restriction, if any
   e. Signs and symptoms of rejection and infection
   f. Important laboratory values (serum creatinine, blood urea nitrogen level, white blood cell count, calcium, and phosphate); with an arteriovenous fistula, do not have blood pressure taken or blood drawn in that arm
2. Long-term follow-up includes teaching the following:
   a. Medical appointment schedule for routine follow-up; plans for telephone communication between appointments
   b. Personal hygiene, prevention of infection, care of minor trauma, contraceptive device, and need for regular dental and eye examinations
   c. Body changes resulting from uremia and long-term corticosteroid therapy, including increased possibility of malignancies
   d. Physical activity levels (daily exercise, avoidance of contact sports, and avoidance of seat belts across the hips) and return to work and other activities
   e. Resources for rehabilitation (including vocational)

Evaluation

Patient Outcome	Data Indicating That Outcome is Reached
Renal function returns.	Renal function findings are normal. Red blood count, hematocrit, and clotting time are normal. There is no further bone resorption or progressive neuropathy. Libido improves; menses, ovulation, and potency return.
Patient is aware of susceptibility to infection and drug side effects.	Patient understands risk of hepatitis from azathioprine, kidney and liver problems with cyclosporine, and risk of infection, osteoporosis, and peptic ulceration from steroids. Patient is aware of increased susceptibility to infection.
Patient and family understand renal transplantation.	Patient and family describe medical plan of care, plan for follow-up, precautions, and any restrictions. Patient and family demonstrate self-care skills.
Patient and family adjust to life after transplantation.	Patient and family return to work and social activities.

References

1. American Dietetic Association: Handbook of clinical dietetics, New Haven, Conn, 1981, Yale University Press.
2. Asscher AW, Moffat DB, and Sanders E: Nephrology illustrated: an integrated text and color atlas, Philadelphia, 1982, WB Saunders Co.
3. Brenner BM and Lazarus JM: Acute renal failure, Philadelphia, 1983, WB Saunders Co.
4. Centers for Disease Control: Tuberculosis in the United States 1985-1986, Atlanta, 1987.
5. Chapman WH et al: The urinary system: an integrated approach, Philadelphia, 1973, WB Saunders Co.
6. Deinhardt F and Deinhardt J, editors: Viral hepatitis: laboratory and clinical science, New York, 1983, Marcel Dekker, Inc.
7. Earle DA, editor, and Levin ML and Quintanilla AP, associate editors: Manual of clinical nephrology, Philadelphia, 1982, WB Saunders Co.
8. Flamenbaum W and Hamburger RJ, editors: Nephrology: an approach to the patient with renal disease, Philadelphia, 1982, JB Lippincott Co.
9. Friedman EA and L'Esperance FA Jr, editors: Diabetic renal-retinal syndrome. Vol 2. Prevention and management, New York, 1982, Grune & Stratton, Inc.
10. Gokal R, editor: Continuous ambulatory peritoneal dialysis, Edinburgh, 1986, Churchill Livingstone.
11. Goodman AG, Goodman LS, and Gilman A, editors: Goodman and Gilman's the pharmacological basis of therapeutics, ed 6, New York, 1980, Macmillan Publishing Co, Inc.
12. Govoni LE and Hayes JE: Drugs and nursing implications, ed 5, Norwalk, Conn, 1985, Appleton-Century-Crofts.
13. Grossman ZD et al: The clinician's guide to diagnostic imaging, ed 2, New York, 1987, Raven Press.
14. Gutch CF and Stoner MH: Review of hemodialysis for nurses and dialysis personnel, ed 3, St Louis, 1979, The CV Mosby Co.
15. Hamburger J, Crosnier J, and Grünfeld JP, editors: Nephrology, New York, 1979, John Wiley & Sons.
16. James JA: Renal disease in childhood, ed 2, St Louis, 1972, The CV Mosby Co.
17. Johns MP: Pharmacodynamics and patient care, St Louis, 1974, The CV Mosby Co.
18. Kass EH and Brumfitt W, editors: Infections of the urinary tract, Chicago, 1978, University of Chicago Press.
19. Klahr S, editor: The kidney and body fluids in health and disease, New York, 1983, Plenum Medical Book Co.

19a. Lancaster L: Core curriculum for nephrology nurses, ANNA, Pitman, NJ, 1987, Anthony J Jannetti, Inc.

20. Larson E, Lindbloom L, and Davis KB, editors: Development of the clinical nephrology practitioner: a focus on independent learning, St Louis, 1982, The CV Mosby Co.
21. Levine DZ: Care of the renal patient, Philadelphia, 1983, WB Saunders Co.
22. Massry SG and Glasscock RJ, editors: Textbook of nephrology, vol 1, Baltimore, 1983, Williams & Wilkins.
23. Muehrcke RC: Acute renal failure, St Louis, 1969, The CV Mosby Co.
24. Paginini EP, editor: Acute continuous renal replacement therapy, Boston, 1986, Martinus Nijhoff Publishing.
25. Papper S and Williams GR, editors: Manual of medical care of the surgical patient, ed 2, Boston, 1981, Little, Brown & Co.
26. Pemberton CM and Gastineau CF, editors: Mayo Clinic diet manual: a handbook of dietary practices, ed 5, Philadelphia, 1981, WB Saunders Co.
27. Rossman I, editor: Clinical geriatrics, ed 2, Philadelphia, 1979, J Lippincott Co.
28. Rowe JW and Besdine RW, editors: Health and disease, Boston, 1982, Little, Brown & Co.
29. Starzl TE et al: Renal homotransplantation. I, Curr Probl Surg, p 3, April 1974.
30. Steinhiser SA and Plawecki HM: OKT3 for treatment of patients with acute renal allograft rejection, ANNA J 14:127, 1987.
31. Tilkian SM, Conover MB, and Tilkian AG: Clinical implications of laboratory tests, ed 4, St Louis, 1987, The CV Mosby Co.
32. Urizar RE, Largent JA, and Gilboa N: Pediatric nephrology: new directions in therapy, New York, 1983, Medical Examination Publishing Co.
33. Van der Hem GK, editor: Nephrology, Amsterdam, 1982, Excerpta Medica.

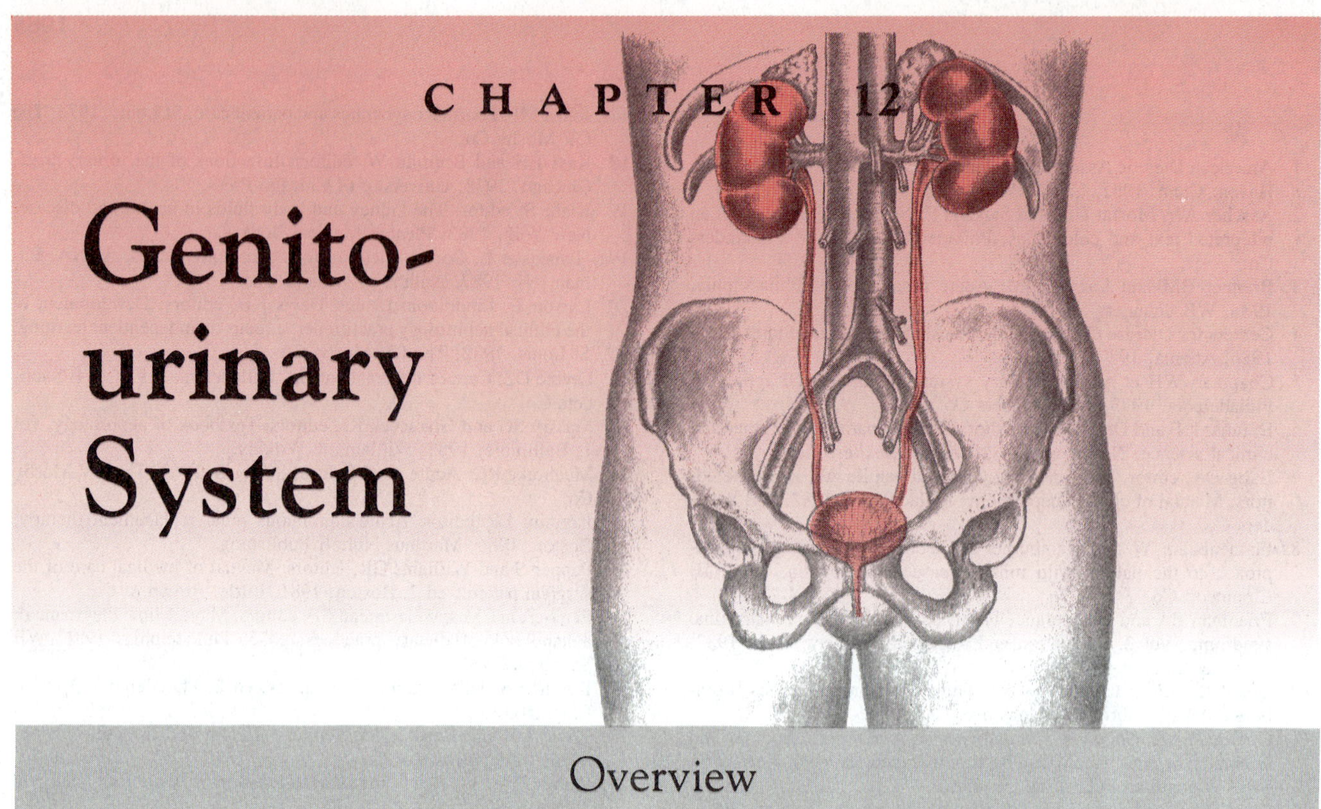

CHAPTER 12

Genitourinary System

Overview

Genitourinary diseases affect the kidneys, ureters, bladder, urethra, or male genitalia. Urologic disorders may result from specific disease states such as infection, hyperplasia, or neoplasia. Other disorders, such as urinary incontinence or male sexual dysfunction, are symptoms rather than specific disease states but also cause significant health problems related to the genitourinary system. For information on the renal system, refer to Chapter 11.

Anatomy, Physiology, and Related Pathophysiology

Urinary Tract Structures

Kidneys. The kidneys are a pair of reddish brown, symmetrically shaped organs located in the retroperitoneal space, adjacent to the vertebral column at spinal levels T12 and L1 to L3 (Figure 12-1). The lateral aspects of the kidneys are smooth and rounded; the medial aspects are marked by a concave surface known as the renal hilus. The renal veins, arteries, nerve plexus, and renal lymphatics are located at this hilus. The renal pelvis attaches to the kidney at the hilus before tapering into the ureters.[24,45]

The weight of the adult kidney varies from 115 to 175 g. Adult women have slightly smaller kidneys than do adult men. The kidney in the infant or young child is smaller than in the adult. However, a child's kidneys occupy a larger proportion of the child's body weight. The normal adult kidney is approximately 11 cm long, 5 to 7 cm wide, and 2 to 3.5 cm thick. The kidneys are remarkably symmetric in size and shape.[45]

A cross section of the kidneys (Figure 12-2) reveals two distinct sections: the renal pelvis and renal parenchyma. Within the renal parenchyma, a cortex and medulla are distinguished using the unaided eye. The renal medulla is characterized by pale, striated conical structures called pyramids. The bases of these pyramids are directed toward the periphery of the kidney; the apices face the renal hilus. The renal pyramids end in papillae that project into a minor calyx. The kidneys normally contain from eight to 18 renal pyramids that drain into four to 13 minor calyces. These minor calyces drain into two or three major calyces that open into the renal pelvis.[24,113]

The renal medulla is bounded by the renal cortex, which appears darker and has a granular rather than striated appearance. Cortical lobules arch over the pyramids within the medulla. Cortical columns dip between the pyramids. The renal cortex is bounded by the true renal capsule, a layer of dense connective tissue loosely adherent to the parenchyma. The kidneys are supported by the perirenal fascia and perinephric fat. The kidneys, along with the superiorly placed adrenals, are enclosed within Gerota's fascia.[24,113]

The renal fossa is bounded superiorly by the diaphragm, laterally by the abdominal musculature, and posteriorly by the quadratus lumborum muscle. Because of the presence of the liver, the right kidney lies lower than the left.[45]

The blood supply of the kidneys arises directly from the abdominal aorta. Typically a single renal artery enters the kidney at the renal hilus. However, duplicate renal arteries may be found and are not considered pathologic. After entering the kidney, the renal artery bifurcates into superior and inferior branches, which further divide into the interlobular

Figure 12-1 Anatomic relation of kidneys to spinal column. **A,** Anterior view. **B,** Posterior view.

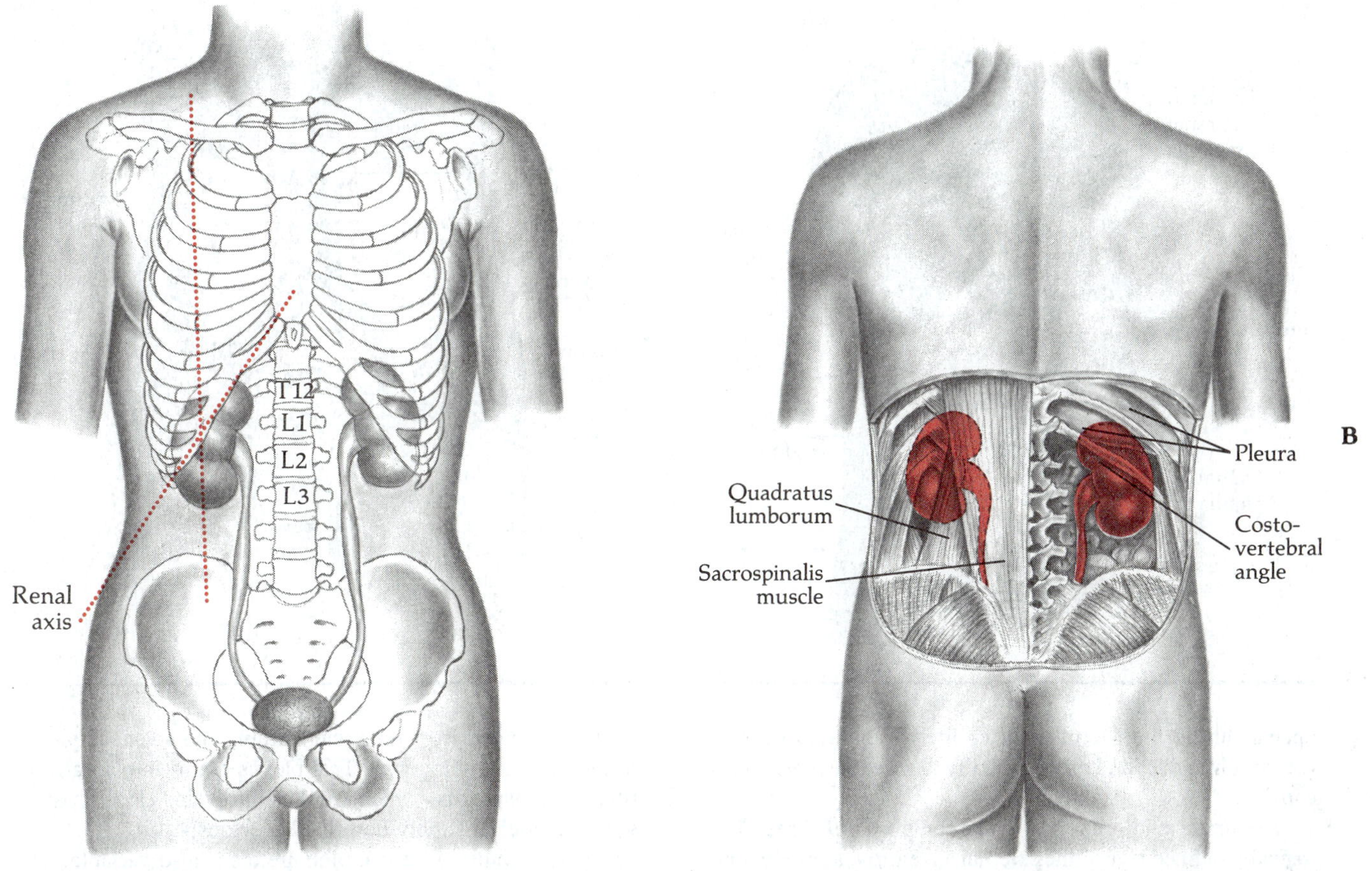

arteries. These vessels and their branches provide the substantial blood supply necessary for renal function.[45]

The veins that drain the kidneys are paired with arterial vessels. The renal veins exiting the kidney empty directly into the inferior vena cava, and their number corresponds to the number of renal arteries present.[95]

Lymphatics adjacent to the renal cortex and medulla drain into para-aortic and para–vena caval lymph nodes. The sensory and motor neurons that innervate the kidneys arise from the dorsal roots of T11 and T12. Autonomic neural control of the kidneys is mediated by fibers from the vagus nerve, splanchnic nerves, semilunar ganglia, and the celiac axis.[45]

The kidneys perform a number of essential functions related to the maintenance of internal homeostasis. These include maintenance of fluid and electrolyte balance and serum pH levels and excretion of the by-products of metabolism.

Renal pelvis and ureters. The renal pelvis and ureters are continuous, thick-walled tubes that originate at the renal hilus and implant into the bladder wall, connecting the kidneys to the bladder. The renal pelvis is a funnel-shaped structure into which the major calyces empty urine for transport to the urinary bladder. After exiting the renal hilus the renal pelvis narrows inferomedially into the ureter.[95]

The ureters are approximately 24 to 30 cm long. The left ureter is slightly longer than the right. The course of the ureters forms an inverted S. After leaving the renal pelvis, the ureters pass medially over the psoas muscle. The ureters then progress medially to the sacroiliac joints before turning laterally to an area near the ischial spines of the pelvis. Finally, the ureters curve back laterally to insert into the bladder base at the trigone muscle.[13,95]

The internal diameter of the ureters varies from 2 to 10 mm. Three areas of anatomic narrowing have clinical implications: the ureteropelvic junction, the area where the ureters cross the iliac arteries, and the ureterovesical junction (Figure 12-3).[45,95]

The ureters and renal pelvis share a common embryologic origin and histologic makeup. The ureter and renal pelvis first

Figure 12-2 Cross section of kidney.

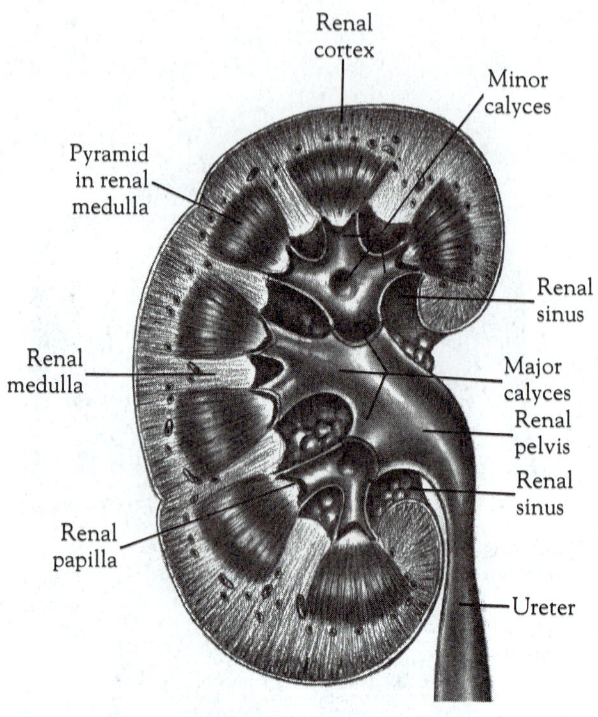

Figure 12-3 Course of ureter with its varying internal luminal sizes.

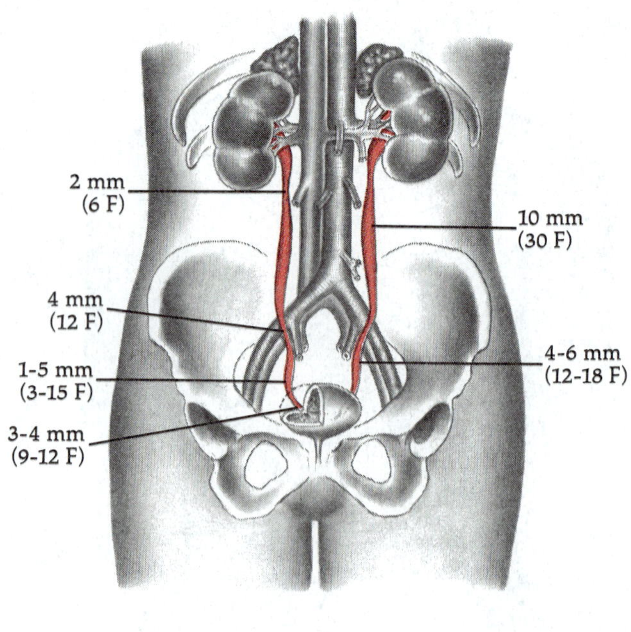

appear during the fourth week of life. They arise from the mesonephric duct and grow cranially to meet the metanephric cap.[95]

The ureter and renal pelvis are composed of three histologically defined layers: the external adventitia, a smooth muscle coat, and an inner mucous membrane. The adventitia is a connective tissue sheath that encircles the renal pelvis and ureters to the level of the ureterovesical junction. The adventitial layer blends into the surrounding retroperitoneal tissue, providing support for the ureters. The exact arrangement of these fibers is not known. Two layers of muscle fibers, an inner longitudinal layer and an outer circular layer, have been described.[113] However, histologic studies of ureteral smooth muscle have disputed this theory.[21] Tanagho[95] and Allen[2] describe the muscle fibers as arranged in bundles that are oriented in a helical or spiral fashion. The muscular tissue layer provides peristaltic activity needed to transport urine from the kidneys to the bladder. The mucous membrane lining the internal ureter is composed of transitional cell epithelium with a supportive lamina propria.[21]

The blood supply of the ureters is variable. The upper portion of the ureter and renal pelvis may receive arterial blood from branches of the renal, gonadal, or adrenal arteries. The pelvic ureters may receive arterial blood from the common iliac arteries, external iliac arteries, deferential arteries in the male, uterine arteries in the female, or the obturator artery. Blood enters the ureters via an arterial plexus located within the outer adventitial layer.[13]

Venous blood from the ureters drains into a venous plexus in the ureteral submucosa. This plexus drains into an adventitial venous plexus, which empties into veins closely paired with the arterial supply described previously.

Lymphatic drainage from the ureters is also variable. The upper ureteral and renal pelvic lymphatic channels empty into para-aortic or renal nodes. The middle and lower ureteral lymphatic channels drain into the common or external iliac nodes.[13]

The nerve supply of the ureters arises from the celiac plexus, mesenteric ganglia, and hypogastric plexus. Although the exact role of the autonomic nervous system in ureteral function remains unclear, the ureter is known to contain a rich supply of sympathetic and parasympathetic nerve receptors.[13]

The primary function of the renal pelvis and ureters is to transport urine from the kidney to the bladder. To accomplish this goal, the ureters must create a peristaltic muscular wave sufficient to drive a bolus of urine from the renal pelvis, through the ureters, and past the ureterovesical junction.[21]

Although the precise mechanisms of ureteral peristalsis remain unclear, it is influenced by mechanical, chemical, and neural stimuli. Generation of a peristaltic wave does not depend on specific neural firing. Like the muscle of the heart, ureteral smooth muscle will continue to rhythmically contract outside the body. In contrast to the heart, no specialized pacemaker has been clearly defined, although the existence of an intrinsic ureteral pacemaker is well established.[13] Multiple pacemaker cells regulating ureteral activity are thought to exist within the renal calyces. The prolonged refractory period of the smooth muscle of the renal pelvis and ureters prevents all calyceal contractions from resulting in ureteral peristaltic waves. The renal pelvis and ureters average two to six peristaltic waves each minute.[13,45]

Ureteral peristaltic waves typically arise within the renal pelvis. They travel in an antegrade direction from the renal pelvis to the ureterovesical junction. During the resting phase, the renal pelvis assumes a conical shape with an area of narrowing at the pelvic-ureteral junction. At this time both the renal pelvis and ureters maintain a low intraluminal pressure of 2 to 5 cm H_2O. Urine enters the ureter from the renal pelvis passively during the resting phase. During a peristaltic wave the pressure rises to 20 to 60 cm H_2O, sufficient to force urine past the ureterovesical junction into the bladder. Only 5% of the total renal pelvic contents is evacuated from the renal pelvis during a peristaltic wave. Once the peristaltic wave is propagated into the ureters, urine is pushed ahead of the wave through the length of the ureter and past the ureterovesical junction into the bladder.[13,45]

An increase in renal output causes greater pelvic distention, which increases both the number of peristaltic waves generated per minute and the proportion of renal pelvic contents transported to the bladder with each contraction.[45]

The ureters are also affected by neural influences. Although it has been demonstrated that the normal ureter continues to contract when removed from the body, the autonomic nervous system does influence ureteral function. The ureters are extensively innervated with α- and β-adrenergic receptors. Stimulation of α-adrenergic receptors causes increased ureteral peristalsis. Stimulation of β-adrenergic receptors results in an inhibition of ureteral peristalsis. The role of the parasympathetic nervous system in ureteral and renal pelvic function is not clearly understood. The parasympathetic nervous system is thought to potentiate ureteral peristalsis directly through cholinergic receptors in the ureteral wall or indirectly through the release of catecholamines.[13]

Ureteral peristalsis is also influenced by various chemical and pharmacologic agents. For example, the administration of epinephrine or catecholamines will, predictably, increase ureteral peristalsis. Increased histamine levels also stimulate ureteral peristalsis. However, the administration of serotonin, which enhances intestinal peristalsis, does not affect ureteral peristalsis. Upper ureteral dilation, which is commonly seen in pregnant women, was once attributed to fluctuations in the serum levels of the sex hormones. Recent investigation has demonstrated that this dilation was caused by mechanical factors rather than hormonal influences. This hypothesis is further supported by the observation that upper ureteral dilation is not seen in women taking oral contraceptives.[45]

Ureterovesical junction and trigone. The ureterovesical junction is of particular interest in any discussion of genitourinary disease because of its importance in preventing vesicoureteral reflux and associated complications. The ureterovesical junction is located near the base of the bladder in the lateral aspects of the trigone muscle. The ureterovesical junction has three components important to its function: the intravesical ureter, the trigone, and the adjacent bladder wall (Figure 12-4).[45,95]

Embryologically, the ureterovesical junction is formed in the seventh week of gestation when the caudal end of the ureter opens into the urogenital sinus. The trigone muscle is formed from the same mesonephric tissue that forms the ureter. The intravesical ureter is further connected to the bladder by a continuous connective tissue sheath. Thus, although the

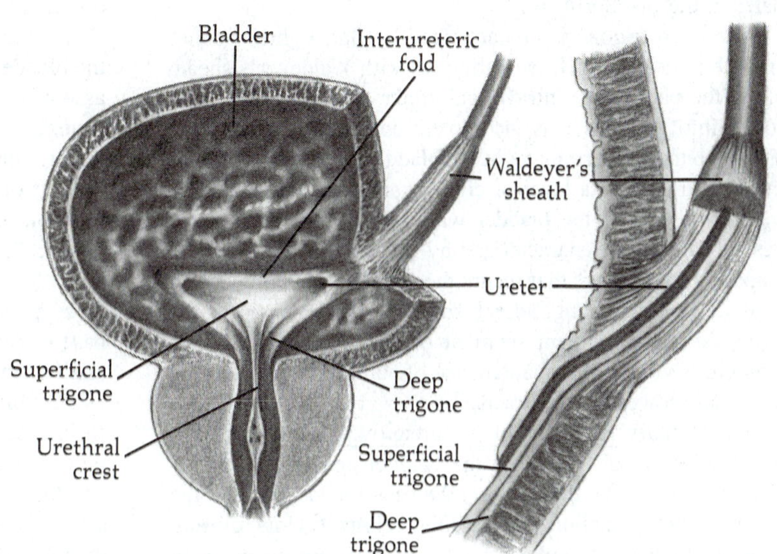

Figure 12-4 Normal ureterotrigonal complex.

intravesical ureter and trigone muscle have different embryologic origins than the bladder, the ureterovesical junction in the fully developed human functions as a single unit to allow for the passage of urine into the bladder while preventing reflux of urine into the upper tracts.[95]

The intravesical ureter enters the bladder at a hiatus in the posterior, lateral aspect of the bladder base and is approximately 1.5 cm long. It is divided into an intramural section surrounded by the detrusor muscle and a submucosal segment that travels under the bladder mucosa. The intravesical ureter terminates at an orifice that opens into the bladder vesicle.[45,95]

The histologic features of the intravesical ureter differ from upper ureteral segments in several ways. The adventitia of the intravesical ureter contains two dense sheaths. The superficial sheath is continuous with the bladder wall. The deep sheath is derived from ureteral adventitia. Between these dense sheaths is a loose connective tissue plane called Waldeyer's sheath. This sheath allows for mobility of the intravesical ureter within the adjacent bladder wall and is of surgical significance when performing ureteroneocystostomy.[45]

The arrangement of smooth muscle fibers also differs in the intravesical ureter. Unlike the upper ureters, the intravesical ureter contains longitudinally arranged fibers and is easily collapsible. The ability of the intravesical ureter to seal itself by collapsing is an important mechanism in the prevention of reflux. Muscle fibers from the intravesical ureter decussate inferiorly to fuse with the superficial trigone and medially to form Mercier's bar.[45,50]

The trigone muscle is another essential component of the ureterovesical junction. The muscle is divided into two parts, the superficial trigone and the deep trigone. The superficial trigone is continuous with muscular fibers from the intravesical ureter. It continues along the bladder base and into the proximal urethra. In the male the trigone terminates at the verumontanum. In the female the superficial trigone terminates at the bladder neck.[152]

The deep trigone is characterized by flat, tightly bound, smooth fiber groups. It is continuous with Waldeyer's sheath along the path of the intravesical ureter. The deep trigone is rolled into a tube that is incomplete on its anterior surface. The deep trigone terminates at the bladder neck and continues into the urethra as a layer of circular smooth muscle.[39,95]

The portion of the bladder wall adjacent to the ureterovesical junction is characterized by circular and longitudinal smooth muscle fibers that secure the ureters within the vesical wall. The outer, longitudinal smooth muscle layer is the strongest, most resilient segment of the bladder wall. This strength is vital to the maintenance of continuity between the upper and lower urinary tracts.[95]

The primary functions of the ureterovesical junction are to allow efflux of urine into the bladder and to prevent reflux of urine into the ureters. During bladder filling the ureterovesical junction maintains a relatively low closure pressure between 8 and 15 cm H_2O. This closure pressure is adequate to prevent reflux of urine from the bladder, which also fills at low pressures. However, the closure pressure is easily overcome by a ureteral peristaltic wave, which generates pressure between 20 and 60 cm H_2O. As the bladder fills and intravesical pressure rises, the intravesical ureter becomes progressively compressed against the adjacent bladder wall. The effect of this compression is to carry the ureteral hiatus outward, thus increasing pressure of the intravesical ureter. This compensatory mechanism prevents reflux of urine even when the bladder is filled with urine. At very high volumes the compression of the intravesical ureter becomes functionally obstructed and interferes with normal ureteral peristalsis.[45,95]

During the voiding phase the ureterovesical junction must generate even greater resistance to prevent reflux into the upper urinary tract. A few seconds before intravesical pressure rises in response to a detrusor contraction, there is a sharp pressure rise within the intravesical ureter. This high closure pressure at the ureterovesical junction is maintained throughout micturition and persists for a brief period after voiding is completed. The sharp increase in pressure was once attributed primarily to the contractile activity of the adjacent bladder wall. However, recent studies have demonstrated that the trigone is primarily responsible for the prevention of reflux during micturition. The marked pressure rise seen immediately before a detrusor contraction is caused by an increase in the tone of the trigone, which pulls the intravesical ureter tightly closed. The trigonal contraction is maintained for approximately 20 seconds after voiding is completed. As expected, no efflux of urine into the bladder occurs during voiding.[95]

Urinary bladder. The urinary bladder is a hollow muscular organ designed to store and expel urine produced by the kidneys. The size and shape of the bladder vary with its state of fullness and with age. When empty, the bladder assumes the shape of a tetrahedron and lies entirely within the lesser pelvis. As the bladder fills, it becomes more spheric in shape and moves upward and anteriorly toward the abdominal cavity.[93,113]

During infancy the bladder is located in the abdomen; even the bladder neck lies above the symphysis pubis. The bladder assumes its place in the pelvis shortly before puberty. The change in position is not caused by migration of the organ; rather, changes in the size and shape of the vesicle and maturation of the pelvic bone result in the change in relative location of the bladder.[45]

The bladder is characterized by two inlets and a single outlet located on the inferior aspect of the organ. Six anatomic areas are seen on gross inspection of the organ: the neck, the base or fundus, the apex, and the superior right inferolateral and left inferolateral surfaces (Figure 12-5).[93]

The bladder neck is the lowest part of the organ and is several centimeters from the lower aspect of the symphysis pubis. The bladder neck is a relatively fixed structure regardless of the volume of urine present in the vesicle or the state of the adjacent rectum. The bladder neck is pierced by the internal urethral orifice. In the male it sits directly superior to the prostate gland; in the female it sits posterior to the vaginal wall.[93]

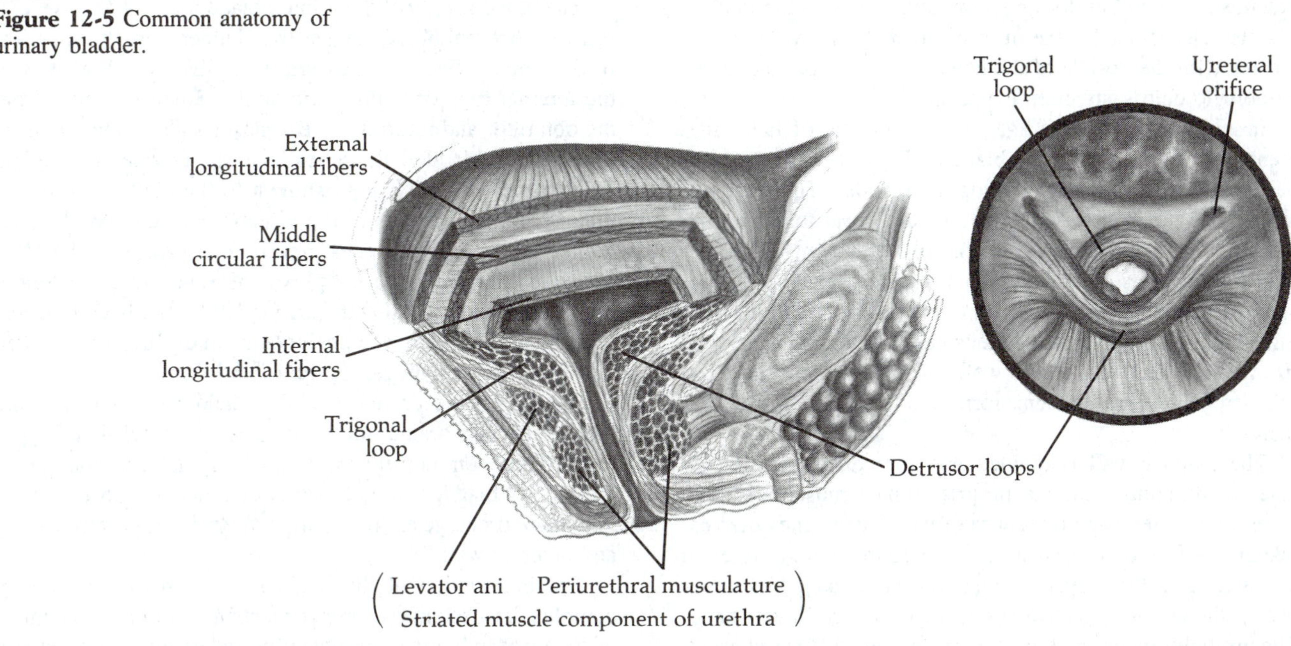

Figure 12-5 Common anatomy of urinary bladder.

The base of the bladder is triangular and oriented posteriorly and downward from the bladder apex. Its borders are rounded and characterized by the junction of the intravesical ureters. In the adult male the bladder is superior to the seminal vesicles and adjacent to the rectum. Denonvilliers' fascia forms an anatomic barrier between the bladder base, rectum, and the vasa deferentia. In adult women the bladder base lies in close proximity to the anterior vaginal wall. Although the female lacks any fascial borders between the bladder and adjacent vagina, the two structures are separate at this point. In contrast, the lower urethra is anatomically continuous with the anterior vaginal wall.[93]

The apex of the bladder is the uppermost surface of the organ and is oriented anteriorly toward the abdominal wall. In the empty bladder of the adult, the apex lies within the pelvis. When the bladder is filled with urine, the apex is pushed upward and anteriorly so it enters the abdominal cavity. The apex is connected to the abdominal wall via the urachus.[93,95]

The superior surface of the empty bladder is bounded laterally by a line extending from the apex to the anterior borders of the intravesical ureters. The posterior border is formed by a line extending between the external borders of the intravesical ureters. In the adult male a reflection of the peritoneum covers the superior surface. When filled, a prevesical pouch is formed that may contain a segment of the small bowel. In the adult female the superior surface of the bladder is separated from the ureters by the ureterovesical pouch.

The inferolateral surfaces of the urinary bladder can be distinguished primarily when the vesicle is empty. They lack any pelvic fascial covering and significantly change shape to accommodate bladder filling. When the bladder reaches capacity, the right and left inferolateral surfaces become a single, convex area lying adjacent to the abdominal wall.

The primary supportive structure of the urinary bladder is the pelvic floor. In addition, the ligaments found adjacent to the bladder are presumed to provide additional support. The true ligaments are thought to play a primary role in maintaining the bladder's position, and the false ligaments are presumed to play a lesser, supplemental role. The arrangement of these ligaments varies between women and men.[93,113]

The true bladder ligaments are dense bands of fascia that arise from the tendinous arch of the peritoneum and connect it with the lateral aspects of the bladder wall. The tendinous arch is a thickening of the peritoneal fascia that lies over the pelvic diaphragm and extends to the symphysis pubis and ischial spines. In the adult male the anterior aspect of this tissue forms the puboprostatic ligaments. The lateral puboprostatic ligaments extend from the anterior end of the tendinous arch to the upper aspect of the prostatic sheath. The medial puboprostatic ligaments extend from the tendinous arch to the back of the pubic bone, near the middle of the symphysis and the back part of the prostatic sheath, forming the retropubic space. In women the analogous structures are the pubovesical ligaments whose attachments are identical to those described in males except that the lower aspects of the ligaments attach to the bladder neck and proximal urethra in contrast to the prostatic sheath. From a neurological perspective the bladder neck may be divided from other bladder surfaces, which are collectively referred to as the bladder body.[93,113]

At the apex of the bladder, the allantois forms the median umbilical ligament or urachus, which is a fibrous cord extending to the umbilicus. Normally, the lower portion of the urachus is patent but does not communicate with the bladder vesicle. Occasionally, the inferior urachal remnant communicates with the vesicle of the bladder; this is not considered pathologic unless infection is present.[93,113]

In addition to the true ligaments, a number of false ligaments are found around the bladder. They are reflections of peritoneum that partially envelop the bladder. The three anterior false ligaments are the median umbilical fold, the medial umbilical fold, and the lateral false ligaments. The median fold extends over the urachal remnant near the bladder apex. The medial umbilical fold covers the remaining umbilical arterial remnants, and the lateral false ligaments extend from the bladder to the side walls of the pelvis. Reflections of sacrogenital peritoneum form the posterior false ligaments.[113]

The bladder wall is divided into four distinct histologic layers: urothelium, lamina propria, tunica muscularis, and outer adventitia. The urothelium of the bladder lines the vesicle and is formed of transitional cell epithelium six to eight layers deep in the empty bladder. As the bladder fills to capacity, the urothelium becomes only two to three layers deep. The urothelium has an associated membrane that is impermeable to water, thus preventing the reabsorption of urine stored in the bladder.[45,68]

Under the urothelium is the submucosal layer, or the lamina propria. The lamina propria is only loosely attached to the urothelium and rich with areolar tissues and elastic fibers. The lamina propria is found throughout the distensible portions of the bladder but is absent in the area of the deep trigone. Here, the mucosal lining of the vesicle is attached directly to the tunica muscularis in this nondistensible portion of the bladder.[45]

Unlike its loose connection with the urothelium, the lamina propria is firmly attached to the tunica muscularis of the bladder. The tunica muscularis is composed primarily of smooth muscle and is called the detrusor. Detrusor muscle cells are arranged in bundles and interspersed within a collagenous framework. A dense autonomic plexus provides autonomic innervation for the detrusor muscle cells. The detrusor muscle is variable in thickness; three layers (inner longitudinal, middle circular, and outer longitudinal) are described. The middle circular and outer longitudinal layers consist of relatively thick muscle cells. They are most prominent in the body of the bladder and terminate at the urethral orifice. Controversy exists whether detrusor muscle bundles of the inner longitudinal layer extend into the proximal urethra. Some investigators argue that the inner longitudinal layer continues into the urethra, forming an outer longitudinal layer of smooth muscle.[39,86] In contrast, others note that continuity between detrusor muscle bundles and urethral smooth muscle bundles is not seen in fetal histologic specimens. They conclude that vesicle smooth muscle and urethral smooth muscle are embryologically separate.[21]

The outermost histologic layer of the bladder is the adventitia. The adventitia is composed of fibroelastic tissue and is loosely connected to the various peritoneal coverings of the bladder described previously.[68]

The blood supply of the urinary bladder arises from several sources. Arterial blood reaches the bladder from the superior, medial, and inferior vesical arteries, which are branches of the internal iliac or hypogastric artery. Small branches from the obturator and inferior gluteal muscles also supply arterial blood to the bladder. Branches from the uterine and vaginal artery supply vascular nourishment to the bladder in the female. Unlike the veins of the kidneys, those of the bladder do not follow arterial routes. Venous drainage from the bladder exits anteriorly into the plexus of Santorini and laterally into a neurovascular sheath surrounded by the lateral vesical ligaments. From here venous blood from the bladder is routed into the inferior hypogastric vein.[45,95]

The lymphatic drainage of the bladder originates in the urothelium and drains into the vesical, external iliac, hypogastric, and common iliac nodes. The lymphatic channels in the urinary bladder are not clearly elucidated. Three areas of lymphatic drainage are postulated: the trigone, posterior wall, and anterior wall.[45,95]

The innervation of the bladder represents a deceptively complex discussion; the precise mechanisms of neural control of the urinary bladder are not fully understood. The sensory innervation of the urinary bladder is poorly understood. Sensory impulses from the urinary bladder are both proprioceptive and exteroceptive. Exteroceptive impulses from the bladder include pain, temperature, and touch. Proprioceptive impulses give the person an awareness of various states of vesical fullness. Morphologic studies in animals have demonstrated the presence of free nerve endings throughout the detrusor muscle with the greatest abundance in the trigone. Tension receptors and stretch receptors have also been noted in the detrusor muscle and presumably play an important role in the awareness of bladder filling. The impulses generated by the sensory receptors are thought to travel in the sensory portion of the pelvic nerve.[45,61]

The motor innervation of the bladder, like all smooth muscle, is provided by the autonomic nervous system. Parasympathetic neural receptors are found throughout the detrusor muscle within the body of the bladder. These receptors are stimulated by acetylcholine and are thus termed cholinergic nerves. Two types of cholinergic receptors are seen in the human body: muscarinic and nicotinic. The bladder contains muscarinic cholinergic receptors. Sympathetic receptors are also found throughout the body of the bladder and are particularly abundant in the bladder neck. The sympathetic nerve endings in the bladder respond to norepinephrine and are called adrenergic nerves. Adrenergic receptors are labeled alpha (α) or beta (β) based on their responses to the various catecholamines found in the body. β-Adrenergic responses are subdivided into β_1 and β_2 types. In the urinary bladder, both α- and β_2-adrenergic receptors are found. The α-adrenergic receptors are most numerous in the bladder neck and trigone; β_2-adrenergic receptors are most abundant in the body of the bladder.[61]

Sympathetic neural signals are routed to the bladder via branches of the inferior hypogastric plexus. The spinal roots of the sympathetic component of the inferior hypogastric are

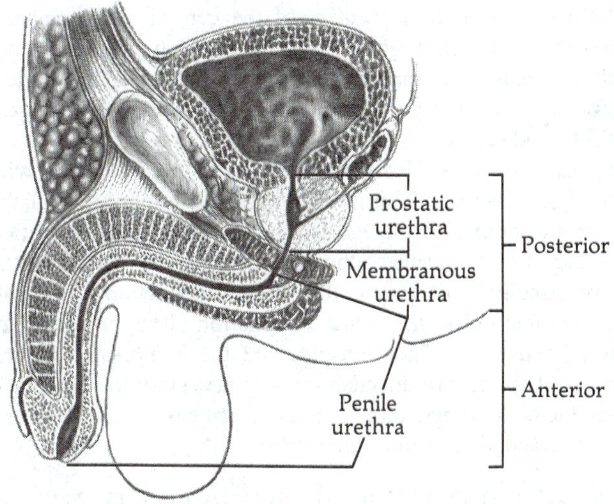

Figure 12-6 Male urethra.

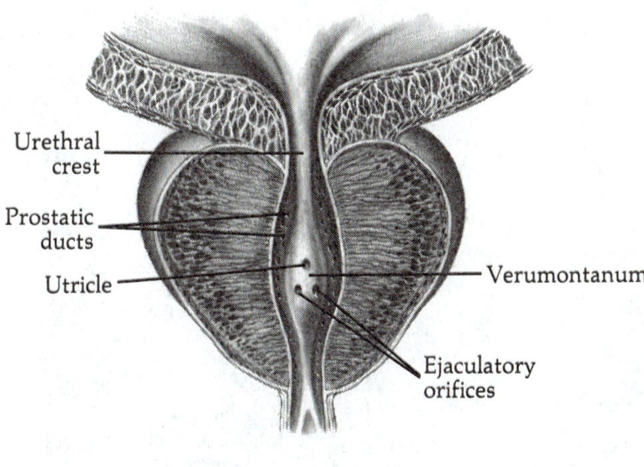

Figure 12-7 Prostatic (posterior) urethra.

at T12, L1, and L2. Parasympathetic neural signals are routed to the bladder via branches of the pelvic nerve. The spinal roots of the parasympathetic component of the pelvic plexus are located in the interomedial gray matter between the dorsal and ventral horns of spinal levels S2 to S4.

Urethra. The urethra extends from the bladder to an external meatus, serves as a conduit for urine expulsion during micturition, and aids in maintaining continence during bladder filling. In the male the urethra also serves as a conduit for semen expelled at ejaculation.[45,113]

The male urethra is approximately 23 cm long and is divided into two parts: anterior and posterior (Figure 12-6). The posterior urethra is subdivided into the prostatic and membranous urethra. The prostatic urethra is approximately 3 cm in length and extends from the bladder neck to the origin of the membranous urethral segment at the apex of the prostate gland. It runs through the prostate vertically, lying nearer the anterior surface of the gland. The posterior floor of the prostatic urethra is elevated at the verumontanum. It tapers inferiorly and superiorly to form the cristae, which are mucous membrane folds that form a depression on the posterior floor known as the prostatic fossa. Secretory ducts from the middle lobe of the prostate enter the urethra at this point (Figure 12-7).[45]

The membranous urethra is 2 to 2.5 cm in length and extends from the apex of the prostate to the bulb of the penis. It pierces the area referred to as the urogenital diaphragm. Striated muscle fibers exist within the wall of the membranous urethra and significantly contribute to sphincteric function in the male. These muscle fibers are arranged in an omega-shaped pattern and are thinnest in the posterior midline. Periurethral striated muscle fibers from the pelvic floor also contribute to striated muscle sphincteric function of the urethra.[42,106] The membranous urethra is the least distensible segment, since it is anchored securely by the triangular ligament. It is the most susceptible to inflammatory urethral stricture.[45,113]

The anterior urethra tunnels the corpus spongiosum of the penis and is divided into the bulbous, pendulous, and glandular urethra. The bulbous and pendulous parts of the urethra together measure 15 cm in length and extend from the distal border of the membranous urethra to the base of the glans penis. The suspensory ligament marks the border between these urethral segments. The bulbous urethra is distinguished by the orifices of the bulbourethral, or Cowper's, glands.[45]

The penile urethra is the most distal segment in the male and terminates at the external meatus. Immediately before the external meatus, the penile urethra is marked by a fusiform dilation called the fossa navicularis. It originates at the corona of the glans and is 2.5 cm in length. The external meatus itself is a vertical slit approximately 8 mm in diameter that lies at the summit of the glans.[45,113]

The microscopic anatomy of the male urethra is characterized by an inner mucous membrane composed of columnar cell epithelium persisting throughout the posterior and anterior urethral segments to the level of the fossa navicularis. Here the urethral mucosa changes to a squamous cell epithelium near the external meatus. A submucosal layer composed of connective tissue and elastic fibers lies under the mucosa. The muscular layer of the urethra is composed primarily of smooth muscle fibers. In the prostatic urethra the smooth muscle fibers are indistinguishable from the adjacent musculature to the level of the verumontanum. Below the verumontanum, the urethral smooth fibers are arranged in an outer circular layer and an inner longitudinal layer. Striated muscle fibers have also been noted in the ventral wall of the prostatic urethra.[21,113]

The arterial blood supply of the male urethra arises from

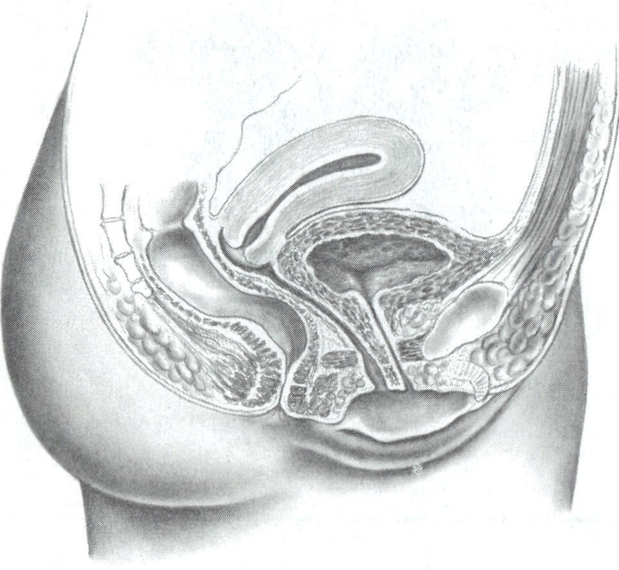

Figure 12-8 Anatomic relations of female urethra.

the urethral artery, which is a branch of the internal pudendal artery. Venous blood from the urethra drains into the deep vein of the penis and the pudendal plexus. The sensory innervation of the urethra is provided by branches of the pudendal nerve. Lymphatic drainage from the male urethra accompanies channels of the glans penis in the anterior segment and empties into the deep subinguinal nodes from the posterior segment.[113]

The female urethra forms a relatively short, straight path when compared with the male urethra (Figure 12-8). In nulliparous adult women the urethra measures 3.5 to 5.5 cm. The female urethra originates at the bladder neck orifice and travels at a 16-degree angle to its external meatus at the vestibule. Striated muscle fibers within the urethral wall are densest in the middle third of the female urethra and deficient in the posterior midline. Periurethral striated muscle fibers of the levator ani also contribute to sphincteric function in the female.[40,113]

Three histologic elements of the female urethra characterize its microscopic anatomy. The inner urethral lumen is lined by columnar epithelium that changes to squamous epithelium near the external meatus. The mucosal layer also contains numerous secreting glands. The muscular lining of the urethra contains an outer sheath of skeletal muscle fibers (the rhabdosphincter), an outer longitudinal layer of smooth muscle bundles, and inner circular layers of smooth muscle bundles. The lower two thirds of the female urethra is fused with the anterior vaginal wall so that the two layers of smooth muscle are indistinguishable. A spongy vascular cushion composed of an extensive venous network and arteriovenous communications lies between the urethral mucosa layer and the muscular layer of the urethral wall.[78,113]

Lower Urinary Tract Function

The bladder and urethra act as a coordinated unit under the influence of multiple centers of the central and peripheral nervous systems. Together with the pelvic floor musculature they form a single functional system called the urethrovesical unit. Lower urinary tract function is divided into two stages, filling and voiding. Bladder filling and storage is characterized by passive filling of the bladder vesicle in conjunction with urethral closure. Micturition is marked by relaxation of the urethral sphincteric mechanism in synchrony with contraction of the smooth muscle of the bladder wall. Knowledge of the two principal components that modulate function of the urethrovesical unit—the neural modulation of the bladder, urethra, and pelvic floor muscles and the components of the urethral sphincteric mechanism—is necessary to understand the factors that maintain continence and ensure complete urinary evacuation during micturition.

Neural Innervation of the Lower Urinary Tract

The neural control of micturition is modulated by three structures—the brain, spinal cord, and peripheral nervous system. Although our knowledge of the neural control of micturition remains incomplete, interest in this area of physiology has increased over the past several decades because of a growing recognition of urinary incontinence as a worldwide health problem.

Brain. Central nervous system influence on lower urinary tract function begins in the cerebral cortex. A detrusor motor area is located in the superiomedial area of the frontal lobe and the genu of the corpus callosum within both hemispheres of the brain.[6] In the experimental animal model, stimulation of the detrusor motor area causes contraction of the bladder, although the net effect of this area in the human is considered inhibitory.[44,63] Distention of the bladder during filling stimulates the detrusor motor area via afferent signals from receptors that travel to the brain via afferents from the pelvic plexus. These afferent signals traverse the spinal cord via reticulospinal tracts. Efferent signals from the detrusor motor area travel to subcortical nuclei in the brainstem (pontine micturition center) to ultimately traverse spinal tracts and synapse on spinal interneurons in the conus medullaris (sacral micturition center).[106]

Volitional control and regulation of basal tone on the pelvic floor musculature and urethral rhabdosphincter also are influenced by the cerebral cortex. A pelvic floor muscle motor area is contained in the sensorimotor cortex and bilaterally in the medial aspect of the cortex.[44,45] The pelvic floor muscles are typical of other skeletal muscle structures in the human and are innervated via the pyramidal tracts of the central nervous system. They are further influenced by the extrapyramidal system.[43] Unlike many muscles of the human, the pelvic floor and rhabdosphincter consist of primarily slow-twitch muscle fibers that are particularly suited for prolonged periods of tone necessary for maintaining urethral closure during bladder filling.[78]

The thalamus is the primary relay center for communication between the cerebral cortex and lower brain centers. Terminal synapses of proprioceptive sensory axons from the detrusor are located in nonspecific intraluminal nuclei of the thalamus. The exact location of the thalamic pathways of detrusor motor function is unclear.[106] The observable effect of the thalamus, then, on the function of the bladder in the human is participation in the brain's net inhibitory influence on micturition in the continent individual.

The basal ganglia are a well-known component of the extrapyramidal tracts and include the caudate nuclei, red nuclei, substantia nigra, putamen, and globus pallidus. Persuasive evidence demonstrates that the basal ganglia exert a direct inhibitory influence on the detrusor muscle.[16,70] Input to the neurons of the basal ganglia is provided by pyramidal cells of the detrusor motor area and pelvic floor muscle motor area in the cerebral cortex. Efferent messages from the basal ganglia are thought to be directed to the cerebral cortex and that area of the brainstem involved with lower urinary tract function.[70]

The limbic system modulates the autonomic nervous system via input to the reticular formation center of the brainstem and hypothalamus.[43] Direct stimulation of the limbic system alters the detrusor reflex,[30] although pathologic ablation of the temporal lobes (including the hippocampus and amygdala) has not been associated with clinically apparent voiding dysfunction in the human.[45]

The hypothalamus consists of a collection of nuclei that regulate the body's internal environment, including neuroendocrine functions and specific sexual behavioral responses. While the hypothalamus is not known to exert any direct influence on bladder function, it is known that bladder distention produces an effect on certain nuclei within the hypothalamus.[101]

The cerebellum is a significant component of the extrapyramidal tract and helps to coordinate voluntary movements and maintain the body's position in space. It affects bladder function by modulation of the detrusor reflex and pelvic floor muscular activity.[106] Cerebellar dysfunction in the clinical setting is associated with detrusor dysfunction.[67]

The brainstem is extremely important in lower urinary tract function. The gray matter of the dorsolateral pons and mesencephalon are the final common pathways to detrusor motor pathways in the spinal cord.[26] The pontine micturition center is of considerable clinical importance and is often referred to as the sphincter coordination center. This label is supported by observations that preservation of bladder and pelvic floor muscle activity is seen in neurologic lesions above the pons, while bladder striated incoordination (dyssynergia) is noted among persons with lesions below the pons and above the sacral micturition center.[14] The pontine micturition center plays a role in the initiation of the detrusor reflex, thus the reference to the act of micturition as a "brainstem reflex."[61]

Spinal cord. The importance of the spinal cord to lower urinary tract function has been demonstrated in both animals and humans. Anatomically separate tracts provide communication between modulatory areas of the brain and pelvic and pudendal nuclei located within the conus medullaris.

The reticulospinal tracts of the lateral columns are involved with motor innervation of the detrusor.[86] Motor innervation of the pelvic floor muscles is mediated via corticospinal tracts. The final synapse within the central nervous system for axons involved with both detrusor and pelvic floor muscle function is in the conus medullaris of the spinal cord. A reflexic inhibitory relationship exists between these systems so that stimulation of pelvic nuclei (involved with motor innervation of the detrusor muscle) results in inhibition of the pudendal nuclei (involved with motor innervation of the pelvic floor nuclei) and vice versa.[106]

In addition to the reticulospinal and corticospinal tracts, two specific areas of the spinal cord are significant to lower urinary tract function. Sympathetic outflow to the urethrovesical unit arises from spinal segments T10 to L1 or L2. Sympathetic outflow to the bladder body promotes relaxation of the detrusor, while sympathetic impulses at the bladder neck are noted to tighten the smooth muscle of the urethra. The significance of this neural modulation to urethrovesical function remains controversial.[44,106]

Spinal segments S2 to S4 are the location of both the pelvic nuclei, which provide motor innervation to the detrusor, and the pudendal nuclei, which provide innervation for the pelvic floor muscles. The pelvic nuclei are located within the interomediolateral portion of the gray matter, and the pudendal nuclei are found more dorsally in the ventromedial portion of the cord.[44] Injury to the sacral micturition center, which is necessary for the bladder to mount a contraction, results in loss of detrusor contractility.

Peripheral nervous system. Two peripheral nerves are significant to urethrovesical function (Figure 12-10, *A*). The pelvic plexus exits the spine at S2, S3, and S4 to supply the bladder wall and proximal urethra with parasympathetic innervation. Stimulation of the pelvic plexus produces detrusor contraction and reflexic inhibition of the pudendal nerve and pelvic floor musculature.[106] Pelvic parasympathetic ganglia terminate on smooth muscle bundles within the detrusor. The parasympathetic ganglia were assumed to be exclusively cholinergic, although recent studies have demonstrated the existence of other neurotransmitter substances within the bladder wall, including adenosine triphosphate (ATP) and vasoactive intestinal polypetide (VIP).[25,45] Neural receptors innervate smooth muscle cells at an approximately 1:1 ratio, thus explaining the discrete neural influence on bladder activity in contrast to visceral muscle in the intestine or stomach.[26]

The plexus nerve, like most peripheral nerves, contains multiple types of fibers. Sympathetic fibers travel via the pelvic plexus to innervate the bladder body, trigone, and bladder neck. Sympathetic innervation of the bladder body is inhibitory in nature; β-adrenergic receptors promote bladder filling and storage by exerting an antagonistic influence on bladder contractility. Sympathetic innervation in the bladder neck is excitatory and mediated by α-adrenergic receptors, although the significance of this neural modulatory mecha-

Figure 12-9 Loops I and II extend from frontal cortex to pelvic nuclei in conus medullaris.

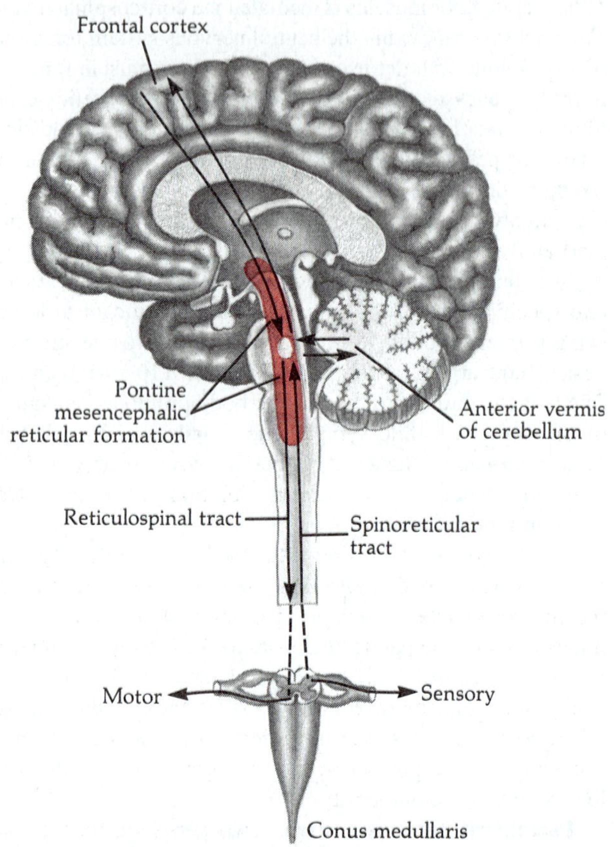

nism remains controversial.[25,44,106] The termination of the pelvic autonomic fibers in the bladder form a microscopic forest that complicates any surgical procedure of the pelvis with the risk of denervation of the urethrovesical unit.

The pudendal nerve also arises from S2 to S4 and exits the spine via the greater sciatic foramen to run with the internal pudendal vessels. It provides somatic and sensory innervation to the pelvic floor musculature.[113]

Bradley's loop concept of innervation. Bradley and his associates[17,45,106] have proposed a conceptual framework of the innervation of the lower urinary tract based on four reflex arcs or loops. Loop I consists of the cerebrocortical areas that modulate detrusor function (Figure 12-9). It originates with the detrusor motor area of the cerebral cortex and extends to the pontine micturition center. Loop II (Figure 12-9) consists of afferent and efferent spinal tracts between the pontine micturition center and detrusor nuclei in the sacral spinal cord. Loops I and II are essential for the maintenance of bladder stability in the human.

Loop III consists of the pelvic and pudendal nuclei and their interneurons (Figure 12-10, *B*). It controls the coordination between the detrusor and pelvic floor musculature. Interruption of loop III results in loss of coordination between detrusor and striated sphincteric activity, and is called detrusor/striated sphincter dyssynergia.

Loop IV consists of the supraspinal and spinal innervation of the pelvic floor musculature. Loop IV provides voluntary control of the striated sphincteric mechanism, which allows the individual to interrupt a urinary stream if desired. Loop IV begins in the sensorimotor cortex and extends to the pudendal nuclei of the conus medullaris. Interruption of spinal segments of loop IV occurs in conjunction with interruption

Figure 12-10 A, Sacral micturition center and peripheral bladder innervations. **B,** Loop III contains pelvic and pudendal nuclei and their interneurons.

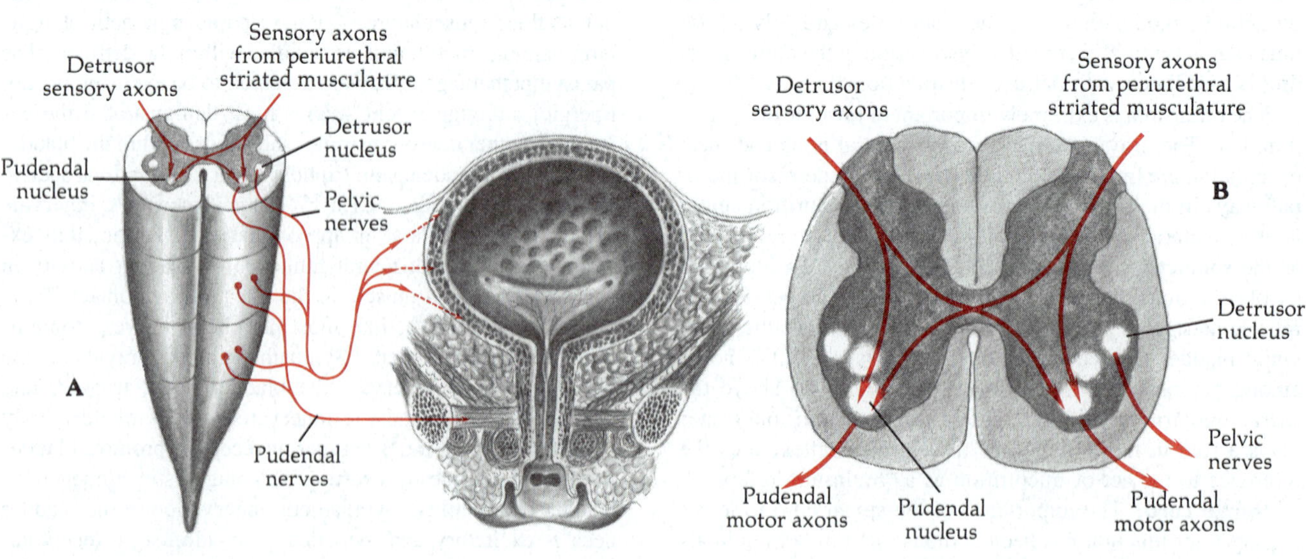

Figure 12-11 Loop IV.

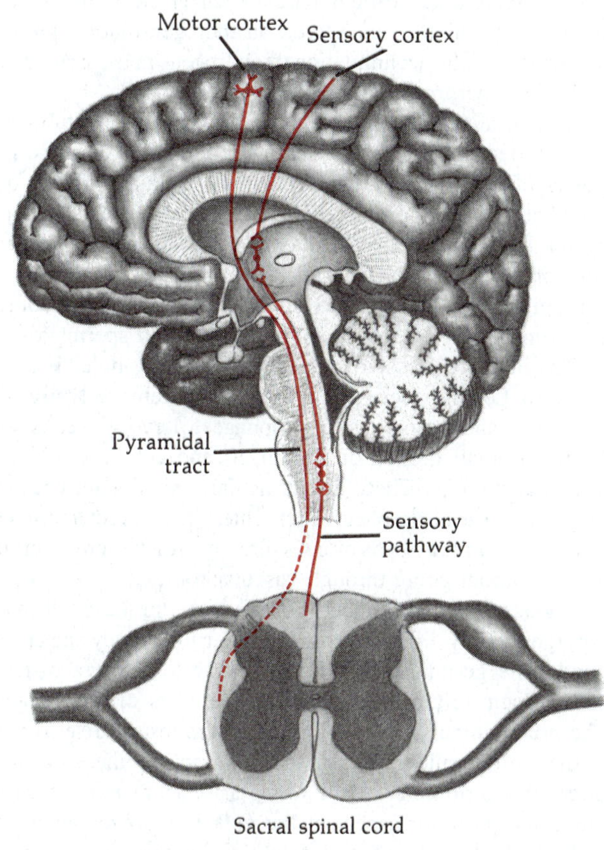

of loops II and III and results in detrusor/striated sphincter dyssynergia.[17,106]

Other modulators of lower urinary tract function. Prostaglandins also play a role in the modulation of urethrovesical function. The bladder produces PGE_2, PGE_1, and PGF_2-alpha. Among these prostaglandins, PGE_2 is predominant and enhances detrusor contractility in conjunction with inhibition of urethral smooth muscle tone. PGF_2-alpha causes increased contractility of both bladder and urethral smooth muscle, but PGE_1 results in only modest increased contractility.[59]

Hormonal regulators of lower urinary tract smooth muscle have not been extensively investigated. Estrogens may exert an indirect influence on detrusor contractility by enhancing the production of prostaglandins.[15] Oxytocin receptors have been documented in the bladder wall of experimental animals and also may exert an influence on smooth muscle contractility in women.

Physiology of Urethral Sphincter Mechanism

The functions of the urethral sphincteric mechanism are to prevent urinary leakage during bladder filling and storage and to allow relatively unobstructed outflow of urine during micturition. A number of components of the urethra and adjacent pelvis contribute to the urethral sphincteric mechanism.

Urethral closure begins with the formation of a watertight seal formed by the epithelial lining of the organ. The plasticity of the urethral epithelium in conjunction with mucosal secretions produced by the urothelial lining produce a remarkably compliant structure that folds and deforms to form a watertight urethral seal in response to extrinsic compression. The effectiveness of this structure's ability to deform into a watertight seal is evident when a Foley catheter is passed without producing dribbling incontinence.[92,100]

A vascular cushion formed by the rich submucosal venous plexus of the urethra also contributes to the urethral sphincteric mechanism. This cushion enhances the pliability of the urethral wall and serves as a transmitter of abdominal pressure along the course of the urethra. Transmission of this abdominal pressure is essential for the urethra to maintain a watertight seal in response to the stress produced by a sudden rise in pressure, for example, coughing, laughing, or physical exertion.[100]

Smooth and skeletal muscle cells within the urethral wall contribute to the sphincteric mechanism by producing active tone during bladder filling and storage. The smooth muscle of the bladder neck and proximal urethra and the fibers of the rhabdosphincter form an area of tension that is transmitted to the pliable urethral mucosa, thereby producing an efficient seal against urinary leakage.[117]

The pelvic floor musculature also contributes to active closure pressure of the sphincteric mechanism. The periurethral striated musculature is formed primarily by the levator ani. It acts as a sling; contraction of the pelvic floor elevates and compresses the proximal urethra and increases urethral resistance to leakage in response to exertion that causes increasing abdominal pressure.[42]

The pelvic floor and its fascial coverings and the pubourethral ligaments in the male and female contribute indirectly to the sphincteric mechanism by maintaining the urethrovesical unit in its proper location in the pelvis. These structures form a hammock that supports the bladder in its proper abdominopelvic position and increases the efficiency of pressure transmission from abdomen to urethra.[42]

Male Genitalia

Scrotum. The scrotum is a cutaneous, fibromuscular sac that is dependent below the pubis bone and houses the testes and lower portion of the spermatic cord. The skin of the scrotum is thin and deeply pigmented and contains abundant sebaceous glands, sweat glands, and hair follicles. The cutaneous layer of the scrotum is bisected by the median ridge or raphe, which extends from the base of the penis to the anus. The skin of the scrotum is further distinguished by rugae. The rugae are formed by parallel dermal muscle fibers and are more clearly seen on younger men, particularly when the testes have retracted because of a certain stimulus. Immediately under the skin is the dartos muscle, which is composed of smooth muscle fibers and elastic tissue. The dartos is a continuation of the suspensory ligament of the penis and superficial fascia of the abdominal, inguinal, and perineal fascia. It sends a sagittal reflection inward, creating an incomplete septum between the median ridge and the radix of the penis, which form the cavities in which the testes lie.[45,113]

The primary functions of the scrotum are to house the testes and provide an adequate environment for the production of sperm. The structure of the dartos allows for considerable variation of scrotal size in response to a variety of stimuli, such as external temperature, physical activity level, and emotions.[45]

Testes. The testes are a pair of ovoid organs that lie in the scrotum. They receive vascular, neural, and lymphatic support from the spermatic cord; the scrotal ligament forms the single scrotal attachment for the testes. Each testis is approximately 4 to 5 cm in length and 2.5 cm in width and weighs from 10.5 to 20 g. The left testis typically lies 1 cm lower than the right.[45,113]

The testes lie under three coverings: the tunica vaginalis, the tunica albuginea, and the tunica vasculosa. The tunica vaginalis arises from the peritoneum and forms a closed sac in which the testis is invaginated. The tunica albuginea is a white, fibrous covering for the testis that helps define the interior architecture of the organ. The posterior border of the tunica albuginea projects into the testis, forming an incomplete vertical septum called the mediastinum testis. From its front and lateral aspects, numerous fibrous projections extend toward the external border of the testis, dividing it into 200 to 300 lobules that contain multiple seminiferous tubules. The tunica vasculosa is the third testicular covering. It consists of a plexus of blood vessels within a framework of areolar tissue extending over the internal aspect of the tunica albuginea and covering its many septa, providing a vascular supply to each lobule.[45,113]

The functional unit of the testicular cortex is the seminiferous tubule. Each lobule of the testis contains one to three (or sometimes more) seminiferous tubules that are 30 to 60 cm of tortuous length with both ends terminating in a relatively short, straight segment called the canaliculus rectus. The seminiferous tubules occupy 75% of testicular mass; their combined length is almost 1 mile.[113]

A seminiferous tubule is formed of stratified epithelium four to eight cells thick with an identifiable internal lumen. The tubules contain Sertoli cells, spermatogenic cells, and an outer basement membrane with a fibrous tunica propria. The Sertoli cells are columnar in shape and extend radially from just within the outer basement membrane toward the tubular lumen. These interesting cells have indefinite cytoplasmic borders; spermatids and spermatocytes may be completely embedded within the cytoplasm of the Sertoli cells. The Sertoli cells are linked in tight junctions that divide the wall of the seminiferous tubule into two parts: a basal compartment containing spermatogonia and spermatocytes and a luminal compartment containing more advanced stages of testicular germ cells. The exact function of the Sertoli cells remains unclear. They are presumed to provide nourishment and succor for the germinal epithelium, help maintain the blood-testis barrier, secrete the testicular fluid seen in the lumen of the seminiferous tubules, and secrete an androgen-binding protein that promotes the accumulation of androgens in the immediate area of the germinal cell epithelium.[3]

The germinal cell epithelium of the seminiferous tubule is characterized by an ever-changing population of maturing stages of spermatic forms. The more primitive forms are found at the outer borders, and more mature forms are found nearer the inner lumen. Spermatogonia are the most immature cell form seen in the spermatic cycle. Other stages of germ cell epithelium seen in the wall of the seminiferous tubules are primary and secondary spermatocytes and spermatids.[3]

The interstitial tissue within the testicular lobules is composed of Leydig's cells, blood vessels, extensive lymphatic channels, and numerous macrophages. Leydig's cells are found in small groups of five to 20 and compose 12% of testicular volume. These are particularly significant because they secrete testosterone, which enters the bloodstream via interstitial capillary beds or goes directly into the seminiferous tubule without going through vascular routes.[3]

The structure and function of the testes in the adult male are significantly different from those during infancy and childhood. The germinal elements of the testes have a distinct embryologic origin from the other elements of the gonads. The nongerminal cell components of the testes arise as part of the mesodermic mass that will develop into the urogenital ridge; the germ cells of the testes arise from the entoderm lining the posterior aspect of the yolk sac. Development of both the germinal cell and somatic elements of the testes begins during the fourth week of life.[72]

From their retroperitoneal position, the testes must descend caudally to the scrotal sac to mature into viable structures away from the high temperature of the internal abdomen. During the third trimester they begin moving down the posterior aspect of the abdomen, bringing their neurovascular sheath with them. By the seventh month of gestation, the testes enter the internal ring of the inguinal canal and move into their extra-abdominal position at or shortly after birth. The complex factors that regulate this migration are still not fully understood.[72]

At birth the testes are composed of small tubules with poorly differentiated components and few identifiable spermatogonia. Interstitial cells are present at birth but regress over the first several weeks of life to a baseline level that persists throughout the pubescent period. During the period between 4 and 10 years of age, the seminiferous tubules slowly increase in tortuosity. Beginning around age 10 a significant increase in the size, number, and mitotic activity of the germ cell epithelium occurs. This process continues until the onset of puberty around age 12 when the interstitial Leydig's cells mature and begin to produce testosterone levels comparable with adult values and active spermatogenesis begins.[3]

The blood supply of the testes is unique, since the temperature of arterial and venous blood must be cooled approximately 2° C from abdominal levels to support spermatogenesis. Cooling arises from interactions between arterial and venous vessels in which a countercurrent heat loss mechanism occurs. In addition, the slow, nonpulsating flow of the spermatic artery aids in cooling the vascular beds of the testes.[3]

The arterial blood supply of the testes arises from the internal spermatic artery, the cremasteric artery, and the deferential, or vasal, artery. The latter are important clinically as collateral circulation of the testes. Venous blood from the testes drains into the pampiniform plexus of the spermatic cord, which empties into the internal spermatic veins.[3]

Because of the unique embryologic origins of the testes, the lymphatic drainage is not into local inguinal or pelvic lymph nodes. Rather, the extensive lymphatic channels of the testes drain into the preaortic lymph nodes.[45]

Three adnexa of the testes are of clinical significance; all are composed of vestiges of the embryonic structures relevant to the formation and migration of the testes and spermatic cord. The appendix testis arises in the groove between the head of the epididymis and the testicular remnant of the müllerian duct. It is subject to torsion and must be differentiated from true testicular torsion, which constitutes a urologic emergency. The appendix epididymidis is a pear-shaped body attached to the epididymal head, which is a remnant of epigenitalis tubules. The organs of Giraldes are a paragenitalis remnant sometimes noted in the lower spermatic cord anterior to the head of the epididymis.[45]

Epididymis and vas deferens. The epididymis and vas deferens are the efferent routes for sperm leaving the testes after completing the spermatogenic cycle. Along with the prostate and seminal vesicles, the epididymis and vas deferens provide transport, storage, and support for maturing sperm as they migrate toward the male urethra.[113]

The epididymis is a sausage-shaped structure approximately 5 cm long that is attached to the posterolateral aspect of the testis. Three anatomic regions of the epididymis are described: the head, or globus major; the body, or corpus; and the tail, or globus minor. The epididymis contains a single compartment, so injury is likely to entirely ablate the function of the organ. The epididymis is covered by the tunica vaginalis on all except the posterior border, where a fascial reflection forms the epididymal sinus.[45,113]

Inside the compartment of the epididymis is a long, tortuous canal with little muscular tone but abundant cilia lining the tubular lumen folded over on itself and tightly packed so that its total length is 4 to 5 cm. The head of the epididymis is directly connected to the efferent ductules, allowing sperm leaving the testis to enter the epididymal tubules via ciliary action. At the tail the tubules have more smooth muscle in their walls as the epididymis opens into the vas deferens.[113]

The vas deferens is a firm, elastic, cylindric tube extending from the termination of the epididymal tail to the ejaculatory duct located near the base of the prostate. The initial segment of the vas deferens is tortuous, although the part of the organ more distal to the testis is straight. From its origin at the epididymal tail, the vas deferens ascends along the posterior wall of the testis adjacent to the medial aspect of the epididymis. The vas then moves upward to the posterior part of the spermatic cord, traversing the inguinal canal to the level of the deep inguinal ring. At this point, the vas deferens leaves the spermatic cord, curves around the lateral aspect of the epigastric artery, and ascends several centimeters to the external iliac artery. The vas then crosses the external iliac obliquely and enters the false pelvis where it becomes a relatively fixed structure attached to the posterior abdominal wall. From this point the vas crosses the ureter and curves at an acute angle to traverse the prostatic base and terminate at the ejaculatory duct (Figure 12-12). The final segment of the vas deferens is characterized by a spindle-shaped dilation of the tube called the ampulla, which is approximately 10 cm long and contains several false pouches or diverticula that may or may not be clinically significant.[113]

The wall of the vas deferens is composed of an innermost mucosal layer, a middle muscular layer, and an outer layer of areolar tissue. The mucosa of the vas is composed of columnar epithelial cells, which, unlike the tubules of the epididymis, are not ciliated. The muscular tunic consists of an inner longitudinal layer, a middle circular layer, and an outer longitudinal layer of smooth muscle cells typical of such structures in the body. The outer layer of areolar tissue con-

Figure 12-12 Anatomic relation of vas deferens to bladder (posterior view).

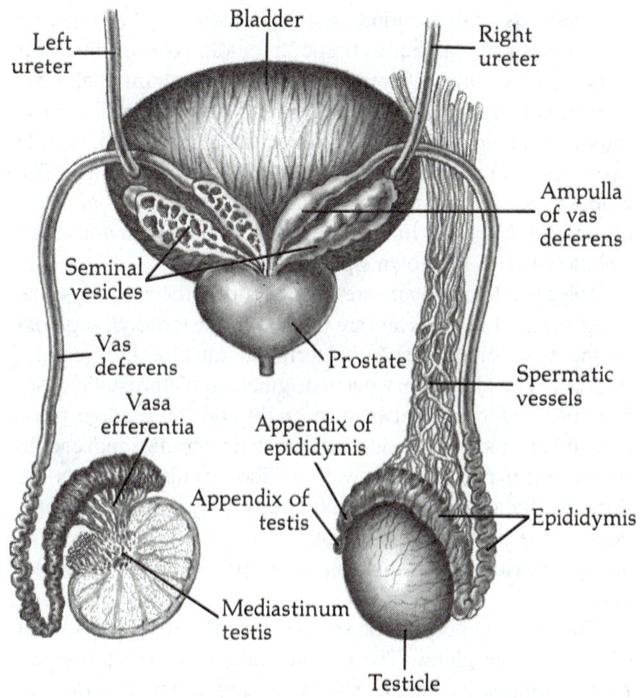

tains the neural, vascular, and lymphatic supply for the vas.[45,113]

The blood supplies of the vas deferens and the epididymis are closely related. The epididymis receives arterial blood from the internal spermatic artery or the deferential artery; the vas deferens receives arterial blood from the deferential artery. Venous blood from the epididymis and lower segments of the vas drains into the pampiniform plexus of the spermatic cord, which becomes the spermatic vein.[45,95]

The motor innervation of the vas deferens arises from the autonomic nervous system. Sympathetic fibers from the hypogastric plexus and parasympathetic fibers from the pelvic nerve modulate the powerful contractile pulses seen in the organ associated with ejaculation. Nerve fibers for pain are also found in the sheaths covering the vas and in the coverings of the epididymis.[3,45]

Lymphatic channels from the epididymis drain into the external iliac and hypogastric nodes. Lymphatic channels from the vas deferens drain into the external and internal nodes.[113]

Seminal vesicles and ejaculatory ducts. The seminal vesicles are a pair of saclike structures that lie between the posterior bladder and the rectum. Each vesicle is 4 cm long; they have a pyramidal shape with the superior end oriented laterally and backward from the base. The structure of the seminal vesicles is formed by a single coiled tube that gives rise to irregularly placed diverticula connected by dense fibrous tissue. The diameter of the tube of the seminal vesicle is 3 to 4 mm, and its length is 10 to 15 cm when uncoiled. The seminal vesicles are directed to the posterior bladder surface near the implantation of the ureters and lie in close proximity to the rectum.[72,113]

The walls of the seminal vesicle are composed of an outer areolar layer of connective tissue, a middle layer of muscular tissue, and a luminal layer of mucosal epithelium characteristic of the organs for sperm transport and maturation. The muscular tunic is formed by inner circular smooth muscle fibers and an outer layer of longitudinal smooth muscle. The mucosal layer consists of columnar epithelium with an abundance of goblet cells in the diverticula of the organ and small stellate cells of unknown significance.[113]

The ejaculatory ducts are located along the median plane of the seminal vesicles and are formed by the terminal segment of the vas deferens and the terminal duct of the seminal vesicles. The ejaculatory ducts originate at the prostatic base, run anteroinferiorly between the right and left median prostatic lobes, pass alongside the prostatic utricle, and end in the posterior urethra. The walls of the ejaculatory ducts are thin and characterized by an outer fibrous layer that terminates beyond the prostatic portion of the ducts, a middle layer of smooth muscle, and an inner layer of columnar epithelial cells.[113]

The blood supply of the seminal vesicles is similar to that of the prostate gland. The primary motor innervation arises from sympathetic fibers. The lymphatic channels from the seminal vesicles drain into the hypogastric, sacral, vesical, and external iliac nodes (Figure 12-12).[95]

Prostate. The prostate is a partly glandular, partly fibromuscular organ that lies at the base of the bladder and surrounds the initial 2 to 3 cm of posterior urethra. The prostate is conical with an anterior and posterior flattening; its average dimensions are 3.4 cm in length, 4.4 cm in width, and 2.6 cm at its greatest thickness. The organ is securely anchored by the puboprostatic ligaments, Denonvillier's fascia, and the adjacent pelvic floor musculature. In addition, the resilient, strong prostatic capsule provides support.[45]

The structure of the prostate has been conceptualized in terms of lobes and zones. Anatomists report that there are no anatomic distinctions among the lobes of the prostate; however, the lobes conceptualized by urologists do have clinical significance. Williams and Warwick[113] conceptualize the prostate in terms of four anatomically distinguishable areas: the base, apex, posterior surface, and superior surface. The base of the prostate is contiguous with the bladder neck area. The urethra pierces the prostate at the base near its anterior border. The apex of the prostate is oriented inferiorly to the base; its surface is contiguous with fascia covering the superior aspect of the external urinary sphincter and transversus perinei muscles. The posterior surface is transversely flat and vertically convex. It is separated from the rectum by the prostatic sheath and loose connective tissue external to this sheath. The superior surface is analogous to the median lobe of the prostate; its inferior border is characterized by a sulcus that is used to mark the border between the right and left lateral lobes.[113]

Clinicians conceptualize the prostate in terms of intraurethral and extraurethral lobes: the intraurethral lobes are the anterior, right and left lateral, and subcervical lobes; the extraurethral lobes are the posterior and median lobes. The anterior lobe undergoes atrophy before pubescence and never becomes hyperplastic. The right and left lateral lobes of the prostate form the lateral walls of the prostatic urethra; they have clinical significance because hyperplasia of the glandular tissue of these lobes produces urinary obstruction and the classic symptoms of benign prostatic hyperplasia. Hyperplasia of the glandular components of the subcervical lobe encroaches on the lumen of the prostatic urethra in an upward fashion. The extraurethral lobes of the prostate gland are not as likely to undergo hyperplasia as are the intraurethral lobes. The posterior lobe lies along the posterolateral wall of the prostate between the apex and ejaculatory ducts. The posterior lobe is of great clinical significance because it is at risk of neoplastic degeneration later in life. The median lobe lies between the seminal vesicles and vesical neck; unfortunately, it is inseparable from the posterior lobe anatomically and is appreciated only in a portion of prostates in adult men.[50]

The microscopic anatomy of the prostate is characterized by glandular components and fibromuscular components. The fibromuscular capsule sends extensions into the interior of the organ, whose apices converge in the posterior urethral surface. The fibromuscular tissue is primarily nonstriated muscle with a relatively small area of skeletal muscle located ventral to and contiguous with the external urinary sphincter. The bulk of muscular tissue is located in the fibromuscular septa found throughout the gland.[113]

The glandular tissue is composed of numerous follicles with frequent papillary elevations that open into long canals seen throughout the organ. These follicles join to form 12 to 20 excretory ducts. The glandular tissue of the prostate is supported by extensions of muscular tissue and delicate areolar stroma that encapsulate a capillary plexus. Three zones of glandular tissue—peripheral, stromal, and glandular—are distinguishable. The peripheral zone contains long branched glands that curve either posteriorly to open into prostatic sinuses or directly into the posterior urethra.[113]

The motor and sensory innervation of the prostate gland arises from the lower segments of the inferior hypogastric plexus. The arterial blood supply of the prostate is derived from branches of the internal pudendal, middle rectal, and inferior vesical arteries. Venous blood from the prostate drains into the periprostatic space and into the internal iliacs or deep penile veins. Lymphatic channels from within the prostate drain into the external iliac nodes or the sacral lymph nodes.[113]

Penis. The penis is a cylindrically shaped organ in its flaccid state that contains two portions: a root that attaches to the perineum and a pendulous portion called the corpus, or body. The root of the penis is attached to the pelvic floor via a continuation of Buck's fascia, the pubic rami (crura of the corpora cavernosa), and the suspensory ligament.[45]

The body of the penis contains three elongated bodies of erectile tissue that are capable of considerable enlargement when they become engorged with blood during tumescence (Figure 12-13). The left and right corpora cavernosa form the majority of the substance of the penile body and lie in close approximation to each other. They are surrounded by an extension of the tunica albuginea containing superficial and deep layers. The superficial layer is composed of longitudinally arranged fibers that surround the two corpora cavernosa as a unit; the deep layer is composed of circularly arranged fibers that encase each corpus separately via a fibrous septum that forms two median grooves of anatomic significance. The larger median groove houses the corpus spongiosum and pendulous urethra; the smaller median groove houses the deep dorsal veins. The corpora cavernosa do not reach the distal end of the penis; instead, they terminate in the proximal portion of the glans.[113]

The corpus spongiosum lies inferior to the corpora cavernosa and is pierced throughout its length by the urethra. It is smaller than the paired corpora cavernosa and is surrounded by a reflection of the tunica albuginea.[113]

The skin of the penis is characterized by its thinness, relatively dark color, and loose connection with the underlying fascia. At the distal portion of the penis, the skin is folded over on itself to form the foreskin covering the glans penis. The glans penis covers the distal portion of the corpora cavernosa and forms their terminal connection. It is pierced by the navicularis fossa of the urethra, which ends at a dorsal slit found on the interior surface of the glans.[113]

The superficial fascia of the penis is characterized by loose areolar tissue and is devoid of fat. A few fibers of dartos muscle from the scrotum are present, as are fibers from the fundiform ligament and the suspensory ligament.[113]

The arterial blood supply of the penis arises primarily from the internal pudendal artery, which branches into the dorsal arteries of the penis to supply the deep structures of the organ. The penile skin also receives arterial blood from the external pudendal and femoral arteries.[45]

The venous drainage of the penis can be divided into deep and superficial groups. The deep veins of the penis drain the erectile bodies via the deep dorsal veins, which empty into the plexus of Santorini and ultimately into the hypogastric

Figure 12-13 Cross section of human penis.

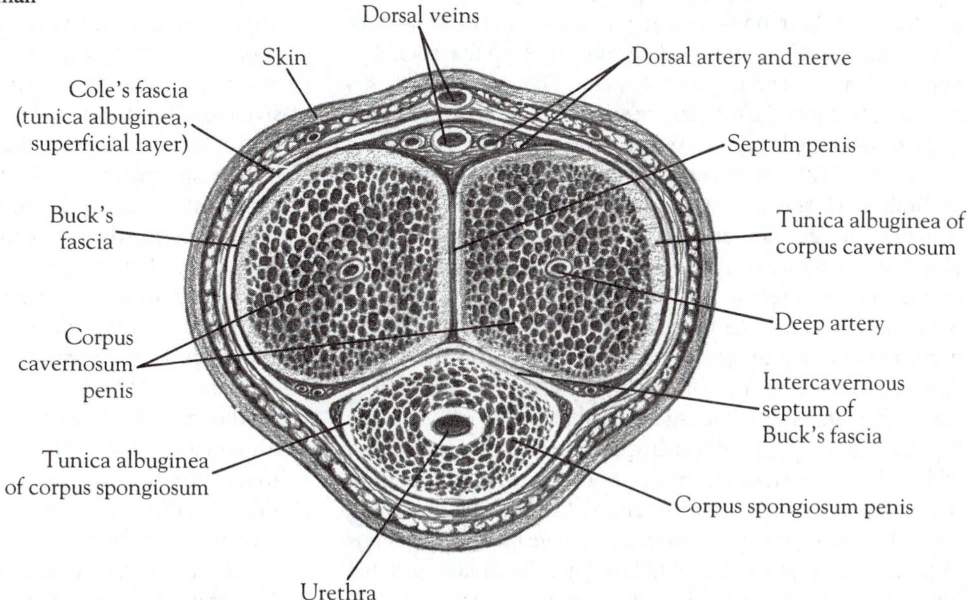

vein. The superficial veins of the penis drain venous blood from the skin via the superficial dorsal penile veins that empty into the saphenous vein.[45]

The lymphatic drainage of the penis is also divided into deep and superficial groups. Deep lymphatic channels of the penis are drained by the subinguinal nodes and the external iliac nodes. Superficial lymphatic channels drain into the superficial inguinal nodes.[45]

The nerve supply of the penis has a somatic and an autonomic component. Sensory innervation of the penile skin arises from the pudendal nerve, which has its roots in spinal segments S2 to S4. Motor innervation to the corpus spongiosum and corpora cavernosa arises from the pelvic nerves, which also have their spinal roots at S2 to S4. Sympathetic fibers from the thoracolumbar spinal cord supply the penile vessels and are particularly evident in the vascular component of the corpus spongiosum.[62]

Male Reproductive Function

Spermatogenesis and hormonal regulation. The testes, epididymis, vas deferens, seminal vesicles, and prostate gland function as a coordinated unit to ensure the production, maturation, and transport of sperm from the male urethra to the female vaginal tract necessary for propagation of the species. Male reproductive functions are regulated by a hormonal axis that consists of certain extrahypothalamic central nervous system centers, the hypothalamus, pituitary, testes, and gonadal-sensitive end organs.[45,54]

Extrahypothalamic central nervous system centers are assumed to play an inhibitory and augmentative role in reproduction. The precise interactions by which brain centers influence the male reproductive hormonal axis are unclear, but a correlation between reproductive function and testicular function is postulated.[45]

The more clearly elucidated hormonal axis governing male reproductive function originates in the hypothalamus, where a luteinizing hormone–releasing hormone (LHRH) is produced and travels to the median eminence of the adenohypophysis via a venous portal system. The presence of this releasing factor in the pituitary results in the direct stimulation of luteinizing hormone (LH) and is thought to stimulate the release of follicle-stimulating hormone (FSH).[45]

Both FSH and LH act at receptor sites in the testes to stimulate the gonadal androgens (primarily testosterone and dihydrotestosterone). LH directly stimulates the Sertoli cells to produce testosterone and stimulate spermatogenesis. FSH is not necessary for the production of testosterone, although it does play a role in spermatogenic testicular function. FSH and LH are released sporadically in response to feedback from the hypothalamic-pituitary-gonadal hormonal axis. When blood levels of the gonadal androgens increase, the production of LHRH in the hypothalamus is inhibited, which suppresses the production of LH by the pituitary. Conversely, decreased serum levels of gonadal androgens stimulate the hypothalamus to produce LHRH so that more LH is produced and excreted into the systemic circulation. The feedback loop for FSH production is not entirely understood; increased levels of testosterone and estradiol exert negative feedback on the production of FSH. In addition, a substance called inhibin, which is produced in the germinal epithelium of the testes, is postulated to inhibit FSH, although its physiologic significance is unclear.[23,54]

The gonadal androgens are essential to the genesis, support, and maturation of spermatozoa. In addition to this direct role in male reproductive function, certain androgens, primarily testosterone and dihydrotestosterone, cause the development and maintenance of the secondary male sex characteristics that characterize pubescence.[23,72]

The process of spermatogenesis occurs within the seminiferous tubule in the testis and is conceptualized in three phases. During the first phase the more primitive spermatogonia enlarge and undergo mitotic divisions into primary spermatocytes that contain 92 chromosomes. The second phase is characterized by two consecutive meiotic divisions accompanied by only one duplication of chromosomes so that the final product of this phase is four spermatids that contain a haploid number of chromosomes suitable for union with the ovum. The third phase of spermatogenesis—spermiogenesis—marks the transformation of spermatid to spermatozoon.[74]

The process of spermiogenesis is relatively slow; it requires 74 days to complete and is divided into four phases. The first phase is the Golgi phase when small granules of hyaluronidase, proteases, and other substances form a single large acrosomal granule enclosed within a vesicle that attaches to the nuclear membrane at the site of the future sperm head. During the second phase a cap appears around the acrosomal vesicle. The two centrioles of the spermatid now begin to move; the proximal centriole assumes a position at the posterior pole of the nucleus opposite the acrosomal sac and the distal centriole sprouts a flagellum consisting of two central microtubules and nine surrounding pairs of microtubules. The distal centriole will become the tail of the future spermatozoon. The third stage of spermiogenesis is the acrosomal phase, in which the developing sperm cell undergoes extensive metamorphosis so that the acrosome, nucleus, flagellum, and cytoplasm assume the characteristic appearance of the mature spermatozoon. During the acrosomal phase a mitochondrial sheath is formed to supply energy for the tail of the mature sperm when it becomes motile after ejaculation. The final stage of spermiogenesis is the maturation phase, which is characterized by the completion of the tail of the spermatozoon and the shedding of excess cytoplasm with the assistance of the Sertoli cells (Figure 12-14).[43,74]

Transport of the sperm from the seminiferous tubule occurs via the muscular activity of the tubules and fluid movement. Although the sperm that enter the epididymis are mature in appearance, they are not yet capable of motility and not yet able to fertilize an ovum. Thus the epididymis also plays a necessary role in the maturation of sperm. The transit time of sperm through the relatively short epididymis is 12 days. The structure of the epididymis allows slow transit resulting

Figure 12-14 Mature spermatozoon cell.

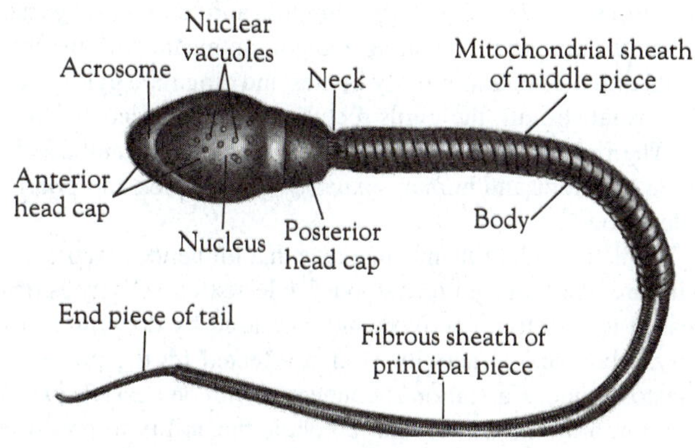

from the slow peristaltic-like activity of the smooth muscle of the organ and the ciliary action of the efferent ductules. During the time spent within the epididymis, sperm gain the potential for motility, although a substance in the tubular fluid prevents sperm from becoming motile before ejaculation. Although the process by which this maturation occurs is not known, the epididymis is thought to play an active role under the influence of the gonadal androgens (primarily testosterone). The probable maturational functions provided by the epididymis are manipulation of the sodium ion, potassium ion, and chloride ion concentrations in the fluid in the epididymal tubule and the secretion of a variety of compounds such as glycerylphosphorylchlorine and glycoproteins, which are thought to enhance maturation of the spermatozoa.[43,45]

The epididymis also serves as a storage compartment for sperm. The cauda epididymidis may store sperm for a period of several weeks, although the storage time in a man who is extremely sexually active is a matter of hours.[45]

After exiting the epididymis the sperm enters the vas deferens in response to smooth muscle contraction associated with ejaculation. Sperm is carried into the ejaculatory ducts where it is mixed with the nutritive secretions of the seminal vesicles. The seminal vesicles do not, as their name implies, serve as storage compartments for sperm; rather, they secrete a mucoid fluid rich with fructose and other nutritive substances into the ejaculatory duct after the vas deferens empties itself of sperm. In addition to their nutritive support, the seminal vesicles add prostaglandins to the ejaculate that are thought to aid in fertilization of the ovum.[43]

The prostate also supports the male reproductive act by adding its secretions to the ejaculate. During ejaculation the prostatic capsule contracts in synchrony with the vas deferens and secretes a thin, milky fluid that contains a variety of substances, including citric acid, calcium, acid phosphate, a clotting enzyme, and profibrinolysin. The pH of this secreted fluid is relatively high (ranging from 6.0 to 6.5), which favors the extended survival of sperm in the acidic environment created by the vaginal mucosa.[43]

The ejaculated semen thus contains fluid from the vas deferens, the seminal vesicles, and the prostate gland, and mucus from the posterior urethral glands, particularly the bulbourethral gland. The pH of the semen is approximately 7.5; the prostatic secretions give the semen a milky appearance, and the seminal vesicle fluid contributes the characteristic mucoid appearance. The normal ejaculate contains 75 million to 400 million sperm cells. After ejaculation a clotting enzyme in the semen interacts with profibrinolysin contributed by the prostate to form a weak coagulum. When this dissolves, the sperm gain their maximal motility as each seeks to fertilize an ovum. Although the sperm cell can survive several months in the male genital ducts, it can survive only 12 to 24 hours in the female genital tract after ejaculation. The relatively short life of sperm in the female genital tract is primarily the result of the acidic nature of the vaginal and fallopian mucosa.[43]

Physiology of erectile activity. The other reproductive function of the male necessary for procreation is the generation and maintenance of an erection to introduce semen into the female genital tract. The penis is primarily an organ of copulation with a secondary function as a conduit for the expulsion of urine during micturition. The erectile activity of the penis depends on complex interactions of neural and vascular events within the context of the psychosocial aspects of male sexuality.[45,113]

An erection of the penis is attained when the cavernous bodies become engorged with blood so the organ assumes a straight line between its root and pendulous portion. Although the corpus spongiosum is involved indirectly with erectile activity, it is the corpora cavernosa that attain the needed volume and rigidity for complete penile erection.[62]

The vascular events that initiate and maintain an erection are arterial infusion, venous constriction, and arteriovenous shunting. During the flaccid state blood is supplied to the corporal bodies by branches of the pudendal arteries and drained via the deep dorsal veins of the penis. Production and maintenance of an erection relies on increased arterial inflow in the penis and constriction of the venous system that drains the cavernous bodies. Arteriovenous shunts are also necessary to modulate tumescence in males. Three types of arteriovenous anastomosis are described; the most abundant and functionally significant occur when the helicine arteries, whose terminal branches open directly into the corpora cavernosa, act as the afferent venous component for the shunting mechanism.[62]

In 1952, Conti[22] argued that von Ebner's polsters are the physiologic regulators of the arteriovenous shunting that occurs during erection. Polsters, or cushions, are formed of longitudinally arranged smooth fibers and areolar tissue that are found in the walls of the penile vasculature. Great variability in the location, extent, and relative proximity of von Ebner's polsters exists. Polsters are also found in the pudendal vessels outside the penis and in other muscular blood vessels such as the carotid, hepatic, renal, and gastric arteries. Therefore the physiologic importance of polsters in erections is questioned. Several alternate theories concerning the nature of polsters exist; the most prominent theory states that these structures are responses to stress and aging that are not seen in neonates but may be observed in varying degrees in the adult male's penis.[61,62]

The generation and maintenance of an erection cannot be explained as a solely vascular event. Rather, penile tumescence requires the coordination of the central nervous system, peripheral nervous system, and neuroendocrine mechanisms. The motor activity of the corpora cavernosa is modulated by the autonomic nervous system, and stimulation of the pelvic nerve produces an erection. The pelvic plexus is only the preganglionic portion of the neural tract; thus infusion of atropine does not ablate an erection. The neurotransmitter substance at the postganglionic nerve in the corpora is unknown. Sympathetic fibers are present in the penile vasculature and are particularly prominent in the corpus spongiosum. Stimulation of sympathetic fibers produces vascular constriction but not erection. The significance of adrenergic fibers in the corpora cavernosa has not been fully appreciated, although they are thought to assume an active role in erectile activity.[62]

The spinal cord is important to male sexual function, since it is the origin of the autonomic outflow for the penis. Since both the sympathetic and parasympathetic nervous systems play a role in erections, injury to the spinal cord produces variations of erectile dysfunction. Injury to the sacral spinal cord is not always connected with impotence. Approximately one third of such patients are able to generate erections using psychogenic stimuli. If the spinal cord is injured, volitional erections are abolished but reflex erections are noted in response to local stimuli.[62]

The brain directly affects penile erections, as well as controlling male sexual behavior. A number of brain centers have been found to influence erectile activity, including the temporal lobes, the gyrus rectus of the cerebral cortex, the cingulate gyrus, the hypothalamus, the mammillary bodies, and the hippocampus. The hippocampus and cingulate gyrus influence emotional responses and communicate with the hypothalamus. The mammillary bodies and cingulate gyrus process visual stimuli; the gyrus rectus processes olfactory stimuli. The precise mechanisms through which the brain affects penile erections and human sexuality are complex and poorly understood.[62]

The neuroendocrine mechanisms that influence erectile activity are also poorly understood. Male sexual activity is decreased by serotonin activity and increased by dopamine activity. Male sexual activity is also affected by the presence of testosterone. Castration is connected with decreased sexual function, although it does not preclude the ability to produce an erection.[62,104]

Wagner[104] has described four phases of erection that combine existing knowledge of erectile physiology. The first is the resting phase, in which the corporal bodies are maintained at a constant volume, and intracavernous pressure and blood flow rate are significantly less than during an erection. The second phase, tumescence, is characterized by an increase in the volume in the cavernous spaces of the penis and a subtle increase in intracavernous pressure. On inspection a small increase in penile length precedes a slight increase in circumference. During the third phase the penis becomes fully erect so that intracavernous pressures will exceed 80 mm Hg. The fourth phase is divided into two segments: a slow and a rapid detumescence stage. During the rapid detumescence phase, rigidity of the penis quickly disappears and is followed by a more gradual loss of blood volume in the corpora cavernosa and a return to the values of the first phase.

Normal Findings

Area of Concern	Normal Adult Findings
Kidney	Overlying skin: edema, bulges, and masses in abdomen absent Palpable only with deep inspiration; may be nonpalpable in obese or muscularly developed persons; smooth, nontender Costovertebral angle tenderness: absent Bruit over costovertebral area or upper abdominal quadrants: absent Transillumination with darkened room and fiberoptic light source: absent
Bladder	Noted as bulge in abdomen when vesicle contains 500 ml or more urine Noted as dull area under suprapubic skin when vesicle is filled with 150 ml or more urine Inspection of voiding act: steady, straight stream, no spraying, no adominal straining; postvoid dribble absent; postvoid residual: less than 20% of total bladder volume *Older adult:* Decreased force of stream compared to younger adult years; absent split stream, spraying, and postvoid dribble
Male genitalia	
Penis	Skin: may be darker than surrounding integument Ulcers, warts, indurated nodules: absent Foreskin: retractable over glans penis; absent in circumcised males Glans penis: hairless, sagittal slit near apex Penile shaft: absent nontender plaques beneath surface in flaccid state

Area of Concern	Normal Adult Findings
	Erect state: even firmness and rigidity over both corpora cavernosa; straight line described between root of penis and glans penis *Older adult:* Decreased rigidity to corpora cavernosa compared to younger adult years; lateral curvature: absent
Scrotum	Skin: rugae; hair bearing and loosely mobile Sebaceous cysts: absent Testes: firm, nontender to gentle palpation; masses: absent *Older adult:* Testes: softer to palpation than in younger adult years Epididymis: palpable as comma-shaped structure on posterior aspect of testes; no tenderness, masses, or nodules Spermatic cord: rolled between thumb and forefinger; vas deferens palpable but nontender Varicocele: absent Transillumination: no edema or solid masses that will transilluminate
Prostate	Posterior aspect of organ accessible beneath anterior rectal wall; two firm, nontender, symmetric, rounded lobes separated by median sulcus (heart shaped and 2.5 cm in length): projects into rectal lumen 1 cm or less Hard, irregular nodes: absent *Older adult:* Increased bogginess noted on digital examination; seen with benign hypertrophy of organ Asymmetric changes in lobe size or discrete nodules: absent

Normal Laboratory Data

Laboratory Test	Normal Adult Values
Acid phosphatase (blood)	Up to 0.8 IU/L; method dependent
Alkaline phosphatase (blood)	Approximately 35-100 IU/L by SMA 12-60; higher in pregnancy
Calcium	
Blood	Up to 30 yr: 8.2-10.5 mg/dl; decreases very slightly in older years
Ionized serum	4.75-5.2 mg/dl
Calculated ionized	3.9-4.8 mg/dl
Urine	Varies with diet; based on average calcium intake of 600-800 mg/24 h, excretion may be 100-250 mg/24 h
Creatinine	
Blood	Male: up to 1.2 mg/dl Female: up to 1.1 mg/dl
Urine	Male: 1-2 g/24 h Female: 0.8-1.8 g/24 h
Creatinine clearance test	Male: 85-125 ml/min/1.73 m^2 Female: 75-115 ml/min/1.73 m^2
Cystine (urine)	Random sample negative
Oxalate (urine)	Up to 40 mg/24 h
Parathormone (blood)	Dependent on individual laboratory and calcium result
Inorganic phosphorus	
Blood	2.5-4.5 mg/dl
Urine	0.9-1.3g/24 h
Sodium	
Blood	135-145 mEq/L
Urine	27-287 mEq/24 h (varies significantly with dietary intake)
Uric acid	
Blood	Male: 3.4-7.0 mg/dl Female: 2.4-6.0 mg/dl
Urine	250-750 mg/24 h
Urea nitrogen	
Blood (BUN)	1-40 yr: 5-20 mg/dl; gradual slight increase subsequently occurs
Urine	6-17 g/24 h
Urinalysis	
Albumin	<20 mg/dl
Bilirubin	Negative
Color	Clear, golden yellow
Glucose	Negative
Hemoglobin	Negative
Ketones	Negative
Microscopic urinalysis	
Bacteria	Negative
Casts	0-4 hyaline casts per low-power field
Crystals	Interpreted by physician
Mucous threads	Negative
Red blood cells	0-5 per high-power field
Squamous epithelial cells	Seen on voided specimen in females; negative on voided specimen in males; negative for catheterized specimens
White blood cells	0-5 per high-power field

Conditions, Diseases, and Disorders

URINARY TRACT DISORDERS

Cystitis

Cystitis is an inflammation of the bladder wall. Many causative agents, including bacteria, viruses, fungi, chemical agents, and radiation exposure, may result in cystitis. The term is often used synonymously with urinary tract infection, although they are not strictly identical. Urinary tract infection is a nonspecific term that may be used to refer to infection anywhere in the urinary tract. Urethritis refers to inflammation of the urethra (see Chapter 15). Pyelonephritis refers to infection of the kidney and renal pelvis (see Chapter 12). Within the context of this discussion, cystitis is used in preference to the more vaguely defined concept of urinary tract infection.

The occurrence of infection in the urinary tract is second only to respiratory tract infections.[88] Infection of the urinary bladder is the most common focus of inflammation in the urinary tract. Women are particularly prone to symptomatic and asymptomatic bacteriuria resulting in cystitis. A study of Jamaican women revealed that 2% of those between 15 and 24 years of age had bacteriuria on culture. Stamey and associates[99] found that the prevalence of bacterial cystitis in women increased approximately 1% to 2% during each subsequent decade of life until reaching 10% among 54- to 64-year-old women. Gaymons and associates[37] corroborated these findings in a prospective study of 1758 Dutch women that revealed a 2.7% prevalence of bacteriuria among those 15 to 24 years of age and 9.3% among those 65 years of age and older. Among the general population, a woman can expect a 10% to 20% chance of having at least one episode of cystitis during her lifetime.[99]

Pregnant women and hospitalized women have an increased incidence of urinary tract infection. Among pregnant women the rate of cystitis is approximately 4% to 6%; studies have demonstrated an incidence of urinary tract infection as high as 30% among hospitalized women.[99]

In addition to a greater susceptibility to bacterial cystitis, women are more likely to have interstitial cystitis than men are. A study in Finland found that the prevalence of interstitial cystitis was 10.6:100,000 with a 10:1 preference of the disease for women.[45] Leach and Raz[86] also report an incidence of 20:100,000 cases of interstitial cystitis among women, with a ratio of 10 cases in women for every case reported among men.

The incidence of cystitis among men has not been extensively studied but is generally thought to occur in only 10% as many men as women. Unlike in women, most cases of bacteriuria in men occur as a result of some known infectious focus such as bacterial prostatitis or urinary calculi.[45]

Clearly, the most significant rate of cystitis, resulting in an alarming incidence of associated morbidity and mortality, is that associated with nosocomial urinary tract infection in the presence of an indwelling catheter. In a prospective study of 1458 patients in the United States, 131 patients acquired 136 urinary tract infections during 1474 indwelling bladder catheterizations. Among those studied, 12 deaths may have been caused by acquired urinary tract infections, and another 10 patients died with a retrospective clinical picture compatible with serious infection, although no conclusive culture data were available. Thus the authors concluded that acquisition of a nosocomial urinary tract infection was associated with a threefold increase in death rate.[85]

Pathophysiology

The pathogenesis of cystitis depends on the causative agent. In this discussion cystitis is divided into three categories:

- Infectious cystitis
  - Bacterial
  - Viral
  - Fungal
  - Tubercular
  - Parasitic
- Chemotherapy- and radiation-induced cystitis
- Inflammatory lesions of the bladder
  - Cystitis cystica
  - Cystitis glandularis
  - Eosinophilic cystitis
  - Cystitis emphysematosa
  - Interstitial cystitis

Bacterial cystitis is the most common form of infectious cystitis. The most common causative pathogen in both women and men is *Escherichia coli*. Other common pathogens include strains of *Klebsiella, Enterobacter, Proteus, Pseudomonas,* and *Serratia;* gram-positive organisms such as staphylococci and streptococci are occasionally seen.[45]

The three routes of bacterial invasion into the bladder are ascension through the urethra, the hematogenous route, and via lymphatic channels; the most common is the ascending urethral pathway. Bacteria are commonly forced into the bladder without necessarily resulting in infection. The determinants of bacterial cystitis depend on the virulence and inoculum size of invasive bacteria and the adequacy of the host's defense mechanisms. Data concerning the number of bacteria needed to produce a bladder infection are based solely on animal studies, which show that an extremely large inoculum (over 1 million) is needed to produce cystitis if host defense mechanisms are not compromised. Fortunately, normal numbers of bacteria that enter the bladder through the urethra are considerably smaller (fewer than 100).[56]

The human body has two primary defense mechanisms that oppose the establishment of infection when bacteria enter the bladder. The first is the urine itself, which is bacteriostatic or bactericidal to the most common pathogens associated with cystitis, such as *E. coli* and a number of other anaerobic bacteria commonly found in urethral flora. The efficiency of this antibacterial activity depends on the size of the bacterial inoculum, the osmolality of the urine, and the concentration of urea nitrogen and ammonium in the urine. A urinary pH of 6.0 or greater adversely affects antibacterial activity, but the presence of specific antibodies in the urine such as IgA and IgG has not been shown to cause significant effects.[56]

The bladder wall is the second line of defense for bacterial invasion from the urethra, bloodstream, or lymphatic route. Inflammatory changes within the bladder wall are apparent within 30 minutes of invasion when polymorphonucleocytes (PMNs) begin to migrate to the bladder mucosa. Within 2 hours the entire mucosal lining is injected by PMNs, and significant antibacterial activity is measurable by the fourth hour. Inspection at 24 hours reveals clumps of PMNs throughout the mucosal lining, and urine culture is negative.[56]

The most important defense against bacterial cystitis is the unobstructed flow of urine throughout the urinary tract and regular, complete evacuation of the bladder. This important concept is the basis of the rationale for clean intermittent catheterization. With regular emptying of the bladder flushes bacteria that would ultimately colonize the urine if allowed to remain within the bladder.[56]

Abnormalities that interfere with natural host defenses against urinary tract infection include the presence of residual urine, which provides an opportunity for bacteria to reproduce and overwhelm other inherent antibacterial mechanisms. Vesicoureteral reflux also compromises the body's defense mechanisms by allowing the spread of bacteria from the urine into the upper tracts and possibly into the renal parenchyma. Urinary calculi are often obstructive to urinary outflow and serve as a nidus for infection during antibiotic therapy. In addition, any disease or circumstance that interferes with the body's immune system decreases the efficiency of the bladder wall's reaction to bacteriuria.[56]

Women are particularly susceptible to bacterial cystitis for a number of reasons. Stamey[99] studied the problem of bacterial cystitis in women and concluded that much of the nomenclature used to describe the condition does not adequately define this condition. He described four bacteriurial states in women: first infection, unresolved bacteriuria during therapy, bacterial persistence, and reinfection (recurrence).

The etiology of first infection is unclear but is presumed to be similar to reinfections. Unlike recurrent episodes of cystitis, bacteria from the first infection are typically sensitive to any antibiotic and are unlikely to recur within a 2- to 3-year period unless other predisposing factors are present.[45]

Unresolved bacteriuria during therapy may arise from several causes. The bacteria may be resistant to the antibiotic chosen for therapy, or selection of a secondary strain may become predominant as the primary form of bacteria is eliminated. In approximately 6% of patients treated, resistant, mutant bacteria develop and proliferate. Renal insufficiency may cause inadequate concentrations of antibiotic in the urinary tract, although the correct agent has been chosen. A staghorn calculus may be large enough to support a critical mass of bacteria too great for antibiotics to resolve.[45]

True bacterial persistence may arise after 5 to 10 days of therapy, resulting in culture-proven nonsterile urine from one of two causes. Men with chronic bacterial prostatitis have a persistent focus for ascending urethral infection from the prostatic ductal system. Women or men with struvite stones in the urinary tract have a site of persistent bacteria even after antibiotic therapy.[45]

Reinfection of the bladder accounts for the majority of occurrences of bacterial cystitis among women. The most common route for bacteria to gain access to the bladder is from the urethra. The colonization of the urethra arises from the vaginal introitus and vestibule rather than from the rectum, as is commonly assumed. Longitudinal studies show that cultures of the vaginal vestibule and distal urethral mucosa are more predictive of recurrent bacterial cystitis than analysis of rectal flora. Ascending infection in the female is particularly problematic because of the relatively short, straight course of the urethra and plentiful flora in the genital area. The relationship between vaginal flora and urethral bacteria is further supported by examining the close anatomic relationship of these two structures, which are confined by the distal labia minora.[99]

The role of sexual intercourse in recurrent urinary infections has been studied repeatedly. Sexual intercourse is associated with an increased incidence of recurrent urinary tract infections, and some women specifically correlate intercourse and recurrence. It is interesting to note that nuns have a 0.4% to 1.6% incidence of urinary tract infection, which is lower than the general population, and that married women have a higher incidence than single women. Although sexual intercourse does not cause bacterial cystitis, it does promote the milking of bacteria into the bladder and can cause minor urethral injury that may result in infection among women predisposed to the condition.[99]

Changes in the urinary tract unique to pregnancy also increase a woman's likelihood for having recurring urinary tract infections or experiencing a first infection of the bladder. The primary urologic change noted with pregnancy is the "physiologic hydroureter of pregnancy," which is the reversible dilation of the ureters and renal pelvis. This dilation often begins as early as the seventh week of gestation and progresses until delivery. The right ureter is more extensively affected than the left, and ureteral peristalsis is significantly slowed after the second month of gestation so that intraureteral volume may be as great as 25 times normal.[8]

Bacteriuria is more common among pregnant women than in nonpregnant women in the same age group. The presence of ureteral dilation may play a role in this increased incidence.

It is known that pregnant women with bacteriuria are at a significantly increased risk (20% to 40%)[74] for developing pyelonephritis and that this risk is dramatically reduced by treating the bladder infection. In addition, catheterization during pregnancy is associated with increased risk of subsequent bacterial cystitis. Although the association between premature delivery and pyelonephritis is well documented, no correlation exists between bacteriuria and premature delivery.[8]

Bacterial cystitis is likely to result in urinary frequency, urgency, and dysuria. Women in particular may complain of suprapubic discomfort and a feeling of pressure in the perineal area. Nocturia and low back pain are also caused by bladder infection. Urge incontinence may take the form of detrusor instability with subsequent painful bladder "spasms" and associated leakage, or it may occur as urethral instability allowing urine passage into the posterior urethra and causing a perception of intense urgency and urinary leakage. Gross hematuria, chills, fever, and flank pain occur only occasionally in the presence of cystitis unless it is also associated with pyelonephritis. Approximately half of patients with significant bacteriuria are asymptomatic.[45] Women with dysuria and frequency who have no bacteriuria or a colony count of fewer than 10,000/ml are typically diagnosed as having an "acute urethral syndrome."[99]

Cystitis caused by fungal infection is much less prevalent than bacterial cystitis, but its incidence and recognition have greatly increased within the past 25 years. The most common fungal infection of the bladder is candidiasis. *Candida* is endemic to the human body and can often be found in the pharynx, stomach, intestinal tract, and vaginal vault (particularly in pregnant women). The increasing incidence of candidal overgrowth is related to the use of antibiotics. Administration of antibiotics is thought to stimulate the production of *C. albicans* by altering the pH of gastrointestinal mucosa, suppressing normal bacterial flora that competes with the fungus for food, and inhibiting polymorphonuclear phagocytosis, which helps the body guard against overgrowth.[77]

The body's defenses against candidal infection of the urinary tract include the presence of normal bacterial flora that inhibit fungal growth and the presence of PMNs in the mucosa of the urethra and bladder, which have marked anticandidal effects. In addition, prostatic fluid in the male is fungicidal, which helps explain the relatively low incidence of candidal cystitis in males compared to females. Cell-mediated immunity and other white blood cells also help the body prevent candidiasis.[77]

Candidal cystitis often occurs in the presence of predisposing factors such as diabetes mellitus, obstructive prostatic enlargement, and pregnancy and is often noted after the patient has undergone antibiotic therapy for bacterial infection. Symptoms are similar to those of bacterial cystitis and include urgency, marked frequency, dysuria, suprapubic pain, and nocturia. Pneumaturia (the expression of gas or air through the urethra during or after micturition) may be seen. The mucosal lining of the bladder is marked by grayish white spots that result in mucosal bleeding if removed. The ureteral orifices may be affected so that cytoscopic findings may resemble tubercular infection of the bladder. In certain cases asymptomatic candidal colonization of the urine without inflammation of the bladder may be seen.[77]

Tuberculosis of the bladder results from the implantation of the tubercle bacilli into the wall, causing an uneven mix of inflamed areas interspersed with normal mucosal segments. The cystoscopic picture of the bladder may resemble interstitial cystitis or candidal infection with patches of inflamed tissue and reddened ureteral orifices. The anterior urethra is not affected by the infection, but the posterior urethra and prostate are heavily involved in men, representing progression from prostate to bladder. The trigone is relatively spared from inflammatory changes, but the dome of the bladder is extensively affected, resulting in a marked loss in capacity.[45]

The primary symptom of tubercular cystitis is marked frequency and urgency. Bladder volume rapidly decreases and may result in irreversible changes in advanced stages of the infection.[45] Urodynamic assessment in advanced cases may reveal poor compliance of the bladder wall and a functional capacity of 60 ml of urine or less.

Although schistosomiasis is relatively rare in the United States, it is relatively common elsewhere in the world. The ova of this parasite enter the bloodstream via penetration of the skin. The veins of the bladder are a popular breeding site for the parasites. The eggs are then extruded into the vesicle for further spread of the parasitic organisms. The healing of the affected areas of the bladder causes thickening and contraction of the bladder wall. Damage of the ureterovesical junction often occurs, resulting in vesicoureteral reflux. Contracted bands mar the bladder and may extend into the lower ureter. Urinary calculi may be present because of urinary stasis and presence of ova in the urine.[90]

Chemotherapy- or radiation-induced cystitis is characterized by inflammatory changes in the bladder wall in the absence of infection. The symptoms are similar to those of infectious cystitis and include urgency, frequency, and suprapubic pain. Detrusor instability and urge incontinence may occur.[49,96]

Although the bladder is relatively resistant to radiation, therapeutic doses greater than 6000 to 7000 rad over a 6- to 7-week period may result in cystitis. The bladder's tolerance to radiation is significantly compromised if schistosomiasis is present. Chemotherapy-induced cystitis may arise from systemic cyclophosphamide (Cytoxan) or intravesical antineoplastic drugs such as mitomycin. Diagnosis is made when symptoms of cystitis are reported in the presence of a normal culture and positive history of exposure to radiation or a chemotherapeutic agent.[49,96]

Cystitis cystica occurs as a result of chronic infection of the bladder or recurrent episodes of cystitis. It is characterized by cysts seen mostly near the base of the bladder and trigone. These cysts are approximately 1 cm in diameter, have a rounded shape, and may extend into the upper urinary tract. The lesions are benign, and the etiology of the condition is unknown. Because of the gross similarities between these lesions and malignancies of the bladder, biopsy is indicated to rule out cancer.[88]

Cystitis glandularis is a relatively rare, potentially premalignant lesion associated with adenocarcinoma of the bladder. This form of cystitis is particularly common among patients with a history of bladder exstrophy and pelvic lipomatosis. Biopsy is done to rule out malignancy, and follow-up examination for potential cancer of the bladder is recommended.[88]

Eosinophilic cystitis is a severe inflammatory lesion of the bladder that is thought to have an allergic etiology. The bladder mucosa is extensively invaded by eosinophils and exhibits multiple polypoid lesions. The associated signs and symptoms of cystitis are particularly severe.[88]

Cystitis emphysematosa is a rare form of bladder inflammation resulting from infection by gas-forming urinary bacteria or (more commonly) vesicoenteric fistula. The condition may also be observed after urologic instrumentation or urodynamic testing using carbon dioxide. Pneumaturia is associated with this form of cystitis.[88]

Interstitial cystitis is a particularly tenacious form of bladder inflammation characterized primarily by the pain it produces. This pain is centered in the suprapubic area and is typically described as burning and constant. Unlike bacterial cystitis, micturition does not typically relieve the pain, which results in marked urgency, frequency, nocturia, and the despair and frustration seen in patients who must cope with chronic, intractable pain.[45]

Interstitial cystitis occurs in both sexes and all age groups; the most commonly affected are adult women. The etiology of interstitial cystitis remains unclear. Causative agents may be viral, fungal, or bacterial. Neurosis has been implicated as the cause of the disease, although it seems likely that any maladaptive coping patterns are a response to chronic pain rather than the origin of the condition. Recent investigation of possible autoimmune dysfunction may elucidate the etiology of this difficult clinical syndrome.[45]

The cystoscopic findings are consistent with a "pancystitis" involving all four layers of the bladder wall, which is typically thickened, injected, and friable. The submucosal layer is swollen and marked by enlarged capillaries and hemorrhagic areas. The venous structures of the bladder are engorged and dilated. White blood cell invasion of the bladder is common and consists mostly of lymphocytes. Filling of the bladder causes pallor of the mucosa and small tears in the lining. The bladder may be lined with small linear scars because of repeated tears in the mucosa related to normal bladder filling.[45]

Diagnostic Studies and Findings

Urine Culture and Sensitivity

Greater than 100,000/ml bacterial colonies on an agar culture plate or tube indicates clinically significant bacteriuria and associated cystitis

Sensitivity discs indicate bacterial sensitivity, intermediate sensitivity, or resistance to a given antibiotic agent

Urine culture negative in other forms of infectious cystitis and cystitis caused by chemotherapy and radiotherapy

Urinalysis

Color: dark yellow or pinkish red, cloudy with or without sediment

Nitrate/nitrite: positive in bacterial cystitis

Glucose oxidase: positive in bacterial infection

Catalase: positive in bacterial cystitis

Microscopic examination: positive for bacteria, fungus, and parasites in the various forms of infectious cystitis; positive for eosinophils in eosinophilic cystitis; greater than 7 WBCs per high-power field in infectious cystitis; red blood cells with or without gross hematuria[45]

Cystoscopy

Red, inflamed bladder wall

Reddened, swollen trigone

Ureteral orifices may be inflamed

Hemorrhagic patches in urothelial lining

Findings for specific inflammatory lesions of the bladder described under "Pathophysiology"

Biopsy

Cystitis cystica: negative

Cystitis glandularis: negative or positive for adenocarcinoma of bladder

Eosinophilic cystitis: extensive infiltration of eosinophils into bladder tissues

Interstitial cystitis: chronic inflammation with extensive invasion of lymphocytes and other white blood cells into submucosa of bladder wall

Urodynamics

Infectious cystitis: urodynamic testing typically contraindicated

Tubercular cystitis: decreased functional capacity with poor compliance of bladder wall; detrusor unstable or areflexic; sensory urgency present

Chemotherapy- or radiation-induced cystitis: sensory urgency with decreased functional capacity; detrusor instability may be present; compliance of bladder wall may be normal or impaired

Interstitial cystitis: marked sensory urgency with decreased functional capacity; detrusor generally stable up to tolerated bladder volume; associated pain may render patient unable to void in testing situation; compliance is typically normal; postvoid residual may be noted

Voiding Cystourethrogram (VCUG)

Cystitis emphysematosa: lucent filling defect consistent with gas in vesicle of bladder with or without extravasation of contrast material into vesicoenteric fistula

Medical Plan

Surgery

Tubercular cystitis: in cases of advanced tubercular cystitis when bladder contraction is irreversible, augmentation cystoplasty may be employed after infection is controlled; colocystoplasty (placing an isolated segment of colon onto the bladder dome in order to enlarge storage capacity) or ileocystoplasty (placing an isolated segment of small bowel on the bladder dome) may be used to restore reasonable bladder storage capacity

Cystitis glandularis: transurethral resection of lesion done because of its premalignant potential[22]

Interstitial cystitis: transurethral resection and fulguration of bladder lesions may give temporary symptomatic relief but remain a controversial form of treatment; denervation procedures (bilateral chordotomy, selective sacral neurectomy, or supratrigonal denervation) may be used to manage chronic pain; irreversibility of these procedures (and their potential side effects) a significant consideration; bladder substitution such as enterocystoplasty or supratrigonal cystoplasty requires extensive resection of detrusor muscle and replacement with an isolated segment of bowel; urinary diversion has been utilized but is considered a final option when all other treatments have failed[41,106]

Medications

Bacterial cystitis

Treatment of choice is oral antibiotic therapy guided by culture and sensitivity data (Table 12-1)

For first-time infections or recurrent infections, short-term therapy with oral antibiotics favored, although single-dose therapy may be used

In more severe cases or when resistant bacteria are identified, parenteral therapy is indicated

For recurrent infections, suppressive antibiotic therapy may be used for 6 mo to 24 mo (Table 12-2); first choice for long-term antibiotic suppression among women with recurrent bacterial cystitis is nitrofurantoin or trimethoprim-sulfamethoxazole

Nitrofurantoin absorbed in upper intestinal tract so that it does not promote mutation of resistant strains of bacteria in intestinal tract; exerts its antibacterial effects on bacteria that have reached bladder

Trimethoprim-sulfamethoxazole will kill pathogens in vaginal vestibule, preventing bacterial invasion of bladder but does alter intestinal flora, which can lead to selection of bacteria resistant to drug

Table 12-1

Bacterial Pathogens Commonly Encountered in the Urinary Tract and Treatment Options

Pathogen	Commonly Effective Antibiotic Agents*
Escherichia coli	Trimethoprim-sulfamethoxazole, ampillicin, norfloxacin, amoxicillin clavulanate (Augmentin), nitrofurantoin, ciprofloxacin
Pseudomonas	Carbenicillin (Geocillin), gentamicin,† norfloxacin, ciprofloxacin
Klebsiella	Cephalexin, tetracycline, trimethoprim-sulfamethoxazole, norfloxacin
Proteus mirabilis	Ampicillin, tetracycline, trimethoprim-sulfamethoxazole, norfloxacin, amoxicillin clavulanate, nitrofurantoin
Morganella morganii	Trimethoprim-sulfamethoxazole, norfloxacin
Serratia	Trimethoprim-sulfamethoxazole, norfloxacin, carbenicillin
Group D *Streptococcus*	Ampicillin, nitrofurantoin, amoxicillin clavulanate
Staphylococcus	Cephalexin, tetracycline, trimethoprim-sulfamethoxazole
Staphylococcus saprophyticus	Cephalexin, trimethoprim-sulfamethoxazole, tetracycline

*Antibiotic therapy is guided by individual culture and sensitivity reports.
†Requires parenteral administration.

Table 12-2

Antibiotic Therapy for Bacterial Cystitis

Type of Therapy	Antibiotic Agents*
Single-dose therapy	Amoxicillin (Amoxil), 3 g Trimethoprim-sulfamethoxazole (Bactrim DS, Septra DS), 1 or 2 double-strength tablets Sulfisoxazole (Gantrisin), 1-2 g
Short-term therapy (5-14 d)	Ampicillin (Amcil), 2 g in 4 divided doses Amoxicillin (Amoxil), 2 g in 4 divided doses Trimethoprim-sulfamethoxazole (Bactrim DS, Septra DS), 1 double-strength tablet bid Nitrofurantoin (Macrodantin), 50-100 mg qid
Suppressive therapy for recurrences (6-24 mo)	Trimethoprim-sulfamethoxazole (Bactrim DS, Septra DS), 1 regular-strength tablet daily Nitrofurantoin (Macrodantin), 50-100 mg/d

Modified from Farrar.[32]
*Antibiotic therapy is guided by individual culture and sensitivity reports.

Fungal infections
  Two drugs, amphotericin B and 5-fluorocystine, are indicated in cases of nonmucocutaneous infection
    Amphotericin B has disadvantages of requiring parenteral administration and significant side effects such as fever, chills, nausea and vomiting, headache, vertigo, and potential nephrotoxicity with prolonged use
    5-Fluorocystine may be administered orally and is effective against *Candida;* side effects include bone marrow depression, potential nephrotoxicity, and eosinophilia
  Production of resistant strains of fungi is problematic[77]
Tubercular cystitis
  Drug therapy must be long term (2 yr recommended), and multiple agents are often more effective than any single medication
  Combination of isoniazid (INH), ethambutol, rifampin, streptomycin, para-aminosalicylic acid (PAS), cycloserine, or kanamycin is indicated[45]
Parasitic cystitis
  Drugs used for schistosomiasis have potentially dangerous side effects and are not approved by the U.S. Food and Drug Administration
  Current drug of choice is nitrofurantoin given over a period of 5 to 7 d
  Early treatment essential for prevention of irreversible urinary changes from drug
Other chemotherapeutic agents may be used to provide symptomatic relief from cystitis caused by infection, chemotherapy, or radiotherapy; anticholinergic agents or antispasmodics such as oxybutynin and propantheline may ameliorate sensory urgency and provide greater functional capacity
  Eosinophilic cystitis
    Antihistamines and oral steroid agents are indicated
    Antibiotic therapy will control related bacteriuria[88]
  Interstitial cystitis
    A variety of pharmacologic agents used; currently antibiotics, oral anti-inflammatory agents, antihistamines, analgesics, and vitamins are used with varying success[86]
    Three intravesical agents (silver nitrate, oxychloresene sodium, and dimethyl sulfoxide) may be used; agents are instilled into vesicle per urethral catheter and retained for approximately 30 min before catheter drainage

General Management

Interstitial cystitis: mechanical bladder distention sometimes used in an attempt to increase functional capacity; performed by an intravesical balloon inflated to patient's systolic blood pressure for 1 to 3 hours; therapeutic mechanism of this procedure is the creation of bladder wall ischemia with subsequent lessening of sensory enervation; complications include rupture of bladder[86]
Caffeine intake should be restricted because its mild irritative effect exacerbates frequency
Citrus juices not effective in lowering urinary pH
Cranberry juice effective in lowering urinary pH only if taken in extremely large quantities
Plentiful fluid intake indicated to encourage movement of pathogens out of urinary tract

NURSING CARE

Nursing Assessment

Suprapubic Area

Tender on palpation

Costovertebral Angle

No tenderness

Voiding Behavior

Frequency, urgency, dysuria, nocturia

Nursing Dx & Intervention

Nursing Diagnosis	Nursing Intervention/Rationale
Altered patterns of urinary elimination	• Encourage copious fluid intake and reassure patient that urinary frequency is temporary. *Adequate fluid intake flushes the urinary system and enhances the body's natural defenses against infectious agents. Although urinary frequency is frustrating, it is essential to provide regular, complete bladder evacuation to rid the urinary tract of pathogens.*
Pain	• Encourage patient to take a warm sitz bath *to relieve suprapubic and lower back pain associated with cystitis.* • Encourage patient to void regularly and not attempt to refrain from micturition when the bladder is acutely infected *to encourage regular, complete bladder evacuation.* • Encourage patient with interstitial cystitis to refrain from urination as long as possible *to allow attainment of maximum possible functional capacity of the bladder. In the case of interstitial cystitis, prolonged times between micturition may improve functional capacity and decrease chronic, debilitating urinary frequency.*

Nursing Diagnosis	Nursing Intervention/Rationale
Noncompliance (medical therapy)	• Encourage patient to continue antibiotic regimen for entire period recommended by health care practitioner *to increase chances of preventing persistent or recurrent urinary tract infection.* • Provide counseling concerning potential side effects of medication and appropriate actions should these effects occur. *Alternative antibiotics may be provided to circumvent side effects, or untoward effects may be simply managed by dietary or other means so that antibiotics are taken for full 10-day course.*
Ineffective individual coping related to interstitial cystitis	• Encourage patient to express feelings of fear, frustration, anger, depression, and desperation concerning the condition.
Knowledge deficit, family (interstitial cystitis)	• Educate family members about the physiologic basis of disease, signs of associated voiding dysfunction, and nature of and typical human responses to chronic pain *to decrease likelihood that family will isolate the patient because of the condition and to elicit family support for patient during therapy to correct the condition.* • Include family members in all discussions of medical, nursing, and surgical interventions *to increase their feelings of involvement in the patient's care.* • Women and men with interstitial cystitis suffer from the adverse effects of a chronic, painful condition associated with discomfort, frustration, disturbances in rest patterns, and social isolation. Sleep patterns are significantly disturbed because of nocturnal voidings that may exceed 12 times in a single night. Attempts at rest during the day are also interrupted by the desire to void and constant feelings of suprapubic pressure and discomfort. • Social isolation results from fear of incontinent episodes or painful interludes between opportunities to void and from lack of empathy on the part of family and friends. Social ostracism may result from false perceptions that the person is simply "unwilling" to postpone micturition or that he has "overindulged" the bladder by "giving in" to even mild sensations of urgency. • Feelings of frustration and inadequacy may be encouraged by uneducated health caregivers who incorrectly perceive the condition as a form of maladaptive behavior.

Patient Education

1. Provide instruction concerning potential risk factors for cystitis, including altered urinary elimination patterns or urinary retention.
2. Provide instruction concerning prevention of recurrence of urinary tract infection, including increased fluid intake, strategies to acidify the urine, and choice of materials for undergarments.
3. Provide instruction concerning expected actions and potential side effects of medications used to treat infection or alleviate symptoms associated with cystitis.

Evaluation

Patient Outcome	Data Indicating That Outcome is Reached
Bacterial cystitis is resolved.	Urine culture is negative 24 hours after completing antibiotic therapy.
Fungal cystitis is resolved.	Fungal culture is negative after completion of antifungal therapy.
Parasitic cystitis is resolved.	There are no ova or parasites in urine. There are no complications, or they have been surgically repaired.
Chemotherapy- or radiotherapy-induced cystitis is symptomatically improved.	Urgency and frequency are decreased. Functional capacity as measured by urodynamic assessment is increased. Nocturia is decreased or absent. Patient subjectively reports decreased symptoms of suprapubic discomfort. Cystoscopic findings are normal.
Inflammatory lesion of the bladder is resolved.	Cystoscopic findings are normal.
Interstitial cystitis is symptomatically improved.	Functional capacity on urodynamic testing is increased. Patient subjectively reports decreased diurnal frequency (every 3 to 4 hours) and decreased nocturia (one or two episodes per night).

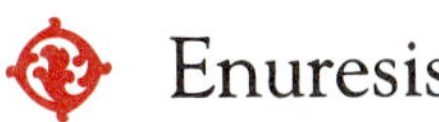

Enuresis

Enuresis is any involuntary micturition past the age when continence should be present. Nocturnal enuresis is defined as bed-wetting past the age of 4 years, and diurnal enuresis may be defined as involuntary voiding while awake.[45,58] Current terminology describes enuresis as inappropriate micturition while asleep; this discussion uses this definition.

Enuresis is classified as either primary or secondary. Patients with primary enuresis have never been dry at night, whereas those with secondary enuresis have been dry for a period of weeks or months before a pattern of bed-wetting begins. The onset of secondary enuresis may be correlated with an identifiable stressor or crisis such as the birth of a sibling or parental divorce.[45,49]

The incidence of enuresis is highest among preschool and school-age children. At 5 years of age, 15% of children are enuretic; the incidence decreases at a rate of 14% to 16% until reaching a rate of 1% to 2% by the age of 15 years. This relatively low incidence persists throughout adulthood.[45]

Enuresis occurs in all cultures and social classes but is more commonly found among children of lower socioeconomic status. Children with enuresis are more likely to be middle children, to have a familial history of bed-wetting, and to come from broken homes. Although the majority of patients with enuresis (85%) have no clinically significant diurnal voiding problems, some patients have daytime urinary frequency, urgency, and possibly urge incontinence. Encopresis (involuntary fecal soiling) is found in 10% to 25% of patients with enuresis.[45]

Pathophysiology

Enuresis is a symptom, not a disease. Multiple factors contribute to its existence, making a single, straightforward explanation of the condition unrealistic. In addition, the condition is difficult to study because of the lack of suitable animal models. Thus the etiology of enuresis remains poorly understood, although a variety of associated abnormalities have been advocated.

Perhaps the most popular theory for enuresis supports the existence of a "maturational lag" of neurologic bladder control resulting in enuresis. Incomplete development of the cortical or subcortical tracts concerned with bladder function is implicated, with resulting alteration in sensations of bladder filling and abnormal sleep patterns leading to abnormal arousal in response to the desire to void or a failure of normal detrusor inhibition. This pattern may or may not be noted during daytime hours. The evidence for this explanation of enuresis is largely circumstantial but nonetheless attractive.[45,58]

Subtle urodynamic abnormalities are noted among patients with enuresis; these include a decreased functional capacity, diurnal urgency, and daytime frequency. Although a subtle form of detrusor instability may be noted among patients who are incontinent only at night, marked instability is found among those with daytime wetting.[58] These findings are purported to implicate an infantile bladder in the absence of neurologic disease. However, such urodynamic findings must be viewed with caution for several reasons. First, the inclusion of children with abnormal daytime voiding patterns with children who have nocturnal voiding problems may be misleading. The presence of urge incontinence during waking hours is clearly connected with detrusor instability and has been named the unstable bladder of childhood, or the nonneurogenic neurogenic bladder. This condition is significantly different from nocturnal enuresis and is associated with recurrent urinary tract infection, uncoordinated external sphincter activity, and upper tract damage in certain cases.[2,11]

Conclusions of maturational lag in enuretic children based on urodynamic data must also be interpreted with caution because of the testing technique. Standard urodynamic testing uses rapid, provocative filling with carbon dioxide or water in a child who is awake or only moderately sedated. Thus the circumstances unique to nocturnal enuresis are not reproduced. This disparity is demonstrated by Whiteside and Arnold,[112] who found that provocative urodynamic testing was clinically useful among enuretic children with diurnal incontinence but was not helpful among patients with nocturnal wetting only. Nielsen and associates[80] examined the relationship between bladder contractions and enuretic episodes. They found that large numbers of contractions were present among children with vesicoureteral reflux (mean of 6.5 to 7.5) and were not all associated with an enuretic episode. Thus the presence of an unstable detrusor alone is not sufficient for enuresis.

Sleep patterns have also been studied among patients with enuresis and have been found to be abnormal. Enuretic children are known to be particularly heavy sleepers. Incontinent episodes typically occur during the transition from deeper to lighter stages of sleep. Enuretic children spend more time in these deeper stages of sleep (stages 3 and 4) when rapid eye movements are absent than do their nonenuretic peers, are more difficult to arouse, and may have greater difficulty suppressing bladder contractions.[45,58]

Some studies have found electroencephalographic abnormalities among enuretic children and subtle developmental delays implying a lag in the functional maturity. However, other studies have disputed these findings.[45,58]

Psychosocial factors have also been implicated in the etiology of enuresis and particularly of secondary enuresis. Proponents of this theory point to the association of enuresis with broken homes and identifiable crises connected with the onset of enuresis in certain cases, such as the birth of a sibling. Significant neuroses are not associated with enuresis, although enuresis may be a component of the symptoms produced by a deeply rooted psychologic or personality disorder. In these cases treatment is directed toward the underlying psychologic disorder rather than the symptom of enuresis.[58]

Familial patterns of enuresis are well documented. Although the incidence of enuresis is 15% among children with no family history of the condition, children whose parents were enuretic have a 44% chance of bed-wetting. The incidence of enuresis among monozygotic twins is significantly increased when one sibling develops the condition.[45]

Allergic causes of enuresis have been reported, although few children ultimately respond to dietary manipulations. Proponents of this theory believe that certain foods irritate the bladder, resulting in decreased functional capacity and an increased likelihood of enuresis.[45,58]

Only a relatively small percentage of enuretic children have significant associated urologic abnormalities in the absence of diurnal incontinence. Detrusor instability is usually subtle, and a detailed urologic workup is rarely beneficial. The most common associated urologic finding among these children is bacteriuria or symptomatic urinary tract infection. Enuretic girls are two to six times as likely to develop cystitis as their nonenuretic peers, although enuretic boys do not have a signficantly increased infection rate.[45,49]

Adult enuresis is defined as enuresis that developed in childhood and persists beyond the age of 15 years, or it may develop spontaneously. Unlike bed-wetting in childhood, adults with enuresis are more likely to have overt urodynamic abnormalities and often have other underlying urologic or neurologic abnormalities.[46]

Diagnostic Studies and Findings

Urodynamic Testing

Children: not recommended unless other voiding abnormalities exist; studies may be normal or reveal decreased functional capacity with sensory urgency and mild or absent detrusor instability; child is often unable to suppress a volitionally induced contraction

Adults: detrusor instability with or without functional outlet obstruction; other abnormalities may be noted

Urinalysis

Normal

Occasional bacteria or white blood cells may be noted

Urine Culture

Normal or asymptomatic bacteriuria among females

Medical Plan

Surgery

No longer considered prudent

Medications

Tricyclic antidepressants, typically imipramine (Tofranil; 25-50 mg hs); have several beneficial actions including anticholinergic activity, α-sympathomimetic activity that increases tone at the bladder neck, and alteration of sleep patterns decreasing amount of time spent in non-REM sleep

General Management

If an allergic component of enuresis is suspected, serial deletions of suspected foods are done; dairy products, egg products, chocolate, carbonated beverages, and cola beverages are common causative agents

NURSING CARE

Nursing Assessment

Abdomen

Normal

External Genitalia

Normal

Voiding Behavior

Normal

Nursing Dx & Intervention

Nursing Diagnosis	Nursing Intervention/Rationale
Altered patterns of urinary elimination	• Use responsibility/reinforcement therapy if both child and parents are motivated. Instruct child to keep a log or calendar of wet and dry nights, and contract goals between nurse, parents, and child for improvement. After a level of improvement is obtained, provide a previously designated reward to child. Encourage patient to develop and record any feelings or emotions that predispose to enuretic episodes. *Responsibility/reinforcement therapy attempts to resolve enuresis by altering the behaviors that lead to bed-wetting. The reward/sanction system may be particularly valuable in child with secondary enuresis.* • Be aware that responsibility/reinforcement therapy is undermined if parental support is lacking or if contracted rewards for improvement are not fulfilled. Counsel parents that strict adherence to the terms of the contract is essential to the program. Assess child's level of maturity to ensure that he or she is capable of fulfilling the contract. Do not perceive failure to remain dry as worthy of punishment.

Nursing Diagnosis	Nursing Intervention/Rationale
	• Use conditioning therapy, which involves an alarm system that senses the presence of urine and triggers a buzzer that awakens the child. Make certain the alarm device is used and functions properly. Instruct child to sleep nude or in relatively lightweight pajamas. Provide a thorough explanation of the use and care of the alarm device and caution that old batteries and device malfunction are associated with ulceration of the skin. Counsel parents that this form of therapy requires approximately 16 weeks before enuresis ceases. • Forewarn parents of the possibility that the use of an alarm system may initially frighten child aroused from a deep stage of sleep. Parents should be available to provide emotional comfort as needed during the first several nights the device is used. *Conditioning therapy attempts to ablate enuresis by behavioral training. The enuretic child or adult is trained to become a nocturnal voider rather than a bed-wetter.* • Provide a thorough explanation of the device and a demonstration on its function.

Patient Education

1. Instruct the patient and family concerning the process and goals of therapy.
2. Provide the patient and family with detailed, easy-to-follow explanations of any devices or written records used to treat enuresis.
3. Provide the patient and family with instruction concerning expected actions and potential side effects of pharmacologic agents used to treat enuresis.

Evaluation

Patient Outcome	Data Indicating That Outcome is Reached
Enuresis is absent.	Patient remains dry every night for a 30-day period.
Recurrences are absent.	Patient does not experience recurrence by the age of 15 years.

Urinary calculi

Calculi are stones that are formed in the urinary tract.

Calculi that pass spontaneously without discomfort present no serious threat to health. However, many urinary calculi are extremely painful, obstructive, and a focus of infection. The problem of urinary calculi must be addressed by both urologists and nephrologists, since stones have both medical and surgical implications. A detailed discussion of medical aspects of urinary calculi is presented in Chapter 11. This discussion focuses on the two primary urologic complications associated with urinary caculi, infection and obstruction, as well as the surgical and electromechanical therapeutic options available to patients.

The incidence of calculi varies significantly with a number of intrinsic factors, such as age, sex, and race, and extrinsic factors, such as geographic location and climate. In the United States the five most common types of urinary stones are calcium oxalate, magnesium-ammonium-phosphate (struvite), uric acid, cystine, and mixed calculi.[45]

The peak incidence of calculus formation is the third to fifth decades of life. Many patients report an onset of symptoms associated with urolithiasis beginning in their twenties; surgical or medical interventions for urinary calculi are most commonly performed in the fifth decade of life. Men are three times more likely to have calculus formation in the upper urinary tract and bladder than are women.[45] The disease is relatively rare among American and African blacks, North American Indians, and native-born Israelis but relatively common among whites and Eurasians.[45]

Throughout the world those persons at greatest risk for urinary calculi live in mountainous areas. The United States, a number of European countries, and Australia have a high incidence of urinary lithiasis, whereas the African and South American countries have a relatively low incidence. The southeastern and arid southwestern United States generally have a higher incidence of calculi than other regions.[45]

Sedentary occupations are associated with an increased incidence of urinary lithiasis. Intake of certain foods can also contribute to stone formation. The patient should be questioned concerning intake of foods containing calcium (dairy products), oxalate (green, leafy vegetables and certain fruits), and purines that are metabolized to uric acid (meat, fish, and poultry).[91] In rare instances medications are responsible for stone disease. Long-term ingestion of calcium carbonate, vitamin D, antacids, megadoses of vitamin C, acetazolamide, probenecid, or triamterene can lead to various types of stone formation.[91]

Pathophysiology

The etiology of calculi formation is complex and incompletely elucidated. Urinary calculi are approximately 97.5% crystalline and 2.5% mucoprotein or glycoprotein matrix and are described by their predominant salt content. To understand the pathophysiologic process of stone formation in the urinary tract, it is necessary to understand basic principles of biologic crystallization. Calculi formation requires the following conditions in the urinary tract. A solution has a given solubility product that is constant. Once this product has been reached, adding further solute (such as calcium oxalate or other stone salt) will not raise its concentration within the solution. Supersaturation occurs when further solute is added to the solute (urine). At a formation concentration the supersaturated solute spontaneously precipitates from the solution, forming the beginning of a potential calculus. Unlike the solubility product, the formation concentration varies with circumstances. Calculus formation requires the initiation of a crystal from precipitation of a stone salt from the urine followed by crystal growth and aggregation. This process requires energy that is obtained from urine in a supersaturation.[33]

Two predisposing epidemiologic factors have been identified in association with an increased likelihood of stone formation: predisposing anatomic or biochemical factors, such as the inherited predisposition for cystinuria or medullary sponge kidney, and environmental factors, such as diet, climate, fluid intake patterns, and occupation.[7]

Several theories have attempted to explain calculus formation in the urinary tract. The *precipitation-crystallization theory* is based on the general principles of biologic crystallization; it delineates four necessary steps for stone formation. The first step is the nucleation phase in which the smallest unit of a crystal is formed in the urine. This nucleus may be of homogenous or heterogeneous form relative to the remaining portion of the calculus. In the second phase the crystal form grows and aggregates into a larger form. For this growth to occur, supersaturation of the urine persists and circumstances allowing a formation concentration to be attained continue. The greater the degree of supersaturation, the greater the rate of stone formation. The third stage of stone formation occurs when the crystal becomes entrapped in the upper urinary tract. Otherwise, the crystal is passed into the urine and no clinically apparent disease occurs. The final stage of the precipitation-crystallization process involves the continued growth of the trapped particle, resulting in clinically significant disease.[34,98]

The *inhibitor lack theory* attempts to explain why some persons form stones and others do not even though both groups excrete urine that is supersaturated with certain substances that inhibit crystallization and subsequent calculi. These substances have been identified as magnesium, pyrophosphate, citrate, mucoproteins, and various peptides.[12]

The *matrix initiation theory* observes the finding that the matrices of calculi in certain persons are mucoproteins that typically act as crystal inhibitors. In this case mucoproteins are hypothesized to contain a qualitative defect that renders them dysfunctional; thus they predispose the person toward calculi formation rather than serve as a crystal inhibitor as they do in normal individuals.[33,106]

The *epitaxy theory* attempts to account for the presence of mixed urinary calculi and the process by which a crystal is formed with layers of different substances. The crystalline lattice of a specific substance is organized in a predictable manner that may closely resemble other crystalline lattices. Certain calculi may have an inner core of uric acid and an outer covering of calcium oxalate. Thus one crystal forms upon the lattice work of a similar substance, resulting in a mixed urinary stone.[34]

Which of these factors relevant to urinary stone formation will prove predominant and which will prove secondary remains to be elucidated. A *final theory* of stone formation will be based on elucidation of the process of biologic crystallization and the role of the kidneys and urinary transport organs for maintaining a crystal- and stasis-free system.[45,106]

The presence of a urinary calculus is typically discovered when the stone becomes entrapped, resulting in the abrupt onset of acute renal or bladder colic. The most common sites of entrapment are a calyx or calyceal diverticulum, the ureteropelvic junction, the segment of ureter at or near the pelvic brim adjacent to the point where the ureter crosses the iliac vessels, the posterior pelvic portion of the ureter in women, and the ureterovesical junction. Of all the areas of anatomic narrowing, the ureterovesical junction is the most difficult for a calculus to pass.[45]

The renal colic typically occurs at night or during the early morning hours when the patient is sedentary. The pain begins in the flank and radiates to the groin and testes in men or the labia majora and broad ligament in women. As the stone moves to the midureter, the pain radiates to the lateral portion of the flank and lower abdomen. As the calculus moves toward the ureterovesical junction, the pain associated with the initial renal colic may recur, associated with irritable voiding symptoms of urinary urgency or urge incontinence. Colic is perceived most intensely as the calculus moves or if it implants at a certain site. Movement of the stone also causes localized pain resulting from obstruction.[45]

Bladder colic is characterized by bladder pain that crescendoes immediately after micturition. A stabbing pain may be felt when changing position, and urinary urgency and urge incontinence are commonly associated.[45]

Because visceral pain such as renal colic is mediated by the autonomic nervous system via the celiac ganglia, nausea and vomiting, intestinal stasis, and ileus may occur. Patients are typically restless as they change position to reduce discomfort. Grunting respirations signaling distress may be present. The pulse and blood pressure may be elevated in response to pain. Fever is rare unless a urinary tract infection is present.[45]

Many urinary calculi pass spontaneously and do not require urologic intervention, but others need prompt attention. The decision to intervene surgically, endoscopically, or via extracorporeal shock wave lithotripsy is based on prevention of the two significant complications of calculi: obstruction and infection.

Obstruction of the urinary tract in the presence of calculi results in adverse changes in renal and ureteral function associated with hydronephrosis. The adverse effects of acute hydronephrosis have been studied in laboratory animals and divided into the following stages. During the first 90 minutes after the onset of obstruction, ipsilateral renal blood flow is dramatically increased and intramural pressure in both ureters rises. In the second stage, lasting from 90 minutes to the end of the fifth hour, renal blood flow to both kidneys decreases while pressure in the ureters remains high in an attempt to compensate for and overcome the obstruction. From the fifth through the eighteenth hour following acute obstruction, renal blood flow in the affected side and intraureteral pressure decrease as compensatory mechanisms are overwhelmed. Intrarenal changes on the affected side include an early rapid redistribution of blood from the medullary to cortical nephrons during the initial period after obstruction. Later, the renal plasma flow, glomerular filtration rate, and tubular function are slowed as kidney function is impaired.[45]

Ureteral peristalsis is also adversely affected by obstruction. The creation of acute obstruction in animal models resulted in an initial rise in ureteral pressure and the frequency of peristaltic waves. However, these compensatory mechanisms were soon overcome, resulting in dilation of the ureters and loss of smooth muscle tone and fibrotic replacement in the ureteral wall.[45]

In humans progressive changes from hydronephrosis include renal pelvic dilation and an initial rise in kidney weight because of renal edema. Parenchymal mass decreases as a result of atrophy and adverse changes in the structure and function of the nephron. If hydronephrosis persists for 8 weeks or more, the parenchymal mass may be dramatically compromised with only a thin shell of tissue remaining around a hydronephrotic, distorted collecting system.[45]

Obstruction may be complicated by infection leading to pyelonephritis. In such cases the infection may become the dominant aspect of the disease, requiring immediate intervention before stone manipulation or surgical removal is attempted. Pyelonephritis is characterized by fever, chills, flank pain, and irritative voiding symptoms. Destruction of parenchymal mass by inflammatory changes and sepsis is a serious complication of the condition. Children with pyelonephritis are especially susceptible to renal scarring with subsequent loss of nephric function.[45,99]

Examination of a patient with calculous pyohydronephrosis may reveal a giant or intermediate-size hydronephrotic kidney or an atrophic kidney. The giant hydronephrotic kidney has a massively dilated collecting system with a thin shell of functioning parenchyma. The surface of the kidney is nodular and densely adherent to adjacent perirenal fat. An atrophic kidney is small because of extensive damage. Only a small mass of parenchymal tissue remains in this kidney, and progressive failure of function is likely. The intermediate-size hydronephrotic kidney is not as large as the giant kidney or as severely compromised in its function as the atrophic kidney. Microscopic examination of this type of kidney reveals more nearly normal nephrons than the other types of infected kidney, although inflammatory damage is present.[45]

Multiple factors influence the decision to attempt endoscopic manipulation or surgical removal of a urinary calculus. The patient's occupation and economic status must be considered when contemplating urologic intervention for a calculus. Persons in certain occupations (for example, a pilot) may subject themselves and others to danger if renal colic occurs during the performance of their jobs.[45]

A stone more than 4 mm in diameter is unlikely to pass through the ureter. Even smaller stones that are securely implanted into the wall of a calyx or ureter are less likely to pass and more likely to be obstructive or cause infection.

Aggressive removal of urinary calculi is considered for any patient who has a single kidney or significant renal insufficiency. Because of age and general health status, however, a patient may be a poor candidate for the anesthesia necessary for calculus manipulation.[45]

Diagnostic Studies and Findings

Kidneys, Ureters, and Bladder (KUB)

Calcifications in urinary tract; calcium phosphate calculi are most densely radiopaque; uric acid stones are radiolucent

Intravenous Pyelogram (IVP)

Filling defects in conjunction with calculus; ureteral dilation on affected side if calculus is obstructive; hydronephrosis may be present with dilation of calyces and renal pelvis; clubbing of calyces in advanced cases of hydronephrosis; signs of pyelonephritis (parenchymal enlargement with impairment of excretion) if calculous pyohydronephrosis is present

Voiding Cystourethrogram (VCUG)

Of limited value in diagnosing bladder calculi, which are appreciated as intravesical filling defect

Retrograde Pyelography

Useful in cases of radiolucent calculi that cannot be localized by routine radiographic studies[45]

Ultrasonography

Presence of calculi

Analysis of Stones

Prominent constituents such as cystine, calcium, oxalate, and uric acid; provides guidance for medical therapy to prevent recurrence

Urine Calcium

Elevated in patients with calcium stones or renal tubular acidosis

Urine Oxalate

Elevated in patients with calcium oxalate stones

Urine Uric Acid

Elevated in patients with uric acid stones

Urinary pH

Acidic in patients with uric acid or cystine stones; alkaline in patients who form calcium phosphate, calcium oxalate, and struvite stones

Urine Culture

Bacteriuria if infection is due to presence of calculi

Antibody-Coated Bacteria

Positive in pyelonephritis

Serum Calcium

Elevated in hyperparathyroidism

Serum Parathormone

Elevated in hyperparathyroidism

Medical Plan

Surgery

Has been mainstay of urologic interventions throughout twentieth century; surgical procedures for removing calculi are nephrolithotomy, pelvolithotomy, and ureterolithotomy; relative incidence of indications for surgical intervention has been greatly limited owing to refinement of percutaneous, ureteroscopic, and extracorporeal therapy

Medications

Anti-infective agents
- Antibiotics guided by urine and blood cultures; pending culture findings: gentamicin, 3-5 mg/kg body weight/d, and ampicillin, 2 g IV q6h

Central nervous system drugs
- Narcotic agents for renal colic

For uric acid stones: allopurinol 200-600 mg/d

For cystine stones: penicillamine

For acidic urine: sodium bicarbonate or potassium citrate or sodium citrate

For calcium stones: potassium acid phosphate or neutral sodium and potassium phosphate

For alkaline urine: ascorbic acid, 1 g/d, or ammonium chloride, 0.3-1 g q4h

General Management

Percutaneous removal of upper urinary tract stones using stone basket or by crushing stones via ultrasonic shock waves, electrohydraulic means, or laser techniques; avoids open surgery but does require invasive percutaneous access into the upper urinary tract

Extracorporeal shock wave lithotripsy uses shock waves to crush calculi into small fragments that can be passed through the urinary tract and expelled into the urine; technique is noninvasive

Chemolysis uses a chemical solution to dissolve urinary calculi by reversing environmental conditions favorable to calculi crystallization and aggregation; a percutaneous tract into the renal pelvis is established and chemolytic solution is used to dissolve calculi

Dietary restrictions for preventive therapy
- To prevent all forms of stones: ensure adequate fluid intake
- To prevent calcium stones: reduction of dietary calcium indicated only in certain patients with abnormal intestinal absorption of calcium (absorptive calciuria); a moderate restriction is recommended (400 to 600 mg/day)[82]
- To prevent oxalate stones: reduce intake of foods high in oxalates, including asparagus, beets, plums, raspberries, rhubarb, spinach, almonds, cashew nuts, cranberries, cocoa, cranberry juice, grape juice, grapefruit juice, Worcestershire sauce
- To prevent uric acid stones: reduce intake of foods high in purines such as organ meats, lean meats, and whole grains

NURSING CARE

Nursing Assessment

Pain

Renal colic or bladder colic; may be severe; flank pain noted with pyelonephritis

Voiding Behaviors

Irritative voiding symptoms

Fever

Elevated if infection is present

Nausea and Vomiting

Associated with renal colic

Nursing Dx & Intervention

Nursing Diagnosis	Nursing Intervention/Rationale
Pain	• Provide pain medications as ordered *to reduce discomfort.* • Minimize environmental noise and activity *to promote rest.* • Observe for intensification of pain, *which may indicate impaction of calculi or increase in obstructive property of calculi.* • Observe for sudden relief of pain, *which may indicate passage of stone through a narrow ureteral segment or across the ureteropelvic or ureterovesical junctions.*
Noncompliance (potential) (medical regimen)	• Instruct patient to strain all urine with proper device *to retain stone particles for laboratory analysis if passed.* • Instruct patient to maintain adequate fluid intake (at least 2.5 L/d) *to reduce urinary concentration of stone-forming salts.* • Reinforce importance of dietary restrictions related to stone formation *to prevent recurrence of calculi disease.*
Altered renal tissue perfusion related to obstruction and renal function compromise	• Observe for renal colic, flank pain, fever, and chills *to detect obstructive uropathy of the urinary tract and prevent renal insufficiency.* • Provide adequate fluid hydration *to prevent loss of renal perfusion resulting from hypovolemia.* • Monitor urinary output *to prevent obstructive uropathy and renal insufficiency.*

Patient Education

1. Provide explanation of analysis of stone, adjunct medical therapy aimed at prevention of recurrence, and associated dietary restrictions.
2. Provide instruction concerning options of treatment should manipulation of stones be indicated.

Evaluation

Patient Outcome	Data Indicating That Outcome is Reached
Spontaneous passage of calculus takes place.	Findings of kidney, bladder, and urine (KUB) are normal. There is no renal colic. Stone is passed in urine and retrieved for analysis.
Calculi do not recur.	Findings of follow-up KUB, 3 to 6 months later, are normal.

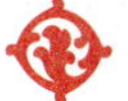

Urinary incontinence

Urinary incontinence is the involuntary leakage of urine after the age of toilet training.

Incontinence is not a disease; it is a symptom that represents a significant health problem and may underlie a serious disease process. Urinary incontinence is a particularly appropriate area of intensive investigation and intervention for nurses who manage patients with genitourinary disease.

The problem of urinary incontinence occurs throughout the life span and is a particularly prevalent and underrated condition among the elderly. The prevalence of urinary incontinence among adults over 65 years of age is approximately 17%.[103] Among nursing home residents the prevalence approaches 50%.[78]

A Welsh study of 1060 women 18 years of age and over revealed that 45% of these women had some degree of incontinence. Symptoms consistent with stress incontinence were reported by 22% of the women, and those of urge incontinence were reported by 10%. A combination of stress and urge incontinence was reported by 14% of those surveyed. In the majority of the women, urinary incontinence was assessed as mild, but 5% related severe enough symptoms to necessitate changing clothing daily. Over 3% of the women reported that urinary incontinence significantly interfered with their daily lives, yet less than half of these had sought medical treatment for the problem.

The prevalence of urinary incontinence in men is less well documented. In the Danish population, 2% of all adults have urinary incontinence severe enough to prompt them to seek medical help. Among men over 65 years of age, 5% suffer from incontinence; among men under 50 years approximately 20% to 25% develop symptoms of obstruction and dribble after voiding because of benign prostatic hypertrophy.[44,47]

Urinary continence in childhood is typically accomplished by 5 years of age. Incontinence most often takes the form of enuresis, which is seen in 15% of all 5-year-olds.[49]

For further information, see Part Three (Incontinence, Urinary Retention, and Altered Patterns of Urinary Elimination).

Pathophysiology

Many classification schemes for urinary incontinence have been proposed. In this discussion, Wheatley's four types of incontinence[110] are used because they offer a simple, comprehensive conceptual framework for this condition. The four types of incontinence are stress urinary incontinence, instability incontinence, overflow or paradoxic incontinence, and constant or extraurethral incontinence.

Stress urinary incontinence occurs when bladder pressure exceeds urethral closure pressure, resulting in leakage of urine in the absence of a detrusor contraction. Although the condition is most common among women, it is also noted among males. The causes of stress urinary incontinence are pelvic relaxation, sphincteric incompetence, or a combination of these factors.[86,100]

Pelvic relaxation, most typically seen in women, occurs when the support structures of the pelvis lose their optimum competence, resulting in descent of pelvic organs. Cystocele describes the protrusion of the bladder into the vaginal space; rectocele describes protrusion of the rectum into the vaginal space. The often used term "urethrocele" is a misnomer; the condition typically refers to hypermobility of the urethra associated with increased abdominal pressure seen during physical examination. Uterine prolapse occurs when the uterus descends into the vaginal space as a result of a loss of normal support mechanisms.[42] Multiparity, aging, and menopause are associated with pelvic relaxation.[110]

Childbirth via vaginal delivery is associated with pelvic relaxation, at least partly because of traction placed on the pelvic ligaments during delivery and denervation of the pelvic floor musculature.[5,97] Other causes of pelvic floor relaxation are associated with pelvic floor muscle denervation. Peripheral neuropathy, as seen in diabetes mellitus, and traumatic and iatrogenic nerve damage resulting from extensive pelvic surgery can cause pelvic floor relaxation. Obesity may exacerbate the condition.[42,100]

Although a causal relationship between pelvic relaxation and stress urinary incontinence remains unestablished, the principal pathophysiologic mechanism is probably loss of normal urethrovesical anatomy. The urethra is no longer maintained in its normal position, resulting in inefficient transmission of abdominal pressures along the urethral length. As a result a precipitous increase in abdominal pressure is not transmitted to the urethral sphincteric mechanism, resulting in a temporary condition when bladder pressure exceeds urethral closure pressure and urinary leakage occurs.

Urethral sphincteric incompetence also causes stress urinary incontinence. Loss of estrogens may result in decreased mucosal secretions and loss of a watertight urethral seal in women. Loss of estrogens also may affect the submucosal vascular cushion, resulting in a loss of efficient urethral compression and urethral closure pressure. Iatrogenic or infectious damage to the urethral lining may result in inefficient coaptation of the urethral wall and loss of a watertight seal.[100,117]

Damage to the neuromuscular components of the urethra results from any process that causes denervation of the pelvic floor musculature or smooth muscle of the proximal urethra. Iatrogenic damage resulting from radical prostatectomy or transurethral resection of the prostate may cause sphincteric incompetence and stress urinary incontinence. Multiple anti-incontinence procedures or Y-V plasty in men or women also may result in sphincteric incompetence and incontinence.[110] Pelvic trauma or metabolic conditions resulting in peripheral neuropathy affecting the pelvis may result in stress urinary incontinence as a result of sphincteric incompetence.[42]

Stress urinary incontinence in a woman often arises because of a combination of sphincteric incompetence and pelvic relaxation. Stress incontinence in a man often results from significant sphincteric incompetence and may be particularly severe.

Instability incontinence is the condition of urinary leakage that occurs when the detrusor contracts at inappropriate times. The concept of instability arises from Hodgkinson, Ayers, and Drukker's description of dyssynergic detrusor activity among women with urinary incontinence.[48] Other terms have been used to describe the condition. Detrusor hyperreflexia is often used synonymously with instability. Nonetheless, the term is defined by the International Continence Society as the occurrence of an uninhibited detrusor contraction in the presence of a known neurologic disease.[51] Other terms, such as detrusor hyperactivity or overactivity, are less commonly used.

Detrusor instability is associated with disease or trauma of the central nervous system. Diseases of the brain typically result in loss of volitional control over detrusor activity with preservation of coordination between the striated sphincter mechanism and detrusor activity. Such diseases include cerebrovascular accidents, parkinsonism, and brain tumors affecting the frontal lobes or cerebellum.[115] Incontinence is preceded by a feeling of urgency followed by an unstable bladder contraction with relaxation of the sphincteric mechanism and evacuation of the bladder. Bladder emptying often is efficient, so urinary tract infections are not typically associated with this condition. The nursing diagnosis associated with this form of incontinence is "Urge incontinence."

Instability incontinence also is associated with neurologic abnormality of the spinal cord above the level of the sacral micturition center (S2-4).[110] Spinal cord injury is the most commonly noted lesion. Nontraumatic lesions include those seen in multiple sclerosis or other demyelinating diseases. Incontinence is not preceded by any sensation of urgency. A detrusor contraction is triggered by bladder filling or other stimulus, and the person is aware of the incontinence via perception of urinary leakage. Detrusor contraction is often associated with contraction of the pelvic floor and rhabdosphincter. This condition is called detrusor-sphincter dyssynergia and is associated with urinary retention, urinary tract infection, and upper tract deterioration.[42] The nursing diagnosis for this form of instability incontinence is "Reflex incontinence."

Nonneuropathic conditions also are associated with detrusor instability. Bladder outlet obstruction has been associated with instability incontinence among men with benign prostatic hypertrophy.[1,4] Irritative bladder disorders caused by bacterial, viral, fungal, or parasitic infection of the bladder have been labeled as a cause of instability incontinence.[110] While these conditions are associated with increased sensations of bladder filling, little evidence supports the supposition that they cause detrusor instability.[10,87] Instability incontinence is associated with bladder irritation caused by bladder calculi and carcinoma of the urothelial lining of the vesicle. The leakage of urine into the posterior seen in stress urinary incontinence has been speculated to cause instability of the detrusor.[9,110] Indeed, detrusor instability is often seen among women with stress urinary incontinence, and the condition is often relieved by surgical correction of the stress incontinence. Nonetheless, other investigators have failed to confirm this association, and the relation of urinary leakage into the posterior urethra remains unclear.[86]

The underlying cause of many cases of instability incontinence is unclear, and the condition is termed idiopathic. Such instability may arise from a psychogenic or behavioral source, or it may be due to subtle neuropathy yet to be elucidated.

Overflow or paradoxic incontinence is the leakage of urine in the presence of a large residual. The two causes of overflow incontinence are deficient detrusor function and bladder outlet obstruction.[110] Deficient detrusor function may result from a variety of causes. Neurologic lesions of the sacral micturition cord such as that noted in myelomeningocele cause an autonomous neurogenic bladder with detrusor areflexia, lack of sensations of urgency, and overflow incontinence. Other central nervous system disorders associated with overflow incontinence are cauda equina syndrome, multiple sclerosis, tabes dorsalis, and poliomyelitis. Peripheral nervous system trauma or abnormalities that compromise parasympathetic innervation of the detrusor muscle also result in overflow incontinence. Examples are herpes zoster, extensive pelvic surgery, pelvic trauma, and diabetes mellitus.[110]

Other factors that result in overflow incontinence and detrusor areflexia are the result of chronic overdistention. The "nurse's bladder," "teacher's bladder," or "librarian's bladder" arises from overdistention of the bladder because of perceived inability to interrupt work for micturition. Acute illness and immobility may also result in deficient detrusor function. Severe constipation or fecal impaction is associated with temporary detrusor failure and overflow incontinence. Certain patients may suffer from urinary retention because of hysterical conversions.

Patients with overflow incontinence may not be aware of their inability to empty the bladder. Symptoms of deficient detrusor function are urgency, frequency, nocturia, and a dribbling, intermittent stream. Urinary tract infection is commonly an associated condition. Low back pain and vague abdominal discomfort may be the result of bladder enlargement.

Bladder outlet obstruction is also a cause of overflow incontinence. Types of bladder outlet obstruction include prostatic enlargement owing to inflammation, benign hypertrophy, or adenocarcinoma. Internal sphincter dyssynergia, bladder neck hypertrophy, and bladder neck contracture are particularly prevalent in men with highly stressful life-styles and may lead to overflow incontinence. Urethral stricture in a man or urethral distortion in a woman may obstruct normal bladder emptying and lead to incontinence.[110]

Patients with bladder outlet obstruction are acutely aware of their problem because of high pressures generated by the detrusor during micturition. Symptoms of bladder outlet obstruction include frequency, nocturia, and poor urinary stream. A dribble after voiding is often noted.

Constant or extraurethral incontinence results when the normal sphincteric mechanism is bypassed, causing failure of urinary storage that is continuous. The causes of extraurethral incontinence are urinary fistula, ectopia, or surgical creation of a conduit for evacuation of urine. Congenital ectopic defects of the urinary tract including urethral duplication, epispadias, and exstrophy are relatively rare and may be associated with severe urinary leakage that may persist even after surgical leakage.[58] Ureteral ectopia is a more common congenital defect and results in a continuous, dribbling discharge superimposed on a normal voiding pattern if the orifice bypasses normal sphincteric mechanisms.[110]

Urinary fistula is most commonly noted among adult women. A fistula is created when tissue between the bladder or urethra and an adjacent structure erodes; the normal sphincteric mechanism is bypassed, resulting in urinary leakage. A fistula between the bladder and vagina is termed vesicovaginal fistula; a fistulous tract between the urethra and vagina is termed urethrovaginal fistula. Symmonds[102] reviewed 800 cases of urinary fistulas seen at the Mayo Clinic over a 30-year period and found that the leading cause of fistula was pelvic surgery. Hysterectomy was the most common procedure associated with the condition. Other causes of fistula include penetrating trauma, radiation therapy, and obstetric complications. In the Mayo Clinic study, only 5% of the patients reviewed developed fistula as a result of obstetric complications. Nonetheless, childbearing is thought to account for the largest incidence of fistulous tracts worldwide.[106]

Diagnostic Studies and Findings

Voiding Cystourethrogram (VCUG)

Stress incontinence: pelvic descent below pubis; urethral excursion and leakage of contrast material with abdominal strain

Instability incontinence: normal or trabeculated narrowing of membranous urethra noted with micturition in presence of detrusor-sphincter dyssynergia; diverticulae, vesicoureteral reflux may be noted in presence of detrusor-sphincter dyssynergia

Overflow/paradoxic incontinence: large capacity, poor filling of proximal urethra with bladder outlet obstruction; failure of bladder neck funneling with detrusor-sphincter dyssynergia; urethral narrowing with stricture

Constant extraurethral incontinence: leakage of contrast material through fistulous tract or from ectopic structure

Urodynamic Testing

Stress incontinence: normal capacity, sensations, and compliance; stable detrusor; explosive flow with low-pressure detrusor contraction during micturition; normal electromyographic (EMG) findings

Instability incontinence: decreased functional capacity; early sensations; normal compliance; unstable detrusor and/or urethra; EMG findings normal or indicative of detrusor-sphincter dyssynergia

Overflow incontinence with deficient detrusor function: large capacity, delayed sensations, abnormally compliant; with detrusor hypotonic or areflexic: urinary stream poor or absent, large residual present after voiding

Bladder outlet obstruction: normal or enlarged capacity; sensations may be delayed; compliance normal or impaired owing to detrusor hypertrophy; detrusor contraction is high pressure with poor urinary flow

Constant incontinence: normal or impaired urine storage with large fistulous tract

Intravenous Pyelogram (IVP)

Constant incontinence: ureteral duplication with ectopic opening below bladder neck or outside urinary tract; extravasation of contrast material in fistula

Retrograde Urethrogram (RUG)

Presence of urethral stricture

Cystoscopy-Urethroscopy

Stress incontinence: normal findings in pelvic relaxation or open bladder neck with sphincteric damage

Overflow incontinence: large capacity in deficient detrusor function; localization of obstruction in some cases

Constant incontinence: ectopia or fistulous tract

Urinalysis and Urine Culture

Instability incontinence: normal findings or presence of bacterial infection

Bladder Biopsy

Instability incontinence: normal findings or presence of transitional cell carcinoma or carcinoma in situ

Medical Plan

Surgery

For stress incontinence

- Vesicourethral suspension; over 100 procedures described in literature; commonly performed types include Marshall-Marchetti-Krantz, Lapides' vesicopexy, Cooper's ligament, Burch's culposuspension
- Artificial urinary sphincter for stress incontinence caused by sphincteric damage; cuff of device placed at bladder neck or proximal urethra, abdominal reservoir positioned, pump mechanism placed in scrotum or fascia of labia

For overflow incontinence

- Transurethral resection of enlarged prostate; open prostatectomy or radical prostatectomy in certain cases
- Correction of urethral stricture by internal urethrotomy or urethral dilation
- Correction of female distortion by open surgical reconstruction

For constant extraurethral incontinence

- Removal or repair of ectopic structures
- Open surgical repair of urinary fistula

Medications

To affect detrusor contractility

- Autonomic drugs
  - Propantheline, up to 150 mg/d in 3 divided doses
  - Oxybutynin, 5 mg bid or tid
- Central nervous system drugs
  - Imipramine, 1.5-2 mg/kg in single dose at bedtime
- Spasmolytic agents
  - Flavoxate, 100-200 mg tid or qid
  - Dicyclomine, 10-20 mg tid or qid

Drugs that increase detrusor activity and tone

- Autonomic drugs
  - Bethanechol, 15-30 mg tid or qid

Drugs used to increase bladder neck tone

- Autonomic drugs
  - Norephedrine or ephedrine (Sudafed S.A.), 1 tablet bid

Drugs used to decrease bladder neck tone

- Autonomic drugs
  - Phenoxybenzamine, 10-30 mg/d in single dose

Drugs used to decrease external muscle tone

- Central nervous system drugs
  - Diazepam, 5-10 mg qid
  - Dantrolene, 25-50 mg/d
  - Baclofen, 5-20 mg tid

NURSING CARE

Nursing Assessment

Bladder

Suprapubic tenderness associated with cystitis; suprapubic and lower abdominal distention in overflow incontinence

Vaginal Vault

Bulge in anterior wall in cystocele associated with pelvic relaxation; discharge in vesicovaginal or ureterovaginal fistula or ureteral ectopia in the vagina or uterus

Nursing Dx & Intervention

Nursing Diagnosis	Nursing Intervention/Rationale
Stress incontinence	• Provide advice concerning urinary containment devices (pads, incontinence briefs) *to assist patient in collecting urinary leakage in a personally and culturally acceptable manner.* • Teach female patient to perform Kegel exercises *to attempt to increase competence of sphincteric mechanism by strengthening pelvic floor muscles.* • Provide α-sympathomimetic medications as directed *to increase competence of sphincteric mechanism by stimulating smooth muscle and vascular components.* • Instruct patient to care for and manipulate pessary device as directed *to alleviate symptom of stress urinary incontinence. A pessary is a nonsurgical means to elevate bladder and urethra to more nearly normal abdominal position.*
Urge incontinence (instability incontinence resulting from any cause other than spinal cord abnormality)	• Place patient on timed voiding schedule *to prevent incontinence by allowing patient to empty bladder voluntarily before uninhibited contraction is triggered.* • Control fluid intake *to ensure adequate fluid intake and attempt to control periods of peak bladder filling. Fluid intake is concentrated during waking hours and severely restricted 2 hours before sleep and during nighttime.* • Provide anticholinergic or antispasmodic medications as directed *to increase bladder capacity and time between timed micturition episodes.* • Provide medications for bladder contractility and teach patient clean intermittent catheterization *to prevent uninhibited contractions that are uncontrollable by other methods. The bladder is pharmacologically paralyzed and emptied via catheterization.*
Reflex incontinence (instability incontinence resulting from spinal cord abnormality above S2-4)	• Provide medication to paralyze bladder contractions; teach patient clean intermittent catheterization *to prevent incontinence and obstructive uropathy associated with detrusor-sphincter dyssynergia.* • Place condom on male patient after sphincterotomy is completed and surgical site healed *to contain urinary leakage. Sphincterotomy is considered a permanent procedure that prevents obstructive uropathy associated with detrusor-sphincter dyssynergia. The unstable detrusor contractions remain.* • Place indwelling urethral or suprapubic catheter as directed *to contain incontinence. Used as a last resort, the indwelling catheter is associated with chronic urinary tract infection and potential upper urinary tract damage.*
Urinary retention (overflow/paradoxic incontinence)	• Teach patient to double void *to encourage complete bladder emptying. Certain patients with deficient detrusor function are able to completely evacuate the bladder if they learn to void, wait 3 to 5 minutes, and void again.* • Teach patient to perform intermittent catheterization as directed *to ensure regular complete bladder emptying and prevent urinary tract infections.* • Place temporary indwelling catheter *to provide temporary drainage for the patient before definitive surgical repair of bladder outlet obstruction.* • Provide medications to decrease urethral resistance or increase detrusor tone *to attempt to increase efficiency of micturition.*
Total incontinence (constant extraurethral incontinence)	• Provide patient with advice concerning urinary containment devices (as temporary solutions before surgical correction or as permanent solutions) *to allow patient to collect urine in a personally and culturally acceptable manner.* The leakage may be severe; options must include anti-incontinence pads, briefs, and adult diapers.
Self-esteem disturbance	• Provide support and encouragement concerning availability of treatment options *to reassure patient that management of this traditionally ignored and culturally embarrassing problem is available. Many patients do not seek care for this problem.* • Provide patient with an opportunity to express feelings related to loss of urinary control and suggest support group if appropriate. *Loss of urinary control is often considered taboo in modern society; support groups such as Help for Incontinent People (HIP) offer networking and support for persons with this condition.*

Patient Education

1. Provide instruction on technique of medication regimens and need for continuous therapy in neuropathic bladder cases.
2. Provide a list of signs and symptoms of urinary tract infection and other conditions requiring medical attention.

3. Provide instructions for intermittent catheterization technique or care of long-indwelling Foley catheter.
4. Provide instruction about the relationship of incontinence to fluid intake, various medications, and compliance with medical and nursing strategies for prevention.

Evaluation

Patient Outcome	Data Indicating That Outcome is Reached
Stress incontinence resulting from pelvic relaxation has been surgically corrected.	Continence is maintained. Residual after voiding is less than 20% of total bladder volume. There is no urinary tract infection.
Stress incontinence has been surgically corrected with placement of artificial urinary sphincter.	Continence is maintained. Sphincter device is functioning. There is no urinary tract infection.
Unstable bladder is adequately managed.	Continence is maintained.
Reflex incontinence is adequately managed.	Continence is maintained or patient is using condom device to collect urine.
Instability incontinence caused by irritative disorder is resolved.	Continence is maintained. Underlying irritative disorder is resolved.
Overflow incontinence in bladder with deficient detrusor function is adequately managed.	Continence is maintained. Residual after voiding is less than 20% of total bladder volume.
Overflow incontinence caused by bladder outlet obstruction is resolved.	Continence is maintained. Obstruction is resolved.
Constant incontinence is resolved.	Continence is maintained. Fistula is closed or ectopia is repaired.

PROSTATE DISORDERS

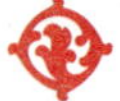 Benign prostatic hypertrophy

Benign prostatic hypertrophy is the progressive enlargement of the prostate gland associated with the aging process. The disease associated with benign prostatic hypertrophy is a result of the obstructive uropathies associated with glandular enlargement rather than a result of the hyperplastic process per se.

Benign prostatic hypertrophy (BPH) is the most common neoplastic growth among men past the fifth decade of life. Autopsy studies have shown that virtually all men over 50 years of age experience an increase in prostatic weight sometimes defined as BPH. However, when histologic changes are scrutinized, only slightly more than half of men are diagnosed with a significant degree of BPH.[45,47]

Because of increasing longevity among individuals in industrialized nations, the incidence of BPH is rising.[45,47] A retrospective study of the male population in the New Haven, Connecticut, area between 1953 and 1961 demonstrated that a man aged 50 had a 10% chance of undergoing corrective surgery for obstructive symptoms from BPH within his lifetime. More current data reveal that a 50-year-old man has a 20% to 25% chance of undergoing surgery for prostatism.[47]

Improvements in the surgical treatment of BPH over the past century have significantly decreased the mortality associated with this condition. In Europe the death rate from prostatic surgery is 0.3% to 1.8%, and the overall death rate from conditions occurring as a result of BPH is 23 per 100,000.[47]

As the number of men in the United States continues to grow, so will the incidence of BPH and the incidence of corrective surgery. Transurethral resection of the prostate (TURP) is the most commonly performed surgical procedure among men over 50 years. In 1983, approximately 290,000 TURP procedures were performed, generating a total medical cost exceeding 1 billion dollars.[107]

Pathophysiology

The etiology and natural history of BPH are not clearly understood. The prostate grows relatively slowly between birth and puberty. During pubescence, rapid growth and maturation continue to a steady state attained at age 20.[53] This steady state lasts to age 45 to 50 when another gradual increase in prostatic size and weight occurs.[107]

Contrary to popular belief, no persuasive evidence exists concerning risk factors for BPH. Sexual activity (or celibacy), tobacco or alcohol use, diabetes, or social factors are not connected with an increased incidence of BPH. Obstructive symptoms of BPH tend to be seen earlier in black men than among white men, and Japanese men have a lower incidence than white men, but the reason for these racial variances is unknown. The two factors necessary for the development of BPH are aging and the presence of functioning testes.[107,114]

The critical role of testicular androgens in BPH is demonstrated by the absence of the condition in males who have undergone castration before puberty and the marked reduction in incidence of BPH among men castrated before 40 years of age. However, the results of castration among men with existing BPH have not produced significant relief of obstructive symptoms in many studies.[107]

Testosterone is the principal hormonal product of the testes. Within the prostate it serves as a precursor for dihydrotestosterone, which is the prominent interstitial androgen that influences prostatic growth. Dihydrotestosterone is known to play a crucial role in normal prostatic growth throughout maturation; however, its role in the development of BPH remains unclear.[107] Wilson and his associates demonstrated that BPH was not produced in a group of male dogs given parenteral dihydrotestosterone. Ironically, spontaneous BPH did develop among some of the control dogs.[115] In human males a gradual decrease in plasma levels of testosterone will logically correspond with a lower level of dihydrotestosterone within prostatic tissue, suggesting that other influences are important in the development of BPH.[107]

Endogenous estrogens have also been implicated in the development of BPH. Walsh and Wilson[105] used a combination of estrogens and dihydrotestosterone to produce BPH in dogs. They found that a combination of androstenediol and dihydrotestosterone produced mild prostatism, and administration of estradiol and dihydrotestosterone produced marked hypertrophy. In human males it is important to note that while plasma testosterone levels are falling off, estradiol and androstenediol levels remain relatively unchanged. Thus, argues Walsh,[107] alteration of the synergy between testosterone and its derivatives and the endogenous estrogens in the male is responsible for the proliferation of BPH, although their role in the generation of prostatism is not established.

Although the development of BPH itself is not harmful, the sequelae produced by this condition cause significant morbidity and may prove fatal. The signs and symptoms of BPH are a result of bladder outlet obstruction resulting from gradual encroachment of the prostatic capsule into the proximal urethra. Early changes include hesitancy initiating micturition, decreased force in urinary stream, diurnal frequency, and nocturia. Compensatory hypertrophy of the detrusor muscle results in trabeculation, diverticula, and hypertrophy of the trigone. Paradoxically, this may produce a reduction in symptoms but does not indicate any objective improvement in bladder outlet obstruction.[94,107]

Later changes produced by bladder outlet obstruction caused by BPH include myogenic decompensation when compensatory hypertrophy is no longer effective. The bladder wall then becomes increasingly noncompliant and hypotonic, resulting in increasing postvoid residuals and greater chance of infection. Increased resistance at the ureterovesical junction results in ureteral dilation and progressive hydronephrosis. Unless infection is present in the upper urinary tract, few symptoms are perceived by the individual, although renal function is impaired. In certain cases incompetence of the ureterovesical junction combined with increased voiding pressure may result in vesicoureteral reflux that compromises the hydrodynamic function of the renal pelvis and ureters and promotes the likelihood of pyelonephritis.[94]

The two primary complications of BPH are urinary tract infection and acute urinary retention. Urinary tract infection results from the presence of postvoid residuals that cause hypoxemia of the bladder wall and decreased resistance to bacterial invasion.[66] Acute urinary retention is a surprisingly common complication of BPH. Epidemiologic studies in Britain revealed that 44% of all men treated for BPH had urinary retention and 54% of those studied experienced at least one episode of acute urinary retention requiring catheterization. Acute urinary retention often results from some other aggravating factor of BPH such as prostatic infarct, or it may be a late result of detrusor decompensation.[47,94]

Diagnostic Studies and Findings

Uroflow with Postvoid Residual

Decreased peak and mean flow and postvoid residual indicate bladder outlet obstruction

Film of Kidneys, Ureters, and Bladder (KUB)

Absence of complicating urinary calculi

Intravenous Pyelogram (IVP)

Hydroureteronephrosis, trabeculation, or diverticula of bladder

Elevation of bladder base resulting from prostatic enlargement

Postvoid residual

Urinalysis and Urine Culture

Will rule out urinary tract infection, a complication of BPH

Cystoscopy

Accurate assessment of degree of prostatic invasion into

proximal urethral lumen and compensatory changes in bladder wall

Cystometrogram, Electromyogram, Flow

Urodynamic studies will accurately assess degree of functional obstruction and severity of detrusor decompensation

Medical Plan

Surgery

Transurethral resection of prostate (TURP) remains most widely used surgical intervention for BPH: a cystoscope is passed down urethra through which a resectoscope is used to remove a portion of the intracapsular tissue

Suprapubic or retropubic prostatectomy (open removal of prostate gland) may be used in selected cases

Cryosurgical technique may be used for patients who are poor risk for anesthesia: an instrument is passed urethrally and the freezing unit placed in the prostatic urethra; liquid nitrogen is passed through the instrument until the prostatic capsule reaches 0° to 10° C, causing slough of prostatic tissue; not as effective as TURP and reserved for select patients

Medications

Antimicrobial therapy indicated if urinary tract infection is present

Exogenous estrogen may be used to reduce progression of prostatic enlargement but is typically contraindicated because of its side effects, which include loss of libido and impotence[95]

General Management

Intermittent self-catheterization may be used in selected individuals to ensure complete bladder evacuation

Urethral catheterization indicated when acute urinary retention occurs

Suprapubic cystostomy may be necessary if a urethral catheter cannot be passed

Avoid all over-the-counter or prescription cold preparations containing α-sympathomimetics (will cause increased tone at bladder neck exacerbating outlet obstruction)

Long-term use of antidepressant drugs will exacerbate urinary retention because of their anticholinergic effects

NURSING CARE

Nursing Assessment

Prostate

Digital examination of rectum will reveal enlargement of all palpable lobes and absence of discrete, hardened nodules

Voiding Behavior

Decreased force of urinary stream

Straining or use of Credé's maneuver to void

Postvoid dribble

Diurnal frequency and nocturia with feelings of incomplete emptying

Nursing Dx & Intervention

Nursing Diagnosis	Nursing Intervention/Rationale
Altered patterns of urinary elimination	• Assess diurnal urinary frequency, force of urinary stream, and incidence of nocturia *to discern the early signs of significant BPH. Early detection may prevent later complications such as infection, urinary retention, and upper tract abnormalities.*
Urinary retention	• Assess fluid intake and urinary output *to ensure adequate urinary output; urine output should approximate fluid intake.* • *Assess force of urinary stream, frequency of urination, and time required to initiate stream; decreased force of stream with increasing urinary hesitancy and frequency are often the first signs of urinary retention.* • Counsel patient to avoid any over-the-counter preparations containing decongestants *to prevent acute urinary retention. The α-sympathomimetics contained in decongestant medications cause increased smooth muscle tone at the bladder neck and increase the degree of bladder outlet obstruction.*
Knowledge deficit (significance of BPH)	• Educate men over 50 years of age about signs and symptoms of BPH *to ensure that they will seek health care as appropriate.* • Educate men who have the signs and symptoms of BPH that spontaneous improved force of urinary stream and decreasing urinary frequency do not indicate improvement in BPH. *Detrusor compensation may improve the symptoms associated with BPH; nonetheless, the obstruction remains and potential complications of this condition (urinary retention, infection, and upper tract abnormalities) persist.*

Patient Education

1. Provide information and assistance in planning a schedule for fluid intake adequate for daily needs, necessity of prompt medical intervention for bladder outlet obstruction, and special instructions for any related drugs taken (e.g., antibiotics).
2. Provide information concerning the true lack of causal relationship between benign prostatic hypertrophy and sexual patterns.

Evaluation

Patient Outcome	Data Indicating That Outcome is Reached
BPH is surgically repaired.	Peak and mean flow on uroflowmetry improve. Postvoid residual is less than 20% of total bladder volume. Urodynamic results demonstrate negative resistance factors. Cystoscopic examination reveals no urethral obstruction. Subjective improvement in voiding symptoms occurs.

Prostatitis

Prostatitis is the inflammation of prostatic acini and surrounding tissue that is particularly pronounced in the periurethral portion of the gland.

Inflammation of the prostate is commonly divided into four types: acute bacterial, chronic bacterial, nonbacterial, and prostatodynia. Each form of prostatitis has a distinctive clinical presentation and is managed differently.[99]

Prostatitis is most commonly observed in males after the onset of pubescence, but rare cases of the disease have been reported among children and infants. Nonbacterial prostatitis (also named prostatosis) is the most common form of the disease. Acute and chronic bacterial prostatitis is less commonly seen. Rarer forms include viral, fungal, parasitic, and allergic prostatitis.[49,76]

Pathophysiology

Acute bacterial prostatitis is caused by the ascent of bacteria via the urethra or the hematogenous route. Acute infection may be precipitated by urethral instrumentation or prostatic massage in the presence of chronic bacterial prostatitis. Common causative pathogens include *E. coli, Proteus, Klebsiella, Pseudomonas,* and *Enterobacter*. An acute episode of prostatic infection is characterized by a sudden onset of fever, chills, myalgia, arthralgia, and general malaise. These symptoms rapidly progress to localized discomfort in the perineal area or low back associated with irritative voiding symptoms including urgency, frequency, nocturia, dysuria, and a persistent burning sensation in the urethra after micturition. Pain in the prostate results in varying degrees of functional bladder outlet obstruction that may cause significant urinary hesitancy or even acute urinary obstruction.[45,49]

Histologic examination of prostatic tissue will reveal diffuse glandular inflammation with edema and hyperemia of the stroma. Abscesses are common and may hemorrhage in severe cases. Polymorphonucleocytes, bacteria, and cellular debris are present within the acini of the gland. Rectal palpation of the prostate reveals an exquisitely tender organ. Vigorous massage is contraindicated because of the associated pain and the danger of bacteremia. Acute bacterial cystitis is typically associated so that urine culture provides an excellent clue to the causative prostatic pathogen. An objective diagnosis of acute bacterial prostatitis is made in the presence of evidence of inflammation on expressed prostatic secretions (over 10 leukocytes per high-power field), positive bacterial culture of this expressed prostatic secretion, positive bacterial cystitis, and an abnormal rectal examination.[45,49]

Chronic bacterial prostatitis commonly occurs as a result of ascending infection from the urethra. The condition may arise following an inadequately treated episode of acute bacterial prostatitis, or it may occur via hematogenous bacterial invasion. However, the precise etiology of chronic bacterial prostatitis remains unclear.[95]

The clinical symptoms of chronic bacterial prostatitis vary widely. Some men have no symptoms of prostatitis other than recurrent urinary tract infections or asymptomatic bacteriuria. More commonly, men with prostatitis note recurring irritative voiding symptoms such as urgency, frequency, dysuria, nocturia, and urethral irritation. Perineal pain, postejaculatory pain, hematospermia, and a mucoid urethral discharge may also be noted.[45]

Rectal palpation of the prostate may reveal the presence of prostatic calculi or may be unremarkable. Histologic examination of the prostate shows moderate inflammatory changes that are less localized than in acute infections. Objective diagnosis of chronic bacterial prostatitis requires the presence of inflammatory cells on microscopic examination of expressed secretion, a positive culture of these secretions, and a nontender gland on rectal examination.[45]

Unlike acute bacterial prostatitis, the chronically infected prostate is relatively resistant to antibiotic treatment because of the poor absorption of non-lipid-soluble substances into the prostatic fluid. The chronically infected prostate has deficient levels of prostatic antibacterial substance. Prostatic calculi may also lower antibiotic susceptibility by serving as a nidus for persistent infection. Thus even extended periods of oral antibiotics may not cure chronic bacterial prostatitis.[45]

Nonbacterial prostatitis is the most common form of symptomatic prostatic inflammation. Although the causative agent of nonbacterial prostatitis has not been identified, chlamydia has been implicated as a possible pathogen. Unfortunately, cultures are difficult to obtain so verification of this suspicion requires further investigation.[29]

The symptoms of nonbacterial prostatitis are similar to those of chronic bacterial prostatitis and include pelvic area pain and irritative voiding symptoms. Objective diagnosis is made by demonstrating the presence of inflammatory cells in expressed prostatic secretions in the presence of negative prostatic secretion and bladder urine cultures. Rectal examination will be normal.[29,45]

Prostatodynia is the presence of symptoms of prostatitis in the absence of physical findings. The etiology of this form of prostatitis is unknown. Objective diagnosis is made by demonstrating negative inflammatory cells in expressed prostatic secretions, negative bacterial culture of these secretions, negative urine cultures in the presence of recurrent perineal pain, and irritative voiding symptoms.[29]

Other forms of prostatitis occur rarely and include viral prostatic inflammation following an upper respiratory infection, tubercular prostatitis, or mycotic prostatitis from blastomycosis, coccidioidomycosis, histoplasmosis, and candidiasis. Symptoms are similar to bacterial prostatitis with the presence of perineal area pain and inflammation of the prostate associated with irritative voiding symptoms.[45]

Complications of prostatitis include acute urinary retention, bladder neck contracture, and obstruction in the presence of chronic inflammation. Cystitis is typically associated with the condition, and epididymitis is not uncommon. Pyelonephritis and bacteremia may be associated with acute infection.[29,45]

Diagnostic Studies and Findings

Intravenous Pyelogram (IVP)

Normal or evidence of bladder neck obstruction with elevation of bladder base (owing to prostatic edema and large postvoid residual)

White Blood Cell (WBC) Count

Acute bacterial prostatitis: 20,000/L

Urinalysis

Bacterial infection: bacteria and WBCs on microscopic examination

Culture: Divided Specimen

Patient is asked to void his first 10 to 15 ml in a sterile cup and switch to another cup without interrupting the urinary stream, where he will collect the next 50 to 100 ml; when voiding is completed, patient is cautioned not to squeeze out the last several drops; prostate is then milked for an "expressed prostatic secretion," or all residual urine is expressed by straining if no secretions are obtained

Three portions are obtained from first container of urine (these represent "urethral discharge"): one portion examined microscopically, one portion used for culture, and remaining portion used for dry mounting on a slide using alcohol

Second container constitutes a midstream urine specimen and is used for routine urine culture and urinalysis

Final specimen is expressed prostatic fluid and is examined microscopically for inflammatory cells and submitted for culture

Bacterial prostatitis diagnosed by presence of over 5000 bacteria/ml with less than 3000 bacteria/ml obtained from bladder and urethral specimens[29]

Urine Culture and Sensitivity

Acute bacterial cystitis: positive
Chronic bacterial prostatitis: positive
Nonbacterial prostatitis: negative
Prostatodynia: negative

Medical Plan

Surgery

Open prostatectomy a possible curative measure but generally contraindicated because of associated side effects, including urinary incontinence and impotence[45,76]

Transurethral resection of prostate effective if all of the affected prostatic tissue is removed; clinical results indicate that approximately one third of patients treated in this manner have complete resolution of symptoms; remaining two thirds have improvement of symptoms or remain the same[29,45]

Medications

Anti-infective agents guided by routine urine culture and sensitivity reports indicated in cases of acute bacterial prostatitis; 30-day course of trimethoprim (Trimpex) or trimethoprim-sulfamethosoxazole (Bactrim DS; 1 tablet po bid) given to prevent occurrence of chronic infection

Mild cases of acute infection may be treated with oral antibiotics

Severe cases require parenteral antibiotic therapy with gentamicin (Garamycin) or tobramycin (Nebcin) and ampicillin (Amcil) until culture sensitivity reports are available or patient is afebrile[49]

Chronic bacterial prostatitis treated by 30 days of double-strength tablets of trimethoprim-sulfamethoxazole (Bactrim DS) given twice daily; tetracyclines may be substituted if patient is allergic to sulfonamides; combination of erythromycin and sodium bicarbonate may be used although results are not uniformly successful[49]

Antipyretics (ASA) often indicated in presence of acute bacterial prostatitis

Stool softeners may lessen discomfort associated with straining with a bowel movement[45]

General Management

Alcohol intake often causes exacerbation of symptoms in prostatitis; should be limited to 2 or 3 ounces per day or deleted from diet totally

Foods that contain chili powder or other "hot" spices are possibly associated with exacerbation of symptoms and are serially deleted from diet to assess their role in relief of symptoms

Dietary manipulation particularly important in management of prostatodynia

Placement of suprapubic catheter or suprapubic needle aspiration of urine indicated in cases of acute urinary retention from acute bacterial prostatitis[45,69]

NURSING CARE

Nursing Assessment

Prostate

Acute bacterial prostatitis: firm gland with assymetry or focal area of enlargement; exquisitely tender to touch

Chronic forms of prostatitis: relatively nontender; may note presence of calculi[99]

Voiding Behavior

Frequency, urgency, dysuria, bladder irritability, difficulty initiating stream

Nursing Dx & Intervention

Nursing Diagnosis	Nursing Intervention/Rationale
Pain	• Force intake of fluid *to decrease irritative voiding symptoms.* • Provide local heat such as sitz bath as prescribed *for symptomatic relief of perineal pain and to encourage urination in patients experiencing discomfort from a distended bladder.* • Note that gentle prostatic massage is contraindicated during acute infection *but may offer relief for chronic prostatitis.* (Massage should be performed no more than once a week.) • Sexual activity may also afford relief in cases of chronic prostatitis.
Altered patterns of urinary elimination related to bladder outlet obstruction	• For acute bacterial prostatitis, monitor intake and output and percuss bladder *to assess for signs of overdistention.* • Provide a warm bath *to encouarge urination by helping relieve discomfort and to relax the pelvic floor musculature.* • If a suprapubic catheter is placed, monitor intake and output *to assess patency of tube.* Securely tape tube to abdomen *to prevent kinking.*
Noncompliance (medical therapy)	• Advise patient to continue antibiotic therapy for the full 30 days *to achieve optimum therapeutic results.*

Patient Education

1. Provide information concerning the prostate's relative resistance to antibiotic therapy.
2. Assure the patient that prostatitis not associated with an increased incidence of adenocarcinoma of the prostate and that prostatitis is not a form of venereal disease.
3. Provide anticipatory guidance on managing acute urinary retention.

Evaluation

Patient Outcome	Data Indicating That Outcome is Reached
Acute bacterial prostatitis is resolved.	There are no bacteria in expressed prostatic secretion. Bacteriuria is not present. Patient is afebrile. Irritative voiding symptoms are absent.
Chronic bacterial prostatitis is resolved.	There are no bacteria in expressed prostatic secretion. Bacteriuria is not present. Irritative voiding symptoms are absent. There are no complications; urinary flow is unobstructed.

Patient Outcome	Data Indicating That Outcome is Reached
Nonbacterial prostatitis or prostatodynia is resolved.	There are no inflammatory cells in expressed prostatic secretions. Irritative voiding symptoms are absent. Perineal pain is absent.

SEXUAL FUNCTION DISORDERS

Epididymitis

Epididymitis is defined as any inflammation of the epididymis; it may be caused by bacteria, viruses, parasites, chemicals, or trauma. Epididymitis is divided into three categories: nonspecific, specific, and traumatic. Complications from this condition include orchitis, testicular infarction, and sterility.[45,49]

Epididymitis is the most common of all intrascrotal lesions. It is almost always unilateral and must be differentiated from testicular torsion, tumor, or trauma.[53] An estimated 600,000 cases occur in the United States each year. In men under 35 years of age, epididymitis is most often associated with sexually transmitted disease. It accounts for 20% of all inpatient admissions in military urology practices. In men over 35 years of age, gram-negative rods associated with some abnormality of the urinary tract or performance of some urologic procedure constitute the most common presentation of the condition. Epididymitis is rare in prepubertal boys.[52]

Pathophysiology

Epididymitis occurs most frequently as a result of reflux of urine or some pathogenic agent through the posterior urethra, prostatic ducts, or seminal vesicles. In rare instances the causative pathogen may reach the epididymis via retrograde lymphatic pathways from the wall of the vas deferens or via hematogenous or metastatic routes. In its earlier stage, epididymitis occurs as a type of cellulitis associated with local pain and edema. In the acute stage the entire hemiscrotum becomes a single erythematous, exquisitely painful mass often associated with an inflammatory hydrocele produced by the tunica vaginalis. Later changes include peritubular fibrosis and occlusion of the epididymis that may result in sterility.[81,95]

Nonspecific epididymitis refers to a group of common pathogens that typically gain access to the organ via urethral-vasal reflux in the presence of infected urine. Bladder outlet obstruction requiring the individual to strain in order to void is a predisposing factor to this condition. Nonspecific epididymitis is a common complication of prostatitis, urethral stricture disease, and seminal vesiculitis. Occasionally a nonspecific epididymitis arises from a septic focus such as a pharyngitis. Reflux of sterile urine into the epididymis has been reported to result in inflammation,[45,49] although others dispute this possibility.[39] Strenuous exercise has also been connected with nonpyrogenic epididymitis.[45]

Nonspecific epididymitis also occurs as a complication of certain urologic procedures, particularly transurethral resection of the prostate and urethral catheterization. Postprocedure epididymitis may occur as late as several months following instrumentation because of the persistence of subclinical amounts of bacteria in the urine. It is significant to note that the rate of epididymitis following transurethral resection of the prostate has dropped from 20% to 4% following the institution of routine prophylactic antibiotics after the procedure. Vasectomy has been advocated as a prophylactic measure for men undergoing prostatectomy, but the efficacy of this intervention remains unproven.[49]

Traumatic epididymitis (also referred to as epididymido-orchitis) arises from straining, with reflux of urine into the organ. The etiology of this form of epididymitis remains unclear. Some argue that the trauma only inflames an already present subclinical inflammation of the epididymis, while others propose that the trauma lessens resistance to some more distant foci of infection, allowing invasion of pathogens into the area.[45]

Specific epididymitis refers to a group of known pathogens that invade the epididymis from a urinary focus or via the hematogenous route. The causative organisms most commonly associated with sexually transmitted epididymitis are *Neisseria gonorrhoeae* and *Chlamydia trachomatis* among heterosexual males and *Escherichia coli* among homosexual males. Prompt, aggressive treatment of these sexually transmitted diseases helps curtail the incidence of subsequent epididymitis as demonstrated by the decreasing incidence of gonococcal epididymitis.[52]

Syphilitic epididymitis may occur more often than has been suspected. This form of epididymal inflammation is typically asymptomatic and connected with the second stage of the disease. Diagnosis of syphilitic epididymitis is presumptive and established when other evidence of syphilis is present while urinary tract infection, prostatitis, and urethritis are absent.[45,52]

Many forms of specific epididymitis have been reported that have spread to the organ via the hematogenous route. In cases of brucellosis, epididymitis may be the initial symptom of the condition. Meningococcal septicemia, pneumococcal pneumonia, *Haemophilus influenzae*, and other bacterial diseases have been associated with epididymal invasion. Various parasites such as amebae, schistosoma, and fungi are known to invade the epididymis.[52]

Tubercular epididymitis arises from involvement of the prostate and is one of the few painless forms of the disease. Tuberculosis of the epididymis produces a thickened, beaded organ on palpation and leads to occlusion of the epididymal lumen.[31]

The most common complication of epididymitis is orchitis so the term "epididymo-orchitis" is used. Infertility is a serious long-term complication of epididymitis. Sterility among men with chronic or recurrent bilateral epididymitis is 40%, and men with unilateral epididymitis have a 25% chance of infertility. Recurrences of epididymitis are particularly likely when the underlying disease process (e.g., prostatitis) remains unresolved.[49]

Diagnostic Studies and Findings

White Blood Cell Count

Generally between 20,000 and 30,000 in an acute episode[95]

Urinalysis

Signs of infection may be present

Urine Culture

Reveals associated bacterial cystitis if present

Urethral Discharge Culture

Reveals associated gonococcal or chlamydial urethritis

Prostatic Secretion Culture

Reveals associated prostatitis

Doppler Stethoscope

Good blood flow rules out torsion of testis

Testicular Radionuclide Scan

Good blood flow rules out torsion of testis

Medical Plan

Surgery

Epididymectomy rarely indicated as a therapeutic measure in chronic or tubercular epididymitis[31]

Medications

Mild to moderate cases: oral anti-infective agents, which may be guided by culture and sensitivity data when appropriate; analgesics (ASA gr X q4-6h) used to manage pain and control fever

Severe cases: hospitalization and broad-spectrum antibiotics; combintation of ampicillin and aminoglycoside given pending results of blood culture

Very severe cases: spermatic cord block with lidocaine or procaine hydrochloride; use of steroids has been advocated but any beneficial anti-inflammatory activity is outweighed by potential side effects[110]

Antiemetic agent may be required to control associated nausea and vomiting during acute epididymitis; antipyretics may be indicated for associated fever

Administration of antiemetics justified in order to prevent progression of nausea to a severe state that threatens fluid and electrolyte balance

General Management

Urethral discharge may be copious and is managed by regular cleansing of meatus with hydrogen peroxide[69]

NURSING CARE

Nursing Assessment

Epididymis

Palpable by rolling contents of spermatic cord between thumb and finger

Early in infection, organ is felt as tender and enlarged; later, becomes indistinguishable because of local inflammation

In chronic epididymitis, organ is firm, nodular, moderately tender

Scrotum

Initial stages of epididymitis: scrotal skin is reddened or normal in appearance; as infection progresses, scrotal skin becomes red and hot to touch

Varicocele a common finding

Moderate to severe cases: significant edema of epididymis and adjacent structures (including testis) causes a large mass in affected hemiscrotum so epididymitis cannot be distinguished; overlying skin dry, flaky, and without its normal rugose appearance; spontaneous rupture may occur; mass is exquisitely tender

Elevation of scrotum may result in relief from pain (Prehn's sign)[49]

Testis

Testis on affected side may be painful and enlarged

Masses or induration possible

Abdomen

Lower quadrant pain perceived on affected side

Nausea and Vomiting

Vomiting may be severe during acute period

Nursing Dx & Intervention

Nursing Diagnosis	Nursing Intervention/Rationale
Pain	• Assess and support the scrotum via an athletic support, a towel placed under the scrotum, or a Bellevue bridge *to relieve discomfort.* • Provide analgesics as ordered *to relieve discomfort.* • Use a sitz bath, local heat, or ice pack as prescribed *to relieve discomfort.* • Provide bed rest during the acute period *to prevent discomfort.* • Inform patient that sexual activity or any strenuous physical activity is contraindicated in even mild cases *to prevent discomfort.*
Potential fluid volume deficit	• Assess and curtail all oral intake *to reduce potential for vomiting.* • Maintain records of intake and output including frequency and amount of vomitus *to assess for fluid volume deficit.* • Administer antiemetics as ordered.
Fear	• Assess and reassure patient that epididymitis is not a malignant process and that the mass effect is due to inflammation.

Patient Education

1. Provide instructions on the risk factors associated with epididymitis: prostatitis, urethritis (particularly gonococcal and chlamydial), cystitis, and unusually strenuous physical activity.
2. Emphasize the need for follow-up care aimed at identifying the underlying causes of epididymitis in certain cases.
3. Provide information on the signs and symptoms as well as the natural history of epididymitis and the importance of seeking care promptly.

Evaluation

Patient Outcome	Data Indicating That Outcome is Reached
Epididymitis is resolved.	There is no pain in affected epididymis. Hemiscrotum is not enlarged. Urethral, prostate, and blood cultures are negative.
There are no recurrences.	Underlying prostatitis, urethritis, cystitis, tuberculosis of the urinary tract, or septic hematogenous focus is resolved.
There are no complications.	Sperm count and motility are normal.

Erectile dysfunction

Erectile dysfunction (impotence) is the inability to produce an erection of the penis of sufficient duration and rigidity to engage in intercourse.

Both psychogenic and organic factors contribute to erectile dysfunction. Treatment is aimed at restoring normal erectile and orgasmic function or mimicking the erect penis by injecting a drug into the phallus or via mechanical or surgically implanted devices. Other forms of male sexual dysfunction manifested as loss of libido, premature ejaculation, or inability to achieve orgasm are discussed in Part Three, Pattern IX, Sexuality—Reproductive.

Sexual dysfunction in the male may be noted anytime after the onset of puberty. The incidence of erectile dysfunction increases with age. The incidence of men who seek treatment for erectile dysfunction during the fourth decade of life is 1.5% of the general population; by the seventh decade of life the incidence has risen to 25% of all males.[71] Although the aging process does not inevitably lead to impotence, sexual activity does generally decrease with age because of a variety of social, cultural, and physical factors. A survey of men revealed that 88% of sexually active males under 20 years of age engage in intercourse at least once each week. During the fourth decade of life the proportion of men reporting intercourse at least once a week declined to 80%. During the sixth decade of life only 50% of the men surveyed reported intercourse on a weekly basis; by the seventh decade only 25% had intercourse each week.[71]

The relative incidence of impotence from psychogenic versus organic causes has received great attention. Some investigators have reported that 90% to 95% of cases of impotence are the result of psychogenic causes.[71,94] However, recent data using more sophisticated diagnostic techniques reveal a greater percentage of men whose erectile dysfunction has organic as well as psychogenic components.[71]

Pathophysiology

A wide variety of organic conditions may cause or be associated with impotence.[106] Within this discussion only some of the more commonly encountered organic causes of impotence are considered. An in-depth discussion of the psychosocial influences and ramifications of this condition is presented in Pattern X.

A number of disease processes are associated with erectile dysfunction. These medical disorders may affect the physiologic processes of erection directly, or they may suppress sexual drive without causing true impotence. The psychosocial implications of illness, particularly a chronic condition, may alter a man's self-image and profoundly affect his sexual identity and sexual behaviors. To understand and treat this complex problem, the nurse or physician must have an understanding of the underlying influences affecting erectile function in each individual.[71]

Endocrine problems may affect male sexual function by altering normal function of the hypothalamic-pituitary-gonadal hormonal axis. The typical result of this problem is hypogonadism, which is potentially reversible. The range of hypogonadism is significant and includes cases of mildly impaired libido and incidences of overt eunuchoidism requiring long-term hormonal replacement.[45,71]

The severity of impotence related to endocrine disorders is based on the age of onset and related symptoms that influence any medical decision to attempt to establish or restore potency in an affected male. Complete prepubertal gonadotropic failure may be expressed as hypogonadotropic eunuchoidism. Kallmann's syndrome, or a specific luteinizing hormone–follicle-stimulating hormone disorder. In all of the above conditions a failure of the production and propagation of gonadotropins is noted prepubertally and persists throughout the patient's lifetime. Abnormal growth patterns, a high-pitched voice, and a lack of secondary sex characteristics are associated with hypogonadism leading to impaired sexual function and infertility. Kallmann's syndrome is associated with significant mental retardation, which may affect the medical approach to treatment of impotence.[71,109]

Partial prepubertal gonadotropic failure produces symptoms similar to those of delayed puberty that actually do stem from an identifiable hormonal deficit rather than normal developmental processes. These males have significantly decreased testosterone levels arising from a deficiency in the production of FSH and LH, or LH only.[71]

Selective postpubertal hypogonadism is associated with a loss of testosterone production and a gradual loss of beard and body hair, declining libido, and resultant impotence and infertility. The eunuchoid aspects of this condition are not as prominent as those associated with prepubertal hypogonadism.[71]

Panhypopituitarism causes erectile dysfunction and a number of other hormonal imbalances. The condition is caused by a lesion that renders the pituitary or hypothalamus functionless or by surgical or traumatic ablation.[71,109]

Several congenital syndromes cause erectile dysfunction along with other medical problems. Prader-Willi syndrome causes neonatal hypotonia, mental retardation, obesity, and hypogonadism. Laurence-Moon-Biedl syndrome is an autosomal recessive disorder that results in retinitis pigmentosa, polydactyly, renal anomalies, cryptorchidism, and erectile dysfunction. Familial cerebellar ataxia is also associated with hypogonadism along with ataxic movements and neural deafness. Other syndromes associated with hypogonadism and impotence include Klinefelter's syndrome, Noonan's syndrome, and Ullrich's syndrome.[71]

Any disease or drug that produces hyperprolactinemia also interferes with the hypothalamic-pituitary-gonadotropic axis and causes erectile dysfunction. Medical conditions associated with hyperprolactinemia include certain hormone-producing tumors, endocrine disorders, and a number of drugs such as estrogen compounds and psychotropic drugs.[71]

Other endocrine-based disorders involving the thyroid or adrenal glands may affect erectile function. Castration has been used since antiquity to decrease libido and ultimately ablate normal male sexual function.[71,109]

Chronic heart disease has been associated with impotence, which may be attributed to the disease processes involved and to the use of certain antihypertensive drugs or digitalis preparations. Men with heart disease that is reasonably well controlled should consider sexual activity reasonably safe. In many of these men erectile dysfunction can be prevented by prudent counseling. Sexual dysfunction may be complicated by the use of antihypertensive or antidepressant medications. Digoxin may also adversely affect sexual function by reducing LH and testosterone levels in the body while raising estradiol. Among those men who undergo heart transplant, erectile dysfunction is a potential complication that may be associated with postoperative immunosuppressions.[104]

Erectile dysfunction is relatively common among men who have chronic renal insufficiency and renal failure. Multiple factors contribute to the problem, related both to the disease process itself and to the use of dialysis as a treatment modality. Impotence is a result of Leydig's cell abnormalities with concomitant decreases in the production of testosterone. Hyperprolactinemia and hyperparathyroidism may further complicate the situation. Erectile dysfunction may worsen after the start of dialysis. Many problems in erectile dysfunction are resolved by renal transplant, although transient impotence may be noted in patients who have ligation of the internal artery to provide a blood supply for the transplanted kidney.[104]

Kass and his associates[55] studied a group of men with chronic obstructive pulmonary disease and found that 19% had problems with sexual function. The incidence of impotence in these men was largely attributed to psychosocial aspects of the disease rather than primary organic sexual dysfunction.

Several neurologic conditions are associated with erectile dysfunction. The presence of erectile dysfunction in spinal cord injury is influenced by the level of the lesion, the presence of spinal shock, and the "completeness" of the injury. Following a traumatic injury to the spinal cord, all erectile activity of the penis is inhibited. The generation of posttraumatic erections is typically associated with cessation of spinal shock. The period of time after which erectile activity reappears following spinal cord injury is highly variable, ranging from 24 hours to 18 months.[71]

Two types of erection are observed in men with spinal cord injury: reflexogenic erections, which are mediated by spinal cord centers, and psychogenic erections, which are mediated by supraspinal sexual centers. The incidence of erections among spinal cord–injured men is 63.5% to 94%, but the incidence of consistently successful erections is 23% to 33%.[71] The relatively low rate of successful potency among men with spinal cord injuries is largely the result of the characteristics of reflexogenic erections, which are relatively brief and respond to a variety of tactile sensations, rendering penile response significantly altered from previous brain-centered control of sexual response.

Ejaculation is relatively rare among men with spinal cord injury. Ejaculation requires smooth coordination between autonomic and somatic impulses. The likelihood of orgasm among patients with complete spinal cord injuries is 3% to 19.7%. Lower spinal cord injury is correlated with an increased likelihood of ejaculation but a relatively low incidence of erections (24.2%).[71]

Multiple sclerosis is another neurologic condition associated with male sexual dysfunction. Demyelination of the lateral horns of the lumbar spinal cord is theorized to be the critical underlying organic explanation for impotence among these men. Approximately 91% of men with multiple sclerosis have significant sexual dysfunction.[71]

Epilepsy involving the parietal lobes of the brain is associated with a higher incidence of impotence than other forms of the disease. In most cases the relative contribution of antiseizure medications to sexual dysfunction is negligible. Many men experience continuing desire for sex with inability to sustain or maintain erections, and fewer experience a loss of libido.[104]

Diabetes mellitus is a causative factor in the development of erectile dysfunction because of a complex interplay of psychologic and organic factors. Erectile dysfunction may be noted near the time a diagnosis of diabetes is established; the diagnosis contributes to psychosocial factors (alterations in self-image and anxiety related to chronic disease) and physiologic factors resulting from insulin deficiency. Sexual dysfunction is generally resolved after the condition is regulated with exogenous insulin.[104]

Later problems related to sexual function in the diabetic male have an insidious onset and are generally progressive. Hormonal factors have been theorized but are not supported by objective evidence. Diabetic neuropathies are often implicated in the genesis of impotence among diabetic men based on indirect evidence linking autonomic nervous abnormalities. Vascular compromise associated with diabetic angiopathy may influence potency by affecting the arterial blood supply of the cavernous bodies of the penis.[71,104]

Various vascular disorders may also lead to male sexual dysfunction by adversely affecting the vascular component of erections. Aortoiliac occlusion leads to erectile impairment in approximately 70% of affected men. Arteriosclerosis is connected with an increased incidence of erectile dysfunction, although a causal link is not always apparent. Peripheral arterial insufficiency most commonly occurs in men over 40 years of age, so other factors of aging may exert an influence. However, it is known that arteriosclerosis is the most common cause of occlusion of the penile artery, which may lead to erectile insufficiency, and that as many as 40% to 50% of men with diagnosed peripheral arterial disease report sexual dysfunction if questioned closely.[57,104]

Many drugs have been associated with erectile dysfunction. Duration, frequency, and dosage of the drug affect the likelihood of impotence or loss of libido and secondary erectile dysfunction. It is essential to assess the use of all drugs including prescribed, over-the-counter, and recreational agents a man may be using.[71]

Endocrine drugs are used in a variety of hormonal abnormalities and may be used to treat cancer. Any exogenous estrogens or progestins ultimately result in impotence if given in sufficient dosages. Anabolic steroids may suppress endogenous steroid levels and cause impotence when the drug is discontinued.[71]

Antihypertensive drugs, particularly the α- and β-adrenergic blocking agents, are associated with impotence, although the exact mechanism of sexual dysfunction may be more closely related to a loss of libido than to lowering of systemic arterial blood pressure.[75] The following antihypertensive drugs are associated with male sexual dysfunction: clonidine (Catapres), guanethidine (Ismelin), hydralazine (Apresoline), monoamine oxidase inhibitors, methyldopa (Aldomet), phentolamine (Regitine), propranolol (Inderal), and reserpine (Serpasil).[71]

Two cardiac agents, digoxin and disopyramide, are commonly linked to male sexual dysfunction. The role of digoxin in erectile function was discussed in Chapter 1; disopyramide is an antiarrhythmic agent with parasympathetic properties that may contribute to erectile difficulties.[71]

The diuretic agents chlorthalidone and spironolactone may cause loss of libido and erectile dysfunction in a few instances. Hydrochlorothiazide is also linked to sexual dysfunction.[71]

Psychoactive drugs affect the central nervous system in many ways that are poorly understood. A significant number of these drugs, including sedatives, amphetamines, antidepressants, and antipsychotic agents, may cause impotence, presumably because of their effects on the central nervous system. The precise mechanisms by which this side effect occurs are not completely understood.[71] These drugs include weight reduction drugs (diethylpropion and phentermine hydrochloride), antidepressant agents (amitriptyline and monoamine oxidase inhibitors), antianxiety/sedative agents (benzodiazapines and glutethimide), and lithium carbonate.[71]

Anticholinergic agents such as propantheline are known to cause impotence as a side effect. Antiparkinson drugs are linked to erectile dysfunction and delayed ejaculation. The immunosuppressive agents are associated with impotence, but the underlying mechanism may be related to chemically induced psychogenic factors and general alterations in metabolism. Indomethacin is related to impotence arising from its antiprostaglandin effects. Metronidazole suppresses libido via some unknown process.[71]

A number of recreational drugs also affect male sexual function. Alcohol has been known to heighten desire while adversely affecting performance. Alcoholism is particularly associated with an increased incidence of impotence. Tobacco use has been linked to erectile dysfunction in several recent studies. Nicotine may cause impotence by causing vasoconstriction of the penile arteries, although the phenomenon requires further study to establish a causal link. Other drugs connected with male sexual dysfunction include amphetamines, barbiturates, opiates, cannabis (the active component of marijuana), and cocaine.[71,104]

A comprehensive discussion of the drugs that affect male sexual function is beyond the scope of this chapter. Inserts in packages of individual drugs are an excellent source for assessing sexual dysfunction as a causative agent when impotence is a problem. However, nurses must be aware that overzealous cautions regarding potential sexual dysfunction are not indicated, since such counseling may itself increase performance anxiety and exacerbate impotence.

Certain surgical procedures of the abdomen, thorax, and genital area may result in temporary failure of erectile function; prostatectomy and ileostomy or colostomy are particularly likely to result in alterations in male sexual function. Of all the forms of prostatectomy, open surgery using a perineal approach is the most likely to produce impotence. Transurethral resection of the prostate, the most common approach to prostatectomy, should not result in impotence but is associated with retrograde ejaculation. An open, communicative relationship with the patient including anticipatory guidance of expected postoperative potency is associated with a dramatically reduced likelihood of complaints of erectile dysfunction following the procedure.[104]

Any extensive surgical procedure involving the lower abdomen may lead to the inadvertent destruction of nerves or blood vessels that supply the cavernous bodies in the penis. The incidence of erectile dysfunction is particularly high in men who undergo ileostomy or colostomy with the attendant alteration in body image. Thus sexual dysfunction in these men may have psychogenic and organic components.[104]

Erectile dysfunction may also arise from local disorders of the penis such as priapism, Peyronie's disease, and abnormal leakage of blood from the corpora cavernosa. Priapism is a prolonged, painful erection caused by the blockage of blood flow from the corpora cavernosa. Underlying causes may be primarily traumatic, neurogenic, vascular, or neoplastic. Some men experience idiopathic episodes of priapism, although the condition has been tentatively linked to alcohol and drug use often noted among these men. Peyronie's disease is an abnormal lateral curvature of the penis that is most likely to occur during the fifth and sixth decades of life. The etiology is unclear; curvature is caused by fibroelastic plaques that form in the penis. The plaques may regress spontaneously, or they may persist despite various treatment methodologies. Impotence often accompanies Peyronie's disease and may be related to abnormal blood flow through the corpora cavernosa. Mechanical defects of the corpora cavernosa may result in low intracavernous pressure, which causes insufficient rigidity for penetration. Potency is restored by surgical repair of the defect.[71,104]

Diagnostic Studies and Findings

Serum Testosterone

Low in impotence because of abnormality of hypothalamic-pituitary-gonadal axis

Serum Prolactin

High when testosterone is abnormally low

Serum FSH

Abnormal when impotence is result of abnormality of hormonal axis

Serum LH

Abnormal when impotence is result of abnormality of hormonal axis

Glucose Tolerance Test

Abnormal in cases of diabetes mellitus

Sacral Evoked Responses

Increased bulbocavernous latency in diabetic males with autonomic neuropathy

Urodynamic Testing

Abnormal sensations of bladder filling on cystometrogram and abnormal urecholine supersensitivity test in males with autonomic neuropathy

Penile Systolic Blood Pressure

Low in cases of vascular impotence

Penile Pulse Volume Recording

Abnormal in cases of vascular impotence

Infusion Cavernosography

Venous leak in cases of vascular impotence[45]

Infusion Cavernosometry

A narrow scalp vein needle is placed into the corpora cavernosus, and saline or contrast medium is injected at a constant or variable rate to maintain a constant intracavernous pressure; detects abnormal cavernous filling or anomalous venous drainage.[61]

Nocturnal Penile Tumescence

Absent nocturnal erections when underlying cause of impotence is primarily organic rather than psychogenic[71]

Snap-Gauge Testing

Breakage of three pressure-sensitive plastic bands indicates sufficient pressure for penetration

Inability to break bands during sleep study indicates erectile dysfunction

Medical Plan

Surgery

Corrective surgery of arterial occlusion or venous drainage anomalies may correct erectile dysfunction

Revascularization of penis may be attempted by isolating epigastric artery and reanastomosing it directly to a corporal body[57]

Penile prosthesis may be implanted to produce sufficient rigidity for penetration and intercourse; semirigid and inflatable devices are available[36,79]

Medications

Testosterone replacement therapy indicated in cases of hypogonadism

Luteinizing hormone–releasing hormone (LHRH), LH, or FSH may be used in males with identifiable abnormalities of the hypothalamic-pituitary-gonadal axis; all other results of hormonal therapy in males with erectile dysfunction are caused by placebo effect[104]

Bromocriptine, zinc, and glyceryl trinitrate have been used to treat erectile dysfunction in selected cases with variable results

Papaverine alone or in combination with phentolamine may be used to produce erections in males with vascular erectile dysfunction; these men are taught to inject the penis themselves[118]

General Management

Mechanical pump systems using a vacuum device such as the Erect-Aid or Correct-Aid may produce erections; a vacuum that encourages blood inflow into the penis is established external to the penis, and a restrictive device is used to discourage venous outflow and thereby produce tumescence

Discontinue use of any recreational drugs associated with erectile dysfunction, including illicit drugs, tobacco, ethanol, and anabolic steroids; alcohol consumption must be controlled to reestablish potency

NURSING CARE

Nursing Assessment

External Genitalia

Normal appearance of penis, scrotum, and perineal area

Normal hair distribution, normal phallic size, bilaterally descended testes except in males with endocrine disorders resulting in hypogonadism, in which cases penis will be small, testes small and abnormally soft or cryptorchid, and hair distribution abnormal or absent

Palpation of penis will reveal hard plaques in Peyronie's disease

Polaroid pictures of penile erection obtained by patient will show penile curvature[71]

Rectal Examination

Loss of anal sphincter tone with absent bulbocavernous reflex in local neuropathy

Absent saddle sensation with certain partial or complete spinal cord injuries[71]

Peripheral Pulses

Decreased or absent in vascular impotence

Neurologic Examination

Abnormal in men with underlying neurologic disease

Nursing Dx & Intervention

Nursing Diagnosis	Nursing Intervention/Rationale
Sexual dysfunction	• Encourage counseling and assistance in seeking appropriate health care *to deal with sexual dysfunction or a surgical procedure likely to alter sexual function because of organic or psychogenic reasons*. Open discussion with physician colleagues and clearly stated politics concerning the nurse's roles and responsibilities in cases of existing or potential dysfunction are needed.
Self-esteem disturbance	• Empathy and opportunities to express feelings are indicated as the patient reintegrates self-concepts following a change in body image. • Male sexuality is deeply rooted in ideals of social, athletic, physical, and sexual performance.

Nursing Diagnosis	Nursing Intervention/Rationale
	Any circumstance that significantly alters self-concepts and threatens self-esteem may adversely affect sexual function. Chronic disease, creation of a surgical stoma, and physical changes resulting from neurologic disease or spinal cord trauma significantly challenge any man's self-image. • Psychologic or psychiatric counseling is often a useful adjunct and may be suggested to a patient after a sufficiently trusting relationship has been established *to reestablish positive, realistic self-concept.*

Patient Education

1. Provide instruction about various implantable prosthetic devices in suitable candidates after consultation with the physician.
2. Instruction of expectations of sexual abilities following specific surgical procedures will help prevent needless loss of sexual function due to anxiety.

Evaluation

Patient Outcome	Data Indicating That Outcome is Reached
Impotence is resolved.	Patient reports increased satisfaction in sexual life and adequate onset, duration, and rigidity of erections.
Penile prosthesis is successfully implanted.	Patient has an operational semirigid or inflatable penile prosthesis. There is no local infection, pain, or erosion.

Medical Interventions and Related Nursing Care

Bladder Neck Suspension

Description and Rationale

Bladder neck suspension is used in women to correct stress urinary incontinence secondary to pelvic relaxation. A number of procedures have been described, including the Marshall-Marchetti-Krantz (MMK) operation, Stamey's vesicopexy, Burch retropubic colposuspension, and Peyrera needle suspension. The restoration of continence is attained via increasing urethral resistance. Other procedures such as repair of urethrocele, cystocele, or enterocele may be performed to promote bladder emptying and optimum detrusor function.

Contraindications and Cautions

1. Bladder neck suspension is contraindicated in cases of severe stress urinary incontinence as a result of urethral sphincter damage.

Preprocedural Nursing Care

1. Preoperative teaching should include information concerning recompensation of detrusor tone and potential for increased difficulty emptying bladder during postoperative period.

NURSING CARE

Nursing Assessment

Abdomen

Redness, edema, and drainage at wound site if abdominal approach used

Perineum

Vaginal discharge
Pain if wound infection present

Voiding Behaviors

Decreased force of urinary stream
Perceptions of incomplete bladder emptying or acute urinary retention

Pain

Dysuria
Pelvic pain
Incisional or abdominal pain

Nursing Dx & Intervention

Nursing Diagnosis	Nursing Intervention/Rationale
Altered patterns of urinary elimination	• Monitor intake and output. • Check urine residuals as directed *to assess for urinary retention.* • Teach intermittent self-catheterization as directed *to prevent urinary retention.* • Teach double-void technique as directed *to prevent urinary retention.*
Fear	• Reasure patient that retention is probably caused by myogenic decompensation of detrusor and that return of normal voiding patterns is expected unless preoperative urodynamics reveal neuropathic bladder.
Pain	• Administer analgesic agents as directed. • Encourage regular bladder emptying during postoperative recuperation *to prevent discomfort from distended bladder.*

Patient Education

1. Explain that return of normal voiding patterns may require time.

Evaluation

Patient Outcome	Data Indicating That Outcome is Reached
Stress urinary incontinence is not present.	Urodynamics are normal. Marshall test is negative.
Bladder emptying is adequate.	Postvoid residual is 20% of total bladder volume or less.

Extracorporeal Shock Wave Lithotripsy

Description and Rationale

Extracorporeal shock wave lithotripsy (ESWL) is an exciting new urologic technology that crushes renal and ureteral calculi without invasion of the body. The patient is given epidural anesthesia and placed in a lithotripter tub with degassed water. The calculi are located via fluoroscopic techniques, and ultrasonic shock waves are used to crush the stone into powder. The fragments are passed in the urine. The entire procedure requires approximately 1 hour.

Contraindications and Cautions

1. Patients unsuitable for epidural or spinal anesthesia may require general anesthesia.
2. Patients unable to cooperate with requirements of positioning may be managed by other approaches.
3. Children may be too small for equipment.

Preprocedural Nursing Care

1. Preoperative teaching is essential to clarify misconceptions concerning this relatively new intervention.

NURSING CARE

Nursing Assessment

Urinary Output and Voiding Behavior

Passage of stone particles
Dysuria; bladder colic

Pain

Renal colic

Temperature

Fever

Nursing Dx & Intervention

Nursing Diagnosis	Nursing Intervention/Rationale
Altered renal tissue perfusion	• Monitor patient for flank pain *to assess potential blockage of urinary transport system by stone fragments.* • Monitor urine for color and consistency *to assess for hematuria.* • Monitor BUN and creatinine *to assess for systemic signs of urinary obstruction.* • Maintain adequate fluid intake and strain urine for passage of stone particles *to prevent urinary stasis and potential upper urinary tract obstruction.*
Altered patterns of urinary elimination	• Monitor output from urethral catheter and observe catheter for kinks *to prevent urinary retention.*
Pain	• Provide analgesics as ordered.

Patient Education

1. Teach techniques for preventing recurrent stone formation, including drugs, diet, and fluid intake.

Evaluation

Patient Outcome	Data Indicating That Outcome is Reached
Stones are not present.	Roentgenogram of kidneys, ureters, and bladder (KUB) and intravenous pyelogram (IVP) are normal.
There is no obstruction.	Patient does not experience pain. IVP is normal.

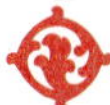

Intrapenile Prosthetic Devices

Description and Rationale

Intrapenile prosthetic devices (IPPs) are used when medical, surgical, or psychologic methods are inadequate to restore erectile function. Placement of a device is completed after thorough investigation of organic and psychogenic stigmata of underlying erectile failure and careful psychologic assessment for suitability of the procedure are completed.

A number of devices are available. Semirigid devices include Small-Carrion, Finney Flexirod, and the Jonas Implant. These devices are generally less expensive than inflatable penile prostheses but more difficult to conceal. The inflatable penile prosthesis allows the penis to remain in a flaccid stage until the device is pumped to produce an erection. These devices are more prone to mechanical difficulties than the semirigid devices.

Contraindications and Cautions

1. IPPs are contraindicated in patients with deep-rooted psychologic abnormalities underlying erectile dysfunction.

Preprocedural Nursing Care

1. Sexual counseling of male patient and partner is essential during both preoperative and postoperative periods.

NURSING CARE

Nursing Assessment

Penis

Redness
Edema
Signs of erosion of prosthetic device

Scrotum and Perineum

Hematoma for 2 to 3 weeks; edema for 24 hours postoperatively
Discharge and hemorrhage from incision

Temperature

Fever

Urinary Output

Normal voiding patterns; catheter drainage rarely needed

Nursing Dx & Intervention

Nursing Diagnosis	Nursing Intervention/Rationale
Pain	• Administer analgesic agents as ordered.
Potential for infection	• Observe penis and scrotum for signs of infection. • Monitor temperature.
Potential impaired skin intregrity	• Observe operative site for signs of erosion—pallid, stretched skin; appearance of device outline at skin surface; and pain—*to assess for erosion of device through skin.*
Self-esteem disturbance	• Offer support and encouragement regarding use of implant. • Reinforce need for patient and partner to have knowledge and understanding of the use of the device.

Patient Education

1. Instruct patient to abstain from sex for 21 days after surgery to allow for adequate healing if semirigid device is used.
2. Instruct patient to inflate Scott inflatable penile prosthesis (IPP) repeatedly before use to encourage formation of fibrous sheath around device.
3. Instruct patient on techniques of concealing semirigid device in clothing.
4. Instruct patient about signs of erosion or infection.
5. Instruct patient *and partner* in inflation and deflation of inflatable penile prostheses.
6. Instruct patient to avoid contact sports or lifting heavy objects for 21 days after IPP is placed.

Evaluation

Patient Outcome	Data Indicating That Outcome is Reached
There is no infection.	Patient is afebrile. Wound healing is normal.
There is no erosion.	Size, color, and contour of penis are normal.
Patient makes an adequate adjustment to the IPP.	Patient *and* partner give subjective report of satisfaction with device. Patient resumes sexual relations with partner. Patient can demonstrate correct technique for inflating and deflating Scott inflatable prosthesis.

Open Prostatectomy

Description and Rationale

Open prostatectomy refers to removal of the prostate with or without the prostatic capsule. Several surgical approaches may be used including suprapubic, transvesical, retropubic, perineal, and transcoccygeal. In the suprapubic or transvesical procedures the prostate is removed through the cavity of the bladder. Retropubic prostatectomy is performed through a low abdominal incision without opening the bladder. The most radical of the open procedures for prostatectomy is the perineal approach in which the incision is made between the scrotum and rectum. The transcoccygeal approach allows better surgical access to the posterior lobes of the prostate. The perineal approach is usually associated with loss of erection, orgasm, and ejaculatory function. It is not uncommon for sexual dysfunction to occur when the prostatic capsule is removed.

The suprapubic and retropubic approaches may be used as open surgical approaches when the gland is too large for transurethral resection; they are not generally used for cancer. In these incidences the capsule is left intact.

Perineal prostatectomy is most often performed for cancer of the prostate when it is confined to the capsule. Some controversy exists regarding the use of radical prostatectomy when the tumor extends through the capsule.

Contraindications and Cautions

1. Small fibrous prostate
2. Presence of cancer (suprapubic, retropubic)

Preprocedural Nursing Care

1. Patient teaching is done, including potential sexual impairment if appropriate.
2. Perineum, external genitalia, abdomen, and upper halves of thighs are shaved the night before surgery.
3. Cleansing enemas are given until clear.

Medical Plan

Medications

Laxatives (stool softeners)
Docusate (Colace), 100 mg/d po
Analgesics prn

General Management

Urethral catheter, suprapubic catheter, and Penrose drain
Intravenous fluids
Clear diet progressing to regular diet
Heat lamp; sitz bath (perineal incision)

NURSING CARE

Nursing Assessment

Incision

Redness; pain; edema; drainage

Temperature

Fever

Pain

Postoperative pain

Urinary Output

Amount of urinary output through urethral catheter or suprapubic catheter
Presence of bright red blood
Stress incontinence (may last for a few days to 6 months)
Urethral stricture

Other Complications

Epididymitis

Sexual Dysfunction

Impotence
Retrograde ejaculation

Nursing Dx & Intervention

Nursing Diagnosis	Nursing Intervention/Rationale
Patient problem: potential hemorrhage	• Observe urine output for color, consistency, volume, and presence of blood clots *to assess for excessive bleeding.* • Maintain catheter traction as directed *to prevent hemorrhage.* • Monitor vital signs *to assess for systemic signs of hemorrhage.*
Potential for infection	• Maintain sterile urinary drainage system *to prevent infection.* • Monitor vital signs to assess for systemic signs of infection.
Altered patterns of urinary elimination	• Assess output through urethral or suprapubic catheter for volume *to prevent urinary retention.* • Observe catheters for kinking and presence of blood clots *to prevent urinary retention.*
Body image disturbance	• Discuss implicatons of removal of prostatic capsule with patient and in consultation with urologist. *Likelihood of altered erectile dysfunction varies significantly with surgical techniques. Altered potential for fertility is expected and must be discussed fully with patient.* • Assist patient in exploring anxiety and fears related to procedure, provide factual information concerning implications of procedure as indicated. *Exploration of feelings of fear and anxiety with reassurance of objective facts related to procedure allows optimum opportunity for patient to regain positive body image.* • Discuss alternative means of sexual expression, such as penile prosthesis, as indicated and in consultation with urologist *to reassure patient of realistic alternatives in cases where erectile dysfunction may occur.*
Potential impaired skin integrity	• Change dressing frequently *to prevent skin irritation from damp dressing.* • Cleanse skin gently and pat dry or use a hair dryer *to dry skin and prevent irritation.* • Apply moisture barrier ointments and skin sealants (Brad Protective Barrier Film; Skin Prep) *to protect the skin.*

Patient Education

1. Discuss incisional care with the patient.
2. Discuss skin protection techniques with the patient if drainage is still continuing at time of discharge.
3. Urine color will not clear up for 4 to 8 weeks, but the patient should notify physician if it changes and becomes bright red with clots.
4. Provide teaching and counseling regarding sexual concerns.

Evaluation

Patient Outcome	Data Indicating That Outcome is Reached
Urinary elimination is normal.	Output is adequate. Color is clear. Patient does not experience pain, burning, or bladder spasms.
Sexual functioning resumes.	Patient is able to obtain an erection. Retrograde ejaculation may occur. Patient is scheduled for or has had a penile prosthesis if indicated.

Open Urologic Surgery

(Nephrectomy, partial nephrectomy, nephrolithotomy, pyelolithotomy, ureterolithotomy, cystectomy)

Description and Rationale

Open urologic surgeries include nephrectomy, partial nephrectomy, nephrolithotomy, pyelolithotomy, ureterolithotomy, and cystectomy. The care of the patient during these procedures is similar, and all involve an open surgical incision. Surgery of the kidney is accomplished through a flank incision, while the operative approach for bladder surgeries is an anterior incision.

Indications for nephrectomy include calculus, hemorrhage, hydronephrosis, hypertension, neoplasms, renal donation, trauma, and vascular disease.[39] Partial nephrectomy is performed to preserve as much renal function as possible in the same conditions that may require nephrectomy. A partial nephrectomy is important when contralateral renal function is impaired. Stones in the kidney, pelvis, or ureter may be removed by an open urologic incision if newer techniques of extracorporeal shock wave lithotripsy (ESWL) and percutaneous ureteroscopic stone removal are ineffective.

Contraindications and Cautions

1. If the condition is bilateral, it is important to preserve total renal function.
2. Nephrostomy drainage may be required following open urologic surgeries through stents or tubes to allow for adequate healing when the potential for wound healing is suboptimal, scar tissue is significant, or reconstructive procedures require splinting.

Preprocedural Nursing Care

1. Preoperative teaching concerns the procedure, presence of catheter, and stents for surgery, and turning, coughing, and leg exercises following surgery.
2. Give nothing by mouth past midnight.

NURSING CARE

Nursing Assessment

Incision

Redness; pain; edema; drainage

Temperature

Fever

Urinary Output

Amount of urinary output through nephrostomy tube or catheter
Presence of bright red blood
Absence of urinary output through catheter

Pain

Incisional; postoperative

Hemorrhage

Incisional; through drains, tubes, or catheter

Nursing Dx & Intervention

Nursing Diagnosis	Nursing Intervention/Rationale
Patient problem: potential hemorrhage	• Assess patient for signs and symptoms of bleeding. • Evaluate all tube drainage for amount, color, and consistency. *Persistent bleeding is noted as bloody or serosanguineous discharge through surgical drains.* • Observe surgical wound for color, warmth, and discharge *to assess for signs of bleeding (bloody discharge through wound with or without separation of borders) and signs of infection (purulent discharge from wound, increasing redness, warmth at operative site).*
Potential fluid volume deficit	• Monitor intake and output, daily weights, and BUN and creatinine levels *to assess for hypovolemia; poor fluid intake, rising BUN and creatinine, and rapid weight loss are potential signs of fluid volume deficit that impair healing and may compromise renal function.*

Nursing Diagnosis	Nursing Intervention/Rationale
Pain	• Provide analgesics as ordered. • Provide medications to decrease detrusor contractility as ordered *to prevent bladder spasms associated with urethral or suprapubic catheterization and surgical manipulation of the lower urinary tract.*
Altered patterns of urinary elimination	• Monitor urinary output through urethral catheter, nephrostomy tube, suprapubic catheter, or other drainage tube *to prevent urinary retention.*
Potential impaired skin integrity	• Use skin barrier (pectin wafer) around Penrose drain or stab wound *to protect skin from potential irritation from discharge.* • Use a sterile drainage wound collection system if drainage is copious *to protect skin from discharge and assess output.* • Maintain sterile dressing changes *to protect skin adjacent to surgical incision from discharge.*

Patient Education

1. Patient education varies with primary etiology; refer to specific discussions of urologic diseases.
2. The patient should be informed about incision care and management of any drains or tubes.

Evaluation

Patient Outcome	Data Indicating That Outcome is Reached
There is no infection.	There are no signs of redness, edema, or inflammation of incision.
Urinary output is adequate.	Urinary output is sufficient. BUN and creatinine levels are normal.
Patient returns to activities of daily living.	Patient is able to manage all presurgical activities, including work and recreational activities.

Percutaneous Nephroscopic Stone Removal

Description and Rationale

Percutaneous nephroscopic stone removal is a nonsurgical technique to treat urolithiasis. A nephrostomy tube is placed percutaneously into the proper calyx under fluoroscopic monitoring, and a dilator system is used to allow insertion of a nephroscope with one or more working channels. Several methods may be used to remove calculi percutaneously. A stone basket may be used to retrieve relatively small calculi. Larger stones may be first broken via ultrasonic lithotripter, laser, or electrolysis. Remaining fragments are then removed via a stone basket or flushed from the collecting system mechanically or physiologically.

Contraindications and Cautions

1. Septicemia should be adequately controlled before percutaneous nephroscopic stone removal is attempted.
2. If obstruction is significant, a nephrostomy tube may be placed with the patient under local anesthesia to facilitate adequate pelvic drainage.

Preprocedural Nursing Care

1. Monitor for signs and symptoms of gram-negative septicemia and septic shock including increased fever, pulse, respirations, and blood pressure followed by hypotension and potential cardiovascular compromise.

NURSING CARE

Nursing Assessment

Pain

Renal colic
Acute flank pain

Temperature

Fever

Urinary Output

Oliguria or anuria in cases of bilateral obstruction

Other Complications

Nausea, vomiting, and ileus secondary to renal colic

Nephrostomy Tube

Hematuria
Frank bleeding

Nursing Dx & Intervention

Nursing Diagnosis	Nursing Intervention/Rationale
Patient problem: potential hemorrhage	• Observe flank for mass and observe nephrostomy tube for amount and characteristics of discharge (color, consistency) *to assess for hemorrhage from affected kidney and urinary transport system.* • Monitor pulse and blood pressure *to assess for systemic signs of hemorrhage.*
Pain	• Administer analgesics as ordered.
Altered patterns of urinary elimination	• Observe output through nephrostomy tube for color consistency and volume *to prevent urinary retention.* • Monitor patency of tubes and irrigate tubes as directed *to prevent urinary retention.*

Patient Education

1. Teach techniques for preventing recurrent stone formation including drugs, diet, and fluid intake.

Evaluation

Patient Outcome	Data Indicating That Outcome is Reached
Hemorrhage is absent.	Urine drainage from nephrostomy tube is clear. Vital signs are within normal limits.
There is no obstruction.	Patient does not experience renal colic. Creatinine and BUN levels are within normal limits.
Infection is absent.	Patient is afebrile. Urine and blood cultures are negative.

Transurethral Resection

Description and Rationale

Transurethral resection (TUR) of bladder tumors, prostatic hyperplasia, and bladder neck fibrosis are common urologic procedures. A resectoscope is inserted through the urethra, and the tissue is removed (resected). The instruments allow excision and coagulation of tissue with continuous flow of an irrigation solution. The anourethral resection of bladder tumors may be indicated for tumors that do not extend through the muscle layer of the bladder and includes radon seed implantation. Transurethral resection of the prostate (TURP) is indicated for benign prostatic hyperplasia when the urethra is being obstructed by tissue. Transurethral resection of the fibrotic bladder neck is used to alleviate obstruction.

Contraindications and Cautions

1. TURP is contraindicated if the prostate gland is more than 40 to 50 g.
2. TURP is contraindicated in the presence of a urinary tract infection.
3. A small-caliber urethra or a urethral stricture may make TUR difficult and an open procedure more appropriate.
4. Physical conditions such as ankylosis of the hip or irreversible scrotal hernia that may interfere with positioning for TUR would be a contraindication.

Preprocedural Nursing Care

1. Preoperative teaching should include the fact that sexual potency is unaffected by retrograde ejaculation but infertility does occur.

Medical Plan

Medications

Analgesics as ordered
Antibiotics
Gentamicin (Garamycin), 3 mg/kg in 3 divided doses per 24 h

General Management

Foley catheter with or without continuous irrigation

NURSING CARE

Nursing Assessment

Bladder and Prostate

Urinary output; presence of clots; adequate drainage of catheter

Hemorrhage; drop in blood pressure; increase in pulse rate
Perforation of bladder; drainage of urine into peritoneal space; fever; pain; peritoneal inflammation
Perforation of prostate; change in blood pressure and respirations; pain; failure of irrigating fluid to return; palpable suprapubic mass

Temperature
Fever

Mental Status
Acute confusion
Restlessness
Changes in behavior

Nursing Dx & Intervention

Nursing Diagnosis	Nursing Intervention/Rationale
Altered patterns of urinary elimination	• Evaluate drainage through Foley catheter frequently; assess for passage of clots *to prevent urinary retention secondary to obstructed catheter.* • Maintain continuous irrigation as ordered *to help prevent obstruction of catheter via blood or other discharge from operative area.* • Irrigate blood clots from bladder and catheter as necessary *to prevent urinary retention.*
Patient problem: potential hemorrhage	• Assess urinary output for color and presence of blood clots *to detect and prevent excessive hemorrhage from operative site.* • Maintain catheter securely in place; maintain any traction placed against catheter as directed *to prevent hemorrhage from operative site.* • Monitor vital signs as indicated *to assess for systemic signs of hemorrhage.*
Pain	• Provide analgesics as ordered. • Provide medications to decrease detrusor contractility as directed *to prevent discomfort associated with bladder spasm.*
Fluid volume excess (potential)	• Observe for signs of cerebral edema: restlessness, confusion, behavioral changes. *Absorption of irrigation fluid through prostatic sinuses may result in fluid volume excess with accompanying electrolyte imbalance (hyponatremia).*
Altered sexuality patterns	• Provide patient with an opportunity to discuss potential issues associated with sexuality after transurethral surgery. *Erectile dysfunction is not expected following transurethral surgery; sexual activity can be resumed 6 to 8 weeks after procedure. Retrograde ejaculations and altered fertility potential are expected.*

Patient Education

1. Encourage the patient to maintain adequate fluid intake and report any signs of incontinence, urinary tract infection (burning, urgency), or inability to void to urologist.
2. Follow-up for bladder tumor resections includes radiation and chemotherapy. Refer to sections on cancer management and interventions.

Evaluation

Patient Outcome	Data Indicating That Outcome is Reached
Vital signs are within normal limits.	There are no signs of infection or hemorrhage.
Urinary elimination is normal.	Urine is clear and yellow. Patient does not experience discomfort or difficulty on voiding.
Sexual function in male is unimpaired.	Patient returns to presurgical sexual pattern.

Urinary Diversion

Description and Rationale

A urinary diversion is any one of a number of surgical procedures that establish an unimpeded flow of urine, usually through a stoma. It is possible to divert the urine at any level in the urinary tract.

Supravesical diversions. Diverting the urine at the level of the kidney is done by nephrostomy or pyelostomy. A nephrostomy is a high urinary diversion involving the placement of a catheter through the renal pelvis and into the renal calyces. Indications for placement of a nephrostomy tube are complete obstruction of the ureter, bypassing a urinary fistula, or irrigation of the renal pelvis. A nephrostomy tube is placed intraoperatively during a pyeloplasty or as an emergency procedure for the relief of kidney or ureteral obstruction.[39] Percutaneous placement of a nephrostomy tube under radiographic or ultrasound control has largely replaced the more traditional method of placement. The Pezzer or mushroom catheter, the Malecot or batwing catheter, or a small-lumen Foley catheter with a 5 cc balloon is used as nephrostomy tubes.[84]

Because of the problems associated with long-term nephrostomy drainage, (infection, stone formation, intermittent hematuria, frank renal hemorrhage, or accidental dislodgment of the tube) it is typically used only as a temporary method of diversion.[106]

A pyelostomy is an opening into the renal pelvis made by catheter placement or by the creation of a stoma. Tube pyelostomy diversion carries equal risk as a nephrostomy; therefore tubeless diversion is substituted whenever possible. A cutaneous pyelostomy is performed infrequently, but is designed for children requiring a high urinary diversion. Because children have less subcutaneous fat and a relatively mobile kidney, it is a comparatively simple technical procedure.[58]

Ureterostomy, another type of supravesical urinary diversion, is done with a tube or stoma. A cystoscope may be used to pass a ureteral catheter up the ureter into the renal pelvis if the ureter is unobstructed or only partially obstructed. A diversion where the ureter is anastomosed to the skin is called a cutaneous ureterostomy.[84] Ureterostomy is appropriate in a patient with thickened dilated ureters when more aggressive urinary diversion surgery is not feasible. A ureterostomy forms a small, flush, pale pink stoma. It is difficult to manage; urinary reflux and infections are common. One or two stomas may be present.[18]

Ureteroenterocutaneous diversions. It is possible to isolate any segment of the healthy intestinal tract caudal to the jejunum for use as a conduit for urine. The isolated intestinal segment serves as a conduit to bridge the gap from ureter to skin when the bladder must be removed or bypassed. Invasive transitional cell carcinoma of the bladder is the most frequent reason for cystectomy in the adult patient.[39]

Urinary diversion using a segment of small intestine is the most common form of permanent urinary diversion. The Bricker ileal conduit was first described in 1950; it is used by isolating a 15 to 20 cm segment of the terminal ileum close to the ileocecal valve.[106] The distal end of the isolated segment is brought out through the right lower abdominal quadrant and everted to form a budded stoma. The ureters are excised from the bladder and implanted near the proximal end of the conduit, which is sutured closed. The conduit is isoperistaltic; urine flows in the same direction as peristaltic waves of the intestine. The ileal conduit is not a storage area; urine passes through quickly without residual.[27]

Jejunum may be used for small bowel permanent diversion if the ileum has been damaged by radiation. Patients with jejunal conduits are prone to a particular electrolyte imbalance called jejunal conduit syndrome, which is characterized by hypochloremic metabolic acidosis with hyperkalemia and hyponatremia.

The principal indications for small bowel urinary diversion are bladder cancer and severe neuropathic bladder dysfunction.[39] Long-term complications of the small bowel diversions are particularly prevalent after the first 5 years. Upper tract deterioration is significant and is associated with the bacteriuria and reflux that characterize the ileal or jejunal conduit.

A segment of large bowel may be isolated to form a urinary conduit. The primary advantage of using a segment of large intestine rather than small is the ability to create a nonrefluxing ureterointestinal anastomosis by tunneling the ureters into the submucosa of the colon. Nonetheless, the large bowel conduit leaves the patient with a stoma and continuous urinary incontinence. In addition, because obstruction at the uretero-enteric anastomosis is a serious complication, the large bowel conduit is used only in select cases.[39]

The ideal urinary diversion has not been developed. It would be an antirefluxing, continent diversion without the electrolyte disturbances that result from urine in prolonged contact with intestinal mucosa. This ideal diversion would have a reservoir with a functional capacity requiring catheterization only two or three times daily.

Continent urinary diversion. A continent urinary diversion provides the patient with an internal reservoir for urine and eliminates the need for an external appliance. There is an abdominal stoma and the patient performs clean intermittent catheterization through the stoma to empty the internal reservoir of urine.

A reservoir for urine constructed from the small intestine was first devised in the 1960s. The urinary Kock pouch involves isolating a 60 to 70 cm segment of the ileum. The mesentery and its blood supply to this isolated segment of ileum is left intact. The middle 40 cm of this segment is split open and folded back on itself to form a reservoir to hold urine. The entrance and exit to this reservoir have a nipple valve constructed by intussusception or telescoping back of the intestine on itself. The ureters are implanted into the proximal nipple valve in an attempt to prevent urine from refluxing up to the kidneys. The distal nipple valve ends in a right-sided abdominal stoma and makes the stoma continent of urine. The reservoir expands in volume with time, and the patient ultimately catheterizes the stoma four or five times a day using a no. 18 to 26 French catheter. The patient wears an absorptive pad or Band-Aid over the stoma to collect the mucus it secretes. In addition, reservoir irrigations are performed at least once daily using a 50 to 60 cc catheter tip or bulb syringe to remove the mucus that has accumulated in the reservoir.[20,35,38]

The ileocecal reservoir is another continent urinary diversion that was developed in the late 1970s. The distal 20 cm of ileum, a segment of the cecum, and part of the ascending colon are isolated, and continuity of the gastrointestinal tract is restored. The ureters are anastomosed into the ascending colon with an antirefluxing tunneling method similar to the one used in the construction of a sigmoid conduit. The ileum forms the outflow tract with a nipple valve for continence and a right lower quadrant abdominal stoma. The cecum and ascending colon form the reservoir for urine. The patient catheterizes the stoma and irrigates the reservoir as with the Kock reservoir.[75]

Continent urinary diversions are an attempt to provide the patient with a more acceptable form of urinary diversion and to make the adjustment to the presence of a stoma easier. Careful patient selection is important. Long-term consequences have yet to be studied.

Contraindications and Cautions

Supravesical diversions

1. Nephrostomy or pyelostomy tube drainage is discouraged in patients with bilateral ureteral obstruction as a result of a malignant disease, because these patients are highly susceptible to serious complications.[39]
2. Cutaneous pyelostomy diversion can be done only in pediatric patients with a large extrarenal pelvis.[58]
3. Adequate methods of securing tube diversions are important to prevent kidney damage or accidental tube dislodgment.
4. Cutaneous ureterostomy is not done if the ureters are of a normal size or poorly vascularized, because stomal stenosis may result. A large adult with a thick abdominal wall may have inadequate ureteral length.[84]

Ureteroenterocutaneous diversions

1. Obesity makes it difficult to construct a good stoma because of tension on the mesentery, which can lead to a flush or retracted stoma and the development of either stomal necrosis in early postoperative phase or subsequent stomal stenosis.
2. A sigmoid conduit is avoided in patients with severe diverticulosis or inflammatory bowel disease.[106]
3. A sigmoid conduit is not advised for the patient needing radical cystectomy and irradiation for bladder cancer, since the altered blood supply to the rectum and the sigmoid colon may negatively affect healing.[39]

Continent urinary diversions

1. The noncompliant patient with a tendency toward psychologic or social problems or the patient with already compromised renal function should not have a continent urinary diversion.
2. The need for postoperative radiation therapy may be related to a higher rate of failure.
3. The patient must be highly motivated to avoid wearing an external appliance.
4. Nipple valve failures can render the diversion incontinent of urine and necessitate a second surgical procedure to revise the intussusception.
5. Electrolyte disorders may result from urine in prolonged contact with intestinal mucosal lining.
6. Risk of malignancy from urine in prolonged contact with intestinal mucosa has not been fully evaluated.

Preprocedural Nursing Care

1. Intensive bowel preparation is started 2 to 3 days before surgery.
2. Preoperative stoma site selection is done by an enterostomal therapy (ET) nurse.
3. Preoperative teaching and consultation with an ET nurse is important.
4. The patient talks to an ostomy visitor if appropriate.

Medical Plan

The following medical plan is for ureteroenterocutaneous diversions.

Medications

Anti-infective agents
- Neomycin (Mycifradin), 1 g po q4h for 4 doses; then 1 g q6h until NPO for surgery (begins 3 days before surgery)
- Erythromycin base (Erythrocin), 1 g po q4h for 3 doses before surgery

Laxative agents
- Castor oil, 0.5 ml/kg po 3 days before surgery

Analgesic/antipyretic agents
- Used for pain and fever prn postoperatively

Mycostatin powder
- Applied to peristomal skin with each pouch change prn for monilial rash

Vitamin
- Vitamin C (ascorbic acid) to maintain acidic urine pH

General Management

Bowel preparation: saline enemas for 2 days before surgery; neomycin retention enemas (200 ml of a 1% solution) the night before and day of surgery if sigmoid conduit is to be performed.

Low-residue diet 2 days before surgery

Clear liquid diet 1 day before surgery

Intravenous fluids during bowel preparation and postoperatively until patient can tolerate food.

NURSING CARE

Nursing Assessment

Incision

Redness, pain, edema, drainage

Hemorrhage

Incisional drains, sumps
Urethral catheter (promotes drainage of operative site)

Urinary Output

Amount and color
Mucus normal in ileal/sigmoid conduit

Sexual Dysfunction (Male)

Erectile dysfunction
Ejaculatory incompetence—if prostate removed

Stoma

Viability
Mucocutaneous border
Edema

Peristomal Skin

Intact
Erythematous
Signs of monilial infection

Intestine

Paralytic ileus, intestinal obstruction, abdominal distention, constipation
Nasogastric suctioning prolonged owing to intestinal anastomosis

Nursing Dx & Intervention

Nursing Diagnosis	Nursing Intervention/Rationale
Altered patterns of urinary elimination	• Assess stoma color and suture line, *to recognize any change in viability or mucocutaneous separation.* • Provide an appropriate pouching system with an antireflux valve and a spout. Connect to bedside drainage and check frequently to prevent tubing from kinking *to prevent urine pooling on skin or refluxing from pouch to stoma.* • Monitor amount and color of urine. If no urine is present in pouch, check all drainage sites (sumps, urethral catheter, Penrose drain) for urine *to determine if there has been an ileal-ureteral leakage or decreased renal function.* • Arrange for enterostomal therapy (ET) nurse to assess stoma and drainage system and *to provide appropriate pouching system.* • Obtain all urine specimens for urinalysis or culture and sensitivity by catheterizing the ileal GI or peripheral conduit (exception: monitoring urine pH).
Altered peripheral tissue perfusion	• Assess blood pressure every 4 hours for 5 to 6 days or until removal of nasogastric suctioning and intravenous fluids. • Apply antiembolic stockings. Remove and reapply daily *to prevent venous stasis and thrombophlebitis.* • Auscultate abdomen for bowel sounds; note any signs of abdominal distention. • Assess stoma for color (i.e., blood supply). Ileal conduit stoma should be bright red and moist; ureterostomy stoma is pale or dark pink. • Assist patient with progressive ambulation. • Encourage patient to turn every 2 hours and to perform leg exercises. • Observe all drains, sumps, and catheters for amount, color, and consistency of drainage. • Monitor intake and output; weigh daily.
Potential for infection	• Provide antibiotics as ordered. • Observe incision for signs of infection: redness, edema, pain, and drainage. Assess patient's skin (under the arms and breasts, groin, perineum) *for monilial infections associated with prolonged antibiotics, intense bowel preparation, and moisture.*
Patient problem: potential hemorrhage	• Observe incisional dressing *for color and amount of drainage.* • Monitor color, consistency, and amount of drainage from nasogastric tube, sumps, urethral catheter, and stoma output *to prevent hypovolemic shock.* • Monitor vital signs for shock.
Ineffective breathing pattern	• Assist patient in turning, coughing, and deep breathing *to counteract effects of general anesthesia.* • Auscultate chest for breath sounds 4 times each day. • Provide analgesics and splinting of abdomen when encouraging patient to deep breathe and cough.

Nursing Diagnosis	Nursing Intervention/Rationale
Constipation	• Monitor patient for first bowel movement. • Auscultate abdomen for bowel sounds each shift. • Observe for signs of paralytic ileus or intestinal obstruction. • Monitor patient for signs and symptoms of peritonitis, which would indicate a leakage or failure of the intestinal reanastomosis: fever, abdominal pain, rebound tenderness, drop in blood pressure, or shallow respirations.
Pain	• Provide analgesics as ordered. • Assist patient in finding comfortable positions.
Body image and personal identity disturbances	• Provide an opportunity for patient and partner to discuss the implications of the surgery, stoma, and external pouch. • Explore the patient's and partner's feelings regarding the presence of the stoma and pouch. • Discuss the presence of the pouch and the inability of detecting it under clothing and how to manage embarrassing leakages and odor.
Potential impaired skin integrity	• Change the pouch whenever it appears to be leaking under the faceplate or when there is an overt leakage. • See pouch change procedure, p. 1150.
Impaired skin integrity	• Assess skin integrity frequently because *rash can occur under the tape or faceplate and on any part of the skin where the pouch lies. Causes of skin rashes may be a leaking appliance, perspiration, allergies to tape, or hair follicle irritation.* • Use lamp with a 60-watt bulb 1 foot away from skin or hair dryer set on cool *to dry the skin.* • Powder the skin on which the pouch lies. *Avoid cornstarch powders, which encourage the growth of monilia.* • Advise patient to make or buy a pouch cover. • Ulcerated area on stoma may occur if stomal opening of the pouch is too small or activities are causing the faceplate to rub or cut into stoma. • Evaluate patient's activities: a different faceplate size or shape may be needed. • Waterlogged skin between opening of the faceplate and the stoma can occur if too much skin is exposed between the stoma and the faceplate and the urine pools on unprotected skin. • Apply lamp or hair dryer to area. • Decrease the size of stomal opening in faceplate; use skin sealant *to waterproof skin.* • Urinary yeast infection on skin surrounding the stoma may extend beyond the faceplate. • Apply nystatin (Mycostatin) powder to the area, blow off the excess powder, and seal this in with a thin coat of a skin sealant. Apply pouch in the usual manner. • Advise patient to drink sufficient fluids and add buttermilk or yogurt to the diet *to help restore normal gut flora.* • Urine crystals may form on the stoma or around the stoma base if the patient has alkaline urine and a predisposition for stone formation. • Swab vinegar on the stoma when changing the pouch *to help dissolve crystals.* • Insert vinegar into the pouch while patient is wearing it. For a minor formation, insert twice a day; for an excessive formation, insert four times a day. • Remove antireflux valves to allow the *vinegar to come into contact with the stoma.* • Monitor urine pH and provide instructions for maintaining an acid urine, including increased fluid intake and ascorbic acid (vitamin C).
Altered sexuality patterns	• Assess patient and partner's readiness to discuss sexual matters. • Discuss the sexual implications of the presence of the stoma, such as feelings of attractiveness, desirability, and worth. • Explain separate nerve pathways for sexual excitement, erection, ejaculation, and orgasm *to point out the effect of cystectomy on erections only.* • Mention sexual counseling, alternative methods of sexual expression, and penile prosthesis or external devices to aid in achieving erections *to assist patient in resuming sexual activity that is fullfilling for him.*

Patient Education

1. Teach the patient how to empty the pouch when it is one-third to one-half full.
2. Instruct the patient on the use of the bedside drainage bag at night.
3. Instruct the patient on pouch change procedure (see box below). This includes treatment of minor peristomal skin irritations and monitoring urine pH.
4. Explain fluid intake requirements—10 to 12 glasses a day to acidify urine.
5. Review dietary considerations in terms of urine odor; fish, eggs, asparagus, and spicy foods can cause a temporary increase in urine odor.
6. Define routine follow-up care for the patient with a urinary diversion, including correct method of obtaining urine for culture (see box, opposite).
7. Provide the patient with ostomy supply and supplier information and availability of community support groups, such as the United Ostomy Association.[28]

Procedure for Urinary Pouch Change

1 Assemble all supplies.
   a. To clean the skin, paper towels, washcloths, or towels may be used. Several of these should be rolled into "wicks" that can be placed on top of the stoma to absorb urine while keeping the peristomal skin unencumbered. Tampons can also be used as wicks. Premoistened towelettes should not be used.
   b. Pouch—a urinary pouch with a precut opening for stoma should be sized large enough to bypass any creases or dimples in the skin around the stoma. A pouch that needs to be cut out before application should be cut to avoid any creases or dimples in the immediate peristomal area. Check for creases or dimples while the patient is sitting and when he is lying down. The outer diameter of the pouch's adhesive faceplate may be trimmed to avoid umbilicus, rib cage, incisions, hip bones, pubic areas, or folds at the waist.
   c. Karaya powder
   d. Skin sealant—protects the skin from the macerating effects of urine and the stripping effects of tape or adhesive. Most skin sealants are a liquid copolymer with alcohol as the vehicle for spreading it. Skin sealants come in spray form, dab-on applicators, or wipes.
   e. Tape—such as Micropore or paper tape. Some patients prefer waterproof tape.
   f. Plastic bag for disposal of used pouches
2. Take off old pouch by unsticking the skin from the pouch's adhesive faceplate. Dispose of used pouch.
3. Wash the stoma and peristomal skin free of mucous and urine with warm water only and let dry.
   a. Soap may leave a residue on the skin and prevent the next pouch from adhering.
   b. Traces of cement or adhesives may be on the skin. Rough cleansing to remove these may do damage to the peristomal skin.
4. Examine the peristomal skin for any signs of redness or irritation. Apply a light dusting of karaya powder to irritated skin.
   a. If the peristomal skin needs to be shaved, use a dry razor over powdered skin. Brush away excess karaya powder.
   b. If irritation is severe, a skin barrier in wafer form may be added to the pouch's adhesive faceplate. Urine will melt the skin barrier and decrease the pouch's seal, but a pouch's adhesive faceplate should not be applied directly over severely irritated skin.
5. Apply a skin sealant to peristomal skin. Keep the stoma "wicked" to absorb urine.
   a. In the presence of skin irritation, a skin sealant will cause a momentary stinging sensation.
   b. If karaya powder was applied to irritated skin, the skin sealant will seal in the karaya powder and, once dry, will provide a skin surface to which the pouch can adhere.
6. Center pouch over stoma and apply to dry skin.
   a. Try to avoid creating any wrinkles or creases in pouch's adhesive faceplate that will encourage urine leakage.
   b. The pouch may be angled straight down or medially for an ambulatory patient to facilitate emptying.
7. Close the pouch's spout.
8. Use the tape to picture-frame the pouch's adhesive faceplate and increase the pouch's wearing time.
9. Check the pH of the urine from the first drops of urine in the freshly changed pouch.
   a. Do not touch the pH paper to the stoma or the skin, since this will give an inaccurate reading.
   b. An acidic urine pH should be maintained, since alkaline urine is more likely to have a foul odor, create crystals on or around the stoma, predispose the patient to kidney stone formation, and provide a medium for infection. An adequate fluid intake or ascorbic acid (vitamin C, 500 mg) four times a day will acidify urine. Acidic urine has a pH of 6.0 or less.

Procedure for Obtaining a Urine Culture from Ileal-Sigmoid Conduit (Single-Lumen Catheterization)

1. Explain procedure to patient.
   a. Catheterizing the stoma is painless because ureteroenterocutaneous stomas have no sensory nerve endings.
   b. Patient should be aware that no urine for culture should be obtained from the pouch itself. This specimen needs to be obtained sterilely.
2. Assemble supplies for reapplying the pouch once the specimen is obtained.
3. Set up equipment for obtaining a urine specimen on a sterile field:
   a. Catheter (may be a no. 12 or 14 French straight catheter)
   b. Betadine swabs (three)
   c. Sterile, water-soluble lubricant
   d. Sterile urine cup
   e. Dry, sterile gauze
   f. Sterile gloves
4. Take off the old pouch.
5. Drape patient with Chux to keep him or her dry.
6. Wipe stoma free of mucous with gauze.
7. Put on sterile gloves.
8. Swab the stoma three times with the Betadine swabs.
9. Let urine run over the stoma to wash away Betadine *or* wipe stoma free of Betadine with dry, sterile gauze. Introducing Betadine into the specimen will kill the bacteria for which the culture is checking.
10. Lubricate the tip of the catheter with water-soluble lubricant.
11. Gently insert the catheter into the stoma about 1½ to 2 inches. Do not force or poke. It is desirable to pass catheter beneath fascia level if possible.
12. Wait until about 5 ml of urine passes through the catheter into the sterile urine cup. To facilitate obtaining specimen, instruct the patient to sit up or turn on one side.
13. Remove the catheter.
14. Reapply the pouch.

Evaluation

Patient Outcome	Data Indicating That Outcome is Reached
There is no infection.	Temperature is within normal range. There are no signs or symptoms of infection. Incision is healed.
Tissue perfusion is normal.	Stoma is red, healthy, moist, and viable. Blood pressure and pulse are within normal limits.
Bowel elimination is normal.	The patient experiences a return to presurgical bowel habits.
Skin integrity is maintained.	Peristomal skin is intact. There are no signs of irritation. Pouch seal is appropriate (3 to 5 days). Women return to presurgical sexual pattern. Men experiencing sexual dysfunction receive counseling regarding erectile dysfunction.
Body image is not disturbed.	The patient adapts to the presence of the stoma and external pouch. The patient recognizes that adaptation is a continuous process.
The patient resumes activities of daily living.	The patient returns to presurgical activities including work and recreational interests. The patient does not change his style of dress.

References

1. Abrams P: Detrusor instability and bladder outlet obstruction, Neurourol Urodynamics 4:317, 1985.
2. Allen TD: The non-neurogenic neurogenic bladder, J Urol 116:638, 1977.
3. Amelar RD and Dubin LE, editors: Male infertility, Philadelphia, 1977, WB Saunders Co.
4. Anderson JT: Prostatism: clinical, radiologic and urodynamic aspects, Neurourol Urodynamics 1:241, 1982.
5. Anderson RS: A neurogenic element to genuine urinary stress incontinence, Br J Obstet Gynaecol 91:41, 1984.
6. Andrew J, Nathan PW, and Spanos NC: Cerebral cortical control of micturition, Proc R Soc Med 58:533, 1968.
7. Andriana RT and Carson CC: Urolithiasis, Clin Symp 38:3, 1986.
8. Andriole VT: Urinary tract infections in pregnancy, Urol Clin North Am 2:485, 1975.
9. Barrington FJF: The nervous mechanisms of micturition of the cat, Q J Exp Physiol 54:177, 1931.
10. Bates CP: The unstable bladder, Clin Obstet Gynecol 5:109, 1978.
11. Bauer SB et al: The unstable bladder of childhood, Urol Clin North Am 7:321, 1980.
12. Baumann JM et al: The role of inhibitors and other factors in the pathogenesis of recurrent calcium containing renal stones, Clin Sci 53:141, 1977.
13. Bergman H, editor: The ureter, New York, 1982, Springer-Verlag, Inc.
14. Blaivas JG: The neurophysiology of micturition: a study of 550 patients, J Urol 127:958, 1982.
15. Borda E et al: Relationship between prostaglandins and estrogens on the motility of isolated rings from the rat urinary bladder, J Urol 129:1250, 1983.
16. Bors E and Comarr AE: Neurological urology, Baltimore, 1971, Williams & Wilkins.
17. Bradley WE, Timm GW, and Scott FB: Innervation of detrusor muscle and urethra, Urol Clin North Am 1:3, 1974.

18. Broadwell DC and Jackson BS, editors: Principles of ostomy care, St Louis, 1982, The CV Mosby Co.
19. Broadwell DC and Sorrells SL: Summary of your urinary diversion, Atlanta, 1983, Emory University.
20. Brogna L and Lakaszawaski M: Nursing management: the continent urostomy, J Enterostom Ther 13:139, 1986.
21. Chisholm GD and Williams ID, editors: Scientific foundations in urology, Chicago, 1982, Year Book Medical Publishers, Inc.
22. Conti G: L'erection du penis human et bases morphologio vascularis, Acta Anat 14:17, 1952.
23. Crockett AT and Urry DL, editors: Male infertility: workup, treatment and research, New York, 1977, Grune & Stratton, Inc.
24. Crouch JE: Functional human anatomy, Philadelphia, 1982, Lea & Febiger.
25. Daniel EE, Cowan W, and Daniel VP: Structural basis for neural and myogenic control of human detrusor muscle, Physiol Pharmacol 61:1247, 1983.
26. DeGroat WE: CNS modulation of detrusor storage, New York, 1986, Presented at Eighth Annual Urodynamic Society Meeting.
27. Dobkin KA: Nursing care of a patient with ileal conduit, J Urol Nurs 4:340, 1985.
28. Dobkin KA: Urinary diversion care plan. In Holloway N, editor: Medical surgical care plans, Springhouse, Pa, 1988, Springhouse.
29. Drach GW: Prostatitis: man's hidden infection, Urol Clin North Am 2:499, 1975.
30. Edvarsdin P and Ursin T: Nervous control of urinary bladder in cats. I. The collecting phase, Acta Physiol Scand 72:157, 1968.
31. Farnell B and Thomas P: Tuberculosis at the epididymis, Can Med Assoc J 128:1296, 1983.
32. Farrar WE: Infections of the urinary tract, Med Clin North Am 67:187, 1983.
33. Finlayson B: Renal lithiasis in review, Urol Clin North Am 1:181, 1974.
34. Finlayson B, Hench LL, and Smith LH, editors: Urolithiasis: physical aspects, Washington, DC, 1972, National Academy of Science.
35. Fowler JE: Continent urinary reservoirs and bladder substitutes in the adult. II. Monographs in urology, 1987.
36. Furlow WL: Use of the inflatable penile prosthesis in erectile dysfunction, Urol Clin North Am 8:181, 1981.
37. Gaymans R et al: A prospective study of urinary tract infections in a Dutch general practice, Lancet 2:674, 1976.
38. Gerber A: The Kock continent ileal reservoir: an alternative to the conventional urostomy, J Enterostom Ther 12:15, 1985.
39. Glenn JF: Urologic surgery, New York, 1983, Harper & Row Publishers, Inc.
40. Gosling JA: The structure of the bladder and urethra in relation to function, Urol Clin North Am 6:31, 1979.
41. Govoni L and Hayes JE: Drugs and nursing implications, Norwalk, Conn, 1982, Appleton-Century-Crofts.
42. Gray ML and Dougherty MC: Urinary incontinence: pathophysiology and treatment, J Enterostom Ther 14(4):152, 1987.
43. Guyton AC: Medical physiology, Philadelphia, 1978, WB Saunders Co.
44. Hald T and Bradley WE: The urinary bladder: neurology and dynamics, Baltimore, 1982, Williams & Wilkins.
45. Harrison JH et al, editors: Campbell's urology, Philadelphia, 1978, WB Saunders Co.
46. Hindmarsh JR and Byrne PO: Adult enuresis: a symptomatic and urodynamic assessment, Br J Urol 52:88, 1980.
47. Hinman JF, editor: Benign prostatic hypertrophy, New York, 1983, Springer-Verlag, Inc.
48. Hodgkinson CP, Ayers MA, and Drukker BH: Dyssynergic detrusor dysfunction in apparently normal females, Am J Obstet Gynecol 87(6):717, 1963.
49. Hurst JW, editor: Medicine for the practicing physician, Boston, 1983, Butterworth Publishers.
50. Hutch JA and Rambo ON: A study of the anatomy of the prostate, prostatic urethra, and the urinary sphincter system, J Urol 104:443, 1970.
51. International Continence Society: The standardization of terminology of lower urinary tract function, Glasgow, Scotland, 1984.
52. Ireton RC and Berger RE: Prostatitis and epididymitis, Urol Clin North Am 11:83, 1984.
53. Isselbacher KJ et al: Harrison's principles of internal medicine, New York, 1980, McGraw-Hill, Inc.
54. Jenkins AD, Turner TT, and Howards SS: Physiology of the male reproductive system, Urol Clin North Am 5:437, 1978.
55. Kass I, Updegraff K, and Muffly RB: Sex in chronic obstructive pulmonary disease, Med Aspects Hum Sex 6:33, 1972.
56. Kay D: Host defense mechanisms in the urinary tract, Urol Clin North Am 2:407, 1975.
57. Kedia KR: Vascular disorders and male erectile dysfunction, Urol Clin North Am 8:153, 1981.
58. Kelalis PP, King LR, and Belman AB, editors: Clinical pediatric urology, Philadelphia, 1985, WB Saunders Co.
59. Klarskov P et al: Prostaglandin type E activity dominates in urinary tract smooth muscle in vitro, J Urol 129:1071, 1983.
60. Kneeland JB: NMR: the new frontier in diagnostic radiology, Adv Surg 18:37, 1984.
61. Krane RJ and Siroky MB: Clinical neurology, Boston, 1979, Little, Brown & Co, Inc.
62. Krane RJ, Siroky MB, and Goldstein I, editors: Male sexual dysfunction, Boston, 1983, Little, Brown & Co, Inc.
63. Reference deleted in proofs.
64. Kuru M.: Nervous control of micturition, Physiol Rev 45:425, 1965.
65. Lapides J: Structure and function of internal vesical sphincter, J Urol 50:341, 1958.
66. Lapides J: Tips on self-catheterization, Urol Dig, p 11, July 1977.
67. Leach GE: Urodynamic manifestations of cerebellar ataxia, J Urol 128:348, 1982.
68. Leeson CR and Leeson TS: Histology, Philadelphia, 1976, WB Saunders Co.
69. Lerner J and Khan Z: Manual of urologic nursing, St. Louis, 1982, The CV Mosby Co.
70. Lewin RJ, Dillard GV, and Porter RW: Extrapyramidal inhibition of the urinary bladder, Brain Res 4:301, 1967.
71. Libertino JA, editor: International perspectives in urology, vol 5, Baltimore, 1982, Williams & Wilkins.
72. Lipschultz LI and Howards SS, editors: Infertility in the male, New York, 1983, Churchill Livingstone, Inc.
73. Lipuma JP et al: Magnetic resonance imaging of the genitourinary tract, Urol Clin North Am 13:531, 1986.
74. Mann R and Lutwak-Mann C: Male reproductive function and semen, Berlin, 1981, Springer-Verlag, Inc.
75. Mansson W: The continent caecal reservoir for urine, Scand J Urol Nephrol Suppl:8, 1985.
76. Meares EM: Prostatitis, Annu Rev Med 30:279, 1979.
77. Michigan S: Genitourinary fungal infections, J Urol 116:390, 1976.
78. Mundy AR, Stephenson TA, and Wein AJ: Urodynamics: principles, practice, and application, Edinburgh, 1984, Churchill Livingstone, Inc.
79. Narayan P and Lange P: Semirigid penile prosthesis in the management of erectile impotence, Urol Clin North Am 8:169, 1981.
80. Nielsen JB et al: Continuous overnight monitoring of bladder activity in vesicoureteral reflux patients. II. Bladder activity types, Neurourol Urodynam 3:7, 1984.
81. Nistal M and Paniagua R: Testicular epididymal pathology, New York, 1984, Thieme Medical Publishers, Inc.
82. Pak CYP et al: Dietary management of idiopathic calcium urolithiasis, J Urol 131:850, 1984.
83. Pfister RC, Newhouse JH, and Hendren WH: Percutaneous pyeloureteral urodynamics, Urol Clin North Am 9:41, 1982.
84. Phipps WJ, Long BC, and Woods NF, editors: Medical-surgical nursing: concepts and clinical practice, St Louis, 1983, The CV Mosby Co.
85. Platt R et al: Mortality associated with nosocomial urinary-tract infection, N Engl J Med 307:637, 1982.
86. Raz S, Editor: Female urology, Philadelphia, 1983, WB Saunders Co.
87. Rees DLP, Wiskham JEA, and Whitfield JM: Bladder instability in women with recurrent cystitis, Br J Urol 50:524, 1978.

88. Resnick MI and Older RA, editors: Diagnosis of genitourinary disease, New York, 1982, Thieme Medical Publishers, Inc.
89. Riff LJ: Bacteremia arising from the urinary tract, Urol Clin North Am 2:521, 1975.
90. Riley TW et al: Use of radioisotopic scan in evaluation of intrascrotal lesions, J Urol 116:472, 1976.
91. Rose BD: Pathophysiology of renal disease, New York, 1981, McGraw-Hill, Inc.
92. Rud T et al: Factors maintaining urethral pressure in women, Invest Urol 17:343, 1980.
93. Sarma KP: Tumors of the urinary bladder, New York, 1969, Appleton-Century-Crofts.
94. Smith AD: Causes and classifications of impotence, Urol Clin North Am 8:79, 1981.
95. Smith DR: General urology, Los Altos, Calif, 1981, Lange Medical Books.
96. Smith PH and Prout GR, editors: Bladder cancer, London, 1984, Butterworth Publishers.
97. Snooks SJ et al: Perineal nerve damage in genuine stress incontinence, Br J Urol 57:522, 1985.
98. Spirnak JP and Resnick MI: Urinary stones, Primary Care 12:735, 1985.
99. Stamey TA: Pathogenesis and treatment of urinary tract infections, Baltimore, 1980, Williams & Wilkins.
100. Staskin DR et al: Pathophysiology of stress incontinence, Clin Obstet Gynaecol 12:357, 1985.
101. Stuart PG et al: Hypothalamic unit activity: visceral and somatic influences, Clin Neurophysiol 16:237, 1964.
102. Symmonds RE: Incontinence: vesicle and urethral fistulae, Clin Obstet Gynecol 27:499, 1984.
103. Thomas TM et al: Prevalence of urinary incontinence, Br Med J 281:1243, 1980.
104. Wagner G and Green R: Impotence, New York, 1981, Plenum Publishing Corp.
105. Walsh PC and Wilson JD: The induction of prostatic hypertrophy in the dog with androstanediol, J Clin Invest 54:1093, 1976.
106. Walsh PC et al, editors: Campbell's urology, Philadelphia, 1986, WB Saunders Co.
107. Walsh PC et al: Tissue content of dihydrotestosterone in human prostatic hyperplasia is not abnormal, J Clin Invest 72:1772, 1983.
108. Watt RR: Nursing management of a patient with urinary diversion, Semin Oncol Nurs 2:265, 1986.
109. Weidman CL and Northcutt RC: Endocrine aspects of impotence, Urol Clin North Am 8:143, 1981.
110. Wheatley JK: Causes and treatment of bladder incontinence, Compr Ther 9:27, 1983.
111. Whitaker R: Clinical application of upper tract urodynamics, Urol Clin North Am 6:137, 1979.
112. Whiteside CG and Arnold EP: Persistent primary enuresis: urodynamic assessment, Br Med J 5954:364, 1975.
113. Williams P and Warwick R: Gray's anatomy, Philadelphia, 1980, WB Saunders Co.
114. Wilson JD: The pathogenesis of benign prostatic hypertrophy, Am J Med 68:745, 1980.
115. Wilson JD, Gloyna RE, and Siiteri PK: Androgen metabolism in the hypertrophic prostate, J Steroid Biochem 6:443, 1975.
116. Yarnell JWG et al: The prevalence and severity of urinary incontinence in women, J Epidemiol Community Health 35:71, 1981.
117. Zinner NR, Sterling AM, and Ritter RC: Role of inner urethral softness in urinary continence, Urology 16:115, 1980.
118. Zorgnotti AW and Lefleur RS: Auto-injection of the corpus cavernosum with a vasoactive drug combination for vasculogenic impotence, J Urol 133:39, 1985.

CHAPTER 13

Infectious Diseases

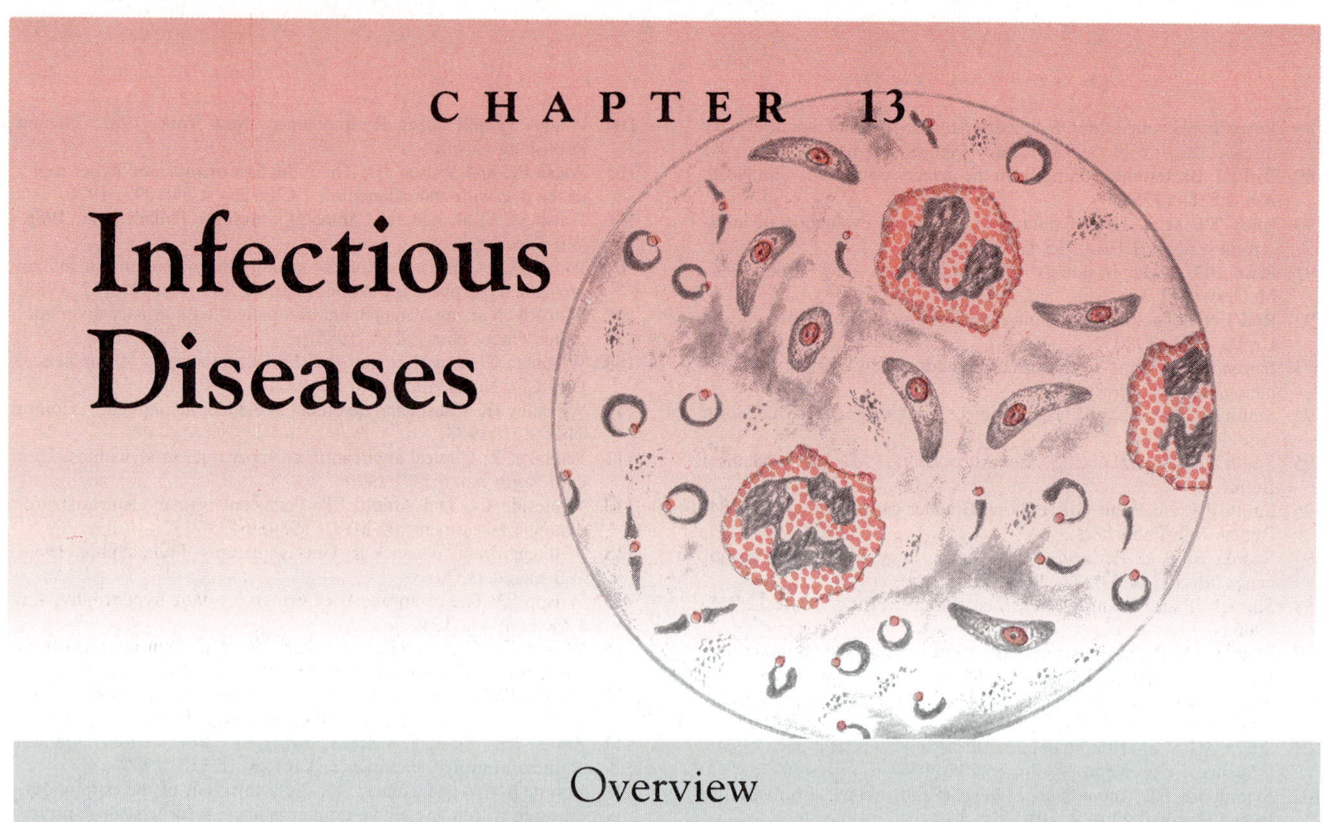

Overview

At the beginning of the nineteenth century no infectious disease was controlled in America. Major efforts in environmental sanitation, advances in immunization and antibiotic therapy, and application of antimicrobial technology to disease agents have resulted in control of many of the dreaded infectious diseases of the past. Today most health professionals in the United States never see cases of the major killers such as yellow fever, cholera, typhus, smallpox, malaria, typhoid fever, or plague. That is not meant to suggest that infectious disease has been eradicated or even controlled. Some infectious diseases, such as hepatitis and acquired immune deficiency syndrome (AIDS) and other sexually transmitted diseases, are increasing in the United States. Others, such as measles and mumps, persist despite the availability of preventive measures. Antibiotic-resistant organisms flourish, and new infectious disease agents continue to be identified. While many of the major killers have been controlled in the United States, these diseases continue to cause death and destruction in other parts of the world, necessitating a vigilant attitude toward them.

Because all infectious diseases have characteristics in common, this overview discusses the following aspects:

- Nature of infectious disease
- Pathogenic agents
- Agent, host, and environmental interaction for disease transmission

Nature of Infectious Disease

Definitions. Contamination, infection, infectious disease, communicable disease, and contagious disease are not synonymous terms. Contamination is merely the presence of a microorganism on an inanimate object, whereas infection is the implantation and successful reproduction of a microorganism on or in the tissue of a human host. If no physiologic response occurs, the organisms have merely colonized the host. The colonized host who also sheds the organisms is a carrier. If physiologic response occurs without overt symptoms, the process is termed a subclinical or inapparent infection. If tissue injury or body responses result in symptoms of illness, an infectious disease is present. Communicable disease is an infectious disease that results from transmission of an infectious microorganism or its products to a susceptible human host either directly or indirectly, through an intermediate animal host, a vector, or the inanimate environment. Contagious diseases are communicable diseases transmitted by direct contact.

Stages of infection. The progression from infection to infectious disease in humans follows definable stages. The duration of the stages and the potential outcomes vary with infectious disease agents and disease processes. A latent stage follows invasion of the cells by a microorganism and lasts until infection is patent and the organism can be shed (i.e., the beginning of communicability). The incubation stage, during which the organism is multiplying, also starts with microorganism invasion and persists until the disease process is present. The disease stage may be asymptomatic (subclinical) or may present overt symptoms. The length of the disease stage is extremely variable, sometimes extending beyond the period of communicability. Resolution of the infectious disease may precede or coincide with termination of the infection. The infectious process may terminate completely or revert to the latent stage. In the latter case intermittent infec-

Figure 13-1 Stages of infection in host.
Modified from Fox.[31]

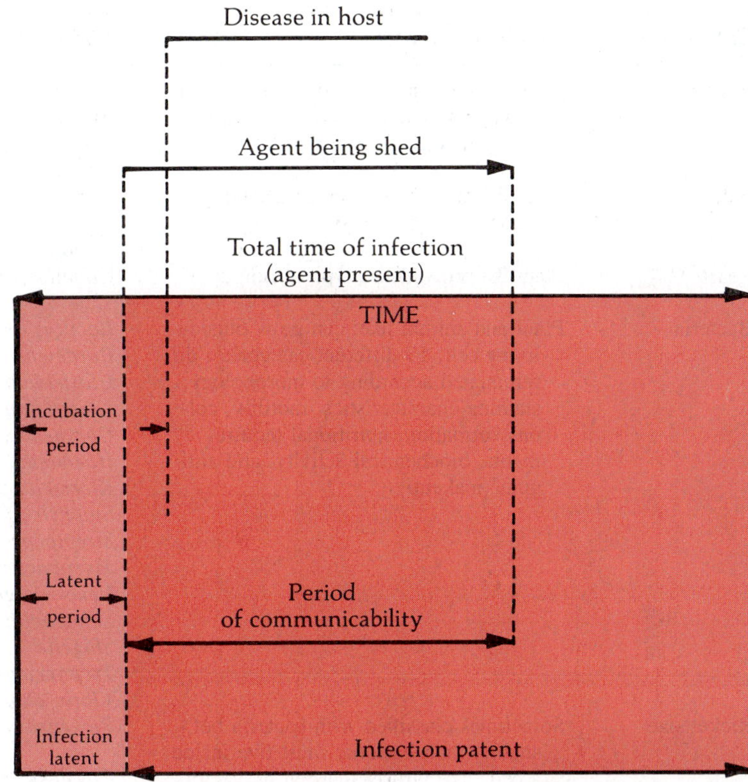

tious disease may result or the host may become a carrier, continuing to harbor and shed the incubating infectious agent.[31] Figure 13-1 depicts the stages of infection in the host.

Spectrum of occurrence of cases. The frequency of occurrence of cases of infectious disease can be characterized as sporadic, endemic, or epidemic. Sporadic refers to occasional and irregular occurrence of cases in a population over a specified period of time. Endemic means that the disease occurs with a constant frequency in a specified population over a definite time period. Epidemic refers to a definite increase in disease incidence over its expected endemic occurrence.

Pathogenic Agents

Infectious diseases have one characteristic in common: a pathogenic agent is necessary to the development of the disease. Although the agent must be present, it is not a sufficient cause for disease; disease development also depends on host susceptibility and pathogen characteristics to be discussed here.

Symbiotic relationships with humans. Pathogenic agents are living parasites, maintaining themselves at the expense of their human host. Parasitic relationships can be differentiated from other types of relationships between living organisms and humans. The human has a constant symbiotic relationship with a normal flora of organisms, some of which are harmless and others of which are pathogenic only under certain conditions. If the relationship benefits both the organism and the human host, as is the case with *Escherichia coli* in the intestinal tract, the relationship is one of mutualism. If the relationship benefits only the organism but causes no harm to the host, it is termed commensalism. Some organisms may have a commensal relationship on one part of the body but become pathogenic elsewhere, as is the case with α-streptococci in the nasopharynx becoming pathogenic to heart valves. Some pathogens that normally have a commensal relationship with the host may produce disease only under conditions of host susceptibility. These pathogens are opportunists, producing opportunistic infections. In addition to establishing one of the symbiotic relationships, many organisms are transient residents on or in the human. These organisms, some of which are pathogenic, are picked up and shed regularly, possibly producing disease in a more susceptible host.

Intrinsic characteristics of agents. One characteristic common to all pathogenic agents is their ability to establish a parasitic relationship in humans. Generally, the greater the

Table 13-1
Characteristics of Categories of Pathogens with Representative Diseases

Category	Characteristics	Pathogen	Diseases
Protozoa	Animal-like, single cell organism; breaks down and absorbs nutrients from host; can grow outside living cells	*Plasmodium*	Malaria
		Entamoeba histolytica	Amebic dysentery
		Giardia	Enteritis
		Trichomonas vaginalis	Vulvovaginitis
Fungi	Plantlike organism; lives on decaying matter	Dermatophytes	Athlete's foot Ringworm
		Histoplasma	Histoplasmosis
Yeasts	Plantlike organism; a type of fungus	*Candida albicans*	Moniliasis Candidiasis
Bacteria	Plant and animal like; can grow outside living cell; 19 different categories; differentiated according to morphology, staining characteristics, motility, colony formation, nutritional requirements, biochemical activity, and antigenic makeup	*Bacillus anthracis*	Anthrax
		Bordetella pertussis	Pertussis
		Clostridium botulinum	Botulism
		Clostridium tetani	Tetanus
		Corynebacterium diphtheriae	Diphtheria
		Haemophilus influenzae	Meningitis
		Klebsiella pneumoniae	Pneumonia
		Staphylococcus aureus	Septicemia
		Streptococcus pyogenes	Strep throat
		Mycobacterium tuberculosis	Tuberculosis
		Neisseria gonorrhoeae	Gonorrhea
		Salmonella typhi	Typhoid fever
		Shigella	Shigellosis
		Treponema pallidum	Syphilis
		Vibrio cholerae	Cholera
Rickettsiae	Sometimes classified with bacteria but smaller than bacteria; must live inside a cell, like viruses; carried by vectors	*Rickettsia rickettsii*	Rocky Mountain spotted fever
		Rickettsia typhi	Typhus
Chlamydiae	Like viruses, can obtain energy only from living cell; sometimes classified with bacteria; spread by person-to-person contact	*Chlamydia trachomatis*	Trachoma Lymphogranuloma venereum
Mycoplasmata	Smallest cellular microbes; sometimes classified with bacteria; can grow outside living cell as can bacteria	*Mycoplasma pneumoniae*	Atypical pneumonia Sinusitis Conjunctivitis
Viruses	Small particles (not classified as living cells); lack ability to produce energy; depend on ribosomes of infected cells for energy production; possess DNA or RNA (not both); replication directed by nucleic acids (RNA or DNA); action: injects RNA or DNA into cell, altering metabolism of host cells; if cells die, all viruses are released at once; if cells do not die, viruses are released one at a time; local reaction: cells undergo hyperplasia or hyperplasia and necrosis; differentiated according to nucleic acid core, according to biologic, chemical, or physical properties, and according to the way they enter the body	Pox virus	Smallpox
		Herpes simplex 1	Cold sores
		Herpes simplex 2	Venereal herpes
		Adenovirus	Pneumonia, conjunctivitis
		Rhinovirus	Colds
		Polio virus	Poliomyelitis
		Hepatitis A; B; non-A, non-B	Hepatitis
		Coxsackievirus	Meningitis
		Enterovirus	Intestinal infection
		Myxovirus parotids	Mumps
		Paramyxovirus	Rubeola
		Rhabdovirus	Rabies
		Orthomyxovirus, types A and B	Influenza
Helminths	Multicellular; large enough to be seen without microscope; migrate within host; induce eosinophilia; unable to multiply in the host; transmitted by ingestion, skin penetration, injection by insects	Nematodes (roundworms, hookworms, and pinworms)	Anemia Anal pruritus
		Trichinella worms	Trichinosis
		Filarial worms	Filariasis
		Cestodes (flatworms and tapeworms)	Anemia
		Trematodes (flukes)	Biliary obstruction Hepatomegaly

Data from Burton[7] and Frobisher.[33]

dose of the pathogen, the greater the risk for disease. Pathogenic agents vary according to observable intrinsic characteristics such as their morphology and chemical composition, their growth requirements, and their viability.

Morphology (size, shape, and structure) of the organism and the chemical composition (nucleic acids, enzyme system, and antigenic proteins) of living agents provide the basis for classification and laboratory identification of specific categories of agents and for differentiation within categories. Morphology alone permits identification of the larger parasitic worms. Identification of the microorganisms depends on knowledge of morphology, colony formation, staining characteristics, nutritional requirements, and the antigenic proteins of specific organisms.

Pathogens can also be differentiated according to their growth requirements. Because they cannot synthesize their own amino acids, they rely on their host to supply their nutritional requirements. Some pathogens, such as bacteria, have a metabolic structure enabling them to sustain themselves outside the human cell for varying lengths of time depending on the organism. Viruses have no metabolic activity and must receive all sustenance for survival from the host cell.

Viability is the ability of the pathogenic agent to survive in an adverse environment by resisting physical, chemical, or thermal agents. Viability is determined by the morphology and chemical composition of various pathogens. The ability of some organisms, such as the tetanus bacilli, to produce spores or to undergo genetic change, as with the antibiotic-resistant strains of bacteria, increases their viability. Antigenic changes in some pathogens, such as the influenza viruses, permit parasitism in previously immune hosts, thus extending the viability of the pathogen.

The microorganisms pathogenic to humans are classified as protozoa, fungi and yeasts, bacteria, rickettsiae, chlamydiae, mycoplasmata, and viruses, in order of decreasing size. A larger group of organisms, also parasitic to humans, are the helminths, or worms. Table 13-1 describes basic characteristics of each of the categories of pathogens with examples of the organisms and diseases they produce.

Effect of agent characteristics on humans.[31,38] Pathogenic agents also vary according to the manner in which they interact with the human host as to their mode of action, infectivity, pathogenicity, virulence, toxigenicity, and antigenicity.

The mode of action may be direct damage to cells by causing hyperplasia, necrosis, and death to the cells; or the action may be through the production of poisonous toxins that cause local or systemic reactions in the host.

Infectivity of the agent is its ability to invade and multiply in the host. It is affected by host defenses and enzymes produced by the organism to facilitate invasiveness. Coagulase, an extracellular enzyme, enables organisms such as staphylococci to clot plasma and form a sticky fibrin layer around themselves to protect against the host's defenses. Another enzyme, streptokinase, lyses or dissolves fibrin clots, allowing streptococci to spread through host tissue. Hyaluronidase causes breakdown of connective tissue and increases tissue permeability of organisms such as streptococci, pneumococci, and clostridia. Collagenase breaks down collagen, allowing deep invasion of organisms such as *Clostridium perfringens* into tendons, cartilage, and bones. Agents have been graded according to their infectivity potential. Poliomyelitis virus is a highly infective agent; rubella virus is an intermediate infective agent; and *M. tuberculosis* is an agent of low infectivity.

Pathogenicity, the ability of an agent to produce disease, depends on the speed with which the agent multiplies, the extent of tissue damage, and the production of a toxin. Agents can be graded according to this characteristic also.[31] Agents causing smallpox and rabies are highly pathogenic, and infection with them generally results in disease. The rubella virus has intermediate pathogenicity, and the poliomyelitis virus has low pathogenicity.

Virulence, or potency, of the pathogenic agent determines the severity of the disease process. It is measured in terms of the number of microorganisms or micrograms of toxin necessary to kill a given host. Gradation of agents according to virulence is possible. The rabies virus is a highly virulent agent; the poliomyelitis virus is intermediate; measles virus is low; and the virus causing the common cold has very low virulence.

The toxigenicity of agents is an important factor in determining virulence. Agent products associated with toxigenicity are hemolysin, leucocidin, and toxins. Hemolysin causes destruction of the host's erythrocytes, and leucocidin destroys leukocytes. Both are factors in the virulence of some streptococci and staphylococci. Agents vary in the amount and destructive potential of the toxins they produce. Some bacteria secrete water-soluble antigenic exotoxins that are quickly distributed by the blood, causing potentially severe systemic and neurologic manifestations. Diseases associated with exotoxins are tetanus, botulism, and diphtheria. Endotoxins make up the cell wall of some bacteria and cause local inflammation and destruction of host tissue. They are weakly toxic, are relatively stable, and are not antigenic. Diseases associated with endotoxins include staphylococcal food poisoning and cholera.

Antigenicity is the ability of a pathogen to induce an immune response in the host. Pathogens vary according to this characteristic. Some have intrinsic antigens (proteins, polypeptides, or polysaccharides) that cause the host to produce antibodies against the antigen. This host response is discussed under immunity.

Agent, Host, and Environment Interaction for Disease Transmission

The ability of a pathogenic agent to produce infectious disease in humans depends on the agent characteristics discussed in the previous section plus an intact chain of transmission. The chain includes a host reservoir, mode of escape from the reservoir, environment conducive to transmission of the pathogen, entry into a new host, and susceptibility of the new host to the infectious disease.

Reservoir. A reservoir is a person, animal, arthropod, plant, soil, or organic substance, alone or in combination, in which an infectious agent lives and multiplies. The agent depends on the reservoir for its reproduction and consequent survival. Humans are the only reservoir for some pathogens, whereas other pathogens require an intermediate animal or chain of animal or inanimate reservoirs. The human reservoir may have a frank or a subclinical infection, or the person may be a carrier.

Escape. The organism escapes from the reservoir at the site of the multiplication of the organism. Portals of exit may be the genitourinary tract, the gastrointestinal tract, the oral cavity, the respiratory tract, open lesions, or mechanical escape of blood. There may be more than one portal of exit for any one disease process. The duration of escape coincides with the period of communicability and varies with each disease. Generally, there is an inverse relationship between the length of the communicable period and the infectivity of the organism. Highly infectious organisms such as the influenza virus have a short duration of escape, whereas the less infective *M. tuberculosis* has a long duration of escape.

The portal of exit determines the mode of transmission and is therefore an important consideration for health workers in contact with infectious agents. An outline* of the types of pathogens usually associated with each portal of exit follows:

- I. Oral and respiratory tracts
  - A. Bacteria
    - 1. Gram-positive cocci (pneumonia, *Streptococcus pneumoniae;* scarlet fever, *S. pyogenes*)
    - 2. Gram-negative cocci (epidemic meningitis, *Neisseria meningitidis*)
    - 3. Gram-positive rods
      - a. Diphtheria *(Corynebacterium diphtheriae)*
      - b. Tuberculosis *(M. tuberculosis)*
    - 4. Gram-negative rods (laryngitis, *H. influenzae;* whooping cough, *B. pertussis*)
    - 5. Spirochetes (Vincent's angina, syphilis)
    - 6. Psittacosis organisms
  - B. Viruses
    - 1. Smallpox
    - 2. Mumps
    - 3. Measles
    - 4. Chickenpox
    - 5. Rabies
    - 6. Myxoviruses
    - 7. Adenoviruses, rhinoviruses
    - 8. Poliovirus
  - C. Fungi (see V)
- II. Intestinal and/or urinary tract
  - A. Bacteria
    - 1. Enterobacteriaceae (typhoid, dysentery)
    - 2. *Brucella* (undulant fever)
    - 3. *Leptospira* (leptospirosis)
    - 4. *Clostridium* (gas gangrene and tetanus; see V)
  - B. Viruses
    - 1. Poliomyelitis
    - 2. Coxsackie
    - 3. ECHO
    - 4. Hepatitis A
  - C. Protozoa
    - 1. *E. histolytica* (dysentery)
    - 2. *Trichomonas hominis* (enteritis)
    - 3. *Giardia lamblia* (enteritis)
  - D. Helminths
    - 1. Hookworm
    - 2. *Ascaris*
    - 3. Pinworms
    - 4. Whipworm
    - 5. Flukes
    - 6. Tapeworms
- III. Genital tract
  - A. Bacteria
    - 1. *Treponema pallidum* (syphilis)
    - 2. *N. gonorrhoeae* (gonorrheal infection)
    - 3. *Haemophilus ducreyi* (chancroid)
    - 4. *Calymmatobacterium granulomatis* (granuloma inguinale)
    - 5. Chlamydiaceae (lymphogranuloma venereum organisms)
  - B. Protozoa
    - 1. *T. vaginalis* (vulvovaginitis)
- IV. Pathogens of humans usually transmitted in blood
  - A. Mainly by sanguiferous arthopods
    - 1. Bacteria
      - a. *Yersinia pestis* (bubonic plague)
      - b. *Pasteurella tularensis* (tularemia)
      - c. *Borrelia* (relapsing fever)
    - 2. Rickettsiae (Rocky Mountain spotted fever, typhus)
    - 3. Viruses
      - a. Yellow and dengue fevers
      - b. Other arboviruses
    - 4. Protozoa
      - a. *Plasmodium* (malaria)
      - b. *Trypanosoma* (trypanosomiasis)
      - c. *Leishmania* (leishmaniasis)
    - 5. Helminths
      - a. Filarias (filariasis)
  - B. Mainly by artificial vectors (e.g., hypodermic needles, syringes, autopsy instruments, surgical instruments, and some blood derivatives [plasma, serum whole blood])
    - 1. Viruses (notably the human immunodeficiency virus [HIV] of AIDS and the hepatitis B[HBV] and non-A, non-B viruses, which may be circulating in the blood at the time the blood is drawn or the instruments used
    - 2. Bacteria that frequently cause bacteremia: *Bru-*

*Adapted from Frobisher.[33]

cella, Salmonella, Streptococcus, Staphylococcus, Neisseria, Pasteurella, Diplococcus, Leptospira, Treponema

V. Pathogens commonly found in the soil
  A. Bacteria
    1. Genus *Clostridium* (anaerobes)
      a. Gas gangrene group
      b. *Cl. tetani* (tetanus)
      c. *Cl. botulinum* (food poisoning)
    2. Genus *Bacillus* (aerobes)
      a. *B. anthracis* (anthrax)
  B. Fungi
    1. *Coccidioides immitis* (coccidiodomycosis)
    2. *H. capsulatum* (histoplasmosis)
    3. *Sporotrichum* (sporotrichosis)
    4. *Blastomyces*
  C. Helminths (see II)

Transmission. The organism may have a single or multiple routes of transmission. In general, the organism may be transmitted directly through person-to-person contact or indirectly through an animate or inanimate vehicle of transmission. Direct contact occurs when there is actual physical contact between the source and the victim as is the case with sexual, fecal-oral, or mucous droplet transmission. Indirect transmission requires that the organism survive outside the human on or in animate or inanimate vehicles. Animate vehicles include animals and vectors. Inanimate vehicles are air, food, water, milk, soil, fomites, or biologic materials. If an inanimate vehicle has the potential of infecting many persons, it is called a common vehicle.[5]

Entry. Portal of entry into a new host corresponds frequently with the portal of exit from the reservoir. Entry may be by ingestion, by inhalation, by percutaneous injection, through the mucous membranes, or across the placenta. The duration of the exposure and the numbers of organisms necessary to start the infectious process in the new host vary with each disease.

Host susceptibility. Susceptibility refers to those host conditions that increase the probability that disease may develop in the host. Susceptibility is affected by specific resistance factors such as the immunologic responses and nonspecific body defenses against disease agents, both of which are discussed in the next section. Host susceptibility is also affected by general human characteristics such as age, sex, ethnic group, and heredity; behaviors regarding eating and personal hygiene; geographic and environmental living conditions; and general health status, including nutritional status, hormonal balance, and the presence of concurrent disease. All of these factors either determine the type of pathogenic agent to which the person is exposed or determine the extent of the host response and resistance to the pathogens. The chain of transmission is summarized in Table 13-2.

Control. Control of infectious disease relies on procedures aimed at breaking the chain of transmission at one or more of its links. The point of the chain most amenable to control varies with the organism and its reservoirs, the disease process, and available technology. Control measures may be directed to killing or altering the virulence of the agent, destroying nonhuman reservoirs and vectors, isolating the infected persons, using precautions with infected body fluids and contaminated inanimate objects, and altering host resistance, defenses, and immunity.

Effective control is also based on monitoring of disease occurrence to facilitate early intervention. Certain diseases must be reported to the local health authority. These are identified in the section on conditions, diseases, and disorders.

Table 13-2
Chain of Transmission of Infectious Disease

Transmission Chain	Factors
Agent (living parasite)	Bacteria, rickettsiae, fungi, chlamydiae, mycoplasmata, viruses, helminths
Reservoir (where agent lives and multiplies)	Humans (frank cases, subclinical cases, carriers) Inanimate organic matter Animals
Portal of exit	Genitourinary tract, gastrointestinal tract, respiratory tract, oral cavity, open lesions, blood
Transmission	Direct: person to person (fecal-oral, sexual, droplet) Indirect: through a vehicle (animate: animal or vector; inanimate: food, water, soil, milk, air, intravenous therapy or catheters)
Modes of entry	Ingestion, inhalation, percutaneous injection, transplacental entry, mucous membranes
Susceptible host	Specific immune reactions Nonspecific body defenses Host characteristics: age, sex, ethnic group, heredity, behaviors Environmental and general health status

Anatomy, Physiology, and Related Pathophysiology[33,36]

Certain anatomic and physiologic characteristics of the human operate to increase resistance to infectious diseases and to fight the infectious process once it occurs. These characteristics can be considered as lines of defense against pathogenic agents. The first two lines are nonspecific to any agent; they result from the body's attempt to prevent the invasion of and to destroy foreign substances. The third line of defense, the immune response, is specific to specific pathogens. In addition to these defenses the human characteristically responds to an infectious process with a change in body temperature.

First Line of Defense: Nonspecific Body Defenses Against Infectious Agents

Mechanical barriers. Certain anatomic characteristics prevent the invasion of microorganisms. These include the intact skin and mucous membranes and oil and perspiration on the skin. Ciliary action in the respiratory tract, reflexes such as coughing and sneezing, and peristalsis in the gastrointestinal tract act to remove an organism before it penetrates tissue. The flushing action of body secretions such as tears, saliva, and mucus further protects against invasion. Compromise in any of these barriers increases susceptibility to invasion of infectious agents.

Chemical barriers. In addition to the mechanical barriers, the chemical composition of body secretions is protective. The pH of saliva, vaginal secretions, urine, and digestive secretions prevents or inhibits growth of some microbes. Bile acts to decrease the surface tension, causing changes in the cell wall of some bacteria. This renders the organisms more digestible by other digestive enzymes. Oil and sweat secretions contain chemicals that are bactericidal to some microbes. The normal flora of microorganisms on the skin and in the intestinal and vaginal tracts is a further means of protection against invasion of pathogenic agents.

Second Line of Defense: Cellular Response

If a microorganism penetrates the first line of body defenses and invades cells, a response is initiated at the cellular level to protect the human cell from death and to prevent further invasion of the microorganism. The cellular response leads to the inflammatory process (the second line of defense).

Mechanisms of cell injury. The cell responds to an invading microorganism in a manner similar to its reaction to nonlethal physical, chemical, or thermal trauma. A biochemical lesion forms within the cell, reflecting a change in one or more cellular metabolic reactions. This may or may not be accompanied by a detectable morphologic change in the cell or impairment of function. The injured cell swells because of its inability to pump out sodium ions. If cellular metabolic activity is severely compromised, intracellular enzymes may digest portions of the cell. The resulting cellular atrophy reduces metabolic demands on the cell. Cell death results if metabolism can no longer be maintained. Enzymes are then released from the dead cell to further dissolve the cellular contents. These enzymes seep into the circulation and are the basis for laboratory tests to detect tissue necrosis in the body. The enzymes also act to stimulate the inflammatory process in surrounding tissue.

Inflammation. Inflammation, an active and aggressive response of tissue to cellular injury, walls off, destroys, or neutralizes infectious agents and prepares the tissue for repair. It involves blood vessels, the fluid and cellular components of the blood, the lymphatic system, and the surrounding connective tissue.

The arterioles, venules, and capillaries dilate, resulting in hyperemia to the injured area. This increases the filtration pressure of the blood and increases permeability of the capillaries, causing a leakage of proteins and of fluid exudate into the interstitial spaces. The leakage of proteins increases the tissue colloid osmotic pressure, further attracting fluid into the interstitial spaces and resulting in visible edema and walling off of the inflamed area from other tissues.

With the leakage of fluid from the blood there is a concomitant slowing of the blood flow resulting in a "pavementing" or margination of leukocytes along the vascular endothelium. Leukocytes emigrate through the endothelium (diapedesis) to the injured tissue, attracted to the tissue by chemicals released by the injured cells or by the enzymes of necrotic cells. These chemicals include histamine, prostaglandins, and plasma kinins. The process of attracting the leukocytes is called chemotaxis.

Leukocytes are the cellular components of the blood associated with the inflammatory response to the infectious process. Leukocytes originate in the bone marrow, where most remain in an immature state until needed during infection. The number of mature leukocytes circulating in the blood is closely controlled to between 4500 and 11,000/mm^3 of blood during noninfection states. Leukocytosis, an abnormal increase in circulating white blood cells, is symptomatic of many bacterial infections. Leukopenia, an abnormal decrease in circulating white blood cells, severely hampers the body's defenses against infectious agents. Leukopenia is characteristic of some adverse drug reactions and of conditions that depress bone marrow production of leukocytes. This latter condition is called agranulocytosis.

Blood leukocytes are differentiated according to their cellular characteristics and according to their various functions. The most numerous are the granulocytes or polymorphonuclear leukocytes with horseshoe-shaped nuclei that become multilobed as the cells age. Most of these cells contain neutrophilic granules in their cytoplasm (neutrophils), but some contain granules that stain with acid dyes (eosinophils), and some have basophilic granules (basophils). The other two cell types, lymphocytes and monocytes, have no granules in their cytoplasm. Table 13-3 outlines types of leukocytes with their characteristics and functions.

The various types of blood leukocytes can be identified and differentiated by hematologic tests, which report each type as a proportion of 100%. An increase in the percentage of one type will result in a decrease in the percentage of the other types even though the actual number of the other types does not change. As the total count of leukocytes increases during an acute bacterial infection, the percentage of polymorphonuclear neutrophils increases with a corresponding decrease in the percentage of mononuclear lymphocytes.

In addition to the circulating blood leukocytes there are mature monocytes called macrophages that are ordinarily fixed in tissue. The tissue macrophage system is referred to as the reticuloendothelial system. Macrophages adhere to tissue in the blood vessels, lymph nodes, spleen, and liver sinuses, destroying infectious agents that enter those systems. Macrophages can become mobile as needed or can produce phagocytosis directly in the involved tissue.

Table 13-3
Differentiation of Leukocytes According to Their Characteristics and Functions

Leukocytes	Characteristics	Functions
Polymorphonuclear or granulocytes	Segmented lobular nucleus and granules in cytoplasm that contain enzymes and antimicrobial particles	
Neutrophils	First at scene of injury; ameboid motion to engulf agents; contain opsonins: substances that coat agent to be ingested; also contain antibacterial chemicals and enzymes; increase markedly during bacterial infections	Phagocytosis: engulf, digest living agents
Eosinophils	Same as above plus contain enzymes that counteract inflammatory process in allergic reactions	Weak phagocytosis
Basophils	Granules contain heparin and histamine	Respond to immunologic reactions
Mononuclear or agranular leukocytes	No granules in cytoplasm	
Lymphocytes	Large, round nuclei with scanty cytoplasm	Antibody production
Monocytes	Abundant cytoplasm and kidney-shaped nuclei; emigrate to site slowly but remain three or four times longer than granulocytes; not a mature cell when released from bone marrow; therefore they divide within injured tissue and increase their metabolic activities there	Phagocytosis

Data from Frobisher.[33]

Phagocytosis is the process of engulfing, digesting, and destroying infectious agents, primarily accomplished by circulating neutrophils and monocytes and tissue macrophages. This process occurs at the site of invasion of an infectious agent into tissue and continues into the lymph and blood circulation if organisms permeate those systems. Intracellular digestion of microorganisms by the phagocytic cells eventually results in further release of enzymes that induce lysis to some of the leukocytes. These dead leukocytes together with dead organisms and fluid from the blood make up the inflammatory exudate.

Four types of inflammatory exudates may be present in or on tissue during inflammation. The serous exudate contains only blood fluid and proteins and is characteristic of edema during early inflammation. Mucinous or catarrhal exudates represent an increase in secretions from inflamed mucous membranes. They may contain live or dead microorganisms. Fibrinous exudates are formed on tissue, particularly mucous membranes, when large amounts of fibrinogen are extravasated into the tissue. Purulent exudates consist of living and dead leukocytes, living and dead microorganisms, fluid exudate from the blood, and the liquefied digestive products of the dead, necrotic tissue. Pus is an example of a purulent exudate. Some inflammatory conditions produce combinations of exudates. A fibrinopurulent exudate, resulting from necrosis of the mucous membrane of the throat, is characteristic of diphtheria.

Inflammation and inflammatory exudates may remain localized, may permeate the tissue, or may spread through the blood or lymph. An abscess is an example of an infection and inflammatory process with purulent exudate in a localized stage. Leukocytes form a wall around the infectious agent in the tissue. The area of abscess deepens into the tissue as more leukocytes are drawn to the area, more organisms are killed, and more necrotic tissue is dissolved. The exudate may eventually be autolyzed and reabsorbed by the body, leading to resolution of the inflammation and abscess. Resolution may leave a cavity or ulcer at the site of the inflammation, may prepare the way for regeneration of cells, or may leave scar tissue. In some cases calcification occurs around the exudate, serving to wall off living infectious agents in the tissue. Such is frequently the case with tuberculosis.

The abscess may rupture or be mechanically ruptured and drained. Rupture of an abscess into a pleural cavity is called empyema; rupture into the peritoneal cavity leads to peritonitis. An abscess may also drain through a sinus or tract to another organ or tissue causing inflammation there. The spread of a purulent inflammatory process diffusely through tissue may result in cellulitis. If the infectious agent enters the bloodstream, bacteremia is present. Septicemia results if a pathogenic agent multiplies or releases toxin in the blood. If the infectious agent enters lymph vessels and initiates inflammation, lymphangitis is present. Lymphadenitis is inflammation of lymph nodes.

Factors affecting the outcome of the inflammatory defense process include host and agent factors. Age, nutritional status, and general health status of the human host greatly affect the person's ability to successfully initiate and resolve an inflammatory process. Agent factors, such as the ability to produce enzymes and fibrin, promote spread of the organism in spite of an aggressive inflammatory defense.

There may be both local and systemic symptoms of inflammation present in the infected human. Local symptoms include erythema, heat, edema, and pain from pressure on nerve endings. A purulent exudate may or may not be visible. Systemic symptoms may include fever and chills, diaphoresis, malaise, and nausea and vomiting. Alterations can be seen in blood leukocyte levels, blood proteins, and the erythrocyte sedimentation rate.

At the cellular level of defense two additional systems of blood and tissue products are important in preventing the spread of invading organisms: the properdin system and cellular interferon. The properdin system is made up of a group of serum components (properidine, magnesium ions, and a complement of 11 interacting proteins) that act as enzymes to inactivate viruses and to directly destroy bacteria. Interferon is a cellular protein produced by cells when viral DNA or RNA is introduced into the cell. Interferon is released by the infected cells and transferred to noninfected cells, thus preventing the spread of the virus to other cells.

Third Line of Defense: Specific Resistance or Acquired Immunity[36,38]

Whereas the first two lines of defense are nonspecific for any one type of infectious agent, the third line of defense, acquired immunity, is a host response to a specific agent. Those agents that have antigenic characteristics are capable of eliciting an immune response in the human host. Not all agents are antigenic or immunogenic. Some agents, although not antigenic by themselves, combine chemically with substances produced by the host to form an antigen that elicits an immune response.

Nature of the immune response. The human immune response has certain general properties. First, antibodies or specific lymphocytes are produced in response to specific antigens. Antigens are the chemical compounds of agents or their toxins that are different from all other chemical compounds. In general, these compounds are proteins, large polysaccharides, or large lipoprotein complexes. Second, the immune system generally recognizes host cells as nonantigenic and thus responds only to foreign proteins or polysaccharides as antigens (autoimmune diseases are an exception to this rule). Third, the immune system remembers the antigens that have invaded in the past. Host cells have a memory for the antigen and respond more rapidly with successive invasions.

Differentiating types of immunity. This section deals with immunity acquired directly as a response to a specific pathogenic and antigenic agent. This can be contrasted with innate immunity that may result from heredity. Acquired immunity can be subdivided into natural immunity (active and passive) and artificial immunity (active and passive). Table 13-4 defines and illustrates these categories of acquired immunity.

Components of the immunologic system. Active acquired immunity results from activity of the body's lymphoid tissue in the lymph nodes, spleen, submucosal areas of the gastrointestinal tract, and bone marrow. Two types of lymphocytes, found in lymphoid tissue and in circulating lymph and blood, are responsible for the immune response. The T lymphocytes, which originate from cells in the thymus gland, are responsible for forming the sensitized lymphocytes important to cellular immunity. The B lymphocytes, originating elsewhere, produce the antibodies important to humoral or antibody-mediated immunity. Both types of immunity may be operative during an infectious process. Figure 13-2 illustrates these two types of immunity.

Stages in the development of immunity. Phagocytosis of an antigenic agent by leukocytes is the first stage in the development of the active immune response. Lymphocytes in the circulating blood, lymph, or tissue exudate recognize the structure of the antigen as different from the body and set up a chain of responses to destroy or neutralize the antigen. The type of response depends on whether T lymphocytes or B lymphocytes or both are operative.

Cell-mediated immunity. The cellular immune response results from the activity of T lymphocytes, which proliferate and are disseminated widely during inflammation. There is a different type of T lymphocyte for each type of antigenic compound. T lymphocytes may attack a specific antigen directly or may secrete chemotactic substances to attract other leukocytes to the area to destroy the antigen. The T lymphocytes differ from other leukocytes in that they are sensitized to a specific type of antigen. This characteristic enables the T lymphocytes to respond more quickly to successive invasions by the specific antigenic agent. Cellular immunity provided by sensitized T lymphocytes persists indefinitely in the host. The cellular response is the basis for skin testing for tuberculosis, which is discussed later in this chapter. Cellular immunity cannot be transferred passively to another host.

Humoral or antibody-mediated immunity. Antibodies are protein molecules produced by the B lymphocytes in response to a specific antigen. First, an antigen stimulates B lymphocytes dormant in lymph tissue. Then lymphocytes specific to the antigen enlarge and divide into plasma cells that produce gamma globulin antibodies. These antibodies circulate from the lymph to the blood and tissue exudate and attach themselves to the specific antigen that stimulated their production. The amount and types of antibodies produced

Table 13-4
Types of Acquired Immunity

	Natural	Artificial
Active	Resistance resulting from natural contact with the pathogenic agent and infection with the agent; may be temporary or permanent	Resistance resulting from injection of dead or attenuated pathogens or toxoids; may be temporary or permanent
Passive	Temporary resistance resulting from transfer of antibodies from mother to infant congenitally, transplacentally, or through colostrum	Temporary resistance resulting from injection of antiserum, antitoxin, or gamma globulins produced in another host

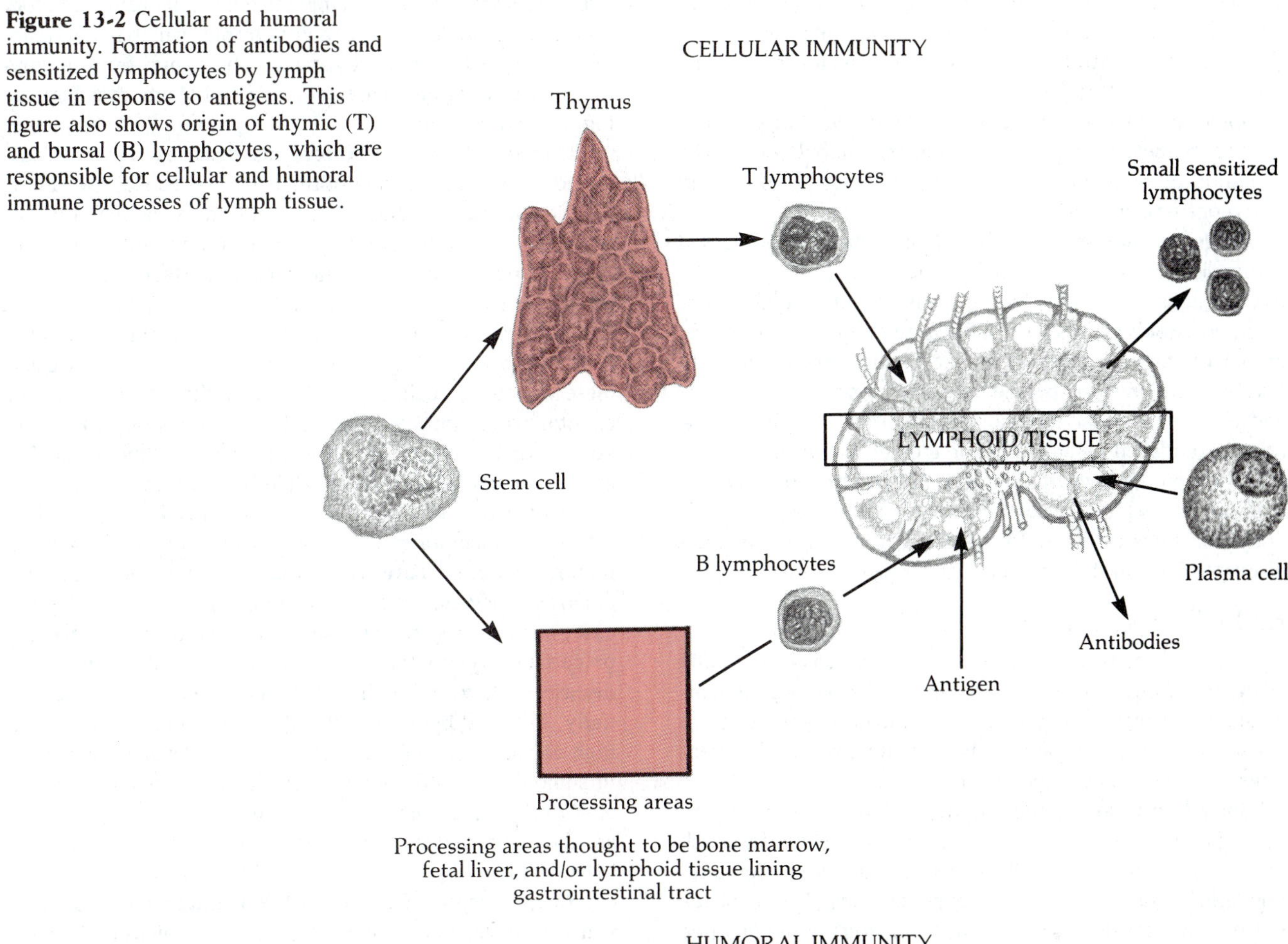

Figure 13-2 Cellular and humoral immunity. Formation of antibodies and sensitized lymphocytes by lymph tissue in response to antigens. This figure also shows origin of thymic (T) and bursal (B) lymphocytes, which are responsible for cellular and humoral immune processes of lymph tissue.

depend on the nature and amount of the antigen, the site of the antigen stimulus, and the number of times a person has been exposed to the specific antigen.

Antibodies have three major activities. The first, although not the major function, is direct attack of the antigen. Through direct attack, antibodies destroy or neutralize antigens through processes of agglutination or clumping of the antigens, precipitation of toxins out of solution, neutralization of antigenic substances, and lysis of the cell wall of the organism. The second major action of antibodies is to activate the complement system of the host. The complement system is composed of nine different enzyme precursors that are normally inactive in the blood. The activated enzymes then attack the antigen directly by lysis, opsonization (attaching to the surface of the antigen to enhance phagocytosis), agglutination, and neutralization. Activated enzymes also promote chemotaxis (by attracting other leukocytes to the area) and inflammation in surrounding tissue. Many diagnostic tests for antibody activity are based on the action of the complement system. The third action of antibodies is to activate the anaphylactic system by releasing histamine in tissue and blood. The resultant inflammation of the area acts to localize the antigenic agent to prevent spread through the body.

There are five classes of antibodies, all with different actions. They are listed here with their major actions and the areas where they are likely to be found:

- IgG: slower to develop during infection but persists for years; activates complement system; attacks antigens; most abundant in blood; crosses placenta
- IgM: first to form during infection; same actions as IgG; found in blood
- IgA: secretory antibody; found in blood and secretions (tears, colostrum, saliva)
- IgE: sensitizing; releases histamine; tissue bound
- IgD: function not clear; found in serum

Not all of the available B lymphocytes form plasma cells to produce antibodies at the time of invasion by an antigen. Some become sensitized and remain dormant so as to be activated quickly with subsequent exposure. These B lymphocytes are called memory cells.

Humoral immunity is faster acting than cellular immunity and is more frequently a factor in resistance to acute bacterial infections. In contrast to cellular immunity, the antibodies in humoral immunity can be transmitted to another human passively, either by artificial injection or by transfer through the placenta or breast milk.

Some few individuals are born without the ability to produce antibodies, a condition called agammaglobulinemia. The condition of producing insufficient antibodies is referred to as hypogammaglobulinemia.

Artificial immunity. Artificial immunity, as discussed earlier, is immunity intentionally induced in a person. In active artificial immunity dead organisms, attenuated organisms, or toxoids are injected in the form of vaccines to induce an active immune response in the human. Such immunity may be temporary or permanent, depending on the disease and vaccine. In passive artificial immunity, antibodies or antitoxins produced by an animal or another human are infused into a person. Passive artificial immunity is temporary, lasting approximately 2 to 3 weeks. Vaccines, antitoxins, and antibody injections available for specific infectious diseases are discussed later in this chapter.

Body Temperature Response[33,38]

A change in body temperature is a characteristic systemic symptom of infectious diseases. The regulation of body temperature and the etiology of fever in infectious diseases are discussed here. Fever patterns associated with specific infectious diseases are described later.

Body temperature regulation. The temperature of the body is regulated primarily by nervous system feedback mechanisms, most of which operate through a temperature-regulating center located in the hypothalamus. The feedback mechanisms consist of heat-sensitive neurons in the preoptic area of the hypothalamus, on the skin, in the spinal cord, and in the abdomen. Signals from the peripheral receptors are transmitted to the posterior hypothalamus, where they are integrated with the receptor signals from the preoptic area. Efferent signals are transmitted from the hypothalamus throughout the body to control heat loss, heat conservation, and heat production.

Heat loss is promoted (1) by stimulation of the sweat glands to cause evaporative heat loss through the skin and (2) by inhibition of sympathetic centers in the posterior hypothalamus, resulting in peripheral vasodilation. Heat conservation is promoted by stimulation of the hypothalamus to send efferent signals for vasoconstriction and abolition of sweating. Heat production is increased in three ways. First, a primary motor center for shivering in the hypothalamus becomes activated as a response to cold. Impulses are transmitted to the anterior motor neurons, which stimulate tone and shivering in skeletal muscle, thus increasing heat production. Heat production can also be increased by stimulation of cellular metabolism by circulating epinephrine and norepinephrine. This means of heat production is more common in infants than adults. A third method of increasing heat production results in a slower response than the first two. Cooling of the preoptic area stimulates release of the thyrotropin-releasing hormone of the hypothalamus. This neurosecretory hormone stimulates release of thyrotropin, which in turn stimulates the production of thyroxine. Thyroxine, from the thyroid gland, acts to increase cellular metabolism, thus increasing heat production.

Etiology of fever in infectious diseases. Fever, a sustained temperature above normal, can be caused by abnormalities of the hypothalamus, brain tumors, dehydration, or toxic substances affecting the temperature-regulating center of the hypothalamus. Certain protein substances and toxins can cause the "set point" of the hypothalamic thermostat to rise. This results in activation of the hypothalamus to conserve heat and to increase heat production. Substances that cause these effects are called pyrogens. In infectious diseases the endotoxins of some bacteria and the extracts of normal leukocytes are pyrogenic. They act to raise the "thermostat" in the hypothalamus, thus raising the body temperature.

Distinct patterns of fever onset and resolution and characteristic temperature curves are associated with different infectious diseases. Fever onset may be abrupt or gradual. A persistent elevation may be maintained throughout the disease, or there may be remissions at specific times of the day or certain days in the illness. Fever associated with some diseases follows a "saddleback" curve with a high fever initially, followed by a few days of remission and then another high elevation. A habitual fever is a low-level fever present in some diseases for years. Intermittent fevers have predictable cycles of paroxysms and remissions. Relapsing fevers are those that recur after apparent recovery. Fevers may resolve suddenly by crisis or gradually by lysis.

For each degree Fahrenheit of temperature elevation there is a 7% increase in body metabolism, necessitating fluid and calorie supplements to meet metabolic needs.

Normal Findings

Refer to specific chapters in this book to obtain normal findings pertinent to each body system.

Areas of Concern	Normal Adult Values
Body temperature: varies with time of day, exercise, room temperature, method of measurement, and accuracy of thermometer	36.3°-37.1° C (97.3°-98.8° F): AM oral 36.8°-37.6° C (98.3°-99.9° F): rectal *Older adult:* More sensitive to changes in environmental temperature
Respiratory rate	12-20/min
Pulse rate	60-90/min

Normal Laboratory Data[7,29,35,47]

Laboratory Test	Normal Adult Values
Complete white blood count (WBC)	4500-11,000/mm^3 *Older adult:* Undocumented decrease with age
Differential WBC	Expressed as a percent of total WBC
Granulocytes	
Neutrophils	62% (range of 60%-70%)
Eosinophils	2.3% (1%-4%)
Basophils	0.4%
Nongranular leukocytes	
Monocytes	5.3%
Lymphocytes	30%
Erythrocyte sedimentation rate (Westergren method)	Men (<50 yr): 0-15 mm/h Women (<50 yr): 0-25 mm/h *Older adult:* Men (>50 yr): 0-20 mm/h Women (>50 yr): 0-30 mm/h
Zeta sedimentation ratio	<50 yr: <55% *Older adult:* >50 yr: 40%-60%
Lactic acid dehydrogenase (LDH)	18-44 yr: 115-200 IU/L 44 yr and up: 115-225 IU/L
Serum albumin	1-31 yr: 3.5-5 g/dl with A/G ratio >1.0; after 40 yr, normal range gradually decreases
Partial thromboplastin time	25-39 sec (usually stated to be within 10 sec of control)
Fibrinogen	Quantitative: 200-400 mg/dl
RBC	Men: 4,600,000-6,200,000/mm^3 Women: 3,900,000-5,900,000/mm^3
Sodium (serum or plasma)	135-145 mEq/L
Potassium (plasma)	3.5-5.0 mEq/L
Chloride (serum)	97-107 mEq/L
Magnesium (serum)	1.2-1.9 mEq/L
Calcium (serum)	1-30 yr: 8.2-10.5 mg/dl *Older adult:* Decreases very slightly
Blood urea nitrogen (BUN)	1-40 yr: 5-20 mg/dl Gradual slight increase subsequently occurs
Fibrin split products	<10 μg/ml
Serum complement C_3	900-2000 μg/ml
Reticulocytes (expressed as a percentage of 1000 RBCs)	0.5%-1.5%
Direct bilirubin	Up to 0.4 mg/dl
Total bilirubin	0.3-1 mg/dl
Serum creatinine	Men: up to 1.2 mg/dl Women: up to 1.1 mg/dl
Coagulation factors	
V	60%-140%
VII	70%-130%
VIII	50%-200%
IX	60%-140%
X	70%-130%
Glycosylated hemoglobin	5.7%-8.8%
Plasma hemoglobin	1-5 mg/dl
Hemoglobin	Men: 15.5 ± 1.1 g/dl Women: 13.7 ± 1.0 g/dl
Hematocrit	Men: 42%-52% Women: 35%-47%
Blood pH	7.35-7.45
Serum iron	42-135 μg/dl
Serum enzymes	
SGOT	8-42 U/L
SGPT	3-30 U/L
CPK	Men: 55-70 U/L Women: 15-57 U/L
Serum aldolase	1.3-8.2 mU/ml
Serum alkaline phosphatase	35-100 IU/L
Blood platelets	150,000-400,000/mm^3
Prothrombin time	10-13 sec
Prothrombin levels	60%-140%
O_2 saturation	95%-99%
Bleeding time	Ivy: 2-7 min Duke: 5 min
CO_2	Arterial: 22-29 mEq/L Venous: 23-30 mEq/L
Po_2	80-95 mm Hg
Pco_2	35-45 mm Hg
Urine output	1500-3000 ml/24 h
Urine specific gravity	1.001-1.035
Urine protein (electrophoresis)	No monoclonal gammopathy detected
Cerebrospinal fluid	
Glucose	50-80 mg/dl in fasting patients
Protein	6 mo and up: approximately 15-50 mg/dl
IgG	0-11% of total protein
Pressure	80-180 mm H_2O
Serum proteins (immunoglobulins)	
IgG	1140 mg/dl (75% of total; range of 564-1765 mg/dl)
IgA	214 mg/dl (10%-15% of total; range of 85-385 mg/dl)
IgM	168 mg/dl (7%-10% of total; range of 40-120 mg/dl)
IgD	0.5-3 mg/dl (<1% of total)
IgE	0.01-0.04 mg/dl (<1% of total)

Conditions, Diseases, and Disorders

There are many schemes in common practice for categorizing infectious diseases. They include categorizing according to the type of pathogenic agent, the mode of transmission, the body system affected, or alphabetical order. The infectious diseases presented here are ordered as to body system, whenever possible, to allow the reader to refer to other body system chapters for additional information on pathophysiology, assessment, diagnostic studies, and nursing diagnoses and interventions pertinent to the system. The exceptions to this scheme are (1) that all communicable diseases for which there is a routine immunization schedule are grouped together even though they have neurologic, skin, or respiratory symptoms; (2) that the nosocomial (hospital-acquired) infections are grouped together although they cross all systems; and (3) that enteric infections are subdivided to include food poisonings, gastroenteritis, and parasitic infections where eggs are ingested or found in the stool even though the diseases may affect other body systems.

VACCINE-PREVENTABLE INFECTIOUS DISEASES

The infectious diseases presented in this section, with the exception of chickenpox, are preventable with routine immunization. These diseases are outlined in Table 13-5.

Chickenpox

Chickenpox (varicella) is an acute, highly communicable viral disease common in childhood and young adulthood. It is characterized by a sudden-onset fever, mild malaise, and a skin eruption that is maculopapular for a few hours and vesicular for 3 to 4 days, leaving a granular scab. Lesions generally occur in successive crops with several stages of maturity present at one time. They are generally more abundant on covered areas of the body, but they may appear everywhere including the scalp, conjunctivae, and upper respiratory tract.

Pathophysiology[5,48]

The varicella-zoster (V-Z) virus, a herpesvirus, enters the body by way of the respiratory mucous membranes and produces systemic disease. As is characteristic of herpesvirus lesions, the skin lesions of chickenpox consist of eosinophilic intranuclear inclusions and contain giant multinucleated cells. The lesions are generally superficial unilocular vesicles, with the fluid containing more polymorphonuclear cells than mononuclear cells. Lesions have been found in the lungs, liver, spleen, adrenal glands, and pancreas. Complications include conjunctival involvement, secondary bacterial infections, viral pneumonia, encephalitis, aseptic meningitis, myelitis, Guillain-Barré syndrome, and Reye's syndrome. Disease is severe in those with deficiencies in cell-mediated immunity. After recovery the virus is believed to remain in the body in an asymptomatic latent stage, possibly localized in the dorsal root ganglia.

Reactivation of the infection with the V-Z virus can occur later in life or during times of altered immune status. It leads to the disease manifestation of herpes zoster, in which there is a localized eruption of vesicles with an erythematous base. The vesicles are restricted to the skin areas supplied by sensory nerves of a single or associated group of dorsal root ganglia.

Diagnostic Studies and Findings[48]

Electron Microscopy or Tissue Culture of Vesicular Fluid from Lesions

Visualization of V-Z virus during first 3 days after eruption

Giemsa-Stained Scrapings from Lesions

Multinucleated giant cells

Immunofluorescence

Increase in long-lasting antibodies 2 weeks after rash

Complement Fixation

Increase in antibodies up to 2 months after infection, with subsequent decrease in antibodies

Medical Plan[5,48]

Medications

Acyclovir (Zovirax) or vidarabine (Ara-A, Vira-A) may be helpful for immunocompromised persons if administered early in the disease

Zoster immune globulin (ZIG) (for high-risk persons only), 125 U/10 kg body weight up to maximum of 625 U IM within 96 h of exposure

General Management

Relief of pruritus

Management of fever

Treatment of complications: encephalitis (see p. 1246), viral pneumonia (see Chapter 2)

Strict isolation of hospitalized patients until all lesions have crusted (see p. 1297)

NURSING CARE

Nursing Assessment

Skin and Mucous Membranes

Lesions in various stages of development; erythematous macules forming over a 4- or 5-day period progress rapidly to vesicles and crusts; start on scalp and trunk and spread in a centrifugal fashion to the extremities; may have lesions on buccal mucosa, palate, or conjunctivae

Body Temperature

Fever: 38° to 39° C (101° to 103° F)

Subjective Symptoms

Headache, anorexia, malaise

Nursing Dx & Intervention

Nursing Diagnosis	Nursing Intervention/Rationale
Impaired skin integrity	• Assess extent of lesions. • Bathe or encourage patient to bathe regularly *to remove exudate*. • Caution patient against scratching lesions *to prevent spread of exudate and potential scarring*. • Ensure smoothness of bed linen and clothing *for comfort*. • Use minimal clothing and bed linens *for comfort*. • Maintain cool room temperature with adequate humidity *for comfort*.
Hyperthermia	• Assess for fever. • Administer antipyretics as ordered *to lower fever*. • Administer tepid sponge baths *to lower fever*.
Pain	• Apply calamine lotion or cornstarch *to relieve itching*.
Potential for infection: patient contacts	• Assess for secondary infection of lesions. • Observe strict isolation of hospitalized patient until all lesions have crusted (see p. 1297) *to prevent transmission to others*. • Refer high-risk patient contacts to a physician for prophylactic treatment with zoster-immune globulin *to prevent transmission of virus to others*.

Patient Education

1. Teach care for the patient at home as described above.

Evaluation

Patient Outcome	Data Indicating That Outcome is Reached
Skin and mucous membrane functions are good, with minimal scarring.	Crusts are shed, and warm, moist natural color returns to skin and mucous membranes.
Complications and infection are absent.	There are no respiratory or neurologic pathologic findings. Body temperature is normal. Infection has not been transmitted to others in the environment.

Tetanus

Tetanus (lockjaw) is an acute neurointoxication induced by the tetanus bacillus growing anaerobically at the site of an injury. It is manifested as tonic rigidity and painful, intermittent tonic spasms of the masseter and cervical muscles and muscles of the trunk and extremities. Abdominal rigidity, a position of opisthotonus, generalized spasms induced by sensory stimuli, and a facial expression known as risus sardonicus are characteristic. Fatality is high.

Pathophysiology[48]

Tetanus spores enter through a trivial or extensive injury to the skin. The anaerobic organism multiplies in the wound, even after the injury has healed, producing a lethal toxin. The

Table 13-5
Childhood Communicable and Immunizable Infectious Diseases

	Chickenpox	Tetanus	Diphtheria	Pertussis (Whooping Cough)
Occurrence	Worldwide; in metropolitan areas 75% of the population has had chickenpox by age 15 yr, and 90% by young adulthood	Worldwide; occurs sporadically and affects all ages; rare in United States with immunization; common among agricultural workers, parenteral drug abusers, and elderly	Formerly a prevalent disease; rare in United States with immunization; affects unimmunized children under 15 yr and adults	Common in children; worldwide; decline in incidence in areas with active immunization programs
Etiologic agent	Varicella-zoster (V-Z) virus, a member of the *Herpesvirus* group	*Clostridium tetani*, the tetanus bacillus (an anaerobic pathogen)	*Corynebacterium diphtheriae*, with many toxigenic strains	*Bordetella pertussis*, the pertussis bacillus
Reservoir	Humans	Intestines of humans and animals	Humans	Humans
Transmission	Direct and indirect contact with droplets from respiratory passages; an extremely contagious disease	Tetanus spores enter body through a wound contaminated with soil and feces; necrotic tissue favors the growth of the bacillus	Direct or indirect contact with exudate from mucous membranes of infected person or carrier; raw milk may also be a vehicle	Direct contact with droplets from respiratory passages
Incubation period	2-3 wk; commonly 13-17 d	3-21 d; commonly 10 d	2-5 d	7-21 d; commonly 7d
Period of communicability	1-2 d before onset of rash and until lesions have crusted over (not more than 6 d after first appearance of vesicles)	Not directly transmitted	Variable; until bacilli have disappeared from discharges and lesions (usually in 2 wk); a carrier may shed bacilli for 6 mo	7 d after exposure to 3 wk after onset; highly communicable in early catarrhal stage before cough; not communicable after 3 wk even though cough may persist
Susceptibility and resistance	General; one attack confers long immunity; second attacks are rare	General; recovery from tetanus does not confer permanent immunity; temporary active immunity provided by tetanus toxoid	Unimmunized children most susceptible; infants born of immune mothers have passive immunity for 6 mo; recovery from clinical disease confers temporary immunity	General; children under 7 yr most susceptible; no passive immunity from mother; attack confers prolonged, but not lifetime, immunity
Report to local health authority	In some areas	Case report required	Case report required	Case report required

Data from Benenson.[5]

toxin (tetanospasmin) reaches the central nervous system by the bloodstream or by centripetal passages along peripheral motor nerves. The toxin binds with central nervous system tissue and spinal motor ganglia. There it interferes with the release of an inhibitory transmitter and induces a hyperexcitability of motor neurons, resulting in tonic rigidity and spasms of facial, cervical, masseter, respiratory, abdominal, and extremity muscles. The bound toxin cannot be neutralized by an antitoxin.

The permanency of pathologic changes in the central and peripheral nervous system in patients who recover has not been determined. Neonatal tetanus generally leaves no permanent neurologic sequelae. Central nervous system findings in fatal cases range from mild congestion to definite hem-

Poliomyelitis	Mumps (Infectious Parotitis)	Rubella (German Measles)	Rubeola (Hard Measles)
Worldwide; commonly in summer and early autumn; highest in children and adolescents but does affect nonimmune adults; United States incidence decreasing with immunization	Occurs commonly in winter and spring; one third of those exposed have subclinical infections; incidence decreasing with immunization	Worldwide and endemic; most common in winter and spring; primarily a disease of children but does occur in unimmunized adolescents and adults	Worldwide; endemic and epidemic occurrences; seen more in adolescents and adults since routine immunization of children
Polio virus, types 1, 2, and 3; all are paralytogenic	A type of paramyxovirus; antigenically related to parainfluenza viruses	Rubella virus	Measles virus, a type of paramyxovirus
Humans, particularly children with subclinical infections	Humans	Humans	Humans
Direct and indirect contact with respiratory discharges and feces; fecal-oral route more common than respiratory transmission	Direct contact with saliva droplets from infected person	Direct or indirect contact with nasopharyngeal secretions of infected persons; transplacental transmission leads to congenital rubella syndrome	Direct or indirect contact with nasal secretions from infected persons; highly communicable
3-35 d; commonly 7-14 d	2-3 wk; commonly 18 d	14-23 d; commonly 16-18 d	Commonly 10 d; 8-13 d until fever; 14 d until rash
Highly communicable during first days after onset of symptoms; virus is in throat secretions in 36 h and in feces in 72 h after infection and remains 1 wk in throat and 6 wk in feces	6 d before parotid symptoms to 9 d after; most communicable 48 h before parotid swelling	From 1 wk before and 4 d after appearance of rash; highly communicable; infants with congenital rubella syndrome may shed virus for months after birth	A few days before fever to 4 d after appearance of rash
General; paralytic infections are rare and risk increase with age; infection confers long-term immunity; second attacks are result of another virus type	General; immunity is lifelong and develops jafter clinical and subclinical disease; placental transfer of antibodies occurs	General; infants born with passive immunity from mother lasting 6-9 mo; one attack confers lifetime immunity for most, but reinfections (mostly asymptomatic) have been documented	General; acquired immunity from infection is permanent; artificial active immunity may not be permanent
Case report required	Case report required in some areas	Case report required	Case report required

orrhage, perinuclear chromatolysis, and perivascular areas of demyelination and gliosis with confluent areas of tissue necrosis in the cerebral hemispheres.

Pathologic changes in other parts of the body result from anoxia caused by respiratory impairment, asphyxial convulsions, toxic degeneration, and inanition. Pulmonary complications are frequent in tracheotomized patients. Changes in striated muscles such as hemorrhage and rupture also occur throughout the body. The risk for further pathologic change increases with duration of the disease. Cardiac, pulmonary, and musculoskeletal complications are common.

Diagnostic Studies and Findings[48]

There are no definitive diagnostic studies. The organism is rarely recovered from the site of the lesion, and there is no detectable antibody response. Clinical findings are important for differential diagnosis.

Tetanus must be differentiated from meningitis, poliomyelitis, encephalitis, rabies, strychnine poisoning, reactions to phenothiazides, tetany, peritonsillar abscess, and peritonitis. Abnormal laboratory and physiologic data include the following:

- Increased spinal pressure
- Moderately elevated WBC count
- Slight decrease in blood platelets and prothrombin time
- Low prothrombin levels, impaired thrombin generation, and increased fibrinolytic activity
- Increased serum enzymes: SGOT (serum glutamic oxaloacetic transaminase), SGPT (serum glutamic pyruvate transaminase), CPK (creatinine phosphokinase), serum aldolase, alkaline phosphatase
- Decreased serum iron and iron-binding capacity
- Metabolic acidoses
- Hypoxemia
- Sinus tachycardia and transient electrocardiograph (ECG) changes
- Electroencephalographic (EEG) changes

Medical Plan[5,48]

Surgery

- Tracheostomy or laryngotracheal intubation as needed to aid respiration
- Surgical care of local lesion by removal of foreign bodies only (debridement or amputation of locus of infection is not indicated)

Medications

- Antitoxin serum therapy (two types)
- Hyperimmune human tetanus immune globulin, 500-6000 U IM (1 dose), or hyperimmune equine or bovine serum, 10,000-20,000 IU IV or IM (1 dose)
- Sensitivity test dose of 0.01-0.05 ml undiluted antitoxin should be administered IM and patient observed for 15-30 min for anaphylactic-type reaction before administering full dose
- Sedative-relaxant therapy
  - Sedatives
    - Thiopental sodium (Pentothal sodium), 0.4% IV drip
    - Phenobarbital (Luminal), 3-5 mg/kg body weight IM, IV, or po q3-6h
    - Paraldehyde (Panal), 0.15 mg/kg IM q4-6h
  - Psychotherapeutic agents
    - Chlorpromazine (Thorazine), 0.5 mg/kg IM or IV q4-8h; 100 mg IV (up to 300 mg/24 h) used for relaxant effect and emergency control of seizures in adults; 25-50 mg po q6h for mild cases
  - Antianxiety agents
    - Meprobamate (Miltown Injectable), 200-400 mg for patients over 5 yr IM q3h
    - Diazepam (Valium), 0.2 mg/kg IM or IV q3-4h; dosage may be increased with severity of seizures up to 9.5 mg/kg/24 h for adults
  - Muscle relaxants
    - Methocarbamol (Robaxin), IM or IV; initial dose of 15 mg/kg; maximal dose of 50 mg/kg/24 h divided into 4-6 doses to be infused at rate of 3 mg/min
    - Neuromuscular block is indicated only in severe cases when above agents are ineffective; agents used include tubocurarine chloride, demethyl tubocurarine chloride, gallamine triethiodide, and succinylcholine chloride; assistive or controlled respiration must be available
- β-Adrenergic blockers
  - Propranolol (Inderal), 0.2 mg aliquots, to total of 2 mg IV for adults or 10 mg q8h intragastric; used for treatment of cardiovascular sympathetic overactivity syndrome
- Active or passive immunization (p. 1293)

General Management

- Intermittent positive-pressure breathing (IPPB)
- Suction of respiratory secretions
- Control of environment to reduce stimulation
- Hyperalimentation, nasogastric feedings, or IV fluids, plus liquid feedings as patient's condition warrants
- Indwelling catheter to control urinary retention
- Physical therapy to prevent contractures and to facilitate return of muscle function and ambulation during convalescence
- Care of vertebral compression fractures
- Control of delayed allergic anaphylactic reactions to antitoxin
- Treatment of local lesions and tetanus prophylaxis in wound management to prevent tetanus
- Aseptic care of umbilical stump and circumcision wound to prevent tetanus

NURSING CARE

Nursing Assessment

Skin

- Pain, tingling at site of injury
- Profuse perspiration

Musculoskeletal Concerns

- Early: stiff neck, tight jaw, incipient stiffness of arms and legs
- Later: locked jaw (trismus); spasms of facial muscles with raising of eyebrows, wrinkling of forehead, and drawing out of mouth corners (risus sardonicus)
- Difficulty in swallowing, rigid muscles

Neurologic Concerns

Early: restlessness, irritability
Later: convulsions; paralysis of one or more cranial nerves in cephalic tetanus

Respiratory Concerns

Dyspnea; asphyxia and cyanosis result from viselike constriction of chest muscles

Urinary Elimination

Urinary retention

Body Temperature

Early: 38° to 40° C (101° to 104° F) or afebrile
Terminal: 43° to 44° C (110° to 112° F)

Bowel Elimination

Constipation

Hematopoietic Concerns

Increased risk for hemorrhage

Cardiovascular Concerns

Arrhythmias
Tachycardia
Hypertension

Nursing Dx & Intervention

Nursing Diagnosis	Nursing Intervention/Rationale
Ineffective airway clearance	• Assess for airway patency. • *Maintain patent airway* by frequent aspiration of secretions and care of tracheostomy or endotracheal tube.
Ineffective breathing pattern	• Observe for signs of respiratory failure in sedated patients; provide respiratory assistance as needed. • Administer oxygen as prescribed *to maintain adequate oxygen intake when breathing is compromised.*
Potential for trauma; potential for suffocation	• Use padded side rails and headboard on bed, padded tongue blade, and removal of dentures *to protect patient from injury in convulsions.* • Provide continuous supervision. • Monitor for signs of internal trauma and hemorrhage. • *To minimize convulsions precipitated by environmental stimuli:* Maintain quiet, nonstimulating environment to reduce seizures. Minimize physical handling of patient during acute stage. • Take vital signs and perform any procedures while patient is in a sedated state *to minimize stimuli.* • Monitor patient closely for anaphylactic reaction to antitoxin therapy. • Provide standby emergency equipment and be prepared to resuscitate and provide life support.
Potential fluid volume deficit	• Administer IV therapy as prescribed. • Monitor intake and output *to ensure intake equal to output.*
Altered nutrition: less than body requirements	• Administer alimentation therapy as prescribed *to provide nutrients not provided orally.*
Urinary retention	• Monitor urinary output, or maintain indwelling catheter *to relieve urinary retention.*
Constipation	• Administer enemas as prescribed *to prevent patient from straining to defecate.*
Decreased cardiac output	• Assess vital signs *to detect tachycardia and hypertension.* • Monitor for symptoms of arrhythmias. • Administer prescribed therapy (see Chapter 1).
Hyperthermia	• Assess for fever. • Sponge patient while patient is sedated *to lower body temperature while minimizing stimuli.*
Potential for infection: patient	• Assess vital signs *to detect signs of secondary infection.* • Use aseptic technique for all invasive procedures *to prevent secondary infection.*
Potential impaired skin integrity	• Turn frequently during convalescence *to avoid pressure.* • Place on air mattress or lamb's wool.
Impaired physical mobility	• Position sedated patient *to maintain proper body alignment.* • Administer range of motion exercises, and supervise gradually increasing movement during convalescence.

Patient Education

1. Teach the public the dangers of tetanus and the advantages of initiating immunization at 2 to 3 months of age and adhering to the recommended immunization schedule (see p. 1295).
2. Remind adults to receive tetanus toxoid vaccine every 10 years in the absence of a wound.
3. Refer persons with skin injuries for tetanus prophylaxis (see p. 1296).

Evaluation

Patient Outcome	Data Indicating That Outcome is Reached
Respiratory function is normal.	Patient is breathing on own without mechanical assistance. There are no periods of cyanosis or labored breathing or signs of pulmonary complications such as pneumonia. Respiratory rate is normal.
Neurologic function is normal.	There are no convulsions. Reflexes, including cough and gag reflexes, are normal.
Neuromuscular function is normal.	Spasms, muscular rigidity, posturing, or spasmodic facial expressions are not present.
Musculoskeletal function is normal.	Fractures, contractures, or prolonged muscle weakness is not present. Mobility returns.
Cardiovascular function is normal.	Heart rate is normal, without tachycardias or arrhythmias. Blood pressure is normal.
Body temperature is normal.	Temperature is normal.
Essential nutrients are part of daily intake.	Patient is able to eat a regular diet during convalescence.
Bowel elimination is normal for individual.	Stools are soft. Abdomen is soft and not distended.
Urinary elimination is normal.	Patient is able to empty bladder completely without assistance. Urine output equals fluid intake.
Integrity of skin and mucous membranes is maintained.	Injuries that may have been sustained during convulsions are healed. There are no decubiti. Skin is warm and moist with good color.
Laboratory studies are within normal limits.	WBC count is normal. Spinal pressure decreases to normal. There is no acidosis. Serum iron and serum enzyme levels are normal. Blood platelet count is normal. Prothrombin time is normal. Prothrombin levels are normal.

Diphtheria

Diphtheria is an acute communicable disease in which a bacterial toxin affects the mucous membranes of the respiratory tract. The disease is manifest as fibropurulent exudative membranes, commonly on the tonsils and pharynx but also on the larynx, nasal passages, skin, conjunctivae, and genitalia, and as systemic symptoms resulting from toxin dissemination.

Pathophysiology[5,48]

Corynebacterium diphtheriae, widely available in the nasopharynx of carriers and persons with inapparent infection, invades and multiplies in the nasopharynx of susceptible persons. The pathogen produces a toxin that is disseminated by the blood and lymph throughout the body. The toxin first causes necrosis of the local tissue, resulting in a fibrinopurulent exudative membrane characteristic of this disease. The membrane appears as grayish membrane patches surrounded by a red zone of inflammation on the tonsils, pharynx, larynx, nasal mucosa, or skin. Edema is present in adjacent and underlying tissue and in the cervical lymph nodes. Laryngeal edema and the extension of the membrane into the trachea, bronchial tree, and alveoli may result in suffocation. Nasopharyngeal diphtheria and laryngeal diphtheria are the most severe types. Nasal diphtheria is mild and marked by one-sided nasal excoriations and discharge. Cutaneous diphtheria lesions are variable and may resemble impetigo.

Disseminated toxin inhibits protein synthesis primarily in the heart, peripheral nerves, and muscle tissue. Effects of toxin absorption appear early and include fatty degeneration, edema, and interstitial fibrosis in the myocardium and in the myelin sheath of peripheral nerves. Damage to peripheral nerves results in peripheral motor and sensory palsies. The spleen and kidneys also may be affected. Otitis media, peritonsillar abscess, and albuminuria are less severe complications. Severe toxemia may result in a life-threatening myocarditis, motor or sensory paralysis, pharyngeal and respiratory paralysis, and pneumonia. ECG changes and an increase in SGOT levels may be present.

Diagnostic Studies and Findings[5,48]

Bacteriologic Examination of Lesions Using Loeffler's Methylene Blue Stain

Positive for *C. diphtheriae*

Test for Toxigenicity by Inoculation of an Animal with Serum from Patient

Necrosis at site of inoculation; animal will become ill if toxin is present in patient's serum

Hemagglutination and Radioimmunoassay

Positive for agglutinating antibodies

Schick Skin Test

0.1 ml of active diphtheria toxin and 0.1 ml of an inactive toxin (for a control) are injected at two different sites on person; read at 24 and 48 hours; increased redness, edema, and flaking of skin at test site between two readings indicate no circulating antitoxin; this is a test for susceptibility

Differential Diagnosis

Rule out acute tonsillitis, septic sore throat, infectious mononucleosis, scarlet fever, Vincent's angina, syphilis, and candidiasis

Medical Plan[48]

Surgery

Tracheostomy

Medications

- Immunologic agents
  - Diphtheria antitoxin administered IM in mild infections and IM and IV (diluted) in severe infections; dosages vary with severity of infection and number of days since disease onset:
    - Tonsillar: 20,000 U
    - Pharyngeal: 20,000-40,000 U
    - Tonsillar and uvular: 40,000 U
    - Nasopharyngeal: 60,000-100,000 U
    - Laryngeal: 20,000 U
    - Laryngeal with other: 20,000-100,000 U
- Corticosteroids
  - May be used to prevent or ameliorate myocarditis
- Anti-infective agents
  - Local application of penicillin solution plus IM antitoxin for cutaneous diphtheria
  - Erythromycin (Robimycin), 50 mg/kg body weight/d for 1 wk for carrier state
- Active or passive immunization for prevention (see p. 1293)
- Prophylaxis for case contacts

General Management

- Laryngeal and tracheal suction
- Intubation
- Nasogastric feedings if pharyngeal paralysis occurs
- Positive-pressure ventilation if respiratory paralysis occurs
- Bed rest with minimal exertion for 4 to 6 weeks
- IV administration of glucose and amino acids if oral feeding is impossible; otherwise, soft diet
- Strict isolation until two nasopharyngeal cultures 24 hours apart are negative; for cutaneous diphtheria, contact isolation (see p. 1297)

NURSING CARE

Nursing Assessment

Body Temperature

Moderately elevated: 38° to 39° C (100° to 102° F)

Head and Neck

Edema of neck and lymph nodes

Nasopharynx

- Presence of edema and gray membranous patches on tonsils, pharynx, larynx, or nasal passages
- Difficulty in swallowing

Breathing Pattern

Noisy, labored; may be sudden obstruction; neck muscle retraction; suprasternal and substernal retraction

Activity Patterns

Restlessness as a sign of impaired oxygenation

Cardiovascular Concerns

Sudden slowing of pulse and beginning irregularity; pallor

Neurologic: Peripheral Nerves

- Palatal paralysis: nasal tone to voice (tenth day)
- Oculomotor paralysis: strabismus (third week)
- Ciliary paralysis: dilation of pupils and blurring of vision (third week)
- Facial paralysis: loss of tone of cheek muscles; flattening of one side of face; inability to blow out cheeks equally (third week)
- Pharyngeal paralysis: difficulty in swallowing; regurgitation of food through nose (third or fourth week)
- Laryngeal paralysis: hoarseness or aphonia (third to fifth week)
- Paralysis or paresis in extremities: weakness, numbness, and tingling in extremities
- Paralysis of diaphragm: difficulty in breathing; cyanosis (fifth or sixth week)

Nursing Dx & Intervention

Nursing Diagnosis	Nursing Intervention/Rationale
Ineffective airway clearance	• Assess for symptoms of obstruction, particularly neck muscle retraction, suprasternal and substernal retraction, dyspnea, and signs of restlessness. • Have tracheostomy tray available; administer tracheostomy care *to maintain patent airway.* • Increase humidity of inspired air; administer oxygen as prescribed.
Decreased cardiac output	• Assess for changes in pulse (rate, rhythm, and quality) and changes in blood pressure. Look for sudden decrease in pulse rate and onset of irregularity and pallor. • Employ complete bed rest *to decrease stress on cardiovascular system.* • Minimize anxiety. • Perform care for cardiac complications as prescribed (see Chapter 1).
Altered nutrition: less than body requirements	• Provide frequent, small feedings of soft foods and liquids as can be swallowed *to maintain adequate intake with impaired swallowing.* Nasogastric feedings may be necessary if patient cannot swallow.
Sensory/perceptual alterations	• Assess for onset of peripheral nerve paralysis as listed under "Nursing Assessment."
Potential fluid volume deficit	• Assess intake and output. • Administer IV fluids, as prescribed, *for patient who cannot swallow.*
Activity intolerance	• Employ complete bed rest for up to 6 weeks *to reduce neurologic and cardiovascular stress.* • Provide total hygiene and feeding *to conserve patient's energy.*
Altered oral mucous membrane	• Assess mouth and throat for edema and gray membranous patches *to report findings and provide early intervention.* • Provide frequent use of mouth rinses; avoid swabbing or any oral hygiene procedure that induces gagging *for comfort.* • Lubricate nostrils in nasal diphtheria with zinc oxide ointment.[48]
Potential for infection: patient contacts	• Employ strict isolation precautions until two nasopharyngeal cultures 24 hours apart are negative *to prevent transmission* (see p. 1297). • Refer patient contacts to a physician for prophylaxis *to prevent acute infection in patient contacts.*
Impaired verbal communication	• Anticipate needs of patient who is unable to communicate because of labored breathing and swallowing *to minimize anxiety and meet basic needs.*
Hyperthermia	• Assess body temperature. • Sponge bathe patient or administer antipyretics as prescribed *to lower body temperature.*

Patient Education

1. Teach the public the dangers of diphtheria and the importance of initiating immunization at 2 to 3 months of age and of adhering to the recommended immunization schedule (see p. 1295).

Evaluation

Patient Outcome	Data Indicating That Outcome is Reached
Body hydration and oxygenation are normal.	Skin, nails, lips, earlobes, and mucous membranes are warm and moist, with natural color. Skin turgor is good. Secretions are thin. Patient is not restless.
Vital signs are within normal limits.	Pulse rate, respiratory rate, blood pressure, and temperature are normal.
Airway clearance and breathing patterns are effective.	The patient can swallow secretions. Breathing is unlabored, with normal rhythm.
Sensory function is normal. Visual tests are positive.	The patient correctly identifies letters on Snellen eye chart from distance of 20 feet. Pupils are normal and reactive.

Patient Outcome	Data Indicating That Outcome is Reached
Touch test is positive.	Patient responds to touch of extremities. There are no feelings of tingling or numbness. Patient feels pinprick, heat, and cold.
Motor function is normal.	Patient moves extremities and changes body position in bed. There are no signs of facial paralysis; patient is able to blow out cheeks equally. Patient can swallow without difficulty. Patient is able to speak coherently, without nasal tone to voice.
Rest and sleep are adequate.	Patient gets adequate sleep: 7 to 9 hours for adult. Bed rest is maintained.
Patient is in a relaxed state while resting.	Facial expression is calm and serene; breathing is regular; there are periods of motionlessness. There is no startle response to stimuli.
Mucous membranes return to prepathogenic state.	There is no secondary infection in nasopharynx. There is no edema, erythema, or membranous patches. Two nasopharyngeal cultures are negative.
There is no infection.	Infection has not been transmitted to others in the environment.

Pertussis
(Whooping cough)

Pertussis (whooping cough) is an acute communicable bacterial infection of the mucous membranes of the tracheobronchial tree, characterized by paroxysms of repeated and violent coughing. Paroxysms are terminated by a prolonged, high-pitched inspiratory whoop and the expulsion of clear, tenacious mucus. This disease is most severe in children under 1 year of age and in persons living in poverty.

Pathophysiology[40,48]

The toxigenic *Bordetella pertussis* bacillus enters the respiratory passages by airborne droplets of respiratory secretions from persons with asymptomatic infections or with clinical disease. The organism reproduces in the mucous membranes of the trachea, bronchi, and bronchioles, producing a toxin that causes necrosis to the ciliated mucosa. There are three stages of the disease: catarrhal, paroxysmal, and convalescent. A serous exudate is produced initially in the catarrhal stage, lasting 1 to 2 weeks. This is followed by a viscid mucopurulent exudate that is irritating to the mucosa. The exudate, which is difficult to expel, initiates severe spasmodic coughing (paroxysms) that may persist for 1 to 2 months. Coughing may also be initiated by toxin stimulation to the central nervous system.

Local necrosis of the tracheal and bronchial epithelium is extensive, with an associated peribronchial and interstitial inflammatory infiltrate. Unexpelled mucous plugs may produce areas of atelectasis and emphysema. Paratracheal and bronchial lymphadenopathy may be present. Edema, congestion, and hemorrhage may occur in lung tissue, and edema and petechial hemorrhages are commonly found in brain tissue. These pathologic findings result from anoxia during the prolonged paroxysms of coughing. Paroxysms may also result in epistaxis, scleral hemorrhage, periorbital edema, vomiting, exhaustion, aspiration, and aspiration pneumonia. Also, umbilical and inguinal hernias and rectal prolapse may result from increased intra-abdominal pressure during paroxysms.

Additional complications include secondary bacterial infections such as otitis media or pneumonia. Convulsions occur in small children as a result of high temperature and anoxia caused by prolonged paroxysms.

A marked hyperleukocytosis and lymphocytosis are characteristic. The WBC count may range as high as 175,000 to 200,000, and lymphocytes increase to 90% in the differential count.

The convalescent stage is characterized by a cessation of whooping and vomiting with a gradual decrease in the number of paroxysms over a 2- to 3-week period. Some patients develop exacerbations of paroxysms of cough, whooping, and vomiting during subsequent respiratory tract infections.

Diagnostic Studies and Findings[5,48]

Direct Fluorescent Antibody Staining of Nasopharyngeal Secretions During Catarrhal Stage

Positive for *B. pertussis*

WBC Count

Leukocytes: 15,000 to 40,000/mm^3; may be as high as 175,000 to 200,000/mm^3

Differential WBC Count

90% lymphocytes

Agglutination Tests

Variable results; of questionable value

Medical Plan[5,48]

Medications

Anti-infective agents
- Erythromycin (Erythrocin), 35-50 mg/kg/24 h po in 4 divided doses for 14 d

Betnesol, 0.075 mg/kg/24 h po
Corticosteroids
Hydrocortisone sodium succinate (Solu-Cortef), 30 mg/kg/24 h for 2 d IM; to be reduced gradually and discontinued by eighth day
Active immunization for prevention (see p. 1293)
Prophylaxis for case contacts

General Management

Suction of respiratory secretions
Ventilatory assistance, if needed
Oxygen administration
Parenteral fluid and electrolyte therapy
Small, frequent feedings
Postural drainage following paroxysms
Respiratory isolation for 3 weeks after onset of paroxysms or 7 days after antimicrobial therapy (see p. 1297)

NURSING CARE

Nursing Assessment

Respiratory Concerns

Catarrhal stage: normal respirations; dry, hacking cough
Paroxysmal stage (after 1 or 2 weeks): paroxysms of cough (40 to 50/24 hours in severe cases) followed by high-pitched inspiratory whoop; vomiting frequently follows paroxysm
Convalescent stage: paroxysms and vomiting become gradually less frequent and prolonged

Mucous Membranes

Catarrhal stage: serous rhinorrhea, sneezing, lacrimation, conjunctivitis
Paroxysmal stage: tenacious mucus; epistaxis

Skin

Color may be cyanotic following paroxysms
Loss of turgor because of dehydration

Body Temperature

Normal or low-grade fever; elevated in secondary infection

Head and Neck

Venous engorgement of face and neck during paroxysms
Scleral hemorrhages and periorbital edema may be present

Neurologic Concerns

Anoxic convulsions

Activity Patterns

Exhaustion following paroxysms

Abdomen

Umbilical or inguinal hernia complications

Nursing Dx & Intervention

Nursing Diagnosis	Nursing Intervention/Rationale
Ineffective airway clearance	• Suction pooled secretions if necessary *to maintain patent airway.*
Ineffective breathing pattern	• Provide oxygen by mask *to restore breathing after paroxysms.* • Assist respiration if necessary *to maintain oxygen.* • Monitor breathing for signs of atelectasis or pneumonia.
Potential fluid volume deficit	• Assess turgor and urinary output for signs of dehydration. • Give frequent, small liquid feedings or parenteral fluids if vomiting is excessive *to maintain adequate fluids.*
Impaired gas exchange	• Assess color and behavior *to detect symptoms of anoxia.* • Administer oxygen as prescribed following paroxysms *to restore circulating oxygen not taken in during paroxysms.*
Activity intolerance	• Provide for rest in a nonstimulating environment *to compensate for exhaustion from paroxysms.*
Potential for injury	• Provide convulsion precautions: padded bed, side rails, and tongue blade *to protect from trauma during convulsions.*
Potential for infection: patient	• Collect nasopharyngeal specimen for fluorescent antibody staining. • Monitor temperature and respiratory status *to detect signs of secondary infection.*
Potential for infection: patient contacts	• Employ respiratory isolation (see p. 1297) for 3 weeks after onset of paroxysms or for 7 days after onset of antimicrobial therapy *to prevent transmission to others.* • Refer patient contacts to a physician *for prophylactic immunization.*

Patient Education

1. Teach the public, particularly the parents of infants, about the dangers of pertussis and the advantages of initiating immunization at 2 to 3 months of age and of adhering to the recommended immunization schedule (see p. 1295).

Evaluation

Patient Outcome	Data Indicating That Outcome is Reached
All cells receive oxygen.	Skin, nails, lips, and earlobes are warm and moist, with natural color.
Respirations are normal.	Breathing pattern, rhythm, rate, and depth are regular.
Laboratory studies are within normal limits.	Oxygen saturation, carbon dioxide, Po_2, and Pco_2 are normal.
Body hydration is normal.	Skin turgor is good; secretions are thin. Urine output equals intake. Urine specific gravity is normal.
There is no evidence of infection.	Blood leukocyte count is normal. Bacterial culture is negative. Breathing patterns are normal. Body temperature is normal. Infection has not been transmitted.
Energy level is adequate.	Patient moves and cares for self at level of development. There is no weakness or malaise. Breathing during activity is regular.

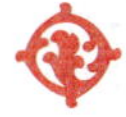

Poliomyelitis

Poliomyelitis is an acute communicable systemic viral disease affecting the central nervous system with variable severity ranging from subclinical infection, to a nonfebrile illness, to an aseptic meningitis, to paralytic disease, and possibly to death.

Pathophysiology[40,48]

Three immunologically distinct polioviruses produce poliomyelitis, an infection that occurs 100 times more frequently in a subclinical form than in clinical disease. The polioviruses are all enteroviruses; that is, they multiply in the intestinal tract and can be recovered from the feces of cases and subclinical cases. Transmission of the virus is primarily by the fecal-oral route and sometimes by direct contact with respiratory secretions.

Once in a susceptible host, the virus multiplies in the lymphoid tissue of the throat and ileum, producing a lymphocytic hyperplasia and follicular necrosis there. A transient viremia follows with subsequent viral invasion of the central nervous system producing cell damage primarily in the anterior horn cells of the spinal cord, in the medulla and pons, in the midbrain, and in the motor area of the precentral gyrus. Damage to the motor neurons results from destruction within the body of the cells. Diffuse chromatolysis of the Nissl substance of the cytoplasm occurs first, followed by nuclear changes and pericellular infiltration of polymorphonuclear leukocytes and monocytes. Damage may be reversible at this point, with complete recovery, or it may progress to necrosis and phagocytosis of the neurons resulting in clinical disease concomitant with the extent and concentration of neuron destruction.

Clinical paralysis results when there is extensive damage to motor neurons associated with any one functional motor group. Skeletal muscle fiber groups atrophy rapidly from absence of innervation from associated destroyed motor neurons. Paralysis is characteristically asymmetric, involving the lower extremities and muscles of respiration and swallowing.

Clinical poliomyelitis may be seen in three phases: a systemic stage, a phase of central nervous system involvement, and the paralytic stage. The onset of the systemic phase is acute, with low-grade fever, headache, nausea, abdominal tenderness, occasional vomiting, and the presence of a mild tonsillitis or pharyngitis. These symptoms subside within 24 to 36 hours, and the infectious process is terminated for about 80% of patients.

A small percentage of patients manifest signs of the second phase within 1 to 4 days, with a higher fever, frontal headache, vomiting, strained anxious expression on the face, dermal hypersensitivity, and hyperhidrosis, particularly around the head and neck. The symptoms may end here or progress to the paralytic stage, with nuchal and spinal stiffness from spasm of back and hamstring muscles, positive spinal fluid findings (protein levels of 80 to 200 mg/dl), hypertension, and paralysis.

Paralysis may affect different parts of the body depending on the area of central nervous system damage, giving rise to the differentiation of types of paralysis as spinal, spinobulbar, bulbar, ataxic, encephalitic, or meningitic. Complications are associated with the areas of muscle paralysis or weakness and the effect on body functioning. They include intercostal and respiratory paralysis, pharyngeal, facial, and palatal paralysis, and paralysis of eye muscles and of the urinary bladder.

Diagnostic Studies and Findings[40,48]

Culture of Feces

Positive for poliovirus 5 days after exposure to 1 to 4 months after exposure

Culture of Nasopharyngeal Secretions

Positive for poliovirus 5 days after exposure to 14 days after disease onset

Neutralization and Complement Fixation Tests

Increase in IgA antibody titer 7 days to 4 months after exposure; antibodies persist for a few years

Differential Diagnosis

Rule out aseptic meningitis, suppurative meningitis, toxic neuronitis, brain trauma, encephalitis, diphtheria, leptospirosis, lymphocytic choriomeningitis, infectious mononucleosis

Medical Plan[48]

Medications

Active immunization for prevention (see p. 1293)

General Management

- Respiratory assistance
- Tracheostomy
- Suction
- Indwelling catheter for urinary bladder paralysis
- Oxygen
- IV fluids; nasogastric feeding
- Complete bed rest
- Hot, moist packs to muscles in spasm
- Passive range of motion exercises for paralytic disease
- Muscle reeducation during convalescence
- Stabilizing prosthesis may be used later in convalescence
- Enteric precautions for 7 days after disease onset (see p. 1298)

NURSING CARE

Nursing Assessment

Systemic Stage

- Body temperature
  - 37° to 38° C (99° to 101° F)
- Abdomen
  - Abdominal tenderness; nausea
- Head and pharynx
  - Erythema of throat and tonsils
  - Headache
- CNS involvement
  - Body temperature
    - 38° to 39° C (100° to 102° F)
  - Abdomen
    - Vomiting
  - Head and neck
    - Strained, anxious expression
    - Frontal headache
- Skin
  - Hypersensitive to touch
  - Profuse perspiration, particularly around head and neck
- Neuromuscular system
  - Pain and stiffness in neck, back, and legs

Paralytic Stage

- All of above plus:
  - Level of consciousness
    - Drowsiness, stupor, or restlessness
  - Neuromuscular concerns
    - Pain and spasm (neck, back, and legs)
    - Hyperactive deep tendon reflexes followed by absence of reflexes
    - Asymmetric paralysis (variable parts of body): legs, arms, abdomen, back, face, urinary bladder, pharyngeal, and respiratory
  - Blood pressure
    - May be elevated
  - Breathing patterns
    - Dyspnea, respiratory stridor
    - Rib cage fixed in inspiration because of spasm of sternocleidomastoid, platysma, and trapezius muscles
    - Movement of diaphragm and intercostal muscles may be absent
  - Head and neck
    - Paralysis of face may be observed by an inability to pull up the corner of the mouth when smiling, flattening on one side, or an inability to close one eye
  - Oropharynx
    - Patient may be unable to stick out tongue; or tongue may deviate to one side
    - Palate and uvula may deviate to one side; voice may have nasal tone
    - Liquid may be regurgitated through nose
    - Difficulty in swallowing
  - Speech
    - Aphonia may be present
  - Urinary elimination
    - Distended bladder
    - No urinary output

Nursing Dx & Intervention

Nursing Diagnosis	Nursing Intervention/Rationale
Ineffective breathing pattern	• Monitor for dyspnea, avoidance of speech, abnormal chest movement, respiratory stridor, or cyanosis *to provide assistance early.* • Initiate ventilatory assistance with respirator or positive-pressure breathing and oxygen as prescribed *to maintain adequate oxygen intake.* • Gradually wean from respirator, as prescribed, during convalescence *to restore respirations to normal patterns.*
Ineffective airway clearance	• Monitor for inability to swallow. • Provide suctioning or tracheotomy care as prescribed *to prevent aspiration of secretions, food, or fluids.* • Feed with nasogastric tube if swallowing is impaired *to prevent aspiration of secretions, food, or fluids.*
Impaired physical mobility	• Position (on a firm mattress with a footboard, with no pillow) in a dorsal or prone position with extremities extended *to maintain perfect alignment.*
Activity intolerance	• Employ complete bed rest in a quiet, nonstimulating environment *to minimize stress on the already compromised system.*
Pain	• Handle and move patient as little as possible. • Support body parts completely when moving patient *to prevent pain.* • Apply hot, moist packs to muscles in spasm *to relax muscles.*
Self-care deficit	• Feed patient, starting with fluids and increasing toward normal diet as tolerated. • Provide frequent oral hygiene *for comfort.* • Bathe patient daily during convalescence; omit bathing during acute stage *to reduce stress.* • Refer for home nursing care if needed at time of hospital discharge *to provide care that patient cannot provide.*
Impaired verbal communication	• Anticipate patient's needs. • Observe and encourage nonverbal communication.
Altered patterns of urinary elimination	• Monitor output *to detect bladder atony and distention.* • Maintain indwelling catheter *to ensure emptying of bladder.* • Provide bladder retraining during convalescence *to increase bladder capacity gradually.*
Potential for infection: patient contacts	• Employ enteric precautions for duration of hospitalization *to prevent spread of fecally shed virus to others* (see p. 1298).

Patient Education

1. Patient teaching depends on the amount of physical function the patient has at discharge.
2. Refer the patient for home nursing and physical and occupational therapy, if necessary.
3. Educate the public to the advantages of immunization during early childhood as recommended (see p. 1293).

Evaluation

Patient Outcome	Data Indicating That Outcome is Reached
There is no infection.	Fecal and nasopharyngeal cultures are negative. Body temperature is normal. Infection has not been transmitted to others.
Blood pressure is normal.	Blood pressure is within normal range.
Breathing pattern is effective.	Breathing pattern, rhythm, and depth are regular. Respiratory rate is normal.
Urinary elimination is normal.	Urine output is normal. Patient empties bladder completely on own during convalescence.
Laboratory studies are within normal limits.	O_2 saturation and carbon dioxide levels are normal.

Patient Outcome	Data Indicating That Outcome is Reached
Patient appears comfortable.	Facial expression is calm and relaxed; posture is normal; muscles are relaxed when patient is resting and motionless.
Patient participates in therapeutic exercise.	Patient participates in muscle-building physical therapy. Mobility is adequate. Patient ambulates independently with mechanical devices if needed.
There is no evidence of deformity resulting from treatment.	Arms, legs, feet, and spine are in good alignment. There are no contractures.
Patient is able to function independently or with assistance when discharged from hospital.	Patient can carry out all activities of daily living. Arrangements have been made for home help if needed.

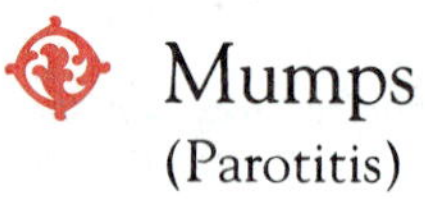

Mumps
(Parotitis)

Mumps (parotitis) is an acute, communicable systemic viral disease characterized by localized unilateral or bilateral edema of one or more of the salivary glands, with occasional involvement of other glands.

Pathophysiology[48]

The paramyxovirus invades and multiplies in the parotid gland or the superficial epithelium of the upper respiratory passages, enters the blood, and subsequently localizes in glandular or nervous tissue. Interstitial tissue edema and infiltration with lymphocytes occur in the affected gland. Cells of the glandular ducts degenerate, producing an accumulation of necrotic debris and polymorphonuclear leukocytes in the lumina, resulting in plugging of the ducts or tubules. The parotid and testes are the glands most frequently involved, but mumps may also affect the pancreas, other salivary glands, ovaries, breast, and thyroid. Meningoencephalitis is a common complication; pericarditis and permanent deafness are less common complications. Testicular atrophy follows mumps orchitis, but sterility is rare. The intensity of symptoms in mumps is variable; at least 30% of infections are asymptomatic. Elevated cerebrospinal fluid protein concentrations are common even in the absence of clinical symptoms of meningoencephalitis. Glucose levels may be depressed.

Diagnostic Studies and Findings[40,48]

Cell Cultures from Saliva, Urine, Cerebrospinal Fluid Specimens (Not Ordinary Procedures)

Positive for virus up to 7 days after onset of infection; in urine up to 2 weeks after infection onset

Serum Amylase Determination

Elevated early in acute illness

Serology: Complement Fixation, Hemagglutination, Neutralization

Fourfold increase in antibody titer between acute and convalescent stages; neutralization is a more time-consuming and expensive procedure

Medical Plan[48]

Medications

Steroids for treatment of orchitis
Analgesics for pain
Active immunization for prevention (see p. 1293)

General Management

Relief of pain with heat or cold applications
Fluid diet until patient tolerates solid food
Support of scrotum (small pillow or Alexander bandage)
Respiratory isolation of hospitalized patients for 9 days after onset of swelling (see p. 1297)

NURSING CARE

Nursing Assessment[48]

Body Temperature

38° to 39° C (100° to 103° F) for 3 or 4 days; higher if orchitis is present

Head and Neck

Variable parotid swelling lasting up to 1 week; severe parotid pain aggravated by eating, particularly sour substances

Parotid gland (or other glands) tender to the touch; hooked lobe of parotid gland (extending under ear lobe) can be palpated

Abdomen

Pain from pancreatitis or oophoritis

Breasts

Inflammation and pain associated with mastitis

Sensory Concerns

Photophobia and headache associated with meningoencephalitis

Unilateral mild transient hearing loss to permanent deafness possible

Testes

Swollen and tender to touch; patient has severe pain

Neuromuscular Concerns

Stiff neck

Convulsion in severe cases

Ataxia

Symptoms of transverse myelitis (rare complication)

Cardiovascular Concerns

Dyspnea, tachycardia, and bradycardia (symptoms of myocarditis; a rare complication)

Urinary Concerns

Symptoms of nephritis (a rare complication)

Skeletal Concerns

Symptoms of arthritis (a rare complication)

Nursing Dx & Intervention

Nursing Diagnosis	Nursing Intervention/Rationale
Pain	• Administer analgesics as prescribed *to relieve pain.* • Give liquid or soft diet as prescribed *to minimize pain with swallowing.* • Apply warm or cold compresses, whichever is more comfortable to patient. • Support scrotum with small pillow or an adhesive tape bridge between the thighs *to minimize pain.*
Anxiety	• *To allay anxiety and concern regarding effects of orchitis,* inform patient that testicular atrophy does not result in impotence and that sterility is extremely rare.[48]
Impaired swallowing	• Encourage liquid or soft bland diet as prescribed. Allow patient to drink from a straw.
Potential for infection: patient contacts	• If patient is hospitalized, employ respiratory isolation for 9 days after onset of swelling *to prevent transmission to others* (see p. 1297).

Patient Education

1. Teach the family to perform nursing care as listed above for the patient who remains at home.
2. Educate the public to the advantages of immunization during childhood (see p. 1293).

Evaluation

Patient Outcome	Data Indicating That Outcome is Reached
Patient appears comfortable.	Facial expression is calm and relaxed. Posture is normal. Muscles are relaxed when patient is resting and motionless. There is no pain in any glandular area. Patient has not developed distress mannerisms.
Patient is not anxious regarding sexual function after orchitis.	Patient discusses any concerns about future sexual functions.
Body hydration and nutrition are normal.	Skin turgor is good. Elimination is adequate. Intake is adequate for needs.
There is no infection or glandular inflammation.	There are no signs of glandular edema or pain. Body temperature is normal. Infection has not been transmitted to others.

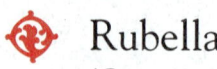

Rubella

(German measles)

Rubella (German measles) is a mild, febrile, highly communicable viral disease characterized by a diffuse punctate macular rash. Symptoms in the prodromal period include low-grade fever, coryza, malaise, headache, lymphadenopathy, and conjunctivitis. Infection during the first trimester of pregnancy may lead to infection in the fetus and may produce a variety of congenital anomalies (the congenital rubella syndrome).

Pathophysiology[40,41,48]

Rubella is a usually mild disease caused by a specific virus that invades and is present in nasopharyngeal secretions, blood, urine, and feces. The virus is transmitted primarily through contact with nasopharyngeal secretions of persons with clinical and subclinical infections 7 days before to 5 days after the appearance of the rash. The virus may also be transmitted transplacentally, producing active infection in the fetus. This may result in death to the fetus or congenital damage (congenital rubella syndrome). Infants born with congenital rubella syndrome generally have the virus in their nasopharyngeal secretions, stools, and urine for up to 1 year after birth, indicating the presence of a chronic infection.

In postnatal rubella the virus invades the lymph glands from the nasopharynx, producing a lymphadenopathy. It subsequently enters the blood, stimulating an immune response that is responsible for the development of the rash. Once the rash appears, the virus can no longer be found in the blood, and prodromal symptoms of a viremia subside. There may be a temporary leukopenia during acute infection. The disease is generally mild, particularly in children. Complications are rare. They include a transitory arthritis, an extremely rare encephalitis, and hemorrhagic manifestations that subside in 2 weeks. In the latter case there is a decrease in blood platelets and an increase in clotting time.

Congenital rubella syndrome is a much more serious manifestation, affecting about 25% of infants born to mothers who were infected with rubella virus during their first trimester. Infection later in the pregnancy carries a lesser risk for congenital damage. The syndrome is characterized by a variety of permanent or transitory defects including cataracts, microphthalmia, microcephaly, mental retardation, deafness, patent ductus arteriosus, arterial or ventral septal defects, congenital glaucoma, retinopathy, purpura, hepatosplenomegaly, neonatal jaundice, and bone defects. There is a high risk for death during the first 6 months, generally from congenital heart disease and sepsis.

The pathologic mechanisms producing the syndrome are not clear, but they appear to be the direct result of viral invasion and infection of developing tissue of the placenta and embryo. One hypothesis is that persistent infection with the virus may lead to mitotic arrest of cells, causing retardation in organ growth. Maternal infection may also result in placental and fetal vasculitis resulting in retarded growth of the fetus. Also, chromosomal breakage has been found in cultured cells from children with congenital rubella syndrome.

The following diagnostic studies, medical plan, and nursing care are for acquired rubella. Congenital rubella is beyond the scope of this chapter.

Diagnostic Studies and Findings[40]

Culture of Pharyngeal Secretions (Also Blood, Urine, or Stool)

- Positive for rubella virus in pharyngeal secretions 7 days before rash in postnatal rubella
- Virus present up to 1 year following birth in congenital rubella syndrome; decreasing with age

Hemagglutination Inhibition (HI)

Complement Fixation (CF)

Solid-Phase Radioimmunoassay (SPRIA)

Medical Plan

Medications

- Antipyretics for temperature control
- Antibiotic treatment of otitis media, an infrequent complication
- Active immunization for prevention (see p. 1293)

NURSING CARE

Nursing Assessment[40,41,48]

Body Temperature

37° to 38° C (99° to 101° F) during 1- to 5-day prodrome in adult and adolescent, subsiding after rash appears

Upper Respiratory Concerns

Coryza, sore throat, cough during prodrome

Head and Neck

Postauricular, postcervical, and occipital lymphadenopathy (small, shotty, and occasionally tender nodes can be palpated during prodrome and a few days after rash fades); mild conjunctivitis and headache possible later complications

Skin

Light pink to red, discrete macular rash, rapidly becoming papular; appearing on the first day of the rash on face and trunk and by the second day on the upper and lower extremities; rash fades within 3 days; purpura is a rare complication, appearing several days to several weeks after the rash

Oral Cavity

Reddish spots, pinpoint or larger, on soft palate during prodrome or on first day of rash (Forchheimer spots)

Musculoskeletal Concerns

Self-limiting polyarthritis possible complication; inflammation and pain in proximal interphalangeal and metacarpophalangeal joints of hand and knee and ankle joints (begins within 5 days of rash and persists for less than 2 weeks)

Neurologic Concerns

Symptoms of complicating encephalitis very rare, occur usually during first few days after rash

Nursing Dx & Intervention

Nursing Diagnosis	Nursing Intervention/Rationale
Pain	• Administer antipyretics and analgesics as prescribed *to relieve pain.*
Anxiety	• Reassure family and patient of the benign nature of this condition.
Potential for infection: patient contacts	• Isolate patient from pregnant women. • If patient is hospitalized, employ contact isolation for 5 days after rash *to prevent transmission to others* (see p. 1297).

Patient Education

1. Educate the public as to the advantage of immunization for rubella during childhood as recommended (see p. 1293).
2. Inform women patients that pregnant women should not be given rubella vaccine and that women should avoid pregnancy for 3 months after receiving rubella vaccine.

Evaluation

Patient Outcome	Data Indicating That Outcome is Reached
There is no infection.	Temperature is 37° C (98.6° F). Joints are not inflamed or tender. There are no signs of encephalitis or purpura. Lymph nodes are not palpable. Skin is free of rash. Infection has not been transmitted.
Laboratory values are within normal limits.	Leukocyte and platelet counts and bleeding time are normal.

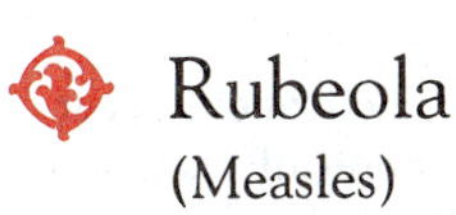

Rubeola

(Measles)

Rubeola (hard measles or red measles) is an acute, highly communicable viral disease manifest as a prodromal fever, conjunctivitis, coryza, bronchitis, Koplik's spots on the buccal mucosa, and a characteristic red blotchy rash. The rash appears on the third to seventh day on the face, becomes generalized, lasts 4 to 7 days, and sometimes ends in a branny desquamation.

Pathophysiology[5,40,41]

The virus of rubeola (measles) is a paramyxovirus that can be found in the blood, urine, and pharyngeal secretions of infected persons. It is transmitted directly and indirectly through contact with respiratory secretions of infected persons during the catarrhal phase of the illness (from 4 days before to 5 days after the onset of the rash). The virus invades the respiratory epithelium and multiplies there. It spreads by way of the lymph system, producing hyperplasia of lymphoid tissue. A primary viremia results and spreads the virus in leukocytes to the reticuloendothelial system. The infected reticuloendothelial cells necrose, an increased amount of virus is released, and a reinvasion of leukocytes with a secondary viremia results. With the secondary viremia the entire respiratory mucosa becomes infected, producing upper respiratory symptoms. Edema of the mucosa may predispose to secondary bacterial invasion and complications such as otitis media and pneumonia.

Within a few days after the occurrence of generalized involvement of the respiratory tract, Koplik's spots appear on the buccal mucosa and a dermal rash develops. The virus appears to invade the cells of the epidermis and oral epithelium, producing histologic changes and stimulating a cell-mediated immune response manifested by the rash. The onset of the rash, following respiratory prodrome, coincides with the production of serum antibodies. Uncomplicated disease lasts 7 to 10 days. There are frequently leukopenia and lymphocytosis. Leukocytosis later in the disease occurs if there is a secondary bacterial infection.

Complications of measles involve the respiratory tract and central nervous system. Pneumonia may result from direct invasion of the virus or by secondary bacterial infection. Encephalitis resulting from direct viral invasion of the brain affects many persons subclinically. Pathologic specimens of brain tissue show demyelination, vascular cuffing, gliosis, and infiltration of fat-laden macrophages near blood vessel walls. Gross evidence of edema, congestion, and petechial hemorrhages can be seen in the brain and spinal cord. Symptoms range from mild to severe. Many patients are left with neurologic sequelae. Rarely, a subacute sclerosing panencephalitis develops several years after infection.

Diagnostic Studies and Findings[41]

Tissue Culture of Secretions from Nasopharynx, Conjunctiva, and Culture of Blood or Urine

Positive for measles virus

Hemagglutination Inhibition

Detects long-lasting antibodies; therefore useful for determining immune status; fourfold increase in antibodies between acute and convalescent stages is diagnostic

Complement Fixation Tests

Detect short-lasting antibodies during and shortly after rash; titer as high as 1:512

Neutralization Tests

Lack of antibodies indicates susceptibility

Medical Plan[5]

Medications

Anti-infective therapy for secondary infections only
Antipyretics for temperature control
Active immunization for prevention (see p. 1293)
Passive immunization for high-risk contacts: immune globulin, 0.25 ml/kg to maximum of 15 ml within 6 d of exposure

General Management

Bed rest during febrile period

NURSING CARE

Nursing Assessment[40,41]

Body Temperature

Up to 40° C (104° F) during prodrome; decrease in 3 to 5 days (when rash appears)

Upper Respiratory Concerns

Hacking cough; coryza within 24 hours of fever, increasing in intensity until rash appears, gradually subsiding within 5 to 10 days

Eyes

Periorbital edema; conjunctivitis, subsiding with appearance of rash; photophobia

Head and Neck

Lymphadenopathy possible

Oral Cavity

Koplik's spots on buccal mucosa, most often opposite second molars; appear 2 to 4 days after onset of prodrome; resemble tiny grains of bluish white sand surrounded by inflammatory areola

Skin

Irregular macules appear on face and neck and in front of and behind the ears 3 to 4 days after onset of prodrome; rash rapidly becomes maculopapular, spreading to trunk and extremities within 24 to 48 hours; at this time it begins to fade from the face; rash is brownish pink in color and irregularly confluent; petechiae or ecchymoses may be present in severe cases; rash fades in 4 to 7 days, leaving a brownish desquamation; acute thrombocytopenic purpura with hemorrhage may be a complication

Neurologic Concerns

Symptoms of an encephalitis, a rare complication, occurring within 2 days to 1 week after onset of rash; secondary elevation of temperature; headaches; seizures; altered state of consciousness

Ears

Otitis media may result as a secondary infection

Abdomen

Symptoms of secondary acute appendicitis

Activity Level

Severe lethargy or prostration after onset of rash may indicate a secondary bacterial infection

Breathing Patterns

Dyspnea may indicate secondary bacterial infection

Nursing Dx & Intervention

Nursing Diagnosis	Nursing Intervention/Rationale
Activity intolerance	• Provide bed rest during febrile period *to conserve energy.*
Potential fluid volume deficit	• Assess skin turgor and urinary output *to detect signs of dehydration.* • Provide adequate oral fluids of a variety that appeals to patient *to maintain adequate fluids.*
Sensory/perceptual alterations (visual)	• Assess patient for photophobia. • Dim lights if photophobia is present *to prevent pain.* • Cleanse eyelids with warm water *to remove crusts or secretions.*
Hyperthermia	• Assess body temperature. • Administer antipyretics as prescribed and give cool sponge baths *to lower body temperature.*
Potential for infection: patient	• Assess for secondary infection: delayed increase in body temperature, ear pain, dyspnea, chest pain, lethargy, and increased coughing. • Protect patient from exposure to bacteria, particularly *Streptococcus, to prevent secondary infection.*
Potential for infection: patient contacts	• If patient is hospitalized, employ respiratory isolation for 4 days after onset of rash *to prevent transmission to others* (see p. 1297).

Patient Education

1. Teach the family to provide care as listed above for the patient who is cared for at home.
2. Educate the public as to the advantage of immunization for rubeola during childhood as recommended (see p. 1293).

Evaluation

Patient Outcome	Data Indicating That Outcome is Reached
There is no infection.	Body temperature is normal. Infection has not been transmitted.
Laboratory studies are within normal limits.	Leukocyte and lymphocyte counts are normal.
There is no secondary otitis media.	There is no pain in ear: tympanic membrane is normal.
There is no secondary pneumonia.	Respiratory rate, rhythm, and depth are normal. Breath sounds are clear.
Skin and mucous membranes are normal.	Skin and mucous membranes are warm and moist, with natural color.

RESPIRATORY INFECTIOUS DISEASES

The respiratory infectious diseases discussed in this section are those acute and chronic respiratory pathologic conditions that are caused by a specific pathogenic agent that is transmitted by inhalation or by direct contact with infectious respiratory secretions. Although diphtheria, pertussis, and measles fit this definition, they are discussed in this chapter under vaccine-preventable infectious diseases. Rheumatic fever and scarlet fever are discussed here, because of their etiologic agent, the group A streptococcus, causing streptococcal throat (Table 13-6). Nonspecific lower respiratory infections such as pneumonia are discussed in Chapter 2. Nonspecific upper respiratory infections such as pharyngitis and tonsillitis are discussed in Chapter 7.

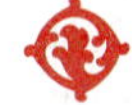

Streptococcal throat, scarlet fever, rheumatic fever

Streptococcal throat is an acute exudative tonsillitis or pharyngitis caused by group A β-hemolytic streptococci. Coincident or subsequent otitis media or peritonsillar abscess may be present. Rheumatic fever, chorea, and acute glomerulonephritis are possible sequelae.

Table 13-6
Overview of Respiratory Infectious Diseases

	Streptococcal Throat	Scarlet Fever	Rheumatic Fever
Occurrence	More common in temperate zones; may be endemic, epidemic, or sporadic in occurrence; highest in late winter or spring; ages 3-15 most often affected; no sex or racial difference		
			Females at greater risk for certain characteristics
Etiologic agent	*Streptococcus pyogenes* (group A streptococcus of approximately 70 serologically distinct types)		
		Three erythrogenic toxins	
Reservoir	Humans	Humans	Humans
Transmission	Direct or intimate contact with patient or carrier; may follow ingestion of contaminated food		
Incubation period	1-3 d	2-4 d (range: 1-7 d)	3-35 d after clinical strep throat (average: 19 d)
Period of communicability	Untreated, uncomplicated cases: 10-21 d; complicated: weeks to months; antibiotic treated: 24-48 h		
Susceptibility and resistance	General; many develop antitoxic or antibacterial immunity to one of the types of streptococci through inapparent infection		Persons who have suffered one attack are predisposed to a recurrent episode following group A streptococcal upper respiratory infections
		Permanent acquired immunity from active disease with type of toxin; second attacks due to different toxin	
Report to local health authority	Epidemics only		

Data from Benenson.[5]

Scarlet fever is a group A β-hemolytic streptococcal disease characterized by a skin rash. It occurs when the infecting strain of streptococcus produces a toxin causing a sensitivity reaction in the infected host. Clinical characteristics may include those of streptococcal sore throat plus enanthem, strawberry tongue, and exanthema.

Rheumatic fever is a sequela of group A streptococcal infection of the upper respiratory tract, occurring in about 2.8% of those having a streptococcal throat infection. The condition is thought to result from an altered immune reaction to the streptococcus. Rheumatic heart disease is a potential complication.

Pathophysiology[40,41,48]

Infection with group A streptococci results in a number of related clinical disease entities such as streptococcal throat, scarlet fever, erysipelas, and nonsuppurative complications such as nephritis and rheumatic fever. The type of disease resulting from group A streptococci depends on the site of tissue invasion, the antigenic characteristics of the infecting strain of streptococcus, and the immune status of the host. There are 60 to 70 serologically distinct strains of group A streptococci, producing a variety of different enzymes and at least three different erythrogenic toxins. These antigenic characteristics determine the type of enzyme-specific and toxin-

Histoplasmosis	Influenza	Legionellosis (Legionnaires' Disease)	Tuberculosis
Worldwide; higher in eastern and central United States; increases with age to 30 yr; no differences by sex; outbreaks in groups with common exposure	Worldwide in pandemics, epidemics, localized outbreaks, and sporadic cases; highest in winter in temperate zones	Europe, United States, and Canada; first recognized in 1977; sporadic cases and outbreaks in summer and autumn; increases with age	Worldwide; mortality and prevalence decreasing in many places; highest in males and poor; most active disease arises from latent infection
Histoplasma capsulatum (a fungus)	Three types of viruses (A, B, and C), each with many strains	*Legionella pneumophila* (a bacteria with subgroups)	*Mycobacterium tuberculosis* and *M. bovis*
Soil around chicken houses, caves harboring bats, and around starling roosts and decaying trees	Humans; some mammals suspected as sources of new strains of viruses	Unknown but probably environmental; organism survives in hot and cold tap water and distilled water for months	Humans; *M. bovis* in diseased cattle
Inhalation of airborne spores	Direct transmission by inhalation of virus in airborne mucous discharge	Common source, airborne transmission suspected	Inhalation of bacilli in airborne mucous droplets from sputum of persons with active disease; less frequent: ingestion or skin penetration
5-18 d after exposure, commonly 10 d	24-72 h	2-10 d, commonly 5-6 d	4-12 wk after exposure or anytime when disease is in latent stage
Not transmitted from person to person	3 d from onset of symptoms	No documented person-to-person transmission	As long as bacilli are in sputum; some are intermittently communicable for years
General; inapparent infections common and result in increasing resistance	Universal; infection produces immunity to a specific strain of virus, but duration of immunity depends on antigenic drift in strain	General; rare in those less than 20 yr; greatest in males, smokers, and immunosuppressed persons	General; highest in children less than 3 yr, those greater than 65 yr, chronically ill, silicone and asbestos workers, and malnourished and immunosuppressed individuals
In some states	Mandatory case report	In some states	Mandatory case report

specific antibodies produced by the host. A host with adequate antibodies against a particular serotype with or without antitoxic immunity may develop no clinical disease if reinfected with the same serotype. A person with antitoxic immunity resulting from previous group A infections but with no antibodies against a particular invading serotype may develop a clinical streptococcal throat. A person with no antitoxic immunity and no antibodies against an invading toxigenic group A streptococcus may develop clinical scarlet fever. In all clinical streptococcal disease a leukocytosis is present.

Streptococcal throat (septic sore throat) results when the streptococcus invades and remains in the lymphoid tissue of the oropharynx, rapidly producing inflammation with edema, erythema, and infiltration with polymorphonuclear leukocytes. The mucosal surfaces, particularly over the tonsils, become ulcerated, releasing a mucopurulent exudate. Cervical lymphadenopathy is present. Severity of symptoms increases with age. Untreated, uncomplicated disease lasts a few days to a week. The streptococcus may invade surrounding tissue producing suppurative complications such as peritonsillar cellulitis and abscess, retropharyngeal abscess, sinus empyema, otitis media, mastoiditis, meningitis, cervical lymphadenitis, pneumonia, and periorbital abscess. Toxin dissemination may result in rheumatic fever or nephritis.

Scarlet fever results if the invading streptococcus releases an erythrogenic toxin stimulating a sensitivity reaction in the host. Dilation of small capillaries and toxic injury of the vascular epithelium may be widespread in the body, particularly in the liver, myocardium, and kidneys. The pathologic changes are most visible on the skin, with an erythematous rash and desquamation, and in the oral cavity, with the strawberry tongue and an enanthem. Hepatocellular damage and destruction of red cells may result in jaundice, increase in bilirubin, mild anemia, and an increase in reticulocytes. In rare situations, toxins may be disseminated in the bloodstream, producing a severe toxic illness. Streptococcus may invade adjacent tissue and the bloodstream, producing a severe septic scarlet fever.

Rheumatic fever is a delayed complication of upper respiratory infection with group A streptococci producing nonsuppurative inflammatory lesions in connective tissue of the heart, joints, subcutaneous tissues, and central nervous system. Symptoms may be present in all or some of those systems. The exact causal mechanism is not known. The following have been hypothesized: (1) there is direct tissue invasion by group A streptococci or by cell wall antigens of the microorganism; (2) streptococcal enzymes, particularly streptolysins S or O, induce tissue injury; (3) antigen-humoral antibody reactions localize in affected tissue; and (4) an autoimmune reaction is operative. The autoimmune theory is supported by the detection of heart-reactive antibodies (HRAs) in the sera of patients with rheumatic heart disease. A genetic predisposition to this disease is suggested by the fact that rheumatic fever consistently affects only 2.8% of those with a clinical upper respiratory streptococcal infection.

Cardiac connective tissue lesions show early fragmentation of collagen fibers, cellular lymphocytic infiltration, and fibrin deposits. These changes are followed by the development of the Aschoff nodule, a perivascular locus of inflammation with an area of central necrosis surrounded by large mononuclear and polymorphonuclear leukocytes. Cardiac findings include pericarditis, myocarditis, and left-sided endocarditis. Valvular lesions begin with edema and cellular infiltration of the leaflets and chordae with small verrucae forming along the closure lines. With healing the valves become thickened and deformed, the valve commissures become fused, and the chordae become shortened. These changes result in valvular stenosis and insufficiency, varying in extensiveness and severity. Carditis may result in long-term disability or death.

Joint lesions are characterized by a fibrinous exudate over the synovial membrane and a serous effusion without joint destruction. Subcutaneous nodules form that resemble the Aschoff nodules described above.

Laboratory tests demonstrate the presence of C-reactive proteins in the blood and an increased erythrocyte sedimentation rate. Electrocardiograms may exhibit an elongation of the P-R interval before the development of symptoms.

A later neurologic sequela of rheumatic fever is Sydenham's chorea. The latent period for this condition may be so long as to occur in the absence of laboratory changes associated with rheumatic fever.

Diagnostic Studies and Findings[29,41,48]

Streptococcal Throat

Culture of Throat Exudate

Positive for group A hemolytic streptococci (10 or more colonies)

Scarlet Fever

Schultz-Charlton Reaction Skin Test

Rash blanches at site of intradermal injection of antitoxin

Dick Skin Test for Susceptibility

Erythema and induration greater than 3 mm within 24 hours of intradermal injection of 0.1 ml exotoxin; reaction is compared with control site where 0.1 ml of a control substance is injected intradermally

Rheumatic Fever

Antistreptolysin O (ASO)

Increase in ASO suggests recent infection with streptococcus; ASO peaks 2 to 5 weeks after strep infection and decreases thereafter; 80% to 85% of patients with rheumatic fever develop ASO titers of 200 Todd U/ml or greater; ASO titers exceeding 1:85 in adults may be diagnostic

Anti-DNAse B (ADN-B) Test

ADN-B develops later and persists longer than ASO; titers greater than 1:85 in adults are diagnostic

Streptozyme Test (a Slide Hemagglutination Test)

Measures five different streptococcal enzymes; titers of 100 to 200 are equivocal; titers greater than 300 indicate recent streptococcal infection

C-Reactive Protein (CRP)

Normally not present in serum
Presence of CRP in serum is diagnostic

Medical Plan[41,48]

Medications

- Anti-infective agents
  - Benzathine penicillin G (Bicillin), 1,200,000 U IM one time for adults
  - Oral penicillin, 250,000 U tid for 10 d, *or*
  - Procaine penicillin (Wycillin), 600,000 U IM for 10 d for severe scarlet fever
  - Erythromycin (Erythrocin, others), 250 mg po qid for 10 d for patients allergic to penicillin
- Antipyretic agents
  - Aspirin, 90-100 mg/kg/d for 2 wk; 60-70 mg/kg/d for subsequent 6 wk for treatment of polyarthritis of rheumatic fever
  - Antipyretics for management of fever

Corticosteroids
Prednisone (Deltasone, others), 40-60 mg/d for 2-3 wk for treatment of carditis, *or*
Methyl prednisone sodium succinate (Solu-Medrol), IV, in severe cases; decrease to complete withdrawal in 3 wk
To prevent recurrent streptococcal infections in postrheumatic fever patients:
Anti-infective agents
Benzathine penicillin G (Bicillin), 1,200,000 U IM q4wk during and following convalescence for life (recommended duration is controversial), *or*
Erythromycin (Erythrocin, others), 250 mg bid po for those allergic to penicillin

General Management

Bed rest during febrile stage of all streptococcal diseases; bed rest for 3 weeks for patients without carditis; for an additional month after carditis is detected
Nonstimulating environment and sedation for patients with chorea
Fluid therapy as indicated
Treatment of heart failure with O_2, salt restriction, diuretics, and digitalis
To prevent transmission to others: secretion precautions of hospitalized patients with an upper respiratory streptococcal infection for 24 hours following initiation of antibiotic therapy

NURSING CARE

Nursing Assessment[41,48]

Body Temperature

38° to 39° C (100° to 103° F)

Pulse

Rapid

Head and Neck

Enlarged, tender cervical lymph nodes
Symptoms of suppurative complications: mastoiditis, otitis media, periorbital abscess, sinus empyema

Oropharynx

Edema, erythema (fiery red to dull red), and petechiae of uvula, tonsils, and posterior oropharynx
Confluent, easily removable mucopurulent exudate
May be suppurative complications

Subjective Symptoms

Pain on swallowing
Headache
Anorexia
Malaise
Chills

Respiratory Concerns

Complications: symptoms of pneumonia (Chapter 2)

Neurologic Concerns

Complications: symptoms of meningitis (described in this chapter)

Scarlet Fever

All of the above plus the following
Skin
Erythematous and punctate rash appearing within 2 days of streptococcal throat, becoming generalized rapidly; appearing first on upper chest and back and then on the lower back, upper extremities, abdomen, and lower extremities
Extensiveness of rash is variable; it may be better felt (like sandpaper) than seen
Petechiae may precede the rash on the lower extremities; more common in skin folds
Desquamation may develop between 5 days to 4 weeks after appearance of the rash, starting on the neck, upper chest, back, fingertips, or toes; skin peels in large sections, particularly on the palms and soles
Flushing of cheeks with circumoral pallor
Oral cavity
Tongue is inflamed and heavily coated at first; after the rash appears, the papillae become swollen and appear as red bumps on a gray background (strawberry tongue); within a few days the tongue peels, first at the tip and margins; by day 6 the tongue is completely denuded, beefy red, moist, and glistening (raspberry tongue); tongue returns to normal by the end of the second week
Enanthem: for a few days around the time of rash appearance on the skin there may be a hemorrhagic rash on the soft palate and anterior pillars of the fossae
Abdomen
Liver may be slightly enlarged and tender
Musculoskeletal concerns
Tender, slightly inflamed, and edematous joints possible

Septic Scarlet Fever

Body temperature
40° to 42° C (104° to 108° F)
Pulse
Rapid and weak
Oropharynx
Throat manifestations more severe but same as those for streptococcal throat and scarlet fever
Ulceration and perforation on uvula, soft palate, and tonsils
Seropurulent or mucopurulent nasal discharge
Excoriations on lips, mouth, and nares

Skin
Rash may be slight to severe
Head and neck
Cervical lymphadenopathy
Mastoid and middle ear pain
Breathing patterns
Labored, due to swelling and occlusion

Toxic Scarlet Fever (Fulminating Scarlet Fever)

Body temperature
41° to 42° C (105° to 108° F)
Pulse
Very rapid
Skin
Heavy punctate or erythematous hemorrhagic rash: bright to purple-red
Vascular concerns
Capillary fragility as seen by hematuria, epistaxis, and hematemesis
Oropharynx
Edema without exudate
Systemic concerns
Intense headache
Vomiting
Cardiovascular concerns
Symptoms of toxic myocarditis
Mental status
Delirium
Irrationality
Coma

Rheumatic Fever (Variable Onset)

Body temperature
Low-grade fever: 38° C (100° F)
Musculoskeletal concerns
Acute onset of mild to severe symptoms of polyarthritis: heat, swelling, redness, and severe tenderness affecting mainly the knees, ankles, elbows, and wrists; migratory, with multiple joint involvement at one time; inflammation subsides in each joint in 1 to 2 weeks; entire episode subsides in 4 weeks
Cardiovascular concerns
Insidious onset of symptoms of carditis within 3 weeks: cardiac enlargement, pericardial friction rubs, congestive heart failure, signs of effusion, tachycardia, gallop rhythm, and diastolic and possibly systolic murmurs
Three types of murmurs associated with acute carditis: (1) high-pitched blowing holosystolic apical murmur of mitral regurgitation, (2) low-pitched apical mid-diastolic flow murmur, (3) high-pitched decrescendo diastolic murmur of aortic regurgitation heard at the secondary and primary aortic areas
Mitral and aortic stenotic murmurs associated with chronic rheumatic valvular disease
Skin
One to two dozen firm, painless, variable in size (3 mm to 2 cm), subcutaneous nodules; usually over bony prominences and tendons; lasting 1 to 2 weeks
Nonpruritic, erythematous macular eruption on the trunk or proximal extremities (erythema marginatum); lesions appear to be a vasomotor phenomenon, moving over the skin with a tendency to advance at the margins and clear at the center; individual lesions clear within hours, but the process persists intermittently for weeks or months
Neurologic concerns
Symptoms of chorea: involuntary, purposeless, rapid motions; irritability; emotional lability; weakness; restlessness; fretfulness; gradually increasing in intensity over a 2-week period, reaching a plateau, and gradually subsiding
Subjective symptoms
Malaise
Abdominal pain

Nursing Dx & Intervention

Nursing Diagnosis	Nursing Intervention/Rationale
Altered oral mucous membrane	• Assess pharyngeal area *to detect hyperemia and exudate.* • Provide frequent oral fluids and oral hygiene *for comfort.* • Provide high humidity in room *for comfort.* • Lubricate lips and nares *for comfort.*
Activity intolerance	• Maintain complete bed rest for scarlet fever and rheumatic fever patients *to prevent complications.* • Provide all care including hygiene and feeding *to conserve patient energy.*
Potential fluid volume deficit	• Assess skin turgor and urine output *to detect signs of inadequate fluid intake.* • Encourage frequent oral fluids as tolerated. • Administer IV fluids as prescribed *to maintain adequate fluids if oral intake is decreased.*
Impaired skin integrity	• Give sponge baths with a solution of sodium bicarbonate or calamine lotion *to relieve pruritus associated with desquamation in scarlet fever.*
Decreased cardiac output	• Assess for symptoms of carditis and congestive heart failure in rheumatic fever patients. • Administer therapy as prescribed (see Chapter 1).

Nursing Diagnosis	Nursing Intervention/Rationale
Impaired physical mobility	• Assess for symptoms of polyarthritis. • Maintain rest of involved joints *to decrease risk of trauma.* • Administer anti-inflammatory agents as prescribed.
Hyperthermia	• Assess body temperature. • Give tepid sponge baths *to reduce fever.* • Administer antipyretics as ordered *to decrease elevated temperature.*
Potential for infection: patient	• Collect pharyngeal secretions for culture. • Administer antibiotics as prescribed.
Potential for infection: patient contacts	• Maintain respiratory secretion precautions of hospitalized patients for 24 hours after antibiotic therapy is initiated (see p. 1297) *to prevent transmission to others.*

Patient Education

1. Oral antibiotics must be taken for prescribed length of time. Follow-up throat cultures may be necessary.
2. Compliance with prescribed long-term antibiotic therapy is necessary to minimize risk for recurrence of rheumatic fever with subsequent streptococcal infections.
3. Upper respiratory infections should be diagnosed and treated promptly in post–rheumatic fever patients.
4. Continued rest during convalescence is necessary for post–rheumatic fever patients.
5. Medical monitoring for cardiac complications is necessary after rheumatic fever.
6. Persons with residual rheumatic valvular disease must follow an antimicrobial regimen whenever they undergo dental or surgical procedures that would increase their risk for bacteremia.

Evaluation

Patient Outcome	Data Indicating That Outcome is Reached
Laboratory values are within normal limits.	Leukocyte count and sedimentation rate are normal. There is no C-reactive protein in serum.
There is no infection.	Cervical lymph nodes are not palpable. There are no subjective symptoms of malaise, abdominal pain, or pain on swallowing. Body temperature is normal. Infection has not been transmitted.
Skin and mucous membranes are normal.	Skin and mucous membranes are warm and moist, with natural color. There is no edema, inflammation, or exudate in oropharynx. Exanthema and enanthem of scarlet fever are not present. Exanthema and subcutaneous nodules of rheumatic fever are not present.
Physical activity patterns are normal.	There is no limitation of joint movement. Patient can move all joints without pain. Patient exhibits purposeful movement, indicating no signs of chorea.
Cardiac function is normal.	Pulse rate is normal. There is no fatigue on exertion. Electrocardiogram is normal. No murmurs are auscultated.

Histoplasmosis

Histoplasmosis is a pulmonary and systemic infection, similar to tuberculosis, resulting from inhalation of the spores of *Histoplasma capsulatum,* which are frequently found in the soil. Infection is common, but overt clinical disease is rare. Five clinical forms of the disease have been recognized.

Pathophysiology[5,41]

Spores of *H. capsulatum,* a fungus, are inhaled when soil containing them is disturbed. A lesion is formed within the lung parenchyma where the spores convert to a yeast phase and are phagocytosed by macrophages. Lesions may also be formed in the hilar or mediastinal lymph nodes as a result of migration of yeast-laden macrophages to those areas. Dissemination and lesion formation may also occur in the spleen and liver. These primary lesions become necrotic at the center, build up a fibrotic capsule, and frequently calcify. In most cases where calcification occurs there is no reactivation of the infection and the host manifests no symptoms except an immune response to histoplasmin.

Four other clinical forms of the disease are possible: acute benign respiratory disease, acute disseminated disease, chronic disseminated disease, and chronic pulmonary disease.

In acute benign respiratory disease the primary pulmonary lesion remains active, resulting in a spreading infiltration pneumonia. In acute disseminated disease, inflammatory and necrotic lesions may result in septic-type fever, hepatosplenomegaly, severe prostration, and death. Chronic disseminated histoplasmosis results when there is extensive invasion by yeast-laden macrophages via the reticuloendothelial system to bone marrow, spleen, liver, and lungs. The inflammatory and necrotic reaction in those tissues is subacute but progressive and may eventually result in death. Chronic pulmonary histoplasmosis is manifest as a progressive emphysema. Fluid-filled cysts surrounded by chronic inflammation progress through stages of caseation necrosis and cavitation, continuing to disseminate the yeast through pulmonary tissue.

The clinical symptoms are quite varied but are generally more severe in infants, immunosuppressed persons, and chronically debilitated persons.

Diagnostic Studies and Findings[41,48]

Sabouraud's Agar Culture; Giemsa- or Wright-Stained Smears of Respiratory Exudate, Blood, or Exudate from Ulcerated Lesions

Positive for *H. capsulatum*

Results are frequently erratic, necessitating the culture of many specimens

Precipitation and Complement Fixation Tests; Agglutination Test

Increase in antibodies within 3 to 4 weeks; fourfold increase suggests disease progression

Agglutinins greater than 1:8 or 1:16 have suggestive diagnostic value

Skin Test

Induration greater than 5 mm in 24 hours indicates past or present infections; not routinely used for diagnosis

Chest Roentgenogram

Acute: transient parenchymal pulmonary infiltrates resembling lobar pneumonia

Chronic: progressively enlarging areas of necrosis with or without cavitation

Medical Plan[41,48]

Medications

- Anti-infective agents
  - Amphotericin B (Fungizone), 5-10 mg initial dose, increasing 10 mg/d until 50 mg is attained; then 50 mg 3 times wk until a total of 2.5 g has been administered; give IV in 500 ml 5% dextrose and water
- Corticosteroids
  - Corticosteroids, 10-20 mg may be mixed with the infusion to minimize the side effects of amphotericin B
- Antihistamines
  - Diphenhydramine (Benadryl), 25-50 mg added to IV to control side effects

NURSING CARE

Nursing Assessment[41,48]

Pulmonary, Acute

- Mild to severe; duration: days to weeks
- Respiratory concerns
  - Pleural and substernal chest pain
  - Dry or productive cough with a metallic tone, suggesting tracheobronchial obstruction
- Subjective symptoms
  - Malaise
  - Weakness
  - Anorexia
- Body temperature
  - Low-grade fever
- Skin
  - Erythema multiforme
  - Erythema nodosum
- Cardiovascular concerns
  - May have complicating symptoms of a pericarditis

Pulmonary, Chronic

- May have above symptoms, progressing over months or years plus
- Respiratory concerns
  - Purulent sputum; hemoptysis
  - Increasing signs of pulmonary insufficiency

Disseminated, Acute

- Abdomen
  - Enlarged liver and spleen
- Body temperature
  - High fever

Disseminated, Chronic

- Symptoms vary depending on site of dissemination
- Abdomen
  - Symptoms of gastrointestinal ulcers, hepatitis, and peritonitis
- Oropharynx
  - Ulcerated lesions in larynx, mouth, nose, or pharynx, resembling epidermoid cancer
- Skin
  - Purpura
- Neurologic concerns
  - Symptoms of meningitis (see p. 1243)
- Respiratory concerns
  - Symptoms of pneumonia (see Chapter 2)
- Cardiac concerns
  - Symptoms of endocarditis (see Chapter 1)

Nursing Dx & Intervention

Nursing Diagnosis*	Nursing Intervention/Rationale
Patient problem: adverse chemotherapeutic response	• Monitor for cyanosis, changes in pulse and respiratory rate, and signs of renal dysfunction *to detect signs of amphotericin toxicity.* • Administer antihistamines and corticosteroids as prescribed. • Encourage fluids high in potassium if nausea and vomiting persist *to replace lost potassium.* • *Prevent phlebitis* by using small-gauge needle for IV line. Agitate IV fluid bag every 15 to 20 minutes while chemotherapeutic agent is being administered to ensure even distribution of drug and fluid in bag and in intravenous line. Give infusion over a 5- to 6-hour period.
Pain	• Frequently reposition the patient *for comfort* during prolonged, painful IV infusions. • Provide diversional activities. • Administer analgesics before IV administration as prescribed *to decrease pain from drug therapy.*

*Other diagnoses depend on extent of dissemination and pulmonary dysfunction (see Chapters 1 and 2) and meningitis (see p. 1240).

Patient Education[5]

1. Inform the patient that medical follow-up for 1 year after treatment to prevent relapses is necessary.
2. Inform the patient that reinfection can be prevented by avoiding infected sites, wearing a protective mask, or sterilizing the site with 3% formalin.

Evaluation

Patient Outcome	Data Indicating That Outcome is Reached
Patient is free of complications from treatment.	There are no signs of phlebitis, renal dysfunction, electrolyte imbalance, pain, or neuritis.
Patient is aware of need for protection from reinfection.	Patient states methods to use to avoid reexposure.
Patient is aware of need for medical surveillance.	Patient states intent to see physician on a regular basis for 1 year after hospitalization.
Breathing patterns are normal.	There is no cough, dyspnea, sputum, or hemoptysis.
Oropharynx is normal.	There are no lesions in mouth, larynx, pharynx, or nose.
Skin is normal.	There is no purpura, erythema multiforme, or erythema nodosum.
Energy levels are adequate.	Patient has energy to carry out all daily activities.
Gastrointestinal function is normal.	Patient does not have abdominal pain. Patient is able to eat all desired foods. Patient is not jaundiced.
There is no infection.	Sputum cultures are negative. Body temperature is normal.

Influenza

Influenza is a generalized, acute, febrile disease associated with upper and lower respiratory infection; it is characterized by a severe and protracted cough, fever, headache, myalgia, prostration, coryza, and mild sore throat. The disease may be indistinguishable clinically from the common cold. Complications include bacterial pneumonia, particularly in elderly and debilitated persons.

Pathophysiology[40,48]

Influenza viruses A, B, or C, each with many mutagenic strains, are inhaled in aerosolized mucous droplets shed from infected persons. The viruses are deposited on and penetrate the surface of upper respiratory tract mucosal cells, producing cell lysis and destruction of the ciliated epithelium. Viral neuraminidase decreases the viscosity of the mucosa, thus facilitating the spread of virus-containing exudate to the lower respiratory tract. An interstitial inflammation and necrosis of the bronchiolar and alveolar epithelium result, filling the alveoli with an exudate containing leukocytes, erythrocytes, and hyaline membrane.

Regeneration of epithelium, following necrosis and desquamation, slowly begins after the fifth day of illness. Regeneration reaches a maximum within 9 to 15 days, at which time mucus production and cilia begin to appear. Before complete regeneration the compromised epithelium is prone to secondary bacterial invasion resulting in bacterial pneumonia usually caused by *S. aureus*.

The initial invasion of the virus can be aborted at the portal of entry if virus-specific secretory antibodies (IgA) are present in mucous secretions and if virus-specific serum antibodies are adequate.

The disease is usually self-limited. Acute symptoms last 2 to 7 days and are followed by a convalescent period of about a week. The disease is important because of its cyclic epidemic and pandemic nature and because of the high mortality associated with pulmonary complications resulting from secondary bacterial pneumonia. This risk is highest in elderly and chronically diseased persons.

Laboratory findings show an elevated sedimentation rate, leukopenia or a slight leukocytosis, and a febrile albuminuria.

Diagnostic Studies and Findings[48]

Tissue Culture of Nasal or Pharyngeal Secretions

Positive for influenza virus

Sputum Culture

Positive for bacteria in secondary infections

Fluorescent Antibody Staining of Secretions

Positive for influenza virus

Hemagglutination Inhibition or Complement Fixation Tests

Fourfold increase in antibody titer between acute and convalescent stages

Medical Plan[5,26]

Medications

- Anti-infective agents
  - Amantadine, 100 mg po bid for duration of epidemic (3-6 wk) for prevention of high-risk persons over age of 9 yr; 100 mg/d po for persons over the age of 65 years (dosage to be reduced further for persons with impaired renal function)
  - Agent-specific anti-infective agents for bacterial complications or for patients with chronic pulmonary disease
- Antipyretics
  - ASA, 600 mg po q4h for adults
- Adrenergic agents
  - Phenylephrine (Neo-Synephrine), 0.25%, 2 drops in each nostril for nasal congestion
- Antitussive agents
  - Terpin hydrate with codeine, 5-10 ml po q3-4h for adults for cough
- Active immunization
  - Vaccine, 0.5 ml IM; must be repeated yearly in the fall for viral strain expected in the winter; recommended for elderly individuals, chronically ill adults, children with chronic heart or pulmonary disease, residents of nursing homes and chronic care facilities, and health care providers with contact with high-risk patients

General Management

Oxygen and IV fluid and electrolytes for complications
Steam inhalation for congestion

NURSING CARE

Nursing Assessment

Body Temperature

Sudden-onset fever (38° to 39° C [102° to 103° F]) that gradually falls and rises again on the third day

Subjective Symptoms

Prostration
Myalgia, particularly in back and legs
Anorexia and malaise
Headache, photophobia, and retrobulbar aching

Respiratory Concerns

Mild at first: sore throat; substernal burning; nonproductive cough; coryza
Later: severe and productive cough; erythema of soft palate, posterior hard palate, tonsillar pillars, and posterior pharynx; increased respiratory rate

Head and Neck

Conjunctivitis may be present
Flushed face
Anterior cervical lymphadenopathy may be present

Complicating Viral Pneumonia

Dyspnea
Cyanosis
Hemoptysis
Crepitant and subcrepitant rales
See Chapter 2

Complicating Bacterial Pneumonia

- Respiratory concerns
  - Same as for viral pneumonia plus purulent or bloody sputum

See Chapter 2
Body temperature
Secondary rise in fever

Nursing Dx & Intervention

Nursing Diagnosis	Nursing Intervention/Rationale
Ineffective airway clearance	• Administer decongestants as prescribed. • Provide cool, humidified air *to liquefy secretions.* • Suction if necessary *to remove secretions.* • Monitor for signs of viral or bacterial pneumonia. • Provide oxygen as prescribed.
Potential fluid volume deficit	• Assess skin turgor and urinary output *to detect dehydration.* • Encourage fluids as much as patient can tolerate (3000 ml for adult). • Administer IV fluids as prescribed *to provide additional fluids required during infection.*
Activity intolerance	• Maintain bed rest for 2 or 3 days after temperature returns to normal. • Provide for diversional activity *to maintain quiet during convalescence.*
Hyperthermia	• Administer analgesic and antipyretic agents as prescribed *to reduce fever.* • Give tepid sponge baths *to reduce fever.* • Provide cool, humidified air *for comfort.*
Potential for infection: patient	• Protect patient from exposure to bacteria. • Monitor for a subsequent increase in temperature accompanied by chest pain, dyspnea, hemoptysis, purulent sputum, or ear pain *to detect secondary infection.* • See discussion of pneumonia in Chapter 2. • Collect sputum specimens for culture.
Potential for infection: patient contacts	• Employ contact isolation for duration of the illness for hospitalized infants and children (see p. 1297) *to prevent transmission of infection to others.*

Patient Education

1. Maintain bed rest for 2 or 3 days after temperature returns to normal.
2. Force fluids.
3. Continue to take antibiotics for duration as prescribed for bacterial complications.
4. Report symptoms of secondary infection (ear pain, purulent or bloody sputum, chest pain, increase in temperature) to physician.
5. High-risk persons should be encouraged to receive influenza vaccine before the start of the flu season.
6. Side effects of amantadine prophylaxis include nausea, dizziness, nervousness, insomnia, and impaired concentration. These disappear when the drug is stopped. These and other side effects, particularly in persons at risk for impaired renal function, should be reported to a physician.

Evaluation

Patient Outcome	Data Indicating That Outcome is Reached
There is no secondary bacterial infection.	Energy returns. There is no otitis media, cyanosis, dyspnea, chest pain, hemoptysis, or mucopurulent sputum. Sputum cultures are negative. Body temperature is normal.
Laboratory values are within normal limits.	Leukocyte count and sedimentation rate are normal.
Airways clearance is effective.	Secretions are clear and thin. There is no cough.
Respirations are normal.	Rate, depth, and rhythm of respirations are normal.

Legionellosis
(Legionnaires' disease)

Legionellosis (Legionnaires' disease) is an acute bacterial infection so named because it caused an outbreak of pneumonia at a convention of American Legionnaires at a Philadelphia hotel. The acute disease is a patchy pulmonary infiltrate and consolidation, with a high fever, malaise, myalgia and headache, nonproductive cough, and a high risk for respiratory failure and death.

Pathophysiology[48]

Inhalation of *Legionella pneumophila* causes two distinct clinical syndromes: Pontiac fever, which resembles influenza, and Legionnaires' disease, with pathologic changes characteristic of lobar pneumonia. In the latter there is a cellular exudate consisting of polymorphonuclear leukocytes and macrophages with extensive necrosis of the exudate and alveolar septa. Bronchi are clear of the necrotic process. Rarely is a purulent sputum produced. The disease progresses rapidly during the first 4 to 6 days of clinical illness. Complications include renal failure, bacteremic shock, and respiratory failure resulting in death to 15% of patients.

Chest radiographs show a patchy pattern of pneumonia and small pleural effusions. There may be a normal or slight leukocytosis, markedly elevated sedimentation rate, hematuria, proteinuria, and laboratory evidence of liver dysfunction.

Diagnostic Studies and Findings[48]

Culture of Blood, Sputum, Pleural Fluid, Lung Tissue

Positive for *L. pneumophila*

Direct Immunofluorescent Stain of Respiratory Secretions

Positive for *L. pneumophila*

Enzyme-Linked Immunosorbent Assay (ELISA) on Urine

Positive for *L. pneumophila* antigen

Indirect Immunofluorescence

Fourfold or greater rise in antibody titer to 1:128 within 21 days of onset of illness

Medical Plan[48]

Medications

Anti-infective agents
- Erythromycin (Robimycin), 0.5-1 g/6 h for adults IV or oral, for 14 d
- Rifampin (Rifomycin, others; as adjunct therapy)

General Management

Assisted ventilation
Oxygen therapy
Temporary renal dialysis
IV fluids and electrolytes

NURSING CARE

Nursing Assessment[48]

Body Temperature

38° to 41° C (102° to 105° F) within a day

Subjective Symptoms

Anorexia
Malaise
Myalgia
Chills
Abdominal pain

Respiratory Concerns

Nonproductive cough
Dyspnea
Tachypnea
Pleuritic chest pain
Rales or rhonchi

Cardiovascular Concerns

Tachycardia
Symptoms of shock

Digestive Concerns

Diarrhea
Sometimes vomiting

Neurologic Concerns

Confusion, slurring of speech, and falling: infrequent symptoms

Elimination

Renal insufficiency
Hematuria

Nursing Dx & Intervention

Nursing Diagnosis	Nursing Intervention/Rationale
Ineffective breathing pattern	• Monitor for signs of respiratory failure; assist ventilation and administer oxygen as prescribed (see Chapter 2).
Altered tissue perfusion	• Monitor for symptoms of shock and report findings *for early intervention.* • Administer vasoactive drugs as prescribed.
Altered patterns of urinary elimination	• Monitor for edema and decreased urine output. Record intake and output *to detect early renal insufficiency.* Assist with dialysis as prescribed.
Potential fluid volume deficit	• Administer IV therapy as prescribed. • Monitor intake and output *to ensure intake equal to output.*
Potential for injury: falling	• Protect a confused, ataxic patient from falls: use side rails; monitor closely *to prevent trauma.*
Hyperthermia	• Assess body temperature. • Bathe with tepid water *to reduce temperature.* • Administer antipyretic agents as prescribed *to reduce temperature.*

Evaluation

Patient Outcome	Data Indicating That Outcome is Reached
Body temperature is normal.	Oral adult temperature is 37° C (98.6° F).
Breathing patterns are normal.	Respiratory rate is normal. There is no dyspnea, cough, rales, or rhonchi.
All cells receive oxygen.	Skin is warm, and color is normal.
Laboratory values are within normal limits.	Leukocyte count, sedimentation rate, urine specific gravity, carbon dioxide, Po_2, and Pco_2 are normal.
Urine elimination is normal.	Urine output is adequate.

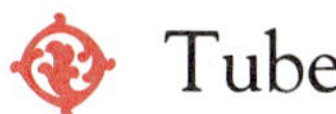

Tuberculosis

Tuberculosis is a chronic pulmonary and extrapulmonary infectious disease acquired by inhalation of a dried-droplet nucleus containing a tubercle bacillus into the alveolar structure of the lung; it is characterized by stages of early infection (frequently asymptomatic), latency, and a potential for recurrent postprimary disease.

Pathophysiology[5,40,41,48]

Tuberculosis infection can be differentiated from tuberculosis disease. Tuberculosis infection is characterized by the presence of mycobacteria in the tissue of a host who is free of clinical symptoms and who demonstrates the presence of antibodies against the mycobacteria. Tuberculosis is manifest as pathologic and functional symptoms indicating destructive activity of mycobacteria in host tissue. Both infection and disease result from tissue invasion by *Mycobacterium tuberculosis, M. bovis,* or a variety of atypical mycobacteria. All are spore formers capable of remaining viable and virulent for long periods of time inside or outside host tissue. *M. tuberculosis*, the tubercle bacillus, is the most frequent etiologic agent in human tuberculosis. Transmission is primarily by inhalation of minute dried-droplet nuclei (each containing a single tubercle bacillus), coughed or sneezed into the air by a person whose sputum contains virulent tubercle bacilli. Less commonly, transmission may occur by ingestion or by invasion of the skin or mucous membranes.

The pathologic condition of the infection and disease occurs in three stages: initial or primary infection, latency, and postprimary disease. In the initial infection the bacilli invade the tissue at the portal of entry, usually the middle or lower zones of the lungs; multiply there over a 3-week period; and create a small inflammatory lesion. Bacilli immediately enter the lymphatic system and are carried to the nearest group of lymph nodes, where they also produce inflammatory lesions. In addition, hematogenous dissemination of bacilli results in a subclinical bacteremia and the production of inflammatory lesions throughout the body. The sites and the extensiveness of the systemic lesions depend on the numbers of disseminated bacilli and the speed with which the host produces an immune response. These early lesions at the portal of entry, in the lymph nodes, and disseminated are referred to as the primary complex.

The extent of inflammatory response at the sites of tissue invasion increases with the number of invading bacilli. Nonspecific cellular resistance permits some phagocytosis of tubercle bacilli, producing suppuration and necrosis in the central portion of the lesion. Bacilli continue to replicate at the periphery of the lesion. This initial or primary infection stage is generally symptom free.

Within 3 to 12 weeks a cellular and humoral immune response can be detected. *Mycobacterium*-specific lymphocytes and antibodies stimulate a fibroblastic response at the periphery of the lesion, resulting in a dense connective tissue enclosure and the formation of a noncaseating granuloma. The focal lesions continue to harbor viable tubercle bacilli, with the potential for reactivation under conditions of decreased host resistance.

The specific immune response results in successful encapsulation of all lesions in 85% to 95%, depending on age, of those persons infected. These people enter the latent stage of the disease and remain disease free for variable periods of time, depending on their ability to maintain specific and nonspecific resistance. The specific immune response does not preclude reinfection with subsequent exposure.

For 5% to 15% of infected persons, host responses are inadequate to contain the infection, and active disease progresses in the portal of entry lesion or in all lesions in the body. Necrosis and cavitation continue in the lesions, forming caseation. The lesions may rupture, spreading necrotic residue and bacilli throughout the tissue and throughout the body. Disseminated bacilli establish new focal lesions that progress through stages of inflammation, noncaseating granulomas, and caseating necrosis.

The disease symptoms vary with the body tissue affected. Extrapulmonary tuberculosis in the meninges, blood vessels, kidneys, bones, joints, larynx, skin, intestines, lymph nodes, peritoneum, or eyes is much less common than pulmonary tuberculosis.

Reactivated disease following latency accounts for most of the active tuberculosis diagnosed today. It occurs most frequently in aged persons and persons with chronic and debilitating disease. Although reactivation may occur in any of the focal lesions, it most commonly occurs in those in the upper lobes or at the apex of the lower lobes of the lungs, forming abscesses and tuberculous cavities at those sites. Untreated reactivated disease has a variable course with many exacerbations and remissions. Complications caused by excessive cavitation are common.

Diagnostic Studies and Findings[5,48]

Sputum Culture

Positive for *M. tuberculosis* within 2 to 3 weeks of active disease; will not be positive during latency

Acid-Fast with Ziehl-Neelsen Stain Smear of Sputum (Cerebrospinal Fluid or Blood in Extrapulmonary Disease)

Positive for acid-fast bacilli

Histologic Examination or Culture of Tissue in Extrapulmonary Disease

Positive for *M. tuberculosis*

Skin Tests: Intradermal Injection of Antigen

PPD: five tuberculin units of purified protein derivative (PPD)

Heaf test: old tuberculin (OT) injected with pressure gun

Mantoux test: PPD or OT injected intradermally

Tine test: OT pressed into skin with tine unit

Vollmer patch test: OT on gauze strip applied to skin

Tuberculin reaction begins 3 to 6 weeks after infection; an area of induration greater than 10 mm in 48 to 72 hours indicates past infection and presence of antibodies; does not indicate active disease; nonspecific reactions during first 48 hours can be overlooked

If reaction is questionable, a second test may be done 1 week later; if the second test is less than significant, person is considered not to have been infected; increase in size of induration greater than 6 mm to a diameter of 10 mm indicates recent tuberculin infection

Pleural Needle Biopsy

Positive for granulomas of tuberculosis; giant cells indicating caseation necrosis

Chest Roentgenogram

Findings may show calcification at the original site, enlargement of hilar lymph nodes, parenchymal infiltrate representing extension of the original site of infection, or the appearance of pleural effusion or cavitation

Not diagnostically definitive of tuberculosis

Medical Plan[5,41,48]

Surgery

Intervention for complications

Resectional procedures for persisting cavitary lesions (less common since antimicrobial therapy)

Surgical intervention for massive hemoptysis, spontaneous pneumothorax, abscess drainage, intestinal obstruction, or ureteral stricture

Medications

A combination of anti-infective agents is recommended: two primary drugs or a primary plus a secondary drug; initial dosages are higher, followed by prolonged therapy at reduced dosages; the combination of drugs used, the dosage, and duration of administration depend on the stage of the infection or disease, the presence of extrapulmonary disease, and the sensitivity of the patient to certain chemotherapeutic agents

Anti-infective agents

- Primary drugs
  - Isoniazid (INH), 10-20 mg/kg/d (up to 300 mg/d) po for 1-2 yr
  - Ethambutol (Myambutol), 15 mg/kg/d po for 1-2 yr; initial dose: 25 mg/kg/d for 2 mo
  - Rifampin (Rifomycin, others), 20 mg/kg/d po for 6 mo to 2 yr

Streptomycin, 30 mg/kg/d IM for 2-3 mo
Secondary drugs
Pyrazinamide (Aldinamide), 20-30 mg/kg/d
Ethionamide (Trecator), 10-30 mg/kg/d
Para-amino salicylic acid (PAS), 0.2 mg/kg/d po for 1-2 yr
Cycloserine (Seromycin), 0.5-1 g/d po in divided doses
Capreomycin (Capastat), 0.75-1 g/d IM for 30 d; twice weekly thereafter
Kanamycin (Kantrex), 1 g/d IM
Viomycin (Viocin), 1 g/d IM
An example of recommended treatment plans
Primary pulmonary tuberculosis
Isoniazid, 300 mg/d po for 9 mo plus
Rifampin, 600 mg/d po for 9 mo *or*
Isoniazid, 300 mg/d po for 18-24 mo plus
Ethambutol, 15-18 mg/kg/d po for 18-24 mo
Chronic pulmonary tuberculosis
Isoniazid, 10-20 mg/kg/d for 18 mo or more, plus
Rifampin, 20 mg/kg/d for 18 mo or more, *or*
PAS, 0.2 mg/kg/d for 18 mo or more, *or*
Ethambutol, 15 mg/kg/d for 18 mo or more
Corticosteroids
May be used in conjunction with the anti-infective agents for overwhelming and life-threatening disease

General Management

After stabilization most patients can be effectively managed on an outpatient basis with monitoring for compliance with drug taking, drug side effects, and patient response to the drug therapy
AFB isolation until antimicrobial therapy is successfully initiated for sputum-positive patients to prevent spread to others (see p. 1298)
Secretion precautions until wounds stop draining for patients with external tuberculosis lesions (see p. 1298)
Skin testing: identify recent converters to tuberculosis skin tests; trace their contacts to identify persons with active disease; isoniazid therapy for 1 year for recent converters and for close household contacts of persons with active disease (not routine for those over 35 years); tuberculosis skin testing is recommended for children at school entry and again at age 14 years
BCG vaccine for those persons who are at high risk for contact with active cases, who are skin test negative, and who are not immunosuppressed (benefits of BCG vaccine are controversial); receiving the vaccine results in a positive skin test

NURSING CARE

Nursing Assessment[48]

Body Temperature

Slight continued elevation with chills and night sweats

Respiratory Concerns

Initially a nonproductive cough
Later mucopurulent secretions
Advanced: hemoptysis; dyspnea on exertion and at rest; rales over apex of lung; chest pain with respiratory movement if pleura is involved; hoarseness with involvement of larynx; dysphagia with pharyngeal involvement; sibilant and sonorous rhonchi

Cardiovascular Concerns

Tachycardia

Subjective Symptoms

History of weight loss
Anorexia
Generalized weakness and fatigue

Assessment of extrapulmonary tuberculosis depends on the system involved. The onset of symptoms is generally insidious, as is the onset of pulmonary tuberculosis.

Tuberculosis Pericarditis

Precordial chest pain, fever, and pericardial friction rubs
Jugular venous distention, hepatic congestion, ascites, and peripheral edema

Tuberculosis Peritonitis

Abdominal pain simulating that of appendicitis
Abdominal distention
Anorexia, vomiting, and weight loss
Night sweats
Abdominal tenderness when palpated
Ascites

Miliary Tuberculosis

More severe symptoms of respiratory involvement: dyspnea, hyperventilation, and cough
Hypoxemia
Spontaneous unilateral or bilateral pneumothorax (manifested by sudden chest pain and breathlessness) and fever
Painful, nodular cutaneous lesions, which may ulcerate, may be present

Tuberculosis Meningitis

Headache, vomiting, fever, and anorexia
Alterations in intellectual function, diminishing levels of consciousness, and neurologic deficits

Cerebrospinal fluid leukocytes of 100 to 400 cells/mm^3 and increase in protein

Tuberculosis Lymphadenitis

Palpable enlargement of supraclavicular and cervical lymph nodes

Osteoarticular Tuberculosis

Pain in joints, aggravated by movement
Swelling, minimal erythema, and tenderness to palpation
Limitation of motion and gross deformities (most common in vertebral column, hip, and knee joints)

Tuberculosis of Gastrointestinal Tract

Symptoms depend on area involved
May have gastrointestinal bleeding, pain, constipation, or diarrhea
Partial or complete obstruction
Perforation with peritonitis

Tuberculosis of Genitourinary Organs

Urgency, frequency, dysuria, hematuria, and pyuria
Salpingitis with lower abdominal pain and infertility
Amenorrhea
Abnormal vaginal discharge or bleeding

Nursing Dx & Intervention

Nursing Diagnosis*	Nursing Intervention/Rationale
Ineffective airway clearance	• Assist patient to turn, cough, and deep breathe every 2 to 4 hours.
Ineffective breathing pattern	• Monitor breathing *to detect dyspnea and signs of pneumothorax.* • Initiate respiratory assistance as needed. Observe sputum for hemoptysis *to detect complications.*
Potential fluid volume deficit	• Force fluids to 2000 to 3000 ml daily unless contraindicated *to provide for increased needs during infection.*
Anxiety	• Explain that tuberculosis is a completely curable condition with proper long-term antimicrobial therapy *to decrease anxiety and promote medication compliance.*
Altered nutrition: less than body requirements	• Maintain high-protein, high-carbohydrate diet with frequent, small feedings *to provide for increased metabolic needs during infection.*
Potential for infection: patient contacts	• Employ AFB isolation until antimicrobial therapy is succesfully initiated for sputum-positive patients (see p. 1298) *to prevent transmission.* • Employ secretion precautions until wounds stop draining for patients with external tuberculosis lesions (see p. 1298) *to prevent transmission.* • Teach hospitalized patient to cough and sneeze into paper tissues and to dispose of tissues properly *to prevent transmission of the organism.*

*There may be other nursing diagnoses if the patient has extrapulmonary tuberculosis complicated with other chronic disease.

Patient Education

1. Teach care of sputum if discharged patient still has positive sputum cultures.
2. Teach handwashing and good hygiene.
3. Drug therapy must be continued uninterrupted for the designated time period. Explain dosage, frequency of administration, and purpose for prolonged treatment.
4. Explain medication's toxic and side effects:
   a. INH: infrequent toxic effects: peripheral neuropathy, convulsions, ataxia, dizziness, optic neuritis; older patients may experience a drug-related hepatitis with fatigue, malaise, and anorexia
   b. Ethambutol: reduced visual acuity with inability to perceive the color green
   c. Streptomycin: skin rash, fever, malaise, vertigo, and deafness; gastrointestinal disturbances and central nervous system symptoms
   d. PAS: toxic reactions more common with this drug and include symptoms of hypersensitivity, hepatic damage, gastrointestinal disturbances, and renal failure
   e. Rifampin: red-orange colored urine common, jaundice, nausea, anorexia, vomiting, diarrhea, cramps, occasional central nervous system disturbances, and hypersensitivity reactions; may interfere with actions of oral contraceptives
   f. Ethionamide: gastrointestinal irritation and symptoms of hepatotoxicity
   g. Pyrazinamide: hepatoxicity
   h. Cycloserine: central nervous system effects including seizures, somnolence, and muscle twitching
5. Report side effects to physician immediately.
6. Emphasize need for periodic reculturing of sputum

during period of therapy: monthly until cultures are negative; then every 3 months for duration of therapy.

7. Report to physician: hemoptysis, chest pain, difficulty in breathing, hearing loss, or vertigo.
8. Maintain adequate fluid and caloric intake.
9. Household and close contacts should be examined at time of treatment of patient and again in 2 to 3 months.

Evaluation

Patient Outcome	Data Indicating That Outcome is Reached
There is no active infection.	Sputum cultures are consistently negative. Roentgenograms show a reduction in the size of cavities and decrease in the thickness of cavity walls. Body temperature is normal. Patient does not experience chills or night sweats.
Laboratory values are within normal limits.	Serum alkaline phosphatase levels, hematocrit, hemoglobin, and leukocyte count are normal. Urine does not contain erythrocytes.
Patient contacts are free of infection.	Contacts do not convert to a positive skin test.
Breathing patterns are normal.	Patient does not experience dyspnea, cough, or pain on breathing.
There is no extrapulmonary disease.	Patient does not manifest the extrapulmonary symptoms described under "Nursing Assessment."

ENTERIC INFECTIOUS DISEASES

A wide range of enteric infectious diseases are caused by bacteria found in contaminated food or water. Food poisoning can be caused by infectious agents that have already multiplied in food (food intoxications such as staphylococcal food poisoning, botulism, and enteric infections) or by bacteria that multiply in the body after ingestion (bacterial and viral gastroenteritis and parasitic enteritis). Food and water can also be sources of *Salmonella* infection, which can produce a variety of clinical entities. Intestinal infections caused by parasitic worms (helminths) are also discussed in this section.

Food poisoning is the generic term applied to illnesses acquired through consumption of food or water contaminated with chemicals, bacteria and bacterial toxins, or organic poisons naturally present in some edible substances. The food poisonings caused by bacteria and bacterial toxins are discussed here. In all cases disease is produced in the host shortly after ingestion of food containing bacteria that have already multiplied in the food. These diseases are not directly communicable. If the bacteria have produced a toxin in the food, the resulting disease in the host is intoxication, as in staphylococcal food poisoning and botulism. If the bacterial cells are antigenic, they produce an infection in the host, such as those caused by *Clostridium perfringens* and *Vibrio parahaemolyticus* (Table 13-7).

Staphylococcal food poisoning

Staphylococcal food poisoning is an enteric intoxication of acute onset. Symptoms are severe nausea, intestinal cramps, vomiting, diarrhea, prostration, and occasionally, subnormal temperature and hypotension. The intensity of the disease depends on the quantity of the ingested toxin and host susceptibility. The duration of the illness is 1 to 2 days, and recovery is generally complete.

Pathophysiology[48]

The ingested enterotoxin acts on the abdominal viscera, creating a sensory stimulus that reaches the vomiting center of the brain by way of the vagus and sympathetic nerves. The action of the enterotoxin on the gastric mucosa produces a patchy hyperemia, erosions, petechiae, and a purulent gastric exudate. Diarrhea results from inhibition of water absorption from the intestinal lumen and from increased transport of fluid into the lumen.

Diagnostic Studies and Findings[48]

Culture of Stomach Contents, Feces, or Suspected Food

10^6 enterotoxin-producing staphylococci per gram of specimen

Enterotoxin Tests

Not routinely available

Table 13-7
Overview of Food Poisoning: Intoxications and Enteric Infections

	Intoxications		Enteric Infections		
	Staphylococcal Food Poisoning	**Botulism**	***Clostridium perfringens***	***Vibrio parahaemolyticus***	***Bacillus cereus***
Occurrence	Widespread and frequent; one of the principal acute food poisonings in United States	Sporadic; family-grouped cases occur	Widespread and frequent in countries with cooking practices that favor growth of organism	Sporadic cases and outbreaks occur in warm months of the year	Outbreaks in Europe and United States
Etiologic agent	Several enterotoxins of staphylococci; stable at boiling temperature	Toxins produced by *Clostridium botulinum* in anaerobic conditions; destroyed by boiling	Type A strains of *C. perfringens (C. welchii)*	*V. parahaemolyticus* (many types)	*Bacillus cereus*, an aerobic spore former that produces two enterotoxins—one heat stable causing vomiting and one heat labile causing diarrhea
Reservoir	Humans; cows with infected udders	Soil, water, and intestinal tract of animals and fish	Soil and gastrointestinal tract of humans and animals	Marine silt, coastal waters, fish, and shellfish	Soil; commonly found in raw, dried, and processed foods
Transmission	Ingestion of food containing staphylococcal toxin, which formed while food was held at room temperature	Ingestion of food in which toxin has formed; generally home-canned vegetables, fruits, and meats; also onions and potatoes cooked and held at room temperature	Ingestion of food, especially meat, contaminated by soil or feces; spores survive normal cooking temperatures, germinate, and multiply during cooking and reheating	Ingestion of raw or undercooked contaminated seafood	Ingestion of food that has been kept at ambient temperatures after cooking, permitting multiplication of the organism
Incubation period	30 min-7 h, usually 2-4 h	12-36 h	6-24 h; usually 10-12 h	4-96 h; usually 12-14 h	1-6 h for disease causing vomiting; 6-16 h for disease causing diarrhea
Period of communicability	Not applicable	Not applicable	Noncommunicable	Noncommunicable	Noncommunicable
Susceptibility and resistance	General; no immune response	General; no immune response	General; no resistance develops from exposure	General	Unknown
Report to local health authority	Prompt report of outbreaks	Report of cases and outbreaks	Prompt report of outbreaks	Report outbreaks	Report cases and outbreaks

Data from Benenson.[5]

Medical Plan

General Management

Oral or IV fluids and electrolytes

NURSING CARE

Nursing Assessment

Digestive System

Acute-onset nausea, vomiting, intestinal cramps, and diarrhea

Vital Signs

Subnormal temperature
Hypotension

Energy Level

Weakness
Prostration

Nursing Dx & Intervention

Nursing Diagnosis	Nursing Intervention/Rationale
Potential fluid volume deficit	• Assess skin turgor and urinary output *to detect signs of dehydration.* • Monitor frequency and characteristics of vomitus and diarrhea. • Encourage small amount of oral fluids as tolerated *to maintain adequate intake.* • Administer IV fluids and electrolytes as prescribed *to replace those lost in vomitus and diarrhea.*

Patient Education

1. Teach food handlers the proper temperatures for maintaining food to prevent another occurrence of food poisoning. Perishable foods should be kept hot (60° C or 140° F) or cold (4° C or 39° F).
2. Persons with purulent lesions of the face, hands, or nose should not handle food.
3. Teach food handlers the importance of handwashing and strict food hygiene and kitchen sanitation.

Evaluation

Patient Outcome	Data Indicating That Outcome is Reached
Body hydration is normal.	Skin turgor is good. Urine output is adequate.
Digestive function is normal.	Stools are soft, formed, and normal colored. Patient tolerates regular diet.
Laboratory studies are within normal limits.	Urine specific gravity is normal. Measurements of sodium, potassium, chloride, magnesium, and calcium in blood are normal.

Botulism

Botulism is a severe neurointoxication with a wide range of neurologic symptoms and severity of symptoms. In the United States 10% of cases under treatment result in death, primarily from respiratory failure. Three types of botulism have been recognized: foodborne, wound, and infant botulism.

Pathophysiology[48]

Clostridium botulinum, a spore-forming anaerobe capable of withstanding boiling, produces a potent toxin in anaerobic conditions. A common source of botulinal toxin is improperly processed canned foods. Less commonly, *C. botulinum* enters the body through a wound and produces toxin in traumatized, necrotic tissue. Ingestion of *C. botulinum* spores does not result in toxin production in adults and children but does cause toxin production in the bowel lumen of some infants, producing infant botulism.

The botulinal toxin is hematogenously disseminated to peripheral cholinergic synapses, where it becomes irreversibly bound. This action blocks the release of acetylcholine, producing impaired autonomic and voluntary neuromuscular transmission and muscular paralysis. Gradual recovery occurs over a period of weeks from the regeneration of terminal motor neurons to reinnervate noncontracting muscle fibers.

Intestinal stasis predisposes to the colonization of any ingested viable spores of *C. botulinum*. Additional toxin is produced in vivo, prolonging the course of the disease.

Complications in hospitalized patients with botulism are similar to those affecting other critically ill paralyzed persons who depend on mechanical support to sustain life.

Diagnostic Studies and Findings[48]

Culture of Feces

Positive for *C. botulinum*

Serum

Positive for toxins; circulating toxins found in about one third hospitalized patients with botulism

Differential Diagnosis

- Electromyography (EMG)
  - Demonstrates a defect in transmission at neuromuscular junction
- Cerebrospinal fluid cultures and chemistries
  - Normal
- Serology
  - Normal

Medical Plan[5,48]

Medications

- Immunologic agents
  - Trivalent (ABE) botulinal antitoxin (not used for infants) administered IV or IM as soon as possible after onset of symptoms
  - Anti-infective agents
  - Penicillin for wound botulism
  - Agent-specific and anti-infective agents for secondary bacterial infection

General Management

- Gastric lavage initially
- Mechanical ventilation in the event of respiratory paralysis
- Suction of secretions
- Intubation or tracheostomy
- Nasogastric feedings
- IV fluid and electrolytes
- Must be reported to local health authority immediately
- All patient contacts known to have eaten the same food should have gastric lavage, high enemas, and cathartics and should be kept under close medical supervision
- Public education
  - Proper home canning methods
  - Boiling all home canned food before eating
  - Not feeding honey to infants under 1 year of age

NURSING CARE

Nursing Assessment[48]

Neurologic Concerns

- Head and neck
  - Abrupt onset, bilateral and symmetric: ptosis, blurred vision, diplopia, dry mouth, dysphagia, dysphonia, dysarthria, nasal regurgitation
- Gastrointestinal concerns
  - Vomiting
  - Diarrhea
  - Constipation
- Respiratory concerns
  - Paralysis of muscles of respiration
- Large muscles
  - Symmetric flaccid paralysis
  - No sensory disturbances, only motor

Temperature and Pulse

Normal

Wound Botulism

Same as above except there are no gastrointestinal symptoms

Nursing Dx & Intervention

Nursing Diagnosis	Nursing Intervention/Rationale
Potential for aspiration	• Provide patent airway. • Suction secretions. • Provide tracheostomy care. • Offer nasogastric tube feedings per protocol *to prevent aspiration of oral fluids.*
Ineffective breathing pattern	• Monitor for signs of respiratory paralysis and oxygen insufficiency. • Initiate mechanical ventilation and oxygen as prescribed. • Monitor patient on respirator for signs of hyperventilation or hypoventilation.
Impaired physical mobility	• Position *to prevent contractures.* • Assist with range of motion exercises *to prevent joint stiffness.*

Nursing Diagnosis	Nursing Intervention/Rationale
Altered nutrition: less than body requirements	• Administer nasogastric tube feeding or alimentation as prescribed. • Offer frequent, small oral feedings as patient tolerates *to maintain adequate intake.*
Fluid volume deficit	• Administer IV fluids as prescribed. • Offer liquids as patient can tolerate.
Bathing/hygiene self-care deficit	• Provide total hygienic care as needed.
Potential for infection	• *To protect patient from a complicating bacterial infection:* Suction *to prevent aspiration of secretions.* Monitor for signs of pneumonia and urinary tract infection. Turn every 2 hours *to prevent pooling of secretions.* Provide skin care and catheter care. Ensure adequate fluid intake. Assess temperature *to detect onset of fever.*

Patient Education[5]

1. Destroy all canned food and containers from same batch that contained the *C. botulinum* by burying deep in soil or boiling 3 minutes before discarding. Commercial canned foods should be submitted for laboratory examination.
2. Contaminated cooking utensils should be sterilized by boiling for 3 minutes before reuse.
3. No questionable canned food should ever be tasted. Foods containing *C. botulinum* do not necessarily have off odors or a spoiled taste.
4. Recommended processing times and temperatures for home canning must be followed to ensure killing of all *C. botulinum* spores. This information is available through state agricultural extension services.
5. Home-canned vegetables and meats should be boiled for 3 minutes to destroy botulinal toxin.
6. No cooked food should be kept at ambient room temperatures. It should be kept hot or should be refrigerated.

Evaluation

Patient Outcome	Data Indicating That Outcome is Reached
Breathing patterns are normal.	Respiratory rate is normal. Respirations are of normal depth. There is no dyspnea. Skin and mucous membranes are warm and moist, with normal color.
Airway clearance is effective.	Airway is open. Secretions are thin and easily coughed up by patient. Patient swallows without difficulty.
There is no secondary infection:	Body temperature is normal.
Respiratory	Secretions are thin. There is no cough, rales, or rhonchi. Breathing patterns are normal.
Urinary	Urinary output is normal.
Skin	Skin is warm and moist. There are no lesions or decubiti.
Neuromuscular function is normal.	Neuromuscular innervation and muscle control are regained. Patient can see, speak, swallow, breathe, cough, and move around at will. Gastrointestinal tract peristalsis is normal.
Laboratory studies are within normal limits.	Blood leukocytes, O_2 saturation, CO_2, Po_2, and Pco_2 are normal. Urine is negative for protein, blood, or bacteria.

Food poisoning: enteric infections

Clostridium perfringens **generally causes a mild intestinal infection characterized by sudden onset of abdominal colic, nausea, and diarrhea. Fever and vomiting are rare.**

Vibrio parahaemolyticus **is a moderately severe intestinal infection characterized by sudden-onset abdominal cramps and watery diarrhea lasting 1 to 7 days. Nausea, vomiting, fever, and headache may be present.**

Bacillus cereus **food poisoning is a gastrointestinal infection characterized by sudden-onset nausea and vomiting or colic and diarrhea, lasting no longer than 24 hours.**

The three enteric infections discussed here are all caused by ingestion of food contaminated with specific bacteria that have already multiplied in the food. Disease is produced in the host shortly after ingestion of the food and is manifest as symptoms of gastroenteritis.

Pathophysiology[5,48]

C. perfringens, a spore former widely distributed in feces, soil, and water, multiplies rapidly in foods that have been cooled and reheated. The organism produces an enterotoxin in the intestinal tract within 6 to 24 hours after ingestion. The enterotoxin acts on the epithelial layer of the ileum, increasing the secretion of sodium, chloride, and fluid and inhibiting the absorption of glucose.

V. parahaemolyticus multiplies in uncooked, contaminated seafood. When ingested, the pathogen directly invades intestinal tissue to produce necrosis, ulceration, possible hemorrhage, and granulocytic infiltration of the mucosa. Disease intensity ranges from asymptomatic to severe; duration ranges from 2 hours to 10 days.

The spores of *B. cereus* survive cooking and multiply in food held at room temperature. One type of enterotoxin that is heat stable attacks the gastric mucosa. Another type, which is heat labile, affects the intestinal mucosa. Thorough reheating of food destroys the heat-labile enterotoxin but not the enterotoxin that causes vomiting.

Diagnostic Studies and Findings[48]

These conditions are most commonly diagnosed by identification of the pathogen in a food or fecal culture.

Quantitative Culture of Food or Fecal Specimen to Estimate Number of Organisms

Greater than 10^5 spores of *C. perfringens* or *B. cereus* per gram of specimen, or positive for *V. parahaemolyticus*

Medical Plan[48]

General Management

Oral fluids if tolerated
IV fluids and electrolytes if needed

NURSING CARE

Nursing Assessment[48]

Digestive Concerns

Acute-onset nausea, abdominal cramping, and diarrhea in *C. perfringens* infections
Diarrhea may be watery and bloody and persist up to 7 days in *V. parahaemolyticus* infections
Acute-onset nausea and vomiting or colic and diarrhea in *B. cereus* infections

Body Temperature

Usually normal

Nursing Dx & Intervention

Nursing Diagnosis	Nursing Intervention/Rationale
Diarrhea	• Obtain stool specimen *for culture to detect pathogen present.* • Provide privacy for patient *to decrease embarrassment.* • Eliminate odors. • *To prevent skin around anal opening from irritation,* wash and lubricate frequently.
Potential fluid volume deficit	• Monitor for symptoms of dehydration and electrolyte imbalance. • Administer frequent liquids as tolerated *to maintain adequate intake.* • Administer IV electrolytes as prescribed *to replace those lost during diarrhea.*

Patient Education[5]

1. Cooked foods should not be held at room temperature; they should be kept hot or should be refrigerated. Reheating should be done rapidly and completely.
2. All seafood should be cooked at a temperature above 60° C (140° F) for 15 minutes.
3. Keep all seafood, raw or cooked, adequately refrigerated before eating.
4. Handle cooked seafood to avoid its contamination with raw seafood or with contaminated seawater.

Evaluation

Patient Outcome	Data Indicating That Outcome is Reached
Digestive wastes are eliminated normally.	Stools are soft and formed. Abdomen is not distended. There is no cramping.
Fluid and electrolyte balance is normal.	Skin turgor is good. Mucous membranes are moist. Urine output is normal. Secretions are thin.
Laboratory studies are within normal limits.	Blood levels of sodium, potassium, chloride, magnesium, and calcium are normal. Urine specific gravity is normal.

Acute bacterial and viral gastroenteritis

***Campylobacter* enteritis is an acute bacterial enteric infection lasting from 1 to 10 days and is considered to be an important cause of "traveler's diarrhea."**

Diarrhea caused by *Escherichia coli* is another cause of "traveler's diarrhea." Three types of pathogenic *E. coli* are capable of producing a self-limited enteritis of varying intensity.

Shigellosis (bacillary dysentery) is an acute bacterial infection of the large intestine with severity ranging from asymptomatic infection to fulminating diarrheal disease and death.

Epidemic viral gastroenteritis is usually a self-limited, mild gastric and intestinal infection lasting 24 to 48 hours. Disease often occurs in outbreaks.

Rotavirus gastroenteritis is a sporadically occurring gastric and intestinal infection of infants and young children ranging in severity from asymptomatic to severe disease and occasionally to death.

Many forms of acute gastroenteritis are caused by ingestion of food and water contaminated with pathogenic agents or by fecal-oral transmission directly or indirectly from an infected person. These infections differ from the food poisonings previously discussed in the following ways:

- The pathogenic agents causing these diseases invade, colonize, and multiply in the human intestinal tract.
- The incubation periods are slightly longer, ranging from 1 day to several weeks.
- Direct and indirect fecal-oral transmission is possible.
- Acquired immunity of varying duration results from many of these infections.

In addition, the predominant manifestation of these diseases is acute-onset diarrhea of varying intensity and duration. The bacterial- and viral-caused gastroenteritises are usually self-limited diseases (Table 13-8).

Pathophysiology[5,40,48]

Bacterial and viral agents that produce gastroenteritis produce pathologic conditions in one of three ways:

- Toxigenic agents, such as some *Shigella* strains and enterotoxigenic *E. coli,* release an enterotoxin that acts on the small intestine to produce a local inflammation and a secretory diarrhea with rapid loss of electrolytes.
- Invasive pathogens, such as *Shigella, Campylobacter,* and invasive strains of *E. coli,* penetrate the small or large intestine, producing cellular destruction, necrosis, and potential ulceration. The diarrheal stools in these conditions frequently contain leukocytes and erythrocytes.
- Some pathogens such as the rotaviruses attach to the mucosal epithelium without invasion. They destroy cells of the intestinal villi, resulting in malabsorption of electrolytes and the potential for electrolyte imbalance.

The general effect of all of the above pathologic conditions is to increase gastrointestinal motility and to increase the secretory rate of fluids and electrolytes into the intestines. The result may be rapid dehydration, electrolyte imbalance, circulatory failure, and death. Fluid and electrolyte loss in other forms of gastroenteritis may develop more gradually or may not occur at all. Infants, small children, and debilitated individuals are at greater risk for severe dehydration.

The attachment of the pathogens to the mucosa may be altered by nonspecific resistance factors in the host:

- The normal bacterial flora of the intestinal tract prevents attachment by competing for attachment sites or by production of volatile organic acids. If the normal flora is diminished as a result of antibiotic therapy or malnutrition, this host defense is ineffective.
- The pH of the gastrointestinal tract impedes the growth of some microbes. Altering the pH through the ingestion of antacids reduces the effectiveness of this defense.
- Normal gastrointestinal motility purges the intestinal tract of many pathogens, and interference with this function increases the risk for invasion of pathogens.

Specific immune responses of varying duration occur in the host following infection with *Shigella,* parvovirus-like agents, rotavirus, and *E. coli.*

Diagnostic Studies and Findings[5,48]

The diagnosis of these conditions relies on identification of the pathogen in a specimen of feces and by a fourfold or greater rise in serum antibody titer between acute disease and convalescence.

Table 13-8
Overview of Acute Bacterial and Viral Gastroenteritis

	***Campylobacter* Enteritis (Traveler's Diarrhea)**	**Diarrhea Caused by *E. coli* (Traveler's Diarrhea)**	**Shigellosis (Bacillary Dysentery)**	**Epidemic Viral Gastroenteritis**	**Rotavirus Gastroenteritis**
Occurrence	Worldwide; common-source outbreaks occur; highest in warmer months	Worldwide; common-source outbreaks occur; high in areas of poor sanitation and during warm months	Worldwide; highest in children under 10 yr old; outbreaks common in crowded living conditions, day care	Worldwide and common; epidemics and outbreaks occur; affects infants and adults	Worldwide; sporadic and in outbreaks; highest in infants and young children
Etiologic agent	*Campylobacter jejuni*	Enterotoxigenic, invasive, or enteropathogenic strains of *E. coli*	From different groups of *Shigella* bacteria, with many strains	Many viruses; Norwalk virus most common	Many types of rotaviruses
Reservoir	Domestic and wild animals and birds	Infected humans, who are often asymptomatic	Humans	Humans	Humans; pathogenicity of animal viruses undetermined
Transmission	Ingestion of water, food, or raw milk contaminated with organism from feces; contact with infected animals or infants; fecal-oral	Fecal contamination of food, water, or fomites; transmitted to infant during delivery; fecal-oral, by hand	Direct or indirect fecal-oral transmission from infected person or carrier, usually by hand	Fecal-oral route; foodborne and waterborne transmission	Fecal-oral; possibly fecal-respiratory
Incubation period	3-5 d; range: 1-10 d	12-72 h	1-7 d; usually 1-3 d	Usually 24-48 h; range: 10-51 h	48 h
Period of communicability	Several days to weeks throughout course of infection; usually 2-7 wk; carriers are rare	Duration of fecal excretion of organism, possibly weeks	During acute infection to 4 wk after illness; carrier state may persist for months	During acute stage and shortly thereafter	During acute stage and shortly thereafter
Susceptibility and resistance	General	Infants very susceptible; duration of acquired immunity unknown	General; more severe in children and elderly and debilitated individuals; strain-specific antibodies develop	General; short-term (14 wk) immunity may follow infection with specific serotypes	By age 2 yr most individuals have acquired antibodies against most serotypes
Report to local health authority	In some endemic areas	Report epidemic only	Mandatory case reporting	Report epidemics; no individual case reports	Report epidemics; no individual case reports

Data from Benenson[5] and Wehrle.[48]

Campylobacter

Direct examination of stool with phase-contrast microscopy
- Positive for leukocytes and erythrocytes and *C. jejuni*

Serology: immunofluorescence or agglutination tests
- Fourfold increase in antibody titer

E. coli Diarrhea

Stool culture
- Positive for enterotoxigenic or invasive strains of *E. coli*

Serology
- Fourfold increase in antitoxic antibodies

Shigellosis

Examination of stool specimen
- Pus cells in specimen

Fecal culture
- Positive for *Shigella*

Epidemic Viral Gastroenteritis

Immune electron microscopy or radioimmunoassay of feces specimen
- Positive for virus

Serologic tests using immune electron microscopy, immune adherence hemagglutination assay, or radioimmunoassay
- Fourfold or greater increase in antibody titer

Rotavirus Gastroenteritis

Electron microscopy or immunologic examination of feces or rectal swabs
- Positive for rotavirus (10^6 per gram of feces)

Serology: complement fixation, ELISA, or immunofluorescent techniques
- Fourfold increase in antibody titer; 80% to 90% of children have detectable antibodies by age 3 years

Medical Plan[5,41,48]

Medications

Agents that suppress intestinal motility are not given for bacterial gastroenteritis

For shigellosis
- Anti-infective agents
  - Trimethoprim-sulfamethoxazole (Septra, Bactrim), 1 tablet (80 mg trimethoprim and 400 mg sulfamethoxazole) q12h for 5 d

For *E. coli* diarrhea
- Anti-infective agents for prevention
  - Trimethoprim-sulfamethoxazole, 160 mg of TMP to 800 mg of SMX/d, or doxycycline (100 mg/d) po for 2 wk before travel to a high-risk area

General Management

IV fluids and electrolyte replacement
- For shock: rapid infusion of 20 to 30 ml/kg of Ringer's lactate, isotonic saline, or similar isotonic solution given within an hour
- For complete rehydration after circulation is restored: glucose electrolyte solution (oral or IV hypotonic electrolyte solutions in amounts equal to estimated fluid loss)

NURSING CARE

Nursing Assessment[5,40,48]

Campylobacter

Gastrointestinal concerns
- Days 1 and 2: nausea, vomiting, abdominal pain
- Days 2 to 4 (sometimes lasts 10 days): foul-smelling, or liquid diarrhea; sometimes 20 or 30 stools per day; blood in stools after day 4
- Day 7: ulcerative colitis may occur

Body temperature
- 38° to 41° C (100° to 105° F)

Neurologic concerns
- Later in course of disease: febrile convulsions

E. coli Diarrhea

Gastrointestinal concerns
- Day 1: vomiting
- Day 2 (lasting 7-10 days): mucoid and bloody diarrhea or profuse watery diarrhea without blood or mucus

Fluids and electrolytes
- Anytime during disease: poor skin turgor, dry mucous membranes, faint pulse, hypotension

Body temperature
- Days 1 and 2: fever possible

Shigellosis

Gastrointestinal concerns
- Day 1: nausea, abdominal pain, colic, vomiting, painful diarrhea
- Days 2 to 5: stools contain blood, pus, and mucus; rectal irritation and tenesmus

Fluids and electrolytes
- Days 2 to 5: loss of turgor, oliguria, hypotension, weak pulse, shock

Body temperature
- Days 1 to 5: 38° to 41° C (101° to 105° F)

Epidemic Viral Gastroenteritis

Gastrointestinal concerns
- Day 1 (lasts 24 to 48 hours): nausea, vomiting, diarrhea, abdominal pain

Body temperature
- Day 1: low-grade fever

Subjective symptoms
- Myalgia

Headache
Malaise

Rotavirus Gastroenteritis

Gastrointestinal concerns
Day 1: vomiting for 48 hours
Days 2 to 8: watery diarrhea, rectal bleeding may occur
Fluids and electrolytes
Days 2 to 8: severe dehydration possible
Body temperature
Day 1: usually low-grade fever (up to 39° C [102° F]); may go higher
Upper respiratory concerns
Anytime during course of disease: pharyngeal exudate, cough, and rhinitis may be present

Nursing Dx & Intervention

Nursing Diagnosis	Nursing Intervention/Rationale
Fluid volume deficit (1)	• Monitor blood pressure, temperature, pulse, and respirations *to detect symptoms of circulatory collapse early.* • Administer IV fluids and electrolytes as prescribed. (Once circulation is stabilized, the initial rate of IV infusion and type of IV electrolytes may be altered to provide for rehydration.) • Continue monitoring *to detect symptoms of dehydration* (oliguria, loss of skin turgor). • Measure all fluid output (emesis, urine, diarrhea). • Measure all intake *to ensure that intake compensates for output.* • Provide oral liquids as tolerated *to ensure adequate intake.*
Diarrhea	• Obtain stool specimens for culture *to identify pathogen.* • Measure watery diarrhea output *to estimate rapidity of fluid loss.* • Cleanse perianal area and lubricate after each diarrheal stool *to prevent irritation of skin.* • Provide adequate air circulation and room deodorization *to remove odors.*
Altered nutrition: less than body requirements	• Provide patient with oral glucose electrolyte solution as soon as patient can take oral fluids. • Oral fluids can usually be tolerated once electrolyte imbalance is corrected. • Gradually add clear fluids and soft foods (milk and cream products should be avoided at first; apple juice and 7-Up are usually well tolerated).
Hyperthermia	• Monitor temperature *to detect fever.* • Sponge with tepid water *to reduce temperature.*
Potential for infection: patient contacts	• Use enteric precautions until three consecutive fecal cultures are negative for infecting organism for *Shigella.* • Use enteric precautions for duration of illness for others *to prevent transmission of the pathogen to others* (see p. 1298).

Patient Education

1. For patients being cared for at home, teach family:
   a. Signs of dehydration and the importance of prompt medical attention should dehydration occur
   b. Measurement of intake and measurement or estimation of output
   c. Maintenance of oral fluid intake equal to output
   d. Types of clear, high-glucose oral fluids that may be tolerated (apple juice; defizzed carbonated beverages such as 7-Up)
   e. Scrupulous handwashing; avoidance of contamination of food
2. Persons with *Shigella* infections should not be permitted to handle food or provide child care until two successive fecal samples or rectal swabs are free of *Shigella* organisms.
3. Child day-care programs should provide for:
   a. Frequent handwashing of workers
   b. Separate areas for food preparation and diaper changing
   c. Separate rooms for children of different age groups
   d. Routine exclusion of children with diarrhea
4. Most acute gastroenteritis can be prevented by:
   a. Thorough handwashing after toileting, handling feces, or contact with animals
   b. Thorough cooking of all food derived from animals, and avoidance of recontamination within the kitchen after cooking
   c. Drinking pasteurized milk and chlorinated water
   d. Maintaining food at hot or cold temperatures

Evaluation

Patient Outcome	Data Indicating That Outcome is Reached
Fluid and electrolyte balance is achieved:	
Circulating fluid is adequate.	Blood pressure and pulse are normal.
Body hydration is normal.	Skin turgor is good. Mucous membranes are moist. Urine output is equal to intake.
Laboratory values are normal.	Blood levels of sodium, potassium, chloride, magnesium, and calcium are normal. Urine specific gravity is normal.
Bowel elimination is normal.	Stools are soft, formed, and brown colored.
There are no signs of infection.	Body temperature is normal.

Acute and chronic parasitic enteritis

Amebiasis (amebic dysentery) is an infection with an ameba. This parasite may form a commensal relationship with the host or invade the intestinal mucosa, producing an enteritis ranging from asymptomatic to fulminating diarrheal and systemic disease. The parasite may persist in the host for years (Table 13-9).

Giardiasis is a protozoan infection of the upper intestinal tract ranging in severity from asymptomatic infection to chronic damage to the duodenal and jejunal mucosa resulting in a malabsorption syndrome (Table 13-9).

Parasitic enteritis is similar in several ways to the bacterial and viral forms of gastroenteritis described on p. 1207, but it may become chronic under some conditions.

Pathophysiology[5,48]

Amebiasis

Ingested cysts of *Entamoeba* develop into trophozoites that penetrate the mucosa and submucosa of the large intestine by mechanical and proteolytic activity. Edema, fibrin formation, and necrosis occur, creating necrotic lesions that may extend laterally in the submucosa, giving a flasklike appearance. These discrete lesions appear primarily in the cecal area, sigmoid colon, and rectum. Hematogenous dissemination may occur to the liver, peritoneum, pleura, lung, pericardium, vagina, cervix, skin, and brain, with microabscesses produced in those tissues. Symptomatic onset may be acute or ill defined, or the infection may be asymptomatic. Untreated persons develop symptoms similar to a chronic persistent colitis. Complications include perforated bowel, hemorrhage, systemic deterioration, anemia, or extraintestinal disease re-

Table 13-9
Overview of Acute and Chronic Parasitic Enteritis

	Amebiasis	Giardiasis
Occurrence	Widespread; higher in areas with poor sanitation, in homosexual communities, and in institutions	Worldwide; more common in children, institutions, and where sanitation is poor
Etiologic agent	*Entamoeba histolytica* (a parasitic ameba)	*Giardia lamblia* (a protozoan)
Reservoir	Humans, usually an asymptomatic carrier	Humans; possibly beaver and other animals
Transmission	Water contaminated with human feces of infected persons; fecal-oral by hand or contaminated food; oral-rectal sexual contact	Ingestion of contaminated water; fecal-oral by hand contamination or by homosexual activity; cysts in water are not killed with chlorine
Incubation period	Variable: 3 d to months; usually 2-4 wk	1-4 wk; average: 2 wk
Period of communicability	As long as cysts are in feces, probably years	Entire period of infection; could persist for months
Susceptibility and resistance	General, although most people harboring the organism do not develop disease	General; asymptomatic carrier rate is high
Report to local health authority	In some endemic areas	Case report in endemic areas

Data from Benenson.[5]

sulting from abscesses in other organs and tissue. Antibody titers increase and persist after infection but do not confer protection against reinfection.

Giardiasis

Ingested cysts of the *Giardia lamblia* protozoan develop into trophozoites that attach by a powerful ventral sucker to the mucosa of the jejunum and ileum without producing an inflammatory response. Diarrhea and malabsorption are thought to occur as a result of mechanical obstruction in the intestinal mucosa. Trophozoites and cysts are both excreted in the stool of ill individuals. Cysts may continue to be excreted for months in untreated persons. The disease is characterized by acute-onset diarrhea that may progress to a chronic intermittent diarrhea with malabsorption of fats and the fat-soluble vitamins. There is no invasion beyond the bowel lumen.

Diagnostic Studies and Findings

Amebiasis[48]

- Microscopic examination of feces, rectal secretions, aspirates of abscesses, or tissue sections
  - Positive for trophozoites or cysts of protozoan
- Serology: agglutination tests
  - Increased titer may persist for some time after infection
- Liver scan
  - Detection of abscesses

Giardiasis[48]

- Examination of feces or duodenal contents
  - Positive for cysts or trophozoites of the *Giardia lamblia* protozoan

Medical Plan

Surgery

- Aspiration of abscesses

Medications[42,48]

- Amebiasis: treatment regimens depend on the severity of the illness and the location and dissemination of the parasite; some combination of the following amebicides and antibiotics is used; the number of drugs and potency of the drug used increase with the severity of the symptoms
  - Anti-infective agents
    - Emetine hydrochloride, 1 mg/kg IM (not to exceed 65 mg/24 h) for 7-10 d; not to be repeated for 8 wk
    - Dehydroemetine, 1.5 mg/kg (not to exceed 80 mg/24 h)
    - Chloroquine (Aralen) (to be used concurrently with one of the above), 0.25 g qid for first day; 0.5 g/24 h for next 14 d (adults)
    - Metronidazole (Flagyl), 750 mg po tid for 10 d (adults)
    - Diiodohydroxyquin (Diodoquin), 650 mg po tid for 20 d (adults)
    - Diloxanide furoate (Furamide), 0.5 g po tid for 10 d (adults)
    - Tetracycline, 250 mg po q6-8h for 10 d (adults)
- Giardiasis
  - Anti-infective agents
    - Quinacrine hydrochloride (Atabrine), 100 mg po tid for 7 d (adults)
    - Metronidazole (Flagyl), 250 mg tid for 7 d (is not currently licensed for giardiasis use)

General Management[5]

- Household and sexual contacts should be examined and treated; pregnant women should be treated only if they show significant symptoms and then should not be given metronidazole or dehydroemetine during the first trimester

NURSING CARE

Nursing Assessment[5,48]

Amebiasis

- Gastrointestinal concerns
  - Nondysenteric colitis: recurring episodes of loose stools; vague abdominal pain; tenesmus; hemorrhoids with occasional rectal bleeding; constipation alternating with diarrhea
  - Dysenteric colitis: intense, intermittent, bloody, mucoid diarrhea
  - Rigid abdomen symptomatic of appendicitis
- Systemic manifestations
  - Signs of dehydration, anemia, or hemorrhage
- Body temperature
  - May have fever and chills
- Skin
  - May have ulceration of perianal area
- Abdomen
  - Enlarged, tender liver (with hepatic abscess)
- Respiratory concerns
  - Expectoration of reddish brown odorless pus suggesting rupture of hepatic abscess to lung

Giardiasis

- Gastrointestinal concerns
  - Acute: explosive, foul-smelling diarrheal stool (frothy appearance with steatorrhea); abdominal cramping and flatulence; nausea (no vomiting)
  - Chronic: intermittent loose stools; increased flatulence and distention; vague abdominal discomfort

Nursing Dx & Intervention

Nursing Diagnosis	Nursing Intervention/Rationale
Diarrhea	• Obtain stool specimen *for examination*. (Specimen obtained within 3 days of a barium enema or of a soapsuds, oil, hypertonic, or water enema cannot be examined.) • Administer amebicide therapy as prescribed. • Observe stool for signs of bleeding *to detect complications*. • Monitor patient *to detect symptoms of perforation, obstruction, or liver disease*.
Potential fluid volume deficit	• Monitor for signs of dehydration. • Encourage oral fluids as tolerated *to prevent dehydration*. • Administer IV line as prescribed. • Measure intake and output and patient's weight *to ensure intake equal to output*.
Potential for poisoning related to chemotherapeutic agent	• Amebicides are toxic. Monitor for symptoms of toxicity to gastrointestinal, cardiovascular, muscular, and neurologic systems.
Activity intolerance	• Enforce restricted activities during amebicide therapy *to decrease additional metabolic demands*.
Potential for infection: patient contacts	• Employ enteric precautions for duration of the infection *to prevent transmission of the pathogen* (see p. 1298).

Patient Education

1. Cyst passers must wash their hands thoroughly after defecating to prevent recontamination or transmission to others.
2. Travelers to areas where the water supply is not chemically treated or protected from sewage contamination should boil all water used in cooking, drinking, or making ice.
3. Relapses after treatment for amebiasis and giardiasis are common. Patient should be monitored by a physician at 6 weeks and 6 months.
4. Household and sexual contacts should seek medical examination and treatment.
5. Patients receiving amebicides should be taught side effects of the drug and the importance of restricting their activities during treatment and of abstaining from alcohol if taking metronidazole (Flagyl).
6. Food supplies should be protected from fly contamination.

Evaluation

Patient Outcome	Data Indicating That Outcome is Reached
There is no infection.	Stool culture is negative for protozoan cysts. There are no signs of hepatic abscesses. There are no skin, vaginal, or lung abscesses or drainage. Body temperature is normal.
Bowel elimination is normal.	Stools are soft, formed, and normal colored. Abdomen is soft and nontender. Liver is normal sized. Bowel sounds are normal.
Body hydration is normal.	Skin turgor is good. Mucous membranes are moist.

Waterborne and foodborne *Salmonella* infections

Salmonellosis is manifested by an acute gastroenteritis and sometimes a septicemia. It is frequently classified as a food poisoning because of the short incubation period following ingestion of food contaminated with *Salmonella*. The greater the number of organisms present in the food, the shorter the incubation period.

Paratyphoid fever is an acute systemic infection manifested by an enteric fever generally of less severity than typhoid fever. Mild and asymptomatic infections occur.

Typhoid fever is an acute enteric fever manifested by a sustained bacteremia, reticuloendothelial involvement, and microabscess formation and ulceration of the distal ileum. Gastrointestinal symptoms generally follow the systemic manifestations. Mild and asymptomatic infections occur. Acute typhoid is less common than other *Salmonella* infection.

Table 13-10
Overview of Waterborne and Foodborne *Salmonella* Infections

	Salmonellosis	Paratyphoid Fever	Typhoid Fever
Occurrence	Worldwide; frequently classified as a food poisoning; small outbreaks in institutions; 2 million cases per year in United States; increasing	Worldwide; sporadic cases and small outbreaks	Worldwide; rare; sporadic cases occur in United States; usually associated with unsanitary conditions
Etiologic agent	2000 serotypes of *Salmonella*, a bacterium	*Salmonella paratyphi* with many serotypes	96 types of *Salmonella typhi* (the typhoid bacillus)
Reservoir	Humans and domestic and wild animals including turtles	Humans	Humans; carriers are common
Transmission	Ingestion of food contaminated with feces from an infected person or animal; ingestion of meat and animal products; handling infected animals; fecal-oral	Ingestion of food, particularly milk contaminated with feces from an infected person or carrier; direct or indirect contact with urine or feces	Ingestion of food or water contaminated with feces or urine from infected person or carrier; sewage-contaminated shellfish; food contaminated with feces carried by flies
Incubation period	6-72 h; usually 12-36 h	1-3 wk	1-3 wk
Period of communicability	Throughout infection; days to weeks; temporary carrier state may continue up to 1 yr	As long as bacilli are in excreta; weeks to months; commonly 1-2 wk after recovery	As long as bacilli are in excreta; first week to 3 months; 2%-5% of cases become permanent carriers
Susceptibility and resistance	General; increased risk for those with achlorhydria, antacid therapy, gastrointestinal surgery, and immunosuppression	General; some immunity follows infection	General; increased risk with gastric achlorhydria; susceptibility usually declines with age; lifelong immunity sometimes follows infection as long as antibiotic therapy was not used
Report to local health authority	Mandatory case report	Mandatory case report	Mandatory case report

Data from Benenson.[5]

Salmonella bacteria multiply in food and water contaminated with feces from an infected person, carrier, or, in the case of salmonellosis, an animal. Person-to-person transmission is least common. Once ingested, the organisms invade and multiply in the gastrointestinal mucosa, producing systemic as well as enteric pathologic findings and symptoms. Four overlapping clinical entities are possible, dependent on the type of *Salmonella* ingested and on host defenses. They are acute gastroenteritis, enteric fever, septicemia with or without localized infection, and asymptomatic carrier state (Table 13-10).

Pathophysiology[5,40,48]

Salmonella organisms ingested in contaminated food or water invade and multiply in deep mucosal layers of the stomach and small intestine, lodging in the lamina propria. An inflammatory response in the tissue with many polymorphonuclear leukocytes produces a gastroenteritis if the *Salmonella* is not *S. typhi* or *S. paratyphi*. The mesenteric lymph nodes become edematous, and the Peyer's patches show edema and superficial ulceration. The disease may be contained here, or the organism may invade beyond the lymph system and be disseminated into the vascular circulation, producing a septicemia or lesions in other organs.

S. typhi and *S. paratyphi* stimulate a mononuclear leukocyte reaction in the lamina propria, facilitating early hematogenous dissemination of the organisms. Disease is manifest as an enteric fever. Invasion of other organs results in lesion formation with disease manifestations dependent on the organ involved. Endocarditis, meningitis, pneumonia, pyelonephritis, osteomyelitis, cholecystitis, and hepatitis may result from the invasion of any type of *Salmonella*.

Complications of gastroenteritis may include intestinal perforation and hemorrhage. Secondary infections such as otitis media, pneumonia, skin infections, and septicemia sometimes occur with all types of *Salmonella*.

A leukocytosis (10,000 to 15,000 WBC/mm^3) is generally

present in the gastroenteritis form of *Salmonella* infections. Leukopenia is present in enteric fevers, although children with typhoid fever sometimes have a leukocytosis.

Thrombocytopenia (50,000 platelets/mm^3) and anemia frequently occur in typhoid fever.

Several nonspecific host defenses affect the type and severity of clinical disease produced by *Salmonella*. Gastric acidity impedes *Salmonella* growth, and persons with hypochlorhydria or achlorhydria or who have had gastric surgery are more susceptible to infection. Normal intestinal peristalsis, intact mucous membranes, and the normal intestinal flora all act to prevent invasion. Anything interfering with these defenses increases the risk for more severe infection.

Cellular and humoral immunity appears also to interfere with invasion of *Salmonella,* and persons with an impaired immune system are more susceptible to systemic disease with *Salmonella*. In addition, systemic focal lesions most commonly appear in those tissues that are damaged or devitalized or in those persons with altered immune systems.

About 2% of acute cases of typhoid fever result in the chronic carrier state (excreting *S. typhi* for 12 months or longer following infection). Subclinical infections or other *Salmonella* disease may also result in the chronic carrier state. Relapse is common in treated and untreated typhoid and paratyphoid fevers.

Diagnostic Studies and Findings[5,48]

Culture of Feces

Positive for *Salmonella* during first week

Culture of Feces and/or Urine

Positive for *S. typhi* or *S. paratyphi* during second week

Culture of Blood

Positive for *S. typhi* or *S. paratyphi* during first week

Serology: Widal Agglutination Test

- Not specific for *Salmonella* organisms and not used for salmonellosis
- Increase in antibody titer to the O antigen after 10 days to 2 weeks
- Titer greater than or equal to 1:160 or fourfold increase to 1:640 by 4 weeks is presumptive
- Initial high antibodies to H antigen suggests past infection
- Gradual increase during acute disease suggests concurrent infection

WBC Count

- Leukocytosis in salmonellosis
- Leukopenia in typhoid and paratyphoid fever

Medical Plan[5,32,40,48]

Medications*

- Anti-infective agents
  - Chloramphenicol (Chloromycetin), 100 mg/kg/d in four divided doses IV or po until defervescence; then 50 mg/kg/d h until a total 14-d course has been completed
  - Ampicillin, 1-2 g IV qid for 2 wk (adults)
  - Ampicillin, 8 g/d po in divided doses for 6 wk for carrier state
  - Trimethoprim-sulfamethoxazole (for organisms resistant to above drugs)
- Corticosteroids
  - Prednisone, 40-50 mg/d for 3 d (adults)
- Large prolonged doses of ampicillin and surgical removal of gallbladder, if it is the site for focal infection, for treatment of carriers

General Management

- IV fluids and electrolytes
- Bed rest
- Hyperalimentation
- Treatment of complications such as perforation and hemorrhage
- Avoidance of antispasmodics, laxatives, and salicylates
- Prevention of carriers from handling food for general consumption
- Typhoid vaccine given in a primary series of two injections, 4 to 6 weeks apart, with boosters in 3 to 5 years; recommended only for those living in or traveling to areas of high endemicity; confers only partial immunity

NURSING CARE

Nursing Assessment[5,40]

Salmonellosis

- Gastrointestinal concerns
  - Acute-onset abdominal pain, diarrhea, nausea, and vomiting persisting for several days
  - Stool is green-brown, slimy, watery, and foul; may contain mucus, pus, or blood
  - Bloody diarrhea more common in children
- Fluids and electrolytes
  - Dehydration may be severe in infants: loss of skin turgor, dry mucous membranes, prostration, circulatory collapse, and death are possible
- Body temperature
  - Low-grade fever to 41° C (105° F); chills; lasting 2 to 7 days

*For typhoid fever and paratyphoid fever (anti-infective agents are not used with salmonellosis unless there is systemic disease).

Neurologic concerns
Vertigo
Skin
May have rose spots on trunk

Typhoid Fever

Gradual onset of symptoms
Body temperature
Stair-step rise in temperature during first week to 40° C (104° F) (slightly lower in morning)
Sustained at 40° C (104° F) for 3 to 4 weeks
Subjective symptoms
Early: headache, malaise, anorexia
Pulse
Slower than expected with fever
Abdomen
Enlarged spleen
Abdominal pain
Distention
Skin
Discrete rose spots that blanch on pressure, on trunk after first week
Secondary skin infections frequently occur
Respiratory concerns
Nonproductive cough
Gastrointestinal concerns
Constipation more common than diarrhea
Acute cholecystitis is a complication
Sensory concerns
May have slight deafness or otitis media
Musculoskeletal concerns
Pain in joints
Urinary tract
Urinary retention
Cardiovascular concerns
Tachycardia, hypotension, and shock if hemorrhage, secondary infection, or septicemia develops
Central nervous system
Delirium to stupor
Personality change
Catatonia
Aphasia

Paratyphoid Fever

Some symptoms of salmonellosis and some of typhoid fever
Body temperature
Acute-onset fever 39° to 40° C (102° to 104° F) spiking to 41° C (105.8° F)
Gastrointestinal concerns
Similar to salmonellosis
Early: nausea and vomiting in children; abdominal pain and diarrhea in adults; abdominal distention; enlarged spleen
Central nervous system
Meningeal symptoms similar to typhoid

Septicemia with Localized Infection

Symptoms depend on site of systemic lesions caused by any of the *Salmonella* organisms
Symptoms of appendicitis, cholecystitis, peritonitis, otitis media, meningitis, pneumonia, osteomyelitis, pyelonephritis, cystitis, and endocarditis (refer to specific chapters for assessment of those conditions)

Septicemia without Localized Infection

Intermittent fever
Chills
Anorexia
Weight loss

Nursing Dx & Intervention

Nursing Diagnosis	Nursing Intervention/Rationale
Potential for infection: patient	• Collect fecal specimens for culture.
Potential for infection: patient contacts	• Employ enteric precautions for duration of diarrhea with salmonellosis *to prevent transmission.* • Employ enteric precautions until three consecutive fecal cultures, after cessation of antibiotic therapy, are negative for *S. typhi* and *S. paratyphi to prevent transmission of pathogen* (see p. 1298).
Salmonellosis	
Diarrhea	• Measure output *so fluids can be replaced equal to output.* • Apply heating pad to abdomen *to help cramping* (antispasmodic agents should be avoided). • Use room deodorizers and adequate ventilation *to remove odors.*
Fluid volume deficit	• Assess *to detect symptoms of dehydration.* • Administer IV fluids and electrolytes as prescribed or clear liquids as tolerated.

Further diagnoses depend on whether bacteremia, septicemia, or systemic focal abscesses are present and where they are located.

Nursing Diagnosis	Nursing Intervention/Rationale
Typhoid Fever and Paratyphoid Fever	
Constipation	• Observe stool *to detect blood.* • Monitor for signs of perforation and hemorrhage *for immediate medical intervention.* • Check for and prevent abdominal distention. • Administer small low enema or glycerin suppositories as ordered (do not give laxatives) to relieve distention.
Altered patterns of urinary elimination	• Monitor for bladder distention. • Measure output *to detect urinary retention.* • Catheterize if necessary *to empty bladder.*
Potential for trauma	• Protect delirious patient from injury with padded headboard and side rails. Supervise closely *to prevent trauma.*
Altered oral mucous membrane	• Assess mucous membranes of mouth. • Provide frequent oral fluids and mouth care *to provide for comfort and to prevent dryness.* • Lubricate lips *to prevent cracking.*
Potential impaired skin integrity	• Provide skin care and frequent position changes *to prevent skin pressure and breakdown.*
Potential fluid volume deficit	• Assess for symptoms of dehydration. • Give oral fluids as tolerated *to maintain adequate intake.* • Administer IV fluids, if prescribed, cautiously *to prevent circulatory overload.*
Activity intolerance	• Maintain bed rest *to reduce metabolic demands.*
Hyperthermia	• Sponge bathe *to reduce temperature* (do not give salicylates because of potential for gastrointestinal hemorrhage).

Patient Education

1. Scrupulous handwashing after defecation and before preparing food is necessary.
2. Carriers must not handle food for consumption by others until six consecutive fecal and urine cultures taken 1 month apart are negative for *S. typhi* and *S. paratyphi*.
3. Family and close contacts should be examined and treated if specimens from them are positive for any *Salmonella* bacilli.
4. All foods of animal origin, including eggs, must be thoroughly cooked; cross contamination of cooked and uncooked foods must be avoided; and foods must be refrigerated below 8° C (46° F) to avoid infection with *Salmonella*.
5. Protect food and water supply from contamination with sewage containing *S. typhi*. Screen food against flies or other mechanical vectors.
6. Frozen meat, particularly poultry, should be defrosted in the refrigerator.
7. All milk should be pasteurized, and water should be chlorinated.
8. Children should be protected from handling pet turtles and should be taught to wash hands after touching any animal.
9. Relapse is common following typhoid and paratyphoid fevers. Recurrence of symptoms should be reported to physician immediately.

Evaluation

Patient Outcome	Data Indicating That Outcome is Reached
There is no infection.	Blood, stool, or urine cultures are negative for *Salmonella*. The patient is mentally alert and oriented and has good concentration. There are no symptoms of complications or secondary infection. There is no pain anywhere. Temperature and pulse are normal.
Laboratory data are normal.	Leukocyte count, hemoglobin, hematocrit, platelets, and blood measurements of sodium, potassium, chloride, magnesium, and calcium are normal.
Bowel elimination is normal for individual.	Stools are soft, formed, and brown. Abdomen is soft and nondistended. There is no abdominal cramping or pain.

Patient Outcome	Data Indicating That Outcome is Reached
Body hydration is normal.	Skin turgor is good. Mucous membranes are moist.
Urinary elimination is normal.	There is no bladder distention. Urine output equals intake.
Digestive function is normal.	Patient eats regular diet and fluids without nausea, vomiting, or abdominal distention.

Intestinal parasitic worm infections

Ancylostomiasis is a chronic debilitating disease manifest as an iron deficiency anemia and hypoproteinemia that result from intestinal blood loss to the hookworm.

Ascariasis, the most common roundworm infection of the small intestine, is a chronic infection producing vague gastrointestinal symptoms and sometimes acute and severe manifestations of infection in other organs, commonly the lung. Bowel obstruction is a potential complication.

Enterobiasis (pinworm) is a mild infection of the cecum and colon producing mild symptoms of anal pruritus.

Strongyloidiasis is a chronic, frequently asymptomatic infection of the duodenum and upper jejunum manifest as a dermatitis in which larvae penetrate the skin, respiratory symptoms caused by migration through the lungs, and gastrointestinal symptoms.

Taeniasis is a mild infection of the small intestine with the adult stage of the large tapeworm. It is manifest as variable gastrointestinal symptoms and loss of weight.

Toxocariasis is a chronic and usually mild infection of young children with systemic and local symptom manifestation depending on the organs and tissues where the nematode has migrated.

Trichinosis is a chronic disease, ranging from asymptomatic to acute, caused by migration of the *Trichinella* larvae to striated muscles where they become encapsulated. Severity of symptoms depends on the number of larvae and the organ system involved.

Trichuriasis is an infection of the cecum and colon resulting in enteritis and potential rectal prolapse.

Helminths, or worms, differ from other agents pathogenic to humans in the following ways: they are large enough to be seen directly; they migrate within the host; their life cycles are more complex; they replicate by means of eggs, which are shed through the feces; and they are capable of producing an eosinophilia. There are three groups of helminths: the nematodes (roundworms), trematodes (flukes), and cestodes (tapeworms). The portal of entry into the host is by ingestion, skin penetration, or injection into the blood by an insect. The portal of entry is not related to group membership.

Trematode (fluke) infections are not commonly found in the United States and therefore are not discussed here. The most common roundworm and tapeworm parasitic enteric infections are discussed (Table 13-11).

Pathophysiology[5,41,48]

The helminths discussed here produce pathologic conditions in the human by one or more of the following ways: feeding on the host's blood, resulting in anemia; feeding on nutrients in the intestinal tract, which deprives the host of those nutrients; growing in numbers or size, which causes blockage in the intestinal tract or ducts in other organs where they have migrated; causing inflammation and necrosis in tissue; or causing an allergic response in tissue with a resulting eosinophilia. The site of their damage depends on their life cycle migratory patterns within the host, which is specific for each type of helminth. The extent of pathologic findings is greatly affected by the number of helminths present in the host. Unless treated, helminths remain for long periods. Reinfection or autoinfection greatly adds to the worm burden in the host, particularly in a host whose defenses are compromised by the presence of the worms, malnutrition, and debilitation.

In both *ancylostomiasis* and *strongyloidiasis* the larvae of the respective hookworm and threadworm, present in the soil, penetrate the host's skin. An erythema and papular vesicular rash appear at the site of the penetration, possibly resulting in a generalized urticaria. The larvae migrate through the blood to the lungs, producing an eosinophilia and transitory respiratory inflammation. From the lungs the larvae migrate to the pharynx and are swallowed to the small intestine. There the hookworms attach and the threadworms burrow in the intestinal mucosa. Localized irritation is manifest as symptoms of burning or colicky abdominal pain and diarrhea. The adult hookworm may remain attached to the intestinal mucosa for as long as 5 years. It ingests 15 ml of the host's blood per worm per day, resulting in weight loss, anemia, and hypoalbuminemia. Eggs from the hookworm pass through the feces as long as the hookworm is attached. The threadworm produces the same pathologic findings as the hookworm, with the additional ability to lay eggs that hatch within the mucosa of the duodenum and upper jejunum. The larvae may be excreted in the feces or may invade the bloodstream directly from the mucosa, reinitiating the life cycle to produce an autoinfection. Septicemia and death may be complications of threadworm infections in immunosuppressed individuals.

In *ascariasis* the eggs of the roundworm are ingested, hatch in the small intestine, penetrate the mucosa, and migrate by way of the blood to the lungs. There they produce inflammation, transitory respiratory symptoms, and an eosinophilia similar to that produced by the hookworm and threadworm. The larvae then penetrate the alveoli and migrate to the pharynx, where they are swallowed to the small intestine. They attach to the mucosa, where they impair digestion and protein absorption. They may also travel to the biliary duct and attach there. The irritating presence of the worms may produce vomiting, abdominal distention, and cramps. Blockage of the biliary duct results in colicky epigastric pain, nausea, and vomiting. Because of the size of these roundworms a large mass may obstruct the bowel lumen.

The roundworms causing *enterobiasis* (pinworm) and *trichuriasis* (whipworm) have simpler life cycles in the human host. Ingested eggs hatch in the small intestine, and larvae migrate directly to the cecum. The tiny gravid female pinworm migrates at night to the perianal area to deposit eggs, which embryonate within 6 hours. Perianal and perineal irritation and pruritus are the only symptoms. Occasionally appendicitis, salpingitis, or ulcerative lesions result from migrating pinworms. Embryonated eggs remain infective on the skin, clothing, and bedclothes for 29 days and may be reingested by the host.

Once in the cecum, the whipworm larvae embed their heads in the mucosa and consume 0.005 ml of blood per worm per day, producing a mild anemia. In 1 to 3 months the adult female worms discharge eggs which are eliminated in the feces.

The roundworms causing *toxocariasis* and *trichinosis* produce more severe systemic pathologic findings because of the ability of the larva to invade and encyst in organs beyond the intestinal tract. In *toxocariasis* eggs from animal feces (particularly puppies) are ingested and hatch in the intestinal tract. The larvae penetrate the intestinal mucosa and migrate through the blood to the eye, skin, liver, lung, kidney, brain, or muscles. The larvae invade those tissues, producing a localized inflammatory reaction and granulomatous nodules. The larvae remain viable in the nodules for years. Systemic manifestations include an eosinophilia ($3000/mm^3$); a leukocytosis ($100{,}000/mm^3$); an increase in IgG, IgM, and IgE antibodies; and an increase in isoagglutinin titers to A and B blood group antibodies. Specific pathologic findings depend on the organ sites of invasion but may include hepatomegaly, an elevated SGOT, respiratory symptoms, blindness and central nervous system manifestations.

In trichinosis the ingested larvae from improperly cooked infected meat attach to the intestinal mucosa within 2 to 3 weeks after infection. The body responds by producing an inflammatory exudate containing polymorphs, eosinophils, lymphocytes, and macrophages. Intestinal symptoms may be present. Each female *Trichinella* releases about 500 larvae over a 2-week period. The adult females are then discharged in the feces. The larvae penetrate into the bloodstream, migrate, and invade striated muscle. There they increase in length 10-fold during a 3-week period. Muscle fibers become edematous, lose their cross-striations, and undergo basophilic degeneration and nuclear proliferation. An acute toxemia results from inflammatory destruction of larvae in the blood. The toxemia subsides when the larvae become encysted in the muscles during the fourth to sixth weeks. Although most infections are subclinical, disease manifestations may be severe, depending on the numbers and sites of invading larvae. Muscles and organs most frequently affected are the intercostal, diaphragm, eye, masseter, neck, pectoral, and limb flexors. Laboratory findings show an eosinophilia and an increase in serum creatinine phosphokinase and lactic dehydrogenase, indicating muscle destruction. Death may result from respiratory failure or pneumonia, myocarditis, or encephalitis caused by the toxemia.

Taeniasis (tapeworm) infections may be local or systemic. If eggs of the pork tapeworm are ingested, they hatch in the intestine, and the larvae penetrate the intestinal mucosa and migrate and form cysts in subcutaneous tissue, striated muscles, or other vital organs. Disease may be severe if larvae localize in the eye, central nervous system, or heart. When larvae from the beef or pork tapeworm are ingested directly, the larvae attach to the intestinal mucosa where they feed and grow. The adult may remain attached for more than 30 years, discharging segments (proglottids) containing eggs into the feces. This form of the disease is less severe than the systemic form.

Diagnostic Studies and Findings[41]

The diagnosis of the parasitic infections where the worm localizes in the intestinal tract is confirmed when eggs or larvae are detected in a fecal specimen or at the anal opening. Toxocariasis and trichinosis are confirmed by biopsy of affected tissue together with the demonstration of elevated serum antibodies.

Ancylostomiasis

- Fecal specimen
  - 1200 hookworm eggs/ml
- Microscopic examination of cultured specimen
  - Positive for larva

Ascariasis

- Fecal specimen
  - Eggs of *Ascaris lumbricoides*

Enterobiasis

- Fecal specimen
  - Adult pinworms
- Transparent adhesive tape to perianal region
  - Eggs can be visualized
  - Five examinations will detect 99% of infections

Strongyloidiasis

- Fecal specimen
  - Motile threadworm larvae; after 24 hours adults may be visualized

Table 13-11
Overview of Intestinal Parasitic Worm Infections

	Strongyloidiasis (Threadworm)	Taeniasis (Tapeworm)	Toxocariasis
Occurrence	Common in warm wet climates; endemic or epidemic where hygiene is poor, particularly in institutions	Particularly high where beef and pork are eaten raw or undercooked; pork tapeworm rare in United States	Worldwide; highest in children 14-40 mo; some infection in adults
Etiologic agent	*Strongyloides stercoralis,* a roundworm (nematode)	*Taenia saginata* (beef tapeworm); *T. solium* (pork tapeworm); cestodes	*Toxocara canis* and *T. cati*, predominantly the former
Reservoir	Humans and dogs	Humans, swine, and cattle	Dogs and cats; almost 100% of newborn puppies are infected
Transmission	Infective larvae in soil penetrate skin, usually the foot, migrate through blood to lungs, migrate up to pharynx, and are swallowed to intestines	Ingestion of inadequately cooked, infected meat; anal-oral transfer from person to person; contaminated food or water with eggs from feces	Direct or indirect transmission of eggs in soil (from animal feces) to mouth
Incubation period	2-3 wk	8-14 wk	Weeks or months
Period of communicability	As long as living worms remain in intestine; up to 35 yr	As long as worm is in intestine; up to 30 yr	Not directly communicable
Susceptibility and resistance	General; no acquired immunity has been demonstrated	General; no resistance follows infection	Adults have lower exposure or decreased susceptibility
Report to local health authority	No	Reportable in some areas	No

Data from Benenson.[5]

Differential white blood cell count
Increase in eosinophils

Trichuriasis

Fecal specimen
Lemon-shaped eggs of whipworm
Sigmoidoscopy
Visualizes adult worms attached to colon wall

Taeniasis

Fecal specimen
Visualizes worm segments (proglottids)

Toxocariasis

Liver biopsy
Toxocara larvae in about 20% of cases
Serology: ELISA
Increase in IgG, IgM, and IgE antibodies

Ancylostomiasis (Hookworm)	Ascariasis (Roundworm)	Enterobiasis (Pinworm)	Trichinosis	Trichuriasis
Endemic in tropic and subtropic areas where disposal of human feces is inadequate	Worldwide and common; in United States, most common in the South; greatest in moist, tropical areas; greatest in children	Worldwide and very high in some areas; most common helminth infection in United States; highest in school- and preschool-aged children and in mothers of infected children	Worldwide in areas where pork is eaten	Common in warm, moist regions
Necator americanus and *Ancylostoma duodenale*, roundworms (nematodes)	*Ascaris lumbricoides*, a common roundworm (nematode)	*Enterobius vermicularis*, roundworm (nematode)	Larvae of *Trichinella spiralis*, an intestinal roundworm (nematode)	*Trichuris trichiura* (human whipworm), a roundworm (nematode)
Humans	Humans	Humans; pinworms of animals not transmitted to humans	Swine, rats, dogs, cats, and many wild animals	Humans
Infective larvae in soil penetrate skin, usually foot, and migrate through blood to intestine; may be ingested directly	Ingestion of infective eggs from soil contaminated with feces	Direct transmission of infective eggs from anus to mouth; indirect transmission through contaminated food, clothing, or dust	Ingestion of inadequately cooked flesh of infected animals	Ingestion of eggs from soil contaminated with human feces
Weeks to months, depending on health status of host	Worms reach maturity 2 mo after ingestion	Life cycle of worms requires 4-6 wk	1-45 d; usually 10-14 d	Indefinite; eggs appear in feces 90 d after ingestion; symptoms may be earlier
Infected persons can excrete larvae for years; larvae remain infective in soil for weeks	As long as mature, fertilized female lives in intestine (10-18 mo); embryonated eggs viable in soil for years	As long as gravid females are depositing eggs on perianal skin; continuous reinfection occurs	Not directly communicable; animal hosts are infective for months	As long as eggs reach the soil, probably years
General; immunity unknown	General	General	General; infection probably results in immunity	General
No	No	No	Mandatory case report	No

Trichinosis

Skeletal muscle biopsy
Trichinella larvae 10 days after exposure
Serology: complement fixation, precipitin, fluorescent antibody
Fourfold increase in antibody titer 2 weeks after infection
Bentonite flocculation
Antibody titer greater than 1:5
Differential WBC count
Increase in eosinophils

Medical Plan[5,41,48]

Medications

Anti-infective agents
Antihelminthic agents are toxic substances and should not be used for small worm burdens

Ancylostomiasis (hookworm)
- Mebendazole (Vermox),* 100 mg bid for 3 d
- Pyrantel pamoate (Antiminth), single oral dose of 11 mg/kg up to total of 1 g/d

Ascariasis (roundworm)
- Mebendazole (Vermox),* 100 mg bid for 3 d
- Piperazine citrate (Antepar), 150 mg/kg initially followed by six doses of 65 mg/kg for 12 h through nasogastric tube for intestinal or biliary obstruction

Enterobiasis (pinworm)
- Mebendazole (Vermox),* 100 mg po one time, or
- Pyrantel pamoate (Antiminth), or
- Pyrvinium pamoate (Povan), or
- Piperazine citrate (Antepar)
- Treatment should be repeated after 2 wk

Strongyloidiasis (threadworm)
- Thiabendazole (Mintezol), 25 mg/kg bid for 2 d, or
- Mebendazole (Vermox),* 100 mg bid for 3 d
- Repeated treatment may be required

Taeniasis (tapeworm)
- Niclosamide (Yomesan), 2 g in one dose (adults)
- Paromycin (Humatin), 1 g q4h min for 4 doses (adults)
- Quinacrine (Atabrine), 800 mg in one dose or 400 mg in two doses; 30 min apart for adults

Toxocariasis
- Diethylcarbamazine (Banocide), 5 mg/kg/d for 2-3 wk
- Thiabendazole (Mintezol), 50 mg/kg/d for 7-10 d (questionable effectiveness; infections recur after treatment)

Trichinosis
- Thiabendazole (Mintezol) (within 24 h of eating infected meat), 25 mg/kg/d for 1 wk
- No treatment available once larvae are in bloodstream and muscle

Trichuriasis
- Mebendazole (Vermox),* 100 mg bid for 3 d po

*Contraindicated during pregnancy.

General Management

- Iron therapy to correct anemias
- Nutritional supplements
- Follow-up examination of stool
- Examination and treatment of contacts

NURSING CARE

Nursing Assessment[41]

Area of Concern	Worm Infection	Assessment
Skin	Ancylostomiasis, strongyloidiasis	Erythematous papular or vesicular eruption at site of invasion (generally soles of feet); may become generalized
	Trichinosis	Petechial rash; periorbital edema
	Toxocariasis	Pallor; nodular skin eruptions
Respiratory concerns	Ancylostomiasis, strongyloidiasis, ascariasis	Transitory cough and irregular respirations (Löffler's syndrome) during migration of larvae
	Trichinosis	During third to sixth week: painful breathing; dysphagia; cough, shortness of breath
	Toxocariasis	Continual cough; rales; rhonchi
Gastrointestinal concerns	Ancylostomiasis, strongyloidiasis	Colicky abdominal pain; diarrhea
	Trichuriasis	Bloody diarrhea; rectal prolapse
	Ascariasis	Vomiting; abdominal distention; cramps; acute abdominal symptoms
	Taeniasis	Mild abdominal discomfort
	Trichinosis	Abdominal discomfort and diarrhea (first week only)
	Toxocariasis	Abdominal pain; hepatomegaly
Musculoskeletal concerns	Trichinosis	Edema and pain in affected muscles, including eye, diaphragm, intercostal, pectoral, masseter, neck, limb flexors, and lumbar muscles
Sensory concerns	Toxocariasis	Strabismus; loss of vision
	Trichinosis	Periorbital edema; subconjunctival, subungual, and retinal hemorrhage; photophobia
Perianal area	Enterobiasis	Pruritus at night; may be localized erythema
Central nervous system	Toxocariasis	Seizures
	Trichinosis	During third to sixth week: symptoms of encephalitis
	Taeniasis (systemic)	Seizures; psychiatric symptoms
Cardiovascular concerns	Trichinosis	Symptoms of myocarditis during fourth to eighth week

Area of Concern	Worm Infection	Assessment
Body temperature	Toxocariasis	Fever throughout infection
	Ancylostomiasis, strongyloidiasis, ascariasis	Fever during migration of larvae through lungs
	Trichinosis	Fever during second week (40° C [104° F]); profuse sweating
Systemic manifestations	Ancylostomiasis, trichuriasis, ascariasis, taeniasis	Anemia; weight loss; impaired growth
	Trichinosis	Weakness and headache persisting for varying periods of time beyond migratory phase of larvae; prostration during acute phase

Nursing Dx & Intervention

Nursing Diagnosis	Nursing Intervention/Rationale
Altered nutrition: less than body requirements related to ancylostomiasis, trichuriasis, ascariasis, taeniasis	• Administer iron and nutritional supplements as prescribed *to replace those absorbed by the parasite*. • Encourage frequent high-protein feedings. (Blood transfusions may be necessary in ancylostomiasis.)
Potential for trauma related to toxocariasis, trichinosis, taeniasis	• Monitor for signs of central nervous system involvement. • Closely supervise these patients *to protect from injury*. • *Protect from injury* during seizures with padded tongue blade, padded headboard, and side rails.
Ineffective breathing pattern related to toxocariasis, trichinosis	• Monitor for signs of pneumonia (see Chapter 2). • Administer oxygen and respiratory assistance if required *to maintain adequate oxygen intake*. • Aid patients to deep breathe *to prevent atelectasis*.
Diarrhea related to ancylostomiasis, strongyloidiasis, trichuriasis, trichinosis, taeniasis	• Monitor diarrhea output *for fluid replacement*. • Collect stool specimen *for laboratory analysis*.
Pain related to ascariasis, trichinosis	• Assess abdomen for bowel sounds, distention, and pain. • Report to physician symptoms of acute abdominal pain and distention that may suggest obstruction *so intervention may be started early*. • Encourage rest *to relieve muscle pain*. • Administer analgesics as prescribed *for pain relief*.
Sensory/perceptual alterations (visual) related to toxocariasis, trichinosis	• Reassure patient that visual symptoms will disappear in 3 months. • Assist patient as needed with mobility *to protect from injury*.
Hyperthermia related to toxocariasis	• Assess body temperature. • Provide tepid sponge baths *to reduce temperature*. • Administer antipyretics as prescribed *to reduce fever*. • Encourage fluids *to compensate for those lost during fever*.

Patient Education

1. Follow-up examination of stools 2 weeks after therapy is necessary in ascariasis, ancylostomiasis, strongyloidiasis, and taeniasis. Monthly examinations for 3 months are necessary for taeniasis.
2. Toxocariasis and strongyloidiasis tend to recur following treatment. Patients should be monitored by a physician.
3. Anemias and protein deficiencies from ancylostomiasis, trichuriasis, ascariasis, and taeniasis may take time to correct. Patients should receive nutrition counseling and be encouraged to take iron and vitamin supplements until deficiencies are corrected.
4. Treatment for enterobiasis should be repeated in 2 weeks following first treatment. Daily machine washing of underwear and bedclothes with hot water is necessary during that time. Thorough handwashing after defecation is also necessary.
5. Family members and close contacts of patients with any of these intestinal parasitic infections should be examined and treated for parasites.

6. Thorough handwashing after defecation is necessary.
7. Treatment of puppies for worms may prevent toxocariasis in humans.
8. Prevent children from eating dirt.
9. Proper cooking of pork to 65.6° C (150° F) is necessary.
10. Home freezing of meat for 3 weeks at −25° C (−13° F) destroys larvae.
11. Employ sewage disposal of contaminated feces. No human feces should be used as fertilizer.
12. Wear shoes in areas where human or animal feces may be on soil.
13. Bury animal feces deep in an area where children do not play.

Evaluation[29]

Patient Outcome	Data Indicating That Outcome is Reached
There is no infection.	Stool specimen is negative for larvae of pinworms or threadworm; negative for eggs of hookworm, ascariasis, and whipworm; negative for tapeworm segments. There is no perianal pruritus. Respiratory patterns are normal without cough, rales, or rhonchi. There is no muscle or abdominal pain. Spleen and liver are not palpable. There are no signs of myocarditis, encephalitis, meningitis, or visual loss. Body temperature is normal.
Bowel elimination is normal.	Abdomen is soft; stools are soft, formed, and normal colored.
All cells receive nutrition.	Energy is at preinfection level. The patient is mentally alert. Growth, development, and weight are normal for person's age. Skin and mucous membranes are warm and moist, with natural color. Skin turgor is good.
Laboratory values are within normal limits.	Leukocyte and eosinophil counts are normal. For toxocariasis and trichinosis, SGOT, CPK, and lactic dehydrogenase levels are normal. For ancylostomiasis, trichuriasis, ascariasis, and taeniasis, hemoglobin, hematocrit, and erythrocyte levels are normal.

Viral hepatitis

Viral hepatitis is an inflammatory primary infection of the liver with at least three distinct clinical forms, each caused by a different hepatitis virus.

Depending on the etiologic agent, the diseases differ in their transmission and in their immunologic, pathologic, and clinical characteristics. Treatment is similar for each disease, but prevention and control vary greatly. Hepatitis may also occur as a secondary infection during the course of diseases caused by the cytomegalovirus, Epstein-Barr virus, herpes simplex virus, varicella-zoster virus, coxsackie B virus, and rubella virus (Table 13-12).

Pathophysiology[17,40,41,48]

Although the etiologic agents, mode of transmission, and course of the disease vary with each type of hepatitis, the pathologic condition produced in the liver is the same with all types. The similarities in pathologic findings for each type are presented first, followed by the variations.

The hepatitis virus, regardless of its mode of transmission, invades, replicates, and produces damage only in the liver. Inflammation and mononuclear cell infiltration in the parenchyma and portal ducts, hepatic cell necrosis, proliferation of Kupffer cells, cellular collapse, and accumulation of necrotic debris in the lobules and portal ducts all act to produce architectural changes in the lobules and portal ducts. The result is disturbance in bilirubin excretion.

Cellular regeneration and mitosis are usually concurrent with hepatocyte necrosis; complete regeneration usually occurs within 2 to 3 months. Failure of the liver cells to regenerate while the necrotic process progresses results in a severe, fulminant, frequently fatal hepatitis. This occurs more often in hepatitis B. Continuation of the inflammatory response and necrosis, also more common in types B and non-A, non-B, results in active chronic or persistent chronic hepatitis. In active chronic hepatitis the necrotic process, fibrosis, and architectural destruction continue throughout the hepatic lobes and portal ducts. In persistent chronic hepatitis the inflammatory process is limited to the portal tracts with little or no evidence of hepatocellular necrosis. There is a great deal of variability in clinical manifestations of hepatitis. All types of hepatitis may be present with or without icterus and may have a clinical severity ranging from subclinical infection to acute fulminating disease. Only hepatitis A does not lead to chronic disease or the chronic carrier state. All types stimulate an antibody response specific to the type of virus causing the disease.

Hepatitis A virus (HAV) is acquired by ingestion of the HAV in food, water, or uncooked shellfish contaminated with feces containing the virus or by direct fecal-oral transmission. The virus localizes in the liver, replicates, enters the bile, and

Table 13-12
Overview of Viral Hepatitis

	Hepatitis A	Hepatitis B	Non-A, Non-B Hepatitis
Occurrence	Worldwide; sporadic and epidemic, with a tendency toward cyclic recurrence; outbreaks in institutions	Worldwide; endemic; highest in homosexual men, parenteral drug abusers, and health care workers	An epidemic form similar to hepatitis A; a posttransfusion form similar to hepatitis B
Etiologic agent	Hepatitis A virus (HAV)	Hepatitis B virus (HBV) Delta agent may coinfect with HBV	More than one viral agent distinct from HAV and HBV (NANB)
Reservoir	Humans and captive primates	Humans and possibly captive primates	Probably similar to hepatitis A and hepatitis B
Transmission	Person to person by fecal-oral route; contaminated food, water, shellfish	Direct and indirect contact with blood, saliva, and semen; sexual contact; perinatal	Same as hepatitis A and hepatitis B
Incubation period	15-50 d; average: 28-30 d	45-180 d; average: 60-90 d	Hepatitis A form: 26-42 d; hepatitis B form: same as hepatitis B
Period of communicability	Latter half of incubation period to 1 wk after onset of jaundice	During incubation period and throughout clinical course of disease; carrier state may persist for years	Unknown
Susceptibility and resistance	Usually affects children and young adults; immunity after infection probably lasts for life; 45% of population has hepatitis A antibodies	All age groups; disease is mild in children; lifetime immunity follows infection	All age groups; degree of immunity following infection is unknown; pregnant women have highest fatality in hepatitis A form
Report to local health authority	Mandatory case report	Mandatory case report	Mandatory case report

Data from Benenson[5] and Mandell.[41]

is carried to the intestinal tract where it is shed in the feces. Fecal shedding occurs late in the incubation period, usually before onset of clinical symptoms. Antibodies develop during acute disease and later during convalescence.

Hepatitis B virus (HBV) is viable in blood and in secretions containing serum (oozing cutaneous lesions) or derived from serum (saliva, semen, vaginal secretions). Transmission may be by one of five routes: direct percutaneous inoculation of infective serum or plasma by needle or transfusion of infective blood or blood products; indirect percutaneous introduction of infective serum or plasma, such as through minute skin cuts or abrasions; absorption of infective serum or plasma through mucosal surfaces, such as those of the mouth or eye; absorption of other potentially infective secretions such as saliva or semen through mucosal surfaces, as might occur following sexual (heterosexual or homosexual) contact; and transfer of infective serum or plasma via inanimate environmental surfaces or possibly vectors. Fecal transmission of HBV does not occur. HBV may be transmitted transplacentally, or the infant may become contaminated with the mother's infective blood at birth.

A viral-like particle called the delta agent has recently been identified. This agent is pathogenic only with HBV, causing coinfection with the HBV or superimposing infection on an inapparent HBV carrier state. Prolongation or an increase in severity of an HBV infection may be due to the delta agent.

Several complex antigen-antibody systems have been identified with the HBV. These will be described subsequently in this section. HBV antigens infect the blood within 30 to 60 days of exposure to HBV and are at their peak before disease onset. They persist for varying lengths of time, and their presence is useful for determining the course of the disease and the carrier state. Antibodies specific for the antigens develop at different times during convalescence. Detection of serum antibodies is useful for predicting the course of the disease and for determining immune status.

Non-A, non-B hepatitis represents more than one clinical disease for which the etiologic agents have not been identified. An epidemic form of the disease appears to be similar to hepatitis A with fecal-oral transmission, shorter incubation period, acute onset, and complete recovery. Another form is similar to hepatitis B with percutaneous transmission, potentially prolonged incubation period, less acute onset, and a great probability of chronicity. It is the most common form

Table 13-13
Standard Nomenclature, Abbreviations, and Characteristics of Hepatitis

Abbreviation	Term	Characteristics and Implications
HAV	Hepatitis A virus	Etiologic agent with one serotype
Anti-HAV	Antibody to HAV	Detectable at onset of symptoms and persists for lifetime; probably confers lifetime immunity
IgM	Immunoglobulin M (antibody to HAV)	The anti-HAV is present early in the infection; it represents current infection and is used to establish the diagnosis; serum levels drop during convalescence and disappear in 4-6 mo
IgG	Immunoglobulin G (antibody to HAV)	The anti-HAV that develops late in the infection and persists for years; its presence in serum indicates past infection and present immunity
HBV	Hepatitis B virus	Etiologic agent of hepatitis B; also called Dane particle
HBsAg	Hepatitis B surface antigen	Previously known as Australian antigen; large quantities detectable in serum 2-7 wk before and during acute clinical disease, during chronic disease, and in carriers; its presence indicates infectious blood
HBeAg	Hepatitis Be antigen	Soluble antigen that correlates with HBV replication; indicates a high titer of HBV in serum and consequent infectivity of serum; it rises 2-7 wk before clinical disease onset and usually drops before acute disease; its persistence is associated with progression to chronic hepatitis; found only in HBsAg-positive serum
HBcAg	Hepatitis B core antigen	Found in liver cells; cannot be detected in sera with present technology
Anti-HBs	Antibody to HBsAG	Rises in serum during convalescence; its presence indicates immunity to HBV from past infection, passive antibody from HBIG, or active immune response from HBV vaccine
Anti-HBe	Antibody to HBeAg	Its presence in serum of person with continuing levels of HBeAg suggests chronic presence of HBV and infectivity of blood
Anti-HBc	Antibody to HBcAg	Increases during clinical disease, peaks during convalescence, and persists for years; presence indicates past infection with HBV
IGM anti-HBc	IGM antibody to HBcAg	Indicates recent infection with HBV; positive for 4-6 mo after infection
IG	Immunoglobulin	Formerly called immune serum globulin (ISG) or gamma globulin; given before and within 2 wk after exposure to HAV and NANB
HBIG	Hepatitis B immune globulin	Contains a higher titer of HB immune globulins than does IG; preferred for use after exposure to HBV
HB vaccine	Hepatitis B vaccine	Inactivated vaccine prepared from carriers of HBsAg; stimulates production of anti-HBs; series of three injections recommended for those at risk for hepatitis B
NANB	Non-A, non-B hepatitis	Diagnosis by exclusion of HAV and HBV
δ virus	Delta virus	Etiologic agent of delta hepatitis; may only cause infection in presence of HBV
δ-Ag	Delta antigen	Detectable in early, acute delta infections
Anti-δ	Antibody to delta antigen	Indicates past or present infection with delta antigen

Data from Centers for Disease Control[17,25] and Mandell.[41]

of posttransfusion hepatitis, possibly because serologic screening for hepatitis B in potential donors has decreased this mode of transmission for hepatitis B.

The identification of serologic markers for type-specific virus antigens and antibodies has been important in the diagnosis, prevention, and control of viral hepatitis. The standard nomenclature and abbreviation with characteristics and implications are presented here for easy reference (Table 13-13).

Diagnostic Studies and Findings[17,40,41,48]

Serum Enzymes

Asparate aminotransferase (AST, SGOT) and alanine aminotransferase (ALT, SGPT)
- At least eight times normal during clinical disease
- Indicators of liver damage
- Peak at onset of jaundice and fall during recovery
- May be 20 to 50 times normal for hepatitis B and 10

to 20 times normal for non-A, non-B hepatitis, persisting at two to five times normal for months

Alkaline phosphatase

One to three times normal

Lactic dehydrogenase (LDH)

One to three times normal

Creatine phosphokinase (CPK)

Normal

Serum Bilirubin

Elevated: measures extent of liver dysfunction

Ratio of direct to indirect fraction—1:1

Prothrombin Time

Normal

Elevated only in severe fulminating hepatitis

VDRL

False positive

Hepatitis A

Stool specimen: immune electron microscopy, radioimmunoassay, or enzyme immunoassay

Positive for HAV 2 to 4 weeks after exposure, remains until onset of clinical disease, then is negative

HAV may be absent from stool by time patient is hospitalized

Serology: radioimmunoassay or ELISA test

Fourfold rise in anti-HAV antibodies between early disease and convalescence

Identification of IgM antibodies during early disease indicates present infection; peak at 3 mo and then drop

IgG peaks after clinical disease and persists for life; high levels indicate past infection and present immunity

Hepatitis B

Serum antigen tests: radioimmunoassay, enzyme immunoassay

HBeAg and HBsAg in serum 1 to 2 weeks after exposure and 2 to 7 weeks before onset of clinical disease; peak and begin to drop during clinical disease

HBsAg remains in serum of chronic carriers for life; positive tests indicate present infection or carrier state

Positive test in carrier with disease symptoms may misdiagnose infection with HAV or NANB

Serum antibody tests: radioimmunoassay

Anti-HBe increases during clinical disease and peaks during convalescence; anti-HBe begins rising during convalescence; both persist and gradually decrease over time; anti-HBs rises rapidly during late convalescence and persists

Carriers are always HBeAg positive and/or HBsAg positive and anti-HBs negative

For screening purposes: anti-HBs greater than 10 RIA sample ratio units indicates immunity

Non-A, Non-B Hepatitis

If above tests are negative in patient with clinical symptoms of viral hepatitis, non-A, non-B is suspected; no serologic test is currently available

Medical Plan[17,40,41,48]

Medications

There is no direct chemotherapeutic treatment for viral hepatitis (there is no evidence that corticosteroids are helpful)

Supportive medications may be used for fulminating hepatitis:

Anti-infective agents

Neomycin (Mycifadrin), 1-1.5 g po q6h until loose stools are achieved

Histamine-receptor antagonist

Cimetidine (Tagamet), 300-500 mg IV q6h or vigorous antacid therapy for gastrointestinal bleeding

Preventive medications may be used for less than 2 mo for preexposure prophylaxis against hepatitis A (HAV) for those traveling to high-risk areas outside tourist routes

Immunologic agent

Immune globulin (IG), 0.02 ml/kg in a single dose IM

For prolonged travel

Immunologic agent

Immune globulin (IG), 0.06 ml/kg IM in a single dose q5 mo

Postexposure prophylaxis within 2 wk of close personal contact with hepatitis A–infected person in the home, day-care center, institution for custodial care, or hospital

Immunologic agent

Immune globulin (IG), 0.02 ml/kg in a single dose IM

Preexposure prophylaxis against hepatitis B (HBV) for high-risk groups (health care workers in contact with blood or blood products, clients and staff of institutions for the mentally retarded, hemodialysis patients, homosexual males, illicit injectable drug users, patients with clotting disorders who receive factor VII or IX concentrates, household and sexual contacts of HBV carriers, classroom contacts of deinstitutionalized mentally retarded carriers, and inmates of long-term correctional facilities)

Prevaccination serologic screening to identify HBV carriers and those already immune; one anti-HBc test will identify both; anti-HBs test will identify those immune but will not identify carriers.

Hepatitis B vaccine (Heptavax-B)

Vaccinate those with negative anti-HBe or negative anti-HBs tests

Three doses of 1 ml vaccine (20 μg/ml) IM at 0, 1, and 6 mo
Hemodialysis patients: three doses of 2 ml vaccine (40 μg) IM at 0, 1, and 6 mo
New HB vaccine (Recombivax HB)
Immunogenicity is comparable to Heptavax)
Three doses (10 μg per dose) 1 ml IM at 0, 1, and 6 mo
Hemodialysis patients: three doses of 2 ml (40 μg) IM at 0, 1, and 6 mo
Do not accept blood from HBsAg-positive donors
Postexposure prophylaxis
Household contacts of patients with acute hepatitis B; health workers who receive needle sticks from HBsAg-positive patients
Hepatitis B immune globulin (HBIG), 0.06 ml/kg IM or 5 ml for adults within 24 hr of exposure (repeat in 1 mo if hepatitis B vaccine is not given at time of exposure) *plus*
Hepatitis B vaccine (Heptavax B, Recombivax HB), 1 ml IM at same time as HBIG in another site (or within 7 d); repeat 1 mo and 6 mo after initial dose
Immune globulin in same dose and schedule if HBIG B unavailable
Sexual contacts should receive HBIG, 0.06 ml/kg IM or 5 ml for adults within 14 d of sexual contact

General Management

For nonfulminating hepatitis
Hospitalization for those with bilirubin concentrations greater than 10 mg/dl or greater than 10 times normal and for those with a prolonged prothrombin time
Bed rest until symptoms subside.
Diet as tolerated: small, frequent, low-fat, high-carbohydrate feedings may be better tolerated.
Symptomatic treatment for nausea (avoid chlorpromazine)
Symptomatic treatment for pain (acetaminophen preferred over aspirin)
All unnecessary medications, particularly sedatives, to be avoided
For fulminating hepatitis
Hospitalization and bed rest
Low-protein diet: 20 to 30 mg protein/day
Enemas
Discontinue any sedatives
IV fluids and electrolytes
Central venous pressure line
Nasogastric tube feedings
Urinary catheter
Fresh frozen plasma to correct coagulation defects

NURSING CARE

Nursing Assessment[40,41]

Preicteric Phase (3 to 10 Days)

Onset
Acute for hepatitis A
Insidious for hepatitis B and non-A, non-B
Subjective symptoms
Malaise, weakness, dull headache, anorexia, intermittent nausea and vomiting, myalgias, chills
Right, upper quadrant abdominal pain
Body temperature
38° to 40° C (100° to 104° F) for hepatitis A
Low-grade fever or normal for hepatitis B and non-A, non-B
Skin
For hepatitis B and non-A, non-B
Urticarial pruritic hives, maculopapular lesions, or fleeting, irregular patches of erythema in some patients
Multiple forearm needle pricks in drug users
Exacerbation of acne
Excoriations with severe pruritus
Musculoskeletal concerns
For hepatitis B and non-A, non-B: mild to moderate, nondeforming polyarticular arthritis: migratory, affecting elbows, wrists, knees, and small joints of hands
Abdomen
Bowel sounds normal
Slightly enlarged, tender liver (9 to 13 cm)
Edges smooth, regular, and firm

Icteric Phase (Bilirubin Greater Than 2.5 mg/dl; Lasts 1 to 3 Weeks)

Skin
Jaundice with or without pruritus may be present or absent; can be observed under the tongue
Eyes
Scleral icterus
Urine
Dark
Stools
May be clay colored
Vital signs
Normal, although there may be a bradycardia with severe hyperbilirubinemia
Subjective symptoms
Nausea and vomiting frequently abate and appetite returns, but symptoms may worsen
Malaise continues
Temperature
Normal or low grade

Complications: Fulminant Hepatitis with Encephalopathy

Level of consciousness
- Patient becomes lethargic and somnolent with personality changes; may show mild confusion, sexual or aggressive activity, loss of usual inhibitions
- Lethargy may alternate with excitability, euphoria, or unruly behavior
- Worsening of the condition leads to stupor and eventual coma
- An early sign is asterixis (the irregular flapping of forcibly dorsiflexed, outstretched hands)

Circulatory system
- Prothrombin time is prolonged: abdominal bleeding; epistaxis; prolonged bleeding from puncture sites; blood in vomitus, stool, or urine; easy bruising

Nursing Dx & Intervention

Nursing Diagnosis	Nursing Intervention/Rationale
Potential fluid volume deficit	• Provide frequent high-carbohydrate fluids as tolerated during acute symptoms. • Administer IV fluids for patients with persistent vomiting or for those with hepatic encephalopathy, as ordered.
Altered nutrition: less than body requirements	• Encourage frequent small feedings as patient tolerates. • Administer nasogastric tube feedings for patients with hepatic encephalopathy and coma.
Activity intolerance	• Maintain bed rest during acute symptoms. (Patients need not be limited in their activity during convalescence.)
Knowledge deficit regarding disease transmission and potential chronicity	• Educate patient about disease and disease transmission. • Emphasize the self-limited nature of most hepatitis but the need for follow-up of liver function tests and serum HBsAg. • Explain precautions.
Potential for infection: patient, patient contacts	• Collect fecal or blood specimens as required. • Employ enteric precautions for 7 days after onset of jaundice for hepatitis A (see p. 1298). • Employ blood and body fluid precautions until patient is HBsAg serum negative for hepatitis B and for the duration of illness for non-A, non-B *to prevent transmission to others* (see p. 1299). • Ensure that all patient contacts, including health care personnel, are protected against hepatitis.
Patient problem: hemorrhage	• Monitor and report signs of gastrointestinal bleeding. • Provide care as warranted by bleeding (see Chapter 8).
Patient problem: encephalopathy	• Monitor and report signs of encephalopathy as were described under "Nursing Assessment." • Monitor and report progression of icterus. • Provide care as warranted by level of consciousness of patient.

Patient Education[41]

1. Follow-up serology in 1 or 2 months is necessary for all hepatitis B patients to determine the presence or absence of HBsAg.
2. Patients should follow precautions with blood and secretions until they are determined to be free of HBsAg. Close personal contacts should be examined and receive HBIG or HB vaccine.
3. HBV carriers should be aware that their blood and secretions are infectious. Close contacts of HBV carriers should receive HB vaccine. Carriers should not share razors or toothbrushes and must be cautious in handling cuts and lacerations. HBV carriers and patients with a history of NANB should not donate blood.
4. Patients caring for themselves at home during the acute stage of the disease should avoid alcohol and any nonprescribed medications, particularly sedatives and aspirin.
5. Severity of symptoms can determine patterns for bed rest and diet. Frequent, small feedings of low-fat, high-carbohydrate foods may be better tolerated, but it is not necessary to limit the diet in any way.
6. Liver function tests should be monitored until normal.
7. Hepatitis A patients must wash hands thoroughly following toileting, must disinfect articles soiled with feces (boil 1 minute), and must not prepare foods for others during symptomatic disease. They should avoid sharing eating utensils, toothbrushes, toys, etc.
8. Sexual activity should be avoided during acute stage of hepatitis B and non-A, non-B. Ideally hepatitis B patients should not resume sexual activity until tests for HBsAg are negative or until partner has received HB vaccine or HBIG if HB vaccine is unavailable.

Evaluation

Patient Outcome	Data Indicating That Outcome is Reached
There is no infection.	Serum HBsAg and HBeAg tests are negative. Close, personal contacts of hepatitis B patients have received HBIG or HB vaccine.
Liver function is normal.	There is no icterus. Patient has full appetite, energy, and no right upper quadrant abdominal pain. Urine and stool are normal colored. There are no changes in personality or level of consciousness.
Liver function tests are normal.	SGPT (ALT), SGOT (AST), alkaline phosphatase, LDH, serum bilirubin, and prothrombin time are all within normal limits.
Patient is knowledgeable about need for follow-up, means of preventing transmission to others, and convalescent self-care.	Items listed in "Patient Education" are met.

INFECTIOUS DISEASES OF THE HEMATOLYMPHATIC SYSTEM

The infectious diseases grouped here produce either primary pathologic findings in the lymphatic system or disseminated infection with lymphadenopathy as part of the clinical picture. Two of the diseases can be transmitted transplacentally with serious consequences to the fetus (Table 13-14).

Mononucleosis

Mononucleosis is an acute viral infectious disease producing a generalized lymph node hyperplasia and characterized by fever, exudative pharyngitis, lymphadenopathy, and splenomegaly.

Pathophysiology[41]

The Epstein-Barr virus (EBV) is transmitted in saliva by prolonged direct contact, probably through kissing with salivary exchange. The pathogen invades B lymphocytes in lymphatic tissue and stimulates the development of a surface membrane antigen on the infected lymphocytes. T lymphocytes actively proliferate in response to the antigen and produce a generalized lymph node hyperplasia. Atypical T lymphocytes infiltrate the spleen, tonsils, lungs, heart, liver, kidneys, adrenal glands, central nervous system, and skin. The circulating T cells are not infective and therefore do not produce necrosis in these systems. Their infiltration causes enlargement, particularly of the spleen, and disturbs functioning of those organs.

The severity of the disease varies from asymptomatic disease (usually in children) to severe systemic and localized organ involvement. Lymphadenopathy, splenomegaly, and exudative pharyngitis are characteristic. More serious manifestations of the disease include hepatitis, pneumonitis, and central nervous system involvement. Rare but serious complications include splenic rupture, hematologic complications (hemolytic anemia, agranulocytosis, thrombocytopenic purpura), pericarditis, and orchitis.

Saliva remains infective for 18 months despite the development of EBV-specific antibodies early in the disease. The virus can be cultured from the throats of 10% to 20% of normal, healthy adults, suggesting that the disease may be contracted from asymptomatic viral shedders.

Diagnostic Studies and Findings[40,41,48]

Differential White Blood Count

Lymphocytes and monocytes greater than 50% with more than 10% being atypical lymphocytes

Leukocyte Count

Normal early in disease; rises to 12,000 to 20,000/mm^3 in second week; occasionally rises to 50,000/mm^3

Serology: Heterophil Agglutination Antibody Tests

Rapid forms of this test are Monospot, Monoscreen, and Monotest, all commercially prepared kits

Heterophil antibody titer greater than 1:40 to 1:128 (depending on the laboratory), usually by the end of the first week; usually disappears by the fourth week, although disappearance may be delayed

May be false negative reactions to this test

If the heterophil antibody test is negative but there is strong clinical evidence for mononucleosis, the following EBV-specific antibody tests may be performed (both IgM antibodies and IgG antibodies are present early in the disease):

EBV-Specific Antibody Tests: Immunofluorescence

Elevated EBV–IgM antibody titers of 1:80 to 1:160; may be false positive reactions; titers drop rapidly after clinical disease

Elevated EBV–IgG antibody: 1:80 is suggestive; persists for life; titer greater than 1:5 suggests immunity

Table 13-14
Overview of Infectious Diseases of the Hematolymphatic System

	Mononucleosis	Cytomegalovirus Infections	Toxoplasmosis	Brucellosis
Occurrence	Worldwide; highest in adolescents and young adults in developed countries; asymptomatic infection in children	Worldwide; many asymptomatic infections; congenital infection may be severe	Worldwide; common in humans, mammals, and birds; many asymptomatic infections; congenital infection may be severe	Worldwide; an occupational disease of those working with infected animals; about 170 cases per year in United States
Etiologic agent	Epstein-Barr virus (EBV), one of the herpesviruses	Cytomegalovirus, one of the herpesviruses	*Toxoplasma gondii,* a protozoan	*Brucella abortus, B. canis, B. melitensis, B. suis*
Reservoir	Humans and possibly primates	Humans	Cats; other mammals and birds are intermediate hosts	Cattle, swine, sheep, horses, and dogs
Transmission	Direct contact with saliva; through blood transfusions	Direct contact with secretions and excretions; through blood transfusions, breast milk, and cervical secretions, and transplacentally	Transplacental if mother has active infection; eating infected meat; water contaminated with cat feces	Contact with blood, tissues, urine, or vaginal discharges of infected animals; ingestion of raw milk from infected animals
Incubation period	4-6 wk	Unknown; 3-8 wk following transfusion; in neonate, 3-12 wk following delivery-produced infection	Unknown; probably between 5-23 d	Variable; 5-30 d
Period of communicability	Prolonged; pharyngeal excretion may persist for years; 15%-20% of adults are carriers	Virus excreted in saliva and urine for months to years	Not directly transmitted except transplacentally; cysts in infected meat remain infective as long as meat is edible and uncooked	Not communicable person to person
Susceptibility and resistance	General; infection confers a high degree of resistance	General; fetuses, immunosuppressed individuals, and those with other chronic disease have more severe symptoms	General, but risk for infection increases with age; immunity after infection persists indefinitely	Children have less severe symptoms; duration of immunity unknown
Report to local health authority	No	No	In some states	Mandatory case report

Data from Benenson.[5]

Liver Function Tests

Serum transaminases (AST [SGOT], ALT [SGPT])
All elevated in hepatic involvement, two to three times upper normal limits
Bilirubin
Elevated if there is hepatic involvement

Throat Culture

Positive for group A hemolytic streptococci in 10% of patients; EBV may be cultured from oropharyngeal secretions; cultures are not routinely available

Platelet Count (in Complications)

Less than 140,000/mm^3 occurs frequently
Less than 1000/mm^3 in severe complications

Medical Plan[40,48]

Surgery

For splenic rupture: surgical removal of the spleen

Medications

Corticosteroids

Prednisone (Deltasone, others), 30 mg/d in divided doses, decreasing for 5 d, for severe neurologic complications, airway obstruction, thrombocytopenic purpura, or hemolytic anemia

General Management

Bed rest during acute stage
Saline throat gargle
Aspirin or acetaminophen for sore throat and fever

NURSING CARE

Nursing Assessment[48]

Prodromal Symptoms

Fatigue
Anorexia
Chilliness
Retro-orbital headache

Body Temperature

Marked elevation, sometimes persisting for 1 to 2 weeks
38° to 41° C (101° to 105° F)
Peaks in afternoon

Head

Photophobia with headache
Periorbital edema

Throat

Painful, exudative tonsillitis
Exudate either white, pasty, and discrete or greenish gray membrane with a bad odor
Inflammation and tonsillar edema may be extreme
Dysphagia

Oral Cavity

Bleeding gums
Palatine petechiae

Lymph Nodes

Cervical adenopathy of posterior cervical chain and anterior cervical, submandibular, and axillary nodes
Nodes are discrete and slightly tender

Abdomen

Splenomegaly
Tenderness of liver

Skin

Jaundice in 5% of patients
Measleslike rash in 5% of patients
Purpura in complicated disease

Respiratory Complications

Symptoms of pneumonia

Neurologic Complications

Symptoms of meningitis or encephalitis

Subjective Symptoms

Fatigue, often becoming chronic

Nursing Dx & Intervention

Nursing Diagnosis	Nursing Intervention/Rationale
Activity intolerance	• Encourage bed rest during acute symptomatic disease *to conserve energy.*
Pain	• Administer analgesics per order or saline gargle for sore throat *to relieve pain.*
Anxiety	• Assist patient in developing a realistic plan for returning to work or school during convalescence *to reduce anxiety.* (The prolonged malaise accompanying this disease may produce anxiety in the patient, particularly college students.)
Patient problem: potential for ruptured spleen	• Monitor for signs of neurologic or purpuric complications *to detect splenic rupture.* • Protect patient from activity *that may risk splenic rupture.*
Hyperthermia	• Monitor body temperature *to detect fever.* • Administer antipyretics. • Bathe with tepid water or alcohol *to reduce high fever.* • Encourage adequate fluid intake *to compensate for increased demands associated with elevated body temperature.*

Patient Education

1. Although complete bed rest is usually unnecessary during acute disease or convalescence, the patient caring for himself at home should be encouraged to rest as symptoms dictate. Convalescence may be as long as 3 to 4 weeks.

2. The patient with splenomegaly should avoid heavy lifting, contact sports, or any activity that may increase the risk of injury to the spleen. Active children must be protected from injury.
3. Report to physician any jaundice, excess bruising or bleeding, or symptoms of abnormal central nervous system functioning.

Evaluation

Patient Outcome	Data Indicating That Outcome is Reached
There is no infection.	Cervical lymph nodes are nonpalpable and nontender. Throat and tonsils are normal colored and not swollen. There is no exudate on tonsils. Patient swallows without pain. Body temperature is normal.
Laboratory findings are within normal limits.	Leukocyte, lymphocyte, and platelet counts, bilirubin level, and serum transaminase (SGOT; SGPT) levels are normal.

Cytomegalovirus infections

Cytomegalovirus infections are extremely common viral infections that are ordinarily asymptomatic. Clinical disease in the adult resembles mononucleosis. Congenital and perinatal acquired infections are serious in the neonate and lead to irreversible central nervous system damage.

Pathophysiology[40,41,48]

The cytomegalovirus (CMV), with several antigenically related strains, is a member of the herpesvirus group and has characteristics common to other herpesviruses. Like the Epstein-Barr herpesvirus, CMV produces a frequently asymptomatic mononucleosis-type infection in children and adults. CMV is similar to herpes types 1 and 2 in that it remains latent in body tissue and has the potential for producing recurrent infection. CMV, like herpes 1 and 2, also crosses the placental barrier and is shed in cervical secretions. Therefore it has the potential for producing congenital infection with severe congenital anomalies and perinatal infection acquired during vaginal delivery. Like herpes 2, the CMV is suspected of having oncogenic properties.

CMV can be found in all body secretions including saliva, blood, urine, semen, cervical secretions, and breast milk, even in the presence of CMV-specific antibodies. Transmission requires prolonged direct contact with secretions. Although the exact mechanism for postnatal transmission is not known, sexual, oral, and blood transfusion transmission is suspected in postnatal acquired infections.

Regardless of the mode of transmission, CMV may invade the cells of most tissues in the body. An inflammatory response with focal tissue destruction, areas of calcification, and hyperplasia of the reticuloendothelial system develops. Typical cellular lesions are characterized by enlarged cells containing intranuclear and cytoplasmic inclusion bodies. These lesions are disseminated widely, particularly in the brain, liver, lungs, kidney, and spleen.

A humoral and cell-mediated anti-CMV antibody response occurs. The response does not appear to alter the course of the spread of the virus from cell to cell or alter the presence of the virus in body secretions. Nor do circulating maternal antibodies in the fetus appear to impede the infectious process or the development of congenital anomalies.

Dependent on the mode of transmission, three different forms of the infection have been identified: congenital, perinatal, and postnatal acquired. All three forms can either be asymptomatic or occur as a mild or severe clinical disease.

Congenital CMV infection is acquired by transplacental transmission, usually resulting from a primary infection the mother acquired during pregnancy. Of infants with congenital infections, 95% are asymptomatic at birth. Maternal antibodies are present in cord blood at birth and the virus can be detected in the infant's urine until age 15 months. In utero viral invasion is most destructive to the developing fetal central nervous system, particularly the cerebellum and cerebral cortex. Neurologic defects such as microcephaly, psychomotor retardation, and severe mental retardation result. The infant born with symptomatic CMV infection also has evidence of a severe generalized infection plus symptoms of organ involvement of the liver, lung, kidney, or eye. This extraneural organ involvement is usually self-limited. If the child lives, there are invariably neurologic sequelae. Congenital CMV infections need to be differentiated diagnostically from toxoplasmosis, rubella, herpes, hemolytic anemias, and bacterial sepsis.

Perinatal infection is acquired at delivery from a serologic-positive mother who had either a primary infection during pregnancy or a reactivation of a latent infection. Cervical secretions of CMV are high during the last trimester, having increased as the pregnancy progressed. Perinatally infected infants develop signs of infection (virus in urine and an antibody response with or without clinical evidence of organ involvement) 4 to 8 weeks following birth. The long-term effects on neurologic development are unknown.

Postnatal acquired infection requires close contact with body secretions containing the virus, usually from an asymptomatic person. Blood transfusions and renal and bone marrow transplants (possibly because of immunosuppression) have been linked with CMV transmission. Sexual transmission and kissing are also suspected as modes of transmission. The disease may be asymptomatic, or there may be symptoms of liver and lung involvement or a mononucleosis-like syndrome. There is no evidence of chronic organ impairment in acquired CMV infections. Primary or reactivation infection can be severe and life threatening in the immunosuppressed individual. Such patients may develop a progressive pneumonitis, hemolytic anemia, purpura, gastrointestinal ulceration, hepatitis, or pericarditis.

Diagnostic Studies and Findings[40,41,48]

Cell Culture of Urine Specimen, Oral Secretions, Cervical Secretions, or Biopsy Tissue

Positive for specific cytopathic effect of CMV
Presence of CMV in infant's urine at birth suggests congenital infection

Biopsy of Liver Tissue

Histologic evidence of typical inclusion bodies

Complement Fixation

Presence of IgG antibody in infant blood during first 6 months represents maternal antibodies; levels persisting after 6 months suggest congenital CMV infection
Fourfold rise in titer in adult or child suggest current infection
Very specific test with few false positive results

Indirect Fluorescent Antibody, Immunofluorescence, Anticomplement Immunofluorescent Test

Presence of IgM in cord blood at birth suggests congenital CMV infection
Elevated titer in adult or child suggest current infection
These tests are more sensitive and detect antibodies earlier in infection

Serum Transaminase (AST)

Elevated in CMV hepatitis but rarely more than 800 U

Platelets

May be as few as $5000/mm^3$

Differential WBC Count

Increase in lymphocytes, many atypical

Differential Diagnosis: Heterophil Agglutination

Negative in CMV (positive in mononucleosis)

Medical Plan[5,40,41,48]

Medications

Results of clinical trials using antiviral drugs, corticosteroids, or immune globulins in treating CMV infections are equivocal

General Management

Transfusion of sedimented RBCs for anemia
Transfusion of platelet-rich plasma for thrombocytopenia
Antipyretics for fever in CMV mononucleosis-like syndrome
Experimental live CMV vaccines currently being evaluated for prevention
Infants born of antibody-free mothers should not receive breast milk from a woman serologically positive for CMV antibodies since the virus may be in the milk

NURSING CARE

Nursing Assessment[40,41,48]

Postnatal Acquired CMV

Body temperature
- Fever lasting 2 to 5 weeks

Skin
- Rubelliform rash

Musculoskeletal concerns
- Migratory polyarthritis in knees, fingers, and toes

Subjective symptoms
- Headache
- Myalgia; malaise
- Nausea (with hepatitis)

Abdomen
- Hepatomegaly and splenomegaly

Respiratory concerns
- Paroxysmal cough or symptoms of pneumonia

Postnatal acquired CMV is usually asymptomatic. When clinical disease is present, the symptoms are variable and similar to mononucleosis without the lymphadenopathy and exudative pharyngitis. Complications include the following:

Respiratory Concerns

Progressive pneumonitis

Neurologic Complications

Sensory and motor weakness; photophobia
Pyramidal tract signs

Cardiac Complications

Symptoms of myocarditis

Eye Complications

Retinitis

Nursing Dx & Intervention

Nursing Diagnosis	Nursing Intervention/Rationale
Potential for infection: patient contacts	• Employ secretion precautions for hospitalized infants known to be shedding the virus *to prevent transmission.* • Women of childbearing age or who are pregnant should wash hands thoroughly after handling diapers of neonates with congenital CMV *to prevent acquiring CMV infection.*

Adults with CMV infections are generally not hospitalized and rarely have symptoms requiring medical intervention. The care of those who do is similar to that of mononucleosis (p. 1230) or is dependent on the complications (pneumonitis, myocarditis, hepatitis, meningoencephalitis, or chorioretinitis).

Toxoplasmosis

Toxoplasmosis is a systemic protozoan infection, ranging from subclinical to severe to chronic. Four different clinical syndromes can be identified depending on where the pathogen localizes in the body. Transplacental transmission results in congenital toxoplasmosis, which may be fatal to the fetus or neonate.

Pathophysiology[40,41,48]

Toxoplasmosis, like the cytomegalovirus (CMV) infections, may be congenital or acquired. Unlike CMV, there is not a risk for perinatal acquired toxoplasmosis. Both forms of toxoplasmosis may be present with clinical patterns ranging from subclinical infection to severe generalized infection (with neurologic and sensory sequelae) to death. Both may occur in latent or recurring forms under conditions of reduced host defenses.

The pathogen producing toxoplasmosis, *Toxoplasma gondii,* is a protozoan that is pathogenic to animals and humans. The pathogen can multiply only in living cells. This parasite exists in three forms: trophozoites, tissue cysts, and oocysts. Trophozoites are capable of invading, multiplying in, and necrotizing all host cells. Trophozoites can remain viable extracellularly in body secretions such as peritoneal fluid, breast milk, urine, saliva, or tears for a few hours to days. They cannot survive drying, heating, freezing, or contact with digestive juices.

Tissue cysts are formed within host cells. A surrounding membrane produced by the pathogen encapsulates up to 3000 organisms. This enables the parasites to maintain their viability for the life of the host in spite of circulating host antibodies. Tissue cysts are responsible for recurrent infection in humans and for transmission of the pathogen from animal reservoirs. Tissue cysts also cannot survive freezing, drying, or heating.

Oocysts are a form in the life cycle of *T. gondii* that occurs only in cats. Oocysts, a noninfectious form, are discharged in the feces of infected cats. Oocysts sporulate in 1 to 21 days in environmental temperatures of 4° to 37° C (39° to 99° F). They can remain infectious in the soil for 1 year, given favorable environmental conditions.

Transmission of *T. gondii* can occur by one of two modes: by ingestion of tissue cysts in uncooked meat or ingestion of sporulated oocysts by hands or food contaminated with cat feces, or by transplacental transmission of trophozoites in maternal circulation during acute infection acquired by the mother during the pregnancy.

In ingestion-acquired toxoplasmosis the capsule surrounding ingested cysts is digested by gastric juices. This permits viable trophozoites to invade intestinal mucosa and to disseminate throughout the body by way of blood and the lymphatics. Organ cell invasion produces foci of necrosis surrounded by intense inflammatory reaction with mononuclear cell infiltration. The spleen, liver, brain, lung, myocardium, and eye are most frequently involved. The development of cysts and tissue calcifications may impair organ functioning.

An early antibody response destroys many parasites before they form tissue cysts and supports cyst formation by the remainder. Thus the infection is limited to its mild or subclinical form for the majority of infected persons. Failure of an immune response, as is the case with immunosuppressed patients or those with debilitating disease, is more likely to result in progressive, life-threatening infection with multiple organ involvement and extensive damage.

Transplacentally transmitted *T. gondii* is disseminated to every organ in the developing fetus, particularly to the brain, heart, lungs, adrenal glands, striated muscle, and eye. Focal necrotic and inflammatory lesions are produced with cyst formation and calcification. Extensive destruction may occur in the central nervous system, affecting the cortex, subcortical white matter, caudate and lenticular nuclei, midbrain, pons, medulla, and spinal cord. Obstruction of the foramina of Monro or the aqueduct of Sylvius may result in an internal hydrocephalus. Microcephalus, hydrocephalus, or varying degrees of central nervous system impairment may occur.

Infection in the eye produces edema and necrosis of the retina, necrosis and disruption of the pigmented layer of the rods and cones, and infiltration of the retina and choroid with inflammatory cells. Granulation tissue and exudate may spread to the vitreous. This chorioretinitis may be manifested within weeks after birth or at some time later in life when the latent infection becomes reactivated.

Maternal infection early in the pregnancy is usually associated with fetal death or severe disease at birth. Infection later in pregnancy results in less severe or no manifestations at birth. Only 11% of maternal infections result in infants damaged at birth. The majority, 60% of infants, are not affected; 29% have subclinical infections that are manifest as neurologic or sensory defects as the infant develops.

Diagnostic Studies and Findings[40,41]

Inoculation of Mice With Specimens from Blood, Spinal Fluid, Lymph Nodes, Muscle Tissue; Morphologic Examination of Mouse Tissue after 4 Weeks

Identification of *T. gondii* cysts or trophozoites in mouse tissue is presumptive evidence of present infection

Electron Microscopic Examination of Tissue Sections or Smears

Identification of trophozoites present during acute infection

Identification of cysts does not differentiate between acute or chronic infection

Indirect Fluorescent Antibody Test or Sabin-Feldman Dye Test

IgG antibodies (1:4) appear within 1 to 2 weeks after acute infection; reach high titers (over 1:1000) in 6 to 8 weeks; and then gradually decline over months or years to titers of 1:4-1:64*

False positive results may follow blood transfusions; fourfold rise in titers or slow decline after the peak is diagnostic

Indirect Hemagglutination Test

Becomes positive for IgG antibodies (1:16) in 2 to 4 weeks; reaches peak (1:1000) in 8 to 16 weeks and stays positive longer (1:16 to 1:64); fourfold rise in titer is diagnostic*

IgM Fluorescent Antibody Test

Detects IgM antibodies (1:10) in 5 days, which peak (1:80) in 2 to 4 weeks; these antibodies decrease (1:10 to 1:40) during convalescence and are negative in 3 weeks to 4 months*

Test is useful for diagnosing acute infection

Radioimmunoassay, Agglutination Tests, and Enzyme-Linked Assay (ELISA)

Detects both IgG and IgM antibodies*

Detects antigen in human sera

Cerebrospinal Fluid

Acquired: glucose and protein normal

*These tests may show false negative results in immunosuppressed hosts.

Medical Plan[41,48]

Medications

Sulfadiazine (or sulfamerazine and sulfamethazine) in combination with pyrimethamine synergistically affects trophozoites but not cysts. Treatment does not prevent recurrence of chorioretinitis. It is indicated for severe, protracted disease, for those with chorioretinitis, for immunosuppressed individuals, and for active infections in newborns. Pyrimethamine is contraindicated for pregnant women.

- Anti-infective agents
  - Sulfadiazine (Suladyne), or triple sulfonamides po for 4 wk, initial dose of 50-75 mg/kg followed by 75-100 mg/d in 2-4 equal doses
  - Pyrimethamine (Daraprim), for 4 wk, initial dose 100-200 mg/d in 2 divided doses for 2 d, followed by 1 mg/kg/d in 2 divided doses (maximum: 25-50 mg/d or every other day)
- Vitamins
  - Folinic acid (calcium leucovorin), IM or po, 2-10 mg/d to prevent bone marrow suppression; 6-10 mg/d if platelets are less than 100,000/mm^3
  - Baker's yeast, three or four cakes per day

General Management

To prevent spread, reject leukocyte or organ donors who are antibody positive

NURSING CARE

Nursing Assessment[40]

Acquired Disease

Ranges from subclinical to a variety of clinical syndromes, occurring singly or in combination (four syndromes outlined below)

- Systemic syndrome
  - Subjective symptoms
    - Weakness and malaise for 6 to 10 days preceding following symptoms
  - Body temperature
    - Fever up to 41° C (106° F)
  - Skin
    - Generalized, bright red or pink, maculopapular rash, blanching on pressure; rash not seen on scalp, palms, or soles
- Respiratory concerns
  - Pneumonitis: coarse rales; dullness over both lung bases; cough, dyspnea, and cyanosis
  - Progresses to prostration and death in 2 to 4 weeks
- Cardiovascular concerns
  - Myocarditis

Neurologic Syndrome

Encephalitis: headache, vomiting, generalized convulsions, ataxia, and transitory confusion
Neurologic sequelae common

Lymph Node Syndrome

Generalized lymphadenopathy: firm, smooth, discrete, movable, enlarged nodes; tender early, painless later; no involvement of overlying skin; self-limiting

Abdomen
Splenomegaly

Eye Syndrome

Chorioretinitis (more frequently associated with congenital infection or recurrence of congenital chorioretinitis); blurred vision, pain, photophobia, loss of central vision, tearing; results in permanent loss of visual acuity

Nursing Dx & Intervention

Nursing Diagnosis	Nursing Intervention/Rationale
	The diagnoses and care of infants born with symptomatic toxoplasmosis depend on the type of anomaly. Care of acutely ill neonates is beyond the scope of this chapter.
Potential for injury	• Monitor for signs of bone marrow depression caused by pyrimethamine: purpura, epistaxis, bleeding at injection site (see "Patient Education") *to report to physician.*
Sensory/perceptual alterations (visual)	• Provide a safe environment for patients with chorioretinitis. Assist patient with interpreting the environment, with personal care, and with ambulation as needed *to prevent injury.* Refer for rehabilitation for vision loss.
Hyperthermia	• Monitor body temperature. • Administer sponge bath and antipyretics, as ordered, *to lower body temperature.*
	For persons with encephalitis, see p. 1246. For persons with pneumonitis or myocarditis, see Chapters 1 and 2.

Patient Education[5,40]

1. Patients treated with pyrimethamine (which depresses bone marrow) should have peripheral blood cell and platelet counts twice a week during therapy. Explain medication regimen, particularly the use of folinic acid and/or baker's yeast to counteract effects of pyrimethamine.
2. Immunocompromised persons and pregnant women can avoid exposure by cooking all meat to 60° C (140° F), washing fruits and vegetables, washing hands thoroughly after handling uncooked meat, wearing gloves while working in soil, and avoiding cat feces. Children's sandboxes should be kept free of cat feces.

Evaluation

	Data Indicating That Outcome is Reached
There are no toxic effects from therapy.	Leukocyte, reticulocyte, and platelet counts and bilirubin level are normal.

Brucellosis

Brucellosis is an acute or subacute systemic bacterial infectious disease of the reticuloendothelial system, with a variety of toxic manifestations that mimic other diseases.

Pathophysiology[5,41,48]

The microorganism causing brucellosis is a bacterium appearing as a coccus, a bacillus, or a coccobacillus, with six species pathogenic to specific animals. Four of the species found in cattle, swine, sheep, buffaloes, goats, horses, and dogs are pathogenic to humans.

Brucella is transmitted to humans by ingestion of infected milk, milk products, or uncooked meat, by skin or conjunctival contact with tissues, blood, urine, vaginal discharges, aborted fetuses, and placentas from infected animals, or by inhalation of airborne *Brucella* organisms in pens or stables.

The transmitted organism invades the lymphatics, bloodstream, and reticuloendothelial system and is disseminated throughout the body. Lesions infiltrated with large mononuclear cells are formed. The lesions may be suppurative or nonsuppurative, depending on the species of infecting *Brucella*. Focal necrotic and granulomatous lesions develop in the endocardium, bones, central nervous system, gallbladder, lungs, spleen, liver, kidneys, and intestinal mucosa. A fatal septicemia is possible.

Brucellosis may be asymptomatic or be manifest as an acute systemic disease, a chronic relapsing disease, or an infection localized in one or more organs. *Brucella* contains an endotoxin that is liberated when the organism dies. The endotoxin may be responsible for the systemic symptoms of pain, fever, and mental changes associated with the disease.

An immune response develops early in the disease and is sustained at low levels for years after acute disease. Antibodies do not prevent reinfection, the development of chronic disease, or relapses of acute symptoms during convalescence. It appears that *Brucella* organisms are able to survive within the phagocytes of the reticuloendothelial system, producing relapses of the disease in spite of high antibody titers. Recovery is usual, but disability may be pronounced.

Diagnostic Studies and Findings[41,48]

Culture of Blood, Lesions, or Exudate

Positive for *Brucella*

Widal Agglutination Test

- Titer greater than 1:80 (preferably 1:160 to 1:320) is presumptive; a fourfold rise to 1:640 1:1280 is diagnostic
- May be false negative in localized brucellosis
- Agglutination antibodies should begin a gradual decrease during convalescence and have faded after 1 year
- Rapid increase suggests a relapse during chronic brucellosis
- Radioimmunoassay (RIA) and enzyme-linked assay (ELISA)
  - IgM rises in first week of infection, peaks at 3 months, and persists into chronic stages at very low levels
  - IgG and IgA rise in 2 to 3 weeks, peak in 6 to 8 weeks, and remain high in chronic disease
  - With relapse there is a sharp rise in IgG and IgM titers

Erythrocyte Sedimentation Rate

Elevated

Differential WBC Count

Relative or absolute lymphocytosis

Skin Test: Intradermal Injection of 0.1 ml Antigen

- Induration and erythema at injection site within 48 hours indicate antibodies from present or past infection
- Of questionable use for diagnosis

Medical Plan[5,48]

Surgery (Depends on Complications)

- Splenectomy
- Drainage of abscesses

Medications

- Adults
  - Anti-infective agents
    - Tetracycline (Achromycin), 2 g/24 h po in four divided doses of 500 mg, plus
    - Dihydrostreptomycin or streptomycin, 1-2 g/24 h po, plus
    - Triple sulfonamides, 4-6 g/24 h po in four divided doses
- In uncomplicated, acute cases, the combined therapy is given for 3 weeks followed by 2 weeks of tetracycline (1-2 g/24 h) alone; for chronic cases or cases with complications, combined therapy is given for 4-6 wk
- Corticosteroids
  - Steroids in severe disease

General Management

- Bed rest in severe and complicated cases
- Additional supportive therapy depending on the complications
- Diet: 3000 to 3700 cal/day; 2 g protein/kg/day

NURSING CARE

Nursing Assessment[5,41,48]

Early: Subjective Symptoms

Gradual-onset weakness and malaise; worsens as day progresses

Acute Stage: Duration 2 to 3 Months

- Body temperature
  - Gradual rise in temperature (38° to 40° C [101° to 104° F]), showing sharp remissions
  - Chills
  - Continues for weeks, declines, and may spike again during a relapse
- Subjective symptoms
  - Myalgia, severe in back and legs

Headache
Insomnia
Pain in joints, particularly hip, knee, ankle, and shoulder

Skin
Heavy perspiration with a disagreeable odor

Gastrointestinal concerns
Indigestion
Diarrhea or constipation
Weight loss
Bleeding

Lymph nodes
Lymphadenopathy: anterior and posterior cervical, axillary; small, firm, discrete, nontender

Oral mucous membranes
Gums become spongy and bleed easily when pressed

Respiratory concerns
Dry cough

Abdomen
Painful, enlarged spleen
Hepatomegaly less common

Mental status
Depression
Hysterical episodes

Complications: Localized Disease of Variable Duration and Outcome

Symptoms of pneumonia and pleurisy, neurasthenia, meningoencephalitis, orchitis, epistaxis, extremely high fever, spondylitis, endocarditis, and vertebral osteomyelitis

Chronic Stage: Duration Greater Than 1 Year

Usually asymptomatic
Low-grade fever
Neuropsychiatric manifestations

Nursing Dx & Intervention

Nursing Diagnosis	Nursing Intervention/Rationale
Pain	• Administer analgesics as prescribed *to relieve pain.* • Position *for comfort.* • Apply heat *to relieve pain in muscles and joints*
Altered oral mucous membrane	• Provide frequent oral hygiene *to prevent secondary infection.* • Observe gums for bleeding.
Activity intolerance	• Maintain bed rest during acute illness; gradually increase activity during convalescence *to conserve energy.*
Potential impaired skin integrity	• Bathe; change position frequently; massage skin over bony prominences *to relieve pressure.* • Provide intermittent pressure mattress *to relieve pressure on skin.*
Altered thought processes	• Monitor for signs of depression or increasing irritability. • Assure patient that these reactions are normal and temporary. • Provide safety, diversional activity, and opportunities for patient to express concerns *to prevent further depression.* • Monitor for changes in mentation or consciousness *to detect complicating encephalitis; report to physician* (see p. 1246).
Altered nutrition: less than body requirements	• Offer frequent food and fluids in a variety that will encourage patient to eat. • Measure intake and output *to ensure adequate intake.* • Provide vitamin supplements and 3000 to 3700 cal/day diet, *which is required because of increased metabolism due to fever.*
Sleep pattern disturbance	• Control the environment *to facilitate sleep.* • Allow patient opportunities *to relieve anxiety* by talking or listening to music before bedtime. • *Provide for relaxation* techniques, such as bathing and massage.
Sensory/perceptual alterations (visual and auditory)	• Monitor for changes *to detect encephalitis and report to physician.* • Continuously monitor patient's safety. • Interpret the environment to the patient *to prevent injury.*
Anxiety	• Encourage patient to express anxiety about prolonged illness and lost work and income *to decrease anxiety.* • Refer to social service or other community agencies *if financial aid is needed.*
Potential for injury	• Monitor for toxic reactions and temporary increase in severity of symptoms, which are sometimes precipitated by antimicrobial therapy. • Note changes in temperature, other vital signs, levels of pain, and mood. • Reassure patient and report changes to physician.

Nursing Diagnosis	Nursing Intervention/Rationale
	• Administer steroids, if ordered. • Observe also for drug reactions such as hearing loss caused by streptomycin or severe diarrhea caused by tetracycline *to report to physician.*
Hyperthermia	• Monitor body temperature. • Bathe patient frequently *to lower body temperature and to remove perspiration.* • Administer oral fluids freely *to compensate for increased needs.* • Maintain comfortable environmental temperature with freely circulating air.

Patient Education[5]

1. Premature resumption of activity during convalescence aggravates symptoms and predisposes to relapses. Convalescence may take 6 to 8 weeks in treated patient.
2. The patient must complete the entire medication regimen.
3. The patient should report to the physician any symptoms recurring after completion of the therapy, since another course of therapy will be required.
4. Duration of acquired immunity from the disease is uncertain. The patient should protect self from exposure and reinfection, and others from exposure:
   a. Drink only pasteurized milk and milk products.
   b. Boil milk if pasteurization is not possible.
   c. Animals suspected to be diseased should be tested and slaughtered if infected. Diseased meat should not be eaten.
   d. Placenta, discharges, and fetus from aborted animals should be handled with care (with gloves).
   e. Farmers, slaughterers, and butchers should handle carcasses or products of potentially infected animals with gloves.

Evaluation

Patient Outcome	Data Indicating That Outcome is Reached
Body temperature is normal.	Oral adult temperature is normal for 2 to 7 days.
Laboratory findings are within normal limits.	Erythrocyte sedimentation rate, differential WBC count, leukocyte count, RBC count, hematocrit, and hemoglobin are normal.
Nutrition and fluids are adequate for body requirements.	Patient has not lost weight, or daily weight is stabilized for body build. Skin color and turgor are good. Mucous membranes are moist. Urinary output equals fluid intake. Stools are soft, formed, and normal colored.
There is no chronic infection.	There is no malaise, weakness, or fatigue. Patient can perform all ADLs without tiring and is mentally alert and attentive. There is no adenitis, arthritis, neurosensory alterations, or signs of other complications.
Patient is aware of needs and able to use resources.	Patient verbalizes intent to take entire course of antimicrobial therapy and to report to physician any recurrence of symptoms. Patient has plans for gradual return to normal activities and has realistic expectations for progress during convalescence. Patient has adequate income to live during convalescence.

NEUROLOGIC INFECTIOUS DISEASES

Meningitis[5,40,48]

Meningococcal meningitis is an acute communicable inflammation of the meninges caused by *Neisseria meningitidis.* It frequently occurs in epidemic form.

***Haemophilus* meningitis is an acute communicable inflammation of the meninges caused by *Haemophilus influenzae.* It is the most common form of bacterial meningitis.**

Pneumococcal meningitis is an acute inflammation of the meninges caused by *Streptococcus pneumoniae.* The meningitis frequently results from an extension of a primary infection in the upper respiratory tract. Patients infected with *S. pneumoniae* have a high risk of fatality.

Viral (aseptic or serous) meningitis is an acute meningeal inflammation that occurs as a sequela to many

viral diseases. The condition is usually self-limited and benign.

Meningitis is an inflammation of the meninges covering the brain and spinal cord. The inflammation may result from an acute infection of the meninges caused by the invasion of bacteria, viruses, fungi, or parasitic worms into the tissues or from the iatrogenic introduction of a substance that is irritating to the meninges. The forms of meningitis discussed in this section are those caused by bacterial and viral invasion.

The invasion may produce a primary or secondary infection. Some bacteria produce a primary focal infection in the meninges. Such is the case with *N. meningitidis* and *H. influenzae,* which cause meningococcal and *Haemophilus* meningitides, respectively. Other bacterial and viral pathogens are capable of producing a secondary infection in the meninges following hematogenous dissemination from a primary focal infection elsewhere in the body. *H. influenzae, S. pneumoniae* (pneumococcal meningitis), many viruses, and other bacteria have this pathogenic potential.

In addition to the differentiation as to primary and secondary infection, two clinical forms of meningitis, suppurative and nonsuppurative, can be identified. Suppurative (purulent) meningitis results from bacterial invasion and is manifest as a characteristic high leukocytosis in cerebrospinal fluid with the majority of the leukocytes being neutrophils. In nonsuppurative (aseptic or serous) meningitis, cerebrospinal fluid leukocytes are less and are primarily made up of lymphocytes. Viruses from an antecedent infection elsewhere in the body are the predominant causes of nonsuppurative meningitis (Table 13-15).

Although many bacteria are capable of producing a sup-

Table 13-15
Overview of Meningitis

	Meningococcal Meningitis	Pneumococcal Meningitis	Haemophilus Meningitis	Viral Meningitis (Aseptic)
Occurrence	Endemic and epidemic; worldwide; greatest during winter and spring; greatest in males, in children less than 5 yr, and in persons in crowded living conditions	Endemic; greatest in infants, elderly persons, and alcoholics; follows pneumococcal pneumonia	Worldwide; most common bacterial meningitis in children 2 mo to 3 yr	Worldwide; epidemics and sporadic cases associated with other infections
Etiologic agent	*Neisseria meningitidis,* with many subgroups	*Streptococcus pneumoniae,* many serotypes	*Haemophilus influenzae,* six serotypes; type B responsible for 90% of *Haemophilus* meningitis	Most viruses produce the syndrome: mumps, herpes, polio, etc.
Reservoir	Humans	Humans; many carriers	Humans	Humans
Transmission	Direct contact with droplets from respiratory passages of infected persons and carriers	Direct and indirect contact with discharges from respiratory passages	Direct contact with droplets from respiratory passages	
Incubation period	2-10 d; usually 3-4 d	1-3 d for pneumonia	2-4 d	
Period of communicability	Until organism is not present in discharges: within 24 h of treatment with sulfonamides	Until organism is not present in respiratory discharges: 24-48 h after antibiotic treatment	Prolonged; until organism is not present in nasal discharge	Depends on virus and associated viral disease
Susceptibility and resistance	Susceptibility to clinical disease is low; many carriers; group-specific immunity of unknown duration follows infection	Infants and elderly most susceptible; immunity for specific type persists for years	Children most susceptible; otitis media may be a precursor; immunity of unknown duration follows infection	
Report to local health authority	Mandatory case report	Only epidemics; no individual case reports	Yes in certain endemic areas	Yes in endemic areas

Data from Benenson.[5]

purative meningitis, the most common forms are *Haemophilus*, meningococcal, and pneumococcal meningitides. They are discussed together, since their pathologic manifestations and symptoms are similar. Viral meningitis will be discussed as a separate disease entity regardless of the viral disease that preceded the meningitis.

Pathophysiology[48]

Bacteria causing the suppurative meningitis being considered here are inhaled in mucous droplets from infected persons or carriers, invade the respiratory passages, and are disseminated by way of the blood to meninges of the brain and spinal cord. The respiratory phase is generally subclinical in meningococcal meningitis, although organisms present in respiratory secretions can be transmitted to another host. The respiratory phase is usually symptomatic in pneumococcal and *Haemophilus* meningitides. The bacteremia produced during dissemination gives rise to toxic manifestations. In the case of meningococcus the organism penetrates and damages vascular endothelium. This results in petechial and purpuric lesions of the skin.

Bacteria in the meninges elicit an inflammatory response and the production of an exudate consisting of leukocytes, fibrin, and bacteria in the subarachnoid space. Cerebrospinal fluid may be thin or thick with plaquelike accumulations. In untreated disease the cerebrospinal fluid may achieve a thickness that interferes with its circulation and reabsorption. An internal or external hydrocephalus may result. Extension of the bacteria into brain tissue may produce a bacterial encephalitis.

Meningococcal infections may be so severe in the systemic stage that they produce an acute meningococcemia that leads to death or the initiation of therapy before meningeal involvement. Meningococcemia may become chronic with toxic symptoms persisting intermittently for weeks or months. Recurrent meningitis is usually of the pneumococcal form and is frequently associated with an undetected skull fracture.

Complications of bacterial meningitis include internal hydrocephalus, deficits of cranial nerve function that lead to blindness and deafness, arthritis, myocarditis, pericarditis, and neuromotor and intellectual deficits. Symptomatic and asymptomatic infection with bacterial meningitis results in a protective immune response of unknown duration.

Aseptic (viral, serous, or nonsuppurative) meningitis is a syndrome generally associated with an existing systemic viral disease, the most common one being mumps. Inflammation and lymphocytic infiltration of the meninges occur with a wide gradient in clinical severity depending on the infectious agent. Toxic and meningeal symptoms are usually less severe than in suppurative meningitis. This form may also progress to clinical encephalitis. The disease is usually self-limited with complete recovery, although patients may experience muscle weakness and malaise during a prolonged convalescence.

Diagnostic Studies and Findings[40,48]

Cerebrospinal Fluid Examination

- Gross appearance
  - Turbid: bacterial
  - Clear: viral (aseptic)
- Leukocytes
  - 500 to 20,000/mm^3: bacterial
  - 10 to 500/mm^3: viral (aseptic)
- Cell types
  - Neutrophils: bacterial
  - Lymphocytes: viral (aseptic)
- Protein
  - Increased for both
- Glucose
  - Low to normal: bacterial
  - Normal: viral (aseptic)

Cerebrospinal Fluid Culture or Gram's Stain or Serologic Techniques (Counterimmunoelectrophoresis, Coagulation, Latex Agglutination, or Fluorescent Antibody Techniques)

- Positive for bacteria
- Absence of bacteria with cerebrospinal fluid cell changes would suggest viral (aseptic) meningitis

Gram's Stain of Scrapings from Petechial Skin Lesions

- Positive for meningococci

Blood Culture

- Positive for *H. influenzae* or *N. meningitidis* (meningococci)

Serology

- Increase in antibody titer with specific viral infections

Medical Plan*

Medications†

- Anti-infective agents
  - Initial therapy until organism is identified
    - Ampicillin, 200 mg/kg/24 h IV, plus chloramphenicol if *H. influenzae* is suspected for patients more than 2 mo of age
  - Definitive therapy: meningococci or pneumococci
  - Ampicillin (Amcill), 200 mg/kg/24 h IV, or chloramphenicol (Chloromycetin), 100 mg/kg/24 h IV to a maximum of 4 g
  - Definitive therapy: *H. influenzae*

*References 5, 12, 15, 16, 21, 48.
†For bacterial meningitis.

Ampicillin or chloramphenicol (Chloromycetin), 100 mg/kg/24 h IV to a maximum of 4 g

All of the above are administered by rapid intravenous infusion; initial dose should be one third of daily dose, the remainder divided into six equal doses; therapy should continue for 5 days after temperature is normal and clinical signs have cleared; barbiturates may be given for seizures

Analgesics for headache and muscle pain (nonnarcotic)

Immunologic agents for prevention of bacterial meningitides

- Meningococcal polysaccharide vaccine against group A and C serotypes for those more than 2 yr of age at risk for epidemic disease; given in single dose (0.5 ml subcutaneously)
  - Routine immunization of civilians not recommended
- Pneumococcal polysaccharide vaccine is available for administration to those at high risk for pneumococcal pneumonia and subsequent systemic complications; persons at risk are those more than 65 yr of age, adults with cardiovascular and chronic pulmonary disease, and liver and renal dysfunction, children with chronic disease and recurrent respiratory disease, and anyone with immunosuppression

Anti-infective agents for meningococcal contacts

- Rifampin (Rifamycin, others), 600 mg bid (adults) for 2 d
- Sulfadiazine, 1 g bid for 3 d for mass prophylaxis during meningococcal epidemics or for close patient contacts if strain is proven susceptible

Anti-infective agents for *H. influenzae* household contacts

- Children and adults (excluding pregnant women):
  - Rifampin, 20 mg/kg/d (maximum daily dose of 600 mg) for 4 days as soon as possible after contact

General Management

Endotracheal intubation
Ventilatory assistance
IV therapy and dopamine if shock is present
Fluid restriction to two thirds of daily needs if excess secretion of ADH
Control of intracranial pressure
Close monitoring for early diagnosis of patient contacts

NURSING CARE

Nursing Assessment[5,40,48]

Subjective Symptoms

Severe throbbing headache
Muscle pains
Stiff neck
Backache
Chills

Body Temperature

38° to 41° C (100° to 106° F), starting in systemic phase

Pulse

May be slow as intracranial pressure increases

Cardiovascular Concerns

Symptoms of shock with increase in intracranial pressure

Level of Consciousness

Alert early in disease but may show delirium progressing to deep coma later

Neurologic Concerns

Reflex changes: absence of abdominal reflexes; absence of cremasteric reflexes in male; alteration of tendon reflexes

Resistance to neck flexion

Brudzinski's sign positive: attempted flexion of neck will elicit flexion of knees and hips

Kernig's sign positive: limitation in angle at which a straight leg may be raised from bed with patient in supine position

• • •

In addition to the above symptoms of meningitis, some symptoms are characteristic of specific forms of the disease:

Pneumococcal

Symptoms of pneumonia or otitis media frequently precede the meningitis

Meningococcal

Petechial and purpuric skin lesions preceded by a rash resembling measles on trunk and extremities

Large ecchymotic lesions on face and extremities in severe disease

Haemophilus

Respiratory concerns
- Symptoms of pneumonia or otitis media frequently precede the meningitis

Chronic Meningococcemia

Musculoskeletal concerns
- Swelling and pain in large joints, particularly knees and ankles

Skin
- Recurrent macular or petechial lesions

Subjective symptoms
- Headache
- Malaise
- Irritability

Body temperature
- Intermittent low-grade fever

Aseptic Meningitis

Symptoms preceding meningeal signs depend on the disease and its etiologic agent; may have parotid swelling of mumps, respiratory or gastrointestinal symptoms, skin manifestations of measles or chickenpox

Nursing Dx & Intervention

Nursing Diagnosis	Nursing Intervention/Rationale
Altered cerebral tissue perfusion	• Monitor patient carefully, particularly after lumbar puncture. • Have patient lie flat for 4 to 6 hours or as ordered after lumbar puncture *to prevent headache.* • Watch for changes in pulse *to detect signs of shock and to report alterations to physician for early intervention.* • Monitor for signs of intracranial pressure throughout course of the disease, e.g., slowing of pulse, increase in blood pressure, decreased level of consciousness, arrhythmic breathing, altered pupillary response, and facial weakness (see Chapter 3 for further neurologic assessment). • Monitor vital signs and neurologic findings every 5 to 30 minutes for patient with intracranial pressure *to detect early changes.* • Report changes to physician immediately. • Avoid any position or movement of patient *to prevent increased intracranial pressure.* • *To prevent increases in intracranial pressure:* Provide for bed rest. Elevate patient's head slightly *to decrease intracranial pressure.* Prevent any sudden or unnecessary movements of patient's head and neck and avoid neck flexion. Assist patient with all activities and movement *to prevent muscle straining.* Administer stool softeners as prescribed (avoid enemas). Instruct patient to exhale while turning or moving in bed. Position to avoid knee or hip flexion. Time nursing procedures to coincide with periods of relaxation or sedation. Avoid unnecessary environmental stimuli. Administer hypertonic agents as prescribed. • Evaluate during convalescence for motor, sensory, and intellectual impairment *in order to refer for rehabilitation.*
Ineffective airway clearance	• Maintain fully patent airway for patient with increased intracranial pressure. • Suction secretions; perform endotracheal care. • Continually supervise patient who has convulsions *to protect from injury.*
Impaired gas exchange	• Monitor blood gases. • Oxygenate before suctioning, and limit suctioning to 10 to 15 seconds for apneic patients *to maintain adequate circulating oxygen.* • Employ mechanical ventilation if necessary. • Continually monitor delirious or convulsive patient *to prevent aspiration.*
Potential for trauma	• Pad bed and provide restraints for delirious patient *to protect from injury.* • Prevent aspiration or injury during convulsions.
Potential fluid volume deficit	• Administer frequent oral or continuous IV fluids *to prevent dehydration.* • Monitor intake and output *to detect signs of fluid retention.* • Restrict IV fluids to two thirds of needs if signs of fluid retention occur.
Altered nutrition: less than body requirements	• Provide high-caloric liquids and nasogastric tube feedings if needed *to provide adequate nutrients to compensate for increased metabolic needs.*
Pain	• Administer analgesics as prescribed. (Do not give narcotics or sedatives that will depress vital functions in patients with increased intracranial pressure.) • Provide moist heat *to relieve muscle aches and pains* (in absence of high fever). • Place blanket roll under knees *to relieve back pain* (in absence of elevated intracranial pressure).
Impaired physical mobility	• Administer range of motion exercises to patient who has no sign of elevated intracranial pressure *to prevent contractures.* • Frequently change position *to prevent contractures and decubiti.*
Feeding and hygiene self-care deficit	• Provide all feeding and hygiene measures for patient *to conserve energy.*

Nursing Diagnosis	Nursing Intervention/Rationale
Altered patterns of urinary elimination	• Assess for retention. • Maintain indwelling catheter if necessary *to empty bladder.*
Hyperthermia	• Take rectal temperature every 2 hours *to detect fever.* • Administer antipyretics as prescribed *to lower body temperature.* • Sponge with tepid water or alcohol in water *to lower body temperature.*
Potential for infection: patient contacts	• Employ respiratory isolation for 24 hours after initiation of antimicrobial therapy for bacterial meningitis *to prevent transmission of pathogen* (see p. 1297). • Employ excretion precautions for duration of hospitalization for viral meningitis *to prevent transmission to others* (see p. 1298).
Potential for infection: patient	• Assist in collection of cerebrospinal fluid specimens *for culture and analysis.* • Record amount and character of cerebrospinal fluid *for correct medical diagnosis.* • Administer IV antibiotics as prescribed *to maintain therapeutic levels of circulating antibiotics.*

Patient Education

1. Anti-infective therapy for bacterial meningitis must be continued as prescribed for 5 days after the temperature returns to normal.
2. Exacerbation of symptoms should be reported to the physician immediately.
3. Convalescence is of variable duration, depending on the severity of the disease. Patients should allow adequate time for recovery before resuming full activities.
4. Recovery is usually complete; however, neurologic sequelae do occur. The patient should be evaluated during convalescence for functional and neurologic deficits, and should participate in rehabilitation if prescribed.
5. Prophylactic measures should be initiated for close patient contacts, as described in the "Medical Plan."
6. Patient contacts should be evaluated medically for early detection and treatment of bacterial meningitis.

Evaluation

Patient Outcome	Data Indicating That Outcome is Reached
Body temperature is normal.	Temperatures are normal for 5 days.
Cerebrospinal fluid findings are normal.	There are less than 30 cells/mm^3. Glucose, protein, and pressure are normal. There are no organisms in cultures. Color is clear.
Blood pressure, pulse, and respirations are normal.	Blood pressure, pulse, and respirations are normal.
All cells receive oxygen.	Blood levels (O_2 saturation, carbon dioxide, and Po_2) are normal.
There is no systemic infection.	There are no skin petechiae or purpura. Blood cultures are negative for bacteria.
Patient returns to premorbid level of consciousness.	Patient is alert, responds appropriately to questions and environmental stimuli, and is oriented to person and place. Patient has memory for recent and past events.
Patient exhibits appropriate motor responses to stimuli.	Pupils are equal and reactive to light. There is no resistance to neck flexion. Straight legs may be raised from the bed with patient in a prone position. Abdominal, cremasteric, and tendon reflexes are normal. Patient is able to walk and carry out all functions without residual weakness or impairment.
Patient does not experience pain.	Patient does not have headache or pain in neck and back.
Infection has not been transmitted to patient contacts.	Hospital personnel and other patient contacts are free of infection.

Encephalitis

Amebic meningoencephalitis is an acute and severe inflammation of the brain and meninges caused by invasion of the tissues by a free-living ameba usually found in water, soil, and decaying vegetation. The disease is frequently fatal.

Mosquito-borne viral encephalitides are a group of acute inflammatory diseases of the brain, spinal cord, and meninges caused by a variety of viruses transmitted to humans through bites from infected mosquitoes.

Infectious viral encephalitides are acute inflammations of the central nervous system that are associated with and sequelae to systemic viral infections; they are commonly caused by the genus *Herpesvirus*.

Whereas meningitis is an inflammation of the meninges covering the brain and spinal cord, encephalitis is an inflammation of the tissues of the brain and spinal cord, resulting in altered function of various portions of these tissues. Encephalitis is frequently accompanied by signs of systemic infection. Clinical disease manifestations range from mild to severe to death, and disease may be followed by temporary or permanent neurologic sequelae or complete recovery.

Like meningitis, encephalitis may result from at least four causes: a toxemia accompanying an infectious disease, an allergic response to microbial antigens, direct invasion of central nervous system tissue by pathogens as a primary focal infection, or direct invasion of central nervous system tissue secondary to hematogenous dissemination from a primary focal infection elsewhere in the body. Direct invasion, either primary or secondary, is usually caused by a virus, a great many of which are capable of producing encephalitis.

The majority of viruses producing encephalitis as a primary focal infection are transmitted by mosquitoes and are discussed together. Encephalitides occurring secondary to other viral diseases are discussed as infectious encephalitis. A rarer form of meningoencephalitis caused by direct invasion by an ameba is also discussed (Table 13-16).

Table 13-16
Overview of Encephalitis

	Amebic Meningoencephalitis	Mosquito-Borne Viral Encephalitides (Equine and St. Louis Encephalitis)	Infectious Viral Encephalitis
Occurrence	Worldwide, but rare; greatest in young persons, in warm climates, and during summer	Warm, moist climates; summer and early fall when mosquitoes are greatest	Worldwide; epidemic and sporadic; associated with other viral diseases
Etiologic agent	*Naegleria fowleri; Acanthamoeba culbertsoni*	A variety of diseases, each caused by a different virus	A variety of viruses, commonly the *Herpesvirus*
Reservoir	Amebae that are free living in water and soil	Birds, rodents, bats, reptiles, and amphibians; differing for each virus	Humans
Transmission	Water infected with *N. fowleri* forced into nasal passages while swimming; *Acanthamoeba* enters a skin lesion	Bite of infective mosquitoes	Direct contact with droplets from respiratory passages or other excretions harboring the virus
Incubation period	3-7 d or longer	5-15 d	Depends on viral disease
Period of communicability	Not communicable person to person	Not communicable person to person; mosquitoes are infective for life	Depends on viral disease
Susceptibility and resistance	Unknown; immunosuppressed persons are susceptible to infection with *Acanthamoeba*	Highest susceptibility to clinical disease is infancy and old age; in endemic areas, adults are immune to local strains of virus because of subclinical infections	Depends on viral disease
Report to local health authority	Only for means of surveillance	Mandatory case report	In select endemic areas

Data from Benenson.[5]

Pathophysiology[5,40,41,48]

Amebic meningoencephalitis. Two types of amebae, *Naegleria* and *Acanthamoeba,* are capable of producing meningoencephalitis in humans. *Naegleria* infection is caused when water containing the pathogen is forced into the nasal passages, usually by diving or swimming in water containing large amounts of organic matter. The organism colonizes and invades the mucosa, travels along olfactory nerves to the meninges and brain, and produces a severe and rapidly fatal fulminating pyogenic meningoencephalitis. *Acanthamoeba* colonizes a skin lesion and travels to the central nervous system along peripheral nerves to produce a meningoencephalitis with a more insidious onset and prolonged course. Immunologic investigations have shown many people to have a natural antibody against these organisms, suggesting that more subclinical than clinical infections may occur.

Mosquito-borne viral encephalitis. A variety of viruses capable of infecting animals and birds can be carried to humans by vector mosquitoes that feed on infected animals. The virus, injected into humans from a mosquito bite, rapidly localizes in the central nervous system and produces congestion, edema, and small hemorrhages in the brain. Neuronal lesions with nerve cell necrosis and destruction and foci of cellular infiltration are widespread throughout the brain and spinal cord. Disease severity depends on the virus and on host resistance factors. Generally, older persons are more severely affected and have the highest fatality. Disease onset may be acute or insidious, depending on the virus involved. Infants generally have a more acute-onset encephalitis than do other age groups. Infants and children are also more likely to develop motor and mental disabilities (seizures, hydrocephalus, and mental retardation) as a sequela to mosquito-borne encephalitis.

An antibody response can be seen within 7 days. Duration of the disease is variable, depending on the virus. Blood leukocyte levels are generally normal or slightly elevated with some viruses. The virus cannot be recovered from blood, secretions, or discharges and is therefore not communicable from person to person.

Infectious encephalitis. A variety of directly transmittable viruses are capable of producing encephalitides either as a concomitant to or as a sequela of clinical viral diseases (e.g., measles, mumps, rubella, and chickenpox) or as a result of a subclinical viral infection such as herpes. In both cases the pathologic manifestations of the encephalitis may result from a postinfection autoimmune response to the virus or from direct invasion of the central nervous system by the virus. Timing of the onset of central nervous system manifestations in relationship to the associated disease symptoms and the ability to isolate the virus from cerebrospinal fluid allow differentiation as to postinfection or direct invasion encephalitis.

Disease onset may be acute or insidious, and disease severity may be mild to severe depending on the virus and the distribution, location, and concentration of the neuronal lesions. Mumps virus usually produces a more benign disease, whereas herpes encephalitis is frequently fatal. Permanent neurologic sequelae are also more common in herpes infections.

Diagnostic Studies and Findings[5,48]

Amebic Meningoencephalitis

- Phase contrast microscopic examination of fresh spinal fluid mount
  - Mobile amebae can be visualized
- Cerebrospinal fluid examination
  - Large number of polymorphonuclear leukocytes; may be RBCs

Mosquito-Borne Viral Encephalitis

- Neutralization, complement fixation, hemagglutination inhibition, fluorescent antibody, or agar gel precipitation
  - Fourfold increase in antibody titer between early disease and convalescence
- Blood count
  - Leukocytes vary with virus: range from 10,000 to 66,000/mm^3
- Cerebrospinal fluid examination
  - Not diagnostic
  - Leukocytes: 50 to 500/mm^3; usually lymphocytes

Infectious Viral Encephalitis

- Complement fixation, hemagglutination inhibition, or neutralization
  - Fourfold decrease in antibody titer between early disease and convalescence
- Cerebrospinal fluid examination
  - Virus isolation
  - Increase in protein: 50 to 150 mg/dl
  - RBCs; leukocytes: 50 to 500/mm^3, predominantly lymphocytes

Medical Plan[40,48]

Medications

- Anti-infective agents
  - Amebic meningoencephalitis: combination of the following drugs (individual dose calculation)
    - Amphotericin B (Fungizone), IV
    - Sulfadiazine, IV
    - Miconazole (Monistat), IV
    - Rifampin (Rifamycin; others), po
  - Mosquito-borne: no specific treatment
  - Infectious viral encephalitides: no specific treatment except for herpes infections; adenine arabinoside (Vidarabine, ara-A), IV 15 mg/kg/24 h for 10 d

General Management

Tracheostomy
Assisted ventilation
Suction
Sedatives for hyperexcitability and seizures
IV fluids and electrolytes
Nasogastric tube feedings

NURSING CARE

Nursing Assessment[40,48]

Body Temperature

39° to 41° C (102° to 105° F)

May be acute-onset fever accompanying central nervous system symptoms, or there may be a 1- to 4-day prodromal period with fever and chills before central nervous system symptoms

Central Nervous System

Signs of meningeal irritation: severe frontal headache, nausea, vomiting, dizziness, nuchal rigidity

Level of consciousness
- Alterations in consciousness: mild listlessness progressing to confusion, stupor, and eventual coma
- May have extreme irritability
- Bizarre behavior with temporal lobe involvement of herpes encephalitis
- Seizures, particularly in infants with postinfectious encephalitis

Neurologic concerns
- Focal neurologic signs
- Aphasia
- Olfactory hallucinations

Motor concerns
- Weakness, accentuated deep tendon reflexes, extensor plantar response
- Ataxia, spasticity, and tremors
- In herpes encephalitis there may be a flaccid paralysis and depression of tendon reflexes with spinal cord involvement and bowel and bladder paralysis
- Postinfectious encephalitis may not manifest motor signs

Regulatory mechanisms
- Excess or deficient antidiuretic hormone secretion
- Increasing hyperthermia

Nursing Dx & Intervention

Nursing Diagnosis	Nursing Intervention/Rationale
Altered cerebral tissue perfusion	• Monitor patient carefully, particularly after lumbar puncture. • Have patient lie flat for 4 to 6 hours or as ordered after lumbar puncture. • Watch for changes in pulse. • Monitor for signs of intracranial pressure throughout course of the disease: slowing of pulse, increase in blood pressure, decreased level of consciousness, arrhythmic breathing, altered pupillary response, and facial weakness (see Chapter 3 for further neurologic assessment). • Monitor vital signs and neurologic findings every 5 to 30 minutes for patient with intracranial pressure. • Report changes to physician immediately. • *To prevent increases in intracranial pressure:* Avoid any position or movement of patient that would increase intracranial pressure. Provide for bed rest. Elevate patient's head slightly. Prevent any sudden or unnecessary movements of patient's head and neck, and avoid neck flexion. Assist patient with all activities and movement to prevent muscle straining. Administer stool softeners as prescribed (avoid enemas). Instruct patient to exhale while turning or moving in bed. Position to avoid knee or hip flexion. Time and space nursing procedures to coincide with periods of relaxation or sedation. Avoid unnecessary environmental stimuli. Administer hypertonic agents as prescribed. • Evaluate during convalescence for motor, sensory, and intellectual impairment *in order to refer for rehabilitation.*
Ineffective airway clearance	• Maintain fully patent airway for patient with increased intracranial pressure. • Suction secretions; provide endotracheal care. • Continually supervise patient having convulsions *to protect from injury.*
Impaired gas exchange	• Monitor blood gases. • Oxygenate before suctioning. Limit suctioning to 15 seconds or less for apneic patient *to maintain adequate circulating oxygen.* • Employ mechanical ventilation if necessary.

Nursing Diagnosis	Nursing Intervention/Rationale
	• Continually monitor delirious or convulsive patient *to prevent aspiration.*
Potential for trauma	• Pad bed and provide restraints for delirious patient *to protect from injury.* • Prevent aspiration or injury during convulsions.
Potential fluid volume deficit	• Administer frequent oral or continuous IV fluids *to prevent dehydration.* • Monitor intake and output *to detect signs of fluid retention.* • Restrict IV fluids to two thirds of needs if signs of fluid retention occur.
Altered nutrition: less than body requirements	• Provide high-calorie liquids and nasogastric tube feedings if needed *to provide adequate nutrients to compensate for increased metabolic needs.*
Pain	• Administer analgesics as prescribed. (Do not give narcotics or sedatives that will depress vital functions in patients with increased intracranial pressure.) • Provide moist heat *to relieve muscle aches and pains* (in absence of high fever). • Place blanket roll under knees *to relieve back pain* in absence of elevated intracranial pressure.
Bathing/hygiene and feeding self-care deficit	• Provide all feeding and hygiene measures for patient.
Altered patterns of urinary elimination	• Assess for retention. • Maintain indwelling catheter if necessary *to empty bladder.*
Hyperthermia	• Take rectal temperature every 2 hours *to detect fever.* • Administer antipyretics as prescribed *to lower body temperature.* • Sponge with tepid water or alcohol in water *to lower body temperature.*
Ineffective breathing pattern	• Monitor closely for signs of respiratory paralysis, and initiate ventilatory assistance as needed.
Sensory/perceptual alterations (visual, auditory, olfactory)	• Monitor for reflex and sensory changes. • Minimize environmental stimuli; give clear, concise explanations to patient. • Clarify stimuli that patient may be misperceiving.
Altered thought processes	• Supervise closely; disoriented patients cannot be responsible for their actions. • Protect from injury with side rails or restraints, if needed. • Monitor for changes in level of consciousness, orientation, and memory. • Reorient the confused patient as appropriate.
Impaired physical mobility	• *To prevent decubiti, footdrop, contractures, and muscle weakness:* Use intermittent-pressure mattress, foot board, and frequent turning of comatose patients. Administer range of motion exercises. Give attention to body alignment. Gradually increase physical activity during convalescence. • Monitor for impaired motor ability during convalescence. • Refer for graded rehabilitation therapy, and reinforce and support patient's relearning efforts on the unit.
Potential for infection: patient contacts	• The viral disease associated with infectious viral encephalitis can be transmitted, and isolation procedures specific for the disease should be instituted (see specific diseases and isolation procedures in this chapter). • Only general principles of asepsis are necessary for amebic meningoencephalitis or mosquito-borne encephalitis.

Patient Education

1. Amebic meningoencephalitis can be prevented by swimming in chlorinated pools only.
2. Mosquito-borne encephalitis can be prevented by environmental control of mosquitoes, particularly through elimination of stagnant pools of water, where they breed, and by wearing protective clothing, screening living quarters, and using repellents.
3. Sequelae of encephalitis include mental deterioration, paralysis, and possible convulsive disorders, particularly in children. Families should be informed of the need for periodic evaluation and long-term physical therapy and of potential resources to help them cope with a handicapped family member.

Evaluation

Patient Outcome	Data Indicating That Outcome is Reached
Cerebrospinal fluid findings are normal.	There are fewer than 30 cells/mm^3. Glucose, protein, and pressure are normal. There are no organisms in cultures. Color is clear.
Vital signs are normal.	Blood pressure, temperature, pulse, and respiration are normal.
All cells receive oxygen.	Blood levels (O_2 saturation, carbon dioxide, and Po_2) are normal.
Motor responses to stimuli are appropriate.	Pupils are equal and reactive to light. There is no resistance to neck flexion. Straight legs may be raised from the bed with patient in a prone position. Patient is able to walk and carry out all functions without residual weakness or impairment.
There is no pain.	Patient does not have headache or pain in neck and back.
Motor function is normal, or patient is participating in therapeutic exercise.	Patient has full range of motion and is increasing in muscle strength and purposeful movement and coordination. Patient is able to or is increasing in ability to ambulate and to carry out all activities of daily living.
Sensory perceptions are normal.	Patient responds appropriately to all stimuli. Visual, hearing, smell, and touch test are positive. There is no hallucinatory behavior.
Mental status is normal.	Patient is oriented to person, place, and time and exhibits recall of recent and past events. Affect is appropriate to environment stimuli. Patient is awake and responds to environmental stimuli. Adults demonstrate cognitive ability, ability to problem solve, concentration, and attentiveness.
Patient or family is aware of needs and able to use resources.	Patient or family of patient with a residual limitation in physical or mental function has been referred for appropriate therapy during convalescence. Family of disabled person has been given an opportunity to express concerns and has been referred for counseling and to support groups if necessary.

INFECTIOUS DISEASES OF THE SKIN

The two diseases discussed in this section are manifested primarily with skin lesions that have potential or actual systemic pathologic findings. They are differentiated from skin infections discussed in Chapter 5 because a distinct pathogen causes each of these conditions (Table 13-17).

Leprosy

Leprosy is a chronic systemic infection characterized by lesions of the skin and mucous membranes, involvement and palpable enlargement of peripheral nerves, and trophic changes in skin, muscle, and bone.

Pathophysiology[41,48]

The exact transmission of the *Mycobacterium leprae* is uncertain. The organism can be found in the skin lesions, nasal passages, blood, and breast milk of infected persons, which suggests that skin contact may not be the only vehicle of transmission. The disease is not highly contagious. Because the incubation period is long, there is speculation that adult-onset disease may actually be acquired in childhood.

The disease is differentiated into two forms, lepromatous and tuberculoid, with borderline classifications representing the clinical expressions between the two distinct forms. The exact clinical expression of the disease may be determined in part by cell-mediated immune responses in the host; a cellular immune response is lacking in persons developing lepromatous leprosy.

Both forms produce progressively destructive granulomatous skin and mucous membrane lesions, which can be differentiated histologically, and sensory and autonomic peripheral nerve damage.

The course of the lepromatous type is progressive and malignant with continual activity of the organism in the lesions that causes an extensive, gradually developing granulomatous condition in the skin and peripheral nerves and a continuous bacteremia. Nerve destruction leads to atrophy of skin and muscles and eventual absorption of small bones with extensive deformity. Erythema nodosum and eye damage, secondary to corneal insensitivity, are possible complications.

The course of the tuberculoid type is benign and less progressive, with few bacteria in the lesions but with acute-onset asymmetric nerve involvement.

Diagnostic Studies and Findings[48]

Microscopic Examination of Stained Tissue from Lesion

Positive for acid-fast bacilli

Biopsy from Periphery of Skin Lesion

Foamy lepra cells plus acid-fast bacilli in lepromatous leprosy

Damage to peripheral nerves in tuberculoid leprosy

Table 13-17
Overview of Infectious Diseases of the Skin

	Leprosy	Erysipelas (Necrotizing Cellulitus)
Occurrence	11 million cases in world; highest in low socioeconomic areas; endemic in some tropic and subtropic areas; increasing in United States	Sporadic; most common in persons over 20 yr and in infants
Etiologic agent	*Mycobacterium leprae* (Hansen's bacillus)	*Streptococcus pyogenes*, group A, with 70 serologically distinct types
Reservoir	Humans; infections has been found in armadillos in Louisiana and Texas	Humans
Transmission	Prolonged intimate contact, agent gains entrance through broken skin and respiratory passages	Direct contact with respiratory secretions of a person infected with organism or with a carrier
Incubation period	3-6 yr; shortest known is 7 mo	1-3 d
Period of communicability	As long as bacilli are present; not communicable after 3 mo of treatment	10-21 d; months in untreated cases with purulent discharge
Susceptibility and resistance	Resistance depends on ability to develop a cell-mediated immunity; children may be more susceptible	General; one attack predisposes person to subsequent attacks; women and those with debilitating conditions more susceptible
Report to local health authority	Mandatory case report	Only outbreaks; no individual case reports

Data from Benenson.[5]

Lepromin Skin Test for Patients with Known Leprosy to Distinguish the Types

Positive test: hard nodule 3 to 4 weeks after intradermal injection; majority of the population shows a positive test
Positive in patients with tuberculoid leprosy
Negative in patients with lepromatous leprosy

Medical Plan[5]

Surgery

Plastic surgery to correct deformities

Medications

Anti-infective agents used in combination
- Dapsone (DDS), 100 mg/d for 6 mo to 2 yr
- Clofazimine, 300 mg once a mo plus 50 mg/d for 6 mo to 2 yr
- Rifampin, 600 mg once a mo for 6 mo to 2 yr

General Management

Counseling to cope with stigma attached to the disease
Orthopaedic aids
Prevention: immunization of close contacts with BCG: prophylactic treatment of contacts with dapsone for 3 years

NURSING CARE

Nursing Assessment[5,48]

Skin

Initial: flat pigmented or erythematoid skin lesions
Lepromatous: symmetric lesions consisting of numerous macules, with diffuse infiltrations and margins shading into the surrounding skin; lesions may be nodular and may ulcerate; they are not anesthetic; usually appear on earlobes, nose, eyebrows, forehead, cheeks, lips, elbows, and fingers; loss of hair, particularly eyebrows
Tuberculoid: asymmetric, circumscribed, dry macules or plaques; always anesthetic

Neurologic Concerns

Peripheral nerves: local or widespread anesthesia; muscle weakness, atrophy, and paralysis; trophic ulcers; disfigurement on extremities resulting from traumatic injury
Eye: photophobia, conjunctivitis, paralysis of eyelids; corneal injury

Upper Respiratory Tract

Nasal stuffiness or obstruction
Epistaxis
Perforated septum
Collapse of nasal bridge

Ulceration in any mucous membrane
Difficulty in breathing or swallowing
Change in timbre of voice

Systemic Concerns

Manifestations of erythema nodosum leprosum: malaise, fever, lymphadenopathy, and arthralgia

Nursing Dx & Intervention

Nursing Diagnosis	Nursing Intervention/Rationale
Noncompliance	• Monitor medication usage and side effects *to facilitate compliance*. (See "Patient Education.")
Body image disturbance	• Refer for or provide long-term support and rehabilitative help needed for patients with disfigurement. (See p. 1751 for additional interventions.)
Potential for infection	• For hospitalized patients with lepromatous leprosy, use contact isolation procedures *to prevent transmission to others* (see p. 1297).

Patient Education[5]

1. Compliance with therapy is necessary. Explain side effects of long-term drug treatment.
2. The patient should report medication reactions to the physician immediately.
3. Household contacts of the patient should be examined every 6 to 12 months for at least 5 years.
4. Assure the patient that continuing with therapy can minimize disfigurement.

Evaluation

Patient Outcome	Data Indicating That Outcome is Reached
Patient is complying with treatment.	Patient is taking prescribed medication and is returning for periodic evaluation. Close contacts are being evaluated.
Patient is aware of needs and able to use resources.	Patient is using rehabilitative or counseling services as needed.

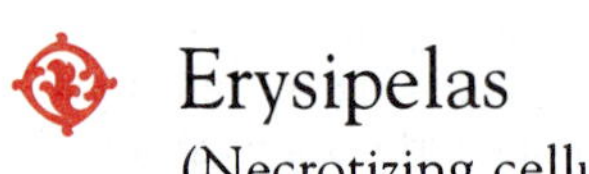

Erysipelas

(Necrotizing cellulitis)

Erysipelas is an acute inflammatory reaction of the superficial lymphatics of the skin accompanied by fever and systemic symptoms.

Pathophysiology[40,41]

Erysipelas is an acute, rapidly progressive inflammatory reaction of superficial lymph vessels. It is frequently associated with previous respiratory or systemic infection with group A streptococcus or with preexisting lymph obstruction. Lymph channels become filled with the streptococci, leukocytes, and fibrin. The inflammation spreads peripherally through the lymph channels, and creates a lesion characteristic of the condition. The infection may remain localized in the dermis, may extend into subcutaneous tissue and form a cellulitis, or may be disseminated into the blood to produce a bacteremia. Leukocytosis is always present. There is a tendency for the condition to recur.

Diagnostic Studies and Findings[41]

There are no tests to diagnose erysipelas definitively, since the group A streptococcus is rarely isolated or cultured from lesion exudate. A history of a streptococcal infection plus the characteristics of the lesion is used for diagnosis.

Medical Plan[41]

Medications

Anti-infective agents
- Mild cases in adult
  - Procaine penicillin (Wycillin), 600,000 U IM once or twice daily, or
  - Penicillin V (V-cillin), 250-500 g po q6h, or
  - Erythromycin (Erythrocin), 0.25-0.5 mg po q6h
- Extensive cases: penicillin G, 600,000-2 million U IV q6h

NURSING CARE

Nursing Assessment[5,40,48]

Skin

Abrupt-onset, hot, stinging, itching of skin
Painful, red, indurated thickening that begins as a small lesion and spreads marginally for 4 to 6 days; margins have a raised, firm, palpable border
Rash on face may have a butterfly distribution; central point of origin may clear as periphery extends; face and legs are common sites; raised portion may contain superficial blebs with clear yellowish fluid

Systemic Symptoms

Fever
May have sore throat, cervical adenopathy, headache, and vomiting

Nursing Dx & Intervention

Nursing Diagnosis	Nursing Intervention/Rationale
Impaired skin integrity	• Administer antibiotics as prescribed *to maintain therapeutic levels of circulating antibiotics.* • Apply cool, sterile saline dressings *to decrease pain.* • Observe for symptoms of systemic spread of infection. • If lesion is on an extremity, elevate and immobilize extremity *to prevent edema.*

Patient Education

1. Patient must take complete course of antibiotic therapy.
2. Report recurrence of pain, erythema, or edema to physician.

Evaluation

Patient Outcome	Data Indicating That Outcome is Reached
There is no infection.	Temperature is normal. Blood leukocyte count is normal. There is no heat, erythema, pain, or edema of skin.

ARTHROPOD-TRANSMITTED FEVERS

The diseases presented in this section are severe systemic infections of the blood caused by pathogens transmitted to humans by infected arthropods. The rickettsial fevers, caused by rickettsiae that are transmitted by infected body lice, fleas, mites, or ticks, are presented first. The mosquito-borne fevers, malaria and dengue, caused by protozoa and viruses, are discussed second. Table 13-18 summarizes arthropod-borne fevers.

Rickettsial fevers: Rocky Mountain spotted fever, epidemic and endemic typhus

Rocky Mountain spotted fever is an acute rickettsial infectious disease transmitted to humans by infected ticks and manifested by severe systemic symptoms and a macular or maculopapular rash. The disease is severe, with a 10% to 20% fatality rate in the untreated. The rate increases with age.

Epidemic typhus is an acute rickettsial infectious disease transmitted from person to person by infected body lice during epidemics. It is characterized by acute-onset, severe systemic symptoms and a macular rash. The fatality rate in untreated individuals is 10% to 40%.

Endemic (murine) typhus is an acute rickettsial infectious disease transmitted to humans by fleas that have fed on infected rats. It is clinically similar to epidemic typhus, but milder, with a fatality rate of 2% in untreated individuals.

There are 10 immunologically distinct, but clinically similar, infectious diseases caused by different types of rickettsiae. These five have occurred in the United States: epidemic typhus, endemic (murine) typhus, Rocky Mountain spotted fever, rickettsialpox, and Q fever. Rocky Mountain spotted fever and endemic typhus occur with the greatest frequency.

Table 13-18
Overview of Arthropod-Transmitted Fevers

	Rickettsial Fevers			Mosquito-Borne Fevers	
	Rocky Mountain Spotted Fever	**Epidemic Typhus Fever (Louse Borne)**	**Endemic Typhus Fever (Flea Borne; Murine Typhus)**	**Malaria**	**Dengue**
Occurrence	United States: spring and summer; in western United States incidence is highest in adult males; in eastern United States, highest in children; two thirds of cases are from North and South Carolina, Virginia, Maryland, Georgia, Tennessee, and Oklahoma	Endemic in underdeveloped areas; epidemics occur; last outbreak in United States in 1921	Worldwide; found in areas where rats are uncontrolled; increases in late summer and autumn; 80 cases/yr in United States	Endemic in tropics and subtropics; acquired by travelers to those areas; 400-800 cases/yr in the United States; increasing possibly due to spread of chloroquine resistance	Endemic in tropical areas; recent epidemics in Central America, Mexico, the Caribbean, and the Rio Grande valley; mosquitoes carrying the virus have been migrating north to United States, although most cases seen in the United States are in travelers to endemic areas
Etiologic agent	*Rickettsia rickettsii*	*Rickettsia prowazekii*	*Rickettsia typhi*	*Plasmodium vivax, P. malariae, P. falciparum, P. ovale*	Flavivirus, four immunologically distinct serotypes (types 1, 2, 3, and 4)
Reservoir	Ticks	Humans	Rats	Humans	Mosquitoes and humans as one reservoir
Transmission	Bite from infected tick	Infected body louse	Infected rat fleas carry agent to humans	Bite from infected female *Anopheles* mosquito, blood transfusion, or congenital	Bite from infected mosquito; *Aedes* species, particularly *A. albopictus*
Incubation period	3-14 d	1-2 wk; average is 12 d	1-2 wk; average is 12 d	Dependent on strain of *Plasmodium* agent; average is 12-30 d; may be as long as 8-10 mo	3-15 d; average is 5-6 d
Period of communicability	Not communicable person to person	Not directly communicable; body louse acquires organism from infected person during febrile illness and for 3 d after fever	Not directly communicable; infected fleas remain so for life (up to 1 yr)	Untreated cases may be a source of mosquito infection for 1-3 yr; stored blood is infected for 16 d	Infected persons are a source of infection for mosquitoes 1 d before and 5 d after disease onset; mosquitoes are infective for the remainder of their lives (1-4 mo)
Susceptibility and resistance	General; infection confers lifetime immunity	General; infection confers long-lasting immunity	General; infection confers immunity; cross-immunity with epidemic typhus	General; tolerance present in adults in endemic areas; black Africans show a natural resistance	General; children have less severe cases; immunity to one subtype of virus follows infection with that type
Report to local health authority	In some states where disease is endemic	Mandatory case report	Mandatory case report	Mandatory case report	Report during epidemics

Data from Benenson.[5]

Although epidemic typhus is rare, it is discussed with endemic typhus because of the clinical similarities (Table 13-18).

Pathophysiology[40,41,48]

The pathophysiology, although not completely understood, appears to be the same for all of these rickettsial infections. Differences in severity of disease manifestations are the result of differences in degree of the pathologic process and not of differences in the process.

Rickettsiae, like viruses, are intracellular parasites that replicate and metabolize only within host cells. The pathogens are carried in the feces of their respective arthropods and are deposited on the skin while the arthropod feeds on humans. Rickettsiae are subsequently rubbed or scratched into the open skin lesion produced by the arthropod bite.

Initially, a local neutrophilic inflammatory response occurs at the site of skin inoculation. Later, mononuclear cells infiltrate and phagocytose the rickettsiae. This local tissue reaction may result in an eschar. The rickettsiae then replicate and are disseminated within mononuclear cells throughout the vascular system.

Once in the blood, rickettsiae invade the cytoplasm of vascular endothelial cells, replicate there, and cause the cells to burst. A rapidly progressive systemic angiitis with severe systemic manifestations develops, heralding the acute onset of these diseases. Vascular endothelial edema, fibrin and platelet deposition, and microthrombi development lead to obstruction and occlusion of small blood vessels with resultant hemorrhage, tissue infarction, and necrosis.

Other vascular changes include increased permeability with perivascular accumulation of neutrophils, macrophages, and lymphocytes, and plasma loss into tissues. The mechanism for this process is unknown. It is hypothesized that the vascular permeability results from an allergic response of the host to the toxin produced by the pathogen.

Vascular lesions are widely disseminated and most frequently affect the skin, myocardium, skeletal muscles, kidneys, and central nervous system. Disease symptoms, following the initial systemic manifestations, result from the localization of the vascular lesions and tissue infarctions and the loss of circulating plasma. A petechial skin rash that becomes purpuric, clouded sensorium, edema, hypotension, and peripheral vascular circulatory collapse are characteristic. Myocardial involvement with symptoms of myocarditis results from the focal vascular lesions plus a diffuse mononuclear cell infiltration. A shift in intracellular water and electrolytes in terminal stages of the disease may result in increases in circulating volume and tissue edema.

Complications include shock, disseminated intravascular coagulation, gangrene of distal extremities and genitalia in cases of severe local thrombosis, renal failure, pneumonia, coma, and death. Fatality generally is associated with delay in diagnosis and treatment rather than with treatment failure.

Both antibiotic therapy and the development of circulating antibodies during the second week of acute disease arrest the progression of rickettsiae but do not completely eradicate them. The pathogen remains latent in cells, and relapses, although uncommon, do occur. Recurrence of epidemic typhus in the form of Brill-Zinsser disease is seen in U.S immigrants who contracted typhus in Europe during World War II.

Neurologic or myocardial sequelae are uncommon in survivors of typhus but are common in survivors of Rocky Mountain spotted fever. Potential sequelae include deafness, disturbances in vision and speech, mental confusion, cardiac arrhythmias, and amputations.

Common laboratory findings include decreased platelets, normocytic anemia, hyponatremia, hypochloremia, and hypoalbuminemia. The WBC count is normal, and liver function tests are normal or slightly abnormal. In disseminated intravascular coagulation there is a thrombocytopenia, hypofibrinogenemia, and prolonged prothrombin and partial thromboplastin times.

Diagnostic Studies and Findings[40,41]

Immunofluorescence of Skin Tissue

Identification of rickettsiae during third or fourth day of Rocky Mountain spotted fever

Weil-Felix Agglutination Test

Does not differentiate Rocky Mountain spotted fever from typhus

Increase in antibody titers can be detected after 7 to 10 days of illness in the untreated but may be delayed for 4 weeks if antibiotic therapy is begun early

Titers decrease rapidly during late convalescence

Strong reaction to *Proteus* OX-19 strain is diagnostic of typhus

Weaker reaction to *Proteus* OX-19 and OX-2 strains is suggestive of Rocky Mountain spotted fever

Complement Fixation

Fourfold rise in antigen-specific antibodies by end of second week

Medical Plan[5,40,41]

Medications

Anti-infective agents

- Tetracycline (Achromycin; others), 25-50 mg/kg/d po in 4 divided doses until patient is afebrile for 48 h, or for 5-7 d, *or*
- Chloramphenicol (Chloromycetin), 50-100 mg/kg/d po in four divided doses until patient is afebrile for 48 h, or for 5-7 d
- Either of above may be given IV in appropriate doses during initial toxic stage
- Doxycycline (Vibramycin), 5 mg/kg po in a single dose is curative for epidemic typhus

Delousing epidemic typhus patients with dusting with an insecticide powder (10% DDT or 1% lindane)
Cardiac glycosides
Digitalis for cardiac decompensation
Narcotic analgesics
Codeine or meperidine (Demerol) for severe headache

General Management*

IV fluids and electrolytes (to be administered cautiously)
Sedation of delirious patients with paraldehyde or chloral hydrate
High-protein, high-calorie diet
Transfusion of serum albumin
Packed red cells for anemia
Oxygen for pulmonary complications
Refrigerated blanket for fever control
Prevention: epidemic typhus patient contacts should be deloused

*Depends on severity of disease and complications.

NURSING CARE

Nursing Assessment[40,41,48]

	Rocky Mountain Spotted Fever	Epidemic Typhus	Endemic Typhus
Onset	Sudden	Sudden	Gradual and less severe
Subjective symptoms	Chills; severe headache; extreme myalgias and arthritic-type pain; prostration	Chills; severe headache; extreme myalgias and arthritic-type pain; prostration	Chills; severe headache; extreme myalgias and arthritis-type pain; prostration
Body temperature	39°-40° C (102°-104° F); AM remissions; fever lysis in 2-3 wk if untreated	40°-41° C (104°-106° F); unremitting; fever lysis in 2-3 wk if untreated	39°-40° C (102°-104° F); fever lysis in 2-3 wk if untreated
Eyes	Injected and suffused conjunctiva; photophobia	Injected and suffused conjunctiva; photophobia	
Skin	Eschar at site of tick bite Macular rash (3-5 mm) on mucous membranes, face, palms, and soles, beginning on third to fifth day; red to purple colored; blanches on pressure; begins on face and extremities; spreads in a centripetal fashion, involving the trunk last; if untreated, rash becomes maculopapular to petechial to purpuric; areas coalesce with possible necrosis and gangrene Jaundice	No eschar Macular rash (3-5 mm) beginning on fourth to seventh day; pink to rose colored; blanches on pressure; begins in axillary folds and upper trunk; spreads to involve the whole body except face, palms, and soles; if untreated, rash becomes maculopapular to petechial to purpuric; areas coalesce with possible necrosis and gangrene	Macular rash (3-5 mm) beginning on fourth to seventh day; pink to rose colored; blanches on pressure; begins on upper thorax and abdomen; remains central in distribution; becomes maculopapular, lasting 4-8 d; rash is more sparse and discrete than in epidemic typhus
Respiratory concerns	Nonproductive cough may be present; rapid respiration	Nonproductive cough may be present	Nonproductive cough may be present
Lymph nodes	Unilateral postauricular adenopathy if bite was on the head		
Abdomen	Hepatosplenomegaly, gastrointestinal distress, anorexia; constipation	Splenomegaly; constipation	
Central nervous system	Mental dullness and lethargy, progressing to delirium, stupor, convulsions, coma, and death; may have focal neurologic signs such as deafness, tinnitus, nuchal rigidity, tremor, vertigo; hallucinations, paranoid behavior, and extreme irritability	Mental dullness and lethargy, progressing to delirium, stupor, convulsions, coma, and death; may have focal neurologic signs such as deafness, tinnitus, vertigo; hallucinations, paranoid behavior, and extreme irritability	Rare to have central nervous system symptoms

	Rocky Mountain Spotted Fever	Epidemic Typhus	Endemic Typhus
Cardiovascular concerns	Early: bradycardia Later: tachycardia, gallop rhythm; hypotension and intractable shock may lead to death	Early: bradycardia Later: tachycardia, gallop rhythm; hypotension and intractable shock may lead to death	Rare to have cardiovascular symptoms
Urinary concerns	Oliguria or anuria in the event of circulatory collapse; incontinence in severely ill	Oliguria or anuria in the event of circulatory collapse; incontinence in severely ill	
Complications	Pneumonia; hemorrhage; iritis; nephritis; hemiplegia; deafness; impaired vision; persistent tachycardia	Pneumonia; otitis media; parotitis	

Nursing Dx & Intervention

Nursing Diagnosis	Nursing Intervention/Rationale
Altered tissue perfusion	• Administer antibiotics as soon as ordered *to prevent vascular damage.* • Regularly check vital signs and intake and output *to detect changes early.* • Monitor for signs of shock: hypotension, cyanosis, tachycardia, absent peripheral pulses, urinary output less than 30 ml/hour. • Administer oxygen *to maintain adequate circulating oxygen.* • Maintain patient in a supine position, and give nothing by mouth *to prevent aspiration.* • Prepare for cardiopulmonary resuscitation. • Maintain indwelling urinary catheter *to monitor output.*
Pain	• Administer analgesics regularly as prescribed *to relieve severe headache.*
Sensory/perceptual alterations (visual and auditory)	• Minimize unnecessary environmental stimuli *to prevent hallucinations.* • Continuously interpret the environment for patient *to prevent confusion.* • Supervise closely *to prevent injury.* • Restrain if necessary *to prevent injury.* • Administer sedatives as prescribed.
Impaired skin integrity	• Turn frequently and position *to prevent pressure over bony prominences or purpuric or necrotic areas.* • Monitor distal extremities, nose, and genitalia *to detect signs of gangrene.*
Potential fluid volume deficit	• Administer IV fluids slowly in enough quantity to maintain 1500 ml/day urine output.
Fluid volume excess	• Monitor IV infusion rate hourly *to prevent overhydration.* • Monitor for edema *to detect overhydration.* • Measure intake and output *to ensure output equal to intake.* • Stop IV line if anuria occurs.
Altered nutrition: less than body requirements	• Offer frequent, small high-protein, high-calorie feedings *to compensate for increased metabolic needs.* • Administer nasogastric feedings if necessary.
Altered oral mucous membrane	• Administer frequent oral hygiene *to prevent parotitis.* • Monitor *to detect hemorrhage* in patients with Rocky Mountain spotted fever.
Altered patterns of urinary elimination	• Monitor intake and output (hourly output should be at least 40 ml) *to detect oliguria and anuria.*
Potential for trauma	• Constantly supervise delirious or convulsing patient *to prevent injury.* • Use padded headboard and side rails *to prevent injury.* • Administer sedatives as prescribed *to decrease uncontrolled muscle activity.*
Activity intolerance	• Provide opportunity for adequate rest until patient's energy returns. • Reassure patient that the loss of energy is temporary *to relieve anxiety.*
Constipation	• Administer small enemas *to relieve constipation* and rectal tube *to relieve flatulence.*
Potential for infection	• Search for ticks in warm, dark areas of patients suspected of having Rocky Mountain spotted fever.

Nursing Diagnosis	Nursing Intervention/Rationale
	• Wear gloves and do not touch ticks with hand *to prevent contamination with tick feces.* • Attached ticks cannot be removed directly but must be induced to release their hold on skin. Apply a drop of kerosene, lighter fluid, gasoline, or alcohol, or barely touch with a hot match. • Remove loosened tick with tweezers or forceps *to prevent contamination with tick feces.* • Disinfect patient's clothing *to kill body lice and ticks.* • Thoroughly bathe patient with epidemic typhus and delouse patient weekly until discharged. Wear gown and gloves when handling patient until delousing is complete *to protect yourself from infestation.*
Hyperthermia	• Monitory body temperature *to detect fever.* • Sponge bathe frequently *to lower and maintain* temperature at 39° C (102° F). • Use refrigerated blankets if necessary *to lower body temperature quickly.*

Patient Education

1. Explain that relapses may occur and recurrence of symptoms should be reported to physician immediately so antibiotic therapy can be resumed rapidly.
2. Tell patient to avoid tick-infested areas, to check body surfaces every 3 to 4 hours for attached ticks if working or playing in infested areas, and to remove ticks in fashion described above.

Evaluation

Patient Outcome	Data Indicating That Outcome is Reached
Body temperature is normal.	Oral adult temperature is 37° C (98.6° F).
All cells receive oxygen.	Skin and mucous membranes are warm, moist, and normal colored. There are no purpuric or necrotic skin lesions. Peripheral pulses are palpable. Blood pressure, pulse, and respirations are normal. Patient is awake and oriented and communicates coherently; sensory and visual perceptions are normal.
Urinary elimination is normal.	Urinary output is between 1500 and 3000 ml/day or equal to intake. There is no edema.
Laboratory findings are within normal limits.	Serum albumin, sodium, and chloride levels are normal. Prothrombin time, partial thromboplastin time, platelets, fibrinogen, and RBC count are normal.
There are no complications.	Pneumonia, renal failure, gangrene, mental or neurosensory sequelae, or cardiac arrhythmias are not present.
Nutrition is adequate for body requirements.	Patient has not lost weight during course of the illness. Energy level is adequate, following convalescence, to enable patient to perform all ADLs. There are no signs of anemia or hypoalbuminemia.

Malaria

Malaria is a severe systemic infection caused by one of four protozoan parasites of the *Plasmodium* genus. The parasite is transmitted to humans through mosquito bites. Disease severity varies with the type of plasmodium causing the infection, with some plasmodia killing more than 10% of untreated individuals. The duration of acute malarial disease is long, sometimes lasting months, with recurrent fever in treated individuals. Relapses occur irregularly for years in untreated persons.

Pathophysiology[41,48]

Four species of plasmodia produce malaria in humans, and more than one species may be present in any given malarial infection. The life cycle of the plasmodium is important to the pathophysiology of the disease. The sexual stage of the cycle occurs only in the intestines of the *Anopheles* mosquito, producing sporozoites that are discharged in mosquito saliva. The asexual development of the pathogen takes place in humans. There are two phases to the asexual cycle within humans, the exoerythrocytic and the erythrocytic. The exoerythrocytic phase begins when plasmodium sporozoites from mosquito saliva are inoculated into human blood and are carried to the liver, where they invade hepatocytes. There they form cystlike structures that rupture and release hundreds of merozoites into the blood when they mature. Once in the blood parasites never reinvade the liver. Two of the species, *P. vivax* and *P. ovale,* may retain some merozoites in the liver in a dormant form. Release of these at a later time causes relapsing malaria. Infection induced by transfusion of blood containing the life cycle form of merozoites does not progress through the exoerythrocytic phase but begins directly with the erythrocytic phase.

The erythrocytic phase of the plasmodium life cycle is responsible for pathologic findings in the human host. Plasmodium merozoites invade select erythrocytes that contain surface receptors that attract the plasmodia. The absence of these RBC receptors in black Africans protects them from symptomatic malaria. Once in erythrocytes the merozoites feed and grow into trophozoites. Trophozoites feed on hemoglobin, metabolizing the globin fraction and depositing the heme fraction as hematin granules into the cytoplasm. Trophozoites sexually segment into numerous merozoites. This causes the erythrocytes to rupture and release merozoites into the circulation, enabling them to reinvade additional erythrocytes within seconds.

The process of erythrocytic invasion, asexual multiplication of the plasmodia, and erythrocytic rupture continues until antibodies develop within the host to control the parasite or until the host is treated with sufficient antimicrobial agents. An antibody response is adequate to limit all malarial plasmodia except *P. falciparum*, which, in the absence of treatment, may overwhelm the host with severe fulminating disease resulting in death.

Symptomatic attacks of chills, fever, and diaphoresis coincide with completion of the erythrocytic life cycle of the plasmodium in humans. The length of time between attacks varies with the *Plasmodium* species: every 42 to 48 hours in *P. vivax*, 48 hours in *P. falciparum,* 50 hours in *P. ovale,* and 72 hours in *P. malariae*.

The erythrocytic activity of the parasite produces the following pathophysiologic changes: fever and its physiologic consequences, hemolytic anemia, tissue hypoxia resulting from anemia and alterations in the microcirculation, and coagulation defects resulting from immunopathologic events.

Fever with marked vasodilation leads to a decrease in effective plasma volume with a resultant orthostatic hypotension and an increased secretion of ADH and aldosterone. Diaphoresis and vomiting that accompany the toxic fever result in fluid and electrolyte loss and possible hyponatremia.

Anemia triggers the spleen to store erythrocytes, resulting in splenomegaly. Anemia also results in tissue hypoxia, particularly in the kidneys, lungs, liver, and central nervous system, with resultant dysfunction to those systems. Erythrocyte invasion also causes erythrocytes to adhere to vascular endothelium, slowing the blood flow and accentuating tissue hypoxia, edema, and vascular pathologic findings and hemorrhage.

The immune response is pathologic as well as protective. Excess immunoglobulin production triggers hypersplenism and plays a role in the further development of anemia and in the development of neutropenia and thrombocytopenia. Laboratory evidence of coagulation defects in some patients can be observed. These include decreases in fibrinogen and platelets (platelets less than 50,000/mm^3), decreases in factors V, VII, VIII, and X, and prolonged prothrombin and partial thromboplastin times.

Specific organ system complications resulting from the previously described pathologic conditions include renal and hepatic failure, pulmonary edema, and central nervous system disturbances resulting from perivascular edema and hemorrhage in the cerebral cortex. Laboratory evidence of renal failure includes proteinuria and increased serum creatinine. Laboratory findings in hepatic failure include increases in serum transaminase and indirect serum bilirubin.

Laboratory findings present in uncomplicated malaria include leukopenia, relative or absolute monocytosis, a normochromic, normocytic hemolytic anemia, decreased platelets, and a false positive VDRL.

Diagnostic Studies and Findings[41,48]

Microscopic Examination of Stained Peripheral Blood Smear Taken at Least Twice Daily, Within 6 to 12 Hours After Chills

Identification of plasmodia in blood

Detection of granular, brownish pigment within monocytes or neutrophils, or identification of parasitized RBC

If more than 5% of RBCs are affected, *P. falciparum* should be suspected

Indirect Fluorescent Antibody

Increase in antibody titer after 1 week of illness

Useful for screening blood donors but should not be relied on for diagnosis

Medical Plan[5,14,41]

Uncomplicated infections with *P. ovale, P. vivax,* and *P. malariae* can be treated in an outpatient setting. Patients infected with *P. falciparum* should be hospitalized.

Medications

Anti-infective agents

- For uncomplicated infection with all species except chloroquine-resistant *P. falciparum*: chloroquine phosphate (Aralen), po, 25 mg/kg (base) administered over 3 d: 15 mg/kg the first day (10 mg initially and 5 mg 6 h later), 5 mg/kg the second day, and 5 mg/kg the third day
- For emergency treatment of severe infections or for persons unable to retain orally administered medications:
  - Chloroquine hydrochloride (Aralen hydrochloride), IM, 200 mg base q6h for 3 d
  - Quinine dihydrochloride, 650 mg (10 gr), diluted in

500 ml of normal saline, glucose, or plasma, administered slowly IV (never push and never give IM); repeat in 6 h (no more than three doses per 24 h)

For infection caused by chloroquine-resistant *P. falciparum:*

Quinine sulfate, po, 25-30 mg/kg/24 h in 3 divided doses for 7-10 d, plus

Pyrimethamine (Daraprim), po, 0.85 mg/kg/24 h in divided doses for 3 d, plus

Sulfadoxine, po, 500 mg qid for 5 d

Prevention of relapses from *P. vivax* and *P. ovale*

Primaquine phosphate, po, 0.25 mg base/kg/d for 14 d (26.3 mg/d for average adult) following treatment with chloroquine phosphate

Chemoprophylaxis for people traveling to areas where malaria is endemic

Chloroquine phosphate (Aralen), po, 300 mg (base) once weekly for 2 wk before entering and 6 wk after leaving an endemic area

NOTE: Those traveling to areas with high risk for acquiring *P. falciparum* malaria, and who are not sensitive to sulfonamides or pyrimethamine and who are not pregnant, can be given one dose of sulfadoxine-pyrimethamine (Fansidar) to have in their possession while traveling to take if symptoms develop. As an alternative to Fansidar for persons allergic to sulfonamides: doxycycline, 100 mg/d po while traveling.

General Management

IV fluids and electrolytes; restrict fluids in cerebral edema; monitor body weight and fluid intake and output

Assisted ventilation and intubation in pulmonary edema

Transfusion of packed RBCs in anemia

Transfusion of whole blood in shock

Corticosteroids in cerebral edema

Heparin, low-molecular weight dextran, or fresh frozen plasma in coagulopathy

Peritoneal or hemodialysis in renal failure

NURSING CARE

Nursing Assessment[41,48]

Prodrome: Subjective Symptoms Lasting 1 to Several Days

Myalgia

Fatigue, malaise

Slight chills

Paroxysms of chills, fever, and diaphoresis

Chill Phase: Skin

Cold, pale skin

Cyanotic nail beds

Severe shaking chills lasting 1 to 2 hours

Fever Phase

Body temperature

Fever of 39° to 41° C (103° to 106° F) lasting 3 to 6 hours, decreasing suddenly by lysis

Vital signs

Tachycardia

Tachypnea

Hypotension

Systemic manifestations

Severe headache, nausea, and vomiting

Cough

Diaphoresis phase

Skin

Profuse sweating

Systemic concerns

Weakness leading to sleep

Between Attacks

Abdomen

Hepatomegaly in *P. vivax* and *P. falciparum*

Splenomegaly in *P. vivax*

Abdominal pain

Lungs

Scattered rales

Systemic concerns

Energy returns to normal between attacks in all but *P. falciparum* infections

Vital signs

Tachycardia persisting between fever episodes

Additional Symptoms in *P. falciparum* Infections

Gastrointestinal concerns

Severe prolonged vomiting and diarrhea leading to dehydration and electrolyte imbalance

Skin

Jaundice resulting from hepatic dysfunction

Neurologic concerns

Delirium, convulsions, coma

Altered intellectual function, behavior changes, focal neurologic signs, positive Babinski's sign, tremors, and hemiparesis

Respiratory concerns

Pulmonary congestion and respiratory distress

Nursing Dx & Intervention

Nursing Diagnosis	Nursing Intervention/Rationale
Potential for infection	• Employ blood and body fluid precautions for duration of illness *to prevent transmission of pathogen* (see p. 1299).
Hypothermia	• Provide hot drinks and application of external heat *to provide comfort.*
Hyperthermia	• Monitor body temperature *to detect fever.* • Administer tepid water or alcohol sponge bath, ice cap to head, and analgesics and antipyretics as ordered *to decrease body temperature.* • Bathe patient and change clothing following diaphoresis *to promote comfort.*
Potential fluid volume deficit	• Monitor body weight, intake and output, and skin *to detect dehydration or overhydration.* • Encourage oral fluids *to ensure adequate intake.* • Administer IV fluids and electrolytes cautiously per protocol.
Potential for trauma	• Palpate gently *to protect patient from splenic rupture.* • Caution patient against lifting heavy objects *to protect from splenic rupture.*
Potential for injury related to chemotherapeutic agent	• Monitor patient receiving IV drugs to detect cardiotoxicity, hypotension, and widening of QRS complex. • Monitor to detect toxic reactions to oral quinine (tinnitus, headache, nausea, altered vision) and for hypersensitivity (bronchospasm, hemolytic anemia, thrombocytopenia).
Altered cerebral tissue perfusion	• Monitor for potentially fatal skin reactions to Fansidar *to discontinue drug immediately.* • Monitor and report changes in level of consciousness, behavior, or neurologic signs. • Protect delirious patient from injury.
Altered cardiopulmonary tissue perfusion	• Monitor for signs of pulmonary edema. • Limit fluid intake if necessary. • Prepare to assist ventilation if needed.
Altered renal tissue perfusion	• Monitor intake and output and body weight *to report edema or urinary output less than intake.* Limit intake *to prevent overhydration.*

Patient Education

1. Patients infected with *P. vivax* or *P. ovale* may still have plasmodia in the liver after treatment; remissions are possible. They should continue with prescribed medication for 14 days following initial treatment and should report recurrence of symptoms immediately.
2. All patients should return for blood examination 4 or 5 days after completion of treatment.
3. Patients should discontinue medications and seek medical help if they experience any reactions.
4. Persons taking doxycycline prophylactically during travel to areas where *P. falciparum* is endemic should be reminded that photosensitivity is possible when taking tetracyclines.
5. Travelers to malaria-endemic countries should follow recommendations for prophylaxis.
   a. Comply with pharmacologic prophylaxis (see "Medical Plan").
   b. Wear clothing that covers as much skin as possible, particularly during the evening and night.
   c. Frequently apply insect repellent on uncovered skin. Products containing *N,N*-diethylmeta-toluamide (Deet) are the most effective.
   d. Sleep only in screened areas and use mosquito netting if necessary.
   e. Stay indoors during the evening and night when the *Anopheles* mosquito is likely to bite.
   f. Use pyrethrum-containing flying insect spray in living and sleeping areas during the evening and night.
6. Chemoprophylaxis is not completely protective. Travelers who develop symptoms should seek medical assistance immediately. Early treatment is most effective and safe.

Evaluation

Patient Outcome	Data Indicating That Outcome is Reached
There is no infection.	No parasites are detetcted in peripheral blood smears 4 or 5 days after treatment.
Body temperature is normal.	Adult oral body temperature is consistently around 37° C (98.6° F) for 4 to 5 days after treatment. Paroxysms of chills and diaphoresis that accompany fever are absent.
Laboratory findings are within normal limits.	Leukocyte, monocyte, erythrocyte, and platelet counts are normal. Coagulation factors V, VII, VIII, and X are normal. Prothrombin time and partial thromboplastin time are normal. Serum transaminase, indirect bilirubin, and creatinine levels are normal. Serum sodium level is normal. Urine protein is normal.
Patient is aware of need for follow-up.	Patient expresses intent to return to physician for follow-up blood cultures
All cells receive oxygen.	Patient is alert and oriented to surroundings, speaks coherently, and has memory for recent and past events; behavior and affect are appropriate to the situation. All neurologic signs are normal.
Respiratory function is normal.	Breath sounds are clear. There is no dyspnea or cyanosis.
Urinary elimination is normal.	Urine output is 1500 to 3000 ml or equal to input. There is no evidence of edema.
Vital signs are normal.	Blood pressure, pulse, and respirations are normal.

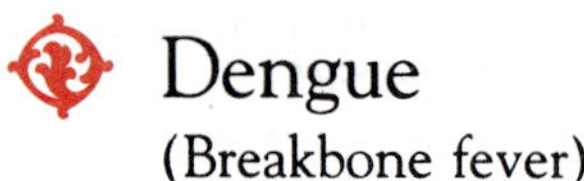

Dengue
(Breakbone fever)

Dengue (breakbone fever) is an acute viral febrile illness of short duration that is transmitted to humans through mosquito bites. The disease has clinical characteristics similar to other arthropod-borne viral fevers such as yellow fever, Colorado tick fever, and Venezuelan equine fever. The risk for dengue is increasing in the southern United States because of movement of infected mosquitoes northward from Mexico. Dengue is presented here as a prototype of the arthropod-borne viral fevers. Two forms of the disease, a benign and a hemorrhagic form, occur.

Pathophysiology[5,41,48]

The pathologic agents producing dengue are four immunologically distinct viruses that require both *Aedes* mosquitoes and humans for their viability. An *Aedes* mosquito that feeds on an infected person during the symptomatic viremic stage of dengue becomes infective after an incubation period of 8 to 10 days. Infective mosquitoes transmit the virus to every person they bite. In tropical and subtropical areas where *Aedes* organisms survive year-round, dengue is an endemic, and sometimes epidemic, disease in the population. Epidemics or disease outbreaks may occur anywhere that *Aedes* mosquitoes are present by the introduction of either infective mosquitoes or persons into the area.

Dengue occurs in two clinical disease forms: classic (benign) dengue and the more severe dengue hemorrhagic fever. Either form may be produced by any of the four viral serotypes. The mechanism for the development of two different dengue diseases is unknown. One hypothesis is that the form of the disease varies with differences in virulence within viral strains. A second hypothesis is that a primary infection with one viral serotype may result in the benign form of the disease but predispose one to an immunopathologic response to a subsequent infection with another serotype resulting in dengue hemorrhagic fever.

The pathologic process is similar in both disease forms although more extensive and life threatening in dengue hemorrhagic fever. Once injected, the virus replicates at the site of inoculation and in local lymphatic tissue. Viruses invade the blood within days, producing a viremia that lasts 4 to 5 days after symptomatic disease onset. The viremia results in endothelial swelling, mononuclear cell infiltration, increased vascular permeability, and perivascular edema. Extravasation of blood from dermal vessels produces a maculopapular or petechial rash. Leukopenia and lymphadenopathy are common. Symptom severity varies in the benign form.

In the hemorrhagic form of the disease, the increased vascular permeability is more severe, with extensive extravasation of blood and fluid into serous cavities and hemorrhage and congestion within many organs, particularly the spleen, liver, kidneys, pleura, and peritoneum. Blood changes include a thrombocytopenia, increase in platelet agglutinability, mild or moderate disseminated intravascular coagulation, and hemoconcentration. A rising hematocrit concentration on the third day of illness is a sign of impending life-threatening hypovolemic shock, the dengue shock syndrome. Vascular and blood component pathologic findings coincide with the development of an immune response and may result from the action of circulating antigen-antibody complexes, the activation of complement, or the release of vasoactive amines.

Laboratory findings in dengue hemorrhagic fever include decreased serum albumin and sodium; decreased platelets, fibrinogen, and coagulation factors V, VII, IX, and X; decreased C3 serum complement; a 20% or greater increase in hematocrit; the presence of fibrin split products in plasma and an increase in prothrombin time; and an increase in BUN and serum transaminase proportional to kidney and liver dysfunction, respectively.

Patients may spontaneously recover from dengue hemorrhagic fever or progress to hypovolemic shock. Untreated shock leads to tissue anoxia, coma, metabolic acidosis, hyperkalemia, and death within 12 to 24 hours.

Virus serotype-specific IgM antibodies develop early during the febrile period of both forms of the disease and persist for 8 weeks. This initial antibody response is followed within 1 or 2 days by a rise in IgG antibodies that persists for more than 40 years and confers lifetime immunity against the specific dengue serotype. Secondary infections with another dengue serotype initiate an early and extremely high IgG antibody response that cross reacts against the infecting serotype, the initial serotype, and other flaviviruses. This immune response is thought to play a role in the pathogenesis of dengue hemorrhagic fever.

Diagnostic Studies and Findings[44]

Animal or Cell Culture of Serum: Plaque Reduction Neutralization Method

- Isolation of dengue virus subtypes
- Takes 1 to 2 weeks for test
- Useful for diagnostic confirmation and epidemiologic surveillance

Neutralization, Hemagglutination Inhibition (HI), Radioimmunoassay (RIA), or Complement Fixation Tests

- Fourfold rise in titer to one serotype in a series of paired sera or single HI titer greater than 1:640 or CF titer greater than 1:32 suggests primary infection
- Single HI titer greater than 1:1280 or CF titer greater than 1:256 without fourfold change suggests secondary infection
- Fourfold change in titer to more than one serotype with HI titer greater than 1:640 or CF titer greater than 1:128 also suggests secondary infection

Medical Plan[5,41,48]

Medications

- Analgesic/antipyretic agents
  - Acetaminophen (Tylenol) (salicylates should not be used), 325-600 mg q4-6h
- Anticoagulants
  - Heparin for disseminated intravascular coagulation

General Management

- IV fluids and electrolytes
- Frequent monitoring of hematocrit
- Shock
  - IV lactated Ringer's solution, 10-20 ml/kg/h, plus plasma or plasma expanders (discontinue IV line when hematocrit decreases to 40% to prevent hypervolemia and pulmonary edema)
  - Central venous pressure line
  - Whole blood transfusions in severe hemorrhage
- Oxygen

NURSING CARE

Nursing Assessment[41,48]

Benign Dengue

- Subjective symptoms
  - Prodome: 12 hours; malaise, anorexia
  - Abrupt onset: chills, severe frontal headache, ocular pain, severe and incapacitating myalgia, arthralgia, and backache
- Throat
  - Mild pharyngitis
- Gastrointestinal concerns
  - Nausea and vomiting
  - Epigastric pain
- Body temperature
  - Fever of 40° C (104° F), unremitting and persisting for 3 to 7 days
  - Diphasic course with "saddle back" temperature curve
- Heart rate
  - Tachycardia for first few days of fever
  - Bradycardia during last days of fever
- Eyes
  - Injected conjunctivae
- Lymph nodes
  - Generalized tender lymphadenopathy
- Skin
  - First 1 or 2 days: transient erythematous flush over face, neck, and upper trunk, disappearing within a day
- Third to fifth day: distinct macular or maculopapular rash on trunk, spreading centrifugally to face and extremities; petechiae on palate, in the axillae, and on the lower extremities at the end of the febrile period
- Subjective symptoms during convalescence
  - Prolonged fatigue and depression
- Laboratory values
  - Leukopenia during febrile period

Hemorrhagic Dengue

- Same symptoms as benign dengue with the following additions:
- Skin and mucous membranes
  - Hemorrhagic symptoms during the febrile period: pos-

itive tourniquet test, purpura, epistaxis, gingival bleeding, hematemesis, melena, and hematuria
Jaundice
Abdomen
Hepatomegaly
Severe epigastric or generalized abdominal pain
Shock phase
Vital signs
Rapid, weak pulse
Hypotension; narrow pulse pressure
Rapid drop in body temperature
Skin
Cool, clammy, edematous skin
Circumoral cyanosis
Laboratory values
Profound thrombocytopenia
Increased hematocrit concentration

Nursing Dx & Intervention

Nursing Diagnosis	Nursing Intervention/Rationale
Altered tissue perfusion	• Monitor vital signs and intake and output *to detect symptoms of hemorrhage and shock.* • Monitor for signs of internal hemorrhage and for signs of shock: hypotension, cyanosis, cold edematous skin, tachycardia, absent peripheral pulses, and urinary output less than 30 ml/hour. (See Chapter 1 for interventions with shock.) • Administer oxygen *to ensure adequate circulating oxygen.* • Discontinue IV line in presence of pulmonary edema.
Pain	• Regularly administer analgesics, as prescribed, during acute symptomatic phase *to relieve pain.* • Frequently reposition patient *for comfort.* • Provide diversional activities as tolerated.
Potential fluid volume deficit	• Give IV fluids and electrolytes or oral fluids as tolerated *to meet additional needs resulting from fever.* • Monitor intake and output for output equal to intake.
Anxiety	• Inform patient that prolonged weakness and depression may extend into convalescence; reassure patient that this is expected and that it will not affect the eventual prognosis.
Hyperthermia	• Monitor body temperature *to detect fever.* • Administer antipyretics (avoid salicylates), tepid sponge baths, and adequate fluids *to decrease body temperature.*
Potential for infection: patient contacts	• Use blood and body fluid precautions for duration of hospitalization *to prevent transmission of pathogens to others.*

Patient Education

1. During illness, the patient must protect self from mosquito vectors to prevent transmission to others.
2. Patient can prevent future infections by protecting self from mosquito vectors with screened living quarters, protective clothing, and insect repellents on exposed skin and clothing when in the proximity of mosquitoes. *Aedes* mosquitoes enter homes and usually bite during the day.
3. Mosquitoes can be controlled around living quarters by eliminating potential breeding places, particularly any water-filled containers.
4. Persons living close to the patient may have been exposed to mosquito vectors infected with dengue. They should be monitored for early diagnosis of dengue.
5. Prolonged weakness and depression are characteristic of the convalescent period.

Evaluation

Patient Outcome	Data Indicating That Outcome is Reached
All cells receive oxygen.	Skin is warm and normal colored; there is no edema, cyanosis, or purpura. Peripheral pulses are strong. Urinary output is 3000 ml or equal to intake.
There is no infection.	There are no signs of internal hemorrhage or dermal bleeding. Vital signs are normal.

Patient Outcome	Data Indicating That Outcome is Reached
The patient appears physically comfortable.	During acute stage, patient rests without signs of pain.
The patient returns to preillness energy level.	During convalescence, patient gradually increases self-care and daily activities.
Laboratory findings are within normal limits.	The following measurements are all in the normal range: hematocrit; platelets; leukocytes; serum albumin; serum sodium; coagulation factors V, VII, IX, X; fibrinogen; serum complement C3; prothrombin time; fibrin split products; serum transaminase; BUN; and blood pH.

Sepsis

Bacteremia refers to the presence of bacteria in the circulating blood as demonstrated by blood culture. It is asymptomatic; it may be transient and abate spontaneously or become sustained, leading to septicemia.

Septicemia is a bacteremia with clinical manifestations of the pathogenic activity of bacteria in the blood. Symptoms vary with the pathogen.

Septic shock is a syndrome of circulatory insufficiency with hypoperfusion of body tissues caused by the effects of pathogenic bacterial toxins on peripheral blood vessels. It frequently results in death.

The infections manifesting a clinical picture consistent with the presence of bacteria or bacterial toxins in circulating blood (and not discussed elsewhere in this section) are grouped under sepsis (Table 13-19).

Table 13-19
Overview of Sepsis

	Bacteremia and Septicemia	Septic Shock
Occurrence	Bacteremia is common and transient; associated with medical procedures on hospitalized patients, colonization and dissemination of normal flora in debilitated persons, or dissemination of bacteria from a locus of infection; sustained bacteremia leads to septicemia	25%-30% of septicemias lead to shock; highest in hospitalized neonates and chronically ill persons
Etiologic agent	Gram-positive bacteria, particularly *S. aureus* and group B streptococci; gram-negative bacteria, particularly *Pseudomonas, Klebsiella, Proteus, E. coli, Serratia,* and *Enterobacter*	75% caused by gram-negative bacteria and their endotoxins; most common bacteria in order of frequency: *E. coli, Klebsiella, P. aeruginosa, Serratia, Enterobacter,* and *Proteus*; 25% caused by exotoxins of gram-positive bacteria, particularly *S. aureus*
Reservoir	Humans	Humans
Incubation period	Variable	Variable
Transmission	Bacteria may be introduced directly into blood as a primary bacteremia or may be secondary to an infection elsewhere in the body	Results from a primary or secondary septicemia
Period of communicability	Not directly transmittable; organism in draining lesions or respiratory secretions may be transmitted	Not directly transmittable
Susceptibility and resistance	Primary: invasive medical procedures increase susceptibility Secondary: urinary tract infections and pneumonia; neonates and elderly persons at greatest risk	Susceptibility greatest in neonates and chronically ill and immunocompromised individuals
Report to local health authority	No	No

Data from Axnick,[3] Benenson,[5] and Wehrle.[48]

Pathophysiology*

Bacteria may enter the blood directly through contaminated needles, catheters, monitoring transducers, or perfusion fluid to produce a primary bacteremia. In this situation there is no evidence of infection elsewhere in the body. About one third of diagnosed bacteremias are primary, and most are caused by gram-negative bacteria that are part of the normal flora of the skin or intestinal tract. Immunocompromised patients are at greatest risk for primary bacteremia. Secondary bacteremia results from dissemination of bacteria from a localized infection at another body site. Usually, clinical symptoms of infection precede the bacteremia. Urinary tract infections with gram-negative bacteria (usually catheter induced), surgical wound infections with gram-positive *Staphylococcus aureus,* and pneumonia (particularly with gram-negative *Pseudomonas*) are the infections that most frequently precede secondary bacteremias. Bacteremia may also be polymicrobial.

Bacteremia may abate spontaneously, or the multiplying bacteria in the blood may overwhelm host defenses and produce a symptomatic septicemia or metastatic bacterial abscesses at other organ sites, particularly in the brain, endocardium, kidneys, bones, and joints. Renal failure and endocarditis are serious complications of untreated, bacteremia-produced metastatic abscesses.

Progression of a bacteremia to septicemia or septic shock depends greatly on host characteristics and defenses. Premature infants, elderly persons, individuals with chronic debilitating diseases (cirrhosis, diabetes, renal disease, collagen diseases), and immunocompromised persons are at greatest risk.

Symptoms of septicemia result from the release of bacterial toxins and enzymes in the blood. In the case of gram-positive *Staphylococcus aureus,* exotoxins and enzymes cause RBC hemolysis, aggregation of platelets, leukocyte destruction, and increase in cell membrane permeability with protein leakage. Gram-negative bacterial endotoxins appear to activate at least four interacting humoral systems responsible for the pathologic findings in septicemia and progression to septic shock.

- Activation of complement results in release of anaphylatoxins that enhance the inflammatory reaction and increase vascular permeability.
- Activation of the coagulation system by stimulation of the conversion of fibrinogen to fibrin results in clotting. Consumption of clotting factors II, V, and VII and platelets may produce clinical bleeding. Other complications include thrombosis with tissue ischemia, necrosis, and organ failure and disseminated intravascular coagulation.
- Activation of the plasmin-fibrinolytic mechanisms lyses fibrin into fibrin-split products, which have anticoagulant properties. This results in prolonged prothrombin time and partial prothrombin time.
- Activation of the bradykinin system is thought to be partially responsible for progression to shock. Bradykinin, a vasoactive peptide, stimulates vasodilation and increased vascular permeability.

Two processes appear to produce skin lesions in septicemia. The lesions may be the result of direct bacterial invasion into dermal vessels with vessel damage and necrosis. They may also be manifestations of the vasoactive effect of toxins.

About 30% of gram-negative and 5% of gram-positive septicemias progress to septic shock. Gram-negative septic shock is more severe with death more likely.

The shock syndrome is precipitated by the complex action of bacterial toxins on peripheral blood vessels and blood components, with an end result of microcirculatory failure and cellular anoxia similar to shock of any cause. The sequence of events is as follows:

- Vasoactive toxins induce spasms of precapillary sphincters and venules, especially in visceral organs. This results in reduced capillary perfusion and hypoxic damage to capillaries as well as organ tissue.
- The precapillary sphincters eventually dilate while the venules remain constricted, causing blood to stagnate in the capillaries, capillary pressure to increase, and fluid to be lost from the vascular system.
- Blood stasis in the capillary bed plus decreasing blood volume potentiates intravascular clotting and impairment of venous return.
- Anoxia to the capillaries causes them to lose their integrity and to release whole blood as well as fluid into the tissues. This further decreases venous return.
- Loss of venous tone with dilation further impairs venous return. The end result is reduced cardiac output, extreme hypotension, further impairment of tissue perfusion with severe tissue anoxia, metabolic acidosis, renal and brainstem dysfunction, heart failure with pulmonary edema, respiratory insufficiency, and potential death.

There is a wide spectrum of cardiovascular and laboratory findings in septic shock depending on the organism and the stage in the progression and on the patient's hemodynamic compensation mechanisms. Initially, the patient may be warm with peripheral vascular dilation and normal or decreased peripheral resistance, normal or increased cardiac output with tachycardia, and respiratory alkalosis and hypotension. Progression of the vascular pathologic conditions leads to higher peripheral resistance, worsening hypotension, acidosis, heart failure, and anuria. Gram-positive septic shock may not progress beyond peripheral vasodilation with no anoxia or acidosis.

Laboratory findings in both gram-positive and gram-negative septicemia and septic shock are as follows:

Hematology

Leukocytes: 15,000 to 30,000/mm^3 (there may be an early leukopenia in gram-negative infections, increas-

*References 34, 36, 40, 41, 42, 48.

ing in 6 to 12 hours; a persistent leukopenia is a poor sign in gram-positive infections)
Differential: increase in neutrophils and decrease in lymphocytes (in elderly persons, the shift may be present without leukocytosis)
Hemoglobin: 10 g/dl in *S. aureus* infections
Hematocrit: less than 30% in *S. aureus* infections
Decrease in platelets (less than 100,000)
Prolonged prothrombin time and partial thromboplastin
Low fibrinogen concentration
Presence of fibrin-split products in the blood

Renal function tests
- Increased BUN greater than two times normal
- Increased serum creatinine greater than two times normal
- Decreased creatinine clearance

Blood electrolytes
- Hyponatremia
- Hypochloremia
- Potassium may be high or low depending on status of kidney function

Arterial blood gases
- Decreased Pco_2 and increased serum lactate early in shock
- Po_2 less than 70 mm Hg and acidosis later

Urine
- High specific gravity
- Albuminuria and hematuria in *S. aureus* infections

Diagnostic Studies and Findings[41]

Blood Culture for Both Anaerobic and Aerobic Bacteria

- Two or three sets of temporally separated blood cultures should be drawn before antibiotics are administered
- One or more cultures positive for bacteria are diagnostic of bacteremia
- Septicemia diagnosed based on positive cultures with clinical evidence of toxicity

Gram Stain

- Differentiates gram-positive from gram-negative bacteria

Limulus Amebocyte Lysate Test on Blood Specimens

- Positive for gram-negative endotoxins

Counterimmunoelectrophoresis or Ouchterlony Gel Diffusion Tests

- Positive for serum antibody to *S. aureus* cell wall antigen
- Tests take only 40 minutes to perform and are useful for rapidly differentiating *S. aureus* from other bacteria

Medical Plan[41,42]

Surgery

- Incision and drainage of any suppurative lesion containing staphylococci
- Removal of intravenous catheter or any foreign body that may be a source of the infection (prosthesis, stitches, etc.)

Medications

- Anti-infective agents
  - Antibiotic therapy depends on type of bacteria that is present in blood or is releasing a toxin from a localized infection elsewhere in the body and on the sensitivity of the organism to the antibiotic; a series of blood cultures should be drawn before antibiotic therapy is initiated
  - Anti-infective agents should be administered IV every 4 to 6 h
  - Combinations of agents may be used in severe disease before culture and sensitivity results are obtained; an effective regimen for bacteremia of unknown etiology is as follows:
    - Gentamicin (Garamycin), 3-5 mg/kg/d IM or IV, plus either
    - Methicillin (Staphcillin), 6-12 g/d IV, or
    - Cephalothin (Keflin), 6-8 g/d IV, plus
    - Carbenicillin (Geopen), 30 g/d IV if *Pseudomonas* is suspected
  - Duration of therapy will be long (2-6 wk dependent on the presence of a primary source of the infection, host defenses, and the response of the pathogen to the antibiotic)
- For treatment of shock
  - Adrenergic agents
    - Dopamine
    - Phenoxybenzamine
    - Isoproterenol (Chapter 1)
  - Corticosteroids
    - Methylprednisone (Medrol), 30 mg/kg as a bolus; repeat at 6-12 h intervals q12-48h
- Control of hemorrhage
  - Fresh frozen plasma if there is a clotting factor deficiency
  - Platelets if thrombocytopenia is present
- Diuretics
  - Mannitol (Osmitrol), 50-100 mg IV in 15%-20% solution, or ethacrynic acid (Edecrin), 25-200 mg/d po
- Heart failure: digitalis (Chapter 1)
- Intravascular coagulation: heparin (Chapter 15)

General Management

- Monitoring of central venous pressure or pulmonary artery pressure
- IV fluids until central venous pressure reaches 10 to 12

cm water or until pulmonary wedge pressure is 12 to 15 mm Hg

Blood volume replaced with blood, plasma, dextran, human serum albumin, or dextrose saline with bicarbonate

Respiratory assistance with nasal oxygen, tracheal intubation, or tracheostomy as required

NURSING CARE

Nursing Assessment[41]

Septicemia

- Body temperature
  - Fever: may be intermittent with wide diurnal variations; high in evening
- Subjective symptoms
  - Chills
  - Prostration
  - Myalgia and headache
  - Hypothermia sometimes present in gram-negative septicemia
- Respiratory system
  - Tachypnea
- Gastrointestinal concerns
  - Nausea
  - Diarrhea
- Skin
  - Petechial, purpuric, papular, pustular, or vesicular skin eruptions depending on type of bacteria present

There will be additional symptoms if septicemia is secondary to a localized infection elsewhere in the body (genitourinary or gastrointestinal tract, skin, or lungs). Symptoms may be insidious in elderly persons (hypothermia, lethargy, confusion).

Septic Shock

- Cardiovascular concerns
  - Tachycardia
  - Hypotension (systolic blood pressure less than 90 mm Hg)
  - Congestive failure
- Respiratory concerns
  - Tachypnea
- Skin
  - Cool, pale, or cyanotic extremities (in gram-positive or early gram-negative septic shock, skin is likely to be warm and flushed)
- Mental status
  - Confusion and disorientation rapidly leading to coma
- Urinary elimination
  - Oliguria (urinary output less than 20 ml/h)
- Abdomen
  - Hepatosplenomegaly in some patients

Nursing Dx & Intervention

Nursing Diagnosis	Nursing Intervention/Rationale
Potential for infection: patient	• Administer IV antibiotic as soon as ordered *because untreated septicemia may rapidly lead to septic shock.* • Monitor for adverse reaction to drugs *and report any immediately to physician.*
Potential for infection: patient contacts	*To prevent transmission to others:* • If the bacteremia or septicemia is secondary to a major skin, wound, or burn infection, maintain contact isolation for duration of the illness. Maintain drainage and secretion precautions for a minor skin wound or burn infection or pulmonary infection for duration of the illness. • Collect at least two blood specimens *for culture and sensitivity tests* before administration of antibiotics.
Altered cardiopulmonary, renal, cerebral, and peripheral tissue perfusion	• Monitor for signs of impending shock: decreased blood pressure, tachycardia, pale cool skin, alteration in consciousness, and urinary output less than 30 ml/hour (for nursing interventions for patients in shock, refer to Chapter 1).
Hyperthermia	• Monitor body temperature *to detect fever.* • Administer tepid water or alcohol sponge baths *to lower body temperature.* • Administer antipyretics as ordered *to lower body temperature.* • Maintain room temperature at 17° to 20° C (63° to 68° F) *to decrease metabolic needs,* particularly during shock.

Refer to Chapter 1 for further interventions for shock patients.

Patient Education

1. Take antibiotics as directed for prescribed length of treatment.
2. Report recurrence of symptoms or side effects of medication to physician immediately.

Evaluation

Patient Outcome	Data Indicating That Outcome is Reached
There is no infection.	Blood cultures are negative for bacteria. Cultures of secretions, excretions, or exudates (from a primary source of infection) are negative for bacteria. Body temperature is normal. There are no skin lesions.
Laboratory findings are normal.	Hematologic findings (leukocyte count, hemoglobin, hematocrit, platelet count, fibrinogen, prothrombin time, and partial thromboplastin time) are within normal limits. Findings of renal function tests (blood urea nitrogen and serum creatinine) are normal. Blood electrolytes (sodium, chloride, and potassium) are normal. Arterial blood gases (Pco_2 and Po_2) are normal. Urine specific gravity is normal. There is no albuminuria or hematuria.
Oxygen reaches all body cells.	Patient is alert and oriented and responds appropriately to environmental stimuli. Skin is warm and of normal color, with no petechiae or purpuric skin manifestations.
Vital signs are normal.	Blood pressure, pulse, and respirations are normal.
Urinary output is normal.	Urinary output is equal to intake.
Gastrointestinal function is normal.	Patient is able to eat regularly without nausea or vomiting. Stools are soft, formed, and of normal color.
Patient is comfortable.	Patient does not have a headache or myalgia. Energy returns to preillness level.

SEXUALLY TRANSMITTED DISEASES

The term "sexually transmitted diseases (STDs)" refers to a large group of disease syndromes that can be transmitted sexually irrespective of whether the disease has genital pathologic manifestations. STD is more encompassing than the previously used "venereal disease" categorization. The STDs, like other infectious diseases, can be classified as to their etiologic agent or according to their disease manifestations. The following pathogens are known or thought to be sexually transmitted[5,37]:

Bacteria: *Neisseria gonorrhoeae; Chlamydia trachomatis; Mycoplasma hominis; Ureaplasma urealyticum; Treponema pallidum; Gardnerella vaginalis; Haemophilus ducreyi; Shigella; Calymmatobacterium granulomatis*

Viruses: Herpes simplex virus; *Papillomavirus;* hepatitis A, B, and non-A, non-B viruses; molluscum contagiosum virus; cytomegalovirus; human immunodeficiency virus (HIV)

Protozoa: *Trichomonas vaginalis: Entamoeba histolytica; Giardia lamblia*

Fungi: *Candida albicans*

Ectoparasites: *Pthirus pubis; Sarcoptes scabiei*

The list of disease syndromes produced by the above pathogens is equally extensive. Many pathogens produce multiple disease syndromes, and many of the disease syndromes may be caused by more than one pathogenic agent. The STDs are grouped in this section according to disease manifestations patients are most likely to present to health care providers. These categories can be seen in Table 13-20. Some of these diseases have been discussed elsewhere in this chapter but are included in the table for completeness. It must be noted that patients with symptoms of a sexually transmitted disease frequently have multiple sexually transmitted diseases and should be evaluated accordingly (Table 13-20).

Gonorrhea and nongonococcal urethritis

Gonorrhea (clap, strain, gleet, dose, jack) is an inflammation of the columnar and transitional epithelium caused by the sexually transmitted gonococcus. Symptoms, course of disease, and severity differ between males and females. Chronic and severe complications may result from untreated infections.

Nongonococcal urethritis is a sexually transmitted urethritis in males (cervicitis and salpingitis in females) caused by an agent other than the gonococcus, most commonly *Chlamydia trachomatis*.

The diseases discussed in this section are manifest as urethritis or cervicitis with an inflammatory pyogenic exudate. Salpingitis and other related sequelae may be present (Table 13-21). Refer to Chapter 10 for a discussion of pelvic inflammatory disease.

Pathophysiology[5,37,39,43]

In *gonococcal infections* the gonococcus attaches to and penetrates columnar epithelium, producing a patchy, inflammatory response in the submucosa with a polymorphonuclear exudate. Affected areas in the male are the urethra, Littre's and Cowper's glands, the prostate, seminal vesicles, and the epididymis. Affected areas in the female include the glands of Bartholin and Skene, the urethra, the cervix, and the fal-

Table 13-20
STD Categories According to Disease Manifestations

Disease Manifestations	STD
Urethritis, cervicitis with an inflammatory pyogenic exudate, salpingitis, and related sequelae	Gonorrhea Nongonococcal urethritis Pelvic inflammatory disease
Ulcerative lesions with systemic dissemination of pathogen	Syphilis Lymphogranuloma venereum Herpes
Ulcerative lesions only	Chancroid Granuloma inguinale (donovanosis)
Nonulcerative lesions	Molluscum contagiosum Condylomata acuminata
Vulvovaginitis	Trichomoniasis Candidiasis *Gardnerella vaginalis* vaginitis
Systemic infections without lesions	Cytomegalovirus Hepatitis Acquired immunodeficiency syndrome (AIDS)
Enteric infections	Giardiasis *Campylobacter* enteritis Shigellosis Amebic dysentery
Pubic infestations (see Chapter 5)	Scabies Pediculosis
Congenital and perinatal infections and anomalies (see specific infection in this chapter)	TORCH organisms (syndrome): *T*oxoplasmosis *O*ther (e.g., syphilis) *R*ubella *C*ytomegalovirus *H*erpes simplex Others Gonorrhea *C. trachomatis* infections Candidiasis Trichomoniasis

Data from Benenson.[5]

lopian tubes. The stratified and transitional squamous epithelia are resistant to the gonococcus; therefore the bladder, upper urinary tract, preputial sac, vulva, vagina, and uterus are infrequently involved. The only exception is prepubescent girls who are susceptible to a gonococcal vulvovaginitis before changes in the vaginal epithelium that accompany puberty. In both sexes primary infections may also affect the pharynx, conjunctivae, and anus. Homosexual males are at risk for primary infections in the anus. Anal infections in females result from an extension of the infection to the anus.

Direct extension of the infection occurs by way of lymph vessels. In the female, extension most frequently occurs unilaterally or bilaterally to the fallopian tubes, bypassing the uterus. It appears that some cell surfaces of gonococci have greater ability to attach to fallopian tube mucosa. Thus not all gonococcal cervicitis leads to salpingitis. Direct extension in the male most frequently occurs to the epididymis.

Localized infection in any of the above areas may produce cysts and abscesses. The infection may infrequently resolve without treatment if an adequate cellular immune response develops and if there is adequate drainage of the purulent exudate containing the organism. More commonly, the inflammatory exudate is replaced with fibroblasts, and fibrous tissue fills the inflamed tissue. Hardening of the fibrous tissue causes strictures of the lumen of the urethra, epididymis, or fallopian tubes. Complete or partial occlusion of the fallopian tubes results in sterility or increased risk for ectopic pregnancy.

Infection of the fallopian tubes may also result in an acute pelvic inflammatory disease. Exudate may be released into the pelvic cavity, causing a severe peritonitis; or the pelvic inflammatory disease may become chronic, with recurrent inflammatory flare-ups that predispose to pelvic inflammation with normal flora organisms.

Between 1% and 3% of gonococcal infections become disseminated in the blood, producing septicemia, arthritis, endocarditis, meningitis, or skin lesions. Most disseminated infections are asymptomatic before the dissemination. Oc-

Table 13-21
Overview of STDs Manifested with Urethritis or Cervicitis

	Gonorrhea	Nongonococcal Urethritis (NGU), Cervicitis
Occurrence	Worldwide; increasing in incidence; highest in 15-30 yr olds and among male homosexuals	Worldwide; increasing more rapidly than gonorrhea; higher in upper socioeconomic brackets
Etiologic agent	*N. gonorrhoeae*, the gonococcus	*C. trachomatis, U. urealyticum, T. vaginalis, C. albicans*
Reservoir	Humans	Humans
Transmission	Contact with exudates from mucous membranes of infected persons, usually by direct contact	Direct contact with exudates
Incubation period	2-7 d	Range of 2 to 35 d
Period of communicability	Months if untreated	Unknown
Susceptibility and resistance	Universal	Universal; no acquired immunity
Report to local health authority	Mandatory case report	No

Data from Benenson.[5]

casionally an extension of salpingitis in a female leads to perihepatitis.

Infection with gonorrhea does result in a short-lived cellular immune response and a longer-lasting humoral immune response, neither of which protects against future infections.

Nongonococcal urethritis and cervicitis are most frequently caused by strains of *Chlamydia trachomatis* that are pathogenic to columnar epithelium in a manner similar to *Neisseria gonorrhoeae*. Symptomatic manifestations are generally less severe than with gonorrhea, with many subclinical infections. Extension of the inflammation into the fallopian tubes with the potential for a pelvic inflammatory disease is a potential complication of infection with *C. trachomatis*. Transmission of the pathogen during birth can result in ophthalmia neonatorum and pneumonia in the neonate. Infection with *C. trachomatis* stimulates a cellular and humoral immune response, neither of which is protective against future infections.

Diagnostic Studies and Findings[10,19]

Culture of Exudate From Urethra, Vagina, or Fallopian Tubes

Positive for *N. gonorrhoeae* or *C. trachomatis* associated with gonorrhea, nongonococcal urethritis, or cervicitis

Microscopic Examination of Gram-Stained Exudate

Positive for gram-negative intracellular diplococci of gonorrhea

Fluorescent Antibody (FA) Stain and Fluorescent Microscopic Examination

Positive for *C. trachomatis*

Enzyme-Linked Immunoabsorbent Assay (ELISA)

Detects *C. trachomatis* antibody reaction in specimen

Complement Fixation Test, Immunofluorescent Test

For systemic gonococcal infections

Fourfold rise in antibody titer between onset of infection and later disease for gonorrhea

Slow-rising titer in sera obtained at 2-week intervals

Medical Plan[5,19,20,24]

Medications

- Anti-infective agents
  - Uncomplicated gonococcal infections in adults
    - Tetracycline (Achromycin; others), 500 mg po qid for 7 d, or
    - Doxycycline hyclate (Vibramycin), 100 mg po bid for 7 d, or
    - Amoxicillin (Amoxil; others), 3 g po, single dose with 1 g probenecid po, or
    - Ampicillin (Amcill; others), 3.5 g po, single dose with 1 g probenecid po, or
    - Aqueous procaine penicillin G, 4.8 million U IM at two sites with 1 g of probenecid po
  - For gonococcal infections with chlamydial infection
    - Amoxicillin or ampicillin (as above), plus tetracycline or doxycycline (as above; tetracycline is effective against *Chlamydia*)
  - For anorectal gonorrhea
    - Aqueous procaine penicillin (as above)
  - For pharyngeal gonorrhea

Tetracycline or aqueous procaine penicillin
For penicillin-allergic patients who cannot tolerate tetracycline or for treatment failures: spectinomycin (Trobicin), 2 g IM in one injection
For treatment failures resulting from penicillinase-producing *N. gonorrhoeae*
Spectinomycin (Trobicin), 2 g IM in one injection, plus
Tetracycline (Achromycin; others) (for *Chlamydia*), or
Cefoxitin (Mefoxin), 2 g IM in one injection plus probenecid, 1 g po, or
Cefotaxime (Claforan), 1 g IM in one injection without probenecid
For pharyngeal infections with penicillinase-producing *N. gonorrhoeae*
Trimethoprim-sulfamethoxazole (Septra, Bactrim), 80 mg trimethoprim and 400 mg sulfamethoxazole po in a single dose of 9 tablets daily for 5 d
For gonococcal infections during pregnancy
Amoxicillin or ampicillin (as described above), or
Spectinomycin (Trobicin), 2 g IM
For disseminated gonococcal infections, excluding meningitis and endocarditis
Aqueous crystalline penicillin G, 10 million U IV/d until improvement, followed by
Amoxicillin (Amoxil), 500 mg, or ampicillin (Amcill; others), 500 mg po qid to complete 7 d of antibiotic treatment, or
Amoxicillin (Amoxil), 3 g, or ampicillin (Amcill; others), 3.5 g po; each with probenecid, 1 g, single dose followed by amoxicillin or ampicillin, 500 mg po qid for 7 d, or
Tetracycline (Achromycin; others), 500 mg po qid for 7 d, or
Cefoxitin (Mefoxin), 1 g IV, or
Cefotaxime (Claforan), 500 mg IV given qid for 7 d, or
Erythromycin (Erythrocin), 500 mg po qid for 7 d
Disseminated gonorrhea with penicillinase-producing *N. gonorrhoeae*
Inpatient:
Ceftriaxone, 1-2 g/d IV until symptoms resolve
Outpatient:
Ceftriaxone, 250 mg/d IM for at least 1 wk of antimicrobial therapy
Nongonococcal urethritis, cervicitis, or rectal infection
Tetracycline (Achromycin; others), 500 mg po qid for 7 d, or
Doxycycline (Vibramycin), 100 mg po bid for 7 d, or
Erythromycin (Erythrocin), 500 mg po qid for 7 d
All sexual partners of patients with gonorrhea or nongonococcal urethritis (or cervicitis) should be examined and treated
All persons treated for gonorrhea or *C. trachomatis* infection should be recultured 4-7 d after completion of treatment. Rectal cultures should be obtained from women treated for gonorrhea
All persons treated for gonorrhea or *C. trachomatis* infection should also be tested for syphilis

NURSING CARE

Nursing Assessment[5,40]

Gonorrhea: Males

2 to 7 days after exposure
Urinary tract
Purulent yellow-white discharge from anterior urethra
Dysuria
Inflammation around urinary meatus
Pain and urinary retention with prostatitis
Severe pain and swelling with epididymitis
Rectum
Pruritus, tenesmus, and discharge (homosexuals)

Gonorrhea: Females

2 to 7 days after exposure: may be asymptomatic
Urinary tract
Dysuria sometimes occurs
Vagina
Purulent discharge (may go unnoticed)
Uterus
Abnormal and painful menses
Symptoms of endometritis
Rectum
Tenesmus
Bloody mucoid diarrhea
Burning and discharge

Gonorrhea: Males and Females

Oropharynx
Pharyngitis possible
Eyes
Conjunctivitis possible
Systemic manifestations (possible)
Septicemia
Endocarditis
Meningitis
Arthritis
Painful vesicular pustular skin lesions on an erythematous base
Petechial skin lesions

Nongonococcal Urethritis: Males

Opaque discharge from urethra
Dysuria
Urethral pruritus

Nongonococcal Cervicitis: Females

Asymptomatic usually

Nursing Dx & Intervention

Nursing Diagnosis	Nursing Intervention/Rationale
Potential for infection: patient contacts	• *To prevent transmission to others:* See "Patient Education" below. Collect specimen for culture. Administer antibiotics as prescribed.
Sexual dysfunction	• See "Patient Education" *to prevent complications of disease.*

See Chapter 10 for care of patients with pelvic inflammatory disease.

Patient Education[10]

1. Avoid sexual activity until follow-up cultures are negative for *N. gonorrhoeae* organisms or until treatment is completed for other organisms.
2. Sexual contacts must be examined and treated to prevent reinfection of the patient.
3. Course of antibiotic therapy must be completed to avoid chronic infection and subsequent complications. If tetracycline is prescribed, it should be taken 1 hour before or 2 hours after meals. Patient should avoid dairy products, antacids, iron, other mineral-containing preparations, and sunlight.
4. Condoms provide some protection.
5. Individuals who are at high risk for reinfection should be screened periodically. All treated patients should return for evaluation 4 to 7 days after completion of therapy.
6. Care should be taken with vaginal or urethral discharges to avoid contamination of eyes.

Evaluation

Patient Outcome	Data Indicating That Outcome is Reached
There is no infection.	Cultures are negative for gonococcus. There is no urethral or vaginal discharge, dysuria, tenesmus, urethral pruritus, or abdominal pain. Menses are normal, with no dysmenorrhea.
There are no chronic complications.	Female is able to conceive. Male is free of urinary retention and pain of epididymitis.
Body temperature is normal.	Oral adult temperature is 37° C (98.6° F).
Laboratory values are within normal limits.	Leukocyte count and sedimentation rate are normal.
The patient complies with recommendations.	Sexual partners have been examined and treated.

Syphilis

Syphilis (lues) is a chronic systemic disease characterized by a primary lesion, a secondary eruption involving skin and mucous membranes, long periods of latency, and late seriously disabling lesions of skin, bone, viscera, central nervous system, and cardiovascular system.

Syphilis is one of several sexually transmitted diseases that have both ulcerative lesions and systemic dissemination. Others are herpesvirus infections and lymphogranuloma venereum (Table 13-22).

Pathophysiology[40,41,48]

Syphilis is a systemic infection of the vascular system characterized by five distinct stages: incubation, primary and secondary stages, latency, and late syphilis. Incubation begins with the penetration of *Treponema pallidum* into intact mucous membranes or abraded skin. Some of the pathogens remain at the site of invasion while others migrate, within hours, to regional lymph nodes, where some remain while others are disseminated throughout the body. *Treponema* can invade and multiply in any organ system, producing lesions wherever the concentration of the microorganism is the great-

Table 13-22
Overview of STDs with Ulcerative Lesions and Systemic Dissemination

	Syphilis	Genital Herpes	Herpes Type 1	Lymphogranuloma Venereum
Occurrence	Worldwide; increasing in incidence; highest in 15-30 yr olds and in males, particularly male homosexuals	Worldwide; increasing rapidly; highest in 15-30 yr olds; most common STD in United States	Worldwide; 70%-90% of adults have antibodies against herpes type 1; primary infection probably occurs by age 5	Worldwide; higher in tropical and subtropical climates
Etiologic agent	*Treponema pallidum,* a spirochete	Herpes simplex virus 2; possibly herpes simplex virus 1	Herpes simplex virus type 1	Several strains of *C. trachomatis*
Reservoir	Humans	Humans	Humans	Humans
Transmission	Direct contact with exudates from lesions on skin and mucous membranes; blood transfusion; congenital	Direct contact with saliva or secretions from mucous membranes and lesions; congenital	Contact with saliva of carriers and active lesions; may be transmitted sexually	Direct contact with open lesions
Incubation period	10 d to 10 wk; usually 3 wk	2-12 d; average of 6 d	2-12 d	4-21 d; usually 7-12 d
Period of communicability	Variable; during primary and secondary stages and in mucocutaneous recurrences; 2-4 yr if untreated	Transient shedding of virus in absence of lesions probably occurs; 7-12 d with lesion	During lesions; virus in saliva found as long as 7 wk after recovery of lesions; transient shedding of virus is common	Variable; weeks to years as long as lesions are present
Susceptibility and resistance	Universal, although only 10% of exposures result in infection; no natural immunity; infection leads to gradually developing resistance to new infections	Universal; immune response does not prevent recurrence	Universal susceptibility	General
Report to local health authority	Mandatory case report	No	No	In some states

Data from Benenson.[5]

est. During this incubation period, blood containing the *Treponema* organisms is infectious.

Vascular pathologic manifestations are the consequence of treponemal tissue invasion at all stages. The inflammatory response in the endothelial tissue produces perivascular infiltration of lymphocytes and plasma cells, resulting in endothelial swelling and an obliterative endarteritis of terminal arterioles and small arteries. Concentric fibroblastic proliferative thickening occurs in the vessels, resulting in eventual foci of tissue necrosis.

The primary stage is characterized by a single lesion at the site of initial invasion containing the *Treponema* and appearing 10 to 90 days after infection. The lesion is firm and hard as a result of intense cellular infiltration accompanied by serum accumulation in connective tissue. The lesion heals spontaneously within 1 to 5 weeks (average of 2 to 3 weeks). A satellite lesion, or bubo, may develop in an inguinal lymph node.

The secondary stage begins as the primary lesion is resolving, lasts 2 to 6 weeks, and is manifested with parenchymal, systemic, and mucocutaneous symptoms that indicate treponemal pathologic manifestations throughout the body. *Treponema* can be recovered from all skin and mucous membrane lesions.

A period of latency, ranging from 1 to 40 or more years, follows the secondary stage. During the first year of latency there may be recurrence of secondary stage manifestations. Subclinical infection with progressive arterial damage continues for some number of infected persons.

About one third of infected, untreated persons manifest symptoms of late syphilis with clinical evidence of degenerative lesions of the cardiovascular and central nervous systems, the skin, and the viscera. These lesions, called gummas, may be the result of a hypersensitive cellular immune response to the *Treponema* in the tissue. Gummas are granulomatous lesions consisting of a necrotic, coagulated center with obliterative endarteritis of small vessels in the tissue. Lesions of late syphilis, including open gummas on the skin, do not contain *Treponema*. They are therefore not infectious.

Disease manifestations of late syphilis depend on the area of arterial lesions and the extent of circulatory insufficiency. Central nervous system disease may be asymptomatic, meningovascular, or parenchymatous. Parenchymatous neurosyphilis can be seen clinically as paresis (resulting from progressive cortical neuron degeneration) or tabes dorsalis (resulting from posterior column degeneration).

Cardiovascular symptoms frequently result from aortic necrosis with resultant aortic insufficiency.

The immune response in syphilis is not completely understood. Humoral antibodies develop early and persist in untreated persons, but they do not seem to alter the course of the disease. The cell-mediated immune response increases during latency. This may account for the lack of progression to late syphilis for a large portion of untreated persons. Antibody levels will gradually decrease in persons treated in primary and secondary stages.

Congenital transmission of *Treponema* may occur at any time during pregnancy, but the fetus does not develop an inflammatory response to the pathogen until around the fifteenth week of gestation. Treatment of infected pregnant women before the fifteenth week may prevent damage to the fetus. Evidence of congenital syphilitic damage includes early malformations, observed at birth or during the first 2 years of life, and later evidence of developmental deformities. Infants with congenital syphilis born to untreated or inadequately treated mothers will have active infection and must be treated.

Diagnostic Studies and Findings[40,41,48]

Dark-Field or Phase-Contrast Microscopic Examination of Exudate or Cells from Lesions or Regional Lymph Nodes

- Positive for *T. pallidum* in primary and secondary stages
- Not useful for latent or tertiary stages

Nontreponemal Serologic Tests: VDRL (Most Common), Kline, Kahn, Hinton, Mazzini Tests; Rapid Plasma Reagin (RPR), Automated Reagin Test (ART), Reagin Screen Test (RST)

- Useful for screening; many false positive results
- Increase in nonspecific antibodies 1 to 3 weeks after appearance of the chancre or 4 to 6 weeks after infection
- Become negative in 6 to 12 months after treatment of primary syphilis; 12 to 18 months after treatment of secondary syphilis
- Serologic tests may not revert to negative if treatment is delayed beyond 2 years

Treponemal Serologic Tests: Fluorescent *Treponema* Antibody Absorption (FTA-ABS); *T. Pallidum* Hemagglutination Assay (TPHA-TP); *T. Pallidum* Immobilization (TPI; Rarely Done); Microhemagglutination Assay (MHA-TP)

- Useful for confirmation of positive screening tests
- Reported as nonreactive, borderline, or reactive
- These tests become reactive earlier in the primary stage and remain reactive longer in latent and late syphilis
- More sensitive and specific but expensive

Medical Plan[20,40]

Medications

- Anti-infective agents
  - Primary, secondary, or early syphilis of less than 1 yr duration: benzathine penicillin G, 2.4 million U IM
  - Of more than 1 yr duration: benzathine penicillin G (Bicillin), 7.2 million U total; 2.4 million U IM weekly for 3 successive wk
  - Patients allergic to penicillin: tetracycline (Achromycin; others), 500 mg po qid for 15 d for infections of less than 1 yr; for 30 d for infections of longer duration (pregnant women should not receive tetracycline)
  - For penicillin-allergic pregnant women: erythromycin (stearate, ethyl succinate, or base), 500 mg po qid for 15 d for infections of less than 1 yr; for 30 d for infections of longer duration (infants born to women treated with erythromycin should be treated with penicillin)

NURSING CARE

Nursing Assessment[40,41,48]

Primary Stage

- Within 10 to 90 days after exposure (average of 21 days); lasts 1 to 5 weeks
- Genitalia
  - Single painless papule erodes to become a hard, painless indurated chancre without an exudate; usually located on the glans penis of the male and on the cervix or external genitalia of the female; may be on the scrotum, anus, rectum, lips, tongue, tonsils, nipple, and fingers
- Inguinal lymph nodes
  - Hard, nonfluctuant, painless, enlarged inguinal lymph node

Secondary Stage

- Within 6 weeks of onset of primary infection; lasts a few days to 1 year
- Skin
  - Local or generalized, papulosquamous, macular, pap-

ular, or pustular rash; bilateral and symmetric, beginning on trunk and proximal extremities; frequently on soles of feet and palms of hands
- Lesions: 3 to 10 mm; nonpruritic
- Condylomata lata: lesions on moist areas coalesce and erode to produce painless, moist, gray-white raised plaques
- Alopecia: nonscarring, temporary hair loss in patches on head and eyebrows

Mucous membranes
- Mucous patches: silver-gray superficial erosion surrounded by red periphery on mucous membranes

Systemic symptoms
- Malaise
- Fever
- Headache

Gastrointestinal concerns
- Epigastric pain or vomiting associated with ulceration

Latent Stage

May have relapses of mucocutaneous symptoms of secondary stage early in latency; otherwise, no symptoms

Late Stage

Symptoms may be manifested in one or more systems

Neurologic concerns
- Asymptomatic
  - No symptoms except leukocytes and protein in cerebrospinal fluid
- Meningovascular symptoms
  - Focal neurologic signs depending on area of lesions
  - Seizures
- Parenchymatous symptoms
  - Paresis: personality changes ranging from minor to severe psychosis; alteration in intellect and judgment; hyperactive reflexes
  - Tabes dorsalis: ataxia, areflexia, paresthesias, bladder disturbance, impotence; sharp, tearing pain
  - Trophic joint changes
  - Optic atrophy with small, irregular pupils that are not reactive to light but respond normally to accommodation

Cardiovascular concerns
- Signs of aortic insufficiency

Skin and mucous membranes
- Gummas: lesions varying from small to large tumorlike masses or ulcers

Nursing Dx & Intervention

Nursing Diagnosis	Nursing Intervention/Rationale
Potential for infection: patient contacts	• Employ drainage and secretion precautions and blood and body fluid precautions for hospitalized patients with primary or secondary syphilis *to prevent transmission of the pathogen.*

Interventions for late-stage syphilitic changes and congenital syphilis are beyond the scope of this chapter.

Patient Education[10,41]

1. All sexual partners should be referred for examination and treatment (sexual contacts up to 3 months preceding primary infection, up to 6 months preceding secondary stage, and up to 1 year preceding latent stage).
2. Sexual activity should be avoided until patient and partners are adequately treated and all lesions are healed.
3. Condoms may prevent future infections.
4. Treated patients should return for follow-up serologic tests 3, 6, 12, and 24 months after therapy.
5. If tetracycline is administered, it must be taken for the full prescribed course. It should be taken 1 hour before or 2 hours after meals. Dairy products, antacids, iron, other mineral-containing preparations, and sunlight should be avoided.
6. A systemic reaction (fever, chills, headache, tachycardia) 1 or 2 hours after onset of antibiotic treatment is due to endotoxin release from dying spirochetes. The condition is benign and self-limited. Bed rest and aspirin help.

Evaluation

Patient Outcome	Data Indicating That Outcome is Reached
There is no infection.	Lesions have cleared. Cerebrospinal fluid is normal. Patient and sexual contacts have been adequately treated with antibiotics. Follow-up serologic tests indicate decreasing antibody titers.

Herpesvirus infections

Herpes simplex is a systemic viral infection characterized by a localized primary lesion, latency, and a tendency to localized recurrence. Two serologically distinct herpes viral agents, 1 and 2, generally produce distinct clinical syndromes. Herpes simplex virus type 2 (HSV-2) is most often implicated in genital herpes.

Both types of herpesvirus infections are summarized with other sexually transmitted diseases with ulcerative lesions and systemic dissemination in Table 13-22.

Pathophysiology[37,41,48]

Two antigenically distinct herpes simplex viruses (HSV), types 1 and 2, are responsible for herpes infections. Both are capable of producing infection in epithelial tissue anywhere in the body, but HSV-1 is most often associated with oral, labial, ocular, or skin herpes above the waist, whereas HSV-2 is implicated in 90% of genital, anal, and perianal herpes or oral herpes associated with genital, oral, or sexual transmission. Infections caused by both types of HSV are discussed in this section because of the potential for sexual transmission of both agents and because both produce essentially the same pathologic findings.

All HSV infections have two characteristics in common:

Once present in tissue, HSV produces a chronic infection initiated with active self-limiting tissue destruction. The lesions heal, but the organism continues to be viable in the body in the presence of circulating antibodies and in the absence of symptomatic disease.

There is a latent period during which the genome of the virus is present in tissue in a nondestructive form. Infectious virions cannot be recovered until the virus becomes reactivated and produces recurrent infectious disease. Active infection, either initial or recurrent, need not be symptomatic.

Initial infection refers to the first infection with the HSV type. Initial infection with HSV-1 usually occurs by age 4 years and is manifest as a clinical or subclinical gingivostomatitis. Initial infection with HSV-2 usually occurs during the ages of sexual activity and is usually manifested by clinical or subclinical genital herpes.

The organism is transmitted by close contact with saliva or genital secretions of persons with active clinical or subclinical infections either directly or by hand.

The transmitted virus invades and replicates in the parabasal and intermediate epithelial cells of mucous membranes or traumatized skin. Intracellular and extracellular edema and cell lysis cause the cells to lose their intercellular bridges and to undergo a ballooning degeneration. Polymorphonuclear cells infiltrate, forming a thin-walled intradermal vesicle on an erythematous base. Multiple grouped vesicles can be visualized at the sites of tissue inoculation. The superficial epithelium collapses and sloughs, leaving single shallow ulcers, or the vesicles may coalesce into large painful ulcers. Crusting may occur on non–mucous membrane ulcers. All ulcers spontaneously granulate without scarring in about 12 days in initial infections.

The virus may enter the lymphatic system, producing localized lesions there. Rarely, the virus is disseminated to visceral organs, particularly the liver, adrenal glands, lungs, or central nervous system, producing discrete focal areas of necrosis in epithelial tissues in those organs. The virus may also be spread to other external body sites by autoinoculation.

Cellular immune response and nonspecific host defenses appear to inhibit dissemination. Circulating humoral antibodies develop but do not appear to be protective against reinfection or recurrent infection.

Following the primary infection the HSV travels along sensory nerve pathways to a sensory nerve ganglion where it remains in a latent stage. The viral DNA is stored in ganglion neurons in the absence of other viral products. The virus is not pathogenic in this form. It appears that the transient viral shedding may occur during this stage.

The exact mechanism for reactivation of the virus to produce recurrence of lesions is not known; but there are two predominant hypotheses. The *ganglion trigger theory* suggests that a stimulus to latently infected ganglion neurons stimulates the replication of the virus in the neurons. The virus migrates along peripheral nerves to reinvade epithelial cells, producing focal and cellular destruction as in initial infections. The *skin trigger theory* proposes that virus replication in the ganglion neurons is continuous, with viruses regularly reaching the epidermis by way of peripheral nerves. Cellular immune responses block the development of a cellular infectious process unless an external stimulus, such as trauma, overwhelms the defenses.

Recurrence of HSV lesions is generally in the area of initial inoculation. Genital recurrence is usually associated with HSV-2 and is usually less severe, lasting 4 or 5 days. Genital recurrence is common in women with asymptomatic cervical lesions. Oral HSV-1 infections frequently recur on the lips. Recurrence of either type may be triggered by another infectious disease, menstruation, emotional stress, and immunosuppression.

Potential complications of herpes infections include neuralgia, meningitis (HSV-1), encephalitis (HSV-2), ascending myelitis, urethral strictures, and lymphatic suppuration. In females there is the possibility of an increased risk for spontaneous abortion and cervical cancer. Neonates may become infected during vaginal delivery. Congenital herpes ranges from subclinical infections to severe infections of the skin, eyes, mucous membranes, visceral organs, or central nervous system. Congenital herpes has a high mortality. Many survivors have ocular or neurologic sequelae.

Diagnostic Studies and Findings[10,48]

Virus Tissue Culture of Specimen from Base of Vesicles Using Fluorescent Antibody or Neutralization Techniques

Identification of type 1 or type 2 viral cytopathogenic effect in tissue culture

Microscopic Examination of Stained Smear from Base of Vesicles

Direct identification of multinucleated giant cells with intranuclear inclusions

Complement Fixation or Neutralization Tests

Fourfold increase in antibody titer in convalescent serum; difficult to differentiate type 1 from type 2

Indirect Immunofluorescence and Radioimmunoassay

IgM antibodies detected in primary and recurrent infections

Medical Plan[20,48]

Surgery

Caesarean delivery before membranes rupture when primary or recurrent genital herpes occurs in late pregnancy

Medications

Anti-infective agents
- For first clinical episode of genital herpes: acyclovir 200 mg po, 5 times daily for 7-10 days, initiated within 6 days of onset of lesions
- For severe infections: acyclovir 5 mg/kg q8h IV for 5-7 d

NURSING CARE

Nursing Assessment

Gingivostomatitis

Initial HSV-1 infection
Oral cavity
- Multiple vesicular and ulcerative lesions on labial and buccal mucosa, tongue, and larynx
- Erythema of gums; excessive salivation
- Infection heals in 7 to 10 days; recurrent infections rare in mouth

Cervical lymph nodes
- Enlarged and palpable

Lips
- Recurrent "cold sore" or "fever blister" preceded by 1 or 2 days of paresthesia; lesions crust and heal within 3 to 10 days

Ocular Herpes

Eyes
- Keratitis and conjunctivitis (unilateral or bilateral)

Lymph nodes
- Periauricular lymphadenopathy

Cutaneous

Skin
- Clustered vesicular lesions anywhere on body
- Deep burning pain; skin edema

Lymph nodes
- Regional lymphadenopathy

Genital Herpes

Genitourinary: females
- Asymptomatic or extensive vesicular lesions with deep ulceration and marked hyperplasia and erythema of cervix, labia, fourchette clitoris (sometimes vagina); may extend to anal area, buttocks, and thighs
- Dysuria, leukorrhea, and marked genital tenderness

Genitourinary: male
- Scattered vesicles over glans, prepuce, and shaft of the penis
- Urinary retention
- Urethritis may occur without genital lesions
- Anal lesions in homosexual males

Inguinal lymph nodes
- Bilateral lymphadenopathy in 50% of initial genital infections

Systemic manifestations
- Fever in initial infections

Oral cavity
- Genital lesions may be sexually transmitted to oral cavity

Nursing Dx & Intervention*

Nursing Diagnosis	Nursing Intervention/Rationale
Pain	• Keep involved area clean and dry *for comfort*.
Potential for infection: patient contacts	• See "Patient Education" below *to prevent transmission to others*. • Employ drainage and secretion precautions for hospitalized patient. • Health care workers must wear gloves when in contact with secretions and lesions *to prevent infection with the pathogen*.

*For genital herpes only.

Patient Education

1. Abstain from sex while lesions are present during initial and recurrent infections. Condoms may offer protection during latency.
2. Pregnant women should inform physician of history of genital herpes.
3. Annual Papanicolaou smears are recommended.

Evaluation

Patient Outcome	Data Indicating That Outcome is Reached
Infection does not spread.	Herpes is not spread to health care workers, newborn infants, or sexual partners of the patient.

Lymphogranuloma venereum

Lymphogranuloma venereum is a systemic, disabling bacterial infection that begins with a small, painless evanescent erosion on the penis or vulva. Regional lymph nodes undergo suppuration, spreading the inflammatory process into adjacent tissue. The disease is disseminated further by way of the lymph system. There are usually systemic symptoms of lymphadenitis and serious complications in untreated individuals.

For an overview of lymphogranuloma venereum with other sexually transmitted diseases characterized by ulcerative lesions and systemic dissemination, see Table 13-22.

Pathophysiology[48]

Lymphogranuloma venereum is a systemic infection produced by mucosal invasion of a number of closely related strains of *Chlamydia*. The disease has three stages: a primary lesion, regional and disseminated lymphadenitis, and late complications resulting from progression of the regional lymphadenitis.

A primary transient nodular or vesicular lesion forms at the site of inoculation. Dissemination of the organism to regional lymph nodes (primarily inguinal lymph nodes) results in lymph node lesions that are initially similar to the inoculation lesion. The lesions are composed of small masses of epithelioid cells with multinucleated cells scattered throughout and a necrotic center filled with polymorphonuclear leukocytes. Satellite lesions are formed in the lymph node, surrounded by a narrow layer of epithelioid cells. The nodes show hyperplasia with an inflammatory cellular infiltration consisting of plasma cells, polymorphonuclear leukocytes, large mononuclear cells, and lymphocytes. Spread of the inflammation throughout the nodes causes the nodes to become matted together and form a large abscess. These abscesses develop in one or more areas along the lymphatic system. Untreated, the abscesses may rupture through the skin or other epithelial surfaces to produce chronic draining sinuses or fistulas. If the condition is not treated, it progresses, producing complications resulting from the impaired lymph and draining sinuses.

Complications include genital elephantiasis and perianal abscesses and fistulas resulting in eventual rectal stricture. Advanced stages of rectal stricture may be manifest as symptoms of painful ileus, distention, complete obstruction, perforation, and peritonitis.

Diagnostic Studies and Findings[5,48]

Cell Culture of Lesion Exudate or Bubo Aspirate

Positive for *C. trachomatis*

Complement Fixation

Antibody titer of 1:16 or higher within 1 to 3 weeks of infection; fourfold rise in titer between early infection and convalescence; nonspecific, since it detects antibodies against all *C. trachomatis* strains

Medical Plan[10]

Surgery

Aspiration of fluctuant lymph nodes as needed (Incision and drainage or excision is contraindicated.)

Strictures or fistulas may require surgery

Medications

Anti-infective agents
- Tetracycline hydrochloride (Achromycin; others), 500 mg po qid for 14 d, or
- Doxycycline (Vibramycin), 100 mg po bid for 14 d, or
- Erythromycin (Erythrocin; others), 500 mg po qid for 14 d, or
- Sulfamethoxazole (Gantanol), 1 g po bid for 14 d (other sulfonamides can be used in equal doses)

NURSING CARE

Nursing Assessment[10,48]

Primary Lesion (Genitalia)

2-3 mm painless, discrete, superficial vesicle or nonindurated ulcer at site of inoculation; frequently unnoticed
Usually on glans or shaft of the penis in males and on the labia, vagina, or cervix in females
May be in the rectum or mouth
Rectal inoculation produces bloody discharge and tenesmus at first; mucopurulent discharge, cramps, and diarrhea later

Regional Lymph Nodes

7 to 30 days after primary lesion
Initially a firm, tender, discrete, movable inguinal lymph node, which later becomes indolent, fixed, and matted; may be unilateral or bilateral; may subside spontaneously or proceed to form an abscess that may rupture to produce a draining sinus or fistula
Female lymph node involvement may be mainly in the pelvic nodes with extension to the rectum and rectovaginal septum

Systemic Symptoms

Fever
Chills
Headache
Joint pains
Anorexia
Abdominal pain
Urinary retention

Complications

Genitalia
Elephantiasis of prepuce, penis, scrotum, or vulva
Rectum
Perianal abscess; rectovaginal, rectovesical, and ischiorectal fistulas
Rectal stricture 1 to 10 years after infection

Nursing Dx & Intervention

Nursing Diagnosis	Nursing Intervention/Rationale
Potential for infection: patient contacts	• Handle exudates with caution *to prevent infection and transmission of the pathogen to others.* • See "Patient Education" below.

Patient Education

1. The sequelae of untreated lymphogranuloma venereum are serious. Patient must complete the prescribed antibiotic regimen and return for evaluation 3 to 5 days after treatment is begun and weekly or biweekly until the infection is entirely healed.
2. Tetracycline should be taken 1 hour before or 2 hours after meals. Dairy products, antacids, iron, other mineral-containing preparations, and sunlight should be avoided.
3. Sexual partners should be examined and treated.

Evaluation

Patient Outcome	Data Indicating That Outcome is Reached
There is no infection.	Lymph nodes are not swollen, hot, or tender. Mucopurulent exudate no longer drains from sinuses. Body temperature is normal.
There are no complications.	Rectum and anal opening are patent. There is no abdominal distention or cramping. Defecation is normal.

Chancroid and granuloma inguinale

Chancroid, also called "soft sore" or "soft chancre," is an acute, localized, autoinoculable bacterial infection of the genitalia. Necrotizing ulceration occurs at the site of inoculation, frequently accompanied by suppuration of regional lymph nodes. Systemic dissemination does not occur.

Granuloma inguinale (donovanosis) is a mildly communicable, chronic and progressive, autoinoculable

bacterial infection of the skin and mucous membranes, external genitalia, inguinal and anal regions, face, and oral cavity. Lesions first appear as small, painless papules or vesicles that become ulcerated and slowly develop into bleeding granulomatous masses. The disease may be difficult to differentiate from carcinoma (Table 13-23).

Pathophysiology[37,48]

Although both chancroid and granuloma inguinale are manifest as ulcerative lesions, their pathophysiologies differ. In *chancroid* the transmitted pathogenic bacteria initially invade genital skin or mucous membranes at sites traumatized by sexual contact. A preexisting abrasion facilitates invasion. A small papule is formed, surrounded by a zone of erythema. This erupts to form a shallow and painful ulcer. The lesions histologically show three layers. The shallow surface layer contains many polymorphonuclear cells, erythrocytes, and necrotic debris. The middle layer is edematous and shows endothelial proliferation of blood vessels. In the deep layer there is dense infiltration of plasma cells and lymphocytes. A purulent exudate results from the extensive necrotic process. The ulcers may enlarge and continue to erode and destroy tissue, or they may become secondarily infected and produce even more rapid destruction of tissue. Fresh lesions may occur from autoinoculation. Extragenital lesions may occur on fingers, tongue, lips, breasts, and eyelids.

Lymphatic dissemination results in a unilateral or bilateral painful inguinal adenitis within 7 to 10 days of the primary lesion. The enlarged lymph gland (bubo) softens, becomes fluctuant, and may rupture spontaneously. Long-term complications include phimosis and urethral fistulas in males. Females are frequently asymptomatic.

The transmission of *granuloma inguinale* is less well understood. The pathogenic bacterium can be found in the rectum of nondiseased patients, suggesting that the organism may be part of the normal gastrointestinal flora of some persons. Lesions may result from autoinfection, possibly following trauma to the genitalia. The pathogen in the lesions is transmitted sexually, but repeated exposure seems to be necessary for transmission. The disease is rare in heterosexual partners of infected persons. Clinical disease is highest in homosexual males.

The organism invades mononuclear endothelial cells and forms a small, painless papule or nodule at the site of dermal invasion. The prickle cell layer becomes thick, and a dense dermal infiltrate containing plasma cells, histiocytes, and polymorphonuclear cells forms in the lesion. The epithelium overlapping the lesion softens, erodes, ulcerates, and then produces a gradually enlarging granulomatous ulcerating lesion that bleeds easily. Pronounced marginal epithelial proliferation may simulate early epitheliomatous changes of cancer. The raised mass of granulation tissue looks more like a tumor than an ulcer. Single or multiple lesions may coalesce, or lesions may spread to contiguous tissue. Lesions have variable clinical appearances depending on the area located, mode of spread, tissue resistance, and texture of the skin. Secondary infection and expanding necrosis in untreated lesions may result in complete genital erosion.

The lesions heal by fibrosis at the same time that tissue destruction is occurring in expanding lesions. Resultant scarring may produce urethral occlusion.

Hematogenous spread of the pathogen to bones, joints, and liver is rare but has been reported. Lymphatic spread is questionable. The inguinal swelling that is sometimes seen with this disease is not a lymphadenopathy, but rather a subcutaneous granuloma.

Table 13-23
Overview of STDs with Ulcerative Lesions

	Chancroid	Granuloma Inguinale (Donovanosis)
Occurrence	Most common in tropical and subtropical climates	Most common in tropical and subtropical climates and in males
Etiologic agent	*Haemophilus ducreyi*, a bacterium	*Calymmatobacterium granulomatis*
Reservoir	Humans	Humans
Transmission	Direct sexual contact with exudate from lesions; indirect transmission is rare	Direct sexual contact with lesions or with organism in rectum of nondiseased carriers
Incubation period	3-14 d	8-80 d
Period of communicability	Until lesions heal (can be weeks)	Duration of open lesions
Susceptibility and resistance	General, but highest in uncircumcised males; no evidence of resistance, although women may have more subclinical infections	No evidence of immunity
Report to local health authority	Mandatory case report	Mandatory case report

Data from Benenson[5] and Wehrle.[48]

Diagnostic Studies and Findings[10]

Chancroid

Culture or microscopic examination of exudate from bubo or lesions
  Positive for *H. ducreyi* bacilli
Ducrey skin test
  Induration of at least 8 mm within 72 hours indicates past infection
  Antibody reaction may persist for years

Granuloma Inguinale

Microscopic examination of scrapings from ulcer margin
  Donovan bodies can be visualized

Medical Plan[10,20]

Surgery

Chancroid: fluctuant lymph nodes should be aspirated through adjacent normal skin (incision and drainage or excision of nodes is contraindicated)

Medications

Anti-infective agents
  Chancroid
    Erythromycin (Erythrocin), 500 mg po qid, or
    Trimethoprim/sulfamethoxazole (Septra; Bactrim), tablet containing 160 mg trimethoprim and 800 mg sulfamethoxazole, po bid for at least 7 d or until ulcers or lymph nodes have healed, or
    Ceftriaxone, 250 mg IM once
  Granuloma inguinale
    Tetracycline (Achromycin; others), 0.5 g po qid for 21 d or until lesions heal, or
    Streptomycin, 0.5 g IM bid for at least 21 d, or
    Chloramphenicol (Chloromycetin), 0.5 g po tid for at least 21 d, or
    Gentamicin (Garamycin), 40 mg IM bid for at least 21 d

NURSING CARE

Nursing Assessment[37,39,48]

Genitalia

Chancroid
  One to 10 primary lesions: inflamed macule/papule/pustule; irregularly shaped and of variable size (1 mm to 2 cm); surrounded by a zone of inflammation; erupts to produce a sharply circumscribed, nonindurated ulcer with a granulating base and ragged edges; abundant, purulent exudate; location: frenulum, prepuce, coronal sulcus, glans and shaft of penis, and urinary meatus in males; cervix, vagina, fourchette, labia, and perianal area in females
  Variations in clinical appearance of lesions
    Follicular pustules rupture and form ulcers
    Dwarf chancroid lesions look like herpes lesions
    Transient chancroid lesion resolves quickly but is followed by an inguinal bubo
    Papular chancroid starts as an ulcer but becomes raised
    Giant chancroid frequently follows rupture of inguinal abscess and grows rapidly
    Phagedenic chancroid, a small lesion, rapidly extends and becomes necrotic and destructive
Granuloma inguinale
  Single or multiple, indurated, sharply defined but irregular papules/nodules; erode to form a beefy, exuberant granulomatous, heaped, clean ulcer, progressing slowly and coalescing with adjacent lesions; serous exudate; location: glans, prepuce, urethra, shaft of penis, and perianal area in males; labia and fourchette in females; lesions bleed easily; if secondarily infected, may have odorous necrotic exudate
  Variations in clinical appearance
    Oral lesions are painful and look like malignancies
    Vaginal and cervical ulcers produce profuse, purulent discharge and irregular bleeding
    Cervical ulcers are soft, friable, irregular, and not well fixed to tissue; resemble cancer
    Male genital ulcers may be hypertrophic and verrucose, destructive and necrotic, discoid (buttonlike), or chronic and indolent
    Inguinal ulcers and ulcers on female genitalia are generally fleshy and exuberant
    Anal ulcers are hypertrophic and verrucose or chronic and indolent

Inguinal Area

Chancroid
  Single, unilateral (can be bilateral), tender, and unilocular lymphadenopathy with overlying erythema
  Suppuration and rupture of fluctuant nodes in 5 to 10 days may occur, leaving a single, large ulcer
Granuloma inguinale
  Rarely any inguinal involvement
  May have a subcutaneous granuloma that suppurates, and mimics a lymphadenopathy

Subjective Symptoms

Chancroid
  Pain
Granuloma inguinale
  Rarely any pain

Nursing Dx & Intervention

Nursing Diagnosis	Nursing Intervention/Rationale
Potential for infection: patient contacts	• See "Patient Education" below *to prevent transmission of the pathogen to others.*

Patient Education

1. Antibiotics must be taken for complete course of treatment.
2. Tetracycline is to be taken 1 hour before or 2 hours after meals. It is not to be taken with dairy products, antacids, iron, or other mineral-containing preparations. The patient should avoid sunlight.
3. The patient should return for evaluation within 3 to 5 days of beginning therapy and weekly or biweekly thereafter until all lesions are healed. Total healing of granuloma inguinale takes 3 to 5 weeks. If treatment is stopped prematurely, lesions may become reactivated.
4. Sexual partners should be examined and treated as soon as possible. Sexual contacts 2 weeks before or after onset of chancroid lesions must be treated. Females may be asymptomatic but should be treated.
5. In chancroid the prepuce should remain retracted during therapy and the lesions should be cleaned three times daily. Retraction is contraindicated if there is preputial edema.
6. Use of condoms may prevent future infections.

Evaluation

Patient Outcome	Data Indicating That Outcome is Reached
There is no infection.	All lesions are healed without scarring.
Patient complies with recommendations.	Sexual partners have been examined and treated. Patient is returning for follow-up examination.

Molluscum contagiosum and condylomata acuminata

Molluscum contagiosum is a viral disease of the skin that results in pearly pink to white papules with a central exudative pore. Multiple lesions appear on the genitalia and clear spontaneously in 6 to 9 months. Children develop lesions on skin elsewhere on the body.

Condylomata acuminata constitute one of the four major categories of virus-produced warts; this category occurs primarily on the genitalia or perineum. The warts appear as single or multiple, soft pink to brown, elongated lesions, usually in clusters and sometimes as large cauliflower-like masses. The warts sometimes heal spontaneously. Malignant transformation has been reported (Table 13-24).

Pathophysiology[5,37,41]

The viruses of both these diseases invade superficial layers of the epidermis, and infect single epithelial cells and stimulate the cells to divide. In the case of condylomata there is excessive proliferation of the prickle cells of the stratum spinosum, constituting the bulk of the wart. There is marked papillomatosis but no hyperkeratosis. Microscopic examination of the infected cells shows aggregates of the virus particles plus basophilic inclusions. In the case of molluscum contagiosum, a central pore containing the virus and exudative material develops in the papules.

Both molluscum papules and genital warts appear as multiple lesions on the external genitalia. Genital warts may also be found in the vagina and cervix of females and anterior urethra of males. Perineal and anal warts in females are generally caused by spread, whereas anal warts in males are associated with anal coitus among homosexuals. Genital warts that resemble skin warts suggest hand-to-genital transmission of another category of skin warts.

Complications from warts occur. Laryngeal papillomatosis may develop in infants born to mothers with vaginal warts. Also, the enlarged size of some warts may lead to difficulty during a vaginal birth. Secondary infection and bleeding of warts are common. Enlarged or giant condylomata of the penis, although benign, may destroy large areas of the penis. Cancer must be ruled out in this situation. Malignant transformation, both invasive and intraepithelial, has been observed in some warts.

Table 13-24
Overview of STDs with Nonulcerative Lesions

	Molluscum Contagiosum	Condylomata Acuminata (Anogenital Warts)
Occurrence	Worldwide; 90% of adults have antibodies; four times higher in prepubertal males	Worldwide
Etiologic agent	A member of the poxvirus group	*Papillomavirus*
Reservoir	Humans	Humans
Transmission	Direct sexual contact and indirect contact	Direct sexual contact
Incubation period	2-7 wk	1-20 mo (usually 4 mo)
Period of communicability	Unknown; probably as long as lesions persist	Unknown; probably as long as lesions persist
Susceptibility and resistance	Usually occurs in small children	General
Report to local health authority	No	No

Data from Benenson.[5]

The papules of molluscum contagiosum clear spontaneously in 6 to 9 months as a result of an immune response. Warts sometimes clear spontaneously, which suggests an immune response.

Diagnostic Studies and Findings

Molluscum Contagiosum: Microscopic Examination of Material in Core of Lesion

Pathognomonic molluscum inclusion bodies can be visualized

Condylomata

Biopsy necessary for definitive diagnosis to rule out malignancy

Rule out condylomata lata of syphilis with serologic test for syphilis

Medical Plan[20]

Surgery

Alternative therapies for warts may include cryotherapy, electrosurgery, or surgical removal (scissors or curette); no treatment should be initiated on cervical warts until results of a Papanicolaou smear are available

Molluscum lesions may resolve spontaneously or be removed by curettage after cryoanesthesia or cryotherapy or by the use of caustic chemicals

Medications

Keratolytic agents

Condylomata acuminata: podophyllin, 10%-25% in compound tincture of benzoin to wart only; to be washed off in 1-4 h; four weekly treatments (not to be used during pregnancy or with urethral, oral, cervical, or anorectal warts)

NURSING CARE

Nursing Assessment

Anogenital Area

Molluscum: multiple papules, 1 to 10 mm, pearly pink to white, with a central pore

Condylomata: multiple or single, soft pink to brown, elongated lesions, usually in clusters; may be in large masses

Nursing Dx & Intervention

Nursing Diagnosis	Nursing Intervention/Rationale
Potential for infection: patient contacts	• See "Patient Education" *to prevent transmission to others.*

Patient Education[10]

1. Sexual partners should be examined and treated.
2. During therapy, the patient should abstain from sex or should use a condom.
3. Follow-up examination should take place 1 month after treatment for molluscum so new lesions can be removed.
4. Follow-up examinations should be done weekly until all warts have been resolved.
5. All women with anogenital warts should have a Pap smear.

Evaluation

Patient Outcome	Data Indicating That Outcome is Reached
There is no infection.	Lesions have been removed or are resolved.
The patient complies with recommendations.	Sexual partners have been examined and treated, if necessary. Females have negative Pap smear.

Vulvovaginitis

Vulvovaginitis is an inflammation of the superficial mucous membranes of the vulva and vagina caused by a number of microorganisms that are frequently part of the normal vaginal flora in adult women. The inflammation is accompanied by a purulent exudate with characteristics that differ with causative agents. The etiologic agents most frequently associated with vulvovaginitis are *Trichomonas vaginalis* (a protozoan), *Candida albicans* (a yeast form of fungus), and *Gardnerella vaginalis (Corynebacterium vaginale, Haemophilus vaginalis)* (a bacterium). They are responsible for trichomoniasis, candidiasis, and *Gardnerella vaginalis* vaginitis, respectively (Table 13-25). In addition, the inflammation can be caused by mechanical irritants, contact allergens, and ectoparasites (pinworms, lice) (Table 13-26).

Pathophysiology[41]

The presence of estrogen in women supports a normal flora of microorganisms in the vagina and anterior urethra. Under certain conditions (alterations in hormonal levels during the menstrual cycle, pregnancy, antibiotic therapy, immunosuppression), imbalance occurs in the normal flora. Certain opportunistic organisms become pathogenic or may be sexually transmitted in large enough numbers to become pathogenic. They colonize on the superficial mucosal layers and produce patches of inflammation and exudate that contain large numbers of the pathogens. The infection rarely extends beyond the endocervix. There is a wide range in severity of infections. Many are asymptomatic. The organism may be transmitted to a male sexual partner who may or may not develop symptomatic urethritis. Reinfection of the female from untreated males is common.

The organisms may be transmitted to an infant during birth. Infections in newborns are generally temporary and are limited to the period before maternal estrogens are metabolized by the newborn.

Certain physiologic changes in the host support the pathogenic growth of different organisms. Trichomoniasis is exacerbated during and after menstruation, whereas bacterial infections such as *G. vaginalis* vaginitis are not associated with hormonal changes during the menstrual cycle. *G. vaginalis* vaginitis is associated with an altered vaginal pH; the organism usually does not grow in the normal acid secretions. Yeast infections, such as candidiasis, are greatly exacerbated preceding menstruation, during pregnancy, and in women taking oral contraceptives. Candidiasis is also exacerbated by the elimination of normal flora bacteria with antibiotic therapy or with any other condition that compromises skin or mucous membrane defenses.

Whereas *Trichomonas* and *Gardnerella* rarely extend beyond the vulvovaginal or anterior urethral area, *Candida* has the potential for producing infection anywhere in the body where normal defenses are altered. *Candida* is part of the normal gastrointestinal, oral, and cutaneous flora of many persons, and it may become pathogenic in those areas. Severe infection with invasion and abscess formation, particularly in the gastrointestinal tract, may lead to hematogenous dissemination of the yeast to other organs. The organism may also be introduced iatrogenically to internal organs through surgical procedures, catheters, or implanted devices and produce multiple microabscesses in infected tissue. The areas most commonly infected are the central nervous system (particularly the meninges), lungs, peritoneum, heart (myocardium, pericardium, and endocardium), endometrium, eyes, ears, joints, oral cavity, esophagus, skin, and nails. Deep tissue infection is more common in patients with neoplastic disease. Cutaneous infections are more commonly associated with skin injury or continual wetting of the skin. *Candida* infections may involve multiple organs and tissue simultaneously, a particular risk for immunosuppressed individuals.

Table 13-25
Vulvovaginitis Caused by a Pathogen

	Trichomoniasis	Candidiasis	*Gardnerella vaginalis* Vaginitis
Occurrence	Worldwide; highest in females 16-35 yr; often accompanies other STDs	Worldwide; fungus is part of normal flora in 50% of women 15-45 yr; most common cause of vaginitis	Worldwide; bacteria are part of normal vaginal flora in many asymptomatic women
Etiologic agent	*Trichomonas vaginalis*, a protozoan	*Candida albicans*, a fungus	*Gardnerella vaginalis (Haemophilus vaginalis, Corynebacterium vaginale)*, a gram-negative coccobacillus
Reservoir	Humans	Humans	Humans
Transmission	Direct and indirect contact with vaginal and urethral discharges; transmitted to infant during birth	Direct and indirect contact with excretions from mouth, skin, vagina, and rectum of infected persons and carriers; transmitted to infant during vaginal delivery	Direct contact with vaginal and urethral discharges
Incubation period	4-20 d; average is 7 d	2-5 d in thrush in newborn	5-7 d
Period of communicability	Duration of infection	Duration of lesions	Duration of infection
Susceptibility and resistance	General, but clinical disease is mainly in females; exacerbated during menstruation and pregnancy	Low level of pathogenicity or high level of natural resistance because many persons have organism but few acquire infection	General, but clinical disease is only in females; many women have the organism, but not all acquire symptomatic infections
Report to local health authority	No	No	No

Data from Benenson[5] and Holmes.[37]

Vaginal candidiasis may be transmitted to the infant during delivery. A common manifestation of such an infection in the newborn is thrush, an infection in the oral cavity. Creamy white, curdlike patches consisting of desquamated epithelial cells, leukocytes, bacteria, keratin, necrotic tissue, and food debris are formed on the oral mucosa. Scraping of the patches leaves a raw, bleeding, painful surface. Thrush may be acquired by adults also.

Diagnostic Studies and Findings[10]

Trichomoniasis

Culture of vaginal secretions
- Positive for *T. vaginalis*

Microscopic examination of saline wet mount of vaginal secretions
- Visualization of motile protozoa

Candidiasis

Culture of vaginal secretions
- Positive for *C. vaginale* in symptomatic women
- Because *Candida* is part of normal oral flora, culture is not useful in thrush

Microscopic examination of Gram's stain or KOH wet mount preparation of vaginal secretions
- Visualization of yeast cells

Gardnerella vaginalis Vaginitis

Culture of vaginal secretions
- Positive for *G. vaginalis* in symptomatic women

Microscopic examination of Gram's stain or KOH wet mount preparation of vaginal secretions
- Identification of "clue" cells

Medical Plan[5,20,41]

Medications

Anti-infective agents
- Trichomoniasis: metronidazole (Flagyl), 2 g po at one time (contraindicated during first trimester of preg-

Table 13-26
Vulvovaginitis of Nonpathogenic Origin

Etiology	Epidemiology	Signs and Symptoms	Diagnostic Studies	Medical Plan
Postmenopausal vaginitis (atrophic vaginitis)	Occurs because of decreased estrogen levels	Thin watery discharge; burning and itching	Direct visual examination	Atrophic changes cannot be reversed but can usually be prevented with hormone therapy
Allergic or irritative vaginitis owing to thermal, chemical, and physical causes	Thermal sources: douching with excessively hot water, wearing nylon undergarments	Redness, burning, and itching of excoriated skin	Direct visual examination; wet smear; detailed history; bimanual examination	Avoidance of source; secondary infection should be treated according to etiology; oral antihistamines for allergic vaginitis, local cortisone ointment; wearing cotton undergarments
	Chemical sources: douche solutions, hygiene sprays, soaps, detergents on undergarments, poor personal hygiene	Increase in type and amount of secretions; rash; burning and itching		
	Physical sources: retained tampon, diaphragm, toilet paper, condom, or pessary	Foul-smelling, serosanguineous, or purulent discharge		

nancy; asymptomatic women should be treated to prevent sexual transmission

Candidiasis

- Nystatin (Mycostatin), one vaginal suppository (100,000 U) qd for 14 d
- Miconazole nitrate 2% vaginal cream (Monistat), one applicator intravaginally at bedtime for 7 d (and applied externally for vulvitis), or
- Clotrimazole: 500 mg tablet intravaginally once

Gardnerella vaginitis

- Metronidazole (Flagyl), 500 mg po bid for 7 d, or
- Ampicillin (Amcill; others), 500 mg po qid for 7 d

Systemic *Candida* infections: amphotericin B (Fungizone), 5-10 mg IV first day, increasing the dosage 5 mg as tolerated to 0.7 mg/kg every other day for 6-10 wk

Prevention

- Sexual partners should be examined and treated
- Treatment of candidiasis during third trimester of pregnancy to prevent oral thrush in newborn

NURSING CARE

Nursing Assessment[41]

Vulvovagina

Trichomoniasis

- Inflammation of vaginal walls and endocervix; punctate hemorrhagic lesions
- Painful coitus
- Copious loose discharge with an odor
- One third of patients have yellow-green discharge with bubbles

Candidiasis

- Pale or erythematous labia; labial excoriations; erythema extending into vagina and toward anus
- Tiny papulopustules beyond main area of erythema
- Severe perivaginal pruritus
- Discharge: thick and adherent, containing curds, or thin and loose; without an odor

Gardnerella vaginalis vaginitis

- Milder symptoms; less erythema
- Mild or moderate discharge; thin white or gray white; uniformly adheres to vaginal walls; 25% have gas bubbles in discharge; fishy or aminelike odor to discharge

Urinary Concerns

Candidiasis

- Dysuria

Trichomoniasis

- Dysuria or frequency

Lymph Nodes

Trichomoniasis

- Inguinal adenopathy possible

Nursing Dx & Intervention

Nursing Diagnosis	Nursing Intervention/Rationale
Pain	• Place cool compresses on perineal area *to relieve itching and burning.* • Provide sitz baths several times a day.
Impaired skin integrity; potential impaired skin integrity	• Administer medications as ordered or teach self-medication *to ensure compliance.* • Advise against scratching *to prevent spread of exudate.* • Avoid use of thermal, chemical, or physical sources of inflammation. • Reinforce good personal hygiene to remove smegma and perspiration *for comfort.* • Pat skin area after washing rather than rubbing with towel.
Potential for infection	• See "Patient Education" *to prevent recurrence and transmission.*

Patient Education[10]

1. Sexual partners, even though asymptomatic, should be referred for treatment.
2. Recurrent infections are common. Patient should return for treatment if symptoms recur.
3. Condoms are protection against reinfection.
4. Alcohol should be avoided until after 3 days following metronidazole therapy.
5. If tetracycline is given for *Gardnerella,* it should be taken 1 hour before or 2 hours after meals. It should not be taken with dairy products, iron, or other mineral-containing preparations. Patient should avoid sunlight.
6. Vaginal suppositories for candidiasis should be stored in a refrigerator. Treatment should continue during menstruation. Sanitary pads can be worn to protect clothing.
7. Teach the patient to wipe from front to back.
8. Instruct the patient not to douche routinely to avoid removal of normal vaginal flora.
9. Instruct the patient to avoid using sprays, soaps, powders, and deodorants.
10. Instruct the patient to wear cotton undergarments to permit free airflow to the perineum and to avoid trapping moisture.
11. Instruct the patient to wash undergarments in mild detergent and to rinse them twice.
12. Instruct the patient to avoid sharing towels and washcloths with others.
13. Instruct the patient to use water-soluble lubricants if necessary before intercourse.
14. Instruct the patient to ensure cleanliness of her sexual partner.

Evaluation

Patient Outcome	Data Indicating That Outcome is Reached
Comfort is achieved.	There is no soreness or itching.
Color and integrity of skin and mucous membrane are good.	There is no vaginal drainage or pruritus or inflammation of vulva and perineum.
Infection and inflammation are controlled.	Patient verbalizes intent to adhere to hygienic treatment and practices as described in "Patient Education." Sexual partners have been treated to minimize risk for reinfection.

NOSOCOMIAL INFECTIONS

Nosocomial describes infections that are hospital acquired in contrast to community acquired. An infection classified as nosocomial is not present nor is the microorganism incubating (unless the organism was acquired during a previous hospitalization) at the time of admission to an inpatient health care facility. Symptoms of the nosocomial infection need not be present during the hospitalization but may become evident after discharge.

Any infectious disease that is transmitted directly or indirectly from person to person has the potential for becoming a nosocomial infection. Infections that develop in a hospital from microorganisms present in normal flora or from normally nonpathogenic microorganisms in the hospital environment and that invade and colonize in a susceptible patient are also considered nosocomial.

A community-acquired infection is one that is present or incubating at the time of hospital admission. The known incubation period of a disease is used to determine whether an infection that becomes symptomatic during or after hospitalization is hospital or community acquired. A disease occurring in the hospital with an unknown incubation period is generally classified as nosocomial. Infections occurring in newborns that are acquired during birth from an infected mother are also classified as nosocomial.[48]

Iatrogenic infections are those arising from treatment or other actions of health care providers. They may be nosocomial or community acquired, depending on where the pathogen was encountered. Many nosocomial infections are iatrogenic. Neither iatrogenic nor nosocomial classifications imply provider negligence or error.[2]

Extent. Reported occurrences of nosocomial infections in the United States range from 3% to 15.5% of hospital discharges, depending on the type of hospital, type of patients, and completeness of the reporting system. On the average, 5% to 7% of people who are admitted to a general hospital acquire a nosocomial infection. The extent of nosocomial infections in hospital personnel has not been quantified. The incidence is thought to be high, especially for tuberculosis and hepatitis.[48]

Nosocomial infection studies report on body sites and the hospital services where infections occur most frequently. The National Nosocomial Infections Surveillance System reported that in 1984, 38.5% of all nosocomial infections involved the urinary tract, 16.6% involved surgical wounds, 17.8% involved the lower respiratory tract, 7.5% were primary bacteremias, 5.8% were cutaneous infections, and 13.8% were other types. Most infections (64%) were caused by a single pathogen, with *E. coli, Pseudomonas aeruginosa,* enterococci, and *Staphylococcus aureus* most often implicated.[23]

Etiology. Certain interacting agent, host, and environmental characteristics of hospitals contribute to the risk for nosocomial infections. A large number of individuals (patients, families, and personnel) are brought together in one small environment. Some of these individuals have community-acquired, overt or subclinical infections. Patient care necessitating close contact with body fluids and excretions increases the risk of transmission of pathogens from person to person and to the hospital environment. Thus a greater variety of microorganisms of greater virulence are likely to be present in hospitals. The increase in antibiotic-resistant strains of bacteria in hospitals is an example of this phenomenon. Hospitals also contain a wide range of potential reservoirs for microorganism growth such as infusion liquids, foods, biologic materials, and equipment.

Patients, already weakened by existing disease or treatment, are susceptible to invasion and infection by normal flora microorganisms, opportunistic organisms in the environment, and pathogens. Use of invasive diagnostic and treatment technologies further increases opportunities for microorganism invasion. Treatments that result in immunosuppression compromise patient resistance and further increase the risk for infection.

Epidemiology of Transmission

Nosocomial infections are transmitted according to the same chain of transmission as described on p. 1157 of this chapter. Select hospital factors associated with the chain are listed below.

Agents: endogenous (part of patient's flora) or exogenous (part of environment)

- Aerobic and anaerobic bacteria, particularly gram-positive *S. aureus,* streptococci, and *Legionella pneumophila*
- Gram-negative bacteria, particularly *E. coli, Proteus, Pseudomonas, Klebsiella, Enterobacter,* and *Serratia*
- Fungi, particularly *Candida* and *Aspergillus*
- Viruses, particularly human immunodeficiency virus (HIV), hepatitis B and non-A, non-B, herpes, cytomegalovirus, varicella, rubella, influenza, and respiratory syncytial virus

Reservoir

- Patients, visitors, health care personnel, equipment, products, or the environment
- Human reservoirs may be frank cases, subclinical cases, or carriers

Portal of exit

- Genitourinary tract
- Gastrointestinal tract
- Respiratory tract
- Skin or mucous membranes
- Blood

Mode of transmission

- Direct contact with secretions, excretions, exudates, or blood in provision of direct patient care, from mother to infant, or from patient to patient
- Indirect contact through handling of specimens, contaminated equipment, infusion fluids, biologic materials, or food or by health care workers' hands

Portal of entry

- Ingestion
- Inhalation
- Percutaneous injection or infusion
- Surgical incision
- Invasive diagnostic procedures

Susceptible host

- Characteristics of hospitalized patients that increase their susceptibility: chronic disease, malnutrition, dehydration, stasis of body fluids, traumatized tissue, leukopenia, preexisting infection, and any condition or treatment that interferes with host defenses and immune responses

Control

Control of nosocomial infections, as with community-acquired infections, relies on efforts to break the chain of transmission at one or more of its links. The point of the chain most amenable to control varies with the microorganism and disease process. General hospital procedures for control are outlined below.

Agent

- Sterilization and disinfection of inanimate reservoirs and vehicles of transmission

Reservoir

- Antibiotic treatment of patients and employees

Limitation of visitors
Policies that encourage ill employees to stay home
Portal of exit and mode of transmission
Isolation procedures and secretion and excretion precautions
Handwashing between patients by personnel
Proper handling of specimens
Environmental air control, sanitation, proper waste disposal, and proper laundry practices
Portal of entry
Protective isolation of high-risk patients
Sterile techniques
Recommended procedures that minimize organism invasion (see recommendation for each body system discussed in this section)
Susceptible host
Nursing procedures that minimize stasis of body fluids (i.e., coughing, turning, ambulating), that prevent compromise in body defenses (i.e., skin and mucous membrane care, hydration, nutrition), and that improve immunologic status (i.e., active and passive immunization of patients and employees)

Hospital infection control also requires systematic monitoring and complete reporting to the hospital infection control committee of *all* infections occurring in the hospital. In addition, select infections must be reported to the local health authority. These infections are identified in the tables in each disease section in this chapter.

The Joint Commission for Accreditation of Healthcare Organizations requires that hospitals have an effective infection-control program in order to qualify for accreditation. The program must contain the following components[48]:

Infection-control committee
Systematic surveillance of nosocomial infections
Employee health program
Isolation policies
In-service education on infection control for employees
Regular procedures for environmental sanitation
Microbiology laboratory
Implementation of accepted infection control procedures in patient care

Urinary Tract Infections[6,48]

The urinary system, except for the distal urethra, is normally sterile. Endogenous or exogenous microorganisms enter the system from devices that enter it or have contact with it. Approximately 75% of nosocomial urinary tract infections have been preceded by urologic implementation, including catheterization. The organisms most frequently associated with urinary tract infections are gram-negative organisms usually found in the colon, including *E. coli, Klebsiella, Proteus, Enterobacter,* group D *Streptococcus, Pseudomonas,* and *Candida*. They are frequently introduced from the hands of health personnel at the time of catheterization. Bacteriuria increases the risk for septicemia and nephritis and should be treated.

Criteria for classification.[2] Urinary tract infections meeting the following Centers for Disease Control (CDC) criteria are classified as nosocomial:

Asyptomatic bacteriuria with colony counts greater than 100,000 organisms/ml urine where patient had had a previous negative culture at a time when the patient was not receiving antibiotics; or colony counts of a new organism greater than 100,000/ml even if patient had previous positive cultures of a different organism
Symptomatic urinary tract infection (fever, dysuria, costovertebral angle tenderness, suprapubic tenderness) with onset after admission and a prior negative urinalysis or present urinalysis with one or both of the following:
- Colony counts greater than 10,000 microorganisms/ml of midstream urine specimen
- Pyuria greater than 10 WBCs per high-power field in an uncentrifuged specimen

Urinary system alterations that increase risk for infection[2]

Obstructions: urethral strictures, calculi, tumors, blood clots
Trauma: injury to abdomen, ruptured bladder
Congenital anomalies: polycystic kidneys, exstrophy of bladder, horseshoe kidney
Disorders of other symptoms: abdominal or gynecologic surgery, rectovesicular fistula, meningomyelocele, spina bifida
Acute or chronic renal failure
Postpartum state
Aging changes, particularly in the female

Procedures that increase risk[2]

Urethral catheterization
- Indwelling (continuous): risk increases greatly after 7 days. A closed system is superior to an open system in delaying colonization of urine. Disconnecting a closed system increases the risk.
- Straight catheterization: less risk than with indwelling catheter. Intermittent urethral catheterization, using clean technique and performed by the patient, has less risk than indwelling catheterization.

External (condom) catheter can cause urinary tract infections, but the risk is less than with urethral catheterization.
Suprapubic catheterization: risk for infection may be lower than for urethral catheterization.
Ureteral catheterization: microorganisms from urethral colonization or contaminated instruments increase the risk for urinary tract infection.
Irrigations: irrigation equipment and solutions have great potential for contamination. Frequent disconnection of system further increases risk for infection.
Urethral dilation: the procedure may introduce bacteria and produce tissue trauma.
Cystometrography: same risks as those with urethral catheterization.
Cystoscopy: septicemia may result if urine is not sterile before the procedure.
Transurethral resection of the prostate: bacteremia may

result if urine is not sterile before the procedure.

Operative procedures on the bladder and kidneys: microorganisms introduced at the time of the procedure or from a subsequent wound infection increase the risk for a urinary tract infection

Urinary diversion procedures: chronic infections are common as a result of colonization of bacteria at the stomal site.

Recommendations for prevention[2,6,8]

Avoid unnecessary catheterization.

Use aseptic techniques for insertion of devices and for opening the drainage system.

Use closed indwelling catheter system in preference to an open system.

Decrease the duration of indwelling catheters.

Use external catheter for males who can empty bladder but cannot control micturition.

Use clean-catch midstream method of collecting urine specimens in preference to catheterization.

Use straight rather than indwelling catheter whenever possible.

Use smallest catheter possible to minimize trauma.

Avoid leg bags in acute care setting.

Obtain specimens by aspirating urine from catheter or sampling port rather than by disconnecting catheter from drainage tubing.

Use silicone catheters rather than latex for long-term catheterization.

Anchor the catheter to stabilize and reduce irritation of the urethra.

Maintain a continual downward flow of urine.

Routinely empty drainage bags, but do not change unless entire closed system is changed. The addition of disinfecting agents in the bag is still controversial.

Use a separate, clean measuring container for each patient.

Gently and regularly clean perineum. Meatal care with antimicrobial agents has not been found to be helpful and in some cases has produced infection.

Avoid irrigations unless obstruction is anticipated. Use continuous irrigation in a closed system in preference to intermittent irrigation in an open system.

Persons with chronic catheterization should receive antibiotic treatment only for clinically apparent pyelonephritis, epididymitis, or bacteremia.

Surgical Wound Infections[2,46,48]

The intact integumentary system provides the first line of defense against the invasion of microorganisms; and any disruption in the integrity of the system increases the risk for infection. The risk is increased with the extensiveness and severity of the disruption of the skin integrity and the length of time until the disruption is repaired. Repair and healing are further influenced by host factors. Postoperative wound infections vary substantially by hospital, suggesting that hospital practices and surgical skill may also greatly affect the occurrence. The incubation period for surgical wound infections is 3 to 8 days after the operation, suggesting that many infections are acquired in the operating suite.

Criteria for classification. A surgical wound is classified as the site of a nosocomial infection if it drains purulent material with or without a positive culture for bacteria.

Alterations in the host that increase risk for infection

Impaired immune response

Age (newborns and elderly individuals)

Diabetes mellitus with accompanying degenerative blood vessel changes

Corticosteroids, which reduce inflammatory response

Chemotherapy, which decreases immune response

Neurologic deficits causing loss of sensation and potential tissue pressure and anoxia

Infection elsewhere in the host

Malnutrition resulting in inadequate nitrogen for tissue repair

Obesity

Presence of *Staphylococcus aureus* on patient, particularly in the anterior nares

Surgical variables that increase risk for infection[2,48]

Class of operation (The risk for infection increases from class I to class IV procedures.)

Class I (clean wound): no break in sterile technique; the gastrointestinal or respiratory tract is not entered; if genitourinary or biliary tract is entered, their contents are sterile

Class II (clean, contaminated wound): gastrointestinal, genitourinary, or respiratory tract is entered with no spillage of contents; minor breaks in technique

Class III (contaminated wound): acute inflammation without pus encountered; spillage from a hollow viscus occurs; trauma from a clean source

Class IV (dirty): pus or a perforated viscus is encountered; trauma from a dirty source

Duration of preoperative stay: prolonged presurgery hospitalization increases the risk for microbial colonization in or on the patient before the surgery.

Location of the surgery: infection increases if surgery is in body areas with impaired circulation or in areas with microorganisms already present.

Surgical technique: delayed wound closure, excess tissue trauma, improper suture tension, excess blood loss, and presence of a drain increase the risk.

Presence of bacteria at closure: the single most common agent causing postoperative wound infections is *S. aureus*, which is part of the normal flora for some people and has been found in the respiratory passages of 21% of operating suite personnel. Other gram-negative bacteria, accounting for 60% of infections, are transient on the hands of hospital employees and may be transmitted after surgery as well as in the operating suite.

Recommendations for prevention[46]

Surveillance and classification: all surgical procedures should be classified and recorded; and surveillance should be maintained on all postsurgical infections by classification. Surgeons should be apprised of their infection rates.

Preoperative preparation: the preoperative hospital stay should be as short as possible. Preexisting bacterial infections, excluding those for which the operation is performed, should be treated and controlled. Malnourished patients should receive oral or parenteral hyperalimentation before elective surgery. The patient should be bathed the night before elective surgery with an antiseptic soap. Hair should not be removed unless it will interfere with the procedure. If hair removal is necessary, it should be done immediately before surgery. Skin preparation includes scrubbing with a detergent solution followed by application of an antiseptic solution, preferably tincture of chlorhexidine, iodophors, or tincture of iodine. The patient should be completely covered with sterile drapes.

Postoperative wound care: use aseptic technique in dressing changes. A drain for an infected wound should be placed in an adjacent stab wound and attached to a closed suction system. Dressings should be changed if wet or if patient has signs of infection. Exudate should be cultured. Personnel must wash hands before and after caring for a surgical wound.

Prophylactic antibiotics: parenteral antibiotic prophylaxis should be started 2 hours before operations that are associated with a high risk of infection. They should be discontinued between 12 and 48 hours after the surgery.

Bacteremia and Septicemia[2,45]

See description of sepsis in this chapter.

Vascular system alterations that increase risk for infection

Thrombophlebitis caused by mechanical or chemical irritation from IV cannula or infusate

Decreased blood volume

Circulatory stasis caused by immobility or pressure

Immunosuppression of host

Vascular changes associated with diabetes, collagen diseases, and other chronic diseases

Procedures that increase risk for cannula-related infection[45]

Type of cannula used for IV therapy (plastic cannulas generally associated with higher rate of infection than steel "scalp vein" cannulas)

Method of insertion: cutdown has greater infection risk than percutaneous insertion

Duration over 48 to 72 hours

Purpose of the cannula: CVP lines are associated with high risk for infection

Microbial contamination of infusion fluid: rare and usually caused by gram-negative bacteria

Recommendations for prevention of secondary bacteremia

Prevention of original underlying infection

Early recognition and treatment of underlying surgical wound, urinary tract, and pulmonary infections

Recommendations for prevention of primary bacteremias induced by intravenous catheters[2,45]

Wash hands before insertion.

Use sterile gloves and antiseptic hand wash for cutdowns or central lines.

Use upper extremity veins; lower extremity veins develop phlebitis more readily.

Use an antiseptic preparation before venipuncture (in declining order of preference: tincture of iodine, chlorhexidine, iodophors, 70% alcohol); avoid quaternary ammonium compounds and hexachlorophene.

Use plastic catheters for cannulation of central veins and steel needles for IV infusions.

Secure catheter and apply sterile dressing.

Inspect daily.

Insert new cannula every 48 to 72 hours.

Change dressing and apply antibiotic ointment every 48 hours.

Change IV tubing every 48 hours and after blood products or lipid emulsions.

Avoid irrigations or blood drawing.

Lower Respiratory Tract Infections[2,6]

As many as 1% to 2% of hospitalized patients develop nosocomial bacterial pneumonias, with 30% of those infected persons dying even with adequate antimicrobial therapy. Certain factors contribute to the risk for pneumonia in hospitalized patients.

The integrity of normal respiratory defense mechanisms may be disrupted, thus permitting the invasion of oropharyngeal normal flora microorganisms into the lung alveoli.

Medical diagnostic and treatment procedures may introduce microorganisms from the oropharynx or from the equipment or solutions into the lower respiratory tract.

Ill persons with altered respiratory clearance mechanisms are susceptible to rapid oropharyngeal colonization of pathogens from the hospital environment, equipment, or the patient's normal flora. The pathogens that frequently colonize in hospitalized patients and are most often associated with nosocomial pneumonia are *Klebsiella, S. aureus, Pseudomonas, E. coli, Enterobacter, S. pneumoniae,* and *H. influenzae*. Opportunistic organisms such as *Candida, Aspergillus,* cytomegalovirus, and *Pneumocystis carinii* cause pneumonia in immunocompromised hosts.

Microbial invasion of lung alveoli can occur from one of three routes:

Aspiration from the oropharynx

Inhalation of aerosolized droplets or gas containing suspended organisms

Lymphohematogenous spread

Aspiration is probably the most frequent route in nosocomial pneumonia.

Criteria for classification. The criteria used by the Hospital Infections Branch of the Centers for Disease Control for classifying nosocomial pneumonia are as follows.[6]

Purulent sputum developing 48 hours or more after admission, or increased production of purulent sputum with recrudescence of fever in a patient hospitalized with pulmonary disease; plus one of the following:

Cough, fever, and pleuritic chest pain, or

Infiltration seen on chest roentgenography or physical findings of infection

An infection present on admission can be classified as nosocomial if it is related to a previous hospitalization.

Host factors that increase the risk for nosocomial pneumonia[2,6]

Airway obstruction caused by tumors, foreign bodies, edema, fluid, or chronic obstructive pulmonary disease

Impairment of mucociliary defenses as a result of dehydration, inhalation of chemical irritants, viral infection, or anticholinergic drugs

Impaired immunologic function

Traumatic injury to respiratory tract or surgery to abdominal or thoracic cavity

Altered swallowing, clearing, or coughing caused by central nervous system disorders; alcoholism; depressed levels of consciousness; dysphagia; nasogastric tubes; anesthesia, sedation, or medications that alter the cough reflex; immobilization

Oropharyngeal colonization of bacteria (Colonization increases with length of hospital stay, prolonged intubation, and preceding antibiotic therapy.)

Smoking

Procedures that increase risk for infection[2,6]

Large-volume nebulizers: the major source of aerosolized bacteria; humidifiers do not have the same risk

Any device or airway that may carry bacteria from the oropharynx to the lower respiratory tract including nasogastric tubes and endotracheal tubes

Ventilation equipment including intermittent positive pressure machines

Administration of oxygen or anesthesia

Pulmonary function testing

Bronchoscopy

Surgical procedures, including lung biopsy and tracheostomy

Recommendations for prevention of nosocomial pneumonia associated with respiratory care equipment[2,6]

Use sterile, adequately disinfected, or disposable breathing circuits (mouthpieces, tubing, cannulae) that come in contact with the patient.

Replace circuitry for patients on continuous assisted or controlled ventilation and on intermittent therapy every 24 to 48 hours. Remove fluid buildup in the tubing.

Use high-efficiency bacterial filters on ventilators and intermittent positive pressure machines between the machine and the patient. Use in-line filters to prevent contamination of internal parts of anesthesia machines and ventilators from patient's exhaled air.

Change, sterilize, or disinfect aerosol-producing equipment between patients and every 24 hours for the same patient. Do not use spinning disc nebulizers.

Use sterile solutions in fluid reservoirs, dispensed under aseptic conditions. Fill water reservoirs at the time needed, not in advance. Unused portions should be discarded every 24 hours at the time the reservoir is sterilized or replaced.

Do not add to fluid levels in nebulizers or humidifiers. If additional fluid is needed, empty reservoir and fill with sterile water.

Use sterile medications in single-use vials for nebulization.

For suctioning, use sterile catheter and sterile glove. Change suction catheter after each use. Use intermittent rather than continuous suctioning.

Recommendations for prevention of nosocomial pneumonia associated with patient risk factors

High-risk surgical patients and patients with impaired chest function should receive[6]:

Preoperative and postoperative therapy to treat any underlying infection.

Preoperative instruction to discontinue smoking.

Preoperative and postoperative instruction and therapy to encourage and stimulate postoperative deep breathing, coughing, movement in bed and early ambulation.

Postoperative interventions to remove secretions and stimulate coughing (i.e. percussion, postural drainage).

Postoperative pain control.

Medical Interventions and Related Nursing Care

 Immunizations

Some infectious diseases are preventable with artificial active immunization. In some cases artificial passive immunization can be used to provide temporary immunity. Clinical considerations for active and passive immunization, general recommendations for administration of vaccines, and a schedule for administration of vaccines for the diseases discussed in the section on vaccine-preventable infectious diseases (p. 1166) will be presented here. (Refer to "Anatomy, Physiology, and Related Pathophysiology" in this chapter for an overview of the development of specific immune responses.)

Clinical Considerations for Active and Passive Immunization[48]

Active immunization. Vaccines used for active immunization are prepared from bacteria or viruses, or their derivatives, that have been modified to stimulate antibody production without causing disease. Modification is accomplished by inactivation or killing of the organism or by alteration of the organism so it retains its antigenicity while losing its virulence (attenuated).

Inactivated vaccines must be given in multiple first doses to stimulate an adequate antibody response, and a periodic booster must be given to maintain serum antibody levels. Attenuated vaccines stimulate lifetime antibody levels with one administration.

Routine immunizations are given according to a schedule that facilitates administration at a time earliest in life when the vaccine will be effective. The health care provider administering the immunization should fully inform the patient or parent of the reason for the immunization, the schedule, side effects that may occur, and actions to take in the event of side effects. Informed consent must be obtained.

Passive immunization. Active immunization is preferred to passive in most situations. Passive immunization with serum antitoxins prepared in animals or with human immune globulins is recommended only for those situations where active immunization procedures have not been developed; exposure has already occurred, leaving insufficient time for active immunization; or concurrent active and passive immunization is required for immediate and future protection.

The use of human immune globulins for passive immunization is preferred to use of serum antitoxins from animals. The risk for anaphylaxis-like reactions and serum sickness is greater when prepared animal sera are used. Anaphylaxis-like reactions affect principally the cardiovascular and respiratory systems, producing dyspnea, asthma, respiratory decompensation, and possible death. These reactions occur in minutes to a few hours after administration of the serum, and they range from mild to severe. The much more common serum sickness reactions develop in 7 to 12 days after injection of the serum, producing mild to severe symptoms of fever, urticaria, or arthralgia. The severity of the symptoms depends on the type of serum and the route of administration (IV administration leads to more severe reactions). Individuals previously sensitized to the serum may react within 1 to 3 days of receiving the serum.

General Recommendations[9]

Multiple dose vaccines. Some vaccines must be administered in more than one dose for full protection. If the intervals between doses are longer than recommended, there is usually not a reduction in final antibody levels. It is therefore unnecessary to restart an interrupted series or to add extra doses.

Simultaneous administration of certain vaccines. Most of the widely used vaccines can be safely and effectively administered simultaneously. Inactivated vaccines can be administered simultaneously at different sites unless the person is known to have experienced past side effects to one or more of the vaccines. In that case the vaccines should be administered on separate occasions. An inactivated vaccine and a live attenuated virus vaccine can be administered simultaneously at different sites.

Hypersensitivity to vaccine components. Vaccine antigens produced in systems or with substrates that contain allergenic substances may cause hypersensitivity reactions and possible anaphylaxis. Antigens grown in eggs of chickens or ducks should not be given to anyone with a history (or questionable history) of allergy to eggs. Influenza vaccine antigens, although produced from viruses grown in eggs, are highly purified and are associated with only rare hypersensitivity reactions. Influenza vaccine should not be administered to anyone with a history of an anaphylactic reaction to eggs.

No hypersensitivity reactions have been reported from administration of live attenuated measles, mumps, or rubella (MMR) vaccine prepared from viruses grown in cell cultures.

Some vaccines that are derived from organisms grown in bacteriologic media frequently produce local or systemic reactions that are not allergenic. These vaccines—including cholera; diphtheria, pertussis, and tetanus (DPT); plague; and typhoid—should not be given to persons who have a history of serious side effects from the vaccine.

Vaccines that contain preservatives or trace amounts of antibiotics, as indicated on the package insert, should not be given to any person with a history of hypersensitivity to those substances.

Contraindications for immunization[9,18]

1. Altered immunity: immunosuppressed persons should not receive live attenuated virus vaccines because of the risk for multiplication of the virus within those persons. Also, individuals living in the same household with an immunocompromised person should not be given oral polio vaccine (OPV) because vaccine viruses are excreted and may be transmitted to other persons.
2. Severe febrile illnesses: although the presence of mild illnesses does not preclude vaccination, immunization should be deferred for those with severe febrile illnesses.
3. Pregnancy: attenuated virus vaccines, particularly MMR, should not be given to pregnant women or women who may become pregnant within 3 months of the vaccination. OPV and yellow fever vaccines may be given if there is a high risk for acquired infection. There is no contraindication for administration of inactivated viral vaccines, bacterial vaccines, or toxoids to pregnant women.
4. Recent administration of immune globulin: live attenuated virus vaccines should not be administered within 3 months of passive immunization. Similarly, immunoglobulins should not be administered for at least 2 weeks after a vaccine has been given. These precautions reduce the risk that high serum levels of immunoglobulins would prevent the development of active acquired immunity.

Table 13-27
Immunization Schedule

	Tetanus	Diphtheria	Pertussis	Polio (Trivalent Oral Polio Vaccine [TOPV])	Measles (Rubeola)	Mumps	Rubella
Vaccine	Toxoid (detoxified toxin)	Toxoid (detoxified toxin)	Killed vaccine	Live attenuated virus	Live attenuated virus	Live attenuated virus	Live attenuated virus
Administration	1. Primary (under 7 yr) One dose diptheria, pertussis, tetanus toxoid (DPT) IM q4-8wk; give three times (2, 4, and 6 mo) Fourth dose 1 yr later (15 mo) Booster: school entry and q10 yr (DT only) 2. Primary (7-65 yr or older) Two doses DT IM separated by 4-8 wk period Third dose 6-12 mo later Booster q10 yr			One dose at 6-8 wk followed by a second dose 6-8 wk later; third dose 8-12 mo later; booster at school entry	Single dose Give combined as MMR; may be administered at 15 mo	Single dose	Single dose
Recommendations	Ideally begin at 2-3 mo of age		Do not give pertussis after 7 yr	Not recommended over 18 yr	Must be given on or after age of 15 mo	All persons over 12 mo with no history of mumps (includes adults)	All persons over 12 mo with no evidence of immunity (includes adults)
Major adverse reactions	Rare: neurologic reactions including neuritis and transverse myelitis		Convulsions; loss of consciousness	Rare: paralysis within 2 mo	Rare: central nervous system reactions (encephalitis)	Rare: encephalomyelitis	In older children and adults, transient arthralgias and arthritis 2 wk after immunization
Less severe reactions	Fever within 24-48 h; soreness, swelling, and redness at injection site; lump may persist for weeks but gradually disappears; may also have urticaria and malaise		Thrombocytopenia	None	Anorexia, malaise, rash, and fever within 7-10 d	Brief, mild fever	Mild rash lasting 1 or 2 d after immunization
Passive immunization	Immune globulin following injury for those without active immunization	Antitoxin for unimmunized contacts with an active case	Hyperimmune pertussis globulin for active cases	None	When active immunization is contraindicated in exposed person, give immune globulin; recommended for all persons born after 1957 with no documentation of disease or vaccine after age 12 mo	Not recommended	Not recommended

Data from Centers for Disease Control.[13,18,22,27]

5. All adverse reactions to vaccines should be reported to the local or state health authority and to the manufacturer of the vaccine.
6. DPT or single-antigen pertussis vaccine is contraindicated if any of the following events occurred after the patient received a vaccine containing pertussis antigen:
   a. Allergic hypersensitivity
   b. Fever of 40.5° C (105° F) or higher within 48 hours
   c. Collapse or shocklike state within 48 hours
   d. Persistent, inconsolable crying lasting 3 hours or more or an unusual, high-pitched cry occurring within 48 hours
   e. Convulsion(s) with or without fever occurring within 3 days of receipt of pertussis vaccine
   f. Encephalopathy (with generalized or focal neurologic signs and/or alterations in consciousness) occurring within 7 days
   g. Children with a history of seizure or other neurologic disorders should be evaluated before vaccine administration

Tetanus prophylaxis in wound management is as follows. Medical treatment regarding the administration of active or passive tetanus immunization after a skin injury depends on the severity of the injury and on the patient's history of active tetanus immunization. Complete active immunization provides long-lasting immunity, so booster injections of toxoid are unnecessary more often than every 5 years in the event of a wound and every 10 years without injury. Serum antitoxin develops rapidly following a toxoid booster in persons who have received at least two doses of tetanus toxoid out of the four doses recommended for primary immunization. In this situation it is important to administer the toxoid within 24 hours of injury.

For persons without a full series of tetanus toxoid in the past and with a wound over 24 hours old, it may be necessary to administer tetanus antitoxic antibodies together with tetanus toxoid. If such passive immunization is to be used, tetanus immune globulin (TIG), 250 U, is recommended rather than antitoxin because TIG provides longer immunity with no undesirable reactions. Toxoid and TIG, given concurrently, should be administered with separate syringes in separate sites. There would no indication for giving TIG without also giving toxoid. The recommendations for tetanus prophylaxis in wound management are described in Table 13-28.

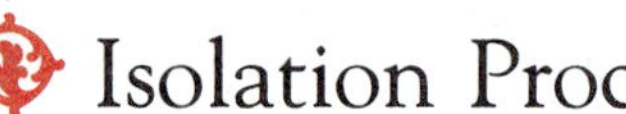

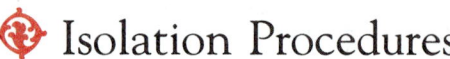

Isolation Procedures

Isolation procedures are designed to prevent the spread of microorganisms among hospitalized patients, personnel, and visitors. Most of the infectious diseases discussed in this chapter have the potential for being transmitted to others. For infections that can be transmitted, the recommended hospital isolation category precautions are specified in this chapter under "Nursing Diagnoses and Interventions." These recommendations were published in 1983 by the Centers for Disease Control (CDC).[11]

The 1983 CDC guidelines provide for two isolation systems: one based on revised categories of isolation and a new system based on disease-specific isolation precautions. The disease-specific isolation system differs from the category system by specifying only the necessary precautions to interrupt the transmission of each disease. Only a single instruction card is used, on which specific precautions may be checked or written.

The category system specifies seven categories of isolation based on the major modes of transmission of infectious diseases. Each disease has been assigned to one of the categories. Precautionary procedures have been specified for each category. Color-coded, category-specific instruction cards are available for use with this system.

Hospitals may choose one of these systems, modify one, or develop their own system. The CDC recommendations are not meant to restrict hospitals or medical and nursing per-

Table 13-28
Recommendations for Tetanus Prophylaxis in Wound Management

	Clean Minor Wounds		All Other Wounds	
History of Tetanus Immunization	**Toxoid (Detoxified Toxin; Td)***	**Tetanus Immune Globulin (TIG)**	**Toxoid (Detoxified Toxin; Td)***	**Tetanus Immune Globulin (TIG)**
Uncertain history or <three doses	Yes	No	Yes	Yes
Three or more doses†				
Last dose within past 5 yr	No	No	No	No
Last dose 5-10 yr ago	No	No	Yes	No
Last dose over 10 yr ago	Yes	No	Yes	No

Data from Centers for Disease Control.[18]
*For children under 7 years, administer DTP (or DT if pertussis vaccine is contraindicated).
†If only three doses of fluid toxoid have been administered, a fourth dose of toxoid, preferably an absorbed toxoid, should be given.

Category-Specific Isolation System

Strict isolation

Strict isolation is an isolation category designed to prevent transmission of highly contagious or virulent infections that may be spread by both air and contact.

Specifications for strict isolation

1. Private room is indicated; door should be kept closed. In general, patients infected with the same organism may share a room.
2. Masks are indicated for all persons entering the room.
3. Gowns are indicated for all persons entering the room.
4. Gloves are indicated for all persons entering the room.
5. Hands must be washed after touching the patient or potentially contaminated articles and before taking care of another patient.
6. Articles contaminated with infective material should be discarded or bagged and labeled before being sent for decontamination and reprocessing.

Diseases requiring strict isolation

Diphtheria, pharyngeal
Lassa fever and other viral hemorrhagic fevers, such as Marburg virus disease*
Plague, pneumonic
Smallpox*
Varicella (chickenpox)
Zoster, localized in immunocompromised patient or disseminated

Contact isolation

Contact isolation is designed to prevent transmission of highly transmissible or epidemiologically important infections (or colonization) that do not warrant Strict Isolation.

All diseases or conditions included in this category are spread primarily by close or direct contact. Thus, masks, gowns and gloves are recommended for anyone in close or direct contact with any patient who has an infection (or colonization) that is included in this category. For individual diseases or conditions, however, 1 or more of these 3 barriers may not be indicated. For example, masks and gowns are not generally indicated for care of infants and young children with acute viral respiratory infections; gowns are not generally indicated for gonococcal conjunctivitis in newborns; and masks are not generally indicated for patients infected with multiply-resistant microorganisms, except those with pneumonia. Therefore, some degree of "over-isolation" may occur in this category.

Specifications for contact isolation

1. Private room is indicated. In general, patients infected with the same organism may share a room. During outbreaks, infants and young children with the same respiratory clinical syndrome may share a room.
2. Masks are indicated for those who come close to patient.
3. Gowns are indicated if soiling is likely.
4. Gloves are indicated for touching infective material.
5. Hands must be washed after touching the patient or potentially contaminated articles and before taking care of another patient.
6. Articles contaminated with infective material should be discarded or bagged and labeled before being sent for decontamination and reprocessing.

Diseases or conditions requiring contact isolation

Acute respiratory infections in infants and young children including croup, colds, bronchitis, and bronchiolitis caused by respiratory syncytial virus, adenovirus, coronavirus, influenza viruses, parainfluenza viruses, and rhinovirus
Conjunctivitis, gonococcal in newborns
Diptheria, cutaneous
Endometritis, group A *Streptococcus*
Furunculosis, staphylococcal in newborns
Herpes simplex, disseminated, severe primary or neonatal
Impetigo
Influenza, in infants and young children
Multiply-resistant bacteria, infection, or colonization (any site) with any of the following:

1. Gram-negative bacilli resistant to all aminoglycosides that are tested. (In general, such organisms should be resistant to gentamicin, tobramycin, and amikacin for these special precautions to be indicated.)
2. *Staphylococcus aureus* resistant to methicillin (or nafcillin or oxacillin if they are used instead of methicillin for testing).
3. *Pneumococcus* resistant to penicillin.
4. *Haemophilus influenzae* resistant to ampicillin (betalactamase positive) and chloramphenicol.
5. Other resistant bacteria may be included if they are judged by the infection control team to be of special clinical and epidemiologic significance.

Pediculosis
Pharyngitis, infectious, in infants and young children
Pneumonia, viral, in infants and young children
Pneumonia, *Staphylococcus aureus* or Group A *Streptococcus*
Rabies
Rubella, congenital and other
Scabies
Scalded skin syndrome, staphylococcal (Ritter's disease)
Skin wound or burn infection, major (draining and not covered by dressing or dressing does not adequately contain the purulent material) including those infected with *Staphylococcus aureus* or group A *Streptococcus*
Vaccinia (generalized and progressive eczema vaccinatum)

Respiratory isolation

Respiratory isolation is designed to prevent transmission of infectious diseases primarily over short distances through the air (droplet transmission). Direct and indirect contact transmission occurs with some infections in this isolation category but is infrequent.

Specifications for respiration isolation

1. Private room is indicated. In general, patients infected with the same organism may share a room.
2. Masks are indicated for those who come close to the patient.
3. Gowns are not indicated.
4. Gloves are not indicated.
5. Hands must be washed after touching the patient or potentially contaminated articles and before taking care of another patient.
6. Articles contaminated with infective material should be discarded or bagged and labeled before being sent for decontamination and reprocessing.

From Centers for Disease Control.[11]
*A private room with special ventilation is indicated.

Continued.

Category-Specific Isolation System, cont'd.

Diseases requiring respiratory isolation
Epiglottis, *Haemophilus influenzae*
Erythema infectiosum
Measles
Meningitis
Haemophilus influenzae, known or suspected
Meningococcal, known or suspected
Meningococcal pneumonia
Meningococcemia
Mumps
Pertussis (whooping cough)
Pneumonia, *Haemophilus influenzae*, in children (any age)

Tuberculosis isolation (AFB isolation)

Tuberculosis isolation (AFB isolation) is an isolation category for patients with pulmonary TB who have a positive sputum smear or a chest X-ray that strongly suggests current (active) TB. Laryngeal TB is also included in this isolation category. In general, infants and young children with pulmonary TB do not require isolation precautions because they rarely cough, and their bronchial secretions contain few AFB, compared with adults with pulmonary TB. On the instruction card, this category is called AFB (for acid-fast bacilli) Isolation to protect the patient's privacy.

Specifications for tuberculosis isolation (AFB isolation)

1. Private room with special ventilation is indicated; door should be kept closed. In general, patients infected with the same organism may share a room.
2. Masks are indicated only if the patient is coughing and does not reliably cover mouth.
3. Gowns are indicated only if needed to prevent gross contamination of clothing.
4. Gloves are not indicated.
5. Hands must be washed after touching the patient or potentially contaminated articles and before taking care of another patient.
6. Articles are rarely involved in transmission of TB. However, articles should be thoroughly cleaned and disinfected or discarded.

Enteric precautions

Enteric precautions are designed to prevent infections that are transmitted by direct or indirect contact with feces. Hepatitis A is included in this category because it is spread through feces, although the disease is much less likely to be transmitted after the onset of jaundice. Most infections in this category primarily cause gastrointestinal symptoms, but some do not. For example, feces from patients infected with "poliovirus" and coxsackieviruses are infective, but those infections do not usually cause prominent gastrointestinal symptoms.

Specifications for enteric precautions

1. Private room is indicated if patient hygiene is poor. A patient with poor hygiene does not wash hands after touching infective material, contaminates the environment with infective material, or shares contaminated articles with other patients. In general, patients infected with the same organism may share a room.
2. Masks are not indicated.
3. Gowns are indicated if soiling is likely.
4. Gloves are indicated if touching infective material.
5. Hands must be washed after touching the patient or potentially contaminated articles and before taking care of another patient.
6. Articles contaminated with infective material should be discarded or bagged and labeled before being sent for decontamination or reprocessing.

Diseases requiring enteric precautions
Amebic dysentery
Cholera
Coxsackievirus disease
Diarrhea, acute illness with suspected infectious etiology
Echovirus disease
Encephalitis (unless known not to be caused by enteroviruses)
Enterocolitis caused by *Clostridium difficile* or *Staphylococcus aureus*
Enteroviral infection
Gastroenteritis caused by
Campylobacter species
Cryptosporidium species
Dientamoeba fragilis
Escherichia coli (enterotoxic, enteropathogenic, or enteroinvasive)
Giardia lamblia
Salmonella species
Shigella species
Vibrio parahaemolyticus
Viruses—including Norwalk agent and rotavirus
Yersinia enterocolitica
Unknown etiology but presumed to be an infectious agent
Hand, foot, mouth disease
Hepatitis, viral, type A
Herpangina
Meningitis, viral (unless known not be caused by enteroviruses)
Necrotizing enterocolitis
Pleurodynia
Poliomyelitis
Tyhoid fever *(Salmonella typhi)*
Viral pericarditis, myocarditis, or meningitis (unless known not be caused by enteroviruses)

Drainage/secretion precautions

Drainage/secretion precautions are designed to prevent infections that are transmitted by direct or indirect contact with purulent material or drainage from an infected body site. This newly created isolation category includes many infections formerly included in Wound and Skin Precautions, Discharge (lesion), and Secretion (oral) Precautions, which have been discontinued. Infectious diseases included

Category-Specific Isolation System, cont'd.

in this category are those that result in the production of infective purulent material, drainage, or secretions, unless the disease is included in another isolation category that requires more rigorous precautions. For example, minor limited skin, wound, or burn infections are included in this category, but major skin, wound, or burn infections are included in Contact Isolation.

Specifications for drainage/secretion precautions

1. Private room is not indicated.
2. Masks are not indicated.
3. Gowns are indicated if soiling is likely.
4. Gloves are indicated for touching infective material.
5. Hands must be washed after touching the patient or potentially contaminated articles and before taking care of another patient.
6. Articles contaminated with infective material should be discarded or bagged and labeled before being sent for decontamination and reprocessing.

Diseases requiring drainage/secretion precautions

The following infections are examples of those included in this category provided they are not (a) caused by multiply-resistant microorganisms, (b) major draining (and not covered by a dressing or dressing does not adequately contain the drainage) skin, wound, or burn infections, including those caused by *Staphylococcus aureus* or group A *Streptococcus,* or (c) gonococcal eye infections in newborns. See Contact Isolation if the infection is one of these three.

Abscess, minor limited
Burn infection, minor limited
Conjunctivitis
Decubitus ulcer, infected, minor or limited
Skin infection, minor or limited
Wound infection, minor or limited

Blood/body fluid precautions

Blood/body fluid precautions are designed to prevent infections that are transmitted by direct or indirect contact with infective blood or body fluids. Infectious diseases included in this category are those that result in the production of infective blood or body fluids, unless the disease is included in another isolation category that requires more rigorous precautions, for example, Strict Isolation. For some diseases included in this category, such as malaria, only blood is infective; for other diseases, such as hepatitis B (including antigen carriers), blood and body fluids (saliva, semen, etc.) are infective.

Specifications for blood/body fluid precautions

1. Private room is indicated if patient hygiene is poor. A patient with poor hygiene does not wash hands after touching infective material, contaminates the environment with infective material, or shares contaminated articles with other patients. In general, patients infected with the same organism may share a room.
2. Masks are not indicated.
3. Gowns are indicated if soiling of clothing with blood or body fluids is likely.
4. Gloves are indicated for touching blood or body fluids.
5. Hands must be washed immediately if they are potentially contaminated with blood or body fluids and before taking care of another patient.
6. Articles contaminated with blood or body fluids should be discarded or bagged and labeled before being sent for decontamination and reprocessing.
7. Care should be taken to avoid needle-stick injuries. Used needles should not be recapped or bent; they should be placed in a prominently labeled, puncture-resistant container designated specifically for such disposal.
8. Blood spills should be cleaned up promptly with a solution of 5.25% sodium hypochlorite diluted 1:10 with water.

Diseases requiring blood/body fluid precautions

Acquired immunodeficiency syndrome (AIDS)
Arthropod-borne viral fevers (for example, dengue, yellow fever, and Colorado tick fever)
Babesiosis
Creutzfeldt-Jakob disease
Hepatitis B (including HBsAg antigen carrier)
Hepatitis, non-A, non-B
Leptospirosis
Malaria
Rat-bite fever
Relapsing fever
Syphilis, primary and secondary with skin and mucous membrane lesions

sonnel from requiring more stringent precautions. Nurses are advised to follow isolation procedures that are operative within their institution of employment and to use the material presented here for reference and clarification. The isolation precautions presented here may also require modification for patients who need constant care or require emergency intervention.

Hospital policy usually designates the personnel responsible for placing a patient on isolation precautions and the personnel who have ultimate authority to make decisions regarding isolation precautions when conflicts arise. All personnel are responsible for complying with isolation precautions to protect themselves, co-workers, patients, and visitors.

Recent research on AIDS transmission (see Chapter 14) has led the CDC to publish recommendations for prevention of human immunodeficiency virus (HIV) transmission in health care settings. The CDC now recommends that all health personnel consistently use "universal blood and body-fluid precautions" with *all* patients, especially those in emergency care settings where the risk of blood exposure is greater and the infection status of the patient is unknown. Portions of these recommendations are reproduced in the box on p. 1300.

Universal Blood and Body Fluid Precautions

1. All health-care workers should routinely use appropriate barrier precautions to prevent skin and mucous-membrane exposure when contact with blood or other body fluids of any patient is anticipated. Gloves should be worn for touching blood and body fluids, mucous membranes, or non-intact skin of all patients, for handling items or surfaces soiled with blood or body fluids, and for performing venipuncture and other vascular access procedures. Gloves should be changed after contact with each patient. Masks and protective eyewear or face shields should be worn during procedures that are likely to generate droplets of blood or other body fluids to prevent exposure of mucous membranes of the mouth, nose, and eyes. Gowns or aprons should be worn during procedures that are likely to generate splashes of blood or other body fluids.
2. Hands and other skin surfaces should be washed immediately and thoroughly if contaminated with blood or other body fluids. Hands should be washed immediately after gloves are removed.
3. All health-care workers should take precautions to prevent injuries caused by needles, scalpels, and other sharp instruments or devices during procedures; when cleaning used instruments; during disposal of used needles; and when handling sharp instruments after procedures. To prevent needlestick injuries, needles should not be recapped, purposely bent or broken by hand, removed from disposable syringes, or otherwise manipulated by hand. After they are used, disposable syringes and needles, scalpel blades, and other sharp items should be placed in puncture-resistant containers for disposal; the puncture-resistant containers should be located as close as practical to the use area. Large-bore reusable needles should be placed in a puncture-resistant container for transport to the reprocessing area.
4. Although saliva has not been implicated in HIV transmission, to minimize the need for emergency mouth-to-mouth resuscitation, mouthpieces, resuscitation bags, or other ventilation devices should be available for use in areas in which the need for resuscitation is predictable.
5. Health-care workers who have exudative lesions or weeping dermatitis should refrain from all direct patient care and from handling patient-care equipment until the condition resolves.
6. Pregnant health-care workers are not known to be at greater risk of contracting HIV infection than health-care workers who are not pregnant; however, if a health-care worker develops HIV infection during pregnancy, the infant is at risk of infection resulting from perinatal transmission. Because of this risk, pregnant health-care workers should be especially familiar with and strictly adhere to precautions to minimize the risk of HIV transmission.

Implementation of universal blood and body-fluid precautions for *all* patients eliminates the need for use of the isolation category of "Blood and Body Fluid Precautions" previously recommended by CDC for patients known or suspected to be infected with blood-borne pathogens. Isolation precautions (e.g., enteric, "AFB") should be used as necessary if associated conditions, such as infectious diarrhea or tuberculosis, are diagnosed or suspected.

Precautions for invasive procedures

In this document, an invasive procedure is defined as surgical entry into tissues, cavities, or organs or repair of major traumatic injuries 1) in an operating or delivery room, emergency department, or outpatient setting, including both physicians' and dentists' offices; 2) cardiac catheterization and angiographic procedures; 3) a vaginal or cesarean delivery or other invasive obstetric procedure during which bleeding may occur; or 4) the manipulation, cutting, or removal of any oral or perioral tissues, including tooth structure, during which bleeding occurs or the potential for bleeding exists. The universal blood and body-fluid precautions listed above, combined with the precautions listed below, should be the minimum precautions for *all* such invasive procedures.

1. All health-care workers who participate in invasive procedures must routinely use appropriate barrier precautions to prevent skin and mucous-membrane contact with blood and other body fluids of all patients. Gloves and surgical masks must be worn for all invasive procedures. Protective eyewear or face shields should be worn for procedures that commonly result in the generation of droplets, splashing of blood or other body fluids, or the generation of bone chips. Gowns or aprons made of materials that provide an effective barrier should be worn during invasive procedures that are likely to result in the splashing of blood or other body fluids. All health-care workers who perform or assist in vaginal or cesarean deliveries should wear gloves and gowns when handling the placenta or the infant until blood and amniotic fluid have been removed from the infant's skin and should wear gloves during post-delivery care of the umbilical cord.
2. If a glove is torn or a needlestick or other injury occurs, the glove should be removed and a new glove used as promptly as patient safety permits; the needle or instrument involved in the incident should also be removed from the sterile field.

From Centers for Disease Control.[28]

References

1. American Public Health Association: Control of communicable diseases in man, ed 13, Washington, DC, 1980, The Association.
2. Association for Practitioners in Infection Control: The APIC curriculum for infection control practice, Iowa, 1981, Kendall/Hunt Publishing Co.
3. Axnick K and Yarbrough M, editors: Infection control: an integrated approach, St Louis, 1984, The CV Mosby Co.
4. Beland IL and Passos JY: Clinical nursing: pathophysiological and psychosocial approaches, ed 4, New York, 1981, Macmillan Publishing Co., Inc.
5. Benenson A, editor: Control of communicable diseases in man, ed 14, Washington, DC, 1985, The American Public Health Association.
6. Bennett JV and Brachman PS, editors: Hospital infections, ed 2, Boston, 1986, Little, Brown & Co.
7. Burton GR: Microbiology for the health sciences, Philadelphia, 1979, JB Lippincott Co.
8. Center for Infectious Diseases: Guidelines for prevention and control of nosocomial infections, Feb 1981, The Center.
9. Centers for Disease Control: Recommendations of the Immunization Practices Advisory Committee (ACIP): general recommendations on immunizations, MMWR 26(81), Feb 22, 1980.
10. Centers for Disease Control: Sexually transmitted diseases treatment guidelines 1982, MMWR 31(35s), Aug 20, 1982.
11. Centers for Disease Control: CDC guideline for isolation precautions in hospitals, HHS pub no (CDC) 83-8314, Atlanta, 1983, The Centers.
12. Centers for Disease Control: Recommendations of the Immunization Practices Advisory Committee (ACIP): update: pneumococcal polysaccharide vaccine usage—United States, MMWR 33(20), May 25, 1984.
13. Centers for Disease Control: Recommendations of the Immunization Practices Advisory Committee (ACIP): adult immunization, MMWR 33(1S), Sept 28, 1984.
14. Centers for Disease Control: Revised recommendations for preventing malaria in travelers to areas with chloroquine-resistant *Plasmodium falciparum,* MMWR 34(14), Apr 12, 1985.
15. Centers for Disease Control: Recommendation of the Immunization Practices Advisory Committee (ACIP): polysaccharide vaccine for prevention of *Haemophilus influenzae* type b disease, MMWR 34(15), Apr 19, 1985.
16. Centers for Disease Control: Recommendation of the Immunization Practices Advisory Committee (ACIP): meningococcal vaccines, MMWR 34(18), May 10, 1985.
17. Centers for Disease Control: Recommendation of the Immunization Practices Advisory Committee (ACIP): recommendations for protection against viral hepatitis, MMWR 34(22), June 7, 1985.
18. Centers for Disease Control: Recommendation of the Immunization Practices Advisory Committee (ACIP): diphtheria, tetanus, and pertussis: guidelines for vaccine prophylaxis and other preventive measures, MMWR 34(27), July 12, 1985.
19. Centers for Disease Control: Chlamydia, MMWR 34(3S), Aug 23, 1985.
20. Centers for Disease Control: Guidelines for treatment of sexually transmitted diseases, MMWR 34(4S), Oct 18, 1985.
21. Centers for Disease Control: Recommendations of the Immunization Practices Advisory Committee (ACIP): update: prevention of *Haemophilus influenzae* type b disease, MMWR *35*(11), Mar 21, 1986.
22. Centers for Disease Control: Recommendation of the Immunization Practices Advisory Committee: new recommended schedule for active immunization of normal infants and children, MMWR 35(37), Sept 19, 1986.
23. Centers for Disease Control: Nosocomial infection surveillance, 1984, MMWR 35(1SS), 1986.
24. Centers for Disease Control: Disseminated gonorrhea caused by penicillinase-producing *Neisseria gonorrhoeae,* MMWR 36(11), Mar 27, 1987.
25. Centers for Disease Control: Recommendations of the Immunization Practices Advisory Committee: update on hepatitis B prevention, MMWR 36(23), June 19, 1987.
26. Centers for Disease Control: Recommendations of the Immunization Practices Advisory Committee (ACIP): prevention and control of influenza, MMWR 36(24), June 26, 1987.
27. Centers for Disease Control: Recommendations of the Immunization Practices Advisory Committee: measles prevention, MMWR 36(26), July 10, 1987.
28. Centers for Disease Control: Recommendations for prevention of HIV transmission in health-care settings, 36(2S), August 21, 1987.
29. Corbett JV: Laboratory tests in nursing practice, East Norwalk, Conn, 1982, Appleton-Century-Crofts.
30. Duke University Hospital Nursing Services: Quality assurance: guidelines for nursing care, Philadelphia, 1980, JB Lippincott Co.
31. Fox, JP, Hall, CE, and Elveback, LR: Epidemiology, man and disease, New York, 1970, Macmillan Publishing Co, Inc.
32. Freitag JJ and Miller LW, editors: Manual of medical therapeutics, ed 23, Boston, 1980, Little, Brown & Co.
33. Frobisher M and Fuerst R: Microbiology in health and disease, ed 13, Philadelphia, 1973, WB Saunders Co.
34. Ganong, WF: Review of medical physiology, ed 11, Los Altos, Calif, 1983, Lange Medical Publication.
35. Garb S: Laboratory tests in common use, ed 6, New York, 1976, Springer Publishing Co.
36. Guyton AC: Human physiology and mechanisms of disease, ed 3, Philadelphia, 1982, WB Saunders Co.
37. Holmes KK and Mardh PA, editors: International perspectives on neglected sexually transmitted diseases, New York, 1983, McGraw-Hill Book Co.
38. Jawetz E, Melnick, JL, and Adelberg EA: Review of medical microbiology, ed 16, Los Altos, Calif, 1984, Lange Medical Publications.
39. King A, Nicol C, and Rodin P: Venereal diseases, London, 1980, Bailliere Tindal.
40. Krugman S and Katz SL: Infectious diseases of children, ed 7, St Louis, 1981, The CV Mosby Co.
41. Mandell GL, Douglas RG Jr, and Benett JE, editors: Principles and practice of infectious diseases, ed 2, New York, 1985, John Wiley & Sons.
42. Merck manual of diagnosis and therapy, ed 14, New Jersey, 1982, Merck & Co., Inc.
43. National Institute of Allergy and Infectious Diseases Study Group: Gonorrhea. In Sexually transmitted diseases 1980: status report, US DHHS, PHS, NIH pub no 81-2213.
44. Rymzo WT Jr et al: Dengue outbreaks in Guanica-Ensenada and Villalba, Puerto Rico, 1972-1973, Am J Trop Med Hyg 25:136, 1976.
45. Simmons BP: Guideline for prevention of intravenous therapy related infections, Oct 1981 (reprinted Feb 1982), Center for Infectious Diseases, Centers for Disease Control.
46. Simmons BP: Center for Disease Control guideline for prevention of surgical wound infections, Infect Control 3:187, 1982.
47. Tilkian SM, Conover MB, and Tilkian AG: Clinical implications of laboratory tests, ed 4, St Louis, 1987, The CV Mosby Co.
48. Wehrle PF and Top FH Sr, editors: Communicable and infectious disease, ed 9, St Louis, 1981, The CV Mosby Co.

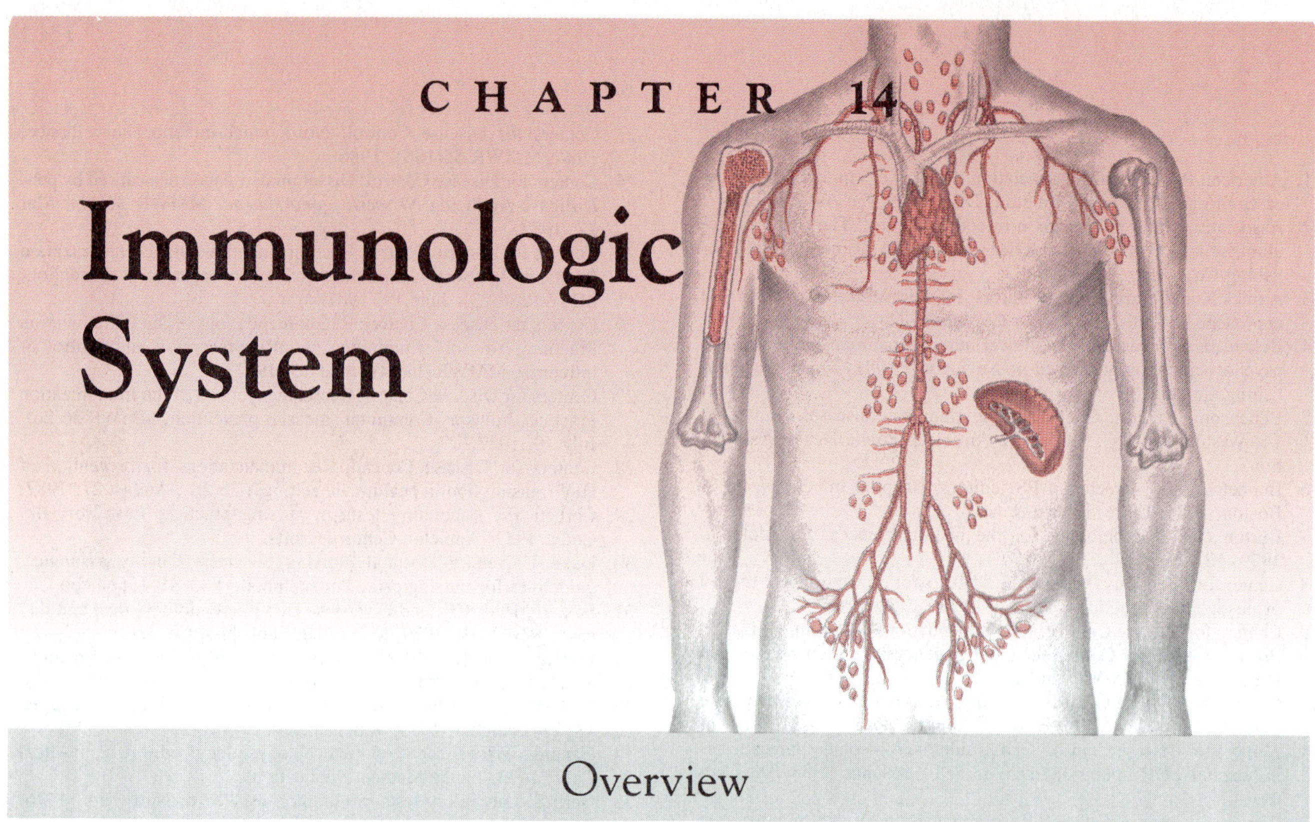

CHAPTER 14

Immunologic System

Overview

The immune system is a highly specialized group of cells and tissues that protects the internal milieu of the host. Immune responses are initiated when cellular components of the system recognize an agent as foreign and attempt to eliminate it. One role of the immune system is defense against invasive microorganisms. A second function is to maintain homeostasis by removing effete or damaged cellular elements from the circulation. Recently it was also discovered that the immune system serves as a surveillance network to guard against the development, growth, and dissemination of tumor cells.

When the immune system responds appropriately to a foreign stimulus, the host's integrity is maintained. If the immune response is too weak or too vigorous, a derangement in homeostasis results. Certain hypersensitivity reactions and autoimmune diseases can occur when the regulatory cells of the immune system do not adequately control effector cell activities. Similarly a depression in immune reactivity caused by regulatory or effector cell dysfunction can result in host susceptibility to recurrent infections and malignant disease.

Knowledge of basic immunology is increasing at a rapid rate and has had a profound influence on medical and surgical practice. Immunomodulatory agents are being widely used to augment immune function in cancer patients and persons with immunodeficiency diseases. Histocompatibility matching and the development of pharmacologic agents that selectively depress immune reactivity have had a major impact on organ transplantation. Since a number of diseases, such as cancer, rheumatoid disorders, and certain hematologic and gastrointestinal problems, have been associated with immunologic changes, therapies involving immunologic manipulation may soon play a pivotal role in all clinical specialty fields.

Anatomy, Physiology, and Related Pathophysiology

Cellular Components and Their Anatomic Organization

The cellular constituents of the immune system include granulocytes, mononuclear phagocytes, and lymphocytes (Figure 14-1). White cells have been grouped into these three general categories on the basis of cell morphology, functional activities, and stem cell derivation.

Cells of the granulocyte series, that is, basophils or mast cells, eosinophils, and neutrophils, are derived from a common bone marrow progenitor cell, the myeloblast. *Basophils* comprise 0.5% to 1% of the circulating white blood cell (leukocyte) population. *Mast cells,* tissue counterparts of the blood basophil, are found adjacent to smooth muscle in the perivascular and peribronchiolar tissues. Mast cells and basophils play an important role in allergic reactions. *Eosinophils* make up 1% to 3% of peripheral blood leukocytes. They accumulate at sites of anaphylaxis and in addition may influence the host response to parasitic infections. *Neutrophils* comprise as much as 70% of the blood leukocyte population. Neutrophils are actively phagocytic cells that leave the vascular compartment and rapidly accumulate within the tissue spaces at sites of inflammation.

Cells of the mononuclear phagocyte series, all originally derived from the bone marrow monoblast, are distributed throughout the body. *Monocytes* comprise approximately 5% of the circulating leukocyte population. Following a brief interval in the blood, monocytes migrate into the tissues where

Figure 14-1 Leukocyte development. All peripheral blood white cells are thought to be derived from common pluripotent bone marrow stem cell that can differentiate into myeloblasts, monoblasts, or lymphoblasts. Replication of these differentiated stem cells serves to replenish blood and tissue leukocyte populations. Mature leukocytes protect host against invasive organisms, participate in removal of particulate material from circulation, and serve as surveillance network to guard against development and dissemination of tumor cells. *DTH*, Delayed-type hypersensitivity.

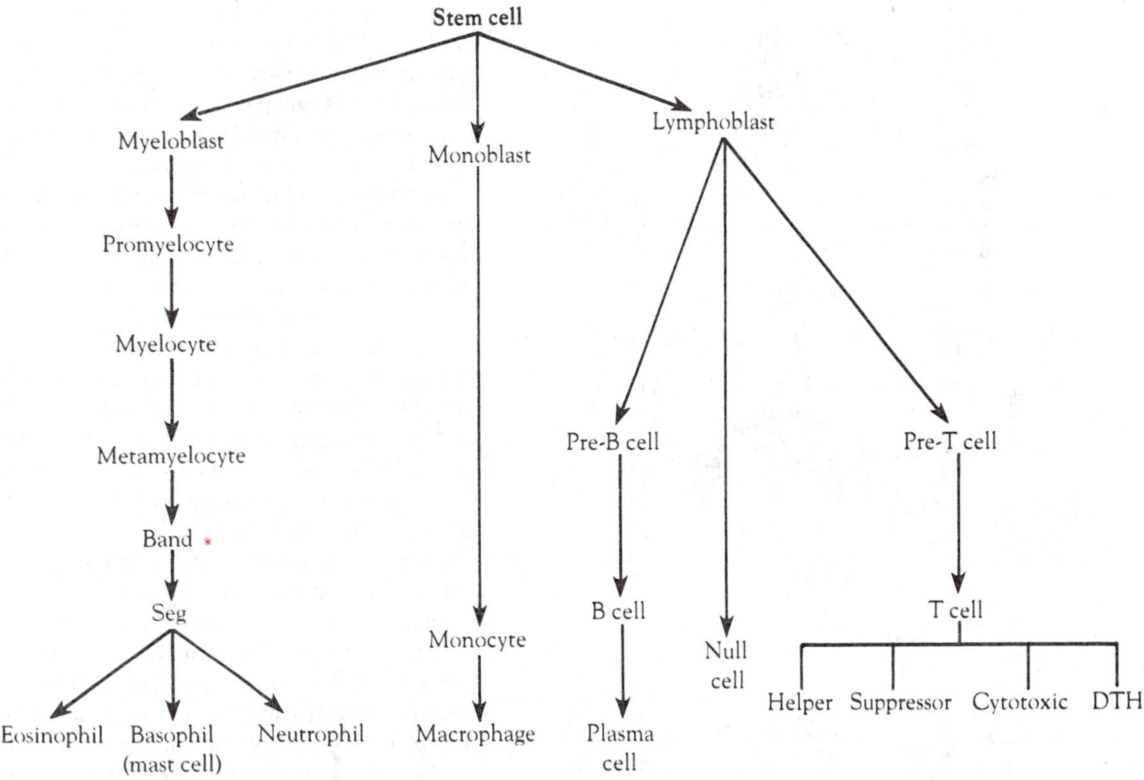

they mature into *macrophages,* the metabolically and functionally mature cells of this series. Macrophages are present in the brain (microglial cells), spleen, and lymphoid tissues. They also line the lung alveoli, the blood sinusoids of the liver (Kupffer cells), and most extravascular tissue spaces. Mononuclear phagocytes help protect the host from invasive organisms, clear tissue debris from sites of tissue injury, and may serve as surveillance cells in antitumor host defense.

Cells of the lymphoid series play a key role in the development of acquired immunity. All *lymphocytes* (T, B, and null cells, which do not have surface markers identifying them as either B or T lymphocytes) are derived from a common bone marrow progenitor cell. Certain immature lymphocytes leave the bone marrow and populate the thymus, where under the influence of thymic hormones they proliferate and differentiate into mature *T lymphocytes*. Other immature lymphocytes proliferate and differentiate into mature *B lymphocytes*. In birds this maturation takes place in an organ called the bursa of Fabricius. No mammalian bursal equivalent tissue has been identified. It is thought that B cell maturation in humans may take place in the bone marrow or in the lymphoid tissues lining the gastrointestinal tract.

After maturation, T and B lymphocytes, now capable of interacting specifically with foreign materials and participating in immune responses, are released into the circulation and populate the peripheral lymphoid tissues, including the spleen, lymph nodes, and tonsils. Mature lymphocytes are also localized in lymphoid tissues directly associated with the mucosal surfaces of the body. Such organized tissues comprise the appendix, Peyer's patches of the ileum, and bronchial-associated lymphoid tissue. The major organs housing the cellular elements of the immune system are illustrated in Figure 14-2.

Nonspecific Immune Mechanisms

Physical and chemical barriers. The first line of defense against invasive organisms is provided by intact skin and mucous membranes. These structures not only serve as a

Figure 14-2 Organization of immune system. Cellular constituents of immune system are derived from bone marrow stem cells. On maturation, these cells are released into peripheral blood and subsequently populate organized tissues of lymphoreticular system.

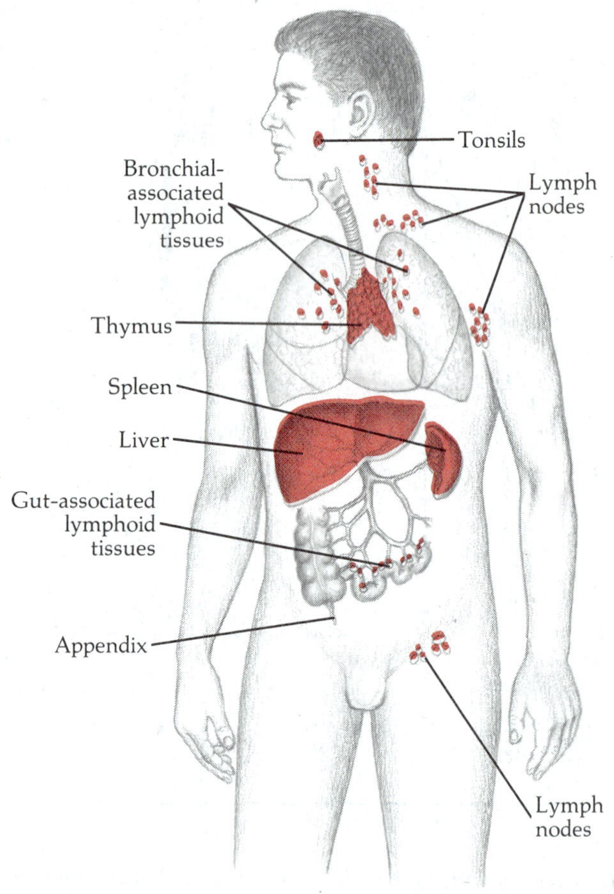

physical barrier to invasion but also provide a chemically unsuitable milieu to support microbial growth. Certain skin and mucosal secretions, such as lactic acid, gastric acid, and lysozyme, have bactericidal properties. Mechanical factors, such as ciliary action in the respiratory tract, also act to protect the host in a nonspecific manner.

Microbial factors. Resident normal flora of the skin and mucous membranes also provide a defense against colonization with pathogenic bacteria. These resident microorganisms suppress growth of infectious agents by competing for essential nutrients, producing growth-inhibiting substances, and altering pH. When normal flora are reduced by antibiotic treatment, a person is more susceptible to infection with pathogenic microorganisms.

Inflammatory response. When a microorganism transcends the physical, chemical, and microbial barriers afforded by the host, or the body is injured by mechanical or chemical means, an inflammatory response is generated. At the onset of inflammation a rapid vasodilation occurs. Within minutes, blood neutrophils accumulate near the site of injury, migrate to the junctional zones between the vascular endothelial cells, and extravasate into the tissue spaces. Neutrophils within an inflammatory site represent the first line of cellular defense against invasive microorganisms.

If neutrophils do not neutralize the inflammatory focus within a few hours, monocytes and lymphocytes begin to accumulate at the site of tissue injury. These cells attempt to localize the inflammatory response, providing a cellular barrier against the migration of the infectious organism into the lymphatic compartment or blood vessels. When neutrophils, lymphocytes, and monocytes neutralize the inflammatory focus, granulation tissue is laid down and inflammation subsides. If the acute inflammatory response is unsuccessful at eliminating the infectious agent or tissue repair is incomplete, chronic inflammation results.

The persistence of an infectious agent during chronic inflammation results in granuloma formation. *Granulomatous lesions* are characterized by accumulations of lymphocytes and macrophages surrounding a central core of foreign material. Fibrotic tissue laid down on the periphery of the granuloma acts as a physical barrier that separates the lesion from surrounding normal tissues.

Accompanying the cellular responses that occur during inflammation are elevations in serum levels of certain proteins. These *acute phase proteins,* which include C-reactive protein and serum amyloid A protein, are used clinically to detect the presence of an infectious or inflammatory process. *C-reactive protein* may play a protective role by activating the complement pathway and influencing certain leukocyte responses. Large increases in the serum concentrations of globular proteins and fibrinogen may also accompany episodes of infection, inflammation, and tissue necrosis. In vitro, an elevation in the levels of these plasma proteins increases the aggregation and precipitation of erythrocytes suspended in plasma. This phenomenon, manifested in the laboratory as an elevation in *erythrocyte sedimentation rate* (ESR), is indicative of an ongoing inflammatory process.

Other serum proteins that play a major role in inflammation include the kinins, vasoactive amines, prostaglandins, and certain complement components (C3a, C4a, and C5a). These factors increase *vasodilation* and induce a widening of the junction between adjacent vascular endothelial cells, thus facilitating the exudation of fluid and cellular elements into the tissue spaces. *Chemotactic factors,* molecules that attract leukocytes toward an inflammatory focus, also contribute to the generation of inflammatory processes. These mediators include bacterial products, certain fluid phase components of the complement system (C5a), and products of stimulated leukocytes.

Lymphoreticular system. When an infectious agent is able to permeate the barriers afforded by the local cellular response that occurs during acute or chronic inflammation, it

Figure 14-3 Lymph node structure. Lymph enters node via afferent lymph vessels, percolates through cortex and medulla, and leaves via efferent lymphatics. Foreign materials are trapped by macrophages in cortex, digested, and presented to lymphoid cells to initiate specific immune response. Superficial cortex is comprised primarily of B lymphocytes clustered into follicles. Interfollicular regions of superficial cortex and bulk of deep cortex are populated by T lymphocytes.

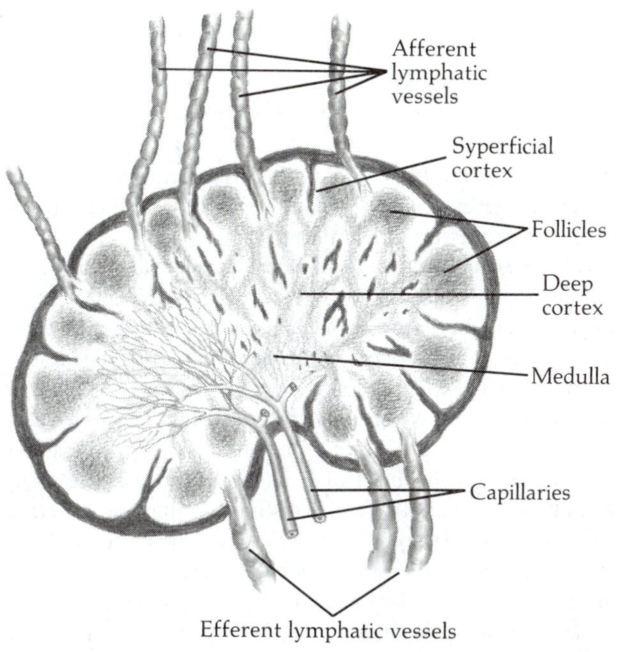

Figure 14-4 Phagocytosis. This multistep process is used by granulocytes, monocytes, and macrophages to remove foreign materials from body. These materials come in contact with digestive enzymes and destructive oxygen metabolites within phagocytic vacuole. Incompletely digested materials, lysosomal enzymes, and toxic oxygen products may be released from cell.

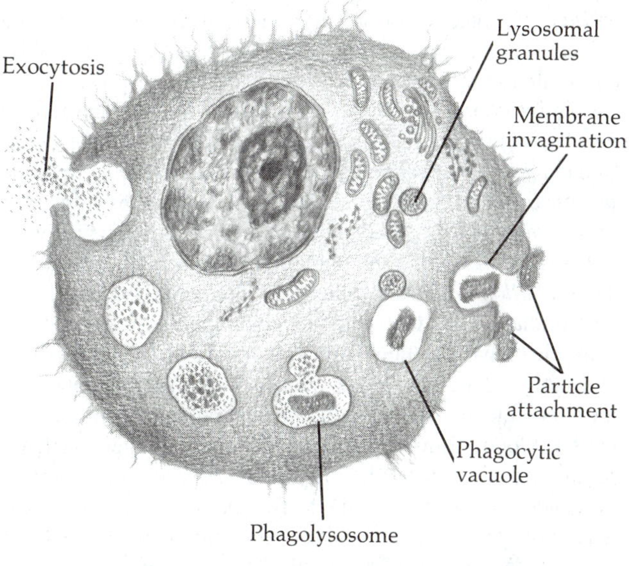

enters the vascular compartment or the lymphatic channels. The lymphoreticular system, comprised of organs housing both tissue macrophages and lymphoid cells, functions to remove bacteria, tissue debris, or tumor cells from the lymph and blood.

When foreign materials enter the lymphatics, they are filtered by, and become lodged within, the lymph nodes (Figure 14-3). Within the nodes they may be engulfed and destroyed by fixed phagocytic cells or, alternatively, may activate a specific immune response. In a corresponding fashion, when a foreign agent enters the blood, it is phagocytosed by macrophages lining the blood sinusoids of the liver and spleen. If these macrophages do not completely destroy or neutralize the foreign material, they present it in a modified form to lymphoid cells, initiating a specific immune response.

Phagocytosis. Granulocytes and mononuclear phagocytes are key cellular participants in the nonspecific immune response. Monocytes and neutrophils that have migrated into an inflammatory site and tissue macrophages that encounter foreign materials within the respiratory, vascular, or lymphatic compartments protect the host largely by their phagocytic capabilities.

Phagocytosis is a multistep process that is initiated by the attachment of a damaged or foreign material to the surface of the phagocytic cell (Figure 14-4). Particle recognition may occur at nonspecific membrane receptors or may be mediated by *opsonic proteins,* such as immunoglobulins and certain complement components that coat particles and facilitate their attachment to specific receptors on phagocytic cells. After particle attachment the cell membrane on the surface of the phagocyte invaginates, encloses the particle, pinches off, and is internalized. The phagocytic vacuole subsequently fuses with lysosomal granules, vacuoles within the cell containing potent hydrolytic enzymes.

During the process of phagocytosis a number of metabolic changes occur within the cell. These include a stimulation in glucose oxidation via glycolysis and the hexose monophosphate shunt and an elevation in oxygen consumption. These metabolic changes are tightly linked to the activities of certain cellular enzymes, NADPH oxidase and glucose 6-phosphate dehydrogenase. Associated with these biochemical events is the increased production of lactic acid, hydrogen peroxide, superoxide anion, hydroxyl radical, and singlet oxygen.

These oxidative products of the *respiratory burst,* in concert with lysosomal granule constituents such as myeloperoxidase, lysozyme, lactoferrin, and granular cationic proteins, are important antimicrobial agents employed by phagocytic cells. Under certain conditions, lysosomal enzymes and toxic oxygen products are released from the phagocytic cell. These events are responsible for much of the tissue damage that occurs in an ongoing inflammatory process.

Specific Immune Mechanisms

Antigenicity. An *antigen* (or immunogen) is a substance capable of evoking an immune response. To qualify as an antigen a molecule must be recognized as foreign by the immune system. Antigens present on bacteria, viruses, molds, and pollens can induce a detectable immune response.

Similarly antigens found on mammalian cells and tissues can be immunogenic. *Autologous antigens* are tissue determinants that under normal conditions do not evoke an immune response. When these "self" antigens are altered by infectious or inflammatory processes, the immune system recognizes its own tissues as "foreign" and produces an autoimmune response. *Alloantigens* are genetically determined antigens that discriminate individuals within a given species. Red cells, for example, have on their surface a number of determinants, including A, B, and Rh antigens, that may precipitate an immunologic reaction following the transfusion of incompatible blood. Similarly human leukocyte antigens (HLA), present on the surface of all nucleated cells, have a profound influence on allograft survival. The human *major histocompatibility complex* (MHC) is a genetic region on chromosome 6 that codes for these human alloantigens. Gene products of the HLA-A, HLA-B, and HLA-C loci appear on all nucleated cells, whereas HLA-D region products are found primarily on lymphocytes, macrophages, epidermal cells, and sperm.

Induction of a specific immune response. Antigen-specific responses are designated as either humoral or cellular immunity (Table 14-1). *Humoral immunity* is mediated by B lymphocytes that synthesize and secrete γ-globulins in response to antigenic challenge. *Cell-mediated immune mechanisms* involve the participation of effector T lymphocytes and macrophages. Humoral immunity can be transferred from an immune to a nonimmune host with cell-free globulin-bearing serum, whereas cellular immunity is transferred with sensitized cells. Although the body's response to an antigenic challenge usually involves both cellular and humoral immune mechanisms, one response may predominate.

A specific immune mechanism involves the participation of T and B lymphocytes that have been genetically programmed to recognize and interact with unique antigenic determinants on a foreign material. A specific immune response is triggered after the clearance of foreign materials from an inflammatory site, the lymph, or the vascular compartment by tissue macrophages. These phagocytic cells internalize and degrade the foreign antigens. The processed antigens are reexpressed on the macrophage surface in a highly immunogenic form for presentation to lymphocytes that continuously circulate through the lymphoid organs. Recognition of antigen by specific receptors on lymphocytes results in their stimulation and sequestration within the tissue.

Table 14-1
Humoral and Cell-Mediated Immune Responses

	Humoral	Cell-Mediated
Effector cells	B lymphocytes	T lymphocytes and macrophages
Regulatory cells	T helper cells and T suppressor cells	T helper cells and T suppressor cells
Effector mechanisms	Elaboration of antibody	Generation of factors that are directly toxic to target cells
Host protection	Against many gram-positive and certain gram-negative bacteria	Against mycobacteria, fungi, protozoa, and tumors

Humoral immunity. When confronted with an antigen, B lymphocytes synthesize and secrete specifically reactive γ-globulins called *antibodies* or *immunoglobulins.* On first exposure to a given antigen, a *primary humoral immune response* is evoked. This response occurs after a lag period of 1 to 7 days during which only trace amounts of specific antibody can be detected. During this induction period, antigen is processed and specific clones of B lymphocytes are stimulated to divide and differentiate ultimately into two different cell types. The first type, *plasma cells,* synthesizes and secretes antibodies. Other B lymphocytes, *memory cells,* remain quiescent until secondary exposure to a given antigen.

The *secondary,* or *anamnestic, response* that occurs after subsequent exposure to a particular antigen has a short lag period, produces high levels of antibody, and is more sustained than the primary response. This memory property of the immune system increases resistance to infection in persons who have been immunized against, or previously infected with, a particular antigen.

The humoral immune response offers protection against many gram-positive and certain gram-negative organisms. Specific antibody generated during a humoral immune response facilitates viral neutralization, enhances bacterial ingestion and destruction by phagocytic cells, and results in activation of the complement system.

When a humoral immune response is generated against soluble antigens, small antigen-antibody complexes form. These *immune complexes* may be rapidly cleared from the circulation by fixed macrophages in the liver and spleen or, alternatively, may be deposited within tissues. Tissue-bound immune complexes can activate the complement system and provoke inflammatory destruction of normal cells.

Regulation of the humoral immune response. Certain antigens are capable of stimulating B cells directly or after

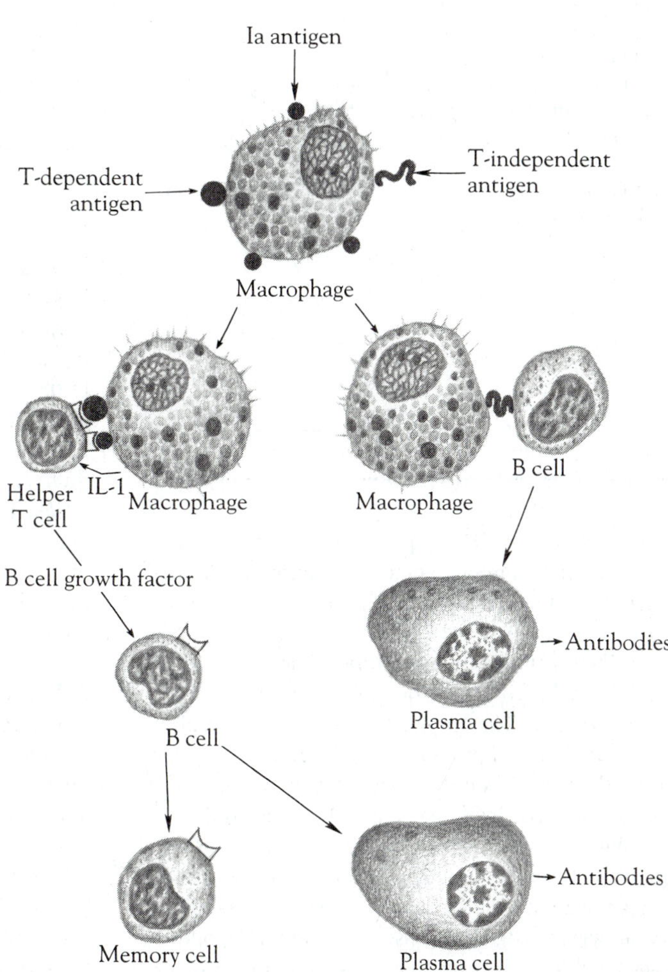

Figure 14-5 Humoral immune responses. Antibody response to T-dependent antigens involves interaction between macrophages, T cells, and B cells. Macrophages ingest foreign materials, reexpress processed antigen on their surface, and present it in context of Ia molecule to T helper cells. T helper cells facilitate B lymphocyte proliferation and differentiation. On primary exposure to given T-dependent antigen, memory cell generation occurs, although little antibody is generated. During anamnestic response, plasma cells synthesize large quantities of specific antibody. Humoral response to T-independent antigens may be macrophage-dependent or independent process. This response generally produces only antibody of IgM class and has little or no memory. *IL-1,* Interleukin 1.

presentation on the macrophage surface. These *T-independent antigens* have a primary structure of repeating identical units.

Most antigens, however, require the activation of a subpopulation of lymphocytes, *T helper cells,* in addition to B lymphocytes, to effect an antibody response. The antibody response to a *T-dependent antigen* is initiated by macrophage presentation of antigen to T helper cells and secretion of interleukin 1, a T cell growth–promoting substance. T helper cells, stimulated in this way, interact with B lymphocytes and promote their growth and differentiation. B cell growth factor, derived from T cells, may play a role in B cell activation (Figure 14-5).

The antibody response to T-dependent antigen is under the control of the major histocompatibility complex (MHC). To interact with antibody-presenting macrophages, helper T cells have to recognize and bind "self" antigens, called Ia antigens, on the macrophage surface. These self antigens are coded for by genes of the HLA region. Similarly, T cell binding to B lymphocytes involves their recognition of a genetically determined marker on the B cell surface.

In addition to T lymphocytes that provide help in the induction of an immune response, certain other T lymphocytes depress immune reactivity. *Suppressor T cells* have an important role in homeostatic control, since they maintain the humoral immune response at a level appropriate for the stimulus. Suppressor T cells are activated during the generation of all immune responses. They limit the immune response by acting at the level of the helper T cell or B lymphocyte (Figure 14-6). The modulatory activity of suppressor T cells may be mediated by direct cell-to-cell contact or, alternatively, may involve the release of suppressor factors.

The relative numbers and functional reactivities of helper and suppressor cells determine the strength and persistence of an immune response. When the delicate balance between T helper and T suppressor cell populations is disrupted, autoimmune or immunodeficiency disease may result. Since helper and suppressor T lymphocytes have distinct surface markers and can be readily discriminated in the laboratory, immune function can be estimated by measuring the T helper/T suppressor cell ratio. Normally a person has roughly twice

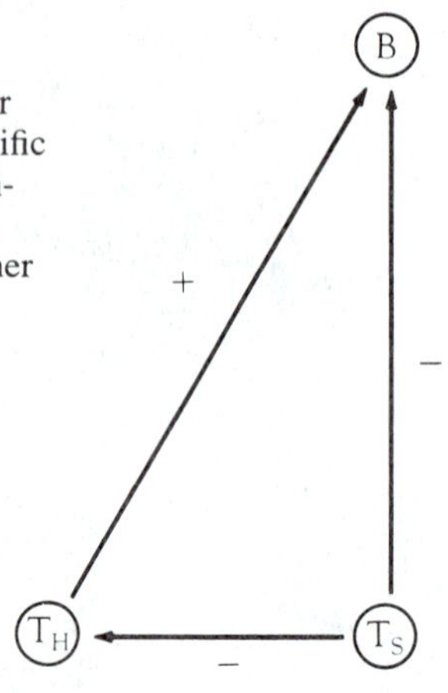

Figure 14-6 Regulation of humoral immune responses. Generation of humoral immune response is facilitated by interaction of T helper (T_H) lymphocytes with antigen-specific B cells. This response can be down-regulated by T suppressor (T_S) lymphocytes that act at level of either T helper or B lymphocyte.

as many T helper cells as T suppressor cells. In contrast, patients with acquired immunodeficiency syndrome (AIDS) frequently demonstrate a T helper/T suppressor cell ratio of 1:1 or less.

Biologic activities of immunoglobulins. The γ-globulin–bearing or antibody-bearing fractions of serum are referred to as *immunoglobulins*. The immunoglobulins are a highly heterogeneous population of proteins, not a singular molecular species. Currently five physicochemical classes of immunoglobulins are recognized: IgG, IgM, IgA, IgE, and IgD.

Immunoglobulin molecules are made up of a four-chain polypeptide (protein) unit consisting of two identical high–molecular weight (heavy) chains and two identical low–molecular weight (light) chains. The immunoglobulins have been assigned to their respective classes on the basis of their heavy chains, gamma (γ), mu (μ), alpha (α), epsilon (ϵ), and delta (δ). There are two different light chain types, kappa (κ) and lambda (λ). A schematic representation of the five major immunoglobulin classes is shown in Figure 14-7.

When a humoral immune response is triggered, one or more classes of antibody may be elaborated. The nature of the antibody response is dependent on the chemical and physical nature of the antigen, route of administration, and immunization history of the host.

IgG is the predominant serum antibody and represents a large proportion of the immunoglobulin found in internal secretions (for example, pleural, synovial, and peritoneal fluids). Specific IgG is produced only in small amounts late in the primary immune response, but it is the major antibody generated during a *secondary challenge* with antigen. The generation of IgG protects the host, since this class of immunoglobulin has a number of biologically significant properties. For example, IgG can neutralize toxins produced by various strains of bacteria and induces the agglutination of infectious organisms, facilitating their uptake by phagocytic cells. In addition, IgG has opsonic activity and can activate complement, resulting in the lysis of certain strains of bacteria. IgG is thought to play a crucial role in neonatal host defense, since it is the only immunoglobulin class to be transferred across the placenta.

IgM, comprising approximately 10% of the serum immunoglobulins, is the first antibody to appear during the *primary immune response*. Exposure to antigen via the respiratory or gastrointestinal tract results in the elaboration of IgM into the external secretions. IgM shares many of the biologic properties of IgG: it can neutralize bacterial toxins, can agglutinate certain microorganisms, and is a potent activator of the complement system.

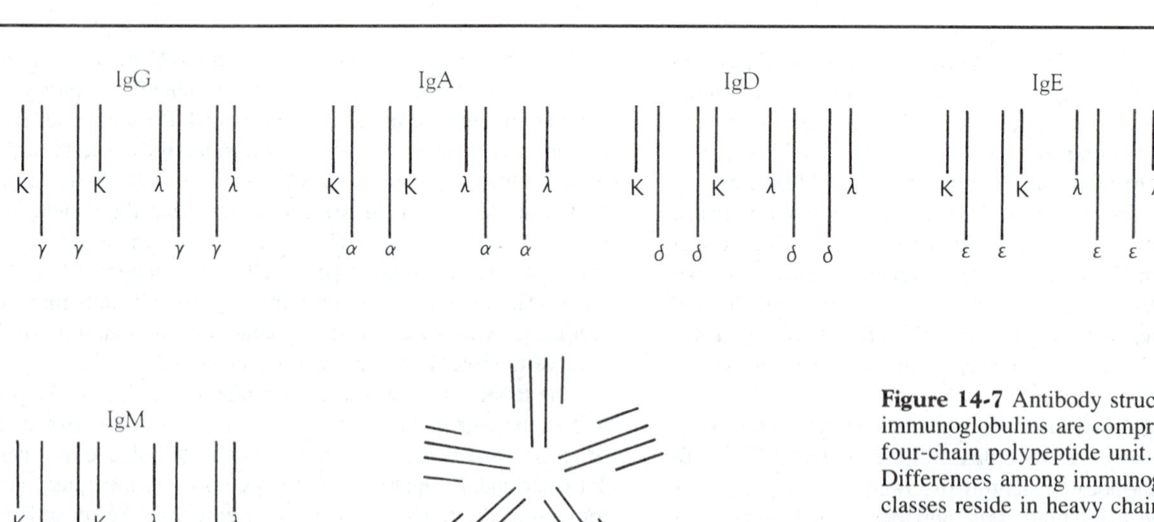

Figure 14-7 Antibody structure. All immunoglobulins are comprised of a four-chain polypeptide unit. Differences among immunoglobulin classes reside in heavy chain structure. IgM, found in serum and external secretions, is pentamer consisting of five identical subunits.
Modified from Unaue.[53]

IgA, comprising only a small proportion of the serum antibody pool, is the predominant immunoglobulin in all *serous* and *mucous secretions*. Secretory IgA interferes with bacterial attachment to mucosal surfaces, impedes colonization, and virtually prevents bacterial penetration into the general circulation. In addition, IgA is capable of neutralizing certain bacterial toxins but does not have opsonic or complement-fixing properties. Secretory IgA in maternal milk affords protection to infants before maturation of their secretory immune system.

IgE antibodies, present in the serum in trace amounts, are found attached to mast cells and basophils. These immunoglobulins play a major role in the generation of anaphylactic reactions. When an *allergen*, a substance capable of inducing an allergic reaction, binds to IgE on the surface of basophils or mast cells, mediators such as histamine, serotonin, and leukotrienes are released. These products stimulate bronchial smooth muscle contraction and precipitate systemic vasodilation. Although IgE is generated in small amounts during conventional humoral immune responses, the physiologic significance of IgE production is not well understood. Evidence suggests that IgE may afford protection against parasitic infections by facilitating eosinophil recognition and destruction of the parasite.

IgD is only a minor component of the serum immunoglobulin pool and is not found in appreciable amounts in external or internal secretions. The biologic function of IgD has not been elucidated.

Cell-mediated immunity. Whereas humoral immune mechanisms afford protection against many gram-positive and certain gram-negative organisms, *cell-mediated immunity is important during host infection with intracellular pathogens such as mycobacteria, fungi, viruses, and protozoa*. Cell-mediated reactions are also elicited as a component of the host response to *tumors* and *tissue transplants*.

Cell-mediated immune responses have been classically characterized as either *delayed-type hypersensitivity* (DTH) or *cytotoxic T lymphocyte* (CTL) reactions (Figure 14-8). CTL reactions play a major role in host defense against tumors, virally infected cells, and allogeneic tissue transplants, whereas DTH reactions are activated by host infection with intracellular pathogens.

Generation of a DTH response involves the participation of macrophages, T helper cells, and DTH-effector T cells. During a primary infection the organisms are ingested by macrophages that process and reexpress antigen on their surface for presentation to helper cells. T helper cells, stimulated by antigen presentation and macrophage release of interleukin 1, induce proliferation of a pool of antigen-specific DTH-precursor T cells. The major portion of these cells remain quiescent until secondary challenge with antigen.

On secondary exposure an anamnestic response develops. Macrophages present processed antigen to antigen-specific T helper cells that rapidly stimulate large numbers of DTH-effector T cells, previously generated by clonal expansion. The activated DTH-effector cells release factors, called lymphokines, that stimulate other cells, particularly macrophages. Most tissue macrophages are incapable of killing intracellular pathogens; however, macrophages activated by exposure to lymphokines are avidly bactericidal.

Figure 14-8 Cell-mediated immune reactions are initiated by macrophage presentation of processed antigen to helper T lymphocytes. Stimulated T helper cells release interleukin 2 *(IL-2)* that activates DTH and cytotoxic T lymphocytes. Targets, such as tumor or virus-infected cells, are lysed directly by cytotoxic T cells. Following infection with intracellular pathogens, activated macrophages are major effector cell population generated. *IL-1*, Interleukin 1.

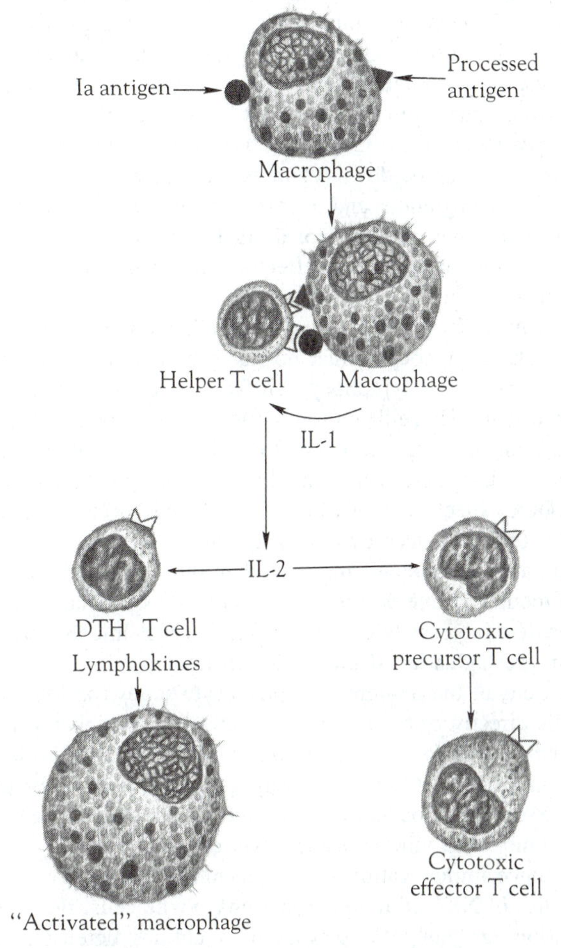

The duration and magnitude of a DTH response are regulated by T suppressor cells. In general, a secondary DTH reaction can be demonstrated within a few hours of antigen challenge, peaks at 24 to 48 hours, and gradually recedes as the inflammatory focus is eliminated. A person's capacity to generate a secondary DTH response can be measured by intradermal injection with a battery of skin test antigens. If, for example, persons with normal immunity and a history of tuberculosis are tested with purified tuberculoid antigen (PPD), they demonstrate a classic wheal-and-flare reaction. This positive response is evidence of a functionally intact cell-mediated immune system.

CTL reactions are mediated by a subpopulation of T lymphocytes known as *cytotoxic T lymphocytes*. These lymphocytes have surface receptors that recognize genetically different MHC markers on allogeneic tissues and mediate tissue rejection. Similarly cytotoxic lymphocytes recognize tumor- and virus-infected host cells as foreign. On primary exposure to genetically different or altered cells, a population of cytotoxic T precursor cells is expanded with the participation of T helper cells. On secondary exposure an anamnestic response is generated. The cytotoxic T lymphocyte, once activated, attaches to its target and lyses it, employing an unknown mechanism. CTL reactions, like all classic immune responses, can be down-regulated by T suppressor cells.

The recognition and destruction of tumor- and virus-infected target cells are not limited to cytotoxic T lymphocytes. Other categories of effector cells include mononuclear phagocytes and natural killer cells.

Natural killer (NK) cells, often called null cells, are large granular lymphocytes that do not bear the classic markers found on B or T lymphocyte surfaces. They bind to and lyse target cells using either an antibody-dependent or independent mechanism. Target cell lysis by NK cells that requires antibody is described as an antibody-dependent cellular cytotoxic (ADCC) mechanism. Killing by NK cells occurs naturally and is not enhanced by immunization. Although NK cells do not have immunologic memory, their functional activities can be modified. Interferons, protein products of stimulated leukocytes, increase NK killing of target cells. In contrast, certain prostaglandins depress NK function.

Cells of the mononuclear phagocyte series can kill target cells directly or by an ADCC mechanism. Peripheral blood *monocytes* and resident tissue *macrophages* exhibit low levels of antitumor activity. Following activation with T lymphocyte–derived products such as γ-interferon, macrophage lysis of tumor- and virus-infected target cells increases.

Since immunization is not generally required for the activities of NK and mononuclear phagocytic cells, these populations are thought to play an important host defense role in early stages of infection and tumor growth, before CTL effector cells have been generated. Interferon, shown experimentally to increase both NK cell and macrophage cytotoxic activities, is being used in clinical trials to treat certain malignancies and immunodeficiency disorders.

Complement system. The complement system is comprised of a series of proteins that when activated serve to amplify an immune response. Activation of the complement system leads to the elaboration of potent inflammatory mediators, facilitates particle opsonization and clearance, and may result in the direct lysis of altered mammalian cells and certain bacteria. The complement system may be activated by a number of immunologic and nonimmunologic stimuli. Complement activation proceeds by two mechanisms, the classical and alternative pathways (Figure 14-9).

The *classical complement pathway* is comprised of 11 distinct proteins. The early-acting components are numbered according to the order of their discovery, and the later-acting

Figure 14-9 Complement activation. Complement activation can proceed by either classical or alternative pathway. Activation of these pathways results in generation of chemotactic factors (C5a), anaphylatoxins (C3a, C5a), and membrane attack complex (C5b6789).

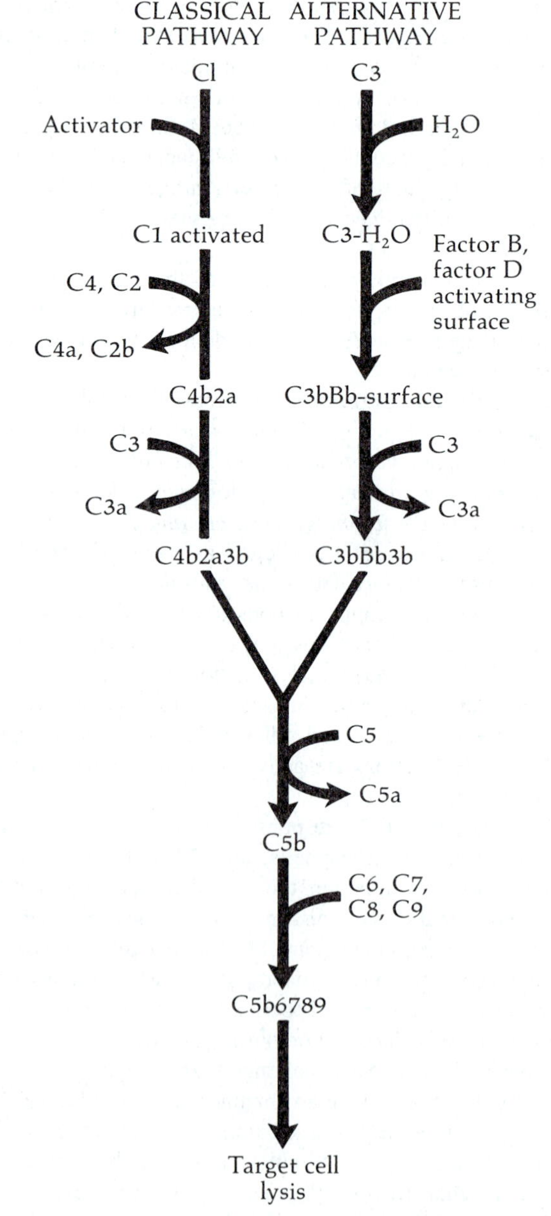

components according to their order of reaction. Thus the sequence of action of these components is C1, C4, C2, C3, C5, C6, C7, C8, and C9. C1 is made up of three distinct proteins, Clq, Clr, and Cls.

The first step of complement activation through the classical pathway involves the interaction of C1 with immune complexes containing IgM or IgG or with antibody-coated particles. When activated, C1, the recognition complex of the classical pathway, cleaves C4 and C2. Two protein fragments subsequently combine and form an active enzyme (C4b2a) that cleaves C3 molecules. C3a generated in this way is a potent anaphylatoxin, a substance capable of stimulating basophils and mast cells and thus provoking release of vasoactive amines. A portion of the C3b fragments elaborated during this cleavage is deposited on the activating surface and facilitates particle attachment to phagocytic cells. Certain other C3b molecules combine with C4b2a to form an enzyme (C4b2a3b) that cleaves C5 into two fragments. C5a released into the fluid phase has both anaphylatoxic and chemotactic properties. C5b has an affinity for membranes and, when deposited on a surface, facilitates the binding of C6 and C7. This trimolecular complex (C5b67) provides a binding site for C8, the complement component responsible for initiating target cell lysis. Although some membrane damage occurs following the formation of the C5b-8 complex, lysis is accelerated by the binding of C9. C5b-9, on the surface of a target cell, is called the membrane attack complex.

Before the generation of specific antibody, the complement system can be activated via the *alternative pathway*. Known activators of the alternative pathway include bacterial lipopolysaccharide, virus-infected cells, yeasts, fungi, and certain bacterial cell walls. The constituents of the alternative pathway include all the classical complement components except C1, C4, and C2. Two other proteins, factor B and factor D, contribute to activation of the alternative pathway.

The alternative pathway is activated with the formation of an enzyme that cleaves C3 molecules. This enzyme (C3bBb), distinct from the classical pathway enzyme (C4b2a), is generated following the spontaneous hydrolysis of C3, which in the presence of factor D cleaves factor B. C3bBb generated in this way and bound to an activating surface (such as a bacterium) is capable of cleaving many more C3 molecules, which results in the generation of C3bBb3b, an enzyme that cleaves C5 into C5a and C5b. The subsequent steps of the alternative pathway are identical to those of the classical pathway and lead to the elaboration of anaphylatoxins, chemotactic factors, and target cell lysis.

Although the complement system protects the host against infectious organisms and may play a role in tumor cell destruction, the uncontrolled activation of this system would result in inflammatory changes and lytic destruction of host tissues. These potentially devastating effects are modulated by a number of control proteins including C1 inhibitor, factors H and I, C4 binding protein, S protein, anaphylatoxin inhibitor, and inhibitors of the membrane attack complex.

Normal Findings[6,9,24,48]

Since certain alterations in immune status appear to be genetically determined, a *family history* of recurrent infections, malignancies, allergies, immunodeficiency, and autoimmune diseases should be elicited.

A detailed *patient history* is an essential component of the immune status profile. In addition to documentation of the patient's age, race, sex, and ethnic background, the following information should be obtained:

- Past history—allergies, childhood and recurrent infections, malignancy, autoimmune disease, primary disorders known to suppress immune function, immunization profile, medications
- Social, occupational, and nutritional habits
- Abnormal signs and symptoms—fever, diaphoresis, rashes, joint pain, unusual masses, lymphadenopathy, overt signs of infection, poor wound healing, eczema, hepatosplenomegaly

Since immunologic and inflammatory diseases can involve many organ systems, a complete physical examination is warranted. Particular attention should be paid to signs of infection (abscesses, persistent lesions, and so on), inflammatory tissue changes, wheezing, joint swelling, and skin integrity.

Alterations in vital signs may indicate the presence of an ongoing inflammatory process. (Geriatric patients, however, frequently demonstrate a reduced febrile response to infection.)

Area of Concern	Normal Adult Findings
Liver	Usually located completely under rib cage; may be palpated just below right costal margin with deep inspiration
Spleen	Not generally palpable
Thymus	Can be detected only by radiologic examination; size varies with age (between birth and 20 years, thymic mass increases; after age 20, thymus progressively decreases in size until age 60, when thymic involution is complete)

Area of Concern	Normal Adult Findings
Lymph nodes (head and neck, axillary, inguinal, epitrochlear)	Generally not palpable; small, nontender nodes may be found in cervical or inguinal chain of persons with history of local infection

Normal Laboratory Data[19,30]

Patient history and physical examination will determine which laboratory tests are indicated. For example:

If a patient has persistent fungal or viral infections, one may suspect a defect in cell-mediated immunity.

A history of gram-positive bacterial infection may indicate a potential humoral immune deficit.

Recurrent infections with organisms that do not elicit a strong antibody response, such as *Pseudomonas aeruginosa* or *Staphylococcus aureus,* are frequently observed in persons with phagocytic cell defects.

When interpreting laboratory data, be aware that certain diseases may alter white cell numbers and functional activities. Other processes may be associated with impaired cell function despite normal leukocyte numbers. Alternatively, perturbations in cell numbers may be observed in association with normal cell function.

Laboratory Test*	Normal Adult Values
White blood cell counts	
Total WBC ($\times 10^3/mm^3$)	5-10
Differential counts (%)	
Segmented (mature) neutrophils	26-60
Band cells (immature neutrophils)	2-20
Lymphocytes	35-40
Monocytes	5-10
Eosinophils	0-7
Basophils	0-1.5
Lymphocyte populations (%)	
Total B cells	5-11
Total T cells	75-90
T helper cells (T_4 positive)†	40-58
T suppressor/cytotoxic cells (T_8 positive)†	19-30
Bone marrow differential cell counts (%)	
Erythroblasts	22.5
Myeloblasts	1.0
Promyelocytes	3.0
Myelocytes	15.0
Metamyelocytes	15.0
Stab cells	15.0
Segmented cells	7.0
Eosinophils	4.0
Basophils	<0.5
Monocytes	2.0

Laboratory Test	Normal Adult Values
Lymphocytes	7.5
Reticular cells	6.5
Plasmacytes	1.0
Megakaryocytes	<0.5
Serum immunoglobulin levels	
IgG (mg/dl)	600-1600
IgM (mg/dl)	50-250
IgA (mg/dl)	80-350
IgE (units/ml)	<125
IgD (mg/dl)	0-30
Autoantibody titers‡	
Anti-DNA	Low levels of antibody or none; units and reference range depend on laboratory and method
Antinuclear antibody (ANA)	Negative at 1:20 dilution
Rheumatoid factor (RF)	Negative
Sjögren's antibody	Negative
Nonspecific indicators of inflammation	
Erythrocyte sedimentation rate (ESR)	<20 mm/hr
C-reactive protein (CRP)	<6 μg/ml
C3 complement (serum)	800-1800 μg/ml
Circulating immune complexes	
C1q binding assay	<25 μg/ml aggregated human γ-globulin (AHGG) equivalents
Raji cell assay	0-12 μg/ml AHGG equivalents

*Many of these analyses are not performed in smaller hospitals. Complete diagnostic workups may be obtained from the immunology laboratory of a major medical center.

†In normal persons the T helper/T suppressor cell ratio is approximately 2:1.

‡A profile of tests to identify and discriminate autoimmune diseases is available in many clinical laboratories. In addition to screening for antinuclear antibody and rheumatoid factor, these panels screen for erythrocyte sedimentation rate and C-reactive protein as nonspecific indicators of inflammation, measure functional complement, and quantitate C3 and C4.

Conditions, Diseases, and Disorders

IMMUNODEFICIENCY DISEASES

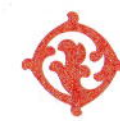

Common variable immunodeficiency

Common variable immunodeficiency (CVID) is an immune disorder of unknown cause that predominantly affects the B cell system. The clinical features include severe depression or absence of plasma cells.

The immunologic feature of acquired hypogammaglobulinemia that is shared with the X-linked form is the marked depression or absence of all five classes of immunoglobulin. Consequently, recurrent bacterial infections are observed in this disorder. Other common features include malabsorption syndromes (usually resulting from *Giardia lamblia* infestation) and an increased incidence of autoimmune and lymphoreticular malignancies. A predilection for autoimmune and neoplastic disease in first-degree relatives of these patients suggests a hereditary influence.

CVID is distinguished by the presence of B lymphocytes. Also, patients with CVID may manifest hyperplasia of lymphoid tissue, including the tonsils, nodes, and spleen. In addition, acquired hypogammaglobulinemia occurs at any age and in both sexes equally.

Pathophysiology

The pathogenesis of acquired hypogammaglobulinemia is unknown. The presence of normal numbers of B cells together with markedly depressed amounts of immunoglobulin suggests that decreased synthesis or release of antibody is the problem. Researchers have suggested that faulty differentiation of the B lymphocyte to the plasma cell may be the primary defect. It is also speculated that this defect occurs as the result of increased T suppressor cell activity or failure of T cell cooperation.[40]

Diagnostic Studies and Findings

B Cell Quantitation and Function

B cells low, normal, or increased; cells clonally diverse and relatively immature; fail to respond to most antigens and mitogens by differentiating into plasma cells; in some patients B cells synthesize but do not secrete immunoglobulin[40]

Immunoglobulin Quantitation

Total greater than 300 mg/dl

T Cell Studies

Levels may be normal or reflect increased numbers of T suppressor cells with decreased numbers of helper cells; B cells are unable to function without T helper cell feedback; generally T cell function deteriorates with time[40]

Lymphoid Tissue Biopsy

Absence of plasma cells in B cell–dependent areas; hyperplasia of lymphoid tissue

Chest Roentgenogram

Chronic lung disease

Sinus Roentgenogram

Chronic sinusitis

Pulmonary Function Tests

Findings abnormal

Malabsorption Studies

Blunting of villi on biopsy; abnormal findings on D-xylose absorption test; lack of normal intestinal enzymes

Stool Examination for Ova and Parasites

Giardia lamblia detected most frequently

Antinuclear Antibody and Other Optional Studies

To detect presence of autoimmune disease or lymphoreticular malignancies; antinuclear antibody present in autoimmune disease

NURSING CARE

Nursing Assessment

Recurrent Infection

Sinusitis; pharyngitis; pneumonia; osteomyelitis; conjunctivitis; abscesses; otitis

Gastrointestinal Tract

Chronic diarrhea; malabsorption

Lymphatic System

Lymphadenopathy; splenomegaly

Presence of Concomitant Autoimmune Disease

Signs and symptoms associated with systemic lupus erythematosus, dermatomyositis, and hemolytic anemia

Presence of Concomitant Neoplastic Disease

Signs and symptoms associated with leukemia, lymphoma, and gastric carcinoma

Nursing Dx & Intervention

Nursing Diagnosis	Nursing Intervention/Rationale
Impaired gas exchange related to recurrent sinopulmonary infections	• Assess respiratory status: monitor rate, rhythm, and quality of respirations, presence of cyanosis, adventitious breath sounds, and restlessness. • Monitor results of sputum cultures and pulmonary function studies (arterial blood gases and so on), and chest roentgenograms. • In collaboration with physician, administer appropriate antibiotics, oxygen therapy, bronchodilators, and chest physiotherapy. Assess effectiveness and note side effects.
Impaired skin integrity related to skin reaction from autoimmune disorder	• In collaboration with physician, administer appropriate topical or systemic medications as ordered and assess patient's response (see Chapter 5). • Monitor skin lesions for evidence of infection. • Assess changes in skin integrity in response to treatment of the underlying humoral deficiency.
Pain related to polyarthritis and infection	• In collaboration with physician, administer appropriate analgesic or anti-inflammatory medication as ordered; assess patient's response and note side effects. • Provide joint support for affected areas throughout the night. • Provide thermal therapy to affected joints as needed. • Assess patient's response to treatment of underlying cause of pain.
Diarrhea related to giardiasis and other intestinal infections	• Monitor intake and output *to assess for volume depletion.* • Monitor for electrolyte imbalances. • Maintain adequate hydration and oral intake as tolerated. • Determine need for tube feeding and parenteral alimentation. • In collaboration with physician, administer appropriate antimicrobial therapy. Assess effectiveness and note side effects.
Altered nutrition: less than body requirements related to malabsorption	• Assess degree of nutritional deficit. • Provide high-protein, high-calorie diet as tolerated. • Provide small, frequent feedings as tolerated. • Encourage family members to provide patient's favorite foods. • Provide vitamin supplements. • Determine need for parenteral nutrition if oral intake is deficient.
Ineffective individual coping	• Assess patient's anxiety related to limited understanding of diagnostic procedures, disease process and prognosis, and therapies employed. • Explain relationship of disease process and rationale for various therapeutic interventions at level appropriate for comprehension and degree of anxiety. • Involve family in care as appropriate. • Encourage patient to verbalize questions, fears, and anxieties.
Potential for infection	• Assess for anorexia, failure to thrive, pain, weakness, and lethargy. • Assess for evidence of infection at sites of invasive procedures. • Assess for breaks in skin integrity, particularly over pressure areas and oral mucosa. • Assess pulmonary status: auscultate lung fields *to determine presence of adventitious breath sounds.* • Maintain optimal nutritional status and fluid intake. • Assess ocular integrity for evidence of conjunctivitis: erythematous, pruritic conjunctiva. • Assess mentation for evidence of central nervous system infection: decreased level of consciousness, headache, and visual disturbances. • Assess for evidence of gastrointestinal infection abdominal pain, fever, and diarrhea. • Monitor temperature and vital signs for evidence of fever and sepsis. • Maintain body hygiene. • Limit environmental stress. • Monitor laboratory data: white blood cell count and differential, erythrocyte sedimentation rate, C-reactive protein, urinalysis, and cultures. • In collaboration with physician, administer appropriate antimicrobial, antipyretic, or analgesic medication. Assess patient's response and monitor for side effects.

Nursing Diagnosis	Nursing Intervention/Rationale
	• Promote pulmonary toilet: breathing exercises, postural drainage, and chest physical therapy. • Maintain normal sleep and rest patterns. • Protect patient from physical injury. • Provide clean environment. • Maintain protective isolation based on hospital policy. • Restrict contact with family and health care providers who have infectious diseases.

Patient Education

1. Teach signs and symptoms of infection.
2. Teach techniques to prevent recurrent pulmonary infection: prophylactic antibiotics, breathing exercises, postural drainage, and chest physiotherapy.
3. Teach the importance of compliance with regular follow-up examinations for γ-globulin level and clinical evaluation.
4. Teach about the avoidance of risk factors associated with infection.
5. Teach principles of good nutrition.
6. Teach facts about and the importance of prescribed medications.
7. Refer the patient for genetic counseling to explain the inheritance pattern.
8. Stress the importance of wearing medical alert identification.

Evaluation

Patient Outcome	Data Indicating That Outcome is Reached
Infection is decreased or gone following chemotherapy.	There are no signs or symptoms associated with recurrent pyogenic infections.
Laboratory data return to normal limits.	IgG, IgE, IgD, white blood cell count, erythrocyte sedimentation rate, and C-reactive protein level are within normal limits. (IgA and IgM may not return to normal limits.) Cultures findings are negative. Urinalysis findings are within normal limits.
Unnecessary complications are avoided.	No live vaccines are administered.

Selective IgA deficiency

Selective IgA deficiency is the presence of serum IgA in quantities less than 10 mg/dl while other immunoglobulins are present in normal amounts.

Selective IgA deficiency is the most common immunodeficiency disease. In the United States the incidence is approximately 1 in 700. Although the disease is most commonly detected during the first decade of life, patients often survive until the sixth or seventh decade. It cannot be diagnosed before 1 year of age because infants may not produce IgA until then.

As discussed previously, IgA is the predominant immunoglobulin of external secretions. Therefore bacterial infections of the respiratory, gastrointestinal, and urogenital tracts are the major clinical manifestations associated with this disorder.

Many affected persons are asymptomatic. Autoimmune disease develops in 25% of those affected. Recently IgG subclass deficiencies were reported in association with IgA deficiency.[40]

Morbidity is associated with recurrent sinopulmonary infections, autoimmune disease, and rarely, neoplastic disease. Spruelike disease may also complicate the disease course.

Pathophysiology

The immunopathogenesis of this disorder is unclear. The presence of normal numbers of IgA B cells suggests that the underlying defect involves decreased synthesis or release of IgA. However, lymphocyte culture studies have demonstrated that IgA B cells synthesize but do not secrete immunoglobulin. Therefore the underlying defect probably occurs in the transformation of the IgA B lymphocyte to the plasma cell. T suppressor mechanisms may influence this process.[20] The presence of antibodies to IgA in as many as 44% of cases of IgA deficiency implies that an autoimmune process is involved as well.[10] See p. 1309 for a description of the role of IgA.

A genetic predisposition has also been postulated. Autosomal recessive and autosomal dominant modes of inheritance have been implicated. IgA deficiency appears with greater than normal frequency in families with a variety of immunodeficiency diseases. In addition, the presence of HLA-A1, HLA-B8, and HLA-DW3 is associated with IgA deficiency and autoimmune disease.[20]

Whatever the cause, the lack of secretory IgA antibody promotes the attachment of infectious microbes at the mucosal surfaces and explains the occurrence of gastrointestinal, urogenital, and sinopulmonary infections. In addition, IgA probably acts to prevent absorption of other foreign proteins such as those in the diet. Its absence may explain the spruelike syndrome associated with selective IgA deficiency.

The deficiency of IgA may not be primary. Instead it may follow the administration of certain drugs such as phenytoin. In this case the decreased serum levels may result from induction of T suppressor cells that interfere with B cell maturation.[40]

Diagnostic Studies and Findings

Ig Quantitation

IgA level less than 10 mg/dl; IgG, IgM, IgD, and IgE normal or increased

Immunization

Normal antibody response

B Cell Quantitation

Normal numbers of B cells, including IgA-bearing lymphocytes

T Cell Studies

Normal findings

Chest Roentgenograms

Pneumonia

Sinus Roentgenograms

Sinusitis

Pulmonary Function Tests

Findings abnormal

Gastrointestinal Studies

Findings abnormal in celiac disease; abnormal D-xylose absorption in malabsorption

Antinuclear Antibody

Positive findings in presence of autoimmune disease

Differential diagnoses that must be excluded include chronic mucocutaneous candidiasis, Nezelof syndrome, and drug-induced IgA deficiency.

Medical Plan

Since no replacement therapy is yet available, treatment is aimed at management of recurrent infections and serial assessment for the presence of autoimmune and neoplastic disease.

Medications

γ-Globulin for selected patients who also demonstrate IgG subclass deficiency

Antibiotic therapy according to system involved and culture results

General Management

Gluten-free diet for celiac disease

Chest physical therapy, breathing exercises, postural drainage, and oxygen therapy as prophylaxis or for treatment of chronic pulmonary disease

Serial sinus and chest roentgenograms and pulmonary function tests to follow the disease course and determine adequacy of treatment

Follow-up for, and treatment of, concomitant autoimmune or neoplastic disease as needed

Administration of IgA-deficient blood products to prevent future antigen-antibody reaction

NURSING CARE

Nursing Assessment

Recurrent Infection

Sinusitis; pneumonia; urogenital infections; gastrointestinal infections

Gastrointestinal Status

Celiac disease

Presence of Concomitant Autoimmune Disease

Signs and symptoms associated with systemic lupus erythematosus, rheumatoid arthritis, dermatomyositis, hemolytic anemia, Sjögren's syndrome[20]

Presence of Concomitant Neoplastic Disease

Signs and symptoms associated with squamous cell carcinoma of the esophagus and lung[20] or thymoma

Nursing Dx & Intervention

The majority of IgA-deficient patients are asymptomatic; the rest may have infections. See Chapter 13 for nursing care related to specific infections.

Patient Education

1. Teach techniques to prevent recurrent pulmonary infection: breathing exercises and postural drainage.
2. Teach methods to prevent recurrent urogenital infection: adequate hydration, intake of fluids (such as cranberry juice) to maintain urine acidity, frequent voiding (every 2 to 3 hours), meticulous perineal care, voiding before and after intercourse, antibiotic prophylaxis, use of condom, and limited exposure to multiple or anonymous sex partners.
3. Teach the patient a gluten-free diet (if celiac disease is present).
4. Teach methods of self-assessment for infection: signs and symptoms associated with sinopulmonary, urogenital, and intestinal infections. Teach the patient to report significant symptoms.
5. Teach the patient the importance of medical alert identification that specifies the need for IgA-deficient blood products.

Evaluation

Patient Outcome	Data Indicating That Outcome is Reached
Number of recurrent sinopulmonary, intestinal, and urogenital infections is decreased.	Serial follow-up indicates decreased incidence of infections.
Complications of recurrent infections are avoided.	Evidence of chronic progressive lung, kidney, and intestinal disease is limited or absent.
Complications associated with IgA deficiency (autoimmune disease, malignancies) are detected early or are absent.	Serial monitoring for autoimmune phenomena and malignancies reveals early disease, or results of studies are negative.

Disorders of complement

Primary deficiency or dysfunction of complement components in the classical pathway increases host susceptibility to infection. In acquired complement disorders, particularly immune complex disease, activation of complement and subsequent inflammatory mediator involvement may cause increased tissue damage.

The classical and alternative complement systems (Figure 14-9) play an integral role in the amplification of nonspecific host defense mechanisms to invading organisms and in clearance of circulating immune complexes from the serum.

Complement proteins are present in the serum in inactive form, and activation leads to biologic activity. Activation occurs in a cascade fashion and is regulated by four complement proteins.

Certain complement components, when activated, generate chemotactic factors, enhancing the accumulation of leukocytes at an inflammatory site. Other components are deposited on the surface of bacteria, enhancing their ingestion by phagocytic cells (osponization). The terminal components (C5 to C9) have the capacity to mediate direct lysis of certain bacteria. Complement attaches to circulating immune complexes, decreasing their solubility and thus increasing their removal from the serum.

Primary complement disorders account for less than 1% of primary immunodeficiencies. Deficiency or dysfunction has been identified for each of the classical complement components; none have been identified in the alternative pathway. Certain of these disorders, especially those late in the cascade, have a benign clinical course, but as many as 5% of these patients have severe *Neisseria* infections.

In contrast, defects involving key complement components that regulate the complement cascade or components early in the cascade may be associated with severe, recurrent infections or autoimmune diseases.

Secondary complement deficiencies arise when a disease process causes decreased synthesis or triggers increased consumption. With increased activation, as occurs in immune complex disease, tissue damage often occurs because of the inflammatory mechanisms modulated by complement.

Pathophysiology

A brief schema of the sequence of activation is shown in Figure 14-10.

Figure 14-10 Sequence of compliment activation.

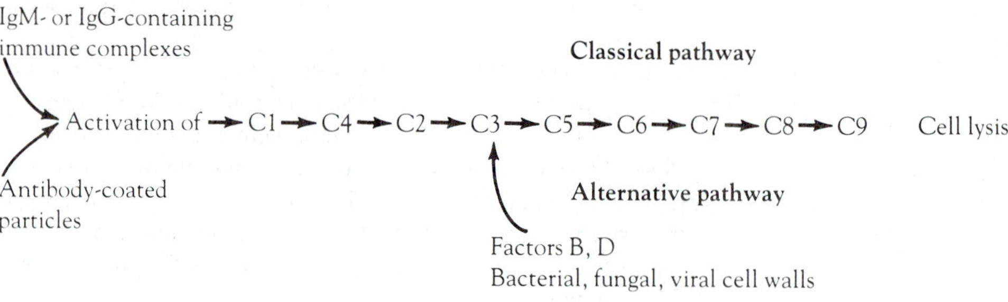

With deficiency or dysfunction in one of the classical complement components, activation of the normal cascade can occur only to the deficient component. Activation of the remainder of the pathway theoretically should not occur. However, because the classical and alternative pathways share the same terminal components, activation through a different regulatory point in the cascade can compensate for the deficiency.

Deficiencies in the C1, C4, and C2 proteins are the most commonly reported. C2 deficiency occurs in 1 in 10,000 persons. Persons with these deficiencies may be in good health and usually do not have difficulties with recurrent infections. When infections do develop, bacterial rather than viral organisms are involved. In addition, as many as 50% of persons with C2 deficiency have autoimmune disease, particularly systemic lupus erythematosus and juvenile rheumatoid arthritis.

Clinically, C3 is one of the most important complement components because of its place in the complement cascade, and C3 deficiency is the most severe disorder identified. Patients with this abnormality have recurrent, fulminant, pyogenic bacterial infections. C3 deficiency may result from a genetic defect in production. Some persons, including those with nephritic factor, have serum factors that continuously activate and thus deplete C3. Other persons lack C3bI, a regulatory protein that prevents continuous consumption of C3 once the alternative pathway is activated.

Terminal complement component deficiencies (C5 through C9) have also been identified. Many affected persons are asymptomatic. Others may manifest an increased incidence of infection with *Neisseria gonorrhoeae* and *N. meningitidis*. Although persons with C9 deficiency have been identified, this abnormality has not been associated with clinical disease. These persons show normal resistance to infection with bacterial, viral, and fungal organisms.

In C5 dysfunction all levels of complement components including C5 are normal, but serum chemotactic and opsonic

Table 14-2
Complement Component Deficiencies and Associated Diseases

Component	Collagen-Vascular Diseases*	Infections†	Other
C1q	+	+	Glomerulonephritis; immunodeficiencies
C1r	+	−	Glomerulonephritis
C1s	+	−	
C4	+	−	
C2	+	+	Glomerulonephritis
C3	+	+	Nephritis
C5	+	+	
C6	+	+	
C7	+	+	
C8	+	+	
C9	−	+	
I‡	−	+	
H‡	−	−	Hemolytic uremic syndrome
Properdin‡	−	−	
C1INH‡	+	+	Hereditary angioedema

*A variety of autoimmune diseases have been described.
†A variety of infective organisms have been identified.
‡Control proteins.

activities are reduced because of a defect in C5 activity. Clinical features of C5 dysfunction resemble those of C5 deficiency. Susceptibility to recurrent infections, particularly of the skin and gastrointestinal tract, is increased.

C1 inhibitor deficiency is also known as hereditary angioedema. C1 inhibitor is a regulatory protein that controls activation of C1. Continuous activation of C1 with resultant depletion of C2 and C4 may be due to a failure of this control protein to "turn off" primary pathway activation once initiated. Possibly deficiency of C1 inhibitor, which also inhibits kinin activation, allows kinin formation with subsequent vascular permeability and tissue edema, leading to angioedema.

Association of primary complement disorders with various autoimmune diseases is common (Table 14-2), although the cause is unknown.

Secondary disorders of complement have multiple pathophysiologic mechanisms. The degree of complement disorder will vary with the severity of the underlying disease process. In extreme protein deficiency states, decreased synthesis results in overall depression of the total complement component quantities resulting in inadequate host defense.

Various disease states may result in increased complement consumption. In fulminant bacterial infections, complement is consumed and production cannot meet demand.

Complement activation is an integral component of the pathophysiology of diseases associated with circulating immune complexes. With involvement of complement, and resultant inflammatory response, tissue damage occurs. Degree of complement activation correlates with activity of disease and is often monitored as an indicator of disease activity or response to therapy.

The following are some of the factors associated with secondary disorders of complement:

- Decreased synthesis
  - Asplenia
  - Sickle cell disease
  - Protein-deficient states
    - Cirrhosis
    - Malnutrition
    - Severe burns
    - Anorexia nervosa
  - Newborns (up to 6 months)
- Increased consumption
  - Acute nephritis
  - Partial lipodystrophy
  - Immune complex diseases, especially systemic lupus erythematosus
  - Bacteremia, endotoxins
  - Dialysis (renal, plasmapheresis, heart-lung)

Diagnostic Studies and Findings

History

Recurrent bacterial infections, especially meningitides; associations with autoimmune disease

Physical Examination

Dependent on disease process

Serum complement protein levels*

- Classical pathway†
  - C1q, 7 mg/dl
  - C1r, 3.4 mg/dl
  - C1s, 3.1 mg/dl
  - C4, 50 mg/dl
  - C2, 2.5 mg/dl
  - C3, 160 mg/dl
  - C5, 8 mg/dl
  - C6, 7.5 mg/dl
  - C7, 5.5 mg/dl
  - C8, 8 mg/dl
  - C9, 5.8 mg/dl
- Alternative pathway
  - Factor B, 20 mg/dl
  - Factor D, 0.2 mg/dl
  - Properdin, 1.5 mg/dl
- Control proteins
  - C1q inhibitor, 12.5 mg/dl
  - C3b inactivator (factor I), 2.5 mg/dl
  - Anaphylatoxin inactivator, 5 mg/dl
  - C4 binding protein, 25 mg/dl
  - S protein, 50 mg/dl
  - Factor H, 50 mg/dl
- CH50, 20 to 40 units/ml‡

Medical Plan

No therapy is available for direct treatment of complement disorders. With primary complement disorders, aggressive management of infections is indicated. Management of hereditary angioedema is discussed elsewhere in this text.

In secondary complement disorders, management of the disease process should restore normal complement levels. The reader is referred elsewhere in this text for management of individual diseases.

Acquired immune deficiency syndrome

Acquired immune deficiency syndrome (AIDS) is characterized by dysfunction of cell-mediated immunity. The cell-mediated immune defect is manifest clinically as the development of recurrent, often severe, oppor-

*C3, C4, and CH50 assays are available in most laboratories. Reference laboratories generally perform other assays. Numbers will be decreased in specific complement deficiency. With control protein abnormalities, succeeding components will be depressed.

†Detects quantity and not functional capacity. Ranges vary among laboratories.

‡Indicative of classical pathway integrity; measures the dilution of serum required to lyse 50% of a standard number of antibody-coated sheep red blood cells; normal values determined within each laboratory.

tunistic infections (such as *Pneumocystis carinii* pneumonia) or unusual malignancies (such as Kaposi's sarcoma).

AIDS was first recognized in homosexual men in 1981. By 1983 the incidence of the disease had reached many diverse populations. However, only when the epidemiology of the disease was clearly defined was a hypothesis formed to explain the pathogenesis of AIDS. It is now understood that AIDS is an infectious disease transmitted via intimate contact with body fluids, blood, or blood products.

April 1984 brought news of a breakthrough in AIDS research. Dr. Robert Gallo of the National Institutes of Health announced his discovery of the probable AIDS virus, a strain of the human T cell leukemia/lymphoma virus (HTLV-3). The original virus was discovered by Gallo in 1980 and is known to induce hematologic malignancies by infecting T cells and altering their genetic structure. A similar virus was previously isolated by French researchers at the Pasteur Institute. In 1987 the virus was renamed human immunodeficiency virus (HIV).

Gallo believes that HIV originated in Africa and traveled via slave trade to Europe, Latin America, and the Caribbean. Subsequently, a new strain of HIV evolved. Gallo says, "The virus may have been in the bush for some time, but with mass migration into cities, crowding and prostitution, what was contained at a low level became a problem."[55] That Kaposi's sarcoma, a connective tissue cancer to which AIDS patients are prone, has been prevalent in Central Africa for decades supports his hypothesis. In addition, AIDS itself is common in that region. How the AIDS virus entered the Unites States is unknown.

The signs and symptoms of AIDS vary greatly. Clinical manifestations depend on the degree of immunosuppression and the particular infection or neoplasm that develops secondarily. Nonspecific constitutional complaints may also occur and are usually exacerbated as the disease progresses.

A syndrome referred to as pre-AIDS, AIDS-related complex (ARC), or chronic lymphadenopathy syndrome has been described. Essentially, it is one way of describing immunosuppression in a person from a high-risk behavior group who has not yet developed the sequelae of recurrent infections and neoplastic disease. As many as 25% of these patients may develop AIDS. Signs and symptoms of ARC include severe fatigue, malaise, weakness, persistent unexplained weight loss, persistent lymphadenopathy, fevers, arthralgias, rigors, nocturnal diaphoresis, and persistent diarrhea. Laboratory tests and other diagnostic measures are important because such observations are nonspecific.

The most recent revision of the surveillance case definition for AIDS by the Centers for Disease Control (CDC) appeared in August 1987.[13] It is based on laboratory evidence of HIV infection. This new definition includes some individuals whose disorder would have previously been diagnosed as ARC.

By far the most common manifestations associated with full-blown AIDS are two life-threatening diseases: Kaposi's sarcoma and *Pneumocystis carinii* pneumonia.

Kaposi's Sarcoma

Named after a turn-of-the-century dermatologist, Kaposi's sarcoma (KS) is a malignant tumor of the endothelium, the layer of epithelial cells that lines the cavity of the heart, blood vessels, lymphoid tissues, and serous cavities. In its most benign form KS is usually limited to the skin, particularly of the lower extremities. Lesions are characteristically soft, vascular, bluish purple, painless areas of discoloration. Lesions may be either macular or papular or may appear as plaques, keloids, or ecchymotic areas. In this classic form the course of the disease is usually indolent with a high rate of survival at 10 years. This form until recently affected only select populations. In the United States these included Jewish and Italian men more than 50 years of age and severely immunocompromised persons such as organ transplant recipients and cancer patients receiving immunosuppressive drug therapy. The disease was rare; fewer than 40 cases were reported to the CDC between 1976 and 1980.

Late in 1980 physicians in New York City began to notice an alarming increase in the number of KS patients. Approximately 30 cases were reported during a period of months.

Two findings were disturbing to investigators. First, KS was identified in apparently healthy persons, not persons with known histories of or predispositions for immunosuppression. Moreover, these patients were sexually active homosexual men between 25 and 50 years of age.

Second, the KS decribed by clinicians was not the classic, chronic form limited to the skin. Rather, the syndrome mimicked the invasive form previously detected only in a population inhabiting Central Africa. It was initially characterized by diffuse cutaneous spread of lesions to the upper extremities and trunk. In addition, multicentric lesions were found in the endothelium of the gastrointestinal tract and other organs such as the lungs, liver, viscera, bones, and lymph nodes. More recent data suggest that, although KS in AIDS patients tends to resemble the aggressive African form, patients have varying degrees of systemic and cutaneous involvement. Possibly the invasiveness of the KS reflects the degree of immunodeficiency.

Diagnosis of KS is based on biopsy of suspect tissue or skin lesions. Before therapy is started, a staging workup is also performed to identify involvement elsewhere and to assist in determining the type and dosage of systemic chemotherapy. Pharmacologic agents used have included vinblastine, vincristine, adriamycin, bleomycin, VP-16 (etoposide), doxorubicin, and interferon. All have been used in various protocols with variable results.

Generally AIDS patients with KS have a milder immunodeficiency. However, severe immunosuppression and invasive KS carry a poor prognosis, although survival rates are longer than for patients with recurrent opportunistic infections. It is interesting to note that many patients who have KS when AIDS is diagnosed ultimately develop opportunistic infections but few individuals who have opportunistic infections at initial AIDS diagnosis later develop KS.[31] Other malignancies that may be associated with AIDS are non-Hodgkin's lymphomas, leukemias, and squamous cell carcinomas of the mouth and rectum.

Pneumocystis carinii Pneumonia

About the same time the CDC began to receive reports of KS, cases of another relatively rare condition, *Pneumocystis carinii* pneumonia (PCP), were reported from San Francisco and Los Angeles. As in the KS cases, patients affected were young homosexual men without known history of immunosuppression.

P. carinii is a one-celled protozoan that is ubiquitous in the environment. Usually a benign flora in the healthy population, it becomes an aggressive pathogen in immunocompromised hosts. Infestation can result in death from respiratory failure. Until the advent of AIDS, PCP was considered a relatively rare complication in cancer patients receiving chemotherapy, transplant patients, and patients with congenital defects of cellular immunity.

Probably spread person-to-person via the respiratory route, this opportunistic organism assaults pulmonary tissue, resulting in diffuse, bilateral interstitial infiltrates and alveolar infiltration by exudates of many clumped organisms, or cysts. PCP is usually slow to manifest itself, and the duration of symptoms varies from 2 weeks to 8 months.

Early symptoms often include increasing dyspnea on exertion, dry cough, and weight loss. Fever is sometimes present. Chest roentgenograms are unremarkable initially, and lung fields are clear to percussion and auscultation. Abnormal findings of pulmonary function studies may be the only way to confirm early suspicions that an infection is brewing. Patients have low Po_2 when arterial blood gases are measured. PCP can be definitively diagnosed only by bronchoscopy with transbronchial lung biopsy or by open lung biopsy.

The later course of PCP can be rapid and associated with clinical findings compatible with respiratory failure. AIDS patients with untreated PCP will develop life-threatening pulmonary insufficiency as a result of extensive pulmonary consolidation.

Two drugs are available to control this disease. The first-line defense is trimethoprim-sulfamethoxazole (Bactrim) given intravenously and later orally. Unfortunately, for as yet unexplained reasons, severe allergic reactions to this sulfa drug occur in many AIDS patients.

Pentamidine isothionate is the second drug of choice. It is administered intramuscularly or intravenously over a minimum of 10 days. Potential complications with this medication include hypotension, hypoglycemia, severe nausea and vomiting, renal insufficiency, hepatotoxicity, bone marrow suppression, and sterile abscesses (from IM injections). Currently research trials are being conducted on an aerosolized form of pentamidine.

In addition, new antibiotic approaches for PCP are being evaluated. These include dapsone-trimethoprim regimens. Dapsone was previously used as the treatment for human leprosy.

Use of the aforementioned drugs usually decreases the mortality associated with PCP. However, AIDS patients tend to clear the organism very slowly despite therapy, and relapses are common. Chances of survival from subsequent episodes of infection are greatly diminished. Therefore prolonged treatment is required in AIDS patients.

Opportunistic Infections

Listed below are a few of an ever-growing number of opportunistic infections associated with AIDS*:

- Protozoal
  - *Pneumocystis carinii* pneumonia
  - Toxoplasmosis
  - Cryptosporidiosis
  - Giardiasis
- Fungal
  - Candidiasis
  - Cryptococcosis
  - Histoplasmosis
  - Coccidioidomycosis
  - Aspergillosis
- Viral
  - Cytomegalovirus (CMV)
  - Progressive multifocal leukoencephalopathy
  - Herpes (HSV)
  - Epstein-Barr virus
- Bacterial
  - *Mycobacterium avium-intracellulare*
  - Miliary mycobacterial tuberculosis
  - Salmonellosis

Despite the variety, these organisms have one commonality: all are intracellular pathogens. As discussed previously, this has significance in that cell-mediated immune defenses are responsible for clearing these organisms. T lymphocytes and macrophages are important cells responsible for this defense. The occurrence of these pathogens in AIDS patients is consistent with findings that the immune deficiency is characterized by dysfunction of T cells.

Antimicrobial drugs are poorly effective against intracellular pathogens because most of these agents are unable to penetrate cell membranes. Thus, if the immune system cells (T cells) responsible for clearing these microbes are not functioning properly, these infections will clear much more slowly, if at all, despite attempts to facilitate a response with currently available pharmacologic agents. This necessitates lifelong therapy for most of the treatable infections such as *Pneumocystis carinii* pneumonia, cryptococcosis, and toxoplasmosis.

A discussion of the most frequently seen opportunistic infections follows.

Oral candidiasis, more commonly known as thrush, pro-

*Most infections are disseminated, tend to recur, and do not respond well to therapy.

duces creamy plaques on the oral mucosa. When these white plaques are removed, bleeding ulcers are revealed. Oral candidiasis occurs in about 75% of ARC and AIDS patients.[4] Treatment involves use of antifungal drugs such as nystatin, clotrimazole, ketoconazole, and amphotericin B for *Candida* esophagitis.

Oral hairy leukoplakia was first identified with AIDS and is a white lesion found predominantly on the lateral margins of the tongue. It does not rub off. It may be smooth, corrugated, or markedly folded and hairy. Studies of the lesion have revealed the presence of Epstein-Barr virus. Current data indicate that more than 75% of patients with hairy leukoplakia develop AIDS, usually with PCP as the first manifestation.[4] No effective treatment is yet available for hairy leukoplakia.

All three types of herpesvirus—type 1 (oral), type 2 (genital), and zoster (shingles)—are found in the AIDS population. Type 2 is the second most prevalent infection next to oral candidiasis.[15] Herpes outbreaks range from mild to disseminated. Treatment is with topical, oral, or intravenous acyclovir. Topically it is effective for all localized outbreaks except perianal ones. Oral administration controls mild cases; intravenous treatment is required for disseminated infections.

Cytomegalovirus (CMV) may affect many organs. Frequently AIDS clinically manifests as retinitis, which ranges from lack of symptoms to near blindness. Also common are pneumonitis and colitis. Treatment is available with intravenous administration of an anti-CMV agent called dihydroxyphenoxymethyl guanine (DHPG) (Gancyclovir). Duration includes a loading dose for 10 days followed by smaller doses and decreased frequency. Retinitis patients respond well to therapy, colitis patients respond only about half the time, and pneumonitis patients do not respond at all.

Neurologic symptoms include headache, changing mental status, seizures, and fever. They may be the result of toxoplasmosis, a brain infection caused by *Toxoplasma gondii*. Treatment is a combination of sulfadiazine and pyrimethamine (Fansidar) administered orally for the lifetime of the patient.

Infection with *Cryptococcus neoformans* can be either disseminated or organ focused. Disseminated cryptococcosis patients undergo a chronic debilitating process characterized by various combinations of fever, pulmonary infiltrates, malaise, and weight loss. Meningitis symptoms may include an insidious personality change, an alteration of consciousness, a debilitating illness, or an acute form of the disease. Amphotericin B, with or without flucytosine (5-FC), via central line for 6 weeks is the standard therapy. Maintenance follows either with amphotericin B weekly or experimentally with high doses of ketoconazole daily.

Chronic, watery, and very profuse or voluminous diarrhea characterizes cryptosporidiosis, an infection of the lining of the gastrointestinal tract by *Cryptosporidium*. Since there is no effective antimicrobial therapy known for this infection, treatment is aimed at controlling the diarrhea. Antimotility drugs may be successful in decreasing the volume or frequency of diarrhea. Supportive therapy includes fluid and electrolyte replacement. Hope for the future lies with spiromycin, an experimental drug that is now undergoing clinical trials.

Mycobacterial infections are present in AIDS patients in both pulmonary and nonpulmonary forms. *Mycobacterium tuberculosis* and *Mycobacterium avium-intracellulare* (MAI) are the usual culprits of infection. *M. tuberculosis* can be effectively treated with standard antituberculosis drugs. Unfortunately, in MAI infection even antituberculosis medications may be only partially effective, if at all. Symptoms such as fever, sweats, fatigue, and anorexia may be somewhat relieved by treatment, but the patient remains infected and cultures retain positive readings throughout treatment. Nonsteroidal anti-inflammatory drugs may alleviate symptoms associated with MAI. Ansamycin (a derivative of rifampin) and clofazimine are being tested for the treatment of MAI.

Autoimmune Phenomena

AIDS may also be associated with several disorders characterized by the development of hemolytic anemia and thrombocytopenia. The significance of these findings is unclear. A possible explanation is that, because of abnormal regulation of immunity in AIDS, the large numbers of B cells and immunoglobulins present may react with self-tissues or blood components. In any case the presence of autoantibodies generally reflects the overall immune system dysfunction that characterizes this disease.

Populations at Risk

AIDS has been identified in diverse populations (Table 14-3). Further dissemination of AIDS outside these groups seems possible considering that its transmission is similar to that of hepatitis B. The incidence of AIDS in these populations sup-

Table 14-3
Groups at Higher Risk for AIDS Because of High-Risk Behaviors

Behavior	AIDS Patients Who Engaged in This Behavior (%)
Homosexual or bisexual male contact since 1977	65
Intravenous needle and/or syringe sharing (heterosexual)	17
Both homosexual or bisexual male contact and IV sharing	8
Heterosexual contact with any of the other groups	4
Blood or blood product transfusion 1978-1985, including hemophilia	2
Neonates born to infected women	1
Initially "undetermined"*	3

Data from AIDS-HIV 1988.[4]
*74% reclassified into other groups after a second interview; others died, could not be relocated, or refused a second interview.

ports the theory that the disease is transmissible via direct contact with body fluids, blood, and blood products of known AIDS patients. In addition, there appears to be a carrier state associated with AIDS transmission. That is, exposure may occur from direct contact with persons who are infected with the virus but remain asymptomatic. Evidence supporting the existence of a carrier state suggests that the incubation period of the AIDS virus may be as long as 10 years.

Most children with AIDS are offspring of high-risk behavior parents and contract the disease in utero, during the birth process, or during the perinatal period. Some children acquire AIDS through transfusions.

Most heterosexual AIDS patients report exposure to members of the high-risk behavior groups. Probably the disease will spread beyond the current risk groups through heterosexual contacts.

The ratio of male to female patients with AIDS varies, but males generally far outnumber females. All races and major ethnic groups are affected. Cases are reported in every state and many foreign countries and territories. The majority of patients are less than 49 years of age; the median age range is 30 to 39.

If death rates are calculated by year of diagnosis, the ultimate mortality associated with AIDS approaches 100%. No one has fully regained immunocompetence. Patients typically die of recurrent infections and malignancies that respond poorly to therapy. Scientific research is aimed at new approaches to antiviral therapies and vaccines that will halt the spread of this life-threatening disease. The focus of current treatment is on control rather than cure.

Pathophysiology

Viruses are generally successful pathogens because of their ability to invade host cells and utilize the metabolism and genetic material of the host cells to produce copies of themselves. HIV, a retrovirus, is no exception. According to Gallo's theory, HIV-3 infects T helper lymphocytes, which are normally present in a ratio of 2:1 over T suppressor cells. When the virus decreases the number of T helper cells, this ratio is reversed and T suppressor mechanisms dominate. Clinical findings are compatible with profound immunosuppression. Because T cell–mediated immunity is important in tumor surveillance and in defense against intracellular pathogens such as viruses, protozoa, mycobacteria, and fungi, deregulation within this component of the body's defensive network results in the development of characteristics of AIDS, such as the following:

- Cutaneous anergy
- Leukopenia
- Lymphopenia
- Decreased T cell function and reactivity
- Reduced or absent T helper cells
- Increased percentage of T suppressor cells
- Depressed natural killer cell activity
- Depressed interferon production by peripheral blood leukocytes
- Normal or increased immunoglobulin levels
- Abnormal immunoglobulin function in some cases
- Normal phagocytic function

Diagnostic Studies and Findings

No test points to a diagnosis of AIDS with 100% accuracy. Laboratory data are nonspecific and merely support a diagnosis of immunosuppression, which can occur for a variety of reasons.

White Blood Cell Count

Depressed

Lymphocyte Count

Depressed

T Cell Studies

T cell numbers and function depressed; delayed hypersensitivity skin test shows decreased or absent response to cutaneous recall antigens (anergy); T helper/T suppressor cell ratio reversed (less than 0.5)

B Cell Studies

B cell numbers and function normal or increased; immunoglobulin levels normal or increased

Natural Killer Cell Activity

Usually depressed

Cultures

Polymicrobial (fungal, viral, protozoal, and bacterial) infections

Tissue Biopsy

Kaposi's sarcoma; *Pneumocystis carinii* pneumonia; lymphoreticular malignancies

Viral Titers

Document exposure to herpes simplex, hepatitis, Epstein-Barr virus, cytomegalovirus; elevated titers may explain panhypergammaglobulinemia

Chest Roentgenogram

Used in initial evaluation of respiratory complaints; pneumonia, pneumonitis, pulmonary infiltrates detected (causative agents determined via culture, bronchoscopy with brushings, or biopsy)

Gallium Scan

Useful in early detection of interstitial pneumonias

Stool for Ova and Parasites

Variety of parasites, including *Giardia lamblia* and *Cryptosporidium*

Neurologic Workup, Cerebrospinal Fluid Analysis, Brain CT Scan, Brain Biopsy, Electromyography, Nerve Conduction Studies, Ophthalmic Examination, Electroencephalogram, Magnetic Resonance Imaging (MRI)

Indicated for evaluation of changes in mentation and fever of unknown etiology; variety of AIDS-associated disorders may be detected, including progressive multifocal leukoencephalopathy, cryptococcal meningitis, encephalitis, organic brain syndrome, and toxoplasmosis

Staging Workup for Kaposi's Sarcoma[19]

Skin: Photographs and biopsies of representative lesions
Nodes: Biopsy of accessible nodes, CT scan of abdomen and pelvis
Gastrointestinal tract: Endoscopy, colonoscopy, and gastrointestinal contrast studies
Lung: Bronchoscopy (if chest roentgenogram shows abnormalities)
Liver: CT scan or radioisotope scan
Bone: Bone scan when alkaline phosphatase level is elevated
See Table 14-4

Bronchoscopy

Pneumocystitis carinii pneumonia (PCP)
Cryptococcal pneumonia

Sputum Induction

Pneumocystis carinii pneumonia (PCP)
Cryptococcal pneumonia

Pulmonary Function Tests

Useful in early detection of interstitial pneumonias

Table 14-4
Staging System of Kaposi's Sarcoma

Stage	Description
I	Cutaneous, locally indolent
II	Cutaneous, locally aggressive with or without regional lymph nodes
III	Generalized mucocutaneous or lymph node involvement
IV	Visceral

Subtypes
A. No systemic signs or symptoms
B. Systemic signs: 10% weight loss or temperature greater than 100° F orally, unrelated to identifiable source of infection, and lasting more than 2 weeks
Generalized: more than upper or lower extremities alone; includes minimal gastrointestinal disease defined as more than five lesions and larger than 2 cm in combined diameters

From Friedman-Kien.[19]

Serologic Antigen Test

Cryptococcosis

Bone Marrow Biopsy

Histoplasmosis disseminated in bone marrow

AFB Stain

Confirmation of *Mycobacterium tuberculosis*

Endoscopy

Disseminated CMV in the gastrointestinal tract
Candida esophagitis

Barium Swallow

Candida esophagitis

KOH Preparation of Yeast

Confirmation of oral thrush

Lumbar Puncture

Cryptococcal meningitis

Ophthalmic Examination

Disseminated CMV causing retinitis

Medical Plan

The goals of the medical plan include rapid detection and treatment of opportunistic infections and neoplastic disease, management of signs and symptoms, and prevention of complications from treatment. The ultimate objective for treatment of AIDS is reconstitution of the immune system. However, all attempts to correct the underlying immune defect, including bone marrow transplantation, have been unsuccessful.

Treatment for individual AIDS patients varies considerably and depends on the degree of immunosuppression and systemic involvement.

Surgery

Placement of a venous access device, such as a Hickman catheter, to facilitate frequent blood drawing, hyperalimentation, transfusions, and administration of chemotherapy
Surgical intervention for treatment of malignancies in certain cases

Medications

Directed at treatment of opportunistic diseases associated with AIDS; experimenting with antiviral and immune modulation therapy
Kaposi's sarcoma
Vinblastine sulfate (Velban), IV, usual dose 0.1-0.2 mg/kg/wk
Adverse reactions: bone marrow suppression, nausea, vomiting, anorexia, diarrhea, constipation, numbness,

paresthesias, peripheral neuritis, rarely alopecia
Vincristine sulfate (Oncovin), IV 1.5-2 mg/m^2/wk
Adverse reactions: neuritic pain, paresthesias, muscle weakness, headache, constipation, leukopenia, alopecia
Above agents administered in combination on an alternating weekly basis
Etoposide (VePesid), IV for 1 hr (oral administration is not recommended), 150 mg/m^2 qd for 3 d every 3-4 wk
Adverse reactions: hypotension, bone marrow suppression, nausea, vomiting, alopecia
Interferon Alfa-2A (Roferon-A), parenteral usual dose 3 million IU qd for 16-24 wk; maintenance 3 million IU 3 times wk
Adverse reactions: nausea, anorexia, diarrhea, fatigue, myalgia, fever, chills, headache
Pneumocystis carinii pneumonia
Two drugs are available to control this disease; first-line defense is trimethoprim-sulfamethoxazole (Bactrim) given IV for average of 2 wk (based on severity of disease), then po as needed for prophylaxis
Trimethoprim (Bactrim) and sulfamethoxazole (Septra), po and IV preparations, usual dose 15 mg/kg/d (in 4 divided doses)
Adverse reactions: nausea, vomiting, anorexia, diarrhea, fever, headache, rash, bone marrow suppression
Pentamidine isothionate, IV (route of choice) 4 mg/kg/d (90 min infusion); parenteral 4 mg/kg/d
Adverse reactions (IV): nausea, vomiting, anorexia, renal toxicity, bone marrow suppression
Adverse reactions (parenteral): same as above plus sterile abscesses at injection site
Aerosolized (experimental) 600 mg/6 ml sterile H_2O (10% absorption)
Adverse reactions: irritation of bronchial tree produces cough, no systemic effects, or
Dapsone and trimethoprim (under evaluation), oral preparation, dapsone 100 mg/d, trimethoprim 15 mg/kg/d (in 4 divided doses)
Adverse reactions: same as for Septra plus decreased erythrocyte life span, which leads to immature hemoglobin (methemoglobin)
Toxoplasmosis
Pyrimethamine (Fansidar), oral preparation, 100 mg loading dose, 25 mg/d
Adverse reactions: anorexia, nausea, vomiting, diarrhea, rash, headache, inhibits folinic acid metabolism (therefore folinic acid is usually given with pyrimethamine)
Sulfadiazine,* oral preparation, 1000 mg q6h
Adverse reactions: anorexia, nausea, vomiting, diarrhea, rash, headache
Clindamycin, po 600-1200 mg q6h; IV 900 mg q8h; usually used for patients intolerant of sulfadiazine; primarily indicated for retinal toxoplasmosis (still experimental for CNS toxoplasmosis)
Adverse reactions: nausea, vomiting, diarrhea, abdominal pain, rash, elevated liver enzyme levels
Candidiasis
Nystatin suspension (mycostatin), 5-10 cm^3 po q6h
Adverse reactions: nausea, vomiting, diarrhea
Clotrimazole lozenges (Mycelex; Lotrimin), 1 lozenge or troche po 5 times daily
Adverse reactions: nausea, vomiting, diarrhea
Ketoconazole (Nizoral), po 200-400 mg/d
Adverse reactions: nausea, vomiting, diarrhea, elevated liver enzymes
Cryptococcosis
Amphotericin B (Fungizone), IV over 4-6 h; requires central line; initial test dose 1 mg in 50 ml fluid over 1 h, then 0.6-0.8 mg/kg/d to total dose of 1.5 g, then 1-3 times/wk; usually mixed with hydrocortisone and heparin and requires premedication with Benadryl, Tylenol, and sometimes Demerol to prevent severe adverse reactions; also indicated for *Candida* esophagitis
Adverse reactions: nausea, vomiting, fever, chills, headache, diarrhea, abdominal cramping, body aches, renal toxicity, hypokalemia
Flucytosine (Ancobon), po, 75-100 mg/kg/d in 4 divided doses administered with amphotericin B
Adverse reactions: nausea, vomiting, diarrhea, bone marrow suppression, renal toxicity, elevated liver enzyme levels
Ketoconazole (Nizoral), po 800-1000 mg/d (high doses for maintenance suppressive therapy)
Adverse reactions: nausea, vomiting, diarrhea, elevated liver enzyme levels
Herpes simplex virus (HSV)/herpes zoster virus (HZV)
Acyclovir sodium (Zovirax), po, IV, and topical preparations; for HSV 200 mg po 5 times/d, or topically for localized outbreaks, except perianally; for HZV 10-15 mg/kg po or IV q6h
Adverse reactions: nausea, headache, rash, bone marrow suppression
Cytomegalovirus
Dihydroxyphenoxymethyl guanine (DHPG) (Gancyclovir), IV for 1 h; requires central line; 2.5-7.5 mg/kg q8h; 10-d loading dose, then maintenance 5 mg/kg 3-5 times/wk
Adverse reactions: nausea, anorexia, diarrhea, muscle aches, disorientation, headache, neutropenia, pruritic rash, thrombocytopenia
Antiviral
Azidothymidine (AZT; Zidovudine; Retrovir), po 200

*Works synergistically with pyrimethamine; therefore the two agents are administered together.

mg q4h; clinical trials still in progress while available to a limited group of patients

Adverse reactions: headache, fever, nausea, anemia, granulocytopenia, leukopenia

General Management

Chest physiotherapy, postural drainage, positioning, and oxygen therapy in conjunction with antimicrobial therapy if needed for pulmonary infections

Reduction of risk factors for infection: malnutrition, exposure to infectious sources or invasive procedures such as contaminated equipment, frequent venipuncture, or Foley catheterization

Maintenance of personal hygiene including optimal skin integrity with intact oral mucosa

Maintenance of adequate hydration, particularly during acute febrile episodes and with administration of nephrotoxic medications or with individuals who have chronic diarrhea

Maintenance of optimal nutritional status with high-calorie, high-protein diet, use of supplemental feedings such as Osmolite and Ensure if needed; parenteral alimentation if necessary

Frequent attempts to maintain patient's orientation and safety (especially fall precautions) in central nervous system disturbances

Physical therapy for immobilized patients; regular program of rest and exercise for ambulatory patients

Administration of analgesics as needed to minimize discomfort and pain; assistance with alternative therapies and selection of distracting measures

Uninterrupted periods of sleep whenever possible

Support services as appropriate: social worker, clergy, psychologist, psychiatrist, clinical nurse specialist, support groups, involvement of significant others (partner and family) in care

As discharge nears, referral to professional support services as well as local support groups for home care and followup

NURSING CARE

Nursing Assessment

As noted earlier, the signs and symptoms of AIDS vary greatly. Clinical manifestations depend on the degree of immunosuppression and the opportunistic infections and neoplasms that develop secondarily. Nonspecific complaints may also occur and are usually exacerbated as the disease progresses. Therefore significant time and energy are devoted to dealing with the multiple needs of this patient population. One way to address these needs is to obtain a thorough baseline assessment from which the appropriate nursing diagnoses can be identified. Some specific examples follow:

- General appearance and disposition
- Cognitive functioning
- Complaints of pain or numbness and tingling
- Ability to ambulate
- Pulmonary status
- Ability to maintain adequate hydration and nutrition
- Skin integrity: note any red-violet raised lesion, white plaques on oral mucosa, rash, or palpable lymph nodes
- Past medical history for
  - Hepatitis
  - Viral infections
  - Fever of unknown origin
  - Sexually transmitted diseases
  - Lymphadenopathy
  - Parasitic infections
- Medications, recreational drugs, allergies
- Psychosocial history
  - Support systems available
  - Financial concerns and responsibilities

Nursing Dx & Intervention

Nursing Diagnosis	Nursing Intervention/Rationale
Impaired gas exchange related to pulmonary infection	• Assess respiratory status: rate, rhythm, and regularity of respirations, use of accessory muscles, presence of adventitious breath sounds on auscultation, cough, and cyanosis. • Maintain patent airway at all times. • Encourage patient to report cough and progressive dyspnea on exertion. • In collaboration with physician, administer oxygen therapy *to help patient breathe and rest more easily.* Assess effectiveness *to determine if oxygen delivery method and flow rate are sufficient to prevent hypoxia or respiratory distress.* • In collaboration with physician, administer appropriate anti-infective medications. Assess effectiveness and side effects *to determine if treatment is adequate.* • Visit patient frequently *to reassure, comfort, and alleviate anxiety or feelings of isolation.* • Obtain sputum specimens as needed *to determine appropriate antibiotic therapy.* • Monitor results of pulmonary function studies. • Provide preprocedural teaching before bronchoscopy, lung biopsy, CT scans, pulmonary function tests, and other procedures *to decrease anxiety and ensure informed consent.*

Nursing Diagnosis	Nursing Intervention/Rationale
	• Provide chest physiotherapy and postural drainage as indicated *to open the airways and mobilize secretions.* • Instruct patient in breathing exercises such as pursed-lip or diaphragmatic breathing and encourage patient to perform them *to decrease respiratory effort required.* • Instruct patient in relaxation techniques *to prevent hyperventilation resulting from anxiety caused by shortness of breath.* • Instruct patient in energy conservation measures during ADLs *to decrease respiratory effort required.* • Encourage patient to stop smoking *to increase resistance to respiratory infections.* • In collaboration with physician, determine need for mechanical ventilation if respiratory status worsens or if patient becomes uncomfortable.
Altered nutrition: less than body requirements related to protracted diarrhea, malabsorption, anorexia, stomatitis	• Assess nutritional status: height and weight, caloric intake, total protein, serum albumin, hematocrit, and hemoglobin level. • Determine need for dietary changes, enteral feedings, and parenteral alimentation. • Provide vitamin supplements for deficiencies. • In collaboration with physician, provide prescribed therapy such as antiemetic agents 30 to 60 minutes before meals *to alleviate nausea and aid patient's food tolerance.* • Provide small, frequent, high-calorie, high-protein feedings *to help patient take in more calories, tolerate food, and regain and maintain weight.* Encourage patient to eat. Have favorite foods brought from home. • Provide or encourage patient to perform frequent oral hygiene *to prevent oral infection and offer comfort.* Correct stomatitis. • Monitor intake and output, daily weight, laboratory values, and skin integrity *to maintain accurate knowledge of nutritional status.*
Diarrhea related to chemotherapy or gastrointestinal infection	• Assess elimination pattern: quality, quantity, and frequency of stool and presence of gross blood, fat, or undigested food. • Monitor intake and output and daily weight *to determine fluid deficit and weight loss.* • Monitor vital signs for evidence of hypovolemia. • Monitor for signs and symptoms associated with fluid and electrolyte imbalances *to determine appropriate replacement therapy.* • Assess perianal skin condition and provide skin care after every stool *to prevent breakdown*; provide application of skin barrier or fecal incontinence bag if necessary. • Monitor stool culture results *to determine appropriate antibiotic therapy.* • In collaboration with physician, administer and assess effectiveness of prescribed antibiotics and antidiarrheal agents *to determine whether treatment is adequate.*
Potential impaired skin integrity related to malnutrition, Kaposi's sarcoma, frequent venipunctures, immobility, or side effects of chemotherapy	• Assess skin integrity: presence of lesions, texture, temperature, moisture, color, vascularity, and evidence of poor wound healing. • Monitor lesions for signs of infection, dissemination, and other abnormal changes *to prevent further skin breakdown.* • Provide or encourage patient to perform meticulous hygiene in involved areas *to prevent infection.* • For stomatitis: perform regular oral care, avoid acidic oral fluids, provide topical viscous anesthetic, and serve bland foods at medium temperatures *to alleviate pain and discomfort.* • Provide or encourage use of mild, hypoallergenic, nondrying soaps for skin cleansing and massage with oils and lotions. • Soak feet and hands in warm water and apply isopropyl alcohol afterward *to prevent or treat fungal infections.* • If Kaposi's lesions are present, assess response to chemotherapy; note changes in size, color, and configuration *to determine if therapy is adequate.* • Avoid trauma to the skin. Do not allow more than 2-hour periods of immobilization. Assist with position change *to prevent pressure sores.* • Encourage mobility within functional limits *to facilitate circulation to extremities and pressure points.* • Implement pressure sore care as indicated. • Use appropriate beds and appliances such as egg-crate mattresses, *to allow pressure relief.*
Pain related to side effects of chemotherapy, infections, frequent venipunctures, or immobility	• Assess pain: location, onset, duration, precipitating or alleviating factors, character, and frequency. Have patient describe intensity on scale of 0 to 10. • In collaboration with physician, provide appropriate anti-inflammatory and analgesic agents. Assess effectiveness and note side effects *to determine whether therapy is relieving patient's pain.*

Nursing Diagnosis	Nursing Intervention/Rationale
	• Consider routine administration as needed for analgesic agents. • Give analgesics with the intent of relieving pain. Suggest that medication will be effective *to stimulate the placebo response.* • Ensure calm environment and quiet, undisturbed rest periods *to allow patient the opportunity to relax.* • Use alternative therapies such as massage, visualization, and meditation, and teach relaxation techniques *to minimize patient's perception of pain.* • Provide diversional activities as tolerated. • Provide thermal therapy for affected muscles and joints as needed *to promote vasodilation.* • Consider placement of venous access device if frequent venipuncture is necessary.
Potential activity intolerance related to weakness, fatigue, arthralgias, myalgias, side effects of therapy, dyspnea, fever, malnutrition, or fluid and electrolyte imbalances	• Assess degree of activity intolerance. • Assist with ADLs as needed. • Encourage regular exercise and rest as tolerated. Confer with physical or occupational therapist *to determine optimal approach.* • Teach patient energy conservation measures and evaluate response to instruction. • Monitor tolerance for visits and phone calls. Suggest limits as appropriate *to conserve energy and reduce environmental factors of intolerance.* • In collaboration with physician, provide appropriate treatment for underlying causes of activity intolerance such as pain, infections, sleeplessness, or malnutrition. Assess effectiveness *to determine if treatment is adequate.*
Anxiety related to diagnosis, fear of death or hospitalization, perception of unknown threat, knowledge deficit	• Assess level of anxiety in terms of behaviors and statements. • Provide atmosphere of individual acceptance. • Provide opportunities for patient to express feelings. • Avoid false reassurances but encourage hope. Inform patient of promising research findings to stimulate positive mental attitude. • Engage in honest, consistent communication with patient. • Provide accurate information about AIDS and related treatment. Include information about diagnostic procedures *to ease fear of the unknown.* • Increase simplicity, concreteness, and repetitions in communications *to ensure that patient hears, absorbs, and understands information.* • Explain features of immediate environment *to allow patient self-control.* • Keep door open and light on at night, visit frequently, and use touch as appropriate *to decrease feelings of isolation and loneliness.* • Assist patient in identifying signs and symptoms of anxiety. Tell him or her your own most positive and effective anxiety-control techniques and encourage patient and significant others to use them. • Encourage patient to participate in care as much as possible *to promote feelings of self-control.* • Involve hospital and community resources *to assist patient and significant others where appropriate.* • Encourage patient to use available resources *to decrease feelings of isolation.* • Assess need and monitor effectiveness of psychopharmacologic intervention *to determine whether therapy is adequate.*
Body image disturbance related to diagnosis, Kaposi's lesions, side effects of chemotherapy, depression, or social stigmatization and isolation	• Assess patient's self-concept in terms of statements and behavior. • Provide atmosphere of acceptance, encourage expression of feelings, and refrain from negative criticism. • Acknowledge change in body image but focus on identifying strengths and accomplishments. Praise appropriately and emphasize functions that have stabilized or improved. • Provide accurate information as indicated *to correct myths and clarify controversial information the patient might have seen, heard, or read.* • Strongly encourage participation in self-care to tolerance, even if tolerance is severely limited, *to enhance self-esteem.* • Have family and significant others bring in clothes, pajamas from home, and personal toileting items and suggest use of makeup for Kaposi's sarcoma lesions, especially facial lesions. • Direct patient to appropriate resources: clergy, social worker, psychologist, psychiatrist, or AIDS clinic counselor. • Encourage patient to participate in AIDS support groups *to decrease feelings of isolation.*

Nursing Diagnosis	Nursing Intervention/Rationale
Knowledge deficit (AIDS disease process, life-style implications, and therapy) related to anxiety, unavailable resources, poor communication skills, or fear	• Assess patient's understanding of disease process, life-style implications, and therapy. • Based on assessment, provide information to patient, significant others, and family on the following topics (see "Patient Education" section): nutrition, rest and activity, stress management, desired and untoward effects of medications, reportable signs and symptoms, infections, community resources, disease process, infection control, and safe sex practices. (Provide written material where available.) • Include significant others and family in teaching sessions whenever possible. • Refer patient to available resources. • Encourage patient and others to be involved in the discharge planning process.
Potential for infection related to immune deficiency, disease process, neutropenia, effects of chemotherapy, malnutrition, frequent venipunctures, immobility, and environmental pathogens	• Assess skin integrity including pressure areas, oral mucosa, rectum, invasive procedure sites (IVs) for evidence of infection or breakdown. • Monitor vital signs, especially temperature, every 4 hours and as needed *to note evidence of fever and signs of infection.* • Monitor laboratory data: WBC count and differential and shifts in these *to note acute stress on the bone marrow or severe bacterial disease.* • Observe strict aseptic technique for all invasive therapies and procedures. • Initiate neutropenic precautions per hospital protocol whenever necessary (usually when absolute neutrophil count is <1000). • Restrict contact with family and health care providers who have infectious diseases. • In collaboration with physician, administer appropriate anti-infective, antipyretic, or analgesic medication. Assess patient's response and monitor side effects *to determine whether therapy is adequate.* • Maintain thorough handwashing before and after patient contact. • Provide clean environment. • Protect patient from physical injury. • Limit environmental stress. • Maintain body hygiene. • Maintain optimal nutritional status and fluid intake. • Maintain normal sleep and rest patterns.
Impaired home maintenance management related to knowledge deficit concerning local resources, activity intolerance, impaired mobility, self-care deficit, inadequate finances, and/or support systems	• Assess patient's knowledge level concerning own needs for care and assistance at home and personal support available. • Refer to social worker for counsel on various forms of financial assistance. • Advise patient about support groups available and encourage patient to participate *to decrease feelings of isolation and loneliness.* • Assess need for equipment at home, such as oxygen, bedside commode, hospital bed, and walker, and arrange for delivery. (Obtain input from patient, significant others, and family.) • Contact professional local support services for home care. • Assess need for transportation home *to ensure smooth transition from hospital to home environment.*
Hyperthermia related to increased metabolic rate, infectious process	• Assess vital signs and temperature every 4 hours (while awake if afebrile) and as needed *to note increases as soon as possible.* • In collaboration with physician, administer acetaminophen, 650 mg, for temperature more than 38.5° C (101.8° F) every 4 hours. • In collaboration with physician, consider alternating acetaminophen with aspirin or ibuprofen every 4 hours if platelet count is adequate *to capitalize on the benefits of different drug actions.* • Give alcohol and water sponge bath for temperature more than 39° C (104° F) or initiate cooling blanket or ice packs *to alleviate fever.* Discontinue cooling blanket or ice packs if patient begins to shiver. • In collaboration with physician, monitor laboratory tests (blood, stool, urine, sputum cultures) and lumbar puncture results *to rule out infectious process.* • Encourage fluid intake as appropriate *to prevent dehydration.* • Assess mucous membranes, skin turgor, sodium, hematocrit, and specific gravity as indicators *to monitor for dehydration.* • Change linen after diaphoretic episodes *to offer comfort.*
Potential for injury related to weakness, medication reactions, neuromuscular changes, dehydration	• Assess risk factors such as weakness, sedation, mental confusion, and diarrhea. • Initiate fall precautions and evaluate need for a fall precaution device (according to hospital protocol). • For all patients and especially those with weakness: Encourage use of call bell or light.

Nursing Diagnosis	Nursing Intervention/Rationale
	Assist with ambulation. Leave belongings within reach. • Evaluate patient for effects of sedation. If patient is drowsy or unsteady, assist with movement. • For patient with mental confusion: Reorient frequently and remind to call for assistance. Check status every 30 minutes and as needed. Restrain as appropriate. • For patient with diarrhea, provide bedside commode and have bedpan within reach. • For patient with orthostasis, monitor for medication effects and check blood pressure.
Patient problem: bleeding related to decreased circulating hemostatic mechanisms	• Assess vital signs every 4 hours and as needed. Note tachycardia, hypotension, pallor, anxiety, and restlessness as signs of internal bleeding. • Assess body surfaces for ecchymosis, petechiae, and hematomas every 8 hours. Monitor urine, stool, and emesis for heme. • Implement safety precautions for patients with low platelet counts (<50,000) *to decrease risk of bleeding*. Avoid using toothbrushes, use electric razors, do not take rectal temperatures, use side rails and fall precautions, avoid IM injections, avoid use of aspirin, and use stool softeners *to prevent rectal bleeding*. • Instruct patient, family, and significant others on safety precautions. • Assess use of experimental drugs such as AZT on admission, and monitor hematologic effects *to note any decrease in bone marrow activity*.
Fatigue related to disease process, weakness, adverse reactions to medication, neuromuscular changes, insomnia, anxiety	• Assess level of fatigue by noting time spent in activity before feeling exhausted. • Assist patient in identifying factors related to fatigue (e.g., anxiety) and his or her best ways of effectively dealing with these. Encourage use *to promote feelings of self-control*. Assist patient in identifying tasks and routines that require less physical and mental effort and determining most productive hours of the day. Assist patient in coordinating a manageable schedule considering these factors *to optimize strength*. Encourage use of schedule. • Encourage rest after activities. • Allow for uninterrupted periods of sleep. • Instruct in energy conservation measures and evaluate response to instruction. • In collaboration with physician, assess need for mild sedative at night *to enhance length and quality of sleep*. Monitor effectiveness *to determine whether therapy is beneficial*.

Patient Education

1. Teach the importance of obtaining up-to-date factual information about AIDS.
2. Teach the importance of meticulous hygiene.
3. Teach the importance of regular oral care before breakfast, after meals, and at bedtime.
4. Teach the patient to avoid accidental injury to skin or mucous membranes and to inspect all wounds for signs of infection.
5. Teach safety precautions when the patient is at risk of bleeding.
6. Teach the patient to limit contact with persons who are infected.
7. Teach the patient that smoking further limits resistance to respiratory infections.
8. Teach methods of self-assessment for recurrent infections.
9. Teach the patient to maintain a balanced program of rest and exercise as tolerated.
10. Teach pursed-lip, diaphragmatic breathing exercises to decrease respiratory effort required.
11. Teach energy conservation measures to decrease effort needed in daily activities.
12. Teach the principles of a balanced diet. Encourage the use of dietary supplements, such as Ensure, for weight gain. Encourage the patient to take a multivitamin daily.
13. Teach the patient to avoid alcohol in excess and other recreational drugs.
14. Teach relaxation technique to ease anxiety.
15. Teach the patient to identify signs and symptoms of anxiety and his or her most positive and effective anxiety-control techniques.
16. Teach the patient safe sexual habits: decrease number of partners; avoid contact with anonymous partners; use condoms; explore alternative sexual activities that limit direct contact with mucous membranes; avoid analingus.
17. Teach the importance and side effects of medications.

18. Teach the patient to refrain from donating blood.
19. Teach the patient about available resources and the importance of using them.
20. Teach the patient that travel outside the United States may increase the risk for amebic infections and may require antibiotic prophylaxis.
21. Teach home care to the family (see box).
22. Teach care of a venous access device if indicated.
23. Teach home hyperalimentation or tube-feeding administration if indicated.
24. Teach the importance of regular follow-up by a physician.
25. Explain that the patient's dentist should be made aware of the infection.
26. Teach the patient to keep a log of medical history (diary of symptoms and treatment).
27. Teach the importance of medical alert identification.

Body Substance Isolation (BSI) Precautions

All patients are considered infected.

In hospital

1. The door to the patient's room need not be closed.
2. Gloves should be worn only if in *direct* contact with specimens, linen, and items or surfaces exposed to blood or body fluids. Gloves need *not* be worn if one is merely conversing with the patient or walking into the room.
3. A mask should be worn if secretions may be aerosolized onto the face during suctioning, oral hygiene, and other procedures. A mask should be worn if a health care worker with a respiratory infection must enter the room of a severely immunosuppressed patient.
4. Protective eyewear should be worn if aerosolization of secretions or blood may contact the conjunctiva (as during suctioning or blood drawing).
5. A gown should be worn if clothing is likely to become contaminated with blood or body fluids, as during bathing of the patient, linen changes, some specimen collections, or dressing changes.
6. Proper isolation technique should be used. Gown and gloves should be removed in the room when used.
7. Specimens should be bagged.
8. Special care in handling contaminated needles is essential. Attempts to recap needles should be avoided, since most needle-stick injuries occur this way. Needles should be disposed of in a puncture-resistant container, which should be sealed before being taken from the room.
9. Handwashing should be performed in the room before and after contact with the patient.
10. Contaminated nondisposable items should be cleaned with soap and water and bagged (using paper bags) for autoclaving. Items that cannot be autoclaved should be washed with soap and water, 10% bleach solution, or other solution recommended in the hospital procedure manual.
11. A private room may be given to patients unable to maintain scrupulous hygiene (those with intractable diarrhea, incontinence, or central nervous system infections leading to altered sensorium).
12. Usually no precautions are needed when handling food trays.
13. Disposable resuscitation equipment (Ambu bags, airways, and so on) should be available at all times.
14. Postmortem handling of the body may include the use of gown and gloves.

At home*

1. Disposable gloves should be worn by family members who come in direct contact with the patient's blood and body fluids.
2. Linen and clothing soiled with secretions or excretions should be washed separately with a 10% bleach solution (¼ cup bleach to 1 gallon water).
3. Dishes and eating utensils do not require separate handling but should be washed in hot, soapy water.
4. Dry waste contaminated with blood or body fluids should be disposed of in a separate container and bagged securely.
5. Any needles used for the administration of medication should be placed in an impervious container before disposal.
6. Meticulous handwashing before and after contact with the patient is essential.

*Recommendations of New York Red Cross Nursing Service.

Evaluation

Patient Outcome	Data Indicating That Outcome is Reached
Optimal respiratory status is maintained.	Arterial blood gases within normal range. There are no symptoms associated with respiratory distress.
Optimal nutritional status is maintained.	Albumin and total protein are within normal limits. Weight is approaching normal for patient's height and build.
Frequency and consistency of stools are within normal limits.	Frequency of stools is reduced and soft consistency returns.
Dermatologic signs and symptoms are improved or controlled.	Skin integrity is intact. Circulation to affected part is uncompromised.
Pain is managed or minimized.	Patient reports that pain is reduced to a tolerable level or resolved. Patient can now perform activities, since pain is controlled.
Activity intolerance is increased.	Patient participates in ADLs. Patient uses energy conservation measures.
Anxiety level is diminished.	Patient verbalizes understanding of own anxiety and demonstrates methods to manage it.
Positive feelings are expressed.	Patient participates in own hygiene and grooming. Patient verbalizes realistic expectations. Patient acknowledges personal strengths.
Knowledge is acquired through individual learning experiences.	Patient verbalizes accurate information about diagnosis and treatment.
New infectious processes are prevented or minimized.	There is no WBC elevation or shift in differential.
Optimal care is managed at home.	Patient demonstrates knowledge of local support systems and resources. Patient completes plans for adequate living arrangements.
Regulation of body temperature is maintained.	Temperature is within normal limits. There is no fever, chills, diaphoresis, or flushing.
Injury is prevented or minimized.	There are no falls or other causes of injury. Patient verbalizes need for assistance with movement.
Bleeding episodes are prevented or minimized.	There are no ecchymoses, petechiae, hematomas, or signs of internal bleeding.
Level of fatigue is decreased.	Patient says that energy level sufficient to maintain usual routine.

INFLAMMATORY DISEASES

Wegener's granulomatosis

Wegener's granulomatosis is a multisystem disorder of unknown cause characterized by diffuse granuloma formation and vasculitis primarily involving the respiratory tract.

Wegener's granulomatosis occurs in both sexes equally. It may appear at any age, with a peak incidence in the fourth and fifth decades of life.

Signs and symptoms may be widespread but usually occur in the upper or lower respiratory tract. For example, a patient may have headache, sinusitis, rhinorrhea, and otitis media. Other manifestations include hearing loss (resulting from recurrent otitis), renal disease, pericarditis, myocarditis, granulomatous lung disease, ocular inflammatory disease, arthralgias, and some dermatologic manifestations associated with vasculitis.

Once considered a fatal disease, Wegener's granulomatosis now has a good prognosis when detected early and treated with cyclophosphamide, which is capable of inducing prolonged remission in most cases. However, extensive renal disease is indicative of a poor prognosis.

Pathophysiology

Any organ may become involved with granuloma formation and vasculitis. Although the immunopathogenesis remains an enigma, these manifestations suggest that delayed-type hypersensitivity or cell-mediated reactions may be involved. Immune complex deposition may also occur.[26]

Histologic features include widespread necrotizing vasculitis of small arteries, venules, arterioles, and some capillaries, together with granuloma formation. Almost all patients have pulmonary involvement. Paranasal sinuses and the nasopharynx demonstrate granuloma formation. Pansinusitis may result in erosion of adjacent bones and septum perforation. Sinuses often become secondarily infected with bacteria. Saddle-nose deformity may be observed as well. Diffuse, bilateral, nodular lesions that tend to cavitate are found in lung tissue. When renal tissue is affected, focal glomerulitis may progress to diffuse proliferative disease.

Diagnostic Studies and Findings

Biopsy of Affected Tissue

Granuloma formation; vasculitic lesions

Complete Blood Count

Mild anemia (normochromic, normocytic); leukocytosis in presence of superimposed infection

Erythrocyte Sedimentation Rate

Elevated during active disease

Serum Protein Electrophoresis

Mild hypergammaglobulinemia (especially IgA)

Differential diagnoses include other vasculitides, connective tissue diseases, infectious and noninfectious granulomatous diseases, pulmonary neoplasia, and lymphomatoid granulomatosis.

Medical Plan

Medications

Antineoplastic agents (used as immunosuppressant)
Cyclophosphamide (Cytoxan), 1-2 mg/kg/d po; dosage adjusted to maintain total WBC at > 3000/mm^3; treatment continued 1 yr after remission is achieved

Corticosteroids
Prednisone; may be added to above regimen if disease course is fulminant; 60 mg recommended as starting dose and should be continued until cyclophosphamide produces therapeutic effect (within 14 d); prednisone should then be tapered and eventually discontinued unless disease course accelerates

NURSING CARE

Nursing Assessment

Respiratory Status

Paranasal sinus pain; purulent or bloody rhinorrhea; nasal mucosa ulceration; septal perforation; saddle-nose deformity; serous otitis media; epistaxis; chronic cough; pleurisy; dyspnea; chest pain; sinusitis; hemoptysis

Ocular Integrity

Mild conjunctivitis; episcleritis; granulomatous sclerouveitis; ciliary vessel vasculitis; proptosis

Skin Integrity

Vasculitic dermatitis

Neurologic Status

Cranial neuritis; mononeuritis multiplex

Renal Status

Hematuria; abnormal urinalysis findings; progressive glomerulonephritis on biopsy

Nursing Dx & Intervention

Nursing Diagnosis	Nursing Intervention/Rationale
Decreased cardiac output related to pericarditis or myocarditis	• Monitor for signs and symptoms of pericarditis and myocarditis: edema, ascites, rales, angina, friction rub, pulsus paradoxus, electrocardiographic changes.
Impaired gas exchange related to sinusitis, chest pain, saddle-nose deformity, or granulomatous lung disease	• Assess degree of impairment: monitor blood gases, note presence of cyanosis or respiratory distress, auscultate lungs for presence of adventitious sounds, monitor chest roentgenograms, and note presence of hemoptysis, epistaxis, and sinus pain; report significant abnormal findings to physician. • Assess response to cyclophosphamide therapy. • In collaboration with physician, institute other interventions (such as oxygen therapy) for related conditions. Assess effectiveness.
Pain related to sinusitis, ocular inflammation, dermatitis, arthralgias, headache, pleurisy, or angina	• Assess pain: location, onset, duration, and precipitating or alleviating factors. Have patient describe intensity on a scale of 0 to 10. • Assess response to cyclophosphamide therapy. • In collaboration with physician, administer appropriate analgesic and anti-inflammatory agents. Assess effectiveness and note side effects.

Nursing Diagnosis	Nursing Intervention/Rationale
Altered renal tissue perfusion related to glomerulonephritis	• Assess renal status: blood urea nitrogen, serum creatinine, blood pressure, urinalysis results, presence of edema, and rapid weight gain *to detect and prevent renal compromise.* • Assess response to cyclophosphamide. • In collaboration with physician, institute appropriate interventions related to treatment of glomerulonephritis (diet, fluids, and so on). Assess effectiveness.
Altered cerebral and peripheral tissue perfusion related to cranial neuritis or mononeuritis multiplex	• Assess degree of neurologic impairment. • Monitor for cranial neuropathy: diplopia, ptosis, headache, and so on. • Monitor for peripheral neuropathy: changes in sensation and motor ability, paresthesias, and so on.
Sensory/perceptual alterations (visual) related to conjunctivitis, episcleritis, or proptosis	• Assess degree of visual impairment. • In collaboration with physician, administer appropriate analgesics and anti-inflammatory medications as ordered. Assess effectiveness. • Assess response to cyclophosphamide therapy. • Provide for patient safety *to protect from injury.*
Potential impaired skin integrity related to vasculitis dermatitis	• Assess skin integrity: texture, lesions, temperature, moisture, color, and vascularity. • Monitor lesions for signs of infection, dissemination, and other abnormal changes. • Provide or encourage patient to maintain meticulous hygiene in involved areas. • Monitor skin for evidence of impaired circulation or necrosis *caused by vasculitis.*
Anxiety	• See p. 1743.
Body image disturbance	• See p. 1751.

Patient Education

1. Teach the importance of and information about cyclophosphamide and steroid therapy.
2. Teach the importance of regular follow-up by a physician.
3. Teach the patient to report significant changes: visual impairment, hematuria, oliguria, pyuria, sinusitis, hemoptysis, dyspnea, and pain.
4. Teach the importance of semiannual eye examinations.
5. Teach the importance of medical alert identification.

Evaluation

Patient Outcome	Data Indicating That Outcome is Reached
Complications and medical crises are avoided.	There are no repeated sinus infections, progressive glomerulonephritis, visual loss, or respiratory insufficiency.
Laboratory findings are within normal limits or improved.	Erythrocyte sedimentation rate and urinalysis findings are within normal limits or improved. Tissue biopsy findings are normal or show decreased evidence of granulomatous and vasculitic changes.

Polyarteritis nodosa
(Periarteritis nodosa)

Polyarteritis nodosa, a multisystem inflammatory disorder of unknown cause, is characterized by necrotizing inflammation of segments of medium and small arteries.

Polyarteritis nodosa is a disease of adulthood and affects two to three men for every woman. The onset and clinical presentation of this disorder vary greatly depending on the location of the arteries affected and the severity of the involvement. Widespread lesions may involve arteries of the heart, abdominal mesentery, kidneys, muscles, and vasa vasorum. Involvement of the central nervous system and pulmonary tissue is unusual.

Although the cause remains an enigma, some evidence suggests that this type of vasculitis may result from immune complex deposition in tissues following exposure to an infectious antigen. The finding of hepatitis B surface antigen (Hb_sAg) in the sera of 30% to 40% of these patients further suggests that this may be true.[26,35]

The prognosis of polyarteritis nodosa is guarded. Renal involvement denotes rapid disease progression. Death often occurs from renal failure, myocardial infarction, heart failure, infection, or gastrointestinal bleeding.

Pathophysiology

The inciting agent that leads to inflammation within the blood vessels is unknown. The inflammatory process is characterized by early infiltration of polymorphonuclear leukocytes. New lesions are often surrounded by older lesions characterized by cells that respond late in the inflammatory reaction—monocytes, lymphocytes, and plasma cells. This suggests that the inflammatory process involved in polyarteritis is chronic, although subjected to repeated insults, perhaps by antigen that is continuously available.[35]

Chronic inflammation within the vessel walls leads to occlusion and necrosis with possible hemorrhage. Blood supply to major organs and other structures diminishes. Tissue ischemia and infarction are the notable outcomes.

Diagnostic Studies and Findings

No specific laboratory tests exist for polyarteritis nodosa. The abnormalities observed depend largely on the organ systems affected. Differential diagnoses include systemic lupus erythematosus, trichinosis, heart failure, and infection.

White Blood Count

Elevated owing to neutrophilia

Erythrocyte Sedimentation Rate

Elevated during acute phase

Angiography

Detects characteristic aneurysms at bifurcation points of arteries in kidneys, mesentery, liver, pancreas, and so on (acute), or narrowing and thrombosis of involved arteries (late)

Tissue Histologic Studies

Necrotizing inflammation of segments of medium and small arteries; aneurysms at areas of arterial bifurcation; invasion of tissue by polymorphonuclear leukocytes and monocytes

Medical Plan

Medications

Corticosteroids
- Prednisone, 40-60 mg to start; tapered gradually

Antineoplastic agents
- Used as immunosuppressants; use controversial and poorly documented but has been successful in some cases, particularly when corticosteroid therapy has failed

NURSING CARE

Nursing Assessment

Nonspecific Manifestations

Fever; weakness; anorexia

Cutaneous

Subcutaneous nodules (5 to 10 mm) along course of arteries in extremities; purpuric, urticarial exanthemata; subcutaneous hemorrhage; ulcerations; livedo reticularis; ischemic changes of distal digits

Muscles

Muscle weakness; myalgias

Joints

Migratory arthralgias

Peripheral Nervous System

Mononeuritis multiplex; paresthesias; hemiparesis

Kidneys

Glomerulitis; glomerulosclerosis; progressive renal failure; hypertension

Eyes

Retinopathy

Gastrointestinal Tract

"Surgical abdomen"; abdominal pain; anorexia; nausea and vomiting; mucosal ulceration and hemorrhage; appendicitis; cholecystitis; hepatitis

Brain

Headache; seizures; papillitis

Testes

Pain; edema

Heart

Coronary arteritis; myocardial ischemia or infarction; pericarditis; congestive heart failure

Nursing Dx & Intervention

Nursing Diagnosis	Nursing Intervention/Rationale
Altered cerebral tissue perfusion related to cerebral arteritis	• Assess for development of headache, changes in sensorium, seizures, and papilledema *to determine presence of cerebral edema, anoxia.* • Perform mental status examination *to assess level of consciousness and overall mentation.* • Perform ophthalmic examination of fundus and disc *to determine presence of cerebral edema.* • Provide for patient's safety *to prevent injury.* • In collaboration with physician, administer treatment for conditions detected during assessment. Assess effectiveness.
Altered renal tissue perfusion related to polyarteritis of kidneys	• Assess for development of glomerulonephritis, renal failure, and hypertension. Monitor blood urea nitrogen, creatinine, hemoglobin, hematocrit, blood pressure, urinalysis results, presence of edema and rapid weight gain, and symptoms associated with hypertension (headache and visual disturbances). Report significant findings to physician. • In collaboration with physician, institute appropriate treatment as ordered. Assess effectiveness.
Altered tissue perfusion (eye) related to retinal arteritis	• Assess for presence of retinopathy *to prevent visual loss.* • Monitor for visual disturbances: changes in acuity, scotomas, etc. • Perform ophthalmic examination *to determine presence of retinal exudates.* • Report significant findings to physician.
Altered tissue perfusion (muscles) related to vasculitis of vessels supplying musculature	• Assess muscle strength to determine weakness, atrophy, etc. • Protect from injury *resulting from muscle weakness.*
Altered gastrointestinal tissue perfusion related to mesenteric arteritis, intestinal mucosal arteritis, or vasculitis in liver, gallbladder, or appendix	• Assess for presence of abdominal pain, anorexia, nausea, vomiting, and findings compatible with gastrointestinal ulceration or hemorrhage, appendicitis, cholecystitis, or hepatitis. • Palpate abdomen *to detect areas of tenderness or pain.* • Perform Hemoccult or guiaic test of stool *to check for gastrointestinal blood loss.* • Report significant findings to physician. • In collaboration with physician, institute appropriate treatment as ordered. Assess effectiveness.
Altered cardiopulmonary tissue perfusion related to coronary arteritis, pericardial arteritis, or vasculitis of pleural sac	• Assess for myocardial ischemia, infarction, pericarditis, pleuritis: Monitor for presence of pleuritis, chest pain. Monitor serial electrocardiograms and chest roentgenograms. Auscultate chest for presence of pericardial friction rub. Monitor serial cardiac enzymes. Monitor vital signs. • Report significant findings to physician. • In collaboration with physician, institute appropriate treatment as ordered. Assess effectiveness.
Impaired physical mobility related to neuritis, paresthesia, paresis, myalgias, or muscle weakness	• Assess degree of physical limitations: perform neuromusculoskeletal assessment. • Provide progressive physical and occupational therapy. Encourage patient's participation. • Provide for patient's safety *to prevent injury.* • Assist with activities of daily living as needed.
Pain related to tissue and organ ischemia resulting from vasculitis	• Assess pain: location, onset, duration, and precipitating and alleviating factors. Have patient describe intensity on scale of 0 to 10. • In collaboration with physician, provide appropriate analgesic agents. Assess effectiveness and note side effects. • In collaboration with physician, institute appropriate other measures relative to the tissues and organs involved. Assess effectiveness.
Impaired skin integrity related to impaired perfusion of cutaneous tissue resulting from peripheral vasculitis	• Assess skin for presence of ecchymosis, purpura, ulcerations, gangrene, and vasculitic lesions. • Monitor lesions for signs of infection, dissemination, and other abnormal changes. • Provide meticulous skin care using mild, nondrying hypoallergenic soaps for cleansing. • In collaboration with physician, provide appropriate treatment for lesions as ordered. Assess effectiveness. • Protect skin from further injury: use paper or cloth tape; apply dressings loosely; avoid venipunctures. • Gently massage skin *to promote circulation to area.*

Nursing Diagnosis	Nursing Intervention/Rationale
Decreased cardiac output related to myocardial ischemia	• Assess for signs and symptoms associated with changes in cardiac output: hypotension, dyspnea, edema, jugular venous distention, rales, and pulse irregularities. • Monitor electrocardiogram for rate, rhythm, and ectopy. • Report significant irregularities to physician. • In collaboration with physician, administer appropriate medication as ordered. Assess effectiveness and note side effects. • Adjust patient's activity *to reduce oxygen demands and provide rest periods.* • Assess response to oxygen therapy and other interventions.
Sensory/perceptual alterations (visual) related to retinopathy resulting from retinal arteritis	• Assess degree of visual impairment. • Provide for patient's safety *to prevent injury.* • Perform regular ophthalmic examinations *to prevent vision loss.*
Anxiety	• See p. 1743
Body image disturbance; altered role performance	• See pp. 1751 and 1765.

Patient Education

1. Explain that many specialists will be involved in care, since this disease is multisystemic.
2. Teach the importance of regular physician follow-up.
3. Teach methods of self-assessment, and emphasize the importance of reporting significant changes to the physician.
4. Teach the method of self-assessment to detect early crises: monitoring blood pressure, pulse, weight, proteinuria, edema, intake, and output. Instruct the patient to report dyspnea, unexplained weight gain, proteinuria, oliguria, hematuria, hypertension, abnormal changes in the eyes, paresis, new pain, and melena.
5. Stress the importance of medications and provide information about them.
6. Emphasize the need for regular eye examinations.
7. Teach alternative methods for pain relief: relaxation techniques, biofeedback, guided imagery, and so on.
8. Teach the patient to keep a log of disease course, treatments, and other disease-related information.
9. Teach the patient to carry medical identification (especially if taking steroids).

Evaluation

Patient Outcome	Data Indicating That Outcome is Reached
Medical crises are prevented.	There is no deterioration of renal function: blood urea nitrogen and creatinine levels and urinalysis results stabilize or improve. Major organ involvement remits.
Signs and symptoms are managed.	Signs and symptoms related to involved organ system(s) diminish or disappear in response to therapeutic maneuvers.
Laboratory values return to within normal limits in response to steroid therapy.	C-reactive protein, erythrocyte sedimentation rate, C3, and C4 are within normal limits.

Giant cell arteritis
(Temporal arteritis)

Giant cell arteritis is an inflammatory disorder of unknown etiology that affects large and medium-sized arteries in the elderly.

Giant cell arteritis affects persons of both sexes older than 50 years of age. It is twice as common in women as men. This disease is rarely seen in blacks. Any artery or the aorta may be involved, but the diagnosis is often made through biopsy of the temporal artery. Patients initially show nonspecific systemic signs, including fever. Morning headaches are frequent. Other clinical findings are related to the arteries involved.

Although the etiology is unknown, the disease may have some basis in immunologic dysfunction similar to that of other vasculitides such as polyarteritis nodosa. Cellular and humoral mechanisms reactive against elastic arterial tissue may play a role.[35]

The prognosis for giant cell arteritis is good, particularly when major vessels are uninvolved. The disease tends to be self-limited in 2 to 5 years, but the threat of blindness makes treatment imperative. Patients respond dramatically to corticosteroid therapy with remission of clinical manifestations and lowering of the erythrocyte sedimentation rate, which can be serially monitored for recurrence of inflammatory episodes.

Pathophysiology

Giant cell arteritis is distinguishable from other vasculitides because small vessels such as arterioles and capillaries are not involved. Histologic characteristics include the accumulation of histiocytes, epitheloid cells, multinucleated giant cells, lymphocytes, and plasma cells in the interna and media adjacent to the internal elastic lamina of medium-sized arteries. The elastic lamina is fragmented and may be absent in some areas. In large arteries and the aorta the media tends to be inflamed, with fragmentation of the elastic fibers. The intima is thickened more than would be expected from age alone. The lesions are spotty and do not involve long stretches of arteries. Thrombosis may occur at inflammation sites.[35]

Diagnostic Studies and Findings

Giant cell arteritis should be suspected in any elderly person who has a fever of unknown origin and an elevated erythrocyte sedimentation rate. It is often associated with polymyalgia rheumatica.

Erythrocyte Sedimentation Rate

Greater than 50 mm/hour

Temporal Artery Biopsy

Positive; demonstrates inflammation of superficial temporal artery

Muscle Enzymes

Normal

Electromyography

Normal

Muscle Biopsy

Normal

Complete Blood Count

Anemia

Medical Plan

Medications

Corticosteroids

Prednisone, 60 mg po tapered for 4 wk until symptoms abate and erythrocyte sedimentation rate returns to normal; maintenance dose 10 mg or less po qd; alternate-day therapy not successful; can be discontinued eventually in most patients; monitor for side effects associated with steroid therapy

NURSING CARE

Nursing Assessment

Temporal Artery

Temporal pain; headache; marked scalp tenderness; intermittent claudication of jaw and tongue

Aorta

Aneurysm; dissection

Internal and External Carotid Arteries and Vertebral Arteries

Transient ischemic attacks

Ophthalmic Artery and Central Retinal Artery

Visual loss (insidious or sudden onset)

Coronary Arteries

Myocardial ischemia and infarction

Iliac and Femoral Arteries

Claudication of lower extremities

Mesenteric Arteries

Abdominal pain; gastrointestinal bleeding; bowel infarction or obstruction

Systemic Signs and Symptoms

Fever; malaise; anorexia

Nursing Dx & Intervention

Nursing Diagnosis	Nursing Intervention/Rationale
Altered cerebral tissue perfusion related to carotid arteritis	• Assess for development of headache, transient ischemic attacks, and other changes in sensorium. Perform mental status examination *to assess mentation*. • Maintain patient's safety *to prevent injury*. • In collaboration with physician, administer appropriate treatment for headache and other symptoms detected during assessment. Assess effectiveness. Assess patient reponse to steroid therapy.

Nursing Diagnosis	Nursing Intervention/Rationale
Altered tissue perfusion (temporal aspect of head) related to temporal arteritis	• Assess for presence of temporal pain, headache, scalp tenderness, and intermittent claudication of jaw and tongue. • Assess patient response to steroid therapy. • In collaboration with physician, administer appropriate analgesics as ordered. Assess effectiveness.
Altered tissue perfusion (eye) related to ophthalmic or central retinal arteritis	• Assess for presence of retinopathy, visual disturbances, and changes in acuity. • Report significant findings to physician.
Altered gastrointestinal tissue perfusion related to mesentery arteritis	• Assess for presence of abdominal pain, anorexia, nausea and vomiting, gastrointestinal ulceration, and hemorrhage. • Palpate abdomen *to detect areas of tenderness.* • Perform Hemoccult or guaiac test of stool *to check for gastrointestinal blood loss.* • Report significant findings to physician. • In collaboration with physician, institute appropriate treatment of above conditions as ordered. • Assess effectiveness.
Altered cardiopulmonary tissue perfusion related to coronary arteritis	• Assess for myocardial ischemia and infarction: monitoring for angina, monitoring of serial electrocardiograms, monitoring of chest roentgenograms, auscultation of heart to determine rate, rhythm, and regularity of pulse, monitoring of cardiac enzymes, monitoring of vital signs. • Report significant abnormal findings to physician. • In collaboration with physician, institute appropriate treatment (oxygen, vasodilators, etc.) as ordered. Assess effectiveness.
Altered peripheral tissue perfusion related to iliac and femoral arteritis	• Assess for claudication: presence of pain during ambulation. Report claudication to physician. • Assess response to steroid therapy.
Impaired physical mobility related to claudication	• Assess degree of impairment. • Encourage regular program of walking distances slowly and Buerger-Allen exercises.
Pain related to myocardial ischemia, temporal arteritis, or claudication	• Assess pain: location, onset, duration, and precipitating and alleviating factors. Have patient describe intensity on scale of 0 to 10. • In collaboration with physician, provide appropriate analgesic agents as ordered. Assess effectiveness and side effects. • Assess response to steroid therapy. • In collaboration with physician, institute appropriate other measures relative to tissues and organs involved. Assess effectiveness.
Sensory/perceptual alterations (visual) related to ophthalmic and retinal arteritis	• Assess degree of visual impairment. • Provide for patient safety *to prevent injury.* • Encourage patient to receive regular ophthalmic examinations *to prevent vision loss.*
Decreased cardiac output related to aortic aneurysm or aortic dissection	• Assess for findings associated with aortic aneurysm. • Assess for findings associated with aortic dissection. • Report significant abnormal findings to physician. • In collaboration with physician, institute appropriate interventions. Assess effectiveness.
Anxiety	• Counsel patient that this disorder is often self-limited and is highly responsive to chemotherapy (see p. 1393).

Patient Education

1. Emphasize the importance of steroid therapy and provide information about it (see p. 1393).
2. Teach the patient complications and crises for which to monitor: transient ischemic attacks, claudication, visual loss, gastrointestinal bleeding, and myocardial infarction.
3. Teach the importance of medical alert identification.

Evaluation

Patient Outcome	Data Indicating That Outcome is Reached
Complications and medical crises are avoided in response to steroid therapy.	There is no evidence of progressive pain, visual loss, aortic aneurysm or dissection, gastrointestinal bleeding, cerebral ischemia, or myocardial infarction.
Laboratory values return to normal in response to steroid therapy.	Erythrocyte sedimentation rate is within normal limits.

Polymyalgia rheumatica

Polymyalgia rheumatica is a well-defined inflammatory disorder of the proximal muscles that usually affects men and women older than 50 years of age.

Polymyalgia rheumatica is accompanied by a highly elevated erythrocyte sedimentation rate and is often diagnosed on the basis of a rapid clinical response to corticosteroid therapy. The onset may be acute or insidious and is associated with pain and morning stiffness in the back and neck, as well as in the pelvic and shoulder girdles. Anorexia, weight loss, fever, and mild anemia may be present as well. Temporal arteritis also develops in many patients.

Pathophysiology

The origin and pathogenesis of polymyalgia rheumatica are unknown. Although elevation of the erythrocyte sedimentation rate is indicative of an inflammatory process, and despite the severe pain associated with the muscle involvement, findings of muscle examinations are normal.

Diagnostic Studies and Findings

Erythrocyte Sedimentation Rate

Elevated (often greater than 100 mm/hour)

Corticosteroid Challenge

Rapid, dramatic response

Creatine Phosphokinase

Normal; to distinguish from polymyositis

Muscle Biopsy

Normal; to distinguish from polymyositis

Serum Protein Electrophoresis

Normal; to distinguish from myeloma

Rheumatoid Factor

Normal; along with absence of synovitis, to distinguish from arthritis

Medical Plan

The goal of the treatment plan is to induce a remission of the disease using low-dose corticosteroid therapy.

Medications

Corticosteroids

Prednisone, 10 mg/d, or equivalent low-dose corticosteroid; larger doses may be employed but are usually tapered rapidly; although some patients are able to discontinue drug after several months, most require prolonged maintenance therapy with small doses

NURSING CARE

Nursing Assessment

Musculoskeletal System

Pain in proximal muscles: shoulder girdle, back, neck and pelvis, unassociated with deformity or synovitis; elevated erythrocyte sedimentation rate; normal creatine phosphokinase level (above findings in combination in elderly patient are classic diagnostic features of polymyalgia rheumatica)

Nursing Dx & Intervention

Nursing Diagnosis	Nursing Intervention/Rationale
Pain related to proximal muscle involvement	• Assess pain: location, onset, duration, and provocative and palliative factors. Have patient rate intensity on scale of 0 to 10. • Assess response to corticosteroid therapy. • Supplement with aspirin or acetaminophen as prescribed. • Administer hot or cold thermal therapy to affected muscles. • Perform limited range of motion exercises as tolerated *to combat stiffness and prevent atrophy from immobilization.*
Activity intolerance related to proximal muscle weakness and pain	• Assess patient's limitations. • Employ interventions listed above *to limit pain.* • Encourage patient to explore alternative methods of performing activities of daily living. • Encourage balanced program of rest and exercise as tolerated.
Anxiety	• Counsel patients that this disorder responds well to steroid therapy; activity intolerance may be short lived.
Altered role performance	• See p. 1765.

Patient Education

1. Teach the importance and side effects of prednisone.
2. Explain that family members may find it difficult to accept the patient's illness, since patients often do not appear to be sick. Encourage honest, open communication between family members. Include the family when giving information about polymyalgia.
3. Teach that temporal (giant cell) arteritis may be a complication of the disease. Alert the patient to associated symptoms, including headache, scalp tenderness, and intermittent claudication of the jaw or tongue.
4. Teach the importance of medical alert identification.

Evaluation

Patient Outcome	Data Indicating That Outcome is Reached
Laboratory findings are within normal limits.	Erythrocyte sedimentation rate is within normal limits.
Pain is relieved or minimized.	Subjective distress is decreased. Objective decrease is based on rating scale.

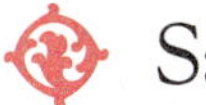

Sarcoidosis

Sarcoidosis is a multisystem granulomatous disorder of unknown cause.

In the United States approximately 34 cases of sarcoidosis per 100,000 persons are diagnosed each year. Cases are equally distributed between both sexes. Although all races and age groups may be affected, sarcoidosis occurs most commonly in adults, especially blacks younger than 40 years of age.

The prognosis of sarcoidosis varies depending on the degree of systemic involvement and the intensity of steroid therapy. Sarcoidosis may be staged according to international standards that are based on chest roentgenograms of patients with pulmonary involvement, the major clinical finding (Table 14-5). The disease is fatal in about 5% of patients. Current research focuses on determining the immunologic pathogenesis of the disease through detailed studies of immune function of cells derived from sarcoid tissue.

Pathophysiology

No single factor has been convincingly identified as the etiologic agent, although several have been proposed: viruses, organic dust, pine pollen, fungi, and beryllium, to name a few. Immune system abnormalities include lymphopenia with decreased T cell numbers, impaired lymphocyte function, anergy, and panhypergammaglobulinemia. Although the exact role of such mechanisms is unknown, these findings suggest a problem of the T cell population and perhaps, more

Table 14-5
Staging, Prognosis, and Treatment of Sarcoidosis

Stage	Chest Roentgenogram	Prognosis	Corticosteroid Therapy
1	Bilateral hilar adenopathy	Resolves in 60% of cases	None
2	Bilateral hilar adenopathy with parenchymal pulmonary infiltration	Resolves in 46% of cases	Yes, to decrease pulmonary fibrosis and relieve symptoms
3	Advanced parenchymal pulmonary infiltration with nodular densities	Resolves in 12% of cases	Same as stage 2

specifically, with lymphokine production. In other granulomatous diseases, such as tuberculosis, granuloma formation occurs as a result of inadequate clearance of a pathogen by macrophages. These macrophages require the help of T cells that secrete lymphokines that, in turn, activate poorly effective macrophages to become aggressive phagocytic cells. The lack of lymphokine secretion may help to explain the granuloma formation in sarcoidosis.

Diagnostic Studies and Findings

Differential diagnoses include tuberculosis, mediastinal lymphoma, and other granulomatous lung diseases.

Delayed-Type Hypersensitivity Skin Test

Absence of response (anergy)

Chest Roentgenogram

Varies from prominent hilar lymphadenopathy to diffuse pulmonary infiltrates with fibrosis

Serum Protein Electrophoresis

Polyclonal hypergammaglobulinemia: usually increased IgG, but IgA and IgM may also be elevated

Kviem Test

Intradermally injected sarcoid tissue suspension; positive in 60% to 80%

Tissue Biopsy

Noncaseating granulomas

C-Reactive Protein

Elevated in associated acute arthritis

Erythrocyte Sedimentation Rate

Elevated in associated acute arthritis

Medical Plan

Medications

Corticosteroids
Prednisone in doses adjusted to relieve symptoms and reverse fibrosis of pulmonary tissue

Optic agents
Methylcellulose eye drops and assorted ophthalmic ointments to treat ocular manifestations

Antiarrhythmic agents
For ventricular ectopy

Treatment of arthritis manifestations varies depending on their severity; salicylates used first, followed by nonsteroidal anti-inflammatory agents, and finally corticosteroids, including intra-articular injections

General Management

Chest physiotherapy, breathing exercises, postural drainage, and oxygen therapy as necessary for prophylaxis or as treatment for chronic pulmonary disease

Serial sinus and chest roentgenograms and pulmonary function studies as necessary to follow disease course and determine adequacy of treatment

Thermal therapy and joint supports for arthritis

NURSING CARE

Nursing Assessment

Constitutional Signs and Symptoms

Malaise; fever; weight loss; anorexia

Pulmonary Status

Parenchymal lesions (in asymptomatic patients or associated with dyspnea and nonproductive cough); pulmonary fibrosis; cough; superinfection; restrictive disease; decreased vital capacity

Skin and Mucous Membrane Integrity

Small skin nodules over face, neck, and extremities; vitiligo; alopecia; erythema nodosum

Ocular Integrity

Blurred vision; lacrimation; ocular pain; conjunctival infection; uveitis; Sjögren's syndrome; iritis

Salivary Gland Status

Nontender enlargement of parotid and other salivary glands

Reticuloendothelial System Status

Lymphadenopathy; bilateral hilar adenopathy; mediastinal or peripheral lymphadenopathy; splenomegaly with or without anemia, leukopenia, and thrombocytopenia

Cardiovascular Status

Arrhythmias: bundle-branch block or ventricular ectopy; cor pulmonale

Hepatic Manifestations

Chronic granulomatous hepatitis: jaundice, hepatomegaly, increased alkaline phosphatase

Musculoskeletal Status

Arthritis (symmetric, migratory); arthralgias (diffuse); muscle weakness, soreness, and wasting (symmetric)

Nursing Dx & Intervention

Nursing Diagnosis	Nursing Intervention/Rationale
Impaired gas exchange related to pulmonary fibrosis, infection, restrictive disease, or parenchymal lesions	• Assess respiratory status: note respiratory rate, rhythm, and quality, presence of hemoptysis, cough, adventitious breath sounds, or dyspnea *to prevent respiratory compromise.* • Monitor results of pulmonary function studies. • Obtain sputum specimens for culture *to determine presence of secondary pulmonary infection(s).* • Reinforce teaching related to proper positioning, body mechanics, and breathing exercises. • In collaboration with physician, administer appropriate respiratory medications and oxygen therapy for treatment of restrictive lung disease or infection. Assess effectiveness and note side effects.
Decreased cardiac output related to arrhythmias or cor pulmonale	• Assess for signs and symptoms associated with decreased cardiac output: hypotension, dyspnea, edema, jugular venous distention, rales, and pulse irregularities. • Monitor electrocardiograms for rate, rhythm, and ectopy. • Report significant electrocardiographic irregularities and other abnormal assessment data to physician. • In collaboration with physician, administer appropriate cardiac medications. Assess effectiveness and note side effects. • Adjust patient's activity *to reduce oxygen demands and provide rest periods.* • Assess response to oxygen therapy and other interventions.
Pain related to ocular discomfort, infection, arthralgias, erythema nodosum, or synovitis	• Assess pain: location, quality, onset, duration, and provocative and palliative factors. Have patient rate pain on scale of 0 to 10. • In collaboration with physician, institute appropriate interventions and administer analgesics based on underlying cause of pain. Assess effectiveness, and note side effects.
Sensory/perceptual alterations (visual) related to Sjögren's syndrome, lacrimation, conjunctivitis, iritis, or uveitis	• Assess degree of visual impairment. • Provide for patient safety *to prevent injury.* • Encourage patient to have regular ophthalmic examinations *to prevent vision impairment.* • In collaboration with physician, administer appropriate ocular medication as ordered. Assess effectiveness.
Altered tissue perfusion (liver) related to hepatitis granulomatous disease	• Assess for hepatic dysfunction: monitor serum glutamic oxaloacetic transaminase, serum glutamic pyruvic transaminase, lactic dehydrogenase, alkaline phosphatase, and total bilirubin. • Monitor for associated jaundice, lethargy, and weakness.
Potential for infection	• Assess for anorexia, failure to thrive, pain, weakness, and lethargy. • Assess for evidence of infection at sites of invasive procedures. • Assess for breaks in skin integrity, particularly over pressure areas and oral mucosa. • Assess pulmonary status: auscultate lung fields to determine presence of adventitious breath sounds *to monitor for respiratory compromise.* • Maintain optimum nutritional status and fluid intake *to prevent malnutrition and dehydration.* • Assess ocular integrity for evidence of conjunctivitis: erythematous, pruritic conjunctivae. • Assess mentation *for evidence of central nervous system infection:* level of consciousness, headache, and visual disturbances. • Assess for evidence of gastrointestinal infection: abdominal pain, fever, and diarrhea. • Monitor temperature and vital signs *for evidence of fever and sepsis.* • Maintain body hygiene. • Monitor laboratory data: white blood cell count and differential, erythrocyte sedimentation rate, C-reactive protein, urinalysis, and cultures *for signs of infection or inflammation.* • In collaboration with physician, administer appropriate antimicrobial, antipyretic, or analgesic medication. Assess patient response. Monitor for side effects. • Promote pulmonary toilet: breathing exercises, postural drainage, and chest physical therapy *to prevent pulmonary infection.*

Nursing Diagnosis	Nursing Intervention/Rationale
	• Protect patient from physical injury. • Provide clean environment. • Maintain protective isolation based on hospital policy. • Restrict contact with family and health care providers who have infectious diseases. • Wash hands before and after contact with patient.
Anxiety	• See p. 1743.
Body image disturbance	• See p. 1751.

Patient Education

1. Teach facts about, and the importance of, prescribed medications.
2. Provide information related to system involvement: assessment and reporting of signs and symptoms.
3. Teach the importance of chest physiotherapy, postural drainage, steroid therapy, and other methods of dealing with pulmonary compromise.
4. Teach signs and symptoms of infections.
5. Teach about the avoidance of risk factors associated with infection.
6. Teach the principles of good nutrition.
7. Teach the importance of medical alert identification.

Evaluation

Patient Outcome	Data Indicating That Outcome is Reached
Pulmonary involvement is reversed.	Chest roentgenogram shows clear or improved lung fields.
Other symptoms are resolved or prevented.	There are no symptoms associated with individual system involvement.
Laboratory findings are within normal limits.	There is positive response to cutaneous recall antigens (anergy is reversed). Serum protein electrophoresis findings return to normal. Kviem test findings are negative.
Medical complications and crises are prevented.	There is no respiratory failure, secondary infection, vision loss, or hepatic failure.

Reiter's syndrome

Reiter's syndrome is a relatively common, chronic, multisystem inflammatory disease characterized by the development of seronegative asymmetric arthropathy that may be associated with urethritis, cervicitis, dysentery, inflammatory eye disease, or mucocutaneous disease involving the penis, oral mucosa, or skin.

Reiter's syndrome has been a subject of worldwide research since the discovery of its link with HLA-B27 in 1973. This finding suggested a genetic predisposition. A search for the environmental factor or factors that act as inciting agents ensued. Although such an agent remains elusive, current data suggest that enteric infection may play a role. Microbes that have been implicated include *Shigella flexneri*, *Shigella dysenteriae*, and *Yersinia enterocolitica*.[26] Venereal infections with *Chlamydia* and *Mycoplasma* have also been associated with Reiter's syndrome.

Based on this evidence it is theorized that patients with a specific genetic background (HLA-B27) may develop Reiter's syndrome following infestation by a variety of microbes. Research continues with the goals of improving its recognition, defining etiologic factors, and ultimately, finding a cure.

The incidence of Reiter's syndrome is difficult to assess for a variety of reasons. Current research indicates that this disease occurs primarily in white males throughout the world. Although it may be detected at any age, it is usually diagnosed in the third decade. Reiter's syndrome may be the most common inflammatory arthropathy detected in young men. The pathogenesis of Reiter's syndrome is unknown.

Diagnostic Studies and Findings

Differential diagnoses include infective arthritis, rheumatic fever, and psoriatic arthropathy.

History

Recent history of dysentery or venereal disease combined with inflammatory monarthropathy or oligoarthropathy, urethritis, cervicitis, and ocular and cutaneous inflammatory changes

Roentgenograms of Musculoskeletal System

Erosive joint changes; juxta-articular osteoporosis; plantar spurs

Erythrocyte Sedimentation Rate

Variable from 1 to 130 mm/hour

HLA Typing

HLA-B27 (this test is costly and unnecessary and is usually performed only as an academic endeavor)

Medical Plan

The goals of the treatment plan include management of signs and symptoms and early detection of disabling complications. This disease has no cure, and current treatment is empiric and inadequate.

Medications

Nonsteroidal anti-inflammatory agents

To treat synovitis and arthralgias; any agent may be tried; one clinician reports success with indomethacin (Indocin), 25-50 mg tid, and phenylbutazone (Butazolidin), 100 mg tid or qid[26]

Corticosteroids

Methylprednisone (Medrol), 40-80 mg intralesionally for arthropathy, tendinitis, etc.

Steroid eye drops or subconjunctival ointments for conjunctivitis

Antineoplastic agents[26]

Azathioprine (Imuran), 0.75-2.5 mg/kg body weight qd for immunosuppression until symptomatic improvement, usually 2-12 wk, then tapered dosage

Methotrexate may be used in cases of severe illness but is not warranted in majority of patients

Anti-infective agents

Use is controversial and varies depending on existing infection

Analgesics and nonsteroidal anti-inflammatory agents

To reduce pain associated with arthritis and ocular inflammation

Optic agents

Methylcellulose eye drops for symptomatic relief of ocular discomfort

General Management

Physical therapy for arthritis complications

Rest to conserve energy during acute exacerbations

Counseling to allay feelings of guilt or anxiety about sexual misconduct

Use of condom to protect patient from postvenereal exacerbation[26]

Discouragement of use of topical steroidal medications for skin involvement, since atrophy may occur

Meticulous skin care of involved areas

Periodic assessment for symptoms associated with uveitis, spondylitis, and cardiac or pulmonary involvement

NURSING CARE

Nursing Assessment

Musculoskeletal Involvement

Arthritis, particularly of weight-bearing joints; tendonitis, especially of Achilles tendon; plantar fasciitis; back pain such as sacroiliitis and ankylosing spondylitis; costochondritis, often manifested as pleuritic chest pain; dactylitis

Genitourinary Involvement

Urethritis; cervicitis; cystitis; balanitis

Gastrointestinal Involvement

Stomatitis; diarrhea: acute passage of bloody, loose stools during 24-hour period, precedes rheumatic syndrome by 1 to 3 weeks

Ocular Involvement

Conjunctivitis; uveitis; optic neuritis; intraocular hemorrhage; blindness (late)

Skin Integrity

Keratoderma blennorrhagica (hyperkeratotic nodules); balanitis: painless, superficial lesions of coronal margins of prepuce and adjacent glands; nails: subungual corny material that accumulates under and may lift nail plate, which becomes yellow and thickened

Cardiovascular Status

Electrocardiogram: increased PR interval, heart block, ST segment changes, abnormal Q waves; palpitations; transient murmurs; pericardial rub; aortic regurgitation

Nursing Dx & Intervention

Nursing Diagnosis	Nursing Intervention/Rationale
Impaired physical mobility related to arthritis	• Assess degree of physical immobility resulting from arthritis. • In collaboration with physician, provide nonsteroidal anti-inflammatory agents. Assess effectiveness.

Nursing Diagnosis	Nursing Intervention/Rationale
	• Encourage patient to rest joints during periods of acute inflammation. Otherwise, encourage program of regular exercise, including range of motion exercises, as tolerated. Confer with physical or occupational therapist *to determine other beneficial interventions.*
Pain related to inflammatory conditions of eye, genitourinary tract, joints, and gastrointestinal tract	• Determine location of pain. • Assess degree of discomfort using subjective data and objective measurement on 0 to 10 rating scale. • In collaboration with physician, provide analgesic agents as ordered. Assess effectiveness and note side effects. • In collaboration with physician, institute other appropriate measures relative to system involved. Assess effectiveness.
Sensory/perceptual alterations (visual) related to conjunctivitis and uveitis	• Assess degree of visual impairment. • Provide for patient's safety *to prevent injury.* • Provide methylcellulose 1% eye drops as needed *to maintain moisture at conjunctival surface.* • Encourage patient to seek evaluation of eye pain which may be caused by corneal abrasion to conjunctivitis. • In collaboration with physician, provide steroidal eye drops and anti-infective agents as ordered. Assess effectiveness.
Impaired skin integrity related to multiple skin lesions	• Assess skin for presence of lesions and hyperkeratotic nodules. • Monitor lesions for signs of infection, dissemination, and other abnormal changes. • Provide or encourage patient to perform meticulous foot care with special attention to nail integrity. • Provide mild, nondrying, hypoallergenic soaps for skin cleaning and encourage their use. • Assess effectiveness of treatment of lesions.
Diarrhea related to gastrointestinal infection	• Assess severity of diarrhea: monitor for passage of bloody stools and quantify output. • Assess for signs and symptoms associated with electrolyte imbalance *caused by malabsorption.* • Provide fluids and encourage adequate fluid intake *to maintain hydration.* • Provide for patient's safety if weakness becomes a problem. • In collaboration with physician, administer appropriate anti-infective agents. Assess effectiveness and note side effects.
Altered patterns of urinary elimination related to urethritis or cystitis	• Assess for signs and symptoms associated with urethritis or cystitis: dysuria, pyuria, hematuria, and fever. • In collaboration with physician, administer appropriate anti-infective agents. Assess effectiveness and note side effects.
Decreased cardiac output related to cardiovascular manifestation of Reiter's syndrome	• Assess patient for presence of palpitations, murmurs, and pericardial rub. • Assess electrocardiogram for prolonged PR interval, heart block, ST segment changes, and abnormal Q waves. • In collaboration with physician, institute appropriate measures based on assessment. Assess effectiveness of specific interventions.
Anxiety	• See p. 1743.
Body image disturbance	• See p. 1751.

Patient Education

1. Teach the importance of reporting symptoms associated with significant complications of Reiter's syndrome: spondylitis, uveitis, ocular hemorrhage, and cardiopulmonary disease.
2. Teach that the use of a condom during sexual activity will limit exposure to venereal disease, which could exacerbate Reiter's syndrome.
3. Teach the importance of physician follow-up to monitor the disease course. The physician should also be consulted for management of acute episodes.
4. Teach facts about and the importance of prescribed medications.
5. Teach the importance of keeping a log of the disease course, treatments, and other disease-related information.
6. Teach the importance of medical alert identification.

Evaluation

Patient Outcome	Data Indicating That Outcome is Reached
Symptoms resolve in response to therapeutic measures.	There are no symptoms associated with individual system involvement.
Pain is relieved or minimized.	There is decrease in subjective distress. Objective decrease is based on rating scale.
Medical crises are prevented.	There are no life-threatening side effects of chemotherapeutic interventions. Blindness, crippling spondylitis, and cardiopulmonary compromise do not occur.
Patient complies with treatment.	Patient verbalizes understanding of importance of compliance, adherence to prescribed regimens, and symptom control.

Sjögren's syndrome

Sjögren's syndrome is a chronic inflammatory disorder of unknown etiology that affects primarily the lacrimal and salivary glands.

The major symptoms of Sjögren's syndrome are keratoconjunctivitis and xerostomia, which result from decreased lacrimal and salivary gland secretion, respectively. The syndrome is often associated with other connective tissue diseases, especially rheumatoid arthritis, systemic lupus erythematosus, and progressive systemic sclerosis (scleroderma). Raynaud's phenomenon is manifested by 20% of patients with Sjögren's syndrome. Middle-aged women with a mean age of 50 years constitute 90% of Sjögren's syndrome patients. All races may be affected. There is evidence that sex hormones play an etiologic role in the disease, and research in this area continues.

Pathophysiology

Biopsy specimens from glandular lesions demonstrate infiltration by lymphocytes, plasma cells, and macrophages, which replace secretory acinar tissue. Anti–salivary duct antibodies have been observed. The factors precipitating such autodestruction of host tissue are unknown. Destruction of tissue results in decreased secretion by involved glands. In addition, dryness of the nose, pharynx, and tracheobronchial tree may occur.

Diagnostic Studies and Findings

Differential diagnoses include Felty's syndrome, Raynaud's phenomenon, chronic thyroiditis, hepatomegaly, chronic active hepatitis, gastric achlorhydria, acute pancreatitis, adult celiac disease, polymyositis, drug-induced xerostomia, irradiation xerostomia, diabetes, sarcoidosis, salivary duct stones, and mumps.

Salivary Scintigraphy

Decreased uptake, concentration, and excretion of intravenous ^{99m}Tc pertechnetate by major salivary glands; measured by means of sequential scintophotographic technique

Sialography

Dilations and other changes such as atrophy within intrasalivary duct system[26]

Labial Salivary Gland Biopsy

Infiltration of tissue by lymphocytes, plasma cells, and macrophages; replacement of acinar tissue

Schirmer Test

Decreased tear production; less than 15 mm of filter strip wetted

Complete Blood Count

Mild anemia; leukopenia

Erythrocyte Sedimentation Rate

Elevated

Serum Protein Electrophoresis

Hypergammaglobulinemia

Rheumatoid Factor

Elevated (90%)

Antinuclear Antibody

Greater than 1:80 (70%) anti–salivary duct antibodies, thyroid antibodies, gastric-parietal cell autoantibodies

Medical Plan

The goals of the treatment plan are to provide palliative measures and prevent complications of this chronic disorder.

Medications

Corticosteroids
- Prednisone; dose titrated for relief of *severe* symptoms; usually administered only late in course of disease when symptoms are unrelieved by supportive approaches

Antineoplastic agents
- Cyclophosphamide; success varies and use is controversial[26]

Optic agents
Artificial tears (0.5% methylcellulose eye drops) as needed

General Management

Avoidance of sour or sweetened drinks or candies
Mouth rinses of 1% methylcellulose
Oral hygiene with frequent brushing, flossing, and fluoride rinses
Regular dental examinations
Regular conjunctival cultures to detect ocular infections

NURSING CARE

Nursing Assessment

Oral Cavity

Xerostomia: dental caries (multiple), oral candidiasis, dysphagia, difficulty chewing, changes in phonation, adherence of food to buccal mucosa, hoarseness, fissures and ulcerations of tongue, buccal mucosa, and lips, frequent ingestion of liquids with meals

Eyes

Conjunctivitis: foreign body sensation, "grittiness," burning, accumulation of thick, ropy strands at inner canthus, decreased tearing, redness, photosensitivity, eye fatigue; pruritus; filmy sensation that interferes with vision; (late) corneal ulceration, vascularization, and opacification

Skin

Dryness

Ears

Recurrent otitis media

Respiratory Tract

Nasal mucosal dryness; epistaxis; bronchitis; pneumonia

Parotid Gland

Episodic, unilateral parotitis (often associated with fever, tenderness, and erythema)

In addition to the above, a relatively small percentage of patients with Sjögren's syndrome show symptoms associated with pancreatitis, hepatomegaly, renal tubular defects, thyroiditis, glomerulonephritis, myositis, and lymphoreticular malignancies.[26]

Nursing Dx & Intervention

Nursing Diagnosis	Nursing Intervention/Rationale
Sensory/perceptual alterations (visual) related to keratoconjunctivitis	• Assess degree of visual deficit. • Administer 0.5% methylcellulose eye drops as needed *to maintain moisture at conjunctival surface*. • Obtain regular cultures of eye *to determine presence of infection*. • In collaboration with physician, administer antimicrobial ointments for ocular infections as needed. • Administer hot or cold therapy to eyes as needed for *pain control*. • Encourage use of sunglasses as needed *to prevent photophobia*. • Encourage patient to have semiannual ophthalmic examinations.
Altered oral mucous membrane related to xerostomia	• Assess oral skin integrity for presence of ulcerations, fissures, and candidiasis. • Provide or encourage patient to perform frequent oral hygiene: brushing, flossing, and fluoride rinses. • Force fluids as tolerated; avoid sour or sweetened liquids. • Encourage semiannual dental examinations.
Pain related to parotitis, conjunctivitis, and otitis	• Assess pain: location, onset, duration, and provocative and palliative factors. Have patient rate intensity on scale of 0 to 10. • In collaboration with physician, administer appropriate analgesics as ordered. • Assess effectiveness, and note side effects.
Impaired gas exchange related to nasal mucosal dryness, bronchitis, and pneumonia	• Assess degree of respiratory impairment: monitor rate, rhythm, and quality of respirations, and monitor for epistaxis, hemoptysis, dyspnea, and cough. • Obtain sputum specimens for culture *to determine presence of pneumonia*. • In collaboration with physician, administer appropriate anti-infective therapy and other respiratory-related medications for treatment of bronchitis or pneumonia; assess effectiveness and note side effects. • Administer saline soaks *for nasal dryness*.
Potential impaired skin integrity related to skin dryness	• Assess skin integrity: color, moisture, lesions, vascularity, etc. • Provide and encourage use of lotions, creams, or ointments *for skin dryness*. • Provide and encourage use of lubricants such as K-Y Jelly *for vaginal dryness*.

Patient Education

1. Teach the use of artificial tears.
2. Teach the importance of obtaining regular eye examinations.
3. Teach the importance of meticulous oral hygiene: frequent brushing of teeth and use of dental floss and mouth rinses.
4. Teach the importance of increasing fluid intake to control xerostomia.
5. Teach the patient to avoid sour or sweetened drinks and candies.
6. Teach the importance of regular dental examinations to detect dental caries and obtain fluoride treatments.
7. Teach self-assessment of the oral cavity for development of lesions, fissures, and ulcerations.
8. Teach the importance and side effects of medications.
9. Teach the importance of regular follow-up to detect presence of underlying autoimmune or neoplastic disease.
10. Teach that the use of unnecessary antibiotics should be avoided (owing to increased incidence of drug allergy, especially to penicillin).
11. Teach that regular application of saline soaks for nasal dryness may be beneficial. Oil-based lubricants should be avoided to limit the risk of lipoid pneumonia.
12. Teach that skin dryness often responds to a variety of lotions, creams, and emollients. Vaginal dryness leading to dyspareunia usually responds to lubricants such as K-Y Jelly.

Evaluation

Patient Outcome	Data Indicating That Outcome is Reached
Pain is relieved or minimized.	Patient reports subjective decrease. Objective decrease is based on rating scale. Patient has fewer subjective complaints of oral and ocular dryness.
Medical complications and crises are avoided.	There is no evidence of corneal abrasions, oral ulcerations, recurrent otitis, or respiratory infections.

Amyloidosis

Amyloidosis is a syndrome characterized by deposition of amyloid (proteinaceous material) in tissues.

Amyloidosis occurs as an acquired or hereditary disorder and may be a primary disease or be associated with a variety of other illnesses. Although its etiology is unknown, at least two observations suggest that amyloidosis represents immunologic dysfunction: the presence of immunoglobulin proteins in amyloid deposits and the syndrome's increased incidence in inflammatory, infectious, and neoplastic diseases.

The term "amyloid," which means starchlike, is a misnomer. The syndrome is actually characterized by the diffuse deposition of insoluble proteinaceous material in the extracellular matrix of one or more organs. The accumulation of amyloid encroaches on parenchymal tissues and compromises organ function. Clinical manifestations of amyloidosis vary widely and depend on the organs involved and the severity with which they are affected. Specific immunotherapy to treat the underlying cause of organ failure is lacking, so treatment is restricted to management of signs and symptoms. For this reason amyloidosis is usually fatal. Renal failure and cardiac diseases are the most frequent causes of death.[26,37]

Types of Amyloidosis[26]

Primary generalized amyloidosis (PGA) occurs in the absence of associated diseases, although most patients exhibit some type of plasma cell dyscrasia. PGA accounts for 50% to 60% of all cases of amyloidosis. Deposits of amyloid are found in mesenchymal tissues of the heart, tongue, carpal tunnel, gastrointestinal tract, peripheral nerves, skin, joints, and skeletal muscle. Although this type of amyloidosis may occur as early as the second decade, the mean age at diagnosis is approximately 60 years. Men are affected more often than women, and whites more than nonwhites. Virtually all patients with classic PGA demonstrate a monoclonal immunoglobulin in their serum or urine and bone marrow plasmacytosis.

Multiple myeloma-associated amyloidosis (MMA) accounts for approximately 30% of cases. In roughly 15% of myeloma patients, clinical findings are consistent with a diagnosis of amyloidosis.[21] Serum and urine paraproteins are found. The clinical symptoms, age at diagnosis, and sexual predilection are similar to PGA. Amyloidosis contributes to early morbidity in myeloma disease.

Secondary generalized amyloidosis (SGA), detected in 10% of the patients, occurs as a result of a variety of long-term or poorly controlled inflammatory, infectious, or neoplastic diseases. Adult and juvenile rheumatoid arthritis may be the most frequent predisposing factor. SGA is also reported in other inflammatory conditions, including ankylosing spondylitis, Reiter's syndrome, psoriatic arthritis, chronic rheumatic heart disease, dermatomyositis, scleroderma, Behçet's disease, and systemic lupus erythematosus.

Neoplastic diseases associated with the development of amyloidosis include gastrointestinal, pulmonary, and genitourinary carcinomas, non-Hodgkin's lymphomas, malignant melanomas, and most frequently, hypernephroma and Hodgkin's disease. Chronic, systemic infections are a significant factor associated with worldwide distribution. Such infectious diatheses include tuberculosis, pyelonephritis, osteomyelitis, inflammatory bowel disease, and chronically infected burns.

In addition to the above types, amyloidosis is also described as a hereditary illness detected with increased frequency in various countries and some well-defined areas of the United States. Neuropathic, nephropathic, and cardiopathic syndromes have been described.

Pathophysiology

Only limited insight has been gained into the pathogenesis of this syndrome. Histologic staining techniques and electron microscopy have provided some clues. Fibers formed from laterally aggregated protein fibrils have been detected in amyloid deposits. Some of these fibrils are apparently derived from free immunoglobulin light chains. In addition, amyloid deposits are further constructed of globular glycoprotein subunits (pentagonal, or "P" components) absorbed from the serum into the fibrillar units.

An explanation for the deposition of the proteinaceous substance has not yet been found. Whatever the reason, accumulation of amyloid in extracellular spaces results in pressure atrophy and eventual necrosis and destruction of underlying tissue. Organ dysfunction and failure are responsible for clinical manifestations. Amyloid deposition occurs in the following areas:

- Articular
  - Glenohumeral junction
  - Synovial villi
- Neurologic
  - Dural blood vessels
  - Autonomic ganglia
  - Spinal nerve roots
  - Peripheral nerves
- Renal
  - Glomeruli
  - Arteriolar walls
  - Tubular basement membranes
- Cardiac
  - All layers of the cardiac walls (predominantly myocardium)
  - Conduction tissue
  - Intramural coronary arterioles
- Pulmonary (any area)
  - Upper nasal passages
  - Vocal cords
  - Tracheobronchial submucosa
  - Parenchyma
- Gastrointestinal (any area)
  - Gingiva
  - Tongue
  - Oropharyngeal muscles
  - Liver
  - Voluntary muscles of upper third of esophagus
  - Diffuse esophageal infiltrates
  - Small bowel
- Integumentary
  - Face
  - Upper trunk

Diagnostic Studies and Findings

Tissue Biopsy

Apple-green birefringence of Congo red–stained tissue specimens under polarization microscopy; tissue from organ suspected to be infiltrated with amyloid preferred, but rectal biopsy findings positive in approximately 80% of cases of generalized amyloidosis[26]

Serum and Urine Electrophoresis

Paraproteins detected in presence of associated plasma cell dyscrasia

Bone Marrow Aspiration and Biopsy

Plasmacytosis in presence of associated multiple myeloma

Medical Plan

The goals of therapy in amyloidosis are to prevent further deposition of amyloid material and to promote or accelerate its resorption.

Surgery

Serial biopsies to determine regression of amyloid deposition

Medications

Antineoplastic agents
- May be used to reduce the serum concentration of amyloid precursor light chains if underlying B cell dyscrasia is present

Colchicine, dimethyl sulfoxide (DMSO), and corticosteroids have met with some success, although their use remains controversial; corticosteroids are used primarily to treat underlying inflammatory or neoplastic disorder

General Management

Plasmapheresis may interrupt dissemination of amyloid precursor light chains (see p. 1397)

Family and patient counseling to assist in coping with fatal illness

Supportive approaches for complications

For congestive heart failure: conservative management; avoid use of digitalis unless closely monitored in hospital setting (usually cardiac amyloid is unresponsive to treatment with digitalis)

For neuropathic hypotension: elastic stockings

For malabsorption syndromes: broad-spectrum antibiotics

For macroglossia: supplemental Keo-Feed gastrostomy feeding; tracheostomy for upper airway obstruction

For respiratory tract amyloidosis: bronchoscopy with curettage of amyloid deposits

For renal failure: dialysis

NURSING CARE

Nursing Assessment

Neurologic Status

Idiopathic, sensorimotor, peripheral neuropathy with autonomic neuropathy; depressed pain and temperature sensation, and motor dysfunction of lower extremities

Cardiovascular Status

Restrictive cardiomyopathy with low-voltage electrocardiogram; chest pain; myocardial infarction; conduction disturbances in absence of other recognized causes

Skin Integrity

Waxy, indurated papules and purpura; skin thickening; "orange-peel" skin; alopecia; periorbital purpura

Joint Integrity

Rheumatoid-like arthritis

Renal Status

Proteinuria; idiopathic nephrotic syndrome

Pulmonary Status

Nasal lesions; vocal cord nodules; bronchiectasis; airway obstruction; wheezing; dyspnea; hilar adenopathy

Gastrointestinal Status

Macroglossia: dysphagia, deglutination, and dysphonia; impaired esophageal peristalsis: gastric accumulation, motility disturbances, hemorrhage, obstruction achlorhydria, and vitamin B_{12} deficiency; small bowel impairment: diarrhea, constipation, malabsorption, hemorrhage, protein-losing enteropathy, perforation, and ischemic necrosis; hepatomegaly without portal insufficiency or hypertension

Nursing Dx & Intervention

Nursing Diagnosis	Nursing Intervention/Rationale
Impaired gas exchange related to amyloid deposition in pulmonary tissue	• Assess degree of respiratory distress: note rate, rhythm, and quality of respirations, auscultate lung fields for presence of adventitious breath sounds, and note use of accessory muscles. • Maintain open airway at all times. • In collaboration with physician, institute appropriate interventions, relative to type and severity of pulmonary compromise. Assess effectiveness.
Decreased cardiac output related to amyloid deposition in cardiac structures and subsequent myopathy and ischemia	• Assess for signs and symptoms associated with decreased cardiac output: hypotension, dyspnea, edema, jugular venous distention, rales, and pulse irregularities. • Monitor electrocardiogram for rate, rhythm, and ectopy. Note in particular presence of ischemia, infarction, and conduction abnormalities. • Report significant electrocardiographic changes and other abnormal assessment data to physician. • In collaboration with physician, institute appropriate interventions (such as oxygenation) relative to type and severity of cardiac compromise. Assess effectiveness and note side effects of medications. • Adjust patient's activity and provide rest periods *to reduce oxygen demands*.
Altered renal tissue perfusion related to amyloid deposition in kidneys	• Assess for renal insufficiency: monitor blood urea nitrogen and creatinine, 24-hour urine for creatinine clearance, blood pressure, urinalysis result, presence of edema and rapid weight gain, and intake and output. • Report significant abnormal findings to physician. • Institute dialysis in event of renal failure.
Altered nutrition: less than body requirements related to amyloid deposition in gastrointestinal tract	• Assess degree of malnutrition: note presence of hypoalbuminemia, hypoproteinemia, negative nitrogen balance, protein and calorie deficit, and weight loss. • Assist physician in determining underlying cause of malnutrition, such as malabsorption, dysphagia, and impaired esophageal peristalsis. • Provide and encourage patient to maintain nutritionally balanced diet. Determine need for parenteral nutrition *to maintain nutritional balance*.

Nursing Diagnosis	Nursing Intervention/Rationale
	• Weigh patient weekly *to detect weight loss.* • In collaboration with physician, institute appropriate interventions relative to underlying causes of malnutrition. Assess effectiveness.
Pain related to arthritis, cardiac ischemia, or gastrointestinal distress	• Assess pain: location, onset, duration, and provocative and alleviating factors. Have patient describe intensity on scale of 0 to 10. • In collaboration with physician, administer appropriate analgesics. Assess effectiveness and note side effects. • In collaboration with physician, institute other appropriate interventions relative to tissues and organs involved. Assess effectiveness.
Sensory/perceptual alterations (tactile) related to peripheral neuropathy	• Assess degree of sensory impairment: perform sensory neurologic examination. • Provide for patient's safety *to prevent injury.* • Discuss loss or alteration with patient and provide appropriate reassurance. • In collaboration with physician, institute appropriate interventions relative to severity of neurologic impairment. Assess effectiveness.
Impaired physical mobility related to peripheral and autonomic neuropathy	• Assess degree of motor impairment: perform motor neurologic examination. • Provide for patient's safety *to prevent injury.* • In collaboration with physician, institute appropriate interventions relative to severity of neurologic impairment. Assess effectiveness.
Potential impaired skin integrity related to amyloid deposition in dermis	• Assess skin integrity: color, temperature, moisture, and presence of lesions. • Protect skin from injury or infection.
Family coping: potential for growth related to poor prognosis	• Assess family's anxiety related to limited understanding of diagnostic procedures, disease process, prognosis, and therapy. • Provide information in areas needed. • Explain relationship of disease process and rationale for various therapies at level appropriate for comprehension and degree of anxiety. • Involve family in care as appropriate. • Encourage family to verbalize questions and anxieties.
Anxiety	• See p. 1743.
Body image disturbance	• See p. 1751.

Patient Education

1. Teach facts about and the importance of managing signs and symptoms and frequent physician follow-up.
2. Teach care and methods of self-assessment relative to the systems involved.
3. Refer the patient and family for counseling to assist in coping with this potentially fatal illness.
4. Teach the importance of medical alert identification.

Evaluation

Patient Outcome	Data Indicating That Outcome is Reached
Pain is relieved or minimized.	There is decrease in subjective distress. Objective decrease is based on rating scale.
Laboratory findings improve.	Paraprotein level detected in serum and urine electrophoresis is decreased.
Medical crises are avoided.	There is no evidence of renal failure, myocardial infarction, paralysis, airway obstruction, or gastrointestinal obstruction.

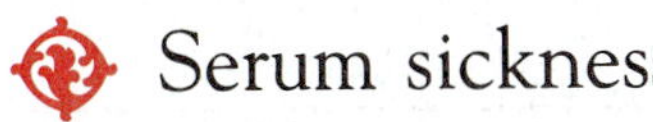

Serum sickness

Serum sickness is a relatively uncommon, acute reaction that was originally noted in persons who had received antisera made from animal sources.

Today serum sickness occurs most commonly after the administration of a variety of drugs, particularly penicillin. However, it may also occur after injection of heterologous antiserum used in the treatment of rabies, venomous snake bites, gas gangrene, botulism, and tetanus.

Serum sickness is characterized by the abrupt onset of a skin rash or urticaria, fever, arthralgias, edema (particularly of the face), and hepatosplenomegaly 7 to 15 days after an inoculation. Its course is self-limited, lasting 1 to 3 weeks. Although complications are rare, vasculitis, glomerulonephritis, and neuropathies may occur secondarily. Serum sickness can develop in anyone. Its severity increases with age. The following agents are known to cause serum sickness[21]:

- Animal serums
- Barbiturates
- Griseofulvin
- Hydralazine
- Insulin
- Iodides
- Mercurial diuretics
- Nitrofurantoin
- Oxyphenbutazone
- Para-aminosalicylic acid
- Penicillins
- Phenylbutazone
- Probenecid
- Procainamide
- Quinidine
- Quinine
- Salicylates
- Streptomycin
- Sulfonamides

Pathophysiology

The basic mechanism responsible for the development of serum sickness is antibody reaction against foreign protein with subsequent immune complex formation. The antigen-antibody complexes are deposited in the endothelium and basement membranes of vessel walls, and the subsequent inflammatory response results in vascular injury, thrombosis, and hemorrhage. Such widespread inflammation accounts for the clinical findings associated with this disease.

Diagnostic Studies and Findings

History

Exposure to inciting agent

White Blood Cell Count

Mild leukocytosis

Erythrocyte Sedimentation Rate

Mildly elevated or within normal limits

Complement (C3 and C4)

Decreased during acute phase

Medical Plan

The goals of treatment include symptomatic relief and prevention of medical crises.

Medications

Before pharmacologic intervention, serum or drug that allegedly caused reaction should be discontinued

Antihistamines
- Contraindicated in acute asthmatic attacks; caution patient to avoid alcohol ingestion, driving, and other hazardous activities; coffee or tea may reduce drowsiness; gum, sour hard candy, or ice chips may relieve dry mouth
- Brompheniramine maleate (Dimetane, Spentane, Veltane), 4-8 mg po tid or qid
- Tripelennamine (Pyribenzamine, Ro-Hist), 25-50 mg po q4-6h
- Diphenhydramine (Benadryl), 25-50 mg po tid or qid; 10-50 mg/d IM or IV to 400 mg maximum

Antipruritic agents
- Cyproheptadine (Periactin), 4-8 mg po q6h
- Chlorpheniramine (Chlor-Trimeton), 2 mg/kg/24 h po in 4 divided doses
- Clemastine (Tavist), 1.34 or 2.68 mg po q8-12h
- Diphenhydramine (Benadryl), 25-100 mg po q6h or 5 mg/kg/d
- Doxepin (Sinequan), 10-30 mg po q8-12h

Corticosteroids
- Prednisone, 10-40 mg/d for 4-5 d; response often remarkable within 24 h

Nonsteroidal anti-inflammatory agents
- May be used to treat accompanying myalgias, arthralgias, or synovitis

NURSING CARE

Nursing Assessment

Skin Integrity

Urticarial rash (often the first sign and starts at site of injection); petechial pruritic rash; erythematous pruritic rash; angioedema of face, lips, glottis, and eyelids; lymphadenopathy (begins in area of injection)

Musculoskeletal Integrity

Arthralgias; synovitis; stiffness; myalgias

Constitutional Signs and Symptoms

Fever; malaise; headache; abdominal pain; nausea and vomiting

Nursing Dx & Intervention

Nursing Diagnosis	Nursing Intervention/Rationale
Impaired skin integrity related to urticaria, pruritic rash, or angioedema	• Assess skin integrity: lesions, texture, temperature, moisture, color, and vascularity. • Monitor lesions for signs of infection, dissemination, and other abnormal changes. • Provide and encourage meticulous hygiene to involved area *to prevent infection.* • Provide and encourage use of mild, nondrying, hypoallergenic soaps for skin cleaning. • Apply antipruritic medication as needed. • In collaboration with physician, administer appropriate antihistamines. Assess effectiveness and note side effects.
Pain related to arthritis and myalgias	• Assess pain: location, onset, duration, and precipitating and alleviating factors. Have patient describe intensity on scale of 0 to 10. • In collaboration with physician, provide appropriate anti-inflammatory and analgesic agents. Assess effectiveness and note side effects. • Administer thermal therapy to affected muscles and joints as needed.

Patient Education

1. Teach side effects of medication.
2. Teach the patient to avoid subsequent exposure to the inciting agent.
3. Teach the patient to request skin desensitization before administration of drugs listed on p. 1353.
4. Teach the importance of medical alert identification.

Evaluation

Patient Outcome	Data Indicating That Outcome is Reached
Laboratory findings are within normal limits.	Erythrocyte sedimentation rate is within normal limits.
Medical crises are prevented.	There is no vasculitis, neuropathy, or glomerulonephritis.
Abnormal clinical findings are resolved in response to therapeutic measures.	Initial signs and symptoms have disappeared.

Systemic lupus erythematosus

Systemic lupus erythematosus (SLE) is a chronic, multisystem, autoimmune, inflammatory disorder characterized chiefly by antibody formation directed against autologous tissues and serum factors.

SLE has no cure. Although its origin remains elusive, increasing evidence suggests that multiple factors—genetic, hormonal, immunologic, and possibly viral—may play a role in the onset and perpetuation of the disease.

In the United States approximately 500,000 persons have this disease. Although virtually anyone may be affected, SLE has a predilection for women of childbearing age. Nine times more women than men are affected. Three times as many blacks as whites have SLE. Late-onset (sixth decade or later) SLE accounts for 12% of cases.

SLE was once considered a fatal illness of young women, but 85% of patients now survive longer than 15 years after diagnosis. This improved prognosis reflects advances in the diagnosis and treatment of the disease. Patients with central nervous system involvement and renal failure have poorer prognoses. Complications, especially infections, associated with the long-term use of steroids used to control the disease also significantly contribute to early mortality.

Despite the significant improvements in the treatment of SLE, it can be a serious and potentially life-threatening illness. Because of this, as well as the recognition that SLE is a prototype of autoimmune disease, it has been a subject of worldwide research.

The cause of SLE remains unknown, but several etiologic factors have been proposed. It is unlikely that any single factor is the cause. Most researchers conclude that SLE is probably caused by an unknown inciting agent coupled with a genetic "lupus diathesis."

Drugs

During the past 30 years many drugs have been implicated in the development of a reversible lupuslike syndrome that includes elevated antinuclear antibody (ANA) titers and well-defined clinical features. Perhaps certain drugs alter tissues to such a degree as to make them act as immunogenic stimuli. Both hydralazine and procainamide can bind to and alter the physical properties of DNA, perhaps enhancing its immunogenicity. There may also be some correlation between an individual's ability to metabolize certain drugs and a predisposition for SLE.[43]

The following outline lists drugs thought to induce lupus-like syndromes.[43] Once these drugs are discontinued, clinical manifestations disappear:

- Definite
  - Hydralazine
  - Procainamide
  - Isoniazid
- Possible
  - Dilantin
  - Chlorpromazine
  - Methyldopa
  - Penicillamine
  - Quinidine
  - Propylthiouracil
  - Practolol
  - Acebutolol
  - Lithium carbonate
- Unlikely
  - Griseofulvin
  - Phenylbutazone
  - Oral contraceptives
  - Gold salts
  - Sulfonamides
  - Penicillin

Pathophysiology

The pathogenesis of SLE is characterized by the development of antibodies directed against "self" tissues, cells, serum proteins, or all of these. The presence of autoantibodies reflects a loss of tolerance, or autoimmunity, and constitutes a serious defect in the regulatory components of the immune system. As discussed on p. 1303, the T lymphocytes are the primary group of white cells responsible for control of the immune response. In SLE the number of T suppressor cells is decreased. In addition, T suppressor cell activity is inhibited. Polyclonal hypergammaglobulinemia occurs as a result, since B cells proliferate unrestrained by normal suppressor mechanisms.

In most SLE patients, antibodies develop directed against native, double-stranded DNA, as well as other antigens. The combination of autoantibodies and autoantigens, or immune complexes, may circulate or be deposited within capillary plexuses, near basement membranes, and in other tissues such as glomeruli, renal interstitia, serosal (pleural, pericardial, or peritoneal) membranes, the choroid plexus, and the vasculature of the lungs. Immune complex formation triggers the inflammatory response, which is the primary mechanism by which tissue destruction and subsequent clinical disease occur. Chronic deposition of immune complexes leads to chronic destruction of host tissue. *The intensity and location of the inflammatory process dictate the severity of the clinical response and organ involvement, respectively.*

A variety of autoantibodies may be detected by serologic assay. Some of these are listed in Table 14-6. Further discussion of the pathogenesis of SLE by systems is summarized here:

Table 14-6
Autoantibodies in SLE

Autoantibody	Clinical Manifestations
Antinuclear Anti–double-stranded DNA (ds-DNA)	Nephritis; vasculitis; pleuritis; pericarditis; synovitis; peritonitis
Antineuronal	Cerebritis; organic brain syndromes; peripheral neuropathies
Anticoagulant	Coagulopathies
Anti-RBC	Anemia
Anti-WBC	Leukopenia; lymphopenia; immunosuppression; infection
Antiplatelet	Thrombocytopenia
Anti–basement membrane	Dermatitis; nephritis

- Musculoskeletal
  - Deposition and accumulation of fibrin along synovial surfaces; arteriolar and venular inflammation; perivascular inflammation; inflammation of tendon sheaths; interstitial inflammation of muscle tissue leading to necrosis, degeneration, and fibrosis (late)
- Gastrointestinal
  - Ulceration of mucosal membranes associated with collagen degeneration and vasculitis; vasculitis leading to infarction, necrosis of tissue, and organ rupture; arteritis of mesenteric circulation
- Renal: "lupus nephritis"
  - Immune complex deposition and inflammation of the glomerular basement membrane and mesangium; glomerular sclerosis
- Hematologic
  - IgG and IgM against erythrocytes (cells destroyed by macrophages and complement); IgM antibodies against leukocytes; antibodies detected against platelets (cells destroyed by splenic macrophages); periarterial fibrosis and inflammatory infiltration of lymph nodes; circulating anticoagulant proteins
- Pulmonary
  - Inflammation of pleura; infiltration of parenchyma; interstitial vasculitis leading to infarction, necrosis, and fibrosis
- Cardiovascular
  - Diffuse vasculitis; inflammation and scarring of SA and AV nodes; inflammation of pericardial sac
- Cutaneous
  - Immune complex deposition and inflammation of dermal-epidermal junctions; vasculitis
- Neurologic
  - Immune complex deposition and inflammation in choroid plexus; antineuronal antibody action

Diagnostic Studies and Findings

Antinuclear Antibody (ANA)

Positive in titers greater than 1:80

Anti–Double-Stranded DNA Antibody (ds-DNA)

Positive in titers greater than 1:80

Rapid Plasma Reagin (RPR) Test

Falsely positive

Fluorescent Treponemal Antibody Absorption (FTA-ABS)

Negative

Complement (C3 and C4)

Decreased during flares, indicative of acute inflammation; otherwise within normal limits

Skin or Muscle Biopsy

Evidence of inflammation with or without tissue necrosis; deposits of immunoglobulin and complement at dermal-epidermal junctions

Kidney Biopsy

Focal or diffuse proliferative nephritis; also membranous or interstitial disease

Complete Blood Count

Pancytopenia or selective deficits; lymphopenia during flare

C-Reactive Protein

Elevated during flares, indicative of acute inflammatory state

Erythrocyte Sedimentation Rate

Elevated during flares, indicative of acute inflammatory state

Coombs' Test

Positive in presence of hemolytic anemia because of autoantibody production against erythrocytes

Coagulation Profile

Prolonged prothrombin time and partial thromboplastin time if circulating anticoagulant antibodies are present

Rheumatoid Factor (RF) (Anti-IgG Antibody)

Usually positive in titer greater than 1:40

Circulating Immune Complexes

Present during flares

Urinalysis

Abnormal casts and sediment associated with renal damage

Antibodies to Single-Stranded DNA (ss-DNA)

May be present in ANA-negative lupus and associated with congenital heart block in lupus patients' neonates

The 1982 revised classification of SLE is based on the 11 criteria defined below. For the purpose of identifying patients in clinical studies, a person should be said to have SLE if any four or more of the 11 criteria are present, serially or simultaneously, during any interval of observation.

Malar rash: fixed erythema, flat or raised, over malar eminences, tending to spare nasolabial folds

Discoid rash: erythematous raised patches with adherent keratotic scaling and follicular plugging; atrophic scarring may occur in older lesions

Photosensitivity: skin rash as result of unusual reaction to sunlight, based on patient history or physician's observation

Oral ulcers: oral or nasopharyngeal ulceration, usually painless, observed by physician

Arthritis: nonerosive arthritis involving two or more peripheral joints, characterized by tenderness, swelling, or effusion

Serositis: pleuritis—convincing history of pleuritic pain or rub heard by a physician or evidence of pleural effusion—*or* pericarditis—documented by electrocardiogram, rub, or evidence of pericardial effusion

Renal disorder: persistent proteinuria greater than 0.5 g/day or greater than 3+ if quantitation not performed *or* cellular casts—may be red cell, hemoglobin, granular, tubular, or mixed

Neurologic disorder: seizures in absence of offending drugs or known metabolic derangements (such as uremia, ketoacidosis, or electrolyte imbalance) *or* psychosis in absence of offending drugs or known metabolic derangements

Hematologic disorder: hemolytic anemia with reticulocytosis *or* leukopenia—less than $4000/mm^3$ total on two or more occasions *or* lymphopenia—less than $1500/mm^3$ on two or more occasions *or* thrombocytopenia—less $100,000/mm^3$ in absence of offending drugs

Immunologic disorder: positive LE cell preparation *or* anti-DNA—antibody to native DNA in abnormal titer *or* anti-Sm—presence of antibody to Sm nuclear antigen *or* false positive serologic test for syphilis known to be positive for at least 6 months and confirmed by *Treponema pallidum* immobilization or fluorescent treponemal antibody absorption test

Antinuclear antibody: abnormal titer of antinuclear antibody by immunofluorescence or equivalent assay at any point in time and in absence of drugs known to be associated with "drug-induced lupus" syndrome

Medical Plan

The goals of the treatment plan include management of signs and symptoms, induction of remission, prevention of untoward complications of therapy, and early recognition of "flares."

Surgery

Joint replacement may be indicated if chronic synovitis and pain have been problematic.

Medications[43]

Nonsteroidal anti-inflammatory agents. Acetylsalicylic acid (aspirin) may be given in a daily oral dosage of 3 to 6 g for adults. Indomethacin (Indocin) is given orally, 25 to 50 mg three or four times a day for adults. The patient should be monitored for evidence of gastrointestinal bleeding.

Anti-infective agents. Hydroxychloroquine (Plaquenil), 200 to 400 mg orally twice a day for adults, or chloroquine, 250 mg orally daily to twice weekly for adults, is given. The patient should be started on therapy slowly. Gastrointestinal intolerance may occur when full doses are used initially. The beneficial effect of these drugs is usually demonstrated within a month or two. Nonsteroidal anti-inflammatory agents should be continued until this time. Retinal toxicity may occur at higher doses, so patients should receive pretreatment and annual ophthalmic examinations.

Corticosteroids. Prednisone (Orasone, Deltasone, Meticorten) is given orally in low doses (15 mg/day), moderate doses (16 to 40 mg/day), or high doses (41 to 120 mg/day). Alternate-day dosage may be instituted as maintenance therapy (see p. 1393). The amounts listed above may be given in divided doses to provide more sustained anti-inflammatory action.

Any amount of prednisone given as a single oral dose in the morning has *less* adrenal suppressing activity than the same amount given in divided doses throughout the day. However, any given amount of this drug, taken in divided doses, has greater lupus-suppressing activity than does the same amount of drug given as a single morning dose.[38] Fever, cutaneous involvement, arthropathy, and serositis are usually managed with 20 to 30 mg of prednisone orally each day. Major organ involvement (cardiac and vascular systems and kidneys) often requires 15 to 20 mg prednisone orally (or intravenous equivalent) every 6 hours until attenuation of disease activity is achieved.

Methylprednisolone (Solu-Medrol, A-methaPred) is given intravenously in a dosage of up to 1000 mg/day for adults. One gram may be administered in divided doses. The use of intravenous therapy is limited to situations of acute exacerbations of the disease or when the patient is unable to tolerate oral administration. Central nervous system involvement (psychosis, grand mal seizures) requires 35 to 40 mg methylprednisolone intravenously every 6 hours. The dose should be doubled if no response is attained in 48 hours.

In addition, bolus or "pulse" steroid therapy may be administered, though its use remains controversial. The usual course involves the intravenous infusion of 1 to 1.5 g of methylprednisolone daily for three doses. Oral medications, which may include up to 60 mg of prednisone daily, may be continued through the treatment episode. Pulse therapy has been used with varying success during acute exacerbations of the disease, involving renal failure and central nervous system and hematologic "crises." This treatment is not without inherent hazards. Sudden death has been reported.

Topical steroids include hydrocortisone (Cortaid), fluocinonide (Lidex), betamethasone dipropionate (Diprosone), flurandrenolide (Cordran), betamethasone valerate (Valisone), and fluocinolone acetonide (Synalar).

Once remission is achieved on moderate to high divided dose therapy, the steroids are gradually tapered (decreased 5 mg per week). After reaching 40 mg, the dose should be consolidated to a single morning dose and tapered to 20 mg/day. The dose is then decreased by 2.5 mg a week until a 10 mg/day schedule is reached. The dose may be further decreased by 1 mg per week until the patient is totally weaned from the drug. If the disease flares while the dose is being decreased, the prednisone will be increased back to the last dosage at which the patient was asymptomatic and laboratory findings were within normal limits.

Alternate-day therapy is usually not successful during acute phases of SLE. Once the disease is under control, the physician may place the patient on an alternate-day schedule (which has less adrenal suppressing activity) using the following protocol[38]:

1. The patient initially receives 2x (x = daily dose) on the "on" day and ¾x on the "off" day.
2. One week later, the "off" day dose is switched to ½x.
3. One week later, the "off" day dose is switched to ¼x.
4. One week later, the "off" day dose is discontinued.

Patients receiving long-term steroid therapy should be assessed for the following signs and symptoms: hyperglycemia, central fat distribution, arrhythmias, hypertension, edema, electrolyte imbalances, violaceous striae, alopecia, glaucoma, cataracts, infections, osteoporosis, myopathies, seizures, gastrointestinal ulceration, and pancreatitis.

In addition, patients should be assessed frequently for signs and symptoms associated with adrenal crisis, particularly when tapering of dosages is begun: sudden fatigue and profound weakness, muscle weakness, arthralgias, fevers, anorexia, dizziness, syncope, dyspnea, lethargy, and hypotension.

Antineoplastic agents. Azathioprine (Imuran) is given in an oral dosage of 150 mg/day to 25 mg thrice weekly for adults. The patient should be monitored for pancytopenia, gastrointestinal distress, skin rash, hepatic toxicity, and hyperuricemia. Cyclophosphamide (Cytoxan, Neosar) is given as 150 mg/day to 25 mg thrice weekly for adults. The patient should be monitored for pancytopenia, cardiotoxicity, gastrointestinal distress, hemorrhagic cystitis, and hyperuricemia. Chlorambucil (Leukeran) is given orally as 10 mg/day to 2 mg thrice weekly for adults. The patient should be monitored for pancytopenia, exfoliative dermatitis, and hyperuricemia.

Other medications. A variety of anti-infective agents may be used to treat infections associated with SLE or immunosuppressive therapy. Treatment of renal disease includes the use of antihypertensive agents and aluminum derivatives. Raynaud's phenomenon may respond to biofeedback or sympatholytic drugs such as guanethidine, nifedipine, reserpine, and tolazoline. Intra-articular steroid injections may prove useful in the alleviation of synovitis and joint pain.

General Management

Plasmapheresis (see p. 1397) has been shown to decrease circulating immune complexes and autoantibodies. After the procedure, which may be done two or three times a week, a rebound effect may be noted. This is characterized by elevated antibody or immune complex titers. To circumvent this problem, a brief course of cytotoxic medication, often cyclophosphamide intravenously, may be administered after the plasmapheresis series. Although the use of plasmapheresis as a therapeutic modality remains controversial, it has been suggested for extremely ill patients who do not respond well to conventional treatment.

Peritoneal dialysis or hemodialysis may be indicated in the treatment of renal insufficiency or failure.

A balanced diet should be encouraged. A weight reduction diet may be indicated for patients receiving steroids. Salt restriction often prevents fluid retention. Vitamins are useful during pregnancy and dieting.

A balance is needed between rest and exercise. Flares probably warrant temporary rest. Otherwise, a regular exercise program should be implemented to increase and maintain strength, endurance, and muscle tone. Aerobic exercises such as walking, swimming, and bicycling are recommended. Jogging should be avoided because it places stress on joints, but swimming is particularly beneficial because it avoids this problem. For patients unable to engage in the aforementioned activities, a regular program of exercise, including range of motion, should be planned with the aid of a physical therapist.

Many patients with SLE cannot tolerate sun exposure. Flares have been associated with photosensitivity. Patients are especially intolerant of type B ultraviolet light. Therefore they should be encouraged to avoid the sun, wear protective clothing, and liberally apply sunscreens with a sun protection factor of 15 or above.

Patients with SLE should not take birth control pills or use intrauterine devices (IUDs). Use of diaphragm and foam is the preferred contraceptive method.

NURSING CARE

Nursing Assessment

Skin and Mucous Membrane

Facial erythema; butterfly dermatitis; alopecia; "lupus hair"—thin unruly hair that fractures easily around frontal hairline; periorbital edema; Raynaud's phenomenon; photosensitivity; oral and nasal ulcers; purpura; petechiae; periungual erythema; leg ulcers; digital gangrene; diffuse, transient rashes; urticarial lesions; livedo reticularis; "discoid" lesions: demarcated, annular, erythematous plaques with atrophy, scaling, and telangiectasia; scale is adherent and "plugs" dilated hair follicles, with classic distribution over sun-exposed areas of skin

Neuropsychiatric Status

"Lupus cerebritis"; encephalitis; aseptic meningitis; progressive multifocal leukoencephalopathy; seizures (usually grand mal); cranial neuropathies: ophthalmoplegias, visual disturbances, papilledema, facial weakness, dysarthria, vertigo, nystagmus, trigeminal neuralgia; cytoid bodies; aphasia; hemiparesis; headache; peripheral neuropathies; anxiety; depression; mania; insomnia; confusion; hallucinations; disorientation; emotional lability; psychosis

Musculoskeletal Integrity

Arthralgias; arthritis: polyarticular, often episodic, may or may not result in deformities; tenosynovitis; synovial Baker's cysts; diffuse myalgias; polyfocal myositis;

Table 14-7
Frequency of Clinical Symptoms in SLE

Symptom	Percent
Fever	83
Weight loss	62
Arthritis, arthralgia	90
Skin	74
Butterfly rash	42
Photosensitivity	30
Mucous membrane lesions	12
Alopecia	27
Raynaud's phenomenon	17
Purpura	15
Urticaria	8
Renal	53
Nephrosis	18
Gastrointestinal	38
Pulmonary	47
Pleurisy	45
Effusion	24
Pneumonia	29
Cardiac	46
Pericarditis	27
Murmurs	23
Electrocardiographic changes	39
Lymphadenopathy	46
Splenomegaly	15
Hepatomegaly	25
Central nervous system	32
Psychosis	15
Convulsions	15
Cytoid bodies	11

From Schur.[43]

steroid-induced osteoporosis, aseptic bone necrosis, or myopathy; pseudothrombophlebitis

Gastrointestinal Status

Dysphagia; gastric and duodenal ulcerations (may also be steroid induced); pancreatitis; hepatomegaly; peritonitis; "acute abdomen"

Hematologic Status

Anemia: autoimmune hemolytic anemia, iron deficiency anemia, chronic anemia; granulocytopenia; leukocytosis; lymphocytopenia; thrombocytopenia; lymphadenopathy; splenomegaly; hepatomegaly; coagulopathies; potential infection

Cardiovascular Status

Diffuse vasculitis; pericarditis; myocarditis; endocarditis; atherosclerosis (also steroid induced); thrombophlebitis; arrhythmias

Pulmonary Status

Pleurisy; pleural effusions; pneumonitis; interstitial fibrosis; decreased pulmonary function; pulmonary hypertension; pulmonary emboli

Renal Status

"Lupus nephritis": focal (mild), diffuse proliferative (severe), membranous, interstitial fibrosis, tubular necrosis; edema; retinopathy; hypertension; anemia; electrolyte imbalances

See Table 14-7

Nursing Dx & Intervention

Because of the multiple systemic effects of SLE, nursing care must be structured to cope with the patient's individual requirements. Therefore nursing care often varies greatly, ranging, for example, from minor application of topical steroids to aggressive pulmonary toilet for an intubated patient. The following is meant to provide a generalized perspective. Refer to other chapters for a detailed approach to systems involved.

Nursing Diagnosis	Nursing Intervention/Rationale
Ineffective breathing pattern related to pulmonary complications	• Assess respiratory status: monitor respiratory rate and rhythm, auscultate lungs for presence of adventitious breath sounds, and monitor for subjective distress (chest pain, dyspnea, etc.) *to detect or prevent respiratory compromise.* • Maintain bed rest during acute phase *to conserve oxygen.* • In collaboration with physician, administer oxygen, analgesics, inhalants, bronchodilators, and steroids as appropriate. • Provide chest physiotherapy and postural drainage *to treat or prevent pneumonia.* • Teach deep breathing exercises and encourage patient to perform exercises as often as needed *to treat or prevent pneumonia.* • Monitor chest roentgenograms and sputum culture results *to detect pneumonia.* • Monitor results of pulmonary studies: VQ scan, pulmonary function tests, lung biopsy, etc.
Decreased cardiac output related to cardiovascular complications	• Assess cardiac status. Auscultate apical pulse for irregularities, presence of murmurs, tachycardia, and bradycardia. Auscultate for pericardial friction rub. Monitor for subjective distress: syncope, palpitations, and dyspnea. Monitor electrocardiographic results. Monitor for presence of peripheral edema. Auscultate lung for presence of rales or rhonchi. Auscultate arterial pulses for presence of bruits. • In collaboration with physician, administer oxygen, steroids, and antiarrhythmic agents if appropriate. Assess patient's response.
Ineffective individual coping related to organic brain syndrome associated with SLE or difficulty dealing with diagnosis and its implications	• Assess changes in neurologic status: orientation, judgment, and intellectual function. • Assess patient's ability to cope. • Assess for suicidal ideation. • Work with patient to identify resources for support and coping mechanisms that have proved helpful in past. • Provide emotional support and attempt to limit patient's fears through frequent explanations of tests and procedures. • Provide patient education (see p. 1361). • Encourage visits by family and friends. • If orientation is problem in hospital, provide familiar articles from home. Provide clock and calendar *to orient patient to time.* • Maintain patient's safety. • Encourage participation in local chapter of Lupus Foundation.

Nursing Diagnosis	Nursing Intervention/Rationale
Altered renal tissue perfusion related to the renal complications	• Assess renal status. Monitor for presence of dyspnea, hypertension, edema, weight gain, anorexia, and nausea. Monitor urinalysis results, blood urea nitrogen, serum creatinine, hemoglobin, hematocrit, and urine and serum electrolytes *to detect or prevent renal compromise*. • Modify diet as indicated *to prevent azotemia*. • In collaboration with physician, administer antihypertensive medications. Assess patient's response. • Monitor for symptoms of electrolyte imbalance.
Impaired physical mobility related to arthritis and general weakness	• Assess degree of limitation: range of motion, joint integrity, presence of pain (location, duration, quality, severity, and precipitating or alleviating factors), deformity, and muscular atrophy. • Perform range of motion exercises as tolerated *to maintain joint integrity*. • In collaboration with physician, administer analgesics according to appropriate and regular time schedules. Assess patient's response. • Administer thermal therapy to muscles and joints *for pain control*. • Confer with physical or occupational therapist *to determine other beneficial interventions*.
Impaired skin integrity related to integumentary manifestations	• Assess skin and mucous membranes: Inspect and palpate noting color, vascularity, lesion size, configuration, and distribution, edema, moisture, temperature, texture, thickness, mobility, and turgor. • Monitor skin lesions *for signs of infection*. • In collaboration with physician, administer topical steroidal or anti-infective creams and ointments as indicated. Assess response. • Provide hypoallergenic, nondrying soaps and mild shampoos. • Encourage use of sunscreen products if patient is photosensitive.
Altered nutrition: less than body requirements, related to anorexia, electrolyte imbalance, or chemotherapy side effects	• Assess nutritional status: Monitor serum protein and albumin values; monitor for evidence of poor wound healing; determine weight loss and compare to ideal body weight. • Encourage balanced diet with supplements if indicated. • Encourage weight reduction diet for patients who have gained weight while taking steroids. • Low-sodium, high-potassium diet may be indicated for patients receiving steroids. • Encourage intake of vitamin supplements for patients who are pregnant or dieting.
Potential activity intolerance related to flare, chronic anemia, arthralgias, and other effects of SLE	• Assess degree of activity intolerance. • Encourage balance between rest and exercise. • Flares warrant temporary rest. • During periods when disease is quiescent, encourage program of regular, aerobic exercise that places as little stress on joints as possible (such as swimming).
Body image disturbance related to multisystem disturbances, including skin changes	• See p. 1751.
Potential for infection	• Assess for anorexia, pain, weakness, and lethargy. • Assess for evidence of infection at sites of invasive procedures. • Assess for breaks in skin integrity, particularly over pressure areas and oral mucosa *to prevent infection*. • Assess pulmonary status: auscultate lung fields to determine presence of adventitious breath sounds *to detect or prevent pneumonia*. • Maintain optimum nutritional status and fluid intake. • Assess ocular integrity for evidence of conjunctivitis: erythematous, pruritic conjunctiva. • Assess mentation for evidence of central nervous system infection: changes in level of consciousness, headache, and visual disturbances. • Assess for evidence of gastrointestinal infection: abdominal pain, fever, and diarrhea. • Monitor temperature and vital signs for evidence of fever or sepsis. • Maintain body hygiene. • Monitor laboratory data: white blood cell count and differential, erythrocyte sedimentation rate, C-reactive protein, urinalysis, and cultures. • In collaboration with physician, administer appropriate antimicrobial, antipyretic, or analgesic medication. Assess patient's response. Monitor for side effects. • Promote pulmonary toilet: breathing exercises, postural drainage, and chest physical therapy. • Maintain normal sleep and rest patterns. • Protect patient from physical injury. • Provide clean environment. • Maintain protective isolation based on hospital policy. • Restrict contact with family and health care providers who have infectious diseases. • Wash hands thoroughly before and after contact with patient.

Patient Education

1. Teach side effects of medications.
2. Teach the importance of avoiding contact with persons who may expose the patient to infection.
3. Teach the importance of frequent assessment for signs and symptoms associated with infection. While steroids are being given, many of these findings are masked, so the slightest change in temperature, wound characteristics, or other parameters should be reported immediately.
4. Teach the importance of skin care. Tell the patient to avoid dryness and use of irritant soaps, shampoos, chemical coloring, or permanent waving of hair. Encourage use of hypoallergenic makeup and wearing wig if there is hair loss. Teach photosensitive patients to avoid sun exposure: limit outdoor activities between 10 AM and 4 PM, wear long sleeves, pants, and hats, and use PABA sunscreen products with a sun protection factor of at least 15.
5. Teach methods to cope with arthralgias and myalgias: range of motion exercises, balance between rest and exercise, use of analgesics and nonsteroidal anti-inflammatory agents, joint supports at night, contacting Arthritis Foundation.
6. Teach the importance of regular follow-up by a physician and the need for blood tests.
7. Teach the importance of recognizing factors that lead to a flare: psychologic and physical stress, use of drugs that induce a lupuslike syndrome (see p. 1355), abrupt cessation of medications, and photosensitivity.
8. Teach warning signs of a flare: fever, chills, excessive fatigue and malaise, nausea, muscle weakness, increased joint pain, chest pain, oliguria, and dysuria—essentially, exacerbation of an old symptom or development of a new one.
9. Teach the importance of maintaining a balanced diet; include restrictions associated with medications.
10. Teach family planning. Pregnancy is usually allowed during remissions with close monitoring. Barrier contraceptives such as a condom or diaphragm are recommended.
11. Teach the importance of keeping a log of the disease course, treatments, and other disease-related information.
12. Teach the importance of obtaining up-to-date information about SLE.
13. Teach the patient to carry medical alert identification.
14. Direct the patient to available resources.

Evaluation

Patient Outcome	Data Indicating That Outcome is Reached
Laboratory findings are within normal limits.	Anti–double-stranded DNA (anti-dsDNA) and antinuclear antibody (ANA) are less than 1:80. Complement (C3 and C4), C1q binding, CH50, complete blood count, white blood cell count, erythrocyte count, hematocrit, hemoglobin level, and platelet count are within normal limits. Prothrombin time and partial thromboplastin time are within normal limits. Urinalysis findings, blood urea nitrogen, and creatinine levels are within normal limits.
Symptoms resolve in response to therapeutic measures.	There are no symptoms associated with individual system involvement.
Patient maintains independence in activities of daily living.	Patient returns to baseline ability to perform activities of daily living.
Pain is relieved or minimized.	There is decrease in subjective distress. Objective decrease is based on rating scale.
Medical crises are prevented.	There are no life-threatening side effects of chemotherapeutic interventions: cardiopulmonary failure, renal failure, sepsis, or psychosis.
Patient complies with treatment.	Patient verbalizes understanding of importance of compliance and adheres to prescribed regimens and methods of symptom control.
No infection occurs.	There are no signs or symptoms associated with infections. Patient says there is no malaise, fatigue, weakness, anorexia, dysuria, or pain. There is no evidence of rhinitis; productive cough; pyuria; erythema, heat, edema, or purulent drainage at wound site(s); breaks in skin integrity; rales; rhonchi; or wheezing. Temperature and vital signs are within patient's normal limits. Culture findings are negative. White blood cell count, erythrocyte sedimentation rate, C-reactive protein, and urinalysis findings are within normal limits.

ALLERGIC DISORDERS

Atopic disease

The term "allergy" was initially used to describe "altered reactivity" and has evolved over the years to refer broadly to any immunologic reaction to a foreign substance that produces detrimental consequences to the body. It is often used interchangeably with atopy.

Atopy is an abnormal immune response mediated by IgE antibody produced against substances that normally occur in the environment. Atopic diseases include anaphylaxis, allergic rhinoconjunctivitis, allergic asthma, atopic dermatitis, gastrointestinal allergy, and occasionally urticaria or angioedema. Allergy to a drug or an insect bite or sting can cause anaphylaxis or hives by an immunologic IgE mechanism in persons with or without other allergic symptoms (atopic or nonatopic).

Atopy appears in approximately 20% of the population and is thought to be inherited through genes linked to HLA antigen haplotypes. The expression of atopy has been linked to multiple factors including hormonal changes, antigen exposure, and concurrent illness. Expression of symptoms can occur at any time during life and varies from mild to life threatening in severity.

Pathophysiology

The genetic defect is thought to be in T suppressor cell modulation, which allows increased or unmodulated production of IgE antibody.

The antigens precipitating the IgE response are restricted to either complete protein antigens with specific carrier and antigenic determinants or low–molecular weight substances that function as haptens by combining with serum or tissue proteins to form a complex. Antigens may be inhaled (tree, grass, or weed pollens, mold spores, dust, animal proteins), ingested (food, drugs), injected (venom, drug), or touched.

On initial exposure the antigen (allergen) is processed by

Figure 14-11 Mediators of immediate hypersensitivity. Interaction of allergen-antibody reaction, complement system, clotting system, and kinin system (→ indicates stimulation; ⊣⊢ indicates inhibition).

From Lawlor, G., et al., editors: Manual of allergy and immunology, Boston, 1981, Little, Brown & Co.

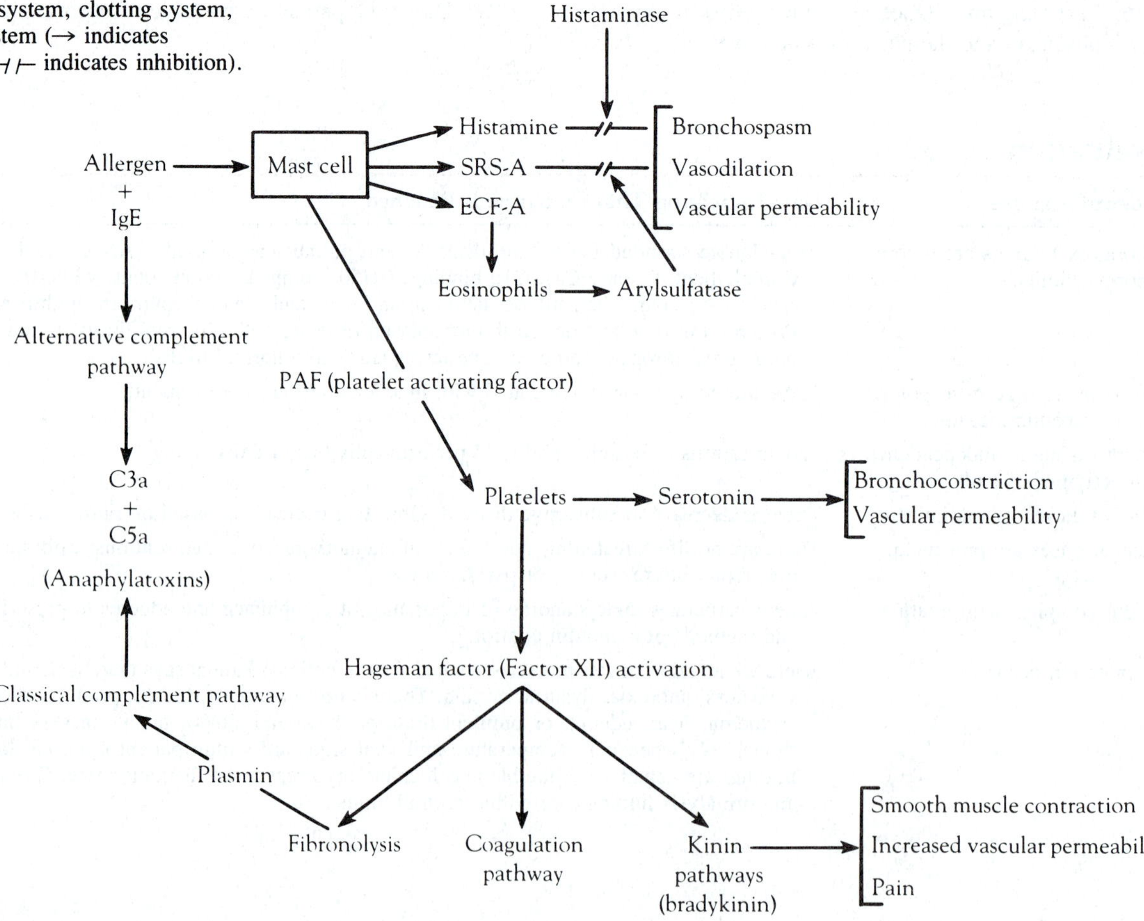

a macrophage and then presented to the appropriately responsive T lymphocyte. Interaction then occurs with B lymphocytes, which, when stimulated, develop into mature plasma cells and secrete the antigen-specific IgE antibody.

Only a very small amount of IgE antibody circulates in the serum. Most IgE is found fixed to the surface of mast cells (fixed in tissue) or basophils (circulating). There may be 5000 to 500,000 IgE molecules on a single mast cell. A mast cell may have a large variety of antigen-specific IgE antibodies on its surface.

Mast cells and basophils contain several potent chemical mediators of inflammation, including histamine, arachidonic acid metabolites such as prostaglandins and leukotrienes C, D, or S, eosinophil chemotactic factors of anaphylaxis (ECF-A), and platelet-activating factor (PAF). Mediators may exert a direct pharmacologic effect or release or activate other mediators potentiating the response. Mediators initiate a sequence of physiologic events in various organ systems that result in such responses as vasodilation, enhanced vasopermeability, smooth muscle contraction, and increased mucus production (Figure 14-11).

On reexposure and entry the antigen binds to IgE antibodies. This causes degranulation of the mast cell and release of the mediators that initiate the pathophysiologic responses. Symptoms of atopic disease are the result of tissue response to the mediators. Symptoms may be generalized (anaphylaxis) or localized (for example, in bronchi, conjunctiva, nasal membranes, skin, or gut). This mechanism of tissue reaction occurs immediately on exposure to the antigen and is identified as a type I anaphylactic or immediate hypersensitivity reaction by the Gell and Coombs nomenclature.

Mast cell mediators are responsible for both the well-known "classic" allergic response, in which symptoms occur immediately upon exposure, as well as the less well-known late phase response in which symptoms begin hours after allergen exposure and result from tissue inflammation and damage.

Anaphylactoid reactions mimic allergic reactions and clinically may be identical to IgE-mediated responses. However, no IgE is involved and symptoms result from direct action on mast cells that causes release of chemical mediators (occurs with dextran and radiocontrast media), prostaglandin activation (occurs with acetylsalicylic acid and some nonsteroidal anti-inflammatory agents), or complement activation (occurs with aggregated IgG). The exact trigger mechanism and pathways of inflammatory responses are not fully understood. However, these reactions are treated in the same manner as anaphylactic reactions. The only clinical difference is that, since IgE is not involved, skin testing is of no value and reactions can occur with the first exposure; prior sensitization is not required.

Diagnostic Studies and Findings

A thorough history is by far the most important diagnostic tool. The physical examination focuses on all areas of potential atopic manifestations. Laboratory studies may be useful in supporting the diagnosis and in monitoring response to therapy but are not in themselves diagnostic.

History

Onset, nature, and progression of symptoms; aggravating and alleviating factors; frequency, time, and duration of symptoms; complete environmental history including occupational, chemical, smoking, animal, and hobby exposures; household description including heating and cooling systems, pets, and bedding; past medical history; medications; family history including atopic history.

Physical Examination

Skin; external ear canal and tympanic membrane; conjunctiva; nasal membranes; naso-oropharynx; chest

Laboratory Studies

Complete blood count
- Within normal limits

Differential
- May have eosinophil percentage, up to 5%

Eosinophil count
- Within normal limits or increased up to 10% (up to 700 cells/mm^3), but range of normal is wide and increases may also occur in other diseases that have similar symptoms

Smears for eosinophils
- Generally predominate in secretions (up to 90% of total) during symptomatic periods

Total serum IgE levels
- Within normal limits or increased (up to 700 U/ml), but there is wide range of normal and increases can also occur in other diseases

Skin testing
- Demonstrates presence of specific IgE antibody; most reliable test for allergy; reliable correlation for inhalants, much less reliable for foods; false positive findings may result from irritant response; false negative findings may result from poor skin response or antihistamines; findings must correlate with history; drug may be hapten or metabolite; testing currently limited to penicillin, horse serum, insulin, and egg-based vaccines

Radioallergosorbent test (RAST)
- Demonstrates presence of specific circulating IgE antibody; less reliable than skin testing (not as sensitive; difficulty in standardization of test and reproducibility of tests among reference laboratories)

Provocative testing
- Specific antigen challenges performed under controlled conditions to demonstrate clinical reactivity

Elimination testing
- Demonstration of clinical sensitivity to antigen by removing and then reintroducing it while monitoring clinical symptoms

Medical Plan

The goals of the treatment plan include symptom management through medications, environmental control, and immunotherapy. Specific plans are discussed with each disease.

Medications

Medications are used to prevent the tissue response and resultant symptoms. The choice of medication is to some extent organ specific, since the tissue response differs in specific organ systems, and these are discussed with the specific allergic disease.

Antihistamines are competitive antagonists of histamine and compete for cell surface receptors. Thus better symptom control is achieved by using the drug on a regular basis or as needed before allergen exposure. Six classes of older antihistamines are available; all have central nervous system and anticholinergic side effects. The side effects, drowsiness and dryness, may limit their use in susceptible patients. Occasionally central nervous system excitation, palpitation, urinary retention, or constipation occurs. A newer H_1 antihistamine that does not cross the blood-brain barrier eliminates these side effects and is now available (terfenadine [Seldane], 60 mg). Topical preparations should be avoided because of the potential for sensitization. They may be given orally or intramuscularly depending on preparation and with dose adjustments to any patient older than 3 months, including pregnant women (who may receive selected antihistamines, including chlorpheniramine).

Cromolyn sodium stabilizes the mast cell membrane, preventing mediator release. It has no known side effects other than occasional sore throat or hoarseness after inhalation. It must be used preventively, either before exposure or on a regular basis. Topical nasal, otic, and bronchial cromolyn preparations are currently available for any age patient; oral administration preparations are undergoing clinical trials. Available agents include the following:

- Intal, via Spinhaler or metered dose inhaler, every 6 hours or as needed before exposure for adult and child older than 6 years
- Nebulizer solution, 1 ampule via nebulizer every 6 hours or as needed before exposure for adult and child older than 2 years
- Nasalcrom, 1 spray every 4 to 6 hours or as needed before exposure for adult and child older than 6 years
- Opticrom, 1 drop in each eye as above

Environmental Control

Environmental control is the preferred method of treatment because complete avoidance of the offending allergen affords total relief of symptoms. Decreasing the amount of allergen exposure will reduce symptom severity. Removal of the offending antigens, especially those of an inhalant perennial nature, often seems to have an ameliorative effect on the progression of disease. The following is a representative list of allergens and possible measures:

- Tree, grass, and weed pollens—air-conditioning, closing bedroom and car windows during pollen season (times of pollination depend on geographic area)
- Mold spores—removal of source (such as plant dirt), application of mold retardant solutions for damp areas (for example, crawl spaces, bathrooms), air filtration by a high-efficiency particulate-arresting (HEPA) filter or electrostatic air cleaner
- House dust and mites—plastic mattress casing, removal of carpets, damp dusting and face masks while dusting, air filtration
- Epidermals (feather, animal protein)—removal of source
- Foods—avoidance
- Drugs—avoidance
- Stinging or biting insects—avoidance

Immunotherapy

The response to immunotherapy with inhaled antigens is well known, but the mechanism is not definitely elucidated. Proposed mechanisms include the following[11]:

- Development of IgG serum "blocking" antibodies
- Induction of tolerance in IgE-producing B cells
- Impairment of T helper cell function
- Restoration of antigen-specific or isotype-specific T suppressor cells or factors
- Decreased IgE synthesis by anti-idiotypic autoantibodies
- Decreased sensitivity of mediator-releasing cells

The major risk of immunotherapy is anaphylaxis from antigen overdose. The clinical efficacy of immunotherapy varies with different antigens, depending on the antigen involved, potency and dose of the antigen preparation, and complete match of antigens used with those clinically important to the patient. For certain antigens, a 95% improvement from baseline may be achieved. Currently the minimum length of therapy is 3 years. Immunotherapy is recommended for inhalant antigens (for example, tree, grass, and weed pollens) and venoms but not for foods. Gradual diminution of symptoms occurs during the therapy. When no further clinical improvement is noted, therapy is discontinued but may be reinstituted over the life span as necessary. Current investigations center on specifically identifying the antigenic components of various allergens and preparing immunotherapy extracts that increase the antigen load, require fewer injections, and minimize adverse effects.

Desensitization for insulin and penicillin requires special protocols performed under close supervision and is done only when medically indicated.

General Management

Although atopy should be considered a chronic illness, adequate patient education and motivation, coupled with a specific medical plan, should enable the patient to manage the disease successfully.

If the inflammatory response is prevented or blocked, sequelae such as fatigue, malaise, and secondary bacterial infections will be minimized.

NURSING CARE

Nursing Assessment

Allergic responses may involve one or more organ systems, and symptoms may range from mild to severe. Symptoms may be episodic or perennial depending on exposures. Assessment must also discriminate among possible concurrent diseases. Specific assessment is discussed with each allergic disease.

Nursing Dx & Intervention

Because of the variable expression of atopic disease, the following is included as part of the comprehensive overview of the disease. Specific interventions are addressed with discussion of each disease.

Nursing Diagnosis	Nursing Intervention/Rationale
Potential for injury related to exposure to antigen	• Obtain complete allergy history and record in appropriate places. • Emphasize potential harm of repeat exposure. • Identify and teach patient the measures to institute if patient is reexposed to antigen. • Emphasize need for medical alert identification.
Potential activity intolerance	• Modify activity prescriptions based on current symptom status, including fatigue. • Encourage full activity schedule for growth and developmental age. Make appropriate medication adjustments and apply environmental control measures.
Potential for infection	• Assess for signs and symptoms of concurrent infection. • Maintain optimal nutritional intake. • Maintain appropriate rest patterns. • Monitor use of medications *to control or eliminate symptoms.*
Personal identity and body image disturbances	• Assess patient for currrent restrictions in life-style and work, adjustment to illness, self-management behaviors, and family's adjustment to illness. • Coordinate with physician and patient modifications in medical, therapeutic prescriptions as indicated.
Anxiety	• Assess patient for current symptoms. • Teach patient methods for achieving symptom control and prevention measures. • See general intervention strategies on p. 1743. • Reassure patient that symptoms can be prevented or controlled.
Altered health maintenance	• Assess patient's and family's knowledge of disease process, relationship to symptoms, and methods of preventing or controlling symptoms. • Provide education *to achieve optimum level of health.*

Patient Education

1. Review the disease process with the patient to assess the accuracy of the patient's understanding.
2. Review with the patient medication use and expected response to therapy.
3. Teach the patient self-responsibility for allergen identification and avoidance measures.
4. Direct the patient to support and educational groups.

Evaluation

Specific criteria are identified with discussion of each atopic disease. The following are general outcome measures for any atopic disease.

Patient Outcome	Data Indicating That Outcome is Reached
Symptoms are resolved in response to therapeutic measures.	There are no symptoms associated with individual system involvement.

Patient Outcome	Data Indicating That Outcome is Reached
Normal activity and exercise are maintained.	Patient performs activities appropriate for growth and developmental age.
Patient is knowledgeable about allergy and its treatment.	Patient and family describe allergy, medical plan of care, environmental control, and other self-care measures.

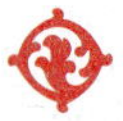

Allergic rhinitis/allergic rhinoconjunctivitis

Allergic rhinitis/allergic rhinoconjunctivitis is a complex of symptoms resulting from an antigen–IgE antibody reaction occurring in the nasal membranes, conjunctiva, or nasopharynx. The antigen is generally inhaled and deposited on the mucous membrane surface. Symptoms may also result from injected or ingested antigen transported to the site.

Approximately 18.6 million infants, children, and adults in the United States have seasonal or perennial allergic rhinitis. An estimated $224 million is spent annually for physician services and $300 million for medications, and some 28 million days each year are lost because of restricted activity or absence from school or work.

Symptoms may develop as early as infancy but can occur at any time throughout the life span. A positive family history may be obtained in the majority of cases. Without intervention, symptoms may remain constant, increase, or diminish over time.

Pathophysiology

With antigen-antibody linkage, mast cell degranulation and chemical mediator release occur, resulting in slower ciliary action, stimulation of mucosal glands, vasomotor instability, leukocyte infiltration (primarily eosinophilic), and tissue edema because of vasodilation and capillary permeability. Histamine is the major mediator of the inflammatory response, although other mediators such as eosinophil chemotactic factor of anaphylaxis (ECF-A), prostaglandins, and leukotrienes participate.

With prolonged exposure, basement membrane destruction and foamy cell formation occur. More chronic and irreversible changes include hyperplasia and thickening of the mucosal epithelium, mononuclear cellular infiltration, and connective tissue proliferation.

Symptoms generally result from inhalant allergen exposure or occasionally, especially in infants, from food ingestion. The inflammatory response may be confined to the nasal membranes or extend to the conjunctiva or oropharynx. Symptoms begin immediately on exposure and may be prolonged because of the late phase reaction.

Acute ocular manifestations may include bilateral conjunctival edema, hyperemia, photophobia, profuse tearing, blurring, and occasional superficial keratitis. With chronic exposure, dryness, itching, and photophobia are more pronounced than hyperemia, and the conjunctivae may appear pale.

Serous otitis occurs because swelling of the eustachian tube meatus prevents normal serous drainage. Although otitis is more prevalent in childhood, any age group may be affected. Decreased hearing and a sensation of fullness or ear popping are common symptoms. In younger children otitis is often asymptomatic, and therefore regular ear examinations are mandatory.

Seasonal inhalant exposures may generate intense, acute symptoms including nasal congestion, paroxysmal sneezing, itching, and clear, watery secretions. When these secretions drain into the pharynx, dry cough or hoarseness may occur. Occasionally epistaxis or headache may be present. Seasonal allergic rhinitis may be confused with viral infection, since the symptoms are similar.

Chronic or perennial exposure generally results in attenuated responses manifested by pressure, congestion, mucoid secretions, and chronic postnasal drip with cough, hoarseness, or recurrent throat clearing. Snoring or obligatory mouth breathing may be present. Perennial allergic rhinitis may be misdiagnosed as vasomotor rhinitis, perennial nonallergic rhinitis, or sinusitis.

Particularly with adults, allergic rhinitis may occur with other nasal diseases. A primary vasomotor response may intensify symptoms. Allergic rhinitis may aggravate existing nasal polyps. Increased sensitivity to nonspecific irritants occurs during an allergic episode. Occasionally secondary bacterial infections occur with prolonged nasal congestion, mucus production, and host fatigue. The sense of smell may diminish but usually remains intact during allergic episodes.

Diagnostic Studies and Findings

See p. 1363.

Skin Tests

Positive responses that correlate with history

Sinus Roentgenograms

Within normal limits; may be necessary to rule out other diseases such as cysts, nasal polyps, infective rhinitis, and structural defects

CT Scan of Sinuses

Rules out other diseases and structural defects

Medical Plan

The goal of the treatment plan is to block symptoms, maintain optimum function, and prevent sequelae such as fatigue, infections, serous otitis, and restricted activity.

Medications

Antihistamines

May be used prn or round the clock; long-acting compounds generally best; tolerance avoided by using different antihistamines; often combined with decongestants; see also p. 1364

Cromolyn sodium, prn before known antigen exposure (cat, dog, dusting) but more effective round the clock; short half-life often requires doses q4-6h or concomitant nocturnal antihistamine; see also p. 1364

Sympathomimetic agents

Topical decongestants: over-the-counter; should not be used for more than 3 consecutive d; useful for severe acute symptoms until other medications take effect

Oral decongestants: agents available (phenylephrine, phenylpropanolamine, pseudoephedrine); may be obtained over-the-counter or by prescription; age-dependent dosage; may be used from 3 mo of age; often used in combination with antihistamines and in long-acting preparations for decreased dosage schedule; must be used with caution in patients with hypertension or glaucoma; blood pressure monitoring needed

Corticosteroids

Topical: excellent for controlling more severe symptoms; must be used on regular basis; prn use ineffective; flunisolide and beclomethasone have no systemic effects, but occasional local effects of stinging, dryness, or irritation may occur; may be used on long-term basis

Flunisolide (Nasalide), 1 spray q8h for adult or child older than 6 yr

Beclomethasone (Vancenase, Beconase), 2 sprays q8h for adult or child older than 12 yr

Decadron (Decadron Turbinaire), 2 sprays q8h for adult; 1-2 sprays bid for child older than 6 yr

Oral: rarely used since advent of topical agents; should be considered only when symptoms are severe and other measures have failed

Ocular: because of side effects, even short-term use severely restricted and closely monitored

Anti-infective agents

Used for secondary bacterial infections; synthetic penicillins, sulfa, or erythromycin generally recommended and should be used for 10 d to 2 wk

Analgesic agents

Used to reduce symptoms of pressure headache until appropriate medications achieve symptom control

Environmental Control

Allergic rhinitis responds dramatically to removal of allergen; see p. 1364 for control of antigen exposure

Immunotherapy

Allergic rhinitis responds well to appropriately designed immunotherapy program; see p. 1364

General Management

Increased fluid intake to liquefy secretions and counter loss from obligatory mouth breathing

Steam or topical nasal saltwater solutions to decrease irritability and help loosen secretions

Encourage antigen-free environment

NURSING CARE

Nursing Assessment

The goal of assessment is to confirm the extent and severity of organ involvement and establish a baseline for later evaluation.

Conjunctival Inflammation

Hyperemia; edema (chemosis) involving either palpebral or bulbar membranes; secretions in palpebral fissures; superficial keratitis; edema; hyperplasia of papillae

Facial Changes

Dark discoloration in orbital-palpebral groove beneath lower eyelids ("allergic shiners"); adenoidal facies consisting of elongated maxilla, narrow chin, gaping expression, possible dental malocclusion, and transverse crease across top of nose

Nasal Membrane Inflammation

Swollen, wet, pale turbinates; mucosal edema; glistening, clear, watery or serous discharge; more variability in chronic disease

Oropharyngeal Inflammation

Nasal secretions; erythema; edema; high-arched palate; overbite

Tympanic Membrane Involvement

Bulging or retracted; prominent bony landmarks or none present; membrane thick, dull, or wrinkled, with gray, pink, amber, slightly yellow, or deep blue color; injected; evidence of fluid levels or bubbles

Nursing Dx & Intervention

Nursing Diagnosis	Nursing Intervention/Rationale
Ineffective breathing pattern	• Assess for obligatory mouth breathing, paroxysmal nocturnal dyspnea, snoring, or sleep apnea that may contribute to "allergic fatigue." • Elevate head of bed to 45 degrees *to facilitate mucus drainage.* • Humidify air as needed. • Monitor medication schedule *to block symptoms adequately.* • Assess environment for presence of offending allergens and remove if possible. • Emphasize importance of nasal breathing.
Altered health maintenance	• Discuss chronicity of disease process and reinforce need to prevent symptoms through medications and environmental control.
Potential for injury	• Emphasize importance of avoiding antigens known to cause severe reactions, and explain potential for severe reactions to people who are likely to have contact with patient. • Adhere strictly to immunotherapy protocols, and monitor patient for 20 minutes after injections.
Potential activity intolerance	• Explain that normal work, exercise, and recreation activities can and should be maintained through medications and environmental control.
Pain	• Identify adequate analgesia for pain relief in collaboration with physician.
Potential for infection	• Assess for signs and symptoms of infective rhinitis, infective otitis, and infective conjunctivitis. • Maintain adequate nutritional intake and appropriate rest. • Discuss rationale for adequately controlling symptoms and self-monitoring for secondary infections.

Patient Education

1. Assess the patient's current knowledge of the disease process and reinforce the concept of self-care and self-management of the disease.
2. Assess the patient's current knowledge of medications, side effects, and rationale for the use of medications, and reinforce the concepts of prophylaxis and prevention of symptoms.
3. Teach the importance of environmental control measures and the patient's responsibility for implementing recommended measures.
4. Teach the patient the importance of monitoring symptom response to therapies, recording any difficulties, new symptoms, and untoward effects, and communicating this on an ongoing basis to those prescribing the therapies.

Evaluation

Patient Outcome	Data Indicating That Outcome is Reached
Symptoms are resolved in response to therapeutic measures.	There are no symptoms associated with inflammatory response or infective process.
Health is maintained at optimum level.	Patient can identify all recommended therapies and provide information related to self-management.
Optimum functional levels are maintained.	Patient engages in normal work, school, or recreational activities without restrictions.

Anaphylaxis

Anaphylaxis results from a systemic IgE-mediated antigen-antibody response. It is an immediate and often life-threatening event in which massive release of mediators triggers a sequence of events in target organs throughout the body, resulting in a variety of symptoms that may include respiratory embarrassment or circulatory collapse.

As with other IgE antigen-antibody reactions, prior sensitization to the antigen must have occurred for anaphylaxis to take place. Anaphylactoid reactions and blood transfusion reactions are mediated by a non-IgE mechanism with the same final common pathway as IgE-mediated reactions. Reactions must be differentiated from vasovagal reactions, syncopal attacks, myocardial infarctions, insulin reactions, hysterical reactions, and shock or respiratory obstruction from other causes.

A history of atopic disease is often not elicited from patients with anaphylaxis. Previous exposures to the offending antigen may or may not have caused an untoward reaction.

Anaphylactoid reactions, through direct mast cell destabilization, immune complex aggregation, or prostaglandin-activating mechanisms, may also cause the release of mediators that results in a systemic reaction clinically similar to anaphylaxis. Anaphylactoid reactions appear frequently in hospital settings. The following are some mechanisms that have been proposed for anaphylactoid reactions:

- Direct mediator release (agents such as dextran and radiopaque dyes)
- Immune complex aggregation (agents such as γ-globulin administered intramuscularly or intravenously)
- Cytotoxic antibody transfusion reactions (agents such as whole blood and cryoprecipitate)
- Prostaglandin-induced (agents such as aspirin and nonsteroidal anti-inflammatory agents)

Anaphylaxis may result from injection of antigen (subcutaneous, intravenous, or intramuscular drugs or venom stings), although enough antigen may be absorbed from the gut (ingested food or drug) or from the respiratory tract (inhaled antigen) to precipitate the reaction. The antigen is distributed via the bloodstream and fixes to IgE antibody on mast cells and basophils, triggering mediator release.

A systemic reaction is any organ involvement away from the site of antigen deposition. Reactions are classified as mild, moderate, or severe and may involve the respiratory tract, cardiovascular system, gastrointestinal tract, or skin (Table 14-8). Symptoms may progress in minutes from mild to severe, or severe reaction may occur without warning. Reactions may occur up to 2 hours after exposure. Reactions that occur immediately are the most life threatening. Resolution of symptoms may be immediate or take several days. Resolution depends on the severity of the reaction, the promptness of medical intervention, and any complications occurring during the reaction. Early recognition and rapid intervention may prevent progression to severe reactions.

Pathophysiology

On reexposure to antigen and its subsequent linkage with IgE antibody, mediator release occurs and affects the end organ responses (Table 14-9).

Almost any drug may precipitate an anaphylactic reaction. Subcutaneous, intramuscular, and intravenous routes provide sufficient antigen for overwhelming systemic reactions. Anaphylaxis produced by insect venom may account for more than 100 deaths annually. Foods may generate an anaphylactic reaction, particularly in adults, although this is not common. The following are some common antigens of anaphylaxis[47]:

- Drugs
  - Proteins (presumably complete antigens)
    - Foreign serum
    - Vaccines
    - Allergen extracts
    - Enzymes

Table 14-8
Potential Symptom Complex of Anaphylaxis

Target Organ	Mild	Moderate	Severe
General status (prodromal)	Malaise; sense of illness	Greater malaise and sense of illness	Deep malaise and strong sense of illness
Skin	Hives; erythema; tingling; warm sensation; itching	Generalized urticaria; flushing; generalized pruritus; periorbital edema	Cyanosis; pallor
Upper respiratory tract	Nasal congestion; sneezing; rhinorrhea; conjunctivitis	Profuse congestion and rhinorrhea	Periorbital edema; obligatory mouth breathing
Upper airway	Fullness in mouth or throat	Edema of tongue, larynx, and pharynx; hoarseness	Stridor; completely occluded airway
Lower airway	Cough	Bronchospasm; dyspnea; cough; wheezing; air trapping	Severe dyspnea; hypoxia; respiratory arrest
Gastrointestinal tract	Cramping	Nausea; vomiting; increased peristalsis	Dysphagia; intense abdominal cramping; diarrhea
Cardiovascular system	Tachycardia	Hypotension; syncope	Coronary insufficiency; cardiac arrhythmias; shock; circulatory collapse
Central nervous system	Anxiety	Intense anxiety; confusion	Seizures; coma

Table 14-9
Physiologic Response to Mediators

Mediator	Effect	End Organ Response
Histamine	Vascular permeability	Edema of larynx, gut, and airways; urticaria
Leukotrienes	Vascular smooth muscle relaxation	Decreased peripheral volume; decreased peripheral resistance
Kalikrein	Vasodilation and vascular engorgement	Decreased blood pressure; bronchospasm
Platelet-activating factor	Increased bronchial smooth muscle tone	Rhinorrhea; bronchorrhea
Others	Mucous gland secretion; irritability of peripheral nerve endings; intestinal smooth muscle tone	Pruritus; gut motility; rhinorrhea; bronchorrhea

- Nonprotein drugs (presumably haptens)
  - Penicillin and other antibiotics
  - Sulfonamides
  - Local anesthetics
  - Hormones
- Venoms
  - Hymenoptera (honeybee, wasp, hornet, yellow jacket)
  - Deerfly
  - Fire ant
- Foods
  - Legumes (especially peanuts)
  - Nuts
  - Berries
  - Seafood
  - Egg albumin

Diagnostic Studies and Findings

The diagnosis is based on a history of signs and symptoms of anaphylaxis immediately after exposure to a likely offending agent, as well as supportive laboratory data.

Complete Blood Count

Within normal limits or increased hematocrit value resulting from hemoconcentration

Blood Chemistries

Within normal limits unless myocardial or renal damage has occurred owing to circulatory collapse

Chest Roentgenogram

Normal appearance or hyperinflation with or without atelectasis; pulmonary edema

Electrocardiogram

Normal unless myocardial damage or hypoxemic changes are present

Skin Tests

Must be done at least 4 weeks after anaphylactic episode to ensure adequate repopulation of IgE antibody; requires extreme caution; usefulness limited to egg-based vaccines, venom, foods, horse serum, insulin, and penicillin

Medical Plan

The goal of the treatment plan is swift, aggressive management of symptoms. Establishment of an airway and maintenance of blood pressure are crucial. Therapy is individualized based on organ involvement and severity of reaction.

Medications

Medications used to counteract effects of mediator release, block additional mediator release, and protect organ system involved; continued until all symptoms have completely resolved; given over sufficient time to prevent further symptom development; withdrawn with careful monitoring

General Management

- Maintained until all symptoms of anaphylaxis are resolved
- Respiratory status
  - Airway maintained in position; suctioning as appropriate
  - Monitoring of laryngeal involvement
  - Airway patency maintained with endotracheal tube or tracheostomy if indicated
  - Arterial blood gas monitoring as indicated
  - Treatment of acidosis, if present; administration of oxygen if hypoxemic
  - Monitoring for bronchospasm, rales, and bronchorrhea by peak flow assessment and physical assessment, and treatment if present
  - Monitoring of pulmonary edema and treatment if present
- Vascular status—blood pressure maintained through volume replacement of vasopressors
- Renal status
  - Monitoring of urine output
  - Treatment of oliguria if present
- Cardiac status
  - Monitoring of electrocardiograms
  - Treatment of arrhythmias if present
- Mental status
  - Monitoring for orientation three times
  - Explanation of therapies
  - Monitoring for seizure activity and coma
- Avoidance of known offending agents mandatory
- Complete drug allergy history before administration of any new drug
- For patient with history of episodes, reemphasis on avoid-

ance of allergens and on labels listing allergy in appropriate places
Parenteral therapy avoided if possible
If parenteral therapy must be instituted, close monitoring needed for first 20 minutes
If parenteral therapy must be instituted, all emergency equipment must be ready to use
Human serum preparations preferred if antiserum indicated
If indicated, skin testing for vaccines, venoms, antivenoms, insulin, and penicillin
Use of pretreatment protocols and close monitoring required in the special circumstances when patients at risk must be exposed (to radiocontrast media, insulin, or penicillin)
Appropriate identification carried by patients at risk and information shared with significant others
Teaching self-administration of epinephrine and subsequent measures to take to patients at risk
Attempts to identify causative agent, and sharing of information with patient

NURSING CARE

Nursing Assessment

Because of multisystem involvement, anaphylactic or anaphylactoid reactions may initially have a variety of manifestations.

Laryngeal Involvement

Hoarseness; stridor; use of accessory muscles; difficulty in speech

Respiratory Status

Dyspnea; substernal tightness; use of accessory muscles; cough

Bronchospasm

Mucus production; rales; wheezing; decreased breath sounds; anxiety; inability to lie supine; evidence of air trapping or atelectasis on chest roentgenogram

Pulmonary Edema

Wet rales at base; frothy clear or blood-streaked secretions

Respiratory Arrest

No air movement

Circulatory Status

Hypotension; weak, thready pulse; tachycardia; oliguria; mental confusion

Cardiac Status

Arrhythmias; tachycardia; cardiac arrest

Central Nervous System Status

Anxiety; malaise; sense of illness; mental confusion; obtundation; coma

Dermal Status

Pruritus; erythema; flushing; urticaria; angioedema; cyanosis; pallor

Gastrointestinal Status

Nausea; vomiting; diarrhea; gastrointestinal cramping

Upper Respiratory Status

Rhinorrhea; congestion; sneezing; conjunctivitis; tearing

Nursing Dx & Intervention

Nursing Diagnosis	Nursing Intervention/Rationale
Ineffective breathing pattern	• In collaboration with physician, maintain airway patency; administer epinephrine, aminophylline, antihistamines, and oxygen; assess and document patient's response. Maintain endotracheal tube or tracheostomy if instituted. • Assess and record ventilation pattern, including rate, rhythm, use of accessory muscles, and length of expiratory phase. • Monitor for mouth breathing and rhinorrhea. • Maintain 45-degree elevation of patient's head if possible. • Assess for laryngeal involvement, including stridor, hoarseness, and difficulty in swallowing or speech.
Impaired gas exchange	• Monitor blood gases in collaboration with physician. • Administer oxygen at indicated rate. • Assess for presence of breath sounds including rales, rhonchi, cough, and wheezing. • Assess for shortness of breath, dyspnea, and substernal tightness. • Monitor fluid replacement and assess for pulmonary overload.
Ineffective airway clearance	• Suction if necessary.
Altered cerebral tissue perfusion	• Assess for symptoms of anxiety, confusion, obtundation, or coma. • In conjunction with physician administer fluid replacement.

Nursing Diagnosis	Nursing Intervention/Rationale
Altered renal tissue perfusion	• Monitor and record intake and output. • In conjunction with physician, administer epinephrine, vasopressors, or fluid as indicated.
Altered gastrointestinal tissue perfusion	• Monitor for nausea, vomiting, abdominal cramping, and diarrhea. Record findings. • In conjunction with physician administer antihistamines as indicated.
Altered peripheral tissue perfusion	• Monitor for cyanosis, pallor, and pulse abnormalities. Record findings. • In conjunction with physician, administer epinephrine, fluids, or vasopressors as indicated.
Altered cardiopulmonary tissue perfusion	• Monitor electrocardiogram for arrhythmias. • In conjunction with physician, administer epinephrine or antiarrhythmic agents as indicated.
Altered tissue perfusion (dermal)	• In conjunction with physician, administer epinephrine or antihistamines as indicated. • Assess for pruritus, erythema, flushing, angioedema, and urticaria. Record findings.
Potential for injury: anaphylaxis related to exposure to inciting agent	• Obtain complete drug allergy history before administering new drug. • Put labels noting allergic drug history in all appropriate places. • Closely monitor patient for 30 minutes after administering new drug. • Closely monitor patient for 20 minutes after administering drug subcutaneously, intramuscularly, or intravenously.

Patient Education

1. Reassure patient during procedures.
2. Explain reason for each procedure.
3. Explain relationship of symptoms to anaphylactic reaction.
4. Explain absolute necessity of avoiding causative agent.
5. Explain patient's responsibility in interactions with care givers.
6. Explain need to carry appropriate identification and to share information when necessary.
7. Provide information on medical alert identification.
8. Teach self-administration of epinephrine and subsequent measures, including oral administration of antihistamine and seeking immediate medical care.

Evaluation

Patient Outcome	Data Indicating That Outcome is Reached
Symptoms resolve in response to therapeutic measures.	Patient is symptom free. Patient expresses feeling of well-being. There is no evidence of urticaria or angioedema or subjective complaint of pruritus or swelling. There is no evidence of rhinoconjunctivitis, asthma, pulmonary edema, or laryngeal edema. Bowel sounds and elimination pattern are normal. Blood pressure and pulse rate are normal. There is no evidence of hypoxia.
Recurrence is prevented.	Patient can identify triggering agent and explain all appropriate avoidance measures.

Food allergy

Food allergy is an IgE-mediated hypersensitivity disease. It may be manifest in the respiratory, integumentary, or gastrointestinal system as rhinitis, asthma, atopic dermatitis, urticaria, nausea, vomiting, diarrhea, or cramps or may result in anaphylaxis. An adverse food reaction is any untoward symptom complex resulting from food ingestion.

Adverse reaction to food is a complex diagnostic problem. There are various causes for adverse food reactions. True food allergy is mediated by IgE antibody (type I hypersensitivity reaction) in sensitized individuals on exposure to the offending antigen. Antibody-antigen linkage occurs and results in mediator release and symptoms.

Food intolerance is any abnormal physiologic response to an ingested food or food additive that is nonimmunologic in nature. Other immunologic mechanisms have been identified in adverse food reactions, including IgA deficiency, cytotoxic responses (type II), immune complex formation (type III), and cell-mediated reactions (type IV). Adverse reactions to foods may have multiple origins, with a variety of nonimmunologic mechanisms resulting in a clinically abnormal host response. An idiosyncratic response in an individual may result in an anaphylactoid reaction, as with ingestion of monosodium glutamate. A metabolic defect such as lactose enzyme deficiency may cause foods to be improperly digested, or a metabolic problem such as diabetes may result in an abnormal response. Toxic responses to spoiled food are well known. Pharmacologic properties such as those of caffeine may exert a direct untoward effect. All these reactions are well documented and reproducible in controlled settings.

Other clinical syndromes are ascribed to foods or food additives, but this cannot be substantiated by reproducible, objective studies. While anecdotal evidence exists to support a relationship between food ingestion and behavior, other causal relationships have not been adequately ruled out. Tension-fatigue syndrome, hyperactivity syndrome, and psychiatric disorders such as mood swings are among the many disorders identified as being linked to food. Similar reports linking foods to rheumatoid arthritis or vasculitis and other physical syndromes also have not been substantiated. Other causes of vomiting, diarrhea, and stool abnormalities must also be excluded.

The prevalence of food allergy is unknown. Estimates range from 0.1% to 7% of the population, with a male/female ratio of approximately 2:1. If one sibling has a documented food allergy, a 50% probability of food hypersensitivity exists in other siblings. Anaphylactic episodes are most common in adults but may occur at any age. Non-immunologic-mediated adverse food reactions have a much higher prevalence than immunologic reactions.

In exquisitely sensitive persons merely inhaling the antigen in cooking odors can precipitate a massive allergic reaction. Reactions are often dose related and may vary with time in the same individual. The foods most commonly associated with allergic reactions are milk, eggs, wheat, and soybeans in children, and fish, shellfish, peanuts, nuts, and seeds in adults, although virtually any food may cause an allergic response. Families of foods may share allergenic features, and thus cross-reactivity among those foods (for example, shellfish) is more common. Because of absorption characteristics, the reaction may be immediate or delayed up to 2 hours after ingestion.

Pathophysiology

As with other antigen–IgE antibody–mediated responses, prior exposure with sensitization in the atopic individual must occur. On reexposure, antigen-antibody linkage occurs with resultant mediator release. For reasons unknown, one end organ may be affected with a localized response, as in urticaria, or loss of sensitivity may occur with time.

Why different individuals become sensitized to particular foods is also unknown. Allergenicity of the protein correlates with its heat-labile or enzyme-resistant properties. Although cooking or digestion may alter the protein, rendering it less allergenic, the altered protein may still precipitate an allergic response. An alteration in the original protein may contribute to false negative skin test findings if the unaltered food is used as the test antigen.

The gastrointestinal tract plays an important role in food allergy. The gut normally reaches maturity by 2 years of age. Before maturation there is a greater likelihood of absorption of food protein prior to complete digestion. Increase in absorption of potentially antigenic substances may also occur in IgA deficiency, malabsorption disease, and chronic inflammatory bowel diseases and after viral, parasitic, or bacterial diseases when the normal protective barriers have been damaged. These clinical syndromes may also contribute to adverse food reactions by decreasing normal flora, decreasing digestive enzymes, bile salts, and other secretions, reducing peristalsis, and interfering with cell renewal.

When the gut mucosal wall is damaged, protein may be absorbed and may precipitate IgE and IgG involvement or immune complex formation. Increased immunologic reactivity involving IgG and immune complex formation may result in enteropathies. Aspiration of milk in infancy may stimulate an IgE host defense response.

Genetic factors, amount of food ingested, food-drug interactions, contaminants, infections, pharmacologic properties, and nonimmunologic mechanisms have all been identified as contributing to adverse food reactions (Table 14-10).

Because of the multiple pathophysiologic mechanisms involved, clinical manifestations of adverse food reactions are widely variable (Table 14-10). Depending on the mechanism, amount, and duration of exposure, symptoms may vary from episodic to chronic and from mild to severe, and consequences may be reversible or irreversible.

Diagnostic Studies and Findings

Diagnostic studies are chosen based on the presentation of the adverse food reaction. The history is by far the most important diagnostic tool. The physical examination focuses on the clinical presentation.

Laboratory tests are chosen based on the suspected mechanism of the adverse food reaction. Cytotoxic testing, sublingual testing, and red blood cell lysis have no proven efficacy in diagnosis and should not be employed.

History

Frequency, duration and seasonality of symptoms; onset, severity, progression, and nature of symptoms; timing between ingestion and symptom onset; amount and nature of provoking food; concomitant illnesses; nutritional history; drug history; atopic history; infectious disease history

Physical Examination

Skin; upper and lower respiratory tract; gastrointestinal tract; oropharynx; weight and height; growth and development; general appearance; vital signs; muscle mass and amount of subcutaneous tissue; texture and amount of hair; hepatomegaly

Table 14-10
Adverse Reactions to Foods

Type	Mechanism	Food (Examples)	Host Response
Type I Hypersensitivity			
Food allergy	IgE antibody–antigen linkage	Shellfish; nuts	Urticaria; angioedema; rhinitis; bronchospasm; nausea; vomiting; diarrhea, anaphylaxis
Metabolic Reactions			
Enzyme deficiencies	Lactase deficiency	Milk	Bloating; diarrhea; cramps
	Glucose 6-phosphate dehydrogenase (G6-PD) deficiency	Fava beans	Hemolytic anemia
	Phenylketonuria	Nutrasweet	Central nervous system changes
Severe chronic inflammatory bowel disease	Loss of enzymes through diarrhea and decreased production	Saccharides	Bloating; diarrhea; cramps; malabsorption
Medication interactions	Monoamine oxidase inhibitors	Cheese	Hypertensive crisis
Celiac disease	Probable type IV reaction	Wheat	Bloating; diarrhea; malabsorption
Gallbladder disease	Decreased bile salts	Fats	Bloating; indigestion; diarrhea; cramping
Diabetes	Decreased insulin	Sugar	Hyperglycemia
Cystic fibrosis	Inadequate pancreatic function	Fats; proteins	Fatty, foul-smelling stools; malabsorption
Natural Pharmacologic Agents			
Psychoactive agents	Direct sympathetic stimulation	Caffeine; theobromine	Central nervous system stimulation
Vasoactive amines (e.g., tryptamine, tyramine)	Direct action on end organ or autonomic stimulation	Cheese; chocolate	Headaches
Food Contamination by Infectious Agents, Microbes, and Toxins			
Bacteria; viruses; parasites; fungi	Endotoxins; neurotoxins; toxic alkaloids; damage to gut wall	Contaminated foods	Nausea; vomiting; diarrhea; bloating; weight loss; liver dysfunctions; headaches; fever; chills
Natural Toxic Agents			
Licorice	Sodium retention	Licorice	Hypertension
Glycoalkaloids	Probable direct blood vessel effect	Green potatoes; lima beans	Angioedema; urticaria
Anaphylactoid Reactions			
Chemical mediator release	Direct action on mast cell	Strawberries; tomatoes	Urticaria; angioedema; diarrhea
Nonimmunologic	Unknown	Tartrazine (FD & C yellow #5)	Urticaria; angioedema; rhinitis; asthma
	Unknown	Sodium metabisulfite	Urticaria; angioedema; rhinitis; asthma; anaphylaxis
	Unknown	Monosodium glutamate	Headache; flush; asthma
Types II, III, and IV Hypersensitivity			
Immune complexes with food antigen	Complement activation	After acute viral gastroenteritis	Diarrhea; cramping
Weiner's syndrome	IgG-antigen complexes; also type IV reaction	Milk	Respiratory symptoms; failure to thrive
Enteropathies	IgG precipitating antibodies	Milk; soy	Gastrointestinal bleeding; malabsorption; diarrhea; cramping
IgA deficiency	Failure to regulate antigen absorption	Variable	Malnutrition; diarrhea; increased with severity of disease

Laboratory Tests

Type I hypersensitivity
- Skin tests
  - May have false positives or negatives; not diagnostic; must be used in conjunction with challenge tests
- Radioallergosorbent test (RAST)
  - May be less sensitive and has more limited panel than skin tests; may also have false positives or negatives; not diagnostic; must be used in conjunction with challenge tests
- Total serum IgE
  - Not specific indicator, not helpful
- Eosinophil count
  - Not specific indicator, not helpful
- Elimination diets
  - Aid in diagnosis by symptom response; used in conjunction with rechallenge; strict elimination diets difficult and cannot be used for more than 7 days
- Food rechallenge
  - Confirms diagnosis; not to be used if there is history of anaphylaxis

Types II, III, and IV hypersensitivity
- Biopsy of involved tissue
  - Demonstrates presence of IgG, IgM, complement activation, or T cell involvement
- Hemagglutination
  - May be present in persons without disease or absent in persons who have disease
- IgA deficiency
  - IgA level
    - Wide range of normal (80 to 350 mg/dl); may be low normal or depressed

Natural pharmacologic agents
- Diet diary and elimination diet
  - Correlates symptoms with suspected agents
- Food rechallenge
  - Confirms diagnosis

Food contamination by infectious agents
- Stool cultures
  - Document infectious agent

Natural toxic agents
- Diet diary and elimination diet
  - Correlate symptoms with suspected agent
- Food rechallenge
  - Confirms history

Anaphylactoid reactions
- Diet diary and elimination diet
  - Correlate symptoms with suspected agent
- Food rechallenge, unless systemic reaction
  - Confirms history

Metabolism
- Disease-specific workup (refer to discussion of specific disease elsewhere in text)

Medical Plan

The goal of the treatment plan is to eliminate the offending food, thus preventing recurrence of symptoms. Types I, II, III, and IV hypersensitivity, reactions to natural pharmacologic agents and natural toxic agents, and anaphylactoid reactions respond completely to elimination of the offending food.

Often symptoms are time limited and resolve without therapy. Choice of medications and supportive therapy are dependent on the nature and severity of symptoms, organ system involved, and mechanism of the reaction.

Medications

Based on severity and nature of symptoms, organ system involved, and mechanism of reaction (Table 14-11)

General Management

Based on nature and severity of symptoms and mechanism of adverse drug reaction; goal of supportive therapy is

Table 14-11
Medications Used in Treatment of Adverse Food Reactions

Mechanism	Potential Organ Involvement	Class of Medication
Type I hypersensitivity	Skin	Antihistamines
Anaphylactoid reactions	Upper respiratory tract	Sympathomimetic agents
Penicillin, drug contamination	Lower respiratory tract	Bronchodilators
Glycoalkaloids	Upper airway; gastrointestinal tract; multiorgan	Corticosteroids
Types II, III, and IV hypersensitivity (IgG-mediated, immune complex, and T cell sensitization, respectively)	Gastrointestinal tract	Topical or oral corticosteroids
	Skin; respiratory tract	Nonsteroidal anti-inflammatory agents
Infectious agents (bacterial, fungal, parasitic, viral)	Multisystemic response; gastrointestinal tract	Anti-infective agents
Metabolic reactions (enzyme deficiencies [cystic fibrosis], chronic inflammatory bowel disease)	Gastrointestinal malabsorption; protein-calorie deficiencies	Enzyme replacement; see specific therapy for disease process

to facilitate healing process; see elsewhere in text for further organ specific-supportive measures

For type I hypersensitivity, anaphylactoid reactions, drug contamination (IgE), glycoalkaloids, and types III and IV hypersensitivity
- See specific therapy for rhinitis, angioedema, and anaphylaxis
- Maintenance of appropriate elimination diet
- Monitoring for further symptom involvement
- High-caloric replacement therapy if needed
- Keeping affected skin dry and clear and preventing further injury
- Restriction of activity while symptoms are acute

For metabolic reactions
- See specific therapy for underlying disease process
- Maintenance of appropriate elimination diet
- Monitoring for further symptom development
- High-caloric replacement therapy as appropriate
- Restricted activity while symptoms are acute

For reactions to natural pharmacologic agents
- Restful, calm, quiet environment
- Restricted activity while symptoms are acute

For reactions to infectious agents
- See specific therapy for underlying disease process
- Analgesics if appropriate
- Adequate hydration
- Restricted food intake until gastrointestinal healing has occurred
- Restricted activity while symptoms are acute

Avoidance of known offending foods mandatory; patient should be taught relationship of foods to symptom development

For patient with history of atopic reaction, reemphasis on avoidance of agent and on labels warning of reaction posted in appropriate places

Emphasis on carrying appropriate identification and sharing information with significant others

For patients at risk, education about self-administration of epinephrine and subsequent measures to take

Patient education about self-monitoring of symptoms using cause-effect approach

Emphasis on patient's responsibility in interactions with care givers

Immunotherapy has no proven efficacy in food allergy

Breast feeding with some maternal dietary restriction and delay in introduction of new foods to prevent or minimize food allergy in infants

NURSING CARE

Nursing Assessment

Response to therapy is based on the underlying mechanism, degree, and length of exposure. The symptom complex may vary among individuals.

Type I Hypersensitivity, Anaphylactoid Reactions, Reactions to Glycoalkyloids

Laryngeal involvement
- Hoarseness; stridor; use of accessory muscles; difficulty in speech

Respiratory involvement
- Dyspnea; substernal tightness; use of accessory muscles; cough

Bronchospasm
- Mucus production; rhonchi; wheezing; decreased breath sounds; anxiety; inability to lie down; evidence of air trapping or atelectasis on chest roentgenogram

Dermal involvement
- Pruritus; erythema; flushing; urticaria; angioedema; cyanosis; pallor

Upper respiratory involvement
- Rhinorrhea; congestion; sneezing; tearing; conjunctivitis

Gastrointestinal involvement
- Nausea; vomiting; bloating; diarrhea; cramping; distention

Anaphylaxis
- All the above

Immunogenic (Type II [IgG], Type III [Circulating Immune Complexes], Type IV [T Cell Sensitization], IgA Deficiency)

Gastrointestinal involvement
- Nausea; vomiting; bloating; distention; diarrhea; cramping; gastrointestinal bleeding; malabsorption; failure to thrive; hepatomegaly

Dermal involvement
- Vasculitic lesion; contact dermatitis; hair thinning

Musculoskeletal involvement
- Muscle mass loss; subcutaneous tissue loss

See IgA deficiency assessment

Infective Agents

Gastrointestinal involvement
- Nausea; vomiting; bloating; distention; diarrhea; cramping; gastrointestinal bleeding; malabsorption

Systemic
- Fever; arthralgias; malaise

Reactions to Natural Pharmacologic Agents

Psychoactive agents
- Central nervous system stimulation
  - Palpitations; anxiety; tachycardia; irritability

Vasoactive amines
- Central nervous system
  - Vascular headaches; migraines

Metabolic Reactions (Cystic Fibrosis, Diabetes, Phenylketonuria, Glucose 6-Phosphate Dehydrogenase Deficiency, Chronic Inflammatory Bowel Disease, Celiac Disease, Gallbladder Disease)

See specific disease process
Gastrointestinal involvement
Nausea; vomiting; diarrhea; cramps; bloating; flatulence; fatty, foul-smelling stools; presence of occult blood in stool; failure to thrive; malnutrition; hepatomegaly; protuberant abdomen
Dermal involvement
Sparse hair; lanugo
Musculoskeletal
Loss of muscle mass; subcutaneous tissue

Nursing Dx & Intervention

The nursing diagnosis and interventions are based on the mechanism of the adverse food reaction and the severity of symptoms.

Nursing Diagnosis	Nursing Intervention/Rationale
Potential for injury	• Obtain complete history of adverse food reactions and put labels specifying history in appropriate places. • Maintain elimination diet. • Teach patient self-management behaviors.
Altered nutrition: less than body requirements (potential)	• Assess current dietary intake for caloric and nutritional requirements. • Teach alternative choices for balanced diet.
Diarrhea	• Monitor intake, output, and weight. • Assess for signs and symptoms of dehydration. • Assess for signs and symptoms of electrolyte imbalance. • Provide fluid supplementation. • Monitor stool for occult blood, character, and pathogens. • Provide adequate hygiene. • Monitor for further symptom development. • In conjunction with physician, administer medication as appropriate.
Activity intolerance	• Restrict activity during acute and convalescent phases.
Pain	• Assess for bloating or other symptoms. • Provide calm, quiet, restful environment. • Maintain hygiene and skin care. • In conjunction with physician, administer analgesics and other medications as needed.
Anxiety	• See general intervention strategies listed on p. 1743. • Teach patient self-care measures such as reading labels, alternative choices, and role in management of disease process.

Patient Education

1. Assess the patient's current knowledge of the disease process and reinforce the concept of self-care and self-management of the disease.
2. Explain that the disease is a chronic one, and reinforce the need to prevent symptoms through avoidance of foods that cause them.
3. Teach the patient the importance of monitoring the response of symptoms to therapies, recording any difficulties, new symptoms, and cause-effect relationships noted, and communicating this on an ongoing basis to those prescribing the therapies.
4. Emphasize the importance of carrying appropriate identification and sharing information with significant others.
5. For patients at risk of anaphylaxis, teach self-administration of epinephrine and subsequent measures to take.

Evaluation

Patient Outcome	Data Indicating That Outcome is Reached
Symptoms resolve in response to therapeutic measures.	Patient is symptom free.
Recurrences are prevented.	Patient can identify causative food and explain appropriate measures to avoid it.

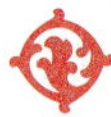

Drug allergy

An adverse drug reaction is any noxious or unintended effect of a drug. True drug allergy is mediated by IgE antibody–antigen interaction. Adverse reactions may also be mediated by other immunologic or nonimmunologic mechanisms.

Adverse drug reactions have steadily increased with the increase in available pharmacologic preparations. Drug allergy is one of the most common iatrogenic problems.

The incidence of adverse reactions is unknown. Three percent of hospitalizations are attributed to adverse drug reactions, and approximately 15% to 30% of hospitalized patients have an adverse drug reaction. Hospitalized patients sometimes receive 10 or more drugs, which obviously increases the risk of adverse drug reaction. The contribution of most additives or contaminants in adverse reactions is unclear, although idiosyncratic responses to tartrazine, sodium metabisulfite, and sodium benzoate have been well described.

Symptoms may affect any organ system of the body and may have a short or protracted course. Symptoms may range

Table 14-12
Adverse Drug Reactions

Reaction	Mechanism	Example
Non-Drug-Related (symptoms dissimilar to expected pharmacologic effects)		
Psychogenic	Vasovagal	Syncope; anxiety
Coincidental symptoms	Disease process itself	Viral rash with antibiotics
Drug-Related in Any Patient (symptoms similar to expected pharmacologic effects)		
Overdose	Increased intake, lowered metabolism, overdose, decreased liver excretion, toxic pharmacologic effect	Digoxin toxicity in elderly
Side effects	Undesirable pharmacologic effect of drug, often unavoidable with normal dose	Sleepiness with antihistamine
Secondary effects	Indirectly related to primary pharmacologic action	Vaginal infection after orally administered antibiotics
Drug interactions	Alter normal physiology of host, e.g., changes in absorption, metabolism, excretion; additive effects	Erythromycin changes liver metabolism and thus slows metabolism of theophylline
Disease-associated effects	Decreased absorption, metabolism, excretion; alteration in metabolic pathways	Digoxin toxicity
Drug-Related in Susceptible Patients (symptoms, except for intolerance, dissimilar to expected pharmacologic response)		
Intolerance	Quantitively greater effect at normal dosages	CNS excitation with pharmacologic dose of adrenergic drug
Idiosyncracy	Qualitatively abnormal response that is different from pharmacologic effects (nonimmunologic)	Adverse response to local anesthetics
Genetic	Lack of enzyme or metabolic pathway	Hemolytic anemic in G6-PD deficiency
Anaphylactoid	Nonimmunologic	Aspirin-induced bronchospasm
Allergy	IgE antigen-antibody	Penicillin allergy
Cytotoxic	Cytotoxic antibody-mediated against cell membranes with involvement of complement, IgG, and IgM	Coomb's test–positive hemolytic anemia
Immune complex	Drug-IgG, IgM-drug immune complexes, complement	Serum sickness, drug-induced lupus
Cell-mediated	T lymphocyte sensitization	Fixed drug eruption, photosensitivity eruptions

from mild to severe, and resolution of symptoms depends on the initiating mechanism, amount of drug, and host response.

Drug and host factors can influence the development of an adverse drug reaction:

Drug factors

- Nature of drug—class; weight; size; metabolites; ability to bind as hapten to protein (generally low molecular weight [500-1000])
- Route of administration—IV, IM, subcutaneous, oral, topical (in descending order of risk)
- Degree of exposure—prolonged course, high doses, and intermittent exposures increase risk; risk increases in first 2 to 3 weeks of therapy

Host factors

- Age—adult at greater risk than child, probably because of total exposures and greater need for drugs
- Sex—no difference except that women at greater risk with muscle relaxants and chymopapain
- Atopic history—no greater incidence but appears to be associated with more severe reactions
- Genetic—may contribute by influencing metabolic pathways or increased mediators
- Prior drug reactions—increased tendency with new drugs

Underlying disease state—may compromise immunologic mechanisms or alter metabolic pathways

Pathophysiology

Adverse drug reactions may be classified according to mechanism of reaction (Table 14-12).

Non-drug-related reactions of the psychogenic type generally occur only with fear of pain, as with the intramuscular or subcutaneous route of administration. Coincidental symptoms are more easily distinguished with knowledge of disease symptoms.

Adverse drug reactions that any patient may experience are the most common and most predictable. Overdosage results in toxic pharmacologic effects of the drug and occurs most commonly in pediatric or geriatric populations with dosage miscalculations or with failure to recognize concurrent drug or host factors that delay the metabolism and excretion of the drug.

Side effects vary among patients and with drugs. They are most commonly seen with drugs that directly or indirectly affect the central nervous system or gastrointestinal system.

Drug interactions are complex, and thoughtful analysis is required before administration of more than one drug. Drug interactions may potentiate, decrease, or negate the desired therapeutic effects and may place the patient at risk of overdose.

Disease-associated effects generally result in toxic overdose as a result of decreased metabolism or excretion. In gastrointestinal diseases, drugs may be poorly absorbed, resulting in lack of therapeutic response.

Intolerance is a common problem. Many patients exhibit increased side effects or gastrointestinal sensitivity to numerous drugs at normal doses.

Idiosyncratic responses of an anaphylactoid nature are nonimmunologic. Direct action on mast cells resulting in release of chemical mediators, prostaglandin activation, or IgG aggregation result in clinical symptoms similar to IgE antibody hypersensitivity. The following are some mechanisms of anaphylactoid reactions:

- Mast cell degranulation (for example, codeine, morphine, radiocontrast media)
- Prostaglandin-induced reactions (for example, dextran and other plasma expanders, aspirin, nonsteroidal anti-inflammatory agents, tartrazine)
- Immune complex aggregation (for example, intramuscular or intravenous γ-globulin)
- Cytotoxic antibody transfusion reactions (for example, mismatched blood transfusions)

In anaphylactoid reactions, prior exposure is not required, the host response may be variable over time, reactions can be produced with minute quantities, and the reaction resolves after the drug is discontinued.

Allergic, IgE antibody mechanisms account for a large proportion of adverse drug reactions because of the frequency with which drugs that fall in this category are prescribed. Some examples are penicillin and synthetic penicillins, sulfonamide antibiotics, sulfonylurea hypoglycemics, thiazide diuretics, carbonic anhydrase inhibitors, insulin and other hormones, egg-based vaccines, enzymes including chymopapain, antitoxins, and allergen extracts. The drug may act directly, it may bind with serum or tissue protein as a hapten, or a metabolite of the drug may be the offending antigen.

The allergic response requires prior exposure, can be reproduced by agents with cross-reacting structures, and can be produced by minute quantities. The reaction resolves after the drug is discontinued.

In cytotoxic or type II hypersensitivity, IgG or IgM antibody activates complement that results in damage to cell membranes. A drug may act as a hapten by binding to a cell surface, a drug-antibody complex may be absorbed to the cell surface, or a drug may change or modify a cell membrane leading to cell destruction.

In circulating immune complex or type III hypersensitivity, drug or drug hapten bound to protein may bind with antibody, forming circulating immune complexes.

In cell-mediated reactions or type IV hypersensitivity, T lymphocytes are sensitized, resulting in skin or organ damage. A drug may elicit symptoms through more than one mechanism, for example, penicillin allergy or serum sickness.

In allergic, cytotoxic, immune complex and cell-mediated reactions the evolution of symptoms often suggests an immunologic mechanism, although the exact mechanism may be impossible to establish and the diagnosis is commonly made on clinical grounds.

Certain medications have been associated with induction of antinuclear antibody (ANA). This may lead to a clinical picture of rashes or arthritis-like symptoms.

Diagnostic Studies and Findings

There are no simple, rapid, and predictable in vitro tests, nor is there safe and reliable in vivo testing for most adverse drug reactions. Demonstration of IgE antibody is limited to selected cases. No test is available for non-drug-related reactions, drug-related intolerance, or anaphylactoid adverse drug reactions. The clinical history is the most important tool in diagnosing adverse drug reactions.

Drug History

All drugs taken by patient within last 2 weeks, including over-the-counter preparations; time between exposure and symptom onset (delay of 7 to 10 days is common); route of administration and duration of treatment; prior drug exposure; onset, progression severity, and nature of symptoms; clinical course after drug is discontinued; concomitant diseases; infectious disease history

Skin Testing

Limited because of lack of knowledge of true antigen-inducing response; available only for penicillin, toxoids, antisera, insulin, ACTH, egg-based protein; must be done under strict protocol with close supervision

Patch Testing

Useful in diagnosing contact sensitivity to topical preparations only

Radioallergosorbent Test (RAST)

Not generally useful for drug allergy
Useful for chymopapain

Enzyme Assays

See specific enzyme deficiency disease, G6-PD

Eosinophil Levels

May be elevated in inflammatory tissue response

Anti-DNA (12%)

May be elevated (single stranded) in certain drug-induced reactions

Antinuclear Antibody (ANA) (1:20)

Speckled or homogeneous pattern

Complete Blood Count with Differential

Leukocytosis in serum sickness

Erythrocyte Sedimentation Rate

May be elevated in inflammatory tissue response

Direct Challenge

Can confirm suspected drug but is generally not done because of potential morbidity and mortality

Medical Plan

The goal of the treatment plan is to eliminate the offending drug and thus prevent further symptoms. Most symptoms respond quickly to removal of the offending drug and resolve without therapy. Choice of medications and supportive therapy is dependent on the nature and severity of symptoms, organ system involved, and mechanism of the reactions.

Medications

See Table 14-13.

General Management

Maintained until resolution of symptoms; see elsewhere in text for organ-specific therapy
Forcing fluids to increase renal clearance of drug
Plasmapheresis to remove circulating immune complexes
Hemodialysis or peritoneal dialysis in severe overdose to remove drug rapidly
Emesis or stomach lavage to remove drug in overdose
Patient with allergic drug reaction should not receive that drug or cross-reacting one, if possible
If drug must be given, informed consent and administration under strict protocol necessary
Always check history before administering a new drug

Table 14-13
Medications Used in Treatment of Adverse Drug Reactions

Mechanism	Potential Organ Involvement	Categories of Medications
Type I hypersensitivity, anaphylactoid reactions	Skin Upper and lower respiratory tract Upper airway Gastrointestinal tract	Antihistamines Sympathomimetic agents Bronchodilators Corticosteroids
Type II, cytotoxic	Gastrointestinal tract, skin	Rarely immunosuppressive agents, e.g., azothiaprine, cyclophosphamide, nonsteroidal anti-inflammatory agents
	Renal	Corticosteroids
	Hematologic	Oral corticosteroids
Type III, immune complex	Vascular, skin, kidney, heart, liver	Nonsteroidal anti-inflammatory agents
Type IV, cell mediated	Skin	Antihistamines, topical corticosteroids

NURSING CARE

Nursing Assessment

Adverse drug reactions have multiple mechanisms. Coincidental symptom assessment varies, since it is based on manifestations of the disease process. Drug-related reactions of overdose toxicity, side effects, intolerance, and secondary effects are related to specific drugs, and knowledge of the drug mechanism makes it possible to identify potential symptoms. In immunologic mechanisms, organ system involvement may also be variable. The reader is referred elsewhere in this text for specific organ assessment.

Type I Hypersensitivity, Anaphylactoid Reactions

See section on anaphylaxis

Type II, Cytotoxic

- Hematologic involvement
  - See assessment for hemolytic anemia, thrombocytopenia, agranulocytosis
- Renal involvement
  - See assessment for interstitial nephritis

Type III, Immune Complex

- Serum sickness
  - See serum sickness assessment
- Drug fever
  - Systemic
    - Low-grade fever, malaise
  - May be associated with serum sickness
    - See serum sickness assessment
  - Vasculitis
    - See vasculitis assessment
- Drug-induced lupus
  - See lupus assessment
- Vasculitis
  - See vasculitis assessment

Type IV, Cell Mediated

- Contact dermatitis
  - See assessment for contact dermatitis
- Photosensitivity eruptions
  - See assessment for photosensitivity eruptions

Nursing Dx & Intervention

Nursing interventions are based on the mechanism and the organ involved. The reader is referred to the discussion of the specific organ involved for the nursing diagnosis and nursing interventions.

Nursing Diagnosis	Nursing Intervention/Rationale
Potential for injury	• Obtain complete drug allergy history before administering new drug. • Put labels concerning allergic drug history in appropriate places. • Closely monitor patient for 30 minutes after administering new drug intramuscularly, subcutaneously, or intravenously. • Maintain emergency equipment and drugs. • Maintain high index of suspicion with patients receiving any medications. • Monitor patient for development of new symptoms during course of medication therapy and for 2 weeks after drug administration ends.
Activity intolerance	• Restrict activity level through acute and convalescent periods.
Anxiety	• Provide explanations of disease process and expected course of symptoms. See also p. 1743.

Patient Education

1. Explain the relationship of symptoms to the adverse drug reaction.
2. Explain the absolute necessity of avoiding use of the causative agent.
3. Explain the patient's responsibility in interactions with care givers.
4. Explain the need to carry appropriate identification and to share information when necessary.
5. Provide information on medical alert identification.

Evaluation

Patient Outcome	Data Indicating That Outcome is Reached
Symptoms resolve in response to therapeutic measures.	Patient is symptom free.
Recurrence is prevented.	Patient can identify causative drug and explain appropriate avoidance measures.

Angioedema (and urticaria)

Angioedema is soft tissue swelling in submucosal or subcutaneous tissues as the result of increased local vascular permeability and serum transudation. Urticarial lesions occur in the upper stratum corneum of the dermis, whereas angioedema lesions occur in the deeper subcutaneous tissues.

Urticaria (discussed in detail in Chapter 5) and angioedema have the same pathophysiologic features. Urticaria is more common; angioedema may be associated with urticaria or may occur independently. Why some patients have urticaria and others have angioedema is not known.

Angioedema may occur anywhere on the skin, but the periorbital area, lips, throat, tongue, larynx, area around joints, and tips of the extremities are the most common sites. Urticaria and angioedema may occur at any age, and as much as 20% of the population may be affected with acute, self-limited episodes. Episodes greater than 6 weeks in duration are defined as chronic. Symptoms may be mild or life threatening, and death may result from laryngeal involvement.

Pathophysiology

With antigen-antibody linkage, mast cell or basophil degranulation and chemical mediator release occur. Histamine and other mediators interact with receptors along the lymphatic, capillary, and venule walls, resulting in dilation, engorgement, and increased capillary permeability with a perivascular mononuclear cell infiltrate in which eosinophils may predominate. This inflammatory response usually resolves within 6

Table 14-14
Mechanisms of Angioedema

Mediator	Example	Proposed Mechanism
Immunologic		
Circulating immune complexes	Autoimmune phenomena	Activation of complement cascade
Cytotoxic antibodies	Transfusion reactions	Activation of complement cascade
Antigen-antibody complexes	Serum sickness reactions; malignancies	Activation of complement cascade
Drugs—directly or as haptens	Opiates; muscle relaxants; dextran	Direct mast cell degranulation
Foods—directly or as haptens	Tomatoes; strawberries; citrus fruits	Direct mast cell degranulation
Chemicals—directly or as haptens	Radiocontrast media; thiamine; bile salts	Direct mast cell degranulation
Drugs	Aspirin; indomethacin	Alteration of arachidonic acid metabolism
Chemical additives	Tartrazine	Alteration of arachidonic acid metabolism
Nonimmunologic		
Pressure	Tight garments; sitting	Unknown
Vibratory	Electric shavers; steering wheels	Unknown; autosomal dominant; genetically transmitted
Solar (five types)	Exposed areas	Unknown except for type IV, production of erythrocytic protoporphyria
Aquagenic	Water contact, regardless of temperature	Unknown
Heat	Direct contact	Unknown
Cholinergic	Heat exposure; emotional stress; vigorous exercise	Release of acetylcholine from cholinergic sympathetic nerve fibers
Cold	Delayed onset (30 minutes to 4 hours)	Autosomal dominant inheritance
	Exposed areas, immediate response	Unknown
	Associated with underlying disease	Presence of abnormal proteins with cold-dependent properties: cold hemoglobins, cryofibrinogens, cold agglutinins, cryoglobulins

hours after insult, although in soft tissues nonpitting edema may be more diffuse and reabsorption of fluid may take up to several days. Complaints of burning pain or tightness are more commonly associated with angioedema than is pruritus.

Other immunologic mechanisms may precipitate the same pathophysiologic response.

Physical or environmental factors may also trigger or exacerbate urticaria and angioedema (Table 14-14). In addition, urticaria and angioedema may occur in different disease states (Table 14-15). In as many as 60% of cases, no causative agent can be identified.

Diagnostic Studies and Findings

History

Exceptionally important: onset; distribution; aggravating and ameliorating factors; time sequencing; food history; past, current, and infective history; contactant or insect exposures; family and atopic history; occupational, hobby, and environmental history; travel

Drug History

Any medications, including over-the-counter and oral contraceptive preparations, may precipitate urticaria and angioedema

Table 14-15
Diseases Association with Angioedema

Type	Proposed Mechanisms
Systemic mastocytosis	Accumulation of mast cells that spontaneously or easily degranulate in dermis, bone marrow, and gastrointestinal tract
Infections: viral parasitic (infectious mononucleosis, hepatitis), rarely bacterial	Circulating antigen-antibody complexes with activation of complement cascade
Endocrinopathies: hyperthyroidism, pregnancy, menses	Unknown
Hereditary angioedema	Autosomal dominant, genetically inherited deficiency or malfunction of C1 esterase inhibitor with activation of complement cascade
Malignancies	In addition to antigen-antibody complexes, interference with C1 esterase inhibitor and resultant activation of complement cascade
Psychogenic	Rarely primary but may be exacerbating factor through hormonal and neural secretory mediators

Clinical Examination

All areas of potential involvement: periorbit, oropharynx, joints, tips of extremities

Tests

See Table 14-16

Table 14-16
Diagnostic Tests for Urticaria and Angioedema

Condition Suspected	Test*
Atopic: food or drug (inhalant or contactant) sensitivity	Elimination of offending agent; daily symptom diary; challenge with suspected foods; skin tests to food or selected drugs; total serum IgE determination; eosinophil count; skin tests or radioallergosorbent tests of suspected antigens
Cutaneous vasculitis or systemic collagen vascular disease	Immunoglobulin analysis; antinuclear antibody; rheumatoid factor; cryoglobulins; cryofibrinogens; complete complement profile; skin biopsy with immunofluorescence
Hereditary angioedema	C4; C2; C3; total hemolytic complement (CH50); C1-esterase inhibitor (immunochemical and functional assays)
Physical urticaria	
Dermatographia	Firm stroke on skin with tongue blade
Cold	Ice cube test; cryoglobulins; cryofibrinogens; VDRL test
Cholinergic urticaria	Exercise challenge; methacholine skin test
Solar urticaria	Exposure to various wavelengths of light; protoporphyrin and coproporphyrin determinations
Pressure urticaria and angioedema	Application of pressure with weights for 10 minutes
Vibratory angioedema	Vibratory stimulation of skin for 4 minutes
Aquagenic urticaria	Tap-water challenge at various temperatures
Infections	Appropriate cultures and x-rays; stool for ova and parasites; hepatitis B antigen and antibody
Urticaria pigmentosa	Test for dermatographia; skin biopsy
Malignancy with angioedema	Total hemolytic complement (CH50); C1; C1-esterase inhibitor
Idiopathic urticaria	Skin biopsy with immunofluorescence

From Fineman, S.: Urticaria and angioedema. In Lawlor, G.J., et al., editors: Manual of allergy and immunology. Copyright 1981 by Little, Brown & Co., p. 210. Used with permission of Little, Brown & Co.
*General screening consists of complete blood count, urinalysis, and erythrocyte sedimentation rate determination.

Medical Plan

The goal of the treatment plan is to prevent symptoms of angioedema. Obviously, with removal of the causative agent, no further therapy is necessary.

Medications

Unless symptoms are mild and sporadic, regular medication therapy is advised. Antihistamines are the drugs of choice. If there is lack of clinical efficacy within one class of antihistamines, response may be obtained from alternatives within the other four classes. Long-acting preparations require less frequent doses. The physician dictates the specific drug protocol. In hereditary angioedema, in addition to treatment of existing symptoms, certain drugs are used to prevent symptoms or treat acute symptoms.

Drugs Used in Hereditary Angioedema

- Hormones
  - Danazol (Danocrine), 200 mg tid; androgen derivative; contraindicated in children and pregnancy
- Hemostatic agents
  - Aminocaproic acid, 3.5 mg qid for adults; antifibrinolytic agent, plasminogen inhibitor
- Tranexamic acid, 1 g tid for adults before dental procedures etc.
- Blood products
  - Fresh-frozen plasma during acute attacks

Drugs Used in Urticaria and Angioedema

- Antihistamines*
  - Cyproheptadine (Periactin), 4-8 mg po q6h
  - Chlorpheniramine (Chlor-Trimeton), 2 mg/kg/24 h po in 4 divided doses
  - Clemastine (Tavist), 1.34 or 2.68 mg po q8-12h
  - Diphenhydramine (Benadryl), 25-100 mg po q6h or 5 mg/kg/d
  - Doxepin (Sinequan), 10-30 mg po q8-12h
- Histamine receptor antagonists*
  - Cimetidine (Tagamet), 300 mg po q6h
  - Ranitidine (Zantac), 150 mg po q12h
  - Famotidine (Pepcid), 20 mg po q12h
  - Hydroxyzine (Atarax), 25 mg po q6h to maximum total of 400 mg
- Adrenergic agents
  - Appear to be of limited value in long-term therapy but may be employed for control of acute symptoms
  - Epinephrine
    - Aqueous (Adrenalin), 0.2-0.3 ml subcutaneously q30 min or 0.01 mg/kg
    - Long-acting (Sus-Phrine), 0.1-0.3 ml subcutaneously q4-6h or 0.005 mg/kg (maximum dose 0.15 ml)
  - Ephedrine (Bronkaid), 20-50 mg q4h or 3 mg/kg/24 h in 4 divided doses

*Available in syrup form; dosage calculated by patient's weight.

- Corticosteroids
  - May be used if symptoms are unresponsive to above therapy but should be limited to lowest possible dose and alternate-day therapy with monitoring of side effects
  - Prednisone (Deltasone, Orasone, Liquid Pred), 2 mg/kg/d up to 100 mg
- Topical agents
  - Sun blockers with sun protection factor of at least 15 (Total Eclipse [15-18], Super Shade [15], Coppertone [15], Pre Sun [20]); used to block ultraviolet light in solar urticaria
  - Mild analgesics for pain associated with swelling

General Management

- Cool compresses to reduce periorbital edema
- Support for involved joints as necessary
- Restricted activity during acute episodes
- Monitoring for full response to medication therapy
- Monitoring to prevent further progression of symptoms
- Avoidance of physical or environmental agents and food or chemical additives
- Endotracheal tube placement or tracheostomy for extensive laryngeal involvement

NURSING CARE

Nursing Assessment

Because angioedema may have multiorgan involvement, careful assessment should be made of all potential organ systems.

Laryngeal Involvement

Hoarseness; stridor; use of accessory muscles; difficulty in speech

Dermal Status

Concurrent urticaria

Ocular Status

Periorbital edema

Gastrointestinal Status

Nausea; vomiting; diarrhea; gastrointestinal swelling

Oropharyngeal Status

Swelling of lip, tongue, and uvula

Articular Status

Swelling at tips of extremities, in soft tissue, and around joints

Nursing Dx & Intervention

Nursing Diagnosis	Nursing Intervention/Rationale
Ineffective breathing pattern	• Maintain endotracheal tube or tracheostomy if instituted. • In collaboration with physician, administer appropriate medications and assess and record patient's response. • Assess and record ventilation pattern including rate, rhythm, and use of accessory muscles. • Assess for presence of laryngeal involvement, including stridor, hoarseness, and difficulty in speech or swallowing. Record if present.
Altered gastrointestinal tissue perfusion	• In collaboration with physician, administer appropriate medications as indicated. • Assess for presence of nausea, vomiting, abdominal cramping, and diarrhea. Record if necessary.
Altered peripheral tissue perfusion	• In collaboration with physician, administer appropriate medications as indicated. • Assess and record involvement in periauricular areas and tips of extremities.
Potential for injury	• Obtain complete history of drug allergies before administering new drug. • Put labels indicating allergic drug history in all appropriate places. • Closely monitor patient for 30 minutes after administering each new drug.

Patient Education

1. Explain to the patient the relationship between symptoms and exposure to the causative agent.
2. Explain the necessity of avoiding use of the causative agent.
3. Explain the patient's responsibility in interactions with health care givers.
4. Explain the need, if appropriate, to carry appropriate identification and to share information when necessary.
5. Provide information on medical alert identification.
6. Teach self-administration, if appropriate, of epinephrine and subsequent measures including oral administration of antihistamine and seeking immediate medical care.

Evaluation

Patient Outcome	Data Indicating That Outcome is Reached
Symptoms resolve in response to therapeutic measures.	Patient is symptom free, with no evidence of soft tissue swelling, joint restriction or subjective feelings of tightness or swelling, hoarseness, or difficulty in swallowing, speech, or air movement. Bowel sounds and elimination pattern are normal.
Recurrence of symptoms is prevented.	Patient can identify triggering agent and explain appropriate avoidance measures. Patient can identify appropriate medications to use, dosage, and length of therapy if symptoms occur. Patient can identify nondrug therapeutic measures to institute if symptoms occur.

Medical Interventions and Related Nursing Care

Bone Marrow Transplantation

Description and Rationale

Bone marrow transplantation (BMT) is the treatment of choice for patients with severe aplastic anemia who are younger than 40 years of age and have a compatible donor. Marrow transplantation is also a treatment modality for severe immunodeficiency disorders, and recently it has been used with increasing success in the treatment of patients with leukemia, lymphoma, and selected solid tumors.

Bone marrow is harvested in the operating room with the donor under general or spinal anesthesia. Multiple aspirations from the posterior iliac crests are performed; if necessary the anterior iliac crests and sternum may be used. A small volume of bone marrow is collected with each aspiration and placed into tissue culture medium containing heparin. This solution is filtered through stainless steel screens to remove bone chips, fat globules, and clots and then is transferred to a blood transfusion bag.

The amount of bone marrow aspirated depends on a number of factors: the donor's weight, the concentration of cells in donated marrow, and the processing procedure employed before the marrow is transfused. If no special processing is done, the volume of marrow obtained is approximately 10 to 15 ml/kg of the recipient's body weight. In the typical adult a volume of 500 to 750 ml of blood and marrow contains 10 to 20 $\times$ 10^9 nucleated marrow cells.[52]

After harvesting, the marrow is either administered intravenously to the recipient through a central venous access device such as a Hickman or Raaf catheter or is cryopreserved and stored for future use. In the latter case, which occurs only with autologous bone marrow transplantation, the harvested marrow may be treated before cryopreservation to eliminate any occult tumor cells that may be present, especially in lymphohemopoietic malignancies. Ex vivo treatment with 4-hydroperoxyclophosphamide (4-HC), an analog of cyclophosphamide, is one method used to treat the marrow. More recently, immunologic approaches using monoclonal antibodies are being tested in clinical trials for diseases such as T cell lymphoma and common acute lymphocytic leukemia (ALL).

Until recently most marrow transplants have involved donors of two types, an identical twin or an HLA-matched, mixed lymphocyte culture (MLC)–compatible sibling. A syngeneic transplant, using marrow from an identical twin, is ideal because the donor is matched with the recipient at all genetic loci.

Transplantation using marrow from anyone other than an identical twin or the patient himself is called an allogeneic transplant. In most allogeneic bone marrow transplants a sibling who matches at HLA-A, -B, -C, and -D loci is the donor. The HLA loci are on a small chromosomal region, and these loci are usually inherited as a unit known as a haplotype. Each parent has two haplotypes, and a child inherits one haplotype from each parent. A 25% probability exists that two siblings will be HLA identical.

A partially matched donor (such as a sibling, parent, or uncle) may be selected when no HLA-identical sibling is available, or an HLA-identical unrelated donor may be used. Preliminary reports using partially matched donors are encouraging, but further investigation in this area is needed.

A third form of bone marrow transplantation, the autologous graft, involves use of the patient's own marrow. As with the identical twin situation, in this circumstance no clinically significant graft-versus-host disease will occur. However, with autologous grafts, tumor cells may be present in marrow harvested during remission; therefore attempts to purge marrow of occult tumor cells before cryopreservation are being investigated. Autologous bone marrow transplants are experimental and are indicated only when a genetically identical donor is not available.

The rationale for bone marrow transplantation is to replace defective or missing host hemopoietic stem cells with healthy stem cells. In the treatment of neoplasm the transplant is done after therapy designed to rid the patient of the tumor. The patient's normal bone marrow is destroyed with high-dose therapy, and the transplant is designed to repopulate the patient's hemopoietic system.

Graft-Versus-Host Disease

Graft-versus-host disease (GVHD) presumably results from the attack of host tissue by immunocompetent donor T lymphocytes. In acute cases the peak onset occurs 30 to 50 days after the transplant.[34] In chronic cases the onset occurs 100 days after the transplant.[50] Tables 14-17 and 14-18 give two systems for the clinical staging of GVHD.

Conditioning Regimen

Pretransplant conditioning regimens include high-dose chemotherapy with or without radiotherapy. The purposes of conditioning are to eliminate defective stem cells, to provide immunosuppression to minimize the possibility of rejection, and to eliminate any residual malignant cells.

The conditioning regimen used before bone marrow trans-

Table 14-17
Proposed Clinical Stage of Graft-Versus-Host Disease According to Organ System

Stage	Skin	Liver	Intestinal Tract
+	Maculopapular rash over 25% of body surface	Bilirubin 2-3 mg/dl	Greater than 500 ml diarrhea/day
+ +	Maculopapular rash over 25%-50% of body surface	Bilirubin 3-6 mg/dl	Greater than 1000 ml diarrhea/day
+ + +	Generalized erythroderma	Bilirubin 6-15 mg/dl	Greater than 1500 ml diarrhea/day
+ + + +	Generalized erythroderma with bullous formation and desquamation	Bilirubin greater than 15 mg/dl	Severe abdominal pain with or without ileus

From Thomas, E.D. Reprinted by permission of the New England Journal of Medicine 292:896, 1975.

plantation varies depending on the disease being treated. The use of multiple-day chemotherapy (with cyclophosphamide, busulfan, or other agents) may or may not be preceded or followed by local or total body irradiation (TBI).

In the case of leukemias or lymphomas, intrathecal methotrexate (approximately 10 mg/m^2) is given for central nervous system prophylaxis before transplantation.

With allogeneic transplants, prophylaxis for graft-versus-host disease includes additional treatment with agents such as methotrexate and cyclosporine A (dosage and route of administration vary). Use of cyclosporine A may continue for several months after marrow transplantation.

The following is an example of a schedule using cyclophosphamide and TBI conditioning. Days before transplant are indicated by negative numbers, with day 0 being the day of transplant.

Monday	Day − 8	Admission
Tuesday	Day − 7	Cyclophosphamide
Wednesday	Day − 6	Cyclophosphamide
Thursday	Day − 5	Rest
Friday	Day − 4	TBI
Saturday	Day − 3	TBI
Sunday	Day − 2	TBI
Monday	Day − 1	TBI
Tuesday	0	Bone marrow infusion

Preprocedural Nursing Care

Immediate concerns are related to the conditioning regimen using chemoradiotherapy. The patient, family, donor, and significant others are instructed on the procedure, its course, and complications.

Radiation. Dosage varies, in general from 800 to 1200 rad. For example, 1000 rad may be given in fractionated doses (250 rad per day). Single-dose whole body irradiation may be used. Typical side effects include nausea, vomiting, diarrhea, erythema of the skin, and parotitis. These side effects are usually of short duration when moderate fractionated radiotherapy is used. With the exception of erythema of the skin, they usually resolve within 7 days.

Cyclophosphamide. Nausea and vomiting may occur 6 to 8 hours after administration of cyclophosphamide and may last 8 to 10 hours. The drug may cause hemorrhagic cystitis in the bladder. Uric acid is released as cells are destroyed, resulting in deposition and accumulation of uric acid crystals in the kidney. Cardiotoxicity is a further problem with cyclophosphamide.

Table 14-18
Overall Clinical Grading of Severity of Graft-Versus-Host Disease

Grade	Degree of Organ Involvement
I	+ to + + skin rash; no gut involvement; no liver involvement; no decrease in clinical performance
II	+ to + + + skin rash; + gut involvement or + liver involvement (or both); mild decrease in clinical performance
III	+ + to + + + skin rash; + + to + + + gut involvement or + + to + + + + liver involvement (or both); marked decrease in clinical performance
IV	Similar to grade III with + + to + + + + organ involvement and extreme decrease in clinical performance

From Thomas, E.D. Reprinted by permission of the New England Journal of Medicine 292:896, 1975.

Medical Plan

Infusion of bone marrow is used to restore defective or missing stem cells. For autologous marrow, blood bags containing approximately 50 ml of cryopreserved marrow are thawed quickly, one at a time, in a basin of warm water at approximately 100° F. The contents of the blood bag are removed using a 50 ml syringe with a 16-gauge needle and then administered rapidly through a central line (double-lumen Raaf catheter or Hickman catheter). A solution of 0.9 normal saline is infused during the procedure. Epinephrine, diphenhydramine, and hydrocortisone are kept at the bedside.

For a syngeneic or allogeneic donation, a standard-type blood bag containing fresh bone marrow just obtained from a donor is transported from the operating room. The donated marrow is administered slowly (over a period of 4 hours) through a Raaf catheter without a filter.

NURSING CARE

Nursing Assessment

Fluid Overload

Increased respiratory rate; dyspnea; rales; rhonchi

Micropulmonary Emboli

Shortness of breath; chest pain; increased heart rate

Reaction to White Cells in Marrow

Chills; fever; urticaria; chest pain

Hematuria

Hemastix-positive urine normal for first 24 hours after bone marrow transplant

Bacterial Contamination of Marrow

Hypotension; fever; shaking chills

Engraftment

No evidence of hematologic recovery 2 to 4 weeks after bone marrow transplant

Infection

Fever; pain; redness; swelling of any site; wound drainage; cough; dyspnea; sore throat; headache; dysuria; frequency; urgency; positive blood culture findings; change in mental status

Anemia

Decreased red blood cell count, hematocrit, and hemoglobin level; excessive fatigue

Stomatitis

Oral soreness; dryness; burning or tingling; taste changes; erythema; ulcerations or patches on oral mucosa

Thrombocytopenia

Petechiae; purpura; bleeding from any body orifice or site of catheter; hemoptysis; hematemesis; hematuria; hematochezia; seizures; change in mental status

Nutritional Status

Anorexia; decreased weight; nausea; vomiting; diarrhea

Psychosocial Status

Anger; depression; frustration; anxiety

Graft-Versus-Host Disease (GVHD)

Mild maculopapular rash; generalized erythroderma with desquamation; increase in serum bilirubin, serum glutamic oxaloacetic transaminase (SGOT), or alkaline phosphatase; abdominal cramping; diarrhea (green, watery); hematochezia

Veno-Occlusive Disease (VOD)

Sudden weight gain; right upper quadrant pain; jaundice; hepatomegaly; ascites; encephalopathy

Nursing Dx & Intervention

Nursing Diagnosis	Nursing Intervention/Rationale
Altered nutrition: less than body requirements related to nausea and vomiting from chemoradiotherapy	• Administer antiemetic drug before treatment and at frequent intervals after treatment as ordered. Choice of drug is largely empiric. Drugs should be administered intravenously. • Consider use of behavioral relaxation techniques. • Provide frequent oral hygiene. • Instruct patient to avoid quick movements while nauseated. • Encourage patient to eat or drink when not nauseated regardless of the time. • Encourage patient to eat slowly and chew thoroughly. • Suggest high-protein, high-calorie diet. • Suggest small, frequent, low-fat meals. • Encourage patient to drink liquids (clear, cool beverages or soups) slowly through a straw before, not during, meals. • Provide patient with beverages or foods that may curb nausea: carbonated beverages such as cola or ginger ale; dry crackers or toast; tart foods such as lemons or sour pickles; ice pops and gelatin desserts. • Instruct patient to avoid favorite foods during periods of nausea. • Instruct patient to avoid lying flat for at least 1 hour after eating.
Hyperthermia	• Maintain adequate hydration. • Administer antipyretics as ordered. • Inform patient that fever usually disappears in 4 to 6 days following total body irradiation.
Pain related to parotitis	• Encourage increased fluid intake. • Encourage frequent oral hygiene. • If xerostomia is present, suggest hard candies, sugarless gums, or commercial product such as Xero-Lube. • Avoid use of irritants such as alcohol or tobacco. • Use measures for oral pain according to physician's order; narcotic analgesics may be required.
Diarrhea related to effects of total body irradiation on gastrointestinal mucosa	• Administer antidiarrheal agents as ordered. • Maintain adequate hydration. • Suggest bland, low-residue diet that is high in potassium. • Instruct patient in meticulous perianal skin care. • Apply soothing lubricant to perianal area after each bowel movement.
Potential impaired skin integrity related to erythema of skin	• Instruct patient to keep skin clean and dry. Use mild soap such as Dove or Dial for bathing, rinse skin well, and pat dry. • Avoid use of perfumed powders or lotions. • Avoid extremes of temperature to skin, that is, hot or cold baths, ice packs, and heating pads. • Avoid pressure from constricting clothing.

Nursing Diagnosis	Nursing Intervention/Rationale
Altered bladder tissue perfusion (hemorrhagic cystitis related to local effect of cyclophosphamide)	• Begin intravenous hydration 4 hours before cyclophosphamide administration and continue for 24 hours after therapy. Intravenous fluids should be administered 1½ to 2 times maintenance rates. • Perform continuous bladder irrigations using three-way Foley catheter if ordered. If patient can void every hour to eliminate toxic products of cyclophosphamide that irritate bladder lining, catheter is unnecessary. • Monitor urine for blood every 4 hours. • Maintain accurate intake and output records.
Altered renal tissue perfusion	• As above, administer hydration fluids. • Check urine output hourly. • Administer furosemide as ordered. • Check urine pH every 4 hours; maintain at or above 7.0. • Administer sodium bicarbonate as ordered. • Administer allopurinol as ordered, if needed. Allopurinol may increase incidence and degree of bone marrow suppression by prolonging half-life of cyclophosphamide.
Decreased cardiac output (potential) related to cardiotoxicity	• Check results of electrocardiogram (ECG) for decreased voltage. (ECG is taken daily while patient is treated with high-dose cyclophosphamide.)
Potential for infection related to leukopenia	• Maintain protective environment. (Reverse isolation protocols vary among centers from simple protective isolation to sterile laminar airflow rooms.) • Monitor white blood cell count and absolute granulocyte count daily. • Monitor vital signs every 4 hours. • Check skin and mucous membranes. • Inspect all body orifices daily *for redness, swelling, and pain.* • Auscultate lungs every 8 hours *for increased or decreased breath sounds, rhonchi, and rales.* • Inspect site of insertion of venous access device for redness, swelling, and pain. • Assess patient for complaints of dysuria and frequency. • Note any change from patient's baseline vital signs, behavior, or appearance. • Encourage turning, coughing, and deep breathing exercises. • Maintain integrity of skin and mucous membranes. (Skin care measures vary among centers from use of povidone-iodine to use of antibacterial soap.) • Maintain meticulous mouth care. (Mouth care varies among centers). • Use strict aseptic technique when changing dressings. • Use strict aseptic technique in intravenous preparation and administration. • Avoid bladder catheterization. • Avoid administering enemas and suppositories and taking rectal temperatures. • Encourage patient to use deodorant rather than antiperspirant. (Axillary sweat glands are blocked by antiperspirants, which may promote infection.) • Obtain surveillance cultures of throat, urine, stool, skin, and other areas as ordered. (Need for surveillance cultures to detect colonization before infection is controversial.) • Maintain dietary restrictions as ordered. (Efficacy of low-bacteria diets has not been established.) • Eliminate stagnant water in patient's room. • Do not allow fresh-cut flowers or plants in patient's room. • Limit number of visitors, and screen them for infection, recent vaccinations, or exposure to communicable diseases. • Provide mask, gloves, and gown for patient when patient leaves room. • Obtain culture and sensitivity tests and Gram's stain of all potential sites of infection per physician's order. • Administer antibiotics on schedule per physician's order. • Monitor vital signs every 4 hours. (Subtle changes may be early sign of septic shock.) • Control fever with tepid sponge baths and acetaminophen. • Maintain adequate hydration of patient.
Patient problem: hemorrhage related to thrombocytopenia	• Monitor platelet count regularly. Risk of bleeding is high when platelet count is less than 10,000 cells/mm^3. • Inspect skin and mucous membranes daily. Monitor for increased bruising tendencies, petechiae, bleeding gums, and epistaxis. • Test stool, urine, and emesis for occult blood. • Note any changes in patient's vital signs or behavior. Changes may indicate intracranial hemorrhage.

Nursing Diagnosis	Nursing Intervention/Rationale
	• After invasive procedures such as bone marrow aspiration and biopsy, monitor site frequently for any oozing of blood. • Avoid giving intramuscular or subcutaneous injections. • Avoid taking rectal temperatures and administering rectal suppositories and enemas. • Encourage adequate fluid intake and use of stool softener to prevent constipation and straining. • Avoid invasive procedures. • Place sign indicating bleeding precautions over patient's bed. • Administer medroxyprogesterone acetate as ordered to control menses. • Instruct patient to avoid cutting, bruising, or bumping self. Eliminate sharp objects in environment. • Instruct patient to use electric razor rather than hand razor. • Instruct patient to wear shoes or slippers—no bare feet while walking. • Instruct patient to use soft-bristled toothbrush. If platelet count is less than 20,000/mm^3, use toothette rather than a toothbrush. • Flossing may be contraindicated. Instruct patient to discontinue if bleeding occurs. • Instruct patient to avoid use of toothpicks. • Discourage patient from having elective dental work. • Teach patient to avoid use of aspirin and products containing aspirin. • Teach patient to avoid use of all beverages containing alcohol. • Instruct patient to avoid blowing the nose forcefully or sneezing forcefully. • If epistaxis occurs, keep patient in sitting position. Application of ice helps to constrict small vessels. Local application of pressure may control bleeding. Nasal packing may be indicated if these measures fail. • Apply topical agents such as thrombin, aminocaproic acid, cocaine, or Gelfoam to bleeding sites per physician's order. • Bleeding in oral cavity may be controlled with iced saline mouth rinses. • Administer irradiated platelet transfusions rapidly as ordered. (Families are encouraged to find donors for blood products.) Monitor posttransfusion platelet counts.
Activity intolerance related to anemia, inadequate nutritional status, disruption of sleep, anxiety, or depression	• Administer irradiated red blood cell transfusions as ordered. • Monitor hemoglobin levels and hematocrit values regularly. • Maintain optimal nutritional status. • Arrange nursing care so patient has uninterrupted periods of rest and sleep, especially during the night. • Encourage progressive activity program as tolerated. • Encourage patient to verbalize feelings and concerns. • Explain reasons for fatigue.
Altered oral mucous membrane related to conditioning regimen or infection	• Implement nursing care for stomatitis based on assessment using grading system developed by Capizzi[12]: Grade 1—generalized erythema of oral mucosa Grade 2—isolated small ulcerations or white patches Grade 3—confluent ulcerations with white patches covering more than 25% of oral mucosa Grade 4—hemorrhagic ulcerations • For grade 1 or 2 stomatitis: 1. Perform oral hygiene regimen every 2 hours while awake and every 6 hours during night, as follows: a. Use normal saline mouthwash if crusts are absent. (One teaspoon of salt in 1 L of sterile water may be used.) If crusts and debris are present, use *either* one part hydrogen peroxide* diluted† with three parts water‡ *or* sodium bicarbonate solution (1 teaspoon mixed in 8 ounces of water.‡). Perform mouth care every 2 hours while patient is awake. Alternate *either* hydrogen peroxide or bicarbonate solution with normal saline. Rinse with normal saline after the use of either. b. Floss gently with unwaxed dental floss every 24 hours; discontinue if bleeding occurs. c. Brush using soft toothbrush and nonabrasive toothpaste, such as Colgate, after each meal and before sleep. d. Removes dentures or partial plates. Replace only for meals. e. Apply lip lubricant such as Vaseline, Blistex, or K-Y Jelly four times a day and as needed.

*Hydrogen peroxide should not be used if the patient has fresh granulation tissue.

†Hydrogen peroxide solutions should be prepared immediately before use, since hydrogen peroxide decomposes rapidly in water.

‡Sterile water or normal saline should be used for mouthwash or dilution of agents when patients are immunosuppressed. Whether using non-sterile solutions for dilution increases the number of infections is unknown.[12]

Nursing Diagnosis	Nursing Intervention/Rationale

2. Use measures for oral pain per physician's order. Suggestions are:
   a. Dyclonine (Dyclone) 0.5% or 1% (available in spray or gargle), 5 to 10 ml every hour
   b. Viscous lidocaine (Xylocaine) 2%, 10 ml every 2 hours
   c. Hydrocortisone (Orabase) or carbamide peroxide (Gly-Oxide) applied to affected sites
   d. "Stomatitis cocktail"—equal parts viscous lidocaine (Xylocaine), diphenhydramine (Benadryl) elixir, and magnesium and aluminum hydroxide mixture (Maalox), 30 ml every 2 to 4 hours
   e. One part diphenhydramine (Benadryl) elixir mixed with one part kaolin and pectin (Kaopectate), every 2 to 4 hours
3. Implement dietary measures including the following:
   a. Instruct patient to avoid abrasive foods such as toast, apples, and celery.
   b. Encourage intake of pureed, bland foods.
   c. Instruct patient to avoid tart or acid foods such as hot beverages or iced drinks.
   d. Instruct patient to avoid spices and vinegar.
   e. Instruct patient to avoid alcohol.
   f. Arrange for dietary consultation.
4. Discourage smoking.
5. Recommend use of artificial saliva for xerostomia. No comparative research on various agents is available.

- For grade 3 or 4 stomatitis:
  1. Obtain samples from suspicious area and culture—one culture for bacteria and one for fungus—per physician's order.
  2. Institute oral hygiene regimen:
     a. Alternate antifungal or antibacterial suspension with warm saline mouthwash every 2 hours while patient is awake and every 4 hours during night.
     b. Do not floss.
     c. Brush gently using toothettes or cotton-tipped applicators.
     d. Remove dentures or bridge. Do not replace for meals.
     e. Apply lip lubricant every 2 hours.
  3. In addition to local measures as indicated for grade 1 and 2 stomatitis, systemic analgesics may be indicated, especially before eating.
  4. Liquid diet may be indicated. If not, use pureed diet. See other measures as indicated in no. 3 for grade 1 and 2 stomatitis.
  5. Discourage smoking.

Altered nutrition: less than body requirements related to inability to ingest or digest food

- Maintain optimum nutritional status.
- Check weight daily.
- Monitor calorie counts.
- Arrange dietary consultation.
- Administer total parenteral nutrition (TPN) as ordered.
- Monitor serum electrolytes daily.
- Check urine for glucose, ketones, and protein.

Patient problem: graft-versus-host disease (GVHD)

- Assess skin integrity daily.
- Assess level of pain and pruritus and administer analgesics and antihistamines as needed.
- Provide meticulous skin care, including daily bath with povidone-iodine and normal saline or other antibacterial solution. Oatmeal baths may be indicated for pruritus.
- Apply creams or lotions (Aquaphor or A & D Ointment with mineral oil) on intact skin *to minimize breakdown*.
- Apply mixture of silver sulfadiazine and nystatin on open areas of skin. (Other creams and ointment such as fluocinonide, hydrocortisone, and petroleum gauze may be used.)
- Explain need to prevent scratching. Use mittens if necessary on infant or child.
- Use Mediscus or other flotation-type bed for patient with extensive skin involvement.
- Use bed cradle *to prevent linens from touching skin* if patient has extensive skin involvement.
- Assist patient frequently with active and passive range of motion exercises.
- Note character and quantity of stool.
- Administer antidiarrheal agent as ordered. (Antidiarrheal agents are usually not helpful in controlling diarrhea with GVHD.)
- Provide meticulous perianal skin care.
- Test all stools for occult blood.
- Permit nothing by mouth as ordered *to allow bowel to rest*.
- Reinstate oral feedings with isosmotic, low-fat, lactose-free beverages as ordered; increase diet as tolerated.

Nursing Diagnosis	Nursing Intervention/Rationale
	• Monitor closely for dehydration, electrolyte imbalance, and weight change. • Auscultate bowel sounds every 8 hours *to monitor for development of ileus.* • Monitor bilirubin and serum glutamic oxaloacetic transaminase (SGOT) levels daily. • Measure abdominal girth twice a day. • Position patient on left side *to decrease pressure on liver.* • Administer drugs (such as steroids, cyclosporin A, methotrexate, and antithymocyte globulin) as ordered according to protocol.
Patient problem: veno-occlusive disease related to fibrous obliteration of small hepatic venules	• Assess for sudden weight gain, right upper quadrant pain, ascites, jaundice, and disorientation. • Measure abdominal girth twice a day at level of umbilicus with patient supine. • Restrict sodium intake as ordered. • Administer all intravenous medication in minimum volume of fluid. • Monitor urine sodium levels. • Monitor blood pressure for orthostatic change daily. • Monitor patient closely for toxic side effects of medications *because of impaired liver function.* • Monitor blood urea nitrogen levels frequently.
Body image disturbance related to alopecia, weight loss, sterility, and so on	• Encourage patient and significant others to verbalize feelings and concerns. • Explore perceived meaning of loss with patient and significant others. • Help patient and significant others recognize that alopecia and weight loss are temporary. • Assist patient to identify methods to improve appearance (such as use of clothing, scarves, hats, or hairpieces). • Assist patient to identify strengths. • Convey attitude of acceptance and understanding. • Emphasize that negative reactions to altered body image are normal and expected. • Consult other health care providers in planning comprehensive approach to patient.
Fear related to uncertain outcome of treatment, threat of death, isolation, treatment protocols, and so on	• Encourage patient and significant others to express feelings and concerns. • Encourage patient and significant others to ask questions *to dispel misconceptions and reduce fear.* • Assist patient to cope with isolation through use of radio, television, tape recorder, or video cassette recorder. • Reinforce and restate information given to patient and significant others *to promote understanding.* • Encourage patient and significant others to discuss hopes for positive outcome.

Patient Education

1. Teach daily care for the central venous access device to maintain the patency of the catheter and prevent infection and bleeding.
2. Explain diet for optimum nutritional status. (Ideally the patient must be able to tolerate 1000 calories a day to be discharged.)
3. Teach measures to prevent the occurrence of infection. Precautions are more rigid during the first 3 months after bone marrow transplantation and are relaxed as the year progresses.
   - Wear face mask when outside home.
   - Avoid contact with young children who attend school.
   - Avoid contact with anyone who has a cold or illness.
   - Avoid crowds; go to grocery stores, theaters, restaurants, and other public places when they are not crowded.
   - Avoid restaurant food for the first 3 months.
   - Wear a mask. (Walks can be taken without wearing a mask, but one should be carried in case of contact with other pedestrians.)
   - Wash hands well before eating, after using the toilet, and after contact with someone who has a cold.
   - Avoid contact with any pets in living quarters for the first 3 months. Do *not* clean litter boxes or come in contact with animal feces.
   - Avoid contact with plants and flowers.
   - Children should not attend school for the first year after a bone marrow transplant.
   - Do not swim in private or public pool for the first year after bone marrow transplant.
   - Maintain good dental hygiene.
   - Do not have immunizations without the physician's approval.
   - Take prophylactic antibiotics as prescribed.
4. Tell the patient to take temperature daily and notify the physician of an elevation 2° above baseline.
5. Tell the patient to report appearance of rash, change in color or consistency of bowel movements, change in color of urine, nausea or vomiting, appearance of pain, dysphagia, and xerostomia.
6. Tell the patient to report cough and dyspnea immediately.

Evaluation

Patient Outcome	Data Indicating That Outcome is Reached
Patient demonstrates proficiency in care of catheter.	Line is patent and site is free from infection.
Patient tolerates diet.	Ideal body weight is maintained.
There is no evidence of active infection.	Patient is afebrile, with no local or generalized findings and a clear chest roentgenogram.
There is no evidence of graft-versus-host disease.	There are no skin, gastrointestinal, or liver abnormalities.
Engraftment is successful.	Peripheral blood counts are in normal range.

Corticosteroids

Synthetic corticosteroids are pharmacologic agents that mimic the effects of the major endogenous glucocorticoid, cortisol. They are used in the treatment of many immunologic diseases because of their potent anti-inflammatory and immunosuppressive effects. Corticosteroids exert their widespread effects by initially binding to a specific cytoplasmic receptor protein that is present in most cells. This complex then enters the nucleus where alteration of the rate of synthesis of specific proteins occurs.

Synthetic corticosteroids should be used with caution in persons with hepatic disease or hypoalbuminemia or in patients who are receiving phenytoin, barbiturates, or rifampin. Lower-dose therapy is recommended in these cases. In addition, care should be exercised in prescribing steroid therapy for persons who are predisposed to or have known histories of diabetes, osteoporosis, peptic ulcer disease, infections, hypertension, psychosis, or coronary artery disease.

A major concern with the use of corticosteroid therapy is suppression of the hypothalamic-pituitary-adrenocortical axis (HPAA). Exogenous steroids provide negative feedback to this mechanism, which promotes total body homeostasis via the regulation of cortisol production. Therefore suppression of the HPAA results in widespread systemic manifestations. To limit this untoward effect, steroids are administered in as low a dosage as possible to control the disease for which they are being prescribed. However to control acute exacerbations of many inflammatory disorders, corticosteroids are usually prescribed initially in relatively high doses (greater than 40 mg daily), so HPAA suppression is unavoidable. Once the disease is under control, the dosage is lowered at a rate of 2.5 to 5 mg per week. *Gradual* tapering of the dosage of corticosteroids is necessary, since the body cannot respond quickly to changes in cortisol levels owing to the initial suppression of the natural HPAA feedback mechanism. It may take as long as 12 months for adaptation to occur when the patient has received high-dose therapy for a month or more.[26] Although useful in controlling many clinical manifestations, steroid therapy is not without inherent dangers. Because these agents exert such widespread systemic effects, their adverse effects are diverse and often complicate the course of the disease for which they are being used.

The type and severity of side effects are dose dependent and related to the duration of therapy. Although alternate-day therapy (single doses every other day) has been associated with fewer side effects, it is not recommended for control of acute disease.

Table 14-19
Comparison of Various Glucocorticoids with Hydrocortisone

Glucocorticoid	Anti-Inflammatory Potency	Equivalent Potency (mg)	Sodium-Retaining Potency	Duration of HPAA Suppression (Hours)
Hydrocortisone	1.0	20	2	12
Cortisone	0.8	25	2	12
Prednisolone	4.0	5	1	24-36
Prednisone	3.5	5	1	24-36
Methylprednisolone	5.0	4	0	24-36
Triamcinolone	5.0	4	0	24-36
Paramethasone	10.0	2	0	24-36
Betamethasone	25.0	0.60	0	More than 48
Dexamethasone	30.0	0.75	0	More than 48

γ-Globulin Therapy

γ-Globulin administration is indicated as replacement therapy for immunodeficiency diseases affecting the humoral or antibody-mediated immune system. Recurrent, severe, sinopulmonary infections are hallmark clinical manifestations of the humoral immunodeficiency diseases. The frequency and severity with which these infections occur assist the clinician in evaluating the effectiveness of γ-globulin therapy. γ-Globulin is also used to provide passive immunity against a variety of infectious agents, such as the hepatitis virus.

For the past 30 years, human immune serum globulin (HISG) has been available for intramuscular administration. Its use has effectively limited both the severity and frequency of infections in antibody immune deficient patients. The usual dose of HISG ranges from 100 to 200 mg/kg/month. Only IgG is present in significant quantities in HISG.

Although untoward side effects are uncommon, rare anaphylactic reactions to the intramuscular injections have been reported. Patients who have such reactions should be treated immediately with epinephrine and antihistamines. Later, therapy may resume, but HISG from a different manufacturer

Table 14-20
Experimental Immunotherapeutic Agents

	Results in Humans		
Agent	**Disease**	**Response**	**Side Effects**
Nonspecific			
BCG (several types)	Malignant melanoma	Regression of dermal metastases after intralesional injection; no effect on visceral metastases; effect on survival rates unknown	Chills, fever, malaise; granulomatous hepatitis, immune complex renal disease; anaphylaxis (rarely) due to antibody formation; persistent BCG infection at injection site in immunodepressed patients; side effects vary, depending on route of administration
	Childhood acute lymphoblastic leukemia	Prolongation of disease-free interval after induction of remission by chemotherapy	
	Lung carcinoma (intrapleural injection)	Prevention of relapse (?)	
	Lymphoma (after radiotherapy)	Prolongation of remission, prevention of relapse (requires confirmation)	
	Colorectal cancer	Increase in disease-free interval (in some patients)	
	Metastatic breast cancer	Increase in survival	
Muramyl dipeptide	—	Results not available	—
C. parvum (heat-killed and formaldehyde-treated)	Malignant melanoma (cutaneous metastases)	Regression of lesions after intralesional injection; effects on survival unknown	Fever (up to 40.5° C), headache, nausea, vomiting; mild hypertension, peripheral vasoconstriction
	Lung cancer (intrapleural)	No effect on survival	
	Other solid tumors, acute leukemia (in combination with other agents or with irradiated leukemic cells)	Trials in progress	
Thymic hormones (thymosin fraction V, facteur thymique sérique [FTS], thymopoietin, thymosin polypeptides α_1, β_1, α_5, α_7, β_3, β_4, and others)	Hereditary deficiencies of cell-mediated immunity	Immunologic normalization, clinical improvement	Allergic reactions (rarely severe)
	Oat cell carcinoma	Increase in survival	
	Other malignancies (e.g., melanoma, in combination with chemotherapy)	Trials in progress	

Modified from Stites.[48]

Table 14-20—cont'd
Experimental Immunotherapeutic Agents

Agent	Results in Humans: Disease	Response	Side Effects
Fetal thymus (13-week) or fetal liver (8-week) transplants	DiGeorge syndrome, severe combined immunodeficiency	Restoration of immune function, reduced infections, increased survival (better success with fetal liver than fetal thymus)	Mild or none
Cultured thymic epithelium; autologous T cells cultured with fetal thymic epithelium	Severe combined immunodeficiency	Restoration of immune function, reduced infections, increased survival	None reported
Immunoglobulins (plasma, immune serum globulins, Cohn fraction V)	Hypogammaglobulinemia, severe combined immunodeficiency, Bruton's disease, complement deficiencies	Temporary improvement in immune function and clinical course; repeated injections required to maintain humoral immunity	None reported
	Malignancies (plasma therapy)	Trials in progress	
Levamisole	Rheumatoid arthritis	Improvement in some	Neutropenia (occasionally severe) in rheumatoid arthritis
	Aphthous stomatitis	Marked improvement	
	Bronchogenic carcinoma	Results controversial	
	Malignant melanoma	No significant increase in survival rates	
	Juvenile periodontitis	Improvement	
	SLE	Trials in progress	
Interferon	Osteosarcoma, lymphomas, myeloma, breast cancer, laryngeal papillomatosis, brain tumors, hairy cell leukemia	Induction of remissions	Occasional leukopenia, anemia, fever, chills, myalgias, rigors
	Herpes infections	Healing of the lesions	
Inosiplex	Herpes labialis, herpes progenitalis, shingles, rhinovirus infection, influenza A infection, cytomegalovirus infection	Marked reduction in duration of illness and severity of symptoms	None reported
	Viral hepatitis (both type A and type B)	Possible effect	
	Subacute sclerosing panencephalitis	Prevention of further deterioration	
	Rheumatoid arthritis	Rapid response in 60% of patients	
Pyrimethamine (antimalarial)	No trials in humans	—	—
Glucan	Metastatic malignancy (intralesional injection)	Prompt tumor cell necrosis and regression of lesions	None reported
Tilorone	Trials in progress	—	—
L-Fucose	No trials in humans	—	—
Synthetic polynucleotides (e.g., poly A·U/poly I·C)	Poly A·U, trial in breast cancer	Increased survival after conventional therapy	—
Specific			
Active specific immunotherapy (tumor antigen in Freund's adjuvant)	Bronchogenic carcinoma (stage I) after chemotherapy	Marked prolongation of survival	Local ulceration at injection site
	Colon carcinoma, breast carcinomas	Trials pending	

Continued.

Table 14-20—cont'd
Experimental Immunotherapeutic Agents

	Results in Humans		
Agent	**Disease**	**Response**	**Side Effects**
Enzyme-treated (neuraminidase) autochthonous tumor cells	Leukemia (in combination with other agents)	Increased survival (in some trials)	None reported
	Stage III breast carcinoma (in combination with BCG)	Trials in progress	
	Malignant melanoma (without concomitant therapy)	Apparent cessation of local tumor growth	
Irradiated tumor cells	Acute leukemia (in combination with BCG or *C. parvum*)	Trials in progress	—
Immune RNA (xenogeneic)	Metastatic renal cell carcinoma	Regression or complete disappearance of metastases in some patients	None reported in phase I studies
Dialyzable leukocyte extracts (transfer factor)	Genetically determined immune deficiency	Dramatic decrease in parasitic, viral, and fungal infections	Remarkably few: severe pain at site of primary or metastatic bone tumors; occasionally hypersensitivity pneumonia if pulmonary metastases are present
	Recurrent infections with a single organism unresponsive to antibiotic therapy: fungal (e.g., *Candida*), viral (e.g., cytomegalovirus, herpes zoster), parasitic (e.g., *Leishmania*), mycobacterial (e.g., lupus vulgaris, *Mycobacterium fortuitum*, progressive BCG infection)	Excellent clinical results, provided proper donors are used and recipients are monitored by appropriate immunologic tests for frequency and amount of administration	
	Malignancies (especially those presumed to be of viral origin), e.g., epidermodysplasia verruciformis with squamous cell carcinoma and osteosarcoma	Clinical improvement, prevention of metastases, prolongation of survival	
	Multiple sclerosis	Decrease in incidence of relapses, especially in mild disease	
Interleukin-2 (IL-2)	Melanoma, renal cell carcinoma, breast, colon, lung, and rectal carcinomas, gastric lymphoma	Trials in progress	IL-2 fever; chills; rigors; decreased renal function; increased creatinine; decreased sensorium; nausea; vomiting; diarrhea; increased uric acid[7]
Lymphokine-activated killer cells (LAK)	Melanoma, renal cell carcinoma, breast, colon, lung, and rectal carcinomas, gastric lymphoma	Trials pending	LAK fever; chills; rigors; hypotension; nausea; vomiting; diarrhea; decreased urinary output; increased creatinine; altered sensorium; increased uric acid[7]
Monoclonal antibodies	Melanoma, lymphoma, leukemia	Trials in progress	Fever; chills; rigors; hypotension; headache; flushing; serum sickness; anaphylaxis; neutropenia; thrombocytopenia[8]
Tumor necrosis factor	Breast, colon, gastric, and lung carcinomas, AIDS, lymphoma	Trials in progress	Fever; chills; headache; fatigue; soreness at injection site; hypotension[9]

should be used following a skin test of HISG from the new lot.

Long-term monthly injections produce local pain. HISG is slowly degraded within the injection sites. The risk of entering the intravenous compartment in infants and malnourished patients is high. In addition, large doses of γ-globulins require multiple injections.

Recently, modified preparations of intravenous immune serum globulin (Gamimmune, Intraglobin) are available. Data indicate that these products are effective as replacement therapy.[18,20,42] Larger doses of γ-globulin may be delivered with greater efficacy. Serum levels of IgG are reached early and maintained longer. In addition, minimum side effects are associated with its administration.

Doses of intravenous γ-globulin preparations range from 100 to 300 mg/kg/month to maintain IgG serum levels at a minimum of 200 mg/dl. The therapy is usually well tolerated,[42] although chills, fever, and transient leukopenia have been reported.[18] Several researchers indicate that intravenous γ-globulin therapy is highly superior, in terms of clinical efficacy, to intramuscularly administered immunoglobulin.[18,20,42] Intravenous γ-globulin therapy appears to be useful for the treatment of patients who require large doses of immunoglobulin, debilitated patients who might not tolerate monthly intramuscular injections, and Wiskott-Aldrich patients who are prone to hemorrhage. It is used routinely in all bone marrow transplant patients and in all patients who have immunoglobulin deficiencies. Resesarch to prolong platelet half-life is under way.

γ-Globulin is used for passive immunization in bone marrow transplant patients to provide passive immunity against a variety of infectious and viral agents. It is also used to protect against the hepatitis virus in the immunocompetent host.

Immunotherapy

Immunotherapy has a role in the treatment of allergic and immune deficiency diseases, some autoimmune disorders, and cancer. In allergic diseases immunotherapy is used to hyposensitize the patient. (Desensitization is discussed elsewhere.) In immunodeficiency disease the aim is to restore absent or deficient products; for example, in X-linked hypogammaglobulinemia, treatment involves administration of γ-globulin. Patients with autoimmune disorders such as systemic lupus erythematosus may benefit from therapeutic plasmapheresis (a type of immunotherapy), with removal of circulating immune complexes. (Immunodeficiency and autoimmune disorders are discussed elsewhere.) Immunotherapy in the treatment of cancer, whether it is the sole form of treatment or used as adjunct therapy, is currently being investigated. There are now some forms of immunotherapy available for the oncology patient. Cancer immunotherapy is manipulation of the immune system to control or eliminate the growth of neoplastic cells.

Table 14-20 lists several immunotherapeutic agents that are being intensively investigated.

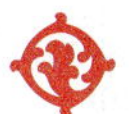

Plasmapheresis

Apheresis is the separation of whole blood into its various components by passage through automated centrifugation devices or membrane filters. After fractionation, certain blood constituents are discarded, while others are returned to the donor. Apheresis can be performed as a therapeutic protocol or to obtain donor blood products.

Plasmapheresis is the procedure by which plasma is selectively removed from whole blood. This experimental therapeutic manipulation is employed in certain diseases to remove an abnormal constituent from the plasma or replenish a deficient plasma factor. During therapeutic plasma exchange, patient plasma is removed and the cellular elements of the blood are reinfused following reconstitution with normal plasma or a suitable colloidal substitute.

Although not many well-controlled scientific studies concerning the therapeutic efficacy of plasmapheresis have been performed, it is being employed to treat a number of immunologic and nonimmunologic disorders. Conditions commonly treated with plasma exchange are outlined in Table 14-21.

Patients treated with plasmapheresis may expect to experience only temporary clinical improvement. Since therapeutic plasma exchange is designed to relieve the manifestations of a clinical disease process without affecting the underlying disorder, repeated treatments are usually indicated. Patients undergoing therapeutic plasma exchange to remove plasma antibodies or circulating immune complexes are

Table 14-21
Disorders Treated with Therapeutic Plasma Exchange

Disorder	Rationale
Autoimmune hemolytic anemia	Removal of antiplatelet antibodies
Myasthenia gravis	Removal of antibodies directed at acetylcholine receptor
Goodpasture's syndrome	Removal of anti–basement membrane antibodies
Multiple sclerosis	Removal of putative antimyelin antibodies
Systemic lupus erythematosus	Removal of circulating immune complexes
Amyloidosis	Removal of immunoglobulin
Thrombotic thrombocytopenia purpura	Replenishment of plasma factor

Table 14-22
Complications of Therapeutic Plasma Exchange

Complication	Nursing Care
Trauma or infection at site of vascular access	Keep entry site clean and dry; inspect regularly for signs of infection
Disequilibrium syndrome (nausea, diaphoresis, lightheadedness, tachycardia, and hypotension resulting from hypovolemia)	Monitor fluid balance and vital signs closely; administer fluids as needed; offer patient orange juice or saltines
Hypokalemia, hypocalcemia (which may predispose to cardiac irregularities)	Monitor electrolyte balance and replace electrolytes as needed
Bleeding owing to temporary depletion of platelets and clotting factors	Maintain safe environment; observe for signs of bleeding or bruising
Temporary paresthesias, muscle twitching, nausea, and vomiting owing to administration of citrated plasma	Provide comfort measures and reassurance; add calcium gluconate to replacement fluids
Anemia owing to hemolysis	Replace erythrocytes in combination with fluids or plasma
Increased risk of infection owing to depletion of certain plasma proteins	Observe for signs of infection
Transient peripheral edema owing to fluid shifts	Symptoms are transient and no further treatment is warranted
Hypothermia owing to infusion of cool fluids	Provide extra blankets; prewarm replacement fluids

treated concomitantly with immunosuppressive drugs to retard the recovery of immunoglobin levels.

Although plasmapheresis is generally believed to be a benign procedure, a number of complications are associated with this treatment. These untoward effects and suggested patient management* are described in Table 14-22.

*References 22, 25, 29, 44, 49, 54.

References

1. Abrams DI: AIDS: clinical update, part 1, Calif Nurs Rev 8:4, 1986.
2. Abrams DI: AIDS: battling a retroviral enemy, Calif Nurs Rev 8:1, 1986.
3. Abrams DI: AIDS: a new direction in therapy, Calif Nurs Rev 9:1, 1987.
4. AIDS-HIV 1988: overview and update, San Francisco, 1988, AIDS Professional Education Project and UCSF Departments of Medicine and Psychiatry, School of Medicine.
5. Barnhardt ER: Physicians desk reference, Oradell, NJ, 1987, Medical Economics Co Inc.
6. Bates B: A guide to physical examination, Philadelphia, 1983, JB Lippincott Co.
7. Bennett J: What we know about AIDS, Am J Nurs 86:1015, 1986.
8. Broder S, editor: AIDS: modern concepts and therapeutic challenges, New York, 1987, Marcel Dekker Inc.
9. Brown MS and Hudak CM: Student manual of physical examination, Philadelphia, 1984, JB Lippincott Co.
10. Buckley RH: Immunodeficiency, J Allergy Clin Immunol 72:627, 1983.
11. Cantani A et al: A three year controlled study in children with pollenosis treated with immunotherapy, Ann Allergy 53:79, 1984.
12. Capizzi RL et al: Methotrexate therapy of head and neck cancer: improvement in therapeutic index by the use of leucovorin "rescue," Cancer Res 30:1782, 1970.
13. Centers for Disease Control: Revision of the CDC surveillance case definition for acquired immunodeficiency syndrome, MMWR 36, 1987.
14. Daeffler R: Oral hygiene measures for patients with cancer, Cancer Nurs 4:29, 1981.
15. Daniels VG: AIDS: the acquired immune deficiency syndrome, ed 2, Boston, 1987, MTP Press Limited.
16. Diem K and Lentner C: Scientific tables, Ardsley, NY, 1970, Geigy Pharmaceuticals.
17. DiJulio J: Treatment of B-cell and T-cell lymphomas with monoclonal antibodies, Semin Oncol Nurs 4:102, 1988.
18. Eibl MM et al: Safety and efficacy of a monomeric, functionally intact intravenous IgG preparation in patients with primary immunodeficiency syndromes, Clin Immunol Immunopathol 31:151, 1984.
19. Friedman-Kien AE and Laubenstein LJ, editors: AIDS: the epidemic of Kaposi's sarcoma and opportunistic infections, New York, 1984, Masson Publishing USA Inc.
20. Fudenburg HH et al, editors: Basic and clinical immunology, ed 3, Los Altos, Calif, 1980, Lange Medical Publications.
21. Harvey AM et al: The principles and practice of medicine, New York, 1976, Appleton-Century-Crofts.
22. Huestis DW: Mortality in therapeutic haemapheresis. Lancet 1:1043, 1983.
23. Jones P, editor: Proceedings of the AIDS Conference 1986, Ponteland, Newcastle upon Tyne, UK, 1986, Intercept.
24. Judge RD and Zuidema GD, editors: Methods of clinical examination: a physiologic approach, Boston, 1974, Little, Brown & Co.
25. Keller AJ, Chirnside A, and Urbaniak SJ: Coagulation abnormalities produced by plasma exchange on the cell separator with special reference to fibrinogen and platelet levels. Br J Haematol 42:593, 1979.
26. Kelley WN et al, editors: Textbook of rheumatology, Philadelphia, 1981, WB Saunders Co.
27. Lab Comp: clinical laboratory user's guide, Stow, Ohio, 1984, Lexi-Comp, Inc.
28. Lawlor G et al, editors: Manual of allergy and immunology, Boston, 1981, Little, Brown & Co.
29. Levy J: Safety and standards in therapeutic apheresis, Plasma Ther 3:195, 1982.
30. Lewis A, editor: Nursing care of the person with AIDS/ARC, Rockville, Md, 1988, Aspen Publishers Inc.
31. Macher AM et al: AIDS diagnosis and management, Research Triangle Park, NC, 1983, Burroughs Wellcome Company.
32. Mahon SM: Taking the terror out of amphotericin B, Am J Nurs 88:960, 1988.
33. Moldawer NP and Figlin RA: Tumor necrosis factor: current clinical status and implications for nursing management, Semin Oncol Nurs 4:120, 1988.
34. Parker N and Cohen T: Acute-graft-versus-host disease in allogeneic marrow transplant, Nurs Clin North Am 18:570, 1983.

35. Petersdorf RG et al: Harrison's principles and practice of internal medicine, vol 1, New York, 1983, McGraw-Hill Book Co.
36. Price DM and Scimeca AM: The epidemic of the 80's: AIDS, Cancer Nurs, p 283, August 1984.
37. Primer on the rheumatic diseases, ed 7, Atlanta, 1973, Arthritis Foundation.
38. Rackel RE, editor: Conn's current therapy, Philadelphia, 1984, WB Saunders Co.
39. Rocklin RE: Clinical and immunologic aspects of allergic-specific immunotherapy in patients with seasoned allergic rhinitis and/or allergic asthma, J Allergy Clin Immunol 72:323, 1983.
40. Rosen FS et al: The primary immunodeficiencies, N Engl J Med 311:235, 1984.
41. Schietinger H: A home care plan for AIDS, Am J Nurs 86:1021, 1986.
42. Schiff RJ et al: Use of new chemically modified intravenous IgG preparation in severe primary humoral immunodeficiency: clinical efficacy and attempts to individualize dosage, Clin Immunol Immunopathol 31:13, 1984.
43. Schur P, editor: The clinical management of systemic lupus erythematosus, New York, 1983, Grune & Stratton Inc.
44. Shumak KH, and Rock GA: Therapeutic plasma exchange, N Engl J Med 310:762, 1984.
45. Simpson C, Seipp C, and Rosenberg S: The current and future applications of IL-2 and adoptive immunotherapy in cancer treatment, Semin Oncol Nurs 4:132, 1988.
46. Sipes C: AIDS: the haunting facts, the human care, Nurs Life 8:33, 1988.
47. Sipes C: Giving amphotericin B in the home, Am J Nurs 88:965, 1988.
48. Stites DP et al, editors: Basic and clinical immunology, Los Altos, Calif 1984, Lange Medical Publications.
49. Sutton DMC et al: Complications of extensive plasma exchange, Plasma Ther 2:19, 1981.
50. Thomas ED: Marrow transplantation for malignant diseases, J Clin Oncol 1:526, 1983.
51. Thomas ED: N Engl J Med 292:896, 1975.
52. Thomas EDL: Marrow transplantation for acute leukemia, Cancer 42:895, 1978.
53. Unaue ER and Benacerraf B: Textbook of immunology, Baltimore, 1984, Williams & Wilkins.
54. Wallace DJ and Klinenberg JR: Apheresis, Chicago, 1984, Year Book Medical Publishers Inc.
55. Wallis C and Thompson D: Knowing the face of the enemy, Time, April 30, 1984, pp 66-67.

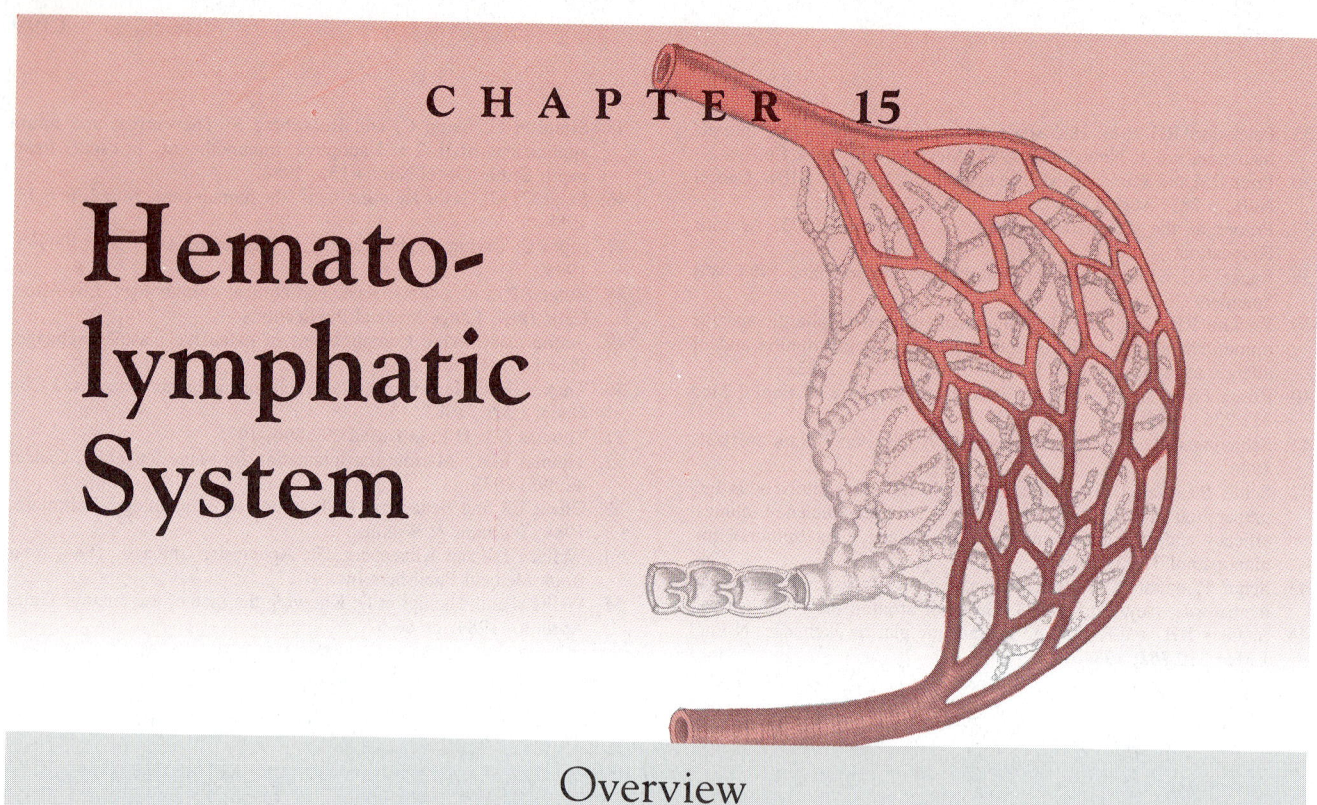

CHAPTER 15

Hemato-lymphatic System

Overview

The hematolymphatic system is composed of blood and blood-forming organs, the bone marrow, spleen, liver, and the lymphatics.

Blood, which circulates continuously through the heart and vascular system, performs numerous vital functions, such as (1) transporting oxygen and absorbed nutrients to cells and waste products, including carbon dioxide, to the kidneys, skin, and lungs; (2) transporting hormones from their origin in the endocrine glands to other tissues; (3) protecting the body from life-threatening microorganisms; and (4) regulating body temperature by heat transfer.

Major characteristics of blood include color (arterial blood is bright red; venous blood is dark red); viscosity (blood is three to four times thicker than water); reaction (the pH is 7.35 to 7.40); and volume (adults have approximately 70 to 75 ml/kg of body weight, or 5 to 6 L).

The four physiologic disturbances likely to occur in the hematologic system are decreased number of cells, overproduction of normal or abnormal cells, defects in the clotting mechanism, and disorders of the spleen. Causative factors may be idiopathic (unknown) or one of the following: dietary deficiencies, malabsorption, drug toxicity, metabolic disorders, hemorrhaging, infection, malignancy, genetic predisposition, or immunologic defects.

The lymphatic system also has numerous functions, including transporting lymph; producing lymphocytes and antibodies; phagocytosis; and absorption of fats and fat-soluble matter from the intestine.

The major characteristics of the lymphatic system are that the formation of lymph is regulated by exchange of fluid between capillaries and tissue spaces; that the muscle pump is responsible for the movement of lymph; and that the amount of lymphoid tissue and the distribution of lymph nodes are related to age. The lymphatic system includes peripheral lymphatics, regional nodes, main lymphatic ducts, and the thoracic duct.

The two basic physiologic disturbances that can occur in the lymphatic system, enlargement and swelling of soft tissues, are usually caused by infection, inflammation, neoplasm, or obstruction.

Anatomy, Physiology, and Related Pathophysiology

Blood, a suspension of particulate matter in an aqueous solution of colloid and electrolytes, serves as a medium of exchange for body cells between themselves and the exterior. It also has protective properties that benefit the body and the blood itself. The liquid portion, plasma, is a suspension of colloid, electrolytes, proteins, and numerous other substances. The particulate matter includes red blood cells (erythrocytes), white blood cells of several types (leukocytes), and platelets (thrombocytes). All of these cells are believed to be derived from a single stem cell, which divides and matures to produce three distinct types of cells with different functions, properties, and characteristics.

Erythrocytes, of which there are approximately 5 million/mm^3 of blood, have as their principal functions transporting oxygen (which attaches to hemoglobin, the iron-containing substance of the cell) to the tissues; transporting carbon dioxide to the lungs; and maintaining normal blood pH through a series of intracellular buffers. Normal hemoglobin is 15 g/

100 ml of blood. Erythrocytes are produced in the red bone marrow and found in the ribs, sternum, skull, vertebrae, and bones of the hands, feet, and pelvis. Numerous nutrients are needed for normal cell formation, including iron, vitamin B_{12}, folic acid, and pyridoxine. The young reticulocytes released from the bone marrow circulate for 4 days while maturing into adult erythrocytes. The average life span of an erythrocyte is 115 to 130 days; dead cells are eliminated by phagocytosis in the reticuloendothelial system, particularly in the spleen and liver.

Hemoglobin is composed of a simple protein called globin and a red compound called heme, which contains iron and porphyrin. Each erythrocyte contains 200 to 300 million molecules of hemoglobin, which combine chemically with oxygen to form oxyhemoglobin. Hemoglobin also combines with carbon dioxide. These two capacities enable the blood to carry oxygen to the tissues and carbon dioxide to the alveoli and thus to the atmosphere.

Total iron in the body ranges from 2 to 6 g, two thirds of which is contained in hemoglobin; the rest is stored in the bone marrow, spleen, and liver. Iron is obtained from such rich dietary sources as liver, oysters, lean meats, kidney beans, green leafy vegetables, apricots, and raisins.

When hemoglobin is phagocytosed in the liver or spleen, it breaks down into its heme and globin factors. The heme's iron is reused by the liver to make fresh hemoglobin, while the porphyrin is converted into bilirubin that is excreted by the body in feces and urine.

Leukocytes, of which there are approximately 5000 to 10,000 per mm^3 of blood, are divided into three major categories: granulocytes, lymphocytes, and monocytes. Granulocytes, which make up 70% of all white blood cells, are produced by the bone marrow and function according to the type of granule: (1) polymorphonuclear leukocytes (PMNs or neutrophils), whose main function is to fight bacterial infections through a process of phagocytosis (foreign particulate matter, or breakdown products from cells, is also digested); these cells are present during the early, acute phase of an inflammatory reaction; (2) eosinophils, which have a similar phagocytic function and are particularly important in digesting bacteria; they appear to play a role in combating allergic reactions; and (3) basophils, which contain many enzymes believed to play a role in combating acute systemic allergic reactions.

Lymphocytes, which are mainly produced in the lymph nodes, make up about 25% of the leukocytes. They are primarily concerned with producing antibodies and maintaining tissue immunity. Monocytes, which are derived from components of the reticuloendothelial system, are responsible for the phagocytosis of dead erythrocytes and leukocytes in the blood. They are also important in the processing of antigenic information.

There are approximately 250,000 to 500,000 thrombocytes/mm^3 of blood. Formed in the bone marrow, they maintain capillary integrity, initiate coagulation, and retract clots.

The lymphoid system includes lymph nodes, spleen, thymus, lymphoid tissue associated with mucosal surfaces, and bone marrow. Lymph nodes, the most numerous component, are present in virtually every area of the body. The most familiar nodes are those palpable in the neck and groin. They serve as filters along the course of lymphatic channels and have a rich blood supply, which is important in transporting lymphocytes. The spleen is a mass of lymphoid and reticuloendothelial cells found under the ribs in the upper left quadrant of the abdomen. Its structure allows close interaction among lymphocytes, macrophages, and materials carried in the bloodstream. The thymus is located in the thorax anterior to the upper part of the heart and great vessels and contains lymphatic follicles and lymphocytes. The bone marrow is considered an important part of the lymphoid system because millions of lymphocytes are scattered throughout it.

The various lymphatic channels in the body drain fluid from organs and tissues, conduct it centrally, and introduce it to the bloodstream via a large vein in the thorax. Many lymphocytes are found in the lymph and are recycled for variable periods of time.

Normal Findings[11]

Area of Concern	Normal Adult Findings
Blood	
Erythrocyte	Biconcave disc when viewed laterally; appears to have lighter center and to be thicker on outer perimeter
Reticulocyte	Young, nonnucleated cells formed in bone marrow; stain gray-blue
Granulocyte	Neutrophil (PMN): faint, pink, acidophilic granules
	Eosinophil: refractive, eosinophilic granules
	Basophil: large blue granules
Lymphocyte	Single, round nucleus; cytoplasm has faintly basophilic, heavily clumped nuclear chromatin pattern
Monocyte	Folded or indented nucleus; often looks lobulated; has clumped nuclear chromatin pattern; cytoplasm is bluish gray or light sky blue
Thrombocyte	Nucleate, disc-shaped fragments of megakaryocytes of the lymphoid system
Lymph nodes	Not normally palpable in adults
Spleen	Located in the left upper outer quadrant; not normally palpable
Thymus	Reticular framework densely infiltrated with lymphocytes arranged in pattern of cortex and medulla

Area of Concern	Normal Adult Findings
Lymphoid tissue associated with mucosal surfaces; that is, gastrointestinal and respiratory tracts	May be distributed diffusely or in nodular aggregates
Bone marrow	Myeloid tissue located only in the ribs, sternum, and at the ends of long bones

Normal Laboratory Data

Laboratory Test	Normal Adult Values
Red blood cell count ($10^6/\mu L$)	Men: 5.11 ± 0.38 Women: 4.51 ± 0.36
Hemoglobin (g/dl)	Men: 15.5 ± 1.1 Women: 13.7 ± 1.0
Hematocrit (%)	Men: 46.0 ± 3.1 Women: 40.9 ± 3
Mean corpuscular volume (MCV)	Men: 90 (80-100) μm^3 Women: 88 (79-98) μm^3
Mean corpuscular hemoglobin (MCH)	Men: 30 (25.4-34.6) pg Women: 30 (25.4-34.6) pg
Mean corpuscular hemoglobin concentration (MCHC)	Men: 34% (31%-37%) Women: 33% (30%-36%)
Reticulocyte count (expressed as % of 1000 RBCs)	0.5%-1.5%
Erythrocyte fragility test	Hemolysis starts at 0.45%-0.39% saline solution Hemolysis complete at 0.33%-0.30% saline solution
Erythrocyte life span determination	Approximately 120 days; half-life, 27-86 days
Serum	
Serum iron level	42-135 μg/dl
Bilirubin	
Direct	Up to 0.4 mg/dl
Indirect	0.8 mg
Total	0.3-1.0 mg/dl
Fecal and urinary urobilinogen	2 hr urinary urobilinogen Men: 0.3-2.1 mg/2 h Women: 0.1-1.1 mg/2 h Results are sometimes expressed in Ehrlich units; 1 mg urobilinogen = 1 EU Fecal: 50-300 mg/24 h
Erythrocyte peroxide hemolysis test	<20% hemolysis
Total white cell count	4500-11,000 cells/mm^3
Granulocytes	
Neutrophils	38-70/mm^3
Eosinophils	50-350/mm^3
Basophils (%)	0-2
Monocytes (%)	1-8
Lymphocytes (%)	15-45
Platelets	150,000-400,000/mm^3
Bleeding time	5 min (Duke) 2-7 min (Ivy)
Coagulation time	8-15 min
Capillary fragility	Presence of less than 5 petechiae in men and less than 10 in women in an area with a 2.5 cm radius

Conditions, Diseases, and Disorders

ERYTHROCYTIC DISORDERS[15]

Two basic pathophysiologic processes can be used to classify all disorders of red blood cells: inadequate numbers of circulating cells (anemia) and increased numbers of circulating cells (polycythemia). Anemias result from insufficient production or defective synthesis, increased destruction, or loss of erythrocytes. Polycythemia results from idiopathic causes or as a compensatory mechanism in response to tissue hypoxia.

Although not a disease per se, anemia is the primary manifestation of many abnormal states, including dietary deficiencies of iron, vitamin B_{12}, and folic acid; hereditary disorders; bone marrow damaged by toxins, radiation, or chemotherapy; renal disease; malignancy; chronic infection; overactive spleen; or bleeding from a tract or organ. The incidence of anemia is high; as much as 50% of the world's population suffers from anemia at any one time.

The major physiologic effect of anemia is to reduce the oxygen-carrying capacity of the blood; thus the symptoms of anemia are the result of tissue hypoxia.

Posthemorrhagic anemia

Posthemorrhagic anemia is a disorder of decreased hemoglobin in the blood caused by traumatically induced hemorrhage.

Acute posthemorrhagic anemia develops as the result of the rapid loss of large quantities of erythrocytes during a hemorrhage, that is, traumatic severance of blood vessels, rupture of an aneurysm, or arterial erosion by a cancerous or ulcerative lesion. The severity of symptoms and the prognosis depend on the rate of bleeding, site of bleeding, and volume of blood loss. The rapid loss of less blood is more dangerous than is the slower loss of more blood.

In general, 20% loss of total blood volume results in vascular insufficiency; 30% loss causes circulatory failure, shock, and coma; with 40% loss death is imminent unless there is immediate and extensive blood value replacement.

Pathophysiology

During the first 24 to 48 hours after hemorrhage, vasoconstriction and loss of plasma volume distort the erythrocyte count, hemoglobin, and hematocrit, which appear high when they are actually quite low. These laboratory tests more accurately reflect the patient's status after intravenous fluids are infused and extracellular fluid moves into the blood vessels. The red blood cell count and hemoglobin usually return to normal in 4 to 6 weeks, with many reticulocytes observed in the blood.

Chronic blood loss anemia, which is caused by bleeding peptic ulcers, menstrual disorders, bleeding hemorrhoids, or gastrointestinal neoplasms, results in continuous loss of erythrocytes and iron. Symptoms and laboratory findings are identical to those of iron deficiency anemia.

Diagnostic Studies and Findings

Erythrocytes

6.1/mm^3 (initial); 4.7/mm^3 (after fluid volume increase)

Hemoglobin

16.5 g/dl (initial); 14.5 g/dl (after fluid volume increase)

Hematocrit

50% (initial); 40% (after fluid volume increase)

Coagulation Time

Decreased

Medical Plan

Surgery

If indicated to control source of bleeding

Medications

Hematinic agents
- Iron supplements when dietary therapy is insufficient: ferrous sulfate (Feosol), 200 mg tid po with meals

General Management

- Initial intravenous fluids noncolloid, contain electrolytes; followed by plasma and/or packed red blood cells as needed to correct cell deficit
- Whole blood may be administered, after typing and crossmatching, to correct fluid volume and cell deficit as needed
- Oxygen by nasal catheter or mask to maintain sufficient oxygenation of circulating blood volume
- Sedation and rest to reduce patient's energy expenditure
- Oral fluids as tolerated to maintain adequate tissue hydration and renal perfusion
- Diet high in protein and iron as basis for erythropoiesis

NURSING CARE

Nursing Assessment

Sensory Function

Restlessness, dizziness, syncope, severe headache

Mental Status

Disorientation

Appearance of Skin

Pallor, diaphoresis, coolness

Level of Comfort

Pain in area of bleeding caused by tissue distention

Fluid and Electrolyte Balance

Thirst

Cardiovascular Function

Rapid, thready pulse
Hypotension

Respiratory Function

Rapid, deep respirations; later become shallow

Nursing Dx & Intervention

Nursing Diagnosis	Nursing Intervention/Rationale
Decreased cardiac output	• Provide rest and anticipate patient's needs *to reduce cardiac workload.* • Monitor apical pulse, heart sounds, orthostatic blood pressure, and respirations *to assess cardiopulmonary function.* • Monitor central venous pressure, breath sounds, and pulmonary artery pressure as indicated *to assess fluid volume and cardiopulmonary function.* • Monitor erythrocyte count, hemoglobin, and hematocrit *to determine effectiveness of blood component therapy and body's compensatory mechanisms.* • Avoid stress (e.g., strong emotions, overexertion, fatigue, coughing, and straining at stool) *to reduce cardiac workload.*
Fluid volume deficit (1)	• Apply ice bag and manual pressure or dressing over site of blood loss *to constrict damaged vessel or tissue and prevent further loss of blood.* • Elevate and immobilize affected body part *to promote blood return to the heart and reduce blood loss at site of damage.* • Estimate blood loss *to determine need for volume replacement.* • Administer intravenous fluid, including blood components, as ordered *to replace lost fluid volume.* • Monitor for transfusion reaction if blood is administered. • Assess patient's response to fluid therapy (i.e., check breath sounds, pulse, and blood pressure) *to avoid circulatory overload.* • Measure intake and output *to determine adequacy of renal function.* Output should be at least 30 ml/hour. • Increase oral fluid intake as tolerated *to maintain tissue hydration and renal perfusion.* • Observe for recurrent bleeding, which may result from dislodgment of clot, increased vascular pressure, or further pathophysiology.
Altered peripheral tissue perfusion	• Place patient on bed rest in semi-Fowler's position *to reduce cardiac workload and enhance systemic circulation.* • Maintain warm environment *to prevent shivering and vasoconstriction.* • Inspect trunk and extremities *for adequacy of circulation.* Skin should be pink, dry, and warm. • Palpate for arterial pulses *to determine patency of peripheral arterial circulation.* • Protect patient from injury (e.g., put up side rails) *to prevent further blood loss.* • Assess level of consciousness and orientation *to determine adequate cerebral circulation.* Patient should be alert and oriented to time, place, and person. • Discourage smoking, *which causes vasoconstriction of peripheral vessels and increased cardiopulmonary activity.* • Encourage exercise, including range of motion exercises, *to promote peripheral circulation.*
Altered nutrition: less than body requirements related to blood loss	• Encourage increased intake of iron and protein foods *to provide nutrients needed for erythropoiesis.* • Administer iron medication as prescribed *to stimulate production of hemoglobin.*
Anxiety related to threat of death	• Assure patient of health care team's knowledge and skill in care of bleeding, as well as availability of blood component therapy and cardiopulmonary support *to reduce fear.* • Sedate or tranquilize patient as needed *to reduce feeling of grave danger and helplessness.*
Fatigue	• Increase activities each day until patient returns to normal functioning. • Help identify temporary adjustments in usual routines *until fatigue is resolved or minimized.*

Patient Education

1. Teach the patient to avoid overexertion, fatigue, and emotional states because they place a strain on the cardiovascular system that may result in respiratory distress, cardiac damage, or impaired peripheral arterial circulation.
2. Instruct the patient to report to the physician serious symptoms, such as pain, dyspnea, extreme fatigue, and blood in urine or feces, because they may signal recurrent internal bleeding.
3. Instruct the patient in maintenance of normal bowel elimination to avoid strain on the cardiovascular system.
4. Teach the importance of regular exercise to maintain adequate peripheral circulation and cardiac and respiratory tone.

5. Teach the patient how to maintain a diet high in iron and protein, with adequate fluid intake, to promote production of erythrocytes and ensure adequate fluid volume.

Evaluation

Patient Outcome	Data Indicating That Outcome is Reached
Vital signs are within normal limits.	Respirations and pulse are within normal limits.
Laboratory studies are within normal limits.	The hemoglobin level and hematocrit are within normal limits.
The patient's vitality is maintained.	The patient is mentally alert, with good concentration and attentiveness. The patient experiences no malaise, fatigue, or weakness.
Color of the skin and mucous membranes is good.	The skin, nails, lips, and ear lobes are warm and moist and have a natural color.
Bowel elimination is normal for the individual.	Stools are soft; the abdomen is soft and nondistended. There is no abdominal pressure or cramping.
Body dehydration is normal.	There is no edema or thirst.
Daily intake includes the essential food groups.	The diet includes foods high in protein and iron.
The patient participates in daily physical activities.	The patient participates in activities such as walking.

Iron deficiency anemia

Iron deficiency anemia is caused by an inadequate supply of iron needed to synthesize hemoglobin.

Iron deficiency anemia, which is high in incidence worldwide and the most prevalent anemia, is caused by inadequate absorption or excessive loss of iron. The disease occurs most frequently in women and young children in underdeveloped countries.

The principal cause of iron deficiency anemia in adults is acute or chronic bleeding secondary to trauma, excessive menses, gastrointestinal tract bleeding (usually chronic and occult), or blood donation. Another cause is inadequate dietary intake of foods high in iron. A third cause is defective absorption caused by malabsorption syndromes, clay-eating (pica), chronic diarrhea, high intake of cereal products with low intake of animal protein, and partial or complete gastrectomy.

Pathophysiology

Iron deficiency anemia is a chronic, microcytic, hypochromic anemia; in other words, the erythrocytes are small and pale because of a low hemoglobin level. Although the total erythrocyte count is only moderately reduced, the serum iron level may drop dramatically.

Diagnostic Studies and Findings

Hemoglobin Level

As low as 3.6 g/dl

Total Erythrocyte Count

Rarely below 3 million cells/dl

Mean Corpuscular Hemoglobin (MCH)

<27 pg

Mean Corpuscular Hemoglobin Concentration (MCHC)

20 to 30 g/dl

Serum Iron Level

As low as 10 μg/dl

Hematocrit

Male: <47 ml/dl
Female: <42 ml/dl

Iron Binding Capacity

Increased

Serum Ferritin Level (One of the Forms in Which Iron is Stored in the Body)

Decreased

Medical Plan

Medications

Hematinic agents (to increase iron available in the blood)
- Ferrous sulfate (Feosol), 0.2 g tid with meals
- Ferrous gluconate (Fergon), 0.3 g bid
- Iron-dextran (Imferon), 100-250 mg/d

Ascorbic acid (as indicated)

General Management

Diet high in iron-rich foods to correct nutritional deficiency

NURSING CARE

Nursing Assessment

In a mild case the patient generally has no symptoms.

Sensory, Neural, and Motor Function

Dizziness
Dysphagia
Numbness
Tingling
Decreased concentration
Headache
Fatigue

Condition of Skin, Hair, and Nails

Sensitivity to cold
Brittle hair and nails (spoon-shaped)

Appearance of Oral Cavity

Atrophic glossitis (tongue inflamed and smooth)
Stomatitis

Cardiovascular Function

Tachycardia

Respiratory Function

Dyspnea on exertion

Nursing Dx & Intervention

Nursing Diagnosis	Nursing Intervention/Rationale
Sensory/perceptual alterations (kinesthetic)	• Provide safe environment *to prevent injury.* • Assist patient with ambulation and changing position, since patient's sense of balance and position may be altered.
Altered oral mucous membrane	• Remove dentures if present *to prevent infection.* • Provide soft food and nonirritating fluids *to decrease discomfort and irritation.* • Provide frequent mouth care *to remove secretions.* • Initiate dental consultation *to correct caries and other sources of irritation or infection.*
Altered nutrition: less than body requirements	• Administer iron medication as ordered *to correct deficiency.* • Monitor laboratory reports *to determine effectiveness of medication.* • Encourage diet high in iron *to correct deficiency.* • Observe for difficulty in swallowing *to determine need for changes in diet or nutritional support.* • Provide small, frequent feedings as indicated by patient's condition.
Impaired skin integrity	• Maintain warm, clean environment *to decrease sensitivity to cold.* • Wash hair with care *to avoid breaking and other damage.* • Provide nail care *to avoid damage.*
Potential activity intolerance	• Help patient plan balance between rest and activity *to reduce cardiac workload.* • Monitor pulse and respirations *to identify signs of increased cardiopulmonary workload, such as tachycardia or dyspnea on exertion.* • Assess patient for headache and decreased concentration, *which may indicate inadequate cerebral oxygenation.*
Fatigue	• Help patient and significant others understand the physiologic basis for fatigue and that it will diminish upon improvement or correction of the iron-deficient state. • Encourage patient to discuss feelings related to fatigue. • Encourage patient to identify behaviors associated with fatigue, such as emotional lability or irritability, and *to understand that they are temporary, caused by the anemic condition.*

Patient Education

1. Explain the need for correct oral hygiene, including regular dental care, to prevent irritation and infection of the oral cavity.
2. Instruct the patient in the maintenance of a diet high in iron to promote the production of healthy erythrocytes.

3. Explain factors in ongoing self-medication with iron supplements, including proper timing, dilution, and awareness of change in the stool color.
4. Explain the importance of continuing all prescribed therapy, even when the patient is feeling well.
5. Explain general hygienic measures (e.g., proper care of hair and nails) to prevent damage and loss.
6. Explain general safety precautions to prevent injury from dizziness.

Evaluation

Patient Outcome	Data Indicating That Outcome is Reached
Laboratory findings are within normal limits.	Red blood cells are normocytic and normochromic. The hemoglobin level, MCV, MCH, MCHC, and serum iron level are within normal limits.
Daily intake includes the essential food groups.	Patient's diet includes foods high in iron.
Body temperature is normal.	Patient feels neither hot nor cold.
Patient can easily ambulate.	Patient avoids contact with stable and moving objects. There is no reported dizziness. Activities of daily living are accomplished without fatigue.
General body cleanliness is maintained.	Hair and nails are clean and not brittle. Mouth is clean, with no ulceration or other oral irritation.

Pernicious anemia

Pernicious anemia is a progressive anemia caused by a lack of intrinsic factor essential for the absorption of vitamin B_{12}.

Pernicious anemia is the most prevalent type of vitamin B_{12} deficiency anemia in the United States. Caused by a deficiency of the intrinsic factor, it is a chronic, progressive, macrocytic anemia that affects adults, mainly men and women over the age of 50, and blue-eyed people of Scandinavian origin.

Pathophysiology

Atrophy of the glandular mucosa of the gastric fundus results in a lack of intrinsic factor. Why this occurs is unknown, but there are several popular explanations: heredity (the disease tends to "run in families"); prolonged iron deficiency, which can cause gastric atrophy; or an autoimmune disorder (90% of patients have autoantibodies that react against gastric cells, and 40% of patients react against the intrinsic factor).

Other anemias in this category result from a lack of vitamin B_{12}, which is caused by inadequate dietary intake and corrected by daily oral administration and a more balanced diet, or caused by poor absorption, which is treated with vitamin B_{12}.

Anemias caused by a deficiency in folic acid are quite common and usually the result of a poor diet, especially one lacking in green leafy vegetables, liver, citrus fruits, and yeast; malabsorption syndromes; or the increased need during the third trimester of pregnancy. Parenteral or oral therapy with folic acid is required. Vitamin C may be used supplementally. The symptoms of this anemia resemble those of pernicious anemia except for the absence of neurologic signs and symptoms.

Diagnostic Studies and Findings

Erythrocyte Count

Below 3 million/dl
Elevated MCV and MCHC
Decreased WBC and MCH

Blood Film

Red blood cells are oval, macrocytic, and hyperchromic

Bone Marrow Biopsy

Increased number of megaloblasts

Bilirubin

Unconjugated forms; usually elevated

Schilling Test

Abnormal urinary excretion of vitamin B

Gastric Analysis

Scanty secretions, elevated pH, and no free hydrochloric acid

Therapeutic Trial with Parenteral Vitamin B_{12}

Large numbers of reticulocytes in blood 4 to 5 days after injection

Hemoglobin

Decreased to 4 to 5 g/dl

Medical Plan[11]

Medications

Lifelong maintenance therapy
Vitamin derivatives (to correct nutritional or metabolic deficiency)
- Cyanocobalamin (Berubigen, Hemocyte, vitamin B_{12}, and others), 100 mg IM 2-3 times/wk until 10 doses are given and remission is obtained
- Cyanocobalamin, 200 mg IM monthly or 100 mg IM every 2 wk (maintenance therapy)
- Folic acid (Folvite), up to 1 mg/d po

Hematinic agents (to correct nutritional deficit)
- Ferrous sulfate (Feosol) or ferrous gluconate (Fergon), 0.3 g tid with meals po as needed

Digestants (to enhance metabolism of vitamins)
- Hydrochloric acid (HCl), 4-10 ml po well diluted in water tid with meals during first weeks of vitamin B_{12} therapy

General Management

Blood transfusions to correct anemia
Nutritious diet, including fish, meat, milk, and eggs to enrich diet deficient in vitamins
Bed rest as needed for rest, recovery, and safety
Physical therapy to prevent complications from impaired motor function

NURSING CARE

Nursing Assessment

Mental Status

Irritability, depression
Poor memory, impaired judgment

Appearance of Skin

Pallor and jaundice, waxy

Oral Cavity

Sore mouth
Smooth, beefy red tongue

Respiratory Function

Dyspnea

Gastrointestinal Function

Weight loss, indigestion, constipation, or diarrhea
Anorexia

Sensory and Motor Function

Tingling, numbness of hands and feet, weakness, fatigue
Disturbed coordination

Cardiovascular Function

Tachycardia
Wide pulse pressure
Palpitations

Nursing Dx & Intervention

Nursing Diagnosis	Nursing Intervention/Rationale
Impaired gas exchange	• Provide bed rest, with side rails up, *to decrease cardiopulmonary workload.* • Monitor pulse, blood pressure, and rate and quality of respirations *to assess adequacy.* • Observe mood, appropriateness of behavior, and orientation *to determine mental status.* • Assist with increased activity *to maintain cardiopulmonary fitness.* • Ask patient to report dyspnea and palpitations. • Monitor laboratory reports *to determine oxygenation of blood.*
Impaired physical mobility	• Provide bed rest with gradual ambulation *to promote safety.* • Provide range of motion exercises progressing to regular exercise *to prevent immobility.* • Use bed cradle or footboard *to prevent footdrop.* • Observe for signs of trauma *caused by unassisted mobility.* • Monitor patient's response to increased activity *to maintain recovery.*
Potential impaired skin integrity	• Observe skin color, warmth, texture, moisture, and intactness. • Apply heat with extreme caution *to avoid burning.* • Maintain skin with proper hygiene *to prevent irritation or damage.*
Altered nutrition: less than body requirements	• Administer vitamin B_{12} and other medications as prescribed *to promote erythropoiesis.* • Encourage diet high in vitamins, iron, and protein *to promote production of healthy erythrocytes.*
Diarrhea; constipation	• Offer small, frequent feedings *to prevent digestive overload.* • Observe for diarrhea or constipation and treat as prescribed *to avoid fluid and electrolyte imbalance and discomfort.*

Nursing Diagnosis	Nursing Intervention/Rationale
Potential for injury related to sensory and motor losses, alteration in mental status	• Use bed rest with side rails up as needed *to prevent patient fatigue and falls caused by weakness.* • Assist with ambulation *to avoid falls.* • Use bed cradle or footboard *to prevent pressure on lower extremities.* • Apply heat with extreme caution *to avoid burning the skin.* • Support patient with patience and reassurance *to reduce irritability and depression.*
Potential for infection	• Instruct patient to avoid contact with people who have infectious diseases. • Encourage and help patient perform respiratory toilet (e.g., deep breathing, turning) *to prevent respiratory infections.* • Promote effective handwashing by patient, staff, and significant others or visitors.

Patient Education

1. Teach precautions in the use of heat therapy devices such as heating pads or hot compresses (patient may have impaired sensitivity to heat and pain), as well as general safety measures.
2. Emphasize general hygiene; that is, skin and oral care.
3. Explain physical therapy activities and general exercise (patient may have possible neurologic damage as a result of the disease).
4. Teach the importance of a diet high in vitamin B_{12}, the use of maintenance therapy with vitamin B_{12}, and the need to maintain this lifelong treatment.
5. Instruct the patient in how to administer intramuscular injections as ordered.

Evaluation

Patient Outcome	Data Indicating That Outcome is Reached
Color of the skin and mucous membranes is good.	The skin, nails, lips, and ear lobes are warm and moist and have a natural color.
Vital signs are within normal limits.	Respirations, pulse, and blood pressure are within normal limits.
Laboratory studies are within normal limits.	Erythrocyte count and serum bilirubin level are within normal limits, red blood cells are normocytic and normochromic.
The patient's vitality is maintained.	Patient is mentally alert, has good concentration, and is attentive. Malaise, fatigue, weakness, or disturbances in the gastrointestinal tract are absent.
Daily intake includes the essential food groups.	Patient's diet is high in iron, protein, and vitamins.
Patient participates in daily physical and therapeutic exercise.	Patient participates in activities such as walking and in therapeutic and range of motion exercises.
There is no evidence of physical injury.	There is no evidence of skin damage or physical sign of an injury. There is no infection.
Patient has a realistic disposition.	Patient smiles appropriately and uses social conversation.

Aplastic anemia

Aplastic anemia is the term most frequently used to describe a decrease in the number of circulating erythrocytes caused by a failure of the bone marrow. It is usually accompanied by agranulocytosis and thrombocytopenia, in which case the condition is referred to as pancytopenia.

Pathophysiology

In half of all diagnosed cases of aplastic anemia, the cause is unknown; in the other half, it results from exposure to a specific toxin. The myelotoxins are (1) agents that always cause damage when given in large doses: radiation (x-rays, radium, radioactive isotopes, etc.), benzene and its derivatives, alkylating agents, and antimetabolites; (2) agents that sometimes cause failure: chloramphenicol (Chloromycetin), sulfonamides, phenytoin, and others; and (3) suspicious agents such as streptomycin, chlorophenothane (DDT), and carbon tetrachloride. The disease also may be immunologic in origin or the result of a severe disease, such as liver failure.

Diagnostic Studies and Findings

Erythrocyte Count

Usually less than 1 million/mm^3; reticulocyte count also low

Leukocyte Count

May be less than 2000/mm^3

Serum Iron

Elevated

Total Iron Binding Capacity

Normal or slightly reduced

Platelet Count

$<30,000/mm^3$

Bone Marrow Biopsy

Marrow fatty with few developing blood cells

Medical Plan

General Management

Immediate removal of the causative agent

Blood transfusions as needed to replace cells

Prevention and treatment of complications such as infection and bleeding with such therapies as antibiotics, corticosteroids, and bone marrow transplantation

NURSING CARE

Nursing Assessment

Energy Level

Progressive fatigue, lassitude, and dyspnea

Intolerance to activity

Possibility of Infection

Fever, "sniffles," sore throat, severe anorexia, ulcerations on mucous membranes, pain and burning with urination

Vascular Status

Petechiae or ecchymosis

Bleeding from gums, hematuria, occult or frank blood in feces

Nursing Dx & Intervention

Nursing Diagnosis	Nursing Intervention/Rationale
Impaired gas exchange	• For hypoxia: Place the patient in a sitting position; observe respiration rate, pulse, and dyspnea; observe skin color and temperature; assist with care; plan rest periods; administer oxygen as needed; monitor laboratory values to improve gas exchange.
Potential fluid volume deficit	• Handle the patient gently, since the patient is predisposed to bleeding. • Give injections only if necessary and apply pressure afterward *to prevent extravasation.* • Observe for changes in vital signs and for bleeding (e.g., urine, stool, gums, or nose) *to identify internal blood loss.* • Avoid constipation *to prevent tissue irritation and possible bleeding.*
Altered nutrition: less than body requirements	• Provide food selection and seasonings when possible *to meet patient preferences.* • Offer small, frequent feedings *to avoid distention and oversatiation.* • Encourage foods that are high in vitamins and protein *to provide essential nutrients.* • Record food intake *to monitor patient's nutritional status.* • Arrange pleasant environment at mealtime *to enhance appetite.* • Provide oral hygiene *to make patient comfortable and enhance taste.* • Monitor body weight and blood studies *to determine adequacy of nutrition.*
Potential impaired skin integrity related to intradermal bleeding	• Apply ice bag or manual pressure *to promote vascular constriction and clotting.* • Handle gently *to avoid trauma.* • Monitor blood studies *to determine status of intravascular volume.* • Avoid use of injections *to prevent extravasation.* • Observe for petechiae and ecchymosis *as signs of intradermal bleeding.*
Potential for infection	• Maintain reverse isolation *to avoid exposure to pathogens.* • Observe for increases in temperature, pulse, and respirations *as signs of infection.* • Observe the patient for "sniffles," sore throat, anorexia, pain on urination, and so on. • Administer antibiotics as needed *to combat specific pathogens.* • Encourage mobility, turning, coughing, deep breathing, and increased fluids *to reduce susceptibility to infection.*

Nursing Diagnosis	Nursing Intervention/Rationale
Fatigue	• Assist with activities of daily living as necessary. • Encourage patient to engage in activities on a progressive basis as fatigue decreases in response to therapy. • Help patient explore feelings associated with fatigue.

Patient Education

1. Teach the patient to maintain a balance between rest and activity.
2. Instruct the patient in how to avoid trauma (e.g., use soft toothbrush and electric razor) to prevent bleeding.
3. Instruct the patient to maintain adequate nutrition and oral hygiene to enhance his or her appetite.
4. Teach the patient how to avoid infection, especially of the respiratory or urinary tract.
5. Teach the patient self-assessment for bleeding, what signs and symptoms to report, and first aid for bleeding.

Evaluation

Patient Outcome	Data Indicating That Outcome is Reached
Color of the skin and mucous membranes is good.	The skin, nails, lips, and ear lobes are warm and moist and have a natural color.
Vital signs are within normal limits.	Respirations, pulse, and blood pressure are within normal limits.
Patient has normal body functioning.	Elimination is adequate. Healing is prompt. Patient's daily weight is stabilized at a normal level for body build. Digestion is good.
Laboratory studies are within normal limits.	Hemoglobin level and hematocrit are within normal limits. Blood leukocyte count is 5000 to 10,000/mm³. No erythrocytes, leukocytes, hemoglobin, etc. are present in the patient's urine. The findings of bacterial culture are negative.
The patient's vitality is maintained.	Patient is mentally alert. Malaise, fatigue, and weakness are absent.
Daily intake includes essential food groups.	Foods high in vitamins and protein are emphasized.
The physical appearance of the patient indicates sufficient rest.	Patient has good concentration and coordination.
Patient participates in daily exercise.	Patient walks, bicycles, or performs some other type of exercise.
Patient's surroundings are safe.	Patient uses safety precautions.
There is no evidence of physical injury.	Patient does not have cuts, abrasions, or other signs of injury.
Patient does not have an infection.	Oral temperature is 37° C (98.6° F). There is no evidence of inflammation, purulent drainage, pain, or aching.

Hemolytic anemia

Hemolytic anemia is a disorder in which the rate of erythrocyte destruction is greatly accelerated.

Pathophysiology

Hemolytic anemia is the result of either an intracorpuscular defect or an extracorpuscular factor. This causes a shortened life span for the erythrocytes, abnormally large numbers of erythrocytes being destroyed by reticuloendoethelial cells, and inadequate replacement of lost cells by the bone marrow.

Intracorpuscular defects include a deficiency in glucose 6-phosphate dehydrogenase (G6-PD) and hereditary spherocytosis. Extracorpuscular factors include trauma, such as burns or surgery; chemical agents or drugs, such as lead poisoning; immune response; infectious organisms, such as infectious hepatitis, mononucleosis, miliary tuberculosis; systemic diseases, such as Hodgkin's disease, leukemia, systemic lupus erythematosus; isoimmune reactions, such as fetalis erythroblastosis; autoimmune disorders; and paroxysmal hemoglobinurias.

Hemolytic anemia may be acute or chronic; hemolytic crises can occur in either form, both of which have the particular danger of acute renal failure.[11,15]

Diagnostic Studies and Findings

Red Blood Cell Count

Normocytic anemia

Reticulocyte Count

Increased

Red Blood Cell Fragility

Increased

Erythrocyte Life Span

Shortened

Bilirubin Level

Increased

Fecal and Urinary Urobilinogen

Increased

Bone Marrow Biopsy

Hyperplasia

Medical Plan

Surgery

Splenectomy if steroids fail to arrest erythrocyte destruction by the spleen

Medications

Corticosteroids to suppress extracorpuscular factors, such as inflammation

Prednisolone (Delta-Cortef, Meti-Derm, others), 10-20 mg qid (used if autoimmune disease is present)

General Management

Eliminate causative factors

Maintain fluid and electrolyte balance for fluid volume

Maintain renal function, using sodium bicarbonate or lactate to alkalize the blood to prevent overload and failure

Combat anemia and shock with careful administration of blood component therapy

NURSING CARE

Nursing Assessment

Appearance of Skin

Jaundice

Level of Comfort

Fever and chills

Back or abdominal pain

Energy Level

Weakness and fatigue

Gastrointestinal Function

Abdominal pain, nausea, and vomiting

Enlargement of liver or spleen

Cholelithiasis

Nursing Dx & Intervention

Nursing Diagnosis	Nursing Intervention/Rationale
Fluid volume deficit (1)	• Increase oral fluid intake *to maintain intravascular fluid volume.* • Give small but frequent drinks *to prevent distention or cardiac overload.* • Monitor intake and output *to determine fluid therapy needs.* • Observe for adequate renal function: color, specific gravity, volume, and pH of urine *to detect failure early.* • Administer intravenous fluids as ordered *to correct volume deficit.* • Administer urine alkalizers as ordered *to promote renal function.* • Administer blood transfusions as ordered *to correct volume deficit.* • Assess skin turgor *to determine adequacy of hydration.*
Impaired physical mobility	• Assist with mobility *to compensate for patient's weakness.* • Provide walker, wheelchair, or cane as needed *to assist patient with mobility.* • Observe for weakness and fatigue *to pace exercise and rest.*

Nursing Diagnosis	Nursing Intervention/Rationale
	• Medicate for back pain as ordered *to relieve discomfort.* • Encourage exercise as tolerated *to increase patient's strength.*
Altered nutrition: less than body requirements	• Provide balanced diet rich in iron and protein *to enhance erythropoiesis.* • Give small, frequent feedings *to prevent distention or satiation.* • Avoid fatty foods *to decrease discomfort and stress on gallbladder.* • Measure body weight *to monitor nutritional status.* • Observe and record food intake *to assess patient's appetite.* • Palpate liver and spleen *to assess for enlargement.* • Observe urine color *to assess liver function; mahogany color indicates dysfunction.* • Monitor laboratory values, especially bilirubin, *to assess liver function.*
Impaired skin integrity	• Provide skin care, such as cool water and lubrication, *for patient's comfort.* • Maintain cool room temperature with adequate humidity *to enhance patient's comfort.* • Expose skin to sunlight *to promote warmth and circulation.* • Advise patient not to scratch skin *to avoid irritation and abrasions.*
Patient problem: discomfort related to back or abdominal pain, fever and chills, nausea and vomiting	• Provide warmth, analgesia, and other pain relief measures as needed and prescribed *to relieve discomfort or at least increase patient's tolerance.* • Administer antipyretics as needed *for temperature control.* • Have blankets, extra clothing, and external sources of warmth such as a heating pad or lighted bed cradle available *to warm patient when chilling occurs.* • Offer antiemetics, carbonated beverages, oral care, and other measures of patient's choice *to reduce incidence of nausea and vomiting.*

Patient Education

1. Instruct the patient in the need for a balance between rest and exercise.
2. Instruct the patient in the need for a well-balanced diet.
3. Teach the patient how to maintain skin cleanliness and integrity.
4. Teach the patient comfort measures.

Evaluation

Patient Outcome	Data Indicating That Outcome is Reached
Skin and mucous membranes have good color.	The skin, nails, lips, and ear lobes are warm and moist and have a natural color.
Vital signs are within normal limits.	Respirations, pulse, and blood pressure are within normal limits.
Laboratory studies are within normal limits.	The red blood cell count, reticulocyte count, red blood cell fragility, erythrocyte life span, and serum bilirubin level are within normal limits. The fecal and urinary urobilinogen levels are within normal limits. The results of bone marrow biopsy are normal, and urine specific gravity and pH are within normal limits.
Body hydration is normal.	Skin turgor and color are good. Patient has thin secretions. Balance between intake and output is maintained.
Daily intake includes essential food groups.	Patient's diet is especially high in iron and protein.
Patient's surroundings are safe and comfortable.	Patient uses safety precautions, especially when ambulating. Room temperature and humidity are appropriate.
Patient maintains general body cleanliness.	Patient's skin is clean, and patient does not complain of itching.

Sickle cell anemia

Sickle cell anemia is a severe incurable anemia that occurs in people who are homozygous for hemoglobin S (Hb S).

Pathophysiology

Sickle cell anemia is the result of a genetic mutation that is transmitted from parent to child. Between 45,000 and 75,000 black people in this country have the disease, and 2.5 million carry the trait. The incidence of the trait is less than 1% in nonblacks and the disease nonexistent.

The erythrocytes of patients with sickle cell anemia contain more Hb S than Hb A, which causes them to assume a sickle or crescent shape when exposed to decreased oxygen tension. These "sickled" cells are then easily destroyed as they enter smaller blood vessels in the body. The sickle cell trait is usually a mild condition found in heterozygous carriers, who have few or no symptoms.

The exact cause of sickling crises is unknown, but two factors have been identified: hypoxia caused by low oxygen tensions (such as climbing to high altitudes, exercising strenuously, or inadequate oxygenation during anesthesia) and elevated blood viscosity caused by a concentration of cells and dehydration resulting from such factors as vomiting, diarrhea, diaphoresis, or diuretics. Occlusion of the microcirculation then occurs, with resultant hypoxia, which causes more sickling. Anoxia leads to infarction and thrombosis in tissues and organs such as the brain, kidneys, bone marrow, and spleen.[11,15]

Many patients die during childhood from cerebral hemorrhage or shock. Some individuals survive into their fifties or older. Progressive renal damage, which eventually causes uremia, results in death.

Diagnostic Studies and Findings

Stained Blood Smear

Sickle cell observed

Sickle Cell Slide Preparation of Blood

Sickling noted after deoxygenation

Sickle-Turbidity Tube Test

When patient's blood is mixed with Sickledex, turbid solution indicates presence of Hg S

Hemoglobin Electrophoresis

Hb S and Hb A indicate presence of sickle cell trait; only presence of Hb S indicates sickle cell anemia

Medical Plan

The medical plan of care is generally supportive: rest, oxygen, intravenous fluids and electrolytes, sedatives, and analgesics; urea therapy via a central venous catheter into the superior vena cava is still somewhat controversial.

NURSING CARE

Nursing Assessment

General

- Integrity of skin
  - Jaundice or pallor
  - Ulceration
- Skeletal integrity
  - Joint swelling
  - Disproportionately long arms and legs, fragility
  - Bone pain
- Development status
  - Delayed sexual maturity
  - Retarded growth
- Gastrointestinal function
  - Enlargement of liver and spleen
- Psychoemotional status
  - Self-esteem disturbance
  - Ineffective family coping
  - Altered family processes
  - Anticipatory grieving
  - Noncompliance with health regimen
  - Powerlessness
  - Hopelessness
  - Self-care deficit in ADLs
  - Altered thought processes

Crisis Complications

- Cardiac function
  - Systolic murmurs
  - Arrhythmias
  - Enlargement
- Respiratory function
  - Dyspnea
  - Acute respiratory distress, that is, shortness of breath, chest pain, and cyanosis
- Sensory and motor function
  - Signs and symptoms of increased intracranial pressure due to cerebral hemorrhaging
- Renal function
  - Signs and symptoms of uremia, such as decreased urinary output and edema

Nursing Dx & Intervention

Nursing Diagnosis	Nursing Intervention/Rationale
Altered cerebral tissue perfusion (potential) related to increased intracranial pressure	• Place the patient on complete bed rest with the head elevated *to reduce energy expenditure.* • Decrease environmental stimuli *to promote rest.* • Change the patient's position slowly *to avoid trauma or excessive energy use.* • Discourage oral stimulants, such as smoking, *to avoid increasing vasoconstriction.* • Monitor neurologic signs, such as level of consciousness, pupillary response, and reflexes, *to detect changes in status.* • Observe for changes in pulse, blood pressure, and behavior *to detect changes in status.*
Altered cardiopulmonary tissue perfusion related to dysrhythmias	• Encourage the patient to rest and avoid strenuous activity *to decrease cardiac workload.* • Advise the patient to avoid oral stimulants, such as smoking, *to avoid vasoconstriction.* • Auscultate apical pulse *to detect dysrhythmias.* • Monitor blood pressure *to assess peripheral circulation.* • Monitor blood studies, especially enzymes and electrolytes, *to evaluate cardiac status and tissue perfusion.*
Altered cardiopulmonary tissue perfusion related to cell sickling	• Auscultate for breath sounds, rate, rhythm, and so on *to assess cardiopulmonary status.* • Monitor blood pressure and pulse *to assess cardiovascular function.* • Monitor blood studies for gas exchange *to determine pulmonary function.* • Observe for headache, nausea, confusion, dyspnea, cyanosis, and so on *as signs of decreased tissue perfusion.*
Altered renal tissue perfusion	• Inspect for edema *as sign of impaired renal function.* • Measure body weight and intake and output *to assess renal status.* • Monitor blood studies for abnormal electrolytes, hematology, and renal function. • Monitor urine studies *for indications of renal function failure.* • Monitor temperature and blood pressure *for signs of infection or fluid retention.* • Observe urine for abnormal color, content, and odor *as signs of infection or bleeding.* • Test urine for protein; *its presence in the urine is a sign of renal failure.* • Maintain adequate fluid intake (oral, intravenous) *to maintain fluid balance and enhance renal perfusion.*
Altered peripheral tissue perfusion	• Place the patient on complete bed rest in a comfortable position. • Remove constrictive clothing *to enhance circulation.* • Maintain room and body warmth *to avoid discomfort or chilling.* • Initiate range of motion exercises; support joints at rest and with movement *to stimulate circulation.* • Inspect extremities *for adequate circulation.* • Palpate for arterial pulses *to assess patency of arterial circulation.* • Monitor blood studies for gas exchange and hematology *as indicators of adequate tissue perfusion.*
Impaired skin integrity related to altered circulation	• Place on bed rest *to decrease resistance to peripheral circulation.* • Elevate affected part *to enhance venous return.* • Implement cleaning procedure, such as with hydrogen peroxide or saline solution, *to remove drainage and necrotic tissue.* • Apply sterile dressing or expose affected area to air *to promote healing.* • Apply heat with lamp or cradle *to enhance circulation and healing.* • Observe response to therapy *to evaluate its effectiveness.*
Pain related to increased intra-abdominal pressure and discomfort	• Place the patient in a sitting position *to increase intra-abdominal space.* • Remove constrictive clothing *to relieve pressure.* • Change the patient's position frequently *to relieve pressure and enhance comfort.* • Give small, frequent feedings *to avoid distention.* • Auscultate for abdominal bowel sounds *to assess gastric motility.* • Monitor for physical dependency on analgesics.
Potential for injury related to fracture	• Change the patient's position frequently with joint support *to avoid trauma.* • Initiate range of motion exercises and physical activity *to maintain muscle tone.* • Encourage the patient to eat foods high in calcium, protein, and vitamins *to enhance bone integrity.* • Observe for pain, swelling, or abnormal alignment *as signs of trauma such as fracture.*

Nursing Diagnosis	Nursing Intervention/Rationale
See "Functional Health Patterns": Cognitive-perceptual; Self-perception/self-concept; Role relationship; Coping–stress tolerance	• Assess patient's stated feelings and behaviors for nursing diagnoses in these functional health patterns. Refer to Part Three for detailed information on assessment factors and nursing interventions.

Patient Education

1. Alert the patient to the need for family testing to determine the presence of Hb S; genetic counseling is available for carriers.
2. Instruct the patient in how to avoid sickle cell crises: avoid altitudes, flying in unpressurized planes, dehydration, cold temperatures, iced liquids, and vigorous exercise; use stress-reduction methods.
3. Explain to the patient that young pregnant women have a high risk of developing pulmonary and/or renal complications.
4. Teach range of motion exercises and encourage regular physical activity to prevent bone demineralization. Explain the need for balance between rest (physical and mental) and activity, such as range of motion and isometric exercises.
5. Teach principles of good nutrition, such as the importance of protein, calcium, vitamins, and adequate fluids; the patient should not have oral stimulants, such as smoking.
6. Alert the patient to the signs and symptoms of increased intracranial pressure, to the need to blow the nose gently, to avoid coughing, and to avoid straining on elimination.
7. Teach the patient to monitor his or her oral intake and urinary output.
8. Advise the patient to avoid trauma and extremes in temperature; patients should not smoke and should protect extremities from injury because of impaired circulation.
9. Teach the patient to monitor urine protein with Combistix or Urostix.

Evaluation

Patient Outcome	Data Indicating That Outcome is Reached
Tissue perfusion is adequate.	The skin, nails, lips, and ear lobes are warm and moist and have a natural color. Vital signs, blood gas values, hemoglobin level, and hematocrit are within normal limits. Electrocardiogram shows a normal tracing.
Fluid-electrolyte balance is adequate.	Skin turgor is good; edema and ascites are not present. Urine specific gravity and blood levels of sodium, potassium, chloride, and calcium are within normal limits.
Nutrition is adequate.	Bone development, posture, and skin turgor are good. Elimination is adequate, and healing is prompt. Diet includes foods high in calcium, protein, and vitamins.
Acid-base balance is maintained.	Blood and urine pH are within normal limits.
Waste elimination is adequate.	Daily fluid output is equal to fluid intake. Blood urea nitrogen and serum creatinine levels are within normal limits. Results of urine protein test are negative. Results of urine specific gravity, creatinine level, and creatinine clearance are within normal limits.
The patient's energy and vitality levels are good.	Patient is mentally alert and has good concentration and attentiveness. Malaise, fatigue, and weakness are absent.
Patient performs adequately in work and play.	Patient can maintain self-care, perform household or work activities, and participate in recreation and sports.
Activity and exercise are adequate.	Patient changes position and body movement frequently (walking, sitting, and standing). Patient participates in daily physical exercise, such as walking, and in range of motion and isometric exercises; patient avoids strenuous exercise.
The patient's surroundings are safe and comfortable.	Patient uses safety precautions. Temperature and humidity level are appropriate. There is no evidence of physical injury or that accidents have occurred.
Patient has physical appearance of comfort.	Posture is normal. Patient has freedom of body movement and expresses comfort.

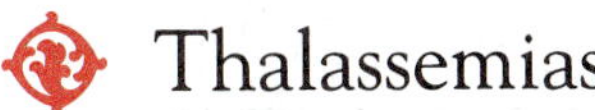

Thalassemias

Thalassemias, another group of chronic hemolytic anemias, are caused by an insufficient number of hemoglobin polypeptide chains, which are necessary for production of hemoglobin.

Pathophysiology

The thalassemias are inherited disorders most frequently affecting people of Mediterranean or Southern Chinese ancestry, as well as American blacks and individuals from Southern Asia and Central Africa. Thalassemia major and intermedia, the more serious anemias, appear in homozygotes; thalassemia minor is milder and appears in heterozygotes. The deficiency in hemoglobin polypeptide chains results in extremely thin, fragile erythrocytes called "target cells." People with thalassemia major do not reach adulthood, while those with the intermedia or minor disorder respond to supportive care.

Diagnostic Studies and Findings

Blood Smear

Target cells and other strangely shaped erythrocytes observed
Pale, nucleated RBCs

Red Blood Cell Count

Decreased

Serum Bilirubin

Greatly elevated

Fecal and Urinary Urobilinogen

Greatly elevated

Fetal Hemoglobin (Hb F)

Elevated; may be as high as 90%

Hemoglobin A (Hb A)

Elevated; may be as high as 6%
(Normal: 1.5% to 3.0%)[6,9]

Medical Plan

The medical plan of care is supportive, such as transfusions of packed red cells on a monthly, bimonthly, and/or "as needed" basis. Splenectomy is necessary if transfused cells are rapidly destroyed by the spleen.

Chelating agents such as diethylenetriamine pentaacetic acid (DTPA) may be used if iron overload results from multiple transfusions.

NURSING CARE

Nursing Assessment

Integrity of Skin

Jaundice
Leg ulcers
Pallor

Gastrointestinal Function

Enlarged spleen and liver
Intolerance of fatty foods and abdominal discomfort

Skeletal Integrity

Cranial bone hyperplasia
Mongoloid appearance
Pathologic fractures

Cardiac Function

Dysrhythmia
Heart failure

Delayed Puberty (Thalassemia Intermedia)

Frequent infections
Bleeding tendency

Nursing Dx & Intervention

Nursing Diagnosis	Nursing Intervention/Rationale
Altered cardiopulmonary tissue perfusion related to dysrhythmia	• Encourage patient to rest and to avoid strenuous activity *to reduce cardiac workload.* • Avoid oral stimulants, such as smoking, *to prevent vasoconstriction.* • Auscultate apical pulse *to assess cardiac function.* • Monitor blood pressure and respirations *to assess peripheral blood flow and pulmonary function.* • Monitor blood studies (i.e., enzymes, electrolytes, and gas exchange) and electrocardiogram *to determine cardiac status.*
Potential impaired skin integrity	• Place the patient on bed rest *to rest the affected part(s).* • Elevate the affected part *to enhance peripheral circulation.* • Implement cleaning procedure, such as with hydrogen peroxide or saline solution, *to remove drainage and necrotic tissue.* • Apply sterile dressing or expose affected area to air *to promote healing.* • Apply heat with lamp or cradle *to promote healing.* • Observe the patient's response to therapy *to evaluate its effectiveness.*

Nursing Diagnosis	Nursing Intervention/Rationale
Pain related to an increase in discomfort from intra-abdominal pressure	• Place the patient in a sitting position *to increase intra-abdominal space.* • Remove constrictive clothing *to relieve pressure.* • Change the patient's position frequently *to relieve pressure and enhance comfort.* • Give small, frequent feedings *to avoid distention.* • Auscultate for abnormal bowel sounds *to assess gastric motility.*
Impaired skin integrity	• Provide skin care, using cool water and lubrication, *to promote hygiene and moisture.* • Maintain cool room temperature with adequate humidity *to enhance comfort.* • Expose the skin to sunlight *to promote warmth and circulation.* • Advise the patient not to scratch the skin *to avoid injury.*

Patient Education

1. Teach the patient to maintain skin cleanliness and integrity and to minimize potential damage from jaundice or stasis ulcer.
2. Teach the patient to observe a balance between rest and activity.
3. Explain to the patient the need to avoid trauma, extremes in temperature, and smoking to protect the extremities from injury caused by impaired circulation.
4. Advise the patient to seek genetic counseling.

Evaluation

Patient Outcome	Data Indicating That Outcome is Reached
Color of the skin and mucous membranes is good.	The skin, nails, lips, and ear lobes are warm and moist and have a natural color.
The patient's body functions are normal.	Vital signs are within normal limits. Elimination is adequate, and healing is prompt.
Laboratory studies are within normal limits.	Blood levels of hemoglobin, serum glutamic-oxaloacetic transaminase, lactic dehydrogenase, creatine phosphokinase, bilirubin, sodium, potassium, and carbon dioxide are within normal limits. Oxygen saturation and urobilinogen levels of feces and urine are within normal limits. Electrocardiogram shows normal tracings.
Patient performs adequately in work and play.	Patient can maintain self-care, perform household or work activities, and participate in recreation and sports.
Patient has physical appearance of comfort.	The patient's posture is normal. Patient has freedom of body movement and expresses comfort.
Patient has general body cleanliness.	Patient's skin is clean. Patient has no ulceration and does not complain of itching.

Polycythemias

Polycythemia is a term used to describe an increase in the number of circulating erythrocytes and the concentration of hemoglobin in the blood.

Pathophysiology

The three forms of polycythemia are:

Polycythemia vera, a myeloproliferative disorder ("overgrowth of bone marrow"), which usually develops in middle age, particularly among Jewish men; the etiology is unknown, but the overproduction of erythrocytes, myelocytes, and thrombocytes results in increased blood viscosity, blood volume, and congestion of tissues and organs with blood.

Secondary polycythemia, a compensatory response to tissue hypoxia in the presence of chronic obstructive lung disease, congenital heart disease, and prolonged exposure to high altitudes (10,000 feet or more).

Relative polycythemia, which is a relative increase in erythrocyte concentration in the presence of plasma loss that is caused by fluid loss and dehydration; specific causes may include insufficient fluid intake, diarrhea, vomiting, burns, or excessive diuretics.

Diagnostic Studies and Findings

Erythrocyte Count

As high as 8 million to 12 million/mm^3

Hemoglobin Concentration

8 to 25 g/dl

Myelocytes

Increase in polycythemia vera

Thrombocytes

Increase in polycythemia vera

Medical Plan

Medications

Antineoplastic agents (to suppress bone marrow function)
- Busulfan (Myleran), 4-8 mg/d po
- Chlorambucil (Leukeran), 4-10 mg/d po
- Radioactive phosphorus P32 (Phosphotope), 6 μCi po; 3-5 μg IV
- Mechlorethamine (Nitrogen mustard), 200-600 μg/kg IV in a single or divided dose

General Management

Venesection (phlebotomy) with emergency removal of 500 to 2000 ml blood until hematocrit reaches 45%, then 500 ml every 2 to 3 months to reduce circulatory overload

Activity and ambulation to prevent circulatory stasis

Pheresis therapy

NURSING CARE

Nursing Assessment

Appearance of Skin

Ruddy complexion

Dusky redness of mucosa

Cardiovascular Function

Hypertension with dizziness, headache, and sense of fullness in head

Congestive heart failure (shortness of breath, orthopnea, etc.)

Thrombus formation, leading to cerebrovascular accident, myocardial infarction, or gangrene of the feet

Bleeding and hemorrhage in gastrointestinal tract, oropharynx, or brain

Gastrointestinal Function

Enlargement of liver and spleen

Signs and symptoms of peptic ulcer

Skeletal Integrity

Signs and symptoms of secondary gout

Nursing Dx & Intervention

Nursing Diagnosis	Nursing Intervention/Rationale
Altered cardiopulmonary tissue perfusion related to increased arterial pressure	• Encourage rest and quiet *to decrease cardiac workload.* • Discourage oral stimulants, such as smoking, *to prevent vasoconstriction.* • Avoid emotional situations, *which tend to increase systemic blood pressure.* • Administer medication as ordered *to promote vasodilatation and/or diuresis.* • Monitor blood pressure *to assess effectiveness of therapy.* • Avoid sodium-rich foods *to reduce fluid retention.*
Altered cardiopulmonary tissue perfusion related to inadequate pulmonary ventilation	• Change the patient's position frequently; sitting is considered best *to enhance lung expansion.* • Encourage coughing and deep breathing *to promote removal of secretions.* • Ambulate as soon as possible *to enhance cardiopulmonary function.* • Observe respiratory rate and auscultate breath sounds etc. *to assess pulmonary function.* • Monitor for cyanosis *as a sign of pulmonary decompensation.* • Assess breath sounds.
Altered peripheral tissue perfusion	• Place on complete bed rest in a slightly sitting position *for patient comfort and decreased energy use.* • Maintain warm environment with room temperature and clothing *to avoid vasoconstriction.* • Initiate range of motion exercises *to enhance circulation.* • Avoid applying heat or cold, tight clothing, and pressure under the knee, *which can impair circulation.* • Inspect extremities for adequate circulation *to assess need for further intervention.* • Monitor blood studies for hematology and gas exchange *as indicators of pulmonary status.* • Monitor peripheral pulses. • Auscultate for abnormal bowel sounds *to assess gastric motility.*

Nursing Diagnosis	Nursing Intervention/Rationale
Impaired physical mobility related to inflammation of the joints	• Prescribe bed rest and joint rest *to reduce inflammation and irritation.* • Administer medications as ordered, such as analgesics and antigout drugs, *to promote comfort.* • Provide soft diet *to reduce necessity of chewing.* • Provide compresses according to patient's tolerance *to reduce swelling and pain.*
Pain	• Place the patient in a sitting position *to promote comfort and increase intra-abdominal space.* • Remove constrictive clothing *to relieve pressure.* • Change the patient's position frequently *to relieve pressure and enhance comfort.* • Give small, frequent feedings *to avoid distention.* • Observe for evidence of favorable response to therapy *to determine need for same or modified intervention.* • Discourage smoking *to avoid vasoconstriction.* • Decrease acidic and gas-forming foods *to avoid distention and flatus.* • Give bland foods, carbonated beverage, and antacids *to relieve gastric distress.* • Provide skin care *to prevent injury and to treat any urticaria or pruritus.*
Ineffective breathing pattern related to thrombus formation	• Encourage patient to perform range of motion and isometric exercises *to promote circulation.* • Administer anticoagulants as ordered *to reduce incidence of clotting.* • Observe for chest pain; dyspnea; coughing; hemoptysis; changes in pulse, respirations, blood pressure, pupillary response, reflexes, and level of consciousness, *which are signs of a pulmonary or cerebral embolism.*
Patient problem: potential for hemorrhage	• Change the patient's position slowly; handle gently *to avoid trauma.* • Place the patient on complete bed rest *to prevent accidents such as falls.* • Brush teeth with soft toothbrush *to avoid injury to mucous membranes.* • Use small-gauge needle for injections; apply pressure *to prevent extravasation.* • Avoid hot liquids, oral stimulants, and straining at elimination *to prevent bleeding.* • Inspect for bleeding in stool, mouth, and nose *to assess need for intervention.* • Observe for signs of increased intracranial pressure *as indication of central nervous system bleeding.* • Monitor blood studies *to detect signs of internal bleeding.*

Patient Education

1. Instruct the patient to protect extremities from injury, such as heat, cold, or pressure.
2. Assist and teach the patient to do range of motion and isometric exercises safely and correctly.
3. Advise the patient to avoid trauma and protect body parts, to use safety precautions, and to use a soft toothbrush.
4. Instruct the patient to balance rest with exercise.
5. Teach the patient to handle stress in a healthy way.
6. Advise the patient of the need to stop smoking and to avoid other oral stimulants.
7. Advise the patient of the need for dietary modification; that is, to use low-sodium, low-acid, and low–gas-forming foods, foods high in alkaline, and foods low in purines.
8. Teach the patient the signs and symptoms of bleeding and thrombus formation, as well as interventions and the need to report findings.

Evaluation

Patient Outcome	Data Indicating That Outcome is Reached
Color of the skin mucous membranes is good.	The skin, nails, lips, and ear lobes are warm and moist and have a natural color.
Vital signs are within normal limits.	Respirations, blood pressure, and temperature are within normal limits.
Laboratory studies are within normal limits.	Red blood cell count and thrombocyte count are within normal limits.
Daily intake includes essential food groups.	Patient's diet includes milk, meat, fruits, vegetables, breads, and cereals as required to control gastric irritation, hypertension, and gout.
Patient has physical appearance of comfort.	Patient is calm, contented, and relaxed. Posture is normal, and patient has freedom of body movement.

Patient Outcome	Data Indicating That Outcome is Reached
Patient frequently changes position and body movement.	Patient walks, sits, and stands.
Patient participates in daily physical and therapeutic exercises.	Patient participates in walking and other mild exercise and performs range of motion and isometric exercises safely and correctly.
Patient's surroundings are safe and comfortable.	Patient uses safety precautions. Temperature and humidity are at an appropriate level.
There is no evidence that accidents have occurred.	There is no evidence of physical injury.

LEUKOCYTIC DISORDERS

Agranulocytosis

Agranulocytosis, also referred to as granulocytopenia or malignant neutropenia, is an acute, potentially fatal blood disorder characterized by (1) agranulocytic angina, a severe, painful, ulcerative infection of the oral mucosa and throat, with symptoms of high fever and severe weakness and (2) severe neutropenia.

Agranulocytosis is a worldwide disorder that affects women more often than men. The onset is usually rapid, and prompt treatment is required. The condition may develop slowly based on drug dosage and duration of effect, such as in response to cancer chemotherapy.

Pathophysiology

Agranulocytosis is most frequently caused by drug toxicity or hypersensitivity from large dose, long-duration drugs such as nitrogen mustard, radiation, and benzenes and drugs that produce individual sensitivity such as certain tranquilizers (chlorpromazine HCl [Thorazine]), antithyroid agents (propylthiouracil), anticonvulsants (phenytoin), and antibiotics (chloramphenicol). It may also develop during the course of diseases such as tuberculosis, uremia, aplastic anemia, multiple myeloma, and overwhelming infection.

Diagnostic Studies and Findings

Leukocyte Count

Leukopenia (500 to 3000 white blood cells/mm^3 with extremely low polymorphonuclear [PMN] cell count of 0% to 2%)

Bone Marrow Biopsy

Absence of PMN leukocytes; maturational arrest of young developing cells

Cultures of Urine and Blood; Ulcerative Lesions in Throat and Mouth

Positive for bacteria

History

Exposure to offending drug, radiation, or chemical

Medical Plan

Medications

Agent-specific anti-infective agent (to treat infection)

General Management

Monitoring of patient's blood cell count to evaluate status
Observation for infection to initiate therapy
Reverse isolation to reduce exposure to pathogens
Bed rest and high-protein, high-vitamin, high-calorie diet to conserve energy and enhance resistance to infection
Granulocyte transfusions to replace deficient cells

NURSING CARE

Nursing Assessment

Energy Level

Severe fatigue and weakness
High fever, severe chills, tachycardia, and prostration

Gastrointestinal Function

Sore throat, ulcerative lesions of pharyngeal and buccal mucosa, and dysphagia
Diarrhea

Cardiac Function

Weak, rapid pulse

Nursing Dx & Intervention

Nursing Diagnosis	Nursing Intervention/Rationale
Altered oral mucous membrane	• Give frequent mouth care; irrigate every 1 to 2 hours *for hygiene and patient comfort.* • Apply ice collar *to reduce pharyngeal swelling.* • Offer anesthetic lozenges, analgesics, and sedatives as ordered *to provide comfort.* • Offer soft, bland foods and protein concentrates *to reduce buccal irritation and increase ease of swallowing.*
Activity intolerance	• Anticipate the patient's needs *to avoid excess energy expenditure.* • Encourage rest and adequate activity *to maintain energy level.* • Place objects within reach while patient is on bed rest *to decrease need for getting out of bed.* • Observe for increasing weakness and dyspnea *to assess need for further intervention, such as oxygen therapy.* • Assess pulse and respirations *to monitor cardiopulmonary function.*
Potential for infection	• Place the patient on bed rest *to conserve energy.* • Enforce reverse isolation *to protect patient from pathogens.* • Provide high-protein, high-vitamin, high-calorie diet *to maintain nutritional status.* • Encourage patient to take fluids *to promote hydration.* • Monitor heart rate, respirations, blood pressure, and temperature *to assess for signs of infection.* • Observe for restlessness and irritability *as possible signs of infection.* • Observe the patient for extreme fatigue, sore throat or mouth, and fever *as signs of infection.* • Observe white blood cell count, *as a marked increase indicates infection.* • Use cooling measures (alcohol rub and tepid baths) *to reduce fever if present.* • Administer antibiotics as ordered *to combat specific pathogens.* • Use enemas and stool softeners as needed *to prevent intestinal stasis as site for infection.* • Provide perineal care *to maintain hygiene and prevent infection.*

Patient Education

1. Teach the patient the use of frequent, thorough oral hygiene to treat or prevent mouth and pharyngeal infection.
2. Explain the need for a diet high in protein, vitamins, and calories with soft, bland foods.
3. Teach the importance of normal bowel elimination.
4. Explain the need to avoid self-medication because of the danger of hypersensitivity.
5. Encourage a balance between rest and activity to prevent fatigue and generalized weakness.
6. Teach avoidance of crowds, people with infectious diseases, and cold or hot environments; also teach signs and symptoms of infection and appropriate interventions.

Evaluation

Patient Outcome	Data Indicating That Outcome is Reached
Patient's body functions are normal.	Vital signs are within normal limits. Elimination is adequate, and healing is prompt.
Laboratory studies are within normal limits.	Leukocyte count is 5000 to 10,000 cells/mm^3. The results of a bone marrow biopsy are normal, and cultures of urine and blood are negative.
The patient's vitality is maintained.	Malaise, fatigue, and weakness are absent.
Patient consumes daily intake of essential food groups.	Patient consumes diet high in protein, vitamins, and calories and eats soft, bland foods as needed; patient drinks adequate fluids.
Bowel elimination is normal for the individual.	Patient's stools are soft.
Patient has frequent changes in position and body movement.	Patient is walking, sitting, and standing.
Patient participates in daily physical exercise.	Patient participates in mild exercise.

Patient Outcome	Data Indicating That Outcome is Reached
Patient's surroundings are comfortable.	Temperature and humidity are appropriate, and patient has a well-ventilated room.
There is no evidence of physical injury.	There is no evidence of complications arising from drugs or treatment.
Infection is gone.	There is no evidence of inflammation, purulent secretions or drainage, pain, or aching.

Leukemia

Leukemia ("white blood") is a usually fatal cancer that involves the blood-forming tissues of the bone marrow, spleen, and lymph nodes. It is characterized by the neoplastic proliferation of leukocytes and their precursors.

Leukemia represents about 3% of cancers detected each year and causes about 4% of cancer deaths, or about 16,000 people annually. Although survival rates have improved since the 1950s, mortality is still high, especially for those with acute leukemias, that is, acute lymphocytic leukemia (ALL), which is responsible for half of all cancer deaths among children.

Although leukemia is considered a disease that strikes children, most cases occur in adults over 55 years of age, except in blacks, whose median age for leukemia ranges from 35 to 54 years. Men develop leukemia slightly more often than do women.

For reasons as yet unknown, the incidence of leukemia is rising. However, several factors have been implicated: chronic, repeated exposure to relatively small doses of radiation; chloramphenicol; exposure to certain chemicals, such as benzene; presence of primary immune deficiency diseases; possible viral etiologies; and a genetic predisposition, such as among siblings or in children with Down's syndrome.

Pathophysiology

Leukemia's major effects on the body are proliferation of large numbers of abnormal, immature leukocytes, accumulation of these cells within the lymph nodes, and eventual infiltration of these cells into tissues all over the body. All organs are eventually involved in the leukemic process.

Leukemias are classified according to the following criteria:

Type of cell and tissue involved: The major type of cells are lymphocytes (lymphocytic leukemia: acute and chronic) and granulocytes (myelocytic: acute and chronic; monocytic: acute and chronic). The acute leukemias are sometimes classified as lymphoblastic, myeloblastic, or monoblastic because of the prevalence of immature cell forms. Lymphocytic leukemia causes hyperplasia of the lymphoid tissue, while myelocytic leukemia causes hyperplasia of the bone marrow and spleen. Ninety percent of all leukemias are lymphocytic.

Course and duration of disease: Acute forms have a rapid onset with progression to death within days or months. The large numbers of leukocytes produced are immature and rapidly cause organ malfunction. Chronic forms have a gradual onset and a slower course. The cells are more mature and function more effectively. Acute leukemia occurs more frequently in children, while chronic leukemia is more prevalent in people 25 to 60 years of age.

Number of leukocytes in blood and bone marrow: If the patient has a normal or lower than normal leukocyte count, the disease is called aleukemic or subleukemic leukemia.

Acute leukemia has its peak incidence in children who are 1 to 5 years of age. There is usually a prodromal period when the child experiences fatigue, headache, sore throat, night sweats, and shortness of breath. These symptoms are followed by severe tonsillitis, ulcerations in the mouth, bleeding from the gums and rectum, bleeding into the skin, and joint and bone pain. The lymph nodes, liver, and spleen enlarge, and severe anemia develops. The patient dies from overwhelming infection or severe hemorrhaging. With treatment the patient may survive 5 years or longer.

Chronic myelocytic leukemia, which is usually found in people 25 to 40 years of age, is characterized by a massive spleen, enlarged liver, and severe pain in the long bones. The onset is usually insidious, with the patient complaining for months or years of weight loss and weakness. Initial signs of disease may be a heavy sensation in the abdomen, a sense of extreme abdominal distention after meals, sternal tenderness, and mild enlargement of the lymph nodes.

Chronic lymphocytic leukemia is found most often in people 50 to 70 years of age, many of whom do not have symptoms for years. Early signs and symptoms are chronic exhaustion, anorexia, swollen lymph nodes, and a slightly enlarged liver and spleen. Anemia, fever, increased susceptibility to infections, and mild bleeding tendencies occur as the disease progresses. Visual disturbances, skin lesions, deafness, otitis media, or Ménière's syndrome may develop. Pain and paralysis result from lymph node pressure on the nerves. Respiratory symptoms result from enlargement of the mediastinal lymph nodes. Late complications include hemolytic anemia and hypogammaglobulinemia.[5,11,17]

Diagnostic Studies and Findings

During its early stages, leukemia may be accidentally found during a routine physical examination that includes blood work.

Leukocyte Count

Elevated (15,000 to 500,000/mm^3 or higher)
"Shift to the left" (presence of large numbers of immature neutrophils); one type of white cell predominates

Bone Marrow Biopsy

Massive number of white blood cells

Blood Smear

Numerous blast cells

Red Blood Cells

Decreased

Platelets

Decreased

Medical Plan[1,12]

The goal of treatment is to stop the proliferation and infiltration of abnormal and immature leukocytes and to obtain as long a remission as possible.

Medications

Dosages are based on body surface area; the following are examples of standard and experimental drugs in use
Acute lymphoblastic leukemia
Antineoplastic agents
Methotrexate (Amethopterin, Mexate), 2.5-5 mg/kg/d po or parenterally
Mercaptopurine (Purinethol, 6-MP), 2.5 mg/kg/d po
Cyclophosphamide (Cytoxan), 40-50 mg/kg IV in divided doses over several days, then adjusted to lower maintenance dosage
Vincristine sulfate (Oncovin, VCR), po 50-100 mg/m^2/d, 1.4 mg/m^2 IV q wk
Cytarabine (Cytosar-U), 2 mg/kg IV for 10 d; raised to 4 mg/kg for maintenance
Thioguanine (6-TG), 2 mg/kg/d po
Asparaginase (Elspar, L-asparagine), 1000 IU/kg/d IV for 10 d, or 6000 IU/m^2 IM intermittently
Carmustine (BCNU), 200 mg/m^2 IV q6 wk
Hydroxyurea (Hydrea), 20-30 mg/kg/d po or 80 mg/kg q3 d
Dactinomycin (Actinomycin D, Cosmegen), 0.015-0.05 mg/kg IV divided dosages over 1 wk; repeat for 3-5 wk
Corticosteroids
Prednisone (Meticorten), 5-80 mg/d
Acute myeloblastic leukemia
Antineoplastic agents
Methotrexate (Mexate), 2.5-5 mg/kg/d po or parenterally
Mercaptopurine (Purinethol, 6-MP), 2.5 mg/kg/d po
Cytarabine (Cytosar-U), 2 mg/kg IV for 10 d; raised to 4 mg/kg for maintenance
Thioguanine (6-TG), 2 mg/kg/d po
Daunorubicin (Cerubidine), 30-60 mg/m^2 IV daily for 3 d or weekly
Carmustine (BCNU), 200 mg/m^2 IV q6 wk
Chronic lymphocytic leukemia
Corticosteroids
Prednisone (Deltasone, Meticorten), 10-100 mg/d po
Antineoplastic agents
Chlorambucil (Leukeran), 4-10 mg/d po
Cyclophosphamide (Cytoxan), 40-50 mg/kg IV individual doses over several d, then adjusted to lower maintenance dosage; po 1-5 mg/kg/d
Triethylenemelamine (TEM), 2.5 mg po for 2-3 d; then 0.5-5 mg weekly for several weeks
Chronic myelocytic leukemia
Antineoplastic agents
Busulfan (Myleran), 4-8 mg/d po
Chlorambucil (Leukeran), 4-10 mg/d po
Mercaptopurine (Purinethol, 6-MP), 2.5 mg/kg/d po
Triethylenemelamine (TEM), 2.5 mg po for 2-3 d; then 0.5-5 mg/wk for several wk
Hydroxyurea (Hydrea), 20-30 mg/kg/d po or 80 mg/kg q3d

General Management

X-ray therapy for the entire body or focused on liver and spleen to suppress bone marrow and reduce organ size
Bone marrow transplants to provide healthy tissue
Transfusions (whole blood, platelets); reverse isolation techniques; antibiotics to treat bleeding and infection
Parenteral fluids to maintain hydration
Medications such as analgesics and hypnotics to relieve patient's discomfort and fear

NURSING CARE

Nursing Assessment

Susceptibility to Infection

Ulcerations of mouth and throat
Signs and symptoms of pneumonia
Signs and symptoms of septicemia
Recurrent infections

Energy Level

Fatigue, lethargy, and weakness

Susceptibility to Bleeding

Gum bleeding, ecchymoses, petechiae, and retinal hemorrhages
Epistaxis

Organ Size

Enlargement of liver, spleen, and lymph nodes

Appearance of the Skin

Pallor

Renal Function

Pain in area of kidneys
Renal insufficiency; that is, decreased urinary output

Sensory and Motor Function

Headache and disorientation
Convulsions (late)
Hemiplegia, aphasia, and other deficits caused by cerebral vascular accident

Gastrointestinal Function

Anorexia, nausea, and vomiting
Weight loss
Abdominal pain

Cardiac Function

Tachycardia
Palpitations

Pulmonary Function

Shortness of breath
Cough

Skeletal Integrity

Bone and joint pain

Nursing Dx & Intervention

Nursing Diagnosis	Nursing Intervention/Rationale
Altered cerebral tissue perfusion	• Place the patient on bed rest with quiet, dim environment *to reduce stimulation.* • Provide safety (e.g., side rails up) *to protect patient from injury.* • Provide emergency equipment, such as padded tongue blade, *in case of convulsion.* • Observe for increased intracranial pressure: vital signs, pupillary response, level of consciousness, reflexes, and orientation *to assess need for intervention.* • Observe the characteristics of the convulsion if it occurs *to aid in diagnosis of irritation site.*
Altered cardiopulmonary tissue perfusion	• Encourage alternate rest and activity as tolerated *to reduce cardiopulmonary workload.* • Count pulse and respirations and auscultate breath sounds and blood pressure *to monitor function.* • Observe for signs of fatigue, lethargy, restlessness, and dyspnea *as indications of inadequate tissue perfusion.*
Altered peripheral tissue perfusion	• Check for bleeding from body orifices or into skin *as signs of decreased clotting activity.* • Handle patient carefully *to avoid injury and possible bleeding.* • Avoid use of injections, constrictive clothing, or other agents *that impair circulation or cause trauma.* • Provide for patient's safety *to prevent injury.*
Altered patterns of urinary elimination (potential)	• Ambulate patient as tolerated *to enhance circulation and elimination.* • Change patient's position frequently *to enhance circulation.* • Encourage patient to take fluids such as carbonated beverages and urine-alkalinizing juices *to maintain normal pH and prevent crystallization.* • Inspect for bleeding and flank pain *as signs of possible obstruction.* • Test pH of urine *to assess effectiveness of fluids and medication.* • Administer allopurinol as ordered *to inhibit uric acid biosynthesis.* • Observe urine studies *to assess renal function.* • Observe blood studies *to detect elevated levels of minerals.*
Pain	• Position patient comfortably in semi-Fowler's position *to enhance pulmonary function.* • Remove constrictive clothing *to relieve pressure.* • Handle gently *to avoid irritation or injury.* • Discuss possible pain and ways to relieve it with patient *to individualize intervention.* • Administer analgesics as prescribed and per the patient's request *to control discomfort.* • Provide oral hygiene and local anesthetic *to relieve oral discomfort.* • Observe effectiveness of pain relief measures *to determine need for further or different interventions.*

Nursing Diagnosis	Nursing Intervention/Rationale
Altered nutrition: less than body requirements related to increased metabolic rate and anorexia	• Provide balanced diet, with emphasis on protein, vitamins, and calories, *to restore nutritional balance.* • Monitor caloric intake *to ensure sufficient intake.* • Give small, frequent feedings; snacks should be soft, bland, and cold *to enhance appetite and prevent distention.* • Encourage patient to make specific food requests *to increase intake.* • Balance rest with exercise *to stimulate appetite.* • Discourage smoking and oral stimulants *that may alter taste or appetite.* • Measure body weight *to monitor nutritional status.* • Use oral anesthetic or antiemetic before eating *to decrease buccal irritation and nausea.* • Encourage patient to take fluids *to maintain hydration.*
Fear	• Approach patient calmly and unhurriedly. • Express empathy, warmth, and friendliness. • Touch patient as appropriate. • Provide frequent contact. • Encourage expression of feelings. • Listen attentively and offer feedback. • Encourage questions. • Provide reliable information. • Encourage problem solving *as a means of resolving specific fears.* • Explore with patient his or her strengths, resources, and normal coping mechanisms *as bases for present and future coping.* • Encourage interaction with significant others (if patient views them as a support system). • Encourage diversional activities *to distract patient from worry and anxiety for at least short periods of time.*
Potential for infection	• Place patient in reverse isolation (may use life island or laminar air flow environment) *to protect from pathogens.* • Encourage rest and limited activity *to prevent fatigue.* • Maintain warm, clean environment *to avoid chilling and exposure to pathogens.* • Encourage increased intake of foods high in protein and fluids *to enhance antibodies and prevent dehydration.* • Teach patient and family proper handwashing, and screen visitors with infections *to prevent exposure to pathogens.* • Monitor vital signs: temperature, pulse, respirations, and blood pressure, *since changes may signal infection.* • Observe the patient for restlessness, temperature elevation, sore throat, "sniffles," chills, skin lesions, and so on *as signs of infection.* • Check blood studies *for evidence of specific pathogens.* • Administer antibiotics as ordered *to treat infection.* • Use cool sponge baths, alcohol rubs, and antipyretic drugs as needed *to reduce fever.* • Administer granulocyte transfusions as ordered *to replace defective WBC and to fight infection.* • Administer γ-globulin as ordered (for chronic lymphocytic leukemia) *to provide protein for antibody formation.*
Patient problem: hemorrhage	• Protect the patient from falls and other injuries *to avoid bleeding.* • Apply pressure over an injection site *to prevent extravasation.* • Prevent constipation; use stool softener, fiber in diet, and fluids *to avoid anal trauma.* • Assess pulse, respirations, blood pressure, level of consciousness, skin color, and so on *to detect signs of internal bleeding.* • Observe the skin for petechiae and ecchymosis *as signs of bleeding.* • Observe for signs of bleeding from mouth, nose, and rectum *to assess need for intervention.* • Monitor blood studies *to detect decreased hematocrit, hemoglobin, and platelets, which indicate actual or potential bleeding.* • Administer transfusions as ordered; whole blood and platelets *to replace loss and enhance clotting.*

Patient Education

1. Advise the patient to avoid situations in which he or she is likely to contract infection, such as inclement weather or crowds.
2. Teach the patient to maintain a clean body and environment.
3. Teach the patient to maintain a well-balanced diet especially high in protein, fiber, and fluids.
4. Instruct the patient to observe for and report signs and symptoms of infection.
5. Instruct the patient to take antibiotics as prescribed.
6. Teach the patient how to maintain a safe environment.
7. Instruct the patient to observe for and report signs and symptoms of bleeding.
8. Teach the patient to avoid tissue damage (e.g., use soft toothbrush, blow nose gently, and avoid constipation).
9. Instruct the patient to maintain a schedule of alternate rest and activity and to avoid overexertion.
10. Instruct the patient to observe for and report signs and symptoms of anemia.
11. Tell the patient to drink large volumes of fluid, especially carbonated beverages and urine-alkalinizing juices.
12. Teach the patient to observe urine for change in color and amount.
13. Teach the patient to use nonaddictive pain relief measures as long as possible; pain will increase with progression of the disease and is likely to increase in amount, intensity, types, and locations.
14. Teach the patient to avoid smoking and oral stimulants and instruct him or her in the need to stimulate appetite and maintain tissue perfusion.
15. Teach the patient to deal with stress and fear in constructive, healthful ways.
16. Be sure that the patient is aware of support resources available: financial, treatment related, and psychosocial.

Evaluation

Patient Outcome	Data Indicating That Outcome is Reached
Color of skin and mucous membranes is normal.	Skin, nails, lips, and ear lobes are warm and moist and have a natural color.
Patient's body functions are normal.	Vital signs are within acceptable limits. Elimination is adequate, and healing is prompt. Daily weight is stabilized at normal level for body build.
Laboratory studies are within normal limits.	Hemoglobin, hematocrit, blood urea nitrogen, and serum creatinine levels are within acceptable limits. Blood and urine pH, urine specific gravity, and creatinine level are within normal limits. Results of a urine protein test are negative.
Patient maintains vitality.	Patient is mentally alert, has good concentration and attentiveness, and experiences less malaise, fatigue, or weakness.
Daily intake includes essential food groups.	Protein, vitamins, and calories are emphasized.
Bowel elimination is normal for patient.	Stools are soft, and the abdomen is soft and nondistended; there is no evidence of bleeding. There is no abdominal pressure.
Daily fluid output is equivalent to fluid intake.	Urine output is 1500 to 3000 ml daily or equivalent to intake.
Patient performs adequately in work and play.	Patient can maintain self-care, perform some household or work activities, and participate in some form of recreation.
Patient has physical appearance of comfort.	Patient is calm and contented and has relaxed facial expression. Posture is normal, and patient has freedom of body movement. Patient expresses comfort and uses pain control methods effectively.
Patient frequently changes position and body movement.	Patient is walking, sitting, and standing.
Patient participates in daily physical exercise and therapeutic exercise.	Patient walks or performs other mild exercises, as well as range of motion and isometric exercises.
Patient's surroundings are clean, safe, and comfortable.	Patient's environment is free from dust, dirt, etc., and room temperature and humidity are appropriate. Patient uses safety precautions.

Patient Outcome	Data Indicating That Outcome is Reached
Patient has a positive attitude toward using available resources.	Patient accepts suggestion of referral.
Patient follows through on referral.	Patient actively seeks assistance and expresses satisfaction.
Patient prevents accidents, physical injury, deformity, infection, and hypersensitivity response.	There is no evidence of physical injury or that accidents have occurred. There is no evidence of deformity resulting from treatment.
Infection is absent.	There is no evidence of inflammation, purulent drainage or secretions, or pain or aching. Oral temperature is 37° C (98.6° F), and blood leukocyte count is 5000 to 10,000/mm³. There are no red blood cells, white blood cells, or hemoglobin casts in urine. Results of the bacterial culture of γ-globulin are negative: 20% or 0.7 to 1.6 g/dl.
Patient uses healthy coping mechanisms.	Patient reaches out to appropriate support systems and expresses feelings of safety.

Multiple Myeloma

Multiple myeloma, a neoplastic disease, strikes men over the age of 40 years twice as often as it does women.

Pathophysiology

Multiple myeloma used to be a relatively rare disorder, but the incidence is increasing. The characteristics of the disease are an abnormal malignant growth of plasma cells; development of single or multiple abnormal plasma cell tumors within the bone marrow; destruction of bone throughout the body; and later dissemination of the disease into the lymph nodes, liver, spleen, and kidneys.

The onset of the disease is usually gradual and often insidious. Many patients experience a presymptomatic period for 5 to 20 years, during which some people experience recurrent bacterial infections, especially pneumonia. This increased susceptibility to infection is believed to be related to disturbed antibody formation caused by plasma cell abnormalities.

Symptoms usually involve the skeletal system, especially the pelvis, spine, and ribs, and produce backache or bone pain that worsens with movement. Some patients sustain a pathologic fracture that causes severe pain. As skeletal destruction increases, the deformities in the sternum and rib cage may develop, with some people losing stature (5 or more inches). Diffuse osteoporosis with a negative calcium balance is also present. As the diseased bones become demineralized, renal stones develop, especially if the patient is on bed rest.

In addition, impaired production of erythrocytes, leukocytes, and thrombocytes occurs, with resultant anemia, bleeding tendencies, and increased danger of infection.

Complications may also be neurologic, such as spinal cord compression and/or renal dysfunction caused by convoluted tubules' blockage by coagulated protein particles.[1,11]

Diagnostic Studies and Findings

Roentgenograms

Diffuse bone lesions, demineralization, and osteoporosis

Bone Marrow Biopsy

Large numbers of immature plasma cells (30% to 95% of cell population)

Blood Studies

High concentration of serum globulin, particularly m-type globulin called Bence Jones protein
Decreased hemoglobin, red blood cells
Increased sedimentation rate
Increased calcium level
Increased total protein

Medical Plan

Medications

Antineoplastic agents (to suppress bone marrow function)
- Melphalan (Alkeran; L-PAM), 6 mg po for 2-3 wk; maintenance 2 mg/d
- Cyclophosphamide (Cytoxan), 40-50 mg/kg IV in divided doses over several d, then adjusted to lower maintenance dosage.

General Management

Reduction of tumor mass by radiation to relieve pressure and pain
Control of pain to enhance patient's comfort
Promotion of adequate ambulation to maintain mobility
Treatment of complications: anemia, infection, hypercalcemia, and spinal cord compression to increase patient's comfort and longevity

NURSING CARE

Nursing Assessment

Skeletal Integrity

Backache or bone pain that worsens with movement
Loss of stature
Signs and symptoms of pathologic fractures

Renal Function

Signs and symptoms of calculi

Energy Level

Weakness, fatigue, dyspnea, bleeding, and infection

Sensory and Motor Function

Spinal cord compression, as evidenced by loss of sensory and motor function

Fluid and Electrolytes

Hypercalcemia, as evidenced by lethargy, polyuria, polydipsia, etc.

Nursing Dx & Intervention

Nursing Diagnosis	Nursing Intervention/Rationale
Chronic pain	• Position the patient for comfort. • Change the patient's position slowly *to prevent trauma.* • Maintain the patient's body alignment *to prevent injury.* • Apply heat *to reduce muscle spasm and swelling.* • Massage gently *to reduce muscle spasm.* • Use firm mattress *to support skeletal structure.* • Encourage rest *to reduce stress on skeletal structure.* • Work with patient on ways to reduce pain, including analgesics, *to intervene most effectively.*
Impaired physical mobility related to musculoskeletal impairment	• Assist with ambulation *to prevent injury.* • Mobilize as necessary using a walker, cane, or wheelchair *to prevent injury.* • Provide range of motion exercises and assistance with turning *to maintain mobility.* • Decrease environmental barriers, such as chairs, tables, or rugs, *to prevent injury.* • Limit distance patient ambulates *to avoid fatigue and injury.* • Observe patient's gait, coordination, and stability *to assess changes in musculoskeletal function.* • Provide trapeze *to assist with movement in bed.* • Help patient turn in bed every 1 to 2 hours *to prevent pulmonary-circulatory stasis and to promote mobility.* • Encourage increased protein and vitamin intake *to enhance mineralization and muscle tone.*
Potential for injury related to falling	• Handle patient gently. • Change patient's position slowly. • Avoid jarring the bed. • Assess body alignment and complaints of pain *as signs of injury.*
Altered patterns of urinary elimination (potential) related to renal calculi	• Provide adequate hydration of 3000 to 4000 ml of fluid per day *to prevent urinary stasis.* • Maintain adequate urinary output *to prevent urinary stasis.* • Ambulate the patient as much as possible *to enhance elimination.* • Encourage a diet low in calcium and phosphorus *to prevent formation of calculi.* • Give urine-acidifying juices *to maintain urinary pH.* • Avoid bicarbonates and carbonated beverages *to maintain slightly acid urine.* • Monitor output, frequency, and urgency; report findings to physician *to detect retention, inflammation, and infection.*
Fluid volume excess; potential fluid volume deficit related to renal calculi and failure	• Monitor intake and compare with output *to identify fluid deficit or excess.*
Activity intolerance	• Place patient in sitting position *to enhance cardiopulmonary function.* • Observe respiration rate and dyspnea *to assess respiratory status.* • Observe skin color and temperature *to assess oxygenation and circulation.* • Assist with care *to provide rest and reduce fatigue.* • Plan rest periods *to control fatigue.* • Monitor laboratory values *to detect inadequate cardiopulmonary function.*

Nursing Diagnosis	Nursing Intervention/Rationale
Impaired physical mobility (potential) related to spinal cord compression	• Maintain body alignment *to prevent injury to vertebrae.* • Support the spine with brace or traction *to avoid injury.* • Place the patient on bed rest as needed *to protect from falls.* • Log roll the patient *to maintain alignment.* • Observe respiratory rate and rhythm *to assess for cervical cord compression.* • Assess motor function, sensation, and reflexes; report findings to physician if abnormalities occur *to detect early signs of compression.*
Altered nutrition: potential for more than body requirements related to hypercalcemia	• Encourage a decrease in intake of foods with calcium, and encourage an increase in fluid intake *to correct imbalance.* • Monitor blood studies *to determine effectiveness of interventions.* • Observe for complaints of constipation, headache, nausea, thirst, weakness, bone pain, and fatigue; report findings to physician, *since these are signs and symptoms of hypercalcemia.*
Altered peripheral tissue perfusion (potential) related to bleeding	• Handle the patient gently *to avoid trauma.* • Give injections only if necessary; apply pressure afterward *to prevent extravasation.* • Observe for change in vital signs or for blood in urine, stool, gums, nose, or skin, *as these are signs of internal bleeding.* • Avoid constipation *to prevent anal irritation and bleeding.*
Potential for infection	• Maintain reverse isolation *to protect patient from pathogens.* • Observe for increases in temperature, pulse, and respirations *to assess for infection.* • Observe the patient for "sniffles," sore throat, anorexia, pain on urination, and so on *to assess for infection.* • Administer antibiotics as ordered *to treat specific pathogens.* • Help patient to turn, cough, and deep breathe *to maintain respiratory function.* • Provide oral, skin, and perineal hygiene *to prevent development of irritation and infection.*

Patient Education

1. Explain the need for good body balance, good body mechanics, and mechanical support, such as a cane or brace.
2. Teach methods of pain control: pain-reducing measures and medications.
3. Teach the importance of drinking adequate fluids and controlling intake of high-calcium foods.
4. Explain the need for a diet high in protein and vitamins.

Evaluation

Patient Outcome	Data Indicating That Outcome is Reached
Color of the skin and mucous membranes is good.	The skin, nails, lips, and ear lobes are warm and moist and have a natural color.
Vital signs are within normal limits.	Respirations, pulse, and blood pressure are within normal limits.
Laboratory studies are within normal limits.	Hemoglobin level and hematocrit are within normal limits; thrombocyte and leukocyte counts are within normal limits. Total protein, albumin, α-globulin, β-globulin, γ-globulin, and calcium levels are within normal limits. Urine pH is within normal limits.
Body hydration is normal.	Skin turgor is good, mucous membranes are moist, and patient is not thirsty.
Daily fluid output is equal to fluid intake.	Urine output is 1500 to 3000 ml. Patient's diet includes foods high in protein and vitamins.
Patient has physical appearance of comfort.	Patient is calm, contented, and has relaxed facial expression. Posture is normal, and patient has freedom of body movement. Patient relaxes muscles when resting and motionless.
Patient verbally expresses comfort.	Patient expresses comfort and uses analgesics effectively.
Patient frequently changes position and body movement.	Patient walks, sits, and stands using assistive devices as needed.

Patient Outcome	Data Indicating That Outcome is Reached
Patient participates in therapeutic exercise.	Patient participates in range of motion and isometric exercises.
Patient's surroundings are safe.	Patient uses safety precautions, such as side rails, low bed, and so on. Patient's movement is not hampered by environmental barriers.
There is no evidence of physical injury.	There is no evidence of pathologic fractures.
Infection is gone.	There is no evidence of inflammation, pain, or aching.

THROMBOCYTIC DISORDERS

Thrombocytopenia

Thrombocytopenia is a term used to describe a platelet count below 200,000/mm^3, which causes (1) spontaneous bleeding into the skin, mucous membranes, internal cavities, and organs, and (2) oozing of blood for long periods of time from lacerations and punctures.

Pathophysiology

The major types of thrombocytopenia are idiopathic thrombocytopenic purpura (ITP) and secondary thrombocytopenic purpura. In ITP platelets are prematurely destroyed (survival decreases from 8 to 20 days to 1 to 3 days). It is believed to be caused by an autoimmune process. The acute form is found mostly in children, whereas the chronic form is found among all ages; it is more common among women. Secondary thrombocytopenic purpura results from diseases such as viral infections, bone marrow failure, infectious mononucleosis, and drug hypersensitivity.

Diagnostic Studies and Findings

Platelet Count

$<$100,000/mm^3

Bleeding Time

Prolonged

Coagulation Time

Normal

Capillary Fragility

Increased

Medical Plan

Surgery

Splenectomy

Medications

Corticosteroids
Prednisone (Deltasone, Meticorten), 10-20 mg po qid

General Management

Platelet transfusions

NURSING CARE

Nursing Assessment

Vascular Integrity

Petechiae, ecchymosis, and easy bruising
Epistaxis
Bleeding from gums and nose

Female Reproductive Function

Heavy menses and bleeding between periods

Sensory and Motor Function

Cerebral hemorrhage, as evidenced by signs and symptoms of increased intracranial pressure
Nerve pain and anesthesia of extremities and/or paralysis

Gastrointestinal Tract

Hematemesis
Melena

Renal Function

Hematuria

Cardiac Function

Tachycardia

Respiratory Function

Dyspnea
Tachypnea

Nursing Dx & Intervention

Nursing Diagnosis	Nursing Intervention/Rationale
Altered cardiopulmonary tissue perfusion	• Place patient on bed rest in a slightly sitting position *to enhance cardiopulmonary function.* • Dress patient warmly and maintain warm room temperature *to enhance vasodilation.* • Remove constrictive clothing *to facilitate chest expansion.* • Discourage smoking and oral stimulants, *which cause vasoconstriction and dyspnea.* • Monitor vital signs and laboratory studies *to determine adequacy of function.* • Observe pulse rate and rhythm, respiration rate and depth, and blood pressure *to determine need for intervention.*
Altered cerebral tissue perfusion	• Observe for signs of increased intracranial pressure: level of consciousness, pupillary response, and reflexes. • Instruct patient to avoid Valsalva maneuver (e.g., coughing or straining at stool) *to decrease potential for bleeding.*
Altered renal tissue perfusion	• Observe color, amount, and presence of red blood cells in urine.
Altered oral mucous membrane	• Remove dentures *to avoid irritation.* • Provide mouth care with soft toothbrush *to minimize tissue trauma.* • Give soft foods and iced liquids *to avoid trauma.* • Observe for bleeding.
Impaired tissue integrity (vaginal mucous membrane)	• Provide perineal hygiene *to promote comfort.* • Count pads used *to determine amount of bleeding.* • Observe amount, color, consistency, and frequency of discharge *to monitor blood loss.*
Impaired tissue integrity (nasal mucous membrane)	• Observe amount, color, and consistency of discharge *to monitor blood loss.* • Position the patient with the head forward and elevated *to stop bleeding.*
Impaired tissue integrity (rectal mucous membrane)	• Observe amount, color, consistency, and frequency of discharge *to monitor blood loss.* • Maintain perianal hygiene *for patient comfort.* • Avoid use of rectal thermometer, enema tube, or other instruments *that might cause bleeding.* • Encourage high-fiber foods and increased fluids *to prevent constipation.* • Test stool for occult blood.
Impaired skin integrity related to intradermal bleeding	• Apply ice bag and/or manual pressure over any bleeding site *to control bleeding.* • Handle gently *to avoid trauma.* • Avoid injections or use of straight razor, *which may cause bleeding.* • Observe for petechiae, ecchymoses, or frank bleeding. • Protect patient from injury by assisting with ambulation and avoiding environmental barriers.
Pain	• Position patient comfortably *to minimize pain and pressure.* • Handle patient gently (massage) *to relax muscles.* • Apply bed cradle, lightweight clothing, and blanket *to relieve pressure.* • Apply heat lamp, cradle pad, hot water bottle, compress, or cold compress bag; do what the patient thinks will make him or her comfortable. • Give analgesics as ordered.

Patient Education

1. Explain the need to stop smoking to avoid impairment of arterial circulation.
2. Teach the patient to avoid mechanical trauma:
   a. General safety precautions
   b. Soft toothbrush
   c. Gentle nose blowing
   d. Stool softeners and maintenance of diet high in roughage and fluids
3. Teach the patient to detect and report signs and symptoms of bleeding.

Evaluation

Patient Outcome	Data Indicating That Outcome is Reached
Vital signs are within normal limits.	Respirations, pulse, blood pressure, and temperature are within normal limits.
Laboratory studies are within normal limits.	Platelet count and bleeding time are within normal limits. Capillary fragility test shows occasional petechiae or none.
Daily intake includes essential food groups.	Diet includes milk, meat, fruits, vegetables, bread, and cereals.
Bowel and bladder elimination are normal.	Stools are soft, and there is no evidence of bleeding.
Patient is mentally alert.	Patient has good concentration.
Patient has physical appearance of comfort.	Posture is normal, and patient has freedom of body movement. Patient changes position and body movement frequently (i.e., walks, sits, and stands).
Patient's surroundings are safe.	Patient uses safety precautions; room temperature and humidity are appropriate.
There is no evidence that an accident or physical injury has occurred.	There are no signs of infection.

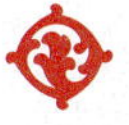

Disseminated intravascular coagulation syndrome

Disseminated intravascular coagulation (DIC) syndrome is a bleeding disorder that results from the blood's increased tendency to clot.

DIC syndrome causes the transformation of fibrinogen to fibrin clot and is often associated with acute hemorrhage. States of physiologic disequilibrium that precipitate this syndrome include hemorrhagic shock, crush syndrome, leukemia, carcinoma, abruptio placentae, septic abortion, incompatible blood transfusion, and endotoxic shock.

Pathophysiology

The result of the physiologic disequilibrium caused by the factors cited previously is a systemic activation of coagulation and fibrinolysis, with diffuse intravascular fibrin formation and deposition of fibrin in the microcirculation. As a consequence of these processes, clots accumulate in the body's capillaries, which are more than 100,000 miles in length. Clotting factors are used at a rate that exceeds their replenishment, with circulating thrombin waiting in the intravascular space for fibrinogen. The excessive thrombin formation greatly decreases the availability of the inhibitor antithrombin III.

Activation of the fibrinolytic system results in fibrin degradation products, which interfere with both platelet function and fibrin clot formation. As a consequence, the patient has a simultaneous, self-perpetuating combination of thrombosis and bleeding.

The kallikrein and complement systems also are activated, resulting in arterial hypotension. Clotting activity is enhanced by kallikrein's activation of factor XII to XIIa. Kallikrein also releases kinins, which increase vascular permeability and vasodilation, thereby further increasing the arterial hypotension.

Activation of the complement system causes not only increased vascular permeability but also lysis of erythrocytes, granulocytes, and platelets; this produces phospholipids, which activate factor XII.

Arteriolar vasoconstriction and capillary dilation result in shunting of blood to the venous side, leaving the dilated capillaries with stagnant blood, which produces metabolic waste and resultant acidity. This results in three concurrent, procoagulating effects in the capillary blood: blood stagnation, the presence of coagulation-promoting substances, and acidosis.

The patient with DIC syndrome bleeds because of increased fibrinolysis, diminished antithrombin III, and consumption of clotting factors. Antithrombin III cannot keep pace with the excessive production of thrombin, which continues to activate the conversion of plasminogen to plasmin, exacerbating the bleeding.

Diagnostic Studies and Findings

Prothrombin Time (PT)

Prolonged

Partial Thromboplastin Time (PTT)

Prolonged

Platelet Count

$<100{,}000/mm^3$

Fibrinogen Level

Decreased

Antithrombin III Level

Decreased

Thrombin Time

Prolonged

Fibrin Degradation Products

Elevated

Plasminogen Levels

Decreased

Plasmin

Present

Medical Plan

Medications

Heparin therapy, 30,000 IV in 24 h; 2500-5000 U q4-8h subcutaneously

General Management

Elimination of the cause
- May require correction of hypovolemia, hypotension, hypoxia and acidosis, or hemostatic deficiencies
- Physiologic disequilibrium, such as septic shock, must also be treated

Administration of depleted factors such as whole blood or fresh-frozen plasma, which contain fibrinogen

Investigational antithrombin III concentrate

NURSING CARE

Nursing Assessment

Vascular Integrity

Bleeding from the nose, gums, and infection sites
Petechiae, purpura, and ecchymosis

Respiratory Function

Tachypnea, dyspnea
Cyanosis or pallor
Basilar rales

Cardiac Function

Dysrhythmias, tachycardia
Hypotension
Gallop rhythm

Renal Function

Decreased urinary output

Sensory and Motor Function

Altered level of consciousness, orientation, and pupillary reaction
Decreased movement and strength of extremities

Mental Status

Fear, anxiety
Restlessness

Nursing Dx & Intervention

Nursing Diagnosis	Nursing Intervention/Rationale
Fluid volume deficit (1)	• Monitor vital signs and level of consciousness *for evidence of acute hemorrhage.* • Administer blood component and intravenous fluids as ordered *to replace fluid loss.* • Apply ice pack and manual dressing over site of blood loss *to promote clotting and slow or stop bleeding.* • Place patient in semi-Fowler's position *to prevent respiratory distress caused by nasal bleeding.* • Avoid using injections or razor *to prevent further bleeding.* • Assess amount, consistency, and frequency of bleeding *to determine need for replacement therapy.* • Monitor laboratory tests *to determine degree of blood loss and effect of treatment.* • Administer heparin as prescribed; apply pressure to injection site for at least 5 minutes *to avoid seepage.* • Assess skin for presence, size, and color of petechiae, purpura, and ecchymosis *to determine degree of bleeding into tissues.* • Check stool, urine, emesis, and sputum for presence of occult and observable blood *to identify presence of gastrointestinal or renal hemorrhage.* • Provide gentle care to skin, oral mucosa, fingernails, and toenails *to avoid further bleeding.*
Impaired gas exchange	• Position patient to facilitate breathing, that is, in semi-Fowler's position, *to reduce pressure on diaphragm and promote chest expansion.* • Encourage patient to take deep breaths *to reduce hyperventilation.*

Nursing Diagnosis	Nursing Intervention/Rationale
	• Provide oxygen therapy as prescribed *to reduce cardiopulmonary workload and to enhance tissue oxygenation.* • Help patient maintain a balance between rest and activity *to decrease oxygen requirement.* • Maintain warm environment *to avoid shivering.* • Monitor respiratory rate and breath sounds *to identify increasing difficulty and assess effectiveness of treatment.* • Assess skin color and temperature *to determine adequacy of tissue oxygenation.*
Decreased cardiac output; altered cardiopulmonary tissue perfusion	• Maintain patient in semi-Fowler's position with legs elevated *to enhance cardiac output and venous return.* • Administer antiarrhythmic drugs as prescribed *to correct dysrhythmias, slow the heart rate, and increase cardiac output.* • Monitor apical, brachial, carotid, radial, femoral, and tibial pulses *to determine pumping action of heart and adequacy of tissue perfusion.* • Administer cardiotonic and vasoconstricting drugs as ordered *to strengthen pumping action of the heart and increase vascular tone.* • Help patient avoid stress as much as possible *to decrease cardiac workload* (e.g., balance rest and activity, avoid straining at stool, use relaxation exercises). • Assess skin color *to determine adequacy of tissue perfusion.* • Monitor laboratory tests, especially blood pH, *to detect acidosis.*
Altered patterns of urinary elimination related to decreased output	• Monitor intake and output, color and consistency of urine, and frequency of voiding *to assess renal function.* • Use Foley catheter and drainage bag as prescribed *to monitor urine production.* • Monitor laboratory studies, including electrolytes, *to determine adequacy of renal function.* • Monitor intravenous and oral fluids *to detect early signs and symptoms of fluid overload, such as shortness of breath, restlessness, confusion, hypertension, and abnormal breath sounds.*
Sensory/perceptual alterations	• Place patient on bed rest with the head elevated *to reduce intracranial pressure and unnecessary activity.* • Decrease environmental stimuli *to lessen stress and distraction or confusion.* • Discourage use of oral stimulants, such as caffeine, *which might increase intracranial pressure.* • Monitor neurologic signs, such as level of consciousness, orientation, pupillary responses, and reflexes *to detect changes early.* • Assess range of motion and strength of extremities *to monitor neurologic status.* • Monitor vital signs for alterations *that would indicate increasing intracranial pressure.* • Report to physician any change in pupillary response, projectile vomiting, or decrease in level of consciousness.
Fear	• Encourage patient to talk about specific fears, *so that each can be dealt with.* • Have patient describe his or her perception of danger and coping skills as a basis *for identifying specific interventions.* • Deal with distorted perceptions of danger, isolation, and so on *to reduce degree of fear.* • Orient patient to environment, including such equipment as drainage tubes, IV lines, hemodynamic monitoring equipment, and mechanical ventilator *to reduce fear of the unfamiliar.* • Assure patient of observation and monitoring by health care providers *to reduce fear of abandonment.* • Avoid startling patient by telling him or her what to expect and when. • Teach patient ways of maintaining some degree of control, such as having access to the call light or bell and asking about his or her status and test results, *to reduce fear of dependence.*
Potential for infection	• Provide meticulous care to open areas, IV sites, and other portals of entry for microorganisms *to prevent contamination.* • Maintain gastric tubes with clean technique, Foley catheter with sterile technique *to avoid nosocomial infection.* • Monitor vital signs, especially temperature, and patient's behavior *to detect infection early.* • Report chills, headache, severe hyperthermia or hypothermia, tachypnea, tachycardia, hypotension, oliguria, confusion, or disorientation to physician, *since these may be indications of septic shock.*

Patient Education

1. Teach the patient and family signs and symptoms of the syndrome, which should be reported immediately to the nurse or physician.
2. Teach the patient to administer heparin therapy subcutaneously.
3. Teach the patient and family to avoid mechanical trauma such as a hard toothbrush, blade razor, rough nose blowing, or contact sports.

Evaluation

Patient Outcome	Data Indicating That Outcome is Reached
Vital signs are within normal limits.	Pulse, respirations, blood pressure, and temperature are within normal limits.
Laboratory studies are within normal limits.	Platelet count, bleeding time, and other relevant parameters are within normal limits.
Bowel and bladder elimination are normal.	There is no evidence of bleeding. Urinary output is sufficient.
Skin integrity is within normal limits.	There are no open wounds. There is no evidence of discoloration, and the skin is warm, dry, and natural in color.
Neurologic function is within normal limits.	Patient is oriented, alert, and calm. Pupillary responses are equal and normal. Patient has adequate movement and strength of extremities.

Hemophilia

Hemophilia is a disorder characterized by impaired coagulability of the blood and a tendency to bleed.

The classic disease is hereditary and limited to males; thus it is an X-linked recessive disease. All daughters of hemophiliac males become carriers, and the son of a female carrier has a 50% chance of being a hemophiliac. Homozygous females with hemophilia (father a hemophiliac, mother a carrier) are extremely rare.

Pathophysiology

Two of the major types of hemophilia are clinically identical: classic hemophilia, or hemophilia A, in which antihemophilic factor VII activity is deficient or absent, and Christmas disease, or hemophilia B, in which factor IX activity is deficient or absent. The degree of bleeding experienced by the patient is related to the amount of factor activity and the severity of the injury. When factor activity levels are below 1%, spontaneous bleeding, hemarthrosis (joint bleeding), and deep tissue bleeding occur. When levels are 5% or higher, bleeding usually results from trauma or surgical procedures, such as at circumcision.

Other less common forms of hemophilia include hemophilia C, a hemorrhagic susceptibility transmitted as an autosomal dominant trait and caused by a lack of clotting factor XI; calipriva, a bleeding tendency caused by a serum calcium deficiency; vascular hemophilia, also called angiohemophilia; and von Willebrand's disease, an autosomal dominant trait in both males and females with factor VIII_{VWF} and VIII_{AHC} deficiency and a platelet adhesion defect.

Diagnostic Studies and Findings

Prothrombin Time (PT)

Normal

Partial Thromboplastin Time (PTT)

Prolonged

Bleeding Time (Platelet Function)

Normal
Prolonged in von Willebrand's disease

Medical Plan

General Management

Replacement of deficient factor
- For hemophilia A, cryoprecipitate containing 8 to 100 U of factor VIII per bag at 12-hour intervals until bleeding ceases
- For hemophilia B, plasma or factor IX concentrate (Konyne or Proplex), given every 24 hours until bleeding ceases

Treatment for the development of antibody inhibitors against the specific coagulation factor

Immunosuppressive agents
Plasmapheresis to remove the inhibitor
Prothrombin complexes, which bypass the inhibitors
Synthetic product OOAVP (1-deamino 8-D arginine vasopressin) administered IV can induce a threefold to sixfold increase in factor VIII activity level

NURSING CARE

Nursing Assessment

Vascular Integrity

Bleeding from nose, gums, lips, tongue, and infection sites
Petechiae, purpura, and ecchymosis
Menorrhagia

Mobility

Hemarthrosis with pain and deformity

Renal Function

Hematuria

Sensory Function and Mental Status

Intracranial bleeding

Hepatic Function

Hepatitis related to infusion of concentrates

Gastrointestinal Function

Melena

Nursing Dx & Intervention

Nursing Diagnosis	Nursing Intervention/Rationale
Fluid volume deficit (1)	• Monitor vital signs and level of consciousness *for evidence of acute hemorrhage.* • Administer blood component therapy as ordered *to control bleeding:* Cryoprecipitate—observe for reactions such as urticaria or hives; administer Benadryl to counteract reaction. Use normal saline to flush cryoprecipitate from bag to remove it from plastic. Include number of bags and amount of solution in intake and output records. Plasma thromboplastin component (PTC) and antihemophilic factor (AHF)—must be refrigerated until use; shake gently for up to 10 minutes and administer over a 5-minute interval; reactions are rare. Prothrombin complexes—high risk of hepatitis; dosage depends on patient's condition. • Apply ice pack to affected joint or traumatized area *to control bleeding.* • Casting may be used *to protect and rest affected joints.* • Administer analgesics *to relieve joint pain.* • Assess amount, consistency, and frequency of bleeding *to determine need for replacement therapy:* Nose, gums, lips, tongue Joints Skin Stool and urine Pad counts • Measure abdominal girth *to detect occurrence of deep bleeding.* • Monitor laboratory tests *to determine degree of blood loss and effect of therapy.* • Avoid trauma, such as falls, bumps, or injections. • Observe for signs and symptoms of hepatitis, such as jaundice, clay-colored stool, mahogany-colored urine, nausea, and abdominal distention.
Sensory/perceptual alterations (potential)	• Place patient on bed rest with head elevated *to reduce intracranial pressure and unnecessary activity.* • Protect head with helmet, and use padded side rails if patient is restless. • Discourage oral stimulants, such as caffeine, *which might increase intracranial pressure.* • Monitor neurologic signs, such as level of consciousness, orientation, pupillary response, and reflexes *to detect changes early.* • Monitor vital signs *for evidence of increasing intracranial pressure.* • Report changes in pupillary response, projectile vomiting, or decrease in level of consciousness to physician.

Patient Education

1. Teach the patient self-administration of factor(s).
2. Instruct the patient to avoid injury, such as that caused by contact sports or use of sharp instruments.

3. Teach the patient to report signs and symptoms of bleeding to a nurse or physician.
4. Encourage the patient to seek genetic counseling if he or she has a hereditary form of hemophilia.

Evaluation

Patient Outcome	Data Indicating That Outcome is Reached
Vital signs are within normal limits.	Pulse, respirations, blood pressure, and temperature are within normal limits.
Laboratory studies are within normal limits.	PT, PTT, bleeding time, and other relevant parameters are within normal limits.
Gastrointestinal function is normal.	There is no evidence of bleeding, and there are no signs or symptoms of hepatitis.
Renal function is normal.	There is no evidence of bleeding.
The skin and skeletal structure are within normal limits.	There is no evidence of bleeding or discoloration and no swelling of the joints; the skin is warm and dry.
Neurologic function is within normal limits.	The patient is oriented, alert, and calm. Pupillary responses are equal and within normal limits.

Plasma Clotting Factors

I. Fibrinogen: precursor of fibrin
II. Prothrombin: precursor of thrombin
III. Thromboplastin: activator of prothrombin
IV. Calcium
V. Plasma accelerator globulin
VII. Serum prothrombin conversion accelerator
VIII. Antihemophilic globulin (AHG)
IX. Christmas factor
X. Stuart-Prower factor
XI. Plasma thromboplastin antecedent (PTA)
XII. Hageman factor
XIII. Fibrin-stabilizing factor
Fletcher factor
Fitzgerald factor

Malignant Lymphomas

Malignant lymphomas are neoplasms of the lymphoid tissue.

Malignant lymphomas include lymphosarcoma, reticulum cell sarcoma, and Hodgkin's disease. Although the cause of these cancers is unknown, a viral etiology is believed responsible for several types, particularly Burkitt's lymphoma (a childhood disease) and Hodgkin's disease. There may also be a genetic factor in Hodgkin's disease.

Non-Hodgkin's lymphomas may be further categorized as follows:

- Lymphocyte malignancies
  - Lymphocytic lymphosarcoma
  - Lymphoblastic lymphosarcoma
  - Reticulum cell sarcoma
  - Burkitt's lymphoma
  - Stem cell lymphoma/immunoblastoma
  - "Mixed" lymphoma
- Histiocytic lymphoma

Pathophysiology

Lymphosarcoma and reticulum cell sarcomas account for about 40% of malignant lymphomas; the incidence increases with age, primarily striking middle-aged people. Early widespread dissemination is common, with oropharyngeal lymphoid tissue, the gastrointestinal tract, and bones frequently affected. The earliest sign is painless lymphadenopathy, usually unilateral and in the neck. The disease spreads via lymphatic channels to other nodes and, in the case of lymphosarcoma, invades the bone marrow. Other organs that may be involved are the skin and nervous system. Pressure and organ obstruction produce symptoms such as abdominal pain, nerve pain, and paralysis. Other patient problems include anemia, fever, sweating, pruritus, weight loss, and malaise. Diagnosis and treatment of these lymphatic malignancies are similar to those of Hodgkin's disease.

 Hodgkin's Disease

A chronic and progressive cancer, Hodgkin's disease primarily affects adults aged 20 to 40 years. Men are affected twice as often as women and boys five times more than girls.

The disease is characterized by the abnormal proliferation of histiocytes called "Reed-Sternberg cells," which eventually replace the normal cellular structure of the lymph nodes and cause areas of necrosis and fibrosis to develop. Malignant reticulum cells are also present.

Hodgkin's disease initially affects one lymph node and then travels by lymphatic channels to nodes throughout the body; it may also appear in the liver and spleen, vertebrae, ureters, and bronchi. Staging of the disease is based on microscopic appearance of the lymph nodes, extent and severity of the disease, and prognosis. Table 15-1 shows one method of staging.

Prognosis for untreated patients is about 5 years; those diagnosed in stage I or II have a 95% cure rate, while those in stages III or IV have a poor prognosis.[1,5,11]

Diagnostic Studies and Findings

Lymph Node Biopsy

Presence of Reed-Sternberg cells

Roentgenogram of Chest

Mediastinal or hilar lymphadenopathy

Blood Studies

Normocytic normochromic anemia

Skin Tests for Tuberculosis

Abnormal reaction

Table 15-1
Staging of Hodgkin's Disease

Stage*	Definition
I	Single lymph node region
II	Two or more node regions limited to one side of the diaphragm
III	Disease on both sides of the diaphragm but limited to the lymph nodes and spleen
IV	Involvement of the bones, bone marrow, lung parenchyma, pleura, liver, skin, gastrointestinal tract, central nervous system, renal, etc.

From Luckmann.[11]
*All stages are subclassified as A or B to describe the absence (A) or presence (B) of systemic symptoms.

Medical Plan[1,11]

Surgery

The tumor that is causing pressure on an organ or nerve is excised

Medications

Antineoplastic agents in combination therapy (see Chapter 16)
- MOPP
  - Mechlorethamine (Nitrogen mustard)
  - Vincristine (Oncovin)
  - Prednisone (Deltasone)
  - Procarbazine (Matulane)
- MVPP
  - Mechlorethamine (Nitrogen mustard)
  - Vinblastine (Velban)
  - Procarbazine (Matulane)
  - Prednisone (Deltasone)

Table 15-2
Karnofsky Performance Scale

Activity Status	Point	Description
Normal activity	10	Normal, with no complaints or evidence of disease
	9	Able to carry on normal activity but with minor signs or symptoms of disease present
	8	Normal activity but requiring effort; signs and symptoms of disease more prominent
Self-care	7	Able to care for self but unable to work or carry on other normal activities
	6	Able to care for most needs but requires occasional assistance
	5	Considerable assistance required, along with frequent medical care; some self-care still possible
Incapacitated	4	Disabled and requiring special care and assistance
	3	Severely disabled; hospitalization required but death from disease not imminent
	2	Extremely ill; supportive treatment, hospitalized care required
	1	Imminent death
	0	Dead

COPP
Cyclophosphamide (Cytoxan)
Vincristine (Oncovin)
Prednisone (Deltasone)
Procarbazine (Matulane)

No specific drug dosages are given for the chemotherapy combinations because (1) doses may change when used in combination; (2) doses differ depending on the patient's physical status, such as white blood cell and platelet counts and Karnofsky scale rating (Table 15-2); and (3) individual drug protocols differ from one institution to another.

General Management

Wide-field megavoltage radiation (3500 to 4000 roentgens over a 4- to 6-week period can be curative for stages I or II)

Combined radiotherapy and chemotherapy for stages III and IV

NURSING CARE

Nursing Assessment

Skin Integrity

Painless swelling of lymph nodes, usually cervical (early sign)

Severe pruritus
Jaundice
Edema and cyanosis of face and neck
Irregular fever, night sweats

Sensory and Motor Function

Bone pain, vertebral compression, fracture, paraplegia, and nerve pain

Respiratory Function

Cough, stridor, dyspnea, chest pain, and pleural effusion
Recent upper respiratory infections
Laryngeal paralysis

Energy Level

Fatigue, malaise (early sign)
Increased susceptibility to infection

Gastrointestinal Function

Splenomegaly and hepatomegaly, with resultant abdominal distention and discomfort
Weight loss, anorexia

Nursing Dx & Intervention

Nursing Diagnosis	Nursing Intervention/Rationale
Impaired skin integrity	• Bathe the patient in cool water or apply cool, moist compresses *to enhance comfort.* • Apply calamine lotion, cornstarch, sodium bicarbonate, and medicated powder *to relieve itching.* • Use a bed cradle and lightweight blankets and clothing *to relieve pressure.* • Lubricate skin with baby oil, bath oil, body lotion, or petrolatum for comfort. • Maintain adequate humidity and cool room *to decrease itching.* • Avoid adhesive, alkaline soap, and local heat, *which irritate the skin.*
Impaired physical mobility (potential)	• Maintain body alignment *to enhance mobility and comfort.* • Move body as a single unit *to prevent injury.* • Provide mechanical support during ambulation *to enhance mobility.* • Observe motor function in extremities; monitor complaints of numbness and tingling; report findings to the physician.
Pain[13]	• For bone pain: position the patient comfortably, change position gradually, and handle the patient gently and in an unhurried manner *to avoid trauma.* • Support affected body part *to prevent pressure.* • Encourage adequate rest *to reduce incidence of pain related to activity.* • Provide pain relief measures based on patient's choice. • Give analgesics as ordered. • For intra-abdominal pressure: place patient in a sitting position; remove constrictive clothing; change patient's position frequently; give small, frequent feedings.
Ineffective breathing pattern related to airway edema[9]	• Place patient in a sitting position *to increase chest expansion.* • Remove constrictive clothing *to relieve pressure on chest.* • Encourage deep breathing *for alveolar expansion.* • Administer oxygen as needed *to provide tissue oxygenation.* • Provide standby emergency equipment *to relieve airway obstruction.* • Inspect chest for respiratory rate and rhythm and symmetric expansion.

Nursing Diagnosis	Nursing Intervention/Rationale
	• Auscultate lungs for abnormal breath sounds, aeration, rales, and rhonchi. • Observe for hoarseness, cough, stridor, pain, and change in skin color (cyanosis). • Monitor blood studies for abnormal gas exchange. • Plan rest periods *to avoid hyperventilation.*
Altered nutrition: less than body requirements	• Provide small feedings of high-calorie, high-protein foods and fluids *to increase nutritional intake.* • Assist with oral care, general hygiene, environmental control (temperature, appearance, odors) *to enhance appetite.* • Identify food preferences and provide them as often as possible *to promote adequate nutritional intake.* • Place the patient in a sitting position after meals *to decrease feeling of fullness.*
Potential for infection	• Have the patient turn, cough, and deep breathe at regular intervals *to prevent respiratory tract infection.* • Encourage fluids and balanced diet *for maintenance of general well-being.* • Maintain reverse isolation *to protect patient from microorganisms.* • Observe the patient for "sniffles," sore throat, anorexia, pain on urination, and increases in temperature, pulse, and respirations, *which indicate infection.* • Administer antibiotics as ordered *to treat infection.*
Hyperthermia	• Apply cool, damp cloth to the patient's face *for comfort.* • Bathe the patient in cool water and apply ice bag or alcohol *to reduce fever.* • Cover with lightweight blankets and clothing *to avoid chilling.* • Maintain cool room temperature *for patient's comfort.* • Increase fluid intake, especially iced liquids, *for hydration.* • Monitor oral temperature level and pattern *to determine need for antipyretics, cooling blanket, or other interventions.*

Patient Education

1. Explain the need to avoid scratching and to correctly care for skin to reduce susceptibility to infection and mechanical skin damage.
2. Teach correct maintenance of body alignment, use of body mechanics and ambulatory aids, and the early symptoms of vertebral compression and paralysis to report to physician or nurse.
3. Teach ways to relieve pain without the use of medications as often as possible; bone, nerve, and abdominal pain is chronic in nature and increases with pressure of disseminated disease.
4. Emphasize the importance of respiratory therapy to prevent or decrease severity of symptoms of mediastinal lymph node enlargement, involvement of lung parenchyma, and invasion of pleura.
5. Teach the need for adequate rest and exercise and a balanced diet.
6. Help the patient make use of coping methods after exploring these with the patient and family.

Evaluation

Patient Outcome	Data Indicating That Outcome is Reached
Color of the skin and mucous membranes is good.	The skin, nails, lips, and ear lobes are warm and moist and have a natural color.
Vital signs are within normal limits.	Respirations, pulse, blood pressure, and temperature are within normal limits.
Laboratory studies are within normal limits.	The hemoglobin level, hematocrit, oxygen saturation, and leukocyte count are within normal limits.
Body hydration is normal.	Skin turgor is good; mucous membranes are moist.
Patient has physical appearance of comfort.	Patient is calm and relaxed. Posture is normal, and patient has freedom of body movement. Patient verbally expresses comfort and ceases previous complaining. Patient uses medications effectively.
Patient's surroundings are comfortable.	Room temperature is appropriate. Humidity level is appropriate, and room is well ventilated.

Patient Outcome	Data Indicating That Outcome is Reached
There is no evidence of physical injury.	There is no evidence of complications arising from drugs, treatment, disease process, or nursing care. The patient uses ambulatory aids effectively.
There is no infection.	There is no evidence of inflammation, pain or aching, or purulent secretions.

Medical Interventions and Related Nursing Care

Blood Transfusions

Infusion of blood may be lifesaving for the patient with anemia caused by acute blood loss whose hemoglobin is less than 10 g. The transfusion immediately increases the body's ability to receive oxygen and avoid severe tissue damage. Transfusions are used less frequently for patients with severe chronic anemia (hemoglobin <6 g) because of potential complications.

Contraindications and Cautions

1. Hemolytic reaction is caused by the administration of mismatched blood.
2. Bacterial reactions are usually caused by contaminated blood.
3. Allergic reactions can occur. Their exact cause is unknown, although in some cases the donor may have ingested drugs or foods to which the recipient is allergic.
4. Circulatory overload results from too rapid an infusion or too great a quantity.
5. Transmission of infectious agents such as hepatitis virus can occur.

Medical Plan

General Management

Medications and other interventions are administered as needed in response to reactions to transfusions.

NURSING CARE

Nursing Assessment

Hemolytic Reaction

Chills and fever
Tachycardia
Nausea and vomiting
Hematuria or oliguria
Headache
Backache
Dyspnea
Cyanosis
Chest pain

Bacterial (Febrile) Reaction

Fever, chills, lumbar pain, headache, malaise, bloody vomitus, diarrhea, or red shock (skin warm, dry, and pink)

Allergic Reaction

Mild edema, hives, bronchial wheezing, or anaphylaxis

Circulatory Overload

Cough, dyspnea, edema, tachycardia, hemoptysis, and frothy pink-tinged sputum
Distended neck veins

Nursing Dx & Intervention

Nursing Diagnosis	Nursing Intervention/Rationale
Potential for injury related to hemolytic reaction	• Discontinue blood transfusions immediately. • Notify the physician and laboratory. • Send remaining blood and sample of the patient's blood to the laboratory *for repeat type and cross-matching*. • Administer intravenous fluids *(to maintain patency of line)*, oxygen, and drugs, such as vasopressor agents, epinephrine, sedatives, and mannitol, as ordered *to manage hemolytic reaction*. • Monitor vital signs. • Insert Foley catheter *to monitor urinary output*. • Provide analgesics, antiemetics, and massage *for patient comfort*.

Nursing Diagnosis	Nursing Intervention/Rationale
Potential for injury related to bacterial reaction	• Discontinue blood; notify the physician. • Send remaining blood and sample of the patient's blood to the laboratory for repeat type and cross-matching. • Monitor vital signs. • Use cooling measures as needed. • Administer intravenous fluids *(to maintain patency of line).* • Insert Foley catheter *to monitor urinary output.* • Administer medications as ordered, such as vasopressors, corticosteroids, broad-spectrum antibiotics, analgesics, and antiemetics, *to manage bacterial reaction.*
Potential for injury related to allergic reaction	• Decrease transfusion flow if mild reaction occurs (mild edema, hives, or bronchial wheezing). • Stop blood if severe reaction occurs (bronchospasm or severe dyspnea) and administer intravenous fluids *(to maintain patency of line).* • Give medications as ordered, such as bronchodilators or epinephrine. • Provide oxygen therapy as needed.
Fluid volume excess	• Slow rate of transfusions, and notify the physician. • Give digitalis as ordered *to enhance cardiac output.* • Prepare for venesection or rotating tourniquets as ordered *to decrease circulating volume.* • Monitor pulse, respirations, blood pressure, and central venous pressure.

Evaluation

Patient Outcome	Data Indicating That Outcome is Reached
Color of the skin and mucous membranes is good.	The skin, nails, lips, and ear lobes are warm and moist and have a natural color.
Vital signs are within normal limits.	Respirations, pulse, and blood pressure are within normal limits. Breathing pattern is regular.
Laboratory studies are within normal limits.	The hemoglobin level, hematocrit, and leukocyte count are within normal limits.
Patient has normal body hydration.	Secretions are thin and mucous membranes are moist. There is no edema.
Daily fluid output is equal to fluid intake.	Urine output is 1500 to 3000 ml daily or equivalent to intake. Patient feels neither hot nor cold.
There is no evidence of physical injury.	There is no evidence of complications arising from drugs, treatments, or nursing care.
There are no signs of infection.	There is no evidence of inflammation, purulent drainage or secretions, or pain or aching.

Bone Marrow Transplantation

For a discussion of bone marrow transplantation, see p. 1385.

Splenectomy

Description and Rationale

Although it serves various important functions, the spleen can be surgically removed from adults without harm. Hypersplenism, the destruction of excessive numbers of blood cells by the spleen, is a major reason for its surgical removal. Another frequent indication is splenic rupture with severe hemorrhage, often caused by trauma. The procedure is relatively simple unless the spleen is greatly enlarged or surrounded by adhesions.[11]

Medical Plan

Surgery

Removal of the spleen

General Management

Parenteral therapy
Analgesia

NURSING CARE

Nursing Assessment

Vascular Function

Signs and symptoms of hemorrhaging and shock

Gastrointestinal Function

Abdominal distention and discomfort
Gastric discharge

Metabolic Activity

Elevated temperature

Pulmonary Functions

Decreased breath sounds
Splinting with respirations
Tachypnea
Atelectasis

Nursing Dx & Intervention

Nursing Diagnosis	Nursing Intervention/Rationale
Altered peripheral or gastrointestinal tissue perfusion (potential) related to hemorrhaging	• Check surgical incision *to determine its condition.* • Apply ice bag and manual pressure or dressing over surgical site *to control bleeding.* • Estimate blood loss *to determine need for replacement.*
Potential fluid volume deficit related to intravascular hypovolemia	• Administer intravenous fluids, including blood, as ordered *to maintain adequate fluid volume.* • Measure intake and output *to assess balance.* • Increase oral fluid intake as tolerated. • Monitor pulse, respirations, and blood pressure.
Potential fluid volume deficit related to fever	• Monitor oral temperature and notify physician if patient becomes febrile. • Apply cool, damp cloth to the face of febrile patient *to promote heat loss by evaporation.* • Bathe the patient in cool water, apply ice bag or alcohol, and cover with lightweight blankets and clothing *to reduce fever.* • Maintain cool room temperature. • Encourage rest. • Increase fluid intake, especially iced liquids.
Potential fluid volume deficit related to nasogastric drainage, paralytic ileus	• Monitor amount, color, and consistency of drainage. • Replace fluids as necessary by intravenous infusion as ordered. • Assess for bowel sounds and abdominal distention. • Ambulate when possible *to promote gastric motility.*
Potential for infection	• Monitor temperature, pulse, respirations, and breath sounds *for early indications of infection.* • Have patient turn, cough, and deep breathe and use incentive spirometry at regular intervals *to maintain ventilatory function.* • Change dressing, using sterile technique. • Encourage fluids, monitor intake and output, and assess urine *to prevent urinary tract infection.*
Pain	• Identify the patient's preferred pain relief measures; implement when feasible. • Apply abdominal binder *for support of dressing and wound.* • Apply warmth, such as with a heating pad, to abdominal area. • Administer medications, such as neostigmine (Prostigmin) and mild analgesics, as ordered *to relieve distention.* • Observe for increased complaints of pain, nausea, vomiting, diarrhea, and abdominal distention, *which indicate dehiscence and obstruction.* • Evaluate effectiveness of pain relief measures.

Patient Education

1. Teach the patient care of the surgical incision.
2. Explain the importance of gradually increasing the level of activity.
3. Emphasize the importance of a well-balanced diet, exercise, rest, and other healthful behaviors.

Evaluation[2]

Patient Outcome	Data Indicating That Outcome is Reached
Color of the skin and mucous membranes is good.	The skin, nails, lips, and ear lobes are warm and moist and have a natural color.
Vital signs are within normal limits.	Respirations, pulse, blood pressure, and temperature are within normal limits.
Laboratory studies are within normal limits.	The hemoglobin level and hematocrit are within normal limits.
Patient has the physical appearance of comfort.	Patient has calm, relaxed facial expression. Posture is normal, and patient expresses comfort.

References

1. American Cancer Society: A cancer source book for nurses, New York, 1981, The Society.
2. Beck WS: Hematology, Cambridge, Mass, 1985, MIT Press.
3. Brown BA: Hematology: principles and procedures, Philadelphia, 1988, Lea & Febiger.
4. Campbell C: Nursing diagnosis and intervention in nursing practice, New York, 1978, John Wiley & Sons, Inc.
5. Cancer Facts and Figures, New York, 1984, American Cancer Society.
6. Donovan CF: Protective isolation, Oncol Nurs Forum 9:50, 1982.
7. Everson LK: Hematologic diseases, New Hyde Park, NY, 1983, Medical Examination Publising Co.
8. Hoogstraten B: Hematologic malignancies, New York, 1986, Springer-Verlag.
9. Kim MJ, McFarland GK, and McLane AM: Pocket guide to nursing diagnoses, St Louis, 1987, The CV Mosby Co.
10. Luby CK and Wood PW: Thrombotic thrombocytopenia purpura, Dimensions Crit Care Nurs 4:209, 1985.
11. Luckmann J and Sorensen KC: Medical-surgical nursing: a psychophysiologic approach, Philadelphia, 1987, WB Saunders Co.
12. Newcom SR and Kadin ME: Hematologic malignancies in the adult, Reading, Mass, 1981, Addison-Wesley.
13. Oncology Nursing Society, Clinical Practice Committee: Guidelines for the nursing care of patients with altered comfort, Oncol Nurs Forum 10:93, 1983.
14. Oncology Nursing Society, Clinical Practice Committee: Guidelines for nursing care of patients with altered ventilation, Oncol Nurs Forum 10:113, 1983.
15. Quick guide to common anemias, Nursing 83 83:24, 1983.
16. Reich PR: Hematology: physiopathologic basis for clinical practice, Boston, 1984, Little Brown & Co.
17. Ungaro PC: Hematology, New Hyde Park, NY, 1985, Medical Examination Publishing Co.
18. Wiley FM and De-Cuir-Walley S: Allogenic bone marrow transplantation for children with acute leukemia, Oncol Nurs Forum 10:49, 1983.
19. Williams WJ: Hematology, New York, 1983, McGraw-Hill Book Co.

CHAPTER 16

Neoplasia

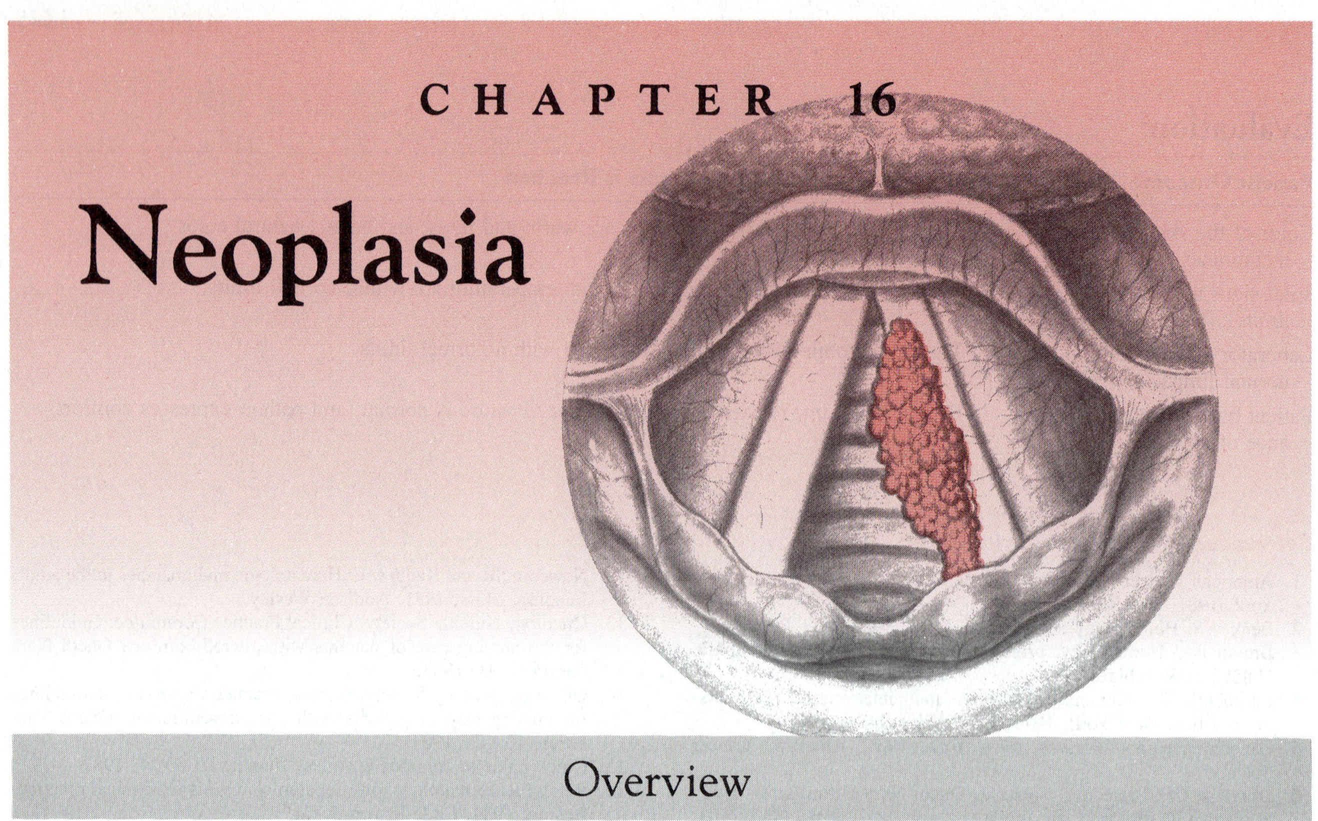

Overview

Cancer is the second most common cause of death in the United States; it kills about 450,000 people annually. Cancer is the leading cause of death in children 3 to 14 years of age, and it is estimated that 870,000 new cases of cancer are diagnosed in Americans every year. Earlier diagnosis and treatment of certain cancers and better health practices have improved the outlook for people with cancer. Three out of eight people whose cancer was diagnosed in 1988 will be alive 5 years later.[5]

Cancer is a universal disease that affects people without regard to race, sex, socioeconomic status, or culture; however, different forms of cancer strike specific age, racial, and sexual groups. For example, cancer mortality increases rapidly with aging; some researchers believe that anyone who lives long enough will eventually develop cancer. Social and environmental factors are thought to explain racial differences in cancer. Both incidence and mortality are higher in blacks than in whites. Although women are more likely than men to develop cancer, more men die of the disease. The sites in men that are associated with the greatest mortality are the lung, colon and rectum, and prostate. In women the leading sites are the breast, lung, colon, and rectum (Figure 16-1).[4] Another interesting variable is heredity. Certain cancers, such as those of the stomach, breast, colon and rectum, uterus, and lung, occur in a familial pattern. Whether this is indicative of "an inherited susceptibility or common exposure to an etiologic factor"[2] is unknown. In addition, certain diseases that are cancer precursors, such as multiple familial polyposis and Gardner's syndrome, seem to be hereditary.

Cancer is probably caused by many interacting factors (initiators and promoters) rather than by a single one, and its development appears to be a multistep process. Some causative agents have been found, and others are suspected. One predisposing factor is chronic irritation, such as frequent, prolonged exposure to sunlight or sustained alcohol consumption. Some benign lesions, such as leukoplakia of the oral cavity, colon and rectal polyps, and pigmented moles, may undergo malignant transformation. People whose cancer is already diagnosed are at risk for later development of the disease at the same or another site. Environmental carcinogens that have been identified include cigarette smoke, asbestos, uranium, asphalt, and aniline dye. Iatrogenic factors that have been implicated are radiation and drugs, for example, diethylstilbestrol (DES), certain cancer chemotherapeutic agents, radioisotopes such as phosphorus (^{32}P) and radium, and immunosuppressive drugs.

Among the factors theorized to cause cancer are (1) oncogenes that are normally dormant but may be activated by external agents and (2) viruses, such as the Epstein-Barr virus (EBV) and hepatitis B virus, which are associated with neoplasms and with impaired immune surveillance.

Anatomy, Physiology, and Related Pathophysiology

In describing the nature and possible causes of cancer, it is important to understand that cancer cells, unlike normal cells, proliferate without organization and often without differentiation. Certain stimuli are believed to initiate this process, which subsequently overpowers the normal control mechanism. The results are uninhibited growth (autonomy), uncontrolled function (anaplasia), and uncontrolled motility,

Figure 16-1 Cancer incidence and deaths by site and sex—1987 estimates.
From American Cancer Society.[4]

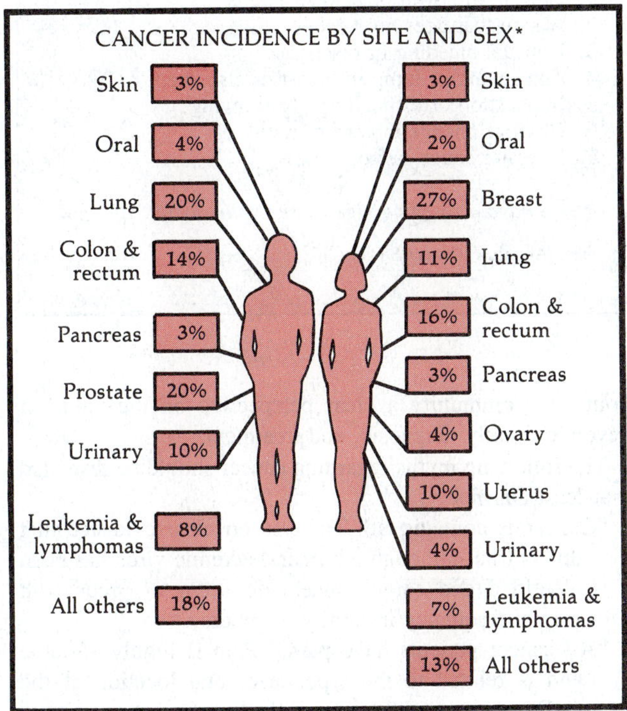

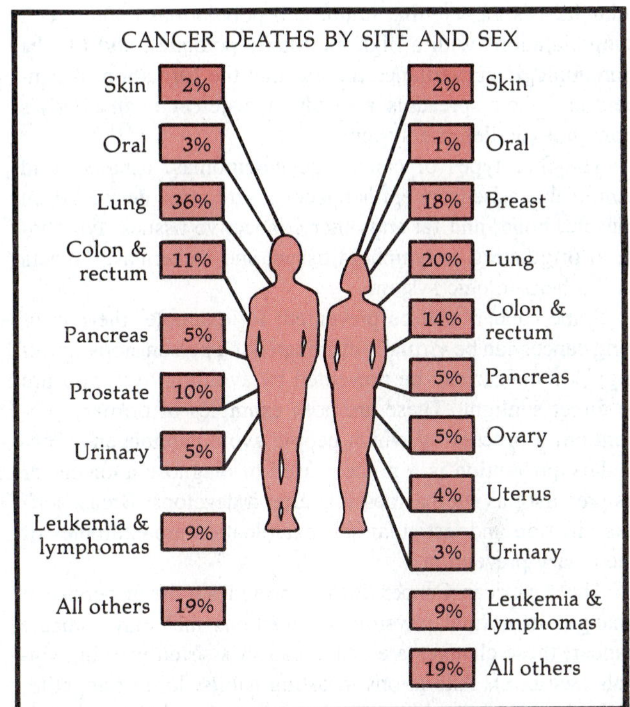

*Excluding nonmelanoma skin cancer and carcinoma in situ.

permitting spread to other parts of the body (metastasis) via blood or the lymphatic system.

Normal cell division occurs in a pattern of sequential events referred to as the cell cycle. The stages of this cycle are mitosis and interphase. Mitosis, the actual growth phase, involves the cytoplasmic and nuclear separation within the cell, which results in two identical daughter cells containing the full complement of genetic information found in the parent cell. The interphase is the "resting stage" between cell divisions.

Neoplasia, a group of "new growth" cells, is the result of cells' unresponsiveness to the normal mechanisms of growth control. Cancer cells exhibit changes in the cytoplasm, including enzyme alterations, chromosome changes, and the production of new proteins via an active anabolic process; mitochondrial changes, increased energy production to meet the neoplasm's increased rate of glucose utilization and lactic acid production; and nuclear changes in which DNA is altered.

Unique characteristics of neoplasms include their having more cells in active reproduction at a given time than do normal tissues, a shorter cell cycle time, and increased doubling time.

Neoplasms are described as benign or malignant. Benign tumors have little or no invasive activity, are generally encapsulated, usually grow more slowly, and are rarely fatal. Malignant tumors not only invade surrounding tissues but also produce metastases. If untreated these tumors usually result in death.

The primary site of a malignant neoplasm is its place of origin, which is sometimes discovered after a secondary or metastatic site has been identified and diagnosed. The secondary site has characteristics similar to those of the primary site. Some people have additional primary sites, which may be different types of cancer presenting different signs and symptoms at the same time (e.g., breast and ovarian cancers).

The malignant neoplasm's ability to invade surrounding tissues and to colonize distant sites is called metastasis. This may occur via direct extension, wherein the neoplasm expands, invades, and destroys normal adjacent tissue. The most frequent route is penetration of the lymphatic system and bloodstream, which enables cancer cells to disseminate throughout the body. Another less common route is penetration of body cavities, for example, dissemination through the cerebrospinal fluid or transabdominal spread within the peritoneal cavity.

There are numerous theories regarding the process of cancer invasion and metastasis. Some of these are (1) the mechanical theory, that the incidence and number of metastases are a function of the number and size of cells and cell groups gaining access to the circulation; (2) the "soil" theory, that metastasis is determined by the environment of the organs and tissues in which cancer cells arrive; (3) the intrinsic cellular factors theory, that tumor cell populations contain cell subpopulations with a high metastatic potential; and (4) the immunologic surveillance theory, that the formation of cancers and their spread is a result of a defect in the body's immunologic defense system.

The four types of cancer are carcinomas, usually solid tumors that arise from epithelial cells; sarcomas, derived from muscle, bone, and fat and other connective tissues; lymphomas, originating in lymphoid tissue; and leukemias, cancers of the hematologic system.

Some cancers can be prevented; for example, the risk of lung cancer can be virtually eliminated if a person stops smoking; skin cancer can be prevented by avoiding overexposure to direct sunlight. These are both examples of primary prevention, a process by which people avoid carcinogens. Secondary prevention is a process used to diagnose a cancer or its precursor as soon as possible after it develops. Breast self-examination and testicular self-examination are examples of secondary prevention.

The American Cancer Society provides a list of persistent changes in normal physiologic functions that may indicate cancer; these changes are called cancer's seven warning signals (see box). Alterations in eating habits, loss of appetite, difficulty in swallowing, or increased constipation or diarrhea should be evaluated. The presence of a lump or nodule anywhere in or on the body (especially if it is painless and slowly increasing in size), bleeding from orifices, unexplained recurrent pain or fever, steady weight loss, and repeated infections are typical signs and symptoms of cancer that must be assessed. The nurse must stress primary and secondary prevention through public education, screening, and early detection activities.

Cancer's Seven Warning Signals

1. Change in bowel or bladder habits
2. A sore that does not heal
3. Unusual bleeding or discharge
4. Thickening or lump in breast or elsewhere
5. Indigestion or difficulty in swallowing
6. Obvious change in wart or mole
7. Nagging cough or hoarseness

If you have a warning signal, see your doctor.

From American Cancer Society.[4]

Psychosocial Aspects of Cancer

Cancer evokes deep fears of pain, suffering, dependence, disfigurement, and death. Indeed, the fear of the disease is often so strong that a person may delay examination and diagnosis in hopes that the signs or symptoms will go away. This lag time between awareness of a problem and seeking medical attention can affect the impact of therapy and the prognosis. Thus awareness of attitudes toward cancer and efforts to influence them in a more hopeful direction through education are an important part of the nurse's role.

Variables that have been identified as shaping attitudes toward cancer are life experiences, especially those related to this disease; parental and cultural values and attitudes toward illness; society's emphasis on youth, health, and beauty; social pressures for early sexual experience, smoking, and other harmful behaviors; and portrayals of people with cancer in the mass media. Positive experiences and hopeful presentations of cancer and its treatment will give the individual, group, or community a clear perspective on the value of prevention, early diagnosis, and treatment.

The following myths regarding cancer should be dispelled or at least clarified:

"Cancer is contagious." There is no clear evidence that this is true, although a human leukemic virus has been identified and some cancers do seem to occur with greater frequency in family members.

"All cancer patients have pain." Pain is highly variable and is related to the type, size, and location of the malignancy as well as the patient's pain tolerance.

"The treatment is worse than the disease because of disfiguring surgery and side effects of chemotherapy." This may be true in patients who are asymptomatic or relatively free of symptoms at the time of diagnosis.

"Sexual activity and other aspects of normal life must be forfeited." This is certainly not true if the patient and significant others are willing to consider modifications in life-style.

"Cancer is a death sentence." There are hundreds of thousands of cured cancer patients (almost 50% of people with cancer) in the United States today. With early diagnosis and treatment, most people with cancer could live long and productive lives.

The most common concerns of cancer patients are fear of alienation from family, friends, or health care providers; mutilation, particularly if surgery is the treatment of choice; vulnerability, dependence, or lack of control; and mortality. The emotional responses of a patient to these and other concerns related to the disease may be feelings of hopelessness, helplessness, guilt, denial, apathy, hostility, self-blame, withdrawal, and a sense of unreality. The nature and severity of these behaviors depend on the patient's usual behavior, attitudes toward illness in general and cancer in particular, the site of the disease, therapeutic options, and the expected outcome. All of these factors must be recognized as influencing the response of the patient and family.

All people with cancer have certain basic needs that transcend their individual responses to cancer. These are:

To know what is happening and talk about its reality with someone who will listen
To participate in decisions affecting how they will live and die
To experience the pain of "feeling bad" rather than having to hide feelings from others

Not to be ignored are the effects of employability and insurability, potential loss of support systems, and the unfamiliarity of terms, procedures, drugs, and other aspects of therapy.

The ways in which patients cope with cancer are as varied as their reactions to the diagnosis. Some of the more positive coping strategies that have been identified and described by researchers include the following:

Seeking more information about the disease and its treatment
Using humor to lighten the situation
Using various distraction techniques
Sharing concerns with others, for example, in self-help groups
Negotiating feasible alternatives, such as treatment options

These coping strategies are generally considered less positive:

Reducing tension and anxiety with excessive drinking, drugs, or dangerous activities
Withdrawing into isolation
Blaming others, the situation, or the Supreme Being
Becoming fatalistic
Blaming self and expressing guilt feelings

The nurse and other health care providers should assess the patient's coping style, evaluate its effectiveness, and intervene when there is increasing distress or a continuing problem.

General nursing interventions that have been identified as helpful to cancer patients during the various stages of the illness include maintaining hope while avoiding false optimism, using a gentle, unhurried manner, expressing caring and concern, and focusing on the patient's strengths rather than weaknesses.

Many patients find self-help groups useful in dealing with the effects of cancer and its treatment. The value of receiving help from another person who has undergone a similar experience is well documented. The functions of such groups are to provide special information and successful coping techniques to people with similar problems, encouragement to maintain prescribed regimens, normalization of a behavior, and education of health care professionals and the public about cancer patients' special needs. The most useful aspects of this approach to coping are believed to be the modeling aspects ("You can do it—I did!") and the observation that helping someone else benefits the helper.

The family of the cancer patient may also need the assistance of health care team members. Factors to be assessed when determining the impact of cancer on the family include the age of the patient and other family members, family dynamics, communication style, family background, and practical matters of concern to the patient and family. Specific nursing interventions that are of value to the family are:

Giving the patient quality care
Communicating frequently with the family
Listening to the family
Making the family comfortable, as by orientation to the institutional setting and policies
Referring the family to other members of the health care team as appropriate
Using touch to comfort family members as appropriate
Preparing the family for home care of the patient
Doing small things that are important to the family, such as rearranging mealtime to permit a special dinner from home

Additional coping strategies that patients and their families may wish to learn about and use include relaxation exercises, meditation, imagery, self-hypnosis, music therapy, and humor. The nurse may serve as teacher or provide referral to resources for instruction in these techniques.

As previously mentioned, disfigurement is a particular concern of cancer patients. A change in body image may be actual (as with mastectomy) or perceived (as with hysterectomy). The visibility of the alteration may not affect the patient's reaction to it; perhaps of more significance is the function of the part or system and the patient's emotional attachment to it.

Patients may react to a change in body image in a variety of ways:

Denying the existence of the change, minimizing its presence, or deemphasizing its importance
Increased perception of phantom sensations
Use of unrealistic goal-setting
Use of inappropriate defenses, such as denial, inappropriate dress, self-imposed isolation, aggression, or dissociation

The nurse should help the patient develop more realistic responses to the change in body image. Some suggestions that may be beneficial to the patient include:

Resumption of prealteration life-style
Confinement of the effect of the disability to the area of loss
Emphasis on assets rather than liabilities
Solicitation of support from others
Reevaluation of personal and professional goals

Another area of concern to patients and their families that may be less readily discussed is sexuality and feelings regarding gender and gender role identity. Many beliefs (cultural, religious, personal, and societal) affect a person's ability to deal with an alteration in sexuality. These have been identified as especially influential:

The duty of a man to satisfy a woman and vice versa
The man as the aggressor and the woman as the passive recipient
The obsession of both sexes with performance
The use of sexual intercourse for procreation

These beliefs, as well as the other attitudes regarding masculine and feminine behaviors, may confuse and depress both the patient and partner. In addition, the symptoms of cancer, such as fatigue, malaise, fever, discharge, and odor, may adversely affect libido and the patient's general view of his or her sexuality. This is further complicated by hospitalization, with the resultant lack of privacy.

The nurse's role in this sensitive area is to assess the patient's readiness to discuss sexual concerns, identify appropriate resources, provide oral and written information that will assist the patient in understanding sexual concerns and possible solutions, and respect the patient and partner's need for privacy.

Unproven methods of cancer treatment pose special challenges for both patient and nurse. These methods, which are touted as providing a high probability of cure, include a variety of machines and devices, drugs and chemicals, nutritional approaches, and psychologic techniques. The characteristics of unproven methods include a promoter with suspect credentials; no controlled studies of the treatment; an unscientific data base; the illusion of classified information; and an emphasis on the patient's freedom of choice and the availability of emotional support. The nurse's role in this domain includes assessing the presence of feelings of helplessness and hopelessness in the patient as well as pressure from family and friends to "keep trying," providing open communication with the patient and family regarding these issues, and providing information about and opportunities to discuss alternative therapies.

The issue of informed consent often presents dilemmas for both the patient and nurse, especially if experimental therapy is being recommended. The nurse should serve as both teacher and advocate for the patient, who may need further explanation of the proposed procedure or protocol, answers to specific questions, or an opportunity to "think out loud." The consent process should include, at the least, the basic steps of explanation of the medical condition, explanation of the nature and purpose of the procedure or protocol, and explanation of the risks, alternatives, and consequences of the procedure or protocol.

If consent is to be informed there must be a patient of legal age and sound mind; a patient capable of cognition and reason; voluntariness; lack of coercion, deceit, or fraud; the right to refuse; comprehensible language; satisfactory answers to the patient's questions; and assurance of privacy and confidentiality.

Whatever the issue, the nurse should assess the patient's comprehension of the consent form, notify the physician if the patient is confused or ambivalent (unless a nursing procedure or protocol is being proposed), respect the individual's freedom of choice, and promote the patient's autonomy and independence in decision making.

This section has included a few of the psychosocial issues confronting the cancer patient. Not discussed here but of equal concern is the experience of dying, which is faced by many cancer patients and their families. The nurse's support during this phase of the illness is invaluable. The hospice movement has been particularly useful to patients and their families who desire terminal care at home.

Meeting the psychosocial needs of the cancer patient and family is one of the greatest challenges facing the nurse. The roles of counselor, teacher, consultant, and resource person are used to their maximum to enhance the patient's and family's coping with this complex of diseases and therapies.

Normal Findings

For assessment of a specific body system, see that chapter.

Area of Concern	Normal Adult Findings	
Respiratory rate	16-20 breaths/min	
Pulse rate	70-82 beats/min	
Blood pressure	18-44 yr	140/90 mm Hg
	45-64 yr	150/95 mm Hg
	65 yr and older	160/95 mm Hg
Temperature	36°-37.5° C (96.8°-99.5° F)	

Normal Laboratory Data

Laboratory Test	Normal Adult Values
Blood	
Glycosylated hemoglobin	5.7%-8.8%
Plasma hemoglobin	1-5 mg/dl
Hemoglobin	Men: 15.5 ± 1.1 g/dl Women: 13.7 ± 1 g/dl
Hematocrit	Men: 42%-52% Women: 35%-47%
Ferritin	Men: 15-200 mg/dl Women: 12-150 mg/dl
pH	Arterial: 7.35-7.45 Venous: 7.32-7.43
Blood urea nitrogen (BUN)	Under 40 yr: 5-20 mg/dl *Older adult:* Gradual slight increase after 40 yr
O_2 saturation	95%-99%
CO_2	Arterial: 22-29 mEq/L Venous: 23-30 mEq/L
Po_2	80-95 mm Hg
Pco_2	Arterial: 35-45 mm Hg Venous: 38-50 mm Hg
Calcium	Under 30 yr: 8.2-10.5 mg/dl *Older adult:* Decreases very slightly in older years
Potassium	3.5-5 mEq/L
Serum creatinine	Men: <1.2 mg/dl Women: <1.1 mg/dl
Glucose	70-105 mg/dl
Cholesterol	140-310 mg/dl

Laboratory Test	Normal Adult Values
Uric acid	Men: 4.2-8 mg/dl Women: 3.2-7.3 mg/dl
Urine	
Specific gravity	1.001-1.035
pH	4.8-7.8
Protein	Negative
Creatinine	Men: 1-2 g/24 hr Women: 0.8-1.8 g/24 hr *Older adult:* Decreases with advancing age as muscle mass diminishes
Creatinine clearance	Men: 85-125 ml/min/1.73 m² Women: 75-115 ml/min/1.73 m²

Conditions, Diseases, and Disorders

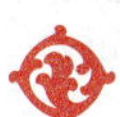

Primary Carcinoma of the Lung

Carcinoma of the lung is an uncontrolled growth of anaplastic cells in the lung. Types are epidermoid (squamous cell), adenocarcinoma, small cell undifferentiated (oat cell), and large cell undifferentiated.

Carcinoma of the lung is the leading cause of death from cancer in men and women in the United States.[4] The incidence among women is steadily increasing, and more blacks than whites develop the disease. More than 90% of people with lung cancer will die of it.

Approximately 80% of lung tumors are linked to cigarette smoking. The people at highest risk began smoking in their teens, inhale deeply, and smoke at least half a pack a day. People who quit smoking have a gradual decline in risk, eventually reaching levels similar to those of nonsmokers.

Another etiologic factor in the development of carcinoma of the lung is occupational exposure to such substances as asbestos, uranium, nickel, and chromate. Air pollutants have not yet been proved a cancer risk factor, but the incidence of the disease is higher in urban populations.[3]

Pathophysiology

The major histologic types of lung cancer are[28]:

- Epidermoid (squamous cell)—the most common, comprising 40% to 50% of all lung tumors; 90% occur in men; tend to be centrally located; often produce bronchial obstruction
- Adenocarcinoma—25% of lung cancers; often peripherally located; a common scar carcinoma that arises in area of fibrosis resulting from previous pulmonary damage; less association with smoking than other types
- Small cell undifferentiated (oat cell)—20% to 25% of lung cancers; usually centrally located; most aggressive, with lymphatic and distant metastases at time of diagnosis; most responsive to chemotherapy
- Large cell undifferentiated—10% of malignant lung tumors; may appear in any part of lung

All types have lymphatic metastasis early in the course of the disease, beginning in the bronchial and mediastinal nodes and extending upward to supraclavicular nodes and downward to nodes below the diaphragm and to the liver and adrenal glands. Distant metastasis via the bloodstream to brain, bones, and contralateral lung may occur.

A chronic cough and wheezing are the most common early symptoms; other symptoms are fatigue, chest tightness, and aching joints. Late but clinically significant signs include hemoptysis, clubbing of the fingers, weight loss, and pleural effusion. Invasion of the superior vena cava causes edema of the neck and face. Phrenic nerve involvement results in paralysis of the diaphragm. A superior sulcus tumor involving the brachial plexus may be manifest as shoulder and arm pain and paresthesias.

The chest lesion may be relatively asymptomatic, with the chief complaint caused by metastatic disease. Metastasis to the brain may result in headache, unsteady gait, and other neurologic signs. Weight loss, jaundice, or anorexia may occur with liver involvement. Localized bony pain or pathologic fractures may accompany skeletal involvement.

Paraneoplastic syndromes may be associated with lung cancer. For example, inappropriate antidiuretic hormone (low serum sodium) or Cushing's syndrome from ectopic adrenocorticotropic hormone production occurs in some patients with small cell cancer. Other syndromes include hypercalcemia, resulting from production of ectopic parathormone-like substance (epidermoid lung cancer); carcinomatous neuropathy and myopathy; dermatomyositis; and hypertrophic pulmonary osteoarthropathy.[28]

Diagnostic Studies and Findings[6]

Chest Roentgenogram (Lateral and Posterior-Anterior Views), Chest Tomography, and Computed Tomographic Scanning

Outline shape, size, and position of lesion

Sputum Collection for Cytology, Bronchoscopy with Biopsy, Brushings, or Washings, and Percutaneous Biopsy under Fluoroscopy

Cells gathered for histologic examination show evidence of malignancy

Scalene Node Biopsy

Evidence of spread to scalene nodes

Mediastinoscopy

Evidence of spread to ipsilateral and contralateral mediastinal lymph nodes

Radioisotope Scanning

Reveals size, shape, and position of lesion

Liver Function Studies and Scans, Brain and Bone Scans

Evidence of metastases

Skin Tests, Absolute Lymphocyte Counts

Evidence of immunocompetence

Medical Plan[28]

Surgery

Lobectomy (see Chapter 2 for details)
Pneumonectomy for centrally located lesions (see Chapter 2)
Segmental and wedge resection based on patient tolerance and absence of spread (see Chapter 2)

Medications

For small cell lung cancer
- Antineoplastic agents
  - Cyclophosphamide (Cytoxan), 40-50 mg/kg IV in individually determined doses over several days and then adjusted to lower maintenance dosage; po 1-5 mg/kg/d
  - Methotrexate (Mexate), 2.5-5 mg/kg/d po or parenterally
  - Doxorubicin (Adriamycin), 60-75 mg/m^2 at intervals of 21 d, or 30 mg/m^2/d for 3 d repeated every 4 wk
  - Vincristine sulfate (Oncovin; VCR), 1.4 mg/m^2 for adults
  - Carmustine (BCNU), 200 mg/m^2 IV q6 wk
  - Procarbazine (Mastulane), 2-4 mg/kg/d po initially and then 4-6 mg/kg/d until maximum response occurs; maintain at 1-2 mg/kg/d
  - Hexamethylmelamine (HXM), in combination therapy; dose individually determined

These agents only slightly useful in non–small cell cancer; partial regression with cisplatin-based regimens (see "Chemotherapy," p. 1495)

General Management

Radiation therapy—sole modality for patient who has clinically resectable lesion but is medically nonoperable and for patient with locally advanced, nonresectable tumor without demonstrable distant metastases but with such symptoms as cough, wheezing, obstructive infection, hemoptysis, pain, dysphagia, or superior vena cava syndrome; may be used preoperatively or postoperatively[6] (see p. 1500)

• • •

The prognosis for people with lung cancer is correlated with tumor cell type. Those with well-differentiated squamous cell cancer have the best chance of survival; those with undifferentiated small cell cancer have the poorest. Peripheral tumors are more curable than central lesions. The presence of lymph node and distant metastases reduces the chance of cure. The stage of disease, patient's performance status, and immunologic state of the patient are important prognostic signs. Patients with gross supraclavicular adenopathy, a malignant pleural effusion, massive local extension, or distant metastases usually survive less than 1 year.

NURSING CARE

Nursing Assessment[22]

Respiratory Function

Chronic cough, nonproductive or productive; wheezing; chest tightness; hemoptysis; dyspnea; hoarseness

Comfort Level

Clubbed fingers; chest pain

Systemic Function

Fatigue; weight loss; edema of neck and face; anorexia; fever

Nursing Dx & Intervention

Nursing Diagnosis	Nursing Intervention/Rationale
Ineffective airway clearance	• Place patient in sitting position and change position frequently *to enhance breathing.* • Encourage coughing and deep breathing with splinting of chest *to relieve congestion.* • Ambulate patient as soon as possible *to increase circulation and chest expansion.* • Encourage fluids *to liquefy secretions.*

Nursing Diagnosis	Nursing Intervention/Rationale
	• Administer oxygen therapy as prescribed *to maintain adequate tissue oxygenation.* • Anticipate patient's needs *to decrease unnecessary energy expenditure.*
Ineffective breathing pattern	• Inspect chest for respiratory rate and rhythm and symmetric expansion *to determine adequacy of pulmonary function.* • Auscultate for abnormal breath sounds, lung aeration, rales, and rhonchi *to detect ventilatory problems.* • Percuss chest for abnormal resonance or decreased diaphragmatic descent *to detect ventilatory problems.* • Monitor blood studies for abnormal gas exchange *to detect inadequate oxygenation.* • Observe for cyanosis and change in amount or character or sputum *as signs of respiratory failure or infection.* • Discourage smoking *to decrease pulmonary workload.*
Impaired physical mobility	• Assist with ambulation; encourage efforts to move about while conserving energy *to promote mobility.* • Move patient as necessary with walker, wheelchair, or cane *to assist with ambulation.* • Minimize environmental barriers *to avoid excess energy expenditure.* • Observe for complaints of weakness, fatigue, abnormal gait, and impaired coordination as indications for promoting immobility *as these may be signs of a progressively deteriorating metastatic condition.* • Encourage range of motion and isometric exercises that can be done in bed *to maintain mobility while conserving energy.*
Pain (chest)	• Remove constrictive clothing *to increase chest expansion.* • Administer respiratory therapy as prescribed *to provide bronchodilation and increased oxygenation of tissues.*
Altered nutrition: less than body requirements	• Provide pleasant surroundings and attractive meal tray *to enhance patient's appetite.* • Postpone feeding when patient is fatigued, *since rest may increase appetite.* • Give small, frequent, nutritious feedings *to avoid patient's overeating at one time and feeling uncomfortable.* • Provide selection of foods *to increase patient's appetite.* • Provide foods at appropriate temperature *to enhance taste.* • Encourage family and friends to bring food *to appeal to patient's preference.* • Season food to patient's taste *to enhance taste.* • Administer antiemetics before meals *to decrease nausea.* • Monitor intake and output and weight *to determine adequacy of nutrition.*
Patient problem: metastasis	• See "Metastatic Disease," p. 1492.

Patient Education

1. Discourage smoking by the patient and family or significant others.
2. Teach the patient to cough productively and to perform breathing exercises and other respiratory therapy as prescribed to maintain pulmonary function.
3. Help the patient ambulate, and instruct the patient in the use of assistive devices such as canes and walkers to maintain mobility.
4. Teach the patient to self-administer medication for pain to maintain comfort.
5. Inform the patient of the need for adequate nutrition (high-calorie, high-protein diet) to maintain energy.
6. Inform the patient of the signs and symptoms of complications or adverse reactions to chemotherapy and/or radiation therapy so that they can be treated immediately.
7. Help the patient identify resources and support systems to help in rehabilitation and maintenance of quality of life.
8. Alert the patient to the signs and symptoms of recurrence or metastatic disease, such as shoulder or arm pain, superior vena cava syndrome, liver disease, and central nervous system changes, so that they can be treated as soon as possible.

Evaluation

Patient Outcome	Data Indicating That Outcome is Reached
Skin and mucous membrane color is normal.	Skin, nails, lips, and earlobes are warm and moist and have natural color.
Vital signs are within normal limits.	Respirations, pulse, and blood pressure are within normal limits.
Laboratory findings are within normal limits.	Blood oxygen saturation, carbon dioxide, Po_2, and Pco_2 are within normal limits.
Blood hydration is normal.	Skin turgor is normal, secretions are thin, and there is no edema.
Body functioning is normal.	Weight is stabilized.
Vitality is good.	There is no malaise, fatigue, or weakness.
Patient has daily intake of essential food groups.	Milk, meat, fruits, vegetables, breads, and cereals are included in daily diet.
Patient is comfortable.	Facial expression is calm, contented, and relaxed. Posture is normal. Patient has freedom of body movement and expresses comfort.

Cancers of the Colon and Rectum

Cancer of the colon and rectum is an uncontrolled growth of anaplastic cells in the colon or rectum. Types are adenocarcinoma, carcinoid tumor, leiomyosarcoma, and lymphoma.

Each year approximately 114,000 new cases of colon or rectal cancer are diagnosed in the United States. These tumors occur almost equally in men and women, usually after 40 years of age.[3]

No definite external etiologic factors have been identified, although dietary habits, such as frequent ingestion of refined carbohydrates, are suspected. Conditions that increase the risk of colorectal cancers include familial polyposis of the colon or rectum, chronic ulcerative colitis, diverticulosis, and villous adenomas of the colon. Exposure to asbestos has also been identified as a possible cause of these diseases.[28]

Pathophysiology[6]

The most common symptom of colorectal cancer is rectal bleeding, followed by changes in bowel pattern (constipation or diarrhea), excessive flatus, distention, cramps, obstruction, and unexplained anemia. The presence of symptoms depends on the location of the tumor. Right-sided colonic lesions may be manifest as unexplained iron deficiency anemia and gastrointestinal tract bleeding. Tumors of the sigmoid are characterized by obstruction from napkin ring growth. Rectal tumors are evidenced by rectal pain, gross rectal blood, and tenesmus with a feeling of incomplete evacuation.

The majority of colorectal cancers are adenocarcinomas; others are carcinoid tumors, leiomyosarcomas, and lymphomas. Regional lymph nodes are involved in at least half of the patients. Most colon cancers spread to periaortic nodes. Anal carcinomas spread into perineal nodes. Distant metastasis is most often to the liver and lungs.

The 5-year survival rate for patients with localized disease is 75% for colon tumors and 70% for rectal lesions. These rates are reduced by half with regional or distant involvement. The earlier the diagnosis and treatment, the more curable the cancer. Even with a large tumor and invasion of adjacent structures, the prognosis is favorable if appropriate treatment is provided. Only the presence of distant metastases precludes the possibility of cure. For early detection the American Cancer Society recommends annual digital rectal examination for all people 40 years or older, an annual stool guaiac test at 50 years or older, and sigmoidoscopy every 3 to 5 years after two initial negative ones 1 year apart.

Diagnostic Studies and Findings[6]

Digital Rectal Examination

Palpation of suspect lesion

Proctosigmoidoscopy with Fiberoptic Scope

Visualization and biopsy of suspect lesion

Barium Enema

Visualization of suspect lesion

Testing of Stool for Occult Blood

Presence of blood may be indicative of ulcerating malignancy

Medical Plan[28]

Surgery

Depends on cancer's location and invasive characteristics
End-to-end anastomosis with or without temporary colostomy
Abdominoperineal resection with permanent colostomy
Transverse colostomy to relieve distal bowel obstruction, with later resection
Oophorectomy in women because of possible ovarian involvement
Resection en bloc of other organs attached to primary tumor, such as small bowel loops, urinary bladder, uterus, and adnexa
Electrocoagulation of tumor transanally (experimental approach)
Ostomy to relieve obstruction

Medications

No proven effective adjuvant therapy; palliation for liver or lung metastases with 5-fluorouracil or floxuridine produces 20% response rate

General Management

Radiation therapy for prevention of local recurrence after surgery, preoperative reduction of tumor, intraoperative sterilization of operative field, and relief of symptoms such as bleeding, discharge, tenesmus, and pain (see p. 1500)

NURSING CARE

Nursing Assessment[22]

Gastrointestinal Function

Right colon—anemia, weight loss, abdominal pain, nausea, and vomiting
Sigmoid—bleeding, obstruction
Left colon—mucous stool, constipation, intermittent abdominal pain
Rectal—bleeding, diarrhea, abdominal and/or low back pain, incomplete evacuation

Nursing Dx & Intervention

Nursing Diagnosis	Nursing Intervention/Rationale
Constipation	• Ambulate patient frequently, and encourage physical exercise *to enhance gastrointestinal (GI) motility.* • Encourage increased intake of high-bulk foods and fluids; give fresh fruits, prune juice, hot coffee, and warm and iced liquids *to increase GI motility.* • Place patient in sitting position *to relieve abdominal pressure.* • Give stool softeners and laxatives *to enhance elimination.* • Administer enemas *to cleanse bowel.* • Measure intake and output *to monitor hydration and quantity of feces.*
Diarrhea	• Provide fluids so intake equals output *to prevent dehydration.* • Cover patient with warm blankets *to prevent loss of body heat.* • Encourage adequate rest *to decrease energy expenditure.* • Discourage oral stimulants, *which increase GI motility.* • Discourage intake of high-bulk foods, *which increase GI motility.* • Give tea, carbonated beverages, clear-liquid or full-liquid diet, and dry crackers *to maintain hydration.* • Administer antidiarrheal drugs as ordered *to control diarrhea.* • Refrain from giving hot or iced liquids, enemas, or laxatives, *which irritate bowel.* • Refrain from inserting rectal tube or taking rectal temperatures, *which irritate bowel.* • Check for impaction; employ caution with pancytopenic patients *to prevent bleeding.* • Auscultate abdomen for abnormal bowel sounds *to assess GI status.* • Measure body weight and intake and output *to monitor hydration and nutrition.* • Monitor blood studies for acid-base and electrolyte abnormalities resulting from loss of electrolytes and acid *caused by diarrhea.* • Be alert for complaints of pain caused by abdominal cramping or anal irritation *which may be precursors to diarrhea.*
Pain related to abdominal distention	• Change patient's position frequently; increase movement if tolerated *to relieve distention.* • Discourage smoking, *which may increase distention.* • Give small, frequent feedings *to prevent further distention.* • Encourage decreased intake of gas-forming foods *to prevent further distention.* • Restrict liquids at mealtime; give warm liquids after meals *to relax abdomen.* • Refrain from giving iced liquids and carbonated beverages, *which increase cramping.*

Nursing Diagnosis	Nursing Intervention/Rationale
	• Avoid use of straws and swallowing of air, *since this causes gas formation in GI tract.* • Give nonprescription drugs, such as simethicone, *to relieve flatus.* • Encourage moderate physical activity *to relieve pressure on abdomen.* • Remove restrictive clothing *to relieve pressure on abdomen.* • Inspect abdomen for distention *to determine need for further intervention.* • Auscultate abdomen for abnormal bowel sounds *to assess effect of therapy.*
Pain related to cramping	• Encourage decreased intake of fatty foods *to decrease formation of flatus.* • Give bland foods *to relieve GI irritation.* • Apply heat to abdomen *to relax abdomen and relieve cramping.* • Involve patient in selection of other pain relief measures *to enhance comfort and patient's participation in care.* • Evaluate effectiveness of pain relief measures *to determine need for further intervention.*
Pain (rectal)	• Position patient comfortably *to relieve pressure.* • Apply warm, moist compress to rectal area, or provide sitz bath *to relax anal sphincter.* • Increase fluid intake to 2000 ml daily *to maintain soft stool.* • Encourage decreased intake of high-bulk food *to relieve GI distention.* • Involve patient in selection of pain relief measures *to enhance comfort.* • Evaluate pain for duration, intensity, and quality *to determine intervention needed.* • Evaluate effectiveness of pain relief measures *to determine need for further intervention.*
Patient problem: bleeding	• Apply ice bag to rectal area *to enhance vasoconstriction.* • Change patient's position slowly *to avoid vascular trauma.* • Cover patient with warm blankets *to maintain warmth and comfort.* • Maintain complete bed rest if bleeding is severe *to avoid excessive blood loss.* • Elevate foot of bed *to maintain blood flow to vital organs.* • Refrain from giving enemas or laxatives, inserting rectal tube, or taking rectal temperature *to avoid tissue trauma and bleeding.* • Estimate blood volume loss *to determine replacement need.* • Monitor blood pressure and blood studies *to determine blood volume.*
Patient problem: metastasis	• See "Metastatic Disease," p. 1492.

Refer to Chapter 8 for postoperative nursing interventions and care of diversions. Refer to "Medical Interventions and Related Nursing Care" for care related to chemotherapeutic and radiation therapy–related nursing interventions.

Patient Education

1. Inform the patient of the need to maintain adequate gastrointestinal function.
2. Instruct the patient in pain relief measures.
3. Explain bowel changes (such as bleeding) the patient should report.
4. Instruct the patient in the care of an ostomy if present.
5. Help the patient plan an adequate and appropriate diet.
6. Help the patient contact resources and support groups, such as the United Ostomy Association.

Evaluation

Patient Outcome	Data Indicating That Outcome is Reached
Vital signs are within normal limits.	Respirations, pulse, and blood pressure are within normal limits.
Laboratory findings are within normal limits.	Blood values for hemoglobin, hematocrit, and potassium are within normal limits.
Body hydration is normal.	Skin turgor is normal. There is no edema. Body functioning is normal. Elimination is adequate. Weight is stabilized at normal level for body build.

Patient Outcome	Data Indicating That Outcome is Reached
Vitality is good.	Patient is not fatigued or weak.
Patient has daily intake of essential food groups.	Diet includes milk, meat, fruits, vegetables, breads, and cereals (as tolerated).
Bowel elimination is normal for patient.	Stools are soft. Abdomen is soft and not distended.
Patient is comfortable.	Facial expression is calm, contented, and relaxed. Posture is normal. Patient expresses comfort and satisfaction. Patient no longer complains. Patient frequently changes position and walks, sits, and stands with normal body movement.
Patient participates in daily physical exercise.	Patient walks and/or participates in other forms of mild exercise.

Carcinoma of the Breast

Carcinoma of the breast is an uncontrolled growth of anaplastic cells in the breast. Types include ductal, lobular, and nipple adenocarcinomas.

Although lung cancer is increasing in prevalence, the breast is the most common site of cancer in women between 25 and 75 years of age. Each year breast cancer is diagnosed in approximately 115,000 women in the United States, and it is the leading cause of death in women 40 to 44 years of age. Breast cancer also develops infrequently in men. Symptoms and treatment are the same for men and women.

Most breast lesions are first detected by a woman during breast self-examination or by her sexual partner. The possibility for cure is 85% for women with localized disease at the time of diagnosis. Half of breast cancers are in the upper outer quadrant, 20% in the central portion, 20% in the medial quadrants, and 10% in the lower outer quadrant.

Risk factors that have been cited in the incidence of breast cancer include previous breast cancer, a family history of breast cancer, nulliparity, or a first pregnancy after 30 years of age. Irradiation, particularly as therapy for postpartum mastitis or as multiple chest fluoroscopies, is believed to contribute to breast cancer development. Obesity and total fat content in the diet, especially animal fat, may be factors. Total lifetime exposure to endogenous estrogen is a major risk factor. This disease is more common among white women, but the incidence among blacks is rising.[3,28]

Pathophysiology[6]

The most common initial sign of carcinoma of the breast is a mass, usually painless. Bloody discharge is more indicative of cancer than is spontaneous unilateral serous nipple discharge in a nonlactating breast. Signs of advanced breast cancer include dimpling of skin, nipple retraction, change in breast contour, fixation to the pectoral fascia or chest wall, edema and erythema of the breast skin, and axillary adenopathy. Dermatitis of the nipple or areola may be indicative of Paget's disease. Important associated findings are described in "Nursing Assessment."

Diagnostic Studies and Findings[28]

Monthly breast self-examination and annual examination by a physician are important for early diagnosis. Mammography offers the potential for the identification of occult breast cancer. The following are current recommendations of the American Cancer Society and the National Cancer Institute:

- Annual or other periodic mammography for asymptomatic women 50 years of age or older
- Annual or periodic mammography for women between 40 and 49 years of age if they are at high risk, that is, have a history of breast cancer, have had prior breast biopsy results of lobular carcinoma in situ or an atypical proliferative process, or have been successfully treated for carcinoma of the ovary or endometrium
- Annual or other periodic mammography in women less than 40 years of age if they have a history of breast cancer or a premenopausal mother or sister with breast cancer, especially if bilateral
- Baseline mammogram for women 35 to 50 years of age

A person of any age with a suspect breast mass should undergo mammography and biopsy.

Other procedures being used or studied as adjuncts in the diagnosis of breast cancer include thermography, ultrasonography, and identification of tumor markers. Biopsy for histologic diagnosis is by needle aspiration, core or cutting needle, or open excision. The histologic type of breast cancer is adenocarcinoma, usually of the duct (in situ, invasive, inflammatory, medullary, mucinous, papillary, scirrhous, or tubular), lobule, or nipple (Paget's disease). In addition to the procedures already cited, the following tests may be used to diagnose this disease:

- Level of estrogen receptor protein, which predicts response to hormonal manipulation of metastatic disease, as well as prognosis for primary cancer
- Level of carcinoembryonic antigen (CEA), which is elevated 6 months to 1 year before other evidence of hepatic involvement is noted
- Gross cystic disease protein (investigational)
- Metastatic evaluation, including bone scanning, liver function studies, brain or computed tomography (CT) scan, and chest roentgenograms

Medical Plan[6,28]

Surgery

Controversial, with various options
Radical mastectomy (rarely used now)
Modified radical mastectomy (total mastectomy with partial axillary dissection) for stages I and II
Lumpectomy, segmental mastectomy, or quadrantectomy with axillary node dissection; primary irradiation of remaining breast tissue
Resection of local recurrences or metastases to opposite breast; stabilization of fractures by orthopedic devices; decompression laminectomy

Medications

As initial treatment before radiation or surgery; as adjuvant for premenopausal patients with axillary node metastases
Hormone therapy with antiestrogens; hormone ablation by oophorectomy
Chemotherapy with cyclophosphamide, methotrexate, 5-FU with or without prednisone, and vincristine; doxorubicin as single agent
Antineoplastic agents
Hormones
Tamoxifen citrate (Nolvadex), 10-20 mg bid (indicated for women who are estrogen receptor protein positive)
Phenylalanine mustard or other alkylating agent
Other antineoplastic agents
Cyclophosphamide (Cytoxan), 40-50 mg/kg IV in divided doses over period of several days, then adjusted to lower maintenance dosage; po 1-5 mg/kg/d
Fluorouracil (5-FU, Adrucil, others), 12 mg/kg IV for 4 d followed by 6 mg/kg on alternate days for approximately 12 d
Methotrexate (Amethopterin; Mexate), 2.5-5 mg/kg/d po or parenterally
Doxorubicin (Adriamycin), 60-75 mg/m^2 at intervals of 21 d; or 30 mg/m^2 on each of 3 successive days repeated q4h
Vincristine sulfate (Oncovin), 1.4 mg/m^2
Vinblastine (Velban), 0.1 mg/kg increased weekly by 0.05 mg/kg up to 0.5 mg/kg
See "Chemotherapy," p. 1495

General Management

For recurrent disease
Radiation therapy for pain control, prevention of pathologic fractures, and control of local soft tissue disease preoperatively or postoperatively (adjuvant), cerebral metastases, and localized symptoms (see p. 1500)
Ablative surgery, such as bilateral oophorectomy, adrenalectomy, or hypophysectomy
Additive therapy with large doses of estrogen, androgen, or progestin (in women more than 10 years past menopause)

• • •

Patients with stage I tumors and no involvement of axillary nodes have a 10-year survival greater than 80%; those with stage II tumors have greater than 60% 10-year survival. If the lymph nodes are involved, the 10-year survival is 30% to 40% in the absence of adjuvant chemotherapy. Recent studies have shown that patients whose cancers are estrogen receptor protein negative have a much poorer prognosis. Patients with stage IV disease have a 10-year survival of less than 10%.

Follow-up care includes early detection of second primary breast cancers and recurrent disease. Breast self-examination, yearly mammography, and physician's examination of the intact breast and nodes are important. Rehabilitation is an essential intervention after primary treatment.

NURSING CARE

Nursing Assessment[6]

Breast Tissue

Presence of mass; bloody discharge; dimpling of skin; nipple retraction; change in breast contour; fixation; edema and erythema; enlarged axillary or supraclavicular nodes

Nursing Dx & Intervention

Nursing Diagnosis	Nursing Intervention/Rationale
Potential impaired skin integrity	• Cleanse skin *to prevent infection.* • Apply warm, moist compress *to promote circulation and drainage.* • Apply antibiotic ointment and sterile dressing if indicated *to prevent or treat infection.* • Expose draining area to air (depends on patient's immunocompetence) *to promote healing.* • Elevate arm *to enhance venous return.* • Observe for increased discharge, skin changes (color, dimpling), swelling, enlarged nodes, and dermatitis *to detect complications early.*

Nursing Diagnosis	Nursing Intervention/Rationale
Body image disturbance	• Encourage patient to discuss feelings and concerns with health care providers and significant others. • Help patient identify, label, and express feelings about the significance of the breasts, treatment modalities, and anticipated prognosis. • Involve other disciplines in planning and managing patient care. • Promote acceptance of a positive, realistic body image.
Patient problem: metastasis	• See "Metastatic Disease," p. 1492.

Patient Education

1. Teach care of skin overlying breast to prevent infection and ulceration.
2. Explain how to assess the body for further breast disease or evidence of spread by performing breast self-examination.
3. Provide information about resources and support systems, such as the Reach to Recovery program of the American Cancer Society.

Evaluation

Patient Outcome	Data Indicating That Outcome is Reached
Vital signs are within normal limits.	Respirations and pulse are within normal limits. There is no respiratory distress.
Body functioning is normal.	Weight is stabilized at normal level for body build. Incision is healed.
Patient is comfortable.	Facial expression is calm, contented, and relaxed. Posture is normal. Patient has freedom of body movement. Patient expresses comfort and satisfaction and demonstrates acceptance of loss of breast. Patient frequently changes position and walks, sits, and stands with normal movement.
Patient shows no evidence of physical injury.	There is no evidence of complications arising from drugs, treatments, or nursing care.
Body image is realistic.	Patient verbalizes realistic sense of self and body image. Patient can look at and touch affected breast.

CANCERS OF THE URINARY TRACT

Renal tumors

Renal cancer is an uncontrolled growth of anaplastic cells of the kidney. Types include hypernephroma, parenchymal tumors, papillary tumors, and nephrotic carcinomas.

Renal cancer usually occurs in people over 40 years of age. It is twice as common in men as in women and has a lower incidence in blacks. Signs and symptoms develop late in the course of the disease; the most common sign is painless, intermittent hematuria.

Pathophysiology

Hypernephroma, or adenocarcinoma of the renal parenchyma, is the most common renal neoplasm in adults. It grows slowly but may metastasize at any stage. Metastasis via the bloodstream results in spread to the lungs, bone, regional lymph nodes, liver, and other visceral organs. Parenchymal tumors infiltrate more rapidly than hypernephroma and have a poor prognosis. Papillary tumors of the renal pelvis (transitional cell, squamous cell, adenocarcinoma) are usually multiple, involving the ureter and often the bladder, as well as lymphatics.

Nephrotic carcinomas are usually large and encapsulated; as many as 50% may perforate the apparently intact capsule. Hematogenous metastasis results from early invasion of renal venules. The neoplasm often extends into the renal vein and vena cava. Distant metastases occur in the lung, lymph nodes, liver, bone, adrenal gland, opposite kidney, brain, and heart (in decreasing frequency).

The kidney is the site of more metastatic than primary tumors. The most frequent sites of origin are the lung and breast.[6,28]

Diagnostic Studies and Findings[28]

Retrograde Pyelogram, Ultrasonography, and Computed Tomography

Visualization of lesion

Cyst Aspiration

Determination of whether process is benign or malignant

Selective Renal Angiography

Clear visualization of renal vascular anatomy

Cystoscopy with Surface Biopsy, Washings for Cell Block, and Papanicolaou Smear

Evidence of malignant cells or tissue

Blood Studies

Normochromic, normocytic anemia; polycythemia in some patients; leukocytosis; hypercalcemia; elevated erythrocyte sedimentation rate

Alkaline Phosphatase, Bilirubin, and Transaminase Levels

Elevated

Prothrombin Time

Prolonged

Urine LDH

Elevated

Medical Plan[6]

Surgery*

Radical nephrectomy
Nephroureterectomy
Palliative nephrectomy for bleeding and pain control
Resection of solitary metastatic site, such as in brain or liver

Medications

Progestins
- Medroxyprogesterone acetate (Provera, Depo-Provera), 2.5-10 mg po or 100-400 mg IM

*See Chapter 12 for postoperative nursing diagnoses and interventions.

Antineoplastic agents
- Cyclophosphamide (Cytoxan), 40-50 mg/kg IV in divided doses over several days, then adjusted to lower maintenance dosage; po 1-5 mg/kg/d
- Vinblastine (Velban), 0.1 mg/kg, increased weekly by 0.05 mg/kg up to 0.5 mg/kg
- Hydroxyurea (Hydrea), 20-30 mg/kg/d po or 80 mg/kg every third day

See "Chemotherapy," p. 1495

General Management

Preoperative radiation therapy
Palliative radiation therapy
Postoperative radiation therapy for patients with high risk of local recurrence
See "Radiation Therapy," p. 1500

• • •

Improved survival rates (5-year survival of 65% for early hypernephroma) have been attributed to thoracoabdominal nephrectomy with node dissection and earlier diagnosis of "incidental" carcinomas. Spontaneous regression has prompted investigational therapy with biologic response modifiers, such as the histamine H_2 antagonist cimetidine.

NURSING CARE

Nursing Assessment

Urinary Function

Painless hematuria; urinary retention

Comfort

Chronic aching pain; renal colic; nerve pain

Systemic Function

Unexplained weight loss; reflex gastrointestinal disturbances, such as nausea and vomiting; fever; hypertension; seizures

Cardiovascular Status

Abdominal bruit; ascites; edema of lower extremities and scrotum; dilated abdominal veins; high-output heart failure

Nursing Dx & Intervention

Nursing Diagnosis	Nursing Intervention/Rationale
Altered patterns of urinary elimination	• Measure intake and output *to monitor for fluid balance.* • Inspect urine for bleeding; check with Hemastix *to detect urinary tract bleeding.* • Inspect abdomen for distention; palpate bladder *to determine bladder emptying.* • Encourage adequate rest and exercise *to maintain general well-being.* • Ambulate patient often *to promote renal circulation and urinary elimination.*

Nursing Diagnosis	Nursing Intervention/Rationale
	• Apply heating pad or hot water bottle *to relax bladder musculature.* • Catheterize only if necessary *to avoid infection.*
Pain	• Be alert for complaints of pain; assess duration, radiation, intensity, and precipitating and relieving factors *to determine appropriate interventions.* • Approach patient unhurriedly; provide reassurance *to relieve fear of causing pain.* • Position patient comfortably, and handle gently *to avoid further discomfort.* • Encourage adequate rest *to relax patient and decrease pain.* • Discuss possible pain-reducing measures, such as guided imagery, relaxation, distraction, and hypnosis, *to enhance medical interventions.* • Administer medications as ordered, such as nonsteroidal anti-inflammatory agents and narcotics, *to control pain.* • For chronic, aching pain, apply heating pad, hot water bottle, or warm, moist compress *to relax muscles and increase circulation.* • For renal colic, increase fluid intake, remove constrictive clothing, and provide sitz bath *to increase hydration, relieve pressure, and relax muscles.* • For nerve pain, apply heat or cold, apply bed cradle, decrease drafts, and massage gently *to promote patient comfort.*
Altered nutrition: less than body requirements	• Estimate required daily calories *to determine goal for patient intake.* • Give small, frequent feedings *to avoid distention.* • Grant special food requests *to promote patient control and enhance appetite.* • Encourage adequate rest *to decrease energy requirement.* • Encourage increased fluid intake to *maintain hydration.* • Supplement protein and caloric intake *to meet nutritional needs.* • Provide mouth care *to promote appetite with oral hygiene.* • Monitor intake and output and temperature *to determine hydration and nutritional status.* • Measure body weight *to monitor nutritional status.* • Administer medications as ordered, such as antiemetics and antipyretics, *to decrease nausea and fever.*
Altered peripheral and cardiovascular tissue perfusion	• Remove constrictive clothing *to prevent pressure on vascular system.* • Raise head of bed *to enhance circulation.* • Elevate extremities without elevating bed at knee gatch or placing pillow under knees *to promote vascular return.* • Apply elastic stockings *to increase venous return.* • Change position frequently *to promote circulation.* • Perform range of motion exercises *to promote circulation.* • Ambulate patient as much as possible *to enhance cardiovascular status.* • Inspect extremities for adequate circulation *to detect problems early.* • Palpate for pulses *to assess arterial status.* • Measure abdominal girth, circumference of extremities, and scrotal size *to determine adequacy of circulation.*
Patient problem: alteration in arterial blood pressure	• Elevate patient's head *to prevent headache.* • Change patient's position frequently *to promote circulation.* • Provide restful, quiet environment *to enhance vasodilation.* • Tell patient to avoid oral stimulants such as caffeine, emotional situations, and smoking *to prevent hypertension.* • Monitor blood pressure *to determine status.*
Patient problem: metastasis	• See "Metastatic Disease," p. 1492.

Patient Education

1. Emphasize need for balanced diet, adequate fluid intake, and high-calorie, high-protein diet.
2. Explain pain-relieving measures, such as exercise, warmth, and analgesics.
3. Discuss changes that should be reported to physician: headache, seizures, fever, blood in urine, increasing pain, increasing edema, and respiratory distress.

Evaluation

Patient Outcome	Data Indicating That Outcome is Reached
Skin and mucous membrane color is normal.	Skin, nails, lips, and earlobes are warm and moist and of natural color.
Vital signs are within normal limits.	Respirations, pulse, blood pressure, and temperature are within normal limits.
Body hydration is normal.	Skin turgor is normal. Secretions are thin. Mucous membranes are moist. There is no edema, ascites, or venous distention.
Patient has daily intake of essential foods.	Diet includes milk, meat, fruits, vegetables, breads, and cereals.
Daily fluid output equals fluid intake.	Urine output is 1500 to 3000 ml daily or equivalent to intake.
Vitality is good.	There is no malaise, fatigue, or weakness.
Patient has physical appearance of comfort.	Patient expresses comfort and satisfaction. Patient ceases to complain.
Patient frequently changes position.	Patient walks, sits, and stands with normal body movement.
Patient participates in therapeutic exercise.	Patient performs range of motion exercises.
Patient's surroundings are safe and comfortable.	Patient uses safety precautions. Temperature, humidity, and ventilation of patient's room are appropriate.
There is no evidence of physical injury.	Patient shows no evidence of complications arising from drugs or treatments.

Carcinoma of the bladder

The bladder is the most common site of urinary tract malignancy.

Cancer of the bladder occurs most often in men between 50 and 70 years of age. In the past 25 years the incidence in men has increased while the incidence in women has decreased; now the prevalence is nearly twice as great in men. The most frequent sign of bladder cancer is hematuria, although some patients are asymptomatic until uretheral obstruction occurs.

The second most common symptom complex is marked urgency, dysuria, and frequency with small volumes of urine in an older patient. Low back pain may be indicative of sacral or lumbar metastases.[28]

Pathophysiology[6]

Ninety percent of bladder tumors are transitional cell carcinoma, 6% to 7% are true squamous cell carcinoma, and only 1% to 2% are glandular cancer. Some of these tumors are undifferentiated. Depth of invasion (stage) is more important than grading in predicting prognosis.

Lymph node involvement is present in half of the patients with deep muscle infiltration and has a poor prognosis. The disappointing long-term survival rate of patients with deeply invasive tumors has led to an integrated form of therapy in which irradiation is followed by cystectomy.

The best way to reduce the incidence is elimination of known carcinogens, especially cigarette smoke.

Diagnostic Studies and Findings[28]

Urine Culture

Sterile urine in patient with symptoms of cystitis

Urinary Tract Cytology

Examination of midmorning specimen or bladder washings to detect abnormal cells

Intravenous Urogram

Dilated ureter or nonfunctioning kidney

Intravenous Pyelogram

Filling defects, halo or dye around base of bladder, flattening or rigidity of bladder wall

Cystoscopy with Multiple Biopsies

Evidence of malignant tissue

Bimanual Examination

Revelation of firm or hard nodularity

Chest and Skeletal Roentgenograms, Bone Scans, and Liver Function Studies

Evidence of metastatic disease

Medical Plan[6]

Surgery

Endoscopic resection and fulguration; cystectomy, prostatectomy and urethrectomy
Cystectomy with urinary diversion*

Medications

Antineoplastic agents
- Thiotepa (Triethylenethiophosphoramide), IV 60 mg initially, usually at 1- to 4-wk intervals
- Cyclophosphamide (Cytoxan), 40-50 mg/kg IV in divided doses over several days, then adjusted to lower maintenance dosage; po 1-5 mg/kg/d
- Doxorubicin (Adriamycin), 60-75 mg/m² at intervals of 21 d, or 30 mg/m²/d for 3 d and repeated q4wk
- Cisplatin (Platinol), 50-80 mg/m² IV q3wk or individually determined dosage

See "Chemotherapy," p. 1495

*See Chapter 12 for care of patient undergoing urinary diversion procedure.

General Management

Hydrostatic pressure from intravesical balloon
Hyperthermia (investigational)
Open diathermy
External radiation—preoperative, radical alone, or palliative for local recurrence and bone pain
See "Radiation Therapy," p. 1500

NURSING CARE

Nursing Assessment[6]

Urinary Function

Hematuria; urgency; dysuria; frequency; azotemia; pelvic mass

Comfort

Low back pain

Nursing Dx & Intervention

Nursing Diagnosis	Nursing Intervention/Rationale
Altered patterns of urinary elimination	• Measure intake and output *to monitor adequacy of elimination.* • Inspect urine for blood; check with Hemastix *to detect bleeding.* • Inspect abdomen for swelling and distention *to determine presence of urinary retention.* • Encourage adequate rest and exercise *to avoid stress-related distention.* • Increase patient's fluid intake *to enhance renal circulation and flush bladder.* • Apply heating pad or hot water bottle to abdomen as ordered *to relax muscles.* • Catheterize patient only if necessary *to avoid infection.* • Monitor blood studies: acid-base balance, hemoglobin level, hematocrit value, blood urea nitrogen, and creatinine level *to assess renal function.* • Monitor urine studies: acid-base balance, creatinine level, specific gravity, and protein level *to assess renal function.*
Pain	• Change patient's position slowly *to avoid injury and strain.* • Place patient in whirlpool bath, or apply heat *to relax muscles.* • Provide safety measures *to avoid injury.* • Administer bladder antispasmodics as ordered *to relieve bladder spasms.* • Discuss possible pain-relieving measures with patient; use those possible *to promote self-care.* • Evaluate effectiveness of pain relief measures *to determine need for further intervention.*
Patient problem: metastasis	• See "Metastatic Disease," p. 1492.

Patient Education

1. Emphasize the need for adequate fluid intake, exercise, and rest.
2. Discuss pain-relieving measures, such as exercise, warmth, safety, and medication.
3. Instruct the patient in self-care if the patient has undergone urinary diversion.

Evaluation

Patient Outcome	Data Indicating That Outcome is Reached
Daily fluid output is equal to fluid intake.	Urine output is 1500 to 3000 ml daily or equivalent to intake.

Patient Outcome	Data Indicating That Outcome is Reached
Laboratory findings are within normal limits.	Blood urea nitrogen, serum creatinine, hematocrit, hemoglobin, and blood pH values are within normal limits. Creatinine clearance and urine creatinine level, pH, and specific gravity are within normal limits; no protein is found in urine.
Patient is comfortable.	Facial expression is calm and relaxed. Patient has freedom of body movement. Patient expresses comfort and ceases to complain.

CANCERS OF THE MALE REPRODUCTIVE SYSTEM

Cancer of the prostate

Cancer of the prostate is a malignant tumor arising from the parenchyma of the prostate gland.

The prostate is the third most common site of cancer in men, accounting for 17% of all male cancers. The incidence and mortality of this cancer are increasing, especially in blacks.[3]

Most prostatic cancers are adenocarcinomas discovered by a physician during rectal examination, which should be done yearly on all men over 50 years of age. These slow-growing tumors arise in the posterior portion of the prostate and eventually involve the entire gland. They spread via the lymphatics throughout the pelvic region and into the pelvic bones.

Early symptoms resemble those of benign prostatic hypertrophy and include weak urinary stream, urinary frequency, dysuria, and difficulty in starting and stopping urination. Some patients initially report pain in the lower back, pelvis, or upper thighs. Bilateral ureteral obstruction with renal insufficiency is not uncommon at the time of diagnosis.[28]

Pathophysiology[6]

The cellular appearance of these adenocarcinomas is a definite glandular pattern with small gland size or lack of papillae in a disorderly connective tissue framework. By the time of diagnosis, most prostatic cancers have already invaded the base of the bladder, seminal vesicles, or perivesicular fascia or moved laterally into the levator ani muscles.

Grading of these tumors—well, moderately, or poorly differentiated—correlates with the prognosis.

Diagnostic Studies and Findings[28]

Digital Rectal Examination

50% of palpable prostatic nodules are cancer

Closed Needle Biopsy via Perineal or Transrectal Route or Open Biopsy

Evidence of malignant cells

Prostatic Acid Phosphatase (PAP)

Elevated in localized disease

Serum Total Acid Phosphatase

Elevated in two thirds of cases of metastatic spread; bone marrow acid phosphatase more accurate indicator

Alkaline Phosphatase

Elevated with bony metastases

Bone Survey, Bone Scan

Detection of bony metastases

Excretory Urogram

Bladder outlet involvement; ureteral obstruction or displacement

Pelvic Computed Tomography Scans

Local extensions; nodal involvement

Lymphangiography

Para-aortic and pelvic node involvement

Medical Plan[6]

Treatment is based on clinical assessment, stage of disease, anticipated tolerance to therapy, morbidity, and expected longevity.

Surgery*

Radical prostatectomy by perineal, retropubic, or transpubic route

Orchiectomy

Medications

Estrogens

Diethylstilbestrol (DES, Stilbestrol), 1.5-15 mg po

Corticosteroids

Prednisone (Deltasone, others), 10-100 mg po

See "Chemotherapy," p. 1495

General Management

Supervoltage radiotherapy for primary treatment, control, palliation (see p. 1500)

*See Chapter 12 for postoperative nursing diagnoses and intervention.

NURSING CARE

Nursing Assessment[20]

Urinary Function

Weak urinary stream; urinary frequency; dysuria; difficulty starting and stopping urination; renal insufficiency (azotemia, decreased output)

Comfort Level

Pain in lower back, pelvis, or upper thighs

Nursing Dx & Intervention

Nursing Diagnosis	Nursing Intervention/Rationale
Urinary retention (potential)	• Measure intake and output *to monitor adequacy of elimination.* • Be alert for patient's complaints of frequency, pain, and urination difficulties *as indications of infection or obstruction.* • Encourage adequate rest and activity *to decrease stress on urinary system.* • Increase patient's fluid intake *to flush renal system.* • Catheterize patient only if necessary *to eliminate urine retention.*
Altered patterns of urinary elimination related to renal insufficiency	• Monitor blood studies: blood urea nitrogen, creatinine, acid-base balance, hemoglobin, and hematocrit *to assess renal function.* • Monitor urine studies: acid-base balance, creatinine, and specific gravity *to assess renal function.* • Inspect for edema *as indication of fluid retention.* • Weigh daily and measure intake and output *to monitor renal function.* • Monitor blood pressure *as indication of fluid retention.* • Test urine for protein *as indication of impaired renal function.*
Patient problem: metastasis	• See "Metastatic Disease," p. 1492.

Patient Education

1. Inform the patient of the need for adequate fluid intake, exercise, and rest.
2. Instruct the patient in pain-relieving measures, such as exercise, warmth, and medication.
3. Tell the patient to notify the physician if signs and symptoms of renal insufficiency appear.

Evaluation

Patient Outcome	Data Indicating That Outcome is Reached
Laboratory findings are within normal limits.	Blood urea nitrogen, hemoglobin, hematocrit, blood pH, and serum creatinine are within normal limits. Creatinine clearance and urine specific gravity, pH, and creatinine are within normal limits; urine test for protein is negative.
Body hydration is normal.	There is no edema.
Fluid output equals fluid intake.	Urine output is 1500 to 3000 ml daily or equivalent to intake.

Testicular carcinoma

Testicular cancer is a malignant neoplastic disease of the testis occurring most frequently in men between 20 and 35 years of age.

The incidence of testicular carcinoma is higher in men with undescended testes (cryptorchidism). The first sign of the disease is usually a small, hard, painless lump in the testicle; symptoms are a sensation of heaviness in the testicle, sudden fluid accumulation in the scrotum, and perineal pain or discomfort.[3]

Pathophysiology[28]

Most testicular tumors are of germ cell origin and are malignant. The basic categories are the seminoma and heterogeneous, nonseminomatous germ cell tumor. Para-aortic lymph node involvement, ureteral obstruction, and pulmonary metastases may be present.[6]

Diagnostic Studies and Findings[28]

Palpation of Testes

Presence of mass

Examination of Breasts

Presence of gynecomastia

Transillumination

Detection of intrascrotal lesions

Abdominal Examination

Palpable mass

Excretory Urogram

Ureteral deviation from para-aortic or paracaval nodal involvement

Radioimmunoassay (RIA)

Elevated serum α-fetoprotein (AFP) and human chorionic gonadotropin (HCG)

Abdominal Computed Tomography Scan

For staging

Chest Roentgenogram and Computed Tomography Scan

To detect metastatic disease

Medical Plan[6]

Surgery

Inguinal exploration and orchiectomy
Bilateral retroperitoneal lymph node dissection

Medications

Antineoplastic agents
- For seminomas
  - Cyclophosphamide (Cytoxan), 40-50 mg/kg IV in divided doses over several days; then adjust to lower maintenance dosage
  - Chlorambucil (Leukeran), 4-10 mg/d po
- For nonseminomas
  - Cisplatin (Platinol), 50-80 mg/m^2 IV q3wk, or dosage individually determined
  - Vinblastine sulfate (Velban), 0.1 mg/kg increased weekly by 0.05 mg/kg up to 0.5 mg/kg
  - Bleomycin sulfate (Blenoxane), 0.25-0.5 U/kg, or 10-20 U/m^2 IV, IM, or subcutaneously 1 or 2 times/wk
  - Dactinomycin (Cosmegen), 0.015-0.05 mg/kg IV divided doses over 1 wk; repeat for 3-5 wk

See "Chemotherapy," p. 1495

General Management

Radiation
- For seminomas—irradiation of retroperitoneal and homolateral iliac nodes to level of diaphragm; may also include mediastinum and supraclavicular node area
- For nonseminomas—occasionally used for localized metastases that cannot be excised and do not respond to chemotherapy

See "Radiation Therapy," p. 1500

• • •

Dramatic responses to single agent and combination drug chemotherapy have made even advanced cases of testicular cancer curable. Radiation therapy is still used for seminomas but has been replaced by chemotherapy for nonseminomatous tumors. Tumor markers (AFP and HCG) are useful not only in early diagnosis but also in follow-up monitoring for recurrent disease.

NURSING CARE

Nursing Assessment[6]

Scrotum

Small, hard, painless lump; sensation of heaviness; fluid accumulation; pain or discomfort

Urinary Function

Renal insufficiency (azotemia); decreased output

Nursing Dx & Intervention

Nursing Diagnosis	Nursing Intervention/Rationale
Pain (scrotal)	• Handle patient gently *to avoid further discomfort.* • Apply heat as ordered with heating pad, hot water bottle, warm moist compress, or warm water bath *to promote circulation and decrease swelling.* • Discuss pain-relieving measures, such as scrotal support and analgesics; implement them as feasible *to further patient comfort.* • Evaluate effectiveness of pain-relieving measures *to determine need for further intervention.*

Nursing Diagnosis	Nursing Intervention/Rationale
	• Be alert for complaints of pain, and assess duration and radiation *to assess effectiveness of intervention*.
Altered patterns of urinary elimination related to renal insufficiency	• Monitor blood studies: blood urea nitrogen, creatinine, acid-base balance, hemoglobin, and hematocrit *to assess renal function*. • Monitor urine studies: acid-base balance, creatinine, and specific gravity *to assess renal function*. • Inspect for hematuria and edema *as evidence of renal status*. • Measure blood pressure *(elevation is indicative of renal insufficiency)*. • Test urine for protein *as evidence of renal insufficiency*.
Patient problem: metastasis	• See "Metastatic Disease," p. 1492.

Patient Education

1. Inform the patient of the need for adequate fluid intake, exercise, and rest.
2. Instruct the patient in the use of pain relief measures, such as exercise and warmth.
3. Tell the patient to notify the physician if signs of respiratory distress or renal insufficiency appear.
4. Emphasize the need for follow-up evaluation at regular intervals.

Evaluation[10]

Patient Outcome	Data Indicating That Outcome is Reached
Vital signs are within normal limits.	Respiratory rate, rhythm, and depth are normal; pulse and blood pressure are within normal limits.
Laboratory findings are within normal limits.	Blood urea nitrogen, hemoglobin, hematocrit, blood pH, oxygen saturation, and serum creatinine are within normal limits. Creatinine clearance and urine specific gravity, pH, and creatinine are within normal limits; findings of urine test for protein are negative.
Body hydration is normal.	There is no edema.
Body functioning is normal.	Elimination is adequate.
Daily fluid output is equal to fluid intake.	Urine output is 1500 to 3000 ml daily or equivalent to intake.
Patient is comfortable.	Facial expression is calm and relaxed. Posture is normal. Patient has freedom of body movement. Patient expresses comfort and ceases to complain.
Patient frequently changes position and has normal body movement.	Patient walks, sits, and stands with normal body movement.

GYNECOLOGIC CANCERS

Cancer of the uterus, both endometrial and cervical (including in situ), accounts for 14% of all female cancers. Cancers of the female genital organs—uterus, ovaries, vulva, and vagina—are second only to breast cancer in causing morbidity and mortality in women.

Cancer of the cervix

Cancer of the uterine cervix is a neoplasm of the uterine cervix that can be detected in the early, curable stage by the Papanicolaou (Pap) test.

Cancer of the uterine cervix has its highest incidence in women who are 35 years of age or older, began sexual activity in puberty, and have had multiple partners. Other risk factors include low socioeconomic status, poor prenatal and postnatal care, and in utero exposure to diethylstilbestrol (DES). Women in urban, industrialized areas and white or Jewish women have a lower incidence of the disease than do those in rural, underdeveloped areas and nonwhites. Celibate women and those in religious groups that encourage male circumcision and monogamy also have a lower incidence. Women with multiple genital infections such as herpes, *Trichomonas* infection, and gonorrhea are at greater risk.

Improved general and genital hygiene and cytologic screening with the Papanicolaou (Pap) smear have contributed to decreased mortality of cervical cancer. The American Cancer Society now recommends that, after two negative Pap tests 1 year apart, women over 20 years who are not at high risk should be tested at least every 3 years. Sexually active women under 20 years should also follow this schedule. Women at risk are encouraged to have a yearly Pap test.

Changes in cells of the cervical epithelium may be present for 10 years before invasive cancer develops. However, a Pap smear can detect even the earliest changes, so regular Pap tests, as well as manual pelvic examinations, are the most important means of reducing mortality from cervical cancer.[3,6]

Pathophysiology[6]

The first sign of uterine cancer is unusual bleeding or vaginal discharge between menstrual periods, after intercourse, or after menopause. When symptoms appear, the cancer has usually progressed beyond its early stages. Squamous cell carcinoma accounts for 95% of all invasive tumors diagnosed, and adenocarcinomas account for most of the rest. Clear cell carcinoma develops in the cervix and vagina of women exposed in utero to DES. Invasive carcinoma of the cervix spreads by direct extension to the vaginal wall, laterally into the parametrium toward the pelvic wall, and anteroposteriorly into the bladder and rectum. Metastases to the pelvic lymph nodes are more common than those to distant nodes.

Diagnostic Studies and Findings[28]

Pathologic Examination of Multiple Cervical Biopsy Specimens by Schiller Test with Endocervical Curettage or Colposcopy; Conization When Colposcopic Examination Unsatisfactory

Evidence of malignant cells by Pap test

Cystoscopy

Establishes normal bladder anatomy

Intravenous Pyelogram

Ascertains that ureters are unobstructed and that kidney and upper collecting system are normal

Lymphangiography

Screening for lymph node metastases

Medical Plan[6]

The clinical stage of the tumor at the time of diagnosis is used to determine therapy and prognosis.

Surgery*

For mild to moderate dysplasia
- Cryocautery
- Thermocauterization
- Laser surgery

For carcinoma in situ
- Simple hysterectomy if patient is beyond childbearing age or does not want more children
- Excision of mucocutaneous junctional tissue and regular examinations for women who wish to have children

For invasive carcinoma
- Total hysterectomy (see p. 1016)

For central recurrent or persistent pelvic cancer
- Pelvic exenteration

Medications

Poor results when patient has far advanced disease

Antineoplastic agents
- Drugs used in combination; dosages of combination drugs individually determined
- Methotrexate (Amethopterin, Mexate, MTX)
  - Bleomycin (Blenoxane)
  - Mitomycin (Mutamycin)
- Cisplatin (Platinol), 50-80 mg/m² IV q3wk or by individually determined dosage

See "Chemotherapy," p. 1495

General Management

Radiation therapy—combination of external and intracavity (radium) therapy; doses determined by tolerance of surrounding organs (rectum, bladder, and small intestine) (see p. 1500)

• • •

The prognosis for stage I (vaginal wall) invasive cancer is similar for pregnant and nonpregnant women, but pregnancy seems to have an unfavorable effect on the prognosis of more advanced disease. Caesarean section is the indicated delivery method for these patients.

There is no proof that postoperative pelvic or para-aortic radiation is effective in improving the prognosis for patients with lymphatic metastases, although further studies are in progress.

More than 55% of treated patients live 5 years. Radical surgery can now be performed safely with limited morbidity. The overall cure rate is 29%.

NURSING CARE

Nursing Assessment[20]

Perineal Hygiene

Unusual bleeding or vaginal discharge; profuse, malodorous discharge

Circulatory Function

Lymphedema

*See Chapter 10 for postoperative nursing diagnoses and interventions.

Level of Comfort

Back and leg pain; inability to lie with leg straightened; feeling of pressure; heavy, aching abdominal pain

Gastrointestinal

Rectal discharge; feeling of pressure

Nursing Dx & Intervention

Nursing Diagnosis	Nursing Intervention/Rationale
Pain	*For abdominal pressure:* • Change patient's position frequently *to relieve pressure.* • Give small, frequent feedings *to avoid abdominal distention.* • Place patient in sitting position *to relieve abdominal pressure.* • Remove constrictive clothing *to relieve pressure.* • Insert rectal tube as indicated *to relieve flatus.* • Auscultate abdomen for abnormal bowel sounds *to assess GI status.* *For back pain, leg pain, or lymphedema:* • Position comfortably, and change position slowly *to avoid injury.* • Maintain body alignment *to avoid injury or muscular stretching.* • Apply heating pad, hot water bottle, or warm, moist compress *to relax muscles and increase circulation.* • Bathe patient in warm water *to relax muscles.* • Massage gently *to promote circulation and relax muscles.* • Encourage adequate rest *to decrease energy expenditure.* • Provide pain relief measure of patient's choice *to promote self-care.* • Be alert for complaints of pain, and assess duration and radiation of pain *to determine need for further intervention.*
Potential impaired skin integrity related to vaginal or rectal infection	• Change dressings or pads frequently *to maintain cleanliness.* • Maintain dry, clean linen and dry skin *to enhance patient's comfort.* • Provide clean clothing *to enhance patient's comfort.* • Observe skin for irritation *to determine need for further intervention.* • Observe quality and quantity of drainage *to determine status of infection.* • Administer antibiotics as ordered *to combat infection.* • Monitor vital signs *to assess systemic response to infection.* • Administer perineal care as indicated *to promote comfort and remove drainage from skin.*
Patient problem: metastasis	• See "Metastatic Disease," p. 1492.

Patient Education

1. Teach the patient to use nonpharmacologic comfort measures whenever possible.
2. Teach the patient ways to avoid unnecessary pain to abdomen, back, legs, and other areas.
3. Emphasize the need to maintain skin hygiene.

Evaluation

Patient Outcome	Data Indicating That Outcome is Reached
Vital signs are within normal limits.	Respirations, pulse, blood pressure, and temperature are within normal limits.
Body is clean.	Skin is clean. There is no unpleasant body odor. Patient feels clean and refreshed.
Patient is comfortable.	Facial expression is calm, contented, and relaxed. Posture is normal. Patient has freedom of body movement. Patient expresses comfort and satisfaction.
Patient does not have infection.	There is no evidence of inflammation, purulent drainage or secretions, pain, or aching. Blood leukocyte count is 4500 to 11,000 cells/mm^3.

 Other gynecologic cancers

Malignant diseases occur in all parts of the female reproductive system. They include cancers of the uterine endometrium, the vagina, the vulva, the ovaries, and the fallopian tubes, as well as gestational trophoblastic neoplasms.

Endometrial cancer. Endometrial cancer is less common than cervical cancer in young women, but the diseases occur with equal frequency in postmenopausal women. Etiologic factors include infertility, late menopause (after 55 years of age), obesity, diabetes, and hypertension. Long-term diethylstilbestrol (DES) therapy may also be a factor. Cancer of the endometrium occurs with higher frequency in urban, white, and Jewish women. The benefits of maintaining an ideal weight and careful management of estrogen therapy for menopause should be emphasized.[3]

The most common initial symptom is intermenstrual or postmenopausal bleeding. The diagnosis of endometrial cancer is based on histologic tissue examination.

The usual treatment for cancer limited to the fundal portion of the uterus is preoperative intracavity radiation therapy followed by total hysterectomy and bilateral salpingo-oophorectomy. External radiation is added to the treatment plan when the cancer extends beyond the fundus.

The 5-year survival rate for patients with early endometrial cancer is greater than 85%. The cure rate drops to 50% when the cancer has metastasized.

Vaginal cancer. Vaginal carcinoma is rarely a primary lesion, although it does occur in both menopausal and postmenopausal women. It is related to in utero DES exposure in younger women. Vaginal cancer is rare in black and Jewish women. The primary signs and symptoms are vaginal spotting and discharge, pain, groin masses, and changes in urinary pattern.

Radiation therapy consists of intracavity irradiation combined with total pelvic external irradiation. Radical surgery includes complete vaginectomy, pelvic node dissection, and anterior exenteration as indicated. Grafting may be used to avoid vaginal stenosis, especially in younger patients.

Vulvar cancer. Fewer than 1% of female genital cancers are found in the vulva. Vulvar cancer occurs most commonly in women who are between 50 and 70 years and in lower socioeconomic strata. Symptoms include vaginal discharge, pruritus, and bleeding.

The leukoplakic changes (whitish, plaquelike or ulcerated lesions) that precede carcinoma can be eliminated by simple vulvectomy. Once carcinoma develops, invasion of the inguinal nodes and the lower vagina is common.

Surgery for this form of cancer may be preventive to remove precancerous lesions (hemivulvectomy or local excision with a wide margin of normal tissue), curative (radical vulvectomy), or palliative (extent depends on the patient's symptoms).

The 5-year survival rate is greater than 80% for women with early, localized lesions but is much lower when nodal or distant metastasis is present.

Ovarian cancer. Ovarian cancer has replaced cervical cancer as the leading cause of death from genital cancer. Its development is closely linked to breast cancer, which suggests abnormal endocrine activity. The peak incidence is between 60 and 80 years of age.

These tumors do not usually produce symptoms until intraabdominal metastasis has occurred, with outward signs such as ascites. Therefore the mortality is high; only 34% of patients survive the disease. When symptoms do occur, they include increasing abdominal girth, weight loss, abdominal pain, dysuria or urinary frequency, and constipation.

Treatment of ovarian cancer consists of hysterectomy and bilateral salpingo-oophorectomy. Radiation therapy and chemotherapy may be used in conjunction with surgery or when the cancer is inoperable.

Cancer of the fallopian tube. Fallopian tube cancer is the rarest of the gynecologic malignancies. It is difficult to diagnose, and diagnosis is usually at time of surgery. Most are adenocarcinomas. Patients are usually in their midfifties when fallopian tube cancer is detected. The most common symptoms are pelvic pain, abnormal vaginal bleeding, and a heavy, watery vaginal discharge. Colicky pain may be associated with bleeding.

Removal of the uterus, fallopian tubes, ovaries, and omentum is the usual treatment. Radiation and chemotherapy have been used postoperatively with some success. Survival rates are as high as 90% with early disease, although the overall 5-year survival rate is 38%.

Gestational trophoblastic neoplasms. The gestational trophoblastic neoplasms include hydatidiform mole, invasive mole (chorioadenoma destruens), and choriocarcinoma. Molar pregnancy, the most common of these tumors, occurs in approximately 1 in 1500 live births in the United States; locally invasive disease develops in 16% of these patients and metastatic disease in 31%. These neoplasms can also develop after abortal, ectopic, and term gestations.

The measurement of human chorionic gonadotropin (HCG) by the β subunit radioimmunoassay test is essential for diagnosis, monitoring of therapy, and follow-up. Early diagnosis is facilitated by amniography and ultrasonography.

Hydatidiform mole is treated with suction curettage when preserving fertility is desirable. Actinomycin D, given prophylactically, reduces the incidence of sequelae when the uterus is larger than the fruit dates, the serum HCG titer is over 100,000 mU/dl, and the ovaries are cystic. Postevacuation monitoring of HCG levels is done weekly for 3 consecutive weeks and then monthly for 6 months or until HCG is undetectable. During this time pregnancy should be avoided. If fertility is not desired, total abdominal hysterectomy is the treatment of choice when the mole is in situ.

Locally invasive mole or choriocarcinoma is diagnosed by elevated HCG level, pelvic angiography, ultrasonography, and curettage. If fertility is desired, intermittent courses of single agent chemotherapy, such as methotrexate with citrovorum rescue or actinomycin D, yield a cure rate of 100%. When fertility is not desired, hysterectomy is the treatment of choice.

Metastasis is most common with choriocarcinoma; the most frequent sites are the lung, vagina, oral cavity, gastrointestinal tract, central nervous system, and liver. The treatment of choice is chemotherapy with a single agent or a combination of drugs. Surgery or adjunctive radiation therapy may be required. The overall survival with metastasis is still good, although the prognosis is poor with metastases to the liver or brain.[6,28]

CANCERS OF THE HEAD AND NECK

Cancers of the head and neck are neoplasms characterized by the uncontrolled growth of anaplastic cells in the larynx, oral cavity, pharynx, or salivary glands.

Although less than 5% of all cancers are neoplasms of the head and neck, they are important because surgical treatment may result in extensive cosmetic deformities and may impair such vital functions as eating and speaking. Patients with head and neck cancers represent 15% of cancer admissions to large medical centers.[3]

The most common site is the larynx, followed by the oral cavity, pharynx, and salivary glands. Etiologic factors for oral and laryngeal cancers include wood dust (nasal cavity cancer), chronic irritation, poor oral hygiene, prolonged heavy use of alcohol, snuff, or tobacco, and Epstein-Barr virus (associated with nasopharyngeal cancer).

Pathophysiology

Most head and neck cancers grow as malignant ulcerations on surface mucosa. The infiltrative, endophytic lesions are more aggressive and difficult to control than the less common elevated, fungating, exophytic growths. The signs and symptoms depend on the location and are as follows:

Oral cavity—swelling or ulcer that fails to heal and bleeds easily

Oropharynx—"silent" area; dysphagia; local pain, pain on swallowing, referred pain to ear, enlarging cervical mass

Hypopharynx—another "silent" area; dysphagia, painful swallowing of food, referred ear pain, or neck mass

Nasopharynx—bloody nasal discharge, obstructed nostril, neurologic problems such as facial pain, diplopia, or hoarseness, conductive deafness

Nose and sinuses—bloody nasal discharge, nasal obstruction, diplopia, facial pain or swelling

Parotid and submandibular glands—painless local swelling, hemifacial paralysis

Larynx—persistent hoarseness, pain, referred ear pain, dyspnea, stridor[6,28]

Diagnostic Studies and Findings[28]

Inspection, Directly and Via Mirror, of Oral Cavity, Nasopharynx, Oropharynx, Larynx, and Hypopharynx

Visualization of suspect lesion

Fiberoptic Aerodigestive Endoscopy

Visualization and biopsy of suspect lesion

Palpation of Cervical Lymphatics

Metastatic nodes hard, oval, or round

Biopsy of Suspect Lesions

Histologic evidence of malignancy

Radiographic Studies for Staging Workup; Plain Films of Skull and Its Base, Sinuses, and Lateral Neck Soft Tissue; Computed Tomography for Staging

Visualization of suspect lesion and metastatic process

Chest Roentgenograms

Presence of metastasis or second primary tumor

Bone Scan

Evidence of metastasis

Anti-Epstein-Barr Virus (EBV) Antibody Titers

Elevation of immunoglobulin G (IgG) and immunoglobulin A (IgA) fairly specific indicators for nasopharyngeal carcinoma

Medical Plan[6]

The goals of treatment for head and neck cancers are eradication of both clinically demonstrated disease and microscopic subclinical disease; maintenance of adequate physiologic function by reversal of present dysfunction and post-treatment dysfunction in the special senses, chewing and swallowing, respiration, and speech; and socially acceptable cosmesis, including sufficient surgical, radiation, plastic surgical, and prosthesis rehabilitation.

Treatment decisions involve a multidisciplinary approach with emphasis on such factors as age, general physical condition, other morbidity (such as extensive dental disease, premalignant mucosa, leukoplakia, erythroplasia, or second primary lesion), habits and life-style, occupation, and the patient's desires.

Surgery (see p. 1504) and radiation therapy (see p. 1500) are the major curative modalities. Chemotherapy is employed as adjuvant therapy or sequentially before radiation or surgery (see p. 1495).

More than 75% of head and neck cancer patients whose treatment fails have the first recurrence in areas above the clavicles. The most common failure pattern is recurrent primary tumor with neck metastasis and subsequent carotid erosion or rupture. Distant metastasis to the lung, bone, and elsewhere occurs in long-term survivors of local or regional disease. Intercurrent disease such as alcoholism or chronic lung disease, accidents, and suicide account for 10% to 30% of deaths.

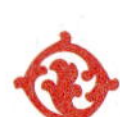

Cancers of the oral cavity

Cancers of the oral cavity are neoplasms that may invade the tongue, buccal mucosa, and hard palate.

Small, localized lesions of the oral cavity may be treated with radiation therapy or surgery or both. Larger lesions may be irradiated before surgical excision. Tumors that spread to cervical lymph nodes require radical neck dissection. Overall survival for carcinoma of the oral cavity is 40% to 65%, depending on site. Early primary lesions have the best prognosis.

NURSING CARE

Nursing Assessment[6]

Oral Cavity Appearance and Function

Leukoplakia (white patch); erythroplasia (red patch); chronic, nonhealing ulcer; localized pain; dysphagia

Lymphatic Function

Enlarged nodes

Nursing Dx & Intervention

Nursing Diagnosis	Nursing Intervention/Rationale
Altered oral mucous membrane	• Provide frequent oral hygiene; use soft brush *to prevent trauma.* • Offer nonirritating (nonacidic) foods *to avoid irritation and discomfort.* • Refrain from giving hot or iced liquids, *which may also irritate membranes.* • Apply local analgesics as needed *to relieve pain and enhance comfort.*
Altered nutrition: less than body requirements	• Feed slowly with small, frequent feedings; provide high-calorie, high-protein diet *to promote adequate nutrition.* • Give clear-liquid, full-liquid, pureed, or soft foods as tolerated in presence of oral irritation and discomfort. • Have suction equipment available *to remove excessive secretions.*
Patient problem: metastasis	• See "Metastatic Disease," p. 1492.

Patient Education

1. Emphasize the need for adequate oral hygiene and dietary management.
2. Discuss signs and symptoms of progressive disease or side effects of treatment that should be reported to the physician.

Evaluation

Patient Outcome	Data Indicating That Outcome is Reached
Mucous membrane color is normal.	Mucous membrane is warm, moist, and of natural color.
Body hydration is normal.	Mucous membranes are moist. Patient is not thirsty.
Body functioning is normal.	Digestion is adequate.
Patient is comfortable.	Facial expression is calm and relaxed. Patient expresses comfort.

 Cancer of the larynx

Cancers of the larynx arise from the epithelial lining of the laryngeal mucous membrane.

Carcinoma of the supraglottic larynx (epiglottis, aryepiglottic folds, arytenoids, and false cords) has a lower incidence than glottic carcinoma; 60% to 65% of laryngeal carcinomas occur in the glottic larynx (true vocal cord). Ninety percent occur in men, with highest incidence in those between 60 and 70 years of age. The early warning sign of progressive hoarseness, caused by a change in the phonating edge of the vocal cord, has led to 5-year survival rates of nearly 80% for localized lesions.[3,28]

Early cancer can be treated by radiation therapy or surgery. Extensive lesions, which cause necrosis of cartilage or glottic extension, require total laryngectomy.[6]

NURSING CARE

Nursing Assessment[6]

Respiratory Function

Hoarseness; dyspnea; stridor; hemoptysis

Gastrointestinal Function

Dysphagia

Level of Comfort

Pain referred to ear (otalgia)

Nursing Dx & Intervention

Nursing Diagnosis	Nursing Intervention/Rationale
Ineffective breathing pattern	• Place patient in sitting position *to enhance chest expansion.* • Encourage deep breathing *to ensure effective ventilation.* • Inspect chest for respiratory rate, rhythm, and expansion *to monitor respiratory status.* • Auscultate for abnormal breath sounds and lung aeration *to monitor respiratory status.* • Palpate and percuss chest *to assess pulmonary function.* • Monitor blood studies *to determine adequacy of gaseous exchange.*
Ineffective airway clearance	• Suction airway as necessary *to remove secretions.* • Provide standby emergency equipment (oxygen and tracheostomy tray) *in case of acute obstruction.* • Provide tracheostomy or laryngectomy care as indicated (see Chapter 7). • Feed slowly with small, frequent feedings *to avoid choking.* • Give clear-liquid, full-liquid, pureed, or soft foods as tolerated *to avoid choking.* • Have suction equipment available *in case of aspiration.*
Pain	• Apply heating pad, hot water bottle, or warm, moist compress *to relieve pain.* • Maintain warm room temperature *to avoid irritation caused by cold air.* • Provide pain relief measure of patient's choice *to enhance self-care.* • Evaluate effectiveness of pain relief measures *to determine need for further intervention.* • Be alert for complaints of pain, and assess duration and radiation *to determine effectiveness of intervention or progression of problem.*
Impaired verbal communication	• Maintain open communication by call light in patient's reach at bedside and use of pad and pencil or Magic Slate. • Ask questions that require a "yes" or "no" answer. • Wait for patient to write responses. • Assist with use of artificial larynx if applicable.
Patient problem: metastasis	• See "Metastatic Disease," p. 1492.

Patient Education

1. Explain methods of maintaining respiratory function, such as deep breathing and use of oxygen; provide a list of emergency resources.
2. Emphasize the need for adequate dietary management.
3. Discuss the value of speech therapy, and put the patient in touch with support groups, such as the Lost Cord Club.
4. Teach the patient methods of managing pain.

5. Discuss signs and symptoms of progressive disease and side effects of treatment that should be reported to the physician.
6. Support instruction in the use of an artificial larynx.

Evaluation

Patient Outcome	Data Indicating That Outcome is Reached
Skin and mucous membrane color is normal.	Skin, nails, lips, and earlobes are warm and moist and have natural color.
Vital signs are within normal limits.	Respiratory rate, rhythm, and depth are normal. Breathing pattern is regular. Patient does not have respiratory distress.
Laboratory findings are within normal limits.	Blood oxygen saturation and carbon dioxide are within normal limits.
Body hydration is normal.	Mucous membranes are moist. Patient is not thirsty.
Body functioning is normal.	Digestion is adequate.
Patient is comfortable.	Facial expression is calm and relaxed. Patient expresses comfort.
Communication is maintained.	Patient expresses himself or herself in clear manner, whether with use of assistive larynx device or on paper.

CANCERS OF THE DIGESTIVE ORGANS AND ENDOCRINE GLANDS

Cancers of the esophagus and stomach account for 4% of all cancers. Unfortunately, many of the early symptoms of these diseases (dysphagia, epigastric discomfort, anorexia, and weight loss) are nonspecific, and therefore affected people often delay seeking treatment. Approximately 6% of cancers detected in the United States affect the digestive and endocrine glands. Some are easily detected because of their location and secretory patterns, whereas others are more difficult to diagnose. The 5-year survival rate varies from 1% for pancreatic carcinoma to 95% for localized thyroid cancer.[3]

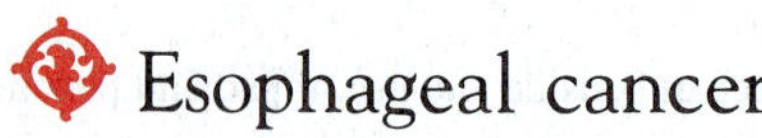

Esophageal cancer

Malignancy of the esophagus usually arises from squamous epithelium and is epidermoid in type.

Esophageal cancer usually occurs in people 50 years of age or older and predominantly in men. It is also more common in the black population. There are indications that esophageal cancers are related to tobacco and alcohol use, nutritional deficiencies, and environmental carcinogens. The highest frequency of esophageal cancers is found in the Caspian Sea area, Transkei in southern Africa, and northern China.

Some of the suggested environmental or nutritional factors in the development of esophageal cancer include nitrosamines or fungi contaminating pickled vegetables or in grains; chronic addiction to morphine, particularly in areas where opium is eaten; tobacco residue; silica fragments associated with millet bran (northern China); and abuse of alcohol. In associating the above suggested carcinogens with esophageal cancer, alcoholism is the one that has a clear relationship with epidermoid carcinoma of the esophagus. Chronic inflammation of the esophagus is also associated with a higher incidence of carcinomas. There is also an association between cancer of the esophagus and squamous cell carcinoma of the oropharynx or larynx, which is probably a result of exposure of the oral cavity, respiratory tract, and esophagus to the same carcinogenic factors.

Pathophysiology

Approximately 50% of esophageal cancers are at the esophagogastric junction (these cancers are generally adenocarcinoma and arise from the stomach rather than the esophagus); 25% are in the upper thoracic esophagus; 17% are in the lower esophagus; and 8% are in the cervical esophagus. The preceding three carcinomas are primarily epidermoid, and a small percentage are adenocarcinomas. Lesions above the piriform sinus are transitional cell lesions, or lymphoepitheliomas.

The epidermoid carcinoma begins as a small mucosal patch that eventually grows, ulcerates, and protrudes into the lumen. Local extension to the recurrent laryngeal nerve or tracheobronchial tree is common. Unfortunately, local extension of the cancer is often present at the time of diagnosis. Metastasis to the local lymph nodes includes those around the hilum of the lung and in the neck. Metastases to the abdominal lymph nodes of the celiac axis occur. Metastases to the liver, lungs, kidney, and bone occur with decreasing frequency. Submucosal spread of the carcinoma does occur. Satellite lesions will occur several inches away from the primary lesion.

The esophageal cancer may be clinically staged as follows[28]:

Stage I: localized tumor involving 5 cm or less of the esophagus; no spreading; no obstruction

Stage II: involves regional lymph nodes, or tumor is greater than 5 cm

Stage III: distant metastases

Carcinoma of the bronchus or stomach will often metastasize to the esophagus. Mediastinal lymph node metastasis from other organ carcinomas may lead to esophageal involvement and symptoms of obstruction. Breast carcinomas may metastasize to the esophagus. Primary adenocarcinoma of the esophagus is rare and should be considered the result of Barrett's esophagus or of spread from an adenocarcinoma of the stomach cardia.

Diagnostic Studies and Findings

Radiography: Barium Studies

Source of upper gastrointestinal bleeding
Tumor outline

Chest Roentgenogram

Pulmonary complications (e.g., fibrosis or fistula)

Endoscopy with Biopsy or Cytology Studies

Tumor invasion
Source of upper gastrointestinal bleeding

Bronchoscopy

Detects bronchial involvement and provides examination of vocal cords

Liver Function Studies

Detect hepatic involvement

Liver Scan: CT Scans of Liver and Chest

Determine tumor size and location and mediastinal involvement

Medical Plan

The major goal may not be to remove the tumor if it is widely metastasized but rather to provide the patient with a way to eat.

Surgery

Adenocarcinoma of gastroesophageal junction treated by surgical resection of esophagus and cardia, a procedure called gastric pull-up

Epidermoid carcinoma may be resected with colon interposition or esophagogastrectomy

Gastrostomy may be done to provide a route for nutrition

Medications

Chemotherapy in conjunction with irradiation or surgery; no one protocol proven effective

General Management

Irradiation, primary form of treatment
Plastic tubes inserted to maintain lumen (Celestin tube)
Relief of obstruction
Prevention of aspiration
Nutritional support

NURSING CARE

Nursing Assessment

Nutritional Status

Dysphagia initially with liquids, progressing to solids and odynophagia; swallowing may be difficult or painful; sensation of food taking longer to go through segments of the chest (i.e., reach the stomach) may be described by the patient

Chest pain, which may indicate local extension of the disease

Weakness
Anorexia
Anemia
Profound weight loss

Pulmonary Status

Bronchopulmonary symptoms include pneumonia, aspiration, or fistula

Hoarseness from involvement of recurrent laryngeal nerve

Upper gastrointestinal bleeding from tumor or from irritation by stagnant food in esophagus

Nursing Dx & Intervention

Nursing Diagnosis	Nursing Intervention/Rationale
Ineffective airway clearance	• Observe patient's ability to swallow liquids and solid foods. • Keep head of bed elevated *to prevent regurgitation and aspiration.* • Encourage patient to refrain from drinking fluids 1 to 2 hours before bedtime. • Provide suction *if patient is unable to manage saliva.*

Nursing Diagnosis	Nursing Intervention/Rationale
Altered nutrition: less than body requirements	• Request nutritional consultation. • Provide patient with meals and fluids that can be tolerated. • Weigh patient daily. • Maintain accurate intake and output records. • Work closely with other health professionals *to provide nutrition*. Some possibilities that may be prescribed include the following: Nasogastric tube Liquid supplements before surgery Celestin tube Small feeding tubes placed during endoscopy Gastrostomy tube Total parenteral nutrition in preparation for surgery Provide nasogastric or gastrostomy care per protocols
Pain	• Provide prescribed analgesia as needed, and document effectiveness.
Ineffective family coping: compromised	• Assist patient and family in dealing with emotional reactions to the disease, treatment, and possible poor prognosis. • Provide opportunities for expression of feelings and concerns. • Recommend that home care be provided after discharge *for assistance with activities of daily living (ADLs)*. • Encourage patient to discuss feelings about possibly not being able to join family members in eating at mealtimes.
Impaired verbal communication	• Encourage patient to use notepad and pencil or Magic Slate if hoarseness from recurrent laryngeal nerve involvement is severe.
Patient problem: metastasis	• See "Metastatic Disease," p. 1492.

Patient Education

1. When a Celestin or plastic tube is used, the patient must sleep with the head of the bed elevated since the gastroesophageal junction is open and reflux can occur. Also, with the plastic tube, the patient should be instructed to swallow small amounts and not to lie down after eating. Semisolid foods can be eaten. The diet may be pureed. If obstruction occurs, sips of commercial meat tenderizer or dilute hydrogen peroxide may be used to break down the food and unblock the tube.
2. Patients and families should be given information on available support groups in their areas (I Can Cope, American Cancer Society, etc.).
3. Patients should be taught to check placement of gastrostomy, residual gastric contents, and type of feeding before providing gastrostomy feeding. They should also be taught to care for the skin and tube.

Evaluation

Patient Outcome	Data Indicating That Outcome is Reached
Nutritional status is maintained.	Patient is comfortable, able to handle secretions, and has sufficient enteral nutrition with a gastrostomy or a plastic (Celestin) tube.
Home care is provided adequately.	Patient and family have available resources mobilized to assist them (home health agency, self-help group, etc.).

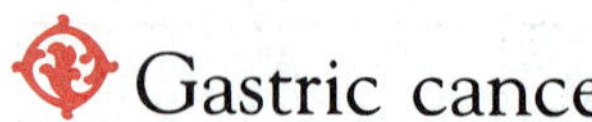

Gastric cancer

Gastric carcinoma refers to malignant neoplasms and tumors found in the stomach. Adenocarcinomas that arise from normal or metaplastic mucosa cells are the most common. Benign neoplasms of the stomach are rare and include leiomyomas and polyps.[30]

The incidence of gastric cancers has significantly decreased in western Europe and the United States. The American Cancer Society[3] estimated approximately 24,700 new cases in 1985. The ACS statistics of gastric cancer deaths decreased in males 59% (22.1 to 9.1 per 100,000) and in females 65% (11.7 to 4.1 per 100,000) from 1952 to the present.[3] In the 1940s gastric cancer was the most common malignant disease in the United States.[11] No apparent change in the incidence of gastric cancer has occurred in Japan, where it accounts for 60% of all cancers in men and 40% of all cancers in women.[31]

Many questions exist about the decline in gastric cancer. The answers to those questions would provide valuable clues in the early diagnosis, treatment, and ultimately prevention of gastric carcinomas. In addition, interesting geographic variations exist. Gastric cancer is higher in the north central and northeast regions of the United States. It is more common in urban than rural areas in England, but this is not true in the United States. Although it is very common in Japan, gastric cancer is less common in Japanese persons in Hawaii and the incidence decreases with each generation. In 1980 Hawaiian Japanese individuals appeared to have the same low incidence rates as native Hawaiians.[30]

Genetic factors may play a role in the development of gastric cancer. Gastric cancers are more frequent in certain families and in persons with type A blood. In the United States, gastric cancer is more common in blacks than whites and in men than women. In Israel the incidence of gastric cancer is two and a half times higher in Jews of northern European backgrounds than Jews of Mediterranean or Asian descent.

The role of dietary factors has been studied to identify foods or soil contaminants that may lead to gastric cancers. Starches, pickled vegetables, and salted fish and meats have been associated with gastric cancers. However, whole milk, fresh vegetables, vitamin C, and refrigeration are inversely associated with gastric cancers.[18] Increased salt consumption is also seen in patients with gastric cancers. Nitrates, which are converted into nitrites, are commonly found in our diet. Compounds formed with nitrites (nitrosamines and nitrosamides) have been carcinogenic in animals. Although not confirmed as a carcinogen in humans, nitrite-forming bacteria are increased in the upper gastrointestinal tract in people with hypochlorhydria and achlorhydria and following gastric surgery. Hypochlorhydria and achlorhydria are often found in patients with pernicious anemia and atrophic gastritis. The reduced acid appears to support or allow colonization of the stomach by the bacteria.

Cold temperatures inhibit the conversion of nitrates to nitrites. Better refrigeration and decreased use of nitrates as food additives might explain the decreased incidence of gastric cancers.[29]

Gastric cancer appears to be higher in individuals with late-onset immunoglobulin deficiency. Patients with celiac sprue with reduced IgA are at greater risk for gastric cancer.[31] Other factors associated with gastric cancer are gastric ulcers, atrophic gastritis, gastric polyps, pernicious anemia, and gastrectomy.

Pathophysiology

The carcinoma found in the stomach is epithelial growth arising from the mucosa membrane. Microscopically the cells resemble intestinal metaplasia and contain goblet cells characteristic of the intestines. The parietal and chief glands of the stomach are seldom seen in gastric tumors. Adenocarcinomas in the stomach have been classified in several ways.

First, according to cellular or extracellular characteristics, carcinomas are referred to as papillary, colloid or mucinous, medullary, and signet ring.[30] Papillary refers to cells forming glandular structures in a papillary form. When excessive mucin secretion and extracellular aggregates are present, the adenocarcinoma is referred to as colloid or mucinous. Medullary is a solid band or a mass of undifferentiated cells. The signet ring adenocarcinoma refers to a well-differentiated adenocarcinoma with large amounts of intracellular mucinous material that compresses the nucleus to an unusual location.

Second, an adenocarcinoma of the stomach may be classified histologically according to the degree of cell differentiation from well differentiated to poorly differentiated.

Unfortunately, the preceding two classifications and their parts are not mutually exclusive. Various cellular characteristics and degrees of differentiation may occur within a tumor. The third classification system reflects the biologic behavior of the tumor and defines gastric carcinomas as intestinal or diffuse.[21] The intestinal type is a glandular tumor, and the diffuse type is composed of single cells or small groups of cells.

The fourth system is an expansion of the intestinal and diffuse definitions and classifies cancers in the stomach as expanding or infiltrating.[23] The expanding (intestinal) type is characterized by a group of cells that are similar, maintain a coherent relationship, and push aside other cells as they grow. The infiltrative (diffuse) class is characterized by deep, wide infiltration by individual tumor cells.

The intestinal type of gastric cancer is associated with intestinal metaplasia and gastritis. The carcinoma tends to be circumscribed, and spread of the disease is through the bloodstream. The liver is a common site of metastasis. The diffuse type of carcinoma is less circumscribed, spreads by way of the lymphatics, and may take the form of linitis plastica, which is a diffuse fibrosis and thickening of the gastric wall.

The most common site of carcinomas is the lower half of the stomach. An exception occurs when gastric atrophy is a precursor to the cancer, and then the lesion tends to be in the upper portion of the stomach.

In early gastric cancers the disease is confined to the mucosa and submucosa. The symptoms with early gastric cancers may be vague and nonspecific. Early gastric cancers have been divided into three types:

Type I: polypoid or protruded
Type II: superficial
IIa: elevated
IIb: flat
IIc: depressed
Type III: excavated

Advanced gastric cancer denotes involvement of the muscular layer of the stomach. Metastases, local and distant, are common. Advanced gastric carcinomas may be a polypoid or fungating mass, diffuse and infiltrating, or ulcerating.

Gastric ulcers have been associated with gastric cancers. This may be a diagnostic issue.[31] Previously radiologically diagnosed gastric ulcers have later been found to be carcinomas. Occasionally a benign gastric ulcer will have a focal carcinoma at a margin. Also, malignant cells may be found at the base of the ulcer as well as at the margin. Most physicians will routinely do a biopsy of gastric ulcers during endoscopy to rule out the presence of gastric carcinoma.

Gastric atrophy and pernicious anemia are associated with achlorhydria. Achlorhydria is a precursor of gastric cancer. Gastric polyps are often found in atrophic mucosa. A polyp may be benign or malignant, and the recommended treatment is removal through an endoscope and histologic examination. Approximately 10% of gastric polyps will be malignant.[31]

Diagnostic Studies and Findings

Hematocrit

Slightly below normal
Patient may have macrocytic or microcytic anemia secondary to decreased iron or vitamin B_{12} absorption

Stool for Occult Blood

Positive for blood

Serum Albumin

Hypoalbuminemia

Plain Chest Roentgenogram

Distance between base of lung and stomach bubble greater than a few millimeters (gastric infiltration)
Mass projecting into gas shadow of stomach
Separation of gas shadow from diaphragm
Absence of gas bubble

Upper Gastrointestinal Series (Barium Swallow)

Polypoid mass
Ulceration surrounded by mass
Thickened, fibrosed gastric wall

Computed Tomography

Thickness of gastric wall
Presence of metastasis (may assist in differentiating between benign and carcinogenic lesion)

Endoscopy and Cytology

Biopsy and cytology specimens examined for cancer cells
Can visualize lesion
- Benign: sharply delineated with a white base and regular margins
- Malignant: gray with irregular margins and "heaped-up" edges[31]

Dye-Spraying Techniques

During endoscopy, spray gastric mucosa with methylene blue; stains intestinalized mucosa; normal or cancerous mucosa uncolored

Liver Function Studies

Abnormal findings may indicate metastasis

Medical Plan

Surgery

Subtotal or total gastrectomy

Medications

Antineoplastic agents
- Combination chemotherapy postoperatively
  - 5-Fluoruracil (5-FU) IV for 5 d q5wk; dosage: 12 mg/kg
  - Methyl-CCNU, po q10wk
  - Doxorubicin (Adriamycin), 60-75 mg/sq m IV at 21-d intervals

See "Chemotherapy," p. 1495

General Management

Radiation therapy in combination with chemotherapy postoperatively (see p. 1500)
Immunotherapy: an investigational treatment at this time (see p. 1499)
Regular follow-up endoscopy procedures (1% to 2% may develop a second primary gastric carcinoma[26])
Symptom management

NURSING CARE

Nursing Assessment

Stomach

Loss of appetite; anorexia
Feeling of fullness with minimum intake
Distaste for meats
Weight loss
Persistent midepigastric pain
Dysphagia

Physical Examination

Tenderness in midepigastrium
Mass in epigastrium (late stage)
Enlarged liver
Positive supraclavicular nodes
Ascites (loss of albumin into gastric lumen)
Acanthosis nigricans (rare)
Signs of metastasis: myeloid metaplasia or primary CNS disease

Nursing Dx & Intervention

Nursing Diagnosis	Nursing Intervention/Rationale
Ineffective individual coping	• Provide opportunities for patient to express feelings about diagnosis and prognosis. • Assist patient in making adaptations or changes in activities and relationships.
Pain	• Provide analgesia for pain as ordered.
Altered nutrition: less than body requirements	• Weigh patient daily. • Maintain intake and output records. • Record symptoms associated with food intake before and after any surgical procedure. • Ensure adequate caloric intake after surgery if dietary alterations must be made (i.e., tube feedings; use of high-calorie liquid supplements).
Ineffective family coping: compromised	• Provide opportunities for expression of feelings (gastric cancers may be diagnosed after metastasis has occurred and prognosis is poor). • Provide information to assist patients and their families in working through their emotional reactions to disease, the treatment, and the prognosis.
Anticipatory grieving	• Support the patient and family during the dying phase. • Identify appropriate resource people for the patient and family; these may include clergy, friends, and lawyers. • Provide list of support groups (I Can Cope; American Cancer Society).
Patient problem: metastasis	• See "Metastatic Disease," p. 1492.

Patient Education

1. Instruct the patient on the rationale for combination therapies of surgery, chemotherapy, and radiation therapy in the treatment of gastric cancers. Provide written information in the form of do's and don'ts during chemotherapy and radiotherapy, sequence of treatment, and potential side effects.
2. Instruct patient regarding the necessity for regular follow-up endoscopies.

Evaluation

Patient Outcome	Data Indicating That Outcome is Reached
Patient can manage pain.	Patient is comfortable and able to relieve pain and symptoms effectively.
Patient adapts to or accepts disease and prognosis.	Patient has mobilized available resources to assist him or her and family in handling the emotional, social, and financial stressors of having cancer. Patient attends "I Can Cope" groups.
Patient complies with medical regimen.	Patient has regular appointments with physician, maintains treatment sequence of drugs and radiotherapy, and reports signs of side effects. Patient uses home care (visiting) nurses to evaluate progress, reinforce teaching, and provide physical care as needed.
Laboratory findings are normal.	Hematocrit and albumin levels are within normal limits. Stools are negative for occult blood. There is no cancer on repeat endoscopy.
Nutritional status is adequate.	Caloric intake is maintained at level patient can tolerate. Weight loss is minimized.

Digestive gland tumors

Carcinomas of the digestive glands are neoplasms that may involve the pancreas, liver, or gallbladder.

Carcinoma of the gallbladder, with its insidious onset, may be diagnosed only during surgery for presumed acute cholecystitis. The only possibility of cure is with complete removal of the gallbladder; often a partial hepatectomy is also required because of early liver invasion. Mortality is as high as 75%; four times as many women as men are dead 1 year after diagnosis.

Carcinoma of the liver is usually metastatic; primary tumors constitute only 1% of hepatic cancer. One primary tumor, hemangiosarcoma of the liver, is a rare disease believed to be caused by vinyl chloride exposure. The risk of hepatocellular carcinoma is about 40 times greater in patients with cirrhosis. Early signs and symptoms of hepatic cancer are often absent or insidious and slow to localize. The most common complaints are vague upper abdominal pain and generalized weakness. Other indications of liver involvement are anemia, anorexia, jaundice, weight loss, pain, and respiratory distress. Obstruction of the portal vein, sometimes occurring suddenly, may cause splenomegaly, esophageal varices, and ascites. Patients may also have fever of unknown origin and dependent edema. Diagnosis is based on laboratory data obtained from a liver profile, scanning, angiography, and biopsy.

The only possibility for cure is lobectomy to remove the diseased tissue. In some major medical centers, liver transplantation is being used as an alternative procedure for eligible patients. If surgery is contraindicated by the extent of the disease or the patient's condition, radiation therapy and chemotherapy via implantable infusion pump may be used. The prognosis is poor, and few patients are alive 5 years after the initial diagnosis.

Carcinoma of the pancreas has increased more than 20% in recent years. The reason for this is unknown, although cigarette smoking and coffee may be causative factors. As in liver and gallbladder disease, the onset is insidious and the diagnosis is made late in the course. Clinical signs indicating the tumor's location include the following:

Head of the pancreas—obstructive jaundice resulting from blockage of the common bile duct

Body and tail of the pancreas—vague abdominal or back pain, progressive weight loss, anorexia, and a variety of gastrointestinal symptoms

Islet cells—hypoglycemia and insulin-shock syndrome, resulting from production of large quantities of insulin

As many as half of these patients have occult blood in the stools. The pain is steady, dull, and aching and unrelated to digestive activity. Because of the vagueness of the signs and symptoms, few pancreatic tumors are diagnosed at a curable stage. The diagnosis is usually based on tomographic scanning, ultrasonography, and biopsy.

Pancreatoduodenectomy (Whipple's procedure) is rarely used because of its high morbidity and mortality, although it has been helpful in cancer of the head of the pancreas. Palliation may be effected with radiation therapy or chemotherapy. The prognosis is extremely poor; only 10% of patients are still alive 1 year after diagnosis.

Salivary gland tumors grow slowly and are often diagnosed late. Complete excision, although difficult to accomplish without producing facial nerve damage, is important to prevent recurrence. If the tumor cannot be removed surgically, radiation therapy may be used to shrink it.

 Endocrine gland tumors

Endocrine gland tumors may occur in the parathyroid, thyroid, or adrenal glands.

Parathyroid tumors are rare. When they do occur, they produce excessive amounts of parathyroid hormone, which causes bony deformities and renal calculi. These tumors are treated by surgical excision.

Carcinoma of the thyroid has its highest incidence (37% of endocrine cancers) in people 25 to 44 years of age. It occurs most frequently in women and in whites. Those at high risk are people who as children received radiation therapy to the neck for such conditions as hypertrophy of the tonsils, adenoids, or lymphatic tissue, enlarged thymus gland, or skin disorders such as acne.

The initial sign of a thyroid tumor is a lump in the gland, which may first be palpated during a routine physical examination. More extensive local involvement causes hoarseness, dysphagia, or dyspnea. Thyroid scanning, ultrasonography, and biopsy are used to diagnose the lesion, which is most commonly papillary carcinoma of the thyroid, a slow-growing, easily removed tumor. Even without total surgical eradication, many patients live 10 to 15 years with few symptoms. The 5-year survival rate is 97% for patients with localized disease and 86% if the disease has spread. Spread is usually to adjacent cervical lymph nodes.

Undifferentiated thyroid cancers are more likely to cause tracheal compression and metastasis to cervical lymph nodes. For these patients treatment is lobectomy or total thyroidectomy and en bloc dissection of lymph nodes. Radioactive iodine (^{131}I) and radiation therapy may also be used.

Neoplasms of the adrenal glands cause changes in body functioning, depending on the affected component. Cortical neoplasms may alter the body's sex characteristics and cause complex steroidal changes, such as Cushing's syndrome. Medullary neoplasms may precipitate attacks of hypertension.

The median age for occurrence is 40 years, although people of any age may be affected. The tumors may be benign or malignant and may be linked with a specific pituitary tumor.

Signs and symptoms, such as pain, distention, and hemorrhage, are usually noted at a late stage, when local extension obstructs or destroys the kidneys. Pheochromocytoma, a tumor of the adrenal medulla, secretes an adrenalin-like substance that causes paroxysmal or sustained hypertension. The diagnosis is based on intravenous pyelography, tomography, ultrasonography, and urinalysis of hormones such as 17-ketosteroid.

Surgical excision, the treatment of choice, necessitates temporary or permanent cortisone replacement therapy. Radiation and chemotherapy may also be used, but since the diagnosis is rarely made before extension of the tumor has occurred, the prognosis is poor.[6,28]

Ovarian and testicular tumors are discussed elsewhere in this chapter.

CANCERS OF BONE AND CONNECTIVE TISSUES

Sarcomas of bone and soft tissue, although relatively uncommon, are of particular interest because of their tendency to occur in young people, their generally poor prognosis, and the major surgery usually required. The prognosis has been improved in recent years by the combination of local surgery and chemotherapy. In addition, in many patients the primary lesion can be successfully treated by more conservative surgical procedures combined with high-dose radiation therapy. However, 60% to 65% of bone cancers are metastatic from other primary lesions and thus are more difficult to treat successfully. In 1987 there were approximately 7400 new cases of these cancers and 4200 deaths.[3]

Bone sarcomas

Bone cancer is a skeletal malignancy occurring as a primary sarcomatous tumor in an area of rapid growth.

People at high risk for development of bone sarcomas are those with Paget's disease of bone, Ollier's disease, multiple exostoses, retinoblastoma, or previous high-dose radiation therapy to bone. Osteosarcoma and Ewing's sarcoma occur most commonly in people under the age of 20 years. This is in contrast to reticulum cell sarcoma, fibrosarcoma, and chondrosarcoma, which occur later in life but with a much wider age distribution.

Pathophysiology[6]

The patient's complaints are initially subtle and intermittent, with gradually increasing severity. An initially painless mass is the most common symptom; others include pain, functional deficit, or pathologic fracture. The pain is usually described as mild and brief and is often associated with a minor injury. It may increase in severity but is often reported as being a localized, dull ache. It usually does not increase with activity or decrease with rest but may be greater at night. This pain rarely responds to simple analgesic medication but requires narcotics for relief.

There may not be any symptoms; if they are present, they are dependent on the size, site, and patterns of local infiltration. The site and extent of pathologic fractures dictate the severity of symptoms. Metastases to regional lymph nodes are uncommon, but systemic illness may be related to pulmonary, visceral, and subcutaneous tissue involvement.[6,28]

Diagnostic Studies and Findings[28]

Roentgenograms of Involved Bones and Soft Tissues

Visualization of suspect lesion

Chest Roentgenogram

Evidence of metastasis

Bone Scan

Evidence of primary lesion or metastasis

Computed Tomography

Evidence of cortical bone destruction

Blood Studies

Increased alkaline and acid phosphatase; increased calcium indicative of bone disease/demineralization

Urine Study

High calcium excretion secondary to hypercalcemia

Medical Plan[6]

Surgery*

- Amputation with limb salvage to degree possible
  - Foot and ankle—below-knee amputation or knee disarticulation
  - Proximal tibia—thigh amputation
  - Distal femur—hip disarticulation
  - Proximal end of femur—modified hemipelvectomy
- En bloc resection for low-grade malignant lesions; reconstruction with bone autografts, cadaver hemografts, or metal or plastic devices

Medications

- Antineoplastic agents
  - Preoperative and postoperative systemic chemotherapy for osteogenic sarcoma; high-dose methotrexate (Amethopterin; Mexate) with leucovorin rescue; doxorubicin (Adriamycin) by intra-arterial perfusion; dosages individually determined
  - Systemic chemotherapy for metastatic disease
- See "Chemotherapy," p. 1495

General Management

- Radiation therapy for treatment of Ewing's sarcoma before surgery (see p. 1500)
- Immunotherapy with interferon (investigational) (see p. 1499)

*See Chapter 4 for postoperative nursing diagnoses and interventions.

Disease-free survival rates for patients whose osteogenic sarcoma is treated with surgery and chemotherapy appear to be greater than 50% at 5 years. Among patients with localized Ewing's sarcoma, the disease-free survival at 5 years is 50% following chemotherapy and radiation therapy.

NURSING CARE

Nursing Assessment[6]

Musculoskeletal Function

Presence of mass; functional deficit; pathologic fracture

Pain

Mild and fleeting; dull and aching; increased at night; not affected by activity or rest; need for narcotics to obtain relief

Systemic Function

Fever; malaise, easy fatigability; anorexia; weight loss

Nursing Dx & Intervention

Nursing Diagnosis	Nursing Intervention/Rationale
Impaired physical mobility	• Assist patient with ambulation; control distance *to avoid injury and fatigue*. • Have patient use walker, cane, or wheelchair as needed as assistive devices *to promote mobility*. • Minimize environmental barriers *to avoid falls*. • Encourage use of involved limb *to maintain function*. • Observe for deficits, weakness, or abnormal gait *as indications of further impairment of mobility*.
Pain	• Change patient's position slowly *to avoid stretching and pressure*. • Provide whirlpool, or use heat applications *to promote relaxation and healing*. • Provide safety *to avoid further injury to patient*. • Discuss possible pain-relieving measures with patient; use those possible *to involve patient in self-care*. • Observe for increasing pain and dysfunction *to determine need for further intervention*. • Discuss "phantom" pain with patient (amputee) and significant other. • Assist with and teach use of patient-controlled analgesic device if ordered. • Administer morphine solution via continuous drip as ordered according to facility policy.
Activity intolerance	• Ambulate patient, or seat patient in armchair *to promote circulation*. • Encourage moderate physical exercise, adequate rest, and performance of range of motion exercises *to maintain activity level and avoid immobility*. • Balance nutritional intake; supplement protein *to increase strength*. • Observe for increased nutritional requirements and weakness *as indications of advancing disease*.
Patient problem: metastasis	• See "Metastatic Disease," p. 1492.

Patient Education

1. Discuss the principles of safe ambulation: wide supportive stance; well-fitting, low-heeled shoes; good body mechanics; and weight bearing on unaffected side.
2. Discuss the principles of good nutrition, especially protein supplementation.
3. Instruct the patient to report changes in respiratory status to health care provider.

Evaluation

Patient Outcome	Data Indicating That Outcome is Reached
Patient is comfortable.	Facial expression is calm and relaxed. Posture is normal. Patient has freedom of body movement. Patient expresses comfort and ceases to complain.
Patient frequently changes position and has normal body movement.	Patient walks, sits, and stands with normal body movement.

Patient Outcome	Data Indicating That Outcome is Reached
Patient participates in therapeutic exercises.	Patient performs range of motion and isometric exercises.
Patient is receiving sufficient rest.	Coordination is good. Patient is not fatigued.
Patient's surroundings are safe.	Patient uses assistive devices such as walker or cane. There is no physical sign of accident having occurred. There is no evidence of complications arising from drugs or treatments.
No deformity has resulted from health treatment.	Hands, feet, limbs, and spine are in good alignment and functional. Patient has little or no pain.

Soft tissue sarcomas

Soft tissue sarcomas are neoplasms that arise in soft tissue, parenchymatous organs, or hollow viscera and include fibrosarcoma, malignant fibrous histiocytoma, liposarcoma, rhabdomyosarcoma, leiomyosarcoma, angiosarcoma, synovial sarcoma, mixed mesenchymal sarcoma, Kaposi's sarcoma, and unclassified or spindle cell sarcoma.

Only among children are soft tissue tumors, especially rhabdomyosarcoma, relatively frequent.[28]

Pathophysiology[6]

A painless mass is the most common initial symptom. Masses in the thigh area are suspect because of the high number of sarcomas occurring there. Advanced local disease is rare except for large tumors arising in the retroperitoneal or pelvic areas. Lymph node metastases are uncommon except in patients with rhabdomyosarcoma, high-grade synovial sarcoma, and epithelioid sarcoma.

Rhabdomyosarcoma arises from the embryonic mesenchymal cells that form striated muscle. It may develop in almost any body site; the most common primary sites are the head and neck, extremities, genitourinary tract, trunk, and orbit. The prognosis depends on the primary site and the stage of the disease (histologic grade), which is in turn based on extent of disease and resectability. Genitourinary lesions generally have the most favorable prognosis, and extremity tumors have one of the worst prognoses.

Kaposi's sarcoma (KS), the malignancy most frequently associated with AIDS, is recorded as the syndrome's initial clinical manifestation in approximately 25% of cases. The epidemic form (EKS) affects primarily homosexual men and may be of greater incidence than noted above, since subsequent malignant and infectious complications (after initial diagnosis) are not reported to the Centers for Disease Control.

The initial manifestations of EKS include nodular, macular, or papular lesions on the skin and mucosal surfaces; fever; weight loss; malaise; anorexia; and diarrhea. The lesions are frequently located on the trunk, arms, head, neck, and oral cavity. Lesions on the head and neck can be especially disfiguring and can cause symptoms of obstruction or compression. Fifty percent of EKS patients have visceral involvement, particularly of the gastrointestinal tract. Pulmonary involvement can lead to progressive respiratory dysfunction and failure. Lymph nodes are often affected; involvement of the brain, liver, pancreas, adrenal glands, spleen, heart, and testes have been noted. Therapy for EKS remains experimental and controversial, with chemotherapy, radiotherapy, and immunotherapy used with varying degrees of success.

Diagnostic Studies and Findings[28]

Radiographic Study of Affected Part (Computed Tomography, Xerography, Arteriography)

Visualization of suspect lesion and vasculature

Chest Tomography or Chest Computed Tomography

Evidence of metastasis

Excisional, Incisional, or Needle Biopsy

Histologic evidence of malignancy

Medical Plan[6]

Surgery

Radical surgical excision—amputation, muscle group resection, radical local excision

Medications

Antineoplastic agents
- Vincristine sulfate (Oncovin), 2 mg/m² for children, 1.4 mg/m² for adults
- Doxorubicin (Adriamycin), 60-75 mg/m² at intervals of 21 d or 30 mg/m² on each of 3 successive d repeated q4wk
- Cyclophosphamide (Cytoxan), 40-50 mg/kg IV or individual doses over several days, then adjusted to lower maintenance dosage; po 1-5 mg/kg qd
- Cisplatin (Platinol), 50-80 mg/m² IV q3wk or by individually determined dosage

See "Chemotherapy," p. 1495

General Management

Radiation therapy—used with more conservative surgery preoperatively and postoperatively (see p. 1500)

NURSING CARE

Nursing Assessment[6]

Body Contours

Painless mass

Sensory and Motor Function

Peripheral neuralgia; paralysis

Vascular Status

Ischemia

Gastrointestinal Function

Bowel obstruction

Urinary Function

Ureteral obstruction

Respiratory Function

Dyspnea

Nursing Dx & Intervention

Nursing Diagnosis	Nursing Intervention/Rationale
Impaired physical mobility	• Assist patient with ambulation; control distance *to avoid stress and fatigue.* • Use walker, cane, or wheelchair as needed *for added support.* • Minimize environmental barriers *to prevent injury.* • Encourage use of involved limb *to maintain tone.* • Observe for deficits, complaints of weakness, and abnormal gait *as evidence of further dysfunction.* • Test for impaired coordination *as evidence of further dysfunction.*
Pain	• Change patient's position slowly *to avoid additional discomfort.* • Support affected part(s) *to prevent strain.* • Place patient in whirlpool, or use heat applications *for muscle relaxation.* • Provide safety measures *to avoid injury.* • Discuss possible pain-relieving measures with patient; use those possible. • Monitor effectiveness of pain relief methods. • Administer analgesics as ordered. • Observe for increases in pain and dysfunction *as signs of need to reevaluate interventions.*
Altered patterns of urinary elimination	• Inspect urine for bleeding *as evidence of inflammation.* • Increase fluid intake to about 2000 ml daily *to flush bladder and hydrate kidneys.* • Monitor intake and output *to determine adequacy of renal function.* • Palpate bladder, and inspect abdomen for distention *as signs of urinary retention.* • Catheterize only if necessary *to relieve retention.*
Constipation	• Place patient in sitting position *to relieve pressure on diaphragm.* • Remove constrictive clothing *to relieve pressure on abdomen.* • Give small, frequent feedings *to avoid distention.* • Insert a rectal tube if necessary *to relieve flatus.* • Auscultate abdomen *for abnormal bowel sounds.* • Inspect abdomen for distention and absence of bowel sounds. • Record bowel movements *to monitor adequacy of bowel function.*
Patient problem: metastasis	• See "Metastatic Disease," p. 1492.

Patient Education

1. Explain the principles of safe ambulation.
2. Discuss the management of disease-related pain.
3. Instruct the patient to report any change in respiratory status and urinary and bowel function.

Evaluation[10]

Patient Outcome	Data Indicating That Outcome is Reached
Body hydration is normal.	There is no edema, ascites, or venous distention.
Body functioning is normal.	Elimination is adequate. Weight is stabilized. Digestion is adequate.
Bowel elimination is normal for patient.	Stools are soft. Abdomen is soft and not distended. There is no abdominal pressure or cramping.
Daily fluid output is equal to fluid intake.	Urine output is 1500 to 3000 ml daily or equivalent to intake.
Patient is comfortable.	Facial expression is calm and relaxed. Posture is normal. Patient has freedom of body movement. Patient expresses comfort.
Patient frequently changes position with normal body movement.	Patient walks, sits, and stands with normal body movement.
Patient participates in therapeutic exercise.	Patient performs range of motion and isometric exercises.
Patient's surroundings are safe.	Patient uses safety precautions.
Patient shows no evidence of accident or physical injury.	There is no physical sign of accident or evidence of complications arising from drugs or treatment.
Patient shows no evidence of deformity resulting from treatment.	Patient's hands, feet, limbs, and spine are in good alignment and functional.

 Cancers of the Central Nervous System

Tumors of the central nervous system are neoplasms of the brain or spinal cord.

Tumors of the central nervous system (CNS) account for more than 2% of annual cancer deaths. Eighty percent of CNS tumors involve the brain, with as many as half of these metastatic from primary cancers of the lung, breast, kidney, melanoma, and gastrointestinal tract; the other 20% involve the spinal cord.

Many CNS tumors occur in children and young adults. In children, brain tumors are second only to leukemia as a cause of death. In contrast to brain tumors in adults, those in children are largely infratentorial and involve the cerebellum, midbrain, pons, and medulla.[28]

Pathophysiology[6]

The majority of CNS tumors are gliomas, which are peculiar because they rarely spread beyond the CNS. There are no known etiologic factors, although childhood tumors are believed to be developmental in origin.

Spinal cord tumors are gliomas (23%), meningiomas or schwannomas (56%), or miscellaneous other forms such as epidermoid and dermoid cysts, hemangioblastomas, and chordomas. These tumors produce symptoms in the body below the level of tumor location in the cord: difficulty in walking, postural disturbances, back pain, and changes in sensation and muscle power. The pain of a spinal cord tumor is worse at night.

Brain tumors in adults are divided as follows:

Gliomas (50%), of which 50% are glioblastomas; occur most often in the cerebrum of people between 40 and 60 years of age

Meningiomas, the most common of nongliomatous tumors; average host age is 50 years; common sites are parasagittal area and anterior part of base of skull

Pituitary adenomas (12% to 18%), which are almost never malignant

Neurilemomas (schwannomas), which are usually benign

Brain tumors in children are divided as follows:

Medulloblastomas (30%)

Astrocytomas (30%) such as optic pathway gliomas

Ependymomas (12%), the most common fourth ventricular tumors

Posterior fossa tumors

Craniopharyngiomas

Pineal tumors

Brain tumors cause nonlocalized signs and symptoms by increasing intracranial pressure. Localized signs and symptoms are caused by direct compression, invasion, or irritation of regions of the brain (see "Nursing Assessment").

Diagnostic Studies and Findings[28]

Physical and Neurologic Examinations

Identification of specific neurologic deficits

Visual Field Examination

Alterations caused by optic nerve lesion

Funduscopic Examination

Alterations caused by optic nerve lesion

Computed Tomography; Skull Roentgenograms

Visualization of suspect lesion

Electroencephalography

Altered tracings in presence of central nervous system lesion

Technetium Pertechnetate Brain Scanning

Visualization of suspect lesion

Cerebral Arteriography

Visualization of suspect lesion

Air Study, Pneumoencephalography, and Ventriculography

Cytologic evidence of malignant lesion

Spinal Fluid Examination

Visualization of suspect cells

Magnetic Resonance Imaging (MRI)

Visualization of suspect lesion

Medical Plan[22]

Surgery

Excision—initial treatment for all intracranial tumors, with removal limited by location of lesion and its invasiveness

Medications

Of limited value because of blood-brain barrier

Antineoplastic agents

Procarbazine (Matulane), 2-4 mg/kg/d po initially, then maintained at 4-6 mg/kg/d until maximum response occurs; maintain at 1-2 mg/kg/d

Carmustine (BiCNU), 200 mg/m^2 IV q6wk

Vincristine sulfate (Oncovin), 2 mg/m^2 for children, 1.4 mg/m^2 for adults

Corticosteroids

Prednisone (Deltasone, others), 10-100 mg po for metastatic brain tumors

See "Chemotherapy," p. 1495

General Management

Radiation therapy—external irradiation for malignant brain tumors; usually postoperative; used when tumor is centrally located and surgery is likely to aggravate it or when vital structures are involved, for example, brainstem tumor, metastatic deposit, uncomplicated pituitary adenoma, or medulloblastoma (see p. 1500)

Combination Therapy

May include surgery, chemotherapy, and radiation therapy

• • •

Despite therapeutic advances, CNS tumors have high morbidity and mortality. About 40% of people with brain tumors can return to a useful life, and another 30% gain good palliation. The neoplasms vary in their aggressiveness and consequently their prognosis. The earlier the diagnosis, the better the patient's chances for maximum restoration of function.

NURSING CARE

Nursing Assessment[6]

Increased Intracranial Pressure

Early headache; nausea and vomiting; decreased level of consciousness; failing vision; changing pupillary response

Localized Signs

Contralateral homonymous hemianopsia; jacksonian seizures or weakness; convulsions; headache; suboccipital tenderness; personality change, such as irritability or bizarre behavior; dizziness; disturbances in gait and balance

Nursing Dx & Intervention

Nursing Diagnosis	Nursing Intervention/Rationale
Sensory/perceptual alterations (visual)	• Anticipate patient's needs, and reassure patient that assistance is available. • Arrange environment *to minimize barriers and avoid injury.* • Illuminate room adequately *to enhance visibility.* • Place objects within sight and reach *to facilitate self-care.* • Provide frequent patient contact *to monitor needs.* • Encourage expression of feelings, listen attentively, and offer feedback *to lower anxiety.* • Reduce demands placed on patient *to avoid added stress.* • Observe for irritability or unusual behavior *as evidence of difficulty with coping.*

Nursing Diagnosis	Nursing Intervention/Rationale
Potential for injury related to increased intracranial pressure	• Maintain complete bed rest *to avoid falls.* • Provide quiet *to reduce stimulation.* • Lower bed height *to avoid injury if patient leaves bed.* • Subdue room lighting *to reduce stimulation.* • Elevate patient's head, and change position slowly *to avoid increased intracranial pressure.* • Discourage oral stimulants *to avoid increased intracranial pressure.* • Refrain from jarring bed and performing nonessential procedures *to keep patient calm.* • Place padded side rails up; place airway or padded tongue blade on bed for use in case of seizure *to avoid injury.* • Inspect eyes for pupillary response, and observe for papilledema *as evidence of increasing intracranial pressure.* • Monitor blood pressure and intracranial pressure as ordered *for early detection of increase.* • Observe for confusion, lethargy, restlessness, vomiting, and complaints of headache and nausea *as signs of increasing pressure.* • Palpate pulse rate and rhythm, and monitor volume *to determine adequacy of cardiovascular function.*
Potential for injury related to falling	• Minimize environmental barriers *to avoid injury.* • Assist patient with mobility *to avoid injury.* • Safeguard patient with side rails when in bed. • Place safety helmet on patient's head *to prevent injury if patient falls.* • Cover bed with netting as needed *to prevent patient leaving bed unassisted.*
Pain related to headache or suboccipital tenderness	• Position patient comfortably. • Massage gently *to relax muscles.* • Provide pain relief measures of patient's choice. • Encourage adequate rest *to prevent decreased tolerance of pain.* • Apply cold, moist compress or ice bag *to relieve pain.* • Assess pain duration, intensity, and quality, and change interventions as necessary.
Patient problem: metastasis	• See "Metastatic Disease," p. 1492.

Patient Education

1. Emphasize the need to avoid injury.
2. Explain ways of adjusting to potential visual changes.
3. Teach the patient to carry out various pain relief measures.
4. Tell the patient and family to report difficulty with mobility or changes in behavior.

Evaluation[10]

Patient Outcome	Data Indicating That Outcome is Reached
Vital signs are within normal limits.	Respirations, pulse, and blood pressure are within normal limits.
Vision is adequate.	Pupillary response and size are normal.
Vitality is good.	Patient is mentally alert and shows good concentration and attentiveness.
Performance of work and play is adequate.	Patient is able to maintain self-care.
Patient ambulates safely.	Patient avoids contact with stable and moving objects when walking.
Patient is comfortable.	Facial expression is calm, contented, and relaxed. Posture is normal. Patient has freedom of body movement. Patient expresses comfort and satisfaction and ceases to complain.
Patient has positive disposition.	Patient smiles appropriately.
Patient's ability to communicate is adequate.	There is no evidence of frustration in communication.
Patient's surroundings are safe.	Safety precautions such as side rails and low bed are used. There is no physical sign or subjective evidence of accident.

CANCERS OF THE SKIN

Basal cell and squamous cell carcinoma

Basal cell carcinoma is a malignant, epithelial cell tumor that begins as a papule and enlarges peripherally. Squamous cell carcinoma is a slow-growing malignant tumor of squamous epithelium.

Skin cancer is the most common human malignancy. An estimated 400,000 cases are discovered each year. The vast majority are the highly curable basal cell and squamous cell carcinomas. These lesions are more common among people with lightly pigmented skin and those at latitudes near the equator. Additional risk factors are excessive exposure to the sun and occupational exposure to coal tar, pitch, creosote, arsenic compounds, and radium.[3]

Pathophysiology

Basal cell carcinoma is usually a pearly gray nodule on the face, neck, or back of the hand.[3] Invasion is usually local, although metastatic disease occurs rarely. The histologic appearance is that of small undifferentiated basal cells with minimum nuclear atypia. Recurrence indicates initial incomplete tumor destruction; however, 90% to 95% of patients are considered cured.[28]

Squamous cell carcinoma is a scaly, slightly elevated lesion with or without a cutaneous horn. With complete tumor destruction, the prognosis is excellent. Tumors more difficult to treat are those arising in a scar, a chronically ulcerated area, or a site of radiation damage or in an immunosuppressed patient. Squamous cell carcinoma can metastasize, with 2% to 3% spreading to regional lymph nodes. The cure rate for this cancer is 75% to 80%.[28]

Diagnostic Studies and Findings[28]

Physical Examination

Careful inspection, particularly of lesions showing biologic activity, such as change in size, shape, or color; bleeding and ulceration seen in more advanced lesions

Simple Shave or Dermal Punch Biopsy

For histologic confirmation of malignancy

Medical Plan[6]

Surgery

Scalpel excision with wide margin of skin and subcutaneous tissue; may be supplemented with split-thickness graft, adjacent flaps, distant pedicles, or free graft

Chemosurgery (Moh's procedure)

Medications

Antineoplastic agents

Fluorouracil (5-FU), topical application to skin bid for several weeks

See "Chemotherapy," p. 1495

General Management

Radiotherapy by beam electron and superficial x rays, especially for cancers around face (see p. 1500)

Cryotherapy—tumor tissue with margin of normal skin frozen to 20° to 40° C by liquid nitrogen; excellent cosmetic results

Electroexcision—use of diathermy for repetitive coagulation and curettage

Lesions greater than 20 cm in diameter, those in such critical areas as the central third of the face, recurrent lesions, and lesions with histologic signs of sclerosis are associated with a poor prognosis. Treatment for cure at the time of initial therapy and frequent examination for at least 2 years are essential.

NURSING CARE

Nursing Assessment[3]

Skin Integrity

Raised, hard, red or red-gray, pearly lesion on forehead, eyelid, cheek, nose, preauricular fold, or lip; scaly, slightly elevated lesion with irregular border; ulceration

Nursing Dx & Intervention

Nursing Diagnosis	Nursing Intervention/Rationale
Impaired skin integrity	• Bathe patient in warm water or apply warm, moist compress *to maintain cleanliness.* • Clean skin with agents appropriate to therapy *to prevent infection.* • Maintain dry skin *to avoid irritation and infection.* • Use paper or transparent tape over dressings *to avoid irritation.* • Observe lesions for change in shape, size, and color and bleeding.
Patient problem: metastasis	• See "Metastatic Disease," p. 1492.

Patient Education

1. Inform the patient of the need for regular physical examinations and self-examination.
2. Inform the patient of the need for careful protection of the skin with use of sunscreens, avoidance of excessive exposure to sun, and limited exposure to ionizing radiation.

Evaluation[10]

Patient Outcome	Data Indicating That Outcome is Reached
Skin is healed.	Skin integrity is maintained without infection or ulceration.
Patient has physical appearance of comfort.	Facial expression is calm and relaxed.
Patient shows no evidence of physical injury.	There is no evidence of complications arising from drugs or treatments.

Malignant melanoma

Malignant melanoma is a skin cancer that is composed of melanocytes.

Seventy-five percent of deaths from skin cancer, an average of 5500 deaths a year, are caused by malignant melanoma. This cancer develops from melanocytes that migrate into the skin, eye, central nervous system, and mucous membranes during fetal development. Only 40% of melanomas develop from nevi; the majority arise de novo from melanocytes.

The exact cause of malignant melanoma is unknown. A hereditary factor is involved in 10% of patients. Other theories suggest possible hormonal factors, ultraviolet light exposure, or an autoimmunologic effect.

Malignant melanoma is easily recognized in its early stages and should be suspected in any patient with a history of change in a preexisting nevus or with a new pigmented lesion that has irregularities such as the following:

- Various shades of brown and black plus red, white, or blue and the half tones of pink or gray
- Notching or indentation of the border and pigment streaming from the lesion's edge
- Loss of skin markings or development of a nodule, especially with erosion or ulceration
- Bleeding of mole or change in color, size, or thickness[3,28]

Pathophysiology[6]

The four distinct forms of malignant melanoma, in order of decreasing incidence, follow:

- Superficial spreading melanoma (70%) occurs anywhere on the body surface. The average patient age is 50 years. The lesion has a haphazard combination of colors and irregular shapes.
- Nodular melanoma (15%) also occurs anywhere on the body surface and has a wide age distribution. It may be small and usually is darkly pigmented. Invasion is usually into the dermis, with resultant lymph node metastasis.
- Acral (extremity) lentiginous melanoma (10%) occurs on palms, soles, nail beds, and mucous membranes. It is usually flat to slightly raised with an irregular pigment pattern and border.
- Lentigo malignant melanoma (5%) is a slowly evolving lesion occurring on exposed surfaces (especially face and hands) of elderly people. It usually undergoes many color changes.

Diagnostic Studies and Findings[28]

Total Excisional Biopsy

Deep margin to include subcutaneous fat preferred; performed to determine presence, type, and stage of malignancy

Punch or Incisional Biopsy

Followed by wide excision if findings are positive; incisional biopsy performed for large lesions and those in areas of cosmetic concern; done to determine presence, type, and stage of malignancy

Measurement of Tumor Thickness and Depth of Invasion

To determine stage of disease

Physical Examination and Symptom- or Organ-Oriented Diagnostic Tests

Ordered as needed to detect metastases in lung, liver, bone, or brain (or anywhere in body); examples are chest roentgenogram, liver function test, and baseline liver and spleen scan

• • •

The prognosis is poorer with increased depth of invasion, lymphatic and vascular invasion, high number of mitotic figures per high-power microscopic field, little or no lymphocytic infiltration at the tumor base, and ulceration. The overall prognosis is better in women.

Medical Plan[6]

Surgery

Wide, deep excision of primary lesion
Regional lymph node dissection

Medications

Antineoplastic agents
- Dacarbazine (DTIC), 2-4.5 mg/kg/d IV for 10 d or 250 mg/m^2/d IV for 5 d
- Tamoxifen citrate (Nolvadex), 10-20 mg bid (morning and evening)

Anti-infective agents
- BCG vaccine, active specific forms used as investigational drug

See "Chemotherapy," p. 1495

General Management

Radiotherapy for palliation of metastases (see p. 1500)
Hyperthermic isolation perfusion

NURSING CARE

Nursing Assessment[6]

Skin Integrity

Dark brown or black pigmentation; ulceration and bleeding; enlarged regional lymph nodes

Nursing Dx & Intervention

Nursing Diagnosis	Nursing Intervention/Rationale
Skin integrity, impaired: actual	• Bathe patient in warm water, or apply warm, moist compresses *to maintain cleanliness*. • Clean skin with agents appropriate to therapy *to prevent infection*. • Maintain dry skin *to avoid irritation and infection*. • Observe lesions for change in shape, size, color, and bleeding.
Patient problem: metastasis	• See "Metastatic Disease," p. 1492.

Patient Education

1. Emphasize the need for regular physical examinations.
2. Inform the patient of the need for meticulous skin care and assessment and the importance of avoiding ultraviolet light.
3. Instruct the patient to report changes such as those in respiratory status, abdominal girth or comfort, mobility, and level of consciousness.

Evaluation

Patient Outcome	Data Indicating That Outcome is Reached
Vital signs are within normal limits.	Respiratory rate, rhythm, and depth and pulse are within normal limits. Breathing pattern is regular.
Patient is comfortable.	Facial expression is calm and relaxed. Posture is normal. Patient expresses comfort and no longer complains.
Patient's surroundings are safe.	Safety precautions, such as side rails, are used.
Patient shows no physical sign of injury.	There is no evidence of accident, physical injury, or complications arising from drugs or treatments.

 Oncologic Emergencies

Oncologic emergencies arise from the impact advanced cancer has on body functioning. As many as 20% of patients develop one or more of these emergent conditions. Among the most serious but most treatable acute conditions that can occur are hypercalcemia, obstruction of the superior vena cava, spinal cord compression, and cardiac distress. Other oncologic emergencies include pleural effusions, sepsis, disseminated intravascular coagulation, syndrome of inappropriate antidiuretic hormone (SIADH), and tumor lysis syndrome.

Hypercalcemia. Hypercalcemia occurs when the bones release more calcium into the extracellular fluid than can be excreted in the urine. This occurs most frequently in patients with multiple myeloma or cancer of the breast, lung, or prostate. In addition, some tumors produce parathyroid hormone or a substance with the same physiologic effects, which include increased resorption of calcium from bone, increased intestinal absorption of calcium, and reduced renal excretion.

The most common cause of hypercalcemia is thought to be bone destruction by invasive metastases. Other causes are tumor production of vitamin D–like substances and osteoclast-activating factors, dehydration, and immobilization.

Excessive calcium can cause bradycardia, increased cardiac contractility, depression of the central and peripheral nervous system (mild lethargy that may progress to coma), fatigue, muscle weakness, anorexia, nausea and vomiting, confusion, or irritability. Interference with reabsorption of water from the distal tubules leads to nocturia, polyuria, and dehydration.

Acute hypercalcemia is treated initially with intravenous saline. Furosemide may also be given intravenously to encourage diuresis. Careful recording of intake and output, monitoring of electrolyte levels, and frequent cardiopulmonary assessment are necessary. Mithramycin inhibits bone resorption of calcium; given as a rapid intravenous infusion at 25 μg/kg body weight, it can lower serum calcium levels in 48 hours.

Steroid administration and restriction of dietary calcium are thought to be of little therapeutic value. Orally administered phosphates and calcitonin injections may be used. Use of vitamin D, thiazides, absorbable antacids, and estrogens should be avoided.

External compression of the superior vena cava. Compression of the superior vena cava can occur slowly or quickly, owing to pressure from an adjacent tumor mass or enlarging lymph node. Most patients with superior vena cava syndrome have bronchogenic cancer; other causes of this syndrome are lymphoma, breast cancer, and gastrointestinal tract metastases.

Prompt diagnosis and treatment are needed to relieve the distressing symptoms, which are progressive shortness of breath, cough, distention of neck veins, and edema of the face and hands. Dilated veins may appear on the upper chest wall. The patient may complain of headache and visual disturbances.

The patient must be kept in Fowler's position. Diuretics may be of some help. However, the obstruction must be relieved to prevent cerebral anoxia, hemorrhage, or strangulation. Radiation therapy is the treatment of choice for this. If the obstruction is not accessible, chemotherapeutic agents such as cyclophosphamide (Cytoxan) can produce good results.

Spinal cord compression. Compression of the spinal cord is extremely dangerous because of the possibility of a permanent neurologic deficit. The usual cause of compression is a tumor, such as lymphoma or cancer of the breast, lung, or prostate, that metastasizes to the bony vertebral body and grows into the epidural space.

Pain, localized in the spinal region or radicular, is almost always an early symptom. The pain may be constant and aggravated by movement or coughing. Relief is usually obtained with morphine, meperidine (Demerol), or an analgesic agent. Bed rest is recommended, and transfer and position change should be done by multiple personnel.

A careful neurologic examination should be performed to check motor and sensory function and the autonomic nerve tracts. Roentgenograms or myelograms should be done immediately to localize the destruction and determine its extent. The prognosis appears to be related to the patient's ability to walk at the time of diagnosis; if he or she is unable to do so, motor function is not recoverable, even with emergency radiotherapy or laminectomy.

Severe or prolonged cord compression can lead to extremity paralysis and loss of sphincter control, which is manifest as difficulty starting urination or as bowel incontinence.

Treatment must be prompt. Corticosteroids, such as dexamethasone, in high doses reduce swelling and inflammation around the cord. Surgical decompression or radiotherapy may be required. Early diagnosis is important for recovery.

Cardiac tamponade. Cardiac tamponade results from excessive amount and pressure of fluid on the pericardial sac, which is a response to metastasis or direct invasion by tumor. The normal diastolic filling is impaired, and stroke volume is reduced. If tamponade is untreated, circulatory collapse occurs.

Signs and symptoms depend on how quickly the fluid accumulates. Frequent signs of tamponade include rapid and weak pulse, distended neck veins during inspiration (Kussmaul's sign), pulsus paradoxus (inspiratory decrease in arterial blood pressure of greater than 10 mm Hg from baseline), ankle or sacral edema, pleural effusion, lethargy, and altered consciousness.

The diagnosis is confirmed with echocardiography and pericardiocentesis; the latter also provides immediate symptomatic relief. Palliative measures, such as surgical construction of a pericardial window, must also be taken; total pericardectomy is usually not practical. Newer techniques include catheter drainage of fluid and instillation of a sclerosing agent, such as tetracycline.

Pleural effusion. See Chapter 2.

Sepsis. This serious condition is exemplified by inadequate tissue perfusion, which results from bacterial invasion of the circulatory system. The most common causative agents, gram-negative bacteria, release an endotoxin from their cell walls, which causes increased capillary permeability and leakage. This in turn causes stagnation of blood, lactic acidosis, a decrease in the circulating blood volume, and decreased cardiac output. Sepsis is the most common cause of death in neutropenic patients. Signs and symptoms of sepsis include fever, chills, restlessness, confusion, tachycardia, hypotension, decreased pulses, cool clammy skin, decreased urinary output, and bleeding from one or more sites, which may be caused by disseminated intravascular coagulation (DIC).

The diagnosis is confirmed by positive blood cultures, the presence of infiltrates on chest roentgenogram, depressed or elevated white blood cell level, metabolic acidosis via arterial blood gas analysis, and a prolonged prothrombin time and partial thromboplastin time. Interventions include monitoring of vital signs, arterial blood gas values, and hemodynamic stability; performance of blood cultures as needed; administration of antibiotics; temperature reduction with antipyretics, ice packs, hypothermia blanket, and so on; and fluid volume replacement.

Disseminated intravascular coagulation (DIC). This imbalance of normal coagulation is always secondary to an underlying cause, such as the release of tissue thromboplastin from tumor cells (e.g., lung and prostate leukemia); sepsis; infection, hemolytic transfusions, or hepatic failure. The pathophysiology is based on the uncontrollable triggering of the internal or external pathway of the clotting cascade, resulting in accelerated coagulation and the formation of excessive thrombin. As long as coagulation occurs, the fibrinolytic system is activated, so that clotting and bleeding continue at a life-threatening pace. Signs and symptoms of DIC include systemic bleeding, ranging from petechiae to hematuria to an acute gastrointestinal hemorrhage; organ dysfunction (e.g., pulmonary emboli, thromboemboli in the extremities, renal failure); decreased blood pressure and pulse; cool, clammy skin; anemia; pallor; and shortness of breath. A diagnosis of DIC is confirmed by the presence of prolonged thrombin time, prothrombin time, and partial thromboplastin time; decreased platelets; decreased fibrinogen; and elevated fibrin-split products. Appropriate interventions include such medical therapies as antibiotics, chemotherapy, heparin, and blood products. The nurse should continuously monitor sites and amount of bleeding and laboratory values, assess adequacy of tissue perfusion, and prevent or minimize bleeding.

Syndrome of inappropriate antidiuretic hormone (SIADH). Antidiuretic hormone, which is normally released from the posterior pituitary in response to increased plasma osmolarity or decreased plasma volume, may be abnormally produced or stimulated as a result of tumor secretion (e.g., small cell lung cancer, lymphoma, and pancreatic and prostate cancers); stimulation by such drugs as vincristine and cyclophosphamide; viral or bacterial pneumonia; or neurologic trauma. The results of this abnormal production or stimulation are excessive water retention and hyponatremia. Signs and symptoms of SIADH include confusion, irritability, weakness, lethargy, headache, hyporeflexia, nausea, vomiting, anorexia, diarrhea, and weight gain without edema. Diagnosis is confirmed by a serum sodium level of less than 130 mEq/L, serum osmolarity of less than 280 mOsm/kg H_2O, and a urine sodium level of more than 20 mEq/L. Medical interventions may include chemotherapy, antibiotics, hypertonic saline (3% to 5% sodium chloride), diuretics, demeclocycline and discontinuation of the causative agent. The nurse should also maintain an accurate intake and output record, restrict fluids as necessary, monitor laboratory reports of fluid and electrolyte balance, and provide safety measures for weak and confused patients.

Tumor lysis syndrome. This metabolic imbalance is caused by the rapid release of such intracellular components as potassium, phosphorus, and uric acid. The patient's risk of developing tumor lysis syndrome increases with the presence of bulky tumors that have a high growth fraction. The syndrome usually begins 1 to 5 days after the initiation of chemotherapy for non-Hodgkin's lymphomas and leukemia. Signs and symptoms include oliguria, anuria, urine crystals, flank pain, hematuria, cardiac dysrhythmias, muscular cramps, tetany, and confusion. The diagnosis is confirmed by elevated serum blood urea nitrogen (BUN), creatinine, potassium, phosphorus, and uric acid and by decreased serum calcium. Medical orders may include administering allopurinol and calcium supplements, giving intravenous fluids with sodium bicarbonate for 3 to 5 days after initiating chemotherapy, and preparing the patient for peritoneal dialysis or hemodialysis.

Metastatic Disease

Metastases are the major cause of death from cancer. The likelihood of a person with cancer developing metastatic disease is increased by the presence of a primary tumor of extended duration; high mitotic rate; trauma, such as tumor biopsy; dead tumor cells; heat; radiation; and chemotherapeutic agents. A metastasis is a tumor that is distant from the primary tumor and occurs as a result of seeding throughout a body cavity, such as the peritoneal or thoracic cavity; mechanical transport via instruments or gloved hands; lymphatic spread; and hematogenous spread. The most common sites of metastases follow:

- The lung, from such primary sites as the colorectum, breast, renal system, testes, and bones
- The liver, from such primary sites as the lung, colorectum, breast, and renal system
- The central nervous system, from such primary sites as the lung and breast
- Bone, from such primary sites as the lung, breast, renal system, and prostate

The nurse should include in her ongoing assessment of a person with cancer an emphasis on early detection of signs and symptoms of metastatic disease. This requires a knowledge of usual sites of spread for specific cancers, as well as sensitivity to patient complaints, changes in laboratory values, and observable alterations in function that indicate metastatic spread.

Nursing diagnoses and interventions appropriate to each of the common metastatic sites follow.

Nursing Dx & Intervention

Nursing Diagnosis	Nursing Intervention/Rationale
Altered cardiopulmonary tissue perfusion related to pulmonary metastasis	• Position patient comfortably, with head elevated, *to promote chest expansion.* • Encourage coughing and deep breathing *to maintain a patent respiratory tract.* • Suction airway as needed *to relieve obstruction caused by secretions.* • Administer vaporized air *to moisten secretions and oxygen to ensure adequate tissue perfusion.* • Encourage adequate rest *to decrease respiratory workload.* • Remove constrictive clothing *to relieve pressure on chest.* • Discourage smoking *to decrease respiratory distress.* • Inspect chest symmetric expansion *to assess respiratory status.* • Auscultate for abnormal breath sounds, voice sounds, rales, and rhonchi *to assess pulmonary function.* • Monitor blood studies *to determine adequate oxygenation.* • Be alert for complaints of pain, cyanosis, dyspnea, confusion, and fatigue, *which indicate increasing respiratory distress.* • Encourage coughing and deep breathing *to clear respiratory tract.* • Monitor respiratory rate and rhythm and pulse *to assess for adequacy of cardiopulmonary function.*
Altered nutrition: less than body requirements related to liver metastasis	• Arrange pleasant surroundings, and provide attractive meal tray *to enhance appetite.* • Postpone feeding when patient is fatigued, as patient is more likely *to eat when rested.* • Give small, frequent feedings *to avoid distention.* • Provide selection of foods *to enhance patient's appetite.* • Provide foods at appropriate temperatures *to make them more appetizing.* • Encourage family and friends *to bring in food of the patient's choice.* • Measure body weight daily *to monitor nutritional status.* • Observe and record food intake *to monitor nutritional status.* • Elevate patient's head *to promote comfort.* • Encourage deep breathing *to relieve feeling of nausea.* • Feed slowly, and provide rest periods *to avoid tiring patient.* • Give bland food or carbonated beverages or hot tea *to relieve nausea.* • Give nonprescription antiemetics or drugs as prescribed *to relieve nausea.* • Observe effectiveness of interventions *to determine need for further intervention.*
Potential for injury related to central nervous system metastasis	• Maintain bed rest *to avoid falls or other trauma.* • Provide quiet environment with subdued lighting *to relax patient.* • Minimize environmental danger by removing furniture, rugs, and other barriers. • Inspect patient for abnormal body movements indicating seizure activity. • Observe for confusion and reduced level of consciousness *as signs of increased intracranial pressure.*
Pain (headache) related to central nervous system metastasis	• Position patient comfortably; change position slowly *to decrease pressure.* • Elevate patient's head *to relieve intracranial pressure.* • Apply cold, moist compress or ice bag *to relieve pressure.* • Massage patient's neck and shoulders *to relax muscles.* • Subdue room lighting *to decrease stimulation.* • Provide quiet and encourage patient to rest *to decrease stimulation.* • Encourage adequate rest *to relieve stress.* • Provide pain relief measure of patient's choice *to promote self-care.* • Be alert for complaints of pain, and assess pain for duration and radiation *to determine intervention needed.* • Evaluate effectiveness of pain relief measures *to determine need for further intervention.*
Hyperthermia related to central nervous system metastasis	• Apply cool, damp cloth to face *to promote evaporative heat loss.* • Bathe in cool water or apply ice bag or alcohol to skin *to decrease body temperature.* • Cover with lightweight clothing. • Maintain cool room temperature *to maintain environment cooler than patient's body.*

Nursing Diagnosis	Nursing Intervention/Rationale
	• Encourage rest. • Give antipyretics as indicated *to decrease temperature.* • Increase fluid intake *to promote hydration.* • Measure temperature and intake and output. • Obtain bacterial cultures as indicated. • Monitor neurologic vital signs.
Pain (bone)	• Maintain body alignment *to prevent muscular stretching.* • Position patient with support (e.g., pillows), change position slowly, and support joints *to avoid fractures.* • Apply heating pad, hot water bottle, warm, moist compress, whirlpool bath, or mentholated ointment *to provide relaxation and relieve pain.* • Exercise gently in range of motion *to maintain muscle tone.* • Massage gently *to relax muscles.* • Be alert for complaints of pain, and assess its duration and radiation *to intervene early.* • Provide pain relief measure of patient's choice, such as relaxation therapy, diversion, or distraction, *to enhance effect of medication.* • Administer pain medications as ordered *to control pain.* • Evaluate pain for intensity and quality *to determine need for further intervention.* • Evaluate effectiveness of pain relief measures *to determine need for same or different intervention.*

Evaluation

Patient Outcome	Data Indicating That Outcome is Reached
Skin and mucous membrane color is normal.	Skin, nails, lips, and earlobes are warm and moist and of natural color.
Vital signs are within normal limits.	Respirations, pulse, blood pressure, and temperature are within normal limits.
Body hydration is normal.	Skin turgor is normal. Secretions are thin. Mucous membranes are moist. There is no edema, ascites, or venous distention.
Patient has daily intake of essential foods.	Diet includes milk, meat, fruits, vegetables, breads, and cereals.
Daily fluid output equals fluid intake.	Urine output is 1500 to 3000 ml daily or equivalent to intake.
Vitality is good.	There is no malaise, fatigue, or weakness.
Patient has physical appearance of comfort.	Patient expresses comfort and satisfaction. Patient ceases to complain.
Patient frequently changes position.	Patient walks, sits, and stands with normal body movement.
Patient participates in therapeutic exercise.	Patient performs range of motion exercises.
Patient's surroundings are safe and comfortable.	Patient uses safety precautions. Temperature, humidity, and ventilation of patient's room are appropriate.
There is no evidence of physical injury.	Patient shows no evidence of complications arising from drugs or treatments.

Medical Interventions and Related Nursing Care

Blood Component Therapy

The goal of blood component therapy is to administer only the component needed by the patient. This minimizes transfusion reactions and increases the number of patients who can benefit from a single unit.

Granulocytes are used to treat granulocytopenic patients with severe infection, particularly those in whom severe bone marrow depression develops during chemotherapy. Granulocytes are collected from a single donor by means of a machine that withdraws donor blood, removes the granulocytes, and returns the rest of the blood to the donor. This procedure, called leukopheresis, requires several hours. Administration of steroids before donation can increase the cell yield.

Although granulocytes can be stored up to 24 hours, immediate transfusion is recommended. Because of the short posttransfusion cell life, frequent transfusions are usually needed; for example, daily for at least 4 days, administered slowly over a 2- to 4-hour period.

The most common untoward reactions are shaking chills and temperature elevation, which are treated symptomatically with acetaminophen 30 minutes before subsequent transfusions and with reduction of the flow rate. Hives are another minor reaction and are usually treated with an antihistamine. Life-threatening reactions include hypotensive response, anaphylactic response, and respiratory reaction. Emergency intervention is necessary.

Platelets are usually given to patients with thrombocytopenia and bone marrow depression resulting from chemotherapy or radiation therapy. Platelet concentrates are obtained through platelet pheresis of a single donor or prepared from units of platelets collected from as many as four to 10 donors. Blood is removed from the donor into a machine with a centrifuge bowl, where platelets are separated, and red cells and plasma are then returned to the donor. The procedure takes 1½ to 2 hours. Pheresis donors may give as many as 12 units of platelets at a time. The platelets should be administered within 24 hours.[6,28]

The nurse is an essential member of the team involved in this therapy; it is often the nurse who identifies the patient's need for blood components, recruits donors, obtains the blood components from the donors, and administers the therapy to the patient.

Chemotherapy

Description and Rationale

Chemotherapy is a relatively new cancer treatment modality, the first patient having been treated with nitrogen mustard in 1942. The use of chemical agents is especially important in the treatment of systemic disease. Researchers continue to discover drugs that kill cancer cells without causing extensive damage to normal tissues. In addition, combinations of chemotherapeutic agents, as well as the combination of chemotherapy with other treatment modalities, have increased the cancer cure rate.

Chemotherapy is used to cure patients, prolong life, increase the disease-free interval, and palliate symptoms, thus improving the quality of life.

Chemotherapeutic agents are highly toxic, attacking all rapidly dividing cells, both normal and malignant. Thus the contraindications and cautions are a reflection of the patient's pretreatment condition, stage of disease, response to therapy, and allergies or sensitivities. The nurse involved in drug administration and monitoring of the patient's responses must have a comprehensive baseline assessment to use in evaluating the patient's condition and ability to tolerate the treatment.

The most commonly used chemotherapeutic agents are listed in Table 16-1. Many others are being developed and tested for possible therapeutic value.[2,6,28]

Depending on the drug's pharmacodynamics, chemotherapy may be administered by a variety of routes: intravenous, oral, central venous catheter, venous access via an implantable access device, intra-arterial, intraperitoneal, intrapleural, intrathecal, or ventricular reservoir. The intramuscular and subcutaneous routes are rarely used. In recent years use of intra-arterial and venous access lines (i.e., Hickman catheter) has become important because of the ease of access to the arterial or venous system for drug delivery, increased patient comfort, and the addition of external or internal pump systems for more continuous infusion of drugs.

NURSING CARE

Nursing Assessment[6,28]

Gastrointestinal

Nausea and vomiting; diarrhea; constipation; stomatitis; esophagitis; anorexia

Dermatologic

Alopecia; dermatitis; changes in skin color; extravasation; hyperpigmentation of nail beds

Hematologic

Anemia owing to decreased RBCs; bleeding owing to thrombocytopenia (petechiae); infection owing to leukopenia

See "Blood Component Therapy," p. 1494

Reproductive

Sterility; amenorrhea; decreased libido

Urinary

Hemorrhagic cystitis, as evidenced by hematuria, burning during urination, and backache; nephrotoxicity, as evidenced by renal failure

Neurologic

Ototoxicity (vertigo, tinnitus, loss of hearing); peripheral neuropathies, as evidenced by muscle weakness; numbness and tingling; jaw pain; absence of deep tendon reflexes

Respiratory

Pulmonary fibrosis, as evidenced by dyspnea, chest pain, or cyanosis

Musculoskeletal

Myalgia; muscle weakness; osteoporosis; gout

Table 16-1
Cancer Chemotherapeutic Agents

Classification	Agents	Mechanism of Action
Alkylating agents	Mechlorethamine (nitrogen mustard); cyclophosphamide (Cytoxan); phenylalanine mustard (Alkeran, L-PAM, Melphalan); chlorambucil (Leukeran); bulsulfan (Myleran); dacarbazine (DTIC); thiophosphoramide (Thiotepa)	Produce breaks in DNA module and cross-linking of strands and thus interfere with DNA replication
Antimetabolites		
Folic acid analog	Methotrexate (MTX)	Competitively inhibit enzymes necessary for cell function and replication
Pyrimidine analogs	5-Fluorouracil (5-FU); floxuridine (FUDR); cytosine arabinoside (Cytosar)	
Purine analogs	6-Mercaptopurine (6-MP); 6-thioguanine (Thioguanine)	
Vinca alkaloids	Vinblastine (Velban); vincristine (Oncovin)	Bind to substances needed for formation of mitotic spindle and thus prevent cell division
Antibiotics	Doxorubicin (Adriamycin); daunorubicin (Daunomycin); bleomycin (Blenoxane); dactinomycin (actinomycin D); mithramycin (Mithracin); mitomycin C (Mutamycin)	Bind with DNA to inhibit DNA and RNA synthesis
Nitrosoureas	Bis-chloroethyl nitrosourea (BCNU); lomustine (CCNU), carmustine/BCNU (BiCNU); streptozocin	Action similar to that of alkylating agents
Hormonal agents		Alter cellular environment
Corticosteroids	Prednisone; prednisolone; methylprednisolone (Solu-Medrol); hydrocortisone (Solu-Cortef); dexamethasone (Decadron)	
Estrogens	Ethinyl estradiol (Estinyl); fosfestrol (Stilbestrol); diethylstilbestrol (DES); diethylstilbestrol diphosphate (Stilphostrol); conjugated estrogens (Premarin)	
Antiestrogens	Clomiphene; nafoxidine; tamoxifen (Nolvadex)	
Androgens	Testosterone; calusterone; fluoxymesterone (Halotestin); nandrolone	
Progestins	17-Hydroxyprogesterone (Delalutin); medroxyprogesterone acetate (Provera); megestrol acetate (Megace)	
Biologic response modifiers	Interferon Alfa-2b	Immune modulation
Miscellaneous agents	Cisplatin diamine dichloride (Platinol); hydroxyurea; L-asparaginase; procarbazine (Matulane); aminoglutethimide (Cytadren); estramustine (Emcyt); etoposide (VP-16); mitotane	

Cardiac

Congestive heart failure, as evidenced by exertional dyspnea, cough, and rales; ECG changes

Hepatic

Jaundice

Emotional and Mood Changes

Depression; anger; withdrawal; preoccupation with self

Nursing Dx & Intervention

Nursing Diagnosis	Nursing Intervention/Rationale
Fluid volume deficit related to nausea and vomiting	• Administer antiemetic (prochlorperazine, thiethylperazine, trimethobenzamide, mitoclopramide, intravenous dexamethasone, or δ-9 tetrahydrocannabinol [THC]) prophylactically before chemotherapy and on a regular schedule after therapy per physician order *to decrease incidence of nausea and vomiting*. • Withhold food and fluids for 4 to 6 hours before treatment *to decrease gastric irritation*.

Nursing Diagnosis	Nursing Intervention/Rationale
	• Provide small feedings and increase fluids *to maintain nutrition and hydration.* • Provide frequent mouth care *to promote patient's comfort.* • Provide clean environment with fresh air and no odors *to reduce noxious stimuli.* • Monitor intake and output, weight, and electrolytes *to avoid dehydration.* • Administer intravenous therapy as ordered *to maintain fluid and electrolyte balance.* • Use relaxation techniques, guided imagery, self-hypnosis, and distraction as indicated *to reduce nausea.*
Constipation	• Offer fluids and foods high in fiber and bulk *to stimulate motility.* • Offer stool softener or laxatives *to stimulate motility.* • Avoid enemas *because they may traumatize the intestinal mucosa.*
Diarrhea	• Offer clear liquids *to prevent dehydration.* • Offer antidiarrheal agent, such as Kaopectate or diphenoxylate (Lomotil), per physician's order. • Maintain good perineal care *to avoid irritation and discomfort.* • Test stools for occult blood *to identify evidence of blood.* • Record number and consistency of stools *to monitor need for further intervention.* • Observe for dehydration and electrolyte imbalance.
Altered oral mucous membrane related to stomatitis	• Encourage good oral hygiene *to promote comfort and prevent infection.* • Discourage spicy or hot foods *to avoid irritation or pain.* • Offer topical agents for relief of pain (lidocaine or dyclonine) per physician's order. • Apply K-Y Jelly to lips *to maintain moisture.* • Offer popsicles *for hydration and comfort.*
Altered oral mucous membrane related to infection	• Administer nystatin oral suspension or suppository or clotrimazole (Mycelex) troche per physician's order *to combat infection.* • Have patient postpone dental work if possible, brush teeth gently, and use toothettes *to avoid further trauma.*
Altered nutrition: less than body requirements related to esophagitis	• Offer bland or pureed foods *to facilitate swallowing.* • Have patient avoid spicy foods, alcohol, and tobacco *to decrease irritation.* • Offer antacids *to counteract gastric acid.*
Altered nutrition: less than body requirements related to increased body requirements	• Identify food preferences *to increase patient's interest in eating.* • Encourage patient to eat *by explaining need to maintain strength.* • Offer small, frequent feedings *to avoid distention.* • Do not rush meals, *so that patient will increase intake.* • Keep room free of odors and clutter *to reduce noxious stimuli.* • Provide meticulous mouth care *to enhance appetite.* • Use enteral feeding tube or total parenteral nutrition if necessary *to maintain nutritional balance.* • Weigh daily *to monitor nutritional status.*
Impaired skin integrity	*For alopecia:* • Help patient plan for wig, scarf, or hat before hair loss. • Offer tourniquet or ice cap preventive therapy based on policy and diagnosis. • Have patient wash and comb remaining hair gently *to decrease hair loss.* • Reassure patient that hair will grow back after therapy. *For dermatitis:* • Use cornstarch, Alpha Keri, calamine lotion, or other agent *to relieve itching.* • Warn against overexposure to sun *to avoid further irritation.* • Keep skin clean and dry *to avoid infection.* *For changes in color of skin or nail beds:* • Assure patient that discoloration will fade with time. • Use nail polish according to patient's wishes *to mask discoloration.* *For jaundice:* • Monitor hepatic enzymes *to determine liver function.* • Assess skin and sclera daily for evidence of increase or decrease in discoloration.
Impaired gas exchange related to anemia	• Have patient change position slowly *to conserve energy.* • Encourage adequate rest *to conserve energy.* • Observe patient for dyspnea and increased weakness *as evidence of further dysfunction.* • Administer oxygen therapy as needed *to increase oxygenation of tissues.* • Monitor hemoglobin and hematocrit *to determine effect of therapy.* • Administer transfusions as ordered *to increase RBC count.*

Nursing Diagnosis	Nursing Intervention/Rationale
Impaired gas exchange related to fibrosis	• Monitor respiratory function with pulmonary function tests. • Note limitation of lifetime dosage of bleomycin. • Assist with pulmonary function studies. • Observe for dyspnea; report to physician as ordered for further interventions.
Altered cardiopulmonary tissue perfusion	• Limit cumulative dosage of doxorubicin.
Potential for infection	• Warn patient to avoid crowds and people with cold, flu, or cold sore. • Use sterile technique whenever needed *to prevent infection.* • Initiate reverse isolation as indicated *to protect patient from pathogens.* • Monitor temperature and leukocyte count; observe skin temperature, color, and odor. • Encourage careful hygiene *to prevent infection.* • Discourage fresh-cut flowers, which may carry *microorganisms.* • Avoid using indwelling catheters or performing rectal procedures or examination. • Administer antibiotics as prescribed *to treat infection.*
Patient problem: bleeding	• Protect patient from injury; e.g., use precautions when shaving with razor blade, do not permit cluttered environment, and do not administer rectal suppositories. • Have patient avoid using aspirin and aspirin products, *which increase clotting time.* • Avoid giving injections; if they are necessary, apply pressure at site for 3 to 5 minutes afterward *to prevent bleeding.* • Use toothettes for oral care *to avoid trauma to mucosa.* • Monitor petechiae, ecchymoses, and stools *for blood.* • Evaluate neurologic status *to identify intracranial bleeding.* • Have nasal packing available should bleeding occur. • Administer platelet transfusions as necessary.
Sexual dysfunction	• Help patient explore alternatives for sterility, such as sperm banking, hormonal therapy during treatment, and postponement of conception and childbearing. • Refer to sexual counselor as needed.
Altered patterns of urinary elimination	• Force fluids *to maintain renal blood flow.* • Monitor blood urea nitrogen, serum creatinine, creatinine clearance, and electrolytes *as indicators of renal function.* • Monitor intake and output and presence of edema. • Administer diuretics as ordered *to enhance renal excretion.* • Encourage foods high in potassium *to prevent diuretic-related hypokalemia.* • Administer normal saline and mannitol before cisplatin therapy per physician's order *to maintain fluid and electrolyte balance.* • Administer allopurinol as prescribed with high fluid intake *to prevent uric acid accumulation in kidneys.* • Encourage patient to empty bladder frequently, especially at night, *to avoid stasis, inflammation, and infection.* • Provide adequate hydration *to maintain renal function.*
Sensory/perceptual alterations (auditory)	• Monitor hearing with baseline and periodic audiograms.
Sensory/perceptual alterations (tactile)	• Assess patient for numbness and tingling in extremities. • Encourage safety, e.g., by prohibiting smoking and having patient observe placement of feet and hands.
Impaired physical mobility	• Monitor calcium level *to determine bone status.* • Provide safety measures *to prevent injury.* • Be alert for complaint of pain over bony area; if patient has such a complaint, maintain bed rest until roentgenograms are taken for fracture. • Use assistive devices for ambulation *to enhance tolerance of activity.* • Encourage range of motion exercise *to maintain mobility.* • Position patient in proper anatomic alignment *to avoid stretching, pressure, or fracture.*
Ineffective individual coping	• Assess coping behavior; determine its effectiveness for patient. • Reassure patient that mood changes are temporary and dose related. • Allow independence in self-care *to maintain patient self-esteem and promote effective coping.* • Maintain supportive, nonjudgmental attitude *to foster patient coping.* • Encourage use of resources, such as support groups, *to assist patient in coping.*

Nursing Diagnosis	Nursing Intervention/Rationale
Patient problem: metastasis	• See "Metastatic Disease," p. 1492.

Patient Education

1. Encourage maintenance of adequate nutrition and hydration.
2. Emphasize the need for self-regulation of medication to control nausea, vomiting, constipation, diarrhea, or itching.
3. Discuss the warning signs of bleeding and infection that the patient should report to a physician.
4. Emphasize the need for thorough personal hygiene and oral care.

Evaluation

Patient Outcome	Data Indicating That Outcome is Reached
Skin and mucous membrane color is normal.	Skin, nails, lips, and earlobes are warm and moist and have natural color.
Vital signs are within normal limits.	Respirations, pulse, blood pressure, and temperature are within normal limits.
Laboratory findings are within normal limits.	Blood urea nitrogen, hemoglobin, hematocrit, blood pH, sodium, potassium, and serum creatinine are within normal limits. Urine creatinine clearance, specific gravity, pH, and creatinine are within normal limits. Blood leukocyte count is 5000 to 10,000 cells/mm^3.
Body hydration is normal.	Skin turgor is normal. Mucous membranes are moist. There is no edema or ascites.
Body functioning is normal.	Elimination is adequate. Healing is prompt. Weight is stabilized.
Vitality is good.	Patient is mentally alert and without malaise, fatigue, or weakness.
Patient has daily intake of essential food groups.	Diet includes milk, meat, fruits, vegetables, breads, and cereals. High-calorie, high-protein foods are included.
Bowel elimination is adequate.	Stools are soft and normal for individual.
Daily fluid output is equal to fluid intake.	Urine output is 1500 to 3000 ml daily.
Hearing is adequate.	Patient performs appropriate actions or gives appropriate verbal response. Audiometry findings are within normal limits.
Touch is adequate.	Patient feels pinprick, heat, cold, and touch.
General body cleanliness is good.	Patient has clean hair, eyes, ears, nose, mouth, skin, nails, teeth, and clothes. Patient has no unpleasant body odor.
Patient's disposition is good.	Patient's conversation is cheerful. Patient smiles appropriately.
Patient's surroundings are clean, safe, and comfortable.	Room is free from dust, dirt, and clutter. Safety precautions, such as side rails and low bed, are in effect. Temperature and humidity are appropriate. Room is well ventilated. No unpleasant odors are noticeable.
Patient has not suffered accidents or physical injury.	There is no physical sign or subjective evidence of accident or injury.
Patient does not have infection.	There is no evidence of inflammation, purulent drainage or secretions, pain, or aching.

Immunotherapy

Description and Rationale

Immunotherapy is still considered an investigational treatment for cancer. Its usefulness in treating a wide variety of tumors is being studied, but its value in improving long-term survival will require many years of evaluation.

The rationale for the use of immunotherapy in cancer care is based on animal studies and clinical observations such as the following:

Postoperative patients are often found to have malignant cells in circulating blood and in operative wound washings but may never receive a diagnosis of cancer.

Among transplant patients who receive immunosuppressant therapy, cancer occurs at a rate at least 80 times that of the general population.

Rapidly progressive recurrent cancer sometimes appears 10 to 20 years after cure.

Patients with congenital or acquired immunologic deficiencies have a greater incidence of cancer than does the general population.

People with faulty immune systems cannot be sensitized to certain chemicals, such as 2,4-dinitrochlorobenzene (DNCB), and are thus classified as anergic. An anergic cancer patient usually has a rapidly growing tumor and a poor prognosis.

The three types of immunotherapy are active, passive, and adoptive. Active therapy involves administration of an antigen to stimulate the patient's immune system, with subsequent development of immunity (antibody).

Specific active immunotherapy stimulates an immune response to a tumor-associated antigen:

Autologous vaccine produced from the patient's own tumor and injected intradermally at various sites

Allogeneic vaccine—a mixture of tumor cells that are of the same type as the patient's but that may be more immunogenetic because they are new to the patient's immune system

Modified tumor cells—cells treated artificially to increase their antigenicity; cells may be irradiated or treated with neuramidinase, a chemical found to stimulate the immune system by removing a coating on tumor cells

Nonspecific immunotherapy stimulates the immune response to a wide variety of antigens, including tumor-associated antigens. Most frequently used in BCG (bacillus of Calmette and Guérin), which has some benefit as local treatment for superficial or subcutaneous melanoma metastases on the extremities. BCG immunotherapy is accomplished by scarification, intradermal injection into the tumor nodule, or a multiple puncture tine technique (which is quicker and causes less discomfort).

Corynebacterium parvulum is a gram-positive anaerobic bacillus also used for nonspecific immunotherapy. Other agents are 2,4-dinitrochlorobenzene (DNCB), pertussis vaccine, MER (methanol-extracted residue of BCG), and bacterial endotoxins.

Passive immunotherapy involves the direct transfer of transient immunity from person to person. Substances used include the antisera of patients with similar tumors, close family members, or associates, and lymphocytes from cured cancer patients; cross-immunization and cross-transfusion are also performed.

Adoptive immunotherapy is based on the transfer of passive immunity and subsequent development of active immunity by the host. Transfer factor and immune RNA are the substances used.

Recent developments in immunotherapy include the synthesis of interferon, a substance discovered as natural body protein that has anticancer growth activity. Having already been proved active against viral diseases such as herpes zoster and hepatitis, interferon is believed to activate the immune system. It has been used with some success in the treatment of lymphomas and other cancers.

Monoclonal antibodies are the result of the genetic fusing of cancer cells with leukocytes to produce specific antibodies, which provide passive immunity and serve as carriers of cytotoxic agents to cancer cells.

Thymic factors or extracts (e.g., thymosin fraction 5 [TF-5] and thymosin alpha 1 [T-1]) have been shown to enhance the immunologic responses in people who have cancer and are in depressed immune states.

Lymphokines, such as interleukin-1 (IL-1) and interleukin-2 (IL-2), are soluble cell products of lymphocytes. IL-2, also known as T cell growth factor, stimulates the expansion of activated T cells and natural killer cells.

Tumor cell vaccines (active immunotherapy) are administered in small intradermal injections and may produce reddened or pruritic injection sites and painful ulcerations. The sites should be washed at least twice a day with soap and water. If excoriation occurs, they may be cleansed with hydrogen peroxide and covered with a dressing. Fever, chills, and general malaise can usually be effectively treated with an analgesic such as acetaminophen.

When BCG is used for nonspecific immunotherapy, an inflammatory reaction occurs at the injection site after the patient becomes sensitized. Intradermal injection may cause fever, chills, and general malaise, as well as localized abscesses and drainage. Pretreatment with antihistamines and acetaminophen is helpful. If symptoms persist, isoniazid (INH) is effective. These same side effects may occur, although with less severity, after tine technique treatment. The lymph nodes that drain BCG may become enlarged and painful; SGOT or alkaline phosphatase levels may rise, and jaundice may appear. These reactions are usually temporary.[6,28]

Radiation Therapy

Description and Rationale

The goal of radiation in the treatment of cancer is the local destruction of malignant cells or their reproductive capability with minimum damage to normal tissue. This treatment modality is used in the prevention, treatment, and palliation of cancer, either alone or with chemotherapy or surgery. Radiation therapy can be administered either externally or internally.

Ionizing radiation is the form used in cancer treatment because it causes cellular damage or alteration. Some examples of such radiation are x rays, gamma rays, electrons, and beta particles. Cells exposed to ionizing radiation undergo the following stages of reaction:

Physical stage—the cells' molecules become agitated and excited

Physiochemical stage—the agitated molecules break into stable molecules and chemically active substances

Chemical stage—chemical reactions take place inside the cell, causing changes in nuclear DNA

Biologic stage—DNA alterations occur, with consequent cell death

The substances used most for radiation therapy include:

X rays—the higher the voltage, the deeper the penetration; for example, high voltage is used for bladder cancer, and low voltage is used for superficial tumors such as skin cancers

Radioactive elements, such as radium and cobalt, which occur in nature

Radioactive isotopes, such as iodine, gold, and phosphorus, which are produced in atomic reactors

External radiation, the treatment of choice for such cancers as early laryngeal cancer, early retinoblastoma, and some brain tumors, is delivered by x ray or radioisotope via sophisticated equipment with refined delivery, such as the linear accelerator. External radiation is also used as adjuvant therapy and for palliation through reduction of tumor mass.

Internal radiation may include temporary or permanent implants, intracavitary or interstitial instillation, or parenteral or oral administration. Specific uses for these forms of therapy are:

Implants (such as radon, iodine, and gold seeds) sutured into the tumor via tubes or needles for cancers of the tongue, lip, breast, and vagina and small bladder tumors

Intracavitary or interstitial instillation via "seeding" with radioactive gamma ray–emitting beads such as radium or cesium for localized but inoperable lung cancers and invasive tumors of the uterus; "afterloading" with an applicator that provides channels through which to place the radioisotope may be used to reduce exposure

Radioactive isotopes administered orally or parenterally for thyroid cancer, chronic leukemia, or myeloma

The nurse involved in the care of patients receiving internal irradiation should avoid radiation damage by adhering to the principles of time (by being efficient but brief), distance (by standing as far as possible from the source), and shielding (by wearing a lead apron or using other precautions as determined by the radiation safety officer).

Radiosensitive cells—those most likely to be adversely affected by radiation—include relatively undifferentiated and rapidly dividing cells such as those of genes, the mucosa of the gastrointestinal tract, and lymphoid tissue. The most radioresistant cells are those originating from the connective tissue. At the cellular level the degree of sensitivity is related to the degree of cell differentiation, rate of mitosis, and mitotic potential. The degree of vascularity and oxygenation are also important in determining tissue responsiveness.

The side or toxic effects of radiation therapy depend on the site of irradiation, the volume of tissue irradiated, the total dosage delivered, and the time frame within which it is administered. Although newer technology has increased the therapist's ability to treat the cancer more precisely, surrounding or underlying healthy tissue may still be damaged.

The dose of radiation that can be delivered to any tumor is limited by the radiation tolerance of the adjacent normal tissues. One method of improving the therapeutic ratio is fractionation of treatment, or dividing the total dosage of radiation into multiple doses. This allows four processes to occur: repair of sublethal tissue damage, repopulation of clonogenic cells, reassortment of cells in the cell cycle, and reoxygenation of hypoxic cells. The best results are achieved with predetermined doses given five times a week for 4 to 6 weeks.

Before initiating therapy the therapist may localize the treatment portals with a stimulator, such as an x-ray machine that produces the geometric factors of actual therapy or computed tomography scanning that defines both the tumor-bearing volume and critical normal structures. The information obtained is used to produce, with computer assistance, an individualized treatment plan.

In combining surgery with radiation, the relative merits of preoperative or postoperative radiation for many cancers are still a matter of controversy. The use of chemotherapy with radiation requires careful monitoring of peripheral blood counts and observation for exacerbation of drug-induced disorders, such as severe dysuria (cyclophosphamide), enhanced mucositis (methotrexate), or carcinogenesis, such as leukemia. Actinomycin D and doxorubicin produce a recall phenomenon in which reactions appear in previously irradiated tissues when the drug is given as late as 1 year after the patient's radiation exposure.

NURSING CARE

Nursing Assessment[6]

Gastrointestinal Tract

Nausea and vomiting; anorexia; taste changes; esophagitis; diarrhea; xerostomia; mucositis; radiation tooth decay

Genitourinary

Urinary frequency; vaginal discharge; amenorrhea; impotence

Skin

Hair loss; dry reaction-reddened area; dry, itchy feeling; moist desquamation—blistering and sloughing of skin surface

Central Nervous System

Headache

Neuromuscular

Transient paresthesia; paresis or paralysis

Cardiovascular

Pneumonitis—dry, hacking cough; dyspnea; pericarditis; chest pain, ECG changes; myocarditis; friction rub

Hemopoietic

Anemia; infection; bleeding

Nursing Dx & Intervention

Nursing Diagnosis	Nursing Intervention/Rationale
Potential fluid volume deficit related to nausea and vomiting	• Administer antiemetic as needed *to control incidence of nausea and vomiting.* • Plan rest periods before and after meals *to enhance patient's appetite.* • Provide small, bland feedings and increased fluids *to maintain nutrition and hydration.* • Offer frequent mouth care *to promote comfort and appetite.* • Provide clean environment with fresh air and no odors *to decrease noxious stimuli.* • Administer intravenous therapy as ordered *to maintain hydration.* • Monitor intake and output, daily weight, and electrolytes *to determine need for further intervention.*
Altered nutrition: less than body requirements related to anorexia and taste changes	• Encourage patient to eat high-calorie, high-protein diet *for maximum nutrition.* • Offer small, frequent feedings *to increase intake.* • Do not rush meals *to increase intake.* • Keep room free of odors and clutter *to reduce noxious stimuli.* • Provide meticulous mouth care *to increase comfort and appetite.* • Use enteral feeding tube or total parenteral nutrition if necessary *to maintain nutritional balance.* • Monitor weight daily.
Altered nutrition: less than body requirements related to esophagitis or rectal mucositis	• Encourage clear liquids and low-residue diet *to increase comfort.* • Offer antidiarrheal agents per physician's order *to control intestinal irritability.* • Maintain good perineal care *to prevent pain, infection, and patient's fear of eating caused by painful bowel movement.* • Test stools for occult blood *to identify intestinal bleeding.* • Record number and consistency of stools *to monitor effect of therapy.* • Observe for dehydration and electrolyte imbalances *to determine need for further intervention.*
Altered oral mucous membrane related to mucositis, xerostomia, or radiation tooth decay	• Encourage good oral hygiene with use of dental floss or Water Pik. • Discourage spicy or hot foods and dry, thick foods, *which increase discomfort.* • Offer topical relief of pain with lidocaine ointment, Aspergum, or ice chips. • Apply K-Y Jelly to lips *to maintain moisture.* • Offer popsicles *to increase comfort and hydration.* • Offer artificial saliva *to moisten mucosa.* • Encourage increased fluid intake with meals *to maintain hydration.* • Use mouth irrigations or sprays, such as half-strength hydrogen peroxide and saline, *for oral hygiene.* • Encourage use of sugarless lemon drops or mints *to promote feeling of freshness.* • Discourage smoking, alcohol, or ginger ale, *which irritate mucosa.* • Assess mouth for dryness, lesions, bleeding, discharge, and tooth decay for specific interventions. • Consult with dentist as needed for dental care, including fluoride therapy, *to prevent further irritation and infection.*
Altered patterns of urinary elimination	• Force fluids *to maintain renal and bladder hydration.* • Encourage patient to empty bladder completely *to avoid distention.* • Catheterize for residual urine as indicated *to avoid distention.* • Administer urinary antiseptics as prescribed *to reduce inflammation.* • Observe for signs of infection, such as burning, cloudy urine, hematuria, and fever, *to determine the need for antibiotics and other interventions.*
Impaired skin integrity	*For alopecia:* • Help patient plan for wig, scarf, or hat before hair loss. • Have patient gently wash and comb remaining hair *to avoid further hair loss.* • Reassure patient that hair will grow back after therapy. *For dermatitis:* • Observe irradiated area daily *to monitor for inflammation or other reactions.* • Apply baby oil or ointment as prescribed: lanolin or Aquaphor *to maintain moisture.* • Keep reddened area dry and aerated *to avoid infection.* • Use cornstarch, A & D Ointment, or hydrocortisone ointment *to relieve dryness and itching.* *For moist desquamation:* • Provide saline soaks, exposure to air, topical vitamins, steroids, or antibiotic ointments *to enhance healing.* • Avoid the use of adhesive tape, *which irritates the skin.* • Assist patient with bathing *to maintain markings.*

Nursing Diagnosis	Nursing Intervention/Rationale
	• Have patient avoid excessive heat, sunlight, tight, restrictive clothing, and soap, *which further irritate damaged skin.* • Provide special skin care to tissue folds such as buttocks, perineum, groin, and axilla, *which may be sites of infection.* • Avoid application of deodorant or after-shave lotion to treated area, *as these may irritate the skin.*
Pain (headache)	• Assess presence and characteristics of headache. • Administer medications such as steroids and analgesics as prescribed. • Offer patient other pain relief measures *if desired.*
Impaired physical mobility related to fatigue and impaired motor function	• Plan frequent rest periods *to avoid fatigue.* • Avoid injury by assisting with ambulation and removing environmental barriers. • Assess reflexes, tactile sensation, and movement in extremities, and report abnormal findings. • Observe for Lhermitte's sign (sensation of electric shock running down back and over extremities), *which is indicative of cervical cord compression.*
Altered cardiopulmonary tissue perfusion related to pneumonitis	• Auscultate lungs, and report signs of pleural rub. • Observe for cough, dyspnea, and pain on inspiration *as evidence of respiratory dysfunction.* • Treat with antibiotics and steroids as prescribed.
Altered cardiopulmonary tissue perfusion related to pericarditis or myocarditis	• Auscultate heart, and report signs of friction rub, arrhythmias, or hypertension. • Observe for chest pain and weakness, *which are indicative of cardiac dysfunction.* • Monitor ECG reports. • Administer drugs as prescribed *to counteract arrhythmias.*
Impaired gas exchange related to anemia	• Encourage adequate rest; alternate rest and activity periods *to avoid stress on respiratory system.* • Observe patient for dyspnea and increased weakness *as signs of further anemia.* • Administer oxygen therapy as needed *to increase oxygenation of tissues.* • Monitor hemoglobin and hematocrit *to determine effectiveness of therapy.* • Administer transfusions as ordered *to increase circulating RBCs.*
Potential for infection	• Warn patient to avoid crowds and people with colds, flu, or cold sore. • Use sterile technique whenever needed *to prevent infection.* • Initiate reverse isolation as indicated *to protect patient from infection.* • Monitor temperature and leukocyte count *to determine need for further intervention.* • Encourage careful hygiene *to prevent infection.*
Sexual dysfunction	*For sterility:* • Help patient explore alternatives such as sperm banking and hormonal therapy. • Refer patient to sexual counselor as necessary. *For vaginal discharge:* • Encourage patient to douche as needed and to perform thorough perineal care. • Observe for redness, tenderness, discharge, or drainage, *which may require further intervention.*
Patient problem: hemorrhage	• Protect patient from injury when shaving or ambulating, *which could cause bleeding.* • Have patient avoid aspirin and aspirin products, *which prolong bleeding.*
Patient problem: metastasis	• See "Metastatic Disease," p. 1492.

Patient Education

1. Discuss the need for skin care such as maintenance of dye markings, avoidance of soap and other ointments, and avoidance of sunbathing or heat applications.
2. Emphasize the need to avoid injury to the skin.
3. Explain the maintenance of adequate nutrition.
4. Explain the patient's "radioactive state," if present, and precautions to be taken.
5. Discuss the management of fatigue and the maintenance of mobility.

Evaluation

Patient Outcome	Data Indicating That Outcome is Reached
Skin and mucous membrane color is normal.	Skin, nails, lips, and earlobes are warm and moist and have natural color.
Vital signs are within normal limits.	Respirations, pulse, blood pressure, and temperature are within normal limits. There is no respiratory distress.
Laboratory findings are within normal limits.	Blood hemoglobin, hematocrit, sodium, potassium, chloride, and pH are within normal limits. Leukocyte count is 5000 to 10,000 cells/mm^3. Urine output is 1500 to 3000 ml daily or equivalent to intake. There are no erythrocytes or leukocytes in urine, and findings of bacterial culture are negative.
Body hydration is normal.	Skin turgor is normal. Secretions are thin. Mucous membranes are moist.
Body functioning is normal.	Elimination is adequate. Healing is prompt. Weight is stabilized. Digestion is good.
Vitality is good.	Patient has no malaise, fatigue, or weakness.
Patient has daily intake of essential food groups.	Diet includes milk, meat, fruits, vegetables, breads, and cereals (as tolerated). High-calorie, high-protein foods are included.
Patient has positive attitude toward food.	Use of salt and spices is not excessive. Patient indicates that foods taste good.
Patient gives physical appearance and verbal expression of comfort.	Facial expression is calm, contented, and relaxed. Patient expresses comfort.
Patient frequently changes position with normal body movement.	Patient walks, sits, and stands with normal body movement.
Surroundings are clean and safe.	Room is free from dust, dirt, and clutter. Safety precautions are in effect. There is no evidence that accident has occurred.
Patient has not suffered physical injury.	There is no evidence of complications arising from treatment.
Patient does not have infection.	There is no evidence of inflammation, purulent drainage or secretions, pain, or aching.

Surgery

(Biopsy/staging, resection, and reconstruction)

Surgery has historically been the treatment of choice for most cancers. A decision to use this therapy is based on analysis of a variety of data, including a thorough history and physical examination; laboratory, radiologic, and other specialized procedures; and biopsy proof of cancer.

A radical surgical approach to operable tumors is no longer routinely used because of an increased variety of surgical procedures and more sophisticated disease staging. The current treatment of choice is excision of the primary tumor and enough surrounding tissue and lymph nodes to offer maximum protection against local recurrence. These are termed curative resections. Palliative resections may be done when there is spread to distant, previously (preoperatively) undetected sites.

A tumor is considered inoperable if it is large or in a difficult-to-reach place or if there is evidence of extensive local growth or metastasis.

Staging operations such as laparotomy may be performed to determine appropriate therapy. Secondary operations may be done for local recurrence. "Second look" operations may be performed in the absence of clinical evidence of recurrent disease, but the effectiveness of this procedure for finding recurrent disease is questionable.

Distant metastasis (e.g. pulmonary or hepatic) may respond to direct surgical resection. Indirect ablative procedures such as adrenalectomy and hypophysectomy may be useful in the palliation of hormonally sensitive cancers of the breast or prostate. Other indirect palliative procedures include cordotomy for relief of intractable pain and ostomy to relieve gastrointestinal obstruction.[6]

Reconstructive surgery of the head and neck, breast, and extremities has become an important aspect of cancer rehabilitation in recent years. For example, the development of maxillofacial prosthodontics has enabled people treated with radical neck dissection to regain cosmetic appearance and the ability to eat and drink in a more natural manner. Breast reconstruction is an option for women whose disease and treatment enable the surgeon to implant a prosthesis or to transplant tissue from other areas of the body.

Whatever the surgery, the patient's nutritional status, both preoperatively and postoperatively, has been found to be significant in the amount of surgery that can be tolerated, recovery from the surgical procedure, and wound healing.

References

1. Aiken S: Family structure and utilization of cancer support groups, Oncol Nurs Forum 9:22, 1982.
2. American Cancer Society: A cancer source book for nurses, New York, 1981, The Society.
3. American Cancer Society: Cancer facts and figures—1985, New York, 1985, The Society.
4. American Cancer Society: Cancer facts and figures—1987, New York, 1987, The Society.
5. American Cancer Society: Cancer facts and figures—1988, New York, 1988, The Society.
6. American Cancer Society, Massachusetts Division: Cancer: a manual for practitioners, Boston, 1982, The Society.
7. Astchega Y and Jacob JG: Providing "safe conduct": helping your patients cope with cancer, Nursing 84 14:42, 1984.
8. Baird S: Decision-making in oncology nursing, Philadelphia, 1988, BC Decker, Inc.
9. Brager B and Yasko J: Care of the client receiving chemotherapy, Reston, Va, 1984, Reston Publishing Co, Inc.
10. Campbell C: Nursing diagnosis and intervention in nursing practice, New York, 1984, John Wiley & Sons, Inc.
11. Cancer statistics, Cancer 31:13, 1981.
12. Concilus E and Bohachick P: Cancer: pericardial effusion and tamponade, Cancer Nurs 1:391, 1984.
13. Coping with cancer: a resource for the health professional, Bethesda, Md, 1980, US Department of Health and Human Services, Public Health Service, National Institutes of Health.
14. Donehower M: Malignant complications of AIDS, Oncol Nurs Forum 14:57, 1987.
15. Doogan RA: Hypercalcemia of malignancy, Cancer Nurs 4:299, 1981.
16. Ellerhorst-Ryan J: Complications of the myeloproliferative system: infection and sepsis, Semin Oncol Nurs 1:244, 1985.
17. Groenwald SL: Cancer nursing: principles and practices, Boston, 1987, Jones & Bartlett Publishers.
18. Joossens JV and Geboers J: Nutrition and gastric cancer, Proc Nutr Soc 40:37, 1981.
19. Kelley PP and Tinsley C: Planning care for the patient receiving external radiation, Am J Nurs 81:338, 1981.
20. Kim MJ, McFarland GK and McLane AM: Pocket guide to nursing diagnoses, St Louis, 1987, The CV Mosby Co.
21. Lauren P: The two histologic main types of gastric carcinoma: diffuse and so-called intestinal type carcinoma. An attempt at a histochemical classification, Acta Pathol Microbiol Scand 64:31, 1965.
22. Luckmann J and Sorensen KC: Medical-surgical nursing: a psychophysiologic approach, Philadelphia, 1987, WB Saunders Co.
23. Ming SC: Gastric carcinoma: a pathobiological classification, Cancer 39:2475, 1977.
24. Nicholson G: Cancer-metastasis, Sci Am 240:66, 1979.
25. Oncology Nursing Society: Cancer chemotherapy guidelines, Pittsburgh, Pa, 1988, The Society.
26. Parks AG and Nicholls RJ: Proctocolectomy without ileostomy for ulcerative colitis, Br Med J 2:85, 1978.
27. Preston FA and Wilfinger C: Memory bank for chemotherapy, Baltimore, 1988, Williams & Wilkins.
28. Rubin P, editor: Clinical oncology for medical students and physicians: a multidisciplinary approach, New York, 1983, American Cancer Society.
29. Shearman DJC and Finlayson NDC: Diseases of the gastrointestinal tract and liver, New York, 1982, Churchill Livingstone.
30. Sleisenger MH and Fordtran JS: Gastrointestinal disease, ed 3, Philadelphia, 1983, WB Saunders Co.
31. Spiro HM: Clinical gastroenterology, New York, 1983, Macmillan Publishing Co.
32. The new immunology: helping the body heal itself, Am J Nurs 87:455, 1987.
33. Toal DR: Tumor cell kinetics and cancer chemotherapy, Am J Nurs 80:1802, 1980.
34. Valentine AS and Stewart JA: Oncologic emergencies, Am J Nurs 83:1281, 1983.
35. Welch-McCaffrey D: When it comes to cancer, think family, Nursing 83 13:32, 1983.
36. Yasko J: Guidelines for cancer care: symptom management, Reston, Va, 1983, Reston Publishing Co.
37. Ziegfeld C: Core curriculum for oncology nursing, Philadelphia, 1987, WB Saunders.

CHAPTER 17

Mental Health

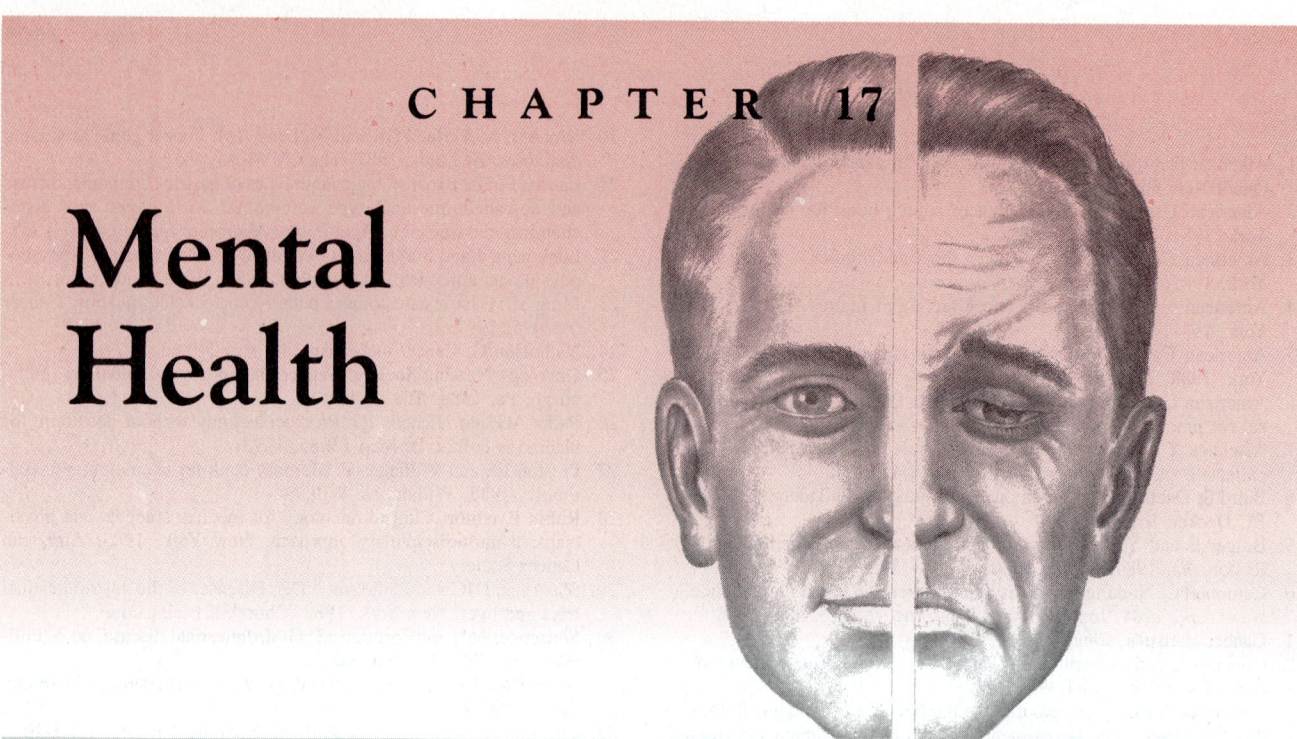

Overview

Mental health is an elusive concept with diverse definitions. Not all theorists identify the same personality traits as indicators of healthy functioning, but their definitions are not necessarily contradictory. The diversity is related to the complexity of human beings and the beliefs each theorist has about human nature. Theorists recognize that biologic, social, and psychologic influences all contribute to healthy personality functioning, but each theorist emphasizes one dimension over the others.

Characteristics of healthy personality functioning compiled from psychoanalytic, interpersonal, and cognitive theories are listed below. The list is not exhaustive and is not in order of importance, but all characteristics are indicators of mental health.

- Positive self-identity
- Awareness of oneself as a psychologically separate individual
- Responsibility for oneself and one's own actions
- Acceptance of emotions and ability to correct faulty ones
- Constructive use of cognitive processes
- Achievement of satisfying interpersonal relationships
- Autonomy, which includes use of self-supports
- Flexibility to adapt to change

When personality growth and development go awry because of psychologic, social, cultural, or biologic influences, the person may become mentally ill. This chapter describes major mental health problems nurses are likely to encounter.

Normal Laboratory Data

Laboratory Test	Normal Adult Values
Serum tests—sequential multiple analyzer with computer (SMAC)	
Triglycerides	
Ages 1-29 yr	10-140 mg/100 ml
Ages 30-39 yr	10-150 mg/100 ml
Glucose	80-120 mg/100 ml
Carbon dioxide (CO_2)	22-34 mEq/L
Calcium (Ca)	4.5-5.5 mg/100 ml
Chloride (Cl)	100-108 mEq/L
Potassium (K)	3.5-5 mEq/L
Sodium (Na)	135-145 mEq/L
Phosphorus (P)	3-4.5 mg/100 ml
Creatine phosphokinase (CPK)	
Males	23-99 U/L
Females	15-57 U/L
Lactic dehydrogenase (LDH)	48-115 IU/L (total)
Serum glutamic oxaloacetic transaminase (SGOT)	5-40 U/ml (Frankel)
Serum glutamic pyruvic transaminase (SGPT)	5-35 U/ml (Frankel)
Alkaline phosphatase	5-13 U/100 ml (King-Armstrong units)

Laboratory Test	Normal Adult Values
Acid phosphatase	1-5 U/100 ml (King-Armstrong units)
Total protein	6-8 g/100 ml
Albumin	3.3-4.5 g/100 ml
Blood urea nitrogen (BUN)	8-20 mg/100 ml
Creatinine	0.6-1.2 mg/100 ml
Uric acid	
Males	4.3-8 mg/100 ml
Females	2.3-6 mg/100 ml
Bilirubin	
Direct	0.1-0.4 mg/100 ml
Total	0.2-0.9 mg/100 ml
Iron	
Males	80-160 μg/100 ml
Females	50-150 μg/100 ml
Urinalysis	
Color	Straw
Appearance	Clear
Specific gravity	1.005-1.030
pH	4.5-8.0
Cells and protein	None
Sugars and acetone	Negative

Conditions, Diseases, and Disorders

 Anorexia Nervosa and Bulimia Nervosa

Anorexia nervosa is a formidable disorder mainly affecting young women and characterized by a determination to lose weight despite emaciation. Bulimia nervosa is characterized by recurrent eating binges, purging, and dieting.

Although anorexia nervosa is usually viewed as an eating disorder and a distorted drive to thinness, these hallmarks are secondary to the desire to achieve a sense of control and the rejection of a mature body.[19] Afflicted persons have a history of being high achievers, compliant pleasers of others, and model children to their parents.

Eating is a source of anxiety for both anorexic and bulimic patients. Some with anorexia never engage in binge eating and purging because of their strong self-discipline; bingers are more impulsive and unable to maintain the strict self-control. The purging behaviors (self-induced vomiting often more than once a day, misuse of diuretics, and overuse of laxatives) are less pervasive in anorexics than bulimics. Anorexics, whether or not they binge, are likely to become emaciated, whereas bulimics are usually nearer their normal weight. Bulimics are more outgoing and sensitive to others and less likely to reject their mature-appearing bodies and feminine roles than the more ascetic anorexics.[19,39]

As the disorders develop, personal relationships tend to become more superficial and distant. Social contacts are avoided because of the fear of being invited to eat and being discovered; purging is also performed out of view of others. The patients are preoccupied with food, meal planning (especially for others), their own caloric intake throughout the day, and methods to avoid eating. Eating—whether it is normal, in tiny quantities, or as much as 20,000 calories—becomes a private endeavor rather than a socially enjoyable activity. The "model child" becomes defiant, aggressive, and irritable when the pattern becomes well ingrained.

Severe physiologic complications result from nutritional deficits and binge-purge behaviors. Some of them are bradycardia, arrhythmia, hypotension, renal changes such as elevated blood urea nitrogen and reduced glomerular filtration rate, electrolyte imbalance such as hypokalemia and hypochloremic alkalosis, and neurologic complications such as convulsions. A decrease in gonadotropins leads to amenorrhea in women and reduced testosterone in men. Skeletal maturation is delayed when anorexia nervosa is tenaciously maintained. A mortality of 5% to 18% is associated with this eating disorder.[1,19,39]

Researchers have limited data on the biochemical factors that may predispose individuals to these disorders. Some of these factors include the neurotransmitters (such as dopamine and serotonin) that increase or inhibit food intake.[28] It is unknown whether these disturbances in the neurotransmitters and other hormonal and neuroendocrinologic abnormalities reflect an underlying biologic pathology or are secondary to the eating disorders.

Anorexia nervosa should be differentiated from other mental disorders such as depression, schizophrenia, hysteria, and obsessive-compulsive disorders. In these disorders weight loss occurs because of lack of interest in food or delusions, not because of a fundamental drive for thinness. Physiologic diseases also need to be differentiated from anorexia nervosa on the basis of a thorough history and physical examination. Such conditions include chronic wasting owing to tumors and hypothalamic diseases and endocrine disorders such as hyperthyroidism, diabetes mellitus, and Addison's disease. An anorexic person does not consult a physician with complaints of weight loss but for treatment of amenorrhea, gastrointestinal disturbances, and disturbances in sleep and concentration. Occasionally she seeks help for emotional disturbances.

Prevalence

The estimated incident range for anorexia nervosa is 1 in 800 to 1 in 100 among adolescents. Approximately 95% are female. The enormous increased rate in incidence especially in the last decade may be partly due to greater medical and public awareness of the disorder. Bulimia nervosa is more difficult to identify in the population because the bulimic person seldom loses more than 20% of her ideal body weight and because it is more possible to hide bingeing and purging behaviors than severely anorexic behavior. When restrictive criteria for the diagnosis (such as purging at least once per week) are used, it has been estimated that 1% to 5% of women and less than 1% of men are bulimic.[1,39]

Population at Risk

The onset of anorexia nervosa ranges from prepuberty to middle age. The incidence is greatest between 12 and 22 years of age and is increasing in older age groups. Until 1976 the disorder was seen almost exclusively in the upper social classes, but it is now observed almost equally in all socioeconomic levels. Recently anorexia has appeared in blacks, mainly from upper-class professional families. A high incidence is observed among models and dancers, especially ballerinas.[19,39]

Hospitalization

Hospitalization is recommended when a person with anorexia nervosa or bulimia evidences severe medical complications such as weight loss of more than 20% of normal body weight and electrolyte and acid-base imbalances resulting from endless cycles of starvation and binge-purges. The patient may continue to deny any physical dangers and need for hospitalization even when emaciated. The fear of losing control looms large in her mind. To decrease resistance, the protective nature of and reasons for hospitalization should be emphasized.

The patient needs to believe that the staff is interested in helping her deal with other areas of her life in addition to her weight. Although steady weight gains are essential before psychotherapy can be initiated, the patient needs to feel supported and nurtured by staff from the beginning. Development of a safe, trusting relationship within a consistently supportive environment provides the patient with a sense of security.

The patient's cooperation may be gained by involving her in the treatment plan and criteria for discharge. Weight gain to 80% of ideal body weight, or stabilization of weight for a nonemaciated patient, should be part of the discharge criteria.

If weight gain does not occur and eating is resisted, nasogastric tube feeding may be prescribed. High-protein and high-calorie feedings are instilled by tube every hour. If the patient begins to drink the liquid diet, tube feedings may be discontinued.[19,28] Daily weight gains of ¼ to ½ pound are generally expected for the emaciated patient, and weight stabilization without gorging-purging behavior is expected for the bulimic patient.

A dietitian is involved in the treatment to discuss food preferences, teach nutrition, and plan a well-balanced diet for the patient. Food intake is limited to regular meals and prescribed snacks, and the family is prohibited from bringing food in and visiting or calling during mealtimes. Close supervision of meals is necessary initially, with a nurse in attendance to monitor food intake. Obsessional discussions of food and power struggles about eating should be avoided. The nurse should be cognizant of the patient's anxiety about eating and weight gain; reassurance that weight gain is being controlled to prevent obesity is vital. Assisting the patient to interpret weight gain or stabilization of weight as a sign of being in control can decrease her sense of powerlessness and lack of control.

The nurse should challenge the patient's misconceptions about her illness and herself by questioning her assumptions and irrational conclusions. As the relationship develops, the nurse helps the patient increase her self-awareness and self-acceptance by encouraging her to clarify her own thinking and trust her own thought processes and self-evaluations.

Since parents may convey to an adolescent daughter that her growing maturity is a threat to the family system, they should be included in the therapy. Goals of family therapy are to decrease patterns of overinvolvement within the family and to strengthen the marital relationship. The therapist encourages new interactional patterns by having each family member accept responsibility for his or her own perceptions and behaviors, listen and respond to messages, and participate in the resolution of conflict.

Psychopathology

Psychoanalytic Theory

Psychoanalytic theorists view anorexia nervosa and bulimia as oral fixations in which eating disturbances and gastrointestinal disturbances can be traced to infancy.[19] Affected persons had anxious, compulsive mothers and continue to have disturbed mother-child relationships.

Oral fixation is the persistent concentration of psychic energy on the objects of the infant developmental phase. The focus is on taking in or spitting out, as evidenced by overeating, rejecting food, smoking excessively, vomiting, and oral conceptions of sexuality. These individuals may hold ascetic views, believing self-indulgence in eating and other behaviors to be sinful and starvation to be superior and saintly.

Interpersonal Theory

Interpersonal theorists believe that anorexia arises because of family relationships. They view the family as an emotionally closed system that "traps" members in intense relationships with one another. Individual ego boundaries and identities of members are blurred. By focusing on the child, parents avoid dealing with their own tensions and conflicts. As the child moves into adolescence and begins to seek independence and autonomy, the parents are unwilling to give up their accustomed pathologic interpersonal patterns of behavior. They become more overcontrolling and demanding, which foils the adolescent's efforts to achieve autonomy.

The parents expect selfless conformity from the child but are emotionally inaccessible; they demand that the child deny and mistrust perceptions that are incongruent with theirs. As the adolescent responds to the parents by offering support and strength, she perceives herself as loved for what she gives rather than for herself. She overorganizes her life to become perfect in her parents' eyes and to assume responsibility for her own physical and emotional safety. These dynamics within the family prohibit maturation of the adolescent to maintain the family's status quo.[57]

Although family characteristics predispose to the development of anorexia, environmental, constitutional, and psychologic factors also enter into the determination of whether a person develops this eating disorder.

Cognitive Theory

Cognitive and behavioral theorists say that the behaviors of the anorexic person are learned. The glorification of thinness in Western society results in attempts to conform to cultural ideals of physical appearance. Thinness is equated with self-control, beauty, and success. Models resembling prepubertal girls in high-fashion magazines are considered elegant beauties. These magazines and other media bombard women with reduction diets, exercises, and recipes.

The preanorexic, who may or may not be slightly overweight, is told by parents, teachers, or friends that she would look much better if she lost a little weight. The positive reinforcement she receives for dieting and losing weight and the pleasure she experiences in her new shape encourage her to lose more. If she happens to eat more than she deems correct, she learns from peers to purge her body by vomiting and misusing laxatives and diuretics. The elation of controlling caloric intake and losing weight leads her to compete with others to be the thinnest in her peer group. She devotes herself to activities related to food, weight, and exercise, with no time or energy left for social relationships and activities. The young woman's perceptions of her body size and self-appraisals are distorted so that low self-worth is related to fatness, and high self-worth to thinness.[21]

Diagnostic Studies and Findings

Serum Test

Sequential multiple analyzer with computer (SMAC); if electrolyte and acid-base values are abnormal, repeat once a day until stable

Electrocardiography

To rule out cardiopathy

Urinalysis

To screen for urinary and systemic abnormalities

Medical Plan

Medications

Doxepin (Sinequan, Adapin), 25 mg bid and hs to decrease anxiety and depression related to eating and sense of lack of control

General Management

Diet

Consultation with dietitian; high-protein and high-calorie diet; for severely emaciated client, 1200-calorie diet gradually increased to 3000-calorie diet

Occupational therapy

Recreational therapy

NURSING CARE

Nursing Assessment

Signs and symptoms of anorexia and bulimia vary from individual to individual; no one experiences all of those listed.

Emotional

Anxiety; depression; lability of mood; irritability; anger

Thought Processes

Denial of hunger; fear of eating and weight gain; mistrust of self and others; low self-esteem; shame at being discovered bingeing and purging; sense of failure even when successful; perfectionism; rejection of feminine role; fear of psychosexual maturation; fear of physical changes, especially the development of secondary sexual traits; lack of interest in sex and opposite sex; impairment in concentration

Power and Control

Powerlessness; struggle for control; helplessness; nonassertiveness

Body Image

Denial of thinness or emaciated appearance; rejection of feminine body; self-loathing; delusions about body size

Fluid Volume

Decreased fluid intake; excessive loss of fluids through (1) induced vomiting (possibly 18 times a day) with finger, toothbrush, or use of emetics such as Ipecac, especially after eating, (2) diarrhea caused by laxatives (up to 50 a day), or (3) diuretics; altered electrolytes such as hypokalemia or hypochloremic alkalosis; muscle weakness; convulsions or muscle tetany; altered kidney function such as elevated blood urea nitrogen; altered cardiac function such as bradycardia or arrhythmias

Skin Integrity

Skeletal prominence; bruised skin; altered circulation with cyanosis of extremities; dry, cracked skin; loss of scalp hair; lanugo on cheeks, neck, forearms, and thighs; peripheral edema; delayed skeletal maturation related to duration of emaciation

Sleep Patterns

Disturbances in sleeping such as insomnia, early morning wakening, and restlessness

Nutrition

Fasting; starvation diet; bingeing (up to 20,000 calories a day with average of 5000); aversion to eating; weight loss to 20% of normal body weight and occasionally to 50%; frequent checking of weight, such as 10 times a day; nausea; bloating of abdomen; grossly distended stomach and duodenum because of bingeing; disposing of meals by feeding to dog and placing in garbage or toilet; hiding food for binges; eating secretly; amenorrhea; esophageal abrasions from vomiting; dental caries, loss of teeth, and buccal erosion because of hydrochloric acid from stomach; diarrhea; constipation; abdominal pain

Social Activities

Sense of social inadequacy and ineffectiveness; insecurity; withdrawal from social relations to isolation; fear of interpersonal closeness

Family Processes

Fear of abandonment and engulfment; overinvolvement of parents; overprotectiveness or lack of protectiveness by parents; denial of family conflict

Nursing Dx & Intervention

Nursing care should be implemented selectively based on severity and type of symptoms and behaviors.

Nursing Diagnosis	Nursing Intervention/Rationale
Anxiety	• Assess for severity of anxiety and events that evoke anxiety. • Begin to develop safe, trusting relationship with patient *to promote security.* Continue to develop relationship through working and termination phases. • Explain treatment plan explicitly *to allay anxiety and decrease resistance.* Review plan with the patient at regular intervals. • Assist patient to identify feelings such as anxiety and to begin to express her emotions *to affirm her right to feelings including anger.* • As patient begins to gain weight or stabilize her weight, help her deal with anxiety (which sometimes reaches panic level). Remain with patient (especially when eating) and teach slow, deep relaxation breathing *to decrease anxiety.* Reinforce relaxation technique. • Administer medication as prescribed. Explain purpose of medication and its effects and side effects *to increase compliance with treatment.*
Ineffective individual coping	• Assess previous coping skills for dealing with events and relationships. • Assist patient to identify emotions that precede bingeing and past alternatives to bingeing or fasting. • Assist patient to identify and participate in healthy coping strategies—such as relaxation techniques, reinterpretation of thoughts and emotions, problem solving, and diversionary activities (watching television, talking to a friend, reading)—*to develop alternatives to dysfunctional eating.* • If patient denies she has eating problem, encourage her to examine difficulties in other areas of life and eventually to relate these to preoccupations with eating *to deal with less anxiety-provoking areas than eating.* • Begin to help patient identify fears associated with starving, bingeing, and purging *to eventually identify issues dealing with loss of control.* • Correct misconceptions about bingeing-purging behaviors; for example, laxatives will not prevent absorption of calories. Teach patient to use problem-solving approach *to examine issues, and to assess possible consequences of choices.* • Encourage patient to implement and evaluate new behaviors *to determine appropriateness of choices.* • Teach patient how to get needs met by herself *to develop self-support* and how to ask others to meet her needs rather than meeting only theirs. • Begin to assist patient to identify and reinforce strengths. Help patient assess abilities and accomplishments realistically using problem-solving approach. Encourage acceptance of abilities and choices patient makes *to begin to feel positive about herself and to develop realistic self-expectations, including an acceptance of limitations and mediocre performance.*

Nursing Diagnosis	Nursing Intervention/Rationale
Altered nutrition: less than body requirements	• Assess patient's eating pattern and food preferences. • Have dietitian discuss nutritional plan and rationale, as well as body's nutritional needs. Teach importance of well-balanced diet that contains wide variety of foods. Encourage patient as able to assume responsibility for planning well-balanced meals *to increase sense of control.* • If patient has been on starvation diet, be alert for gastric dilation if refeeding is rapid. *To prevent this,* 1200- to 1500-calorie, well-balanced diet, sometimes divided into more than three feedings, may be prescribed initially. • Teach patient to eat slowly *to taste and enjoy food.* • *To allow more supervision,* have patient eat alone rather than in unit dining room. When patient develops control over eating, encourage eating in dining room with others. • *To prevent vomiting* permit patient's use of bathroom only if accompanied by staff for 1 to 2 hours after eating. • Explain nasogastric feedings and rationale in matter-of-fact yet sensitive, supportive manner. (Nasogastric feedings may be prescribed if patient does not gain or electrolyte balance is viewed as unsafe.) After each instillation of high-protein, high caloric fluid (such as Isocal), observe patient for at least 30 minutes *to prevent vomiting.* If patient is willing, allow drinking of feeding instead of instilling in tube. • Inform patient that abdominal discomfort or bloating will be experienced with increased food intake and that symptoms will disappear. • *To allay patient's fears of becoming obese,* inform her that uncontrolled weight gain is not the goal. With assistance of dietitian, teach patient weight-maintenance diet. • Explain that, as caloric intake is increased, the amount will not make patient fat *to assure her that metabolism is slowed as protective mechanism during a starvation diet.* • Avoid getting into obsessional discussions of food and diet with patient. Avoid casual conversation about your eating preferences and habits. • Avoid power struggles over food *to prevent reenactment of food struggles at home.* • Encourage good oral hygiene *to prevent oral disease from vomiting and malnutrition.* • Begin to help patient identify role low weight plays in patient's life (for example, as way of avoiding dealing with frightening adolescent issues). Continue to explore meaning of weight loss, expectation and reality of weight loss, and restrictions in areas of life resulting from preoccupation with food *to increase self-awareness.* • Monitor patient's weight as prescribed, possibly daily, but prevent patient from indiscriminate frequent self-weighing. Remain nonjudgmental about weight gains and losses. (Weight monitoring will continue with less frequency.)
Body image disturbance	• Assess patient's feeling about self and body. • Encourage patient to wear loose clothing *to avoid focus on body size and weight gain.* Encourage patient to give "skinny" wardrobe away *to avoid longing for thinness and relapsing.* Suggest new life-style for patient in nonthreatening way. • Begin to correct patient's distorted perceptions about body size. Assist patient to perceive body size correctly and accept appearance. • Encourage patient to accept positive self-appraisals and take pride in appearance. • As patient gains more mature-appearing body, explore meanings of sexuality and feminine role *to assist in dealing with sexual identity issues including menses.* Encourage self-acceptance.
Potential fluid volume deficit	• Assess and monitor fluid intake and output because of dieting and purging behavior. • Maintain adequate hydration. • Monitor vital signs as prescribed and as deemed advisable. • Administer replacement fluids and electrolytes such as potassium if indicated and as prescribed *to correct or prevent electrolyte imbalances as evidenced from blood work and from such symptoms as bradycardia, arrhythmias, weakness, and elevated temperature.* • Limit physical activity initially *to decrease stress on body,* such as stress on cardiac function when arrhythmias and muscle weakness are present.
Potential impaired skin integrity	• Assess patient's skin condition as affected by altered nutritional state. Teach patient that skin conditions such as bruises, loss of scalp hair, lanugo, and dry skin are related to malnutrition. • Encourage good skin hygiene. Instruct patient to use body lotion *to alleviate dry skin.* • Attend to skin lesions and bruises as indicated *to prevent infection.*
Powerlessness related to life-style of helplessness	• Assess patient's sense of lack of control about treatment plan and sense of helplessness in relation to her life. • Convey to patient that treatment plan is developed *to help and protect and not to control her.* • Encourage patient, when able, to make decisions about her treatment regimen *to provide a sense of control and to increase self-confidence.*

Nursing Diagnosis	Nursing Intervention/Rationale
	• Begin to teach patient how to become assertive with others and, as able, with parents. Emphasize that patient can assume responsibility for herself and that she is not responsible for others' happiness or discomfort. • Help patient to practice assertiveness skills and critique them together *to learn how to assess her behavior realistically.* • Help patient identify her wants and choose not to binge or starve. • Teach patient to function in ambiguous situations *to learn how to deal with conflict and unclear situations*—for example, by negotiating, assessing importance of issue, or clarifying issue with others.
Constipation	• Assess frequency and consistency of stools and use of medications including laxatives. • If patient is accustomed to laxative abuse, provide high-fiber diet and adequate fluid intake *to prevent constipation.* • Administer a laxative or enema as prescribed for reduced bowel activity because of laxative abuse. • Teach methods for adequate elimination, such as diet, fluid intake, and proper exercise. (See also p. 1662.)
Sleep pattern disturbance	• After assessing patient's sleep pattern, explore methods that have been conducive to sleep in past *to reinforce healthy methods.* • If applicable, explain that malnourishment contributes to sleep disturbances. • Teach relaxation routines that promote sleep, including warm baths, quiet activities such as reading and watching television, and breathing techniques.
Social isolation	• Assess patient's level of social isolation and circumstances related to discomfort with others. • As medical condition stabilizes, suggest that patient participate in activities with other patients. • Encourage occupational therapy *to develop skills such as crafts and sewing.* • Encourage development of enjoyable minor personal activities *to replace focus on exceptional ones.* • Encourage recreational therapy such as group games and participation in graded exercise program. • Assist patient to deal with free periods *to learn to enjoy relaxing times.* • Assist patient to identify and discuss discomfort in social interactions. • Encourage patient to assess social interactions and to pursue satisfying ones. • Emphasize personal satisfaction in social interactions and activities rather than perfectionism. • Encourage patient, as able, to initiate contact with friends *to engage in activities patient enjoys with friends.*
Altered family processes	• Assess family's knowledge of eating disorder and interaction patterns with patient. • Discourage family from discussing patient's dietary intake, bringing in food, or phoning during mealtimes *to avoid power struggles about eating.* • Assist parents to understand illness without blaming each other. • In family sessions help parents and patient become aware of parents' overprotectiveness and overinvolvement. • Begin to help family members alter their interactional patterns—for example, by speaking for self only and not for others and by responding to one another's messages *to foster relationships that encourage autonomy of family members.*

Patient Education

1. Reinforce the use of problem-solving technique to correct misconceptions of self and performance.
2. Teach planning of well-balanced weight-maintenance diet.
3. Reinforce compliance with the medical regimen.
4. Teach assertiveness skills.
5. Reinforce the need for continued psychotherapy.

Evaluation

Patient Outcome	Data Indicating That Outcome is Reached
Patient establishes normal eating habits and achieves increased sense of self-control.	Patient participates actively in making decisions about treatment plans. Patient makes decision not to binge or starve. Patient views weight-maintenance diet as evidence of self-control. Patient states that preoccupation with food has diminished. Patient identifies and accepts relationships between preoccupation with eating and problems in other areas of life.
Patient achieves weight gain or weight stabilization near ideal body weight.	Patient perceives body size accurately and states acceptance of more mature-appearing body. Patient makes plans to engage in new life-style without continual concerns about losing weight.
Patient implements problem-solving approach to dealing with issues.	Patient practices problem-solving approach in dealing with issues such as feminine role, sexuality, and control. Patient develops more realistic expectations for self and performance.
Patient demonstrates ease in interpersonal relationships by assertive behaviors and ability to initiate interactions with others.	Patient practices assertiveness when interacting with family and friends. Patient verbalizes increased self-confidence during interactions with family. Patient initiates and engages in relaxing activities with friends and family. Patient verbalizes awareness and increased acceptance of her own needs and wants.
Patient makes plans to continue treatment after discharge.	Patient states actions of medicine and plans to self-administer medicine as ordered. Patient schedules appointment to continue counseling after discharge.

PSYCHOACTIVE SUBSTANCE USE DISORDER

Psychoactive substance use disorders are those in which maladaptive behaviors result from regular use of mood-altering chemical substances that affect the central nervous system and adversely affect health.

Such substances include depressants, stimulants, hallucinogens, and analgesics. Some substances, such as alcohol, over-the-counter drugs, and medically prescribed drugs, are obtained legally; others, such as cocaine and marijuana, are obtained illicitly.

Substance use disorders are divided into two general classes: *psychoactive substance abuse* and *psychoactive substance dependence*. Psychoactive substance abuse is the pathologic use of mood-altering chemicals that continues for at least 1 month and often impairs work or social functioning. Psychoactive substance dependence is a more severe form of chemical use that involves an impaired ability to control use and has adverse consequences when the dosage is reduced or discontinued.[1] Excessive time and energy are spent obtaining the substance and recovering from the consequences with an inability to fulfill social and occupational responsibilities. Dependence, which may be mild to severe or in remission, is evidenced by tolerance for the chemical and/or withdrawal symptoms when the drug is discontinued.[1]

Types of dependence on chemicals include the following[62]:

Tolerance. Drug dosage must be increased progressively to reproduce the original physical and psychologic effects.

Physiologic dependence. Physiologic changes that occur with repeated use result in withdrawal symptoms when the dose is reduced or discontinued abruptly.

Psychologic dependence. Feelings of pleasure and satisfaction are experienced with drug use. These produce intense cravings for repetitive use of the substance.

Psychoactive substance abuse and dependence most commonly begin during adolescence and young adulthood. Persons between 18 and 25 years of age are the heaviest users of illegal chemicals.[8] Vulnerability to abuse is greater among the drugs that have the greatest addictive power (such as cocaine, heroin, and morphine) than the least addictive drugs (such as caffeine and nicotine). However, the least addictive chemicals can also become severe problems.[31] The reasons for becoming involved with chemical substances are many and include influence of peers, rebellion against parents and society, and attempts to bolster self-esteem. Most young adults are able to discontinue use as they take on the responsibilities of adulthood, but some may become chronic abusers.

Substance abuse and dependence or addiction may also be associated with relief of pain, especially among immature, easily frustrated persons, those with psychic disorders, and those with countercultural life-styles. Viewing substances as a way for coping with life stresses and experiences is one factor in continued abuse.[1,9]

Since chemical substances affect the central nervous system, abuse may cause transient or permanent brain dysfunction and other physical illnesses. Deterioration of physical health is caused in part to inadequate diet, poor personal hygiene, and inattention to physical disorders. Infections such as hepatitis and septicemia can occur when substances are administered with contaminated needles. In addition, the transmission of autoimmune deficiency syndrome (AIDS) via intravenous injections of drugs has become an increasing threat to substance users. Since the potency and purity of illicitly obtained substances are often unknown, fatal overdoses and toxic reactions occur.[9,62]

The mood-altering effects of substances may cause erratic, impulsive, and irresponsible behavior. Relationships with family and friends become disturbed and are sometimes severed. The alcohol or drug habit may drain the financial resources of the person's family. The person may also engage in criminal behaviors to support the use of substances or violate laws when in an intoxicated alcohol or drug state (for example, causing an automobile accident).

Changes in occupational and scholastic functioning occur with substance abuse. The person loses interest in job or school activities, fails to strive to achieve, and is less able to perform tasks.[1,9]

Table 17-1 lists some commonly used types of chemical

Table 17-1
Effects of Intoxication and Withdrawal of Substances

Drug	Usual Route of Administration	Use
Opiates		
Opium	Oral; sniffed; smoked	Analgesic, antidiarrheal
Morphine	Oral; injected	Analgesic
Diacetylmorphine (heroin)	Injected; sniffed; smoked	Analgesic (illegal)
Hydromorphone (Dilaudid)	Oral; injected	Analgesic
Meperidine (Demerol)	Oral; injected	Analgesic
Propoxyphene (Darvon)	Oral; injected	Analgesic
Codeine	Oral; injected	Analgesic; antitussive
Methadone	Oral; injected	Detoxification of opiates
Depressants		
Alcoholic beverages (e.g., liquor, beer, wine)	Oral	Tension relief; analgesic
Sedative-hypnotics		
Barbiturates		Anesthetic; anticonvulsant; sleep
Amobarbital (Amytal)	Oral; injected	
Secobarbital (Seconal)	Oral; injected	
Pentobarbital (Nembutal)	Oral; injected	
Other		
Meprobamate (Equinal, Miltown)	Oral	Anti-anxiety; sedation
Diazepam (Valium)	Oral; injected	Anti-anxiety; anticonvulsant
Glutethimide (Doriden)	Oral	Hypnotic
Chloral hydrate (Noctec and others)	Oral	Hypnotic
Stimulants		
Cocaine	Oral; smoked; sniffed; injected	Local anesthetic
Amphetamine (Benzedrine, Dexedrine)	Oral; injected	Narcolepsy; attention deficit disorder; weight control
Methylphenidate (Ritalin)	Oral	Attention deficit disorder with hyperactivity
Phenmetrazine (Preludin)	Oral	Weight control
Hallucinogens		
Lysergic acid diethylamide (LSD)	Oral	None
Phencyclidine (PCP)	Oral; smoked; injected	Animal tranquilizer
Mescaline	Oral	None
Psilocybin	Oral	None
Cannabis sativa		
Marijuana, hashish	Oral; smoked	Stimulant and sedative (illegal drug)

substances, their uses, and intoxication and withdrawal effects.[1,9,62]

Between 5% and 10% of the employed population in the United States suffer from alcoholism with an estimated 13% of adults having abused alcohol at some period of their lives. An estimated 3% to 7% of the employed use some type of illicit drug.[1,48] The annual cost for health care, absences from work, and decreased productivity of workers related to alcohol and drugs is approximately $70 billion. Almost half of work fatalities and injuries are due to alcohol abuse.[48] At least half of automobile accidents involve alcohol use by the driver or a pedestrian. Aside from the damage the alcohol does to the one who abuses it, family stresses with marital and family dysfunction occur.

Intoxication Effect	Withdrawal Effect
Euphoria with tranquility; emotional lability; drowsiness; clouding of consciousness; psychomotor retardation; slow, shallow respiration; constricted pupils; decreased muscle tone; with circulatory collapse and cyanosis, dilated pupils; coma; possible death	Runny nose; watery eyes; severe anxiety to panic; gooseflesh; hot and cold flashes; yawning; irritability; loss of appetite; muscle cramps; tremors; nausea and vomiting; tachycardia; hypertension; increased respirations and temperature; insomnia; after 24 hours diarrhea and dehydration; symptoms peak 48 to 72 hours after last dose
Slurred speech; lack of coordination; unsteady gait; talkativeness; euphoria or depression; emotional lability; impaired attention	Hyperactivity; tremors; psychomotor agitation; hypertension; tachycardia; irritability or depression; impaired attention and memory; illusions (misinterpretation of stimuli); hallucinations, auditory or visual; disorientation; delusions; delirium; orthostatic hypotension; convulsions
Slurred speech; irritability; impaired attention, memory, and judgment; emotional lability; talkativeness; lack of coordination; confusion; tremors; cold, clammy skin; dilated pupils (with barbiturates, constricted pupils)	Nausea and vomiting; weakness; hypertension; tachycardia; orthostatic hypotension; gross tremors; agitation; disorientation; anxiety; nightmares; visual hallucinations; hyperthermia; delirium; convulsions; coma
Psychomotor agitation; mood lability; hypervigilance; tachycardia; hypertension; dilated pupils; perspiration and chills; impaired judgment; psychotic symptoms; insomnia; tremors; confusion; convulsions; possible death	Fatigue; depression; disturbed sleep; apathy; cravings; possible agitation after prolonged use
Tachycardia; hypertension; hyperthermia; dilated pupils; hyperreflexia; nausea; visual hallucinations; extreme emotional lability; poor time perception; feeling of depersonalization; psychic numbness; psychosis; violent outbursts; amnesia; convulsions; possible death	None reported; flashbacks occur for 5 days and longer after use of PCP, with catalepsy, agitation, and unpredictable violent outbursts
Panic; depression; disorientation; hallucinations; delusions; flashbacks; psychotic symptoms; apathy; impaired attention and judgment	Irritability; insomnia; loss of appetite; tremors; perspiration; nausea

Alcohol abuse/alcohol dependence

***Alcohol abuse* consists of a pattern of daily intake of large amounts of alcohol. *Alcohol dependence* involves daily intake of large amounts, excessive drinking limited to weekends, or periods of abstinence with binges lasting for weeks or months.**

Tolerance and physical and psychologic dependence are experienced, usually with an unawareness of any lack of control.[1]

This discussion focuses on alcohol because it appears to be abused more than other chemicals. Use of alcohol is accepted at social gatherings and business meetings and as part of cultural and religious celebrations such as marriages and births. About 70% of the adult population consumes at least one drink during a 1-year period, but about 1 in 10 will become a problem drinker.[1,62] Among the many reasons for dependence on alcoholic beverages are stress, family- and work-related problems, economic difficulties, and feelings of social inadequacy. Some mental disorders also increase the risk for alcoholism, such as early behavioral problems in children, antisocial personality disorder in adults, and depression. In some instances, depression may be the result of alcoholism rather than its precipitant. Genetic factors have been implicated in the development of alcoholism, but the specific significance is unclear.[1,24] Alcoholism in a parent increases the risk of offspring even when the child is adopted by nonalcoholic parents. Biologic sons of parents with alcohol problems have a three to four times greater possibility of developing alcoholism than sons of nonalcoholic parents. The social constraints against alcoholism and lower tolerance level in women may account for the lower prevalence rates among this sex, although the incidence in women is rising.[24,50]

A careful assessment of the drinking patterns and use of other chemicals by all patients, including those being treated for other conditions, is essential.[47] Attention must be given to abuse of multiple drugs, since a person found to be dependent on one substance is probably also dependent on others that potentiate or inhibit the effects of the first. Although it is common for patients to deny use or minimize the amount they consume, a nonjudgmental attitude will help the nurse elicit the necessary information.

A person who drinks moderately experiences minor symptoms during the 24 hours after the last drink. These include irritability, anxiety, a slight increase in heart rate and blood pressure, gastric irritation, and restless sleep.[9,62] A person who consistently consumes large amounts of alcohol over a long period is likely to develop a more severe withdrawal syndrome characterized by agitation, tachycardia, hypertension, tremors, anorexia, abdominal cramps, insomnia, sweating, and blushing. Memory lapses (blackouts) concerning events that occurred while the person was drinking may occur. A minority of persons have seizures, typically grand mal, within 48 hours after the last drink. Delirium tremens may occur 72 to 96 hours after the person's last drink.[47] Symptoms of delirium tremens include confusion, disorientation, delirium, frightening hallucinations that are usually visual, illusions in which stimuli are misinterpreted, nightmares, diaphoresis, and elevated temperature. The mortality for persons with delirium tremens is approximately 10%; death is often caused by hyperthermia or cardiovascular collapse. If adequate preventive treatment is instituted during the early signs and symptoms of alcohol withdrawal, delirium tremens will not develop.

Some physiologic problems of chronic alcoholism are the following[62]:

- Cardiovascular system
  - Anemia
  - Hypertension
  - Tachycardia
  - Arrhythmias
  - Cardiomegaly
  - Edema
- Liver
  - Hepatomegaly
  - Edema
  - Ascites
  - Cirrhosis
- Gastrointestinal system
  - Gastritis
  - Esophagitis
  - Duodenal and gastric ulcers
  - Nausea
  - Malabsorption syndrome
  - Pancreatitis
  - Colitis
- Neurologic system
  - Fatigue
  - Depression
  - Irritability
  - Memory and learning deficits
  - Tremors
  - Polyneuropathy that typically occurs in feet first
  - Wernicke-Korsakoff syndrome
- Immune impairment and infection
- Fetal alcohol syndrome

Alcoholic Family

Family members may initially accept drinking alcoholic beverages and occasional drunkenness as normal social behavior. However, as the frequency of use increases, the problem drinking begins to have detrimental effects on the drinker and family members. The drinker's personality changes with severe mood swings, he may be arrested for driving while intoxicated, and engage in mental and physical abuse especially of family members; his employment behavior may change, with decreased productivity, frequent absences, and tardiness.[9,42] Family relationships deteriorate, and family members feel trapped between the sober and intoxication phases of the alcoholic. They experience shame, anger, confusion, and guilt. Family conversations are increasingly focused on the alcohol-dependent behavior and issues related to it. Family members unconsciously engage in enabling behaviors to protect the family reputation and keep the family secret. Such behaviors include making excuses to friends and employers, attempting to keep the alcoholic out of trouble, and sometimes buying liquor for the alcoholic. The person with a drinking problem offers alibis for his behavior or is unwilling to discuss it. If the spouse threatens to leave or no longer make excuses, the alcohol-dependent person may promise never to touch another drop. These promises are usually broken. The family may feel locked into dysfunctional behaviors or may sever their relationship with the drinker.

Chemical Dependence Among Health Professionals

Chemical dependence among health professionals such as nurses and physicians is estimated to be two to three times greater than that in the general population; yet only recently has the severity of the problem been recognized by colleagues.[41] State nurses' associations have established peer assistance programs to guide nurses into treatment and provide support during the recovery phase. These programs often depend on volunteer nurses to assist their colleagues into rehabilitation programs.[23]

Diagnostic Studies and Findings

Serum: SMAC

To screen for systemic abnormalities (see preceding page for possible pathologic conditions)

Urinalysis

To screen for urinary and systemic abnormalities

Electrocardiogram

To screen for cardiopathy

Chest Roentgenogram

To screen for pulmonary infection and cardiac disease

Medical Plan

Medications

Antianxiety agents

Diazepam (Valium), 20 mg po stat and q3h if necessary to prevent or decrease serious withdrawal symptoms of alcohol; intramuscular administration is generally avoided because of slow and erratic absorption; for elderly or adolescent, 5 mg po stat and q3h if necessary to decrease or prevent withdrawal symptoms; drug acts to reduce anxiety and seizure and promotes drowsiness and hypotension

Vitamins

Megadose, multivitamin and multimineral supplement, 1 tablet po with meals; because of malnutrition generally seen in alcoholism, improvement in nutritional status is essential

General Management

Bland diet; introduction of regular diet as able to tolerate

NURSING CARE

Nursing Assessment

Emotional

Anxiety; emotional lability; depression

Thoughts

Denial of alcoholism; guilt; shame; sense of inadequacy; impairment of judgment and memory; suicide ideation (correlation exists between alcoholism and suicide)

Physical

Type of drinking pattern established; duration and amount of last alcohol consumed; irritability to psychomotor agitation; demanding behavior; memory lapses (blackouts); tachycardia; hypertension; increased respirations; tremors; fatigue; nausea and vomiting; anorexia; abdominal cramps; insomnia; elevated temperature; illusions; hallucinations (most frequently visual, sometimes auditory); seizure potential

Social and Occupational

Argumentativeness with family, friends, and co-workers; aggressiveness with others; tardiness at work; work absences because of "not feeling well"; sensitivity to criticism; mistakes at work

Nursing Dx & Intervention

Nursing Diagnosis	Nursing Intervention/Rationale
Patient problem: alcohol withdrawal	• Assess time and amount of the last alcohol consumed and kinds of other chemicals used; assess for potential seizures, such as tremors, elevated vital signs, and agitation. • Minimize the number of people attending the patient *to prevent excitement;* provide quiet environment *to decrease stimuli and decrease possibility of agitation, anxiety, and belligerence resulting from CNS stimulation in withdrawal.* • Administer diazepam as needed and in collaboration with the physician *to prevent agitation and seizures* (because of patient's tolerance to sedative effects of alcohol, larger doses are needed than for nonalcoholic patients). • Briefly explain effects of medicine • Evaluate effects of medicine. • Provide physical protection in bed as needed, such as side rails and mechanical restraints *to protect patient from harm.* • If suicidal ideation exists, assess its seriousness. See also the discussion of suicide for nursing intervention. • Maintain light in the room, especially at night, *to decrease the possibility of misinterpreting environmental stimuli.*
Fluid volume excess	• Assess and record fluid intake and output. • Avoid forcing fluids *to prevent overhydration,* since alcohol initially exerts antidiuretic effect. • Monitor blood pressure, pulse, and respirations hourly or more often if needed, until stable *to detect increases resulting from agitation and other complications of withdrawal.* • Monitor temperature every 4 hours *to detect signs of infection.* • Observe for infection (for instance, respiratory) resulting from low resistance.
Impaired physical mobility related to perceptual and cognitive impairment	• Assess orientation and motor stability. • Maintain bed rest until patient is cognitively oriented and physically stable and vital signs are normal *to prevent patient from falling.* • Assist patient to ambulate as needed and when permitted.
Bathing/hygiene self-care deficit	• Assess abilities to participate in self-care activities. • Assist patient with bathing and personal hygiene as needed *to promote comfort.* • Observe for infections, bruises, and broken skin when providing care *to prevent or treat skin lesions or infections.*
Altered nutrition: less than body requirements	• Assess nutritional intake. • Help to ensure adequate nutritional diet in collaboration with the physician and dietitian *to counteract the effects of inadequate diet and malabsorption of nutrients.* • Offer bland food for gastric distress. Antacids may be prescribed *to decrease distress.* • Administer vitamin as ordered with meal *to decrease nutritional deficits.* • Teach patient essentials of nutritionally balanced diet and importance of compliance *to prevent or alleviate malnutrition.*
Ineffective individual coping	• Assess types of situations or interactions in which patient resorts to alcohol. Assess other coping strategies. • Establish supportive, nonjudgmental relationship *to promote a decrease in the sense of guilt.* • Assist patient to identify feelings of anxiety and relate them to stress-producing situations. • Help patient identify healthy methods for coping with anxiety instead of relying on alcohol. Methods include problem solving, relaxation techniques (such as slow, deep breathing), and diversionary activities (such as physical exercise and watching television). • Teach assertiveness skills and evaluation of effects of skills *to increase self-esteem.* • Encourage patient to learn to ask for support and to deal with positive and negative responses. • Assist the patient in developing skills to refuse alcohol in social situations *to help in learning to socialize without the use of alcohol.* Refer patient to Alcoholics Anonymous *to obtain support for nondrinking behavior and prevent relapse.* • Correct patient's misconceptions about physiologic, psychologic, and social effects of alcohol. • Encourage patient to examine consequences of drinking behavior on self, family, and social and work functioning and to identify alternative behaviors *to increase patient's sense of adequacy when engaged in nondestructive behaviors.*
Altered family processes	• Assess family's knowledge of patient's alcoholism and enabling behaviors. • Assist patient and family members to identify expectations of one another within the family and their willingness to meet these expectations.

Nursing Diagnosis	Nursing Intervention/Rationale
	• Assist each to listen and respond to the others and to learn to compromise on or negotiate differences. • Begin to teach family members not to blame themselves *to prevent them from believing they caused the abuse.* • Refer family for counseling if indicated. • Suggest attendance at Al-Anon for spouse and Alateen for children *to deal with painful feelings such as a false sense of guilt, rage, and disloyalty.*

Patient Education

1. Reinforce healthy coping behaviors for dealing with anxiety.
2. Teach the use of self-support and support from others.
3. Reinforce the importance of a nutritionally balanced diet.
4. Teach the patient to accept responsibility for his own behavior and sobriety.

Evaluation

Patient Outcome	Data Indicating That Outcome is Reached
Recovery from withdrawal symptoms of alcohol is uncomplicated.	Vital signs are stable. Patient performs self-care activities. Patient responds appropriately to people and other stimuli. Patient eats regular, well-balanced meals.
Patient demonstrates knowledge of adverse effects of alcohol.	Patient describes physiologic effects of prolonged alcoholism. Patient discusses psychologic effects of alcohol. Patient discusses social effects of alcohol on self and others.
Patient is aware of alternative behaviors for coping with stress-producing situations.	Patient practices relaxation techniques and engages in physical exercise. Patient practices assertiveness skills and evaluates their effects on self and others. Patient practices refusal of alcoholic beverages in social situations.
Patient demonstrates ability to obtain support from family and others.	Patient verbalizes awareness of needs and is able to ask for support. Patient listens and responds to family members. Patient contacts Alcoholics Anonymous and begins to attend meetings.

Cocaine abuse/cocaine dependence

Cocaine abuse and cocaine dependence are the use of any of several different types of preparations from the coca plant, which is a highly addictive illicit psychoactive substance.

Although classified as a narcotic, cocaine is an amphetamine-like stimulant.[1,4] Cocaine abuse is a pathologic pattern of use that impairs psychologic, social, and occupational functioning; cocaine dependence is associated with progressive tolerance (requiring increasing doses to produce the pleasurable effect) with persistent cravings for the substance. Whether physiologic dependence exists is still controversial because it does not produce the severe withdrawal symptoms experienced with other substances; however, psychologic addiction is extremely high because of euphoric effects and strong cravings for the substance. One pattern of use is episodic: several days of nonuse are interspersed with use of sometimes high doses in a single 48-hour period. Another pattern is chronic or almost daily use, when low or high doses are used on successive days.

Depending on the type of preparation, cocaine may be chewed, smoked, inhaled, or injected intravenously. Since the mid-1980s, crack, a highly purified, concentrated cocaine alkaloid, has become the drug of choice because of its availability and popularity.[4] It is a white, rock-hard substance prepared from cocaine hydrochloride powder and is smoked, usually in a water pipe, or inhaled. When it is smoked or inhaled as crack, the effects are more immediate and intense than the euphoria of intravenous cocaine and is therefore the most addictive form. The immediate euphoria is short lived, lasting for a few minutes to about 30 minutes followed by extreme depression, which creates the compulsion to use it again to regain the pleasurable feelings.

Polydrug abuse must be considered, since other drugs—such as alcohol, marijuana, and opiates such as heroin—are also used in combination with cocaine. These other substances are sometimes used to relieve the agitation, insomnia, and depression associated with cocaine or to prolong its euphoric effects.

Aside from the euphoria in which feelings of inferiority disappear, other effects of the drug are psychomotor agitation, confusion, anxiety, paranoid ideation, impaired judgment, and impaired social or occupational functioning. Physiologic symptoms include headache, tachycardia, palpitations, hypertension, tremors, pupillary dilation, diaphoresis or chills, and nausea. Especially with high doses, the person may experience chest pain, convulsions, small strokes that cause brain damage from high blood pressure, myocardial infarctions, and death, often from cardiac arrhythmias or respiratory paralysis. Lethal convulsions can occur within 1 hour after use.[4,54]

Because the quality and purity of the cocaine are often unknown, serious consequences are possible. Some medical problems from contaminated needles used for intravenous administration are hepatitis, skin infections, septicemia, and acquired immune deficiency syndrome (AIDS). Snorting or inhaling cocaine injures nasal mucous membrane with ulceration and bleeding, and when minute particles of cocaine remain on nasal tissue, erosion of the nasal septum may occur, requiring surgical repair. Damage to the vocal cords with permanent hoarseness and lung impairment occur when cocaine is inhaled, especially with chronic use.

Some psychologic changes are loss of ambition and drive and deterioration of relationships with all energies directed toward obtaining more cocaine. Malnutrition with severe weight loss results from not eating, and self-care activities such as bathing and grooming deteriorate with chronic use.

Few thorough studies have been performed to determine with clarity the withdrawal effects of cocaine. Depression, suicidal ideation, insomnia, irritability, confusion, anxiety, and paranoid features may be evident for several hours to about 6 days after termination, with milder symptoms occurring for longer time periods. Cravings for the drug persist and can continue to reemerge indefinitely.[54]

Among cocaine abusers, several studies have found that many persons have mood disorders, with 30% having a depressive condition and a high proportion have personality disorders.[54] Difficulties in self-concept, interpersonal relationships, and sense of identity and feelings of emptiness are some motivations for cocaine use, although they are maladaptive coping strategies.

Reasons for hospitalization include the inability to terminate cocaine use, the presence of severe symptoms such as severe depression and medical problems, the absence of an adequate support system in the community, and repeated outpatient failures.

Prevalence

Although cocaine abuse and dependence in the general population was 0.2% in a study completed in 1983,[1] it is increasing rapidly in use. An estimated 22 to 25 million persons have experimented with cocaine at least once, and 4 to 5 million are regular users.[4,54] Since 1976 there have been a 200% increase in emergency room cocaine-related deaths and a 500% increase in cocaine-related admissions to government treatment centers.

Population at Risk

Cocaine is prevalent among the affluent and the poor, with crack enjoying a rapid increase in popularity because of its availability and low price (small amounts cost less than $10). According to the National Institute on Drug Abuse surveys, about 4% of high school seniors have used crack at least once and about 17% have tried cocaine.[4]

Tolerance for the illegal substance causes the dose to increase, and the habit becomes extremely expensive to maintain. To support it, the person engages in illegal activities such as violent crimes, robberies, prostitution, and drug dealing.

Medical Plan

Medications

Antidepressant such as trazodone (Desyrel), 50 mg po tid, to treat severe symptoms of depression and possibly counter the physiologic cocaine effects; if bipolar disorder exists, lithium may be prescribed to counter the euphorigenic effects of cocaine

General Management

Group therapy
Recreational therapy

NURSING CARE

Nursing Assessment

Emotion

Depression, anxiety, sense of worthlessness, irritability, sense of emptiness

Physiologic

Headache, nausea, disturbed sleep, agitation, lethargy, confusion, malnutrition, fatigue

Thoughts/Activities

Suicidal ideation, denial, impaired concentration and judgment, psychomotor agitation

Social and Occupational

Deterioration in social behavior, interpersonal difficulties, impairment in occupational or student role

Nursing Dx & Intervention

Nursing Diagnosis	Nursing Intervention/Rationale
Patient problem: cocaine withdrawal	• Assess patterns and amount of cocaine use including type of cocaine, route of administration, and time of last dose. Assess use of other street drugs and prescribed and over-the-counter drugs. • Assess physical and mental condition. • If suicidal ideation exists, assess its seriousness (see also p. 1545 for nursing intervention). • Restrict visitors during the first week of hospitalization *to prevent stimulation and possible stresses associated with visitors and to prevent reintroduction of drugs.* • Obtain urine specimens at intervals, as ordered, for drug testing. • Administer medication as ordered *to decrease severe symptoms associated with termination of cocaine, such as depression.* • Encourage patient to disclose experiences including emotional and physical discomforts with drug use *to begin self-awareness of problems arising from abuse.* • Provide information on cocaine and other psychoactive substances as indicated *to increase patient's knowledge of effects and adverse consequences and to correct misconceptions.*
Ineffective individual coping	• Assess types of discomforts patient has in various social and occupational or school situations and strategies used to cope. • Establish supportive, nonjudgmental relationship *to promote trust and comfort.* • Assist patient to identify stress-provoking situations *to help increase awareness of areas of discomfort.* Help patient identify healthy coping strategies *to reinforce strengths.* • Teach assertiveness skills rather than reliance on cocaine *to increase patient's self-confidence and comfort in social and work situations.* Techniques include role playing and confrontation with feedback in group therapy setting. • Encourage patient to ask for help from others in group therapy *to begin reaching out to others for help.* • Teach patient relaxation techniques, such as muscle relaxation and slow, deep breathing *to manage stress.* • Encourage participation in recreational therapy *to expend energy, decrease stress, and develop leisure-time interests.* • Encourage patient to anticipate postdischarge stressors *to begin to develop strategies for managing them.* • Because termination of substance abuse increases patient's free time, assist patient to develop a schedule of enjoyable non-drug-related activities *to prevent a sense of emptiness and anxiety related to free time.* • Connect patient with self-help groups such as Cocaine Anonymous while in hospital *to act as transition for continuation after discharge.* • Work with patient to learn how to deal with person who may pressure him or her to use cocaine, how to say no to use, and how to avoid places where drugs are available *to develop a life-style free of drugs and to increase self-supports.*
Altered nutrition: less than body requirements	• Assess nutritional intake and observe for signs of malnutrition. • Ensure adequate nutrition in collaboration with physician and dietitian *to counteract effects of inadequate diet.* • Provide a bland diet and antacids as ordered *to decrease gastric discomfort.* • Teach essentials of a nutritionally balanced diet *to prevent or alleviate malnutrition.*
Altered family processes	• Assess family's knowledge of patient's drug use and quality of family relationships. • Teach family about cocaine and its consequences *to provide information and correct misconceptions.* • Help patient and family members to identify and discuss problem areas, including feelings of anger, and help them begin to resolve difficulties *to improve relationships and develop realistic expectations of each other.* • Refer family members for counseling, if indicated, and self-help groups such as Al-Anon or Nar-Anon *to learn how to deal with effects of patient's substance abuse.*

Patient Education

1. Reinforce healthy coping behaviors for dealing with stress.
2. Teach the use of self-supports and supports from others including participation in self-help groups
3. Teach the patient a relapse-preventive life-style.

Evaluation

Patient Outcome	Data Indicating That Outcome is Reached
Patient had an uncomplicated termination from cocaine.	Patient demonstrates drug-free state verbally, and urine tests during hospitalization are drug free. Patient eats regular, well-balanced meals.
Patient demonstrates knowledge of effects and consequences of cocaine dependence.	Patient describes psychologic and physiologic effects and consequences of cocaine use. Patient discusses effects of cocaine use on self and significant others.
Patient demonstrates evidence of practicing healthy coping techniques for dealing with stress-producing situations.	Patient practices relaxation techniques. Patient practices assertiveness skills and evaluates their effects on self and others. Patient practices techniques for avoiding cocaine-related situations. Patient develops an enjoyable non-drug-related activity schedule to manage free time.
Patient demonstrates participation in relationships with family and in a self-help group.	Patient contacts Cocaine Anonymous and attends meetings. Patient participates in dealing with conflicts in the family and in shared activities.

SCHIZOPHRENIC DISORDERS

A diagnosis of schizophrenia is made if the person exhibits continuous signs of marked behavioral impairment in the areas of work, social relationships, and self-care activities for at least 6 months, including a minimum of 1 week of psychotic symptoms such as delusions, hallucinations, and grossly inappropriate affect. The following types of schizophrenia are identified in DSM-III-R[1]: disorganized, catatonic, paranoid, undifferentiated, and residual.

The symptoms the person develops are the best solutions he or she is capable of at the time to restore a sense of equilibrium. The presentation of schizophrenia that follows is not specific to a diagnostic type but deals with dysfunctional behaviors that are common to persons with schizophrenia.

Schizophrenia

Schizophrenia is a disorder in which a person exhibits psychotic symptoms, including disturbances in perceptions, thought, affect, and psychomotor behaviors during an acute phase. The person's social and psychologic abilities are impaired.[1,2]

Schizophrenia is characterized by the following:

Thoughts
- Associations—irrational, illogical, and bizarre
- Delusions—false beliefs that are usually negative, persecutory, and injurious; may be grandiose
- Ideas of reference—belief that events or conversations are related to the individual or have special significance to him (for example, that others are making negative comments about him)
- Thought broadcasting—belief that others can hear the person's thoughts
- Loosening of associations—irrational, illogical, and bizarre thoughts (for example, shifts from one to another unrelated or obliquely related idea)
- Incoherence—incomprehensibility, inability to think or express thoughts in a clear, orderly manner
- Poverty of content—paucity of ideas and thoughts; vague, repetitive, overly concrete ideas
- Information processing and attention—limited ability to process incoming information with slow reaction time; impaired ability to select relevant from irrelevant aspects of communication
- Projection—disowning of perceived or actual attributes of self while attributing them to someone or something in the environment

Perception
- Hallucinations—false sensory perceptions with no external stimulus; auditory is most frequent form of perceptual disturbance; voices may be negative, insulting, or commands; especially in chronicity, voices may be friendly and helpful; visual hallucinations occur occasionally in acute phase and involve seeing nonexistent things such as insects or people; smell (olfactory), taste (gustatory), and touch (tactile) are less common
- Illusions—misidentification or distortion of stimulus

Affect
- Blunting—reduction of affective, emotional expression
- Flatness—impoverishment of emotional reactivity; emotionally dull, cold, colorless; monotonous voice
- Apathy—apparent absence of emotions
- Inappropriateness—incongruence between emotions and content or ideas (for example, laughing in response to news of death of significant other)

Activity level
- Psychomotor activity—decreased reaction to environment; stereotypic, purposeless movement such as rocking or pacing

Spontaneity and activity—markedly decreased activity to withdrawal; repetitive, stereotypic activity; apathy; immobility

Posture—rigid, inappropriate, manneristic

Other

Self-identity—impairment or loss of ego boundaries; impairment of self-identity

Volition—impaired ability to will self to act; disturbance in goal-directed activities

Role behaviors—impairment in work and social roles; lack of social skills

Personal appearance—neglect

The onset of schizophrenia may be slow and insidious or sudden. In some persons the onset is preceded by a significant external event such as loss of a friend, marriage, or leaving home; in others the onset is not related to an identifiable external event. External events, if identified, are insufficient to evoke a psychosis if the internal processes such as relatedness to self and environment are not impaired.

Psychotic symptoms are present during the active phase. The person loses contact with reality.[2] Behaviors are unpredictable, in part because the person responds to internal processes such as hallucinations and delusions. He may hear voices that order him to protect himself from the evil and harmful world. Projection, the externalization of rejected, undesirable thoughts, feelings, and behaviors onto others, is a common defense mechanism. The secondary processes of mental integration that is based on logic and the reality principle deteriorate and give way to the primary processes of illogical, disorganized mental activity of the unconscious system that is normal during infancy.

Although some persons recover completely a majority have residual effects of the schizophrenic process with acute relapses. Vulnerability to stressors generally remains and may trigger relapses.[2] The impairments they have limit their ability to cope with social and psychologic experiences, such as interactions with others and social problem-solving. Long-term rehabilitation programs are needed to identify the deficiencies and to teach appropriate coping strategies.[56] By actively involving families of patients in psychoeducational and support groups, the patient relapse rate is decreased significantly.[55]

Prevalence

In Europe and Asia the prevalence of schizophrenia ranges from 0.2% to 1%. The criteria some researchers in the United States have used are broader than those used by others, producing an estimated U.S. rate of 2%.[1,20]

Population at Risk

The onset of schizophrenia usually occurs during adolescence and young adulthood. The disease is almost equally distributed between males and females. A relationship appears to exist between social class and schizophrenia; the prevalence is greatest in low-status socioeconomic groups and in poor neighborhoods of large cities.[1] Whether schizophrenia-prone persons are products of these environments or drift toward inner cities when they lose economic and social status is unknown.

Responses of Nurses to Schizophrenics

Schizophrenia is a chronic disorder in which the person appears cold, distant, and apathetic. Response to therapy is extremely slow, and obvious signs of success are few. The schizophrenic is emotionally unnourished and is unnourishing to the nurse and others around him. Nurses often find it easier to withdraw from the withdrawn schizophrenic than to experience a sense of helplessness, hopelessness, and inadequacy in dealing with the patient. The nurse needs to establish small goals with the patient such as having the patient speak to her, share an activity, or ask to have a need or want met. If unrealistic goals are established, the nurse is bound to experience frustration and hopelessness. If the goal is attainable, specific, and immediate, the nurse's frustration is reduced.

Psychopathology

The discussion of the psychopathology of schizophrenia is preceded by a brief presentation of genetic and biologic hypotheses.

A genetic predisposition to the development of schizophrenia has been proposed because of the familial transmission observed in some children and relatives of those with the disorder; however, no specific gene has been identified. Many biologic abnormalities have been linked to schizophrenia such as structural abnormalities of the brain (e.g., cortical atrophy, viral infections, autoimmune disturbances) and alterations in the neurotransmitters serotonin, norepinephrine, and dopamine.[36]

Dopamine has been the focus of research for a long time as a prominent factor involved in schizophrenia. The overabundance of dopamine may cause some symptoms such as delusions and hallucinations.[36] Part of the evidence is based on the effects of the antipsychotic medicines that block dopaminergic activity, although the specific pathways of change are unclear. However the abnormalities in dopamine do not account for the great variety of symptoms evidenced in schizophrenia. The complexity of even defining schizophrenia clearly makes it imperative to examine how a broad range of social and environmental stressors interact with genetic and biologic susceptibilities to produce the disorder.

Psychoanalytic Theory

The functions of the ego include the ability to differentiate the self from objects in the environment, reality testing, organization of affect, and development of cognitive processes such as perception, thinking, remembering, and learning. The organizing processes operate in integrating the id, ego, and superego and in differentiating the self from objects outside the self.

Since the functions of the ego develop in stages, traumatic experiences do not affect all functions adversely. Those functions affected negatively are subject to regression to an earlier phase of development and reflected in symptoms. Since the secondary processes of cognition that are reflected in abstract, logical thinking develop later in the person's development, these are among the first to be lost. The person regresses to the early primary processes of infancy, including memory traces, lack of differentiation between subjective imagery and reality, and illogical connections between experiences.[44]

The ego, as mediator of the id's instinctual drives, libido and aggression (death instinct), neutralizes the aggressive energy and puts the energy into the service of itself. The ego uses the energy to maintain the various ego functions. If aggression is unneutralized, disorganization occurs when the person entertains angry thoughts or acts on them. When aggression is deneutralized, the person has a low tolerance for his own aggressive feelings and a tendency toward acting out violently.[44] The aggressive energy regresses to an instinctual drive, is no longer available to maintain some of the ego functions, especially the cognitive processes, and consequently plays a role in the initiation of schizophrenic symptoms.

Interpersonal Theory

Interpersonal theory stresses that the personality develops through relationships with others. Sullivan[59] assumed that the mother of the future schizophrenic is more intensely anxious than the average mother. Because she transmits anxiety to the infant, severe anxiety experienced as dread and terror is evoked in the infant. To avoid overwhelming panic and with few resources, the infant attempts to get rid of the discomfort by dissociating from it as a "not-me" experience. The infant with excessive "not-me" experiences is vulnerable to future excessive anxiety.[59] Although dissociation serves to protect the person from extremely uncomfortable experiences, it also prevents him from recalling, examining, and correcting perceptions of these experiences and limits his capacity to deal with future ones. To avoid the sense of terror, the person urgently gets rid of situations that may evoke anxiety without determining whether the event is frightening and what aspect of it is. No learning can take place when the person is busy defending against anxiety.

Regression occurs when the feelings of self are compromised and weakened. The self-system is actively warding off or decreasing anxiety, and the dissociated experiences are no longer available for learning. Since complex cognitive processes of thinking, learning, and remembering are compromised, the person reverts to earlier modes of experiencing such as the momentary reverie of infancy or the distorted thinking of the young child in which illogical connections are made between experiences. The severity of the schizophrenic processes is related to the strength of the self-system and the degree of regression to more primitive functioning of the infant or young child.[2,59]

Cognitive Theory

Although all human beings are biologically predisposed to think illogically at times, to be self-destructive, and to experience inappropriate feelings, a seriously ill person may have a greater predisposition to disordered thinking. The person underestimates his abilities and emphasizes problems. Because past traumatic events are exaggerated, the person overreacts to even minor problems.[5] Even when new information makes possible a different perspective, the person resists and continues to think about the self and others illogically.

Thinking and emotional disturbances are also related to social learning. The child is taught to please his parents even when the directive appears illogical and begins to accept directives without thinking. When told often enough that he is worthless to himself and to others, he accepts the idea. Self-defeating beliefs are rigidly held and become strongly habituated patterns of thinking, feeling, and acting.[5]

Medical Plan

Medications

Haloperidol (Haldol)

For severely disturbed patient: 5 mg bid by tablet or concentrate to manage symptoms of psychotic disorders; for acute agitation: 2 mg IM prn; for elderly disturbed patient: 2 mg bid by tablet or concentrate; major initial side effect is orthostatic hypotension; in addition to the adverse effects of extrapyramidal symptoms, neuroleptic malignant syndrome (NMS), a potentially fatal disorder, has been reported with antipsychotic medicines; major clinical manifestations of NMS are muscular rigidity, tachycardia, diaphoresis, labile blood pressure with hypotension and hypertension, cardiac dysrhythmia, dyspnea, hyperpyrexia, and coma

General Management

Occupational therapy to make possible participation in activities and to decrease problems

Recreational therapy to make possible participation in exercises, development of skills in group activities, and learning of leisure activities

NURSING CARE

Nursing Assessment

Thoughts

Disturbance in orientation to person, place, and time; retarded thought processes; impaired ability to process incoming information; blocking of thoughts; autistic thinking, i.e., inability to distinguish between reality and fantasy; suspiciousness; distorted, illogical thinking;

false beliefs, such as of being persecuted or poisoned; projection, i.e., disowning aspects of self while ascribing them to something or someone in environment; poor judgment; fear of rejection and of interpersonal and physical closeness; lack of trust; vulnerability to stress

Perception

Appearance of listening to voices observed as movement in vocal cords and lips and head and facial movement

Affect

Anxiety; loneliness; depression; apathy; colorless speech and monotonous voice; incongruity between emotional responses and idea; hostility

Activity

Withdrawal from relationships and contact with others; impairment in goal-directed activity; purposeless movement such as pacing and mannerisms; unpredictable behavior that may be related to delusions or hallucinations; agitation; impairment or absence of social skills; poor work history

Self-Care

Neglectfulness; lack of motivation; impairment in bathing, grooming, and hygiene

Nutrition

Unawareness of hunger or thirst; apathy to food at mealtime; fear of eating, for example, belief that food is poisoned

Sleep

Disturbed sleep patterns; reluctance to go to bed at night or inability to awaken in morning

Nursing Dx & Intervention

Nursing Diagnosis	Nursing Intervention/Rationale
Social isolation related to alterations in mental illness	• Assess degree of withdrawal and types of preoccupations patient has. • Begin to establish a trusting relationship *to provide sense of security for patient.* • Maintain appropriate physical distance when with patient *to decrease any sense of terror of physical closeness.* • Speak slowly to patient, using brief statements *to increase patient's ability to process information and understand.* • Visit patient frequently for brief time periods *to demonstrate concern and to decrease fears of interpersonal closeness.* • Tell patient when you are leaving and let him know when you will return. • Avoid pushing a nonverbal patient to respond to questions *to prevent further withdrawal.* • Comment on neutral subjects, such as patient's immediate environment (e.g., items in the room, activities of others in the room, pictures in a shared magazine). • As you and patient are able to tolerate longer time periods together, increase time gradually *to help patient begin working on issues.* • If patient becomes increasingly agitated and distracting techniques are unsuccessful, medication may be administered in collaboration with physician *to decrease agitation.* Briefly explain reason for medication and its major effects and side effects to the extent that patient is able to comprehend. • Teach social skills *to help patient interact, initiate a conversation, or make requests,* since these skills are often impaired. • Teach patient that others have responsibilities for interactions and that patient is responsible only for his own behavior. Assist patient to elaborate on and build on strengths *to encourage patient to identify and accept skills.* • Teach patient assertiveness skills and encourage practice of them; examine attempts to be assertive *to help patient become aware of successes,* even if attempts were awkward. • Help patient to attend and participate in occupational therapy as prescribed *to promote skills and interests.* • As patient is able to tolerate interactions with others, encourage recreational therapy *to gain skills in various activities, to expend energy through exercise, and to learn leisure activities.*
Altered thought processes	• Assess level of distractibility, delusional thinking, and ability to process incoming stimuli. • Orient patient, as needed, to person, place, and time *to correct disorientation.* • Listen attentively to patient, listening for themes, feeling tones, or reality-oriented phrases or thoughts *to increase patient's willingness to relate to another human being.* Do not pretend understanding, but comment on understandable conversation. • Assist patient, as able, to elaborate on reality-oriented ideas. • Assist patient *in correcting misconceptions about environment, self, and experiences* through recall of events and use of problem solving.

Nursing Diagnosis	Nursing Intervention/Rationale
	• Do not encourage patient to repeat false beliefs, arguing with him or agreeing with him, *to avoid reinforcing ideas of reference and delusions*. "I find that hard to believe" may be appropriate comment. • Assist patient to examine what he was experiencing before delusional thoughts began. Attempt to assist patient to identify thoughts and feelings toward himself *to determine if patient was feeling threatened*. Gradually assist patient *to recognize and correct delusional content of thoughts and feelings*. • When patient shows signs of anxiety or expresses discomfort, change topic *to decrease anxiety*. If patient is able to discuss an anxiety-provoking topic, help him identify his feelings (awareness of feelings will evolve slowly). • Administer medication as ordered. If you suspect patient is not swallowing tablets, concentrates may be administered in collaboration with physician. • Briefly explain reason for medication, as well as its effects and side effects. Inform patient of possible sleepiness and dizziness, especially when standing up. Caution patient to stand up slowly *to prevent falling*. • Observe patient closely *to detect effects and side effects of medication* and report to physician for dose adjustments as needed. Check vital signs four times a day initially. • As patient is able to comprehend, teach effects and side effects of medication and reasons for medication *to increase potential for compliance*.
Sensory/perceptual alterations (auditory)	• Assess for perceptual distortions such as hallucinations. • When patient is observed moving lips and vocal cords or cocking head as if listening, ask him, "Do you hear voices?" or "Who is talking to you?" Use distractive techniques such as involving patient in conversation or activity if patient is unable to examine reality of voices. If "voices" are chronic, teach patient to hum or whistle to prevent him from using vocal cords for "voices" *to increase his sense of control*. • Gradually assist patient to examine thoughts and feelings just before hallucinations. Help patient recognize eventually that he expects to hear voices. Accept patient's protests and denials as his understandings now. Slowly encourage patient to accept a connection between thoughts or feelings and expectation of voices *to be aware that he has ability to control his experiences and correct thoughts and feelings about himself*. Continue examination of hallucinatory experience.
Altered nutrition: less than body requirements	• Assess nutritional intake and misconceptions about food. • When patient is suspicious of food, emphasize that food is nutritious and has not been tampered with; have patient participate in choosing foods and liquids *to decrease suspiciousness*. Obtain patient's attention and suggest eating *to decrease preoccupations or hallucinations*. If necessary, direct patient to take each mouthful—for example, "Take a spoonful. Now eat it." • Offer fluids between meals *to maintain hydration*. • Teach the ingredients and importance of good nutrition when patient is able to process information.
Bathing/hygiene and dressing/grooming self-care deficits	• Assess abilities and impairments in self-care activities. • Assist patient with bathing, grooming, and personal hygiene as needed. • Wash patient if he is unable to bathe himself or to follow directions such as "Wash your left arm" *to maintain skin integrity*. • Offer each article of clothing to put on, and direct patient to complete grooming and hygiene care. Assist patient as needed. • Encourage patient to initiate self-care activities as able. • Acknowledge patient's self-care activities *to encourage him to identify and eventually accept appearance and positive characteristics*.
Sleep pattern disturbance	• Assess sleep patterns and fears about sleeping. • If patient has fears of going to sleep, assist him to talk about them *to begin to correct misconceptions*. • Offer warm milk *to assist sleeping*. • Encourage slow, deep breathing while focusing on number "1" *to promote relaxation*. • If helpful, turn the radio to soothing music at low volume *to decrease panic or fears*. • Discourage naps during the day *to enhance restful sleep at night*.

Patient Education

1. Teach beginning skills in use of problem-solving technique.
2. Reinforce the patient's strengths.
3. Teach social skills.

4. Discuss the use of social supports and resources in community, such as continuing care programs in community or mental health centers.
5. Teach compliance with medication therapy and encourage continuation of counseling.

Evaluation

Patient Outcome	Data Indicating That Outcome is Reached
Patient no longer has psychotic symptoms.	Patient is oriented to person, place, and time. Patient states that he no longer hears "voices." Patient uses problem-solving method to correct misconceptions. Patient performs self-care.
Patient participates in social activities with staff and other patients.	Patient initiates activities with others. Patient spends less time alone in unit. Patient says that he enjoys participating in some of the planned activities.
Patient complies with medication regimen.	Patient describes effects and side effects of medication and refers to handout on drug information as needed. Patient has developed system to keep track of self-administration of medication. Patient states action he will take when adverse effects of medication are experienced.
Patient plans to continue counseling after discharge.	Patient has made appointment with health professional for counseling after discharge. Patient has visited day care center and plans to attend regularly after discharge.

MOOD DISORDERS

The affective disorders have been renamed mood disorders in the DSM-III-R[1] to reflect more accurately the essential features of the diagnostic category. Mood is an emotional reaction that is sufficiently intense to affect the person's entire psychic state. The two major moods are manic and depressive patterns of disturbances. Another way of classifying mood disorders is as bipolar or unipolar. A person with a bipolar disorder has experienced one or more manic and depressive episodes, whereas a person with a unipolar disorder has experienced at least one or more episodes of depression with no manic phase. The manic and depressive manifestations of the disorders are compared in Table 17-2.[1,3,11]

The bipolar disorders are discussed here first with a focus on manic behavior. This is followed by a presentation of depression.

Bipolar disorders

The bipolar disorders include at least one manic episode and usually one or more depressive episodes. The manic phase is characterized by grandiosity, excessive excitement, flight of ideas, and psychomotor overactivity; the depressive phase is characterized by a sense of despair, retarded thinking, and psychomotor retardation or agitation.

Three major types of bipolar disorders, as well as another cyclic condition that is milder, are included in the DSM-III-R.[1]

Bipolar disorder, mixed. Both manic and major depressive episodes are involved currently, intermixed or alternating rapidly.

Bipolar disorder, manic. The episode currently or in the past fulfills the criteria for the manic episode.

Bipolar disorder, depressed. The current or past symptoms meet the criteria for a major depressive episode, with at least one previous manic episode.

Cyclothymia. Numerous milder manic and depressive symptoms are present for at least 2 years but do not achieve the severity of a major depressive or manic episode.

Manic Behaviors in Bipolar Disorders

Manic behavior is excessive mental and physical activity.[1] Thought is accelerated and expansive; mood is labile with rapid sequences of euphoria, irritability, depression, elation, and rage; and physical activity is excessive with boundless energy, little need for sleep, constant motion, and assaultiveness in response to limit setting. Persons in manic states have pressured speech and flight of ideas and are self-indulgent, impatient, humorous, extroverted, friendly, impulsive, and distractible. They appear to have unlimited self-confidence and self-assurance as they propel their energy outward into the environment. The levels of mood disturbance vary from mild to severe with psychotic features.

Prevalence

The prevalence of bipolar disorders, although difficult to estimate is 0.4% to 2% in the adult population. Cyclothymia is reported to be between 0.4% and 3.5%.[1,51] To make a more accurate diagnosis, a careful history of previous symptoms must be identified rather than focusing only on the current acute episode.

Table 17-2

Comparison of Manic and Depressive Phases

Mania	Depression
Elation, expansiveness, irritability	Melancholia, sense of despair
Inappropriate laughing, joking, punning	Tearfulness, crying
Accelerated, sharpened thinking, flight of ideas	Retarded thinking, impaired attention and concentration
Unlimited self-confidence	Lack of self-confidence
Overoptimism	Pessimism, hopelessness
Loquacity	Decreased talkativeness
Exhibitionism	Inhibition
Extroversion to environment	Introversion
Rapid shift to aggression toward environment	Self-destructiveness
Gregariousness	Social withdrawal
Hedonism	Limited or absence of pleasure
Licentiousness	Limited or absence of sexual interest
Reduced need for sleep	Insomnia or hypersomnia
Unlimited energy	Fatigue, psychomotor retardation
Appetite ravenenous but "no time" to eat	Appetite decreased or lost
Flight from superego	Submission to superego

Population at Risk

The findings of recent epidemiologic studies conducted in the United States indicate an even distribution of bipolar disorders in men and women.[1]

Relatives of those with the disorder are a higher risk for developing mood disorders than persons in the general population, with a rate of 6% for first-degree biologic relatives as compared with 1% to 2% in the general population.[51] Bipolar disorders are more likely to occur in the upper socioeconomic class than in poor or lower strata, which helps to explain why these individuals are generally treated in private health facilities.

The onset of manic episodes is generally in people between the ages of 20 and 25, with new cases appearing after age 50.[1,29] The first depressive episode may occur 10 years later. The onset of each phase can be sudden—especially in mania, in which symptoms escalate within several hours; however, both phases can have slower onsets. The episodes in the bipolar disorders occur irregularly but may also alternate regularly, as seen with those having seasonal patterns (mania in the spring and summer and depression in the fall and winter).[1,11] They may be separated by symptom-free periods or follow each other with no appreciable interval between them. The average duration for untreated manic moods is 6 months and for untreated depressive moods is 9 months. Modern treatment methods including medicines have obscured the phases and blurred the development of symptoms.[29]

Biologic factors contribute to the development of bipolar disorders; however, because of the complex interactions in the brain, it is difficult to identify the pathology clearly. Because of the high prevalence of bipolar and cyclothymic disorders among relatives of those with manic symptoms, genetic factors such as the dominant X-chromosome may be a contributor to the condition. Some research efforts are directed toward identifying factors that alter the metabolism of the neurotransmitters such as norepinephrine, serotonin, and dopamine, which play a role in regulating mood and behavior.[29,51,60] Others include study of electrolyte disturbances, cortisone metabolism, and circadian biologic rhythms. The biologic disturbances are supported by the effectiveness of the medication lithium in preventing recurrence of symptoms. However, the importance of stressful environmental events preceding the onset of manic symptoms—possibly interacting with biologic predispositions to precipitate the symptoms—cannot be dismissed.

Behaviors associated with the manic phase overlap with those of other psychiatric conditions and, when mild, those of nonpathologic deviations of normal behavior. Bipolar disorder should be differentiated from schizophrenia, personality disorders, unipolar depressions, and drug states. Drugs such as steroids, for example, cortisone and amphetamines, can produce elation. Organic disease such as multiple sclerosis must also be ruled out.

Levels of Manic Mood Disturbances

Hypomania is a pathologic state that is less severe than mania. The person has intensified energy, a stable elated mood, self-indulgence, distractibility, pressured speech, poor judgment, and increased motor activity.[3] Hypomanic persons radiate good health, appear tireless, and are humorous and friendly to the point of being unacceptably personal with others. Their intolerance to limit setting is observed as irritability or anger.

Mania or acute mania is a more intense and disturbed level in which propriety and discretion are absent. Persons in this state tease and joke, often making others the butt of their jokes. Their good humor can change rapidly to vicious anger. They flit from one activity to another without ever completing anything. Talk may be incessant, since impulses are expressed in words with flight of ideas proceeding to incoherence and clang association (mental association between dissociated ideas made because of similarity in sounds of words used to describe the ideas). These persons have delusions of grandeur concerning their wealth and power and have lost control of their behavior, but they do not have severe disturbances of self-identity as in schizophrenia.

Persons with delirious mania or psychosis evidence all of the symptoms of the previous levels plus loss of contact with reality. Speech is incoherent, activity is constant and purposeless, and delusions and hallucinations are present. At times incontinence of urine and feces occurs.[3]

Interactions with manics, and less so with hypomanics, are stressful to others because of their exploitative behaviors, which include the following:

Manipulating the self-esteem of others by praise and deflation
Striking exploitatively at vulnerable areas
Projecting responsibility onto others
Testing limits of rules by trying to extend them
Alienating others, especially family members

Psychopathology

Psychoanalytic Theory

Persons with bipolar disorders have an oral-dependent character and the basic psychopathologic characteristic of unipolar depressives: the introjection of anger and hostility. Depression is repressed hostility, and mania, a defensive behavior, is a massive denial of depression. Manic behavior is a flight from the superego with an abatement of ego restraints, whereas depressed persons submit to the superego.

The apparent warmth and social responsiveness of persons with bipolar disorders may be related to satisfying early relationships with their mothers. However, these persons are unable to master the intrapsychic separation-individuation processes of development to become separate individuals with a sense of self-identity. Psychoanalysts think that biologic factors operate in the alternating moods of manic-depressives, since the condition recurs in successive generations.[17,29]

Interpersonal Theory

The family environment is extremely important in the development of manic depression. The mother enjoys her relationship with the helpless, dependent infant but attempts to control the independent and rebellious strivings of the toddler with threats of abandonment. As the young child develops, the mother or both parents expect compliance and conformity to extremely high standards of behavior and achievements to improve the family's social position and reputation rather than to instill a sense of self-achievement and pride in the child. The child receives favoritism and special attention because of either his superior ability to achieve or his greater effort to please and to remain dependent. The child grows into adulthood learning to use others for unlimited help and support, yet fears competitiveness and confrontation because he is afraid to alienate others. Mania is an escape from the burdens of the duty-bound self into superficial liveliness and freedom. Although these persons appear warm and sincere in interpersonal relations, they are shallow and nonempathetic.[3]

Cognitive Theory

According to Beck,[38] manic and hypomaniac persons, in contrast to depressive persons, unrealistically evaluate their efforts as decidedly positive and their accomplishments as impressive. The euphoria they experience because of their inflated evaluations of their superiority and superb performance drives them into uninterrupted motion. When questioned about their inaccurate self-appraisals and fantasies, they become inappropriately angry or belligerent.

Medical Plan

Medications

Lithium carbonate (Lithane, Eskalith),* 300 mg po qid or 600 mg po tid to treat manic symptoms and prevent recurrence; lithium citrate syrup may be ordered initially instead of tablets *to ensure that medicine is swallowed*

General Management

Occupational therapy
Recreational therapy as condition permits
Regular diet with normal sodium intake; sometimes high-carbohydrate supplements are ordered

NURSING CARE

Nursing Assessment

The mental and physical activities of manic persons vary with the severity of the mood disturbance.

Physical Activity

Hyperactivity (moving rapidly from one activity to another, bustling about, restlessness, pacing, fidgeting); limited ability to complete tasks owing to distractibility; eyes bright; face flushed; head erect; animated facial expression; increased metabolism; unrestrained playfulness and mischievousness; uninhibited activity (singing, dancing, and so on); expansive gesturing; dramatic self-expression in movement; colorful appearance (wearing bright colors, jewelry); telephone abuse (calls at all hours); acting out of impulses; sexual acting out without discretion; alcohol abuse; giving money and possessions away; assaultiveness, especially when requests are denied and limits are set; violation of rules; abusiveness; destruction of belongings or bedclothes to be busy; violent motor excitement in severely disturbed

Thought Processes

Enhanced sensory acuity (stimulated by other people, objects, and environment); flight of ideas (skipping from one idea to another without completing any); distractibility; expansive, vivid, intense thoughts; impaired judgment; intact memory and orientation to person, place, and time (except when severely disturbed); lack of motivation to change based on "feeling well"; self-

*Serum lithium level determination is made before initiating lithium therapy, especially if the patient was formerly receiving medication. Normally no lithium is present without medication. After therapy is initiated, serum levels are examined frequently (for example, every other day until level has stabilized and just before a lithium dose). Therapeutic serum lithium levels are 0.6 to 1.2 mEq/L. Toxic symptoms may occur at slightly more than or even at therapeutic levels. Early signs of lithium intoxication are diarrhea, vomiting, drowsiness, polyuria, and weakness. If hypothyroidism occurs with lithium treatment, thyroid supplement eliminates the condition.

confidence, self-centeredness; enthusiasm; self-will; overvaluing of abilities and performance; projection of responsibility onto others; loose associations evidenced in incoherence; paranoid ideation (emerges from anger); arrogance; haughtiness; vengeful ideas; criticism of others; delusions of grandeur (false beliefs of power, wealth, achievements; wish-fulfilling type); clang association of thoughts (words with similar sounds but no relation of meaning, such as ring, ding, and ling); loss of contact with reality; clouded consciousness; visual and auditory hallucinations when severe

Communication

Loquacity to logorrhea; pressured rapid speech; speaking with vigor, excitement, animation, emphasis; flowery, witty, loud, lewd, or pompous speech; superficial content; manipulativeness (pleas and threats, praise and deflation, ingratiating manner, excuses, bargaining, demanding, deception, verbal abuse, trying to extend limits)

Affect

Labile mood (elation, euphoria, exhilaration, irritability, anger, laughter, cheerfulness, tearfulness, tremulousness, depression, sadness)

Social Interactions

Appearance of warmth and likability; entertaining, humorous affect; joking, making others the butt of joke; fear of interpersonal intimacy; meddling; interference with and intrusion in others' interaction; attempts to dominate others; exploitation of others' vulnerable areas; destructiveness in group interactions

Self-Care

Obliviousness concerning infections and other physical illness as disturbance increases; neglect of personal needs and grooming

Nutrition

Decrease in appetite but no major weight loss; dehydration possible with hyperactivity

Family Processes

Promises to partner made and broken; demeaning of family with anger and blame; family conflicts and instability; spouse perceives patient as spiteful, lacks understanding and knowledge of condition, and has diminished self-esteem

Nursing Dx & Intervention

Nursing care should be implemented selectively based on severity of symptoms and presenting behaviors. Nurses need to be alert to their own responses to these patients and their behavior. These patients can evoke frustration and anger in nurses because of their hyperactivity, verbal abuse, and attempts to manipulate staff.

Nursing Diagnosis	Nursing Intervention/Rationale
Patient problem: hyperactivity	• Assess degree of hyperactivity. • Provide quiet, nonstimulating environment *to prevent escalation of excitement*. • If patient is highly excited, restrict him from the general patient population areas *to avoid stimulation and the possibility of aggression toward others and abuse by other patients*. • Explain restrictions simply and make use of distractibility. • Begin to develop a supportive relationship through consistent, frequent interpersonal exchanges. • Administer medication as prescribed *to begin treatment of mania*. • Be certain patient swallows oral medication; *to set limits*, do not allow patient to bargain to take medication later. • Monitor for effects and possible adverse reactions to medication *to prevent toxicity*. • Teach effects and side effects of medication when condition stabilizes and patient is able to hear instruction *to increase compliance*. • Teach importance of maintenance dose of medication and ongoing compliance (be aware that patient is concerned about losing sense of well-being). • As excitement begins to decrease, involve patient in gross motor activities such as walking and exercise. Be aware that activities often increase excitement rather than produce tranquility and fatigue. • *To set firm, consistent limits on behavior*, give short explanation as needed. Staff members need to understand and conform to uniform limits. Encourage patient, when able, to set own limits of behavior consistent with treatment goals. • Allow patient opportunity to express anger about restriction in an appropriate way; if anger is inappropriate, use distraction *to change focus*. • Gradually help integrate patient into general unit milieu; be alert for overstimulation.

Nursing Diagnosis	Nursing Intervention/Rationale
Potential for violence: self-directed or directed at others	• Assess potential for aggressiveness and suicide potential. • Be alert for possible physical aggression against other patients and staff. If patient is in general unit area, remove him from situation, giving short, firm directions *to provide a "time out."* • Use distraction before aggressiveness escalates. • Protect patient from other patients' aggressiveness and pranks *to prevent him from being verbally or physically abused.* • If necessary, obtain an order for medication as needed (for example, haloperidol) *to decrease aggressiveness.* • Evaluate patient for suicide potential. If patient is suicidal, institute precautions. • Encourage patient, when able, to identify and accept angry feelings *to increase self-understanding.* • Encourage use of a problem-solving approach *to relate feelings to events that evoked them and develop appropriate ways to resolve issues.* • Help patient to attend occupational therapy activities and recreational activities when ready and as prescribed. • Provide opportunities to talk about activities *to resolve problem areas.* • Encourage patient to identify enjoyable activities. • Direct patient to appropriate activities, such as punching bag or exercise, *to discharge energies.*
Altered thought processes	• Assess orientation to time, place, and person (usually it is intact) and type of thought disturbances. • Listen for themes in flight of ideas and clarify them with patient (for example, "Are you saying you're . . . ?") *to help patient focus thoughts.* • Allow some digressions and then bring patient back to topic *to increase logical development of ideas without criticism.* • Observe closely for increased excitement *to intervene before serious escalation occurs.* • Slowly help to decrease patient's resistance to accept responsibility *to avoid threat to self-esteem.* • Help decrease patient's resistance to accepting responsibility slowly *to prevent threat of self-esteem.* • Assure patient that it is all right to make mistakes *to encourage patient to accept responsibility for positive and negative events.* • Help patient examine distortions in thinking and correct them without negating patient's self-esteem. • Teach patient to use problem-solving approach *to develop alternative ways for dealing with situations and to evaluate possible consequences.*
Impaired verbal communication	• Assess patient's communication patterns and content. • When patient's speech is pressured, rapid, and loud, respond in soft, assertive voice, make short statements, and speak slowly *to help calm patient.* • Respond to appropriate humor, but be careful not to escalate excitement and hostility. • When patient is able, explore inappropriate humor. For example, when humor is inconsistent with content, assist patient to express himself directly. • Let patient know what you will do and will not do in interactions and in the treatment plan when patient makes requests *to maintain consistent limits.* • Maintain limits even when requests appear reasonable *to be firm and consistent.* • Schedule frequent brief sessions with patient during an acute phase—for example, 15 minutes—*to begin to develop a relationship.* Increase length of sessions as excitement decreases and patient is able to use the time. • When patient verbally strikes out at you, help patient identify underlying feelings. If patient continues, communicate your discomfort and let patient know that you will leave if abuse continues. Leave if patient does not stop. • Teach assertiveness skills *to give patient sense of control and influence.*
Ineffective individual coping	• Assess adaptive strategies to deal with mood disorder and problem-solving abilities. • As patient is able, assist to identify frequency, duration, and type of mood changes *to learn to detect subtle changes and patterns indicating mood disturbances.* • Encourage patient to accept appropriate feelings of sadness and happiness. • Assist patient to deal with stressors in healthy ways and to accept strengths and resources. • Teach patient about illness and treatment *to deal with chronicity and cyclic nature of illness and to increase self-awareness and compliance with treatment regimen.*
Bathing/hygiene and dressing/grooming self-care deficit	• Assess patient's ability to attend to self-care activities psychologically. • Help patient with activities of daily living and hygiene activities (which patient may ignore because "pressed for time"). • During hygiene activities, observe for skin integrity and infections *to identify health problems.*

Nursing Diagnosis	Nursing Intervention/Rationale
	• Give clear, concise directions to patient *to carry out in self-care activities;* use patient's distractibility constructively *to help patient attend to care.* • Allow patient, as able, to make decisions in self-care activities *to promote independence.* • Teach patient good hygiene and grooming practices as needed.
Sleep pattern disturbance	• Assess patient's inability to sleep and have quiet periods. If needed, obtain order for sedative or neuroleptic agent (haloperidol) *to promote sleep or relaxation.* • As patient is able, help identify methods that produce rest and sleep. • Teach relaxation exercises such as deep breathing *to induce sleep.*
Altered nutrition: less than body requirements	• Assess eating patterns and food and fluid intake. • When patient is highly excited, provide food in small unbreakable containers or finger foods *to eat while standing or pacing.* If necessary, provide food in liquid form. • Ensure that patient's fluid intake is more than 1000 ml *to prevent lithium toxicity.* • Teach patient importance of good nutrition with normal sodium and fluid intake. • If oral intake of fluids is to be restricted before medical treatments such as surgery or laboratory tests, inform physician so intravenous fluids can be given *to prevent dehydration and lithium toxicity.* • Have dietitian provide additional information on diet as needed.
Social isolation	• Assess patient's level of hyperactivity and effects of the environment on mood. • When patient is highly excited restrict him from other patients in unit *to prevent overstimulation.* • Convey your accessibility by your presence and comments. • As patient's excitement decreases, gradually permit patient on unit for brief periods of time *to adapt to stimulation and less structure.* • Participate in and observe interactions with other patients. Provide feedback on interactions with other patients and staff *to increase patient's awareness of behavior.* • Help patient work through difficulties in interactions. • Encourage patient to begin making contact with friends. • Teach patient healthier coping strategies and interpersonal skills.
Altered family processes	• Assess family interactions, reactions to patient, and knowledge of illness. • Allow patient's spouse and other family members to talk about experiences, including feelings, with patient. They often think patient is spiteful and willful in hurting them rather than ill. • Teach spouse and other family members about the illness, its cyclic nature, and its treatment *to support patient's compliance with medical regimen.* • Help patient and family identify unhealthy interactions such as hostility, blaming, and talking for each other, *to help them change these behaviors.* • Remain neutral; avoid siding with a family member. • Encourage members to talk about effects of illness on entire family *to learn to deal with these issues.* • Help all family members to recognize need for continued family therapy, if appropriate, after patient leaves hospital.

Patient Education

1. Teach the patient about the chronic and cyclic nature of the illness and the importance of complying with the medical regimen.
2. Teach the patient the signs of increasing mood disturbances in depressive and manic behaviors.
3. Reinforce the patient's awareness of the effects and adverse effects of the medicine and the need for regular assessments of serum lithium levels (for example, at 1- to 2-month intervals when stabilized).
4. Teach the patient the importance of a normal diet and an adequate daily fluid intake.

Evaluation

Patient Outcome	Data Indicating That Outcome is Reached
Patient attains persistent mood level nearing healthy state for self.	Patient carries on normal conversation with others. Patient accepts realistic limits and delays. Patient sits quietly for periods of time. Patient is able to engage in an activity for long periods of time. Patient carries out his own self-care activities.
Patient demonstrates knowledge of illness.	Patient verbalizes knowledge of illness. Patient identifies patterns of own mood changes. Patient states symptoms that indicate beginning of own manic and depressive phases.
Patient demonstrates knowledge of treatment.	Patient verbalizes knowledge of effects and side effects of prescribed medicine. Patient states knowledge of accurate self-administration of prescribed medicine and importance of compliance. Patient states importance of daily sodium and fluid intake to prevent adverse effects of medication. Patient verbalizes importance of regular serum lithium tests.
Patient demonstrates importance of continued counseling.	Patient makes arrangements to continue counseling to work on personal issues and family relationships. Patient continues to work on listening skills with spouse and other family members.

Depressive disorders

Depression is an abnormal mood state in which a person characteristically has a sense of worthlessness and despair, morbid thoughts, and psychomotor retardation or agitation.

Depression is the polar opposite of mania and as such occurs as one phase of the bipolar disorder. It frequently occurs as a unipolar disorder, in which a person experiences only depressive symptoms. To be diagnosed as a major depressive episode, symptoms of depressed mood and loss of interest in most or all activities must be intense and continuous for at least 2 weeks.

The common diagnostic categories of unipolar depression listed in DSM-III-R[1] are listed below:

Major depression, single episode. Severe symptoms of depression and loss of interest in the environment last for at least 2 weeks and typically more than 6 months, especially if untreated. Impaired thinking, hopelessness, and psychomotor retardation or agitation are present. The person has had no manic episodes and has only one episode of depression with a return to premorbid functioning.

Major depression, recurrent. The person has two or more episodes of intense symptoms with a separation between episodes of at least 2 months and without any previous manic states. If a seasonal pattern exists (e.g., depression occurring in fall and winter,) this is specified.

Dysthymia. This is a chronic, milder depressive disturbance than the above with a duration of at least 2 years.

Prevalence

Depression is the single most frequently occurring psychiatric condition in the general population. The occurrence of major depressions in women ranges from 9% to 26%, and in men, from 5% to 12%, with the milder form, dysthymia, being very common.[1] The age of onset of depression is usually in the twenties, but it may begin in childhood, in infancy, and in old age.

Population at Risk

Some categories of individuals are more susceptible to depression than others. Women are commonly at greater risk for depression than men, although in children the occurrence may be equal among both sexes. The disorder has been found to be 1.5 to 3 times more common among first-degree biologic relatives than the general population.[1]

The increased prevalence in women is partly caused by the traditional socialization practices of women, which reinforce their sense of dependence, compliance, and emotional vulnerability. What is viewed as a personal problem may be a social one in which women are "trained" to accept victimization in a patriarchal society.[21] Depressive symptoms in the elderly are often missed or incorrectly attributed to organic disorders. Although mild depression evidenced in sulkiness, withdrawal from social activities, and restlessness is common among adolescents because of maturational crises, their more severe depressions may not be identified.[1]

Types of Depression

Depression may be primary or secondary to other factors, such as a medical or another mental disorder or use of medicine and other chemicals. The primary type of depression is an underlying component of the syndrome rather than superimposed on an existing condition. Depression may range in severity from mild to psychotic, with only one acute episode or with recurrent episodes that become chronic.[1]

The most frequent precipitating events are psychosocial stressors including potential or actual losses.[1] In some persons a lifelong pattern of many mild depressive episodes is unnoticed until severe symptoms develop in response to a seemingly mild stressor.

Biologic changes are present in unipolar depressions as they are in the bipolar manic-depressive episodes. The increased incidence of depression in families indicates a genetic predisposition to the mood disorder. An imbalance in one or more neurotransmitters in the brain is thought to exist.[51] The positive response of most depressive patients to antidepressants is probably due to an increase in the neurotransmitters norepinephrine and/or serotonin, possibly by changes in the receptor sites in the brain.

Degrees of Depression

Mild depression is often undiagnosed. Those with severe depression are easier to identify. Some symptoms of mild and severe depression, differentiated by Arieti and Bemporad,[3] are listed below:

- Mild
  - Unpleasant feelings about self and the environment
  - Self-sacrificing, especially in relation to giving to others
  - Inhibition of normal pleasurable activities
  - Inhibition of spontaneous behavior
  - Extra effort needed to concentrate
  - Preoccupation with trivial failures and underestimating ability
  - Pessimistic outlook toward life
  - Self-reproach and irritability for not living up to an ideal standard
  - Dependence on others for gratification
  - Somatic symptoms
- Severe
  - Utter despair and hopelessness
  - Sense of emptiness
  - Unrelieved sense of guilt and feeling of worthlessness
  - Severe immobility or agitated behavior that is purposeless and lacks conscious control
  - Catastrophic expectations
  - Lack of interest in self and environment
  - Retarded thought processes to process and respond to stimuli
  - Retardation of bodily processes
  - Preoccupation with bodily functions
  - Delusional thinking that becomes severe when contact with reality is greatly impaired or lost

Psychopathology

Psychoanalytic Theory

Psychoanalysts theorize that persons experience ambivalent feelings of love and hate toward a former love object. Psychic energy (libido) is withdrawn from the lost object; hate or aggression felt for the love object is turned inward toward the self. The person then feels worthless, guilty, and depressed.[17]

Interpersonal Theory

Interpersonal theorists believe that depressive patterns develop within an interpersonal context and may begin in childhood. The child introjects an exaggerated sense of duty and responsibility. The duty and responsibility along with dependence on others are often emphasized by parents so that the child is unaware of self and his own resources. The inability to live up to parents' expectations provokes anxiety in the child; the anxiety becomes guilt, self-criticism, and lowered self-esteem. The child may experience many mild episodes of depression throughout life with no identifiable major stressor.[3]

Cognitive Theory

Cognitive and behavioral theorists are similar in their belief that depression is a consequence of faulty logic. Persons blame themselves for actual or perceived loss of an object and become self-critical and self-rejecting. They generalize their feelings of self-blame to viewing themselves as failures, inferior, and helpless and as having bleak futures. Successes and achievements are disowned. Behaviorists view depression as a consequence of negative reinforcement or no reinforcement of positive, successful behavior.[6]

Diagnostic Studies and Findings

Dexamethasone Suppression Test (DST)

Dexamethasone, 1 mg administered orally at bedtime, and on the following day specimens obtained for serum cortisol at 4 PM and 11 PM (if outpatient, 4 PM specimen only); serum cortisol greater than 5 μg/100 ml at either 4 or 11 PM is indicative of depression (administration of dexamethasone, a synthetic steroid similar to cortisol, suppresses the adrenal corticotropin hormone in most normal persons); NOTE: this test is experimental, with false negatives and false positives; positive DST findings have also been present in other mental disorders[25,60]; weakness and nausea may occur as mild side effects from dexamethasone

Medical Plan

Medications

Amitriptyline (Elavil), 50 mg tid po (rarely doses to 300 mg/d); for elderly and adolescent patients, 10 mg tid and 20 mg at hs; when depression lifts, single dose at hs; although sedative effect occurs after initiation of therapy, antidepressant effect may be delayed 3 or 4 weeks

If depression is part of bipolar disorder, along with the antidepressant may be prescribed:

- Lithium carbonate, 300 mg tid po; serum lithium levels must be assessed frequently until condition is stabilized, then at 1- to 2-mo intervals, to determine therapeutic serum levels and current toxic levels; blood is drawn for testing just before administration of next lithium dose; therapeutic serum lithium levels are 0.6 to 1.2 mEq/L; if bipolar disorder, observe closely to identify rapid change to manic phase

General Management

Electroconvulsive therapy, *only* if patient does not respond to antidepressant or if suicidal risk is severe[18]
Occupational therapy
Recreational therapy

NURSING CARE

Nursing Assessment

The severity and types of symptoms vary with each patient, with no one symptom experienced by all with depression.

Affect

Extreme sadness; despair; painful dejection; tearfulness; irritability; anxiety; feeling of emptiness

Activities

Low energy; fatigue; lack of ability or motivation to perform tasks; slow movements; eyes downcast and avoidance of eye contact; agitated, purposeless behavior evidenced by pacing and restlessness; substance abuse such as alcohol

Self-Care

Lack of interest and energy to perform activities of daily living such as bathing, dressing, and hygiene

Nutrition

Lack of appetite or interest in food (occasionally increased appetite); indigestion; weight loss, usually not critical but may be when condition is very severe or psychotic

Bowel Elimination

Constipation

Sleep Pattern

Inability to fall asleep, especially with anxiety, or waking early in morning; restless sleep; hypersomnia, occasionally to most of day owing to fatigue or withdrawal

Power

Sense of lack of power or control; hopelessness, usually greatest when awakening in the morning; helplessness; feeling that nothing patient can do will make a difference

Self-Harm

Seriousness of suicidal risk: suicidal thoughts and threats, previous self-harming behavior, statements indicating intent and development of a plan (see also discussion of suicidal behavior, p. 1545)

Thought Processes

Morbid thoughts; worry; narrow and repetitive range of thoughts; forgetfulness and inability to concentrate; self-rejection and criticism of self and others; somatic complaints; delusions about body and environment, especially bizarre in severe depression; negative view of self, environment, and the future; failures exaggerated; achievements disowned; paranoid ideation

Communication

Impaired ability to process and respond to verbal stimuli; slow thinking; slow speech; low voice; monotonous tone; limited ability to concentrate

Social Interactions

Withdrawal from social interactions and activities because of sense of unworthiness; limited social skills; loneliness; apathy concerning others

Nursing Dx & Intervention

Nursing care should be implemented selectively based on severity of symptoms and presenting behaviors.

Nursing Diagnosis	Nursing Intervention/Rationale
Potential for violence: self-directed or directed at others	• Assess for suicidal thoughts and self-destructive behaviors. • Institute suicide precautions: safe environment, removal of harmful objects, and close observation *to prevent suicidal attempts.* • Begin to establish trusting, supportive relationship *to let patient know you care and are concerned.* • Continue close observation as depression lifts, since patient has energy, and as depression deepens, when patient still has energy to attempt suicide; observe for verbal and nonverbal clues to self-harm. • Administer medication as ordered. • Briefly describe the medicine's effects and side effects initially. • When patient has improved, teach effects of medications and importance of compliance *to counteract depressive symptoms.*
Impaired verbal communication	• Assess ability to attend to and process communications. • Address patient by name *to obtain his attention.*

Nursing Diagnosis	Nursing Intervention/Rationale
	• Speak slowly, using short sentences *to increase patient's ability to attend to and comprehend words.* • Give concrete directions. • *To develop relationship,* schedule frequent, brief (10-minute) therapeutic periods daily so they are tolerable to both patient and nurse; schedule longer sessions as patient is able to tolerate more.
Ineffective individual coping	• Assess strengths and coping strategies. • When patient is agitated, accept pacing and inability to sit still. • *To let patient know of your presence,* say, for example, "I am here and want to help you." • Teach diversionary techniques when restless such as an activity *to decrease emotional discomfort;* encourage patient to practice them *to help strengthen patient's healthy strategies for dealing with inappropriate feelings.* • Help patient, as able, to identify positive attributes about himself *to begin to accept self realistically.* • Teach assertiveness techniques *to give patient sense of control.*
Bathing/hygiene and dressing/grooming self-care deficit	• Assess patient's psychologic ability and interest to care for self physically. • Assist patient with activities of daily living as needed. • Acknowledge in a matter-of-fact manner patient's accomplishments *to recognize patient's efforts to perform self-care activities.* • Encourage patient to be aware of and accept improved appearance *to enhance self-esteem.*
Altered nutrition: less than body requirements	• Assess and monitor adequacy of nutritional and fluid intake and assess difficulties eating. • Do not give patient opportunity to avoid eating or taking fluids. • Remain with patient during meals *to assist with eating as needed.* If patient is nauseated, offer a bland diet and, if needed, prescribed antacids *to decrease gastric discomfort.* • Offer small, frequent meals if patient has difficulty eating. • If patient is receiving lithium, ensure adequate liquid and normal sodium intake *to prevent toxicity.* • Teach patient about well-balanced nutritional meals and adequate fluid intake.
Constipation	• Assess and monitor bowel elimination. • Administer laxatives as ordered and if needed *to assist in elimination.* • Teach patient to include roughage in diet, drink adequate amounts of fluids, and exercise *to prevent constipation.* • If patient is receiving lithium, be alert for diarrhea *to identify toxicity.*
Altered patterns of urinary elimination	• Assess for urinary hesitance, frequency, and output. • Inform patient that an antidepressant may cause urine retention and inhibition of urinary response. • Teach patient to concentrate and apply pressure on area above pubic bone *to begin urinary flow.*
Sleep pattern disturbance	• Assess sleep patterns and feeling of restfulness after sleep. • Assist patient, as able, to identify past successful methods for promoting sleep *to reinforce implementation of positive behaviors.* • Give warm milk at bedtime *to promote relaxation.* • If patient is unable to sleep after 30 minutes, suggest that patient get out of bed and assist patient in diversionary activities. • *To correct misconceptions,* inform patient that insufficient sleep will not endanger health. • Teach patient to develop a relaxing routine before bedtime *to promote readiness for sleep.* • Teach patient to breathe slowly and deeply while focusing on number "1" with exhalation *to learn relaxation.* • If patient has hypersomnia, encourage patient to get out of bed and participate in simple diversionary activities *to counteract immobility.*
Altered thought processes related to psychologic conflicts and psychomotor retardation	• Assess thought processes and quality of cognition. • *To interrupt ruminations,* suggest diversionary activities if attempts to help patient focus on topics appropriately fail. • Assist patient in monitoring subject change *to make decisions about changing subject a conscious choice.* • Encourage patient to think about self and experiences realistically *to identify and accept positive attributes.* • Teach problem-solving methods, including evaluating possible consequences of alternative solutions *to learn effective methods of resolving issues.* • Teach assertiveness skills to help patient express self *to let others know needs and desires.* • Help patient to anticipate problems that may be encountered after discharge *to identify possible responses to issues and consequences of each.*

Nursing Diagnosis	Nursing Intervention/Rationale
Powerlessness	• Assess level and types of powerlessness patient experiences. • Allow patient to be dependent initially *to increase comfort and decrease stress.* • Communicate to patient your hopes for patient's future *to reinforce strengths.* • Identify patient's self-supports and support system of family and friends to reinforce resources. • Identify and reinforce realistic goals for patient's future *to increase a positive outlook.* • Teach patient to ask for and accept help from others *to increase a sense of control.* • Teach patient how to accept others' refusals to give help without feeling rejected, guilty, or self-critical *to reinforce the idea that refusals are not rejections of patient.*
Social isolation	• Assess degree of isolation and discomforts patient experiences with others. • Identify patient's interests and skills, as patient is able. • Participate initially with patient in simple social activities such as looking at pictures and commenting about them *to increase interest in the environment.* • Recognize patient's efforts to socialize with others *to reinforce healthy behaviors.* • Structure patient's activities with input from patient as able, and give patient copy of the plan. • Encourage patient to make changes in plan or participate in developing his own goals for care *to increase patient's participation in treatment plan.* • Assist patient in developing interests and social skills *to increase self-confidence.* • Encourage attendance and participation in occupational therapy *to share in structured activity.* • Reinforce attendance at recreational therapy *to promote enjoyment of activities and development of social and physical skills.* • Encourage family to be supportive of patient's efforts to interact with them. • Assist patient to learn adaptive skills for interaction with family and others *to relate in healthy ways.* • Help patient and family members listen and respond to one another's messages; teach them how to resolve conflicts *to develop healthier communication patterns.*

Patient Education

1. Reinforce a problem-solving approach to correct faulty thinking.
2. Teach the use of support systems for help; for example, write down the crisis center's name and telephone number or names of significant others who could be called on to help.
3. Reinforce the use of self-supports and resources.
4. Review the effects and side effects of medication, the importance of taking medicine as prescribed, and the importance of reporting adverse effects to the physician.
5. If the patient is receiving lithium, reinforce the need to monitor serum lithium levels as prescribed by the physician.
6. As the termination of nurse-patient relationship nears, review the patient's progress and teach the patient to deal with loss of the relationship to learn to deal with other losses.

Evaluation

Patient Outcome	Data Indicating That Outcome is Reached
The patient demonstrates relief of symptoms.	The patient verbalizes positive feelings about self. The patient expresses enjoyment in participating in activities. The patient initiates interactions with others. The patient sleeps soundly and awakens rested.
The patient demonstrates use of problem solving to correct thinking.	The patient consciously monitors and corrects misconceptions about self and others.
The patient evidences knowledge of depression and of the importance of continued treatment.	The patient verbalizes an awareness of depressive thoughts and feelings and of the importance of obtaining help early. The patient states effects, side effects, and methods of self-administration of medication. The patient has made plans to continue counseling.

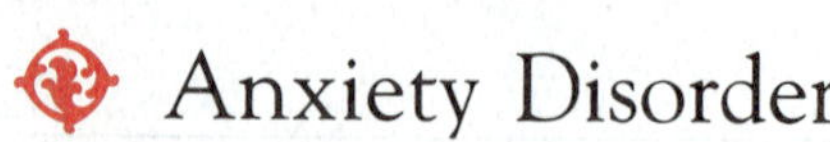

Anxiety Disorders

Anxiety disorders are a group of disturbances in which anxiety is the predominant symptom experienced or defended against (that is, avoiding the anxiety-provoking object).[1]

Anxiety is a subjective experience that can be inferred by observing the person's behavior and physiologic responses and by subjective reports. Apprehension, dread, and intense alertness to an unspecified source of danger are symptoms of anxiety. Unlike fear that is a response to an actual object or event, anxiety is a response to no specific source or actual object. The categories of anxiety disorders listed in the DSM-III-R[1] are in the following sections.

Prevalence

The findings in recent studies reported in the DSM-III-R[1] indicate that anxiety disorders occur frequently in the general population.

Population at Risk

Generalized anxiety disorder is found equally in men and women; obsessive-compulsive disorder and social phobia are more common in men; and simple phobia and panic disorder are found more frequently in women.

A hereditary predisposition is believed to be a factor in at least some anxiety disorders. The incidence of panic, phobic, and obsessive-compulsive disorders is more frequent among first-degree biologic relatives of those with these disorders than in the general population.[1,6]

Psychologic and interpersonal factors that predispose a person to anxiety disorders include early psychic trauma such as separation anxiety in childhood, pathogenic parent-child relationships, pathogenic family patterns, disturbed interpersonal relationships, and loss of social supports. Other experiences that may contribute to the disorders include threats to one's values, stressors that interfere with achievement of important goals, and exhaustion of adaptive coping resources.[1,6]

The person may experience chronic anxiety that is punctuated at intervals by acute anxiety attacks, that is, panic states. These panic attacks are sudden and intense and may subside in a few minutes or last an hour or more. The person may have them several times a day, once a week, or less than once a month. The attacks occur during the day or night. The person may awake from a sound sleep with intense apprehension or terror. During the attack the person has fears of imminent death or physical catastrophe. Other fears include humiliation or appearing foolish and stupid. The fears arise in the absence of any apparent cause such as marked physical exertion or a life-threatening event.

Perceptions and interpretations of threatening situations influence how a person responds. Some react disproportionately to the threat by panicking or use nonadaptive defenses such as repression, denial, displacement, and somatization. Some use chemicals such as alcohol. The response is related in part to the person's ego strengths and the types of coping strategies used.

In addition to anxiety disorders, anxiety occurs in other mental disorders such as somatization disorders, schizophrenic disorders, psychophysiologic conditions, and various depressive disorders.[1]

Organic disorders must be ruled out, since symptoms of these disorders can be confused with symptoms of anxiety. For examples, in cardiopulmonary disorders, symptoms may include angina pectoris, palpitations, and breathing difficulties. Endocrine disorders such as hyperthyroidism are characterized by rapid pulse, perspiration, tremors, and restlessness. Some medicines such as epinephrine, antidepressants, thyroid tablets, and dextroamphetamine produce symptoms associated with anxiety.

Psychopathology

Psychoanalytic Theory

In psychoanalytic theory, anxiety, an intrapsychic phenomenon, develops as an automatic response to the ego's perception of a traumatic situation, that is, the ego's inability to master or discharge the overwhelming influx of stimuli. It initially develops in infancy when the ego is too weak and immature to deal with the stimuli. As the young child learns to anticipate dangerous stimuli that originate usually from the id (drives) but also from external situations, he reacts to avoid trauma. The maturing ego uses psychic energy (libido) to cope with dangerous events. The dangers and concomitant anxiety are characteristic of situations children face, particularly during the first 6 years of life, and persist throughout life in varying degrees and to an excessive degree in psychoneurotic conditions. Intrapsychic conflicts are present in all psychoneurotic anxiety.[10]

The ego, the reality principle of the personality, attempts to neutralize the energy of the dangerous id by dealing with anxiety rationally and by developing healthy adaptive strategies, including identification and sublimation. When the ego is unsuccessful in dealing with anxiety adaptively, it overuses defense mechanisms. Less healthy defenses and their overuse require continuous expenditure of psychic energy and decrease the ego's strength. Since repression is part of all defense mechanisms, repressed experiences are functionally separate from the ego but continue to operate unconsciously by falsifying or distorting reality.[10]

Interpersonal Theory

In interpersonal theory, anxiety is viewed as developing within an interpersonal context. It is transmitted from the mother in infancy; later it is a response to real or imagined threats to the person's self-system. Anxiety is experienced as apprehension and discomfort, which the person attempts to avoid by developing defensive strategies. The self-system begins to develop to protect the person by excluding painful, threatening experiences from awareness. However, as the organization of the self-system becomes more complex in late childhood, experiences that provoked severe anxiety are out of awareness of or dissociated from the rest of the personality. The person is unable to examine dissociated experiences, correct distortions, and integrate these experiences into the personality. The dissociated material impairs the person's ability to perceive, remember, and think rationally. Persons are able to increase awareness of self and the environment when they integrate dissociated material into their personality.[13]

Cognitive Theory

Severe anxiety or panic is a sudden, overwhelming reaction to a perceived threat that is viewed as overpowering. Unlike depression, which is related to actual or perceived loss, anxiety is related to anticipated loss.

At the core of severe anxiety are faulty cognitive patterns that evoke a sense of vulnerability and helplessness because the person magnifies weaknesses and catastrophizes actual or imaginary threats to the self.[6] An anxious person has impaired ability to examine repetitive, dangerous thoughts logically and evaluate them objectively. He may generalize dangers to almost any other stimulus or perceived changes in his world. Anxiety evoked in response to an initial danger is also evoked in response to the generalizations. The person responds automatically to dangerous thoughts and their generalizations without examining their validity, which leads the person to feel trapped in overwhelming situations. Correction of faulty thinking initiates appropriate emotional responses to perceived dangers that do not negate feelings about the self.[5,6]

Medical Plan

Medications

Alprazolam (Xanax), 0.5 mg po tid as an initial dose that may be increased cautiously to a maximum total daily dose of 4 mg, in divided doses for severe anxiety; 0.25 mg po bid for elderly patients; the action of the medication, a central nervous system depressant, is to decrease symptoms of anxiety; when anxiety levels decrease, dosage is decreased gradually, since convulsions may occur after abrupt discontinuation, especially of high doses

General Management

Occupational therapy
Recreational therapy

NURSING CARE

Nursing Assessment

Not all dysfunctional responses are experienced by all anxious persons.

Affect

Apprehension; dread; terror; tearfulness; sobbing; irritability; anger; helplessness; frustration; sometimes laughter; nervousness

Thoughts

Scattering of thoughts or focus on details; preoccupation with self, behavior, and bodily functions; lack of confidence in abilities; low self-esteem; worry; anticipation of adversity; jealousy; envy of others; lack of control to effect or influence outcome; impaired sense of responsibility for self and behavior; sense of worthlessness and rejection by others; distractibility; indecisiveness; vacillation, especially in conflict; forgetfulness; somatization

Communication

Stuttering; blocking; rapid, pressured speech; selective inattention to stimuli observed in limited ability to hear; frequent requests, for example, in hospital for water, medication, information on physician's visit, or laboratory tests; repetitive questioning about treatments, procedures, activities, and so on; petty complaining

Physical

Dizziness; light-headedness; hyperventilation; chest pain; difficulty breathing; palpitation; perspiration; weakness; heartburn; flushing or pallor of face; tachycardia; muscle ache, especially in the neck and back; jitteriness; tremulousness; restlessness to agitation; pacing; dry mouth; dilated pupils; blurred vision; darting eyes; headache; accident proneness; impaired sexual functioning

Nutrition

Increased (occasionally decreased) appetite; nausea; belching

Bowel and Bladder Elimination

Diarrhea or occasionally constipation; urinary urgency and frequency

Sleep Pattern

Insomnia; difficulty falling asleep; restless or interrupted sleep

Social Interactions

Discomfort interacting with others because of fear of rejection or humiliation; decreased social activities because of fear of failure, especially in competitive activities

Nursing Dx & Intervention

Before severely anxious patients can learn, anxiety levels must be reduced. Anxiety is contagious, affecting others by increasing their anxiety. Nurses need to be aware of their responses to anxiety and how they deal with their own feelings to be able to intervene therapeutically with patients. They can use changes in their anxiety level as indicators of changes in a patient's anxiety.

Nursing Diagnosis	Nursing Intervention/Rationale
Anxiety	• Assess anxiety level and how it is manifested. • Provide a nondemanding, comfortable environment *to decrease stressors.* • Begin to establish a supportive, safe relationship *to prevent threats to self-esteem.* • Allow temporary dependence. • Remain with patient during panic attack *to decrease terror.* • Acknowledge painfulness of patient's feelings *to convey understanding of his sense of helplessness.* • Listen to patient's somatic complaints initially and slowly help patient relate it to anxiety level *to connect somatic symptoms with anxiety.* • Inhibit patient's ventilation of feelings if escalation to a nonconstructive level occurs; change focus, for example, to comfort measures, such as offering juice, *to decrease overwhelming discomfort.* • Instruct patient to breathe slowly and deeply; breathe with patient as needed *to demonstrate technique.* • Briefly explain that breathing slowly at regularly scheduled times and when anxiety increases will help patient *to learn to relax and increase the oxygen supply and energy.* • Administer medication as ordered. Teach effects and side effects of medication including need for gradual discontinuation of medication *to promote informed participation in and compliance with medical regimen.* • Teach patient to monitor his own restlessness and engage in diversionary activities such as exercise, walking, and table tennis, *to decrease anxiety and to develop a sense of control over feelings.* • Encourage patient to identify and realistically accept strengths and weaknesses *to develop self-supports.*
Altered thought processes related to psychologic conflicts	• Assess cognitive abilities and effects of anxiety on thought processes. • Speak calmly, using patient's name frequently *to obtain patient's attention.* • Give clear, concise directions *to ensure that patient is able to comprehend.* • Assist patient to identify any thoughts had just before anxiety experience *to connect cognitions to anxiety.* • Begin to help patient to correct misconceptions about experiences before anxiety using problem-solving approach *to alter emotional reaction of anxiety.* • Teach patient to become aware of automatic thoughts when anticipating negative experiences and to examine evidence *to learn to monitor own thoughts.* • Teach patient to reframe events, for example, to think of boss as a "purring kitten" instead of a "growling lion" and to redefine anxiety as a pleasant, exciting sensation *to learn to think positively and decrease anxiety.* • Teach patient to anticipate realistically possible negative and positive outcomes of anxiety-evoking events *to learn how to implement remedial actions as needed.* • Assist patient to accept abilities *to influence events.* • Teach patient to set realistic goals *to prevent a decrease in self-confidence by failure to achieve unrealistic goals.* • Teach patient to ask for help in work and home situations *to prevent patient from viewing self as weak or incompetent.*
Impaired verbal communication	• Assess skills and type of impaired communication. • Initially answer repetitive questions simply and concisely *to help patient decrease anxiety.* • Inform patient of plans and schedules and write them down so patient can refer to the paper *to assist in remembering, thereby increasing a sense of security.* • As patient is able, help identify anxiety when patient questions repetitively, has petty complaints, stutters, and blocks *to increase awareness of emotional state.* • Suggest that patient speak more slowly when stuttering. Encourage patient to breathe slowly and deeply *to increase energy, decrease stuttering and blocking, and be able to complete sentences.* • Inform patient that saying "I stutter when I get excited or uncomfortable" to others may help him *to decrease stuttering and embarrassment.* • State matter-of-factly that patient will remember blocked material later *to acknowledge patient's strength and abilities.*

Nursing Diagnosis	Nursing Intervention/Rationale
Altered nutrition: potential for more or less than body requirements	• Assess nutritional and fluid intake and relationship to anxiety state. • Monitor food and fluid intake. • If needed, obtain order for soft, bland diet to decrease belching and nausea; small, more frequent meals may be advisable *to decrease gastric distress*. • Administer medication such as antacid as ordered and needed *to decrease nausea and belching*. • Teach good nutrition and ways to increase or decrease caloric intake as needed. Delay weight reduction diet until condition is stable and patient has sense of control of own life.
Altered patterns of urinary elimination	• Assess and monitor urinary difficulties such as urgency and frequency. • Help patient, as able, to relate urinary difficulty to anxiety level. • Inform patient that urinary difficulty will diminish as patient becomes more comfortable. • Encourage adequate fluid intake.
Diarrhea or constipation related to anxiety and stress	• Assess bowel habits and their relationship to anxiety level. • Administer antidiarrheal medication (such as diphenoxylate) as ordered and indicated *to manage diarrhea*. • For constipation, encourage adequate diet and fluid intake and exercise. Obtain temporary order for laxative if indicated *to obtain relief*. • Teach patient importance of adequate fluid intake, roughage in diet, and exercise, along with routine for bowel elimination to prevent constipation.
Sleep pattern disturbance related to psychologic stress	• Assess sleep patterns such as restlessness, ability to fall asleep, and morning waking pattern. • If patient is able to identify previously used adaptive methods to promote sleep, reinforce these *to strengthen effective coping strategies*. • If needed, teach patient how to develop a fixed evening routine, such as warm bath, watching television, and reading *to promote sleep*. • Assist patient to practice focusing on breathing slowly and deeply *to promote relaxation*. • Encourage patient to listen to tape recordings on relaxation when settled in bed *to decrease ruminations*.
Social isolation	• Assess abilities, fears, and difficulties interacting with others. • Identify patient's social skills and activities enjoyed in past and encourage patient to accept them *to promote self-confidence*. • Encourage participation in occupational and recreational therapies for enjoyment, development of skills, and physical stimulation *to increase confidence in social activities and interactions*. • Teach patient that responsibility in social activities is shared and that successes or failures are not entirely patient's. • Teach assertiveness skills and practice them with patient *to increase self-confidence*. • Teach patient to accept positive feelings about interactions with significant others, and help patient examine interactions in which patient expects rejection or disapproval *to identify evidence and resolve the issue*. • Help patient accept strengths, abilities, and imperfections *to encourage patient to accept self*.

Patient Education

1. Reinforce knowledge of antianxiety medications, especially effects that impair alertness and dangers of abrupt discontinuation.
2. Reinforce self-management strategies for decreasing anxiety, such as relaxation techniques, physical activities, and diversionary activities.
3. Teach the patient to deal realistically with issues to be faced immediately after discharge.

Evaluation

Patient Outcome	Data Indicating That Outcome is Reached
Patient evidences relief of severe symptoms.	Patient practices relaxation techniques and engages in diversionary activities to relieve anxiety. Patient is able to relate anxiety to physical sensations and incorrect thinking. Patient uses problem-solving approach to correct misconceptions about events and self. Patient verbalizes sense of increased confidence in ability to perform tasks and interact with others. Patient is able to fall asleep more easily than in past and awaken feeling rested.

Nursing Diagnosis	Nursing Intervention/Rationale
Patient demonstrates knowledge of medication and importance of compliance with treatment plan.	Patient describes effects and side effects of medicine, including danger of abrupt discontinuation. Patient develops system to ensure accurate self-administration of medicine as prescribed after discharge. Patient schedules appointment with health professional to continue counseling after discharge.

PERSONALITY DISORDERS

Personality disorders are a category of conditions in which a person evidences enduring personality traits that are inflexible and maladaptive. These traits are stable patterns of perceiving, thinking, feeling, and relating to the person's world and self.[1] The inflexibility of the personality may remain unnoticed until adaptation to environmental changes or pressures is expected.

The borderline personality disorder is discussed here because its occurrence is increasing and its management creates difficulties for health professionals in all settings.

Borderline personality disorder

Borderline personality disorder is a condition in which the person exhibits enduring patterns of behavior that do not change with experiences.[1] The person may appear to function adequately until exposed to personal or environmental stressors.

Behaviors associated with borderline personality disorder are intolerance to frustration, impulsivity in which the person acts destructively toward self and others, substance abuse, and instability of affect, with anger the prominent expression rather than anxiety or depression. Anger and hostility are expressed in irritability, sarcasm, demandingness, and projection of feelings onto others. The borderline personality is vulnerable to brief, mild psychotic episodes that are triggered by stress.

Although the person forms intense relationships, he has difficulty with intimacy and maintaining close relationships; he shifts from idealizing to devaluing others. Being unable to hold an integrated view of self and others with degrees of good and bad, the borderline personality splits objects and thus holds compartmentalized, polarized views of either positiveness or negativeness at any one time.[34] Because of feelings of loneliness and emptiness, the borderline personality avoids being alone and spends most of his time in the presence of others. His relationships are strongly dependent, masochistic, sadistic, and manipulative. Through manipulation he exploits others to gain control and support.[32,34]

Distorted perceptions are related to self-centeredness and inability to empathize with others. Denial is a common ego defense against uncomfortable feelings and relevant past experiences.

When the person is questioned about or confronted with his contradictory actions and feelings, he uses denial and projection to avoid awareness of himself and his behavior.

Hospitalization

The decision to hospitalize a person with a borderline personality disorder is usually based on a crisis, severe anxiety or panic, self-destructive acts including suicidal threats, or transient psychosis.

While in the hospital the patient provokes conflict and tension among staff members.[22] Contradictory views of the patient held by staff lead to strong disagreement about the patient and his behavior. The strong emotional reactions evoked in the staff by the patient, countertransference, confirm the patient's projections. Some staff members receive positive projections from the patient and may respond in a nurturing, permissive way; other staff members receive negative projections from the patient and may respond in a punitive, controlling, and hostile manner. The nurse needs to be aware that the flattery and criticism are ego defenses used by the patient in his shifting projections of the self.[34,46]

An understanding of the dynamics of the condition and open communication among staff members with regular staff meetings are essential to implement consistent care.

The hospital structure can provide the patient with a sense of security and protection. However, care must be taken not to overwhelm the borderline personality with too much nurturing and closeness because this evokes feelings of suffocation from which the patient needs to escape. Setting limits consistently and nonpunitively establishes expectations of responsibility and accountability for the patient. Since the borderline personality's tolerance for frustration is low, he responds to limit setting with hostility and rage. The nurse helps the patient examine the factors leading to the hostility, explore alternative responses, and handle feelings. The nurse clearly communicates the patient's behaviors that will and will not be permitted; for example, verbal expressions of anger may be allowed but not physical ones.[32]

Prevalence

Borderline personality disorder is a commonly occurring condition in the general population, with an estimated incidence of 15%.[1,22] Some health professionals think the prevalence is increasing, possibly because society is becoming less structured and there is increasing emphasis on individualism and violence.

Population at Risk

The borderline personality disorder begins in childhood or adolescence; however, the diagnosis is not applicable to those before the age of puberty, and a clearer clinical picture of the borderline personality emerges in middle or late adolescence.[1,34] The diagnosis is more common in women. Symptoms frequently overlap with other disorders, especially those within the personality disorder classification. Borderline personality disorder is most difficult to differentiate from the histrionic, narcissistic, and antisocial personality disorders, since they are all characterized by impulsivity, dramatization, and emotionalism.

The presence of organicity in this disorder remains unclear. In some cases the disorder appears to be purely psychogenic; in others a minimal degree of organic involvement, such as minimal brain dysfunction and neurologic deficits, may contribute to the symptoms.[34]

Motivation for psychotherapy is low, and dropout rates are high. When the patient's stress decreases, motivation for continuing in therapy frequently declines until the next crisis. Expected outcomes of therapy are increased adaptability in interpersonal relationships and to environmental events and increased openness in communications with others.

Psychopathology

Conceptualizations of the borderline personality disorder have been developed most clearly and extensively by psychoanalytic theorists. The interpersonal and cognitive theorists have not specifically addressed this disorder. Without an understanding of the dynamics of the borderline personality, it is difficult to intervene therapeutically to interrupt the psychopathologic condition.

Psychoanalytic Theory

The borderline personality has impaired development of object relations that have been conceptualized in the separation-individuation process. In this process, which occurs from 4 to 36 months of age, the child develops a sense of self as a psychologically separate object with clear boundaries differentiating him from other objects in the environment. In the identity of self the child has integrated stable inner images of himself and other objects as having both good and bad qualities. He has the ability to function independently, that is, without his mother's presence.[27,30]

In the borderline personality the separation-individuation process is arrested during the rapprochement phase, which occurs between 16 and 24 months of age. The rapprochement phase occurs concomitantly with the anal phase of development during which aggression and ambivalence are experienced in response to the powerful parent figures. Issues of dependence and independence and control are intertwined with fears of abandonment, loss of love, or engulfment (being "swallowed up") by the mother. The toddler with his growing autonomy experiences conflicts between the desire to be separate and omnipotent and the wish to have needs magically fulfilled. His feelings and wishes are still poorly differentiated from what he perceives as his mother's; he believes his thoughts and feelings are similar to his mother's as evidenced by her meeting his needs. The mother's empathetic understanding is viewed by the toddler as reading his mind.[27]

The anger and aggression of this period are unstructured and outside of ego control; no cohesive, integrated mental images of self and others have emerged within the personality. The split in mental images of good or bad precludes the development of evocation of memories and past experiences. In the borderline personality the images of self and others are predominantly bad. The arrest in this developmental phase in the borderline personality is generally attributed to the mother who rewards clinging, regressive behaviors and withdraws and is unavailable when the child shows healthy development. Constitutional and other environmental factors may contribute to the arrest of the child's development in this phase.[34]

Medical Plan

Medications

Oxazepam (Serax), 15 mg po bid and hs; for elderly, 10 mg po bid and hs to reduce symptoms such as anxiety, agitation, irritability, and anxiety associated with depression (choice of medication may vary according to the presenting symptoms); oxazepam causes drowsiness and occasionally dizziness; its mean half-life is 8.2 h; since abrupt discontinuation may result in seizurelike symptoms, gradual reduction is advised

NURSING CARE

Nursing Assessment

Signs and symptoms vary in type and severity among patients.

Emotions

Anger; hostility; depression; anxiety; emptiness; loneliness; emotional shallowness

Thoughts and Actions

Denial of contradictory feelings; denial of responsibility for behavior; intolerance of stress ad frustration; demandingness; acting out of tensions and feelings; poor judgment; projection of hostile feelings onto others; misinterpretation of stimuli; impaired problem solving; sense of inadequacy and insecurity; ambivalence; polarized views of others as good or bad; sense of specialness; masochistic and sadistic behavior; destructive behavior toward self and others

Communication

Demanding; sarcasm; criticism; verbally striking out at others' vulnerabilities; manipulativeness by evoking rescue fantasies in some individuals or hostility with subsequent counterattacks from others; evoking disagreements and competitive behaviors among others

Nursing Dx & Intervention

Nursing care should be implemented selectively based on severity and type of behavior. Since hospitalization is likely to be brief and change is slow, usually interventions only begin to have positive effects on the patient's healthy adaptation.

Nursing Diagnosis	Nursing Intervention/Rationale
Ineffective individual coping	• Assess level of functioning and coping strategies. • Begin to develop trusting relationship with patient without being too nurturing or overinvolved *to prevent fears of engulfment.* • Involve patient in treatment plan by having him identify how he wants you and other staff members to help him *to avoid trying to anticipate needs and meeting them magically.* • Communicate routines and expectations in a matter-of-fact way *to provide structure for patient.* • Encourage patient to describe events that lead to impulsive behaviors, including thoughts and actions in events *to help patient become aware of personal contributions in events.* • Be alert to patient's omissions of own behaviors and focus on others *to prevent patient from projecting difficulties onto others.* • Help patient correct distortions in perceptions, thought process, and definitions of an event *to begin using problem-solving approach.* • Encourage patient to identify and evaluate consequences of impulsive behaviors *to learn, for example, how they achieved or did not achieve desired outcome.* • Assist patient to examine and evaluate possible alternative behaviors *to achieve a satisfying outcome.* • Ask patient what help he wants in controlling or preventing impulsive behaviors *to increase self-responsibility.* • If patient is unable to control impulsivity, use diversionary techniques (such as escorting patient to quiet area, taking him for a walk, or changing subject) *to prevent or interrupt unacceptable behaviors.* • After patient is calmer, encourage discussion of details of both issue and patient's feelings *to use problem-solving approach for dealing with situation and to examine possible consequences of alternative responses.* • Inform patient what behaviors are permitted and set limits consistently to provide a sense of security *to communicate clearly to patient what behaviors will not be permitted.* • Be alert to self-destructive acts; take suicide threats and minor suicidal acts seriously, even if manipulative. If indicated and in collaboration with physician, institute suicide precautions. • Administer any medication ordered by physician *to decrease disturbing symptoms;* observe for adverse reactions such as an increase in hostility; teach patient the medication's effects and possible side effects. • Teach patient to use relaxation techniques, such as slow deep breathing and focus on breathing or the number "1" *to decrease panic and promote sleep and relaxation.* Listening to quiet, "easy-listening" music on the radio can have a hypnotic effect. • Avoid an empathetic understanding of patient's thoughts and feelings. Since patient may conclude that you can read his mind; ask him to tell you his thoughts *to help him recognize the reality of his separateness.* • Matter-of-factly point out inconsistencies or contradictions in patient's actions and expressions of thoughts and feelings *to increase patient's awareness of his behavior.* • Keep in mind that patient's negative and positive appraisals of others are his defenses *to be alert to patient's playing one staff member against another.* • When patient complains about another staff member, encourage him to talk with that person *to work his problems out rather than tell you.* • Hold regular staff meetings *to clarify or modify treatment plans, reinforce need for consistency, and support one another.* • Assess whether patient is able to accomplish requested task; assist him as needed to complete task. • Have the patient evaluate his own behaviors realistically *to encourage patient to accept his strengths.*

Patient Education

1. Teach the patient to monitor responses to events by thinking before acting out and using diversionary techniques.
2. Teach the patient to focus on his own behavior in situations rather than on others only.

3. Teach the importance of compliance with the medical regimen and long-term psychotherapy.

Evaluation

Patient Outcome	Data Indicating That Outcome is Reached
Patient demonstrates reduction in symptoms	Patient begins to monitor his own behavior to control impulsive behavior. Patient is able to state needs and accept delays. Patient verbalizes decrease in uncomfortable feelings. Patient begins to use problem-solving approach to deal with issues.
Patient evidences acceptance of need for continuing treatment.	Patient verbally recognizes the value of examining his own behavior. Patient states effects and side effects of medication and knowledge of accurate self-administration after discharge. Patient makes plans to continue counseling by scheduling appointment after discharge.

ADAPTIVE AND MALADAPTIVE BEHAVIOR

Two conditions, potential for self-harm and crisis, are presented in this section. Although these related conditions are not classifications of mental disorders, they have serious implications for mental health. Crisis intervention services arose from suicide prevention programs of the 1950s and 1960s.[14] Preventive strategies are emphasized in both. In potential for self-harm the immediate goal is prevention of suicide; in crisis intervention a goal is prevention of the maladaptation of mental illness. Alternative effective coping responses are sought when intervening in these conditions.

Stressors play an important part in the development of dysfunctional responses. DSM-III-R[1] takes into account psychosocial stressors (ranging in influence from "none" to "catastrophic" depending on severity) as contributors to the development or exacerbation of dysfunctional behaviors. Therapeutic interventions are directed toward fostering adaptive rather than maladaptive responses. Adaptation is the ability to mobilize the resources needed to make changes in the self or in the external environment to cope effectively with stress. Maladaptation is the inability to mobilize the necessary resources to manage stress.

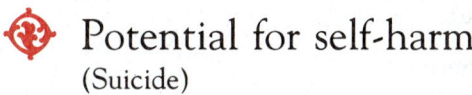

Potential for self-harm

(Suicide)

Suicide is a self-harm act to terminate one's life. The term can be broadly categorized to include completed suicide, suicide attempt, and suicide ideas.

Completed suicide is the cessation of life resulting from self-destructive behavior, whereas attempted suicide is an apparently life-threatening act that does not result in death.[43] Persons with suicidal ideas are preoccupied with thoughts of ending their lives and may indicate these directly or indirectly by behavior such as making a final will or saying "Others would be better off without me." The term "suicide" does not explain the cause of death but only the mode of death or the presence of life-threatening thoughts and acts.

The seriousness of suicidal acts and thoughts is related to the lethality and intent. Lethality of an act or contemplated act is ranked from zero to high depending on its destructiveness and reversibility. Suicide attempts by firearms and hanging are highly lethal, whereas ingesting 15 aspirin is not. Sometimes ignorance of the consequences of a method enters into the lethality; that is, persons who lack information may incorrectly choose a method that is or is not fatal.[26]

Intent to commit suicide is a determination to end one's life. Extremes of intent range from absolute determination to none. The degree of intent is difficult to assess accurately, since people exaggerate or deny their intent to kill themselves. Some persons may state a strong desire to commit suicide in order to manipulate others, with no intention of committing suicide. Others deny their intentions even though they have well-formulated plans and serious intent to kill themselves. All threats and attempts must be taken seriously.

Families are often reluctant to admit that a member engaged in self-destructive acts or intended suicide because of the stigma attached to such behaviors. Religious beliefs and cultural norms in many countries prohibit self-destructive behaviors, viewing them as "sinful" or disgraceful.[26]

Accidental suicides occur for a variety of reasons. A "suicidal gesture" used as a manipulative ploy to gain favors and influence others may inadvertently result in death. Conditions that cloud consciousness such as chronic pain, organic disease, dysfunctional states (panic, severe depression, psychosis, and high stress), and drugs may lead to unintentional self-destructive behavior. For example, persons with severe pain may take repeated doses of analgesics until they no longer remember if or how much medicine was ingested. Psychotic suicides in depression or schizophrenia may be in response to delusional ideas or hallucinatory orders to punish the self through self-destructive behaviors.[3]

Some suicidal acts are conscious, logical decisions persons

make when they believe life is less desirable than death. These persons have no hope that their life circumstances will change, and they carefully plan and carry out their suicides. Altruistic suicides are carried out for the welfare of others and are often viewed as honorable acts.[26]

Health professionals must take the perspective of the person with suicidal ideation and behaviors rather than superimpose their own beliefs on the person regardless of whether the behaviors are manipulative ploys or serious attempts in response to mild or severe stressors. All suicidal thoughts and acts must be taken seriously and responded to appropriately.

Prevalence

The official statistics on attempted and completed suicides are highly unreliable and underestimated owing to negative attitudes in the United States. Unless the evidence clearly points to suicide, other causes are stated on medical records and death certificates. A reported suicide figure in 1982 was 30,000, with suicide attempts estimated at 10 times that figure.[43] In recent years suicide has ranked among the 10 leading causes of death in industrial countries.

Population at Risk

Many people have had at least fleeting thoughts of killing themselves at some point in their lives or know someone who has attempted self-harm. Women are four times more likely than men to attempt suicide, but more men succeed at it. In 1982 the suicide rate for the 15- to 25-year-old age group was 12.2 per 100,000 with eight to 10 attempts for every completed act.[43]

Separation from and death of loved ones, divorce, loss of health, loss of jobs and money, and serious illness are powerful factors in suicide. The suicide rate increases with advancing age; midlife and old age are particularly difficult periods, with those aged 60 and older in 1980 making up 16% of the population but 23% of the suicide victims.[43]

Persons whose significant others have committed suicide or who have attempted suicide themselves in the past are more prone to suicide. The suicide may be related to a significant date such as an anniversary, a birthday, or becoming the same age as the lost person. A history of previous suicide attempts is an important predictor of future suicidal behavior; many of those who successfully complete a suicide have attempted suicide previously.[26]

Family disruptions affect younger family members more than older ones. Conflicts and arguments within the family create suicidal pressures on members. The potentially suicidal member is often isolated within the family and becomes the scapegoat.

Sequelae in the Family

Family members, loved ones, and friends of those who commit suicide are survivor-victims of suicide. They are tortured by guilt, shame, hatred, and confusion for years after the episode. Obsessional thoughts about the death and the search for reasons are often attempts to relieve self-blame. Significant others may deny that the cause of death was suicide despite the evidence and may continue to believe that the death was accidental or due to natural causes.

The survivors need help to alleviate their emotional distress and prevent the development of maladaptive coping techniques such as suicide or abnormal grief responses for years after the death. Crisis counseling for survivor-victims needs to be available to prevent or reduce the harmful effects of the suicide.[26]

Psychopathology

Psychoanalytic Theory

Psychoanalytic theorists view suicide from the psychopathology of depression. Ambivalent feelings of love and hate experienced toward the lost love object are withdrawn from the object, and the hate or aggression are turned inward toward the self. Suicide is the extreme response of self-hatred. The self-destructive act is carried out as self-punishment with the hope of gaining forgiveness from the sadistic component of the developing superego.[17]

Interpersonal Theory

In interpersonal theory, suicide stems from depression in which the person believes that it is better to die than to suffer emotional pain and emptiness. Through self-punishment the person hopes to gain relief from guilt, feelings of helplessness, and failure. Often through self-destructive behavior the person gains relief from negative self-feelings and, if he survives, may begin to improve.[3]

Suicide in children is markedly different from that in adults. Before 9 years of age, children have no concept of the permanence and irreversibility of death. The rarity of suicide in children is due to their cognitive immaturity to plan and implement it. When suicide occurs, it may be related to fears of punishment, especially by parents. Adolescents attempt suicide because of self-hatred and losses, especially of love objects; some do so as a desperate cry for help, often to others beyond their family. In some adolescents coercive manipulation is involved to obtain revenge or peer approval.[3]

Delusions and hallucinations in psychotic persons reinforce and support self-redemption and forgiveness through the self-punishment of suicide.

Cognitive Theory

Petrie and Chamberlain[45] found in their own and others' studies that suicidal behavior and ideation are not significantly related to depression per se but that hopelessness is the important explanatory variable in suicide. These studies support Beck's finding that persons experiencing hopelessness and negative views of their future are at high suicidal risk. Depressed persons with hope are less likely to engage in suicidal behavior.

Hopeless persons see no escape from their unbearable feelings and situation. The sense of no escape gives rise to suicidal ideas and behavior as the only solution and as an end to emotional distress.

Beck and others[7] state that realistic problems related to environmental factors such as work and school performance, loss of job by the head of the family, and unsatisfying interpersonal relationships may contribute to a person's hopelessness and wish to end it all. It is true that the expectation of regaining a lost loved one, wealth, status, or health is unrealistic unless the person is able to accept alternative solutions. Persons who view suicide as the only solution may carry it out in a logical rational manner or may perform it as a highly illogical response to a situation.

The nurse should be aware that the tranquility and peacefulness observed in a formerly distressed or agitated person might not be a sign of improvement but rather a sign of having made a decision and plans to commit suicide.

Medical Plan

Medications

Amitriptyline (Elavil) for depression or personality disorder to decrease symptoms of hopelessness and suicidal ideation; 50 mg po bid for adults; 10 mg po tid for elderly or adolescents; if there is suspicion that patient is not swallowing pills or is hoarding them, IM medication may be substituted

Chlorpromazine (Thorazine) for psychotic disorders to reduce symptoms and distress of psychotic conditions; 25 mg po qid for adults; 25 mg po bid for elderly and adolescents; IM or liquid may be substituted if patient is not swallowing pills

General Management

Suicide precautions

Seclusion if deemed necessary for patient's protection

Electroconvulsive therapy may be necessary to prevent completion of suicide act if the threat of suicide is strong and the patient does not respond to antidepressive medication

NURSING CARE

Nursing Assessment

Signs and symptoms will vary among individuals.

Violence*

Instability or changes in life situation; thoughts that life is not worthwhile; presence, duration, and strength of self-harm thoughts; contemplation of ways of harming or killing self; development of well-formulated plans; strength of motive or serious intent to follow through with plans; availability of chosen suicide method; factors, such as family, religion, and additional stress, that may push person toward or deter suicide; previous thoughts and attempts of suicide along with intent and lethality of attempts or ideas; loss of significant other through suicide

Power and Control

Hopelessness; inability to influence or alter interpersonal or life situation

Affect

Sadness or depression; inappropriate feelings such as laughter; anger; distress; tranquility once decision and plan are finalized

Thoughts

Negative view of the future; humiliation (for example, feeling of being a failure); perceived or actual recent losses, stressors, or changes; ambivalence; fantasies about how others may react (for example, "They'll be sorry"); vengeful thoughts; delusions or auditory hallucinations of sin, self-punishment, and atonement

Communication

Comments such as saying good-bye instead of good night, "I won't be seeing you again," or "Next time you see me I'll be riding in a hearse"; informing family or spouse of whereabouts of important papers, such as insurance papers, bankbooks, and will; threats of suicide as a cry for help or to manipulate interactions

Activities

Making or changing will; increasing life insurance; visiting or phoning relatives and friends for intense conversations; giving away prized possessions; demonstrating increased concern or care for others; buying tools needed to implement suicide, such as a gun, rope, or prescription refills; acting out behavior; writing a farewell note

Social Interactions

Perceived or actual lack of support from others; loss of valued relationships through separation, divorce, death, or romantic breakups

Family Process

Dysfunctional patterns of interactions such as conflict, arguments, and blaming; others not perceiving and responding to needs or wishes

*These may be used for a graded level of assessment to determine potential for self-harm.

Nursing Dx & Intervention

Although the environment should be made as safe as possible by removing any materials suicidal patients might use to harm themselves, it is not possible to make the environment completely suicide proof.[12] The importance of developing a concerned, supportive interpersonal relationship with the patient cannot be overemphasized.

When working with suicidal patients, even when they are manipulative, nurses need to be aware of and manage their own feelings while empathizing with the patients' point of view. Nursing care should be implemented selectively based on seriousness of symptoms and presenting behaviors.

Nursing Diagnosis	Nursing Intervention/Rationale
Potential for violence: self-directed	• Assess level of hopelessness and seriousness of suicidal ideations and intent. • Begin to establish supportive relationship with patient *to demonstrate concern and worth of patient.* • Institute precautions such as removing all harmful objects from environment (glass containers, drugs, belts, shoe laces, and so on), and closely observe patient (initially one-to-one observation day and night if necessary; later, observation every 15 minutes and frequent interactions while awake; and eventually hourly checks) *to decrease opportunities for self-harm and ensure safety of patient.* • Allow patient to keep more possessions as deemed safe and as precautions become less stringent *to provide reasonable restrictions that promote the well-being of patient.* • Continue close observation with knowledge of patient's whereabouts when on unit. • While suicide precautions are in effect, engage patient, as able, in simple activities such as exercises or looking at magazines *to promote the relationship and encourage interest in the environment.* • Evaluate patient's condition frequently at first and at least once a day *to determine his mood and potential for self-harm.* • Observe for changes in patient's mood, such as calmness or tranquility, as a possible prelude to suicide. • Administer medication with a simple explanation, including a description of possible side effects, such as orthostatic hypotension and drowsiness. When condition improves, teach patient about effects and side effects of medication, and leave opportunities to ask questions *to encourage knowledgeable participation in treatment plan.*
Powerlessness	• Assess patient's sense of helplessness and ability to control self and life situations. • As patient is able, explore experiences that contributed to sense of helplessness *to help patient begin to explore factors.* • During interactions, convey sense of hope in patient's abilities to maintain control of his behavior. • Convey to patient that you are there to help control behavior if he is unable to do so for himself *to provide relief and a sense of security.* • Teach assertiveness skills *to begin to increase patient's confidence in himself and learn how to let others know his needs.* • Help patient deal with uncomfortable feelings in situations *to begin to develop healthy coping strategies.*
Altered thought processes	• Assess abilities to think logically and to problem solve. • Convey acceptance of patient and take suicidal ideation seriously *to demonstrate respect and concern for patient.* • Assist patient to identify meaning of suicide threats (or attempts) and what patient expected to happen to himself and others *to help patient become aware of experiences that led to self-harm behaviors.* • Examine losses and stressors that evoked self-harm behaviors *to begin a problem-solving approach to correct illogical thoughts.* • Help patient recall and identify reasons for living *to examine experiences when life was better than it is currently.* • Avoid reinforcing delusions and hallucinations; assist patient to examine experiences before delusions or hallucinations *to help patient gradually connect thoughts and feelings with development of false beliefs and perceptions.* • Teach patient how to anticipate future issues and to develop methods other than suicide for handling them.
Impaired verbal communication	• Assess ability and willingness to talk about suicide and other issues. • Help patient identify how he decided to stop sharing information and problems with others *to identify blocks in communication.* • If patient denies suicidal intent, ask patient what he was experiencing at the time.

Nursing Diagnosis	Nursing Intervention/Rationale
	• If patient says suicidal behavior was an accident, help him identify ways to prevent future "accidents." • Encourage patient to identify people he thinks he can share ideas with *to connect him with a support system.* • Assist patient to decide whom he wants to share information with on self-harm behaviors: what information and how to share it. Use role playing to rehearse the telling. Assist patient to deal with those he does not wish to share information with *to help him accept that he has a right to choose not to tell others.*
Ineffective individual coping	• Assess coping strategies to deal with stressors and life situations. • Examine appropriateness of patient's emotional responses to events, using problem-solving approach *to reinforce healthy adaptive behaviors.* • When patient shows signs of increased tension, encourage slow, deep breathing *to help decrease tension.* Teach patient to practice relaxation techniques daily.
Social isolation	• Assess abilities and comfort level in interactions with others. • Assist patient to identify enjoyable interactions with others *to help recall details of pleasurable experiences.* • Encourage patient to identify and accept social skills. • Help patient to identify feelings of social inadequacies and begin to help to correct these; provide names of community resources *to assist with correcting these after discharge.*
Altered family processes	• Assess relationships among family members. Identify interaction patterns. • Assist family members to identify and begin to deal with thoughts and feelings about the self-harm behaviors *to correct misconceptions and inappropriate feelings such as shame and guilt.* • Assist patient and family members to listen and respond to each other *to improve communication patterns for greater understanding.* • Assist family members to identify positive aspects of relationships, such as warmth and caring, as they interact *to help each member accept those aspects and to reinforce these behaviors.* • Suggest continued counseling for family members, if needed, *to work through the crisis successfully.*

Patient Education

1. Reinforce alternative solutions and methods for handling situations instead of suicide: identification of feelings and thoughts when the patient experiences loss of control and asks for help, reaching out to supports within the family and among friends, problem-solving approach, and self-supports and strengths.
2. Have the patient write down names, addresses, and phone numbers of the local suicide prevention center and 24-hour help lines. Encourage the patient to use them day or night to obtain support or to talk with someone when the therapist is not available.
3. Reinforce the need for continued counseling or psychotherapy, and emphasize that this is a sign of strength rather than weakness.
4. Review the effects and side effects of medicine.
5. Review possible ways of dealing with situations after discharge. Help the patient learn to share or avoid sharing aspects of suicide and hospitalization with others.

Evaluation

Patient Outcome	Data Indicating That Outcome is Reached
Patient demonstrates ability to manage stressors without resorting to suicide.	Patient verbalizes coping strategies for dealing with issues. Patient evidences increased self-assurance in behavior. Patient verbalizes desire to live and states plans for resolving similar problems in future.
Patient develops plans to increase satisfaction by changing his life situation.	Patient is able to use self-supports. Patient identifies and voices acceptance of supportive social network. Patient sets aside time for leisure activities. Patient identifies more realistic goals for performance in work and play.
Patient plans to continue treatment plan after discharge.	Patient states accurate information about actions and self-administration of medication. Patient verbalizes commitment to continue counseling and makes appointment.

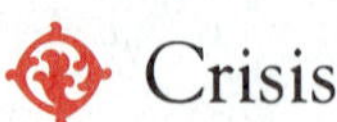

Crisis

A crisis is a temporary personality disorganization with an acute emotional state when habitual problem-solving abilities are inadequate and can result in maladjustment or growth in the personality. It is accepted generally as a normal response produced by a threatening external event rather than a pathologic state.

The person may be in a vulnerable state because of efforts to deal with hazardous events before the crisis reaction. Despite being in a state of moderate anxiety or depression, the person is able to mobilize resources to cope, although possibly at a reduced level, with the initial stressors.[26] However, when an overpowering experience, the precipitant, occurs, it produces the disorganizing effect of a crisis reaction. For example, the initial stressor may be a surgical procedure that produces a vulnerable state, and the crisis-precipitating event may be the knowledge that the excised tumor was cancerous. Sometimes a person experiences just one stressor of sufficient force to precipitate the crisis.

An acute crisis is a subjective state of psychologic and physical disorganization in which the person experiences a temporary loss of control. This is called a panic state. Since emotional reactions to the stimulus are overwhelming and nonintegrated, the cognitive processes such as assessing, thinking, decision making, and judging are inoperative.[53] Thinking is scattered, with no ability to attend to anything or fix on one narrow point[61]; affectional ties to others are severely disrupted or severed so that the person feels isolated. The person is immobilized or moves about aimlessly.

Korner[53] differentiates between two types of crisis on the basis of the person's prior life experiences: an exhaustion and a shock crisis. In an exhaustion crisis the person has coped effectively under emergency conditions for a long time and reaches a point of exhaustion when all energy and resources have been spent. In a shock crisis the person is overwhelmed by an explosive release of emotions in response to a sudden external change. Too much has happened unexpectedly and rapidly for the person to assimilate and integrate the excess stimuli. Nursing interventions for these two crisis types differ. A person in exhaustion crisis is unable to gain control over emotions and is apathetic to interpersonal contact or intervention techniques. A benign, supportive environment is essential for the person to regain energy slowly before attempting to deal with the crisis. A person in shock crisis is open to change and highly motivated to accept help in resolving it.

Although theoretically it is possible to isolate the phases in crises—vulnerable state, precipitating event, acute crisis, and reorganization—they overlap in reality. A crisis is conceived as lasting 4 to 6 weeks but may be much longer or shorter depending on the type of precipitating event, the level of stress experienced, the person's coping repertoire, and social supports.

Prevalence

Crisis situations occur episodically throughout a person's lifetime because of normal developmental stages and the demands associated with anticipated life situations. In addition, unanticipated crisis situations occur during the life span. Many crises do not come to the attention of health professionals but are resolved with the help of family, friends, or the clergy. Since crises are time limited, the person may successfully deal with them or maladaptively resolve them so that precrisis functioning level is not regained[14,53]

Population at Risk

From birth to death a person is exposed to crisis situations that are anticipated and predictable or unanticipated and accidental. Anticipated crises, which are described as maturational or developmental, are somewhat inconsistent with the assumptions of crisis theory that threatening events are external rather than internal. Unanticipated crises are unexpected traumatic events that may occur at any stage of life.[14]

According to Erikson[15] the eight developmental phases are basic trust versus mistrust; autonomy versus shame and doubt; initiative versus guilt; industry versus inferiority; identity versus role confusion; intimacy versus isolation; generativity versus stagnation; and ego integrity versus despair. The identity crisis of adolescents has been given considerable attention because of their rapid physiologic and cognitive changes and high vulnerability to stress. Parents who have difficulty dealing with their children in this age group may themselves be experiencing midlife crises in the generativity versus stagnation phase of development. The elderly, who are in the ego integrity versus despair phase of development, are particularly susceptible to crisis because of decreases in physical and cognitive functioning, roles, and sense of purpose.

A person who has not resolved the conflicts engendered in previous phases of development may find the expectations of the current phase fraught with stress and may have a greater predisposition in crises.[26]

The expected transitional life crises, such as toilet training, beginning or changing schools, entering or retiring from the work force, marriage, parenthood, the "empty nest" syndrome when children leave home, and death of parents, produce upheavals in roles and status and necessitate adaptation to new conditions.

Unanticipated events may affect individuals, communities, and countries.[26] They include natural catastrophic events, such as tornadoes, floods, and earthquakes, and man-made catastrophes, such as economic depressions, unemployment, and bank failures. Loss of a job and money creates a crisis not only for the person experiencing the loss but also for the family members, who are suddenly faced with changes in life-style and status.

Loss or threatened loss of a loved one through an untimely death or reduced capacity to function because of an accident or illness creates havoc for all involved. Although death of any loved person is stressful, the loss of a child or young adult is especially shocking to survivors. Unanticipated traumatic stress occurs in "victim crisis," in which physically or emotionally aggressive acts are perpetrated on a person. These include persecution of an individual or group and violent crimes such as assault, rape, and murder. The crisis situation can have a lifelong effect because of the intense emotional trauma and possible irreversible physical disability such as paralysis or loss of an extremity. The person may have flashbacks in which the violence or aggressiveness of the precipitating event is reexperienced. This can happen in persons who have successfully resolved the crisis issues.

In some instances a preexisting psychopathologic condition, such as schizophrenia or anxiety disorder, in a person or family is a contributing variable to a crisis reaction. The person's lowered tolerance to stressors, personal and social resources, and inadequate coping skills impair his ability to resolve crises successfully.

Approaches to Crisis Intervention

Generally persons experiencing crises have healthy personalities, and interventions are focused on the current crisis situation. Even when an underlying psychopathologic condition exists, interventions remain issue oriented to alleviate the crisis situation; the patient can be referred later to other resources for further help. If treatment is continued to deal with problems other than those related to the crisis, interventions are no longer viewed as crisis ones.

General goals of crisis intervention are to reinforce interpersonal assets, to resolve the crisis event, to connect with social supports in the family and/or community, and to integrate the crisis experience into the personality. A minimum expectation of crisis intervention is the person's return to a precrisis level of functioning.

There are two general approaches in crisis intervention: generic and individual.[14] The generic approach involves the use of brief, supportive interventions focused on the characteristic phases (such as that of grief) of the crisis experience. Little or no attention is directed toward the patient's personality dynamics. Nonprofessionals or paraprofessionals, such as trained volunteers at a 24-hour hotline or crisis center, usually use the generic approach. Although this approach is effective for some persons, dangers may exist when individual personality differences are not considered.

The individual approach is also focused on the current issues but has a more in-depth view in which the personality of the individual is considered. Stressors before the precipitating event, previous coping behaviors, and reactivated conflicts that contribute to the current reactions are identified, and how the individual's behavior contributed to worsening a threatening situation is evaluated. Resolution includes not only relief of symptoms but also development of effective coping skills to deal with similar situations in the future.

Korner[53] presented three general approaches useful in crisis intervention. The first is the free discharge of emotions such as despair, anxiety, and anger. If anger is the only emotion expressed, it may be nonconstructive when used to deny fear and emotional pain, but it is constructive when it counteracts the feelings of helplessness. A second approach is the enhancement of the patient's cognitive processes, thus providing a sense of control. The patient is helped to remember details of the event, including painful ones, and to correct misconceptions. A third approach allows the patient to experience security and hope through a supportive relationship to reduce anxiety (which leads to increased disorganization of the personality). The supportive approach is particularly useful in exhaustion crisis, when the person must regain energy before beginning to deal with the crisis. These approaches overlap to some extent, and all three are useful with a given patient depending on his or her needs at different phases of crisis intervention.

Since a crisis has built-in time limits, the nurse takes an active role to discover what kind of help the patient wants, to establish concrete, achievable goals. The nurse assists the patient in acute crisis in the following ways:

- Allows the patient to be dependent initially, satisfying basic needs such as directing the patient to a chair, giving a drink, and providing a damp washcloth for face
- Provides the patient with opportunities to express emotions in his own way (as long as they are nondestructive) within a safe, supportive relationship
- Increases use of cognitive processes by helping the patient review details of stressful events and, if appropriate, by providing factual information related to the event to correct misperceptions and to expand the patient's perspective
- Assists the patient to examine alternative choices and possible consequences of each choice
- Encourages the patient to identify social supports in the family and community
- Helps the patient deal with initial reactions to the crisis situation such as emotional upsets and to accept and integrate the crisis experience into his personality

Support for Nurses Involved in Crisis Intervention

Because of their intense involvement with patients in crisis, nurses experience high levels of pressure and stress. The need for a fast, accurate assessment and rapid intervention requires a great expenditure of energy and can be emotionally and cognitively exhausting. Nurses continually involved in crisis interventions with patients need their own support system to deal with their responses to emotion-laden situations and to receive emotional nourishment.

Psychopathology

Psychoanalytic Theory

In psychoanalytic theory crisis is viewed as occurring in persons who have low stress tolerance and inadequate skills to deal with stressors. These persons may have been unsuccessful in resolving conflicts of early development and have not established a clear self-identity. The goals of therapy include working through unresolved conflicts related to the crisis situation and rebuilding and strengthening defenses through an intensive, long-term psychotherapeutic relationship.[61]

Interpersonal Theory

According to interpersonal theory, persons are influenced by others and their environment throughout their lives. Persons who have excluded a significant number of anxiety-provoking experiences from awareness are less able to respond to events, since these dissociated processes are no longer accessible to consciousness. These persons may have decreased ability to assess new situations, especially stressful ones, and respond to them adequately. The goals of therapy are helping the patient to perceive the situation accurately, resolve reactivated conflicts, and develop skills to deal with the situation and future stressful events. Therapy is a growth-producing experience for the patient.[2,61]

Cognitive Theory

In cognitive or learning frameworks crisis is considered to be a result of sensory overload that interrupts the cognitive processes of perceiving, thinking, decision making, and evaluating. The overload may be related to a perceived or actual bombardment with stressful stimuli the person is unable to process logically. The person's definition of the situation determines whether it is interpreted as a crisis or as a challenging, exciting experience. Thus the person's definition also determines the person's response and methods of dealing with the situation. Intervention is directed toward correcting cognitive distortions, learning new skills to resolve the problem, unlearning inappropriate thinking patterns, and reinforcing gratifying patterns of behavior.[7,61]

Medical Plan

Medications

Trazodone (Desyrel) for depression; 50 mg tid po; has high sedative action and low anticholinergic action to manage depressive symptoms such as guilt, worthlessness, and despair

or

Alprazolam (Xanax) for anxiety; 0.5 mg tid po for adults; 0.25 mg tid po for elderly; belongs to benzodiazepine class of drugs; to decrease symptoms of severe anxiety and/or anxiety associated with depression

General Management

Occupational and recreational therapy after initial acute phase if patient is hospitalized and there are no contraindicating medical conditions

NURSING CARE

Nursing Assessment

Persons may seek help 1 to 2 weeks after the precipitating event; however, some do so immediately after the onset of an acute crisis. These persons ask for assistance in a variety of health care facilities such as hospital emergency rooms, community agencies, including mental health centers, and private physicians' offices. Acute crisis often affects hospitalized patients and their families as the result of a change in the seriousness of an illness, discovery of a poor prognosis, family responses to the patient's illness or death, or family difficulties unrelated to the ill member.

In crisis, rapid assessment is necessary and intervention often begins before the assessment has been completed. Each person responds to crisis in an individual way.

Affect

Severe anxiety to panic; depression; anger; apathy; tearfulness to convulsive crying; feeling of alienation; emptiness; motionless state; temporary lowered self-esteem

Thoughts

Paralysis of cognitive processes; impaired recall of crisis event; misinterpretation of events; forgetfulness; blocking; confusion; indecisiveness; frustration; conflicting thoughts; denial; guilt; psychophysiologic symptom complaints; suicidal or homicidal thoughts

Power and Control

Helplessness; hopelessness; vulnerability; lack of control

Activities

Paralysis or aimless, automatic behavior; agitation; tremors; stiffness of body as if trying to hold self together; clenched fists; contorted facial features; limpness of body, sometimes with impaired balance; impaired performance of tasks; regressive childlike behaviors such as tantrums

Sleep Patterns

Impaired sleep; inability to sleep; restless sleep; hypersomnia

Nutrition

Change in eating pattern, such as overeating or inability to eat; picking at food; nausea; vomiting

Social Interactions

Withdrawal from social support network; loosening of ties with loved ones

Nursing Dx & Intervention

Nursing care should be implemented selectively based on seriousness of symptoms and presenting behaviors. Because of the time limits of crisis, patients may be seen for only one or as many as 10 sessions.

Nursing Diagnosis	Nursing Intervention/Rationale
Anxiety related to situational and maturational crises	• Assess emotional state rapidly to determine level of anxiety. • Observe patient closely for appearance, dress, general demeanor, and muscle tightness *to identify signs of distress and comfort.* • Provide quiet, calm environment *to avoid increasing anxiety.* • Convey concern and caring through temporarily taking charge of activities *to reduce panic and loss of control;* for example, direct patient to comfortable chair and provide comfort measures such as drink and tissues. • Address patient by name and speak calmly in concise sentences *to obtain patient's attention.* • If exhaustion crisis is present, be supportive and giving *to help patient regain energy.* • Encourage patient to express feelings *to discharge emotions rather than keep them bottled up inside.* • If patient is crying, help to identify and clarify feelings (such as despair, anger, or hopelessness) during or after this expression; for example, say "Tell me what you're feeling as you're crying" *to become aware of meaning of emotions.* • Administer medication if ordered and as needed *to relieve emotional discomfort.* Briefly inform patient of effects and side effects, such as drowsiness and lightheadedness. More fully discuss effects and side effects when patient is calm if medication is to be continued. Emphasize the need for medical follow-up care. • Acknowledge physical signs of discomfort and ask patient to identify emotional experience *to connect bodily sensation with feeling state.* • When patient is able, identify previous painful emotions and successes in dealing with them *to reinforce positive coping techniques.* • Teach relaxation techniques, such as slow, deep breathing, diversionary activities, and sharing feelings with others, *to help patient develop ways to deal with current feelings.* • If patient is in hospital, encourage participation in occupational therapy as ordered *to provide diversionary activity and learn new skills.* (If there is no physical or emotional contraindication, recreational therapy may also be ordered *to reduce anxiety, expend excess energy, and teach new skills.*)
Ineffective individual coping related to situational or maturational crises	• Assess type of crisis (for example, anticipated or unanticipated), precipitating event, duration of crisis and coping abilities. • Assess for suicide ideation; if needed, institute suicide precautions. • Clarify perceptions of issues and events before the crisis. • When the patient with exhaustion crisis is able, identify various stressors along with their patterns, and explore coping strategies used in the past. Reinforce healthy methods for dealing with those stressors *to support successful behaviors and increase patient's confidence in his abilities.* • If crisis is developmental, identify specific issues and assist patient to resolve them *to learn to deal with developmental tasks and accept self.* If crisis was unanticipated, assist patient to begin to resolve issues related to both crisis and underlying conflict reactivated because of crisis events *to understand meaning of current crisis and integrate this new understanding into the personality.* • In problem solving, help patient explore possible consequences of various choices *to evaluate potential impact of decisions.* • Provide factual information, as appropriate, *to alter and broaden patient's perspective on issues*—for example, knowledge of crisis phases, tasks of developmental stage, and factors related to crisis situation. • Assist patient in identifying behaviors that contributed to or exacerbated the threatening situation *to help patient become aware of noneffective forms of behavior*—for example, accumulation of large debts before loss of employment. Help patient anticipate similar future events and identify ways of coping *to increase a sense of security and decrease apprehension about recurrence of crisis.* • Assist patient to begin to deal with long-term impact of crisis events such as cancer, changes in body image (for example, facial disfigurement and mastectomy), and birth of an imperfect baby. • Assess whether basis exists for physical complaints such as headache and abdominal pain. Medication, such as an analgesic or antacid, may be ordered for symptomatic relief. • Help patient identify relationship between physical symptoms and emotional state *to increase understanding of his maladaptive coping strategies.*

Nursing Diagnosis	Nursing Intervention/Rationale
Powerlessness	• Assess level and source of helplessness and aspects of events that provoked those feelings. • Convey to patient a realistic sense of optimism and hope that alternative ways of viewing and dealing with issues exist. • Assist patient to recall and accept previous and current successful coping strategies *to increase confidence in his abilities and a sense of control over self.* • Teach assertiveness skills and practice these with patient *to increase self-concept and abilities to be direct in making requests of others.*
Sleep pattern disturbance	• Assess type of sleep disturbances patient is experiencing and how patient is attempting to manage them. • Assist patient in talking about problems—such as fears of dying, anxieties, and dangers—that interfere with sleep *to begin helping patient resolve these issues.* • Teach patient to establish a routine before bedtime such as reading, watching television, or taking a warm bath *to promote relaxation and sleep.* If patient is afraid of being alone, suggest having someone stay with him in hospital or at home. • Encourage patient to practice slow, deep breathing and listen to relaxation tapes *to promote sleep.*
Altered nutrition: less than body requirements	• Assess fluid and food intake, eating difficulties, and changes in patterns. • Explore relationship between emotional discomfort and changes in eating pattern *to identify impact of crisis and connection between the two.* • Help patient identify strategies for dealing with eating difficulties in the past. Assist patient in identifying helpful methods for meeting nutritional requirements, such as planning soft bland food, frequent small meals, and adequate fluid intake *to decrease discomforts of eating.* • Inform patient that, as emotional state returns to near normal, usual eating patterns can be reestablished *to offer hope that disturbance is temporary.*
Social isolation related to alterations in mental status	• Assess interpersonal assets and current state of social supports. • Help patient identify persons viewed as supportive *to begin to reconnect with significant others.* • Discuss how supportive person(s) can be helpful now and how patient can share problems *to encourage patient to use available resources.* • If useful, ask patient to role play, sharing problems and asking for help *to increase confidence in asking for support.* • If patient is in an emergency room or a community agency and alone, arrange to have someone drive him home (if he will not be hospitalized). If patient lives alone, encourage staying at someone else's home or having someone stay with patient *to alleviate fears of being alone and to reduce stress.* • Identify community resources, write down names, addresses, and phone numbers, and encourage patient to use them *to obtain immediate emergency services as needed.*

Patient Education

1. To relieve any embarrassment the patient may be experiencing, teach the patient to accept emotional expressions during the acute crisis as a normal response to the stressor.
2. Reinforce the use of self-supports and support from significant others.
3. Reinforce the use of a problem-solving approach to deal with stressors.
4. Teach the importance of follow-up care after discharge.

Evaluation

Patient Outcome	Data Indicating That Outcome is Reached
Patient evidences return to pre-crisis level of functioning.	Patient verbalizes awareness of events leading to crisis. Patient practices use of problem-solving approach to deal with crisis and related issues. Patient asks for and receives support from significant others. Patient describes his ability to cope with changes in his life situation. Patient sleeps peacefully at night and awakens rested. Patient no longer experiences physical manifestations of crisis reactions.
Patient demonstrates knowledge of treatment pain.	Patient describes effects and side effects of medicine. Patient accurately states information about self-administration of prescribed medicine after discharge. Patient makes plans to continue treatment after discharge.

Medical Interventions and Related Nursing Care

The major therapeutic interventions for psychiatric disturbances are counseling and drug therapy. Counseling techniques have been discussed in detail throughout this chapter. Specific pharmacologic interventions have been presented with each disorder. The specific categories and classes of pharmacologic agents used for psychiatric disturbances include antidepressants, tranquilizers, and sedative-hypnotics.

References

1. American Psychiatric Association: Diagnostic and statistical manual of mental disorders, revised ed 3, Washington, DC, 1987, American Psychiatric Association.
2. Arieti S: Interpretation of schizophrenia, ed 2, New York, 1974, Basic Books, Inc, Publishers.
3. Arieti S and Bemporad J: Severe and mild depression: the psychotherapeutic approach, New York, 1978, Basic Books, Inc, Publishers.
4. Beattie M: Crack: the facts, Center City, Minn, 1987, Hazelden Foundation.
5. Beck AT: Cognitive therapy and the emotional disorders, New York, 1976, New American Library, Inc.
6. Beck AT and Emery G: Anxiety disorders and phobias: a cognitive perspective, New York, 1985, Basic Books, Inc, Publishers.
7. Beck AT et al: Cognitive therapy of depression, New York, 1979, Guilford Press.
8. Bennett G, Vourakis C, and Woolf DS, editors: Substance abuse: pharmacologic, developmental, and clinical perspectives, New York, 1983, John Wiley & Sons, Inc.
9. Bratter TE and Forrest GG: Alcoholism and substance abuse: strategies for clinical intervention, New York, 1985, Macmillan, Inc.
10. Brenner C: An elementary textbook of psychoanalysis, revised ed 1, Garden City, NY, 1974, Doubleday & Co, Inc.
11. Brenners DK, Harris B, and Weston PS: Managing manic behavior, Am J Nurs 87:620, 1987.
12. Busteed EL and Johnstone C: The development of suicide precautions for an inpatient psychiatric unit, J Psychosoc Nurs Ment Health Serv 21(5):15, 1983.
13. Chapman AH: The treatment techniques of Harry Stack Sullivan, New York, 1978, Brunner/Mazel, Inc.
14. Cohen LH, Claiborn WL, and Specter GA, editors: Crisis intervention, ed 2, New York, 1983, Human Sciences Press, Inc.
15. Erikson E: Childhood and society, ed 2, New York, 1963, WW Norton & Co, Inc.
16. Esman AH, editor: The psychology of adolescence: essential readings, New York, 1975, International Universities Press, Inc.
17. Fenichel O: The psychoanalytic theory of neurosis, New York, 1945, WW Norton & Co, Inc.
18. Frankel FH: The use of electroconvulsive therapy in suicidal patients, Am J Psychother 38:384, 1984.
19. Garfinkel PE and Garner DM: Anorexia nervosa: a multidimensional perspective, New York, 1982, Brunner/Mazel, Inc.
20. Goldstein MJ: Psychosocial issues, Schizophr Bull 13:157, 1987.
21. Greenspan M: A new approach to women and therapy, New York, 1983, McGraw-Hill Book Co.
22. Gunderson JG: Borderline personality disorder, Washington, DC, 1984, American Psychiatric Press, Inc.
23. Harakal BM: What the SNAs are doing in Ohio, Am J Nurs 82:582, 1982.
24. Helzer JE: Epidemiology of alcoholism, J Consult Clin Psychol 55:284, 1987.
25. Hirshfield RMA, Koslow SH, and Kupler DJ: The clinical utility of the dexamethasone suppression test in psychiatry, JAMA 250:2172, 1983.
26. Hoff LA: People in crisis: understanding and helping, ed 2, Menlo Park, Calif, 1984, Addison-Wesley Publishing Co.
27. Horner AJ: Object relations and the developing ego in therapy, New York, 1979, Jason Aronson, Inc.
28. Kaplan AS and Woodside DB: Biological aspects of anorexia nervosa and bulimia nervosa, J Consult Clin Psychol 55:645, 1987.
29. Kolb LC and Brodie HKH: Modern clinical psychiatry, ed 10, Philadelphia, 1982, WB Saunders Co.
30. Mahler MS, Pine F, and Bergman A: The psychological birth of the human infant, New York, 1975, Basic Books, Inc, Publishers.
31. Mann GA: The dynamics of addiction, revised ed 1, Minneapolis, 1987, Johnson Institute, Inc.
32. Mark B: Hospital treatment of borderline patients: toward a better understanding of problematic issues, J Psychosoc Nurs Ment Health Serv 18(8):25, 1980.
33. Meissner WW: The schizophrenic and the paranoid process, Schizophr Bull 7:611, 1981.
34. Meissner WW: The borderline spectrum, New York, 1984, Jason Aronson, Inc.
35. Meissner WW: Psychotherapy and the paranoid process, New York, 1986, Jason Aronson, Inc.
36. Meltzer HY: Biological studies in schizophrenia, Schizophr Bull 13:77, 1987.
37. Michelson L, and Ascher LM, editors: Anxiety and stress disorders: cognitive-behavioral assessment and treatment, New York, 1987, Guilford Press.
38. Millman HL, Huber JT, and Diggins DR, editors: Therapies for adults, San Francisco, 1982, Jossey-Bass, Inc, Publishers.
39. Mitchell JE and Eckert ED: Scope and significance of eating disorders, J Consult Clini Psychol 55:628, 1987.
40. Mullahy P and Mellinek M: Interpersonal psychiatry, New York, 1983, Spectrum Publications, Inc.
41. Naegle MA: Creative management of impaired nursing practice, Nurs Administration Q 9(3):16, 1985.
42. Nathan PE and Skinstad A: Outcome of treatment for alcohol problems: current methods, problems, and results, J Consult Clin Psychol 55:332, 1987.
43. National Institute of Mental Health: Useful information . . . suicide, Rockville, Md, 1986, US Department of Health and Human Services.
44. Pao P: Schizophrenic disorders: theory and treatment from a psychodynamic point of view, New York, 1979, International Universities Press, Inc.
45. Petrie K and Chamberlain K: Hopelessness and social desirability as moderator variables in predicting suicidal behavior, J Counseling Clin Psychol 51:485, 1983.
46. Platt-Koch LM: Borderline personality disorder: a therapeutic approach, Am J Nurs 83:1666, 1983.
47. Powell AH and Minick MP: Alcohol withdrawal syndrome, Am J Nurs 88:312, 1988.
48. Quayle D: American productivity: the devastating effect of alcoholism and drug abuse, Am Psychol 38:454, 1983.
49. Sanger E and Cassino T: Eating disorders: avoiding the power struggle, Am J Nurs 84:31, 1984.

50. Schuckit MA: Biological vulnerability to alcoholism, J Consult Clin Psychol 55:301, 1987.
51. Simmons-Alling S: New approaches to managing affective disorders, Arch Psychiatr Nurs 1:219, 1987.
52. Small IF et al: Electroconvulsive treatment: indications, benefits, and limitations, Am J Psychother 40:343, 1986.
53. Specter GA and Claiborn WL, editors: Crisis intervention, vol 2, New York, 1973, Behavioral Publications, Inc.
54. Spitz HI and Rosecan JS, editors: Cocaine abuse: new directions in treatment and research, New York, 1987, Brunner/Mazel, Inc.
55. Strachan AM: Family intervention for the rehabilitation of schizophrenia: toward protection and coping, Schizophr Bull 12:678, 1986.
56. Strauss JS: Discussion: what does rehabilitation accomplish? Schizophr Bull 12:720, 1986.
57. Strober M and Humphrey LL: Familial contributions to the etiology and course of anorexia nervosa and bulimia, J Consult Clin Psychol 55:654, 1987.
58. Sullivan HS: The interpersonal theory of psychiatry, New York, 1953, WW Norton & Co, Inc.
59. Sullivan HS: Schizophrenia as a human process, New York, 1962, WW Norton & Co, Inc.
60. Tirrell C and DeForest D: Neuroendocrine factors in affective disorders, Arch Psychiatr Nurs 1:225, 1987.
61. Umana RF, Gross SF, and McConville MT: Crisis in the family: three approaches, New York, 1980, Gardner Press, Inc.
62. Wiener MB and Pepper GA: Clinical pharmacology and therapeutics in nursing, ed 2, New York, 1985, McGraw-Hill Book Co.
63. Weiner RD: Electroconvulsive therapy: contemporary issues, Carrier Foundation Letter, no 105, March, 1985.

PART TWO

Diagnostic Procedures

Cardiovascular system

Ambulatory electrocardiography (Holter monitor), 1576
Cardiac catheterization, 1588
Digital vascular imaging (DVI) (digital subtraction arteriography), 1589
Electrocardiogram (ECG, EKG), 1576
Electrophysiologic studies (bundle of His), 1576
Exercise stress test (EST), 1605
^{125}I fibrinogen uptake (radioactive fibrinogen uptake, RFU), 1584
Phlebography (venography), 1591
Plethysmography, 1577
Scintigraphic blood pool imaging (multiple-gated blood pool), 1589
Scintigraphy (radionuclide arteriography), 1589
Scintigraphy (technetium-99m pyrophosphate myocardial imaging), 1589
Scintigraphy (thallium-201 imaging), 1589
Ultrasonography, 1578

Respiratory system

Arterial blood gas analysis, 1593
Barium swallow, 1572
Bronchography, 1571
Chest roentgenogram, 1569
Computerized tomography (CT), 1584
Fiberoptic bronchoscopy, 1562
Gastric lavage, 1567
Lung biopsy, 1579
Lymph node excision and scalene node biopsy, 1580
Mantoux test (tuberculin skin testing), 1587
Mediastinoscopy, mediastinotomy, thoracoscopy, 1562
Pleural biopsy, 1579
Pleural fluid examination (diagnostic thoracentesis), 1566
Pulmonary arteriography, 1589
Pulmonary function testing, 1599
Schick test, 1587
Sputum examination (direct method), 1565
Sputum examination (indirect method), 1566
Testing for fungal diseases, 1587
Ultrasonography, 1578
Ventilation/perfusion lung scan, 1582

Neurologic system

Brain biopsy, 1579
Brain scan, 1582
Caloric test, 1598
Cerebral arteriography, 1588
Cerebrospinal fluid studies, 1567
Cisternography, 1582
Computerized tomography, 1584
Discogram, 1576
Echoencephalogram, 1598
Electroencephalogram (EEG), 1577
Electromyogram (EMG), 1577
Lumbar venography, 1591
Muscle and nerve biopsy, 1580
Myelogram, 1575
Nerve conduction velocity determination, 1577
Pneumoencephalogram (PEG), 1597
Positron emission tomography (PET), 1585
Sella turcica/skull films, 1569
Spinal films, 1569
Ventriculography, 1571

Musculoskeletal system

Arteriography, 1588
Arthrogram, 1576
Arthroscopy, 1565
Bone scan (scintigraphy), 1583
Computerized tomography (CT), 1584
Discogram, 1576
Electromyogram (EMG), 1577
Magnetic resonance imaging (MRI), 1585
Muscle and nerve biopsy, 1580
Musculoskeletal films, 1569
Myelogram, 1575
Nerve conduction velocity determination, 1577
Synovial biopsy, 1580

Integumentary system

Culture, 1586
Cytology, 1586
Diascopy, 1586
Electron microscopy, 1586
Gram stain, 1586
Patch test, 1587
Scrapings, 1586
Side lighting, 1586
Skin and tissue biopsy, 1581
Thermography, 1587
Wood's light, 1586

Eye

Computerized tomography, 1584
Direct ophthalmoscopy, 1560
Fluorescein arteriography (and photography), 1588
Gonioscopy, 1560
Indirect ophthalmoscopy, 1560
Lacrimal system testing, 1560
Provocative testing, 1561
Pupil dilation, 1560
Slitlamp examination, 1560
Tonometry, 1598
Ultrasonography, 1578
Visual field screening, 1561

Ear, nose, and throat

Caloric test, 1598
Direct laryngoscopy, suspension laryngoscopy, indirect laryngoscopy, 1562
Electrocochleography, 1577
Mastoid films, 1569
Otoscopy, 1561
Pharyngoscopy, 1562
Rhinoscopy, 1561
Sinus films, 1569
Specific audiometric and hearing testing, 1599
Transillumination, 1561

Gastrointestinal system

Acid perfusion test (Bernstein test), 1605
Barium enema, 1572
Barium swallow, 1572
Celiac and mesenteric arteriography, 1590
Colonoscopy, 1563
Computerized tomography (CT), 1584
Endoscopic retrograde cholangiopancreatography (ERCP), 1573
Endoscopy, 1563
Esophageal acidity test (pH monitoring), 1605
Esophageal manometry, 1605
Esophagogastroduodenoscopy, 1563
Fecal fat, 1568
Fecal occult blood, 1568
Fecal urobilinogen, 1568
Gastric acid stimulation test, 1567
Gastric analysis (basal gastric secretion test), 1566
Hypotonic duodenography, 1573
Intravenous cholangiography (IVC), 1573
Liver biopsy, 1581
Liver or spleen scan, 1583
Oral cholecystography (OCG), 1572
Percutaneous transhepatic cholangiography, 1573
Peritoneal fluid analysis, 1567
Postoperative cholangiography or T-tube cholangiography, 1573
Proctosigmoidoscopy, 1564
Splenoportography (transsplenic portography), 1574
Ultrasonography, 1578
Upper gastrointestinal and small bowel series (UGI and SB series), 1572

Endocrine and metabolic system

Arteriography, 1588
Computerized tomography (CT), 1584
Endocrine studies of hormones, 1593
Sella turcica/skull films, 1569
Thyroid biopsy, 1579
Thyroid uptake and scan, 1582
Thyroid-releasing hormone stimulation test (TRH, TRF test), 1582
Ultrasonography, 1578
Vena caval catheterization, 1589
Visual field screening, 1561

Female reproductive system

Renal system

Genitourinary system

Infectious diseases

Immunologic system

Hematolymphatic system

Neoplasia

Visualization Studies

Direct Ophthalmoscopy

Description. Examiner uses an ophthalmoscope to view the retinal surface and inner structures of eye. Pupils are usually dilated, and examination takes place in dark room. Retinal structures and vessels are magnified 15 times.

Indications. Used for diagnosis and visualization of the optic disk, arteries, veins, retina, choroid, and media and for evaluation of significant ocular and systemic disease. About half the fundus may be seen.

Complications. Caution should be used when dilating the pupil of a patient with a shallow anterior chamber to avoid precipitating an attack of angle-closure glaucoma. Soft contact lenses should be removed before pupil dilation, and dilation should not be performed if an implanted intraocular lens was placed during cataract surgery.

Nursing care. Indicate both the duration of effect of the medication used to dilate the pupil and the limitation in vision.

Indirect Ophthalmoscopy

Description. Examiner wears a head-mounted binocular instrument. The patient is supine, usually with dilated pupils. The examiner stands 30 inches away and holds a convex lens over the patient's eye for focusing. The image is magnified four to five times; a greater visual field can be viewed than with direct ophthalmoscopy. A scleral depressor (blunt rod) may be used to compress the eyeball so ora serrata (tissue behind the iris) can be viewed.

Indications. Permits detection and evaluation of minimal elevations of the sensory retina and retinal pigment epithelium, which are not evident with direct ophthalmoscopy. Useful in the detection of opacities in the media.

Complications. None.

Nursing care. Assure the patient that mild or no discomfort will be experienced if a scleral depressor is used. Inform the patient about side effects of the medication.

Gonioscopy

Description. A corneal contact lens (goniolens) is placed over an anesthetized cornea to permit viewing of anterior chamber angles with a microscopic lens, mirror, or contact lens combined with a prism, since the opaque sclera and corneoscleral limbus prevent direct inspection of the angle of the anterior chamber.

Indications. Assists in distinguishing between angle-closure glaucoma and open-angle glaucoma. It has also been used in the development of an effective surgical procedure for congenital glaucoma and in the diagnostic and therapeutic evolution of many types of secondary glaucoma.

Complications. None.

Nursing care. None except explaining the procedure to the patient.

Slitlamp Examination

Description. The examiner views corneal layers, anterior chamber, lens, and anterior vitreous through a microscope that magnifies these structures up to 20 times. A thin slit of light permits scrutiny of anterior structures for lesions or trauma.

Indications. Used to detect the depth of the abnormality.

Complications. None.

Nursing care. None.

Pupil Dilation

Description. Short-acting, topical medication is used for pupil dilation to facilitate examination of the fundus with direct or indirect ophthalmoscopy. Mydriatic (adrenergic) drugs such as phenylephrine 2.5% (Neo-Synephrine, Mydfrin) dilate the pupil but do not inhibit accommodation. Mydriatic drug may be combined with cycloplegic drug (which inhibits accommodation) such as tropicamide 0.5% (Mydriacyl) to enhance and maintain pupil dilation.

Indications. Diagnosis and evaluation of significant ocular and systemic disease.

Complications. May be contraindicated for patients with shallow anterior chamber, certain intraocular lens implants, or vascular hypertension or who are taking MAO inhibitors or tricyclic antidepressants.

Nursing care. Remove contact lenses before instillation. Warn the patient that blurred vision and photophobia may last for 3 to 6 hours after examination.

Lacrimal System Testing

Description

Basic secretion test. Topical anesthetic is administered to the eyeball before a filter paper is inserted. The anesthesia reduces lacrimal output to allow measurement of the tear production of accessory glands in eyelid.

Dacryocystography. A radiopaque medium such as Pantopaque is injected through the punctum and canaliculus into the lacrimal sac, and is followed by roentgenography.

Dacryoscintigraphy. Sodium pertechnetate (^{99m}Tc) in a dilute solution is instilled in each conjunctival sac, followed by a scintigram taken with a gamma camera to indicate its passage through the lacrimal drainage system.[20]

Dye disappearance.[20] A dye, 0.25% to 2% fluorescein in alkaline solution or rose bengal, is instilled topically into the conjunctival sac to stain the Bowman's membrane and the stroma of the cornea. The stain can be intensified if a 2% cocaine ophthalmic solution is instilled into the eye or if the eye is illuminated with a cobalt blue filter to stimulate fluorescence.

Rose bengal staining. A drop of 1% or 2% solution is placed in conjunctival sac. The 2% solution demonstrates loss of corneal and conjunctival epithelium in keratoconjunctivitis sicca; the 1% solution is valuable in demonstrating conjunctival and corneal epithelial cell loss and degeneration. Patients with a deficiency of the aqueous portion of tears have punctate staining of the lower two thirds of the cornea and bright red staining of bulbar conjunctiva in the area corresponding to the palpable aperture.

Schirmer's test. A strip of filter paper, 3.5 × 0.05 cm, placed in the conjunctival cul-de-sac of the lower lid for 5 minutes. A 10- to 15-mm length of paper wetted with tears is considered normal. More than 25 mm of moistened paper indicates excessive tearing.

Indications. Used to determine the adequacy and patency of the lacrimal system; it can demonstrate obstruction or overproduction of tears.

Fluorescein is instilled in the eye for a variety of diagnostic tests. It demonstrates breaks in the epithelium and the dilution that occurs when anterior aqueous humor escapes from a postoperative fistula, penetrating wound, or conjunctival bleb following glaucoma surgery. It is also used to demonstrate areas of contact between the lens and the cornea and sclera in the fitting of contact lenses. The rate of disappearance through the nasolacrimal passages (normally 1 minute) estimates their patency.

Rose bengal dye is usually used to demarcate devitalized conjunctival epithelium in keratoconjunctivitis sicca, since it stains devitalized cells better than fluorescein does.

Complications. Dyes stain soft contact lenses, so the lenses should be removed before the dye is instilled. Because it is possible for fluorescein to become contaminated with *Pseudomonas* spp., it should be instilled with either a single-dose container or a strip of sterile filter paper saturated with the dye.

Nursing care. None, other than explaining the procedure to the patient.

Provocative Testing

Description. Used for patients with mildly elevated intraocular pressure (IOP), those who have optic nerve changes or field defects without elevated IOP, and those with shallow anterior chambers and compromised anterior angles. Their results are not definitive but may distinguish potentially glaucomatous persons from others.

Water drinking test. In the morning, the fasting patient drinks approximately 1 L of water as fast as possible (within 2 to 4 minutes). The IOP is measured before and at 15-minute intervals for 45 minutes. Normal eyes show an IOP increase of 3 to 5 mm Hg. An increase of 8 mm Hg is indicative of glaucoma.

Dark room test (for narrow-angle glaucoma). The patient sits in a dark room for 60 minutes to dilate pupils. An IOP increase of 7 to 8 mm Hg is indicative of iris bunching into and blocking of anterior angle flow.

Mydriatic testing. One eye is dilated at a time (under careful supervision), and the pupil is constricted when the test is ended. IOP increase of 8 mm Hg is indicative of glaucoma.

Indications. These tests are indicated in patients with an intraocular pressure of 21 mm Hg or more, a coefficient outflow of less than 0.18, a ratio of intraocular pressure to coefficient outflow facility greater than 100, optic nerve changes suggestive of glaucoma, and field changes suggestive of glaucoma.[20]

Complications. None.

Nursing care. None, other than explaining the study to the patient.

Visual Field Screening

Description

Central field tangent screen. Central vision covers approximately 50 degrees of patient's central vision, 25 degrees in each direction from the central fixation point. A black screen (1 m^2) is placed 1 m from eye. Blind spots are outlined by using a 1- to 3-mm white target placed on a board. A normal blind spot is 13 to 18 degrees temporal from central fixation. Abnormal isolated spots (scotomas) or confluent areas can be identified. Nasal areas are usually lost first.

Automated perimetry. Various automatic machines (such as Goldmann perimeter) measure both central and peripheral fields.

Indications. Method of assessing function of retinal periphery by measuring the peripheral field of vision. It is indicated as part of a routine vision screening or as part of a diagnosis of visual problems or deterioration.

Complications. None.

Nursing care. None, other than explaining the study to the patient.

Otoscopy

Description. Inspection of the external auditory canal and middle ear. The largest speculum that will fit comfortably in the patient's ear is inserted to a depth of 1 to 1.5 cm to inspect the auditory canal from the meatus to the tympanic membrane.

Indications. Any discharge, scaling, excessive redness, lesions, foreign bodies, or cerumen can be noted. The tympanic membrane is inspected for landmarks, color, contours, and perforations. The direction of the light can be varied to see the entire tympanic membrane and anulus.[25]

Complications. None.

Nursing care. None.

Rhinoscopy

Description. Inspection of the nasal cavity using a nasal speculum and a light. The patient's head should be held erect to examine the vestibule and inferior nasal turbinate, and tilted back to visualize the middle meatus and turbinate.[25]

Indications. Color, discharge, masses, lesions, and swelling of the turbinates may be noted, and the septum inspected for alignment, perforation, bleeding, and crusting.

Complications. None.

Nursing care. None.

Transillumination

Description. This examination is performed in a completely darkened room. A small, bright light is placed lateral to the nose just beneath the medial aspect of the eye to transilluminate the maxillary sinuses. The patient's hard palate should be illuminated through the patient's open mouth. To transilluminate the frontal sinuses, the light is placed against the medial aspect of each supraorbital rim. A dim, red glow should show just above the eyebrow.

Indications. Pain or sinus tenderness, suspicion of sinus infection. Absence of a glow indicates that the sinus is filled with secretion or is absent.[25]

Complications. None.

Nursing care. None.

Pharyngoscopy

Description. The instrument producing bright illumination is held in the patient's mouth to visualize nasopharynx when the instrument is turned upward, and hypopharynx and larynx when turned downward.

Indications. Detection of abnormalities of the oropharynx or nasopharynx, and evaluation of symptoms of infection or abscess.

Complications. None.

Nursing care. None.

Direct Laryngoscopy, Suspension Laryngoscopy, Indirect Laryngoscopy

Description

Direct laryngoscopy. Direct examination of the larynx under local or general anesthesia, performed by introducing a laryngoscope into the patient's mouth over the tongue; the tongue is raised, the patient's neck is slowly extended, and the laryngoscope is passed over the posterior portion of the epiglottis and raised to expose the vocal cords.

Suspension laryngoscopy. Essentially the same as direct laryngoscopy, but an attachment holds the laryngoscope so the examiner can use both hands; usually used in conjunction with a microscope, which provides magnification and binocular vision.

Indirect laryngoscopy. The most common way to examine the larynx; usually performed in the physician's office; the patient sits upright in a chair, and a laryngeal mirror is used to visualize the larynx; the method can be used for biopsy or excision of a polyp.

Indications. Hoarseness, burning in throat, dysphagia, dyspnea, muffled voice.

Complications. None except that the gag reflex is abolished. The usual care must be taken to prevent aspiration.

Nursing care. The patient may return from the study with an intravenous line, which can be discontinued as soon as the patient can take fluids. Observe the patient for respiratory distress for the first 2 to 4 hours. If the patient had a local anesthetic administered before the procedure, be aware that the gag reflex may be absent until the anesthetic wears off. Humidified oxygen provides additional moisture to the patient's airway.

Fiberoptic Bronchoscopy

Description. This procedure, performed with the patient under local anesthesia, permits direct inspection of the larynx, trachea, and bronchi. The flexible fiberoptic bronchoscope is the preferred instrument because it is better tolerated by patients and permits improved visualization of distal subsegmental airways. The fiberoptic bronchoscope, which has an external diameter between 3 and 6 mm, is inserted through the patient's nose or mouth. General anesthesia may be used for this procedure if necessary.

Indications. Collection of secretions for cytologic or bacteriologic examination; tissue biopsy for examination; cells and secretions via a brush biopsy technique; this procedure involves using a small brush inserted through the bronchoscope to brush the tissue walls. Location and biopsy of tumors; bleeding locations; removal of foreign bodies or heavy, blocking, mucous plug secretions; implantation of radioactive gold seeds for tumor treatment.

Complications. Bronchospasm, increased sputum production, productive mild bronchitis, sore throat, hoarseness.

Nursing care. The patient should receive nothing by mouth for 8 hours before the procedure and should be given a preprocedure sedative medication. Any dental prostheses should be removed. In the examination area, the patient's mouth, throat, and tongue will be sprayed with a topical anesthetic. An oxygen catheter should be placed in one nostril and remain there throughout the procedure. Lidocaine jelly is generally used as the bronchoscope lubricant; this suppresses the patient's cough and gag reflexes. After the procedure the patient should be carefully watched and positioned until the full gag and swallowing reflexes return. Patency of the patient's airway and the swallowing reflex should be evaluated, and the patient should be assessed for severe complications such as bronchospasms.

Mediastinoscopy, Mediastinotomy, Thoracoscopy

Description. Surgical endoscopy procedures in which a biopsy is taken from a tumor in the upper mediastinum, the pleura, or the lung. They are also used to determine if metastasis has occurred.

Mediastinoscopy. The incision is made in the suprasternal notch, and the scope is passed through that incision to biopsy tissue from the upper mediastinum.

Mediastinotomy. The incision is made above the third rib along the sternal border. Lung biopsy may also be done by this technique.

Thoracoscopy. This is indicated to obtain a biopsy from a peripheral lesion of the lung or pleura. The incision site, along the lateral or anterior chest wall, depends on the location of the lesion.

Indications. Diagnosis of primary or secondary mediastinal disease; evaluation of metastasis to mediastinal nodes in primary lung carcinoma.

Complications. Hemorrhage, pneumothorax, infection, left recurrent laryngeal nerve damage.

Nursing care. For all procedures the patient receives a general anesthetic; therefore all preoperative procedures apply. Postoperatively the patient should be observed for pneumothorax, cardiac arrhythmias, and bleeding. A drainage chest tube is frequently used after the thoracoscopy procedure.

Esophagogastroduodenoscopy

Description. Permits visual examination of the esophagus, stomach, and upper duodenum. Dentures are removed. A local anesthetic is sprayed into the mouth and throat. An endoscope is passed through the mouth and swallowed. Saliva may need to be suctioned if the patient is unable to allow it to flow out the side of the mouth adequately. A mouth guard should be used to protect the teeth. The patient's head is repositioned throughout the procedure to facilitate movement of the endoscope.

The procedure is contraindicated in patients with recent ulcer perforation, large aortic aneurysms, cardiac disease or a recent myocardial infarction, and Zenker's diverticulum.

Indications. Useful in diagnosing inflammatory disease, ulcers, tumors, structural abnormality, and Mallory-Weiss tears.

Complications. Complications include the following perforations: cervical esophagus perforation: pain on swallowing and neck movements; thoracic esophagus perforation: substernal or epigastric pain that increases with respirations and trunk movements; diaphragmatic esophageal perforation: shoulder pain and dyspnea; gastric perforation: abdominal or back pain, cyanosis, fever, or pleural effusion.

Other signs of complications include difficulty in swallowing, persistent pain, fever, black stools, or hematemesis.

Nursing care. Give nothing by mouth for 6 to 12 hours before the procedure; during an emergency procedure a nasogastric tube is used to aspirate gastric contents. Explain the procedure to the patient and obtain a signed consent form. Before the procedure, have the patient remove any dentures or partial plates. Monitor blood pressure, pulse, and respirations. Anxiety and fear of procedure are expected, and the patient should be given emotional support throughout the procedures; sedatives and analgesics may be used to help the patient relax. Fluids and foods should be withheld until the gag reflex returns.

Endoscopy

Description. Direct visualization of the lining of a hollow viscus via an endoscope—a long, flexible tube with a cable-like cluster of glass fibers that transmits light and returns an image to the scope's optical head; used to diagnose a variety of gastrointestinal disorders and allowing for biopsy of lesions through the scope.

Indications. Useful in diagnosing inflammatory disease, ulcers, tumors, structural abnormality, and Mallory-Weiss tears.

Complications. Complications include cervical esophagus perforation (pain on swallowing and neck movements); thoracic esophagus perforation (substernal or epigastric pain that increases with respirations and trunk movements); diaphragmatic esophageal perforation (shoulder pain and dyspnea); and gastric perforation (abdominal or back pain, cyanosis, fever, or pleural effusion). Other signs of complications include difficulty in swallowing, persistent pain, fever, black stools, or hematemesis.

Nursing care. Give nothing by mouth for 6 to 12 hours before the procedure; during an emergency procedure a nasogastric tube is used to aspirate gastric contents. Explain the procedure to the patient and obtain a signed consent form. Before the procedure, have the patient remove any dentures or partial plates. Monitor blood pressure, pulse, and respirations. Anxiety and fear of the procedures are expected, and the patient should be given emotional support throughout them; sedatives and analgesics may be used to help the patient relax. Fluids and foods should be withheld until the gag reflex returns.

Colonoscopy

Description. The patient is placed in the left lateral decubitus position, and a well-lubricated colonoscope is inserted through the anus. Air is inserted to help the physician visualize the mucosa and to facilitate advancement of the colonoscope. Occasionally position changes are required to assist advancement of the scope at the descending-sigmoid colon junction and splenic flexure. Barium studies should be made after the colonoscopy, or thorough bowel preparation is required for good visualization of mucosa. Specimens for cytology and histology may be obtained as well as for biopsy.

Contraindications to the procedure include pregnancy, ischemic bowel disease, acute diverticulitis, peritonitis, toxic megacolon of ulcerative colitis, fulminant granulomatous colitis, and irradiation colitis.

Indications. Used to examine the colon and rectum to diagnose inflammatory bowel disease, including ulcerative colitis and granulomatous colitis. Polyps can be removed through the colonoscope. The colonoscope is also helpful in diagnosing or locating the source of lower gastrointestinal bleeding. A biopsy of lesions suspected to be malignant may also be performed; biopsies may also be advisable for patients with ulcerative colitis or Crohn's disease.

Complications. Complications include perforation of the bowel. Signs and symptoms include abdominal pain and distention, rectal bleeding, fever, and mucopurulent drainage. If the bowel is fixed—secondary to irradiation, surgical adhesions, or inflammatory disease—the physician may have difficulty during the procedure.

Nursing care. Bowel preparation is required for visualization of the mucosa. Colon electrolyte lavage preparations (Colyte, Go-lyte) may be used.

Patients need instructions for mixing the solution. Avoid all solid food and sugar the day of the prep. Alternatively, the bowel should be cleansed with laxatives and enemas; be careful in patients with ulcerative colitis and granulomatous colitis, since laxatives can exacerbate the disease (special protocols are required for this patient group). Avoid soapsuds enemas in all patients, since this irritates the mucosa.

The procedure is uncomfortable and embarrassing, so be supportive. Let the patient know that flatus is from air inserted during the procedure and cannot be controlled. A sedative may be given to help the patient relax.

Proctosigmoidoscopy

Description. Examination of the sigmoid colon, rectum, and anal canal. The sigmoidoscope and proctoscope may be rigid metal instruments or flexible scopes inserted for visualization of the mucosa; a biopsy may be performed. Examination usually includes a digital examination of anus and anal canal.

Patients often dread the proctosigmoidoscopy examination because of the embarrassing and uncomfortable positioning and the discomfort caused by the rigid instrument. Patients are placed in a knee-chest position on a tilting table. Although the procedure can be done with the patient in a left lateral position, it is important to elevate the right buttocks; most physicians prefer to use a tilting table and the knee-chest position for best visualization.

A proctoscope may be used to examine the rectum and anus, but when a sigmoidoscope is removed slowly, the rectum and anal canal can be viewed, thereby eliminating the need for a proctoscope.

Indications. Changed bowel habits, rectal bleeding, weight loss, anemia, stools positive for occult blood.

Complications. Complications include possible bowel perforation (see the discussion of colonoscopy); decreased blood pressure, pallor, diaphoresis, and bradycardia are signs of vasovagal stimulation and require immediate notification of the physician.

Nursing care. Preparation varies with the expected diagnosis; clear liquid diets for 48 hours and a small sodium biphosphate enema may be used.

Cystoscopy and Panendoscopy

Description. The cystoscope and panendoscope are instruments that allow direct visualization of the bladder and urethra. Cystoscopy and panendoscopy may be performed while the patient is under general or spinal anesthesia; in other cases, a local anesthetic, consisting of a lubricant jelly impregnated with lidocaine, is used.

The patient is placed in the lithotomy position. Sterile equipment is used; surgical gowns, gloves, and masks are typically used. A single sheath through which both cystoscope and panendoscope will be passed is inserted into the bladder via the urethra, with adequate lubrication. A telescope is then passed through the sheath while the bladder is being filled with fluid. Using a fiberoptic system within the cystoscope, the urologist visualizes the internal architecture of the bladder including the bladder neck, urothelial lining, and ureteral orifices. Bladder tumors, trabeculation, and inflammatory changes within the internal mucosa are assessed via cystoscopy. A panendoscope is used to view the bladder neck, prostatic urethra (in a male), external urinary sphincters, and anterior urethra.

Fluid is infused into the bladder throughout the procedure. Infusion is stopped and the bladder drained when it becomes filled with 300 to 500 ml of fluid.

Cystoscopic and panendoscopic examination may be combined with radiographic diagnostic studies such as a retrograde pyelogram or with therapeutic procedures, such as transurethral resection of bladder tumor or prostate.

The patient should experience minimal discomfort following the procedure if it is performed gently and with adequate lubrication.

Indications. Hematuria, dysuria, tumor or polyp removal or biopsy.

Complications. Mild dysuria and transient hematuria should disappear within the first 48 hours after the procedure. The patient should be able to void normally after a routine cystoscopic examination.

Nursing care. If a general or spinal anesthetic is used, the patient will be sent to the recovery room after the procedure and should be closely monitored for potential postanesthesia complications, such as a low-grade fever ($\leq$ 38° C [101° F]), for 24 to 48 hours.

Pelvic Endoscopy

Description. Visualization and examination of pelvic and abdominal viscera with a high-intensity fiberoptic light source.

Indications. The procedure is performed when a hysterosalpingography suggests tubal abnormality and the patient does not become pregnant. It is also performed before certain surgical procedures, such as a tuboplasty, and may reveal the presence of unsuspected tubal or ovarian disease, such as peritubal adhesions and endometriosis.

Complications. None.

Nursing care. None.

Colposcopy

Description. Examination of the cervix and vagina with a colposcope—a stereoscopic binocular microscope with various levels of magnification.

Indications. To evaluate the vascular pattern, intercapillary distance, surface pattern, color, tone, opacity, clarity, demarcation, and extent of a lesion. To differentiate between inflammatory atypia and neoplasms or between invasive and noninvasive cervical lesions, and to enable follow-up.

Complications. None.

Nursing care. Prepare the patient for the vaginal examination. Show her the colposcope and inform her that it will not be inserted into her vagina. Inform her beforehand if a biopsy is to be performed.

Culdoscopy

Description. Visual examination of female pelvic viscera by means of an endoscope inserted through the posterior vaginal fornix. The patient is usually sedated, and a general anesthetic is not used. The procedure is performed with the patient in the knee-chest position. If necessary, CO_2 may be instilled into the peritoneal cavity to allow better visualization of the pelvic organs.

Indications. Investigation of infertility. It determines gross anatomic and pathologic conditions, i.e., congenital abnormalities or the sequelae of traumatic or inflammatory processes.

Complications. None.

Nursing care. Explain to the patient that once the endoscope is removed, she will be required to exhale as forcefully as possible to force out intraperitoneal air; this maneuver will minimize shoulder pain when she sits up.

Culdotomy

Description. With the patient under general anesthesia, the posterior vagina is excised, with entry into a cul-de-sac for visual and manual examination. Operative procedures that can be performed with this technique include salpingectomy for ectopic pregnancy and tubal ligation.

Indications. To diagnose obscure pelvic disease or perform certain surgical procedures.

Complications. If the patient has a history of salpingitis with possible cul-de-sac adhesions, intestinal perforation is a potential complication.

Nursing care. Provide routine preoperative and postanesthetic recovery care. Explain to the patient that she may experience sensations of pelvic fullness and pressure. Instruct the patient not to put anything into her vagina, including douches and tampons, and not to have sexual intercourse until permitted by a physician.

Hysteroscopy

Description. Direct visual examination of the cervical canal and uterine cavity through a hysteroscope, a fiberoptic instrument; procedure most often performed with the patient under spinal anesthesia.

Indications. To examine the endometrium, secure a specimen for biopsy, remove an intrauterine device, or excise cervical polyps.

Complications. Perforation of the uterus (usually at the fundus), bleeding, infection.

Nursing care. The patient should be maintained in a flat position for 8 hours after the procedure.

Laparoscopy

Description. With the patient under general anesthesia, the abdominal and pelvic organs are visualized and examined with a laparoscope inserted through a small incision in the abdominal wall; the abdomen is insufflated with carbon dioxide to enhance visualization. The procedure usually lasts 10 to 15 minutes.

Indications. Therapeutic procedures may also be performed, including removal of peritubular adhesions, sterilization through fulguration of oviducts, and laser treatment for endometriosis.

Complications. Bleeding from a puncture injury, misplacement of gas, thermal burns.

Nursing care. Provide routine presurgical and postanesthetic care. Inform the patient that she may experience a sore throat from intubation and a sore chest from insufflation of her abdomen. These sensations usually disappear within 48 hours.

Arthroscopy

Description. Insertion of a specially designed endoscope through an incision at a certain point, often the knee. By means of lenses and lights on the scope, the tissues are examined. The arthroscope also permits the removal of loose bodies, pieces of torn cartilage, and biopsy of the synovium if desired. The procedure is performed in an outpatient surgical or operative suite.

Indications. To determine the condition of the joint, tissues, cartilage, meniscus (of knee), and ligaments. It is most frequently performed on the knee and shoulder, and less often on the hip, elbow, ankle, and other joints.

Complications. Possible joint swelling after the procedure and at times some bleeding into the joint. Infection is also possible.

Nursing care. Explain to the patient about the skin preparation, application of a tourniquet to decrease blood flow, sterile draping, and administration of a local anesthetic to one or more areas before insertion of the arthroscope into the joint. After the procedure, instruct the patient about applying a compression dressing and ice around the joint to lessen bleeding and edema. Caution the patient to avoid excessive joint use for 24 to 48 hours, and explain that weight bearing is permitted after knee arthroscopy. Use of other joints varies with the purpose and extent of the arthroscopic repair or procedure done. Instruct the patient regarding signs of infection, restrictions or limitations of joint use, and the time to return to the physician. Mild analgesics may be prescribed for postprocedural discomfort or pain.

Body Fluid Examination

Sputum Examination (Direct Method)

Description. The microbiologic evaluation of sputum is vitally important in the evaluation of the respiratory system. The two laboratory procedures commonly performed with sputum examination are microscopic Gram stain and culture and sensitivity.

Direct method. Voluntary coughing to produce sputum specimen. With this procedure, early morning specimens are sent on three consecutive days. It is most important to ensure that a sputum and not a saliva specimen has been obtained.

Sputum induction. This technique may be used if voluntary coughing does not produce a specimen. With this technique the patient is instructed to breathe for several minutes using a heated, nebulized mist of distilled water or a sodium chloride solution. Following this nebulization the sputum collection technique as described is performed.

Indications. Evaluation of pneumonias, suspected malignancies.

Complications. None.

Nursing care. The sputum should be collected in a wide-mouthed, sterile container with a tightly fitting lid and should be transported immediately to the laboratory.

Instruct the patient to brush teeth and gargle before the collection of the specimen. Instruct the patient to expectorate any postnasal secretions and spit them out. Instruct the patient to take a deep breath to the lungs' full capacity and then to exhale the air with an expulsive deep cough. The specimen should be coughed directly into the sterile, wide-mouthed container. Note the color, consistency, odor, and amount of the sputum. Number the specimens serially for each of the 3 days.

Sputum Examination (Indirect Method)

Description. One of two indirect methods may be used.

Nasotracheal suctioning. This technique is used to obtain specimens from the trachea via a catheter that has been passed transnasally.

Transtracheal aspiration. This technique may be preferred over nasotracheal suctioning. The specimens are better, but the patient may have discomfort. The technique involves puncture and needle aspiration. The needle is inserted through the cricothyroid membrane and the mucosal layer of the trachea.

Indications. Evaluation of pneumonias or suspected malignancies.

Complications

Nasotracheal suctioning. Hypoxemia.

Transtracheal aspiration. Subcutaneous or mediastinal emphysema and cervical infections at the site of the aspiration.

Nursing care

Nasotracheal suctioning. Assist the patient to a sitting position. The nurse or physician passes a catheter through the patient's nose into the trachea to suction tracheobronchial secretions. Oxygen should be administered during the procedure. Cardiac response and the patient's oxygenation should be monitored.

Transtracheal aspiration. Set up sterile procedural equipment, including gloves, gauze sponges, large-bore intracatheter needle, 10 cc syringe, sterile specimen cup, local anesthetic with needles and syringe, and iodophor for skin cleansing. Prepare the patient for high-flow supplemental oxygen during the procedure. Position the patient in a supine position and hyperextend the patient's neck by placing a pillow under the shoulders. Administer oxygen, assist the physician, and monitor the patient's cardiovascular and respiratory status during the procedure. After the procedure, light pressure should be placed over the site for at least 3 to 5 minutes. Continue to assess the patient for postprocedural complications. Anaerobic culture specimens are best sent to the laboratory in the aspirating syringe after all excess air has been expelled.

Pleural Fluid Examination (Diagnostic Thoracentesis)

Description. A needle is inserted through the chest wall into the pleural space for the purpose of removing pleural fluid.

Indications. May be performed therapeutically to drain off fluid and relieve lung congestion, and also diagnostically to collect pleural fluid for examination in patients with symptoms of inflammation, infection, or malignancy.

Complications. Hemothorax, pneumothorax, air embolism, subcutaneous emphysema.

Nursing care. Instruct the patient regarding the procedure. Advise the patient not to move suddenly, cough, or breathe deeply during the procedure. Record baseline vital signs. Assist with positioning the patient comfortably. After the procedure, monitor the patient's vital signs and respiratory status for any complications.

Gastric Analysis (Basal Gastric Secretion Test)

Description. Measures basal secretion under fasting conditions by aspirating stomach contents through a nasogastric tube, with the patient in supine, left lateral decubitus, and right lateral decubitus positions.

Histamine may be injected to stimulate flow. Normal values are 0.2 to 3.8 mEq/hr for females; 1 to 5 mEq/hr for males. High values may indicate a duodenal or jejunal ulcer; depressed values may indicate gastric carcinoma or benign gastric ulcer; absence of gastric secretion indicates pernicious anemia; markedly high levels indicate Zollinger-Ellison syndrome.

Indications. Indicated for patients with anorexia, weight loss, and epigastric pain.

Complications. None.

Nursing care. The patient must be relaxed and isolated from sensory stimulations of foods. (Gastric acid secretions are increased by external factors, including the sight and smell of food and psychologic stress.) The patient should have nothing to eat for 12 hours and no smoking for 8 hours. The following drugs should be withheld for 24 hours: antacids, anticholinergics, cholinergics, alcohol, cimetidine, ranitidine, reserpine, adrenergic blockers, and adrenocorticosteroids.

To prevent contamination of gastric contents with saliva, the patient should be instructed to expectorate excess saliva rather than swallow it.

Check the location of the catheter for placement. Paroxysms of coughing or cyanosis may indicate a catheter in the trachea. Arrhythmias may develop during intubation. Clamp the catheter during removal to prevent aspiration from fluids in the lumen. Sore throats following intubation may be treated with soothing lozenges, viscous lidocaine (Xylocaine), or benzocaine (Cetacaine) spray.

Gastric Acid Stimulation Test

Description. Normally follows basal gastric secretion test. A drug, usually pentagastrin, is given to stimulate gastric acid output; specimens are collected every 15 minutes for 1 hour. Normal values are 11 to 21 mEq/hr for females and 18 to 28 mEq/hr for males.

Indications. Clinical diagnosis of the following is indicated by certain results of gastric acid secretion:

Duodenal ulcers: high values
Zollinger-Ellison syndrome: markedly high values
Gastric carcinoma: low values
Pernicious anemia: achlorhydria (low acid levels are considered normal in patients over 60 years of age)

Complications. Side effects of pentagastrin include abdominal pain, nausea, vomiting, flushing, transitory dizziness, faintness, and numbness of extremities. Check the patient's history for hypersensitivity to pentagastrin.

Nursing care. Same as for gastric analysis.

Gastric Lavage

Description. The procedure includes an early morning suctioning of gastric contents once a nasogastric tube has been properly placed. The timing of the procedure is early morning because it is assumed that the patient swallows sputum at night while sleeping and in the early morning with morning coughing. The gastric contents are sent to the laboratory for sputum analysis.

Indications. This technique, although infrequently used, may be helpful in the diagnosis of patients with suspected tuberculosis or lung cancer. It is perhaps most valuable in patients who may be unable to cooperate, such as young children and the acutely ill.

Complications. None.

Nursing care. The patient should be given nothing by mouth after midnight. A nasogastric (NG) tube is inserted through the patient's nose. Suction is applied to the NG tube with a large syringe, and the gastric contents are removed. The contents are placed in a specimen container and are sent immediately to the laboratory. The NG tube is removed.

Peritoneal Fluid Analysis

Description. Examines a sample of peritoneal fluid obtained by paracentesis. Normally, peritoneal fluid is sterile, odorless, clear to pale yellow, and less than 50 ml, with no red blood cells, bacteria, or fungi. Normal values: white blood count—less than 300 mg/μl; protein—0.3 to 4.1 g/dl; glucose—70 to 100 mg/dl; amylase—138 to 404 amylase U/L; ammonia—less than 50 μg/dl. Alkaline phosphatase: male over 18 years—90 to 239 U/L; female under 45 years—76 to 196 U/L; female over 45 years—87 to 250 U/L.

Indications. To determine the composition of ascitic fluid, to assist in diagnosis of hepatic or other systemic disease, or to detect abdominal trauma.

Complications. Perforation of an abdominal organ or vessels. Signs include those for hemorrhage and shock, increasing pain, and abdominal tenderness.

Patients with severe hepatic disease should be observed for signs of hepatic coma, which may be from loss of sodium and potassium with accompanying hypovolemia. Observe the patient for mental changes, drowsiness, and stupor.

Nursing care. Record baseline vital signs, weights, and abdominal girth measurements for comparisons with posttest results. Consent forms are generally required. The patient should void immediately before the procedure to prevent injury to bladder. The patient is usually sitting with feet flat on the floor and the back supported; if the patient cannot tolerate this, use a high Fowler's position.

Check vital signs every 15 minutes during the procedure and compare with baseline values; note signs of dizziness, pallor, perspiration, and increased anxiety. Rapid aspiration may induce hypovolemia and shock; in such a case, slow the rate of aspiration.

After the test has been completed, monitor vital signs frequently (every 30 minutes for 2 hours; every hour for next 4 hours; every 4 hours for 24 hours). Weight and abdominal girth should be measured and compared with baseline.

Cover the site with a sterile dressing. If the site continues to drain, requiring frequent dressing changes, consider application of a skin barrier and a pouch for collection of drainage and accurate measurement of output.

Monitor urinary output for 24 hours and observe for hematuria. Observe the patient closely for signs of hypovolemic shock if large amounts were aspirated.

Cytologies

Description. Body secretions collected and examined for cells, which are stained and evaluated; examples are the Papanicolaou smear and examinations of cervical discharge, sputum, gastric washings, pleural fluid, and urinary washings.

Indications. Suspected malignancies, infection, inflammation.

Complications. None, usually.

Nursing care. Explain purpose of test. Assist with individual procedures.

Cerebrospinal Fluid Studies

Description

Lumbar puncture. Insertion of needle into the lumbar subarachnoid space to obtain cerebrospinal fluid for examination and to detect spinal subarachnoid block. The needle is inserted in the L3-L4 interspace.

Lateral cervical puncture. Insertion of a needle into the C1-C2 interspace through to the subarachnoid space to obtain cerebrospinal fluid. The needle is inserted perpendicular to the neck with the patient in a supine position.

Cisternal puncture. Insertion of a short-beveled needle immediately below the occipital bone into the cisterna magna to obtain cerebrospinal fluid. It can be inserted simultaneously with lumbar puncture to demonstrate subarachnoid block.

Ventricular puncture. Insertion of a ventricular needle (in adults and older children) through burr holes into the lateral ventricle.

Indications. The lumbar puncture, or spinal tap, is a common neurologic test performed to measure cerebrospinal fluid pressure, remove cerebrospinal fluid for visualization and laboratory analysis, inject medications (i.e., spinal anesthesia, intrathecal injection of antibacterial agents) or contrast media, and determine the degree of subarachnoid block by means of spinal dynamics.

A cisternal puncture may be performed if a subarachnoid block is present, if a lumbar puncture is contraindicated, to reduce intracranial pressure, to perform encephalography, and to introduce air or a contrast medium for myelography.

A ventricular puncture is indicated if a lumbar or cisternal puncture is contraindicated, for injection of contrast medium into an infant's ventricles to determine the type of hydrocephalus, for removal of cerebrospinal fluid, for injection of air or oxygen to localize a tumor, and as a preliminary to ventricular drainage.

Complications. Infection, leakage of cerebrospinal fluid, dysuria, headache, nausea, and vomiting. Signs of meningeal irritation are increased intracranial pressure and convulsions.

Nursing care. Position the patient on a firm surface and maintain the spine in a horizontal position. Assist in obtaining a manometer reading of cerebrospinal fluid pressure.

If a subarachnoid block is suspected, a Queckenstedt test is performed. Place the blood pressure cuff around the patient's neck and inflate to 20 mm Hg pressure (or compress jugular veins) for 10 seconds. Obtain manometer pressure readings at 10-second intervals until the pressure stabilizes. Keep the patient flat in bed (or on side) for 4 to 6 hours after procedure. Force fluids, unless contraindicated. Monitor vital signs and neurologic signs frequently. The procedure should be performed with *extreme* caution when intracranial pressure is elevated.

Vaginal Smears

Description. Vaginal examination is performed, and vaginal secretions are placed on a slide with 1 drop of normal saline placed on one side and 1 drop of 10% to 20% potassium hydroxide (KOH) on the other side.

Indications. *Trichomonas vaginalis* can be observed at the saline end of the slide, and *Candida albicans* at the KOH side; other organisms can also be identified with this procedure.

Complications. None.

Nursing care. Prepare the patient for a vaginal examination and assist with the procedure.

• Fecal Examination

Fecal Fat

Description. Qualitative (random sample) and quantitative (72-hour collection) tests are used. Qualitative tests identify undigested muscle fibers and various fats, and quantitative tests can confirm steatorrhea. Fecal lipids normally are less than 20% of excreted solids or less than 7 g/24 hr.

A sudan stain can be made on a sample to test for presence of fat.

Indications. Steatorrhea—excessive secretions of fecal lipids—may be observed in some malabsorption syndromes.

Complications. None.

Nursing care. Have the patient avoid alcohol ingestion for 72 hours before and during stool collection, and maintain a high-fat diet, 100 g/day for 72 hours before and during collection.

Avoid use of waxed collection containers, since wax can become incorporated into the stool and distort results. The specimen container must be refrigerated.

Avoid use of azathioprine, kanamycin, bisacodyl, cholestyramine, neomycin, colchicine, aluminum hydroxide, calcium carbonate, potassium chloride, and mineral oil, since they inhibit absorption of fats or affect chemical digestion, producing inaccurate results.

Fecal Urobilinogen

Description. Determines the amount of urobilinogen (result of breakdown of bilirubin by intestinal flora) excreted in urine and feces.

Random stool specimen required. Normal values are 50 to 300 mg/24 hr. Low levels may indicate hepatocellular jaundice from cirrhosis or hepatitis or extrahepatic disorders such as tumors obstructing bile flow. Low levels are also seen in aplastic anemia with depressed erythropoiesis. Elevated levels are found in hemolytic jaundice, thalassemia, and hemolytic pernicious anemia.

Indications. May be used as an indicator of hepatobiliary and hemolytic disorders.

Complications. None.

Nursing care. May be a 2-hour afternoon specimen or a 24-hour collection. If possible avoid the following for 2 weeks before stool collection: broad-spectrum antibiotics, which inhibit bacterial growth in the colon and may inhibit fecal urobilinogen levels; sulfonamides, which react with the reagents used in the test; salicylates, which in large doses can raise fecal urobilinogen levels. Stool container must be light resistant, since urobilinogen breaks down to urobilin on exposure to light. Keep in mind that serum bilirubin and urine urobilinogen can be measured easily.

Fecal Occult Blood

Description. Procedure consists of a patient collecting three separate stool specimens. Their color usually indicates the site of bleeding (e.g., melena is common with esophageal or gastric bleeding; a dark maroon color may indicate a lesion below the ligament of Treitz; and bright red may be from a low rectal carcinoma or hemorrhoids).

Indications. Used to detect gastrointestinal bleeding and as a screening test for colorectal cancer.

Complications. None.

Nursing care. With guaiac-impregnated pad tests (Hemoccult, HemoFec, Colo-Screen), discuss with the patients how to collect the stool specimen. Have the patient avoid red meats, poultry, fish, turnips, and horseradish for 48 to 72 hours before the test begins and throughout the collection period.

Withhold iron preparations, bromides, iodides, rauwolfia derivatives, indomethacin, colchicine, salicylates, and phenylbutazone for 48 hours before collection begins and throughout the test. If the patient is taking steroids, the accuracy of test may be affected. Do not collect during menses, since false positive results may be obtained. Ascorbic acid can interfere with the accuracy of the test and should be withheld 48 hours before the collection period begins.

With HemoQuant tests, explain to the patient how to use the collection device included in HemoQuant kits. Have the patient avoid ingesting aspirin and red meat for 48 to 72 hours before the test begins and during the collection period.

• Roentgenograms

Chest Roentgenogram

Description. Gives information regarding the anatomic location and abnormalities of the heart, great vessels, and lungs. Routine views in a cardiac series are posterior-anterior (PA), lateral, right anterior oblique (RAO), and left anterior oblique (LAO). Roentgenograms are also used to determine the position of the heart (normal is situs soltis: left thoracic heart); cardiothoracic size (normal is less than 50% of the internal dimensions of the thorax); cardiac silhouette (thorax, aorta, ventricular chambers, atrial chambers, pulmonary artery); presence of calcifications (visualized in great vessels and on valves); lung fields (used to determine normal distribution of pulmonary blood flow); increase of pulmonary congestion; presence of pulmonary hypertension; and presence of pleural effusions.

The normal chest roentgenographic examination includes PA and lateral views (as shown in Figure 1). In young, healthy individuals or in asymptomatic persons only the PA view is used for screening. A lateral view should be obtained if disease is suspected or if the individual is over 40 years old. Chest roentgenograms in the upright position are preferred so that the abdominal viscera does not push up on the diaphragm.

Indications. Chest roentgenograms are evaluated for normal structure, position, and outlines, the presence of fluid lines, foreign bodies, infiltration, and abnormal shadows. An anterior oblique view may be used to visualize the thymus in immune disorders.

Complications. None.

Nursing care. Explain the procedure. Inquire if the patient is pregnant. All neck jewelry or garments containing metal clasps, buttons, or ornaments must be removed. The patient should be wearing a hospital gown.

Musculoskeletal Films

Description. Examination of musculoskeletal tissues by means of roentgenographic exposure.

Indications. To determine injury, fracture, degeneration, inflammation, or neoplasm in one or more musculoskeletal tissues.

Complications. None.

Nursing care. Explain to the patient the purpose of the examination. Caution radiologic technicians to move the patient carefully and to support the joints above and below the affected tissues to prevent additional discomfort or trauma.

Sella Turcica/Skull Films

Description. Simple roentgenographic study of the skull. AP and lateral views are most frequently ordered to detect configuration, density, and vascular markings of skull. Initial roentgenographic evaluation of the pituitary gland begins with high-quality skull films that focus on the sella turcica, the bony structure in which the pituitary gland is located.

Indications. Skull films provide important data about vascular abnormalities, the shape and size of the cranial and facial bones, the presence of fractured skull bones, degenerative changes (i.e., bone erosion), unusual calcifications (e.g., tumors or chronic subdural hematomas), the position of the pineal body, investigation for cranial masses, Cushing's disease workup, hypopituitary workup, and precocious puberty.

Complications. None.

Nursing care. Instruct the patient regarding the procedure.

Spinal Films

Description. Simple roentgenographic study of different spinal regions: cervical, thoracic, lumbar, or sacral. Anterior, posterior, and lateral views are most common.

Indications. Spinal roentgenograms are taken when there has been trauma, pain, or sensory or motor impairment to the back or vertebral column. Roentgenograms of the spine usually include anterior, posterior, and lateral views to pinpoint fractures of the irregularly shaped vertebrae. Abnormal findings of spinal roentgenography include vertebral dislocation or fracture, bone erosion, unusual calcification, collapsed vertebrae and wedging, spondylosis, and spurs.

Complications. None.

Nursing care. Instruct the patient regarding the procedure.

Mastoid Films

Description. Roentgenograms of temporal bone. If mastoiditis is present, characteristic findings are clouding of the mastoid air cells and decalcification of bony walls between the cells.

Indications. A thick purulent discharge from the ear, low-grade temperature, a dull ache behind the ear.

Complications. None.

Nursing care. None.

Sinus Films

Description. Roentgenograms taken to diagnose sinusitis by determining clouding or possible fluid levels in sinuses.

Figure 1 Normal PA and lateral chest roentgenogram. Note no abnormal bony prominences, heart of normal size, sharp costophrenic angles, lung fields clear, diaphragms visible throughout except against heart border, mediastinum midline with bronchial structures visible, and breast shadows.

Courtesy R. Keith Wilson, M.D., Baylor College of Medicine, Houston, Texas.

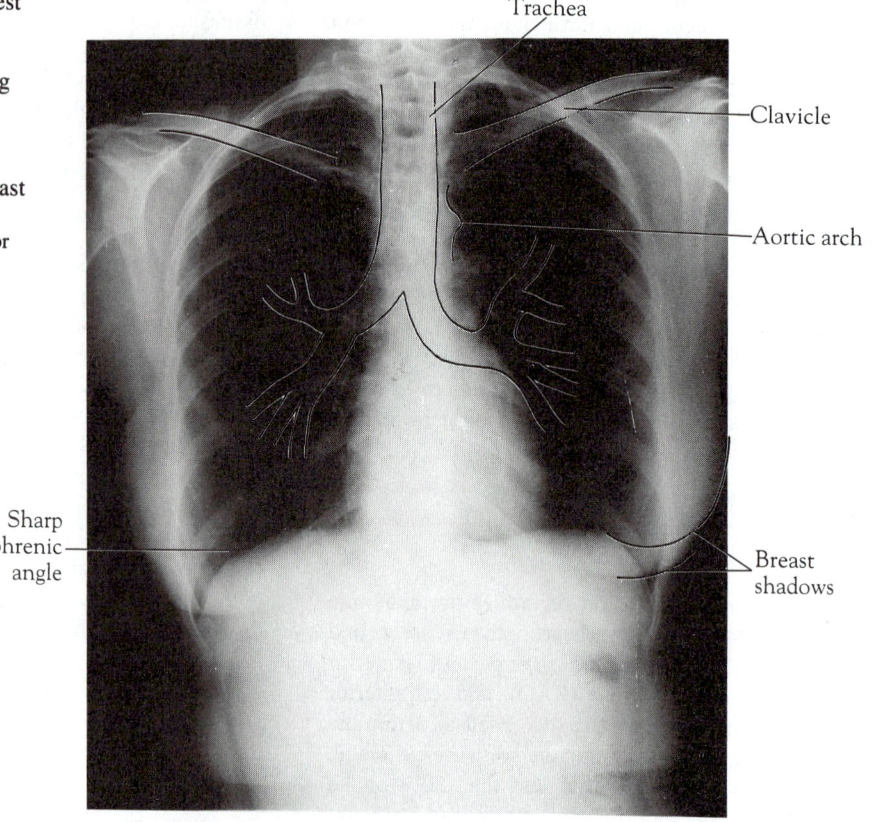

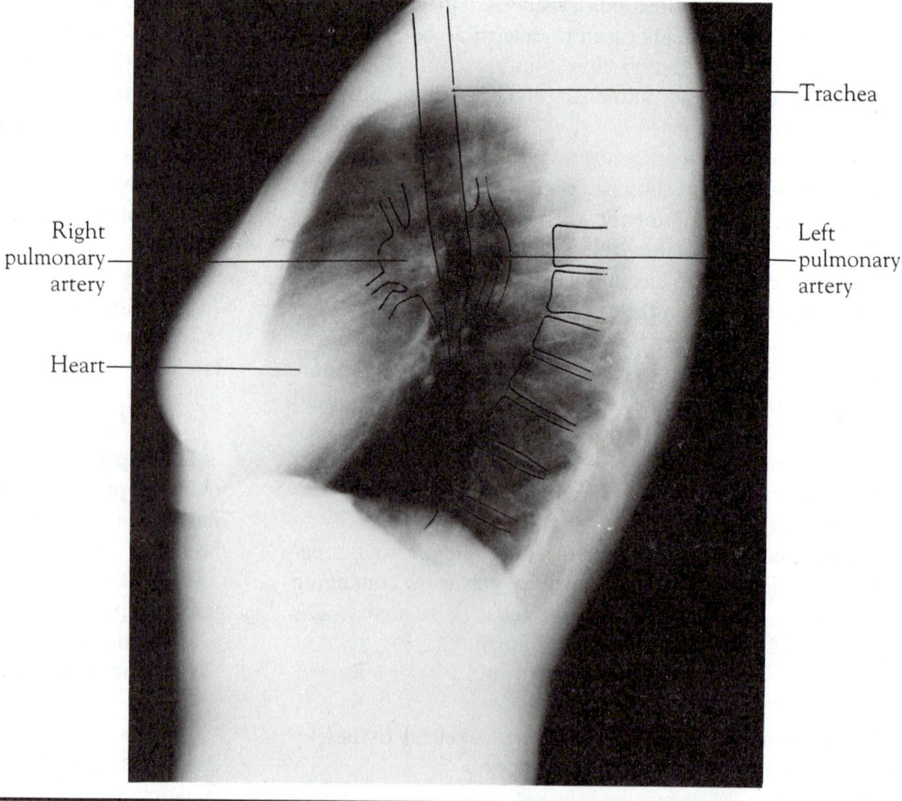

The usual views include Waters' view (orbits, frontal and maxillary sinuses, and nasal septum); Caldwell view (frontal sinuses, ethmoid air cells between each orbit, nasal septum, and petrous portion of temporal bone); and the lateral view (sphenoid sinus and posterior wall of frontal sinuses).

Indications. Headache, facial pain, low-grade temperature, a feeling of fullness or pressure in the face or sinus area.

Complications. None.

Nursing care. None.

Mammography, Xeromammography

Description. Mammography is soft tissue roentgenography of the breast with low-energy roentgenographic and high-contrast film. Xeromammography is the use of a dry photoelectric process to make roentgenograms of soft tissues of the breast. The roentgenographic image is recorded on an electrostatically charged plate. The image is transferred to plastic-coated paper by pressing the plate and the paper together and exposing them to heat. All of this is performed automatically in a commercial processor.

Indications. Annual routine screening is recommended for women 35 to 40 years and older. It assists in the diagnosis of breast masses, tumors, and abnormalities.

Complications. None.

Nursing care. Ensure that the patient does not have powder, lotion, or ointment on her breasts. Explain the procedure.

Kidneys, Ureters, Bladder (KUB)

Description. Roentgenographic film of kidneys, ureters, and bladder without contrast material. It is important as a scout film when performing an intravenous pyelogram and as a diagnostic study to determine the presence of radiopaque calculi.

Indications. To determine the size and location of kidneys and radiopaque stones.

Complications. None.

Nursing care. Preparation is not standardized. An IVP prep is used when KUB is performed as part of this extensive roentgenographic study. In other situations, no preparation is indicated.

• Contrast Studies

Contrast Radiography

Description. Examination of an area of the body with a contrast medium during a roentgenographic study. Barium sulfate is one form of a contrast medium; meglumine diatrizoate is another form and can be injected or given intravenously or through a tube or catheter. Other commercial agents are available.

Single-contrast studies use barium alone, whereas double-contrast studies use barium and air.

In addition to roentgenography (passage of radiation through the patient to create a roentgenogram), cineradiography, fluoroscopy, and video are used in many of these procedures. Cineradiography is a rapid-sequence roentgenographic procedure that films motion; fluoroscopy is the projection of roentgenograms onto a screen or fluoroscope, permitting continuous observation of motion.

Indications. Examination of soft and bony tissues of the body; diagnosis of certain pathologic conditions that requires the visualization of details not revealed by plain film radiography.

Nursing care. Barium as a contrast material precludes effective use of fiberoptic endoscopy for several hours and of arteriography for 24 to 48 hours.

The patient with a colostomy should be instructed to irrigate after the barium procedure is concluded and should repeat the irrigation the next morning. If upper gastrointestinal series or small bowel follow-through has been performed, the patient should irrigate after the last delayed spot film (approximately 6 hours after ingestion). The patient with an ileostomy should never receive a laxative or an enema before or after a barium study. Clear liquid for 48 hours before the procedure and forced fluids afterward are sufficient. Healthy patients may want to take a mild laxative.

Complications. Barium retained in intestine may harden and cause an obstruction or fecal impaction. Before giving meglumine diatrizoate, check for hypersensitivity to iodine, seafood, and contrast media. Symptoms of an allergic reaction include nausea, vomiting, flushing, urticaria, sweating, and rarely anaphylaxis. An intraductal injection may be accompanied by tachycardia and fever.

Ventriculography

Description. A ventriculogram depends on the injection of air or positive contrast medium via a ventricular puncture directly into the lateral cerebral ventricles. The procedure is performed in the operating room under strict aseptic technique. Following the ventricular puncture, cerebrospinal fluid is gradually removed and replaced with air or a positive contrast medium, and roentgenograms are taken.

Indications. Indications for a ventriculogram include determination of patency of the ventricular system, localization of a brain tumor, and detection of cerebral anomalies.

Complications. Nausea and vomiting, headache, increased intracranial pressure, respiratory distress, seizures, air embolus shock.

Nursing care. General anesthesia may be required for young pediatric patients. Observe for signs and symptoms of intracranial or subdural hematoma (especially in patients with noncommunicating hydrocephalus). Frequently monitor vital signs and neurologic signs. Keep the patient flat in bed for 24 to 48 hours after the procedure. Encourage fluids. Keep accurate intake and output records. Institute seizure precautions after the procedure for 24 hours.

Bronchography

Description. Radiopaque contrast medium is inserted into the lumina of the trachea and bronchial tree. Bronchography is being used more and more infrequently.[6] The advent of fiberoptic bronchoscopy has rendered fewer lesions inaccessible to direct vision. More precise methods for diagnosing a pulmonary lesion include bronchoscopic brush, forceps biopsy, and transthoracic needle puncture.

Indications. Diagnosis and evaluation of pulmonary lesions.

Complications. None.

Nursing care. Give nothing by mouth for 8 hours before procedure. Assess allergies to the anesthesia agent or contrast media. Assess for dental prosthesis. Approximately 1 hour before the procedure, administer barbiturate medication with atropine to decrease anxiety and secretions. To lessen the patient's discomfort during the procedure, the throat may be sprayed with 0.5% tetracaine or a similar substance. Oxygen and suction should be available during the process. After the procedure the patient should be evaluated for gag and cough reflex and tissue oxygenation. Food and water should be withheld until the gag reflex returns. Following the procedure the patient should be encouraged to cough. If the cough is inadequate, postural drainage may be needed.

Barium Swallow

Description. Examination of the pharynx and esophagus on a fluoroscope after ingestion of barium sulfate.

Indications. Used to diagnose or detect hiatal hernia, achalasia, diverticulum, varices, strictures, ulcers, tumors, motility disorders, and polyps.

Complications. Retained barium may harden and cause an impaction or obstruction.

Nursing care. Required fasting after midnight. Once the mixture is ingested, the patient is placed in various positions. The esophagus is also examined fluoroscopically during swallowing of the solution. Barium swallow is contraindicated in patients with an intestinal obstruction. A laxative may be given to facilitate the expulsion of barium (unless otherwise noted); also, have the patient increase fluid intake.

Upper Gastrointestinal and Small Bowel Series (UGI and SB Series)

Description. Fluoroscopic examination of the esophagus, stomach, and small intestine after ingestion of barium sulfate; as barium passes through the system, fluoroscopy outlines mucosal contours. Spot films are used to record significant findings. Follow-up spot films after 6 hours can provide some evaluation of gastrointestinal motility. The procedure is contraindicated in patients with intestinal perforations and intestinal obstructions.

Indications. Useful in detecting or diagnosing hiatal hernias, diverticulum, varices, ulcers, strictures, tumors, regional enteritis (also called granulomatous ileitis or Crohn's ileitis), and motility disorders.

Complications. Retained barium may cause a fecal impaction or obstruction.

Nursing care. The patient is given nothing by mouth past midnight, and a mild laxative may be ordered. The patient should also increase fluid intake and maintain a low-residue diet for 2 or 3 days before test. Smoking should be avoided from midnight before the test and throughout procedure. Anticholinergics and narcotics are withheld for 24 hours before the study if intestinal motility is of concern. Laxatives are used following the procedure to assist in expulsion of barium.

Oral Cholecystography (OCG)

Description. Roentgenographic examination of the gallbladder. Contrast medium given the evening before the test. Iopanoic acid is usually used, but other commercial contrast media are available. The abdomen is examined fluoroscopically to evaluate gallbladder opacification. Spot films are taken of significant findings. Fat stimulus may also be used during the roentgenographic procedure. Fluoroscopy is then used to observe emptying of the gallbladder. Spot films are taken as indicated.

The procedure is not performed in the presence of severe renal or hepatic disease or jaundice.

Indications. Evaluation of gallbladder disease.

Complications. Diarrhea commonly occurs; nausea, vomiting, abdominal cramps, or dysuria occurs in rare cases.

Nursing care. The diet before the test includes a lunch meal containing fats and a fat-free evening meal. Check the patient for allergies to iodine, seafood, or contrast media before giving tablets—iopanoic acid, 3 g, given as one tablet with a total of 240 ml (8 oz) of water. Check any emesis or diarrheal stools for undigested tablets.

The large intestine is generally cleansed by an enema the morning of the test.

Barium Enema

Description. Instillation of barium sulfate or barium sulfate and air through the anus into the large intestine. A barium enema should precede a barium-swallow upper gastrointestinal series with small bowel follow-through. Once this was the most effective means of identifying colon carcinomas above the level of sigmoidoscope; colonoscopy examinations are now effectively used for visualization of the entire large intestine.

Barium enemas are contraindicated in patients with fulminant inflammatory bowel disease, toxic megacolon, suspected perforations, and suspected obstructions. Caution should be used for patients with acute inflammatory bowel disease, ischemic bowel disease, acute fulminant bloody diarrhea, and pneumatosis cystoides intestinalis.

Indications. Used as one method of diagnosing colorectal cancer and inflammatory bowel disease. It will also detect polyps, diverticula, and other changes in the colon and rectum.

Complications. Retained barium may cause fecal impaction or obstruction.

Nursing care. Careful bowel preparation is necessary to cleanse the bowel of fecal material. An ileostomy patient has no large intestine and requires only clear liquid for 24 to 48 hours as a "bowel" preparation; the site of the colostomy will determine the preparation.

Patients with suspected inflammatory bowel disease (ulcerative colitis or granulomatous colitis) should not be given a routine preparatory kit for barium enemas. The condition can be greatly exacerbated by irritants and may require surgical intervention; check with the physician.

Laxatives are required (unless otherwise stated) to facilitate the removal of barium.

Intravenous Cholangiography (IVC)

Description. Provides better visualization of the biliary ducts than does oral cholangiography, which is useful in gallbladder disease. IVC involves roentgenographic and tomographic studies after intravenous infusion of a contrast medium. Fluoroscopy spot films are made every 10 minutes until visualization of the bile ducts is satisfactory, which may take 25 to 40 minutes; tomograms are then made. Films and tomograms are repeated 2 to 2½ hours later, when maximal opacification of the gallbladder has occurred. (This would be unnecessary in patients with cholecystectomies.) Delayed films of the gallbladder may be taken at 4 and 24 hours. IVC should precede any barium studies, since retained barium clouds roentgenograms.

Indications. Generally indicated in patients with right upper quadrant or epigastric pain after cholecystectomy. Pain suggests biliary tract disease.

Complications. Hypersensitivity reactions.

Nursing care. The diet should be low residue the day before the test with an evening meal high in simple fats (milk, cream, eggs, butter); the patient should be given nothing to eat after midnight. Check with the patient for a history of hypersensitivities to iodine, seafood, and contrast media. A fatty meal may be given so that, with fluoroscopy, emptying may be viewed.

Bowel preparations used to cleanse the colon are contraindicated in patients with hyperthyroidism, severe renal or hepatic disease, tuberculosis, or hypersensitivity to iodine.

Hypotonic Duodenography

Description. Barium sulfate and air instilled through an intestinal catheter for fluoroscopic examination of the duodenum. Intravenous infusion of glucagon or intramuscular injection of propantheline bromide is used to induce duodenal atony. A catheter is inserted through the nose and into the stomach while the patient is sitting; in a supine position under fluoroscopy, a catheter is advanced into the duodenum.

Administration of anticholinergics is contraindicated in the presence of severe cardiac disorders or glaucoma.

Indications. Demonstrates small duodenal lesions and tumors at the head of the pancreas.

Complications. Retained barium may cause fecal impaction or obstruction.

Nursing care. Explain the procedure to the patient. A laxative may be needed after the procedure to facilitate the expulsion of barium.

Percutaneous Transhepatic Cholangiography

Description. Fluoroscopic examination of biliary ducts after the injection of iodinated contrast medium directly into the biliary tree. The liver is punctured by a thin, flexible needle, and contrast medium is injected as the needle is slowly withdrawn. Contrast medium slowly flows through the biliary ducts, outlining the biliary tree. The catheter used to inject the dye is sometimes left in place to drain the biliary tree.

Percutaneous transhepatic cholangiography is contraindicated in patients with cholangitis, severe ascites, uncorrectable coagulopathy, and hypersensitivity to iodine.

Indications. Helps to distinguish between obstructive and nonobstructive jaundice. With mechanical obstruction of the biliary tree the procedure helps to determine the location, the extent, and often the cause.

Complications. Hypersensitivity reactions, peritonitis, bleeding.

Nursing care. Check with the patient for a history of hypersensitivity to iodine, seafood, or contrast media. Check the patient for normal bleeding, clotting, prothrombin times, and platelet count.

The patient should remain in bed for 6 hours after the procedure. Check vital signs frequently (every 15 minutes for 1 hour, every 30 minutes for the next 2 hours, every hour for 4 hours after that, and then every 4 hours). Check the injection site for bleeding, swelling, and tenderness. Check for signs of peritonitis: chills, a temperature of 38° to 39° C (102° to 103° F), abdominal pain, tenderness, distention.

Postoperative Cholangiography or T-Tube Cholangiography

Description. Contrast medium is injected through a T-tube, and the flow of medium outlining biliary tree can be visualized with fluoroscopy. This is performed 7 to 10 days following a cholecystectomy or common bile duct exploration in which a T-tube has been left in the common bile duct to facilitate drainage.

Indications. To evaluate the patency and size of ducts and to identify calculi, strictures, neoplasms, or fistulas in the ductal system.

Complications. Sepsis, hypersensitivity reactions.

Nursing care. Some physicians have the T-tube clamped for 24 hours before the procedure to eliminate air bubbles in the tube. A cleansing enema to evacuate large intestine may be ordered. Check with the patient for allergies to iodine, seafood, and contrast media.

The T-tube may be removed after the procedure. A sterile dressing is applied. Note the amount and characteristics of any drainage. If frequent dressing changes are required, consider application of a sterile skin barrier and drainable pouch. Monitor the patient for signs and symptoms of sepsis.

Endoscopic Retrograde Cholangiopancreatography (ERCP)

Description. Roentgenographic examination of the pancreatic duct and hepatobiliary ductal system by injection of a contrast medium into the duodenal papilla. Endoscopy is performed, and the duodenal papilla located. A cannula filled with contrast medium is passed through the endoscope, into the duodenal papilla and ampulla of Vater. The pancreas is visualized first with injection of dye and then fluoroscopically; then the cannula is repositioned for injection of additional contrast medium, allowing for visualization of the hepatobiliary tree. Tissue biopsy or fluid for histology may be obtained before the endoscope is removed. Some centers are able to perform sphincterotomy and to snare and remove stones.

ERCP is contraindicated in patients with acute pancreatitis, pancreatic pseudocysts, strictures or obstruction of the esophagus or duodenum, cholangitis, infectious disease, or cardiorespiratory disease.

Indications. To diagnose cancer of the duodenal papilla, pancreas, or biliary ducts; to detect calculi or stenosis of ducts; and to evaluate obstructive jaundice.

Complications. Cholangitis and pancreatitis may develop. Signs of cholangitis include fever, chills, and hyperbilirubinemia; late symptoms may include hypotension and gram-negative septicemia. Pancreatitis may be indicated by upper left quadrant pain, tenderness, elevated serum amylase, and transient hyperbilirubinemia.

Nursing care. Assess the patient for a history of hypersensitivity to iodine, seafood, or contrast media.

Frequent vital sign checks are indicated when the patient returns to the floor (every 15 minutes for 4 hours; every hour for the next 4 hours; and then every 4 hours for 48 hours). Check for voiding, since urinary retention may be a side effect of anticholinergics. Monitor the patient for bleeding after the procedure.

Splenoportography (Transsplenic Portography)

Description. Cineradiographic study of the splenic veins and portal system. It generally provides a cleaner definition of the venous system than does superior mesenteric arteriography (which offers the advantage of outlining the splenic and portal veins during reverse blood flow and has fewer complications). Splenoportography may result in excessive bleeding, requiring transfusions and occasionally a splenectomy.

Splenic pulp pressure is measured before the dye is injected by attaching a spinal manometer filled with normal saline to a sheath inserted in the spleen. Normal splenic pulp pressure is 50 to 180 mm H_2O (or 3.5 to 13.5 mm Hg). Contrast medium is injected into the splenic pulp.

This procedure is contraindicated in patients with ascites, uncorrectable coagulopathy, splenomegaly secondary to infection, hypersensitivity to iodine, or markedly impaired liver or kidney function.

Indications. Used to diagnose or assess portal hypertension and to stage cirrhosis.

Complications. Hypersensitivity reactions, bleeding.

Nursing care. Assess the patient for a history of allergies to iodine, seafood, or contrast media. Frequent assessment of vital signs is required after the procedure (every 15 minutes for 1 hour, every 30 minutes for the next 2 hours, and then every hour for 4 hours). Check for bleeding, swelling, and tenderness at the site of injection.

The patient should remain on the left side for 24 hours to minimize risk of bleeding. An additional 24 hours of bed rest is recommended. Hematocrit levels may be obtained every 8 to 12 hours until values have stabilized.

Intravenous Pyelogram (IVP), Intravenous Urogram, Excretory Urogram

Description. Contrast-enhanced roentgenographic study that provides detailed anatomic information about the urinary tract. Clues to kidney function are provided by assessment of the organ's ability to concentrate and excrete contrast material. Information concerning the transport of urine through the ureters is provided by use of sequential films after a contrast medium is injected. Compression over ureters may be used to provide additional detail. Assessment of bladder function is made by obtaining films of the vesicle filled with contrast material (after asking the patient to void). IVP is performed after adequate preparation and after a KUB is done.

The patient is placed in a slight Trendelenburg's position or supine, and contrast material is injected intravenously. Serial films of kidneys, ureters, and the bladder are obtained over a period of time. The entire examination requires approximately 30 minutes.

Radiation doses for IVP vary widely, ranging from approximately 1047 mR (milliroentgens) to 1465 mR.[4] A nephrotomogram may be performed as part of the IVP to provide a more detailed reproduction of anatomic detail by focusing on a specific plane of the kidney rather than a nonspecific picture of the entirety of the kidneys.

Because of the risk of hypersensitivity reactions and potential renal failure secondary to IVP, a number of relative contraindications should be considered before completing the study. These include (1) a history of allergic reaction when given intravenous iodine-bound contrast material and (2) patients at higher risk for dehydration, including elderly persons and patients with severe diabetes mellitus, multiple myeloma, or renal insufficiency.[15]

Indications. Evaluation of renal masses, cysts, ureteral obstruction, retroperitoneal tumors, renal trauma, and bladder abnormalities; evaluation of renal disease and hypertension.

Complications. Hypersensitive reactions and acute renal failure. Observe for allergic reactions such as urticaria, rhonchi, and shortness of breath. Acute renal failure is a rare but serious complication of IVP. Observe urinary output (at least 30 ml/hour) while ensuring adequate fluid intake.[15]

Nursing care. Explain procedure to patient and ensure that patient has no allergies to iodine. After procedure, encourage increased fluid intake to ensure excretion of contrast.

Whitaker and Pfister Tests

Description. The Whitaker test is performed by placing a nephrostomy tube percutaneously into the pelvis of the affected kidney. A urethral catheter is also placed to measure bladder pressure. Sterile water, saline, or radiographic contrast material is perfused through the nephrostomy tube via a pump at a specific rate. Continuous-pressure monitoring is used to detect the presence of ureteral obstruction with the bladder empty and full.[30]

The Pfister test is similar to the Whitaker test, except that a 20-gauge spinal needle is used in place of a nephrostomy tube, and intermittent rather than continuous pressure monitoring is used to assess ureteral obstruction.[21]

Indications. Performed to assess ureteral obstruction when other methods (IVP, Lasix-enhanced renogram) fail to diagnose clearly or to rule out any obstruction.

Complications. Bleeding and infection.

Nursing care. Vital signs should be monitored regularly for the first 24 hours after testing. Temperature is an important parameter in the assessment of febrile urinary tract infection.

Retrograde Pyelogram (RPG)

Description. Provides a detailed anatomic description of the ureter and renal pelvis. It is performed in conjunction with cystoscopy because it requires placement of a 4 or 5 French ureteral catheter within the ureter to be studied. Radiographic contrast material is then injected into the collecting system via gravity infusion or by syringe, and roentgenographic images are obtained.

Indications. Evaluation of renal disease, obstruction, or trauma.

Complications. Pyelonephritis and overdistention of renal collecting system, which may result in extravasation of contrast medium leading to pain and fever. The reaction is typically transient; effects should disappear within 48 hours.

Nursing care. The patient should be closely observed for signs of infection (flank pain, fever, chills) for a 24- to 48-hour period after testing.

Retrograde Urethrogram (RUG)

Description. Provides a detailed description of urethral anatomy. It is made by injecting contrast material in a retrograde manner into the urethra via a catheter-tipped syringe or a Brodny clamp. The patient is typically placed in a supine position, and oblique films are taken.

Indications. Evaluation of trauma or stricture.

Complications. Urethritis, cystitis.

Nursing care. The patient should be encouraged to force fluids for a 24-hour period after testing. Mild dysuria should cease within 24 hours of testing.

Cystogram, Voiding Cystourethrogram (VCUG)

Description. Provides a detailed picture of bladder anatomy; also, vesicoureteral reflux is assessed by visualizing the area over the ureters and right and left renal pelves. A voiding cystourethrogram provides information given by a cystogram along with images of the urethra during the voiding phase of bladder function. A cystogram is performed by infusing a roentgenographic medium intravesically under fluoroscopic monitoring. A voiding cystourethrogram is made in the same manner. Urethral images during voiding are obtained by removing the catheter and asking the patient to void while under the fluoroscope.

Indications. Assessment of bladder function.

Complications. Because cystogram and VCUG require placement of an indwelling catheter, cystitis is a potential complication.

Nursing care. The patient should be encouraged to force fluids for 24 hours following testing. Urinary frequency or mild dysuria should disappear completely within 24 hours.

Hysterosalpingography

Description. Injection of radiopaque contrast material, such as iodized oil or water-soluble material, through the cervix so that it fills the cervical canal and body of the uterus, flows through the fallopian tubes, and spills into the peritoneal cavity. The procedure should be performed no sooner than 6 weeks after delivery, abortion, or dilation and curettage.

The patient should be screened for contraindications to the procedure, including active pelvic inflammatory disease, vaginitis, cervicitis, or severe systemic illness.

Indications. Most commonly, to determine whether infertility is caused by an anatomic defect. It can also be used to confirm tubal occlusion and investigate the cause of dysmenorrhea, postmenopausal bleeding, or repeated abortion.

Complications. None.

Nursing care. The patient may experience pelvic pain resulting from spillage of contrast material; manage as indicated. If indicated by the physician, assist the patient to walk for 30 minutes after the procedure until another film is taken.

Myelogram

Description. A roentgenographic procedure in which a needle is inserted into a disc space below the spinal cord, and 2 to 6 ml of spinal fluid is removed. A radiopaque solution is injected and distributed to the various tissues and structures to be examined, and roentgenograms are taken frequently. A water-soluble radiopaque solution is absorbed into the cerebrospinal fluid rather rapidly, but an oil-based solution must be removed by tilting the patient while observing the image monitor until the solution moves to the needle tip, from which it is withdrawn into a syringe. It is important that all or most of the solution be removed because even small amounts of retained solution may lead to persistent postmyelogram headaches and possibly adhesive arachnoiditis.

Indications. Aids in the diagnosis of spinal stenosis or obstruction within the spinal canal caused by a ruptured or herniated nucleus pulposus. It also detects distortion of spinal cord, spinal nerve roots, and the subarachnoid space.

Complications. Complications vary depending on whether a water-soluble agent, metrizamide (Amipaque), or an oil agent, iophendylate (Pantopaque), is used. With metrizamide, the patient may have nausea, vomiting, or headache and possible seizures, chest pain, dysrhythmias, and speech disorders. With iophendylate, common complications include headache, meningeal and nerve root irritation, and adhesive arachnoiditis.

Nursing care. The patient is allowed a clear liquid breakfast and then is given nothing by mouth. Any possible allergy to iodine is determined, and a mild sedative (diazepam, 10 mg) may be given. The patient must lie flat in bed for 8 to 12 hours if oily iophendylate was used, and fluids are forced to replace the cerebrospinal fluid. After the use of metrizamide the head of the patient's bed may be raised and fluids forced. If the patient complains of a headache, lowering the bed to the flat position is usually sufficient to relieve the pain. Mild analgesics may be ordered for persistent pain. Observe the patient for the other side effects already described.

Discogram

Description. A roentgenographic procedure similar to a myelogram, in which radiopaque solution is injected into a disc space (L3-L5 areas) and roentgenograms are taken.

Indications. To determine the condition of the disc spaces.

Complications. Possible development of discitis.

Nursing care. Explain to the patient that a radiopaque solution will be injected into the disc and roentgenograms will be taken. After the procedure, neurologic checks are performed, and mild analgesics may be required for pain. Monitor vital signs frequently.

Arthrogram

Description. Through use of a radiopaque solution, fluoroscopy, and multiple roentgenograms, any tissues not normally seen by roentgenograms are visualized. A needle is inserted into the joint; its position is verified by fluoroscopic examination. A radiopaque solution is injected into the joint, and the needle is removed. The site is sealed with collodion. The patient is asked to move the joint through its range of motion while roentgenograms are taken. The radiopaque solution is usually rapidly absorbed into the joint fluids.

Indications. To outline the structures of the joint capsule being studied and to aid in the diagnosis of injuries to the joint muscles, ligaments, cartilage, or bursa.

Complications. Joint swelling after the procedure, soreness or pain, and crepitus (noise on joint movement).

Nursing care. Explain to the patient that skin around the joint will be cleansed with an antiseptic and that a local anesthetic will be administered. After the procedure, instruct the patient in applying a compression bandage and ice around the joint to lessen edema. Explain that the joint should be held at rest for 12 or more hours and that use is then dependent on the findings of the arthrogram. Mild analgesics can be prescribed for pain.

• Electrodiagnostic Studies

Electrocardiogram (ECG, EKG)

Description. Electrical representation of myocardial activity. It is used to determine the presence of abnormal transmission of heart impulses through the conduction tissue of heart muscle (see p. 14 for normal findings).

Indications. Chest pain; to evaluate cardiac disturbance; for routine diagnostic study during physical examinations and preoperatively.

Complications. None.

Nursing care. Explain the procedure. Ensure electrical safety measures.

Ambulatory Electrocardiography (Holter Monitor)

Description. A portable recorder, worn by the patient, magnetically records cardiac activity continuously while the patient is going about usual activities. The tapes are scanned by electrocardioscanners, and areas of interest can be printed out in real time.

Indications. Used to detect ECG rhythm disturbances that may occur over an extended period of time, to evaluate effectiveness of antiarrhythmic drug therapy, and to evaluate chest pain episodes. It is also capable of recording ECGs over a 24- to 48-hour period.

Complications. None.

Nursing care. Explain the procedure. Instruct the patient in the care of electrodes at home and about the importance of keeping a diary of symptoms or activities at times designated by the physician.

Electrophysiologic Studies (Bundle of His)

Description. Involves insertion of a catheter via the peripheral vein into the right atrium and right ventricle (right heart catheterization).

Indications. To detect atrioventricular conduction disturbances, diagnose syncope, and assist in selection of antiarrhythmic agents.

A-V interval (atrioventricular). Conduction time from the low right atrium through the AV node to the His bundle. Normal is 60 to 125 msec.

H-V interval (His-ventricle). Conduction time from the proximal His bundle to the ventricular myocardium. Normal is 35 to 55 msec.

P-A interval. Conduction time from the beginning of the P wave to the beginning of the A defection. Normal is 20 to 40 msec.

Sinus node disease. Sinus node exit block; depression of sinus node automaticity.

Atrioventricular block. Mobitz II.

Intraventricular block. Bifascicular block.

Tachycardias. Supraventricular tachycardia with a rate of more than 200 beats per minute associated with symptoms, or with recurrent bouts that are refractory to therapy.

Accessory pathway tachycardias. Wolff-Parkinson-White syndrome.

Ventricular tachycardia. Tachycardia caused by irritable ventricular foci firing repetitively.

Unexplained syncope. Cardiac arrest patients resuscitated from sudden cardiac death.

Contraindications include arrhythmias that will be difficult to treat because of an underlying cardiac disorder, e.g., acute myocardial infarction, class IV heart failure, severe aortic stenosis.

Complications. Arrhythmias, phlebitis, pulmonary emboli, hemorrhage, cardiac perforation.

Nursing care. Obtain informed consent. Explain that the procedure will last 1 to 3 hours and that the patient will be awake and may feel slight pressure. Instruct the patient to report any discomfort. Permit nothing by mouth for 6 hours before the procedure. After the procedure, check vital signs every 15 minutes for 1 hour, then every 4 hours for 24 hours. Check the insertion site for bleeding every 30 minutes to 1 hour for 8 hours.

Electroencephalogram (EEG)

Description. An electroencephalogram (EEG) provides a graphic record of brain wave activity. Generally, between 17 and 21 electrodes are attached with collodion to the patient's head at corresponding areas over the prefrontal, frontal, temporal, parietal, and occipital lobes. After the electrodes are attached, the patient is instructed to remain quiet with the eyes closed and is informed of the need to refrain from talking or moving unless otherwise required (the patient is asked to hyperventilate for a short period during the test to accentuate abnormalities).

The brain waves recorded during an EEG are called alpha, beta, delta, and theta rhythms. *Alpha* rhythms occur in the adult at 8 to 13 cycles/sec and are most prominent in the occipital leads. Apprehension and anxiety can decrease the frequency of the alpha waves. *Beta* wave forms are prominent in the frontal and central areas and occur at a rate of 18 to 30 cycles/sec. Beta rhythm indicates normal activity, when an individual is alert and attentive with the eyes open. *Delta* wave forms indicate serious brain dysfunction or deep sleep. This rhythm occurs at a rate of less than 4 cycles/sec. *Theta* wave forms occur at a rate of 4 to 7 cycles/sec and come primarily from the temporal and parietal areas. Theta rhythm indicates drowsiness or emotional stress in adults.

Complications. None.

Nursing care. Stimulants such as coffee, tea, and cola are not permitted for 8 hours before the procedure. The adult patient should have minimal sleep (i.e., 4 to 5 hours) the night before the procedure.

Electromyogram (EMG)

Description. Surface electrodes or monopolar electrodes measure and record electrical properties of skeletal muscle and nerve conduction. Electrical activity is picked up by a needle electrode inserted into the muscle and displayed on a cathode-ray oscilloscope. Also, EMG needles or hooked wire electrodes are placed directly into the external urinary sphincter, or ECG patches are placed over perianal sphincter to measure the activity of pelvic floor musculature.

Indications. To aid in the diagnosis of myopathies and muscle responses to electrical stimuli. It may be performed in the patient's room, depending on the number of muscles to be studied. It measures electrical activity of the external, striated urinary sphincter in response to bladder filling and storage and to micturition.

Complications. None.

Nursing care. Explain to the patient that a small needle will be inserted into one or more muscles to be studied and that the muscle will be stimulated with a small electrical impulse. The results will be recorded on a graph. Explain to the patient that the procedure may cause some minor discomfort when the needle is inserted but otherwise is not painful.

Nerve Conduction Velocity Determination

Description. Study of nerve conduction velocity calculated by division of the distance between proximal and distal points by the time required for the electrical stimulus to travel between those two points.

Indications. To diagnose neuromuscular problems.

Complications. None.

Nursing care. Explain that this study may be performed in conjunction with the electromyogram (EMG) and uses the same machine.

Electrocochleography

Description. Permeatal transtympanic electrode placement in contact with the promontory of the cochlea to record acoustically evoked potentials from the cochlea. Three distinct evoked potentials can be recorded: cochlear microphonic potential, summating potential, and vestibulocochlear nerve compound action potential.

Indications. Measures auditory function; aids in the differential diagnosis of auditory disorders (i.e., vestibulocochlear nerve disorders); provides the prognosis for auditory disorders.

Complications. Potential vertigo, middle ear infection, perilymph leak.

Nursing care. None.

Electronystagmography

Description. Graphic recording and measurement of electrical potentials of eye movements during spontaneous, positional, or calorically evoked nystagmus. Intensity, frequency, and speed of the fast and slow components of nystagmus are recorded.

Indications. To assess and evaluate neurologic disorders.

Complications. None.

Nursing care. Instruct the patient to keep the eyes open during the procedure.

Plethysmography

Description. Measures venous flow in limbs by recording changes in volume and vascular resistance. There are two types: digital plethysmography (to evaluate digital pulse volume) and venous occlusion plethysmography (to evaluate arterial responses to temporary block of the venous system). A pneumatic cuff is applied to a limb to occlude venous return. Two electrodes are applied to the limb, and a very weak electrical current is passed through it. The resistance of the limb to the current is measured and recorded on graph paper.

Indications. Used to detect deep vein thrombosis in the leg and to screen patients at high risk for thrombophlebitis.

Complications. None.

Nursing care. Explain the procedure, and assist the patient into a position to promote venous drainage of the limb to be studied.

Ultrasound

Ultrasonography

Description. The ultrasound machine uses high-frequency waves (5000 to 20,000 Hz) to detect vibrations reflected from soft tissues of varying density. The vibrations (echoes) are converted into electrical potential and displayed on an oscillograph. The A-scan machine registers varying acoustic densities as spikes on linear tracing; the B-scan registers a two-dimensional "picture."

Ultrasonography is a painless procedure that is useful in evaluating soft tissues and does not involve the use of roentgen rays. A transducer, which is able to transmit and to receive high-frequency sound waves, is placed against the patient's body. The sound waves, which cannot be heard by the human ear, are bounced off the tissues inside the body. Tissues of different densities echo the sound in different ways. The echoes are received by the machine and are translated into an image on a TV screen.

In dehydrated patients, ultrasound can fail to define boundaries between organs and tissue structures because of a deficiency of body fluids.

Indications. Ultrasonography is useful for assessment of almost all body systems.

Eye. For the eye ultrasonography is useful for diagnosing intraocular tumors, retinal detachment, and fibrous tissue proliferation. The examiner holds the probe (attached to machine) over the patient's eyelid. For the thyroid ultrasonography reveals diffuse or localized enlargements of the gland and differentiates between cystic or solid lesions. For the lungs and pericardium ultrasound has limited usefulness in evaluation of the lungs because sound beams are not transmitted well by air-containing tissue. Ultrasonographic examination is useful to detect pericardial effusion and fluid-containing or solid tissue lesions.

Gastrointestinal ultrasonography

Gallbladder and biliary system. Ultrasonography of the gallbladder and biliary system can be used if cholecystography is inconclusive or does not adequately visualize the gallbladder. It is useful in confirming cholelithiasis, diagnosing acute cholecystitis, and distinguishing between obstructive and nonobstructive jaundice. Sincalide, a hormonal analogue, may be given to cause the gallbladder to contract and expel bile. It allows an evaluation of gallbladder function.

Liver. Ultrasonography of the liver is indicated for patients with jaundice of unknown cause, since it helps to distinguish between obstructive and nonobstructive jaundice. It can be used in a screening or diagnostic test for hepatocellular disease and hepatic metastases. It can also be used after abdominal trauma to detect a hematoma and define cold spots found on liver scans.

Spleen. Ultrasonography of the spleen is used to demonstrate splenomegaly, to evaluate changes in splenic size, to evaluate the spleen following abdominal trauma, and to clarify cold spots found on scans of the spleen. CT scans often provide more information on splenomegaly than ultrasonography does.

Pancreas. Ultrasonography of the pancreas is used to detect anatomic abnormalities such as pseudocysts and pancreatic carcinomas. It detects alterations in size, contour, and parenchymal texture of the pancreas.

Renal and genitourinary tracts. Ultrasonography of these tracts is a noninvasive way to identify a dilated collecting system, calculi, cysts, perirenal collections of blood, pus, lymph, urine, solid masses, and kidney size.

Ultrasonography of kidneys. The patient is placed in the prone position. An outline of the kidneys is obtained and marked on the skin. Serial scans are then made 1 to 2 cm apart perpendicular to the longitudinal axis. Additional views may be obtained with the patient in a supine position, which helps elucidate the kidneys' relative position to other abdominal organs.

Ultrasound-guided biopsy of kidney. Ultrasonic examination may be combined with placement of a biopsy needle to define makeup of a renal or juxtarenal mass. Routine ultrasonographic examination of the affected kidney is completed first. The mass is then located and marked on the skin. With use of sterile drapes, gloves, and a local anesthetic, the biopsy needle is placed into the mass, and a tissue sample is withdrawn. Aspiration of a renal cyst may be performed in a similar manner.

Ultrasonography of bladder and ureters. Ultrasonography of a distended bladder provides some detail of vesical outline and may be used to evaluate the diverticulum. Abdominal ultrasound detects the presence of ureteral dilation, although normal ureters may not be completely visualized. It is typically combined with examination of the kidneys.

Ultrasonography of testes. This is used to differentiate solid and cystic masses. In addition, torsion of the testes is assessed by Doppler ultrasound techniques, which assess both testicular morphology and blood flow.

Ankle pressure. Doppler ultrasound is used to measure systolic blood pressure in distal arteries, to amplify audible sounds of peripheral pulses, and to measure blood flow velocity along the course of an artery. Ankle systolic pressure should be equal to or greater than brachial systolic pressure—0.45 to 0.75 mm Hg (ankle/brachial index).

Complications. None.

Nursing care. Explain the procedure to the patient. For gastrointestinal ultrasonography, the patient is allowed nothing by mouth 8 to 12 hours before the procedure to reduce bowel gas. For gallbladder ultrasound give the patient nothing to eat for 8 to 12 hours before the procedure. The patient should have a fat-free meal the evening before the test (which allows bile to accumulate in the gallbladder).

Side effects of sincalide include abdominal cramping, tenesmus, nausea, dizziness, sweating, and flushing; sincalide should not be given during pregnancy.

For bladder ultrasound, because of the necessity of distending the bladder to evaluate it, the patient will wish to void immediately after the examination.

Echocardiogram

Description. Noninvasive method of evaluating internal structures and motion of heart. The ultrasound beam penetrates cardiac structures, which reflect "echo" waves that travel back to the transducer to form images.

There are several modes: M-mode, or one-dimensional; two-dimensional, cross-sectional, real-time motion; and Doppler, in which continuous wave combined with pulse ultrasound gives an image of heart pulse and indicates the direction of blood flow within the heart.

Indications. Echocardiograms are used to determine internal dimensions of ventricles, the size and motion of the intraventricular septum and posterior wall of left ventricle, valve motion and anatomy, the presence of pericardial fluid, the direction of blood flow, and the presence of blood clots and myomatous tumors.

Complications. None.

Nursing care. None other than explaining the procedure to the patient.

Biopsies

Brain Biopsy

Description. Removal of a small brain tissue sample, usually accomplished during intracranial surgery.

Indications. Useful in the evaluation of neurologic disorders.

Complications. Bleeding, infection.

Nursing care. Frequent monitoring of vital signs and neurologic signs.

Thyroid Biopsy

Description. Sterile aspiration of thyroid tissue. It is often performed to help determine if surgery is needed, since it is a relatively simple, effective way of ascertaining if a thyroid nodule is malignant.

Indications. Differentiates between benign and malignant nodules; assists in the diagnosis of subacute thyroiditis in atypical cases, Hashimoto's disease, or multinodular goiter.

Complications. Puncture of the esophagus or trachea.

Nursing care. Support during procedure; assessment for esophageal or tracheal puncture.

Lung Biopsy

Description and indications. Lung biopsy may be performed in one of four ways. The purpose of all techniques is to obtain a tissue sample for histologic evaluation.

Transbronchial biopsy. This biopsy is taken with the fiberoptic bronchoscope from the bronchial area of concern.

Nursing care. See the discussion under fiberoptic bronchoscope.

Percutaneous needle biopsy with aspiration. In this procedure fluids and cells are aspirated into the syringe through a long, 18- to 20-gauge needle inserted percutaneously under fluoroscopic control into the suspected lesion. When the needle is in the lesion, the syringe is generally rotated to obtain a tissue specimen. This procedure is used most often if malignancy is suspected. A contraindication to needle aspiration is an uncooperative patient.

Nursing care. The procedure is performed with the patient under local anesthesia after the skin has been disinfected and a sterile field has been prepared. The patient is instructed to hold his breath for 15 to 30 seconds during the procedure. The aspirated material is sent for cytologic examination and for stains and cultures of microorganisms. The major postprocedural complication is pneumothorax. Therefore careful respiratory assessment is indicated.

Percutaneous biopsy with a cutting needle. Three procedure options are possible: a punch biopsy with a Vim-Silverman needle; a high-speed drill biopsy with trephine–lung biopsy drill; a suction excision biopsy with an Abrams needle or a modification of the Abrams needle. The cutting needle procedure is indicated when the patient has diffuse pulmonary infiltrates. These techniques have significant complications and therefore are not usually done until other diagnostic procedures have failed to identify the problem.

Nursing care. These procedures are performed with the patient under local anesthesia and after a sterile field has been prepared. Major complications include hemorrhage and pneumothorax. Careful postprocedural assessment is indicated.

Open lung biopsy or exploratory thoracotomy. This is an invasive procedure used to confirm a suspected diagnosis of lung or chest disease by obtaining lung specimens. The chest is opened through a standard thoracotomy incision, and the lung is inspected and biopsied. An open lung biopsy is indicated only after other investigative procedures have not clearly identified the patient's problem.

Nursing care. General anesthesia is used. A chest tube connected to water-seal drainage is used for 1 to 2 days after surgery because of the surgically induced pneumothorax. Several days of postprocedural chest roentgenograms are normally ordered. The procedure may have several major complications, including postoperative respiratory failure, emphysema, and chronic bronchopleural fistula.

Pleural Biopsy

Description. A small tissue sample is taken by special biopsy needle from the parietal pleura. It may be necessary to collect tissue samples from several different spots. Although some authorities advocate pleural biopsy every time a thoracentesis is performed, others claim that it should be done only when granulomatous disease or malignancy is suspected.

Indications. Evaluation of pulmonary disease.

Complications. Rare, but include pneumothorax, hemothorax, and intercostal nerve injury.

Nursing care. Position the patient as for thoracentesis. Monitor vital signs and assess the patient for symptoms of complications.

Lymph Node Excision and Scalene Node Biopsy

Description. Excision of peripheral lymph node or biopsy of a palpable scalene node. The incision and biopsy are performed in the supraclavicular scalene region.

Indications. Performed to assess immunologic function in suspected immunodeficiency diseases and to stage certain malignancies.

Complications. Bleeding, erythema, infection at site.

Nursing care. Provide an occlusive dressing. Check the surgical site for bleeding, erythema, or purulent drainage.

Bone Marrow Aspiration and Biopsy

Description. Needle biopsy of marrow performed after entering marrow cavity of sternum, iliac crest, posterosuperior iliac spine, spinous process, rib, or tibial head. Bone marrow cellularity is determined.

Indications. Evaluation of the immune and hematolymphatic systems, useful in differential diagnosis of thrombocytopenia, leukemia, granulomatous disease, and aplastic, hypoplastic, or megaloblastic anemias.

Complications. Bleeding, infection at site.

Nursing care. Exert immediate pressure over the biopsy site. Apply an occlusive dressing. Check the biopsy site for bleeding, erythema, or purulent drainage. Maintain bed rest for 1 hour. Administer analgesics as needed.

Muscle and Nerve Biopsy

Description. Removal of a small muscle or nerve tissue sample for histologic, histochemical, ultrastructural, or biochemical studies.

Indications. Aids in the diagnosis of myopathies such as muscle atrophy, degeneration, or inflammation and determines the extent of damage to myelinated and unmyelinated nerve fibers.

Complications. Mild soreness or stiffness of muscle or nerve that has undergone biopsy.

Nursing care. Explain to the patient that the procedure will be performed with the patient under local anesthesia in the operating suite. After the procedure, encourage the patient to move the affected area and to walk (if the leg or foot is involved) to prevent stiffness. Provide analgesics if required. Monitor for bleeding or infection at the site. If sutures are used, remove them in 7 to 10 days.

Synovial Biopsy

Description. Biopsy of the synovium by means of a special needle. The biopsy specimen is sent for histologic examination.

Indications. Aids in the differential diagnosis of various forms of arthritis.

Complications. Joint effusion or hemorrhage into the joint.

Nursing care. Explain to the patient that the biopsy is performed after the skin is cleansed with antiseptic solutions and a local anesthetic is administered (occasionally a synovial biopsy is taken during open surgery). After the procedure, apply a small compression dressing and an elastic bandage around the joint. Caution the patient to restrict joint use for 24 hours to prevent hemorrhage or effusion.

Bladder, Prostate, Urethra Biopsies

Description. Biopsy specimens from a bladder, urethra, or prostate may be obtained with a cystoscopic/panendoscopic system. A resectoscope, which uses an electrically activated wire loop or a tubular cold knife, is positioned over the lesion, and a specimen is obtained. It is important to ensure that the bladder is relatively full when a specimen is obtained to prevent inadvertent damage to normal mucosal folds. Transrectal or transperineal needle biopsies are often taken in conjunction with cystoscopic examination. In other cases, biopsies may be taken in the clinic with use of a local anesthetic only.

A transperineal biopsy is performed by injecting a local anesthetic into the skin of the perineum, over the area where the needle will enter. A finger in the rectum is used to guide the needle toward the area in question. The procedure may be repeated several times to ensure an adequate biopsy.

A transrectal biopsy requires no anesthesia. Preparation includes cleansing enemas to decrease the likelihood of introducing intestinal bacteria into the bloodstream or prostatic tissue. Prophylactic antibiotics are also indicated. When obtaining the specimen, the tip of the needle is placed on the examining finger and advanced gently to an area over which the biopsy is to be obtained. The needle is then pushed, and a biopsy is taken. The procedure may be repeated several times.

Indications. Hematuria, pain, suspected malignancy.

Complications. Hematuria. The primary complication of transrectal biopsy (the more commonly performed of the two techniques described) is sepsis from perforation of the bowel.

Nursing care. Postprocedural care is similar to that of routine cystoscopic examination. Mild dysuria may be seen with hematuria during the first 48 hours following the procedure. If a general anesthetic is used, low-grade fever may occur over the first 24 to 48 hours after the procedure. Hematuria may recur 5 to 7 days after the procedure. The patient should be assured that the lesion is healing and that such hematuria is normal; the patient should not experience dysuria or a significant frequency of urination at this time. Fever and chills must be reported to the physician at once. A prophylactic antibiotic regimen must be strictly adhered to after the transrectal needle biopsy.

Renal Biopsy

Description. In a renal biopsy a small piece of tissue is obtained via a special needle (percutaneous) or through a surgical incision (open). Roentgenography of the kidney, ureter, or bladder, intravenous urography, and ultrasonography may be used to locate the kidney for biopsy.

The absolute contraindications to renal biopsy are a solitary kidney or irreversible hemorrhagic tendencies. The relative contraindications are an uncooperative patient, a suspected renal tumor or cysts, gross sepsis, very small kidneys, horseshoe kidney, ectopic kidney, severe hypertension, massive obesity, severe spinal deformity, and pregnancy.

Indications. Indications include persistent proteinuria, nephrotic syndrome, unexplained hematuria, and controlled therapeutic trials of new drugs.

Complications. Bleeding from the biopsy site, i.e., microscopic or gross hematuria, perirenal hematoma, retroperitoneal hematoma, arteriovenous fistula in the kidney, passage of clots, ureteric colic from a clot; hypotension; anemia; local infection; pain; perforation of other nearby structures.

Nursing care. Before the procedure, prepare the patient for the possibility of pain during the procedure. The patient should cooperate by holding his breath on command. Explain that 24 hours of bed rest is needed after the biopsy, and that some hematuria is normal in the first 24 hours.

Record baseline vital signs. Review the chart for hemoglobin and hematocrit levels, platelet count, prothrombin time, and bleeding and clotting times. Review the type and cross-match report for two units of blood. Review the outcome of any test for pregnancy.

Explain the reason for the biopsy and the need for observation after the biopsy. Explain that for several days the patient should avoid contact sports; lifting or heavy exercise; wrestling; riding bicycles, horses, and snowmobiles; and swimming. Normal activities can be resumed gradually after 48 to 72 hours. Explain the need to call the physician if there is any hematuria, draining from the biopsy site, persistent fever, or pain.

Measure output carefully and collect the voidings individually. Watch for hematuria. Check for microscopic hematuria, which is invariably present in the first two specimens. The urine may appear pink. Report profuse or persistent hematuria. If no hematuria occurs in the first 24 hours, bathroom privileges can be instituted for the next 24 hours.

A tight dressing is applied to the biopsy site. Check the dressing for bleeding. Apply external pressure for 30 minutes by having the patient lie prone with a sandbag placed directly on the biopsy site. Measure the blood pressure, pulse, and respirations every 15 minutes for 4 hours and then every 4 hours for 24 hours.

Ensure adequate hydration of 1000 to 2000 ml to ensure a good urine flow. Monitor the hematocrit 3 to 6 hours after biopsy. Any decrease from the prebiopsy level suggests perirenal bleeding.

Give a nonaspirin analgesic agent for mild pain after the anesthesia wears off, as ordered by the physician. Report severe loin pain.

Brush Biopsy of Renal Pelvis and Calyces

Description. A ureteral catheter with a steel guide wire is placed using a cystoscope as a guide. The catheter is then removed, and a steel or nylon brush is inserted to the level of lesion to obtain a biopsy. The specimen is then smeared on slides and prepared with a 95% ethanol solution. After the specimen is obtained, the renal pelvis is irrigated with normal saline.[8]

Indications. Allows urologist to obtain a tissue biopsy from the renal pelvis or calyces without an open surgical incision to assist in the diagnosis of renal disease.

Complications. Irritation of the renal system because of manipulation.

Nursing care. Postprocedural care is similar to that of routine cystoscopic examination. A low-grade fever may be noted. Flank pain secondary to ureteral manipulation is not uncommon and should disappear within 48 hours. Fevers greater than 38° C (101° F) and severe flank pain should be reported to physician.

Skin and Tissue Biopsy

Description. The lesion is marked, and the area is infiltrated with lidocaine. A small circular punch or scalpel is used to obtain tissue to determine cell histology.

Indications. For evaluation of abnormal lesions or tissue. The biopsy can be incisional (surgical excision of tumor section), excisional (removal of entire growth), or aspiration (removal of small tumor plug or fluid). Frozen section involves freezing questionable tissue removed during surgery for microscopic study.

Complications. Infection, bleeding at site.

Nursing care. Cleanse the site with an antibacterial solution. Give the patient information regarding the procedure. Apply direct pressure over the area to stop the bleeding (sutures may be used for areas larger than 3 cm). Apply a bandage.

Liver Biopsy

Description. Percutaneous biopsy of liver tissue. With the patient lying down, a needle is inserted into the liver, and a small amount of tissue is withdrawn to establish a pathologic and microscopic picture of the liver cells.

Indications. Abnormal liver function; hepatomegaly or hepatosplenomegaly of unexplained origin; suspected malignancy of the liver; suspected systemic or infiltrative disease, such as sarcoidosis.

Complications. Hemorrhage.

Nursing care. Permit nothing by mouth after midnight before the biopsy. Have the patient void before the biopsy. Instruct the patient to lie on his right side for 4 to 6 hours after the biopsy to keep pressure on the site. Monitor the vital signs frequently for 4 to 6 hours. Maintain bed rest for 24 hours after the biopsy.

Cervical Biopsy

Description. Biopsy of cervical epithelium and shallow layer of underlying stroma to diagnose malignant invasion.

Indications. Class IV or V Pap smear.

Complications. Bleeding.

Nursing care. Prepare the patient for a vaginal examination. After the procedure, give the patient a perineal pad, and inform her that spotting will occur.

Endometrial Biopsy

Description. Biopsy of endometrial uterine lining. It is generally performed on the first day of menses of premenopausal patients and anytime in postmenopausal patients. A tissue specimen may be obtained by a Gravlee jet washer (isotonic saline solution is forced through an intrauterine cannula, flushing endometrial cells into an external collecting reservoir) or a Nova curette (a curette attached to a syringe scrapes the endometrium, and cell samples are drawn into the syringe).

Indications. Suspected endometrial carcinoma.

Complications. None.

Nursing care. Prepare the patient for a vaginal examination. Explain that she may experience cramping because of dilation of the cervix during the procedure. Teach and assist her with relaxation and breathing techniques. Give the patient a perineal pad after the procedure. Ensure that menstrual data is noted on the laboratory specimen slip for the pathologist.

Cervical Conization (Cone Biopsy)

Description. Surgical removal of cervical tissue in the shape of a cone for diagnosis or for treatment of cervical infection or carcinoma in situ. It is performed by a physician with a cold knife scalpel. The procedure is frequently called cold knife conization (CKC) or cryosurgery.

Indications. Treatment of cervical infection or carcinoma in situ.

Complications. Bleeding.

Nursing care. After the procedure assist the physician with removal of vaginal packing, usually within 24 hours. Give perineal care with an antiseptic solution and change the perineal pad every 4 hours and as needed. Instruct the patient to avoid coitus, douching, or tampons for 6 weeks or until directed by the physician; report excessive bleeding (if it lasts longer than 7 to 10 days); avoid constipation; maintain good perineal hygiene; and report signs of infection to physician.

• Radioisotope Studies and Scans

Brain Scan

Description. Intravenous injection of a small amount of radioactive substance (e.g., technetium-99). The head is then scanned with a special sensing device to pick up areas of concentrated uptake.

Indications. Assessment of neurologic disease, brain tumors, headache, coma, intracerebral hemorrhage.

Complications. None.

Nursing care. Obtain a careful history regarding any existing allergies, particularly to iodine. Assure the patient that the procedure is painless, the radioactive substance is harmless, and there will be no after effects.

Cisternography

Description. Injection of a radioisotope into the subarachnoid space through a cisternal or lumbar puncture. The head is then scanned at regular intervals to determine the amount of time it takes for the radioisotope to clear from the circulating cerebrospinal fluid.

Indications. To assess the circulation of the cerebrospinal fluid.

Complications. As for cisternal or lumbar puncture.

Nursing care. As for cisternal or lumbar puncture.

Thyroid Uptake and Scan

Description. Tracer doses of ^{131}I, ^{123}I, or ^{99m}Tc pertechnetate are given. A scanner is then passed over the gland to record graphically the amount of radioactive iodine taken up by the gland over a period of time (e.g., 6, 8, or 24 hours). Pregnancy is a contraindication.

Indications. Not used for routine screening, but rather to answer specific questions regarding the localization of functioning or nonfunctioning thyroid tissue; it gives evidence of gland size and function.

Complications. None.

Nursing care. Assess for dietary intake of iodine, for administration of iodine-containing medications, and for the use of antithyroid drugs before the test, since test results may be affected by any ingestion of these.

Thyroid-Releasing Hormone Stimulation Test (TRH Test, TRF Test)

Description. T_3 (liothyronine), 75 mg, is given daily for 7 days. Radioiodine uptake by the thyroid gland is measured before and after the test. Uptake should be 50% or less of the pretest uptake.

Indications. To distinguish hyperthyroid conditions from the euthyroid state.

Complications. None.

Nursing care. The test may be dangerous for elderly patients, weakened patients, or patients with heart disease. Careful monitoring is required.

Ventilation/Perfusion Lung Scan

Description. A scanning device records the pattern of pulmonary radioactivity after the inhalation or intravenous injection of gamma ray–emitting radionuclides (such as xenon-133), thus providing visual images of the distribution of blood flow in the lungs.

Indications. The major indications for this procedure are to evaluate a pulmonary thromboembolism and to study preoperative lung function.

Complications. None.

Nursing care. None, other than explaining the procedure to the patient.

Radionuclide Imaging of Breast

Description. Evaluation of breast image after intravenous injection of radioactive substance.

Indications. Breast masses or tissue abnormalities.

Complications. None.

Nursing care. None, other than explaining the procedure to the patient.

Bone Scan (Scintigraphy)

Description. Roentgenographic procedure in which a radioisotope, usually technetium-99 (^{99}Tc–sodium pertechnetate) is injected intravenously. The radioisotope is picked up on a special scanning camera as it is passed over the musculoskeletal tissues of the body from head to foot, and a picture of the isotope's distribution in the bony tissues is developed. The scan takes about 1 hour and is painless.

Indications. Aids in the diagnosis of bony metastatic lesions and traumatic, inflammatory, or infectious conditions of musculoskeletal tissues. The scan will show the injured or diseased tissues as darker or "hot" areas on the scan pictures as much as 3 to 6 months earlier than roentgenograms can reveal the condition.

Complications. None usually, although infrequently a hematoma, redness, or edema may develop at the site of the injection.

Nursing care. Explain to the patient that the radioisotope will be injected intravenously 1 to 3 hours before the scan is to be performed and that he or she will be required to drink several glasses of water or tea during the waiting period to aid in excreting the radioisotope that is not absorbed by bone tissue. After the patient returns to the unit, check the injection site for redness or edema.

Liver or Spleen Scan

Description. Injection of a radioactive colloid (e.g., technetium-99m), which concentrates in the reticuloendothelial cells through phagocytosis. Kupffer cells in the liver take up to 80% to 90%, spleen takes 5% to 10%, and bone marrow takes 3% to 5%.

Indications. Used to screen patients for hepatic metastases, cirrhosis, and hepatitis. It also assists in identifying focal lesions such as tumors, cysts, and abscesses, and may demonstrate splenic infarct, hepatomegaly, and splenomegaly. It is also used to evaluate liver and spleen following abdominal trauma.

Complications. None.

Nursing care. The patient will need to know he will be asked to lie very still and placed in several positions. He should also know that the procedure will not be painful, with the exception of the intravenous injection.

Some patients will have a reaction to a stabilizer added to the colloid; observe for anaphylaxis or for pyogenic response.

Do not schedule the patient for more than one radionuclide scan on one day. Radionuclides administered in other studies may interfere with liver-spleen imaging.

Renal Scan (DTPA, DMSA Scan)

Description. Provides a functional assessment of glomerular filtration rate (GFR) and effective renal plasma flow (ERPF). The DTPA scan also provides an assessment of the ureters and bladder. Renal scans expose patients to less radiation than does IVP. A DMSA scan provides an assessment of individual kidney function.

Other radionuclides such as hippurate and radioxenon have been used for renal scans[11] but are no longer widely used.

The DTPA scan is used primarily to assess upper urinary tract obstruction. Radionuclide is injected in an intravenous bolus and sequential images are obtained. A 30-second film is taken to assess cortical blood flow; a 1-minute image and two images are obtained at 5, 10, 15, and 20 minutes. The bladder and ureters are included in the DTPA scan. It assesses GFR and ERPF and provides differential renal function.

Indications. To assess urinary tract obstruction because the radionuclide used is affected by diuretics. Furosemide is typically utilized, and the change in renal excretion rate is quantified. Delays in excretion indicate obstruction.[11]

The DMSA scan is useful in assessing functional renal cortical mass[11]; the radionuclide used in DMSA scanning is taken up by renal tubule so that functional cortical mass can be quantified. As with the DTPA scan, an intravenous bolus of radioisotope is administered, and delayed images are obtained. It is indicated in cases of suspected renal scarring, assessment of segmental renal ischemia, and suspected intrarenal mass.

Complications. None.

Nursing care. Requires no preparation. Patients exposed to significantly less radiation than required by IVP; however, since a radioisotope is injected and excreted by the kidneys, the patient may continue to excrete radionuclide after the study is completed. Pregnant women are advised not to care for these patients during the initial 24 hours after testing.

Nuclear Cystogram (Radionuclide Cystogram)

Description. Performed in a manner similar to roentgenographic cystography except that normal saline with a dose of a pertechnetate radionuclide is used instead of an iodine-bound contrast solution. Like roentgenographic cystography, the study requires no preparation.

An indwelling catheter is passed into the bladder via the urethra. Normal saline is infused into the bladder, and radionuclide is injected into the solution during bladder filling. It may be performed in place of a roentgenographic cystogram because the patient is exposed to less radiation; however, a nuclear cystogram does not provide the anatomic detail seen with standard cystography.

Indications. Measures certain parameters of bladder function.

Complications. Cystitis.

Nursing care. The patient should be encouraged to force fluids for a 24-hour period following the test and informed that mild dysuria and urinary frequency should disappear completely within this time period.

^{125}I Fibrinogen Uptake (Radioactive Fibrinogen Uptake, RFU)

Description. A noninvasive procedure involving the injection of a small amount of a radioisotope and then the passing of a scanning camera over the involved area beginning 2 hours later. The procedure is used to detect the presence or enlargement of a deep vein thrombosis. Readings are taken on succeeding days following administration of the radioactive tagged fibrinogen. Serial readings are taken on succeeding days following administration of the radioisotope. A 20% increase in uptake in one area over a 24-hour period is considered positive.

Indications. Deep vein thrombosis.

Complications. None.

Nursing care. Explain the procedure to the patient.

• CT and MRI Scans

Computerized Tomography (CT)

Description. Computerized tomography (CT) scanning was introduced in the early 1970s. CT scans use a roentgenray beam and a computer to provide very accurate images of thin cross sections (0.8 to 1.3 cm) of the body.[3]

The CT scanner has many advantages: it is safe and painless; there is a very small amount of radiation exposure; data can be collected in early stages of the dysfunction; and it reduces the need for more invasive diagnostic procedures.

Figure 2 CT scan printouts. CT brain scan differentiates between gray and white brain matter.
From Ballinger.[1]

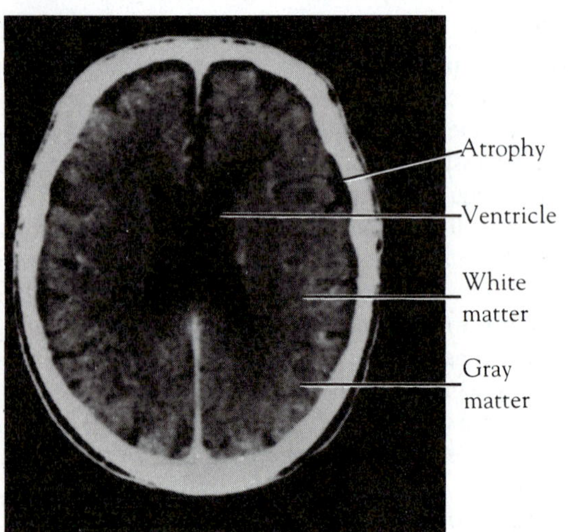

During the CT scan procedure the patient lies on a table with the body part to be studied inside the scanner's opening. The scanner then is moved to various angles and rotated slowly around the patient's body as repeated roentgenograms are taken. This information is recorded on a computer printout, and film prints (i.e., hard copy) of these visual images are taken. The scan usually is completed in 10 to 45 minutes. Cross-sectional, horizontal, or sagittal plane roentgenographic images are translated by a computer and displayed on an oscilloscope. These images are much sharper, more sensitive, and clearer than conventional roentgenograms. The CT scan takes pictures of small layers or "slices" of the tissues being examined (Figures 2 and 3).

CT scanning is contraindicated during pregnancy.

Indications. Useful in diagnosing disorders of multiple body systems.

Brain. Head trauma, cerebrovascular disturbances, hydrocephalus, abnormal brain development, identification of space-occupying lesions, metastatic tumors, and brain abscesses.

Endocrine. CT of sella turcica, adrenal glands, and abdomen is indicated in the following: presence of adrenal adenoma, diabetes-related tumors, Cushing's disease workup, hypopituitary workup, and precocious puberty workup.

Figure 3 CT scan of female patient. On this transverse scan through upper chest, bilateral breast shadows are evident. Heart, pulmonary arteries, and main bronchi are also visible.
Courtesy R. Keith Wilson, M.D., Baylor College of Medicine, Houston, Texas.

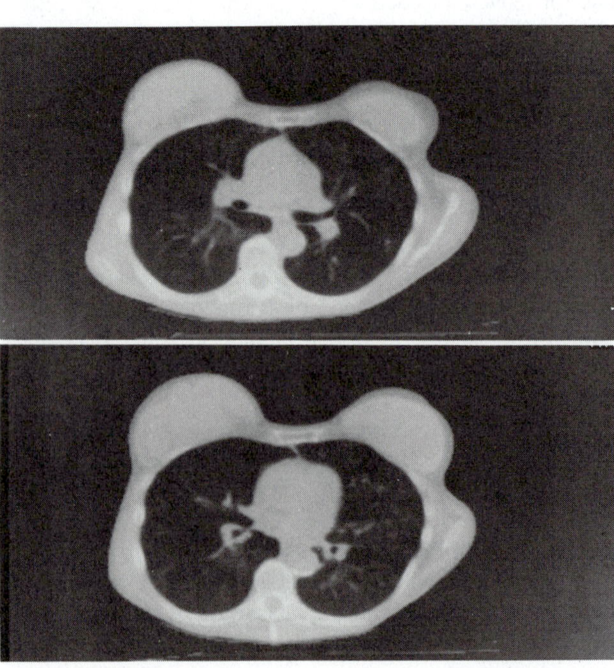

Eye. Diagnosis of eye disorders. It contrasts orbital contents and tumors because of difference in tissue density.

Respiratory system. Identifies exact morphologic characteristics of a chest lesion.

Renal and genitourinary systems. Determines kidney size, cysts, abscesses, masses, hematomas, and collecting system dilation. It is particularly valuable in defining abnormalities of the renal parenchyma. It provides an estimate of the density of masses and has the potential to differentiate solid tissue masses from cystic or hemorrhagic structures. Varying densities are displayed as Hounsfield units: normal renal parenchyma measures 80 to 100 Hounsfield units, and density of a cyst is lower whereas solid tumors have a density similar to that of renal parenchyma. CT scanning is also used in evaluation of adrenal masses. It is a useful technique for evaluating masses (tumors) of pelvic contents and lymphatic enlargement that may be the result of metastatic invasion. Pelvic abscesses may be elucidated by CT scanning of that area; it may elucidate any mass effect that causes distortion of bladder.

Gastrointestinal system. In the biliary tract and liver CT scanning can be used to identify focal points found on nuclear scans as solid, cystic, inflammatory, or vascular. A biopsy may be necessary to distinguish between metastatic or primary tumors or to rule out malignancy. CT scanning can also identify hematomas after abdominal trauma. It is used to determine if the cause of jaundice is obstructive or nonobstructive.

CT scanning and ultrasound are both effective in biliary tract and liver diagnosis. A CT scan proves to be better in obese patients or patients whose liver is located high under the rib cage, since bone and excessive fat hinder ultrasound transmission. Contrast medium is also used during CT scanning to intensify vascular structures and liver parenchyma, aiding in visualization of the biliary tract. A general CT scan of the abdomen is valuable in defining the relationship of organs and identifying the presence of tumors. In the pancreas, CT scanning is used to diagnose pancreatic carcinoma and pancreatitis and to distinguish between pancreatic disorders and disorders of the retroperitoneum.

Complications. None.

Nursing care. Explain to the patient that he will lie flat on a narrow table, which will be moved inside a round opening of the scanner. The scanner will make a clicking sound as it moves around and along the patient. The scan will take 10 to 60 minutes, depending on whether or not some parts only or the entire body is scanned. The patient must lie still without moving during the scan. A radiopaque solution may be given to outline the blood vessels more clearly if needed, although the majority of CT scans are made without such an agent. Occasionally a sedative may be required to calm a nervous or restless patient.

If contrast medium is to be used, assess the patient for allergies to iodine, seafood, or contrast media. Barium studies should be made at least 4 days before the CT scan or barium obscures the film. The contrast media excreted in bile used in earlier diagnostic studies may interfere with biliary tree detection.

The patient is given nothing to eat past midnight before the test.

Positron Emission Tomography (PET)

Description. Intravenous injection of deoxyglucose with radioactive fluorine. The head is scanned, and a color-composite picture is obtained. Various shades of colors indicate levels of glucose metabolism.

Indications. Assists in the diagnosis and differentiation of neurologic disorders.

Complications. None.

Nursing care. Same as for a CT scan.

Magnetic Resonance Imaging (MRI)

Description. Magnetic resonance imaging (MRI), also termed nuclear magnetic resonance (NMR) imaging, is a technique of tomography based on the magnetic behavior of protons (hydrogen nuclei) in body tissues.[9,29] The scanner produces images when protons are placed in a strong external magnetic field and then are subjected to short computer-programmed pulses of additional energy in the form of radiofrequency waves. When placed in the magnetic field, positively charged nuclei and negatively charged electrons align uniformly. Short pulses of radiofrequency waves are then applied, which tip the atoms out of their magnetic alignment, causing uniform spinning (resonance) of the nuclei. When the radiofrequency wave is stopped, the atoms realign uniformly with the magnetic field and emit tissue-specific signals that are based on realignment time and the relative proton density (water content) of nuclei. These signals are then monitored, processed, and displayed as a high-resolution image by the MRI computer.

Indications. MRI is indicated for detecting a variety of neurologic disorders, including central nervous system (CNS) malignancies, CNS degenerative disorders (e.g., Alzheimer's disease), brain edema, spinal cord edema, spinal lesions, ischemic-infarcted areas of the CNS, arteriovenous malformations, congenital anomalies, and hemorrhagic areas of the CNS and spinal cord.[14]

MRI is an excellent aid for the diagnosis of musculoskeletal conditions because MRI clearly differentiates various types of tissues such as bones, fat, and muscles. It produces clear images of soft tissues such as tumors, nucleus pulposus, and blood vessels. Individual cells may be defined. It also aids in the detection of renal masses, especially in distinguishing simple cysts from those complicated by hemorrhage. It is used to detect and stage neoplasms.

Complications. MRI is a noninvasive and painless procedure that does not expose the patient to any known risks and has no known complications.

Nursing care. The patient should be instructed that MRI is a painless procedure with no known risks. Explain to the patient that he will lie flat on a narrow table inside a round opening of a large magnet and should lie still during the scan. A description of the equipment and procedure should be given. The patient also should be informed that a soft humming sound and the on-off pulses of the radiofrequency waves will be heard. The patient should be instructed to remove all metal objects, since the strong magnetic field may damage jewelry and watches.

A careful assessment of any existing ferromagnetic implants (e.g., pacemakers, metallic orthopedic devices) or known foreign bodies (e.g., metallic splinters or fragments) must be made before the procedure because these objects produce image deformation. MRI also may move some metallic devices (e.g., metal intracranial aneurysm clips); therefore patients with such implants or foreign bodies cannot be exposed to MRI.

Skin Testing

Many skin diseases can be diagnosed by physical examination alone—through observation of changes in normal findings (see pp. 479-480) and through identification of primary or secondary lesions and their arrangement and usual distribution (see pp. 481-483).

The patient should undress and be examined completely to determine the presence of lesions on clothed areas of the body. The oral mucosa, anogenital area, scalp, and nails also frequently provide clues to the diagnosis. Good lighting, preferably daylight, is essential. A thorough history is also important in assessing physical findings.

The following areas should be included in a dermatologic history:

- Usual care of skin, hair, and nails
  - Products used
  - Sun-exposure patterns
  - Cleaning regimens
  - Home remedies or preparations
- Dermatologic history
  - Skin sensitivities
  - Allergic skin reactions
  - Tolerance to sunlight
  - Increased or decreased sensitivity to stimuli
- Family history
  - Dermatologic diseases or disorders (acute, chronic, intermittent, and allergic)
  - Genetic-related allergic conditions, such as asthma or hayfever
- Present dermatologic problem
  - Temporal sequence: date of onset, sequence of lesion occurrence and development, and date of recurrence
  - Symptoms
  - Apparent cause
  - Seasonal or climate variations
  - Exposure to drugs, environmental toxins, or chemicals
  - Relationship to stress or leisure activity
  - Factors that make the condition worse or better
  - Ways with which the patient is adjusting to the problem
- Medications
  - Topical or systemic
  - Prescribed or over the counter
- Travel history
  - Where, when, length of stay
  - Exposure to diseases
  - Contact with travelers

The following studies are commonly used for diagnostic purposes.

Scrapings

Description. The area is cleansed with alcohol and air dried so that superficial fine dry scale is apparent. The scale is scraped with a sharp scalpel and gathered on a glass slide or in a blood collection tube. Nail and hair clippings are also used. Scrapings are covered with 10% KOH (potassium hydroxide) and examined microscopically for the presence of mycelia in fungal infections. The fungus appears as branching, threadlike elements.

Indications. Fungal conditions of skin.

Complications. None.

Nursing care. None.

Diascopy, Side Lighting, Wood's Light, Gram Stain, Culture, Electron Microscopy, Cytology

Description

Diascopy. The lesion is covered with a glass slide or piece of clear plastic to determine whether dilated capillaries or extravasated blood is causing redness of lesion.

Side lighting. A beam of light is directed from the side over the lesion to reveal minor elevations or depressions in the lesion. This helps determine the configuration and degree of eruption.

Wood's light. The skin is viewed in a darkened room under ultraviolet light with wavelength of 360 nm ("black light"). Certain disease-producing fungi and bacteria show a characteristic color.

Gram stain. Exudate from the lesion is smeared onto a glass slide and stained with gentian or crystal violet. The violet is washed off, and the smear is flooded with iodine solution, which is then washed off. The smear is then flooded with 95% alcohol and counterstained with safranin red dye. The stain will differentiate gram-negative from gram-positive bacteria based on their ability to pick up one or both of the two stains.

Culture. For pustular lesions a swab sample is placed in a broth culture media. For chronic bacterial and fungal infections, a biopsy specimen is used for culturing. Cultures are incubated or refrigerated and observed for fungal or bacterial growth.

Electron microscopy. A glass slide smear of vesicular fluid or crusted tissue is viewed under an electron microscope to determine the presence of a virus.

Cytology. Cellular material is scraped from the base of the vesicle and stained with Wright's or Giemsa stain, or a clean glass slide is touched to the surface of the lesion so cells can adhere to it. The cells are sprayed with a fixative and viewed microscopically after staining. Multinucleated giant cells are present in herpes simplex, herpes zoster, and varicella. Pemphigus is diagnosed by the presence of typical acantholytic cells.

Indications. Dermatologic lesions.

Complications. None.

Nursing care. None.

Patch Test

Description. The suspected allergen is applied to the skin under a nonabsorbent adhesive patch and left for 48 hours. A positive test consists of erythema with some induration and occasional vesicle formation. Some reactions do not occur until after the patch is removed from the site.

Indications. Sensitivity to allergens.

Complications. None, although itching or burning may occur.

Nursing care. Instruct the patient to leave the patch on, to keep the area dry, and to return for inspection of the site in 48 hours. Instruct the patient to remove the patch if itching or burning develops before 48 hours and to return for inspection of the site. Reinspect the site at 72 hours.

Thermography

Description. Measures and plots areas of localized elevation of skin temperature over inflammatory or malignant lesions; takes photographs of infrared radiation (heat) coming from any part of the body. For breast thermography the patient is placed in a draft-free room at a temperature of about 20° C (68° F). Clothing above the waist is removed, and the patient waits for about 15 minutes until the skin cools before infrared photographs are taken.

Indications. Presence of dermatologic lesions that are inflamed or suspected of being malignant.

Complications. None.

Nursing care. Explain to the patient that the room will be cool.

Allergy Skin Testing

Description. An antigen is introduced by scratching or pricking the skin surface or by intradermal injection.

Indications. Sensitivity to allergens.

Complications. Erythema at site; hypersensitivity, including anaphylaxis.

Nursing care. Check for erythema at the site of antigen introduction after 20 minutes. Observe for potential anaphylactic reactions following antigen introduction. Antihistamines may be administered as a comfort measure.

Schick Test

Description. This is a test to determine the presence or absence of a significant quantity of diphtheria antitoxins in the blood. The presence of these antitoxins indicates an immunity to diphtheria.

Indications. For susceptibility to diphtheria.

Complications. None.

Nursing care. Draw 0.1 ml of purified diphtheria toxin dissolved in human serum albumin into a tuberculin syringe. In a second syringe draw up 0.1 ml of inactivated diphtheria toxoid to be used as a control in the other arm (to rule out any sensitivity to culture proteins). Attach 26- or 27-gauge 1.25 cm (½ inch) needles to both syringes. Clean the volar surfaces of both forearms. Intradermally inject the toxin on one forearm and the toxoid in the other forearm. Carefully record which was injected in each arm. Examine the areas at 24 and 36 hours.

A positive reaction is indicated when the site of the toxin injection begins to redden in 24 hours. The redness, swelling, and tenderness continue until it reaches maximum size—usually 3 cm in diameter at the end of 1 week. The skin at the injection site may flake, and the center may appear as a dark pigmented spot. The area of the toxoid injection should show no reaction. With a negative result there is no flaking or erythema at either injection site.

Mantoux Test (Tuberculin Skin Testing)

Description. Two types of tuberculin are currently being used for testing: old tuberculin (OT) and purified protein derivative (PPD). The PPD is the preferred tuberculin preparation because its strength is standardized and tests with the same dose are comparable.

Contraindications for testing include any rash, allergic dermatitis, scabies, current reactions to smallpox vaccinations, or previous BCG vaccine.

Indications. Provides evidence of whether the tested individual has been infected, either past or present, with *Mycobacterium tuberculosis*.

Complications. None.

Nursing care. Each type of multiple puncture unit is slightly different. Carefully read the manufacturer's instructions regarding the administration of the test. A positive reaction for all brands consists of the formation of separate papules at each of the puncture sites or a large papule over the entire area. Refer to the manufacturer's instructions regarding specific interpretation.

Testing for Fungal Diseases

Description. For patients suspected of having coccidioidomycosis, skin tests are available from lysates of both the mycelial (coccidioidin) and the spherule (spherulin) forms. Skin tests with either form are highly specific and become positive 3 to 4 weeks after infection and 12 to 20 days after the onset of clinical illness. An intradermal injection is given.

Indications. Respiratory or other systemic symptoms that may indicate infection with coccidioidomycosis.

Complications. None.

Nursing care. Explain the purpose of the test to the patient. Observe the injection site for a reaction: erythema, swelling, or hardening at the site.

Delayed-Type Hypersensitivity (Anergy) Testing (Cell-Mediated Immunity Testing)

Description. Measures the capacity to generate a delayed-type hypersensitivity (DTH) response. The patient is injected intradermally with four common soluble recall antigens (for example, PPD, *Candida* spp., *Trichophyton* spp. and tetanus) and examined for induration and erythema after 48 hours. Most young, healthy persons respond positively to at least one antigen. Reactivity may decline with age and with protein- and calorie-deficiency states.

Indications. Suspected immunodeficiency or protein-calorie deficiency.

Complications. None.

Nursing care. Check for local erythema and induration at 48 hours.

Arteriographic (Angiographic) and Venographic Studies

Arteriography or venography consists of the infusion of a radiopaque substance into the arterial or venous system, followed by a series of roentgenograms that allow visualization of the vessel systems and assist in the diagnosis of any abnormalities.

Arteriography and venography may be used in many body systems. In addition to those described here, selective arteriography may also be performed to localize possible tumors of the parathyroid, adrenal, and pancreatic glands, and a procedure similar to arteriography may be used to perform serial venous sampling to obtain hormone levels.

Cerebral Arteriography

Description. Cerebral arteriography requires the infusion of a radiopaque substance into the cerebral arterial system; during infusion of the contrast medium, a series of roentgenograms is taken for visualization of the extracranial and intracranial vessels. To outline the anterior, middle, and posterior cerebral arteries and returning venous circulation, the injection is made into the carotid system. If visualization of the vertebral-basilar system in the posterior fossa is needed, the injection is made into the vertebral artery.[3]

There are two approaches (open or closed) to performing the arteriography. The *open* method is performed in the operating room and involves the surgical exposure of the internal carotid before injection of the contrast substance. After the procedure, the incision is sutured and dressed. The actual procedure and aftercare are the same as those for the closed method. The *closed* method involves injection of the contrast medium directly into the carotid or vertebral arteries or indirectly (injection of the carotid or vertebral vessels by way of the femoral, brachial, subclavian, or axillary artery).[3] Following the injection a series of roentgenographs is taken for visualization of arterial and venous circulations.

Contraindications include the following: anticoagulant therapy, age, recent embolic or thrombotic occurrences, sensitivity to the contrast medium, and severe liver, thyroid, or kidney disease.

Indications. Identification of cerebral circulatory anomalies (e.g., aneurysm, hematoma) and their site and size, and visualization of cerebral arteries and veins.

Complications. Complications generally occurring during or shortly after the procedure include seizures, stroke, allergic reactions (to dye), thrombosis, hemiparesis, visual disturbances, pulmonary emboli, and dysphasia.

Nursing care. Observe the puncture site for hematoma or hemorrhage. Frequently monitor vital signs and neurologic signs during and after procedure. Observe for signs of allergic dye reactions.

Fluorescein Arteriography (and Photography)

Description. A 10% solution of sodium fluorescein injected into the antecubital vein is relayed to retinal arteries in 10 to 16 seconds and to veins in 25 seconds. The pupils are dilated with short-acting cycloplegics in combination with a mydriatic. An ophthalmoscope with a blue filter can show the entire diameter of vessel, whereas ordinary ophthalmoscopy provides only a surface view.

Photography. Black and white film with appropriate filters should be used in a camera that takes rapid-sequence photographs from 9 to 30 seconds after injection of fluorescein. The patient and examiner are seated at a table opposite each other, each looking into the camera.

Indications. Eye disorders.

Complications. Subcutaneous leakage of dye causes local burning. A patient may experience a brief hot flash or nausea. A temporary yellowish discoloration of sclera may occur until the dye is excreted in the urine (within 48 hours).

Nursing care. Inquire about previous allergies to fluorescein (the allergic response is usually hives and itching). Inform the patient what to expect in terms of the effects of mydriatic or cycloplegic medications.

Cardiac Catheterization

Description. An invasive procedure involving insertion of a radiopaque catheter via the peripheral artery or vein into the heart. It is used to determine the anatomy of heart chambers, valves, great vessels, and coronary arteries; ventricular wall thickness and motion; hemodynamic functions of the heart by pressure recordings of heart chambers and great vessels and pressure gradients across the valves; ventricular function and cardiac output; degree of valve competence; and intracardiac oxygen saturations. It also selectively visualizes the heart, coronary arteries, and great vessels by recording serial roentgenograms (angiograms).

Indications. Symptoms of angina pectoris, myocardial infarct, or other cardiac dysfunction.

Complications. Myocardial infarction, arrhythmias, hematoma or hemorrhage at the insertion site, reaction to contrast medium, infection, pulmonary edema, cardiac tamponade.

Nursing care. Obtain informed consent. Explain that the procedure will last 2 to 4 hours, that the patient may feel pressure during insertion of the catheter and a hot flushing sensation or nausea with injection of contrast medium, that the patient should cough when instructed by the physician, and that the patient will receive medication if chest pain occurs and may be given nitroglycerin to dilate coronary vessels.

Determine any allergies or hypersensitivity to shellfish, iodine, or other contrast media. After the procedure check the vital signs every 15 minutes, decreasing in frequency. Keep the patient flat in bed for 6 to 8 hours with a pressurized dressing over the puncture site. Check the dressing and surrounding area for bleeding, pain, and swelling. Check the peripheral pulses, color, warmth, and feeling of the extremities distal to the insertion site. Give pain medication as indicated. Encourage fluid intake for first 6 to 8 hours to assist in the elimination of contrast medium.

Digital Vascular Imaging (DVI) (Digital Subtraction Arteriography)

Description. An invasive procedure using a computer system and fluoroscopy with an image intensifier to permit complete visualization of the arterial supply to a specific area.

Indications. Carotid and renal artery disease, pulmonary embolism, aneurysms, thrombotic and embolic disease of the great vessels, coarctation of the aorta.

Complications. Arrhythmias, reaction to contrast medium, infection, bleeding at site.

Nursing care. Obtain informed consent. Explain that the procedure will last 1 to 2 hours and that the patient will be requested to hold his breath for 10-second intervals. This can be done on an outpatient basis, and may cause certain sensations. After the procedure, check the vital signs immediately and as ordered. Check site for bleeding. Instruct the patient to observe the site for infection and/or bleeding and to drink a minimum of 1 L of fluid on the day of the procedure.

Scintigraphy (Radionuclide Arteriography)

Description. Gives information regarding myocardial perfusion and contractility through the use of radionuclide imaging. The procedure involves injecting a radioisotope and passing a scanning camera over the patient repeatedly.

Indications. Poor myocardial perfusion or contractility.

Complications. None.

Nursing care. Explain the procedure. Obtain informed consent. Reassure the patient that the radiation exposure involved is less than with a chest roentgenogram; caution the patient to remain quiet and still during the study.

Scintigraphy (Technetium-99m Pyrophosphate Myocardial Imaging)

Description. Tracer isotope is injected 2 to 3 hours before the procedure, and scanning takes 30 to 60 minutes, during which time a scanning camera is passed repeatedly over the patient in several positions: anterior, left anterior oblique, right anterior oblique, and left lateral.

Indications. To detect recent myocardial infarction and the extent of its damage; "hot spots" appear within 12 hours of the infarct and disappear after 1 week.

Complications. None.

Nursing care. Explain the procedure. Obtain informed consent. Inform the patient that he may eat lightly before the study but should not smoke or drink alcoholic or caffeine-containing beverages for 3 hours before the test.

Scintigraphy (Thallium-201 Imaging)

Description. "Cold spot" myocardial imaging used in conjunction with a bicycle ergometer or treadmill stress ECG test to diagnose ischemic heart disease.

Indications. To assess myocardial perfusion (myocardial blood flow) and to evaluate the patency of grafts after bypass surgery; also used in conjunction with exercise stress testing in the diagnosis of coronary artery disease (stress imaging).

Complications. None.

Nursing care. If performed in conjunction with EST, instruct the patient to avoid tobacco, alcohol, or unprescribed medication for 24 hours before the study and to take nothing by mouth for 3 hours before the test. NOTE: If chest pain, shortness of breath, or a drop in blood pressure develops, stress imaging should be halted.

Scintigraphic Blood Pool Imaging (Multiple-Gated Blood Pool)

Description. Involves injection of human serum albumin or RBCs tagged with the isotope technetium-99m pertechnetate. A scintillation camera records several pass images of the isotope as it passes through the ventricle. Imaging can be "gated" to systolic and diastolic events of the cardiac cycle. The normal left ventricular ejection fraction is 55% to 65%. The procedure is contraindicated in pregnancy.

Indications. Used to evaluate regional and global ventricular performance and to detect aneurysms of the left ventricle and areas of hypokinesis and dyskinesis.

Complications. None.

Nursing care. Explain the procedure. Obtain informed consent. Determine if the patient is pregnant. The patient may eat and drink before the procedure. Inform the patient that the blood-labeling agent is given intravenously.

Pulmonary Arteriography

Description. A radiopaque dye is injected rapidly into the pulmonary circulation by various routes: one or more systemic veins, or the chambers of the heart, or directly into the pulmonary arteries. After the rapid injection a series of roentgenograms is taken.

Indications. To detect pulmonary emboli and a variety of congenital and acquired thromboembolic lesions.

Complications. Hematoma development; occasionally, frank hemorrhage or thrombus formation; infection at the catheter insertion site.

Nursing care. Before the procedure, determine any allergies to radiopaque dye. After the procedure the patient must be observed for hematomas or inflammation around the injection site, absence of peripheral pulses, or complaints of numbness or pain.

Vena Caval Catheterization

Description. In vena caval catheterization a radiopaque catheter is introduced into the vena cava through the femoral vein. The catheter is guided into the vena cave with fluoroscopic assistance. Venous samples are obtained from different sites along the vena cava for catecholamine determination.

Patients with pheochromocytoma should receive alpha blockers before the procedure to prevent catecholamine relase and hypertensive crisis.

Indications. The procedure is performed to assist the surgeon to localize the pheuchromocytoma, and rule out bilateral or multiple tumors.

Complications. Pulmonary embolus, hematoma formation at catheter insertion site.

Nursing care. Before the procedure, give alpha blockers as prescribed. Have a cardiac arrest cart available. A physician or nurse should accompany the patient with a supply of intravenous phentolamine.

After the procedure, assess vital signs every 15 minutes for an hour, every 30 minutes for another hour, and every hour twice after that. Observe the affected extremity for color, temperature, edema, and pedal pulses to observe for postoperative loss of perfusion. Observe for hematoma formation, and notify the physician if any occur. Keep the patient flat in bed for 4 hours with no bending at the hip.

Celiac and Mesenteric Arteriography

Description. Contrast medium is injected into the celiac, superior mesenteric, or inferior mesenteric artery for visualization of the vasculature. Superselective arteriography permits a detailed visualization of a particular area. As the contrast medium is injected, serial roentgenograms outline abdominal vessels in arterial, capillary, and venous phases of perfusion.

A radiologist inserts a needle into the femoral artery. A guide wire is passed through the needle into the aorta, and the needle is then removed. An arteriographic catheter is inserted over the guide wire, and placement is checked roentgenographically and fluoroscopically before the guide wire is removed. The catheter, under fluoroscopy, is advanced into one of the three arteries; placement is checked, and an automatic injection of contrast medium is attached. A rapid sequence of serial films is taken as the medium is injected. The catheter is repositioned for superselective visualization.

Indications. Can be used for locating gastrointestinal bleeding and for treating bleeding by either infusion of vasopressin at the site or injection of embolic material to form a clot. The embolic material includes aminocaproic acid (Amicar) clot or gelatin sponge (Gelfoam). It is also used to evaluate cirrhosis and portal hypertension, vascular damage after abdominal trauma, intestinal ischemia, and vascular abnormalities. It may be used in evaluating tumors (distinguishing between benign and malignant) when other tests are inconclusive.

Complications. Bleeding, hematoma formation, or infection at the catheter's insertion site.

Nursing care. Assess the patient for sensitivities to iodine, seafood, and contrast media. Blood work should include hemoglobin, hematocrit, clotting time, prothrombin time, activated partial thromboplastin time, and platelet count. The patient should remain flat in bed for at least 12 hours. Check the puncture site frequently for bleeding and hematoma; a sandbag is often used for 2 to 4 hours to prevent bleeding.

Monitor the vital signs as ordered—usually every 15 minutes for 1 hour, every 30 minutes for 2 hours, and then every hour for 4 hours or until the patient is stable. Depending on the patient's reactions to the test and the potential problems of bleeding, this pattern may change. Monitor the peripheral pulses by observing vital signs. Compare pulses in each foot. Also observe the leg (of the puncture site) for color and temperature and compare with the alternate leg if unsure of changes.

Notify the physician about continued or excessive bleeding, changes in the peripheral pulse and temperature, and color changes. Also notify the physician if vital signs change significantly.

Renal Arteriography and Venography

Description. Provides information concerning arterial and venous blood supply to the kidneys.

Arteriography. A preprocedure antianxiety or narcotic injection is given. The patient is taken to a radiologic suite, and an additional local anesthetic is given in the area over the femoral artery. The patient is placed in a supine position, and a femoral puncture is performed. An opaque catheter is then passed from the femoral artery to the aorta and into the desired renal artery under fluoroscopy. A radiopaque contrast material is then injected into the renal artery. (If passage into the aorta via the femoral artery is not feasible, the axillary artery may be used as an alternative.)

Rapid roentgenographic images are used to assess the three phases of the arteriogram: the arterial phase lasts 2 to 4 seconds and provides a detailed outline of the principal renal arteries; the nephrogenic phase is seen as a marked opacification of the renal parenchyma, lasting 15 to 20 seconds; and the venous phase is of limited value because of the kidney's ability to extract and excrete contrast material (principally useful in assessing arteriovenous shunting).

Digital subtraction arteriography (DSA) is a new method of imaging that allows visualization of the kidney's arteries using a significantly smaller dose of contrast material than does the standard technique. It has the advantage of being rapid and relatively noninvasive, compared with standard techniques so it can be performed on an outpatient basis with an IVP. Limitations include poorer visualization of peripheral renal artery branches.[30]

Venography. To perform this procedure, a percutaneous catheter is placed into the right femoral vein and advanced to the opening of the renal vein. Contrast material is injected, and the catheter is then directed upward to enter the contralateral (right) renal vein. The procedure is repeated. Imaging may be enhanced by injecting 6 to 10 μg of epinephrine into the renal artery followed by renal venography 10 seconds later.

Indications. Indications for arteriography include palpable renal masses, potential renovascular hypertension, and renal trauma; it is also used to determine the suitability of renal donors.[8]

Indications for venography include renal vein thrombosis, renovascular hypertension, elucidation of renal cell carcinoma, and various congenital abnormalities of the renal veins.

Complications. The two major complications are bleeding at the site of the arterial puncture and allergic reactions to the contrast material.

Nursing care. Pedal pulses and capillary filling of the nail beds of the foot should be assessed before the procedure. After the renal arteriogram is completed, the femoral puncture site should be assessed regularly (every 1 to 2 hours) for hematoma or external bleeding. Assessment of capillary refill and the affected foot's appearance is indicated. Vital signs and signs of allergic reaction to the contrast material should be assessed frequently (every 1 to 2 hours). Signs of allergic reaction include pruritus, wheezing, dyspnea, and flushed skin.

Phlebography (Venography)

Description. Invasive procedure used to identify and locate venous thrombi. It involves injection of a radiopaque dye (technetium-99 microaggregated albumin) into the venous system of the affected extremity followed by serial roentgenograms. Abnormal filling of the vein indicates a positive finding that thrombosis exists.

Indications. Deep vein thrombosis.

Complications. Reaction to the contrast media, subcutaneous infiltration of dye, embolism caused by dislodgment of the thrombus.

Nursing care. Explain that the procedure may take from 30 minutes to an hour and that a warm flushed sensation may be felt with the injection of the dye. No preprocedure fasting is required.

Lumbar Venography

Description. Injection of contrast medium to visualize epidural venous plexus. The catheter is inserted percutaneously into the femoral vein and then guided into the internal iliac vein or ascending lumbar vein.

Indications. When performed for neurologic or musculoskeletal conditions, lumbar venography aids in outlining the blood supply to or through a tumor or other structure under study and thereby aids in the preoperative assessment and determination of possible operative treatment. The study can be made as an outpatient procedure.

Complications. Bleeding, hematoma formation, infection at the catheter's insertion site.

Nursing care. Monitor the site for signs of hemorrhage or infection. Immobilize the affected extremity for 12 hours after the procedure.

Lymphangiography

Description. Radiopaque medium introduced via a tiny catheter into the peripheral lymphatics to allow visualization of the deep femoral, iliac, and periaortic lymph nodes. Dye is injected locally into the hands and feet via small incisions, and roentgenograms are taken immediately after the injection and 24 hours later.

Indications. Swelling of lymph nodes; suspected malignancy, such as lymphoma, Hodgkin's disease.

Complications. Hypersensitive reaction to the contrast material; inflammation at the infection sites.

Nursing care. Inform the patient about the procedure. Obtain informed consent. Encourage fluids after the procedure to flush the dye. Inform the patient that a bluish tint to the skin and urine will disappear within a few weeks.

Blood Studies

Blood Studies

Blood studies are a key diagnostic indicator, and are used to assist in the diagnosis of almost every body system. Studies specific to each body system and normal values are found in each chapter. Following, however, are some descriptions of blood studies that require any special nursing care, utilized for hematolymphatic, immune, and neoplastic disorders. Also included is a discussion of arterial blood gas analysis.

The following blood studies are used to diagnose a wide variety of disorders:

Red cell count determines the number of red blood cells (RBCs) in 1 mm^3 of blood.

White cell count determines the number of white blood cells (WBCs) in 1 mm^3 of blood.

Differential count determines the percentage of various types of WBCs.

Platelet count determines the number of platelets in 1 mm^3 of blood.

Hemoglobin concentration determines the amount of hemoglobin in a given volume of blood.

Hematocrit determines the percentage of blood composed of RBCs.

Mean corpuscular volume (MCV) determines the size and volume of each RBC.

Mean corpuscular hemoglobin (MCH) determines the hemoglobin content in RBCs of average size.

Mean corpuscular concentration (MCHC) determines the amount of hemoglobin in packed RBCs (hemoglobin of 100 ml RBCs).

Reticulocyte count determines the effectiveness and speed of RBC production and the responsiveness of bone marrow to decreased circulating RBCs.

Erythrocyte life span determination estimates the rate at which RBCs tagged with chromium-51 disappear from circulation. The patient and a normal subject with comparable blood type are injected with tagged cells.

Erythrocyte fragility test measures the rate at which RBCs burst in hypotonic solutions of varied concentrations.

Direct Coombs' test is used to examine RBCs for the presence of antibodies (agglutinins) that damage RBCs, but will not cause clumping or hemolysis.

Indirect Coombs' test is used to identify antibodies to RBC antigens.

Serum iron level is the amount of iron found in a sample of blood.

Bleeding time is measured by making a small stab wound in the earlobe or forearm. The time it takes to stop the bleeding is noted, and a measurement is made of the rate at which a clot is formed. The patient must not take aspirin for at least 5 days before the test. The patient is also advised not to drink alcoholic beverages before the test.

Coagulation time is the time required for blood to form a solid clot in a foreign surface such as glass test tube.

Capillary fragility is determined by the tourniquet test; positive or negative pressure is applied to various areas of the body, and the relative number of petechiae is noted.

Therapeutic trial with parenteral vitamin B_{12} requires that the patient be given intramuscular injections of vitamin B_{12} for 10 days. Blood work and the patient's subjective feeling of well-being are evaluated.

Schilling test measures the absorption of radioactive vitamin B_{12} before and after parenteral administration of intrinsic factor; it may be a three-stage procedure.

Bilirubin test requires that a venous sample be collected for measuring the total amount of bilirubin. Differentiation of conjugate and unconjugate levels can also be determined.

Serologic tests are frequently used to help determine the causative pathogens in fungal diseases and atypical pneumonia. The outcome of the test depends on the development of antibodies to the organism in the patient's serum that can be detected by agglutination, complement fixation, or precipitation reactions when the serum is exposed to a specific antigen. Examples are the fungal antibody tests that detect coccidioidomycosis, blastomycosis, and histoplasmosis.

HLA typing requires that a venous blood specimen be collected for use in the identification of HLA-A, HLA-B, HLA-C histocompatibility antigens. It is used for screening patients and potential donors for tissue transplantation.

Immunofluorescence (IF) is measured after the serum or tissue specimen is viewed microscopically. An indirect IF test demonstrates that the serum of a patient with pemphigus or bullous pemphigoid contains specific antibodies that bind to different areas of the epithelium. In the direct IF test, a skin sample shows characteristic patterns for specific diseases.

In vitro leukocyte function tests are used to evaluate patients with recurrent infections and suspected immunodeficiency diseases. Normal values are determined in each laboratory.

Lymphocyte stimulation requires that lymphocytes be incubated with a particular antigen or mitogen (polyclonal activator), and the cell proliferation determined. Alterations may be seen in genetic or acquired immunodeficiency states.

Cytotoxicity. Lymphocytes are incubated with tumor cells or virally infected cells, and target cell lysis is measured. In the absence of any antibody, natural killer (NK) cell function measured. If the donor has been sensitized to a target cell in vivo, a secondary cytotoxic T lymphocyte (CTL) response can be determined.

Chemotaxis. Phagocytic cells are incubated in a chamber that permits cells to migrate through a filter toward a chemoattractant. When samples from the patient are incubated with standard chemotactic factors, chemotactic capabilities of phagocytic cells are assessed. Alternatively one can intubate normal phagocytes with patient serum to test the ability of that serum to generate chemotactic factors.

Phagocytosis. Particle uptake assays measure phagocytic cell function or the opsonizing capacity of the patient's serum. To assess phagocyte function, the patient's monocytes or neutrophils are incubated with test particle in the presence of normal human serum. To examine opsonization, normal phagocytic cells are incubated with particles in the presence of the patient's serum. Phagocytosis can be assessed by direct visualization or use of radiolabeled particles.

Bactericidal activity. Phagocytic cells are incubated with appropriately opsonized bacteria and then washed and lysed. The number of live intracellular bacteria is then determined.

NBT dye reduction. Phagocytic cells are incubated with particles in the presence of oxidized nitroblue tetrazolium (NBT). On stimulation of respiratory burst activity, reducing equivalents are generated and NBT is converted into deep blue insoluble precipitate. NBT dye reduction does not occur in certain patients with genetic phagocytic cell defects.

Chemiluminescence. Phagocytes are incubated with opsonized particles, and light emission is measured in a spectrophotometer. During phagocytosis, normal monocytes and neutrophils generate highly unstable oxygen intermediates that emit light during decay to the ground state. Chemiluminescence is reduced in patients with certain phagocyte dysfunctions.

Tumor markers

Acid phosphatase
- Increased in prostatic cancer
- Increased in some primary bone malignancies, multiple myeloma

Alkaline phosphatase
- Increased in metastatic cancer to bone and liver, osteogenic sarcoma, myeloma, and Hodgkin's lymphoma with bone involvement

Alphafetoprotein (AFP)
- Increased in hepatocellular cancers; choriocarcinoma; teratoma; embryonal cell tumors of testis and ovary; some pancreatic, stomach, colon, and lung tumors

Carcinoembryonic antigen (CEA)
- Increased in colon cancer

Also seen in lung, pancreas, stomach, breast, head and neck, and prostate cancers
Chorionic gonadotropin (beta subunit) (B-HCG)
Increased in hydatiform mole, choriocarcinoma, testicular teratoma
Ectopic HCG production by some cancers of pituitary gland, stomach, pancreas, lung, colon, and liver
Pancreatic oncofetal antigen (POA)
Positive in large percentage of pancreas tumors
Placental alkaline phosphatase (PAP)
Increased in a variety of tumors

Hormones
Adrenocorticotropic hormone (ACTH)
Increased in ectopic-ACTH producing tumors (especially small cell lung cancer), adrenal carcinoma, adenoma
Androstenedione
Increased in ectopic ACTH-producing tumors, ovarian tumors
Antidiuretic hormone (ADH)
Increased in brain tumors, systemic malignancies with ectopic ADH production
Calcitonin
Increased in medullary carcinoma of thyroid, some lung and breast tumors, colon cancer, and GI malignancies
Estrogens, total
Increased in estrogen-producing ovarian tumors, some testicular tumors, and adrenal cortical tumors
Estrogen (Estradiol) receptor assay
60% of breast cancer characterized by estrogen receptors
Glucagon
Decreased in some pancreatic tumors
Growth hormone (LGH)
Increased in ectopic secretion by some stomach and lung tumors
Parathyroid hormone (LPTH)
Increased squamous cell or epidermoid lung cancers and renal cell
Progesterone
Increased in some ovarian tumors
Progesterone receptor assay
May be useful in predicting tumors likely to respond to hormonal manipulations
17-Ketogenic steroids
Increased in adrenal adenoma and carcinoma, ectopic ACTH syndrome
17-Ketosteroids
Increased in adrenal tumors, testicular tumors, interstitial cell tumors, androgenic ovarian tumors
Testosterone
Increased in some adrenocortical tumors, gonadotropin-producing extragonadal tumors

Enzymes
Amylase
Increased in some lung and ovarian tumors
Amylase isoenzymes
Increased in some bronchogenic or serous ovarian tumors
Lactic dehydrogenase (LDH) and LDH isoenzymes
Increased in extensive carcinomatosis and malignant processes; acute leukemia
Leucine aminopeptidase (LAP)
Increased in pancreatic cancer with liver metastases
Lysozyme
Increased in acute monocytic or myelomonocytic leukemia and chronic myeloid leukemia
Serum gamma glutamyl transpeptidase (SGGT)
Increased in some cases of renal cell cancer and liver metastases
Serum glutamic oxaloacetic transaminase (SGOT)
Increased in liver metastases
Serum glutamic pyruvic transaminase (SGPT)
Increased in some liver cancers

Proteins (immunoglobulins produced by lymphocytes and plasma cells)
IgA
IgO
IgE
IgG
IgM

Endocrine Studies of Hormones

Provocative endocrine testing is classified as either stimulation or suppression studies. Evaluation of secretory reserve by a *stimulation* test is useful for diagnosing hypofunction and for detecting impaired secretory reserve. *Suppression* tests are useful for diagnosis of hyperfunction because the hyperfunctioning gland by definition is not operating under normal control mechanisms.

Table 1 lists tests according to the hormone being evaluated. These tests are associated with specific procedures dependent on the laboratory capabilities of the institution. Injection of some hormones (e.g., TRH) may produce a warm, flushed feeling. The nursing care includes education of the patient about the purpose, procedure, and possible side effects and support of the patient during the procedure. The insulin tolerance test will cause profound and purposeful hypoglycemia, requiring a nurse in attendance at all times. When the physician terminates the test, intravenous glucose (10% D/W; 20% D/W; 50% D) is infused immediately and is followed by a high-protein meal.

Arterial Blood Gas Analysis

Description. Arterial blood gas analysis is the most direct method to assess the patient's oxygen and blood gas status.

Indications. The procedure is indicated for any patient who is seriously ill or injured, whose respiratory status and metabolic balance are in question. Most commonly, arterial blood gases are required for patients with hypoxemia or desaturation secondary to altered ventilatory patterns from any cause.

Arterial blood gas collection procedure

1. Gather the equipment: a 2- or 3-ml syringe with a 25-gauge needle; a 10-ml glass or disposable syringe with

Table 1
Hormone Tests

Hormone	Stimulation	Suppression
Antidiuretic hormone (ADH)	Water deprivation Nicotine	Saline infusion Pitressin
Growth hormone (GH)	Insulin tolerance test Arginine tolerance test Levodopa Exercise stimulation test	Glucose tolerance test
Thyroid-stimulating hormone (TSH)	Thyrotropin-releasing hormone (TRH)	Triiodothyronine Thyroxine
Prolactin (PRL)	Insulin tolerance test Chlorpromazine TRH	Levodopa
Adrenocorticotropic hormone (ACTH)	Insulin tolerance test (hypoglycemia will occur) Corticotropin-releasing hormone (CRH)	Dexamethasone Metyrapone
Luteinizing hormone (LH)	Luteinizing-releasing hormone (LRH)	Testosterone Estrogen
Follicle-stimulating hormone (FSH)	Clomiphene	
Triiodothyronine (T_3)	TSH	T_3
Thyroxine (T_4)		T_4
Cortisol	ACTH CRH Insulin tolerance test Arginine tolerance test	Dexamethasone Metyrapone
Aldosterone	ACTH	Salt loading/volume expansion Spironolactone
Norepinephrine	Histamine Tyramine Glucagon	Phentolamine
Progesterone	Human menopausal gonadotropin (HMG) Human chorionic gonadotropin (HCG)	Provera Progesterone
Testosterone	HMG HCG	Testosterone
Parathyroid hormone (PTH)	PTH infusion	Calcium infusion
Glucose	Glucagon	Insulin tolerance test Tolbutamide
Insulin	Glucose tolerance test (GTT) Leucine Fructose	Prolonged fast
Gastrin	Pentagastrin Calcium infusion High-protein, high-carbohydrate meal	Cimetidine

a 20- or 21-gauge needle (21- or 23-gauge for children); rubber stopper or Luer-Lok cap, 1 ml sodium heparin (1:1000), lidocaine (Xylocaine) or procaine, alcohol swab or iodophor prep, gauze pads, and basin with crushed ice and water.

2. Heparinize the 10 ml glass syringe by using the 20- or 21-gauge needle and drawing up 0.5 ml of heparin into the syringe to wet the cylinder and plunger; then discard the heparin as much as possible by holding the syringe upright and expelling the heparin and air bubbles. Recover the needle and lay it aside.
3. Position the patient in either a sitting or supine position and explain the procedure.
4. Locate the arterial puncture site: possible sites include the radial artery, brachial artery, and femoral artery (Figure 4). Vessel criteria include the following:
   a. Collateral blood flow: the radial artery has excellent collateral flow; the brachial artery has reasonable collateral flow; and the femoral artery has no collateral blood flow.
   b. Vessel accessibility: it is easier to palpate, stabilize, and puncture superficial vessels than it is to work with deep ones. The more distal an artery, the more superficial it is.
   c. Periarterial tissue: muscles, tendon, and fat are reasonably insensitive to pain. Bone periosteum and nerves are very sensitive. Therefore choose a site that avoids close sensitive structures or parallel veins. The sites of choice are first, radial; second, brachial; third, femoral.

Figure 4 Arterial blood gas sites. **A,** Radial artery. **B,** Brachial artery. **C,** Femoral artery.

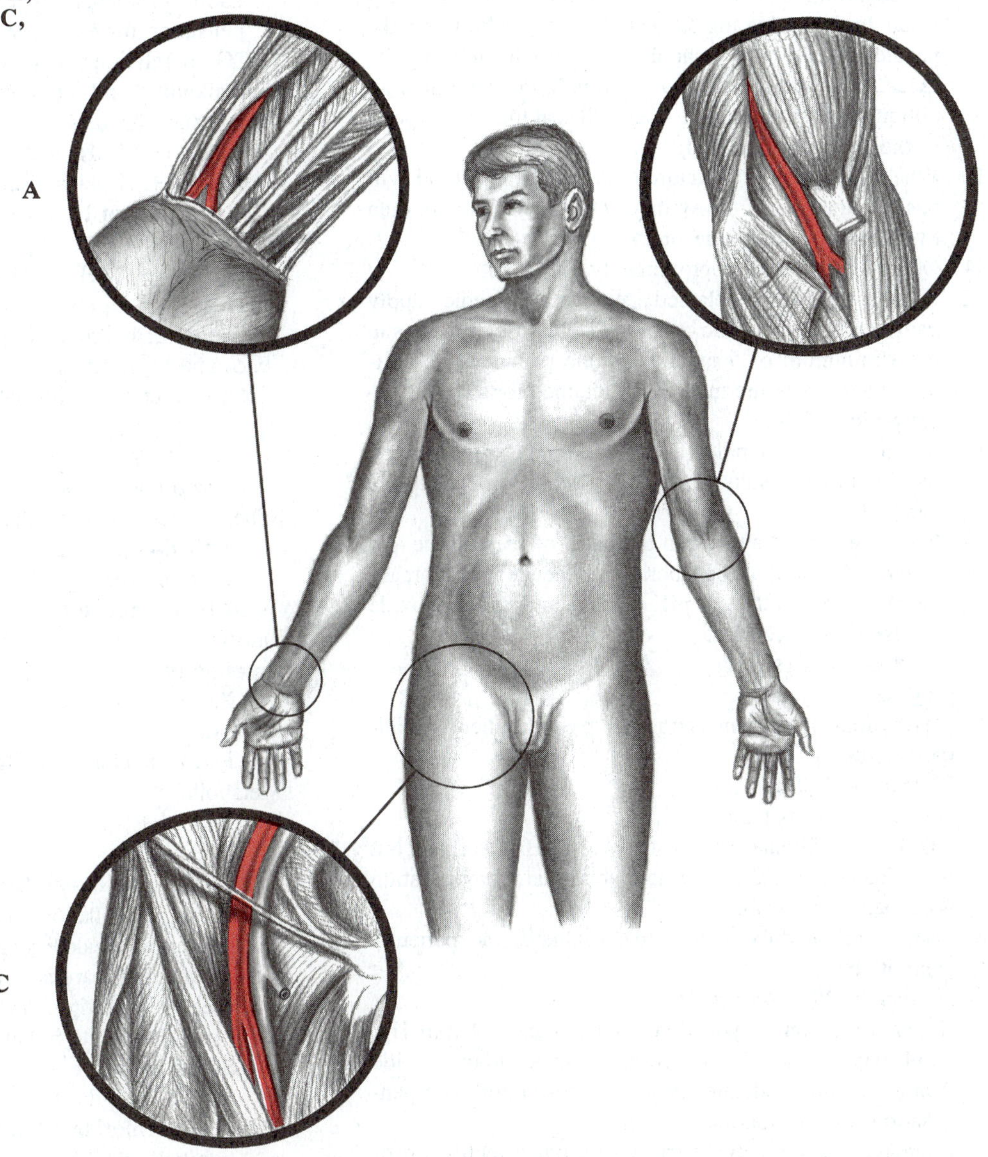

5. When using the radial artery, perform the Allen test. This will evaluate the collateral blood supply. The technique is as follows:
   a. Instruct the patient to close his fist tightly.
   b. Obliterate both radial and ulnar nerves simultaneously.
   c. Instruct the patient to relax his hand (not fully); watch for blanching of palm and fingers.
   d. Remove obstructing pressure from only the ulnar artery and observe for capillary refill and flush of hand (within 15 seconds). This refill response, which is a positive Allen test, verifies that the ulnar artery alone is capable of supplying the entire hand.
   e. If the Allen test is negative, do not use the radial artery for arterial puncture.
   f. If the patient is unconscious or uncooperative, a similar response to the closed fist can be obtained by placing the patient's hand up in the air until blanching occurs; obliterate the arteries, lower the hand, and release pressure over the ulnar artery.

NOTE: The remaining procedure assumes that the radial artery has been chosen for arterial puncture:

6. Donning gloves, palpate the radial artery to locate a spot where maximum pulsation is felt.
7. Clean the area with iodophor prep, then with alcohol swab.
8. The skin may then be injected with an anesthetic agent using the small syringe with a 25-gauge needle.
9. With one hand locate the radial pulse proximal to the area cleaned. This will provide landmark information.

Keeping the fingers of the one hand on the pulse, insert the heparinized needle and syringe into the radial artery distal to the palpating fingers. The angle between the needle and the artery should be approximately 45 degrees. This makes the hole through the arterial wall oblique so that the muscle fiber will seal the hole as soon as the needle is removed.

10. When the artery is punctured, the pulsating blood will push up the hub of the syringe. Do not make more than two attempts at any one site.
11. Obtain a sample of approximately 3 to 5 ml.
12. After the blood is obtained, remove the needle, apply gauze, and use firm and continuous pressure over the site for a minimum of 5 minutes. If the patient is on anticoagulants, pressure must be maintained for a much longer period of time.
13. Remove all air bubbles from the syringe (this will affect blood gas results) and apply a rubber stopper to the needle tip.
14. Place the capped syringe in the basin of crushed ice and water and send it to the laboratory. The ice will decrease the alterations of the true pH, oxygen, and carbon dioxide levels of the specimen.

Blood gas analysis[18,23]

Step by step analysis

1. pH (hydrogen ion concentration): assess patient's acid-base status
   Normal = 7.35 to 7.45
   Acidosis = Less than 7.35
   Alkalosis = Greater than 7.43 (when pH is normal, but when $Paco_2$ and HCO_3^- are both abnormal, compensation is probably occurring)
2. $Paco_2$ (carbon dioxide tension): evaluates the patient's ventilation
   Normal = 35 to 45 mm Hg
   Hyperventilation (hypocarbia) = Less than 34 mm Hg; this means that there is excessive loss of carbon dioxide
   Abnormal value indicates there is no respiratory compensation for a metabolic problem
   Decreased values may be caused by hyperventilation or ventilation-perfusion inequality
   To evaluate for respiratory acidosis and alkalosis and for compensation due to metabolic acidosis and alkalosis
3. $Paco_2$ in relation to pH
   ↑ $Paco_2$ + ↓ pH = Acidemia of respiratory origin
   ↑ $Paco_2$ + ↑ pH = Respiratory retention of carbon dioxide to compensate for metabolic alkalosis
   ↓ $Paco_2$ + ↑ pH = Alkalosis of respiratory origin
   ↓ $Paco_2$ + ↓ pH = Respiratory elimination of carbon dioxide to compensate for metabolic acidosis
4. Bicarbonate (HCO_3^-): This is the metabolic component
   Normal = 16 to 24 mEq/L (infant), 21 to 28 mEq/L (arterial, children and adults), 22 to 27 mEq/L (venous, children and adults)
   Alkalosis = Greater than 26 mEq/L
   Acidosis = Less than 22 mEq/L
   A normal value indicates that there are no primary metabolic problems and that there is no metabolic compensation for a respiratory problem
5. HCO_3^- in relation to pH: To evaluate for metabolic acidosis and alkalosis and for compensation due to respiratory acidosis and alkalosis
   ↓ HCO_3^- + ↓ pH = Acidemia of metabolic origin
   ↓ HCO_3^- + ↑ pH = Renal retention of hydrogen ion or elimination of HCO_3^- to compensate for respiratory alkalosis
   ↑ HCO_3^- + ↑ pH = Alkalosis of metabolic origin
   ↑ HCO_3^- + ↓ pH = Renal retention of HCO_3^- or elimination of hydrogen ion
6. Pao_2 and O_2 saturation
   Pao_2 saturation: Normal = 80 to 95 mm Hg
   60 to 70 mm Hg (newborn)
   O_2 saturation: Normal = 95% to 99%
   These values may be due to hypoventilation, shunting, ventilation-perfusion inequality, or a reduction of inspired oxygen

Acid-base imbalance[22]

Alkalosis

Respiratory
- ↓ $Paco_2$ + ↓ HCO_3^- = Patient attempting to compensate
- ↓ $Paco_2$ + Normal HCO_3^- = No patient compensation

Metabolic
- ↑ HCO_3^- + ↑ $Paco_2$ = Patient attempting to compensate
- ↑ HCO_3^- + Normal $Paco_2$ = No patient compensation

Clinical signs of alkalosis: dizziness, tingling of fingers and toes, muscle weakness or muscle spasm, muscle twitching, sweating, cardiac arrhythmia, shallow respirations, nausea or vomiting, tachypnea, tremor, or convulsion

Fluid and electrolyte imbalances
- ↓ Serum sodium
- ↑ Serum chloride
- ↓ Serum chloride (if alkalosis is due to gastric suctioning)
- ↓ Potassium

Acidosis

Respiratory
- ↑ $Paco_2$ + ↑ HCO_3^- = Patient attempting to compensate
- ↑ $Paco_2$ + Normal HCO_3^- = No patient compensation

Metabolic
- ↓ HCO_3^- + ↓ $Paco_2$ = Patient attempting to compensate
- ↓ HCO_3^- + Normal $Paco_2$ = No patient compensation

Clinical signs of acidosis: headache, slowness in responding to questions, hand tremor when patient is instructed to extend arms, confusion, drowsiness, Kussmaul respirations, nausea or vomiting, tremor, confusion, tachycardia, coma

Fluid and electrolyte imbalances
↓ Serum sodium
↓ Serum chloride
↑ Serum potassium

Complications.[10] Hematoma from multiple attempts at puncture or from inadequate pressure to the site after arterial stick; ischemia of an extremity secondary to thrombus after the procedure; adjunct nerve damage secondary to incorrect technique.

Nursing care. Explain the procedure fully before attempting technique. Assist the physician in administering a local anesthetic if indicated before obtaining arterial blood gases. Following procedure, apply direct pressure over the puncture site for at least 5 minutes to prevent hematoma or bleeding into the tissues. Carefully and systematically analyze the blood gas results according to the assessment guidelines. Monitor the patient's response to actual or potential blood gas acid-base imbalances to include the following:

Mental state: depression or stimulation of the central nervous system
Respiratory status: breathing pattern and depth and quality of respiration
Cardiovascular response: pulse rate, rhythm, and quality
Fluid and electrolyte status: disorders, such as vomiting and diarrhea, that could cause the imbalance; the patient's responses secondary to fluid and electrolyte imbalances

• Urodynamic Studies

Uroflowmetry

Description. Determines the rate, time, and volume of urinary flow. This study requires no catheterization; the patient voids into a device that measures the characteristics of bladder elimination. Results are displayed in graph form.

Indications. Aids in the diagnosis and description of ureteral, urethral, and bladder function.

Complications. None.

Nursing care. The patient should force fluids and refrain from voiding for 2 hours before testing in order to have at least 300 ml of urine in the bladder.

Urethral Pressure Studies

Description. These studies measure urethral resistance to urinary outflow. The catheter is pulled through the urethra at a given rate while water or carbon dioxide is infused through several side ports. A specialized catheter may be placed at the external urinary sphincter to measure the urethral response to bladder filling/storage and micturition.

Indications. Aids in the diagnosis of bladder disorders.

Complications. Cystitis.

Nursing care. Instruct the patient to watch for signs of cystitis (frequency of urination and mild dysuria), which should disappear within the first 24 hours after testing.

Cystometry

Description. Evaluates the two phases of bladder function: filling/storage and expulsion/micturition. One or more catheters is placed in the bladder urethrally or suprapubically. The bladder is then filled with liquid contrast material (water or a roentgenographic material) or carbon dioxide. The patient is asked to report sensations of an urgency to void or a bladder fullness. The study is completed by asking the patient to void voluntarily.

Indications. Bladder, micturition disorders.

Complications. Cystitis.

Nursing care. Instruct the patient to watch for signs of cystitis (frequency of urination, dysuria), which should completely disappear within the first 24 hours after testing.

Cystometry with Pharmacologic Testing

Description. Two comparative cystometrograms are performed before and 30 minutes after administration of a certain drug. The most commonly used drugs are bethanechol chloride (Urecholine) and propantheline bromide (Pro-Banthine).

Indications. Bethanechol is used to assess "denervation" (neuropathic changes in bladder function) as opposed to functional voiding abnormalities. Propantheline is used to assess the clinical response of detrusor overactivity to an anticholinergic agent.

Complications. Bethanechol may cause nausea and vomiting, hypotension, and shock. Atropine is given subcutaneously as an antidote if needed. Propantheline may cause hypotension, hypertension, tachycardia, angina, and atrial or ventricular fibrillation; physostigmine salicylate is given parenterally as an antidote if needed.

Nursing care. Vital signs should be monitored every 15 to 30 minutes for a 2-hour period after testing.

Loopogram

Description. Water-soluble contrast material is instilled into the urostomy stoma via a small catheter. The filling is observed under fluoroscopy, and a roentgenogram is taken. The loop is then drained and the catheter removed; the procedure takes about 10 minutes.

Indications. Assesses length and emptying ability of the ileal/sigmoid conduit; also assesses presence of stricture, reflux angulation, or obstruction.

Complications. None.

Nursing care. Provide the patient with a replacement urinary pouch, since it will be removed during the test.

• Miscellaneous Studies

Pneumoencephalogram (PEG)

Description. Involves the injection of air, helium, or oxygen into the lumbar subarachnoid space after intermittent removal of the cerebrospinal fluid by lumbar puncture. This procedure allows for the roentgenographic visualization of the ventricular space, basal cisterns, and subarachnoid space overlying the cerebral hemispheres of the brain.[3]

The procedure is performed with the patient in a sitting position. Following the lumbar puncture, a small amount of cerebrospinal fluid (about 5 ml) is withdrawn and replaced with an equal amount of air, helium, or oxygen. Serial roentgenograms are taken to visualize the ventricular system. Contraindications to the PEG include infection at the puncture site and clinical evidence of significantly increased intracranial pressure (i.e., an ICP greater than 15 mm Hg).

Indications. Include localization of intracranial lesions, visualization of the ventricular system and subarachnoid space, and detection of cerebral atrophy.

Complications. Postprocedural complications can include nausea and vomiting, headache, increased intracranial pressure, respiratory distress, seizures, air embolus, and shock.

Nursing care. Keep the patient flat in bed for 12 to 24 hours after the procedure. Force fluids, unless contraindicated. Maintain accurate intake and output records. Frequently monitor the vital signs and neurologic signs. (Many patients will be febrile for as long as 36 to 48 hours after the procedure.) If indicated, administer analgesics as ordered by the physician.

Echoencephalogram

Description. An echoencephalogram is a noninvasive diagnostic technique that records sonic pulses from cerebral structures by reflection of ultrasonic impulses directed through the patient's skull and back toward the source. These pulses then are recorded and projected onto an oscilloscope screen.[3]

The procedure is performed by placing an ultrasonic transducer on the skull's midaxis in the temporoparietal region. The waves produced are called M-echos, which then are recorded and projected on a screen to provide a graphic representation of the distance from the reflecting surface to the source of the ultrasonic beam.[32] Pictures of these M-echo waves may become a permanent part of the patient's record. The procedure takes only several minutes, and the reliability of the results depends on the skill of the technician. Abnormal shifts of the midline structures are recorded in millimeters, and a shift of 3 mm or more in the adult is considered abnormal.

Indications. Useful in determining ventricular size and cerebral midline shifts.

Complications. None.

Nursing care. None.

Tonometry

Description. Several types of instruments (tonometers) measure intraocular pressure; all of them indent the globe and measure the force (or weight) necessary to cause the indentation.

Schiötz tonometer. This hand-held instrument has a curved footplate that is rested on the cornea. A local anesthetic is instilled into each eye. The patient lies supine and is asked to stare straight ahead. The examiner holds the lids open. As the tonometer is placed on the corneal surface, a scale reading is taken from the instrument and converted with a chart to pressure in mm Hg.

Applanation tonometer. This machine measures the force required to flatten rather than indent the central cornea. It is more accurate than the Schiötz tonometer. A spring tension knob records the pressure, and a local anesthetic is used.

Noncontact tonometer. This machine uses a rapid puff of air to exert and register pressure. It does not require any anesthetic and is very accurate except in higher-pressure ranges. It cannot be used for patients with corneal edema or those with irregular optic interface.

Indications. For measurement of intraocular pressure; for routine screening of glaucoma and diabetes; for assessment of penetrating injuries.

Complications. None, although there is a risk of cross contamination if the tonometer is not sterilized properly between patients.

Nursing care. Sterilize the tonometer daily, and clean it before each use. Inquire about corneal injuries or abrasions. Assure the patient that no discomfort will be experienced.

Caloric Test

Description. Stimulation of the semicircular canals by introduction of either water or air (above or below body temperature) into the external auditory canal. Water below body temperature causes endolymphatic fluid to flow in a downward direction when directed against the tympanic membrane. The injection of cold water into the ear causes maximal stimulation of the semicircular canals and causes nystagmus and falling reactions in 10 to 20 seconds in the normal individual. Warm caloric tests have given reactions opposite to those induced by cold water tests. Specific tests include the following.

Caloric test for vestibular function. Cold or hot water is injected into the external auditory canal with the patient lying down and the head elevated at 30 degrees. The patient is observed for nystagmus.

Hallpike caloric test. Hot or cold water is injected into the external auditory canal. The time interval from the beginning of water flow to the end of visible nystagmus is recorded.

Nelson caloric test. Small amounts of ice water are injected into the external aural canal while the patient is in a supine position with the head tilted 30 degrees forward or in a sitting position with the head tilted 60 degrees backward. The patient is observed for nystagmus.

Indications. The caloric test indicates whether the labyrinth is reacting normally and is hypoactive or hyperactive, or whether no labyrinthine response is present[16]. In patients who complain of dizziness, vertigo, unsteadiness, or nystagmus, it is important to know whether the labyrinth is functioning normally.

Complications. None.

Nursing care. Maintain bed rest, with the head of the

bed elevated 20 to 30 degrees until subjective symptoms disappear. The patient is given nothing by mouth 6 hours before the procedure.

Specific Audiometric and Hearing Testing

Description. The following are some of the tests used to determine hearing loss.

Weber's test. The handle of a lightly vibrating tuning fork is placed in the middle of the forehead. Tones should normally be heard equally in both ears.

Rinne's test. The normal ear hears a tuning fork about twice as long by air conduction as by bone conduction, when a softly struck tuning fork is placed behind the ear on the mastoid process, and in front of the same ear.

Schwabach test. The examiner and patient hear tones equally when a tuning fork is alternately placed on the patient's and the examiner's mastoid processes.

Pure tone test. A series of tones is volume-calibrated at different frequencies (400 to 3000 Hz). The speech threshold represents the loudness at which a person with normal hearing can perceive a tone. Both air and bone conduction are measured for each ear, and the results are graphed. With normal hearing, the line is plotted at 0 dB.

Speech audiometry. A person with normal hearing hears and correctly repeats 95% of the words transmitted by the examiner.

Impedance audiometry. Disorders of the middle ear are detected, thereby determining the degree of tympanic membrane and middle ear mobility. An impedance audiometer is used. One end is a probe with three small tubes inserted into the external canal, and the other end attaches to an oscillator. One tube delivers a low tone of varying intensity, the second contains a microphone, and the third has an air pump. A normal tympanic membrane reflects minimal sound waves and produces a low-voltage curve on the graph.

Tympanometry. A tympanometer, with the impedance audiometer, measures the tympanic membrane's compliance with air pressure variations in the external canal and determines the degree of negative pressure in the middle ear.

In addition to these tests, patients may be tested to differentiate sensory (cochlear) hearing losses from neural (acoustic nerve) hearing losses. These tests include recruitment, sensitivity to small increases in intensity, and pathologic adaptation.

Recruitment is the ability to hear loud sounds normally despite a hearing loss or an abnormal increase in the perception of loudness. This is absent in neural hearing losses and present in sensory hearing losses. It can be demonstrated by having the patient compare the loudness of sounds in the affected ear with the loudness of sounds in the normal ear. In sensory hearing losses the sensation of loudness in the affected ear increases more with each increment in intensity than it does in the normal ear. In neural hearing losses the sensation of loudness in the affected ear increases less with each increment in intensity than it does in the normal ear. This is called *decruitment*.[16]

Sensitivity to small increments in intensity can be determined by having a patient listen to a continuous tone of 20 dB and then briefly and intermittently increasing the intensity. Patients with neural hearing losses, as well as those with normal hearing, cannot detect small changes in intensity. On the other hand, a patient with a sensory hearing loss can easily perceive these changes.

Pathologic adaptation, or tone decay, is found when a person cannot continue to hear a constant tone above the hearing threshold. The findings are mildly abnormal with sensory losses and severely abnormal with neural losses.

Indications. To diagnose hearing impairment.

Complications. None.

Nursing care. None.

Pulmonary Function Testing

Simple Spirometer

Description. The simple spirometer is a basic office tool used to measure the presence and severity of disease in large and small airways and to distinguish between obstructive and restrictive patterns. It is most commonly used to measure VC, IC, ERV, T_V, IRV, $FEF_{200\text{-}1200}$, and $FEF_{25\%\text{-}75\%}$. There are two types of spirometers: volume and flow. Both of these types are commonly computerized. Two of the most common are the water seal and dry rolling seal spirometers. The volume measurement spirometer is most common. This type works so that as the individual exhales or inhales into the mouthpiece, water or air already in the spirometer is displaced, causing the pen to touch the rotating drum and record the pattern. The presence and severity of respiratory dysfunction are determined by comparing observed values with those predicted for a normal person considering age, sex, height, weight, and race.

Spirometer with Gas Dilution

Description. The spirometer with gas dilution is used to measure the following:

FRC (functional residual capacity)
RV (residual volume)
RV/TLC ratio (residual volume/total lung capacity)
D_LCO (oxygen diffusing capacity of the lung)

The purpose of the technique is to measure the rate of diffusion. The measurement of lung volumes is by either the helium-dilution technique or the nitrogen-washout technique. In the *helium-dilution technique* the patient rebreathes a known concentration of diluted helium through the spirometer mouthpiece until the helium concentration in the spirometer and the patient's lungs are equal. The helium concentration in the spirometer and the volume of gas can then be used to calculate the patient's FRC. In the *nitrogen-washout technique* the patient breathes 100% O_2 from one source and exhales the expired gas into the spirometer.

Body Plethysmography

Description. Plethysmography is used to measure the following:

R_{aw} (airway resistance)
G_{aw} (airway conductance)
FRC (VTG = FRC shutter is closed at end of expiration)

The plethysmograph is an air-tight chamber in which the patient sits. The patient is seated in the air-tight chamber, is fitted with nose clips, and is instructed to breathe through the mouthpiece, which is connected to a transducer. To calculate VTG, the patient is instructed to pant into the mouthpiece while keeping the cheeks rigid and glottis open. This provides the pressure readings for the VTG calculator. The R_{aw} and G_{aw} may be mathematically calculated as the patient breathes rapidly and shallowly.

Pulmonary Function Tests*

Test	Description	Significance
Lung Volume Tests†		
VC = Vital capacity (VC = ERV + V_T + IRV)	This capacity test combining more than one lung volume is the maximum amount of air that can be expired slowly and completely following a maximum inspiration. Response values of this test, as well as all other pulmonary function tests, are directly dependent on patient's effort. From VC other pulmonary function values may be calculated, including ERV, IRV, V_T, and IC.	A decrease in VC may be caused by a loss of distensible lung tissue, as seen in bronchiolar obstruction, pulmonary edema, pneumonia, atelectasis, pulmonary restriction, surgery, pulmonary congestion, or by depression of the respiratory center in the brain.
FRC = Functional residual capacity (FRC = ERV + RV)	This capacity test combining more than one lung volume is the volume of air remaining in the lungs at the end of normal expiration. Open- or closed-circuit techniques of body plethysmography are used to measure concentrations of a gas (either helium or nitrogen); from this the FRC can be calculated. This is actually calculated measurement of airway resistance.	The values help to differentiate obstructive from restrictive diseases. An increased FRC represents hyperinflation, which is seen with bronchiolar obstruction, emphysema, or asthma. An increased FRC results in muscular and mechanical inefficiency. A decreased FRC may be seen in diseases that occlude the alveoli such as pneumonia, and in fibrosis, asbestosis, or silicosis.
ERV = Expiratory reserve volume	This single-volume calculation is the maximum amount of air that can be exhaled following a resting expiratory level.	Although the ERV (approximately 25% of VC) has no diagnostic value, it must be calculated so that the RV can be calculated.
IRV = Inspiratory reserve volume	This single-volume calculation is the maximum amount of air that can be inspired following a normal inspiration.	
RV = Residual volume (RV = FRC − ERV)	This single-volume measurement is the volume of air remaining in the lungs at the end of maximal expiration. This is measured indirectly by subtracting the ERV from the FRC.	This value helps to differentiate restrictive from obstructive diseases. An increased RV indicates that despite maximal expiratory effort the lungs still contain an abnormally large amount of air. This may be seen in patients with emphysema or chronic bronchial obstruction. The RV usually decreases with restrictive lung disease.
IC = Inspiratory capacity (IC = V_T + IRV)	This calculated measurement is a capacity test involving more than one lung volume. It is the largest volume of air that can be inspired in one breath from the resting expiratory level.	IC normally composes approximately 75% of the VC. Changes in the IC usually parallel increases or decreases in VC. Other than its use in postoperative care, this value is not commonly measured.
TLC = Total lung capacity (TLC = FRC + IC) or (TLC = VC + RV)	This capacity test combining more than one lung volume is the volume of air contained in the lung at the end of a maximal inspiration. The TLC is a derived calculation.	TLC differentiates obstructive from restrictive diseases. It may be decreased in pulmonary edema, atelectasis, neoplasms, pulmonary congestion, pneumothorax, or thoracic restriction. TLC may be increased in bronchiolar obstruction with hyperinflation and in emphysema.

*Normal values for pulmonary tests vary depending on the patient's age, sex, weight, and race.
†To best interpret these tests see Figures 5 and 6.

Figure 5 Lung volume measurements. All values are approximately 25% less in women. *TLC*, Total lung capacity; V_T, tidal volume; *FRC*, functional residual capacity; *IC*, inspiratory capacity; *IRV*, inspiratory reserve volume; *ERV*, expiratory reserve volume; *RV*, residual volume; *VC*, vital capacity.

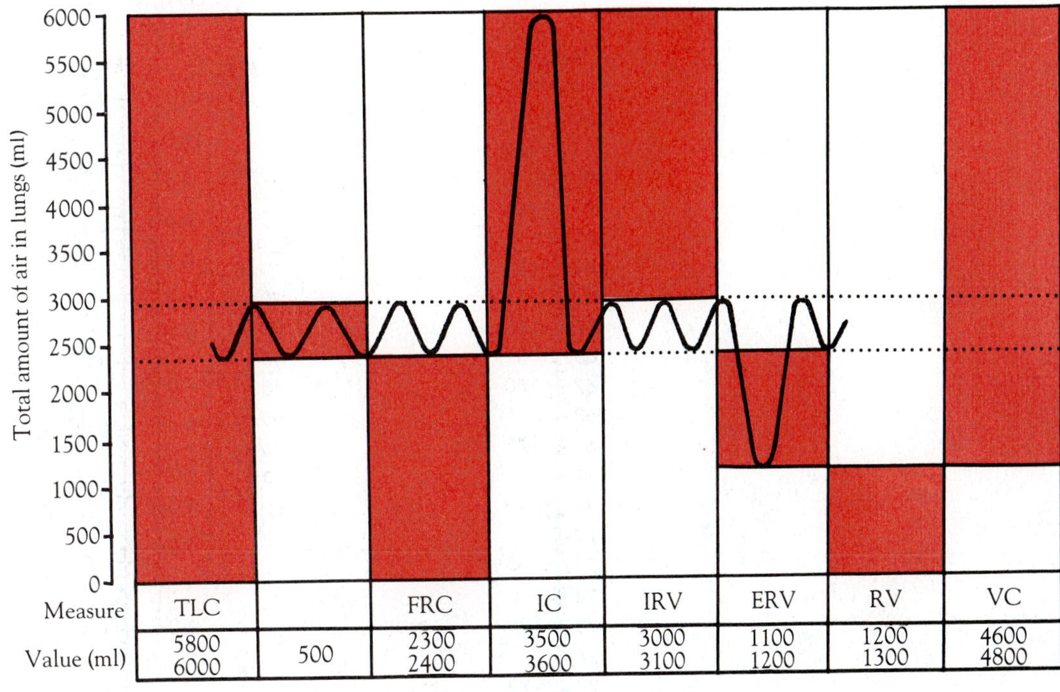

Measure	TLC		FRC	IC	IRV	ERV	RV	VC
Value (ml)	5800 6000	500	2300 2400	3500 3600	3000 3100	1100 1200	1200 1300	4600 4800

Test	Description	Significance
RV/TLC Ratio = Residual volume/Total lung capacity ratio (RV/TLC × 100)	This is a statement of the fraction of the TLC that can be defined as RV, expressed as a percentage.	Values greater than 35% are seen in patients with emphysema or chronic air trapping.
Ventilation Tests		
V_T = Tidal volume	This single-volume measurement is the volume of air inspired or expired during each respiratory cycle. This is measured at the bedside by a simple spirometer for 1 minute. The total is then divided by the rate (the number of breaths per minute) to determine the average V_T.	Decreased or increased V_T may occur in various pulmonary disorders. V_T should be considered in relation only to arterial blood gases and respiratory rate and minute volume.
V_E = Minute volume	This is the total volume of air inspired or expired in 1 minute. It is determined by measuring the inspired or expired air over several minutes and dividing by the number of minutes. It may also be measured easily at the bedside by simple spirometry.	This value must be considered in conjunction with arterial blood gases. V_E increases in response to hypoxia, hypercapnia, acidosis, and exercise. It is most commonly used in exercise testing.
V_D = Respiratory dead space	This is the volume of the lungs that is ventilated but not perfused by pulmonary capillary blood flow. This includes the conducting airways, or anatomic dead space, and the nonfunctioning alveoli, or alveolar dead space.	The measurement of V_D provides important information regarding the status of the functional lung capacity. It is used primarily for exercise testing.

Figure 6 Spirometric standards for males and females.
From Morris.[19]

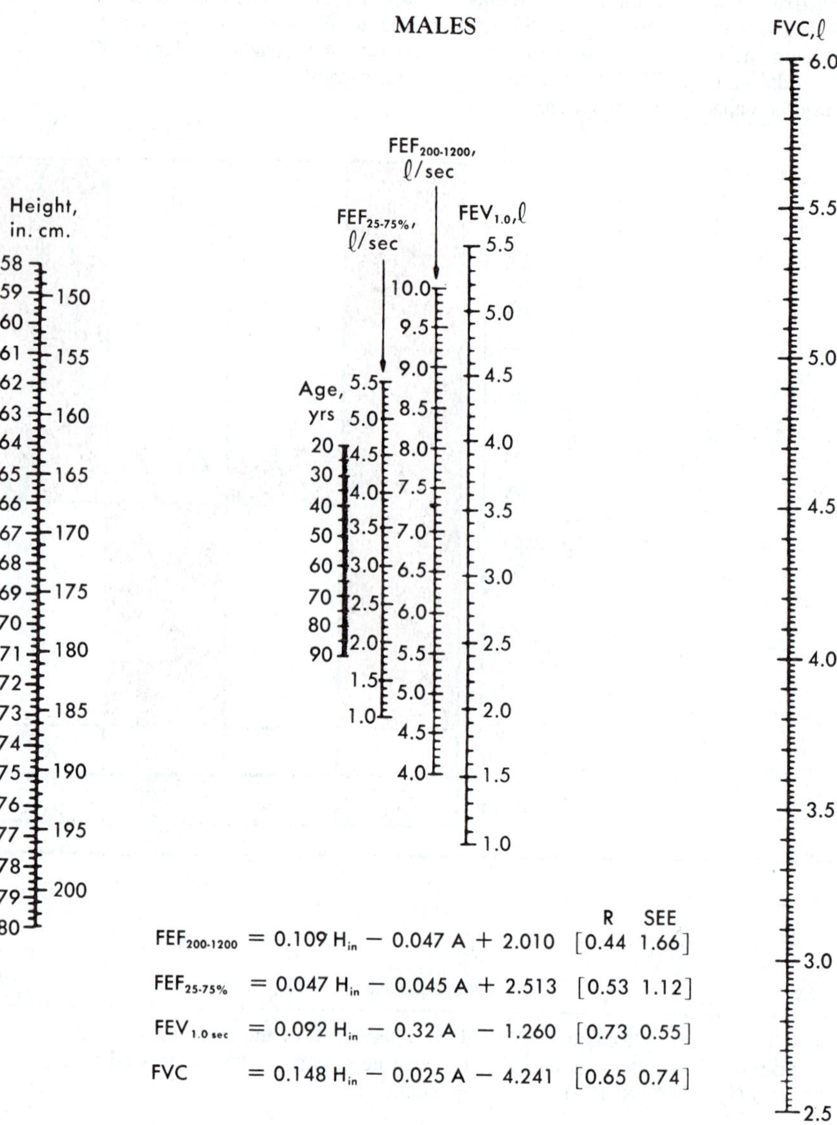

Test	Description	Significance
$\dot{V}_A$ = Alveolar ventilation $\dot{V}_A = (V_T - V_D)\,f$ f = respiratory rate	This is the volume of air that participates in gas exchange in the lungs.	The adequacy of $\dot{V}_A$ can be determined only by arterial blood gas studies. It is used primarily for exercise testing.
Pulmonary Spirometry Tests		
FVC = Forced vital capacity	This is the volume of air that can be expired forcefully and rapidly after maximal inspiration. The measurement is made directly by spirometer.	The FVC is normally equal to the VC. FVC may be reduced in chronic obstructive diseases, whereas the VC may appear close to normal. The FVC is decreased in restrictive diseases also. The test's validity depends largely on the individual's effort and cooperation.

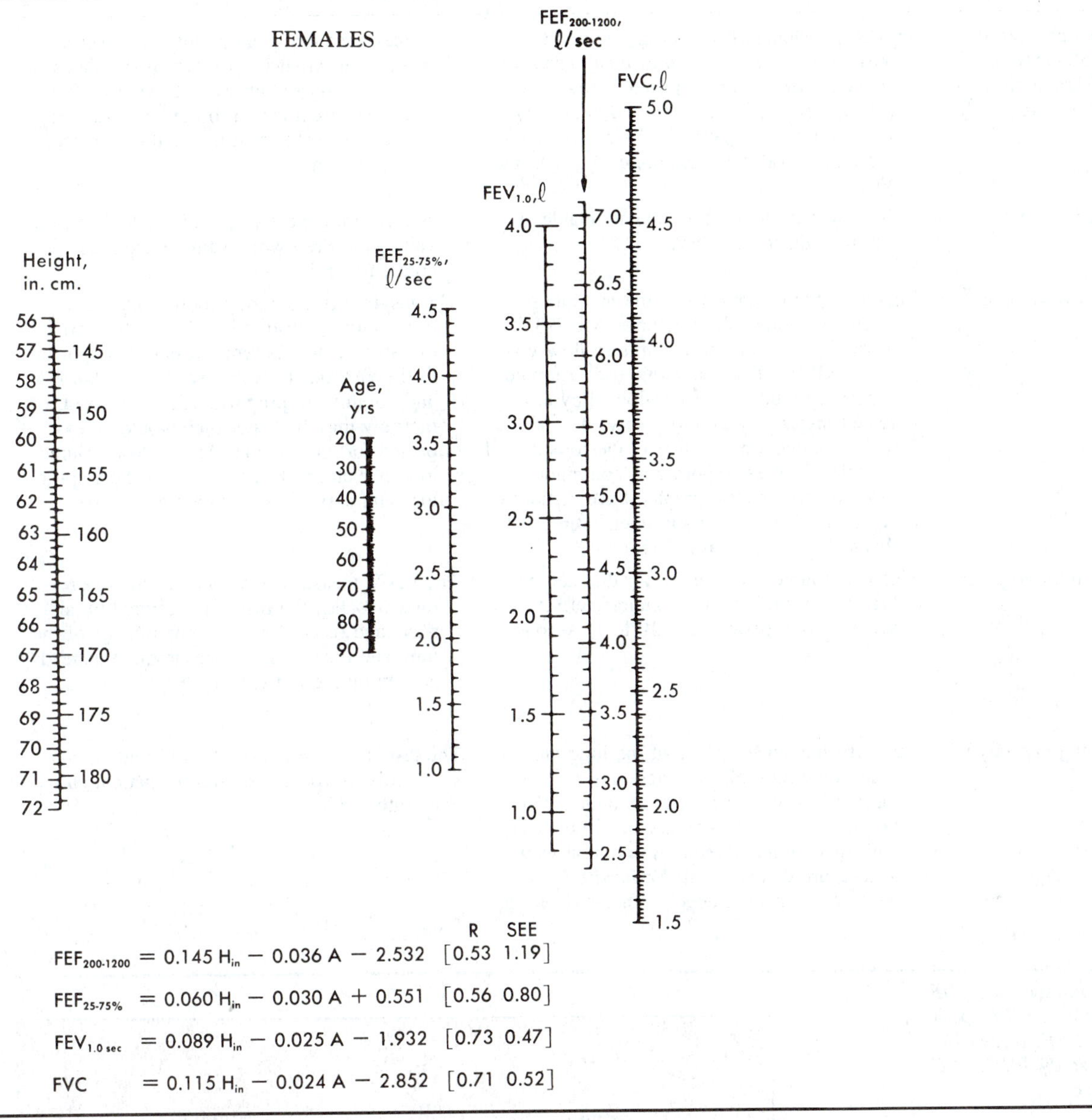

Test	Description	Significance
FEV_T = Forced expiratory volume timed	This is the volume of air expired over a given interval during the performance of an FVC. The interval (T) is stated as a subscript to FEV. For example, $FEV_{0.5}$ indicates the interval is 0.5 second, and in FEV_1 the interval is 1 second. FEV_T is a calculated measurement by spirometer. After 3 seconds, FEV should equal FVC.	FEV_T is the most common screening test for detection of obstructive airway disease, in which the finding is a reduced response.
FEV% = FEV_T/FVC ratio × 100 (usually FEV_1/FVC%)	This is the percentage of the measured FVC that a given FEV_T represents.	By measuring the expiratory flow over time the severity of obstruction can be assessed. FEV% or a reduced ratio is decreased in obstructive lung disease. It usually remains within normal limits for persons with restrictive disease unless there is some type of secondary problem.

Test	Description	Significance
$FEF_{25\%-75\%}$ = Forced expiratory flow, 25%-75% or MMEF = Maximum midexpiratory flow rate	This is the average flow during the middle 50% of an FEV. It was previously known as the maximum midexpiratory flow rate (MMEF or MMF). Its reported value provides a picture of peripheral airways resistance. This value is then compared with the VC.	This measures the average flow rate over a given interval. It is an index of the status of the medium-sized airways. Decreased flow rates, when compared to the VC, are seen in early stages of obstructive diseases such as emphysema.
PEFR = Peak flow	This is the maximum flow rate attainable at any time during an FEV.	This measurement is of questionable diagnostic value. Children with asthma have a decreased PEFR.
F-V loop = Flow-volume loop	This is a graphic analysis of the maximum forced expiratory flow volume (MEFV) followed by a maximum inspiratory flow volume (MIFV). This technique uses a forced expiratory vital capacity followed by a forced inspiratory vital capacity. It is actually another way to display the forced vital capacity. Curves, reported as continuous loops on spirometric graphs, have distinctive sizes and shapes. The spirometry report of this technique is seen in Figure 7.	The inspiratory flow may show evidence of upper airway obstruction. With obstructive disease the flow is reduced out of proportion to the volume. In restrictive disease the flow and volume are proportionally decreased, or the flow may be better than would be expected for the volume. As the flow-volume loop is examined, the shapes of the inspiratory and expiratory sides are analyzed.
MVV = Maximum voluntary ventilation	This is the largest volume of air that can be breathed per minute by voluntary effort. The actual testing period lasts 10 to 15 seconds.	The MVV measures the status of the respiratory muscles, the resistance offered by airways and tissues, and the compliance of the lung and thorax. This measurement depends greatly on the individual's effort.
Gas Exchange		
DL_{CO} = Diffusing capacity of CO	The diffusing capacity rate of the lung provides a measure of the lung's gas exchange mechanism. It assesses the amount of functioning pulmonary capillary bed in contact with functioning alveoli. A common way to measure this is the *single-breath Krogh method:* the patient deeply inhales (from the	The test is used primarily to differentiate various disease processes and for patient care monitoring.

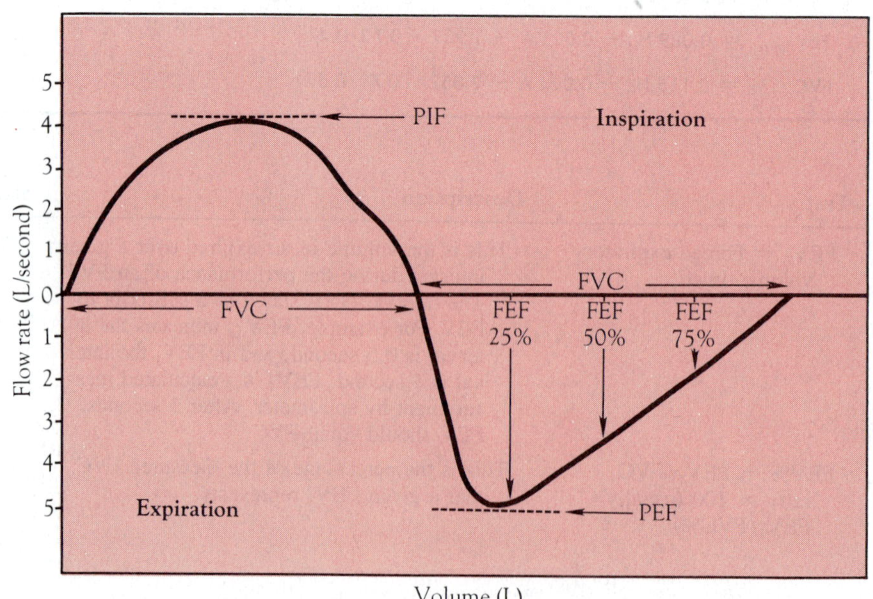

Figure 7 Flow-volume loop. *PIF,* Peak inspiratory flow; *PEF,* peak expiratory flow; *FEF,* forced expiratory flow at *x*% FVC; *FVC,* forced vital capacity.

Test	Description	Significance
	residual volume level) a mixture of air containing 0.3% carbon monoxide and 10% helium gas, holds his breath for 10 seconds, and then exhales. The carbon monoxide levels are then remeasured.	
R_{aw} = Airway resistance G_{aw} = Airway conductance	R_{aw} is the pressure difference required for a unit flow change. G_{aw} is the flow generated per unit of pressure drop in the airway. It is the reciprocal of R_{aw}. Measurements are made with a body plethysmograph. They are taken at the same time as FRC.	R_{aw} increases in an acute asthmatic attack, emphysema, or other obstructive diseases. The calculations are most useful in evaluation of the qualitative response to various bronchodilators.

Exercise Stress Test (EST)

Description. Examines cardiovascular response to exercise. It is also used to detect and quantify ischemic heart disease, to determine patients considered at risk, and to determine cardiovascular fitness preceding exercise programs. The test consists of raising, in gradual increments, the exercise level on a motorized treadmill while the ECG is being monitored. Blood pressure and heart electrical activity are also measured, and expired gases can be collected, O_2 consumption and saturation monitored, and samples collected for blood gas determinations. Key end points during exercise may define physiologically the causes of the patient's symptoms.

Indications. Differential diagnosis of chest pain; determination of workload level (exercise) when symptoms of ischemia occur; evaluation of therapy for angina; evaluation of patients who have multiple risk factors for coronary artery disease; evaluation of exercise-induced arrhythmias.

Complications. Recent myocardial infarction (4 to 6 weeks) (but such patients may perform submaximal EST before discharge from hospital); rapid ventricular or atrial arrhythmia; heart failure; severe aortic stenosis; blood pressure greater than 170/100 mm Hg before the onset of exercise; complete A-V block.

Nursing care. Explain the procedure, stressing the need for the patient to report any symptoms during and after the procedure. Instruct the patient to dress comfortably in shorts or gym clothes and tennis shoes. Instruct the patient not to eat for 1 hour before the test. During the procedure, monitor blood pressure, heart rate, ECG changes such as ST elevation or depression and arrhythmias. Observe for symptoms such as chest pain or pressure, shortness of breath, fatigue.

Esophageal Manometry

Description. Measures upper and lower esophageal sphincter pressure. A manometric catheter containing a small pressure transducer along its length is swallowed. Baseline measurements are taken, and then pressures are recorded before, during, and after swallowing. Peristaltic contractions are recorded.

Indications. Used to evaluate patients for achalasia, diffuse spasm of esophagus, and esophageal scleroderma.

Normal values are baseline pressure—20 mm Hg; relaxation pressure—18 mm Hg. Peristaltic pressure appears as a series of high-pressure peaks.

Complications. None.

Nursing care. Provide ice water for swallowing during the procedure.

Acid Perfusion Test (Bernstein Test)

Description. Evaluates esophageal mucosa. Two solutions (saline and acidic) are dripped through a nasogastric tube. The presence of pain with the acidic solution indicates esophagitis. This test is contraindicated in patients with esophageal varices, congestive heart failure, acute myocardial infarction, and other known cardiac disorders.

Indications. Patients with gastric reflux often have symptoms of epigastric or retrosternal pain that radiates to the back or arms. The test is used to distinguish between the chest pain of esophagitis and the chest pain of cardiac disorders.

Complications. None.

Nursing care. If the patient continues to complain of pain or burning after the test, antacids may help to relieve discomfort.

Esophageal Acidity Test (pH Monitoring)

Description. Evaluates competence of lower esophageal sphincter by measuring intraesophageal pH with an electrode attached to a manometric catheter.

Indications. Will indicate gastric reflux. Normal value: pH of esophagus is 6.0 or higher. The 24-hour monitoring involves the patient writing down all the activities performed during that period.

Complications. None.

Nursing care. Antacids, anticholinergics, cholinergics, adrenergic blockers, cimetidine, ranitidine, and reserpine should be withheld for 24 hours before the test. If these medications are not withheld, note this on the laboratory request sheet.

Papanicolaou Test (Pap Test)

Description. Simple smear method of examining exfoliative cells, particularly malignant and premalignant conditions of the cervix. Desquamated cells from the cervical epithelium are obtained during a pelvic examination, stained, and examined under a microscope. Histologic classification includes class I through class V.

Class I—normal cells
Class II—atypical cells

Class III—mild dysplasia
Class IV—severe dysplasia, suspicious cells
Class V—carcinoma cells

Indications. For routine gynecologic examination screening for malignant or premalignant conditions of the cervix.

Complications. None.

Nursing care. Prepare the patient for a vaginal examination and verify that the patient has not douched or inserted any vaginal medications for 24 hours before the procedure. Obtain an accurate history, including the date of the last Pap test and results; date of the last menstrual period (LMP); frequency and duration of periods; amount of bleeding with the periods; method of contraception; hormonal drugs; and presence and color of vaginal discharge, pain, or itching. Give the patient a perineal pad after the procedure to absorb any bleeding.

Tubal Insufflation (Rubin Test)

Description. Assesses patency of fallopian tubes by insufflation with carbon dioxide, which is introduced through tight-fitting cannula inserted through the cervical os at pressures up to 200 mm Hg. If the tubes are open, gas enters the abdominal cavity, and recorded pressure falls below 180 mm Hg. High-pitched bubbling can be heard through the abdominal wall with the stethoscope as gas escapes from the tubes. Shoulder pain from diaphragmatic irritation also indicates that gas has escaped into the abdominal cavity. Kymographic tracing shows pressure changes and may indicate tubal obstruction, spasm, or a leak in the system.

Indications. Inability to conceive.

Complications. None.

Nursing care. Be prepared to assist the patient with the cramping pain, dizziness, nausea, and vomiting that may occur after the procedure. Explain that shoulder pain (if present) is caused by an insufflation of gas and will subside.

Erectile Dysfunction Studies

Description and indications. Monitors nocturnal penile tumescence and snap-gauge devices are designed to determine whether cases of erectile dysfunction are caused by psychogenic or organic disease and to assess the efficiency of an erection. Endocrine disorders that may affect erectile activity are investigated by determining serum levels of FSH, LH, and testosterone and by physical examination. Vascular disorders are diagnosed via infusion cavernosgraphy, which reproduces an erection via mechanical means, or by vascular studies of the arterial or venous supplies of the penis—including internal pudendal arteriography, venography, or penile blood pressure or pulse volume assessment. Neurologic disorders that may contribute to erectile dysfunction are diagnosed by a variety of methodologies including physical examination, electromyography, nerve conduction, and evoked potential studies. The effect of drugs on erectile dysfunction may be determined by altering drug regimens and observing the effects on tumescence.

Complications. None.

Nursing care. None, except providing a supportive atmosphere.

References

1. Ballinger PW: Merrill's atlas of radiographic positions and radiologic procedures, ed 6, St Louis, 1985, The CV Mosby Co.
2. Bates B: A guide to physical assessment, ed 4, Philadelphia, 1987, JB Lippincott Co.
3. Davis JE and Mason CB: Neurologic critical care, New York, 1979, Van Nostrand Reinhold Co.
4. Emmett JL and Witten DM: Clinical urography, Philadelphia, 1971, WB Saunders Co.
5. Fishman AP, editor: Pulmonary diseases and disorders, New York, 1980, McGraw-Hill Book Co.
6. George RB, Light RW, and Matthay RA, editors: Chest physiology, New York, 1983, Churchill Livingstone.
7. Gray LP: Deviated nasal septum: incidence and etiology, Ann Otol Rhinol Laryngol (suppl 50):3, 1978.
8. Harrison JH et al: Campbell's urology, Philadelphia, 1978, WB Saunders Co.
9. Hickey J: The clinical practice of neurological and neurosurgical nursing, Philadelphia, 1981, JB Lippincott Co.
10. Hirsch J and Hannock L: Mosby's manual of clinical nursing procedures, St Louis, 1981, The CV Mosby Co.
11. Kelalis PP, King LR, and Belman AB: Clinical pediatric urology, Philadelphia, 1985, WB Saunders Co.
12. Kendall AR and Karafin R: Urology: Goldsmith's practice of surgery, Philadelphia, 1983, Harper & Row.
13. Kim MJ, McFarland GK, and McLane AM, editors: Pocket guide to nursing diagnoses, ed. 3, St Louis, 1989, The CV Mosby Co.
14. Kintzel K, editor: Advanced concepts in clinical nursing, ed 2, Philadelphia, 1977, JB Lippincott Co.
15. Lerner J and Khan Z: Manual of urologic nursing, St Louis, 1982, The CV Mosby Co.
16. Maran AGD and Stell PM, editors: Clinical otolaryngology, Oxford, Eng, 1979, Blackwell Scientific Publications, Inc.
17. Merritt HH: A textbook of neurology, ed 6, Philadelphia, 1979, Lea & Febiger.
18. Miller LG and Kazemi H: Manual of clinical pulmonary medicine, New York, 1983, McGraw-Hill Book Co.
19. Morris JF, Roski WA, and Johnson LC: Spirometric standards for healthy nonsmoking adults, Am Rev Respir Dis 103:57, 1971.
20. Newell FM: Ophthalmology: principles and concepts, ed 6, St Louis, 1986, The CV Mosby Co.
21. Pfister RC, Newhouse JH, and Hendren WH: Percutaneous pyeloureteral urodynamics, Urol Clin North Am 9:41, 1982.
22. Robinson S and Russo P, editors: Providing respiratory care: nursing photobook, Springhouse, Pa, 1979, Intermed Communications.
23. Rokosky JS: Assessment of altered respiratory function, Nurs Clin North Am 16:198, 1981.
24. Saunderson RG and Kurth CC: The cardiac patient, ed 2, Philadelphia, 1983, WB Saunders Co.
25. Seidel HM et al: Mosby's guide to physical examination, St Louis, 1987, The CV Mosby Co.
26. Thorn GW et al, editors: Harrison's principles of internal medicine, ed 8, New York, 1977, McGraw-Hill Book Co.
27. Tilkian SM, Conover MB, and Tilkian AG: Clinical implications of laboratory tests, St Louis, 1987, The CV Mosby Co.
28. Tucker SM et al: Patient care standards, ed 4, St Louis, 1988, The CV Mosby Co.
29. Urdang L, editor: Mosby's medical and nursing dictionary, ed 2, St Louis, 1987, The CV Mosby Co.
30. Whitaker R: Clinical application of upper tract urodynamics, Urol Clin North Am 6:137, 1979.
31. Williams ID and Johnston JH: Paediatric urology, London, 1982, Butterworth & Co.
32. Yousmans JR, editor: Neurological surgery, vol 6, Philadelphia, 1982, WB Saunders Co.

PART THREE

Nursing Diagnoses

FUNCTIONAL HEALTH PATTERN

I

Health Perception–Health Management

 Altered Health Maintenance

Altered health maintenance is the inability to identify, manage, and/or seek out help to maintain health.

Altered health maintenance can be caused by a variety of physical, psychologic, social, and situational factors.[16,18] This nursing diagnosis is encountered in persons with mental retardation,[17] chemical addiction, emotional disorders, inadequate finances, inadequate information, and in persons consciously choosing not to engage in primary health prevention.

The 1980 ANA Social Policy Statement[2] clearly identified health maintenance as a responsibility of the nursing profession. This responsibility affects every nurse-patient encounter. As such, the nursing diagnosis Altered Health Maintenance transcends disease-related categories and requires development by nurses in all facets of nursing practice. A listing of the related factors and defining characteristics currently developed for the nursing diagnosis Altered Health Maintenance is presented below. The related factors have been clustered into categories, and defining characteristics are listed for each general category. Since the diagnosis encompasses such an extensive population, the remainder of this chapter focuses on a specific related factor: failure to assume responsibility for primary prevention.

Related Factors

- Alteration in cognitive ability (pathologic causes)
  - Lack of or significant alteration in communication skills
  - Lack of ability to make deliberate and thoughtful judgments
  - Perceptual/cognitive impairment
  - Complete or partial lack of gross and/or fine motor skills
  - Ineffective individual coping
  - Unachieved developmental task
  - Ineffective family coping[18]
- Alteration in cognitive ability (addictive behaviors)
  - Perceptual/cognitive impairment related to alcohol and/or drugs
- Inadequate resources
  - Inadequate finances
  - Inadequate or limited insurance
  - Inadequate material resources
- Inadequate information
  - Inadequate knowledge
- Emotional difficulties
  - Dysfunctional grieving
  - Ineffective coping
  - Depression
- Failure to assume responsibility for primary prevention
  - Conflicting information
  - Inadequate time and energy
  - Health beliefs and motives inconsistent with desired behavior
  - Lack of personal autonomy
  - Inaccessibility of information and services
  - Desired behavior poses conflict with social norms
  - Value conflict

Defining Characteristics

- Lack of knowledge regarding basic health practices
- Lack of adaptive behaviors to internal/external environmental changes

Inability to take responsibility for meeting basic health practices
Lack of health-seeking behavior
Lack of expressed patient interest in improving health behaviors
Impaired personal support system

Need for alcohol or drugs directing behavior

Lack of equipment, financial, and/or other resources

Unable to answer questions correctly
Verbalizes inaccurate information

Verbalizes discrepancies in content from different informational sources
Illiteracy
Does not have access to or use television, radio, or newspaper

Diet high in saturated fats and cholesterol
Diet high in salt
Diet low in fiber
Lack of regular exercise
Obesity
Cigarette smoking
Failure to manage stress
Failure to have periodic medical examinations

Nursing Interventions[1,7,15,19-23]

Patient Goal	Nursing Intervention
General Public	
Receive consistent, accurate information.	• Use mass media, printed material, closed-circuit television, and teaching methods requiring patient interaction. • Provide positive reinforcement.
Assume responsibility for primary health maintenance.	• Provide information. • Use problem-solving techniques. • Use assertiveness training. • Help clarify values* and establish personal health goals.
High-Risk Individuals	
Use behavior modification techniques.	• Use self-monitoring,* guided practice and reinforcement, contracting,* cuing,* and tailoring.* • Help establish patterns of environmental control.
Use cognitive restructuring.	• Encourage positive self-control of preferences.* • Use relaxation training, biofeedback, meditation, imagery, and thought-stopping.*
Use support systems.	• Encourage participation in reference groups.* • Provide information on community resources. • Use small group discussion and support groups.*

*These nursing interventions are discussed in the section on noncompliance.

Principles and Rationale for Nursing Interventions

A sick role implies certain rights and obligations that can be briefly summed up[14]:

1. Sick persons are exempt from certain social responsibilities.
2. They cannot be expected to take care of themselves.
3. They should want and do everything to get well.
4. They should seek medical advice and cooperate with medical experts.

This concept of sick-role behavior provides a description of the role assumed during an acute period of illness and, with minor modification, chronic illness. The concept does not adequately explain the behavior of persons who are at risk of developing an illness. Baric[4] compared and contrasted the concept of sick-role behavior to the at-risk role (Table 1).

The primary goal for an individual with altered health maintenance is to establish behavior patterns that maintain health. Nursing interventions are designed to provide large numbers of individuals with a cue or message identifying the behaviors necessary to maintain health and to provide individuals at high risk with the specific information on how to modify the behavior.

Messages appropriate for the general public need to be kept simple, identifying a global theme while avoiding complex, specific behavior.[12,13] Some evidence supports increased effectiveness of the message with professional reinforcement.

Primary prevention is the responsibility of the "healthy individual" who generally has limited contact with the health care system. A large percentage of health information is acquired from mass media, sources known for persuasive messages, fictionalization, and opinion. Personal encounters with a health care professional may take place, but they are infrequent, irregular, and generally during an acute health crisis. Receptiveness to information not directly related to the acute crisis is limited.

Table 1
Comparison of Sick Role and At-Risk Role

Sick Role	At-Risk Role
1. Duties—must want to get well, try to get well, and seek and follow medical advice. Advantages—exempt from social responsibilities; it is legitimate to expect help from others.	1. Duties—must continue to fulfill social obligations; must change some existing behavior without help or social recognition.
2. Sick role is legitimized by society.	2. At-risk role is not formally recognized by society; behavior change depends on the individual.
3. Payoff (return to usual role) will occur in limited time.	3. Payoff (possibility of avoiding or minimizing disease) in distant future and often unrecognized.
4. Positive reinforcement for sick role behaviors.	4. New behavior not formally reinforced by medical profession or society; rather, society is a continual source of stimuli to revert to prior behavior.
5. Symptoms decrease with sick-role behaviors.	5. Symptomless—relies on abstract beliefs or statistical probability.
6. Person not held responsible for illness.	6. Person held responsible for behavior.

Modified from Baric, L: Recognition of the "at-risk" role: a means to influence health behavior, 1969, International Seminar on Health Education, 1970, Hamburg, Federal Republic of Germany.

Nursing interventions to assist the general public in health maintenance should communicate clear, concise, and meaningful information. In addition, positive reinforcement of health information by a nurse validates the significance of the health message. Such positive reinforcement could occur during routine activities, such as contact with visitors by nurses in acute care facilities, with families by nurses in home health care agencies,[9] at work and school settings by occupational and school health nurses, and by professionals speaking to lay groups.

In addition to providing information and positive reinforcement, nurses can identify persons at high risk for specific diseases.[3] For example, persons who smoke are at high risk for developing both cancer and heart disease. These high-risk individuals require general information and information related to methods of behavioral alteration. Specifically, they would benefit from learning behavior modification and cognitive restructuring techniques. They need encouragement and assistance to strengthen their social support. Persons with altered health maintenance and those with noncompliance require changes in their behavior. Many of the nursing interventions listed are discussed in the section on noncompliance (specify) and are so indicated.

Evaluation

Patient Outcome	Data Indicating That Outcome is Reached
Responsible for health maintenance	Personal health goals identified Appropriate decisions Problem-solving strategies Desired health goals attained
Controls antecedents and consequences of targeted behavior	Behavior modification techniques used Specific behavior plan to alter targeted behavior Multiple personal reinforcers identified
Controls thoughts related to targeted behavior	Cognitive restructuring technique Personal preference in relaxation techniques identified
Uses social support and alternative resources	Community resources used Sources of long-term support identified

Noncompliance (Specify)

Noncompliance is a person's informed decision not to adhere to a therapeutic recommendation.

The health belief model has been demonstrated to have a statistically significant relationship with compliance and has been very popular, both clinically and in research. The health belief model[18,22,23] is based on the patient's perceptions rather than those of the health care professional. This model assumes that an individual will cognitively decide to choose a goal based on the attractiveness of the goal to the individual, the patient's estimation of his ability to attain the goal, and the occurrence of a cue. Basically, the health belief model states that motivation = reward − (perceived cost + barriers). The health belief model has several components: motivation, value of illness threat reduction, probability of threat reduction, and modifying and enabling factors. However, the health belief model does not appear to be predictive of compliance.[18] That is, the measured beliefs do not always precede the behavior, but rather behavior can be changed before a change in beliefs.

Much has also been learned about compliance by observing the effects of different approaches to the treatment of noncompliance. For instance, Sackett and Haynes[37] found behavioral approaches to the management of noncompliance more effective than patient education, increasing convenience, and reducing the expense of treatment. They reported increased compliance with the use of the behavioral methods of self-monitoring, tailoring, and reinforcement. Another behavioral approach rigorously tested is contracting, or a systematic arrangement for granting a reward in return for performance of a specific behavior. Steckel[41] has clearly identified the efficacy of contracting in altering the compliance of patients with hypertension, diabetes, and arthritis.

Related Factors

Alteration in cognition*
- Inadequate knowledge
- Alteration in thought process[13,46]
- Inability to read or write
- Sensory deficits

Alteration in perception[5]
- Inadequate motivation
- Alteration in affective state[3,8,47]
- Conflict to value system[10]
- Belief in therapy but inability to change behavior[43]

Inadequacies in social system
- Inadequate social support[13,14]
- Inadequate resources[9,18]

Deficits in health care system
- Complexity of regimen[7,39]
- System inadequacy[13]
- Nontherapeutic relationship with health care professional[11,13,20]

*References 3, 18, 28, 33, 40, 42.

Defining Characteristics

Behavior indicative of failure to adhere by direct observation or statements by patient or significant others
Objective tests (physiologic measures, detection of markers)
Evidence of development of complications
Evidence of exacerbation of symptoms
Failure to keep appointments
Failure to progress
Inability to set or attain mutual goals

Has never been taught
Unable to answer questions accurately
States, "I don't know"
Does not want information
Makes inaccurate statements
Holds myths and fantasies to be true
Information has not been updated by new knowledge

Disturbance in recent or remote memory
Inability to solve problems
Inability to concentrate
Inability to follow directions
Presence of psychopathology

Illiteracy
Neuromuscular deficits

Hearing deficit
Visual deficit

Does not perceive illness or risk to be serious
Does not feel susceptible to the risk or effects of the illness
Does not feel vulnerable in terms of the risk
Does not believe in the efficacy of therapy
Prefers illness to treatment
Cultural beliefs are opposed to prescribed regimen

Behavioral denial
Verbal denial
Depression
Anger
Fear and anxiety

Agrees that behavior is desirable but "not for me" or "not now"
Identifies desired behavior as being of low priority

History of making behavior change but returning to undesirable behavior
Has made repeated attempts to do something but cannot

Significant other does not:
1. Possess accurate information
2. Believe in the efficacy of therapy
3. Have the necessary time, energy, or resources
4. Perceive support of the health care regimen as part of his role responsibilities

Failure of social systems to provide necessary support

Financial difficulty
Lack of personal energy
Inadequate transportation
Lack of proper material or equipment

Patient perceives regimen as too complex
Therapy effective for one health problem is contraindicated for coexisting health problem

Complaints of failure to provide specific and comprehensive information
Failure of individual members of the health care team to endorse behavioral change
Failure of the system to provide:

1. Accurate feedback
2. Adequate follow-up referral
3. Specifics on how to make a behavioral change

Verbalizes dissatisfaction with the professional
Inconsistent caregivers

Nursing Interventions

Patient Goal	Nursing Intervention
Alteration in Cognition	
Demonstrate accurate performance of specific health-related behavior.	• Offer patient education, accommodating for personality characteristics, coping styles,[26,27] and locus of control.[24,35,45] • Engage in discussion. • Correct patient misconceptions. • Provide reminders. • Encourage self-monitoring. • Help the person use a structured method of remembering and performing routine aspects of the therapeutic regimen (a fishing tackle box to set up medications). • Teach problem-solving skills. • Help the patient use resources appropriately (Meals on Wheels). • Provide information in multiple forms (written, audiotapes, pictures). • Ensure printed material is at appropriate reading level.
Alteration in Perception	
Engage in behaviors consistent with goals of therapeutic regimen.	• Engage in discussion groups. • Inform about reference groups.[4,16,17,31] • Participate in values clarification techniques. • Use reminders. • Provide cues. • Use prompts. • Encourage self-monitoring. • Use applied analysis of behavior. • Use framing. • Assist with shaping behavior.
Inadequacies in Social System	
Use alternative sources of social support. Engage in activities to strengthen and/or maintain coping ability.	• Provide alternative sources of support and resources. • Offer assertiveness training. • Involve appropriate social support. • Encourage participation in reference group. • Use problem solving. • Assist with goal setting. • Use imagery. • Use relaxation therapies. • Use thought-stopping.
Deficits in Health Care System	
Report that the health care system recognizes and provides for individual needs and abilities.	• Use foot-in-the-door strategy. • Demonstrate graduated regimen. • Use tailoring. • Use self-monitoring. • Provide opportunities for negotiation. • Use reinforcement. • Use contracting. • Simplify the regimen. • Provide referral.

Principles and Rationale for Nursing Interventions

Comprehensive Program

A. Organizational components
   1. Consistent care
   2. Appointment times
   3. Waiting time
   4. Reminders
   5. Allied health workers
B. Educational components
   1. Methods
      a. Individual instruction
      b. Lecture
      c. Programmed learning
      d. Skill development
      e. Simulation and games
      f. Inquiry learning
      g. Audiovisual modalities
   2. Process[6]
      a. Repetition
      b. Primacy
      c. Organization
      d. Specificity
      e. Brevity
      f. Readability
C. Behavioral techniques
   1. Cues
   2. Reminders
   3. Self-monitoring
   4. Applied analysis of behavior
D. Cognitive restructuring
   1. Assertiveness training
   2. Problem solving
   3. Thought-stopping
E. Maintenance
   1. Stress reduction
   2. Regular exercise
   3. Involvement of significant others

Sequencing of Strategies

Sequencing of strategies is intended to maximize the impact of the professional in the minimum time necessary to attain compliance. Once the diagnosis of noncompliance has been made, strategies can be sequenced from the easiest to the more complex.[37] Easily adjusted factors include attention and supervision (i.e., increasing the length of the visit or decreasing the interval between appointments), modification of the regimen (see discussion on tailoring), and use of allied health members. If noncompliance continues to be a problem, the behavioral and cognitive strategies should be enforced.

Values clarification. "Values clarification is the process of examining alternatives and deciding what is important to you."[44] It is a process that assists an individual to increase consistency between beliefs and actions. The following steps or tasks are necessary to the process of values clarification[34]:

1. Choosing freely
2. Choosing from alternatives
3. Choosing after consideration of the consequences
4. Prizing and cherishing
5. Publicly affirming
6. Acting on one's choice
7. Acting repetitively and with consistency

Numerous tools enable a patient to progress through the process as outlined. An example of a values clarification technique is the "pie of life." A patient is asked to cut a pie (circle) into slices that represent his current activity. He is then asked to slice a second pie into slices representing what he would really like to be doing. As differences in the circles become apparent, the patient is able to clearly see the discrepancy between doing and believing. The patient is ready to begin work on decreasing the differences between what is actually occurring and what he wants to occur.

The purpose of values clarification is to provide the patient with an experience that allows him to explore beliefs about a specific aspect of his life. Once the patient has been helped to identify the discrepancies between intellectual beliefs and actual behavior, he will be better able to make a choice about future behavior.

Reminder, prompts, cue. A reminder[13,15,25,29] is a stimulus that serves as the antecedent for a desired behavior. A variety of reminders have been successfully used to improve compliance. Written reminders, as well as telephone calls, serve equally well as appointment reminders. Medication reminders, calendars, reminder systems, and special packaging have all been shown to be effective.

Reminders are most effective for problems of forgetting. Their effectiveness decreases rapidly over a short time, and some evidence suggests that a combination of reminders even further increases the effectiveness of this technique.

Self-monitoring. Self-monitoring is the process of recording one's own behavior to allow specific behavioral patterns to become observable.[13,31] Behavioral patterns can effectively be identified by recording the specific behavior (smoking, overeating) in relation to specific variables (time, environment, persons). Through discussion the professional can guide the patient to identify the antecedents and consequences of the behavior (e.g., nibbling was at its height when dinner was late, the children were noisy, and the individual was hungry). Behavior can be changed by identifying alternatives to the identified antecedents and consequences. Planning with the patient to change conditions that are associated with the behavior changes the antecedents to the behavior and therefore the behavior. Self-monitoring identifies the when, where, how, and frequency of a behavior.

Various authors have pointed out that behavior changes, once recording or observation starts (even before any deliberate change has been planned), and that the benefits of self-monitoring are self-limiting (i.e., they do not continue much beyond the period of recording). Some evidence also suggests that observing one's behavior rather than an outcome is more effective in achieving compliance (e.g., eating behaviors rather than weight change).

Applied analysis of behavior. Applied analysis of behavior[2] is the combination of self-recording, functional analysis, and tailoring. Applied analysis of behavior is a five-step process:

1. Identify target behavior.
2. Patient records the behavior.
3. Patient learns pattern identification and explores feelings, perceptions, and barriers.
4. Alternative behaviors are developed as a result of the analysis.
5. Effectiveness of alternatives is evaluated, and they are locked into place.

This behavioral technique has been recommended in particular for increasing medication compliance.

Thought-stopping. "Thought-stopping or covert assertion is a cognitive technique in which the client deliberately and consciously develops a method to reduce or obliterate negative, unproductive thoughts that can lead to unwanted emotions and a perception of helplessness."[12] Thought-stopping is a five-step process:

1. Stressful thoughts are identified in terms of their frequency and effect on the patient.
2. The stressful thought is imagined.
3. Deliberate interruption of the thought occurs.
4. Alternative behaviors are developed as a result of the analysis.
5. Effectiveness of alternatives is evaluated, and they are locked into place.

To demonstrate the impact of this cognitive technique on compliance, consider the following example: "I just can't make it without a cigarette." The thought itself is a cue to the behavior of smoking. Deliberately blocking that thought and replacing it with an alternate thought changes the antecedent or cue to the behavior. "I am really proud of myself. I find deep breathing much more relaxing than a cigarette."

Tailoring. Tailoring[18] is the process of fitting the prescribed regimen and intervention strategies to an individual's life-style, value system, and circumstances (e.g., the modification of a standard 2 g sodium diet to include particular favorites). Modification of this kind decreases the life-style changes being requested of the patient and demonstrates to the patient that his needs are recognized and that compromise is possible.

Graduated regimen implementation. Graduated regimen implementation,[13,32] or shaping, is the process of introducing components of the regimen sequentially as the patient successfully masters prior steps in the sequence. The steps are graded in order of difficulty to the patient. This technique is helpful for a patient who is overwhelmed or has had an experience with a regimen and "just can't do it."

Contracting. "Contract is a systematic arrangement for granting a reward in return for performance of a specific behavior."[41] A contract has three elements:

1. The desired behavior
2. The consequences of a behavior (reward)
3. Identification of roles

A contract does not challenge an individual to live up to its terms but rather is made knowing that the patient will be successful in meeting its terms. A contract can be written or verbal; however, there is evidence that the written contract has a higher success rate in terms of increasing compliance.*

Foot-in-the-door is a strategy borrowed from marketing in which the patient is asked to participate in some aspect of the therapy that she "can't" refuse, such as a request to read a one-page brochure or acceptance of a telephone call by a nurse 1 week following their initial contact. This continual contact keeps the individual in touch with the health care system, and other innocuous changes can gradually be introduced without alienating the patient.

*References 2, 8, 13, 19, 41, 43.

Evaluation[13,30]

Patient Outcome	Data Indicating That Outcome is Reached
Accurate performance of specific health-related behavior	Accurate knowledge of specific health-related behavior Verbalization, in concrete terms, of plan to carry out desired health-related behavior Verbalization of errors or misconceptions in prior thoughts and/or behavior Ability to compensate for problems with memory, vision, and/or hearing by using alternative materials or resources
Behaviors consistent with goals of therapeutic regimen	Active participation in therapy Freedom to express feelings and beliefs Goals and priorities consistent with therapeutic regimen
Uses alternative resources and social support	Through discussion, identification of help obtained from alternative sources of support Verbalization of behavioral plan to deal with social situation that opposes therapeutic regimen
Engages in activities to strengthen and/or maintain coping ability	Use of specific cognitive therapy and identification of times when it was effective and times when it was not Requests for more information related to specific therapy
Reports that health care system recognizes and provides for individual needs and abilities	Use of available resources Acceptance of referral Active contribution to establishment of goals, priorities, and methods of evaluation Positive intention Noncompliance reported, with the expectation of further negotiation or assistance

 Potential for Infection

Potential for infection is the state in which an individual is at increased risk for being invaded by pathogenic organisms.

The risk of infection can be present because of the state of the individual's resistance to potentially invading environmental or normal flora organisms and because of increased exposure to pathogens in the environment.

Because of the nature of this nursing diagnosis, it can be applied to more than one individual at a time. For example, persons who have a potential for infection may be close personal contacts of an infected person, the health care professionals caring for infected individuals, an entire patient care unit, a classroom, a workforce, or a geographic community.

Risk Factors[2,4,5,14-19]

Pathophysiologic

Inadequate primary defenses
- Broken or burned skin
- Traumatized tissue
- Decreased ciliary action
- Stasis of body fluids
- Decreased secretions or changes in pH of secretions
- Altered enzyme activity
- Altered peristalsis
- Altered cough, blink, or sneeze reflex
- Alterations in protective normal flora organisms

Inadequate secondary defenses
- Decreased hemoglobin
- Leukopenia
- Suppressed inflammatory response
- Immunosuppression
- Agranulocytosis
- Dysfunction of the thymus and lymphatic system

Inadequate acquired immunity
Tissue destruction caused by existing infectious process, altered circulation, or trauma
Chronic disease
Malnutrition
Premature rupture of amniotic membranes
Spinal cord injury
Loss of consciousness
Impaired oxygenation

Treatment Related

Invasive procedures: surgery, catheterization, IV monitoring or fluid administration
Infusions of blood and fluids
Pharmaceutical agents
Inadequate or prolonged use of antibiotics
Forced immobility
Contaminated equipment associated with respiratory therapy
Artificial rupture of amniotic membranes
Fetal monitoring
Immunosuppression
NPO orders
Radiation therapy
Dialysis
Chemotherapy
Organ transplant

Developmental

Age (infancy, childhood, older ages)
Menarche, childbearing, menopause

Situational (Personal)

IV drug abuse
Unsafe sexual practices
Postpartum period
Inadequate knowledge to avoid exposure to pathogens
Poor hygiene practices
Inadequate food and fluid intake
Bites (animal, insect, human)
Stress
Inadequate clothing, shelter
Smoking practices

Situational (Environmental)

Increased environmental exposure to pathogens resulting from occupation or living situation
Increase of pathogens in the environment; contamination of food, water, hard surfaces, or any vector for transmission
Inadequate control of vectors in the environment
Inadequate sanitation and control of sewage and solid wastes
Behaviors of others in the environment that increase the risk for transmission of the pathogens
Inadequate community immunization levels

Defining Characteristics[2,4,15-18]

Because this diagnosis reflects a condition of being at increased risk for infection, all the previously listed risk factors are also defining characteristics. That is, the characteristics that must be present for the diagnosis of "potential for infection" are the risk factors. For example, the individual receiving an invasive procedure or who has been pharmacologically immunosuppressed or has been exposed to trauma has the potential for infection. Combinations of the risk factors are also likely to increase the potential.

In addition, certain observable characteristics identify the actual presence of pathogens in an individual or identify the individual's response to the pathogen. These represent defining characteristics of potential for infection for patient's contacts. These include:

- Detection of viable pathogens or their eggs in body secretions, excretions, or exudates (urine, feces, blood, mucous secretions, mucous membrane or dermal lesion exudates, semen, gastric contents, cerebrospinal fluid)
- Systemic responses suggesting infection with a pathogen
  - Elevated body temperature
  - Leukocytosis
  - Increase in serum antibodies

Nursing Interventions

Patient Goal	Nursing Intervention
Individual in the community will experience no infection.	• Assess for the presence of risk factors (primarily developmental and situational). • Ensure adequate immunization of individuals of all ages. • Teach family how to maintain adequate nutrition, hydration, rest, and hygiene. • Educate about proper use of antibiotics and other anti-infective agents. • Educate about proper personal and environmental hygiene. • Educate how to protect from infected vectors in the environment. • Educate regarding safe sexual practices. • Educate regarding the hazards of sharing needles. • Educate regarding safe food-handling practices.
Hospitalized patient will experience no infection.	• Assess for the presence of risk factors (pathophysiologic and treatment related). • Obtain cultures as ordered and report results. • Assess vital signs and body secretions, excretions, and exudates for signs of infection; report abnormalities. • Monitor hydration and electrolyte balance. • Monitor changes in WBC count. • Observe for signs of superinfection in patients receiving antimicrobial therapy. • Avoid invasive procedures if possible. • Use strict aseptic technique when performing invasive procedures. • Discontinue invasive lines as soon as possible. • Wear gloves when handling infective secretions, excretions, and exudates and when drawing blood. • Wash hands before and after contact with patient. • Prevent patient's exposure to infected visitors or staff. • Use isolation procedures as indicated (see Chapter 13). • Turn patient frequently; instruct in deep breathing and provide skin care for immobilized, bed-bound, or postsurgical patients. • Follow recommendations for prevention of nosocomial infections as described in Chapter 13. • Ensure that staff members caring for patient do not work when they have an infectious disease. • Provide for patient's discharge as soon as possible to minimize risk of colonization of pathogens from hospital environment.
Infection will not be transmitted to patient's contacts.	• Initiate universal blood and body secretion precautions and other procedures as indicated (see isolation procedures in Chapter 13). • Detect and report new infections as early as possible so that treatment and isolation may be initiated. • Dispose of contaminated equipment, body fluids, and dressings as required. • Report to the local health authority those infections that must be reported by law (see Chapter 13). • Participate in follow-up of patient contacts if necessary to ensure that they are examined and treated. • Protect pregnant nursing personnel from contact with selected infections (rubella, cytomegalovirus, toxoplasmosis, herpes). • Ensure that high-risk patient care staff have been immunized against hepatitis B virus (see Chapter 13). • Educate patient, family, community groups, and patient care staff about importance of handwashing, environmental hygiene, and other personal behaviors to prevent spread of pathogens. • Participate in community immunization programs to provide immunizations to high-risk populations (see Chapter 13). • Educate pregnant women to prevent or seek early treatment for infections that can be transmitted to the fetus. • Participate in public education programs regarding safer sexual practices. • Participate in providing community education programs for safe food handling, water purification, and avoidance of vectors that normally carry pathogens. • Support public health programs aimed at environmental control of vectors and general environmental sanitation; report to public health officials any infractions against sanitation codes.

*References 1-3, 5-13, 20, 21.

Principles and Rationale for Nursing Interventions

A *potential* nursing diagnosis describes an altered state that may occur in the absence of intervention. The desired outcome for the person is that the potential state does not occur. With the diagnosis of potential for infection, the patient goals all refer to prevention of infection in persons in various health states. The first goal specifies that individuals in the community who are at risk will experience no infection. The nurse may intervene with these persons in their home and in outpatient clinics. Prevention of community-acquired infections to these persons requires nursing interventions that identify the specific risk factors affecting persons and help them to reduce the risk factors and/or promote their general health status and resistance.

The goal that the hospitalized patient will experience no infection implies the setting for intervention. This goal also assumes that the patient will have greater alterations in general health status and resistance and will be at increased risk because of these alterations, the hospital environment, and medical procedures and treatments. Prevention of hospital-acquired (nosocomial) infections requires nursing interventions that promote resistance in sick individuals while also minimizing invasion of pathogenic agents during medical procedures.

Prevention of infection in population groups is a nursing challenge in the hospital as well as in the community. Pathogenic organisms are readily transmitted in the hospital and institutional environments to patient care staff, visitors, and other patients. Pathogenic organisms are transmitted in the community to persons in direct contact with infected individuals and to the community at large through environmental contamination. In both situations nursing interventions are aimed at control of contact with infective secretions, excretions, and exudates by detecting and treating infected persons early; minimizing contamination in the environment; and raising the immunity levels of the population.

Evaluation

Patient Outcome	Data Indicating That Outcome is Reached
Individuals in the community will experience no infection.	Individuals have received recommended immunizations for their age. Individuals can describe health behaviors that increase their resistance to infections. Individuals can describe health practices that decrease their exposure to pathogens. Individuals take antibiotics as prescribed.
Hospitalized patient will experience no infection during or immediately after hospitalization.	Vital signs are within normal limits. Cultures of body secretions, excretions, and exudates are negative for colonized pathogens. WBC count is within normal limits. Invasive lines are discontinued as soon as possible. Surgical wounds have healed without signs of infection.
Infection will not be transmitted to patient's contacts in the hospital or in the community.	Patient contacts have been examined and treated for infection. High-risk patient care staff is immunized against rubella and hepatitis B. Patient care staff members wash hands between patient visits and follow universal blood and body secretion procedures with all patients. Patient care staff remains free of signs of infection. All segments of the community are adequately immunized. Incidence of congenital anomalies and infections associated with maternal infections decreases in the community. Incidence of immunizable childhood infectious diseases, food-borne illness, and sexually transmitted diseases decreases in the community.

Potential for Injury

(Potential for trauma; potential for poisoning; potential for suffocation)

Potential for injury is the state in which an individual is at risk of injury as a result of environmental conditions interacting with the individual's adaptive and defensive resources.

Potential for trauma is the accentuated risk of accidental tissue injury, e.g., wound, burn, or fracture.

Potential for poisoning is the accentuated risk of accidental exposure to or ingestion of drugs or dangerous products in doses sufficient to cause poisoning.

Potential for suffocation is the accentuated risk of accidental suffocation (inadequate air available for inhalation).

The diagnostic label *potential for injury* includes three subcomponents accepted by the North American Nursing Diagnoses Association (NANDA): trauma, poisoning, and suffocation. However, these are merely examples of the broader label. Therefore the discussion that follows is presented from a theoretical perspective and does not specifically include trauma, poisoning, and suffocation.

The injury process requires interaction of human factors (the host), energy sources (the agents), and physical and sociocultural factors (the environment).

Injury Model

	Human Factors (Host)	Energy Sources (Agents)	Physical-Sociocultural Factors (Environment)
Preevent Phase			
Event Phase			
Postevent Phase			

Preevent: those events and factors before the injury; the interaction of these factors leads to the injury.
Event: during the injury process; the physical response, the intensity of the energy, and the environmental situation.
Postevent: following the injury; the body's response to the energy source, the final energy dose, and the emergency care provided by those in the environment.

Host, or human, factors include variables that pertain specifically to the person being considered. Examples include the individual's age, physical condition, eyesight, muscle strength, mental ability, fatigue level, growth and development, personal habits and values, stress level, blood alcohol level, and dexterity. Host factors also include the individual's ability to cope with an unexpected energy source that may cause harm. These factors are essentially the individual's resistance characteristics.

Agent factors are the energy sources that challenge the individual's resistance characteristics and actually cause the injury. These include mechanical and gravitational (e.g., falls), thermal (e.g., burns), radiant (e.g., sunburn), chemical (e.g., poisoning), electrical (e.g., electrical shock), and lack of oxidation (e.g., drowning).

Environmental factors may be divided into two areas: physical and sociocultural. Examples of physical environmental factors are defective or unsafe equipment, hazardous road conditions, and exposure to solid, liquid, or gaseous poisons. Sociocultural environmental factors include unsupervised small children, lack of knowledge to establish a safe environment, family stress, and lack of knowledge regarding developmental ability.

To establish the nursing diagnosis *potential for injury,* one must consider the collective interrelationship of host, agent, and environmental factors. The diagnosis may then be defined as the interaction between the individual (the host), the energy source (the agent), and the environment (physical and sociocultural) that imposes a risk for physical harm to the individual.

Risk Factors[11]

Host Factors (Internal Factors)

Biologic and physiologic
- Age (under 40 years, over 60 years)
- Gender (males more than females)
- Chronic diseases
- Current disabilities, especially musculoskeletal, visual, hearing, and sensory
- Metabolism and nutritional status, especially calcium deficiency
- Fatigue
- High chemical substance or alcohol blood level

Mental/psychologic
- Mental disorders
- Orientation
- Temperament/mood
- Irritability, anger
- Emotional state/lability
- Personal stresses
- Social adjustment
- Altered levels of consciousness
- Aggressiveness/social deviance

Psychomotor
- Developmental level inappropriate for task or environment
- Skill/performance capabilities
- Muscle strength and coordination

Cognitive
- Experience
- Judgment
- Education (safety and general)

Behavioral
- Attitude
- Beliefs
- Habits
- Motivation
- Preoccupation

Environmental Factors (External Factors)

Physical factors
- Mechanical
  - Defective or unsafe vehicle
  - Excessive speeds
  - Nonuse or misuse of safety belts
  - Nonuse or misuse of headgear for bicycle or motorcycle riders
  - Unsafe road or road-crossing conditions
  - Play near vehicle pathways (driveways, laneways, railroad tracks)
  - Dangerous machinery and appliances

Sharp-edged toys
Slippery floors (wet or highly waxed)
Furniture with sharp edges, projections, or glass
Unanchored rugs
Bathtub without hand grip or antislip equipment
Unsteady furniture
Inadequately lit rooms
Unsturdy or absent stair rails
Unanchored electrical wires
Litter or liquid spills on floor or stairways
Unprotected open windows or stairs
Use of cracked dishes or glasses
Knives stored uncovered
Guns or ammunition stored unlocked
Fireworks or gunpowder
Absence of designated play areas
Shoes without traction

Thermal
Playing with matches, candles, or cigarettes
Highly flammable children's toys or clothing
Smoking in bed or near oxygen
Grease waste collected on stoves
Contact with intense cold
Pot handles facing toward front of stove
Hot water heater set higher than 54.5° C (130° F)
Lack of smoke detectors
Potential igniting gas leaks
Delayed lighting of gas burner or oven
Experimenting with chemicals or gasoline
Unscreened fires or heaters
Improperly stored combustibles or corrosives (matches, oily rags, lye, gasoline)

Chemical
Large supply of drugs in home
Medicines stored in unlocked cabinets accessible to children
Hazardous products placed or stored within reach of young children
Lack of childproof caps
Products not stored in properly labeled storage container or space
Availability of illicit drugs potentially contaminated by poisonous additives
Flaking, peeling paint or plaster
Chemical contamination of food or water
Unprotected contact with heavy metals or chemicals
Paint, lacquer, etc. in poorly ventilated areas or without effective protection
Presence of poisonous vegetation
Presence of atmospheric pollutants
Contact with acids or alkalies

Radiant
Overexposure to sun, sunlamps, or radiotherapy

Electrical
Overloaded fuse boxes
Lack of safety plugs or appliance outlets
Unused extension cords plugged in
Worn electrical cords
Electrical appliances and cords near water
Overloaded electrical outlets

Lack of oxidation
Household gas leaks
Fuel-burning heaters not vented to outside
Pacifier hung around infant's neck
Pools without structural barriers
Toys with cords
Pillow or plastic sheet placed in infant's crib
Propped bottle placed in an infant's crib
Vehicle running in closed garage
Children playing with plastic bags or inserting small objects into mouth or nose
Discarded or unused refrigerators or freezers without doors removed

Sociocultural factors
Lack of parental awareness of hazards
Lack of safety education
Fatalistic attitude about injuries
Lack of knowledge of developmental stages
Negligent, abusive, or overprotective childrearing practices
Lack of parental supervision
Lack of resources to establish safe environment (knowledge, finances)
Presence of family stress (marital, financial, health)
Inadequate community emergency medical services response
Lack of public education (first aid, CPR)
Lack of community safety programs (water safety, lifeguards, crossing guards, building codes)

Nursing Interventions

Patient Goal	Nursing Intervention
Host Factors	
Engage in strategies to prevent injury.	• Teach and counsel patient about strategies and countermeasures to prevent injury: Prevent the creation of the hazard. Reduce the amount of the energy source created. Prevent the release of the energy source that already exists. Modify the rate or spatial distribution of the energy from its source. Separate, in time or in space, the hazard or energy source and person or object to be protected. Separate the energy source by physical barrier. Modify the basic qualities of the energy source.

Patient Goal	Nursing Intervention
	Increase resistance to damage from energy source. Counter damage already done by energy source. Repair and rehabilitate injured individual.
Identify variables leading to increased susceptibility.	• Inform that injury is more likely to occur in individuals under 40 or over 60 years of age. • Inform that injury is more likely to occur in males than in females.
Identify biologic and physiologic factors that increase risk of injury.	• Perform assessment. • Provide information regarding disease processes or physiologic conditions that increase risk of injury. • Provide alteration strategies to adapt physical environment to the patient's physiologic state.
Identify psychomotor variables that increase risk of injury.	• Conduct assessment of developmental level of individual. • Provide educational information regarding safety strategies appropriate for individual. • Assess skill competence and performance capabilities of individual. • Assess muscle strength and coordination capabilities. • Provide strategies to protect individual from potential injury. • Assess and provide alteration strategies to increase self-protective capabilities for individual.
Identify mental and psychologic variables that may increase risk of injury.	• Assess mental impairment or decision-making ability that may interfere with individual's ability to protect self from injury. • Provide protective interventions that will protect individual from injury. • Monitor mood and temperament, which may increase risk of injury. • Assess individual's stress patterns, which may increase risk of injury. • Assess personal and social adjustments, which may increase risk of injury. • Provide protective interventions if necessary to prevent injury.
Identify behavioral factors that increase risk of injury.	• Identify individual's habits or aggressive acts that place the individual at higher risk for injury. • Assess social deviance or effect of TV violence, which may place individual at high risk for injury. • Attempt to identify variables that affect individual behavior. • Provide education and passive protection that will protect individual from injury. • Assess for lack of motivation regarding injury protection. • Where possible, provide passive protection.
Evaluate cognitive ability to prevent injury.	• Assess experience and judgment in individual's ability to determine and maintain adequate injury prevention strategies. • Assess educational needs in area of safety education and injury prevention.
Agent Factors	
Use appropriate countermeasures to prevent injury from specific energy sources.	• Provide education relevant to strategies and countermeasures. • Provide prevention strategies that will protect individual from injury.
Identify appropriate safety factors that protect the individual from injury.	• Provide information regarding product design and characteristics: restraining devices, safety caps, barriers separating the individual from the hazard (stairs, windows, pools, streets).
Environmental Factors	
Identify physical environmental risks that increase potential of injury.	• Assess physical risks in the environment. • Provide education and structural recommendations to decrease injury risk. • Assess task demand and provide protective intervention where necessary. • Provide education regarding home hazards and methods to decrease injury potential.
Identify social environmental risks that increase potential of injury.	• Assess parental expectations for child's behavior. Where appropriate, provide educational information congruent with growth and developmental level. • Perform assessment of parental attitude toward injury prevention strategies. • Where appropriate, provide information regarding injury potential and alternative prevention strategies. • Assess components of family socioeconomic status that may place family in stress situation and thus increase injury risk. • Assess child-rearing practices and provide alteration strategies to assist parents. • Assess potential for family abusive behavior (see further intervention strategies under Potential for Violence: Self-Directed or Directed at Others).
Identify family structure factors that may increase the potential of injury.	• Assess family structure and potential family stresses such as income, physical, and emotional situation of family members that may increase family risk to injury.

Principles and Rationale for Nursing Interventions

The nursing care for this nursing diagnosis is directed toward the host, agent, and environmental factors that potentially lead to injury. The intent of the interventions is preventive and not curative. Because of this, many of the interventions are either educational or include strategies to alter the environment or the individual's position in the environment. Injury prevention is a very complex process that takes place in an equally complex environment. Attention to prevention requires careful evaluation of the individual, the environment, and the agents with which the individual may come in contact.

Host Factors

Host factors deal with the human aspects of the injury process. Specific physiologic, biologic, psychomotor, psychologic, and behavioral factors must be considered as goal statements of potential for injury. The condition of the individual as it relates to each of these variables is assessed and determined if an area of risk is present.

Agent Factors

The injurious agent first must be identified. Then the countermeasures may be determined. The patient needs instruction to protect himself from the injury agent. Countermeasures may be passively or actively applied; their purpose is to protect the patient from the injury mechanism.

Environmental Factors

Injury may also be caused by factors in the environment such as the physical environment, social environment, and family. Each of these factors requires a special assessment to determine areas of stress or concern. Often injury occurs because the demand for performance outweighs the individual's ability to perform. In such cases the environmental factors must be readjusted to meet the individual's ability to perform the tasks.

Evaluation

Patient Outcome	Data Indicating That Outcome is Reached
Host Factors	
Accurate appraisal of susceptibility factors	Valid appraisal of age and gender factors that indicate increased risk of injury Appropriate steps to protect self or patients at high risk from injury
Appropriate recognition of biologic and physiologic factors that increase risk of injury	Identification of chronic diseases or physiologic conditions that increase risk of injury Protective strategies to alter risk potential Modification of environment to increase safety potential
Appropriate assessment of psychomotor variables that increase risk of injury	Appropriate assessment of developmental capabilities and recognition of injury risk Protective steps to prevent injury Accurate assessment of skill competence and performance ability Strategies to increase skill performance or to protect self from injury potential Exercise or training program to meet task demand Protective devices to separate self from potential injury source Accurate recognition of fatigue state, which may lead to potential injury Appropriate steps to prevent injury
Accurate assessment of mental and psychologic variables that increase risk of injury	Recognition of variables (mental, mood, temperament, stress, irritability, hostility) that may increase risk of injury Seeking new methods to express emotions that will not increase injury potential Demonstration of methods to decrease risk of injury
Appropriate behavioral response pattern to decrease risk of injury	Recognition of habits, aggressive behavior, and motivations that may increase injury potential Seeking new knowledge and skill to decrease potential risk Demonstration of methods that decrease risk of injury
Accurate assessment of cognitive ability to decrease risk of injury	Accurate assessment of own ability, experience, judgment, and education to reduce injury risk Seeking new information and skill to decrease deficit areas Use of new knowledge and skill to decrease injury risk
Agent Factors	
Appropriate use of countermeasures to protect self from injury	Knowledge of countermeasures to reduce potential of injury Use of appropriate countermeasures Knowledge and use of safety devices and approved products that decrease risk of injury
Environmental Factors	
Ability to reduce environmental physical risks of injury	Accurate assessment of exposure to environmental risks such as home products, hazardous materials, hazardous surfaces, and unprotected areas Knowledge to reduce environmental physical risk Altering physical environment to reduce risk of injury

Patient Outcome	Data Indicating That Outcome is Reached
Ability to reduce environmental social risks of injury	Recognition of social variables, such as childrearing practices, child supervision, and discipline practices, that may increase risk of injury Seeking instruction to modify childrearing practices where appropriate Seeking support to intervene when stress or knowledge limits adult's ability to provide safe environment for childrearing Acknowledgment of own limitations regarding ability to cope with social environmental stress Seeking new knowledge and skill to cope with environmental social stress

 Health-Seeking Behaviors (Specify)

Health-seeking behaviors is the state in which a person in stable health is actively seeking ways to alter personal health habits and/or the environment to move toward optimum health. (*Stable health* status is present when the person has achieved age-appropriate illness prevention measures and reports good or excellent health and when signs and symptoms of disease, if present, are controlled.)

Motivation for the maintenance or expansion of a person's state of wellness manifests itself at different levels. Illness prevention motivation occurs when individuals in a health state are aware of personal, public, or environmental risks that jeopardize their state of well-being. Others are concerned about such public threats as sexually transmitted diseases, infectious diseases, criminal assaults, or bombardment by modern life stressors. They seek community services and education for assistance. The mass media have increased public awareness of certain prevalent problems such as alcoholism, AIDS, family violence, or some forms of cancer, and people want to know what they can do to prevent such afflictions. Still others are concerned about industrial pollution, nuclear waste products, or ultraviolet rays. They are motivated to prevent exposure and illness for themselves as well as the general population. People are generally motivated to change their self-care habits when they are convinced that the effort will deter or eliminate a specific threat.

Beyond the prevention of illness, people wish to maintain their present satisfactory health state to ensure that they can continue to function successfully in their daily activities. Functional capacity incorporates physical, emotional, cognitive, spiritual, and social performance. Individuals engage in health-seeking behaviors to enhance their self-esteem, their appearance, or their physical capacity to work; to avoid discomfort and pain; and to recreate or maintain independence. Aging individuals are often concerned about dietary or exercise efforts that will help them maintain an independent functional status. People frequently engage in activities that promise to raise their participation level so that they can work, relate to other people, and live to their satisfaction. Still others wish simply to improve or excel in the physical, psychosocial, or spiritual realm. They are directed toward a level of mastery or self-actualization and are willing to explore greatly different or vigorous approaches to attain a peak level of wellness and fulfillment. Variables that typically affect motivation to seek and carry through with health improvement behaviors are the perceived threat of a particular disease or problem, the perceived benefits of taking action, the lack of interference with a present life-style, situational barriers (real or imagined) that might impose on a person, public (e.g., mass media campaigns) or private support for taking action, sense of self-efficacy (i.e., a sense of confidence that a person can complete the proposed actions successfully), and the individual's personal definition of health.

Individuals or groups in a health-seeking mode may exhibit a variety of behaviors. They may ask for information, outright assistance, advocacy, or support. They may exhibit frustration with present circumstances, fear of the future, or confusion about a specific concern. They may express concern about themselves, a loved one, or their entire community. They may display great self-confidence or exhilaration with the idea of impending change or self-improvement.

Related Factors*

Fear of disease or illness
Desire to maintain functional status
Cultural beliefs and norms; personal and family values
Increased awareness through public education (media, magazines) for optimum health state
Professional prescription, advice, or encouragement
Fear of pain

Defining Characteristics*

Expressed or observed desire to seek a higher level of wellness
Stated or observed unfamiliarity with wellness community resources
Verbalized or observed lack of knowledge in health promotion behaviors
Expressed or observed desire for increased control of health practices
Expression of concern about current environmental conditions on health status

*Adapted from North American Nursing Diagnosis Association, 1988 Ballot.

Nursing Interventions

Patient Goal	Nursing Intervention
Clarify health goals.	• Assess the patient for: Definition of health Perceived threat(s) to health Description of goals the patient wishes to attain Perceived barriers to goal(s) Perceived benefits of taking action Perceived public or private support Sense of self-efficacy Any incapacities or barriers to health-seeking behavior • Review assessment information with patient. • Restate patient goal(s) with patient.
Achieve current accurate knowledge on subject of interest.	• Assess patient for present level of knowledge on given subject. • Identify supplemental areas for learning and share them with patient. • Review new material with patient and request patient's evaluation of the usefulness of the new information.
Participate in identifying strategies for meeting goals.	• Assess patient's perception that goal is attainable. • Review any incongruities between nurse's and patient's perception(s). • Identify specific strategies (behaviors) patient must enact to attain goal(s). • Establish a schedule or time frame for goal attainment (goal attainment may be identified in increments over a time). • Describe goal attainments in measurable or behavioral terms (e.g., Mrs. M will lose 3 pounds by (date); Mr. G will identify three specific stressful incidents at work on his next visit). • Identify specific behaviors that will precede or accompany each increment and review them with patient. • Review nurse's and patient's perceptions about attainability of goal(s).
Develop self-monitoring behaviors.	• Assess patient's comprehension of goal attainments. • Assess patient's motivation to follow specific attainments. • Work with patient to design a record-keeping system or a means of describing/reporting progress to self, support system, and nurse.
Engage in self-rewarding behaviors.	• Review benefits of health-seeking activity with patient and include possible side benefits (e.g., feeling more energetic, improved sleeping). • Urge patient to note benefits during progress. • If patient wishes, devise a "reward" as increments are attained.
Identify social support for reinforcement of health-seeking behaviors.	• Review family, loved ones, and peer support for patient's activities (e.g., purchasing prepared food for diet, transportation to exercise facility).
Differentiate between negative and positive influences and factors on self.	• Ask patient to monitor negative/positive influences and discuss them with family. • Continue education about potential negative factors.
Expand involvement in state of well-being.	• Continue education and discussion about healthful life patterns that extend beyond patient's current interests (goals). • Assess patient's motivation to expand health-seeking concerns. • Assist patient with translating wishes into options for healthful living.

Principles and Rationale for Nursing Interventions

A person who expresses or exhibits health-seeking behaviors may wish to pursue an urgent, short-term issue (e.g., acquisition of knowledge about AIDS prevention) or an elaborate long-term plan for high-level wellness. Nursing interventions rest heavily on careful assessment of the patient's goals, perceptions, and values. It is important to recognize incongruities between the nurse's wishes for the patient and the patient's own wishes. Carrying out a health care activity requires commitment and well-entrenched convictions from the patient. The patient will be more receptive to education and support when it is clear that his goals and the nurse's goals are not in conflict.

Goal attainment is best acquired in small increments (e.g., weight loss, stress reduction). The patient is rewarded with more immediate and frequent accomplishments if assisted in breaking down ambitious goals into small ones. Once the short-term, more immediate goals have been attained and the patient is feeling confident, further education and encouragement may lead to other health-seeking behaviors.

Evaluation

Patient Outcome	Data Indicating That Outcome is Reached
Patient's goals met	Measurable or behavioral goals achieved (e.g., final weight loss achieved; specific stressors identified and eliminated; reports for aerobic classes four times a week for 8 weeks without fail)
Maintains normal growth and development status	Reports that life-style is satisfactory and that daily living patterns are within control and are fulfilling
Continues to monitor health progress in all aspects of life	Seeks further information and education about wellness Expresses motivation to continue or expand health-seeking behaviors

FUNCTIONAL HEALTH PATTERN

II

Nutritional-Metabolic

Altered Nutrition: Potential for More Than Body Requirements

Altered nutrition: potential for more than body requirements is the state in which an individual is at risk of experiencing an intake of nutrients that exceeds metabolic needs.

Nutrition is defined as the sum of all processes by which a living organism receives and uses nutrients for growth, maintenance, and repair of the body. Nutrients include proteins, carbohydrates, fats, vitamins, minerals, and water.

Individuals who are at risk for more nutrition than the body requires benefit from primary prevention regarding overweight or obesity. Overweight is defined as 10% above the desirable weight for individuals according to their height and body build. Obesity is defined as 20% to 25% above the desirable weight according to height and body build. These two definitions assume a normal muscle/fat ratio.

Risk Factors[15]

Hereditary predisposition
Excessive energy intake during late gestational life, early infancy, and adolescence
Frequent, closely spaced pregnancies
Dysfunctional psychologic conditioning in relation to food
Membership in lower socioeconomic group
Reported or observed obesity in one or both parents*
Rapid transition across growth percentiles in infants and children
Reported use of solid food as major food source before 5 months of age
Observed use of food as reward or comfort measure
Reported or observed higher baseline weight at beginning of pregnancy
Dysfunctional eating patterns
- Pairing foods with other activities; concentrating food intake at end of day
- Eating in response to external cues, such as time of day or social situation
- Eating in response to internal cues other than hunger, such as anxiety

Nursing Interventions[8,15,21,30]

Patient Goal	Nursing Intervention
Alter patterns of food and fluid intake.	• Discuss with patient the relationship between food intake, exercise, and obesity. • Discuss risks of obesity: increased incidence for diabetes mellitus, hypertension, and atherosclerosis. • Determine patient motivation for changing eating habits. • Determine patient's ideal body weight. • Develop method for patient to keep daily record of intake. • Determine desirable weekly weight loss. • Encourage patient to write down realistic weekly goals for food intake and exercise and to display them in a location where they can be reviewed daily.
Increase energy expenditure.	• Help patient to participate in at least one energy-expending activity three times a week. • Ask patient to chart weekly weights.

Principles and Rationale for Nursing Interventions

Two patient goals are derived from the assessment data: alter patterns of food and fluid intake and increase energy expenditure.

The patient needs to understand the relationship among food and fluid intake, energy expenditure, and weight gain. Since the patient is at risk, he also must understand the consequences of obesity. When designing a plan for altering intake patterns and increasing energy expenditure, the nurse and patient need to develop a realistic plan. To design a realistic plan, the patient's ideal body weight for age and body size is determined. Next, a review of the patient's typical day is helpful to identify what food and fluid patterns can be altered and when exercise can be planned. A plan is derived with weekly goals for the patient to meet. A reward system also is included in the plan when goals are accomplished.

The growth and development of the patient needs to be considered. For example, an expectant mother needs a diet adequate in nutrients for herself and the fetus. For a breast-fed infant, parents use weight gain as the criterion for adequacy of feeding. For a bottle-fed infant, parents use this same criterion rather than whether the infant finishes all feedings. Infants and children should not be forced to eat, since this may contribute to overeating. Children should be offered well-balanced meals in an environment free from distractions such as television and be encouraged to eat at their own pace. Food should not be used as reward or punishment for children because this practice may cause compulsive eating. While growing up, the child needs to learn the foods in a balanced diet, as well as the importance of physical activity. When the child becomes an adolescent and begins taking responsibility for foods eaten, he will have a sufficient knowledge base about nutrition and exercise from which to make decisions. Adolescents and adults also need to balance food intake with physical activity. The hormonal change that occurs during puberty requires a change in eating and activity patterns. Likewise, after 50 years of age hormonal changes again necessitate reassessment of one's food intake and activity balance.

Instruction on how to prevent overweight and obesity is facilitated when all family members are present to discuss eating patterns and the meaning of food to them. If this is not possible, at least those individuals responsible for selecting food and preparing meals need to learn about overweight prevention practices. Sometimes this is the same person, but in some cultures one person selects food for another to prepare. Potential obesity caused by hormonal imbalances or hypothalamic disorders must be treated with specific medical or surgical regimens. This treatment protocol is carried out in conjunction with a balance between food intake and exercise.

Evaluation

Patient Outcome	Data Indicating That Outcome is Reached
Alters intake patterns and increases energy expenditure	Maintains ideal body weight for age and body size Can explain dietary and exercise plans for maintaining ideal body weight

 Altered Nutrition: More Than Body Requirements

Altered nutrition: more than body requirements is the state in which an individual is experiencing an intake of nutrients that exceeds metabolic needs.

Related Factor

Excessive intake in relationship to metabolic need[15]

Defining Characteristics[15]

Weight 10% over ideal for height and frame
Weight 20% over ideal for height and frame
Triceps skinfold greater than 15 mm in men and 25 mm in women
Sedentary activity level
Reported or observed dysfunctional eating patterns
- Pairing food with other activities
- Concentrating food intake at the end of the day
- Eating in response to external cues, such as time of day or social situation
- Eating in response to internal cues other than hunger
- Reported excess in food intake
- Reported little or no physical exercise

Nursing Interventions[15,21,30]

Patient Goal	Nursing Intervention
Reduce body weight.	• Weigh patient. • Determine patient's desire to reduce body weight. • Determine patient's ideal body weight. • Determine patient's triceps skinfold measurements. • Set a realistic plan with the patient to include reduced food intake and increased energy expenditure. • Have the patient post the goal for weight loss in a strategic location. • Discuss eating a balanced diet. • Ask patient to keep a diary of what, when, and where he eats to evaluate changes that need to be made in life-style. • Reward patient for attaining goals, and encourage patient to use an internal reward system when goals are accomplished. • Provide a list of support groups for weight loss, such as Overeaters Anonymous or TOPS (Take Off Pounds Sensibly).

Principles and Rationale for Nursing Interventions

One patient goal is derived from the assessment data: reduce body weight.

Comparing the patient's current weight with the ideal body weight provides baseline data from which realistic goals can be set. Triceps skinfold thickness provides data about the body's fat stores. Motivation for weight reduction comes from within the person. The person must want to lose weight before a program can be successful. Learning the hazards of obesity may be a motivator. These hazards include atherosclerosis, hypertension, and diabetes mellitus. The patient should write down realistic goals and post them in strategic places, such as on the refrigerator door, pantry door, or bathroom mirror. A goal of 1 to 2 pounds a week frequently is suggested as a starting point. This goal is based on the fact that 1 pound of adipose tissue has the energy potential of 3500 calories. Reducing caloric intake by 500 calories for 7 days theoretically yields a weight loss of 1 pound. In conjunction with decreased caloric intake, the patient needs to begin an exercise program and work toward a goal. The goal can be *minutes* of exercise or activity or *distance* (walking, jogging, swimming). These goals also should be written down and posted in strategic places.

Patients need to examine their eating patterns and behaviors. To assist them, they can keep a diary of what they eat, when they eat, where they eat, and the circumstances around which they eat. This activity will provide a data base for both the adequacy of nutrients eaten and the psychosocial conditions of eating. What one eats reveals how well balanced the diet is. Meats, fruits, vegetables, milk, cereals, and bread are needed daily for essential nutrients. To decrease food intake, a person can drink an 8-ounce glass of water before eating and use a smaller than usual plate so that the smaller serving will not look small. The person should eat slowly, chew thoroughly, and think about the taste and smell of the food. While eating, the patient should avoid any other activity, such as reading or watching television. Recommended low-calorie snacks are carrots, celery, and apples, which satisfy the oral need for chewing and provide needed vegetables and fruits. Water and low-calorie soft drinks also are recommended.

When a person eats is important as well. One person may skip breakfast, work through lunch, snack while preparing dinner, and eat dessert while watching television. The caloric intake should be subdivided throughout the waking hours. Instead of eating while watching television, the person can do something else with the hands and chew sugar-free gum. Where a person eats includes the type of restaurant as well as which room at home. Fast-food restaurants provide filling food quickly, but it often is high in carbohydrates. Excessive consumption of foods from fast-food restaurants may contribute to obesity. The room where a person chooses to eat is important when reducing caloric intake. Eating in only one place, such as the dining room table or kitchen, is helpful.

The circumstances around which the person eats poses the most difficult data collection problem. This includes the motivation for eating, the external and internal cues, such as anxiety, stress, fear, anger, peer pressure, loneliness, and depression. Some overeating problems are due to psychologic factors. Psychologic counseling or support groups such as Overeaters Anonymous and TOPS (Take Off Pounds Sensibly) may be needed to identify and deal with the problem. Behavior modification is another strategy used for reinforcement and cue elimination.

Surgical procedures may be considered for an obese person who is unsuccessful in repeated weight reduction attempts or whose health is jeopardized by the obese state. An intestinal bypass (jejunoileal bypass) decreases absorptive surfaces of the jejunum. Preoperatively the patient requires counseling about causes of obesity and the consequences of this type of surgery. Postoperative care is similar to that for patients undergoing abdominal surgery.

Evaluation

Patient Outcome	Data Indicating That Outcome is Reached
Reduced body weight	Firm muscles Subcutaneous fat sufficient to pad bones and muscles; triceps skinfold measurement within normal limits (see Altered Nutrition: Less Than Body Requirements) Daily weight stabilized at normal level for body build Diet includes meat, milk, fruits, vegetables, and breads
Aware of learning needs	The patient can explain: 1. Reason for obesity 2. Dietary plan for weight reduction 3. Exercise plan for weight reduction 4. Plans for follow-up care

Altered Nutrition: Less Than Body Requirements

Altered nutrition: less than body requirements is the state in which an individual experiences an intake of nutrients insufficient to meet metabolic needs.

Related Factors

Inability to ingest or digest food or absorb nutrients because of biologic, psychologic, or economic factors[15]

Defining Characteristics[14,15,21]

Loss of weight with adequate food intake
Body weight 20% or more under ideal for height and frame
Reported inadequate food intake less than Recommended Daily Allowance (RDA)
Weakness of muscles required for swallowing or mastication
Reported or evidence of lack of food
Lack of interest in food
Perceived inability to ingest food
Aversion to eating
Reported altered taste sensation
Satiety immediately after ingesting food
Abdominal pain with or without pathology
Sore, inflamed buccal cavity
Capillary fragility
Abdominal cramping
Diarrhea and/or steatorrhea
Hyperactive bowel sounds
Pale conjunctiva and mucous membranes
Poor muscle tone
Excessive hair loss
Lack of information; misinformation
Misconceptions
Decreased triceps skinfold
Decreased midarm circumference
Decreased midarm muscle circumference

Alteration in smell
Chronic sputum production
Decreased appetite
Inability to chew
Dysphagia
Self-care deficit
Electrolyte imbalance
Decreased serum albumin
Decreased serum transferrin or iron-binding capacity
Decreased lymphocyte count
Dry, scaly, inelastic skin
Pallor of the oral mucosa

Nursing Interventions*

Patient Goal	Nursing Intervention
Increase intake of nutrients.	• Weigh patient daily. • Auscultate bowel sounds during each shift. • Assess skin turgor. • Assess patient's ability to chew and swallow. • Assess for nausea and vomiting; identify causes and eliminate when possible. • Calculate intake and output during each shift; intake of 2400 ml is recommended unless patient requires fluid restriction. • Monitor daily calorie count. • Monitor skinfold measurements. • Monitor laboratory data: albumin, lymphocytes, and electrolytes. • Medicate as ordered to reduce nausea and pain before eating. • Provide foods in the form appropriate for patient: general diet, mechanical soft, blenderized, formula via nasogastric or gastrostomy tube, or total parenteral nutrition via subclavian vein as ordered by physician. • Consider patient's food preferences as governed by personal choices and cultural and religious preferences. • Provide oral care before meals and as needed. • Provide rest periods as needed. • Ensure that patient is in a sitting position before eating or feeding. • When patient feeds self: Serve food at its appropriate temperature. Ensure patient is comfortable and can reach necessary utensils for eating. Provide adaptive/assistive devices. • When patient is fed by mouth: Serve food at its appropriate temperature. Ensure patient is comfortable. Allow patient sufficient time between bites. Talk with the patient during the meal. • When patient is fed by nasogastric (NG) or nasoduodenal tube: Ensure proper placement of tube. Add blue or green food coloring to feeding to detect aspiration. Ensure feeding at room temperature. Flush periodically with full-strength cranberry juice followed by water. • When nasogastric tube is used: Aspirate gastric contents to determine the amount of the last feeding still in stomach. If aspirated contents is less than 50 ml, proceed with the feeding. • When continuous feeding is used: Refill feeding bag every 4 hours. Check gravity drip rate or pump rate every hour. • When the patient is fed by total parenteral nutrition: Check infusion rate every hour or infusion pump rate every hour. Monitor blood glucose and urinary glucose and acetone every 6 hours. Change dressing daily, using sterile technique; inspect insertion site. Monitor patient's temperature every 4 hours. • Provide high-calorie feedings between meals or six small feedings daily.
Identify factors that contribute to inadequate nutritional intake:	
Socioeconomic	• Problem-solve with patient and family to identify socioeconomic factors contributing to inadequate nutrition.

*References 5, 6, 8, 15, 21, 30.

Patient Goal	Nursing Intervention
	• Determine with patient and family appropriate strategies to use to solve problems. • Use referrals to other members of the health care team as needed (dietitian, social worker, community health nurse).
Psychologic	• Discuss with patient perceptions of factors interfering with ability or desire to eat. • Discuss with patient strategies useful to improve nutrition. • Refer patient for additional therapy as needed.
Gain knowledge of nutritional needs.	• Assess learning needs of patient and family. • Determine their understanding of the reason for altered nutrition. • Teach types of menus to be used. • Teach foods to avoid. • Determine their understanding of the plan for follow-up treatment. • Teach them reason for vitamin and mineral supplements to be taken. • Provide them with names and phone numbers of personnel in community agencies.

Principles and Rationale for Nursing Interventions

Three patient goals are derived from assessment data: increase intake of nutrients, identify factors contributing to alterations in nutrition, and gain knowledge of nutritional needs.

The patient's height and weight are compared with tables of ideal weight for the height. Bowel sounds are assessed to determine if peristalsis is present. Skin turgor provides data on amount of subcutaneous fat and on fluid balance. Physiologic causes of altered nutrition are ruled out as possible causes of inadequate nutrition. These include difficulty in chewing or swallowing and presence of nausea or vomiting.

Nausea and vomiting can be lessened with small amounts of cool liquids (cola, ginger ale, Jello, water). Cleaning the mouth and blowing the nose after vomiting eliminates nauseous tastes and smells. Alteration of medicines should be considered to prevent nausea and vomiting. Rectal administration of medication rather than oral may help. The vomiting center stimulation is decreased by slow deep breathing through the mouth, removal of unpleasant sights and smells, and eating and drinking slowly.

Fluid intake as well as calorie intake must be calculated to determine nutrition adequacy.

Skinfold measurements include triceps skinfold, midarm muscle circumference, and midarm circumference. Triceps skinfold thickness gives data about fat stores, and arm circumference provides data about protein stores. The site measured for both the skinfold thickness and arm circumference is at the midpoint between the shoulder (acromial process) and the elbow (olecranon) of the nondominant arm. The average of three measurements is recorded. Measurement is made by pinching the skin and measuring its thickness with calipers. The arm circumference is measured at the same place on the arm. Midarm muscle circumference (cm) = mean arm circumference (cm) − (0.314 × triceps skinfold thickness [mm]). The standards for these anthropometric measurements are in the evaluation section. Serum albumin values are no longer useful after an infusion of albumin to maintain intravascular pressure. Visceral protein depletion is indicated when total lymphocyte count falls below 1500 cells/mm^3 (Table 1).[14]

For patients who eat a general diet, the nurse considers cultural or religious food preferences. Offering patients some selection in the food gives them a feeling of control in their lives. When meals are served, patients need to feel as comfortable as possible, which may require oral hygiene, position change, or medication. They need to be able to reach their food, and some patients may require assistance with cutting food or opening containers. A pleasant eating environment free from unpleasant aromas enhances eating, as does an appropriate temperature for the food.

Before eating, the patient must be comfortable and in the optimum position. The patient also is encouraged to rest, receives medications for nausea or pain, and is offered oral care as needed before eating. Regardless of whether patients feed themselves or are fed, they need to be in an upright position. When the feeding is accomplished via nasogastric (NG) or nasoduodenal tube, the nurse adds food coloring to the formula so that any aspiration of the feeding can be detected quickly. The feeding tubing is flushed with full-strength cranberry juice to prevent protein buildup in the tube. Flushing the tube with water is necessary to provide water to the patient as well as to flush the tube. Before NG tube feedings, the nurse aspirates gastric contents to determine the amount of feeding left in the stomach. When more than 50 ml is obtained, the feeding should be delayed. After consultation with the physician, the nurse administers all the nutrients through the subclavian vein via total parenteral nutrition (TPN). TPN

Table 1

Serum Assessments in Malnutrition

	Serum Albumin (g/dl)	Lymphocytes (per ml^3)
Mild deficit	3.0-3.5	1500-1800
Modest deficit	2.1-3.0	900-1500
Severe deficit	2.1	900

is used when the gut cannot be used; it contains 50% glucose, protein, electrolytes, vitamins, and trace elements. When a high concentration of glucose is given, the nurse must monitor blood glucose and urinary glucose and acetone to determine the possible presence of glycosuria. Regular insulin is given in consultation with the physician to move the glucose into the cells when blood glucose or urinary glucose is found to be high. Since sepsis is a complication of TPN, the patient's temperature is monitored every 4 hours.

Evaluation

Patient Outcome	Data Indicating That Outcome is Reached
Adequate nutrition	Good bone and tooth development Erect body posture Good skin turgor Clear skin and eyes Firm muscles Triceps skinfold: men, 12.5 mm; women, 16.5 mm Midarm circumference: men, 29.3 cm; women, 25.8 cm Serum albumin: 3.5-5 g/dl or 53% of total protein Lymphocytes: 1800-3000 mm^3 or 30% of leukocyte per ml^3 blood Midarm muscle circumference: men, 26.2 cm; women, 19.7 cm Adequate elimination Prompt healing Weight at normal level for body build Growth of 3-5 inches annually for children Mental alertness Energy to perform activities of daily living Absence of malaise, fatigue, and weakness Includes meats, fruits, vegetables, and breads in daily diet
Identifies factors that contributed to inadequate nutritional intake	Identifies strategies to improve nutrition Uses referrals to health team members as needed
Gains knowledge of nutritional needs	Patient and family can explain: 1. Reason for altered nutrition 2. Actions to avoid it 3. Types of menus to be used 4. Any necessary dietary alterations (foods to include and avoid) 5. Community agencies to be contacted for assistance 6. Medication program to be followed: state dosage, action, and side effects of prescribed drugs; list over-the-counter drugs to avoid

Ineffective Breastfeeding

Ineffective breastfeeding is the state in which a mother, infant, and/or family member experiences dissatisfaction or difficulty with the breastfeeding process.

The increase in breastfeeding in recent years is related to many factors. Consumer concerns with alterations in lifestyle, increased health-seeking behaviors, and reemergence of family values, particularly related to parenting and bonding with infants, has contributed to an increase in breastfeeding. With the increase in delayed pregnancies and distance from families, women have turned for assistance to support groups such as La Leche League.[19,25,28]

Difficulties with breastfeeding are consistently reported as the most significant problem in the postpartum period. Ineffective breastfeeding can negatively impact family processes and functioning by interfering with integration of the infant into the family unit, accommodation of new parenting roles, maintenance of the marital bond, and parent-infant bonding. It is therefore important for nurses to intervene by supporting and promoting behaviors that contribute to a positive breastfeeding experience.

Related Factors*

Prematurity
Infant anomaly
Maternal breast anomaly
Previous breast surgery
Previous history of breastfeeding failure

*Adapted from North American Nursing Diagnosis Association, 1988 Ballot.

Infant receiving supplemental feedings with artificial nipple
Poor infant sucking reflex
Nonsupportive partner or family
Knowledge deficit
Interruptions in breastfeeding
Severe anxiety
Competition of father with infant for breast

Defining Characteristics*

Unsatisfactory breastfeeding process
Actual or perceived inadequate milk supply

*Adapted from North American Nursing Diagnosis Association, 1988 Ballot.

Infant inability to attach onto maternal nipple properly
No observable signs of oxytocin release (lack of let-down reflex)
Nonsustained sucking at the breast
Suckling at only one breast per feeding
Nursing less than seven times in 24 hours (during neonatal period)
Persistence of sore nipples beyond the first week of life
Maternal reluctance to put infant to breast as necessary
Infant exhibiting fussiness or crying within the first hour after breastfeeding; unresponsive to other comfort measures
Infant arching and crying at breast, resisting latching on
Inadequate weight gain in infant
Infant has fewer than eight wet diapers per day

Nursing Interventions

Patient Goal	Nursing Intervention
Provide adequate milk supply for infant weight gain.	• Assist mother to assume the most comfortable position for her when nursing: side-lying or sitting. • Instruct mother to: Feed baby on demand. Compress areola and nipple area to ensure that it is soft enough for the baby to latch on; if not, express some milk to soften by partially emptying ducts. Gently compress nipple while inserting breast into infant's mouth to ensure that infant's mouth compresses milk-collecting sinuses in areola. Alternate breasts once during the feeding process. Allow infant to release nipple naturally after nursing or break suction of baby's mouth on nipple by placing finger inside mouth between gums. Burp baby in an upright position after nursing at each breast. • Inform mother that total feeding time can range from 20 minutes to 1 hour.[20] • Explain that supply of milk is related to demand and that: Giving formula only decreases breast milk supply. There is no need to supplement with formula (unless indicated by physician to increase infant's fluid volume, as in treatment for physiologic jaundice). Maternal fluid and nutrient intake requirements are increased with breastfeeding. • Assess maternal intake and output and ensure adequate hydration. • Encourage patient to drink fluids immediately before and during breastfeeding. • Discuss adjustments of dietary intake to meet infant's needs: Maintain well-balanced, high-protein diet. Avoid foods that cause infant distress (colicky, crying, wakeful); do not arbitrarily omit foods usually eaten. • Explain that it may be necessary to keep infant awake during feedings by unwrapping blankets and gently rubbing back or feet. • Explain importance of calming infant who cries and arches back before or during feeding: Swaddle infant snugly. Burp and rub back. Stroke eyebrows gently to promote vagal response and calming effect. Offer pacifier until infant is calm. Warm crib or bassinet with heating pad; then remove it before placing infant prone. • Remind mother that one way to tell if baby is receiving enough milk is to listen for swallowing when sucking. • Explain that adequate intake and nutrition is judged by six to eight wet diapers per day, that baby sleeps 1 to 2 hours between feedings, and that infant is gaining enough weight by the time of newborn examination with first visit to health care provider.
Engage in normal breastfeeding process that is satisfying to mother, infant, and family.	• Encourage family and friends to assist with household chores, shopping, and meal preparation. • Explain mechanisms of let-down reflex and that this often occurs shortly after infant begins to nurse.

Patient Goal	Nursing Intervention
	• Explain that milk normally leaks: From one breast while nursing on the other During coitus When hearing own (or other) infant crying • Assess breasts for hardness, tenderness, pain, and redness. • Discuss treatment for engorged breasts and have patient: Demonstrate these techniques. Place warm towel pack on breast for 15 minutes. Massage from outer breast to areola. Manually express breast or nurse infant. • Apply small amount of hydrous lanolin to nipples to prevent dryness and cracking; explain that this does not need to be washed off before each feeding. • Explain the need for and importance of planned rest periods for mother (these are best taken during the infant's sleep period). • Discuss with mother the potential adjustments to be made by father. • Encourage mother to discuss and share feelings regarding breastfeeding with spouse, especially if father demonstrates signs of competition with infant for breast or for attention in general. • Encourage mother to be aware of time spent with infant and breastfeeding and need to plan time with other children. • Explore value of breastfeeding with mother in terms of physiologic and psychologic rewards. Be sensitive to clues that mother does not like breastfeeding and may even express guilt for not meeting her own and others' expectations. • Support mother in decision to discontinue breastfeeding and explain that this will not adversely affect infant bonding or outcome.

Principles and Rationale for Nursing Interventions

The goals of the nursing interventions for ineffective breastfeeding are to ensure appropriate infant weight gain in a normal breastfeeding process that is satisfying to the mother, infant, and family.

A positive breastfeeding experience enhances and facilitates maternal-infant bonding, delivers protective antibodies to the infant, decreases infant weight loss in the immediate neonatal period, and contributes to overall infant well-being. In addition, an adequate supply of breast milk can help to prevent physiologic jaundice in the newborn. Note that "breast milk jaundice" is not caused by an inadequate milk supply but is attributed to a substance in the milk of some mothers that inhibits the hepatic enzyme glucuronyl transferase, which prevents the conjugation of bilirubin and its ultimate excretion.

Evaluation

Patient Outcome	Data Indicating That Outcome is Reached
Adequate milk supply for infant weight gain is established and maintained.	Infant maintains appropriate progressive weight gain. Mother demonstrates breastfeeding techniques without difficulty. Infant has six to eight wet diapers daily.
Breastfeeding process is satisfying to mother, infant, and family.	Breasts are not engorged. Infant sleeps 1 to 2 hours after being fed. Father is supportive of breastfeeding by assisting in household and child caretaking activities. Siblings demonstrate adaptive behaviors to mother's breastfeeding, e.g., not interrupting process and showing positive disposition.

Potential for Aspiration

Potential for aspiration is the state in which an individual is at risk for entry of gastric secretions, oropharyngeal secretions, or exogenous food or fluids into tracheobronchial passages because of dysfunction of normal protective mechanisms.

Aspiration occurs most often when the patient is in an altered state of consciousness resulting from seizure, drugs, alcohol, anesthesia, acute infection, or shock.

Risk Factors*

Reduced level of consciousness
Depressed cough and gag reflexes
Presence of tracheostomy or endotracheal tube
Underinflated tracheostomy/endotracheal tube cuff
Gastrointestinal tubes
Nasogastric tube feedings
Bolus tube feedings; medication administration
Situation hindering elevation of upper body
Supine position
Esophageal disease; hiatal hernia
Increased gastric residual
Decreased gastrointestinal motility
Impaired swallowing
Facial, oral, or neck surgery or trauma
Wired jaws
Impaired mastication
Inattentiveness to process of selecting, chewing, and swallowing food

*Adapted from North American Nursing Diagnosis Association, 1988 Ballot.

Defining Characteristics*

Reduced level of consciousness
Depressed cough and gag reflexes
Impaired swallowing
Impaired mastication

*Adapted from North American Nursing Diagnosis Association, 1988 Ballot.

Nursing Interventions

Patient Goal	Nursing Intervention
Do not aspirate food, fluid, or other substances into tracheobronchial passages.	• Monitor patient closely for respiratory rate, effort, and quality. Vesicular breath sounds should be heard over distal lung fields. • Avoid triggering gag mechanism when performing care activities, especially mouth care. • Confirm that patient has received nothing by mouth for several hours before surgery. • For patient with diminished swallowing reflex, elevate head of bed when giving oral fluids and encourage patient to take only small sips. • Assess and document amount of secretions present, patient's level of consciousness, and ability to handle (swallow) secretions effectively. • Test patient's gag reflex to identify whether it is diminished. • Identify contributing factors, such as oral surgery with jaw wiring, nasogastric tube feedings, or facial trauma. • Provide for suction equipment at patient's bedside. • Suction as often as necessary to remove secretions and maintain patent airway. • Elevate head of bed and patient's head during tube feedings and for 30 minutes after tube feeding is stopped. • For patients with reduced level of consciousness, ensure head of bed is elevated, unless contraindicated. • If patient is receiving tube feedings, ensure proper placement of tube before initiating feeding, as well as checking for residual. • Add food coloring to tube feeding; when suctioning, aspiration of tube feeding can be detected. • If secretions are thick or inspissated, ensure adequate humidification to help liquefy them. • If patient has a tracheotomy, ensure that cuff is inflated when patient eats or receives ventilatory assistance. • Monitor patient closely if eating for evidence of adequate swallowing with no gagging or emesis. • If patient is confused, remind him to chew and swallow. • Participate in public education about the risk of aspirated food in public places, and teach the Heimlich maneuver. • Perform the Heimlich maneuver when appropriate. • Instruct patient or significant other in method of cutting wires if jaw is wired. Keep wire cutters at patient's bedside. • Instruct patient with wired jaws to avoid the use of alcohol and mind-altering substances.

Principles and Rationale for Nursing Interventions

The nurse should frequently assess patient for vesicular breath sounds to ensure potential systemic oxygenation. Bronchial or bronchovesicular breath sounds over distal lung fields may indicate that aspiration has occurred. The nurse should take appropriate actions to reinstate normal breathing.

Evaluation

Patient Outcome	Data Indicating That Outcome is Reached
Aspiration prevented	Breath sounds heard over all lung fields Appears well oxygenated; blood gases within normal limits Shows no sign of air hunger

Impaired Swallowing

Impaired swallowing is the state in which an individual has decreased ability to pass fluids and solids voluntarily from the mouth to the stomach.

Related Factors[15]

Neuromuscular impairment, e.g., decreased or absent gag reflex, decreased strength or excursion of muscles involved in mastication, perceptual impairment, or facial paralysis

Mechanical obstruction, e.g., edema, tracheostomy tube, or tumor

Fatigue

Limited awareness

Reddened, irritated oropharyngeal cavity

Defining Characteristics[15]

Observed evidence of difficulty in swallowing, e.g., stasis of food in oral cavity or coughing and choking

Evidence of aspiration

Nursing Interventions*

Patient Goal	Nursing Intervention
Maintain adequate nutrition and hydration.	• Assess gag and cough reflexes. • If no gag reflex found, give food and fluid by feeding tube or parenterally. • Auscultate breath sounds. • Assess ability to swallow. • Provide rest periods before and after eating. • Determine patient's food preferences. • Encourage patient to wear properly fitted dentures. • Assist patient to 90-degree sitting position during meals and for 30 minutes after meals. • Have suction at the bedside ready for use. • Assist with oral hygiene before and after eating. • Add green or blue food coloring to liquids during the initial trials for feeding. • Progress patient slowly from swallowing own saliva, then to thick juice or nectar, semisolids, pureed diet, soft diet, and regular diet. • Place food in the unaffected side of the mouth. • Massage over the throat prn as patient swallows. • Measure intake and output. • Discontinue use of feeding tube when patient is receiving adequate nutrition by mouth.
Communicate knowledge of self-care.	• Involve patient and family in feeding process. • Supervise family members feeding patient. • Teach Heimlich maneuver to family members for use in an emergency.

*References 5, 6, 8, 15, 21, 30.

Principles and Rationale for Nursing Interventions

Two goals are derived for the patient with impaired swallowing: maintain adequate nutrition and hydration and communicate knowledge of self-care.

Before a patient with impaired swallowing eats or drinks, his gag and cough reflexes must be assessed, since these are the protective reflexes to prevent aspiration into the lungs. If these reflexes are absent, the patient should not be fed by mouth at this time; alternative routes such as feeding tubes or parenteral nutrition should be used. Breath sounds are assessed to determine if aspiration has occurred previously. Next the patient is asked to swallow saliva so that the musculature can be observed. Before attempts at eating, the patient should be allowed to rest because fatigue can impair swallowing. The patient's food preferences should be considered to facilitate patient cooperation. If the patient wears dentures, they should fit properly and be used at each meal.

For meals the patient should be seated at a 90-degree angle to allow gravity to assist in the peristaltic motion. A suction machine should be ready for use at the bedside in case the patient chokes. Oral hygiene is important before feeding to stimulate salivation and after feeding to clean the oral cavity. Green or blue food coloring added to the liquids will help determine if the patient is aspirating. The consistency of the food is progressed gradually from liquids to solids. Massaging over the throat may be necessary to stimulate the laryngopharyngeal muscles. Food is placed on the unaffected side of the mouth to facilitate movement to the back of the mouth. Some patients may benefit from the placement of food on the back of the tongue to assist in swallowing. These patients are fed slowly and in an environment without distraction such as television, radio, or visitors. They need to concentrate on swallowing until the behavior is learned again. Tilting the head forward 45 degrees keeps the esophagus patent to facilitate swallowing. The mouth is inspected frequently to ensure food is being swallowed rather than collected in the cheeks.

A record of intake and output should be maintained to evaluate hydration. If the patient was previously being fed by an alternative route, that method should continue until the patient is able to take adequate nutrition by mouth.

The patient and family need knowledge of how to assist the patient to eat at home. When the patient requires feeding, the family should practice in the hospital. To prevent choking, the family members must know how to perform the Heimlich maneuver on the patient. If a suction machine will be required at home, the family members will need instruction on how to use it. The family may require instruction on what foods to serve and how to prepare them. Finally, they need to know the plan for follow-up care.

Evaluation

Patient Outcome	Data Indicating That Outcome is Reached
Maintains nutrition and hydration	Patient swallows without gagging or choking. Intake is 2000 ml daily.
Explains knowledge of self-care	Family members assist patient with eating. Family members demonstrate Heimlich maneuver and can state their plan of action if patient chokes. Patient and family members select nutritious foods.

Altered Oral Mucous Membrane

Altered oral mucous membrane is the state in which an individual experiences damage to the tissue layers of the oral cavity.

Related Factors[15]

Pathologic conditions of oral cavity (radiation to head and/or neck)
Dehydration
Trauma
Chemical (acidic foods, drugs, noxious agents, alcohol)
Mechanical (ill-fitting dentures, braces, and endotracheal, nasogastric, or surgery tubes)
NPO instructions for more than 24 hours
Ineffective oral hygiene
Mouth breathing
Malnutrition
Infection
Lack of or decreased salivation
Medication

Defining Characteristics[15]

Coated tongue
Xerostomia (dry mouth)
Stomatitis
Oral lesions or ulcers
Lack of or decreased salivation
Leukoplakia
Edema
Hyperemia
Oral plaque
Oral pain or discomfort
Desquamation
Vesicles
Hemorrhagic gingivitis
Carious teeth
Halitosis

Nursing Interventions[6,8,15,30]

Patient Goal	Nursing Intervention
Maintain a comfortable and functional oral cavity.	• Assess patient's teeth, gums, oral mucosa, lips, and tongue. • Measure intake and output. • Provide oral hygiene (brushing, flossing, mouthwash); irrigate lesions as ordered. • Lubricate lips. • Administer local anesthetics as ordered before mealtime. • Serve food and fluids at appropriate temperatures; avoid extreme temperatures (hot or cold) when they cause discomfort. • Change texture of food to soft or puree when necessary. • Maintain intravenous or oral fluids as ordered. • Discourage smoking and use of alcohol.
Communicate knowledge of self-care.	• Assess what the patient and family already know. • Provide information about: Reasons for alteration in oral mucous membrane Importance of dental hygiene for all family members Review of medications and treatments ordered for home use Plan for follow-up care

Principles and Rationale for Nursing Interventions

Two patient goals are derived from assessment data: maintain a comfortable and functional oral cavity and communicate knowledge of self-care.

The patient's lips, tongue, gums, and oral mucosa are assessed for moisture, color, texture, and presence of debris and infection. The teeth are checked for color, shine, and debris. Intake is measured to ensure adequacy, and the patient is encouraged to drink fluids when necessary. The toothbrush used should have soft bristles of equal length. A commercial toothpaste or sodium bicarbonate may be used. The brushing motion is in small circles or sweeping motion moving downward from the gums. The tongue should be brushed as well.

Oral care for the unconscious patient is performed with the patient in a side-lying position and the head of the bed elevated at least 30 degrees to prevent aspiration. The brushing procedure is the same as for the alert patient. Rinsing is done using a large syringe and oral suction. When the patient has an oral airway in place, it is changed or cleaned. Dentures and bridges require soaking and brushing daily. After brushing, the mouth is rinsed. Commercial mouthwashes are not recommended because they contain alcohol, which is painful; instead, saline solution or water can be used. Hydrogen peroxide when used 1:2 or 1:4 with water acts well as a germicide to destroy bacteria chemically and clean mechanically. Its bubbling action removes film from tongue and teeth. Glycerin swabs tend to dry mucous membranes and are recommended only daily for clean, healthy mouths. Open lesions are irrigated with a pulsating jet stream of water or with saline in a small syringe. A gauze pad wrapped around the finger moistened with saline or water also can be used.

Fluid and food intake decreases when it causes pain. Relief of the pain can be accomplished by changing the temperature of the fluid or food to tepid or to warm, or the texture of the food to soft or pureed. Foods to avoid include fried foods, spicy foods, citrus fruits, crusty foods, and foods of extreme temperatures. Local anesthetics, per physician's orders, are useful before mealtime to provide temporary pain relief to increase intake. These include lidocaine (Xylocaine) viscous 2%; 0.5 aqueous Benadryl solution and Maalox; or equal parts of 0.5 aqueous Benadryl solution and Kaopectate. The patient swishes the solution and then swallows or expectorates. When lidocaine is swallowed, however, it may affect the gag reflex.[6] The patient is encouraged to avoid smoking and alcoholic beverages because they irritate the mucosa and act as drying agents.

The nurse assesses the patient's and family's knowledge to determine what content to teach. Prevention of alteration of oral mucous membranes is very important. The patient and family need to review their dental hygiene practices. Children benefit from visits to the dentist every 6 months after the age of 2 years. Fluoride supplements are helpful for children. They will need help brushing their teeth until age 6, but it is important for children to develop the recommended dental hygiene practices. Infants who are put to bed with a bottle should receive a bottle of water rather than juice or milk. The infant who is teething needs safe objects to put in the mouth. Adults require annual visits to the dentist. Daily brushing and flossing with sufficient fluids and adequate nutrition will help prevent dental caries.

Evaluation

Patient Outcome	Data Indicating That Outcome is Reached
Maintains adequate nutrition and hydration	Moist oral mucous membranes, coral color Able to drink and chew without discomfort Lack of halitosis
Explains knowledge of self-care	Patient and family can explain: 1. Reasons for alteration in oral mucous membrane 2. Plan for dental hygiene for all family members 3. Medications and treatment for home use 4. Plan for follow-up care

Potential Fluid Volume Deficit

Potential fluid volume deficit is the state in which an individual is at risk of experiencing vascular, cellular, or intracellular dehydration.

Risk Factors[15]

Extremes of age
Extremes of weight
Excessive losses through normal routes (diarrhea)
Loss of fluid through abnormal routes (indwelling tubes)
Deviations affecting access to, intake of, or absorption of fluids (physical immobility)
Factors influencing fluid needs (hypermetabolic states)
Knowledge deficiency related to fluid volume
Medications (diuretics)
Increased fluid output
Urinary frequency
Thirst
Altered intake
Hyperventilation
Clinical evidence of body fluid or blood loss through artificial orifices, lumens, wounds, or drainage tubes

Nursing Interventions[6,8,15,30]

Patient Goal	Nursing Intervention
Achieve fluid replacement.	• Monitor vital signs. • Weigh patient. • Assess skin turgor. • Assess oral mucous membranes. • Measure intake and output. • Assess and describe drainage from wounds. • Monitor electrolyte values. • Keep oral fluids at the bedside within patient's reach; encourage fluid intake. • Maintain tube feedings as ordered. • Maintain intravenous fluids and electrolytes as ordered. • Maintain total parenteral nutrition as ordered. • Administer medication as ordered to prevent fluid losses: antiemetics, antidiarrheals. • Evaluate therapeutic, adverse, and toxic effects of medications given.
Communicate knowledge to maintain fluid balance.	• Assess what patient and family already know. • Provide information concerning: Actions to prevent actual deficit Reasons for treatments What foods and fluids to consume What foods and fluids to avoid

Principles and Rationale for Nursing Interventions

Two goals for the patient with potential fluid volume deficit are to achieve fluid replacement and to communicate knowledge to maintain fluid balance.

Changes in vital signs expected in a potential fluid volume deficit are a gradual increase in the pulse as the heart pumps faster to circulate blood and a gradual decrease in blood pressure as fluid is lost from the intravascular spaces. A decrease in the patient's weight may indicate fluid loss. Loss of skin turgor occurs as fluid moves from the interstitial spaces. Dry oral mucous membranes may indicate dehydration. A change in the fluid balance could indicate a fluid deficit when output exceeds intake. The patient requires fluids to replace those lost. Along with the fluid losses, the patient may have electrolyte imbalances, particularly of sodium and potassium.

If oral fluids are tolerated, they should be kept within the patient's reach. Intravenous fluids can provide water, glucose, electrolytes, and vitamins. Albumin may be given intravenously, per physician's order, to provide protein to maintain oncotic pressure. Total parenteral nutrition is frequently ordered by the physician when prolonged fluid therapy is required, since it supplies additional calories in the form of 50% dextrose as well as proteins, electrolytes, vitamins, and water. Nasogastric tube feeding is another means of providing fluids along with nutrients. Data on body weight and daily fluid balance must be obtained.

The patient needs not only replacement fluids, but also treatment for the source of the fluid loss. Loss from vomiting can be lessened by discontinuing oral intake of fluids and food, in addition to changing medications that cause vomiting as a side effect. When medications causing vomiting cannot be discontinued, administration of antiemetics as ordered by the physician should be considered. Drainage from abnormal routes is difficult to stop. At times the drainage is necessary and must be replaced with fluids. Profuse diaphoresis also requires fluid replacement until the cause can be treated and fluid balance regained. Diarrhea is arrested by discontinuing oral intake and administering drugs as ordered to slow peristalsis.

The second goal is to communicate knowledge of fluid balance. Family members need to know the types of fluid replacements to use. For example, milk and milk products should be withheld from individuals with diarrhea. Clear liquids, such as ginger ale, apple juice, beef broth, and popsicles, are the fluids of choice. Family members need to know the purpose, frequency of administration, and side effects of medications to be taken. They can keep a record of the intake and output to evaluate fluid balance.

Evaluation

Patient Outcome	Data Indicating That Outcome is Reached
Achieves fluid replacement	Vital signs within normal limits Good skin turgor Moist mucous membranes Absence of thirst Balanced intake and output Blood: Sodium: adult, 135-145 mEq/L Potassium: 3.5-5.0 mEq/L; add approximately 0.2 to normal range if serum is sampled rather than plasma; pediatric ranges sometimes reported as slightly higher than adult levels Chloride (serum): full-term infant, 96-106 mEq/L; children and adults, 97-107 mEq/L
Communicates knowledge of fluid balance	Patient and family can explain: 1. Actions to prevent actual loss 2. Foods and fluids to consume 3. Foods and fluids to avoid 4. Medications and treatments for home use 5. Plan for follow-up care

Fluid Volume Deficit (1)

Fluid volume deficit (1) is the state in which an individual experiences vascular, cellular, or intracellular dehydration related to failure of regulatory mechanisms.

Related Factor

Failure of regulatory mechanism[15]

Defining Characteristics[15]

Failure of regulatory mechanism
- Dilute urine
- Increased urine output
- Sudden weight loss
- Possible weight gain
- Hypotension
- Decreased venous filling
- Increased pulse rate
- Decreased skin turgor
- Decreased pulse volume and pressure
- Increased body temperature
- Dry skin
- Dry mucous membranes
- Hemoconcentration
- Weakness
- Edema
- Thirst

Nursing Interventions[5,8,15,30]

Patient Goal	Nursing Intervention
Maintain adequate fluid and electrolyte balance.	• Measure vital signs. • Assess capillary refill time. • Measure intake and output. • Weigh patient. • Monitor electrolyte values. • Measure urine specific gravity. • Monitor hemoglobin and hematocrit. • Assess oral mucous membranes. • Assess skin turgor. • Measure abdominal girth when ascites is present. • Administer intravenous or oral fluids as ordered by physician. • Administer electrolytes as ordered. • Administer regulating hormones as ordered (e.g., insulin, vasopressin).
Communicate knowledge of self-care.	• Assess what patient and family already know. • Provide information concerning: Cause of this fluid deficit and how to prevent recurrence Reasons for treatments Foods and fluids to consume Purpose, frequency of administration, and side effects of medications ordered by physician for patient to take at home • When patient is going home to receive total parenteral nutrition as ordered by physician, have family demonstrate how to change tubing and fluid bags as well as what to do when problems arise. • Review the plan for follow-up.

Principles and Rationale for Nursing Interventions

Two patient goals are derived from the assessment data: maintain adequate fluid and electrolyte balance and communicate knowledge of self-care.

In the area of assessment interventions, vital sign changes can indicate fluid losses. An elevated body temperature also may occur with a fluid loss. The pulse rate increases, reflecting the heart trying to circulate adequate blood volume. Blood pressure frequently drops because of a shift in fluid out of the intravascular spaces. Slowed capillary refill time indicates decreased venous filling. Intake and output are monitored because a change in fluid balance may signal a fluid loss when the output exceeds intake. Changes in weight indicate fluid volume changes. For example, a weight gain may occur in the patient with ascites, and a weight loss may occur in the patient with excessive urine output. Because both these patients have decreased intravascular fluid volume, they both have a fluid volume deficit. Along with fluid losses, the patient may have electrolyte losses, particularly sodium and potassium. Urine specific gravity increases in many conditions as a result of hypoperfusion of kidneys, leading to oliguria. Elevated hemoglobin and hematocrit indicate hemoconcentration. Dry oral mucous membranes may indicate a fluid deficit. Loss of skin turgor occurs as fluid moves from the interstitial spaces. Abdominal girth measurements increase as ascites develops.

Fluids and electrolytes are replaced in consultation with the physician by an intravenous route in the form of blood or blood products and/or glucose in water or saline with electrolytes. When long-term therapy is needed, total parenteral nutrition is used as ordered to provide concentrated glucose and proteins for calories and positive nitrogen balance, respectively. Regulatory hormones are replaced as ordered to regain balance, such as insulin and antidiuretic hormone (ADH) (Pitressin).

The nurse assesses learning needs of the family to determine what content to provide. The patient and family may need instructions about nutrition. They will need to know the purpose, frequency of administration, and side effects of medications ordered by the physician to be taken at home. Return demonstration will be needed by the family who will care for a patient receiving intravenous fluids at home.

Evaluation

Patient Outcome	Data Indicating That Outcome is Reached
Maintains adequate fluid and electrolyte balance	Good skin turgor Moist mucous membranes Balanced intake and output

Patient Outcome	Data Indicating That Outcome is Reached
	Blood pressure: 160/95 (over 65 years) 150/95 (45-65 years) 140/95 (18-44 years) Pulse: 70-80/min Blood (see Potential Fluid Volume Deficit) Serum osmolality: 280-300 mOsm/kg water Hemoglobin (g/dl): Men 15.5 ± 1.1 Women 13.7 ± 1.0 Hematocrit (%): Men 46.0 ± 3.1 Women 40.9 ± 3 Urine Specific gravity: range of 1.001-1.035; adult on normal fluid intake, 1.016-1.022; specific gravity decreases with increasing age Osmolality: 250-900 mOsm/kg for random specimens
Communicates knowledge of self-care	Patient and family are able to explain: 1. Reasons for fluid deficit 2. Foods and fluids to consume to prevent recurrence 3. Purpose, dosage, and side effects of medications ordered by physician 4. Plan for follow-up care

Fluid Volume Deficit (2)

Fluid volume deficit (2) is the state in which an individual experiences vascular, cellular, or intracellular dehydration related to active loss.

Related Factor

Actual loss[15]

Defining Characteristics[15,21,23]

Decreased urine output
Concentrated urine
Output greater than intake
Sudden weight loss
Decreased venous filling
Increased serum sodium
Hypotension
Thirst
Increased pulse rate
Decreased skin turgor
Decreased pulse volume and pressure
Change in mental status
Increased body temperature
Dry skin
Dry mucous membranes
Weakness
Hemoconcentration
Decreased central venous pressure
Pulmonary capillary wedge pressure less than 6 mm Hg

Nursing Interventions*

Patient Goal	Nursing Intervention
Maintain adequate fluid and electrolyte balance.	• Measure vital signs. • Measure central venous pressure or pulmonary capillary wedge pressure. • Assess capillary refill time. • Measure intake and output. • Monitor electrolyte values. • Measure urine specific gravity. • Monitor hemoglobin and hematocrit. • Assess oral mucous membranes. • Assess skin turgor. • Administer intravenous or oral fluids as ordered by physician.

*References 5, 6, 8, 15, 21, 23, 30.

Patient Goal	Nursing Intervention
	• Administer electrolytes as ordered by physician. • Administer blood, blood products, or plasma expanders as ordered by physician. • Administer medications as ordered to prevent further fluid losses (antiemetics, antidiarrheals). • Cover wounds according to protocol.
Communicate knowledge of self-care.	• Assess what patient and family already know. • Provide information concerning: Cause of this fluid deficit and how to prevent recurrence Reasons for treatments Foods and fluids to consume The purpose, frequency of administration, and side effects of medications ordered by the physician for the patient to take at home • When patient is going home to receive total parenteral nutrition as ordered by the physician, have family demonstrate how to change tubing and fluid bags as well as what to do when problems arise. • Review the plan for follow-up.

Principles and Rationale for Nursing Interventions

Two patient goals are derived from the assessment data: maintain adequate fluid and electrolyte balance and communicate knowledge of self-care.

In the area of assessment interventions, vital sign changes can indicate fluid losses. An elevated body temperature also may occur with a fluid loss. The pulse rate increases, reflecting the heart trying to circulate adequate blood volume. Blood pressure frequently drops because of a shift in fluid out of the intravascular spaces. Slowed capillary refill time indicates decreased venous filling. Intake and output are monitored because a change in fluid balance may signal a fluid loss when the output exceeds intake. Along with fluid losses, the patient may have electrolyte losses, particularly sodium and potassium. Urine specific gravity increases in many conditions as a result of hypoperfusion of kidneys, leading to oliguria. Elevated hemoglobin and hematocrit indicate hemoconcentration. Dry oral mucous membranes may indicate a fluid deficit. Loss of skin turgor occurs as fluid moves from the interstitial spaces.

Next, treatment is initiated to reduce and stop the fluid loss: stop hemorrhage, treat burns, and give drugs as ordered to halt diarrhea or vomiting. Fluids and electrolytes are given as needed to restore those lost. Fluids may include crystalloids, blood, blood products, and plasma expanders.

The nurse assesses learning needs of the family to determine what content to provide. The patient and family may need instructions about nutrition. They will need to know the purpose, frequency of administration, and side effects of medications ordered by the physician to be taken at home. Return demonstration will be needed by the family who will care for a patient receiving intravenous fluids at home.

Evaluation

Patient Outcome	Data Indicating That Outcome is Reached
Maintains adequate fluid and electrolyte balance	Good skin turgor Moist mucous membranes Absence of thirst Balanced intake and output Clearing of mentation Blood pressure: 160/95 (over 65 years) 150/95 (45-65 years) 140/95 (18-44 years) Pulse: 70-80/min Blood (see Potential Fluid Volume Deficit) Serum osmolality: 280-300 mOsm/kg water Hemoglobin (g/dl): Men 15.5 ± 1.1 Women 13.7 ± 1.0 Hematocrit (%): Men 46.0 ± 3.1 Women 40.9 ± 3

Patient Outcome	Data Indicating That Outcome is Reached
	Urine Specific gravity: range of 1.001-1.035; adult on normal fluid intake, 1.016-1.022; specific gravity decreases with increasing age Osmolality: 250-900 mOsm/kg for random specimens
Communicates knowledge of self-care	Patient and family are able to explain: 1. Reasons for fluid deficit 2. Foods and fluids to consume to prevent recurrence 3. Purpose, dosage, and side effects of medications ordered by physician 4. Plan for follow-up care

Fluid Volume Excess

Fluid volume excess is the state in which an individual experiences increased fluid retention and edema.

Related Factors[15]

Compromised regulatory mechanism
Excess fluid intake
Excess sodium intake

Defining Characteristics[15]

Edema
Effusion (pleural, pericardial)
Anasarca (generalized massive edema)
Weight gain
Shortness of breath, orthopnea
Intake greater than output
Third heart sound
Pulmonary congestion on roentgenogram
Abnormal breath sounds: crackles (rales)
Change in respiratory pattern
Change in mental status
Decreased hemoglobin, hematocrit
Blood pressure changes
Central venous pressure changes
Pulmonary artery pressure changes
Jugular venous distention
Positive hepatojugular reflex
Oliguria
Specific gravity changes
Azoturia
Altered electrolytes
Restlessness and anxiety

Nursing Interventions[5,6,8,15,30]

Patient Goal	Nursing Intervention
Regain fluid balance.	• Measure vital signs. • Measure central venous pressure or pulmonary artery pressure. • Weigh patient. • Measure intake and output. • Measure specific gravity. • Monitor electrolyte, albumin, urea nitrogen, creatinine, hemoglobin, and hematocrit values. • Assess skin turgor and inspect skin for redness and edema. • Measure abdominal girth. • Auscultate breath sounds. • Administer drugs as ordered: diuretics, albumin. • Evaluate the therapeutic, adverse, and toxic effects of drugs given. • Restrict sodium and fluid as ordered. • Position patient in semi-Fowler's position. • Administer oxygen as ordered by physician.
Avoid complications of fluid excess.	• Inspect skin continuously for redness. • Reposition patient frequently. • Perform passive or active range of motion several times each day. • Apply elastic stockings. • Encourage patient to cough and deep breathe.
Communicate knowledge of self-care.	• Assess what patient and family already know. • Provide information concerning: Reasons for fluid excess

Patient Goal	Nursing Intervention
	Reasons for treatments Dietary alterations required, such as low-sodium diet Purpose of drugs ordered for home use Ways to support peripheral circulation Plan for follow-up care

Principles and Rationale for Nursing Interventions

The three goals for the patient with fluid volume excess are to regain fluid balance by removing excess fluid and treating the underlying cause, to prevent complications of fluid excess, and to communicate knowledge of self-care.

Changes in vital signs may include a full, bounding pulse and elevated blood pressure because of an increase in the intravascular volume. Central venous pressure or pulmonary artery pressures also may be elevated, indicating an increased fluid volume. A change in fluid balance may indicate a fluid excess when intake is greater than output. Urine specific gravity increases in any condition, causing hypoperfusion of the kidneys and leading to oliguria. Electrolytes, blood urea nitrogen, and creatinine may be elevated with fluid excess. Hemoglobin and hematocrit may be low because of hemodilution. Skin turgor may be edematous as a result of excessive interstitial fluid. An increased abdominal girth indicates development of ascites. Auscultation for breath sounds may be decreased from fluid in the lung.

Therapy to remove excess fluid is based on the cause of the problem. In accordance with physician orders, diuretics are given for excessive fluid caused by inadequate circulation, albumin is given to provide protein to pull fluid into the intravascular space so that it can be excreted by the kidneys, dialysis is used in renal failure when diuretics and albumin are inappropriate, thoracentesis is used to remove fluid from the pleural space, and paracentesis is used to remove fluid from the abdomen. In addition to removing fluid, treatment also includes restricting sodium and fluid intake to prevent further fluid excess. A balance is maintained between providing fluid and restricting sodium.

While administering treatment for fluid excess, the nurse protects edematous parts of the body from prolonged pressure, injury, and extremes of hot and cold. When excess fluids compromise respiratory effort, the nurse can place the patient in a semi-Fowler's position and administer oxygen as ordered by the physician. Skin is inspected for redness and blanching. The patient's position is changed every 1 or 2 hours to prevent pressure on edematous areas. Active or passive range of motion is done to prevent contractures and improve venous return. Application of elastic stockings provides support to veins and prevents venous stasis. Thirst becomes a problem because oral intake is limited but the patient is thirsty. Chewing gum or sucking hard candy may stimulate enough saliva to reduce the patient's thirst. There is a psychologic advantage for the patient when the nurse puts the small amount of oral fluid allowed in a small (medicine) cup rather than a standard-size cup.

To communicate a knowledge of self-care, the nurse determines what the patient and family already know. They need to understand the cause of the fluid volume excess. Many patients require dietary alterations of low sodium or altered protein intake. Persons who buy the food and prepare the meals need written information on appropriate menus. They need to read labels of food for sodium content. Information about medications to be taken includes the purpose, frequency of administration, and side effects. The patient needs to know how to support peripheral circulation. This includes applying elastic stockings before rising and avoiding crossed legs and standing for long periods. The feet and legs need to be inspected daily for edema and redness to prevent pressure sores.

Evaluation

Patient Outcome	Data Indicating That Outcome is Reached
Regains fluid balance	Blood pressure (upper limits): 160/95 (over 65 yr) 150/95 (45-65 yr) 140/95 (18-44 yr) Respiration: 12-20/min Blood (see Potential Fluid Volume Deficit) Hemoglobin (g/dl): Men 15.5 ± 1.1 Women 13.7 ± 1.0 Hematocrit (%): Men 46.0 ± 3.1 Women 40.9 ± 3

Patient Outcome	Data Indicating That Outcome is Reached
	Albumin 3.2-5.6 g/dl blood Potassium 3.5-5 mEq/L Sodium 135-145 mEq/L BUN 8-20 mg/dl Creatinine 0.6-1.2 mg/dl Good skin turgor Balanced intake and output Clearing of mentation Absence of edema
Communicates knowledge of self-care	Patient and family can explain: 1. Reasons for fluid volume excess 2. Dietary alterations 3. Medication and treatments for home use 4. Plan for follow-up care

 Potential Impaired Skin Integrity

Potential impaired skin integrity is the state in which the individual's skin is at risk of being adversely altered.

Risk Factors[15]

External (environmental)
- Hyperthermia or hypothermia
- Chemical substance
- Mechanical factors
  - Shearing forces
  - Pressure
  - Restraint
- Radiation
- Physical immobilization
- Excretions and secretions
- Humidity

Internal (somatic)
- Medication
- Altered nutritional state (obesity, emaciation)
- Altered metabolic state
- Altered circulation
- Altered sensation (anesthesia, paresthesia, pruritus)
- Altered pigmentation
- Skeletal prominence
- Developmental factors
- Alterations in skin turgor (change in elasticity)
- Psychogenic factors
- Immunologic deficit

Nursing Interventions*

Patient Goal	Nursing Intervention
Maintain intact skin.	• Inspect skin for color and integrity. • Palpate skin for temperature, turgor, elasticity, and moisture. • Palpate peripheral pulses; check capillary refill time. • Teach patient and family members to inspect skin daily for reddened areas, broken skin, and bruised areas, blisters, and swelling; include how healthy skin appears and actions to take when abnormalities are found. • Monitor laboratory values and report abnormalities: Hemoglobin, hemotocrit Blood glucose Blood urea nitrogen Creatinine Albumin Bilirubin Electrolytes Arterial blood gases • Monitor drugs patient is taking, especially steroids and estrogen. • Keep patient's skin clean and dry. • Provide balanced diet and adequate fluids. • Assess patient's and family's knowledge of a balanced diet and teach as necessary.

*References 5, 6, 8, 15, 21, 30.

Patient Goal	Nursing Intervention
	• Inform individuals with altered pigmentation to wear long-sleeved shirts or blouses and hats to shield the skin. • Tell children and adults playing and working in the sun to wear protective clothing, to apply a sun screen lotion, or to limit exposure time. • Inform individuals receiving radiation to blot dry their skin rather than rub. • Lubricate dry skin with lotion or oil. Blisters or redness may occur from ill-fitting clothes or shoes; have person pad skin with bandage and clothing or change shoes until blister or redness subsides. • When itching is a problem, encourage individual not to scratch; pressing the area or applying ice decreases the sensation and does not damage the skin. A cool environment is soothing as opposed to a warm environment. Other soothing measures include lubricating the skin with oil or lotion and taking a tub bath containing oatmeal powder, potassium permanganate, or corn starch at 32° to 38° C (89.6° to 100.4° F). When other methods are unsuccessful, give antihistamines as ordered by a physician.
Maintain circulation to the skin.	• Provide for active or passive exercise. • Change position every 2 hours, or ambulate patient if possible. • Use a turning sheet when moving patient. • Use heel protectors as needed. • Massage pressure points after turning. • *Do not massage legs.* • Teach patient or family to turn patient. • Use egg-crate, air-filled, or foam mattress and pillows as needed. • When feet swell, use support stockings and periodic leg elevation. Reduction in sodium and fluids may also be indicated to decrease swelling.

Principles and Rationale for Nursing Interventions

Two patient goals are derived from the assessment data: maintain intact skin and maintain circulation to the skin.

The nurse assesses the skin for color and integrity to identify any areas of impairment. Further skin assessment includes temperature, turgor, elasticity, and moisture because loss of these factors places the patient at risk for skin impairment. Peripheral pulses are palpated and capillary refill time is assessed to determine tissue perfusion to the extremities. The nurse teaches the patient and family to perform this assessment so that they can detect problems early. Laboratory values are monitored to detect abnormalities that might affect the skin, e.g., renal failure, liver failure, anemia, and diabetes mellitus. Certain drugs make the skin more susceptible to impairment, e.g., estrogen and steroids. Patients who are taking these drugs need to be especially protective of their skin.

The skin is kept clean and dry to remove bacteria and prevent maceration from excessive moisture. Eating an adequate diet that includes protein for tissue vitality and vitamin C for collagen formation is important. Moisture of the skin is maintained internally by the intake of adequate fluids and externally by lubricating the skin. Protection of the skin includes wearing clothing appropriate for the outdoor temperature and humidity. Patients should avoid behaviors that constrict circulation; e.g., they should not smoke because tobacco causes vasoconstriction and not wear constrictive clothing. When itching is a problem, the patient should be in a cool environment to decrease the perception of itching. The patient should be encouraged to press the area that itches rather than scratching to decrease itching without damaging the skin. Keeping the patient's nails short will limit the damage to the skin when scratching does occur. The patient and family can be active participants when they are taught to maintain the skin and prevent skin impairment.

Circulation to the skin is maintained by moving, turning, and exercising. Using a turning sheet when moving a patient up in bed or to a side-lying position avoids the shearing force to the patient's buttocks. Heel protectors also are useful to reduce the shearing force on the heels as the patient moves about in bed. Massaging pressure points after turning stimulates circulation to those points previously receiving the body's pressure. The legs of a patient who is confined to bed are *not* massaged because the massage may dislodge a blood clot, creating an embolus. A pressure-relieving mattress is useful for a patient confined to bed. Applying elastic bandages facilitates venous return and is useful to prevent swelling of the feet.

Evaluation

Patient Outcome	Data Indicating That Outcome is Reached
Maintains intact skin	Skin dry with natural color Moist, adequate turgor with no breaks in skin integrity Intake of balanced diet reported Behaviors required to maintain skin integrity verbalized by patient and family
Maintains circulation	Skin warm; peripheral pulse present and strong

Impaired Skin Integrity

Impaired skin integrity is the state in which the individual's skin is adversely altered.

Nurses maintain the skin integrity of patients to ensure the body's first line of natural defense. The diagnosis of impaired skin integrity is appropriate when the patient has impairment of the epidermis or dermis. When impairment extends into the subcutaneous tissue, the diagnosis of tissue impairment is used.

Related Factors[15]

External (environmental)
- Hyperthermia or hypothermia
- Chemical substance
- Mechanical factors
  - Shearing forces
  - Pressure
  - Restraint
- Radiation
- Physical immobilization
- Excretion and secretions
- Humidity

Internal (somatic)
- Medication
- Altered nutritional state (obesity, emaciation)
- Altered metabolic state
- Altered circulation
- Altered sensation
- Altered pigmentation
- Skeletal prominence
- Developmental factors
- Immunologic deficit
- Alterations in skin turgor (change in elasticity)
- Excretions and secretions
- Psychogenic factors
- Edema

Defining Characteristics[15]

Disruption of skin surface
Destruction of skin layers
Invasion of body structures

Nursing Interventions*

Patient Goal	Nursing Intervention
Regain skin integrity.	• Inspect area of impaired integrity for healing. • Monitor leukocytes. • Ambulate patient if possible. • Change position every 2 hours. • Use pressure-relieving mattress, e.g., egg-crate, foam, or air-filled mattress and pillows. • Cover areas of impaired skin integrity as ordered with dressings, ointments, etc. • Administer intravenous fluids as ordered. • Administer anti-infective agents as ordered. • Maintain sterile technique when caring for wounds. • Provide balanced diet as ordered: high in calories and proteins, iron, and vitamins.
Maintain intact skin.	• See nursing interventions for Potential Impaired Skin Integrity.
Achieve comfort.	• Reduce itching sensation. • Encourage patient to discuss feelings about impaired skin integrity and body image changes. • Use distraction techniques for pain relief. • Administer local and systemic analgesics as ordered. • Evaluate the therapeutic, adverse, and toxic effects of drugs given.

*References 5, 6, 8, 15, 21, 30.

Patient Goal	Nursing Intervention
Communicate knowledge of self-care.	• Assess what patient and family need to learn. • Provide information concerning: Prevention of skin integrity alterations How to change dressing and apply topical medication Purpose, frequency of administration, and side effects of medication Dietary intake to promote wound healing How to achieve comfort and relieve pain

Principles and Rationale for Nursing Interventions

Four goals are derived for the patient with impaired skin integrity: regain skin integrity, maintain intact skin, achieve comfort, and communicate knowledge of self-care.

Skin integrity is regained by protecting the skin from further damage and by promoting wound healing. The size and color of the area of impairment are documented to evaluate healing. Protection of the skin is provided when pressure is relieved from the dependent part of the body by turning or ambulating the patient or by using a pressure-relieving mattress. Skin integrity can be impaired by infections, as indicated by an elevated leukocyte count, foul-smelling odor, or purulent drainage from the wound. Covering the areas of impaired skin and giving anti-infective agents as ordered serve to treat existing infections by interrupting the growth of microorganisms.

Healing is promoted by adequate oxygen and blood supply along with nutrients to support tissue growth. These nutrients include protein and carbohydrate to maintain a positive nitrogen balance. Iron and vitamins A, B complex, C, D, and E also are required. The age of the patient is a factor in wound healing because children normally heal more rapidly than adults. Elderly persons often heal more slowly because of decreased fibroblastic activity and impaired circulation. Patients receiving steroids have delayed wound healing because these drugs depress the inflammatory response, which occurs before wound healing.

Relief of pain and itching promotes comfort. This itching sensation is felt at varying stages of tissue repair. The normal response is to scratch the area, but one gentle scratch can infect an area. Repeated scratching in one area can further damage the epidermis. Cold applied to the itch can anesthetize the area for a short time. The patient's nails must be clipped short and kept as clean as possible. The patient can be encouraged to press on the itching area rather than scratch. This pressing briefly interrupts the sensory (afferent) nerve impulse without damaging the epidermis. Distraction techniques may be effective to relieve itching perception.

Another aspect of comfort for some patients is psychologic. Impaired skin integrity can disfigure a person, resulting in a disturbance in self-concept (refer to Self-Perception–Self-Concept). The patient should verbalize feelings about the body image change and consider how to cope with the reactions of others to this change.

The nurse instructs the patient and family on actions to prevent skin impairment and to continue treatment of the impaired skin after discharge. Time should be made for the family and patient to perform return demonstrations on dressing changes and to ask questions about the treatment schedule.

Evaluation

Patient Outcome	Data Indicating That Outcome is Reached
Regain skin integrity	Skin intact Skin warm with dry, natural color No reports of pain or itching from involved area(s)
Communicates knowledge of self-care	Patient/family can explain: 1. Cause and prevention of altered skin integrity 2. Medications and treatment for home use 3. Dietary intake to promote wound healing 4. Plan for follow-up care

Impaired Tissue Integrity

Impaired tissue integrity is the state in which an individual experiences damage to mucous membranes or corneal, integumentary, or subcutaneous tissue.

The diagnosis of impaired tissue integrity is appropriate for the patient who has impairment of the corneas, mucous membrane (other than oral mucous membranes), and the subcutaneous tissue. This diagnosis also is appropriate for a patient who has a pressure sore, defined as tissue trauma occurring over a bony prominence and resulting from sustained pressure and other contributing factors.[9] Likewise, impaired tissue integrity applies to a patient with corneal abrasion or ulceration.

Related Factors[15]

Altered circulation
Nutritional deficit or excess
Fluid deficit or excess
Knowledge deficit
Impaired physical mobility
Irritants
  Chemical (including body excretions and secretions, medications)
  Thermal (temperature extremes)
  Mechanical (pressure, shear, friction)
  Radiation (including therapeutic radiation)

Defining Characteristics[9,15,21]

Damaged or destroyed tissue (cornea, mucous membrane other than oral, and subcutaneous with integumentary involvement)
Cornea: pain, photophobia, decreased vision, lacrimation, blepharospasm
Subcutaneous tissue: redness over a bony prominence that does not disappear within 10 to 15 minutes; exposure of the dermis; serous or purulent drainage from subcutaneous tissue

Nursing Interventions[5,8,9,15,21]

Patient Goal	Nursing Intervention
Regain tissue integrity.	• Assess skin integrity daily. • Monitor albumin and leukocyte levels. • Ensure balanced diet with adequate fluid intake up to 2400 ml daily. • Keep skin clean and dry blot skin, never rub. • Use pressure-relieving mattress, e.g., egg-crate, foam, or air-filled mattress, and pillows. • Massage skin over bony prominences each time position is changed. • Change position at least every 2 hours. • Keep linens free of wrinkles. • Apply topical medications as ordered. Apply wet-to-dry dressings as ordered. *Corneal tissue:* • Examine the cornea. • Maintain patches over eyes when there is no drainage from the eye. • Administer atropine or scopolamine as ordered. • Administer topical or systemic steroids and antibiotics as ordered.
Communicate knowledge of self-care.	• Instruct patient and family on the following: Care of the lesion Purpose and side effects of medications How to prevent tissue damage Plans for follow-up care

Principles and Rationale for Nursing Interventions

Two patient goals are derived from the assessment data: regain tissue integrity and communicate knowledge of self-care.

When subcutaneous tissue is impaired, it requires assessment to determine the extent of impairment. The color and size of the damaged area are documented for evaluation of healing. Monitoring leukocyte and albumin levels indicates the patient's nutritional status. A positive nutritional balance, especially protein, is needed for tissue growth and repair. Also, an increased leukocyte level may indicate an infection, which is treated by topical or systemic antibiotics as ordered. The lesions are kept clean and dry to prevent further tissue damage. Massaging the skin around the lesions stimulates circulation to the area. Undue pressure is treated by using pressure-relieving mattresses, changing the patient's position frequently, and smoothing out wrinkled sheets. Topical ointments are ordered to treat local infections as well as to stimulate the granulation of tissue. At times wet-to-dry dressings are used to debride the lesion.

When the cornea is damaged, the nurse assesses the eye for drainage, photophobia, and reports of pain. Patches are not used when the eye is draining because, if the drainage remains in the eye, it could become infected. A patch may be placed over the eye when no drainage is noted, especially when the patient reports photophobia. Atropine or scopolamine are given to dilate the pupil to rest the ciliary body and iris. Antibiotics and steroids are given as ordered to treat the inflammatory processes.[21]

Evaluation

Patient Outcome	Data Indicating That Outcome is Reached
Regains intact tissue	For subcutaneous tissue, tissue and skin intact Skin color and temperature consistent with unaffected skin For cornea, vision returned to previous status, without photophobia No reports of pain or itching in involved area
Communicates knowledge of self-care	Patient and family can explain: 1. Causes and prevention of impaired tissue integrity 2. Medications and treatments for home use 3. Dietary intake to promote wound healing 4. Plan for follow-up care

 Potential Altered Body Temperature

Potential altered body temperature is the state in which an individual is at risk for failure to maintain body temperature within normal range.

Risk Factors[15]

Extremes of age
Extremes of weight
Exposure to cool/cold or warm/hot environments
Dehydration
Inactivity or vigorous activity
Medications causing vasoconstriction or vasodilation, altered metabolic rate, or sedation
Inappropriate clothing for environmental temperature
Illness or trauma affecting temperature regulation

Nursing Interventions[15,21]

Patient Goal	Nursing Intervention
Maintain normal body temperature.	• Measure vital signs. • Assess capillary refill time. • Assess skin color, temperature, and turgor. • Inspect oral mucous membranes. • Provide fluids. • Measure fluid intake and output.

Principles and Rationale for Nursing Interventions

One patient goal is derived from the assessment data: maintain normal body temperature.

For patients at risk, the nurse collects data to determine the adequacy of their thermoregulatory system. This is accomplished by monitoring temperature, pulse, blood pressure, and respiration for changes over time. Capillary refill time may slow with a reduced body temperature. Skin color becomes reddened and warm during abnormally high temperatures and pale and cool or cold during abnormally low temperatures. Poor skin turgor and dry oral mucous membranes may indicate dehydration. Fluids maintain the normal balance and replace insensible fluid losses as well as losses from perspiration. Consult principles and rationale for the nursing diagnoses of hypothermia and hyperthermia.

Evaluation

Patient Outcome	Data Indicating That Outcome is Reached
Maintains body temperature	Body temperature within normal limits Capillary refill time: 3 to 5 seconds Skin warm and dry with normal color

Ineffective Thermoregulation

Ineffective thermoregulation is the state in which the individual's temperature fluctuates between hypothermia and hyperthermia.

Related Factors[15]

Trauma or illness
Immaturity
Aging
Fluctuating environmental temperature

Defining Characteristics[15]

Fluctuations in body temperature above or below the normal range
See also defining characteristics for hypothermia and hyperthermia.

Nursing Interventions

See nursing interventions for hypothermia and hyperthermia.

Evaluation

See evaluation for hypothermia and hyperthermia.

Hyperthermia

Hyperthermia is the state in which an individual's body temperature is elevated above his or her normal range.

Related Factors[15]

Exposure to hot environment
Vigorous activity
Medications and anesthesia
Inappropriate clothing
Increased metabolic rate
Illness or trauma
Dehydration
Inability or decreased ability to perspire

Defining Characteristics[15]

Increase in body temperature above normal range
Flushed skin
Warm to touch
Increased respiratory rate
Tachycardia
Seizures or convulsions

Nursing Interventions[5,8,15,21]

Patient Goal	Nursing Intervention
Maintain normal temperature.	• Measure vital signs. • Assess skin temperature and color. • Monitor white blood cells, hemoglobin, and hematocrit values. • Cover patient with sheet only. • Apply ice bag covered with a towel to the axilla and/or groin. • Give a tepid sponge bath. • Increase air circulation by using a fan in patient's room. • Encourage fluid and food intake. • Measure intake and output. • Maintain intravenous fluids as ordered. • Encourage frequent oral hygiene. • Administer antipyretics as ordered. • Place patient on a hypothermia blanket as ordered.

Principles and Rationale for Nursing Interventions

A single goal is derived for the patient with hyperthermia: maintain normal temperature.

Vital signs are taken as needed to evaluate whether the goal is met. During hyperthermia the temperature is elevated as a result of any of the causes listed under related factors. The heart, pulse, and respiratory rates are elevated because the metabolic rate increases during a fever. The temperature of the skin is warm and the skin appears flushed because of vasodilation of the peripheral blood vessels. An increased white blood cell count may indicate an infection as a cause of the fever. An elevated hemoglobin or hematocrit value suggests dehydration. The patient is covered lightly with a sheet to prevent chilling, since shivering will further increase the metabolic rate. Extra bedding is removed so that body heat will not be retained. An ice bag covered with a towel is applied to the axilla and/or groin to facilitate heat loss by conduction. The purpose of the towel is to change the temperature of the ice from cold to cool. Cold ice might induce shivering, which increases heat production. A tepid bath reduces fever by evaporation of heat. Using a fan in the patient's room increases air circulation, which reduces body heat by convection. Fluids are given to replace those lost by insensible water loss and perspiration. Oral hygiene is important because the oral mucous membranes easily become dehydrated. Food intake also is important to meet the patient's increased metabolic needs. Antipyretics reduce fever through action on the hypothalamus. A hypothermia blanket facilitates loss of body heat through conduction.

Evaluation

Patient Outcome	Data Indicating That Outcome is Reached
Maintains normal body temperature	Body temperature normal Skin temperature warm Skin color normal

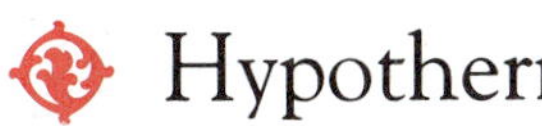

Hypothermia

Hypothermia is the state in which an individual's body temperature is reduced below the normal range.

Hypothermia has been arbitrarily defined as a core body temperature of less than 35° C (95° F) and can be considered mild, moderate, or severe. Mild hypothermia ranges from 33° to 36° C (91.4° to 96.8° F), moderate hypothermia from 30° to 33° C (86° to 91.4° F), and severe hypothermia from 27° to 30° C (80.6° to 86° F).

Although used historically as a treatment modality for a variety of disorders because of the resultant decrease in metabolic rate and endocrine functions, hypothermia as discussed here relates to accidental or unintentional hypothermia and the need for its prompt recognition and treatment.

Related Factors*

Exposure to cool or cold environment
Illness, trauma
Inability or decreased ability to shiver
Malnutrition
Inadequate or wet clothing
Consumption of alcohol
Medications causing vasodilation
Loss of subcutaneous fat
Cardiovascular insufficiency
Decreased metabolic rate
Physical immobility
Physical illness (e.g., hypothyroidism)
Exposure to windy or wet environment

Defining Characteristics*

Reduction in body temperature below normal range
Cool skin
Mental confusion
Decreased pulse and respiration
Shivering
Pallor
Slow capillary refill
Tachycardia
Hypertension
See p. 1655 for associated effects of hypothermia

Rewarming Methods for Hypothermia

Passive rewarming

Removal from environmental exposure
Insulating material (e.g., blankets)

Active external rewarming

Immersion in heated water
Electric blankets
Heated objects (e.g., water bottle)

Active core rewarming

Intragastric balloon
Colonic irrigation
Mediastinal irrigation via thoracotomy
Hemodialysis
Peritoneal dialysis
Extracorporeal blood rewarming
Inhalation rewarming

Modified from Reuler J.B.: Hypothermia: pathophysiology, clinical settings, and management. Annals of Internal Medicine. 1978, vol. 89, p. 525.

*Adapted from North American Nursing Diagnosis Association, 1988 Ballot.

Nursing Interventions[7,22,27]

Patient Goal	Nursing Intervention
Regain normal body temperature.	• Accurately assess patient's temperature, using a low-recording thermometer if necessary. • Assess and document any symptoms, e.g., undue fatigue, weakness, confusion, apathy, impaired coordination, slurred speech, shivering, and skin color. • Question patient about recent activities, e.g., heavy activity in wet cold weather, elderly person living alone in a cool environment, or poor nutritional status. • Monitor patient's vital signs closely to detect bradycardia, hypotension, metabolic acidosis, and respiratory difficulties if body temperature should continue to fall. • Place patient on cardiac monitor and handle patient carefully, since defibrillation often occurs if the myocardium is cooled. • Remove any wet or cold clothing and replace with warm, dry garments or warmed blankets. • Give patient warm fluids if alert and able to swallow. • Ensure that appropriate laboratory studies are drawn, including arterial blood gases, and ensure that laboratory knows patient's actual temperature so that necessary factorial adjustment can be made. • In collaboration with physician, administer warmed intravenous fluids or needed medications, keeping in mind that delayed metabolism will occur when patient is warmed. • Depending on severity of hypothermia, assist with rewarming. Possibilities include (see box on p. 1653): Passive rewarming Active external rewarming Active core rewarming • Assess patient's respiratory status and color of nail beds, since bronchopneumonia is a typical complication.
Develop awareness of prevention of hypothermia.	• Teach patients about the dangers of alcohol, the role of nutrition, and the need for warm clothing in efforts to prevent future hypothermic episodes. • Assess patient's nutritional status, and ensure that patient's caloric intake is adequate to maintain body temperature. • Assess for any underlying condition that may precipitate hypothermia and require treatment, e.g., diabetes, myxedema, or anorexia nervosa. • Teach about the early warning signs of hypothermia, since the condition can be reversible if it is identified and treated early enough. • Establish support systems for the elderly to compensate for isolation.

Principles and Rationale for Nursing Interventions[22,27]

Hypothermia is a nursing diagnosis with many causes and physiologic consequences that can complicate accurate diagnosis and intervention. Unfortunately, hypothermia is often unrecognized and appropriate treatment is delayed, since the thermometer may be incorrectly used or may not register the patient's actual temperature if it is below the lowest number on a standard thermometer. However, recognition of the scope of the problem is increasing and new advances in therapy are being discovered, such as core rewarming. The aging of the population and the increase in the number of homeless persons, as well as the popularity of winter sports, are factors that necessitate a thorough understanding of the symptoms of hypothermia. Trauma victims also frequently become hypothermic, since treatment rooms are kept cool and the victim is uncovered while being treated.

The most obvious consequence of hypothermia is a decrease in the basal metabolic rate, falling to 50% of normal at 28° C (82.4° F). Shivering, which is the most obvious early symptom of the lowering of the core temperature, is an attempt by the muscles to provide a large amount of heat, with associated vasodilation, increased blood flow, and delivery of warmed blood to the core.[27] Partly in response to shivering in the early stages of hypothermia and partly because of sympathoadrenal stimulation, early symptoms are tachycardia and a gradual decline in heart rate and cardiac output as temperature falls. The principles governing heat loss are critical to the understanding of hypothermia: conduction, convection, radiation, and evaporation of water.

Evaluation

Patient Outcome	Data Indicating That Outcome is Reached
Achieves and maintains appropriate body temperature	Experiences no serious complications, e.g., ventricular fibrillation, postwarming hypoglycemia, volume depletion, or overmedication after rewarming Understands how hypothermia developed and how to prevent it in the future, including need for adequate caloric intake, how to dress appropriately, and effects of inactivity and alcohol on body temperature

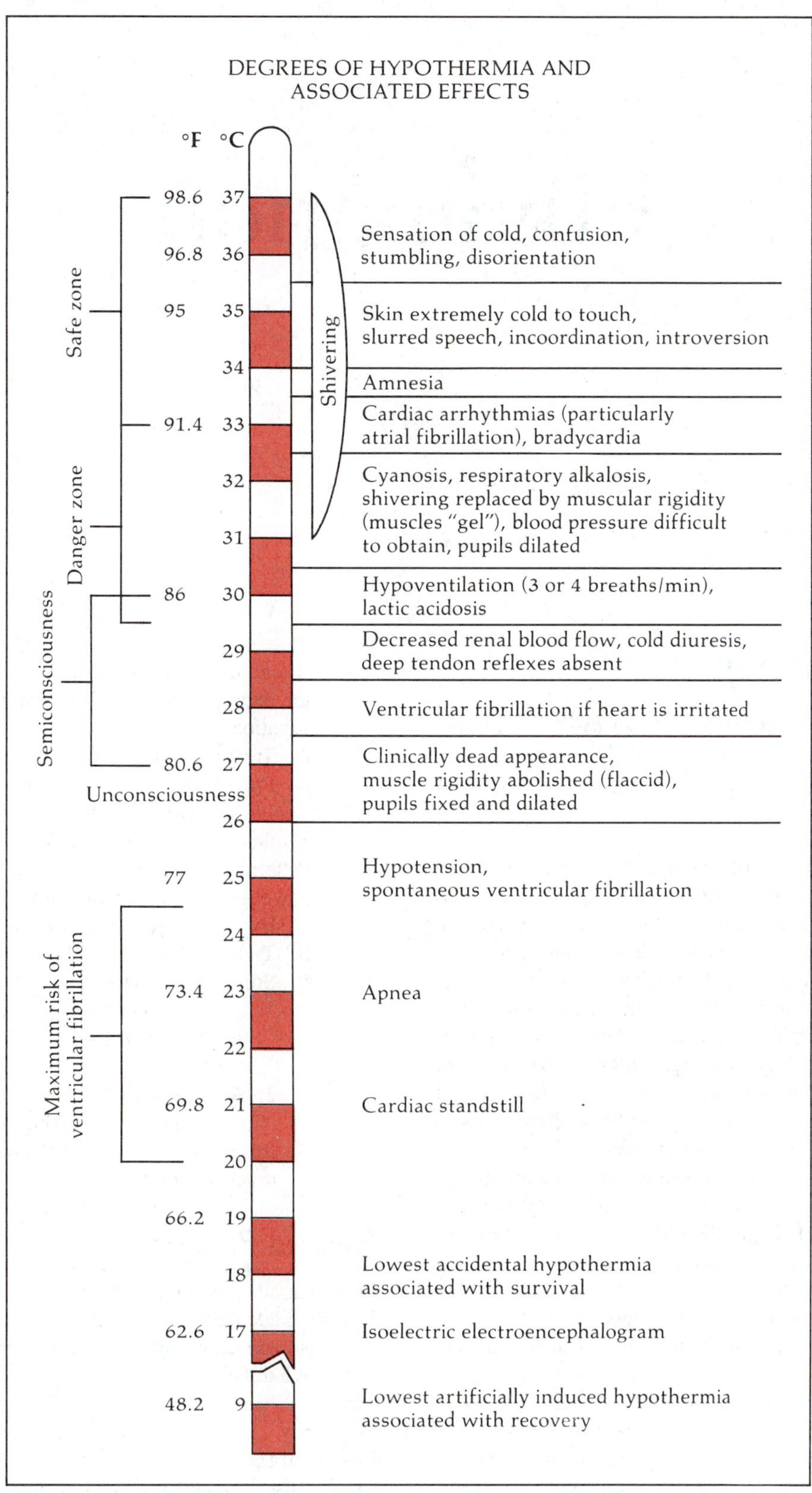

Reprinted with permission from Hospital Practice. From Matz Robert: Hypothermia: measures and countermeasures, Hospital Practice 21:1A, January 30, 1986, p.47. Illustration by Mr. Albert Miller.

FUNCTIONAL HEALTH PATTERN

III

Elimination

 Constipation

Constipation is the state in which an individual experiences a change in normal bowel habits characterized by a decrease in frequency and/or passage of hard, dry stools.

Since constipation may be a symptom of some underlying disease as well as a functional health problem, a medical evaluation, including abdominal and rectal examinations, should be done to exclude organic causes. "Constipation associated with weight loss, abdominal pain, or fresh rectal bleeding, particularly in the elderly, should alert the doctor to possible serious organic disease."[9] "Patients with constipation of recent onset, sudden aggravation of existing constipation with recent abdominal pain, or the passage of blood and mucus in the stools should always be subjected to sigmoidoscopy and barium enema examination."[1]

Although patients usually diagnose constipation themselves, its true nature is very elusive. Five categories and eight subcategories of diagnostic indicators reflect the complexity of normal elimination and constipation[5]:

I. Signs and symptoms
   A. Description of constipated stool
      1. Character: qualities of the stool, color, consistency
      2. Amount: amount of stool
      3. Frequency: lapse of time between stools
   B. Feelings and sensations: physical feelings and sensations associated with constipation, e.g., stomachache, bloating

II. Etiology: contributing factors, e.g., diet, fluids, inadequate exercise, medications, change in routine

III. Attending behaviors: consistent use of measures for the express purpose of alleviating or preventing constipation
   A. Treatment: measures taken to relieve constipation
   B. Prevention: measures taken to prevent constipation

IV. Health behaviors: health behavior influencing normal elimination, diet, fluid intake, exercise

V. Patterning: behaviors related to the production of a bowel movement, including toilet routine
   A. Expected frequency of bowel movement(s)
   B. Time of day of bowel movement(s)
   C. Stimulus behaviors
      1. Actions taken to stimulate a bowel movement, short term, within the hour, e.g., drinking hot water
      2. Actions in daily routine that result in a bowel movement, e.g., eating breakfast
   D. Response to reflexes: behaviors in response to the urge to defecate

Related Factors

Less than adequate fluid intake
Less than adequate dietary intake and bulk
Less than adequate physical activity; immobility
Personal habits
Lack of privacy
Pregnancy
Emotional status
Chronic use of medication and enemas
Pain on defecation
Diagnostic procedures
Neuromuscular impairment

Table 1
Nonprescription Drug Therapy to Relieve Constipation

Generic (Trade) Name	Dosage and Administration	Comments
Bulk-Forming Agents		
Karaya gum	Oral: 5-10 g daily, taken with water	Nonprescription
Methylcellulose, carboxymethylcellulose (Cologel, Hydrolose)	Oral: 4-6 g daily	Nonprescription
Mantago (psyllium) seed	Oral: 2-5 to 30 g daily; add to water and drink rapidly	Nonprescription
Polycarbophil	Oral: 4-6 g daily	Nonprescription
Psyllium hydrocolloid (Effersyllium) Psyllium hydrophilic (Konsyl) Pscilloid (L A Formula, Metamucil, Modane Bulk)	Oral: 1 round tsp (7 g) or 1 packet; add to glass of water and drink rapidly and then follow with second glass of water; repeat 1 or 2 times daily if necessary	Nonprescription
Stimulant (Irritant) Cathartics		
Blacodyl (Biscolax, Dulcolax, various others)	Oral: 10 mg, up to 30 mg may be given to clear gastrointestinal tract Rectal: 10 mg	Nonprescription; initial response in 6 to 12 hr; do not take within 60 min of milk or antacids; rectal administration effective in 15 min
Cascara sagrada (Bileo-Secrin, Cas-Evac)	Oral: 200-400 mg of extract; 0.5-1.5 ml of fluid extract or 5 ml of aromatic extract	Nonprescription; one of the mildest of the stimulant cathartics
Castor oil	Oral: 15-60 ml	Nonprescription; castor oil is degraded to ricinoleic acid, which is the active drug
Castor oil, emulsified (Neoloid)	Oral: 30-60 ml	Nonprescription; mint flavored; turns alkaline urine pink
Damron (Anavac, Danvac, Dorbane, Modane, Weslax)	Oral: 75-150 mg	Nonprescription; turns alkaline urine pink
Glycerine suppositories	Rectal: 3 g	Nonprescription; effective in 15 to 30 min
Phenolphthalein (Chocolax, Exlax, Feen-A-Mint)	Oral: 30-270 mg daily	Nonprescription; turns alkaline urine pink
Senna, whole leaf	Oral: 0.5-2 g or 2 ml of senna fluid extract	Nonprescription
Sennosides A and B (Glysennid)	Oral: 12-24 mg at bedtime	Nonprescription
Saline Cathartics		
Magnesium hydroxide (Milk of magnesia)	Oral: 10-15 ml (concentrated) or 15-30 ml (regular)	Nonprescription
Magnesium sulfate (Epsom salt)	Oral: 15 g in glass of water	Nonprescription
Monosodium phosphate (Sal Hepatica)	Oral: 5-20 ml with water	Nonprescription
Sodium phosphate	Oral: 4 g in glass of warm water	Nonprescription
Sodium phosphate with sodium biphosphate (Phospho-Soda)	Oral: 20-40 ml in glass of cold water	Nonprescription
Lubricants		
Mineral oil (Agoral, Plain; Kondremul, Plain; Neo-Cultol; Petrogalar, Plain)	Oral: 15-30 ml at bedtime	Nonprescription; to ease strain of passing hard stools; should not be used regularly because the fat-soluble vitamins (A, D, E, and K) are not absorbed; response in 1-3 days
Fecal Softeners		
Dioctyl calcium sulfosuccinate (Surfak)	Oral: 50-360 mg daily	Nonprescription
Dioctyl sodium sulfosuccinate (Colace, Comfolax, D-D-S, various others)	Oral: 50-360 mg	Nonprescription

From Clark.[3]

Musculoskeletal impairment
Weak abdominal musculature
Chronic obstructive lesions
Decreased activity level
Use of laxatives

Defining Characteristics

Frequency less than usual pattern
Hard formed stool
Palpable mass
Reported feeling of pressure in rectum
Reported feeling of rectal fullness
Straining at stool
Abdominal distention
Abdominal pain
Appetite impairment
Back pain
Headache
Interference with daily living (consequence)

Nursing Interventions

Patient Goal	Nursing Intervention
Describe health behaviors that prevent constipation in relation to diet, fluid, and exercise.	• Provide instruction for: Appropriate use of bulk in diet Adequate daily fluid intake Appropriate level of exercise for age and physiologic status
Establish a program to repattern bowel elimination.	• Provide instruction for understanding: Role of stimulus behaviors Recognition and attention to stimulus behaviors, e.g., warm fluids on arising Importance of immediate response to defecation urge Effective position for defecation • Assist with implementation of new health behaviors relative to good bowel habits, including diet, fluids, exercise, and emotional equilibrium.
Take oral laxatives and enemas when other measures are ineffective.	• Provide instruction for appropriate use of oral laxatives (see Table 1). • Assess and monitor side effects of medications. • Assess and monitor laxative and enema use.

Principles and Rationale for Nursing Interventions

Health behaviors, such as a well-balanced diet, adequate fluid intake, and exercise, are essential to the promotion of normal bowel functioning. A diet adequate in dietary fiber provides bulk and keeps the stool soft through the mechanism of water absorption. The fiber acts as a bulking agent through its water-binding properties. This mechanism increases the speed at which the stool passes through the intestines. The increased speed decreases the amount of water absorbed by the large intestine, and the stool remains soft and bulky. Some high-fiber foods are whole-grain cereals and breads, leafy vegetables, and raw and cooked fruits. Fruits such as bananas, prunes, dates, figs, and rhubarb are good laxatives as well as being high in fiber.[12]

In health, body fluids (water and electrolytes) are constantly being metabolized and must be replaced to maintain normal processes. In health, normal fluid intake should be about 2500 ml per day. Of this amount approximately 1000 ml is obtained from water in food, 300 ml from oxidation, and 1200 ml as liquid. These fluids enter the intestines each day, along with saliva, gastric secretions, pancreatic juices, and bile to comprise total body fluids of 9 to 10 L for absorption of nutrients and electrolytes. In health, most of this fluid is reabsorbed; only about 100 ml of water is excreted in feces.[8]

Exercise in any form is essential for total body functioning and well-being. Normal defecation depends on adequate muscular strength in the abdominal and pelvic muscles. People who are sedentary, immobile, or debilitated from illness benefit from conditioning exercises to strengthen the muscles of the abdomen and pelvic floor. Lack of tone in abdominal muscles can be best corrected by doing sit-ups. These should be done with knees bent and arms flexed behind the head, so as not to put undue strain on the back. Isometric contraction of perineal muscles and the pelvic tilt strengthen muscles of the pelvic floor. Walking briskly for at least 15 minutes a day is the easiest overall exercise.[2] Exercise in the form of strenuous activity is related to preventing the incidence of constipation.

Persons can be educated to use health behaviors for maintaining bowel function that are familiar and have proved helpful, such as a cup of hot liquid before breakfast, prune juice, or other measures. Many of these measures are based on stimulating physiologic processes and have sound bases for their effectiveness. The practice of drinking warm fluids on arising, for example, sets in motion the duodenocolic, gastrocolic, gastroileal, enterogastric, and defecation reflexes.

When feces are forced into the rectum, the process of defecation is normally initiated, including reflex contraction of the rectum and relaxation of anal sphincters.[4] However, before actual defecation occurs, the conscious mind takes over voluntary control of the external sphincter and either inhibits it to allow the process to occur or further contracts it if the moment is not socially acceptable. When contraction of the external sphincter is maintained, the defecation reflex stops after several minutes and will not return until an additional amount of feces enters the rectum, which may not happen for several more hours.

When the time is more convenient for the person to defecate, defecation reflexes can usually be initiated by taking a deep breath to force the diaphragm downward and then contracting the abdominal muscles to increase abdominal pressure, thereby forcing feces into the rectum to initiate new reflexes. However, it should be noted that reflexes initiated this way are never as effective as those that arise naturally. For this reason, people who inhibit their natural reflexes often become severely constipated.[4]

Stress and tension can interfere with normal bowel elimination, especially in an already stressful hospital environment. Stimulation of the sympathetic nervous system inhibits gastrointestinal activity, slowing the peristaltic waves yet innervating the internal anal sphincter at the same time. Therefore, during a time of stress, movement is delayed temporarily, but incontinence can occur. Thus, in addition to including measures to decrease stress and ensuring adequate privacy, it is important to provide enough time for a bowel movement. In the acute care setting, treatments and tests are frequently scheduled so closely that the person has no relaxed uninterrupted time for a bowel movement. This situation can be very serious for a person with constipation who has succeeded in developing a satisfactory schedule of elimination, only to have it thoughtlessly disrupted during a hospitalization.[8] This problem can be minimized by making sure that hospitalized patients participate in decision making and planning related to their care.

The most physiologically effective position for defecation is a squatting position in which the pressure of the thighs increases the intraabdominal pressure and thus aids expulsion of the stool. Most adults can achieve this position by leaning forward while sitting on the toilet, but children and short people may find it comfortable to use a footstool to raise their thighs when using the toilet. Some elderly people who find it difficult to use a low seat use an elevated toilet seat to get off the toilet without assistance. A higher toilet seat often means that their feet barely touch the floor; they may therefore need a footstool to flex knees and hips for effective defecation.

Enemas are used when lower bowel and rectal evacuation are indicated in the management of a fecal impaction or to prepare a patient for endoscopic and radiographic tests and surgery. Enemas should not be used regularly for the treatment of constipation. The normal saline enema is the safest, most effective, and best tolerated. Large volumes of normal saline solution, when correctly administered, cleanse the rectum and sigmoid colon with little mucosal irritation or disturbance in fluid and electrolyte balance. Disposable oil-retention enemas are frequently used in small volumes to soften a fecal impaction. Removal of the impaction is easily achieved if the oil-retention enema is followed by a normal saline enema after 4 to 6 hours. Disposable hypertonic saline solution enemas (Fleet) are safe and frequently used. They contain a mixture of sodium phosphates and citrates. They are easy to self-administer and are disposable. They act by drawing water into the lumen from the body in significant quantities so that adequate fluid and electrolyte balance is maintained.[11]

Evaluation

Patient Outcome	Data Indicating That Outcome is Reached
Describes health behaviors that prevent constipation in relation to diet, fluid, exercise; contributing factors when known; and methods to reduce contributing factors	Explains importance of well-balanced diet, including importance of eating breakfast Describes importance of bulk in diet through ingestion of dietary fiber and bran Names six readily available foods high in fiber Discusses importance of including 8 to 10 glasses of fluid in daily intake Recognizes and integrates daily exercise into life-style (15-minute walk/day minimum amount) Describes individual stimulus behaviors (e.g., warm fluids on arising, prune juice) that are helpful in initiating bowel movement Expresses importance of responding to defecation urge when it arises naturally Understands physiology of defecation Names conditions that promote normal bowel functioning as well as those that contribute to development of constipation
Bowel repatterning program to establish normal bowel functioning	Eliminates regular use of laxatives or enemas Attends to defecation urge when it arises naturally Consumes well-balanced diet, including sufficient fiber and laxative foods Relates following process of bowel repatterning: 1. Eats large breakfast; sits on toilet 10 minutes 2. Establishes relaxing environment (diversional activities, reading, listening to music) 3. When defecation urge occurs, responds to it so it does not weaken
Oral drug therapy to produce bowel movement within 12 to 24 hours	Takes oral laxative correctly Understands desired effects of medication Makes correct decision if prescribed therapy is no longer effective

 Perceived Constipation

Perceived constipation is the state in which an individual makes a self-diagnosis of constipation and ensures a daily bowel movement through use of laxatives, enemas, and suppositories.

Individuals develop a set of expectations regarding their bowel evacuation patterns based on their past experiences as well as family beliefs and practices. Failure to evacuate on a daily basis is the most common contributor to perceived or imagined constipation. Many individuals expect to have a bowel movement on arising or immediately after breakfast. This physiologic and emotional ritual signals the beginning of a healthy day. Concern over the failure to evacuate may result in regular concerted efforts to defecate (straining), abdominal discomfort, and a growing preoccupation with the failure. Use or abuse of laxatives is a typical solution for this concern. Laxatives may be consumed until the person has established a satisfactory elimination pattern and is convinced that regular laxative intake is mandatory. The person may discover that constipation only worsens, since chronic laxative abuse may lead to an atonic colon musculature, decreased awareness of the presence of stool in the rectum, and finally authentic constipation.

If a careful assessment has established that real constipation does not exist, further assessment of beliefs, life-style changes, self-treatment measures, and the degree of concern must precede any nursing intervention. Intervention involves an alteration of beliefs and possibly long-standing self-care practices. This may not be easily accomplished until the nurse and the patient are fully enlightened about the origins of this problem.

Related Factors*

Cultural/family health beliefs
Lack of information about normal processes
Impaired thought processes
Long-term expectations and habits

Defining Characteristics*

Expectation of daily bowel movement with resulting overuse of laxatives, enemas, and suppositories
Expected passage of stool at same time every day

*Adapted from North American Nursing Diagnosis Association, 1988 Ballot.

Nursing Interventions

Patient Goal	Nursing Intervention
Modify belief about need for daily evacuation.	• Assess patient for: Present beliefs about elimination practices Influence of others (family, peers) who contribute to beliefs Alterations in life-style that would contribute to elimination pattern alterations Food consumption: frequency (timing), quantity, quality (variety/content) Fluid consumption: frequency, quantity Exercise/mobility habits Sleep patterns Access to privacy Recent illnesses, treatments, medication Presence of other problems/symptoms Boredom, loneliness, isolation Flatus, distention, abdominal discomfort • Help patient identify beliefs and convictions about present bowel habits. • Support patient's right and need to have convictions. • Identify life-style alterations that might contribute to elimination changes and discuss connections and mechanisms causing bowel habit alterations with patient. • Establish with patient a normal bowel elimination pattern (e.g., every 2-3 days). • Clarify with patient what is viewed as a normal pattern. • Describe signs and symptoms of constipation (e.g., difficult, painful passage of stool; failure to evacuate beyond the established normal time; hard stool; lower abdominal discomfort or a feeling of fullness in the rectum; marked distention). • Support patient's efforts to monitor difference between real and perceived constipation.
Explore life-style changes that will promote healthy, regular elimination.	• Assess patient's willingness and interest in altering eating, fluid intake, mobility, or exercise habits. • If numerous alterations are needed, proceed slowly and establish priorities according to patient's wishes. • Acknowledge possibility that life-style changes and ensuing elimination routines may alter slowly. • Enlist support of family or peers to assist patient with change.

Patient Goal	Nursing Intervention
Decrease reliance on laxatives.	• Suggest substituting natural bulk and fiber from fruits, grains, and vegetables for laxative being consumed. • Acknowledge possibility that reduction in use of a laxative may be gradual if there is heavy consumption at present or if patient needs time to relinquish or alter convictions. • If gradual reduction of laxative use is necessary, establish a schedule with patient. • Be prepared to provide support in future to review patient's concerns and progress.

Principles and Rationale for Nursing Interventions

Assessment of the patient's beliefs and degree of concern about bowel habits is as important as any intervention that follows. Concern about bowel habits may be coupled with other concerns about aging, illness, or physical deterioration. A preoccupation with defecation might be an indicator of boredom or mental alterations that lead to a fixation on this daily event. A mere confrontation with facts and a new regimen may leave the patient confused, suspicious, and ultimately noncompliant if his beliefs and convictions about the body and its functions are not fully explored and acknowledged. The nurse must be prepared to expect changes in the patient or for the patient to accept the idea of change very slowly. The patient must believe that control of his body is being maintained and that giving up an ingrained habit will not be a health risk.

Evaluation

Patient Outcome	Data Indicating That Outcome is Reached
Experiences regular, comfortable bowel movements	Attains previously identified "normal" elimination schedule Notes absence of discomfort and straining at defecation Reports absence of distention, flatus, or intense feelings of rectal fullness before defecation Reports that stools are soft, brown, and regular in caliber
Is not dependent on laxatives	Reports taking laxatives rarely Describes variety of bulk and fiber foods eaten daily to support regular bowel habits
Expresses acceptance of present bowel habits	Verbalizes comfort with present bowel habits

Colonic Constipation

Colonic constipation is the state in which an individual's pattern of elimination is characterized by a hard, dry stool that results from a delay in passage of food residue.

Dietary and fluid consumption and exercise alterations are the major contributors to changes in stool consistency. The chronic nature of delayed, painful fecal passage can create a major disruption in an individual's life. Assessing and changing the life-style patterns that affect elimination patterns may be complicated and slow to occur.

Related Factors*

Inadequate fluid intake
Changes in dietary intake
Inadequate fiber in diet
Missed meals, change in mealtimes
Inadequate physical activity
Immobility
Lack of privacy
Emotional disturbances
Chronic use of medications, laxatives, and enemas
Stress
Change in daily routine
Metabolic problems (e.g., hypothyroidism, hypocalcemia, hypokalemia)

*Adapted from North American Nursing Diagnosis Association, 1988 Ballot.

Defining Characteristics*

Decreased frequency of bowel elimination
Hard, dry stool
Straining at stool
Painful defecation
Abdominal distention
Palpable mass
Rectal pressure
Headache; appetite impairment
Abdominal pain
Blood with stool

*Adapted from North American Nursing Diagnosis Association, 1988 Ballot.

Nursing Interventions

Patient Goal	Nursing Intervention
Repattern bowel elimination.	• Assess history and chronicity of bowel elimination pattern. • Assess physical states that may contribute to constipation (e.g., immobility, medications). (See also Constipation.) • Provide instruction for: Appropriate use of bulk in diet Adequate daily fluid intake Appropriate level of exercise for age and physiologic status Recognition and attention to stimulus behaviors, e.g., warm fluids on arising Importance of immediate response to defecation urge Effective position for defecation Well-supported sitting or squatting position (elevation of feet on footstool while seated on toilet) Exercises to strengthen abdominal muscles (See Constipation.) Maneuvers to ease defecation (e.g., rotate and pivot upper body while seated on toilet) Provision of privacy and adequate time to allow for defecation • Assist patient with planning for and carrying out dietary, exercise, and other life-style changes. • Assist patient with gradual reduction of laxative or enema usage. • Institute regular bowel evacuation program if patient is severely impaired.

Principles and Rationale for Nursing Interventions

Careful assessment of dietary, medication, fluid consumption, and exercise patterns and potential must precede any intervention. Long-standing habits of eating and mobility must be altered slowly with full commitment from the patient to be effective. Both nurse and patient must be aware of changes that cannot occur and ready to work for an improved lifestyle within the constraints of chronicity. Dietary bulk should include about 6 to 10 g of fiber each day, but fiber must be added slowly to avoid abdominal cramping and flatus.[3] Adequate fluids (2500 ml/day) must accompany fiber intake. Fluids that stimulate diuresis (e.g., coffee, colas) should not be included as part of the required intake. The purchasing and preparation of food must be explored, in addition to consideration of the patient's preferences, before changes can be planned. Sedentary individuals can begin an exercise program by walking 15 to 20 minutes every day. Walking with other people not only increases physical activity, but also may be a social stimulus.

Multiple stressors or emotional disturbances that result in life-style upheavals may require referral or prolonged counseling before a routine can be reestablished. Medical intervention may be needed to stabilize endocrine disorders or other illnesses that disrupt daily routines, mobility, or dietary practices. When patients are irreversibly impaired, the nurse and patient must work together to plan for a bowel retraining program that incorporates abdominal exercises, positioning techniques, and constant elimination monitoring and supervision. Laxatives and enemas may have to be used for some patients to assist with regulation of elimination.

Evaluation

See evaluation section for Constipation.

Diarrhea

Diarrhea is the state in which an individual experiences a change in normal bowel habits characterized by the frequent passage of loose, fluid, unformed stools.

Consistency is a more reliable indicator of diarrhea than frequency, since there is general agreement that loose or watery stools are abnormal.[10] "Quantitatively, diarrhea is defined as the passage of over 200 g of stool per day containing 70% to 90% water. . . . Normal stool is 60%-80% water, and an increase in daily rectal water excretion of 100 to 200 ml will markedly alter the frequency and consistency of bowel movements."[2] Acute diarrhea is usually self-limiting, lasting 24 to 48 hours, whereas chronic diarrhea persists for several weeks or is intermittently present for several weeks.

Doe and Barr[4] consider the volume of diarrhea fluid an important indicator of the mechanism of the diarrhea. Stools of high volume, often exceeding 1 L a day, suggest a small intestinal origin for the diarrhea, whereas a small stool volume suggests a colonic origin, as does the presence of bright blood and mucus. The authors associated tenesmus and urgency with rectal inflammation, periumbilical colicky pain with small intestines, and lower abdominal pain on the left side as colonic in origin.

Related Factors

Acute Diarrhea

Diet alteration
Improper cooking
Spoiled food
Drug reaction
Infection
Ingestion of toxins

Chronic Diarrhea

Lactase deficiency
Laxative abuse
Stress and anxiety
Inflammatory bowel disease
Irritable bowel syndrome
Cancer of colon
Chemotherapeutic agents
Radiation
Gastrointestinal surgery
Malabsorption diseases

Defining Characteristics

Abdominal pain
Cramping
Increased stool frequency
Increased frequency of bowel sounds
Loose, liquid stools
Urgency
Change in color of stool

Nursing Interventions

Patient Goal	Nursing Intervention
Achieve relief of symptoms.	• Provide instructions for: Use of antidiarrheal medications Modifications of diet Perirectal skin care • Assess/monitor hydration. • Assess/monitor body weight.
Take prescribed medications.	• Provide instructions for use of antidiarrheal medications. • Assist with implementation of medication taking as part of activities of daily living. • Assess/monitor side effects of medications.
Decrease number of episodes of diarrhea.	• Provide instructions for: Use of food and elimination diary Personal hygiene measures, e.g., handwashing techniques

Principles and Rationale for Nursing Interventions

The goals of nursing care include prevention, treatment, health teaching, and repatterning of bowel elimination. Prevention begins with a determination of the etiology or mechanism of the diarrhea; maintenance of fluid, electrolyte, and nutritional status; and assessment of the need for health teaching.

Treatment of acute diarrhea is focused on management of symptoms, elimination of the offending agent, and physician referral when indicated. Antidiarrheal drugs are not recommended for routine use in acute infectious diarrhea, since they may delay the natural eradication of the infection.[4] Physician referrals should be made when specific drug therapy is needed, when the diarrhea persists for more than 3 days, when the stool contains blood or has the appearance of steatorrhea, and when patients admit to fecal incontinence. Diarrhea associated with the use of anti-infective agents is normally alleviated when the offending agent is withdrawn. However, some persons continue to have diarrhea associated with cramps, tenderness, and fever because of an overgrowth of anaerobic organisms and/or the presence of their toxins. Physician consultation is suggested, since the individual may have developed pseudomembranous colitis. Tube feeding–induced diarrhea can be controlled by the use of Metamucil or by adjusting the type of tube feeding. Lactose-intolerant individuals will experience immediate relief when all lactose is removed from their diet. Although this may seem a simple solution, the actual implementation of a lactose-free diet is complicated by the presence of powdered whey and nonfat dry milk in many food products, including crackers, cookies, cereals, and sausages. Maintaining an adequate fluid and caloric intake may be difficult in more severe cases of diarrhea, and hospitalization for intravenous replacement of fluid and electrolytes might be required.

The type of health teaching required is unique to the situation and the patient. Initially, sufficient information should be given to the patient and family to help them understand the nature of the problem, treatment objectives, and rationale for laboratory studies, drugs, and supportive care. The patient's history and results of microbiologic studies provide a guide for other patient education programs designed to improve safe handling of food, handwashing techniques, and understanding of the mechanisms of disease transmission at home and when traveling in foreign countries.

Persons with chronic diarrhea associated with irritable bowel syndrome may benefit from individual and group counseling and from learning stress reduction techniques, such as systematic relaxation. It is important to remember that an individual's bowel elimination pattern is a reflection of the total life process and is not comprised of isolated physiologic events.

Evaluation

Patient Outcome	Data Indicating That Outcome is Reached
Number and consistency of stools within normal limits	No more than three bowel movements per day Stool is formed and easy to pass
Adequate dietary intake	Skin well hydrated Urinary output maintained at 50 ml/hour Body weight stabilized within normal limits
Pain relief	No complaints of abdominal pain or discomfort
Decrease in episodes of fecal incontinence	Seeks medical consultation for evaluation of fecal incontinence Keeps a record of incontinent episodes
Perirectal skin normal in appearance	Absence of areas of redness, itching, and irritation in perirectal area
Plans to take medications	Schedules taking medications as part of daily activities
Reports side effect of medications to health professional	Verbalizes actions, dosages, and side effects of medications
Understands mechanism of diarrhea	Describes factors associated with diarrhea Lists two changes in health practices that will affect bowel elimination pattern, e.g., washing hands after use of toilet and reading labels on food products to avoid ingestion of lactose

Bowel Incontinence

Bowel incontinence is the state in which an individual experiences a change in normal bowel habits characterized by involuntary passage of stool.

Persons at high risk for becoming incontinent are the elderly, persons with a low level of awareness, patients with a longstanding dependence on suppositories, individuals with neurologic abnormalities regardless of age, diabetic patients with neuropathy, patients with chronic diarrhea, persons with a history of rectal surgery, especially hemorrhoidectomy, and those with a history of trauma to the lumbosacral area.

Fecal incontinence is often functionally disabling.[5,7] Social isolation and depression may occur as individuals attempt to cope with odor and continence aids by remaining at home. Patients in long-term care agencies also tend to withdraw from social interaction as they attempt to deal not only with the incontinence but also with the reactions of personnel who continually face the unpleasant task of "cleaning up."

Related Factors

Autoimmune diseases such as myasthenia gravis
Central nervous system disruptions such as stroke
Cognitive-perceptual impairment
Demyelinating diseases
Depression
Diarrhea
Fecal impaction
Loss of sphincter control
Musculoskeletal involvement
Neuromuscular involvement
Severe anxiety
Spinal cord injuries (transient or permanent)

Defining Characteristics

Involuntary passage of stool
Embarrassed conduct
Fecal odor
Stained clothing
Stained bed linens
Decrease in social interaction
Washed underwear

Nursing Interventions

Patient Goal	Nursing Intervention
Eliminate or reduce episodes of incontinence.	• Reduce or eliminate contributing factors when possible. • Teach alternate contraction and relaxation of pelvic floor muscles. • Ingest foods and fluids consistent with bowel elimination program.
Prevent skin breakdown.	• Wash area, rinse, and dry after each incontinent episode.
Eliminate fecal contents regularly, usually every other day.	• Implement bowel retraining program: Initiate when bowel sounds return and ileus is resolved. Establish evacuation schedule consistent with patient and family preferences. Teach patient and family use of laxatives and stool softeners to aid timing of defecation.
Promote self-esteem, personal integrity, and social functioning.	• Use incontinence aids temporarily until elimination pattern is established. • Change clothes immediately after an incontinent episode.

Principles and Rationale for Nursing Interventions

Bowel management programs are designed to reduce the unpredictability of fecal incontinence and provide individuals with more security from episodes of incontinence. Reestablishment of continence through a successful bowel training program and the assistance of supportive, understanding nurses who provide privacy and an unhurried atmosphere are the key elements in the treatment of incontinence. The type of bowel retraining program selected for a patient depends on the etiology of the incontinence and the preferences of the patient and family. Retraining a cord-injured patient is delayed until bowel sounds have returned and paralytic ileus is resolved.

Evaluation

Patient Outcome	Data Indicating That Outcome is Reached
Amount and number of stools are within normal limits	Regular evacuation of bowel contents Rare episodes of incontinence
Perirectal skin normal in appearance	Absence of areas of redness, itching, and irritation in perirectal area
Reestablishes patterns of social interaction	Engages in social activities Engages in planning future goals Free of odor

Altered Patterns of Urinary Elimination

Altered patterns of urinary elimination are states in which the individual experiences a disturbance in urine elimination.

The diagnosis of altered patterns of urinary elimination is a broad, nonspecific description of voiding dysfunction that predates the more specific conditions of functional, reflex, stress, urge, and total incontinence and urinary retention.

A disturbance in urinary elimination patterns implies an alteration in the filling, storage, or evacuation function of the lower urinary tract. Altered patterns of urinary elimination is a descriptive diagnosis applicable to a variety of dysfunctional voiding states. The diagnosis remains useful despite the acceptance of six more specific diagnoses that address voiding disturbances. Altered patterns of urinary elimination is useful when describing a form of voiding disturbance not classified as incontinence or urinary retention or when a case of incontinence remains unclassified. Following the diagnostic label with a colon (:) and a brief description of the voiding dysfunction is a useful strategy for applying the diagnosis to various dysfunctional voiding states. These include urinary frequency without incontinence, urinary infrequency, hesitancy of urination, urinary urgency without incontinence, dysuria, and nocturnal enuresis.

Related Factors[2,10,20]

Incontinence (see specific diagnoses)
- Functional
- Reflex

- Stress
- Urge
- Total
- Stress urinary
- Overflow/paradoxic
- Instability
- Extraurethral/continuous
- (See Chapter 12.)

Urinary retention
Urinary tract infections
- Bacterial cystitis
- Fungal cystitis
- Parasitic cystitis
- Chemotherapy-induced cystitis
- Radiotherapy-induced cystitis
- Interstitial cystitis
- Cystitis glandularis
- Cystitis cystica
- Eosinophilic cystitis
- Cystitis emphysematosa
- Pyelonephritis

Inflammation of testis/epididymis
Inflammation of prostate
- Acute bacterial prostatitis
- Chronic bacterial prostatitis
- Nonbacterial prostatitis
- Prostatodynia

Inflammation of urethra
- Gonococcal urethritis
- Nongonococcal urethritis

Urethral syndrome
Bladder outlet obstruction
- Prostatic enlargement
  - Benign prostatic hypertrophy
  - Prostatic cancer
- Urethral stricture
- Female urethral distortion

Bladder diverticula
Paraurethral diverticula
Urinary fistulas
- Vesicovaginal
- Urethrovaginal
- Vesicoenteric
- Vesicocutaneous
- Ureterovaginal

Urinary ectopia
- Bladder exstrophy
- Hypospadias
- Epispadias
- Ureteral ectopia

Neuropathic bladder dysfunction
- Autonomous neurogenic bladder
- Reflex neurogenic bladder
- Motor paralytic neurogenic bladder
- Sensory paralytic bladder
- Uninhibited neurogenic bladder

Urinary calculi
- Ureteral
- Bladder

Psychogenic states
- Depression
- Attention seeking
- Regression
- Anxiety
- Confusion
- Disorientation
- Hysterical conversions

Constipation
Fecal impaction
Impaired physical mobility
Fluid volume state
- Fluid volume deficit: dehydration
- Fluid volume excess
  - Water intoxication
  - Syndrome of inappropriate antidiuretic hormone secretion

Polyuria

Defining Characteristics[20]

Failure to store urine (incontinence)
Failure to eliminate urine (urinary retention)
Urinary frequency (voids more often than every 2 hours)
Urinary infrequency (voids less often than every 6 hours during waking hours)
Dysuria
Strangury
Split stream or spraying stream
Urinary urgency
Urinary hesitancy
Nocturia
Nocturnal enuresis

Nursing Interventions[13,26-28]

Patient Goal	Nursing Intervention
Resolve incontinence. Contain incontinence. Maintain skin integrity.	(See nursing interventions for Functional, Reflex, Stress, Urge, and Total Incontinence.)
Reestablish normal voiding pattern.	• Assess patient's current fluid intake and urinary output. • Ask patient to keep voiding diary for 7-day period.

Patient Goal	Nursing Intervention
	• Determine symptoms associated with this alteration of urinary elimination patterns: incontinence, dysuria, strangury, urinary urgency, urinary hesitancy, feelings of incomplete bladder emptying. • Assess patient's medications that affect urinary elimination. • Assess strategies patient is currently employing to cope with altered urinary elimination patterns. • Institute a timed voiding schedule with fluid volume control. Have patient void by the clock every 2 to 4 hours as appropriate. Ask patient to keep voiding diary at intermittent periods after initiation of timed voiding schedule, including fluid intake. Devise appropriate fluid intake schedule based on current fluid intake and recommended daily needs (approximately 2000 to 2500 ml for adult). • Consult physician concerning referral to mental health care professional for altered urinary elimination patterns secondary to behavioral or psychogenic causes. • Consult physician concerning referral to endocrinologist for altered urinary elimination patterns secondary to inappropriate antidiuretic hormone secretion or other fluid electrolyte imbalance caused by hormonal abnormality.
Prevent or resolve urinary tract infection.	• Assess types of urinary tract infections patient experiences and presence of pain and burning on urination. • Determine if infection is associated with hematuria; fever; testicular, perineal, or scrotal pain; or vaginitis. • Assess identifiable factors that place patient at increased risk for urinary tract infection: feelings of incomplete bladder emptying, sexual activity, history of urinary calculi, or history of known neurogenic bladder dysfunction or incontinence. • Assess coping strategies, including medically prescribed regimens, patient uses to deal with urinary tract infections. • Assess type of infections patient is currently experiencing. Determine if this is first infection or one of several recurrent infections. (See Chapter 12.) • Establish voiding routine of every 2 hours as needed. Postponing voiding is contraindicated in presence of active bacterial, fungal, or parasitic cystitis. • Encourage adequate fluid intake of approximately 2000 to 2500 ml/day. • Provide patient with appropriate expectations for reduction and ablation of symptoms after anti-infective medications are begun. Counsel patient concerning appropriate time to contact physician (typically 72 hours after anti-infective medication is begun) for possible alteration of medication regimen if symptoms persist. • Advise patient of importance of adherence to anti-infective medication regimen to reduce likelihood of recurrence or persistence of infection. • Teach patient principal side effects of anti-infective medications: nausea and diarrhea. Advise patient to take antibiotics with meals to reduce nausea and to ingest yogurt, buttermilk, or other appropriate dairy products with active cultures to restore normal intestinal flora. • Teach patient to recognize allergic reactions to medications (rash, urticaria) and when to consult physician concerning discontinuing medication. • Teach women proper perineal hygiene: wipe from urethral meatus to anal area rather than the opposite. • Teach women to avoid underwear made of synthetic materials that may trap fluid against the perineum. Recommend all-cotton undergarments and avoidance of synthetic materials in swimwear. • Teach patient strategies for lowering urinary pH (ascorbic acid) as appropriate to prevent recurrence of urinary tract infections. Advise patient that a large daily intake of cranberry juice (1000 ml or greater) is required to lower urinary pH significantly. • Consult physician concerning appropriateness of long-term prophylactic or suppressive anti-infective medications for recurrent urinary tract infections. • Advise patient to take prophylactic or suppressive anti-infective medication at bedtime. • Contact physician if symptoms of infection occur. • Consult physician concerning appropriateness of self-start therapy for recurrent urinary tract infections. • Consult physician for appropriateness of postcoital therapy for recurrent urinary tract infections.

Principles and Rationale for Nursing Interventions

Altered urinary elimination patterns arise from excessively frequent or infrequent episodes of urination. Abnormal bladder function, such as that seen in incontinence and urinary retention, abnormal fluid intake, or altered bladder sensory states, may produce an altered pattern of micturition. Chronic bladder overdistention may predispose the individual to delayed perceptions of bladder filling and ultimately to urinary retention and deficient detrusor muscle function.[10] Prolonged urinary frequency predisposes the individual to early perceptions of bladder filling and decreased functional capacity.

The causes of urinary frequency are inflammation of the lower urinary tract, frequent micturition as a behavior, excessive fluid intake, and endocrine disorders, including diabetes mellitus and diabetes insipidus, that produce polyuria and polydipsia.[14] The causes of infrequent micturition are behavioral postponement of urination, urinary retention because of lower urinary tract dysfunction, or diseases producing oliguria or anuria.[14] A voiding diary that includes fluid intake and urinary output assists the health care professional in the assessment of the cause of altered urinary elimination patterns.[22] Establishing a routine of controlled fluid intake and timed voiding habits in conjunction with care for the physiologic or psychogenic causes of the voiding dysfunction is the best approach to this often persistent condition.

Urinary tract infections alter urinary elimination patterns by producing inflammation of the urinary tract. The most common form of urinary tract infection is cystitis; in addition, the condition is often associated with infection of the upper urinary tract and ureters (see Chapters 11 and 12). Postponement of urination is not recommended in this condition because routine, complete bladder evacuation is a useful defense mechanism against microbial invasion of the urinary system.[21,27] Adequate fluid intake promotes regular bladder evacuation and serves to flush the urinary system of pathogens and associated debris.[27,28]

Anti-infective therapy remains the cornerstone of care for urinary tract infection. Patients are taught side effects and allergic reactions of medications. Certain anti-infective medications may be taken with meals to reduce nausea or stomach upset. Diarrhea occurs with anti-infective medications because of a reduction in normal intestinal flora. Use of yogurt or other dairy products with active cultures containing common intestinal flora assists in resolving diarrhea.

Recurrent urinary tract infections are managed by strategies designed to prevent recurrences as well as measures designed to ablate a current infection. Using proper perineal cleansing and choosing rapid-drying undergarments are advocated in the prevention of recurrent infections.[26] Ingestion of cranberry juice or oral intake of ascorbic acid has been tentatively recommended as a strategy to lower urinary pH. An acidic urine is advocated because it exerts an antibacterial effect against certain strains of bacteria. The ingestion of cranberry juice is not recommended because of the unrealistically large quantities required to produce significant urinary pH reduction.[13]

Alternate forms of anti-infective medication therapy may be used when recurring urinary tract infections occur. Prophylactic medication is used for recurrent urinary tract infections, whereas suppressive medications are used when pathogenic persistence occurs. A single dose is typically given at bedtime so that the highest serum level is attained while the patient experiences prolonged retention of urine during sleep.[27]

Self-start therapy offers two advantages. The strategy allows the patient to begin therapy quickly after recognizing symptoms of urinary tract infection and reduces the cost of multiple visits to a physician's office or clinic. The patient is provided with a home urine collection system for cultures and a prescription that allows him to begin anti-infective agent therapy immediately. The principal limitations of the strategy are the need for meticulous follow-up placed on the patient and for reasonable accuracy in recognizing the symptoms of infection.[28]

Postcoital therapy for urinary tract infections is used for women who experience cystitis following coitus. These women are provided with adequate antibiotics for a prophylactic dosage of medication after coitus. Successful therapy requires a well-established correlation between coitus and urinary tract infection occurrences and meticulous compliance with the medication regimen.[28]

Evaluation

Patient Outcome	Data Indicating That Outcome is Reached
Resolves incontinence Contains incontinence Maintains skin integrity	(See evaluations for Functional, Reflex, Stress, Urge, and Total Incontinence.)
Urinary elimination patterns within normal ranges	Diurnal voiding patterns: 2 to 4 hours during waking hours Nocturia limited to two times or less nightly Fluid intake: 2000 to 2500 ml/day
Resolves or prevents urinary tract infection	Sterile urine in urine culture No symptoms of urinary tract infection

Functional Incontinence

Functional incontinence is the state in which an individual experiences an involuntary, unpredictable passage of urine.

The diagnosis Functional Incontinence occasionally may be a distinct entity or may be a complicating factor in the presence of one or more other forms of incontinence.

Establishing the diagnosis Functional Incontinence is complex because the interaction between cognitive, locomotor, and environmental factors and the pathophysiologic aspects of incontinence remains unclear.[7] For example, the relationship between cognitive impairment and detrusor muscle instability still is not clear, since the International Continence Society's definition of instability implies that the person being tested is attempting to inhibit micturition.[15] No such statement can be made with confidence if the individual undergoing testing has significant short-term memory loss and dementia. Thus, it is best to apply the diagnosis of functional incontinence most often in conjunction with other forms of incontinence unless urodynamic data exist to rule out physiologic bladder dysfunction contributing to urinary leakage.

Related Factors[20]

Altered environment
Activity intolerance
Impaired adjustment
Anxiety
Impaired verbal communication
Ineffective individual coping
Urge incontinence
Stress incontinence
Total incontinence
Urinary retention
Impaired physical mobility
Sleep pattern disturbance
Social isolation
Depression
Despair

Defining Characteristics[20]

Loss of urinary control, typically associated with urinary urgency
Inability to reach toilet facility in time
Loss of recognition of sensations or signs of impending micturition

Nursing Interventions[2,5,20]

Patient Goal	Nursing Intervention
Restore continence.	• Assess patient's current voiding pattern. • Assess factors associated with incontinent episodes, including environmental factors and patient's cognitive function and physical mobility. • Assess other forms of urinary incontinence associated with functional incontinence. • Establish timed voiding schedule with fluid intake control. (See Urge Incontinence.) • Alter environment to maximize access to toilet facilities. Provide bedside toilet facility or urinal. Provide toilet facility that may be reached with minimum number of steps and without necessity of using stairs. Provide patient with assistance choosing toilet device as needed. Consider following criteria when choosing a toilet seat: *Accessibility*. Device should be firmly anchored to floor with rubber grips. Toilet should have side arms to help support patient while sitting down. Height of chair should be adjustable to allow patient to place both feet and heels firmly on floor while using the device. Width of chair may be a constraint for obese patients. *Convenience of cleaning*. Device should be easily disassembled to empty. *Comfort*. As assessed by patient, padded seat may enhance comfort. *Cost*. • Teach patient to clean and empty device on routine basis; white vinegar or Urikleen is used to clean and deodorize receptacle. • Teach patient to use incontinent devices or systems as needed to control urinary leakage between trips to toilet. (See Total Incontinence and Stress Incontinence.) • Provide telephone or intercom access for patient at commode side. • Help patient formulate plans for bladder management during outings. Outings should be determined in consultation with patient and significant others and may include trips to shops and restaurants or visits to friends and relatives. Accompany patient on one or more such outings as feasible. • Consult physician concerning feasibility and appropriateness of biofeedback or training to enhance bladder control.
Maintain skin integrity.	• Assess condition of patient's perineal skin. • Assess strategies, including routine hygiene habits and products patient is using to protect perineal skin from irritation caused by urinary leakage.

Patient Goal	Nursing Intervention
	• Provide skin care to areas exposed to urinary leakage using regular hygiene routine: Wash skin once daily with soap and water. Dry thoroughly using hair dryer at low or warm setting with fan at lowest speed. Use skin sealant or moisture barrier to protect skin between washings. • Teach patient and family to perform skin care and to recognize common skin rashes, as well as indications for contacting health care professional regarding rashes, inflammation, or skin infections.

Principles and Rationale for Nursing Interventions

Strategies to reestablish continence among persons with functional incontinence are designed to overcome the cognitive, mobility, and environmental factors that contribute to urinary leakage. A timed voiding schedule with fluid intake control is designed to reestablish a pattern of voiding and prevent inappropriate (incontinent) micturition episodes.

Providing a toilet that is easily accessible minimizes impaired physical mobility. A nighttime toilet seat precludes the necessity of the patient attempting to awaken sufficiently and walk to the bathroom.[2] A telephone or intercom system at the commode allows the patient to contact others in the home or other helpers if needed.[5,20]

Provision of plans for bladder management during outings allows patients to engage in anticipatory management of a problem and increases their confidence as they seek to increase social contacts. Accompanying patients on a trial outing may increase confidence for continued social activities and provides added support while newly learned strategies for bladder control are attempted.

Behavioral strategies attempt to resolve functional incontinence by combining biofeedback of detrusor and/or pelvic floor muscle activity, timed voiding, and maintenance of a voiding/incontinence diary. Favorable results have been reported using this methodology, although the individual strategies of the program that exert these beneficial effects remain to be elucidated.[5]

Recurrent urinary leakage threatens to impair the integrity of affected skin. Use of an appropriate skin care regimen provides routine cleaning, thorough drying, and moisture barriers that help protect integumentary integrity. (See Total Incontinence.)

Evaluation

Patient Outcome	Data Indicating That Outcome is Reached
Restores continence	Regular, complete bladder emptying is achieved without intermittent urinary leakage. Access to toilet allows evacuation of urine during daytime and nighttime hours.
Contains continence	Urinary leakage is contained. Patient and family demonstrate adequate knowledge of incontinent containment device or system.
Maintains skin integrity	Skin exposed to urinary leakage remains without rash or lesions. Patient and family demonstrate adequate knowledge of care routine for skin affected by urinary leakage and indications for contacting physician concerning skin lesions.

Reflex Incontinence

Reflex incontinence is the state in which an individual experiences an involuntary loss of urine, occurring at somewhat predictable intervals when a specific bladder volume is reached.

Reflex incontinence is distinguished from urge incontinence by the absence of sensations and differing etiology. The diagnosis probably arises from the term *reflex incontinence* used by the International Continence Society[15] to denote incontinence caused by neurologic abnormality. This form of incontinence arises from complete spinal cord injury or abnormality above sacral segments 2 to 4.[11]

Establishment of the diagnosis reflex incontinence requires the presence of a known neurologic deficit and documentation of bladder contraction (often described as *spastic*) in the absence of sensations.[20] Since the underlying abnormality is an unstable detrusor muscle, the value of establishing unique nursing diagnoses for each form of instability incontinence remains controversial.

Related Factors[2,23]

Neurologic abnormalities
- Complete spinal cord injury above sacral micturition center
- Cerebellar ataxia
- Amyotrophic lateral sclerosis
- Multiple sclerosis
- Spinovascular disease

Spinal cord tumor
Myelomeningocele (greatest in first years of life)
Autonomic dysreflexia
Neuropathic sphincter: detrusor sphincter dyssynergia
Urinary retention
Obstructive uropathy
Urinary tract infection
Trabeculation of bladder with poor bladder wall compliance
Bladder diverticula
Hydronephrosis
Upper urinary tract deterioration
Renal insufficiency

Defining Characteristics[20]

Uncontrolled urinary leakage associated with detrusor muscle instability and absent sensations of urgency
Absent sensations of bladder filling
Detrusor sphincter dyssynergia and intermittent urinary stream

Nursing Interventions[12]

Patient Goal	Nursing Intervention
Restore continence. Prevent urinary tract infection.	• Assess patient's current urinary elimination pattern and incidence of incontinence. • Determine stimuli that cause bladder emptying in addition to reaching a certain intravesical volume. • Assess for presence of diaphoresis, dizziness, or palpitations with voiding. (See Chapter 12.) • Monitor patient's current fluid intake (amount and time). • Begin clean intermittent catheterization program with appropriate autonomic drugs (propantheline or oxybutynin) or spasmolytic drugs (flavoxate or dicyclomine) under physician's direction: Teach catheterization using clean, rather than sterile, technique unless latter is specified by physician. Teach patient to wash hands. Use clean or sterile catheter; water-soluble lubricant is necessary for men and advisable for women. May wash perineum with soap and water or a prepackaged towelette. Lubricate catheter and gently insert into urethra; bladder is drained completely. Teach patient to withdraw catheter slowly to ensure adequate evacuation of urine. Pinch catheter on removal from urethra to prevent spillage of urine. Wash catheter immediately with cold tap water and later with warm, soapy water. Rinse thoroughly. Store catheters in clean, dry container suitable for carrying in purse or pocket. Catheters are never stored in any solution because of infection risk. • Establish catheterization schedule in accordance with patient's schedule, approximately every 4 to 6 hours as needed during waking hours. Sleep is not typically interrupted for intermittent catheterization. • Teach patient and family members catheterization procedure as feasible. • Maintain fluid intake at approximately 200 ml/day. Fluid intake control may be used to minimize nighttime urinary output. (See Urge Incontinence.) • Monitor patient for side effects of medications: dry mouth, blurred vision, dizziness, weakness, or tachycardia if cardiac disease is present. Consult physician concerning altering pharmacologic regimen if incontinent episodes occur between catheterizations. • Teach patient signs of urinary tract infection: sudden change in continence between catheterizations, fever, flank pain, hematuria, or change in character or odor of urinary output. • If clean intermittent schedule is not feasible or successful, use urinary containment devices or indwelling Foley catheter. • Use condom catheter and drainage system for males who have undergone transurethral sphincterotomy. Condom should have following features: Availability in appropriate size Adequate comfort as perceived by patient Adequate drainage characteristics, including resistance to occlusion by twisting Adherence to penis, forming watertight seal without tourniquet effect Relative ease of application for patient or family • Teach patient and significant others to apply device as feasible and to care for drainage system. • Use other urinary containment devices (pads, diapers, incontinent briefs) as indicated. (See Total Incontinence.) • Maintain skin integrity when using incontinent containment devices. • Use indwelling Foley catheter drainage of bladder as directed by physician.

Patient Goal	Nursing Intervention
	• Insert appropriate size and type of catheter for long-term use. Suprapubic cystostomy may be used as alternative to urethral catheter. Foley catheter should be made of inert or hydrophilic material. • Choose appropriate drainage system for daytime and nighttime use. Daytime system should be reasonably concealed in clothing and comfortable against leg or thigh. Cloth sleeve is best for drainage bag. Nighttime drainage system should contain a minimum of 2000 ml. • Teach patient to clean drainage bags regularly with vinegar and water solution. • Maintain adequate fluid intake of 2000 to 2500 ml. Fluid intake control is not indicated when indwelling Foley catheter is used. • Consult physician if patient is incontinent around catheter. Consider use of drugs to decrease detrusor muscle instability before increasing size of Foley catheter. • Do not overfill catheter balloon. • Teach patient and family indications for contacting health care professional concerning indwelling Foley catheter use (signs of urinary tract infection, untoward drug reactions, decreasing urinary output). • Teach patient and family to assess catheter daily to ensure adequate drainage. • Change the catheter as needed, approximately every 30 days.

Principles and Rationale for Nursing Interventions

The goals of management of reflex incontinence are the restoration of continence and prevention of urinary tract infection and associated complications. Bladder training is not feasible in these patients. The neurologic abnormality underlying reflex incontinence is centered in the spinal reflex arcs.[11,20] Attempts at cortical retraining will not be successful.

Autonomic or spasmolytic drugs are used to convert the bladder to a low-pressure storage vesicle that can be regularly emptied through a clean intermittent catheterization (CIC) program. Medications are closely monitored for side effects and may have to be altered periodically because of development of tolerance or untoward effects. The rates of infection and upper urinary tract abnormality associated with this strategy are minimal compared to patients who experience chronic urinary retention.[12] Nonetheless, long-term prophylactic medication is often used in an attempt to prevent colonization of the urinary tract with pathogens.[28]

A significant reason for failure of a pharmacologic-CIC program is noncompliance. Compliance to the regimen may be maximized by carefully tailoring the catheterizations around the patient's daily schedule. Teaching others in the patient's environment to catheterize provides the patient with other resources for catheterization if needed.

Transurethral sphincterotomy is a surgical strategy designed to reduce sphincteric resistance and prevent urinary retention (see Chapter 12). The incontinence will persist after sphincterotomy, and a condom device is used to contain urinary leakage.[2] This strategy for coping with reflex incontinence is restricted to males because no acceptable condom device exists for female patients.

The long-term indwelling catheter is considered a last resort for patients with reflex incontinence. Long-term catheter drainage is associated with significant urinary tract complications, including infection, upper tract dilation and deterioration, and renal insufficiency. Complications associated with the catheter may be minimized with careful care of the system. The choice of catheter material is important. Inert or hydrophilic materials are purported to reduce urethral irritation. Choosing a catheter with a large internal lumen relative to the external French size will minimize the likelihood of the catheter becoming clogged with urinary sediment. Choosing an appropriate drainage system allows optimum patient comfort and prevents urinary stasis caused by filling of an inadequately sized bag.

Bacteriuria is inevitable in the presence of a long-term indwelling Foley catheter. A suprapubic cystostomy site may be chosen by the physician instead of urethral catheterization in an attempt to create a cleaner insertion site and prevent complications associated with infection. The goal of care is not prevention of bacteriuria; rather, care is aimed at preventing symptomatic urinary tract infections and serious related urologic conditions.[28] Long-term use of prophylactic antibiotics are not indicated because resistance may develop, requiring the use of intravenous anti-infective agents when symptomatic urinary tract infections occur. Maintenance of adequate fluid intake assists in the prevention of serious urinary tract infections by flushing the urinary system of sediment. Maintaining a patent catheter through regular assessment of urinary drainage and routine changes, as well as use of an adequately sized drainage bag, also prevents stasis. Routine cleansing of the drainage bag may help prevent serious urinary tract infection by preventing bacterial overgrowth and colonization of the bladder.

Incontinence around the Foley catheter may indicate a catheter that is no longer patent or persistent detrusor muscle instability. Increasing the catheter size is not indicated unless routine clogging of the catheter is a known problem. Consulting the physician concerning use of a drug to decrease detrusor instability may be adequate to prevent incontinence. Increasing the size of the retention balloon is contraindicated, since this is associated with irritation of the bladder outlet and may lead to exacerbation of detrusor instability.[2]

Evaluation

Patient Outcome	Data Indicating That Outcome is Reached
Attains continence	Maintains continence between catheterizations Is dry at night or successfully uses urinary containment device or system while asleep
Contains urinary leakage	Reports no leakage from containment device or system No symptoms of urinary tract infection Foley catheter in place and draining into adequately sized drainage bag No urinary leakage around Foley catheter
Prevents urinary tract infection	No symptoms of urinary tract infection Sterile urine in urine culture

Stress Incontinence

Stress incontinence is the state in which an individual experiences a urine loss of less than 50 ml, occurring with increased abdominal pressure.

This nursing diagnosis arises from descriptions of stress incontinence or stress urinary incontinence in which urinary leakage is associated with physical exertion.[10,15,28,29] The International Continence Society[15] defines stress incontinence as a symptom or sign. The *symptom* of stress incontinence is the patient's subjective report of urinary leakage on physical exertion; the *sign* of stress incontinence is the objective confirmation of the symptom in a clinical or laboratory setting. *Genuine stress incontinence* is a urodynamically proved condition in which urinary leakage occurs when intravesical (bladder) pressure exceeds urethral closure pressure in the absence of a detrusor muscle contraction.

The limitation of stress incontinence to volumes less than 50 ml is an attempt to differentiate stress incontinence from total incontinence. The use of volume as a distinction to differentiate these conditions is certainly vulnerable to criticism. A better differentiation could be made by recognizing the difficulty of distinguishing incontinence by symptoms such as the magnitude of urinary leakage. Other classification systems avoid this problem by distinguishing stress urinary incontinence from extraurethral (continuous or constant) incontinence. Under such a system, stress incontinence would be defined as the leakage of urine on physical exertion caused by increased abdominal pressure, whereas extraurethral incontinence would be defined as the leakage of urine that occurs when the normal sphincteric mechanism is bypassed. Unfortunately, under the current schema, overlapping related factors and defining characteristics will be noted between stress incontinence and total incontinence.

Related Factors[1,10,19,25,29]

- Forms of pelvic relaxation
  - Cystocele
  - Rectocele
  - Enterocele
  - Urethrocele
  - Uterine prolapse
- Risk factors of pelvic relaxation
  - Multiple vaginal deliveries
  - Aging and menopause
  - Peripheral neuropathies
  - Trauma to pelvic support structures
  - Iatrogenic pelvic floor denervation
- Obesity
- Gravid uterus
- Sphincteric incompetence
  - Trauma to sphincteric mechanism
  - Iatrogenic trauma to sphincteric mechanism
    - Multiple anti-incontinence procedures
    - Radical prostatectomy
    - Transurethral prostatectomy (rare)
  - Congenital sphincteric incompetence
    - Myelomeningocele
    - Spina bifida
    - Sacral agenesis
    - Spinal dysraphism
- Urinary frequency
- Urinary urgency
- Urge incontinence
- Functional incontinence
- Nocturia

Defining Characteristics[15,20]

- Reported urinary leakage associated with physical exertion (increased abdominal pressure)
- Observed urinary leakage associated with increased abdominal pressure
- Urinary leakage when urodynamically assessed bladder pressure exceeds urethral pressure in absence of detrusor contraction

Nursing Interventions

Patient Goal	Nursing Intervention
Contain continence.	• Determine causes of incontinence and any association with coughing, laughing, sneezing, or abdominal strain. • Assess urgency associated with incontinence. Determine if element of urge incontinence is related, and identify stressors that produce these symptoms. (See Urge Incontinence.) • Assess severity of incontinence and frequency that urinary leakage requires a change of clothing. • Determine frequency of voiding, if patient is nocturic, and how often desire to void interrupts sleep each night. • Monitor patient's current fluid intake pattern (volume and time). • Assess coping strategies, including drugs or mechanical devices, patient currently employs to cope with urinary leakage. • Assess risk factors for this patient (e.g., number of vaginal deliveries, status of estrogen production or replacement, relation to climacteric, previous surgical procedures, conditions related to peripheral neuropathies). • Provide patient with incontinent containment device or system. Absorbent pads are usually sufficient. Pad is evaluated on the basis of following criteria: *Absorbency*. Devices with Superabsorbents are typically the most absorbent of all pads; often a less absorbent device is adequate in cases of mild to moderate leakage. *Wetness protection*. Outer waterproof lining should protect clothing from urinary leakage. *Size*. Pads should be easily concealed in clothing. *Comfort*. This is assessed by patient. • Teach female patient to do Kegel's exercises to strengthen circumvaginal muscles (CVMs) through resistive and endurance maneuvers.[10] Instruct patient to: Empty bladder. Lie down in comfortable position with knees elevated 20 degrees. Relax completely. Tighten CVMs with abdominal and thigh muscles relaxed. Patient will need help isolating the CVMs. Ask patient to visualize vagina and contract only those muscles that press against pubic bone as if they were stopping the urinary stream. Tighten muscles quickly and hold for 10 seconds. Relax completely for 10 seconds and repeat procedure. Begin with 10 repetitions and increase regimen to 30 repetitions over three sessions per week. Advise patient to increase repetitions in increments of five until goal is attained. • Provide female patient with appropriate pessary device in consultation with or under direction of physician. Teach patient care of pessary device, including appropriate hygiene and necessity of regular follow-up to change device as indicated. • Administer sympathomimetic medications (pseudoephedrine) as directed. • Inform patient of availability of surgical options to correct stress incontinence as indicated, and encourage patient to speak with appropriate health care professional.

Principles and Rationale for Nursing Interventions

Conservative treatment for stress incontinence is typically recommended for a mild to moderate disorder. Stress incontinence is not typically associated with serious urologic complications. It is important to remember that the treatment of stress incontinence is based on the patient's perceptions of the condition as a significant social or hygienic problem. Providing a patient with a suitable pad to contain incontinence is often an acceptable solution for the condition, whereas other persons will seek more definitive solutions.

Kegel[18] is credited for originating an exercise regimen to strengthen the pelvic floor muscles to control stress incontinence in women. The exercises are designed to strengthen the striated portion of the sphincteric mechanism and may play a role in alleviation of pelvic descent caused by muscle weakness. Balloon devices have been used, but their contribution to the success of exercise remains unclear.

The pessary device alleviates stress incontinence by mechanically alleviating pelvic descent and loss of anatomic relationships of the urethrovesical unit. Voiding is not obstructed when the pessary is placed correctly, and adequate care prevents common hygienic problems associated with use of a pessary.[3,10]

Alpha-sympathomimetic medications are available in several over-the-counter preparations. Such drugs are effective in cases of stress incontinence because they increase tone at the smooth muscle component of the sphincteric mechanism. In addition, sympathomimetics may contribute to sphincteric closure through a vascular effect at the urethral submucosa.[11]

Many patients with more severe urinary leakage may undergo surgical correction of stress incontinence. Evaluation of a patient for surgical repair is done by a urologist or gynecologist and includes urodynamic assessment. (See Chapter 12 for a description of the care of patients undergoing urethral suspension procedures.)

Evaluation

Patient Outcome	Data Indicating That Outcome is Reached
Contains continence	No longer perceives urinary leakage as uncontrolled problem
Restores continence	Increases in abdominal pressure no longer accompanied by urinary leakage Resolves urinary urgency and urge incontinence Diurnal frequency every 3-4 hours Experiences nocturia no more than two times per night

Urge Incontinence

Urge incontinence is the state in which an individual experiences involuntary passage of urine, occurring soon after a strong sense of urgency to void.

Urge incontinence arises from the International Continence Society's (ICS) designation.[15] The ICS subdivides the concept into two forms of urge incontinence. *Motor* urge incontinence is associated with detrusor muscle instability; *sensory* urgency is associated with hypersensitivity (irritative) disorders of the bladder. (See Chapter 12.)

The physiologic mechanism underlying urge incontinence is detrusor muscle instability. Nonetheless, cognitive, functional, and logistic components of the patient and environment influence whether incontinence occurs. A patient who is alert, ambulatory, and familiar with the environment may be able to prevent urinary leakage by use of the pelvic floor muscles until a toilet is reached. A person who is confused, immobile, or unfamiliar with the location of a nearby toilet is more likely to experience incontinence. Thus, the diagnosis urge incontinence is not mutually exclusive of functional incontinence.

Related Factors[10,20,22,29]

- Neurologic disease/trauma
  - Cerebrovascular accident
  - Brain tumor
  - Parkinsonism
  - Alzheimer's disease
  - Multiple sclerosis
  - Incomplete suprasacral spinal cord injury
  - Closed head injury
- Bladder outlet obstruction
  - Prostatic enlargement
    - Benign prostatic hypertrophy
    - Prostatic adenocarcinoma
    - Prostatitis
  - Bladder neck hypertrophy
  - Bladder neck contracture
  - Bladder neck dyssynergia
- Irritative bladder disorders
  - Cystitis
    - Bacterial
    - Viral
    - Fungal
    - Parasitic
    - Chemotherapy induced
    - Radiotherapy induced
  - Bladder wall tumor
  - Bladder calculi
- Stress incontinence
- Age (childhood or elderly)
- Altered thought processes
- Altered state of mobility
- Unfamiliar environment
  - Lack of knowledge of toilet facilities
  - Toilet facilities unavailable
  - Lack of access to toilet
- Anxiety
- Impaired physical mobility
- Impaired verbal communication
- Sleep pattern disturbance related to nocturia

Defining Characteristics[20]

- Urinary leakage associated with marked sensation of urge to void
- Inability to reach toilet in time
- Urinary urgency
- Urinary frequency (voids more often than every 2 hours)
- Nocturia (awakened by desire to void more than once per night)

Nursing Interventions[20,24]

Patient Goal	Nursing Intervention
Restore urinary continence.	• Assess related factors that predispose toward urge incontinence: neurologic disease or trauma, bladder outlet obstruction, irritative bladder disorders, stress incontinence. • Determine if patient is in high-risk age group for condition.

Patient Goal	Nursing Intervention
	• Assess associated related factors for urge incontinence: physical or cognitive impairment, environmental alterations. • Assess patient's access to toilet facilities and approximate transit time to nearest toilet facility, considering the patient's physical mobility limitations, if any. • Determine patient's current daytime urinary elimination patterns (frequency of urination, number of incontinent episodes per day). • Ask if patient experiences nocturia, enuresis, or incontinence before reaching toilet. • Check patient's current fluid intake pattern (volume and time). • Determine specific circumstances that patient and family identify as predisposing toward urge incontinence. • Assess current coping strategies, including drugs or medical treatments, patient uses to deal with urge incontinence. • Have patient maintain timed voiding schedule of approximately every 2 hours during the day. Schedule must be individualized in consultation with patient and family. Progress to every 3 to 4 hours as feasible. • Instruct patient to control fluid intake. Patient should receive approximately 2000 to 2500 ml/day. Recommended schedule: 1100 to 1600 ml between breakfast and dinner; 900 ml after dinner until 2 to 4 hours before bedtime. Small amount (100 to 200 ml) may be given at night as needed to swallow oral medications. • Consider administration of autonomic drugs (propantheline or oxybutynin) or spasmolytic drugs (flavoxate or dicyclomine) under physician's direction to increase functional bladder capacity if urinary frequency and urge incontinence persist despite timed voiding schedule with fluid intake control. • Institute bladder drill therapy regimen in consultation with physician. Instruct the patient to postpone urination for 1½ hours during waking hours even if incontinence occurs in the interim. As continence is attained for this period, increase increment between voidings by ½ hour until a goal of 3 to 4 hours is reached. Negotiation of goals concerning bladder drill therapy must occur in conjunction with patient and family. • If attempts at timed voiding and fluid control schedules and bladder drill therapy fail, consult physician concerning institution of significant pharmacologic relaxation of the detrusor muscle with intermittent catheterization schedule. • Begin clean intermittent catheterization program and teach patient and family members as soon as feasible. Catheterization should be accomplished approximately every 4 to 6 hours. Sleep patterns are not usually interrupted for catheterization. (See Reflex Incontinence.) • Monitor patient for side effects of autonomic or spasmolytic drugs (blurred vision, constipation, dry mouth, weakness, tachycardia in presence of existing cardiac disease). • If attempts to control urge incontinence fail, consult physician concerning use of indwelling Foley catheter. • Alter patient's environment in following ways to promote restoration of continence: Provide portable urinal as feasible. Assess home environment for access to toilet facility. Climbing stairs to the toilet is not feasible for patients with limited mobility. Provide for bedside toilet facility for nocturic voiding needs. Because of nighttime awakening, urinal or bedside commode is needed for patients with limited physical mobility or potential altered cognition. Allow patient to sit up to use toilet whenever possible; bedpans or diapers should be employed as a final resort rather than for convenience.
Prevent urinary tract infections.	• Assess patient for history of urinary tract infections, their frequency, and any association with fever or hematuria. • Assess coping strategies, including pharmacologic agents, patient currently uses to deal with infections. • Determine if patient thinks that bladder is completely emptied and if patient uses specific strategies (e.g., double voiding, self–intermittent catheterization, Credé's maneuver) to ensure complete bladder emptying. • Assess efficiency of bladder emptying by maintaining accurate record of fluid intake and urinary output. • Measure postvoiding residuals at least three times using straight catheter or ultrasound assessment within 5 minutes of voiding. • Encourage adequate fluid intake, 2000 to 2500 ml/day. • Consider recommendation for acidification of urine. One gram of ascorbic acid may be given each day under a physician's direction. Note that intake of even substantial quantities of cranberry juice will not significantly lower urinary pH.

Principles and Rationale for Nursing Interventions

The overriding goal of treating any patient with altered urinary elimination patterns is the prevention of incontinence and the assurance of complete, regular bladder emptying. A timed voiding schedule is used in an attempt to prevent urinary leakage precipitated by bladder filling to a threshold volume. Oral fluid control is used to ensure adequate intake and encourage maximum urinary output while the patient is awake, maximally mobile, and engaged in activities of daily living. Fluid intake is severely restricted just before bedtime in an attempt to minimize altered sleep patterns caused by nocturia.

Autonomic or spasmolytic drugs are used to increase functional bladder capacity and decrease urinary frequency.[11] They are adjunct measures to the timed voiding and fluid control schedule and should not be used as a substitute. Urinary residuals may increase with these agents, and assessment of postvoiding residual is essential.

Bladder drill therapy is a strategy designed to eliminate detrusor muscle instability or bladder hypersensitivity through behavioral means. The patient is taught to postpone urination for increasingly longer periods until an optimum routine of urinary frequency (every 3 to 4 hours) during waking hours is attained. Sleep patterns are not interrupted for bladder therapy regimens. Success of such a program is optimized by intensive support of persons undergoing bladder drill therapy. Goals for therapy should be determined by both patient and nurse. It is probably best to begin with a relatively modest goal of voiding every 1½ hours and working toward a 3- to 4-hour interval between voiding at ½-hour increments.[10,16,17]

Pharmacologic relaxation of the bladder can be attained by careful use of autonomic or spasmolytic drugs.[11] The goal of pharmacologic therapy is to decrease detrusor contractions significantly and convert the bladder to a low-compliance storage compartment for urine suitable for routine emptying using catheterization. Bladder evacuation through clean intermittent catheterization is employed to ensure regular, complete vesicle emptying. This strategy is typically used if the patient fails other means of therapy because of significant urinary retention or persistent incontinence.

An indwelling Foley catheter is used when conservative management, as well as surgical options in selected patients, have failed and the incontinence continues to be a significant health and hygiene problem as perceived by the patient and/or family.[23] (See Urinary Retention.)

Control of the environment is needed to maximize the chances of success of a fluid control and timed voiding program. Accessibility of toilet facilities is essential for the patient to establish a reasonable voiding schedule that does not unduly interfere with other activities of daily living. It is important to remember that the goal is control of incontinence; a timed voiding and fluid control program is a coping strategy and not a curative measure for urge incontinence.

Prevention of urinary tract infection and associated urologic abnormalities is accomplished by ensuring that the patient completely empties the bladder on a regular schedule. Persistent residual urine is a significant risk factor for recurrent urinary tract infections with their associated complications. (See Chapters 11 and 12.)

Evaluation

Patient Outcome	Data Indicating That Outcome is Reached
Restores continence	Symptoms of urge incontinence are absent. Symptoms of urinary urgency and urinary frequency remain present, but incontinent episodes are absent. Patient and family describe goals and process of timed voiding schedule with fluid intake control. Urodynamic tracings indicate restoration of normal functional bladder capacity, normal report of sensations of filling, and stable detrusor function. Patient and family demonstrate adequate knowledge of continence containment device. Patient reports dryness between intermittent catheterizations. Foley catheter is in place; patient reports no leakage around catheter. Patient has rapid and adequate access to toilet facilities in hospital, extended care, and/or home environment.
Prevents urinary tract infections	No symptoms of urinary tract infection are present. Urine cultures show sterile urine.

Total Incontinence

Total incontinence is the state in which an individual experiences a continuous and unpredictable loss of urine.

Total incontinence is partly analogous to extraurethral incontinence, as described by the International Incontinence Society (ICS),[15] and to severe genuine stress incontinence.

Total incontinence is caused by urinary ectopia or a fistulous tract through which urine leaks, bypassing the normal sphincteric mechanism. Because of the limited definition of stress incontinence to volumes of 50 ml or less, the diagnosis total incontinence also applies to cases of severe stress incontinence caused by significant sphincteric incompetence.

Related Factors[2,19,20]

Urinary fistula
- Vesicovaginal
- Ureterovaginal
- Urethrovaginal
- Urethrocutaneous

Urinary ectopia
- Ectopic ureter that bypasses sphincteric mechanism
- Bladder exstrophy
- Urethral duplication

Surgically created stomas
- Ileal conduit
- Sigmoid conduit
- Ureterostomy
- Pyelostomy
- Vesicostomy

Sphincteric incompetence
- Iatrogenic
  - Multiple anti-incontinence procedures
  - Y-V plasty
- Trauma to sphincteric mechanism
- Congenital sphincteric incompetence
  - Epispadias
  - Absent urethra (associated with cloacal deformity)
  - Spina bifida
  - Myelomeningocele
  - Sacral agenesis
  - Spinal dysraphism
- Urinary tract infection
- Functional incontinence

Defining Characteristics

Continuous urinary leakage imposed on otherwise normal voiding pattern
Continuous urinary leakage with failure of urinary storage
Unawareness of incontinence
Refractory to pharmacologic or behavioral treatment

Nursing Interventions

Patient Goal	Nursing Intervention
Contain continence.	• Determine when incontinence occurs and if patient is ever dry. • Assess conditions (if any) that make leakage more or less severe. • Determine if leakage is ever associated with sensation of urgency. • Assess patient's normal voiding patterns. Determine if continuous urinary leakage occurs in addition to "regular" voiding pattern or if incontinence is severe enough to have replaced micturition. • Determine origin of urinary leakage: urethra, vagina, or other opening. • Assess whether urinary tract infections are associated with leakage and whether hematuria or fever is present. • Provide patient with urinary containment device or system to cope with incontinence. Evaluate products using following criteria: Absorbency Ease of application, use Ability to conceal in clothing Comfort Patient's desires, preferences Cost • Consider following devices: Pads should adhere to the patient's underclothing and remain well concealed in clothing. Pads should have water-resistant backing to prevent leaking through device onto clothing. Absorption may be relatively limited; products containing Superabsorbents hold maximum amount. Adult briefs combine a pad with a brief specifically designed to hold pad in place. Absorbency is typically greater than with pads. Application of system may be more difficult than with pads, particularly in patients with limited mobility. Certain devices are equipped with panel that opens in front, using Velcro strips for patients confined to wheelchair. System should be easily concealed in clothing and have outward appearance of normal underclothing. Briefs should be constructed of breathable material with comfort comparable to regular undergarments. Condom catheters (See Reflex Incontinence.) Adult diapers are typically reserved for particularly severe cases of incontinence or for persons confined to bed. Devices are very absorbent and relatively easy to apply, but they are difficult to conceal in clothing and often are considered uncomfortable to wear. Patient acceptance of diapers is often problematic because of social stigma attached to "wearing diapers."

Patient Goal	Nursing Intervention
	Urinary pouching system is option of choice for patients with total incontinence caused by surgical diversion. This system requires enterostomal therapy (ET) nurse to design and place pouch for urinary containment. System provides watertight drainage device connected to a drainage bag so that absorbency is not an issue. System may be more difficult to apply than other prepackaged devices. Device should be relatively simple to conceal under clothing and comfortable. Patient acceptance is typically high because of interaction with the ET nurse. (See Chapter 12.) • Consult physician concerning definitive plan for repairing fistulous tract, implanting artificial urinary sphincter device, or removing ectopic urinary segment.
Maintain skin integrity.	• Assess condition of patient's perineal skin. • Assess strategies, including routine hygiene habits, and products patient is currently using to protect perineal skin from irritation caused by urinary leakage. • Provide skin care to areas exposed to urinary leakage using regular hygiene routine: Wash skin once daily with soap and water. Dry thoroughly using hair dryer at low or warm setting with fan at lowest speed. Use skin sealant or moisture barrier to protect skin between washings. • Teach patient and family to perform skin care and to recognize common skin rashes, as well as indications for contacting health care professional regarding rashes, inflammation, or skin infections.

Principles and Rationale for Nursing Interventions

Because the normal sphincteric mechanism is bypassed or ablated, total incontinence is refractory to routine management with treatment modalities such as timed voiding, fluid control, bladder drill, physiotherapy, or pharmacologic manipulation. Urinary containment devices are the immediate treatment of choice. For certain patients who are suitable surgical candidates, incontinence is resolved by surgical closure of a fistulous tract or resection of an ectopic urinary structure. For others who are not surgical candidates or for whom a urinary diversion has been accomplished as a lifesaving measure, urinary containment is a permanent management strategy.

Skin care is essential for the patient with total incontinence. The goal of skin care is to prevent loss of integrity. Routine cleaning is followed by careful and thorough drying. Skin sealants or moisture barriers form a protective barrier to protect the integument from urine; sealants with an alcohol base are not used on a patient who does not have intact skin because the solution will cause severe discomfort.[4]

Evaluation

Patient Outcome	Data Indicating That Outcome is Reached
Contains continence	Urinary leakage around continent pad, diaper, or brief is absent. Urinary leakage from condom catheter system is absent. Urinary leakage from urinary pouch system is absent.
Maintains skin integrity	Skin rashes, lesions, inflammation, and infection are absent. Patient and family accurately describe routine for providing skin care to areas exposed to constant urinary leakage. Patient and family accurately describe indications for contacting health care professional concerning loss of skin integrity.

Urinary Retention

Urinary retention is the state in which the individual experiences incomplete emptying of the bladder.

Two factors contribute to urinary retention: deficient detrusor muscle function and bladder outlet obstruction. Urinary retention may manifest as an acute state requiring immediate intervention or as a chronic condition. The symptom of urinary retention is not necessarily harmful to the individual. A person requires treatment for urinary retention when potentially harmful sequelae of the condition, such as urinary tract infection and upper tract dilation, threaten to compromise renal function.

Related Factors[6,10,11,29]

Bladder outlet obstruction
- Prostatic enlargement
  - Benign prostatic hypertrophy

Prostatic cancer
Prostatitis
Bladder neck hypertrophy
Bladder neck dyssynergia
Bladder neck contracture
Urethral stricture
Female urethral distortion
Detrusor sphincter dyssynergia
Urethral trauma
Deficient detrusor function
Chronic overdistention
Infrequent voiding
Sensory paralytic bladder
Diabetes mellitus
Incomplete spinal cord injury
Pelvic trauma
Sacral spinal cord injury
Cauda equina injury
Cauda equina syndrome
Tabes dorsalis
Polio
Multiple sclerosis
Herpes zoster
Cannabis ingestion
Constipation/fecal impaction
Prolonged bed rest
Hysterical conversions
Drugs
Propantheline
Oxybutynin
Methantheline
Flavoxate
Dicyclomine
Ganglion-blocking agents
Tricyclic antidepressants
Phenothiazines
Antiparkinsonian agents
Calcium channel blockers
Instability incontinence
Urinary tract infections
Pyelonephritis
Bladder overdistention
Bladder trabeculation
Hydronephrosis
Upper urinary tract deterioration
Renal insufficiency

Defining Characteristics[20]

Urinary frequency
Small voided volumes
Intermittent or poor urinary stream
Nocturia
Overflow incontinence
Postvoiding dribble
Absence of micturition with suprapubic pain or pressure
Postvoiding residual greater than 25% of total bladder volume

Nursing Interventions

Patient Goal	Nursing Intervention
Resolve acute urinary voiding.	• Relieve urinary retention by employing straight urethral catheterization or introduction of indwelling catheter as directed. • Institute intermittent catheterization or maintain indwelling catheter as appropriate. (See Reflex Incontinence.)
Resolve urinary retention.	• Assess patient's current diurnal voiding patterns. • Assess quality of patient's voided stream. • Determine patient's awareness of feelings of incomplete emptying. • Assess maneuvers (if any) patient is using to cope with urinary retention. Determine if patient strains or uses Credé's maneuver to assist voiding. • Teach patient to double void to enhance complete bladder emptying. Patient should void normally, then wait on the toilet for approximately 5 minutes and attempt to void again. Use of abdominal straining or Credé's maneuver may be used to enhance bladder evacuation. • Teach patient to void using a timed schedule. Patient should void every 3 to 4 hours when awake regardless of absence or of desire to urinate. Sleep patterns are not typically interrupted for timed voiding schedule. • Consult physician concerning use of bethanechol chloride to stimulate detrusor muscle contractility for patients with deficient detrusor function or phenoxybenzamine for patients with increased sphincteric resistance.
Establish regular, complete bladder emptying using mechanical means to manage urinary retention.	• Teach patient and family members to perform intermittent catheterization. (See Reflex Incontinence.) • Teach patient to perform intermittent catheterization after micturition. Teach patient to keep diary or log of voided volume versus volume catheterized, and provide parameters for returning to physician for alteration of catheterization schedule as needed. • Teach patient to maintain long-term indwelling catheter. (See Reflex Incontinence.)

Patient Goal	Nursing Intervention
Prevent urinary tract infection.	• Assess for presence of current urinary tract infections. • Determine if constipation is present and if patient has routine bowel program. • Assess strategies, including medically prescribed ones, patient uses to manage urinary tract infections. • Teach patient to completely empty bladder on regular basis. • Provide patient with bowel program, including dietary manipulation (increased fluid intake with dietary fiber and bulk), stool softeners, and/or enemas in consultation with physician. • Consult physician concerning use of long-term antibiotic prophylaxis for patients with chronic urinary retention as appropriate.

Principles and Rationale for Nursing Interventions

Acute urinary retention represents an immediate threat to the patient experiencing the condition. Urethral or suprapubic catheterization is used to relieve immediate bladder overdistention. Severe suprapubic pain and pressure sensations arise because of bladder overdistention. Following relief of immediate urinary retention, the nurse clarifies causative factors of voiding insufficiency and institutes a care plan to prevent recurrent acute urinary retention and manage chronic incomplete bladder emptying.

Timed voiding and double voiding are attempts to maximize the individual's ability to empty the bladder. *Double voiding* attempts to allow a brief resting period followed by an attempt to empty remaining urine through a second bladder contraction. *Timed voiding* is a preventive strategy as well as treatment modality for urinary retention. Chronic bladder overdistention is avoided by retraining the patient to void at regular intervals. The strategy is most effective among patients with moderate to severe bladder sensory deficit and minimum to mild motor deficit.

Bethanechol chloride is designed to increase bladder contractility by action at the neuromuscular junctions of the detrusor muscle. Phenoxybenzamine is designed to decrease sphincteric resistance to urinary outflow by antagonistic action at the bladder neck and urethral smooth muscle. These drugs may assist in bladder evacuation among patients with deficient detrusor function or bladder outlet obstruction caused by bladder neck smooth muscle overactivity.[11]

The goal of intermittent catheterization or indwelling catheterization for patients experiencing urinary retention is to ensure regular, complete bladder emptying, thus preventing the complications associated with the condition. Urinary tract infection still is a prominent complication, and these strategies are used primarily when more definitive methodologies prove inadequate.[10]

The likelihood of urinary tract infection is enhanced by urinary stasis and subsequent ischemia of the bladder wall. Regular, complete bladder emptying through intermittent catheterization is one strategy to prevent this condition.[12] Prevention of constipation also may help in the prevention of urinary tract infection. Bacteriuria is inevitable in the presence of a long-term indwelling catheter; this strategy is primarily used as a temporary measure to relieve urinary retention unless other strategies have failed to resolve the condition.

Evaluation

Patient Outcome	Data Indicating That Outcome is Reached
Resolves urinary retention	Urinary frequency and nocturia absent Overflow incontinence absent Postvoiding residual less than 20% of total bladder volume
Manages urinary retention	Postvoiding residual less than 20% of total bladder volume Overflow incontinence absent
Prevents urinary tract infection	Urine cultures negative Symptoms of urinary tract infections absent

FUNCTIONAL HEALTH PATTERN

IV

Activity-Exercise

 Potential Activity Intolerance

Potential activity intolerance is the state in which an individual is at risk of experiencing insufficient physiologic or psychologic energy to endure or complete required or desired daily activities.

Yura and Walsh[15] define the human need for activity as "a behavior or action requiring an expenditure of energy by the person with volition and intent." The need is further described as one that contributes to a person's survival. The potential inability to tolerate activity can threaten a person's well-being.

Definitions of potential activity intolerance address the presence of risk factors in distinguishing this diagnosis from that of activity intolerance. Potential activity intolerance can be viewed as an indication that a person is at risk for developing physical or psychologic blocks to participation in an expected or desired activity.[3] Whereas some authors distinguish the risk factors and etiology from the defining characteristics, Gordon[5] views the defining characteristics and risk factors as being the same. She describes potential activity intolerance as "a useful category to describe the presence of risk factors for abnormal response to energy-consuming activities."[6]

The proceedings of the seventh conference on classification of nursing diagnoses[11] support Gordon's view. Assessment data that had been classified as defining characteristics in the proceedings of the fifth and sixth conferences[8,9] are now classified as risk factors.

Risk Factors[1-3,5,7,10-13]

History of previous intolerance to activity
Fatigue, weakness
Sedentary life-style
Deconditioned status (prolonged bed rest, inactivity)
Presence of chronic or progressive disease (e.g., chronic obstructive pulmonary disease, multiple sclerosis, coronary artery disease, arthritis)
Presence of circulatory or respiratory problems
More than 15% overweight
Pain
Inexperience with activity
Expresses concern about ability to perform the activity
Expresses lack of interest in the activity
Refuses to participate in prescribed activities

Nursing Interventions[3-5,10,14,15]

Patient Goal	Nursing Intervention
Participate in activities that promote optimum well-being.	• Assess patient's past and present activity pattern. • Assess type, intensity, duration, and frequency of each patient activity. • Determine physiologic response to activity. • Determine psychologic response to activity. • Assess risk factors for potential activity intolerance.

Patient Goal	Nursing Intervention
	• Provide patient with information about desired or required daily activities. • Assist patient in selecting activities that are enjoyable and can be integrated into life-style. • Assist patient in identifying risk factors that reduce activity tolerance. • Encourage patient to participate in activities that promote an increase in activity tolerance within therapeutic limits. • Identify organized activities and exercise programs in which patient might want to participate. • Encourage family and significant others to support patient and to participate in activities and exercise programs with patient.

Principles and Rationale for Nursing Interventions

The person who is at risk for experiencing an inability to tolerate activity requires support and guidance in choosing activities that will promote optimum well-being. The patient's physiologic and psychologic response to particular activities must be taken into consideration when developing an appropriate plan for the patient's participation in required or desired activities.

The patient should be given information that will assist in identifying those activities that are therapeutic and enjoyable and within the patient's physiologic capabilities.[4] Information about factors that might interfere with the patient's ability to tolerate activity can help the patient to make changes that will promote activity tolerance. If the patient lacks the motivation to participate in required or desired activities on a regular basis, support can be elicited from significant others and through organized activity or exercise programs.

Evaluation

Patient Outcome	Data Indicating That Outcome is Reached
Demonstrates benefits of participating in regular activities	Describes benefits of regularly engaging in activity Specifies activities that promote physiologic and psychologic well-being Participates in required and desired activities in recommended manner Controls those factors that could inhibit activity tolerance
Appreciates need to participate in required and desired activities	Expresses desire to participate in recommended activities Willingly participates in self-care, exercise, and leisure activities Plans activities with persons who can support participation in activities that will enhance well-being

Activity Intolerance

Activity intolerance is the state in which an individual has insufficient physiologic or psychologic energy to endure or complete required or desired daily activities.

The definitions for activity intolerance proposed by other authors contribute to further understanding of the concept. Campbell's definition[2] is presented in terms of the degree of activity that can be tolerated, i.e., minimum, mild, and moderate activity tolerance. Her definitions are as follows:

> Minimum activity tolerance: the inability to tolerate any physical activity without the presence of discomforts. . . . Mild activity tolerance: the ability to tolerate only a very limited amount of physical activity without the presence of discomforts. . . . Moderate activity tolerance: the ability to tolerate a moderate, but not a full day of physical activity without the presence of discomfort.

Gordon[6] defines activity intolerance in terms of "abnormal responses to energy-consuming body movements involved in required or desired daily activities." Four levels of endurance are specified that, when used with the diagnostic label, describe an individual's response to specific activities. Gordon[7] also supports using activity intolerance, when appropriate, "in describing the etiology for problems such as self-care deficit, perceived sexual dysfunction, impaired home maintenance management, or social isolation."

The diagnostic label of activity intolerance implies inability to engage in and endure a required or desired physical activity as a result of functional, structural, or situational limitations. Physical activity encompasses all activity that requires the expenditure of energy. *Functional* limitations include those factors reflecting altered or impaired physiologic functioning. The energy expenditure required to perform the activity may be more than the individual has to expend. *Structural* limitations that can lead to activity intolerance are associated with an impairment or alteration of the anatomic structure. The extent of the structural impairment or alteration influences the degree to which the individual's mobility is restricted and the consequent effect on his ability to tolerate activity. *Situational* limitations that can alter an individual's tolerance for activity include factors relevant to the person's cognitive and emotional status and environment.

The diagnosis of activity intolerance is made in relation to a specified etiology or related factor. The related factor can be a functional, structural, or situational limitation that an individual experiences.

Related Factors[2,4,9,10]

- Functional limitations
  - Generalized weakness
  - Decreased mobility or immobility
  - Imbalance between oxygen supply and demand
- Structural limitation
  - Decreased mobility or immobility
- Situational limitations
  - Lack of knowledge
  - Lack of motivation
  - Deconditioning (related to life-style)
  - Lack of support

Defining Characteristics[1,4-6,9,10]

- Decrease in activity (self-care, exercise, leisure)
- Avoidance of activity
- Verbal report of fatigue or weakness
- Cardiovascular response to activity
  - Bradycardia
  - Inappropriate tachycardia
  - Dysrhythmia
  - Decrease in pulse strength
  - Decrease in systolic pressure
  - Excessive increase in systolic pressure
  - Excessive increase in diastolic pressure
- Respiratory response to activity
  - Dyspnea
  - Excessive increase in rate
  - Decrease in rate
  - Irregular rhythm
- Skin in response to activity
  - Pallor
  - Cyanosis
  - Excessive redness
  - Cool
  - Dry with strenuous activity
- Posture
  - Drooping of shoulders or head
  - Decrease in muscle tone and strength
- Equilibrium
  - Ataxia
  - Dizziness
- Emotional status
  - Lack of interest in activity
  - Fearful of activity

Nursing Interventions[1-5,11,12,14]

Patient Goal	Nursing Intervention
Participate in activities that enhance physiologic well-being.	• Assess patient's past and present activity pattern. Determine past activities (self-care, exercise, and leisure) engaged in; intensity, duration, and frequency of each activity; and how these activities were tolerated. Determine present activities and how these are tolerated. • Assess physical impediments. Determine if any physical impediments restrict participation in particular activities. Determine if any physical impediments prevent active participation in activities. • Assess physiologic status. Determine if there is any change in physiologic status when engaging in activity. Cardiovascular response: note heart rate and rhythm; pulse strength; blood pressure. Respiratory response: note rate, depth, and rhythm of respirations. Skin: note color, signs, temperature, moistness. Posture: note signs of muscle fatigue. Equilibrium: note gait, fine and gross movements. • Assess emotional status. Determine if there is any change in emotional status before or when engaging in activity. Determine if patient is fearful of harming himself. • Provide patient information about activities in which to participate. • Assist patient in interpretation of activity/exercise prescription. • Seek consultation with physician, exercise physiologist, and occupational and physical therapists as necessary. • Assist patient in identifying factors that reduce activity tolerance (inadequate sleep, medication, treatments, environmental conditions). • Engage immobile patient in passive exercise regimen. • Assist patient with structural limitations to adapt self-care, exercise, and leisure activities to meet needs. • Provide assistance to patient as needed, encouraging independence in performing activities. • Encourage patient to engage in self-care, exercise, and leisure activities that he can tolerate. • Guide patient in increasing activity within therapeutic limits.

Patient Goal	Nursing Intervention
Develop activity/rest pattern supporting increased tolerance of activity.	• Discuss with patient usual activity/rest pattern; suggest ways to modify an ineffective pattern. • Discuss the importance of increasing activity tolerance. • Encourage patient to participate in planning daily rest periods and activity periods. • Adjust medication and treatment schedule to support adequate rest. • Teach patient to monitor response to activity and to alter activity when signs and symptoms of anoxia or excessive fatigue are present. • Encourage patient to increase active participation gradually in self-care, exercise, and leisure activities. • Encourage patient to adhere to activity/rest schedule that best promotes increase in activity tolerance.
Use support of family, friends, and health care providers in adjusting activity/rest pattern to meet need for activity.	• Provide patient and significant others with information about importance of establishing therapeutic activity/rest pattern. • Review schedule of daily activities of significant others and identify with them how it can be altered to support fulfillment of patient's needs. • Encourage patient and significant others to participate in planning mutually agreeable daily schedule of activity/rest periods. • Facilitate expression of patient and significant others' concerns regarding proposed schedule. • Identify support available from health care providers if need arises to revise or alter schedule. • Encourage family and friends to support patient in efforts to meet need for activity.

Principles and Rationale for Nursing Interventions

The initial nursing assessment provides the opportunity to collect data relevant to an individual's ability to engage in activity and his response to activity. The identification of factors contributing to an inability to tolerate activities (the related factors) and the presence of signs and symptoms that reflect this inability (the defining characteristics) lead to a nursing diagnosis of activity intolerance.

In the preceding section, goals and nursing interventions supporting goal achievement were specified. Although the goals and interventions are presented in general terms, it is assumed that these will be adapted and expanded according to the needs of each individual. The general physiologic and emotional status of the individual, as well as the optimum therapeutic level of activity that should be attained, must be a primary consideration in planning nursing care.

An activity-exercise prescription must be tailored to each patient's needs and abilities. The data gathered in the assessment phase of the nursing process and the consequent identification of the goal should be validated with the patient. In reviewing the patient's past and present activity pattern, as well as the patient's physiologic and emotional status related to participation in activity and exercise, information can be shared to assist the patient in identifying activities that will enhance physiologic well-being.

To ensure a patient's adherence to a recommended activity-exercise pattern, it is important that the pattern can be integrated into the patient's life-style.[13] The patient should be assisted in developing and implementing an activity/rest schedule that supports an increased tolerance of activity. The schedule should incorporate the patient's requirements for medications and treatments, as well as participation in self-care and leisure activities. The patient should be taught to monitor responses to activity and to adjust the activity-exercise schedule as needed.

The patient's own life-style incorporates the life-styles of family, friends, and significant others. It may be necessary for family members to alter or revise their daily activities to support a therapeutic activity/rest schedule for the patient. Support of family and friends can be essential in assisting the patient to adhere to an activity/rest pattern that will promote optimum participation in therapeutic activities and exercise.

Evaluation

Patient Outcome	Data Indicating That Outcome is Reached
Absence of weakness during or after engaging in activity	No verbal report of fatigue or weakness after engaging in activity Increased participation in self-care, exercise, and/or leisure activities Erect posture Desire to engage in activity
Optimum level of mobility	Active participation in self-care, exercise, and leisure activity Verbalizes need for active and/or passive exercise and participation as able Adapts activities to meet requirements
Evidence of balance between oxygen supply and demand	Heart rate, rhythm, and quality within therapeutic limits Blood pressure within therapeutic limits Respiratory rate, rhythm, and depth within therapeutic limits Skin color, temperature, and moistness appropriate for amount and intensity of activity Absence of ataxia, dizziness, and confusion

Patient Outcome	Data Indicating That Outcome is Reached
Knowledge of importance of and intensity, duration, and frequency of various activities	Describes benefits of engaging in activity Specifies recommended intensity, duration, and frequency of various activities Participation in activities in recommended manner
Appreciation of need to participate in activities	Expresses desire to engage in activities Willing participation in self-care, exercise, and leisure activities
State of being physiologically conditioned to participate regularly in activities	Cardiovascular and respiratory status supports participation in activities Regularly engages in variety of activities
Uses support of significant others to achieve and maintain therapeutic levels of activity	Identifies persons available to support efforts to enhance activity tolerance Plans activities with those persons who can assist in achieving optimum activity tolerance Seeks advice of health care providers as needed Maintains therapeutic activity schedule

Impaired Physical Mobility

Impaired physical mobility is the state in which an individual experiences a limitation of ability for independent physical movement.[9]

It should be clear from the definition of impaired physical mobility that this diagnosis could be appropriately applied in a wide variety of situations (e.g., an unconscious trauma patient, a stroke patient with residual weakness of one side of the body, or even the person who has sustained an exercise-related injury of bone, joint, or muscle). Immobility can affect all major body systems. The major possible consequences of immobility include effects on the following*:

- Muscular system (decreased muscle mass, or atrophy; decreased muscle strength; decreased endurance; contractures)
- Skeletal system (fibrosis and ankylosis of joints, osteoporosis)
- Cardiovascular system (increased workload of the heart, decreased exercise tolerance, postural hypotension, venous stasis, thrombus and embolus formation)
- Respiratory system (decreased respiratory rate, decreased chest expansion, decreased tidal volume, impairment of coughing mechanism, atelectasis, pneumonia, respiratory acidosis)
- Nervous system (perceptual changes, altered sensation, autonomic lability, peripheral nerve palsy)
- Digestive system (anorexia, constipation)
- Integumentary system (decubitus ulcer, increased heat loss through skin)
- Urinary system (urinary stasis, urinary retention, renal calculi, proteinuria)
- Metabolism (negative nitrogen balance, negative calcium balance, decreased metabolic rate)
- Psychosocial functioning (sensory deprivation, role changes, decreased problem-solving ability, body image distortions, changes in sleep patterns, mood changes)

*References 1, 7, 8, 10-15, 18-20.

Related Factors[2,3,6,9]

Intolerance to activity
Decreased strength and endurance
Pain or discomfort
Perceptual or cognitive impairment
Certain physical disorders or states
- Cranial lesion or disease
- Central nervous system disorders
- Muscular conditions
- Neuromuscular junction disease
- Connective tissue disorders
- Peripheral neuropathies
- Joint and bone disorders

Depression
Severe anxiety
Schizophrenic disorders
Paranoid disorders
Substance use disorders
Restrictive or suppressive therapeutic regimens
- External devices (casts, splints, traction, braces, intravenous tubing, cardiac monitors, ventilators)
- Pharmacologic agents (sedatives, anesthetics)
- Trauma or surgical procedure
- Bed rest

Advanced age

Defining Characteristics[2,3,6,9]

Internal
- Inability to move purposefully within physical environment, including bed mobility, transfer, and ambulation
- Reluctance or refusal to attempt movement

Constancy of body posture in relation to gravity
Decreased physical activity
Limited range of motion
Decreased muscle strength, control, and/or mass
Impaired coordination
Impaired perception of position or presence of body parts
Perceived inability to move

External
Imposed restrictions of movement (mechanical or medical protocol restrictions)

Nursing Interventions*

Patient Goal	Nursing Intervention
Maintain normal musculoskeletal functioning during bed rest.	• Teach and monitor active range-of-motion exercises for all joints; should be performed at least two to three times daily (each movement should be performed at least twice during each exercise period). • Perform passive range-of-motion exercises for patient if previous intervention is not possible; same frequency as for previous intervention. • Teach and monitor isometric and isotonic exercises. • Assist patient with position change *at least* every 2 hours. • Assist patient to maintain proper body alignment, using supportive devices as necessary. • Encourage self-care activities. • Consider referral to physical therapist.
Exhibit minimum cardiovascular alterations during bed rest.	• Teach and monitor leg exercises. • Teach patient to exhale through mouth while exercising or moving in bed. • Teach patient to avoid straining while defecating. • Assist patient with frequent position changes. • Apply elastic stockings. • Teach patient to avoid compression of veins.
Maintain normal respiratory functioning during bed rest.	• Teach and monitor deep breathing and coughing regimen. • Assist patient with frequent position changes. • Teach and monitor use of incentive spirometer. • Encourage increased activity level. • Encourage increased fluid intake.
Maintain normal nervous system functioning during bed rest.	• Assist patient to function at the highest possible cognitive level. • Avoid use of positions that put prolonged pressure on nerves. • Assist patient with frequent position changes.
Maintain normal digestive functioning during bed rest.	• Provide small, frequent meals containing desired foods. • Encourage increased activity level. • Provide companionship during meals, if desired by patient. • Encourage increased bulk and fluids in diet. • Assist patient to assume a sitting position for defecation, if possible. • Provide privacy for defecation. • Offer bedpan after meals, especially after breakfast. • Obtain order for stool softener, if indicated. • Provide foods that are natural laxatives, e.g., prunes. • Obtain order for laxative, suppository, or enema; give only if absolutely necessary.
Maintain healthy integument during bed rest.	• Assist patient with position change *at least* every 2 hours. • Inspect susceptible areas of skin (e.g., areas over bony prominences) for condition at each position change. • Gently massage area over bony prominences at each position change. • Keep skin clean and dry but lubricated. • Provide pressure-equalizing or pressure-reducing equipment, if indicated (e.g., alternating-pressure mattress). • Avoid shearing force when moving patient. • Encourage well-balanced diet with adequate fluids, protein, and vitamin C.
Maintain normal urinary functioning during bed rest.	• Encourage increased fluid intake. • Provide foods and fluids that acidify urine (meats, fish, nuts, cereals). • Encourage increased activity level. • Assist patient to assume sitting position for urination, if possible.

*References 4, 5, 7, 11, 13, 16, 17.

Patient Goal	Nursing Intervention
	• Provide privacy for urination. • Assist patient with frequent position changes. • Try nursing measures to relieve urinary retention, if present; sound of running water, pouring warm water over perineum (of females), having females contract and release perineal muscles. • Perform catheterization as last resort (per physician's order and using strict sterile technique).
Maintain normal psychosocial functioning during bed rest.	• Provide meaningful interactions with patient. • Encourage family and/or significant other(s) to visit patient. • Provide meaningful sensory input. • Encourage use of glasses and/or hearing aid if needed. • Provide time-orienting devices (clocks, calendars, newspapers). • Encourage self-care activities. • Encourage responsibility for decision making about own care. • Encourage ventilation of feelings about illness and immobility. • Provide meaningful diversions for patient. • Provide uninterrupted periods for sleeping. • Maintain deliberate use of touch in providing nursing care.

Principles and Rationale for Nursing Interventions[11,13,17]

Nursing interventions directed toward the goal of maintaining normal musculoskeletal functioning during bed rest are related to several scientific principles, including the maintenance of joint mobility, muscle tone, and growth-producing stress on bones caused by exercise.

Nursing interventions related to the goal of exhibiting minimum cardiovascular alterations during bed rest are based on such important principles as the maintenance of peripheral resistance, the prevention of venous stasis, a decrease in the use of the Valsalva maneuver, and a decrease in pressure exerted on the veins.

The goal of maintaining normal respiratory functioning during bed rest suggests several essential nursing interventions. Rationales underlying these interventions include moistening of secretions, mobilization of secretions, improved respiratory gas exchange, strengthening of abdominal and respiratory muscles, and stimulation of deeper breathing.

Principles underlying the nursing interventions related to maintaining normal nervous system functioning during bed rest are promotion of high-level cognitive functioning and prevention of pressure and damage to nerves.

Nursing interventions directed toward maintaining normal digestive functioning during bed rest are based on several principles, including stimulation of appetite, stimulation of peristalsis, use of the gastrocolic reflex, and prevention of constipation.

The goal of maintaining a healthy integument during bed rest is a challenge for nursing. Nursing interventions designed to meet this goal are based on the principles of prevention of prolonged pressure, increased circulation to area, and maintenance of skin turgor and elasticity.

Principles underlying the nursing interventions directed toward maintaining normal urinary functioning during bed rest include maintaining muscle tone, increasing urinary volume, maintaining acidity of urine, and using gravity to allow more complete emptying of the bladder.

Two principles basic to the nursing interventions related to maintaining normal psychosocial functioning during bed rest are increasing sensory stimulation and promoting healthy interaction patterns.

Evaluation[11,13,17]

Patient Outcome	Data Indicating That Outcome is Reached
Normal musculoskeletal function	Maintains usual range of motion in all body joints Maintains muscle mass and strength Participates actively in self-care activities
Minimum cardiovascular alterations	Normal heart rate (60 to 100 beats/minute) and blood pressure (100 to 140 mm Hg systolic, 70 to 90 mm Hg diastolic) Maintains normal venous return No evidence of venous compression No evidence of thrombus or embolus
Normal respiratory function	Clear lungs on auscultation Normal tidal volume (approximately 500 ml) Normal chest expansion No evidence of atelectasis

Patient Outcome	Data Indicating That Outcome is Reached
	No evidence of pneumonia No evidence of respiratory acidosis
Normal nervous system function	Oriented to time, person, and place Normal peripheral nerve functioning (no abnormal pain or tingling present)
Normal digestive fuction	Maintains usual weight Maintains usual bowel elimination habits No evidence of fecal impaction
Normal integument	Intact skin No evidence of pressure (pallor, redness, increased warmth, or tenderness in involved area)
Normal urinary function	Adequate urine output (at least 1500 mg/day) No evidence of renal calculi No evidence of urinary retention
Normal psychosocial function	Maintains relationships with family and/or significant other(s) Participates actively in decisions about own care Verbalizes fears, concerns, and other feelings Accepts support from others Uses defense mechanisms constructively

Potential for Disuse Syndrome

Potential for disuse syndrome is the state in which an individual is at risk for deterioration of body systems as the result of prescribed or unavoidable inactivity.

The physiologic and psychologic alterations from potential for disuse syndrome can have a dramatic and negative effect on a healthy individual's ability to function and an even more injurious effect on an already ill or debilitated person.

Risk Factors*

Paralysis
Mechanical immobilization
Prescribed immobilization
Severe pain
Altered level of consciousness
Physical or mental illness

*Adapted from North American Nursing Diagnosis Association, 1988 Ballot.

Nursing Interventions

Patient Goal	Nursing Intervention
Do not experience disuse syndrome.	• Assess and document patient's risk factors for skin breakdown and effects of immobilization on other body systems. • Plan and implement passive and active range of motion exercises. • Consult with physical therapist as appropriate. • Instruct and encourage patient in use of isometric exercises and use of idle body parts, e.g., eyes. • Assess need for air or fluid flotation bed or provide convoluted foam mattress. • Frequently turn and position patient comfortably to prevent contractures. • Assess skin frequently; whenever turning patient, monitor for possible breakdown or abrasions related to traction and other devices. • If appropriate, place patient on kinetic treatment table to maintain motion and circulation. • Assess lungs frequently and promote coughing and deep breathing to prevent atelectasis. • Assess nutrition and fluid status to maintain adequate balance; prevent muscle and skin breakdown; promote normal bladder and bowel elimination. • Assess need for stool softener or bulk laxative, and administer as needed per physician's order. • Teach patient to move in bed without increasing intrathoracic pressure to decrease cardiac work-load. • Consult with physician regarding prophylactic use of anticoagulants to prevent thrombus formation. • Ensure that patient receives excellent hygiene: skin, hair, and mouth care.

Patient Goal	Nursing Intervention
	• Plan and implement a pain management protocol, if necessary, to allow patient to move comfortably and exercise enough in bed to achieve therapeutic goals. • Assess and maximize available support resources for meeting emotional needs, and stimulate intellectual faculties. • Provide frequent interaction to maintain sensory stimulation. • Ensure that patient has clock, calendar, radio, and television and assist in reality orientation as necessary. • If patient mobilization can be improved assist with planning and implementing progressive rehabilitation regime to increase strength and bodily functions incrementally.

Principles and Rationale for Nursing Interventions[8,9,11,18,22]

Immobility results in negative or deleterious effects on every body system, as well as on the patient's psychosocial equilibrium. Studies have shown that enforced bed rest, even with young healthy individuals for short periods, can cause distorted sensations and bodily discomforts. Patients who are elderly and debilitated are at great risk for orthostatic hypotension, muscle wasting and atrophy, contractures, dependent edema, atelectasis, thrombus formation, loneliness, boredom, and sensory deprivation.

A serious effect is the decrease in the autonomic nervous system's ability to equalize the blood supply when a person who has been lying down for a time stands up. This results from two factors: loss of general muscle tone and decreased efficiency of the orthostatic neurovascular reflexes, although the problem is thought to originate in the autonomic rather than the central nervous system. Patients also experience changes in vascular resistance and hydrostatic pressure and have an increased cardiac output and stroke volume when recumbent. Other changes in homeostatic metabolic equilibrium cause significant problems with bodily functions and systems.

Evaluation

Patient Outcome	Data Indicating That Outcome is Reached
Does not experience disuse syndrome	Body systems maintained in normal function Psychosocial equilibrium maintained

Fatigue

Fatigue is the overwhelming sense of exhaustion and decreased capacity for physical and mental work, regardless of adequate sleep or rest.

Fatigue can be a particularly severe and long-standing problem for certain patients, including those with rheumatic or immune diseases.

Related Factors*

Altered biochemical factors
Overwhelming psychologic or physical demands (perceived or actual)
Increased energy expenditures to perform activities of daily living (ADLs)
Excessive role demands
Conflicting role demands
Sleep pattern disturbance
Pain and discomfort
Decreased metabolic states
Environmental stressors (e.g., noise, humidity, heat, excessive light, allergens)
Physical illness (e.g., hypothyroidism, cancer, chronic obstructive pulmonary disease, AIDS)
Psychiatric illness (e.g., depression)
Inadequate nutrition
Immobility

*Adapted from North American Nursing Diagnosis Association, 1988 Ballot.

Defining Characteristics*

Verbalization of fatigue or lack of energy
Inability to engage in usual activities
Irritability
Lethargy
Emotional lability
Impaired ability to concentrate
Listlessness
Disinterest in surroundings
Decreased performance of tasks
Injury prone
Decreased libido
Apathy
Increased physical complaints

Nursing Interventions

Patient Goal	Nursing Intervention
Have sufficient energy to engage in ADLs or adapt to decreased energy levels.	• Assess patterns of fatigue. • Ensure that patient has complete physical workup to determine if there are physical or mental causes. • Assist patient to identify factors related to fatigue and strategies for dealing with them. • Assist patient to identify more effective energy expenditure. • Assess support systems and resources available. • Identify specific tasks that patient is unable to perform. • Administer treatments or medications to relieve discomfort (e.g., pain, itching). • Enhance patient's ability to rest and sleep by means of mild sedatives, warm bath, massage, and quiet environment. • Provide supportive listening for irretrievable functional losses. • Engage in systematic exercise routine. • Assess nutritional habits and alter those that contribute to fatigue. • Consult with physical therapist to develop incremental physical exercise program. • Evaluate new or added stressors (e.g., new baby, ill family member, financial burdens, multiple competing demands). • Assist patient to identify: Tasks and routines that require less physical and mental effort Most productive hours of day • Encourage rest after activities. • Allow for uninterrupted periods of sleep. • Instruct in energy conservation measures and evaluate response to instruction.

Principles and Rationale for Nursing Interventions[5,7,9]

A major focus of care for fatigue should be to assist the patient to conserve as much energy as possible and to increase energy resources. For patients with active disease processes, adequate rest is vital. The patient should participate in the planning process. If fatigue is a new symptom, physical and psychiatric illnesses should be ruled out; this should include both physiologic and psychologic testing. Nursing care should also focus on enhancing strategies to increase patient energy resources.

Evaluation

Patient Outcome	Data Indicating That Outcome is Reached
Experiences no fatigue	Engages in ADLs in productive manner Reports improvement in mental outlook Reports ability to complete all ADLs to own satisfaction Able to concentrate Is injury free Verbalizes understanding of need for nutritionally sound diet Engages in adequate rest and sleep
Adapts to decreased energy level	Able to seek support for incomplete ADLs

Self-Care Deficit

(Bathing/hygiene; dressing/grooming; feeding; toileting)

Bathing/hygiene self-care deficit is the state in which an individual experiences an impaired ability to perform or complete bathing and hygiene activities.

Dressing/grooming self-care deficit is the state in which an individual experiences an impaired ability to perform or complete dressing and grooming activities.

Feeding self-care deficit is the state in which an individual experiences an impaired ability to perform or complete feeding activities.

Toileting self-care deficit is the state in which an individual experiences an impaired ability to perform or complete toileting activities.

The impaired ability to perform self-care may be temporary or permanent. It occurs as a result of decreased motor or cognitive function. These in turn may be related to a physiologic or psychologic health problem. In some instances, physical restraint, such as being in a cast to treat a bone fracture, impairs self-care. The ability to perform these activities independently provides the individual with a sense of control, which contributes to a healthy self-concept.

These activities of daily living (bathing/hygiene, dressing/grooming, feeding, toileting) are learned and become habitual, usually having a certain pattern or sequence. They are principally affected by the functional health status of the individual, but social and situational factors also play a part. The functional health status has three components that are assessed in determining the diagnosis of self-care deficit: the age-related biologic status, developmental task status, and disease (if present) and its treatment.[1]

Age-related factors that may affect basic self-care are most often portrayed in elderly persons. Developmental task assessment relates to maturational factors, including knowledge, skill, and motivation. Pathologic states caused by trauma or disease may alter structure and function and thus compromise self-care ability in all age groups. The treatment may also impose limitations (e.g., being in a cast for a fracture, restricted by bed rest). Being functionally dependent, i.e., requiring assistance from others in the activities of bathing/hygiene, dressing/grooming, feeding, and toileting, affects the individual's morale, self-esteem, and sense of dignity. These are human needs that contribute to the quality of life.

Table 1
Classification of Functional Levels of Self-Care*

Level	Behavioral Indicator
0	Independent; able to initiate and complete activity for self
1	Requires minimum assistance; may use equipment but manages it alone; does at least 75% of work
2	Requires moderate assistance, supervision, or teaching; does approximately 50% of work
3	Requires extensive assistance from another person *and* equipment or devices; does less than 25% of work
4	Dependent on caregivers, total care; does not participate actively

*Use of this scale to indicate level of dependence/independence further defines functional deficit and guides nursing intervention. Self-care deficits exist for levels 1 through 4.

Related Factors[4,8-10]

Intolerance to activity
Decreased strength and endurance
Pain, discomfort
Perceptual or cognitive impairment
Neuromuscular impairment
Musculoskeletal impairment
Depression, severe anxiety

Defining Characteristics[3-10]

Bathing/Hygiene (Levels 0 to 4)*

Inability to wash body or body parts
Inability to obtain or get to water source
Inability to regulate temperature or flow

Dressing/Grooming (Levels 0 to 4)

Impaired ability to put on or take off necessary items of clothing
Impaired ability to obtain or replace articles of clothing
Impaired ability to fasten clothing
Inability to maintain appearance at satisfactory level

Feeding (Levels 0 to 4)

Inability to bring food from receptacle to mouth
Inability to cut food

Toileting (Levels 0 to 4)

Unable to get to toilet or commode
Unable to sit on or rise from toilet or commode
Unable to manipulate clothing for toileting
Unable to carry out proper toilet hygiene
Unable to flush toilet or empty commode

*See Table 1 for levels.

Nursing Interventions*

Patient Goal	Nursing Intervention
Achieve or maintain behavioral control.	• Assess with patient his strengths and weaknesses; discuss what behavioral activities he can do for himself. • Assess factors in home and work setting that support or hinder self-care. • Explore the use of assistive devices that can help the patient become more self-sufficient. • Encourage or allow patient to do as much as possible for himself. • Observe for evidence of readiness to increase amount of self-care.

*References 5, 8, 9, 11, 13, 18.

Patient Goal	Nursing Intervention
	• Provide help, supervision, and teaching as necessary to improve self-care. • Act as patient advocate to increase sensitivity of others to effects of their actions on the patient.
Achieve or maintain cognitive control.	• Plan care with patient; validate conclusions with him. • Discuss any changes in patient's condition with him. • Inform of anticipated effects of therapy. • Assist in relating concerns to physician.
Achieve or maintain decisional control.	• Discuss daily routines with patient; allow him a voice in scheduling functional activities. • Consult with patient in making choices about his treatment; do not plan activities without his knowledge. • Evaluate outcomes of care with patient.
Bathing/Hygiene*	
Achieve or maintain responsibility for bathing/hygiene congruent with level of self-care ability.	• 0, Independent: praise and encourage to maintain independence. • 1, Minimum assistance: may provide care to one area, e.g., back. • 2, Moderate assistance: prepare bath, provide back, leg and foot care, comb hair. • 3, Extensive care: provide majority of bath, hair care, and oral care. • 4, Dependent, total care: provide complete bath and hygiene care.
Dressing/Grooming*	
Achieve or maintain responsibility for dressing/grooming congruent with level of self-care ability.	• 0, Independent: praise and encourage to maintain independence. • 1, Minimum assistance: help with buttons, zippers, shoelaces. • 2, Moderate assistance: Provide help with clothing on lower extremities, with shoes, with fasteners. • 3, Extensive assistance: provide help with putting on all of clothing; do not hurry; allow patient to make choices in order of activity, makeup, etc., if able; comb hair, shave. • 4, Dependent, total care: dress/groom patient.
Feeding*	
Achieve or maintain responsibility for feeding congruent with level of self-care ability.	• 0, Independent: praise and encourage to maintain independence. • 1, Minimum assistance: cut or prepare food as necessary. • 2, Moderate assistance: arrange tray, prepare food; encourage patient to feed self. • 3, Extensive assistance: feed patient as necessary (patient may have some difficulty with chewing or swallowing and require special diet); encourage patient to eat, allow adequate time, use pleasant manner. • 4, Dependent, total care: feed patient through manner prescribed (may be tube feeding or parenteral therapy); have equipment available for emergencies, e.g., suctioning.
Toileting*	
Achieve or maintain responsibility for toileting congruent with level of self-care ability.	• 0, Independent: praise and encourage to maintain independence. • 1, Minimum assistance: provide needed support or equipment for patient to manage own toileting; be prompt in responding to patient's request. • 2, Moderate assistance: respond promptly to patient's request; assist with needed equipment. • 3, Extensive assistance: provide and position toilet equipment; anticipate toileting needs; clean patient, rearrange clothing or bedding; be prompt, nonjudgmental. • 4, Dependent, total care: if possible, develop routine to stimulate or anticipate urination or defecation such that it may be controlled or expected at a certain time; promptly clean patient, rearrange clothing and bedding.

*Numbers before nursing interventions refer to functional levels of self-care; see Table 1.

Principles and Rationale for Nursing Interventions*

Lack of the ability to perform the necessary activities of daily living independently prolongs a patient's stay in an acute care facility. *Functional dependency* in the elderly is a major contributing factor to placement in long-term care facilities. Changes in the health status, particularly long-lasting musculoskeletal and perceptual/cognitive impairment, are the bases for formation of self-care deficits. However, independence in self-care can be influenced by factors and resources in the environment, and these should be assessed. Such factors and resources include not only assistive devices, but also household arrangements and access to transportation, shops, and professional services. Social support systems, including family, friends, and neighbors, should be evaluated, as should the possibility of home care. At the same time the nurse should be aware that these resources also generate demands on the

*References 2, 6, 7, 9, 11, 12, 15-18.

individual, when, where, and how long it will take to eat, bathe, and dress. The patient and family should be involved in this appraisal.

The primary goal is that the basic human needs be met. Requiring assistance from others in these activities affects the individual's morale, self-esteem, and sense of dignity. The loss of the ability to perform a functional task and the loss of respect, threatened or real, that may accompany that loss may have a devastating effect on the sense of self of the individual. One expects to be in control of one's simplest functions and of the appropriateness of the time and place of their occurrence; when this control is lost, one is ashamed of oneself.[15] A personal judgment of failure is made and the ego is threatened; it is even more telling when one's failure is witnessed by others. Lack of participation in activities of daily living and verbal responses indicating lack of control over activities and outcomes, associated with negative affective responses (withdrawal, pessimism, submissiveness, undifferentiated anger), indicate the diagnosis of powerlessness.[11]

The interventions of the nurse or caregiver and her attitudes are essential in determining the responses and outcomes of self-care deficits in body functions. The perception of situational control is a key variable for the morale of the individual.[2,16] The outcome will also be affected by the specific nature of the deficit and whether it is temporary or long term. For example, individuals who are temporarily restrained by intravenous tubing and have to be fed by others may feel uncomfortable and prefer not to eat. On the other hand, the sudden traumatic deficits of accident-related quadriplegia and the progressive deficits that sometimes accompany growing older present more serious problems that may eventually threaten the ego.

Evaluation

Patient Outcome	Data Indicating That Outcome is Reached
Has control over physical activities and environment as much as capable	States realistic appraisal of own self-care ability States realistic appraisal of factors in home or work setting Initiates and completes as much of care as physically possible
Knows and understands what is happening; maintains sense of self-esteem and self-worth	Takes active interest in own care; asks questions, shares own values, helps to prioritize care Verbalizes positive feelings about self; does not express feelings of insecurity, worthlessness
Makes choices concerning care; influences others	Sets reasonable goals for self; takes physical strength and endurance into account Sets specific time for performing activities but also shows respect for goals and time constraints of nursing staff; negotiates
Bathing/Hygiene*	
0, Independent	Initiates and completes own bath; clean body, hair, nails, teeth; no offensive odors (applies to all levels)
1, Minimum assistance	Does approximately 75% of the work
2, Moderate assistance	Does approximately 50% of the work
3, Extensive assistance	Does less than 25% of work; may perform light hygiene with some assistive devices, e.g., electric toothbrush
4, Dependent, total care	No participation; bath and hygiene completed by caregivers
Dressing/Grooming*	
0, Independent	Initiates and completes own dressing and grooming appropriately
1, Minimum assistance	Initiates dressing activity, dresses appropriately; does majority of work; pleased with appearance
2, Moderate assistance	Does approximately 50% of the work
3, Extensive assistance	Does less than 25% of the work
4, Dependent, total care	No active participation; dressed and groomed by caregivers
Feeding*	
0, Independent	Initiates and completes feeding self; no help
1, Minimum assistance needed	Completes feeding self; does approximately 75% of work
2, Moderate assistance needed	Feeds self satisfactorily with supervision; does approximately 50% of work
3, Extensive assistance needed	Feeding completed with assistance; client does less than 25% of work
4, Dependent, total care needed	Ingests diet when fed

*Numbers refer to functional levels of self-care; see Table 1.

Patient Outcome	Data Indicating That Outcome is Reached
Toileting*	
0, Independent	Performs toileting activities for self; clean, no odors
1, Minimum assistance	Goes to bathroom, cleans self; may need support getting to and from bathroom; may use bedpan or urinal by self at night if placed conveniently; continent
2, Moderate assistance	Requests bedside commode, bedpan, or urinal when needed; able to transfer to same and to complete elimination; may need assistance with cleaning
3, Extensive assistance	Uses equipment provided; may have occasional episodes of incontinence
4, Dependent, total care	Toileting care initiated and completed by caregivers

*Numbers refer to functional levels of self-care; see Table 1.

Diversional Activity Deficit

Diversional activity deficit is the state in which an individual experiences decreased stimulation from, interest in, or engagement in recreational or leisure activities.

Philosopher Arthur Schopenhauer wrote that "the two foes of human happiness are pain and boredom."[1] Nursing has devoted much of its efforts to the treatment of pain but very little to the alleviation of boredom. A deficit in diversional activity often is manifested by reports of boredom by patients whose usual forms of activity are interrupted by illness, disability, or life changes. Boredom is especially prevalent in those persons whose illnesses extend for a long time, those who are hospitalized or otherwise institutionalized, or those who spend many hours in health treatment situations.

For many individuals their self-expression is linked closely to their leisure activities. Frye and Peters[4] see the "relaxed freedom of self chosen activity in unobligated time (as) . . . a good frame of reference for seeing oneself as one truly is."

Diversion encompasses those activities that are recreational and are pursued during leisure time for the purpose of personal amusement or satisfaction. Leisure is the time that is free from obligations. In keeping with the highly individual nature of this phenomenon, a diversional activity deficit is a personally defined dissatisfaction with a lack of sufficient leisure-time recreational activities.

Related Factors

Personal factors
- Problematic time management
- Lack of specification of desired diversions
- Depression
- Apathy
- Fatigue
- Impaired mobility
- Impaired sensory functions
- Lack of knowledge
- Lack of exposure or orientation to diversional activity

Environmental factors, home-based patients
- Limited finances
- Lack of transportation
- Social isolation
- Fear of neighborhood crime

Environmental factors, patients in treatment centers
- Lack of space
- Lack of resources
- Lack of knowledge of treatment center routines

Defining Characteristics[2,3,5-7]

Little or no unobligated time or increase in amount of unobligated time
No pattern of leisure activities
Preillness leisure activities impossible since illness
No postillness substitute activities defined
Unavailability of resources for identified leisure activities
Confined space
Perception of impossibility of leisure activities
Perception of time passing slowly
Statement of desire for something to do
Statement of boredom
Daytime napping
Disinterest in television viewing
Energy level sufficient for recreational activities but no participation in such activities
Restlessness
Flat affect
Frequent yawning
Hostility
Inattentiveness
Overeating or decreased eating

Nursing Interventions

Patient Goal	Nursing Intervention
Describe usual pattern of diversional activities.	• Assess usual activity routines before illness: Amount of unobligated time Leisure activities: type amount, and resources used Knowledge of recreational options • For persons with excessive stress and little unobligated time, suggest that they record their schedule of activities for 1 week. • Let patient know rationale, i.e., that usual pattern is a baseline for planning. • Maintain nonjudgmental response to patient report. • Elicit details of amount of time spent in diversional activity, location, and resources.
Identify changes in ability to engage in usual diversional activities, *or* identify problems perceived with usual pattern of activities. (Consider etiology of problem to choose one outcome or the other.)	• Assess usual activity routines since illness, hospitalization, or life change: Amount of unobligated time Leisure activities: type, amount, and resources used Degree of confinement Energy level (sufficient for diversional activities?) Desire for activity Mental status • Focus on patient's perceptions of present situation. • Avoid leading questions. • Encourage patient to consider changes in desire, available time, energy level, space, and other constraints.
Choose one usual diversional activity to continue, *and/or* identify usual diversional activity that may be adapted to new constraints, *and/or* identify new diversional activity that may be started.	• Whenever possible, encourage patient to continue with these activities that were meaningful to him. • Encourage creativity in choices. • Help person with busy schedule to prioritize activities. • Encourage patient to identify activity; avoid suggestions unless patient unable to think of possibilities. • If necessary, prompt patient thinking with suggestions of categories of activities, e.g., music, games, arts, crafts, physical exercise, toys, reading, writing, change of scene, change of routine, companionship, video programs, talking, productive chores (sorting, cleaning, etc.). • Remember that diversional activities should be personally meaningful. • Focus on the positive more than negative ("You can do this" rather than "You can't do that"). • Orient patient to options available within the system, e.g., recreational therapy programs. • After patient makes choice, if appropriate, validate with medical team patient capabilities to engage in chosen activity.
List resources needed for chosen activity.	• Maintain emphasis on personal choice. • Be careful not to assume what patient needs for chosen activity.
Identify means to obtain needed resources.	• Consider what can be obtained within the system, what could be provided by family and friends, what are vital to activity, and what can be adapted from available options. • If necessary, teach time management or stress management strategies.
Engage in chosen diversional activity.	• Support patient in chosen activity. • Adapt environment as necessary. • Provide positive feedback.
Express satisfaction with chosen activity.	• Evaluate patient's perception of chosen activity. • Allow for change of plans if activity unsatisfactory.

Principles and Rationale for Nursing Interventions

Because diversional activities have meaning, purpose, and value for the individual, the determination of a deficit in those activities is highly personal. The amount of time spent idly and the point at which boredom occurs vary greatly. Therefore, to study diversion and diagnose a deficit in this area, a patient's own preillness or pre–life change schedule of activities must be a baseline for comparison with the postillness or post–life change schedule. A person who has a definite set of hobbies or recreational activities may experience more of a deficit when they become impossible than a person who normally engages in few activities.

To maintain the personal meaning of a new or adapted diversional activity, the nurse must avoid planning the activity for the patient; rather, interventions should be geared to assisting the patient to identify a meaningful activity. Often patients in hospitals cannot think of alternative activities, nor do they consider the possiblity of developing new methods of expression. The social structure of hospitals is such that patients have little say in establishing routines. Their world becomes small and detail oriented. In these cases the nurse can educate patients as to the possibilities for change in the routine. A focus on the positive possibilities rather than on the negative aspects of their situation will allow for more creativity in choosing a diversional activity. This same focus on the positive options should be applied in interventions with homebound patients who have an excess of unobligated time and with persons who have diversional deficits because of schedules with too little unobligated time.

Creativity is another principle guiding nursing intervention. Possibilities for diversional activities are as numerous as the creative mind allows. Creativity means considering options beyond the common three: reading, watching television, and doing crossword puzzles. The creative mind sees ways to adapt resources to meet diversional needs. For the immobilized patient who misses a daily workout in the gym, exercises that can be done in bed, such as squeezing a rubber ball, may be a welcomed diversional activity. Children's toys can be adapted to adult needs. Introducing two bored patients gives each of them companionship. The list is limited only by the confines of the imagination.

Evaluation

Patient Outcome	Data Indicating That Outcome is Reached
Describes usual pattern of diversional activities	Indicates time free from obligations Lists activities that are self-chosen Relates the what, where, when and how of diversional activities
Identifies changes in ability to engage in usual diversional activities, *or* identifies problems perceived with usual pattern of activities	Can realistically list changes in situation Compares present situation to past
Chooses one usual activity to continue, *or* identifies usual activity that may be adapted, *or* identifies new diversional activity	Makes a personal choice Sees possibilities of continuation of activity within constraints, *or* is able to see old activity in new light, *or* lists other interests that could be tried Can use a problem-solving approach to changed situation
Lists resources needed for chosen activity	Gets involved in details of activity chosen Exhibits an action orientation
Identifies means to obtain needed resources	Takes responsibility for choice Uses problem-solving approach
Engages in chosen diversional activity	Is seen actually doing something Fits activity into daily routine Makes choices as to when activity occurs Establishes new pattern that decreases idle time
Expresses satisfaction with chosen activity	No reports of boredom Discusses activity Shows increase of interest in self

Impaired Home Maintenance Management

Impaired home maintenance management is the inability to maintain independently a safe, growth-promoting immediate environment.

The overall nursing goal for impaired home maintenance management is to enable the patient to continue living at home as long as it is safe and desirable.[12] High-risk populations include physically and mentally handicapped patients, dependent children, the frail elderly, and chronically ill patients. Adaptation of the home for health care is also relevant to this diagnosis.

To facilitate discharge and effective long-term care, nurses in the hospital, when planning discharge need to look beyond the identified patient to assess the family and home environment. Whether this is an acutely ill, chronically ill, newly disabled, or terminally ill person going home, the family will be the principal caregivers. Ideally, planning is done before the patient is discharged to train the caregivers in the techniques of patient care and to adapt the home as a workplace to provide necessary nursing care.[9] The social roles of family members may also need to be permanently adapted to compensate for patient handicap or susceptibility caused by illness. Success or failure of home placement may also hinge on the structural characteristics of the dwelling and the supports available in the community for both family respite and professional services.[15] Training for self-care and adaptation, including home management, may be needed for newly disabled persons or those who become disabled over time with a chronic illness.[5] A typical example is the patient with severe arthritis who lives at home. The home care nurse works as a part of the multidisciplinary team to assist the family and patient to adapt their home and roles to allow maximum independence for the disabled member.[15]

Related Factors

- Individual/family characteristics
  - Disabled by acute illness, injury, or congenital anomaly
  - Chronic debilitating disease
  - Impaired sensory functioning
  - Impaired cognitive or emotional functioning
  - Change in family composition
- Insufficient knowledge
  - Lack of socialization (role model and/or emigration)
  - Unfamiliarity with neighborhood resources
  - Lack of training in adaptation of home maintenance skills
- Insufficient family organization and planning
- Insufficient finances
- Dysfunctional grieving
- Inadequate social support system
  - Insufficient amount
  - Insufficient quality
  - Impaired family member
- Inadequate dwelling and/or furnishings
  - Overcrowding
  - Lack of adaptation of home structure or furnishings
  - Structural defects
  - Lack of equipment or aids for home care by disabled individual
- Inadequate community resources
  - Insufficient community environmental sanitation or control of environmental contaminants or pollutants
  - Lack of community professional and paraprofessional home care services

Defining Characteristics[2,11,12,14]

Subjective (Stated by Patient or Household Member)

- Expresses difficulty in maintaining the home in a comfortable, safe, and hygienic manner
- Expresses difficulty in supporting personal growth of family members
- Requests assistance with home maintenance management
- Describes outstanding debts or financial crises that impede home maintenance management
- Expresses ignorance in how to provide environment conducive for patient care
- Expresses exhaustion or inability to keep up the home
- Discusses dissatisfaction with dwelling because of overcrowding or lack of personal space
- Complains that furnishings are inadequate to maintain order or support healthful living patterns
- Shows nurse defects in structure or utilities and expresses inability to have them repaired
- Expresses lack of knowledge about community resources
- Expresses that environmental factors negatively affect ability to maintain the home
- Expresses frustration that known resources are unavailable or insufficient in community

Objective (Observed by Nurse)

- Presence of disease or disability necessitating adaptation of home maintenance
- Lack of knowledge of caregiver
- Overtaxed family members
- Inadequate support system
- Apparent lack of economic resources
- Disorganized home
- Knowledge of home maintenance inconsistent with current environment
- Home lacking personal items and attempts at decoration
- Presence of indoor pets that are not housebroken
- Disorderly surroundings
- Unavailable cooking utensils, linen, or clothes because of insufficient supply or being unwashed
- Accumulation of dirt, food waste, or hygienic waste
- Offensive odors
- Inadequate lighting
- Inappropriate household temperature and/or insufficient ventilation
- Presence of vermin or rodents
- Repeated hygienic disorders, infestations, or infections
- Lack of necessary equipment or aids
- Overcrowding for available space
- Presence of structural barriers
- Unrepaired defects in structure or utilities
- Characteristics of neighborhood making it difficult for effective home maintenance
- Inadequate or contaminated water or sewage supply

Nursing Interventions

Patient Goal	Nursing Intervention
Participate in appropriate discharge planning.	• Document discharge plan after assessing needs with patient and family. • Teach patient and family as appropriate. • Identify appropriate referrals using multidisciplinary team. • Establish realistic plan for home management involving patient and family members.
Identify factors perceived as making it difficult to maintain the home.	• Ask each member to identify how the home is different now and how long they think it has been unsatisfactory. • Systematically identify factors that impede meeting household standard. • Have members state what factors in the home affect their health and in what way. • Compare patient's perceptions with nurse's observations. Share nurse's observations.
Recognize what daily maintenance can be realistically performed.	• Discuss what each member now does and how often. Discuss possible role changes. • Differentiate hygienic factors that are esthetic from ones that negatively impact on health. • Listen nonjudgmentally to realities of home situation.
Use current support system and participate in developing plan to supplement family resources.	• Identify members of current support system and assess their capabilities. • Discuss community resources for daily home maintenance. • Mutually develop plan of care to increase supports consistent with family values.
Use community resources in efficient, appropriate manner.	• Initiate referrals for supplementation of daily home maintenance. • Investigate community resources for long-term maintenance. • Review with support system members how to use nurse as continuing resource.
Adapt the home and/or life-style to promote maximum health and safety	• Discuss specific life-style and home changes that will promote health. • Discuss rearranging furnishings for cleaning and safety. • Reinforce changes by discussing positive impact. Praise attempts at adaptation. • Review with family plan to respond to emergencies. • Assist family to complete home safety assessment and follow up on deficits found.
Repair structural defects.	• Discuss relationship of defects to health. • Discuss possible disease caused by defects. • Investigate alternative ways to have repairs made within financial capabilities of family. • Support attempts to obtain repairs.
Obtain and appropriately use equipment facilitating home maintenance.	• Determine equipment and supplies needed, identify sources, and obtain. • Teach appropriate use and maintenance of equipment. • Review means of maintaining sufficient supplies.
Manage home maintenance adequately.	• Arrange for additional support regularly or periodically for caregiver respite. • Have caregiver and family establish mutually agreeable standard of cleanliness and order that is safe. • Teach caregiver to support maximum independence of patient. • Observe for increased level of health secondary to cleaner home environment. When observed, compliment on changes.
Increase awareness of impact of neighborhood on home maintenance.	• Identify factors in community that negatively affect client's ability to maintain home. • Identify local resources that work to promote changes. Encourage family participation. • Assist family to assess safety of neighborhood and periodically consider their housing options.

Principles and Rationale for Nursing Interventions

Impaired home maintenance management is rarely the reason a patient seeks nursing care in the home. However, in the nursing assessment of the patient, family, support system, dwelling, and community the nurse may identify current home maintenance management as a barrier to either healthful living or to providing nursing care.[1,6,13] Necessary adaptations of the structure or furnishings for home care may be missing. Aids that could increase the patient's independence may be lacking. Intervention for this diagnosis may take precedence over others to create a workplace for safe care or to prevent injury of the patient or family. The home maintenance practices and facilities may be adequate for a family with healthy members but may be hazardous for a patient.

Impaired home maintenance management may also be secondary to other nursing diagnoses or even a sign of their presence. For example, one objective sign of dysfunctional grieving is failing to participate in home maintenance tasks until the home is unsafe or unhygienic. Other diagnoses in which impaired home maintenance management may be a sign are altered parenting and ineffective individual or family coping. Impaired home maintenance may also be part of the etiology of another nursing diagnosis, such as potential for injury, especially the subcategories of potential for poisoning (if garbage is not removed or food is stored under unsafe conditions), or potential for trauma (if necessary home repairs are not done).

Several excellent tools developed for the assessment of the family and the home environment are printed in the community health literature.[5] Reutter[17] describes a tool that assesses the family using Orem's self-care nursing framework and also includes the collection of environmental data. Gordon[10] includes an assessment guide that addresses the nursing diagnosis of impaired home maintenance management in her text.

When assessing for the nursing diagnosis of impaired home maintenance management, the nurse must consider the individual, family, dwelling, and the community. The key observation is of the dwelling itself and its organization, cleanliness, and safety for both daily living and patient care. Observation for signs of provision for personal growth and individuality of family members is also necessary. The following parameters should be considered:

1. What is the individual patient's physical or mental status? Is there a disease or disability present that may impede home maintenance?
2. What is the home situation?
   a. Type of housing unit
   b. Location of housing unit
   c. Condition of housing unit
   d. Number of occupants in unit
3. What is the patient's "standard" of home maintenance?
4. What is the patient's perception of ability to maintain the home?
5. What support system is available and what are its capabilities?
6. What community resources are available to enable the patient to remain in the home situation?
7. Are financial resources adequate to maintain the home?
8. What equipment is needed to facilitate adaptation?
9. Are there structural deficits or barriers that make home maintenance difficult?
10. What effect does the neighborhood or community have on the patient's ability to maintain the home?

A safe, hygienic environment that offers social and physical stimulation for personal growth and development is the baseline sought for each identified patient. Failure to achieve this goal is associated with an imbalance in compensation by the patient, family, and/or community or a deficit in the dwelling or surrounding environment. The dwelling may be unsuitable for the patient and family, in need of adaptation, or situated in a community that is unsafe or unhealthy for the patient.

Support may also be the home care nurse and other professionals in the community who provide social stimulation and refer the patient to appropriate resources. People are often unaware of community services until they have a need for them. The consumer movement and health education campaigns by local, state, and federal governments and professional organizations have had some impact increasing the public's knowledge of health practices and resources available in their communities. Many communities have homemaker services, extended payment plans for winter heating bills, institutional temporary respite care for the disabled, and other programs to assist families to maintain disabled members at home.

The community also contributes to the quality of life of its residents through its environmental health and sanitation programs. This support is especially important to community members who are disabled or sick. For instance, no matter how well the person maintains and adapts the home, if the building codes are not enforced and pest control not done on a community-wide basis, the home will not be hygienic or safe. In addition, disabled people may be especially susceptible to pollutants that the general population can tolerate. An example is a person with emphysema living where there is smog.

Lack of knowledge of community resources was mentioned previously. A person may also be unaware of how to maintain a safe, hygienic home or how to provide a growth-stimulating environment because of developmental status, impaired cognitive functioning, or lack of role models. A very young person with few social supports may not have the necessary experience in caring for a dwelling to keep it clean or control pests. Another person may not know that a baby has poor internal temperature control and needs extra warmth in cold weather. Alternatively, elderly persons may not realize their declining ability to sense cold and may fail to keep themselves warm enough at night.

Impaired cognitive functioning is a problem for both mentally retarded adults and patients with organic brain dysfunctions. The health care trend of deinstitutionalization may have led to their placement in the community without the supports and training they need for home maintenance management. However, many programs demonstrate how these patients can learn to care for themselves and their homes through training and continuing support in halfway houses, group homes, or foster homes.

Evaluation

Patient Outcome	Data Indicating That Outcome is Reached
Feasible discharge plan	Patient and family identify documentation of needs. Nurse documents learning after patient teaching.

Patient Outcome	Data Indicating That Outcome is Reached
	Nurse makes appropriate referrals. Nurse documents discharge plan and forwards copy with referrals.
Accurate assessment of factors associated with home maintenance	Home maintenance is defined as a health problem. Each member states personal standard of home maintenance. Each member contributes in identification of factors that impede home maintenance. Family verbalizes financial constraints. Nurse shares validation and discrepancies observed with family.
Realistic assessment of family members' capacity for daily maintenance	Current roles are stated and possible role changes discussed. Hygienic factors are differentiated.
Accurate assessment of support system and development of realistic plan	Patient shares perception of support system and its strengths and weaknesses. Need for outside help is defined. Patient states what resources are available after nurse shares knowledge of available resources. Nurse and patient develop plan of care.
Appropriate and efficient use of community resources	Contact with resources is initiated. Deficits in support are compensated. Support system members use nursing services appropriately.
Adaptation of home and/or lifestyle to promote health	Unsafe objects are removed. Patient relates change to improvement of health status. Patient participates as able in performance of activities of daily living and home maintenance. Patient remains at home as long as feasible and desirable.
Completion of repairs to structural defects	Patient states relationship between defects and maintaining healthy, safe home. Patient and family seek help from community resources for repair of and financial help in eliminating structural defects. Observation of repairs is made.
Appropriate use of equipment and supplies	Equipment and supplies are obtained. Equipment is used appropriately. Patient verbalizes how to obtain future supplies and how to arrange for repair of equipment.
Adequate home maintenance management	Additional support is obtained. Client and household members mutually determine standard of cleanliness for home. Family maximally participates in home maintenance. Family discusses roles in maintaining cleaner, safer environment. Patient and family express satisfaction with home situation. Nurse observes clean, safe, growth-promoting environment.
Awareness of impact of neighborhood on home maintenance	Patient verbalizes factors negatively affecting home maintenance. Patient identifies neighborhood improvement resources; at least one family member participates. Patient and family verbalize factors that would lead to changing residence.

 Ineffective Airway Clearance

Ineffective airway clearance is the state in which an individual is unable to clear secretions or obstructions from the respiratory tract to maintain airway patency.

Related Factors[7]

Decreased energy and fatigue
Tracheobronchial
- Infection
- Obstruction
- Secretion

Perceptual/cognitive impairment
Trauma

Defining Characteristics[1,2,3,7,8]

Abnormal breathing sounds: crackles (rales), rhonchi, wheezes
Changes in rate or depth of respiration
Tachypnea
Cough, effective or ineffective, with or without sputum (indicates irritant or secretion is stimulating cough reflex; thus cough is both sign of as well as treatment for ineffective airway clearance)
Cyanosis (bluish discoloration of skin and mucous membranes; late sign of hypoxia, not observed until oxygen saturation has fallen below 78%)

Dyspnea
Fever
Nasal bogginess (edema of the mucous membranes in the nasal cavity)
Altered speech (edematous sinuses cause nasal sounding speech; dyspnea may interrupt speech while patient catches breath; total airway obstruction causes inability to speak)
Increased anterior-posterior diameter of chest
Prolonged expiratory phase of respiration through pursed lip breathing
Use of accessory muscles for breathing
Choking or gasping
Noisy respirations
Nasal flaring
Anxiety
Fearfulness
Hemoptysis

Nursing Interventions*

Patient Goal	Nursing Intervention
Maintain airway patency.	• Auscultate lungs. • Determine rate and depth of respirations. • Assess use of accessory muscles. • Inspect color of skin, mucous membranes, and nail beds. • Monitor arterial blood gases and hemoglobin. • Monitor tidal volume and vital capacity. • Monitor sputum color, consistency, and amount. • Perform head tilt to remove tongue from obstructing the airway. • Perform Heimlich maneuver to remove foreign object. • Prepare equipment for bronchoscopy if patient aspirated solid material. • Suction mucus and secretions from airways. • Provide humidification to airways as ordered. • Administer oxygen as ordered. • Provide mechanical ventilation as ordered. • Provide oral care as needed for patient who is coughing. • Plan rest periods of at least 1 hour during day. • Assist in decreasing fear or anxiety. • Encourage patient to breathe deeply and cough each hour while awake. • Encourage fluid intake to thin secretions if patient is not fluid restricted. • Assist patient to appropriate position for postural drainage. • Use percussion and vibration to dislodge pulmonary secretions. • Turn and position patient every 2 hours. • Administer medications as ordered: corticosteroids, bronchodilators, anti-infectives, decongestants, and antibiotics. • Evaluate therapeutic, adverse, and toxic effects of medication given. • Discourage patient and family from smoking.
Achieve physical and psychologic comfort.	• Place warm, moist compresses over painful sinuses. • Elevate head of bed to facilitate gravity drainage of sinus and reduce work of breathing. • Provide oral care as needed for patient who is coughing productively.
Communicate knowledge of self-care.	• Assess what patient and family need to learn. • Provide information concerning: How to prevent recurrence of airway obstruction How to perform diaphragmatic and pursed-lip breathing Purpose of drugs taken at home, frequency of administration, and side effects Smoking cessation Eating balanced meals with adequate fluids Performing bronchial hygiene and productive coughing techniques Changing daily activities to decrease oxygen demands Plans for follow-up

*References 1, 2, 3, 7, 8, 11.

Principles and Rationale for Nursing Interventions

Three goals are derived for the patient with ineffective airway clearance: maintain airway patency, provide comfort, and communicate knowledge of self-care.

The nurse auscultates the patient's lungs for crackles (rales), rhonchi, and wheezes to determine airway patency. The rate and depth and use of accessory muscles are assessed to determine the work of breathing. The nurse inspects the color of skin, mucous membranes, and nail beds because these are the best locations to observe cyanosis. Arterial blood gases and hemoglobin are monitored to determine the adequacy of oxygen-carrying capacity as well as acid-base balance. Tidal volume indicates the amount of air moved with each breath, whereas the vital capacity measures the amount of air exhaled after a maximum inhalation. Both the tidal volume and the vital capacity can decrease when the airway is not patent. The nurse observes color, consistency, and amount of sputum because pulmonary irritants or infections often cause an increased mucus production. Changes in the color or consistency of sputum may indicate the presence of an infection, such as a change from thin white sputum to thick yellow sputum. Humidified oxygen is given to supplement environmental oxygen and to prevent drying of mucous membranes.

When the cause of upper airway obstruction is the tongue or a foreign object, the patient requires immediate care to clear the obstruction. When a foreign body is suspected, the nurse determines if the patient can speak to distinguish an occluded airway from another condition, such as myocardial infarction. The person with an occluded airway will be unable to speak. To dislodge the obstruction, the nurse uses the *Heimlich maneuver:* four quick back blows to the patient between the scapula followed by abdominal thrusts. To deliver the abdominal thrusts, the nurse stands behind the patient and places both hands at the patient's diaphragm, grabs the right fist with the left hand, and gives a sudden, strong upward thrust against the abdomen. This pressure compresses the lungs, forcing the object into the mouth to clear the airway. This procedure can be done with the patient supine and the nurse kneeling astride and facing the patient. The nurse places the heel of one hand just above the umbilicus and places the other hand atop the first. A quick upward thrust is delivered against the abdomen to dislodge the object. The back blows and abdominal thrusts are continued until the obstruction is relieved or advanced life support is available. The airway is suctioned to remove excess secretions.

Ineffective airway clearance related to laryngospasm occurs most frequently in infants and children. It requires prompt care also but is placed in order of priority after obstruction by foreign object or tongue. Initially, the airway is opened using the head tilt with forward displacement of the mandible. An oropharyngeal airway is inserted followed by artificial ventilation by mouth-to-mouth means or inflation bag. A medical treatment of laryngospasm is administration of a paralytic drug followed by orotracheal intubation. If this action is inadequate and the patient is unconscious, the nurse, in collaboration with the physician, inserts an esophageal obturator airway. An emergency tracheostomy is performed by a physician as a last resort to open the airway. Once the airway is opened, the patient is placed in an upright position and encouraged to breathe deeply. Humidified oxygen is given as ordered.

When the cause of lower airway obstruction is edema or excessive mucus and secretion production, the airways are cleared by effective coughing. The patient is instructed to sit up as high as possible to facilitate chest expansion. Then the patient inhales slowly and deeply to dilate airways and force air behind the mucus and secretions. The patient exhales forcibly until the cough reflex is stimulated. Endotracheal stimulation is used to produce coughing when the patient is too weak to cough. Coughing is necessary but does require work that can fatigue the patient. The nurse determines the frequency of coughing needed by patients to clear the airways but not to tire them unnecessarily. Along with coughing, postural drainage is recommended to allow gravity to drain secretions from segmental bronchi. Percussion and vibration are used to dislodge pulmonary secretions. The patient who is obese, has unstable vital signs, or has extreme dyspnea may not be able to tolerate postural drainage.

To maintain comfort, the nurse encourages frequent oral and nasal hygiene for the patient who has a productive cough. The patient should blow the nose gently to remove mucus. Nostrils may be cleaned with moistened cotton-tipped applicators. Since coughing can cause fatigue and can interfere with sleep, the patient needs planned rest periods of at least 1 hour. After receiving treatments for airway clearance and medications, the patient can be encouraged to sleep. A dyspneic, apprehensive patient may need to talk with the nurse about fears and anxieties related to breathing.

Evaluation

Patient Outcome	Data Indicating That Outcome is Reached
Maintains patent airway	Arterial blood gases normal for patient Skin, nails, lips, and earlobes natural color Breath sounds clear bilaterally Normal respirations
Communicates knowledge of self-care	Patient and family can explain: 1. Reason for ineffective airway clearance

Patient Outcome	Data Indicating That Outcome is Reached
	2. Actions to avoid it 3. Medications and treatments for home use 4. Plan for follow-up care

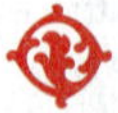

Ineffective Breathing Pattern

Ineffective breathing pattern is the state in which an individual's inhalation and/or exhalation pattern does not enable adequate ventilation.

Related Factors[7]

Neuromuscular impairment
Pain
Musculoskeletal impairment
Anxiety
Decreased energy and fatigue
Inflammatory process
Decreased lung expansion
Tracheobronchial obstruction

Defining Characteristics[1,2,3,7,8]

Dyspnea
Shortness of breath
Tachypnea
Fremitus
Abnormal arterial blood gases
Cyanosis
Cough
Nasal flaring
Respiratory depth changes
  Shallow respirations
  Cheyne-Stokes respirations
  Hyperventilation
Assumption of three-point position
Pursed-lip breathing or prolonged expiratory phase
Increased anterior-posterior diameter of chest
Use of accessory muscles
Altered chest excursion (paradoxic breathing or flail chest)
Orthopnea
Bradypnea
Tachycardia
Bounding pulse
Rising blood pressure
Reduced vital capacity

Nursing Interventions[3,5,8,11]

Patient Goal	Nursing Intervention
Maintain adequate ventilation.	• Assess respiratory rate and depth. • Auscultate breath sounds. • Monitor arterial blood gases. • Measure tidal volume. • Assess skin and nail color. • Monitor chest roentgenogram reports. • Encourage patient to deep breathe and cough. • Encourage use of incentive spirometry as ordered. • Suction airway as needed using sterile technique. • Turn patient frequently. • Elevate head of bed unless contraindicated (as in spinal cord injury). • Perform chest physiotherapy. • Monitor air bubbling down chest tube into underwater seal chamber; milk chest tube as necessary. • Administer oxygen as ordered. • Assist patient with activities of daily living as necessary. • Schedule frequent rest periods.
Achieve comfort.	• Splint patient's chest during coughing. • Use mild sedatives and small doses of meperidine (Demerol) or codeine to control pain as ordered by physician. • Unless patient is intubated, encourage him to discuss fears of inadequate ventilation. • Change patient's position frequently and position comfortably. • Plan periods of rest for at least 1 hour. • Achieve pain relief by distraction, mental imagery, meditation, physical pressure on the painful site, massage, and relaxation.

Patient Goal	Nursing Intervention
Communicate knowledge of self-care.	• Assess what patient and family need to know. • Review reasons for ineffective breathing patterns. • Make referral for ventilatory equipment to be used in the home. • Review reason for medications and treatments ordered for home use. • Review plan for follow-up care.

Principles and Rationale for Nursing Interventions

Three goals are derived for the patient with ineffective breathing pattern: maintain adequate ventilation, achieve comfort, and communicate knowledge of self-care.

To accomplish the first goal, the nurse assesses the respiratory rate and depth, which frequently are rapid and shallow because a related factor is interference with the inhalation or exhalation of air. When the patient is breathing rapidly and shallowly, the breath sounds are diminished. Auscultation also detects crackles and rhonchi, which may indicate an inflammatory process. Arterial blood gases are monitored to determine the effect the ineffective breathing pattern has had on alveolar-capillary gas exchange. Also, blood gases are used to evaluate the effectiveness of oxygen therapy. Tidal volume is the measurement of the amount of air exhaled during a normal breath. When the breathing pattern is ineffective, the tidal volume is reduced. The skin and nail bed color often are pale when the patient's breathing pattern does not allow adequate ventilation. Chest roentgenograms indicate the amount of chest expansion, as well as areas of inflammation, consolidation, and obstruction. The patient is encouraged to breathe deeply and cough to expand the chest and mobilize secretions. Encouraging the use of incentive spirometry is one way for the patient to deep breathe. When the patient's secretions cannot be removed by coughing, the nurse can use sterile techique to suction secretions from the airways. The patient is turned frequently to mobilize secretions by gravity and to facilitate ventilation. Raising the head of the bed assists ventilation by removing the pressure of the abdominal contents away from the diaphragm. Chest physiotherapy (percussion and vibration) is performed to help mobilize secretions. When the patient's treatment includes use of chest tube to reexpand the lung, the nurse maintains the water seal, monitors the air bubbling, and maintains the patency of the tube by milking it. The nurse also observes and records the drainage from the chest tube. Oxygen is administered as ordered to maintain a normal arterial level. The patient may require assistance with activities to daily living and frequent rest periods to conserve energy and reduce the oxygen demand.

When pain is the factor related to the ineffective breathing patterns, the patient goal of comfort is necessary. Patients who have a chest or an abdominal incision experience less pain when coughing when they splint the incision with a pillow. Medicating the patient for pain 20 to 30 minutes before coughing, turning, or chest physiotherapy provides comfort during these interventions to improve ventilation. Alternative forms of pain relief are also beneficial, such as distraction and mental imagery.

Finally, the patient and family require instruction about how to prevent the ineffective breathing pattern from recurring. Also, they need to know how to use ventilatory equipment, the purpose and side effects of medications prescribed, and the plans for follow-up care. They need to be well informed so that they can carry out the plan of care after discharge.

Evaluation

Patient Outcome	Data Indicating That Outcome is Reached
Maintains adequate ventilation	Arterial blood gases: pH: 7.35-7.45 Po_2: 80-95 mm Hg (lower for patient with chronic obstructive pulmonary disease) Pco_2: 35-45 mm Hg (lower for patient with COPD) O_2 saturation: 95%-99% Chest rises symmetrically on inhalation and falls symmetrically on exhalation No use of accessory muscles Respiratory rate: 12-20/min
Communicates knowledge of self-care	Patient and family can explain: 1. Reasons for ineffective breathing 2. Medication and treatment for home use 3. Plan for follow-up care

 Impaired Gas Exchange

Impaired gas exchange is the state in which an individual experiences an imbalance between oxygen uptake and carbon dioxide elimination at the alveolar-capillary membrane gas exchange area.

Related Factors[7]

Altered oxygen supply
Alveolar-capillary membrane changes
Altered blood flow
Altered oxygen-carrying capacity of blood

Defining Characteristics[1,2,3,7,8]

Confusion
Somnolence
Restlessness
Irritability
Inability to move secretions
Hypercapnia
Hypoxia
Polycythemia (a compensatory mechanism)
Increased anterior-posterior diameter of chest
Hyperresonance on chest percussion
Tachycardia, arrhythmias
Anxiety
Dyspnea
Cyanosis
Decreased mental acuity
Tachypnea
Widened alveolar-arterial gradient
Three-point position
Pursed-lip breathing with prolonged expiratory phase

Nursing Interventions[2,3,7,8]

Patient Goal	Nursing Intervention
Maintain adequate ventilation.	• Auscultate breath sounds. • Measure vital signs. • Monitor cardiac rhythm. • Monitor arterial blood gases and hemoglobin. • Monitor chest roentgenogram reports. • Administer humidified oxygen as ordered. • Suction airway as needed using sterile technique. • Encourage patient to cough and deep breathe when not receiving mechanical ventilation. • Administer drugs as ordered: bronchodilators, antihistamines, anti-infectives, expectorants, and corticosteroids. • Evaluate therapeutic, adverse, and toxic effects of drugs given. • Turn patient at least every 2 hours. • Elevate head of bed. • Administer packed cells or whole blood as ordered; observe for adverse reaction to blood administration.
Achieve physical and psychologic comfort.	• Explain care being given and being planned. • If patient not intubated, encourage verbalization of feelings. • Provide back rub and position change frequently. • Provide oral hygiene. • Provide pain relief with independent nursing measures and with medications as ordered. • Provide planned periods of rest for at least 1 hour.
Communicate knowledge of self-care.	• Assess what patient and family need to know. • Provide information about pursed-lip breathing and diaphragmatic breathing. • Discover reason for impaired gas exchange and its prevention in the future. • Know actions, side effects, dosage, and frequency of administration for all medications ordered by physician. • Plan referral for ventilatory equipment to be used in the home. • Alter daily activities as necessary to decrease oxygen demand.

Principles and Rationale for Nursing Interventions

Three goals are derived for the patient with impaired gas exchange: maintain adequate ventilation, achieve physical and psychologic comfort, and communicate knowledge of self-care.

When auscultating breath sounds, the nurse may hear crackles (rales), indicating fluid in the alveoli. Decreased or absent breath sounds may indicate collapsed alveoli. A temperature elevation may indicate an inflammatory process. Tachycardia frequently accompanies hypoxemia. Assessing the respiratory rate and depth will reflect the amount of air being moved and the work of breathing. Cardiac rhythms are monitored because hypoxia is associated with dysrhythmias. Arterial blood gases are monitored to evaluate the alveolar-capillary gas exchange as well as the effectiveness of oxygen therapy. Chest roentgenograms will indicate the areas of obstruction, consolidation, and inflammation. Sterile technique is used to suction the airways to maintain airway patency so that oxygen can be delivered to the alveoli. Another intervention to clear airways is encouraging the patient to deep breathe and cough. Medications are given to dilate the bronchi (bronchodilators), to interrupt the inflammatory process (antihistamines, anti-infectives, corticosteroids), and to facilitate productive coughing (expectorants). The patient is turned to facilitate ventilation. The head of the bed is elevated so that the weight of the abdominal contents will not rest against the diaphragm, thus decreasing the work of breathing. Whole blood or packed cells are given to increase the oxygen-carrying capacity.

To help patients achieve comfort, the nurse explains all care being given and allows patients to verbalize their feelings about their state of health. Back rubs and position changes will provide physical comfort. Planning frequent rest periods also are important. Pain relief using independent methods (imagery, relaxation techniques, etc.) and/or using pain medication will facilitate rest and comfort.

Before discharge the patient and family need instruction on how to prevent impaired gas exchange in the future. Also, they must know how to use ventilatory equipment, the purpose and side effects of medications prescribed, and the plans for follow-up care. They need to discuss how to alter their lifestyles as needed because of chronic gas exchange impairment.

Evaluation

Patient Outcome	Data Indicating That Outcome is Reached
Maintains adequate ventilation	Arterial blood gases (see Ineffective Breathing Pattern) Hemoglobin: 12-14 g/dl (women) 14-16 g/dl (men) Effortless breathing No use of accessory muscles Respiratory rate: 12-20/min Perform activities of daily living without becoming short of breath
Communicates knowledge of self-care	Patient and family can explain: 1. Reasons for impaired gas exchange 2. Medication and treatment for home use 3. Plan for follow-up care

Decreased Cardiac Output

Decreased cardiac output is the state in which the blood pumped by an individual's heart is sufficiently reduced that it is inadequate to meet the needs of the body's tissues.

Cardiac output is the amount of blood ejected from the left ventricle each minute and normally ranges from 4 to 8 L. Cardiac output is a function of the stroke volume (amount of blood ejected per contraction) and the heart rate (number of contractions per minute).[5]

Related Factors[7]

Mechanical
- Alteration in preload
- Alteration in afterload
- Alteration in inotropic changes in heart

Electrical
- Alterations in rate
- Alterations in rhythm
- Alterations in conduction

Structural

Defining Characteristics[5,7,8]

Variations in hemodynamic readings
Arrhythmias (ECG changes)
Fatigue
Jugular vein distention*
Cyanosis (pallor of skin and mucous membranes)
Oliguria
Anuria
Decreased peripheral pulses
Cold clammy skin
Rales†
Dyspnea†
Orthopnea†
Restlessness
Change in mental status†
Syncope†
Vertigo†
Edema, dependent*

*Occurs with right ventricular failure.
†Occurs with left ventricular failure.

Cough*
Frothy sputum*
Abnormal heart sounds (e.g., gallop rhythm)*

*Occurs with right ventricular failure.
†Occurs with left ventricular failure.

Weakness
Liver engorgement and tenderness†
Ascites†
Tachycardia
Angina

Nursing Interventions*

Patient Goal	Nursing Intervention
Restore cardiac output.	• Assess vital signs frequently according to patient's condition. • Monitor cardiac rhythm continuously. • Initiate prompt treatment of life-threatening arrhythmias per protocol: Cardiopulmonary resuscitation Appropriate drug therapy as ordered Prepare for insertion of pacemaker • Monitor hemodynamic parameters: Pulmonary artery pressures Central venous pressures Cardiac output • Measure intake and output. • Monitor intravenous fluids with electrolytes as ordered. • Administer antiarrhythmic drugs as ordered. • Administer inotropic drugs as ordered by physician. • Observe cardiac enzyme values, electrolyte values (especially potassium), and arterial blood gases. • Observe for therapeutic, adverse, and toxic effects of drugs given. • When intra-aortic balloon pump is inserted by physician, assess heart rate, mean arterial pressure, and pulmonary capillary wedge pressure, heart rhythm and regularity (especially R waves), urine output, skin color, peripheral perfusion, and mental status.
Reduce heart workload.	• Assist patient to semi-Fowler's position. • Maintain patient on complete bed rest according to policy. • Perform activities of daily living for patient. • When able to get out of bed, permit patient to use bedside commode. • Measure intake and output to monitor fluid balance. • Administer stool softener as ordered. • Administer diuretics as ordered. • Administer oxygen as ordered. • Encourage deep breathing and coughing. • Administer nitrates as ordered. • Administer hypnotics or analgesics as ordered to provide rest. • Administer morphine as ordered. • Observe for therapeutic, adverse, and toxic effects of drugs given. • Provide a restful, quiet environment. • Evaluate patient's tolerance to activities of daily living; monitor for hypotension and arrhythmias. • Administer drugs as ordered: antiarrhythmics, inotropics, diuretics, and potassium. • Evaluate the therapeutic, adverse, and toxic effects of drugs given.
Communicate knowledge of self-care.	• Assess patient's current knowledge and provide information as needed. • Provide information concerning: Prevention of recurrence Risk factors to avoid Pathophysiology of illness Medication uses, side effects, and frequency of administration Stress management techniques Physical activity program Dietary alterations Guidelines for resuming sexual relations Guidelines for returning to work

*References 1, 2, 3, 7, 8, 10, 11.

Principles and Rationale for Nursing Interventions

Three goals are derived for the patient with decreased cardiac output: restore cardiac output, reduce workload of the heart, and communicate knowledge of self-care.

The goals of care vary with the acuity of the problem. To restore cardiac output, the causative condition must be corrected. Assessment data the nurse collects to meet this goal include the following:

Auscultating the heart
Measuring the heart rate and blood pressure
Palpating pulses
Identifying the rhythm of the heart through the ECG pattern
Measuring the pressures of the right atria, pulmonary artery, and pulmonary capillary wedge through a pulmonary artery catheter
Measuring cardiac output and urinary output
Measuring daily body weight

The nurse is aware of laboratory data, including electrolytes, cardiac enzymes, arterial blood gases, hemoglobin, and hematocrit. Under physician orders the nurse administers medications to maintain cardiac output and monitors the therapeutic effects and side effects of these drugs. When preload is reduced because of decreased volume, the nurse administers intravenous fluids as ordered. Per physician orders antiarrhythmic drugs are given to stabilize the rhythm, inotropic drugs are given to increase the force of contractility, and electrolytes are given to correct imbalances and facilitate contractility.[10] An intra-aortic balloon is inserted by the physician to increase oxygen supply to the myocardium, decrease left ventricular work, and improve cardiac output. Assessment of the patient with balloon pump therapy includes monitoring heart rate, mean arterial pressure, pulmonary capillary wedge pressure, heart rhythm and regularity, urine output, skin color, peripheral perfusion, and mental status.[5]

To reduce the workload on the patient's heart, the nurse intervenes to meet physical and psychologic needs. Oxygen is provided as ordered to ensure an adequate supply for the myocardium. Pain medication is given based on protocol for comfort as needed. Morphine is a preferred drug because it not only relieves pain, but also provides peripheral vasodilation to reduce venous return.[5] Diuretics and vasodilators are given to reduce systemic vascular resistance. The patient is asked to reduce physical activity by resting in bed in a semi-Fowler's or Fowler's position or in a chair. This position also reduces the patient's work of breathing, which decreases the workload of the heart. The patient's hygiene activities are performed for him. Specific times of rest are planned throughout the day. As the patient improves, a progressive activity schedule is implemented. The physician may prescribe stool softeners to prevent straining during defecation. The diet is changed as needed. Frequently caffeine and sodium are restricted. Small meals require less work by the heart.

To meet psychologic needs, the nurse attempts to reduce the patient's stress and anxiety. A quiet, pleasant environment relieves stress. The patient is encouraged to discuss feelings and is given as much information as possible. Relaxation techniques are taught to reduce tension (see Ineffective Individual Coping).

To achieve awareness of learning needs, the nurse first assesses what the patient and family already know. They need to know what caused the decrease in cardiac output and how to avoid its recurrence. The patient and family will need to know actions and side effects of medications. Life-style changes will require regular exercise of at least 30 minutes three times a week. Dietary alterations are needed to restrict sodium or cholesterol. It is important to consider the patient's cultural food preferences when adapting dietary alterations to fit the life-style. When obesity is a problem, the patient needs to understand that extra weight increases the heart's workload. Smoking adds a burden to the heart by causing vasoconstriction.

Evaluation

Patient Outcome	Data Indicating That Outcome is Reached
Maintains adequate cardiac output	Normal sinus rhythm Heart rate within 20 beats of normal Blood pressure upper limits: 140 mm Hg systolic 90 mm Hg diastolic 30-40 mm Hg pulse pressure Clear breath sounds bilaterally Alert, oriented Absence of angina Urinary output at least 30 ml/hr Skin warm, dry Peripheral pulses present and strong (normal for patient) Able to perform activities of daily living
Communicates knowledge of self-care	Patient and family can explain: 1. Reasons for decreased cardiac output and how to prevent it 2. Dietary alterations

Patient Goal	Nursing Intervention
	3. Exercise program 4. Stress management activities 5. Medication uses and side effects 6. Plan for follow-up care

Altered (Specify Type) Tissue Perfusion (Renal, Cerebral, Cardiopulmonary, Gastrointestinal, Peripheral)

Altered tissue perfusion (renal, cerebral, cardiopulmonary, gastrointestinal, peripheral) is the state in which an individual experiences a decrease in nutrition and oxygenation at the cellular level because of a deficit in capillary blood supply.

Related Factors[7]

Interruption of arterial flow
Interruption of venous flow
Exchange problems
Hypervolemia
Hypovolemia

Defining Characteristics*

Skin temperature: cold extremities
Skin color
- Dependent, blue or purple
- Pale on elevation, and color does not return on lowering
- Diminished arterial pulsation

Skin quality: shining
Lack of lanugo
Round scars covered with atrophied skin
Gangrene
Slow-growing, dry, thick brittle nails
Claudication
Blood pressure changes in extremities
Bruits
Slow healing of lesions
Renal
- Edema
- Decreased urinary output
- Hypertension

Cerebral
- Decrease in consciousness
- Restlessness
- Altered thought processes
- Memory loss

Cardiopulmonary
- Low systolic and diastolic blood pressure readings
- Cold clammy skin
- Slow capillary filling
- Tachycardia
- Angina
- Tachypnea

Gastrointestinal
- Abdominal distention
- Positive guaiac findings of stool
- Nausea or vomiting
- Thirst

Peripheral
- Edema
- Pain
- Numbness, tingling
- Muscle weakness
- Diminished sensitivity to pressure, temperature, and tissue trauma

*References 1, 2, 3, 5, 7, 8.

Nursing Interventions*

Patient Goal	Nursing Intervention
Maintain tissue perfusion and cellular oxygenation.	• Assess vital signs and peripheral pulses. • Assess skin color and temperature. • Inspect extremities and abdomen for edema. • Assess level of consciousness and memory. • Auscultate bowel sounds. • Monitor arterial blood gases and hemoglobin.

*References 1, 2, 3, 8, 10, 11.

Patient Goal	Nursing Intervention
	• When giving anticoagulants, monitor clotting times. • Measure intake and output. • Position extremities to facilitate circulation: elevation for venous problems, downward for arterial problems. • Change position frequently. • Encourage regular active or passive exercise. • Administer drugs as ordered to improve circulation: anticoagulants, vasodilators. • Evaluate therapeutic, adverse, and toxic effects of drugs given. • Administer oxygen as ordered. • Encourage balanced diet with adequate iron.
Reduce metabolic needs.	• Encourage alternate periods of rest and activity. • Protect extremities from extreme temperatures. • Discuss stress reduction strategies.
Communicate knowledge of self-care.	• Assess what patient and family need to know. • Provide information concerning: Changes required in activities of daily living Maintaining reduction in metabolic needs Assessing skin and peripheral circulation daily Purpose, frequency of administration, and side effects of medication Safety needs for patients taking anticoagulants Providing balanced diet Taking action to prevent recurrence of altered tissue perfusion Plans for rehabilitation

Principles and Rationale for Nursing Interventions

Three goals are derived for the patient with altered tissue perfusion: maintain tissue perfusion and cellular oxygenation, reduce metabolic needs, and communicate knowledge of self-care.

Nursing actions to maintain tissue perfusion are based on the cause of the alteration. Elevation of the affected extremity is appropriate when venous circulation is altered, since this position uses gravity to facilitate return of blood toward the heart. Likewise, elevating both legs is helpful when the patient has hypovolemic shock to facilitate blood flow from the lower extremities to the trunk. Conversely, arterial circulation is hindered by prolonged elevation of lower extremities because the normal flow of arterial blood is downward. The flat position is best for long periods. The patient needs a firm bed to prevent hip flexion allowed on a soft mattress. Flexion of the hip may compromise circulation to the legs. The patient must also select chairs carefully. The knees must not be bent at more than a 90-degree angle, and the popliteal space must not press against the chair seat. Active and passive exercises as well as walking stimulate blood flow to the legs. External pressure on the legs is reduced by not crossing legs, not wearing tight clothing on the legs, and not sitting for prolonged periods. Drug administration may include heparin or dihydroxycoumarin as prophylaxis against blood clotting per physician's order. Vasodilators are given, as ordered by physician, for arterial spasm and to improve general circulation. Cellular oxygenation is promoted by maintaining tissue perfusion. In acute conditions, however, supplemental oxygen may be ordered. Anemia needs to be treated per physician's orders to maximize oxygen transport.

Cellular metabolic needs are reduced by alternating periods of rest and activity. The patient needs to protect affected extremities from trauma and infection, which increase metabolic needs. Extremities need to be warm without becoming overheated. To accomplish this, heating pads, time spent in hot tubs, and exercise must be used in moderation. Fear, worry, and anxiety can increase the metabolic needs of tissue. To the extent possible, the patient needs to use stress reduction strategies to prevent detrimental physical effects of these psychologic states.

To achieve awareness of learning needs, the nurse discusses with the patient and family the actions needed to maintain tissue perfusion and decrease metabolic demands. Activities of daily living may need to be changed. The need for rehabilitation also will vary depending on the site and extent of altered perfusion. Safety needs to be emphasized for the patient taking anticoagulants. This includes watching for signs of bleeding from the gums, rectum, and skin. The patient and family should be informed about the anticoagulation properties of aspirin and cautioned against using it in combination with other anticoagulants. A well-balanced diet is important to provide sufficient glucose for adenosine triphosphate formation. Family members need to discuss action needed to prevent recurrence of this problem. This may include smoking cessation, dietary alterations, stress reduction strategies, and exercise programs.

Evaluation

Patient Outcome	Data Indicating That Outcome is Reached
Maintains adequate tissue perfusion	All pulses palpable Extremities warm and normal color Vital signs normal for patient Bowel sounds present 1500-3000 ml output or equivalent to intake Alert with recent memory normal Hemoglobin (g/dl) Men: 15.5 ± 1.1 Women: 13.7 ± 1.0 Partial thromboplastin time: 25-39 seconds (usually stated to be within 10 seconds of control) Arterial blood gases pH: 7.35-7.45 Po_2: 80-95 mm Hg Pco_2: 35-45 mm Hg O_2 sat: 95%-99%
Communicates knowledge of self-care	Patient and family can explain: 1. Reasons for altered tissue perfusion 2. Medication and treatments for home use 3. Dietary and activity modification 4. Safety precautions 5. Follow-up treatment regimen

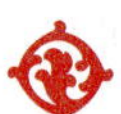

Dysreflexia

Dysreflexia (autonomic dysreflexia) is the state in which a person with a spinal cord injury at the seventh thoracic vertebra (T7) or above experiences or is at risk for a life-threatening uninhibited response of the nervous system to a noxious stimulus.

Autonomic dysreflexia was first described in 1890 and continues to be a problem in the care of patients with spinal cord injuries and those undergoing rehabilitation.

Related Factors*

Bladder distention or spasm
Catheter insertion or irrigation
Obstructed catheter
Bowel distention
Bowel stimulation
Traction of viscera during surgery
Manipulation of perineum
Sexual stimulation or intercourse
Cystometric examination or cystogram
Uterine contractions

*Adapted from North American Nursing Diagnosis Association, 1988 Ballot.

Defining Characteristics*

Paroxysmal hypertension (sudden periodic elevated blood pressure with systolic pressure greater than 140 mm Hg and diastolic greater than 90 mm Hg)
Bradycardia or tachycardia (pulse rate less than 60 or more than 100 beats/minute)
Diaphoresis (above injury)
Red splotches on skin (above injury)
Pallor (below injury)
Headache (diffuse pain in different portions of head and not confined to any nerve distribution area)
Chilling (shivering accompanied by sensation of coldness or pallor of skin)
Conjunctival congestion (excessive amount of blood or tissue fluid in conjunctiva)
Horner's syndrome (contraction of pupil, partial ptosis of eyelid, enophthalmos, and sometimes loss of sweating over affected side of face; caused by paralysis of cervical sympathetic nerve trunk)
Paresthesia (abnormal sensation, e.g., numbness, prickling, tingling; increased sensitivity)
Pilomotor reflex (gooseflesh formation when skin is cooled)
Blurred vision
Chest pain
Metallic taste in mouth
Nasal congestion

*Adapted from North American Nursing Diagnosis Association, 1988 Ballot.

Nursing Interventions

Patient Goal	Nursing Intervention
Experience less frequent *and* less severe attacks of dysreflexia.	• Develop awareness for signs and symptoms of dysreflexia and ensure that other staff and patient are aware of symptoms and precipitating factors. • Assess patient for history of previous attacks of dysreflexia and possible causes. • Assess and monitor bowel and bladder elimination patterns to prevent distention. • Observe urinary catheters for kinks and obstructions; ensure patency and change catheter per routine. • Check cautiously for fecal impaction if necessary and relieve promptly with suppository or enema. • Minimize manipulation and stimulation when performing procedures involving bladder and bowel. • Be aware that early symptoms can include pounding headache, sweating, and blotching of skin of face and thorax. • If symptoms occur, stop any procedure being performed and prepare to assist with treatment. • Monitor blood pressure and pulse continuously until symptoms subside. • Administer antihypertensive or α-adrenergic blockers as ordered. • Prop patient up to counteract hypertension with orthostatic hypotension in attempt to reduce headache. • Reassure patient and take measures to promote comfort.
Assist with identification of symptoms and causes.	• Instruct patient about syndrome so that awareness is developed about possible causes and early symptoms experienced. • Arrange for patient to wear *Medic-Alert* bracelet.

Principles and Rationale for Nursing Interventions[1,3,4]

Autonomic dysreflexia results most frequently from distention of pelvic viscera (bladder, colon, rectum) and less frequently from manipulation of the renal pelvis and intestines during surgery, uterine contractions during labor, skin stimulation, and other proprioceptive stimuli below the level of the lesion. Sensory impulses from pelvic viscera reach the spinal cord by way of pelvic parasympathetic, hypogastric, and pudendal nerves, and cutaneous sensations enter through peripheral and dorsal nerve roots. These afferent impulses ascend along spinothalamic tracts and dorsal columns. At segmental levels these impulses may cause reflex motor response. With reflex motor outflow through neurons in the lateral horns, sensory impulses may cause vasoconstriction below the level of the spinal cord lesion (in the splanchnic vascular bed, kidney, skin, legs), with resultant elevation of the blood pressure, pilomotor spasm, and sweating.[3]

Evaluation

Patient Outcome	Data Indicating That Outcome is Reached
Experiences fewer and less severe episodes of dysreflexia	Blood pressure and heart rate return to normal. Usual bowel and bladder elimination patterns are maintained. Headache subsides. Patient participates in avoiding or minimizing bowel and bladder distention. Patient recognizes symptoms and notifies health care professional.

Altered Growth and Development

Altered growth and development is the state in which an individual demonstrates deviations in norms from his or her age group.

Dysfunctional children are those whose developmental disability or disabilities interfere with their growth and who progress at a significantly slower rate in acquiring motor, adaptive, communication, and social skills than normal children in their peer group.[11] Altered growth and development may occur in an infant who appears to be normal at birth but later suffers from maladaptive family relationships and other harmful environmental conditions.[6] In the child with developmental vulnerability, the effects of stress might result in developmental delays when the child's coping mechanisms become maladaptive.[10] Labeling a child with a specific disability should not be considered an indication about the true extent of the disability or the level of services needed. Rather, the child's relative ability to function is the most appropriate factor to consider.[7] Although children who have significant delays probably will attain a lower final level of cognitive development, the rate of development and the extent of the limitations will vary with the characteristics of each condition.[3]

Related Factors*

Prenatal
- Maternal chronic or acute disease
- Maternal malnutrition
- Maternal age
- Maternal exposure to teratogens

Fetal distress during intrapartum period
Prematurity
Asphyxia in neonatal period
Genetic abnormality
Metabolic disorder
Birth defects
Neonatal disease
- Kernicterus
- Sepsis
- Respiratory distress syndrome
- Immature circulatory system

Persistent, chronic health problem
Suboptimum parent-infant attachment
Infant cues difficult to interpret; little interaction
Disadvantaged social situation; poverty
Lack of stimulation in environment
Parental feelings of guilt, anger, or rejection toward child with significant health problems
Serious illness or injury in older child
Psychologic or emotional trauma in older child: abuse, traumatic separation, or loss

*References 1, 2, 6, 7, 10, 13, 17.

Defining Characteristics*

Altered physical growth inappropriate for age
Low birth weight
Irritable, unpredictable infant temperament
Impairment in adaptive functioning
Requires significant deviation from care provided for most children
Listlessness, decreased responses
Flat affect
Inability to perform self-care or self-control activities appropriate for age
Delay or difficulty in performing skills (motor, social, expressive) typical of age group
Observations in older children:
- Persistent clumsiness
- Unusually withdrawn
- Unable to participate in peer group situations
- Extremely aggressive
- Any sign of grand mal or petit mal seizures
- Persistent inappropriate or unexpected behavior

*References 5, 7, 8, 10, 11, 15.

Nursing Interventions*

Patient Goal	Nursing Intervention
Attain maximum level of coping and adaptation to process of daily living and to development of good health.	• Conduct initial and ongoing health assessments of infant or child appropriate to age. • Perform age-appropriate developmental screening test. • Avoid potential physical problems caused by developmental delay. • Prevent dehydration. • Ensure proper diet and exercise to avoid constipation. • Prevent nutritional deficit. • Assess for signs of increased intracranial pressure. • Assess for seizure disorder. • Prevent or minimize upper respiratory tract infections. • Prevent skin breakdown. • Assist parents and caregivers in coping with developmentally delayed child. • Assist caregivers in being able to understand and predict child's day-to-day behaviors. • Help caregivers to see and relate to child as a child. • Help parents adjust to unexpected crisis at their own pace. • Do not offer too much information at one time. • Clarify all terminology (mental retardation, developmental delay, etc.). • Remain nonjudgmental as parents make choices for their child and themselves. • Provide anticipatory guidance, especially for certain high-stress periods: initial diagnosis, start of schooling, and reaching ultimate attainment. • Provide support to parents while they gather strength and resources to adjust. • Assist parents in locating services that might be available to child and/or family.

References 2, 4, 12, 13, 15-17.

Patient Goal	Nursing Intervention
	• Provide parents with opportunities to ventilate feelings in safe environment. • Facilitate progress toward independent functioning, recognizing that pace differs from the norm. • Act as case manager, coordinating multidisciplinary team of medical management, school services, therapies, and social workers. • Facilitate infant/child becoming integrated and accepted member of family and community.

Principles and Rationale for Nursing Interventions

Children with altered growth and development are vulnerable to health problems, and therefore services to provide adequate prevention and early detection are essential. Many of these conditions, often with secondary complications, may be prevented or reduced through early detection services. The incidence and severity of these conditions can be altered with the availability of such services.[7] It is essential to deliver and ensure comprehensive health and development services to the infant or child who exhibits developmental delay, as well as to the family.[2] Health professionals must use a developmental approach to health and habituation. They must view the delayed child as a whole, existing within the context of a family, and not from the narrow perspective of their own area of specialization.[6] The idea that the parents of a developmentally delayed child may suffer from chronic sorrow should be accepted by health professionals as an expected response to a tragic situation. When health professionals apply principles of normalization, they humanize the environment for the developmentally delayed child. By doing this, they help to establish a normal rhythm to the child's life.

Evaluation

Patient Outcome	Data Indicating That Outcome is Reached
Attains maximum level of health and adaptation to process of daily living	Health assessments made regularly Maintains state of good health Parents able to maintain child in home Therapeutic goals and activities integrated into normal daily interactions with infant or child Unwarranted secondary disabilities prevented Parents able to view themselves as child's greatest resource Has modified goals and expectations for mastering developmental tasks

FUNCTIONAL HEALTH PATTERN

V

Sleep-Rest

 Sleep Pattern Disturbance

Sleep pattern disturbance is the state in which disruption of sleep time causes discomfort or interferes with an individual's desired life-style.

Sleep has been identified as a basic human need.[10] Bahr[2] states, "The phenomenon of sleep has the potential for relieving an individual of stress and responsibility when a break is needed to recharge the person's spirit, mind and body; or, it can remain maddeningly aloof when it is needed the most." Henderson[5] has described the inability to rest and sleep as "one of the causes, as well as one of the accompaniments, of disease."

Sleep is a complex physiologic phenomenon influenced by pathophysiologic, physical, psychologic, environmental, and maturational factors. Sleep patterns are highly individual, and their natural pattern should be assessed for each individual. The cyclic pattern of sleep stages for rapid eye movement (REM) and non-REM sleep and the circadian rhythmic synchronization of sleep are influenced by chronic and acute illness, stress, age, pain, medications, hospitalization, sensory overload and deprivation, and life-style disruptions. Because of this complexity, the nursing management of the patient with a diagnosis of sleep pattern disturbance requires a holistic approach.

Related Factors[3,8]

- Major categories
  - Fragmented sleep
  - Circadian desynchronization
- Pathologic factors
  - Impaired oxygen transport
    - Cardiopulmonary disease
    - Peripheral arteriosclerosis
  - Impaired bowel or bladder elimination
  - Impaired metabolism
    - Hyperthyroidism
    - Hepatic disorders
  - Sleep apnea
- Physical factors
  - Immobility imposed by traction, casts, or restraints
  - Inadequate physical exercise
  - Pain
  - Pregnancy
- Psychologic factors
  - Stress
  - Anxiety
  - Fear
  - Depression
  - Psychiatric disorders
  - Life-style disruptions
- Environmental factors
  - Hospitalization
  - Unfamiliar or uncomfortable sleep environment
  - Rapid time zone change (jet lag)
  - Frequent changes in sleep schedule
  - Medications/drugs (e.g., tranquilizers, barbiturates, monoamine oxidase inhibitors, amphetamines, hypnotics, antidepressants, antihypertensives, sedatives, anesthetics, steroids, decongestants, caffeine, alcohol)
- Maturational factor: age

Defining Characteristics

Verbal complaints of difficulty in falling asleep
Awakening earlier or later than desired
Interrupted sleep
Verbal complaints of not feeling well rested
Changes in behavior and performance
- Increasing irritability
- Restlessness
- Disorientation
- Lethargy
- Listlessness

Physical signs
- Mild, fleeting nystagmus
- Slight hand tremor
- Ptosis of eyelid
- Expressionless face

Thick speech with mispronunciation and incorrect words
Dark circles under eyes
Frequent yawning
Changes in posture
Related to fragmented sleep:
- Decreased sleep time occurring in one block of time
- Daytime sleepiness
- Fatigue
- Sleep deprivation
  - Less than one-half normal total sleep time
  - Decreased slow-wave or REM sleep
- Frequent awakenings
- Decreased arousal threshold
- Agitation or mood alteration

Related to circadian desynchronization:
- Sleep out of synchronization with biologic rhythms, resulting in sleeping during daytime and awakening at night
- Anxiety and restlessness
- Decreased arousal threshold

Nursing Interventions

Patient Goal	Nursing Intervention
Describe factors that contribute to sleep pattern disturbance.	• Educate patient and significant others about sleep and rest needs and about factors that contribute to sleep pattern disturbances (e.g., pain, fear, stress, immobility, decreased activity, impaired oxygen transport, pregnancy, urinary frequency, medication, unfamiliar environment; see related factors.) • Facilitate patient expression of emotional factors that may be interfering with normal sleep. • Offer emotional support and continuity of care providers.
Verbalize increased satisfaction with rest and sleep patterns.	• Assess normal sleep pattern and any history of sleep disturbance or illness that may affect sleep or any sedative/hypnotic use. • Promote normal sleep activity while hospitalized. • Assess sleep effectiveness by asking patient how sleep in hospital compares to that at home. • Promote comfort, relaxation, and a sense of well-being; relieve pain. • Eliminate stressful situations before bedtime; use of stress relaxation techniques may be helpful. • Minimize awakenings; allow for at least 90-minute sleep cycles. Continually assess need to awaken patient, particularly at night; distinguish between essential and nonessential nursing tasks. • Organize nursing care to allow for maximum amount of uninterrupted sleep while ensuring close monitoring of patient's condition. • Monitor physiologic parameters without awakening patient whenever possible. • Inform patient about when you will awaken him during night so as not to startle patient. • Coordinate awakenings with other departments (e.g., respiratory therapy, laboratory, radiology). • Minimize noise, particularly related to staff and equipment. • Reduce level of environmental stimuli that may cause sensory overload. • Plan nap times to assist in equilibrating normal sleep time; early morning naps may be beneficial in promoting REM sleep.[8] • Be aware of effects of commonly used medications on sleep, since many sedative and hypnotic medications decrease REM sleep. Do not withhold sedative and analgesic medications; rather, use drugs that minimally disrupt sleep to complement comfort measures, reducing dosages gradually as medication becomes no longer necessary. Diuretics may interrupt sleep by increasing number of awakenings and should not be scheduled at bedtime. • Offer tryptophan-containing foods (e.g., milk) to promote sleep.[6] • Assess for signs of sleep deprivation (e.g., confusion, hallucinations, restlessness, combativeness, paranoia). Be aware that best treatment for sleep deprivation is prevention. • Document amount of uninterrupted sleep per shift in hospitalized patients. • Promote staff attitude that sleep is essential and should be encouraged. Assess unit for sleep-reducing stimuli and work to reduce them.
Demonstrate optimum balance of rest and activity.	• Assist patient to maintain normal day/night cycles by decreasing lighting, noise, and sensory stimulation at night and assessing need to awaken patient at night. • Do not schedule routine procedures at night.

Patient Goal	Nursing Intervention
	• Be aware that cardiac arrhythmias can be precipitated because of decreased arousal threshold secondary to desynchronization. • If desynchronization occurs, plan for resynchronization by maintaining constancy in day/night pattern for at least 3 days (may require 5 to 12 days to reacclimatize). Plan for activities during day to stimulate wakefulness, and use comfort measures (position of comfort, warm blankets, back rub, etc.) to promote sleep at night. During resynchronization, fatigue, malaise, and decreased ability to perform tasks typically are found.[8] • Administer hypnotics as ordered, and monitor their effectiveness.

Principles and Rationale for Nursing Interventions

Sleep occurs in two distinct stages, REM and non-REM, as determined by the electroencephalogram (EEG), electro-oculogram (EOG), and electromyogram (EMG). In addition, non-REM sleep has four stages. Stage 1 is a transitional stage between sleep and wakefulness. During stage 2 the individual becomes progressively more relaxed. A young adult typically spends 50% to 60% of total sleep time in non-REM stages 1 and 2. Non-REM stages 3 and 4 are characterized by slow-frequency delta waves on the EEG and are differentiated by the relative percentage of these waves. Non-REM stages 3 and 4, the deeper stages of sleep, comprise about 20% of total sleep time. These are the restorative stages of sleep during which much protein synthesis and energy conservation occurs.

During REM sleep, or paradoxic sleep, there are bursts of eye movements seen on the EOG. The large muscles of the body become functionally paralyzed. EEG activity increases so that there is a resemblance to the waking state. REM sleep comprises 20% to 25% of the total sleep time and is the stage during which the individual is most difficult to awaken. The many functions of sleep are only theorized by researchers in the field.[9]

Sleep is cyclic. At its onset the individual normally progresses through repetitive cycles, beginning with non-REM stages 1 through 4 and then back again to stage 2. From stage 2, REM sleep is entered. Stage 2 is then reentered and the cycle repeats. These cycles occur at approximately 90-minute intervals, so that four or five cycles are normally completed in the sleep period.[4]

Illness can decrease the amount, quality, and consistency of sleep. Sleep is often interrupted or fragmented, altering the normal stages and cycles and producing dysfunctional sleep. With frequent interruptions the patient spends more time in the transitional stages (non-REM 1 and 2) and less time in the deeper stages of sleep (non-REM 3 and 4, REM). Thus, total sleep time and/or selective deprivation of the deeper stages of sleep can occur.[8]

Sleep is normally synchronized with the circadian rhythm; thus, sleep normally occurs at the low phase of the circadian cycle. Sleep that is desynchronized is rated as poor in quality. Irritability, restlessness, daytime hypersomnolence, fatigue, tiredness, depression, anxiety, and decreased accuracy of task performance are characteristic effects of desynchronized sleep.[8] Barbiturates, sedatives/hypnotics, and analgesic medications may add to sleep disorders by promoting the lighter stages of sleep (non-REM 2) and/or further decreasing non-REM stages 3 and 4 and REM sleep.[6] Knowledge of the effects of these drugs on sleep will assist the nurse to use them more effectively in patient care.

Evaluation

Patient Outcome	Data Indicating That Outcome is Reached
Sleeps for a time approximating patient's normal time	Total sleep time typically is between 6 and 9 hours for adults. Patient's normal time is reached consistently, as evidenced by daily record of sleep.
Completes sleep cycles of 90 minutes without interruption	Awakenings are limited to essential ones only.
Experiences minimum awakenings during bulk sleep time	Environmental distractions are eliminated. Sleep environment provides for patient safety and comfort.
Sleeps mostly during low cycle of circadian rhythm	Medication schedule promotes bulk sleep time and sleep cycles of at least 90 minutes. Patient and significant others report satisfactory sleep and activity pattern. Patient does not exhibit signs of sleep deprivation (disorientation; irritability; hyperactivity; fatigue; sleepiness; delusions; hallucinations; decreased integration and personal effectiveness; decreased memory, judgment, and reasoning).

FUNCTIONAL HEALTH PATTERN

VI

Cognitive-Perceptual

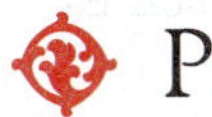 Pain

Pain is the state in which an individual experiences and reports the presence of severe discomfort or an uncomfortable sensation.

The diagnostic category of pain concerns the phenomenon of pain and the nurse's role as a patient advocate in its management. Pain is an abstract concept; it is an invisible yet complex personal experience. Pain is defined by the International Association for the Study of Pain as "an unpleasant sensory and emotional experience associated with actual or potential tissue damage or described in terms of such a damage."[3]

Even in similar situations, the pain experience varies from individual to individual and includes sensory and affective components. It is described in terms of both the sensation of pain and the distress or degree of suffering that an individual experiences. Feldman[12] describes the total pain response as being "determined by such factors as threshold, tolerance, attention to pain, action of pain relievers, counterirritation measures (such as heat or cold), summation, expectations, and perceptions." These factors help determine an individual's perception of pain, response to the pain, effectiveness of the pain control measures, and tendency to report pain.

McCaffery[24] defines pain as "whatever the experiencing person says it is, existing whenever he says it does." Pain means different things to different people. An individual may have difficulty describing the pain to others because pain is a personal experience. Pain expression can be influenced by sex and cultural norms. Women in the United States are permitted to express their pain more freely than men. Individuals with chronic pain may learn to cover up their pain. Therefore, pain expression is not always an accurate indication of pain.

Pain is further described according to its duration. *Acute pain* is intense and generally lasts less than 6 months. It provides a warning to the individual of actual or potential tissue damage and resolves when healing occurs. *Chronic pain* is generally characterized by lasting longer than 6 months. The pain can be either continuous or intermittent and as intense as acute pain. Chronic pain does not serve as a warning of tissue damage (see Chronic Pain).

This discussion provides an overview of the pain phenomenon to address pain's wide spectrum.

Related Factors*

Injuring agents
- Biologic
  - Disease
  - Inflammation
  - Ischemia
- Chemical
  - Cytotoxic agents
  - Electrolyte imbalance
  - Endocrine dysfunction
  - Noxious agents
- Physical
  - Trauma
  - Temperature extremes
- Psychologic
  - Anxiety
  - Distress
  - Fear
  - Stress
  - Tension

*References 2, 5, 6, 17, 19, 22, 25, 27, 31.

Defining Characteristics*

Guarding, protective behavior
Hands placed over painful area
Autonomic response (with acute pain only); may have periods of physiologic adaptation and potential for shock:
- Diaphoresis
- Pallor
- Changes in blood pressure (accentuated in patients with hypovolemia and unstable hemodynamics), pulse rate, stroke volume, respiratory rate and depth, muscle tone
- Dry mouth
- Pupillary dilation

Change in appetite
Weight change
Fatigue
Preoccupation with pain
Self-focusing
Shortened attention span
Altered time perception

*References 4, 7, 14, 16-19, 25, 29, 31.

Impaired thought processes
Facial mask of pain (lackluster eyes), "beaten look," fixed or scattered movement, grimace
May or may not verbalize:
- Pain descriptors (may deny them)
- Fear, anxiety, anger, helplessness, depression, hopelessness, suicidal thoughts
- Hope that pain will end (or possibly that pain may persist, with chronic pain)
- Frustration at lack of treatment
- Increased irritability, feelings of being a burden, feelings of guilt, anger at others

Does not verbalize anger at caretakers when dependent
Disturbed sleep pattern with difficulty falling asleep; awakens from sleep because of pain
Altered ability to continue previous activities
Social isolation
Family or marital dissonance
Reduced sexual activity
Uses unproved remedies or visits "quacks"
Discontinues or reduces employment
Financially dependent on external sources if pain prolonged

Nursing Interventions*

Patient Goal	Nursing Intervention
Verbalize information about pain experience.	• Assess patient's pain status incorporating following information: Nurse and patient have perceptions of pain based on past experiences, cultural influences, and other factors. Patient may assume that nurse is aware of how patient is experiencing pain so may not readily offer information about it. Patients will provide honest information if they know that this information will be used to help control their pain. People need reassurance that their complaints of pain are believed and that nurse will continue to provide control interventions. Patient may not offer information about pain experience because of desire to be "good patient." Meaning of pain for each patient influences that person's response to pain. Pain can cause fatigue; therefore a complete pain assessment is not always practical. Eliciting information on changes since last pain assessment may help conserve patient's energy. • Incorporate following factors in assessment of patient's pain status: Location/characteristics Onset Frequency Intensity, using 0-5 scale: 0, not present; 5, very intense Quality Precipitating factors Effective pain control measures Ineffective pain control measures Desired interventions Pain expression style (stoic, verbal, crying, moaning) Movement (guarding, favoring posture) Muscle tone Emotional distress Impact on quality of life Effect of pain on daily activities Activities affected or eliminated because of pain Effect on sleep/wake pattern Effect on energy level

*References 1, 2, 6, 7, 10-12, 14, 16, 23, 25, 28, 29, 32-34.

Patient Goal	Nursing Intervention
	Effect on sexual activity Effect on relations with others Effect on feelings of self-worth Medication use Use of health care system
Identify strategies that eliminate or control pain.	• Explore strategies that have been successful in past. • Identify strategies that patient values as essential for pain reduction. • Assess patient's willingness to incorporate nonpharmaceutical pain control measures. • Instruct patient on pain reduction strategies as pain experience dictates (for short attention span in acute pain, give brief explanations; for chronic pain, provide more detail). • Administer medication per physician's orders and protocol using appropriate delivery system. Monitor effectiveness at frequent intervals. Graphically record pain assessment data. Provide physician with evidence of need to change medication. Provide or instruct patient in importance of regular doses around clock. Intervene at onset of pain. • Implement remaining strategies for this patient goal as indicated by patient condition and pain status. • Position for comfort. • Encourage attention to proper posture and alignment. • Immobilize or rest affected area. • Provide distraction. • Suggest and instruct patient in relaxation techniques: short simple techniques with nurse directing for acute pain; more complex techniques for chronic pain. • Help patient use imagery to the extent he or she is able to concentrate: use image patient has actually experienced; one at a time, and employ all senses. • Employ hypnotic strategies: Blocking awareness of pain Substitution of painful feeling Displacement of pain sensation • Use counterstimulation: pressure, massage, vibration, heat/cold, external analgesics, transcutaneous nerve stimulation. • Provide music therapy. • Pace activities and plan activities ahead of time. • Provide touch. • Attempt interventions several times before judging success. • Provide supportive environment. • Give positive suggestions regarding feelings of comfort. • Determine realistic pain control goals with patient. • Identify emotional responses from patient. • Assess which pain reduction strategies patient finds helpful. • Use several pain reduction strategies.
Identify and reduce activities that precipitate or enhance pain.	• Help patient to identify activities that may enhance or precipitate pain. • Discuss strategies to prevent or reduce precipitation or enhancement of pain. • Discuss strategies to avoid these activities within patient's life-style. • Encourage family members to help patient prevent precipitation of painful event. • Encourage patient to keep daily log to help identify other activities that precipitate or enhance pain.
Incorporate interventions to reduce or eliminate pain.	• Assess patient's ability to implement interventions into present life-style. • Discuss life-style modifications that may be necessary. • Assess patient's desire and ability to change these aspects of his or her life. • Help patient identify measures to implement life-style modifications. • Provide referrals or information on community resources.
Set realistic goals.	• Assess patient's ability to project realistically impact of pain in all areas of life. • Encourage patient to set priorities and plan ahead. • Ask patient to identify one or two realistic goals to achieve each day. • Discuss progress in goal attainment. • Teach patient that realistic goal setting can aid in reducing fatigue, anxiety, and depression. • Instruct patient in goal setting to normalize life-style and place pain on periphery of life.

Patient Goal	Nursing Intervention
Verbalize positive feelings about self.	• Assess patient's perception of his progress in goal attainment. • If patient is unable to return to work, help identify meaningful ways to fill time and promote positive feelings of self-worth during free hours. • Provide patient with positive reinforcement for activities focused away from pain. • Assist patient in developing normalizing strategies for activities encountered in daily life. • Educate patient on community resources for prevention or reduction of problems related to job retraining, financial assistance, etc. • Inform patient of importance of maintaining communication with all health professionals. • Assess need for referrals for family or individual counseling, financial needs, or sexual concerns. • Encourage gradual reentry into family, society, and work activities; set realistic goals for reentry. • Provide positive reinforcement for achievements. • Discuss patient and family feelings regarding role changes. • Assess patient's ability to identify strengths and weaknesses and to build on strengths.

Principles and Rationale for Nursing Interventions

Nursing interventions are derived from information elicited during pain assessment. The information may or may not give clues to the source of the pain. Knowing the etiology is helpful, but not essential, in selecting appropriate nursing interventions.

At times the nurse may be able to modify or act directly on the factors that cause pain. At other times, however, the etiology is unknown. The expected patient outcomes are appropriate for any individual in pain, but the emphasis may differ for patients in acute or chronic pain. The interventions are directed at achieving the expected patient outcomes and are not specific for either acute or chronic pain.

The pain assessment includes both subjective and objective data. The depth of the assessment varies according to the individual's pain status, the situation, setting, and the nurse's expertise. The frequency of the assessments varies according to individual needs. The data can be recorded on a flowsheet or a graph to identify trends. Some patients are able to assist in monitoring their pain and keeping a diary of their pain experience.

To treat pain effectively, the patient (and nurse) must be able to identify strategies that eliminate or control pain. Strategies that were effective in the past may be continued or adapted for the current situation, e.g., breathing techniques to aid in relaxation with a woman who has had Lamaze preparation before childbirth. How an individual copes with pain is usually enduring. The nurse should help the patient identify the style of pain coping he typically uses. This may help the individual understand why some strategies are more effective. Additional interventions can be tried and their effectiveness evaluated. The patient should be instructed that using several strategies allows more options and may provide better pain control.

A pain assessment flowsheet or a diary of pain kept by the patient will help to identify activities that precipitate or enhance pain. Nursing care should be planned when the patient feels the pain is best controlled. A subjective pain rating scale is helpful. A daily log will help patients identify pain-producing activities. The nurse and family can help the patient evaluate the significance of these activities to determine if they can be modified or eliminated.

Realistic goal setting is important for both acute and chronic pain. The goals related to acute pain have a shorter deadline. All goals should be realistic for the individual and measurable. The nurse and patient should mutually determine the goals and evaluate goal achievement regularly. Goals should be progressed as healing occurs and/or the patient begins to adjust to the pain. Goal progression is an essential component of coping with the chronic pain.

Pain affects all aspects of an individual's existence. There may be deterioration of relationships with significant others, resulting in social isolation and loss of support systems. Many feelings can occur as an individual attempts to cope with acute or chronic pain. Patients can be anxious, depressed, and angry all at the same time. Pain disrupts basic life activities that are essential for positive feelings about self. If the patient is able to perceive control over the pain and focus on aspects of life other than pain, a more positive view of self will prevail.

Evaluation

Patient Outcome	Data Indicating That Outcome is Reached
Identifies strategies that eliminate or control pain	Demonstrates ability to differentiate between strategies that are effective and ineffective Applies previous strategies that have controlled pain Uses variety of pain control strategies
Incorporates interventions to reduce or eliminate pain	Fatigue controlled Returns sleep pattern toward normal or adapts to changes in sleep pattern Returns activity toward normal or modifies activity to control pain

Patient Outcome	Data Indicating That Outcome is Reached
	Uses pain control strategies appropriately Attention span returned to or approaching prepain status Reduction or absence of guarding, protective behavior Verbalizes increased control over pain Social and family interactions approaching prepain status Incorporates life-style modifications Uses community resources or referrals appropriately
Sets realistic goals	Goals realistic for pain experience Sets priorities for achievement of goals Identifies short-term achievable goals and implements goal progression after accurate evaluation of previous goal attainment Moves toward resumption of previous life-stlye or modifies life-style according to limitations imposed by pain experience Able to control or reduce fatigue, anxiety, and depression
Verbalizes positive feelings about self	Builds on personal strengths Reenters family, society, and work activities at level consistent with pain experience No longer revolves life around pain experience Verbalizes increased control over self Incorporates effective coping strategies

Chronic Pain

Chronic pain is the state in which an individual experiences pain that continues for more than 6 months in duration.

Chronic pain may be associated with a disease or injury but has continued beyond the normal healing time. In some cases the pain may be caused by progressive or destructive disease processes (cancer, arthritis). Sometimes the pain does not have an identifiable cause. It is important to remember that even though a cause is not identified, the pain still exists. Individuals with chronic pain may not show outward evidence of pain. The patient's subjective statements about pain need to be assessed.

Chronic pain can be continuous or intermittent and can be as intense as acute pain. Habituation of the autonomic response occurs so that the fight-or-flight response is no longer present. Chronic pain does not serve as a warning of tissue danger. In rheumatoid arthritis, for example, joint pain may still be present when the disease process is no longer active because of the structural damage that has already occurred in the joint. The reason for some forms of chronic pain may not be known. Chronic pain does not necessarily serve a purpose. Fortin (in Kim et al.[12]) provides a vivid description of the effects of chronic pain:

> Eventually the debilitating effects of the chronic pain experience and loss of coping reserves alters the individual's perceptions, personality and social functioning. As the person changes, the environment to which he responds changes; that is, personal variability in pain sensation and psychophysiologic responses become intrinsically woven into the situational milieu. Problems of altered self-esteem, social identity, changes in roles and social interaction, and the responses that feed back into the problems, depression, anxiety, and irritability become integral to the chronic pain experience.

Fortin suggests a beginning model for viewing chronic pain. Acute pain has traditionally been viewed from a sensory-reactive model, which does not encompass the chronic pain experience. Fortin uses the gate control theory to depict the psychophysiologic aspects of pain and describes the psychosocial aspects using an interactional approach. Viewing these models together, Fortin has reformulated a model for describing chronic pain and defines the model as (Kim et al.[12]):

> an integrated pattern of sensory, sentience and interactive components. Sensory refers to the quality and intensity of the pain sensation. Sentience refers to the motivational and affective qualities of the experience. Interactive refers to the simultaneous interaction between the individual and the environment. It is suggested that in the experience of chronic pain, these forces act collectively to repattern the person and the environment in a transactional process.

Related Factors[4,13]

Disbelief of others that pain exists
Lack of support systems
Fear about addiction
Monotony
Fatigue
Lack of knowledge about pain control measures
Poor self-concept
Past experiences of poor pain control
Overactivity
Helplessness/hopelessness
Overweight

Defining Characteristics

Verbal report or observed evidence of pain experienced for more than 6 months

Guarding, protective movements
Habituation of autonomic response
Change in appetite
Weight changes
Fatigue
Preoccupation with pain
Self-focusing
Shortened attention span
Altered time perception
Impaired thought processes

Nursing Interventions*

Patient Goal	Nursing Intervention
Verbalize information about pain experience.	• Assess patient's pain status (see Pain). • Incorporate factors in assessment of patient's pain status (see Pain).
Identify strategies that control pain.	• See Pain. • Implement remaining strategies for this patient goal as indicated by patient condition and pain status. • Provide therapeutic positioning. • Encourage attention to proper posture and alignment. • Rest affected area. • Provide distraction. • Instruct patient in relaxation techniques or guided imagery. • Use hypnotic strategies. • Provide music therapy. • Use counterstimulation: pressure, massage, vibration, heat/cold, external analgesics, transcutaneous nerve stimulator. • Pace activities and plan activities ahead of time. • Provide touch. • Attempt interventions several times before judging success. • Provide supportive environment. • Determine realistic pain control goals with patient. • Identify emotional responses from patient. • Assess which pain reduction strategies patient finds helpful. • Use several pain reduction strategies.
Identify activities that enhance pain.	• Help patient to identify activities that may enhance pain. • Discuss strategies to reduce enhancement of pain. • Discuss strategies to avoid these activities within patient's life-style. • Encourage family members to help patient prevent enhancing painful event. • Encourage patient to keep daily log to help identify other activities that enhance pain.
Incorporate interventions to reduce pain.	• See Pain.
Set realistic goals.	• Assess patient's ability to project realistically impact of pain in all areas of life. • Teach patient to discriminate between pain that is normal and pain that is abnormal. • Encourage patient to set priorities and plan ahead. • Ask patient to identify one or two realistic goals to achieve each day. • Discuss progress in goal attainment. • Teach patient that realistic goal setting can aid in reducing fatigue, anxiety, and depression. • Instruct patient in goal setting to normalize life-style and place pain on periphery of life. • Use quota-setting principles for achieving exercise goals when behavioral barriers exist.
Verbalize positive feelings about self.	• Assess patient's perception of progress toward goal attainment. • If patient unable to return to work, help identify meaningful ways to fill time and promote positive feelings of self-worth. • Reinforce behaviors that decrease the risk of medical, social, and financial problems. • Provide patient with positive reinforcement for activities focused away from pain. • Assist patient in developing normalizing strategies for activities encountered in daily life. • Educate patient on community resources for prevention or reduction of problems related to job retraining and financial assistance. • Inform patient of importance of maintaining communications with all health professionals. • Assess need for referrals for family or individual counseling, financial needs, or sexual concerns.

*References 3-5, 7-11, 13-25.

Patient Goal	Nursing Intervention
	• Encourage gradual reentry into family, society, and work activities; set realistic goals for reentry. • Assist patient in effective transition to retirement if work is no longer a realistic option. • Use support groups. • Provide positive reinforcement for achievements. • Discuss patient and family feelings regarding role changes. • Assess patient's ability to identify strengths and weaknesses and to build on strengths. • Implement appropriate activity/exercise plan for physical condition. • Assess feelings regarding pain, suffering, and spiritual well-being. • Encourage open communication between patient and family. • Help patient and family understand effects of pain experience on each family member. • Reinforce each person's role in helping patient cope with pain experience.
Avoid use of life-threatening, unproven remedies.	• Inform patient and family about identification of unproven remedies. • Instruct patient in dangers of unproven remedies: they can be life threatening, expensive, and can serve as a substitute for ongoing health care. • Assist patient in exploring feelings regarding unproven remedies. • Counsel patient in determining how to respond to individuals who suggest unproven remedies. • Provide patient with community resources to assist in identification of unproven remedies. • Do not remove unharmful unproven remedies from patient (patient may have faith in this remedy not found in other treatments).
Maintain weight or move toward normal weight index for height and frame.	• Instruct patient about effects of pain on nutrition and influence of proper nutrition on health status. • Instruct patient on need for balanced diet to maintain ideal weight for height and frame. • Obtain dietitian referral. • Assess motivation toward obtaining proper nutrition and achievement of ideal weight. • If underweight for height and frame, refer to Altered Nutrition: Less Than Body Requirements. • If overweight for height and frame, refer to Altered Nutrition: More Than Body Requirements.

Principles and Rationale for Nursing Interventions

To determine which interventions should be incorporated into the nursing care plan, the nurse must first consider the pain assessment information and relate this to current knowledge derived from pain theories. The pain assessment information may or may not give clues to the source of pain. Knowing the related factors is helpful in selecting appropriate interventions. Since pain is a subjective experience perceived by the individual, the nurse must elicit information from the patient about the pain experience. The frequency of assessment is individualized.

To treat pain, the patient must be able to identify strategies that are effective in controlling pain. Any previously used interventions that were effective in controlling this pain should be continued. Interventions unfamiliar to the patient should also be attempted and assessed using a subjective rating scale. Using more than one intervention may provide better pain control.

Activities that enhance pain should be identified. By keeping a daily diary of activities and pain ratings, the patient may be able to identify pain enhancers. Once identified, methods to modify or reduce the activity can be explored. The importance of the activity to the individual should be addressed. If the activity has little meaning or value, the patient may readily avoid it, but interventions are needed to maintain the activity if it is meaningful to the person.

Throughout the pain management process, realistic goal setting is important. Goals should be mutually determined by the patient and nurse. Goals should be measurable and achievable. After achievement, another goal is identified. Goal progression continues until the final outcome is reached. Frequently a multidisciplinary team is working with the patient in chronic pain. All team members should be aware of established goals so that all goals are consistent in working toward the final outcome and the health care regimens required for goal attainment remain realistic.

The patient may acquire a positive view of self as he perceives control over pain and is able to focus on aspects of life other than pain. At this point, nonpain behaviors are reinforced. The patient focuses on relationships with family, friends, work, society, and God. The individual takes self-responsibility for pain management and learns to use the health care system appropriately.

The use of unproven remedies poses a special problem for persons with chronic pain. Individuals need to feel comfortable discussing their use of unproven remedies. The nurse can provide comfort by remaining nonjudgmental. The nurse needs to provide information about the expense of some forms of unproven remedies and that some forms may be life threatening. The patient can then make informed decisions. It can be easy to reject current health care when pain relief is not found and an unproven remedy proclaims pain relief abilities.

Weight problems frequently occur when chronic pain is present. Many patients find that loss of appetite occurs during severe episodes of pain. If a patient has decreased mobility, yet appetite is unchanged, he is at risk of gaining weight. Interventions for weight problems should be implemented as early as possible.

Chronic pain is multidimensional. It affects every aspect of life and the significant individuals in the person's life. Interventions are geared toward improving the quality of life through pain control.

Evaluation

Patient Outcome	Data Indicating That Outcome is Reached
Identifies strategies that control pain Incorporates interventions to reduce pain Sets realistic goals Verbalizes positive feelings about self	See evaluation for Pain.
Avoids use of life-threatening, unproven remedies	Identifies dangers of life-threatening, unproven remedies Verbalizes knowledge of resources to assist in identification of unproven remedies Seeks support to avoid using life-threatening, unproven remedies Maintains contact with health care system
Maintains weight at or moves toward normal weight index for height	Incorporates strategies for weight gain or weight loss Uses resources within family, community, and health care agency as warranted Adjusts weight to identified goal

Sensory/Perceptual Alterations (Specify) (Visual, Auditory, Kinesthetic, Gustatory, Tactile, Olfactory)

Sensory/perceptual alterations (visual, auditory, kinesthetic, gustatory, tactile, olfactory) is the state in which an individual experiences a change in the amount or patterning of incoming stimuli accompanied by a diminished, exaggerated, distorted, or impaired response to such stimuli.

Understanding the definition of sensory/perceptual alteration is enhanced by viewing and defining the concept of perception. The following definition is stated as a serial order of emergent behaviors. This technique is described as a method for defining abstract concepts.[9]

An individual with physiologic, psychologic, and sociocultural sets who has certain assumptions, motivations, and expectations encounters a concrete situation.

Stimuli bombard one or more of the sense organs. Categories of senses:

Exteroreceptors (distance senses)

1. Vision
2. Audition

Proprioceptors (near senses)

1. Tactile sense
2. Taste (gustatory)
3. Smell (olfactory)

Interoceptors (deep senses)

1. Kinesthetic (muscle, bone, joint sense)
2. Vestibular (sense of balance)
3. Visceral (hollow organ sense)

Sense organs transduce the stimuli (transduction is the sensory transformation of raw stimulus data into informational messages/nerve impulses).

Nerve impulses are relayed to the brain and reticular activating system (RAS), which creates an arousal state.

Impulses are automatically forwarded, or impulses are selected, reorganized, and modified based on perceptual set, past experience, present needs, and future goals and then forwarded (transformation).

Meaningful impulses are integrated, and a percept is formed.

The resulting percept may have a direct or indirect effect on subsequent emotions and behavior.

An alteration in sensory perception occurs when an interruption occurs at or during one or more of the steps set forth in the operational definition. The extent and severity of the alteration depend on the point or points of interruption and the etiologic nature of the interruption. The classification of related factors also spells out persons at risk for an alteration in sensory perception.

Related Factors[6]

- Altered environments (excessive or insufficient stimuli)
  - Therapeutically restricted (isolation, intensive care, bed rest, traction, continuing illness, incubator)
  - Socially restricted (institutionalization, homebound, aging, chronic illness, dying, infant deprivation)
  - Stigmatized (mentally ill, retarded, handicapped)
  - Bereaved
- Altered sensory reception, transmission, or integration
  - Neurologic disease, trauma, or deficit
  - Altered states of sense organs
  - Inability to communicate, understand, speak, or respond
  - Sleep deprivation
  - Pain
- Chemical alteration
  - Endogenous (electrolyte imbalance, elevated blood urea nitrogen, elevated ammonia, hypoxia)
  - Exogenous (central nervous system stimulants/depressants, mind-altering drugs)
- Extreme anxiety or panic (narrowed perceptual fields caused by anxiety)

Defining Characteristics[3,5,6,10]

- Changes in thought processes
  - Disorientation in time, place, or person
  - Disordered sequencing in thought, time, or events
  - Altered abstraction or conceptualization
  - Change in problem-solving abilities
  - Bizarre thinking
  - Hallucinations
  - Hypersuggestibility
- Changes in attention span
  - Diminished concentration
  - Daydreaming
  - Restlessness
  - Increased distractibility
  - Inability to follow flow of conversation
- Emotional lability
  - Rapid mood swings
  - Exaggerated responses
  - Ambivalence
  - Apathy
  - Flat affect
  - Emotional detachment
  - Anger
  - Depression
  - Fear
  - Irritability
  - Anxiety
- Changes in routine patterns or habits
  - Change in behavior pattern
  - Change in response to stimuli
  - Altered communication patterns
  - Change in sleeping patterns
  - Altered eating habits
- Changes in sensory capabilities
  - Vision
    - Diminished visual capacity
    - Visual distortion
    - Photosensitivity
  - Audition
    - Hypersensitivity/hyposensitivity
    - Auditory distortion
    - Distortion of verbal messages
  - Tactile sense
    - Hyperesthesias/hypoesthesias
    - Inability to tell nature of object by touch
  - Taste
    - Increased taste sensitivity
    - Diminished sense of taste
    - Altered taste sense
    - Loss of appetite
  - Smell
    - Diminished sense of smell
    - Hypersensitivity to odor
    - Distortion of odor
  - Kinesthetic sense
    - Motor incoordination
    - Inability to tell where body parts are located
    - Paralysis
    - Muscular weakness, flaccidity, rigidity
    - Surgical joint replacement
  - Vestibular sense
    - Diminished sense of balance
  - Visceral sense
    - Feelings of emptiness, hollowness
- Presence of any of related factors associated with diagnosis
- Changes in percept characteristics
  - Distortion of color, hue, intensity, light, or size
  - Distortion of environment
  - Growth of inanimate objects
  - Failure to notice stimuli
  - Disregard of normally "important" percepts

Nursing Interventions

Patient Goal	Nursing Intervention
Prevention	
Enhance ability to identify factors that increase risk for sensory/perceptual alteration.	• Assess patient for risks and potential risks for alteration (see related factors). Present resulting risk profile to patient when possible.
Identify ways to reduce risks of alteration.	• Provide strategies for reduction or elimination of identified related factors (e.g., altering sleep pattern to reduce sleep deprivation; altering drug habits; rearranging environment).
Identify stimuli needed for daily functioning.	• Explore source, type, amount, and patterns of stimuli needed by patient for optimum functioning.
Identify methods for maintaining adequate stimuli in environment.	• Provide strategies for maintaining adequate amounts of meaningful stimuli in identified therapeutically or socially restricted environments (e.g., introducing pattern and structure in environment, orienting features, noise control, presence of familiar objects and persons).
Acute Care[1-4,13,14]	
Prevent injury.	• Maintain safety precautions (bed rails up, bed lowered, sharp objects out of reach, call bell in reach).
Decrease or eliminate presence of defining characteristics.	• Restore sensory/perceptual function by implementing following interventions. • Assess stimuli present in environment: intensity, quantity, quality, repetitiveness, movement, change, novelty, incongruity, clarity, and ambiguity. • Alter environmental factors to increase meaningful stimuli and decrease extraneous stimuli: Use orienting features (e.g., clocks, calendars, windows, name tags, favorite objects). Maintain verbal contact, eye contact, and touch. Reduce unnecessary traffic, personnel, and noise. Structure routines. Structure input by giving clear, concise explanations of surroundings, treatments, and procedures. Allow frequent short visits by significant others. • Orient to reality: Address by name; introduce self frequently; regularly state time and place. Explain and allow participation when possible in all tasks and treatments. Interpret sights, sounds, and smells present in environment. Explain routines and policies. • Obtain feedback or perception of events and objects; clarify misperceptions. • Assist in clarifying reality (see Altered Thought Processes for more detailed intervention with hallucinations and delusions).
Chronic Care[3,5,7,10,11]	
Maintain orientation to surroundings.	• Use reality orientation techniques: Address by name; orient to time. Point out surroundings; identify self. Structure input with concrete, concise explanations. Maintain eye contact. Reinforce behavior that is reality oriented (e.g., responding to meaningful comments). • Provide meaningful stimuli and reduce extraneous stimuli in environment: Keep clocks and calendars in view; make use of windows and outdoors. Observe holidays and significant occasions. Provide structured routines. Place familiar objects in plain sight. Structure experiences that make use of all senses.
Increase appropriate social interaction.	• Arrange physical environment to encourage interaction (open spaces, circles instead of rows); increase mobility with wheelchairs, walkers, carts, etc. • Encourage exploration of surroundings; encourage verbalization of experiences, desires, and thoughts. • Set up interactions with others in structural settings with defined purpose. • Encourage reminiscence. • Encourage decision making. • Use small group sessions to widen interaction.

Principles and Rationale for Nursing Interventions

Perceptual adequacy and accuracy are necessary prerequisites to enable nurses and patients to engage in mutual goal setting and exploration of means for goal achievement.

The nursing diagnostic category Sensory/Perceptual Alterations is an encompassing one. Alterations range from mild to severe; manifestations can be acute or chronic; age of affected persons ranges from infancy to old age. Thus many specific nursing interventions depend on individual patient characteristics, identified related factors for a particular patient, and defining characteristics for the patient.

Nursing care is divided into three major modes: prevention, acute care, and chronic care. Prevention requires careful assessment of the patient's environment for risk factors. Patient education plays a major role. Once a pattern of defining characteristics appears and a diagnosis of sensory/perceptual alteration is made, the alteration may be classified as acute or chronic.

Acute alterations tend to be abrupt in onset and temporary in nature. The degree of alteration is usually severe and dramatic in presentation of defining characteristics (e.g., sudden confusion and disorientation, rapid large mood swings, bizarre behavior). Etiologies for acute alterations include trauma, drug intoxication, sudden sensory loss (blindness, deafness), acute pain, panic, and placement in intensive care units or recovery rooms.

Chronic alterations are progressive in onset and are subject to recurrence because of the long-term or permanent nature of the related factors. The degree of alteration may range from mild to severe, and defining characteristics may be subtle and ambiguous. When chronic alterations are left untreated, defining characteristics become more clear-cut and overt. Etiologies for chronic alterations typically include socially restricted environments (e.g., nursing homes, children's homes, prisons), declining sensory equipment, neurologic disease, chronic pain, prolonged immobility, social isolation, and chronic illness.

In all cases the ultimate goal is to promote, maintain, and restore optimum contact with reality. Nursing interventions are aimed at preventing, reducing, or eliminating related factors and defining characteristics.

Evaluation

Patient Outcome	Data Indicating That Outcome is Reached
Prevention	
Identifies related factors	States related factors Recognizes self-risk profile
Identifies risk reduction methods	States or demonstrates use of strategies for reduction or elimination of identified risk factors
Identifies daily stimulus needs	States source, type, amount, and patterns of usual daily stimulation Recounts life-style and role patterns
Identifies stimulus maintenance methods	Verbalizes or demonstrates use of strategies for maintaining and altering environment Lists changes planned for or already made
Acute Care	
No injury sustained	No physical or reported evidence of injury
Decrease in or elimination of defining characteristics	Increased ability to test reality Orientation to person, place, and time Absence of hallucinations and delusions Stabilization of emotions Increased participation in care Accurate perception of stimulus input, as evidenced by verbal feedback and appropriate behavior Appropriate responses to environment Absence of bizarre behavior Increased decision-making and problem-solving abilities Lowered anxiety levels
Chronic Care	
Oriented to surroundings	Oriented to person, time, and place Can recall past and present events Can verbalize future plans No evidence of confusion Communicates meaningfully; responds appropriately to questions and cues; initiates interaction
Increases appropriate social interaction	Increases interaction time Makes interaction meaningful

Patient Outcome	Data Indicating That Outcome is Reached
	Verbalizes about time spent with others Verbalizes plans for future outings and social times Verbalizes choices for dyadic and group plans

 Unilateral Neglect

Unilateral neglect is the state in which an individual is perceptually unaware of and inattentive to one side of the body.

Associated with brain damage on the contralateral side, most often right cerebral hemisphere lesions (e.g., cerebrovascular accidents[9]), unilateral neglect is frequently accompanied by hemiplegia, hemiparesis, or hemianopia.[3,10]

The patient typically fails to complete one side of drawings, dress or groom the affected side of the body, or eat food from one half of a tray and may not respond to commands from someone standing in the unattended space.[1,2,14] In more severe forms patients may not realize that they are paralyzed or may not recognize their own limbs on the affected side.[2,12]

Although manifestations of unilateral neglect tend to be most pronounced in the first few weeks following the cerebral damage, some deficits may persist for months or years.[7] Symptoms tend to resolve slowly and may complicate patient rehabilitation.[4] Certainly the behavior of patients with unilateral neglect presents a challenge for nursing management.

Related Factors[3,6,8,10]

Effects of disturbed perceptual abilities, e.g., hemianopia
One-sided blindness
Neurologic illness or trauma
Hemianesthesia
Hemiparesis
Hemiplegia
Anosognosia

Defining Characteristics[2,3,8,11,12]

Consistent inattention to stimuli on affected side
Inadequate self-care
Absence of positioning or safety precautions in regard to affected side
Does not look toward affected side
Leaves food on plate on affected side
Does not recognize limbs on affected side as belonging to self
Fails to complete drawings (drawing does not include affected side)

Nursing Interventions*

Patient Goal	Nursing Intervention
Have realistic awareness of perceptual deficit.	• Explain to patient that one side is being neglected; repeat as needed. • Encourage patient to share perceptions. • Provide realistic feedback.
Be protected from injury.	• Provide safe environment: Regularly orient patient to environment. Remove excess furniture and equipment. Provide good lighting. Place call bell and frequently used objects on unaffected side within easy reach. Keep side rail up on affected side. • Supervise or assist to transfer and ambulate: Protect neglected side during activities; teach patient to assume this responsibility. Teach patient to check position of limbs on affected side to prevent unfelt trauma. • Note perceptual deficit on patient record and in patient's room to inform caregivers.
Demonstrate decrease in deficit and/or adaptation to deficit.	• Assess regularly for degree of deficit and adaptation to deficit. • Assess contributing factors.
Acquire knowledge and skill in adaptive coping with deficit.	• *Initially,* assist compensation for perceptual deficit by arranging environment within patient's perceptual field, e.g., place frequently used items on unaffected side. • *After initial stress,* promote conscious attention to neglected side: Place frequently used items on affected side. Position patient so affected side is in view. Talk to patient from affected side.

*References 2, 4, 5, 7, 8, 12-14.

Patient Goal	Nursing Intervention
	• Spend time with patient manipulating affected side and encouraging patient to use it. Have patient handle ignored limbs with unaffected side. Increase stimulation to affected side by touching or massage with scented lotion. Use visual and verbal communication regarding limb placement on affected side. • Teach patient to scan affected side. • Place clock or some frequently used item on side of deficit to help establish pattern of scanning. • Use "cueing" to affected side to increase awareness of that side: Mark red line in margin of books on affected side. Attach small bells to limbs of affected side. • Place food tray toward unaffected side. • Teach patient to rotate plate periodically. • Encourage patient to perform activities of daily living (ADLs), e.g., toothbrushing in front of mirror. Supervise and give feedback. • Decrease confusing stimuli: Avoid relocation. Maintain constancy of caregivers and consistent routine for self-care. Explain procedures and treatment well in advance. • Include family in rehabilitation process so that they understand, support, and can continue it in home environment.

Principles and Rationale for Nursing Interventions

Initially, nursing management for the patient with unilateral neglect is oriented toward provision of safety and assistance in developing a realistic awareness of the perceptual deficit. Structuring the environment to decrease hazards is essential for the patient who typically ignores or underestimates the disability during this period.[7,14] An established plan of care and assistance with ADLs by consistent caregivers can do much to decrease the confusion and disorientation that results from distortions in perception.[13] The nurse can assist the patient to understand and acknowledge the condition by encouraging the patient to share perceptions and by providing realistic feedback in response.

Active rehabilitation focuses on decreasing the deficit and increasing the patient's ability to manage self-care. This is accomplished by helping the patient organize and interpret his experiences and environment. Verbal and visual cues to decrease neglect of the affected side have demonstrated effectiveness in enhancing perceptual functioning.[7,12] An environment that provides high levels of meaningful sensory stimulation is also effective.[5,7] Specific activities that involve attention directed to the affected side can increase awareness and use of that side.[2] Involvement of the family in the rehabilitation process facilitates their understanding and support in both hospital and home environments.

Evaluation[5,7,8,13]

Patient Outcome	Data Indicating That Outcome is Reached
Reduction or resolution of deficit	Absence or reduction of defining characteristics indicating presence of unilateral neglect
Realistic awareness of perceptual deficit	Verbalization of realistic estimation of degree of deficit; does not ignore or underestimate
Protection from injury	Accidents prevented or minimized No physical or reported evidence of injury
Adequate knowledge and skill in adaptive coping strategies	Responds to verbal and/or visual cues to decrease neglect of affected side; scans and protects affected side Compensates for perceptual loss Demonstrates increased participation and independence in ADLs Verbalizes feeling of progress in regard to perceptual deficit

 Knowledge Deficit (Specify)

Knowledge deficit is the state in which specific information is lacking.

Knowledge deficit has been defined as an inability to state or explain information or demonstrate a required skill related to disease management procedures, practices, or self-care health management.[2] Knowledge deficit occurs frequently, usually for one of four reasons:

1. The patient may have entered a new health condition (e.g., pregnancy), be undergoing newly prescribed treatments or diagnostic tests, be taking new medications, or beginning a new developmental phase (e.g., adolescence, parenthood, old age). If one has not experienced these states before or learned about them from others in the culture, knowledge deficit is possible.

2. Some patients may not have access to information or know where to seek it; others may have providers who are not interested in teaching them or whom they cannot understand because of cultural or language differences. This lack of an open, information-flowing relationship with a provider often exacerbates inevitably misinterpreting information or forgetting it because of disuse or lack of reinforcement for correct use.

3. Temporary or permanent deficits in ability to learn often have a physiologic base and may preclude removal of knowledge deficits through instructional means. High blood urea nitrogen concentration, low oxygenation of the blood, chemical substances (e.g., alcohol, drugs), brain damage from trauma or cerebrovascular accident, mental retardation, or to a lesser extent fatigue are examples, as are limitations caused by immature developmental stage.

4. Lack of motivation to learn, often accompanied by anxiety and coupled with lack of adherence to a health care regimen, is another typical reason for knowledge deficit.

The standard by which to judge the adequacy of knowledge (and thus absence of a deficit) is changing rapidly as more self-care is required, not only to assist those with chronic illness, but also to contain health care costs in general and to maintain patients in their normal social settings. Sometimes knowledge deficit is defined by a legal standard, as in informed consent. It also must be noted that knowledge is the lowest level of cognitive learning—recalling or remembering information as opposed to applying and synthesizing information in problem solving. In general, it has been found that removal of knowledge deficits is insufficient for most significant health behavior changes. Attitudinal change, a higher level of understanding, and practiced behavioral sequences with adequate reinforcement are necessary. Much health teaching is still knowledge oriented, probably because it is much easier to teach information than it is to change behavior.

Related Factors

Need to make sense of life-threatening diseases
Underdeveloped or inappropriate cognitive level
Low level of formal education, possibly including illiteracy
Lack of orientation to future
Lack of emotional stability in patient, family, or environment, often linked to chaotic or irresponsible behavior
Inadequate economic resources
Irrational beliefs
Lack of belief in efficacy of treatment
Denial regarding diagnosis
Ineffective coping regarding diagnosis or treatment
Inadequate self-confidence
Self-defeating attitudes
Impaired practitioner/patient communication
Depression and excessive anxiety
Fantasies that one is immune from harm; denial of need for knowledge
Altered locus of control
Social isolation restricting sources of information
Lack of awareness by health care providers of body of knowledge important to patients
Lack of appropriate cultural focus in available information
For patients on ongoing regimen, past experiences and learning, including misinformation
New stressor in patient's life
Impairment of neurologic and perceptual functioning; abnormal physiology regarding blood oxygenation or clearance of waste products from body; impaired thinking caused by drugs and/or alcohol
In community, lack of access to information, self-defeating attitudes, lack of a custom, or lack of open communication between health care providers and patients

Defining Characteristics

Verbalization of problem, which can point out lack of knowledge or perception of inability to cope
Inaccurate or no follow-through of instructions
Inadequate performance of test or task
Inappropriate or exaggerated behaviors (e.g., hysterical, hostile, agitated, apathetic)
Occurrence of preventable and undesired event (e.g., premature readmission)
Inability to make decision about own care
Not seeking needed services
Infant or child not meeting developmental norms because of actions of caregiver
Living with a health problem, below level of potential wellbeing
Overdependence on others for self-care
Request for information
Inability to repeat and comprehend correctly information taught
Inability to demonstrate correctly skills previously taught
Inability to care for self after discharge

Nursing Interventions

Patient Goal	Nursing Intervention
Increase knowledge or decrease cognitive deficit in such areas as self-care; decision making regarding health; enhancing life processes such as birth, development, and death; and activities related to health care regimens.	• Check that communities and institutions provide freely available information through reading materials, hotlines, mass media, health fairs at work sites and schools, etc. • At every provider/patient interaction, assess for knowledge deficit. • Talk to patient's significant other to obtain evidence of knowledge deficit. • Use patient's theories about his illness as a starting point for teaching, and continually seek patient's perceptions. • During interactions, check frequently to see if patient understands. • See if patient accepts diagnosis. • Simplify information to conform to patient's terms, thought patterns, and daily routines. • Give explicit directions. • Be accessible to patient when he has a question; this may require new structures of care (e.g., a diabetes education center). • Demonstrate to patient and family how to use information. • Reinforce correct use of information, and ensure that others in patient's natural environment do the same. • Teach patient how to set up system of cues in the environment to remember health actions. • Teach patient how to rehearse mentally a necessary health action. • Teach patient how to use rewards for positive health behaviors. • Call patient to remind him, show support, and see if he has questions. • Make certain patient is actively involved in decisions about own care. • Provide opportunities for patient to gain sense of control over illness. • Offer peer support network and opportunity for patient to watch others successfully mastering health care problems. • Ask patient if he is satisfied with care. • Use practice of knowledge and skill, perhaps with role playing, until patient feels confident and has met the standard. • Use special teaching approaches to deal with neurologic learning deficits. • After procedure, offer opportunity for reflection about what happened. • Provide instruction in multiple modalities (visual, experimental, written, discussion) so that patient will remember it in various ways. • Provide materials for patient to take so that he can review and use the new knowledge. • Provide motivators by appealing to patient's interests and future uses of new knowledge.
Become a self-sufficient user and obtainer of health care knowledge.	• Teach with a questioning, discussion, application of knowledge, and feedback approach. • Teach patient and family to use self-care protocols and instructional packages when appropriate. • Teach patient how to find and use sources of knowledge and social support in the community. • If available, help patient learn to use computerized monitoring systems (e.g., those providing diabetic persons with running summary of food and medication requirements met for the day).

Principles and Rationale for Nursing Interventions

Essentially all evidence of knowledge deficit is more or less indirect. With assessment, the nurse sets up situations in which the quality of the inference obtained from verbalizations or behaviors is as strong and direct as possible: ask the patient directly or set up an unobtrusive test. Since most meaningful health behaviors require knowledge, motivation, and skill, it is important in the assessment to seek evidence in each of these areas to obtain as complete a diagnosis as possible. This means data gathered must be both objective, to determine adequacy of present knowledge and behaviors, and subjective, which is the source of crucial information about the patient's motivation, sense of self-efficacy, frame of reference, and cognitive schemata.

A diagnosis of knowledge deficit means the evidence gathered does not meet the standard of adequate knowledge. However, the nurse must be certain that the standard is justified and that the nurse intends to provide an opportunity for the patient to learn.

In general, nursing goals include helping the patient attain the knowledge and skills needed through the teaching and learning process. This includes assessing readiness, planning realistic goals, developing a teaching plan using appropriate multiple verbal, behavioral, and audiovisual instructional strategies, and evaluation of learning and reteaching when necessary.[4]

Active involvement of the patient is essential, as is practice of the thoughts and behaviors to be learned. For many, psychologic support and follow-up are important, along with a feeling of personal reward, sometimes developed through a contract with the provider, and involvement of the family. Instruction provides models for behavior, cues for correct responses, corrective feedback, and problem-solving strategies.

Social support provides an opportunity for patients to clarify their situation and obtain new information. It also helps in development of a cognitive schema, or way of conceptualizing their situation, and ways of coping that they had not considered. Teaching is not only a focused intervention to deal with a particular knowledge deficit. It is also an integral part of the everyday provider/patient relationship, with the goal of making patients independent regarding health in their natural environments.

Patient education usually cannot assist with development of basic learning skills. In this day of required self-care, however, it is important to help patients become as independent as possible in recognizing and resolving their own knowledge deficits. The questioning, discussing, application, and feedback approach is most likely to develop not only knowledge but greater satisfaction, improved compliance, more complete learning, and ability to think about the problem or goal.

Learning in health care settings as they exist at present has many constraints for adequate knowledge and skill development. This has occurred in part because what was reimbursed and therefore rewarded were medical procedures, not adapted patients. At the same time it is clearly possible to alter delivery of care so that teaching and learning are expected and rewarded components of care and consistent over sufficient periods so that complex learning can occur. Diabetes education and detection centers and oncology centers are examples of these new organizations of services in which education and learning are central. Also, examples of tools used for assessment can be found in various sources, e.g., knowledge and behavior assessment in diabetes,[1] assessment of self-efficacy in diabetes,[3] and assessment of patient management of an asthma episode.[5]

Evaluation

Patient Outcome	Data Indicating That Outcome is Reached
Adequate knowledge and skill to support needed self-care activities, including procedures, medications, when to seek care, and use of appropriate community resources	Has adequate knowledge to carry out health care regimen Can explain how and why to take action or perform skill Takes appropriate action when necessary and can explain appropriate reasoning process Uses knowledge to lessen discomfort and side effects and enhance efficacy of medical and nursing procedures and treatments Can function on health regimen with minimum guidance from health care practitioner for appropriate period
Use of knowledge in health care decision satisfactory to patient (e.g., whether to have surgery, what types of regimens are agreeable)	Can describe how to assess benefits and costs of particular health action Can describe why decision was made; is prepared to follow through with required treatment activities Has accurate expectations of likely outcomes of health care actions
Knowledge of how to guide own and others' development in area of health	Monitors body and mental state for signs and symptoms of illness Acts on basis of realistic expectations in guiding development of self and others
Competent to carry out health care activities necessary to well-being	Can describe how to use verified health knowledge in daily living Moves ahead to take health actions when satisfied they are worthwhile Decrease in symptoms and indicators of disease state and increase in indicators of health
Knowledge to cope adequately with health stresses	Knows where to obtain sources of health care information efficiently and does so when needed Can describe problem-solving process to deal successfully with injury, threatening diagnosis, or persistent symptom, including what is causative and what is controllable Describes how action met personal standards of adequate coping Develops sense of mastery and self-efficacy regarding particular health behavior Avoids overreactions, feelings of helplessness, and depression caused by inadequate knowledge and skill

Altered Thought Processes

Altered thought processes is the state in which an individual experiences a disruption in cognitive operations and activities.

As nursing diagnoses, altered thought processes and sensory/perceptual alterations are closely aligned. Many of the defining characteristics and nursing interventions are similar. This is to be expected because perception and thought are both higher-order cognitive processes. Because the two processes are internal and highly interrelated, an alteration in either process is likely to produce an alteration in the other. (See Sensory/Perceptual Alterations.)

Carpenito[2] makes a distinction between the two diagnoses on the basis of etiology. She states that sensory/perceptual alterations result from environmental, sensory, physical, or motor alterations. Altered thought processes are seen as stemming from personality and mental disorders. This may serve as a viable distinction, although it should be noted that both diagnoses share some common ground (e.g., chemical alteration). Based on this distinction, Carpenito[2] offers the following definition of altered thought processes: "A state in which an individual experiences a disruption in such mental activities as conscious thought, reality orientation, problem-solving, judgment, and comprehension related to coping disorders."

A disruption in thought processes, whether in the area of comprehension, judgment, memory, problem solving, or other aspects, creates a disruption in the way one perceives reality. Thus one's thinking processes become non-reality-based, the critical defining characteristic for this nursing diagnosis. Additional defining characteristics assist in the evaluation of the severity of non-reality-based thinking and the extent of altered thought processes.

Related Factors[2,4,8,12]

- Physiologic changes
- Biochemical changes
- Genetic predispositions
- Psychologic conflicts
- Impaired judgment
- Ineffective coping
- Loss of memory
- Sleep deprivation
- Substance abuse
- Mental disorders and illnesses

Defining Characteristics[2,5,8,13]

- Disruption of thinking process
  - Disorientation in time, place, person, circumstances, or events
  - Disordered sequencing of thought
  - Impaired ability to think abstractly
  - Impaired ability to solve problems and make decisions
  - Impaired reasoning ability
  - Impaired ability to grasp ideas
  - Impaired ability to calculate
  - Concretizing of ideas
- Memory disruption
  - Memory deficit
  - Changes in remote, recent, and immediate memory
  - Confabulation
- Changes in attention span
  - Distractibility
  - Difficulty concentrating
  - Inability to follow flow of conversation
- Emotional changes
  - Feelings of worthlessness
  - Extreme sadness
  - Mistrust
  - Guilt
  - Anxiety
  - Lability
  - Exaggerated response
  - Fear of others, of losing control, of falling apart
  - Decreased or shallow affect
  - Apathy
- Inaccurate interpretation of stimuli
  - Hallucinations
  - Delusions
  - Ideas of reference
  - Obsessions
- Changes in routine patterns and habits
  - Altered sleep pattern
  - Insomnia
  - Too much sleep
  - Change in grooming habits
  - Change in eating habits
  - Change in motor activity: repetition, agitation
  - Hypervigilance
  - Inappropriate social behavior
- Bizarre thinking, as noted by language use
  - Inappropriate use of global pronouns and global adjectives
  - Evidence of automatic thinking: universal "you know," assumption that listener knows omitted details
  - Circumstantiality: inability to get to the point
  - Lack of verbal distinction between thoughts, feelings, and actions
  - Use of indirect statements, extensive use of modifiers and qualifiers
  - Overgeneralization
  - Imputing intentions to others
  - Loose connection of ideas
  - Use of neologisms

Nursing Interventions*

Patient Goal	Nursing Intervention
Prevent physical injury to self and others.	• Maintain patient safety. • Prevent suicide and aggression. • Assess for suicide potential (history, plans for self-harm, verbalization of desire to die, disposal of possessions, viewing self in past tense). • Institute suicide precautions as indicated.

*References 2, 4, 6, 8, 10-14.

Patient Goal	Nursing Intervention
	• Assess potential for aggressive behavior. • Identify early signs of aggressive behavior. • Remove environmental factors that contribute to aggression. • Promote individual control: set limits on destructive behavior; encourage verbalization and safe acting-out behaviors within limits; allow choice within constraint; use seclusion if indicated. • Help patient set limits on own behavior: substitute verbalizations and physical activity for behavioral acting out; set incremental goals; recall and repeat successful ways of coping.
Reduce anxiety or stress.	• Approach in calm, nurturing manner: use calm level voice, lower tone, and familiar terms; avoid sudden movements; compose facial expression. • Provide physical and emotional structure as needed (physical: environment altered to provide for safety and comfort; emotional: prediction of feelings and occurrences, imaging of situations that evoke safety and comfort).
Enhance realistic, constructive interpretations of reality.	• Explore patient's representation of reality by analyzing language behavior: Listen intently to patient's verbal and nonverbal communication. Analyze communication for generalizations and distortions. • Assist patient in clarifying representation of reality: Clarify generalizations ("Nobody pays any attention to what I say." Clarify who specifically. Ask, "What specifically do you say?"). Elicit deletions in communication ("I am scared." Scared about what?). Clarify nominalistic statements. Change statements of event into statements of process ("I hate my relationship with my wife." Explore "relating" as process versus "relationship" as event.). Challenge distortions of control ("Steve makes me act up." Repeat statement with emphasis on "Steve makes?" Explore how that is possible.). Challenge distortions that impute intentions to others ("The doctor hates me." Analyze basis for statement: "What was said or done that makes you feel your doctor hates you?"). • Use reality orientation where indicated: Orient to person, time, and place. Use direct terminology, clear sentence structure. Avoid generalization. Use terms that help patient maintain individuality (e.g., "I" instead of "we"). Avoid vagueness, asides, and whispered comments. Have patient focus on real things and people.
Increase ability to relate with others positively.	• Provide group process situations that allow patients to experience relating in controlled setting. • Encourage validation of thoughts and feelings. • Encourage patient to ask for wants and to express feelings. • Help patient examine effect of behavior on others. • Help patient recognize use of and need for personal space and distance.
Enhance responsibility for self-care.	• Provide opportunity for patient to contribute to own treatment plan. • Encourage acceptance of responsibility for actions and interactions. • Encourage acceptance of responsibility for seeking help, following treatment plans, and changing behaviors.

Principles and Rationale for Nursing Interventions

The goal of nursing intervention for patients with altered thought processes is to improve the individual's ability to define and communicate reality. This goal is achieved primarily through a patient/nurse dyadic interaction or small group process. Such encounters frequently occur in, but need not be limited to, mental health care settings. Nursing intervention strategies are aimed at reducing or eliminating related factors and/or defining characteristics.

Thought and language are closely tied and interrelated.[3] Therefore it is logical to assume that altered thought processes are reflected in the patient's language behavior. The nursing interventions are based on this link between cognitive processes and language.

Paradoxically, the same cognitive processes that allow survival, growth, and change can also block growth, inhibit change, and produce limitations in living. Through the cognitive processes (thought, perception, memory, judgment) one creates one's own unique representation or model of reality. That model is bounded by physical, social, and psychologic factors that make each representation unique.

Three major mechanisms are used in a person's model making: generalization, deletion, and distortion.[1] *Generalization* is the process by which elements from an experience structure themselves to represent a category; the experience is an example of this category. For example, one generalizes from the experience of being cut that knives are sharp and must be used with care. This is a useful and necessary coping skill. If, however, one were to refuse to use knives at all or even to have knives in the house as a result of being cut, the generalization has become limiting.

Deletion is a process of selective attention to certain parts of an experience (e.g., the ability to read while the television is on). Deletion allows one to manage the world and not be overwhelmed. However, one can also use deletion in ways that are limiting (e.g., not hearing compliments about accomplishments and hearing only criticism).

Distortion is a process of experience shifting. It allows one to interpret experience under a different set of circumstances or to project an experience into the future (e.g., fantasizing). Distortion can also be limiting if experiences are shifted in a limiting fashion (e.g., compliments about accomplishments might be heard but shifted to mean that the person giving the compliment must want something).

These three mechanisms work together to create a person's model of reality. An altered cognitive process disrupts or distorts this model. These alterations can be detected by viewing the individual's model of reality, as expressed symbolically in language behavior. Exploration of the patient's use of generalization, deletion, and distortion can clarify his reality model. Limiting uses of generalization, deletion, and distortion can then be challenged. This allows patients to broaden their models of reality.

Evaluation

Patient Outcome	Data Indicating That Outcome is Reached
Safety maintained: no injury to self or others	No reported or physical evidence of injury to self or others Absence or decrease in violent response Absence or decrease in suicidal behavior Ability to control own behavior
Anxiety and stress reduced	Verbal statement that patient feels less anxious Physical signs of stress and anxiety decreased or absent
Model of reality realistic and constructive	Verbalizations clearer, more well rounded (decrease in generalizations, deletions, nominalistic statements, distortions of control, distortions of intent) Oriented to environment, self, time, and space Decrease in or absence of hallucinations and delusions Increased signs of problem solving and abstraction
Ability to relate with others positively	Functions as group member: expresses thoughts and feelings; makes wants and needs known to group; uses group response as guide to monitoring behavior Increased interaction with others Appropriate interaction process observed
Assumes responsibility for self-care	Makes contribution to treatment plan Follows through on assumed responsibility Seeks increasing responsibility for own activity and behavior Increase in self-monitoring

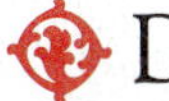 Decisional Conflict (Specify)

Decisional conflict is the state of uncertainty about courses of action to be taken when choice among competing actions involves risk, loss, or challenge to personal life values. (Specify means identifying the focus of conflict, e.g., choices regarding health, family relationships, career, finances, or other life events.)

Related Factors*

Knowledge deficit (lack of relevant information)
Identified consequences equally desirable/undesirable
Conflicting or unclear values and beliefs
Lack of experience or interference with decision making
Lack of problem-solving skills
Indecisive behavior pattern
Support system deficit
Low self-esteem disturbance
Interference in decision-making process
Perceived threat to value system

*Adapted from North American Nursing Diagnosis Association, 1988 Ballot.

Defining Characteristics*

Expressed or unexpressed distress about choices available
Verbalization of undesirable consequences of alternatives being considered
Vacillation between alternative choices

*Adapted from North American Nursing Diagnosis Association, 1988 Ballot.

Delayed decision making
Self-focusing
Physical signs of stress or tension (increased heart rate, increased muscle tension, restlessness)
Questioning personal values and beliefs while attempting to make decision
Expresses concern about inadequate knowledge base to make choice

Nursing Interventions

Patient Goal	Nursing Intervention
Make informed decisions in appropriate time frame.	• Promote decision making in accord with patient's values/beliefs. • Provide time for patient and family to discuss options privately. • Explore expectations and roles of significant others related to decisional conflict. • Assess urgency to determine time frame. • Support decision making in face of unknown consequences. • If appropriate, provide for psychiatric clinical nurse specialist.
Verbalize feelings of acceptance for decisions made.	• Assist patient to identify how past conflicts have been managed. • Encourage patient to verbalize concerns or feelings of distress about choices to be made. • Support patient for decisions made, especially if unexpected consequences occur.
Develop realistic perceptions about potential consequences of choices of action.	• Provide accurate and consistent information to patient to prevent conflicting messages. • Answer questions openly and honestly about condition and possible consequences of treatment. • Evaluate pros and cons of potential consequences of decision making. • Assist patient to identify coping skills and situational and environmental factors. • Ensure that patient and family are provided with as much information as possible about alternatives and consequences of each choice of action.

Principles and Rationale for Nursing Interventions

The patient needs an adequate knowledge base about the decision-making process and possible alternatives and consequences. This knowledge should be free of the bias of health care providers. The patient should be encouraged to verbalize feelings and perceptions about his value system and to explore alternatives available.

Evaluation

Patient Outcome	Data Indicating That Outcome is Reached
Makes informed decision	Engages in informed decision making Identifies and assesses available alternatives Recognizes consequences of available alternatives Makes decision(s) congruent with personal values and life-style Can continue to make decisions when consequences are uncertain Seeks support as needed, when decision making falters

FUNCTIONAL HEALTH PATTERN

VII

Self-Perception–Self-Concept

 Fear

Fear is the feeling of dread related to an identifiable source that an individual validates.

Fear is the response aroused by a person's perception of a real external threat. Fear can be viewed as a "client-expressed or client-confirmed response of apprehension or dread of the presence of a recognized, usually external, threat or danger to one's limb, autonomy, self-image, or community with others."[2] Physiologic reactions to fear and anxiety include increased heart rate, blood pressure, and respirations; urinary frequency and urgency; dilated pupils; and dry mouth.

Related Factors[3]

Definable, specific danger
Powerful unmet needs
Natural dangers (e.g., sudden noise, loss of physical support, height, pain)
Sensory impairment
Language barrier
Knowledge deficit
Lack of social support in threatening situation
Learned response, as by conditioning or identification
Environmental stimuli

Defining Characteristics[2,3]

Differentiated emotional response to definable specific danger
Increased tension, jittery
Apprehension
Scared, frightened
Terrified, panic
Increased alertness
Concentration on danger
Fight behavior (aggression)
Flight behavior (withdrawal)
Pupil dilation
Increased respiratory and heart rates
Goal-directed behavior facilitated (during mild or moderate fear)
Organization of person enhanced to flee or flight danger
Increased muscle tension
Diaphoresis

Nursing Interventions[1,2,4]

Patient Goal	Nursing Intervention
Reduce or prevent fear.	• Help patient to identify danger that is causing fear; use indirect and open-ended questions. • Assist patient in identifying major response pattern to danger—fight or flight. • Encourage verbalization, when timing is appropriate, about: Feelings experienced Perception of danger Perception of ability to cope with danger Questions about progress and/or outcome of diagnoses or treatment • Help patient use most appropriate approach to cope with present fear: Clearly identify danger. Use strategies to avoid danger. Use strategies to work around danger. Develop alternative goals, resources, etc. Engage in problem-solving activities to cope with danger. Facilitate realistic or alternative perception of danger. • Help patient identify strengths and adaptive skills to cope with fear(s): Scrutinize types of learning involved. Gain more constructive facts about the feared situation. Engage in stimulus exposure or systematic desensitization to reduce and eliminate fear. • Avoid situations that could aggravate the fear and related feelings: Give careful explanations of what is to happen to patient in health care setting. If fear cannot be reduced, make appropriate referrals. Involve and provide information to patient's family and/or friends.

Principles and Rationale for Nursing Interventions

The nursing diagnosis of fear is formulated from a synthesis of data, which are collected by means of clinical assessment. Assessment parameters for consideration for fear include the following:

Identify and observe for definable specific dangers.

What behavioral and physiologic changes indicating fear are present?

How does the patient perceive the danger and describe the discomfort?

Identify maladaptive or adaptive coping responses to fear.

What strategies has the patient used to cope with past fear?

What resources are available to deal with the fear?

Determination of the diagnosis of fear is based on the presentation of a set or cluster of defining characteristics. The defining characteristics manifested by a client are useful in determining the nursing diagnosis. Not all characteristics need be present at a given time. To complete the nursing diagnosis, the nurse then adds, when possible, the identified etiology, or related factor, to the diagnostic label of fear. An example is fear related to knowledge deficit.

Evaluation

Patient Outcome	Data Indicating That Outcome is Reached
Reduction or absence of fear	Absence or reduction of defining characteristics indicating presence of fear (e.g., tension, apprehension, fright, panic, overalertness) Blood pressure and heart rate within normal range Relaxed muscles Normal pupil size

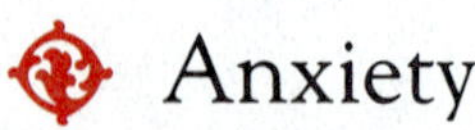

Anxiety

Anxiety is a vague, uneasy feeling, the source of which is often nonspecific or unknown to an individual.

In describing the effects of anxiety, one can differentiate between mild and moderate anxiety, which increase one's capabilities, and severe or extreme anxiety, in which capabilities and structures are paralyzed or overworked.[1] Physiologic changes, such as the release of epinephrine, can cause such manifestations as anorexia, urinary urgency, shifts in blood pressure, temperature, and menstrual flow, increased heart rate, and increased respiration. Observational capacity is increased in mild anxiety, whereas in moderate anxiety the perceptual field is somewhat narrowed but attention is directed to the situation of concern. In severe anxiety attention is focused on scattered detail, whereas in extreme anxiety the detailed focus is blown out of proportion or the speed of focusing on scattered details is increased. In mild anxiety the person is aware, is alert, and perceives connections between elements of a situation. In moderate anxiety the person does not notice peripheral details. In severe and extreme anxiety the person displays dissociating tendencies, failing to notice what goes on in a situation. In mild and moderate anxiety the person can learn; "i.e., is able to observe, describe, analyze, formulate meanings and relations, validate with another person, test, integrate, use the learning product."[1] In severe and extreme anxiety learning is diminished and the person seeks means of reducing the discomfort of anxiety.

One model of anxiety identifies predisposing factors—genetic endowment; present needs, thoughts, feelings, and resources; and past experiences—that affect the actual internal or external stimuli the person then cognitively evaluates as a threat.[19] The central nervous system is aroused and anxiety is felt. The sympathetic reaction appears to prepare the body for a flight-or-fight reaction in most persons. With perception of the threat in the cortex, the sympathetic branch of the autonomic nervous system is stimulated and the adrenal glands activated. Epinephrine is released. Blood flows to the central nervous system, muscle, and heart from the stomach and intestines. The heart beats faster, blood pressure rises, breathing becomes more rapid, and blood glucose levels increase.

Two types of anxiety are state and trait anxiety.[18] *State* anxiety is a transitory condition varying in intensity and fluctuating over time. *Trait* anxiety is a stable personality characteristic that predisposes a person's response and intensity in reactions to stress. When a person has a relatively high level of trait anxiety, he will tend to perceive a greater danger in situations that threaten the self than do persons who have lower levels of trait anxiety and consequently respond with higher levels of state anxiety.

Related Factors[6,8,9,12,19]

Perceived or actual threat to personal security pattern
Perceived or actual threat to core/essence of personality
Perceived or actual threat to self-concept
Perceived or actual threat to value system, beliefs, or ideals
Perceived or actual threat to meaningful interpersonal relationships/patterns and belonging
Adverse interpersonal relationships
Perceived or actual threat to biologic integrity
Perceived or actual failure of adaptive coping skills
Perceived or actual threat to physical safety
Unmet needs
Perceived or actual threat to ability to meet physiologic needs
Interpersonal transmission/contagion
Perceived or actual threat to goal achievement
Situational or maturational crises
Perceived or actual threat to stable environment
Perceived or actual change in role functioning
Perceived or actual change in socioeconomic status
Unconscious conflict
Arousal of both positive and negative evaluative thoughts
Perceived, actual, or anticipated disapproval by significant others
Empathic linkage with significant other
Terminal illness or potential death
Adverse influences (especially in childhood)
- Absence of love from significant other(s)
- Absence of respect from significant other(s)
- Criticism by significant other(s)
- Rejection by significant other(s)
- Disapproval by other person(s)

Defining Characteristics*

Mild Anxiety

Mild, vague, diffuse, objectless, apprehensive response to threat
Mild, vague, diffuse, objectless, apprehensive response to threat to personality core
Slight discomfort or tension
Slight uneasiness
Irritability
Restlessness
Repetitive questioning
Attention seeking
Belittling
Misunderstandings
Increased alertness
Enhanced problem-solving ability
Increased awareness and perception
Increased learning
Increased involvement in activities approved by others (especially during childhood)
Tension-relieving behaviors
- Lip chewing
- Finger tapping
- Foot shuffling
- Nail biting

Moderate Anxiety

Moderate, vague, diffuse, objectless, apprehensive response to threat
Moderate, vague, diffuse, objectless, apprehensive response to threat to personality core
Moderate discomfort or tension
Moderate uneasiness
Moderate feeling of diffuseness
Shakiness
Rattled

*References 1, 5, 6, 8-10, 12, 15-17, 19.

Pacing
Increased verbalizations
Increased alertness
Moderate sense of isolation
Slightly lowered self-esteem
Slight sense of worthlessness
Narrowing of perceptual field
Selective inattention
Increasing concentration on problem situation
Increased concentration on sensory data relevant to problem
Increased learning
Increasingly engaging in activities that elicit approval from significant others (especially during childhood)
Voice tremors
Change in voice pitch
Increased heart rate
Increased respiratory rate
Increased muscle tension
- Trembling
- Hand tremors
- Facial tension

Diaphoresis
Urinary frequency
Urinary urgency
Somatic complaints
Sleeplessness

Severe Anxiety

Severe, vague, diffuse, objectless, apprehensive response to threat
Severe, vague, diffuse, objectless, apprehensive response to threat to personality core
Sense of impending doom
Severe uneasiness
Severe discomfort, distress, tension
Dissociation of anxious feelings from self
Denial of existence of uncomfortable feelings
Painful sense of helplessness and inadequacy
Severe feeling of being in hostile environment
Moderately low self-esteem
Moderate sense of worthlessness
Moderate feeling of powerlessness
Uncertainty
Severe sense of isolation
Severe feeling of diffuseness
Inability to learn
Purposeless activity
Ineffective functioning
Difficult and/or inappropriate verbalizations
Reduced range of perception
- Inability to concentrate
- Focus on scattered or small details
- Selective inattention
- Inability to see connections between events or details

Lack of clear comprehension of immediate situation
Hyperventilation
Tachycardia
Urinary frequency
Urinary urgency
Nausea
Headache
Dizziness
Insomnia

Extreme Anxiety (Panic)

Extremely severe, vague, diffuse, objectless, apprehensive response to threat
Extremely severe, vague, diffuse, objectless, apprehensive response to threat to personality core
Extremely severe discomfort, tension
Extremely severe uneasiness
Severe shakiness
Severe hyperactivity
Immobility
Extreme sense of helplessness and inadequacy
Extreme feeling of isolation
Extreme feeling of diffuseness
Extreme sense of being in a hostile environment
Severely lowered self-esteem
Severe worthlessness
Severe powerlessness
Extreme uncertainty
Inability to communicate
Unintelligible communication
Inability to learn
Disruption of perceptual field
- Distortion or unrealistic perception of situation
- Enlargement of detail

Feeling of personality disintegration
Mental disorders
Dilated pupils
Pallor
Vomiting
Sleeplessness

Nursing Interventions*

Patient Goal	Nursing Intervention
Experience reduced anxiety.	• Assess for presence and level of anxiety. • Observe for perceived or actual threats to: Personal security pattern Core or essence of personality Self-concept Value system, beliefs, or ideals • Determine signs and symptoms (defining characteristics) indicating presence of anxiety. • Determine level of anxiety present. • Listen to patient's description of state of discomfort. • Identify maladaptive and adaptive current responses to anxiety. • Identify strategies used by patient in past to cope with anxiety. • Determine what strengths and resources are available to cope with anxiety: problem-solving skills, decision-making skills, significant others, religion, professional assistance, recreational activities, hobbies, etc. • For patient with severe or extreme anxiety: Employ comfort measures (e.g., warm bath, restful environment). Keep in calm, nonstimulating milieu: remove any stress or threat; limit contact with other anxious patients. Use short, simple sentences. Use calm, firm tone of voice. Administer tranquilizers or sedatives as prescribed. Observe for and institute needed protective measures. Use nonverbal behavior (e.g., quiet physical presence or touch) to offer reassurance. Avoid asking patient to make decisions. Avoid probing for cause of anxiety. Avoid interpreting behavior or confrontation. • Develop constructive, positive interpersonal relationship with patient: Be empathetic. Convey unconditional positive regard. Be congruent. • Intervene early to prevent escalation of anxiety to severe or extreme levels. • Use active listening skills. • Facilitate patient's participation in recreational and diversional activities aimed at decreasing anxiety: Group singing or instrumental groups Simple games Housekeeping chores Grooming Routine tasks Walking or jogging Simple concrete tasks Swimming • Remain calm: Avoid reciprocal anxiety. Recognize own anxiety. Develop control over own responses. • Encourage ventilation of feelings when ready; permit crying. • Offer brief and clear information about experiences during hospitalization. • Offer, clarify, and validate information as needed. • Offer reassurance. • Convey attitude that there is hope and that a constructive resolution can be found. • Prevent further escalation of anxiety by *avoiding* threats, indifference, rejection, judgmental attitude, impatience, unrealistic demands, insincerity, and focusing on weakness. • Mutually develop daily schedule of activities, incorporating patient's strengths, abilities, preferences, and goals. • During short-term hospitalization, offer additional support and assistance in dealing with anxiety on admission, on about the fifth day, and on notification of discharge.

*References 2-7, 10, 11, 13, 14, 20.

Patient Goal	Nursing Intervention
Recognize anxiety, develop insight, and use adaptive coping strategies.	• If anxiety is at mild or moderate levels, help patient to: Recognize presence of anxiety by providing feedback on characteristics indicating anxiety and asking questions such as, "Are you uncomfortable right now?" Explore similarity between present and past experiences. Ask questions such as, "Have you felt like this before? What was happening to you then? What did you do to reduce your discomfort?" Identify thoughts or expectations before becoming anxious. Identify relationship between anxiety and consequent adaptive or maladaptive responses. Clarify nature of threat to self. Develop adaptive strategies to reduce anxiety. Problem-solve. Evaluate results of strategies used. Seek and implement alternatives for results that were unsuccessful. • Reduce any secondary gains from maladaptive strategies used in coping with anxiety. • Permit patient to set pace in solving problems. • Reduce negative expectations. • Facilitate development of constructive and optimistic view of existence, especialy if view is distorted, closed, or deadened. • Facilitate choice of effective, objective environmental interventions to cope with anxiety, especially if patient is already optimistic, open to new experiences, and flexible. • Encourage participation in new interests and hobbies. • After establishing relationship with patient and extreme or severe anxiety has been reduced: Encourage social activities despite reluctance and fears. Attend activities with patient initially. Permit patient to leave if anxiety is greatly increased. Gradually encourage attendance independent of staff support. • Use role playing to deal with anxiety-provoking situations. With children, try role-play strategies using puppets, dolls, or other playthings; art; or play requiring large motor activities. • Teach patient to: Recognize constructive aspects of mild or moderate anxiety in learning, growth, and movement toward self-actualization. Recognize personal characteristics indicating presence of anxiety. Describe present state of anxiety. Analyze current expectations, goals, beliefs, and values versus what is preceived as actually happening. Develop assertive communication skills. Develop problem-solving and decision-making skills. Use progressive muscle relaxation. Increase repertoire of strategies to reduce severe anxiety; talking or being in presence of someone; simple, concrete tasks; walking; noncompetitive sports; professional assistance.

Principles and Rationale for Nursing Interventions

Anxiety varies among persons in its intensity depending on severity of threat, perception by the person, previous and current coping skills, and success or failure of the person's efforts to cope with the feelings of discomfort experienced in anxiety. Coping mechanisms can be either adaptive or maladaptive. Disturbed or maladaptive coping strategies include inability to make choices, rigidity and repetition, alienation, withdrawal, conflict, extreme denial, distortion of awareness of the situation, acting out, depression, moderate to severe aggression, somatizing, and seeking secondary gains. Adaptive strategies for dealing with anxiety include learning more about the confronting situation, problem solving, increasing self-understanding, and seeking and engaging in constructive outlets for emotions.

In anxiety the security pattern, the foundation on which the patient distinguishes himself from the environment, is threatened. These threats can be directed toward anything the patient holds essential to that central core or security pattern, whether a threat to physical safety, the ability to meet physiologic needs, or the ability to meet higher-level needs (e.g., self-esteem, belonging, meaning, freedom, patriotism, goal achievement).

Evaluation

Patient Outcome	Data Indicating That Outcome is Reached
Reduction of anxiety	Absence or reduction of defining charactistics indicating presence of anxiety
Anxiety recognized, insight developed, and adaptive coping strategies used	Recognition of anxiety in self Demonstration of insight about cause of anxiety Use of adaptive coping strategies to reduce anxiety Use of mild or moderate anxiety for personal change or growth

Hopelessness

Hopelessness is the subjective state in which an individual sees limited or no alternatives or personal choices available and is unable to mobilize energy on own behalf.

The inability to mobilize energy, or state of inactivity, that occurs in hopelessness results in dependence on others and a concomitant lowering of self-esteem.[4] Some authors describe a relationship between hopelessness and goal attainment.[2,17] Motivation (action) to achieve a goal is related to the individual's perception of the probability of attaining the goal and the perceived significance of the goal. When experiencing hopelessness, the individual believes that the future holds little promise and that plans will not achieve goals. A passive acceptance of the future and inability to determine personal goals result.

Brandt[3] describes a process by which hopelessness evolves from powerlessness, a perception that one's behavior cannot affect an outcome. The perception of inability to achieve outcomes through personal actions results in helplessness. The individual who feels helpless is hesitant to initiate actions and develops negative expectations for the future. Inability to cope with the present and the belief that the future will not improve result in hopelessness.

Related Factors[2,4,6,8,9]

Prolonged restriction of activity resulting in isolation
Deteriorating physiologic condition
Deteriorating mental condition
Terminal illness
Sudden event disruptive to life pattern
Long-term stress
Abandonment
Perceived significant loss, e.g., loved one, youth, influence, opportunity
Belief that stress, event, or illness is uncontrollable
Loss of belief in transcendent values or God
Series of failures to reach desired goal
Persistent cognitive errors, i.e., negative ideas of self, world, and future
Life-style of helplessness

Defining Characteristics*

Passivity
Decreased verbalization
Apathy
Verbal expressions of despondency
Lack of initiative or motivation
Decreased response to stimuli
Nonverbal cues of withdrawal from others, e.g., turning away from speaker, closing eyes
Decreased appetite
Increased sleep
Fatigue or lethargy
Lack of participation in self-care
Verbalization of low self-esteem
Verbalization of lack of control over self and environment
Isolating self from others
Inability to identify specific feelings
Expressions of psychologic discomfort, e.g., tenseness, irritability, sensation of lump in throat
Expressed loss of gratification from roles or relationships
Absence of sense of continuity between past, present, and future
Verbal or nonverbal expressions of negative future expectations
Lack of personal goals
Impaired decision making

*References 4, 6, 7, 8, 11-13, 16.

Nursing Interventions[2-4,6-16]

Patient Goal	Nursing Intervention
Express hope for future.	• Assist patient to meet self-care needs: Monitor patient's strengths and abilities (cognitive, psychologic, physiologic) to perform self-care.

Patient Goal	Nursing Intervention
	Assist patient gradually to assume responsibility for own care through teaching and support. Implement self-care activities to meet needs that patient is unable to meet. Involve significant others in care of patient. Encourage patient involvement in decision making about self-care activities. Provide positive reinforcement and acknowledgment for successful attempts at self-care. • Lessen patient's isolation: Initiate contact with patient. Build trust through consistency and reliability. Designate same staff, as possible, to work with patient. Furnish opportunities for patient to spend time with others; gradually increase amount of time and number of persons. Determine patient's current support system. With patient, identify options for increasing support system. Encourage visits and activities with significant others. • Encourage expression of feelings: Develop trusting relationship with patient. Encourage expression of feelings verbally or nonverbally (e.g., writing, drawing). Facilitate expression of feelings through active listening, open-ended questions, and reflection. Assist patient to identify (name) feeling being experienced. Assist patient to identify reason for living by focusing on concrete feelings and ideas. Express empathy while communicating belief that patient can act contrary to way he feels. Communicate belief that patient has or can learn needed coping skills. With patient, identify persons with whom feelings can be shared. Assist patient to recognize and describe feeling of hopelessness and its related thoughts. Assist patient to direct thoughts beyond present to future. Help patient regain spiritual self. Observe for suicidal intent, e.g., sudden changes in mood or behavior, theme of death in conversation, giving belongings away. • Assist patient to increase self-esteem: Convey unconditional positive regard for patient. Assist patient to identify current and potential strengths and abilities. Encourage patient to continue to carry out roles and relationships that reinforce positive feelings. Assist patient to develop skills that contribute to mastery of environment. Support positive self-statements of patient. Provide recognition for patient's success and accomplishments. Demonstrate and teach assertive skills. Focus on present and future; discourage rumination on past. Encourage patient's participation in treatment decisions. Encourage patient's participation in treatment modalities that offer support and opportunities for success. • Help patient control or influence self and environment: Encourage independent behavior. Provide relevant information about illness and treatment. Provide opportunity for patient input into health care decisions. Allow patient to ask questions. Teach patient how to distinguish between controllable and uncontrollable events. Help patient to develop and revise realistic goals. Demonstrate and teach patient problem-solving skills. Expand patient's coping repertoire. Demonstrate and teach effective communication techniques. Provide opportunities in which patient can succeed and experience control. Assist patient to evaluate performance realistically. Provide positive reinforcement for patient's success in problem solving, coping, and control. Use cognitive therapy techniques to correct cognitive errors.

Principles and Rationale for Nursing Interventions

Hope is an expectation of achieving a goal. A hopeful patient believes that there is a way out and that changes can be managed with help.[13] Hopefulness has been positively correlated with health status and quality of life, even in chronic or terminal illness.[1,3,5,13,15] In addition, hopefulness is influenced by others.[1,13,17] Therefore the concept of hopefulness is pertinent to the practice of nursing; i.e., a nurse can affect health care outcomes through positively influencing a patient's hopefulness.

Nursing interventions designed to facilitate the patient's ability to identify a variety of alternatives, mobilize energy and resources, determine personal goals, and initiate effective actions to meet goals will overcome feelings of hopelessness. A patient's hopelessness can be abated by involvement in his health care, interaction with significant others, expression of feelings, enhancement of self-esteem, and control over self and the environment.[3,16]

Evaluation

Patient Outcome	Data Indicating That Outcome is Reached
Express hope for future.	Maintains adequate self-care Accepts assistance from others when appropriate Establishes support system Maintains sustaining relationships Identifies feelings experienced Verbalizes feeling of hopefulness and related thoughts Verbalizes future expectations Verbalizes feelings of adequacy Develops realistic self-esteem Develops adequate role mastery and coping skills Participates in health care and other life decisions Sets realistic goals Verbalizes increased ability to control or influence self and environment

Powerlessness

Powerlessness is the perception that one's own action will not significantly affect an outcome; a perceived lack of control over a current situation or immediate happening.

McFarland, Leonard, and Morris[11] define power "as the generalized capacity or potential to get others to do something one wants them to do and which they would not ordinarily do otherwise." Although power can be abused, these authors point out that power has a positive aspect and exists within the context of interpersonal relationships.

One can identify five bases for personal social power[3]:

Expert power—based on skill or knowledge

Reward power—based on ability to give positive rewards to others

Referent power—based on personal characteristics with which another person identifies

Legitimate power—based on the right to be influential over others

Coercive power—based on the ability to administer punishment

Miller[13] states, "The greater the individual's expectation to have control and the greater the importance of the desired outcomes to the individual, the greater the perceived powerlessness experienced when the individual does not, in fact, have control." Powerlessness can be situationally determined and related to locus of control, a long-term tendency to perceive situations in a certain way.[13] Powerlessness also can be seen as a variety of alienation and described as a sense of low control rather than a sense of mastery over events.[2] A sense of powerlessness arises from an individual's belief that outside forces such as chance govern what happens in life and that personal resources are not available to influence consequences of one's own actions and control of one's situation.

Related Factors*

Institutional environment and staff behavior
- Stripping of personal possessions
- Excessive surveillance
- Assault on privacy
- Lack of individuation
- Castelike separation from persons in authority
- Misuse of rewards
- Misuse of punishment
- Staff monopoly of scarce or strategic resources
- Misuse of power, authority, or force
- Absolute power of staff to structure conditions of negotiation
- Deployment or blocking of resources by staff

Situational crises

Parental influences and parenting styles

Social conditions

Peer influences

Repeated interpersonal failures and problems

Actual or potential loss of significant other

*References 2, 8-10, 13, 14, 17, 19, 22.

Lack of available or accessible social and personal resources
- Lack of ability to reward a favor
- Lack of ability to extort a concession or do without
- Belief in lack of control over resources

Altered state of physical wellness
Loss of independent role
Hospitalization
Alterations in mental status
Loss of autonomy
Weak ego identity
Spoiled identity/stigma
Hostile environment
Delay or distortion in accomplishing developmental tasks
Developmental changes
Perception of authority figures as distant or unapproachable
Alterations in schedule
Lack of knowledge
Lack of participation in decision making
Excessive threatening experiences
Unsupportive environment
Battering relationship
Lack of belief in ability to do a task or engage in a behavior
Lack of parental role model

Defining Characteristics*

Verbal expression of having no control or influence over situation
Verbal expression of having no control or influence over outcome
Verbalizes feelings of loss of control and powerlessness
Low orientation to learning control-relevant information
Lack of knowledge about own illness
Inability to seek information about care

*References 1, 8, 9, 14, 17, 19.

Low orientation to achievement in control-relevant area
Verbal expression of having no control over self-care
Frustration about inability to perform previously mastered activities
Doubtful about role performance
Low planned use of health services
Acknowledges failure readily
Expresses feelings of inadequacy
Rationalizes failure
Displays aggression when goal achievement frustrated
Devalues desired goal when achievement frustrated
Apathy
Passivity
Resignation
Aimlessness
Lack of participation in decision making
Feelings of depression
Anxiety
Restlessness and uneasiness
Sadness or crying
Inappropriate aggression
Low self-esteem
Resentment
Mistrust of others
Overly dependent on others
Fears alienation from caregivers
Fluctuating or low energy levels
Asks many questions or no questions
Loss of control over environment
Loss of control over self-functioning and personal behavior
Inappropriate or immature coping abilities for developmental stage
Projects blame on others and environment
Inability to influence others
Seeks immediate rewards in favor of long-term goals

Nursing Interventions*

Patient Goal	Nursing Intervention
Control or influence outcomes in current situations.	• Assess patient's powerlessness by asking these questions: Does the patient belong to a high-risk group? Women? Elderly? Educationally/economically disadvantaged? The chronically ill or handicapped? Ethnic/racial minorities? Are perceived or actual abilities to influence personal outcome and control the situation present? Are there verbal expressions of: Having no control or influence over situation? Having no control or influence over outcomes? Feelings of loss of control and powerlessness? Does the patient experience characteristics such as lack of decision making? Lack of knowledge about illness and treatment? Withdrawn? Are coping strategies currently or previously used? Are environmental factors, staff behaviors, or other related factors present? Excessive surveillance? Assault on privacy? Lack of individuation? Does patient believe he or she has ability to accomplish given task or do given behavior (level of self-efficacy)?

*References 1, 4-7, 10, 12-15, 17-22.

Patient Goal	Nursing Intervention
	• Make change within institutions or residential settings: Decrease surveillance of patient unless essential for safety. Minimize rules and regulations; permit patient input in his or her development. Enhance individuality and autonomy. Increase patient control over rewards. Preserve privacy; increase territorial rights. Allow patient to wear own clothes. Prevent a castelike separation between staff and patients. Vary setting and routine of daily activities based on patient input. Do not block patient's attainment and use of resources (within limits of safety). Do not use coercion. Support patient's efforts to increase resources, e.g., benefits that can be shared with other patients or allies who can be mobilized. Decrease dependency on staff; encourage independent behavior. Maintain patient's sense of dignity; permit exploration of environment. Be less directive and overprotective. Foster personal powerfulness by putting bedside stand, call light, telephone, etc. within reach. Promote active involvement in appropriate decision making in activities of daily living. Involve patient in other decision-making opportunities and planning own care. Provide patient with positive and predictable events, e.g., group experiences. Provide opportunities for engagement in meaningful activities. • Help patient reduce feelings of powerlessness: Help patient recognize and describe powerlessness; identify the behavior with patient. Help patient separate controllable from uncontrollable events. Help patient set realistic goals. Teach patient to problem-solve and try out alternative coping strategies. Help patient identify personal preferences, wants, feelings, values, and attitudes. Help patient identify ability to do specific behavior. Help patient identify and use strengths and potential; identify improvement in condition. Encourage verbalization of feelings and concerns about feelings of powerlessness. Improve self-esteem. Provide situations in which patient can succeed and experience control. Assess patient's perception and knowledge of treatment program, encouraging expression of views *before* giving information. Assess internal versus external locus of control before patient teaching. For those with internal locus of control, provide information that gives patient a sense of control, using different strategies of content presentation. For those with external locus of control, provide structured approaches, teach in small increments, and involve in determining readiness for learning. Provide needed information. Encourage patient to ask questions; reinforce right to ask questions. Help patient seek and master relevant health information. Help patient use health care personnel. Help patient develop long-term valued health goals and take fewer risks. Restore energy imbalance. Teach assertive communication skills. Allow patient to assume more complicated decision making when ready. Provide positive reinforcement and acknowledgment for active participation in own care. Help patient develop increased internal locus of control by encouraging participation in sensitivity training, behavior modification, brief psychotherapy, encounter groups, community action programs; altering perception of life situation; using behavioral rehearsal and role playing; rewarding manifestations of internality; challenging external locus of control–oriented verbalizations; examining possible outcomes of alternative approaches. Facilitate improvement in life circumstances—returning to work, constructive significant other interactions, successful therapy experiences, constructive family interactions, role models. Involve significant others in care of patient within realm of capability. Sensitize significant others to importance of their reactions. Build trusting relationship; be consistent and dependable. Use active listening. Refer for family therapy as appropriate. Refer to self-help group as appropriate.

Principles and Rationale for Nursing Interventions

A patient with a high *internal* locus of control perceives that his or her life and circumstances are controlled primarily by self-determined activity, actions, and characteristics. A patient with a high *external* locus of control, on the other hand, perceives his life and circumstances to be primarily controlled by external events, e.g., fate, chance, luck, powerful people, or unpredictability caused by the complexity of situations. Increased external locus of control reflects a sense of helplessness[16] and a general expectancy of powerlessness.

Powerlessness can cause difficulty in learning control-relevant information and can be enhanced by involving the patient in making decisions about content to be included in patient teaching programs. Locus of control can influence one's ability to use control-relevant information.[13] Therefore it is important to assess the degree of powerlessness before patient teaching and provide information that gives patients with an internal locus of control a sense of control, using different strategies of content presentation. For those with an external locus of control, the nurse should provide structured approaches, teach in small increments, and involve them in determining what aspects of health care they are ready to learn.

A patient's powerlessness can be diminished by power rebuilding, augmenting, or improving power resources—physical strength, psychologic stamina, support networks, self-concept, energy, knowledge, motivation, and a belief system (hope). Effective coping strategies must be preserved, augmented, and developed. Effective coping strategies result in a decrease in uncomfortable feelings, generation of hope, enhancement of self-esteem, maintenance of positive interpersonal relationships, and maintenance of or improvement in the state of coping.

Evaluation

Patient Outcome	Data Indicating That Outcome is Reached
Controls or influences outcomes in current situations	Verbalization of ability to control or influence situation and outcomes
	Verbalization of feelings of powerfulness
	Seeking control-relevant information
	Knowledge about control-relevant situation
	Adequate role-functioning and coping skills
	Feelings of adequacy
	Goal-directed behavior
	Hope
	Involvement in decision making
	Appropriate mood
	Welcoming assistance from others when needed but not overly dependent
	Working toward long-term goals
	Sense of responsibility over behavioral outcomes
	Holding self responsible when appropriate; no projecting of blame on environment

Body Image Disturbance

Body image disturbance is the disruption in the way an individual perceives his body image.

Body image disturbance refers to difficulties experienced in the perceptions one has of one's own appearance or of one's body functions, as well as difficulties with the accompanying beliefs and values. The body image includes both physiologic and psychologic factors, is both conscious and unconscious, depends on both internal and external factors, and is both reality bound and influenced by fantasy. Body image is a very dynamic process, is a highly individual concern, and is an important influence of behavior. Body image disturbances can potentially occur in a variety of illnesses. These can include congenital or hereditary conditions (e.g., Down syndrome, orthopaedic deformities, cleft lip), traumatic accidents resulting in scarring, illnesses affecting body structure and functioning (e.g., metastatic carcinoma), dermatologic conditions, or surgical procedures (e.g., abdominal hysterectomy).

Related Factors[7,13,14]

Change in body function
Change in body structure
Cognitive difficulties
Perceptual difficulties
Inability to adjust to body changes
Inability to integrate body changes
Lack of adequate coping skills
Change in social expectations
Change in cultural values
Rigid ideals about appearance and body function
Low self-esteem
Mental illness (e.g., depression)

Lack of self-confidence
Inadequate knowledge about social norms related to appearance
Social prejudices about handicapping conditions
Inability to adapt to limitations
Peer criticism or ostracism
Identification with others whose bodies are considered ideal
Spiritual difficulties

Defining Characteristics[1,10,12,13]

Change in life-style
Fear of rejection by others
Focus on past strength, function, or appearance
Negative feelings about body
Feelings of helplessness, hopelessness, or powerlessness
Feelings of depersonalization and/or derealization
Feelings of grandiosity relating to physical size and strength
Preoccupation with change or loss
Extension of body boundary to incorporate environmental objects
Personalization of part or loss by name
Depersonalization of part or loss by use of impersonal pronouns
Refusal to verify actual change
Missing body part
Actual change in structure and/or function
Not looking at body part
Not touching body part
Hiding or overexposing body part
Trauma to nonfunctioning part
Change in social involvement
Change in ability to estimate spatial relationship of body to environment
Inability to discriminate stimuli from inside or outside self (loss of ego boundaries)
Inability to accept change in body wall
Inability to accept change in body boundaries (e.g., stroke patient who is unaware of paralysis despite efforts to make him conscious of it)
Disruption in activities of daily living (ADLs)
Grieving
Verbalizations about difficulties accepting lost body function or structure
Verbalizations about difficulties in adjusting to limitations
Aggression
Low frustration level

Nursing Interventions*

Patient Goal	Nursing Intervention
Maintain positive, accepting, and realistic body image.	• Assess patient's perception of body image by asking these questions: What aspects of his or her body does he or she find pleasing? Not pleasing? How are changes perceived in relation to society's norms? How are changes in body function or structure being integrated, and what is impact on attitudes and feelings? What strengths, potentials, social resources, or community resources are available to patient? • Explore with patient how he or she came to perceive his or her body image as negative (as in past experiences with significant others). • Acknowledge and give positive reinforcement whenever patient attempts to improve personal body image (e.g., improved hygiene, wearing makeup, wearing new clothes, wearing cosmetic devices after disfiguring surgery). • Help patient to accept realistically and value his or her present physical self. Stress that certain physical characteristics of a person cannot be changed but that a person has other, more important, positive strengths unique to that individual. List these strengths with patient. • Teach patient ways he or she might go about improving body image (e.g., how to dress, apply makeup, perform exercises to improve physical tone, use cosmetic devices). • Resolve grief. • Encourage attendance in self-help groups. • Prepare patient for possible experiences that might be encountered as consequence of physical limitations. • Be nonjudgmental. • Demonstrate empathy and unconditional positive regard. • Assist significant others to understand impact of limitations. • Offer supportive counseling. • Offer physical assistance as needed (e.g., stoma care). • Direct patient to community resources for needed assistance. • Explore with patient how overt body changes will be discussed with others. • Mutually set realistic goals with patient regarding body image. • Assist in developing self-confidence and maintaining it.

*References 1, 2, 11, 12, 15, 17.

Patient Goal	Nursing Intervention
Accept body wall or body boundary change and incorporate change into body image and self-concept.	• If patient has had an amputation, mastectomy, colostomy, or cerebrovascular accident and is experiencing a body boundary disturbance because of change in body wall or body boundary: Encourage patient to verbalize feelings of concern, anger, anxiety, loss, and fear over change in body wall or body boundary. Encourage patient to verbalize and explore feelings regarding what impact missing body part or changed body boundary has had on assuming ADLs (family, work, social relationships). Encourage patient to look at and touch changed body wall or body boundary area. Ask patient to verbalize feelings after performing these behaviors. Encourage patient to assume normal social activities as soon as possible without hiding or overexposing changed body wall area. Reinforce to patient the reality of changed body wall or body boundary area and that it may or may not be permanent. Encourage patient to use rehabilitative and physical therapy services to improve functioning of affected body wall or body boundary area. Encourage patient to use cosmetic services available for disfiguring surgery and mechanical devices for improved functioning of affected body boundary area. Encourage patient to use support services or reference groups in community (e.g., visit by a former colostomy, mastectomy, or stroke patient). Facilitate interaction with patient who has successfully adjusted to similar difficulties.
Reintegrate ego functions and boundaries so that they are congruent with reality and self-concept.	• When ego boundaries become distorted and patient no longer can discriminate between inside and outside stimuli, the following interventions should be used: Provide patient with structured, quiet, nonstimulating environment. As the person's ego strength improves, increase environmental stimuli. Help patient to discriminate between real and unreal environmental and internal stimuli. Encourage patient to verbalize feelings and anxieties over his or her distorted perceptions of reality. Reinforce and maintain the patient's contact with reality. Engage patient in reality-oriented activities. Encourage patient to participate in all treatment modalities (pharmacologic therapy, individual or group therapies, etc.). Discuss therapeutic benefits of these modalities. When patient has regained control of ego boundaries, encourage patient to examine critically and evaluate what caused him or her to experience a disturbance in body boundaries.

Principles and Rationale for Nursing Interventions

To assist the patient effectively, the nature of the threat to the patient's body function and structure and the meaning the patient attaches to this threat must be adequately assessed. The more central the change is to a person's sense of self, the greater the potential for difficulties in body image. Knowledge of coping abilities and supportive resources are essential in designing nursing interventions. Assistance with the normal grieving process can prevent dysfunctional grieving and facilitate a more rapid adjustment to the change. Self-esteem is preserved when the patient is encouraged to use remaining skills and develop ways to adjust to changes encountered. Social support will facilitate an adequate adjustment to the loss. Knowledge about community resources augments coping skills.

To incorporate the change into the self-concept, feelings encountered must be worked through and resolved. Resources and services that can preserve appearance or aid in adjusting to a physical limitation foster successful coping and reduce body image disturbances. Readjustment of one's body image is gradual, so time is needed to resolve the feelings encountered.

When ego boundaries become distorted, it is essential that the distortions and accompanying feeling states be explored with the patient at an appropriately timed level of tolerance. A supportive, structured, and calm environment and approach, along with a gradual assistance in differentiating reality from nonreality, will allow the patient to regain control of his ego boundaries. Again, time is needed to experience and fully accept changes in the structure or function of the body so that a satisfactory body image can be achieved.

Evaluation[3,5]

Patient Outcome	Data Indicating That Outcome is Reached
Positive, accepting, and realistic body image	Decrease in manifestation of defining characteristics Positive expression of acceptance of body image

Patient Outcome	Data Indicating That Outcome is Reached
	Understands how negative body image possibly developed in relation to growth and development and social, cultural, and interpersonal experiences Uses problem-solving skills with subsequent strategies that promote and maintain positive body image Assumes usual social interactions Engages in appropriate role functions Engages in appropriate recreational activities Verbalizes acceptance of limitations Demonstrates effort to improve appearance Maximizes use of remaining strengths Demonstrates resolution of grief Expresses satisfaction with social support available
Body wall or body boundary change accepted and incorporated into body image and self-concept	Decrease in manifestation of defining characteristics Positive expression of the acceptance and reality of changed body wall or body boundary area Ability to look at, touch, and discuss with others changed body wall or body boundary area Describes impact the changed body wall or body boundary has had on assumption of ADLs and in family work and social relationships Uses appropriate cosmetic or mechanical devices as well as reference support groups Uses all available treatment modalities to improve functioning of affected body wall or body boundary area
Reintegration of ego functions and boundaries so that they are congruent with reality and self-concept	Decrease in manifestation of defining characteristics Improvement in mental functioning (absence of or decrease in psychosis and regressive behaviors) Discrimination between environmental stimuli and external stimuli

Personal Identity Disturbance

Personal identity disturbance is the inability to distinguish between the self and nonself.

Personal identity is the component of self-concept that refers to how a person recognizes himself as a unique being, separate from the rest of the world. In psychoanalytic theory it concerns a person's ability to distinguish self from nonself. In Freudian terminology it is a person's ego. Personal identity formation is greatly influenced by an individual's developmental needs, capabilities, consistent role models, identifications, and successful ego defenses. Its development starts in early infancy when the child begins to differentiate self from the environment. Through this differential process the child begins to experience separateness and uniqueness from the rest of the world. It is through personal identity that one recognizes what belongs to self. If this process of differentiation does not occur (e.g., if a pathologic symbiotic relationship exists between the child and mother, from which the child never learns or experiences separateness and autonomy from the mother), the person's ego becomes fused, or undifferentiated. The person then loses a sense of coherent self with a resultant inability to actualize abilities. There are accompanying feelings of confusion and indecisiveness.

Related Factors

Poor ego differentiation
Faulty resolution of Oedipus or Electra complexes
Biochemical body changes
Identification with inappropriate person
Negative role model
Overidentification
Pathologic symbiotic relationship with significant other

Defining Characteristics

Feelings of confusion, uncertainty
Indecisiveness about one's sense of self, purpose, and direction in life
Feelings of anxiety, dissatisfaction, depression, and confusion over one's sexual identity and sexual preference
Distorted or blurred ego boundaries
Dependent behaviors
- Inability to make decisions
- Fear of making changes
- Uncertainty
- Inability to articulate one's feelings
- Clinging to others

Sexual behaviors and/or mannerisms that are in conflict with one's sexual preference
Lack of self-confidence
Depression
Indecisiveness

Nursing Interventions

Patient Goal	Nursing Intervention
Develop and maintain positive concept of personal identity.	• Encourage patient to verbalize concerns and anxieties regarding personal identity. • Help patient develop problem-solving skills and subsequent strategies that will facilitate achieving sense of personal identity. • Encourage patient to take responsibility for personal behavior and to take risks in exploring new behaviors. • Encourage participation in peer group activities and in development and maintenance of meaningful interpersonal relationships. • Provide therapeutic environment that will foster patient's sense of personal self. • Teach patient principles of normal growth and development. Emphasize that certain phases of development (e.g., adolescence) are accompanied by *normal* crises in personal identity.
Achieve satisfaction with own sexual identity and sexual preference.	• Encourage patient to verbalize anxieties concerning sexual identity and sexual preference for companionship. In nonjudgmental manner support patient in choice of sex role. • Explore with patient meanings of being a man or woman. Stress that sexuality is only one component of a person's identity. • Encourage patient to explore positive and negative consequences as perceived in making decision to assume particular sexual role. Stress that decision is a personal choice, but that consequences of the choice must be accepted.

Principles and Rationale for Nursing Interventions[2,5,6]

The concept of personal identity in relation to psychosexual development has been addressed by Freud, Erikson, and Sullivan. Each perceived personal identity as evolving on a developmental continuum, with successful resolution resulting in the development of integrated psycho-social-sexual behaviors. If the process of a person's psychosexual development is interfered with, several problems may result, e.g., unsucccessful resolution of Oedipus or Electra complexes, verbalizations of feelings of uncertainty, dissatisfaction, and confusion about sexual identification and preference.

When examining personal identity from a nonpsychoanalytic framework, one realizes that personal identity concerns can sometimes be associated with developmental life crises. For example, in adolescence the individual experiences personal identity concerns (Who am I? What direction is my life taking?) In midlife, persons become concerned with what accomplishments they have made in life. Concerns of this nature are normal, but if the person becomes overly anxious, resolution of problems may require professional intervention. Providing a therapeutic, nonjudgmental environment assists the patient in expressing feelings about self-identity openly. Teaching coping skills and providing opportunities for taking personal responsibility for one's own behavior in successful situations will increase self-confidence.

Anxieties and concerns about sexual identity must be resolved so that the patient can gain a healthy sense of self. Opportunities for the patient to explore consequences of choice in behavior must be explored.

Evaluation

Patient Outcome	Data Indicating That Outcome is Reached
Development and maintenance of a positive concept of personal identity	Decrease in manifestation of defining characteristics Positive acceptance of self Problem-solving skills with subsequent strategies that can promote and maintain development of personal identity Understanding of what are considered to be normal crises in growth and development associated with personal identity issues
Satisfaction with sexual identity and sexual preference	Decrease in manifestation of defining characteristics Acceptance of sexual identity and sexual preference Understanding of the consequences in choice of particular sexual identity and sexual preference

Self-Esteem Disturbance

(Situational low self-esteem; chronic low self-esteem)

Self-esteem disturbance is a disruption in the way an individual perceives his self-esteem.

Situational low self-esteem is negative self-evaluation and feelings about self that develop in response to a loss or change in an individual who previously had a positive self-evaluation.

Chronic low self-esteem is long-standing negative self-evaluation or feelings about self or one's capabilities.

Self-esteem disturbance is a disruption in the estimate one places on oneself, including one's self-worth, self-approval, self-confidence, and self-respect. Self-esteem is the evaluative component part of self-concept. The terms *self-concept* and *self-esteem* are often used interchangeably yet are defined differently by various authorities. Self-concept consists of four selves: physical self (body image), psychologic self (personal identity, self-esteem), social self (role performance), and moral self (spiritual beliefs and values). Variables that influence a person's self-concept and that can produce tension and stress, resulting in subsequent anxiety and eventual disorganization of a person's self-concept, are physical and personality characteristics present at birth, family and environmental factors, and emotional-social-cultural interactive experiences. How a person develops self-esteem depends on the number of repetitive positive experiences encountered in interactions with significant others in the environment. Sullivanian theory stressed the importance of the parental relationship and the reflected appraisal the child receives from parents. Rogers[14] states:

> The state of a person's self-esteem is not the product of a single issue or happening but is formed gradually over time. Therefore the collapse of self-esteem is not something which is reached in a day or even a month. It is the cumulative result of a long succession of failures. . . . Self-esteem represents the reputation a person has acquired within himself.

Persons with high self-esteem feel significant and confident and capable of achieving desired goals, whereas those with lowered self-esteem may be less confident.

Related Factors

Self-Esteem Disturbance

Repeated negative interpersonal experiences with significant others
Cognitive/perceptual difficulties
Inadequate social support
Early loss of parent or significant other
Traumatic developmental experiences
Excessive ridicule by others
Inability to adjust to body function alterations
Inability to adjust to body structure losses
Inadequate knowledge to cope with life stressors
Inadequate positive feedback
Lack of problem-solving skills
Unresolved emotionally traumatic experiences
Multiple stressors encountered over limited time
Unrealistic self-expectations
Depression
Negative interpretations of life events, e.g., assuming guilt

Situational Low Self-Esteem*

Major loss
- Loss of body part/function
- Loss of significant other
- Loss of job/work/role
- Loss of pet
- Loss of material goods
- Loss of reputation

Major life change or stress
- Divorce/marriage
- Prison term
- Addition or loss of family member
- Failure in school
- Financial burden
- Promotion/demotion
- Adolescent adjustments
- Sexual difficulties
- Hospitalization
- Occupational change

Environmental factors
- Disasters
- Poverty
- Change in living conditions or residence
- Discrimination
- Acculturation

See also Self-Esteem Disturbance.

Chronic Low Self-Esteem*

Long-standing, pernicious, nebulous fixated life response
Maladroit survival mechanisms
Insular life-style pattern
See also Self-Esteem Disturbance.

Defining Characteristics†

Feelings of hopelessness, helplessness, powerlessness, despair, guilt, inferiority, inadequacy, failure, defeatism, frustration, disappointment, worthlessness, and isolation
Expression of suicide intention with accompanying feelings of sadness, loss, depression, anxiety, and anger

*Adapted from North American Nursing Diagnosis Association, 1988 Ballot.
†References 2, 4, 6-8, 10, 11, 12.

Frequent expression of body aches and pains and overconcern with somatic woes
Perception of minimum strengths and assets with refusal to accept positive feedback
Denial of past and present successes and accomplishments
Frequent ruminations of past problems
Fear of handling change, making decisions, taking risks, expressing anger, and relating to others
Feelings of self-deprecation, inadequacy, and self-dislike; judging self harshly and punitively
Self-accusation
Appearance of signs of depression: psychomotor retardation, retarded thought processes, lack of energy, etc.
Slouched or drooping posture
Anorexia or obesity
Withdrawal from activities and interpersonal-social relationships
Decrease in sexual relationships and drive
Decrease in motivation and spontaneous behavior
Inability to communicate one's needs and concerns, to defend oneself, and to confront and overcome difficulties
Homicidal and/or suicidal behavior
Inability to initiate, follow through, or complete task in timely fashion
Inability to assume responsibilities for self-care
Inability to accept and/or extreme sensitivity to criticism
Avoiding situations of self-disclosure; tending to assume passive, nonparticipatory roles; tending to be "wallflower" in social situations
Misperception and misinterpretation of real self from self-ideal
Nonparticipation in therapy
Lack of eye contact
Lack of energy
Lack of attention to appearance
Lack of initiative in problem solving
Verbalizing difficulty in coping with tasks
Depreciative comments about self
Difficulties in job performance
Reluctance to engage in social interactions
Limited friendship network
Timid
Seclusive
Isolated play habits (children)
Inability to face new situations
Difficulties in school
Behavioral problems
Hesitant to ask for help
Pessimistic
Unassertive
Resentful of others who are well
Lack of confidence in one-to-one or group interactions
Self-blame

Situational Low Self-Esteem*

Episodic negative self-appraisal
Self-negative verbalization
Expressions of shame/guilt and evaluating self as unable to handle situations and events
Difficulty in making decisions
See also Self-Esteem Disturbance.

Chronic Low Self-Esteem*

Long-standing low self-evaluations and feelings about self and self-capabilities
Frequent lack of success in work or other life events
Hesitant to try new things and situations
Alienated from community resource network
Passive
Ruminations about past problems
Withdrawal
See also Self-Esteem Disturbance.

*Adapted from North American Nursing Diagnosis Association, 1988 Ballot.

Nursing Interventions*

Patient Goal	Nursing Intervention
Self-Esteem Disturbance	
Improve and maintain a constructive level of self-esteem.	• Communicate acceptance of the patient as a worthwhile, trusted human being who has intrinsic value. • Show genuine interest in and concern for patient. Spend time with patient in groups and in one-to-one relationships. • Avoid judgmental attitudes when working with patient. Do not criticize or belittle patient's feelings, actions, or ideas. • Assist patient in developing attitude of not always having to be perfect to feel adequate and good about oneself. Point out that patient is as worthy as anyone else despite imperfections. • Encourage patient to identify strengths, assets, and potential and how they are currently being used. • Help patient to list current and past successes.

*References 1-3, 6, 10, 11, 13, 14.

Patient Goal | **Nursing Intervention**

- Encourage patient to identify and participate in experiences he finds satisfying and rewarding.
- Encourage patient to develop new interpersonal and social skills and to initiate activities in which patient will be reasonably successful.
- Encourage patient to participate in various treatment modalities (e.g., group or family therapy) in which support, acceptance, and concern of others are major emphases, and in which patient learns that he is not alone in experiencing fears and failures.
- Teach patient assertive techniques and communication skills:
  - Use of "I" statements
  - Conveying clear expectations of others
  - Use of negotiation as viable tactic
  - Use of body posture, facial expression, and tone of voice consistent with verbal communication
  - Remaining firm but gentle and unyielding when appropriate
- Encourage patient to accept responsibility for personal opinions and behavior and to evaluate their outcome in relation to options available.
- Encourage patient to identify disappointments and dissatisfactions. In turn, have patient develop constructive problem-solving steps, with action behaviors and realistic time frames and goals to lessen or correct these problem areas successfully. Encourage patient to use this same approach when confronted with future problems.
- Offer supportive, positive, and genuine comments and feedback to patient when appropriate. Focus on specific changes in behavior and appearance when making these statements. Offer positive reinforcers for actual achievements. Avoid false praise.
- Maintain therapeutic environment that will foster patient's level of self-esteem. Emphasis should be on helping patient recognize that self-respect is first related to one's ability to respect self and then to respect and understand others.
- Increase social opportunities for interaction.
- Identify activities in which patient can be successful, and offer positive feedback.
- Encourage attractive grooming habits.
- Work through expressed fears and anxieties.
- Assist in developing problem-solving skills.
- Assist in increasing self-awareness.
- Identify previously used and successful coping skills.
- Assist patient to assess stressors realistically.
- Encourage participation in support or activity groups.
- Assist patient in expressing positive statements about self and eliminating self-derogatory statements:
  - Listen to statements.
  - Help patient to reappraise statements cognitively and make more positive statements.
- Review appropriate social activities with patient:
  - Assist patient in becoming aware of effect of constructive social experiences in building self-esteem.
  - Encourage involvement in positive social experiences.

Situational Low Self-Esteem

Patient Goal: Improve and maintain constructive level of self-esteem.

- Explore with patient the reason for loss, stress, or environmental factor causing low self-esteem.
- Develop strategies for coping with loss, stress, or environmental factors causing low self-esteem.

See also Self-Esteem Disturbance.

Chronic Low Self-Esteem

Patient Goal: Improve and maintain constructive level of self-esteem.

- Encourage self-support strategies for caregivers.
- Develop expectation in caregiver for possibly slow improvement.
- Plan for change in small increments.
- Identify life-style patterns that affect self-esteem and strategies for coping.
- Assist patient in identifying family and community resources for assisting with improving self-esteem.
- Refer patient to interdisciplinary colleagues for assistance in identifying needed resources.
- Refer to therapist if indicated.

See also Self-Esteem Disturbance.

Principles and Rationale for Nursing Interventions[9,11]

In examining the etiology of how a person develops low self-esteem, one realizes that it occurs through repeated negative experiences and attacks on self-worth, self-respect, self-confidence, and self-appraisal systems.

Maslow postulated that all people have a need to esteem or value themselves and that positive values about self help persons seek and deal with their environmental experiences constructively. A person with a low value of self tends to perceive environmental stimuli as negative and threatening. In turn, the ability to deal with environmental experiences positively is disrupted in an effort to ward off further threats to an already damaged self-esteem. Positive self-esteem can be a powerful resource in enabling a patient to participate in care, engage confidently in interpersonal communications, gain accurate feedback from others, and enhance the ability to cope successfully in role demands.

The patient with a self-esteem disturbance can feel worthless and unable to cope with daily stressors or achieve desired outcomes for self. Thus it is important to provide a supportive but reality-oriented environment in which a patient can engage in a variety of activities and therapies that allow for successful and constructive experiences to aid in the development of a positive self-esteem. For patients with situational low self-esteem the nurse uses a problem-solving approach to help them deal with cause and effect. For patients with chronic low self-esteem the nurse should recognize and accept chronicity, expect progress in small increments, seek support for the self, and be familiar with resources to provide referrals.

Evaluation

Patient Outcome	Data Indicating That Outcome is Reached
Improvement and maintenance of a constructive level of self-esteem	Decrease in manifestation of defining characteristics Acceptance of self-worth, self-respect, self-approval, and self-confidence Improvement in personal appearance (hygiene and grooming) Improvement in psychologic test scores that measure self-concept and self-esteem (e.g., Tennessee Self-Concept Scale) Demonstrates problem-solving skills with subsequent strategies that can promote and maintain positive level of self-esteem Identification and use of existing strengths, assets, and successes Recognition of value and use of various treatment modalities (e.g., group and family therapy) Appropriate assertive behaviors and communication skills Engages in age-appropriate activities Increased social contacts and friendship networks Expressed satisfaction with own achievements Takes initiative for new learning tasks Demonstrates adequate involvement in relevant job performance Displays appropriate mood Displays confidence in self Grooms self appropriately Engages in positive talk about self Expresses satisfaction with functional ability in preferred life roles

FUNCTIONAL HEALTH PATTERN

VIII

Role-Relationship

 Anticipatory Grieving

Anticipatory grieving is the state in which an individual grieves before an actual loss.

Anticipatory grieving is the initiation and actual process of grieving that takes place when anticipating a significant loss, before the significant loss actually takes place. The significant loss can refer to the potential death of a significant person who is facing terminal illness, the potential loss of a limb in upcoming surgery, the potential loss of a friend who is planning to move away, or anticipation of one's own impending death.[4] The anticipation of a significant loss requires that an individual deal with the consequences of the loss before the loss actually occurs.[9] The process of anticipatory grieving can help a person adjust to the loss before its occurrence. It can also decrease the intensity of the grieving after the actual loss occurs.[14]

Anticipatory grieving may be functional or dysfunctional for an individual or family depending on the manner in which it is experienced and responded to by others in the environment.[10] Determination of the diagnosis of anticipatory grieving is based on the timing of grief.

Related Factors[13,14]

Perceived potential loss of significant person
Perceived potential loss of significant animal
Perceived potential loss of prized material possession(s)
Perceived potential loss of body part(s) or function(s)
Perceived potential loss of physiopsychosocial well-being
Perceived potential loss of social role
Perceived potential developmental or role-transition loss(es)
Perceived impending death of self

Defining Characteristics[13,14]

Normal grieving initiated on anticipation of a significant loss
Denial of potential loss
- Shock
- Disbelief
- Avoiding focusing on loss

Physiologic symptoms
- Decreased muscular power
- Feeling of emptiness in stomach
- Tightness in throat
- Choking sensation
- Shortness of breath
- Sighing
- Perspiration
- Flushed face
- Exhaustion
- Changes in eating habits, e.g., decreased appetite

Internal preoccupation
Disinterest or difficulty in carrying out activities of daily living
Anger
Hostility or irritability toward others
Guilt
Self-accusation of negligence
Sorrow
Weeping
Feelings of loss and loneliness
Emotional distance from others
Sense of unreality
Alterations in sleep patterns
Social isolation and inhibition
High ambivalence
Altered communication patterns
- Speech pressure
- Reduced communication

Alterations in activity level
  Psychomotor retardation
  Restlessness with inability to engage in organized activities
  Withdrawal
Altered libido

Decreased acceleration of grieving, increased defense mechanisms as death or loss approaches
Hope for preventing loss
Realization or resolution of impending death or loss

Nursing Interventions*

Patient Goal	Nursing Intervention
Participate in constructive anticipatory grief work.	• Encourage description of perceptions of potential loss. • Encourage verbalization of fears and concerns. • Recognize influence of past problem-solving abilities on current and future coping. • Recognize influence of following factors on coping: Previous experience with illness Socioeconomic background Educational preparation Cultural beliefs Spiritual beliefs • Monitor: Length of time since learning of potential loss Past experience with loss, illness, and death Current sources of social support (family, friends, church) Disruptions in current life-style related to anticipated loss (finances, living arrangements, transportation) • Recognize that patient and significant others may differ in stage of grieving they are experiencing. • Acknowledge to patient and significant others that pattern of their past relationships with each other will be similar to their relationships as they experience anticipated loss. • During stage of shock and disbelief: Provide quiet environment. Allow for use of denial and other defense mechanisms. Avoid reinforcement of denial. Avoid confronting patient or significant others when they are experiencing distorted perceptions. Provide opportunity for expression of emotions. Provide assurance that it is normal to experience intense feelings and reactions. Avoid defensive and judgmental responses to criticisms of health care providers. Do not encourage use of antianxiety medications. Do not force decisions. Enlist support from others (e.g., family, friends, clergy). • During stage of developing awareness of potential loss: Encourage expression of feelings with relatives and friends. Facilitate contact with nursing staff and other health team members to correct misinformation about cause of loss. Facilitate exploration of available options. Support verbalizations about possible body image changes. Offer hope for ability to cope with anticipated loss. Encourage and teach good health habits. Encourage persons experiencing similar anticipated losses to consider spending time together to share mutual fears, feelings, and concerns. Evaluate need for referral to resources (e.g., Social Security representatives, legal consultants, support groups). • During stage of developing awareness of potential loss of significant other: Provide significant others with ongoing information of patient's diagnosis, prognosis, and plan of care. Encourage significant others to describe their desires and information needs in caring for patient. Facilitate significant other's assistance with patient's physical care. Facilitate flexible visiting hours and include younger children when appropriate. Help patient and significant others to share mutual fears, concerns, plans, and hopes with each other. Promote imaging of future. Encourage patient and significant others to explore impact of their lives on each other and to visualize lives of unborn descendants. Suggest letter writing as

*References 1-3, 5-9, 11, 12, 13, 15, 16.

Patient Goal	Nursing Intervention
	means for conveying thoughts, wishes, and concerns to significant others as they experience future developmental milestones. Offer hope to patient and significant others that they will have quality time together. Help significant others to understand that patient's verbalizations of anger should not be perceived as personal attacks. Encourage significant others to maintain their own self-care needs for rest, sleep, nutrition, leisure activities, and time away from patient. Facilitate patient's and significant others' discussion of final arrangements (e.g., funeral services, burial wishes, organ donation, desire for autopsy). Teach patient and significant others to recognize and trust decisions that "feel" right to them in relation to their coping with impending losses. • During period of mourning for anticipated loss: Help patient accept reality of impending loss. Provide information as sought. Allow for reminiscence about anticipated loss. Encourage expression of feelings (e.g., crying). Facilitate discussion of both negative and positive aspects of anticipated loss. Foster environment in which loss can be experienced within spiritual context. Provide guidance regarding availability of community resources. • During period of mourning before death of loved one: Promote discussion of what to expect when death occurs. Encourage significant others and patient to share their wishes about family members being present with patient at death. Avoid judgmental responses to choices made. Help significant others to accept that choosing to be absent at death does not indicate a lack of love or caring for patient. Discuss indicators of impending death as appropriate. Provide comforting measures for patient; encourage significant others to assist if they wish. Encourage significant others to maintain verbal communication and touch with their loved one, even though patient may not respond. Provide as much privacy as possible for significant others to be alone or with patient when death is imminent.

Principles and Rationale for Nursing Interventions

The perception of an anticipated loss is a subjective one. Past problem-solving abilities, previous experience with illness, socioeconomic background, educational preparation, and cultural and spiritual beliefs are factors that influence the way in which an individual copes with an anticipated loss. The ultimate outcome of how a person copes with anticipated loss is influenced by the subjective meaning of the loss.[1,3,9]

The stage of shock and disbelief in anticipatory grieving is characterized by attempts to "protect oneself against the overwhelming stress by raising the threshold" of recognition of the painful feelings evoked. Denial is the most frequently used means of coping at this time.[9]

The stage of developing awareness of the potential loss includes "acute and increasing awareness of the pain and anguish of the loss."[9] Feelings of anxiety, helplessness, and hopelessness may be expressed, as well as hope that some action can be taken to prevent the anticipated loss.[14] Anger and guilt may be directed toward oneself or others. Cultural patterns influence the expression of these feelings.[16]

The period of mourning is a time in which "support and sustenance" is helpful as the reality of the impending loss becomes more evident. There may be an increased preoccupation with the personal experience of the anticipated loss and an increased need to talk with others about the meaning of the loss.[9]

Evaluation[11,13,14]

Patient Outcome	Data Indicating That Outcome is Reached
Participates in constructive anticipatory grief work	Discusses thoughts and feelings related to anticipated loss Verbalizes information needs Uses appropriate resources (e.g., friends, clergy, support groups, legal consultants, Social Security representatives) Involvement in mutual decision making related to anticipated loss Maintains constructive interpersonal relationships Significant others able to meet ongoing care needs

 Dysfunctional Grieving

Dysfunctional grieving is a maladaptive process that occurs when grief is intensified to the degree that the person is overwhelmed, remains interminably in one phase of grieving, and demonstrates excessive or prolonged emotional responses to a significant loss.

Normal grieving is the process by which a person adapts to a significant loss. This adaptation, which can last up to 1 year, includes[12]:

Emotional emancipation from the significant loss
Readjustment to the environment
Development of new relationships and emotional investment in new objects to restructure a new life and to achieve personal reorganization

Dysfunctional grieving represents a distortion of normal grieving. In dysfunctional grieving the normal process of grieving is delayed or prolonged or the emotions experienced are excessive or distorted. The "person becomes stuck in one phase of grieving, demonstrating excessive emotional reactions or excessive length of time in a phase."[12]

Dysfunctional grieving can thus be defined as[5]:

> The intensification of grief to the level where the person is overwhelmed, resorts to maladaptive behavior, or remains interminably in the state of grief without progression of the mourning process toward completion. . . . [It] involves the processes that lead to stereotyped repetitions or extensive interruptions of healing.

Dysfunctional grieving may be manifested as unresolved grief, which is associated with "severe reactions to separation, unexplained somatic responses, specific medical diseases, and altered relationships with friends, relatives, and others."[8]

Related Factors[7,12]

Perceived or actual loss of significant person
Perceived or actual loss of significant animal
Perceived or actual loss of prized material possession(s)
Perceived or actual loss of body part(s) or function(s)
Perceived or actual loss of physiopsychosocial well-being
Perceived or actual loss of social role(s)
Perceived or actual development or role-transition loss(es)
Multiple previous or concurrent losses
Previous unresolved or interlocking grief reactions
Lack of adequate social supports
Difficulty or inability in expressing feelings freely
Unresolved guilt related to deceased person
Sudden, untimely, unexpected death or loss
Prolonged or stressful anticipated loss
Unrevealed secrets or unfinished business with deceased person
Loss sustained when confronted with important tasks or need to sustain others emotionally
Previous pattern of delayed or dysfunctional grief reactions
Secondary gain from others to maintain grieving
Powerful but silent contracts with deceased person
Overidentification with deceased person
Dysfunctional grieving process of parents
Unconscious family maneuvers to alleviate guilt or control fate

Defining Characteristics[7,12]

Arrested or excessive time in any stage of normal grieving
Excessive, distorted, exaggerated, and/or delayed emotional reaction
Prolonged or excessive denial of loss
Extreme difficulty in concentration and/or pursuit of tasks
Prolonged developmental regression
Maladaptive behavior interfering with life functioning
Continuous reliving of past experiences
Excessive idealization of lost person
Severely impaired self-esteem
Excessive self-blame or self-reproach
Protracted withdrawal
Protracted symptoms similar to those of dead person
Protracted hyperactivity or irritability
Stereotyped, repetitious behaviors
Being overwhelmed by protracted grief
Severe feelings of loss of identity
Loss of interest in and planning for future
Resurrection-of-the-dead syndrome
Unabated searching behavior or yearning for lost object
Feeling or behaving as if loss occurred yesterday
Inability to remove material possessions of deceased person
Psychosomatic conditions
Social withdrawal or isolation
Engaging in self-detrimental activities
Unusual dependency
Expansive, adventurous overactivity without sense of loss
Prolonged depression, agitated depression
Irrational despair, severe hopelessness
Suicidal thoughts and fantasies
Extremely labile affect
Extreme anger or hostility
Furious, persistent hostility toward specific persons
Prolonged guilt
Protracted apathy
Inappropriate affect
Excessive ambivalence along with inability to deal with it
Prolonged panic attacks
Intense separation anxiety
Schizophrenic-like features
Refusal to follow prescribed treatment regimen, especially in clients with chronic mental illness

Nursing Interventions*

Patient Goal	Nursing Intervention
Demonstrate absence of delayed, excessive, or distorted emotional reactions.	• Monitor patient's perception of: Current adaptation Responses from significant others Social network Past life experiences Past problem-solving skills • Evaluate influence of denial on patient's participation with recommended treatments. • Assess possible needs met by denial. • Observe for responses by health care providers that may be reinforcing maladaptive denial. • Point out reality in nonthreatening manner without arguing with patient or significant others. • Present patient with increasing facts. • Monitor for suicidal ideation/intent. • Clarify and offer missing factual information. • Defer teaching related to adaptation to loss until patient demonstrates decrease in denial. • Facilitate constructive working through of expression of feelings: Demonstrate tolerance for expression of negative feelings. Support verbalizations of ambivalence. Facilitate contact with people who can openly express feelings. Assist patient to understand possible reasons for feelings. • Provide opportunity for patient to describe experiences that preceded current loss. • Point out universality of need for normal grieving. • Encourage description of future expectations.
Experience resolution of dysfunctional grieving.	• Encourage description of current and anticipated problems related to loss. • Monitor for suicidal ideation/intent. • Offer hope for successful adaptation to loss. • Assist patient in proceeding through phase in which he or she is locked: Demonstrate tolerance, patience, and empathy. Permit open expression of feelings without becoming defensive. Assist patient to understand reasons for feelings. Reassure patient that feelings of guilt are part of normal grieving. Assist patient to work through feelings of guilt. Encourage patient to talk and reminisce about loss. Correct misinformation about loss. Facilitate review of positive and negative aspects of loss. • Evaluate need for referral to resources, e.g., brief psychotherapy, support groups, or family therapy. • Promote patient's recognition of past and present strengths that can be used for coping with current loss. • Promote description of possible strategies for coping with current loss. • Consider use of role playing to facilitate patient's awareness of possible alternatives and consequences of decisions. • Facilitate contact with others who have successfully adapted to similar loss. • For inpatients, promote use of weekend and daytime passes (based on individual assessment of patient). • Promote coordination of resources to help patient: Develop new skills. Make readjustments in life-style. Make new emotional investments. • Provide guidance about available community resources.

*References 2, 3, 7, 8, 11, 12, 14.

Principles and Rationale for Nursing Interventions

Delayed emotional reactions to loss are often unpredictable. Sometimes postponement of the reaction to a loss occurs when an individual initially has to deal with difficult tasks or when an individual helps to maintain the morale of others immediately after the loss.[10] The use of denial as an attempt to adjust to the effects from a loss can contribute to a patient's experiencing delayed emotional reactions. The patient's significant others and health care providers may also use denial to cope with their feelings of helplessness and frustration in emotionally charged situations. Although denial initially serves to minimize the anxiety-producing aspects of a loss, its "inconsistency with reality makes it a very brittle defense."[2] Suicidal ideation and intent may occur as the patient begins to come face to face with the reality of a loss. When the patient begins to experience negative feelings, they are frequently directed at the nurse and other caregivers: "It is only within the safety of a trusting relationship that communication can be encouraged and feelings expressed."[3]

The resolution of dysfunctional grieving allows the patient to place the past in its proper perspective. The development of new coping strategies assists the patient to find meaning in the present.[8] The person who is experiencing dysfunctional grieving may benefit from contacts with resources that "mediate a hopeful, positive, healthy balance which will encourage the patient to move forward."[14] Reflection on the disruptions of previous goals leads to the development of new goals. Contact with others who have adapted to similar losses is visible proof that grief can be resolved.

Evaluation[7]

Patient Outcome	Data Indicating That Outcome is Reached
Demonstrates absence of delayed emotional reactions	Acknowledges awareness of loss Verbalizes thoughts and feelings related to loss
Experiences resolution of dysfunctional grieving	Participates in recommended treatment modalities Develops goals that are congruent with loss Identifies alternate plans for meeting goals that were significant before loss Participates in activities of daily living Begins to participate in role responsibilities (e.g., job)

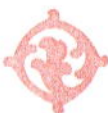

Altered Role Performance

Altered role performance is a disruption in the way an individual perceives his role performance.

Problems associated with role functioning include role insufficiency, role distance, interrole conflict, intrarole conflict, and role failure.

Role insufficiency occurs whenever an individual has difficulty in the cognizance and/or performance of a role or of the sentiments and goals associated with the role behavior as perceived by the self or by significant others.[8]

Role distance implies that an individual demonstrates both instrumental and expressive behavior appropriate to his role, but these behaviors differ significantly from prescribed behaviors for the role.[10]

Interrole conflict occurs when the individual demonstrates instrumental and expressive behaviors incompatible with the expected behaviors for his role as a result of occupancy of one or more roles that require incompatible expected behaviors.[10]

Intrarole conflict occurs when the individual demonstrates instrumental and expressive behaviors incompatible with the expected behaviors for his role as a result of incompatible expectations from one or more persons in the environment concerning the expected behavior.[10]

Role failure occurs when there is an absence of feelings or expressive behavior and/or a lack of action or instrumental behaviors.[10]

Each of these role-functioning problems can develop in relation to developmental transitions (e.g., moving from adulthood to old age), situational transitions (e.g., the addition of a family member), and health-illness transitions (e.g., going from a well state to an acute or chronic illness state).

The functionalist and interactionist approaches are major perspectives of roles and role performance. The functionalists view roles as somewhat fixed in society and see them as reinforced by negative or positive reinforcements from others. The interactionists view society as providing the framework within which the person interacts with others, interprets behavior, and then constructs his role response. Social action and role performance may be best "construed not simply as learned responses but as an organizing and interpreting of cues in one's environment."[3]

Related Factors[9]

Absence of significant role models
Cognitive difficulties
Changes in values and beliefs
Lack of time management skills
Inadequate role socialization
Perceptual difficulties
Mental illness
Developmental transitions
Negative self-perception
Situational transitions
Cultural discrepancies
Health-illness transition
Conflict situations
Physical limitations

Defining Characteristics*

Feelings of grief, loss, powerlessness, anger, anxiety, depression, and withdrawal
Lack of knowledge of role
Change in self-perception of role
Change in others' perception of role performance
Dislike of role
Ambivalence of role
Denial of role
Failure to assume role (role failure)
Behaviors that are appropriate for role but that differ from prescribed behaviors for role (role distance)
Behaviors that are incompatible with expected role because of occupancy of one or more roles that require incompatible expected behaviors (interrole conflict)
Behaviors that are incompatible with expected role because of incompatible expectations from one or more persons in environment concerning expected behavior(s) (intrarole conflict)
Change in physical capacity to resume role
Change in usual patterns or responsibility
Lack of knowledge of how to perform role (role insufficiency)
Behaviors that contradict others' expectation of role performance
Behaviors that contradict self-expectation of role performance
Lack of knowledge on how to perform role
Verbalizations of inadequate role performance

*References 2, 4, 5, 7, 8, 10.

Nursing Interventions

Patient Goal	Nursing Intervention
Develop role mastery.	• Determine which type of role-functioning problem patient is experiencing: role insufficiency, role disturbance, interrole conflict, intrarole conflict, or role failure. • Determine condition(s) predisposing patient to problematic role-functioning behavior: developmental, situational, or health-illness transition. • Encourage patient to verbalize feelings, concerns, fears, and anxieties associated with assuming a particular role. • Help patient to assess what impact this new role will have when assuming present and future roles. • Once type of role-functioning problem has been identified, use: Role clarification. Place emphasis on what role entails in terms of behavior, sentiments, costs, and rewards, and whether significant other reinforces role negatively or positively. Role taking. Place emphasis on helping patient imaginatively assume position or point of view of another person taking on new role. Role modeling. Place emphasis on helping patient enact and play out new role so that he or she can understand and emulate intracacies of behavior associated with new role. Role rehearsal. Place emphasis on helping patient fantasize, imagine, and mentally enact how encounter might take place and how new role might evolve and develop. Reference groups. Place emphasis on exposing patient to other individuals or groups who have successfully assumed role mastery of new role. • Provide therapeutic environment that will allow for opportunities to learn and practice new role behaviors. Help patient practice with feedback the role behaviors he has failed to assume or perform before. • Identify and provide role models. • Provide assistance in obtaining necessary knowledge and skills for role performance. • Use role playing to practice newly acquired role behaviors. • Assist patient in resolving any conflicts regarding role. • Praise and reinforce approximations of expected role performance. • Be nonjudgmental. • Identify and support strengths and capabilities related to adequate role performance. • Encourage self-monitoring of changes in role behavior. • Facilitate increase in self-awareness. • Support and enhance patient's belief in self-worth and self-efficacy.

Principles and Rationale for Nursing Interventions[1,2,4,6,7]

In formulating appropriate intervention strategies for altered role performance, the nurse assesses the type of role disturbance and the patient's perception of self. For example, is the patient satisfied with present role performance? What would the patient like to change? What are the perceived consequences of this change? Role performance is partly learned. Therefore learning opportunities need to be made available to the patient. Empathy and a supportive environment assist the patient in making maximum behavioral changes. Working through excessive feeling states permit the patient to direct energy and focus on the necessary behavioral changes and learning requirements for more satisfactory role performance.

Evaluation

Patient Outcome	Data Indicating That Outcome is Reached
Develops mastery of newly acquired or assumed roles	Decrease in manifestation of defining characteristics Positively expresses acceptance of new role Verbalizes understanding of appropriate cognitive, instrumental, and expressive behaviors, goals, and sentiments associated with role Describes impact new role will have in assuming other role behaviors Demonstrates use of various role supplementation strategies, with resultant ability to perform role without difficulty Demonstrates problem-solving skills with subsequent strategies that can promote and maintain mastery of newly acquired role and possible future roles

Social Isolation

Social isolation is aloneness experienced by an individual and perceived as imposed by others and as a negative or threatened state.

Social isolation can also be defined as the state in which the individual has a need or desire for contact with others but is unable to make that contact because of physiologic, biologic, or sociocultural factors.[3] Social isolation is a negative state of aloneness.

Human relationships are important to mental and physical well-being. Social isolation, the lack of human companionship, death or absence of parents in early childhood, sudden loss of love, and chronic human loneliness are significant contributors to premature death and abnormal human functioning.[11]

To realize the consequences of social isolation, it is important to understand relevant personality theory. A number of personality theorists—Adler, Freud, Horney, Sullivan, Erikson, and Fromm—contributed to an understanding of this diagnosis. Sullivan developed the interpersonal theory of personality. He believed that an individual cannot exist apart from relationships with other people.[7]

Social isolation can be a result of faulty development in the life span. The psychologic ramifications are multiple. If an individual does not learn to cope with the stress and anxieties of life in a healthy manner, he may end up with grave psychologic difficulties.

Often it is difficult to separate completely biologically related factors of isolation from psychologic ones because a biologic cause can lead an individual to exhibit psychologic manifestations of isolation. Conversely, a psychologic cause can lead to a biologic outcome. Moreover, sociocultural etiologies of social isolation overlap the psychologic and biologic causative factors.

Related Factors[10]

Psychologic
- Emotional illness (extreme anxiety, depression, paranoia, phobias, psychosis)
- Inability to engage in satisfying personal relationships
- Delay in accomplishing developmental tasks
- Immature interests
- Obesity, anorexia, bulimia
- Drug or alcohol addiction
- Alterations in physical appearance

Physiologic
- Altered state of wellness
- Drug or alcohol addiction
- Obesity, anorexia, bulimia
- Cancer
- Hospitalization or terminal illness
- Physical handicaps (paraplegia, amputation, arthritis, hemiplegia)
- Incontinence (embarrassment, odor)
- Sensory loss

Sociocultural
- Death of significant other
- Divorce
- Extreme poverty
- Moving into another culture
- Alternative life-styles
- Loss of usual means of transportation
- Unaccepted social values
- Inadequate personal resources
- Single parent

Defining Characteristics[3,10]

Absence of supportive significant other(s): family, friends, group
Sad, dull affect
Inappropriate or immature interests and activities for developmental age or stage
Uncommunicative
Withdrawn
No eye contact
Preoccupation with own thoughts; repetitive, meaningless actions
Projects hostility in voice and behavior
Seeks to be alone or exists in subculture
Evidence of physical and/or mental handicap or altered state of wellness

Obesity
Anorexia
Paraplegia
Shows behavior unaccepted by dominant cultural group
Feelings of uselessness
Doubts about ability to survive
Expresses feeling of aloneness imposed by others
Expresses feelings of rejection
Experiences feelings of difference from others
Expresses values acceptable to subculture but unable to accept values of dominant culture
Inadequacy in or absence of significant purpose in life
Altered thought processes
Agoraphobia
Inability to meet expectations of others
Insecurity in public
Excessive sleeping
Expresses interests inappropriate to developmental age or stage
Self-absorbed
Sleep disturbances
Inability to make decisions
Change in nutritional intake (overeating or anorexia)
Paranoia
Mistrust
Hallucinations: auditory, visual, kinetic
Feelings of inferiority
Depersonalization
Feelings of otherness
Lack of attention

Nursing Interventions[1-7,10-14,17,19]

Patient Goal	Nursing Intervention
Experience less negative state of aloneness.	• Establish trust. • Assess social history. • Identify limitations and barriers in ability to form meaningful relationships with others. • Discuss feelings of loneliness. • Explain relationship between loneliness and unmet intimacy needs. • Encourage verbalization of loneliness. • Discuss potentials for meaningful relationship to decrease loneliness. • Identify with patient possible social outlets. • Promote increased self-esteem. • Explore ways of reaching out to others. • Assess and assist with balancing independence and dependence in family roles. • Encourage involvement in peer groups, social activity, or evening out at least weekly. • Support individual experiencing loss. • Validate normalcy of grieving. • Encourage support group participation for widows and widowers. • Use grandparent programs, day care centers (for children and elderly), retirement communities, house sharing, pets, and telephone contacts to decrease isolation. • Recognize and use churches as valued resource. • Encourage physical closeness (touch). • Help identify and obtain transportation options. • Identify diversional activities that decrease feelings of loneliness. • Assist with development of alternate means of communication, if sensory impairment exists. • Identify and suggest solutions for physical impairments that affect body image (ostomy, cancer odor, incontinence, disfiguring surgery). *Elderly:* • Introduce self and call patient by name. • Establish trust and mutual respect. • Locate and inform about neighborhood social groups and self-help groups specific to patient's needs. • Teach family and older person about process of aging. • Encourage patient to select and perform productive activities that promote self-esteem. • Teach problem-solving techniques. • Encourage selection of activities that broaden social network and facilitate personal growth. • Find ways to maintain life-style that allows personal freedom. • Provide interpreters to assist the elderly Hispanic or other non-English-speaking person to locate appropriate social support resources. • Determine upper and lower levels of mentally disabled patient's functional capacity. • Thoroughly assess social history of mentally disabled patient. • Evaluate physical health problems. • Identify social supports available to mentally disabled patient. • Assess diet and exercise. • Teach self-management skills before inpatient discharge and do weekly follow-up after discharge.

Patient Goal	Nursing Intervention
	• Assess onset, frequency, and impact of manifestations of Alzheimer's disease. • Teach caregiving relatives ways to deal with difficult or inappropriate behavior. • Provide ongoing support to caregiving relatives and encourage social relationships outside family group. • Encourage pets for therapeutic interaction.

Principles and Rationale for Nursing Interventions

The formation of effective human relationships affects the health and well-being of all patients. Therefore it is essential that the nurse assess carefully the patient's social history when limitations or barriers are found in the ability to form relationships with others. Since social isolation is a subjective state, all inferences made regarding a person's feelings of aloneness must be validated.[3] The nurse must possess skilled interview and communication techniques to effectively help patients identify and overcome social isolation.

It is important for the nurse to discuss any feelings of loneliness the patient expresses. Loneliness is the result of unmet intimacy needs. After a therapeutic nurse/patient relationship is established, these feelings can be discussed and ways of meeting intimacy needs explored. To do this effectively, nurses must accept and deal with any of their own feelings of loneliness. Possible etiologies of social isolation must be explored with the patient in an open, direct, and supportive manner. Problem-solving techniques need to be discussed and taught to the patient, with the ultimate decision-making process focusing on the patient to promote behavioral change. Follow-up care is absolutely necessary for the patient's continued support and accomplishment of the outcomes desired.

Isolated older persons pose a complex problem for nursing care because the likelihood that they will seek assistance depends on several factors.[15] A painful physical disorder that cannot be ignored is more likely to lead the individual to seek help. Second, the more isolated older persons are, the less likely they are to seek help. Third, the social support resource must be familiar and acceptable to the person. Last, unsuccessful, uncaring, or inappropriate experiences with the social resources will discourage older persons from seeking future contact.

The elderly person often lacks the social skills to find supports and use referral services. It is important to increase the patient's awareness of appropriate resources that best meet his specific needs. The nurse can help develop adequate communication and assertiveness skills to facilitate the use of available social resources to decrease social isolation. Encouraging the elderly person to accept the need for a broader support system can be challenging. The nurse must establish mutual respect and trust to promote continued self-esteem and openness to outside resources. Family members can often assist in this process. The patient, however, must be encouraged to make his own decision to maintain pride and self-respect, unless the patient is cognitively incapable of making appropriate decisions. Peer groups and other social organizations close to the patient can also help increase awareness of and openness to social support resources.

Cultural differences also affect the social isolation of the elderly. Separation from their extended family, low expectations of service providers, language differences from those of the larger population, limited education, language deficits, and noncitizen status are other barriers that contribute to lack of knowledge of social service resources. The nurse must assess for the presence of these barriers and find ways to promote social interaction.

The chronically mentally disabled elderly face longstanding isolators, including broken family relationships and community ties, limited social coping skills, limited education, and limited employability.[15] These patients need complex multidisciplinary intervention guided by the nurse.

Evaluation

Patient Outcome	Data Indicating That Outcome is Reached
Identifies causes of feelings of isolation	Verbalizes fears, limitations, and barriers to interaction with others Verbalizes feelings of loneliness Recognizes need for intimacy Admits concerns about low self-esteem Verbalizes negative experiences in past that may have ended relationships
Verbalizes and demonstrates ways to promote meaningful relationships	Desire to increase meaningful relationships Increased self-esteem Participates in routine activities as inpatient Talks to others Approaches others to socialize Plans to join social peer group or activity at least once a week

Patient Outcome	Data Indicating That Outcome is Reached
	Increased social skills Admits fears and concerns regarding social interaction Participates in support group Recognizes need for personal freedom and growth Ability to function as part of group
Identifies activities that provide diversion and stimulate interest and self-esteem	Lists at least five activities that provide enjoyment and increased self-worth Participates in one or more of these activities at least biweekly Positive feeling elicited from these activities Increased feelings of involvement

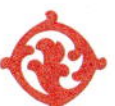

Impaired Social Interaction

Impaired social interaction is the state in which an individual participates in an insufficient or excessive quantity or ineffective quality of social exchange.

A person exhibiting impaired social interactive behavior may have a personality impairment, may have been environmentally deprived, may be socially backward, or may be physically impaired. The related factors are similar to those for the nursing diagnosis Social Isolation, but the behavior exhibited in impaired social interaction could be considered less severe in psychiatric terms.

Children who are physically separated from parents often have difficulty in forming attachments to others in their adult life.[1,3,10] Severe adult depression, dependency, psychosis (social isolation), various neuroses (impaired social interaction), and suicide all have been frequently reported among individuals who suffer early parental loss.

Any way in which a child finds to cope may become a permanent characteristic in the child's adult personality. The child may learn to cope neurotically by using irrational means. Alternately, the child may learn to cope normally by using rational means in a home where there is security, trust, love, respect, tolerance, and warmth.[5] The person who is likely to become neurotic is one who has experienced the culturally determined difficulties in an accentuated form, primarily through childhood experience.[6]

Physical deprivation and/or physical ailments can cause social isolation, pathologic disorders, and impaired social interaction in individuals. Physical deprivation can be viewed as removal of an individual from social supports, e.g., loss of parents, institutionalization, and loss of physical functioning.

Related Factors[9]

Knowledge/skill deficit about ways to enhance mutuality
Communication barriers
Low self-concept
Absence of available significant others or peers
Limited physical mobility
Therapeutic isolation
Sociocultural dissonance
Environmental barriers
Altered thought processes
Inappropriate social behavior
Chemical addiction

Defining Characteristics[9]

Verbalized or observed discomfort in social situations
Verbalized or observed inability to receive or communicate satisfying sense of belonging, caring, interest, or shared history
Observed use of unsuccessful social interaction behaviors
Dysfunctional interaction with peers, family, and/or others
Family report of change of style or pattern of interaction

Nursing Interventions

Patient Goal	Nursing Intervention
Increase social interactive skills.	• Establish trust. • Assess social history. • Identify limitations and barriers in ability to form meaningful relationships with others. • Promote increased self-esteem. • Explore ways of appropriately reaching out to others. • Assess and assist with balancing independence and dependence in family roles. • Encourage involvement in peer groups, social activity, or evening out at least weekly. • Assist with development of alternative means of communication if sensory impairment exists. • Identify and suggest solutions for physical impairments that affect body image.

Patient Goal	Nursing Intervention
	• Support and encourage participation in normal social activities. • Encourage involvement in work, social, or therapeutic group. • Discuss rejection, coping skills, and ways to promote group involvement. • Facilitate conversation between peers. • Encourage expression of feelings regarding social interaction. • Encourage making choices in day-to-day activities. • Give positive reinforcements and praise for social interactions. • Teach social skills and problem-solving techniques.

Principles and Rationale for Nursing Interventions

A major cause for impaired social interaction is the inability to communicate effectively. This inability can be partly caused by feelings of inadequacy. The nurse must be attuned to a patient's feelings of inadequacy. This is often difficult because people exhibit their inadequacies by different and varying forms of communication, e.g., overtalkativeness, silence, anger, or hostility.

Nursing interventions for this patient are similar to intervening with a socially isolated individual; however, one must keep in mind that the person who is interactively impaired is not as severely impaired as one who is socially isolated. This means that the nurse has a better base from which to begin.

Often, social impairment is not perceived by the patient as a problem for himself. The nurse needs to establish a trusting relationship to deal with the issues with the patient, the family, and friends.

Possible causal factors related to impaired social interaction must be explored with the patient in an open, direct, and supportive manner. Problem-solving techniques need to be discussed and taught to the patient, with the ultimate decision-making process focusing on the patient to promote behavioral change. Follow-up care is absolutely necessary for the patient's continued support and accomplishment of the outcomes desired.

Evaluation

Patient Outcome	Data Indicating That Outcome is Reached
Demonstrates increased ability to cope with social interaction	Verbalizes feelings and needs for social interaction Engages in social activities without feeling anxious or embarrassed Verbalizes/demonstrates increased self-esteem Reaches out to others Verbalizes desire to be independent Demonstrates independent social interactions Verbalizes desire to have peer group Demonstrates ability to function interactively in peer group Develops alternate means of communication if sensory impairment present Verbalizes positive or improved body image Verbalizes knowledge of rejection (if it exists) and ways to cope Makes choices in social interactions Demonstrates social skills Demonstrates problem-solving ability

 Altered Family Processes

Altered family processes is the state in which a family who normally functions effectively experiences a dysfunction.

The family has been described as a "human group with significant emotional bonds, usually living together in the same household."[16] Functions of the family include the following[20]:

Reproduction
Socialization (education of the young)
Protection and safety
Economic security (provision of food and shelter)
Conferral of roles
Social contact
Sexual fulfillment
Conferral of status
Belongingness, love, and affection
Physiologic needs
Recreation
Religious needs

In disturbed families several factors apparently cluster at the same time. "A combination of events produce symptomatic behavior in one or more members of a given family."[7]

Characteristics of a functional family include the following[11,17]:

- Homeostatic balance is maintained along with flexibility.
- The family is able to adapt to external (environmental) and internal (developmental) stress or changes.
- Levels of authority are not blurred; family hierarchy is fair and clear.
- Emotional contact is maintained between family members and across generations.
- Emotional problems are viewed as a product of the family as a whole, not blamed entirely on one family member.
- Overcloseness (fusion-enmeshment) is avoided.
- Distance (disengagement) is avoided or not used to solve problems.
- Problems between two family members (spouses, spouse and child, children) are resolved by the two people. A third person is not involved to take sides or become triangulated.
- Individual differences are encouraged to promote growth.
- Preservation of a positive emotional climate is encouraged.
- Children have age-appropriate expectations, responsibility within the family; parents negotiate openly with their children for age-appropriate privileges.
- Each spouse functions within his or her respective role, and spouses maintain a balance of effective expression, rational thought, caretaking, object orientation, and relationship focus.

Altered family processes can be viewed as the lack of one or more of these characteristics.

Related Factors[2,15]

- Situation transition and/or crises
  - Poverty
  - Disaster
  - Relocation
  - Economic crisis
  - Change in family roles
  - Conflict
  - Breach of trust between members
  - Social deviance by family member
- Development transition and/or crises
  - Birth of infant with defect
  - Loss of family member
  - Gain of new family member
- Pathophysiologic factors
  - Illness of family member
    - Discomforts related to illness symptoms
    - Change in member's ability to function
    - Time-consuming treatments
    - Disabling treatments
    - Expensive treatments
    - Psychiatric illness
  - Trauma
    - Surgery
    - Loss of body part or function

Defining Characteristics[2,15]

- Family system unable to meet physical needs of its members
- Family system unable to meet emotional needs of its members
- Family system unable to meet spiritual needs of its members
- Parents who do not demonstrate respect for each other's view on childrearing practices
- Parents who do not respect children's age-appropriate abilities
- Inability to express or accept wide range of feelings
- Inability to express or accept feelings of members
- Family unable to meet security needs of its members
- Inability of family members to relate to each other for mutual growth and maturation
- Family uninvolved in community activities
- Inability to accept help appropriately
- Rigidity in function, rules, and roles
- Family that does not demonstrate respect for individuality and autonomy of its members
- Family inability to adapt to change and deal with traumatic experience constructively
- Family that fails to accomplish current and past developmental tasks
- Ineffective family decision-making process
- Family enmeshment
- Family disengagement
- Fixed triangulation
- Blurred hierarchical system
- Members who use distance to maintain homeostasis
- Use of member scapegoating
- Spouses who do not maintain balance in relationship
- Failure to send and receive clear messages
- Inappropriate boundary maintenance
- Inappropriate or poorly communicated family rules, rituals, or symbols
- Impaired communication
- Unexamined family myths
- Inappropriate level and direction of energy

Nursing Interventions*

Patient Goal	Nursing Intervention
Reduce or resolve family dysfunction.	• Assess family structure and role relationships. • Listen attentively and promote trust. • Encourage verbalization of needs/crisis/fears. • Assist member to problem-solve. • Discuss ability to adapt in various situations. • Ascertain with member strengths and weaknesses of family's ability to adapt. • Identify stressors. • Identify overt and covert rules. • Assess degree of interdependence and bonding among members. • Teach coping skills and ways to decrease stress. • Reassure that some family conflict is healthy. • Encourage members to set goals mutually for providing reciprocal needs. • Assess ability to give and receive love. • Discuss sexuality. • Identify spiritual supports and make referrals if needed. • Discuss child-rearing practices, beliefs, and discipline techniques. • Encourage open communication between parents and children. • If child is acting out: Evaluate if parenting is ineffective. Evaluate if one parent is consistent and stronger and one is inconsistent and lenient. Evaluate if parents are locked in triangle with acting-out child. Explain that person who sets rule must be present to enforce it. If two-parent household, divide areas of responsibility for allowances, bedtime, etc., so it is clear with whom child must negotiate. Encourage parent to control emotion; maintain calmness and ability to think clearly. Help parent to determine consequences of child's disobedient behavior calmly. When acting out occurs, help parent carry out consequences without fail. After child's behavior is controlled, nurse may form third person in triangle to keep focus of problem between spouses. • Teach communication techniques. • Encourage verbalization of each member's feelings and concerns about potential or actual crisis. • Identify immediate stressors. • Discuss possible solutions through use of problem-solving techniques. • Teach problem-solving techniques and ways to prevent or reduce situation. • Validate cause of stressors. • Evaluate effectiveness of problem-solving skills (immediate and over time). • Give positive reinforcement for constructive family behaviors. • Provide opportunities for family to give or participate in the care of hospitalized family member.
Reduce or resolve family crisis.	• Identify if crisis is situational or developmental. • Discuss impact of crisis on all members. • Discuss role adjustment, ability to adapt, and expectations of other members. • Encourage family to ventilate feelings regarding effectiveness of their problem-solving skills. • Provide ongoing support or appropriate referral after crisis. • Role-play possible situations and ways of dealing constructively with crisis. • Reinforce feeling of satisfaction or closeness resulting from working together rather than anger and disruption.

*References 2-4, 7, 8, 13, 16, 21.

Principles and Rationale for Nursing Interventions[9,20,23,24]

Assessment of the family may be difficult because often not all members are available to interact with the nurse. It is of utmost importance that nurses provide early intervention for families at risk because altered family processes, e.g., relationship problems and communication barriers, can be prevented. The nurse should become attuned to the family's environment so that she or he can exchange information with the family system. Three major categories for family assessment are described in the Calgary Family Assessment Model: structural, developmental, and functional.[25]

Structural: who is in the family and what is the connection among household members versus those outside the family

- Internal structure
  - Family composition
  - Rank order
  - Subsystem (delineated by generation, sex, interest, or function)
  - Boundary (defines who participates and how)
- External structure
  - Culture
  - Religion
  - Social class status and mobility
  - Environment
  - Extended family
- Effective tool (genogram)

Developmental: how this family came to be at this stage in its developmental life cycle
- Developmental stage family is in
- Tasks requiring completion during this developmental stage

Functional: details of how individuals actually behave in relation to one another
- Instrumental functioning (routine, mechanical activities of daily living)
- Expressive functioning
  - Emotional communication
  - Verbal communication
  - Nonverbal communication
  - Circular communication
  - Problem solving
  - Roles
  - Control
  - Beliefs
  - Alliances/coalitions

Facilitating change within the family system is the primary goal in family work; thus a thorough knowledge of change theory is essential.[24] The role of nursing in the care of families also includes teaching and helping families to develop adaptive skills. For example, careful family assessment is necessary to intervene effectively when the crisis is a chronically ill individual in the family. Family roles must be revised and strengths and weaknesses identified. Dysfunctional coping mechanisms must be replaced with effective ones. Family members can be supportive of each other by communicating needs and adapting roles to meet reciprocal physical, emotional, spiritual, and mutual respect needs.

The nurse can help the family identify and work toward mutual goals by becoming involved with the family from the onset of the health care situation. For instance, if the family is dealing with painful news, the nurse can acknowledge that the news was unfavorable, encourage and listen to angry or distraught family members, recognize the need to discharge feelings, and facilitate the family's awareness of the nurse's ability to assist in identifying coping strategies. Regular patient/nurse interactions, particularly at crisis times, are necessary to reinforce stress-reducing techniques and problem-solving efforts. Giving choices helps the family feel the important need of control over what is happening. The nurse can often assist best by being the liaison between other health care professionals involved in the care of the family. Later, helping the family examine realistic approaches or expectations of the situation provides structure and support despite the disequilibrium being experienced.

The process of review of the negative experience can help the family sort out what has happened and help them verbalize fears. Guilt feelings may surface and can be dealt with realistically at this time.

Family participation in the care of an ill family member helps meet the needs of closeness, love, sharing, and order in their lives. Separation is extremely threatening and causes pain and anxiety. Even small tasks can be of great comfort to the hospitalized member and the other family members. Family members should be given the opportunity to participate whenever hospitalization occurs.

Preparation for resuming family interactions after a crisis must be made and ongoing follow-up provided. Families lacking nursing support after having received it before flounder and may again become ineffective. Follow-up at 1, 3, and 6 months helps them make the transition to independent role relationships within the family system and provides a time for evaluating the coping mechanisms they are using.

Another important nursing role is to provide family therapy by a qualified family therapist, who has usually had additional education in this area, or intervention that helps clients solve problems now and in future crises. This involves identifying how the family obtains and uses information from the environment.[16] Evaluating the family's ability to seek and use help gives clues to the ability of the family to resolve problems. Dysfunctional families do little or no negotiating when problem solving. The family's cognitive capacity—their ability to appraise a situation realistically and competently and their own capabilities in relation to it—depends on their openness and their respect for each other's unique capabilities.[16] The nurse must help the family adapt to change, deal with the crisis constructively, accomplish developmental tasks, readjust roles to accommodate situational and developmental crises, and use problem-solving techniques. If difficulty is observed with either the family's or the individual's ability to function in the family system when the problem is an acting-out adolescent, an anorexic member, a young person with bulimia, or a violent or sexually abusing member, family therapy is indicated and referral to a qualified family therapist necessary. A family unable to negotiate rules effectively or demonstrating continued enmeshment, disengagement, fixed triangulation, use of distance to maintain homeostasis, or scapegoating also needs family therapy.

Evaluation

Patient Outcome	Data Indicating That Outcome is Reached
Mutual support in family	Effective communication of physical, emotional, and spiritual needs Adapts roles to meet reciprocal needs Mutual respect Belongingness, love, and affection Sexual fulfillment Provision of protection and safety Coping mechanisms
Ability to negotiate	Effective discussion and agreement about rules Openness to others Verbalizes values involved in negotiation Ability to accept help appropriately
Family cohesiveness	Verbalizes/demonstrates emotional bonding Verbalizes boundaries Verbalizes/identifies mutual interest Effective decision-making as a unit
Ability to adapt to change	Deals constructively with crisis Accomplishes developmental tasks Readjusts roles to situational or developmental crises Problem-solving techniques Verbalizes need for continued guidance at 1, 3, and 6 months Ability to seek help if family ineffective in crisis

Potential Altered Parenting; Altered Parenting

Potential altered parenting and altered parenting are states in which the ability of nurturing figure(s) to create an environment that promotes the optimum growth and development of another human being is at risk of being altered or is altered.

Major influences on parental behavior include the following[22]:

Parent's care by his or her own mother
Endowment or genetics of parents
Practices of the culture
Relationships within the family
Experiences with previous pregnancies
Planning, course, and events during pregnancy

Several factors stimulate parents to want to care for their infant. Some of the factors are parent initiated, e.g., seeing their infant as a duplication of themselves. Some of the factors are infant produced and are called care-eliciting behaviors.[22] The infant responds to the care given by quieting, feeding or sucking, and smiling. These behaviors encourage the parent to continue to satisfy the infant's needs. If this positive reciprocal interaction does not occur, both infant and parent suffer.

The lack of an available or effective role model can also influence an individual's ability to learn acceptable parenting skills. Individuals are the result of their parents' upbringing.[20] Attitudes, moral standards, manners, ways of thinking, and patterns of behavior are absorbed by the child from his social environment.[1] Thus the individual integrates a concept about parenting primarily from those behaviors learned from parents. If the parental role model is unavailable or ineffective, the individual may have difficulty being an effective parent.

The presence of outside stressors (a new family location, lack of supportive persons, or a financial or legal crisis) impinge on the individual's ability to parent effectively in high-risk situations.[21,27] The type and degree of problems seem to be related to several common variables. These include the family's coping abilities in crises, health problems, other stress situations, as well as quality of interaction.

One must learn how to become a successful parent, and knowledge of the child's emotional development is the parent's greatest asset.[20] There are three main types of parenting styles: authoritative, authoritarian, and permissive.[9] *Authoritative* parents set firm rules, use reason and explanation when directing the child, encourage competence, and exhibit personal warmth, concern for, and interest in the child. One study[9] found that children of authoritative parents were more responsible, active, successful in schoolwork, and popular with peers. In contrast, *authoritarian* parents were more dominating and punitive and had unrealistically high or low standards. *Permissive* parents were lax and exhibited little control. Both authoritarian and permissive parenting practices were found to shield the child from the opportunity to engage in vigorous interaction with people.

Ginott[14] identifies parents' goals in relation to children and suggests methods of achieving those goals. He discusses 10 areas in which parent and child interact and can either successfully develop their relationship, foster child development, and effectively solve problems or fail to communicate, become frustrated, and hinder development of the parent-child relationship and the child's self-esteem.

The related factors for potential altered parenting and altered parenting are listed together because of overlap. The defining characteristics, nursing interventions, and evaluation sections are presented separately to define further specific characteristics, interventions, and evaluation for each.

Related Factors[8,23]

Lack of available role model
Ineffective role model
Physical abuse of nurturing figure
Psychosocial abuse of nurturing figure
Lack of support from significant other(s)
Unmet social maturation needs of parenting figures
Unmet emotional maturation needs of parenting figures
Interruption in bonding process (maternal, paternal, other)
Perceived threat to own survival (physical or emotional)
Mental and/or physical illness
Presence of stress (e.g., financial or legal problems)
Family relocation
Change in family unit
Lack of knowledge
Limited cognitive functioning
Lack of role identity
Lack of appropriate response of child to relationship
Multiple pregnancies
Unrealistic expectations for self, infant, or partner
Alcoholism
Cultural practices
Absence of infant care behaviors
Chronic fatigue
Congenital anomaly
Prematurity
Inability to show humanness as a parent
Absence of acceptance
Inability to show love
Inability to set clear objectives
Extreme authoritarianism
Extreme permissiveness
Lack of respect for child/adolescent
Lack of responsiveness to infant/child/adolescent
Depression
Inability to facilitate learning for child
Lack of psychologic space
Ineffective communication skills
Negative self-concept
Inappropriate release of anger
Lack of trust
Frequent family conflict

Defining Characteristics*

Potential Altered Parenting

Infancy to preschool

Lack of parental attachment behaviors
  Inappropriate visual, tactile, and auditory stimulation
  Negative identification of characteristics of infant/child
  Negative attachment of meanings to characteristics of infant/child
Constant verbalization of disappointment in gender or physical characteristics of infant/child
Verbalization of resentment toward infant/child
Verbalization of role inadequacy
Disgust at body functions of infant/child
Does not ask to hold, talk to, or ask questions about infant
Affect sad, angry, or without expression
Does not hold infant to neck or face
Does not spontaneously rock, stroke, or kiss infant
Absence of eye-to-eye contact
Visits or calls hospitalized infant less than every other day
Noncompliance with health appointments for self and/or infant/child
Frequent accidents
Frequent illness
History of child abuse or abandonment by primary caretaker
Verbalizes desire to have child call parent by first name despite traditional cultural tendencies
Care provided by multiple caretakers without consideration for needs of child
Compulsive seeking of role approval from others

School age

Demonstrates extreme authoritarian or permissive parenting style
Demonstrates arbitrary rules and enforcements
Provides poor model of prosocial behavior
Demonstrates lack of respect in conversing with child
Expresses anger inappropriately; attacks child's personality or character
Self-defeating patterns (bribes, sarcasm)

Adolescence

Refuses to accept adolescence as developmental stage
Unable to give "silent love"
Hassles, harangues adolescent
Unable to demonstrate verbalized values
Dictates adolescent's life

Altered Parenting

Infancy to preschool

Abandonment
Runaway
Cannot control child

*References 8, 9, 16, 17, 21, 23, 27.

Evidence of physical trauma
Evidence of psychologic trauma
Does not assume en face position despite encouragement
Refuses to hold infant
When infant placed in arms, muscles become tense; does not touch infant; looks away
Repeated negative comments about infant
Predominant affect sad, angry, expressionless
Conflicting attitudes
Inconsistent behaviors
Insists infant has a defect or problem, when none is present†
Distorted perceptions of childrearing
Absence of reciprocal behaviors between parent and infant
Father and child show signs of frustration and emotional distress
Predominance of own needs
Does not talk to infant
Does not want to feed infant at delivery
Inappropriate caretaking behaviors (toilet training, sleep, rest, feeding)
Inappropriate or inconsistent discipline practices
Growth and development lag
Child receives care from multiple caretakers without consideration for his needs
Inattention to infant/child needs

School age
Abandonment
Runaway
Cannot control child
Evidence of physical trauma
Evidence of psychologic trauma
Verbalizes or demonstrates nonacceptance of child
Absence of response to, reading to, or sincere interest in and attention to child
Denies child psychologic space for early tries and failures
Unable to praise efforts and achievements
Uses destructive rather than constructive criticism
Uses words that create hate and resentment

Adolescence
Abandonment
Runaway
Cannot control child
Evidence of physical trauma
Evidence of psychologic trauma
Ignores adolescent's feelings and thoughts
Refuses to negotiate with adolescent

Nursing Interventions*

Patient Goal	Nursing Intervention
Potential Altered Parenting	
Infancy to preschool	
Maintain satisfactory/adequate parenting role.	• Listen attentively. • Sit down, talk with parent. • Validate, offer feedback. • Provide nonthreatening environment. • Encourage role playing. • Assist with identification of strengths, weaknesses, and resources. • Identify disturbing topics. • Observe nonverbal communication. • Provide reality orientation. • Assist with values clarification. • Provide positive reinforcement for adequate parenting behaviors. • Foster self-esteem and positive self-concept. • Observe contact behaviors. • Assess affect. • Demonstrate/assist with chosen feeding method. • Touch, share concerns. • Point out rooting and sucking reflexes. • Answer questions. • Provide consistent nurse for mother and baby. • Promote trust relationship. • Provide father or significant other with opportunities to feed infant. • Avoid gender-specific behavior. • Set goals with patient for infant care. • Assist with feeding.

*References 2-5, 7, 10, 16, 17, 20, 21, 29, 31, 36, 37.

Patient Goal	Nursing Intervention
	• Provide information and teaching needs (e.g., what to expect from the infant, reflexes, feeding, infant care, role change, time management after discharge, rest and nutrition needs for self and infant). • Encourage individual responsibility for amount of time spent with infant (open visitation). • Assess family structure and roles and support system. • Discuss concerns regarding new parenting role. • Teach stress reduction techniques. • Demonstrate and observe parents' bathing, shampoo, cord care, diapering, handling, and positioning infant in crib. • Teach recognition of infant illness. • Discuss need for rest. • Prepare for feeling of disorganization first month at home. • Refer to appropriate resources (e.g., the Public Health Nurse or Social Services). • Assess self-confidence in patients' parenting role. • Teach to be sensitive to signals of distress. • Explain importance of skin contact (closeness, touching, cuddling). • Teach to talk, listen, sing with, and respond verbally to infant/child. • Provide space for gross motor activity.
School age Maintain satisfactory/adequate parenting role.	• Review developmental stage of child. • Encourage reading and learning about emotional development of children. • Explain importance of seeing self as real person with real feelings. • Encourage positive enjoyment of child. • Explain importance of reading to and responding to child verbally. • Explain importance of challenging but not overwhelming child. • Explain importance of psychologic space for early tries and failures. • Encourage parent to serve as emotional mirror to reflect feelings of child. • Explain importance of conversing with child based on respect and skill at deciphering hidden messages. • Explain importance of praising efforts and achievements. • Explain use of constructive rather than destructive criticism. • Reinforce fact that verbally expressing anger is acceptable as long as it does not attack child's personality or character. • Explain importance of avoiding self-defeating patterns (threats, bribes, promises, sarcasm, sermons). • Explain importance of trust as the basis of parent-child relationship. • Teach to listen with sensitivity to feelings and thoughts. • Explain importance of avoiding words that create hate and resentment. • Explain importance of role modeling, consideration, and civility. • Explain importance of some flexibility in daily routines. • Teach importance of not using abandonment as stimulus to get cooperation. • Explain importance of support and sympathy. • Encourage parents to respect own and each other's sexual roles. • Explain authoritative parenting: sets firm rules and uses reason and explanation when directing child versus authoritarian and permissive parenting. • Discuss discipline techniques: consistency, firm but fair rules, and consequences. • Encourage attendance at parenting classes and groups. • Discuss importance of mutual respect between parent and child. • Assess ability to balance independence and limit setting for child. • Encourage need for close contact despite age of child. • Teach about play and toys appropriate for age. • Discuss necessity and ability to provide food, comfort, and closeness appropriate for age of child.
Adolescence Maintain satisfactory/adequate parenting role.	• Review developmental stage of adolescence. • Reinforce adolescence as stage of turmoil, turbulence, stress, and storm. • Teach parent to expect and learn to tolerate rebellion. • Explain importance of silent love. • Teach ways to differentiate between acceptance and approval. • Avoid hassling to change beliefs and values. • Encourage parents to model continuously by living those values. • Explain importance of sharing ideas, knowledge, and experience open-endedly.

Patient Goal	Nursing Intervention
Altered Parenting	
Infancy to preschool	
Promote adequate parenting behaviors.	• Listen attentively. • Foster trust relationship. • Encourage verbalization of childhood experiences. • Encourage discussion of self-concept and self-esteem. • Reduce anxiety. • Teach stress management techniques. • Discuss infant's birth as needed. • Identify any interruption in attachment process. • Encourage verbalization of feelings when with infant (sadness, fear, repulsion). • Point out positive characteristics of infant. • Discuss parents' own relationship as couple. • Discuss change resulting from parenthood. • Discuss couple's problem-solving capabilities. • Discuss goals for attainment of parenting skills. • Reinforce all positive parenting behaviors. • Provide ongoing follow-up and support system during first month after discharge. • Stress importance of improving self-esteem and self-concept. • Refer to clinical nurse specialist, social worker, or psychologist as needed. • Encourage attendance at parenting classes and groups. • Assist parents to become effective problem solvers. • Sit down and discuss child's developmental stage, any physical abnormalities or delays, and emotional concerns. • Collaborate and discuss with physician treatment plans, discharge dates, patient goals, and appropriate referrals. • Set goals with parent for attaining beginning or improved parenting skills. • Demonstrate appropriate behaviors to meet infant or child's physical and emotional needs. • Reinforce fact that feelings of guilt, anger, and depression over abnormality are normal and may last 4 to 6 months. • Discuss coping mechanisms. • Assess and foster social support systems. • Include significant other(s) in modeling behavior. • Observe behaviors over several days. • Facilitate learning of reciprocal behaviors for mutual satisfaction. • Reinforce all positive parenting behaviors. • Encourage touch, holding, relaxation. • Teach parents infant stimulation techniques. • Provide ongoing follow-up during first month after discharge, and minimally at 3, 6, and 12 months. • Initiate protective services intervention if maladaptive parenting behaviors observed. • Encourage stress reduction by appropriate venting of anger. • Use Brazelton Neonatal Scale to demonstrate infant's capabilities. • Use Carey Temperament Questionnaire to identify annoying infant behaviors.
School age	
Promote adequate parenting behaviors.	• Discuss feelings about being a parent. • Review developmental stage. • Identify stressors in parent-child relationship. • Identify activities parent and child engage in and frequency of activities. • Identify reasons for nonacceptance of child. • Evaluate ability to show sincere interest in and give attention to child. • Set goals for improving parenting skills together. • Explain authoritative discipline style. • Explain importance of using constructive rather than destructive criticism. • Explain communication techniques and identify blocks to communication. • Evaluate if undercontrolling or overcontrolling child and set goals to improve.
Adolescence	
Promote adequate parenting behaviors.	• Listen attentively. • Assist parent to identify conflict or problem. • Evaluate parents' knowledge of adolescence. • Review developmental stage of adolescence.

Patient Goal	Nursing Intervention
	• Examine parents' own experience as adolescents (negative feelings, guilt, anger, role model). • Identify parents' goal in their relationship with adolescent. • Suggest family counseling to facilitate communication and problem-solving abilities. • Discuss authoritative discipline techniques. • Identify style of discipline and effectiveness.
Alcoholism	
Identify and resolve parenting problems resulting from alcoholism.	• Refer to appropriate health care and voluntary resources to deal with problem of alcoholism (Alcoholics Anonymous, alcohol treatment programs). • Provide accepting environment, trust. • Encourage verbalization of fears regarding parenting. • Provide support system (e.g., Alcoholics Anonymous). • Reinforce fact that recovery process takes time; set realistic goals. • Encourage parent to show love verbally and physically to child. • Discuss role modeling; teach how. • Discuss acceptable discipline techniques. • Encourage giving praise and recognition to child often. • Provide ongoing follow-up at least monthly to discuss parenting concerns.

Principles and Rationale for Nursing Interventions

Potential Altered Parenting

Parenting behaviors are assessed during different developmental stages: at the time of delivery, at 1 week, at several months or years, or during adolescence. Finely tuned assessment skills are necessary to identify critical factors appropriate for each developmental stage. Valid assessments can be made only after more than one or two parent-infant interactions.[8,21]

To work with parents, the nurse must first convey a genuine concern for each individual in the new family. The establishment of a trust relationship is necessary before learning can occur. Many new parents are fearful, unsure of what their role and responsibilities are, and have expectations of themselves in that role.

The birth of a normal, healthy baby after a planned pregnancy and successful labor and delivery helps begin the process of parenting. However, frequently the pregnancy is not planned, the labor and delivery do not meet the expectations of the individuals, or the infant has some problem. Even a slight problem may augment fears that the parents had up to this point. The parents are vulnerable and need careful attention. It is important to prevent threat to the parents' self-image. This includes generating anxiety associated with inability to meet one's own or one's spouse's expecations in the parenting role or feelings of failure if the infant does not meet the parents' expectations.

To foster the "taking in role," parents must be given responsibility for their infant.[31] This means that within minutes after delivery the parents must have the opportunity to unwrap, touch, hold, and feed their infant. This maternal sensitive and paternal engrossment period facilitates instinctive cues and begins the attachment process.[22] Mercer[26] acknowledges that "early interaction [with the infant] serves as an immediate reward, providing the woman with relief and joy."

The nurse must make every effort to point out the positive aspects of the infant and answer questions during this time. Johnson[19] points out that "in progressive institutions, both parents and children are being included as essential members of the treatment team, since it is apparent that their involvement in the plan directly influences the outcome." Thus providing closeness at birth, as well as later in the child's life, facilitates nurturing. In the infant the attachment process is stimulated. This is a reciprocal process between parent and infant.

Once the initial contact has been made between parents and infant, identification with and claiming of the infant can begin. Again, it is the responsibility of the nurse to provide consistent care, e.g., mother-baby care, a system in which one nurse per shift takes care of the mother *and* the baby through the postpartum hospitalization, to promote trust. Likewise it is important to provide accurate information to the parents about the infant, assess parenting problems, or deal with potential problems when teaching the parents what to expect from their infant.

Ideally this is begun in prenatal classes when the parents' image of the anticipated infant is forming. Pointing out that infants focus on and respond to the human face and voice within the first week of life makes the parents aware of the need for sensory and auditory stimulation. The infant has basic needs: food, air, water, elimination, comfort, closeness, and safety. Positive feeding experiences provide the basis for reciprocal satisfaction of needs for parent and infant. For example, parents need to be told that the infant's cry can be irritating, but it is a communication of need. Ongoing reinforcement of positive parenting behaviors provides the mechanism for support and helps ensure continued mutually satisfying experiences for parent and infant.

The caretaking role is usually thought of as the primary parenting role. Demonstration of bathing, hair washing, cord care, diapering, handling, and positioning the infant in a crib is best accomplished in a nonthreatening environment. New parents feel insecure and often frightened at the thought of providing this care on the first or second postpartum day. Asking the parents to participate in the care, to the extent that they desire, in a supportive manner inspires confidence. Reinforcement on subsequent days provides them with a chance to develop the parenting skills they may have been most frightened of. Fathers and other significant persons in the family system need special encouragement to learn these skills. Validation with the parents and praise before discharge from the hospital reinforce their successful achievement of parenting goals. This interaction facilitates a supportive environment for maintaining the health of the infant.

Altered Parenting

Parents who display actual parenting alterations need expert help. Careful identification of the cause of the parenting problem may take several interactions or observation periods. Often, when caring for patients in an acute care setting, there is little time to accomplish the necessary change of behavior. Identification and implementation of a plan of action must be made as soon as possible.

The parents and the nurse need to establish mutual goals to change parenting behaviors effectively. These goals primarily focus first on identification of the cause for maladaptive attachment behaviors. Once a trust relationship is formed, the history of the parent, including childhood experiences with parents and role models, must be discussed. Parents who were abused as children are more prone to abuse their children.[19] The nurse's responsibility in child abuse is to assess carefully any maladaptive parenting behaviors that might seem connected to physical injuries and to report these to the appropriate child protective services department.

Emotional abuse or neglect is more difficult to determine. The child's basic needs are physical care and protection, affection and approval, stimulation and teaching, discipline and control that are consistent and appropriate to the child's age, and opportunity and encouragement to acquire gradual autonomy.[36] If the parent is indifferent, ignores the child, or refuses to give emotional warmth, the child does not grow and develop normally and emotional needs are not met.

If the unmet social or emotional needs stem from a specific risk situation such as prematurity or congenital anomaly, nursing interventions need to be specific to that problem. "High risk parents and their children are particularly susceptible to problems in their reciprocal behaviors."[19]

Many of these infant problems can cause emotional difficulties for parents. Parental behaviors indicative of grief and mourning, extreme guilt, or depression over having produced such a child may become apparent. These feelings interfere with the parent's ability to respond positively to the infant. Teaching stress reduction techniques may be essential for the parent to cope.

Another problem may be unrealistic expectations of self or child. Providing the parent with knowledge of the developmental stage of the child, realistic expectations, and comfort, play, and learning needs will promote the ability to parent effectively. Assessment and discussion of appropriate discipline techniques must also be included. If the parents are either very young or relatively old, their developmental level and self-concept needs must be considered when analyzing solutions.

The child who is cared for by many caretakers may not form adequate attachments. Withdrawal or poor self-esteem may be seen in the child. Careful family assessment, including thorough knowledge of child development, is essential.

Parents who are alcoholic need help for themselves as well as their children. Careful attention is required to communicate in a nonthreatening manner with alcoholic parents. They view themselves as dual failures, to themselves as well as to their children. Effective nursing care must be provided. A sensitive, caring approach with mutual goal setting is essential.

Evaluation

Patient Outcome	Data Indicating That Outcome is Reached
Potential Altered Parenting	
Positive feelings about own parenting role	Identifies strengths and weaknesses in own parenting; focuses on strengths Communicates concerns clearly Shares troublesome memories from own childhood parenting experience Verbalizes desire to learn more about parenting role Verbalizes knowledge of developmental stage Verbalizes that stress reduction techniques are used *Infancy* Reviews birth experience Ventilates concerns regarding individual performance during labor and delivery *School age* Verbalizes feelings of self-worth Identifies supports *Adolescence* Verbalizes any frustration over turmoil/stress in dealing with ups and downs of adolescent Identifies solutions for and approaches to frustration

Patient Outcome	Data Indicating That Outcome is Reached
Constructive interpersonal relationship with offspring	*Infancy* Demonstrates en face position Fingertip touches infant's face and body Proceeds to finger and palm touch Expresses joy or other appropriate emotions Demonstrates positive attitude toward child Brings infant to own neck and face Talks to infant Asks questions about infant Makes positive statements about infant Verbalizes knowledge of and preferred method of feeding infant Verbalizes desire to breast-feed if preferred Demonstrates comfortable positions for feeding Verbalizes knowledge of rooting and sucking reflexes Verbalizes feelings of adequacy during feeding Asks questions about frequency and amount of feeding Verbalizes knowledge of sleep/wake cycles Exhibits eye-to-eye contact Verbalizes knowledge that infant's burp, falling asleep, and relaxation in arms after feeding indicates satisfying experience Demonstrates ability to comfort infant during or after feeding Verbalizes preparations for infant homecoming and necessary supplies Identifies roles in family Discusses taking on of new role(s) in family Verbalizes feelings of role adequacy Verbalizes coping mechanisms for stress Calls physician if infant shows signs of illness Verbalizes knowledge and demonstrates ability to bathe, shampoo, provide cord care, diaper, handle, and position infant in crib Verbalizes need to nap when infant sleeps during first month Expresses satisfaction with infant or acceptance of infant's limitations Verbalizes ability to assume new or modified roles in family system Provides food, comfort, and closeness for child Child receives care from one or two primary caretakers *School age* Verbalizes knowledge of developmental stage Verbalizes feelings of self-worth Identifies supports Demonstrates authoritative parenting style Demonstrates humanness Verbalizes positive enjoyment of child Responds to child appropriately Reads to child at least every other day Challenges but does not overwhelm child Allows psychologic space Verbalizes comfort and mutual respect in conversing with child Praises child's efforts and achievements Demonstrates constructive criticism Verbalizes anger and frustration appropriately Demonstrates trust in parent-child relationship *Adolescence* Verbalizes any frustration over turmoil or stress in dealing with ups and downs of adolescent Identifies solutions for and approaches to frustration Differentiates between acceptance and approval Avoids hassling to change beliefs and values Demonstrates values cited in own life Shares ideas in "consultant" manner
Altered Parenting	
Admission of unmet social or emotional needs	Identifies childhood experiences that affect parenting behaviors Identifies fears about infant/child/adolescent and self Reality orientation

Patient Goal	Nursing Intervention
	Verbalizes need to work to improve parenting skills Verbalizes that stress reduction techniques are used *School age* Acceptance of child Interest in and attention to child Authoritative parenting style Constructive criticism Effective communication techniques *Adolescence* Identifies conflict/problem Attends family counseling if set as goal for improving parenting ability Authoritative parenting style Verbalizes feelings of frustration
Knowledge of developmental stage and realistic expectations of infant/child/adolescent	Knowledge of risk situation Knowledge of basic needs of infant/child/adolescent appropriate to developmental stage Appropriate discipline techniques
Attachment behaviors to infant/child/adolescent	Assumes en face position Holds infant in relaxed manner Constructive comments about infant/child/adolescent Appropriate affect; able to show sadness if discussing abnormality, but when interacting with infant, shows pleasure and smiles Expresses concerns about mothering/fathering behaviors Changes diapers; disgust over body excretions absent Verbalizes a plan for dealing with inconsistencies Comprehension of any physical defect or abnormality Realistic perceptions of childrearing Ability to deal constructively with stress, feelings of guilt, or depression Knowledge of resources and supports Reciprocal behaviors with infant/child Infant/child receives care from one or two primary caretakers Ability to interact and accomplish mutual goal with adolescent
Admission of parenting problems related to alcoholism	Verbalizes fears and feelings of failure in parenting role Willingness to seek professional help for alcoholism Discusses disease with family and children Mutual goals for improving parenting skills with family Attends Alcoholics Anonymous Recognizes child's/adolescent's need for increased self-worth Verbal and physical expressions of love to child/adolescent Role model to child/adolescent Consistent appropriate discipline for developmental age Praises child's/adolescent's successes

Parental Role Conflict

Parental role conflict is the state in which a parent experiences role confusion and conflict in response to crisis.

The crisis in parental role conflict can be related to a situation such as moving to a new location, financial or legal crisis, or change in health status of a family member that affects the parental role. The crisis may complicate or interfere with the coping mechanisms that were effective before the crisis. The parents may express feelings of inadequacy to provide for the child's needs; caretaking routines may be disrupted; and the parents may be concerned with changes in their role, family functioning, family communication, and family health.

Related Factors*

Separation from child because of chronic illness
Intimidation with invasive or restrictive modalities (e.g., isolation, intubation), specialized care centers, policies
Home care of child with special needs (e.g., apnea monitoring, postural drainage, hyperalimentation)
Change in marital status

*Adapted from North American Nursing Diagnosis Association, 1988 Ballot.

Interruptions of family life caused by home care regimen (treatments, caregivers, lack of respite)

Defining Characteristics*

Expression of concerns or feelings of inadequacy to provide for child's physical and emotional needs during hospitalization or in the home

*Adapted from North American Nursing Diagnosis Association, 1988 Ballot.

Expression of concerns about changes in parental role, family functioning, family communication, or family health

Expression of concerns about perceived loss of control over decisions relating to child

Demonstrated disruption in caretaking routines

Reluctant to participate in normal caretaking activities even with encouragement and support

Verbalization or demonstration of feelings of guilt, anger, fear, anxiety, and/or frustrations about effect of child's illness on family process

Nursing Interventions

Patient Goal	Nursing Intervention
Express feelings of adequacy in providing for child's physical and emotional needs.	• Maintain open communication with parents regarding their perception of caretaking activities. • Be sensitive to clues that parents feel burdened by child caretaking activities. • Encourage parents to discuss concerns, feelings, and their responses to crisis. • Facilitate discussion to identify specific source of conflict. • Assist parents to put label on feelings so feelings can be dealt with. • Encourage parents to participate in child caretaking activities based on their readiness to participate, understanding of disease process, and manual skill to perform tasks. • Give parents choices over decisions relating to child as much as practical, ranging from timing/scheduling of activities/procedures to choices in therapeutic modalities. • Praise parents for participation in caretaking activities. • Assist and support parents to list issues, concerns, and action plans to enhance scheduling and procedure for caretaking routines. • Support parents' plans to maintain or return to previous (precrisis) roles with other siblings. • Identify maladaptive responses to crisis, facilitate parents' discovery of same, and assist and support them to demonstrate adaptive behaviors.
Delineate adjustments in role in response to crisis.	• Assess role changes of all family members. • Support interactive discussion between parents and/or health care provider to identify roles before and since onset of crisis. • Identify role conflicts. • Validate cues of significant other. • Clarify expectations about roles. • Support parents in performance of new roles. • Compliment new role-taking behavior. • Assist parents to modify new role as needed. • Reinforce feedback of other parent. • Reevaluate parents' new role. • Maintain open communication with parents regarding their perception of caretaking activities. • Be sensitive to clues that parents feel burdened by child caretaking activities, and make adjustments to promote a positive sequence in assimilation of child care tasks.

Principles and Rationale for Nursing Interventions

The goals of nursing interventions for parental role conflict are to support and promote parental behaviors that are indicative of role identity functioning and conflict resolution. Parental confusion or conflict in response to crisis is resolved as adaptive coping behaviors are developed to meet the parents' needs as well as those of other family members. Encouraging parents to participate in child care as well as to make appropriate decisions about the health and welfare of their children in a supportive environment will help them to remediate their response to the current crisis and to potential future crises. Achievement of goals in caring for the parent would be evidenced by their self-reported feelings of adequacy and demonstrated ability to exercise control in caretaking and other family routines.

Evaluation

Patient Outcome	Data Indicating That Outcome is Reached
Parents' roles clearly defined with no evidence of conflict in response to crisis	Demonstrate positive, therapeutic reorganization of caretaking routines to facilitate crisis resolution Express realistic action plans in adjusting their roles, family functioning, and family communication in response to crisis

 Impaired Verbal Communication

Impaired verbal communication is the state in which an individual experiences a decreased or absent ability to use or understand language in human interaction.

Communication is a dynamic, complex, continuous series of reciprocal events through which messages are exchanged, primarily to produce a response from a person or a group. Communication includes all modes of behavior used by a person, consciously or unconsciously, to affect another person. Thus communication is an integral part of interpersonal relationships. The types and quality of relationships, as well as what happens to a person in his environment, is determined to a large extent by communication.[16] A person's communication pattern is the particular sequence of communication behaviors practiced over time by that person.

All persons experiencing emotional disorders encounter problems in interpersonal relationships. Communication and interpersonal relationship difficulties can be related factors, defining characteristics, manifestations, or consequences of an emotional disorder.

Related Factors[9]

Developmental or age-related stage(s)
Mechanical impairment(s)
Physical condition(s)
Severe physical or psychosocial stress(es)
Extreme anger
Severe anxiety or panic
Moderate to severe depression
Significant impairment of perception
Unrealistic or inadequate self-concept
Cultural differences
Faulty communication skills

Defining Characteristics[9]

Disorientation
Too little or too much attention to stimuli
Speech impediments
Physical conditions
Inability to speak dominant language
Inability or reluctance to speak
Disregard for speaker
Reliance on nonverbal communication
Inability to organize words
Inappropriate selection of words
Use of unfamiliar words
Inconsistent nonverbal messages
Message inappropriate to context
Excessive or insufficient verbiage
Ill-timed message
Inadequate listening skills
Disparity of punctuation
Absent or inappropriate feedback
Discordant information
Disconfirmation
Absence of gratification
Inability or reluctance to express feelings
Withdrawal from interaction
Unrestrained or inappropriate emotional expression
Imaginary or false perceptions
Incongruent communication styles
Lack of assertive skills

Nursing Interventions

Patient Goal	Nursing Intervention
Reduce or resolve impaired communication.	• Reduce or increase environmental stimuli. • Encourage patient to seek assistance in correcting, modifying, or preventing physical conditions that interfere with communication. • Teach patient to identify and focus on relevant stimuli. • Encourage interaction with others. • Assist patient in increasing or modifying language skills. • Assist in correction of faulty perception. • Teach and support patient's use of appropriate communication techniques.

Patient Goal	Nursing Intervention
	• Teach and support patient's use of assertive communication skills. • Teach and encourage expression of feelings. • Increase self-esteem. • Teach and encourage use of stress reduction techniques. • Help patient examine effects of behavior. • Increase awareness of strengths and limitations in communicating with others. • Point out discrepancies in nonverbal behaviors. • Point out discrepancies in verbal and nonverbal behavior. • Point out discrepancies in message sent and context within which it is sent. • Help patient develop understanding of dynamics of relationships. • Describe, demonstrate, and encourage use of active listening skills. • Request patient to ask for feedback when communicating with others. • Assist and encourage patient efforts to accept positive and negative feedback. • Assist patient in mastering tasks appropriate for age or developmental level. • Demonstrate and support responsibility for communication. • Use facilitative communication techniques in interacting with patient (e.g., reflection, focusing, validation, silence, summarizing, clarification, open-ended questions, stating observations, confrontation, exploring, providing feedback).

Principles and Rationale for Nursing Interventions

The overall goal for the patient with impaired communication is to reduce or resolve impaired communication. Subgoals or short-term goals can include the following:

Attend to appropriate input.

Transmit clear, concise, understandable messages.

Use congruent analogue/nonverbal and digital/verbal communication.

Send and receive feedback.

Experience gratification from communication.

The nurse/patient relationship provides the vehicle for nursing care and is the major tool of the psychiatric nurse. The effectiveness of this relationship depends on the strength of the communication process.[6] Therefore it is essential for the nurse to become more aware of the complexity of the communication process.

The nurse ascertains a patient's pattern of communication through analysis of clinical data acquired from history taking, interaction, and observation. The objective in assessing the communication pattern is to obtain data about how, when, where, what, and with whom the patient communicates. Specific details assessed include the components of the communication process, the variables affecting the communication process, and the characteristics manifested.

To evaluate whether communication is effective or impaired, it is necessary to understand the communication process. Communication has no beginning or end. The events in communication are in dynamic interaction. Successful communication is characterized by the following elements[1-23]:

Both the sender and receiver have the physical ability to receive, analyze, and send messages.

The relationship between the sender and receiver is considered in all components of the communication process.

Selective attention is given to appropriate input.

Both the digital/verbal and the analogic/nonverbal form of communication are employed.

The sender selects and organizes words to best describe the intended meaning of the message.

The sender and receiver have similar meanings for words.

All channels of nonverbal communication are synchronized.

Nonverbal behavior is consistent with verbal communication.

The message sent is appropriate to the context.

The message is complete, i.e., not overloaded with or insufficient in information.

The timing of the message is appropriate to its content and the context.

The receiver listens actively.

The sender and receiver agree on the punctuation of a communication sequence.

Feedback is requested and accepted.

Feedback is relevant to the persons and context, clearly stated, and appropriately timed.

The sender is able to correct the information or message.

Both the sender and the receiver assume responsibility for their communication.

Concordant information is established between the sender and receiver.

Both the sender and the receiver attain confirmation and gratification.

Evaluation

Patient Outcome	Data Indicating That Outcome is Reached
Demonstrates successful communication	Attendance to appropriate input: Oriented to person, place, and time Selects and responds to relevant stimuli Perception accurate Absence or control of physical symptoms Clear, concise understandable messages: Absence of speech impediments Selects and organizes words appropriate to receiver and context Speaks dominant language Uses effective communication techniques Uses appropriate amount of verbiage Expresses feelings appropriately Congruent nonverbal and verbal communication: Expresses congruent nonverbal behaviors Expresses congruent verbal and nonverbal behavior Balances use of verbal and nonverbal behavior Sends and receives feedback: Listens actively Examines effects of behavior on others Asks for and receives feedback Sends feedback to others Experiences gratification from communication: Reports satisfaction from communication Reports sense of high self-esteem Reports or shows willingness to assume responsibility for communication Sends and receives confirmation when communicating

Potential for Violence: Self-Directed or Directed at Others

Potential for violence: self-directed or directed at others is the state in which an individual experiences behaviors that can be physically harmful either to the self or others.

The causes of human violence are complex and remain unclear. By definition the term *violence* means an act of destructiveness. Violence is not an emotion. Violence can be viewed as a result of several psychologic (emotional), biologic, and sociologic influences.[14] No one theory explaining these influences is more valid than the other. Moreover, a combination of theories is often employed to explain the etiology of violent behavior because the potential for violent behavior needs to be assessed on an individual basis.

Risk Factors[2,3,8]

Psychologic
- Physical abuse in family
- Panic states
- Drug or alcohol abuse
- Depression
- Increase in stressors within short time
- Physical immobility
- Real or perceived threat to self
- Fear of the unknown
- Response to catastrophic event
- Misperceived messages from others
- Response to dysfunctional family through developmental stages
- Dysfunctional communication patterns

Physiologic/biologic
- Organic brain syndrome
- Temporal lobe epilepsy
- Toxic reaction to medication
- Toxic reaction to alcohol
- Hormonal imbalance
- Alteration in biochemical functioning leading to depression or manic-depressive illness
- Physical trauma (result of accidents or battering)

Sociocultural
- Environmental controls
- Response to dysfunctional family
- Dysfunctional communication pattern

Defining Characteristics[2,3,8]

Antisocial behavior
Rage reactions
Suicidal behavior
Homicidal behavior
Child abuse
Battering of spouse
Loss of control
- Physical assault
- Forceful damage of inanimate objects
- Forceful injury to others
- Injury to self

Body language
- Clenched fists
- Clenched jaw
- Rigid posture
- Tautness indicating intense effort to control
- Agitation
- Increased motor activity
- Pacing

Hostile threatening verbalizations
Possession of destructive means (gun, knife, other weapon)
Self-destructive behavior resulting in minimum injury
Suspicion of others
Paranoid attitude
Delusions
Hallucinations
Perception of self as worthless or hopeless
Perception of environment as frightening or hostile
Poor impulse control
Provocative behavior
- Argumentative
- Dissatisfied
- Overreactive
- Hypersensitive
- Poor impulse control

Vulnerable self-esteem
Increasing anxiety levels
Fear of self or others
Inability to verbalize feelings
Repetition of verbalizations, e.g. continued complaints, requests, demands
Minimum tolerance to anxiety or stress
Surface appearance of overcontrol, inhibition
Proneness to action rather than words
Inability to remember all or part of recent or past events
Disconnected thoughts
Disorientation to time, place, and person
Staring eye contact or avoidance of eye contact

Nursing Interventions*

Patient Goal	Nursing Intervention
Reduce or eliminate potential for violent behavior.	• Assess and monitor: History of previous homicides, physical or verbal assaults, or suicide attempts Relationships with significant persons and factors in environment that could trigger violent response Conscious awareness of hostile or violent feelings Life experiences that create resentment and bitterness Family history of severe and emotional deprivation History of alcohol or drug use or abuse Inability to control behavior following drug or alcohol ingestion Exposure to violent person History of repeated frustrations History of psychiatric treatment Self-concept in relation to others History of medical problems (e.g., epilepsy, head injuries, brain tumor) Family violence Nurse's feelings regarding violent behavior Abnormal diagnostic studies performed in conjunction with physician's orders: thyroid function, electroencephalogram, computed tomography scan, electrolyte levels, blood gases, blood alcohol levels, blood glucose, drug levels (blood, urine, gastric), renal function Medical history (may be obtained from physician's medical history): epilepsy, head injury, brain disease, hormonal balance, alcohol abuse, drug abuse, insomnia • Encourage patient to talk rather than act out physically. • Use positive reinforcers when patient has reduced or not used profanity for 1 day. • Reward positive behavior by complimenting or spending extra time with patient. • Function as role model: Be calm. Verbalize feelings.

*References 2, 3, 5, 8-10, 14-16.

Patient Goal	Nursing Intervention
	Demonstrate positive interpersonal relationships. Discuss importance of caring about self and others. • Do not threaten patient's self-esteem or sense of control. • Assist with external controls when needed: Remove easily accessible items that could be used as weapons. Do not confront patient with issue of control. When possible, allow patient to make decisions about own actions if not currently being harmful to others; explain what will happen if acting out or violence occurs (security will be called, additional personnel will be called, medications may be used). • Help patient maintain control by discussing frustrations, thus decreasing physical and verbal aggression. • Ensure patient that he will be assisted in controlling violent impulses. • Set limits for each aggressive episode. • Place patient in seclusion if dangerous to self or others. • If seclusion is necessary, maintain safety. • Remove individual from situation if environment is contributing to aggressive behavior; use least amount of control needed (e.g., ask others to leave and take individual to a quiet room). • When using seclusion, institutional policy will provide specific guidelines. The following are general: Observe patient every 15 minutes. Search patient to remove harmful objects before secluding. Check seclusion room to see that safety is maintained. Offer fluids and food periodically. When going into seclusion room, have sufficient staff present. Explain precisely what is happening and why; give patient a chance to cooperate. Assist patient in toileting and personal hygiene. • Assist in verbalization of depressed feelings. • Assist in finding alternatives to deal with depressed feelings.
Experience less precipitating factors.	• Provide and document accurate information concerning relationship of physiologic alteration and disturbing feelings or thoughts. • Provide short, concise, honest statements concerning hospital routines and procedures. • Remove excess equipment. • Decrease noise volume. • Use same personnel. • Discuss rationale for fear, if known, if patient can verbalize. • Identify available support systems. • Allow patient to verbalize feelings about hospital environment. • Allow patient to arrange personal belongings to promote sense of security. • Reinforce reality during each interaction; orient patient to time, place, and person. • Provide calendar and clock for patient's room. • Set realistic day-to-day goals. • Give short, consistent statements when explaining case. • In collaboration with physician, begin medical regimen to counteract effects of toxic medication. • Remove any medications patient may have brought. • Present alternative physical ways to deal with family and community frustrations. • Demonstrate genuine caring, support, and respect when helping family members integrate violent experience. • Listen and provide empathy when patient discusses pain and trauma of family. • Have person role-play family communication with personnel and practice problem-solving techniques. • Discuss how communication can be misperceived by others. • Provide frequent 10-minute interactions rather than one 30-minute interaction. • Give feedback on positive changes in communication pattern. • Administer medications as prescribed. • Provide trusting relationship with patient to help patient feel more comfortable: Be honest, clear, concise during interactions. Recognize that defensive, manipulative behavior has meaning for patient. Maintain stable physical environment. Establish short-term goals; use contracts (e.g., spending a certain amount of time with patient); follow through.

Patient Goal	Nursing Intervention
	• Help to decrease agitation in patient if it occurs: Allow physical activity to channel aggression in accordance with patient's ability. Administer medications as prescribed by physician. Interact with patient on one-to-one basis. Do not touch patient until you explain what procedure or rationale is for such an intervention. Allow patient to maintain personal space. Use calm nonverbal and verbal behavior.

Principles and Rationale for Nursing Interventions

The nurse must provide controls to prevent violent behavior. Setting limits, seclusion, and restraints (chemical and physical, which are not often used today) are all methods of controlling behavior if the patient loses control. The nurse must understand that the potentially violent patient often has low self-esteem, may be lonely, and may feel hopeless. Thus it is of utmost importance to establish trust and rapport by approaching calmly and allowing personal space. Helping the patient think and talk about his problems can correct distorted perceptions and ideas. The violent, threatening patient fails and believes violence to be the sole exit from his stress-bound box of life. The patient is unable to perceive any alternatives other than violence. Complex, long-term supportive or deterrent measures may be required.

Because fear is a possible source for violent behavior, the nurse must help to eliminate the patient's fears. One way to decrease fear is to discuss it and try to find ways to eliminate or deal with it. The nurse can also help to control the environment by minimizing noise and traffic (by other patients or visitors) and by carefully explaining procedures that require equipment or medication.

A person who commits a violent act frequently has tremendous feelings of guilt and remorse. Those family members or staff who witnessed or were victims of the violent behavior also need time to verbalize their feelings, fears, and anger. How a person sees and interprets the surrounding world is crucial to the future eruption of violent behavior.[12]

The nurse must encourage and allow verbal expressions of anger. The key to prevention of violent aggression is finding out what precipitates feelings of anger, frustration, or rage. Then, after careful discussion, the nurse and patient can find ways to decrease or eliminate the related factors and develop alternative coping mechanisms. Encouraging physical expenditure of energy by exercise, unit jobs, games, or discussion helps decrease anxiety and increase self-esteem.

Parents who feel aggressive tendencies toward their child must learn to deal constructively with their feelings and retain control. Teaching the parents stress reduction techniques and realistic expectations of their child by discussing growth and development in detail helps them recognize and deal with frustrations in childrearing. Also, finding acceptable alternate coping mechanisms for those frustrating times is essential in preventing aggressive violence. This must be done on an individual basis for each parent. Trust is again essential to work effectively toward changing behavior.

Nurses who work with abusive families must first work through their own feelings and be nonjudgmental and accepting of the family members as persons. The nurse must be able to use confrontation when necessary. Parents who abuse their children generally have not received the love or nurturing they needed as children and actually lack a basic trust in people. Their basic needs have not been met. Consequently the parents place unrealistic expectations on the child; the child cannot meet these expectations and in turn becomes neglected or abused. The parent is looking for gratification of needs from the child instead of the reverse—providing the child with these needs. The role of the nurse is to provide support and education for the parents to understand themselves, motivation for behavioral change, and strategies for interacting effectively with others. Parent modeling is equally important for abusive adults. Lay therapists who go into the home and provide a warm parent model for the abusing parent have been found to help reduce the tendency for future abuse and neglect. Intensive work with the nurse, psychiatric clinical nurse specialist, psychotherapist, caseworker, and lay therapist is required for any hope of changing behavior.

The etiology of spouse abuse is similar to that for child abuse. Each spouse may have a tremendous amount of unmet needs, and violence occurs when spouses fail to meet each other's needs. The victim of this abuse must understand that the behavior might not change until the violent person seeks help. The victim may need to get out of the situation. This is a long process and requires maximum support from the nurse.

Evaluation

Patient Outcome	Data Indicating That Outcome is Reached
Demonstrates self-control	Body relaxed Eye contact when communicating Verbalizes precipitating factors to incident Verbalizes feelings of hopelessness, loneliness, and decreased self-esteem Verbalizes and demonstrates alternatives to violent, aggressive behavior Allows trusted person to approach boundaries of personal space Knowledge of rationale for limit setting or seclusion, if required Verbalizes fears Desire to control self Admits remorse or guilt
Verbalizes specific aggressive behavior, feelings of anger, and hostility	Verbalizes sources of anger, frustration or rage Verbalizes stress tolerance capacity Recognizes perceptual distortions resulting from anger Knowledge of physiologic or chemical causes of alterations in behavior (if appropriate) Desire to control aggressive behavior Identifies and demonstrates appropriate aids to decrease anger and hostility (physical exercise, visual imagery, relaxation techniques)
Displays no overt or covert dangerous behavior	Verbalizes feelings of anger and hostility rather than acting out physically Participates in therapy Ability to cope effectively in conflict situations or role play Verbalizes supports
Uses adaptive coping mechanisms in conflict situation	Knowledge of alternative ways to deal with aggressive feelings in role playing Ability to maintain self-control Uses thought processes rather than physical response Has perception of violence; acceptable versus unacceptable in own value system Verbalizes feelings when self-esteem is threatened Ability to cope effectively with threats to self-esteem Identifies constructive ways to increase power Identifies supportive person(s) or groups in environment

FUNCTIONAL HEALTH PATTERN

IX

Sexuality-Reproductive

 Sexual Dysfunction

Sexual dysfunction is the state in which an individual experiences a change in sexual function that is viewed as unsatisfying, unrewarding, or inadequate.

Dysfunctional sexual response patterns can be primarily psychogenic, organic, or secondary to illness, psychologic disorders, or stress. The identification of disruption in one of the three phases (orgasm phase disorders, excitement phase disorders, desire phase disorders) is critical when considering focused sex therapy interventions. Self-report of sexual problems is insufficient evidence of actual dysfunctional sexual response patterns. When dysfunctional sexual response patterns are not in evidence, self-reports of sexual problems and dissatisfaction most often have etiologic roots in psychiatric disorders or relationship problems rather than primary dysfunctional sexual responses. Situational sexual response systems, avoidance and phobic responses, and situational inhibition are most often sexual problems not associated with medical problems.[6]

As a general rule, a primary sexual symptom that has "always" been present is more likely to be psychogenic than a secondary disorder that occurs after a period of good functioning, especially in the absence of trauma and stress.[6]

Organic causes should be suspected in a person whose sexual functioning has been normal for a significant period, especially when there is deterioration of ejaculatory functions or orgasm becomes delayed.[6,9]

Sexual disorders frequently associated with organic causes are as follows[6]:

Impotence
Dyspareunia
Vaginismus
Unconsummated marriage
Low or absent libido
Secondary anorgasmia in males and females
Secondary premature ejaculation
Secondary retarded ejaculation

Sexual dysfunction can be a disruption of extreme variation in sexual behavior. It is defined further by an identifiable disturbance of a phase in the sexual response pattern and excessive pain and phobic avoidance of sex (both simple and panic). Sexual dysfunction, as an extreme variation of sexual behavior, is defined by the object, animate or inanimate, required for sexual arousal and release; its habitual use; and a disregard for the rights, damage, pain, fear, and sensitivities when the object is animate.

Sexual dysfunction as an extreme variation of sexual behavior, often called sexual deviations, by virtue of its long-standing and habitual characteristics, is most often psychogenic with roots in psychic conflict and early conditioning. The behavior (e.g., voyeurism, exhibitionism, pedophilia) often brings the individual in conflict with the law; or family members are implicated, as in incest, when the child comes to the attention of the health professional.

A framework of categorizing the broad nursing diagnoses of sexual dysfunction into subdiagnoses is used here. Each subdiagnostic category is described separately regarding the related factors and some defining characteristics. Since multiple subdiagnoses can be made, it is important to make a differential diagnosis.

Related Factors[1-7,9,10]

Biopsychosocial alteration of sexuality
- Ineffectual or absent role models
- Physical abuse
- Psychosocial abuse (e.g., harmful relationships)
- Vulnerability
- Misinformation or lack of knowledge
- Values conflict
- Lack of privacy
- Lack of significant other

Altered body structure or function: pregnancy, recent childbirth, drugs, surgery, anomalies, disease process, trauma, radiation

Possible lowered hormonal functioning as a process of aging, compensating fear of failing sexual prowess

Transitory life experience (e.g., loss of spouse, loss of self-esteem)

Organic brain disease

Complex and severe psychologic disorders with primary character disorder; disturbed social relations
- Marked cognitive set justifying object choice and behavior, claiming it is nonharmful to immature individuals
- History of victimization as child (sexual, physical)
- Primary social networks and family that overlooks, condones indirectly, or supports behavior

Sexual trauma: rape, sexual exploitation (chronic, delayed, silent)

Concern about Sexual Functioning without Disruption of Sexual Response Pattern (Secondary to Organic and/or Psychosocial Causes)

Common organic factors
- Pregnancy, childbirth
- Mild infections of genitourinary tract and genitals (epididymitis, trichomoniasis)
- Disease states (heart attack, back surgery)
- Drugs or medication

Common psychosocial causes
- Unrealistic expectations of self and others
- Inadequate sexual techniques and poor communications
- Religious beliefs or cultural taboos
- Diminished interest and attachment to present sexual object
- Preoccupation with demanding and/or stressful activity
- Disruption and/or lack of comfort and privacy
- Lack of desired sex object (e.g., isolation imposed because of travel, imprisonment)
- Age changes (e.g., in appearance, social functioning)
- More serious psychologic disorders (obsessional disorders, affective disorders, psychotic disorders)
- More serious, complex relationship issues (pathologic spouse, parental transference problems, incompatible marriage)

Pain (Pre- and Post-Orgasm/Ejaculatory Phase)

Organic causes
- Genital muscle spasm
- Infection in urinary tract (prostatitis, vesiculitis, herpes)
- Painful gynecologic conditions (pelvic inflammatory disease, endometriosis, hymenal remnants, ovarian pathology, ectopic pregnancy, lower bowel disease, herpes)
- Conditioned, voluntary painful spasm of perineal muscles of internal reproductive organs; secondary to psychologic problems, can range from minor to severe; neurosis and relationship problems

Functional Pain/Disgust (Dyspareunia)

Organic causes (Pain is more often organic than psychogenic; therefore, organic causes must be ruled out.)

Psychogenic causes (There are usually complex and moderate to severe intrapsychic and relationship problems. Pain provides defense against pleasure.)
- Hypochondriac reaction to hormonal shifts
- Pain: hysterical, depression syndrome
- Intractable schizophrenia
- Functional genital muscle spasm
- Brutal sexual assault; intercourse; foreign object

Phobic Avoidance of Sexual Experience (Simple/Complex)

Associated with panic disorders (hypothesized to panic threshold, as if alarm is on; overreacts to hazards and separations)

Simple sexual phobia (conditioning and neurotic conflicts)

Sexual trauma (rape, sexual exploitation, sex stress situations)

Paraphilias

Extreme variation of sexual behavior and object of sexual arousal without regard for welfare of object: nonhuman objects, suffering or humiliation of oneself or another, children or nonconsenting person(s)

Pedophile—object: infant, child, adolescent

Rapist—object: female, male

Sexual arousal dependent on inanimate objects, parts of body, animals, or particular ritualized acts; causes conflict within subject or with partner or society at large
- Most common are:
  - Fetishism (article of women's clothing)
  - Transvestism (cross dressing)
  - Frotteurism (rubbing against another)
  - Exhibitionism (displaying genitals in public)
- Others:
  - Telephone scatology (lewdness)
  - Necrophilia (corpse)
  - Partialism (body parts)
  - Zoophilia (animals)
  - Coprophilia (feces)
  - Klismaphilia (enemas)
  - Urophilia (urine)
- Other variations of sexual behavior, act dominated:
  - Sexual masochism (hypoxyphilia: sexual arousal through partial strangulation, beatings, etc.)
  - Sexual sadism (whipping, beating another)
  - Voyeurism (peeping)

Gender Identity Disorders

Nonacceptance of biologically determined sexuality; nonacceptance of socially determined sex role

Ego-Dystonic Homosexuality

Conflict over preference for sexual gratification from same-sex partner

Defining Characteristics

Verbalization of problem
Alterations in achieving perceived sex role
Actual or perceived limitation imposed by disease and/or therapy
Conflicts involving values
Alteration in achieving sexual satisfaction
Inability to achieve desired satisfaction
Seeking of confirmation of desirability
Alteration in relationship with significant other
Change of interest in self and others
Concern about sexual functioning without disruption of sexual response pattern (secondary to organic and/or psychosocial causes)
- Concern over sexual functioning because of sudden minor alterations in responsiveness (e.g., time it takes to achieve sexual satisfaction)
- Questions regarding sexual practices (e.g., amount, exertion, should erection be encouraged)
- Confusion, anxiety toward expression of sexual drive
- Confusion over intensity of response
- Concern over adequacy in meeting sexual desire of partner
- Confusion over object of sexual arousal (same for male and female)

Disruption of sexual response pattern: orgasm/ejaculation phase
- Men
  - Premature ejaculation (inadequate control of ejaculation reflex)
  - Retarded ejaculation (delayed or absent)
  - Partial retarded ejaculation; inhibition of emission phase only; no pleasure
  - Retarded ejaculation
  - Premature ejaculation
- Women
  - Inhibited orgasm (delayed or absent orgasm, missed orgasm)
  - Insufficient stimulation

Disruption of sexual response pattern: excitement phase
- Men
  - Impotence
  - Disturbance of sexual pleasure
  - Diminished excitement
- Women
  - Vaginal dryness
  - Painful coitus
  - Disturbance of sexual pleasure

Disruption of sexual response pattern: desire phase
- Total loss of desire
- Loss of desire in specific situations only
- Chronic, low sexual desire

Pain (pre- and post-orgasm/ejaculatory phase)
- Pain before sex (prevents entry or ejaculation)
- Perineal pain (muscle spasm)
- Vaginal spasms after penis has entered
- Postorgasmic uterine spasms

Functional pain (dyspareunia)
- Pain on entry (deep thrusting)
- Vaginismus

Phobic avoidance of sexual experience (simple/complex)
- Phobic avoidance of sexual experience and sexual arousal

Extreme variations of sexual behavior and object of sexual arousal without regard for the welfare of object
- Pedophile
  - Expression of primary sexual interest in infant, child, and/or adolescent by an adult male or female
  - Hypersexual activity with underaged persons
  - Compulsion for involvement with immature sex object
  - Focusing on one object at a time or on a group of children
  - Involvement in pornography purchases and/or production
  - Prefers to be alone (however, can be involved in work activities that either provide contact with immature individuals or time to pursue sexual activities with immature individuals or time to pursue sexual activities with one underaged person)
  - Uses bribes, coercion, and intimidation with object
  - Potentially violent; potentially homicidal
  - Marriage of convenience (cover); or marriage to have access to child
  - May be in clandestine social relationships with other pedophiles
  - More males than females as perpetrators
  - History of legal confrontation for involvement with immature individuals
  - Intelligence often average to above average
- Rapist
  - Requires absolute control of the object
  - Uses force
  - Inflicts physical abuse; can result in murder
  - Justifies actions
  - Blames victim
  - Expresses high level of psychologic abuse (displays disqualifying degrading behavior)
  - Requires power, control, and/or aggression for sexual arousal
  - Experiences disruption of excitement phase with impotence and disruption frequently
  - Experiences orgasm phase with partial ejaculation frequently

Nursing Interventions

Patient Goal	Nursing Intervention
Psychosocial Factors	
Achieve more flexibility in attitudes regarding self and others around sexual functioning.	• Counsel around expectations of self and others. • Counsel around partnership issues. • Educate about sexual techniques and interpersonal communication. • Provide stress reduction instruction.
Reduce cognitive interference that distracts and lessens sexual responsiveness.	• Use cognitive-behavioral approach to stop disruptive cognitive operations.
Reduce critical self-observations; reduce dissociation.	• Alter beliefs regarding performance and adequacy. • Provide training for moving into images of self, increasing awareness of kinesthetic responses, and reducing self-imagery that dissociates feeling states.
Enhance kinesthetic, erotic experience.	• Reinforce prescribed sensation-enhancing exercises with self and partner. • Assist to explore means of intensifying sensations. • Assist patient in identifying techniques to block disruptive thoughts.
Reduce unconscious, intrapsychic conflicts with self and in relationships.	• Counsel patient or couple: work through unconscious hostility to opposite sex; work through guilt regarding pleasure; work through interpersonal problems (e.g., withholding and power plays).
Reduce chronic, delayed reactions to sexual trauma.	• Focus counseling on chronic, delayed reactions to sexual trauma.
Reduce primary organic source of pain.	• Educate in carrying out necessary medical interventions to reduce underlying disease process.
Reduce conditioned, painful voluntary muscle response (secondary to psychologic problems).	• Refer to sex therapist for biofeedback and counseling for psychologic problems.
Reduce underlying psychologic conflicts.	• Refer to counseling and sex therapy.
Reduce avoidance behavior.	• Refer for differential diagnosis of simple/complex phobic response with drug therapy or sex therapy and desensitization.
Organic Factors	
Understand organic issues or illness states' impact on sexual functioning.	• Educate regarding physical illness, illness process, treatment interventions (e.g., drugs). • Reframe distorted beliefs regarding sexual functioning given illness and treatment. • Provide information necessary to enhance functioning (educational materials, counseling, and focused exercises).
Reduce stress regarding sexual response disruption that is reversible and secondary to organic issues.	• Provide accurate information regarding the temporary disruption caused by organic impairment. • Instruct to modify attitudes to accommodate needed behavior change. • Counsel partner or couple.
Reduce stress and institute viable alternatives when disruption is not reversible because of organic problem.	• Counsel and educate patient and sexual partner regarding prosthetics, implants, techniques, and attitudes or beliefs regarding sexual expression.
Resolve past sexual trauma.	• Focus counseling on reactions to sexual trauma.
Pedophile/Rapist	
Prevent further sexual assaults.	• Report to authorities.
Reduce reliance on object, act, for sexual arousal.	• Refer to experienced counselor: confront behavior and its impact on others; drug intervention; individual/family counseling; hypnotherapy, age regression; concerted efforts to have perpetrator identify with victim; management of secondary psychiatric problems; specific strategies to reduce reliance and arousal potential of fantasies, objects, and acts. • Enhance positive regard for victim and self. • Increase arousal and interest in normal sexual practice.

Patient Goal	Nursing Intervention
Gender Identity Disorder in Child/Adolescent	
Reduce intense dissatisfaction in ego-dystonic homosexuality.	• Refer for special evaluation and treatment; counseling to negotiate acceptance of deep-seated conflict; surgery.
Reduce conflict through clarification and free choice.	• Refer for psychotherapy; deal with significance, fear, and interest in homosexuality. • Demonstrate nonbiased, nonjudgmental approach to patient. This can only be done once nurse examines beliefs, feelings, and regard for homosexuality before embarking on counseling.

Principles and Rationale for Nursing Interventions[1-10]

When a behavioral matrix such as sexual functioning becomes a problem, the characteristics of the problem must be understood by the objective evidence as well as the subjective data. The closer the objective evidence coincides with a definitive etiology, the more apt the specific intervention will be.

The following sequencing of data illustrates decisions in the evaluation of defining characteristics and in terms of broad considerations or related factors.

Does the patient have a disruption of sexual response patterns?

If normal functioning present, consider psychiatric diagnosis.

If no psychiatric problems exist, provide education and reassurance.

If psychiatric diagnosis made, differentiate problems, then provide appropriate psychiatric treatment (or refer).

If abnormal functioning present, diagnosis: organic or psychogenic.

If organic, make medical diagnosis. Is it a treatable medical problem that will result in correction, or is it nontreatable? If treatable, consider sexual rehabilitation, counseling, penile implant.

If psychogenic, check etiology. If it is a major psychologic cause, consider long-term therapy. If it is a minor and moderate psychologic cause, consider sex therapy.

If sexual problem is secondary to other psychiatric disorder (e.g., stress, depression, panic disorder, severe marital discord, substance abuse, major mental or emotional illness), consider appropriate psychiatric treatment.

Sexual dysfunction as a diagnosis provides a broad spectrum of general data with a broad array of related factors. When these factors are considered, second- and third-order levels of assessment are required for specifying the particular type of sexual dysfunction and its relationship to important biopsychosocial parameters. In addition, particular types of intervention must be evaluated as to their impact physically, psychologically, and interpersonally. Assessment and differential diagnosis as well as specialized-assessment diagnostic skill are necessary given the complexity of the functional disorder. Collaboration with other professionals as well as the nurse's specialized expertise are required both for differential diagnostic activities and for particular intervention modes.

Concern about Sexual Functioning

When the related factor is organic, nursing care focuses on educating the client and counseling about misconceptions that provoke anxiety and depression. Since sexual functioning most often involves a partner, nursing intervention is also directed at the appropriate partner.

For example, consider a husband recovering from a mild heart attack. The husband and wife are hesitant to resume their sexual relationship for fear the husband will have a heart attack. Sexual desire is present, as are sexual arousal and orgasmic experiences. For these people a causal connection between the energy expended in the sexual act and heart attack has been determined. Information and experience in monitoring exertion with concomitant signs (pulse rate, chest pain) become important for the husband. This is usually done through gradual increments in physical activity. Involvement of the wife provides experience for her as well as an opportunity for them to open up communication between them. Unrealistic expectations can be revealed and countered. In addition, the couple can become comfortable exploring, relaxing, and finding less strenuous methods for enjoying their sexual relationship.

When the related factors are psychologic and secondary to organic causes, education and counseling are the primary interventions. This is particularly true when the problems are minor. Severity of the primary psychologic and relationship problems is determined in part by assessment of the psychologic makeup of the person and/or couple and the critical interactional components of the relationship.

Some medical interventions greatly alter body structure as well as impinge on the physiology of penile erection and erotic responses; therefore special attention has to be paid to the process of the patient gaining acceptance of the body image changes. Partners need support and counseling during periods of adjustment.

Vaginal dryness that impedes the enhancement of sexual excitement may be related to estrogen deficiency, most often associated with menopause. When hormonal replacement is contraindicated or not desired, lubricants can greatly reduce the problem.[6,9] Nursing care is influenced according to whether the medical problem is reversible. With reversible problems, nursing care supports the patient and partner until the reestablishment of sexual functioning. If they are irreversible, rehabilitative efforts and counseling are the modes of intervention.

Removing a sexual complaint can escalate anxiety by exposing other human demands of relating (e.g., commitment, intimacy). Problems in these personal areas are masked through many symptoms of dysfunction. The symptoms may be viewed as defenses for the individual. At times in complex relationship problems the partner with the complaint may be a foil for the more severe psychologic problems of the nonsymptomatic partner. When the symptom is removed, there is an imbalance in the relationship, and the partner's underlying psychologic difficulties are revealed.

In general, the nurse should determine if the disorder has an organic or a psychogenic cause. If there is doubt, the nurse should refer for more specialized evaluation. If organic and psychogenic causes are established, as well as their primary and secondary relationships, the nurse uses one of the following nursing interventions most appropriate to the causes and the level of sexual behavior issues: education, general counseling around personal and relationship issues, focused exercises to alter cognitive sets and physical behavior that impede sexual and erotic behaviors, and inclusion of the partner.

Evaluation[1,3-6]

Patient Outcome	Data Indicating That Outcome is Reached
Separation of attitudes toward sexual functioning that have been linked to organic illness	Sex not confused with organic issues; response to educative information and necessary medical regimen Concern over sexual functioning (self-report) diminishes
Cognitive shifts in restrictive expectations toward self and others	No unrealistic expectations Relaxation Loss of concern over sexual functioning
Understanding of impact of medical treatment and illness on phases of sexual response	Acceptance of temporary problem or irreversibility with no evidence of depression, avoidance, or self-recrimination
Participation in educational counseling programs for reduction of depression and anxieties surrounding illness and enhanced relationship with sexual partner	Techniques to compensate for restrictions Sense of pleasure and gratification in sexual response Physiologic measurements of increased penile circulation Disease process under control
Reduction of psychologic, behavioral patterns that affect phases of sexual response pattern	Alteration in beliefs and attitudes restrictive to sexual behavior and sense of pleasure Alteration in internal thought processes that restrict sexual behavior and sense of pleasure: reduction in disruptive imagery; reduction of negative internal dialogue; increased sense of erotic sensations and how one individual enhances and controls excitement and arousal
Nonreliance on children, violent exploitive sexual actions, or special objects and acts for sexual arousal	Reduction of deviant fantasies associated with sexual arousal; absence of exploitive acts; increased positive, caring sex with another
Resolution of intrapsychic conflicts	Self-report of more comfort, acceptance of self Increased positive experiences with opposite sex/sex partner
Resolution of conflicting interpersonal relationship with sexual partner	Increased sense of erotic sensations Divorces and leaves partner Working through role and dependency issues with partner Increased pointed conversations between partners Increased ease and flexibility in exploring reciprocal, sexually desirable experiences
Resolution of conflict over gender and sexual orientation	Satisfied with gender, sex role, sexual orientation, and choice

Altered Sexuality Patterns

Altered sexuality patterns are states in which an individual expresses concern regarding his or her sexuality.

An altered sexuality pattern is one in which the individual expresses concern regarding sexuality because of actual or perceived difficulties, limitations, or changes in sexual behavior. This is contrasted with the nursing diagnosis of sexual dysfunction, in which the individual experiences a change in actual function that is viewed as unsatisfying, unrewarding, or inadequate. The focus of altered sexuality patterns is with the individual's concerns about sexuality, which may or may not be associated with changes in sexual function (dysfunction).

Related Factors

Knowledge/skill deficit about alternative responses to health-related transitions, altered body function or structure, or illness or medical treatment
Lack of privacy
Lack of significant other
Ineffective or absent role models
Conflicts with sexual orientation or variant preferences
Fear of pregnancy or of acquiring sexually transmitted disease
Impaired relationship with significant other
Body image disturbances

Defining Characteristics

Reported difficulties, limitations, or changes in sexual behaviors or activities
Impaired expression of one's sexuality
Expression of fear of potential limitations of sexual performance

Nursing Interventions

Patient Goal	Nursing Intervention
Express satisfaction with sexuality.	• Facilitate communication with patient and partner. • Explore health-related transitions, altered body function or structure, and illness or medical treatment. • Correct any misconceptions. • Obtain and relate information that is specific to condition: Side effects of pharmacologic agents Normal aspects of aging Postsurgical adjustments, especially after surgery on sexual organs or ostomy Post–myocardial infarction adjustments • Explore issues related to physical setting or environment where sexual activities are usually performed, including attention to visual and auditory factors, privacy, furniture, and ambient temperature. • Encourage patient to accept sexual orientation and/or to seek psychologic counseling if this is source of conflict. • Determine if fear of pregnancy or fear of acquiring sexually transmitted disease is contributing factor to patient's altered sexual pattern. Provide related information and clarify any misconceptions. • Encourage discussion about other factors that may have impaired relationship with significant other. • See nursing interventions for Sexual Dysfunction.

Principles and Rationale for Nursing Interventions

The focus of the nursing interventions is to assist the patient to identify the source of concerns that result in an altered sexuality pattern and to remediate problems by clarifying misconceptions and learning correct information. (See interventions for Sexual Dysfunction for appropriate rationales.)

Evaluation

Patient Outcome	Data Indicating That Outcome is Reached
Resumes normal patterns of sexuality and sexual activity	Verbally expresses satisfaction with sexuality Implements adaptive behaviors to accommodate any health-related transitions, altered body functions or structures, and illness or medical treatment Describes having appropriate environment in which to engage in sexual activity See Sexual Dysfunction for appropriate evaluation criteria.

Rape-Trauma Syndrome

(Compound reaction; silent reaction)

Rape-trauma syndrome is forced, violent sexual penetration against the victim's will and consent. The trauma syndrome that develops from this attack or attempted attack includes an acute phase, or disorganization of the victim's life-style, and a long-term process of life-style reorganization.

Rape trauma syndrome is the acute and long-term psychosocial process of reintegration that occurs as an aftermath of forcible rape or attempted forcible rape.[1] The syndrome is influenced by the type of rape activity: forcible, nonconsenting, sexual exploitation, or sex-stress situation. The legal definition of rape varies from state to state; however, the issues generally addressed include lack of consent, force or threat of force, and sexual penetration. The clinical definition of rape trauma—the focus of this nursing diagnosis—is the stress response pattern of the victim following forced, nonconsenting sexual activity. The rape trauma syndrome of somatic, cognitive, psychologic, and behavioral symptoms is an active stress reaction to a life-threatening situation.[1]

The trauma to the victim results from that person being confronted with the life-threatening and highly stressful situation of rape and sexual abuse. The crisis or reaction that results is in the service of self-preservation. It is the nucleus around which an adaptive pattern may be noted.[1]

What is traumatizing to a rape victim (in all types of rape) is that her life is in jeopardy and she is helpless in the situation. Forcible rape, an act forced on a victim (usually female) by an assailant (usually male), is viewed as an act of violence expressing power, aggression, conquest, degradation, anger, hatred, and contempt.[11] Hilberman[9] characterizes rape as the "ultimate violation of the self, short of homicide, with the invasion of one's inner and most private space, as well as loss of autonomy and control." Hilberman argues that it is the person's self, not an orifice, that has been invaded and that the core meaning of rape is the same for a virgin, a housewife, a lesbian, and a prostitute.

A study of motivational intent of the offender indicates that rape behavior involves a hierarchy of life issues such as power, anger, and sexuality. On the basis of clinical data on 133 convicted rapists and 92 adult victims, Groth, Burgess, and Holmstrom[6] viewed rape as complex and multidetermined, and they addressed issues of hostility (anger) and control (power) more than passion (sexuality). Subdivisions of these categories include the power-assertive rapist, who perceives rape as a means of expressing his virility and dominance; the power-reassurance rapist, who uses the act of rape to resolve doubts about his sexual adequacy; the anger-retaliation rapist, who seeks revenge by degrading and humiliating women; and the anger-excitation rapist, who derives sexual excitement from inflicting pain and punishing his victim. In pair or group rape the motive of seeking male camaraderie has been suggested, and the motive of a sense of entitlement to sexual services has been observed in data on father-daughter incest,[8] wife rape,[13] and date situations.[4]

Analysis of the dynamics and method of operation of the rapist helps to explain what specific aspects have terrorized and victimized the person. Style of attack has been found to contain characteristics classified as blitz, in which the victim is quickly subdued and propelled into the assault[4]; con, in which the victim is approached verbally and then betrayed and assaulted[4]; and surprise, in which the rapist waits and targets a victim or sneaks up on and surprises her.[7]

Sexual Exploitation

Rape trauma syndrome falls within the general category of sexual traumas. Two additional sexual traumas were identified in the study in which rape trauma syndrome was reported.[10] A differential diagnosis needs to be made regarding the additional two sexual traumas.

A second group of sexual assault victims, most of whom were children and young adolescents, were categorized as accessory-to-sex victims. In this type of sexual assault victims are pressured into sexual activity by a person or persons who stand in a power position over them through age or authority. Victims are unable to make a responsible decision of consent because of their level of personality or cognitive development or their learned rules of behavior. The emotional reaction of the victim results from being pressured into sexual activity and from the tension to keep the activity secret. The offender gains access to the victim in several ways: offering material rewards (candy, money); offering psychologic rewards (attention, interest, affection); or misrepresenting moral standards ("It's okay to do this—your mother and I do it").[2]

This trauma syndrome is often characterized by a gradual, social and psychologic withdrawal from usual life activities. This withdrawal is most apt to occur when the sexual activity is repeated with the same person over an extended time. Physical symptoms of trauma may be evidenced through changes in motor behavior and signs of infection. Such overall signs and symptoms are especially prominent when the victim has been pressured into secrecy by the offender. The burden of carrying the secret creates considerable tension, and the victim feels constantly on guard to maintain the secret.[2]

Sex-Stress Situation

A third group of sexual trauma situations results from a sexual encounter in which both parties initially consent to sexual activity. The person for whom the sexual situation produces the most anxiety usually brings the situation to the attention of the nurse. The situation usually includes two consenting people for whom something "goes wrong" during the sexual activity; or there may be anxiety about the results of the sexual activity (pregnancy, infection, disease).[4]

Related Factors

Rape Trauma Syndrome: Nonconsenting Forcible Rape

1. Type of rape
   Force/threat
   Damage/physical
2. Age
3. Demand for cognitive/behavioral assimilation of experience (how the process proceeds)
   Surprise
   Death threat
   Physical penetration
   Physical injury
   Immobilization
   Attributions for cause of rape
   Self-appraisal of response to rapist or victim, mastery
   Stored sounds, smells, images, sensations
4. Major coping behaviors employed to handle assault
5. Demand for cognitive/behavioral assimilation of disclosing experience to others
   Response of judicial/police system
   Response of immediate social support system
6. Prior psychosocial issues
   Prior victimization
   Prior stress experiences
   Social network response
   Major coping behaviors

Rape Trauma Syndrome: Compound Reaction

Factors 1 to 6 with particular emphasis on:

Major defenses and coping mechanisms employed to handle the exploitation

Characteristics of the social support system
- Excessive blame
- Excessive worry, reinforcement of victim role
- Amount of physical violence
- Coping mechanism to master rape
- Quality of support system
- Older age of victims

Prior psychosocial issues
- Attachment to perpetrator
- Degree of political, personal, and financial power of victimizer over victim
- Chronic history of abuse, self-deprecation
- Limited sense of alternatives
- Limited psychologic capacities
- Socialization (delayed labeling of experience[s] as rape because of prevailing sense of social milieu holding victim responsible, deserving and provoking sexual abuse)
- Primary use of dissociative and avoidant defenses and coping behaviors during time of sexual exploitation and through disclosure process, plus perception of self vis-à-vis social support system, seem most important

Rape Trauma Syndrome: Delayed Reaction

Factors 1 to 6 with particular emphasis on dissociative defenses and avoidant coping behavior

Factors contributing to compound reaction also contribute to delayed reaction

Rape Trauma Syndrome: Silent Reaction

Type of rape (particular attention to the threat/fear of violence used to control and the distortion of sense of self, sense of right, wrong, responsibility, perpetrated)

Disclosure
- Confrontation by self/others of sexual exploitation
- Police/judicial proceedings
- Immediate social support system
- Peer and school reaction

Demand for cognitive/behavioral assimilation of experience (how process proceeds)
- Betrayal
- Sorting out responsibility
- Dealing and subtle threats, coercion, distortion
- Blurring of aggressive/sexual impulses
- Stress reaction to disclosure
- Stored sounds, smells, images, sensations

Major coping mechanisms employed to handle exploitation

Prior psychosocial issues; prior victimization

Fears retaliation

Denies importance of rape to avoid deeper personal reactions: shame, guilt, etc.

Attachment to offender before abuse

Psychologic problems

Source of powerlessness

Socialization; woman to bear humiliation alone

Use of defenses; dissociation of affect from memory of rape

Defining Characteristics

Somatic reactions
- Physical trauma: cuts and bruises on neck, throat, breasts, thighs, legs, arms
- Physical trauma to genitals
- Gastrointestinal irritability
  - Stomach pains
  - Nausea
  - Change in appetite
- Skeletal muscle tension, headaches, fatigue
- Sleep disturbance reactions
- Genitourinary disturbances
  - Vaginal discharges
  - Rectal bleeding
  - Burning in urination
  - Itching

Psychologic/behavioral reactions
- Disturbance of mood: depressed, anxious
- Cognitive disruption: confusion, failure of memory, indecisiveness

- Self-appraisal: fear, embarrassment, humiliation, self-blame
- Fear of violence toward self and others
- Desire for revenge
- Intrusive thoughts, nightmares, daymares
  - Replication of the victimization
  - Thoughts of the rape
  - Mastery dreams of overcoming assailant
- Phobic reactions
  - Avoidance of sex
  - Avoidance of people
  - Avoidance of crowds
  - Avoidance of being alone
- More severe psychologic reactions
  - Ideas of reference
  - Psychotic states
  - Severe acting out
- Dysfunctional coping
  - Alcohol, drugs
  - Promiscuity, prostitution
- Suicidal behavior, homicidal behavior
- Self-blame, low self-esteem
- Restrictive and avoidance behaviors
- Fear that something is wrong with sexual organs

Social reactions

- Dependence on others
- Work or school failure, withdrawal
- Avoidance of close or family relationships; social isolation
- Disruption of couple's relationship
- Social stigmatization
- Constant moves to deal with anxiety and fear

Additional aspects

When patient presents herself as psychotic or sexually promiscuous, has psychosomatic complaints, avoids sexual relationships, or has sudden social withdrawal and alcohol and drug abuse, evaluation should be done to rule out sexual trauma diagnoses. These major behavioral deviations often mask sexual trauma, either because prior psychiatric problems are exacerbated by trauma or because these other syndromes defend against sexual event.

There is also a group of victims who do not reveal to others that they have been raped (silent reaction). This population appears different from those with delayed reactions in that total event is not dissociated and repressed; rather, there is memory of event, but emotional reaction and its assimilation are not addressed, nor is event disclosed to others.

Characteristics associated with silent reaction

- Marked anxiety in personal interviews with long periods of silence, blocking of associations, minor stuttering, and physical distress
- Reported extreme irritability or actual avoidance of relationships with men
- History of extreme change in sexual behavior
- History of sudden onset of phobic reactions: fear of being alone, going outside, being inside alone
- Persistent loss of self-confidence and self-esteem; self blame
- Suspiciousness
- Frequent dreams of violence and nightmares

Nursing Interventions

Patient Goal	Nursing Intervention
Reduce immediate negative reactions to rape experience and disclosure.	• Provide safety Provide effective, considerate physical examination; necessary prescriptions; repair of injuries. Establish close relationship with safe person to provide for catharsis with attention to correction of distorted premises regarding self-blame. Establish self-control over person and decisions. Establish supportive social network. Counsel regarding stress response images, sounds, smells, sensations that provoke anxiety; relaxation exercises. Counsel immediate family, spouse, or partner.
Gain support for criminal judicial experience.	• Ensure careful preservation of evidence; reporting. • Assign to rape crisis. • Counsel regarding exacerbation of earlier crisis symptoms with prolonged investigative procedures and court appearances. • Continue counseling of important family member, spouse, or partner. • With children, use particular photographic strategies to provide evidence of physical injury from penetration (vaginal and anal).
Achieve reduction of any prolonged symptoms.	• Provide counseling and focused therapy for: Prolonged anxiety reactions associated with specific flashback phenomena Reframing of descriptive belief patterns • Provide couples counseling where conflict and restriction in sexual activity occurs. • Provide careful examination and follow-up on physical injuries and symptoms.
Reinstate life plan.	• Enhance positive attachment(s) to people and life goals. • Encourage and participate in interactive discussion with a focus on the future.

Principles and Rationale for Nursing Interventions

In the acute phase of rape trauma syndrome there is a great deal of disorganization in the victim's life-style. This disorganization is evidenced as follows.[1]

In *impact reactions* one of two styles of reaction is generally noted: the expressed style, in which feelings of fear, anger, and anxiety are shown through such behavior as crying, sobbing, smiling, restlessness, and tenseness, or the controlled style, in which feelings are masked or hidden and a calm, composed, or subdued affect is noted.[3]

In the first several weeks after a rape the following acute *somatic manifestations* may be evident:

Physical trauma, which includes general soreness and bruising from the physical attack in various parts of the body (e.g., throat, neck, breasts, thighs, legs, arms)

Skeletal muscle tension, which includes tension headaches and fatigue, as well as sleep pattern disturbances and complaints of hyperalertness, feeling edgy and nervous

Gastrointestinal irritability, which includes stomach pains, appetite disruption, and nausea

Genitourinary disturbance, which includes gynecologic symptoms of vaginal discharge, itching, burning on urination, and generalized pain; also, symptoms from sexual penetration of the mouth and rectum

A wide gamut of *emotional reactions* may be expressed and include fear, humiliation, embarrassment, anger, revenge, and self-blame. Fear of physical violence and death is usually the primary affect experienced during the rape.

The long-term process of reorganization is the second phase of the rape trauma syndrome. Although the time of onset varies from victim to victim, this phase often begins several weeks after the assault or identification of the rape. Various factors affect the coping behavior of victims, e.g., ego strength, social network support, and the way people treat them as victims.[3] The following characteristics are noted:

Motor activity. There generally is an increase in motor activity, especially changing residence and taking trips. Victims also turn for support to family members not necessarily seen daily as well as to friends, associates, and colleagues.

Dreams and nightmares. Intrusive thoughts of the rape break into the victim's conscious mind as well as during sleep (nightmares). Three types of nightmares may be reported: replication of the state of victimization and helplessness; symbolic dreams, which include a theme from the rape; and mastery dreams, in which the victim is powerful in assuming control. Nonmastery dreams dominate until the victim is recovered.

Traumatophobia. Fears and phobias are common characteristics following rape. The phobia develops as a defensive reaction to the circumstances of the rape. Some common phobias include fear of indoors, fear of outdoors, fear of being alone, fear of crowds, fear of people behind them, and sexual fears.

The nursing care of the rape trauma victim is based on four models of nursing intervention: biologic, social, cognitive-behavioral, and psychologic.[12]

Biologic Model of Intervention

During the acute phase following the assault, the nurse should carefully review any somatic alteration in the body system such as the following: circulatory system (flushing, perspiration, feeling hot or cold, headaches); respiratory system (breathing style, sighing respirations, rapid breathing, dizziness); gastrointestinal system (abdominal pain, nausea, lack of appetite, constipation); genitourinary system (urinary frequency, interference with sexual functioning).

On the follow-up it is essential for the nurse to document carefully the nature and intensity of the symptoms over a 24-hour period. The somatic side effects of any medication prescribed need to be distinguished from the somatic aftereffects of the assault. For example, the nausea and vomiting from antipregnancy medication should significantly decrease when the medicine is stopped. It is important to check if nausea is from an emotional reaction to thinking about the rape. Similarly, itching and vaginal discharge may be a result of the heavy dose of antibiotics and should decrease on completion of the medication. A careful note should be made that the patient is taking the correct amount prescribed. Physical symptoms after 5 days should be carefully investigated, since the therapeutic regimen of medication is usually completed by then. Minor tranquilizers and sleeping medication should not be routinely prescribed without a careful assessment of the patient's needs.

The victim should have a gynecologic and medical follow-up appointment after she completes her first menstrual period following the assault. All victims, male and female, should have blood test for syphilis and a culture for sexually transmitted diseases taken during a 4- to 6-week follow-up visit. The referral and follow-up is a primary nursing intervention and may be made to either a nurse practitioner or physician.

Social Model of Intervention

This nursing intervention makes explicit use of the victim's social network. The goal of using family and friends of the victim is to strengthen the victim's self-confidence to help her resume a normal style of living. Whether or not the victim chooses to tell family and friends about the rape is not the point, but rather that the victim seeks support from the network.

The victim is encouraged to resume a normal style of activity according to her ability to pace the activities. The longer a victim avoids a normal activity such as school or work, the greater the difficulty in trying to return to it.

An important nursing intervention is to encourage the victim to seek out understanding people to talk to about any concerns. The victim often has specific decisions to make and seeks advice about issues such as whether to press charges against the rapist, whether to quit work, or how to tell people about the incident. It is important for the victim to have an active involvement with a social network and environment to resume a somewhat normal life-style. Repairing estranged family and social relationships is encouraged to provide the victim with additional emotional support during this time.

Cognitive-Behavioral Model of Intervention

The focus of the cognitive-behavioral model is on the belief patterns the victim holds regarding rape and sexual assault, as well as on desensitizing the person to the behavior that results from the assault, specifically the phobic reactions. Identifying the belief patterns (why the victim thinks the rape occurred) provides the nurse with a measurement of the victim's attribution of blame. For example, if the victim believes women are raped because of the way they dress, she will need to be educated as to the myths about rape. If the victim believes that rapists stalk victims and therefore anyone may become a victim, attention can be placed on increasing safety tactics for the prevention of invasion from predators.

One goal of this intervention is to deflate the fears, stresses, and anxieties the victim experiences after the assault and to help inflate the victim's own self-esteem and self-confidence in dealing with the world again. The victim has the potential to reach her previous level of adaptive functioning and to strengthen capabilities to feel secure again.

The nursing intervention is aimed at desensitizing the victim to the memory of the rape. Talking about the painful parts gives the victim psychologic control over the memory and strips it of its power to distress the victim. The victim is encouraged to master her fears, i.e., to think back over the very frightening situation with support from the nurse and friends. Gradually, this method desensitizes the victim so that the thoughts can gradually enter the mind without the terrifying reactions. This technique may be used with the physical setting or other circumstances of the assault.

As the nurse talks with a victim, it is essential to help the victim make psychologic connections between the symptoms and the rape trauma. Although repression may be a protective process, it absorbs valuable psychic energy necessary for the victim to settle the crisis.

A common fear of victims and their families is that the offender will retaliate in some manner or that he will try to harm the victim in some other way. If concrete data exist that the offender is harassing the victim, the police can be notified to help in the matter. In some cases the victim is threatened by the defendant's family, and in such cases the judge may be explicit in condemning such behavior and in stating the sanctions for the assailant if such behavior continues. Retaliative behavior can be quite frightening to the victim.

Psychologic Model of Intervention

During the acute phase the nurse should carefully review mental functioning in terms of impaired attention, poor concentration, poor memory, changes in outlook, and future planning, and emotional reaction in terms of irritability, mood changes, dream disturbance, and changes in relationships with family and friends.

Talking with the victim during the impact phase, or as close as possible to the actual time of the rape, is essential to help repair the emotional damage inflicted on the victim. This intervention also attempts to minimize the psychologic aftereffects of the rape by providing emotional support of a nonjudgmental nature. Talking with the victim helps to establish an alliance and provides an opportunity for assessing the impact of the assault and the victim's reactions.

The overwhelming impulse of the victim is to avoid dealing with the experience. In such situations the nurse encourages the victim to talk about the rape and supports any fearful reaction by saying that the fear is a natural reaction to the danger to which the victim was exposed.

Talking about the assault and bearing the accompanying distressing feelings are essential steps in the total process of settling the crisis and mastering the experience. The treatment goals for the victim are to reestablish a normal style of living and to restore a sense of equilibrium. This means the victim must come to terms intellectually and viscerally by acknowledging the impact of the rape on her life and incorporating it as a stressful memory in the total life experience. The meaning of the assault must be talked about and thought about. The feelings, which may be accompanied by various physical and emotional manifestations, must be experienced. In this way the victim can diminish the painful impact of the experience.

Evaluation

Patient Outcome	Data Indicating That Outcome is Reached
Absence of stress response symptoms	Verbalizes: Normal sleep patterns Ability to think and talk of event without excessive signs of distress Absence of flashbacks and intrusive thoughts
Return to physical functioning	Absence of physical symptoms; repair and rehabilitation from physical injury
Return to physiologic functioning, balance, and flexibility	Memory intake Positive self-regard Absence of mood disturbance and depression Physical energy for learning and solving problems
Return to social functioning	Return to critical role activities at work and as family member Comfortable in sex role Comfortable in social situations Reasonable sense of safety and caution in strange situation, at night, and with people

FUNCTIONAL HEALTH PATTERN

X

Coping–Stress Tolerance

 Ineffective Individual Coping

Ineffective individual coping is the impairment of adaptive behaviors and problem-solving abilities of a person in meeting life's demands and roles.

Given the very broad definition of coping, several models are available to understand this nursing diagnosis. These include a self-regulating system in which coping is one of the processes; a transactional system with coping and cognitive appraisal mediating between the environmental and stress encounters and the outcomes; a focus on the emotional processes alone; methods that describe coping as a process of the ego; those that describe coping patterns as a response to threats or disease. For a further discussion of stress research, see Lowery.[24]

Related factors also arise from the theories and research presented. Defining characteristics represent the signs and symptoms in the person experiencing ineffective individual coping. Outcomes refer to behaviors or end states the nurse wants for the patient. It is a basic assumption that a person copes in the most effective way possible given the genetic, developmental, biologic, and situational context. The Grant Study of Adult Development[43] supports the idea that a person's efforts to cope are complex and that to label the use of certain mechanisms as pathologic is not useful. Therefore the characteristics presented are broad concepts. As the diagnosis becomes more specific in terms of being related to certain factors, the defining characteristics in turn are more defined. For example, potential ineffective individual coping related to inadequate appraisal of an illness/treatment situation could have such characteristics as lack of knowledge about the illness and treatment, anger, and rejection of surgery as an alternative treatment.

Some nursing diagnoses are related to coping in specific situations: pain; potential for injury, poisoning, suffocation, or trauma; posttrauma response; and rape-trauma syndrome. Anticipatory and dysfunctional grieving are related to concepts of mourning; a large body of research literature describes the stages of this process, which is also a coping process.

Interventions can be developed from the theory and designed for specific related factors to reduce, eliminate, or modify defining characteristics. For the nurse to intervene creatively, a broad understanding of theories, the nursing process and diagnosis, and the patient is vital.

Related Factors*

Situation/context
- Lack of adequate resources
- Sociocultural stressors
- Treatment available
- Exhaustion of available treatments

Stress/event/illness
- Loss of loved one
- Threat of life
- Threat to security (e.g., lack of employment)
- Life cycle/stage of development
- Pain

*References 5, 8, 11, 12, 14, 19, 21-23, 26, 30, 31, 33, 36, 38, 40.

Competition
Multiple repetitive stressors over time
Change
Delays
Overload, daily problems
Time limitations
Conflict arising from incompatible motives or goals

Impaired self-efficacy/self-concept
Powerlessness
Impaired competency
Impaired vigor
Lack of perceived control

Lack of social support

Physical/psychologic impairment
Memory loss
Sensory/perceptual impairment
Nervous system impairment
Disease process
Previous psychiatric treatment
Personality disorder
Complications

Inaccurate appraisal of stress/event/illness
Inability to make valid appraisal of situation
Inability to recognize source of threat
Inability to redefine or interpret threat correctly
Inability to find meaning for event
Inability to identify skills, knowledge, and abilities to cope with threat
Lack of clear realistic goals or outcomes
Unresolved memories of past threats or negative experiences

Inadequate response repertoire
Difficulty in expressing feeling, especially anger, guilt, or fear
Use of behavior destructive to self or others, e.g., attempting suicide, aggressive acts toward others, use of alcohol and other drugs
Inability to seek out or to learn new skills and knowledge needed to resolve stress/event/illness
Inability to deal with tangible consequences of stress/event/illness
Increasing emotional responsiveness or lack of objective responsiveness
Defensive avoidance of dealing with threatening situations
Lack of assertive behaviors
Impaired communication skills
Lack of palliative skills

Inappropriate deployment of coping resources
Inability to develop alternative goals, plans, actions, and rewards
Lack of ability to transfer knowledge and skills to actual problem resolution
Giving up hope and spiritual values
Social withdrawal
Difficulty in using problem-solving skills and decision-making skills
Concerns and/or fears about initiating action
Lack of appropriate coping response because no cognitive cue to action available
Lack of supportive social network
Overuse/underuse of certain responses

Defining Characteristics*

Overdependence on significant others, professional help, or institutions
Nonproductive life-style
Nonperformance of activities of daily living
Lack of functioning in usual social roles
Continuance of escape-avoidance behavior
Purposelessness
Unhappiness
Lack of future orientation
Self-absorption
Inflexibility
Hypervigilance pattern
Defense avoidance pattern
Unconflicted change pattern
Unconflicted inertia pattern
Clear, frequent expressions of pessimism
Unconcerned and detached from usual social supports
Refusal or rejection of help
Hopelessness
Quality of life not acceptable to person
Excessive use of denial

*References 5, 7, 8-11, 14, 17, 19, 22, 23, 28, 30, 39, 40, 43, 44.

Nursing Interventions*

Patient Goal	Nursing Intervention
Develop awareness of emotional reactions to stress/event/illness.	• Give empathetic responses to expressions of feelings to encourage acceptance of these feelings in self. • Elicit what patient fears or what causes anger or depression. • Give feedback about behavior observed and feelings expressed. • Assist in identifying feelings with names that are acceptable and understandable to patient.

*References 1-4, 7, 11, 12, 19, 20-23, 25-27, 29-31, 33-35, 37, 38, 41, 43, 46.

Patient Goal	Nursing Intervention
	• Assist in developing ideas about relationship of patient's emotional state and consequent thought patterns and behaviors.
Develop objective appraisal of stress/event/illness.	• Explore perception of event by encouraging description. • Provide factual information about threatening stimulus. • Provide preparatory information to patients undergoing new procedures and experiences. Describe sounds, smells, tastes, and appearances. Explain causes of sensations. Give information about how long pain, procedure, or treatment will last. • Raise questions, encourage data gathering, and promote attitude of openness to new information. • Avoid evaluative statements when providing information. • Work through unresolved memories of past events; image-based reconstruction. • Encourage medical, social work, legal, and other consultation to assist in interpretations. • Make referral for spiritual counseling as way to assist patient in finding meaning for situation.
Develop coping responses to emotional reactions to stress/event/illness.	• Assist patient in reduction of anxiety by use of recreational and diversional activities as well as working through feelings of anxiety. • Foster constructive outlets for anger and hostility by teaching warning signs of outbursts, ways to gain self-control, and ways to express anger appropriately. • Assist patient to work through denial or other defensive mechanisms or to understand and accept these as coping response useful at some time. • Teach patient to observe for coping responses of defensive avoidance and hypervigilance, which may impede decision making. • Encourage attitude of realistic hope as way to deal with feelings of helplessness. • Teach relaxation techniques. • Teach effect of negative self-reflections and derogatory ideas on emotional reactions. • Foster expression of feelings through open communication.
Develop coping responses to objective features of stress/event/illness.	• Assist in identifying and making changes in health behaviors that are necessary because of stress. • Serve as role model and/or social support when helping patient perform activities of daily living.
Develop plans and actions in response to stress/event/illness.	• Teach patient skills involving problem solving, decision making, assertive communication, goal setting, evaluation, study, palliative coping, and relaxation. • Assist in identifying coping responses patient is using and other possible coping responses. • Engage patient in role rehearsal and mental imagery for active social role participation. • Encourage socialization and social support. • Teach patient to monitor self for noneffective thoughts about self or maladaptive behaviors. • Explore past situations in which effective coping behaviors were demonstrated. • Assist in biofeedback by giving information about pulse and blood pressure as patient uses relaxation technique. • Provide constructive tasks to perform and ignore responses that are nonproductive and interfering.
Evaluate impact of coping response on objective aspects, emotional distress level, and plans and actions.	• Confront patient about impaired judgment when appropriate. • Assist patient in determining reasonable goals. • Provide feedback to patient and assist in eliciting feedback from others. • Assist patient in developing cues for self to indicate whether he or she is reacting automatically or objectively. • Give patient conceptual model for understanding event or treatment regimen: model of emotion, model of stress.

Principles and Rationale for Nursing Interventions

A self-regulating system has been proposed as a response to illness.[2,28] The three states, or processes, have feedback loops and are described briefly as:

Input stage (interpretation process). For example, a stimulus arouses a pain sensation and the emotion of fear. Concrete, affective, and conceptual memories are activated, resulting in interpretations of the experience/illness.

Coping stage (process). Plans and actions are made to deal with the emotional reactions and with the objective features of the illness/problem.

Monitoring stage (appraisal process). The outcomes of the actions are compared with the goals set.

Obtaining feedback regarding emotional reactions and behavioral actions is also important. An unstable self-regulating system would demonstrate behaviors characterized by inconsistency, unevenness, purposelessness, distress, unhappiness, and threats.

Various authors describe a transactional, multivariant, multiprocess system to explain how the person and environment interact.[8-12,14,21-23,30] "Coping 'refers' to the person's cognitive and behavioral efforts to manage (reduce, minimize, master or tolerate) the internal and external demands of the person-environment transaction that is appraised as taxing or exceeding the person's resources."[30] Regulation of the emotions and management of the person-environment are the two functions of coping in this model.

Coping is the result of appraisals made by the person. A primary appraisal evaluates the negative and positive effects on the self, one's goals or values, and commitments. In addition, a determination of possible actions is done, which is a secondary appraisal.

Actions or coping may be problem focused. Examples are confrontation, information seeking, direct actions, seeking others, and other problem-solving strategies. Examples of emotion-focused coping strategies are distancing self-control, escape avoidance, imagery-rehearsal, and vigilance.

Among life situations, health problems are particularly demanding of emotional coping resources.[8] The threat to the self is great. The dependence on others for assistance of all types is increased. Therefore particular attention needs to be given to planning for the emotional reactions.

The immediate and long-term effects of the patient's appraisal and coping processes are the outcomes. One research study identifies some immediate effects as disgusted, angry, or pleased/happy; quality of encounters as satisfactory/unsatisfactory; and physiologic responses.[23] Long-term effects are noted as an increase or decrease in social functioning, in psychologic well-being, and in various illnesses.

Fear is one of the primary emotions in ineffective individual coping. For example, in the illness/treatment environment the patient experiences many naturally occurring situations in which fear can be treated by nurses (e.g., impending surgery, making discharge plans, receiving medicine). Treatment in the form of new information can be introduced at the point of habituation of the emotion and when the need to escape/avoid is less intense. Support and interventions to reduce the fear are implied initially as the person avoids/escapes. The treatment can be the activation of fear through confrontation, systematic desensitization, flooding, etc., and the introduction of information that does not match the person's memory structure.[7]

Another model identifies five decision and coping patterns in response to threats and/or life-threatening disease.[17,39] They are:

- Unconflicted inertia—refusing to notice a threat; taking no protective actions; making misjudgments about threat
- Unconflicted change—having awareness of threat; wanting to take protective action; having no awareness of consequences of protective actions that could mean loss, pain, or conflict
- Defensive avoidance—having selective inattentiveness to threat; taking action to shift decision making to another or to rationalize or procrastinate
- Hypervigilance—being overwhelmed by the threat; committing self to one action, then another, with little understanding of consequences; experiencing panic
- Vigilance—effective problem solving

Crisis intervention[1,31] as a form of brief psychotherapy focuses on the precipitating event as the patient is assisted to establish the meaning of event for self, to maintain relationships with family and friends, to reestablish emotional balance, and to identify coping mechanisms to respond to the situation. As the patient and therapist work together to maximize the patient's growth potential, initially the emphasis is on the emotional response. The therapist uses such skills as asking open-ended questions, reflecting, paraphrasing, pausing, using minimum encouraging remarks, giving "I" messages, and labeling the emotions being expressed.

An important area of stress-coping intervention focuses on preventing or reducing stress response by preparatory information. Providing sensory information, assisting in reappraisal of concerns toward a positive view, and providing alternative plans are effective.[30,32,45,46]

Working with hostages, prisoners of war, and other survivors, Segal[36] proposed the five Cs as ways to face crises:

- *Communication* is called the lifeline for survival, offering relief by putting feelings into words, by realizing others have similar experiences, and by learning one's reactions are natural.
- *Control,* or taking charge of one's life, is encouraged by reestablishing the daily routines and by using every opportunity to reestablish or exert control.
- *Conviction,* or giving purpose to pain or the search for meaning, is vital. To view stress as a challenge and an opportunity is more healing.
- *Clear conscience,* or a shedding of self-blame, is essential to the management of the human tendency to blaming self with consequent hopelessness and depression.
- *Compassion,* or healing through helping others, has a beneficial effect.

A treatment for impending stress called *stress inoculation training* is based on cognitive theory and involves three phases: conceptualization; skills acquisition; and application, follow-through, and rehearsal.[27,39] Patients are assisted in analysis of their stress-related problems to understand the relationships among feelings, thoughts, and behavior. Automatic thoughts and feelings are disclosed. Patients then are taught several coping techniques, which generally include relaxation training, problem-solving training, cognitive restructuring, and guided self-dialogue. Finally, the therapist provides opportunities to practice the skills using imaginal and behavioral rehearsal as well as the real-life situations. (For more specific information on the techniques or skill development, see the references for the relaxation,* biofeedback, problem solving, cognitive restructuring, self-dialogue, and imaginal and behavioral rehearsal.[6,15])

In a stress-buffering model using previously discussed coping theories, coping assistance is given by others in areas of behavior and cognition to deal with stress from the situation and the emotions.[41] Applied to nursing, the model offers four

*References 6, 13, 15, 16, 30, 42.

areas in which interventions can be developed. Modes of assistance in the area of behavior and the situation include removing the stress from the patient (e.g., giving medication for pain), removing the patient from the stress (e.g., "Let's go outside"), or suggesting ways to change the situation to make it less stressful (e.g., advice on how to perform a procedure with less pain; "Be sure not to look at the needle"). Another area is behavior and the emotions in which the nurses offer food, drink, rest, quiet, and human touch (e.g., "Here, have a cup of coffee"; "Go ahead and have a good cry; I'll stay"). Third, assistance is given in areas of situation and cognition (e.g., the nurse gives new information about the stress or diverts attention from the threat). The last area of interventions is assisting the patient in cognitively altering his or her emotional state (e.g., teaching relaxation, meditation, desensitization).

Evaluation*

Patient Outcome	Data Indicating That Outcome is Reached
Accurate appraisal of stress/threat/illness	Valid appraisal Recognizes source of stress Uses new facts and/or knowledge to redefine threat/cognitive model of stress-coping Finds meaning for the event Identifies skills, knowledge, and abilities within self to cope with threat Clear, realistic goals
Adequate response repertoire	Appropriate expression of feelings No behaviors destructive to self or others Seeks new knowledge and skills to resolve stress/event/illness Decreased emotional responsiveness Increased objectivity and ability to problem-solve Assertiveness Adequate communication skills to convey needs and plans Skills to reduce anxiety, aggressive feelings, etc.
Appropriate deployment of coping resources	Develops alternative goals, plans, actions, and rewards Uses knowledge and skills learned in past or in training sessions to achieve problem resolution Uses support system and/or development of supportive network Uses hope and spiritual values Uses problem-solving and decision-making skills Initiates action Cognitive cues to indicate appropriate actions Appropriate use of others and professional help
Personal meaning given to stress/threat/illness	Expresses that pain/suffering is not without meaning Views event/illness as opportunity to grow
Communication maintained with significant others, including health professionals	Appropriate use of professional help Talks with others about stress/threat/illness Joins mutual support groups
Social roles and contributions reestablished	Productive life-style Performs activities of daily living Performs usual social and work roles Seeks ways to help another

*References 11, 12, 23, 28, 30, 39.

 Defensive Coping

Defensive coping is the state in which an individual experiences a falsely positive self-evaluation based on a self-protective pattern that defends against underlying perceived threats to positive self-regard.

Defensive coping can be manifested in a variety of ways. A defensive reaction is one in which the individual responds to stressors by demonstrating behaviors indicative of an unrealistic or falsely positive self-evaluation. This serves to defend against perceived threats to personal safety and security. The individual struggles to reach a state of psychic equilibrium and unsuccessfully resolves the crisis by developing an unrealistically positive sense of self-esteem. The resultant behaviors are not perceived as socially acceptable by others, and the response of others to the individual may further stimulate the development of more socially aggressive maladaptive behaviors. Any number of combinations of the defining characteristics can be manifested by the individual who experiences defensive coping. Generally the individual denies any obvious problems or weaknesses and blames others for personal shortcomings. Failures are rationalized, and hypersensitivity to the slightest criticism tends to affect interpersonal communications. Subsequent difficulties ensue as a superior attitude, intellectualization, and ridicule of others erode existing relationships and prohibit the establishment of new ones.

Related Factors*

Repeated negative past experiences
Cognitive/perceptual difficulties
Excessive ridicule by others
Unresolved emotionally traumatic experiences
Multiple stressors
Negative interpretation of life events
Inadequate coping strategies
Inadequate social relationships
Psychiatric disorders
Lack of realistic goals for self
Lack of insight into behavior
Learned family behavior pattern
Victim of abusive/dysfunctional parents (e.g., alcholic family syndrome)

*Adapted from North American Nursing Diagnosis Association, 1988 Ballot.

Defining Characteristics*

Denial of obvious problems/weaknesses
Projection of blame/responsibility
Rationalization of failures
Defensiveness; hypersensitivity to slight criticism
Grandiosity
Superior attitude toward others
Difficulty establishing or maintaining relationships
Hostile laughter or ridicule of others
Difficulty in reality-testing perceptions
Lack of follow-through or participation in treatment or therapy
Intellectualization
Seeking special attention or privilege
Attention-seeking behavior
Refuses or rejects assistance from others
Domineering, authoritative
Autocratic management style
Exaggerated self-importance
Avoidance of intimacy
Difficulty in accepting praise
Criticizes readily
Aggressiveness; "bullies" others
Haughty
Abject self-righteousness
Perceived omnipotence

*Adapted from North American Nursing Diagnosis Association, 1988 Ballot.

Nursing Interventions

Patient Goal	Nursing Intervention
Experience increased feelings of security and worthiness and decreased feelings of defensiveness.	• Assess self-concept and underlying reasons for behavior. • Help patient identify behavior and concomitant consequences. • Teach problem-solving skills to help patient cope with identified stressors. • Use matter-of-fact, nonjudgmental approach. • Be aware of personal response to patient's behavior and maintain neutral approach. • Teach assertive behavior techniques to replace aggressive behavior. • Set consistent limits on behavior. • Refer to group therapy. • Refer to family therapy or other therapy groups. • Model appropriate personal interactions for patient, and provide positive feedback when appropriate. • Provide appropriate social skills training. • Use role-playing techniques to model appropriate social interactions. • Monitor deficits in social skills as specifically as possible. • Teach active listening skills. • Identify and use interpersonal strengths.

Principles and Rationale for Nursing Interventions

The focus of nursing interventions for defensive coping is to assist patients to understand the origins of their behavior and work through them so that positive interrelationships can be established and maintained with others. Socially acceptable behaviors are promoted that result in positive feedback and therefore become self-perpetuating as secondary gains for inappropriate behavior are removed. Achievement of goals in caring for these patients is evidenced by their self-reported feelings of increased security and worthiness and decreased feelings of defensiveness.

Evaluation

Patient Outcome	Data Indicating That Outcome is Reached
Engages in appropriate interpersonal interactions	Uses assertive communication style Is not overly critical of others Does not engage in attention-seeking behavior Demonstrates use of coping skills when experiencing stress Demonstrates realistic sense of self

Ineffective Denial

Ineffective denial is the unconscious attempt of an individual to disavow the knowledge or impact of a problem that can threaten or jeopardize his or her health.

Coping adequately and effectively with health problems and their potential or actual consequences is an ongoing process involving the interplay of several factors. One key factor is the interpretation of the event or illness and the perceived consequences for the individual. The actual threat of an illness may not be matched by a reality-based perception and interpretation by the patient. What may be a threatening, anxiety-provoking illness to one person may not necessarily be so for another person. Previous coping skills, self-confidence, and ability to deal with emotions constitute a second set of factors. A history of successful previous coping, effective coping skills, a positive self-concept, and the ability to deal constructively with the emotions created by a stressor such as illness all mitigate the response to illness. Finally, the environment, including social resources, is critically important in shaping a patient's coping response to a major illness. When this overall adaptive coping process falters and becomes less effective, or the stressors become increasingly threatening, ineffective coping responses may come into play. Among these is ineffective denial.

Related Factors*

Fear of consequences of health problem (treatment, pain, unknown, death, hospitalization, stigma)
Overwhelming stressors
Overwhelming feelings (anxiety, anger, depression)
Negative past experiences
Sense of invincibility
Lack of knowledge
Chronic avoidance pattern
Cultural factors
Lack of social support network
Personal/family value system and beliefs
Learned response pattern
Inadequate coping skills
Lack of adequate resources (money)

Defining Characteristics*

Delays seeking medical attention
Refuses medical attention
Does not perceive/admit consequences of signs or symptoms
Does not admit fear of invalidism or death
Displaces source of symptoms
Minimizes signs or symptoms
Displaces fear of impact of health problem
Displays inappropriate affect
Avoids acceptance of loss of body part or function
Changes in daily life-style patterns (escape behaviors)
Changes in interpersonal relationships
Self-absorption

*Adapted from North American Nursing Diagnosis Association, 1988 Ballot.

Nursing Interventions

Patient Goal	Nursing Intervention
Seek and accept appropriate treatment for health problem.	• Assess seriousness of situation and whether continuation of denial will be harmful to patient's life or well-being. • Assess patient's level of denial and readiness to accept reality of situation. • Determine level of fear and other emotions. • Assess support system. • Assess level of knowledge about subject and consequences of health problem. • Determine cultural and personal values related to health care or specific problem.

Patient Goal	Nursing Intervention
	• Assess and use patient's previous coping strategies and patterns. • Ensure patient and family have all appropriate information and objective appraisal regarding diagnoses, treatment, and consequences. • Provide supportive atmosphere for patient, without becoming angry or blaming patient for denial. • Provide psychologic support person to meet and discuss diagnosis with patient (social worker, counselor, clinical nurse specialist). • Develop with family and other caregivers a timetable for introduction of reality. • Encourage trusted family member or close friend to talk gently but openly with patient regarding need for treatment. • Assist patient in developing awareness of usual cognitive and emotional responses to health problem. • Gradually point out behaviors exhibited by patient that contradict reality of situation. • Incorporate cultural patterns and resources into intervention strategies.

Principles and Rationale for Nursing Interventions

The nurse needs to conduct a thorough assessment to intervene in denial so as not to destroy the patient's defense mechanisms. Assessment of family members is imperative to identify the extent to which they support the denial. The nurse needs to intervene in denial at an appropriate level, based on urgency of the situation. Also, the nurse must ensure that the staff and other caregivers are aware of cultural differences.

Evaluation

Patient Outcome	Data Indicating That Outcome is Reached
Demonstrates adequate coping skills in dealing with health problem	Copes adequately and realistically with health problem Seeks medical attention Compliant with medical/treatment regime Verbalizes understanding of health problem and consequences Exhibits appropriate emotional response to significance of health problem Health state improved

Impaired Adjustment

Impaired adjustment is the state in which an individual is unable to modify his or her life-style or behavior in a manner consistent with a change in health status.

Longman[6] defines adjustment as "the modification of attitudes or behavior to meet the demands of life effectively, such as carrying on constructive interpersonal relations, dealing with stressful or problematic situations, handling responsibilities, or fulfilling personal needs and aims." Impaired adjustment is the inability to adapt to the stressful and problematic aspects of a change in health status. The individual with impaired adjustment experiences difficulty handling responsibilities and fulfilling personal needs and goals. The inability to modify attitudes and behaviors after a change in health status interferes with one's initiating and maintaining constructive relationships with family, peers, and society.

Related Factors[8,9]

Disability requiring change in life-style
Impaired cognition
Loss of previous physical abilities
Loss of previous mental abilities
Fluctuations of exacerbation and remission of illness
Progression of disability, despite adherence to recommended regimen
Treatment side effects, discomforts, and risks
Sensory overload
Assault to self-esteem
Altered locus of control
Incomplete grieving
Lack of predictability of future
Alteration in self-care, family, and/or work roles
Inadequate support systems
Inadequate, dwindling financial resources
Increased confinement and social isolation
Significant others alternating between overprotection and rejection

Defining Characteristics[9]

Verbalization of nonacceptance of health status change
Nonexistent or unsuccessful ability to be involved in problem solving or goal setting
Lack of movement toward independence
Extended period of shock, disbelief, or anger regarding health status change
Lack of future-oriented thinking

Nursing Interventions[1-4,7-12]

Patient Goal	Nursing Intervention
Resolve feelings of loss related to change in health status.	• Promote ongoing therapeutic alliance with patient. • Validate and encourage expression of feelings of distress related to changes. • Recognize likelihood of emotional responses (e.g., high anxiety, anger, guilt, helplessness, sadness, withdrawal, crying). • Provide opportunity for expression of fears of disease and death. • Avoid conveying trivialization of patient's fright and distress. • Encourage patient and significant others to share mutual feelings of loss related to patient's change in health status. • Avoid curtailment of expressions of loss by patient and family. • Promote discussion of impact of change in health status on social life of patient and family. • Recognize influence of premorbid personality and past coping mechanisms on patient's current adaptation. • Avoid contributing to infantilization by assuming that patient is more helpless than he actually is. • Avoid conveying blame to patient for current health problems. • Provide information and instruction based on assessment of learning readiness. • Encourage patient to identify individual learning needs. • Provide factual information regarding disability, treatment, and prognosis. • Recognize influence of age of onset, previous family functioning, and severity of illness on patient's and family's understanding of impact of illness. • Teach patient and family to differentiate between denial of *presence* of change in health status and denial of *possible limitations*. • Generate hope by assisting patient to identify previous coping behaviors and support systems used for past problem solving. • Collaborate with patient to develop individually tailored health care regimen. • Assess for possible correlation between perceived beliefs of family and patient's willingness to participate in plan of care. • Teach family to elicit *patient's* perceptions of difficulties as opposed to *their* possible interpretations and explanations. • Assist patient to examine personal responses to current threatening situation. • Recognize varying degrees of role disruption that might be experienced (e.g., occupational, family, sexual). • Recognize influence of compulsory retirement on adaptation. • Avoid judgmental attitudes, criticism, or belittling of feelings, actions, or ideas. • Encourage identification of current remaining personal strengths and intact roles. • Explore patient's perceptions of how changed health status and treatment will affect life-style. • Support patient's spiritual beliefs (to extent that these do not interfere with plan of care). • Assist patient to develop problem-solving skills in relation to disappointments and dissatisfactions.
Modify life-style to experience maximum control and independence within limits imposed by changed health status.	• Teach patient to understand and manage feelings of rage that may accompany recognition of powerlessness. • Collaborate with other staff to assist in determining what will aid in control and management of patient's health status change. • Avoid overdependence on interventions (e.g., relaxation techniques, biofeedback) that may increase focus on symptoms rather than problems causing patient's distress. • Recognize influence of cultural factors on patient's participation with health care system and compliance with treatments. • Facilitate compromise when patient's identified goals differ from goals developed by health care providers. • Actively orient patient and family to planned health care regimen. • Assess for possible correlation between family's willingness to support patient's changed life-style and patient's ability to adapt to change in health status. • Avoid making value judgments concerning patient's family. • Facilitate communication of topics by patient and family that are not related to patient's health status (e.g., current events, family activities, hobbies, recreational interests). • Reinforce patient's recognition of self-help tips. • Encourage patient to maintain sense of control. Make decisions related to specific aspects of care. Evaluate treatments and therapies in terms of goals patient hopes to achieve. Share observations of physical status and progress with caregivers. Ensure accountability for select aspects of care (e.g., active range of motion, wiping secretions from tracheostomy, irrigating colostomy).

Patient Goal	Nursing Intervention
	• Teach patient strategies for active involvement with health care providers in decision-making issues. • Promote patient's development of plans for modification in life-style, including self-monitoring activities (e.g., blood pressure, diet, rest, activity patterns).
Assume responsibility for using personal and social resources to assist in ongoing health management.	• Assist patient to develop plan for stress management, possibly including engaging in self-control therapies (e.g., relaxation exercises, use of imagery). • Teach patient to develop effective coping skills in relation to perceptions of family, caretakers, and society to change in health status. • Consistently convey value of patient's self-directive behavior. • Encourage patient and family to explore resources (e.g., Medicare, Medicaid, Crippled Children's Programs, Social Security Disability Insurance). • Refer patient and family to self-help organizations for assistance with ongoing informational needs, advocacy issues, and current developments in treatment and research.

Principles and Rationale for Nursing Interventions

The patient who experiences a change in health status is faced with losses that may range from mild to severe. Acknowledgment of these losses and appropriate grieving for them are components for successful adjustment to the health changes. The patient's family must grieve as well as the patient.[8] Communication of "genuine acknowledgment and appreciation of the frightening or destructive situation" facing the patient assists him to discuss fears and be able to grieve.[12] The types and intensity of emotions a patient experiences during illness reveal much about his or her perception of what is happening "to the fate of cherished values, commitments, and other sources of meaning in life."[12]

Kasch[7] states that "helping patients develop functional coping strategies necessarily involves focusing on the way in which patients perceive, interpret, and interact with the environment. . . . Nurses can use communication to provide patients with a positive set of beliefs about themselves which may significantly influence a patient's perceptions of his or her ability to influence the environment." Strategies and components described by hospitalized chronically ill patients include[2]:

Evaluating effectiveness of therapies and treatments

Actively participating in information sharing and decision making about their care

Needing to maintain control over their situation by learning what home remedies worked and what their bodies would tolerate in terms of diet, drugs, treatment, and activity

Seeking specific types of information and benefiting from knowledge that has direct application to solving their specific problems

Successful development and implementation of plans for ongoing stress management are indicators of the patient's ability to use personal resources. Patients who experience a change in health status frequently need formalized help beyond that provided by the health team.[8] Both patients and families benefit from being provided with information on self-help groups, as well as being given lists of other available community support groups and resources. Self-help and support groups can also assist patients and families in coping with the stigmatizing that occurs with certain health problems.

Evaluation[9]

Patient Outcome	Data Indicating That Outcome is Reached
Resolves feelings of loss related to change in health state	Acknowledges losses that accompany change in health status Makes plans for future that are congruent with change in health status Redefines individual, social, and cultural values based on recognition of change in health status
Modifies life-style to experience maximum control and independence within limits imposed by changed health status	Seeks help from and cooperates with assistance of competent caregivers Demonstrates self-care practices that are within prescribed regimen Verbalizes recognition that choice of self-care practices can influence outcome of change in health status
Assumes responsibility for using personal and social resources to assist in ongoing health management	Uses strengths and potential to engage in maximally independent and constructive life-style Uses available community resources and support networks

Posttrauma Response

Posttrauma response is the state of an individual experiencing a sustained, painful response to an unexpected, extraordinary life event(s).

Posttrauma response (PTR) is characterized by a range of emotional responses, from fear and anger to flashbacks and emotional numbing. PTR affects combat veterans and victims and survivors of rape, kidnapping, automobile accidents, natural and man-made disasters, and any experience that may pose a threat to one's emotional and/or physical survival or that of loved ones.[1]

PTR is a process with acute and long-term phases.[3] In the acute phase the individual may experience shock and disbelief followed by intense fear and anxiety. Some victims are highly emotive, whereas others appear calm and subdued, giving the impression of coping well.

In the long-term phase, which begins within a few days to several months after the traumatic event, the individual may have flashbacks (revisualizations of the traumatic scene that seem real),[4] intrusive thoughts, and nightmares in which the event is reenacted. Victims may be preoccupied with the traumatic event and may have difficulty concentrating on work or other matters of daily living. Some remain in denial about the event and develop an emotional numbing, which may lead to total amnesia for the event.[1,9,17]

Those who survived disasters in which others died or were seriously injured may feel helpless, guilty for being spared, and ashamed that they did not do enough to save others.[17] In their efforts to cope with these feelings, some PTR patients abuse drugs and/or alcohol, which may aggravate the symptoms. Interpersonal relationships are impaired, and the victim becomes increasingly alienated from pretrauma activities and commitments.

Related Factors*

Disasters (e.g., flood, fire, earthquake)
Participation in combat
Rape
Assault
Torture
Kidnapping
Catastrophic illness
Accidents
Preexisting emotional disorders (e.g., depression)
Previous experience of trauma (e.g., child abuse, abandonment, illness, injury, assault)
Interpersonal isolation; social withdrawal
Limited community supports

*References 1, 3, 8, 9, 13, 14, 16, 17.

Defining Characteristics*

Flashbacks of traumatic event triggered by visual, auditory, and olfactory stimuli
Nightmares
Intrusive thoughts
Impaired concentration, memory, and cognition
Emotional numbing, including amnesia for and confusion about event
Denial of impact of trauma
Generalized fear and anxiety (related to possibility of trauma recurring as well as nonrelated experiences)
Guilt
Impaired interpersonal relationships
Social withdrawal
Impaired occupational functioning
Withdrawal from activities and commitments
Alcohol and drug abuse
Helplessness
Hopelessness
More common in children and adolescents:
- Posttraumatic play and reenactment
- Impaired time orientation for traumatic event and related events
- Limited view of future
- Fear of dying young

*References 1-5, 9, 10, 12, 16, 17.

Nursing Interventions*

Patient Goal	Nursing Intervention
Maintain structural/physiologic integrity of body systems.	• Provide prescribed medical treatment and nursing care relevant to patient's physiologic needs. • Monitor vital signs, intake and output, and range of motion. • Allow patient to focus on recovery and rehabilitation of physical health while medical status is compromised. • Introduce discussion of emotional impact of trauma as patient demonstrates readiness. • Increase patient's responsibility for activities of daily living (ADLs) as physical tolerance allows. • Discuss and teach self-care needs corresponding with physical strengths and limitations. • Explain to patient and family that as physical recovery progresses, more extreme emotional responses may occur.

*References 2, 3, 5, 7-12, 15, 17, 18.

Patient Goal	Nursing Intervention
	• Assist patient to deal with altered physical status; help patient verbalize feelings of loss, inadequacy, low self-esteem, and distorted body image.
Experience decreased flashbacks, nightmares, and intrusive thoughts.	• Encourage patient to talk about traumatic event and how it interferes with current life goals. • Accept patient's fears associated with thoughts and revisualizations; provide understanding response that acknowledges how real these thoughts seem. • Teach relaxation techniques (e.g., progressive relaxation, deep breathing, imagery). • Expose patient to other calming activities (e.g., listening to soothing music, drinking warm milk, taking walks before bedtime). • Encourage structured time during day and involvement in meaningful activities to reduce opportunity for intrusive thoughts.
Integrate traumatic experience and accept impact on life.	• Encourage patient to talk about traumatic event and to express feelings of fear, anxiety, sadness, confusion, and guilt. • Make referral for individual or group psychotherapy. • State expectations for dress, attendance at meals, meetings, and other activities. • Discourage patient from using feelings about trauma as excuse to avoid responsibility for ADLs and life goals. • Allow patient time out from activities as needed, but encourage discussion of feelings that trigger need to withdraw. • Contact community resources (e.g., Survivors of Trauma, Victims Assistance) and encourage patient to use these resources.
Maintain involvement with family, friends, and other social supports.	• Arrange family meetings while patient is hospitalized to discuss how family can provide support and assistance. • Encourage involvement in unit activities, occupational rehabilitation, and hobbies. • Offer support through frequent one-to-one contact to encourage patient to discuss fears and anxiety about interpersonal relationships. • Discuss with family and significant others the meaning of patient's withdrawal; empathize with their pain and confusion while encouraging them to maintain involvement with patient.
Confront problem of alcohol and drug abuse.	• Refer for psychiatric evaluation and psychoactive drug treatment. • Refer for individual or group psychotherapy. • Refer to Alcoholics Anonymous (AA) or Narcotics Anonymous (NA). • Encourage family support and involvement in Al-Anon or other survivor support groups. • Maintain drug-free environment except for prescribed, therapeutic medications. • Encourage patient to avoid social contact with drug abusers or alcoholics who may encourage substance abuse. • Encourage patient to talk about uncomfortable feelings that patient tries to avoid through drugs and alcohol. • Discuss and teach alternatives to drug and alcohol abuse that may provide patient with a more satisfying state of well-being (e.g., spiritual renewal, physical exercise, yoga, meditation).

Principles and Rationale for Nursing Interventions

Before the victim of PTR can work through the emotional reactions to the trauma, he must be assisted to a state of physiologic equilibrium. Denial is a healthy, necessary, and expected reaction in the initial posttrauma period and should not be discouraged.[2] The patient will focus energies on following the necessary medical regimen to recover from injuries sustained and begin to assess the long-term physical impairment. Rushing in to explore the patient's feelings about the trauma may only contribute to the use of pathologic denial and impair future emotional adjustment. The nurse must be sensitive to the patient's cues of readiness to discuss feelings, realizing that each person has a different ability to be emotionally expressive.[7]

Flashbacks, nightmares, and intrusive thoughts are the most disturbing symptoms of PTR. The patient needs the opportunity to describe the traumatic event in detail, even if it involves an increase in anxiety. Providing a safe, trusting environment in which the patient can talk will permit gradual acceptance of the impact of the trauma.[7,9] The patient can then begin to integrate feelings about the trauma into his lifestyle. As new coping strategies are learned, the patient will not limit activities and responsibilities. Relaxation techniques and other self-calming measures increase a sense of control and decrease fears.[5,10]

Most who suffer from PTR will benefit from supportive psychotherapy, usually focused on the traumatic event and conducted over 6 to 12 sessions.[9] Some patients with a preexisting mental health disorder may need ongoing, insight-oriented psychotherapy to help them integrate the complex emotions about the trauma with other life problems. Involvement with others who have suffered from traumatic experiences helps the patient learn new ways of coping, feel less isolated, and feel more useful to others with similar struggles.[18] The family and significant others of the PTR patient are also victims in that they often feel helpless to respond.[8] Being sensitive to their frustration, as well as giving information, will help them maintain the emotional support and attentiveness that the loved one needs. If the patient has an already established support network, he will benefit from regular contact with them. The patient who has been socially isolated and estranged from family will need encouragement to seek out support groups that are safe and nonthreatening. Interpersonal contact provides a healing effect on the victim that advances recovery and return to all areas of life.[7,11,15]

In despair, the PTR patient may turn to drugs and alcohol to medicate against overwhelming anxiety and disturbing thoughts.[12] The patient needs to understand how substance abuse can aggravate symptoms so that he can choose safer, drug-free ways of coping. Involvement in AA, NA, and Al-Anon for the family provides support, information, and encouragement to deal with the drug's effect on the patient's life, and on the family. Appropriate psychoactive drugs, prescribed by a specialist and administered judiciously, will help the patient tolerate anxiety and will assist in the control of flashbacks while discouraging dependence on the medication.[6,12]

Evaluation

Patient Outcome	Data Indicating That Outcome is Reached
Resolves physiologic changes suffered in trauma	Follows medical regimen, including nutritional, physical, and other prescribed therapies Keeps scheduled medical appointments Responsible use of prescription drugs for physical needs Involvement in rehabilitation services
Adapts to altered body image	Verbalizes feelings about physical limitations and self-image Accepts limitations of physical injuries through involvement in appropriate exercise and activity Learns new methods of self-care through use of services for handicapped persons Able to request assistance from professionals and significant others
Restores cognitive abilities	Absence of flashbacks, nightmares, and intrusive thoughts for increasingly longer periods (several hours to several days) Converses and concentrates on wide range of topics and interests Performs necessary ADLs and work-related tasks consistently Sleeps several hours each night without nightmares or intrusive thoughts Appears less anxious when discussing trauma
Improves interpersonal relationships	Interacts daily with family and significant others Initiates contact with family and significant others Verbalizes need for support from others and expresses satisfaction Offers support to others who are in need Expresses feelings of comfort with work colleagues and people in social situations
Manages anxiety through various means	Uses relaxation techniques daily Organizes schedule to include time out for restful, calming activities (e.g., listening to music, reading, taking walks) Verbalizes feelings to therapist, group members, and significant others
Abstains from drugs and alcohol	Attends AA and/or NA meetings two or three times each week Participates in non–drug-centered social activities Develops social relationships with others who are abstaining from or do not abuse drugs and alcohol Seeks out support of appropriate others when desire to abuse is strong Uses prescription drugs only as ordered Expresses satisfaction with improved cognitive, physical, and emotional state
Develops integrated perspective of trauma on life experiences	Discusses meaning of trauma to developmental tasks and social, occupational, and personal goals Adapts goals for present and future according to impact of trauma Resolves feelings of guilt and shame Expresses hope for future Empathizes with victims of other or similar traumas Volunteers as counselor or support person for victims of trauma Renews involvement in religious or spiritual growth activities Shares personal learning with others through informal and formal channels

 Family Coping: Potential for Growth

Family coping: potential for growth is the effective managing of adaptive tasks by a family member who is involved with the patient's health challenge and who is now exhibiting desire and readiness for enhanced health and growth in regard to self and in relation to the patient.

The family's ability to manage effectively the adaptive tasks required by an altered health status in one of its members may be viewed as a coping response indicating the potential for movement to a different stage of development or growth. Readiness for enhanced understanding of the roles and contributions of each family member and acceptance of the required changes resulting from the challenge suggest that the family can use problem-solving techniques to deal with the current situational stresses and to devise preventive measures to maintain the family system's stability.

Whereas early work related to stress theories and coping focused on the individual, recent research into the effect of stress on family systems indicates that many of the concepts apply to both. Perception of the event, role relations, expectations, value orientation, and situational support are concepts that can be applied in family assessment during crises. These concepts form a construct relating to family constellations, which can be assessed separately from the coping strategies usually used.[13] Nine family tasks related to the ability to cope with stress have been identified[15]:

- Owning up to the stress situation
- Redefining the family identity
- Referring to successful past coping strategies
- Exploring alternative solutions
- Organizing responses
- Attempting new responses
- Reaching decisions by consensus
- Responding to the outcomes of the decisions
- Performing family self-evaluation

One model of family adjustment and adaptation to stress suggests that the three factors of demands on the family, family resources, and the family's perspective of the situation interact in successive phases of adjustment, restructuring, and consolidation. This produces an outcome that is indicative of the family's ability to cope productively.[20] Thus a situation that produces stress within the family system offers an opportunity to strengthen the family and produce growth instead of compromising or disabling the family's ability to cope.

Related Factors*

Basic needs of family/individual members sufficiently gratified
Adaptive tasks related to situation effectively addressed
Goals relating to self-actualization of family/individual members surfacing
Family developmental stages
- Courtship
- Marriage
- Childbirth and young children
- Middle marriage and school-age children
- Children leaving home
- Retirement and old age

Situational crises
- Illness of family member
- Changes in situational supports (e.g., job, friends, extended family, natural disaster)

*References 4, 9, 10, 18, 19, 22.

Defining Characteristics*

Attempts to describe growth impact of situation on values, priorities, goals, or relationships
Movement toward health-promoting and enriching life-style that supports and monitors maturational processes
Auditing and negotiation of treatment programs
Choice of experiences that optimize wellness
Interest in contacting others experiencing similar situations

*References 4, 8, 16, 18, 19, 21.

Nursing Interventions[1,5,13,14,18]

Patient Goal	Nursing Intervention
Actualize growth potential of situation.	• Identify changes in family dynamics resulting from situation. • Identify changes in individual family members resulting from situation. • Discuss goals and experiences that maximize growth potential with family/individual members. • Provide information as needed to enable family/individual members to develop new goals and methods of achieving them. • Facilitate development of new methods of goal attainment.
Develop broader base of support.	• Identify individual or family readiness to accept support from additional sources. • Refer individual or family to appropriate resources. • Initiate contact, if necessary. • Follow up to ensure sustained contact and appropriateness of assistance.

Principles and Rationale for Nursing Interventions

Facilitating the family's potential for growth begins with an assessment of the changes that have resulted from the situation produced by one or more related factors. These changes may be seen in the dynamics of the family as roles and relationships are altered and new patterns of interactions are required[10] or in the attitudes, values, and goals of the individual family members.[21] Discussions with individual family members and the family as a whole provide validation that the family system has been changed as a result of the current situation and that new goals and strategies are appropriate. The use of teaching strategies to provide new information about goals, alternative methods of achieving them, and support for attempting new behaviors recognizes that the family members are ready for problem-solving activities and learning.[5,14]

Supporting the family's efforts to develop its own expanded base of both physical and emotional resources reinforces the potential for growth as the family moves toward decreased dependency on health care professionals. Referrals to appropriate community services and appropriate follow-up contacts ensure the family's ability to continue moving toward its goals.

Evaluation

Patient Outcome	Data Indicating That Outcome is Reached
Actualizes growth potential of situation	Verbalizes changes in family roles/relationships Verbalizes changes in individual attitudes, values, and goals Chooses new individual or family goals Chooses new strategies to meet goals Chooses experiences that foster growth
Develops broader base of support	Verbalizes interest in contacting others experiencing similar situations Contacts additional persons or groups when referred Develops additional relationships for physical or emotional support Sustains contact with additional sources

Ineffective Family Coping: Compromised

Ineffective family coping: compromised is insufficient, ineffective, or compromised support, comfort, assistance, or encouragement, usually by a supportive primary person (family member, close friend). The patient may need this to manage or master adaptive tasks related to his or her health challenge.

When a family demonstrates an inability to maintain its usual patterns of functioning as a result of internal or external stressors, its coping abilities are said to be compromised. These behaviors may take the form of insufficient or ineffective support, comfort, assistance, or encouragement to the identified patient by the primary significant person(s) in the family constellation. Such behaviors are usually the result of inadequate physical, psychologic, cognitive, or behavioral resources.[5,16]

Whereas functional families allow for individual views, experiences, and values during stress situations, families whose abilities to cope are compromised appear to require more conformity to expected behavior and become more rigid in response to the situation.[3] Boundaries between the family and outside social systems become less permeable, and coalitions form between family members.[19] The focus of much of the anxiety and fear in a family with compromised coping skills centers on a need to find a cause or learn the rules that will provide guidance for appropriate behavior in the situation.[3] In many instances, particularly when the family has dealt with a chronic illness or a member with a long-term disability, the resources needed to continue to function have been depleted.[1]

Related Factors[5,8,11,14,16]

Inadequate or incorrect information or understanding by family member(s)
Temporary preoccupation by significant family member(s)
- Inability to cope with own emotional conflict
- Inability to perceive needs of identified patient
- Inability to act effectively to meet needs of identified patient

Role changes resulting in temporary family disorganization
Concurrent situational or developmental crises
Limited support received from identified patient
Prolonged illness or disability that exhausts coping abilities
Economic problems (inflation, unemployment, lack of insurance)
Unrealistic expectations of significant family member(s) by identified patient
Unrealistic expectations of identified patient by significant family member(s)
Lack of mutual decision-making skills
Rigid or inappropriate boundaries within family
Inversion of normal power hierarchies
Coalitions of family members

Defining Characteristics[5,6,11,16]

Concern or complaint by patient about response(s) of family member(s)

Family member(s):

- Verbalize fear, anxiety, and/or anger
- Verbalize inadequate understanding or knowledge base
- Engage in destructive bickering
- Make direct or subtle appeal for help
  - Assistance with communication
  - Permission to express feelings
  - Permission to leave bedside of patient
  - Reassurance that illness is not his or her fault
- Unable to make decision together
- Refuse to assist with patient's care
- Attempt assistive or supportive behaviors with ineffective results
- Display absence of verbal or nonverbal interaction
- Display disproportionate protective behavior
- Tend to interfere with necessary nursing or medical interventions
- Display sudden outburst of emotions without apparent cause or show emotional lability
- Form coalitions

Nursing Interventions[1,6,8,14,16]

Patient Goal	Nursing Intervention
Develop adequate understanding of health challenge.	• Provide adequate and correct information to patient and family. • Discuss "sick role" with patient and family. • Encourage family to have realistic perception based on accurate information. • Discuss usual reactions to health challenges (e.g., anxiety, dependency, depression). • Monitor areas in which knowledge or understanding is inadequate in relation to situation. • Encourage patient and family member(s) to discuss expectations of each other in situation.
Experience increasing comfort.	• Maintain as much privacy as possible. • Provide alternative to patient's room for family discussions. • Encourage patient and family members to verbalize feelings (e.g., loss, guilt, anger, relief). • Use communication techniques to confirm legitimacy of both positive and negative feelings, e.g., reflecting feelings ("You seem frightened"), presenting reality ("Many people feel angry in situations like this").
Cope with changes in family structure and dynamics.	• Assist family to assess situation, including both strengths and weaknesses. • Assist family to identify changes in relationships. • Assist family members to recognize role changes needed to maintain family integrity. • Assist family member to assume new roles as needed. • Involve family members in care of patient as much as possible. • Encourage family members to seek additional sources of help in adjusting to changes in family processes: friends, clergy, other professional health care providers.

Principles and Rationale for Nursing Interventions

Many of the interventions appropriate for helping the family whose coping skills are compromised center on providing sufficient information. Validation of feelings and perceptions of the situation can relieve anxiety to the extent that the learning of new coping strategies may be effective.[1] The nurse should provide information about the extent of the illness of a family member and the probable long-range effects on both the individual and the family system. This information can aid in developing realistic expectations about the positive and negative changes that must occur to maintain functioning.

Evaluation

Patient Outcome	Data Indicating That Outcome is Reached
Develops adequate understanding of situation	Verbalizes need for more information or clearer understanding of situation Demonstrates understanding of information given Discusses changes in patient and family resulting from situation
Experiences increasing comfort	Displays decreased levels of anxiety Verbalizes perception that environment is supportive Verbalizes feelings to health care professionals and other family members
Copes with changes in family structure and dynamics	Identifies changes in family roles and dynamics Recognizes roles needed to maintain family integrity Assumes new roles as necessary to maintain family integrity Participates effectively in care of patient Seeks help in adjusting to changes in family structure and dynamics from appropriate sources

 Ineffective Family Coping: Disabling

Ineffective family coping: disabling is the behavior of a significant person (family member, other primary person) that disables his or her capacities and the patient's capacities to address effectively tasks essential to either person's adaptation to the health challenge.

The coping abilities of a family may be diagnosed as disabling when the behaviors of individual family members or of the family system become destructive in response to either internal or external stressors.[5] Behavior of a significant family member that interferes with the abilities of the identified patient and/or other family members to adapt effectively to the health challenge may also be considered disabling to the family system.[16]

Related Factors[2,3,5,16,24]

Significant person with chronically unexpressed feelings (e.g., guilt, anxiety, hostility, despair)
Dissonant discrepancy of coping styles used to deal with adaptive tasks
Highly ambivalent family relationships
Arbitrary handling of family's resistance to treatment (tends to solidify defensiveness as it fails to deal adequately with underlying anxiety)
High-risk individual(s) or family
Characteristics of parent(s)
- Single
- Adolescent
- Abusive
- Emotionally disturbed
- Substance abuser
- Terminally ill
- Acute disability or accident

Unwanted characteristics or handicaps of child
- Of unwanted pregnancy
- Of undesired sex
- With undesired characteristics
- Physically handicapped
- Mentally handicapped
- Hyperactive
- Terminally ill

Separation from nuclear family
Lack of extended family
Inadequate knowledge base or incorrect information
Economic problems (inflation, unemployment)
Change in composition of family unit
History of ineffective relationships (e.g., abusive with parents)
Lack of mutual decision-making skills
Rigid or inappropriate boundaries within family
Inversion of normal power hierarchies
Coalitions of family members

Defining Characteristics[2,5,16,19,24]

Neglectful care of patient (e.g., basic human needs, illness treatment)
Distortion of reality (e.g., regarding patient's health problem, including extreme denial about its existence or severity)
Intolerance
Rejection
Abandonment
Desertion
Psychosomatic tendency
Taking on illness signs of patient
Unwise decisions and actions by family (e.g., that are detrimental to economic or social well-being of family members)
Unresolved emotions (e.g., agitation, depression, aggression, hostility)
Impaired restructuring of meaningful life for self (e.g., as result of impaired individualization; prolonged overconcern for patient)
Neglectful relationships with other family members
Patient's development of helpless, inactive dependence
Verbalization of abuse by family member(s)
Presence of any serious symptom(s) over protracted period
Poor communication processes within family (e.g., those that are negative, blaming, critical, often concrete in thinking, and poor in affective expressions)
Family problems (e.g., role deficiencies and reversals, generational boundaries, disengagement, enmeshment)

Nursing Interventions*

Patient Goal	Nursing Intervention
Achieve accurate understanding of conflict in coping styles.	• Assist family member(s) to verbalize perceptions of individual coping styles and areas of conflict. • Assist family member(s) to identify alternative coping behaviors that minimize conflict. • Identify areas of conflict in coping styles among family members.
Develop alternate coping strategies.	• Assist family member(s) to focus on present feelings and behaviors. • Clarify communications between family members. • Emphasize positive aspects of present coping strategies.

*References 6, 9, 16, 18, 20, 21.

Patient Goal	Nursing Intervention
	• Assist family member(s) to practice alternative coping behaviors through relabeling, role playing, contracting, etc. • Monitor coping strategies of family members. • Reinforce positive use of new coping strategies.
Improve level of complementarity in role relationship.	• Assist family member(s) to verbalize needs and expectations of relationships. • Assist family member(s) to identify strengths and weaknesses in relation to assuming expected roles. • Assist family member(s) to discuss areas where individual strengths, needs, and expectations complement each other. • Assist family member(s) to identify needs and expectations not being met. • Assist family member(s) to identify strategies to develop complementary role relationships. • Assist family member(s) to practice new strategies. • Reinforce positive strategies and improved complementarity in role relationships.

Principles and Rationale for Nursing Interventions

An understanding of the ways each family member is attempting to cope with the stressors created by any given situation is essential to introducing change in the family system.[12] Members of a disabled family are usually experiencing sufficient anxiety to restrict their ability to view the behavior of others realistically. Thus one of the first goals must be helping the family as individuals or as a group to focus on how the current situation is affecting the identified patient and each member.[24] As various attempts to cope are identified, the patient and family members begin to identify the areas of conflict.

Once coping strategies have been identified and the areas of conflict assessed, the patient and other family members can be introduced to other behaviors that will decrease the potential for conflict within the family structure.[18] A psychoeducational approach has been suggested in which a cognitive basis for behavior is presented for understanding the behavior of family members. This approach allows the family to develop a framework from which to view the behavior of its members and to establish realistic goals for changes in coping strategies.[22] In working with members of disabled families, however, it is essential to use experiential techniques of a highly affective nature (e.g., role playing) with extreme caution. If the members of a severely disabled family are pushed to speak against each other in a way that allows escalation of the conflict, explosiveness probably will occur. Also, the invisible loyalties within the family may create sufficient denial in an attempt to ward off further deterioration of the family so that further treatment is not possible.[24]

Families that are disabled frequently have extreme problems with role deficiencies and reversals. Boundaries between the family members and between the family and society may be rigid and impermeable.[19] It is necessary, therefore, to aid the family in identifying the role expectations of each other and to assess strengths and weaknesses in fulfilling the required roles in a functional family.[24]

Evaluation

Patient Outcome	Data Indicating That Outcome is Reached
Achieves accurate understanding of conflict in coping styles	Verbalizes perceptions of coping styles and areas of conflict Identifies alternative coping behaviors that may minimize conflict
Develops alternative coping strategies	Incorporates alternative coping behaviors in adapting to health challenge Continues to use positive coping strategies in stressful situations
Improves level of complementarity in role relationships	Verbalizes individual needs and expectations of family relationships Identifies strengths and weaknesses in adapting to health challenge Discusses complementary nature of strengths, needs, and expectations of relationships Identifies areas where needs and expectations are not being met Identifies strategies to aid in developing complementary role relationships Incorporates alternative strategies in relationships

FUNCTIONAL HEALTH PATTERN

XI

Value-Belief

 Spiritual Distress (Distress of the Human Spirit)

Spiritual distress (distress of the human spirit) is disruption in the life principle that pervades a person's entire being and that integrates and transcends one's biologic and psychosocial nature.[5]

Tubesing[7] believes that all stress-related illness is fundamentally a spiritual disorder, "often growing from a conflict of values, beliefs and goals," and that differences in stress levels may be determined by the answers persons give to a series of spiritual questions. He proposed that beliefs serve to organize individuals' lives and help them make decisions about how to use their time and focus their energies. "The bottom line of the spiritual dimension of stress is how we 'spend' ourselves."[7]

Recognition of some of the assumptions underlying the concept of spiritual distress is a prerequisite to understanding its potential usefulness as a nursing diagnosis. Two major assumptions are that individuals experience spiritual health and that nurses are able to recognize spiritual health and its deviations (i.e., a person's need for spiritual help). Spiritual health can be defined as "a state of well-being and equilibrium in that part of a person's essence and existence which transcends the realm of the natural and relates to the ultimate good."[9] The premise that people have a need for transcendence provided the stimulus for developing an instrument to measure spiritual well-being, the Spiritual Well-Being Index (SWB).[6]

"The need for transcendence refers to reaching beyond oneself, with the outcome being a sense of well-being that we experience when we find purposes to commit ourselves to."[4] Spiritual well-being refers to a psychologic-experiential dimension arising from an underlying state of spiritual health and is an expression of this state. Spiritual well-being is conceptualized as a continuous rather than dichotomous variable, with many factors influencing the degree of spiritual well-being.

Related Factors

Separation from religious and cultural ties
Challenged belief and value systems
Sense of meaninglessness or purposelessness
Remoteness from God or supreme being
Disrupted spiritual trust
Moral or ethical nature of therapy
Sense of guilt and shame
Intense suffering
Unresolved feelings about death
Anger toward God or supreme being
Intense physical pain

Defining Characteristics[8,9]

Expresses concern with meaning of life or death or any belief system
Anger toward God or supreme being
Questions meaning of suffering
Verbalizes inner conflict about beliefs
Verbalizes concern about relationship with deity
Questions meaning for own existence
Unable to participate in usual religious practices
Seeks spiritual assistance
Questions moral or ethical implications of therapeutic regimen
Gallows humor

Displacement of anger toward religious representatives
Nightmares or sleep disturbance
Alteration of behavior or mood evidenced by anger, crying, withdrawal, preoccupation, anxiety, hostility, apathy, etc.
Loss of or separation from God and/or institutionalized religion
Experience of evil or disillusionment
Sense of failing God; the recognition of one's own sinfulness
Lack of reconciliation with God
Perceived loneliness of spirit
Experiences disturbance in belief system:
- Questions credibility of belief system
- Discouraged
- Unable to practice usual religious rituals
- Ambivalent feelings (doubts) about beliefs
- Sense of spiritual emptiness

Nursing Interventions

Patient Goal	Nursing Intervention
Experience less powerlessness and loneliness related to separation from religious and cultural ties.	• Take time to listen and be open to patient's expressions of loneliness and powerlessness. • Discuss and assess patient's religious and cultural background. • Refer to spiritual advisor of patient's choice. • Provide contact with people with similar cultural background, especially those who have coped with similar situations. • Prepare patient for religious rituals of choice. • Provide an atmosphere conducive to patient's culture and/or religion (e.g., provide religious/cultural articles and objects, prayer pamphlets, audio tapes with spiritual and cultural prayers and songs). • Help patient pray if patient expresses this need. • Share appropriate religious readings that convey a message of hope in dealing with loneliness and doubt, if patient is open and ready. • Express to patient that feeling of loneliness is normal.
Clarify beliefs and values.	• Values clarification[4]: Have patient get in touch with self through use of prayer and/or meditation. Have patient make lists of what is important and how much time is spent on things that are important and not important. Delineate long- and short-term goals. Plan short-term tasks to meet short-term goals. Suggest that patient imagine self asking God, friend, or inner advisor to help clarify doubts and to ask what the person should do and be. Have patient act on advice from inner advisor. • Provide opportunity for patient to meet with spiritual advisor.
Find meaning and purpose in life, illness, and suffering.	• Be available to listen to and be empathetic to patient's feelings. • Suggest and teach use of meditation and centering. • Use religious and/or other readings (e.g., Frankl's *Man's Search for Meaning*[2]) that describe others who have found meaning in difficult situations. • Help patient to put problems into wider perspective. • Have patient select and write down positive labels for each stressor of life. • Aid patient in replacing negative thoughts and labels with positive ones. • Assist patient to find in illness a means to grow and develop depth in understanding life. • Assist patient to take risks and make commitment to something or someone. • Assist patient to do some type of volunteer activity, even something as simple as writing letters to a lonely person.
Experience feelings that God will help to endure and relieve suffering.	• Assure patient that nurse will be available to support patient in times of suffering. • If comfortable to do so, offer to pray with patient in times of suffering. • If patient is comfortable with your touch, hold patient's hand or place your hand gently on patient's arm or other part of body that is causing pain. If patient desires, form a praying team; while touching, pray for God's healing presence. Other members of health team and person close to patient might be included in the praying team. Ask them to pray in a way that is comfortable in asking for God's healing of patient's suffering. After about 5 minutes of prayer conclude with simple closing prayer. While praying, have patient imagine presence of a loving God healing part of body that is painful, injured, or diseased.
Decrease sense of anger with God, self, and others.	• Develop trust with patient by listening and by being present and responsive to patient's needs. • Mention to patient that anger towards God is normal (or typical) part of process of healing past hurts. • Help patient get in touch with feelings of anger.

Patient Goal	Nursing Intervention
	• Help patient share feelings of anger with self or trusting friend. • Problem-solve ways to express and relieve anger properly. • Use prayer and imagery to heal past hurts. • Express that God accepts and loves people for who they are. • Encourage patient to adopt attitude of gratitude for getting deeper insights into life.
Increase relationship with God.	• Be present and available to patient. • Offer to obtain for patient religious articles that could aid in praying or other religious activities. • Teach simple quieting and relaxation skills so patient can relax and experience presence of God. • Offer to pray with patient. • Suggest need to find God's presence in self and others. • Remind patient that many people have experienced remoteness from God (give appropriate examples of people in religious stories and writings). • Refer to clergy if patient agrees.
Experience sense of forgiveness and decreased sense of guilt by healing past hurts and transgressions.	• Be open and present when patient is willing to share past hurts and guilt. • Suggest use of reflective prayer and keeping journals to analyze past hurts. • Teach patient use of centering prayer and healing of memory prayers. • Have patients imagine themselves sharing with a loving God their painful memories and hurts, ask God to take hurt away, heal them, and allow themselves to be filled with love.
Reduce fear of death.	• Be open, present, and empathetic to patient's feelings about death. • Support patient's beliefs of an afterlife in presence of a loving God. • Have patient visualize own death while relaxing and meditating; include in the image being in presence of God and past friends and family who have died. • Refer patient to clergy or other spiritual advisor for religious rites. • Refer patient to religious writings that support concept of afterlife.

Principles and Rationale for Nursing Interventions

Since separation from religious and cultural ties is a factor contributing to spiritual distress, interventions that enhance or provide contact with a religion or culture may help alleviate the problem. The first step in this intervention entails taking time to listen to the patient's feelings and to assess the patient's religious and cultural background. The subsequent interventions are directed toward the nurse providing persons (spiritual advisors and/or cultural representatives), religious and cultural objects, and resources for religious and cultural rituals. Providing a personal contact with a cultural representative who has coped with a similar problem may help the patient to identify with the representative and may provide a role model for coping. Helping patients to pray, if they desire this, and providing readings that convey a message of hope can also decrease feelings of separation from religious and cultural ties and subsequent loneliness.

Another contributing factor to spiritual distress is having a challenged or unclear belief and value system. This is especially true when a patient is suffering or is having a moral or ethical conflict. Helping a patient to clarify beliefs and values could help in this situation. Values clarification is one method designed for that purpose. These interventions provide a simple method of values clarification that includes relaxation and imagery from the perspective of the patient's faith system. A patient who does not believe in God can bring problems to an imaginative friend or an inner advisor. Advice from a spiritual advisor who is from the patient's faith system could also bring peace of mind.

A typical symptom of spiritual distress is struggling with the meaning and purpose of life and questioning the meaning and purpose of suffering and illness. A nurse is often present and available when that happens. Assisting a patient in that situation would begin with helping the patient feel comfortable with expressing those feelings. Once patients are able to articulate their doubts and feelings to another person, they often are able to see their problem more clearly and put the problem into better perspective. Meditation and prayer can help a patient get in touch with feelings and provide a sense of calm. Providing examples of other people who were able to find meaning and purpose under adverse conditions could provide hope, inspiration, and examples of how to cope with life's difficulties. Other cognitive techniques, such as refuting negative thoughts and looking for positive aspects of diversity (i.e., growth in understanding life), will help a patient be less depressed and discouraged because people often feel the way they think. Finally, volunteer activity and helping other people can help clear the mind of problems, provide perspective, and help to transcend everyday existence.

Since suffering is often associated with a depressed spirit and a questioning of meaning and purpose, helping a patient to cope with the suffering or to decrease the suffering could help to lift the spirit. Just the presence of another individual can help a patient cope with suffering. Nurses can convey to a patient who is suffering that they will be available when needed. Gently touching a patient who is suffering can also convey a message of support in a nonverbal way. For many people who suffer, prayer is a way of coping. Helping a patient to pray in a form acceptable to the patient is important. Bringing in significant others to pray with the patient and using imagery to enhance the prayer are other ways of showing that the patient is not alone in his suffering.

Typical symptoms of spiritual distress also may include anger with and alienation from God, self, and others. The interventions in this case are designed to decrease or to understand the feeling of anger. Other interventions can help the patient to develop and increase a relationship with God and thereby decrease the sense of alienation. The first steps in helping the patient to cope with anger are to develop a trusting relationship and to convey the message that anger is a normal or typical response. If the patient realizes that anger is a common feeling and that God is accepting of that anger, then the patient might not have as much guilt. Sharing the anger with another individual will help the patient obtain a perspective on the anger. Problem-solving methods to express and relieve the anger in an acceptable way are positive actions that will help channel the anger. Prayer and imagery processes can often be used to heal past hurts that were the initial reason for the anger and alienation.[3] Part of the process of healing past hurts and decreasing the anger is helping the patient to realize that one can grow and learn from adversity.

Increasing a relationship with God is often accomplished through prayer.[1] Some patients who are spiritually depressed, however, are unable to pray. For them, some type of passive prayer process might be needed. Having patients just let the presence of God be with them without trying to think or say anything is a way of passive prayer. Helping them to pray by providing religious objects and a quiet atmosphere or by actually praying with them could be helpful for patients having difficulty praying. Providing stories of holy people who also had difficulty praying at times will encourage patients, provide an example, and help them to understand that they are not alone in feeling that way. Referral to a spiritual advisor of the patient's choice might also be appropriate at this time.

Obviously a patient's faith system must be taken into consideration for any interventions. A patient who does not believe in God or a supreme being could benefit from techniques not religiously oriented (e.g., relaxation; meditation on life; quieting and uplifting music; allowing patient to express and share feelings, values, and beliefs in a nonjudgmental way).

Although the lack of reconciliation and the feeling of guilt from past hurts and transgressions are defining characteristics of spiritual distress, they could also be contributing factors. The sense of guilt and hurt can weigh a patient down and depress the spirit. Experiencing a sense of forgiveness can relieve these feelings. Sharing past hurts and guilts with another person is one way of reconciling life's transgressions and obtaining a perspective on them. Many faith systems have special rituals for dealing with guilt. A spiritual advisor of the patient's faith system could be of help. Reflective prayer and journaling are also effective ways in helping a patient to obtain a perspective and understanding of past hurts. For those patients who have a belief in God, sharing their past hurts and memories in a prayer and imagery process (guided by a nurse and/or spiritual advisor comfortable in this process) could bring a sense of healing and forgiveness.

Unresolved feelings about death and the fear of death also may distress the spirit. Many faith systems have beliefs about death and an afterlife that could be comforting to a patient. Supporting and reinforcing these beliefs are important. Referring to a spiritual advisor of the patient's choice is appropriate, especially for religious rites. Having patients visualize their own death while they are in a relaxed or meditative state could also help to resolve fears about death and help them prepare for death. Patients should be comforted if they are able to visualize their death in the presence of a loving God (supreme being) and/or friends and family who have died. For patients who do not have a belief in an afterlife, assuring them of the nurse's presence is important.

Evaluation*

Patient Outcome	Data Indicating That Outcome is Reached
Sense of control related to religious and cultural ties	Identification of available religious and cultural resources Comfort in religious and cultural rituals and objects Low score on loneliness scale[6]
Clear beliefs and values	Delineation of short- and long-term goals Plans to meet these goals Values clarification complete
Sense of purpose and meaning in illness	Positive thoughts about life and self High score (40-60) on Existential Well-Being (EWB) scale of Spiritual Well-Being Index (SWB)[7] Participates in volunteer activity
Relief from and/or acceptance of suffering	Feeling that God will help relieve and/or endure suffering Sense of comfort and peace

*These suggested outcome criteria are based on treating the previously listed related factors and defining characteristics of spiritual distress. Some of the outcomes are rather abstract and exist as a matter of degree. Quantifiable outcomes are presented when possible.

Patient Outcome	Data Indicating That Outcome is Reached
Relief of anger toward God, self, and others	Understanding of God's will High score (40-60) on Religious Well-Being (RWB) scale of SWB Feeling that God and others love and accept them for who they are
Closeness with God	Ability to pray and/or meditate Satisfaction in prayer and/or meditation High score (40-60) on RWB scale of SWB
Sense of forgiveness	Sharing of past hurts and guilt Acceptance of forgiveness from God and others Sense of God's and others' love
Decreased fear of and/or acceptance of death	Ability to image and talk about death without undue anxiety

References

Altered health maintenance

1. Altman D and King A: Approaches to compliance in primary prevention, Compliance Health Care 1:55, 1986.
2. American Nurses' Association: Nursing: a policy statement, Kansas City, Mo, 1980, The Association.
3. Anderson S and Bauwens E, editors: Chronic health problems: concepts and application, St Louis, 1981, The CV Mosby Co.
4. Baric L: Recognition of the "at-risk" role: a means to influence health behavior, 1969, International Seminar on Health Education. In Behavior change through health education: problems of methodology: reports on fundamental research in health education, Hamburg, Federal Republic of Germany, 1970.
5. Bausell R and Pruit R: Cholesterol knowledge, avoidance, and monitoring among the American public, Heart Lung 15:543, 1986.
6. Becker M and Mauman L: Sociobehavioral determinants of compliance with health and medical care recommendations, Med Care 13:10, 1975.
7. Becker MH et al: A new approach to explaining sick role behavior in low-income populations, Am J Public Health 84:250, 1974.
8. DiMatteo MR and DiNicola DD: Achieving patient compliance: the psychology of the medical practitioner's role, New York, 1982, Pergamon Press.
9. Flynn JB and Giffin PA: Health promotion in acute care setting, Nurs Clin North Am 19:239, 1984.
10. Fritz W: Maintaining wellness: yours and theirs, Nurs Clin North Am 19:263, 1984.
11. Goorasser SC and Craft BJG: The patient's approach to wellness, Nurs Clin North Am 19:195, 1984.
12. Gottlieb N and Green L: Life events, social networks, lifestyle, and health: an analysis of the 1979 national survey of personal health practices and consequences, Health Educ Q 11:91, 1984.
13. Green L et al: Health education planning: a diagnostic approach, Palo Alto, Calif, 1980, Mayfield Publishing Co.
14. Jaco EG: Patients, physicians and illness, New York, 1958, Free Press.
15. Kar S et al: A psychosocial model of health behavior: implications for nutrition education, research and policy, Health Values: Achieving High Level Wellness 7:2, 1983.
16. Kim MJ and Moritz DA: Classification of nursing diagnoses: proceedings of the third and fourth national conferences, St Louis, 1982, The CV Mosby Co.
17. Kim MJ, McFarland GK, and McLane AM, editors: Classification of nursing diagnoses: proceedings of the fifth national conference, St Louis, 1984, The CV Mosby Co.
18. Kim MJ, McFarland GK, and McLane AM: Pocket guide to nursing diagnoses, ed 2, St Louis, 1987, The CV Mosby Co.
19. Langlie J: Social networks, health beliefs, and preventive health behavior, J Health Soc Behav 18:244, 1977.
20. Lovvorn J: Types of preventive health cues given to high-risk individuals, Heart Lung 10:3, 1981.
21. McAlister A et al: Behavioral science applied to cardiovascular health: progress and research needs in the modification of risk-taking habits in adult populations, Health Educ Monogr 4:45, 1976.
22. Rosenstock IM: What research in motivation suggests for public health, Am J Public Health 50:3, 1960.
23. Shultz C and Smith M: Lifestyle assessment: a tool for practice, Nurs Clin North Am 19:271, 1984.

Noncompliance (specify)

1. Baer CL: Compliance: the challenge for the future, Top Clin Nurs 7:77, 1986.
2. Barofsky I, editor: Medication compliance: a behavioral management approach, Thorofare, NJ, 1977, Charles B Slack Inc.
3. Bartlett E: Behavioral diagnosis: a practical approach to patient education, Patient Counsel Health Educ 4:29, 1982.
4. Bebbington PE: The efficacy of Alcoholics Anonymous: the elusiveness of hard data, Br J Psychiatry 128:572, 1976.
5. Becker M: The health belief model and sick role behavior, Nurs Digest 35, 1978.
6. Bennett A, editor: Communications between doctors and patients, London, 1976, Oxford University Press.
7. Blackwell B: Patient compliance, N Engl J Med 289:249, 1973.
8. Blumenthal J et al: Continuing medical education: cardiac rehabilitation: a new frontier for behavioral medicine, J Cardiac Rehab 3:637, 1983.
9. Brand F, Smith R, and Brand P: Effect of economic barriers to medical care on patients' noncompliance, Public Health Rep 92:72, 1977.
10. Brown N et al: The relationship among health beliefs, health values, and health promotion activity, West J Nurs Res 5:1550, 1982.
11. Davis M: Variations in patients' compliance with doctors' advice: an empirical analysis of patterns of communication, Am J Public Health 58:274, 1968.
12. Davis M, Eshelman E, and McKay M: The relaxation and stress reduction workbook, Richmond, Calif, 1980, Harbinger Publications.
13. DiMatteo M and DiNicola D: Achieving patient compliance: the psychology of the medical practitioner's role, New York, 1982, Pergamon Press.
14. Dracup K and Meleis A: Compliance: an interactionist approach, Nurs Res 31:31, 1982.
15. Gabriel M, Gagnon JP, and Bryan C: Improved patient compliance through use of daily drug reminder chart, Am J Public Health 67:968, 1977.
16. Garb J and Stunkard AJ: Effectiveness of a self help group in obesity control: a further assessment, Arch Intern Med 134:716, 1974.
17. Gussow Z and Tracy GS: The role of self help clubs in adaptation to chronic illness and disability, Nurs Digest 6:23, 1978.
18. Haynes RB, Taylor DW, and Sackett HD, editors: Compliance in health care, Baltimore, 1979, The Johns Hopkins University Press.
19. Herje P: Hows and whys of patient contracting, Nurse Educ, Jan-Feb 1980, p 30.
20. Hulka B et al: Communication, compliance, and concordance between physicians and patients with prescribed medications, Am J Public Health 66:847, 1976.
21. Ice R: Long-term compliance, Phys Ther 65:1832, 1985.
22. Janz N and Becker M: The health belief model: a decade later, Health Educ Q 11:1, 1984.
23. Kasl S: The health belief model and behavior related to chronic illness, Health Educ Monogr 2:433, 1974.
24. Kirscht J: Perceptions of control and health beliefs, Can J Behav Sci 4:225, 1972.
25. Liberman P: A guide to help patients keep track of their drugs, Am J Pharm 29:507, 1972.
26. Lipowski Z: Psychosocial aspects of disease, Ann Intern Med 71:1197, 1969.
27. Lipowski Z: Physical illness, the individual and the coping process, Psychiatr Med 291:91, 1970.
28. Lowe M: Effectiveness of teaching as measures by compliance with medical recommendations, Nurs Res 19:59, 1970.
29. Lowther NB: How to increase compliance in hypertensives, Am J Nurs 81:963, 1981.
30. Marston MV: Compliance with medical regimens: a review of the literature, Nurs Res 19:312, 1970.
31. Nessman D, Carnahan J, and Nugent C: Increasing compliance: patient operated hypertension groups, Arch Intern Med 140:1427, 1980.
32. Oldridge N: Compliance and exercise in primary and secondary prevention of coronary heart disease: a review, Prev Med 11:56, 1982.
33. Powers M and Wooldridge P: Factors influencing knowledge, attitudes, and compliance of hypertensive patients, Res Nurs Health 5:171, 1982.
34. Raths L, Harmin M, and Simon S: Values and teaching, Columbus, Ohio, 1966, Charles E Merrill Publishing Co.
35. Rotter JB: Generalized expectancies for internal vs. external control of reinforcement, Psychol Monogr 80(609), 1966.
36. Ryan P: Strategies for motivating life style change, J Cardiovasc Nurs 1:54, 1987.
37. Sackett D and Haynes R, editors: Compliance with therapeutic regimens, Baltimore, 1976, The Johns Hopkins University Press.
38. Sackett D et al: Randomized clinical trial of strategies for improving

medication compliance in primary hypertension, Lancet 79:18, 1975.
39. Schwartz D: Medication errors made by elderly chronically ill patients, Am J Public Health 52:2018, 1963.
40. Sechrist K: The effect of repetitive teaching on patients' knowledge about drugs to be taken at home, Int J Nurs Studies 16:51, 1979.
41. Steckel S: Patient contracting, New York, 1982, Appleton-Century-Crofts.
42. Tirrell B and Hart L: The relationship of health beliefs and knowledge to exercise compliance in patients after coronary bypass, Heart Lung 9:487, 1980.
43. Ureda J: The effect of contract witnessing on motivation and weight loss in a weight control program, Health Educ Q 7:163, 1980.
44. Uustal D: Searching for values, Image 9:15, 1977.
45. Wise T, Hall W, and Wong O: The relationship of cognitive styles and affective status to post-operative analgesic utilization, J Psychosom Res 22:513, 1978.
46. Wolanin MO and Phillips LF: Confusion: prevention and care, St Louis, 1981, The CV Mosby Co.
47. Yanagida E, Streltzer J, and Siemsen A: Denial in dialysis patients: relationship to compliance and other variables, Psychosom Med 43:271, 1981.

Potential for infection

1. Association for Practitioners in Infection Control: The APIC curriculum for infection control practice, Dubuque, Ia, 1981, Kendall/Hunt Publishing Co.
2. Benenson AS, editor: Control of communicable diseases in man, ed 14, Washington DC, 1985, The American Public Health Association.
3. Bennett JV and Brachman PS, editors: Hospital infections, ed 2, Boston, 1986, Little, Brown & Co.
4. Burton GR: Microbiology for the health sciences, Philadelphia, 1979, JB Lippincott Co.
5. Carpenito LJ: Nursing diagnosis: application to clinical practice, ed 2, Philadelphia, 1987, JB Lippincott Co.
6. Centers for Disease Control: CDC guidelines for isolation precautions in hospitals, HHS Pub No (CDC) 83-8314, Atlanta, 1983, The Centers.
7. Centers for Disease Control: Recommendation of the Immunization Practices Advisory Committee (ACIP): Postexposure prophylaxis of hepatitis B, MMWR 33(21), 1984.
8. Centers for Disease Control: Recommendations of the Immunization Practices Advisory Committee (ACIP): Adult immunization, MMWR 33(1S), 1984.
9. Centers for Disease Control: Guidelines for treatment of sexually transmitted diseases, MMWR 34(4S), 1985.
10. Centers for Disease Control: Recommendation of the Immunization Practices Advisory Committee (ACIP): New recommended schedule for active immunization of normal infants and children, MMWR 35(37), 1986.
11. Centers for Disease Control: Recommendations of the Immunization Practices Advisory Committee (ACIP): Update on hepatitis B prevention, MMWR 36(23), 1987.
12. Centers for Disease Control: Recommendations for prevention of HIV transmission in health-care settings, MMWR 36(2S), 1987.
13. Center for Infectious Diseases: Guidelines for prevention and control of nosocomial infections, Atlanta, 1981, Centers for Disease Control.
14. Fox JP, Hall CE, and Elveback LR: Epidemiology, man and disease, New York, 1970, Macmillan Publishing Co, Inc.
15. Ganong, WF: Review of medical physiology, ed 11, Los Altos, Calif, 1983, Lange Medical Publications.
16. Grimes D: Nursing diagnosis: injury, potential for infection, and potential for transmission of infectious agents to others, 1984, Unpublished manuscripts submitted to NANDA Diagnosis Review Committee.
17. Guyton AC: Human physiology and mechanisms of disease, ed 3, Philadelphia, 1982, WB Saunders Co.
18. Jawetz E, Melnick JL, and Adelberg, EA: Review of medical microbiology, ed 16, Los Altos, Calif, 1984, Lange Medical Publications.
19. Kim MJ, McFarland GK, and McLane AM: Pocket guide to nursing diagnoses, ed 2, St Louis, 1987, The CV Mosby Co.
20. Simmons BP: Guideline for prevention of intravenous therapy related infections, Atlanta, 1982, Center for Infectious Diseases, Centers for Disease Control.
21. Simmons BP: Centers for Disease Control guideline for prevention of surgical wound infection, Infect Control 3(3), 1982.

Potential for injury (trauma, poisoning, suffocation)

1. Baker S: Medical data and injuries, Am J Public Health 73:733, 1983.
2. Baker S, O'Neill B, and Karpf R: The injury fact book, Lexington, Mass, 1984, DC Heath & Co.
3. Benner L Jr: Accident theory and accident investigators, Hazard Prevention 13:18, 1977.
4. Centers for Disease Control: MMWR 32, 1983.
5. Clark D and MacMahon B, editors: Preventive medicine, ed 2, Boston, 1981, Little, Brown & Co.
6. Encyclopaedia Britannica Inc: Webster's third new international dictionary, unabridged, Chicago, 1981, G & C Merriam Co.
7. Gordon J: The epidemiology of accidents, Am J Public Health 39:504, 1949.
8. Haddon W: On the escape of tigers: an ecological note, Am J Public Health 60:2229, 1970.
9. Haddon W: Advances in the epidemiology of injuries as a basis for public policy, Public Health Rep 95:411, 1980.
10. Healthy people: the Surgeon General's report on health promotion and disease prevention: background papers, DHEW-PHS Pub No 79-55071A, Washington, DC, 1979, US Government Printing Office.
11. Kim MJ, McFarland GK, and McLane AM: Pocket guide to nursing diagnoses, ed 2, St Louis, 1987, The CV Mosby Co.
12. Last J, editor: Maxcy-Rosenau: public health and preventive medicine, ed 11, New York, 1980, Appleton-Century-Crofts.
13. Mechanic D: Handbook of health, health care, and the health professions, New York, 1984, The Free Press.
14. National Safety Council: Accident facts, Chicago, 1983, National Safety Council.
15. Robertson L: Injuries: causes, control strategies, and public policy, Lexington, Mass, 1983, Lexington Books.
16. Whitefield R, Zador P, and Fife D: Expected mortality from injuries, Washington DC, 1984, Insurance Institute for Highway Safety.
17. Wintemute G, Mohan D, and Teret S, editors: Injury prevention in developing countries, Baltimore, 1984, The Johns Hopkins University Press.

Health-seeking behaviors

1. American Nurses' Association: Nursing: a social policy statement, Kansas City, Mo, 1980, The Association.
2. Bowers A and Thompson J: Clinical manual of health assessment, ed 3, St Louis, 1988, The CV Mosby Co.
3. Brubaker BH: Health promotion: a linguistic analysis, Adv Nurs Sci 5:1, 1983.
4. Bruhn JG et al: The wellness process, Community Health 2(3):209, 1977.
5. Butler FR: Minority wellness promotion: a behavioral self-management approach, J Gerontol Nurs 13:22, 1987.
6. Cottrell RR et al: Health behavioral change and the college personal health class: a multifaceted approach, J Am Coll Health 36:283, 1988.
7. Duffey ME: Health promotion in the family: current findings and directives for nursing research, J Adv Nurs 13:109, 1988.
8. Dunn HL: High level wellness, Thorofare, NJ, 1977, Charles B Slack.
9. Ford AB et al: Health and function in the old and very old, J Am Geriatr Soc 36:187, 1988.
10. Hall BA and Allen JD: Sharpening nursing's focus by focusing on health, Nurs Health Care 7:315, 1986.
11. Horgan PA: Health status perceptions affect health-related behaviors, J Gerontol Nurs 13:30, 1987.
12. Kim MJ, McFarland GK, and McLane AM: Classification of nursing diagnoses: proceedings of the fifth national conference, St Louis, 1984, The CV Mosby Co.
13. Laffrey SC and Crabtree MK: Health and health behavior of persons with chronic cardiovascular disease, Int J Nurs Stud 25:41, 1988.

14. Laffrey SC, Loveland-Cherry CJ, and Winkler SJ: Health behavior: evolution of two paradigms, Public Health Nurs 3(2), 1986.
15. Maslow AH, editor: New knowledge in human values, New York, 1959, Harper & Bros.
16. Pender NJ: Health promotion in nursing practice, ed 2, Norwalk, Conn, 1987, Appleton & Lange.
17. Rauckhorst LM: Health habits of elderly widows, J Gerontol Nurs 13:19, 1987.
18. Smith JA: The idea of health: a philosophical inquiry, Adv Nurs Sci 3:43, 1981.
19. Travis JW: Wellness workbook for helping professionals, Mill Valley, Calif, 1981, Wellness Associates.

Nutritional-metabolic pattern

1. Awe WC, Fletcher WS, and Jacob SW: The pathophysiology of aspiration pneumonitis, Surgery 60:232, 1966.
2. Bartlett JG and Gorbach SW: The triple threat of aspiration pneumonia, Chest 68:560, 1975.
3. Bristow G: Accidental hypothermia, Can Anaesth Soc J 31:S52, 1984.
4. Cameron JL and Juidema GD: Aspiration pneumonia, JAMA 219:1194, 1972.
5. Campbell C: Nursing diagnosis and intervention in nursing practice, New York, 1978, John Wiley & Sons, Inc.
6. Carpenito LJ: Nursing diagnosis: application to clinical practice, Philadelphia, 1983, JB Lippincott Co.
7. Carroll SM: Validation of the defining characteristics of the nursing diagnosis hypothermia, Unpublished master's thesis, Houston, 1987, The University of Texas Health Science Center.
8. Gettrust K, Ryan S, and Engelman D, editors: Applied nursing diagnosis: guides for comprehensive care planning, New York, 1985, John Wiley & Sons, Inc.
9. Gosnell D: Assessment and evaluation of pressure sores, Nurs Clin North Am 22:399, 1987.
10. Guyton AC: Textbook of medical physiology, ed 7, Philadelphia, 1986, WB Saunders Co.
11. Hoffman LA: Airway management for critically ill patients, ASN 87:39, 1987.
12. Hudak CM, Gallo BM, and Lohr T, editors: Critical care nursing, ed 3, Philadelphia, 1982, JB Lippincott Co.
13. Hurley M: Classification of nursing diagnoses: proceedings of the sixth conference, St Louis, 1985, The CV Mosby Co.
14. Kennan RA and Blackburn GL: Clinical nutritional assessment of the hospitalized patient, Surg Rounds, Oct 1981, p 34.
15. Kim MJ, McFarland GK, and McLane AM: Pocket guide to nursing diagnoses, ed 2, St Louis, 1987, The CV Mosby Co.
16. Knipper JS: Minimizing the complications of tracheal suctioning, Focus Crit Care 13:23, 1986.
17. Konstantinides NN and Shronts E: Managing the basics, Am J Nurs 1312, 1983.
18. Korones S: High-risk newborn infants, ed 4, St Louis, 1986, The CV Mosby Co.
19. Lawrence R: Breastfeeding: a guide for the medical profession, St Louis, 1985, The CV Mosby Co.
20. L'Esperance C and Frantz K: Time limitation for early breastfeeding, J Obstet Gynecol Neonatal Nurs, Mar-Apr 1985, p 114.
21. Luckmann J and Sorenson K: Medical-surgical nursing, ed 3, Philadelphia, 1987, WB Saunders Co.
22. Matz R: Hypothermia: mechanisms and countermeasures, Hosp Pract 21:45, 1986.
23. McLane, A, editor: Classification of nursing diagnoses: proceedings of the seventh conference, St Louis, 1987, The CV Mosby Co.
24. Metheny NA, Eisenberg P, and Spies M: Aspiration pneumonia in patients fed through nasoenteral tubes, Heart Lung 15:256, 1986.
25. Neifert M and Seacat J: A guide to successful breastfeeding, Contemp Pediatr 3:26, 1986.
26. Phipps WM, Long BC, and Woods NF: Medical-surgical nursing, ed 3, St Louis, 1987, The CV Mosby Co.
27. Reuler JB: Hypothermia: pathophysiology, clinical settings, and management, Ann Intern Med 89:519, 1978.
28. Riordan J: A practical guide to breastfeeding, St Louis, 1983, The CV Mosby Co.
29. Shoemaker W, Thompson W, and Holbrook P, editors: Textbook of critical care, Philadelphia, 1984, WB Saunders Co.
30. Taylor C and Cress S: Nursing diagnosis cards, Springhouse, Pa, 1987, Springhouse Corp.
31. Tinker J and Rapier M, editors: Care of the critically ill patient, New York, 1983, Springer-Verlag.
32. Treloar DM and Stechmiller J: Pulmonary aspiration in tube-fed patients with artificial airways, Heart Lung 13:667, 1984.
33. Tucker SM et al: Patient care standards: nursing process, diagnosis, and outcome, ed 4, St Louis, 1988, The CV Mosby Co.
34. Wynne JW and Modell J: Respiratory aspiration of stomach contents, Ann Intern Med 87:466, 1977.

Constipation

1. Banks S and Marks IN: The aetiology, diagnosis and treatment of constipation and diarrhea in geriatric patients, S Afr Med J 51:409, 1977.
2. Clark CC: Enhancing wellness: a guide for self-care, New York, 1981, Springer.
3. Clark J, Queener S, and Burke-Karb V, editors: Pharmacological basis of nursing practice, ed 2, St Louis, 1986, The CV Mosby Co.
4. Guyton AC, editor: Textbook of medical physiology, Philadelphia, 1976, WB Saunders Co.
5. Kim MJ, McFarland G, and McLane AM, editors: Classification of nursing diagnoses: proceedings of the fifth national conference, St Louis, 1984, The CV Mosby Co.
6. Kim MJ, McFarland GK, and McLane AM: Pocket guide to nursing diagnoses, ed 2, St Louis, 1987, The CV Mosby Co.
7. McLane AM: Classification of nursing diagnoses: proceedings of the seventh conference, St Louis, 1987, The CV Mosby Co.
8. Narrow BW and Busehle KB, editors: Fundamentals of nursing practice, New York, 1982, John Wiley & Sons Inc.
9. Rutter K and Maxwell D: Diseases of the alimentary system: constipation and laxative abuse, Br Med J 2:997, 1976.
10. Thompson JM et al, editors: Clinical nursing, St Louis, 1986, The CV Mosby Co.
11. Weiner MB et al, editors: Clinical pharmacology and therapeutics in nursing, New York, 1979, McGraw-Hill Book Co.
12. Zimring JG: High-fiber diet versus laxatives in geriatric patients, NY State J Med, Dec 1976, p 2223.

Perceived constipation; colonic constipation

1. Benson S: Simple chronic constipation: pathophysiology and management, Postgrad Med 57:55, 1975.
2. Ebersole P and Hess P: Toward healthy aging: human needs and nursing response, ed 2, St Louis, 1985, The CV Mosby Co.
3. Ellickson EB: Bowel management plan for the homebound elderly, J Gerontol Nurs 14:16, 1988.
4. Hurley ME, editor: Classification of nursing diagnoses: proceedings of the sixth conference, St Louis, 1986, The CV Mosby Co.
5. Kim MJ, McFarland GK, and McLane AM, editors: Classification of nursing diagnoses: proceedings for the fifth national conference, St Louis, 1984, The CV Mosby Co.
6. Kim MJ, McFarland GK, and McLane AM: Pocket guide to nursing diagnoses, ed 2, St Louis, 1987, The CV Mosby Co.
7. Maas M and Buckwalter KC, editors: Nursing diagnosis and intervention for the elderly, Menlo Park, Calif, Addison-Wesley Publishing Co. In press.
8. McLane AM, editor: Classification of nursing diagnoses: proceedings of the seventh conference, St Louis, 1987, The CV Mosby Co.
9. McShane RE and McLane AM: Constipation: consensual and empirical validation, Nurs Clin North Am 20:801, 1985.
10. McShane RE and McLane A: Constipation: impact of etiological factors, J Gerontol Nurs 14:31, 1988.
11. Pearson LJ and Kotthoff ME: Geriatric clinical protocols, Philadelphia, 1979, JB Lippincott Co.
12. Thompson JM et al, editors: Clinical nursing, St Louis, 1986, The CV Mosby Co.

Diarrhea

1. Bolin TD, Davis AE, and Duncombe VM: A prospective study of persistent diarrhea, Aust NZ J Med 12:22, 1982.
2. Bond JH: Office-based management of diarrhea, Geriatrics 37:52, 1982.

3. Chernoff R and Dean JA: Medical and nutritional aspects of intractable diarrhea, J Am Dietet Assoc 76:161, 1980.
4. Doe WV and Barr GD: Acute diarrhea in adults, Austr Family Physician 10:438, 1981.
5. Hobsley M: Dumping and diarrhea, Br J Surg 68:681, 1981.
6. Kim MJ, McFarland GK, and McLane AM: Pocket guide to nursing diagnoses, ed 2, St Louis, 1987, The CV Mosby Co.
7. McLane AM, editor: Classification of nursing diagnoses: proceedings of the seventh conference, St Louis, 1987, The CV Mosby Co.
8. Pentland B and Pennington CR: Acute diarrhea in the elderly, Age Aging 9:90, 1980.
9. Ravdin JI and Guerrant RL: Infectious diarrhea in the elderly, Geriatrics 38:95, 1983.
10. Read NW et al: A clinical study of patients with fecal incontinence, Gastroenterology 76:747, 1979.
11. Thompson JM: Clinical nursing, St Louis, 1986, The CV Mosby Co.
12. Thompson WG and Heaton KW: Functional bowel disorders in apparently healthy people, Gastroenterology 79:283, 1980.
13. Tilson MD: Pathophysiology and treatment of short bowel syndrome, Surg Clin North Am 69:1273, 1980.

Bowel incontinence

1. Cornell SA et al: Comparison of three bowel management programs during rehabilitation of spinal cord injured patients, Nurs Res 22:321, 1973.
2. Dickinson VA: Maintenance of anal incontinence: a review of pelvic floor physiology, Gut 19:1163, 1970.
3. Habeeb MC and Kallstrom MD: Bowel program for institutionalized adults, Am J Nurs 76:606, 1976.
4. Kim MJ, McFarland GK, and McLane AM: Pocket guide to nursing diagnoses, ed 2, St Louis, 1987, The CV Mosby Co.
5. Leigh RJ and Turnberg LA: Faecal incontinence: the unvoiced symptom, Lancet, June 12, 1982, p 1349.
6. McLane AM, editor: Classification of nursing diagnoses: proceedings of the seventh conference, St Louis, 1987, The CV Mosby Co.
7. Read NW et al: A clinical study of patients with fecal incontinence, Gastroenterology 76:747, 1979.
8. Rudy EB: Advanced neurological and neurosurgical nursing, St Louis, 1984, The CV Mosby Co.

Altered patterns of urinary elimination; functional, reflex, stress, urge, and total incontinence; urinary retention

1. Anderson RS: A neurogenic element to urinary genuine stress incontinence, Br J Obstet Gynecol 91:41, 1984.
2. Benta S et al: Rehabilitation nursing: a core curriculum, Evanston, Ill, 1987, Rehabilitation Nursing Institute.
3. Bhatia NN, Bergman A, and Guning JE: Urodynamic effects of a vaginal pessary in women with stress urinary incontinence, Am J Obstet Gynecol 147:876, 1983.
4. Broadwell DC and Jackson BS: Principles of ostomy care, St Louis, 1982, The CV Mosby Co.
5. Brocklehurst JC: Urology in the elderly, London, 1984, Churchill Livingstone Inc.
6. Burton TA: Urinary retention following cannabis ingestion, JAMA 242:351, 1979.
7. Castleden CM, Duffin HM, and McGrowther CW: Dementia and locomotor problems associated with incontinence, Paper presented at the International Continence Society Meeting, Bristol, Eng, Sept 1987.
8. Dougherty MC and Bishop KR: Circumvaginal (CVM) muscle exercise instruction, Gainesville, 1987, University of Florida.
9. Dougherty MC et al: Effect of exercise on the circumvaginal muscles (CVM), Neurourol Urodynamics 6:189, 1987.
10. Gray ML and Dougherty MC: Urinary incontinence—pathophysiology and treatment, J Enterostomal Ther 14:152, 1987.
11. Hald T and Bradley WE: The urinary bladder: neurology and dynamics, Baltimore, 1982, Williams & Wilkins.
12. Horsley JA, Crane J, and Reynolds MA: Clean intermittent catheterization: CURN project, New York, 1982, Grune & Stratton Inc.
13. Howe SM and Bates P: The cranberry juice cure: fact or fiction: AUAA J 8:13, 1987.
14. Hurst JW: Medicine for the practicing physician, Boston, 1983, Butterworth Publishers.
15. International Continence Society: Standardisation of terminology of lower urinary tract function, Glasgow, UK, 1984, Department of Physics and Bioengineering.
16. Jarvis GJ: A controlled trial of bladder drill and drug therapy in the management of detrusor instability, Br J Urol 53:565, 1981.
17. Jarvis GJ and Millar DR: Controlled bladder drill for detrusor instability, Br Med J 281:1322, 1980.
18. Kegel A: Progressive resistance exercises in the functional restoration of the perineal muscles, Am J Obstet Gynecol 56:238, 1948.
19. Kelalis PP, King LR, and Belman AB: Clinical pediatric urology, Philadelphia, 1985, WB Saunders Co.
20. Kim MJ, McFarland GK, and McLane AM: Pocket guide to nursing diagnoses, ed 2, St Louis, 1987, The CV Mosby Co.
21. Lapides J et al: Clean intermittent self catheterization in the treatment of urinary tract disease, J Urol 107:458, 1972.
22. Mundy AR: The unstable bladder, Urol Clin North Am 12:317, 1985.
23. Mundy AR, Stephenson TP, and Wein AJ: Urodynamics: principles, practice and application, London, 1984, Churchill Livingstone Inc.
24. Physician's desk reference, Oradell, NJ, 1987, Medical Economics.
25. Snooks SJ et al: Perineal nerve damage in genuine stress incontinence, Br J Urol 57:422, 1985.
26. Sorenson KC and Luckman J: Basic nursing, Philadelphia, 1979, WB Saunders Co.
27. Stamey TA: Pathogenesis and treatment of urinary tract infections, Baltimore, 1980, Williams & Wilkins.
28. Walsh PC et al: Campbell's urology, Philadelphia, 1986, WB Saunders Co.
29. Wheatley JK: Causes and treatment of bladder incontinence, Compr Ther 9:27, 1983.

Potential activity intolerance

1. Bulechek GM and McCloskey JC, editors: Nursing interventions: treatments for nursing diagnoses, Philadelphia, 1985, WB Saunders Co.
2. Carrieri VK, Lindsey AM, and West CM, editors: Pathophysiological phenomena in nursing: human responses to illness, Philadelphia, 1986, WB Saunders Co.
3. Doenges M and Moorhouse M: Nurse's pocket guide: nursing diagnoses with interventions, Philadelphia, 1984, FA Davis Co.
4. Gordon M: Assessing activity tolerance, Am J Nurs 76:72, 1976.
5. Gordon M: Manual of nursing diagnosis, 1986-1987, New York, 1987, McGraw-Hill Book Co.
6. Gordon M: Nursing diagnosis: process and application, ed 2, New York, 1987, McGraw-Hill Book Co.
7. Gould MT: Nursing diagnoses concurrent with multiple sclerosis, J Neurosurg Nurs 15:339, 1983.
8. Hurley ME: Classification of nursing diagnoses: proceedings of the sixth conference, St Louis, 1986, The CV Mosby Co.
9. Kim MJ, McFarland GK, and McLane AM: Classification of nursing diagnoses: proceedings of the fifth national conference, St Louis, 1984, The CV Mosby Co.
10. Kim MJ, McFarland GK, and McLane AM: Pocket guide to nursing diagnoses, ed 2, St Louis, 1987, The CV Mosby Co.
11. McLane AM: Classification of nursing diagnoses: proceedings of the seventh conference, St Louis, 1987, The CV Mosby Co.
12. Miller JF, editor: Coping with chronic illness: overcoming powerlessness, Philadelphia, 1983, FA Davis Co.
13. Sanderson RG and Kurth CL: The cardiac patient: a comprehensive approach, Philadelphia, 1983, WB Saunders Co.
14. Snyder M: Independent nursing interventions, New York, 1985, John Wiley & Sons Inc.
15. Yura H and Walsh MB: The nursing process: assessing, planning, implementing, evaluating, ed 5, Norwalk, Conn, 1988, Appleton & Lange.

Activity intolerance

1. American Heart Association, The Committee on Exercise: Exercise testing of individuals with heart disease or at high risk for its development, Dallas, 1975, The Association.
2. Campbell C: Nursing diagnosis and intervention in nursing practice, New York, 1978, John Wiley & Sons Inc.
3. Campbell C: Nursing diagnosis and intervention in nursing practice, ed 2, New York, 1980, John Wiley & Sons Inc.

4. Carpenito LJ: Nursing diagnosis: application to clinical practice, ed 2, Philadelphia, 1987, JB Lippincott Co.
5. Gordon M: Assessing activity tolerance, Am J Nurs 76:72, 1976.
6. Gordon M: Manual of nursing diagnosis, 1986-1987, New York, 1987, McGraw-Hill Book Co.
7. Gordon M: Nursing diagnosis: process and application, New York, ed 2, 1987, McGraw-Hill Book Co.
8. Kim MJ, McFarland GK, and McLane AM: Classification of nursing diagnoses: proceedings of the fifth national conference, St Louis, 1984, The CV Mosby Co.
9. Kim MJ, McFarland GK, and McLane AM: Pocket guide to nursing diagnoses, ed 2, St Louis, 1987, The CV Mosby Co.
10. McLane AM: Classification of nursing diagnoses: proceedings of the seventh conference, St Louis, 1987, The CV Mosby Co.
11. Miller JF, editor: Coping with chronic illness: overcoming powerlessness, Philadelphia, 1983, FA Davis Co.
12. Orem DE: Nursing concepts of practice, ed 2, New York, 1980, McGraw-Hill Book Co.
13. Pender N: Health promotion in nursing practice, Norwalk, Conn, 1982, Appleton-Century-Crofts.
14. Yura H and Walsh M, editors: Human needs and the nursing process, New York, 1978, Appleton-Century-Crofts.

Impaired physical mobility

1. Basmajian JV and Kirby RL, editors: Medical rehabilitation, Baltimore, 1984, Williams & Wilkins.
2. Carpenito LJ: Handbook of nursing diagnosis, ed 2, Philadelphia, 1987, JB Lippincott Co.
3. Creason NS et al: Validating the nursing diagnosis of impaired physical mobility, Nurs Clin North Am 20:669, 1985.
4. Gates SJ: Helping your patient on bedrest cope with perceptual/sensory deprivation, Orthop Nurs 3:35, 1984.
5. Goad S: Clinical application of the motor impairment concept, Rehabil Nurs 8:30, 1983.
6. Gordon M: Manual of nursing diagnosis, 1986-1987, New York, 1987, McGraw-Hill Book Co.
7. Jacobs MM and Geels W, editors: Signs and symptoms in nursing: interpretation and management, Philadelphia, 1985, JB Lippincott Co.
8. Jeffrey DL: The hazards of reduced mobility for the person with a spinal cord injury, J Rehabil 52:59, 1986.
9. Kim MJ, McFarland GK, and McLane AM: Pocket guide to nursing diagnoses, ed 2, St Louis, 1987, The CV Mosby Co.
10. Kottke FJ, Stillwell GK, and Lehmann JF, editors: Krusen's handbook of physical medicine and rehabilitation, ed 3, Philadelphia, 1982, WB Saunders Co.
11. Kozier B and Erb G, editors: Fundamentals of nursing: concepts and procedures, ed 3, Menlo Park, Calif, 1987, Addison-Wesley Publishing Co.
12. Mazess R and Whedon GD: Immobilization and bone, Calcif Tissue Int 35:265, 1983.
13. Murray RB and Zentner JP, editors: Nursing concepts for health promotion, ed 3, Englewood Cliffs, NJ, 1985, Prentice-Hall, Inc.
14. St. Pierre D and Gardiner PF: The effect of immobilization and exercise on muscle function: a review, Physiother Can 39:24, 1987.
15. Sandler H and Vernikos J: Inactivity: physiological effects, Orlando, Fla, 1986, Academic Press.
16. Snyder M, editor: A guide to neurological and neurosurgical nursing, New York, 1983, John Wiley & Sons, Inc.
17. Sorensen KC and Luckmann J, editors: Basic nursing: a psychophysiologic approach, ed 2, Philadelphia, 1986, WB Saunders Co.
18. Stewart NJ: Perceptual and behavioural effects of immobility and social isolation in hospitalized orthopedic patients, Nurs Papers 18:59, 1986.
19. Tyler ML: The respiratory effects of body positioning and immobilization, Respir Care 29:472, 1984.
20. Winslow EH: Cardiovascular consequences of bed rest, Heart Lung 14:236, 1985.

Potential for disuse syndrome

1. Allman RM et al: Pressure sores among hospitalized patients, Ann Intern Med 105:337, 1986.
2. Altman P and Fisher K, editors: Research opportunities in nutrition and metabolism in space, Contract No. NASW 3924, Washington DC, 1986, National Aeronautics and Space Administration.
3. Baird S: Development of a nursing assessment tool to diagnose altered body image in immobilized patients, Orthop Nurs 4:47, 1985.
4. Beland IL and Passos JY, editors: Clinical nursing, ed 4, New York, 1981, Macmillan Publishing Co.
5. Bennett-Canlini S: The kinetic treatment table: a new approach to bed rest, Orthop Nurs 4:61, 1985.
6. Bohachick PA: Pulmonary embolism in neurological and neurosurgical patients, J Neurosci Nurs 19:191, 1987.
7. Brower P and Hicks D: Maintaining muscle function in patients on bed rest, Am J Nurs 72:1250, 1972.
8. Carnevali D and Brueckner S: Immobilization—reassessment of a concept, Am J Nurs 70:1502, 1970.
9. Deitrick JE, Whedon D, and Shorr E: Effects of immobilization upon various metabolic and physiologic functions of normal men, Am J Med 4:3, 1948.
10. Delisa JA et al: Stroke rehabilitation. II. Recovery and complications, AFP 26:143, 1982.
11. Downs F: Bed rest and sensory disturbances, Am J Nurs 74:434, 1974.
12. Drayton-Hargrove S and Reddy MA: Rehabilitation and long-term management of the spinal cord injured adult, Nurs Clin North Am 21:599, 1986.
13. Herbison G and Talbot J, editors: Final report phase IV: research opportunities in muscle atrophy, Contract No. NASW-3728, Washington, DC, National Aeronautics and Space Administration.
14. Hirschberg G, Lewis L, and Vaughan P: Rehabilitation: a manual for the care of the disabled and elderly, ed 2, Philadelphia, 1976, JB Lippincott Co.
15. Hirschberg G, Lewis L, and Vaughan P: Promoting patient mobility, Nursing 77:42, 1977.
16. Konikow NS: Alterations in movement: nursing assessment and implications, J Neurosurg Nurs 17:61, 1985.
17. Lentz M: Selected aspects of deconditioning secondary to immobilization, Nurs Clin North Am 16:729, 1981.
18. Levy T and Talbot J: Research opportunities in cardiovascular deconditioning, Contract No. NASW-3616, Washington, DC, 1983, National Aeronautics and Space Administration.
19. Moser K and Fedullo P: Venous thromboembolism, Chest 83:117, 1983.
20. Myllynen P et al: Deep venous thrombosis and pulmonary embolism in patients with acute spinal cord injury: a comparison with nonparalyzed patients immobilized due to spinal fractures, J Trauma 25:541, 1985.
21. Ng L and McCormick K: Position changes and their physical consequences, Adv Nurs Sci 4:13, 1982.
22. Olson E et al: The hazards of immobility, Am J Nurs 67:780, 1967.
23. Sheppard RJ: Physiology and biochemistry of exercise, New York, 1982, Praeger Publishers.
24. Tompkins E: Effect of restricted mobility and dominance on perceived duration, Nurs Res 29:333, 1980.
25. Tyler M: The respiratory effects of body positioning and immobilization, Respir Care 29:472, 1984.

Fatigue

1. American Nurses' Association and Arthritis Health Professions Nursing Task Force: Outcome standards for rheumatology nursing practice, Kansas City, Mo, 1983, The Association.
2. Freal JE, Kraft GH, and Coryell JKS: Principles of prioritizing symptomatic fatigue in multiple sclerosis, Arch Phys Med Rehabil 63:135, 1984.
3. Johanson BC et al: Standards for critical care, St Louis, 1988, The CV Mosby Co.
4. Lansbury J: Clinical appraisal of the activity index as a measure of rheumatoid activity, Arthritis Rheum 11:599, 1968.
5. McLane AM, editor: Classification of nursing diagnoses: proceedings of the seventh conference, St Louis, 1987, The CV Mosby Co.
6. Meenan RF, Liang MH, and Hadler NM: Social Security disability and the arthritis patient, Bull Rheum Dis 33:1, 1983.
7. Miller JF: Coping with chronic illness: overcoming powerlessness, Philadelphia, 1983, FA Davis Co.

8. Monroe LF: Psychological and physiological differences between good and poor sleepers, J Abnorm Psychol 72:255, 1976.
9. Pigg JS, Driscoll PW, and Caniff R: Rheumatology nursing: a problem oriented approach, New York, 1985, John Wiley & Sons Inc.
10. Pigg JS and Schroder PM: Frequently occurring problems of patients with rheumatic diseases: the ANA outcome standards for rheumatology nursing practice, Nurs Clin North Am 19:697, 1984.
11. Potempa K et al: Chronic fatigue, Image: J Nurs Scholarship 18:165, 1986.
12. Riddle PK: Chronic fatigue and women: a description and suggested treatment, Women Health 7:37, 1982.
13. Stepanski EJ et al: Sleep fragmentation and day time sleepiness, Sleep 7:18.

Bathing/hygiene, dressing/grooming, feeding, or toileting self-care deficit

1. Carnevali DL et al: Diagnostic reasoning, Philadelphia, 1984, JB Lippincott Co.
2. Chang BL: Generalized expectancy, situational perception, and morale among institutionalized aged, Nurs Res 27:316, 1978.
3. Chinn PL, editor: Advances in nursing theory development, Rockville, Md, 1983, Aspen Systems Corp.
4. Gordon M: Manual of nursing diagnosis, 1986-1987, New York, 1987, McGraw-Hill Book Co.
5. Gordon M: Nursing diagnosis: process and application, ed 2, New York, 1987, McGraw-Hill Book Co.
6. Instruments for measuring nursing practice and other health care variables, vol 1, DHEW Pub No HRA 78.53, Washington DC, 1981, US Government Printing Office.
7. Kim MJ, McFarland GK, and McLane AM, editors: Classification of nursing diagnoses: proceedings of the fifth national conference, St Louis, 1984, The CV Mosby Co.
8. Kim MJ, McFarland GK, and McLane AM: Pocket guide to nursing diagnosis, ed 2, St Louis, 1987, The CV Mosby Co.
9. Loxley CM and Cress SS: The pocket guide to clinical nursing process for the adult medical-surgical client, New York, 1987, The Miller Press.
10. McLane AM: Classification of nursing diagnoses: proceedings of the seventh conference, St Louis, 1987, The CV Mosby Co.
11. Miller JM: Coping with chronic illness: overcoming powerlessness, Philadelphia, 1983, FA Davis Co.
12. Panicucci CL: Functional assessment of the older adult in the acute care setting, Nurs Clin North Am 18:355, 1983.
13. Power DJ and Craven RF: ALS and aging: a case study in autonomy and control, Image: J Nurs Scholarship 15:22, 1983.
14. Roy C Sr, editor: Introduction to nursing: an adaptation model, Englewood Cliffs, NJ, 1976, Prentice-Hall Inc.
15. Rubin R: Body image and self-esteem, Nurs Outlook, June 1968, p 10.
16. Ryden MB: Morale and perceived control in institutionalized elderly, Nurs Res 33:130, 1984.
17. Yura H and Walsh M, editors: Human needs and the nursing process, Norwalk, Conn, 1982, Appleton-Century-Crofts.
18. Yura H and Walsh M: The nursing process, ed 4, Norwalk, Conn, 1983, Appleton-Century-Crofts.

Diversional activity deficit

1. Bartlett J: Familiar quotations, ed 14, Boston, 1968, Little, Brown & Co.
2. Carpenito LJ: Nursing diagnosis: application to clinical practice, ed 2, Philadelphia, 1987, JB Lippincott Co.
3. Doenges M and Moorhouse M: Nurses' pocket guide: nursing diagnoses with interventions, Philadelphia, 1985, FA Davis Co.
4. Frye V and Peters M: Therapeutic recreation: its theory, philosophy, and practice, Harrisburg, Pa, 1972, Stockpole Co.
5. Gordon M: Manual of nursing diagnosis, 1986-1987, New York, 1987, McGraw-Hill Book Co.
6. McLane AM, editor: Classification of nursing diagnoses: proceedings of the seventh conference, St Louis, 1987, The CV Mosby Co.
7. Smith MJ: Duration experience for bed-confined subjects: a replication and refinement, Nurs Res 28:139, 1979.

Impaired home maintenance management

1. American Nurses' Association: A conceptual model of community health nursing, Kansas City, Mo, 1986, The Association.
2. Carpenito L: Nursing diagnosis: application to clinical practice, Philadelphia, 1987, JB Lippincott Co.
3. Clemen-Stone S, Eigsti D, and McGuire S: Comprehensive family and community health nursing, New York, 1987, McGraw-Hill Book Co.
4. Coombs EM: A conceptual framework for home nursing, J Adv Nurs 9:157, 1984.
5. Davis AJ: Disability, home care, and the caretaking role in family life, J Adv Nurs 5:475, 1980.
6. Doenges M, Jeffries M, and Moorhouse MF: Nursing care plans: Nursing diagnosis in planning patient care, Philadelphia, 1984, FA Davis Co.
7. Doenges M and Moorhouse M: Nurses' pocket guide: nursing diagnoses with interventions, Philadelphia, 1985, FA Davis Co.
8. Fortinsky R, Granger E, and Seltzer GB: The use of functional assessment in understanding home care needs, Med Care 19:489, 1981.
9. Fralic M: Simultaneous imperatives (editorial), J Nurs Adm 14:9, 1984.
10. Gordon M: Nursing diagnosis, New York, 1982, McGraw-Hill Book Co.
11. Kim MJ, McFarland G, and McLane A: Pocket guide to nursing diagnoses, ed 2, St Louis, 1987, The CV Mosby Co.
12. Kim M and Moritz DJ, editors: Classification of nursing diagnoses, New York, 1982, McGraw-Hill Book Co.
13. Kozier B and Erb G: Fundamentals of nursing: concepts and procedures, Reading, Mass, 1987, Addison-Wesley Publishing Co.
14. Lederer J et al: Care planning pocket guide: a nursing diagnosis approach, Menlo Park, Calif, 1986, Addison-Wesley Publishing Co.
15. Martin N, Holt N, and Hicks D: Comprehensive rehabilitation nursing, New York, 1981, McGraw-Hill Book Co.
16. Mundinger M: Home care controversy, Rockville, Md, 1983, Aspen Systems Corp.
17. Reutter L: Family health assessment: an integrated approach, J Adv Nurs 9:391, 1984.

Ineffective airway clearance; ineffective breathing pattern; impaired gas exchange; decreased cardiac output; altered (specify type) tissue perfusion

1. Campbell C: Nursing diagnosis and intervention in nursing practice, New York, 1978, John Wiley & Sons Inc.
2. Carpenito LJ: Nursing diagnosis: application to clinical practice, Philadelphia, 1983, JB Lippincott Co.
3. Gettrust K, Ryan S, and Engelman D, editors: Applied nursing diagnosis: guides for comprehensive care planning, New York, 1985, John Wiley & Sons, Inc.
4. Guyton AC: Textbook of medical physiology, ed 6, Philadelphia, 1981, WB Saunders Co.
5. Hudak CM, Gallo BM, and Lohr T, editors: Critical care nursing, ed 3, Philadelphia, 1982, JB Lippincott Co.
6. Hurley ME, editor: Classification of nursing diagnoses: proceedings of the sixth conference, St Louis, 1985, The CV Mosby Co.
7. Kim MJ, McFarland GK, and McLane A: Pocket guide to nursing diagnoses, ed 2, St Louis, 1987, The CV Mosby Co.
8. Luckmann J and Sorenson K: Medical-surgical nursing, ed 3, Philadelphia, 1987, WB Saunders Co.
9. McLane A, editor: Classification of nursing diagnoses: proceedings of the seventh conference, St Louis, 1987, The CV Mosby Co.
10. Palmer P: Advanced hemodynamic assessment, Dimensions Crit Care 1:139, 1982.
11. Taylor C and Cress S: Nursing diagnosis cards, Springhouse, Pa, 1987, Springhouse Corp.

Dysreflexia

1. Guttman L and Whitteridge D: Effects of bladder retention on autonomic mechanisms after spinal cord injuries, Brain 70:361, 1947.
2. Head H and Riddoch G: The automatic bladder, excessive sweating and some other reflex conditions in gross injuries of the spinal cord, Brain 40:188, 1917.
3. Kewalramani LS: Autonomic dysreflexia in traumatic myelopathy, Am J Phys Med 59:1, 1980.
4. Kurnick NB: Autonomic hyperreflexia and its control in patients with spinal cord lesions, Ann Intern Med 44:678, 1956.

5. Lindan R et al: Incidence and clinical features of autonomic dysreflexia in patients with spinal cord injury, Paraplegia 18:285, 1980.
6. Mathias CJ et al: Plasma catecholamines during paroxysmal neurogenic hypertension in quadriplegic man, Circ Res 39:204, 1976.
7. Naftchi NE et al: Hypertensive crisis in quadriplegic patients, Circulation 57:336, 1978.
8. Niederpruem MS: Autonomic dysreflexia, Rehabil Nurs 9:29, 1984.

Altered growth and development

1. Brown C, editor: Infants at risk: pediatric round table 5, Skillman, NJ, 1981, Johnson & Johnson Baby Products Co.
2. Early Intervention: Concerns of a Career in Nursing Symposium, Washington, DC, 1986, National Center for Clinical Infant Programs.
3. Guralnick M and Bennett F: The effectiveness of early intervention for at-risk and handicapped children, Orlando, Fla, 1987, Academic Press.
4. Haynes U: Teaching mental retardation nursing, Am J Nurs 75:626, 1975.
5. Haynes U: A developmental approach to casefinding among infants and young children, Rockville, Md, 1980, US Department of Health, Education and Welfare.
6. Haynes U: Holistic health care for children with developmental disabilities, Baltimore, 1983, University Park Press.
7. Healy A: The needs of children with disabilities: a comprehensive view, Iowa City, 1983, University of Iowa.
8. Kim M, McFarland G, and McLane A: Pocket guide to nursing diagnoses, ed 2, St Louis, 1987, The CV Mosby Co.
9. Krajicek M and Tearney A: Detection of developmental problems in children, Baltimore, 1977, University Park Press.
10. Mott S, Fazekas N, and James S: Nursing care of children and families, Menlo Park, Calif, 1985, Addison-Wesley Publishing Co.
11. Mullikin R and Buckey J: Assessment of multihandicapped and developmentally disabled children, Rockville, Md, 1983, Aspen Publications.
12. Olshansky S: Chronic sorrow: a response to having a mentally defective child, Social Casework 43:190, 1962.
13. Powell M: Assessment and management of developmental changes and problems in children, ed 2, St Louis, 1981, The CV Mosby Co.
14. Sasserath V, editor: Minimizing high-risk parenting: pediatric round table 7, Skillman, NJ, 1984, Johnson & Johnson Baby Products Co.
15. Stone N: Approaches to management of the handicapped infant, J Fam Pract 4:217, 1977.
16. Tudor M: Nursing intervention with developmentally disabled children, Matern Child Nurs 3:25, 1978.
17. Woolraich ML: The practical assessment and management of children with disorders of development and learning, Chicago, 1987, Year Book Medical Publishers Inc.

Sleep pattern disturbance

1. American Nurses' Association: Social policy statement, Kansas City, Mo, 1980, The Association.
2. Bahr R: Sleep-wake patterns in the aged, J Gerontol Nurs 9:534, 1983.
3. Carpenito LJ: Nursing diagnosis: application to clinical practice, Philadelphia, 1987, JB Lippincott Co.
4. Freemon F: Sleep research, Springfield, Ill, 1972, Charles C Thomas, Publisher.
5. Henderson V: Basic principles of nursing care, New York, 1969, Macmillan Inc.
6. Lerner R: Sleep loss in the aged: implications for nursing practice, Gerontol Nurs 8(6):323, 1982.
7. Miller J: Coping with chronic illness: overcoming powerlessness, Philadelphia, 1984, FA Davis Co.
8. Sanford S: Sleep and the cardiac patient, Cardiovasc Nurs 19(5):19, 1983.
9. Schirmer M: When sleep won't come, J Gerontol Nurs 9(1):16, 1983.
10. Yura H and Walsh MB: Human needs and the nursing process, New York, 1978, Appleton-Century-Crofts.

Pain

1. Bailey LM: Music therapy in pain management, J Pain Symptom Management 1:25, 1986.
2. Beland IL and Passos JY: Clinical nursing: pathophysiology and psychosocial approaches, ed 4, New York, 1981, Macmillan Publishing Co, Inc.
3. Bonica JJ: The need for a taxonomy of pain, Pain 6:247, 1979.
4. Bonica JJ and Ventagridda V, editors: Advances in pain research and therapy, vol 2, New York, 1979, Raven Press.
5. Bourbannais F: Pain assessment: development of a tool for the nurse and the patient, J Adv Nurs 6:277, 1981.
6. Bray CH: Altering the patient's experience through education, AORN J 43:672, 1986.
7. Carpenito LJ: Nursing diagnosis: application to clinical practice, Philadelphia, 1983, JB Lippincott Co.
8. Chapman RC and Turner JA: Psychological control of acute pain in medical settings, J Pain and Symptom Management 1:9, 1986.
9. Copp LH, editor: Perspectives on pain, Edinburgh, 1985, Churchill Livingstone, Inc.
10. Cotanch PH, Harrison M, and Roberts J: Hypnosis as an intervention for pain control, Nurs Clin North Am 22:699, 1987.
11. Crocker CG: Acute postoperative pain: cause and control, Orthop Nurs 5:11, 1985.
12. Feldman HR: Psychological differentiation and the phenomenon of pain, Adv Nurs Sci 50:50, 1984.
13. Fordyce W: Behavioral methods for chronic pain and illness, St Louis, 1976, The CV Mosby Co.
14. Guyton AC: Human physiology and mechanisms of disease, ed 3, Philadelphia, 1982, WB Saunders Co.
15. Hendler NH, Long DM, and Wise TN, editors: Diagnosis and treatment of chronic pain, Boston, 1982, John Wright/PSG Inc.
16. Infante MC and Mooney NE: Interactive aspects of pain assessment, Orthop Nurs 6:31, 1987.
17. Jacox A: Pain: a source book for nurses and other health professionals, Boston, 1977, Little, Brown & Co.
18. Kim MJ, McFarland GK, and McLane AM, editors: Classification of nursing diagnoses: proceedings of the fifth national conference, St Louis, 1984, The CV Mosby Co.
19. Kim M, McFarland G, and McLane A: Pocket guide to nursing diagnoses, ed 2, St Louis, 1987, The CV Mosby Co.
20. Kim M and Moritz D: Classification of nursing diagnosis: proceedings of the third and fourth national conferences, New York, 1982, McGraw-Hill Book Co.
21. Lipton S, editor: Persistent pain: modern methods of treatment, New York, 1980, Grune & Stratton, Inc.
22. Lutz WJ: Helping hospitalized children and their parents cope with painful procedures, J Pediatr Nurs 1:24, 1986.
23. Mastrovito RC: Psychogenic pain, Am J Nurs 74:514, 1974.
24. McCaffery M: Nursing management of the patient with pain, Philadelphia, 1979, JB Lippincott Co.
25. McLane A: Classification of nursing diagnoses: proceedings of the seventh national conference, St Louis, 1987, The CV Mosby Co.
26. Meinhart NT and McCaffery M: Pain: a nursing approach to assessment and analysis, Norwalk, Conn, 1983, Appleton-Century-Crofts.
27. Ng LKY and Bonica JJ, editors: Pain discomfort and humanitarian care: proceedings of the national conference, New York, 1980, Elsevier/North-Holland.
28. NIH Consensus Development Conference: The integrated approach to the management of pain, J Pain Symptom Management 2:35, 1987.
29. Paice JA: New delivery systems in pain management, Nurs Clin North Am 22:715, 1987.
30. Pomerleau OF and Brady JP, editors: Behavioral medicine: theory and practice, Baltimore, 1979, Williams & Wilkins.
31. Porth C, editor: Pathophysiology: concepts of altered health states, Philadelphia, 1982, JB Lippincott Co.
32. Snyder M: A guide to neurological and neurosurgical nursing, New York, 1983, John Wiley & Sons Inc.
33. Talbert RL: Pharmacotherapeutic modification of the stress response: analgesics, Crit Care Q 7:27, 1985.
34. Wallace KG and Hays J: Nursing management of chronic pain, J Neurosurg Nurs 14:185, 1982.
35. Wright SM: The use of therapeutic touch in the management of pain, Nurs Clin North Am 22:705, 1987.

36. Zabrowski M: Cultural components in response to pain, J Social Issues 8:16, 1952.

Chronic pain

1. Bailey LM: Music therapy in pain management, J Pain Symptom Management 1:25, 1986.
2. Bonica JJ and Ventagridda V, editors: Advances in pain research and therapy, vol 2, New York, 1979, Raven Press.
3. Bulechek GM and McCloskey JC: Nursing interventions treatments for nursing diagnoses, Philadelphia, 1985, WB Saunders Co.
4. Carpenito LJ: Nursing diagnosis: application to clinical practice, Philadelphia, 1983, JB Lippincott Co.
5. Copp LA, editor: Perspectives on pain, Edinburgh, 1985, Churchill Livingstone Inc.
6. Cotanch PH, Harrison M, and Roberts J: Hypnosis as an intervention for pain control, Nurs Clin North Am 22:699, 1987.
7. Fordyce W: Behavioral methods for chronic pain and illness, St Louis, 1976, The CV Mosby Co.
8. Gaston-Johansson F and Asklund-Gustafsson M: A baseline study for the development of an instrument for the assessment of pain, J Adv Nurs 10:539, 1985.
9. Hendler, NH, Long DM, and Wise TN, editors: Diagnosis and treatment of chronic pain, Boston, 1982, John Wright/PSG, Inc.
10. Infante MC and Mooney NE: Interactive aspects of pain assessment, Orthop Nurs 6:31, 1987.
11. Jacox A: Pain: a source book for nurses and other health professionals, Boston, 1977, Little, Brown & Co.
12. Kim, MH, McFarland GK and McLane AM, editors: Classification of nursing diagnoses: proceedings of the fifth national conference, St Louis, 1984, The CV Mosby Co.
13. Kim M, McFarland G, and McLane A: Pocket guide to nursing diagnoses, St Louis, 1984, The CV Mosby Co.
14. Kim M, McFarland G, and McLane A: Pocket guide to nursing diagnoses, ed 2, St Louis, 1987, The CV Mosby Co.
15. Lamb SL and Barbaro NM: Neurosurgical approaches to the management of chronic pain syndromes, Orthop Nurs 6:23, 1987.
16. McCaffery M: Nursing management of the patient with pain, Philadelphia, 1979, JB Lippincott Co.
17. McGuire DB: Advances in control of cancer pain, Nurs Clin North Am 22:691, 1987.
18. McLane A, editor: Classification of nursing diagnoses: proceedings of the seventh conference, St Louis, 1987, The CV Mosby Co.
19. Meinhart NT and McCaffery M: Pain: a nursing approach to assessment and analysis, Norwalk, Conn, 1983, Appleton-Century-Crofts.
20. NIH Consensus Development Conference: The integrated approach to the management of pain, J Pain Symptom Management 2(1)35, 1987.
21. Paice, JA: New delivery systems in pain management, Nurs Clin North Am 22:715, 1987.
22. Snyder M: A guide to neurological and neurosurgical nursing, New York, 1983, John Wiley & Sons Inc.
23. Wallace KG and Hays J: Nursing management of chronic pain, J Neurosurg Nurs 14:185, 1982.
24. Wright SM: The use of therapeutic touch in the management of pain, Nurs Clin North Am 22:705, 1987.
25. Zabrowski M: Cultural components in response to pain, J Social Issues 8:16, 1952.

Sensory/perceptual alterations (specify)

1. Aiello J: The concept of sensory deprivation, Aust Nurs J 7:38, 1978.
2. Ashworth P: Sensory deprivation: the acutely ill, Nurs Times 75:330, 1979.
3. Carpenito LJ: Nursing diagnosis: application to clinical practice, Philadelphia, 1983, JB Lippincott Co.
4. Hahn K: Using 24 hour reality orientation, J Gerontol Nurs 6:130, 1980.
5. Hart L, Reese J, and Fearing M, editors: Concepts common to acute illness: identification and management, St Louis, 1981, The CV Mosby Co.
6. Kim MJ, McFarland GK, and McLane AM: Pocket guide to nursing diagnoses, ed 2, St Louis, 1987, The CV Mosby Co.
7. Kratz C: Sensory deprivation in the elderly, Nurs Times 75:330, 1979.
8. Mitchell P and Loustau A: Concepts basic to nursing, New York, 1981, McGraw-Hill Book Co.
9. Peplau H: Theory: the professional dimension, Unpublished paper, 1972.
10. Perreault J: Assessing for perceptual clarity: closing the gap between theory and practice, Rehabil Nurs 10:28, 1985.
11. Smith M: Changes in judgment duration, Nurs Res 24:93, 1975.
12. Voelkel D: A study of reality orientation and resocialization groups with confused elderly, J Gerontol Nurs 4:13, 1978.
13. Woods N and Falk S: Noise stimuli in the acute care area, Nurs Res 23:144, 1974.
14. Wyness M: Perceptual dysfunction: nursing assessment and management, J Neurosurg Nurs 17:105, 1985.

Unilateral neglect

1. Bisiach E and Luzzatti C: Unilateral neglect of representational space, Cortex 14:129, 1978.
2. Booth K: The neglect syndrome, J Neurosurg Nurs 14:38, 1982.
3. Cutting J: Study of anosognosia, J Neurol Neurosurg Psychiatry 41:548, 1978.
4. Denes G et al: Unilateral spatial neglect and recovery from hemiplegia, Brain 105:543, 1982.
5. De Young S: The neurologic patient—a nursing perspective, Englewood Cliffs, NJ, 1983, Prentice-Hall Inc.
6. Girotti F et al: Oculomotor disorders in cortical lesions in man: the role of unilateral neglect, Neuropsychologia 21:543, 1983.
7. Gordon WA et al: Perceptual remediation in patients with right brain damage: a comprehensive program, Arch Phys Med Rehabil 66:353, 1985.
8. Kim MJ, McFarland GK, and McLane AM: Pocket guide to nursing diagnoses, ed 2, St Louis, 1987, The CV Mosby Co.
9. Levine DN et al: Left spatial neglect: effects of lesion size and premorbid brain atrophy on severity and recovery following right cerebral infarction, Neurology 36:362, 1986.
10. Meienberg O, Harrer M, and Wehren C: Oculographic diagnosis of hemineglect in patients with homonymous hemianopia, J Neurol 233:97, 1986.
11. Plourde G and Sperry RW: Left hemisphere involvement in left spatial neglect from right-sided lesions, Brain 107:95, 1984.
12. Riddoch MJ and Humphreys GW: The effects of cueing on unilateral neglect, Neuropsychologia 21:589, 1983.
13. Wolanin MO and Phillips LRF: Confusion: prevention and care, St Louis, 1981, The CV Mosby Co.
14. Wyness MA: Perceptual dysfunction: nursing assessment and management, J Neurosurg Nurs 17:105, 1985.

Knowledge deficit

1. Bloomgarden T et al: Randomized, controlled trial of diabetic patient education: improved knowledge without improved metabolic status, Diabetes Care 10:263, 1987.
2. Gordon M: Manual of nursing diagnosis, New York, 1982, McGraw-Hill Book Co.
3. Grossman HY, Brink S, and Hauser ST: Self-efficacy in adolescent girls and boys with insulin-dependent diabetes mellitus, Diabetes Care 10:324, 1987.
4. Redman BK: The process of patient education, ed 6, St Louis, 1988, The CV Mosby Co.
5. Taggart VS et al: Adapting a self-management education program for asthma use in an outpatient clinic, Ann Allergy 58:173, 1987.

Altered thought processes

1. Bandler R and Grindler J: The structure of magic, Palo Alto, Calif, 1975, Science and Behavior Books Inc.
2. Carpenito LJ: Nursing diagnoses: application to clinical practice, Philadelphia, 1983, JB Lippincott Co.
3. Chomsky N: Language and mind, New York, 1968, Harcourt-Brace-Jovanovich.
4. Dubovsky S and Weissberg M: Clinical psychiatry in primary care, Baltimore, 1978, Williams & Wilkins.
5. Hurley ME, editor: Classification of nursing diagnoses: proceedings of the sixth conference, St Louis, 1986, The CV Mosby Co.
6. Kaplan HI and Sadok BJ, editors: Comprehensive textbook of psychiatry, vol 2, Baltimore, Md, 1985, Williams & Wilkins.

7. Kim MJ, McFarland GK, and McLane AM, editors: Classification of nursing diagnoses: proceedings of the fifth national conference, St Louis, 1984, The CV Mosby Co.
8. Kim MJ, McFarland GK, and McLane AM: Pocket guide to nursing diagnoses, ed 2, St Louis, 1987, The CV Mosby Co.
9. Kim M and Moritz D: Classification of nursing diagnoses: proceedings of the third and fourth national conferences, New York, 1982, McGraw-Hill Book Co.
10. Knowles R: Disputing irrational thoughts, Am J Nurs 81:735, 1981.
11. Murphy GE: A conceptual framework for the choice of interventions in cognitive therapy, Cognitive Ther Res 9:127, 1985.
12. Pincus J and Tucker G: Behavioral neurology, New York, 1974, Oxford University Press.
13. Schroder P: Nursing intervention with patient with thought disorders, Perspect Psychiatr Care 17:32, 1979.
14. Schwartsman S: The hallucinating patient and nursing intervention, J Psychiatr Nurs Mental Health Services 13:23, 1975.

Decisional conflict (specify)

1. Anger D and Anger DW: Dialysis ambivalence: a matter of life and death, 76:276, 1976.
2. Bayles BH: The value of life—by what standard? Am J Nurs 80:2226, 1980.
3. Beard BH: Fear of death and fear of life, Arch Gen Psychiatry 21:373, 1969.
4. Gilligan C, editor: In a different voice, Cambridge, Mass, 1982, Harvard University Press.
5. Gordon M, editor: Manual of nursing diagnosis, 1986-1987, New York, 1987, McGraw-Hill Book Co.
6. Janis IL and Mann L: Decision making: a psychological analysis of conflict, choice, and commitment, New York, 1977, The Free Press.
7. McLane AM, editor: Classification of nursing diagnoses: proceedings of the seventh conference, St Louis, 1987, The CV Mosby Co.
8. Scannell M: Decisional conflict, Unpublished manuscript, Boston, 1987, Boston College.
9. Tauer KM: Promoting effective decision-making in sexually active adolescents, Nurs Clin North Am 18:275, 1983.

Fear

1. Hartfield M, Cason D, and Cason G: Effects of information about a threatening procedure on patients' expectations and emotional distress, Nurs Res 31:202, 1982.
2. Kim M, McFarland G, and McLane A editors: Classification of nursing diagnoses: proceedings of the fifth national conference, St Louis, 1984, The CV Mosby Co.
3. Kim M, McFarland G, and McLane A: Pocket guide to nursing diagnoses, ed 2, St Louis, 1987, The CV Mosby Co.
4. McCaul K: Sensory information, fear level, and reactions to pain, J Pers 48:494, 1980.

Anxiety

1. Burd S and Marshall M, editors: Some clinical approaches to psychiatric nursing, New York, 1966, The Macmillan Co.
2. Durham R and Turvey A: Cognitive therapy vs behavior therapy in the treatment of chronic general anxiety, Behav Res Ther 25:220, 1987.
3. Gelder M: Psychological treatment for anxiety disorders: a review, J R Soc Med 79:230, 1986.
4. Jennings B and Sherman R: Anxiety, locus of control, and satisfaction in patients undergoing ambulatory surgery Milit Med 152:206, 1987.
5. Kim M, McFarland G, and McLane A, editors: Classification of nursing diagnoses: proceedings of the fifth national conference, St Louis, 1984, The CV Mosby Co.
6. Kim M, McFarland G, and McLane A: Pocket guide to nursing diagnoses, ed 2, St Louis, 1987, The CV Mosby Co.
7. Lindsay W et al: A controlled trial of treatment for generalized anxiety, Br J Clin Psychol 26(pt 1):3, 1987.
8. May R: The meaning of anxiety, New York, 1977, WW Norton Co.
9. May R: The meaning of anxiety, New York, 1979, Pocket Books.
10. Meldman M, McFarland G, and Johnson E: The problem-oriented psychiatric index and treatment plans, St Louis, 1976, The CV Mosby Co.
11. Moss V: The effect of music on anxiety in the surgical patient, Periop Nurs Q 3:9, 1987.
12. Nash E: An overview of the concept of anxiety from various perspectives . . . , S Afr Med J (Suppl), Oct 26, 1985, p 5.
13. Neal M et al: Nursing care planning guides for psychiatric and mental health care, Monterey, Calif, 1981, Wadsworth Health Sciences.
14. Rakel R: Assessing the efficacy of antianxiety agents, Am J Med 82:1, 1987.
15. Rogers C: Counseling and psychotherapy, Boston, 1942, Houghton-Mifflin Co.
16. Rogers C: On becoming a person: a therapist's view of psychotherapy, Boston, 1961, Houghton-Mifflin Co.
17. Rogers C: Client-centered therapy: its current practice, implications, and theory, Boston, 1965, Houghton-Mifflin Co.
18. Spielberger CD: Anxiety and behavior, New York, 1966, Academic Press.
19. Stuart G and Sundeen S: Principles and practice of psychiatric nursing, ed 3, St Louis, 1987, The CV Mosby Co.
20. Teasdale K: Giving reassurance to anxious patients, Prof Nurs 2:112, 1987.

Hopelessness

1. Atwood J and Hinds P: Heuristic heresy: application of reliability and validity criteria to products of grounded theory, West J Nurs Res 8:135, 1986.
2. Beck A: Thinking and depression, Arch Gen Psychiatry 9:324, 1963.
3. Brandt B: The relationship between hopelessness and selected variables in women receiving chemotherapy for breast cancer, Oncol Nurs Forum 14:35, 1987.
4. Campbell L: Hopelessness, J Psychosoc Nurs 25:18, 1987.
5. Craig H and Edwards J: Adaptation in chronic illness: an eclectic model for nurses, J Adv Nurs 8:397, 1983.
6. Helm S: Nursing care of the depressed patient: a cognitive approach, Perspect Psychiatr Care 22:100, 1984.
7. Hickey S: Enabling hope, Cancer Nurs 9:133, 1986.
8. Kim M, McFarland G, and McLane A: Pocket guide to nursing diagnoses, ed 2, St Louis, 1987, The CV Mosby Co.
9. McFarland G and Wasli E: Nursing diagnoses and process in psychiatric mental health nursing, Philadelphia, 1986, JB Lippincott Co.
10. McGee R: Hope: a factor influencing crisis resolution, Adv Nurs Sci 6:34, 1984.
11. Miller J: Coping with chronic illness: overcoming powerlessness, Philadelphia, 1973, FA Davis Co.
12. Miller J: Inspiring hope, Am J Nurs 83:22, 1985.
13. Rideout E and Montemuro M: Hope, morale and adaptation in patients with chronic heart failure, J Adv Nurs 11:429, 1986.
14. Schultz J and Dark S: Manual of psychiatric nursing care plans, ed 2, Boston, 1986, Little, Brown & Co.
15. Stoner C: Learned helplessness: analysis and application, Oncol Nurs Forum 12:31, 1985.
16. Stoner M and Keampfer S: Recalled life expectancy information, phase of illness and hope in cancer patients, Res Nurs Health 8:269, 1985.
17. Stotland E: The psychology of hope, San Francisco, 1969, Jossey-Bass Inc.

Powerlessness

1. Arakelian M: An assessment and nursing application of the concept of locus of control, Adv Nurs Sci 3:25, 1980.
2. Campbell A and Converse P, editors: The human meaning of social change, New York, 1972, Russell Sage.
3. Cartwright D, editor: Studies in social power, Ann Arbor, 1959, The University of Michigan Press.
4. Chang B: Generalized expectancy, situational perception, and morale, Nurs Res 27:316, 1978.
5. Fuchs J: Use of decisional control to combat powerlessness . . . the patient with end stage renal disease on dialysis, ANNA J 14:11, 1987.
6. Grotstein J: The psychology of powerlessness: disorders of self-regulation and interaction regulation as a newer paradigm for psychopathology, Psychoanal Inquiry 6:93, 1986.
7. Hall B and VanServellen G: The effect of a self-help group on feelings of hopelessness and helplessness, West J Nurs Res 6:169, 1984.

8. Kim M, McFarland G, and McLane A, editors: Classification of nursing diagnoses: proceedings of the fifth national conference, St Louis, 1984, The CV Mosby Co.
9. Kim M, McFarland G, and McLane A: Pocket guide to nursing diagnoses, ed 2, St Louis, 1987, The CV Mosby Co.
10. Lawrance L and McLeroy K: Self efficacy and health education, J Sch Health 56:317, 1986.
11. McFarland G, Leonard H, and Morris M: Nursing leadership and management: contemporary strategies, New York, 1984, John Wiley & Sons Inc.
12. Meldman M, McFarland G, and Johnson E: The problem-oriented psychiatric index and treatment plans, St Louis, 1976, The CV Mosby Co.
13. Miller J: Coping with chronic illness: overcoming powerlessness, Philadelphia, 1983, FA Davis Co.
14. Neal M et al: Nursing care planning guides for psychiatric and mental health care, Monterey, Calif, 1981, Wadsworth Health Sciences.
15. Rothlis J: The effect of a self-help group on feelings of hopelessness and helplessness, West J Nurs Res 6:172, 1984.
16. Rotter J: Generalized expectancies for internal versus external control of reinforcement, Psychol Monogr Gen Appl 80:1, 1966.
17. Schmidt M: Exchange and power in special settings for the aged, Int J Aging Hum Dev 14:157, 1981-1982.
18. Schultz R and Hanusa B: Long term effects of control and predictability-enhancing interventions: findings and ethical issues, J Pers Soc Psychol 36:1194, 1978.
19. Seeman M: Alienation studies, Annu Rev Sociol 1:91, 1975.
20. Sheppard K: Powerlessness: a nursing diagnosis, Dimens Oncol Nurs 1:17, 1985.
21. Slimmer et al: Perceptions of learned helplessness, J Gerontol Nurs 13:33, 1987.
22. Wallerstein J: Children of divorce: report of a ten year follow up of early latency-age children, Am J Orthopsychiatry 57:199, 1987.

Body image disturbance

1. Brunner LS and Suddarth DS, editors: The Lippincott manual for nursing practice, ed 3, Philadelphia, 1982, JB Lippincott Co.
2. Carlson C, editor: Behavioral concepts and nursing interventions, Philadelphia, 1970, JB Lippincott Co.
3. Chinn P, editor: Advances in nursing theory development, Rockville, Md, 1983, Aspen Systems Corp.
4. Falon G and Rozin P: Sex differences in perceptions of desirable body shape, J Abnorm Psychol 94:102, 1985.
5. Fitts WH: The self-concept and self-actualization, Nashville, Tenn, 1971, Dede Wallace Center.
6. Franzoi S and Sheilds S: The body esteem scale: multidimensional structure and sex differences in a college population, J Pers Assess 48:173, 1984.
7. Hawkins R and Turrell S: Desirable and undesirable masculine and feminine traits in relation to student's dieting tendencies and body image dissatisfaction, Sex Roles 9:705, 1983.
8. Janelli L: The realities of body image, J Gerontol Nurs 12:23, 1986.
9. Kim M, McFarland G, and McLane A: Pocket guide to nursing diagnoses, ed 2, St Louis, 1987, The CV Mosby Co.
10. Kim MJ, and Moritz DA, editors: Classification of nursing diagnoses: proceedings of the third and fourth national conferences, New York, 1982, McGraw-Hill Book Co.
11. MacElveen-Hoehn P and McCorkle R: Understanding sexuality in progressive cancer, Semin Oncol Nurs 1:56, 1985.
12. McCLoskey JC: How to make the most of body image theory in nursing practice, Nursing 76 6:68, 1976.
13. McFarland G and Wasli E: Nursing diagnoses and process in psychiatric mental health nursing, Philadelphia, 1986, JB Lippincott Co.
14. Noles S, Cash T, and Winstead B: Body image, physical attractiveness, and depression, J Consult Clin Psychol 53:88, 1985.
15. Price B: Body image: keeping up appearances, Nurs Times 82:58, 1986.
16. van der Velde C: Body images of one's self and of others: developmental and clinical significance, Am J Psychiatry 142:527, 1985.
17. Yura H and Walsh MB, editors: Human needs and the nursing process, Norwalk, Conn, 1983, Appleton-Century-Crofts.

Personal identity disturbance

1. Chinn P, editor: Advances in nursing theory development, Rockville, Md, 1983, Aspen Systems Corp.
2. Erikson EH: Childhood and society, ed 2, New York, 1963, Norton.
3. Fitts WH: The self-concept and self-actualization, Nashville, 1971, Dede Wallace Center.
4. Kim M, McFarland G, and McLane A: Pocket guide to nursing diagnoses, ed 2, St Louis, 1987, The CV Mosby Co.
5. Strachey J, editor: The standard edition of the complete psychological works of Sigmund Freud, London, 1962, Hogarth Press.
6. Sullivan HS: The interpersonal theory of psychiatry, New York, 1953, Norton.
7. Wilson HS and Kneisl CR: Psychiatric nursing, Menlo Park, Calif, 1979, Addison-Wesley Publishing Co.

Self-esteem disturbance; situational low self-esteem; chronic low self-esteem

1. Brandon N: The psychology of self-esteem, Los Angeles, 1969, Nash.
2. Brunner LS and Suddarth DS, editors: The Lippincott manual for nursing practice, ed 3, Philadelphia, 1982, JB Lippincott Co.
3. Chinn, P, editor: Advances in nursing theory development, Rockville, Md, 1983, Aspen Systems Corp.
4. Coopersmith S: The antecedents of self-esteem, San Francisco, 1967, Freeman.
5. Fitts WH: The self-concept and self-actualization, Nashville, Tenn, 1971, Dede Wallace Center.
6. Kim M, McFarland G, and McLane A, editors: Classification of nursing diagnoses: proceedings of the fifth national conference, St Louis, 1984, The CV Mosby Co.
7. Kim M, McFarland G, and McLane A: Pocket guide to nursing diagnoses, ed 2, St Louis, 1987, The CV Mosby Co.
8. Kim MJ and Moritz DA, editors: Classification of nursing diagnoses: proceedings of the third and fourth national conferences, New York, 1982, McGraw-Hill Book Co.
9. Maslow AH: Motivation and personality, New York, 1954, Harper & Brothers.
10. McFarland G and Wasli E: Nursing diagnoses and process in psychiatric mental health nursing, Philadelphia, 1986, JB Lippincott Co.
11. Miller J: Coping with chronic illness: overcoming powerlessness, Philadelphia, 1983, FA Davis Co.
12. Roy C Sr, editor: Introduction to nursing: an adaptation model. Englewood Cliffs, NJ, 1976, Prentice-Hall Inc.
13. Taylor MC Sr: The need for self-esteem. In Human needs and the nursing process, Norwalk, Conn, 1982, Appleton-Century-Crofts.
14. Yura H and Walsh MB, editors: Human needs and the nursing process, Norwalk, Conn, 1983, Appleton-Century-Crofts.

Anticipatory grieving

1. Benoliel J: Loss and terminal illness, Nurs Clin North Am 20:439, 1985.
2. Bower F, editor: Nursing and the concept of loss, New York, 1980, John Wiley & Sons Inc.
3. Carlson C and Blackwell B, editors: Behavioral concepts and nursing interventions, ed 2, Philadelphia, 1978, JB Lippincott Co.
4. Clayton P et al: Anticipatory grief and widowhood, Br J Psychiatry 122:47, 1973.
5. Collison C and Miller S: Using images of the future in grief work, Image 19:9, 1987.
6. Derdiarian A: Informational needs of recently diagnosed cancer patients. II. Methods and description, Cancer Nurs 10:156, 1987.
7. Derdiarian A; Informational needs of recently diagnosed cancer patients, Nurs Res 35:276, 1987.
8. Dracup K and Breu C: Using nursing research findings to meet the needs of grieving spouses, Nurs Res 27:212, 1978.
9. Engel G: Psychological development in health and disease, Philadelphia, 1968, WB Saunders Co.
10. Fulton R and Gottsman D: Anticipatory grief: a psychosocial concept reconsidered, Br J Psychiatry 137:45, 1980.
11. Gerety E and Caley J: A nurse-led encouragement group for families of terminally ill patients, Unpublished raw data, 1983.
12. Hampe S: Needs of the grieving spouse in a hospital setting, Nurs Res 24:113, 1975.

13. Kim M, McFarland G, and McLane A: Pocket guide to nursing diagnoses, ed 2, St Louis, 1987, The CV Mosby Co.
14. McFarland G and Wasli E: Nursing diagnoses and process in psychiatric mental health nursing, Philadelphia, 1986, JB Lippincott Co.
15. Welch D: Anticipatory grief reactions in family members of adult patients, Issues Ment Health Nurs 4:149, 1982.
16. York C and Stichler J: Cultural grief expressions following infant death, Dimens Crit Care Nurs 4:120, 1985.

Dysfunctional grieving

1. Bower F, editor: Nursing and the concept of loss, New York, 1980, John Wiley & Sons Inc.
2. Carlson C and Blackwell B, editors: Behavioral concepts and nursing interventions, ed 2, Philadelphia, 1978, JB Lippincott Co.
3. Cheny R: Emotional adaptability to disability, Rehabil Nurs 9:36, 1984.
4. Fulton R and Gottsman D: Anticipatory grief, Br J Psychiatry 139:79, 1981.
5. Horowitz M, Wilner N, and Marmare C: Pathological grief and the activation of latent and self images, Am J Psychiatry 137:1157, 1980.
6. Hospice education program for nurses, DHHS Pub No HRA 81-27, Washington DC, 1981, US Government Printing Office.
7. Kim M, McFarland G, and McLane A: Pocket guide to nursing diagnoses, ed 2, St Louis, 1987, The CV Mosby Co.
8. Lewis K: Grief in chronic illness and disability, Rehabil Nurs 9:8, 1984.
9. Lindemann E: Symptomatology and management of acute grief, Am J Psychiatry 101:141, 1944.
10. Lindemann E: Beyond grief: studies in crisis intervention, New York, 1979, Jason Aronson.
11. Martocchio B: Grief and bereavement, Nurs Clin North Am 20:327, 1985.
12. McFarland G and Wasil E: Nursing diagnoses and process in psychiatric mental health nursing, Philadelphia, 1986, JB Lippincott Co.
13. Melges F and DeMaso D: Grief-resolution therapy: reliving, revising, and revisiting, Am J Psychother 34:51, 1980.
14. Stewart T and Shields C: Grief in chronic illness: assessment and management, Arch Phys Med Rehabil 66:447, 1985.

Altered role performance

1. Browder D et al: Movement training: when trainer initiated reinforcement and self-monitoring are not enough, Int J Rehabil Res 9:363, 1986.
2. Brunner LS and Suddarth DS, editors: The Lippincott manual for nursing practice, ed 3, Philadelphia, 1982, JB Lippincott Co.
3. Hardy M and Conway M: Role theory: perspectives for health professionals, New York, 1978, Appleton-Century-Crofts.
4. Kim M, McFarland G, and McLane A: Pocket guide to nursing diagnoses, ed 2, St Louis, 1987, The CV Mosby Co.
5. Kim MJ and Moritz DA, editors: Classification of nursing diagnoses: proceedings of the third and fourth national conferences, New York, 1982, McGraw-Hill Book Co.
6. Linville P: Self-complexity as a cognitive buffer against stress-related illness and depression, J Pers Soc Psychol 52:66, 1987.
7. McFarland G and Wasli E: Nursing diagnoses and process in psychiatric mental health nursing, Philadelphia, 1986, JB Lippincott Co.
8. Meleis A: Role insufficiency and role supplementation, Nurs Res 24:264, 1975.
9. Monti P et al: Social perception and communication skills among schizophrenics and nonschizophrenics, J Clin Psychol 43:97, 1987.
10. Roy C Sr, editor: Introduction to nursing: an adaptation model, Englewood Cliffs, NJ, 1976, Prentice-Hall Inc.

Social isolation

1. Barth R: Social and cognitive treatment of children and adolescents, San Francisco, 1986, Jossey-Bass Inc.
2. Bowlby J: Attachment and loss. Vol 1. Attachment, New York, 1969, Basic Books Inc.
3. Carpentio LJ: Nursing diagnosis: application to clinical practice, ed 2, Philadelphia, 1987, JB Lippincott Co.
4. Dunlop BD: Need for and utilization of long-term care among elderly Americans, J Chronic Dis 29:75, 1976.
5. Freedman AM, Kaplan H, and Sadock BJ, editors: Comprehensive textbook of psychiatry, Baltimore, 1975, Williams & Wilkins.
6. Gunter L: Do nurses have the power to cause, prevent and cure "social breakdown syndrome"? J Gerontol Nurs 6:648, 1977 (editorial).
7. Hall CS and Lindzey G: Theories of personality, ed 2, New York, 1970, John Wiley & Sons Inc.
8. Horney K: Neurotic personality of our times, New York, 1937, WW Norton Co.
9. Horney K: Our inner conflicts, New York, 1945, WW Norton Co.
10. Kim M, McFarland G, and McLane A: Pocket guide to nursing diagnoses, ed 2, St Louis, 1987, The CV Mosby Co.
11. Lynch JJ: The broken heart, New York, 1977, Basic Books Inc.
12. Mahon NE: Developmental changes and loneliness during adolescence, Top Clin Nurs 5:66, 1983.
13. Meize-Grochowski R: An analysis of the concept of trust in the nursing literature, J Adv Nurs 9:563, 1984.
14. Pasquali EA et al: Mental health nursing: a biocultural approach, St Louis, 1981, The CV Mosby Co.
15. Rathbone-McCuan E and Hashimi J: Isolated elders, Rockville, Md, 1982, Aspen Systems Corp.
16. Schuster CS and Ashburn SS: The process of human development, Boston, 1980, Little, Brown & Co.
17. Savishinsky J: Pets and family relationships among nursing home residents, Marriage Fam Rev 8:109, 1985.
18. Spitz RA: The derailment of dialogue: stimulus overload, action cycles, and the competition gradient, J Am Psychoanal Assoc 12:752, 1964.
19. Stuart GW and Sundeen SJ: Principles and practice of psychiatric nursing, ed 3, St Louis, 1986, The CV Mosby Co.
20. Wright LM: A symbolic tree: loneliness is the root, delusions are the leaves, J Psychiatr Nurs 13:30, 1975.

Impaired social interaction

1. Bowlby J: Attachment and loss. Vol 1. Attachment, New York, 1969, Basic Books, Inc.
2. Crocket MS: Exploring peer relationships, J Psychosoc Nurs 22, 1984.
3. Freedman AM, Kaplan H, and Sadock BJ, editors: Comprehensive textbook of psychiatry, Baltimore, 1975, Williams & Wilkins.
4. Goetz T and Dweck C: Learned helplessness in social situations, J Pers Soc Psychol 39:246, 1980.
5. Hall C and Lindzey G: Theory of personality, ed 2, New York, 1970, John Wiley & Sons, Inc.
6. Horney K: Neurotic personality of our times, New York, 1937, WW Norton Co.
7. Kim M, McFarland G, and McLane A: Pocket guide to nursing diagnoses, ed 2, St Louis, 1987, The CV Mosby Co.
8. Mussen P: Carmichael's manual of child psychology, ed 3, New York, 1970, John Wiley & Sons Inc.
9. Putallaz M and Gottman J: An interactional model of children's entry into peer groups, Child Dev 52:986, 1981.
10. Spitz RA: The derailment of dialogue: stimulus overload, action cycles, and the competition gradient, J Am Psychoanal Assoc 12:752, 1964.

Altered family processes

1. Bradt J and Moynihan C, editors: Systems therapy, Washington DC, 1972, The Groome Child Guidance Center.
2. Carpenito LJ: Nursing diagnosis: application to clinical practice, ed 2, Philadelphia, 1987, JB Lippincott Co.
3. Craven RF and Sharp BH: The effects of illness on family functions, Nurs Forum 11:186, 1972.
4. Cromwell RE and Peterson GW: Multisystem-multimethod family assessment in clinical contexts, Fam Process 22:147, 1983.
5. D'Agostino A, editor: Family, church and community, New York, 1961, PJ Kennedy & Sons.
6. Fogarty T: Triangles, Family 2:165, 1975.
7. Foley VD: An introduction to family therapy, New York, 1974, Grune & Stratton Inc.
8. Ford FR: Rules: the invisible family, Fam Process 22:135, 1983.

9. Framo J, editor: Family interaction, New York, 1972, Springer Publishing Co.
10. Green CP: Assessment of family stress, J Adv Nurs 7:11, 1982.
11. Guerin P, editor: Family therapy theory and practice, New York, 1976, Gardner Press.
12. Haley J: Uncommon therapy: the psychiatric techniques of Milton H. Erickson, M.D., New York, 1973, WW Norton Co.
13. Haley J: Problem solving therapy, San Francisco, 1987, ed 2, Jossey-Bass, Inc.
14. Jackson D, editor: Communication, family, and marriage, Palo Alto, Calif, 1968, Science & Behavior Books.
15. Kim M, McFarland G, and McLane A: Pocket guide to nursing diagnoses, ed 2, St Louis, 1987, The CV Mosby Co.
16. Leavitt MB: Families at risk: nursing assessment and strategies for the family at risk, Philadelphia, 1982, JB Lippincott Co.
17. Minuchin S: Families and family therapy, Cambridge, Mass, 1979, Harvard University Press.
18. Otto HA: Criteria for assessing family strength, Fam Process 2:329, 1963.
19. Satir V: Conjoint family therapy, Palo Alto, Calif, 1964, Science & Behavior Books.
20. Schuster CS and Ashburn SS: The process of human development: a holistic approach, Boston, 1980, Little, Brown & Co.
21. Stuart GW and Sundeen SJ: Principles and practice of psychiatric nursing, ed 3, St Louis, 1986, The CV Mosby Co.
22. Walsh F: Normal family processes, New York, 1982, The Guilford Press.
23. Wilson HS and Kneisel CR: Psychiatric nursing, Palo Alto, Calif, 1983, Addison-Wesley Publishing Co.
24. Wright LM and Leahey M: Nurses and families: a guide to family assessment and intervention. Philadelphia. 1984. FA Davis Co.

Potential altered parenting; altered parenting

1. Bernhardt KS and Bernhardt DK: Being a parent, Toronto, 1970, University of Toronto Press.
2. Bettelheim B: Love is not enough, New York, 1950, The Free Press.
3. Bettelheim B: Dialogues with mothers, New York, 1962, The Free Press.
4. Bossard JH: The sociology of child development, New York, 1954, Harper & Brothers Publishers.
5. Brazelton TB: Toddlers and parents, New York, 1974, Delacorte Press/Seymour Lawrence.
6. Campbell C: Nursing diagnosis and intervention in nursing practice, New York, 1984, John Wiley & Sons Inc.
7. Carew JV: Experience and the development of intelligence in young children at home and in day care, Monogr Soc Res Child Dev 187:45, 1980.
8. Carpentio LJ: Nursing diagnosis: application to clinical practice, ed 2, Philadelphia, 1987, JB Lippincott Co.
9. Cohen S and Cominskey TJ, editors: Child development: contemporary perspectives, Itasca, Ill, 1977, FE Peacock.
10. Curry MA: Maternal attachment behavior and mother's self-concept: the effect of early skin-to-skin contact, Nurs Res 31:73, 1982.
11. Erikson EH: Childhood and society, New York, 1963, WW Norton Co.
12. Gesell A: The child from five to ten, New York, 1946, Harper & Brothers, Publishers.
13. Gesell A: Studies in child development, New York, 1948, Harper & Brothers, Publishers.
14. Ginott HG: Between parent and child, New York, 1965, The Macmillan Co.
15. Ginott HG: Between parent and teenager, New York, 1969, The Macmillan Co.
16. Graybill D: Relationship of maternal child-rearing behaviors to children's self-esteem, J Psychol 100:45, 1978.
17. Greenberg S: Right from the start, Boston, 1978, Houghton-Mifflin Co.
18. Honig AS: The gifts of families: caring, courage and competence, Syracuse, NY, 1981, ERIC Document Reproduction Service.
19. Johnson SH: High-risk parenting: nursing assessment and strategies for the family at risk, ed 2, Philadelphia, 1986, JB Lippincott Co.
20. Katz B: How to be a better parent, New York, 1953, The Ronald Press.
21. Kim M, McFarland G, and McLane A: Pocket guide to nursing diagnoses, ed 2, St Louis, 1987, The CV Mosby Co.
22. Klaus MH and Kennell JH: Parent-infant bonding, ed 2, St Louis, 1981, The CV Mosby Co.
23. Ludington-Hoe S: How to have a smarter baby, Toronto, 1987, Bantam Books.
24. McGillicuddy-DeLisi AV: Parental beliefs about developmental processes, Hum Dev 25:192, 1982.
25. Mercer RT: Nursing care for parents at risk, Thorofare, NJ, 1977, Charles B Slack Inc.
26. Mercer RT: A theoretical framework for studying factors that impact on the maternal role, Nurs Res 30:73, 1981.
27. Mercer RT: Relationship of psychosocial and perinatal variables to perception of childbirth, Nurs Res 32:202, 1983.
28. Perry SE: Parents' perceptions of their newborn following structured interactions, Nurs Res 32:208, 1983.
29. Richard M, editor: The integration of a child into the social world, London, 1974, Cambridge University Press.
30. Roberts FB: Infant behavior and the transition to parenthood, Nurs Res 32:213, 1983.
31. Rubin R: Attainment of the maternal role. I. Processes, Nurs Res 16:237, 1967.
32. Segal J: The mental health of the child: program reports of the National Institute of Mental Health, Rockville, Md, 1971, National Institute of Mental Health.
33. Siefert K et al: Perinatal stress: a study of factors linked to the risk of parenting problems, Health Soc Work 18:107, 1983.
34. Swan RW and Stavros H: Childrearing practices associated with the development of cognitive skills of children in low socioeconomic areas, Early Child Dev Care 2:23, 1973.
35. Triplett JL and Arbeson SW: Working with children of alcoholics, Pediatr Nurs, Sept-Oct 1983, p. 317.
36. Trowell J: Emotional abuse of children, Health Visitor 56:252, 1983.
37. Ventura JN: Parent coping behaviors, parent functioning and infant temperament characteristics, Nurs Res 31:269, 1982.
38. White B: Educating the infant and toddler, Lexington, Mass, 1988, Lexington Books.
39. Wong DL and Whaley LF: Clinical handbook of pediatric nursing, St Louis, 1981, The CV Mosby Co.

Parental role conflict

1. Algren C: Role perception of mothers who have hospitalized children, Child Health Care 14(1), 1985.
2. Anderson J and Chung J: Culture and illness: parent's perceptions of their child's long term illness, Nurs Papers 19:40, 1982.
3. Anthony C and Koupernik C: The child in his family: the impact of disease and death, New York, 1973, John Wiley & Sons, Inc.
4. Ayer A: Is partnership with parents really possible? Am J Matern Child Nurs 3:107, 1978.
5. Carter M et al: Parent environmental stress in pediatric intensive care units, Dimens Crit Care Nurs 4:180, 1985.
6. Chan J and Leff P: Parenting and chronically ill child in the hospital: issues and concerns, Child Health Care 11:9, 1982.
7. Debuskey M: The chronically ill child and his family, Springfield, Ill, 1970, Charles C Thomas, Publisher.
8. Ferraro A and Longo D: Nursing care of the family with a chronically ill, hospitalized child: an alternative approach, Image 16:77, 1985.
9. Freiberg K: How parents react when their child is hospitalized, Am J Nurs 72:1270, 1972.
10. Hardgrove C: Parents and children in the hospital: the family's role in pediatrics, Boston, 1972, Little, Brown & Co.
11. Hayes V and Knox J: The experience of stress in parents of children hospitalized with long term disabilities, J Adv Nurs 9:333, 1984.
12. Nobbs N and Perrin J: Issues in the care of children with chronic illness, San Francisco, 1985, Jossey-Bass Inc.
13. Holmes K: My child is in the hospital, Parents Magazine, 1980, p 42.
14. Home care for children with serious handicapping conditions, Washington, DC, 1984, Public Health Service, US Department of Health and Human Services.

15. Hymovich D: Parents of sick children, their needs and tasks, Pediatr Nurs 2:9, 1976.
16. Hymovich D: Assessing the impact of chronic childhood illness on the family and parent coping, Image 13:71, 1981.
17. Jackson P, Braadham R, and Burwel H: Child care in the hospital a parent/staff partnership, Am J Matern Child Nurs 3:104, 1978.
18. Jay S: Pediatric intensive care: involving parents in the care of their child, Matern-Child Nurs J 6:195, 1977.
19. Johnson SH: High risk parenting, Philadelphia, 1979, JB Lippincott Co.
20. Meadow J: The captive mother, Arch Dis Child 44:362, 1969.
21. Meleis A: Role insufficiency and role supplementation: a conceptual framework, Nurs Res 24:264, 1975.
22. Miezio P: Parenting children with disabilities: a professional source for physicians and a guide for parents, New York, 1983, Marcel Dekker Inc.
23. Mintzer D et al: Parenting an infant with a birth defect, Psychoanal Study Child 39:561, 1984.
24. Mishel M: Parent's perception of uncertainty concerning their hospitalized child, Nurs Res 32:324, 1983.
25. Morrow N and Johnson R: Coping strategies used by parents during their child's hospitalization in an intensive care unit, Child Health Care 14:14, 1985.
26. Roy M Sr: Role cues and mothers of hospitalized children, Nurs Res 16:178, 1967.
27. Whaley L and Wong D: Nursing care of infants and children, ed 3, 1987, St Louis, The CV Mosby Co.
28. Wright and Leahey: Nurses and families, Philadelphia, 1984, FA Davis Co.

Impaired verbal communication

1. Edwards B: Drawing on the right side of the brain, Los Angeles, 1979, JP Tarcher Inc.
2. Edwards B and Brilhart J: Communication in nursing practice, St Louis, 1981, The CV Mosby Co.
3. Hall E: The hidden dimension, New York, 1966, Doubleday & Co.
4. Heidt P: Effect of therapeutic touch on anxiety level of hospitalized patients, Nurs Res 30:32, 1981.
5. Hein E: Communication in nursing practice, ed 2, Boston, 1980, Little, Brown & Co.
6. Heineken J: Treating the disconfirmed psychiatric client, J Psychiatr Nurs Ment Health Services 21:21, 1983.
7. Kaplan H, Freedman A, and Sadock B, editors: Comprehensive textbook of psychiatry, vol 1, Baltimore, 1980, Williams & Wilkins.
8. Kasch C: Role of strategic communication in nursing: theory and research, Adv Nurs Sci 7:56, 1984.
9. Kim M, McFarland G, and McLane A: Pocket guide to nursing diagnoses, ed 2, St Louis, 1987, The CV Mosby Co.
10. Lewis G: Nurse-patient communication, ed 3, Dubuque, Ia, 1978, William C Brown Co, Publishers.
11. McFarland G, Leonard H, and Morris M: Nursing leadership and management: contemporary strategies, New York, 1984, John Wiley & Sons, Inc.
12. Pimental P: Alterations in communications: bio-psycho-social aspects of aphasia, dysarthria, and right hemisphere syndromes in the stroke patient, Nurs Clin North Am 21:321, 1986.
13. Rubin R et al: Communications research: strategies and sources, 1985, Wadsworth Publishing.
14. Ruesch J: Disturbed communication, New York, 1972, WW Norton Co.
15. Ruesch J: Therapeutic communication, ed 2, New York, 1973, WW Norton Co.
16. Satir V: People making, Palo Alto, Calif, 1972, Science and Behavior Books.
17. Springer S and Deutsch G: Left brain, right brain, San Francisco, 1981, WH Freeman & Co.
18. Taylor A et al: Communicating, ed 4, 1986, Englewood Cliffs, NJ, Prentice-Hall, Inc.
19. Tedesco-Carreras P: Communicating with difficult patients, Imprint 33:36, 1986.
20. Watzlawick P, Beavin J, and Jackson D: Pragmatics of human communication, New York, 1967, WW Norton Co.
21. Weiss S: The language of touch, Nurs Res 28:76, 1979.
22. Wilmot W: Dyadic communication, ed 3, New York, 1986, Random House.
23. Wilson H and Kneisl C: Psychiatric nursing, Menlo Park, Calif, 1979, Addison-Wesley Publishing Co.

Potential for violence: self-directed or directed at others

1. Bavolek S: A handbook for understanding child abuse and neglect, ed 2, Eau Claire, Wis, 1985, Family Development Resources Inc.
2. Campbell C: Nursing diagnosis and intervention in nursing practice, New York, 1984, John Wiley & Sons, Inc.
3. Carpenito LJ: Nursing diagnosis: application to clinical practice, ed 2, Philadelphia, 1987, JB Lippincott Co.
4. Dollard J et al: Frustration and aggression, New Haven, Conn, 1939, Yale University Press.
5. Fawcett J: Dynamics of violence, Chicago, 1972, American Medical Association.
6. Fromm E: The anatomy of human destructiveness, New York, 1973, Holt, Rinehart & Winston, Inc.
7. Garbarino J: The psychologically battered child, San Francisco, 1986, Jossey-Bass Inc.
8. Kim MJ, McFarland GK, and McLane AM: Pocket guide to nursing diagnoses, ed 2, St Louis, 1987, The CV Mosby Co.
9. Kolb LC: Modern clinical psychiatry, ed 10, Philadelphia, 1982, WB Saunders Co.
10. Liebert RM, Neale JM, and Davidson ES: The early window: effects of television on children and youth, New York, 1973, Pergamon Press.
11. Lorenz K: On aggression, New York, 1966, Harcourt, Brace & World, Inc.
12. May R: Power and innocence: a search for the sources of violence, New York, 1972, WW Norton Co.
13. Office for Children, Youth and Families: Annual report to the governor and the legislature on the Wisconsin Child Abuse and Neglect Act, Madison, Wis, 1985, Division of Community Services, Department of Health and Social Services.
14. Stuart GW and Sundeen SJ: Principles and practice of psychiatric nursing, ed 3, St Louis, 1986, The CV Mosby Co.
15. Warner CG and Braen GR: Management of the physically and emotionally abused: emergency assessment, intervention and counseling, Norwalk, Conn, 1982, Appleton-Century-Crofts.
16. Wilson HS and Kneisl CR: Psychiatric nursing, Menlo Park, Calif, 1983, Addison-Wesley Publishing Co.

Sexual dysfunction

1. Burgess AW, editor: Child pornography and sex rings, Lexington, Mass, 1984, Lexington Books.
2. Burgess AW, editor: Psychiatric nursing in the hospital and the community, ed 4, Englewood Cliffs, NJ, 1985, Prentice-Hall, Inc.
3. Burgess AW et al: Child molestation: assessing impact in multiple victims. Part I, Orlando, Fla, 1987, Grune & Stratton, Inc.
4. Finkelhor D: Child sexual abuse, New York, 1984, The Free Press.
5. Groth AN: Men who rape: the psychology of the offender, New York, 1979, Plenum Press.
6. Kaplan HS: The evaluation of sexual disorders: psychological and medical aspects, New York, 1983, Brunner/Mazel, Inc.
7. Kaplan HS: Sexual aversion, sexual phobias, and panic disorders, New York, 1987, Brunner/Mazel, Inc.
8. Masters WH and Johnson VE: Human sexual inadequacy, Boston, 1970, Little, Brown & Co.
9. Meyer J, Schmidt C, and Wise T, editors: Clinical management of sexual disorders, Baltimore, 1983, Williams & Wilkins.
10. Zimmerman ML et al: Art and group work: interventions for multiple victims of child molestation. Part II, Orlando, Fla, 1987, Grune & Stratton Inc.

Rape-trauma syndrome

1. Burgess AW and Holmstrom LL: Rape trauma syndrome, Am J Psychiatry 131:981, 1974.
2. Burgess AW and Holmstrom LL: Sexual trauma of children and adolescents: pressure, sex and secrecy, Nurs Clin North Am 10:551, 1975.
3. Burgess AW and Holmstrom LL: Coping behavior of the rape victim, Am J Psychiatry 133:413, 1976.

4. Burgess AW and Holmstrom LL: Rape: crisis and recovery, Bowie, Md, 1979, Brady Co.
5. Burgess AW and Holmstrom LL: Rape: sexual disruption and recovery, Am J Orthopsychiatry 49:648, 1979.
6. Groth AN, Burgess AW, and Holmstrom LL: Rape: power, anger and sexuality, Am J Psychiatry 134:1239, 1977.
7. Hazelwood RR: A behavioral interview of the rape victim, FBI Bulletin.
8. Herman J and Hirschman L: Families at risk for father-daughter incest, Am J Psychiatry 138:967, 1981.
9. Hilberman E: The rape victim, Washington DC, 1976, American Psychiatric Association.
10. Holmstrom LL and Burgess AW: Assessing trauma in the rape victim, Am J Nurs 75:1288, 1975.
11. Holmstrom LL and Burgess AW: Sexual behavior of assailants during reported rape, Arch Sexual Behav 9:427, 1980.
12. Lazare A, editor: Outpatient psychiatry, Baltimore, 1979, Williams & Wilkins.
13. Russell DEH: Rape in marriage, New York, 1982, Macmillan Co.

Ineffective individual coping

1. Aguilera DG and Messick JM: Crisis intervention: theory and methodology, ed 5, St Louis, 1986, The CV Mosby Co.
2. Berkowitz L, editor: Advances in experimental social psychology, New York, 1980, Academic Press.
3. Birren JE and Livingston J, editors: Cognition, stress, and aging, Englewood Cliffs, NJ, 1985, Prentice-Hall, Inc.
4. Brown MA: Social support, stress, and health: A comparison of expectant mothers and fathers, Nurs Res 35:72, 1986.
5. Coleman JC, Morris CG, and Glaros AG: Contemporary psychology and effective behavior, Glenview, Ill, 1987, Scott, Foresman & Co.
6. Davis M, Eshelman ER, and McKay M: The relaxation and stress reduction workbook, ed 2, Oakland, Calif, 1982, New Harbinger Publications.
7. Foa EB and Kozak MJ: Emotional processing of fear: exposure to corrective information, Psychol Bull 99:20, 1986.
8. Folkman S and Lazarus RS: An analysis of coping in a middle-aged community sample, J Health Soc Behav 21:219, 1980.
9. Folkman S and Lazarus RS: If it changes, it must be a process: study of emotion and coping during three stages of a college examination, J Pers Soc Psychol 48:150, 1985.
10. Folkman S and Lazarus RS: Stress process and depressive symptomatology, J Abnorm Psychol 95:107, 1986.
11. Folkman S et al: Appraisal, coping, health status, and psychological symptoms, J Pers Soc Psychol 50:571, 1986.
12. Folkman S et al: Dynamics of a stressful encounter: cognitive appraisal coping, and encounter outcomes, J Pers Soc Psychol 50:992, 1986.
13. Fren M, Fehring R, and Kartes S: Reducing the stress of cardiac catheterization by teaching relaxation, Dimens Crit Care Nurs 5:108, 1986.
14. Gentry WD, editor: The handbook of behavioral medicine, New York, 1984, The Guilford Press.
15. Greenberg JS: Comprehensive stress management, Dubuque, Ia, 1983, WC Brown.
16. Griffin W, Ling I, and Staley D: Stress management groups, J Psychosoc Nurs 23:31, 1985.
17. Janis IL and Mann L: Decision making: a psychological analysis of conflict, choice and commitment, New York, 1977, The Free Press.
18. Kemper TD: How many emotions are there? Wedding the social and the automatic components, Am J Sociol 93:263, 1987.
19. Kim MJ, McFarland GK, and McLane AM: Pocket guide to nursing diagnoses, ed 2, St Louis, 1987, The CV Mosby Co.
20. King KB: Psychological aspects of critical care, Heart Lung 14:579, 1985.
21. Lazarus RS: Psychological stress and the coping process, New York, 1966, McGraw-Hill Book Co.
22. Lazarus RS and Folkman S: Stress, appraisal and coping, New York, 1984, Springer Publishing Co.
23. Lazarus RS et al: Stress and adaptational outcomes: the problem of confounded measures, Am Psychol 40:770, 1985.
24. Lowery B: Stress research: some theoretical and methodological issues, Image 19:42, 1987.
25. Martelli MF et al: Stress management in the health care setting: matching interventions and coping styles, J Consult Clin Psychol 55:201, 1987.
26. McNett SC: Social support, threat, and coping responses and effectiveness in the functionally disabled, Nurs Res 36:98, 1987.
27. Meichenbaum D: Stress inoculation training, New York, 1985, Pergamon Press.
28. Meichenbaum D and Jaremko ME, editors: Stress reduction and prevention, New York, 1983, Plenum Press.
29. Miller BK: Teaching biofeedback techniques in critical care, Dimens Crit Care Nurs 4:314, 1985.
30. Monat A and Lazarus RS, editors: Stress and coping: an anthology, New York, 1985, Columbia University Press.
31. Moos RH and Schaeffer JA: Coping with life crises: an integrated approach, New York, 1986, Plenum Press.
32. Moss RC: Overcoming fear: a review of research on patient, family instruction, AORN J 43:1107, 1986.
33. Pollock SE: Human responses to chronic illness: physiologic and psychosocial adaptation, Nurs Res 35:90, 1986.
34. Roberts JG et al: Analysis of coping responses and adjustment: stability of conclusions, Nurs Res 36:94, 1987.
35. Rutter M: Psychosocial resilience and protective mechanisms, Am J Orthopsychiatry 57:316, 1987.
36. Segal J: Winning life's toughest battles, New York, 1986, McGraw-Hill Book Co.
37. Sideleau BF: Irrational beliefs and interventions, J Psychosoc Nurs 25:18, 1987.
38. Slaby AE and Glickman AS: Adapting to life-threatening illness, New York, 1985, Praeger Publishers.
39. Speilberger CD and Sarason I, editors: Stress and anxiety: a source book of theory and research, New York, 1986, Hemisphere Pubishing Corp.
40. Stoll BA, editor: Coping with cancer stress, Dordrecht, 1986, Martinus Nijhoff.
41. Thoits PA: Social support as coping assistance, J Consult Clin Psychol 54:416, 1986.
42. Turk DC, Meichenbaum D, and Genest M: Pain and behavioral medicine: a cognitive behavioral perspective, New York, 1983, The Guilford Press.
43. Vaillant GE: Adaptation to life, Boston, 1977, Little, Brown & Co.
44. Viney LL: Expressions of positive emotion by people who are physically ill: is it evidence of defending or coping? J Psychosom Res 30:27, 1986.
45. Wallace LM: Psychological preparation as a method of reducing the stress of surgery, J Hum Stress 10:62, 1984.
46. Wilson-Barnett J: Interventions to alleviate patients' stress: a review, J Psychosom Res 28:63, 1984.

Defensive coping

1. Chinn P, editor: Advances in nursing theory development, Rockville, Md, 1983, Aspen Systems Corp.
2. McFarland GK and Wasli EL: Nursing diagnoses and process in psychiatric mental health nursing, Philadelphia, 1986, JB Lippincott Co.
3. Roy C Sr: Introduction to nursing: an adaptation model, Engelwood Cliffs, NJ, 1976, Prentice-Hall Inc.
4. Tucker SM et al: Patient care standards: nursing process, diagnosis, and outcome, ed 4, St Louis, 1988, The CV Mosby Co.
5. Wilson HS and Kneisl CR: Psychiatric nursing, Menlo Park, Calif, 1979, Addison-Wesley Publishing Co.
6. Yura H and Walsh MB: Human needs and the nursing process, Norwalk, Conn, 1982, Appleton-Century-Crofts.

Ineffective denial

1. Bartle SH: Denial of cardiac warnings, Psychosomatics 12:74, 1980.
2. Breznitz S, editor: The denial of stress, New York, 1983, International Universities Press.
3. Croog SH, Shapiro DS, and Levine S: Denial among male heart patients: an empirical study, Psychosom Med 33:385, 1971.
4. Freud A: The ego and the mechanisms of defense, New York, 1946, International Universities Press.
5. Hackett TP and Cassem NH: Development of a quantitative rating scale to assess denial, J Psychosom Res 18:93, 1974.
6. Weinstein EA and Kahn RI: Denial of illness, Springfield, Ill, 1955, Charles C Thomas, Publisher.

Impaired adjustment

1. Beglinger JE: Coping tasks in critical care, Dimens Crit Care Nurs 2:80, 1983.
2. Forsyth GL, Delaney KD, and Gresham ML: Vying for a winning position: management style of the chronically ill, Res Nurs Health 7:181, 1984.
3. Friedman-Campbell M and Hart CA: Theoretical strategies and nursing interventions to promote psychological adaptation to spinal cord injuries and disability, Neurosurg Nurs 16:335, 1984.
4. Fuchs J: Use of decisional control to combat powerlessness, Am Nephrol Nurs Assoc 14:11, 1987.
5. Gentry WD et al: Type A/B difference in coping with acute myocardial infarction: further considerations, Heart Lung 12:212, 1983.
6. Goldenson R, editor: Longman dictionary of psychology and psychiatry, New York, 1984, Longman, Inc.
7. Kasch C: Communication, adaptation, and the restoration of psychosocial competence: helping patients cope with chronic renal failure, Am Nephrol Nurs Assoc J 11:14, 1984.
8. Kerson TS and Kerson LA: Understanding chronic illness, the medical and psychosocial dimension of nine diseases, New York, 1985, The Free Press.
9. Kim MJ, McFarland GK, and McLane AM: Pocket guide to nursing diagnoses, ed 2, St Louis, 1987, The CV Mosby Co.
10. Miller P et al: Indicators of medical regimen adherence for myocardial infarction patients, Nurs Res 34:268, 1984.
11. Ott CR et al: A controlled random study of early cardiac rehabilitation: the Sickness Impact Profile as an assessment tool, Heart Lung 12:162, 1983.
12. Rosen JC and Solomon LJ, editors: Prevention in health psychology, Hanover, NH, 1985, Universtiy Press of New England.

Posttrauma response

1. American Psychiatric Association: Diagnostic and statistical manual of mental disorders, DSM III-R, Washington DC, 1987, The Association.
2. Breznitz S, editor: The denial of stress, New York, 1983, International Universities Press.
3. Burgess A and Holstom L: Rape trauma syndrome, Am J Psychiatry 131:981, 1974.
4. Burnstein A: Post-traumatic flashbacks, dream disturbances, and mental imagery, J Clin Psychiatry 46:374, 1985.
5. Cook J and Fontaine K: Essentials of mental health nursing, Reading, Mass, 1987, Addison-Wesley Publishing Co.
6. Falcon S et al: Tricyclics: Possible treatment for post-traumatic stress disorder, J Clin Psychiatry 46:379, 1985.
7. Field W, editor: The psychotherapy of Hildegard E. Peplau, Austin, 1979, University of Texas.
8. Figley C, editor: Trauma and its wake, New York, 1984, Brunner/Mazel Inc.
9. Horowitz M: Stress-response syndromes, New York, 1976, Jason Aronson Inc.
10. Kim M, McFarland G, and McLane A: Pocket guide to nursing diagnoses, ed 2, St Louis, 1987, The CV Mosby Co.
11. Lynch J: The broken heart: the medical consequences of loneliness, New York, 1977, Basic Books Inc.
12. Mellman T and Davis G: Combat-related flashbacks in post-traumatic stress disorder: phenomenology and similarity to panic attacks, J Clin Psychiatry 46:379, 1985.
13. Pitts F: Editorial, J Clin Psychiatry 46:373, 1985.
14. Rutter M: Psychosocial resilience and protective mechanisms, Am J Orthopsychiatry 57:316, 1987.
15. Sullivan H: The interpersonal theory of psychiatry, New York, 1953, WW Norton Co.
16. Terr L: Chowchilla revisited: the effects of psychic trauma four years after a school bus kidnapping, Am J Psychiatry 140:1543, 1983.
17. Wilkinson C: Aftermath of a disaster: the collapse of the Hyatt Regency Hotel skywalk, Am J Psychiatry 140:1130, 1983.
18. Yalom I: The theory and practice of group psychotherapy, New York, 1975, Basic Books, Inc.

Family coping: potential for growth; ineffective family coping: compromised; ineffective family coping: disability

1. Anderson JM: The social construction of illness experience: families with a chronically ill child, J Adv Nurs 6:427, 1981.
2. Anderson JZ and White GD: An empirical investigation of interaction and relationship patterns in functional and dysfunctional nuclear families and stepfamilies, Fam Process 25:407, 1986.
3. Beavers J et al: Coping in families with a retarded child, Fam Process 25:365, 1986.
4. Burr WR et al, editors: Contemporary theories about the family. Vol 1. Research based theories, New York, 1979, The Free Press.
5. Carpenito LJ: Nursing diagnosis: application to clinical practice, Philadelphia, 1983, JB Lippincott Co.
6. Clements IM and Buchanan DM, editors: Family therapy: a nursing perspective, New York, 1982, John Wiley & Sons, Inc.
7. Cole DA: Out-of-home child placement and family adaptation: a theoretical framework, Am J Ment Defic, 91:226, 1986.
8. Doer BC and Jones JJ: Effects of family preparation on the state anxiety of CCU patients, Nurs Res 28:316, 1979.
9. Getty C and Humphrys W: Understanding the family: stress and change in American family life, Norwalk, Conn, 1981, Appleton-Century-Crofts.
10. Gilliss L: The family as a unit of analysis: strategies for the nurse researcher, Adv Nurs Sci 5:50, 1983.
11. Griffith JL and Griffith ME: Structural family therapy in chronic illness, Psychosomatics 28:202, 1987.
12. Group for the Advancement of Psychiatry: A family affair: helping families cope with mental illness, New York, 1986, Brunner/Mazel Inc.
13. Hall J and Weaver B, editors: Nursing of families in crisis, Philadelphia, 1974, JB Lippincott Co.
14. Hymonovich DP: The chronicity impact and coping instrument: parent questionnaire for use by clinicians and researchers, Nurs Res 32:275, 1983.
15. Kaslow FW, editor: The international book of family therapy, New York, 1982, Brunner/Mazel Inc.
16. Kim MJ, McFarland GK, and McLane AM: Pocket guide to nursing diagnoses, ed 2, St Louis, 1987, The CV Mosby Co.
17. Knafl KA and Grace HK: Families across the life cycle: studies for nursing, Boston, 1978, Little, Brown & Co.
18. Lego S, editor: The American handbook of psychiatric nursing, Philadelphia, 1984, JB Lippincott Co.
19. Lewis JM: Family structure and stress, Fam Process 25:235, 1986.
20. McCubbin H and Patterson J, editors: Systematic assessment of family stress: resources and coping, St Paul, 1981, University of Minnesota.
21. Minuchin S and Fishman HC: Family therapy techniques, Cambridge, Mass, 1981, Harvard University Press.
22. Steinglass P: Psychoeducational family therapy for schizophrenia: a review essay, Psychiatry 50:14, 1987.
23. Streff MB: Examining family and growth and development: a theoretical model, Adv Nurs Sci 3:61, 1981.
24. Weitzman J: Engaging the severely dysfunctional family in treatment: basic considerations, Fam Proc 24:473, 1985.

Spiritual distress (distress of the human spirit)

1. Davidson G and Macdonald M: Anyone can pray, New York, 1983, Paulist Press.
2. Frankl V: Man's search for meaning, Boston, 1963, Beacon Press.
3. Linn D and Linn M: Healing life's hurts: healing memories through five stages of forgiveness, New York, 1978, Paulist Press.
4. McKay M et al: Thoughts and feelings, the art of cognitive stress intervention, Richmond, Calif, 1981, New Harbinger Publications.
5. McLane AM, editor: Classification of nursing diagnoses: proceedings of the seventh conference, St Louis, 1987, The CV Mosby Co.
6. Peplau L and Perlman D, editors: Loneliness: a sourcebook of current theory, research and therapy, New York, 1983, John Wiley & Sons Inc.
7. Tubesing DA: Stress, spiritual outlook and health, Specialized Pastoral Care J 3:17, 1980.
8. Waterhouse J: Spiritual distress. In Nursing diagnosis: application to clinical practice, Philadelphia, 1983, JB Lippincott Co.
9. Yura H and Walsh MB, editors: Human needs and the nursing process, Norwalk, Conn, 1982, Appleton-Century-Crofts.

APPENDIX

Conversion Factors to International System of Units (SI Units)

Conversion Factors (SI Units)

Component	Normal Range in Units as Customarily Reported	Conversion Factor	Normal Range in SI Units, Molecular Units, International Units, or Decimal Fractions
Biochemical Components of Blood*			
Acetoacetic acid (S)	0.2-1.0 mg/dL	98	19.6-98.0 μmol/L
Acetone (S)	0.3-2.0 mg/dL	172	51.6-344.0 μmol/L
Albumin (S)	3.2-4.5 g/dL	10	32-45 g/L
Ammonia (P)	20-120 μg/dL	0.588	11.7-70.5 μmol/L
Amylase (S)	60-160 Somogyi units/dL	1.85	111-296 U/L
Base, total (S)	145-160 mEq/L	1	145-160 mmol/L
Bicarbonate (P)	21-28 mEq/L	1	21-28 mmol/L
Bile acids (S)	0.3-3.0 mg/dL	10	3-30 mg/L
		2.547	0.8-7.6 μmol/L
Bilirubin, direct (S)	Up to 0.3 mg/dL	17.1	Up to 5.1 μmol/L
Bilirubin, indirect (S)	0.1-1.0 mg/dL	17.1	1.7-17.1 μmol/L
Blood gases (B)			
P_{CO_2} arterial	35-40 mm Hg	0.133	4.66-5.32 kPa
P_{O_2} arterial	95-100 mm Hg	0.133	12.64-13.30 kPa
Calcium (S)	8.5-10.5 mg/dL	0.25	2.1-2.6 mmol/L
Chloride (S)	95-103 mEq/L	1	95-103 mmol/L
Creatine (S)	0.1-0.4 mg/dL	76.3	7.6-30.5 μmol/L
Creatinine (S)	0.6-1.2 mg/dL	88.4	53-106 μmol/L
Creatinine clearance (P)	107-139 mL/min	0.0167	1.78-2.32 mL/s
Fatty acids (total) (S)	8-20 mg/dL	0.01	0.08-2.00 mg/L
Fibrinogen (P)	200-400 mg/dL	0.01	2.00-4.00 g/L
Gamma globulin (S)	0.5-1.6 g/dL	10	5-16 g/L
Globulins (total) (S)	2.3-3.5 g/dL	10	23-35 g/L
Glucose (fasting) (S)	70-110 mg/dL	0.055	3.85-6.05 mmol/L
Insulin (radioimmunoassay) (P)	4-24 μIU/ml	0.0417	0.17-1.00 μg/L
	0.20-0.84 μg/L	172.2	35-145 pmol/L
Iodine, BEI (S)	3.5-6.5 μg/dL	0.079	0.28-0.51 μmol/L
Iodine, PBI (S)	4.0-8.0 μg/dL	0.079	0.32-0.63 μmol/L
Iron, total (S)	60-150 μg/dL	0.179	11-27 μmol/L
Iron-binding capacity (S)	300-360 μg/dL	0.179	54-64 μmol/L
17-Ketosteroids (P)	25-125 μg/dL	0.01	0.25-1.25 mg/L
Lactic dehydrogenase (S)	80-120 units at 30 °C	0.48	38-62 U/L at 30 °C
	Lactate → pyruvate		
	100-190 U/L at 37 °C	1	100-190 U/L at 37 °C
Lipase (S)	0-1.5 U/ml (Cherry-Crandall)	278	0-417 U/L

From Tilkian, S.M., Conover, M.B., and Tilkian, A.G.: Clinical implications of laboratory tests, ed. 3, St. Louis, 1983, The C.V. Mosby Co.
*This is a selected (not a complete) list of biochemical components. The ranges listed may differ from those accepted in some laboratories and are shown to illustrate the conversion factor and the method of expression in SI molecular units. For a more complete listing, see Henry, J.B., editor: Todd-Sanford-Davidsohn clinical diagnosis and management by laboratory methods, ed. 16, Philadelphia, W.B. Saunders Co.

Continued.

Conversion Factors (SI Units)—cont'd.

Component	Normal Range in Units as Customarily Reported	Conversion Factor	Normal Range in SI Units, Molecular Units, International Units, or Decimal Fractions
Lipids (total) (S)	400-800 mg/dL	0.01	4.00-8.00 g/L
Cholesterol	150-250 mg/dL	0.026	3.9-6.5 mmol/L
Triglycerides	75-165 mg/dL	0.0114	0.85-1.89 mmol/L
Phospholipids	150-380 mg/dL	0.01	1.50-380 g/L
Free fatty acids	9.0-15.0 mM/L	1	9.0-15.0 mmol/L
Nonprotein nitrogen (S)	20-35 mg/dL	0.714	14.3-25.0 mmol/L
Phosphatase (P)			
Acid (units/dL)	Cherry-Crandall	2.77	0-5.5 U/L
	King-Armstrong	1.77	0-5.5 U/L
	Bodansky	5.37	0-5.5 U/L
Alkaline (units/dL)	King-Armstrong	1.77	30-120 U/L
	Bodansky	5.37	30-120 U/L
	Bessey-Lowry-Brock	16.67	30-120 U/L
Phosphorus, inorganic (S)	3.0-4.5 mg/dL	0.323	0.97-1.45 mmol/L
Potassium (P)	3.8-5.0 mEq/L	1	3.8-5.0 mmol/L
Proteins, total (S)	6.0-7.8 g/dL	10	60-78 g/L
Albumin	3.2-4.5 g/dL	10	32-45 g/L
Globulin	2.3-3.5 g/dL	10	23-35 g/L
Sodium (P)	136-142 mEq/L	1	136-142 mmol/L
Testosterone: Male (S)	300-1,200 ng/dL	0.035	10.5-42.0 nmol/L
Female	30-95 ng/dL	0.035	1.0-3.3 nmol/L
Thyroid tests (S)			
Thyroxine (T_4)	4-11 μg/dL	12.87	51-142 nmol/L
T_4 expressed as iodine	3.2-7.2 μg/dL	79.0	253-569 nmol/L
T_3 resin uptake	25%-38% relative uptake	0.01	0.25%-0.38% relative uptake
TSH (S)	10 μU/mL	1	$<10^{-3}$ IU/L
Urea nitrogen (S)	8-23 mg/dL	0.357	2.9-8.2 mmol/L
Uric acid (S)	2-6 mg/dL	59.5	0.120-0.360 mmol/L
Vitamin B_{12} (S)	160-950 pg/mL	0.74	118-703 pmol/L
Hematology Values*			
Red cell volume (male)	25-35 mL/kg body weight	0.001	0.025-0.035 L/kg body weight
Hematocrit	40%-50%	0.01	0.40-0.50
Hemoglobin	13.5-18.0 g/dL	10	135-180 g/L
Hemoglobin	13.5-18.0 g/dL	0.155	2.09-2.79 mmol/L
RBC count	4.5-6 × 10^6/μL	1	4.6-6 × 10^{12}/L
WBC count	4.5-10 × 10^3/μL	1	4.5-10 × 10^9/L
Mean corpuscular volume	80-96 μm^3	1	80-96 fL

*The International Committee for Standardization in Hematology recommends that the numbers remain the same but that the units change, so that hemoglobin is expressed as grams per deciliter (g/dL) even though other measurements are expressed as units per liter (U/L).

Index

C

D

E

J

K

O

P

Q

R

T